HARRISON'S Volume 1

PRINCIPLES OF INTERNAL MEDICINE

THIRTEENTH EDITION

THIRTEENTH EDITION

HARRISON'S
PRINCIPLES OF INTERNAL MEDICINE

Volume 1

Editors

KURT J. ISSELBACHER, A.B., M.D.

Mallinckrodt Professor of Medicine, Harvard Medical School; Physician and Director, Cancer Center, Massachusetts General Hospital, Boston

EUGENE BRAUNWALD, A.B., M.D., M.A. (Hon.), M.D. (Hon.)

Hersey Professor of the Theory and Practice of Physic, Harvard Medical School; Chairman, Department of Medicine, Brigham and Women's Hospital, Boston

JEAN D. WILSON, M.D.

Charles Cameron Sprague Distinguished Chair and Professor of Internal Medicine; Chief, Division of Endocrinology and Metabolism, The University of Texas Southwestern Medical Center, Dallas

JOSEPH B. MARTIN, M.D., Ph.D., F.R.C.P. (C), M.A. (Hon.)

Professor of Neurology and Chancellor, University of California, San Francisco

ANTHONY S. FAUCI, M.D.

Director, National Institute of Allergy and Infectious Diseases; Chief, Laboratory of Immunoregulation; Director, Office of AIDS Research, National Institutes of Health, Bethesda

DENNIS L. KASPER, M.D.

William Ellery Channing Professor of Medicine, Harvard Medical School; Chief, Division of Infectious Diseases, Beth Israel Hospital; Co-Director, Channing Laboratory, Brigham and Women's Hospital, Boston

McGRAW-HILL, Inc.
Health Professions Division

New York St. Louis San Francisco Colorado Springs Auckland Bogotá Caracas Hamburg Lisbon London
Madrid Mexico Milan Montreal New Delhi Paris San Juan São Paulo Singapore Sydney Tokyo Toronto

Note: Dr. Fauci's work as editor and author was performed outside the scope of his employment as a U.S. government employee. This work represents his personal and professional views and not necessarily those of the U.S. government.

Foreign Language Editions
CHINESE (Twelfth Edition)—McGraw-Hill Book Company-Singapore, © 1994
FRENCH (Twelfth Edition)—Flammarion, © 1992
GERMAN (Tenth Edition)—Schwabe and Company, Ltd., © 1986
GREEK (Twelfth Edition)—Parissianos, © 1994 (est.)
ITALIAN (Twelfth Edition)—McGraw-Hill Libri Italia S.r.l. © 1992
JAPANESE (Eleventh Edition)—Hirokawa, © 1991
PORTUGUESE (Twelfth Edition)—Editora Guanabara Koogan, S.A., © 1992
SPANISH (Twelfth Edition)—McGraw-Hill/Interamericana de Espana, © 1992

This book was set in Times Roman by Monotype Composition Company. The editors were J. Dereck Jeffers and Stuart D. Boynton. The indexer was Irving Tullar; the production supervisor was Roger Kasunic; the designer was Marsha Cohen; R. R. Donnelley & Sons Company was printer and binder.

Library of Congress Cataloging-in-Publication Data

Harrison's principles of internal medicine—13th ed./editors,
  Kurt J. Isselbacher . . . [et al.]
      p.   cm.
    Includes bibliographical references and index.
    ISBN 0-07-032370-4 (1-vol. ed.) : 98.00 — ISBN 0-07-911169-6 (2
  vol. ed. set) : 127.00 — ISBN 0-07-032371-2 (bk. 1). — ISBN
  0-07-032372-0 (bk. 2)
      1. Internal medicine.   I. Harrison, Tinsley Randolph, 1900–
  II. Isselbacher, Kurt J.   III. Title: Principles of internal
  medicine.
      [DNLM: 1. Internal Medicine.   WB 115 P957 1994]
  RC46.H333 1994
  616—dc20
  DNLM/DLC
  for Library of Congress   93-47393
                                                          CIP

A SALUTE TO ROBERT G. PETERSDORF

By The Editors Of Harrison's.

We dedicate this thirteenth edition of *Harrison's Principles of Internal Medicine* to Robert G. Petersdorf. Dr. Petersdorf became an editor of Harrison's in 1968 for the preparation of the sixth edition and served as Editor-in-Chief of the tenth edition. He was a powerful force for seven editions and more than 20 years in establishing the pivotal role of this book in the education of students, residents and practitioners of medicine.

Dr. Petersdorf is a graduate of Brown University and of Yale University Medical School. His graduate training included residencies in medicine at Yale and at the Peter Bent Brigham Hospital and a research fellowship at Johns Hopkins. As Chair of the Department of Medicine at the University of Washington he fashioned one of the truly great departments of internal medicine in the nation, with well-balanced and great strengths in education, clinical care, and research. His interests and contributions broadened steadily and he served successively as the first President of the newly merged Brigham and Women's Hospital in Boston, as Vice Chancellor for Health Sciences and Dean of the School of Medicine, University of California, San Diego, and most recently as President of the Association of American Medical Colleges.

Dr. Petersdorf has, from the beginning of his career, made notable and outstanding contributions in a number of areas in the field of Infectious Disease. He carried out a series of classic studies on the pathogenesis of fever, on pneumococcal meningitis and infective endocarditis, and on the chemoprophylaxis and epidemiology of gram-negative infections, especially of the urinary tract.

NOTICE

Medicine is an ever-changing science. As new research and clinical experience broaden our knowledge, changes in treatment and drug therapy are required. The editors and the publisher of this work have checked with sources believed to be reliable in their efforts to provide information that is complete and generally in accord with the standards accepted at the time of publication. However, in view of the possibility of human error or changes in medical sciences, neither the editors, nor the publisher, nor any other party who has been involved in the preparation or publication of this work warrants that the information contained herein is in every respect accurate or complete. Readers are encouraged to confirm the information contained herein with other sources. For example and in particular, readers are advised to check the product information sheet included in the package of each drug they plan to administer to be certain that the information contained in this book is accurate and that changes have not been made in the recommended dose or in the contraindications for administration. This recommendation is of particular importance in connection with new or infrequently used drugs. Readers should also consult their own laboratories for normal values.

ABBREVIATED CONTENTS

CONTENTS

PART SIX
INFECTIOUS DISEASE

Section 1: Basic Considerations in Infectious Disease

Section 2: Clinical Syndromes—Community Acquired

Section 3: Clinical Syndromes—Nosocomial Infections

Section 4: Bacterial Disease: General Considerations

Section 5: Diseases Caused by Gram-Positive Bacteria

Section 6: Diseases Caused by Gram-Negative Bacteria

PART THIRTEEN
ENDOCRINOLOGY AND METABOLISM

Section 1: Endocrinology

Section 2: Disorders of Intermediary Metabolism

COLOR PLATES

ATLAS OF DERMATOLOGY *Stephen F. Templeton / Thomas J. Lawley*

1 Common skin diseases and lesions

A1-1 Acne vulgaris A1-2 Acne rosacea A1-3 Psoriasis A1-4 Atopic dermatitis A1-5 Dyshidrotic ezcema A1-6 Seborrheic dermatitis A1-7 Stasis dermatitis A1-8 Allergic contact dermatitis A1-9 Lichen planus A1-10 Pityriasis rosea A1-11 Vitiligo A1-12 Alopecia areata A1-13 Urticaria A1-14 Epidermoid cysts A1-15 Seborrheic keratoses A1-16 Keloids A1-17 Cherry hemangiomas

2 Cutaneous neoplasms

A2-18 Actinic keratoses A2-19 Keratoacanthoma A2-20 Basal cell carcinoma A2-21 Squamous cell carcinoma A2-22 Kaposi's sarcoma A2-23 Mycosis fungoides A2-24 Non-Hodgkin's lymphoma A2-25 Metastatic carcinoma

3 Pigmented lesions—benign and malignant

A3-26 Nevus A3-27 Dysplastic nevi A3-28 Superficial spreading melanoma A3-29 Lentigo maligna melanoma A3-30 Nodular melanoma A3-31 Acral lentiginous melanoma

4 Infectious disease and the skin

A4-32 Impetigo contagiosa A4-33 Folliculitis A4-34 Erysipelas A4-35 Herpes simplex A4-36 Varicella A4-37 Herpes zoster A4-38 Verrucae A4-39 Molluscum contagiosum A4-40 Oral hairy leukoplakia A4-41 Pseudomembranous oral candidiasis A4-42 Tinea corporis A4-43 Tinea cruris A4-44 Tinea versicolor A4-45 Scabies A4-46 Erythema chronicum migrans A4-47 Rocky Mountain spotted fever A4-48 Disseminated gonococcemia A4-49 Fulminant meningococcemia A4-50 Primary syphilis A4-51 Secondary syphilis A4-52 Secondary syphilis A4-53 Condylomata lata A4-54 Chancroid A4-55 Condylomata acuminata

5 Immunologically mediated skin disease

A5-56 Systemic lupus erythematosus A5-57 Discoid lupus erythematosus A5-58 Dermatomyositis A5-59 Dermatomyositis A5-60 Scleroderma A5-61 Scleroderma A5-62 Erythema multiforme A5-63 Erythema nodosum A5-64 Vasculitis A5-65 Pemphigus vulgaris A5-66 Dermatitis herpetiformis A5-67 Bullous pemphigoid

6 Skin manifestations of internal disease

A6-68 Acanthosis nigricans A6-69 Pretibial myxedema A6-70 Sarcoid A6-71 Neurofibromatosis A6-72 Coumarin necrosis A6-73 Pyoderma gangrenosum

ATLAS OF ENDOSCOPIC FINDINGS

A7-1 Normal esophagus A7-2 Peptic regurgitant esophagitis A7-3 Ulcerated squamous cell carcinoma A7-4 Moniliasis of the esophagus A7-5 Barrett's metaplasia of the esophagus with an adenocarcinoma A7-6 Normal body of the stomach with rugal folds A7-7 Large, benign lesser curve gastic ulcer A7-8 Gastric polyp A7-9 Arteriovenous malformation of the gastric mucosa A7-10 Normal pylorus A7-11 Normal duodenal bulb A7-12 Duodenal ulcer A7-13 Normal papilla of Vater A7-14 Periampullary carcinoma A7-15 Endoscopic papillotomy A7-16 Normal colon A7-17 Colonic adenomatous polyp A7-18 Multiple small colonic adenomatous polyps A7-19 Colon adenocarcinoma A7-20 Crohn's colitis A7-21 Severe ulcerative colitis A7-22 Kaposi's sarcoma involving the colon A7-23 Colonic varices A7-24 Normal appearing ileal pouch

ATLAS OF FUNDOSCOPIC EXAMINATION

A8-1 Normal optic nerve and retina A8-2 Central retinal artery occlusion A8-3 Central retinal vein occlusion A8-4 Early papilledema A8-5 Drusen of the optic nerve head A8-6 Anterior ischemic optic neuropathy A8-7 Primary optic atrophy A8-8 Angioid streaks A8-9 Retinitis pigmentosa A8-10 Band keratopathy A8-11 Glaucomatous optic disk with secondary atrophy A8-12 Diabetic retinopathy with microaneurysms A8-13 Proliferative diabetic retinopathy A8-14 Cytomegalovirus retinitis in AIDS A8-15 Retinal arteriovenous malformation in the Wyburn-Mason syndrome A8-16 Kayser-Fleischer ring in Wilson's disease.

ATLAS OF HEMATOLOGY

A9-1 Normal blood smear A9-2 Megaloblastic anemia A9-3 Liver disease A9-4 Iron deficiency anemia A9-5 Thalassemia intermedia A9-6 Sickle cell anemia A9-7 Traumatic hemolysis A9-8 Spur cell anemia A9-9 Uremia A9-10 Hereditary spherocytosis A9-11 Immunohemolytic anemia A9-12 Myeloid metaplasia A9-13 Normal granulocyte (A); normal monocyte and lymphocyte (B) A9-14 Normal eosinophil (A); basophil (B) A9-15 Normal granulocyte precursors in marrow A9-16 Neutrophils with toxic granulation A9-17 Band with Döhle body A9-18 Hypersegmentation A9-19 Chediak-Higashi anomaly (A); Pelger-Huët anomaly (B) A9-20 Reactive lymphocytes A9-21 Chronic granulocytic leukemia A9-22 Leukemic cell in acute promyelocytic leukemia A9-23 Chronic lymphocytic leukemia A9-24 Leukemic cells in acute lymphoblastic leukemia A9-25 Hodgkin's disease A9-26 Non-Hodgkin's nodular lymphoma A9-27 Multiple myeloma

LIST OF CONTRIBUTORS

ELIAS ABRUTYN, M.D.

Professor and Associate Chairman, Medicine, and Vice-Dean for Veterans Affairs, Medical College of Pennsylvania; Chief, Infectious Diseases, Veterans Administration Medical Center, Philadelphia

RAYMOND D. ADAMS, B.A., M.A., M.D., M.A. (Hon.), D.Sc. (Hon.), M.D. (Hon.)

Bullard Professor of Neuropathology, Emeritus, Harvard Medical School; Consultant Neurologist, Massachusetts General Hospital; Emeritus Director, Eunice K. Shriver Research Center, Boston; Médicin Adjoint L'Hôpital, Cantonale de Lausanne, Lausanne

MICHAEL J. AMINOFF, M.D.

Professor of Neurology; Director, Clinical Neurophysiology Laboratories, University of California, San Francisco

MICHAEL A. APICELLA, M.D.

Professor and Head, Department of Microbiology, University of Iowa College of Medicine, Iowa City

GORDON LEE ARCHER, M.D.

Professor of Medicine and Microbiology/Immunology and Chairman, Division of Infectious Diseases, Medical College of Virginia, Virginia Commonwealth University, Richmond

ARTHUR K. ASBURY, M.D.

Ruth Wagner Van Meter and J. Ray Van Meter Professor of Neurology; Vice Dean for Research, University of Pennsylvania School of Medicine and Hospital of the University of Pennsylvania, Philadelphia

K. FRANK AUSTEN, M.D.

Theodore Bevier Bayles Professor of Medicine, Harvard Medical School; Chairman, Department of Rheumatology and Immunology, Brigham and Women's Hospital, Boston

ROBERT AUSTRIAN, M.D., D.Sci. (Hon.)

John Herr Musser Professor and Chairman Emeritus, Department of Molecular and Cellular Engineering, University of Pennsylvania School of Medicine, Philadelphia

BERNARD BABIOR, M.D., Ph.D.

Head, Division of Biochemistry, Department of Molecular and Experimental Medicine and Member, Division of Hematology and Oncology, Department of Medicine, Scripps Clinic and Research Foundation, La Jolla

KAMAL F. BADR, M.D.

Professor of Medicine, Emory University; Chief, Division of Nephrology, Atlanta Veteran's Medical Center; Attending Physician, Emory University Hospital, Atlanta

DONALD S. BAIM, M.D.

Associate Professor of Medicine, Harvard Medical School; Chief, Interventional Cardiology Section, Beth Israel Hospital, Boston

ANN SULLIVAN BAKER, M.D.

Associate Professor of Medicine, Harvard Medical School; Director, Infectious Diseases Service, Massachusetts Eye and Ear Infirmary; Physician, Infectious Disease Service, Massachusetts General Hospital, Boston

ANDREA BALLABIO, M.D.

Associate Professor, Institute for Molecular Genetics and Human Genome Center, Baylor College of Medicine, Houston

KENNETH J. BART, M.D., M.P.H.

Director, National Vaccine Program, Office of the Assistant Secretary of Health, Department of Health and Human Services, Rockville

ROBERT C. BAST, Jr., M.D.

R. Wayne Rundle Professor of Medicine and Director, Duke Comprehensive Cancer Center, Duke University Medical Center, Durham

M. FLINT BEAL, M.D.

Associate Professor of Neurology, Harvard Medical School; Assistant Neurologist, Massachusetts General Hospital, Boston

ARTHUR L. BEAUDET, M.D.

Professor, Institute for Molecule Genetics and Departments of Pediatrics and Cell Biology, Baylor College of Medicine; Investigator, Howard Hughes Medical Institute, Houston

JOHN E. BENNETT, M.D.

Head, Clinical Mycology Section, Laboratory of Clinical Investigation, National Institute of Allergy and Infectious Diseases, National Institutes of Health, Bethesda

ANDREW BERCHUCK, M.D.

Associate Professor, Division of Gynecologic Oncology, Duke University Medical Center, Durham

MICHAEL S. BERNSTEIN, M.D.

Assistant Professor of Medicine and Anesthesia, Division of Pulmonary and Critical Care Medicine, University of California at San Francisco Medical Center, San Francisco

DANIEL G. BICHET, M.D.

Associate Professor of Medicine, University of Montreal; Director, Clinical Research Unit, Hôpital du Sacre-Coeur de Montréal, Montreal

DAVID R. BICKERS, M.D.

Professor and Chairman, Department of Dermatology, Case Western Reserve University School of Medicine; Director, Department of Dermatology, University Hospitals of Cleveland, Cleveland

EDWIN L. BIERMAN, M.D.

Professor of Medicine and Head, Division of Metabolism, Endocrinology and Nutrition, University of Washington School of Medicine, Seattle

NEIL R. BLACKLOW, M.D.

Richard M. Haidack Professor of Medicine and Chairman, Department of Medicine, University of Massachusetts Medical School, Worcester

MARTIN J. BLASER, M.D.

The Addison B. Scoville Professor of Medicine; Director, Division of Infectious Diseases and Professor of Microbiology and Immunology, Vanderbilt University School of Medicine; Staff Physician, Veterans Affairs Medical Center, Nashville

JEAN L. BOLOGNIA, M.D.

Associate Professor of Dermatology, Department of Dermatology, Yale University School of Medicine, New Haven

LAWRENCE F. BORGES, M.D.

Associate Professor of Surgery (Neurosurgery), Harvard Medical School; Associate Visiting Neurosurgeon, Massachusetts General Hospital, Boston

RICHARD C. BOUCHER, Jr., M.D.

Professor of Medicine and Director, Division of Pulmonary Diseases, Critical Care and Occupational Medicine, University of North Carolina at Chapel Hill; University of North Carolina Hospitals, Chapel Hill

AUBREY E. BOYD III, M.D.

Professor of Medicine and Neuroscience; Chief, Division of Endocrinology, Diabetes, Metabolism and Molecular Medicine, New England Medical Center, Boston

WALTER G. BRADLEY, D.M., F.R.C.P.

Professor and Chairman, Department of Neurology, University of Miami School of Medicine, Miami

HUGH R. BRADY, M.D., Ph.D., F.R.C.P.I.

Assistant Professor of Medicine, Harvard Medical School; Chief, Renal Section, Brockton/West Roxbury Veteran's Affairs Medical Center; Associate Physician, Brigham and Women's Hospital, Boston

DAVID L. BRAFF, M.D.

Professor of Psychiatry, University of California at San Diego; Director of Psychiatry, UCSD Medical Center, San Diego

KENNETH D. BRANDT, M.D.

Professor of Medicine and Head, Rheumatology Division, Indiana University School of Medicine, Indianapolis; Director, Multipurpose Arthritis and Musculoskeletal Diseases Center, Indiana University School of Medicine, Indianapolis

EUGENE BRAUNWALD, A.B., M.D., M.A. (Hon.), M.D. (Hon.), Sc.D. (Hon.)

Hersey Professor of the Theory and Practice of Medicine, Harvard Medical School; Chairman, Department of Medicine, Brigham and Women's Hospital, Boston

IRWIN M. BRAVERMAN, M.D.

Professor, Department of Dermatology, Yale University School of Medicine, New Haven

JAMES L. BREELING, M.D.

Associate Chief, Medical Service, West Roxbury VA Medical Center, Boston

JOEL G. BREMAN, M.D., D.T.P.H.

Deputy Chief, Malaria Branch, Division of Parasitic Diseases, National Center for Infectious Diseases, Centers for Disease Control and Prevention, Atlanta; Visiting Lecturer, Harvard School of Public Health, Boston

BARRY M. BRENNER, M.D., A.M. (Hon.), D.Sc. (Hon.), D.M.Sc. (Hon.)

Samuel A. Levine Professor of Medicine, Harvard Medical School; Senior Physician and Director, Renal Division, Brigham and Women's Hospital, Boston

KENNETH R. BRIDGES, M.D.

Assistant Professor of Medicine, Harvard Medical School; Brigham and Women's Hospital, Boston

KAREN THATCHER BRITTON, M.D., Ph.D.

Professor of Psychiatry, University of California at San Diego, La Jolla

CLAIRE V. BROOME, M.D.

Associate Director for Science, Centers for Disease Control and Prevention, Atlanta

MARTIN M. BROWN, M.A., M.D., M.R.C.P.

Senior Lecturer in Neurology, St. George's Hospital Medical School, London

MICHAEL S. BROWN, M.D.

Paul J. Thomas Professor, Department of Molecular Genetics, The University of Texas Southwestern Medical Center, Dallas

ROBERT H. BROWN, Jr., M.D., D.Phil.

Associate Professor, Harvard Medical School; Associate Neruologist and Director, Cecil B. Day Laboratory for Neuromuscular Research, Massachusetts General Hospital, Boston

H. FRANKLIN BUNN, M.D.

Professor of Medicine, Harvard Medical School; Senior Physician and Director, Hematology Research, Brigham and Women's Hospital, Boston

RONALD M. BURDE, M.D.

Isidor Tachna Professor and Chairman, Department of Ophthalmology; Ophthalmologist and Neuro-ophthalmologist, Albert Einstein College of Medicine/Montefiore Medical Center, New York

JOAN R. BUTTERTON, M.D.

Clinical and Research Fellow, Infectious Diseases Unit, Massachusetts Gneral Hospital, Boston

STEPHEN B. CALDERWOOD, M.D.

Associate Professor of Medicine, Harvard Medical School; Chief, Infectious Diseases Unit, Massachusetts General Hospital, Boston

CHARLES B. CARPENTER, M.D.

Professor of Medicine, Harvard Medical School; Director, Laboratory of Immunogenetics and Transplantation, Brigham and Woman's Hospital, Boston

BRUCE R. CARR, M.D.

Paul C. MacDonald Professor and Director, Division of Reproductive Endocrinology, Department of Obstetrics and Gynecology, The University of Texas Southwestern Medical Center, Dallas

VERNE S. CAVINESS, Jr., M.D., Ph.D.

Joseph P. and Rose F. Kennedy Professor of Child Neurology and Mental Retardation, Harvard Medical School; Chief, Pediatric Neurology Service, Massachusetts General Hospital, Boston

WALLACE A. CLYDE, Jr., M.D.

Professor of Pediatrics and Microbiology, University of North Carolina, Chapel Hill

FREDRIC L. COE, M.D.

Professor of Medicine and Physiology and Chief, Nephrology Program, University of Chicago Pritzker School of Medicine, Chicago

ALAN S. COHEN, M.D.

Distinguished Professor of Medicine and Rheumatology; Director, Arthritis Center at Boston University School of Medicine, Boston University School of Medicine, Boston

WILSON COLUCCI, M.D.

Associate Professor of Medicine, Harvard Medical School; Physician, Brigham and Women's Hospital

PATRICIA C. COME, M.D.

Associate Professor of Medicine, Harvard Medical School; Harvard Community Health Plan, Boston

JOEL D. COOPER, M.D.

Professor of Surgery and Head, Section of General Thoracic Surgery, Washington University School of Medicine; Barnes Hospital, St. Louis

MAX D. COOPER, M.D.

Professor of Medicine, Pediatrics and Microbiology and Howard Hughes Medical Institute Investigator, University of Alabama at Birmingham, Birmingham

LAWRENCE COREY, M.D.

Professor of Laboratory Medicine, Microbiology and Medicine, University of Washington, Seattle

MARK A. CREAGER, M.D.

Associate Professor of Medicine, Harvard Medical School; Director, Vascular Diagnostic Laboratory, Brigham and Women's Hospital, Boston

RONALD G. CRYSTAL, M.D.

Webster Professor of Medicine, Cornell University Medical College; Attending Physician, New York Hospital; Chief, Division of Pulmonary and Critical Care Medicine, New York Hospital-Cornell Medical Center, New York

JOHN J. CUSH, M.D.

Associate Professor of Internal Medicine, Rheumatic Diseases Division University of Texas Southwestern Medical Center at Dallas, Dallas

CHARLES A. CZEISLER, Ph.D., M.D.

Associate Professor of Medicine, Harvard Medical School; Physician and Director, Laboratory for Circadian and Sleep Disorders Medicine, Brigham and Women's Hospital, Boston

THOMAS M. DANIEL, M.D.

Professor of Medicine and International Health, Center for International Health, CWRU School of Medicine, Cleveland

GILBERT H. DANIELS, M.D.

Associate Professor of Medicine, Harvard Medical School; Physician and Co-Director, Thyroid Clinic, Massachusetts General Hospital, Boston

ROBERT B. DAROFF, M.D.

Gilbert W. Humphrey Professor and Chairman, Department of Neurology, Case Western Reserve University School of Medicine; Director, Department of Neurology, University Hospitals of Cleveland; Neurology Service, Cleveland Veteran's Administration Medical Center, Cleveland

JOHN R. DAVID, M.D.

Richard Pearson Strong Professor and Chairman, Department of Tropical Public Health, Harvard School of Public Health, Boston

CHARLES EDWARD DAVIS, M.D.

Professor of Pathology and Medicine, School of Medicine, University of California, San Diego; Director, Microbiology Laboratory, UCSD Medical Center, San Diego

KENNETH DAVIS, M.D., F.A.C.R.

Professor of Radiology, Harvard Medical School; Department of Neuroradiology, Massachusetts General Hospital, Boston

ROBERT L. DERESIEWICZ, M.D.

Instructor in Medicine, Harvard Medical School; Associate Physician, Brigham and Women's Hospital, Boston

ROBERT J. DESNICK, Ph.D., M.D.

Professor and Chairman, Department of Human Genetics, Mount Sinai School of Medicine; Attending Physician, Mount Sinai Hospital, New York

MARC A. DICHTER, M.D., Ph.D.

Professor of Neurology and Pharmacology, University of Pennsylvania School of Medicine and Graduate Hospital, Philadelphia

JULES L. DIENSTAG, M.D.

Associate Professor of Medicine, Harvard Medical School; Associate Physician, Massachusetts General Hospital, Boston

ALAN R. DIMICK, M.D.

Professor of Surgery, University of Alabama at Birmingham; Director, Burn Center, University of Alabama Hospital, Birmingham

CHARLES A. DINARELLO, M.D.

Professor of Medicine, Tufts University School of Medicine; Division of Geographic Medicine and Infectious Diseases, New England Medical Center, Boston

ROBERT G. DLUHY, M.D.

Associate Professor of Medicine, Harvard Medical School; Associate Program Director of the Clinical Research Center, Brigham and Women's Hospital, Boston

RAPHAEL DOLIN, M.D.

Charles A. Dewey Professor of Medicine; Chair, Department of Medicine, University of Rochester School of Medicine and Dentistry, Rochester

DANIEL B. DRACHMAN, M.D.

Professor of Neurology and Neurosciences and Director, Neuromuscular Unit, The Johns Hopkins University School of Medicine, Baltimore

JEFFREY M. DRAZEN, M.D.

Parker B. Francis Professor of Medicine, Harvard Medical School; Chief, Pulmonary Division, Brigham and Women's and Beth Israel Hospitals, Boston

JOHANNA T. DWYER, D.Sc., R.D.

Professor of Medicine and Community Health, Tufts University School of Medicine; Professor of Nutrition, Tufts University School of Nutrition; Senior Scientist, USDA Human Nutrition Research Center on Aging, Tufts University; Director, Frances Stern Nutrition Center, New England Medical Center Hospital, Boston

VICTOR J. DZAU, M.D.

William G. Irwin Professor of Medicine and Chief, Division of Cardiovascular Medicine, Stanford University School of Medicine; Stanford University Hospital, Stanford

BARRY I. EISENSTEIN, M.D.

Professor of Medicine, Indiana University School of Medicine; Vice President, Lilly Research Laboratories, Indianapolis

VIRGINIA L. ERNSTER, Ph.D.

Professor and Chair, Department of Epidemiology and Biostatistics, University of California, San Francisco

KENNETH H. FALCHUK, M.D.

Associate Professor of Medicine, Harvard Medical School; Physician, Brigham and Women's Hospital, Boston

FERRIC C. FANG, M.D.

Assistant Professor of Medicine and Pathology, University of Colorado Health Sciences Center; Director, Clinical Microbiology Laboratory, University Hospital, Denver

ANTHONY S. FAUCI, M.D.

Director, National Institute of Allergy and Infectious Diseases; Chief, Laboratory of Immunoregulation; Director, Office of AIDS Research, National Institutes of Health, Bethesda

MURRAY J. FAVUS, M.D.

Professor of Medicine, Sections of Endocrinology and Nephrology, Department of Medicine, University of Chicago Pritzker School of Medicine, Chicago

THOMAS F. FERRIS, M.D.

Nesbitt Professor and Chairman, Department of Medicine, University of Minnesota; University of Minnesota Hospital and Clinics, Minneapolis

BERNARD N. FIELDS, M.D.

Adele Lehman Professor of Microbiology and Molecular Genetics, Professor of Medicine and Chairman, Department of Microbiology and Molecular Genetics, Harvard Medical School, Boston

HOWARD L. FIELDS, M.D., Ph.D.

Professor of Neurology and Physiology and Vice Chairman, Department of Neurology, University of California, San Francisco

GREGORY A. FILICE, M.D.

Associate Professor of Medicine and Chief, Infectious Disease Section, University of Minnesota VA Medical Center, Minneapolis

ROBERT W. FINBERG, M.D.

Associate Professor of Medicine, Harvard Medical School; Chief, Laboratory of Infectious Diseases, Dana-Farber Cancer Institute, Boston

STUART C. FINCH, M.D.

Professor of Medicine, University of Medicine and Dentistry of New Jersey-Robert Wood Johnson Medical School and the Cooper Hospital/University Medical Center, Camden

J. STEPHEN FINK, M.D.

Associate Professor, Harvard Medical School; Assistant Neurologist, Massachusetts General Hospital, Boston

DANIEL W. FOSTER, M.D.

Donald W. Seldin Distinguished Chair in Internal Medicine and Chairman, Department of Internal Medicine, The University of Texas Southwestern Medical Center, Dallas

MICHAEL M. FRANK, M.D.

Professor and Chairman, Department of Pediatrics, Duke University Medical Center; Professor of Medicine, Department of Medicine, Duke University Medical Center, Durham

ARNOLD S. FREEDMAN, M.D.

Assistant Professor of Medicine, Harvard Medical School; Division of Tumor Immunology, Dana-Farber Cancer Institute, Boston

STANLEY D. FREEDMAN, M.D.

Clinical Professor of Medicine, University of California at San Diego; Head, Division of Infectious Diseases, Scripps Clinic and Research Foundation, La Jolla

MICHAEL FREISSMUTH, M.D.

Lecturer, Department of Pharmacology, University of Vienna, Vienna

GERALD H. FRIEDLAND, M.D.

Director, AIDS Program, Yale University School of Medicine, New Haven

HARVEY MICHAEL FRIEDMAN, M.D.

Chief, Infectious Disease Division, Department of Medicine, University of Pennsylvania School of Medicine, Philadelphia

LAWRENCE S. FRIEDMAN, M.D.

Associate Professor of Medicine, Harvard Medical School; Associate Physician, Massachusetts General Hospital, Boston

PAUL J. FRIEDMAN, M.D.

Professor of Radiology, University of California, San Diego

WILLIAM F. FRIEDMAN, M.D.

J.H. Nicholson Professor of Pediatrics (Cardiology) and Executive Chairman, Department of Pediatrics, University of California, Los Angeles School of Medicine; University of California, Los Angeles Medical Center, Los Angeles

LAWRENCE A. FROHMAN, M.D.

Edmund F. Foley Professor and Head, Department of Medicine, University of Illinois at Chicago, Chicago

RAYMOND L. HINTZ, M.D.

Professor of Pediatrics and Head, Division of Pediatric Endocrinology, Stanford University School of Medicine, Stanford

MARTIN S. HIRSCH, M.D.

Professor of Medicine, Harvard Medical School; Massachusetts General Hospital, Boston

FRED HOCHBERG, M.D.

Associate Professor of Neurology, Harvard Medical School; Neurologist, Massachusetts General Hospital, Boston

GARY S. HOFFMAN, M.D.

Chairman, Department of Rheumatic and Immunologic Diseases, Cleveland Clinic Foundation, Cleveland

JOHN H. HOLBROOK, M.D.

Professor of Internal Medicine, University of Utah School of Medicine, Salt Lake City

MICHAEL F. HOLICK, Ph.D., M.D.

Professor of Medicine, Physiology and Dermatology; Chief of Endocrinology, Diabetes and Metabolism; Director of the General Clinical Research Center, Boston University School of Medicine, Boston

KING K. HOLMES, M.D., Ph.D.

Professor of Medicine and Director, Center for AIDS and Sexually Transmitted Diseases, University of Washington School of Medicine, Seattle

RANDALL K. HOLMES, M.D., Ph.D.

Chairman, Department of Microbiology and Immunology, Uniformed Services University of the Health Sciences, Bethesda

THOMAS H. HOSTETTER, M.D.

Professor of Medicine, University of Minnesota School of Medicine; Director, Division of Renal Disease, University Hospital, Minneapolis

LYN J. HOWARD, B.M., D.Ch., F.R.C.P.

Professor of Medicine and Associate Professor of Pediatrics; Head, Division of Clinical Nutrition, Albany Medical College, Albany

HOWARD HU, M.D., M.P.H., Sc.D.

Assistant Professor of Medicine, Harvard Medical School; Associate Physician, Channing Laboratory, Brigham and Women's Hospital, Boston

GARY W. HUNNINGHAKE, M.D.

Professor of Internal Medicine and Director, Pulmonary and Critical Care Medicine, University of Iowa College of Medicine, Iowa City

EDWARD P. INGENITO, M.D., Ph.D.

Assistant Professor of Medicine, Harvard Medical School; Director, Medical Intensive Care Unit, Brigham and Women's Hospital, Boston

ROLAND H. INGRAM, Jr., M.D.

Professor of Medicine, Emory University School of Medicine; Chief of Medicine, Emory-Crawford Long Hospital, Atlanta

CHARLES E. IRWIN, Jr., M.D.

Professor of Pediatrics; Director, Division of Adolescent Medicine, Department of Pediatrics School of Medicine, University of California, San Francisco, San Francisco

KURT J. ISSELBACHER, M.D.

Mallinckrodt Professor of Medicine, Harvard Medical School; Physician and Director, MGH Cancer Center, Massachusetts General Hospital, Boston

MARK E. JOSEPHSON, M.D.

Professor of Medicine, Harvard Medical School; Director, Harvard-Thorndike Electrophysiology Institute and Arrhythmia Service, Beth Israel Hospital, Boston

LEWIS L. JUDD, M.D.

Mary Gilman Marston Professor and Chairman, Department of Psychiatry, University of California at San Diego, La Jolla

LEE M. KAPLAN, M.D., Ph.D.

Assistant Professor of Medicine, Harvard Medical School; Assistant in Medicine, Gastrointestinal Unit, Massachusetts General Hospital, Boston

DENNIS L. KASPER, M.D.

William Ellery Channing Professor of Medicine, Harvard Medical School; Chief, Division of Infectious Diseases, Beth Israel Hospital; Co-Director, Channing Laboratory, Brigham and Women's Hospital, Boston

LLOYD H. KASPER, M.D.

Professor of Medicine, Neurology and Microbiology, Dartmouth Medical School, Hanover

SATISH KATHPALIA, M.D., F.A.C.P.

Associate Professor of Medicine, University of Illinois School of Medicine; Attending Physician, Renal Division, Department of Medicine, Michael Reese Hospital and Medical Center, Chicago

DONALD KAYE, M.D.

Klinghoffer Professor and Chairman, Department of Medicine, The Medical College of Pennsylvania, Philadelphia

GERALD T. KEUSCH, M.D.

Professor of Medicine and Chief, Division of Geographic Medicine and Infectious Diseases, New England Medical Center Hospitals, Boston

MICHAEL B. KIMMEY, M.D.

Associate Professor of Medicine and Director of GI Endoscopy, University of Washington School of Medicine, Seattle

LOUIS V. KIRCHHOFF, M.D.

Associate Professor of Internal Medicine and Staff Physician, Department of Veterans Affairs Medical Center, Iowa City

J. PHILLIP KISTLER, M.D.

Associate Professor of Neurology, Harvard Medical School; Associate Neurologist and Director of Stroke Service, Massachusetts General Hospital, Boston

HARVEY G. KLEIN, M.D.

Chief, Department of Transfusion Medicine, Clinical Center, National Institutes of Health, Bethesda

JAMES P. KNOCHEL, M.D.

Professor of Internal Medicine, The University of Texas Southwestern Medical Center; Chairman, Department of Medicine, Presbyterian Hospital, Dallas

HOWARD K. KOH, M.D.

Associate Professor of Dermatology, Medicine, and Public Health; Co-Director, Skin Oncology Program; Director, Cancer Prevention and Control Center, Boston University Schools of Medicine and Public Health, Boston

ANTHONY KOMAROFF, M.D.

Professor of Medicine, Harvard Medical School; Director, Division of General Medicine, Brigham and Women's Hospital, Boston

STANLEY J. KORSMEYER, M.D.

Professor, Howard Hughes Medical Institute, Washington University School of Medicine, Saint Louis

WILLIAM J. KOVACS, M.D.

Associate Professor of Medicine, Division of Endocrinology, Vanderbilt University School of Medicine, Nashville

STEPHEN M. KRANE, M.D.

Persis, Cyrus, and Marlow B. Harrison Professor of Medicine, Harvard Medical School; Physician and Chief, Arthritis Unit, Massachusetts General Hospital, Boston

DONALD KUFE, M.D.

Professor of Medicine, Harvard Medical School and Dana-Farber Cancer Institute, Boston

HELENA KUIVANIEMI, M.D., Ph.D.

Research Assistant Professor, Department of Biochemistry and Molecular Biology, Jefferson Medical College of Thomas Jefferson University, Philadelphia

J. THOMAS La MONT, M.D.

Chief, Section of Gastroenterology, The University Hospital, Boston

LEWIS LANDSBERG, M.D

Irving S. Cutter Professor and Chairman, Department of Medicine, Northwestern University Medical School; Physician-in-Chief, Northwestern Memorial Hospital, Chicago

ROBERT F. GAGEL, M.D.

Professor of Medicine and Chief of Endocrinology Section, The University of Texas, M.D. Anderson Cancer Center, Houston

JOHN I. GALLIN, M.D.

Director, Division of Intramural Research, National Institute of Allergy and Infectious Diseases, National Institutes of Health, Bethesda

ROBERT C. GALLO, M.D.

Chief, Laboratory of Tumor Cell Biology, National Cancer Institute, National Institutes of Health, Bethesda

MARC B. GARNICK, M.D.

Associate Clinical Professor of Medicine, Dana-Farber Cancer Institute and Harvard Medical School; Vice President for Clinical Development, Genetics Institute, Cambridge

JEFFREY A. GELFAND, M.D.

Sara Murray Jordan Professor and Vice Chairman, Department of Medicine, Tufts University School of Medicine; Associate Physician-in-Chief, New England Medical Center, Boston

JAMES L. GERMAN III, M.D.

Professor of Pediatrics, Cornell University Medical College; Director, Laboratory of Human Genetics, New York Blood Center, New York

BRUCE C. GILLILAND, M.D.

Professor of Medicine, Professor of Laboratory Medicine and Adjunct Professor of Microbiology, and Associate Dean, Clinical Affairs, University of Washington School of Medicine, Seattle

ALFRED G. GILMAN, M.D., Ph.D.

Raymond Willie Distinguished Chair in Molecular Neuropharmacology; Department of Pharmacology, The University of Texas Southwestern Medical Center, Dallas

SID GILMAN, M.D.

Professor and Chairman, Department of Neurology, University of Michigan, Ann Arbor

RICHARD J. GLASSOCK, M.D.

Professor and Chairman, Department of Internal Medicine, University of Kentucky College of Medicine, Lexington

ROBERT M. GLICKMAN, M.D.

Herrman Ludwig Blumgart Professor of Medicine, Harvard Medical School; Physician-in-Chief, Beth Israel Hospital, Boston

MARK A. GOLDBERG, M.D.

Assistant Professor of Medicine, Harvard Medical School; Associate Physician, Brigham and Women's Hospital, Boston

ARY GOLDBERGER, M.D.

Associate Professor of Medicine, Harvard Medical School; Physician, Beth Israel Hospital, Boston

DAVID W. GOLDE, M.D.

Professor of Medicine, Cornell University Medical College; Professor of Molecular Pharmacology and Therapeutics, Sloan-Kettering Division of the Cornell Graduate School of Medical Sciences; Member, Attending Physician, and Head, Division of Hematologic Oncology, Memorial Sloan-Kettering Cancer Center, New York

LEE GOLDMAN, M.D.

Professor of Medicine, Harvard Medical School; Vice-Chairman, Department of Medicine and Chief, Division of Clinical Epidemiology, Brigham and Women's Hospital, Boston

JOSEPH L. GOLDSTEIN, M.D.

Paul J. Thomas Professor and Chairman, Department of Molecular Genetics, The University of Texas Southwestern Medical Center, Dallas

RAJ K. GOYAL, M.D.

Rabb Professor of Medicine, Harvard Medical School; Chief, Division of Gastroenterology, Beth Israel Hospital, Boston

JOHN W. GRAEF, M.D.

Associate Clinical Professor of Pediatrics, Harvard Medical School; Director, The Lead/Toxicology Clinic, The Children's Hospital, Boston

HARRY B. GREENBERG, M.D.

Professor of Medicine and Microbiology and Immunology, Stanford University Medical Center, Stanford

NORTON J. GREENBERGER, M.D., M.A.C.P.

Peter T. Bohan Professor and Chairman, Department of Medicine, University of Kansas Medical Center, Kansas City

JOHN S. GREENSPAN, B.D.S, Ph.D., F.R.C.Path.

Professor and Chairman, Department of Stomatology, University of California School of Dentistry, San Francisco

JAMES E. GRIFFIN, M.D.

Professor of Internal Medicine, The University of Texas Southwestern Medical Center, Dallas

J. McLEOD GRIFFISS, M.D.

Professor of Lab Medicine and Medicine, University of California at San Francisco VA Medical Center, San Francisco

ROBERT C. GRIGGS, M.D.

Edward A. and Alma Vollertsen Rykenboer Professor of Neurophysiology, Professor of Neurology and Medicine, and Chairman, Department of Neurology, University of Rochester School of Medicine and Dentistry, University of Rochester Medical Center, Rochester

WILLIAM GROSSMAN, M.D.

Dana Professor of Medicine, Harvard Medical School; Chief, Cardiovascular Division, Beth Israel Hospital, Boston

JOHN H. GROWDON, M.D.

Professor of Neurology, Harvard Medical School; Neurologist and Director, Memory Disorders Unit, Massachusetts General Hospital, Boston

SUBHASH C. GULATI, M.D., Ph.D.

Associate Professor of Medicine, Cornell University Medical College; Associate Member and Associate Attending Physician, Memorial Sloan-Kettering Cancer Center, New York

VLADIMIR HACHINSKI, M.D.

Richard and Beryl Ivey Professor and Chairman, Department of Clinical Neurological Sciences, University of Western Ontario, University Hospital, London, Ontario

BEVRA HANNAHS HAHN, M.D.

Professor of Medicine, Department of Medicine; Chief of Rheumatology, University of California, Los Angeles, Los Angeles

ROBERT I. HANDIN, M.D.

Associate Professor of Medicine, Harvard Medical School; Director, Hematology Oncology Division, Brigham and Women's Hospital, Boston

H. HUNTER HANDSFIELD, M.D.

Professor of Medicine, University of Washington School of Medicine; Director, STD Control Program, Seattle-King County Department of Public Health, Seattle

STEPHEN L. HAUSER, M.D.

Betty Anker Fife Professor and Chairman, Department of Neurology, University of California, San Francisco

BARTON F. HAYNES, M.D.

Director, Arthritis Center; Chief, Division of Rheumatology and Immunology; Frederic M. Hanes Professor of Medicine; Director, Basic Research, Center for AIDS Research, Duke University School of Medicine, Durham

STEVEN C. HERBERT, M.D.

Associate Professor of Medicine, Harvard Medical School; Physician, Brigham and Women's Hospital, Boston

I. CRAIG HENDERSON, M.D.

Professor of Medicine; Chief of Medical Oncology; Director, Clinical Oncology Program, Moffitt-Long Hospitals, San Francisco

CHARLES B. HIGGINS, M.D.

Professor of Radiology and Chief, Magnetic Resonance Imaging, University of California School of Medicine, San Francisco

H. CLIFFORD LANE, M.D.

Clinical Director, National Institute of Allergy and Infectious Diseases, National Institutes of Health; Chief, Clinical Molecular Retrovirology Section, Laboratory of Immunoregulation, National Institute of Allergy and Infectious Diseases, NIH, Bethesda

THOMAS J. LAWLEY, M.D.

Professor and Chairman, Department of Dermatology, Emory University School of Medicine, Atlanta

ALEXANDER R. LAWTON III, M.D.

Edward C. Stahlman Professor in Pediatric Physiology and Cell Metabolism; Professor of Pediatrics and Microbiology; Head, Division of Pediatric Immunology and Rheumatology, Vanderbilt University School of Medicine, Nashville

J. MICHAEL LAZARUS, M.D.

Associate Professor of Medicine, Harvard Medical School; Senior Physician and Director of Clinical Services, Nephrology Division, Brigham & Women's Hospital, Boston

ROBERT SAMUEL LEBOVICS, M.D., F.A.C.S.

Chief, Otolaryngology, National Institute on Deafness and Other Communication Disorders, National Institutes of Health, Bethesda

RICHARD T. LEE, M.D.

Assistant Professor of Medicine, Harvard Medical School; Director, Noninvasive Cardiac Laboratory, Brigham and Women's Hospital, Boston

PHILLIP I. LERNER, M.D.

Professor of Medicine, Case Western Reserve University School of Medicine; Chief, Division of Infectious Diseases, The Mount Sinai Medical Center, Cleveland

NORMAN G. LEVINSKY, M.D.

Wade Professor and Chairman, Department of Medicine, Boston University School of Medicine; Physician-in-Chief, Boston City Hospital and Boston University Medical Center Hospital, Boston

MATTHEW E. LEVISON, M.D.

Professor of Medicine and Chief, Division of Infectious Diseases, Medical College of Pennsylvania, Philadelphia

RICHARD W. LIGHT, M.D.

Professor of Medicine, University of California, Irvine; Physician, Veterans Administration Hospital, Long Beach

CHRISTOPHER H. LINDEN, M.D., F.A.C.E.P.

Associate Professor of Medicine; Associate Director, Toxicology Service and Associate Clinical Director, Department of Emergency Medicine, University of Massachusetts Medical Center, Worcester

PETER E. LIPSKY, M.D.

Professor of Internal Medicine and Microbiology; Director, Rheumatic Diseases Division; Director, Harold C. Simmons Arthritis Research Center, The University of Texas Southwestern Medical Center at Dallas, Dallas

LEO X. LIU, M.D., D.T.M.H.

Assistant Professor of Medicine, Harvard Medical School; Division of Infectious Diseases, Department of Medicine, Beth Israel Hospital, Boston

BERNARD LO, M.D.

Professor of Medicine; Director, Program in Medical Ethics; Co-Director, Robert Wood Johnson Clinical Scholars Program; Physician, Moffitt-Long Hospitals, University of California, San Francisco

RICHARD M. LOCKSLEY, M.D.

Associate Professor of Medicine and Microbiology and Immunology and Chief, Division of Infectious Diseases, Department of Medicine, University of California, San Francisco

DAN L. LONGO, M.D.

Director, Biological Response Modifiers Program, Division of Cancer Treatment, National Cancer Institute, Frederick Cancer Research and Development Center, Frederick

FREDERICK H. LOVEJOY, Jr., M.D.

William Berenberg Professor of Pediatrics, Harvard Medical School; Associate Physician-in-Chief, The Children's Hospital, Boston

SHEILA A. LUKEHART, Ph.D.

Research Associate Professor, Department of Medicine, Division of Infectious Diseases, University of Washington School of Medicine, Seattle

LAWRENCE C. MADOFF, M.D.

Assistant Professor of Medicine, Harvard Medical School; Channing Laboratory, Brigham and Women's Hospital; Division of Infectious Diseases, Beth Israel Hospital, Boston

JAMES HARVEY MAGUIRE, M.D.

Associate Professor of Medicine, Harvard Medical School; Physician, Brigham and Women's Hospital, Boston

HENRY J. MANKIN, M.D.

Edith M. Ashley Professor of Orthopaedic Surgery, Harvard Medical School; Chief, Orthopaedic Services, Massachusetts General Hospital, Boston

JOSEPH B. MARTIN, M.D., Ph.D., F.R.C.P. (C), M.A. (Hon.)

Professor of Neurology and Chancellor, University of California, San Francisco

JOEL B. MASON, M.D.

Assistant Professor, Divisions of Clinical Nutrition and Gastroenterology; Scientist, USDA Human Nutrition Research Center on Aging, Tufts University, Boston

HENRY MASUR, M.D.

Chief, Critical Care Medicine Department, National Institutes of Health, Bethesda

ROBERT J. MAYER, M.D.

Professor of Medicine and Clinical Director, Department of Medicine, Dana-Farber Cancer Institute, Boston

JOHN D. McCONNELL, M.D.

Associate Professor of Surgery, Division of Urology, The University of Texas Southwestern Medical Center, Dallas

E. R. McFADDEN, Jr., M.D.

Argyl J. Beams Professor of Medicine and Director, Division of Pulmonary and Critical Care Medicine, Case Western Reserve University School of Medicine, Cleveland

JAMES E. McGUIGAN, M.D.

Chairman, Department of Medicine, University of Florida College of Medicine, Gainesville

NANCY K. MELLO, Ph.D.

Professor of Psychology, Department of Psychiatry (Neuroscience), Harvard Medical School, Boston; Co-Director, Alcohol and Drug Abuse Research Center, McLean Hospital, Belmont

JERRY R. MENDELL, M.D.

Professor and Chairman, Department of Neurology, The Ohio State University College of Medicine, Columbus

JOHN MENDELSOHN, M.D.

Winthrop Rockefeller Chair in Medical Oncology and Chairman, Department of Medicine, Memorial Sloan-Kettering Cancer Center

JACK H. MENDELSON, M.D.

Professor of Psychiatry (Neuroscience), Harvard Medical School, Boston; Co-Director, Alcohol and Drug Abuse Research Center, McLean Hospital, Belmont

RICHARD A. MILLER, M.D.

Associate Professor of Medicine, University of Washington School of Medicine; Chief, Infectious Disease Section, Seattle VA Medical Center, Seattle

JOHN D. MINNA, M.D.

Professor of Medicine and Pharmacology and Director, Simmons Cancer Center, The University of Texas Southwestern Medical Center, Dallas

JEROME H. MODELL, M.D.

Professor of Anesthesiology, College of Medicine, University of Florida; Senior Associate Dean for Clinical Affairs; Associate Vice President for University of Florida Health Science Center Affiliations, Gainesville

J. P. MOHR, M.D.

Sciarra Professor of Clinical Neurology, College of Physicians and Surgeons of Columbia University Neurological Institute, New York

STEPHEN MORSE, Ph.D.

Director, Division of Sexually Transmitted Diseases Laboratory Research, National Center for Infectious Diseases, Centers for Disease Control and Prevention, Atlanta

KENNETH M. MOSER, M.D.

Professor of Medicine, School of Medicine, University of California at San Diego; Director, Pulmonary/Critical Care Division, UCSD Medical Center, San Diego

ARNOLD M. MOSES, M.D.

Professor of Medicine and Director, Clinical Research, Unit, State University of New York Health Science Center, Syracuse

HARALAMPOS M. MOUTSOPOULOS, M.D.

Professor and Head of Medicine, Department of Internal Medicine, University of Ioannina Medical School, Ioannina, Greece

ROBERT F. MUNFORD, M.D.

Professor of Internal Medicine and Microbiology, University of Texas Southwestern Medical Center, Dallas

DANIEL M. MUSHER, M.D.

Chief, Infectious Disease Section, Veterans Affairs Medical Center; Professor of Medicine and Professor of Microbiology and Immunology, Baylor College of Medicine, Houston

ROBERT J. MYERBURG, M.D.

Professor of Medicine and Physiology and Director, Division of Cardiology, University of Miami School of Medicine, Miami

LEE M. NADLER, M.D.

Professor of Medicine, Harvard Medical School; Division of Tumor Immunology, Dana-Farber Cancer Institute, Boston

THEODORE ELLIOT NASH, M.D.

Senior Scientist, Laboratory of Parasitic Diseases, National Institutes of Health, Bethesda

LAURENCE NEEDLEMAN, M.D.

Associate Professor of Radiology and Associate Director, Division of Diagnostic Ultrasound, Thomas Jefferson University Hospital, Philadelphia

THOMAS B. NUTMAN, M.D.

Senior Investigator, Laboratory of Parasitic Diseases, National Institute of Allergy and Infectious Diseases, National Institutes of Health, Bethesda

JOHN OATES, M.D.

Professor and Chairman, Department of Medicine, Vanderbilt University School of Medicine; Physician-in-Chief, Vanderbilt University Hospital, Nashville

JERROLD M. OLEFSKY, M.D.

Professor of Medicine and Head, Division of Endocrinology and Metabolism, School of Medicine, University of California at San Diego, La Jolla

ANDREW B. ONDERDONK, Ph.D.

Associate Professor of Pathology, Harvard Medical School; Director, Clinical Microbiology Laboratory, Brigham and Women's Hospital, Boston

STUART H. ORKIN, M.D.

Leland Fikes Professor of Pediatric Medicine, Harvard Medical School; Children's Hospital, Boston

ROBERT A. O'ROURKE, M.D.

Charles Conrad Brown Distinguished Professor of Medicine, The University of Texas Health Science Center at San Antonio; Director of Cardiology, The University of Texas Health Science Center Teaching Hospitals, San Antonio

DARWIN L. PALMER, M.D.

Professor of Medicine and Chief, Division of Infectious Diseases, University of New Mexico School of Medicine, Albuquerque

JOSEPH E. PARRILLO, M.D.

James B. Herrick Professor of Medicine, Rush Medical College; Chief, Section of Cardiology; Chief, Section of Critical Care Medicine and Medical Director, Rush Heart Institute, Rush-Presbyterian-St. Luke's Medical Center, Chicago

RICHARD C. PASTERNAK, M.D.

Assistant Professor of Medicine, Harvard Medical School; Director of Preventive Cardiology and Cardiac Rehabilitation, Massachusetts General Hospital, Boston

PETER L. PERINE, M.D.

Professor of Epidemiology, Center for AIDS and STD, University of Washington, Seattle; Professor of Tropical Public Health and Medicine Emeritus, Uniformed Services University of the Health Sciences, Bethesda

ELIOT A. PHILLIPSON, M.D.

Sir John and Lady Eaton Professor of Medicine and Chair, Department of Medicine, University of Toronto; Physician-in-Chief, Mount Sinai Hospital, Toronto

GERALD B. PIER, Ph.D.

Associate Professor of Medicine, Harvard Medical School; Channing Labatory, Brigham and Women's Hospital, Boston

DANIEL K. PODOLSKY, M.D.

Associate Professor of Medicine, Harvard Medical School; Chief, Gastrointestinal Unit, Massachusetts General Hospital, Boston

RONALD J. POLINSKY, M.D.

Senior Associate Director, Human Pharmacology, Drug Safety Department, Sandoz Research Institute, Sandoz Pharmaceuticals Corporation, East Hanover, New Jersey

RONALD E. POLK, Pharm.D.

Professor of Pharmacy and Medicine, School of Pharmacy, Medical College of Virginia, Virginia Commonwealth University, Richmond

MATTHEW POLLACK, M.D.

Professor of Medicine, Uniformed Services University of the Health Sciences, F. Edward Hebert School of Medicine, Bethesda

JOHN T. POTTS, Jr., M.D.

Jackson Professor of Clinical Medicine, Harvard Medical School; Physician-in-Chief, Massachusetts General Hospital, Boston

LAWRIE W. POWELL, M.D.

Professor of Medicine, The University of Queensland; Director, Queensland Institute of Medical Research, Brisbane

DARWIN J. PROCKOP, M.D.

Professor and Chairman, Department of Biochemistry and Molecular Biology, Jefferson Medical College of Thomas Jefferson University; Director, Jefferson Institute of Molecular Medicine, Philadelphia

AMY PRUITT, M.D.

Assistant Professor of Neurology, University of Pennsylvania School of Medicine and Graduate Hospital, Philadelphia

LOUIS J. PTÁČEK, M.D.

Department of Neurology, The University of Utah School of Medicine, Salt Lake City

JOEL M. RAPPEPORT, M.D.

Professor of Medicine, Yale University School of Medicine; Director, Bone Marrow Transplantation Program, Yale New Haven Hospital, New Haven

NEIL H. RASKIN, M.D.

Professor of Neurology, University of California, San Francisco

C. GEORGE RAY, M.D.

Professor and Chairman, Department of Pediatrics, St. Louis University School of Medicine, St. Louis

SHARON LEE REED, M.D.

Associate Professor of Pathology and Medicine and Associate Director, Microbiology Laboratory, Division of Infectious Diseases, UCSD Medical Center, San Diego

ANTONIO J. REGINATO, M.D.

Head, Division of Rheumatology; Professor of Medicine, Cooper Hospital/University Medical Center, University of Medicine and Dentistry of New Jersey/Robert Wood Johnson Medical School at Camden, Camden

RICHARD C. REICHMAN, M.D.

Professor of Medicine and Head, Infectious Disease Unit, University of Rochester School of Medicine and Dentistry, Rochester

NEIL M. RESNICK, M.D.

Assistant Professor of Medicine, Harvard Medical School; Chief, Division of Gerontology, Brigham and Women's Hospital; Geriatric Research Education and Clinical Center, Brockton-West Roxbury Veterans Administration Medical Center, Boston

HERBERT Y. REYNOLDS, M.D.

Chairman, Department of Medicine and J. Lloyd Huck Professor of Medicine, The Pennsulvania State University; University Hospital, The Milton S. Hershey Medical Center, Hershey

STUART RICH, M.D.

Professor of Medicine and Chief, Section of Cardiology, University of Illinois at Chicago College of Medicine, Chicago

GARY S. RICHARDSON, M.D.

Instructor in Medicine, Harvard Medical School; Associate Physician, Brigham and Women's Hospital, Boston

HAL B. RICHERSON, M.D.

Professor of Internal Medicine, University of Iowa College of Medicine; University of Iowa Hospitals and Clinics, Iowa City

JAMES M. RICHTER, M.D.

Assistant Professor of Medicine, Harvard Medical School; Chief, Gastrointestinal Clinic, Massachusetts General Hospital, Boston

R. PAUL ROBERTSON, M.D.

Professor of Medicine and Cell Biology; Director, Division of Diabetes, Endocrinology and Metabolism, University of Minnesota, Minneapolis

ALLAN H. ROPPER, M.D.

Professor of Neurology, Tufts University School of Medicine; Chief, Division of Neurology, St. Elizabeth's Medical Center, Boston

IRWIN H. ROSENBERG, M.D.

Professor of Medicine, Nutrition and Physiology; Director, USDA Human Nutrition Research Center on Aging, Tufts University, Boston

LEON E. ROSENBERG, M.D.

President, Bristol-Myers Squibb Pharmaceutical Research Institute, Princeton

WENDELL F. ROSSE, M.D.

Florence Reynaud McAlister Professor of Medicine and Medical Research, Duke University School of Medicine; Duke University Medical Center, Durham

DANIEL ROTROSEN, M.D.

Medical Office, Laboratory of Host Defenses, National Institute of Allergy and Infectious Diseases, National Institutes of Health, Bethesda

JODI ROY, M.S., R.D.

Frances Stern Nutrition Center, New England Medical Center Hospital, Boston

ARTHUR H. RUBENSTEIN, M.D.

Lowell T. Coggeshall Professor; Chairman, Department of Medicine, University of Chicago Pritzker School of Medicine, Chicago

JEREMY N. RUSKIN, M.D.

Associate Professor of Medicine, Harvard Medical School; Director, Cardiac Arrhythmia Service, Massachusetts General Hospital, Boston

ARTHUR I. SAGALOWSKY, M.D.

Professor of Urology and Surgical Director of Renal Transplantation, The University of Texas Southwestern Medical Center, Dallas

MATTHEW SAMORE, M.D.

Instructor in Medicine, Harvard Medical School; New England Deaconess Hospital, Boston

JAY P. SANFORD, M.D.

Professor of Internal Medicine, University of Texas Southwestern Medical School; Dean Emeritus, Uniformed Services University of the Health Sciences, Dallas

DAVID A. SCHEINBERG, M.D., Ph.D.

Chief, Leukemia Service, Memorial Sloan-Kettering Cancer Center, New York

I. HERBERT SCHEINBERG, M.D.

Senior Lecturer in Medicine, College of Physicians and Surgeons, Columbia University; Senior Research Associate, St. Luke's/Roosevelt Hospital, New York

W. MICHAEL SCHELD, M.D.

Professor of Internal Medicine and Neurosurgery and Associate Chair for Residency Programs, University of Virginia School of Medicine, Charlottesville

ALAN L. SCHILLER, M.D.

Irene Heinz Given and John LaPorte Given Professor and Chairman of Pathology, Mount Sinai School of Medicine; Chairman of Pathology, The Mount Sinai Hospital, New York

ROBERT T. SCHOOLEY, M.D.

Professor of Medicine and Head, Infectious Disease Division, University of Colorado Health Sciences Center, Denver

JOHN SPEER SCHROEDER, M.D.

Professor of Medicine (Cardiology), Stanford University School of Medicine; Stanford Hospital, Stanford

ANNE SCHUCHAT, M.D.

Medical Epidemiologist, Meningitis and Special Pathogens Branch, Division of Bacterial and Mycotic Diseases, National Center for Infectious Diseases, Centers for Disease Control and Prevention, Atlanta

MARC A. SCHUCKIT, M.D.

Professor of Psychiatry, School of Medicine, University of California at San Diego; Director, Alcohol Research Center, San Diego Veteran's Administration Medical Center, La Jolla

PETER H. SCHUR, M.D.

Professor of Medicine, Harvard Medical School; Department of Rheumatology, Brigham and Women's Hospital, Boston

DAVID S. SEGAL, Ph.D.

Professor of Psychiatry, University of California at San Diego, La Jolla

JULIAN I. SEIFTER, M.D.

Associate Professor of Medicine, Harvard Medical School; Physician, Brigham and Women's Hospital, Boston

ANDREW P. SELWYN, M.D.

Associate Professor of Medicine, Harvard Medical School; Director of Cardiac Catheterization, Brigham and Women's Hospital, Boston

PETER A. SELWYN, M.D., M.P.H.

Associate Professor of Internal Medicine, Epidemiology and Public Health, and Associate Director, AIDS Program, Yale University School of Medicine, New Haven

MARY-ANN SHAFER, M.D.

Professor of Pediatrics; Associate Director, Division of Adolescent Medicine, Department of Pediatrics, School of Medicine, University of California, San Francisco

GORDON C. SHARP, M.D.

Curators' Professor and Michael Einbender Distinguished Professor of Medicine; Director, Division of Immunology and Rheumatology; Director, Arthritis Center; Director, Missouri Arthritis Rehabilitation Research and Training Center; Associate Chairman for Research, Department of Internal Medicine, University of Missouri-Columbia School of Medicine; Director, Antinuclear Antibody Laboratory, University of Missouri Hospital & Clinics, Columbia

ELIZABETH M. SHORT, M.D.

Associate Chief Medical Director for Academic Affairs, Department of Veteran's Affairs, Washington, DC

GEORGE R. SIBER, M.D.

Associate Professor of Medicine, Harvard Medical School; Director, Massachusetts Public Health Biologic Laboratories, Jamaica Plain

WILLIAM SILEN, M.D.

Johnson and Johnson Professor of Surgery, Harvard Medical School; Surgeon-in-Chief; Beth Israel Hospital, Boston

FRED E. SILVERSTEIN, M.D.

Professor of Medicine and Director, Gastrointestinal Endoscopy Fellowship Training, University of Washington School of Medicine, Seattle

KARL L. SKORECKI, M.D., F.R.C.P.(C)

Director, Division of Nephrology, Department of Medicine and Pediatrics, University of Toronto, Toronto

THOMAS L. SLAMOVITZ, M.D.

Professor and Vice Chairman, Department of Ophthalmology and Professor of Neurology and Neurosurgery, Albert Einstein College of Medicine/Montefiore Medical Center, New York

CHRISTOPHER A. SLAPAK, M.D.

Assistant Professor of Medicine, Harvard Medical School and Dana-Farber Cancer Institute, Boston

JAMES B. SNOW, JR., M.D.

Director, National Institute on Deafness and Other Communication Disorders, National Institutes of Health, Bethesda

ARTHUR J. SOBER, M.D.

Associate Professor of Dermatology, Harvard Medical School; Associate Chief of Dermatology, Massachusetts General Hospital, Boston

FRANK E. SPEIZER, M.D.

Edward H. Kass Professor of Medicine, Harvard Medical School; Co-Director, Channing Laboratory, Brigham and Women's Hospital, Boston

ANDREW SPIELMAN, SD

Professor of Tropical Public Health, Harvard School of Public Health, Boston

WALTER E. STAMM, M.D.

Professor of Medicine, University of Washington School of Medicine; Head, Infectious Diseases, Harborview Medical Center, Seattle

ALLEN C. STEERE, M.D.

Professor of Medicine and Chief, Rheumatology/Immunology, New England Medical Center and Tufts University School of Medicine, Boston

ROBERT S. STERN, M.D.

Professor, Department of Dermatology, Beth Israel Hospital, Boston

DENNIS L. STEVENS, M.D., Ph.D.

Professor of Medicine, University of Washington School of Medicine, Seattle; Chief, Infectious Diseases, VA Medical Center, Boise

GENE H. STOLLERMAN, M.D.

Professor of Medicine and Public Health, Boston University; University Hospital, Boston

RICHARD M. STONE, M.D.

Assistant Professor of Medicine, Harvard Medical School and Dana-Farber Cancer Institute, Boston

STEPHEN E. STRAUS, M.D.

Chief, Laboratory of Clinical Investigation, National Institute of Allergy and Infectious Diseases, National Institutes of Health, Bethesda

DAVID H.P. STREETEN, M.D.

Professor of Medicine and Head, Section of Endocrinology, State University of New York Health Science Center, Syracuse

ROBERT A. SWERLICK, M.D.

Associate Professor, Department of Dermatology, Emory University School of Medicine, Atlanta

RUP TANDAN, M.D., M.R.C.P.

Associate Professor of Neurology, University of Vermont College of Medicine; Attending Neurologist, Medical Center Hospital of Vermont, Burlington

JOEL D. TAUROG, M.D.

Associate Professor, Department of Internal Medicine and Investigator, Harold C. Simmons Arthritis Research Center, The University of Texas Southwestern Medical Center; Attending Physician, Parkland Memorial Hospital, Sale Lipshy University Hospital, Veterans Administration Medical Center, Dallas

BAYU TEKLU, M.D.

Professor and Chairman, Department of Internal Medicine, College of Medicine, King Saud University, Abha Branch; Consultant Physician, Asir Central Hospital, Saudi Arabia

STEPHEN F. TEMPLETON, M.D.

Assistant Professor of Dermatology and Pathology, Emory University School of Medicine, Atlanta

E. DONNALL THOMAS, M.D.

Professor of Medicine Emeritus, University of Washington; Member, Fred Hutchinson Cancer Research Center, Seattle

LUCY STUART TOMPKINS, M.D.

Associate Professor of Medicine (Infectious Diseases and Geographic Medicine) and Microbiology and Immunology, Stanford University School of Medicine; Director, Clinical Microbiology Laboratory, Stanford University Medical Center, Stanford

PHILLIP P. TOSKES, M.D.

Professor of Medicine and Chief, Division of Gastroenterology, University of Florida, Gainesville

GERARD TROMP, M.D.

Research Assistant Professor, Department of Biochemistry and Molecular Biology, Jefferson Medical College of Thomas Jefferson University, Philadelphia

E. P. TRULOCK, M.D.

Associate Professor of Medicine, Washington University School of Medicine; Barnes Hospital, St. Louis

KENNETH L. TYLER, M.D.

Associate Professor of Neurology, Medicine and Microbiology, University of Colorado Health Sciences Center; Chief, Neurology Service, VA Medical Center, Denver

DAVID VALLE, M.D.

Professor of Pediatrics and Molecular Biology and Genetics, Johns Hopkins University School of Medicine; Investigator, Howard Hughes Medical Institute, Baltimore

MAURICE VICTOR, M.D.

Professor of Medicine (Neurology), Dartmouth Medical School, Hanover; Distinguished Physician of the Veterans Administration, White River Junction

JAMES F. WALLACE, M.D.

Professor of Medicine, University of Washington School of Medicine; Associate Physican-in-Chief, University of Washington Medical Center, Seattle

RICHARD J. WALLACE, Jr., M.D.

Chairman, Department of Microbiology, University of Texas Health Center, Tyler

PETER D. WALZER, M.D.

Professor of Medicine, University of Cincinnati College of Medicine; Chief, Infectious Disease Section, VA Medical Center, Cincinnati

LEONARD WARTOFSKY, M.D.

Professor of Medicine and Physiology, Uniformed Services University of the Health Sciences; Chairman, Department of Medicine, Washington Hospital Center, Washington, DC

CARL V. WASHINGTON, Jr. M.D.

Assistant Professor of Dermatology, Emory University School of Medicine, Atlanta

STEVEN E. WEINBERGER, M.D.

Associate Professor of Medicine, Harvard Medical School; Associate Chairman for Education, Department of Medicine, and Clinical Director, Pulmonary and Critical Care Division, Beth Israel Hospital, Boston

LOUIS WEINSTEIN, M.D., Ph.D.

Senior Physician (Emeritus), Department of Medicine, Brigham and Women's Hospital

ROBERT A. WEINSTEIN, M.D., F.A.C.P.

Professor of Medicine and Program Director, Joint University of Illinois/University of Chicago Infectious Disease Fellowship Training Program, Department of Medicine, Michael Reese Hospital and Medical Center, Chicago

PETER F. WELLER, M.D.

Associate Professor of Medicine, Harvard Medical School; Division of Infectious Diseases, Department of Medicine, Beth Israel Hospital, Boston

MICHAEL R. WESSELS, M.D.

Associate Professor of Medicine, Harvard Medical School; Associate Physician, Beth Israel Hospital; Division of Infectious Diseases, Channing Laboratory, Brigham and Women's Hospital, Boston

NICHOLAS J. WHITE, M.B., B.S., B.Sc., M.R.C.P.

Wellcome Mahidol University, Oxford Tropical Medicine Research Programme, Faculty of Tropical Medicine, Mahidol University, Bangkok

RICHARD J. WHITLEY, M.D.

Loeb Eminent Scholar in Pediatrics and Professor of Pediatrics, Medicine and Microbiology, University of Alabama at Birmingham, Birmingham

GRANT R. WILKINSON, Ph.D.

Professor of Pharmacology, Vanderbilt University School of Medicine, Nashville

GORDON H. WILLIAMS, M.D.

Professor of Medicine, Harvard Medical School; Chief, Endocrine-Hypertension Division, Brigham and Women's Hospital, Boston

JEAN D. WILSON, M.D.

Charles Cameron Sprague Distinguished Chair and Professor of Internal Medicine; Chief, Division of Endocrinology and Metabolism, The University of Texas Southwestern Medical Center, Dallas

BRUCE U. WINTROUB, M.D.

Professor and Chairman, Department of Dermatology, University of California at San Francisco; Associate Dean, UCSF/Mt. Zion Medical Center, San Francisco

SHELDON M. WOLFF, M.D.

Endicott Professor and Chairman, Department of Medicine, Tufts University School of Medicine; Physician-in-Chief, New England Medical Center, Boston

BEVERLY WOO, M.D.

Assistant Professor of Medicine, Harvard Medical School; Physician, Brigham and Women's Hospital, Boston

ALASTAIR J. J. WOOD, M.B.Ch.B., FRCP (Edin)

Professor of Medicine and Professor of Pharmacology, Vanderbilt University School of Medicine; Attending Physician, Vanderbilt University Hospital, Nashville

THEODORE E. WOODWARD, M.D., M.A.C.P.

Professor of Medicine Emeritus, University of Maryland School of Medicine and Hospital, Baltimore

ROBERT L. WORTMANN, M.D.

Professor and Chairman, Department of Medicine, East Carolina University School of Medicine; Chief Medical Service, Pitt County Memorial Hospital, University Medical Center of Eastern Carolina-Pitt County, Greenville

SHIRLEY H. WRAY, M.D., Ph.D., F.R.C.P.

Associate Professor of Neurology, Harvard Medical School; Director, Unit for Neurovisual Disorders, Department of Neurology, Massachusetts General Hospital, Boston

PAUL W. WRIGHT, M.D.

Professor of Family Practice, University of Texas Health Center, Tyler

JOSHUA WYNNE, M.D.

Professor of Internal Medicine and Chief, Division of Cardiology, Wayne State University School of Medicine; Chief, Section of Cardiology, Harper Hospital, Detroit

KIM B. YANCEY, M.D.

Senior Investigator, Dermatology Branch, National Cancer Institute, National Institutes of Health, Bethesda

JAMES B. YOUNG, M.D.

Professor of Medicine, Northwestern University Medical School; Attending Physician, Northwestern Memorial Hospital, Chicago

DORI F. ZALEZNIK, M.D.

Assistant Professor of Medicine, Harvard Medical School; Hospital Epidemiologist, Beth Israel Hospital, Boston

conventional units in parentheses. In most instances, the interconversion between SI and conventional units is straightforward. However, it is imperative that readers consult their own laboratory for normal values. Perhaps the greatest potential danger inherent in the existence of the two systems is in the interpretation of plasma glucose and plasma calcium levels, but caution should be observed in the interpretation of all laboratory values.

In view of the requirements for continuing education for licensure and relicensure, as well as the emphasis on certification and recertification, a revision of the *Pre-Test Self-Assessment and Review* will be published with this edition. It consists of several hundred questions based on *Harrison's*, along with answers and explanations for the answers. In addition, the *Companion Handbook* that was pioneered as a supplement to the 11th edition of *Harrison's* is being updated and will appear shortly.

One of the strengths of *Harrison's* is the close-knit relationship among the editors. In that context, we are delighted to welcome as a new editor Dr. Dennis L. Kasper, who possesses great depth and expertise in all aspects of infectious diseases. Dr. Kasper is Chief of the Infectious Diseases Division at the Beth Israel Hospital in Boston and serves as Co-Director of the Channing Laboratory, which is associated with the Brigham and Women's Hospital. He is also Professor of Medicine at the Harvard Medical School. We welcome Dr. Kasper as both a new editor and distinguished colleague.

We also wish to express our appreciation to our many associates and colleagues, who, as experts in their fields, have helped us with constructive criticism and helpful suggestions: Robert Alpern, Jon Astor, JudyAnn Bigby, Troyen Brennan, Neil A. Breslau, Bruce Bristrian, Charles Carpenter, Richard Davey, William Dec, William P. Dillon, Robert Dluhy, Jeffrey Drazen, Stuart J. Eisendrath, Judy Falloon, Christopher Fanta, Robert A. Fishman, David W. Foster, Patricia Fraser, Jonas Galper, Alan M. Gelb, Donald Goldmann, Stephen Goldring, Linnie Golightly, Christine Grady, James E. Griffin, Rachel Haft, Robert Handin, Seigo Izumo, Joseph H. Keffer, Arthur Kleinman, Anthony Komaroff, H. Clifford Lane, Russell K. Laros, Jr., Richard M. Locksley, Joseph Loscalzo, Carlos Luciano, James Maguire, Robert Mayer, Walter O'Donnell, Tristram G. Parslow, Dolores M. Peterson, Lynn Peterson, Michael Polis, Kenneth Ryan, Frank Sacks, Jay P. Sanford, Paul Sax, Michael Seiden, Egilius Spierings, Chirstopher Stowell, Daniel Vlock, Robert Walker, Steven Weinberger, Michael Wessels, Alison Wichman and Edward Yeh.

This book could not have been edited without the dedicated help of our coworkers in the editorial offices of the individual editors. We are especially indebted to: Dorothy Binford, Marie Bullock, Martha Cassin, Hilda Gardner, Christy K. Gonzales, Brenda H. Hennis, Leslie LaPiana, Julie McCoy, Jaylyn Olivo, Lucy Renzi, Kathryn A. Saxon, and Elin Woodger.

Finally, we continue to be indebted to two outstanding members of the McGraw-Hill organization: J. Dereck Jeffers, Editor-in-Chief, and Stuart Boynton, Development Editor. They are an effective team who have given the editors constant encouragement and sage advice, and have been of enormous help in bringing this edition to fruition in a timely manner.

THE EDITORS

PREFACE

Since the first edition of *Harrison's Principles of Internal Medicine* was published nearly 50 years ago, each subsequent edition has built upon the solid clinical foundation and scientific advances occurring in the interim. In the present 13th edition of *Harrison's*, the Editors have extensively revised the text to reflect important advances in our understanding of the biology and pathophysiology of disease and at the same time to build appropriate links between the extraordinary advances in basic science and clinical medicine, and to emphasize these advances while retaining those facts which, while not new, remain clinically useful and important. Every chapter in the 13th edition has been revised or substantially rewritten, and major new ones have been added. In this preface, we cannot describe all of these revised sections. However, we would like to call to the reader's attention some of the most important ones:

Part One, "Introduction to Clinical Medicine," contains new chapters dealing with medical ethics and the impact of social factors on disease, including the effects of age, gender, genetic background, geography, and ethnic origin. These factors importantly influence the incidence and clinical expression of human disease. Examples of women's health issues discussed in Chap. 5 include screening for ischemic heart disease and discussions of osteoporosis and immunologically mediated diseases in women. Important medical disorders during pregnancy are dealt with in a new Chap. 6. A new Chap. 8, "Geriatric Medicine," describes age-related changes in each organ system and their clinical consequences. There is also a detailed discussion of the management of common geriatric conditions, including intellectual impairment, mobility, incontinence, and iatrogenic drug reactions. Two timely chapters (9 and 10) focus on cost awareness and the quantitative aspects of medicine.

Part Two, "Cardinal Manifestations of Disease," remains the mainstay of this edition, and serves as a comprehensive introduction to clinical medicine. Major patient symptoms are reviewed by organ systems and correlated with specific disease states—the basis of differential diagnosis. The 13th edition also contains chapters on headache, back and neck pain, fever, including fever of unknown origin, and disturbances of smell, taste, and hearing. There is an entirely new and extensively rewritten chapter on diarrhea and constipation, as well as a completely new chapter on jaundice.

Part Three, "Genetics and Disease," has been extensively updated, including a new chapter on genes and neoplasia.

Part Four, "Clinical Pharmacology" and Part Five, "Clinical Nutrition," have been reorganized and updated. The chapters on clinical pharmacology include principles of drug therapy and a new chapter on adverse reactions to drugs. Up-to-date coverage of the physiology and pharmacology of the autonomic nervous system explores its key role in many disease states and the various ways in which drugs interact with this system. Included here also is an updated chapter on G proteins and the regulation of second messengers.

Coverage of nutrition in clinical medicine encompasses nutritional requirements, the assessment of nutritional status, important eating disorders such as anorexia nervosa and bulimia, and obesity. New discussions are presented on diet therapy, including enteral and parenteral nutrition.

A primarily etiologically oriented review in Part Six, "Infectious Disease," has been extensively revised and updated under the aegis of our new editor, Dennis L. Kasper. Here the reader will find the latest approaches to the diagnosis, prevention, and treatment of bacterial, viral, and fungal infections and parasitic infestations. New chapters include "Infections (Excluding AIDS) in Injection Drug Users," "Infections in the Immunocompromised Host," and "Infec-

tions of Skin, Muscle, and Soft Tissues." There have also been major revisions of chapters covering host-organism interaction, the laboratory diagnosis of infectious diseases, septicemia and septic shock, nosocomial infections, and molecular mechanisms of bacterial pathogenesis. There is an important and up-to-date chapter on the human retroviruses.

We believe that the chapter on HIV disease and AIDS by Anthony S. Fauci and H. Clifford Lane is one of the most comprehensive and up-to-date treatises on AIDS. It covers the areas from the natural history and epidemiology to a scholarly treatise on the immunopathogenic mechanisms of HIV disease. In addition, the chapter contains both an organ system by organ system approach as well as an infection breakdown of the major complications of HIV disease.

The core of *Harrison's*, disorders of the organ systems, encompasses Parts Seven through Fourteen, and includes succinct accounts of the pathophysiology of the major human diseases, with emphasis on disease manifestations, diagnostic procedures, differential diagnosis, and treatment strategies. This comprehensive review of organ system disorders includes new chapters on electrocardiography, with excellent new illustrations on the electrocardiographic recognition of acute myocardial infarction. There are updated chapters on cystic fibrosis, lung transplantation, glomerulopathies associated with multisystem diseases, acid-peptic disease (with special focus on *H. pylori*), acute and chronic hepatitis, and liver transplantation.

The section on hematology and oncology includes chapters on oncogenes and tumor suppressor genes, with thorough discussions of p53, the tumor suppressor gene most commonly lost or mutated in human cancers. There is an important new chapter on cancer therapy, with emphasis on immunotherapy and the potential role of gene therapy. There are also new chapters on disorders affecting multiple endocrine systems, porphyrias, and gout. The chapter on diabetes includes a discussion of the impact of tight control on the development of diabetic complications.

In the Part Fourteen, "Neurological Diseases," there are new chapters on the impact of neurobiology on both neurology and psychiatry. There is also a detailed tabulation of the recent molecular genetic discoveries in neurology. There are new chapters on clinical electrophysiology, demyelinating diseases like multiple sclerosis, bacterial meningitis and brain abscess, viral diseases of the central nervous system, and disorders of the autonomic nervous system. For the first time there is a chapter on chronic fatigue syndrome, an entity which has created great interest because of its relationship to psychosomatic medicine.

Finally, Part Fifteen, "Environmental and Occupational Hazards," has been expanded and reorganized.

In the 12th edition of *Harrison's*, the editors decided to identify laboratory data using the International System (SI) of units for clinical laboratory values, plus the conventional system of laboratory nomenclature used in most hospitals in the United States. We felt this was important, since SI units are in frequent use in many countries other than the United States. In the 12th edition and in the present 13th edition, we have listed the SI units first and the conventional units in parentheses for all measurements except blood pressure, which is given only in millimeters of mercury, and for those measurements in which the numbers are the same for both systems. As the readers of the medical literature may be aware, in 1992 the *New England Journal of Medicine*, having previously endorsed SI units, decided to "retreat" to the use of only conventional units. However, the *Harrison's* editors have concluded that, at least for the 13th edition, we should continue to use the SI units, with

1 THE PRACTICE OF MEDICINE

THE EDITORS

WHAT IS EXPECTED OF THE PHYSICIAN The practice of medicine combines both science and art. The role of science in medicine is clear. Technology based on science is the foundation for the solution to many clinical problems; the dazzling advances in biochemical methodology and in biophysical imaging techniques that allow access to the remotest recesses of the body are the products of science. So too are the therapeutic maneuvers which increasingly are a major part of medical practice. Yet skill in the most sophisticated application of laboratory technology or the use of the latest therapeutic modality alone does not make a good physician. The ability to extract from a mass of contradictory physical signs and from the crowded computer printouts of laboratory data those items which are of crucial significance, to know in a difficult case whether to "treat" or to "watch," to determine when a clinical clue is worth pursuing or when to dismiss it as a "red herring," and to estimate in any given patient whether a proposed treatment entails a greater risk than the disease are all involved in the decisions which the clinician, skilled in the practice of medicine, must make many times each day. This combination of medical knowledge, intuition, and judgment is the *art of medicine*. It is as necessary to the practice of medicine as is a sound scientific base.

The editors of the first edition of this book defined what is expected of the physician. Their words ring as true now as they did then.

No greater opportunity, responsibility, or obligation can fall to the lot of a human being than to become a physician. In the care of the suffering he needs technical skill, scientific knowledge, and human understanding. He who uses these with courage, with humility, and with wisdom will provide a unique service for his fellow man, and will build an enduring edifice of character within himself. The physician should ask of his destiny no more than this; he should be content with no less.

Tact, sympathy and understanding are expected of the physician, for the patient is no mere collection of symptoms, signs, disordered functions, damaged organs, and disturbed emotions. He is human, fearful, and hopeful, seeking relief, help and reassurance. To the physician, as to the anthropologist, nothing human is strange or repulsive. The misanthrope may become a smart diagnostician of organic disease, but he can scarcely hope to succeed as a physician. The true physician has a Shakespearean breadth of interest in the wise and the foolish, the proud and the humble, the stoic hero and the whining rogue. He cares for people.

THE PATIENT-PHYSICIAN RELATIONSHIP It may be trite to emphasize that physicians need to approach patients not as "cases" or "diseases" but as individuals whose problems all too often transcend the complaints which bring them to the doctor. Most patients are anxious and frightened. Often they go to great ends to convince themselves that illness does not exist, or unconsciously they set up elaborate defenses to divert attention from the real problem that they perceive to be serious or life-threatening. Some patients use illness to gain attention or to serve as a crutch to extricate themselves from an emotionally stressful situation; some even feign physical illness. Whatever the patient's attitude, the physician needs to consider the terrain in which an illness occurs—in terms not only of the patients themselves but also of their families and social backgrounds. All too often medical workups and records fail to include essential information about the patient's origins, schooling, job, home and family, hopes and fears. Without this knowledge, it is difficult for the physician to gain rapport with the patient or to develop insight into the patient's illness. Such a relationship must be based on thorough knowledge of the patient and on mutual trust and the ability to communicate with one another.

The direct, one-to-one patient-physician relationship which traditionally has characterized the practice of medicine is changing, primarily because of the changing setting in which medicine is being practiced. Often the management of the individual patient requires the active participation of a variety of trained professional personnel as well as several physicians. In most instances, health care is a team effort. The patient can benefit greatly from such collaboration, but *it is the duty of the primary physician to guide the patient through an illness.* To carry out this increasingly difficult task, this physician must have some familiarity with the techniques, skills, and objectives of specialist physicians as well as colleagues in the fields allied to medicine. In giving the patient an opportunity to receive all the benefits of the important advances of science, the primary physician must, in the last analysis, retain responsibility for the major decisions concerning diagnosis and treatment.

Increasingly, patients are cared for by groups of physicians, clinics, hospitals, or health-maintenance organizations (HMOs) rather than by individual, independent practitioners. There are many potential advantages in the use of such organized medical groups, but there are also drawbacks, the chief of which is the *loss of the concept of the physician who is primarily and continuously responsible.* It is essential that even in the group setting each patient have a physician who has an overview of the patient's problems and who maintains familiarity with the patient's reaction to his or her illness, to the drugs given, and to the challenges that the patient faces. Moreover, because a number of physicians may, at any one time, contribute to the care of a particular patient, accurate and detailed medical records are essential to patient care.

The modern hospital poses a particularly intimidating environment for most patients. Lying in a bed surrounded by air jets, buttons, and lights; invaded by tubes and wires; beset by the numerous members of the health care team—nurses, nurses' aides, physicians' assistants, social workers, technologists, physical therapists, medical students, house officers, attending and consulting physicians, and many others; transported to special laboratories and x-ray chambers replete with blinking lights and strange sounds, it is little wonder that patients lose their sense of reality. In fact, the physician is often the only tenuous link between the patient and the real world. A strong personal relationship with the physician is essential in order to sustain the patient in such a stressful situation.

Many influences in contemporary society have the potential of leading to the impersonalization of medical care. Some of these have been mentioned already and include (1) vigorous efforts to reduce the escalating costs of health care, (2) the increasing reliance on technologic advances and computerization for many aspects of diagnosis and treatment, (3) the increased geographic mobility of both patients and physicians, (4) the growing number of health-maintenance organizations, in which the patient may have little choice in selecting a physician, (5) the need for more than a single physician to be involved in the care of most patients who are seriously ill, and (6) an increasing reliance by patients to express their disappointments with the health care system by legal means (i.e., by malpractice litigation). Given these changes in the medical care system, maintaining the humane aspects of medical care and the empathetic qualities of the physician is a major challenge. It is now more important than ever that the physician consider each patient to be a unique individual deserving of humane treatment, regardless of personal or financial circumstances.

The American Board of Internal Medicine has defined humanistic qualities as encompassing integrity, respect, and compassion. Availability, the expression of sincere concern, the willingness to take the time to explain all aspects of the patient's illness, and an attitude of being nonjudgmental with patients who have lifestyles, attitudes, and values different from those of the physician and which he or she may in some instances even find repugnant are just a few of the characteristics of the humane physician. Every physician will, at times, be challenged by patients who evoke strongly negative (and occasionally strongly positive) emotional responses. Physicians should be alert to their own reactions to such patients and situations and consciously monitor and control their behavior so that the patients' best interests remain the principal motivation for their actions at all times.

The famous statement of Dr. Francis Peabody is even more relevant today than when delivered more than a half century ago:

The significance of the intimate personal relationship between physician and patient cannot be too strongly emphasized, for in an extraordinarily large number of cases both the diagnosis and treatment are directly dependent on it. One of the essential qualities of the clinician is interest in humanity, for the secret of the care of the patient is in caring for the patient.

CLINICAL SKILLS   History taking   The written history of an illness should embody all the facts of medical significance in the life of the patient. If the history is recorded in chronologic order, recent events should be given the most attention. Likewise, if a problem-oriented approach is used, the problems that are clinically dominant should be listed first. Ideally, the narration of symptoms or problems should be in the patient's own words. However, few patients have sufficient powers of observation or recall to give a history without some guidance from the physician, who must be careful not to suggest the answers to the questions being posed. Often a symptom which has concerned a patient has little significance, while a seemingly minor complaint may be of considerable importance. Therefore, the physician must be constantly alert to the possibility that any event related by the patient, however trivial or apparently remote, may be the key to the solution of the medical problem.

An informative history is more than an orderly listing of symptoms. Something is always gained by listening to patients and noting the way in which they talk about their symptoms. Inflections of voice, facial expression, and attitude may betray important clues to the meaning of the symptoms to the patient. In listening to the history, the physician discovers not only something about the disease but also something about the patient.

With experience, the pitfalls of history taking become apparent. What patients relate for the most part consists of subjective phenomena colored by past experience. Patients obviously differ widely in their responses to the same stimuli and in their coping mechanisms. Their attitudes are variably influenced by fear of disability and death and by concern over the consequences of their illness to their families. Sometimes the accuracy of the history is affected by language or sociologic barriers, by failing intellectual powers that interfere with recall, or by disorders of consciousness that make them unaware of their illness. It is not surprising, then, that even the most careful physician may at times despair of collecting factual data and be forced to proceed with evidence that represents little more than an approximation of the truth. It is in obtaining the history that the physician's skill, knowledge, and experience are most clearly in evidence.

The family history serves several functions. First, in rare single-gene defects a positive family history of a similarly affected individual or a history of consanguinity may have important diagnostic implications. Second, in diseases of multifactorial etiology that have a familial aggregation, it may be possible to identify patients at risk for disease and to intervene prior to development of overt manifestations. For example, recent weight gain may be a more ominous development in a woman who has a family history of diabetes than in one who does not. In certain situations the family history has major implications for preventive medicine. When a diagnosis of a hereditary condition known to predispose to cancer is made, it is the physician's obligation to follow up this possibility carefully in the patient, to survey the family, and to educate them about the need for long-term follow-up.

However accurate and complete, the medical history does much more than provide facts of critical importance. The very act of taking the history provides the physician with the opportunity to establish or enhance the unique bond that is the basis for the critically important patient-physician relationship. An effort should be made to place the patient at ease, regardless of the circumstances of the encounter. The patient should, at some point, have the opportunity to tell his or her own story of the illness without frequent interruption and, when appropriate, should receive expression of interest, encouragement, and empathy from the physician. It is often enlightening to develop an appreciation of the patient's own perception of the illness, the patient's expectations of the physician and the medical care system, and the financial and social implications of the illness to the patient. The confidentiality of the patient-physician relationship should be emphasized, and the patient should be given the opportunity to identify those aspects of the history which he or she wishes not to be disclosed to anyone else.

Physical examination   Physical signs are the objective and verifiable marks of disease and represent solid, indisputable facts. Their significance is enhanced when they confirm a functional or structural change already suggested by the patient's history. At times, the physical signs may be the only evidence of disease, especially when the history has been inconsistent, confused, or lacking altogether.

The physical examination should be performed methodically and thoroughly, with due regard for the patient's comfort and modesty. Although attention has often been directed by the history to the diseased organ or part of the body, the examination of a new patient must extend from head to toe in an objective search for abnormalities. Unless the examination procedure is systematic, important parts of it may be omitted, a common error even among the most skilled clinicians. The results of the examination, like the details of the history, should be recorded at the time they are elicited, not hours later when they are subject to the distortions of memory. Many inaccuracies stem from the careless practice of writing or dictating notes long after the examination has been concluded. Skill in physical diagnosis is acquired with experience, but it is not merely technique that determines success in eliciting signs. The detection of a few scattered petechiae, a faint diastolic murmur, or a small mass in the abdomen is not a question of keener eyes and ears or more sensitive fingers but of a mind alert to these findings. Skill in physical diagnosis reflects a way of thinking more than a way of doing. Physical findings are subject to change. Just because the examination is normal on one occasion does not guarantee that this will be the case on subsequent examinations. Likewise, abnormal findings may disappear in the course of illness. It is important, therefore, to repeat the physical examination as frequently as the clinical situation warrants.

Laboratory tests   The increase in the number and availability of laboratory tests has resulted in increasing reliance on these studies in the solution of clinical problems. It is essential, however, to bear in mind the limitations of such procedures, which by virtue of their impersonal quality and complexity often gain an aura of authority regardless of the fallibility of the tests themselves, of the individuals doing or interpreting them, or of their instruments. More important, the accumulation of laboratory data cannot relieve the physician from the responsibility of careful observation and study of the patient. Physicians also must weigh carefully the hazards and expense involved in the laboratory procedures they order. Moreover, laboratory tests are rarely ordered and reported singly. Rather, they are produced as "batteries." Some laboratories now perform batteries of 24 and even 40 tests. The various combinations of laboratory tests are often useful. For example, they may provide the clue to such nonspecific symptoms as generalized weakness and increased fatigability by revealing abnormalities of hepatic function together with elevated levels of serum IgG, which, in turn, would suggest the diagnosis of chronic liver disease. Sometimes a single abnormality, such as an elevated serum calcium level, points to a specific disease, such as hyperparathyroidism.

The thoughtful use of screening tests should not be confused with indiscriminate laboratory testing. The use of screening tests is based on the fact that a group of laboratory determinations can be carried out conveniently on a single specimen of blood at relatively low cost. Biochemical measurements, together with simple laboratory examinations such as blood count, urinalysis, and sedimentation rate, often provide the major clue to the presence of a pathologic process. At the same time, the physican must learn to evaluate occasional abnormalities among the screening tests that may not necessarily connote significant disease. There is nothing more wasteful and unproductive than an in-depth workup following a report of an isolated laboratory abnormality in a patient who is otherwise well. Among the more than 40 tests that are performed on many patients, one or two are often slightly abnormal. If there is no suspicion of an underlying illness, these tests are ordinarily repeated to ensure that the abnormality does not represent a laboratory error. If an abnormality is confirmed, it is important to distinguish a minor one (less than two standard deviations) from a major one (more than two standard deviations). Even in the case of the latter, the decision of whether to proceed with further workup is a test of the physician's clinical judgment.

Imaging techniques The past two decades have seen the arrival of ultrasonography, a variety of scans that employ isotopes to visualize organs heretofore inaccessible, computed tomography with its varying permutations, magnetic resonance imaging, and positron emission tomography. Aside from opening up new diagnostic vistas, this new technology benefits patients because it has frequently supplanted invasive techniques that require surgical biopsy or the insertion of tubes, wires, or catheters into the body—procedures that are often painful and sometimes risky. While the enthusiasm for noninvasive technology is understandably justified, all too often the results of these tests have not been validated properly before they are disseminated as clinical dogma. Moreover, the expense entailed in performing these imaging tests is often substantial and is not always considered when ordering them. Nevertheless, these examinations should be used judiciously, preferably in lieu of, not in addition to, the invasive maneuvers they are meant to replace.

THE DIAGNOSIS OF DISEASE Clinical diagnosis requires both aspects of logic—analysis and synthesis—and the more difficult the clinical problem, the more important is a logical approach to it. Such an approach requires that the physician list carefully each problem suggested by the symptoms and physical and laboratory findings and seek answers to each. Most physicians attempt consciously or unconsciously to fit a given problem into one of a series of syndromes. *The syndrome is a group of symptoms and signs of disordered function related to one another by means of some anatomic, physiologic, or biochemical peculiarity.* It embodies a hypothesis concerning the deranged function of an organ, organ system, or tissue. Congestive heart failure, Cushing's syndrome, and dementia are examples. In congestive heart failure, dyspnea, orthopnea, cyanosis, dependent edema, engorged neck veins, pleural effusion, rales, and hepatomegaly are known to be connected by a single pathophysiologic mechanism—insufficiency of the cardiac pump mechanism. In Cushing's syndrome, moon facies, hypertension, diabetes mellitus, and osteoporosis are recognized effects of excess glucocorticoids acting on many target organs. In dementia, deterioration of memory, incoherent thinking, impaired language functions, visual-spatial disorientation, and faulty judgment are related to destruction of the association areas of the cerebrum.

A syndrome usually does not identify the precise cause of an illness, but it narrows the number of possibilities and often suggests certain special clinical and laboratory studies. The derangements of each organ system in humans are reducible to a relatively small number of syndromes. The diagnosis is simplified greatly if a clinical problem conforms neatly to a well-defined syndrome, because only a few diseases need to be considered in the differential diagnosis. In contrast, the search for the cause of an illness that does not conform to a syndrome is more difficult because a much greater number of diseases have to be considered. Even here an orderly approach which proceeds from symptom to sign to laboratory findings will usually result in the diagnosis.

CARING FOR THE PATIENT Patient care begins with the development of a personal relationship between the patient and the physician. In the absence of a sense of trust and confidence on the part of the patient, the effectiveness of most therapeutic measures is diminished. In many instances, when there is confidence in the physician, reassurance is the best treatment and is all that is needed. Likewise, in those cases which do not lend themselves to easy solutions and for which no effective treatment is available, a feeling on the part of the patient that the physician is doing all that is possible is one of the most important therapeutic measures that can be provided. An important aspect of clinical decision making and patient care involves the "quality of life," a subjective assessment of what each patient values most. Such an assessment requires detailed, sometimes intimate knowledge of the patient, which can usually be obtained only through deliberate, unhurried, and often repeated conversation. In situations where complete freedom from signs and symptoms of disease is impossible, enhancement of the quality of life is the major goal of therapy.

Assessing the outcome of treatments Clinicians generally use *objective* and readily measurable parameters to judge the outcomes of a therapeutic intervention. For example, findings on physical or laboratory examination—such as the level of blood pressure, the patency of a coronary artery on an angiogram, the size of a mass on a radiologic examination, or the titer of an antibody—can provide information of critical importance. However, patients usually seek medical attention for *subjective* reasons; they wish relief from pain, to preserve or regain function, and to enjoy life. Although these goals are often nebulous and differ among individuals, the field of "medical outcomes research" has suggested that a patient's health status or quality of life can be separated into a number of categories, including bodily comfort, physical activity, social activity, personal and professional role function, sexual function, cognitive function, sleep, vitality, and overall perception of health. Function in each of these important areas can be assessed by means of structured interviews or specially designed questionnaires. However, in a less formal way these categories also provide useful parameters by which the physician can judge the patient's view of his or her disability and the response to treatment, particularly of chronic illness. The intelligent practice of medicine requires consideration and integration of both objective and subjective outcomes.

Drug therapy With each succeeding year, more drugs are released, every one with the hope and the promise that it is an improvement over its predecessor. Although the pharmaceutical industry must be given most of the credit for advances in drug therapy, it is also true that many new drugs have only a marginal advantage over the agents they are aimed to replace. The barrage of new information with which practitioners are deluged does little to provide a clear picture of clinical pharmacology; on the contrary, to most physicians new drugs are confusing. With some exceptions, however, the approach to a new drug should be one of caution. Unless the new agent is established beyond doubt to be a real advance, it is wiser to use agents the efficacy and safety of which have been well established.

Care of the elderly   Over the next several decades, the practice of medicine will be greatly influenced by the health care needs of the elderly, whose numbers are increasing rapidly. It is estimated that in the United States the population over age 65 will almost triple over the next 30 years. It is therefore essential that we understand and appreciate the physiologic processes associated with aging; the different responses of the elderly compared with younger patients to common diseases or disease mechanisms such as acute infections, hyperthyroidism, and uncontrolled diabetes mellitus; and disorders that occur commonly with aging such as depression, dementia, urinary incontinence, and falls. The elderly have more trouble with medications in large part due to altered pharmacokinetics and pharmacodynamics. Adverse reactions increase steadily above age 50. In the elderly, commonly used drugs such as digoxin have prolonged half-lives in part because of the decreased renal function that accompanies aging and in part because tissues such as the central nervous system become more sensitive to certain drugs, such as the benzodiazepines and narcotics.

Diseases in men versus women   There are significant gender differences in diseases that afflict both men and women. These have not been clearly evident because in the past most epidemiologic studies and clinical research have been carried out in adult men rather than women. There is now increasing evidence that in ischemic heart disease, mortality rates are higher in women. Hypertension is more prevalent in African-American women than in their male counterparts; diseases involving the immune system such as lupus erythematosus, multiple sclerosis, and primary biliary cirrhosis occur more frequently in women; and women have a greater longevity than men. The reason for these differences is not yet clear, and it is all too evident that more research in women's health issues is badly needed.

Iatrogenic disorders   An *iatrogenic disorder* occurs when the deleterious effects of a therapeutic or diagnostic regimen produce pathology independent of the condition for which the regimen is given. No matter what the clinical situation, it is the responsibility of the physician to use powerful therapeutic measures wisely, with due regard to their action, potential dangers, and cost. Every medical procedure, whether diagnostic or therapeutic, has the potential for harm, but it would be impossible to afford the patient the benefits of modern scientific medicine if reasonable steps in diagnosis and therapy were withheld because of possible risks. *Reasonable* implies that the physician has weighed the pros and cons of a procedure and has concluded that it is advisable or essential for the relief of discomfort or the cure or amelioration of disease. For example, the use of glucocorticoids to arrest progressive systemic lupus erythematosus may produce Cushing's syndrome. In this instance, the benefits usually exceed the untoward side effects. However, much harm can result when the deleterious effects of a procedure or a drug exceed any possible advantages that might have been anticipated. Examples include the dangerous or fatal drug reactions that occasionally follow the use of antibiotics given for minor respiratory infections, the gastric hemorrhage or perforation caused by glucocorticoid administration for mild arthritis, and the occurrence of fatal liver disease that may follow needless transfusions of blood or plasma.

However, the harm that a physician can do to a patient is not limited to the imprudent use of medication or procedures. Equally important are ill-considered or unjustified remarks. Many a patient has developed a cardiac neurosis because the physician ventured a grave prognosis on the basis of a misinterpreted finding of a heart murmur on auscultation. Not only the treatment itself but the physician's words and behavior are capable of causing injury.

The physician must never become so absorbed in the disease as to forget the patient who is its victim. As the science of medicine advances, it is all too easy to become so fascinated by the manifesta-

tions of disease that one disregards the ailing person's fears and concerns about suffering and death, job and family, the cost of medical care, and the specter of economic insecurity. Treatment of a patient consists of more than the dispassionate confrontation of a disease. It embodies also the expression of warmth, compassion, and understanding.

Informed consent   In an era of rapidly advancing technology, patients will require diagnostic and therapeutic procedures that are painful and that pose some risk. These include all surgical procedures, e.g., biopsies of tissues, endoscopy, radiographic maneuvers involving the insertion of catheters, and many others. In most hospitals and clinics, patients undergoing such procedures are required to sign a form consenting to them. More important, however, is the notion that the patient must understand clearly the risk entailed in these procedures; this is the definition of *informed consent*. It is incumbent on the physician to explain to the patient, in a clearly understandable manner, the procedures which he or she faces. By doing this conscientiously, much of the dread of the unknown that is inherent in hospitalization will be mitigated.

Accountability   Throughout the world, physicians, once licensed to practice medicine, have not had to account for their actions except to their peers. In the United States, however, during the past two decades there have been increasing demands for physicians to account for the way in which they practice medicine by meeting certain standards prescribed by federal and state governments. The hospitalization of patients whose health care is reimbursed by the government (Medicare and Medicaid) and other third parties is subjected to utilization review. This means that the physician must defend the cause for and duration of a patient's hospitalization if it falls outside certain "average" standards. In some instances, a second opinion is necessary before a patient can have elective surgery. The purpose of these regulations is to contain spiraling health care costs. It is likely that this type of review will be extended to all phases of medical practice and will alter the practice of medicine even more profoundly.

Physicians also may be expected to give account of their continuing competence by mandatory continuing education, patient-record audit, recertification by examination (time-limited certification), or relicensing. While these measures probably enhance the physician's factual knowledge, there is no evidence that they have a similar effect on the quality of practice.

Practice guidelines   Physicians are faced with a large, often bewildering array of potentially useful diagnostic techniques and therapeutic measures from which to choose as they deal with individual patients. The intelligent and cost-effective practice of medicine consists of selecting those most appropriate to a particular patient and clinical situation. To aid physicians and other care-givers in making these selections, professional organizations and government agencies are developing formal clinical practice guidelines. These guidelines may be viewed as double-edged swords. On the one hand, when they are current and properly applied, they can provide a useful framework for managing patients with particular diagnoses or symptoms. They also offer practice standards that protect patients—particularly those with inadequate health care benefits—from receiving substandard care. They can also protect conscientious caregivers from inappropriate charges of malpractice, and they can protect society from the excessive costs associated with the overuse of medical resources. On the other hand, clinical guidelines tend to oversimplify the practice of medicine. Different groups with differing perspectives may develop divergent recommendations regarding issues as basic as the need for a periodic sigmoidoscopy in middle-aged persons. Furthermore, guidelines do not—and cannot be expected to—take into account the complex interplay between genetic and environmental influences that are responsible for the uniqueness of each individual and of his or her illness. The practice of medicine strictly according to guidelines carries with it the danger of transforming medicine from a learned profession rooted in the biologic and behavioral sciences to a technical vocation. The challenge for the physician is to accept and incorporate into clinical practice the valuable recommendations offered by the knowledgeable individuals who prepare clinical practice guidelines without accepting them blindly or being inappropriately constrained.

Cost-effectiveness in medical care As the cost of medical care continues to rise, it is becoming necessary to establish stringent priorities in the expenditure of money for health care. In some instances, preventive measures offer the greatest return for the expenditure; outstanding examples include vaccination, immunization, reduction in accidents and occupational hazards, improved environmental control, and biochemical and molecular biologic screening of newborns. For example, the detection of phenylketonuria by newborn screening may result in a net saving of many thousands of dollars.

As resources become increasingly constrained, it will be necessary to weigh the justification of performing costly procedures that provide only a limited life expectancy against the pressing need for more primary care for those persons who do not have adequate access to medical services. At the level of the individual patient, it is important to reduce costly hospital admissions as much as possible if total health care is to be provided at a cost that most can afford. This, of course, implies and depends on a close cooperative effort between patients, their physicians, their employers, third-party carriers, and government, along with constant surveillance of those types of procedures which can be conducted safely and effectively on an ambulatory basis. Equally important in reducing total health care expenditures is the need for individual physicians to know the cost of medicines that they prescribe and to monitor both the cost and effectiveness of those drugs. In the last analysis, the medical profession should provide leadership and guidance to the public in matters of cost control, and physicians must take this responsibility seriously without being or seeming to be self-serving. It is important, however, that the socioeconomic aspects of health care delivery not be permitted to interfere with the concern of physicians for the welfare of their patients. The patient must be able to rely on the individual physician as his or her principal advocate in matters of health care.

Research and teaching The title *doctor* is derived from the Latin *docere*, ''to teach,'' and the physician should share information and medical knowledge with others and be willing to teach what he or she has learned to colleagues as well as to students of medicine and related professions. The practice of medicine is dependent on the sum total of medical knowledge, which in turn is based on an unending chain of scientific discovery, clinical observation, analysis, and interpretation. Advances in medicine depend on the acquisition of new information, i.e., on research, which must often involve patients; improved medical care requires the transmission of this information. As part of broader societal responsibilities, the physician should encourage patients to participate in ethical and properly approved clinical investigations if they do not impose undue hazard, discomfort, or inconvenience.

Incurability and death No problem is more distressing than that presented by the patient with an incurable disease, particularly when premature death is inevitable. What should the patient and family be told, what measures should be taken to maintain life, and how is death to be defined?

Although some would argue otherwise, there is no ironclad rule that the patient must immediately be told ''everything,'' even if the patient is an adult and the head of a family. How much the patient is told should depend on the patient's ability and capacity to deal with the possibility of imminent death; often this capacity grows with time, and whenever possible, gradual rather than abrupt disclosure is the best strategy. This decision also may take into consideration the patient's religious beliefs, financial and business status, and to some extent the wishes of the family. The patient must be given an opportunity to talk with the physician and ask questions. Patients may find it easier to share their feelings about death with their physician, who is likely to be more objective and less emotional than family members.

One thing is certain; it is not for you to don the black cap and, assuming the judicial function, take hope away from any patient . . . hope that comes to us all.

William Osler

Even when the patient directly inquires, ''Doctor, am I dying?'' the physician must attempt to determine whether this is a request for information, a demand for reassurance, or even an expression of hostility. Most would agree that only open communication between the patient and the physician can resolve these questions and guide the physician in what to say and how to say it.

The physician should provide or arrange for emotional, physical, and spiritual support and must be compassionate, unhurried, and open. There is much to be gained by the laying on of hands. Pain should be adequately controlled, human dignity maintained, and isolation from family avoided. The last two in particular tend to be overlooked in hospitals, where the intrusion of life-sustaining apparatuses can so easily detract from attention to the whole person and encourage concentration instead on the life-threatening disease. The physician also must prepare to deal with guilt feelings on the part of the family when a member becomes gravely or hopelessly ill. It is important for the doctor to reassure the family that everything possible has been done.

The President's Committee for the Study of Ethical Problems in Medicine defined death as (1) irreversible cessation of circulatory and respiratory function or (2) irreversible cessation of all functions of the entire brain, including the brainstem. Clinical and electroencephalographic criteria permit the reliable diagnosis of cerebral death. According to the criteria adopted by the staff of the Massachusetts General Hospital and the Harvard Committee on Brain Death, death occurs when all signs of receptivity and responsivity are absent, including all brainstem reflexes (pupillary reactions, ocular movement, blinking, swallowing, breathing), and the electroencephalogram is isoelectric. Occasionally, intoxications and metabolic disorders may simulate this state; hence the diagnosis requires expert evaluation. Under the aforementioned circumstances, to continue with heroic, highly costly supportive measures merely for the purpose of preserving cardiac function is against the best interests of patient, family, and society. In such instances, the dilemma of continuing care could be avoided if the medical profession, in accord with social sanction, can be brought to redefine life and death by these criteria.

The following guidelines are deserving of consideration:

1 The diagnosis of brain death, based on the preceding criteria, should be corroborated by another physician and confirmed by clinical examination and EEG, repeated one or more times.

2 The family should be informed of the irreversibility of loss of brain function but should not be requested to ratify the decision whether the medical treatment should be discontinued. An exception to this limited decision-making power of the family might apply where the patient has directed the family that he or she wishes them to make the decision.

3 The physician, after consultation with a professional colleague, may withdraw supportive measures, assuming that nothing more can be offered.

4 The possibility that such patients may become sources of organs for grafting should not enter into the aforementioned decisions, although prior to the cessation of heart action the family may be asked whether this would be their wish, or the family may suggest that organs be used for this purpose. In many states, laws now require physicians to request organ donations. A question arises when the patient has indicated in advance a wish to be an organ or tissue donor whether the family must be approached, since many believe the patient's prior wishes carry overriding weight. This issue is controversial.

''Do not resuscitate'' orders and cessation of therapy When carried out in a timely and expert manner, cardiopulmonary resuscitation is often useful in the prevention of sudden, unexpected death.

However, unless there are reasons to the contrary, it should not be carried out when it merely prolongs life in a patient with terminal, incurable disease. The decision not to resuscitate a patient and decisions about the intensity of therapy and, indeed, whether or not treatment is to be delivered or continued to patients who are incurably and terminally ill must be reviewed frequently and must take into consideration any unexpected changes in the patient's condition. In this context the administration of fluids and food are considered therapies that may be withdrawn or withheld. These decisions also must take into account both the underlying medical condition and the wishes of the patient or, if these cannot be or have not been ascertained directly, those of a close relative or other surrogate who can be relied on to transmit the patient's feelings and to be guided by the patient's best interests and wishes. The patient's autonomy—whether the choice is to continue or discontinue treatment or to be resuscitated in the event of a cardiopulmonary arrest—is paramount. The courts have ruled that competent patients may be able to refuse therapy and that an incompetent patient's previously stated wishes regarding life support should be respected. The issues involving death and dying are among the most difficult in medicine. In approaching them rationally and consistently, the physician must combine both the art and the science of medicine.

2   ETHICAL ISSUES IN CLINICAL MEDICINE

BERNARD LO

Physicians frequently confront ethical issues in clinical practice that are perplexing, time-consuming and emotionally draining. Experience, common sense, and simply being a good person do not guarantee that physicians can identify or resolve ethical dilemmas. Knowledge about common ethical dilemmas is also essential.

FUNDAMENTAL ETHICAL GUIDELINES

In patient care, physicians should follow two fundamental but frequently conflicting ethical guidelines: respecting patient autonomy and acting in the patient's best interests.

RESPECTING PATIENT AUTONOMY   Competent, informed patients have the right to be free of unwanted medical interventions. They may exercise their self-determination by refusing recommended interventions and choosing among the available alternatives.

Informed consent   Physicians are required to obtain patients' agreement to care and to provide them with pertinent, comprehensible information about the nature of the proposed care, the alternatives, the risks and benefits of each, and the likely consequences. At the same time, physicians must avoid overwhelming patients with medical jargon, complicated explanations, or too much information at once. Informed consent involves more than obtaining patients' signatures on consent forms; physicians also need to discuss options with patients, educate them about their condition, answer questions, and help them deliberate. Patients and physicians need to share decision-making. Physicians have expertise about the benefits and risks of each option, which must be weighed according to patients' values and goals.

Nondisclosure of information   Physicians may consider withholding a serious diagnosis, misrepresenting it, or limiting discussions of prognosis or risks because they fear that a patient will develop severe anxiety or depression or reject needed care. Patients should not be forced to receive information against their will. Surveys show,

however, that most people want to know their diagnosis and prognosis, even if they are terminally ill. Without such information, patients cannot make informed decisions. Generally physicians should provide relevant information, while offering empathy and hope and helping patients cope with bad news.

Emergency care   Informed consent is not required when patients cannot give consent and delaying treatment would place their life or health in peril. People are presumed to want such emergency care, unless they have indicated otherwise.

Futile interventions   Respect for patient autonomy does not entitle patients to insist on whatever care they want. Physicians are not obligated to provide futile interventions that offer no physiologic benefit or have no prospect of achieving the goals of care. For example, cardiopulmonary resuscitation would be futile in a patient with multisystem failure that is worsening despite maximal therapy. But physicians should be wary of using the term "futile" in looser senses to justify unilateral decisions to withhold interventions because they believe the probability of success is too low, the patient's goals inappropriate, or the costs too high. If patients insist on "futile" care, physicians should check for misunderstandings and unaddressed psychosocial issues. Discussions with an ethics committee may also be helpful.

ACTING IN THE BEST INTERESTS OF PATIENTS   The guideline of *beneficence* requires physicians to take actions for patients' benefit, not just to avoid harming them. Laypeople do not possess medical expertise and may be vulnerable because of their illness. Thus patients rely on physicians to provide sound advice and to promote their well-being. Physicians encourage such trust. For these reasons, physicians have a fiduciary duty to act in the best interests of their patients. The guideline of "do no harm" forbids physicians from providing ineffective therapies or from acting selfishly or maliciously. This precept, while often cited, provides only limited guidance, because many beneficial interventions also have serious risks.

CONFLICTS BETWEEN BENEFICENCE AND AUTONOMY   Patients' refusals of care may thwart their own goals or cause them serious harm. For example, a young man with asthma may refuse mechanical ventilation for reversible respiratory failure. Physicians can approach such conflicts using a series of questions.

1 *What is the patient's diagnosis and prognosis?* Resolving ethical issues requires sound medical information.
2 *Is the patient competent and informed?* Simply to accept such refusals, in the name of respecting autonomy, would fail to show caring. Physicians can elicit patients' expectations and concerns, correct misunderstandings, and try to persuade them to accept beneficial therapies. If disagreements persist after discussions, the patient's informed choices and view of best interests should prevail.
3 If the patient lacks decision-making capacity, two further questions need to be asked. *Has the patient provided advance directives?* Trustworthy advance directives should be respected. *Who is the appropriate surrogate for the patient?* The following section addresses these latter two questions.

PATIENTS WHO LACK DECISION-MAKING CAPACITY

Patients may not be able to make informed decisions because of illness or the effects of medications. Such patients may not express any choices, or their uninformed decisions may jeopardize their health. Generally surrogates need to make decisions for such patients.

ASSESSING CAPACITY TO MAKE MEDICAL DECISIONS   All adults are considered legally competent unless declared incompetent by a court. In practice, however, physicians usually determine that patients lack the capacity to make health care decisions and arrange for surrogates to make them, without involving the courts. By definition, competent patients can express a choice and appreciate the medical situation, the nature of the proposed care, the alternatives, and the risks, benefits, and consequences of each. Their choices should be consistent with their values and should not result from delusions or hallucinations. Assessing decision-making capacity is difficult when patients can understand some important aspects of their situation but not others. Psychiatrists may help in hard cases because they are skilled at interviewing mentally impaired patients and can identify treatable depression or psychosis. When impairments are fluctuating or reversible, decisions should be postponed if possible until the patient recovers decision-making capacity.

CHOICE OF SURROGATE Physicians routinely ask family members to serve as surrogates, presuming that they know the patient's preferences and have the patient's best interests at heart. While most patients want their family members to be surrogates, some may prefer a close friend. Patients' designation of surrogates for health care decisions should be respected. In a few cases, the courts have already named a surrogate for the patient.

STANDARDS FOR SURROGATE DECISION MAKING **Advance directives** These are statements by competent patients that indicate (1) what interventions they would refuse or accept or (2) who should serve as surrogate if they lose decision-making capacity. Following advance directives respects patients' autonomy.

Oral conversations are the most frequent form of advance directives. While such conversations are generally followed in clinical practice, casual or vague comments may not be trustworthy.

Living wills direct physicians to withhold or withdraw life-sustaining interventions if the patient becomes terminally ill and incapable of making decisions. Generally patients may refuse only interventions that "merely prolong the process of dying." In some states, living wills also apply in persistent vegetative states or allow patients to appoint surrogates.

The durable power of attorney for health care allows patients to appoint surrogates to make health care decisions if they lose decision-making capacity. It is more flexible and comprehensive than the living will, applying whenever the patient is unable to make decisions.

Physicians should encourage patients to provide advance directives and to discuss their preferences with family members or surrogates. In discussions with patients, physicians can ensure that advance directives are informed, up-to-date, and address likely clinical scenarios. The federal Patient Self-Determination Act requires hospitals to inform patients of their right to make health care decisions and to provide advance directives.

Substituted judgment In the absence of clear advance directives, surrogates and physicians should try to decide as the patient would under the circumstances, using all information that they know about the patient. While such substituted judgments try to respect the patient's values, they may be problematic. Surrogates may be mistaken about the patient's preferences, particularly when they have not been discussed explicitly. In some cases, so little is known about the patient's values that substituted judgments would be mere speculation.

Best interests When the patient's preferences are unclear or unknown, decisions should be based on the patient's best interests. Best interests are controversial, especially when quality as well as duration of life are considered. Judgments about quality of life are appropriate if they reflect the patient's own values. Bias or discrimination may occur, however, if others project their values onto the patient. For instance, most patients with chronic illness rate their quality of life higher than their family members and physicians do.

Legal issues Physicians need to know pertinent state laws regarding patients who lack decision-making capacity. A few state courts allow life-sustaining treatments to be withheld only if patients have provided written advance directives or very specific oral ones.

Problems Disagreements may occur among potential surrogates or between the physician and surrogate. Physicians can remind everyone to base decisions on what the patient would want, not what they would want for themselves. Consultation with the hospital ethics committee or with another physician often helps resolve disputes. Such consultation is also helpful when patients have no surrogate and no advance directives. The courts should be used as a last resort when disagreements cannot be resolved in the clinical setting.

DECISIONS ABOUT LIFE-SUSTAINING INTERVENTIONS

While medical technology can save lives, it can also prolong the process of dying or be imposed against patients' wishes. Competent, informed patients may refuse life-sustaining interventions. Such interventions may be withheld from patients who lack decision-making capacity on the basis of advance directives or decisions by appropriate surrogates. Patients need not be terminally ill or comatose. Courts have ruled that foregoing life-sustaining interventions is neither suicide nor murder.

MISLEADING DISTINCTIONS People commonly draw distinctions that are intuitively plausible but prove untenable on closer analysis.

Extraordinary and ordinary care Some physicians are willing to forego "extraordinary" or "heroic" interventions, such as surgery, mechanical ventilation, or renal dialysis, but insist on providing "ordinary" ones, such as antibiotics, intravenous fluids, or feeding tubes. However, this is not a logical distinction. All medical interventions, however, have both risks and benefits. Any intervention may be withheld, if the burdens for the individual patient outweigh the benefits.

Withdrawing and withholding interventions Many people feel more responsible for a patient's death if they withdraw an intervention than if they had withheld it. Such reluctance to withdraw treatments needs to be acknowledged. There is no logical distinction, however, between the two acts. Reasons that justify withholding interventions also justify withdrawing them, and additional reasons may emerge after starting treatment: it may prove unsuccessful or new information about the patient's preferences or condition may become available. Patients and surrogates might not start potentially beneficial treatments if they could not be discontinued later.

DO NOT RESUSCITATE (DNR) ORDERS Because cardiopulmonary resuscitation (CPR) must be initiated emergently, decisions to withhold it need to be discussed in advance. While CPR can restore people to vigorous health, it can also disrupt a peaceful death, particularly one that is anticipated. After CPR is attempted on a general hospital service, only 14 percent of patients survive to discharge, and even fewer in certain subgroups. Standard practice is to initiate CPR unless a DNR order has been made. To prevent misunderstandings, DNR orders should be written, not given orally. DNR orders are appropriate if the patient or surrogate requests them or if CPR would be futile. "Slow" or "show" codes that merely appear to provide CPR are deceptive and therefore unacceptable. Strictly speaking, a DNR order signifies only that CPR will be withheld. Concerns that DNR orders may cause other care to be withheld inappropriately need to be worked out among the health care team.

ASSISTED SUICIDE AND ACTIVE EUTHANASIA Proponents of these controversial acts believe that competent, terminally ill patients should have control over the end of life and that physicians should help them end their suffering. Opponents assert that life is sacred, that suffering can generally be relieved in other ways, that abuses are inevitable, that such actions are outside the physician's proper role, and that current prohibitions should continue. Whatever their personal views, physicians need to respond to patients' inquiries with compassion and concern. Physicians need to elicit and address any underlying problems, such as unrelieved suffering, loss of control, or depression. Distress usually can be relieved more effectively and patients in turn may withdraw their requests for these acts. Patients need to be reassured that life-prolonging interventions will not be imposed against their wishes.

CARE OF DYING PATIENTS Relieving pain in terminal illness and alleviating dyspnea when patients forego mechanical ventilation enhances patient comfort and dignity. Spending time with dying patients, listening to them, and paying attention to their psychological distress can ease their suffering. In some cases, relief of symptoms may require doses of narcotics or sedatives that may suppress

to be uncommon among blacks residing in rural Africa. Environmental factors may also play a role in the pathogenesis of hypertension in blacks, in that a high level of social stress, instability, and occupational insecurity may worsen hypertension. Other ethnic differences in the control of blood pressure include the correlation between insulin resistance or hyperinsulinemia and hypertension in whites but not in blacks or Pima Indians, a group with a very high incidence of hyperinsulinemia (see below). Cerebrovascular complications of hypertension (particularly intracerebral hemorrhage) are more frequent in African-Americans than in other ethnic groups.

Diabetes mellitus The prevalence of non-insulin–dependent diabetes mellitus is approximately twice as high in African-Americans and Native Americans as in whites. It is especially high in the Pima Indians, approximately half of whom now develop this disease by age 35. This prevalence has increased dramatically during the past 30 years and appears to parallel the increase in obesity in this population during this period. On the other hand, insulin-dependent diabetes mellitus occurs less frequently in African-Americans than in whites and is apparently even less common among blacks born and residing in Africa.

Coronary and cerebral arterial disease In the United States, the age-adjusted mortality rates for stroke and sudden death are higher in blacks than in whites; the rates for symptomatic coronary artery disease are also higher in black women than white women. Such racial differences are probably related to the aforementioned higher prevalence among African-Americans of hypertension and diabetes mellitus, both of which are major risk factors for coronary and cerebral atherosclerosis. These differences may also be related to cultural factors, such as the high prevalence of obesity in African-American women. Indeed, coronary artery disease is quite uncommon in South African blacks, who tend to be lean and who may be protected by a low-fat, low-sodium diet. Coronary vascular disease is also less common in Asians than in white Americans, especially in Asians living in their native lands, probably because they have lower circulating levels of total cholesterol and low-density lipoproteins.

Neoplastic disease Overall, cancer is somewhat more frequent in blacks than whites in the United States. In particular, deaths caused by cancer of the esophagus and stomach, pancreas, lung, cervix, and prostate are more common in African-Americans. Some of these variations may be related to differences in smoking, diet, and alcohol consumption. However, when adjustments are made for the stage of the disease at the time of diagnosis, these interracial differences diminish. Hepatocellular carcinoma occurs more frequently in Chinese and Southeast Asians and those residing in sub-Saharan Africa, while colorectal, breast, and prostate cancers are less common in Asian than in white Americans.

Tuberculosis Both the prevalence and incidence of tuberculosis are approximately twice as high in blacks as in whites. At first, these differences were ascribed to overcrowding, poor nutrition, and other consequences of economic deprivation. However, the fact that blacks are infected about twice as frequently as whites when exposed under comparable conditions to *M. tuberculosis* in prisons and nursing homes suggests that genetic factors also play a role—perhaps a dominant role. Consonant with this concept, tubercle bacilli grow faster in macrophages harvested from black than from white subjects.

Osteoporosis Both osteoporosis and one of its principal complications, vertebral fractures, occur more frequently in women than in men and in white than in black women. The latter observation correlates with bone density, which is greater in black (and Polynesian) than in white women. These differences may be explained, in part, by the hormonal and metabolic changes that occur during puberty, a time when black women undergo substantially greater increases in vertebral bone density than do white women. On the other hand, Asians have lower bone densities than whites.

Gastrointestinal disorders Both cancer of the stomach and cirrhosis occur more frequently in Hispanics than in whites; which may be related to a high incidence of alcoholism in Hispanics. Lactose intolerance is more common in Africans, African-Americans, Asians,

and Mexicans than in whites. Episodic bouts of peritonitis, a cardinal manifestation of familial Mediterranean fever, occur predominantly in persons of Sephardic Jewish, Armenian, and Arabic ancestry. Inflammatory bowel disease is more common in the Jewish population.

Arthritis and connective tissue disorders Since the histocompatibility antigen HLA-B27 is found more often in white populations, disorders linked to this antigen, such as ankylosing spondylitis and Reiter's syndrome, are more prevalent among whites. In contrast, systemic lupus erythematosus and polymyositis are more common and usually more severe in blacks.

CONCLUSIONS Appropriate understanding and consideration of demographic and ethnic factors in dealing with the individual patient is of diagnostic as well as therapeutic importance. As the practice of medicine and the postgraduate training of physicians grow highly specialized, consideration of these factors is frequently underemphasized. A broad view of the context of the illness is important.

REFERENCES

BOWMAN JE, MURRAY RF JR: *Genetic Variation and Disorders in Peoples of African Origin*. Baltimore, Johns Hopkins University, 1990

CRUICKSHANK JK, BEEVERS DG: *Ethnic Factors in Health and Disease*. Boston, Wright, 1989

FRASER PA: Epidemiology of rheumatic diseases in selected non-European populations, in *Oxford Textbook of Rheumatology*, PJ Maddison et al (eds). Oxford, Oxford University, 1993, in press

KEIL JE et al: Mortality rates and risk factors for coronary disease in black as compared with white men and women. N Engl J Med 329:73, 1993

LEIGH H, REISER MF: *The Patient: Biological, Psychological and Social Dimensions of Medical Practice*, 3d ed. New York, Plenum, 1992.

Report of the Secretary's Task Force on Black and Minority Health. U.S. Department of Health and Human Services, vol. I, Executive Summary. Washington DC, 1985

4   THE IMPACT OF SOCIAL FACTORS ON DISEASE

VIRGINIA L. ERNSTER

Marked variations in health exist among different subgroups of the population, and social factors are major determinants of disease occurrence and survival. Broadly interpreted, social factors include *socioeconomic status, culture and acculturation, religion, and psychosocial factors* (e.g., life events, social mobility, and social networks), as well as aspects of the environment that are the result of human activity. The focus here is on the influence of socioeconomic status (SES) and racial/ethnic factors on health indicators in the United States. Though individual physicians have limited impact on the social world of patients, it is critical to recognize the role of SES and racial/ethnic factors in determining environmental exposures, behavioral risk factors, access to health care, and compliance with recommended regimens, all of which influence disease etiology and prognosis.

The key points of this chapter are that (1) marked improvements have occurred in mortality and life expectancy during this century; (2) individuals of lower SES experience greater morbidity and mortality than individuals of higher SES; (3) the differences in disease occurrence and survival across racial/ethnic groups diminish considerably or disappear entirely once SES is controlled; and (4) behavioral risk factors play a major role in disease etiology but do not entirely explain differences in disease prevalence across SES and racial groups.

IMPROVEMENTS IN MORTALITY AND LIFE EXPECTANCY In 1900, approximate life expectancies at birth in the United States were

TABLE 4-1   Life expectancy in years at birth by race and sex, United States 1900–1989

	White		Black	
	Male	Female	Male	Female
1900	46.6	48.7	32.5	33.5
1940	62.1	66.6	—	—
1950	66.5	72.2	58.9	62.7
1960	67.4	74.1	60.7	65.9
1970	68.0	75.6	60.0	68.3
1980	70.7	78.1	63.8	72.5
1987	72.2	78.9	65.2	73.6
1988	72.3	78.9	64.9	73.4
1989	72.7	79.2	64.8	73.5

SOURCE: U.S. Department of Health and Human Services: Advance report of final mortality statistics, 1989. CDC Monthly Vital Statistics Report 40:1, 1992.
U.S. Department of Health and Human Services: *Health United States and Prevention Profile 1989.* DHHS Pub No(PHS)90-1232, Hyattsville, MD, 1990.

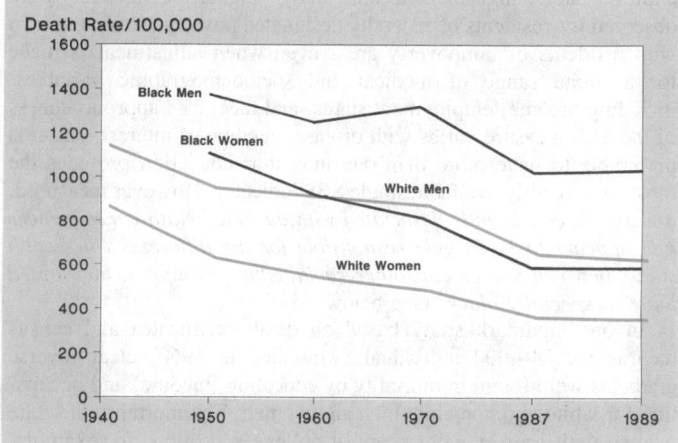

FIGURE 4-1   Death rates per 100,000, 1940–1989, for white and black men and women, age-adjusted to the 1940 U.S. population. *(From U.S. Department of Health and Human Services: Advance report of final mortality statistics, 1989. CDC Monthly Vital Statistics Report 40:1, 1992.)*

47 years for white men, 49 for white women, 32 for black men, and 34 for black women. In less than a century, those figures have increased by nearly 60 percent for whites and doubled in blacks. By 1989, average life expectancy at birth approximated 73 and 79 years, respectively, for white men and women and 65 and 74 years for black men and women (Table 4-1). These gains in life expectancy are the result of declines in age-adjusted mortality rates (Fig. 4-1). Improved environmental conditions in the first half of the century led to declines in infectious diseases and resulted in improvements in infant and early childhood survival. Infant mortality rates have continued to decline largely because of improvements in medical care; between 1950 and 1989, rates decreased from 27 to 8 per 1000 births among whites and from 44 to 18 per 1000 births among blacks. Simply put, at the turn of the century 30 percent of children died before the age of 5 years compared with only 2 percent today. Since the mid-1960s, most of the decline in mortality rates has been due to reductions in death from cardiovascular disease and stroke, affecting primarily the older age groups. Age-adjusted death rates from cardiovascular disease have declined by more than 40 percent since 1970; between 1980 and 1988 alone, age-adjusted ischemic heart disease mortality rates in the population aged 35 and older declined 24 percent—from 588 to 449 per 100,000. Whereas life expectancy at birth increased 8 percent between 1950 and 1980, life expectancy at age 45 increased by 12 percent. By 1988, 12 percent of the U.S. population was over the age of 65, compared with only 4 percent in 1900.

Although overall trends are positive, there was a slowing of life expectancy gains in blacks compared with whites in the mid-1980s

and there remains a continuing gap in life expectancy between blacks and whites and a twofold excess in infant mortality among blacks. The male-female gap in life expectancy has widened and then narrowed during this century, a trend that correlates with the adoption of cigarette smoking first by men and later by women (see Chap. 5). Among whites, life expectancy was on average 2 years longer for women than men in 1900, 8 years longer in 1970, and 6 years longer in 1989. Nonetheless, for all of the leading causes of death in the United States, there is a male excess in the ratio of male-to-female age-adjusted death rates; the excess is more than twofold for deaths due to accidents, suicide, chronic liver disease and cirrhosis, homicide, and HIV-infection (Table 4-2).

HIGHER MORTALITY AND MORBIDITY IN LOWER SOCIOECO-NOMIC GROUPS   Numerous population-based studies demonstrate that, despite dramatic improvements over time in life expectancy and death rates for all major subgroups of the population, SES is still a major determinant of health status. The existence of overall mortality differentials by occupational status is especially well documented in the United Kingdom, and social class differences in mortality there may be widening.

Socioeconomic status is measured in various ways, including education, income, occupation, population density, nature of residence, and combined indices. Different measures of SES are not

TABLE 4-2   Ratio of age-adjusted death rates* for the leading causes of death by sex and race: United States 1989†

All causes	Male to female	White men to white women	Black men to black women	Black to white	Black men to white men	Black women to white women
Heart disease	1.9	1.9	1.6	1.4	1.3	1.6
Malignant neoplasms	1.5	1.4	1.8	1.3	1.5	1.2
Cerebrovascular diseases	1.2	1.2	1.2	1.9	1.9	1.9
Accidents and adverse effects	2.6	2.6	3.1	1.3	1.4	1.2
Motor vehicle accidents	2.4	2.3	3.2	1.0	1.1	0.8
All other	3.0	3.0	3.0	1.7	1.8	1.8
Chronic obstructive pulmonary diseases	1.8	1.8	2.3	0.8	0.9	0.7
Pneumonia and influenza	1.7	1.6	2.0	1.5	1.6	1.3
Diabetes mellitus	1.1	1.1	0.9	2.3	2.0	2.3
Suicide	4.1	4.1	5.2	0.6	0.6	0.5
Chronic liver disease and cirrhosis	2.3	2.4	2.4	1.7	1.7	1.7
Homicide and legal intervention	3.6	2.9	5.0	6.6	7.6	4.5
Human immunodeficiency virus infection	8.7	14.6	5.0	3.3	3.1	9.0
All causes	1.7	1.7	1.8	1.6	1.6	1.6

* Per 100,000 population, age-adjusted to the 1940 U.S. population.
† SOURCE: U.S. Department of Health and Human Services: Advance report of final mortality statistics, 1989. CDC Monthly Vital Statistics Report 40:1, 1992

entirely interchangeable; in one study, higher death rates were observed for residents of federally designated poverty areas compared with residents of nonpoverty areas even when adjustment is made for a broad range of medical and sociodemographic variables, including income, employment status, and race. The appropriateness of the SES measure varies with disease outcome of interest, and it is preferable to have more than one indicator; education provides the most valid readily available single SES indicator. However measured, *low SES is consistently associated with adverse health consequences and appears to be largely responsible for the differences in health status between whites and other racial/ethnic groups in the United States, especially blacks* (see below).

In one landmark study based on death certificates and census records for 340,000 individuals who died in 1960, clear inverse gradients were found in mortality by education, income, and occupation for white and nonwhite men and women. The mortality of white women with four or more years of college education, for example, was only 71 percent of the overall rate for white women, whereas those with less than five years of education had a mortality ratio of 127 percent. Similarly, remaining life expectancy for white women aged 25 with at least one year of college education was almost 10 years greater (56.4 years) than for those with less than five years of schooling. Likewise, in Alameda County, California, death rates in individuals with inadequate family income were twice as high as in those with adequate income. Findings in other areas of the United States and in other developed countries have been similar. Even the onset of the decline in coronary heart disease rates among white women occurs earliest in those areas with the highest average income, education, and occupational levels. Similarly, the 1960 Matched Records Study and the National Health and Nutrition Examination Survey (NHANES I) showed that the decline in heart disease mortality among men between 1960 and 1971-84 was sharpest for those with more years of education.

Morbidity is also inversely related to income. In the United States in 1988, 23 percent of individuals whose family income was less than $10,000 reported limitation of activity due to chronic conditions compared with only 8 percent of those whose income was $35,000 or greater (Table 4-3). Other analyses using a combination of education and income to measure social class show that most preventable morbidity and functional limitation in the U.S. population before age 75 occurs in the lower SES strata. The adverse effect of income on disability is apparent even among children. In 1980, the average number of disability days was 9 for children whose families had annual incomes of $5000, compared with 4 for those whose families had incomes of $25,000 or more, and the incidence of lower respiratory illness among infants is inversely related to educational level of the head of household. Patients of lower SES (whether measured by income, occupation, or education) also have longer and more costly hospitalizations.

A notable exception to the inverse gradient between SES and disease is the fact that the incidence of breast cancer is higher in upper SES groups. However, the inverse gradient of social class correlates with many seemingly unrelated causes of disease, e.g., heart disease death rates, survival of patients with coronary artery disease following cardiac catheterization, incidence and survival for many cancers, visual impairment, childhood accidents, overall childhood mortality, and prevalence of migraine headache. Known risk factors account for some of these patterns but not for the broad effects across disparate conditions. To cite just one study, even after control for baseline medical characteristics related to survival of patients with coronary artery disease, those with annual household incomes of $40,000 or greater were about half as likely to die within 5 years of entering the study as patients with lower incomes.

Considering that about one in eight Americans lives in a family whose income is below the poverty level as defined by the federal government, and realizing that nearly one in four children under age 6 falls into this category, social inequity represents a compelling challenge for the nation's health.

TABLE 4-3   Limitation of activity due to chronic conditions by family income, United States, 1988

Family income, $	Percent of population
<10,000	23.2
10,000–14,999	15.4
15,000–19,999	13.1
20,000–34,999	10.7
≥35,000	8.1

SOURCE: U.S. Department of Health and Human Services: *Health United States and Prevention Profile 1989.* DHHS Pub No(PHS)90-1232, Hyattsville, MD, 1990.

Attention is being given to understanding the reason for the impressive relationship of SES to disease. Differences in disease severity are explained only in part by differences in the prevalence of known risk factors across SES groups, even in the United Kingdom, where a national health system diminishes inequities in health services. Gradients in health status correlate with relative privilege, even among individuals whose absolute levels of income or occupation indicated they are not deprived. In Britain, for example, among individuals in nonmanual occupations who are homeowners, mortality is lower in those with two cars when compared with those with only one car. Nearly two-thirds of the variation in mortality rates among member nations of the Organization for Economic Cooperation and Development may be attributable to *within*-country differences in income distribution, i.e., the relative gap between rich and poor. Similarly, across the 12 countries of the European Community, income distribution correlates with life expectancy.

DIFFERENCES IN DISEASE OCCURRENCE AND SURVIVAL ACROSS RACIAL/ETHNIC GROUPS   Mortality rates have traditionally been presented in the United States for all races combined or for whites and blacks (or nonwhites) separately (Table 4-2). Overall age-adjusted mortality rates are 60 percent higher for blacks, with notable excesses for cerebrovascular diseases, diabetes mellitus, and homicide. Lung cancer incidence rates are 50 percent higher, and rates for AIDS are three times higher in blacks, although there is considerable variation by sex, age, and risk group. An examination of U.S. deaths for 1980-86 from 12 causes considered preventable by medical intervention (tuberculosis, cervical cancer, Hodgkin's disease, rheumatic heart disease, hypertensive heart disease, acute respiratory disease, pneumonia and bronchitis, influenza, asthma, appendicitis, hernias, and cholecystitis) found that mortality rates for the 12 causes combined were 4.5 times higher in blacks than whites, with highest relative differences for tuberculosis, hypertensive heart disease, and asthma. In New York's Harlem, where the population is 96 percent black, the age-adjusted overall mortality rate for the period 1979-81 was more than twice that of U.S. whites; in the population under age 65, the ratio of deaths in Harlem to the number expected was 2.9 for men and 2.7 for women, and black men in Harlem were less likely to survive to age 65 than men in Bangladesh. National morbidity data are consistent with the mortality data. In 1988, 16 percent of blacks compared with 13 percent of whites reported limitation of their activity due to chronic conditions.

Attempts are now being made to collect national mortality and morbidity data for racial/ethnic groups other than whites and blacks. However, the actual disease experience of a group is accurate only if the coding of race/ethnicity is accurate. Moreover, broad categories such as "Hispanic," "Asian," or "Native American" include diverse populations with diverse disease risks. For example, Mexican-Americans appear to have a low risk of cerebrovascular disease, whereas Puerto Ricans have a high risk of stroke, so that statistics for "Hispanics" should not be based on the combined experience. Some precise ethnic categories, particularly for Asians and Pacific Islanders, may have too few individuals for reliable calculation of cause-specific death rates. Finally, increasing interracial admixture makes traditional racial categories less meaningful.

Recognizing these limitations, attempts have been made to characterize the disease experience of minorities in the United States. The results indicate that (1) overall death rates are lowest among Asians; (2) blacks have the highest overall death rates for all age groups except ages 15 to 24, when rates are slightly higher for American Indian/Alaskan Natives; (3) in all age groups under 65, death rates among whites and Hispanics are intermediate between those of Asians and blacks; (4) in young people aged 15 to 24, blacks are seven times more likely and Hispanics and American Indians are three to four times more likely to die of homicide than Asians and whites; (5) in the age groups under 45, injury rates are particularly excessive among American Indian/Alaskan Natives; (6) in the age groups 25 to 64, heart disease rates in blacks are much higher, and rates in Hispanics and especially in Asians are considerably lower than those of whites; and (7) among the population 65 years and older, cancer death rates among Asians, American Indians, and Hispanics are only half or less those of whites, and death rates in blacks are about 20 percent higher than in whites.

Racial/ethnic differences in rates for many diseases are due to differences in socioeconomic status. When SES is controlled, black/white differences in the incidence of some but not all cancers, such as invasive cervical cancer and lung cancer in men, are reduced or disappear. In fact, overall cancer rates are higher in blacks in the United States, but when adjusted for SES rates are higher in whites than in blacks. Though black women have lower survival from breast cancer than white women, race is not significant if SES is controlled. Similarly, although infant mortality rates are twice as high among normal birthweight black babies, no differences are found in comparisons of normal birthweight infants born to black and white college-educated parents. Furthermore, no significant differences have been found in overall mortality or in coronary heart disease mortality by race *within* the low (less than eight years of education and lower occupational group) or high (some college education and occupation of proprietor or professional) SES groups. Differences in heart disease rates across occupational groups in the United States are much greater than differences between blacks and whites. It is of particular concern that social class disparities, as measured by income, are widening.

In addition to social class, other sociocultural factors undoubtedly affect health-related behaviors and outcomes. Even when income, health status, age, sex, and history of chronic disease are taken into account, blacks in the United States have fewer ambulatory visits and are less likely to see a physician, suggesting disadvantages in access to care. In one study, black patients with ischemic heart disease underwent coronary angiography and coronary artery bypass grafting less often than whites, even when age, sex, income, source of payment, primary diagnosis, and the number of secondary diagnoses were controlled. Among Medicare patients, sex- and age-adjusted incidence of coronary artery bypass grafting were about three times higher among whites in 1986 and were not related to admission rates for acute myocardial infarction. Even among college-educated parents, blacks are more likely than whites to have low birthweight babies, which accounts for the higher overall black infant mortality in this group, despite the similarity in mortality rates for normal birthweight infants. Yet in the face of SES adversity, cultural factors may play a protective role. U.S.-born Hispanic infants, with the exception of those of Puerto Rican descent, have infant mortality rates similar to those of whites, i.e., about half those of blacks.

Of course, many racial differences in morbidity and mortality cannot be explained by SES, culture, or racism. Hypertensive end-stage renal disease rates in blacks are higher than in whites, adjusting for age, prevalence of hypertension, diabetes mellitus, and education level. On the other hand, malignant melanoma is more common in whites. It is obviously important to distinguish between genetic and social differences in disease risk across racial/ethnic groups.

KNOWN RISK FACTORS EXPLAIN ONLY PART OF THE DIFFERENCES Differences in health status across SES and racial groups are partially explained by differences in the distribution of known disease risk factors. Cigarette smoking, the leading cause of preventable death in the United States, shows a strong inverse relationship

TABLE 4-4 Prevalence of cigarette smoking in persons aged 25 and over, by sex, race, and education, United States, 1987

Education, years	Men		Women	
	White	Black	White	Black
<12	45.3	49.4	37.0	35.0
12	34.6	43.6	29.4	28.1
13–15	28.0	32.4	26.2	27.2
≥16	17.4	20.9	16.4	19.5
Total	30.6	41.9	27.0	28.6

SOURCE: U.S. Department of Health and Human Services: *Health United States and Prevention Profile 1989.* DHHS Pub No(PHS)90-1232, Hyattsville, MD, 1990.

to SES. In the population 18 years of age and older, 37 percent of men and 27 percent of women with less than a high school education were smokers in 1990, compared with only 14.5 percent and 12 percent, respectively, of college graduates (Table 4-4). By the year 2000 smoking prevalence among those with a high school education or less is projected to be about 30 percent, whereas it will be less than 10 percent among college graduates. In California, between 1984 and 1989, smoking, infrequent use of seat belts, not exercising outside of work, being overweight, and hypertension were more common among women with a high school education or less compared to those with more education (Table 4-5). Self-reports of mammogram screening and having had a Pap smear within the previous year are also positively associated with income. Finally, the proportion of children vaccinated for measles, rubella, diphtheria-tetanus-pertussis, poliomyelitis, and mumps is 15 to 20 percent higher among white children (Table 4-6).

For many diseases, however, controlling for differences in known risk factors does not eliminate differences across SES and racial groups. Controlling for serum cholesterol, systolic blood pressure, smoking, physical activity, body mass, and other factors accounted for only about 60 percent of the differential in coronary heart disease mortality across different employment grades in the British Civil Services. Similarly, adjustment for age, smoking, body weight, blood pressure, and serum cholesterol levels accounted for only a modest proportion of the elevated risks of heart disease death among the least educated men and women aged 45 to 74 in the National Health and Nutrition Examination Survey (NHANES). Approximately a third of excess mortality in blacks is due to identified risk factors and a third to family income, leaving a third unexplained. On the other hand, lower cardiovascular disease mortality has been observed among Mexican-American compared with non-Hispanic white men, despite higher cardiovascular risk factors.

Still, behavioral and other avoidable risk factors account for a large part of differences in disease status in all SES groups, even

TABLE 4-5 Prevalence of behavioral risk factors* by education level in California ages 35–44, 1984-89

Risk factor	Men		Women	
	≤ High-school, %	> High-school, %	≤ High-school, %	> High-school, %
Current smoking	40.7	25.6	30.1	19.1
Irregular/nonuse of seatbelts	29.6	17.8	20.9	10.9
No exercise outside of work	39.4	14.4	31.9	20.2
Overweight	33.1	19.6	21.6	14.1
Hypertension	13.1	20.0	15.9	10.9
Chronic drinking	13.9	12.8	4.0	2.5
Drinking and driving	6.7	5.2	1.1	1.3

* Based on responses to telephone interviews conducted as part of the CDC's ongoing Behavioral Risk Factor Survey. N = 10,650 California participants during 1984-89.
SOURCE: Ackermann SP et al: Cancer screening behaviors among U.S. women: breast cancer 1987–1989, and cervical cancer, 1988–1989. MMWR 41:17, 1992.

TABLE 4-6 Vaccination of children aged 1 to 4 for selected diseases, by race, United States, 1985

	% of population	
	White	All other
Measles	63.6	48.8
Rubella	61.6	47.7
DTP*	68.7	48.7
Polio	58.9	40.1
Mumps	61.8	47.0

* Diphtheria-tetanus-pertussis.

SOURCE: U.S. Department of Health and Human Services: *Health United States and Prevention Profile 1989.* DHHS Pub No(PHS)90-1232, Hyattsville, MD, 1990.

among the elderly. Priority areas for health promotion (individual behaviors), health protection (environmental and regulatory measures), and prevention (counseling, screening, immunization, or chemoprophylactic intervention in clinical settings) are documented in *Healthy People 2000: National Health Promotion and Disease Prevention Objectives.* In this landmark reference, the health consequences and current status of the U.S. population are reviewed, and goals are proposed for the year 2000. Attempts to promote healthy lifestyles among the socially disadvantaged deserve high priority. Unfortunately, such efforts may not be a high priority for the individuals in greatest need. Intensive education about risk factors (tobacco, diet, alcohol, drugs) is needed but will have little impact unless accompanied by adequate income, employment, and housing.

Disadvantaged segments of our population have yet to approximate the purported maximum lifespan, and attempts to change established behavioral risk factors, while critically important, will not be sufficient to improve morbidity for the population as a whole. Improvements in socioeconomic status and recognition of the continuing impact of race and/or racism on health outcomes are fundamental to achieving that goal.

REFERENCES

Mortality, morbidity, and socioeconomic status

EPSTEIN AM et al: Do the poor cost more? A multihospital study of patients' socioeconomic status and use of hospital resources. N Engl J Med 322:1122, 1990

FELDMAN JJ et al: National trends in educational differentials in mortality. Am J Epidemiol 129:919, 1989

KAPLAN GA et al: Socioeconomic status and health, in *Closing the Gap: The Burden of Unnecessary Illness*, RW Amler, HB Dull (eds). New York, Oxford University, 1987, pp 125–129

KITAGAWA EM, HAUSER PM (eds): *Differential Mortality in the United States: A Study in Socioeconomic Epidemiology.* Cambridge, MA, Harvard University, 1973

MARMOT MG et al: Social/economic status and disease. Ann Rev Public Health 9:111, 1987

PAPPAS G et al: The increasing disparity in mortality between socioeconomic groups in the United States, 1960 and 1986. JAMA 329:103, 1993

SMITH GD et al: The Black report on socioeconomic inequalities in health 10 years on. Br Med J 301:373, 1990

WILKINSON RG: National mortality rates: The impact of inequality? Am J Public Health 82:1082, 1992

WILLIAMS RB et al: Prognostic importance of social and economic resources among medically treated patients with angiographically documented coronary artery disease. JAMA 267:520, 1992

Disease occurrence and survival by race/ethnicity

BARKER JC: Cultural diversity—Changing the context of medical practice, In Cross-cultural Medicine—A Decade Later. West J Med 157:248, 1992

BLENDON RJ et al: Access to medical care for black and white Americans. JAMA 261:276, 1989

GOLDBERG KC et al: Racial and community factors influencing coronary artery bypass graft surgery rates for all 1986 Medicare patients. JAMA 267:1473, 1992

GURALNIK JM: Educational status and active life expectancy among older blacks and whites. JAMA 329:110, 1993

KEIL JE et al: Does equal socioeconomic status in black and white men mean equal risk of mortality? Am J Public Health 82:1133, 1992

McCORD C, FREEMAN HP: Excess mortality in Harlem. N Engl J Med 322:173, 1990

NAVARRO V: Race *or* class or race *and* class: Growing mortality differentials in the United States. Int J Health Serv 21:229, 1992

SCHOENDORF KC et al: Mortality among infants of black as compared with white college-educated parents. N Engl J Med 326:1522, 1992

SCHWARTZ E et al: Black/white comparisons of deaths preventable by medical intervention: United States and the District of Columbia 1980–1986. Int J Epidemiol 19:591, 1990

US DEPARTMENT OF HEALTH AND HUMAN SERVICES: *Health, United States, 1990.* Hyattsville, MD, National Center for Health Statistics, 1991

WENNEKER MB, EPSTEIN AM: Racial inequalities in the use of procedures for patients with ischemic heart disease in Massachusetts. JAMA 261:253, 1989

WHITTLE JC et al: Does racial variation in risk factors explain black-white differences in the incidence of hypertensive end-stage renal disease? Arch Intern Med 151:1359, 1991

Socioeconomic status and race

DAVEY SMITH G et al: The magnitude and causes of socio-economic differentials in mortality: Further evidence from the Whitehall study. J Epidemiol Community Health 44:265, 1990

OTTEN MW JR et al: The effect of known risk factors on the excess mortality of black adults in the United States. JAMA 263:845, 1990

PIERCE JP et al: Trends in cigarette smoking in the United States. Projections to the Year 2000. JAMA 261:61, 1989

---

5 WOMEN'S HEALTH

ANTHONY L. KOMAROFF / BEVERLY WOO

In recent years, there has been a growing appreciation that the health problems of women require increased attention. Although certain diseases that occur primarily in women (e.g., breast cancer) have been the subject of considerable research, most illnesses that can affect men and women have not been as well studied in women. Many research studies of disease prevention and pathophysiology have included only male subjects; the findings may not be generalizable to female subjects. There are poorly understood differences in the expression of diseases in the two sexes. For example, several immunologically mediated diseases occur predominantly in women, for reasons that are uncertain. Furthermore, women receive different care than men for health problems that are common to both sexes. Finally, there are differences in morbidity and mortality between men and women. The causes for these differences are only partly understood.

This chapter summarizes some of the issues regarding the health of women that require special attention. Detailed discussions of specific diseases (those that occur predominantly or exclusively in women, as well as those that are not gender-specific) are found in other chapters.

PREVENTION Primary and secondary prevention are crucial elements in improving health. One general risk factor, cigarette smoking, has been well studied in women. In the United States during the 1930s, over 50 percent of men vs. only 20 percent of women smoked. By 1960, the rate had stayed about level in men but had risen to over 30 percent in women. In 1990, 28 percent of men vs. 23 percent of women were regular smokers. Thus, over the past 60 years there has been a sharp decline in smoking among men but not among women. "Low-yield" cigarettes are marketed heavily to women; however, the risk of myocardial infarction is equal for users of "low-yield" and higher-yield brands. Although it is of obvious importance to diminish smoking rates in both men and women (see Chap. 393), different interventions and educational strategies aimed at women may well be required.

Particularly in the past decade, a large number of important case-control and prospective cohort observational studies have been published that concentrate on the prevention of disease in women. A prime example is the Nurses' Health Study, in which more than 100,000 women have been followed prospectively. In this study, women aged 34–45 who used one to six aspirins per week had a 25 percent lower rate of developing a first myocardial infarction than women who reported no aspirin use, a statistically significant difference after adjusting for known cardiovascular risk factors. The study also found that postmenopausal estrogen therapy is associated with a

40 to 50 percent reduction in deaths due to ischemic heart disease (IHD), a finding supported by several case-control studies, as well.

At the same time, the major prospective, randomized controlled trials of primary prevention of cardiovascular disease—the Multiple Risk Factor Intervention Trial (MRFIT), the Physician's Health Study of aspirin and beta-carotene, the Cholesterol-Lowering Atherosclerosis Study (CLAS), the Helsinki Heart Study, and the Lipid Research Clinics Coronary Primary Prevention Trial—have included only male subjects. This is because cardiac endpoints are more common in men, allowing smaller and less costly studies. Now that these studies have contributed valuable information about several interventions in men, it becomes more important to perform studies in women, since IHD is the most common cause of death in women. Indeed, large randomized trials in women now are being organized by the United States National Institutes of Health to study the benefits and risks of postmenopausal hormone replacement therapy, and the value of low-dose aspirin and antioxidants in preventing cardiovascular disease and cancer in healthy women.

GENDER DIFFERENCES IN DISEASE Obviously, some conditions and diseases occur exclusively (or nearly exclusively) in women—e.g., the menopause and various breast and gynecologic disorders (see Chaps. 340, 341). In this chapter, we seek primarily to highlight some interesting gender differences in diseases that occur in both women and men.

Ischemic heart disease Many persons think of IHD as primarily a problem of men, perhaps because men have about twice the total incidence of cardiovascular morbidity and mortality of women from ages 35–84. However, in the United States, IHD is the leading cause of death among women as well as men; nearly 400,000 women die annually from IHD (Table 5-1). This mortality rate is five- to sixfold higher than the mortality rate for either lung or breast cancer, the two most common causes of death from cancer in women. On average, women develop IHD 10 years later than men and have myocardial infarction and sudden death 20 years after men.

LDL cholesterol levels and the ratios of total/HDL cholesterol are lower for women than men until age 60 to 70 years. In all age groups, HDL cholesterol levels are, on average, about 10 mg/dL higher in women than men. Some studies suggest that in women HDL cholesterol is more closely related to IHD risk than LDL cholesterol level.

There is a growing body of knowledge about IHD risk factors in women. However, more information is needed about the relative power of these risk factors and whether interventions can change an individual's risk. Large observational studies suggest that, in women,

obesity is an independent risk factor for nonfatal myocardial infarction and IHD mortality. As mentioned earlier, smoking is an important risk factor for IHD in women. Current use of oral contraceptives is associated with a two- to fourfold increase in the risk of myocardial infarction, independent of other known risk factors, in older premenopausal women. Past use of oral contraceptives does not appear to affect the risk of myocardial infarction. In women who use oral contraceptives, smoke, and have hypertension, the risk of myocardial infarction is especially high.

IHD presents differently in men and women. In the Framingham cohort, myocardial infarction was the first manifestation of IHD in 43 percent of men vs. 29 percent of women. In contrast, angina pectoris was the presenting symptom of IHD in 55 percent of women vs. 39 percent of men. The exercise ECG appears to have a lower specificity for IHD in women than men.

Finally, it has been suggested that women, particularly African-American women, have higher risks of morbidity and mortality than men following a myocardial infarction, coronary artery bypass graft surgery, and percutaneous transluminal coronary angioplasty. Whether this is true after adjusting for age and severity of disease remains uncertain. While women and men apparently experience a similar *relative* benefit with thrombolytic therapy following an acute myocardial infarction, the mortality rates remain higher in women.

Hypertension Although population-based epidemiologic studies in the United States show a higher prevalence of uncontrolled hypertension in men compared to women, the overall prevalence of hypertension (uncontrolled plus successfully treated) is about equal or slightly higher in women. The prevalence of hypertension appears to be the same for white women and men; however, African-American women have a higher prevalence of hypertension than African-American men. The risk of cardiovascular diseases that is attributable to hypertension appears to be the same or greater in women as compared to men, among the largely white subjects in the Framingham Study.

Immunologically mediated diseases Several diseases thought to be immunologically mediated—e.g., rheumatoid arthritis, systemic lupus erythematosus, multiple sclerosis, Graves' disease, and thyroiditis—occur much more frequently in women than in men. Although it is not entirely clear why this is so, estrogens appear to play an important role in pathogenesis. In animal models of rheumatoid arthritis, lupus, and multiple sclerosis, for example, the females of the species are predominantly affected.

Osteoporosis Endogenous levels of estrogen appear to play an important role in osteoporosis. The risk of osteoporosis in postmenopausal women is much greater than in men of the same age, and postmenopausal estrogen supplementation is associated with a decreased incidence of osteoporosis. The mechanisms by which estrogen exerts its protective effects remain to be fully elucidated.

Psychological disorders Depression, anxiety disorders, bulimia, and anorexia nervosa are diagnosed more often in women. However, there is a disagreement as to whether the actual prevalence of these disorders is different in the two sexes. Men may be more reluctant to bring emotional problems to the attention of a physician and may develop substance abuse disorders in response to underlying depression and anxiety more often, causing the former but not the latter to be diagnosed. Similarly, physicians may be more prone to diagnose mood or anxiety disorders when the patient who seeks medical care for vague symptoms with no obvious organic basis is a woman.

Social factors may account for the greater prevalence of some disorders in women. It has been suggested that the traditionally subordinate role of women in society may have generated a greater sense of vulnerability in women than in men. Bulimia and anorexia nervosa are believed, at least in part, to be an exaggerated distortion of the 20th century Western ideal of female beauty: the lean woman.

In addition, it is possible that biological factors, including hormonally influenced neurochemical changes, may also play a role in what may be the greater prevalence of psychological disorders and eating

---

TABLE 5-1 Death rates (per 100,000) for the leading causes of death in U.S. women, 1988

Age 25–34 Total: 74.0	Age 45–54 Total: 350.9	Age 65–74 Total: 2056.1	All ages Total: 826.9
1. Motor vehicle accidents (11.6)	*1.* Breast cancer (45.3)	*1.* Ischemic heart disease (453.1)	*1.* Ischemic heart disease (194.4)
2. Homicide (7.3)	*2.* Ischemic heart disease (36.8)	*2.* Lung cancer* (164.1)	*2.* Cerebrovascular disease (72.0)
3. Suicide (5.7)	*3.* Lung cancer* (35.0)	*3.* Cerebrovascular disease (137.3)	*3.* Lung cancer* (36.8)
4. Nonmotor vehicle accidents (5.0)	*4.* Cerebrovascular disease (17.4)	*4.* Breast cancer (109.4)	*4.* Breast cancer (33.5)

* Cancer of respiratory and intrathoracic organs, predominantly lung cancer.
SOURCE: Adapted from National Center for Health Statistics. *Vital Statistics of the United States, 1988.* Volume II, Mortality, Part A. Washington: Public Health Service, 1991. DHHS Publication No. (PHS)91-1101, pp. 40–52.

disorders in women. For example, the limbic system and hypothalamus, areas of the brain thought to subserve appetite, satiety, and emotion, have recently been shown to contain estradiol and testosterone receptors.

Alcohol abuse   Blood alcohol levels are higher in women than in men after drinking equivalent amounts of alcohol (adjusted for body weight). This greater bioavailability of alcohol in women is probably due to decreased gastric "first pass metabolism" of alcohol, associated with lower activity of gastric alcohol dehydrogenase. On average, alcoholic women drink less than alcoholic men but exhibit the same degree of impairment. In addition, alcoholic women are more likely than alcoholic men to abuse tranquilizers, sedatives, and amphetamines. These findings have important implications in women for suggested "safe" levels of drinking with regard to driving and other activities.

Women alcoholics have a higher mortality rate than both nonalcoholic women and alcoholic men. Compared to men, women also appear to develop alcoholic liver disease and other alcohol-related diseases with shorter drinking histories and lower levels of alcohol consumption.

HIV infection   This is a major health issue for women (as it is for men). There is a rapidly growing number (and percentage) of women who are HIV-infected but who do not yet have AIDS. An anonymous survey of the prevalence of HIV infection, the Sentinel Hospital study, found that as many as 8 percent of women in some urban areas who were felt not to be at high risk for HIV infection were, in fact, HIV-positive.

In the United States, AIDS is now the leading cause of death in young African-American women. Eleven percent of the reported cases of AIDS in the United States are in women, and the rate of increase in the incidence of AIDS is greater for women than men. About half of AIDS cases in women are associated with intravenous drug use and the other half appear to result from infection acquired by heterosexual transmission. A recent study indicates that death occurs sooner after the diagnosis of AIDS in women than in men. Worldwide, during the 1990s, an estimated 3 million women will die of AIDS.

The presentation of HIV infection in women has some special features. Vaginal candidiasis and pelvic inflammatory disease are prominent. Other sexually transmitted diseases as well as preneoplastic and neoplastic disease occur more frequently, and with greater severity, in HIV-infected women than in uninfected women.

Violence against women   During the past 20 years, there has been a growing awareness of the enormous problem of violence against women, particularly involving family members and social acquaintances.

Rape has recently been redefined in many statutes as "nonconsensual sexual penetration of an adolescent or adult obtained by physical force, by threat of bodily harm, or when the victim is incapable of giving consent by virtue of mental illness, mental retardation, or intoxication." Epidemiologic studies in the United States suggest that at least 20 percent of adult women have experienced sexual assault during their lifetimes. Nearly 100,000 cases of rape are reported annually in the United States, and this undoubtedly represents only a fraction of the actual number of cases. Adult women are much more likely to be raped by a spouse, ex-spouse, or acquaintance than by a stranger.

In addition, every year in the United States more than 2 million women receive severe physical injury and more than 1000 women are killed by their current or former male partner. Domestic violence is the most common cause of physical injury in women, exceeding all injuries due to rape, mugging, and auto accidents combined. Surveys of women seeking medical care for any reason in internal medicine and emergency room practices have reported that the prevalence of domestic violence is an astonishing 15–20 percent. Domestic violence is a major health problem in women from all age, ethnic, and socioeconomic groups.

Women who have been raped or injured, as well as women who have been molested during childhood, frequently seek medical care for headaches, sleep and eating disorders, abdominal or pelvic pain, vaginal discharge, or musculoskeletal symptoms. They may also present to physicians with depression, suicidal ideation, and substance abuse. Given this indirect presentation of the consequences of violence, and the high prevalence of violence, clinicians should readily consider the possibility of violence in patients with vague symptoms and psychological disorders.

The immediate treatment of rape and domestic violence is focused on assessing and treating physical injury, providing emotional support, evaluating and dealing with the risks of sexually transmitted infection and pregnancy, assessing the safety of the patient and other family members, and documenting the patient's history and findings on physical examination. In addition to dealing with the medical and psychological issues, appropriate care includes providing information about legal services, shelters and safe houses, hotlines, support groups, and counseling services.

GENDER DIFFERENCES IN RESEARCH   As noted earlier, relatively few women have been involved in studies of the prevention and pathophysiology of major diseases that involve both women and men. The same is also true for research related to treatment. Over $30 billion of pharmaceuticals are sold each year in the United States, and the great majority are used by women. Yet most clinical pharmacologic studies involving diseases that occur frequently in both sexes have been conducted in men. Even clinical pharmacologic studies in animals often concentrate on the males of the species. Two reasons are commonly given for conducting most clinical pharmacologic studies in men. First, cyclic hormonal changes in females could make experiments more difficult to control and interpret. Second, particularly with new drugs, concern about unsuspected pregnancy and subsequent teratogenic effects have discouraged the recruitment of female subjects.

Those studies that have included women indicate that there are clinically significant differences in the way women respond to a number of frequently prescribed pharmaceuticals, including sedative-hypnotics, antidepressants, antipsychotics, anticonvulsants, and beta-adrenoceptor blockers. Some studies have found that women have a higher frequency of adverse drug reactions than men, even after adjusting for several factors, including age, number of drugs being administered simultaneously, and duration of hospitalization. Women have more drug-induced gastrointestinal disturbances and cutaneous allergic reactions than men. Other studies suggest that the efficacy of many drugs may be lower in women. For example, women may be less responsive than men to antidepressant drugs. As another example, it has been shown that women require lower doses of neuroleptics than men to control schizophrenia. The reasons for these differences are not clear. Estrogens may reduce drug clearance via the cytochrome P450 oxidase system, an observation that could be of great practical importance given that millions of women regularly use estrogens. In some instances, drug pharmacokinetics may change during the menstrual cycle. For example, there is reasonable evidence that some anticonvulsants and lithium may be metabolized more rapidly in the premenstrual period, resulting in an increased frequency of premenstrual ("catamenial") seizures and increased symptoms of bipolar disorder, respectively, in women treated with these drugs.

DIFFERENCES IN THE MEDICAL EVALUATION OF MEN AND WOMEN   In recent years, there has been growing evidence that gender, as well as race, may be an important factor in determining the care a patient receives. This has been most extensively studied with regard to IHD and end-stage renal disease. With regard to gender, several studies indicate that women with known IHD or with symptoms that might be secondary to IHD are less likely to undergo coronary angiography and revascularization. Further research is needed to determine why these gender differences exist. For example, do clinicians think that such procedures are of lesser benefit or greater risk in women (and, if so, on what basis do they take this position)? Are women less likely than men to ask about or consent to these diagnostic and therapeutic procedures? Finally, is the current use of coronary angiography and revascularization at the optimal level, in women and men?

Inequalities based on gender and race also have been observed with regard to the treatment of end-stage renal disease in the United States as well as other countries. Women with this condition are only 70 percent as likely to receive dialysis compared to men. In addition, women receiving long-term dialysis have only 75 percent the chance that men have of receiving a kidney transplant. The result of these two gender-related differences in care is that women aged 45 to 60 years receive a transplant less than half as often as men of the same age and race. Biological factors do not appear to explain these differences. Further research is needed to determine what role the beliefs of patients or doctors may play in creating this difference in the utilization of technology related to end-stage renal disease, and whether these beliefs are valid.

MORBIDITY AND MORTALITY IN WOMEN There are substantial differences in the rates of morbidity and mortality between men and women. A number of psychosocial and biological factors have been identified that clearly influence these differences, but much remains to be learned.

Morbidity Women may well experience greater morbidity than men. In 1980, females experienced a 26 percent higher rate of restricted activity and a 40 percent higher rate of bed disability adjusted across all ages. Women also make more visits to physicians, particularly for acute self-limited illnesses. The age-adjusted male/female ratio of the frequency of acute conditions of different types is summarized in Table 5-2. Except for injuries, acute conditions are diagnosed more frequently in women than men. It is unclear whether these differences in the incidence of acute conditions, and the associated increased disability and utilization of medical care, reflect real differences in the prevalence of morbidity, differences in concern about and reporting of symptoms, or differences in care-seeking behavior following the development of symptoms. Interestingly, in children less than age 15, it is the males that have higher rates of acute conditions, acute disability, and physician visits.

Mortality differences As shown in Table 5-1, among young women in the United States almost half of all deaths are violent and are due to accidents, homicide, and suicide. During the middle years, breast cancer is a slightly more common cause of death than IHD and lung cancer. In women between ages 65 and 74, IHD and lung cancer overtake breast cancer as the leading causes of death. Across the entire age spectrum IHD is the leading cause of death in women by a substantial margin.

In the developed nations, women live longer than men. In the United States, the current average life expectancy from birth is 78.8 years for females, and 72.0 years for males. Although there are more male fetuses conceived than female fetuses, females have a survival advantage when compared to males, in all age groups both before and after birth. As shown in Table 5-3, age-adjusted death rates for the 15 leading causes of death in the United States are all greater in men than in women. From age 15 to 44 years, males are more than twice as likely to die than females.

TABLE 5-3 Ratio of age-adjusted death rates for the 15 leading causes of death, United States, 1988: Male/Female

Rank	Cause of death	Male/female ratio
1	Diseases of the heart	1.9
2	Malignant neoplasms	1.5
3	Cerebrovascular diseases	1.2
4	Accidents	2.7
5	Chronic obstructive pulmonary diseases	2.0
6	Pneumonia and influenza	1.7
7	Diabetes mellitus	1.1
8	Suicide	4.0
9	Chronic liver disease and cirrhosis	2.3
10	Nephritis, nephrotic syndrome, and nephrosis	1.5
11	Atherosclerosis	1.3
12	Homicide	3.3
13	Septicemia	1.3
14	Infant perinatal conditions	1.3
15	Human immunodeficiency virus infection	8.6

SOURCE: Adapted from: *MMWR* (40)494, 1991.

Social factors and women's health Gender differences in morbidity and mortality may be explained in part by psychosocial factors such as socially defined gender roles, poverty, participation in the workforce, health insurance, and lifestyle factors.

In the past 30 years in the United States there has been a "feminization of poverty"—a rapid growth in the relative percentage of people in female-headed households who are living in poverty. One-third of families headed by women currently live in poverty, and the fraction is greater than one-half for African-American and Latino women. Almost a fifth of women over age 65 live below the poverty level. Lack of adequate health insurance is a major problem for many women, especially minority women, poor and low-income women, and women of reproductive age. Women in general are more likely than men to have low-paying, part-time, nonunion jobs that do not provide health insurance. Women are more likely than men to lose health insurance, as a consequence of being divorced or widowed.

Women's increasing participation in the workforce could affect their health, although data on this question are limited and controversial. The 20th century has witnessed a striking social change in this regard. Whereas at the beginning of the century only about 20 percent of U.S. women were in the workforce, that figure has risen to about 75 percent, and is expected to continue to rise. Fewer than 10 percent of U.S. families currently consist of a father working outside the home and a mother working at home caring for children.

As discussed earlier, gender differences in lifestyle can explain some differences in morbidity and mortality. Substance abuse (including not only illicit drugs but also cigarettes and alcohol), reckless driving, and armed physical conflict (military and civilian) are more common in men. Men die from homicide approximately four times as often as women. These factors account for a part of the higher mortality rate in men, compared to women, particularly in the adolescent and young adult age groups.

Biological factors influencing morbidity and mortality There also may be biological differences that contribute to the greater longevity of women. The most obvious is the exposure to estrogen that most women experience for about 40 years of their lives. As discussed earlier, premenopausal women are "protected" from IHD, perhaps related to high estrogen levels or other factors. It is hoped that further research on biological differences between the sexes will produce much-needed knowledge in this area.

CONCLUSION Research has demonstrated important differences in the natural history, prevention, evaluation, and treatment of diseases in men and women. Studies are urgently needed of the important health problems of women mentioned above, as well as others not mentioned, including lung, breast, and other major cancers of women;

TABLE 5-2 Incidence of acute conditions for males and females, United States, 1980

Type of condition	Male/female ratio*
Infective and parasitic diseases	0.88
Respiratory conditions	0.81
Digestive conditions	0.92
Injuries	1.39
All other acute conditions, excluding pregnancy-related ones	0.66

* Calculated as incidence per 100 persons per year, adjusted for age.
SOURCE: Adapted from Verbrugge & Wingard, 1987; and Jack SS: Current estimates from the National Health Interview Survey: United States, 1980. In *Vital and Health Statistics*, Ser. 10, No. 139, National Center for Health Statistics, DHHS Publ. (PHS) 82-1567, 1982.

common disorders such as dysmenorrhea and premenstrual syndrome; contraception; and infertility.

REFERENCES

ANASTOS K et al: Hypertension in women: What is really known? Ann Intern Med 115:287, 1991

AYANIAN JZ, EPSTEIN AM: Differences in the use of procedures between women and men hospitalized for coronary heart disease. N Engl J Med 325:221, 1991

BLUME SB: Women and alcohol. A review. JAMA 256:1467, 1986

BLUMENTHAL SJ et al: *Towards a Women's Health Research Agenda. Findings of the Scientific Advisory Meeting.* Washington, Bass and Howes, Inc. 1991

COUNCIL ON SCIENTIFIC AFFAIRS, AMERICAN MEDICAL ASSOCIATION: Violence against women. Relevance for medical practitioners. JAMA 267:3184, 1992

FIEBACH NH et al: Differences between women and men in survival after myocardial infarction. Biology or methodology? JAMA 263:1092, 1990

GIJSBERS VAN WIJK CMT et al: Symptom sensitivity and sex differences in physical morbidity: A review of health surveys in the United States and the Netherlands. Women and Health 17:91, 1991

MANSON JE et al: A prospective study of aspirin use and primary prevention of cardiovascular disease in women. JAMA 266:521, 1991

MINKOFF HL, DEHOVITZ JA: Care of women infected with the human immunodeficiency virus. JAMA 266:2253, 1991

RODIN J et al: Women's health. Review and research agenda as we approach the 21st century. Amer Psychol 45:1018, 1990

VERBRUGGE LM, WINGARD DL: Sex differentials in health and mortality. Women & Health 12:103, 1987

6   MEDICAL DISORDERS DURING PREGNANCY

THOMAS F. FERRIS

Pregnancy may be complicated by chronic disease or a new illness. In the past, many disorders were considered contraindications to pregnancy, but now, with appropriate care, excellent outcomes for both mother and child are the rule.

HYPERTENSION

Systemic vascular resistance is reduced in pregnancy. In spite of a 40 percent increase in cardiac output during the second trimester, blood pressure falls (usually to 100/70 mmHg or lower). Although a modest rise may occur during the last month of normal pregnancy, an increase in systolic pressure of 30 mmHg or diastolic pressure of 15 mmHg at any time during gestation is abnormal. Perinatal mortality increases with blood pressure levels that would be normal in nonpregnant women. For example, when mean arterial blood pressure (diastolic plus one-third of the pulse pressure) is 90 mmHg or higher during the second trimester, there is greater risk for stillbirth, fetal growth retardation, and preeclampsia.

Hypertension during pregnancy usually has one of four causes: (1) preeclampsia (toxemia), (2) chronic essential hypertension, (3) gestational hypertension, or (4) renal disease.

PREECLAMPSIA (TOXEMIA)   Preeclampsia is a disease of late pregnancy in which hypertension is associated with hepatic, neurologic, hematologic, or renal involvement. Rapid development of edema, particularly of the face and hands, along with a rise in blood pressure, usually signals the onset of this condition. Jaundice and abnormal liver function may be present. Hyperreflexia, visual disturbances, and headache indicate neurologic involvement and convulsions indicate the presence of eclampsia. Hematologic manifestations of preeclampsia include thrombocytopenia with elevated lactate dehydrogenase (LDH), microangiopathic hemolytic anemia, and thrombocytopenia. In fulminant preeclampsia, disseminated intravascular coagulation may cause a reduction in plasma fibrinogen and elevated circulating fibrin degradation products (Chap. 316).

Proteinuria indicates renal involvement, and since the glomerular filtration rate (GFR) increases by about 50 percent in normal gestation, a reduction in GFR heralds the onset of preeclampsia even with normal levels of blood urea nitrogen (BUN) and serum creatinine. Indeed, a BUN of 6.4 mmol/L (18 mg/dL) or a creatinine of 90 μmol/L (1 mg/dL) during pregnancy may reflect a 50 percent decline in GFR. In preeclampsia, urate clearance decreases, because of increased proximal tubular reabsorption of urate, which in turn is probably due to the reduction of vascular volume. Hyperuricemia usually precedes the rise in serum creatinine and BUN; in fact, a plasma uric acid above 270 μmol/L (4.5 mg/dL) in a hypertensive pregnant woman suggests preeclampsia. Volume contraction is similar to that in some other hypertensive states in which venoconstriction causes capillary pressure to rise, with expansion of interstitial volume at the expense of intravascular volume.

Fibrin deposits in the glomeruli, with characteristic swelling of the glomerular endothelial cells, are evident in renal biopsies; peripheral necrosis with fibrin deposits in the sinusoids may be present in the liver. Tomographic scanning techniques (CT or MRI) reveal hypodense areas consistent with small cerebral infarctions in approximately half of the women with eclampsia.

An abnormality in endothelial integrity may be the cause of the widespread fibrin deposits. Increased synthesis of two vasodilator prostaglandins—prostaglandin E_2 (PGE$_2$) and prostacyclin (PGI$_2$)—may explain the vasodilation and resistance to angiotensin II in normal pregnancy. In preeclampsia, synthesis of PGI$_2$ decreases, and sensitivity to angiotensin II increases, and the balance that normally exists between the platelet aggregatory and vasoconstrictor effects of thromboxane A_2 (produced by platelets) and the counteracting antiaggregatory and vasodilating effects of PGI$_2$ (produced by endothelial cells) may be lost, contributing to hypertension and platelet aggregation. The likelihood of preeclampsia may be reduced in women at risk when low-dose aspirin (an inhibitor of thromboxane A_2 synthesis) is administered throughout pregnancy.

Management   Once preeclampsia is diagnosed, hospitalization is indicated, since the disease can rapidly progress to eclampsia, characterized by convulsions. The definitive treatment of preeclampsia and eclampsia is delivery of the conceptus, which should be carried out promptly if fetal size and maturity are adequate. If the fetus is immature, bed rest, restriction of sodium intake to 2 g/d or less, and antihypertensive therapy are indicated. Beta blockers, calcium antagonists, hydralazine, and central sympathetic antagonists are all useful agents. Angiotensin converting enzyme (ACE) inhibitors are *contraindicated in pregnancy* since they increase the risk for fetal loss.

If an immediate reduction in blood pressure is needed, as in other forms of severe, uncontrolled hypertension (Chap. 209), several agents are useful. These include intravenous hydralazine (10-mg doses every 15 minutes until the desired effect is maintained); 500 mg alpha-methyldopa over 30 minutes; and labetalol, 1 mg/kg IV, followed by a continuous infusion of 20 mg/h. Obstetricians have long relied upon intravenous magnesium sulfate, which has mild antihypertensive properties and which increases synthesis of PGI$_2$ by endothelial cells.

CHRONIC ESSENTIAL HYPERTENSION   Like normal women, women with chronic essential hypertension experience a reduction in peripheral resistance during pregnancy. Indeed, a "normal" blood pressure may be obtained for the first time during pregnancy. Women with chronic hypertension are at higher risk for preeclampsia. Careful monitoring for proteinuria and of serum creatinine and uric acid are important in detecting the onset of this complication. There is no evidence that pregnancy has an adverse effect on the course of chronic essential hypertension. Thus antihypertensive medication (other than ACE inhibitors) should be continued throughout pregnancy in women with essential hypertension. Alpha-methyldopa has been used extensively in pregnancy, and children born to mothers who have taken this drug throughout pregnancy develop normally.

GESTATIONAL HYPERTENSION Hypertension that develops late in pregnancy (with no evidence of preeclampsia) and disappears after delivery is termed gestational hypertension. Usually women with this condition are overweight; others have a family history of hypertension, eventually develop chronic essential hypertension later in life, and have a high incidence of recurrence during subsequent pregnancies. Attention must be directed toward detecting increases in urinary protein and serum uric acid, creatinine, or BUN, since these remain normal in gestational hypertension and become elevated in preeclampsia. A beta blocker or alpha-methyldopa are usually effective in lowering blood pressure.

RENAL DISEASE

The increase in GFR during normal pregnancy is due to a rise in renal plasma flow without a concomitant rise in glomerular pressure. However, in renal disease, any rise in GFR depends on an elevation in glomerular pressure, which can increase proteinuria and worsen the underlying disease. Hypertension becomes more severe during pregnancy in most women with chronic renal disease, and proteinuria increases in approximately 20 percent. Since autoregulation of renal blood flow may be impaired in renal disease, any increase in blood pressure is more apt to raise glomerular pressure. The development or worsening of hypertension during pregnancy in patients with renal disease may be due to preeclampsia superimposed on renal disease.

It is desirable to maintain blood pressure below 120/80 mmHg in pregnant women with chronic renal disease. Twenty-four-hour urine protein excretion should be assessed throughout pregnancy, and an increase in proteinuria with no clinical evidence of toxemia usually reflects elevated glomerular pressure. Antihypertensive drugs other than ACE inhibitors should be utilized.

Many women have had successful pregnancies after renal transplantation. Although these patients receive chronic immunosuppressive therapy throughout gestation, the incidence of congenital malformations does not appear to be increased.

If systemic lupus erythematosus (SLE) (Chap. 284) is quiescent for 12 to 18 months prior to conception, pregnancy does not appear to activate the disease. In nonpregnant women, flare-ups of lupus nephropathy are usually associated with extrarenal manifestations of the disease, i.e., arthritis, rash, and fever, accompanied by a reduction in serum complement and a rise in anti-DNA antibodies. In contrast, pregnant women with SLE may manifest an increase in blood pressure and proteinuria along with a reduction in renal function in the absence of extrarenal manifestations. The renal exacerbations may be due to superimposed preeclampsia or the effect of hypertension on the nephropathy, since there is no clinical evidence of lupus activity and no increase in anti-DNA antibodies. This is an important distinction because these women may be treated inappropriately with higher doses of glucocorticoids or immunosuppressive agents (which may exacerbate hypertension) when antihypertensive therapy or delivery (depending on gestational age and maternal condition) is indicated instead. Conversely, women with active SLE who could be treated with glucocorticoids are often delivered inappropriately early for the mistaken diagnosis of preeclampsia.

CARDIAC DISEASE

As noted above, pregnancy is associated with a reduction in systemic vascular resistance. Normally, increases occur in stroke volume, heart rate, and cardiac output; these changes often produce systolic (flow) murmurs and third heart sounds. The rise in cardiac output exceeds the increase in oxygen consumption, so the arteriovenous oxygen difference falls. Four cardiac disorders are adversely affected by pregnancy: (1) valvular heart disease, (2) primary pulmonary hypertension, (3) the Eisenmenger syndrome, and (4) the Marfan syndrome.

VALVULAR HEART DISEASE (See also Chap. 201) The increased cardiac output associated with pregnancy may cause deterioration in women with *mitral stenosis*. If severe mitral stenosis is identified *prior* to pregnancy, valvulotomy should be carried out before conception, if possible. Asymptomatic pregnant women with mitral stenosis require close observation but not definitive therapy. However, if symptoms of pulmonary congestion develop, diuretics and restriction of activity are indicated. Atrial fibrillation should be treated with oral digoxin to slow the ventricular rate. Thromboembolism associated with mitral stenosis requires anticoagulation with intravenous heparin; warfarin is *contraindicated* in pregnancy because of its teratogenic effects. A closed mitral valvulotomy (surgical or, preferably, by balloon mitral valvuloplasty) can be carried out during pregnancy, when symptoms of mitral stenosis are severe; open-heart surgery is associated with an increase in fetal loss.

Mitral regurgitation is usually well tolerated during pregnancy, presumably because peripheral resistance is lower. Aortic stenosis is a contraindication for pregnancy until the lesion has been corrected. A maternal mortality of 15 percent has been reported in women with critical aortic stenosis.

Artificial heart valves in pregnant women are associated with many problems. It is mandatory to continue full anticoagulation in patients with mechanical valvular prostheses. Warfarin is contraindicated because of its teratogenic effects; heparin is preferable but may cause bleeding and fetal loss. Tissue valves are less thrombogenic, but their limited durability in young adults is a serious disadvantage. Therefore in women with serious valvular heart disease every effort should be made to allow pregnancy to go to completion prior to valve replacement, and subsequent pregnancies avoided once a mechanical valve has been implanted.

In women with prosthetic valves, antibiotic prophylaxis with agents effective against genitourinary organisms is mandatory during the peripartum period.

PULMONARY HYPERTENSION AND EISENMENGER SYNDROME (See Chaps. 225 and 199) Pulmonary hypertension of all causes is a strong contraindication for pregnancy. If moderate or severe pulmonary hypertension (systolic pulmonary artery pressure >45 mmHg) is detected during the first trimester, termination of the pregnancy is advisable. In women with congenital heart disease, pulmonary hypertension, and a right-to-left shunt, i.e., the Eisenmenger syndrome, both maternal and fetal mortality are high, the latter increasing with the severity of maternal cyanosis.

MARFAN SYNDROME (See Chap. 351) Cardiovascular manifestations of the Marfan syndrome include mitral valve prolapse, mitral and aortic valve abnormalities, and aortic regurgitation due to enlargement of the aortic root. When the aortic root diameter measured by echocardiography exceeds 40 mm, the risk of aortic dissection and rupture during pregnancy is increased. Women with the Marfan syndrome, especially those with a dilated aortic root, should avoid pregnancy; however, if such women become pregnant and refuse abortion, beta-adrenoceptor blocker therapy should be instituted to reduce the force of myocardial contraction and the resultant shear stress on the aorta.

OTHER FORMS OF CARDIAC DISEASE In the absence of pulmonary hypertension, atrial septal defect (p. 1040) is well tolerated by pregnant women, although the risk of fetal loss is increased. Patients with ventricular septal defect (p. 1041) without pulmonary hypertension also tolerate pregnancy well, but this lesion may be complicated by infective endocarditis, so antibiotic prophylaxis at the time of delivery is mandatory. Mitral valve prolapse (p. 1058), which is common among pregnant women, does not appear to complicate the pregnancy, nor does pregnancy complicate prolapse, although antibiotic prophylaxis is warranted. Women with hypertrophic cardiomyopathy (p. 1092) generally tolerate pregnancy well; indeed, the gestational hypervolemia may be associated with a reduction of the intraventricular pressure gradient and thus ameliorate symptoms. Because of its poor prognosis, chronic dilated cardiomyopathy (p. 1090) accompanied by heart failure is a contraindication to pregnancy.

Peripartum cardiomyopathy, a form of acute dilated cardiomyopathy that may be associated with a myocarditis, appears around the time of delivery, most frequently during the first 6 weeks postpartum, is sometimes associated with preeclampsia, and may actually be caused by pregnancy (p. 1090). Infant mortality is high if congestive heart failure ensues, and maternal mortality may be as high as 30 percent within the first few months. About one-third of patients show functional recovery and the remaining third have persistent severely impaired left ventricular function. Subsequent pregnancies should be avoided.

Premature atrial or ventricular systoles during pregnancy can be treated by the elimination of stimulants, avoidance of excessive fatigue, and reassurance. Drug therapy should be avoided, if possible, but cardioversion has been used safely for tachyarrhythmias during pregnancy.

PULMONARY EMBOLISM (See also Chap. 226)

In pregnancy all of the coagulation factors are increased, except factors XI and XIII, and antithrombin III, a major inhibitor of coagulation, is reduced. Pulmonary embolism occurs about once in 750 pregnancies. Because of the immediate need to prevent embolism and the other long-term complications of deep vein thrombosis (DVT), it is important to recognize the latter. DVT may occur during pregnancy owing to compression of the iliac veins by the enlarged uterus as well as changes in the coagulation and fibrinolytic systems that favor thrombosis. This complication also occurs in the postpartum period. Impedance plethysmography and Doppler ultrasonography are noninvasive nonradiologic techniques useful in documenting DVT. When pulmonary embolism is suspected, perfusion lung scanning can be accomplished with smaller quantities of isotope, and pulmonary angiography can be carried out if the abdomen is shielded. Despite the potential small hazard of fetal irradiation posed by these latter procedures, it is extremely important to diagnose pulmonary embolism.

Anticoagulant therapy is indicated in pregnant women with DVT to prevent pulmonary embolism. Heparin, which does not cross the placenta and therefore does not cause fetal complications, can be administered at a dose of 1000 units per hour by continuous infusion until early during labor. Protamine can then be used to reverse the drug's effects, and heparin can be restarted within 2 h of delivery and continued for 3 to 4 days after which subcutaneous heparin or oral warfarin therapy may be instituted for 6 months. When venous thrombosis or pulmonary embolism occur in the early postpartum period, heparin treatment should be instituted for 7 to 10 days, followed by warfarin for about 3 months.

DIABETES MELLITUS (See also Chap. 337)

From a metabolic standpoint, pregnancy resembles starvation—that is, blood sugar and amino acids are low while plasma free fatty acids, ketones, and triglycerides are increased. Plasma glucose is 0.8–1.1 mmol/L (15 to 20 mg/dL) lower after an overnight fast than in nonpregnant women; when fasting lasts longer than 12 h, plasma glucose may fall to 2.2–2.5 mmol/L (40 to 45 mg/dL) while plasma hydroxybutyrate and acetoacetate levels rise to levels two to four times higher than in nonpregnant women. As a consequence, ketoacidosis develops in the absence of striking hyperglycemia in pregnant diabetics. Maternal insulin and glucagon do not cross the placenta, but acetoacetate and beta-hydroxybutyrate are readily transferred and oxidized by the fetal brain and liver.

In spite of the fetal demand for glucose, pregnancy is also a diabetogenic state by virtue of the development of insulin resistance. Elevation of several hormones in pregnancy may be responsible for insulin resistance, including progesterone, estrogen, prolactin, and human placental lactogen.

Pregnancy in diabetics is associated with a higher perinatal mortality (3 to 5 percent vs. 1 to 2 percent in nondiabetic women) and a higher incidence of congenital anomalies (6 to 12 percent vs. 2 to 3 percent in nondiabetics). Glucose control, particularly during organogenesis, reduces the incidence of congenital anomalies. Counseling should emphasize the importance of home monitoring of glucose levels and the need to adjust the insulin dose to maintain fasting blood sugar at a normal level and postprandial glucose no higher than 7.8 mmol/L (140 mg/dL). Glycosylated hemoglobin should also be monitored during pregnancy. Ultrasound evaluation of the fetus should be carried out during the second trimester, and alpha-fetoprotein levels should be assessed in the 20th week to detect neural tube defects.

Women with diabetic nephropathy have an excellent chance of a normal pregnancy, with perinatal survival of approximately 90 percent. As with other renal diseases, hypertension can worsen late in pregnancy, with increased proteinuria and decreased creatinine clearance that represents either superimposed preeclampsia or a rise in glomerular pressure. There is no evidence that pregnancy worsens diabetic nephropathy, but care of pregnant women with diabetic nephropathy requires management by obstetricians skilled in high-risk pregnancies, neonatologists, diabetologists, and nephrologists. Hypertension should be treated as described earlier in this chapter.

GESTATIONAL DIABETES The insulin resistance of normal pregnancy may also contribute to gestational diabetes in women in whom the capacity for insulin secretion is not sufficient to meet the increased insulin demands of pregnancy. The overall prevalence of gestational diabetes is between 1 and 3 percent. An important reason for recognizing the disorder early is that it induces excessive fetal insulin secretion, which in turn can cause fetal macrosomia and increase the risk for birth trauma and the need for cesarean section.

There are no universally accepted criteria for the diagnosis or screening for gestational diabetes if the fasting glucose is normal. The 1990 Workshop-Conference on Gestational Diabetes recommended the screening of pregnant women with normal fasting blood sugar levels between the 24th and 28th weeks of gestation using a 50-g oral glucose load. If the 1-h glucose level exceeds 7.8 mmol/L (140 m/dL) a 100-g oral glucose test is performed after an overnight fast. Gestational diabetes is defined as any two of the following values: 1 h >10.5 mmol/L (>190 ng/dL), 2 h >9.2 mmol/L (>165 ng/dL), and 3 h >8.0 mmol/L (>145 ng/dL). In contrast, the American College of Obstetricians and Gynecologists recommends screening only for women at high risk, namely women over age 30; women with previous macrosomic, malformed, or stillborn infants; and those with obesity, hypertension, or glycosuria.

Gestational diabetes is treated with diet; if fasting glucose remains elevated insulin therapy should be started. Following delivery, carbohydrate tolerance may return to normal, but 30 percent or more of women with gestational diabetes develop diabetes mellitus within 5 years of pregnancy.

THYROID DISEASE (See also Chap. 334)

The diagnosis of thyroid disease in pregnancy is complicated by the increases in thyroid size, radioactive iodine uptake, basal metabolic rate, and thyroxine-binding globulin during normal pregnancy. Plasma T_3 and T_4 are elevated, but free T_3, T_4, and thyroid-stimulating hormone (TSH) remain normal, while the T_3 resin uptake is in the hypothyroid range. Maternal thyrotoxicosis occurs about once in 500 pregnancies, and the diagnosis may be difficult because the increase in cardiac output, tachycardia, skin warmth, and heat intolerance typical of pregnancy can mimic hyperthyroidism. Values of T_4 above 154 mmol/L (12 μg/dL) with a resin T_3 uptake in the euthyroid range (25 to 35 percent) suggests hyperthyroidism in a pregnant woman. Pregnant women can tolerate mild degrees of hyperthyroidism without difficulty, and thyrotoxicosis does not increase fetal loss. Gestation does not worsen thyrotoxicosis; indeed, hyperthyroidism is often more easily controlled during pregnancy. The treatment of gestational thyrotoxicosis involves a choice between antithyroid drugs and ablative surgery. Propylthiouracil is the drug of choice, since methimazole may cause aplasia cutis in the fetus. Maternal T_4 concentration should be maintained in the upper range of normal, using as low a dose of propylthiouracil as possible. Since this drug crosses the placenta and blocks fetal synthesis of thyroxine, fetal goiter occasionally develops due to stimulation of fetal TSH. When surgery is planned for the treatment of thyrotoxicosis, propylthiouracil should be administered preoperatively to control the hyperthyroid state.

Hypothyroidism during pregnancy should be treated with hormone replacement as in the nongravid state.

DISORDERS OF CALCIUM METABOLISM (See also Chap. 357)

Although serum calcium normally falls in pregnancy because of the decrease in serum albumin, the concentration of ionized calcium remains unchanged. Parathyroid hormone (PTH) levels increase in pregnancy with no change in phosphate clearance. This increase in PTH may be the cause of the higher plasma 1,25-dihydroxyvitamin D in pregnancy, resulting in an increase in intestinal calcium absorption and hypercalciuria. Urinary calcium excretion is approximately 7.5 mmol/d (300 mg/d), compared with 2.5 mmol/d (100 mg/d) in nonpregnant women, and urinary calculi develop in about one of 2000 pregnancies. When hyperparathyroidism with hypercalcemia occurs during pregnancy, the neonate may exhibit tetany because of the suppression of fetal PTH secretion.

HEMATOLOGIC DISORDERS

During pregnancy, plasma volume increases more than does red cell mass, so that a fall in hemoglobin concentration of 10 to 20 g/L (1 to 2 g/dL) is usual. Two potential causes of anemia during pregnancy are deficiencies of iron or folate. Since the developing fetus utilizes these substances in large amounts, these deficiencies may be prevented by providing iron and folate supplements. Pregnancy also results in a leukocytosis that can sometimes reach 18,000 per cubic millimeter.

Sickle cell anemia (Chap. 306) may be complicated by pregnancy, and vasoocclusive crises become more frequent, particularly during labor and the postpartum period. The risks for spontaneous abortion, prematurity, and neonatal death are high.

Thrombocytopenia in pregnancy is most often due to preeclampsia, although sepsis and idiopathic thrombocytopenic purpura may also be responsible. In the last-named condition, antiplatelet antibodies cross the placenta and can cause thrombocytopenia in the fetus as well. Cesarean section is indicated if the fetal platelet count obtained by percutaneous umbilical cord sampling performed at 36 to 37 weeks is less than 50,000 per milliliter.

Stillbirth, often associated with placental venous thrombosis, occurs in women with the so-called lupus anticoagulant (Chap. 284), an immunoglobulin that binds to negatively charged phospholipids and interferes with vitamin K–dependent coagulation factors. The lupus anticoagulant is actually more apt to cause thrombosis than bleeding, and treatment with low dose aspirin and prednisone throughout pregnancy may reduce the rate of fetal loss.

Disseminated intravascular coagulation may occur due to abruptio placentae, a retained dead fetus, amniotic fluid embolism, saline induced abortion, or fulminant preeclampsia and can be cured by treating the underlying cause.

GASTROINTESTINAL AND LIVER DISEASES

Nausea and vomiting occur in approximately 90 percent of women between the 6th and 16th weeks of pregnancy. When severe, the problem can be treated with oral dimenhydrinate, 50 to 100 mg every 4 h, or D-oxylamine, 12.5 mg every 4 h. In its severe form *hyperemesis gravidarum* can cause dehydration that requires parenteral feeding. Heartburn, which may be due to relaxation of the lower esophageal sphincter, is usually responsive to treatment with antacids and H-2 receptor blocking agents.

Pregnancy in women with inflammatory bowel disease may be uncomplicated, but it is difficult to anticipate the course in advance. Most patients do well but in some the pregnancy may exacerbate the disease; rarely the pregnancy may need to be terminated. If the disease is active at the time of conception, the incidence of spontaneous abortion is higher than in normal pregnancy.

Although pregnancy is associated with supersaturation of the bile with cholesterol, the incidence of cholelithiasis in a first pregnancy does not appear to be increased. However, the risk for this complication increases with multiparity. Serum triglycerides and cholesterol are elevated during pregnancy; although serum bilirubin remains normal, there is a striking rise in alkaline phosphatase (which originates from the placenta) that may reach a peak 2 to 4 times normal at term.

Although total serum protein concentration declines by approximately 20 percent in midpregnancy because of a decrease in albumin, hepatic synthesis of other plasma proteins increases. In a normal pregnancy, serum gamma-glutamyl transpeptidase and serum lactate dehydrogenase (LDH) are increased, whereas serum aminotransferases and aspartate aminotransferase are normal.

Intrahepatic cholestasis of pregnancy usually appears in the third trimester and is manifested by pruritus, with bilirubin levels usually less than 100 μmol/L (6 mg/dL). Although bilirubin levels usually remain in the range of 34 to 86 μmol/L (2 to 5 mg/dL), there is a striking increase in alkaline phosphatase. The cholestasis and pruritus disappear promptly after delivery, but the syndrome may recur with subsequent pregnancies. Aside from pruritus, the mother does not suffer any adverse effect. However, there appears to be an increase in stillbirths thought to be secondary to the toxicity of bile acids to the fetus. Therefore, fetal surveillance should be carried out once the diagnosis of intrahepatic cholestasis of pregnancy is established. Treatment of pruritus consists of antihistamine and cholestyramine, 4 g four times a day.

Acute fatty liver of pregnancy, with histologic changes showing hepatocytes with increased microvesicular fat and fibrin deposits in the hepatic sinusoids, may occur late in pregnancy and may be associated with preeclampsia. Serum bilirubin may exceed 170 μmol/L (10 mg/dL), and AST and ALT are in the range of 5 to 8 μkat/L (300 to 500 U/L). Prothrombin time may be prolonged, and disseminated intravascular coagulation may cause depressed fibrinogen levels, an increase in fibrin degradation products, and thrombocytopenia. Maternal deaths may occur, but this condition is usually ameliorated following delivery.

Hepatitis B (Chap. 266) during pregnancy increases prematurity and fetal death with a high risk of transmission to the infant, particularly in mothers who are HBe antigen-positive at the time of the delivery. Women who are HBs antigen-positive and HBe antigen-negative transmit the disease less frequently. Approximately 5 to 10 percent of infants infected with hepatitis B acquire the disease by the transplacental route. Infants born to mothers with hepatitis B should be treated with both hepatitis B immune globulin and hepatitis B vaccine.

The severity of viral hepatitis A is not altered by pregnancy and the risk of transmission to the neonate is small.

INFECTIONS

Infectious diseases constitute serious risk to both the pregnant woman and the fetus.

BACTERIAL INFECTIONS Urinary tract infections (see Chap. 90) are the most common type of bacterial infection in pregnancy. Asymptomatic bacteriuria occurs in up to 7 percent of pregnancies.

Physiologic changes in pregnancy such as hormone-induced dilatation of the urinary tract, hydroureter, and vesicoureteral reflux predispose to asymptomatic bacteriuria, and one-third of patients with these conditions develop pyelonephritis, usually during the last trimester. Since over 75 percent of pregnancy-associated acute pyelonephritis can be avoided by treating asymptomatic bacteriuria, screening for bacteriuria at the first prenatal visit is recommended. *Escherichia coli* is the most commonly isolated organism, and treatment for asymptomatic bacteriuria for 3 days with ampicillin, cephalexin, nitrofurantoin, or sulfisoxazole is appropriate, although the last drug should not be used during the final month of gestation because it may cause jaundice in the infant.

Intrauterine infection occurs in up to 4 percent of pregnancies and is associated with increased morbidity and mortality in the prenatal period. Intraamniotic infection is most common when ascending infection follows rupture of the membranes, but it is also seen with intact membranes, especially in preterm labor. Infection is usually polymicrobial, involving both aerobes and anaerobes, genital mycoplasmas, *Gardnerella vaginalis*, and group B streptococci. Since early clinical signs may be subtle, diagnosis requires a high degree of suspicion. Clinical clues include fever, maternal or fetal tachycardia, uterine tenderness, foul-smelling amniotic fluid, and leukocytosis. Delivery of the fetus is indicated. Antibiotic therapy should begin during labor, rather than afterward. Antibiotics with broad coverage are indicated, such as ampicillin and gentamicin.

Postpartum infections remain the most common cause of maternal mortality in the United States. The majority of deaths are related to postpartum endometrial infections complicated by pelvic abscess, peritonitis, or pelvic thrombophlebitis. Rates of endometritis vary from 1 to 3 percent after vaginal delivery and from 6 to 18 percent after cesarean section. Endometritis should be suspected when a patient has a fever after delivery. Few patients exhibit all of the classical manifestations such as fever, abdominal pain, malaise, and purulent or foul-smelling lochia. Work-up should include complete blood count, blood cultures, and a genital tract culture. The most common bacterial pathogens responsible for postpartum endometritis are group B streptococci, mixed anaerobic and aerobic organisms, *E. coli*, and *Staphylococcus aureus*. Treatment depends upon the organism cultured, but broad-spectrum antibiotics or combinations such as ampicillin, an aminoglycoside, and clindamycin are usually used.

Group B *Streptococcus* (Chap. 103) has become a major cause of postpartum bacteremia, accounting for 10 to 20 percent of blood culture isolates from women admitted to obstetrical services. Although most of these patients have an uncomplicated course following appropriate antibiotic therapy, complications such as endocarditis and meningitis are occasionally seen. In contrast to bacteremia with no identifiable source, most severe Group B *Streptococcus* infections in pregnancy are associated with an identifiable source such as endometritis or a urinary tract infection.

Listeria monocytogenes (see Chap. 105) is another bacterial infection which has specific pregnancy-related morbidity. Infection can occur at any time during pregnancy, but is most common during the third trimester. Symptoms are frequently suggestive of a urinary tract infection, but urine cultures are sterile. Diagnosis is made by a positive blood culture. Clinical severity of infection can range from a mild febrile to severe illness. This infection can precipitate labor and result in premature birth of a dead or infected infant.

Neisseria gonorrhoeae (see Chap. 110) can be transmitted from mother to infant in utero, during delivery, or in the postpartum period. The most common clinical problem caused by this transmission is gonococcal conjunctivitis of the newborn. Conjunctival installation of a 1% aqueous solution of silver nitrate is effective in preventing blindness caused by this infection. Congenital syphilis (see Chap. 133) occurs by infection of the fetus in utero. Transmission of *Treponema pallidum* to the fetus, most common in the early stages of syphilis, can occur at any time during pregnancy. Infection of the fetus before the fourth month is rare. Syphilis can have severe effects on the offspring, including stillbirth, neonatal disease, or latent infection.

VIRAL INFECTIONS These are of major concern during pregnancy because of the consequences to the fetus. Since transplacental transmission may occur, maternal infections with cytomegalovirus (CMV), rubella, varicella zoster, and herpes simplex virus have the greatest teratogenic potential, particularly during the first trimester. Perinatal infection can result from transmission of the virus to the infant during passage through an infected uterine cervix.

CMV infection (see Chap. 146) is the most common cause of congenital viral infection. The virus is ubiquitous; 35 to 100 percent of the adult population have evidence of prior infection, with the highest prevalence among lower socioeconomic groups. CMV is usually acquired by the oral-respiratory route, through sexual contact, or by blood transfusion. CMV infection establishes a lifelong latent infection in the host which can be reactivated later by immunosuppression. Rates of cervical infection with CMV increase in later stages of pregnancy. Although during pregnancy CMV can be shed with no evidence of clinical disease in the mother, high numbers of CMV in the cervix suggest the neonate is at risk during birth. Approximately 1 to 2 percent of all newborn infants in the United States are infected with CMV in utero, but the vast majority of these are normal. Clinically apparent congenital infections are most common in the first infant of mothers with primary infection during pregnancy. CMV disease occurs in infants whose mothers are not immune. Cytomegalic inclusion disease is characterized by jaundice, hepatosplenomegaly, a petechial rash, and multiple system and organ involvement. Other manifestations range from subtle neurologic sequelae to severe microcephaly.

Rubella (see Chap. 156) can have severe outcomes in the fetus, including fetal death and premature delivery, if the mother is infected during early pregnancy. A variety of congenital defects are caused by rubella, including cataracts, cardiac abnormalities, deafness, and mental retardation. Fetal abnormalities are greatest when maternal rubella occurs during the first trimester, with 80 percent of children affected; the percentage falls to about 25 percent when infection occurs at the end of the second trimester. Congenital infection can be diagnosed prenatally by detecting rubella IgM antibody in fetal blood under ultrasound guidance. In places where immunization programs have been widely used, the problem has been eliminated. The vaccine can be administered during pregnancy without harm to the fetus. Infection during pregnancy with varicella zoster virus (VZV) represents a health risk to the mother (see Chap. 144). There is nearly a 10 percent risk for severe pneumonia. Early antiviral therapy should be instituted if there is any suspicion of chickenpox-related pneumonia. Although most infants born to VZV-infected mothers are normal, there is a risk to the unborn child of developing congenital teratogenic infection.

Infection of the newborn with herpes simplex virus (HSV) can range from mild localized infection to fatal dissemination (see Chap. 143). Retrograde infection or birth through a maternal genital tract infected with HSV-2 can result in serious disseminated neonatal infection.

OTHER INFECTIONS OF PREGNANCY *Vulvovaginal candidiasis* (see Chap. 166) is more common in pregnant than nonpregnant women. High estrogen levels apparently encourage growth of this organism. Infection rates increase as the gestational period progresses, with up to 55 percent of third-trimester women being colonized and with symptomatic disease developing in the majority of those colonized.

Toxoplasmosis (see Chap. 177) causes symptoms in only 10 to 20 percent of women infected during pregnancy. Unfortunately, the fetus is at risk whether or not the mother is symptomatic. Transmission to the fetus can occur transplacentally or at birth. One-third of infants born to mothers infected during pregnancy become infected. The risk for congenital infection is greater when maternal infection occurs during the third trimester than the first, although the risk of spontaneous abortion is highest when infection is acquired in the first trimester.

Most infected newborns have no symptoms at birth but develop symptoms, particularly chorioretinitis, by adolescence. Less-common manifestations include strabismus, epilepsy, and psychomotor retardation. Toxoplasmosis does not cause fetal malformation.

HUMAN IMMUNODEFICIENCY VIRUS INFECTION

Approximately 80 percent of women with AIDS are of childbearing age. The incidence of infection with HIV will increase in women in the United States during the 1990s (see also Chap. 279). Worldwide, particularly in developing countries, HIV infection is predominantly spread heterosexually with the male-to-female ratio in certain countries approaching 1. The majority of the current cases of AIDS among women in the United States are those who are intravenous drug users (IVDUs) or who are the heterosexual partners of IVDUs. The geographic distribution of HIV infection among women closely parallels the geographic distribution of HIV infection among IVDUs, with the highest incidence in the Northeast and Southeast seaboard states and Puerto Rico. In New York City, approximately 10,000 women of childbearing age developed AIDS by 1993.

EFFECT OF HIV INFECTION ON PREGNANCY Although earlier studies suggested that HIV-positive women were at a higher risk of delivering infants with an unfavorable outcome, at the present time accumulating evidence indicates that HIV infection alone does not impose a significant negative effect on pregnancy outcome, particularly when the infection is in the asymptomatic stage. Further, an acceleration of HIV disease during pregnancy is uncommon and may be due to other factors associated with confounding issues present in the women most likely to be infected such as IV drug use and inadequate access to prenatal care.

Primary infection is generally associated with a burst of viremia with or without an acute HIV syndrome, the latter occurring in approximately 50 to 70 percent of individuals following initial infection. It is unclear what effect this burst of viremia has on the pregnancy itself or the chances of the fetus becoming infected during the pregnancy, if a previously uninfected mother develops a primary infection during the pregnancy.

TRANSMISSION OF HIV TO THE FETUS/INFANT The rate of transmission of HIV from mother to fetus/infant averages approximately 30 percent, with a range of 13 percent in a European collaborative study to 45 percent in Central Africa (see Chap. 279). Higher rates of transmission have been associated with the symptomatic stage in the mother and with low maternal CD4+ T lymphocyte counts. Although infection of the fetus can occur throughout pregnancy, it is felt that maternal transmission occurs most commonly during the perinatal period. Nonetheless, caesarean sections are not currently recommended unless there are other obstetrical reasons for doing so. Postnatal transmission from mother to infant has been documented, and colostrum and breast milk have been implicated. Where possible, breast feeding by an infected mother should be avoided.

TREATMENT OF HIV INFECTION DURING PREGNANCY Despite the fact that the effects of the commonly employed antiretroviral drugs on the pregnant woman and the fetus have not been fully delineated, most physicians treat HIV-infected pregnant women according to the same guidelines as for nonpregnant HIV-infected individuals. Treatment and/or prophylaxis of opportunistic infections should also be approached according to existing guidelines for HIV-infected patients except for those situations in which a drug is clearly contraindicated in pregnancy.

NEOPLASTIC DISEASES

Transmission of leukemia or lymphoma to the fetus has not been reported, and there is no clear evidence that pregnancy adversely affects the course of any type of malignancy; however, it is possible that the high estrogen levels of pregnancy accelerate the course of breast cancer.

Deciding whether the pregnancy should be terminated in women with neoplastic disease requires judgment about whether the pregnant state presents a significant obstacle to effective therapy and whether the fetus will be harmed as a result of such therapy. Although most antineoplastic agents are potentially teratogenic or cause fetal wastage, many healthy full-term infants have been born despite active maternal chemotherapy at the time of conception or during the first trimester. Thus while it would be safer to avoid fetal exposure, the decision to terminate a pregnancy must take into account the parents' desire to have a child. Pregnant women with leukemia who are given the usual chemotherapy for this condition have done surprisingly well; in some studies maternal survival rates have been 100 percent, and the incidence of congenital abnormalities in the newborn is less than 10 percent.

REFERENCES

BARRON WM, LINDHEIMER MD: *Medical Complications in Pregnancy.* St. Louis, Mosby-Year Book Publishers, 1991

BRIGGS GG, FREEMAN RK, YAFFE SJ: *Drugs in Pregnancy and Lactation*, 3d ed. Baltimore, Williams & Wilkins, 1990

BURROW GN, FERRIS TF: *Medical Complications During Pregnancy*, 4th ed. Philadelphia, Saunders, 1994, in press

NANDA D, MINKOFF HL: HIV in pregnancy—transmission and immune effects. Clin Obst Gyn 32:456, 1989

SELWYN PA et al: Prospective study of human immunodeficiency virus infection and pregnancy outcomes in intravenous drug users. JAMA 261:1289, 1989

---

7 ADOLESCENT HEALTH PROBLEMS

CHARLES E. IRWIN, JR / MARY-ANN SHAFER

APPROACH TO THE ADOLESCENT PATIENT

Adolescence is the period between childhood and adulthood. This period is usually defined by rapid onset of biological and psychological growth and development prior to or at the second decade of life and terminating before age 20. Major social and environmental factors influence the onset, duration, and termination of adolescence. Over the next decade, the numbers of adolescents will increase, adolescents will include more ethnic and racial minorities than the general population, and the adolescent population will become more impoverished, thereby decreasing their access to health care. Currently, the adolescent population in the United States is the group least likely to have health insurance. Physicians need a careful understanding of the biological and psychosocial changes of adolescence, the associated environmental changes, and the legal and ethical issues that affect the provision of health care services to adolescents.

BIOLOGICAL MATURATION Puberty (See also Chaps. 339 and 340) Puberty is defined as the biological processes that ultimately lead to reproductive capacity. The onset and tempo of puberty vary by sex, population group, and individual. During puberty, major alterations in the hormonal regulatory systems in the central nervous system, gonads, and adrenals cause changes in skeletal growth and in body composition and the acquisition of secondary sexual characteristics. The mechanisms responsible for the initiation of puberty through activation of the hypothalamic-pituitary-gonadal axis remain undefined.

The sexual maturity ratings (SMRs) of Marshall and Tanner are helpful in monitoring the development of secondary sexual

TABLE 7-1   Sexual maturity rating for females*

A Pubertal development in size of female breasts
  Stage 1: Prepubertal. Elevation of the papilla only.
  Stage 2: Breast bud stage. A small mound of breast tissue is formed by
    the elevation of the breast and papilla. Areolar diameter enlarges.
  Stage 3: Further enlargement of breast and areola with no separation of
    their contours.
  Stage 4: Projection of the areola and papilla to form a secondary mound
    above the level of the breast.
  Stage 5: Adult. The breasts resemble those of a mature female. The
    areola has recessed to the general contour of the breast.

B Pubertal development of female pubic hair
  Stage 1: Prepubertal. There is no pubic hair.
  Stage 2: Sparse growth of long, slightly pigmented, downy hair, straight
    or only slightly curled, primarily along the labia.
  Stage 3: The hair is considerably darker, coarser, and more curled, and
    spreads sparsely over the junction of the pubes.
  Stage 4: The hair, now adult in type, covers a smaller area than in the
    adult and does not extend onto the medial surface of the thighs.
  Stage 5: Adult. The hair is adult in quantity and type, with extension
    onto the thighs.

*Modified from van Wieringen JC et al: *Growth Diagrams*. Gronigen, Neth., Woplter-Noorhoff Publishing, 1971.

characteristics of pubertal maturation, which are the somatic manifestations of adrenal and gonadal activity. These ratings correlate more closely with bone age than chronologic age. The SMRs for girls are based upon breast and pubic hair development, each in five stages (Table 7-1). The ratings for boys are based upon genital and pubic hair development each also in five stages (Table 7-2).

The mean age of onset of puberty for girls as defined by breast budding is 11.2 ± 1.6 years, whereas the mean age of onset for boys as defined by enlargement of testes is 11.6 ± 1.1 years. The mean age of menarch in the United States is 13.3 ± 1.3 years, and the mean age for spermarche is between 13.5 and 14.5 years. The average duration of puberty for girls is 4 years with a range of 1.5 to 8 years, and the average duration of puberty for boys is 3 years with a range of 2 to 5 years. Even though the timing and duration of the events vary, each adolescent follows an orderly sequence in somatic growth and development (Figs. 7-1 and 7-2). Monitoring these events through a careful history and physical examination is helpful in identifying medical conditions that become manifest during adolescence (Table 7-3).

Skeletal growth (See also Chap. 332)   The pubertal height spurt accounts for approximately 25 percent of final adult height and occurs at an average age of 12 years for girls (SMR 2–3) and 14 years for

TABLE 7-2   Sexual maturity ratings for males*

A Pubertal development in size of male genitalia
  Stage 1: Prepubertal. Penis, testes, and scrotum are of childhood size.
  Stage 2: The scrotum and testes enlarge with testicular measurement
    greater than 2.5 cm in length (testicular volume, 4–7 mL). Penis
    usually show no growth. Scrotal skin reddens or darkens.
  Stage 3: Further growth of testes (testicular volume, 8–10 mL) and
    scrotum with enlargement of penis, mainly in length.
  Stage 4: Continued growth of the testes (testicular volume, 10–15 mL)
    and scrotum with increased size of the penis, especially in breadth.
  Stage 5: Adult. The genitalia are adult in size (testicular volume, 20–25
    mL) and shape.

B Pubertal development of male pubic hair
  Stage 1: Prepubertal. Pubic hair is absent.
  Stage 2: Sparse growth of long, slightly pigmented, downy hair, straight
    or only slightly curled, primarily at the base of the penis.
  Stage 3: The hair is considerably darker, coarser, and more curled. The
    hair spreads sparsely over the junction of the pubes.
  Stage 4: The hair, now adult in type, covers a smaller area than in the
    adult and does not extend onto the medial surface of the thighs.
  Stage 5: Adult. The hair is adult in quantity and type, with extension
    onto the thighs.

*Modified from van Wieringen JC et al: *Growth Diagrams*. Gronigen, Neth. Woplter-Noorhoff Publishing, 1971.

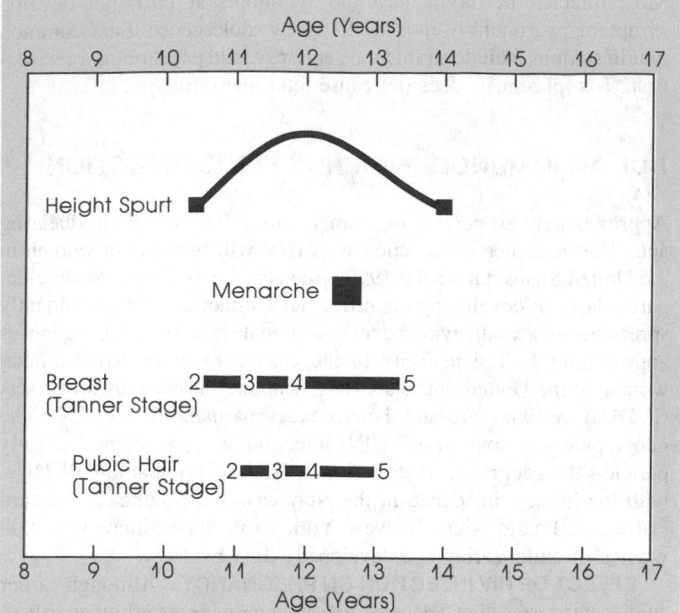

FIGURE 7-1   Pubertal events in females.

boys (SMR 3–4). During this spurt, females gain 9.0 cm ± 1.03 cm/year and reach a final mean adult height of 163 cm at 16 years; males gain 10.3 ± 1.54 cm/year and reach a final mean adult height of 177 cm at 18 years. Assessment of skeletal growth during adolescence should be done through a height velocity curve with consideration of the sexual maturity rating. Bone age can be determined through the utilization of hand roentgenograms.

Changes in body composition   Weight gain during the growth spurt accounts for 40 percent of ideal body weight. Lean body mass increases in males from 80 to 90 percent and decreases in girls from 80 to 75 percent. In males mean body fat increases from 4.3 to 11.2 percent by late puberty and is distributed primarily in the truncal area. In females, mean body fat increases from 15.7 to 26.7 percent and is deposited in the pelvic, breast, upper back, and arm areas. Shortly after the growth spurt is completed, muscle mass peaks and is greater in boys than in girls.

FIGURE 7-2   Pubertal events in males.

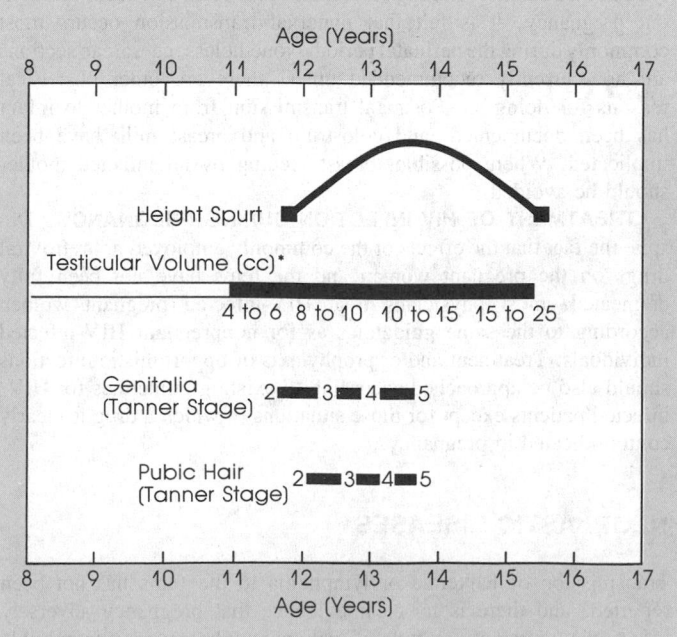

TABLE 7-3 Relation between development of features of maturation and sexual maturity ratings (SMR)*

Clinical feature	SMR
Hematocrit rise (male)	2–5
Alkaline phosphatase peak (male)	3
Alkaline phosphatase peak (female)	2
Adolescent hormonal levels (rise in estrogen for females, testosterone for males)	2–5
Peak height velocity (male)	3–4
Peak height velocity (female)	2–3
Usual timing of menarche	3–4
Slipped capital femoral epiphysis	2–3
Acute worsening of idiopathic adolescent scoliosis	2–4
Osgood-Schlatter disease	3
Appearance of "normal" gynecomastia	2–3
Usual appearance of acne vulgaris	2–3
Increased levels of serum uric acid in males	2–5

*After Daniel WA.

Cardiorespiratory changes At puberty heart rate decreases and stroke volume, cardiac output, and blood pressure increase. The lungs increase in size. The male larynx, under the influence of androgens, develops an acute 90-degree angle in the anterior thyroid cartilage, and the male vocal cords are three times the length of those in females. These changes account for the deepening of vocal quality.

PSYCHOLOGICAL DEVELOPMENT Adolescence is often viewed as a tumultuous period (Table 7-4). However, most adolescents pass through puberty without disruption in their lives. The clinician must assess whether psychosocial development of the adolescent is normal. The adolescent is confronted with a series of changes, which,

if mastered, allow function as an adult. These changes include separation from the family, maturation of sexual identity, planning for education and career, and development of the capacity for intimacy. Adolescents also undergo cognitive changes with behavioral and social sequelae. The functional and cognitive changes do not necessarily correlate with physical maturation. The early adolescent (ages 10 to 13) tends to focus on the physical changes in his/her body and may have concerns about the maturational process.

Middle adolescence (ages 14 to 16 years) is the period of rapid cognitive growth when formal operational thinking emerges. Adolescents begin to understand abstract concepts and may question the judgment of adults. The individual then shifts from the egocentric world of the early adolescent to the sociocentric world of the middle and late adolescent and begins to modulate impulsive behavior.

Late adolescence (ages 17 to 21 years) is the period of establishment of personal identity with intimate relationships and a function in society. The late adolescent views life in a more sociocentric view, characteristic of adulthood. The late adolescent may be altruistic, and conflicts with the family and society may center on moral issues rather than egocentric considerations.

Families can facilitate adolescence by providing a graduated increase in independence and in responsibilities. Adolescents need both individuality and involvement with family and society to facilitate development of identity and of rational competence. Clinicians should support this process by encouraging adolescents to make their own appointments, assisting the chronically ill adolescent in assuming more responsibility for his/her health care, and encouraging parents to decrease their role in clinical management issues.

PSYCHOLOGICAL CHANGES ASSOCIATED WITH PUBESCENCE Hormones and behavior Specific behavioral changes are

TABLE 7-4 Biopsychosocial development during adolescence

Characteristics	Impact
EARLY ADOLESCENCE (Age 10 to 13 Years)	
Onset of puberty, becomes concerned with developing body	Major questions concerning normality of physical maturation; often concerned about the stages of sexual development and how the process relates to peers of same gender. Masturbation begins.
Begins to expand social radius beyond family and concentrate on relationships with peers	Encourage some external responsibilities alone in consultation with parents, i.e., visit with health care provider, contacts with school counselors.
Cognition is usually concrete	Concrete thinking requires dealing with most health situations in a simple, explicit manner using visual and verbal cues.
MIDDLE ADOLESCENCE (Age 14 to 16 Years)	
Pubertal development usually complete and sexual drives emerge	Explores ability to attract opposites. Sexual behavior and experimentation (same and opposite sex) begin. Masturbation increases.
Peer group sets behavioral standards, although some family values persist	Peer group affects compliance, and peers rather than parents offer key support.
Conflicts over independence	Increased assumption of independent action, together with continued need for parental support and guidance; able to discuss and negotiate changes in rules; ambivalence on part of adolescent in discussion and negotiation.
Cognition begins to be abstract	Begins to consider full range of possibilities with poor ability to integrate into real life because of immaturity and incomplete cognitive development.
LATE ADOLESCENCE (Age 17 to 21 Years)	
Physical maturation complete. Body image and gender role definition are secured	Begins to feel comfortable with relationships and decisions regarding sexuality and preference. Individual relationships become more important than peer group.
Narcissism declines; there is a process of giving and sharing	More open to specific questioning regarding behavior.
Idealistic	Idealism may lead to conflicts with family and other authority figures.
Emancipation is nearly secured	With emancipation, more awareness about consequences of person actions.
Cognitive development is complete	Most are capable of understanding a full range of options for health issues.
Functional role begins to be defined	Often interested in significant discussion of life goals because this is the primary function of this stage.

*After Shafer MAB, Irwin CE, Jr.

associated with puberty and its timing. Androgens have been implicated in this process. During peak height velocity (stages 3 to 4), boys tend to have more conflict with their mothers, and as boys complete puberty mothers tend to defer more to their sons. Girls also tend to have more conflict with their mothers and to decrease interactions with their fathers. Other activities associated with changes in androgens include heterosexual behavior. Boys with rising levels of testosterone tend to initiate sexual intercourse and are reported to be more impatient, irritable, and aggressive. Rising levels of adrenal androgens correlate with increased masturbatory activity and heterosocial behavior in girls.

Timing of maturation Timing of puberty is associated with psychological and behavioral sequelae. Earlier physical maturation in girls is associated with more dissatisfaction with their bodies, lower self esteem, and general unhappiness. Early-developing girls also receive less support from peer groups and may associate with older adolescents. The earlier developing girl initiates sexual behavior earlier than her age peers, experiences an early identity crisis, has greater interest in independence and decision making and tends to have more behavioral problems and less interest in academic activities. For boys, early physical maturation is also associated with earlier initiation of sexual behavior, but late maturation in boys seems to be more often associated with negative psychological sequelae. The late-maturing boy tends to have a negative self-concept and body image and an increased frequency of identity crises.

ENVIRONMENTAL CHANGES Social environment Changes in the social environment during the second decade may affect health status. The family tends to provide less supervision and allow for more freedom in choices regarding free time, often providing the adolescent an opportunity to engage in risky behaviors. Schools are transformed from supportive elementary schools to the large, impersonal, and unstructured environments of middle/junior high schools, high schools and colleges. Work environments provide even less supervision and on-the-job guidance for the adolescent. With the economic crisis of the 1990s fewer nurturing programs are available for youth after school, and the increase in poverty has had a negative effect on the health status of children.

Legal environment The law in most states requires consent of a parent for medical care for children younger than 18. In general, the involvement of parents is not a barrier to the provision of health services, but some sensitive health issues (e.g., sexual behavior and substance use) may interfere with access to health care for adolescents. The Mature Minor Doctrine generally allows adolescents to seek health care independently if they are capable of understanding the risks and benefits of the proposed treatment and therefore capable of informed consent. There is generally little risk of liability in providing health care to the older mature minor (14 years or older) if the care is for the adolescent's benefit or is an emergency. In many states adolescents can seek care without parental permission for sensitive issues such as sexually transmitted diseases, contraception, pregnancy, substance use, and some mental health problems. Adolescents may also be treated without parental permission if the condition is an emergency and a delay in treatment would be detrimental to well being. Emancipated minors (adolescents who live away from home, are no longer subject to parental control, are economically self-supporting, are married, or are members of the military service) may also consent to their own health care.

MORBIDITY AND MORTALITY

The concept that adolescence is the healthiest period of life is based on measures of mortality and morbidity that do not include functional assessment of health status or the effects of behaviors initiated during adolescence on adult mortality and morbidity.

Mortality Mortality rates are low, but since 1985, there has been an increase in mortality for adolescents and young adults. Mortality (per 100,000) increases from 28 10 to 14 year olds to 88 15 to 19

year olds to 115 20 to 24 year olds. Most adolescent mortality is due to violence, particularly motor vehicle accidents, homicide, and suicide. In 1988, injuries accounted for most deaths between ages 10 and 24, and mortality rates for males are double those of females. Ethnic groups differ in respect to the cause of death: black males of 15 to 19 years old have a fivefold greater rate of homicide and the lowest life expectancy of all adolescents. In contrast, white male adolescents have higher suicide and motor vehicle accident death rates. Unintentional injuries account for more than half of deaths in the second decade. Risky driving habits account for half of fatal crashes, and adolescent drivers have the highest rates of motor vehicle fatalities. Alcohol is also implicated in other fatal injuries including bicycle, boating, skateboard, and swimming accidents. Suicide is responsible for 13 percent of deaths between ages 15 and 24. Native American males have higher rates, and black adolescents have lower rates of suicide. Between ages 15 and 24 homicide accounts for 14 percent of deaths. Homicide is the leading cause of death in late black male adolescents and young adults, accounting for 40 percent and 37 percent of the deaths, respectively. Adolescents in impoverished metropolitan areas are more likely victims of homicide. Cardiovascular diseases account for 1.4 to 4.8 deaths and malignancies for 3.1 to 5.7 deaths per 100,000 persons aged 10 to 24.

Morbidity Most morbidity during adolescence originates from substance abuse, sexual activity, and accidents. Additional causes include mental health problems and those associated with changes in the skeletal and reproductive systems.

Skeletal system (See also Chap. 332) Rapid growth of the long bones and closure of the epiphyses by age 21 are associated with several orthopedic problems. Slipped capital femoral epiphyses occurs primarily at the time of rapid growth spurt and is more common in the obese. Osgood-Schlatter disease (osteochondrosis of the tibial tuberosity) and idiopathic scoliosis are disorders of adolescence, and neoplasms of osseous origins peak during adolescence. Fractures due to injuries are also common throughout adolescence.

Female reproductive health problems Reproduction health problems are a common cause of morbidity in young women.

ANOVULATORY CYCLES (See also Chap. 340) Dysfunctional uterine bleeding (DUB) is common. Primary DUB results from anovulatory cycles, i.e., oscillations of estrogen levels that lack the characteristic LH surge and subsequent corpus luteum development, progesterone production, and endometrial maturation of a mature cycle. Without progesterone, the endometrial lining becomes thickened and fragile, resulting in intermittent sloughing and irregular, frequently excessive menstrual bleeding. The differential diagnosis includes pregnancy, disorders of coagulation, and disorders of the vagina, cervix, uterus and ovary. Anovulatory cycles may persist for 5 years following menarche.

DYSMENORRHEA Dysmenorrhea, both primary and secondary, is a major complaint of menstruating adolescents and a major cause of school absenteeism. Primary dysmenorrhea is due to prostaglandin-stimulated myometrial contractions during ovulatory cycles. Secondary dysmenorrhea is associated with pelvic infections, intrauterine and extrauterine pregnancy, intrauterine devices and congenital anomalies. Primary dysmenorrhea is treated by suppressing production of the prostaglandins and/or inhibiting ovulation. If the girl fails to respond to oral contraceptives and prostaglandin inhibitors, further evaluation must be undertaken.

SEXUALLY TRANSMITTED DISEASES (STD) (See also Chap. 80) Sexually active adolescents have the highest rates of STD of any age group in the United States. Complications include cervical intraepithelial neoplasia, pelvic inflammatory disease, ectopic pregnancy, infertility, genital cancers, and AIDS. As of September 1992, 912 cases of AIDS have been diagnosed in 13 to 19 year olds and 9270 cases in the 20- to 24-year-old cohort. The extent of HIV seroprevalence in adolescents is unknown. When one STD is diagnosed, the clinician must screen for other STDs.

Male reproductive health problems (See also Chap. 339) Testicular masses and varicoceles may become evident during puberty. Most varicoceles are discovered during a routine physical examination. Surgical repair may be indicated to enhance fertility and in the following situations: genital discomfort, testicular volume loss, abnormal semen analysis, or abnormal luteinizing hormone-releasing hormone stimulation test. Testicular cancer is rare in adolescents, but teaching young adults and adolescents to perform self testicular examinations may increase early identification of tumors.

RISK-TAKING BEHAVIORS

SUBSTANCE USE AND ABUSE Adolescent use of substances has declined in the United States since the 1970s. In 1991, only 29 percent of high school seniors reported illicit substance abuse at any time. The declining rates of marijuana and cocaine use have been accompanied by an increasing perception of harm associated with these substances. Rates of lifetime use of LSD and heroin among high school seniors have remained essentially stable at 9 percent and 1 percent respectively, and only 1.5 percent of high school seniors report use of crack cocaine. Nevertheless, lifetime alcohol and tobacco use approximated 88 percent and 63 percent, respectively, among high school seniors in 1991. Binge drinking (the consumption of at least five drinks or more in a row at least once in the past 2 weeks) was reported by 30 percent of high school seniors and by 43 percent of college students. Substance abuse during adolescence has major negative health consequences in adulthood. Girls consistently report greater use of cigarettes, whereas males have a higher use of alcohol. Approximately 18 percent of adolescents leave high school as smokers, and 14 percent of college students are regular smokers. The lower rates of cigarette smoking in boys may be due to the increase in use of smokeless tobacco (snuff and chewing tobacco).

Surveys may underestimate the true prevalence of substance use, but it is clear that patterns of substance use vary by region, age, gender, and ethnicity. Substance use generally increases with age. Native American adolescents have the highest prevalence rates for cigarettes, alcohol, and most illicit drugs, followed by rates for whites, Hispanics, African-Americans, and Asian-Americans.

UNINTENTIONAL INJURIES Injuries, particularly motor vehicle accidents, account for more than half of deaths in adolescents, and hospitalization for injury accounts for the largest number of hospital days. Alcohol, high speed, and reckless behavior play important roles in these injuries, and are also implicated in injuries with bicycles, skateboards, swimming, and boating. Males outnumber females by greater than 2 to 1 in all injury situations.

SEXUAL BEHAVIOR Adolescents now initiate heterosexual behavior earlier than cohorts of previous generations. By age 15, 26 percent of white females and males, 24 percent of black females, and 69 percent of black males experience coitus. These figures increase by age 19 to 76 percent of white females, 85 percent of white males, 83 percent of black females and 96 percent of black males. White adolescent females report more frequent sexual intercourse and more partners than their age-related black cohorts. Adolescent females with earlier menarche begin to have intercourse earlier than those with a later menarche. Adolescents who initiate sexual behavior early tend to have more sexual partners and are more likely to acquire a sexually transmitted disease or become pregnant. Use of contraceptives among adolescents is increasing, but fewer than half of sexually active adolescents use condoms. Reported rates of unprotected heterosexual anal intercourse are from 12 percent to 26 percent. Reliable data on same-sex behavior during adolescence are not available, but rates may approximate 5 to 10 percent. Retrospective data from adult homosexual and bisexual men indicate that half of these men initiated same-sex sexual behavior by age 16.

Overall birth rates have declined over the past decade; however, the number of births to unmarried adolescent females has increased, and there were an estimated 416,170 abortions in adolescents in 1988. Sexually transmitted diseases are more frequent among sexually active adolescents than any other age group in the United States.

COVARIATION OF RISK BEHAVIORS The onset of one risk behavior is associated with a greater likelihood for initiation of another in the near future. The association between alcohol abuse and injury is well established. Other activities that predispose to injury include reckless driving and failure to use seat belts and helmets.

The strongest evidence for covariation is in substance abuse, sexual activity, and delinquent behavior. The major risk for initiation of cigarette, alcohol, and marijuana use is by age 20 and for illicit substance use is by age 21. Young adults who have not used these substances are unlikely to do so thereafter. During early and middle adolescence, less serious substance use predicts subsequent use of more serious substances. Alcohol use precedes marijuana use, and marijuana use precedes other illicit drugs (including psychedelics, cocaine, heroin, and nonprescribed stimulants, sedatives, and tranquilizers). In girls, cigarette use is predictive of subsequent substance use. The influence of alcohol and tobacco use on subsequent marijuana use is independent of age. The earlier adolescents begin using marijuana the more likely the use of other illicit substances. Substance use is also correlated with delinquent behavior, early sexual debut, and less effective contraceptive use.

MENTAL HEALTH PROBLEMS

Approximately 10 percent of adolescents have symptoms of psychological distress. Psychiatric conditions that may begin in childhood include anxiety and panic disorders, personality disorders, schizophrenia, suicide, and eating disorders. Three common problems encountered by the primary care physician during adolescence are suicide, depression, and eating disorders.

SUICIDE Suicide is the fourth leading cause of death in early adolescence (10 to 14 years old) and the second leading cause in late adolescence and young adulthood. The greatest increase in rates of suicide during the past 20 years is among 15- to 24-year-old males. Suicide is relatively uncommon before puberty and increases after age 16 with most occurring among 18 to 24 year olds. White and Native American late adolescents boys and young men have the highest rates of suicide. The relation between male sex and substance abuse and conduct disorders may be responsible for this predominance. For every completed suicide, there may be 50 to 120 attempted suicides with a female preponderance. Differences in methods may be responsible for the sex differences between fatal and attempted suicides. Methods for fatal suicide include firearms, hanging, and jumping from heights. Drug ingestion, which rarely causes fatality, is the most common method for suicide attempts in adolescents.

Etiology of suicide Common factors in suicidal adolescents include a history of suicide in family members, alcohol and substance abuse, conduct disorders, depressive disorders, anxiety states, and knowing someone who has committed or attempted suicide. Precipitating factors include acute stress, trouble with the law, trouble at school such as cheating or being truant, substance abuse, pregnancy or fear of pregnancy, hypochondriasis, social isolation, and anxiety. In occasional girls perfectionism and anxiety about academic performance (in the presence of average intelligence) or environmental change appear to be causal. Many suicide victims are intoxicated at the time of death.

Recognition of the at-risk suicidal adolescent Recognition of the suicidal or depressed adolescent may be difficult. The most common underlying psychiatric factor in suicidal adolescents is depression, manifested by feelings of hopelessness, low self-esteem, despair, and somatic complaints. In the younger adolescent, depressive equivalents of school problems and acting out behavior may include legal problems. The younger adolescent may also have difficulty in characterizing his/her feelings. In the older adolescent, substance abuse is more common. Injured adolescents should be queried about the cause of the injury to rule out suicidal behavior. Adolescents with a family history of suicide, a history of psychiatric disorders, or a past history of suicidal behavior need to be screen for suicide risk.

A depressed adolescent contemplating suicide generally welcomes the opportunity to communicate his/her feelings.

Once a suicidal adolescent is identified, an extensive evaluation is required to assess the problem. Comprehensive workup should include evaluation of the adolescent, the family, and the family together with the adolescent. Parents and/or guardians should be informed immediately about the suicidal behavior. Confidentiality is immaterial in the face of potential suicide. Suicidal intent is as important as the lethality of the method. Many adolescents have little knowledge of lethality. Evaluation should focus on mental health disorders in the family, past history of mental health problems in the adolescent, sexual abuse, and sexual behavior including same-sex behavior, since homosexual adolescents appear to be at greater risk for suicide. All suicidal adolescents need evaluation by a psychiatrist as soon as possible.

In emergencies, the physician must decide if outpatient or inpatient care is appropriate. If immediate treatment is needed, psychiatric consultation is sought when the patient is stable medically. If the patient is medically stable, the clinician must decide whether he/she is at ongoing risk for suicide. Some programs recommend hospitalization for all suicidal adolescents, and hospitalization is always advisable for the following groups: (1) those still intent on suicide; (2) those with previous suicide attempts; (3) all males; (4) all severely depressed patients; (5) those impaired by substance abuse; (6) those whose attempt was with a lethal method (e.g., firearm, hanging, or jumping from high place); and (7) those without a supportive environment at home or through residential care.

When the patient is discharged, the clinician needs to monitor the compliance with the mental health treatment program and to query the family about the availability of firearms at home. Adolescents who are depressed or suicidal are difficult to engage in treatment programs and a follow-up appointment with the primary care physician is the best way to monitor compliance. If the adolescent fails to keep the appointment, the physician should telephone and reschedule it.

Depression (See also Chap. 389)   Depression is the most common feature in patients who attempt suicide. The prevalence of major depressive disorders in adolescence is between 4 to 6 percent with a slight preponderance of females to males. The diagnostic criteria for depression during adolescence are the same as in adulthood (Table 7-5) and include changes in mood and relationships, cognitive functioning and bodily functioning. Depressive equivalents in the adolescent include hypochondriasis, substance abuse, decrements in school functioning, problems with the law, and major family conflicts.

EATING DISORDERS (See also Chap. 74)   Eating disorders generally have their onset in postpubertal adolescents, and adolescents may fulfill the DSM-IIIR criteria for anorexia nervosa or bulimia nervosa prior to the completion of puberty (Table 74-1). Adolescents with subclinical eating disorders may need the same treatment as adolescents with full-fledged disorders. The warning signs of emerging eating disorders are listed in Table 7-6 and include major body image problems, difficulty establishing autonomy from the family, perfectionism, and family history of eating disorders including obesity.

TABLE 7-5   DSM-III-R criteria for diagnosis of major depression*

Diagnosis requires symptom 1 or 2 and at least four other symptoms for a 2-week period

1 Depressed or irritable mood
2 Diminished interest or pleasure
3 Weight loss or weight gain
4 Insomnia or hypersomnia
5 Psychomotor agitation or retardation
6 Fatigue or loss of energy
7 Feelings of worthlessness or excessive guilt
8 Decreased concentration or indecisiveness
9 Thoughts of death, suicidal ideation, or suicide attempt

*After American Psychiatric Association, p 217.

TABLE 7-6   Possible warning signs for anorexia nervosa or bulimia nervosa*

Anorexia nervosa	Bulimia nervosa
EATING AND RELATED BEHAVIORS	
Caloric intake < 100 kcal/d	Binge eating > twice/week
Calorie counting	Eating used as coping strategy
Denial of hunger cues	Fasting or restrictive dieting
Extreme physical activity	Feels lack of control over eating
Fasting or restrictive dieting	Frequent meal skipping
Feels controlled by food	Frequent sweets, starches, cravings
Food avoidances or hoarding	Frequent thoughts about food
Food seen as good or bad	Guilt after eating/secret eating
Frequent meal skipping	Purging behavior
Frequent thoughts about food	Regular alcohol use
	Wide variation in caloric intake
BODY IMAGE AND BODY SATISFACTION	
Body image disturbance	Current or previous obesity
Fear of weight gain	Fear of weight gain
Previously overweight	Overconcern with weight/shape
Thinness as valued goal	Thinness as valued goal
Weight goal < 85% expected weight	Unrealistic weight goal
HEALTH STATUS	
Amenorrhea (< 3 months w/no menses)	Bloating/nausea/abdominal pain
	Constipation
Bloating/nausea	Frequent weight fluctuations
Cold intolerance	Irregular menses (< 21 days or > 45 days)
Constipation	
Weight < 85% expected weight	
PERSONAL FUNCTIONING	
Delayed psychosexual development	Depressed affect
Depressed affect	Negative self-identity
Individuation difficulties	Perfectionistic
Negative self identity	Poor coping with life event
Perfectionistic	Recent withdrawal from friends
Poor coping with life events	Substance use/early sexual activity
Recent withdrawal from friends	
ENVIRONMENTAL INFLUENCES	
Enmeshed or overinvolved family	Chaotic or uninvolved family
Family history of obesity, eating disorder, or weight focus	Family history of obesity, eating disorder, weight or fitness focus
Few close friends	High achievement expectations
High achievement expectations	Participation in body-focused activity
Participation in body-focused activity	

*Adapted from Adams LB, Shafer MA.

While the eating patterns in many adolescents appear abnormal, and adolescent girls commonly have dissatisfaction with weight and shape and some fear of gaining weight, these feelings and fears are extreme in the adolescent with an eating disorder.

Anorexia nervosa (See also Chap. 74)   Anorexia now involves approximately 1 percent of white girls between ages 14 and 24 (Table 7-6), generally from middle to upper socioeconomic families. The disorder also occurs in Asian-Americans, African-Americans, Hispanics, and Native Americans. Approximately 5 to 10 percent of cases are boys, but the disorder in boys may be more severe and associated with gender disturbances.

The disorder generally begins shortly after the completion of puberty, but some girls develop the disease after graduation from high school when they begin college or employment. The cause is unclear. Some adolescents appear to have the onset with the increased deposition of adipose tissue with puberty and concern generated by parents and peers. Hypothalamic abnormalities may occur prior to weight loss; up to 40 percent of girls with anorexia nervosa have secondary amenorrhea prior to weight loss. The psychological profile is one of low self-esteem, high anxiety, and normal cognitive functioning. Generally, the girls are overachievers and perfectionists.

Associated psychiatric illnesses include depression and other affective disorders. The families tend to be enmeshed: overprotective, rigid, and with little ability to resolve conflicts. Subpopulations at risk include ballet dancers and gymnasts.

The findings depend on the degree and method of starvation. The weight should be measured with the adolescent undressed and in a gown after voiding. Laboratory data are generally not helpful except when vomiting has led to hypokalemia and metabolic alkalosis. With amenorrhea, LH and FSH levels are prepubertal, and serum estradiol levels are low. In boys, serum testosterone level is low. Triiodothyronine levels are low, and cortisol, endorphins, and cholesterol are elevated with an increase in high-density lipoproteins. ST-segment depression on exercise stress testing and prolonged QT intervals have been reported. These findings have been associated with ventricular tachycardia in adults with anorexia nervosa.

Successful treatment begins with early diagnosis and development of a comprehensive medical and psychiatric regimen. Mortality rates range from 2 to 10 percent in the 10 years following diagnosis. Early intensive therapy appears to improve the prognosis.

Bulimia nervosa (See also Chap. 74) Bulimia nervosa is diagnosed by the criteria listed in Table 7-7. The prevalence is approximately 2 to 5 percent of females and less than 1 percent for males. Individual patients may have both anorexia nervosa and bulimia nervosa at the same time or alternate between the two syndromes. The cause is not clear. Individuals with mild disease may function fairly well, whereas others are disabled by repeated binging, purging, suicide attempts, and substance abuse.

The typical patient is a middle to late adolescent who begins bulimic behavior to lose weight. Complaints include fatigue, bloating, or irregular menses, and sore throat or hoarseness secondary to vomiting. Most do not mention purging or binging behavior unless specifically queried. Physical findings include bilateral swelling of the parotid glands and calluses or scars on the dorsum of fingers used to induce vomiting. Teeth enamel may be lost to the acidic nature of vomitus. Reflex esophagitis, aspiration pneumonia, and cardiac abnormalities secondary to hypokalemia can occur. Use of syrup of ipecac to induce vomiting can also cause cardiotoxicity. Metabolic alkalosis and an elevated serum amylase may be present. Once the diagnosis is made, the effect of binging and purging must be dealt with prior to dealing with the underlying psychopathology. Pharmacotherapy may be helpful.

THE CLINICAL VISIT OF THE ADOLESCENT

TRANSITION INTERVIEW Establishing an effective doctor-patient relationship with the adolescent is a formidable task for the physician whose practice is primarily with adults. A transition interview for the adolescent and family helps to define the relationship between the physician and the emerging adult. Areas to be emphasized include the necessity for the physician to interview and examine the adolescent privately and the need for the patient to generate his/her own questions including initiating appointments. Normal adolescence and the continuing need for some decisions to be made with familial guidance and support should be discussed. The payment mechanisms and responsibility for fees should be clarified. During this interview, the physician should inquire about the adolescent's previous source of health care and request authorization to contact the former physician.

CONFIDENTIALITY Fundamental to any doctor-patient relationship is confidentiality. All adolescents need to be able to discuss all matters with the physician openly, honestly, and confidentially, and the physician must provide assurance of the confidential nature of all information. Prior to queries about sexual behavior or substance use, it may be useful to restate the confidential nature of the questioning. With life-threatening behaviors or diseases (e.g., suicidal behavior or management of chronic disease), the physician generally has the right to intervene including identification of a parent, guardian, or supportive adult to assist in the management.

GATHERING THE HISTORY History taking should be guided by the developmental stage of the patient (Table 7-4). The adolescent may not disclose his/her primary concern until a secure and confidential relationship has been established. General screening should be undertaken for the major health-damaging behaviors of adolescence, including sexual activity, substance use, vehicle use, depression and its equivalents, and dietary changes suggestive of an eating disorder. Distinguishing between risk-taking behaviors that are temporary, even though dangerous, and those that are pathologic is a challenge. This judgment requires assessing the effects of risky behavior on the health status and the motivation for engaging in them and determining whether normal psychosocial development is impaired. Figure 7-3 summarizes the biopsychosocial and environmental factors that increase vulnerability for initiating risky behaviors. Male sex, positive

FIGURE 7-3 Principal factors in risk-taking behaviors. (Adapted from Irwin and Millstein.)

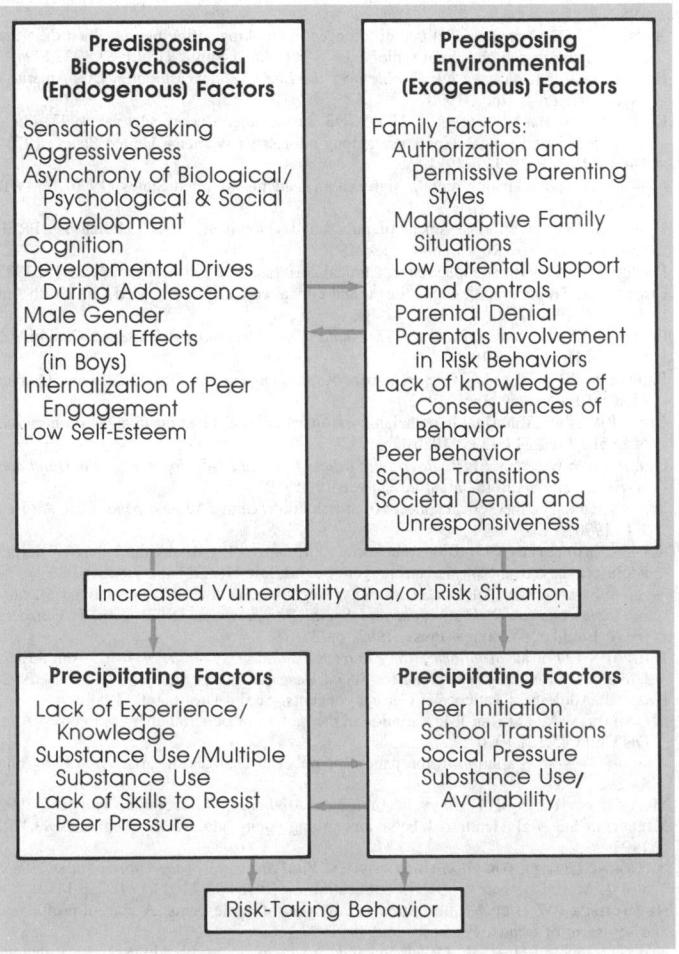

Predisposing Biopsychosocial (Endogenous) Factors	Predisposing Environmental (Exogenous) Factors

Sensation Seeking
Aggressiveness
Asynchrony of Biological/Psychological & Social Development
Cognition
Developmental Drives During Adolescence
Male Gender
Hormonal Effects (in Boys)
Internalization of Peer Engagement
Low Self-Esteem
	Family Factors:
	  Authorization and Permissive Parenting Styles
	  Maladaptive Family Situations
	  Low Parental Support and Controls
	  Parental Denial
	  Parentals Involvement in Risk Behaviors
	Lack of knowledge of Consequences of Behavior
	Peer Behavior
	School Transitions
	Societal Denial and Unresponsiveness

Increased Vulnerability and/or Risk Situation

Precipitating Factors	Precipitating Factors
Lack of Experience/Knowledge Substance Use/Multiple Substance Use Lack of Skills to Resist Peer Pressure	Peer Initiation School Transitions Social Pressure Substance Use/Availability

Risk-Taking Behavior

TABLE 7-7 DSM-III-R criteria for diagnosis of bulimia nervosa*

A Recurrent episodes of binge eating (rapid consumption of a large amount of food in a discrete period).
B A feeling of lack of control over eating behavior during binges.
C The person regularly engages in self-induced vomiting, use of laxatives or diuretics, strict dieting or fasting, or vigorous exercise to prevent weight gain.
D A minimum average of two binge-eating episodes a week for at least 3 months.
E Persistent overconcern with body shape and weight.

* After American Psychiatric Association, pp 68–69.

attitudes toward risky behaviors, lack of parental supervision, contact with peers engaging in the behavior, and multiple school transitions are associated with an increased propensity for risky behaviors. The physician should be specific in questioning about individual behaviors, their frequency and their intensity. One behavior may serve as a warning sign for another risky behavior. For example, early substance abuse correlates with early sexual activity.

Frequently, adolescents do not want to disclose current behavior, and the physician may query instead about general risk-taking and the behavior of peer groups. The physical signs associated with risky behaviors are similar to the signs and symptoms in adult patients, but the behavioral consequences of risky behaviors may have a greater effect on the adolescent, including more family conflicts, impaired academic performance, unwise peer relationships and activities, and changes in extracurricular activities.

Immunization history needs to be reviewed. Previously immunized adolescents who received a complete series of immunizations prior to 5 years of age need to receive a second measles vaccination. This immunization may be for measles alone or MMR (measles, mumps, and rubella). Adolescents who have never been immunized and those for whom the immunization history is not available should receive a three-dose primary series of Td (tetanus, diptheria) and OPV (oral poliovirus) and a two-dose primary series of MMR. Hepatitis B vaccine should be given to sexually active adolescents.

The physical examination and laboratory assessment are guided by the general complaints and the associated physical stigmata of risky behaviors.

REFERENCES

ADAMS LB, SHAFER MA: Early manifestations of eating disorders in adolescents: Defining those at risk. J Nutr Ed 20:307, 1988

AMERICAN PSYCHIATRIC ASSOCIATION: *Diagnostic and Statistical Manual of Mental Disorders*, 3d ed, revised. Washington DC, The American Psychiatric Association, 1987

BACHMAN JAG et al: Racial/ethnic differences in smoking, drinking and illicit drug use among American high school seniors, 1976–89. Am J Public Health 81:372, 1991

BLUMENTHAL SJ, KUPFER DJ: *Suicide over the Life Cycle*. Washington DC, American Psychiatric Press, Inc., 1990

CENTERS FOR DISEASE CONTROL: HIV/AIDS Surveillance Report, October 1992, 11
——: Premarital sexual experience among adolescent women—United States, 1970–1988. MMWR 39:929, 1991
——: Weapon-carrying among high school students—United States, 1990. MMWR 40:681, 1991

COPELAND KC et al: Assessment of pubertal development. Ross Laboratories PREP series. Columbus, Ross Laboratories, 1986

DANIEL WA: Growth at adolescence: Clinical correlates. Semin Adolesc Med 1:15, 1985

ENGLISH A: Treating adolescents: Legal and ethical considerations. Med Clin North Am 74:1097, 1990

FELDMAN SS, ELLIOTT GR: *At the Threshold: The Developing Adolescent*. Cambridge, Harvard University, 1990

FRIEDMAN SB et al (eds): *Comprehensive Adolescent Health Care*. St. Louis, Quality Medical Publishing, Inc., 1992

GOLD PW et al: Abnormal hypothalamic-pituitary-adrenal function in anorexia nervosa. N Engl J Med 314:1335, 1986

GREULICH WW, PYLE SI: *Radiographic Atlas of Skeletal Development of the Hand and Wrist, 2d ed*. Stanford, Stanford University, 1959

IRWIN CE JR: The theoretical concept of at-risk adolescents. Adolesc Med: State Art Rev 1:1, 1990
——, MILLSTEIN SG: Biopsychosocial correlates of risk taking behavior during adolescence: Can the physician intervene? J Adolesc Health Care 7:82S, 1986
——, SHAFER MA: Adolescent sexuality: Negative outcomes of a normative behavior, in *Adolescents at Risk: Medical and Social Perspectives*, DE Rogers, E Ginzberg (eds). Boulder, Westview Press, 1992, pp 35–79

JOHNSTON LD et al: *Monitoring the Future Substance Use Data for 1991*. Ann Arbor, University of Michigan Institute for Social Research: Press release, 27 January 1992

KASS EJ: Adolescent varicocele: Current concepts. Semin Urol 6:140, 1988

MARSHALL WA, TANNER JM: Variation in the pattern of pubertal changes in boys. Arch Dis Child 45:13, 1970
——, ——: Variation in the pattern of pubertal changes in girls. Arch Dis Child 44:291, 1969

MCANARNEY ER et al: *Textbook of Adolescent Medicine*. Philadelphia, Saunders, 1992

MILLSTEIN SG et al: Health risk behaviors among young adolescents. Pediatrics 89:422, 1992

NATIONAL CENTER FOR HEALTH STATISTICS: *Vital Statistics of the United States, 1988*, Vol 2, Mortality, part A. DHHS publication no (PHS) 91-1101, 1991, pp 14–38

NEWACHECK PW et al: Health insurance coverage of adolescents: A current profile and assessment of trends. Pediatrics 90:589, 1992

NOTTELMANN ED et al: Developmental processes in early adolescence: Relations between adolescent adjustment problems and chronologic age, pubertal stage and puberty-related hormones. J Pediatr 110:473, 1987

PALLA B, LITT IF: Medical complications of eating disorders in adolescents. Pediatrics 81:613, 1988

SHAFER MAB, IRWIN CE JR: The adolescent patient, in *Rudolph's Pediatrics*, 19th ed, A Rudolph (ed). Norwalk, Appleton and Lange, 1991, pp 39–81

SHAFFER D et al: Preventing teenage suicide: A critical review. J Am Acad Child Adolesc Psychiatry 27:675, 1988

STYNE D, GRUMBACH MM: Disorders of puberty in males and females, in *Reproductive Endocrinology*, SS Yen, RB Jaffee (eds). Philadelphia, W. Saunders, 1991, pp 511–54

TANNER JM, DAVIES PSW: Clinical longitudinal standards for height and weight velocity for North American Children. J Pediatr 107:317, 1985

UDRY JR: Biological predispositions and social control in adolescent sexual behavior. Am Soc Rev 53:709, 1988

US OFFICE OF TECHNOLOGY ASSESSMENT: *Adolescent Health, Volume III, Crosscutting Issues in the Delivery of Health and Related Services*, OTA-H-467, Washington DC, 1991

US PREVENTIVE SERVICES TASK FORCE: *Guide to Clinical Preventive Services: An Assessment of the Effectiveness of 169 Interventions*. Baltimore, Williams & Wilkins, 1989

8 GERIATRIC MEDICINE

NEIL M. RESNICK

Of all the people who have ever lived to age 65, more than half are now alive. This statistic has important demographic and economic implications, and its impact on medical care is also substantial.

BIOLOGY OF AGING

Numerous theories have been proposed to explain the biologic mechanisms of aging, but all have inherent difficulties. Moreover, most are not mutually exclusive, and at present there is no evidence for a *single* mechanism of aging. Instead, aging is likely to have multiple and interacting causes that are probably different in cells and organs that are postmitotic (such as neurons, cardiac, and skeletal muscle cells) as compared to those with renewable tissues (such as bone marrow, skin, and gastrointestinal cells). For example, damage due to free radicals might be more ominous in a nonreplicating organ, such as the nervous system, than in a continuously replicating organ such as bone marrow, and the mechanisms required to cope with such damage may also be differentially affected by age.

As interest in population-based, organism-based, and organ-based theories of aging has waned, interest in cellular models has increased for several reasons: (1) cells grown in culture universally senesce; that is, after a finite series of doublings they cease to replicate although they perform most metabolic functions and remain alive up to a year or longer; (2) the number of replications prior to senescence is directly proportional to the maximum lifespan of the species; (3) the number of cell doublings is inversely related to the age of the donor; (4) cells taken from patients with premature aging syndromes (e.g., Werner's and progeria) exhibit decreased lifespans in vitro.

Although the mechanism(s) responsible remain elusive, potentially important insights into aging have emerged from studies of cellular aging. For example, the failure of senescent cells to replicate in the presence of growth factors is associated with failure to induce the c-*fos* gene and with a block in the late G_1 phase of the cell cycle. This block can be overcome by fusing senescent cells with those from immortal cell lines. In addition, the block is associated with secretion of statin (a 57-kDa protein) and expression of a still uncharacterized protein located in the outer surface of the plasma membrane. When added to younger cells, this protein blocks DNA synthesis and replication at the same, late G_1 phase of the cell cycle.

Another factor implicated in cellular senescence is retinoblastoma gene product, an inhibitor of cell proliferation, that can be inactivated only by phosphorylation. Failure to induce kinases may be a general feature of aging cells, leading to alterations in phosphorylation such that they become unable to deactivate gene products that inhibit cell proliferation. There is no evidence that important genes coding for specific peptides are routinely deleted or inactivated during aging. However, noncoding DNA sequences, which may be important for cell division or transcription regulation, might be affected. There is also little consistent data that aging affects RNA transcription.

Many mechanisms previously postulated to be involved in aging have not been substantiated, such as somatic mutation (in which aging is due to cumulative spontaneous mutations), error catastrophe (in which aging results from errors in the synthesis of proteins) and intrinsic mutagenesis (in which aging is the result of ongoing DNA rearrangements). Other mechanisms, such as free radical damage, alterations in DNA methylation, and telomere attrition, remain the subjects of active investigation.

PRINCIPLES OF GERIATRIC MEDICINE

From a physiologic standpoint, aging can be described as the progressive constriction of the homeostatic reserve of every organ system. This decline, often referred to as *homeostenosis*, is evident by the third decade and is gradual and progressive although the rate and extent of decline vary. The decline of each organ system (Table 8-1) appears to occur independently of changes in other organ systems and is influenced by diet, environment, and personal habits, as well as by genetic factors.

TABLE 8-1 Selected age-related changes and their consequences

Organ/system	Age-related physiologic change*	Caused by age-related physiologic change	Caused by disease, not age
General	↑ Body fat	↑ Volume of distribution for fat soluble drugs	Obesity
	↓ Total body water	↓ Volume of distribution for water soluble drugs	Anorexia
Eyes/ears	Presbyopia	↓ Accomodation	
	Lens opacification	↑ Susceptibility to glare	Blindness
	↓ High-frequency acuity	Difficulty discriminating words if background noise is present	Deafness
Endocrine	Impaired glucose	↑ Glucose level in response to acute illness	Diabetes mellitus
	↓ Thyroxine clearance (and production)	↓ T_4 dose required in hypothyroidism	Thyroid dysfunction
	↑ ADH, ↓ renin, and ↑ aldosterone		↓ Na^+, ↑ K^+
	↓ Testosterone		Impotence
	↓ Vitamin D absorption and activation	Osteopenia	Osteoporosis, osteomalacia
Respiratory	↓ Lung elasticity and ↑ chest wall stiffness	Ventilation/perfusion mismatch and ↓ P_{O_2}	Dyspnea, hypoxia
Cardiovascular	↓ Arterial compliance and ↑ systolic BP →LVH	Hypotensive response to ↑ HR, volume depletion, or loss of atrial contraction	Syncope
	↓ β-adrenergic responsiveness	↓ Cardiac output and HR response to stress	Heart failure
	↓ Baroreceptor sensitivity and ↓ SA node automaticity	Impaired blood pressure response to standing, volume depletion	Heart block
Gastrointestinal	↓ Hepatic function	Delayed metabolism of some drugs	Cirrhosis
	↓ Gastric acidity	↓ Ca^+ absorption on empty stomach	Osteoporosis, B_{12} deficiency
	↓ Colonic motility	Constipation	Fecal impaction
	↓ Anorectal function		Fecal incontinence
Hematologic/immune system	↓ Bone marrow reserve(?)		
	↓ T cell function	False-negative PPD response	Anemia
	↑ Autoantibodies	False-positive rheumatoid factor, antinuclear antibody	Autoimmune disease
Renal	↓ GFR	Impaired excretion of some drugs	↑ Serum creatinine
	↓ Urine concentration/dilution (see also ''Endocrine'')	Delayed response to salt or fluid restriction/overload; nocturia	↓ ↑ Na^+
Genitourinary	Vaginal/urethral mucosal atrophy	Dyspareunia, bacteriuria	Symptomatic UTI
	Prostate enlargement	↑ Residual urine volume	Urinary incontinence; urinary retention
Musculoskeletal	↓ Lean body mass, muscle		Functional impairment
	↓ Bone density	Osteopenia	Hip fracture
Nervous system	Brain atrophy	Benign senescent forgetfulness	Dementia, delirium
	↓ Brain catechol synthesis		Depression
	↓ Brain dopaminergic synthesis	Stiffer gait	Parkinson's disease
	↓ Righting reflexes	↑ Body sway	Falls
	↓ Stage 4 sleep	Early wakening, insomnia	Sleep apnea

* Changes generally observed in healthy elderly subjects free of symptoms and detectable disease in the organ system studied. The changes are usually important only when the system is stressed or other factors are added (e.g., drugs, disease, or environmental challenge); they rarely result in symptoms otherwise. Abbreviations: T_4 = thyroxine, BP = blood pressure, HR = heart rate, ADH = antidiuretic hormone, GFR = glomerular filtration rate.

Several important principles follow from these facts: (1) Individuals become more dissimilar as they age, belying any stereotype of aging; (2) an *abrupt* decline in any system or function is always due to disease and not to "normal aging"; (3) "normal aging" can be attenuated by modification of risk factors (e.g., increased blood pressure, smoking, sedentary lifestyle); and (4) "healthy old age" is not an oxymoron. *In fact, in the absence of disease, the decline in homeostatic reserve causes no symptoms and imposes few restrictions on activities of daily living regardless of age.*

Appreciation of these facts may make it easier to understand the striking increases that have occurred in life expectancy. Average life expectancy is now 17 years at age 65, 11 years at age 75, 6 years at age 85, 4 years at age 90, and 2 years at age 100. Moreover, the bulk of these years is characterized by a lack of significant impairment (Table 8-2)—only 35 percent of people over age 85 are impaired in any activity required for daily living, and only 20 percent reside in a nursing home. Yet, as individuals age they are more likely to suffer from disease, disability, and the side effects of drugs all of which, when combined with the decrease in physiologic reserve, make the older person more vulnerable to environmental, pathologic, and pharmacologic challenges.

The following concepts underlie the remainder of the chapter:

1. The onset of a new disease in the elderly (usually defined as over age 75 to 80) generally affects an organ system made vulnerable by prior physiologic and pathologic changes. Because this organ system often differs from the diseased organ system in the young, disease presentation in the elderly may be atypical. For example, less than one-fourth of older patients with hyperthyroidism present with goiter, tremor, and exophthalmos; more likely are atrial fibrillation, confusion, depression, syncope, and weakness. Significantly, because the "weakest link" is so often the brain, the lower urinary tract, or the cardiovascular or musculoskeletal system, a limited number of presenting symptoms predominate—acute confusion, depression, incontinence, falling, and syncope—no matter what the underlying disease. Thus for the most common geriatric syndromes, regardless of the presenting symptom, the differential diagnosis is often largely similar. The corollary is equally important: The organ system usually associated with a particular symptom is less likely to be the source of that symptom in older individuals than in younger ones. Compared with middle-aged individuals, for example, acute confusion in older patients is less often due to a new brain lesion, depression to a psychiatric disorder, incontinence to bladder dysfunction, falling to a neuropathy, or syncope to heart disease.

2. Because of impaired physiologic reserve, older patients often present at an earlier stage of their disease. For example, heart failure may be precipitated by mild hyperthyroidism, cognitive dysfunction by mild Alzheimer's disease, urinary retention by mild prostatic enlargement, and nonketotic hyperosmolar coma by mild glucose intolerance. Paradoxically, therefore, treatment of the underlying disease may be easier because it is often less advanced at the time of presentation. A corollary is that drug side effects can occur with drugs and drug doses unlikely to produce side effects in younger people (Chap. 67). For instance, an antihistamine may cause confusion, diuretics may precipitate urinary incontinence, digoxin may induce depression even with normal serum levels, and over-the-counter sympathomimetics may precipitate urinary retention in men with mild prostatic obstruction.

3. Since many homeostatic mechanisms may be compromised concurrently, there are usually multiple abnormalities amenable to treatment, and small improvements in each may yield dramatic benefits overall. For instance, cognitive impairment in patients with Alzheimer's disease may be exacerbated by hearing or visual impairment, depression, heart failure, and electrolyte imbalance. Similarly, urinary incontinence can be worsened by fecal impaction, medications, and excess urinary output. In each case, substantial functional improvement can result from treating the contributing factors even if—as in Alzheimer's disease—specific treatment is not possible.

4. Many findings that are abnormal in younger patients are relatively common in older people—e.g., bacteriuria, premature ventricular contractions, low bone mineral density, impaired glucose tolerance, and uninhibited bladder contractions. However, they may not be responsible for a particular symptom but only be incidental findings that result in missed diagnoses and misdirected therapy. For instance, the finding of bacteriuria should not end the search for a source of fever in an acutely ill older patient, nor should an elevated random blood sugar—especially in an acutely ill patient—be incriminated as the cause of neuropathy. On the other hand, certain other abnormalities must not be dismissed as due to old age—e.g., there is no anemia, impotence, depression, or confusion of old age.

5. Because symptoms in older people are often due to multiple causes, the diagnostic "law of parsimony" often does not apply. For instance, fever, anemia, retinal embolus, and a heart murmur prompt almost a reflex diagnosis of infective endocarditis in a younger patient but may reflect aspirin-induced blood loss, a cholesterol embolus, insignificant aortic sclerosis, or a viral illness in an older patient.

6. Because the older patient is more likely to suffer the adverse consequences of disease, treatment—and even prevention—may be equally or even more effective. For instance, the benefits of thrombolysis and beta-blocker therapy after a myocardial infarction are as impressive in older patients as in younger ones; and treatment of hypertension, and immunization against influenza and pneumococcal pneumonia, are more effective in older patients. In addition, prevention in older patients often must be seen in a broader context. For instance, although efforts to increase bone density may be futile in older patients, fracture still may be prevented by interventions that improve balance, strengthen legs, treat contributing medical conditions, repair nutritional deficits, remove adverse medications, and reduce environmental hazards.

HISTORY TAKING IN ELDERLY PATIENTS Most older patients are able to provide a reliable medical history; however, a multitude of complaints may make obtaining a history more difficult. If the patient is unable to comprehend or communicate, data should be sought from family, friends, and caregivers. The history should include drug ingestion, a dietary history, history of falling, of incontinence, and of depression and anxiety.

Advance directives All older patients should be asked whether they have drafted advance health care directives, and, if they have, a copy should be placed in the record. Such directives may consist of a health care proxy or durable power of attorney for health care, in which patients designate a surrogate decision-maker who makes health care decisions if the patient cannot; and/or a living will or medical directive, in which patients specify their desires for treatment in specific situations if they cannot communicate at the critical time.

Whether or not the patient has formally drafted these directives, it is useful to indicate in the record who should make health care decisions if the patient is no longer able to do so. Patients should then be encouraged to discuss with the physician as well as the designated proxy their feelings about resuscitation, intubation, feeding

---

TABLE 8-2 Life expectancy and number of remaining years free of dependency in ADL*

Age	Life expectancy*, av		Disability-free years remaining	
	Men	Women	Men	Women
65–69	13	20	9	11
70–74	12	16	8	8
75–79	10	13	7	7
80–84	7	10	5	5
≥85	7	8	3	3

* For independent noninstitutionalized elderly men and women in Massachusetts. Longevity and disability-free longevity are surprisingly long and must be incorporated into treatment decisions. ADL = activities of daily living. av = average. All figures rounded to nearest year. See text for more recent data on longevity alone.
SOURCE: Katz S et al: Active life expectancy. N Engl J Med 309:1218, 1983.

tubes, hospitalization, etc. in their current state of health and possible future declining states of health. The early elicitation of a patient's preferences and values can often help both physicians and families in subsequent difficult decisions by giving surrogate decision-makers the sense that they are doing as the patient would have wanted.

PHYSICAL EXAMINATION Certain features of the examination should receive special attention, depending in part on clues from the history. Weight and postural blood pressure should be measured at each visit. Vision and hearing should be checked; if hearing is impaired, excess cerumen should be removed from the external auditory canals. Denture fit should be assessed, and the oral cavity should be inspected with the dentures removed. Although thyroid disease becomes more common with age, the sensitivity and specificity of related findings are substantially lower than in younger individuals; consequently, the physical examination can rarely corroborate or exclude thyroid dysfunction in older patients. The breasts should not be overlooked, since older women are more likely to have breast cancer and less likely to do breast self-examination. In auscultating the chest, the physician must recall that the presence of a fourth heart sound in an elderly person does not imply significant cardiac disease. The systolic murmur of aortic sclerosis is common and may be difficult to differentiate from aortic stenosis.

In inactive patients and those with fecal or urinary incontinence, one should check for fecal impaction. In patients with urinary incontinence—especially men—a distended bladder must be looked for, since it may be the only finding in urinary retention; perineal sensation and the bulbocavernosus reflex also should be tested. Patients who fall should be observed standing up from a chair, walking 10 feet, turning, returning, and sitting again; abnormalities of gait and steadiness on standing should be evaluated with the patient's eyes open and closed and in response to a sternal push. It should be appreciated that "frontal release signs" (e.g., "snout," "glabellar," or palmomental reflexes) and absent ankle jerks and vibratory sense in the feet may be normal in the elderly.

MENTAL STATUS EXAMINATION In addition to evaluating mood and affect, some form of cognitive testing is desirable in all elderly patients, even if it involves only checking different components of the history for consistency. People with mild degrees of dementia usually retain their social graces and may mask intellectual impairment by a cheerful and cooperative manner (Chap. 25). Thus, the examiner should always probe for content. For patients who follow the news, one can ask what stories they are particularly interested in and why; the same applies to reading, social events—even the "soap operas" on television.

If there is any suspicion of a cognitive deficit after this kind of conversational probing, further questioning is indicated. An examination that tests only orientation as to person, place, and time is insufficient to detect mild or moderate intellectual impairment. As a quick screen, simply assessing orientation and asking the patient to draw a clock with the hands at a set time (e.g., 10 min before 2:00) can be very informative regarding cognitive status, visuospatial deficits, ability to comprehend and execute instructions in logical sequence, and presence or absence of perseveration. For slightly more detailed examinations, many practical mental status tests are available. The most widely used is the Mini-Mental Status Examination of Folstein (Chap. 25), which provides a numerical score that can be obtained in 5 to 10 min. Regardless of the test employed, the total score is less useful diagnostically than is knowledge of the specific domain of the deficit. As a general rule, disproportionate difficulty with immediate recall (e.g., of a list of three items) suggests depression, while predominant difficulty with recalling the items 5 min later suggests dementia. For patients with deficits of attention—recognized by inability to spell simple words backwards, repeat five digits, or recite the months of the year backwards—delirium is probably present, and the accuracy of the remainder of the test is dubious. However, the test can be interpreted accurately only in the context of a comprehensive evaluation.

EVALUATION OF FUNCTIONAL CAPACITY A clear description of the patient's degree of fitness or functional incapacity based on both medical and psychosocial problems is essential. The functional assessment includes determination of the patient's ability to perform basic activities of daily life (ADL), which are those needed for personal self-care, as well as the ability to perform more complex tasks required for independent living, the instrumental activities of daily living (IADL). ADLs include bathing, dressing, toileting, feeding, getting in and out of chairs and bed, and walking. IADLs include shopping, cooking, money management, housework, using a telephone, and traveling outside the home. For frail patients, an assessment in the home by a trained observer may be required, but for most patients a questionnaire dealing with these activities can be completed by the family or patient. In either case, the physician must determine the cause of any impairment and whether it can be treated. The assessment should conclude with determination of the socioeconomic circumstances and social support systems.

Since disease can present atypically in the elderly, acute functional decline may represent the first sign of serious acute illness. *Thus, acute functional decline presenting as the onset or worsening of falls, confusion, depression, or incontinence should prompt immediate medical evaluation.*

MANAGEMENT OF COMMON GERIATRIC CONDITIONS

Diseases more common in the elderly are covered elsewhere in the text. The medical problems discussed below do not usually present as clear-cut organ-specific diagnoses and are most common in the frail elderly, especially those over 80 years of age.

INTELLECTUAL IMPAIRMENT The predominant causes of impaired mentation in older patients are delirium, dementia, and depression. Each condition is covered elsewhere in the text in detail (Chaps. 25 and 389), but their management in the elderly is discussed here.

The most important first step is to search for and correct all factors that may contribute to cognitive impairment. Evidence of dangerous behavior also should be sought (e.g., leaving the stove on, wandering, and getting lost) and plans should be devised to deal with it. Although there is no specific pharmacologic treatment for Alzheimer's disease, this does not mean that the physician has no further role in treating the patient and family. In addition to discontinuing all nonessential medications and treating new intercurrent illness, the physician should help the family and patient predict and deal with the disease; indeed, the family often needs the physician's support more than the patient does.

Community services should be suggested as needed. Support groups such as the Alzheimer's Association often are of value to the family and help them to anticipate problems. Signs of patient abuse by an overstressed caregiver should be watched for. Legal counsel should be recommended to help the patient and family devise plans for ongoing management and ultimate disposition of assets.

Finally, the onset of disruptive behavior should always prompt a search for new illness or medication. Exacerbation of cognitive dysfunction may occur with mild infections (e.g., subungual toe abscess or pressure ulcer); with "therapeutic" levels of many drugs; with use of nonprescribed drugs or alcohol; with modest abnormalities of serum sodium, calcium, or thyroxine; with borderline nutritional deficiencies; and even with the development of fecal impaction, urinary retention, pain, or change in environment, particularly in frail older patients. However, if a cause is not found and behavior does not respond to environmental manipulation, low doses of an antipsychotic medication may be helpful (e.g., haloperidol 0.25 to 2 mg per day orally; see below).

DEPRESSION Depression of significant degree occurs in 5 to 10 percent of community-dwelling elderly but is often overlooked. At highest risk are individuals with recent medical illness (e.g., stroke), bereavement, lack of social supports, recent nursing home admission, or psychiatric history (including alcohol abuse). The diagnosis requires the presence of a depressed mood for at least two consecutive weeks plus at least four of the following eight signs: sleep disturbance, lack of interest, feelings of guilt, decreased energy, decreased concentration, decreased appetite, psychomotor agitation/retardation, and suicidal ideation. Also helpful diagnostically are a personal or family history of depression and past response to an antidepressant. It is essential to bear in mind that depression in older patients is often caused or contributed to by drugs or a systemic illness.

Treatment For the hospitalized patient in whom acute depression delays recovery or rehabilitation—when correction of medical and pharmacologic contributing factors is ineffective and there is no prior history of mania or major depression—methylphenidate, 5 to 10 mg at 8 A.M. and noon (to avoid insomnia) is often very effective, with benefits discernible within a few days. For many patients with major depression, there is no ideal antidepressant drug. All are about equally effective, but the side effects differ (see below and Chap. 389). Consequently, one should become familiar with one or two agents for patients with psychomotor retardation (e.g., desipramine, fluoxetine) and for those with agitation (e.g., nortriptyline or trazodone). Because of its potent anticholinergic and orthostatic side effects, amitriptyline should be avoided whenever possible in older patients. Initial low dosages should be increased slowly to avoid serious side effects; low doses of each medication (e.g., doxepin, 10 to 50 mg daily; desipramine, 25 to 75 mg daily) are often effective in the elderly. Careful follow-up is required to anticipate and minimize anticholinergic side effects, orthostatic hypotension, sedating effects, confusion, bizarre mental symptoms, cardiovascular complications, and drug overdose with suicidal intent. Adverse drug reactions should not be assumed to be due to the aging process.

Cautious use of the monoamine oxidase inhibitors is sometimes of benefit when other antidepressants are ineffective. Monoamine oxidase inhibitors should not be used in combination with the cyclic compounds. Electroconvulsive therapy has been successful and is usually well tolerated by elderly patients who remain severely depressed despite drug treatment.

URINARY INCONTINENCE **Transient incontinence** (Table 8-3) Because urinary continence requires adequate mobility, mentation, motivation, and manual dexterity—in addition to integrated control of the lower urinary tract—problems outside the bladder can result in incontinence.

1 *Delirium.* A clouded sensorium impedes recognition of both the need to void and the location of the nearest toilet; once delirium clears, incontinence resolves.
2 *Infection.* Symptomatic urinary tract infection commonly causes or contributes to incontinence; asymptomatic infection does not.

TABLE 8-3 Classification of incontinence

TRANSIENT

Delirium/confusional state
Infection—urinary (symptomatic)
Atrophic urethritis/vaginitis
Pharmaceuticals
Psychological, especially depression
Excessive urine output (e.g., CHF, hyperglycemia)
Restricted mobility
Stool impaction

ESTABLISHED

Detrusor overactivity
Detrusor underactivity
Urethral obstruction
Urethral incompetence

SOURCE: Adapted from Resnick NM: Urinary incontinence in the elderly. Medical Grand Rounds 3:281, 1984.

TABLE 8-4 Medications that can potentially affect continence

Type of medication	Examples	Potential effects on continence
Potent diuretics	Furosemide	Polyuria, frequency, urgency
Anticholinergics	Antihistamines, trihexyphenidyl, benztropine, dicyclomine, disopyramide	Urinary retention, overflow incontinence, delirium, impaction
Psychotropics		
Antidepressants	Amitriptyline, desipramine	Anticholinergic actions, sedation
Antipsychotics	Thioridazine, haloperidol	Anticholinergic actions, sedation, rigidity, immobility
Sedatives/hypnotics	Diazepam, flurazepam	Sedation, delirium, immobility
Narcotic analgesics		Urinary retention, fecal impaction, sedation, delirium
Alpha-adrenergic blockers	Prazosin, terazosin	Urethral relaxation (stress incontinence in women)
Alpha-adrenergic agonists	Decongestants	Urinary retention in men
Calcium channel blockers	All	Urinary retention
Alcohol		Polyuria, frequency, urgency, sedation, delirium, immobility
Vincristine		Urinary retention

SOURCE: Resnick NM: Geriatric medicine and the elderly patient, in *Current Medical Diagnosis and Treatment*, LT Tierney et al (eds). Norwalk, Appleton & Lange, 1993 (in press).

3 *Atrophic urethritis/vaginitis.* Atrophic urethritis/vaginitis, characterized by the presence of vaginal telangiectasia, petechiae, erosions, erythema, or friability, commonly contributes to incontinence in women and responds to a short course of low-dose estrogen or vaginal estrogen creams.
4 *Pharmaceutical.* The drugs most commonly causing transient incontinence are listed in Table 8-4.
5 *Psychologic.* Depression and psychosis are uncommon but treatable causes.
6 *Excess urine output.* Excess urine output may overwhelm the ability to reach a toilet in time. Causes include diuretics, excess fluid intake, and metabolic abnormalities (e.g., hyperglycemia, hypercalcemia, diabetes insipidus); nocturnal incontinence may result from mobilization of peripheral edema.
7 *Restricted mobility.* If mobility cannot be improved, access to a urinal or commode may restore continence. (See Immobility below.)
8 *Stool impaction.* This is a common cause of urinary incontinence, especially in hospitalized or immobile patients. Although the mechanism is unknown, a clue to its presence is the coexistence of both urinary and fecal incontinence. Disimpaction restores continence.

Established incontinence (Table 8-3) The causes of established incontinence include irreversible functional deficits, such as end-stage Alzheimer's disease, and intrinsic lower urinary tract dysfunction. Lower urinary tract dysfunction should be sought after transient causes have been excluded.

DETRUSOR OVERACTIVITY This disorder (uninhibited bladder contraction) accounts for two-thirds of geriatric incontinence in both sexes, regardless of whether patients are demented. Detrusor overactivity can be diagnosed presumptively in a woman when leakage occurs in the absence of stress maneuvers or urinary retention and is preceded by the abrupt onset of an intense urge to urinate that cannot be forestalled. In men, the symptoms are similar, but since detrusor overactivity coexists with urethral obstruction, urodynamic testing should be done if prescription of a bladder relaxant is planned. Because detrusor overactivity also may be due to bladder stones or tumor, the abrupt onset of otherwise unexplained urge incontinence—especially if accompanied by perineal/suprapubic discomfort or sterile hematuria—should prompt cystoscopy and cytologic examination.

The cornerstone of treatment is behavioral therapy. Patients should be instructed (or "prompted" if they are demented) to void every 1 to 2 h while awake and to suppress urgency in between; once daytime continence is restored, the interval between voiding can be progressively increased. When drugs are necessary, they should be added to these regimens and monitored to avoid inducing urinary retention. Effective drugs include anticholinergics (e.g., propantheline, 7.5 to 30 mg four to six times daily), oxybutynin (2.5 to 5 mg three or four times daily), imipramine or doxepin (25 to 100 mg at bedtime), and calcium channel blockers (in doses used for cardiac disease).

Indwelling catheterization is rarely indicated for detrusor overactivity. If all measures fail, an external collection device or protective pad or undergarment may be required.

STRESS INCONTINENCE This disorder, the second most common cause of established incontinence in older women (it is rare in men), is characterized by symptoms and evidence of *instantaneous* leakage of urine in response to stress. Leakage is worse or occurs only during the day unless another abnormality (e.g., detrusor overactivity) is also present. On examination, with the bladder full and the perineum relaxed, instantaneous leakage upon coughing strongly suggests stress incontinence, especially if it reproduces symptoms and if urinary retention has been excluded by a postvoiding residual determination; a several-second delay suggests that leakage is instead caused by an uninhibited bladder contraction induced by coughing.

Surgery is the most effective treatment with a cure rate of approximately 85 percent. For women who can comply, pelvic muscle exercises are an option for mild to moderate stress incontinence; if not contraindicated, an alpha-adrenergic agonist (e.g., phenylpropanolamine) is also helpful in such cases, especially if combined with estrogen. Occasionally, a pessary or even a tampon (for women with vaginal stenosis) provides some relief.

URETHRAL OBSTRUCTION Rarely present in women, urethral obstruction (due to prostatic enlargement, urethral stricture, bladder neck contracture, or prostate cancer) is the second most common cause of established incontinence in older men. It can present as dribbling incontinence after voiding, urge incontinence due to detrusor overactivity (which coexists in two-thirds of cases), or overflow incontinence due to urinary retention. Renal ultrasound is recommended to exclude hydronephrosis in men whose postvoiding residual volume exceeds 100 to 200 mL; in older men for whom surgery is planned, urodynamic confirmation of obstruction is usually required.

Surgical decompression is the most effective treatment for obstruction, especially if there is urinary retention. For a nonoperative candidate, intermittent or indwelling catheterization is used; a condom catheter is contraindicated when urinary retention is present. For a man with prostatic obstruction who is not in retention, treatment with an alpha-adrenergic antagonist (e.g., prazosin, 1 to 2 mg two to four times daily) may relieve symptoms, and the 5α-reductase inhibitor finasteride may partially relieve obstruction in a third or more of patients.

DETRUSOR UNDERACTIVITY Whether idiopathic or due to sacral lower motor nerve dysfunction, this is the least common cause of incontinence (<10 percent of cases). When it causes incontinence, detrusor underactivity is associated with urinary frequency, nocturia, and frequent leakage of small amounts. The elevated postvoiding residual volume (generally over 450 mL) distinguishes it from detrusor overactivity and stress incontinence, but only urodynamic testing (rather than cystoscopy or intravenous urography) differentiates it from urethral obstruction in men; such testing usually is not required in women, in whom obstruction is rare.

For the patient with a poorly contractile bladder, augmented voiding techniques (e.g., double voiding or applying suprapubic pressure) are often effective; pharmacologic agents (e.g., bethanechol) are rarely effective. If further emptying is needed or for the patient with an acontractile bladder, intermittent or indwelling catheterization is the only option. Antibiotics should be used for symptomatic upper tract infection or as prophylaxis for recurrent symptomatic infections only in a patient using intermittent catheterization; they should not be used as prophylaxis with an indwelling catheter.

FALLS Falls are a major problem for elderly people, especially women. Thirty percent of community-dwelling elderly fall each year; and one out of four of those who fall has serious injuries, including fractures in 5 percent. Falls are the sixth leading cause of death for older people and a contributing factor in 40 percent of admissions to nursing homes. Resultant hip problems and fear of falls are major causes of loss of independence. Nonetheless, falling must *not* be viewed as accidental, inevitable, or untreatable.

Causes of falls Balance and ambulation require a complex interplay of cognitive, neuromuscular, and cardiovascular function, and the ability to adapt rapidly to an environmental challenge. Balance becomes impaired and sway increases with age. The resulting vulnerability makes the older person predisposed to fall when challenged by an additional insult to *any* of these systems. Thus, a seemingly minor fall may be due to a serious problem, such as pneumonia or a myocardial infarction.

Much more commonly, however, falls are due to the complex interaction between a variably impaired patient and an environmental challenge. While a warped floorboard may pose little problem for a vigorous, unmedicated, alert person, it may be sufficient to precipitate a fall and hip fracture in the patient with altered balance, muscle tone, and cognition. Thus, falls in older people are rarely due to a single cause, and effective prevention entails a comprehensive assessment of the patient's intrinsic deficits (usually diseases and medications), the routine activities, and the environmental obstacles.

Intrinsic deficits are those that impair sensory input, judgment, blood pressure regulation, reaction time, and balance and gait (Table 8-5). Medications and alcohol use are among the most common, significant, and reversible causes of falling. Other treatable contributors include postprandial hypotension (which peaks 30 to 60 min after a meal), insomnia, urinary urgency, and peripheral edema (which can burden impaired leg strength and gait with an additional 5 to 10 pounds).

Environmental obstacles are listed in Table 8-6. Since most falls occur in or around the home, a visit by a visiting nurse, physical therapist, or physician often reaps substantial dividends.

Complications of falls and treatment The risk of falling and consequent injury, disability, and potential institutionalization can be reduced by modifying where possible those factors outlined above and in Tables 8-5 and 8-6.

Subdural hematoma is a treatable but easily overlooked complication of falls that must be considered in any elderly patient presenting with new neurologic signs, including confusion alone, even in the absence of a headache. Dehydration, electrolyte imbalance, pressure sores, and hypothermia also may occur and endanger the patient's life following a fall.

IMMOBILITY The main causes of immobility are weakness, stiffness, pain, imbalance, and psychological problems. Weakness may result from disuse of muscles, malnutrition, electrolyte disturbances, anemia, neurologic disorders, or myopathies. The most common cause of stiffness in the elderly is osteoarthritis; however, Parkinson's disease, rheumatoid arthritis, gout, pseudogout, and antipsychotic drugs such as haloperidol may also contribute. Pain, whether from bone (e.g., osteoporosis, osteomalacia, Paget's disease, metastatic bone cancer, trauma), joints (e.g., osteoarthritis, rheumatoid arthritis, gout), bursa, or muscle (e.g., polymyalgia rheumatica, intermittent claudication, or "pseudoclaudication"), may immobilize the patient.

Imbalance and fear of falling are major causes of immobilization.

TABLE 8-5   Intrinsic risk factors for falling and possible interventions

Risk factor	Interventions Medical	Rehabilitative or environmental
Reduced visual acuity, dark adaptation, and perception	Refraction; cataract extraction	Home safety assessment
Reduced hearing	Removal of cerumen; audiologic evaluation	Hearing aid if appropriate (with training); reduction in background noise
Vestibular dysfunction	Avoidance of drugs affecting the vestibular system; neurologic or ear, nose, and throat evaluation, if indicated	Habituation exercises
Proprioceptive dysfunction, cervical degenerative disorders, and peripheral neuropathy	Screening for vitamin B_{12} deficiency and cervical spondylosis	Balance exercises; appropriate walking aid; correctly sized footwear with firm soles; home safety assessment
Dementia	Detection of reversible causes; avoidance of sedative or centrally acting drugs	Supervised exercise and ambulation; home safety assessment
Musculoskeletal disorders	Appropriate diagnostic evaluation	Balance-and-gait training; muscle-strengthening exercises; appropriate walking aid; home safety assessment
Foot disorders (calluses, bunions, deformities, edema)	Shaving of calluses; bunionectomy; treatment of edema	Trimming of nails; appropriate footwear
Postural hypotension	Assessment of medications; rehydration; possible alteration in situational factors (e.g., meals, change of position)	Dorsiflexion exercises; pressure-graded stockings; elevation of head of bed; use of tilt table if condition is severe
Use of medications (sedatives: benzodiazepines, phenothiazines, antidepressants; antihypertensives; others: antiarrhythmics, anticonvulsants, diuretics, alcohol)	Steps to be taken: 1. Attempted reduction in the total number of medications taken 2. Assessment of risks and benefits of each medication 3. Selection of medication, if needed, that is least centrally acting, least associated with postural hypotension, and has shortest action 4. Prescription of lowest effective dose 5. Frequent reassessment of risks and benefits	

SOURCE: After Tinetti and Speechley.

TABLE 8-6   Environmental factors affecting the risk of falling in the home

Environmental area or factor	Objective and recommendations
All areas	
Lighting	Absence of glare and shadows; accessible switches at room entrances; night light in bedroom, hall, bathroom
Floors	Nonskid backing for throw rugs; carpet edges tacked down; carpets with shallow pile; nonskid wax on floors; cords out of walking path; small objects (e.g., clothes, shoes) off floor
Stairs	Lighting sufficient, with switches at top and bottom of stairs; securely fastened bilateral handrails that stand out from wall; top and bottom steps marked with bright, contrasting tape; stair rises of no more than 6 in; steps in good repair; no objects stored on steps
Kitchen	Items stored so that reaching up and bending over are not necessary; secure step stool available if climbing is necessary; firm, nonmovable table
Bathroom	Grab bars for tub, shower, and toilet; nonskid decals or rubber mat in tub or shower; shower chair with handheld shower; nonskid rugs; raised toilet seat; door locks removed to ensure access in an emergency
Yard and entrances	Repair of cracks in pavement, holes in lawn; removal of rocks, tools, and other tripping hazards; well-lit walkways, free of ice and wet leaves; stairs and steps as above
Institutions	All the above; bed at proper height (not too high or low); spills on floor cleaned up promptly; appropriate use of walking aids and wheelchairs
Footwear	Shoes with firm, nonskid, nonfriction soles; low heels (unless person is accustomed to high heels); avoidance of walking in stocking feet or loose slippers

SOURCE: After Tinetti and Speechley.

changes occur in skeletal muscle. At the cellular level, intracellular ATP and glycogen concentrations decrease, rates of protein degradation increase, and contractile velocity and strength decline, while at the whole-muscle level, atrophy, weakness, and shortening are seen. Pressure sores are a third serious complication; mechanical pressure, moisture, friction, and shearing forces all predispose to their development. As a result, within days of being confined to bed, the risk of postural hypotension, falls, and skin breakdown rises. Moreover, these changes usually take weeks to months to reverse.

Management The most important step is preventive—to avoid bedrest whenever possible. When it cannot be avoided, several measures can be employed to minimize its consequences. Patients should be positioned as close to the upright position as possible several times daily. Range of motion exercises should begin immediately, and the skin over pressure points should be inspected frequently. Isometric and isotonic exercises should be performed while the patient is in bed, and whenever possible patients should assist their own positioning, transferring, and self-care. As mobility becomes feasible, graduated ambulation should begin.

If a pressure ulcer develops, the multiplicity of topical therapies underscores the fact that no single one is clearly more effective than others. Surgical debridement may be required for severely undermined lesions. A special mattress (e.g., foam or static air mattress) or air-fluidized bed or water bed may be required for the very debilitated patient.

In addition to treating all identified factors that contribute to immobility, consultation with a physical therapist should be sought. Installing handrails, lowering the bed, and providing chairs of proper height with arms and rubber skid guards may allow the patient to be safely mobile in the home. A properly fitted cane or walker may be helpful.

IATROGENIC DRUG REACTIONS For several reasons, older patients are two or three times more likely to have adverse drug reactions (Chap. 67). Drug clearance is often markedly reduced. This

Imbalance may result from general debility, neurologic causes (e.g., stroke; loss of postural reflexes; peripheral neuropathy due to diabetes mellitus, alcohol, or malnutrition; and vestibulocerebellar abnormalities), orthostatic or postprandial hypotension, drugs (e.g., diuretics, antihypertensives, neuroleptics, and antidepressants), or may occur following prolonged bed rest. Psychologic conditions such as severe anxiety or depression also may contribute to immobilization.

Consequences The hazards of bed rest in the elderly are multiple, serious, quick to develop, and slow to reverse. Deconditioning of the cardiovascular system occurs within days and involves fluid shifts, fluid loss, decreased cardiac output, decreased peak oxygen uptake, and increased resting heart rate. Perhaps even more striking

is due to a decrease in renal plasma flow and glomerular filtration rate and a reduced hepatic clearance. The last is due to a decrease in activity of the drug-metabolizing microsomal enzymes and an overall decline in blood flow to the liver with aging. The volume of distribution of drugs also is affected, since the elderly have a decrease in total body water and a relative increase in body fat. Thus, water-soluble drugs become more concentrated, and fat-soluble drugs have longer half-lives. In addition, serum albumin levels decline, especially in sick patients, so that there is a decrease in protein binding of some drugs (e.g., warfarin, phenytoin), leaving more free (active) drug available.

In addition to impaired drug clearance, which alters pharmacokinetics, older patients have altered responses to similar serum drug levels, a phenomenon known as altered pharmacodynamics. They are more sensitive to some drugs (e.g., opiates, anticoagulants) and less sensitive to others (e.g., beta-adrenergic agents). Finally, the older patient with multiple chronic conditions is likely to be taking several drugs, including nonprescribed agents. Thus, adverse drug reactions and dosage errors are more likely to occur, especially if the patient has visual, hearing, or memory deficits.

Precautions to avoid drug toxicity DRUG SELECTION AND ADMINISTRATION Before initiating treatment, the physician should first ensure that the symptom requiring treatment is not itself due to another drug. For example, antipsychotic agents can cause symptoms that mimic depression (flat affect, restlessness, and pacing); such symptoms should prompt lowering of the dose rather than initiation of an antidepressant. In addition, drug therapy should be employed only after nonpharmacologic means have been considered or tried and only when the benefit clearly outweighs the risk.

Once pharmacotherapy has been decided upon, it should begin at less than the usual adult dosage (although many elderly patients require full doses), and the dose should be increased slowly. The dosage schedule should be kept as simple as possible and the number of pills should be kept as low as possible. Serum drug levels are often useful in older patients, especially for monitoring drugs with narrow therapeutic indices such as phenytoin, theophylline, quinidine, aminoglycosides, lithium, and psychotropic agents such as nortriptyline. However, toxicity can occur even with "normal" therapeutic levels of some drugs (e.g., digoxin, phenytoin).

SEDATIVE-HYPNOTICS The effects of sedative-hypnotics persist much longer in the elderly and have been associated with confusional states, falls, fractures, driving accidents, and incontinence. The long acting agents in particular (e.g., flurazepam and diazepam) should be avoided whenever possible; however, even the shortest-acting benzodiazepines (e.g., triazolam) may have adverse effects. If nonpharmacologic treatment of insomnia is unsuccessful, short-term use of an intermediate-acting agent whose metabolism is not affected by age (e.g., oxazepam, 10 to 30 mg/d) may be useful.

ANTIBIOTICS Serum creatinine is not a good index of renal function in old people; however, when it is elevated special care must be taken with the administration of drugs normally excreted by the kidneys. Concentrations of relevant antibiotics should be measured directly.

CARDIAC DRUGS In older patients, digitalis, procainamide, and quinidine have prolonged half-lives and narrow therapeutic windows; toxicity is common at the usual dosages. For example, digoxin toxicity—especially anorexia, confusion, or depression—can occur even with therapeutic digoxin levels.

ANTIDEPRESSANTS AND ANTIPSYCHOTICS These agents can produce anticholinergic side effects in old people (e.g., confusion, urinary retention, constipation, dry mouth). This can be minimized by switching to a nonanticholinergic agent (e.g., fluoxetine or trazodone) or one with less anticholinergic effect (e.g., desipramine). In general, the least potent agents for psychosis (e.g., chlorpromazine) have the most sedating and anticholinergic effects and are the most likely to induce postural hypotension. By contrast, the most potent antipsychotic agents (e.g., haloperidol) have the least sedating, anticholinergic, and hypotensive side effects but cause extrapyramidal side effects, including dystonia, akathisia, rigidity, and tardive dyskinesia. Thus all of these agents are potentially toxic. Moreover, since both depression and agitation often remit spontaneously, cautious discontinuation of these drugs should be considered periodically.

GLAUCOMA MEDICATIONS Both topical beta-blockers and carbonic anhydrase inhibitors can cause systemic side effects. The latter can cause malaise and anorexia independent of the induced metabolic acidosis.

ANTICOAGULANTS Elderly patients benefit from anticoagulation as much as do younger individuals but are more vulnerable to serious bleeding. Hence, more careful monitoring and less aggressive anticoagulation are advisable.

AVOID OVERTREATMENT Drugs are not necessarily indicated in some common clinical situations. For instance, antibiotics need not be given for asymptomatic bacteriuria unless obstructive uropathy, other anatomic abnormalities, or stones are also present. Ankle edema is often due to venous insufficiency, drugs such as NSAIDs or some calcium antagonists, or even inactivity or malnutrition in chairbound patients. Diuretics are usually not indicated unless edema is associated with heart failure. Fitted, pressure gradient stockings are often helpful. Finally, since older patients generally tolerate aspirin and other NSAIDs less well than do younger patients, localized pain should be treated when possible with local measures such as injection, physical therapy, heat, ultrasound, or transcutaneous electrical stimulation (see Chap. 11).

PREVENTION

Much can be done to prevent the progression and even the onset of disease in older people. Dietary inadequacies in the elderly should be corrected; for the patient with inadequate sun exposure and intake of vitamin D, a daily multivitamin capsule is recommended. Tobacco and alcohol use should be minimized, since the benefits of discontinuing these accrue even to individuals over age 65. The importance of reviewing all of a patient's medications and discontinuing them whenever feasible cannot be overemphasized.

The benefits of treating both isolated systolic hypertension and combined systolic and diastolic hypertension in ambulatory elderly have now been documented. Treatment reduces the risk of stroke and the risk of death due to cardiovascular causes in this age group. Conclusive results have been achieved using *low doses* of a thiazide-like diuretic (e.g., chlorthalidone, 12.5 to 25 mg/d) as the first step (alone effective in almost half of patients) and adding low-dose reserpine (0.05 to 0.1 mg/d) or atenolol (25 to 50 mg/d) only as needed. Benefits were dramatic, side effects were minimal, cost was trivial, and concerns about potential toxicity were not borne out.

Because of the prevalence, functional impact, and ease of treatment, glaucoma should be screened for, and visual and auditory impairment should be corrected. Dentures should be assessed for their fit, and oral lesions beneath them should be detected.

A Papanicolaou test should be done in women who have not had one before, since the incidence of both preventable cervical carcinoma and associated death increases with age, especially in this group. Immunizations (for influenza, pneumococcal pneumonia, tetanus) should be current because of the established benefit of prophylaxis in the elderly. PPD testing should be done on residents of chronic care facilities and on those at high risk of tuberculosis; those who have recently converted probably should be treated. Since responsiveness wanes with age, the test, if negative, should be repeated in a week to increase the chances of detecting all exposed patients. Screening mammography is indicated every 1 to 2 years at least until age 75 and thereafter if a positive finding would result in therapeutic intervention. The relative risks and benefits of low-dose aspirin and (for women) estrogen replacement therapy have not yet been elucidated sufficiently to warrant routine use, but they should be considered on an individual basis.

Exercise should be encouraged not only because of its beneficial effects on blood pressure, cardiovascular conditioning, glucose home-ostasis, bone density, and functional status, but also because it may improve mood and social interaction, reduce insomnia and constipation, and prevent falls. Spinal flexion exercises should be avoided in patients with osteopenia; consultation with a physical therapist may be helpful.

Measures should be taken to prevent falling, as outlined in Tables 8-5 and 8-6. Counseling about driving is important, especially for patients with cognitive impairment. But perhaps the most valuable procedure for prevention of disease in old people is to take a careful history, focusing not only on the "chief complaint" but also on common and often hidden conditions such as falls, confusion, depression, sexual dysfunction, and incontinence. In addition, one should always identify the complications for which the specific patient is at risk and take steps to avert them. For instance, a patient with cognitive impairment who smokes is at risk not only for lung cancer but also for starting a fire, and a patient who requires narcotics is at risk for fecal impaction, delirium, urinary retention, and confusion. Community-dwelling patients who are at highest risk of rapid deterioration and institutionalization and who should be monitored more closely include those over age 80, those who live alone, those who are bereaved or depressed, and those who are intellectually impaired.

REFERENCES

Biology of aging

ARKING R: *Biology of Aging: Observations and Principles*. Englewood Cliffs, NJ: Prentice-Hall, 1991

JOHNSON TE, LITHGOW GJ: The search for the genetic basis of aging: The identification of gerontogenes in the nematode *Caenorhabditis elegans*. J Amer Geriatr Soc 40:936, 1992

GOLDSTEIN S: Replicative senescence: The human fibroblast comes of age. Science 249:1129, 1990

Functional assessment

LACHS MS et al: A simple procedure for general screening for functional disability in elderly patients. Ann Intern Med 112:699, 1990

Dementia, delirium, depression

NIH CONSENSUS DEVELOPMENT PANEL: Diagnosis and treatment of depression in late life. JAMA 268:1018, 1992

FRANCIS J: Delirium in older patients. J Amer Geriat Soc 40:829, 1992

HOWELL T, WATTS DT: Behavioral complications of dementia: A clinical approach for the general internist. J Gen Intern Med 5:431, 1990

KATZMAN R, ROWE JW (eds): *Principles of Geriatric Neurology*. Philadelphia, Davis, 1992

SIU A: Screening for dementia and assessing its causes. Ann Intern Med 115:122, 1991

Urinary incontinence

RESNICK NM, OUSLANDER JG (eds): National Institutes of Health Consensus Development Conference on Urinary Incontinence. J Am Geriatr Soc 38:263, 1990

URINARY INCONTINENCE GUIDELINE PANEL: Urinary incontinence in adults: Clinical practice guideline. AHCPR Publication No. 92-0038. Rockville, MD, 1992

Falls/Immobility

TINETTI ME, SPEECHLEY M: Prevention of falls among the elderly. N Engl J Med 320:1055, 1989

WASSON JH et al: The prescription of assistive devices for the elderly. J Gen Intern Med 5:46, 1990

Geriatric pharmacology

MONTAMAT SC et al: Management of drug therapy in the elderly. N Engl J Med 321:303, 1989

SALZMAN C: *Clinical Geriatric Psychopharmacology*, 2d ed. Baltimore, Williams & Wilkins, 1992

Prevention

AMERY A, SCHAEPDRYVER AD: Introduction: The European Working Party on High Blood Pressure in the Elderly. Am J Med 90(Suppl 3A):3, 1991

HAYWARD RSA et al: Preventive care guidelines: 1991. Ann Intern Med 114:758, 1991

SHEP COOPERATIVE RESEARCH GROUP: Prevention of stroke by antihypertensive drug treatment in older persons with isolated systolic hypertension. Final results of the Systolic Hypertension in the Elderly Program (SHEP). JAMA 265:3255, 1991

Miscellaneous

HARRIS J: The treatment of cancer in an aging population. JAMA 268:96, 1992

LIBOW LS, STARER P: Care of the nursing home patient. N Engl J Med 321:93, 1989

MORLEY JE et al: Nutrition in the elderly: ULCA conference. Ann Intern Med 109:890, 1988

PRINZ PN et al: Sleep disorders and aging. N Engl J Med 323:520, 1990

RESNICK NM, GREENSPAN SL: "Senile" osteoporosis reconsidered. JAMA 261:1025, 1989

9   COST AWARENESS IN MEDICINE

LEE GOLDMAN

COSTS OF HEALTH CARE IN THE UNITED STATES

Health care expenditures in the United States are now about $900 billion per year. Through the 1980s and early 1990s, these expenditures rose at a rate of more than 10 percent per year, which exceeded the rates of inflation and of growth in the gross national product (GNP). As a consequence, the percentage of the GNP that is spent on health care increased from about 7 percent in 1970 to 9 percent in 1980 and is expected to be nearly 15 percent in 1995. As a percentage of the GNP, medical care expenditures in the United Kingdom are about four percentage points lower than in the United States. In Canada, expenditures as a percentage of GNP were similar to the United States until about 1970 but now are about two percentage points lower. Much of the difference between the United States and Canada is explained by higher physician fees rather than by a higher per capita use of services. The United States also spends substantially more on the administrative costs of health care than Canada or Great Britain.

The reasons for the increase in health care costs are multifactorial. The aging of the population and the availability of new diagnostic and therapeutic advances have increased the demand for health care. Furthermore, between 1970 and 1990, the supply of physicians in the United States increased from about 150 to 240 per 100,000 population. This increase in physicians provided Americans with easier access to medical services but raised concerns that a possible oversupply of physicians in portions of the country could contribute to an excessive escalation in costs. The costs of care are especially influenced by decisions regarding hospital admission and surgery and by decisions affecting the use of intensive care units, life-sustaining treatments, and long-term care facilities. Efforts at cost-containment have attempted to identify unnecessary services, such as routine preoperative electrocardiograms in healthy young patients, or situations in which extraordinary expenses occur, such as in the last 6 months of life. Although some services may represent "fat" in the health care system, it is likely that any future reduction in unnecessary care may be more than counterbalanced in costs by growth in the number and age of the population and by continued advances in technology.

Despite these rising costs, an estimated 31 million Americans, or about 13 percent of the population, do not have health care insurance of any kind, even though nearly half are in households in which someone is employed. This lack of insurance coverage and access to health care is often blamed for the fact that the United States, despite its high expenditures on health care, ranks about twentieth in the world in infant mortality and is not in the top ten in life expectancy.

HEALTH INSURANCE   Traditional fee-for-service insurance reimburses the hospital and the physician for services rendered but frequently does not cover preventive care. Even when insurance provides coverage for a service, the patient may be responsible for an initial "deductible" and a copayment, which is usually a fixed percentage of the entire amount charged.

Patients who must pay such out-of-pocket charges for some of their medical care seek less care than those whose care is fully covered by insurance. In the working poor this may result in reduced utilization of services and in an increase in the prevalence of serious disease. When adults of all socioeconomic classes lose health insurance coverage, they may use fewer medical services; as a result, their health status tends to decline.

Most alternatives to traditional fee-for-service medical care require enrolled persons to prepay a fixed premium, which, except when a relatively small copayment is required, usually covers acute, chronic, and preventive medical services and sometimes covers medications and other health care needs. Prepaid plans have varying organizational and financial structures. Early on in their development, staff-model HMOs were among the most popular formats. In this model, groups of salaried physicians practiced physically together in one or a few central facilities to provide prepaid care. In recent years, independent practice associations (IPAs) have shown the most rapid growth. IPAs provide prepaid care to the patient by contracting with office-based practitioners who agree to see patients on a prenegotiated fee schedule. To balance the normal fee-for-service incentives and control utilization, IPAs employ various forms of administrative controls and review. The rate of hospitalization can be reduced among enrollees in HMOs, and HMOs have been among the leaders in attempts to reduce hospital costs and lengths of stay.

REIMBURSEMENT OF HOSPITALS AND PHYSICIANS In 1983, Medicare introduced a system of prospective reimbursement using diagnosis-related groups (DRGs), whereby hospitals were paid a predetermined sum based on the patient's principal diagnosis, procedures, complications, and comorbidities regardless of the costs or charges that were actually generated by the hospital stay (Table 9-1). This reimbursement system was designed to reward hospitals for being more efficient, and hospitals could actually be paid more than their costs. In the first few years after the introduction of the DRG system, many hospitals, especially the large teaching hospitals, reported substantial operating surpluses. In response, Medicare kept the rate of annual increase in reimbursement below the rate of increase in hospital costs, and the extra payments for teaching hospitals were reduced. While the prospective reimbursement system has undoubtedly stimulated efficiency, it also has raised concerns about the practice of discharging patients prematurely or transferring them to other institutions if the projected cost of caring for them exceeds the expected reimbursement.

Since the introduction of federal prospective reimbursement, the number of inpatient hospital days has decreased. This reduction has been accompanied by a marked increase in ambulatory services, including a shift to the outpatient arena of services that previously were delivered only on an inpatient basis. This shift should lower the cost of delivering an individual unit of service, such as the cost of a

TABLE 9-1 Example of diagnosis-related groups (DRGs) for prospective payment by Medicare

DRG no.	Name	Approximate Medicare reimbursement for a large urban teaching hospital in 1992, $
89	Simple pneumonia and pleurisy with complications or comorbid conditions	5,000
121	Acute myocardial infarction with complications, discharged alive	6,800
148	Major small or large bowel procedure with complications or comorbid conditions	13,000
106	Coronary artery bypass surgery with catheterization on same admission	23,000

SOURCE: Prospective Payment Assessment Commission.

TABLE 9-2 Physician reimbursement: The relative value scale versus traditional fee for service

Average Medicare reimbursement	Method of calculating reimbursement	
	Traditional fee for service, $*	Relative value scale, $†
Office visit, limited service, established patient	23	22
Initial hospital consultation, comprehensive service	75	83
Repair of sliding inguinal hernia	524	335
Coronary artery bypass, three grafts	3700	2225

* Defined as an individual physician's customary fee for service, limited to a prevailing fee by third-party insurers.
† A service-specific reimbursement based on the resource inputs required to perform a service, including the physician's work involved and specialty differences in practice expenses and costs related to training. Reimbursements are also adjusted to account for local differences in the cost of practice.

breast biopsy, but the overall cost of medical care will rise if, for example, the breast biopsy is performed on an ambulatory basis *and* the inpatient resources that the breast biopsy patient would have used are now consumed by new services such as the treatment of a cancer patient with bone marrow transplantation.

Physician payment Methods of physician payment also have been revised. Physician reimbursement in the United States, whether by Medicare or by private insurers, traditionally was a direct payment based on the doctor's "usual and customary" fee. In recent years, the rate of annual increase in fees has been fixed by the payor so that relative payments really reflect fee patterns from a decade or more ago. Because of concerns that this traditional approach had led to inequities in reimbursement and especially to underreimbursement for nonprocedural tasks such as office visits, recent analyses have considered the resource inputs of physicians' services, including time, intensity, practice costs, and the investment in training, to propose a new and fairer approach to physician reimbursement. These analyses have been incorporated into a new Medicare reimbursement system for physicians using the *relative value scale* (Table 9-2), which is based on the concept that payment rates for medical services should, as with other economic "goods," reflect the costs of producing those services. This change suggests that procedural tasks were being reimbursed at rates exceeding those of nonprocedural tasks that require comparable time, skill, and experience. Medicare's new relative rates are similar to preexisting fee schedules in Canada.

Proponents of changes in the reimbursement system hope that more equitable pay for cognitive tasks will reduce the incentive to perform procedures and increase the incentive for physicians to spend more time with patients, including time for discussion of such issues as health screening, health promotion, and disease prevention. Opponents of a change in the physician reimbursement system argue, among other issues, that changes in the reimbursement system may limit access and fail to take into account the extent to which patients may value some services more than others. Although the consequences of this change in the reimbursement system will not be known for some time, the physician's diagnostic and therapeutic recommendations should be guided by the goal of promoting maximal well-being for the patient, tempered by an awareness of the relative cost that must be incurred to reap this benefit.

Control of health care costs Two different approaches have been suggested to control health care costs: regulation and competition. Regulations, such as per diem rate setting, attempt to control costs by setting and enforcing practice or reimbursement standards. Other regulatory means of attempting to reduce costs include mandatory second opinions prior to elective hospitalization or surgery, but such programs usually do not save more than the costs of administration of the programs themselves. It is vital that physicians work closely with third-party payors, government agencies and commissions, and regulatory bodies such as the Joint Commission on Accreditation of Health Care Organizations that have assumed increasing responsibilities for setting reimbursement rates and for determining performance standards and conditions for payment.

The competitive approach encourages hospitals and providers to bid in a free-market atmosphere, in which consumers will presumably make rational choices based on the perceived cost and quality of the available alternatives. Insurance plans that utilize deductibles and copayments reflect this approach. It also has been proposed that physicians who practice inexpensively should be rewarded financially, but if physicians are paid to perform fewer services, the quality of care may suffer.

The reimbursement system differs in different countries. In the United Kingdom, for example, the National Health Service insurance program covers hospital and physician reimbursement on a non-fee-for-service basis, although patients can pay privately for services outside the system. Patients often must endure long delays for nonemergency procedures. In Canada, hospitals are paid an annual lump sum, and most physicians are paid on a fee-for-service basis via a fee schedule that is negotiated between the medical societies and the provincial governments. Private insurance, by law, can cover only services such as long-term care and dental care that are not covered by public insurance. New technology has diffused less rapidly in Canada, and the rates at which many procedures are performed are lower, but may not be less optimal, than in the United States. In Canada, delays for elective services have not been a major problem, life expectancy is higher than in the United States, and the prestige and relative income of physicians is analogous to those in the United States.

COSTS AND COST-EFFECTIVENESS

The costs of medical care include direct costs, such as the salaries of health personnel, and indirect costs, such as utilities, maintenance, and mortgage payments. Some costs are fixed (i.e., they do not vary with the volume of services provided), and other costs are variable (i.e., they depend on volume). For example, consider a situation in which a new instrument to perform a blood chemistry test costs $1000 and will last for 1 year. Also assume that each individual chemical analysis has an incremental cost of $10 in reagents, personnel time, and other resource inputs. If the laboratory utilizes the instrument to analyze 100 specimens in a year, the average cost per specimen is $20 ($10 each in fixed and variable costs), but if it analyzes 10,000 specimens, the average cost per specimen is $10.10 ($0.10 in fixed costs and $10.00 in variable costs) because the fixed costs are spread over more specimens.

The charges for medical services do not necessarily correspond to the true costs of providing the services. This occurs in part because the costs are difficult to measure and in part because charges are usually fixed regardless of volume, while costs vary with volume. Most analyses of cost and cost-effectiveness in medicine are based on charges rather than on true costs.

The net costs for a health care program include the costs of providing the program, costs that are generated by adverse side effects of treatment, and costs for treating disease that would not have occurred if the patient had not lived longer as a result of the original treatment. From these costs, the savings in health care, rehabilitation, or custodial costs due to prevention or alleviation of disease are subtracted to determine the net cost. For example, consider a program to perform mammography in women over age 40. The program would have its own direct costs related to advertising, screening, mammography, physician visits, breast biopsy, etc. Some women would have false-positive mammograms and would receive unnecessary breast biopsies. Other women would live longer as a result of early diagnosis and treatment of breast cancer, but they might develop other illnesses, such as coronary disease, in the interim. If they developed conditions such as Alzheimer's disease, the custodial costs

might be substantial. However, these costs would be countered by savings from hospitalizations for advanced cancer and by a potential increase in productive wage-earning years.

In all analyses of costs, it is important to consider *when* the costs will be incurred and *when* the effects in health benefits may be realized. Present dollars or health benefits are considered to have greater worth than a promise of future dollars or health benefits for several reasons. Other events may intercede so that a projected future cost or benefit may never occur, and there is always the possibility that money spent now will not achieve the desired effect at some time in the future. Furthermore, another illness may intervene, or there might be better ways to spend the money in the future. The principle by which future dollars and benefits are less highly valued than known immediate costs and benefits is termed *discounting*. It is independent of monetary inflation. By this concept, it is preferable to spend $1000 today to prevent someone from dying today than it is to spend $1000 today in the expectation that someone will not die 10 years from now.

It is unusual for any program simultaneously to achieve the greatest possible benefit and have the lowest possible cost. Instead, one usually either determines the desired benefit and then finds the lowest cost needed to achieve it or determines the resources available and then finds the greatest possible benefit that can be achieved.

Analyses of cost-effectiveness commonly examine the ratio of cost to effectiveness, i.e., the number of dollars required to save a life or a year of life. Such analyses are relevant to medicine because interventions only rarely both save lives and reduce costs. Hence it is important to estimate the tradeoff of costs for gains in health. Two strategies with the same ratio may have quite different absolute costs and absolute benefits. For example, a program that saves 100 lives for $100,000 has the same cost-effectiveness ratio as one that saves 1000 lives for $1 million, but the absolute costs and absolute benefits vary tenfold. The choice between these two programs may depend on how much money is available to spend. In assessing any program, it is important to measure incremental costs and effects rather than average costs and effects. For example, consider two programs to reduce death from lung cancer. If, on average, program A costs $100 million to save 100,000 years of life (average of $1000 per year of life) and program B costs $200 million to save 100,100 years of life (about $2000 per year of life), the *incremental* cost of program B versus program A is $1 million per year of life saved.

SOCIETAL ISSUES IN COSTS It is rare to find a medical intervention, such as measles vaccination programs, that both saves lives and reduces overall costs because the savings from disease prevention more than outweigh the expenses of the treatment itself. More commonly, medical practices that are truly of benefit also cause an associated increase in medical care costs. Among the more cost-effective examples is coronary artery bypass surgery in patients with left main coronary artery disease, which costs under $10,000 per year of life saved.

The shift of services from the inpatient to the outpatient setting or from the hospital to the home generally reduces the expense of delivery of that aspect of medical care. For example, home dialysis is less expensive than dialysis in an outpatient center, which in turn is less expensive than dialysis in a hospital. Similarly, the administration of parenteral nutrition and intravenous antibiotics at home and the home care for patients with AIDS have greatly reduced the need for hospitalization for conditions in which skilled nursing care is otherwise not required. However, a by-product of this strategy is an increased percentage of severely ill hospital inpatients who require more intensive and expensive care than the less sick patients who otherwise might have occupied hospital beds.

To date, society has been reluctant to make ethical decisions regarding the amount of cost appropriate for any particular net benefit. Neither medicine nor society is accustomed to placing a dollar value on a life or a year of life. In many analyses, however, the projected annual costs of approximately $35,000 to $45,000 (in 1995 dollars) for renal dialysis for 1 year of useful life have been used as a benchmark of how much the United States is willing to spend to save a year of life, because such a program is supported with tax dollars and presumably is a reasonable reflection of national priorities.

The physician has a unique responsibility. On the one hand, the physician must serve as an advocate for the individual patient and recommend the course of action most likely to be beneficial to the patient. The overriding nature of the patient-physician relationship is the cornerstone of humane medical care. On the other hand, physicians must understand the costs as well as the benefits of medical interventions so that they can choose from among the wide range of options. The physician must serve as the advocate for providing the best options to the individual patient and should know which options are of little or no value or are more likely to do harm than good. The physician must, with the assistance and consent of the patient and the family, set priorities for the patient's management within any limits or restrictions imposed by society; such limits may be expressed, for example, in a finite number of dollars available for the treatment of a specific illness. In addition, physicians have a broad role in determining health costs. Individually and through various professional organizations, physicians have a responsibility to help set national priorities, based on their appreciation of the finite resources available for health care and their knowledge of the relative benefits and costs of various diagnostic and therapeutic options in particular types of patients. Inappropriate attempts to reduce costs, such as limiting Medicaid payments for effective medications, are counterproductive in that they worsen health and ultimately lead to increased overall costs.

HEALTH SCREENING *Screening* refers to the performance of a medical evaluation and/or diagnostic tests in asymptomatic persons in the hope that early diagnosis may lead to improved outcome. For such persons, it was initially assumed that a periodic health examination, often accompanied by multiphasic diagnostic testing, is beneficial. However, there is no definitive information regarding the value of such an approach and even less information regarding which aspects yield results that are worth the costs incurred. In fact, there is no universally accepted approach to screening in the asymptomatic adult, given the uncertainties about the benefits and cost-effectiveness of each intervention. Nevertheless, the recommendations in Table 9-3 represent a reasonable set of guidelines for the periodic health assessment of asymptomatic adults.

Another issue in screening concerns the choice of which routine tests to perform in a patient who is about to undergo an operation or who is admitted to the hospital. For example, routine preoperative chest radiography is not indicated in persons without signs, symptoms, or risk factors for pulmonary or cardiac disease. Routine preoperative electrocardiography is generally recommended in any person with cardiac signs or symptoms and in men over age 40 and women over age 50 because of the age-related increase in asymptomatic cardiac disease and the likelihood that the preoperative tracing may be helpful for comparison should any cardiac problems arise during the perioperative period. In these situations, appropriate tests must be performed to investigate specific symptoms and signs. In terms of screening tests for asymptomatic conditions, those tests and procedures which have not been performed under the guidelines in Table 9-3 normally should be performed while the patient is under medical care.

HEALTH PROMOTION AND DISEASE PREVENTION Health promotion and disease prevention require investment of time, energy, and resources in the hope that the yield in terms of improved health warrants this investment. Unfortunately, there is limited information on the effectiveness of health promotion and disease prevention efforts. Interventions that result in a specified *relative* reduction in adverse outcomes have a greater *absolute* effect in higher-risk populations. For example, the same relative reduction in serum cholesterol will be of greater absolute benefit in persons with higher serum cholesterol levels or other unfavorable risk factors. In general, interventions to alter risk factors have a diminishing effect as risk factors decrease in severity.

Both patients and society commonly expect physicians to play a leadership role in health promotion and disease prevention. Patients

expect and desire their physicians to make recommendations regarding physical activity, diet, and other lifestyle issues, and physicians often fail in this regard. If physicians do not become involved, patients seek advice elsewhere, risking the possibility that fads or other erroneous sources may influence their choices.

When physicians become actively involved in health promotion, patients respond frequently and make appropriate behavior changes. For example, a physician's encouragement to increase physical activity, especially if combined with explicit suggestions, is likely to lead to changes in behavior so that the time spent by the physician appears to be cost-effective. Advice by a physician that a patient

---

TABLE 9-3 Guidelines for preventive medical services*

	Age of person	
19–39 years	40–64 years	65+ years

HISTORY

Every 1 to 3 years[†]: diet; physical activity; tobacco, alcohol, drugs; sexual practices	Same as 19–39 years	Every year: same as 19–39 years; and also functional status and symptoms of transient ischemia attacks

PHYSICAL EXAMINATION

Every 1 to 3 years: height, weight, blood pressure	Every 1 to 3 years: height, weight, blood pressure, breast	Every year: as for 40–64 years and also hearing and visual acuity
High risk: oral cavity, thyroid, breast, testes, skin	High risk: oral cavity, thyroid, skin, carotids	High risk: as for 40–64 years (but every year)

LABORATORY

Pap smear (every 1–3 years), total cholesterol	Pap smear (every 1–3 years), mammogram (every 1–2 years after age 50), total cholesterol	Mammogram (every 1–2 years until age 75), thyroid indices (women), dipstick urinalysis, total cholesterol
High risk: fasting glucose, rubella antibodies, VDRL, urinalysis, *Chlamydia* testing, gonorrhea culture, HIV testing, hearing, PPD, ECG, mammogram, colonoscopy	High risk: fasting glucose, VDRL, urinalysis, *Chlamydia* testing, gonorrhea culture, HIV testing, hearing, PPD, ECG, fecal occult blood/sigmoidoscopy/colonoscopy, bone mineral content	High risk: fasting glucose, PPD, ECG, Pap smear (every 1–3 years), fecal occult blood/sigmoidoscopy/colonoscopy

SPECIAL COUNSELING

Injury prevention, dental health	Injury prevention, dental health, skin protection from ultraviolet light, discussion of aspirin therapy in men and estrogen replacement in women	As for 40–64 years and also glaucoma testing
High risk: hemoglobin testing, skin protection from ultraviolet light		

IMMUNIZATIONS

Tetanus-diphtheria booster every 10 years	As for 19–39 years except not measles-mumps-rubella	Tetanus-diphtheria booster (every 10 years) influenza (every year), pneumococcal
High risk: hepatitis B, pneumococcal, influenza (every year), measles-mumps-rubella		High risk: hepatitis B

* Except for the visit itself, the frequency is at clinical discretion unless otherwise specified.
† With counseling for any high-risk behaviors.
SOURCE: Adapted from U.S. Preventive Services Task Force (*Guide to Clinical Preventive Services.* Baltimore, Williams & Wilkins, 1989), whose official report lists full details, including the definition of high-risk situations.

should lose weight or discontinue smoking is successful in only a small minority of cases, but it is an excellent first step toward health promotion and disease prevention (Chap. 393).

Physician-directed dietary interventions commonly lower the serum cholesterol level by as much as 10 percent. Drug treatment may be more effective but is more expensive. For example, treatment with lovastatin in men for the primary prevention of coronary heart disease costs more than $50,000 per year of life saved except in very high risk persons. Treatment strategies for hypertension are more cost-effective; the approximate cost of screening and treating hypertension, given the average medication compliance rates and treatment with a generic beta-adrenergic antagonist, ranges from a projection of about $15,000 per year of life saved for a patient with a diastolic blood pressure of 105 mmHg or higher to about $25,000 to $30,000 for a person with a diastolic blood pressure of 95 to 104 mmHg. Costs would be higher with more expensive medications, although the cost could be warranted if a reduction in side effects led to an improvement in an individual's quality of life.

Immunizations, including pneumococcal and influenza vaccination in elderly and high-risk patients, are effective ways to reduce disease and its associated costs. Guidelines for immunizations in adults are indicated in Table 9-3 (see also Chap. 82).

DIAGNOSTIC TESTING   As detailed in Chap. 10, diagnostic tests are valuable only to the extent that they provide new, *incremental* information that cannot be obtained less expensively from the history, physical examination, or other less expensive tests. Although these tests may often be of psychological benefit in reassuring the patient or the physician, they commonly generate redundant information, often result in a needless expense, and may entail risk. For example, in the evaluation of left ventricular function, the physician must decide whether a two-dimensional echocardiogram is sufficient or the more precise but more expensive measurement by radionuclide ventriculography is worthwhile. The physician faces analogous choices when deciding whether to obtain both an abdominal ultrasound examination and an abdominal CT or, in a different case, whether CT and MRI of the head are both required.

Ideally, each test should be ordered in sequence only to the extent that it is expected to add to the data available. However, this iterative approach can be expensive in hospitalized patients, where the sequencing of tests may lead to delays in scheduling and performing them. In these situations, the expense of the additional days of waiting may more than offset the savings from possibly avoiding a particular test. Usually, careful consideration of the problem by a physician is one of the most cost-effective ways to evaluate the patient. Expert consultation may be more cost-effective and helpful than ordering more diagnostic tests. Although interventions designed to reduce test utilization have met with variable success, those which have been successful have generally included educational components, full endorsement by locally respected leaders, and frequent reinforcement.

TREATMENT CHOICES   In choosing among various treatments, physicians try to enhance the likelihood of an optimal outcome. It is important to consider whether an equivalent outcome could be achieved at a lower cost. For example, generic medications may be substituted for more expensive brand-name counterparts. Similarly, outcome is not usually compromised by interventions designed to encourage the use of less expensive antibiotic regimens. Endorsement by the medical profession of restricted indications for procedures such as pacemaker implantation and tonsillectomy have led to decreased utilization without any detectable reduction in life expectancy or quality of life. Whenever possible, diagnostic and therapeutic options should be subjected to strict evaluation of both benefit and cost-effectiveness, and physicians have responsibility to assist in such evaluations and to learn from their results.

INDIVIDUALIZATION

As already stated, the physician has a moral and legal responsibility to serve as an advocate for the patient, within the limits set by society. This requires an individual approach to the patient and an understanding of how the available resources of the health care system can best be applied to the person and the problem at hand. Nevertheless, the physician and the patient must recognize that expensive medicine is not necessarily better medicine, and physicians should not be induced by financial incentives to order tests that are not necessary.

Special consideration revolves around the use of expensive procedures in medical care, such as liver, heart, and bone marrow transplantation. In these situations, the limited availability of donors makes it necessary to choose the best possible recipients from among a wide range of potential candidates and to "ration." Although rationing is not pleasant, physicians have often responded well in situations with limited resources. For example, when faced with a reduction in intensive care unit availability, physicians are usually successful at maintaining normal admission rates for patients who most require intensive care so that little, if any, adverse effects occur in those excluded from intensive care.

There is marked variability in the rates at which various procedures are performed in different geographic areas, even though there are no obvious differences in the types or ages of patients. To date, little difference in health care outcomes can be detected despite wide differences in the rates of various procedures. These variations may in part be related to patients' preferences and in part to differing beliefs among physicians regarding optimal medical care choices. When the records of patients who have undergone such procedures are reviewed to determine how the indications for their procedure compared with the standards recommended by experts, a substantial proportion of procedures are deemed inappropriate. However, so far there is no close correlation between the percentage of cases deemed inappropriate and the rate at which the procedure is performed in a given location. There is no definitive evidence that high rates of performance can be equated with a high rate of unnecessary use.

The variations in rates of utilization, the proportion of cases in which some procedures seem not to be necessary, and the ability of physicians to respond to situations in which rationing is necessary suggest that in many situations the quality of medical care and the likelihood of a favorable outcome can be maintained while lowering costs. Society, with the input of physicians, must exercise this role without compromising the physician's responsibility to the individual patient and without restricting access on the basis of sex, socioeconomic status, or ethnic background.

REFERENCES

DETSKY AS, NAGLIE IG: A clinician's guide to cost-effectiveness analysis. Ann Intern Med 113:147, 1990

ENTHOVEN A, KRONICK R: A consumer-choice health plan for the 1990s: Universal health insurance in a system designed to promote quality and economy. N Engl J Med 320:29, 1989

FUCHS VR, HAHN JS: How does Canada do it? A comparison of expenditures for physicians' services in the United States and Canada. N Engl J Med 323:884, 1990

GOLDBERGER AL, O'KONSKI MS: Utility of the routine electrocardiogram before surgery and on general hospital admission: Critical review and new guidelines, in *Common Diagnostic Tests: Use and Interpretation*, 2d ed, HC Sox Jr (ed). Chicago, American College of Physicians, 1990, pp. 67–78

GOLDMAN L: Cost-effective strategies in cardiology, in *Heart Disease*, 4th ed, E Braunwald (ed). Philadelphia, Saunders, 1992, pp 1694–1707

HAYWARD RSA et al: Preventive care guidelines: 1991. Ann Intern Med 114:758, 1991

HEMENWAY D et al: Physicians' responses to financial incentives: Evidence from a for-profit ambulatory care center. N Engl J Med 322:1059, 1990

HSIAO WC et al: Assessing the implementation of physician-payment reform. N Engl J Med 328:928, 1993

—— et al: Special report: Results and policy implications of the resource-based relative-value study. N Engl J Med 319:881, 1988

IGLEHART JK: The American health care system. N Engl J Med 326:962, 1992

LEVY JM et al: Impact of the Medicare fee schedule on payments to physicians. JAMA 264:717, 1990

REDELMEIER DA, FUCHS VR: Health expenditures in the United States and Canada. N Engl J Med 328:772, 1993

SCHWARTZ WB, MENDELSON DN: Hospital cost containment in the 1980s: Hard lessons learned and prospects for the 1990s. N Engl J Med 324:1037, 1991

WOOLHANDLER S, HIMMELSTEIN DU: The deteriorating administrative efficiency of the U.S health care system. N Engl J Med 324:1253, 1991

10 QUANTITATIVE ASPECTS OF CLINICAL REASONING

LEE GOLDMAN

The process of clinical reasoning is poorly understood but is based on factors such as experience and learning, inductive and deductive reasoning, interpretation of evidence that itself varies in reproducibility and validity, and intuition that often is difficult to define. In an effort to improve clinical reasoning, a number of attempts have been made to analyze quantitatively the many factors involved, including defining the cognitive approaches that clinicians apply to difficult problems, devising computerized decision support systems that are designed to emulate certain features of decision making, and applying decision theory to understand how judgments should be reached. While each of these approaches has advanced the understanding of the diagnostic process, all have practical and/or theoretical problems that limit their direct applicability to the care of the individual patient.

Nevertheless, these preliminary attempts to apply the rigor and logic inherent in the quantitative method have provided significant insights into the process by which clinical reasoning is accomplished, have identified ways in which the process may be improved, and have made it possible to minimize certain features of the workup that are not cost-effective. Thus, while clinical reasoning cannot be reduced to probabilities or numbers, attempts at quantitative analysis of the process may improve the ways in which the problems of individual patients are approached and solved.

In a simplified model, quantitative clinical reasoning includes five phases. The *first* consists of an investigation of the chief complaint through key questions that are included in the history of the present illness (Table 10-1). These questions are supplemented by the past medical history and by a physical examination that emphasizes detailed investigation of potential key organ systems. In the *second* phase, the physician may select from an array of diagnostic tests, each with its own accuracy and usefulness for investigating the possibilities raised in the differential diagnosis. Since each test has its costs, and some entail risk and discomfort as well, the physician must ask whether the history and physical examination are sufficiently diagnostic before ordering tests. *Third*, the clinical data must be integrated with test results to estimate the likelihood of conditions in the differential diagnosis. *Fourth*, the comparative risks and benefits of further diagnostic and therapeutic options must be weighed to reach a recommendation for the patient. In the *fifth* and final phase, this recommendation is presented to the patient, and after appropriate discussion of the options, a therapeutic plan is initiated. Each of the five steps in this simplified model of the clinical reasoning process can be analyzed individually.

HISTORY AND PHYSICAL EXAMINATION It originally had been assumed that physicians begin investigating a patient's chief complaint by obtaining a comprehensive history, which includes many, if not most, of the questions included in a full review of systems, and by performing an all-inclusive physical examination. However, experienced clinicians begin to form hypotheses based on the chief complaint

and on the responses to initial questioning, and they ask further questions in a sequence that allows them to evaluate the initial hypotheses and, if necessary, shorten or amend the list of possibilities. Only a limited number of diagnostic hypotheses can be entertained at any one time, and information is used to build a case for or against the most likely. In such a way, high-priority questions are selected from the almost limitless number that might be asked, and these specific questions are incorporated into the history of the present illness. Often, a key response, such as a history of melena, will be selected, a list of potential explanations for it will be formulated, and this list will then be trimmed, based on the response to more probing questions, so that a principal diagnosis can be selected and then tested. This process, termed *iterative hypothesis testing*, is an efficient approach to diagnosis and is preferable to attempts to gather every conceivable piece of information prior to formulating a differential diagnosis.

Advocacy of iterative hypothesis testing does not argue against the need for a systematic, thorough, and complete history of the present illness, past medical history, review of systems, family history, social history, and physical examination. For example, if a patient presents with abdominal pain, the physician should gather information regarding its location and quality as well as the factors that precipitate and/or relieve it. The physician then asks questions relating to the diagnoses that may be suspected based on the response to the initial questions. If the pain is suggestive of pancreatitis, the clinician would ask about alcohol intake, the use of thiazide diuretics or glucocorticosteroids, symptoms suggestive of concomitant gallbladder disease, a family history of pancreatitis, and questions aimed at uncovering the possibility of a posterior penetrating ulcer. Alternatively, if the discomfort seems more typical of reflux esophagitis, a different sequence of questions would be triggered. The use of iterative hypothesis testing encourages the physician to elicit detailed information in high-yield areas, without forgoing a systematic and thorough approach to the patient. Findings on the history and physical examination should influence each other. The history focuses the physical examination on certain organs, and findings on physical examination should encourage more detailed review of certain systems.

As physicians proceed through this reasoning process with both the history and physical examination, a variety of issues may influence the accuracy of the decision-making process. First is the potential for some historical information or physical findings to be poorly reproducible, either because the patient's responses vary or because different physicians elicit information differently or vary in the way they interpret the answers. The careful use of clear and, when possible, precise questions can increase the reproducibility and validity of the medical history but still cannot eliminate all variability.

When assessing the reproducibility of findings on the physical examination, two observers frequently agree that an uncommon abnormality such as an enlarged spleen is not present but agree less often when one of them thinks that it is present in a patient in whom it would not usually be expected. This principle can best be demonstrated by understanding that some agreement always occurs by chance, and the likelihood of chance agreement is higher if the finding is either very common or very uncommon. For example, if two physicians each consider 90 percent of patients to be abnormal in some manner, such as having a systolic heart murmur, they will agree 81 percent of the time by chance alone. In some studies of the reproducibility of common signs and symptoms, such as an enlarged liver, actual agreement rates have not been substantially better than chance. Disagreement rates may be reduced by emphasizing physical examination skills during medical training, by looking for other correlative physical findings, and by learning how physical findings correlate with the results of diagnostic tests. Therefore, when a clinician notes an unexpected and somewhat subjective abnormality for which there may be a high rate of interobserver disagreement, such as an unexpectedly enlarged spleen, other abnormalities that may often be associated with it, such as hepatomegaly or lymphadenopathy,

TABLE 10-1 Phases of clinical reasoning and decision making

1 Investigation of the complaint by means of clinical examination (history and physical examination)
2 Ordering of diagnostic tests, each with its own intrinsic accuracy and usefulness
3 Integration of clinical findings with test results to assess diagnostic probabilities
4 Weighing of comparative risks and benefits of alternative courses of action
5 Determination of patient's preferences and development of a therapeutic plan

should be sought to increase the likelihood that the spleen would be expected to be abnormal. In some situations, ordering a diagnostic test, such as an abdominal ultrasound, to assess the finding more objectively should be considered if the test is sufficiently reliable.

These comments about the factors that limit the reproducibility and validity of the medical history and physical examination do not denigrate their critical importance in clinical reasoning. Rather, they emphasize that care and diligence in the application of these skills are necessary. For example, careful auscultation of the heart during various bedside maneuvers (see Chap. 188) has been shown to be remarkably accurate in determining the cause of systolic murmurs.

When physicians use the history and the physical examination to arrive at a diagnosis, they are rarely certain of it. Therefore, it would be better to assess the likelihood of the diagnosis in terms of probabilities. All too frequently this probability is not expressed as an actual percentage but rather in such terms as "nearly always," "commonly," "sometimes," or "rarely." Since different physicians may assign different probabilities to the same terms, these imprecise words frequently lead to major misunderstandings among physicians or between the physician and the patient. Physicians should be as rigorous and quantitative as possible in their assessments, and when feasible, a quantitative expression of probability should be used. For example, rather than saying that it is unlikely that a radiographic pattern is indicative of a carcinoma of the colon, it would be preferable, if possible, to provide a more precise indication of the probability of carcinoma with this radiographic pattern. A 10 to 15 percent probability of carcinoma may be interpreted as "unlikely" but from a clinical perspective usually warrants further evaluation because of the serious consequences of missing a potentially resectable tumor.

Although such quantitative estimates would be desirable, they usually are not available in practice. Even experienced physicians often are unable to estimate accurately the likelihood of particular conditions. There is a tendency to overestimate the likelihood of relatively uncommon conditions, and physicians are especially poor at quantifying probabilities that are very high or very low. For example, a physician may not know whether the probability of bacterial meningitis or of another disease that could be diagnosed by a lumbar puncture in a patient with a severe headache is 1 in 20 or 1 in 2000. In both situations, the probability is low, but the decision as to whether a lumbar puncture should be performed may depend on this estimate.

As was emphasized in Chap. 1, the history and physical examination have other important purposes. They allow the physician to evaluate the emotional status of the patient and to understand how the present problems fit into the context of the patient's social and family life, and they encourage the development in the patient of confidence in the physician, which is so necessary for reaching an agreement on the coming plan of action.

DIAGNOSTIC TESTS: INDICATIONS, ACCURACY, AND USEFULNESS A diagnostic test should be ordered for specified clinical indications, be sufficiently accurate to be efficacious for such indications, and be the least expensive and/or risky of the available efficacious tests. No diagnostic test is totally accurate, and physicians often have difficulty interpreting test results. It is therefore critical to understand several commonly used terms in test analysis and epidemiology, including prevalence, sensitivity, specificity, positive predictive value, and negative predictive value (Table 10-2).

Although reports of the accuracies of diagnostic tests are commonly expressed in terms of positive and negative predictive values, these calculated values are dependent on the prevalence of the disease in the population being studied (Table 10-3). A test with a particular sensitivity and specificity has different positive and negative predictive values when used in groups of patients that have different prevalences of disease. For example, a mildly abnormal alkaline phosphatase level in a young adult with a known lymphoma suggests hepatic involvement by the tumor (i.e., it is likely to be a *true positive*), while the same alkaline phosphatase level as part of a routine screening

TABLE 10-2 Definitions of commonly used terms in epidemiology and decision making

Test result	Disease state		
	Present		Absent
Positive	a (true positive)		b (false positive)
Negative	c (false negative)		d (true negative)
Prevalence (prior probability)	= $(a + c)/(a + b + c + d)$		= all patients with the disease/all patients tested
Sensitivity	=	$a/(a + c)$	= true-positive test results/all patients with the disease
Specificity	=	$d/(b + d)$	= true-negative test results/all patients without the disease
False-negative rate	=	$c/(a + c)$	= false-negative test results/all patients with the disease
False-positive rate	=	$b/(b + d)$	= false-positive test results/all patients without the disease
Positive predictive value	=	$a/(a + b)$	= true-positive test results/all positive test results
Negative predictive value	=	$d/(c + d)$	= true-negative test results/all patients with negative results
Overall accuracy	= $(a + d)/(a + b + c + d)$		= true-positive + true-negative test results/all tests

battery of blood tests in an asymptomatic person of the same age is unlikely to be due to tumor (i.e., in this setting it is more likely to be a *false positive*).

Although the sensitivity and specificity of a test do not depend on the prevalence (or percentage of patients being tested who have the disease), they do depend on the spectrum of patients in whom the test is being evaluated. For example, measurement of a prostate-specific antigen for diagnosing carcinoma of the prostate (see Chap. 323) will appear to have a nearly perfect sensitivity and specificity if the diseased population has a palpable prostate nodule and an elevated serum acid phosphatase level while the nondiseased population is composed of normal medical students. If, however, without changing the prevalence of disease in the population being tested, the spectrum of the diseased and nondiseased patients is altered by including patients with other characteristics (i.e., if the population of patients with carcinoma of the prostate were composed principally of those without palpable nodules and with stage 1 disease, while the population without carcinoma of the prostate included elderly men with marked benign prostate hypertrophy), the sensitivity and specificity of the test would change dramatically. In the latter situation, the sensitivity and specificity of the prostate-specific antigen are not only lower than in the first example, because the spectrum of diseased and nondiseased patients has been changed, but more important, they may be so low that the test is of limited clinical value. This example also demonstrates the methodologic problems encountered when applying data from one study to a different type of patient or when pooling data from studies of different subsets of patients.

In some situations, uncertainty about the sensitivity and specificity of the test in the type of patient being assessed may limit its clinical value. Since the physician rarely knows (or can know) the population on which every test that is ordered has been standardized, the results provide information that is far less decisive than usually thought. Furthermore, it may be quite difficult to distinguish random laboratory errors from test results that might be falsely positive or negative because of coexistence of a process that can affect the test, such as the finding of an elevated level of CK in a patient who has undergone strenuous exercise and is being evaluated for chest pain.

Because no single value or cutoff point of an individual test can be expected to have both a perfect sensitivity and a perfect specificity,

TABLE 10-3   How the positive and negative predictive values of the same test vary depending on the prior probability of disease

INTERPRETATION OF TEST RESULT WHEN 10% OF PATIENTS TESTED HAVE THE DISEASE (PRIOR PROBABILITY = 10%)

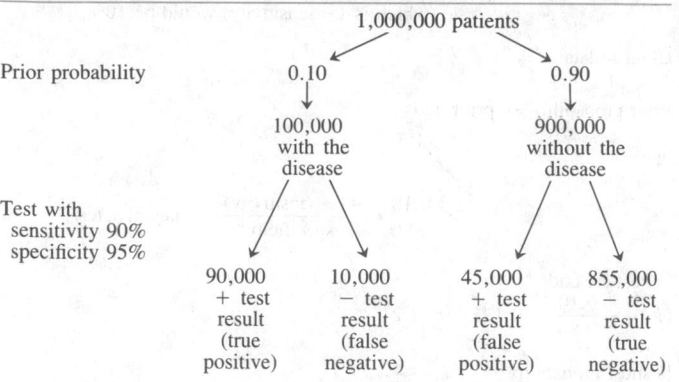

The probability of disease in a patient with a positive test result (positive predictive value) = 90,000/135,000 = 67%

The probability of no disease in a patient with a negative test result (negative predictive value) = 855,000/865,000 = 99%

INTERPRETATION OF TEST RESULT WHEN 50% OF PATIENTS TESTED HAVE THE DISEASE (PRIOR PROBABILITY = 50%)

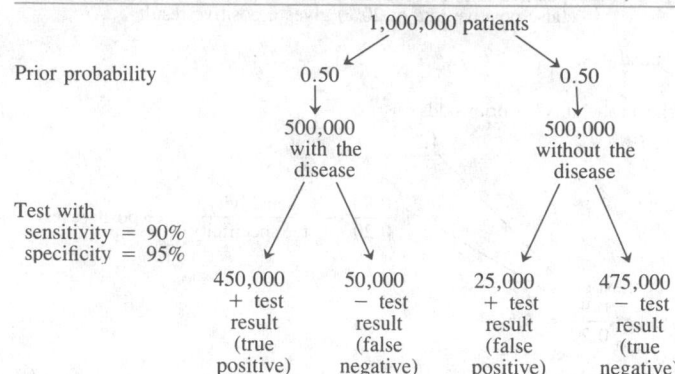

The probability of disease in a patient with a positive test result (positive predictive value) = 450,000/475,000 = 95%

The probability of no disease in a patient with a negative test result (negative predictive value) = 475,000/525,000 = 90%

it is often necessary to determine which value or cutoff point is the most appropriate to guide decision making. A graph (Fig. 10-1) of the test's *receiver operating characteristic curve*, which displays the inevitable trade-off between emphasizing a high sensitivity, such as defining an exercise electrocardiogram as abnormal if it shows ≥0.5 mm of ST-segment depression, versus emphasizing a high specificity, such as defining an exercise electrocardiogram as abnormal only if it shows ≥2.0 mm of ST-segment depression, can help the clinician understand the implications of various definitions of a "positive" test result. Such a graph demonstrates that different definitions of normal versus abnormal may be appropriate depending on whether one wishes to rule in the disease via a positive result on a test that has a high specificity or to exclude the disease via a negative result on a test that has a high sensitivity. Different tests may have different sensitivities and specificities, and better tests may have both a higher sensitivity and a higher specificity than poorer tests.

FIGURE 10-1 The inherent trade-off between sensitivity and specificity. For any diagnostic test, an increase in sensitivity will be associated with a decline in specificity. The closer this curve comes to the upper-left-hand corner, the more useful the test; the closer to the broken line, the less useful it is. When deciding on the cutoff between normal versus abnormal, one must determine what sensitivity and specificity are most useful clinically.

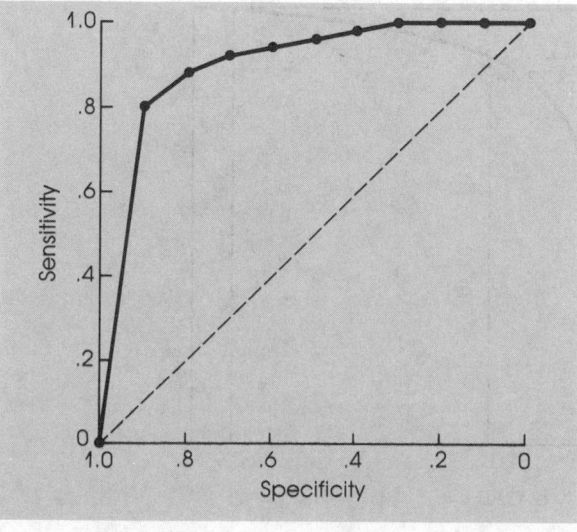

One example of a sensitive test is an enzyme-linked immunosorbent assay (ELISA) to test for the presence of antibodies to human immunodeficiency virus type 1 (HIV-1). This relatively inexpensive test has a high sensitivity for detecting HIV-1 antibodies but is not sufficiently specific to be used as the basis for making a firm diagnosis. Thus, if the ELISA assay is positive, it is commonly repeated. Confirmation of the diagnosis of HIV-1 antibody positivity requires a western blot, or an equivalently specific test, to exclude the possibility of a false-positive ELISA assay (see Chap. 279). A common example of a reasonably specific test would be an electrocardiogram to diagnose acute myocardial infarction. While the precise specificity depends on the spectrum of patients being tested, the presence of new ST-segment elevations exceeding 1.0 mm in two or more electrically contiguous leads in patients who present to an emergency department with prolonged acute chest pain consistent with myocardial ischemia is sufficiently specific, i.e., sufficiently unlikely to be a false-positive result, that admission to an intensive care unit is virtually always recommended. However, this test is not sensitive, and if admission to the unit were restricted to patients with this electrocardiographic finding, almost half of patients with myocardial infarctions presenting to hospital emergency departments would be missed.

To optimize the clinical value of a diagnostic test, it is helpful to obtain local experience with it; often its value will differ from that reported in the literature. Reports of the efficacy of a test should emphasize its accuracy when compared with an independent standard, and the test must be evaluated in a spectrum of patients with varying severities of the disease in question and in patients who have conditions that are part of the same differential diagnosis. The reproducibility of the test should be known, and the "normal limits" of the test should be clear and appropriate. In some instances, the test or procedure required to establish the validity of a diagnostic test is so risky that only a skewed sample of patients is included in a study, as, for example, in the analysis of the usefulness of the abdominal CT scan in patients with suspected pancreatic carcinoma. If patients with "negative" CT scan results never come to laparotomy or postmortem examination, neither the sensitivity nor specificity of the CT scan for pancreatic carcinoma can be assessed. In such situations, an estimated value of the diagnostic test may be inaccurate because it has not been validated.

INTEGRATION OF CLINICAL DATA AND TEST RESULTS   Although, as we have seen, neither clinical data nor test results may be entirely accurate, the integration of the two can lead to better diagnostic predictions than either alone. By knowing the probability

TABLE 10-4   Example of the use of Bayesian analysis to integrate the pretest probability with the test result to calculate a posttest probability

Example 1: Prior probability of disease = 25%; a test with a sensitivity (true-positive rate) of 90% and a specificity of 80% (which implies a false-positive rate of 20%) gives a positive result

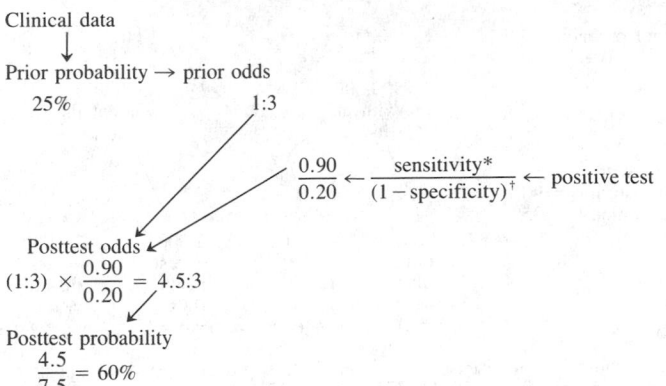

Example 2: Same pretest probability and test, but now the test gives a negative result. Here the true-negative rate would be 80% and the false-negative rate (which is 1 − sensitivity) would be 10%.

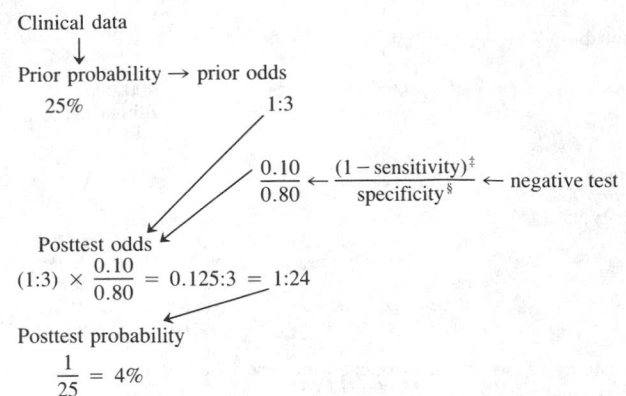

* Sensitivity = probability of a positive test result in a patient with the disease
† (1 − specificity) = probability of a positive test result in a patient without the disease

‡ (1 − sensitivity) = probability of a negative test result in a patient with the disease.
§ Specificity = probability of a negative test result in a patient without the disease.

that the patient has a particular condition before a test is performed (the prior, or pretest, probability), and by knowing the sensitivity and the specificity of the test, the posttest probability can be calculated. A common mathematical technique for integrating clinical data and a test result is the odds-likelihood form of Bayesian analysis (Table 10-4). A pretest probability can be expressed as odds (as in a horse race, for example) and multiplied by the likelihood ratio (which is the sensitivity of the test divided by 1 minus the specificity of the test) to yield the posttest odds, which may be transformed back into a posttest probability. This approach can be employed in any situation in which the physician can use clinical findings to estimate a pretest diagnostic probability and integrate this with the result as well as the sensitivity and specificity of the diagnostic test. Many clinical situations may be so complex that it is not practical to estimate the

prior probabilities of all likely diagnoses or to know the sensitivities and specificities of each of the tests that might be performed individually or in sequence. Nevertheless, attempts in this direction will stimulate critical thinking, expose uncertainties, and generate ideas for original investigations or a review of past experiences to facilitate the application of Bayesian analysis to the integration of clinical data and laboratory tests.

The results of Bayesian analyses often can be expressed in graphic form, such as the value of exercise electrocardiograms for predicting the presence of coronary artery disease (Fig. 10-2; also see Chap. 203). This series of curves also demonstrates how to consider a test whose result may be in the "gray zone" rather than clearly positive or clearly negative.

One of the key assumptions inherent in most such analyses is that

FIGURE 10-2   How the exercise tolerance test affects the probability of coronary artery disease. The before-test probability of coronary artery disease (CAD) will be modified by the result of the exercise electrocardiogram to yield an after-test probability of CAD. Note that the finding of <1 mm of ST-segment depression will reduce the probability of CAD, whereas ≥1 mm of ST-segment depression will increase the probability. For example, if a patient with a before-test probability of CAD of 90 percent (about that of a middle-aged man with typical anginal symptoms) had 2 to 2.49 mm on ST-segment depression on exercise testing, the after-test probability of CAD would be

99.5 percent. In contrast, the same exercise test result in a patient with 30 percent before-test probability of CAD (about that of a patient with atypical anginal symptoms) would yield an after-test probability of about 90 percent. In an asymptomatic patient, with a before-test probability of about 5 percent, the same exercise test result would yield an after-test probability of 53 percent. Thus the same test yields different after-test probabilities in patients with different before-test probabilities. *(Adapted, with permission of the New England Journal of Medicine, from RD Rifkin, WB Hood, Bayesian analysis of electrocardiographic exercise stress testing. N Engl J Med 297:684, 1977.)*

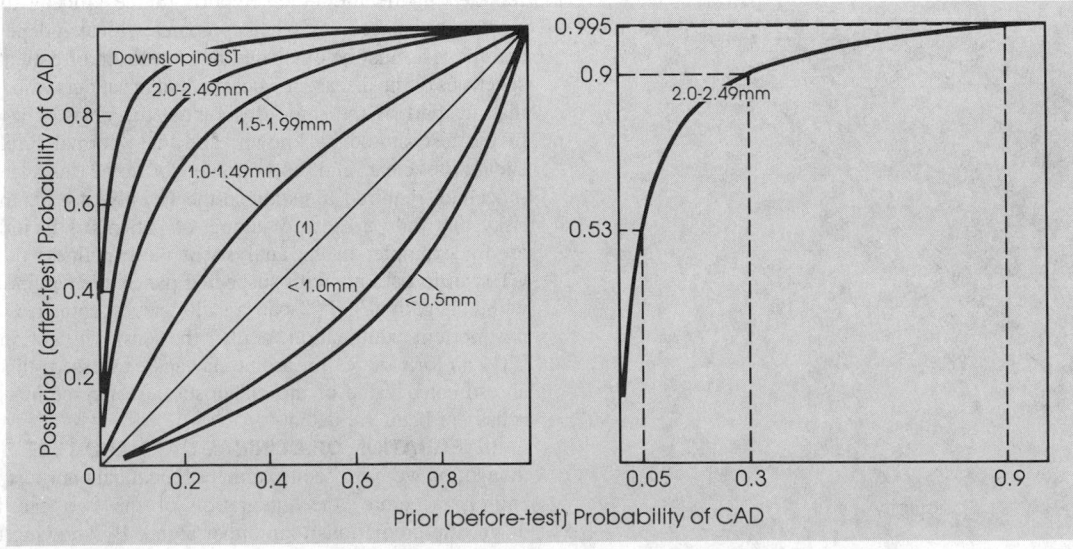

the correlation between the pretest probability and the test result is no greater than expected by chance. If the diagnostic test simply duplicates information that has already been obtained by the clinical examination, it will not have any additional benefit for predicting whether or not the disease is present. For example, in trying to determine whether or not a patient with carcinoma of the colon has hepatic metastases, the finding of jaundice on physical examination should be a strong predictor. The degree of hyperbilirubinemia also can be measured, but the bilirubin level in a patient with clinical jaundice does not add substantial *independent* information to that obtained by a careful physical examination. When integrating a diagnostic test with clinical information, the test is helpful only when it adds incremental information to what can be inferred based on the history and physical examination and on prior, less costly or less risky diagnostic tests. If a diagnostic test (such as a retrograde cholangiogram in a patient with hyperbilirubinemia) provides information that cannot be inferred directly, it is less likely that its results are associated with pretest probabilities to an extent greater than would be expected by chance.

A diagnostic test has an impact on the evaluation of a specific patient only if it changes the diagnostic probability to the extent that the new probability dictates a change in the diagnostic strategy or therapeutic plans or if the test serves as part of a sequence of tests that moves the probability across such a threshold. An example is a patient suspected of having a pulmonary embolism, with an estimated probability of 50 percent based on clinical data alone. Performing a "low probability" pulmonary ventilation-perfusion scan may reduce the probability of pulmonary embolism, but if the goal is to exclude pulmonary embolism with the highest possible degree of certainty, a pulmonary angiogram would be required (Chap. 226).

Because diagnostic tests often do not provide important new information even when their results are accurate, several questions should be considered in deciding when to order diagnostic tests. First, how likely is the disease in question? Second, what would be the clinical consequences if the diagnosis were missed or if the patient were mistakenly treated for a disease that is not present? Third, what is the likelihood that the diagnostic test will change the probability sufficiently to have an effect on either diagnosis or therapy? The physician should consider the probabilities, the risks, the likelihood and costs of obtaining new information, and the adverse consequences of delay, because observation and follow-up are always among the available diagnostic options.

Since the establishment of valid diagnostic probabilities is a cornerstone to clinical reasoning, accumulated clinical experience, often in the form of computerized data banks, has been used to generate statistical approaches for improving diagnostic predictions. In such research, it is common to begin by identifying individual factors that have a univariate correlation with the diagnosis in question. Then these univariate correlates may be included in a multivariate analysis to determine which of them are significant independent predictors of the diagnosis. Some analyses may identify the important predictive factors and then assign them "weights," which can be transformed to calculate a probability. Alternatively, the analysis may result in a limited number of categories of patients, each with a discrete probability of the diagnosis.

These quantitative approaches to the estimation of various diagnostic probabilities, which are often termed "prediction rules," are especially helpful if they are in a format that is readily usable by the clinician and if they have been validated prospectively on a sufficient number and spectrum of patients. For example, by carefully defining the key historical questions, findings on physical examination, and electrocardiographic abnormalities that might predict the probability of acute myocardial infarction among emergency department patients with chest pain, a protocol was devised and shown in prospective validation testing to have the same sensitivity as physicians for identifying infarction and at the same time to have a significantly higher specificity.

For such prediction rules to be useful to the clinician, they must be derived from relevant patient populations and use tests that are reproducible and readily available so that the results can be extrapolated to local medical practice. Since only a minority of published prediction rules have adhered to rigid criteria as to the number and spectrum of patients examined and their prospective validation, most are not yet suitable for routine clinical application. Furthermore, many prediction rules cannot evaluate the probability of each of the diagnoses or outcomes that the clinician must consider.

COMPARING RISKS AND BENEFITS: DECISION ANALYSIS

Inherent in the concept that probabilities can guide decision making is the assumption that one can arrive at a reasonable threshold by knowing the relative risks (or costs) and benefits of various options and deciding at what probability this ratio changes to favor an alternative strategy. Decision analysis is an organized process for evaluating such situations and identifies the key issues and problems.

One problem with applying decision-analysis techniques to difficult clinical problems is that the decision analysis is no better than the data on which it is based. In some instances, an attempted decision analysis of a complex clinical problem may yield no more information than that the critical data required for the analysis are missing and that more research in the field needs to be performed. In addition, when clinicians are uncertain about diagnostic or therapeutic strategies, formal analyses may indicate that the differences in outcome among various strategies are very small. In such cases, the formal analysis may have such inherent error that it is not definitive. Even when decision analysis is potentially helpful, it may not be feasible to complete the detailed estimations and calculations within the time constraints of bedside decision making. Nevertheless, the value of the analytic approach to decision making is that it integrates available data, mandates rigorous thinking, and exposes areas of uncertainty or ignorance.

Decision analysis depicts graphically two types of issues in the decision-making process: first, the decisions (or choices) available to the physician and, second, the probabilities of all the events that may result from each decision. To illustrate how this process works, consider a very simplified decision analysis of whether to use an intravenous thrombolytic agent in a patient with a suspected acute myocardial infarction (see Chap. 202). Figure 10-3 depicts the simplified decision tree for this problem. The square box or "node" labeled *A* indicates a decision that the physician must make. The circular nodes, labeled *B* through *O*, indicate where different outcomes, each of which has an estimatable probability, could occur. In this analysis, the initial choices were to treat the patient with an intravenous thrombolytic agent or not to treat. The use of such an agent may or may not result in serious complications of therapy, especially bleeding and intracranial hemorrhage.

Each of the possible outcomes for a patient is typically assigned a "utility," which is the relative preference for the outcome, where 1.0 is a perfect outcome and 0 is the worst possible outcome. Each terminal branch of the decision tree is assigned the utility corresponding to its outcome, and the "expected value" of each terminal branch is calculated by multiplying its probability by its utility. To calculate the "expected value" of each of the two possible courses of action (see Fig. 10-3, node *A*), the expected values of each of the terminal branches that originate from it would be summed. The preferred course of action is the one which, when all possible outcomes are considered, including the risks and benefits of therapy, yields the highest expected value, which is the sum of the product of the probability multiplied by the utility for each of its possible outcomes.

In performing any decision analysis, the relevant probabilities must be known or estimated, a process that sometimes requires guesswork. Next, utilities could be assigned to each of these outcomes. A major practical limitation of decision analysis is the subjective judgment often required to estimate utilities. It is also difficult to adjust future years of life for their quality in any numerical fashion, e.g., in considering how treatment complications, such as an intracranial hemorrhage, or the advantages of treatment, such as congestive

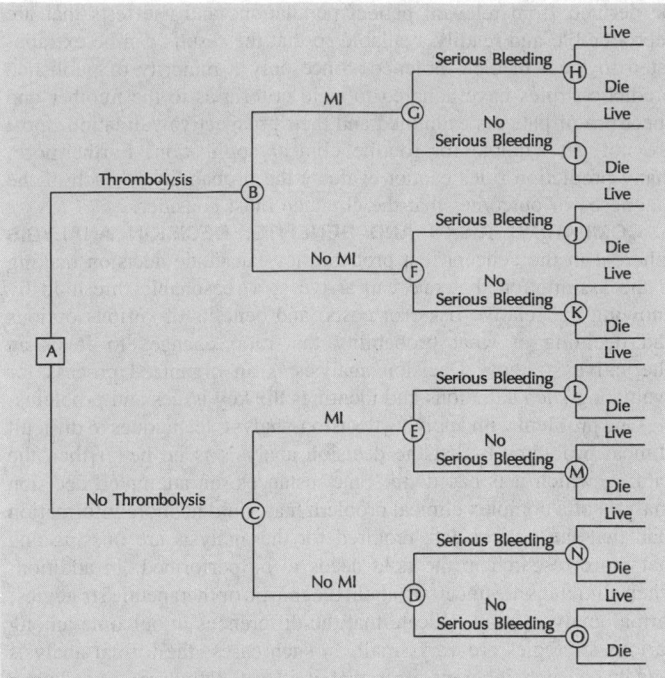

FIGURE 10-3 Simplified decision tree for the decision of whether or not to use an intravenous thrombolytic agent in a patient with a suspected acute myocardial infarction. The square node represents the decision point, and the round nodes denote chance events (see text for details).

heart failure averted because an infarction was smaller, affect the quality of future years of life.

The results and usefulness of a decision analysis depend on the probabilities and utilities that are used in the calculation, and it is imperative for decision analyses to include a *sensitivity analysis*, in which various estimates for each probability are included in the analysis to determine if the conclusions would be changed. For example, in the analysis in Fig. 10-3, some range of probabilities must be assumed for the risk of serious bleeding complications and for the likelihood that any particular patient is having an acute myocardial infarction. Because of the impressive benefit of thrombolysis for improving survival in patients with acute myocardial infarctions, decision analyses have shown treatment to be the preferred option even when an acute myocardial infarction is not certain and even in most elderly patients. If the conclusions of an analysis were altered by relatively minor changes in the assumptions on which it was based, the analysis would not be sufficiently reliable to become the basis for decision making.

Decision analysis sometimes demonstrates a clear and dramatic advantage with one particular option. In other circumstances, there may be little difference between two options; either option may be reasonable, or secondary issues that cannot be taken into account in the formal analysis, such as the patient's feelings about taking risks or the recent local experience with particular interventions, should be the final determinants in the decision. Physicians who perform a decision analysis therefore must determine the probabilities of each of the possible events by reviewing the pertinent patient experience at their own institution or practice or by reviewing the pertinent literature. Even when the outcome of the analysis seems clear, the physician or the patient may believe that the situation in question is

an exception to the rule. Furthermore, even the best analyses, like all clinical intuition, are based on assumptions that may be open to debate.

In the preceding example, dealing with whether or not to use a thrombolytic agent in a patient with a suspected acute myocardial infarction, decision analysis indicated the preferred strategy in terms of outcome but did not consider the costs at which such benefits might be achieved. In determining health policy, a formal cost-effectiveness analysis can be performed to determine how many dollars must be spent to achieve a unit of benefit, often defined as a life saved, a year of life saved, or a quality-adjusted year of life saved, in which the years are adjusted to take into account the quality of life during that time. For example, in 1994 dollars, 1 year of in-center hemodialysis can be estimated to cost about $35,000 to $45,000 per quality-adjusted year of life saved; this figure includes only the direct medical costs and not indirect costs related to issues such as time lost or travel or any benefits in terms of a patient's ability to work. In some situations, the ability of the patient to maintain gainful employment may offset some or all of the direct medical expenses. In other situations, such as with pneumococcal vaccine, the savings from episodes of pneumonia that are averted may more than offset the cost of the vaccine in high-risk persons.

ETHICS AND PATIENT INPUT　In both quantitative and nonquantitative clinical reasoning, the physician must consider ethical issues as well as the patient's values and preferences. While a detailed discussion of these issues is beyond the scope of this chapter, it is important to emphasize that patients' preferences for alternative therapies may not agree with the preferences that the physicians propose on the basis of their own clinical judgment or the results of a decision-analysis approach. For example, many patients with carcinoma of the larynx may prefer radiation therapy, with a lower cure rate but a higher likelihood of maintaining speech, to extirpative surgery. It is imperative that physicians assess those characteristics of life which the patient prizes most (the elusive "quality of life") prior to basing controversial decisions solely on quantitative approaches, the physicians' own subjective impressions of the likely medical benefits, their own personal preferences, or their assumptions about the patient's preferences. While quantitative analyses may apply to groups of patients, judgment must be exercised when adapting them to the individual patient. Therefore, the final plan should reflect an agreement between a well-informed patient and a sympathetic physician who has detailed knowledge of the relevant medical issues and of the impact of the various possible outcomes on the specific patient.

REFERENCES

AMERICAN COLLEGE OF PHYSICIANS: Guidelines for counseling postmenopausal women about preventive hormone therapy. Ann Intern Med 117:1038, 1993

GABLE CB et al: Pneumococcal vaccine: Efficacy and associated cost savings. JAMA 264:2910, 1990

GARNICK MB: Prostate cancer: Screening, diagnosis, and management, Ann Intern Med 118:804, 1993

GOLDMAN L et al: A computer protocol to predict myocardial infarction in emergency department patients with chest pain. N Engl J Med 318:797, 1988

KASSIRER JP: Diagnostic reasoning. Ann Intern Med 110:893, 1989

LEMBO NJ et al: Bedside diagnosis of systolic murmurs. N Engl J Med 318:1572, 1988

MANDEL JS et al: Reducing mortality from colorectal cancer by screening for fecal occult blood. N Engl J Med 328:1365, 1993

SACKETT DL et al: *Clinical Epidemiology: A Basic Science for Clinical Medicine*, 2d ed. Boston, Little, Brown, 1991

SLOAND EM et al: HIV testing: State of the art. JAMA 266:2861, 1991

SOX HC JR (ed): *Common Diagnostic Tests: Use and Interpretation*, 2d ed. Philadelphia, American College of Physicians, 1990

section 1 Pain

11 PAIN: PATHOPHYSIOLOGY AND MANAGEMENT

HOWARD L. FIELDS / JOSEPH B. MARTIN

The task of medicine is to preserve and restore health and to relieve suffering. Understanding pain is essential to both these goals. Because pain is universally understood as a signal of disease, it is the most common symptom that brings a patient to a physician's attention. The function of the pain sensory system is to detect, localize, and identify tissue-damaging processes. Since different diseases produce characteristic patterns of tissue damage, the quality, time course and location of a patient's pain complaint, and the location of tenderness provide important diagnostic clues and are used to evaluate the response to treatment.

THE PAIN SENSORY SYSTEM

Pain is an unpleasant sensation localized to a part of the body. It is often described in terms of a penetrating or tissue-destructive process (e.g., stabbing, burning, twisting, tearing, squeezing) and/or of a bodily or emotional reaction (e.g., terrifying, nauseating, sickening). Furthermore, any pain of moderate or higher intensity is accompanied by anxiety and the urge to escape or terminate the feeling. These properties illustrate the duality of pain: It is both sensation and emotion. When it is acute, pain is characteristically associated with behavioral arousal and a stress response consisting of increased blood pressure, heart rate, pupil diameter, and plasma cortisol levels. In addition, local muscle contraction (e.g., limb flexion, abdominal wall rigidity) is often seen and may produce secondary tenderness.

THE PRIMARY AFFERENT NOCICEPTOR A peripheral nerve consists of the axons of three different types of neurons: primary sensory afferents, motor neurons, and sympathetic postganglionic neurons (Fig. 11-1). The cell bodies of primary afferents are located in the dorsal root ganglia in the vertebral foramina. After emerging from its cell body, the primary afferent axon bifurcates to send one process into the spinal cord and the other to innervate bodily tissues. Primary afferents are classified by their diameter, degree of myelination, and conduction velocity. The largest-diameter fibers, A-beta, respond maximally to light touch and/or moving stimuli; they are present primarily in nerves that innervate the skin. In normal individuals, the activity of these fibers does not produce pain. There are two other classes of primary afferents: the small-diameter myelinated (A-delta) and the unmyelinated (C fiber) axons (see Fig. 11-1). These fibers are present in the nerves to the skin and to deep somatic and visceral structures. Some tissues, such as the cornea, are innervated only by A-delta and C afferents. Most A-delta and C afferents respond maximally only to intense (painful) stimuli and produce pain when they are electrically stimulated; this defines them as *primary afferent nociceptors* (*pain receptors*). The ability to detect painful stimuli is completely abolished when A-delta and C axons are blocked.

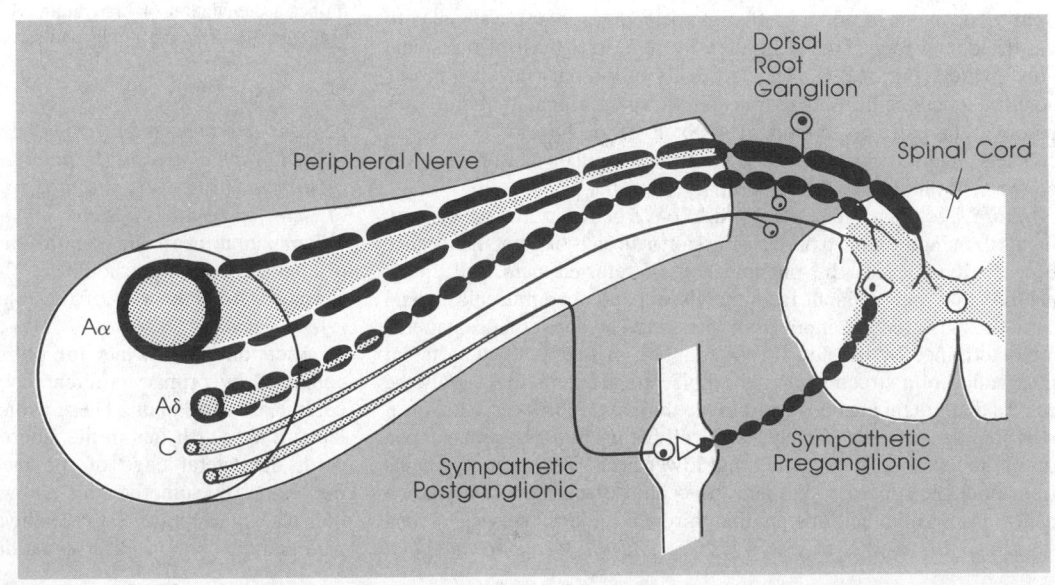

FIGURE 11-1 Components of a typical cutaneous nerve. There are two distinct functional categories of axons: primary afferents with cell bodies in the dorsal root ganglion and sympathetic postganglionic fibers with cell bodies in the sympathetic ganglion. Primary afferents include those with large-diameter myelinated (A-β), small-diameter myelinated (A-δ), and unmyelinated (C) axons. All sympathetic postganglionic fibers are unmyelinated.

Individual primary afferent nociceptors can respond to several different types of noxious stimuli. For example, most nociceptors respond to heating, intense mechanical stimuli such as a pinch, and application of irritating chemicals.

Sensitization   When intense, repeated, or prolonged stimuli are applied, if tissue is damaged or if inflammation is present, the threshold for activating primary afferent nociceptors is lowered and the frequency of firing is higher for all stimulus intensities. This process, called *sensitization*, produces a situation in which stimuli that are normally innocuous can produce pain. Sensitization is a clinically important process that contributes to tenderness, soreness, and hyperalgesia. A striking example of sensitization is sunburned skin in which severe pain can be produced by a gentle slap on the back or a warm shower.

Compared with superficial structures (e.g., skin, cornea), most deep tissues are relatively insensitive to noxious mechanical or thermal stimuli under normal conditions. In contrast, when affected by a disease process with an inflammatory component, deep structures such as joints or hollow viscera characteristically become exquisitely sensitive to mechanical stimulation. Inflammatory mediators such as bradykinin, some prostaglandins, and leukotrienes can activate and/or sensitize primary afferents. (For example, in experimental arthritis produced by Freund's adjuvant, A-delta and C joint afferents are sensitized, and many become active even without mechanical or thermal stimuli.)

Most A-delta and C afferents innervating viscera are completely insensitive in normal noninjured, noninflamed tissue. That is, they cannot be activated by known mechanical or thermal stimuli and are not spontaneously active. However, in the presence of inflammatory mediators, these afferents become sensitive to mechanical stimuli. Such afferents have been termed *silent nociceptors*, and their characteristic properties may explain how under pathologic conditions the relatively insensitive deep structures can become the source of severe and debilitating pain and tenderness.

Nociceptor-Induced Inflammation   One important concept to emerge in recent years is that afferent nociceptors also have a neuroeffector function. Most nociceptors contain polypeptide mediators that are released from their peripheral terminals when they are activated (Fig. 11-2). An example is substance P, an 11 amino acid peptide. Substance P is released from primary afferent nociceptors and has multiple biologic activities. It is a potent vasodilator, degranulates mast cells, is a chemoattractant for leukocytes, and increases the production and release of inflammatory mediators. Interestingly, depletion of substance P from joints reduces the severity of experimental arthritis. Primary afferent nociceptors are not simply passive messengers of threats to tissue injury but also play an active role in tissue protection through these neuroeffector functions.

CENTRAL PATHWAYS FOR PAIN   **The spinal cord and referred pain**   The axons of primary afferent nociceptors enter the spinal cord via the dorsal root. They terminate in the dorsal horn of the spinal gray matter (Fig. 11-3). The terminals of primary afferent axons contact spinal neurons that transmit the pain signal to brain sites involved in pain perception. The axon of each primary afferent contacts many spinal neurons, and each spinal neuron receives convergent inputs from many primary afferents.

From a clinical standpoint, the convergence of many sensory inputs to a single spinal pain-transmission neuron is of great importance because it underlies the phenomenon of referred pain. All spinal neurons that receive input from the viscera and deep musculoskeletal structures also receive input from the skin. The convergence patterns are determined by the dorsal root ganglion that supplies the afferent innervation of a structure. For example, the afferents that supply the central diaphragm are derived from the third and fourth cervical dorsal root ganglia. Primary afferents with cell bodies in these same ganglia supply the skin of the shoulder and lower neck. Thus sensory inputs from both the shoulder skin and the central diaphragm converge on pain-transmission neurons in the third and fourth cervical spinal segments. *Because of this convergence and the fact that the spinal*

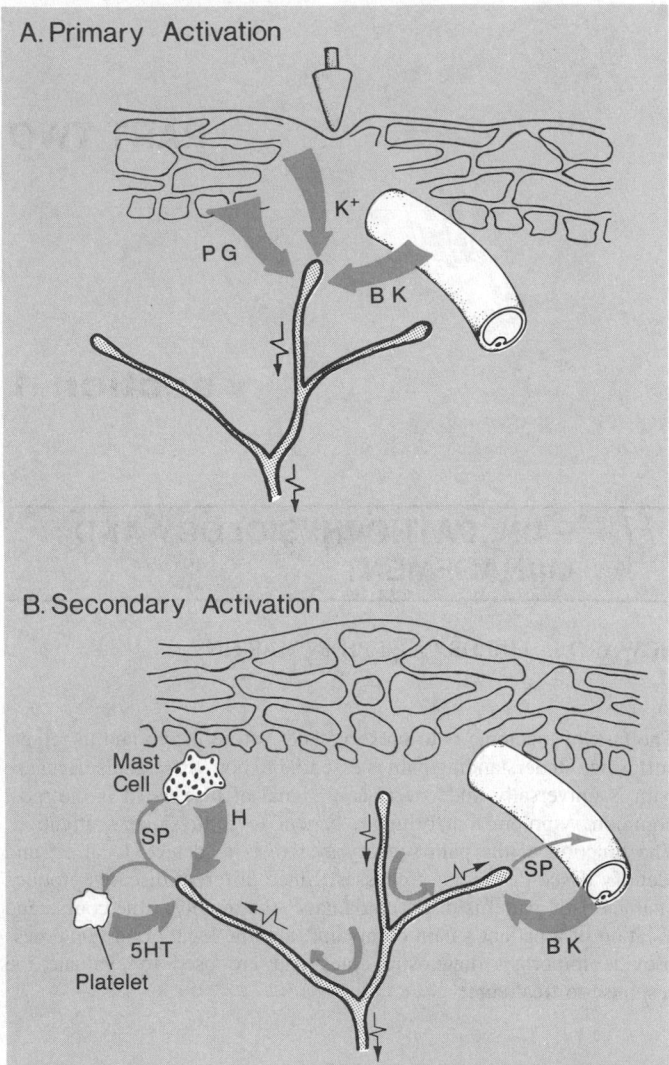

FIGURE 11-2   Events leading to activation, sensitization, and spread of sensitization of primary afferent nociceptor terminals. *A*. Direct activation by intense pressure and consequent cell damage. Cell damage leads to release of potassium (K^+) and to synthesis of prostaglandins (PG) and bradykinin (BK). Prostaglandins increase the sensitivity of the terminal to bradykinin and other pain-producing substances. *B*. Secondary activation. Impulses generated in the stimulated terminal propagate not only to the spinal cord but also into other terminal branches, where they induce the release of peptides, including substance P (SP). Substance P causes vasodilation and neurogenic edema with further accumulation of bradykinin. Substance P also causes the release of histamine (H) from mast cells and serotonin (5HT) from platelets.

neurons are most often activated by inputs from the skin, activity evoked in spinal neurons by input from deep structures is mislocalized by the patient to a place that is roughly coextensive with the region of skin innervated by the same spinal segment. For example, inflammation near the central diaphragm is usually reported as discomfort near the shoulder. This spatial displacement of pain sensation from the site of the injury that produces it is known as *referred pain*.

Ascending pathways for pain   A majority of spinal neurons contacted by primary afferent nociceptors send their axons to the contralateral thalamus. These axons form the contralateral spinothalamic tract which lies in the anterolateral white matter of the spinal cord, the lateral edge of the medulla, and the lateral pons and midbrain. The spinothalamic pathway is crucial for pain sensation in humans. Interruption of this pathway produces permanent deficits in pain and temperature discrimination.

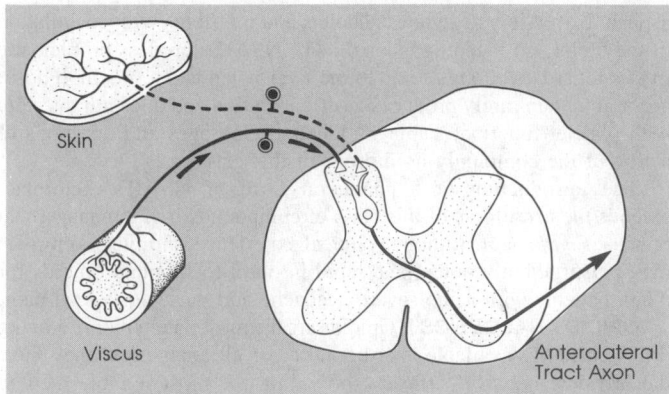

FIGURE 11-3 The convergence-projection hypothesis of referred pain. According to this hypothesis, visceral afferent nociceptors (S) converge on the same pain-projection neurons as the afferents from the somatic structures in which the pain is perceived. The brain has no way of knowing the actual source of input and mistakenly "projects" the sensation to the somatic structure.

One major target area for spinothalamic tract axons is the ventrobasal region of the thalamus (Fig. 11-4). Spinothalamic tract axons connect to thalamic neurons that project to somatosensory cortex. This pathway from spinal cord to thalamus to somatosensory cortex appears to be particularly important for the sensory aspects of pain, i.e., its location, intensity, and quality. Spinothalamic tract axons also connect to medial thalamic regions linked with the frontal cortex and the limbic system. This pathway is thought to subserve the affective or unpleasant emotional dimension of pain.

PAIN MODULATION The pain produced by similar injuries is remarkably variable in different situations and in different people. For example, athletes have been known to sustain serious fractures with only minor pain, and Beecher's classic World War II survey revealed that many men were unbothered by battle injuries that would

have produced agonizing pain in civilian patients. Furthermore, even the suggestion of relief (placebo) has a significant analgesic effect. On the other hand, many patients find even minor injuries (such as venipuncture) unbearable, and the expectation of pain has been demonstrated to induce pain *without a noxious stimulus.*

The powerful effect of expectation and other psychologic variables on the perceived intensity of pain implies the existence of brain circuits that can modulate the activity of the pain-transmission pathways. Although there are probably several circuits that can modulate pain, only one has been studied extensively. This circuit has links in the hypothalamus, midbrain, and medulla, and it selectively controls spinal pain-transmission neurons through a descending pathway (see Fig. 11-4).

There is good evidence that this pain-modulating circuit contributes to the pain-relieving effect of narcotic analgesic medications. Each of the component structures of the pathway contains opioid receptors and is sensitive to the direct application of opioid drugs. Furthermore, lesions of the system reduce the analgesic effect of systemically administered opioids such as morphine. Along with the opioid receptor, the component nuclei of this pain-modulating circuit contain endogenous opioid peptides such as the enkephalins and beta-endorphin.

The most reliable way to activate this endogenous opioid-mediated modulating system is by prolonged pain and/or fear. There is evidence that pain-relieving endogenous opioids are released following operative procedures and in patients given a placebo for pain relief.

Pain modulation is bidirectional. Pain-modulating circuits not only produce analgesia but are also capable of increasing pain. Both pain-inhibiting and pain-facilitating neurons in the medulla project to and control spinal pain-transmission neurons. Since pain-transmission neurons can be activated by modulatory neurons, it is theoretically possible to generate a pain signal with no peripheral noxious stimulus. Some such mechanism could account for the finding that pain can be induced by suggestion alone and may provide a framework for understanding how psychological factors can contribute to chronic pain.

FIGURE 11-4 *A.* Transmission system for nociceptive messages. Noxious stimuli activate the sensitive peripheral ending of the primary afferent nociceptor by the process of transduction (1). The message is then transmitted over the peripheral nerve to the spinal cord, where it synapses with cells of origin of the two major ascending pain pathways, the spinothalamic and spinoreticulothalamic. The message is relayed in the thalamus to both the frontal (F Cx) and the somatosensory cortex (SS Cx). *B.* Pain-modulation network. Inputs from frontal cortex and hypothalamus (Hyp.) activate cells in the midbrain, which control spinal pain-transmission cells via cells in the medulla.

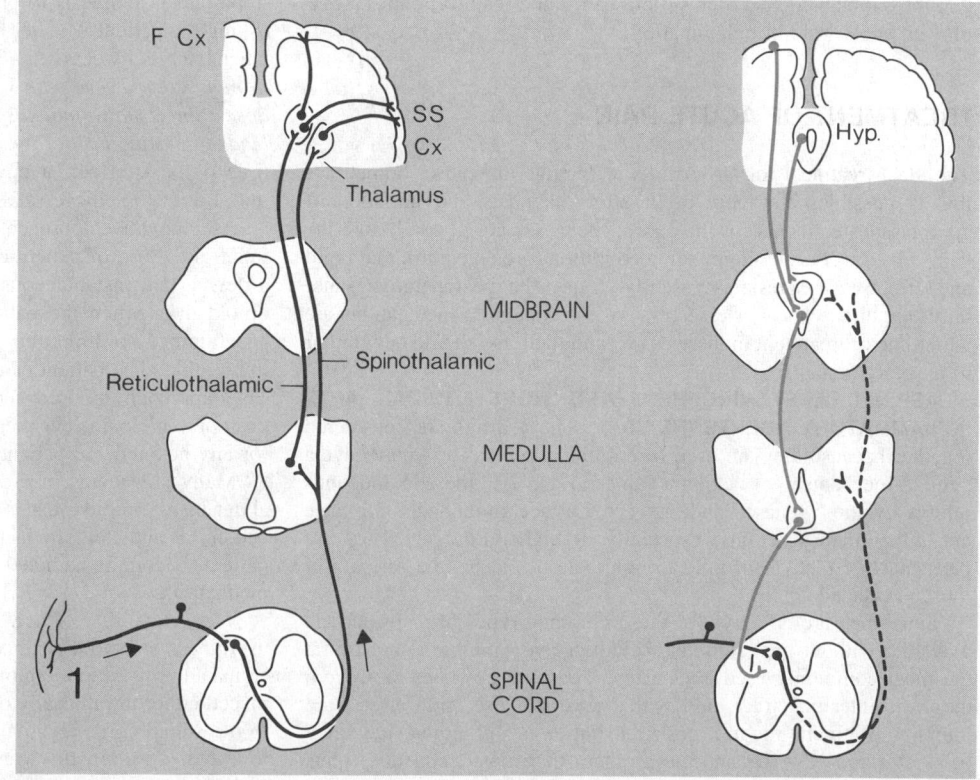

A   B

NEUROPATHIC PAIN   The normal nervous system transmits coded signals that result in pain. Thus lesions of the peripheral or central nervous system may result in a loss or impairment of pain sensation. Paradoxically, damage or dysfunction of the nervous system can produce pain. For example, damage to peripheral nerves, as occurs in diabetic neuropathy, or to primary afferents, as in herpes zoster, can result in pain that is referred to the body region innervated by the damaged nerves. Though rare, pain also may be produced by damage to the central nervous system, particularly the spinothalamic pathway or thalamus. Such neuropathic pains are often severe and are notoriously intractable to standard treatments for pain.

Neuropathic pains typically have an unusual burning, tingling, or electric shock–like quality and may be triggered by very light touch. These features are rare in other types of pain. On examination, a sensory deficit is characteristically present in the area of the patient's pain.

A variety of mechanisms contribute to neuropathic pain. Damaged primary afferents, including nociceptors, become highly sensitive to mechanical stimulation and begin to generate impulses in the absence of stimulation. Damaged primary afferents also may develop sensitivity to norepinephrine released by sympathetic postganglionic neurons. Interestingly, spinal pain-transmission neurons cut off from their normal input may become spontaneously active. Thus both central and peripheral nervous system changes may contribute to neuropathic pain.

Sympathetically maintained pain   A certain percentage of patients with peripheral nerve injury develop a severe burning pain (causalgia) in the region innervated by the nerve. The pain typically begins after a delay of hours to days or even weeks. The pain is accompanied by swelling of the extremity, periarticular osteoporosis, and arthritic changes in the distal joints. A similar syndrome called *reflex sympathetic dystrophy* can be produced without obvious nerve damage by a variety of injuries, including fractures of bone, soft tissue trauma, myocardial infarction, and stroke. Although the pathophysiology of this condition is poorly understood, the pain can be relieved within minutes by blocking the sympathetic nervous system. This implies that sympathetic activity activates nociceptors even if they are not obviously damaged. These results also suggest that the sympathetic nervous system can, under some circumstances, play an active role in inflammation.

TREATMENT OF ACUTE PAIN

The ideal treatment for any pain is to remove the cause. Sometimes this is possible, but more often after diagnosis and initiation of appropriate treatments for the cause, there is a lag period before the pain subsides. Furthermore, some conditions are so painful that rapid and effective analgesia is essential (e.g., the postoperative state, burns, trauma, cancer, sickle cell crisis). Analgesic medications are a first line of treatment in these cases, and their use should be familiar to all practitioners.

ASPIRIN, ACETAMINOPHEN, AND NONSTEROIDAL ANTI-INFLAMMATORY AGENTS (NSAIDs)   These drugs are considered together because they are used for similar problems and may have a similar mechanism of action (Table 11-1). All these compounds inhibit cyclooxygenase, and, except for acetaminophen, all have anti-inflammatory actions, especially at higher dosages. They are particularly effective for mild to moderate headache and for pain of musculoskeletal origin.

Since they are effective for these common types of pains and are available without prescription, cyclooxygenase inhibitors are by far the most commonly used analgesics. They are absorbed well from the gastrointestinal tract, and with occasional use, side effects are minimal. With chronic use, gastric irritation is a common side effect of aspirin and NSAIDs and the problem that most frequently limits the dose that can be given. Gastric irritation is most severe with aspirin, which may cause erosion of the gastric mucosa, and because

aspirin irreversibly acetylates platelets and interferes with coagulation of the blood, GI bleeding is a risk. The NSAIDs are less problematic in this regard. Although toxic to the liver when taken in a high dose, acetaminophen rarely produces gastric irritation and does not interfere with platelet function. Table 11-1 lists the dosages and durations of action of the commonly used drugs of this class.

The introduction of a parenteral form of NSAID, ketorolac, extends the usefulness of this class of compounds in the management of acute severe pain. Although clinical experience is limited, ketorolac may be sufficiently potent and rapid in onset to supplant opioids for many patients with acute severe headache and musculoskeletal pain.

OPIOID ANALGESICS   Opioids are the most potent pain-relieving drugs currently available. Furthermore, of all analgesics, they have the broadest range of efficacy, providing the most reliable method for rapidly relieving pain. Although side effects are common, except for respiratory depression, they are usually not serious and can be reversed rapidly with the narcotic antagonist naloxone. The physician should not hesitate in patients with acute severe pain to use opioid analgesics. Table 11-1 lists the most commonly used opioid analgesics.

Opioids produce analgesia by actions in the central nervous system. They activate pain-inhibitory neurons and directly inhibit pain-transmission neurons. Most of the commercially available opioid analgesics act at the same opiate receptor (mu receptor), differing mainly in potency, speed of onset, duration of action, and optimal route of administration. Although the dose-related side effects (sedation, respiratory depression, pruritus, constipation) are similar among the different opioids, some side effects are due to accumulation of nonopioid metabolites that are unique to individual drugs. One striking example of this is normeperidine, a metabolite of meperidine. Normeperidine produces hyperexcitability and seizures that are not reversible with naloxone. Normeperidine accumulation is much greater in patients with renal failure.

The most rapid relief with opioids is obtained by IV administration; relief with oral administration is significantly slower. Common acute side effects include nausea, vomiting, and sedation. These effects are dose-related, and there is great variability among patients in the doses that relieve pain and produce side effects. Because of this, initiation of therapy requires titration to optimal dose and interval. The most important principle is to provide adequate pain relief. This requires asking the patient whether the drug has relieved their pain and, if so, when the relief wears off. *The most common error made by physicians in managing severe pain with opioids is to prescribe an inadequate dose. Since many patients are reluctant to complain, this practice leads to needless suffering.* In the absence of sedation at the expected time of peak effect, a physician should not hesitate to repeat the initial dose to achieve satisfactory pain relief.

An innovative approach to the problem of achieving adequate pain relief is the use of patient-controlled analgesia (PCA). PCA requires a device that instantaneously delivers a programmed IV dose of an opioid drug when the patient pushes a button. The device can be programmed to limit the total hourly dose so that overdosing is impossible. The patient can then titrate the dose to the optimal level. This approach is used most extensively for the management of postoperative pain, but there is no reason why it should not be used for any hospitalized patient with persistent severe pain.

Many physicians, nurses, and patients have a certain trepidation about using opioids that is based on an exaggerated fear of patients becoming addicted. In fact, there is a vanishingly small chance of patients becoming addicted to narcotics as a result of their appropriate medical use.

The availability of new routes of administration has extended the usefulness of opioid analgesics. Most important is the availability of spinal administration. Opioids can be infused through a spinal catheter placed either intrathecally or epidurally. By applying opioids directly to the spinal cord, regional analgesia can be obtained at a relatively low total dose. In this way, such side effects as sedation, nausea, and respiratory depression can be minimized. This approach has been used extensively in obstetrical procedures and for lower-

TABLE 11-1 Drugs for relief of pain

NONNARCOTIC ANALGESICS: USUAL DOSES AND INTERVALS

Generic name	Dose, mg	Interval	Comments
Acetylsalicylic acid	650 PO	q 4 h	Enteric-coated preparations available
Acetaminophen	650 PO	q 4 h	Side effects uncommon
Ibuprofen	400 PO	q 4–6 h	Available without prescription
Naproxen	250–500 PO	q 12 h	Delayed effects may be due to long half-life
Fenoprofen	200 PO	q 4–6 h	
Indomethacin	25–50 PO	q 8 h	Gastrointestinal side effects common
Ketorolac	15–60 IM	q 4–6 h	Available for parenteral use (IM)

NARCOTIC ANALGESICS: USUAL DOSES AND INTERVALS

Generic name	Parenteral dose, mg	PO dose, mg	Comments
Codeine	30–60 q 4 h	30–60 q 4 h	Nausea common
Oxycodone	—	5–10 q 4–6 h	Usually available with acetaminophen or aspirin
Morphine	10 q 4 h	60 q 4 h	
Morphine sustained release		60–180 bid to tid	Oral slow-release preparation
Hydromorphone	1–2 q 4 h	2–4 q 4 h	Shorter acting than morphine sulfate
Levorphanol	2 q 6–8 h	4 q 6–8 h	Longer acting than morphine sulfate; absorbed well PO
Methadone	10 q 6–8 h	20 q 6–8 h	Delayed sedation due to long half-life
Meperidine	75–100 q 3–4 h	300 q 4 h	Poorly absorbed PO; normeperidine a toxic metabolite
Butorphanol	—	1–2 q 4 h	Intranasal spray
Fentanyl	—	—	Transdermal patch

ANTICONVULSANTS AND ANTIARRHYTHMICS

Generic name	PO dose, mg	Interval
Phenytoin	300	daily/qhs
Carbamazepine	200–300	q 6 h
Clonazepam	1	q 6 h
Mexiletine	150–300	q 6–12 h

TRICYCLIC ANTIDEPRESSANTS

Generic name	Uptake blockade 5HT	NE	Sedative potency	Anticholinergic potency	Orthostatic hypotension	Cardiac arrhythmia	Average dose, mg/day	Range, mg/day
Doxepin	+ +	+	High	Moderate	Moderate	Less	200	75–400
Amitriptyline	+ + + +	+ +	High	Highest	Moderate	Yes	150	25–300
Imipramine	+ + + +	+ +	Moderate	Moderate	High	Yes	200	75–400
Nortriptyline	+ + +	+ +	Moderate	Moderate	Low	Yes	100	40–150
Desipramine	+ + +	+ + + +	Low	Low	Low	Yes	150	50–300

body postoperative pain. Opioids also can be given intranasally (butorphanol), rectally, and transdermally (Fentanyl), thus avoiding the discomfort of frequent injections in patients who cannot be given oral medication.

OPIOID AND CYCLOOXYGENASE INHIBITOR COMBINATIONS When used in combination, opioids and cyclooxygenase inhibitors have additive effects. Because a lower dose of each can be used to achieve the same degree of pain relief and their side effects are nonaddictive, such combinations can be used to lower the severity of dose-related side effects. It is important to recognize that fixed-ratio combinations of an opioid with acetaminophen carry a special risk. Dose escalation as a result of increased severity of pain or decreased opioid effect as a result of tolerance may lead to levels of acetaminophen that are toxic to the liver.

CHRONIC PAIN

PATIENT EVALUATION Managing patients with chronic pain is intellectually and emotionally challenging. The patient's problem is often difficult to diagnose; such patients are demanding of the physician's time and often appear emotionally distraught. Although it is always possible that a rare or obscure bodily disease is the cause of the pain, the traditional medical approach of seeking an obscure organic pathology is usually unhelpful. On the other hand, psychologi-

cal evaluation and behaviorally based treatment paradigms are frequently helpful, particularly in the setting of a multidisciplinary pain-management center.

There are several factors that can cause, perpetuate, or exacerbate chronic pain. First, of course, the patient may simply have a disease that is characteristically painful for which there is presently no cure. Arthritis, cancer, migraine headaches, fibromyalgia, and diabetic neuropathy are examples of this. Such diseases may be sufficient to explain chronic pain without invoking other factors. Second, there may be neural and somatic perpetuating factors that are initiated by a bodily disease and may persist after that disease has resolved. Examples include damaged sensory nerves, sympathetic efferent activity, and painful reflex muscle contraction. Finally, a variety of psychological conditions can exacerbate or even cause pain.

There are certain areas to which special attention should be paid in the medical history. Because depression is the most common emotional disturbance in patients with chronic pain, they should be questioned about their mood, appetite, sleep patterns, and daily activity. A simple standardized questionnaire, such as the Beck Depression Inventory, can be a useful screening device. It is important to remember that major depression is a common, treatable, and potentially fatal illness.

Other clues that a significant emotional disturbance is contributing to a patient's chronic pain complaint are the pain occurs in multiple unrelated sites; a pattern of recurrent, but separate, pain problems beginning in childhood or adolescence; pain beginning at a time of emotional trauma, such as the loss of a parent or spouse; a history of physical or sexual abuse; and past or present substance abuse.

On examination, special attention should be paid to whether the patient guards the painful area and whether certain movements or postures are avoided because of pain. Discovering a mechanical component to the pain can be useful both diagnostically and therapeutically. Painful areas should be examined for deep tenderness, noting whether this is localized to muscle, ligamentous structures, or joints. Chronic myofascial pain is very common, and in these patients, deep palpation may reveal highly localized trigger points that are firm bands or knots in muscle. If injection of local anesthetic into these trigger points relieves the pain, it supports the diagnosis. A neuropathic component to the pain is indicated by evidence of nerve damage, such as sensory impairment, exquisitely sensitive skin, weakness and muscle atrophy, or loss of deep tendon reflexes. Evidence suggesting sympathetic nervous system involvement is the presence of diffuse swelling, changes in skin color and temperature, and hypersensitive skin and joint tenderness compared with the normal side. Relief of the pain with a sympathetic block is diagnostic.

A guiding principle in evaluating patients with chronic pain is to assess both emotional and organic factors before initiating therapy. Addressing these issues together, rather than waiting to "rule out" organic causes of the pain, improves compliance in part because it assures patients that a psychological evaluation does not mean that the physician is questioning the validity of their complaint. Even when an organic cause for a patient's pain can be found, it is still wise to look for other factors. For example, cancer patients with painful bony metastases also may have pain due to nerve damage and significant depression. Optimal therapy requires that each of these factors be looked for and treated.

TREATMENT OF CHRONIC PAIN   Once the evaluation process has been completed and the likely causative and exacerbating factors identified, an explicit treatment plan should be developed. An important part of this process is to identify specific and realistic functional goals for therapy, such as getting a good night's sleep, being able to go shopping, or returning to work. A multidisciplinary approach which utilizes medications, counseling, physical therapy, nerve blocks, and even surgery may be required to improve the patient's quality of life. This may require referral to a pain clinic; however, this is not necessary for all chronic pain patients. For some, pharmacologic management alone can provide significant help.

Antidepressant medications   The tricyclic antidepressants (see Table 11-1) are extremely useful for the management of patients with chronic pain. Although developed for the treatment of depression, the tricyclics have a spectrum of dose-related biologic activities that include the production of analgesia in a variety of clinical conditions. Although the mechanism is unknown, the analgesic effect of tricyclics has a more rapid onset of action and occurs at a lower dose than is typically required for the treatment of depression. Furthermore, patients with chronic pain who are not depressed obtain pain relief with antidepressants. There is evidence that tricyclic drugs potentiate opioid analgesia, so they are useful adjuncts for the treatment of severe persistent pain such as occurs with malignant tumors. Table 11-2 lists some of the painful conditions that respond to tricyclics. Tricyclics are of particular value in the management of neuropathic pains such as painful diabetic neuropathy and postherpetic neuralgia, for which there are few other therapeutic options.

The tricyclics that have been shown to relieve pain have significant side effects. Unfortunately, some of the newer antidepressants such as fluoxetine (Prozac) that have fewer and less serious side effects have not been shown to provide pain relief.

Anticonvulsants and antiarrhythmics   (See Table 11-1)   These drugs are useful primarily for patients with neuropathic pain. Phenytoin (Dilantin) and carbamazepine (Tegretol) were first shown to relieve the pain of trigeminal neuralgia. This pain has a characteristic brief, shooting, electric shock–like quality. In fact, anticonvulsants seem to be helpful largely for pains that have such a lancinating quality.

TABLE 11-2   Painful conditions that respond to tricyclic antidepressants
Postherpetic neuralgia*
Diabetic neuropathy*
Tension headache*
Migraine headache*
Rheumatoid arthritis[†]*
Chronic low back pain[†]
Cancer

* Controlled trials demonstrate analgesia.
[†] Controlled studies indicate benefit but not analgesia.
SOURCE: Fields, 1987, p 291.

Antiarrhythmic drugs such as low-dose lidocaine and mexiletine (Mexitil) seem to be effective for pains that respond to anticonvulsants, as well as other conditions, including postoperative and burn pain. These drugs block the spontaneous activity of primary afferent nociceptors that appears when they are damaged. They should be considered for use in patients with pain associated with damage to peripheral nerves.

Chronic opioid medication   The long-term use of opioids is accepted for patients with pain due to malignant disease. Although its use for chronic pain of nonmalignant origin is highly controversial, it is clear that for many such patients opioid analgesics are the only option available for obtaining effective relief. This is understandable since opioids are the most potent and have the broadest range of efficacy of any analgesic medications. Although addiction is rare in patients who first use opioids for pain relief, some degree of tolerance and physical dependence are likely to occur with long-term use. Therefore, before embarking on opioid therapy, other options should be explored, and the limitations and risks of opioids should be explained to the patient. It is also important to point out that some opioid analgesic medications have mixed agonist-antagonist properties (e.g., pentazocine and butorphanol). From a practical standpoint, this means that they may worsen pain by inducing an abstinence syndrome in patients who are physically dependent on other opioid analgesics.

With long-term outpatient use of orally administered opioids it is desirable to use long-acting compounds such as levorphanol, methadone, or sustained-release morphine (see Table 11-1). The pharmacokinetic profile of these drugs enables prolonged pain relief, minimizes side effects such as sedation that are associated with high peak plasma levels, and, perhaps, reduces the likelihood of rebound pain associated with a rapid fall in plasma opioid concentration. Constipation is a virtually universal side effect of opioid use and should be treated expectantly.

It is worth emphasizing, in conclusion, that many patients, especially those with chronic pain, seek medical attention primarily because they are suffering and because only physicians have access to the medications required for their relief. Clearly, it is a primary responsibility of all physicians to attempt to minimize the physical and emotional discomfort of their patients. Familiarity with pain mechanisms and analgesic medications is an important step toward accomplishing this aim.

REFERENCES

ARNER S: Intravenous phentolamine test: Diagnostic and prognostic use in reflex sympathetic dystrophy. Pain 46:17, 1991

BASBAUM AI, FIELDS HL: Endogenous pain control systems: Brainstem spinal pathways and endorphin circuitry. Ann Rev Neurosci 7:309, 1984

FIELDS HL (ed): Pain Syndromes in Neurology. London, Butterworth, 1990

———: Pain. New York, McGraw-Hill, 1987

GLAZER SAB, PORTENOY RK: Systemic local anesthetics in pain control. J Pain Symptom Manage 6:30, 1991

MAX MB et al: Effects of desipramine, amitriptyline, and fluoxetine on pain in diabetic neuropathy. N Engl J Med 326:1250, 1992

MELZACK R, CASEY KL: Sensory, motivational, and central control determinants of pain, in International Symposium on the Skin Senses, DR Kenshalo (ed). Springfield, Ill, Charles C Thomas, 1968, p 423

Rowbotham MC et al: Both intravenous lidocaine and morphine reduce the pain of postherpetic neuralgia. Neurology 41:1024, 1991

Wall PD, Melzack R (eds): *Textbook of Pain*. New York, Churchill Livingstone, 1989

Willis WD (ed): *Hyperalgesia and Allodynia*. New York, Raven Press, 1992

Willis WD, Coggeshall RE: *Sensory Mechanism of the Spinal Cord*. New York, Plenum Press, 1991

12 CHEST DISCOMFORT AND PALPITATION

LEE GOLDMAN / EUGENE BRAUNWALD

CHEST DISCOMFORT

Chest discomfort is one of the most frequent complaints for which patients seek medical attention; the potential benefit (or harm) resulting from the proper (or improper) assessment and management of the patient with this complaint is enormous. Failure to recognize a serious disorder, such as ischemic heart disease, may result in the dangerous delay of much-needed treatment, while an incorrect diagnosis of a potentially hazardous condition such as angina pectoris is likely to have harmful psychological and economic consequences and may lead to unnecessary cardiac catheterization. There is little relation between the severity of chest discomfort and the gravity of its cause. Therefore, a frequent problem in patients who complain of chest discomfort or pain is distinguishing trivial complaints from coronary artery disease and other serious disorders (Table 12-1).

PATHOPHYSIOLOGY   Discomfort due to myocardial ischemia Discomfort due to myocardial ischemia occurs when the oxygen supply to the heart is deficient in relation to the oxygen need. Oxygen consumption is closely related to the physiologic effort made during

---

TABLE 12-1   Some causes of chest discomfort

I **Cardiac**
  A Coronary artery disease
  B Aortic stenosis
  C Hypertropic cardiomyopathy
  D Pericarditis

II **Vascular**
  A Aortic dissection
  B Pulmonary embolism
  C Pulmonary hypertension
  D Right ventricular strain

III **Pulmonary**
  A Pleuritis or pneumonia
  B Tracheobronchitis
  C Pneumothorax
  D Tumor
  E Mediastinitis or mediastinal emphysema

IV **Gastrointestinal**
  A Esophogeal reflux
  B Esophogeal spasm
  C Mallory-Weiss tear
  D Peptic ulcer disease
  E Biliary disease
  F Pancreatitis

V **Musculoskeletal**
  A Cervical disk disease
  B Arthritis of the shoulder or spine
  C Costochondritis
  D Intercostal muscle cramps
  E Interscalene or hyperabduction syndromes
  F Subacromial bursitis

VI **Other**
  A Disorders of the breast
  B Chest wall tumors
  C Herpes zoster

---

contraction, and coronary venous blood is normally much more desaturated than that draining other areas of the body. As a consequence, the removal of more oxygen from each unit of blood, which is one of the adjustments commonly utilized by exercising skeletal muscle, is already employed in the heart in the basal state. Therefore, the heart must rely primarily on an increase in the coronary blood flow for obtaining additional oxygen.

The blood flow through the coronary arteries is directly proportional to the pressure gradient between the aorta and the ventricular myocardium during systole and the ventricular cavity during diastole but is also proportional to the fourth power of the radius of the coronary arteries. A relatively slight alteration in coronary luminal diameter below a critical level can produce a large decrement in coronary flow, provided that other factors remain constant. Coronary blood flow occurs primarily during diastole, when it is unopposed by systolic myocardial compression of the coronary vessels.

When the epicardial coronary arteries are narrowed critically (>70 percent stenosis of the luminal diameter), the intramyocardial coronary arterioles dilate in an effort to maintain total flow at a level that will avert myocardial ischemia at rest. Further dilatation, which normally occurs during exercise, is therefore not possible. Hence any condition in which increased heart rate, arterial pressure, or myocardial contractility occurs in the presence of coronary obstruction tends to precipitate anginal attacks by increasing myocardial oxygen needs in the face of a fixed oxygen supply.

By far the most frequent underlying cause of myocardial ischemia is organic narrowing of the coronary arteries secondary to coronary atherosclerosis (see also Chap. 203). A *dynamic* component of increased coronary vascular resistance, secondary to spasm of the major epicardial vessels (often near an atherosclerotic plaque) or more frequently to constriction of smaller coronary arterioles, is present in many, perhaps the majority, of patients with chronic angina pectoris. There is no evidence that systemic arterial constriction or increased cardiac contractile activity (rise in heart rate or blood pressure or increase in contractility from liberation of catecholamines or adrenergic activity) due to emotion can precipitate angina unless there is also organic or dynamic narrowing of the coronary vessels. Acute thrombosis superimposed on an atherosclerotic plaque is frequently the cause of unstable angina and acute myocardial infarction.

Aside from conditions that narrow the lumen of the coronary arteries, the only other frequent causes of myocardial ischemia are disorders such as valvular aortic stenosis (Chap. 201) or hypertrophic cardiomyopathy (Chap. 205), which cause a marked disproportion between the coronary perfusion pressure and the heart's oxygen requirements. Under such conditions, the rise in left ventricular systolic pressure is not, as in hypertensive states, balanced by a corresponding elevation of aortic perfusion pressure. Epidemiologic studies indicate that chest pain is no more common in patients with mitral valve prolapse than in those without it.

An increase in heart rate is especially harmful in patients with coronary atherosclerosis or with aortic stenosis, because it both increases myocardial oxygen needs and shortens diastole relatively more than systole, thereby decreasing the total available perfusion time per minute. Tachycardia, a decline in arterial pressure, thyrotoxicosis, and diminution in arterial oxygen content (such as occurs in anemia or arterial hypoxia) are precipitating and aggravating factors rather than underlying causes of angina.

Discomfort due to pericarditis The visceral surface of the pericardium ordinarily is insensitive to pain, as is the parietal surface, except in its lower portion, which has a relatively small number of pain fibers carried in the phrenic nerves. The pain associated with pericarditis is believed to be due to inflammation of the adjacent parietal pleura. These observations explain why noninfectious pericarditis (e.g., that associated with uremia and with myocardial infarction) and cardiac tamponade with relatively mild inflammation are usually painless or accompanied by only mild pain, whereas infectious pericarditis, being nearly always more intense and spreading to the neighboring pleura, is usually associated with pain (Chap. 206).

Vascular causes of chest pain   *Aortic dissection* develops as a result of a subintimal hematoma, which may start either because a tear has developed in the intima of the aorta or because of bleeding into the vasa vasorum. Antegrade movement of this hematoma can compromise major branches off the aorta, while retrograde spread can occlude a coronary artery, disrupt the aortic valve annulus, or rupture into the pericardial space.

Pulmonary emboli   These commonly originate from thrombi in the venous circulation, especially in the lower extremities. Venous thrombosis is usually related to stasis or slowing of blood flow because of inactivity or impedance to venous return, to damage in the vessel wall, or to alterations in the coagulation system. When thrombi from any source embolize to the pulmonary arterial circulation, they can cause not only mechanical obstruction but also vasoconstriction and elevated pulmonary vascular resistance related to the release of humoral factors, such as histamine, serotonin, and prostaglandins. As a result, hypoxemia and, occasionally, right-sided heart failure can ensue, and an acute fall in cardiac output can lead to sudden death. The acute pain from massive pulmonary emboli is thought to be related to pulmonary hypertension and to distention of the pulmonary artery. Infarction of a segment of the lung that is adjacent to the pleura commonly irritates the pleural surface and causes chest discomfort hours or even days later (see Chap. 226).

Other pulmonary causes of chest discomfort   A variety of diseases of the lung can cause chest discomfort. Pleural pain, which is usually brief, sharp pain that is precipitated by inspiration, is very common and generally results from stretching of an inflamed parietal pleura.

Gastrointestinal causes of chest discomfort   Esophageal pain includes *esophageal reflux* and *esophageal spasm*. Esophageal discomfort usually results from chemical (acid) irritation of the esophageal mucosa because of acid reflux or spasm of the esophageal muscle. Injury of the esophagus, such as in a Mallory-Weiss tear that is caused by severe vomiting, can cause severe acute chest pain (Chap. 251).

Occasionally, other gastrointestinal diseases, including *peptic ulcer disease, biliary disease,* and *pancreatitis*, may present with chest discomfort as well as abdominal discomfort.

Neuromusculoskeletal causes of chest discomfort   Neuromusculoskeletal chest discomfort can be caused by *cervical disk disease* because of compression of nerve roots, by *arthritis of the shoulder or spine*, or by *costochondritis*, which is an inflammation of the costochondral junctions. Inflammation of the subacromial bursa or, less commonly, the supraspinatus or deltoid tendon may cause pain that radiates to the chest. *Intercostal muscle cramps* may occur throughout the chest. Anterior scalene and hyperabduction syndromes also can cause chest discomfort.

Other causes of chest discomfort   A variety of *disorders of the breast*, including inflammatory breast disease, benign and malignant tumors, and mastodynia, can cause chest discomfort, usually in association with local abnormalities of the breast. *Chest wall tumors*, including metastases from other organs or malignant disease in the ribs, also can present as chest discomfort. The pain of *herpes zoster* may antedate the typical rash by a day or more, making early diagnosis difficult (see Chap. 144).

DIFFERENTIAL DIAGNOSIS   The key issue in the evaluation of the patient with chest discomfort is to distinguish potentially life-threatening conditions such as coronary artery disease, aortic dissection, and pulmonary embolism from other causes of chest discomfort. Even patients who have brief episodes of pain and are otherwise in apparently excellent health may have intermittent myocardial ischemia or even recurrent pulmonary emboli.

The radiation of pain arising in the thoracic viscera can usually be explained by known neuroanatomic relationships (see Chap. 11). Pain impulses which enter one cord segment may spill over and excite nearby cord segments.

The chest discomfort of myocardial ischemia, most commonly from coronary artery disease but also occasionally from the other causes of ischemia noted above, is angina pectoris. Myocardial ischemia from coronary atherosclerosis is more common in patients who have hypercholesterolemia, diabetes mellitus, hypertension, obesity, or who smoke cigarettes (Chap. 208). Toxins, including cocaine ingestion or withdrawal of chronic exposure to nitroglycerin, can cause sufficient coronary vasoconstriction to result in myocardial ischemia, and cocaine also can cause myocardial infarction.

Angina pectoris is usually described as a heaviness, pressure, or squeezing, or as a sensation of strangling or constriction in the chest, but also may be described as aching, burning, or even as indigestion. Some patients steadfastly deny pain but will admit to a discomfort or unusual feeling or may complain of difficulty in breathing.

Typically, angina pectoris develops gradually during exertion, after heavy meals, and with anger, excitement, frustration, and other emotional states; it is not precipitated by coughing, respiratory movements, or other motion. When angina is induced by walking, it often forces the patient to stop or to reduce speed. Angina occurs most typically in the substernal region, anteriorly across the midthorax; it may radiate to or rarely occur alone in the interscapular region, in the arms, shoulders, teeth, and abdomen. It rarely radiates to below the umbilicus, to the back of the neck, or to the occiput. The more severe the attack, the greater is the radiation from the substernal areas to the left arm, especially its ulnar aspect. Although the radiation of chest discomfort to the left arm increases the likelihood that myocardial ischemia or infarction is present, impulses from the skin and from visceral structures, such as the esophagus and heart, converge on a common pool of neurons in the posterior horn of the spinal cord. Their origin may be confused by the cerebral cortex; hence almost any condition capable of causing chest discomfort may induce radiation to the left arm. Also, stimulation of one of the thoracic nerves that also innervates the heart by, for example, protrusion of an intervertebral disk may be misinterpreted as pain originating from the heart.

When the history is atypical, as is often the case, the correct diagnosis of angina pectoris may be aided by noting that the pain disappears more rapidly (usually within 5 min) and more completely when sublingual nitroglycerin is used. The demonstration that the time required for a given exercise to produce pain is consistently and considerably longer when it is undertaken within a few minutes after a sublingual nitroglycerin pill than after a placebo may, in some instances, represent powerful clinical evidence for the diagnosis of angina pectoris. Angina is rarely relieved within a few seconds of lying down, nor is it precipitated by stooping forward.

Myocardial infarction is usually associated with a discomfort similar in quality and distribution to that of angina but of longer duration (usually 30 min) and usually of greater intensity. In contrast to angina, the pain of myocardial infarction is not rapidly relieved by rest or by coronary dilator drugs and may require large doses of narcotics. It may be accompanied by diaphoresis, nausea, and hypotension (see Chap. 202).

The physical examination in patients with myocardial ischemia frequently is totally normal. However, myocardial ischemia can cause a third or fourth heart sound because of an impairment of myocardial contraction or relaxation. Ischemic papillary muscle dysfunction can cause transient mitral regurgitation and its associated murmur. Myocardial infarction and, less commonly, severe and generalized ischemia can cause congestive heart failure.

The chest discomfort from myocardial ischemia that is caused by aortic stenosis, hypertrophic cardiomyopathy, and nonatherosclerotic causes of coronary artery disease is generally similar to that of angina pectoris from coronary atherosclerosis. However, the physical examination will usually reveal classic findings of an aortic systolic murmur in patients with aortic stenosis (see Chap. 201) and will reveal dynamic outflow obstruction in many patients with hypertrophic cardiomyopathy (see Chap. 205).

Pericarditis can cause pain in several locations (see Chap. 206). Since the central part of the diaphragm receives its sensory supply from the phrenic nerve (which arises from the third to fifth cervical segments of the spinal cord), pain arising from the lower parietal pericardium and central tendon of the diaphragm is felt characteristically at the tip of the shoulder, the adjoining trapezius ridge, and the neck. Involvement of the more lateral part of the diaphragmatic pleura, supplied by branches from the sixth to ninth intercostal nerves, causes pain not only in the anterior part of the chest but also in the upper part of the abdomen or corresponding region of the back, sometimes simulating the pain of acute cholecystitis or pancreatitis.

Pericardial pain commonly has a pleuritic component; i.e., it is related to respiratory movements and aggravated by cough and/or deep inspiration, because of pleural irritation. It is sometimes brought on by swallowing, because the esophagus lies just behind the posterior portion of the heart, and is often altered by a change of body position, becoming sharper and more left-sided in the supine position and reduced when the patient sits upright, leaning forward. It is frequently referred to the neck and lasts longer than the pain of angina pectoris.

In some patients, however, pericardial pain may be described as a steady substernal discomfort that can mimic the pain of acute myocardial infarction. The mechanism of this steady substernal pain is not certain, but it may arise from marked inflammation of the relatively insensitive inner parietal surface of the pericardium or from irritated afferent cardiac nerve fibers lying in the periadventitial layers of the superficial coronary arteries. Occasionally, both pleuritic and steady pain may be present simultaneously.

Patients with marked *right ventricular hypertension* may have exertional pain which is quite similar to that of angina. This discomfort probably results from relative ischemia of the right ventricle brought about by the increased oxygen needs and by the elevated intramural resistance, with reduction of the normally large systolic pressure gradient which perfuses this chamber.

The pain due to *acute dissection of the aorta* (Chap. 210) or to an expanding aortic aneurysm results from stimulation of nerve endings in the adventitia. The pain usually begins abruptly, reaches an extremely severe peak rapidly, is felt in the center of the chest and/or in the back depending on the site of the dissection, lasts for hours, and requires unusually large amounts of analgesics for relief. Patients commonly describe a true pain rather that the vague discomfort that is sometimes described with myocardial ischemia. The pain is not aggravated by changes in position or respiration.

The pain resulting from *pulmonary embolism* (Chap. 226) may resemble that of acute myocardial infarction, and in massive embolism it is located substernally. In patients with smaller emboli, the pain is located more laterally, is pleuritic in nature, and may be associated with hemoptysis.

Pleural pain from fibrinous pleurisy or any pneumonic process is very common. It generally results from stretching of inflamed parietal pleura and is similar in character to the pleural pain of pericarditis (see above). Pneumothorax and tumors involving the pleural space also may irritate the parietal pleura and cause pleural pain; the latter is sharp, knifelike, superficial in quality, and its aggravation by each breath and by coughing distinguishes it from the deep, dull, relatively steady pain of myocardial ischemia. Substernal discomfort also frequently occurs in the presence of *tracheobronchitis;* it is commonly described as a burning sensation accentuated by coughing.

The pain of *mediastinal emphysema* (Chap. 228) may be intense and sharp and may radiate from the substernal region to the shoulders; often a distinct crepitus is heard. The pain associated with *mediastinitis* and *mediastinal tumors* usually resembles that of pleuritis but is more likely to be maximal in the substernal region, and the associated feeling of constriction or oppression may cause confusion with myocardial infarction.

The several *abdominal disorders* which may at times mimic anginal pain may usually be suspected from the history. Esophageal pain commonly presents as a deep thoracic burning discomfort, which is the hallmark of acid-induced pain. Intake of aspirin, alcohol, or certain foods typically exacerbates this burning discomfort, and the discomfort may be relieved promptly by antacids or even by one or two swallows of food or water. Patients may have accompanying dysphagia, regurgitation of undigested food, or weight loss. The symptoms of a hiatus hernia tend to be exacerbated by lying down, and all forms of acid-peptic disease may be worse in the early morning when acidic secretions are not neutralized by food. Esophageal spasm, which may be induced by reflux of gastric acid into an esophagus in which the mucosa has been previously irritated, can cause a squeezing pain that may be indistinguishable from myocardial ischemia and that may even have a similar pattern of radiation. Pain resulting from gastric or duodenal ulcer (Chap. 252) is epigastric or substernal, usually commences about 1 to $1\frac{1}{2}$ h after meals, and is usually relieved in several minutes by antacids or milk.

The discomfort caused by acute cholecystitis is more commonly described as an ache, which may be epigastric or substernal. It most commonly tends to occur an hour or so after meals and not in relation to exertion.

The presence of an abdominal disorder, such as a hiatus hernia or a duodenal ulcer, does not constitute proof that the patient's chest pain is related to it. Such disorders are frequently asymptomatic and are not at all uncommon in patients who also have angina pectoris.

Musculoskeletal pain   The *costochondral and chondrosternal articulations* are the most common sites of anterior chest pain. Objective signs in the form of swelling (Tietze's syndrome), redness, and heat are rare, but sharply localized tenderness is common. The pain may be darting and last for only a few seconds or may be a dull ache enduring for hours or days. An associated feeling of tightness due to muscle spasm (see below) is frequent. *Pressure on the chondrosternal and costochondral junctions and on the pectoralis muscles is an essential part of the examination of every patient with chest pain* and will reproduce the pain arising from these tissues. A large percentage of patients with costochondral pain, especially those who also have minor and innocent T-wave alterations, are erroneously labeled as having coronary disease.

Pain secondary to *subacromial bursitis, biceps tendonitis*, and *arthritis of the shoulder and spine* may be precipitated by motion but not by general exertion. Pain arising in the chest wall or upper extremity may develop as a result of muscle or ligament strains brought on by unaccustomed exercise and felt in the costochondral or chondrosternal junctions or in the chest wall muscles. Other causes are *osteoarthritis* of the dorsal or thoracic spine and *ruptured cervical disk disease*. Pain in the left upper extremity and precordium may be due to compression of portions of the brachial plexus by a cervical rib or by spasm and shortening of the scalenus anticus muscle because of high fixation of the ribs and sternum. Deep breathing, turning or twisting of the chest, and movements of the shoulder girdle and arm may elicit and duplicate the pain of which the patient complains. The pain may be very brief, lasting only a few seconds, or aching and persist for hours. The duration is therefore likely to be either longer or shorter than untreated angina pectoris, which usually lasts for only a few minutes.

Emotional disorders are also commonly associated with chest pain. Usually, the discomfort is experienced as a sense of "tightness," sometimes called "aching," and occasionally it may be sufficiently severe as to be designated a pain of considerable magnitude. Since the discomfort may be described as a tightness or constriction and is often localized at least in part beneath the sternum, it is not surprising that this type of discomfort is frequently confused with that of myocardial ischemia. Ordinarily, it lasts for a half hour or more, is unrelated to exertion, and with slow fluctuation of intensity. The association with fatigue or emotional strain is usually clear, although this may not be volunteered by the patient. Associated hyperventilation can cause innocent changes in the T waves and ST segments, which can be confused with coronary artery disease.

APPROACH TO THE PATIENT WITH CHEST DISCOMFORT   A detailed and *meticulous history* of the behavior of the pain is the cornerstone of the evaluation. The location, radiation, quality, intensity, and duration of the episodes are important. Even more so is the story of the aggravating and alleviating factors. A history of intense aggravation by breathing, coughing, or other respiratory movements will usually point toward the pleura and pericardium or mediastinum as the site, although chest wall pain is likewise affected by respiratory motion. Similarly, a pain that regularly appears on rapid walking, or with other exertion such as sexual activity, and vanishes a few minutes after stopping suggests the diagnosis of angina pectoris, although a similar story will occasionally be obtained from patients with skeletal disorders.

While data from the history are of cardinal importance in the assessment of chest discomfort, physicians should not be misled into overreliance on any single feature. For example, acute myocardial infarction sometimes presents with pain that may be described as burning or even as sharp and may not be principally located in the substernal area.

A thorough *physical examination* can provide important clues to the cause of chest discomfort. Blood pressure should be checked in both arms if aortic dissection is being considered. Examination of the skin may reveal cyanosis, which suggests hypoxemia from either diminished cardiac output or impaired respiratory function, or xanthelasthma, which would suggest hyperlipidemia and associated coronary disease. The finding of lymphadenopathy suggests a tumor. The examination of the chest wall should include both inspection and palpation to search for costochondritis and other musculoskeletal abnormalities. Lung examination may reveal a pleural rub, signs of pneumonic consolidation, or evidence of congestive heart failure. The physical examination may be totally normal in persons with severe myocardial ischemia, but it also may demonstrate abnormalities of vital signs, a third or fourth heart sound, or mitral regurgitation from papillary muscle dysfunction. Aortic stenosis will be accompanied by its typical murmur (Chap. 201). The cardiac examination also should search for an increased pulmonic second sound that may indicate elevated pulmonary artery pressure, such as is found in pulmonary embolism, and the pericardial friction rub that strongly suggests pericarditis. A careful upper abdominal examination may be the first clue to peptic ulcer disease or cholecystitis.

Critical information can often be obtained by attempts to produce or alleviate the pain, such as with nitroglycerin. Careful palpation of the chest wall, subacromial bursa, deltoid tendon, abdomen, and other structures may be very helpful if it reproduces the chest discomfort. Shoulder and arm motion commonly reproduces pain related to these structures. However, the finding that such maneuvers can cause chest discomfort does not mean that such musculoskeletal diseases are the cause of the presenting complaint unless one can be sure that the patient's syndrome is reproduced precisely. Alternatively, the demonstration that a localized pain can be completely relieved by infiltration of a local anesthetic will be conclusive in convincing both the patient and the physician. Evaluation of the patient at the time of a spontaneous episode, such as with an electrocardiogram during pain, is also extremely helpful.

APPLICATION OF THE PRINCIPLES OF CLINICAL REASONING

The assessment of the probability of the various causes of chest pain requires the integration of multiple pieces of data, because no single clinical feature can be considered decisive. Each of the conditions that can cause chest discomfort can have varied presentations, and the diagnostic tests upon which physicians often rely can also have false-positive or false-negative results. Thus the principles of clinical reasoning (Chap. 10) should be applied to the evaluation of the patient with chest discomfort.

History and physical examination   The information obtained from a careful medical history and physical examination can be used to develop a differential diagnosis of the causes of chest discomfort in an individual patient, to rank these diagnostic possibilities, and often to assign approximate percent probabilities to them. Although the various causes of chest discomfort have typical characteristics, these characteristics must be interpreted in light of the prior probability that a person with a given age and sex and with a particular past medical history would have such a cause of chest discomfort. For example, the possibility of angina pectoris as a cause of precordial or substernal discomfort must be seriously considered in a middle-aged man with coronary risk factors such as hypercholesterolemia

and smoking, even if the description of the discomfort is not perfectly typical for angina pectoris. Conversely, when a 20-year-old woman describes the onset of new discomfort in a way that is seemingly classic for angina pectoris, such a diagnosis is relatively unlikely because the prior probability of ischemic heart disease, given her age and sex, is so low.

Although it is not always possible to assign numerical probabilities to the various causes of chest discomfort in an individual patient, experienced clinicians either implicitly or explicitly assess the relative likelihoods of various potential explanations for any chest discomfort syndrome to help guide their future diagnostic evaluations and therapy. For example, a middle-aged or elderly man with typical characteristics for angina pectoris has about an 80 to 85 percent probability of having hemodynamically significant coronary artery disease. By comparison, the same man with a history of chest discomfort that has some characteristics that are typical for angina pectoris but other characteristics that are atypical will have a probability of important coronary disease ranging from about 30 to 60 percent. Even persons with chest pain that is decidedly unlikely to represent coronary disease still have some finite possibility of coronary disease, which may range from exceedingly unlikely in a young woman to the 10 percent range in a middle-aged man with many coronary risk factors.

Diagnostic tests   Although myocardial ischemia commonly is associated with electrocardiographic changes (Chap. 203), many patients have normal tracings between attacks, and some may even be normal during an episode of pain. However, depression of the ST segments, caused by myocardial ischemia, typically occurs during exertion and is accompanied by anginal discomfort; moreover, electrocardiographic evidence of myocardial ischemia may occur at rest and with or without accompanying chest discomfort. The finding of flat or down-sloping ST-segment depressions of 0.1 mV or greater during an attack of pain substantially increases the likelihood that the pain is anginal in origin. Exercise electrocardiography will show ischemic changes in about 50 to 80 percent of persons with symptomatic coronary disease but also in about 10 to 15 percent of patients who do not have coronary disease. The accuracy of ambulatory ischemia monitoring in the general population is less clear. Exercise thallium scintigraphy (Chap. 190) will demonstrate a perfusion defect in about 75 to 85 percent of patients with angina pectoris and will be falsely positive in about 10 percent of patients who have chest discomfort from noncoronary causes.

The evaluation of patients with suspected pulmonary embolism should usually focus on the documentation of deep venous thrombosis (Chap. 226) and the evaluation of pulmonary perfusion with a lung scintigram and/or pulmonary arteriography (Chap. 216). Aortic dissection is often suggested by the routine chest radiograph, and the diagnosis may be established by echocardiography (especially transesophageal echocardiography), computed tomography, or magnetic resonance imaging. Aortography is the definitive test, but because of its invasiveness, it is usually reserved for situations in which the suspicion of dissection is moderate or high and definitive anatomic documentation or localization is needed, often because of the need to consider a surgical repair.

Esophageal or peptic ulcer diseases can often be diagnosed by an upper gastrointestinal roentgenogram. Esophageal manometry and measurement of lower esophageal sphincter pressure are useful in identifying esophageal spasm. The Bernstein acid perfusion test, in which an attempt is made to reproduce the pain by infusing hydrochloric acid into the esophagus, can help establish acid reflux as the cause of pain (Chap. 251).

Integration of clinical data and test results   It is often useful to subdivide patients into those with an *acute* onset of a new or worsened chest pain syndrome versus those with more *chronic* pain. Acute chest pain, with a duration of minutes to hours prior to the patient's presentation to a physician, could be caused by many of the entities described in this chapter and would be especially suspicious for acute myocardial infarction, aortic dissection, pulmonary embolism, biliary colic, or acute musculoskeletal trauma. In many situations, the patient may have had prior pain that was similar to but less severe than the current discomfort; this prior pain may be an important clue to recurrent problems such as biliary colic or esophageal spasm. Some, but certainly not all, patients with acute myocardial infarctions will have had a prior history of angina pectoris.

Accumulated data from large numbers of patients who have presented to emergency departments with acute chest pain can aid the assessment of the probability that an individual is having an acute myocardial infarction. By integrating information from the history, physical examination, and electrocardiogram, such empirically derived algorithms have been able to predict which patients are having acute myocardial infarctions more accurately than are the physicians who actually saw the patients in the emergency department. For example, a person without a history of known coronary disease is unlikely to be having an acute myocardial infarction if the electrocardiogram is normal and the chest pain does not radiate to the neck or left shoulder or arm. Although no algorithm can be considered a perfect predictor that can be used in a vacuum, physicians have the opportunity to improve patient management by incorporating such information into their decision-making.

In patients with chronic or recurrent chest pain, the prior pain pattern is usually very helpful in establishing the current diagnosis. For patients with recurrent myocardial ischemia, a worsening of a stable pain pattern may herald unstable angina pectoris (Chap. 203). Unlike acute chest pain, where decision-making revolves around the need for immediate hospitalization and electrocardiographic monitoring to avoid sudden death, chronic chest pain, unless indicative of unstable angina pectoris, may be clarified by outpatient diagnostic testing, such as exercise electrocardiography and exercise thallium scintigraphy.

Although exercise electrocardiography and exercise thallium scintigraphy are of value in distinguishing between cardiac and noncardiac causes of chest discomfort, the results must be interpreted in light of the prior probability of coronary artery disease, which is the probability

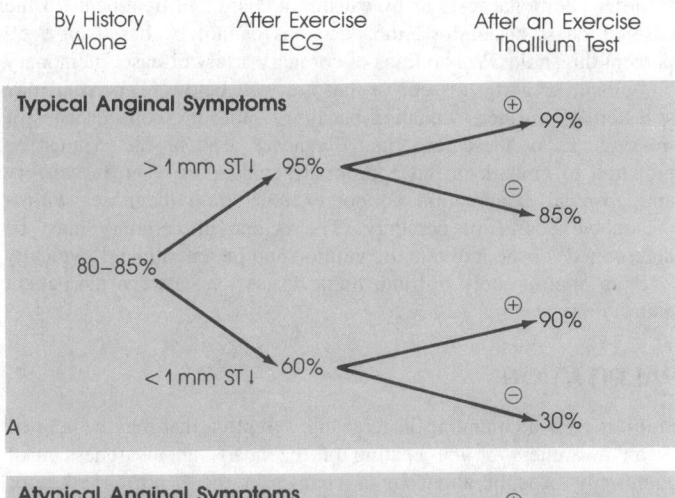

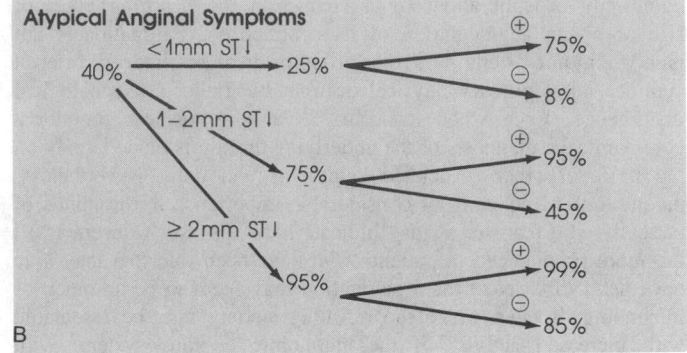

FIGURE 12-2 Approximate probability of coronary artery disease before and after noninvasive testing of a patient with typical (*A*) and atypical (*B*) angina pectoris. The percentages demonstrate how the sequential use of an exercise electrocardiogram and an exercise thallium test may affect the probability of coronary artery disease. (*From L Goldman, in W Branch, Jr (ed): The Office Practice of Medicine, 2d ed, Philadelphia, Saunders, 1987.*)

FIGURE 12-1 The curves show the posterior (after-test) probability as a function of the prior (before-test) probability for positive versus negative exercise thallium scintiscans, defined as a perfusion defect that is produced by exercise and resolves with rest. The before-test probability could be estimated from the clinical presentation or could be a postexercise electrocardiogram probability derived from Fig. 10-2 (p. 46). (*From L Goldman, in W Branch, Jr (ed): The Office Practice of Medicine, 3rd ed, Philadelphia, Saunders, 1994.*)

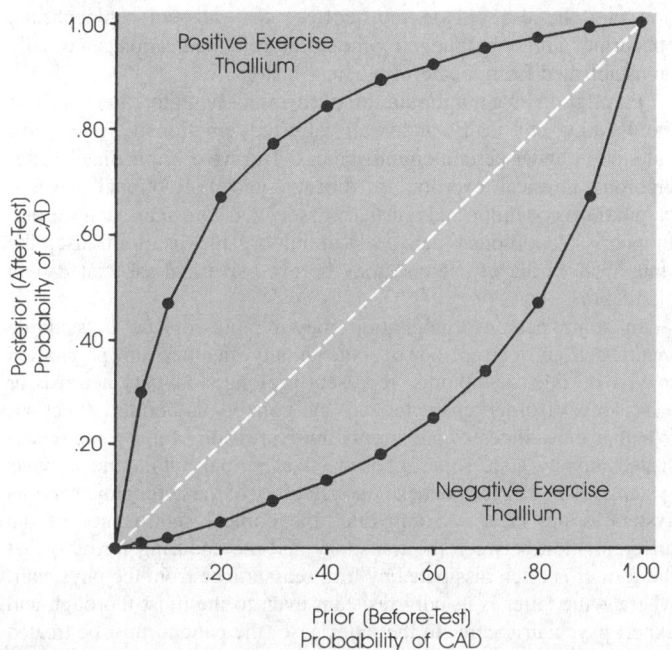

that the patient has coronary disease based on the presenting clinical characteristics, age, and sex (see Fig. 10-2, p. 46). Since exercise thallium scintigraphy appears to provide information that is correlated with the standard exercise electrocardiogram no more than would be expected by chance, it can provide additional independent information (Chap. 10) and further change the probability of coronary artery disease (Fig. 12-1). If absolute diagnostic knowledge is required, cardiac catheterization with coronary angiography serves as the gold standard, i.e., the test that is considered definitive regarding the presence or absence of coronary disease, even though the presence of anatomic disease does not guarantee that the coronary stenoses are causing the chest discomfort.

A sequence of consistently negative cardiologic test results reduces the probability of coronary artery disease to below 10 percent in patients with atypical chest discomfort. However, even after a normal exercise electrocardiogram and exercise thallium scintigram, the probability of coronary disease will still be about 30 percent in a middle-aged or elderly patient with a typical history of angina pectoris (Fig. 12-2). By recognizing the potential change in probabilities that can be obtained with positive and negative results of the diagnostic tests that are planned, the physician can decide whether these potential changes in probability are sufficient to warrant the test. For example, the physician should commonly decide that a patient with typical angina pectoris and a positive exercise electrocardiogram does not require an exercise thallium scintigram to *diagnose* coronary disease, although under some circumstances it might aid in the estimation of the patient's subsequent prognosis.

A useful test result is commonly one that moves the likelihood of a diagnostic possibility across a threshold, so the test result would lead to a change in management, either by influencing the decision to order additional tests or by causing a change in treatment. In the case of chest discomfort, the decisions cannot be based on a 50 percent threshold: Probabilities of coronary artery disease, pulmonary embolism, or aortic dissection that are well below 50 percent may still demand further evaluation because of the dire consequences of missing one of these important diagnoses. The physician must be prepared to embark on an appropriate evaluation when the history and physical examination do not exclude these diagnoses with a reasonable degree of certainty. The degree of certainty must be determined for the individual condition and patient at hand, typically after an appropriately full and frank discussion between the patient and the physician.

PALPITATION

Palpitation is a common, disagreeable symptom that may be defined as an awareness of the beating of the heart, an awareness most commonly brought about by a change in the heart's rhythm or rate or by an augmentation of its contractility. Palpitation is not pathognomonic of any particular group of disorders; indeed, often it signifies not a primary physical disorder but rather a psychological disturbance. Even when it occurs as a more or less prominent complaint, the diagnosis of the underlying disease is made largely on the basis of other associated symptoms and data. Nevertheless, palpitation is frequently of considerable importance in the minds of patients, who fear that it may indicate heart disease. Concern is all the more pronounced in patients who have been told that they *may* have heart disease; to them palpitation may seem to be an omen of impending disaster. Since the resulting anxiety may be associated with increased activity of the autonomic nervous system, with consequent increases of the cardiac rate and rhythm and the vigor of contraction, the patient's awareness of these changes may then lead to a vicious cycle, which may ultimately be responsible for incapacitation.

Palpitation may be described by the patient in various terms, such as "pounding," "fluttering," "flopping," and "skipping," and in most cases it will be obvious that the complaint is of a sensation of disturbed heartbeat. The sensitivity to alterations in cardiac activity among different individuals varies widely. Some patients seem to be unaware of the most serious and chaotic dysrhythmias; others are seriously troubled by an occasional extrasystole. Patients with anxiety states often exhibit a lowered threshold at which disorders of rate and rhythm result in palpitation. The awareness of the heartbeat also tends to be more common at night and during introspective moments but is less marked during activity. Patients with organic heart disease and chronic disorders of cardiac rate, rhythm, or stroke volume tend to accommodate to these abnormalities and are often less sensitive than normal persons to such events. Persistent tachycardia and/or atrial fibrillation may not be accompanied by continuous palpitation, in contrast to a sudden, brief alteration in cardiac rate or rhythm, which often causes considerable subjective discomfort. Palpitation is particularly prominent when the precipitating cause for increased heart rate or contractility or arrhythmia is recent, transient, and episodic. Conversely, in emotionally well-adjusted individuals, palpitation commonly becomes progressively less disconcerting as it becomes more chronic.

PATHOGENESIS OF PALPITATION   Under ordinary circumstances, the rhythmic heartbeat is imperceptible to the healthy individual of placid or even average temperament. Palpitation may be experienced by normal persons who have engaged in strenuous physical effort or have been aroused emotionally or sexually. This type of palpitation is physiologic and represents the normal awareness of an overactive heart—i.e., a heart that is beating at a rapid rate and with an increased contractility. Palpitation due to overactivity of the heart also may occur in certain pathologic states, e.g., fever, acute or severe anemia, or thyrotoxicosis.

When palpitation is heavy and regular, it is usually caused by an augmented stroke volume. Pathologic states, such as aortic regurgitation or a variety of hyperkinetic circulatory states (e.g., anemia, arteriovenous fistula, and thyrotoxicosis) should be considered, as well as the benign so-called idiopathic hyperkinetic heart syndrome. Palpitation also may occur immediately after the onset of cardiac slowing, as with the sudden development of complete atrioventricular block, or upon the conversion from atrial fibrillation to sinus rhythm. Unusual movements of the heart within the thorax are also frequently the mechanism of palpitation. Thus the ectopic beat and/or the compensatory pause may be appreciated, since both are associated with alterations in cardiac motion.

IMPORTANT CAUSES OF PALPITATION (See also Chap. 198)
Extrasystoles   In most cases the diagnosis will be suggested by the patient's story. The premature contraction and postpremature beat are often described as a "flopping," or the patient may say that it feels as if "the heart were turning over." The pause following the premature contraction may be felt as an actual cessation of the heartbeat. The first ventricular contraction succeeding the pause may be felt as an unusually vigorous beat and will be described as "pounding" or "thudding."

When extrasystoles are numerous, clinical differentiation from atrial fibrillation can be made by any procedure that will bring about a definite increase in the ventricular rate. In persons without serious underlying heart disease, the extrasystoles usually diminish in frequency and then disappear at increasingly rapid heart rates, whereas the ventricular irregularity of atrial fibrillation increases.

Tachycardias   These conditions, which are considered in detail in Chap. 198, are common and medically important causes of palpitation. Ventricular tachycardia, one of the most serious arrhythmias, rarely is manifested as palpitation; this may be related to the abnormal sequence, and hence impaired coordination and vigor, of ventricular contraction. If the patient is seen between attacks, the diagnosis of ectopic tachycardia and its type will have to depend on the history, but the precise diagnosis can be made only when an electrocardiogram and observations on the effect of carotid sinus pressure are made during the episode. The mode of onset and offset gives the most important lead in distinguishing sinus from one of the various forms of ectopic tachycardias. Ectopic rhythms characteristically begin instantaneously, while sinus tachycardia has a more gradual onset and ending over seconds or minutes. Continuous ambulatory (Holter) electrocardiography and asking the patient to record the time of onset and cessation of the palpitations in a diary are extremely helpful in determining the cause of this symptom.

Other causes   These include thyrotoxicosis (Chap. 334), hypoglycemia (Chap. 338), pheochromocytoma (Chap. 336), fever (Chap. 16), and drugs. The relationship between the development of palpitation and the use of tobacco, coffee, tea, alcohol, epinephrine, ephedrine, aminophylline, atropine, or thyroid medication can usually be established from a careful medical history.

Palpitation as a manifestation of the anxiety state   Persons who are healthy physically and well adjusted emotionally may have palpitation under certain circumstances. During or immediately after vigorous physical exertion or during sudden emotional tension, palpitation is common and is usually associated with sinus tachycardia. In poorly conditioned persons without organic heart disease, the sinus tachycardia of exercise may be excessive and associated with palpitation.

In some persons, palpitation may be one of the outstanding manifestations of an episode of acute anxiety. In others, the palpitation may, with other symptoms, represent prolonged anxiety neurosis or a lifelong disorder characterized by volatile autonomic function. Whether these illnesses are simply an expression of a chronic, deep-seated anxiety state superimposed on a normal autonomic nervous system or whether they depend on instability of the autonomic nervous system is not clear. At any rate, the clinical significance of the differentiation between the transitory and the enduring forms is that the former is often dissipated by firm reassurance from the physician, whereas the latter is usually resistant even to the most thorough and expert psychiatric care. In the latter case, the patient must be treated

TABLE 12-2   Items to be covered in history of patient with palpitation

Does the palpitation occur:	If so, suspect:
As isolated "jumps" or "skips"?	Extrasystoles
In attacks, known to be of abrupt beginning, with a heart rate of 120 beats per minute or over, with regular or irregular rhythm?	Paroxysmal rapid heart action
Independent of exercise or excitement adequate to account for the symptom?	Atrial fibrillation, atrial flutter, thyrotoxicosis, anemia, febrile states, hypoglycemia, anxiety state
In attacks developing rapidly though not absolutely abruptly, unrelated to exertion or excitement?	Hemorrhage, hypoglycemia, tumor of the adrenal medulla
In conjunction with the taking of drugs?	Tobacco, coffee, tea, alcohol, epinephrine, ephedrine, aminophylline, atropine, thyroid extract, monoamine oxidase inhibitors
On standing?	Postural hypotension
In middle-aged women, in conjunction with flushes and sweats?	Menopausal syndrome
When the rate is known to be normal and the rhythm regular?	Anxiety state

with most carefully planned psychological support and tranquilizing medications. This chronic form of palpitation is known by various names such as *Da Costa's syndrome, soldier's heart, effort syndrome, irritable heart, neurocirculatory asthenia,* and *functional cardiovascular disease*. Aside from palpitation, the chief symptoms are those of an anxiety state.

Physical examination usually reveals the typical findings of the hyperkinetic syndrome. These include a left parasternal lift, a precordial or apical systolic murmur, a wide pulse pressure, rapidly rising pulse, and excessive perspiration. The electrocardiogram may display minor depressions of the ST segment and inversion of T waves and so occasionally lead to a mistaken diagnosis of coronary disease; this is particularly likely to occur when these findings are associated with complaints by the patients of an aching feeling of substernal tightness, commonly present in emotional stress. The presence of any kind of organic disease is one of the most common causes of the underlying anxiety which frequently precipitates this functional syndrome. Thus, even when a patient presents undoubted objective evidence of organic cardiac disease, the possibility that a superimposed anxiety state may be responsible for the symptoms described above should be considered. Palpitation associated with organic cardiac disease is nearly always accompanied by arrhythmia or tachycardia, whereas the symptom may exist with regular rhythm and with a heart rate of 80 beats per minute or less in patients with the anxiety state. An anxiety state, in contrast to heart disease, causes a sighing type of dyspnea. Also, pain localized to the apex, either brief and lancinating in character or lasting for hours or days and accompanied by hyperesthesia, is due usually to an anxiety state, not to structural cardiac disease. Giddiness due to this syndrome usually can be reproduced by hyperventilation or by change from the recumbent to the erect posture.

The *treatment* of the anxiety state with palpitation is difficult and depends on removal of the cause. In many instances a thorough examination of the heart and a statement that it is normal will suffice. Instructions to take more rather than less physical exercise will reinforce these statements. When the anxiety state is a manifestation of chronic anxiety neurosis or related emotional disorder, the symptoms are more likely to persist.

Table 12-2 summarizes the main points of information to be ascertained in the history in elucidating the significance of palpitation. The recording of an ambulatory electrocardiogram and the precise temporal correlation of the cardiac rate and rhythm with the presence of palpitation are extremely useful in the identification or exclusion of an arrhythmia if the symptom does not occur when the patient is under direct observation. The effectiveness of antiarrhythmia treatment also can be assessed objectively in this manner, without the necessity of relying only on the patient's subjective symptoms. Beta-adrenergic blockade with propranolol, beginning with 40 mg/d in divided doses, and ranging as high as 400 mg/d, or with equivalent doses of longer-acting beta-adrenergic antagonists can be extremely effective in patients with palpitation and sinus rhythm or sinus tachycardia.

One point merits special emphasis. *As a rule, palpitation produces anxiety and fear out of all proportion to its seriousness*. When the cause has been accurately determined and its significance explained to patients, their concern is often ameliorated and may disappear entirely.

REFERENCES

GOLDMAN L et al: A computer protocol to predict myocardial infarction in emergency department patients with chest pain. N Engl J Med 318:797, 1988

KOTLER TS, DIAMOND GA: Exercise thallium-201 scintigraphy in the diagnosis and prognosis of coronary artery disease. Ann Intern Med 113:684, 1990

LAM HGT et al: Acute noncardiac chest pain in a coronary care unit: Evaluation by a 24-hour pressure and pH recording of the esophagus. Gastroenterology 102:453, 1992

POZEN MW et al: A predictive instrument to improve coronary care unit admission practices in acute ischemic heart disease: A prospective multicenter clinical trial. N Engl J Med 310:1273, 1984

RUSTGI AK, CHOPRA S: Chest pain of esophageal origin. J Gen Intern Med 4:151, 1989

RUTHERFORD JD, BRAUNWALD E: Chronic ischemic heart disease, in *Heart Disease*, 4th ed, E. Braunwald (ed). Philadelphia, Saunders, 1992, p 1292

SOX HC JR. et al: The role of exercise testing in screening for coronary artery disease. Ann Intern Med 110:456, 1989

WOLF MA: Palpitations and disturbances of cardiac rhythm, in *Office Practice of Medicine* 3rd ed, WT Branch Jr (ed). Philadelphia, Saunders, 1994

13   ABDOMINAL PAIN

WILLIAM SILEN

The correct interpretation of acute abdominal pain is one of the most challenging demands made of any physician. Since proper therapy may require urgent action, the luxury of the leisurely approach suitable for the study of other conditions is sometimes denied. Few other clinical situations demand greater experience and judgment, because the most catastrophic of events may be forecast by the subtlest of symptoms and signs. Nowhere in medicine is a meticulously executed, detailed history and physical examination of greater importance. The etiologic classification in Table 13-1, although not complete, forms a useful frame of reference for the evaluation of patients with abdominal pain.

The diagnosis of "acute or surgical abdomen" so often heard in emergency wards is not an acceptable one because of its often misleading and erroneous connotation. The most obvious of "acute abdomens" may not require operative intervention, and the mildest of abdominal pains may herald the onset of an urgently correctable lesion. Any patient with abdominal pain of recent onset requires early and thorough evaluation with specific attempts at accurate diagnosis.

SOME MECHANISMS OF PAIN ORIGINATING IN THE ABDOMEN
Inflammation of the parietal peritoneum The pain of parietal peritoneal inflammation is steady and aching in character and is

TABLE 13-1 Some important causes of abdominal pain

PAIN ORIGINATING IN THE ABDOMEN

A Parietal peritoneal inflammation
   1 Bacterial contamination, e.g., perforated appendix, pelvic inflammatory disease
   2 Chemical irritation, e.g., perforated ulcer, pancreatitis, mittelschmerz
B Mechanical obstruction of hollow viscera
   1 Obstruction of the small or large intestine
   2 Obstruction of the biliary tree
   3 Obstruction of the ureter
C Vascular disturbances
   1 Embolism or thrombosis
   2 Vascular rupture
   3 Pressure or torsional occlusion
   4 Sickle cell anemia
D Abdominal wall
   1 Distortion or traction of mesentery
   2 Trauma or infection of muscles
E Distention of visceral surfaces, e.g., hepatic or renal capsules

PAIN REFERRED FROM EXTRAABDOMINAL SOURCE

A Thorax, e.g., pneumonia, referred pain from coronary occlusion
B Spine, e.g., radiculitis from arthritis
C Genitalia, e.g., torsion of the testicle

METABOLIC CAUSES

A Exogenous
   1 Black widow spider bite
   2 Lead poisoning and others
B Endogenous
   1 Uremia
   2 Diabetic ketoacidosis
   3 Porphyria
   4 Allergic factors (C′1 esterase inhibitor deficiency)

NEUROGENIC CAUSES

A Organic
   1 Tabes dorsalis
   2 Herpes zoster
   3 Causalgia and others
B Functional

located directly over the inflamed area, its exact reference being possible because it is transmitted by somatic nerves supplying the parietal peritoneum. The intensity of the pain is dependent on the type and amount of foreign substance to which the peritoneal surfaces are exposed in a given period of time. For example, the sudden release into the peritoneal cavity of a small quantity of *sterile* acid gastric juice causes much more pain than the same amount of grossly contaminated neutral fecal material. Enzymatically active pancreatic juice incites more pain and inflammation than does the same amount of sterile bile containing no potent enzymes. Blood and urine are often so bland as to go undetected if exposure of the peritoneum has not been sudden and massive. In the case of bacterial contamination, such as in pelvic inflammatory disease, the pain is frequently of low intensity early in the illness until bacterial multiplication has caused the elaboration of irritating substances.

So important is the rate at which the irritating material is applied to the peritoneum that cases of perforated peptic ulcer may be associated with entirely different clinical pictures dependent only on the rapidity with which the gastric juice enters the peritoneal cavity.

The pain of peritoneal inflammation is invariably accentuated by pressure or changes in tension of the peritoneum, whether produced by palpation or by movement, as in coughing or sneezing. Consequently, the patient with peritonitis lies quietly in bed, preferring to avoid motion, in contrast to the patient with colic, who may writhe incessantly.

Another of the characteristic features of peritoneal irritation is tonic reflex spasm of the abdominal musculature, localized to the involved body segment. The intensity of the tonic muscle spasm accompanying peritoneal inflammation is dependent on the location of the inflammatory process, the rate at which it develops, and the integrity of the nervous system. Spasm over a perforated retrocecal appendix or perforated ulcer into the lesser peritoneal sac may be minimal or absent because of the protective effect of overlying viscera. As in pain of peritoneal inflammation, a slowly developing process often greatly attenuates the degree of muscle spasm. Catastrophic abdominal emergencies such as a perforated ulcer have been repeatedly associated with minimal or occasionally no detectable pain or muscle spasm in obtunded, seriously ill, debilitated elderly patients or in psychotic patients.

Obstruction of hollow viscera The pain of obstruction of hollow abdominal viscera is classically described as intermittent, or colicky. Yet the lack of a truly cramping character should not be misleading, because distention of a hollow viscus may produce steady pain with only very occasional exacerbations. Although not nearly as well localized as the pain of parietal peritoneal inflammation, some useful generalities can be made concerning its distribution.

The colicky pain of obstruction of the small intestine is usually periumbilical or supraumbilical and is poorly localized. As the intestine becomes progressively dilated with loss of muscular tone, the colicky nature of the pain may become less apparent. With superimposed strangulating obstruction, pain may spread to the lower lumbar region if there is traction on the root of the mesentery. The colicky pain of colonic obstruction is of lesser intensity than that of the small intestine and is often located in the infraumbilical area. Lumbar radiation of pain is common in colonic obstruction.

Sudden distention of the biliary tree produces a steady rather than colicky type of pain; hence the term *biliary colic* is misleading. Acute distention of the gallbladder usually causes pain in the right upper quadrant with radiation to the right posterior region of the thorax or to the tip of the right scapula, and distention of the common bile duct is often associated with pain in the epigastrium radiating to the upper part of the lumbar region. Considerable variation is common, however, so that differentiation between these may be impossible. The typical subscapular pain or lumbar radiation is frequently absent. Gradual dilatation of the biliary tree, as in carcinoma of the head of the pancreas, may cause no pain or only a mild aching sensation in the epigastrium or right upper quadrant. The pain of distention of the pancreatic ducts is similar to that described for distention of the common bile duct but, in addition, is very frequently accentuated by recumbency and relieved by the upright position.

Obstruction of the urinary bladder results in dull suprapubic pain, usually low in intensity. Restlessness without specific complaint of pain may be the only sign of a distended bladder in an obtunded patient. In contrast, acute obstruction of the intravesicular portion of the ureter is characterized by severe suprapubic and flank pain which radiates to the penis, scrotum, or inner aspect of the upper region of the thigh. Obstruction of the ureteropelvic junction is felt as pain in the costovertebral angle, whereas obstruction of the remainder of the ureter is associated with flank pain which often extends into the corresponding side of the abdomen.

Vascular disturbances A frequent misconception, despite abundant experience to the contrary, is that pain associated with intra-abdominal vascular disturbances is sudden and catastrophic in nature. The pain of embolism or thrombosis of the superior mesenteric artery or that of impending rupture of an abdominal aortic aneurysm certainly may be severe and diffuse. Yet, just as frequently, the patient with occlusion of the superior mesenteric artery has only mild continuous diffuse pain for 2 or 3 days before vascular collapse or findings of peritoneal inflammation appear. The early, seemingly insignificant discomfort is caused by hyperperistalsis rather than peritoneal inflammation. Indeed, absence of tenderness and rigidity in the presence of continuous, diffuse pain in a patient likely to have vascular disease is quite characteristic of occlusion of the superior mesenteric artery. Abdominal pain with radiation to the sacral region, flank, or genitalia should always signal the possible presence of a rupturing abdominal aortic aneurysm. This pain may persist over a period of several days before rupture and collapse occur.

Abdominal wall Pain arising from the abdominal wall is usually constant and aching. Movement, prolonged standing, and pressure accentuate the discomfort and muscle spasm. In the case of hematoma of the rectus sheath, now most frequently encountered in association with anticoagulant therapy, a mass may be present in the lower quadrants of the abdomen. Simultaneous involvement of muscles in other parts of the body usually serves to differentiate myositis of the abdominal wall from an intraabdominal process which might cause pain in the same region.

REFERRED PAIN IN ABDOMINAL DISEASES Pain referred to the abdomen from the thorax, spine, or genitalia may prove a vexing diagnostic problem, because diseases of the upper part of the abdominal cavity such as acute cholecystitis or perforated ulcer are frequently associated with intrathoracic complications. A most important, yet often forgotten dictum is that the possibility of intrathoracic disease must be considered in every patient with abdominal pain, especially if the pain is in the upper part of the abdomen. Systematic questioning and examination directed toward detecting the presence or absence of myocardial or pulmonary infarction, pneumonia, pericarditis, or esophageal disease (the intrathoracic diseases which most often masquerade as abdominal emergencies) will often provide sufficient clues to establish the proper diagnosis. Diaphragmatic pleuritis resulting from pneumonia or pulmonary infarction may cause pain in the right upper quadrant and pain in the supraclavicular area, the latter radiation to be sharply distinguished from the referred subscapular pain caused by acute distention of the extrahepatic biliary tree. The ultimate decision as to the origin of abdominal pain may require deliberate and planned observation over a period of several hours, during which time repeated questioning and examination will provide the proper explanation.

Referred pain of thoracic origin is often accompanied by splinting of the involved hemithorax with respiratory lag and decrease in excursion more marked than that seen in the presence of intraabdominal disease. In addition, apparent abdominal muscle spasm caused by referred pain will diminish during the inspiratory phase of respiration, whereas it is persistent throughout both respiratory phases if it is of abdominal origin. Palpation over the area of referred pain in the abdomen also does not usually accentuate the pain and in many instances actually seems to relieve it. The frequent coexistence of thoracic and abdominal disease may be misleading and confusing, so differentiation may be difficult or impossible. For example, the patient with known biliary tract disease often has epigastric pain during myocardial infarction, or biliary colic may be referred to the precordium or left shoulder in a patient who has suffered previously from angina pectoris. For an explanation of the radiation of pain to a previously diseased area, see Chap. 11.

Referred pain from the spine, which usually involves compression or irritation of nerve roots, is characteristically intensified by certain motions such as cough, sneeze, or strain and is associated with hyperesthesia over the involved dermatomes. Pain referred to the abdomen from the testicles or seminal vesicles is generally accentuated by the slightest pressure on either of these organs. The abdominal discomfort is of dull aching character and is poorly localized.

METABOLIC ABDOMINAL CRISES Pain of metabolic origin may simulate almost any other type of intraabdominal disease. Here several mechanisms may be at work. In certain instances, such as hyperlipemia, the metabolic disease itself may be accompanied by an intraabdominal process such as pancreatitis, which can lead to unnecessary laparotomy unless recognized. C′1 esterase deficiency associated with angioneurotic edema is also often associated with episodes of severe abdominal pain. Whenever the cause of abdominal pain is obscure, a metabolic origin always must be considered. Abdominal pain is also the hallmark of familial Mediterranean fever (Chap. 293).

The problem of differential diagnosis is often not readily resolved.

The pain of porphyria and of lead colic usually is difficult to distinguish from that of intestinal obstruction, because severe hyperperistalsis is a prominent feature of both. The pain of uremia or diabetes is nonspecific, and the pain and tenderness frequently shift in location and intensity. Diabetic acidosis may be precipitated by acute appendicitis or intestinal obstruction, so if prompt resolution of the abdominal pain does not result from correction of the metabolic abnormalities, an underlying organic problem should be strongly suspected. Black widow spider bites produce intense pain and rigidity of the abdominal muscles and of the back, an area infrequently involved in disease of intraabdominal origin.

NEUROGENIC CAUSES Causalgic pain may occur in diseases that injure nerves of sensory type. It has a burning character and is usually limited to the distribution of a given peripheral nerve. Normal stimuli such as touch or change in temperature may be transformed into this type of pain, which is also frequently present in a patient at rest. A helpful finding is the demonstration that cutaneous pain spots are now irregularly spaced, and this may be the only indication of an old nerve lesion underlying causalgic pain. Even though the pain may be precipitated by gentle palpation, rigidity of the abdominal muscles is absent, and the respirations are not disturbed. Distention of the abdomen is uncommon, and the pain has no relationship to the intake of food.

Pain arising from spinal nerves or roots comes and goes suddenly and is of a lancinating type (see Chap. 15). It may be caused by herpes zoster, impingement by arthritis, tumors, herniated nucleus pulposus, diabetes, or syphilis. Again, it is not associated with food intake, abdominal distention, or changes in respiration. Severe muscle spasm, as in the gastric crises of tabes dorsalis, is common but is either relieved or is not accentuated by abdominal palpation. The pain is made worse by movement of the spine and is usually confined to a few dermatome segments. Hyperesthesia is very common.

Psychogenic pain conforms to none of the aforementioned patterns of disease. Here the mechanism is hard to define. The most common problem is the hysterical adolescent or young person who develops abdominal pain and who frequently loses an appendix or other organs because of it. Ovulation or some other natural event that causes brief mild abdominal discomfort may sometimes be experienced as an abdominal catastrophe.

Psychogenic pain varies enormously in type and location but usually has no relation to meals. It is often at its onset markedly accentuated during the night. Nausea and vomiting are rarely observed, although occasionally the patient reports these symptoms. Spasm is seldom induced in the abdominal musculature and, if present, does not persist, especially if the attention of the patient can be distracted. Persistent localized tenderness is rare, and if found, the muscle spasm in the area is inconsistent and often absent. Restriction of the depth of respiration is the most common respiratory abnormality, but this is in the nature of a smothering or choking sensation and is part of an anxiety state. It occurs in the absence of thoracic splinting or change in the respiratory rate.

APPROACH TO THE PATIENT WITH ABDOMINAL PAIN There are few abdominal conditions that require such urgent operative intervention that an orderly approach need be abandoned, no matter how ill the patient. Only those patients with exsanguinating hemorrhage must be rushed to the operating room immediately, but in such instances, only a few minutes are required to assess the critical nature of the problem. Under these circumstances, all obstacles must be swept aside, adequate access for intravenous fluid replacement obtained, and the operation begun. Many patients of this type have died in the radiology department or the emergency room while awaiting such unnecessary examinations as electrocardiograms or films of the abdomen. *There are no contraindications to operation when massive hemorrhage is present.* Although exceedingly important, this situation fortunately is relatively rare.

Nothing will supplant an orderly, painstakingly *detailed history,* which is far more valuable than any laboratory or roentgenologic examination. This kind of history is laborious and time-consuming, making it not especially popular, even though a reasonably accurate diagnosis can be made on the basis of the history alone in the majority of cases. Recent studies of computer-aided diagnosis of abdominal pain indicate that this technique provides no advantage over clinical assessment alone. In cases of *acute* abdominal pain, a diagnosis is readily established in most instances, whereas success is not so frequently achieved in patients with *chronic* pain. Since the irritable bowel syndrome is one of the most common causes of abdominal pain, the possibility of this diagnosis must always be kept in mind (see Chap. 256). The *chronological sequence of events* in the patient's history is often more important than emphasis on the location of pain. If the examiner is sufficiently open-minded and unhurried, asks the proper questions, and listens, the patient will usually provide the diagnosis. Careful attention should be paid to the extraabdominal regions which may be responsible for abdominal pain. An accurate menstrual history in a female patient is essential. Narcotics or analgesics should be withheld until a definitive diagnosis or a definitive plan has been formulated, because these agents often make it more difficult to secure and to interpret the history and physical findings.

In the examination, simple critical inspection of the patient, e.g., of facies, position in bed, and respiratory activity, may provide valuable clues. The amount of information to be gleaned is directly proportional to the *gentleness* and thoroughness of the examiner. Once a patient with peritoneal inflammation has been examined brusquely, accurate assessment by the next examiner becomes almost impossible. For example, eliciting rebound tenderness by sudden release of a deeply palpating hand in a patient with suspected peritonitis is cruel and unnecessary. The same information can be obtained by gentle percussion of the abdomen (rebound tenderness on a miniature scale), a maneuver which can be far more precise and localizing. Asking the patient to cough will elicit true rebound tenderness without the need for placing a hand on the abdomen. Furthermore, the forceful demonstration of rebound tenderness will startle and induce protective spasm in a nervous or worried patient in whom true rebound tenderness is not present. A palpable gallbladder will be missed if palpation is so brusque that voluntary muscle spasm becomes superimposed on involuntary muscular rigidity.

As in history taking, there is no substitute for sufficient time spent in the examination. It is important to remember that abdominal signs may be minimal but nevertheless, if accompanied by consistent symptoms, may be exceptionally meaningful. Signs may be virtually or actually totally absent in cases of pelvic peritonitis, so careful *pelvic and rectal examinations are mandatory in every patient with abdominal pain*. The presence of tenderness on pelvic or rectal examination in the absence of other abdominal signs must lead the examiner to consider such important operative indications as perforated appendicitis, diverticulitis, twisted ovarian cyst, and many others.

Much attention has been paid to the presence or absence of peristaltic sounds, their quality, and their frequency. Auscultation of the abdomen is probably one of the least rewarding aspects of the physical examination of a patient with abdominal pain. Severe catastrophes, such as strangulating small intestinal obstruction or perforated appendicitis, may occur in the presence of normal peristalsis. Conversely, when the proximal part of the intestine above an obstruction becomes markedly distended and edematous, peristaltic sounds may lose the characteristics of borborygmi and become weak or absent even when peritonitis is not present. It is usually the severe chemical peritonitis of sudden onset which is associated with the truly silent abdomen. Assessment of the patient's state of hydration is important. The hematocrit and urinalysis permit an accurate estimate of the severity of dehydration so that adequate replacement can be carried out.

Laboratory examinations may be of enormous value in assessment of the patient with abdominal pain, yet with but a few exceptions they rarely establish a diagnosis. Leukocytosis should never be the single deciding factor as to whether or not operation is indicated. A white blood cell count greater than 20,000/mm³ may be observed

with perforation of a viscus, but pancreatitis, acute cholecystitis, pelvic inflammatory disease, and intestinal infarction may be associated with marked leukocytosis. A normal white blood cell count is by no means rare in cases of perforation of abdominal viscera. The diagnosis of anemia may be more helpful than the white blood cell count, especially when combined with the history.

The urinalysis is also of great value in indicating to some degree the state of hydration or to rule out severe renal disease, diabetes, or urinary infection. Determination of the blood urea nitrogen, blood sugar, and serum bilirubin levels also may be helpful. The serum amylase determination is overrated. Since many diseases other than pancreatitis, e.g., perforated ulcer, strangulating intestinal obstruction, and acute cholecystitis, may be associated with very marked increase in the serum amylase, great care must be exercised in denying an operation to a patient solely on the basis of an elevated serum amylase level. The determination of the serum lipase may have a somewhat greater accuracy than the serum amylase.

Plain and upright or lateral decubitus roentgenograms of the abdomen may be of the greatest value. They are usually unnecessary in patients with acute appendicitis or strangulated external hernias. However, in cases of intestinal obstruction, perforated ulcer, and a variety of other conditions, films may be diagnostic. In rare instances, barium or water-soluble medium examination of the upper part of the gastrointestinal tract may demonstrate partial intestinal obstruction which may elude diagnosis by other means. If there is any question of obstruction of the colon, oral administration of barium sulfate should be avoided. On the other hand, barium enema is of inestimable value in cases of colonic obstruction and should be used with greater frequency where the possibility of perforation does not exist.

Peritoneal lavage is a safe and effective diagnostic maneuver in patients with acute abdominal pain. It is of special value in patients with blunt trauma to the abdomen, in whom evaluation of the abdomen may be difficult because of other multiple injuries to the spine, pelvis, or ribs and in whom blood in the peritoneal cavity produces only a very mild peritoneal reaction. In the absence of trauma, peritoneal lavage has been replaced by ultrasound and laparoscopy. Ultrasonography has proved to be useful in detecting an enlarged gallbladder or pancreas, the presence of gallstones, an enlarged ovary, or a tubal pregnancy. Laparoscopy is especially helpful in diagnosing pelvic conditions such as ovarian cysts, tubal pregnancies or salpingitis, and acute appendicitis. Radioisotopic scans (HIDA) may help differentiate acute cholecystitis from acute pancreatitis. A computed tomography (CT) scan may demonstrate an enlarged pancreas or a ruptured spleen, but it should be used only for *specific* questions such as these.

Sometimes, even under the best of circumstances with all available auxiliary aids and with the greatest of clinical skill, a definitive diagnosis cannot be established at the time of the initial examination. Nevertheless, despite lack of a clear anatomic diagnosis, it may be abundantly clear to an experienced and thoughtful physician and surgeon that on clinical grounds alone operation is indicated. Should that decision be questionable, watchful waiting with repeated questioning and examination will often elucidate the true nature of the illness and indicate the proper course of action.

REFERENCES

DAVIES AH et al: Ultrasonography in the acute abdomen. Br J Surg 78:1178, 1991

LEE PWR: The plain x-ray in the acute abdomen: A surgeon's evaluation. Br J Surg 63:763, 1976

LEEK BF: Abdominal and pelvic visceral receptors. Br Med Bull 33:163, 1977

SILEN W: *Cope's Early Diagnosis of the Acute Abdomen*, 18th ed. London, Oxford Press, 1991

SUTTON GC: How accurate is computer-aided diagnosis? Lancet 2:905, 1989

VALMAN HB: Acute abdominal pain. Br Med J 282:1858, 1981

14   HEADACHE

NEIL H. RASKIN

Few of us are spared the experience of head pain during our lifetimes; indeed, severe, disabling headache is reported to occur at least annually by 40 percent of individuals worldwide. This incidence occurs whether subjects live in large urban environments or in rural villages. The mechanism generating such "benign" headaches may be activated by stress and anxiety, but emotional factors are not necessary for the symptom to occur. The more severe the headache, the more likely it is to be associated with nausea and to be experienced as a pulsing or pounding discomfort; photo- and phonophobia are also more likely to be reported. Moreover, there does not appear to be any utility in having headache; most sufferers report the contrary.

Since headache is a ubiquitous symptom, it may properly be regarded as a *normal* aspect of living; it then follows that the mechanism for such a common phenomenon is more likely to be ordinary than extraordinary. This "ordinary" headache-generating mechanism appears to be influenced by hereditary factors that may "turn up the gain," resulting in susceptibility to more frequent or more severe head pain. The term *migraine* is used nowadays to refer to such a mechanism, in contrast to its prior usage referring to an aggregation of certain symptoms.

Headache is usually a benign symptom and only occasionally is the manifestation of a serious illness, such as brain tumor or giant cell arteritis. The first issue to resolve in confronting the patient who complains of headache is to make the distinction between benign and more ominous causes.

GENERAL CONSIDERATIONS   The quality, location, duration, and time course of the headache and the conditions that produce, exacerbate, or relieve it should be carefully reviewed with the patient.

Ascertaining the *quality* of cephalic pain is occasionally helpful. Most headaches are dull, deeply located, and of aching character. Superimposed on such nondescript pain may be other pain elements that have greater diagnostic value. It is useful to clarify to the patient that it is of interest to learn about *all* the pain elements that have been experienced regardless of their frequency or intensity. A throbbing quality and tight muscles about the head, neck, and shoulder girdle are common nonspecific accompaniments of headache, suggesting that intra- and extracranial arteries and skeletal muscle surrounding the head and neck are activated by a generic head pain–generating mechanism. It was formerly believed that tight "hat-band" headaches indicated anxiety or depression, but investigations have not supported this view. Jabbing, brief, sharp cephalic pain, often occurring multifocally (ice picklike pain), is the signature of a benign disorder.

Pain *intensity* seldom has diagnostic value—in the head or in any other somatic location. From the therapeutic perspective, it is, of course, the single aspect of pain that is most important. Physicians should be cautious about assessing pain intensity by visually inspecting a patient. People respond to pain in a variety of ways that range from overt histrionic behavior to stoicism. Inquiries as to how pain disturbs day-to-day function may extract more useful information. *Response to placebo medication or procedures produces no useful information—* either diagnostic or therapeutic. It simply identifies a "placebo responder," about 30 percent of the population. There is no evidence that placebo responders have lower pain levels than nonresponders or do not really have pain. Patients entering emergency departments with the most severe headache of their lives usually have migraine. Meningitis, subarachnoid hemorrhage, and cluster headache also produce intense cranial pain. Contrary to common belief, the headache produced by a brain tumor is not usually particularly or distinctively severe.

Data regarding *location* of headache may be informative. If the source is an extracranial structure, as in giant cell arteritis, the correspondence with the site of pain is fairly precise. Inflammation of an extracranial artery causes pain and extensive tenderness localized to the site of the vessel. Lesions of paranasal sinuses, teeth, eyes, and upper cervical vertebrae induce less sharply localized pain, but one that is still referred in a regional distribution that is quite constant. Intracranial lesions in the posterior fossa cause pain that is usually occipitonuchal, and supratentorial lesions most often induce fronto-temporal pain.

Duration and *time-intensity* curves of headaches are particularly useful. A ruptured aneurysm results in head pain that peaks in an instant, thunderclaplike; much less often, unruptured aneurysms may signal their presence in the same way. Cluster headache attacks reach their peak over 3 to 5 min, remain at maximal levels for about 45 min, and then taper off. Migraine attacks build up over hours, are maintained for several hours to days, and are characteristically relieved by sleep. Sleep disruption is characteristic of headaches produced by brain tumors.

Headaches that bear a relationship to certain biologic events or to physical environmental changes are essential data for triage of patients. The following exacerbating phenomena make the benign nature of the syndrome highly probable: provocation by red wine, sustained exertion, organic odors, hunger, lack of sleep, weather change, and menses. The association of diarrhea with attacks (Table 14-1) is pathognomonic of a benign disorder (migraine). The cessation or amelioration of headache during pregnancy, especially the second and third trimesters, is also pathognomonic of migraine. Patients with continuous benign headaches often observe a pain-free interlude of several minutes upon awakening before head pain commences. This phenomenon occurs with other centrally mediated pain syndromes, such as thalamic pain, but does not occur among patients with somatic disease as the cause of pain. In attempting to elicit this information, patients commonly respond negatively to initial inquiries in the mistaken belief that because the relationships are not consistent, the validity of the observation is in question. Activation of the mechanism by red wine and hunger, for example, is *always* inconsistent, for reasons that are unclear. It is important to make this context clear to the patient or else valuable information may be lost, resulting in unnecessary neuroimaging.

A history of amenorrhea or galactorrhea should lead one to question whether the polycystic ovary syndrome or a prolactin-secreting pituitary adenoma is the source of headache. Headache arising *de novo* in a patient with known malignancy suggests either cerebral metastases or carcinomatous meningitis. When there is striking accentuation of pain with eye movement, a systemic infection and particularly meningitis should be seriously considered. Head pain appearing abruptly after bending, lifting, or coughing can be the clue to a posterior fossa mass or the Arnold Chiari malformation. Orthostatic headache arises after lumbar puncture and also occurs with subdural hematoma and benign intracranial hypertension. The

TABLE 14-1   Symptoms accompanying severe migraine attacks in 500 patients

Symptom	Percentage affected
Nausea	87
Vomiting	56
Diarrhea	16
Photophobia	82
Visual disturbances	36
Fortification spectra	10
Photopsia	26
Paresthesias	33
Scalp tenderness	65
Lightheadedness	72
Vertigo	33
Alteration of consciousness	18
Seizure	4
Syncope	10
Confusional state	4

SOURCE: NH Raskin, *Headache*, 2d ed, New York, Churchill Livingstone, 1988.

eye itself is seldom the cause of acute orbital pain if the sclerae are white and not injected; a "red eye" is the sign of ophthalmic disease. Similarly, acute sinusitis nearly always declares itself through a dark green, purulent nasal exudate.

The analysis of facial pain requires a disparate approach. Trigeminal and glossopharyngeal neuralgia are common causes of facial pain, especially the former. "Neuralgias" are painful disorders characterized by paroxysmal, fleeting, often electric shocklike episodes that are caused by demyelinative lesions of nerves (the trigeminal or glossopharyngeal nerves in cranial neuralgias) that result in the activation of a CNS pain-generating mechanism. However, the most common cause of facial pain by far is dental; provocation by hot, cold, or sweet foods is typical. The application of a cold stimulus will repeatedly induce dental pain whereas in neuralgic disorders a refractory period usually occurs after the initial response so that pain cannot be repeatedly induced. The presence of refractory periods can nearly always be elicited in the history so that patients need not be put through a painful experience.

Mealtimes offer the physician an opportunity to gain needed insight into the mechanism of a patient's facial pain. Is it the chewing, the swallowing, or the taste of the food that elicits pain? Chewing points toward trigeminal neuralgia, temporomandibular joint dysfunction, or giant cell arteritis ("jaw claudication"), whereas swallowing *and* taste provocation points toward glossopharyngeal neuralgia. Pain upon swallowing is common among patients with carotidynia (facial migraine, see below) because the inflamed, tender carotid artery abuts the esophagus during deglutition.

Many patients with the complaint of facial pain do not describe stereotypic syndromes, in parallel with most painful conditions; such patients have sometimes had their syndromes categorized as "atypical facial pain" as if this were a well-defined clinical entity. There is only scant evidence that nondescript facial pain is caused by emotional distress, as has sometimes been alleged. Vague, poorly localized, continuous facial pain is *characteristic* of the condition that may result from nasopharyngeal carcinoma and other somatic diseases; a burning painful element often supervenes as deafferentation occurs and evidence of cranial neuropathy appears. Occasionally, the cause of a pain problem cannot be resolved promptly, necessitating periodic follow-up until further clues appear (and they usually do). "Facial pain of unknown cause" appears to be a more reasonable tentative diagnosis than "atypical facial pain."

PAIN-SENSITIVE STRUCTURES OF THE HEAD   The most common type of pain is that resulting from activation of peripheral nociceptors in the presence of a normally functioning nervous system, as in the pain resulting from scalded skin or appendicitis. Another type of pain is the result of injury or activation of the peripheral or central nervous system. Headache, formerly believed to originate peripherally, may originate from either mechanism. Headache may arise from dysfunction, displacement, or encroachment upon pain-sensitive cranial structures. The following are sensitive to mechanical stimulation: the scalp and aponeurotica, middle meningeal artery, dural sinuses, falx cerebri, and the proximal segments of the large pial arteries. The ventricular ependyma, choroid plexus, pial veins, and much of the brain parenchyma are pain-insensitive. On the other hand, electrical stimulation near midbrain dorsal raphe cells has resulted in migrainelike headaches. Thus most of the brain is insensitive to electrode probing, but a particular midbrain site is nevertheless a putative locus for headache generation.

Sensory stimuli from the head are conveyed to the central nervous system via the trigeminal nerves for structures above the tentorium in the anterior and middle fossae of the skull and via the first three cervical nerves for those in the posterior fossa and infradural structures. The ninth and tenth cranial nerves supply part of the posterior fossa and refer pain to the ear and throat.

Headache can occur as the result of (1) distention, traction, or dilation of intracranial or extracranial arteries; (2) traction or displacement of large intracranial veins or their dural envelope; (3) compression, traction, or inflammation of cranial and spinal nerves; (4) spasm, inflammation, and trauma to cranial and cervical muscles; (5) meningeal irritation and raised intracranial pressure; and (6) perturbation of intracerebral serotonergic projections. By and large, intracranial masses cause headache when they deform, displace, or exert traction on vessels, dural structures, or cranial nerves at the base of the brain; this often happens long before intracranial pressure rises. Such mechanical displacement mechanisms do not explain the headaches resulting from cerebral ischemia, or from benign intracranial hypertension after the pressure is reduced, or the headaches that are so common in febrile illnesses and systemic lupus erythematosus. Perturbation of intracerebral serotonergic projections has been posited as a possible mechanism for these phenomena.

PRINCIPAL CLINICAL VARIETIES OF HEADACHE

Normally there is little difficulty in diagnosing the headache of glaucoma, purulent sinusitis, bacterial meningitis, and brain tumor because of the clues provided by the associated symptoms and signs. Headache alone is nondescript. It is when headache is chronic, recurrent, and unattended by other important signs of disease that the physician faces a challenging but ultimately gratifying medical problem. The headache syndromes described below should be considered (see Table 14-2).

MIGRAINE   The term *migraine* stems from Galen's usage of *hemicrania* to describe a periodic disorder comprising paroxysmal blinding hemicranial pain, vomiting, photophobia, recurrence at regular intervals, and relief by dark surroundings and sleep. Hemicrania was later corrupted into low Latin as *hemigranea* and *migranea*; eventually the French translation, *migraine*, gained acceptance in the eighteenth century and has prevailed ever since. The passage of time has proved this to be a misleading designation for a condition manifested by lateralized head pain in less than 60 percent of those affected. Furthermore, undue emphasis on the dramatic features of migraine has often led to the illogical conclusion that periodic headache lacking such features is not migrainous in mechanism. It has become clear that severe headache attacks, regardless of cause, are more likely to be described as throbbing and associated with vomiting and scalp tenderness. Milder headaches tend to be nondescript—tight, bandlike discomfort often involving the entire head—the profile of "tension headache." These differing clinical profiles of headaches that are not caused by an intracranial structural anomaly or systemic disease probably represent different points on a continuum rather than disparate clinical entities. Whether a single common mechanism underlies these varying headache profiles is not entirely clear and remains to be investigated further. A working definition of migraine offered here is benign recurring headache and/or neurologic dysfunction usually attended by pain-free interludes and almost always provoked by stereotyped stimuli. It is by far more common in women; there is a hereditary predisposition toward attacks; and the cranial circulatory phenomena that attend attacks appear to be secondary to a primary CNS disorder.

Clinical subtypes   The designation *classic migraine* (migraine with aura) denotes the syndrome of headache associated with characteristic premonitory sensory, motor, or visual symptoms; *common migraine* (migraine without aura) denotes one in which there is no focal neurologic disturbance preceding the occurrence of headache. However, the latter is by far the most frequent clinical problem, and focal neurologic disturbances are more common during headache attacks than as prodromal symptoms. Focal neurologic disturbances without headache or vomiting have come to be known as *migraine equivalents* or *accompaniments* and appear to occur more commonly in patients between the ages of 40 and 70 years. The term *complicated migraine* has generally been used to describe migraine with dramatic focal neurologic features, thus overlapping with classic migraine; it has also been used to connote a persisting neurologic deficit that is a residuum of a migraine attack.

TABLE 14-2 Common types of headaches

Type	Usual site	Age and sex	Clinical features	Life profile
Migraine, with or without aura	Frontotemporal, uni- or bilateral.	All ages; highest incidence in children and young adults. Female > male in adults. Female = male in children.	Onset after awakening; quelled by sleep. Provoked by menses, odors, foods. Stops after 2d trimester of pregnancy. Duration: 6 h to 2 days.	Cycles of several months to years. Less frequent and less severe with aging.
Cluster headache	Lateralized, orbital or temporal.	All ages above 10; peaks at 30–50. Mainly men (90%). Provoked by alcohol.	Periodic attacks. 1–2 attacks per day, commonly awakens from sleep. Duration: 45 min. Associated with red eye and stuffy nose homolaterally.	Daily attacks for 6 weeks with annual recurrence of bout.
Tension headache	Generalized.	All ages; principally young adults. Female preponderance.	Nondescript, tight bandlike discomfort continuously. Exacerbations provoked by factors similar to migraine.	Cycles of several years.
Brain tumor	Variable.	All ages, both sexes.	Interrupts sleep, unrelieved by sleep. Exacerbated by orthostatic changes. Steadily worsening pain; may be preceded by days to weeks of nausea and vomiting.	Monophasic illness lasting weeks to months.
Giant cell arteritis	Lateralized, temporal or occipital.	Over 55 years, either sex.	Marked scalp tenderness with superimposed jabbing and jolting pain. Deep, intermittent throbbing. Associated with malaise and morning stiffness and pain in shoulders and hips.	Monophasic illness lasting weeks to months.
Lumbar puncture headache	Bifrontal and/or bioccipital.	Over 10 years, either sex.	Orthostatic; head pain present with patient sitting or standing and disappears in prone or supine positions.	Arises 1–2 days after lumbar puncture and persists for 3–4 days.

COMMON MIGRAINE   Benign periodic headache of several hours duration, often attributed to "tension" by its sufferers, is the most liberal way of circumscribing common migraine. The fallacy intrinsic to most of the traditional definitions is that they are acceptable definitions of severe attacks but do not include those patients with more modest degrees of head pain; thus, pain unilaterality, attendant nausea or vomiting, positive family history, responsiveness to ergotamine, and scalp tenderness in varying combinations have been alleged to establish a diagnosis of migraine. However, each of these occur in roughly 60 to 80 percent of patients as *dependent* variables, and the validity of using such clinical features to diagnose migraine has never been established. Common migraine is the most frequent headache type reported by patients and includes the now anachronistic concept of periodic tension headache.

CLASSIC MIGRAINE   The most common premonitory symptoms reported by migraineurs are visual, arising from dysfunction of occipital lobe neurons. Scotomas and/or hallucinations occur in about one-third of migraineurs and usually appear in the central portions of the visual fields. A highly characteristic syndrome occurs in about 10 percent of patients; it usually begins as a small paracentral scotoma, which slowly expands into a "C" shape. Luminous angles appear at the enlarging outer edge, becoming colored as the scintillating scotoma expands and moves toward the periphery of the involved half of the visual field. It eventually disappears over the horizon of peripheral vision, the entire process consuming 20 to 25 min. This phenomenon never occurs *during* the headache phase of an attack and is pathognomonic for migraine, never having been described in association with a cerebral structural anomaly. It is commonly referred to as a *fortification spectrum* because the serrated edges of the hallucinated "C" seemed to Dr. Hubert Airy to resemble a "fortified town with bastions all round it"; "spectrum" is used in the sense of an apparition or specter.

BASILAR MIGRAINE   Symptoms referable to a disturbance in brainstem function such as vertigo, dysarthria, and diplopia occur as the only neurologic symptoms of the attack in about 25 percent of patients (Table 14-1). Bickerstaff called attention to a stereotyped sequence of dramatic neurologic events often comprising total blind-

ness and sensorial clouding that is common among but not restricted to adolescent women. These episodes begin with total blindness accompanied or followed by admixtures of vertigo, ataxia, dysarthria, tinnitus, and distal and perioral paresthesia. In about one-quarter of patients, a confusional state supervenes. The neurologic symptoms usually persist for 20 to 30 min and are generally followed by a throbbing occipital headache. The basilar migraine syndrome is now known to occur in children as well as in adults over age 50. Sensorial alterations may last for as long as 5 days and may take the form of confusional states that may be mistaken for psychotic reactions.

CAROTIDYNIA   The carotidynia syndrome, sometimes called lower half headache or facial migraine, is more prominent among an older population of patients, with peak incidence in the fourth through sixth decades. Pain is usually reported to be located at the jaw or neck, although sometimes periorbital or maxillary pain occurs; it may be continuous, deep, dull, and aching, and becomes pounding or throbbing episodically. There are often superimposed sharp, ice picklike jabs. Attacks occur one to several times per week, each lasting several minutes to hours. Tenderness and prominent pulsations of the cervical carotid artery, and soft tissue swelling overlying the carotid, are usually present homolateral to the pain; many patients also report throbbing ipsilateral headache concurrent with carotidynia attacks as well as interictally. Dental trauma is a common precipitant of this syndrome. Carotid artery involvement in the more traditional forms of migraine appears to be common as well; over 50 percent of patients with frequent migraine attacks are found to have carotid tenderness at several points homolateral to the cranial side preponderantly involved during their attacks.

Pathogenesis   Modern orientations toward migraine began with the publication by Liveing in 1873 of the first major treatise devoted to the subject of migraine, *A Contribution to the Pathology of Nerve Storms*. Liveing believed that the analogy of migraine to epilepsy was obvious, and that the clinically apparent circulatory phenomena that occurred during migrainous attacks were secondary to cerebral discharges, or "nerve storms." Attention was focused on the vascular features of migraine by Graham and Wolff in the 1930s who showed that the administration of ergotamine reduced the amplitude of the pulsations of the temporal artery in patients with headache and that this effect was often, but *not consistently*, associated with a decrease in head pain. Because of these observations and other less substantial lines of evidence, it was widely held for many years that the headache phase of migrainous attacks was caused by extracranial vasodilatation and that neurologic symptoms were produced by intracranial vasoconstriction, the "vascular" hypothesis of migraine. A barrage of publications by Wolff and his coworkers followed in support of this hypothesis so that observations made during the 1940s nonresonant with it were ignored.

K. S. Lashley, neuropsychologist at Harvard, in 1941 was among the first to chart in detail his own migrainous fortification spectrum at brief intervals. He was able to estimate that the evolution of his own scotoma proceeded across the occipital cortex at a rate of 3 mm/min. He speculated that a wavefront of intense excitation followed by a wave of complete inhibition of activity were propagated across the visual cortex. Uncannily, in 1944, the phenomenon that has come to be known as *spreading depression* was described by a Brazilian physiologist, Leão, in the cerebral cortex of laboratory animals. It is a slowly moving (2- to 3-mm/min) potassium-liberating depression of cortical activity, preceded by a wavefront of increased metabolic activity that can be produced by a variety of experimental stimuli, including hypoxia, mechanical trauma, and the topical application of potassium.

These observations, striking in retrospect, could not possibly be incorporated into the aforementioned vascular model of migraine, which had been tenaciously grasped by the medical community. However, observations made over the past decade in Copenhagen have rendered untenable an hypothesis invoking a primary vascular mechanism, and lend support to the possibility that spreading depression, or more likely a neuronal phenomenon with similar characteristics, is important to the mechanism of classic migraine.

The pathogenesis of migraine as it is currently understood can be partitioned into three phases. The first is brain (stem) generation; the second may be expressed as "vasomotor activation" wherein arteries both within and outside brain may contract or dilate; the third is activation of cells of the medullary trigeminal nucleus caudalis (the brain's head and face pain-processing mechanism) and the subsequent release of vasoactive neuropeptides at vascular terminations of the trigeminal nerve. This last phase provides a reasonable mechanism for the soft-tissue swelling and tenderness of blood vessels that attend migraine attacks. It seems clear that activation of any of the phases is *sufficient* for headache production, and that one phase may appear to dominate in a particular migrainous syndrome. For example, the evolution of the fortification spectrum is probably entirely neurogenic, requiring only first phase activation (see below).

Regional cerebral blood flow studies have shown that in patients with classic migraine there is, during attacks, a modest cortical hypoperfusion that begins in the visual cortex and spreads forward at a rate of 2 to 3 mm/min. The decrease in blood flow averages 25 to 30 percent (too little to explain symptoms) and progresses anteriorly in a wavelike fashion independent of the topography of cerebral arteries. The wave of hypoperfusion persists for 4 to 6 h, appears to follow the convolutions of the cortex, and does not cross the central or lateral sulcus, progressing to the frontal lobe via the insula. Subcortical perfusion is normal. Contralateral neurologic symptoms appear during temporoparietal hypoperfusion; at times hypoperfusion persists in these regions after symptoms cease. More often frontal spread continues as the headache phase begins. A few patients with classic migraine show no flow abnormalities; an occasional patient has developed focal ischemia sufficient to cause symptoms. However, focal ischemia does not appear *necessary* for focal symptoms to occur. During common migraine, no flow abnormalities are seen. The cerebral blood flow changes are probably the manifestation of a derangement in cerebral neuronal function; moreover, these cortical events require a "generator," presumably within the brainstem.

Neuromagnetic activity has been detected in the temporooccipital cortex of migraineurs during headache episodes. Spontaneous, long-duration (1- to 8-s) biphasic signals have been observed, consistent with a primary neuronal origin of migraine.

Pharmacologic data converge on serotonin receptors. About 35 years ago, methysergide was found to antagonize certain peripheral actions of serotonin (5-hydroxytryptamine) and was introduced as the first drug capable of preventing migraine attacks through stabilization of the mechanism. Subsequently, it was found that platelet levels of serotonin fall consistently at the onset of headache and that migrainous episodes may be triggered by drugs that release it. Such changes in circulating levels proved to be pharmacologically trivial, however, and interest in the humoral role of serotonin in migraine declined. Currently, there is renewed interest due almost entirely to the introduction of a new drug, sumatriptan, that is remarkably effective for migraine attacks. Of still greater interest is that sumatriptan is a designer drug, synthesized to activate selectively a particular subpopulation of serotonin receptors.

There are four main families of 5-hydroxytryptamine receptors—types 1, 2, 3, and 4—within each family of which receptor subtypes have been found. Sumatriptan interacts with serotonin 1A receptors and especially with 1D receptors. By contrast, dihydroergotamine, another drug that is highly effective in aborting migraine attacks, is most potent as an agonist of serotonin 1A receptors and is an order of magnitude less potent at 1D receptors. After systemic administration, dihydroergotamine in brain is found in highest concentrations in the midbrain dorsal raphe. The dorsal raphe is a good candidate for the generator of migraine and the main site of drug action; the highest concentration of serotonin receptors in brain tissue is found there. They are mainly of the 1A variety, but 1D receptors also are present.

As mentioned earlier, electrical stimulation near dorsal raphe neurons can result in migrainelike headaches. There are projections from the dorsal raphe that terminate on cerebral arteries and alter cerebral blood flow. There are also major projections from the dorsal raphe to important visual processing way stations, including the lateral geniculate body, superior colliculus, retina, and visual cortex. These various projections are the anatomic and physiologic matrices for the circulatory and visual characteristics of migraine. The dorsal raphe cells stop firing during deep sleep, and sleep is known to ameliorate migraine; the antimigraine drugs also stop the firing of the dorsal raphe cells through a direct or indirect agonist effect (Figure 14-1). The shutdown of an inhibitory system might be expected to enhance or stabilize neurotransmission, and there is evidence that this indeed occurs.

Migraine may represent, therefore, a hereditary perturbation of serotonergic neurotransmission. Such perturbation may underlie many types of head pain; ordinary periodic headaches may be the "noise" of the normally functioning system.

Treatment   Several nonpharmacologic treatments have been advocated in recent years, but the most rigorously controlled trials have shown no benefit without concomitant drug treatment. Thus, the mainstay of therapy is the judicious use of one or more of the many drugs that are relatively specific for migraine.

ACUTE TREATMENT   In general, an adequate dose of whichever agent is chosen should be used at the onset of an attack. If additional medication is requested in 30 to 60 min because symptoms return or have not abated, the initial dose should be increased for subsequent attacks. Drug absorption is impaired during migrainous attacks because of reduced gastrointestinal motility. Delayed absorption occurs in the absence of nausea and is related to the severity of the attack and not its duration. Therefore, when oral agents fail, the major considerations revolve about rectal ergotamine, subcutaneous sumatriptan, parenteral dihydroergotamine, and intravenous chlorpromazine and prochlorperazine.

For patients with a prolonged buildup of headache, oral agents may indeed suffice. When aspirin and acetaminophen fail, the addition of butalbital and caffeine to these analgesics is highly effective; ibuprofen (600 to 800 mg) and naproxen (375 to 750 mg) are often useful. Isometheptene compound, 1 to 2 capsules, is effective for

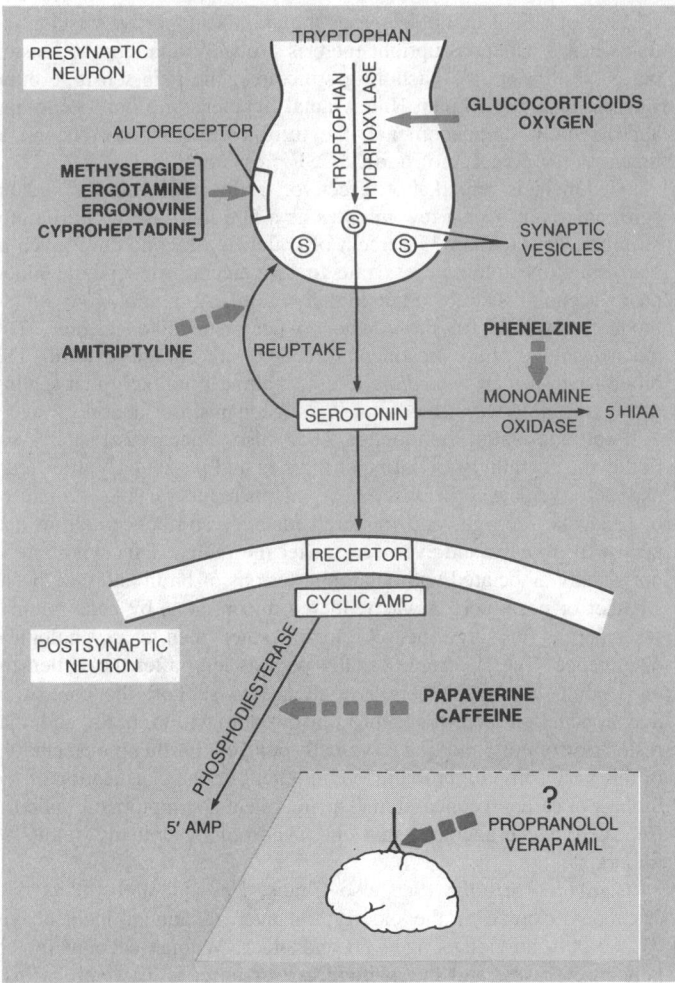

FIGURE 14-1 The actions of the antimigraine drugs at brainstem and forebrain synapses. The solid arrows indicate stimulative or agonist properties and the segmented arrows indicate inhibitory properties. (*From NH Raskin, Headache, 2d ed, New York, Churchill Livingstone, 1988.*)

mild-to-moderate "stress headaches." When these measures fail, more aggressive therapy should be considered.

A subnauseating dose of ergotamine, if possible, should be determined; a dose that provokes nausea—probably a centrally mediated side effect—is too high and may intensify head pain. The average oral dose is 3 mg (three 1-mg ergotamine-caffeine tablets); the average dose of the 2-mg suppository is one-half (1 mg). Many patients use one-quarter of a suppository (0.5 mg) with an optimal result. Sumatriptan may be given as an oral 100-mg dose or a 6-mg subcutaneous dose; there is a high recurrence rate because of the short half-life of this drug (2 h), so that a second dose may be necessary.

Dihydroergotamine is available presently only as a parenteral preparation. Peak plasma levels of dihydroergotamine are achieved 45 min after subcutaneous dosing, 30 min after intramuscular administration, and 3 min following intravenous dosing. If an attack has not already peaked, subcutaneous or intramuscular administration of 1 mg suffices for about 90 percent of patients. A common intravenous protocol is the mixture of prochlorperazine, 5 mg and 0.5 mg dihydroergotamine (they are miscible), administered over 2 min.

When patients' headache profiles transform into a chronic daily headache syndrome, opiate-type analgesics should be restricted to 2 days out of 7. The mainstay of therapy for these patients is daily amitriptyline (30 to 100 mg) or nortriptyline (40 to 120 mg). For recalcitrant individuals, valproate (500 to 2000 mg) or phenelzine (45 to 90 mg) may be necessary.

PROPHYLAXIS A substantial number of drugs are now available that have the capacity to stabilize migraine; they must be taken daily. When to implement this approach is contingent on the frequency of attacks and how well acute treatment is working. At least two or three attacks monthly could signal this approach. There is usually a lag of 2 weeks or so before an effect is seen, which may be the time necessary to down-regulate serotonin receptors. The major drugs and their daily dosage used in this setting are propranolol (60 to 240 mg), amitriptyline (30 to 100 mg), valproate (500 to 2000 mg), verapamil (120 to 480 mg), phenelzine (45 to 90 mg), and methysergide (4 to 12 mg). Phenelzine and methysergide are usually reserved for more recalcitrant patients because of serious potential side effects. Phenelzine is a monoamine oxidase inhibitor; therefore, tyramine-containing foods, decongestants, and meperidine are contraindicated. Methysergide may cause retroperitoneal or cardiac valvular fibrosis when it is used for more than 8 months, so monitoring is required for patients using this drug; the risk of the fibrotic complication is about 1:1500 and is likely to reverse after the drug is stopped.

The probability of success with any one of the antimigraine drugs is of the order of 60 to 75 percent; if one drug is assessed each month, there is the high likelihood that effective stabilization will be achieved within a few months. The large majority of patients are successfully managed with propranolol or amitriptyline; for more urgent resolution, valproate, methysergide, or phenelzine can be implemented. Once effective stabilization is achieved, the drug is continued for 5 to 6 months and then slowly tapered to assess its continued need. Many patients are able to discontinue medication and experience fewer and less severe attacks for long periods of time, suggesting that these drugs may alter the natural history of migraine.

CLUSTER HEADACHE Recognition of this clinical entity has been retarded by a variety of confusing names lent to this condition, including *Raeder's syndrome*, *histamine cephalalgia*, and *sphenopalatine neuralgia*. *Cluster headache* is now firmly established as a distinctive syndrome whose recognition is important since it is likely to be responsive to treatment. The episodic type, the most common, is characterized by one to three short-lived attacks of periorbital pain per day over a 4- to 8-week period, followed by a pain-free interval that averages 1 year. The chronic form, which may begin *de novo* or several years after an episodic pattern has become established, is characterized by the absence of sustained periods of remission. Each type may transform into the other. Men are affected more commonly than women in a proportion of 7–8:1; hereditary factors are usually absent. Although most patients begin experiencing headache between the ages of 20 and 50 years, the syndrome may begin as early as the first decade and as late as the eighth decade. The cluster syndrome is genetically, biochemically, and clinically different from migraine; propranolol and amitriptyline are largely ineffective. Lithium is beneficial for the cluster syndrome and ineffective in migraine. Nevertheless, the two disorders occasionally blend into one in occasional patients, suggesting that their mechanisms bear some degree of commonality.

Clinical features Periorbital, or less commonly, temporal pain begins without warning and reaches a crescendo within 5 min. It is often excruciating in intensity and is deep, nonfluctuating, and explosive in quality; only rarely is it pulsatile. Pain is strictly unilateral and usually affects the same side in subsequent months. Attacks last from 30 min to 2 h; there are often the associated symptoms of homolateral lacrimation, reddening of the eye, nasal stuffiness, lid ptosis, and nausea. Alcohol provocation of attacks occurs in about 70 percent of patients and ceases when the bout remits; this on-off vulnerability to alcohol is pathognomonic of the cluster headache syndrome. Only rarely do foods or emotional factors activate the mechanism, in contradistinction to migraine.

There is an uncanny periodicity of attacks in at least 85 percent of patients. At least one of the daily attacks of pain recurs at about the same hour each day for the duration of a cluster bout. This clock mechanism is set for the nocturnal hours in about 50 percent of the cases, and in such circumstances pain usually awakens patients within 2 h of falling asleep.

Pathogenesis There are no consistent cerebral blood flow changes attending attacks of pain. Perhaps the strongest evidence pointing to a central mechanism is the "periodicity"; reinforcing this conclusion is the observation that the autonomic symptoms that accompany the pain are bilateral, more severe on the painful side. The hypothalamus may be the site of activation in this disorder. The posterior hypothalamus contains cells that regulate autonomic functions and the anterior hypothalamus contains cells (the suprachiasmatic nuclei) that serve as the principal circadian pacemaker in mammals. Activation of both is necessary to explain the symptoms of cluster headache. The pacemaker is modulated serotonergically via dorsal raphe projections. The tentative conclusion may be reached that both migraine and cluster headache may result from abnormal serotonergic neurotransmission, albeit at different loci.

Treatment The most satisfactory treatment is the administration of drugs to prevent cluster attacks until the bout is over. The major prophylactic drugs are prednisone, lithium, methysergide, ergotamine, and verapamil. Lithium (600 to 900 mg daily) appears to be particularly effective for the chronic form of the disorder. A 10-day course of prednisone, beginning at 60 mg daily for 7 days and rapidly tapering, appears to actually curtail the mechanism of a bout for many patients. When ergotamine is implemented, it is most effective when given 1 to 2 h before an expected attack; for patients with a single nocturnal episode, 1 mg ergotamine in suppository formulation taken at bedtime may be all that is necessary. Patients must be educated regarding the early symptoms of ergotism when ergotamine is used daily; a weekly limit of 14 mg should be adhered to.

For the attacks themselves, oxygen inhalation (9 L/min via a tight mask) is the most effective modality; 15 min inhalation of 100 percent oxygen is often necessary. The self-administration of intranasal lidocaine, either 4% topical or 2% viscous, to the most caudal aspect of the inferior nasal turbinate can deliver a sphenopalatine ganglionic block that is usually remarkably effective for the termination of an attack. Sumatriptan, 6 mg subcutaneously, will usually shorten an attack to 10 to 15 min.

TENSION HEADACHE "Tension" headache is usually bilateral and occipitonuchal or bifrontal in localization. The sensation described by patients includes fullness, tightness, or pressure (as if the head is surrounded by a band or in a vise), on which waves of aching pain are superimposed. The onset of pain is more gradual than in classic migraine, but commonly a throbbing "vascular" type of headache is described. Tension headaches may occur acutely under conditions of emotional duress or intense worry and may last for hours or a day or two.

There is no evidence that the origin of the pain is sustained muscle activity. On the other hand, elicitation in some patients of headache after the administration of amyl nitrite, a vasodilator, or after histamine, indicates that there is a close link between tension headaches and migraine.

Treatment For the common everyday headache due to fatigue, acute stress, or excessive use of alcohol or tobacco, the physician may recommend therapy with aspirin, 0.6 g, or acetaminophen, 0.6 g given every 4 to 6 h. Chronic headaches falling into the common migraine or tension category are much more difficult to manage.

OTHER HEADACHE SYNDROMES **Lumbar puncture headache** Headache following lumbar puncture usually begins within 48 h but may be delayed for up to 12 days. Its mean incidence is about 30 percent. Head pain is dramatically positional; it begins when the patient sits or stands upright; there is relief upon reclining or with abdominal compression. The longer the patient is upright, the longer the latency before head pain subsides. It is worsened by head shaking and jugular vein compression. The pain is usually a dull ache, but may be throbbing; its location is occipitofrontal. Nausea and stiff neck often accompany headache, and occasional patients report blurred vision, photophobia, tinnitus, and vertigo. The symptoms resolve over a few days but may on occasion persist for weeks to months.

Loss of CSF volume decreases the brain's supportive cushion, so that when a patient is upright there is probably dilation and tension placed on the brain's anchoring structures, the pain-sensitive dural sinuses, resulting in pain. Intracranial hypotension often occurs but appears to be epiphenomenal; the full-blown syndrome occurs, at times, in the presence of normal CSF pressure.

Treatment is remarkably effective. Intravenous caffeine sodium benzoate given over a few minutes as a 500-mg dose will promptly terminate headache in 75 percent of patients; a second dose given in 1 h brings the total success rate to 85 percent. An epidural blood patch accomplished by injection of 15 mL of homologous whole blood rarely fails for those who do not respond to caffeine. The mechanism for these treatment effects is not straightforward. The blood patch has an *immediate* effect, making it unlikely that sealing off a dural hole with blood clot is its mechanism of action.

Postconcussion headaches (See also Chaps. 291 and 380) Following seemingly trivial head injuries and particularly after rear-end motor vehicle collisions, many patients report varying admixtures of headache, vertigo, and impaired memory and concentration that persist for months and even years after the injury. This syndrome is not usually associated with anatomic lesions of brain and may occur whether or not a person was rendered unconscious by head trauma. In general, this is a neurobiologic rather than a psychological disturbance. The syndrome usually persists long after the settlement of pending lawsuits. There is evidence to support the contention that concussion perturbs neurotransmission within brain and that restoration of this condition is typically delayed. Further understanding of this very common problem is contingent on the clarification of the biology of cerebral concussion. The treatment is symptomatic support. Repeated encouragement that the syndrome eventually remits is important.

Giant cell arteritis (See also Chaps. 291 and 380) This is a common disorder of the elderly; its average annual incidence is 77:100,000 individuals aged 50 and older. Women account for 65 percent of cases, and the average age of onset is 70 years, with a range of 50 to 85 years. The involvement of cranial arteries by an inflammatory process may result in blindness in 50 percent of patients if glucocorticoid treatment is not instituted; indeed, the ischemic optic neuropathy induced by giant cell arteritis is the major cause of rapidly developing bilateral blindness in the patient over 60 years of age.

The most common initial symptoms are headache, polymyalgia rheumatica, jaw claudication, fever, and weight loss (see Chap. 291). Headache is the dominant symptom and often appears in a setting of malaise and muscle aches. Head pain may be unilateral or bilateral and is located temporally in 50 percent of patients but may involve any and all aspects of the cranium. Pain usually appears gradually over a few hours before peak intensity is reached; occasionally, it is explosive in onset. The quality of pain is only seldom throbbing; it is almost invariably described as dull and boring with superimposed episodic ice picklike lancinating pains similar to the sharp pains that appear in migraine. Most patients can recognize that the origin of their head pain is superficial, external to the skull, rather than originating deep within the cranium (the pain site for migraineurs). Scalp tenderness is present, often to a marked degree; brushing the hair or resting the head on a pillow may be impossible because of pain. Headache is usually worse at night and is often aggravated by exposure to cold. Reddened, tender nodules or red streaking of the skin overlying the temporal arteries is found in highest frequency in patients with headache, as is tenderness of the temporal, or less commonly, the occipital arteries. Curiously, temporal artery biopsy not infrequently coincides with the cessation of headache.

The erythrocyte sedimentation rate (ESR) is often but not always elevated; a normal ESR does not exclude giant cell arteritis. A temporal artery biopsy and the initiation of prednisone at 80 mg daily for the first 4 to 6 weeks should be instituted when clinical suspicion is high. Patients with migraine often report amelioration of their headaches with prednisone so that one must be cautious about interpreting the therapeutic response. Contrary to widespread notions, the prevalence of migraine among the elderly is substantial, considerably higher than giant cell arteritis.

Cough headache One of the male-dominated (4:1) syndromes, it is characterized by transient, severe head pain upon coughing, bending, lifting, sneezing, or stooping. Head pain persists for seconds to a few minutes. Many patients date the origins of the syndrome to a lower respiratory infection accompanied by severe coughing or to strenuous weight-lifting programs. Headache is usually diffuse but is lateralized in about one-third of patients. The incidence of serious intracranial structural anomalies causing this condition is about 25 percent; the Arnold-Chiari malformation is a common cause. Magnetic resonance imaging is indicated for most of these patients. The benign disorder may persist for a few years; it is inexplicably and remarkably ameliorated by indomethacin at doses ranging from 50 to 200 mg daily.

Many patients with migraine note that attacks of headache may be provoked by *sustained* physical exertion, such as during the third mile of a 5-mile run. Such headaches build up over hours, distinctly different from the cough headache syndrome. The term *effort migraine* has been used for this syndrome to avoid the ambiguous term *exertional headache*.

Coital headache Another male-dominated (4:1) syndrome, attacks occur periorgasmically, are very abrupt in onset, and subside in a few minutes if coitus is interrupted. These are nearly always benign events and usually occur sporadically; if they persist for hours or are accompanied by vomiting, subarachnoid hemorrhage must be excluded through a CSF examination and CT scanning.

Brain tumor headache About 30 percent of patients with brain tumors consider headache to be their chief complaint. The head pain syndrome is nondescript; a deep, dull aching quality, of moderate intensity, occurs intermittently, is worsened by exertion or change in position, and is associated with nausea and vomiting. This pattern of symptoms results from migraine far more often than from brain tumor. Headache disturbs sleep in about 10 percent of patients. Vomiting that precedes the appearance of headache by weeks is highly characteristic of posterior fossa brain tumors.

Headache caused by systemic illness There is hardly any illness that is never manifested by headache; however, some illnesses are *characteristically* associated with headache. These include infectious mononucleosis, systemic lupus erythematosus, chronic pulmonary failure with hypercapnia (early morning headaches), Hashimoto's thyroiditis, glucocorticoid withdrawal, oral contraceptives, ovulation-promoting medications, inflammatory bowel disease, many of the HIV-associated illnesses, and the acute blood pressure elevations that occur in pheochromocytoma and in malignant hypertension. The last two examples are the exceptions to the generalization that hypertension per se is a very uncommon cause of headache; diastolic pressures of at least 120 mmHg are requisite for hypertension to cause headache.

APPROACH TO THE PATIENT WITH HEADACHE Entirely different diagnostic possibilities are raised by a patient who presents with the first severe headache ever and a patient who has had recurrent headache over many years. In the first instance, the probability of finding a potentially serious cause is considerably greater than in the second; some of the causes that should be considered include meningitis, subarachnoid hemorrhage, epidural or subdural hematoma, glaucoma, and purulent sinusitis. In general, acute, severe headache with stiff neck and fever means meningitis and without fever means subarachnoid hemorrhage; when confronted with such a patient, lumbar puncture is mandatory. Acute persistent headache and fever is often the manifestation of an acute systemic viral infection; if the neck is supple in such a patient, lumbar puncture may be deferred. There is always the possibility of a first attack of migraine, but fever would be a rare associated feature.

When the signature of migraine has not clarified the cause of recurring headache, one should consider the investigation of cardiovascular and renal status by blood pressure and urine examination; eyes by fundoscopy, intraocular pressure measurement and refraction; the cranial arteries by palpation; the cervical spine by the effect of passive movement of the head and imaging; and the nervous system by neurologic and psychological evaluation.

The adolescent with chronic daily frontal or holocephalic headache represents a special type of problem. Extensive diagnostic batteries are most often unrevealing, including the psychiatric assessment. Fortunately, the headaches tend to stop after a few years so that structured analgesic support can enable these teenagers to move through secondary school and enter college. By the time they reach the late teens, the cycle has usually ended.

The relationship of head pain to depression is not straightforward. Many patients in chronic daily pain cycles become depressed, a not unreasonable sequence of events; moreover, there is a greater-than-chance coincidence of migraine with both bipolar (manic depressive) and unipolar depressive disorders. Studies of large populations of depressed patients do not reveal headache prevalence rates that are different from the general population. The physician should be cautious about assigning depression as the cause of recurring headache; drugs with antidepressant actions are effective in migraine also.

Finally, a note on recurring headache that may be pain-driven. Temporomandibular joint dysfunction is an example; in general, it produces preauricular pain that is associated with chewing food. The pain may radiate to the head but is not easily confused with headache per se. On the other hand, headache-prone patients may observe that headaches are more frequent and severe in the presence of a painful temporomandibular joint problem. Similarly, headache disorders may be activated by the pain attending otological or endodontic surgical procedures. Treatment of the headache problem is largely ineffectual until the cause of the primary pain problem is dealt with. Thus pain about the head as the result of somatic disease or trauma may reawaken an otherwise quiescent migrainous mechanism.

REFERENCES

BICKERSTAFF ER: Basilar artery migraine. Lancet 1:15, 1961

BLAU JN: Migraine: Theories of pathogenosis. Lancet: 339:1202, 1992.

BOLES DB: Visual field effects of classical migraine. Brain Cogn 21:181, 1993

COUCH JR: Headache to worry about. Med Clin North Am 77:141, 1993

DECHANT KL, CLISSOLD SP: Sumatriptan. Drugs 43:776, 1992

GOADSBY PJ, EDVINSSON L: The trigeminovascular system and migraine—Studies characterizing cerebrovascular and neuropeptide changes seen in humans and cats. Ann Neurol 33:48, 1993

GOADSBY PJ, GUNDLACH AL: Localization of ³H-dihydroergotamine-binding sites in the cat central nervous system: Relevance to migraine. Ann Neurol 29:91, 1991

HARDEBO JE: Subcutaneous sumatriptan in cluster headache—A time study of the effect on pain and autonomic symptoms. Headache 33:18, 1993

HUGHES RL: Identification and treatment of cerebral aneurysms after sentinel headache. Neurology 42:1118, 1992

JENSEN R et al: Muscle tenderness and pressure pain thresholds in headache—A population study. Pain 52:193 1993

JOHNS D: Benign sexual headache within a family. Arch Neurol 43:1158, 1986

LANCE JW: *Mechanism and Management of Headache*, 5th ed. London, Butterworth Scientific, 1993

———: Headaches related to sexual activity. J Neurol Neurosurg Psychiatry 39:1226, 1976

MOSKOWITZ MA et al: Pain mechanisms underlying vascular headaches. Rev Neurol (Paris) 145:181, 1989

OLESEN J: Cerebral and extracranial circulatory disturbances in migraine: Pathophysiological implications. Cerebrovasc Brain Metab Rev 3:1, 1991

RANDO TA, FISHMAN RA: Spontaneous intracranial hypotension. Neurology 42:481, 1992

RASKIN NH: Pharmacology of migraine. Prog Drug Res 34:209, 1990

———: Lumbar puncture headache:. A review. Headache 30:197, 1990

———: *Headache*, 2d ed. New York, Churchill Livingstone, 1988

RASMUSSEN BK, OLESEN J: Symptomatic and nonsymptomatic headaches in a general population. Neurology 42:1225, 1991

SJAASTAD O: *Cluster Headache Syndrome*. London, Saunders, 1992

STANG PE et al: Incidence of migraine headache: A population-based study in Olmsted County, Minnesota. Neurology 42:1657, 1992.

VINKEN PJ, BRUYN GW, KLAWANS HL (eds): *Handbook of Clinical Neurology*, vol 48: Headache. Amsterdam, Elsevier Science, 1986

15 BACK AND NECK PAIN

HENRY J. MANKIN / LAWRENCE F. BORGES

ANATOMY AND PHYSIOLOGY OF THE LOWER PART OF THE BACK

The bony spine is anatomically divisible into two parts. The *anterior* part consists of a series of cylindrical vertebral bodies connected to one another by the intervertebral disks and held tightly together by the anterior and posterior longitudinal ligaments. The *posterior* part consists of more delicate elements that extend from the vertebral body as pedicles and broaden posteriorly to form laminae, which together with ligamentous structures form the vertebral canal. The posterior elements are joined to adjacent vertebrae by two small facetal synovial joints which allow a modest degree of motion between any two segments but in aggregate produce a rather extensive range (Fig. 15-1). Stout transverse and spinous bony processes project laterally and posteriorly and serve as the attachments of muscles which move, support, and protect the vertebral column. The stability of the spine depends on two types of support: that provided by the bony articulations (principally by the diskal joints and the synovial articulations of the posterior elements) and a second type provided by the ligamentous (passive) and muscular (active) supporting structures. The ligamentous structures are quite strong, but because neither they nor the vertebral body–disk complexes have sufficient integral strength to resist the enormous forces acting on the column during even simple movements, voluntary and reflex contractions of the sacrospinalis, abdominal, gluteal, psoas, and hamstring muscles afford much of the stability.

The vertebral and paravertebral structures are innervated by branches of the segmental spinal nerves that exit the neural foramina at each spinal level. The sinuvertebral nerve, which is considered the major sensory nerve supply to the structures of the lumbar spine, arises from the spinal nerve prior to its division into an anterior and posterior ramus. The sinuvertebral nerve reenters the spinal canal through the intervertebral foramen to provide sensory innervation to the posterior longitudinal ligament, external portions of the posterior annulus fibrosus, anterior dura, dura of the nerve root sleeve, and epidural veins, all within the spinal canal. The other major nerve supply to the spinal and paraspinal structures arises from the posterior primary ramus. The posterior primary ramus of the spinal nerve further divides into medial and lateral branches. Together these nerves supply the posterior parts of the spine, including the facet joints, as well as the paraspinal muscles and fascia. In addition, the upper three lumbar spinal nerves provide cutaneous sensation to the skin of the low back.

FIGURE 15-1 *Left:* Superior view of a stripped lumbar vertebra. *Right:* Lateral view of two articulated lumbar vertebrae. B = body; SC = spinal canal; IVF = intervertebral foramen; IF = inferior articular facet; SF = superior articular facet; P = pedicle; TP = transverse process; SP = spinous process; L = lamina. *(Adapted from DB Levine, in Arthritis and Allied Conditions: A Textbook of Rheumatology, 10th ed, DJ McCarty (ed). Philadelphia, Lea & Febiger, 1985.)*

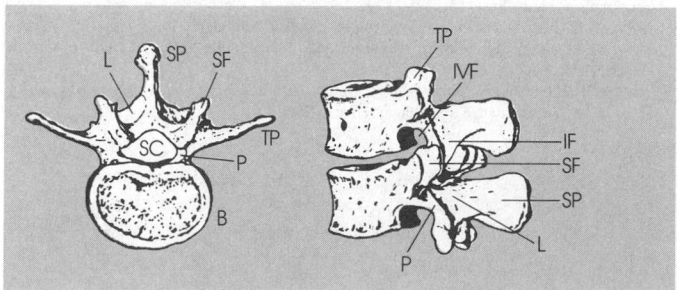

The parts of the back that possess the greatest freedom of movement, and hence are most frequently subject to injury, are the lumbar and cervical regions. In addition to the voluntary motions required for bending, twisting, and other movements, many actions of the spine are reflex in nature and are the basis of posture.

GENERAL CLINICAL CONSIDERATIONS

TYPES OF LOW BACK PAIN Four types of pain may be differentiated: local, referred, radicular, and that arising from secondary (protective) muscular spasm.

Local pain is caused by any pathologic process that impinges on or irritates sensory endings. Involvement of structures that contain no sensory endings is painless. The central, medullary portion of the vertebral body may be destroyed by tumor, for example, without evocation of pain, whereas cortical fractures or tears and distortions of the periosteum, synovial membranes, muscles, annulus fibrosus, and ligaments are often exquisitely painful. The latter structures are innervated by afferent fibers of the posterior primary rami and the sinuvertebral nerve. Although painful states are often accompanied by swelling of the affected tissues, this may not be apparent if a deep structure of the back is the site of disease. Local pain is often described as steady but may be intermittent, varying considerably with position or activity. The pain may be sharp or dull and although often diffuse is always felt in or near the affected part of the spine. Reflex splinting of the spine segments by paravertebral muscles is frequently noted and may produce deformity or postural abnormality. Certain movements or postures that alter the position of the injured tissues aggravate the pain. Firm pressure or percussion on superficial structures in the region involved usually evokes tenderness, which is of aid in identifying the site of the abnormality.

Referred pain is of two types: that projected from the spine into regions lying within the area of the lumbar and upper sacral dermatomes and that projected from the pelvic and abdominal viscera to the spine. Pain due to diseases of the upper part of the lumbar spine is usually referred to the anterior aspects of the thighs and legs; that from the lower lumbar and sacral segments is referred to the gluteal regions, posterior thighs, calves, and sometimes feet. Pain of this type, although of deep, aching quality and rather diffuse, tends at times to be superficially projected. In general, the referred pain parallels in intensity the local pain in the back. In other words, maneuvers that alter local pain have a similar effect on referred pain, though not with such precision and immediacy as in radicular, or "root," pain. Referred pain may be confused with pain from visceral disease, but the latter is usually described as "deep" and tends to radiate from the abdomen through to the back. Also, visceral pain is usually unaffected by movement of the spine, does not improve with recumbency, and may be modified by the activity of the involved viscus. An important exception to this is pain caused by an aortic aneurysm. A slowly enlarging aortic aneurysm may erode the anterolateral spine and produce discomfort that changes with movement or recumbency.

Radicular, or "root," *pain* has some of the characteristics of referred pain but differs in its greater intensity, distal radiation, circumscription to the territory of a root, and the factors which excite it (Table 15-1). The mechanisms are principally distortion, stretching, irritation, and compression of a spinal root, most often central to the intervertebral foramen. In addition, it has been suggested that in patients with spinal stenosis the "lumbar claudication" pattern may be due to a relative ischemia associated with compression. Although the pain itself is often dull or aching, various maneuvers which increase the irritation of the root or stretch it may greatly intensify the pain, eliciting a lancinating quality. Nearly always the radiation of pain is from a central position near the spine to some part of the lower extremity. Cough, sneeze, and strain are characteristic evocative maneuvers, but since they may also jar or move the spine, they may aggravate local pain as well. Forward bending with the knees extended

TABLE 15-1 Anatomic localization of pain referred by lumbar and sacral roots

Root	Region
L1, L5	Inguinal
L2	Lateral thigh
L2, L3	Anterior thigh
L3	Knee
L4	Anterior shin
L5, S1	Lateral calf
L5, S1	Posterior calf
L5	Dorsum of foot
S1	Heel
S1	Lateral foot
L5 ganglion	Anterior leg/foot

or "straight-leg raising" in disease of the lower part of the lumbar spine excites radicular pain on the basis of stretch; jugular vein compression, which raises intraspinal pressure and may cause a shift in the position of or pressure on the root, may have a similar effect. Irritation of the fourth and fifth lumbar and first sacral roots, which form the sciatic nerve, causes pain that extends mainly down the posterior aspects of the thigh and the posterior and lateral aspects of the leg. Typically, this pain radiation—which is termed *sciatica*—stops at the ankle and is associated with sensations of tingling or numbness—*paresthesias*—that radiate more distally into the foot. Tingling, paresthesias, and numbness or sensory impairment of the skin, soreness of the skin, and tenderness along the nerve also may accompany classic sciatic pain, and on physical examination, reflex loss, weakness, atrophy, fascicular twitching, and occasionally stasis edema may occur if the motor fibers of the anterior root are involved.

Pain resulting from muscular spasm is usually mentioned in relation to local pain, but the anatomic or physiologic basis is more obscure. Muscle spasm associated with many disorders of the spine can produce significant distortions of the normal posture; as a result, chronic tension in muscles may give rise to a dull and sometimes cramping ache. In this instance, one can feel the tautness of the sacrospinalis and gluteal muscles and demonstrate by palpation that the pain is localized to these structures.

Other pains often of undetermined origin are sometimes described by patients with chronic disease of the lower part of the back. Unilateral symptoms of drawing, pulling, cramping sensations (without involuntary muscle spasm), tearing, throbbing, or jabbing pains, or feelings of burning or coldness are difficult to interpret but, like paresthesias and numbness, should always suggest the possibility of nerve or root disease.

In addition to assessing the character and location of the pain, one should determine the factors that aggravate and relieve it, its constancy, and its relationship to recumbency and such stereotypical movements and maneuvers as forward bending, cough, sneeze, and strain. Frequently, the most important lead comes from the knowledge of the mode of onset and circumstances that initiated the pain. It cannot be overemphasized that a careful history provides the cornerstone of an accurate diagnosis. Inasmuch as many painful afflictions of the back are the result of injury incurred during work or in an accident, the possibility of exaggeration or prolongation of pain for purposes of compensation or other personal reasons, or because of hysteria or malingering, must always be kept in mind.

EXAMINATION OF THE LOWER PART OF THE BACK

Inspection of the normal spine shows a dorsal kyphosis and lumbar lordosis in the sagittal plane, which in some individuals may be exaggerated (swayback). Patients with spinal disorders may demonstrate excessive curvature, flattening of the normal lumbar arch, presence of a gibbus (a short, sharp, kyphotic angulation usually indicative of a fracture or congenital abnormality), lateral curvature

and/or rotation (scoliosis), pelvic tilt or obliquity, or asymmetry of the paravertebral or gluteal musculature. In severe sciatica, one may observe that the affected limb is held with the hip and knee flexed, presumably to reduce tension on the irritated part.

The spine, hips, and legs should be observed during certain motions, but no advantage accrues from trying to find out how much pain the patient can endure. It is more important to assess when and under what conditions the pain commences. Normally, the motion of forward bending produces flattening and reversal of the lumbar lordotic curve and exaggeration of the dorsal curve. With ruptured lumbar disks or lesions that involve the posterior ligaments, articular facets, or sacrospinalis muscle, protective reflexes prevent stretching of these structures; as a consequence, the sacrospinalis muscles remain taut and limit motion in the lumbar part of the spine, causing forward bending to occur at the hips and at the lumbar-thoracic junction. With disease principally affecting the spinal roots or the lumbosacral joints, forward bending occurs in such a way as to avoid tensing the hamstring muscles, which puts undue leverage on the pelvis. In unilateral "sciatica," with its increased curvature toward the side of the lesion, the lumbar and lumbosacral motions are splinted, and bending is mainly at the hips; at a certain point the knee on the affected side is flexed to relieve hamstring spasm, and tilting of the pelvis occurs to slacken the lumbosacral roots and sciatic nerve.

With lumbosacral lesions and sciatica, passive lumbar flexion in the supine position causes little pain and is not limited as long as the hamstrings are relaxed and the sciatic nerve is not stretched. With lumbosacral and lumbar spine disease (e.g., arthritis), passive flexion of the hips is free, whereas flexion of the lumbar spine may be impeded and painful. Passive straight-leg raising (possible in most normal individuals up to 80 to 90° except in those who have unusually tight hamstrings), like forward bending with the knees extended in the standing posture, places the sciatic nerve and its roots under tension, thereby producing pain. It also may cause an anterior rotation of the pelvis around a transverse axis, increasing stress on the lumbosacral joint, and thus causing pain if this segment is arthritic or otherwise impaired. Consequently, in diseases of the lumbosacral joints and lumbosacral roots, this movement is limited on the affected side and to a lesser extent on the opposite side. Evocation of such a response (pain and limitation of movement during flexion of the hip when the knee is extended) is known as *Lasègue's sign* and is considered to be a useful test of this condition. Straight-leg raising also may be tested by having the patient extend the knee while seated. This maneuver produces the same extent of sciatic nerve stretch as the Lasègue sign but does not stress the lumbosacral joint and thus may identify true nerve root irritation more accurately. A positive contralateral straight-leg raising sign is believed by some to be a sign of a more extensive lesion, such as an extruded disk fragment in the axilla of the nerve, rather than a simple prolapse or protrusion. It is important to remember, however, that the evoked pain is always referred to the diseased side, no matter which leg is flexed.

Hyperextension is best evaluated with the patient standing or lying prone. If the condition causing back pain is acute, it may be difficult to extend the spine in the standing position. A patient with lumbosacral strain or disk disease can usually extend or hyperextend the spine without aggravation of pain. If the lesion is in the upper lumbar segments or if an active inflammatory process, fracture of the vertebral body, or a very tight canal (vertebral stenosis) is present, hyperextension may be markedly limited.

Palpation and percussion of the spine are the last steps in the examination. It is preferable to palpate first those regions which are the least likely to evoke pain. At all times the examiner should know what structures are being palpated (see Fig. 15-2). Localized tenderness is seldom pronounced in disease of the spine because the involved structures are so deep that they rarely give rise to surface tenderness. However, spinal disease may give rise to intense spasm in the paraspinal muscles which could result in local tenderness. Mild superficial and poorly localized tenderness signifies only a disease process within the affected segment of the body, i.e., dermatome.

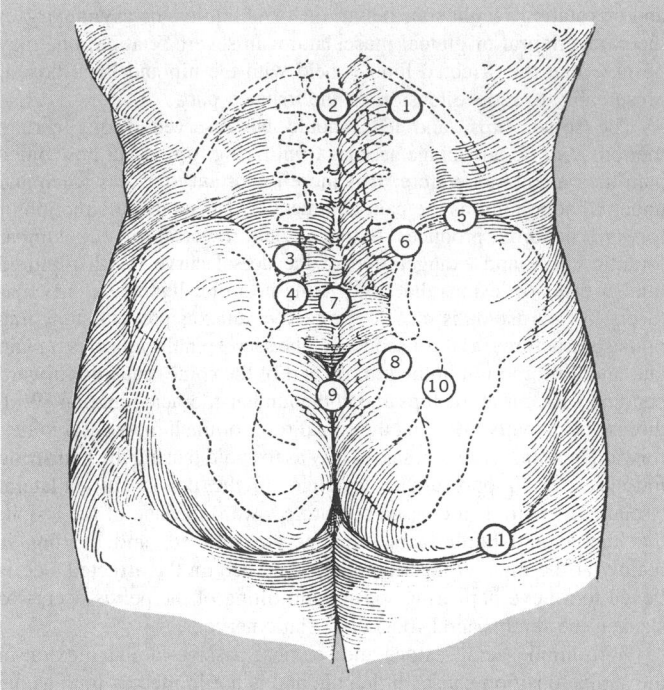

FIGURE 15-2 (1) Costovertebral angle. (2) Spinous process and interspinous ligament. (3) Region of the articular fifth lumbar to the first sacral facet. (4) Dorsum of sacrum. (5) Region of iliac crest. (6) Iliolumbar angle. (7) Spinous processes of fifth lumbar to first sacral vertebrae (tenderness = faulty posture or occasionally spina bifida occulta). (8) Region between posterior superior and posterior inferior spines. Sacroiliac ligaments (tenderness = sacroiliac sprain, often tender with fifth lumbar to first sacral disk). (9) Sacrococcygeal junction (tenderness = sacrococcygeal injury, i.e., sprain or fracture). (10) Region of sacrosciatic notch (tenderness = fourth to fifth lumbar disk rupture and sacroiliac sprain). (11) Sciatic nerve trunk (tenderness = ruptured lumbar disk or sciatic nerve lesion).

Tenderness over the costovertebral angle often indicates renal disease, adrenal disease, or an injury to the transverse processes of the first or second lumbar vertebra. Hypersensitivity on palpation of the transverse processes of the other lumbar vertebrae as well as the overlying sacrospinalis muscles may signify fracture of the transverse process or a strain of muscle attachments. Tenderness of a spinous process or aggravation of pain by the jarring of gentle percussion may be nonspecific but frequently indicates the presence of a disk lesion at the site deep to it, inflammation (as in disk space infection), or fracture. Tenderness in the region of the articular facets between the fifth lumbar and first sacral vertebrae is consistent with disease of a lumbosacral disk (Fig. 15-2). It is also frequent in rheumatoid arthritis.

In palpation of the spinous processes, it is important to note any deviation in the lateral plane (this may be indicative of fracture or arthritis) or in the anteroposterior plane. A "step-off" forward displacement of the spinous process may be an important clue to the presence of a spondylolisthesis one segment below the displaced level.

Abdominal, rectal, and pelvic examination and assessment of the status of the peripheral vascular system are important parts of the examination of the patient with complaints in the lower back and should not be omitted. They may provide evidence for vascular, visceral, neoplastic, or inflammatory disorders which may extend to the spine or cause pain to be referred to this region. Finally, a careful neurologic examination should be performed, with special attention given to motor, reflex, and sensory changes, particularly in the lower extremities. It is especially important when performing the neurologic examination to attempt to identify a pattern of nerve root involvement.

Table 15-2 correlates the motor and reflex components of each of the lumbar roots. It is important to note that isolated lesions of the L2 root do not usually cause identifiable weakness on examination. The L2 root provides innervation to the thigh adductors. However, dysfunction of more than just the L2 root is usually necessary to produce actual weakness in these muscles (see "Protrusion of Lumbar Intervertebral Disks," below).

SPECIAL LABORATORY PROCEDURES Useful laboratory tests, depending on the nature of the problem and the circumstances, include a complete blood count, erythrocyte sedimentation rate (especially helpful in screening for infection or myeloma), measurement of serum calcium, phosphorus, alkaline phosphatase, acid phosphatase, prostate-specific antigen (see Chap. 323) (the last two mentioned are of importance if one suspects metastatic carcinoma from the prostate), serum immunoelectrophoresis, and tests for rheumatoid factor. Roentgenograms of the lumbar part of the spine in the anteroposterior, lateral, and oblique planes should be obtained in every patient with low back pain and sciatica. Special spot views or stereoscopic or laminographic films may provide further information in certain cases. Bone scans are of particular aid in revealing some fractures and neoplastic and inflammatory lesions.

The most sensitive noninvasive imaging modality for examining the spine and paraspinal tissues is magnetic resonance imaging (MRI). Standard MRI scans are performed in the sagittal and axial planes. They provide remarkable anatomic detail of the vertebral bodies, disks, spinal canal, nerve roots, spinal cord, and paraspinal soft tissues. The high-field-strength instruments (1.5 T) often provide more detailed images of the spine than do the lower-field-strength instruments. In select instances, intravenous contrast (gadolinium) may allow additional anatomic details to be visualized (see Chap. 365). Initial MRI scans of the spine should be done without contrast infusion. This is particularly important when the scan is being performed to assess for metastatic disease in the spine. In this situation, contrast medium may actually obscure the difference between tumor tissue and normal vertebral body. Several important caveats surround the use of MRI scans. MRI does not provide an accurate assessment of bone detail in the spine. Computed tomography (CT) is a superior method of evaluating details of spinal bone structure and would be the preferred method of identifying a subtle fracture. Furthermore, MRI scans are so sensitive that they often reveal anatomic abnormalities that are clinically meaningless. Therefore, the data derived from an MRI scan *must* be interpreted by an experienced clinician who also has evaluated the patient's clinical problem.

Despite the sensitivity of the MRI scan, examination of the spinal canal with a contrast medium—myelography—continues to be important, particularly in the assessment of benign degenerative disease of the spine. When a myelogram is performed, a sample of cerebrospinal fluid should always be removed for cytologic and chemical examination prior to the instillation of the contrast medium. Except for special circumstances, a water-soluble contrast medium should be used for myelography. Water-soluble contrast medium is less irritating to the neural structures, is associated with a lower incidence of arachnoiditis, and does not have to be removed from the subarachnoid space because it is systemically absorbed and excreted by the kidneys. In addition, myelography should always include CT

TABLE 15-2 Motor examination of lumbar and sacral roots

Root	Muscle	Reflex
L1	—	—
L2	—	—
L3	Quadriceps, iliopsoas	Knee absent
L4	Anterior tibialis	Knee reduced
L5	EHL,* EDB†	—
S1	Foot evertors, gastrocnemius	Ankle reduced

* EHL = extensor hallicus longus.
† EDB = extensor digitorum brevis.

scanning of the affected area of the spine. CT/myelography can often provide the best definition of subtle compression of nerve roots by herniated disks or osteophytes.

Injection of contrast medium directly into the intervertebral disk (diskograms) has waxed and waned in popularity over the years and remains controversial. The technique of this procedure is more complicated than that of CT/myelography and carries a risk of infection of the disk.

Confirmation of proximal motor and sensory nerve and root disease can be obtained by nerve conduction studies, H and F responses, and electromyography (see Chap. 382).

PRINCIPAL CONDITIONS THAT GIVE RISE TO DISABLING PAIN IN THE LOWER PART OF THE BACK

CONGENITAL ANOMALIES OF THE LUMBAR SPINE One of the most common disorders is a failure of fusion of the laminae of the neural arch (spina bifida) of one or several of the lumbar vertebrae or of the sacrum. Hypertrichosis or hyperpigmentation in the sacral area may betray the condition, but in most patients the spine defect remains entirely occult until disclosed by x-ray. The anomaly has greater potential for causing pain if accompanied by malformation of vertebral joints, and usually the pain is induced by injury. Other congenital anomalies that affect the lower lumbar vertebrae, such as asymmetric facetal joints, abnormalities of the transverse processes, sacralization of the fifth lumbar vertebra (in which L5 is firmly fixed to the sacrum), or lumbarization of the first sacral vertebra (in which the first sacral segment resembles a sixth lumbar), are rarely the cause of specific symptomatology.

Spondylolysis consists of a bony defect probably caused by trauma to a congenitally abnormal segment in the pars interarticularis (a segment near the junction of the pedicle with the lamina) of the lower lumbar area. The defect is best visualized on oblique projections or with CT. In some individuals the defect is bilateral. In the circumstance of either a single injury or repeated minor injuries, the vertebral body, pedicles, and superior articular facets slip anteriorly, leaving the posterior elements behind. This latter abnormality, known as *spondylolisthesis*, more often results in symptoms, often proportional to the degree of forward slip. The patient may complain of pain in the low back radiating into the thighs, and a limitation of motion may be noted. Often tenderness is elicited near the segment which has "slipped" forward (most often L5 on S1 or occasionally L4 on L5), and one can feel a "step" on deep palpation of the posterior elements of the segment above the spondylolisthetic joint. In moderately severe displacements the pelvis is sometimes rotated and hip flexion limited by hamstring spasm. A variety of usually minor neurologic deficits indicative of radiculopathy may be present. In exceptionally severe degrees of spondylolisthesis the trunk may be shortened and the abdomen protuberant, both the result of the extreme forward displacement of L5 on S1.

TRAUMATIC AFFLICTIONS OF THE LOWER PART OF THE BACK Trauma constitutes the most frequent cause of acute low back pain, and such injured patients should be evaluated very carefully. In severe acute injuries that involve fracture or dislocation of the vertebral segments, the examining physician must be careful to avoid further damage, particularly to the neural structures. Tests of mobility and forceful manipulations should be avoided until a diagnosis has been made and adequate measures have been instituted for the proper care of the patient. A patient complaining of back pain and inability to move the legs may have a fractured spine. The neck should not be flexed, nor should the patient be allowed to sit up. (See Chap. 381 for further discussion of spinal cord injury.)

Sprains, strains, and derangements The terms lumbosacral *sprain* and *strain* are often used loosely by patients and their physicians and do not clearly relate to a known anatomic lesion. The authors prefer the term *low back derangement* or *strain* for minor, self-limited injuries usually associated with lifting a heavy object, a fall, or a sudden deceleration, as may occur in an automobile accident. Occasionally, these syndromes are more chronic in nature, suggesting that diskal or arthritic factors may play a role. The patients with low back derangement are often acutely discomfited and may assume unusual postures related to spasm of the sacrospinalis muscles. The pain is usually confined to the lower back and is usually relieved by rest and analgesic medication within a few days. More extensive or longer-lasting problems, formerly classified as sacroiliac strain or sprain, are now known to be due in most instances to disk disease (see below).

Vertebral fractures Most fractures of the lumbar vertebral body result from flexion injuries and consist of anterior wedging or compression. With more severe trauma the patient may sustain a fracture dislocation, "bursting" fracture, or asymmetric fracture involving not only the body but the posterior elements as well. The initiating trauma which causes fractures of the vertebrae is usually a fall from a height (in which case the calcanei also may be fractured), sudden deceleration in an automobile accident, or other major violence. When fractures occur with minimal trauma (or even spontaneously), the bone is presumed to have been previously weakened by some pathologic process. Most of the time, particularly in older individuals, the cause of such an event is senile or postmenopausal osteoporosis (see Chap. 358), but there may be other underlying systemic disorders such as osteomalacia, hyperparathyroidism, hyperthyroidism, multiple myeloma, metastatic carcinoma, and a large number of local conditions that may play a role in weakening the vertebral body. Spasm of the lumbar muscles, limitation of motion of the lumbar segments, and the roentgenographic appearance of the damaged vertebra (with or without neurologic abnormalities) are the basis for the clinical diagnosis. The pain is usually immediate, though occasionally it may be delayed in onset for a few days, and the patient may develop a mild paralytic ileus or urinary retention during the acute period.

Fractures of the transverse processes are almost always associated with severe injury to the paravertebral muscles, principally the psoas. A significant retroperitoneal hemorrhage may be present (identified on CT or MRI) which can result in a marked depression in the hematocrit and, in extensive fractures, hypovolemic shock. Such injuries may be diagnosed by the finding of deep tenderness at the site of the injury, local muscle spasm on one side, and limitation of all movements which stretch the lumbar muscles. Radiologic evidence (especially CT or MRI) provides the final confirmation. Fractures of multiple transverse processes, although seemingly trivial, should be the object of considerable concern, and the patient should be carefully watched for internal hemorrhage.

Protrusion of lumbar intervertebral disks This condition is the major cause of severe chronic or recurrent low back and leg pain. It is most likely to occur between the fifth lumbar and first sacral vertebrae and, with lessening frequency, between the fourth and fifth lumbar, the third and fourth lumbar, the second and third lumbar, and, rarely, between the first and second lumbar vertebrae. Rare in the thoracic portion of the spine, it is next most frequent between the sixth and seventh and fifth and sixth cervical vertebrae. The cause is usually a flexion injury, but in many cases no trauma is recalled. Degeneration of the posterior longitudinal ligaments and the annulus fibrosus, which occurs in most adults of middle and advanced years, may have taken place silently or have been manifested by mild, recurrent lumbar ache. A sneeze, lurch, or other trivial movement may then cause the nucleus pulposus to prolapse, pushing the frayed and weakened annulus posteriorly. In more severe cases of disk disease, the nucleus may protrude through the annulus or become extruded to lie as a free fragment in the vertebral canal.

The fully developed syndrome of ruptured lumbar intervertebral disk consists of backache, abnormal posture, and limitation of motion of the spine (particularly flexion). Nerve root involvement is indicated by radicular pain, sensory disturbances (paresthesias, hyper- and hyposensitivity in dermatome pattern), coarse twitching and fasciculation, muscle spasms, and impairment of a tendon reflex. Motor abnormalities (weakness and muscle atrophy) also may occur but are usually less prominent than the pain and sensory disorder. Since herniation of the intervertebral lumbar disks most often occurs between the fourth and fifth lumbar vertebrae and the fifth lumbar and first sacral vertebrae with irritation and compression of the fifth lumbar and first sacral roots, respectively, it is important to recognize the clinical characteristics of lesions of these two roots. *Lesions of the fifth lumbar root* produce pain in the region of the hip, groin, posterolateral thigh, lateral calf to the external malleolus, dorsal surface of the foot, and the first or second and third toes. Paresthesias may be in the entire territory or in only the distal parts of these territories. The tenderness is in the lateral gluteal region and near the head of the fibula. Weakness, if present, involves the extensor of the great toe and less often of the foot. The knee and ankle reflexes are seldom altered, although occasionally the ankle jerk is moderately depressed. Walking on the heels may be more difficult, because of weakness of dorsiflexion of the foot, and more uncomfortable than walking on the toes. In *lesions of the first sacral root* the pain is felt in the midgluteal region, posterior part of the thigh, posterior region of the calf to the heel, and the plantar surface of the foot and fourth and fifth toes. Tenderness is most pronounced over the midgluteal region (sacroiliac joint), posterior thigh area, and calf. Paresthesias and sensory loss are mainly in the lower leg and outer toes, and weakness, if present, involves the flexor muscles of the foot and toes, evertors of the foot, abductors of the toes, and hamstring muscles. The ankle reflex is diminished or absent in the majority of cases. Walking on the toes is more difficult, because of weakness of plantar flexors, and more uncomfortable than walking on the heel. With lesions of either root there may be limitation of straight-leg raising during the acute, painful stages.

Degeneration of the intervertebral disk without frank extrusion of a fragment of disk tissue may give rise to low back pain, or the disk may herniate into the adjacent vertebral body, giving rise to a Schmorl's node, usually visualized by x-ray. Such cases often show no signs of nerve root involvement, though the back pain may be referred to the thigh and leg.

The rarer *lesions of the fourth and third lumbar roots* give rise to pain in the anterior part of the thigh and knee, with corresponding sensory loss. The knee jerk is diminished or abolished. An inverted Lasègue sign (pain with hypertension of the limb in relation to the trunk, best elicited with the patient in the prone position) is often positive when the third lumbar root is affected.

The lumbar disk syndromes are usually unilateral. Occasionally, with massive derangements of the disk or with the extrusion of a large, free fragment into the canal, the symptoms and signs are bilateral. Often one side is affected more than the other, and the pain and motor and sensory changes may be associated with paralysis of the sphincters. The pain of lumbar disk disease is variable and may be mild or severe. There may be back pain with little or no leg pain, and occasionally the patient experiences leg pain with little or no discomfort in the back. Some patients present with evidence of multiple disk ruptures affecting both cervical and lumbar segments, suggesting a diffuse disorder of the connective tissue of the disks, possibly including both the annulus fibrosus and the nucleus pulposus.

When all components of the syndrome are present, the diagnosis is easy; when only one part is present (particularly backache), it may be difficult, especially if there has not been a clearly remembered initiating traumatic event. Since similar symptoms may occur without demonstrable disk rupture, other diagnostic procedures are required. Plain roentgenograms usually show no abnormality or at most a narrowing of the intervertebral space, sometimes more on the side of the rupture. Traction spurs, which are indicative of disk degeneration, may be present; in extreme cases, there may be a "vacuum" disk sign, in which a gas-density shadow is present in the intervertebral space, usually on lateral roentgenogram. CT transverse images with or without contrast media sometimes show the herniated disk very clearly, and at times the MRI will demonstrate a remarkably sharp

image of cauda equina or nerve root compression by a bulging or extruded disk fragment. Less frequently than in the past do clinicians resort to myelography to demonstrate the disk herniation. The CT/myelogram remains the most reliable of the studies for demonstrating nerve root compression from disk herniation, and many surgeons are loathe to consider laminectomy without such a study. Occasionally, the electromyogram is helpful in showing denervation of paravertebral and leg muscles (see Chap. 382).

It should be noted in evaluating patients with herniated disks that epidural or intradural tumors of the spinal canal may produce a syndrome similar to that of ruptured disk. These lesions may present with unremitting pain even with bed rest and predominant sphincter disturbances even early in the course (see Chap. 381).

OTHER CAUSES OF LOW BACK PAIN AND SCIATICA   In a sizable number of patients, disk-rupture types of symptoms occur, but the problem has a different cause. Often these patients have had multiple operations for diskogenic disease with or without arthrodesis of the lumbar vertebrae, but the pain and disability have not remitted. The indications for the original surgery may have been questionable, with only a disk bulge noted on CT, MRI, or myelogram and no definite neurologic signs. To explain these chronic pain states, a number of pathologic entities have been introduced, some of uncertain status. Entrapment of one or more nerve roots may be the consequence not only of a disk rupture but also of spondylotic spurs with variable stenosis of the lateral recess and intervertebral canal, hypertrophy of apophyseal facets, or a more nebulous cause.

The syndrome that is caused by spondylotic spurs and stenosis of the lateral recess and intervertebral foramen has not been clearly distinguished from that of ruptured disk. Known variously as vertebral stenosis, lumbar claudication, degenerative spinal stenosis, and narrow canal, the cause appears to be related principally to an encroachment on roots of the cauda equina by bony excrescences usually attributed to osteoarthritis but possibly related to spondylolisthesis, old trauma, Paget's disease, or a congenital abnormality of the shape or size of the canal. Many of these patients are elderly, and the pattern must be clearly distinguished from the claudicatory pain associated with peripheral vascular disease. The pain, often bilateral along the sciatic distribution, becomes increasingly severe with standing and walking and is relieved by a short period of rest. Although some of the patients have no physical findings, motor, reflex, and sensory changes may be present. Some patients find sleeping in recumbency difficult and must sleep in a chair.

The *facet syndrome* is closely related to the above but tends to be unilateral. Reynolds et al. have reported 22 cases in which a lumbar monoradiculopathy had simulated a ruptured disk: 16 had an L5 radiculopathy, 3 an S1 radiculopathy, and 3 an L4 radiculopathy. Coexisting back pain was present in 15 of the cases. No disk rupture was found by myelography. At operation, the spinal root was compressed against the floor or roof of the intervertebral canal by an enlarged superior or inferior facet. Foraminotomy and facetectomy relieved the symptoms in 12 of the 15 operated cases.

Lumbar adhesive arachnoiditis with radiculopathy has waxed and waned over the years as an entity employed to explain low back pain persisting after treatment. Most often it is considered in patients who have had multiple lumbar operations and myelograms and are left with backache and leg pain in combination with mild to moderate motor, sensory, and reflex changes. On surgical exploration, the arachnoidal membrane is thickened and opaque, adherent to dura, and tightly bound to pia and roots. The contrast medium during myelography does not fill the root sheaths and tends to be irregularly loculated. Disk rupture, multiple Pantopaque myelograms, operative procedures, infection, and subarachnoid hemorrhage, in various combinations, are factors that favor its development. Treatment is unsatisfactory; lysis of adhesions and epidural steroid injections have been of only limited value.

In patients with persistent chronic low back pain and sciatica after failed disk surgery or due to spondylitic spurs, spondylolysis, facetal joint degeneration, or arachnoiditis, some surgeons have attributed the disability in part, at least, to "instability" of the lumbar segments and the perpetuation of the pain to excessive or abnormal movements of the lumbar vertebral segments. For such patients, spinal fusion is occasionally advocated and can in certain circumstances provide a measure of relief. A posterior arthrodesis of the fourth and fifth lumbar segments to the sacrum may reduce motion at these parts and decrease pressure on the nerve roots associated with abnormal movements. More often than not, however, the patient continues to have pain (although often reduced in degree), and the procedure should not be regarded as a panacea. The authors rarely advocate such an operative intervention, unless clear anatomic evidence exists for a mechanical problem that could be alleviated by stabilization of the spine.

ARTHRITIS Arthritis of the spine is a major cause of backache, cervical pain, and occipital headache.

Osteoarthritis (See also Chap. 296) This more frequent type of osteoarthritic spinal disease occurs usually in later life and may involve any part of the spine. It is most prevalent in the cervical and lumbar regions, however, and the exact location determines the localization of the symptoms. Patients often complain of pain centered in the spine that is increased by motion and is almost invariably associated with complaints of stiffness and limitation of motion. There is a notable absence of systemic symptoms such as fatigue, malaise, and fever, and the pain usually can be relieved by rest. The severity of the symptoms often bears little relation to the radiologic findings; pain may be present when there are minimal findings on an x-ray, and conversely, marked osteophytic overgrowth with spur formation, ridging, and bridging of vertebrae can be seen in asymptomatic patients in middle and later life. Osteoarthropathic changes in the cervical spine and to a lesser extent in the lumbar spine may by their location compress roots or even the cauda equina or spinal cord, giving rise to the spondylitic form of radiculopathy or myelopathy (see Chap. 381).

Rheumatoid arthritis and ankylosing spondylitis (See also Chaps. 285 and 289) Arthritic disease of the spine takes two distinct forms, ankylosing spondylitis (the more common) and rheumatoid arthritis.

Patients with *ankylosing spondylitis* (also called Marie-Strümpell arthritis) are usually young men who complain of mild to moderate pain which early in the course of the disease is centered in the middle or lower back and on occasion radiates to the back of the thighs. The symptoms may be vague at first, and the diagnosis may be overlooked for a considerable period. Although the pain is often intermittent, the finding of limitation of movement is constant and progressive and over a period of time tends to dominate the picture. Early in the course this finding is described as "morning stiffness" or increasing stiffness after periods of inactivity, and it may be present long before radiologic changes are manifest. Limitation of chest expansion, tenderness over the sternum, and decreased motion and flexion contractures of the hips also may be present early in the course. The radiologic hallmarks of the disease are periarticular destructive changes and subsequent obliteration of the sacroiliac joints, development of syndesmophytes on the margins of the vertebral bodies, followed by bridging by bone to produce the characteristic "bamboo spine." The entire spine becomes immobilized, often in a flexed position, and usually the pain then subsides. Patterns of restricted movement, indistinguishable from those of ankylosing spondylitis, may accompany Reiter's syndrome, psoriatic arthritis, and chronic inflammatory bowel diseases. Patients with these disorders rarely show the joint manifestations of peripheral rheumatoid arthritis, and seldom do they display involvement of the hips or knees. The rheumatoid factor is usually absent, but the sedimentation rate is often rapid, and many of the patients are found to have an HLA-B27 antigen.

Occasionally, ankylosing spondylitis is complicated by progressively destructive vertebral lesions. This complication should be suspected whenever the pain returns, after a period of quiescence, or becomes localized. The etiology of these lesions is not known, but they may represent an exaggerated healing response to fracture or excessive production of fibrous inflammatory tissues. Rarely they may result in collapse of a segment of the spine and compression of the spinal cord. Another complication of severe ankylosing spondylitis is bilateral ankylosis of the ribs to the spine, which, coupled with a decrease in the height of axial thoracic structures, causes marked impairment of respiratory function.

Spinal rheumatoid arthritis tends to be localized to the cervical apophyseal joints and atlantoaxial articulation; the pain, stiffness, and limitation of motion are then in the neck and back of the head. Unlike ankylosing spondylitis, rheumatoid arthritis is rarely confined to the spine, and it does not lead to significant degrees of intervertebral bridging. Because of major affection of other joints, the diagnosis is relatively easy to make, but significant involvement of the neck may be overlooked. In the advanced stages of the disease, one or several of the vertebrae may be displaced anteriorly, or a synovitis of the atlantoaxial joint may damage the transverse ligament of the atlas, resulting in forward displacement of the atlas on the axis, i.e., atlantoaxial subluxation. In either instance, serious and even life-threatening compression of the spinal cord may occur gradually or suddenly (see Chaps. 285 and 381). Lateral roentgenograms in flexion and extension, performed cautiously, are sometimes necessary to visualize dislocation or subluxation.

OTHER DESTRUCTIVE DISEASES **Neoplastic, infectious, and metabolic diseases** Metastatic carcinoma (breast, lung, prostate, thyroid, kidney, gastrointestinal tract), multiple myeloma, and non-Hodgkin's and Hodgkin's lymphomas are the malignant tumors which most frequently involve the spine. Since the primary site may be overlooked or asymptomatic, the presenting complaint in such patients may be pain in the back. The pain tends to be constant and dull and is often unrelieved by rest. Indeed, it may be worse at night. Radiographic changes may be absent early in the disease, but when they appear, usually they are manifest as destructive lesions in one or several vertebral bodies with little or limited involvement of the disk space, even in the face of a compression fracture. A ^{99m}Tc diphosphonate bone scan is helpful in demonstrating "hot spots," indicating areas of increased blood flow and reactive bone formation associated with destructive, inflammatory, or arthritic lesions. It should be noted, however, that myeloma and sometimes metastatic thyroid carcinoma may fail to show increased activity on a bone scan.

Infection of the vertebral column is usually the result of pyogenic organisms (staphylococci or coliform bacilli) or, somewhat less commonly today, the tubercle bacilli. Patients complain of pain in the back of subacute or chronic nature that is exacerbated by motion but not materially relieved by rest. There is limitation of motion, tenderness over the spine of the involved segments, and pain with jarring of the spine, such as occurs with walking on the heels. Usually, these patients are afebrile and often do not have a leukocytosis, although the erythrocyte sedimentation rate is almost invariably elevated. Radiographs may demonstrate narrowing of a disk space with erosion and destruction of the two adjacent vertebrae. A paravertebral soft tissue mass evident on contrast CT or MRI may be present, indicating an abscess, which may in the case of tuberculosis drain spontaneously at sites quite remote from the vertebral column. In addition to a bone scan, a gallium scan is sometimes helpful in identifying a soft tissue inflammatory or infectious lesion even when overt bone destruction is not visible in x-rays.

Special mention should be made of the spinal *epidural abscess* (usually staphylococcal), which necessitates urgent surgical treatment. The symptoms are a localized pain, occurring spontaneously, aggravated by percussion and palpation. The patient is febrile and usually has severe radicular complaints, often bilateral, progressing rapidly to a flaccid paraplegia (see Chap. 381). Chronic drug abusers are particularly prone to this problem. Patients with AIDS also have been noted to have increased incidence of epidural abscess and of pyogenic and granulomatous osteomyelitis.

In metabolic bone diseases (hyperparathyroidism, osteoporosis, or osteomalacia), a considerable degree of loss of bone substance may occur without any symptoms whatsoever. Many patients with such conditions do, however, complain of aching in the lumbar or thoracic area. This is most likely to occur following an injury, sometimes trivial in nature, which leads to collapse or wedging of a vertebra. Certain movements greatly enhance the pain, while certain positions relieve it. One or more spinal roots may be involved. Paget's disease of the spine is readily identifiable on x-ray and is often painless. The disease may, however, lead to compression of the spinal cord or roots because of encroachment on the canal or foramina by the pagetoid bone. The recognition of these bone disorders is discussed in some detail elsewhere (Chaps. 358 and 361).

In general, patients thought to have neoplastic, infectious, or metabolic disease of the spine should be thoroughly evaluated by means of radiographs, bone scans, CT or MRI scans, and appropriate laboratory studies (see above). One of the most useful studies is measurement of bone density by dual-beam photon absorbitometry or quantitative digital radiography.

REFERRED PAIN FROM VISCERAL DISEASE
The pain of disease of the pelvic, abdominal, or thoracic viscera is often felt in the region of the spine; i.e., it is referred to the posterior parts of the spinal segment that innervates the diseased organ. Occasionally, back pain may be the first and only sign. The general rule is that pelvic diseases are referred to the sacral region, lower abdominal diseases to the lumbar region (centering around the second to fourth lumbar vertebrae), and upper abdominal diseases to the lower thoracic spine (eighth thoracic to the first and second lumbar vertebrae). Characteristically, local signs or stiffness of the back are not elicited, and motion may be of full range without augmentation of the pain. However, some positions, e.g., flexion of the lumbar area of the spine in the lateral recumbent position, may be more comfortable than others.

Low thoracic and upper lumbar pain in abdominal disease Peptic ulceration or tumor of the wall of the stomach and of the duodenum most typically induces pain in the epigastrium (see Chaps. 252 and 275); but if the posterior wall is involved, and particularly if there is retroperitoneal extension, the pain may be felt in the region of the spine. The pain may be central in location or more intense on one side, or it may be felt in both locations. If very intense, it may seem to encircle the body. It tends to retain the characteristics of pain from the affected organ; e.g., if due to peptic ulceration, it appears about 2 h after a meal and is relieved by food and antacids.

Diseases of the pancreas (peptic ulceration with extension to the pancreas, cholecystitis with pancreatitis, cyst, or tumor) are apt to cause pain in the back, being more to the right of the spine if the head of the pancreas is involved and to the left if the body and tail are implicated.

Diseases of retroperitoneal structures, e.g., lymphomas, sarcomas, and carcinomas, may evoke pain in the adjacent part of the spine with some tendency toward radiation to the lower part of the abdomen, groin, and anterior thighs. A secondary tumor of the iliopsoas region on one side often produces a unilateral lumbar ache with radiation toward the groin, labia, or testicle; there also may be signs of involvement of the upper lumbar spinal roots. An aneurysm of the abdominal aorta may induce pain which is localized to this region of the spine but may be felt higher or lower, depending on the location of the lesion.

Sudden appearance of obscure lumbar pain in a patient receiving anticoagulants should arouse suspicion of retroperitoneal bleeding.

Lumbar pain with lower abdominal diseases Inflammatory diseases of segments of the colon (colitis, diverticulitis) or tumor of the colon cause pain which may be felt in the lower part of the abdomen between the umbilicus and pubis, in the midlumbar region, or in both places. If very intense, the pain may have a beltlike distribution around the body. A lesion in the transverse colon or first part of the descending colon may be central or left-sided, and its level of reference to the back is to the second to third lumbar vertebrae. If the sigmoid colon is implicated, the pain is lower, in the upper sacral region and anteriorly in the midline suprapubic region or left lower quadrant of the abdomen.

Sacral pain in pelvic (urologic and gynecologic) diseases The pelvis is seldom the site of a disease which causes obscure low back pain, although gynecologic disorders may manifest themselves in this manner. Of painful pelvic lesions, less than a third are due to inflammatory disease; other more hypothetical entities, such as relaxation of uterine supporting structures, retroversion of uterus, pelvic varicosities, and adnexal edema, have been largely discredited. Recently, CT, MRI, or diagnostic laparoscopy has been recommended as a valuable supplement to rectal and pelvic examinations, sigmoidoscopy, and intravenous pyelography for patients with obscure pelvic pain. The importance of psychiatric illness in the majority of undiagnosed cases has been stressed.

Menstrual pain itself may be felt in the sacral region. It is rather poorly localized, tends to radiate down the legs, and is often described as cramplike. The most important source of chronic back pain from the pelvic organs, however, is thought to be the uterosacral ligaments. Endometriosis or carcinoma of the uterus (body or cervix) may invade these structures, while malposition of the uterus may cause traction on them. The pain is localized centrally in the sacrum below the lumbosacral joint but may be more on one side than the other. In endometriosis, the pain begins during the premenstrual phase and often continues until it merges with menstrual pain. Malposition of the uterus (retroversion, descensus, and prolapse) is thought by some to lead to sacral pain, especially after the patient has been standing for several hours. One may observe the effect of postural influences here as when a fibroma of the uterus pulls on the uterosacral ligaments. Carcinomatous pain due to involvement of nerve plexuses is continuous and becomes progressively more severe; it tends to be more intense at night. The primary lesion may be overlooked on pelvic examination. Papanicolaou smears, pyelogram, CT scan, and laparoscopy are the most useful diagnostic procedures. X-ray therapy of these tumors may produce sacral pain from necrosis of tissue and injury to nerve roots. Low back pain with radiation into one or both thighs is common in the last weeks of pregnancy.

Chronic prostatitis, evidenced by prostatic discharge, burning and frequency of urination, and sometimes a reduction in sexual potency, may be attended by a nagging sacral ache; it may be mainly on one side, with radiation into one leg if the seminal vesicle is involved on that side. Carcinoma of the prostate with metastases to the lower part of the spine is another more common cause of sacral or lumbar pain. It may be present without urinary frequency or burning. Spinal nerves may be infiltrated by tumor cells, or the spinal cord itself may be compressed if the epidural space is invaded. The diagnosis is established by rectal examination, imaging studies and bone scans of the spine, and measurement of acid phosphatase (particularly the prostatic phosphatase fraction) and prostate-specific antigen. Lesions of the bladder and testes are usually not accompanied by back pain. When the kidney is the site of disease, the pain is ipsilateral, being felt in the flank or lumbar region.

Visceral derangements of whatever type may intensify the pain of arthritis, and the presence of arthritis may alter the distribution of visceral pain. With disease of the spine in the lumbosacral region, for example, distention of the ampulla of the sigmoid by feces or a bout of colitis may aggravate the arthritic pain. In patients with arthritis of the cervical or thoracic spine, the pain of myocardial ischemia may radiate to the back.

OBSCURE TYPES OF LOW BACK PAIN AND THE QUESTION OF PSYCHIATRIC DISEASE
The practitioner is frequently consulted by persons who complain of low back pain of obscure origin. Usually the disorder is benign in nature and results from some minor derangement, muscular strain, or diskal prolapse. This is particularly true for those lesions which are of acute onset, aggravated by motion, and relieved by rest. Considerably more difficult are patients with chronic pain, especially those who have had prior back surgery or chronic visceral disease or those who have severe and progressive pain in which neoplasia or infection is considered.

Even when exhaustive studies have been performed, there remains a group of patients in whom no anatomic or pathologic lesion can be found. These patients generally fall into two categories: those with "postural" back pain and those with psychiatric illness.

"Postural" back pain Some slender asthenic young individuals complain of a vague pain in the back, diffuse in nature, and most frequently noted with prolonged sitting or standing. Similarly, some obese middle-aged patients describe a discomfort in the back, either thoracic or lumbar in location. The physical examination in these patients is negative except for slack musculature and what may be best termed "poor posture." Imaging studies and laboratory evaluation usually show no abnormalities, and characteristically, the pain is relieved by bed rest. Exercises to strengthen the paraspinal and abdominal muscles are sometimes therapeutic.

Psychiatric illness Low back pain may be encountered in compensation hysteria and malingering, in chronic anxiety states or depression, and in many individuals whose symptoms and complaints do not fall within any category of psychiatric illness. It is important to be certain that pain in the back in such patients does not signify disease of the spine and adjacent structures, and all such patients should be studied carefully. However, even when organic factors are found, the pain may be exaggerated, prolonged, or woven into a pattern of invalidism or disability because of coexistent psychological factors, especially when there is the possibility of secondary gain (notably compensation for a work-related injury) (see Chap. 11).

PAIN IN THE NECK AND SHOULDER

It is useful to distinguish three major categories of painful disease—of the spine, brachial plexus (thoracic outlet), and shoulder. Although pain in these three regions of the body may overlap, the patient can usually indicate the site of origin.

Cervical spine Pain arising from the cervical spine is felt in the neck and back of the head (though it may often be projected to the shoulder, arm, and even forearm and hand), is evoked or enhanced by certain movements or positions of the neck, and is accompanied by tenderness and limitation of motions of the neck.

Osteoarthritis of the cervical spine may cause pains which radiate into the back of the head, shoulders, and arms on one or both sides of the thorax. Coincident involvement of nerve roots is manifested by paresthesias, sensory loss, weakness, or deep tendon reflex change. Should bony ridges form in the spinal canal (spondylosis), the spinal cord may be compressed (see Chap. 381). A myelogram, CT, or MRI may reveal the degree of encroachment on the spinal canal (narrowing of the canal to less than 11 mm in the anteroposterior diameter) at the level at which the spinal cord is affected. Difficulty may be experienced in distinguishing the syndrome associated with spondylosis with or without disk rupture and spinal cord dysfunction from primary neurologic diseases (syringomyelia, amyotrophic lateral sclerosis, or tumor) with an unrelated osteoarthritis of the cervical portion of the spine, particularly at the fifth to sixth and sixth to seventh cervical vertebrae, where the disk spaces are often narrowed in the adult. The newer imaging studies such as CT or MRI are helpful in this regard. A painful injury to ligaments and muscles after an accident in which the neck is forcibly extended and flexed (e.g., "whiplash" injury to spine) may be a difficult diagnostic problem, particularly if the patient has some ostensible spurring and especially if in the course of the injury a cerebral concussion has occurred. If the pain is persistent and limited to the neck, imaging studies will sometimes prove that the problem is due to disruption of a disk, but it is often complicated by psychological factors.

Thoracic outlet Pain resulting from abnormalities of the thoracic outlet is experienced in and around the shoulder in the supraclavicular region or between the shoulders, is induced by the performance of certain tasks and by certain positions, and is associated with tenderness of structures above the clavicle. There may be a palpable abnormality above the clavicle (aneurysms of the subclavian artery, tumor, cervical rib). The combination of circulatory symptoms and signs referable to the lower part of the brachial plexus, manifested in the hand by obliteration of pulse when the patient holds a full breath with the head tilted back or turned (Adson's test), unilateral Raynaud's phenomenon, trophic changes in the fingers, and sensory loss over the ulnar side of the hand with or without interosseous atrophy complete the clinical picture. Roentgenograms and other imaging studies showing a cervical rib, deformed thoracic outlet, or superior sulcus tumor of the lung (Pancoast's syndrome) corroborate disease in this location. Electromyography and conduction studies along the plexus from points stimulated above and below the clavicle and studies of arterial and venous circulation (venograms, noninvasive Doppler techniques) are especially helpful in evaluating this problem.

Shoulder Pain localized to the shoulder region is often worse at night and may be associated with local tenderness over the shoulder. The pain is characteristically aggravated by abduction, internal rotation, and extension. Most often shoulder lesions are in the form of a tendonitis or bursitis (sometimes calcific) usually affecting the supraspinatus tendon, the adjacent subdeltoid bursa, or the biceps tendon; occasionally, the lesion is more extensive and consists of a rupture of the rotator cuff, in which case the patient may have weakness on abduction and forward flexion. In some such patients there is an adhesive capsulitis, leading to profound limitation of motion, designated as a "frozen shoulder." Partial cuff tears, impingement of the cuff under the acromion, and slight subluxations produce a variety of symptoms about the shoulder particularly with exercise or maintaining the arm in abduction for long periods of time. The pain of shoulder disease may at times radiate into the arm or hand, but the sensory, motor, and reflex changes which indicate disease of nerve roots, plexus, or peripheral nerves are absent.

RUPTURED CERVICAL DISKS One of the most common causes of neck, shoulder, and arm pain is disk herniation in the lower cervical region. As with rupture of the lumbar disks, the complete syndrome includes the disorder of spinal function and evidence of neural involvement. It may develop after trauma, either major or minor (sudden hyperextension of the neck, diving injuries, forceful manipulations, etc.). Virtually every patient exhibits a diminution in range of motion of the neck (often accompanied by intensification of pain). Hyperextension is the movement that most consistently aggravates the pain, although one occasionally sees patients whose principal limitation is in flexion. Rotation and lateral movements are often moderately restricted by pain. With laterally situated disk lesions between the fifth and sixth cervical vertebrae, the symptoms and signs are referred to the sixth cervical roots. The full syndrome is characterized by pain felt at the trapezius ridge, tip of the shoulder, anterior upper part of the arm, radial forearm, and often in the thumb; paresthesias and sensory impairment or hypersensitivity in the same regions; tenderness in the area above the spine of the scapula and in the supraclavicular and biceps regions; weakness in flexion of the forearm; and diminished to absent biceps and supinator reflexes (triceps retained or exaggerated). When the protruded disk lies between the sixth and seventh cervical vertebrae, the seventh cervical root is involved. Under these circumstances, in the patient with the complete syndrome, the pain is in the region of the shoulder blade, pectoral region and medial axilla, posterolateral upper arm, elbow and dorsal forearm, index and middle fingers, or all the fingers; tenderness is most pronounced over the medial aspect of the shoulder blade opposite the third to fourth thoracic spinous processes, in the supraclavicular area and triceps region; paresthesias and sensory loss are most pronounced in the second and third fingers or tips of all the fingers; weakness is seen in extension of the forearm, in the extension of the wrist, and in the hand grip; the triceps reflex is diminished to absent, and the biceps and supinator reflexes are preserved. Either of these syndromes may be incomplete in that only one of several of the typical findings (e.g., pain) is present. Usually the patient states that cough, sneeze, and downward pressure on the head in the hyperextension position exacerbate pain and that traction (even manual) tends to relieve it.

Unlike lumbar disks, the cervical ones, if large and centrally situated, may result in compression of the spinal cord (central disk, all the cord; paracentral disk, part of the cord). The central disk is often nearly painless, and the cord syndrome may simulate a degenerative disease (amyotrophic lateral sclerosis, combined system disease). A common error is to fail to think of a ruptured disk in the cervical region in patients with obscure symptoms in the legs. The diagnosis of ruptured cervical disk should be confirmed by the same laboratory procedures that were mentioned under "Spondylosis," above.

OTHER CONDITIONS   Metastases to the cervical spine are fortunately less common than to other parts of the vertebral column. They are frequently painful and the cause of disordered root function. Compression fractures or extension of the tumor posteriorly may lead to rapid development of quadriplegia.

Shoulder injuries (rotator cuff), subacromial or subdeltoid bursitis, the frozen shoulder (periarthritis or capsulitis), tendonitis, and arthritis may develop in patients who are otherwise well, but these conditions are also frequent in hemiplegics or in individuals suffering from coronary heart disease. The pain is often severe and extends toward the neck and down the arm into the hand. The dorsum of the latter may tingle without other signs of nerve involvement. Vasomotor and arthropathic changes may also occur in the hand (shoulder-hand syndrome, reflex dystrophy), and after a time, osteoporosis and atrophy of cutaneous and subcutaneous structures occur (Sudeck's atrophy or Sudeck-Leriche syndrome). These conditions fall more within the province of orthopedics than of medicine and are not discussed here in detail. The physician, however, must know that they can often be prevented by proper exercises.

The *carpal tunnel syndrome*, with paresthesias and numbness in palmar distribution of the median nerve and aching pain which extends up into the forearm, may be mistaken for disease of the shoulder or neck. Similarly, other less common forms of nerve entrapment may involve the ulnar, radial, or median nerves and lead to a mistaken diagnosis of brachial plexus lesion or cervical syndrome. Electromyography and conduction studies are especially helpful in such conditions (Chap. 382).

MANAGEMENT OF BACK AND NECK PAIN

Without doubt, the preventive aspects of back pain are important. There would be far fewer back problems if adults kept their trunk muscles in optimal condition by regular exercise such as swimming, bicycle riding, walking briskly, running, or calisthenic programs. A weight-reduction diet and a regular exercise program to strengthen abdominal and paraspinal muscles are frequently very beneficial for patients with chronic low back discomfort. Morning is the ideal time, since the back of the older adult tends to stiffen during the night because of inactivity. This happens regardless of whether a bed board or a stiff mattress is used. Sleeping with the back hyperextended and sitting for long times in an overstuffed chair or a badly designed auto seat commonly cause difficulties for the patient with low back problems. It is estimated that pressures between disks are increased 200 percent by changing from a recumbent to a standing position and 400 percent by sitting slumped in an easy chair. Correct sitting posture lessens this. Long trips in a car or plane without change in position put maximal strain on disk and ligamentous structures in the spine. Lifting from a position of flexed trunk, as in removing a suitcase from the trunk of a car, is dangerous (always lift with the object close to the body). Sudden strenuous activity without conditioning and warm-up also is likely to cause trouble to disks and their ligamentous envelopes (the most common sources of back pain).

Muscular and ligamentous strains and minor disk prolapses are usually self-limited, responding to simple measures in a relatively short period of time. The basic principle of therapy is rest in a recumbent position for several days to weeks. When weight bearing is resumed, a light lumbosacral support is occasionally helpful in continuing the immobilization until the patient is restored to full health. Physical measures such as heat, cold, diathermy, or massage

are of limited value; of considerably greater importance are active exercises to both reduce the spasm and improve muscle tone. Analgesic medication should be given liberally during the first few days: codeine, 30 mg, and aspirin, 0.6 g, or pentazocine, 50 mg, propoxyphene, 65 mg, or meperidine, 50 mg. Muscle relaxants are often a valuable adjunct, particularly in that such drugs as diazepam, 8 to 40 mg in divided doses, may make bed rest more tolerable. If an inflammatory component is suspected, indomethacin, 75 mg/d (in divided doses), ibuprofen, 600 mg three or four times daily, or naproxen, 375 to 500 mg once or twice daily, may be helpful.

In the treatment of a clearly diagnosed acute or chronic rupture of a lumbar or cervical disk, complete bed rest is essential, at least initially, and analgesic medication may be required. Traction is of little value in lumbar disk disease, and it is best to permit the patient to find the most comfortable position. Cervical traction with a halter may be of considerable benefit to patients with cervical disk syndrome. It can be administered with the patient in recumbency or, after sufficient improvement to allow ambulation, can be performed intermittently in the erect, slightly forward flexed position using special equipment. During the recumbent phase of treatment of lumbar disk disease, exercises to reduce spasm, muscle relaxants, and anti-inflammatory agents as described above may be of considerable value. After 2 to 3 weeks in bed, the patient can be allowed to slowly resume activities, usually with the protection of a brace or light spinal support. Exercise programs designed to increase the strength of the abdominal and paraspinal muscles are helpful at this point. The patient may suffer some minor recurrence of the pain but be able to carry on his or her usual activities, and eventually most individuals will recover. If the pain and neurologic findings do not disappear on prolonged, conservative management, or if the patient suffers frequently recurring acute episodes, administration of epidural glucocorticoid may be indicated. For only those patients who fail to improve with a long trial of conservative care or those whose symptoms are worsening at a rapid rate, surgical management may be considered. This should always be preceded by a CT, MRI, and/or myelogram to localize the lesion (and rule out the presence of intra- or extradural tumors). The surgical procedure most often indicated is a partial hemilaminectomy with excision of the disk involved. Arthrodesis of the involved segments is indicated only in cases in which there is extraordinary instability usually related to an anatomic abnormality (such as spondylolysis) or in the cervical region when an extensive laminectomy has rendered the spine unstable. The result of conservative management of patients with diskal disease and sciatica is that approximately 80 percent improve at the end of 4 weeks regardless of whether traction, exercises, manipulation, or corset, or some combination thereof, is used. Therefore, only a small number of patients should be considered to require surgery.

Spondylosis of the cervical spine, if painful, is helped by bed rest and traction; if signs of spinal cord involvement are present, a collar to limit movement may lead to improvement. Decompressive laminectomy or anterior fusion is reserved for severe instances of the disease with advancing neurologic symptoms. The shoulder-hand syndrome may benefit from stellate ganglion blocks or ganglionectomy, but the basic treatment is physiotherapy, with or without medication, and surgical procedures are measures of last resort.

The management of patients with thoracic outlet syndrome is complex and requires first a careful study to be certain that the cause of the lesion is really a mechanical encroachment of the brachial plexus in the interspace between the clavicle and first rib. Exercises to reduce the tension in this region are mainly designed to strengthen the clavicular musculature and improve posture, thus opening the outlet. Many patients benefit from change of work circumstances, and for women with pendulous breasts, a better-designed brassiere is sometimes helpful. Nonsteroidal anti-inflammatory agents are sometimes beneficial, as are muscle relaxants such as diazepam. If the patient's difficulties are intractable or the root compression causes neurologic deficits, exploration of the anterior scalene triangle with resection of the first rib usually gives excellent results.

REFERENCES

BATES D, RUGGIERI P: Imaging modalities for evaluation of the spine. Radiol Clin North Am 29:675, 1991

BELL GR, PARKMAN RH: The conservative treatment of sciatica. Spine 9:54, 1984

BOGDUK N: The innervation of the lumbar spine. Spine 8:286, 1983

BUCHANAN JR ET AL: A comparison of the risk of vertebral fracture in menopausal osteopenia and other metabolic disturbances. J Bone Joint Surg 70:704, 1988

BUNDSCHUH CV et al: Epidural fibrosis and recurrent disk herniation in the lumbar spine: MR imaging assessment. AJR 150:923, 1988

CAPUTY AJ, LEUSSENHOP AJ: Long-term evaluation of decompressive surgery for degenerative lumbar stenosis. J Neurosurg 77:669, 1992

DEYO RA, DIEHL AK: Measuring physical and psychosocial function in patients with low back pain. Spine 8:635, 1983

ELGHAZAWI AK: Clinical syndromes and differential diagnosis of spinal disorders. Radiol Clin North Am 29:651, 1991

EL-KHOURY GY, RENFREW DL: Percutaneous procedures for the diagnosis and treatment of lower back pain: Diskography, facet-joint injection, and epidural injection. AJR 157:685, 1991

FRYMOYER JW: Back pain and sciatica. N Engl J Med 318:291, 1988

GRABIAS SL: The treatment of spinal stenosis. J Bone Joint Surg 62A:308, 1988

GRANT R ET AL: Metastatic epidural spinal cord compression. Neurol Clin 9:825, 1991

LEE C, DEAN BL: Contrast-enhanced magnetic resonance imaging of the spine. Top Magn Reson Imaging 3:41, 1991.

MASARYK TJ et al: High-resolution MR imaging of sequestered lumbar intervertebral disks. AJR 150:1155, 1988

MANELFE C: T1 imaging of degenerative processes of the spine. Curr Opin Radiol 4:63, 1992

MODIC MT, ROSS JS: Magnetic resonance imaging in the evaluation of low back pain. Orthop Clin North Am 22:283, 1991

——— et al: Imaging of degenerative disk disease. Radiology 168:177, 1988

MURPHY RW: Nerve roots and spinal nerves in degenerative disk disease. Clin Orthop 129:46, 1977

PLEATMAN CW, LUKIN RR: Lumbar spinal stenosis. Semin Roentgenol 23:106, 1988

REYNOLDS AV et al: Lumbar monoradiculopathy due to unilateral facet hypertrophy. Neurosurgery 10:480, 1982

RISCH SV et al: Lumbar strengthening in chronic low back pain patients—Physiologic and psychological benefits. Spine 18:332, 1993

WILSON ES, BRILL RF: Spinal stenosis: The narrow lumbar canal syndrome. Clin Orthop 122:244, 1977

section 2 Alterations in body temperature

16 FEVER, INCLUDING FEVER OF UNKNOWN ORIGIN

JEFFREY A. GELFAND / CHARLES A. DINARELLO / SHELDON M. WOLFF

Fever is an elevation of body temperature above the normal circadian variation as the result of a change in the thermoregulatory center, located in the anterior hypothalamus. A normal body temperature is maintained, despite environmental variations, due to the ability of the thermoregulatory center to balance heat production by the tissues, notably muscles and the liver, with heat dissipation. With fever, the balance is shifted to increase the core temperature. *Hyperthermia* is an elevation of body temperature above the hypothalamic set point due to insufficient heat dissipation (e.g., as is seen in exercise, perspiration-inhibiting drugs, hot environment, etc.).

While the "normal" temperature in humans has been said to be 37°C (98.6°F) based on Wunderlich's original observations over 120 years ago, the overall mean temperature for normal individuals aged 18 to 40 years is actually 36.8 ± 0.4°C (98.2 ± 0.7°F), with a nadir at 6 A.M. and a zenith at 4 to 6 P.M. The maximum normal oral temperature at 6 A.M. is 37.2°C (98.9°F), and the maximum normal oral temperature at 4 P.M. is 37.7°C (99.9°F), both defining the 99th percentile for normal individuals. Using these criteria, *an A.M. temperature greater than 37.2°C (98.9°F) or a P.M. temperature greater than 37.7°C (99.9°F) would define a fever*. Rectal temperatures are generally 0.6°C (1°F) higher. Lower esophageal temperatures closely reflect core temperature. The temperature of a freshly passed urine specimen is close to rectal values. The normal 24-h circadian temperature rhythm is associated with temperatures varying typically by 0.5°C (0.9°F) but occasionally as much as 1°C between the A.M. nadir and the P.M. peak. This morning low and evening high pattern is usually preserved in febrile diseases but is abolished in hyperthermia. In menstruating women, the A.M. temperature is generally lower in the 2 weeks prior to ovulation, rising to about 0.6°C (1°F) with ovulation, until menses occur. There may even be a seasonal variation in body temperature. Finally, such physiologic alterations as postprandial state, pregnancy, endocrine factors, and age may alter baseline temperatures.

PYROGENS Substances that cause fever are called *pyrogens* and may be either exogenous or endogenous. *Exogenous pyrogens* are from outside the host, whereas endogenous pyrogens are produced by the host, generally in response to initiating stimuli usually triggered by infection or inflammation. The majority of exogenous pyrogens are microorganisms, their products, or toxins. The best characterized exogenous pyrogen is the heterogeneous group of molecules common to all gram-negative bacteria referred to as *endotoxin* (lipopolysaccharide, LPS). LPS is found in the outer membrane of all gram-negative bacteria and comprises a lipid A and polysaccharide core, linked to an "O-polysaccharide" side-chain composed of repeating units of sugars which vary for each specific gram-negative organism. Gram-positive organisms also produce potent exogenous pyrogens. These include lipoteichoic acid, peptidoglycan, and various exotoxins and enterotoxins. In vivo, LPS is capable of producing fever in humans with as little as 1 ng/kg; while there are no in vivo data in humans, gram-positive cell wall constituents generally require a 2 to 3 log higher amount of material by weight when compared with LPS to induce the production of endogenous pyrogens in vitro. In general, exogenous pyrogens act primarily by inducing the formation of endogenous pyrogens by stimulation of the host's cells, generally monocytes and macrophages. However, the distinction between exogenous and endogenous pyrogens is sometimes blurred. For example, LPS may act directly on endothelial cells in the brain to generate fever, whereas many endogenous products result in the release of endogenous pyrogens, thereby causing fever. Such endogenous substances include antigen-antibody complexes with complement, complement cleavage products, steroid hormone metabolites, bile acids, and some cytokines.

Endogenous pyrogens are polypeptides produced by a variety of host cells, particularly monocytes/macrophages. Endogenous pyrogens, produced either systemically or locally, gain entrance to the circulation and produce fever at the level of the thermoregulatory center of the hypothalamus.

It was originally thought that there was a single endogenous pyrogen, or EP. The standard experimental model utilized injection of leukocyte supernatants or sera of febrile rabbits into normal rabbits. It was then realized that there are two leukocyte EPs, *interleukin 1α* (IL-1α) and *interleukin 1β* (IL-1β). They share a common molecular weight of approximately 17.5 kDa, have only 26 percent amino acid sequence homology, and bind to the same receptors. Originally thought to be produced only by phagocytic cells, IL-1α or IL-1β is produced also by endothelial cells, B lymphocytes, natural killer cells, fibroblasts, smooth-muscle cells, keratinocytes, and glial cells. Because of the ubiquitous production of these and other interleukins, cell-derived inflammatory polypeptides, and growth-promoting peptides, the more general term *cytokine* has been adopted to refer to these substances. Cytokines are regulatory polypeptides produced by a large variety of nucleated cells. Cytokines are produced by monocytes/macrophages, lymphocytes, endothelial cells, hepatocytes, epithelial cells, keratinocytes, and fibroblasts, as well as other cells. Cytokines typically act locally, initiating autocrine (self-stimulating) or paracrine (stimulating nearby) effects. Cytokines, when found in the circulation, are usually present in picogram per milliliter concentrations.

The major pyrogenic cytokines appear to be IL-1β, IL-1α, tumor necrosis factor α (TNFα), tumor necrosis factor β (TNFβ, lymphotoxin), interferon α (IFNα), and interleukin 6 (IL-6). When endogenous pyrogens IL-1α, IL-1β, TNFα, and IL-6 have been administered intravenously to humans, chills and fever occur within 1 h. IL-1α and IL-1β are the most pyrogenic, with febrile responses of 39°C taking place with doses of 10 to 30 ng/kg body weight. At doses of 100 ng/kg, higher fevers and rigors have been observed. TNFα produces chills and fever at 39°C at somewhat higher doses (50 to 100 ng/kg). IL-6 is the least pyrogenic of the three cytokines, producing fever of 39°C at 1 μg/kg. IFNα and IFNγ have been administered primarily by the subcutaneous route, and therefore chills and fever occur after 3 to 4 h. On a weight basis, the interferons are less potent than IL-1 or TNF and similar to IL-6.

HYPOTHALAMIC CONTROL OF TEMPERATURE   The metabolic rate of humans consistently produces more heat than is necessary to maintain core body temperature at 37°C, assuming a neutral environment. Body temperature is controlled by the hypothalamus. Neurons in both the preoptic anterior hypothalamus and posterior hypothalamus receive two kinds of signals—one from peripheral nerves that reflect receptors for warmth and cold and the other from the temperature of the blood bathing the region. These two signals are integrated by the thermoregulatory center of the hypothalamus to maintain normal temperature. In addition, there are clusters of neurons in the preoptic/anterior hypothalamus supplied by a rich and highly permeable vascular network with reduced blood-brain barrier function. The specialized vascular network is called the *organum vasculosum laminae terminalis* (OVLT). It is likely that the endothelial cells of the OVLT release arachidonic acid metabolites when exposed to endogenous pyrogens from the circulation. Arachidonic acid metabolites, largely prostaglandin E$_2$ (PGE$_2$), then presumably diffuse into the preoptic/anterior hypothalamic region and initiate fever. It is possible that PGE$_2$ or other arachidonic acid products induce a second messenger such as cyclic AMP, which in turn raises the thermoregulatory set point. PGE$_2$ is the most potent of the fever-producing arachidonic acid derivatives when injected directly into the hypothalamus and is believed to mediate the rise in the thermoregulatory set point. With the new, higher "thermostatic setting," signals go to various efferent nerves, particularly those sympathetic fibers innervating the peripheral blood vessels, which in turn initiate vasoconstriction and promote heat conservation. The thermoregulatory center also sends signals to the cerebral cortex, initiating behavioral changes such as seeking a warm environment, clothes, special posturing. With the shunting of blood from the periphery, as well as behavioral changes, body temperature usually rises 2 to 3°C; if the hypothalamus calls for more heat, shivering (involuntary muscle contraction) is also triggered to increase heat production. The combination of heat conservation and increased heat production continue until the temperature of the blood bathing the

anterior hypothalamic neurons matches the new "setting." At that point, the hypothalamus maintains the new febrile temperature (Fig. 16-1).

If the hypothalamic set point is reset downward by the disappearance of stimulating endogenous pyrogens or by the inhibition of local prostaglandin synthesis by cyclooxygenase inhibitors such as aspirin, ibuprofen, or acetaminophen, then vasodilation and sweating dissipate heat through radiation and conduction from the skin. Behavioral changes also may be triggered, such as the removal of insulating clothing or bedding. There are also endogenous antipyretic substances. These include arginine vasopressin, adrenocorticotropin, α-melanocyte stimulating hormone, and corticotropin-releasing hormone, each of which appears to alter the ability of endogenous pyrogens to stimulate prostaglandin production.

Several peptides only modulate responses in febrile diseases. These are the cytokine antagonists and inhibitory cytokines. The IL-1 receptor antagonist (IL-1Ra) is a 23- to 25-kDa protein that blocks the binding of IL-1 to its receptors. Whereas IL-1Ra blocks the hypotensive effects of IL-1 and gram-negative and gram-positive bacteremia in experimental animals, in human volunteers it failed to prevent fever in response to minute doses of LPS. Peak molar concentrations of IL-1Ra may exceed those of IL-1β by 100-fold, but these levels tend to occur 1 h after the IL-1β peak and may be part of the recovery process.

Endogenously produced binding proteins for TNF are produced by cleavage of the extracellular domains of the two TNF receptors. Circulating levels of these two soluble TNF receptor fragments (TNFR type I and TNFR type II) are higher than circulating levels of TNF. In addition, cytokines that inhibit the production of the major pyrogens IL-1 and TNF include transforming growth factor β (TGFβ), IL-4, and IL-10. There is very little information regarding the role of these cytokines in modulating the febrile response.

BIOLOGIC ACTIVITIES OF IL-1, TNF, AND IL-6   It is important to distinguish between the critical physiological roles of local IL-1 and TNF and the high systemic blood levels often seen with severe and life-threatening diseases. IL-1 and TNF mediate local phagocytic cell emigration and activation and the release of lipid-derived mediators such as PGE$_2$, thromboxane, and platelet-activating factor (PAF). IL-1 induces IL-8 synthesis, which in turn is a potent neutrophil and monocyte chemotactic factor. IL-8 stimulates the release of enzymes from neutrophils, further enhancing the host's attack on invading microbes. Vasodilation, the induction of adhesive glycoproteins, T and B lymphocyte activation, and enhanced phagocytic cell killing are directly or indirectly mediated by these pyrogenic cytokines. The acute phase response is stimulated, resulting in changes in protein synthesis in the liver. Serum albumin levels decrease, and the production of acute phase proteins, including antiproteases, complement components, fibrinogen, ceruloplasmin, ferritin, and haptoglobin, is increased. C-reactive protein, which in turn binds to damaged and necrotic cells and some microorganisms, may increase 1000-fold. Serum amyloid A (SAA) protein also may increase markedly and be deposited in various organs to cause secondary amyloidosis. Serum iron and zinc levels are decreased, depriving invading microbes of these critical growth factors. Although IL-1 and TNF can induce these hepatic changes, IL-6 is thought to be the prime mediator of the acute phase response.

Both IL-1 and TNF act synergistically to mediate local and systemic inflammatory effects. Amounts that cause little inflammation individually produce refractory hypotension and multiorgan system failure in combination. Suppression of either of these two cytokines may have a significant therapeutic effect by blocking this synergistic toxicity. Furthermore, IL-1–induced activation of T and B cells is greater at 39°C than at 37°C. Both IL-1 and TNF increase loss of mean body mass and cause anorexia, contributing to the cachexia of chronic febrile states. IL-1 and TNF are found in the circulation only briefly but nevertheless induce IL-6. IL-6 levels correlate better with the amount of fever and other pathologic findings in a variety of infectious diseases than IL-1 or TNF because of the persistence of

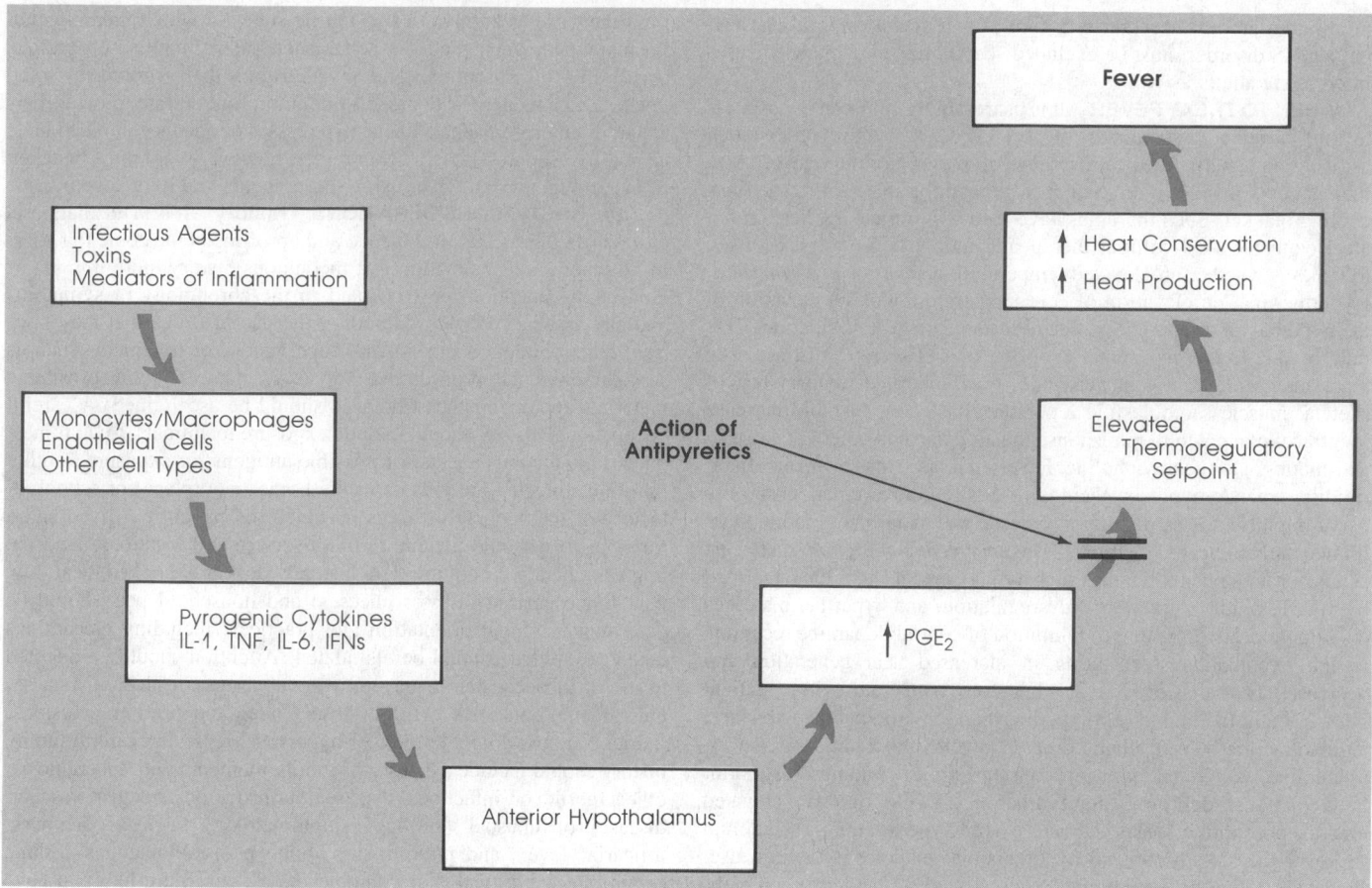

FIGURE 16-1 Chronology of events required for the induction of fever.

IL-6 in the circulation. Unlike IL-1 and TNF, however, there is little or no evidence that IL-6 is a lethal cytokine.

WHY FEVER? Fever has been present for hundreds of millions of years in evolutionary terms. Fish, amphibians, and reptiles develop fever. When fish are injected with bacterial endotoxin or gram-negative bacteria, they raise their body temperature by swimming to warmer water. When lizards are injected with bacteria or pyrogens, they generate fever by basking in the sun to raise their core temperature to "febrile" levels. In many situations, the elevation of body temperature increases survival. The growth and virulence of several bacterial species are impaired at high temperatures, and fever therapy was used to treat neurosyphilis before antibiotics were available. Type III pneumococci are particularly sensitive to high temperature and at 41°C grow poorly and may autolyze. Inhibiting fever in rabbits infected with type III pneumococci increases the mortality rate. Temperatures in the febrile range appear to increase the phagocytic and bactericidal activity of neutrophils and the cytotoxic effects of lymphocytes. Thus fever probably enhances the ability to survive infection. The fact that there are redundancies among the pyrogens (IL-1β, IL-1α, TNF, IL-6, interferons) suggests that it is beneficial to preserve a number of pathways for eliciting this response.

However, there are considerable "costs" to the host in addition to discomfort. For each elevation of body temperature of 1°C, there is an increase in O_2 consumption of 13 percent and increased caloric and fluid requirements. The increased metabolic demand may stress the fetus during pregnancy and patients with marginal cardiac or cerebral vascular supply. IL-1 and TNF accelerate muscle catabolism, leading to a loss of body weight and negative nitrogen balance. Essentially, skeletal muscle is utilized as an energy source, with liberation of amino acids for gluconeogenesis and for the synthesis of acute phase proteins and formation of clones of immune cells. Fever reduces mental acuity and can produce delirium and stupor.

Children are prone to develop seizures with fevers, particularly if there is a prior history of seizures. A single episode of fever ≥37.8°C (100°F) in the first trimester of pregnancy doubles the risk of neural tube defects in the fetus.

ACCOMPANIMENTS OF FEVER Not surprisingly, many of the associated features of fever can be reproduced by infusions of purified cytokines, including back pain, generalized myalgias, arthralgias, anorexia, and somnolence. These symptoms may be reduced by cyclooxygenase inhibitors. *Chills*, a sensation of cold occurring in most fevers, are part of the central nervous system (CNS) response to the thermoregulatory "set point" calling for more heat. A *rigor*, a profound chill, with piloerection ("goose flesh") associated with teeth chattering and severe shivering, is common in bacterial, rickettsial, and protozoal diseases and in influenza (but not in other viral diseases). Sepsis, systemic infections such as leptospirosis, brucellosis, rat bite fever, and endocarditis, malaria, and the intermittent sepsis seen with abscesses may all produce rigors, as can lymphomas, leukemias, renal cell carcinoma, and hepatoma. Rigors are also common with drug-induced fevers. *Sweats* occur with the activation of heat loss mechanisms, either due to antipyretics, reaching the new "thermal ceiling," or to the elimination of the febrile stimulus. The intermittent administration of antipyretics may exaggerate swings of temperature, leading to chilliness, discomfort, and exhaustion. Hypothalamic reflexes trigger sweating, allowing rapid dissipation of heat by evaporative loss.

Alterations of mental status and convulsions are common in the very young and very old and patients with dementia, hepatic failure, and chronic renal failure. There may be a progression from irritability to delirium to frank obtundation. This usually clears with the fever.

Febrile convulsions in infants and children less than 5 years old typically occur particularly at the onset of febrile disease and are more common at higher temperatures (>40°C). Febrile convulsions in children are not necessarily a sign of significant cerebral disease, but a CNS disorder must be excluded. Fever may precipitate seizures in epileptic adults as well.

WHEN TO TREAT FEVER   It is distressingly common in hospitals to find "routine," "standing," or "prn" orders for antipyretics (such as acetaminophen) for a temperature above an arbitrary level or to find patients awake, alert, but most uncomfortable, shivering on a cooling blanket. Such therapies have their appropriate application but are frequently used without therapeutic rationale. The first decision to make is whether an elevated temperature is *fever* or *hyperthermia*. Hyperthermia, an elevation of core temperature without elevation of the hypothalamic set point, is due to inadequate heat dissipation. This may be due to environmental exposure or to two rare, distinct drug reactions. *Malignant hyperthermia* is an inherited abnormality of skeletal muscle sarcoplasmic reticulum that causes a rapid increase in intracellular calcium in response to halothane and other inhalational anesthetics or to succinylcholine. Fever, increased muscle metabolism, rigidity, rhabdomyolysis, acidosis, and cardiovascular instability occur rapidly. Cessation of anesthesia and dantrolene sodium are immediately indicated therapies. The *neuroleptic malignant syndrome* can occur with phenothiazines such as haloperidol and is characterized by muscle rigidity, autonomic dysregulation, and hyperthermia. This disorder appears to be due to inhibition of central dopamine receptors in the hypothalamus, resulting in increased heat generation and decreased heat dissipation. A high core temperature in a patient with a high likelihood of hyperthermia (environmental exposure, anticholinergic or neuroleptic drugs, tricyclic antidepressants, succinylcholine, halothane) with appropriate clinical findings (dry skin, hallucinations, delirium, pupil dilation, muscle rigidity, elevated creatine phosphokinase) is characteristic of hyperthermia. The attempt to lower the already normal hypothalamic set point is of little use. Physical cooling with sponging, cooling blankets, and even ice baths should be initiated immediately, in conjunction with appropriate pharmacologic agents (such as dantrolene for malignant hyperthermia and the neuroleptic malignant syndrome or physostigmine for tricyclic antidepressant overdose). With hyperpyrexia (fever $\geq 41°C$), antipyretics are clearly indicated, and physical cooling while "resetting" the hypothalamic set point with antipyretics will speed the process. Antipyretics also suppress the constitutional symptoms that accompany fever (myalgias, chills, headache, etc.). However, with "low-grade" or moderate temperatures, there is little evidence that fever is harmful or that antipyretic therapy is beneficial. Exceptions include the aforementioned situations of children with febrile seizures, pregnant women, and patients with impaired cardiac, pulmonary, or cerebral function. Temperature is often suppressed needlessly, and "routine" antipyretic orders may obscure the important clinical information to be gained from following the upward, or downward, course of a temperature. In addition, NSAIDs and glucocorticoids may mask the inflammatory features of a localized infection, preventing its detection and even encouraging its spread. In addition, the drugs themselves may cause side effects. Aspirin is to be avoided in children with viral diseases because of the possibility of Reye's syndrome, which occurs in association with influenza and varicella and occasionally with enteroviruses. In addition, the antiplatelet and even antiphagocytic effects of aspirin have led to the general use of acetaminophen. Acetaminophen is a poor cyclooxygenase inhibitor in peripheral tissue and thus lacks anti-inflammatory activity; in the CNS, acetaminophen is oxidized, converting it to an active cyclooxygenase inhibitor, thus explaining its antipyretic effect. Ibuprofen may be safe for children, with possibly greater temperature reduction and duration of effect at similar doses as acetaminophen. Ibuprofen does not appear to pose a risk of Reye's syndrome, but the caveat about bacterial infections remains. Other NSAIDs, particularly indomethacin and naproxen, are also useful as antipyretics.

Glucocorticoids are potent antipyretics. They inhibit PGE_2 synthesis by inhibiting phospholipase A_2 and block both mRNA transcription for IL-1 and TNF and translation of these cytokines. The potent immunosuppressive and antiphagocytic effects of glucocorticoids limit their use as antipyretics to febrile states in which inflammation is a major pathogenic factor—such as bacterial meningitis, tuberculous pericarditis, or vasculitis. The severe rigors that accompany some fevers can be reduced with meperidine, morphine sulfate, prochlorperazine, or chlorpromazine. These two classes of agents combined have an additive suppressive effect on rigors; however, care must be taken to avoid hypotension when using these agents singly or together.

DIAGNOSTIC CONSIDERATIONS   History   It is in the diagnosis of a febrile illness that the science and art of medicine come together. In no other clinical situation is a meticulous history more important. Painstaking attention must be paid to the chronology of symptoms and any associated drugs, including the use of drugs that may have been taken without a physician's supervision, or treatments such as surgical or dental procedures. The exact nature of any prosthetic materials and/or implanted devices should be ascertained. A careful occupational history should include exposure to animals, toxic fumes, potential infectious agents, or possible antigens, or exposure to other febrile or infected individuals in the home, workplace, or school. A history of the geographic areas in which the patient has lived and a travel history should include military service and locations. Unusual hobbies, dietary proclivities (such as raw or poorly cooked meat, raw fish, unpasteurized milk or cheeses) and household pets should be determined. Sexual orientation and practices, including precautions taken or omitted, should be elucidated. Attention should be directed to use of tobacco, marijuana, intravenous drugs, or alcohol, trauma, animal bites, and tick or other insect bites and prior transfusions, immunizations, drug allergies, or hypersensitivities. A careful family history should include a history of family members with tuberculosis, other febrile or infectious diseases, arthritis or collagen vascular disease, or unusual familiar symptomatology such as deafness, urticaria, fevers and polyserositis, bone pains or anemias. Ethnic origin may be critical. For example, blacks are more likely to have hemoglobinopathies. Turks, Arabs, Armenians, and Sephardic Jews are more likely to have familial Mediterranean fever.

Patterns of fever   The widespread use of antipyretics, glucocorticoids, and antibiotics can alter fever patterns so that "classic" fever patterns are not seen. Some patterns are clinically useful, however. Whereas the circadian temperature pattern is preserved and in fact exaggerated with most fevers, a reversal of this pattern may be seen with typhoid fever and disseminated tuberculosis. Temperature-pulse dissociation (relative bradycardia) is seen with typhoid fever, as well as brucellosis, leptospirosis, some drug fevers, and many factitious fevers. Bradycardia in the presence of fever also may signify cardiac conduction abnormalities, as with acute rheumatic fever, Lyme disease, viral myocarditis, or valve ring abscess complicating bacterial endocarditis.

Fever may be sustained, intermittent, remittent, or relapsing. A *sustained* fever is one in which temperature elevation is persistent, with minimal variation. With *intermittent* fever, there is an exaggeration of the normal circadian rhythm; when this variation is extremely large, the fever is termed *hectic* or *septic*. When hectic fevers occur daily, the term *quotidian* is sometimes used. With *relapsing* fevers, febrile episodes are separated by intervals of normal temperature; when paroxysms occur on the first and third days, the fever is called *tertian*. *Plasmodium vivax* causes tertian fevers. *Quartan* fevers are associated with paroxysms on the first and fourth day and are seen with *P. malariae*. Other relapsing fevers are seen with *Borrelia* infections and rat bite fever. Both are associated with days of fever followed by a several-day afebrile period and then relapses of days of fevers. Pel-Ebstein fever, with fevers lasting 3 to 10 days followed by afebrile periods of 3 to 10 days, is classic for Hodgkin's disease and other lymphomas. Another characteristic fever is that of cyclic neutropenia, in which fevers occur every 21 days and accompany the neutropenia. *Intermittent, hectic,* and *septic* fevers are common with deep-seated or systemic infections, malignancy, and drug fevers. *Remittent* fever, in which the temperature falls each day but not to normal is typical for tuberculosis, viral diseases, many bacterial infections, and noninfectious causes of fever. It should be emphasized that newborns, the elderly, patients with chronic renal or hepatic failure, and patients on glucocorticoids or with bacteremic shock may fail to generate fever altogether, and in these individuals, *hypothermia* may be a sign of severe infection.

Physical examination   A meticulous physical examination should be repeated on a regular basis. All the vital signs are relevant. Temperature may be taken orally or rectally, but the specific site used should be kept consistent. Axillary temperatures are notoriously unreliable, as are oral temperatures obtained after recent hot or cold drinks, smoking, or hyperventilation.

In some cases, patients are thoroughly examined at the time of initial evaluation, but the diagnostic emphasis then shifts to laboratory data and other diagnostic procedures. Particular attention should be paid to daily physical examination, sometimes more often, until the diagnosis is certain and the anticipated response has been achieved. Special attention should be paid to the skin, lymph nodes, eyes, nailbeds, cardiovascular system, chest, abdomen, musculoskeletal system, and nervous system. Rectal examination is imperative. The penis, prostate, scrotum, and testes should be examined carefully, and the foreskin, if present, retracted. Pelvic examination is part of every complete physical examination of a female.

Laboratory tests   There are few signs and symptoms in medicine with as many diagnostic possibilities as fever. If the history, epidemiologic circumstances, or physical examination suggests more than a simple viral illness or streptococcal pharyngitis, then laboratory testing is indicated. The tempo and complexity of the workup will depend on the pace of the illness, diagnostic considerations, and the immune status of the host. If findings are focal or if the history, epidemiologic considerations, or physical examination suggests certain diagnoses, the laboratory examination can be focused. If fever is undifferentiated, the "diagnostic nets" must be cast farther, and certain guidelines are then indicated, which follow.

CLINICAL PATHOLOGY   Workup should include a complete blood count, a differential count performed manually or with an instrument sensitive to the identification of eosinophils, juvenile or band forms, toxic granulations, and Döhle bodies, the last three suggestive of bacterial infection. Neutropenia may be seen with some viral infections, particularly parvovirus B19, drug reactions, systemic lupus erythematosus (SLE), typhoid, brucellosis, and infiltrative diseases of the bone marrow, including lymphoma, leukemia, tuberculosis, and histoplasmosis. Lymphocytosis may be seen with typhoid, brucellosis, tuberculosis, and viral disease. Atypical lymphocytes are seen with many viral diseases, including Epstein-Bar virus (EBV), cytomegalovirus (CMV), human immune deficiency virus (HIV), dengue, rubella, varicella, measles, viral hepatitis, serum sickness, and toxoplasmosis. Monocytosis is seen in typhoid, tuberculosis, brucellosis, and lymphoma. Eosinophilia may be found in hypersensitivity drug reactions, Hodgkin's disease, adrenal insufficiency, and certain metazoan infections. If the febrile illness appears severe or prolonged, the smear should be examined carefully, and an erythrocyte sedimentation rate (ESR) should be performed. Urinalysis, with examination of urinary sediment, is indicated. It is axiomatic that any abnormal fluid accumulation (pleural, peritoneal, joint, etc.), even if previously sampled, merits reexamination in the presence of undiagnosed fever. Joint fluids should be examined for crystals. Bone marrow biopsy (not simple aspiration) for histopathology (as well as culture) is indicated when marrow infiltration by pathogens or tumor cells is possible. Stool should be inspected for occult blood; an inspection for fecal leukocytes, ova, or parasites also may be indicated.

CHEMISTRY   Electrolytes, glucose, blood urea nitrogen, and creatinine determinations should be done. Liver function tests are usually indicated if the cause of fever does not point to another organ. Additional chemistries (creatine phosphokinase, etc) can be added as the workup progresses.

MICROBIOLOGY   Smears and cultures of the throat, urethra, anus, cervix, and vagina should be obtained in appropriate situations. Sputum evaluation (Gram stain, AFB stain, cultures) is indicated for any patient with fever and cough. Blood cultures and cultures of abnormal fluid collections and urine are indicated when fever is thought to be more than uncomplicated viral illness. Cerebrospinal fluid should be examined and cultured if meningismus, severe headache, or mental status changes are present.

RADIOLOGY   A chest x-ray is usually part of the evaluation for any significant febrile illness.

In most patients with fever, the history, physical examination, and initial screening laboratory studies lead to a diagnosis, or the patient recovers spontaneously. In the latter case, a viral illness is usually considered the source of the fever. When fever continues for 2 to 3 weeks, during which time repeat physical examinations and laboratory tests are unrevealing, patients are provisionally diagnosed as having fever of unknown origin (FUO).

FEVER OF UNKNOWN ORIGIN   *Fever of unknown origin* (FUO) was defined by Petersdorf and Beeson in 1961: (1) fevers higher than 38.3°C (101°F) on several occasions, (2) a duration of more than 3 weeks, and (3) failure to reach a diagnosis after 1 week of inpatient investigation. While this classification has stood for more than 30 years, Durack and Street have proposed a new classification of FUO: (1) "classical FUO," (2) nosocomial FUO, (3) neutropenic FUO, and (4) HIV-associated FUO (Table 16-1).

Classic FUO   This category corresponds closely to the prior definition of FUO and is modified only with regard to the prior requirement for 1 week's study in hospital to encompass three outpatient visits or 3 days in the hospital without a cause having been determined. In our opinion, 2 weeks of fever is sufficient to entertain the diagnosis when other criteria have been met.

Nosocomial FUO   Nosocomial FUO is used when fever of ≥38.3°C (101°F) occurs on several occasions in a hospitalized patient receiving acute care and in whom infection was not present or incubating on admission. Three days of investigation, including at least 2 days' incubation of cultures is the minimum duration for this diagnosis. In hospitalized patients, occult nosocomial infections, infected intravascular lines, recurrent pulmonary embolism, transfusion-related viral infection, and drug fever are possible diagnoses. In this setting, the approach is to focus on sites where occult infections

TABLE 16-1   Categories of FUO*

	Nosocomial	Neutropenic	HIV-associated	Classic
Patient circumstance	Hospitalized, acute care, no infection when admitted	Has ≤500 neutrophils/mm^3 or anticipated 1 to 2 days	Confirmed HIV-positive	All others with fevers ≥3 weeks
Duration of illness while under investigation	3 days[†]	3 days[†]	3 days[†] or 4 weeks as outpatient	3 days[†] or 3 outpatient visits
Examples of cause	Septic thrombophlebitis, sinusitis, *C. difficile* colitis, drug fever	Perianal infection, aspergillosis, candidemia	MAI, tuberculosis, non-Hodgkin's lymphoma, drug fever	Infections, malignancy, inflammatory diseases, drug fever

* All require fevers ≥ 38.3°C (101°F) on several occasions.
[†] Includes at least 2 days' incubation of microbiology cultures
SOURCE: After Durack and Street.

TABLE 16-2   Classic FUO in adults

Authors	Years of study	No. of cases	Infections (%)	Neoplasms (%)	Collagen vascular diseases (%)	Miscellaneous (%)	Undiagnosed (%)
Petersdorf and Beeson	1952–57	100	36	19	13	25	7
Jacoby and Swartz	1957–71	128	40	20	15	17	8
Howard et al.	1969–76	100	37	31	19	8	5
Larson et al.	1970–80	105	30	31	16	10	12
Knockaert et al.	1980–89	199	22.5	7	21.5*	26.5*	22.5*

* Authors' raw data retabulated to conform to prior diagnostic categories.

might be sequestered (such as the sinuses of intubated patients, infections of prosthetic devices) or on nosocomial complications such as acalculous cholecystitis, *Clostridium difficile* toxin in the stool (if diarrhea is present), and drug reactions. Blood cultures are mandatory. Appropriate diagnostic maneuvers include ultrasonography and computed tomography (CT) of the abdomen, indium 111–labeled white blood cell or immunoglobulin scans, sinus x-rays, and the cessation of suspect drugs.

Neutropenic FUO This is defined as fever of ≥38.3°C (101°F) on several occasions in a patient with less than 500 neutrophils per cubic millimeter (or expected to fall below that level within 1 to 2 days). The diagnosis of neutropenic FUO is invoked if a specific cause is not identified after 3 days of investigation, including at least 2 days' incubation of cultures. Neutropenic patients are susceptible to focal bacterial and fungal and bacteremic infections and to infections involving catheters, including septic thrombophlebitis, as well as to perianal infections. *Candida* and *Aspergillus* infections are common. Viral infections due to herpes simplex or CMV are sometimes causes of FUO in this group. While the duration of illness is far shorter in these patients, the consequences of untreated infection may be catastrophic.

HIV-associated FUO This disorder is defined by fever of ≥38.3°C (101°F) on several occasions over a period of more than 4 weeks for outpatients or more than 3 days' duration in the hospital in a patient with HIV infection. This diagnosis is invoked if 3 days of appropriate investigation, including 2 days' incubation of cultures, reveals no source. In this group of patients, HIV infection alone may be a cause. *Mycobacterium avium intracellulare* (MAI), toxoplasmosis, CMV, tuberculosis, *Pneumocystis carinii*, salmonellosis, cryptococcosis, histoplasmosis, non-Hodgkin's lymphoma, and importantly, drug fever are all possible causes.

Adaptation of these categories of FUO on a wide scale in the literature would allow a more rational compilation of data regarding these disparate groups. In the remainder of this chapter, the discussion will be focused on classic FUO, unless otherwise designated.

CAUSES OF CLASSIC FUO Table 16-2 summarizes the findings of a number of large studies of FUO since the advent of the antibiotic era. Coincident with the widespread use of antibiotics, increasingly useful diagnostic technologies, both noninvasive and invasive, have been developed. Newer studies reflect not only changing patterns of disease but also the impact of diagnostic techniques that make it possible to eliminate many patients with specific illness from the FUO category. The ubiquitous use of microbiologic cultures and widespread use of potent broad-spectrum antibiotics may have decreased the number of infections causing FUO. The wide availability of ultrasonography, CT, and magnetic resonance imaging (MRI) has enhanced detection of occult neoplasms and lymphomas that previously were thought to be FUO. Likewise, the widespread availability of highly specific and sensitive immunologic testing has reduced the numbers of undetected cases of SLE and other autoimmune diseases. Several generalizations can be however. Infections remain the leading cause of FUO. Tuberculosis, especially extrapulmonary tuberculosis, remains an important cause. Prolonged mononucleosis syndromes with EBV, CMV, or HIV are considerations, sometimes confounded by delayed antibody responses. Intraabdominal abscesses, sometimes poorly localized, and renal, retroperitoneal, and paraspinous abscesses continue to be difficult to diagnose. Osteomyelitis, especially where prosthetic devices have been implanted, and infective endocarditis must be considered. Although true culture-negative infective endocarditis is rare, one may be misled by slow-growing organisms of the HACEK group (*Haemophilus aphrophilus*, *Actinobacillus actinomycetemcomitans*, *Eikenella corrodens*, *Kingella kingii*) or by fungal, chlamydial, or rickettsial infections. Prostatitis, dental abscesses, sinusitis, and cholangitis continue to be sources of occult fever.

Fungal disease, most notably histoplasmosis involving the reticuloendothelial system, may cause FUO. FUO with headache should prompt examination of spinal fluid for *Cryptococcus neoformans*. Malaria continues to be a cause of FUO, particularly when nonsynchronized. Malaria may result from transfusion, the failure to take prescribed prophylaxis, or drug resistance.

In most early series, neoplasms were the next most common cause of FUO, after infections (Table 16-3). In a series by Knockaert and associates, of 199 patients studied between 1980 and 1989, the percentage of FUO due to malignancy was reduced, a decrease attributed to the improvement in diagnostic technologies. This does not diminish the importance of suspecting neoplasia in the initial diagnostic evaluation of a patient with fever. This series noted a large number of patients with diseases such as temporal arteritis, adult Still's disease, drug-related fever, and factitious fever. In most series, undiagnosed FUOs account for approximately 10 percent of cases. The general category of "collagen vascular diseases" is used somewhat loosely to apply not only to SLE and temporal arteritis but also to systemic rheumatologic or vasculitic diseases such as polymyalgia rheumatica and adult Still's disease.

Many diseases have been grouped in the various studies as "miscellaneous." At the top of this list are the granulomatous diseases, including sarcoidosis, Crohn's disease, and granulomatous hepatitis. Additional diagnoses include drug fever, erythema multiforme, pulmonary embolism, factitious fever, familial Mediterranean fever (FMF), Behçet's syndrome, Fabry's disease, and Whipple's disease (now attributed to a bacillus named *Tropheryma whippelii*).

Drug fever must be considered in anyone with prolonged fever. Any febrile pattern may be seen, and both relative bradycardia and hypotension are uncommon. Eosinophilia and/or rash are seen in only one-fifth of such patients. Fever usually begins 1 to 3 weeks from the start of the drug and remits 2 to 3 days after the drug is stopped. Virtually all classes of drugs cause fever, but antimicrobials (especialy β-lactam antibiotics), cardiovascular drugs (e.g., quinidine), antineo-

TABLE 16-3   Malignancies that commonly cause FUO

Hodgkin's disease
Non-Hodgkin's lymphoma
Leukemia (includes preleukemic and aleukemic phases)
Renal cell carcinoma
Hepatoma

TABLE 16-4   Causes of FUO lasting more than 6 months

	Percent of cases
No cause determined	19
Miscellaneous	13
Factitious	9
Granulomatous hepatitis	8
Neoplasm	7
Still's disease	6
Infection	6
Collagen-vascular disease	4
Familial Mediterranean fever	3
No fever*	27

* No acutal fever observed during 2 to 3 weeks inpatient observation; includes patients with exaggerated circadian rhythm.
SOURCE: From a study of 347 patients referred to the National Institutes of Health from 1961 to 1977 with a presumptive diagnosis of FUO >6 months (Aduan et al).

plastic drugs, and CNS drugs (e.g., phenytoin) are especially common as causes.

It is axiomatic that as the duration of fever increases, the likelihood of an infectious cause decreases (Table 16-4). In a series of 347 patients referred to one of us (S.M.W.) at the National Institutes of Health from 1961 to 1977, only 6 percent had infection. A significant number (9 percent) had *factitious fevers*, due either to false elevations of temperature or self-induced disease. A substantial number of these factitious cases were young women in the health professions. It is worth noting that 8 percent of the patients with prolonged fevers had granulomatous hepatitis, some of whom had completely normal liver function studies, and 6 percent had adult Still's disease. After prolonged investigation, 19 percent had no specific diagnosis. A total of 27 percent either had no actual fever observed during the weeks of inpatient observation or had an exaggerated circadian temperature rhythm without chills, elevated pulse, or other abnormalities. A differential diagnosis for classic FUO in adults is offered in Table 16-5. While this list is restricted to the United States, the frequency of global travel underscores the need for a detailed travel history.

Specialized diagnostic studies in classic FUO   Certain specific diagnostic maneuvers become critical in dealing with prolonged fevers. If factitious fever is suspected, numbered thermometers should be used, temperature-taking should be supervised, and simultaneous urine and body temperatures should be measured. Any tissue removed in prior relevant surgery should be reexamined; slides should be requested and, if need be, the "paraffin blocks" of fixed pathologic material should be reexamined and additional special studies performed. Any relevant x-rays should be requested and reexamined; reviewing prior reports may be insufficient. Serum should be set aside in the laboratory as soon as possible and retained for future examination of rising antibody titers. *Febrile agglutinins* is a vague term that normally means, in most laboratories, serologic studies for salmonellosis, brucellosis, and rickettsial diseases. They are seldom useful, of low sensitivity, and variable specificity. Rising titers for *Brucella* are usually diagnostic, but false-positive titers may occur in typhoid fever, tularemia, and yersinial infections. Infection with *B. canis* may be missed with standard antibody tests for *Brucella*. *Salmonella* infection elevates antibody titers to the H and O antigens. High titers of antibody to the O antigen persist for years and may reflect previous infection or immunization. Specific antirickettsial titers should be requested for diagnosing Rocky Mountain spotted fever and Q fever. Multiple blood cultures, no less than three, rarely more than six, should be obtained. These should be cultured in the laboratory for at least 2 weeks to ensure growth of HACEK-group organisms. Lysis-centrifugation blood culture techniques should be employed in cases where prior antimicrobial therapy or fungal or atypical mycobacterial infection is suspected. Blood culture media should be supplemented with L-cysteine or pyridoxal to assist in the isolation of nutritional variant streptococci. It should be noted that sequential cultures positive for multiple organisms may be found when fever is caused by self-injection of contaminated substances. Urine cultures, including

cultures for mycobacteria, fungi, and CMV, are indicated. Liver biopsy, even in the absence of abnormal liver function studies, should be considered and pursued if the diagnosis remains elusive. Specimens should be cultured for mycobacteria and fungus. Likewise, bone marrow biopsy (not simple aspiration) should be performed for histology and culture. The blood smear should be examined for malaria, babesia, trypanosomes, leishmania, and *Borrelia*.

In an FUO workup, an ESR should be obtained. Striking elevation of the ESR and anemia of chronic disease are frequently seen in association with giant cell arteritis or polymyalgia rheumatica, common causes of FUO in patients over 50 years of age. Still's disease is also suggested by elevations of ESR, leukocytosis, and anemia and is often accompanied by arthralgias, polyserositis (pleuritis, pericarditis), lymphadenopathy, splenomegaly, and rash. Antinuclear antibody should be measured to rule out other collagen vascular diseases. Another cause of extremely high ESR may be a "false-positive" ESR, from a "cold agglutinin" with a broad thermal amplitude. The ESR is a nonspecific test that depends on certain serum proteins, most notably fibrinogen, that interfere with the zeta-potential that keeps erythrocytes from clumping. When fibrinogen levels go up, the zeta-potential is inhibited, erythrocytes clump, and the ESR is high. A cold agglutinin, by binding to the erythrocyte, can produce a "false-positive" agglutinin that mimics an acute phase response; cold agglutinins may be seen with *Mycoplasma* and EBV infection and lymphomas.

With rare exceptions, the intermediate-strength purified protein derivative (PPD) skin test should be done for tuberculosis in patients with classic FUO. Concurrent controls should be performed. The CMI test (Connaught Labs, Swiftwater, Pa.) is an especially effective control. It should be kept in mind that a negative PPD skin test in the face of negative controls may be seen with miliary tuberculosis, sarcoidosis, Hodgkin's disease, malnutrition, or AIDS. Noninvasive procedures should include an upper gastrointestinal contrast study with small-bowel follow-through and barium enema to include the terminal ileum and cecum. Chest x-rays should be repeated if new symptoms arise. In some cases it may be necessary to do pulmonary function studies. A diminished carbon monoxide diffusing capacity (DL_{CO}) may be present in restrictive lung diseases such as sarcoidosis, even in the face of a normal chest x-ray. In such cases, transbronchial biopsy may prove diagnostic. It may be advisable to perform flexible colonoscopy, since colon carcinoma is a cause of FUO, and these tumors easily escape detection by ultrasound and CT.

CT scan of the chest and abdomen should be performed. If a spinal or paraspinal lesion is suspected, MRI is preferred. MRI may be superior to CT in demonstrating intraabdominal abscesses and aortic dissection, but the comparative utility of MRI and CT in FUO is unknown. At present, it would appear that the use of abdominal CT should be the routine, unless there is a more specific indication for MRI. Ultrasonography of the abdomen is useful for the investigation of the hepatobiliary tract, kidneys, spleen, and pelvis. An echocardiogram also may be useful for bacterial endocarditis, pericarditis, nonbacterial thrombotic endocarditis, and atrial myxomas. Transesophageal echocardiography is especially sensitive for these lesions.

Radionuclide scanning procedures using technetium (Tc) 99m sulfur colloid, gallium (Ga) citrate, or indium (In) 111–labeled leukocytes or immunoglobulin may be useful in identifying and/or localizing inflammatory processes. Technetium bone scans should be undertaken to look for osteomyelitis or bony metastases; gallium scans may be used to identify sarcoidosis or *P. carinii* in the lungs, or Crohn's disease in the abdomen. ^{111}In-labeled white blood cell scans may be used to locate abscesses. ^{111}In-labeled immunoglobulin scanning also shows promise in this regard. With both gallium and indium WBC scans, false-positive and false-negative findings are common.

Biopsy of the liver and bone marrow should be considered routine in the workup of FUO if the studies mentioned above are unrevealing or if fever is prolonged. It goes without saying that areas of suspected abnormality should be pursued for pathologic examination, where

TABLE 16-5   Diseases causing FUO in adults in the United States

Infections
A Localized pyogenic infections
  Appendicitis
  Cat-scratch disease
  Cholangitis
  Cholecystitis
  Dental abscess
  Diverticulitis/abscess
  Lesser sac abscess
  Liver abscess
  Mesenteric lymphadenitis
  Osteomyelitis
  Pancreatic abscess
  Pelvic inflammatory disease
  Perinephric/intrarenal abscess
  Prostatic abscess
  Sinusitis
  Subphrenic abscess
  Suppurative thrombophlebitis
  Tuboovarian abscess
B Intravascular infections
  Bacterial aortitis
  Bacterial endocarditis
  Vascular catheter infections
C Systemic bacterial infections
  Brucellosis
  Campylobacter
  Gonococcemia
  Legionella
  Leptospirosis
  Listeriosis
  Lyme disease
  Melioidosis
  Meningococcemia
  Rat bite fever
  Relapsing fever
  Salmonellosis
  Syphilis
  Tularemia
  Typhoid
  Vibriosis
  Yersinia
D Mycobacterial infections
  MAI
  Other atypical mycobacteria
  Tuberculosis
E Fungal infections
  Aspergillosis
  Blastomycosis
  Candidiasis
  Coccidioidomycosis
  Cryptococcosis
  Histoplasmosis
  Mucormycosis
  Paracoccidioidomycosis
  Sporotrichosis
F Other bacteria
  Actinomycosis
  Cat-scratch disease
  Nocardiosis
  Whipple's bacillus
G Rickettsial infections
  Cat-scratch disease/bacillary angiomatosis (*Rochalimaea henselae*)
  Ehrlichiosis
  Murine typhus
  Q-fever
  Rickettsialpox
  Rocky Mountain Spotted Fever
H Mycoplasma
I Chlamydial infections
  LGV
  Psittacosis
  TWAR
J Viral infections
  Colorado tick fever
  Coxsackie group B
  CMV
  Dengue
  EBV
  Hepatitis A, B, C, D, and E
  HIV
  LCM
  Parvovirus B-19

K Parasitic
  Amebiasis
  Babesia
  Chagas' disease
  Leishmaniasis
  Malaria
  Pneumocystis carinii
  Strongyloides
  Toxoplasmosis
  Toxocariasis
  Trichinosis
L Presumed infections, agent undetermined
  Kawasaki's disease (mucocutaneous lymph node syndrome)
  Kikuchi's disease (necrotizing lymphadenitis)
Neoplasms
A Malignant
  Colon
  Hodgkin's lymphoma
  Immunoblastic lymphadenopathy
  Kidney
  Leukemia
  Liver
  Lymphomatoid granulomatosis
  Malignant histiocytosis
  Non-Hodgkin's lymphoma
  Pancreas
  Sarcoma
B Benign
  Atrial myxoma
  Renal angiomyolipoma
Collagen vascular diseases/hypersensitivity diseases
Adult Still's disease
Behçet's disease
Erythema multiforme
Erythema nodosum
Giant cell arteritis/polymyalgia rheumatica
Hypersensitivity pneumonitis (e.g., "metal fume fever," "farmer's lung," "air-conditioner lung")
Hypersensitivity vasculitis
Mixed connective tissue disease
Polyarteritis nodosa
Relapsing polychondritis
Rheumatic fever
Rheumatoid arthritis
Systemic lupus erythematosus
Takayasu's aortitis
Weber-Christian disease
Wegener's granulomatosis
Granulomatous diseases
Crohn's disease
Idiopathic granulomatous hepatitis
Midline granuloma
Sarcoidosis
Miscellaneous diseases
Aortic dissection
Drug fever
Gout
Hematomas
Hemolytic diseases/hemoglobinopathies
Laennec's cirrhosis
Postmyocardial infarction syndrome
Recurrent pulmonary emboli
Subacute thyroiditis (deQuervain's)
Tissue infarction/necrosis
Inherited and metabolic diseases
Adrenal insufficiency
Cyclic neutropenia
Deafness, urticaria and amyloid
Fabry's disease
Familial Mediterranean fever
Hyperimmunoglobulinemia D and periodic fever
Type V hypertriglyceridemia
Thermoregulatory disorders
A Central
  Brain tumor
  Cerebrovascular accident
  Encephalitis
  Hypothalamic dysfunction
B Peripheral
  Hyperthyroidism
  Pheochromocytoma
Factitious fevers
"Afebrile" FUO (<38.3°C)
Habitual hyperthermia (exaggerated circadian rhythm)

SOURCE: After RK Root, RG Petersdorf, in JD Wilson et al (eds): *Harrison's Principles of Internal Medicine*, 12th ed. New York, McGraw-Hill, 1991.

practical. Where possible, a section of the tissue block should always be retained for further sections or stains. The polymerase chain reaction (PCR) technology makes it possible to identify and speciate mycobacterial DNA in paraffin-embedded, fixed tissues. Thus, in some cases, it is possible to diagnose long-fixed pathologic tissues retrospectively. In a patient over age 50 (occasionally younger) with the appropriate symptoms and laboratory findings, "blind biopsy" of one or both temporal arteries may yield a diagnosis of arteritis. If present, tenderness or decreased pulsation should guide the location of the biopsy. Lymph node biopsy may be helpful if nodes are enlarged, but inguinal nodes are often palpable and seldom diagnostically useful.

Exploratory laparotomy has been performed when all other diagnostic procedures failed, but modern imaging and guided-biopsy techniques have largely replaced laparotomy.

THERAPEUTIC APPROACH TO THE FEBRILE PATIENT The advantages and disadvantages of antipyretic therapy have been discussed earlier in this chapter. More specific therapy is directed on the basis of the differential diagnosis for a given patient, the relative probabilities of these diagnoses, the risks of not treating, and the risks of treatment itself.

Sepsis is defined as evidence of infection with a systemic response. *Sepsis syndrome* refers to a systemic response sufficient to produce organ dysfunction, and *septic shock* is the sepsis syndrome with documented hypotension. In a nonimmunocompromised adult with sepsis, gram-positive infection, gram-negative rod infection, and meningococcal infection can be "covered" by a variety of antibiotic combinations, including imipenem, ticarcillin/clavulanate, or a third-generation cephalosporin. Suspicion of a methicillin-resistant *Staphylococcus aureus* would dictate the addition of vancomycin. If the patient has had a splenectomy, then ampicillin/sulbactam, ceftriaxone, cefotaxime, or cefuroxime would be indicated. Suspicion of *Legionella* would dictate the addition of erythromycin (possibly with rifampin) or, alternatively, clarithromycin or azithromycin. In appropriate settings, rickettsia should be suspected, and either doxycycline or chloramphenicol would be indicated. If septic shock is present without an evident source, the differential diagnosis should include meningococcemia, staphylococcal and streptococcal toxic shock syndromes and, rarely, gram-negative bacteremia. A combination of high-dose penicillin and penicillinase-resistant synthetic penicillins (nafcillin, oxacillin) would "cover" these cocci; a third-generation cephalosporin would treat the gram-negative bacteremia. If a typhoidal syndrome is suspected, then a fluoroquinolone such as ciprofloxacin or ofloxacin would be indicated. Intravenous penicillin should be used if leptospirosis is suspected. Suspected endocarditis should be treated with either penicillin, oxacillin/nafcillin, or vancomycin, plus gentamicin, depending on the type of patient and the suspected origin of infection. In IV drug users, methicillin-sensitive or -resistant *S. aureus* and gram-negative bacilli also would be considerations.

Patients with neutropenic FUO may be treated by a variety of empirical protocols, which usually combine an aminoglycoside plus antipseudomonal β-lactam antibiotic or, alternatively, imipenem or ceftazidime alone. Vancomycin should be added if intravenous catheter-associated infection is suspected. If vancomycin is included and fever continues, the addition of amphotericin B should be considered.

Empirical therapy for nosocomial FUO must be guided by the clinical situation. While empirical antibiotic therapy might be indicated, it should be remembered that complications of drug therapy, including *C. difficile* colitis and drug fever, may be causes.

The treatment of HIV-associated FUO depends on many factors and is discussed in Chap. 279. MAI, CMV, drug fever, and HIV itself are probably the most common causes of FUO, after *P. carinii*, cryptococcosis, toxoplasmosis, tuberculosis, and bacterial sinusitis have been ruled out. Discontinuing or changing drugs is often necessary, and empirical therapy for these infections may be indicated.

The emphasis in patients with classic FUO is on continued observation and examination, with the avoidance of "shotgun" empirical therapy. Empirical therapy for endocarditis, for example,

should be avoided unless there are specific reasons to invoke this diagnosis beyond fever. Every patient with FUO should have an exhaustive examination to prove, or disprove, tuberculosis. If the PPD skin test is positive, or if granulomatous hepatitis or other granulomatous disease is present with anergy (and sarcoid seems unlikely), then a therapeutic trial with isoniazid and rifampin (or possibly three drugs) should be undertaken, usually for up to 6 weeks. A failure of the fever to respond over this period should suggest an alternative diagnosis.

A dramatic response to aspirin and NSAIDs may be seen with rheumatic fever and Still's disease. The effect of glucocorticoids on temporal arteritis, polymyalgia rheumatica, and granulomatous hepatitis are equally dramatic. Colchicine is highly effective in preventing attacks of FMF but is of little use once an attack is well under way. The ability of glucocorticoids and NSAIDs to mask fever while permitting the spread of infection dictates that their use be avoided unless infection has been largely ruled out and unless inflammatory disease is both probable and debilitating or threatening.

When no underlying source is identified after prolonged observation (>6 months), the prognosis is generally good, however vexing to the patient. Under such circumstances, debilitating symptoms are treated with NSAIDs, and glucocorticoids are the last resort. It is axiomatic that the initiation of empirical therapy does not dictate the end of the diagnostic workup; rather, it commits the physician to continued thoughtful reexamination and evaluation. Patience, compassion, equanimity, and intellectual flexibility are indispensable attributes for the successful clinician dealing with FUO.

REFERENCES

Fever: pathophysiology

ATKINS E: Fever: Historical aspects, in *Interleukin-1, Inflammation, and Disease*, Bomford R, Henderson B (eds). New York, Elsevier Science Publishers, 1989, pp 3–15

CANNON JG et al: Circulating interleukin-1 and tumor necrosis factor in septic shock and experimental endotoxin fever. J Infect Dis 161:79, 1990

DINARELLO CA: Interleukin-1 and interleukin-1 antagonism. Blood 77: 1627, 1991

——, WOLFF SM: Pathogenesis of fever, in *Principles and Practice of Infectious Diseases*, 3d ed, GL Mandell et al (eds). New York, Wiley, 1990, pp 462–467

—— et al: New concepts on the pathogenesis of fever. Rev Infect Dis 10:168, 1988

MACKOWIAK PA et al: A critical appraisal of 98.6°F, the upper limit of the normal body temperature, and other legacies of Carl Reinhold August Wunderlich. JAMA 268:1578, 1992

MILUNSKY A et al: Maternal heat exposure and neural tube defects. JAMA 268:882, 1992

Fever of unknown origin

ADUAN R et al: Prolonged fever of unknown origin. Clin Res 26:558A, 1978

—— et al: Factitious fever and self-induced infection. Ann Intern Med 90:230, 1979

DATA FL, THORNE DA: Gastrointestinal tract radionuclide activity on In-111 labeled leukocyte imaging: Clinical significance in patients with fever of unknown origin. Radiology 160:635, 1986

DINARELLO CA, WOLFF SM: Fever of unknown origin, in *Principles and Practice of Infectious Diseases*, 3d ed, GL Mandell et al (eds). New York, Wiley, 1990, pp. 468–479

DURACK DT, STREET AC: Fever of unknown origin—reexamined and redefined, in *Current Clinical Topics in Infectious Diseases*, JS Remington, MN Swartz (eds). Cambridge, MA, Blackwell, 1991

GRANOWITZ EV et al: Interleukin-1 receptor antagonist production during experimental endotoxaemia. Lancet 338:1423, 1991

HOWARD P JR et al: Fever of unknown origin: A prospective study of 100 patients. Tex Med 73:56, 1977

HUGHES WT et al: Guidelines for the use of antimicrobial agents in neutropenic patients with unexplained fever. J Infect Dis 161:381, 1990

ISAAC B et al (eds): *Unexplained Fever*. Boca Raton, CRC Press, 1991

JACOBY GA, SWARTZ MN: Fever of undetermined origin. N Engl J Med 289:1407, 1973

KNOCKAERT DC, VANNESTE LJ: Fever of unknown origin in the 1980s. Arch Intern Med 152:51, 1992

LARSON EB, FEATHERSTONE HJ: Fever of undetermined origin: Diagnosis and follow-up of 105 cases, 1970–80. Medicine 61:269, 1982

MEYERS SP, WIENER SN: Diagnosis of hematogenous pyogenic vertebral osteomyelitis by magnetic resonance imaging. Arch Intern Med 151:683, 1991

PETERSDORF RG, BEESON PB: Fever of unexplained origin. Medicine 40:1, 1961

ROSENBERG MR, GREEN M: Neuroleptic malignant syndrome. Arch Intern Med 149: 1927, 1989

ROWLAND MD, DEL BENE VE: Use of body computed tomography to evaluate fever of unknown origin. J Infect Dis 156:408, 1987

RUBIN RH et al: ¹¹¹In-labeled nonspecific immunoglobulin scanning in the detection of focal infection. N Engl J Med 321:935, 1989

SABBOOR SA et al: Detection of mycobacterial DNA in sarcoidosis and tuberculosis with polymerase chain reaction. Lancet 339:1012, 1992

SCHMIDT KG et al: Indium-111 granulocyte scintigraphy in the evaluation of patients with fever of undetermined origin. Scand J Infect Dis 19:339, 1987

SIMON HB, WOLFF SM: Granulomatous hepatitis and prolonged fever of unknown origin: A study of 13 patients. Medicine 52:1, 1973

SMITH JW: Southwestern internal medicine conference: Fever of undetermined origin: Not what it used to be. Am J Med Sci 292:56, 1986

WEINSTEIN L: Clinically benign fever of unknown origin: A personal retrospective. Rev Infect Dis 7:692, 1985

WILSON ME: A World Guide to Infections: Diseases, Distribution, Diagnosis. New York, Oxford University Press, 1991

WOLFF SM et al: A syndrome of periodic hypothalamic discharge. Am J Med 36:956, 1964

———— et al: Unusual etiologies of fever and their evaluation. Annu Rev Med 26:277, 1975

section 3   Nervous system dysfunction

17   FAINTNESS, SYNCOPE, AND SEIZURES

JOSEPH B. MARTIN / JEREMY RUSKIN[1]

Episodic faintness, light-headedness, and reduced alertness are frequently difficult to distinguish, tending to shade into one another. The difference between faintness and frank syncope is often only quantitative. Types of episodic weakness, such as myasthenia gravis, cataplexy, and familial periodic paralysis, which cause striking reduction of muscular strength but no impairment of consciousness, should be set apart (see Chaps. 386 and 387). Seizures, an important cause of altered consciousness, usually differ from syncope, but in some instances distinguishing the two may be difficult. The features that distinguish seizures from syncope are discussed at the end of this chapter and in Chap. 367.

SYNCOPE AND FAINTNESS

Syncope comprises a generalized weakness of muscles, with loss of postural tone, inability to stand upright, and a loss of consciousness. The term *faintness*, in contrast, refers to lack of strength, with sensation of impending loss of consciousness (*presyncope*). At the beginning of a syncopal attack the patient is nearly always in the upright position, either sitting or standing [the Stokes-Adams attack (see Chap. 197) is exceptional in this respect]. Usually the patient is warned of the impending faint by a sense of "feeling bad." A sense of giddiness and movement or swaying of the floor or surrounding objects ensues. The senses become confused; the patient yawns or gapes, there are spots before the eyes, vision may dim, and the ears may ring. Nausea and sometimes vomiting accompany these symptoms. There is a striking pallor or ashen gray color of the face, and very often the face and body are bathed in cold perspiration. In some patients, a deliberate onset may allow time for protection against injury; in others, the occurrence of syncope is sudden and without warning.

The depth and duration of unconsciousness vary. Sometimes the patient is not completely oblivious of the surroundings, or there may be profound coma with complete lack of awareness and of capacity to respond. The patient may remain in this state for seconds to minutes or even as long as half an hour. Usually the patient lies motionless with skeletal muscles relaxed, but a few clonic jerks of the limbs and face may occur shortly after the beginning of the unconsciousness. In some situations there may be a brief tonic-clonic seizure. Sphincter control is usually maintained. The pulse is feeble or cannot be felt, the blood pressure may be low to undetectable, and breathing may be almost imperceptible. Once the patient is in a horizontal position,

gravitation no longer hinders the flow of blood to the brain. The strength of the pulse may then improve, color begins to return to the face, breathing becomes quicker and deeper, and consciousness is regained. There is usually an immediate recovery of consciousness. Some patients may, however, be keenly aware of physical weakness, and rising too soon may precipitate another faint. In other patients, particularly those with transient tachyarrhythmias, there may be no residual symptoms following the initial syncope. Headache and drowsiness, which, with mental confusion, are the usual sequelae of a convulsion, do not follow a syncopal attack.

ETIOLOGY   The list of causes in Table 17-1 is based on established or assumed physiologic mechanisms. The more common types of faint are reducible to a few simple mechanisms. Syncope results from a sudden impairment of brain metabolism usually brought about by hypotension with reduction of cerebral blood flow.

Several mechanisms subserve circulatory adjustments to the upright posture. Approximately three-fourths of the systemic blood volume is contained in the venous bed, and any interference with venous return may lead to a reduction in cardiac output. Cerebral blood flow may still be maintained, as long as systemic arterial vasoconstriction occurs, but when this adjustment fails, serious hypotension with resultant cerebral underperfusion to less than half normal results in syncope. Normally, the pooling of blood in the lower parts of the body is prevented by (1) pressor reflexes which induce constriction of peripheral arterioles and venules, (2) reflex acceleration of the heart by means of aortic and carotid reflexes, and (3) improvement of venous return to the heart by activity of the muscles of the limbs. Placing a normal person on a tilt table to relax the muscles and tilting upright slightly diminish cardiac output and allow the blood to accumulate in the legs to a slight degree. This may then be followed by a slight transitory fall in systolic arterial pressure and, in patients with defective vasomotor reflexes, may be a means of producing faints.

TYPES OF SYNCOPE   **Vasodepressor (vasovagal) or neurocardiogenic syncope**   This form of syncope is the common faint that may be experienced by normal persons. It is frequently recurrent and commonly precipitated by emotional stress (especially in a warm, crowded room), fear, extreme fatigue, injury, or pain. Many episodes, however, occur without obvious antecedent cause. In its classic form, vasodepressor neurocardiogenic syncope comprises a constellation of symptoms including hypotension, bradycardia, nausea, pallor, and diaphoresis. Syncope typically occurs in the setting of diminished venous return which leads to reduced stroke volume and a reflex increase in sympathetic activity. In susceptible individuals, this increase in sympathetic activity causes cardiac hypercontractility and excessive stimulation of ventricular mechanoreceptors (afferent vagal C fibers), which, in turn, leads to sympathetic withdrawal and activation of the parasympathetic nervous system via a centrally mediated vasomotor reflex. The net result is a vicious cycle of inappropriate peripheral vasodilatation and relative bradycardia leading to progressive hypotension and syncope which can be reversed by assumption of supine posture and elevation of the legs. Orthostatic

---

[1] Raymond D. Adams was senior author of this chapter in an earlier edition.

TABLE 17-1 Causes of recurrent weakness, faintness, and disturbances of consciousness

I **Circulatory (reduced cerebral blood flow)**
  A Inadequate vasoconstrictor mechanisms
    1 Vasovagal (vasodepressor)
    2 Postural hypotension
    3 Primary autonomic insufficiency
    4 Sympathectomy (pharmacologic, due to antihypertensive medications such as methyldopa and hydralazine, or surgical)
    5 Diseases of central and peripheral nervous systems, including autonomic nerves (Chaps. 379 and 383)
    6 Carotid sinus syncope (see also "Bradyarrhythmias," below)
    7 Hyperbradykininemia
  B Hypovolemia
    1 Blood loss—gastrointestinal hemorrhage
    2 Addison's disease
  C Mechanical reduction of venous return
    1 Valsalva maneuver
    2 Cough
    3 Micturition
    4 Atrial myxoma, ball valve thrombus
  D Reduced cardiac output
    1 Obstruction to left ventricular outflow: aortic stenosis, hypertrophic subaortic stenosis
    2 Obstruction to pulmonary flow: pulmonic stenosis, primary pulmonary hypertension, pulmonary embolism
    3 Myocardial: massive myocardial infarction with pump failure
    4 Pericardial: cardiac tamponade
  E Arrhythmias (Chaps. 197 and 198)
    1 Bradyarrhythmias
      a Atrioventricular (AV) block (second- and third-degree), with Stokes-Adams attacks
      b Ventricular asystole
      c Sinus bradycardia, sinoatrial block, sinus arrest, sick-sinus syndrome
      d Carotid sinus syncope (see also inadequate vasoconstrictor mechanisms, above)
      e Glossopharyngeal neuralgia (and other painful states)
    2 Tachyarrhythmias
      a Episodic ventricular tachycardia with or without associated bradyarrhythmias
      b Supraventricular tachycardia without AV block
II **Other causes of weakness and episodic disturbances of consciousness**
  A Altered state of blood to the brain
    1 Hypoxia
    2 Anemia
    3 Diminished carbon dioxide due to hyperventilation (faintness common, syncope seldom occurs)
    4 Hypoglycemia (episodic weakness common, faintness occasional, syncope rare)
  B Cerebral
    1 Cerebrovascular disturbances (cerebral ischemic attacks, see Chap. 368)
      a Extracranial vascular insufficiency (vertebral-basilar, carotid)
      b Diffuse spasm of cerebral arterioles (hypertensive encephalopathy)
    2 Emotional disturbances, anxiety attacks, and hysterical seizures

stress induced by prolonged upright tilt testing at 60 to 80° is a sensitive technique for reproducing syncope in many patients with this syndrome. The use of low-dose isoproterenol infusion enhances the sensitivity of upright tilt testing but may lead to false-positive tests when used in high doses. Because of the critical role of beta-adrenergic stimulation and hypercontractility in this syndrome, effective prophylaxis can usually be achieved with the use of beta-adrenergic receptor blocking agents or disopyramide. Since neurocardiogenic syncope usually occurs in patients with normal left ventricular systolic function, the use of these agents is usually well tolerated. Other pharmacologic agents which have been used to treat neurocardiogenic syncope include theophylline, scopolamine, and ephedrine. Cardiac pacing alone is rarely indicated or effective in the prevention of neurocardiogenic syncope. However, this modality may be necessary in a small minority of patients in whom profound bradycardia or asystole predominates over peripheral vasodilatation as the primary mechanism of syncope.

Postural hypotension with syncope This type of syncope affects persons who have a chronic defect in, or variable instability of, vasomotor reflexes. The fall in blood pressure on assumption of upright posture is due to a loss of vasoconstriction reflexes in resistance and capacitance vessels of the lower extremities. Though the character of the syncopal attack differs little from that of the vasovagal or vasodepressor type, the effect of posture is its cardinal feature; sudden arising from a recumbent position or standing still are precipitating circumstances.

Postural syncope tends to occur under the following conditions:

1 In otherwise normal persons who for some unknown reason have defective postural reflexes (this may be familial). In such individuals, fainting may occur when they are tilted on a table. Under such circumstances it has been found that the blood pressure at first diminishes slightly and then stabilizes at a lower level. Shortly thereafter, the compensatory reflexes suddenly fail and the arterial pressure falls precipitously.
2 In *primary autonomic insufficiency* and in the *dysautonomias*. At least three syndromes have been delineated:

ACUTE OR SUBACUTE DYSAUTONOMIA In this disease an otherwise healthy adult or child develops over a period of a few days or weeks a partial or complete paralysis of the parasympathetic and sympathetic nervous systems. Pupillary reflexes are lost, as are lacrimation, salivation, and sweating, and there is impotence, paresis of bladder and bowel musculature, and orthostatic hypotension. The CSF protein is increased. Sensory and motor nerve fibers are demonstrably intact, but nonmedullated autonomic ones have degenerated. Recovery occurs within a few months, possibly hastened by prednisone therapy. The disease is believed to represent a variant of acute idiopathic polyneuritis, akin to Guillain-Barré syndrome.

CHRONIC POSTGANGLIONIC AUTONOMIC INSUFFICIENCY This is a disease of middle-aged and elderly individuals who gradually develop chronic orthostatic hypotension, sometimes in conjunction with impotence and sphincter disturbances. Upon standing for 5 to 10 min, the blood pressure decreases at least 35 mmHg and the pulse pressure narrows, both without increase in pulse rate, pallor, or nausea. Men are more often affected than women. The condition is relatively benign and seemingly irreversible.

CHRONIC PREGANGLIONIC AUTONOMIC INSUFFICIENCY In this condition, orthostatic hypotension with variable anhidrosis, impotence, and sphincter disturbances is combined with a disorder of the central nervous system. The disorders include (1) tremor, extrapyramidal rigidity, and akinesia (Shy-Drager syndrome), (2) progressive cerebellar degeneration, some instances of which are familial, and (3) a more variable extrapyramidal and cerebellar disorder (striatonigral degeneration). These syndromes lead to disability and often death within a few years (see Chaps. 371 and 379.)

The differentiation of the chronic peripheral postganglionic and central preganglionic insufficiency is based on pathologic and pharmacologic evidence. In the postganglionic type, neurons of the sympathetic ganglia degenerate, whereas in the central type, the lateral horn cells of the thoracic spinal cord degenerate. In the postganglionic peripheral type, the resting levels of norepinephrine are subnormal because of failure to release norepinephrine from postganglionic endings, and there is hypersensitivity to injected norepinephrine. In the central type, resting levels of norepinephrine are normal. On standing, unlike the reaction in the normal individual, there is little, if any, rise in norepinephrine levels in either type. And in both types, the levels of plasma dopamine β-hydroxylase (the enzyme that converts dopamine to norepinephrine) are subnormal.

The distinction between the various types of orthostatic hypotension has therapeutic significance. In the peripheral postganglionic type, the most effective treatment is 9α-fluorohydrocortisone (oral dose 0.1 to 0.2 mg/d) and salt loading to increase blood volume, supplemented by mechanical devices to prevent pooling of blood in the legs and lower trunk (g suit). However, salt together with mineralocorticoids may induce serious supine hypertension, and the dose of the drug must be adjusted for this. For the central preganglionic type, there has been greater success with use of a sympathomimetic amine such as tyramine (which releases norepinephrine from intact postganglionic endings) supplemented by a monoamine oxidase inhibitor (to prevent destruction of the amine) and possibly propranolol. Levodopa has been effective in some cases. In the postganglionic type, judicious use of phenylephrine or ephedrine may be beneficial. Initial reports of the effectiveness of indomethacin in chronic orthostatic hypotension have not been substantiated.

OTHER CAUSES OF POSTURAL SYNCOPE   (1) After physical deconditioning, e.g., after prolonged illness with recumbency, especially in elderly individuals with reduced muscle tone. (2) After a sympathectomy that has abolished vasopressor reflexes. (3) In diabetic, alcoholic, and other neuropathies; syringomyelia; and diseases of the nervous system which cause muscular atrophy and paralysis of vasopressor reflexes. The most common form of neurogenic orthostatic hypotension is that which accompanies diseases of the peripheral nervous system. Diabetic polyneuropathy, beriberi, amyloid polyneuropathy, and the Adie syndrome are examples. Usually the orthostatic hypotension is associated with disturbances in sweating, impotence, and sphincter difficulties. Presumably the lesion involves postganglionic, nonmedullated fibers in peripheral nerves. (4) In patients receiving antihypertensive and vasodilator drugs as well as those who may be hypovolemic because of diuretics, excessive sweating, or adrenal insufficiency.

Micturition syncope, a condition usually seen in the elderly during or after urination, particularly after arising from the recumbent position, is probably a special type of vasodepressor syncope. It has been suggested that release of intravesicular pressure causes sudden vasodilatation, augmented by standing, and that vagally mediated bradycardia is a contributory factor.

Hyperbradykininemia   Deficient kinin-inactivating enzymes with apparently normal sympathetic function may result in symptoms of faintness or syncope on assumption of upright posture. Hyperbradykininemia causes arteriolar and venular dilatation, giving rise to postural hypotension and syncope with tachycardia. The pathophysiology of this condition remains uncertain. Treatment with beta-receptor antagonists has been beneficial.

Syncope of cardiac origin (cardiac syncope)   Cardiac syncope results from a sudden reduction in cardiac output, caused most commonly by a cardiac arrhythmia. In normal individuals, slow ventricular rates, but above 35 to 40 beats per minute, and fast ones not exceeding 180 beats per minute do not reduce cerebral blood flow, especially if the person is in the supine position. However, changes in pulse rate outside these limits may impair cerebral circulation and function. Upright posture, cerebrovascular disease, anemia, and coronary, myocardial, or valvular disease all reduce the tolerance to alterations in rate.

High-degree atrioventricular block is one of the most common arrhythmias that leads to fainting, and syncopal episodes associated with this arrhythmia are known as the *Stokes-Adams-Morgagni syndrome*. The etiology of disturbances in atrioventricular conduction is considered elsewhere (Chap. 197), but in patients with these attacks the block may be persistent or intermittent and is often preceded or followed by disturbed conduction in one or more of the three fascicles through which the ventricles are normally activated. When the block is high-grade or complete and the pacemaker below the block fails to function, syncope occurs. Stokes-Adams attacks occur usually without more than a momentary sense of weakness, the patient suddenly losing consciousness. After cardiac standstill of more than several seconds, the patient turns pale, falls unconscious, and, as in other types of fainting, may exhibit a few clonic jerks. With longer periods of asystole, the ashen gray pallor gives way to cyanosis, stertorous breathing, fixed pupils, incontinence, and bilateral Babinski signs. While recovery following a Stokes-Adams attack is usually prompt and complete, prolonged confusion and neurologic signs due to cerebral ischemia may occur in some patients, and permanent impairment of mental function may occasionally result, although focal neurologic signs are rare. Cardiac faints of this type may recur several times a day. Commonly the heart block is transitory, and the ECG taken later may not show any arrhythmia. In some patients, ventricular tachycardia or fibrillation may follow a period of asystole, resulting in syncope or sudden death.

Disorders of sinus node automaticity or sinoatrial conduction also may result in asystole or bradycardia of sufficient severity to cause presyncope or syncope. This disorder is most frequently detected with ambulatory ECG monitoring. Findings consistent with a diagnosis of sinus node dysfunction include symptomatic sinus pauses (>3 s) resulting from sinus arrest or sinoatrial block and severe unexplained sinus bradycardia (<40 beats per minute). The *bradycardia-tachycardia syndrome* is a common form of sinus node dysfunction in which syncope generally occurs as a result of marked sinus pauses following termination of paroxysmal supraventricular tachycardia. In occasional patients with syncope and suspected sinus node dysfunction in whom the diagnosis is not established by ambulatory ECG recording, electrophysiologic testing may be helpful in unmasking diagnostic abnormalities.

Recurrent paroxysmal tachyarrhythmias also may cause presyncope and syncope as a result of a sudden reduction in cardiac output. The magnitude of tachycardia-induced hypotension is dependent on the interaction of several variables, including the rate and mechanism of the tachycardia, the type and severity of underlying cardiac disease, the patient's posture and activity level at the onset of the tachycardia, the sensitivity of the tachycardia to catecholamines, and the integrity of compensatory autonomic reflexes. Supraventricular tachyarrhythmias are not commonly associated with syncope. However, even in the absence of structural heart disease, the combination of extremely high heart rates and loss of atrial transport may impair cardiac filling and output sufficiently to cause loss of consciousness. These tachycardias result most commonly from the occurrence of paroxysmal atrial flutter, atrial fibrillation, or reentry involving the atrioventricular node or accessory pathways which bypass part or all of the atrioventricular conduction system. Patients with the Wolff-Parkinson-White syndrome are susceptible to several forms of supraventricular tachycardia, the most dangerous of which is atrial fibrillation with rapid antegrade conduction to the ventricles over an accessory atrioventricular connection which may result in syncope and, in rare instances, sudden death. When supraventricular tachycardia is suspected as a cause of syncope, electrophysiologic testing is indicated to define the mechanism and pathway of the tachycardia and to facilitate the selection of an effective antiarrhythmic intervention (see also Chap. 197).

Paroxysmal ventricular tachycardia is a relatively common cause of syncope, particularly in patients with structural heart disease. Typically, the tachycardias are rapid and associated with abrupt loss of consciousness without premonitory symptoms. More often than not the patient is unaware of palpitations, and recovery following an episode is usually prompt and complete without residual neurologic or cardiac sequelae. The occurrence of unexplained syncope in a patient with structural heart disease is a potentially ominous finding and merits careful evaluation. The presence of pathologic Q waves on the ECG indicative of a prior transmural myocardial infarction is strongly associated with ventricular tachycardia as a cause of syncope in patients with ischemic heart disease. Other forms of heart disease such as hypertrophic and dilated cardiomyopathy, right ventricular dysplasia, and the long-QT-interval syndromes are also frequently associated with paroxysmal ventricular tachycardia and syncope.

In another form of cardiac syncope, the heart block is reflexive and is due to irritation of the vagus nerves. Examples of this phenomenon have been observed in patients with esophageal diverticula, mediastinal tumors, gallbladder disease, carotid sinus disease, glossopharyngeal neuralgia, and pleural and pulmonary irritation. However, in these conditions, reflex bradycardia is more commonly of the sinoatrial than the atrioventricular type.

Cardiac syncope also may result from *acute massive myocardial infarction*, particularly when associated with cardiogenic shock. *Aortic stenosis* often sets the stage for exertional syncope, most commonly by limiting cardiac output in the face of peripheral vasodilatation, with resultant myocardial and cerebral ischemia and occasionally arrhythmias. *Idiopathic hypertrophic subaortic stenosis* also may lead to exertional syncope because of intensified obstruction and/or ventricular arrhythmias (Chap. 205). In *primary pulmonary hypertension*, a relatively fixed cardiac output and bouts of acute right ventricular failure may be associated with syncope (Chap. 204). However, vagal reflexes may be involved in this condition as well as in the syncope that occurs with *pulmonary embolism*. Ball-valve thrombus in the left atrium, left atrial myxoma, or thrombosis or malfunction of a prosthetic valve may produce sudden mechanical obstruction of the circulation and syncope. *Tetralogy of Fallot* is the congenital cardiac malformation most commonly responsible for syncope. In this condition, systemic vasodilatation, perhaps associated with infundibular spasm, greatly increases the right-to-left shunt and produces arterial hypoxia, which leads to syncope (Chap. 199).

Carotid sinus syncope The carotid sinus is normally sensitive to stretch and gives rise to sensory impulses carried via the nerve of Hering, a branch of the glossopharyngeal nerve, to the medulla oblongata. Massage of one or both of the carotid sinuses, particularly in elderly persons, causes (1) a reflex cardiac slowing (sinus bradycardia, sinus arrest, or even atrioventricular block), the so-called vagal type of response, and (2) a fall of arterial pressure without cardiac slowing, the so-called depressor type of response. Both types of carotid sinus response may coexist.

Syncope due to carotid sinus sensitivity may be initiated by turning of the head to one side, by a tight collar, or, as in a few reported cases, by shaving over the region of the sinus. Spontaneous attacks also may occur. The attack nearly always begins when the patient is in an upright position, usually when standing. The period of unconsciousness seldom lasts longer than a few minutes. Full consciousness is regained immediately. Most reported cases have been in men. In a patient displaying faintness on compression of one carotid sinus, it is important to distinguish between the benign disorder (hypersensitivity of one carotid sinus) and a much more serious condition—atheromatous narrowing of the opposite carotid or of the basilar artery (see Chap. 368).

Other forms of vasovagal syncope have been described. Exceptionally intense pain of visceral origin may inhibit cardiac action through vagal stimulation, e.g., cardiac standstill during an attack of gallbladder colic, a lesion of the esophagus or mediastinum, bronchoscopy, pleural or peritoneal taps, intense vertigo from labyrinthine or vestibular disease, and needling of body cavities. Occasionally, a patient with a severe migraine attack will sustain a syncopal episode.

Vagal and glossopharyngeal neuralgia Occasionally this induces a reflex type of fainting. Again, the sequence is always pain, then syncope; in this instance the pain is localized to the base of the tongue, pharynx or larynx, tonsillar area, and ear. It may be triggered by pressure at these sites. Section of the appropriate branches of the ninth or tenth cranial nerve relieves the condition. The cardiovascular effects are attributable to excitation of the dorsal motor nucleus of the vagus via collateral fibers from the nucleus of the tractus solitarius.

Tussive syncope (laryngeal vertigo) This is a rare condition that results from a paroxysm of coughing, usually in men with chronic bronchitis. After hard coughing the patient suddenly becomes weak and loses consciousness momentarily. The intrathoracic pressure becomes elevated and interferes with the venous return to the heart, as does the Valsalva maneuver (exhaling against a closed glottis).

Syncope associated with cerebrovascular disease This is usually caused by partial or complete occlusion of the large arteries in the neck. Physical activity may then critically reduce blood flow to the upper part of the brainstem, causing abrupt loss of consciousness (see Chap. 368).

PATHOPHYSIOLOGY OF SYNCOPE The loss of consciousness in each type of syncope is caused by reduction of oxygenation to those parts of the brain which subserve consciousness. There are demonstrable reductions in cerebral blood flow, cerebral oxygen utilization, and cerebrovascular resistance. If the ischemia lasts only a few minutes, there are no lasting effects on the brain. Prolonged ischemia may result in necrosis of brain tissue in the border zones of perfusion between the vascular territories of the major cerebral arteries.

In a patient with faintness or syncope attended by bradycardia, one has to distinguish that due to failure of neurogenic reflexes from

that due to a cardiogenic (Stokes-Adams) attack. The ECG is decisive, but even without it, the Stokes-Adams attacks can be recognized clinically by their longer duration, by the greater constancy of the slow heart rate, by the presence of audible sounds synchronous with atrial contractions, by atrial contraction (A) waves in the jugular venous pulse, and by marked variation in intensity of the first sound despite the regular rhythm (Chap. 197).

DIFFERENTIAL DIAGNOSIS OF CONDITIONS INVOLVING EPISODIC WEAKNESS AND FAINTNESS BUT NOT SYNCOPE **Anxiety attacks and the hyperventilation syndrome** These symptoms are discussed in Chap. 389. The giddiness of anxiety is frequently interpreted as a feeling of faintness without actual loss of consciousness. Such symptoms are not accompanied by facial pallor and are not relieved by recumbency. The diagnosis is made on the basis of the associated symptoms, and part of the attack can be reproduced by hyperventilation. Two of the mechanisms known to be involved in the attacks are reduction in carbon dioxide as a result of hyperventilation and the release of epinephrine. Hyperventilation results in hypocapnia, alkalosis, increased cerebrovascular resistance, and decreased cerebral blood flow.

Hypoglycemia When severe, hypoglycemia is usually traceable to a serious disease, such as a tumor of the islets of Langerhans or advanced adrenal, pituitary, or hepatic disease, or to excessive administration of insulin. The clinical picture is one of confusion or even a loss of consciousness. When mild, as is usually the case, hypoglycemia is often of the reactive type (Chap. 338), occurring 2 to 5 h after eating, and is not usually associated with a disturbance of consciousness. The diagnosis depends on the history and the documentation of reduced blood sugar during an attack.

Acute hemorrhage Acute hemorrhage, usually within the gastrointestinal tract, is an occasional cause of syncope. In the absence of pain and hematemesis, the cause of the weakness, faintness, or even unconsciousness may remain obscure until the passage of a black stool.

Cerebral transient ischemic attacks Such attacks occur in some patients with arteriosclerotic narrowings or occlusion of the major arteries of the brain. The main symptoms vary from patient to patient and include dim vision, hemiparesis or sudden drop attacks, numbness of one side of the body, dizziness, and thick speech. In any one patient all attacks are of identical type and indicate a temporary deficit of function in a certain region of the brain due to inadequate circulation (see Chap. 368).

Hysterical fainting Fainting usually occurs under dramatic circumstances. The attack is unattended by any outward display of anxiety. The evident lack of change in pulse and blood pressure or color of the skin and mucous membranes distinguishes it from the vasodepressor faint. The diagnosis is based on the bizarre nature of the attack in a person who exhibits the general personality and behavioral characteristics of the hysteric.

Type of onset When the attack begins over the period of a few seconds, carotid sinus syncope, postural hypotension, sudden atrioventricular block, asystole, or ventricular tachycardia is likely. When the symptoms develop gradually during a period of several minutes, hyperventilation or hypoglycemia should be considered. Onset of syncope during or immediately after exertion suggests aortic stenosis, idiopathic hypertrophic subaortic stenosis or excessive bradycardia, and, in elderly subjects, postural hypotension. Exertional syncope is seen occasionally in persons with aortic insufficiency and with severe occlusive disease of cerebral arteries. In patients with ventricular standstill or ventricular fibrillation, loss of consciousness occurs several seconds later, followed rapidly by cessation of electroencephalographic activity and then often by brief clonic muscle contractions.

Position at onset of attack Epilepsy and syncopal attacks due to hypoglycemia, hyperventilation, or heart block are likely to be independent of posture. Faintness associated with a decline in blood pressure (including carotid sinus attacks) and with ectopic tachycardia usually occurs only in the sitting or standing position, whereas faintness resulting from orthostatic hypotension is apt to set in shortly after change from the recumbent to the standing position.

Associated symptoms Symptoms such as palpitation may be present when the attack is due to anxiety or hyperventilation, to ectopic tachycardia, or to hypoglycemia. Numbness and tingling in the hands and face are frequent accompaniments of hyperventilation. Genuine convulsions during the attack may occasionally occur with heart block, asystole, or ventricular tachycardia. When *duration of attack* is very brief, i.e., a few seconds to a few minutes, carotid sinus syncope or one of the several forms of postural hypotension is most likely. A duration of more than a few minutes but less than an hour suggests hypoglycemia or hyperventilation.

SPECIAL METHODS OF EXAMINATION In many patients who complain of recurrent weakness or syncope but who do not have a spontaneous attack while under observation, an attempt to reproduce attacks is of great assistance in diagnosis.

When hyperventilation is accompanied by faintness, the pattern of symptoms can be reproduced readily by having the subject breathe rapidly and deeply for 2 to 3 min. This test is often of therapeutic value also, because the underlying anxiety tends to be lessened when the patient learns that the symptoms can be produced and alleviated at will simply by controlling breathing.

Among other conditions in which the diagnosis is commonly clarified by reproducing the attacks are carotid sinus hypersensitivity (massage of one or the other carotid sinus), orthostatic hypotension and orthostatic tachycardia (observations of pulse rate, blood pressure, and symptoms in the recumbent and standing positions), and tussive syncope (by inducing the Valsalva maneuver). In all these instances, the crucial point is not whether symptoms are produced (the procedures mentioned frequently induce symptoms in healthy persons) but whether the exact pattern of symptoms that occurs in the spontaneous attacks is reproduced in the artificial ones. Continuous ambulatory ECG monitoring may be extremely useful in identifying an arrhythmia responsible for the syncopal episode, particularly in patients with frequently recurring symptoms. Monitoring is most helpful if it shows that the syncopal episode is characterized by a bout of asystole, extreme bradycardia, or tachyarrhythmia.

In cases of recurrent syncope of unknown cause in which ambulatory ECG monitoring is unrevealing, the use of intracardiac electrophysiologic techniques with programmed stimulation can be helpful in detecting cardiac rhythm abnormalities and in establishing effective treatment. During stimulation, up to two-thirds of such patients can be shown to have rapid ventricular tachycardia, His bundle conduction delays, atrial flutter, sick-sinus syndrome, or hypervagotonia. The technique is particularly useful in patients with ischemic heart disease and prior myocardial infarction, a common clinical setting for recurrent ventricular tachycardia. The diagnostic yield of electrophysiologic testing is lower with patients with nonischemic heart disease and patients with structurally normal hearts than with patients with ischemic heart disease. Recently, the signal-averaged surface ECG has proved to be useful in identifying patients with unexplained syncope who are likely to have ventricular tachycardia induced by electrophysiologic study.

Head-up tilt testing is a useful provocative technique for the diagnosis of vasodepressor syncope. Upright tilt to a maximum of 60 to 70° usually precipitates symptomatic hypotension or syncope within 10 to 30 min in patients with this syndrome. In normal subjects, passive tilting to 60° causes a small decrease in systolic blood pressure and an increase in diastolic blood pressure and heart rate. Recently, tilt testing has been used in conjunction with electrophysiologic testing to assess the efficacy of prophylactic pacing in selected patients with vasodepressor syncope and to evaluate the impact of posture on the hemodynamic consequences of some tachyarrhythmias.

The electroencephalogram may be helpful in differentiating syncope from seizures. In the interval between epileptic seizures it may show some degree of abnormality in 40 to 80 percent of cases. In the interval between syncopal attacks it should be normal.

TREATMENT In most instances fainting is relatively benign. In dealing with patients who have fainted, the physician should think first of those causes of fainting which constitute a therapeutic emergency. Among them are massive internal hemorrhage and myocardial infarction, which may be painless, and cardiac arrhythmias. In elderly persons, a sudden faint, without obvious cause, should arouse the suspicion of complete heart block or a tachyarrhythmia, even though all findings are negative when the patient is seen.

Patients seen during the preliminary stages of fainting or after they have lost consciousness should be placed in a position which permits maximal cerebral blood flow, i.e., with head lowered between the knees, if sitting, or in the supine position. All tight clothing and other constrictions should be loosened and the head turned so that the tongue does not fall back into the throat, blocking the airway. Peripheral irritation, such as sprinkling or dashing cold water on the face and neck or the application of cold moist towels, is helpful. If the temperature is subnormal, the body should be covered with a warm blanket. Since emesis is frequent, aspiration should be prevented. The head should be turned to the side and nothing given by mouth until the patient has regained consciousness. Patients should not be permitted to rise until the sense of physical weakness has passed and should be watched carefully for a few minutes after rising.

The *prevention* of fainting depends on the mechanisms involved. In the usual vasovagal faint of adolescents, which tends to occur in periods of emotional excitement, fatigue, hunger, etc., it is enough to advise the patient to avoid such circumstances. In postural hypotension, patients should be cautioned against arising suddenly from bed. Instead, they should first exercise their legs for a few seconds and then sit on the edge of the bed and make sure they are not light-headed or dizzy before starting to walk. Sleeping with the headposts of the bed elevated on wooden blocks 8 to 12 in high and wearing a snug elastic abdominal binder and elastic stockings are often helpful. Drugs of the ephedrine group may be useful if they do not cause insomnia. If there are no contraindications, a high intake of sodium chloride, which expands the extracellular fluid volume, may be beneficial.

In the syndrome of chronic orthostatic hypotension, special mineralocorticoid preparations (fludrocortisone acetate tablets, 0.1 to 0.2 mg/d in divided doses) have given relief in some cases. Binding of the legs (g suit) and sleeping with head and shoulders elevated are helpful.

The treatment of carotid sinus syncope involves first of all instructing the patient in measures that minimize the hazards of a fall (see below). Loose collars should be worn, and the patient should learn to turn the whole body, rather than the head alone, when looking to one side. Atropine or the ephedrine group of drugs should be used, respectively, in patients with pronounced bradycardia or hypotension during attacks. If atropine is not successful, a demand pacemaker should be inserted into the right ventricle. Radiation or surgical denervation of the carotid sinus has apparently yielded favorable results in some patients, but it is rarely necessary. Once it has been concluded that the attacks are due to a narrowing of major cerebral arteries, some of the surgical measures discussed in Chap. 368 must be considered.

The treatment of the various cardiac arrhythmias which may induce syncope is discussed in Chap. 197. The treatment of hypoglycemia is found in Chap. 338.

The chief hazard of a faint in most elderly persons is not the underlying disease but fracture or other trauma due to the fall. Therefore, patients subject to recurrent syncope should cover the bathroom floor and bathtub with rubber mats and should have as much of their home carpeted as is feasible. Especially important is the floor space between the bed and the bathroom, because faints are common in elderly persons when walking from bed to toilet. Outdoor walking should be on soft ground rather than hard surfaces, and the patient should avoid standing still, which is more likely than walking to induce an attack.

SEIZURES

A *brain seizure* or *convulsion* is defined as an abrupt alteration in cortical electrical activity manifested clinically by a change in consciousness or by a motor, sensory, or behavioral symptom. Seizures, which may be due to a variety of causes, become important in the differential diagnosis of syncope when the episode occurs with minimal or no warning and results in only a brief loss of consciousness. *Epilepsy* (discussed in Chap. 367) is the term used to describe recurrent seizures present over months or years, often with a stereotyped clinical pattern.

CLINICAL CHARACTERISTICS OF SEIZURES A detailed account of the types of seizures, of their pathophysiology, and of their treatment is found in Chap. 367. The purpose here is to recount briefly the varieties of seizures that occur and to outline their clinical presentation, particularly with respect to their distinction from syncope. A single seizure may occur during the course of many medical illnesses; its importance derives from the fact that it signifies involvement of the central nervous system by the disease process.

Partial seizures (focal seizures) The appearance of focal motor or sensory manifestations provides clinical documentation of the localization of the cerebral lesion. Deviation of the eyes and head to one side (aversive seizure) usually points to an irritative focus in the opposite prefrontal region. A Jacksonian seizure begins as a clonic movement in one portion of the body, often the thumb, the corner of the mouth, or the great toe, and spreads to adjacent muscular groups over a few seconds or minutes. The seizure may progress to involve the entire side or become generalized with attendant loss of consciousness. Jacksonian seizures almost always are accompanied by an abnormal interictal EEG.

Complex partial seizures (temporal lobe or psychomotor seizures) These differ from simple partial seizures. They may begin with an aura that arises from discharges in the autonomic, visceral, and olfactory portions of the temporal lobe and limbic system and are often associated with behavioral or complex motor movements for which the patient is amnesic after the attack. Subjective experiences of the aura include hallucinations (olfactory, gustatory, visual, or auditory), illusions (spatial distortions, shrinkage, or angulation), aberrations in cognition (déjà vu, a sense of familiarity; jamais vu, a sense of unfamiliarity; or recurrent memory), and affective changes (anxiety, fear, and, very rarely, rage). The seizure may terminate with only the subjective component or may progress to the motor phase, which is often evident by repetitive motor acts such as smacking the lips, swallowing, undressing, and incoherent or dysphasic speech.

Tonic-clonic (grand mal) seizure The abrupt presentation, without warning, of a generalized motor seizure is one of the most common indications of involvement of the cerebral cortex by a disease process. Grand mal seizures usually begin with opening of the eyes and mouth, flexion and abduction of the arms, and extension of the legs. The *tonic* phase of the seizure is often heralded by contraction of the respiratory muscles resulting in a vocalization. These motor signs are followed by closure of the jaw, often with laceration of the tongue, respiratory arrest with plethora and cyanosis, and urinary or, less commonly, fecal incontinence. The tonic phase of the seizure, which usually persists for only 15 to 30 s, is followed immediately by the *clonic* phase, characterized by violent rhythmic muscular contractions affecting the whole body, including the muscles of respiration. Eye movements, facial grimacing, and persistence of respiratory apnea are evident. The clonic movements subside in amplitude and frequency, and the seizure terminates, usually within 1 to 2 min. Normal respiration resumes, and the patient falls asleep; arousal may occur in a few minutes, but lethargy, fatigue, and postseizure (postictal) confusion are common and may persist for several hours. Postictal headache is also common.

The generalized seizure occurring in the course of a major medical illness signifies involvement of the central nervous system by the disorder and requires careful assessment and investigation. Such a seizure may accompany high fever, hyponatremia, metabolic acidosis, alcohol or drug withdrawal, and renal or liver failure, indicating the presence of a *metabolic encephalopathy* without requiring the postulation of another separate neurologic illness. The determination that a metabolic encephalopathy may be responsible is dependent on documentation of the systemic illness and careful attention to the exclusion of an additional infectious, vascular, or neoplastic lesion in the nervous system. Central nervous system evaluation should include a careful history, a detailed neurologic examination searching for focal neurologic deficit, and, in many cases, electroencephalography computed tomography (CT) or MRI. If infection is suspected, an examination of the cerebrospinal fluid is mandatory. Recurrent seizures (status epilepticus) indicate a serious compromise of cerebral cortical function and require vigorous treatment to prevent hypoxic damage to the brain and, following termination of the seizures, a thorough investigation of the cause.

An isolated generalized seizure occurring in an otherwise healthy, asymptomatic patient when observed by family or other bystanders is not difficult to distinguish from syncope. More difficult to assess is the circumstance of sudden loss of consciousness occurring without warning and unwitnessed by an observer or an akinetic "drop-seizure." The latter may be indistinguishable from syncope. Postictal confusion or drowsiness, injury such as laceration of the tongue, urinary or fecal incontinence, or muscle soreness suggests that a convulsion has occurred. One common clinical presentation is the sudden occurrence of a brief clonic seizure during a minor surgical or dental procedure. The patient is usually in a seated position, and the episode is considered to be due to cerebral ischemia associated with systemic hypotension and bradycardia accompanying vasovagal syncope. There are usually only two or three clonic movements, without a prior tonic phase, and recovery is rapid without postictal symptoms. Such patients should have a neurologic examination and an EEG and, if these are normal, be treated with reassurance and not given anticonvulsants. There is no evidence to indicate an underlying cerebral lesion in such patients.

Generalized seizures may be preceded by a specific warning or *aura*, and attention to these symptoms may be important in aiding in the localization of the seizure focus and can assist in distinguishing the episode from syncope. Tingling or numbness in one extremity points to involvement of the parietal lobe, and visual or auditory sensations suggest occipitotemporal localization. However, as mentioned, tingling in both hands or a variety of visual "greying out" phenomena may precede syncopal episodes. More complex psychological and cognitive sensations may accompany temporal lobe seizures and also transient cerebral ischemic attacks (see Chap. 368), but in the latter symptoms usually persist for many minutes or hours.

Absence (petit mal) seizures Absence seizures, in contrast to grand mal, are noted for their brevity and for the degree of loss of awareness accompanied by minimal motor manifestations. They are abrupt in onset and are often evident only by a stare or cessation of ongoing behavior; they may be accompanied by fluttering of the eyelids or by a few facial twitches. Full recovery occurs in 5 to 10 s, and the episode may go unnoticed by the patient, the family, or the teacher. Loss of postural tone (atonic or akinetic seizure) with falling is uncommon but, when present, requires distinction from syncope. The EEG is diagnostic in such cases, consisting of three-per-second spike and wave discharges. This condition, which indicates a specific generalized disorder of cerebral electrical activity, is responsive to specific drug treatments (see Chap. 367).

DIFFERENTIAL DIAGNOSIS OF SEIZURES AND SYNCOPE Syncope must be distinguished from disturbances of cerebral function caused by a seizure. A seizure may occur day or night, regardless of the position of the patient; syncope rarely appears when the patient is recumbent, the only common exception being the Stokes-Adams attack. The patient's color may not change in seizures, though there may be cyanosis; pallor is an early and invariable finding in all types of syncope, except chronic orthostatic hypotension and hysteria, and it precedes unconsciousness. Seizures are often heralded by an aura, which is caused by a focal seizure discharge and hence has brain-localizing significance. It is usually followed by rapid return to normal or by loss of consciousness. The onset of syncope is usually more deliberate and without aura. Injury from falling is frequent in a seizure and rare in syncope for the reason that only in seizures are protective reflexes abolished instantaneously. Tonic-convulsive movements with upturning eyes are a feature of seizures and usually do not occur with syncope, although, as stated above, brief tonic clonic seizure-like activity can accompany fainting episodes. The period of unconsciousness tends to be longer in seizures than in syncope. Urinary incontinence is frequent in seizures and rare in syncope. The return of consciousness is prompt in syncope, slow after a seizure. Mental confusion, headache, and drowsiness are common sequelae of seizures; physical weakness with a clear sensorium characterizes the postsyncopal state. Repeated spells of unconsciousness in a young person at a rate of several per day or month are more suggestive of epilepsy than of syncope. No one of these points will absolutely differentiate a seizure from syncope, but taken as a group and supplemented by electroencephalograms, they provide a means of distinguishing the two conditions.

REFERENCES

ABI-SAMRA F et al: The usefulness of head-up tilt testing and hemodynamic investigations in the workup of syncope of unknown origin. PACE 11:1202, 1988

ALMQUIST A et al: Provocation of bradycardia and hypotension by isoproterenol and upright posture in patients with unexplained syncope. N Engl J Med 320:346, 1989

BROOKS R et al: Evaluation of the patient with unexplained syncope, in *Cardiac Electrophysiology*, DP Zipes and J Jalife (eds). Philadelphia, Saunders, 1990

CHEN MY et al: Cardiac electrophysiologic and hemodynamic correlates of neurally mediated syncope. Am J Cardiol 63:66, 1989

DAY SC et al: Evaluation and outcome of emergency room patients with transient loss of consciousness. Am J Med 73:15, 1982

DELGADO-ESCUETA AV et al: The treatable epilepsies (2 parts). N Engl J Med 308:1508 and 1576, 1983

DiMARCO JP et al: Approach to the patient with syncope of unknown cause. Mod Concepts Cardiovasc Dis 52:11, 1983

EAGLE KA et al: Evaluation of prognostic classifications for patients with syncope. Am J Med 79:455, 1985

ECTOR H et al: Bradycardia, ventricular pauses, syncope, and sports. Lancet 1:591, 1984

EWING DJ et al: The natural history of diabetic autonomic neuropathy. Q J Med 49:95, 1980

GRUBB BP et al: Differentiation of convulsive syncope and epilepsy with head-up tilt testing. Ann Int Med 115:871, 1991

HICKLER R: Fainting, in *Signs and Symptoms*, 6th ed, RS Blacklow (ed). Philadelphia, Lippincott, 1977, chap 33

JOHNSON RH, SPAULDING JMK: *Disorders of the Autonomic Nervous System*. Philadelphia, Davis, 1974

KAPOOR WN et al: Diagnostic and prognostic implications of recurrences in patients with syncope. Am J Med 83:700, 1987

——— et al: A prospective evaluation and follow-up of patients with syncope. N Engl J Med 309:197, 1983

KENNY RA et al: Head-up tilt: A useful test for investigating unexplained syncope. Lancet 1:1352, 1986

LEE JE et al: Episodic unconsciousness, in *Diagnostic Approaches to Presenting Syndromes*, JA Barondess (ed). Baltimore, Williams & Wilkins, 1971, pp 133–167

McLEOD JG, TUCK RR: Disorders of the autonomic nervous system. 1. Pathophysiology and clinical features. Ann Neurol 21:419, 1987

———, ———: Disorders of the autonomic nervous system: 2. Investigation and treatment. Ann Neurol 21:519, 1987

POLINSKY RJ et al: Pharmacologic distinction of different orthostatic hypotension syndromes. Neurology 31:1, 1981

RICHARDS AM et al: Syncope in aortic valvular stenosis. Lancet 1:1113, 1984

SILVERSTEIN MD et al: Patients with syncope admitted to medical intensive care units. JAMA 248:1185, 1982

STREETER DHP et al: Hyperbradykininism: A new orthostatic syndrome. Lancet 2:1048, 1972

SUTHERLAND JM, EADIE MJ: *The Epilepsies*, 3d ed. Edinburgh, Churchill Livingstone, 1980

WEISSLER AM, WARREN JV: Syncope and shock, in *The Heart*, 4th ed, JW Hurst et al (eds). New York, McGraw-Hill, 1978, p 705

WINTERS SL et al: Signal averaging of the surface QRS complex predicts inducibility of ventricular tachycardia in patients with syncope of unknown origin: A prospective study. J Am Coll Cardiol 10:775, 1987

YOUNG RR et al: Pure pandysautonomia with recovery: Description and discussion of diagnostic criteria. Brain 98:613, 1975

18   DIZZINESS AND VERTIGO

ROBERT B. DAROFF

Dizziness is a common and often vexing symptom. Patients use the term to encompass a variety of sensations, including those which seem semantically appropriate (e.g., lightheadedness, faintness, spinning, giddiness, etc.) and those which are misleadingly inappropriate, such as mental confusion, blurred vision, headache, tingling, "walking on cotton." Moreover, some patients with gait disturbances and no abnormal cephalic sensations will describe their problem as "dizziness." A careful history is necessary to determine exactly what a patient who states, "Doctor, I'm dizzy," is experiencing.

After eliminating the misleading symptoms such as confusion, "dizziness" usually means either *faintness* (analogous to the feelings that precede syncope) or *vertigo* (an illusory or hallucinatory sense of environmental or self-movement). In other instances, neither of these terms accurately describes a patient's symptoms, and the explanation may only become apparent when the neurologic examination reveals spasticity, parkinsonism, or other ambulation disturbances as the cause of the complaint. Operationally, dizziness is classified into four categories: (1) faintness, (2) vertigo, (3) miscellaneous head sensations, and (4) gait disturbances.

FAINTNESS Fainting (syncope) is a loss of consciousness secondary to cerebral ischemia, more specifically ischemia to the brainstem (see Chap. 17). Prior to the actual faint, there are often prodromal symptoms (*faintness*) reflecting ischemia to a degree insufficient to impair consciousness. The sequence of symptoms is reasonably stereotyped and includes increasing lightheadedness, visual blurring proceeding to blindness, diaphoresis, and heaviness in the lower limbs progressing to postural sway. The symptoms increase in severity until consciousness is lost or the ischemia is corrected, often by assuming the recumbent position. True vertigo almost never occurs during the presyncopal state.

The causes of faintness are described in Chap. 17 and include the multiple etiologies of decreased cardiac output, postural (orthostatic) hypotension, and mimics such as vertebrobasilar insufficiency and seizures.

VERTIGO Vertigo is a hallucination of self- or environmental movement, most commonly a feeling of spinning, usually due to a disturbance in the vestibular system. The end organs of this system, situated in the bony labyrinths of the inner ears, consist of the three semicircular canals and the otolithic apparatus (utricle and saccule) on each side. The canals transduce angular acceleration, while the otoliths transduce linear acceleration and static gravitational forces, the latter providing a sense of head position in space. The neural output of the end organs is conveyed to the vestibular nuclei in the brainstem via the eighth cranial nerve. The principal projections from the vestibular nuclei are to the nuclei of cranial nerves III, IV, and VI, the spinal cord, the cerebral cortex, and the cerebellum. The vestibuloocular reflex (VOR) serves to maintain visual stability during head movement and depends on direct projections from the vestibular nuclei to the sixth cranial nerve (abducens) nuclei in the pons and, via the medial longitudinal fasciculus, to the third (oculomotor) and fourth (trochlear) cranial nerve nuclei in the midbrain (see Fig. 26-1). These connections account for the nystagmus (to-and-fro oscillation of the eyes) which is an almost invariable accompaniment of vestibular dysfunction. The vestibulospinal pathways assist in the maintenance of postural stability. Projections to the cerebral cortex, via the thalamus, provide conscious awareness of head position and movement. The vestibular nerves and nuclei project to areas of the cerebellum (primarily the flocculus and nodulus) which modulate the VOR.

The vestibular system is one of three sensory systems subserving spatial orientation and posture; the other two are the visual system (retina to occipital cortex) and the somatosensory system that conveys peripheral information from skin, joint, and muscle receptors. The three stabilizing systems overlap sufficiently to compensate (partially or completely) for each other's deficiencies. Vertigo may represent either physiologic stimulation or pathologic dysfunction in any of the three systems.

Physiologic vertigo This occurs when (1) the brain is confronted with a mismatch among the three stabilizing sensory systems, (2) the vestibular system is subjected to unfamiliar head movements to which it has never adapted, such as in seasickness, or (3) unusual head/neck positions, such as the extreme extension when painting a ceiling. Intersensory mismatch explains carsickness, height vertigo, and the visual vertigo most commonly experienced during motion picture chase scenes; in the latter, the visual sensation of environmental movement is unaccompanied by concomitant vestibular and somatosensory movement cues. *Space sickness*, a frequent transient effect of active head movement in the weightless zero-gravity environment, is another example of physiologic vertigo.

Pathologic vertigo This results from lesions of the visual, somatosensory, or vestibular systems. Visual vertigo is caused by new or incorrect spectacles or by the sudden onset of an extraocular muscle paresis with diplopia; in either instance, central nervous system compensation rapidly counteracts the vertigo. Somatosensory vertigo, rare in isolation, is usually due to a peripheral neuropathy which reduces the sensory input necessary for central compensation when there is dysfunction of the vestibular or visual systems.

The most common cause of pathologic vertigo is vestibular dysfunction. The vertigo is frequently accompanied by nausea, jerk nystagmus, postural unsteadiness, and gait ataxia.

LABYRINTHINE DYSFUNCTION This causes severe rotational or linear vertigo. When rotational, the hallucination of movement, whether of environment or self, is directed away from the side of the lesion. The fast phases of nystagmus beat away from the lesion side, and the tendency to fall is toward the side of the lesion.

When the head is straight and immobile, the vestibular end organs generate a tonic resting firing frequency which is equal from the two sides. With any rotational acceleration, the anatomic positions of the semicircular canals on each side necessitate an increased firing rate from one and a commensurate decrease from the other. This change in neural activity is ultimately projected to the cerebral cortex, where it is summed with inputs from the visual and somatosensory systems to produce the appropriate conscious sense of rotational movement. After cessation of movement, the firing frequencies of the two end organs reverse; the side with the initially increased rate decreases, and the other side increases. A sense of rotation in the opposite direction is experienced; since there is no actual head movement, this hallucinatory sensation is *vertigo*. Any disease state that changes the firing frequency of an end organ, producing unequal neural input to the brainstem and ultimately the cerebral cortex, causes vertigo. The symptom can be conceptualized as the cortex inappropriately interpreting the abnormal neural input from the brainstem as indicating actual head rotation. Transient abnormalities produce short-lived symptoms. With a fixed unilateral deficit, central compensatory mechanisms ultimately diminish the vertigo. Since compensation depends on the plasticity of connections between the vestibular nuclei and the cerebellum, patients with brainstem or cerebellar disease have diminished adaptive capacity, and symptoms may persist indefinitely. Compensation is always inadequate for severe fixed bilateral lesions despite normal cerebellar connections; these patients are permanently symptomatic.

Acute unilateral labyrinthine dysfunction is caused by infection, trauma, and ischemia. Often, no specific etiology is uncovered, and the nonspecific term *acute labyrinthitis* or, preferably, *acute peripheral vestibulopathy* is used to describe the event. It is impossible to determine whether a patient recovering from the first bout of vertigo will have recurrent episodes.

Acute bilateral labyrinthine dysfunction is usually the result of toxins such as drugs or alcohol. The most common offending drugs are the aminoglycoside antibiotics.

TABLE 18-1 Differentiation of peripheral and central vertigo

Sign or symptom	Peripheral (labyrinth)	Central (brainstem or cerebellum)
Direction of associated nystagmus	Unidirectional; fast phase opposite lesion*	Bidirectional or unidirectional
Purely horizontal nystagmus without torsional component	Uncommon	Common
Vertical or purely torsional nystagmus	Never present	May be present
Visual fixation	Inhibits nystagmus and vertigo	No inhibition
Severity of vertigo	Marked	Often mild
Direction of spin	Toward fast phase	Variable
Direction of fall	Toward slow phase	Variable
Duration of symptoms	Finite (minutes, days, weeks) but recurrent	May be chronic
Tinnitus and/or deafness	Often present	Usually absent
Associated central abnormalities	None	Extremely common
Common causes	Infection (labyrinthitis), Ménière's, neuronitis, ischemia, trauma, toxin	Vascular, demyelinating, neoplasm

* In Ménière's disease, the direction of the fast phase is variable.

Schwannomas involving the eighth cranial nerve (*acoustic neuroma*) grow slowly and produce such a gradual reduction of labyrinthine output that central compensatory mechanisms prevent or minimize the vertigo; auditory symptoms of hearing loss and tinnitus are the most common manifestations. While lesions of the brainstem or cerebellum can cause acute vertigo, associated signs and symptoms usually permit distinction from a labyrinthine etiology (Table 18-1). Rarely, an acute lesion of the vestibulocerebellum may present with monosymptomatic vertigo indistinguishable from a labyrinthopathy.

Recurrent unilateral labyrinthine dysfunction, in association with signs and symptoms of cochlear disease (progressive hearing loss and tinnitus), is usually due to Ménière's disease. When auditory manifestations are absent, the term *vestibular neuronitis* denotes recurrent monosymptomatic vertigo. Transient ischemic attacks of the posterior cerebral circulation (vertebrobasilar insufficiency) almost never cause recurrent vertigo without concomitant motor, sensory, visual, cranial nerve, or cerebellar signs.

Positional vertigo is precipitated by a recumbent head position, either to the right or to the left. Benign paroxysmal positional vertigo (BPPV) is particularly common. Although the condition may be due to head trauma, usually no precipitating factors are identified. It generally abates spontaneously after weeks or months. The vertigo and accompanying nystagmus have a distinct pattern of latency, fatigability, and habituation that differs from the less common central positional vertigo (Table 18-2) due to lesions in and around the fourth ventricle. Moreover, the pattern of nystagmus in BPPV is often distinctive. The lower eye displays a large-amplitude torsional nystagmus, and the upper eye has a lesser degree of torsion combined with upbeating nystagmus. If the eyes are directed to the upper ear, the vertical nystagmus in the upper eye increases in amplitude.

Positio*nal* must be distinguished from positio*ning* vertigo. The latter is provoked by head movement rather than head position and is a feature of *all* vestibulopathies, central or peripheral. Since vertigo increases with rapid head movements, patients tend to hold their heads still.

Vestibular epilepsy, vertigo secondary to temporal lobe epileptic activity, is rare and almost always intermixed with other epileptic manifestations.

TABLE 18-2 Benign paroxysmal positional vertigo (BPPV) and central positional vertigo

Features	BPPV	Central
Latency*	3–40 s	None: immediate vertigo and nystagmus
Fatigability[†]	Yes	No
Habituation[‡]	Yes	No
Intensity of vertigo	Severe	Mild
Reproducibility[§]	Variable	Good

* Time between attaining head position and onset of symptoms.
[†] Disappearance of symptoms with maintenance of offending position.
[‡] Lessening of symptoms with repeated trials.
[§] Likelihood of symptom production during any examination session.

Psychogenic vertigo, usually a concomitant of agoraphobia (fear of large open spaces, crowds, or leaving the safety of home), should be suspected in patients so "incapacitated" by their symptoms that they adopt a prolonged housebound status. Despite their discomfort, most patients with organic vertigo attempt to function. Organic vertigo is accompanied by nystagmus; a psychogenic etiology is almost certain when nystagmus is absent during a vertiginous episode.

EVALUATION OF PATIENTS WITH PATHOLOGIC VESTIBULAR VERTIGO The evaluation depends on whether a central etiology is suspected (see Table 18-1). If so, magnetic resonance imaging (MRI) of the head or, if unavailable, computed tomography (CT), with emphasis on the posterior fossa, is mandatory. Such an examination is rarely helpful in cases of recurrent monosymptomatic vertigo with a normal neurologic examination. Typical BPPV requires no investigation after the diagnosis is made (see Table 18-2).

Vestibular function tests serve to (1) demonstrate an abnormality when the distinction between organic and psychogenic is uncertain, (2) establish the side of the abnormality, and (3) distinguish between peripheral and central etiologies. The standard test is electronystagmography (ENG), where warm and cold water (or air) is applied, in a prescribed fashion, to the tympanic membranes, and the slow-phase velocities of the resultant nystagmus from the right and left ears are compared. A velocity decrease from one side indicates hypofunction ("canal paresis"). An inability to induce nystagmus with ice water denotes a "dead labyrinth." Some institutions have the capability of quantitatively determining various aspects of the vestibuloocular reflex using computer-driven rotational chairs and precise oculographic recording of eye movements.

Treatment of acute vertigo consists of bed rest and vestibular suppressant drugs such as antihistaminics (meclizine, dimenhydrinate, promethazine), centrally acting anticholinergics (scopolamine), or a tranquilizer with GABA-ergic effects (diazepam). If the vertigo persists beyond a few days, most authorities advise ambulation in an attempt to induce central compensatory mechanisms, despite the short-term discomfiture to the patient. Chronic vertigo of labyrinthine origin may be treated with a systematized exercise program to facilitate compensation.

Prophylactic measures to prevent recurrent vertigo are variably effective. Antihistamines are commonly utilized. Ménière's disease may respond to a very low salt diet (1 g/day). The unusual examples of persisting (beyond 4 to 6 weeks) BPPV respond dramatically to specific exercise programs.

There are a variety of surgical procedures for all forms of refractory chronic or recurrent vertigo, but these are only rarely necessary.

Miscellaneous head sensations This designation is used, primarily for purposes of initial classification, to describe dizziness which is neither faintness nor vertigo. However, cephalic ischemia or vestibular dysfunction may be of such low intensity that the usual symptomatology is not clearly identified. For example, a small decrease in blood pressure or a slight vestibular imbalance may cause sensations different from distinct faintness or vertigo but which may be identified properly during provocative testing techniques. Other causes of dizziness in this category are hyperventilation syndrome, hypoglycemia, and the somatic symptoms of a clinical depression. All these patients should have normal neurologic examinations and vestibular function tests.

Gait disturbances Some individuals with gait disorders complain of dizziness despite the absence of vertigo or other abnormal cephalic sensations. The causes include peripheral neuropathy, myelopathy, spasticity, parkinsonian rigidity, and cerebellar ataxia. In this context, the term *dizziness* is being used to describe disturbed mobility. There may be mild associated lightheadedness, particularly with impaired sensation from the feet or poor vision; this is known as *multiple-sensory-defect dizziness* and occurs in elderly individuals who complain of dizziness only during ambulation. Decreased position sense (secondary to neuropathy or myelopathy) and poor vision (from cataracts or retinal degeneration) create an overreliance on the aging vestibular apparatus. A less precise, but sometimes comforting, designation is *benign dysequilibrium of aging*.

EVALUATION OF THE DIZZY PATIENT The most important diagnostic tool is a careful history focused on the meaning of "dizziness" to the patient. Is it faintness? Is there a sensation of spinning? If either of these is affirmed and the neurologic examination is normal, appropriate investigations for the multiple etiologies of cephalic ischemia or vestibular dysfunction are undertaken.

When the source of the dizziness is uncertain, provocative tests may be helpful. These office procedures simulate either cephalic ischemia or vestibular dysfunction. Cephalic ischemia is obvious if the dizziness is duplicated during orthostatic hypotension. Further provocation involves the Valsalva maneuver, which decreases cerebral blood flow and should reproduce ischemic symptoms.

The simplest provocative test for vestibular dysfunction is rapid rotation and abrupt cessation of movement in a swivel chair. This always induces vertigo which the patients can compare with their symptomatic dizziness. The intense induced vertigo may be unlike the spontaneous symptoms, but shortly thereafter, when the vertigo has all but subsided, a lightheadedness supervenes which may be identified as "my dizziness." When this occurs, the dizzy patient, originally classified as suffering from "miscellaneous head sensations," is now properly diagnosed as having mild vertigo secondary to a vestibulopathy.

Patients with symptoms of positional vertigo should be appropriately tested (see Table 18-2); positional testing is more sensitive with special spectacles that preclude visual fixation (Frenzel lenses).

A final provocative test, requiring the use of Frenzel lenses, is vigorous head shaking in the horizontal plane for about 10 s. If nystagmus develops after the shaking stops, even in the absence of vertigo, vestibular dysfunction is demonstrated. The maneuver can then be repeated in the vertical plane. If the provocative tests establish the dizziness as a vestibular symptom, the previously described evaluation of vestibular vertigo is undertaken.

Hyperventilation is the cause of dizziness in many anxious individuals; tingling of the hands and face may be absent. Forced hyperventilation for 1 min is indicated for patients with enigmatic dizziness and normal neurologic examinations. Similarly, depressive symptoms (which patients usually insist are "secondary" to the dizziness) must alert the examiner to a clinical depression as the *cause*, rather than the effect, of the dizziness.

Central nervous system disease can produce dizzy sensations of all types. Consequently, a neurologic examination is always required even if the history or provocative tests suggest a cardiac, peripheral vestibular, or psychogenic etiology. Any abnormality on the neurologic examination should prompt appropriate neurodiagnostic studies.

REFERENCES

BRANDT T: Man in motion: Historical and clinical aspects of vestibular function. *Brain* 114:2159, 1991

DELL'OSSO LF et al: Nystagmus and saccadic intrusions and oscillations, in *Neuro-Ophthalmology*, 2d ed, JS Glaser (ed). Philadelphia, Lippincott, 1990, chap 11

LEIGH RJ, ZEE DS: *The Neurology of Eye Movements*, 2d ed. Philadelphia, Davis, 1991, chaps 2 and 10

SMITH GDP et al: Post-exertion dizziness as the sole presenting symptom of autonomic failure. Brit Heart J 69:359, 1993

TROOST BT: Dizziness and vertigo, in *Neurology in Clinical Practice*, WG Bradley et al (eds). Boston, Butterworth-Heinemann, 1991, chap 17

———, Patton JM: Exercise therapy for positional vertigo. Neurology 42:1441, 1992

19 DISTURBANCES OF VISION AND OCULAR MOVEMENTS

SHIRLEY H. WRAY / THOMAS L. SLAMOVITS / RONALD M. BURDE

THE HUMAN VISUAL SYSTEM

The visual system functions to form color images instantly over a wide range of background illumination. In addition, the image is placed simultaneously on the foveas of both eyes, producing a three-dimensional construct of the image (stereopsis).

Light entering the eye is focused first by the cornea, which has a fixed refractile power throughout adult life, and then by the lens, which can change focal length to form a sharp image on the retina. The variation in lens shape allows objects to be seen clearly at both near and far distances. Focusing an image on the retina is called *refraction*, and optical aberrations can be corrected by spectacles or contact lenses.

The lens is fully pliable at birth. It becomes more spherical when the zonules arising from the ciliary body relax, allowing an increase in its refractive power and a clear near image. With age the lens becomes less malleable, its protein changes, and by the fifth decade it can no longer focus near objects. This accommodative loss (presbyopia) leads to the need for reading glasses. Progressive change in lenticular protein with age also can cause opacification and impaired vision (cataract).

The retina is a multilayered structure lining the posterior wall of the globe. Light reaches the retina after passing through the cornea, aqueous humor, lens, and vitreous humor. Light also must pass through all layers of the retina to reach the photoreceptor cells. Photoreceptors are specialized neurons whose most distal segment consists of a stack of membranes containing wavelength-specific photopigments (vitamin A congeners) connected to a neuron-specific protein. The particular photopigment and the structural anatomy of the cell (whether rod or cone) determine its function. Since each photoreceptor connects with multiple ganglion cells, the photoreceptor cell participates in more than one function.

The retina is divided into a system of rods, dealing with light detection and motion, and a system of cones, dealing with higher visual function (acuity and color perception). Rods contain one photopigment (rhodopsin) and are achromatic; cones contain one of three photopigments (red, blue, yellow) which respond to chromatic stimuli producing color vision. Incoming light is perceived by the photoreceptors as present or absent. The signals are then integrated by a network of neurons, including horizontal, bipolar, and amacrine cells, before reaching the ganglion cells. In the periphery of the retina (containing mostly rods) there is considerable convergence of information; hundreds of thousands of rods influence the response of one ganglion cell. In the foveamacular area, which subserves central vision, there is much less convergence, and for some bipolar cells there is a one-to-one relationship: one photoreceptor is connected to one bipolar cell to one ganglion cell.

Ganglion cells are of several types, each with specialized functions. Large ganglion cells, A cells (M cells, phasic), project to the magnocellular layers of the lateral geniculate body. They respond to contrast and motion. Small ganglion cells, C cells (P cells, tonic), project to the parvocellular layers of the lateral geniculate nucleus and deal with chromatic stimuli (chromaticity). Ganglion cell axons project to the brain through the optic nerve, optic chiasm, and optic tracts. The majority of axons project to the lateral geniculate body. Axon collaterals, which form proximal to the lateral geniculate body, project to suprachiasmatic nucleus of the hypothalamus, pupillomotor centers in the pretectum, and to ocular, sensory, and motor centers in the superior colliculus. Second-order neurons in the lateral geniculate nucleus project to the occipital cortex via the optic radiations.

The image formed by the retina is inverted and reversed. The temporal retina images the nasal visual field, while the nasal retina images the temporal field. Similarly, the superior retina perceives the inferior visual field and the inferior retina the superior field.

The fovea-macula projection (papillomacular bundle) is the major ocular-cortical outflow. The central 5° of retina is subserved by 25 to 27 percent of the axons, and the central 20° by 90 percent of the axons. The temporal field axons (nasal retina), which account for 52 percent of axons in the optic nerve, cross in the chiasm to project to the contralateral lateral geniculate nucleus, where they synapse and project to the striate cortex in the occipital lobe.

CLINICAL ASSESSMENT OF DISTURBANCES OF VISION

ACUITY Acuity is a perceptual response of a subject to a stimulus of minimal magnitude. There are many different types of visual acuity in addition to that determined by the standard Snellen chart, such as resolution, orientation, motion, color, contrast sensitivity, and stereopsis. Visual disturbances are characterized by subnormal visual acuity (less than 20/20 Snellen acuity; see below) and by abnormalities of visual field, color vision, contrast sensitivity, and depth perception. A corrected visual acuity of less than 6/60 metric (20/200 conventional) bilaterally constitutes legal blindness. Refractive errors (myopia, hyperopia, astigmatism) commonly cause subnormal visual acuity and must be assessed for by measuring *best corrected* (i.e., best refracted) visual acuity. A pinhole can be used for a reasonable approximation of best corrected visual acuity. Visual acuity at distance is measured with a Snellen chart [normal 6/6 m (20/20 ft)]. In the fractional denotation—e.g., 6/60 metric (20/200 conventional)—the numerator 6 (or 20) stands for the testing distance (in meters or feet), and the denominator 60 (or 200) stands for the test letter's size normally seen at that denominator distance. Near acuity is measured with a near card (Jaeger chart). Bifocals or near spectacles must be worn by presbyopes (who have difficulties with accommodation) when testing near vision.

COLOR VISION Acquired color vision abnormalities in red/green perception usually imply optic neuropathy. Bedside testing may consist of gross recognition or comparison of prime colors or the use of a series of color charts (Ishihara pseudoisochromatic or American Optical Hardy-Rand-Rittler plates). Color desaturation tests rely on a comparison of the subjective perception of a colored target (e.g., red bottle top) in the right and left eyes or in the nasal and temporal half-fields of a single eye. The test detects unilateral or hemianopic abnormalities.

CONTRAST SENSITIVITY Testing of this acuity requires manipulation of both contrast and spatial frequency by measuring the minimum contrast necessary to see patterns of various sizes. Contrast sensitivity plates (Arden or American Optical) can be used at the bedside.

STEREOPSIS There is a linear relationship between stereoacuity and Snellen visual acuity. Individuals with normal 6/6 (20/20) vision in each eye and binocular fixation (no manifest strabismus) have an average stereopsis of 40 seconds of arc. Stereoacuity is reduced with decreasing acuity down to 6/60 (20/200), at which level monocular and binocular responses become identical. The Titmus stereoacuity test is used in children and adults who have been corrected for presbyopia and is suitable for bedside use. This linearity may not exist in the presence of optic nerve damage even if visual acuity returns to normal.

VISUAL FIELDS   It is possible to perform a visual field test using any perceptual stimulus. The bedside exam is performed by confrontation. Two types of "formal" field testing are in common use:

1. On *kinetic perimetry* (Goldmann, tangent screen), the patient is instructed to look at a central fixation target while test objects of varying brightness and size (white or chromatic) are moved from the periphery toward the fixation point until the patient signals that the test object is visualized. The normal field using white objects is approximately 90° temporally, 50° nasally, 50° superiorly, and 65° inferiorly. Concentric contraction of the visual field binocularly to less than 10° constitutes legal blindness.

2. On *automated static perimetry* (Humphrey, Octopus), the patient fixes on a central target in a hemisphere with a homogeneous white background while a nonmoving light of fixed size and brightness is presented at various points in the hemisphere. Brightness is increased until the patient recognizes the presence of the stimulus above background. Thus static perimetry measures brightness sensitivity of various retinal points.

Visual field defects are localizable on the basis of the anatomy of the visual pathway. Retinal and optic nerve lesions affect one of three types of nerve fiber bundles, leading to blind spots (scotomas) termed (1) central/cecocentral, (2) arcuate, or (3) radial. Loss of nerve fibers between the optic nerve and macula (maculopapillary bundle) leads to central or cecocentral scotomas, i.e., involving the center of the visual field or extending between the center and the physiologic blind spot (cecum) (Fig. 19-1*D* and *E*). Temporal retinal lesions above and below the maculopapillary bundle or those involving the superotemporal or inferotemporal optic nerve affect the *arcuate* bundles and cause inferonasal or superonasal visual field defects, respectively. Because such field defects abut the horizontal midline, they are at times referred to as *altitudinal* (Fig. 19-1*B*). Lesions involving the nasal retinal or optic nerve fibers (radial nerve fiber bundle defects) lead to inferotemporal and superotemporal visual field defects that extend toward the physiologic blind spot (Fig. 19-1*A*).

Retinal field defects frequently correspond to lesions seen with the ophthalmoscope, i.e., areas of infarction, inflammation, or degenerative change. Macular lesions produce central scotomas. Retinitis pigmentosa usually produces constricted fields and equatorial ring scotomas.

Discrete lesions, frequently ischemic, primarily in the anterior optic nerve may produce *arcuate field defects*. Such lesions include anterior ischemic optic neuropathy, glaucoma, and optic atrophy secondary to papilledema. The central/cecocentral scotoma is a specific and common sign of optic nerve disease. It occurs in a variety of conditions both intrinsic (demyelinating, infiltrative, metabolic-toxic) and compressive in nature.

At the chiasm, the visual afferents become divided into a right and left half so that the right brain sees left visual space and the left brain sees right visual space. A discrete vertical midline is the hallmark of all visual pathway disorders at or posterior to the chiasm. A chiasmal lesion most often causes bitemporal hemianopsia (Fig. 19-2*B*), but several different patterns can occur: junctional scotoma, superior or inferior bitemporal quadrantanopsia, or monocular temporal hemianopsia. Each type can occur with chiasmal compression due to a pituitary tumor, craniopharyngioma, or aneurysm. Pseudochiasmal or ocular syndromes that can mimic chiasmal lesions include tilted optic discs, drug toxicity (chloroquine), sector retinitis pigmentosa, and bilateral retinal detachments. A mass in the retrochiasmatic region impinging on or displacing the optic tract results in homonymous hemianopsia of two types: an incongruous homonymous hemianopsia or a complete homonymous hemianopsia.

Homonymous field defects due to lesions of the anterior optic radiation tend to be incongruous. Those due to damage to the

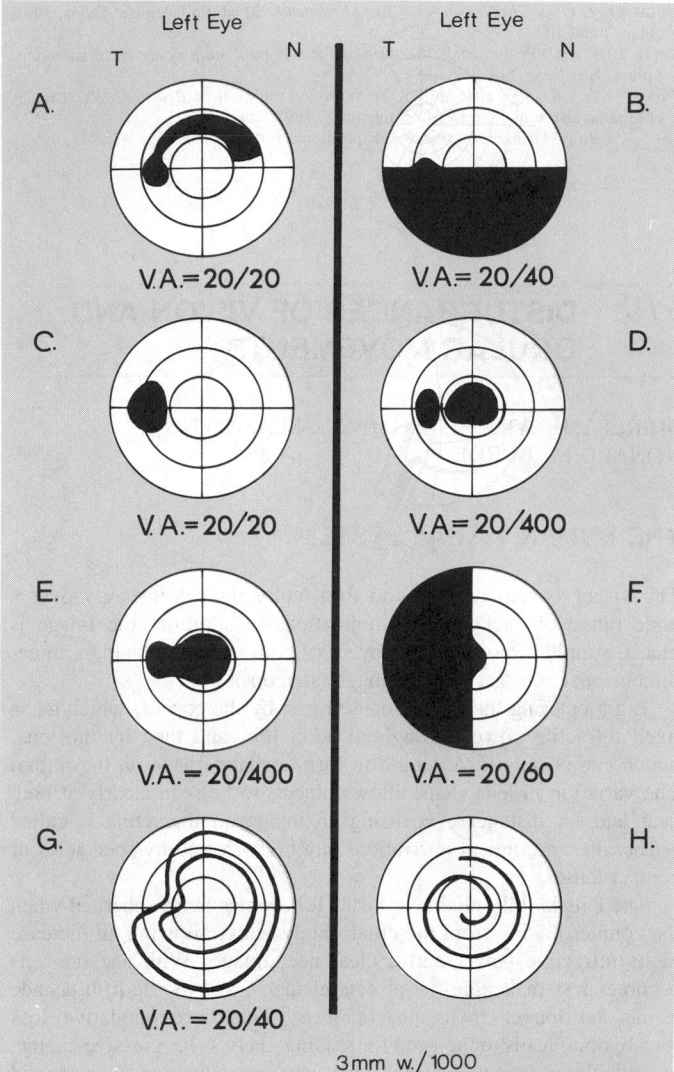

FIGURE 19-1   Types of monocular visual field loss in left eye. *A*. Superior arcuate scotoma (inferior nerve fiber bundle defect). *B*. Inferior altitudinal field defect respecting the horizontal meridian (superior nerve fiber bundle defect). *C*. Enlargement of the blind spot in the left eye. *D*. Central scotoma, normal blind spot. *E*. Centrocecal scotoma. *F*. Temporal hemianopsia respecting the vertical meridian but with involvement of central vision. *G*. Generalized constriction of the visual field to 2 isopters. *H*. Nonorganic "corkscrew" field defect to 1 isopter. *(From Wray, 1985; by permission.)*

radiations close to the visual cortex are congruous. (Congruity is said to be present when the edge of the field defect in each eye is identical in shape.) Depending on its site, the lesion may involve only the upper or lower fibers of the radiation and thus cause a lower or upper quadrant defect in the opposite half-field; e.g., temporal lobe radiation lesion causes "pie in the sky" (Fig. 19-2*E*), whereas a parietal lobe radiation lesion causes "pie on the floor" (Fig. 19-2*G*). A complete hemianopic defect to bilateral simultaneous visual stimulation (attention defect) may, however, be the only detectable sign of visual dysfunction in lesions of the parietal area. Left temporoparietal lesions are associated with defective recognition of visual symbols, alexia, and agraphia; lesions of the right temporoparietal area are manifested by impaired judgment of spatial relationships, as in topographic agnosia and constructional apraxia (see Chap. 27).

Destruction of the visual cortex of one occipital lobe produces a contralateral congruous homonymous hemianopsia. This is the most common type of cortical field defect and is frequently the result of embolic occlusion of the posterior cerebral artery. Other patterns of visual loss permit precise localization of the deficit. These defects

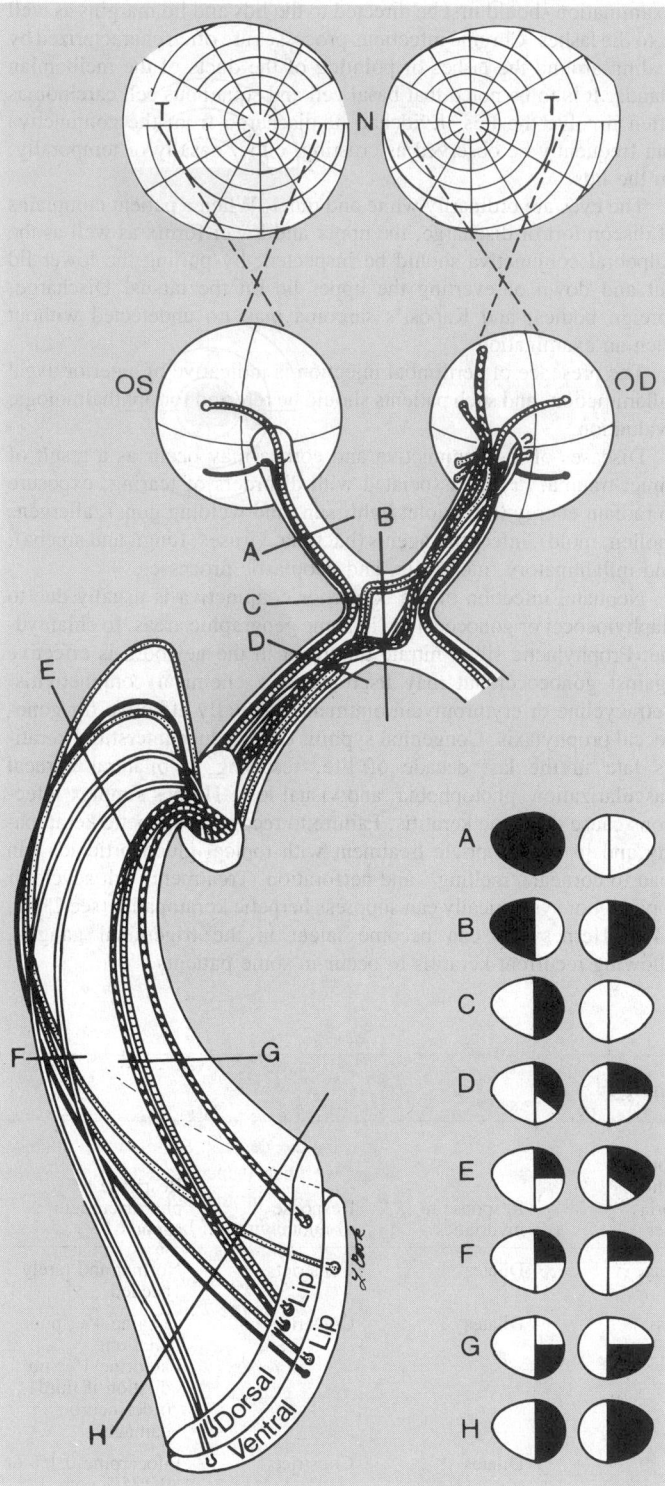

FIGURE 19-2 Nerve fiber anatomy of the visual pathways from retina to occipital cortex. The effect of the fields of vision produced by lesions at various points along the optic pathway is shown on the right. *A.* Complete blindness in left eye. *B.* Bitemporal hemianopsia. *C.* Nasal hemianopsia of left eye. *D* and *E.* Right incongruous homonymous hemianopsia. *F* and *G.* Right upper and lower homonymous quadrantanopsia. *H.* Complete right homonymous hemianopsia. *Courtesy of DD Donaldson. (From Wray, 1985; by permission.)*

PUPILLARY EXAMINATION   Normal pupillary responses consist of prompt, symmetric constriction (miosis) on exposure to light or on attempted near convergence. Diminished response to a direct light stimulus, combined with a normal consensual pupillary response following stimulation of the contralateral eye, is termed a *relative afferent pupillary defect* (RAPD). The RAPD is an important objective sign of ipsilateral optic neuropathy. The best way to elicit the RAPD is to perform a swinging flashlight test (Fig. 19-3). Anisocoria (unequal pupil size) and abnormal pupillary reflexes are two clinically important pupillary abnormalities. Comparing pupil size in the dark and in room light and observing direct light responses help to determine whether the smaller or larger pupil is the abnormal one. With parasympathetic anisocoria, the difference in pupil size will be accentuated in room light, since the affected (large) pupil constricts subnormally. With oculosympathetic paresis, the anisocoria is more marked in dim light because the affected (small) pupil dilates subnormally.

FIGURE 19-3   Swinging flashlight test demonstrates a right relative afferent pupillary defect (RAPD) in a patient with a traumatic right optic neuropathy. The patient is fixating on a distant target to avoid near effort and related accommodative miosis. *A.* Pupils in a dimly lit room. *B.* Flashlight illuminates right eye, leading to minimal direct constriction of right pupil and minimal consensual constriction of left pupil. *C.* Flashlight is swung to the left eye, causing obvious pupillary constriction directly on left and consensually on right. *D.* Flashlight is again swung to right eye, leading to bilateral pupillary dilation—a result of the right optic nerve conduction deficit.

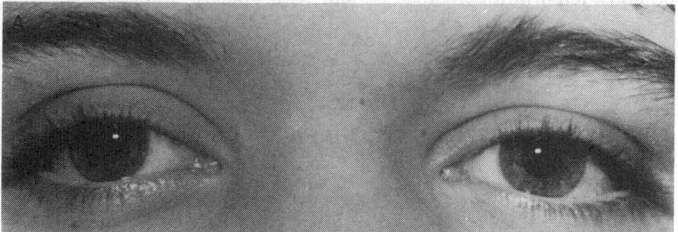

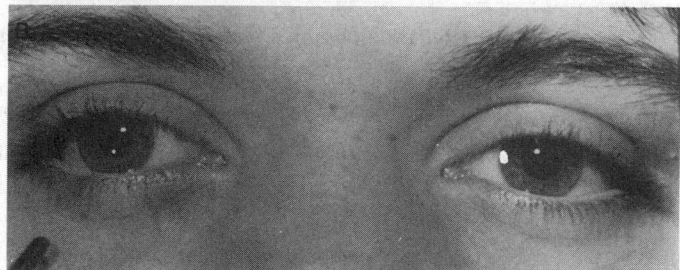

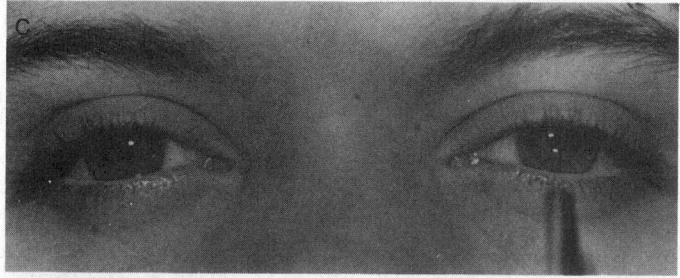

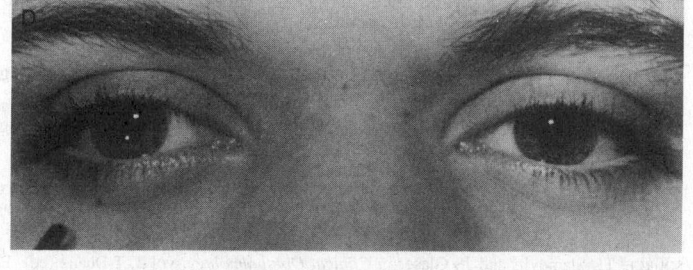

are congruous homonymous hemianopic scotoma, congruous homonymous hemianopsia sparing the temporal crescent, or, rarely, a monocular field defect due to loss of the temporal crescent, bilateral homonymous hemianopsia, bilateral altitudinal scotoma, cortical blindness, and tunnel or keyhole vision.

Isolated chronic pupillary dilation (mydriasis) is almost never caused by a lesion in the oculomotor nerve; it may be constitutional (physiologic, "benign"), pharmacologic (induced by local instillation of mydriatics), traumatic, or a result of a parasympathetic lesion at or distal to the ciliary ganglion (tonic pupil, Adie's pupil). The diagnostic workup utilizes changes in pupil size in response to topical agents (Table 19-1).

Unilateral mydriasis with impaired direct-light and near response, ipsilateral ptosis, and extraocular muscle paresis of the superior, medial, and inferior rectus and inferior oblique muscles constitutes an oculomotor nerve palsy. Unilateral miosis with normal direct-light response and mild ipsilateral ptosis constitutes an oculosympathetic lesion or Horner syndrome. The diagnosis of the Horner pupil can be confirmed by pharmacologic testing (Table 19-1).

Light-near dissociation (LND) of the pupillary response is bilateral and characterized by an impaired response to light with an intact response to near vision. When LND is bilateral and symmetric, it occurs with dorsal midbrain lesions (hydrocephalus, pineal region tumors). Argyll-Robertson pupil is a special form of LND caused by syphilis; the pupils are miotic and usually irregular in shape. LND also can occur in diabetes mellitus. LND accompanied by bilaterally poor vision is generally due to anterior visual pathway disease. Unilateral LND is most commonly seen in patients with ipsilateral retinal or optic nerve disease. Bilateral pupillary enlargement with subnormal direct and near responses occurs with pharmacologic blockade, botulism, or diphtheria. Bilaterally miotic pupils are produced by the use of parasympathomimetics for glaucoma; a pontine lesion (pinpoint pontine pupils) or narcotic (heroin) overdose should be considered in a comatose patient with bilateral miosis.

OCULAR DISEASES

THE CONJUNCTIVA AND CORNEA Diseases of the conjunctiva and cornea can produce loss of visual acuity, pain, and discharge.

Examination should first be directed to the lids and lid margins as well as to the lashes. Chronic infectious processes are often characterized by scaling around the lashes or pointing of the ducts of the meibomian glands. It is to be noted that basal cell and squamous cell carcinomas often involve the lids. Evidence of discharge from the conjunctiva can frequently be observed as crusting, either nasally or temporally, on the lids.

The eyes are ordinarily white and quiet. When a patient complains of discomfort or discharge, the upper and lower fornix as well as the palpebral conjunctiva should be inspected, by pulling the lower lid out and down or everting the upper lid on the tarsus. Discharge, foreign bodies, and Kaposi's sarcoma may go undetected without such an examination.

The presence of perilimbal injection is indicative of anterior uveal inflammation, and such patients should be referred for ophthalmologic evaluation.

Diseases of the conjunctiva and cornea may occur as a result of direct trauma, drying associated with disorders of tearing, exposure to radiant energy (ultraviolet light, sun, and welding guns), allergens (pollen, mold), infectious agents (bacteria, viruses, fungi, and ameba), and inflammatory, metabolic, and neoplastic processes.

Neonatal infection of the cornea or conjunctiva is usually due to staphylococci or gonococci or, in some geographic areas, to chlamydiae. Prophylactic silver nitrate treatment in the newborn is effective against gonococci but may itself cause a chemical conjunctivitis. Tetracycline or erythromycin ointment is equally effective for gonococcal prophylaxis. Congenital syphilis can produce interstitial keratitis late in the last decade of life, resulting in bilateral corneal vascularization, photophobia, and visual loss. Herpes simplex infections cause dendritic keratitis. Failure to recognize herpetic keratopathy and its inappropriate treatment with topical glucocorticoids can lead to corneal "melting" and perforation. Treatment with acyclovir topically or systemically can suppress herpetic keratopathy (see Chap. 143). Herpesvirus can become latent in the trigeminal ganglia, allowing recurrent keratitis to occur in some patients.

TABLE 19-1   Characteristics of pupils encountered in neuroophthalmology

	General characteristics	Responses to light and near stimuli	Room condition in which anisocoria is greater	Response to mydriatics	Response to miotics	Response to pharmacologic agents
Essential anisocoria	Round, regular	Both brisk	No change	Dilates	Constricts	Normal and rarely needed
Horner's syndrome	Small, round, unilateral	Both brisk	Darkness	Dilates	Constricts	Cocaine 4%, poor dilation; Paredrine 1%, no dilation if third-order neuron damage
Tonic pupil syndrome (Holmes-Adie syndrome)	Usually larger* in bright light; sector pupil palsy, vermiform movement Unilateral or, less often, bilateral	Absent to light, tonic to near; tonic redilation	Light	Dilates	Constricts	Pilocarpine 0.1% or 0.125% constricts; Mecholyl 2.5% constricts
Argyll Robertson pupils	Small, irregular, bilateral	Poor to light, better to near	No change	Poor	Constricts	
Midbrain pupils	Middilated; may be oval; bilateral	Poor to light, better to near (or fixed to both)	No change	Dilates	Constricts	
Pharmacologically dilated pupils	Very large†, round, unilateral	Fixed‡	Light		No‡	Pilocarpine 1% will not constrict
Oculomotor palsy (nonvascular)	Middilated (6–7 mm), unilateral (rarely bilateral)	Fixed	Light	Dilates	Constricts	

* Tonic pupil may appear smaller following prolonged near-effort or in dim illumination; affected pupil is initially large, but with passing time gradually becomes smaller.
† Atropinized pupils have diameters of 8 to 9 mm. No tonic, midbrain, or oculomotor palsy pupil ever is this large.
‡ Pupils may be weakly reactive, depending on interim after instillation.
SOURCE: TL Slamovits and JS Glaser in *Clinical Ophthalmology*, vol 2, T Duane (ed). Philadelphia, Lippincott, 1988

Adenovirus infection is the leading cause of keratoconjunctivitis in adults; it is usually self-limiting and benign. In sexually active young adults, inclusion conjunctivitis is common. In developing countries, trachoma and onchocerciasis are leading causes of corneal scarring and blindness.

Chronic indolent amebic ulcers of the cornea can occur in soft contact lens wearers who have a break in the corneal epithelium; such ulcers are difficult to treat. However, this complication is rare in those who remove and clean contact lenses daily. Debilitated patients can develop keratitis due to gram-negative bacteria (*Klebsiella, Pseudomonas*) or fungi. Malnutrition and avitaminosis A can lead to conjunctival and corneal scarring with keratinization (xerosis) and severe visual loss.

Keratoconjunctivitis also can occur in patients with Stevens-Johnson syndrome (Chap. 52), Wegener's granulomatosis (Chap. 291), rheumatoid arthritis (Chap. 285), atopic dermatitis (Chap. 51), and cicatricial pemphigoid (Chap. 53). These processes are often associated with corneal ulceration. Band keratopathy is caused by corneal deposition of calcium salts, especially within the palpebral fissure (Fig. A8-10). It occurs as a result of chronic inflammation (keratouveitis) or of systemic hypercalcemia (see Chap. 357).

Corneal clouding is prominent in G_{MI} gangliosidosis (Chap. 349), in certain of the mucopolysaccharidoses (Chap. 349), and in aminoaciduria [cystinosis (Chap. 352)]. In Wilson's disease (Chap. 348) and in chronic biliary cirrhosis, copper deposits form a golden-brown ring (Kayser-Fleischer ring) (Fig. A8-16) in the cornea at the level of Descemet's membrane. Corneal drug deposition may occur following systemic use of chloroquine, phenothiazine, gold, silver, or amiodarone.

THE LENS AND CATARACTS Opacification of the normally clear and transparent crystalline lens is termed a *cataract*. Visual symptoms are blurred vision, glare, altered color perception, and monocular diplopia. *Congenital* cataracts occur as a complication of intrauterine rubella, herpes simplex, herpes zoster, syphilis, and cytomegalic inclusion disease. The majority are idiopathic or inherited. Acquired cataracts result from trauma, radiation, drugs, metabolic disorders, ocular inflammatory disorders, or aging (senile cataract). Cataracts develop earlier in patients with diabetes mellitus (type I and type II) and in some patients with a strong family history of cataract formation. Metabolic disorders complicated by cataract include galactosemia (Chap. 354), chronic hypercalcemic states (Chap. 357), Fabry's disease, Wilson's disease (Chap. 348), and Lowe's syndrome (Chap. 244). More than a third of patients with myotonic dystrophy have multicolored crystalline opacities scattered throughout the lens. Cataracts also may be associated with chromosomal disorders; with the Alport, cri-du-chat, Conradi, Crouzon, and Down syndromes; and with gonadal dysgenesis. Inflammatory ocular diseases, and drugs and toxic substances such as haloperidol, glucocorticoids, and iron also can cause cataracts. Cataract extraction is performed by removing the lens nucleus and cortex from within the lens capsule. In most adults, a plastic lens is then implanted within the capsule.

The zonules holding the lens may be broken in one region, allowing the lens to move eccentrically, often leaving its edge in the pupillary axis (subluxation), or totally broken, allowing the lens to move into the anterior chamber or into the vitreous cavity (luxation). The most common cause of subluxation or luxation is trauma. Others include homocystinuria (Chap. 352), Marfan's syndrome, spherophakia, and sulfite oxidase insufficiency.

UVEAL DISEASES The uvea consists of the iris and ciliary body anteriorly and the choroid posteriorly. Anatomically, the choroid has three layers of vessels and a cellular matrix including pigmented cells. Common diseases of the uvea are inflammatory or neoplastic. Inflammation can involve the iris (iritis), ciliary body (cyclitis), or choroid (choroiditis) or any combination of the three (uveitis). Uveitis causes photophobia, ocular discomfort, and visual blurring. Chronic uveitis can cause cystoid macular edema with decreased central acuity, cataract formation, and secondary glaucoma. The most common form of uveitis is idiopathic. Systemic diseases causing uveitis include pauciarticular juvenile rheumatoid arthritis (rheumatoid factor nega-

tive), juvenile nevoxanthogranuloma, rheumatoid arthritis, sarcoidosis, Lyme disease, and relapsing polychondritis. Treatment of uveitis (dependent on severity) includes cycloplegic drops and glucocorticoids (topically or systemically) and sometimes immunosuppressive drugs (chlorambucil, azathioprine, cyclophosphamide, and cyclosporin A).

Ocular malignant melanoma is a primary neoplastic disease of the choroid. Choroidal involvement also occurs as a result of metastases (lung, breast, prostate) and in association with lymphoma of the central nervous system (reticulum cell sarcoma)—conditions that are sometimes responsive to low-dose radiation.

RETINAL DISEASES Retinal abnormalities are best seen by performing a dilated fundus examination. Retinal diseases involving the macula cause distortion of straight lines (metamorphopsia), loss of central acuity, and visual field abnormalities. Nonmacular retinal disorders cause scotomata involving the peripheral or paracentral visual field, correlating with the site of retinal pathology. Retinopathies can be due to diseases of the retinal vessels, neurosensory retina, or the retinal pigment epithelium.

Retinal vasculopathies These changes occur in many systemic conditions. In hypertensive retinopathy, the severity of retinal changes correlates closely with the level of systemic hypertension (see Chap. 209). Grade I consists of arteriolar narrowing; grade II includes arteriovenous nicking, minimal exudation, and splinter hemorrhages; grade III includes retinal edema, hemorrhages, and cotton-wool spots (focal ischemia in the nerve fiber layer); grade IV includes grade III changes plus papilledema, often with a macular star produced by deposition of cellular debris (hard exudates). Hypertensive retinopathy can be seen with all forms of hypertension—essential and secondary. Cotton-wool spots, a common feature of malignant hypertension, also may occur in anemia, leukemia, collagen vascular disease, dysproteinemia, infective endocarditis, and diabetes mellitus. They are the most common ophthalmic lesions in acquired immunodeficiency syndrome (AIDS) (see Chap. 279). Other ocular manifestations of AIDS include cytomegalovirus (CMV) retinitis (Fig. A8-14) and toxoplasmic and fungal retinal infections. Nonretinal ocular manifestations of AIDS include optic neuropathy, Kaposi's sarcoma of the conjunctiva, and orbital lymphoma.

Diabetic retinopathy is classified into two groups: (1) background retinopathy (Fig. A8-12), characterized by microaneurysms, dot-blot hemorrhages, cotton-wool spots, hard exudates, intraretinal microvascular shunt vessels, and venous beading, sometimes with related macular edema, and (2) proliferative retinopathy (Fig. A8-13), characterized by neovascularization, proliferation of fibrous tissue into the vitreous cavity, and eventually traction retinal detachments with visual loss (see Chap. 337). Panretinal photocoagulation is beneficial in maintaining vision in early proliferative retinopathy. The progression of diabetic retinopathy correlates best with the concentration of hemoglobin A_{lc}, reflecting the long-term metabolic control. The lower the hemoglobin A_{lc} concentration, the slower is the progression. The acute induction of so-called tight control is often associated with a short-term aggravation of the retinopathic process (e.g., insulin infusion pump or multiple injection regime).

Other proliferative retinopathies Somewhat similar retinal vascular changes ("sea fan" proliferation) occur in sickle cell diseases (S-S, S-C, S-Thal) and in the retinopathy of prematurity. In sickle cell disease focal photocoagulation is helpful. Focal retinal cryotherapy is of benefit in a subset of infants with acute retinopathy of prematurity.

Retinopathy of prematurity (ROP) Retinopathy of prematurity (formerly retrolental fibroplasia) is now classified according to the following criterion: *location* (zones I to III), *extent* (hours of the clock), *stage* (1 to 5), and plus disease (marked vascular shunting). Risk factors for the development of ROP are birth weight and gestational age. Neonates less than 28 weeks and weighing less than 1250 g are especially at risk. Initial fundus examination of these infants should be at 4 to 6 weeks, with subsequent examinations determined by the fundus findings or every 2 to 3 weeks until maturity. Care must be taken in dilating the eyes of these patients owing to the potential side effects of mydriatics and cycloplegic drops. A large multicenter trial has demonstrated the efficacy of transscleral cryotherapy in decreasing the incidence of retinal detachment and retinal folding from 43 to 22 percent in patients with stage 3 + ROP with plus disease. Currently, the effectiveness of laser ablation is being studied.

Occlusive retinal vasculopathies   Permanent blindness occurs with *infarction* of the inner retina due to occlusion of the central retinal artery (CRA). Funduscopic examination shows rectangular "box car" segmentation of venous blood flow and an opaque white retina due to axoplasmic stasis in ganglion cell axons. A central cherry-red spot is due to visualization of the choroid in the macular area devoid of axons (Fig. A8-2). CRA occlusion may be embolic (ipsilateral internal carotid artery, aorta, or heart) or thrombotic due to giant cell arteritis, arteriosclerosis, collagen vascular disease, or hyperviscosity states. CRA occlusion is an ophthalmic emergency. Treatment may include ballotement of the globe, retrobulbar anesthetic block, and paracentesis of aqueous humor in an attempt to move embolic material into peripheral arterioles.

Monocular transient blurring of vision (amaurosis fugax) lasting seconds to minutes may herald CRA occlusion but, more important, may be a precursor of a stroke. Most cases of amaurosis fugax are caused by presumed embolic phenomena. In younger patients a cardiac source is more likely, but with increasing age carotid atheromatous disease becomes a more frequent source. Depending on the physical examination, these patients require an evaluation of the aortic arch and carotid circulation as well as the heart (see Chap. 368). Based on recent studies, patients in both North America and Europe with high-grade stenosis (>70 percent) benefit from carotid endarterectomy by reducing the risk of subsequent stroke by 33 to 66 percent as compared with patients on medical therapy.

Central (Fig. A8-3) and branch retinal vein occlusion may occur spontaneously or in association with hypertension or elevated intraocular pressure. Venous stasis retinopathy mimics early vein occlusion with venous dilatation, hemorrhages, and cotton-wool spots; it is due to impaired retinal perfusion produced by severe carotid occlusive disease and Takayasu's disease. Systemic coagulopathies such as thrombocytopenia, disseminated intravascular coagulopathy, and systemic lupus erythematosus with circulating anticoagulants (cardiolipin) may cause retinal hemorrhages, clotting in the submacular choriocapillaris, choroidal hemorrhages, and detachment of the retina. Perivenous sheathing occurs in primary retinal vasculitis (Eales disease), leukemia, and optic nerve demyelination. Fundus changes may be the mark of an abused child presenting with multiple retinal hemorrhages (subhyaloid lakes, blot and flame hemorrhages) and cotton-wool spots. This retinopathy is caused by severe shaking or choking of the child.

Retinal vascular anomalies are rare and among them are to be found retinal telangiectasia (Coat's disease), retinal angiomatosis [von Hippel-Lindau syndrome (Chap. 378)], direct arteriovenous connections (Wyburn-Mason syndrome), miliary aneurysms, cavernous retinal hemangiomas.

Nonvascular diseases of the retina   These include infections such as congenital and acquired toxoplasmosis, herpes retinitis, and *Monilia* and nematode infestations. Inflammatory diseases of the outer retina and choroid include the presumed ocular histoplasmosis syndrome, acute multifocal placoid pigment epitheliopathy, serpiginous retinopathy, "bird-shot" chorioretinopathy, multiple evanescent white dot syndrome, and neoplastic diseases such as retinoblastoma.

Retinal degenerative disease   These may involve the retinovitreal interface with focal capillary sclerosis and hole formation (lattice degeneration) or may appear as isolated areas of retinovitreal adhesion and vitreous liquefaction (syneresis) leading to retinal traction, retinal horseshoe-shaped tears, and detachment. Lightning-like flashes and/or an acute vitreous hemorrhage producing a spiderweb-like shadow and blurred vision may herald detachment. These patients must be examined by an ophthalmologist utilizing an indirect ophthalmoscope. Emergency surgery (laser, cryotherapy) is required to seal the tears. Degeneration of the outer retina and pigment epithelium is characteristic of retinitis pigmentosa (Fig. A8-9) which occurs in

sporadic, X-linked, autosomal recessive, and autosomal dominant forms. Several mutations have been shown to be associated with the genetic forms of retinitis pigmentosa. Some involve point mutations in rhodopsin, which may present as either an autosomal dominant or autosomal recessive phenotype. Symptoms are loss of night vision, progressive concentric contraction of the visual field, and eventually, loss of central vision.

Multisystem disorders   Several disorders may cause retinal degeneration, including abetalipoproteinemia (Bassen-Kornzweig syndrome, Chap. 344), neuronal ceroid lipofuscinosis (Batten-Mayou disease), Refsum's disease (Chap. 383), certain mucopolysaccharidoses, and the Kearns-Sayre syndrome (Chap. 385).

Certain lysosomal storage diseases, including G_{M1} and G_{M2} gangliosidosis and the sphingolipidoses, affect ganglion cell function, leading to blindness; cherry-red spots are invariably present (Chap. 349). Toxic retinopathy may follow the use of phenothiazine derivatives, especially thioridazine (Mellaril), chloroquine, and hydroxychloroquine. Long-term therapy with these agents should be monitored at regular intervals with static perimetry or kinetic perimetry with red and white targets.

DISEASES OF THE RETINAL PIGMENT EPITHELIUM   Bruch's membrane is a multilayered structure formed by the choriocapillaris and the pigment epithelium of the retina. With aging, the pigment epithelium may accumulate intracellular material, leading to age-related macular degeneration. Visual loss is slowly progressive, associated with metamorphopsia, and rarely causes less than 6/120 (20/400) Snellen acuity. A second type of age-related macular degeneration can occur in the paramacular foveal area and cause visual loss. It results from degeneration of Bruch's membrane with the formation of large or small breaks in its integrity and subretinal neovascularization. Subsequent exudation and hemorrhage cause a further elevation of the sensory or pigment epithelium of the retina. Visual loss is often acute and catastrophic in nature, decreasing acuity to less than 6/120 (20/400) with a large central scotoma that is defined by the anatomic detachment. Laser ablation of the neovascular net may delay blindness. Angioid streaks are large breaks in Bruch's membrane (Fig. A8-8). They are associated with Paget's disease, acromegaly, pseudoxanthoma elasticum, sickle cell disease, and severe myopia.

DISEASES OF THE OPTIC NERVE

The optic disc is the exit site of all retinal ganglion cell axons. The axons leave the globe in the optic nerve by passing through the lamina cribrosa. Just posterior to the lamina, the nerve fibers become myelinated. The blood supply of the nerve head is primarily derived from choroidal and posterior ciliary branches of the ophthalmic artery.

GLAUCOMA   Glaucoma is characterized by progressive field loss due to nerve damage from elevated intraocular pressure. It is an important cause of blindness worldwide and in the United States occurs in 1 to 2 percent of patients above age 60. The disease may be asymptomatic with painless, slow loss of peripheral and paracentral visual fields. Early detection depends on a routine eye examination with intraocular pressure measurement (tonometry), funduscopy with attention to optic disc appearance, and visual field testing. In the normal eye, the optic cups are symmetric and the neural rim is pink (Fig. A8-1). In glaucoma, either localized notching or generalized enlargement of the optic cup can be seen (Fig. A8-11). The rim, although thinned, remains pink until late. The central optic cup diameter can be compared with the diameter of the disc, and a ratio of the horizontal and vertical dimensions can be recorded. The normal cup-disc ratio is less than 0.2 to 0.3. Vertical disparity in one or both eyes is an early sign of glaucoma. Glaucoma is often asymmetric, and the finding of asymmetry of the cup-disc ratio implies glaucoma. Early visual field loss includes nonspecific constriction and small paracentral scotomas. Eventually, arcuate nerve fiber bundle defects develop with a characteristic *nasal step* (e.g., arcuate bundle defect extending to the nasal horizontal raphe forms a steplike configuration on kinetic visual field testing). The papillomacular bundle and acuity are spared until late in the disease. Intraocular pressure reflects the balance between the production and outflow of aqueous humor, and the normal range is 2.09 ± 0.33 kPa (15.8 ± 2.5 mmHg) measured by applanation tonometry. (Schiotz tonometers measure intraocular pressure by indentation of the cornea, whereas most tonometers measure by planating the corneal surface, hence applanation.)

Glaucoma is an appellation for many disease states. It results from decreased outflow of aqueous humor through the pupil, trabecular meshwork, and Schlemm's canal, leading to elevated intraocular pressure. Chronic or *primary open-angle glaucoma*, the most common of adult glaucomas, is asymptomatic and detected only by routine eye examination. It is associated with a relative obstruction to aqueous outflow through the trabecular meshwork and is of unknown cause. Treatment includes the use of topical agents including cholinergic (pilocarpine, carbachol, echothiophate) or adrenergic agonists (epinephrine dipivefrin) or antagonists, i.e., beta-adrenergic blockers (timolol, levobunalol, betaxolol). If topical agents do not reduce the intraocular pressure satisfactorily, systemic carbonic anhydrase inhibitors (acetazolamide or methazolamide) are added. Laser trabeculoplasty or filtration surgery, to improve aqueous outflow, is indicated when medical therapy fails.

Secondary open-angle glaucoma may develop in patients with ocular inflammatory or neoplastic disease, with mature cataracts or elevated episcleral venous pressure, or during a course of long-term glucocorticoid therapy, either topical or systemic.

Angle-closure glaucoma occurs when the iris blocks egress of aqueous humor through the trabecular meshwork. In the primary form, an anatomic abnormality of the eye leads to pupillary block and obstruction of the trabecular meshwork. An acute rise in intraocular pressure occurs, with dilation of the pupil causing severe eye and face pain, nausea, vomiting, colored halos around lights, and loss of visual acuity. Conjunctival hyperemia, corneal edema, and a fixed middilated pupil are common signs. Urgent reduction of the intraocular pressure is best accomplished by the use of hyperosmotic agents, including oral glycerine and sorbitol or intravenous mannitol. Laser or surgical iridotomy is curative in most cases.

Secondary angle-closure glaucoma can occur when the lens or ciliary body becomes swollen, pushing the iris against the trabecular meshwork or sealing the iris to the trabecular meshwork as a result of the formation of a neovascular network. This process occurs in patients with diabetic retinopathy, advanced ocular ischemic syndrome due to severe occlusive carotid disease, or inflammatory adhesions (synechiae).

OPTIC NEUROPATHIES   Diseases of the optic nerve cause acuity loss, subjective color and brightness desaturation, changes in contrast sensitivity, and visual field loss. There is almost always a relative afferent pupillary defect (RAPD) with a unilateral or asymmetric optic nerve process. (Fig. 19-3). Papilledema (optic disc edema secondary to elevated intracranial pressure) and infiltration of the optic nerve sheath cause visual dysfunction late in the course of the disease. In acute optic neuropathy the optic disc may be normal or swollen. In chronic optic neuropathy the disc is swollen or pale (atrophy).

Optic neuritis most commonly afflicts patients in their twenties or thirties, women more than men, and can either be a primary demyelinating disease of unknown etiology or associated with past, present, or future manifestations of multiple sclerosis (see Chap. 373). Acute optic neuritis is usually unilateral. There is acute visual acuity or visual field loss, an RAPD, and more than 90 percent of the time ocular pain, typically exacerbated by eye movement. In the acute phase, the nerve appearance is normal (retrobulbar optic neuritis) in two-thirds or swollen (anterior optic neuritis or papillitis) in one-third of cases. Of patients with acute optic neuritis, about half have brain abnormalities on MRI consistent with demyelination. Prognosis for visual acuity recovery is excellent, even without treatment, but some residual visual dysfunction generally persists, such as abnormal

color vision or visual field or contrast sensitivity. Within a decade and a half of the onset of acute optic neuritis, about three-quarters of women and one-third of men will develop multiple sclerosis.

Treatment of acute idiopathic or demyelinating optic neuritis with oral prednisone in standard doses alone is not indicated because it appears to increase the risk of subsequent episodes of optic neuritis. Treatment with intravenous methylprednisolone (1 g/d for 3 days) followed by a short course of oral prednisone does not appear to increase recurrence risk and, compared with no treatment, hastens reversal of visual loss. However, methylprednisolone therapy only leads to slightly better vision after 6 months in adults, and therefore, the appropriateness of treatment has to be weighed for the individual patient. Treatment benefit may be greater when visual loss is relatively more profound (worse than 20/40) within the first week of onset of visual symptoms.

Anterior ischemic optic neuropathy (AION) occurs most often in patients over 40 years of age. Typically, sudden visual loss and altitudinal field loss occur, i.e., a superior or inferior visual field defect with one border along the horizontal midline, associated with disc swelling due to infarction of the nerve head (Fig. A8-6). It occurs in two forms: (1) nonarteritic (median age 56 years), in which the risk factors are diabetes mellitus in younger patients and hypertension in older patients, and (2) an arteritic (giant cell arteritis) variety (median age 74 years). Symptoms of giant cell arteritis (anorexia, malaise, proximal arthralgia, myalgia, headache, and jaw claudication) and an elevated erythrocyte sedimentation rate are indications for prompt systemic glucocorticoid therapy and a temporal artery biopsy. Untreated, arteritic ischemic optic neuropathy may affect the contralateral eye and cause blindness in 40 percent of cases.

Compression (intrinsic or extrinsic) of the optic nerve causes insidious progressive acuity and field loss. The disc may be normal, swollen, or atrophic (Fig. A8-7). Intrinsic tumors include optic nerve sheath meningioma and glioma. In Graves' ophthalmopathy, the optic neuropathy is due to compression of the nerve in the orbital apex by the enlarged extraocular muscles. Benign or malignant orbital tumors, metastatic lesions, tumors arising from the adjacent paranasal sinuses and middle cranial fossa, and giant pituitary adenomas can each lead to compressive optic neuropathy.

Infiltrative and toxic optic neuropathies are rare. Progressive disc swelling and visual loss characterize infiltration by inflammatory disease (sarcoidosis), infection (cryptococcosis), or neoplasia (leukemia, lymphoma, metastatic carcinoma). Toxic agents (methanol, ethambutol) cause a more acute visual loss with normal or swollen discs, whereas nutritional amblyopias are associated with a more insidious course.

Leber hereditary optic neuropathy   This condition, which affects males primarily (Western populations), is transmitted mitochondrially, i.e., through the female line. Leber's hereditary optic neuropathy probably represents the pure neurologic end of the spectrum of the encephalomyelopathies in contrast to Kearns-Sayre's syndrome (progressive external ophthalmoplegia, pigmentary retinopathy, and cardiac conduction block), which is midspectrum. At least six mutations in the DNA of mitochondria have been identified. Between 50 and 60 percent have a mitochondrial point mutation at the nucleotide position 11,778, where there is a guanine-adenine substitution. This converts a highly conserved arginine to a histidine in complex I of the mitochondrial redox system. This is believed to cause a relative metabolic deficiency, but how or why this produces the clinical complex is uncertain.

This mutation can be demonstrated using *Mae* III or *Sfa* NI restriction probes. The 11,778 mutation has not been found in healthy human beings. As mentioned previously, at least five other mutations have been found. Pedigree studies have demonstrated that 50 percent of men and 20 percent of women who have inherited the 11,778 defect develop an optic neuropathy. This penetrance cannot be explained on the basis of heteroplasmy, and it has been suggested that the mitochondrial DNA mutation can only be expressed when matched with a specific X chromosome allele.

Leber hereditary optic neuropathy is characterized by rapid loss of central vision during early adult life. Both eyes are affected either simultaneously or sequentially. The visual fields contain scotomas that are initially central and rapidly become cecocentral in location. In acute Leber hereditary optic neuropathy, the ophthalmoscopic findings are (1) circumpapillary telangiectatic microangiopathy, (2) swelling of the nerve fiber layer around the disc, and (3) absence of leakage from the disc or peripapillary region on fluorescein angiography with arteriovenous shunting present in the area of telangiectatic vessels. Late in the course of the disease, optic atrophy develops. About 15 percent of patients recover useful vision in one or both eyes many years after the ictus; however, those with the 11,778 mutation have been reported to have a uniformly poor visual prognosis.

Papilledema Optic disc swelling resulting from elevated intracranial pressure (Fig. A8-4) is typically bilateral, often asymmetric, and associated with transient visual loss lasting seconds (visual obscurations) and horizontal diplopia. Optic atrophy, impaired vision, and field loss may ensue if papilledema becomes chronic. Increased intracranial pressure may be caused by mass lesions, inflammatory disease, or idiopathic pseudotumor cerebri (benign intracranial hypertension), but the immediate obligation is to exclude an intracranial mass lesion with appropriate neuroimaging tests (see Chap. 369).

Pseudopapilledema Pseudopapilledema is usually due to congenital disc anomalies, giving rise to apparent rather than true disc swelling. Small or absent optic cups, abnormal branching of the major retinal vessels, and calcific excrescences [optic disc drusen (Fig. A8-5)] may be seen.

DISORDERS OF EYE MOVEMENT

Disorders of eye movement in the adult usually present with diplopia. The diagnostic approach to determine the cause is based on a series of specific questions and a step-by-step analysis of the eye movements to establish first whether the double vision is monocular or binocular. If diplopia is present with one eye covered, the patient has monocular diplopia. Monocular diplopia almost never signals a neurologic disorder but is most often due to an optical problem (refractive error, keratoconus, or cataract). It may be psychogenic or functional. Binocular diplopia resolves with occlusion of vision to either eye and is due to ocular misalignment, whether caused by disorders of the ocular motor nerves, of the myoneural junction (myasthenia gravis; see Chap. 386), or of the extraocular muscles themselves. Myasthenia gravis can usually be diagnosed with the edrophonium or prostigmine test. Restriction of extraocular muscle function can result from inflammation (orbital myositis), infiltration (thyroid ophthalmopathy or metastatic disease), or entrapment (blowout fracture of the orbital floor). Restriction of movement of the globe can be confirmed with a positive forced duction test. Topical proparacaine is used to anesthetize the eye, especially over the insertion of the rectus muscles to be manipulated. While the patient looks in the direction of gaze limitation, the physician, using a cotton-tipped applicator or toothed forceps, attempts to move the globe in the direction of gaze deficit. The inability to overcome the eye movement limitation signifies the presence of a restrictive process.

Once restrictive disease and myasthenia gravis are excluded, the major cause of binocular diplopia is a cranial nerve lesion. The type of binocular diplopia—horizontal, vertical, or oblique—provides clues in determining which muscle is affected. A red glass test allows a more exact documentation of the type of diplopia.

ISOLATED OCULAR MOTOR NERVE PALSIES Oculomotor nerve (third cranial nerve) The oculomotor (third nerve) nuclear complex is a compact midline structure in the rostral midbrain containing somatic motor and visceral nuclei. Motor neurons project ipsilaterally to the medial rectus, inferior rectus, and inferior oblique muscles and contralaterally to the superior rectus muscle. One central caudal nucleus innervates the levator palpebrae superioris bilaterally. Axons from the visceral nuclei project ipsilaterally as the pregangli-

onic, parasympathetic outflow to the sphincter of the pupil and the ciliary ganglion, controlling pupillary sphincter function and accommodation. A complete lesion of the nucleus of the oculomotor nerve (e.g., midbrain infarction) would be expected to produce a unilateral third nerve palsy, paralysis of the contralateral superior rectus muscle, and bilateral ptosis. Subnuclear (i.e., partial nuclear) or fascicular (i.e., intramesencephalic) oculomotor lesions lead to partial third nerve palsies with single or multiple extraocular muscle weakness with or without pupillary involvement. High-resolution magnetic resonance imaging (MRI) of the midbrain, especially with gadolinium enhancement, may demonstrate such focal lesions, which usually are vascular or metastatic in origin.

The fascicular portion of the third nerve courses through the red nucleus and ventral mesencephalon to emerge in the interpeduncular fossa. It then runs forward beneath the posterior cerebral artery and lateral to the posterior communicating artery, pierces the dura, and enters the cavernous sinus. The pupillary fibers travel superficially in the dorsomedial portion of the nerve. At the superior orbital fissure, where the nerve enters the orbit, it divides into a superior branch (supplying the levator and superior rectus) and an inferior branch (supplying medial and inferior rectus, inferior oblique, and pupillomotor fibers).

A complete third nerve lesion causes ptosis and inability to turn the eye upward, downward, or inward. At rest, the eye is deviated down and temporally. The iris sphincter may be involved or spared, as determined by pupillary size and reactivity.

Lesions at various sites along the course of the nerve from the nucleus to the muscle give characteristic patterns of loss of function. As the fascicles of the third nerve traverse the midbrain, they pass through important structures that enable precise localization of fascicular third nerve palsies. Aside from isolated partial third nerve palsies with or without pupillary involvement, four syndromes can be recognized. When the third nerve palsy is accompanied by involvement of the red nucleus, a contralateral cerebellar ataxia and slow "rubral" tremor occur—Claude syndrome. If the oculomotor nerve is damaged as it traverses the cerebral peduncle, a contralateral hemiparesis results—Weber syndrome. More extensive lesions (tumor or infarct) may affect the third nerve, red nucleus, and cerebral peduncle—Benedikt syndrome—and additionally cause vertical gaze palsy—Nothnagel syndrome.

After the third nerve leaves the brainstem, it is susceptible to meningeal processes (infection, tumor, blood) or compression. When the nerve is compressed against the tentorial edge, petroclinoid ligament, or clivus by the uncus of the temporal lobe during cerebral herniation, the pupil fibers are affected first, and the pupils dilate and become unresponsive to light. Compression of the third nerve by aneurysm (posterior communicating artery or posterior cerebral artery) produces an acute, total, isolated painful third nerve palsy and a dilated nonreactive pupil. Initial pupil sparing can be found in 8 to 15 percent of aneurysms, but pupillary involvement usually occurs within 5 to 7 days. Prompt consideration of cerebral angiography and surgery is indicated in all third nerve palsies with pupil involvement at all ages.

Within the cavernous sinus, the oculomotor nerve may be compressed by aneurysm or tumor (pituitary tumor, meningioma, nasopharyngeal carcinoma), or the nerve may be affected by thrombosis, local infection, or inflammation. Pain in the face and paresis of the abducens and/or trochlear nerves also may be present.

Pupillary sparing (normal size and reflex response) is the hallmark of an isolated painful third nerve palsy due to microinfarction in association with diabetes mellitus, hypertension, or collagen vascular disease. Patients over age 50 with an isolated third nerve palsy and pupil sparing without signs of subarachnoid hemorrhage can be followed expectantly. Recovery following microinfarction of the nerve is usually complete within a 3-month follow-up period. In the absence of recovery, the patient should be reinvestigated.

Head trauma, with or without skull fracture, is also a major cause of oculomotor nerve palsy. Mild head trauma causing a third nerve palsy, however, should suggest the presence of a tumor at the base of the skull.

Aberrant regeneration of the third nerve may occur after trauma, aneurysm, congenital third nerve palsy, and migraine. The clinical signs of aberrant regeneration often include abnormal lid movements, most commonly lid elevation with attempted ipsilateral adduction or depression of the eye. If aberrant regeneration is encountered without a history of preceding oculomotor palsy (primary aberrant regeneration), then slowly growing intracavernous mass lesions (meningioma, carotid aneurysm, etc.) are likely, although sometimes no cause can be found.

Isolated lesions (trauma, neurofibroma) of the branches of the third nerve produce partial third nerve palsies involving the structures innervated by the superior or inferior branch.

Trochlear nerve (fourth cranial nerve) The neurons of the fourth nerve nucleus lie dorsally in the rostral brainstem at the level of the inferior colliculi, contiguous to the caudal end of the oculomotor complex. The axons run dorsally and decussate in the anterior medullary velum (the roof of the fourth ventricle), where they are vulnerable to head trauma. The nerve exits the brainstem dorsally, crosses the superior cerebellar artery, runs forward in the cavernous sinus, and enters the orbit through the superior orbital fissure to innervate the superior oblique muscle.

A superior oblique palsy causes vertical diplopia with hypertropia and excyclotorsion of the eye. Many patients compensate for this by adapting a head tilt toward the uninvolved side (i.e., a patient with a right superior oblique palsy will often have a left head tilt). Some patients who have a congenital fourth nerve palsy may be asymptomatic until later in life, when the ability to fuse is lost. Such patients generally have a head tilt documented on childhood and adult photographs.

Damage to the trochlear nerve nucleus by intrinsic brainstem disease (medulloblastoma, ependymoma, metastatic tumor, multiple sclerosis, arteriovenous malformation) cannot be readily distinguished from fascicular nerve palsies. Paresis of the superior oblique muscle with pontine lesions can be obscured by associated conjugate or internuclear gaze defects. In such patients, recognition of a trochlear nerve palsy becomes possible only after the horizontal gaze difficulties have resolved.

Bilateral trochlear nerve pareses may occur with fascicular involvement of both trochlear nerves in the anterior medullary velum by compression, ischemia, hemorrhage, and, most commonly, trauma. Computed tomography (CT) and MRI aid in the topographic diagnosis of such lesions. Neuroimaging has demonstrated an intrinsic lesion in the mesencephalon producing a trochlear paresis and contralateral Horner's syndrome. This is consistent with the known anatomy, in which the sympathetic pathways run through the dorsolateral tegmentum of the mesencephalon adjacent to the trochlear fascicles.

Head trauma, especially blunt frontal injury (motorcycle accidents, vertex blows), is the most common cause of unilateral and bilateral trochlear nerve palsy. Contracoup forces transmitted to the brainstem by the free tentorial edge may injure the nerves in the anterior medullary velum. The second most common cause of a trochlear nerve palsy is ischemic neuropathy, often associated with small-vessel disease such as diabetes (mononeuritis multiplex). Recovery usually occurs within 3 months. Trochlear nerve palsies are also observed with tentorial meningioma, pinealoma, sphenoid sinusitis, encephalitis, and migraine. Management is usually conservative, using vertical prism glasses or unilateral patching to alleviate symptoms. A variety of surgical procedures on the superior oblique or inferior oblique muscle can be performed if conservative treatment is unsatisfactory.

Abducens nerve (sixth nerve) The abducens nucleus is located beneath the floor of the fourth ventricle and lateral to the midline of the pons at the junction of the pons and medulla. The genu of the facial nerve curves over the dorsal and lateral surfaces. The medial longitudinal fasciculus lies adjacent and medial to it. The abducens nucleus contains motor neurons that innervate the ipsilateral lateral rectus muscle and a pool of interneurons whose axons cross the

midline and ascend in the medial longitudinal fasciculus to reach the contralateral oculomotor subnucleus innervating the medial rectus muscle of the opposite eye. The abducens nucleus thus participates in control of horizontal gaze.

The abducens nucleus is susceptible to abnormalities of development or injury in early life. Mobius syndrome consists of a disturbance of horizontal eye movements and facial diplegia. Many cases of Mobius syndrome display a horizontal gaze palsy rather than a simple lateral rectus paralysis, suggesting a failure of development of the abducens nuclei. In cases where only a lateral rectus weakness is apparent, the lesion may be in the abducens nerve or lateral rectus muscle. Failure of normal development of the abducens nucleus is also associated with Duane retraction syndrome; there is an absence of motor neurons innervating the lateral rectus muscle, but preservation in the abducens nucleus of interneurons projecting via the contralateral medial longitudinal fasciculus to the contralateral third nerve subnucleus of the medial rectus muscle. It is postulated that during the developmental stage in these patients, oculomotor neurons intended for various muscle groups innervated by the third cranial nerve are misdirected and innervate the lateral rectus muscle. As a result, patients with Duane syndrome often have a complete abduction deficit but preserved adduction on the affected side. The accompanying retraction of the globe and palpebral fissure narrowing on adduction are due to cofiring of muscles innervated by the oculomotor nerve due to the aberrant developmental oculomotor innervation.

The fascicular portion of the sixth nerve traverses the pons ventrally, laterally, and caudally and passes medial to the olivary nucleus, to exit the brainstem in a groove between the pons and the medulla. The proximity of the sixth nerve nucleus and its fascicular portion to the motor nucleus of the facial nerve, facial nerve fascicle, vestibular nucleus, and descending sympathetic fibers within the brainstem explains the association of sixth nerve deficits with a multitude of disease states.

Causes of nuclear and fascicular sixth nerve lesions include pontine and cerebellar tumors, Wernicke's encephalopathy, and demyelinating disease. Infarction of the pons is an important cause of fascicular sixth nerve palsies, and infarction of the medial inferior pons may produce an ipsilateral abducens palsy, ipsilateral facial weakness, and contralateral hemiplegia—Millard-Gubler syndrome.

After emerging from the brainstem, the nerve runs along the face of the bony clivus to penetrate the dura below the crest of the petrous bone to enter the cavernous sinus. The sixth nerve is not situated within the sinus wall, like the third and fourth cranial nerves, but instead lies within the body of the sinus itself. It enters the orbit through the superior orbital fissure within the annulus of Zinn to innervate the lateral rectus muscle. A sixth nerve palsy causes an inward deviation of the eye and paresis of abduction. Causes of sixth nerve palsy include infarction, aneurysm, tumor, trauma, leptomeningitis, and multiple sclerosis. Papilledema is usually present with a sixth nerve palsy due to raised intracranial pressure. However, despite improved diagnostic techniques, many cases of monocranial nerve palsy remain unexplained (idiopathic).

MULTIPLE OCULAR MOTOR NERVE PALSIES The localization of lesions that cause combinations of third, fourth, or sixth nerve palsies depends on accurate assessment of the various combinations of associated neurologic deficits.

Lesions producing ophthalmoplegia involving the functions of more than one ocular motor nerve and associated with pain or hypesthesia in the distribution of the trigeminal nerve (fifth nerve) can be localized depending on the extent of fifth nerve involvement. The lesion is at the superior orbital fissure or anterior cavernous sinus region if only the first division of nerve V is involved, at the middle to posterior cavernous sinus region if the first (V1) and second (V2) divisions are involved, and in the parasellar region if all three divisions are involved. If the ipsilateral optic nerve is affected, the lesion must be in the orbital apex. Causes of these syndromes include nasopharyngeal carcinomas, granulomatous inflammatory processes (pseudotumor of the orbit or "Tolosa Hunt" syndrome), and lymphoma. Pituitary tumors, meningiomas, chordomas, and other, rarer tumors can produce cavernous sinus–orbital apex syndromes. The diagnosis is aided by neuroimaging of the suspected area, including the nasopharynx.

SUPRANUCLEAR DISORDERS   The bedside diagnosis of brainstem disorders is aided by an understanding of the neuroanatomy of ocular motor control. There are two classes of eye movements, rapid or saccadic movements and slow or pursuit movements. Both systems alter the direction of gaze (eye position in space). Rapid eye movements are used to bring new images onto the fovea. Pursuit eye movements are used to hold the object's image stationary on the moving retina.

Saccadic eye movements are tested by observation of eye movements on command, refixation saccades between two targets, and quick phases of optokinetic nystagmus and/or vestibular stimulation. Saccades and quick phases share the same immediate premotor neural circuitry within the brainstem. The descending pathways transmitting saccadic signals for gaze control are part of a corticobulbar pathway with connections between visual, frontal, and brainstem structures. All decussate in the midbrain to terminate in the contralateral pontine paramedian reticular formation (PPRF) in the brainstem, just rostral to the sixth nerve nucleus. Pursuit eye movements are tested by observation of the eyes tracking a target horizontally and vertically. Three visual cortical areas in the temporal-occipital junction are concerned with control of pursuit eye movements. They are the middle temporal and medial superior temporal cortex and the fundus of the superior temporal cortex. Pursuit pathways descend ipsilaterally to the dorsal lateral pontine nuclei, the Purkinje P cells in the cerebellar flocculus, to the vestibular nuclei and onward to the final common brainstem pathway, the PPRF.

Direct vertical gaze requires bilateral cortical activation. The rostral PPRF acts as the first brainstem center from which fibers project to the pretectal rostral interstitial nucleus of the median longitudinal fasciculus, which is the final vertical gaze center. Paralysis of horizontal and vertical gaze can be produced by lesions affecting cortical, mesencephalic, and pontine centers and their projections. Destruction of the ocular motor nuclei, fascicles, or nerves as well as myasthenia gravis can mimic a gaze palsy. Isolated upward gaze paralysis (Parinaud syndrome) and isolated downward gaze or complete vertical gaze paralysis are produced by lesions involving the mesencephalon and pretectum. Tumors in the region of the pineal gland produce Parinaud syndrome or the sylvian aqueduct syndrome; ocular signs include a supranuclear paralysis of upward gaze, light-near dissociation of the pupils, convergence paresis, skew deviation, and convergence retraction nystagmus. Brainstem infarction is possibly the only cause of selective paralysis of downward gaze, and is caused by occlusion of a single perforating vessel, the posterior thalamosubthalamic paramedian artery.

Degenerative diseases, e.g., progressive supranuclear palsy (see Chap. 371), may selectively or primarily involve the supranuclear structures of the brainstem. Vertical saccades are affected first, being slow and then small. Eventually there is complete loss of voluntary vertical refixations. With chronicity, the horizontal eye movements become similarly affected. Convergence may be impaired. The disease may progress to total ophthalmoplegia. Other degenerative diseases—Huntington chorea, abetalipoproteinema, amyotrophic lateral sclerosis, and olivopontocerebellar degeneration—may be associated with a supranuclear disorder of vertical as well as horizontal gaze. Supranuclear vertical gaze disorders also occur in multiple sclerosis, Whipple's disease, syphilis, brucellosis, tetanus, encephalitis, neurofibromatosis, and tuberculoma, as well as brainstem trauma, including neurosurgical procedures.

Opsoclonus is a striking disorder of saccadic eye movements reflecting the presence of unwanted saccades. It consists of involuntary, arrhythmic, multidirectional, high-amplitude, conjugate back-to-back saccades. The eye movements are usually continuous and persist during sleep. Opsoclonus can occur with encephalitis, trauma, intracranial tumors, hydrocephalus, thalamic hemorrhage, and toxic and metabolic encephalopathies. It occurs as a paraneoplastic or remote effect of neuroblastoma in children and, less commonly, of other carcinomas (ovary, lung, breast) in adults (Chap. 328). Paraneoplastic opsoclonus is accompanied by the presence of antibodies (anti-Purkinje cell or anti-Rhi) in the blood and spinal fluid.

INTERNUCLEAR OPHTHALMOPLEGIA   Clinically, internuclear ophthalmoplegia (INO) is characterized by (1) paresis or paralysis of adduction of the ipsilateral eye on attempted horizontal gaze to the contralateral side and (2) horizontal jerk nystagmus in the contralateral abducting eye. Typically, convergence is intact if the lesion does not extend to the mesencephalon; gaze-evoked vertical nystagmus on upward gaze is frequent. Unilateral INO is due to interruption of the ipsilateral medial longitudinal fasciculus (MLF) after fibers have crossed from the interneurons of the contralateral abducens nucleus projecting to the ipsilateral medial rectus subnucleus. Unilateral internuclear ophthalmoplegia is most commonly due to multiple sclerosis in young adults and to vascular infarction in the elderly. Prognosis for full recovery is good.

Bilateral INO is usually due to brainstem glioma in children and to multiple sclerosis in adults. Myasthenia gravis can mimic both unilateral and bilateral INO.

NYSTAGMUS AND OTHER ENTITIES THAT MIMIC NYSTAGMUS   Nystagmus is a repetitive, to-and-fro movement of the eyes. Pendular nystagmus consists of smooth sinusoidal oscillations, and jerk nystagmus consists of slow drift alternating with corrective quick phases. Normal subjects develop nystagmus in response to vestibular and optokinetic stimuli.

Normally, the vestibular, optokinetic, and pursuit systems each act to hold images steady on the retina, and a neural integrator allows maintenance of eccentric positions of gaze. Disorders of these systems create nystagmus. Identification of the cause of nystagmus requires historical information—especially about drug use (anticonvulsants, haloperidol, lithium) or alcohol abuse—and a complete ocular motor evaluation. The most important clinical types of nystagmus are discussed below.

Congenital nystagmus   Congenital nystagmus is a pendular or jerk nystagmus that remains horizontal in all positions of gaze, is dampened by convergence, and is associated with better vision at near rather than far distances. Patients with congenital nystagmus often have afferent visual system dysfunction.

Labyrinthine-vestibular nystagmus   Disease of the vestibular system causes constant-velocity slow-phase drifts with corrective quick phases that create a "saw-tooth" jerk nystagmus. By convention, the side of the nystagmus is designated by the direction of the quick corrective saccade (fast phase). Vestibular nystagmus may be due to a peripheral or central lesion. In peripheral vestibular disease, the nystagmus is usually of mixed type. For example, in benign positional nystagmus, a mixed vertical-torsional nystagmus is common. In unilateral labyrinthine destruction, a mixed horizontal-torsional nystagmus occurs. Peripheral vestibular nystagmus is suppressed by fixation and exacerbated by changes in head position. Peripheral nystagmus is often associated with severe vertigo, nausea, vomiting, and oscillopsia. Disturbances of central vestibular connections are associated with a central imbalance between semicircular canal inputs and disruption of ascending vestibular or cerebellovestibular connections. Mixed nystagmus can be caused by peripheral labyrinthine or central vestibular disease. Purely bilateral vertical (upbeat, downbeat), torsional, or horizontal nystagmus can only occur with central vestibular disease. Central vestibular nystagmus is poorly suppressed by fixation but exacerbated or induced by changes in head position (Chap. 18).

Four forms of primary position vestibular nystagmus have anatomic localizing value: downbeat, upbeat, horizontal, and torsional nystagmus. Downbeat nystagmus in the primary position and accentuated on lateral gaze occurs with cervicomedullary junction disorders, such as Arnold-Chiari malformation and basilar invagination; in multiple sclerosis, brainstem infarction, cerebellar atrophy, hydrocephalus, metabolic disorders, and familiar periodic ataxia; or as a toxic side effect of anticonvulsant drugs. Lesions associated with primary position upbeat nystagmus are in the tegmentum of the rostral medulla and caudal pons; causes include infarction, demyelination, myelinolysis, and diffuse infiltration with glioma. Horizontal primary position nystagmus is rare and is usually due to peripheral vestibular disease.

Primary position torsional nystagmus is common in the lateral medullary syndrome. With this lesion, the nystagmus may be horizontal or mixed with both torsional and vertical components. Typically, the horizontal nystagmus beats away from the side of the medullary infarction with the eyes in a primary position but beats ipsilaterally when gaze is directed toward the lesion. Vertical nystagmus, if present, is usually upbeating.

Gaze-evoked nystagmus Gaze-evoked nystagmus implies a weakness in holding the eyes in an eccentric position due to a defect in the integrator in the brainstem. It is commonly caused by drugs such as sedatives or anticonvulsants. Asymmetric but conjugate horizontal gaze-evoked nystagmus occurs with unilateral cerebellar disease and cerebellopontine-angle tumors such as acoustic neuroma or meningioma.

REFERENCES

BECK RW et al: A randomized controlled trial of corticosteroids in the treatment of acute optic neuritis. N Engl J Med 326:581, 1992

BURDE RM et al: *Clinical Decisions in Neuro-ophthalmology*, 2nd ed. St. Louis, Mosby, 1992

CRYOTHERAPY FOR RETINOPATHY OF PREMATURITY COOPERATIVE GROUP: Multicenter trial of cryotherapy for retinopathy of prematurity. Arch Ophthalmol 106:471, 1988

DUANE T (ed): *Clinical Ophthalmology*. Philadelphia, Lippincott, 1988

GLASER JS: *Neuroophthalmology*, 2nd ed. Philadelphia, Lippincott 1989

HUMPHRIES P et al: On the molecular genetics of retinitis pigmentosa. Science 256:804, 1992

LEIGH RJ, ZEE DS: *The Neurology of Eye Movements*, 2nd ed. Philadelphia, Davis, 1991

MILLER NR: *Walsh and Hoyt's Clinical Neuroophthalmology*, 4th ed. Baltimore, Williams & Wilkins, 1982

NATHANS J: Rhodopsin: Structure, function, and genetics. Biochemistry 31:4923, 1992

NIKOSKELAINEN EK: Leber hereditary optic neuropathy. Curr Opin Ophthalmol 2:531, 1991

NORTH AMERICAN SYMPTOMATIC CAROTID ENDARTERECTOMY TRIAL COLLABORATORS: Beneficial effect of carotid endarterectomy in symptomatic patients with high-grade carotid stenosis. N Engl J Med 325:445, 1991

OPTIC NEURITIS STUDY GROUP: The clinical profile of optic neuritis: Experience of the optic neuritis treatment trial. Arch Ophthalmol 109:1673, 1991

QUIGLEY HA: Open-angle glaucoma. N Engl J Med 328:1097, 1993

20 DISTURBANCES OF SMELL, TASTE, AND HEARING

JAMES B. SNOW, JR. / JOSEPH B. MARTIN

SMELL The sense of smell determines the flavor and palatability of food and drink. It serves along with the trigeminal system as a monitor of inhaled chemicals, including dangerous substances such as natural gas, smoke, and air pollutants. Although qualitative sensations of smell are subserved by the olfactory neuroepithelium, many substances are capable of producing somatic sensations of coolness, warmth, and irritation through the trigeminal, glossopharyngeal, and vagal afferents in the nose, oral cavity, tongue, pharynx, and larynx. The sense of smell should be considered as one of several chemosensory systems, since most chemical substances initiate olfactory, trigeminal, and taste perceptions.

The *olfactory neuroepithelium* is located in the superior part of the nasal cavities. It contains an orderly arrangement of bipolar olfactory receptor cells, microvillar cells, sustentacular cells, and basal cells. The dendritic process of the bipolar cell has a bulb-shaped knob or vesicle that projects into the mucous layer and bears six to eight cilia. The receptor sites for odorant molecules are located on the cilia. The microvillar cells are located adjacent to the receptor cells on the surface of the neuroepithelium. The sustentacular cells, unlike their counterparts in the respiratory epithelium, are not specialized to secrete mucus. Their function is unknown. The basal cells are progenitors of other cell types in the olfactory neuroepithelium, including the bipolar receptor cells. There is a regular turnover of the bipolar receptor cells, which function as the primary sensory neurons. In addition, with injury to the cell body or its axon, the receptor cell is replaced by a differentiated basal cell which reestablishes a central neural connection. *Hence these primary sensory neurons are unique among sensory systems in that they are regularly replaced and regenerate after injury*.

The unmyelinated axons of the receptor cells form the fila of the olfactory nerve, pass through the cribriform plate, and terminate within spherical masses of neuropil, termed *glomeruli*, in the olfactory bulb. The glomeruli are a focus of a high degree of convergence of information, since many more fibers enter than leave them. The main second-order neurons are the mitral cells. The primary dendrite of each mitral cell extends into a single glomerulus. Axons of the mitral cells project along with the axons of adjacent tufted cells to the limbic system, including the anterior olfactory nucleus, the prepiriform cortex, the periamygdaloid cortex, the olfactory tubercle, the nucleus of the lateral olfactory tract, and the corticomedial nucleus of the amygdala. Cognitive awareness of smell requires stimulation of the prepiriform cortex or the amygdaloid nuclei.

Odorants are absorbed into the mucus overlying the olfactory neuroepithelium, diffuse to the cilia, and reversibly bind to membrane receptor sites. The process causes conformational changes in the receptor proteins which induce a chain of biochemical events that results in generation of action potentials in the primary neurons. Intensity appears to be coded by the amount of firing in the afferent neurons. Indeed, a clear relationship exists in humans between psychophysical measures of intensity and the magnitude of the evoked potential from the olfactory neuroepithelium. The discovery of a large family of receptor genes suggests that there may be specific receptors for each odorant.

Disturbances of the sense of smell Disturbances of the sense of smell are caused by conditions that interfere with the access of the odorant to the olfactory neuroepithelium (transport loss), injure the receptor region (sensory loss), or damage central olfactory pathways (neural loss).

Transport olfactory loss can result from swollen nasal mucous membrane in acute viral upper respiratory infections, bacterial rhinitis and sinusitis, and allergic rhinitis, with structural changes in the nasal cavity such as deviations of the nasal septum, polyps, and neoplasms. It is also likely that abnormalities of mucus secretion in which the olfactory cilia are immersed could result in a loss of olfactory sensitivity.

Sensory olfactory losses are caused by destruction of the olfactory neuroepithelium by viral infections, neoplasms, the inhalation of toxic chemicals, drugs that affect cell turnover, and radiation therapy to the head. *Neural olfactory losses* occur in head trauma, with or without fracture of the base of the anterior cranial fossa or cribriform plate area; Parkinson's disease, Alzheimer's disease, Korsakoff's psychosis, and vitamin B_{12} deficiency; neoplasms of the anterior cranial fossa; neurosurgical procedures; administration of neurotoxic agents (e.g., ethanol, amphetamines, topical cocaine, aminoglycosides, tetracycline, cigarette smoke); and in some congenital disorders such as Kallmann's syndrome. Other endocrine disorders, including Cushing's syndrome, hypothyroidism, and diabetes mellitus, can affect smell perception.

From the psychophysical point of view, disturbances of the sense of smell may be categorized by either the patient's complaint or the objective sensory measurements as *total anosmia* (general anosmia)—

inability to detect any qualitative olfactory sensations; *partial anosmia*—ability to detect some, but not all, qualitative olfactory sensations; *specific anosmia*—loss of ability to appreciate only one or a very limited number of odorants; *total hyposmia* (general hyposmia)—decreased sensitivity to all odorants; *partial hyposmia*—decreased sensitivity to some odorants; dysosmia (cacosmia or paraosmia)—distortion in the perception of an odor, i.e., the perception of an unpleasant odor when a pleasant odorant is being presented or the perception of an odor when there is no odorant in the environment; *total hyperosmia* (general hyperosmia)—increased sensitivity to all odorants; *partial hyperosmia*—increased sensitivity to some odorants; and *agnosia*—inability to classify, contrast, or identify odor sensations verbally, even though the ability to distinguish between odorants or to recognize them may be normal.

CLINICAL EVALUATION   The history of the onset and development of the disturbance of the sense of smell may be of paramount importance in making an etiologic diagnosis. Unilateral anosmia is rarely a complaint. Only by separate testing of smell in each nasal cavity can it be recognized. Bilateral anosmia, on the other hand, does bring patients to medical attention. Anosmic patients usually complain of a loss of the sense of taste even though their taste thresholds may be within normal limits. In actuality, they are complaining of a loss of flavor detection, which is mainly an olfactory function. Flavor appreciation depends on the olfactory detection of volatile substances in food and beverages as well as the sense of taste. The physical examination should include a complete examination of the ears, upper respiratory tract, and head and neck. A neurologic examination emphasizing the cranial nerves is essential. CT scans of the head with enhancement are required to rule out neoplasms of the anterior cranial fossa, unsuspected fractures of the anterior cranial fossa, paranasal sinusitis, and neoplasms of the nasal cavity and paranasal sinuses.

The sensory evaluation of olfactory function is necessary for corroboration of the patient's complaint, evaluation of the efficacy of treatment, and determination of the degree of permanent impairment. The first step in the sensory evaluation is to determine the degree to which qualitative sensations are present. For this assessment, a smell identification test is used that consists of a 40-item, forced-choice, microencapsulated odor, scratch-and-sniff paradigm. For example, one of the items reads, "This odor smells most like (a) chocolate, (b) banana, (c) onion, or (d) fruit punch," and the patient is instructed to answer one of the alternatives. The test is highly reliable (short-term test-retest reliability $r = 0.95$) and is sensitive to age and sex differences (Fig. 20-1). It is an accurate quantitative determination of the relative degree of olfactory deficit. Persons with a total loss of smell function score in the range of 7 to 19 out of 40. The average score for total anosmics is slightly higher than that expected on the basis of chance because of the inclusion of some odorants which act by trigeminal stimulation.

The second step is to establish a detection threshold for the odorant phenyl ethyl alcohol, using a graduated stimulus. Sensitivity for each side of the nose is determined with a detection threshold for phenyl ethyl methyl ethyl carbinol. Nasal resistance is measured with anterior rhinomanometry for each side of the nose.

Techniques have been developed to biopsy the olfactory neuroepithelium, but in view of the widespread degeneration of the olfactory neuroepithelium and intercalation of respiratory epithelium in the olfactory area of adults with no apparent olfactory dysfunction, biopsy material must be interpreted cautiously.

DIFFERENTIAL DIAGNOSIS   At the present time, there are no psychophysical methods to differentiate sensory from neural olfactory losses. Fortunately, the history of the disease provides important clues to the cause. The leading causes of olfactory disorders are head trauma and viral infections. Head trauma is a more frequent cause of anosmia in children and young adults, and viral infections are more important causes of anosmia in older adults.

Cranial trauma is followed by uni- or bilateral impairment of smell in 5 to 10 percent of cases. Frontal injuries and fractures disrupt the

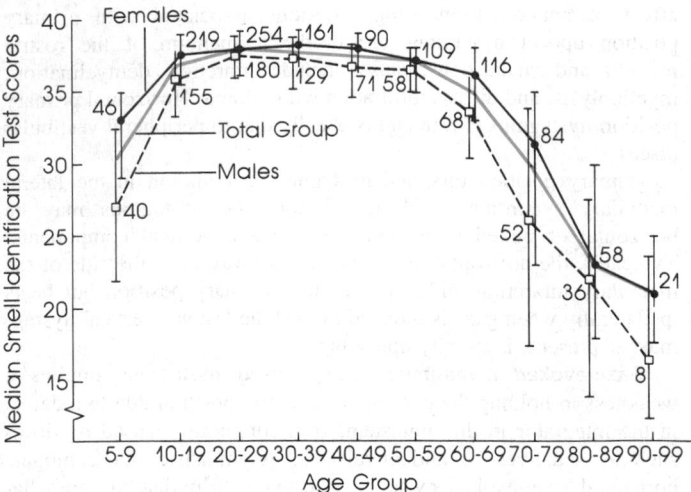

FIGURE 20-1 Smell identification test. Scores for a group of male and female subjects 5 to 99 years in age are shown. *(Reprinted with permission from RL Doty et al. Copyright 1984 by the AAAS.)*

cribriform plate and olfactory axons which perforate it. Sometimes there is an associated cerebrospinal fluid (CSF) rhinorrhea resulting from a tearing of the dura overlying the cribriform plate and paranasal sinuses. Anosmia also may follow blows to the occiput. Once traumatic anosmia develops, it is usually permanent; only about 10 percent of patients ever improve or recover. Perversion of the sense of smell may occur as a phase in the recovery process.

Viral infections destroy the olfactory neuroepithelium, and it is replaced by respiratory epithelium. Congenital anosmias are rare but important. Kallmann's syndrome is a neuronal migration defect for which the X-linked gene (KAL) has been cloned. It is characterized by congenital anosmia and hypogonadotropic hypogonadism (see Chap. 331). The hypothalamic and olfactory bulb defects result from failure of migration from the olfactory placode of olfactory receptor neurons and neurons synthesizing gonadotropin-releasing hormone. Anosmia also can occur in albinos. The receptor cells are present but are hypoplastic, lack cilia, and do not project above the surrounding supporting cells.

Meningioma of the inferior frontal region is the most frequent neoplastic cause of anosmia; rarely, anosmia can occur with glioma of the frontal lobe. Occasionally, pituitary adenomas, craniopharyngiomas, suprasellar meningiomas, and aneurysms of the anterior part of the circle of Willis extend forward and damage olfactory structures. These tumors and hamartomas also may induce seizures with olfactory hallucinations, indicating involvement of the uncus of the temporal lobe.

Dysosmia, subjective distortions of olfactory perception, may occur with intranasal disease that partially impairs smell or may represent a phase in the recovery from a neurogenic anosmia. Most dysomic disturbances consist of disagreeable or foul odors, and they may be accompanied by distortions of taste. Dysosmia is associated with depression.

TREATMENT   Therapy for patients with transport olfactory losses due to allergic rhinitis, bacterial rhinitis and sinusitis, polyps, neoplasms, and structural abnormalities of the nasal cavities can be undertaken rationally and with a high chance of improvement. Allergy management, antibiotic therapy, topical and systemic glucocorticoid therapy, and operations for nasal polyps, deviation of the nasal septum, and chronic hyperplastic sinusitis are frequently effective in restoring the sense of smell.

There is no treatment with demonstrated efficacy for sensorineural olfactory losses. Fortunately, spontaneous recovery often occurs. Zinc and vitamin therapy are advocated by some. Profound zinc deficiency can undoubtedly result in losses and distortion of the sense of smell, but it is not a clinical problem except in very limited geographic areas. Vitamin therapy has mainly been in the form of vitamin A. The epithelial degeneration associated with vitamin A deficiency can cause anosmia, but vitamin A deficiency is not a common clinical problem in the United States.

TASTE Many patients with a loss of olfactory sensitivity also complain of a loss of the sense of taste. On psychophysical testing, most of these patients have normal detection thresholds for taste. Disturbances of the sense of taste are far less frequent than disturbances of the sense of smell.

The taste receptor cells are located in the taste buds, spherical groups of cells arranged like the segments of a citrus fruit. At the surface, the taste bud has a pore into which microvilli of the receptor cells project. Taste buds have a similar appearance wherever they are located. Unlike the olfactory system, the receptor cell is not the primary neuron. Instead, gustatory afferent nerve fibers contact individual taste receptor cells.

The sense of taste is mediated through the facial, glossopharyngeal, and vagal nerves. The gustatory system consists of at least five receptor populations. Taste buds are located in the foliate papillae along the lateral margin of the tongue, in the fungiform papillae throughout the dorsum of the tongue, in the circumvallate papillae at the junction of the dorsum and the base of the tongue, and in the palate, epiglottis, larynx, and esophagus. The chorda tympani branch of the facial nerve subserves taste from the anterior two-thirds of the tongue. The posterior third of the tongue is supplied by the lingual branch of the glossopharyngeal nerve. Afferents from the palate travel with the greater superficial petrosal nerve to the geniculate ganglion and thence via the facial nerve to the brainstem. The internal branch of the superior laryngeal nerve of the vagus nerve contains the taste afferents from the larynx including the epiglottis and esophagus.

The central connections of the nerves terminate in the brainstem in the nucleus of the tractus solitarius. The fibers of the chorda tympani and greater superficial petrosal nerves go to the cephalic portion of the nucleus. The glossopharyngeal gustatory fibers go to the middle, and the superior laryngeal nerve fibers go to the caudal portion of the nucleus. The central pathway from the nucleus of the tractus solitarius projects to the ipsilateral parabrachial nuclei of the pons. Two divergent pathways project from the parabrachial nuclei. One ascends to the gustatory relay in the dorsal thalamus, synapses, and continues to the cortex of the insula. There is also evidence for a direct pathway from the parabrachial nuclei to the cortex. (Olfaction and taste appear to be unique among sensory systems in that at least some fibers bypass the thalamus.) The other pathway from the parabrachial nuclei goes to the ventral forebrain, including the lateral hypothalamus, substantia innominata, central nucleus of the amygdala, and the stria terminalis.

Tastants gain access to the receptor cells through the taste pore. Four classes of taste are recognized: sweet, salt, sour, and bitter. Individual gustatory afferent fibers almost always respond to a number of different chemicals. Response patterns of gustatory afferent axons can be grouped into classes based on the stimulus chemical that produces the largest response. For example, for sucrose-best response neurons, the second-best stimulus is almost always sodium chloride. The fact that individual gustatory afferent fibers respond to a large number of different chemicals led to the *across-fiber-pattern* theory of gustatory coding, while the best-stimulus analysis led to the concept of *labeled* afferents. It appears that labeled fibers are important for establishing gross quality, but the across-fiber pattern within a best-stimulus category, and perhaps among categories, is needed for discriminating chemicals within qualities. For example, sweetness may be carried by sucrose-best neurons, but the differentiation of sucrose and fructose may require a comparison of the relative activity among sucrose-best, salt-best, and quinine-best neurons. As with olfaction and other sensory systems, intensity appears to be encoded by the quantity of neural activity. A family of taste receptors has recently been cloned.

Disturbances of the sense of taste Disturbances of the sense of taste are caused by conditions that interfere with the access of the tastant to the receptor cells in the taste bud (transport loss), injure receptor cells (sensory loss), or damage gustatory afferent nerves and central gustatory pathways (neural loss).

Transport gustatory losses result from xerostomia due to many causes, including Sjögren's syndrome, heavy-metal intoxication, and bacterial colonization of the taste pore. The salivary milieu of the receptors may prove to be important to diverse causes of gustatory loss.

Sensory gustatory losses are caused by inflammatory and degenerative diseases in the oral cavity; a vast number of drugs, particularly those which interfere with cell turnover such as antithyroid and antineoplastic agents; radiation therapy to the oral cavity and pharynx; viral infections; endocrine disorders; neoplasms; and aging.

Neural olfactory losses occur with neoplasms, trauma, and operations in which the gustatory afferents are injured. Taste buds degenerate when their gustatory afferents are transected but remain when their somatosensory afferents are severed.

CLINICAL MANIFESTATIONS From the psychophysical point of view, disturbances of the sense of taste may be categorized by either the patient's complaint or the objective sensory measurements as *total ageusia*—inability to detect the qualities of sweet, salt, bitter, or sour; *partial ageusia*—ability to detect some of but not all the qualitative gustatory sensations; *specific ageusia*—inability to detect the taste quality of certain substances; *total hypoguesia*—decreased sensitivity to all tastants; *partial hypogeusia*—decreased sensitivity to some tastants; and *dysgeusia*—distortion in the perception of a tastant, i.e., the perception of the wrong quality when a tastant is presented or the perception of a taste when there has been no tastant ingested. Confusions of sour and bitter are common and, at times, may be semantic misunderstandings. Frequently, however, they have physiologic or pathophysiologic bases.

It may be possible to differentiate between the loss of flavor recognition in patients with olfactory losses who complain of a loss of taste as well as smell by asking if they are able to taste sweetness in sodas, saltiness in potato chips, etc.

Patients who complain of loss of taste should be evaluated psychophysically for gustatory function in addition to being evaluated for olfactory function. The first step is to perform suprathreshold whole-mouth taste testing for quality, intensity, and pleasantness perception with sucrose, citric acid, caffeine, and sodium chloride. In the quantification of the sense of taste, detection thresholds are obtained by applying graduated dilutions to the tongue quadrants or by whole-mouth sips. Finally, suprathreshold magnitude estimation may be used to shed further light on the patient's complaint. Electric taste testing (*electrogustometry*) is used clinically to identify taste deficits in specific quadrants of the tongue.

Biopsy of the foliate or fungiform papillae for histopathologic study of taste buds remains experimental but holds promise of shedding light on the categorization of taste disorders.

DIFFERENTIAL DIAGNOSIS As with olfaction, psychophysical methods for differentiating transport, sensory, and neural gustatory losses are not available. Once there is objective evidence of a disorder of taste, it is important to establish, as is done in other neurologic deficits, an anatomic diagnosis before proceeding to an etiologic diagnosis. The history of the disease often provides important clues to the cause. For example, absence of taste on the anterior two-thirds of the tongue associated with a facial paralysis indicates that the lesion is proximal to the point of junction of the chorda tympani branch with the facial nerve in the mastoid.

TREATMENT Therapy for gustatory losses remains limited. Artificial saliva benefits some patients with a disturbed salivary milieu. Treatment for bacterial and fungal infections of the oral cavity is appropriate and may be helpful. Withdrawal of drugs affecting cell turnover is usually helpful if the patient's general condition permits. Zinc and vitamin therapy for gustatory losses is advocated by some but lacks demonstrated efficacy. No therapeutic strategies exist for the sensorineural disorders of taste.

HEARING Hearing occurs by air conduction and bone conduction. In air conduction, sound waves reach the ear by propagation in air, enter the external auditory canal, and set the tympanic membrane in motion, which in turn moves the malleus, incus, and stapes. Movement of the footplate of the stapes causes pressure changes in the fluid-filled inner ear eliciting a traveling wave in the basilar membrane of the cochlea. Hearing by bone conduction occurs when the sounding source, in contact with the head, results in vibration of the bones of the skull, including the temporal bone, producing a traveling wave in the basilar membrane. In either case, the traveling wave moves from the base to the apex of the cochlea. Hairs (stereocilia) of the hair cells of the organ of Corti, which rests on the basilar membrane, are imbedded in the tectorial membrane and are deformed by the traveling wave. A point of maximal displacement of the basilar membrane determined by the frequency of the stimulating tone occurs with each traveling wave. High-frequency tones cause maximal displacement of the basilar membrane near the base of the cochlea. As the frequency of the stimulating tone decreases, the point of maximal displacement moves toward the apex of the cochlea.

The inner and outer hair cells of the organ of Corti have different innervation patterns, but both are mechanoreceptors. The outer hair cells have an internal organization that is in certain respects similar to muscle cells. Not only does the organ of Corti respond to acoustic stimulation, it also produces acoustic energy that can be detected in the external auditory canal with sensitive microphones. These otoacoustic emissions occur spontaneously and can be evoked by acoustic stimulation. The sources of this acoustic energy are the outer hair cells.

Motility of outer hair cells occurs with mechanical (acoustical) and electrical stimulation, iontophoretically applied acetylcholine, and changes in their internal and external ionic milieu and is modulated by stimulation of the efferent olivocochlear bundle.

The outer hair cells are capable of slow and fast motility. Slow elongation and contraction occurs with increased intracellular calcium in the presence of ATP, the application of acetylcholine, and changes in the ionic environment (increased potassium, which depolarizes the cell), while rapid motility occurs with mechanical (acoustic) and direct-current electrical stimulation. The electrokinetic membrane is located in the outer or lateral wall of the outer hair cell. Fast contractile activity occurs with changes in the membrane potential. The electromotility is driven by a novel and perhaps unique membrane-based force generator which can achieve audible frequencies.

The motility of the outer hair cells alters the micromechanics of the inner hair cells and thereby satisfies the long-sought cochlear amplifier required to explain the exquisite sensitivity and frequency selectivity of the cochlea.

A resting direct-current potential, the *endocochlear potential*, exists in the scala media and at the stereocilia end of the hair cells. It is generated by the stria vascularis. It is present whether there is acoustic stimulation or not. It has a magnitude of 80 mV, not unlike the intracellular potential, but its polarity is positive within the endolymph relative to the perilymph. It increases the potential differential at the stereocilia end of the hair cell, which undoubtedly is of importance in transduction.

As the traveling wave moves along the basilar membrane, the stereocilia are deformed and several receptor potentials are produced: the cochlear microphonic and the positive and negative summating potentials. It is thought that these receptor potentials arise at the apical end of the stereocilia. It may be that the summating potentials are generated largely by the inner hair cells and the cochlear microphonic is generated by the outer hair cells. The summating potential represents a direct-current shift that approximates the "envelope" of the acoustical stimulus. The cochlear microphonic potential is an alternating-current response that faithfully represents the frequency and intensity of the stimulating tone.

The current concept of cochlear transduction is that displacement of the tips of the stereocilia allows potassium to flow into the cell, resulting in its depolarization. The potassium causes calcium channels near the base to open and allow calcium to enter the cell. The calcium ions stimulate transmitter release. The action potential in the eighth nerve occurs 0.5 ms after the onset of the cochlear microphonic. This latency is taken as evidence for release of an as yet unidentified neurotransmitter at the hair cell and cochlear nerve dendrite interface. Each of the cochlear nerve neurons can be activated at a frequency and intensity specific for that cell. This phenomenon of the characteristic or best frequency occurs at each point of the central auditory pathway: dorsal and ventral cochlear nuclei, trapezoid body, superior olivary complex, lateral lemniscus, inferior colliculus, medial geniculate body, and auditory cortex. At low frequencies, individual auditory nerve fibers can respond more or less synchronously with the stimulating tone. At higher frequencies, phase-locking occurs so that neurons take turns in responding to particular phases of the cycle of the sound wave. Intensity is encoded by the amount of neural activity in individual neurons, the number of neurons that are active, and the specific neurons that are activated.

Disturbances of the sense of hearing   A loss of hearing can result from lesions in the external auditory canal, middle ear, inner ear, or central auditory pathways. Lesions in the external auditory canal or middle ear cause conductive hearing losses, while lesions in the inner ear or eighth nerve cause sensorineural hearing losses.

Conductive hearing losses result from obstruction of the external auditory canal by cerumen, debris and foreign bodies, swelling of the lining of the canal, and stenosis and neoplasms of the canal. Perforations of the tympanic membrane, as in chronic otitis media, disruption of the ossicular chain, as occurs with necrosis of the long process of the incus in trauma or infection, fixation of the ossicles as in otosclerosis, and fluid, scarring, or neoplasms in the middle ear also result in conductive hearing losses. *Sensory hearing losses* are due principally to damage to the hair cells of the organ of Corti caused by intense noise, viral infections, ototoxic drugs, fractures of the temporal bone, meningitis, cochlear otosclerosis, Ménière's disease, and aging. Neural hearing losses are due mainly to cerebellar angle tumors such as acoustic neuromas but also may result from any neoplastic, vascular, demyelinating, infectious, or degenerative disease or trauma affecting the central auditory pathways.

CLINICAL EVALUATION OF HEARING   The physical examination should evaluate the external ear canal and tympanic membrane. Careful inspection of the nose, nasopharynx, and upper respiratory tract is indicated. The other cranial nerves should be carefully evaluated. Conductive and sensorineural hearing losses can be differentiated by comparing the threshold of hearing by air conduction with that elicited by bone conduction. Testing the hearing by air conduction is accomplished by presenting the stimulus in air. Hearing by air conduction is affected by the patency of the external auditory canal, the efficiency of the middle ear, and the integrity of the inner ear, eighth nerve, and central auditory pathways. Testing the hearing by bone conduction is accomplished by placing the stem of a vibrating tuning fork or an oscillator of an audiometer in contact with the head. Hearing by bone conduction bypasses the external auditory canal and middle ear and tests the integrity of the inner ear, eighth nerve, and central auditory pathways. If air-conduction thresholds are elevated and bone-conduction thresholds are in the normal range, the lesion causing hearing loss is in the external auditory canal or middle ear. If both air-conduction and bone-conduction thresholds are elevated, the lesion is in the inner ear, eighth nerve, or central auditory pathways. Of course, conductive and sensorineural hearing losses can coexist, in which case both the air-conduction and bone-conduction thresholds are elevated, but in this case, air-conduction thresholds are elevated more than bone-conduction thresholds.

The Weber and Rinne tuning fork tests are used to differentiate conductive from sensorineural hearing losses. The Weber tuning fork test may be performed with a 256- or 512-Hz fork. The Rinne tuning fork test is most sensitive in detecting mild conductive hearing losses if a 256-Hz fork is used. Weber's test is performed by placing the stem of a vibrating tuning fork on the head in the midline and asking the patient whether the tone is heard in both ears or better in one ear than in the other. With a unilateral conductive hearing loss, the tone is perceived in the affected ear. With a unilateral sensorineural hearing loss, the tone is perceived in the unaffected ear. Rinne's test compares the ability to hear by air conduction with the ability to hear by bone conduction. The tines of a vibrating tuning fork are held near the opening of the external auditory canal, and then the stem is placed on the mastoid process. The patient is asked to indicate whether the tone is louder by air conduction or bone conduction. Normally, a tone is heard louder by air conduction than by bone conduction. With a conductive hearing loss, the bone-conduction stimulus is perceived as louder than the air-conduction stimulus. With sensorineural hearing losses, both air-conduction and bone-conduction perceptions are reduced, but the air-conduction stimulus is perceived as louder, as it is in normal hearing. The combined information from the Weber and Rinne tests permits a tentative conclusion as to whether a conductive or sensorineural hearing loss is present.

Measurement of hearing Quantification of hearing loss is obtained with an audiometer, an electronic device that allows the presentation of specific frequencies at specific intensities to each ear by either air or bone conduction. The testing is done in a sound-attenuated chamber, and masking, usually with broad-spectrum noise, is presented to the nontest ear so that responses are based on perception from the ear under test. Frequencies from 250 to 8000 Hz are used in clinical testing. The responses are measured in decibels. A decibel (dB) is equal to 10 times the logarithm of the ratio of the acoustic power required to achieve threshold in the patient to the acoustic power required to achieve threshold in a normal hearing person. An *audiogram* is a plot of intensity in decibels versus frequency.

The audiometric pattern of hearing loss is often of diagnostic value. Conductive hearing losses usually have a fairly equal threshold elevation for each frequency. Conductive hearing losses with a large mass component, as is often seen in middle ear effusions, have a greater elevation of thresholds in the higher frequencies. Conductive hearing losses with a large stiffness component, as in fixation of the footplate of the stapes in early otosclerosis, have a greater elevation of thresholds in the lower frequencies. In general, sensorineural hearing losses tend to have a greater threshold elevation at each higher frequency. Interesting exceptions to this generalization are noise-induced hearing loss, in which the loss at 4000 Hz is greater than it is at higher frequencies, and in Ménière's disease, particularly in the early stages of the disease, where thresholds are elevated more in lower than in higher frequencies.

Speech audiometry provides essential additional information. The *spondee threshold* is defined as the intensity at which speech is recognized as a meaningful symbol and is obtained by presenting through an audiometer two-syllable words with an equal accent on each syllable. The intensity at which the patient can repeat 50 percent of the words correctly is the spondee threshold and usually approximates the average threshold at the speech frequencies (500, 1000, and 2000 Hz). Once the spondee threshold is determined, the discrimination or word-recognition ability is tested by presenting one-syllable words at 25 to 40 dB above the spondee threshold. The words are phonetically balanced (PB) in that the phonemes (speech sounds) occur in the list of words at the same frequency that they occur in ordinary conversational English. An individual with normal hearing can repeat 90 to 100 percent of the PB words correctly. Likewise, individuals with a conductive hearing loss do well in discrimination testing. On the other hand, patients with a sensorineural hearing loss have a loss of discrimination attributable to the loss of peripheral analysis of sound in the inner ear or eighth nerve. With a lesion in the inner ear, the discrimination is moderately affected, usually in the 50 to 80 percent range, while with neural lesions, the discrimination is severely affected, often in the 0 to 50 percent range.

The discrimination testing may then be done at higher intensities than 25 to 40 dB above the spondee threshold to determine the performance-intensity function. A deterioration in discrimination ability at higher intensities suggests a lesion in the eighth nerve or central auditory pathways.

Tympanometry measures the impedance of the middle ear to sound. A sounding source and microphone are introduced into the ear canal with an airtight seal. The amount of sound that is absorbed through the middle ear or reflected from the middle ear is measured at the microphone. In conductive hearing losses, more sound is reflected than in the normal middle ear. The pressure in the ear canal can be increased or decreased from atmospheric pressure. Normally, the middle ear is most compliant at atmospheric pressure. With a negative pressure in the middle ear, as with eustachian tube obstruction, the point of maximal compliance occurs with negative pressure in the ear canal. With discontinuity of the ossicular chain, no point of maximal compliance can be obtained. Tympanometry is particularly useful in the identification and diagnosis of middle ear effusions in children.

During tympanometry, an intense tone (80 dB above the hearing threshold) elicits contraction of the stapedius muscle. The change in compliance of the middle ear with contraction of the stapedius muscle can be detected. The presence or absence of this *acoustic reflex* is important in the anatomic localization of facial nerve paralysis. The presence or absence of *acoustic reflex decay* helps differentiate sensory from neural hearing losses. In neural hearing loss, the reflex adapts or decays with time.

In order to evaluate a patient with a loss of hearing, the minimum audiologic assessment should include the measurement of pure tone air-conduction and bone-conduction thresholds, spondee threshold, discrimination score, performance-intensity function, tympanometry, acoustic reflexes, and acoustic-reflex decay. This information provides a comprehensive screening evaluation of the whole auditory system and allows one to determine whether further differentiation of a sensory (cochlear) from a neural (retrocochlear) hearing loss is indicated.

In addition to these tests, testing for recruitment, the short increment sensitivity index, tone decay, Békésy audiometry, and auditory brainstem evoked responses (ABR) help differentiate sensory from neural hearing losses. Of these, ABR is the most powerful means of differentiating the site of sensorineural hearing loss (see Chap. 366). In response to sound, five distinct waves can be recorded with computer averaging from scalp surface electrodes. Poor or absent waveforms, abnormal latency of waves, and abnormal interwave latency are evidence of lesions in the eighth nerve and brainstem. In addition, ABR is valuable in situations in which patients cannot or will not give reliable voluntary thresholds. It is also used to measure auditory function in neonates and young children and to monitor the integrity of the auditory nerve and brainstem in various clinical situations, including intraoperatively and in determination of brain death.

Otoacoustic emissions can be measured with sensitive microphones inserted into the external auditory canal in infants, children, and adults. The emissions may be spontaneous or evoked with sound stimulation. The presence of otoacoustic emissions indicates that the outer hair cells are intact and can be used as important evidence in distinguishing sensory from neural hearing losses. Otoacoustic emissions are particularly robust in infants.

The measurement of otoacoustic emissions can be done rapidly and with limited technical expertise in newborns. This technique promises to become the preferred method of screening neonates for hearing impairment. Currently, early identification of hearing impairment depends on the use of high-risk registries and testing of high-risk infants with ABR. High risk is indicated by a family history of hearing impairment, prenatal infection, prematurity, low birth weight, neonatal anoxia, a low Apgar score, neonatal jaundice, and neonatal infection. Unfortunately, 50 percent of infants with profound hearing impairment are not identified by use of ABR in high-risk infants. In the United States, the average age of identification of profound hearing impairment is 2½ years.

The natural acquisition and development of language depend on hearing language. The critical period for language acquisition is the first 2 years of life. Therefore, the early identification of hearing impairment in infants is of the greatest importance so that amplification with a hearing aid and special education can commence within the first several months of life.

In addition to the universal screening of infants for hearing impairment, the hearing should be assessed in all children before the first formal educational experience (preschool or kindergarten). Hearing also should be measured in the late teenage period when otosclerosis and noise-induced hearing loss begin to appear and in the sixth decade of life when presbycusis makes its appearance. Known causes of hearing impairment in addition to the risk factors already mentioned are meningitis, head trauma, middle ear infections and effusions, administration of ototoxic drugs (e.g., salicylates, quinine and its synthetic analogues, aminoglycoside antibiotics, loop diuretics such as furosemide and ethacrynic acid, and cancer chemotherapeutic agents such as *cis*-platinum), and noise exposure. At any time in life when one of these hearing risks is encountered, an audiologic assessment should be carried out.

Ten million Americans have noise-induced hearing loss, and 20 million are exposed to hazardous noise in their employment. Noise-induced hearing loss results from recreational as well as occupational activities and begins in adolescence, particularly among boys as they begin to engage in high-risk activities, such as wood and metal working with electrical equipment and target practice and hunting with small firearms. All internal-combustion and electric engines, including snow and leaf blowers, snowmobiles, outboard motors, and chain saws, require protection of the user with hearing protectors such as ear plugs or fluid-filled ear muffs. Virtually all noise-induced hearing loss is preventable through education, which should begin before the teenage years.

Programs of industrial conservation of hearing are required when the exposure over an 8-h period averages 85 dB on the A scale. Workers in such noisy environments can be protected with preemployment audiologic assessment, the mandatory use of hearing protectors, and annual audiologic assessments.

CLINICAL ASSESSMENT OF A COMPLAINT OF HEARING LOSS In evaluating patients who complain of loss of hearing, associated symptoms of tinnitus, vertigo, difficulty with balance, earache, otorrhea, and aural fullness should be sought along with a careful reconstruction of the history of evolution of the hearing deficit. A sudden onset of unilateral hearing loss, with or without tinnitus, may represent a viral infection in the inner ear. Gradual progression in a hearing deficit is common with otosclerosis, noise-induced hearing loss, acoustic neurinoma, or Ménière's disease. In the latter case, intermittent tinnitus and vertigo are usual. Hearing loss can occur with demyelinative lesions in the brainstem.

One in 1000 infants is born with profound hearing impairment. At least 50 percent of congenital deafness has a genetic basis. A larger number of such individuals develop hereditary hearing impairment in childhood and later in life. Between 70 and 80 percent of hereditary hearing impairment is autosomal recessive, and between 15 and 20 percent is autosomal dominant. Less than 5 percent is X-linked. Approximately 25 percent of hereditary hearing impairment occurs in syndromes in which other organ systems are affected. Greater progress has been made in finding the genes for syndromes of hereditary deafness because of the ease of making the determination of the hereditary basis of the hearing impairment. The gene for Waardenburg's syndrome (failure of melanocytes to migrate from the neural crest, resulting in deafness and pigmentary and integumentary changes) type 1 has been mapped to chromosome 2, and the gene for Usher's syndrome (deafness, vestibular loss, and blindness due to retinitis pigmentosa) type 2 has been mapped to chromosome 1. The genes for one form of Alport's syndrome (deafness and glomerulonephritis leading to renal failure), albinism, and neurofibromatosis type 2 (bilateral acoustic neurinomas) have been found. The first nonsyndromic deafness gene has been found in a Costa Rican kindred with an autosomal dominant hearing impairment on the long arm of chromosome 5. It is likely that most forms of hearing impairment will be found to have a genetic basis, including the predisposition to noise-induced hearing loss and presbycusis.

Between 30 and 35 percent of individuals over 65 years of age have a hearing loss that is sufficiently great to require a hearing aid.

Presbycusis is characterized by a loss of discrimination for phonemes, recruitment (abnormal growth of loudness), and particular difficulty in understanding speech in noisy environments.

Tinnitus is defined as the perception of a sound when there is no sound in the environment. It may have a buzzing, roaring, or ringing quality and may be pulsatile (synchronous with the heartbeat). Tinnitus is usually associated with a conductive or sensorineural loss of hearing. The pathophysiology of tinnitus is not well understood. The cause of the tinnitus can usually be determined by finding the cause of the associated hearing loss. Tinnitus may be the first symptom of a serious condition such as a vestibular schwannoma. Pulsatile tinnitus requires evaluation of the vascular system of the head to exclude vascular tumors such as glomus jugulare tumors, aneurysms, and stenotic lesions.

DIFFERENTIAL DIAGNOSIS Many patients with sensorineural hearing losses should have the vestibular system evaluated with electronystagmography and caloric testing (see Chap. 18). Most patients with conductive hearing losses should have CT of the temporal tones. Patients with unilateral or asymmetric sensorineural hearing losses should have magnetic resonance imaging of the head with gadolinium enhancement.

PREVENTION Conductive hearing losses may be prevented by prompt and appropriate antibiotic therapy of adequate duration for acute otitis media and by reventilation of the middle ear with tympanostomy tubes in middle ear infusions lasting 6 weeks or longer. Loss of vestibular function and deafness due to aminoglycoside antibiotics can largely be prevented by careful monitoring of serum peak and trough levels. Noise-induced hearing loss can be prevented by avoidance of exposure to loud noise or by regular use of ear plugs or fluid-filled muffs to attenuate intense sound. Vaccination of infants against type B *Haemophilus influenzae* meningitis will prevent a major cause of acquired deafness, as has immunization for measles, mumps, and rubella.

TREATMENT Most patients with conductive hearing losses can have the middle ear reconstructed using procedures such as tympanoplasty after chronic otitis media and trauma and stapedectomy for otosclerosis. Tympanostomy tubes allow the prompt return of hearing to normal in children and adults with middle ear effusions. Hearing aids are effective and well-tolerated for patients with conductive hearing losses. Patients with mild, moderate, and severe sensorineural hearing losses are regularly rehabilitated with hearing aids of varying configuration and strength. However, the problem of understanding conversation with a hearing aid in noise remains. Hearing aids have been improved to provide greater fidelity and have been miniaturized. High-frequency emphasis, needed for many sensorineural hearing losses, has been achieved principally by venting the ear mold and with filters. The augmentation of soft sounds and the nonamplification of intense sounds has been achieved. Digital hearing aids lend themselves to programming for the individual, and multiple and directional microphones at the ear level help some with difficulty of hearing with a hearing aid in noisy surroundings. Since all hearing aids amplify noise as well as speech, the only absolute solution to the problem found so far is to place the microphone closer to the speaker than the noise source. This arrangement is not possible with a self-contained, cosmetically acceptable device. It is cumbersome and requires a user-friendly environment.

In many situations, including lectures and the theater, hearing-impaired persons benefit from assistive devices that are based on the principle of having the speaker closer to the microphone than any source of noise. Assistive devices include infrared and FM transmission as well as an electromagnetic loop around the room for transmission to the individual's hearing aid. Hearing aids with telecoils also can be used with properly equipped telephones in the same way.

Cochlear implants are neural prostheses which convert sound energy to electrical energy and which can be used to stimulate the auditory division of the eighth nerve directly. Cochlear implants consist of electrodes that are inserted into the cochlea, speech processors that extract acoustical elements of speech for conversion to electric currents, and a means of transmitting the electrical energy through the skin. Most commonly for this purpose an induction coil is held over an implanted induction coil with magnets in each coil. In most causes of profound hearing impairment, the auditory hair cells are lost, but the ganglionic cells of the auditory division of the eighth nerve are preserved. Cochlear implants are appropriate for children and adults with hearing impairment that is so profound that they are not able to obtain any help with a hearing aid in understanding speech. Worldwide, more than 7000 deaf individuals, 1300 of whom are children, have had cochlear implants. They experience sound which helps with speech reading and allows some open-set word recognition. It is anticipated that improvements in the electrode design and speech processors will permit further improvement in understanding speech. The implant also allows the recipient to hear and identify environmental sounds and distinguish between men's and women's voices. It is also a help in modulating the person's own voice.

For individuals who have had both eighth nerves destroyed by trauma or bilateral acoustic neurinomas, a brainstem auditory implant has been placed into the cochlear nucleus on a limited, experimental basis. Recipients of the brainstem implant derive benefit similar to those with the cochlear implant.

The treatment of tinnitus is particularly problematic. The frequency range and intensity of tinnitus can often be matched with the use of an audiometer. Relief of the tinnitus may be obtained by masking it with background music. Hearing aids also are helpful in tinnitus suppression, as are tinnitus maskers, devices that present a sound to the affected ear which is more pleasant to listen to than the tinnitus. The use of a tinnitus masker is often followed by several hours of inhibition of the tinnitus.

COMMUNICATING WITH HARD-OF-HEARING INDIVIDUALS First of all, unnecessary noise should be eliminated or reduced. The radio and television should be turned off. Persons with hearing impairment depend on speech reading. They should be allowed to see the face of the speaker at all times. Speaking directly into the ear is occasionally helpful, but usually more is lost in communication than gained when the speaker's face cannot be seen. The lighting of the face of the speaker should be considered. The hard-of-hearing person should sit with his or her back to the window so that the light will be on the speaker's face. Speech should be slow enough to make each word distinct, but overly slow speech is distracting and loses contextual benefits. Although speech should be in a loud, clear voice, one should be aware that in sensorineural hearing losses in general and in elderly hard-of-hearing persons in particular, recruitment (the ability to hear loud sounds normally loud) may be troublesome. Above all, optimal communication cannot take place without both parties giving it their full and undivided attention.

REFERENCES

ALBERTI PW, RUBEN RJ (eds): *Otologic Medicine and Surgery*. New York, Churchill Livingstone, 1988

BALDWIN CT et al: An exonic mutation in the HuP2 paired domain gene causes Waardenburg's syndrome. Nature 355:637, 1992

BALLENGER JJ: *Diseases of the Nose, Throat, Ear, Head and Neck*, 14th ed. Philadelphia, Lea & Febiger, 1991

BROWNELL WE et al: Evoked mechanical responses of isolated cochlear outer hair cells. Science 227:194, 1985

COLE P: Upper respiratory airflow, in *The Nose: Upper Airway Physiology and the Atmospheric Environment*, DF Proctor, IB Anderson (eds). Amsterdam, Elsevier, 1982, pp 163–189

DOTY RL: A review of olfactory dysfunctions in man. Am J Otolaryngol 1:57, 1979

——— et al: Smell identification ability: Changes with age. Science 226:1441, 1984

———: Presence of both odor identification and detection deficits in Alzheimer's disease. Brain Res Bull 18:597, 1987

———: Olfactory dysfunction in Parkinsonism: A general deficit unrelated to neurological signs, disease stage or disease duration. Neurology 38:1237, 1988

FRANCO B et al: A gene deleted in Kallmann's syndrome shares homology with neural cell adhesion and axonal path-finding molecules. Nature 353:529, 1991

GETCHELL TV et al: *Smell and Taste in Health and Disease*. New York, Raven Press, 1991

JERGER JR: *Modern Developments in Audiology*, 2d ed. New York, Academic Press, 1973

KACHAR B et al: Electrokinetic shape changes of cochlear outer hair cells. Nature 322:365, 1986

KEMP DT: Stimulated acoustic emissions from within the human auditory system. J Acoust Soc Am 64:1386, 1978

KONIGSMARK BW: Hereditary diseases of the nervous system with hearing loss, in *Handbook of Clinical Neurology*, PJ Vinken, GW Bruyn (eds). Elsevier, Amsterdam, 1975, vol 22, chap 23, pp 499–526

LEVINE SB, SNOW JB: Pulsatile tinnitus. Laryngoscope 97:401, 1987

LIM DJ: Functional structure of the organ of Corti: A review. Hearing Res 22:117, 1986

LOWELL MA et al: Biopsy of human olfactory mucosa: An instrument and a technique. Arch Otolaryngol 108:247, 1982

NAKASHIMA T et al: Structure of human fetal and adult olfactory neuroepithelium. Arch Otolaryngol 110:641, 1984

NORGREN R: The gustatory system in mammals. Am J Otolaryngol 4:234, 1983

RINTELMAN WF: *Hearing Assessment*. Baltimore, Baltimore University, 1979

RUBEN RJ et al: *Genetics of Hearing Impairment*. New York, New York Acad Science, 1991

SNOW JB, TELIAN SA: Sudden deafness, in *Otolaryngology*, 3rd ed, MM Paprella et al (eds). Philadelphia, Saunders, 1991, pp 1619–1628

——— et al: Central auditory imperception. Laryngoscope 87:1450, 1977

———: Clinical problems in chemosensory disturbances. Am J Otolaryngol 4:224, 1983

TALAMO BR et al: Pathological changes in olfactory neurons in patients with Alzheimer's disease. Nature 337:736, 1989

21 PARALYSIS AND MOVEMENT DISORDERS

JOHN H. GROWDON / J. STEPHEN FINK*

Impairments of motor function may be subdivided into (1) paralysis due to lesions of corticospinal, corticobulbar, or brainstem descending (subcorticospinal) neurons, (2) abnormalities of movement and posture due to disease of the extrapyramidal motor system, (3) apraxic or nonparalytic disturbances of purposive movement due to involvement of the cerebral hemispheres, (4) abnormalities of coordination (ataxia) due to lesions in the cerebellar system, including its inputs and outputs, and (5) paralysis due to disorders of the motor unit, including bulbar or spinal motor neurons, neuromuscular junction, and muscle. This chapter reviews signs and symptoms that result from lesions of lower motor neurons, descending corticospinal and other tracts, and the extrapyramidal system. It also includes consideration of apraxic disorders. The cerebellar system is discussed in Chap. 22. Signs and symptoms that result from lesions of the neuromuscular junction and muscle are discussed in Chaps. 385 and 386.

FUNCTIONAL ANATOMY OF PRINCIPAL MOTOR TRACTS AND THE MOTOR UNIT

PYRAMIDAL SYSTEM The motor area of the cerebral cortex includes that part of the precentral convolution which contains Betz cells (area 4 of Brodmann, the *primary motor cortex*) (see Fig. 27A), but it also includes the premotor areas which extend rostrally into area 6 and the adjacent cortex along the banks of the cingulate cortex. In the primary motor cortex, the muscle groups of contralateral face, arm, trunk, and leg are somatotopically organized, with those of the face being at the lower end of the precentral convolution and those of the leg being in the paracentral lobule on the medial surface of the cerebral hemisphere. The parts of the body capable of the most delicate movements have, in general, the largest cortical representation. In humans, the premotor areas include the *premotor cortex*, located over the lateral surface of the hemispheres immediately rostral to the primary motor cortex, and the *supplementary motor area*, located on the medial surface of the hemisphere, rostral to the premotor cortex. The premotor areas are also organized somatotopically and appear to be important in the planning of volitional movements.

Neurons in cortical layer V of the primary motor cortex, the supplementary motor area, the premotor cortex, and the postcentral

*The authors acknowledge the contributions of Robert R. Young, coauthor in the 11th edition.

somatosensory cortex (areas 1, 2, 3, 5, and 7) contribute axons to the pyramidal system. The chief element of the pyramidal system, the corticospinal tract, is the only direct connection between the cortex and spinal cord. Corticospinal fibers descend in the internal capsule, where they intermingle with those destined to end in the striatum, globus pallidus, substantia nigra, red nucleus, and reticular substance, as well as others ascending from the thalamus. Fibers destined for cranial nerves separate in the midbrain and cross the midline to the contralateral cranial nerve nuclei. These fibers form the corticomesencephalic, corticopontine, and corticobulbar tracts and are included in the pyramidal system of motor neurons because they have functions similar to those of the corticospinal tract. The decussation of the corticospinal tract at the lower end of the medulla is variable. Most of the crossing fibers come to occupy a position in the posterolateral part of the lateral funiculus to form the lateral corticospinal tract; a few fibers cross to form an anterior funiculus. A small number of fibers, 10 to 30 percent, do not cross but descend ipsilaterally as the uncrossed corticospinal tract in the anterior funiculus of the spinal cord. Axons that travel in the lateral corticospinal tract terminate on (1) neurons of the dorsal horn, (2) interneurons in the intermediate zone of spinal gray matter, particularly those innervating distal muscles, and (3) motor neurons located dorsolaterally in the anterior horn. The corticospinal tract in the anterior funiculus terminates bilaterally on motor neurons located in the ventromedial anterior horn; these neurons innervate axial muscles. Most corticospinal tract neurons have direct connections with a small number of functionally related muscles, in some cases to muscles that are antagonistic (flexors and extensors of the same joint). The corticospinal tract is particularly important for the performance of highly fractionated movements (e.g., those involving the digits).

BULBOSPINAL SYSTEMS In addition to the pyramidal (corticospinal and corticobulbar) tract, the spinal gray matter receives axons from two groups of descending pathways from the brainstem. Major contributions to the *ventromedial system* come from the lateral and medial vestibulospinal tracts originating in the lateral and medial vestibular nuclei, the reticulospinal tract originating in the reticular formation of the medulla and pons, and the tectospinal tract originating in the superior colliculus of the midbrain. Neurons originating in the raphe nuclei of the medulla (containing serotonin), in the region of the locus coeruleus in the dorsal brainstem (containing norepinephrine), and in the interstitial nucleus of Cajal also contribute axons to the ventromedial brainstem descending system. These descending ventromedial axons terminate largely on motor neurons located in the ventromedial anterior horn that innervate axial and proximal muscles; this pool of motor neurons is important in the maintenance of posture and balance. Neurons in the red nucleus of the midbrain contribute axons to the rubrospinal tract, which is the major component of the *dorsolateral system* of brainstem descending pathways. Other fibers in this system originate in the ventrolateral pontine tegmentum and the caudal raphe nuclei. Like the corticospinal tract in the lateral funiculus, the dorsolateral system terminates in the lateral portion of the intermediate zone and on motor neurons located dorsolaterally in the anterior horn; these motor neurons innervate distal muscles of the limbs.

ANATOMY AND PHYSIOLOGY OF THE MOTOR UNIT Each motor nerve cell, through extensive arborization of the terminal part of its fiber, comes into contact with hundreds of muscle fibers; together they constitute the motor unit. Motor neuron excitability is modulated by segmental afferent and suprasegmental descending pathways. Descending corticospinal axons are believed to release excitatory amino acids (aspartate and glutamate) as neurotransmitters. Afferent modulation of motor unit activity is provided, in part, by axons of dorsal root ganglia cells which innervate most lamina of the dorsal horn, the intermediate zone, and some motor neurons directly. Substance P and glutamate are released by the primary afferent neurons and can modulate the gain of the reflex arc. Release of gamma-aminobutyric acid (GABA) and the neuropeptide enkephalin from interneurons in the dorsal spinal cord gray matter increases presynaptic inhibition of primary afferent neurons. The amino acid glycine is the major postsynaptic inhibitory neurotransmitter and is released by interneurons in the intermediate and ventral gray matter and Renshaw cells. Blockage of glycine receptors by strychnine or glycine release by tetanus toxin produces hyperreflexia. Descending serotonin and catecholamine pathways modulate spinal cord reflex mechanisms and flexor reflex afferents.

Motor nerve fibers of each anterior spinal root intermingle with those from adjacent roots and join to form plexuses and, ultimately, peripheral nerves. Innervation of muscles proceeds from corresponding segments of the spinal cord, and each large muscle is supplied by two or more roots. A single peripheral nerve contains several roots and usually provides the complete motor innervation of a muscle or group of muscles. For this reason, the distribution of paralysis due to disease of the anterior horn cells or anterior roots differs from that which follows a lesion of a peripheral nerve. Acetylcholine is the excitatory neurotransmitter released by axon terminals of anterior horn cells at the neuromuscular junction.

Muscle tone and tendon reflexes depend on muscle spindles and their afferent fibers. A tap on a tendon, by stimulating muscle spindles, activates stretch receptors which transmit impulses to alpha motor neurons in the spinal cord. The result is the familiar brief muscle contraction or tendon reflex. All variations in force and type of movement are determined by differences in the number and size of motor units called into activity, the frequency of their firing rates, and the patterns of activity in different muscles. Feeble movements recruit few units; the number and size of motor units increase in a stereotyped fashion with stronger movements. Motor units involved in tonic contractions have muscle fibers known as type I that are rich in oxidative enzymes and mitochondria; those controlling phasic contractions innervate muscle fibers that have anaerobic metabolism (type II fibers) (see also Chap. 382). When a motor neuron becomes diseased, as in progressive muscular atrophy, its axon may manifest increased irritability, and all the muscle fibers that it controls may discharge sporadically, in isolation from other units. The result of the contraction of one or several such units is a muscular twitch, or *fasciculation*, which can be observed visibly and recorded in the electromyogram (EMG). If the motor neuron or its axon is destroyed, all the muscle fibers to which it is attached undergo profound denervation atrophy. As a result, individual muscle fibers become hypersensitive to acetylcholine and contract spontaneously, although they are unresponsive to nerve impulses. Isolated activity of individual muscle fibers is called *fibrillation;* it is so fine that it cannot be seen through the intact skin and can be recorded only as a short-duration spike potential in the EMG (see Chap. 382).

All motor activity, even of the most elementary reflex type, requires the cooperation of several muscles. Analysis of a relatively simple movement, such as clenching the fist, affords some idea of the complexity of the underlying neural arrangements. In this act, the primary movement is a contraction of the flexor muscles of the fingers, the flexor digitorum sublimis and profundus, the flexor pollicis longus and brevis, and the adductor pollicis brevis. These muscles act as *agonists*, or *prime movers*, in this act. In order for flexion to be smooth and forceful, finger extensor muscles act as *antagonists* and must relax at the same rate at which the flexors contract. The muscles which flex the fingers also tend to flex the wrist, and since that weakens the grip, muscles which extend the wrist must be brought into play to prevent its flexion. The action of the wrist extensors is *synergic*, and these muscles are called synergists in this particular act. The elbow and shoulder must be stabilized by appropriate flexor and extensor muscles, which serve as *fixators*. The coordination of agonists, antagonists, synergists, and fixators involves reciprocal innervation and is managed entirely by segmental spinal mechanisms with guidance from proprioceptive input. Only the agonist movement in a voluntary act is believed to be initiated at a cortical level. There are many other basic motor activities, such as the maintenance of certain postures and stepping movements, where agonists and antagonists contract simultaneously (see Chap. 22). In general, the more delicate the movement, the more precise is the coordination between agonist and antagonist muscles.

CLINICAL MANIFESTATIONS OF MOTOR SYSTEM DISEASES

When applied to voluntary muscles, *paralysis* means loss of contraction due to interruption of one or more motor pathways from the cortex to the muscle fiber. It is preferable to use *paresis* for slight and *paralysis* or *plegia* for severe loss of motor strength. Motor paralysis may result from lesions of upper motor neurons (corticospinal, corticobulbar, or subcorticospinal neurons) or of the motor unit. In addition to weakness, impaired facility of movement is an important functional deficit.

PARALYSIS DUE TO DISEASES OF PYRAMIDAL AND SUBCORTICOSPINAL NEURONS Corticospinal paralysis may be due to lesions in the cerebral cortex, subcortical white matter, internal capsule, brainstem, or spinal cord. Lesions confined to one of these anatomic locations without damaging adjacent parts of the brain are rare but afford an opportunity to assess pure pyramidal tract function. In cases of unilateral pyramidal tract damage in the medulla, for example, initial paralysis may be striking, but there is a remarkable degree of recovery of motor function in the affected contralateral arm and leg, leaving only an extensor plantar reflex (Babinski's sign) and impaired fine finger movement. The extent of recovery is surprising and may be due to preservation of a few fibers in the pyramid or to preservation of lateral brainstem pathways. This picture of pure pyramidal tract damage is much different from the extensive deficits that generally accompany most spastic hemiplegic syndromes. In clinical practice, most lesions of the upper motor neurons interrupt descending fibers from the cerebral cortex (corticospinal, corticorubral, corticostriatal, corticopallidal, corticopontine, and corticoreticular) and from the brainstem (reticulospinal, vestibulospinal, and rubrospinal). These lesions produce the classic upper motor neuron syndrome consisting of weakness, hyperactivity of tendon reflexes, and spasticity (Table 21-1).

With corticospinal lesions in humans, the distribution of the paralysis varies with the lesion site, but there are certain common features. Paralysis due to a lesion of upper motor neurons always involves a group of muscles, never individual muscles. In general, hand, arm, and leg muscles are most affected after a corticospinal lesion; of the cranial musculature, only the lower face and tongue are involved to any significant degree. Whatever volitional movement remains, the maximum effort is attained more slowly than in the normal limb, fewer motor units are recruited, and the frequency of their discharge is reduced. Corticospinal paralysis never involves all the muscles on one side of the body, even with a complete hemiplegia. Movements that are invariably bilateral, such as those of the eyes, jaw, pharynx, larynx, neck, thorax, and abdomen, are usually unaffected.

Acute lesions of the corticospinal and subcorticospinal motor system below the medulla, such as the cervical cord, produce a distinctive picture of total paralysis and areflexia known as *spinal shock*. After a few days to weeks, flaccidity subsides, muscular tone reappears, and the affected limbs become spastic; paralysis persists unchanged. *Spasticity* is a feature of all lesions of the motor system at cerebral, capsular, midbrain, and pontine levels. Spasticity is defined as a motor disorder characterized by a velocity-dependent increase in tonic stretch reflexes ("muscle tone") with exaggerated tendon jerks; it is one component of the upper motor neuron syndrome. Spasticity is related to excessive activity of motor neurons that are released from inhibition consequent to lesions of the corticospinal or descending brainstem pathways. With supraspinal lesions, certain spinal neurons are more active than others; the arm is maintained in a pronated, flexed position and the leg in an adducted, extended position. Attempts to extend the arm or flex the leg passively will elicit increasing resistance which abruptly subsides (*clasp-knife phenomenon*). When the limb is left in the new position, the resistance reappears (*lengthening and shortening reactions*). With combined lesions of corticospinal and other suprasegmental tracts, sustained resistance to movement (*hypertonus*) is more common than the clasp-knife type of spasticity. Upper motor neuron lesions also release the nocifensive spinal flexion reflexes, including Babinski's sign, and diminish or abolish the cutaneomuscular abdominal and cremasteric reflexes. Other signs of corticospinal or upper motor neuron lesions include exaggerated stretch and cutaneous reflexes in cranial as well as in limb and trunk muscles. If the corticospinal lesions are bilateral, there is *pseudobulbar paralysis* (dysarthria, dysphonia, and dysphagia with bifacial paralysis) accompanied by forced crying and laughing. Prolonged flexor and extensor spasms occur with lesions of the spinal cord; they are due to a release of cutaneous reflexes from suprasegmental modulation.

Spasticity is present with paresis as well as paralysis and can add to disturbances of voluntary movements. In general, all attempts by the patient to move the hemiparetic extremities appear to be hampered. Discrete movements of individual fingers and finely coordinated movements of the hand are lost, but voluntary control over proximal muscles is generally maintained. Synergies of movements eventually appear. For example, in the upper extremity a flexion synergy consisting of finger flexion, wrist flexion and pronation, elbow flexion, and shoulder elevation and abduction is produced in a slow, stereotyped fashion upon attempted grasp of an object. Attempts to push with the hand result in a weak pronation of the hand, extension or flexion of the fingers, extension of the wrist and elbow, adduction of the upper arm, and lowering of the shoulder. In the lower extremity the extensor synergy (thigh adduction, thigh and knee extension, and plantar flexion of the toes and foot) is more powerful than the flexor synergy of hip abduction, hip and knee flexion, and dorsiflexion and inversion of toes and foot. A bias toward extensor synergy facilitates weight bearing and walking, which are eventually achieved by nearly all hemiplegic patients. These synergies indicate that there is a diminution in voluntary anterior horn cell activation (the negative effect of a motor lesion) and excessive reflex and synergistic discharges in the same motor neuron pools (the positive effects of the lesion). Strong-willed effort to move the paretic limb also may evoke symmetric associated (mirror) movements in the normal limb.

In spasticity, where the neurons responsible for excitation of the extensor muscles of the leg and flexors of the arm are overactive, it is not known whether there is a functional excess of excitatory neurotransmitters or a deficiency of inhibitory transmitters or both. Current evidence indicates that drugs that decrease spasticity act at the spinal cord level to alter neurotransmitter function. Baclofen slows conduction in the spinal cord reflex arc, perhaps by interfering with the release of excitatory neurotransmitters, including glutamate and substance P, from primary afferent neurons. GABA and glycine interneurons are thought to be underactive in spasticity. Diazepam facilitates GABA-mediated presynaptic inhibition of primary afferent excitatory transmitter release, and enhanced glycinergic neurotransmission suppresses spasticity.

TABLE 21-1   Differences between paralysis due to lesions of upper versus lower motor neurons

Upper motor neuron paralysis	Lower motor neuron paralysis
Muscle groups affected diffusely, never individual muscles	Individual muscles may be affected
Atrophy slight	Atrophy pronounced, 70 to 80% of total bulk
Spasticity with hyperactivity of the tendon reflexes	Flaccidity and hypotonia of affected muscles with loss of tendon reflexes
Extensor plantar reflex, Babinski's sign	Plantar reflex, if present, is of normal flexor type
Fascicular twitches not produced	Fasciculations may be present
	EMG reveals reduced numbers of motor units and fibrillations

PARALYSIS DUE TO DISEASES OF THE MOTOR UNIT Damage to the lower motor neurons can produce paresis or paralysis as a direct result of physiologic block or destruction of anterior horn cells or their axons in anterior roots and nerves. The signs and symptoms of the lower motor neuron syndrome vary according to the location of the lesion: The most important question for clinical purposes is whether sensory changes coexist with muscular weakness. The combination of flaccid areflexic paralysis and sensory loss usually indicates involvement of mixed motor and sensory nerves or damage to both anterior and posterior roots. If sensory changes are absent, the lesion must be situated in the gray matter of the spinal cord, in the anterior roots, in a purely motor branch of a peripheral nerve, or in motor axons alone. The distinction between nuclear (spinal) and anterior root (radicular) lesions may at times be impossible to make.

If all or practically all peripheral motor nerves supplying a muscle are destroyed, voluntary, postural, and reflex movements are abolished. The muscle becomes soft and yields excessively to passive stretching, a condition known as *flaccidity*. Muscle tone—the slight resistance that normal relaxed muscle offers to passive movement—is reduced (*hypotonia* or *atonia*). The denervated muscles undergo extreme atrophy and lose 70 to 80 percent of their original bulk within 4 months. The reflex reaction of the muscle to sudden stretch, as by tapping its tendon, is lost. If only a few motor units in the muscles are affected, partial paralysis will ensue. With partial denervation, EMG evidence of fibrillations also may be obtained. Clinical features that distinguish lower motor and upper motor neuron lesions are summarized in Table 21-1.

APRAXIC OR NONPARALYTIC DISORDERS OF MOTOR FUNCTION Loss of learned movements can simulate paresis of a limb, even though the pyramidal tract and spinal cord motor units are intact. This condition is called *apraxia* and is defined as a disorder of learned movement that is not due to weakness, incoordination, sensory loss, or failure to comprehend commands. A failure to execute a designated action while retaining the ability to carry out the individual movements upon which such an act depends is the main feature of apraxia. A clinical test of motor deficits of this type is to observe a series of self-initiated actions such as using a comb, a razor, a toothbrush, or a common tool or gesturing, e.g., waving goodbye, saluting, shaking the fist as though angry, or blowing a kiss. These actions are usually elicited by a verbal command or a request to imitate the examiner. Of course, failure to follow a spoken or written request may be due to an aphasia that prevents understanding of what is asked or to an agnosia that prevents recognition of the tool or object to be used. But when these difficulties are excluded, there remains a peculiar motor deficit in which the patient appears to understand but has lost the memory of how to perform a given act, especially if it is called for in an unnatural setting. The patient may have the idea of what to do but cannot translate the idea of the sequence of movements into a precise, well-executed act. An apraxic deficit may be evident both after a spoken command and in requests to imitate the gestures of the examiner. Sometimes these two conditions may be dissociated; the patient, while not aphasic, cannot execute a gesture to a spoken command but can still imitate the act if it is called forth by gesture. Also, if merely given the tool, the patient may use it properly in an automatic fashion.

To understand the anatomic basis of apraxia, it is necessary to appreciate that the production of complex motor behavior results from association among several cortical brain areas. The motor response of right-handed (and most left-handed) persons to a command requires the integrity of the left parietal and temporal lobes, especially the region around the left supramarginal gyrus, and their connection with the left premotor regions for control of the right hand. Information flows through the corpus callosum from the left to the right motor cortex for control of the left side of the body. Disconnection of the supramarginal area from motor areas of the right hemisphere (most commonly by lesions of the midcallosum, dominant frontal association cortex, or posterior parietal lobe) results in apraxia of left limbs when tested by response to verbal commands.

EXAMINATION SCHEME FOR MOTOR PARALYSIS AND APRAXIA The first step in examination is to inspect the paralyzed limb, taking note of its posture and whether there are signs of muscular hypertrophy, atrophy, or fascicular twitchings. Slight atrophy may be due to disuse from any cause, i.e., pain, fixation as the result of a cast, or any type of paralysis. Pronounced atrophy usually occurs only with denervation of several weeks' or months' duration. The patient is then called on to move each muscle group, and the power and facility of movement are graded and recorded. The Medical Research Council scale provides a useful clinical measure of weakness:

0 = no contraction
1 = trace contraction
2 = active movement with gravity eliminated
3 = active movement against gravity
4 = active movement against gravity and resistance
5 = normal power

The examiner then determines the range of passive movement and the degree of resistance encountered moving all the joints. This provides information concerning alterations of muscle tone, i.e., hypotonia, spasticity, and rigidity. Dislocations, diseased joints, and ankyloses also may be revealed by these same maneuvers. The tendon reflexes are then tested. The usual routine is to try to elicit the jaw jerk (increased in pseudobulbar palsy) and the biceps, triceps, quadriceps, and Achilles tendon reflexes. Two cutaneous reflexes are then tested, the abdominal and plantar reflexes.

If there is no evidence of upper or lower motor neuron disease, but motor acts are nonetheless imperfectly performed, one should look for a disorder of postural control associated with cerebellar incoordination or consider that rigidity with abnormalities of posture and movement may be due to disease of the basal ganglia. In the absence of these disorders, the possibility of an apraxic disorder may be investigated by watching the patient's own movements and those called forth by specific command and gesture.

DIFFERENTIAL DIAGNOSIS OF PARALYSIS The diagnostic consideration of paralysis may be simplified by the following subdivisions, which relate to the location and distribution of weakness. Paralysis may result from dysfunction of upper motor neurons (corticospinal, corticobulbar, and subcorticospinal neurons) or of the motor unit (bulbar and spinal motor neurons, neuromuscular junction, and muscle). In general, the presence or absence of atrophy of muscles in a monoplegic limb can assist the clinician to arrive at an anatomic and clinical diagnosis.

Monoplegia It is necessary to determine carefully the distribution of muscle weakness. For example, patients who complain of weakness of one extremity often have unnoticed weakness in another limb, and the condition is actually hemiplegia or paraplegia. A comprehensive physical examination should be conducted in order to determine whether there is weakness of all the muscles in a limb or only isolated muscle groups. The examination also should exclude nonparalytic conditions such as ataxia, sensory disturbances, mechanical limitation resulting from arthritis, the rigidity of parkinsonism, or pain in an extremity; such conditions are often interpreted by the patient as weakness.

PARALYSIS WITH LITTLE OR NO ATROPHY The most frequent cause of monoplegia without muscular wasting is a lesion of the cerebral cortex; diseases that interrupt the corticospinal tract at the level of the internal capsule, brainstem, or spinal cord rarely cause monoplegia because corticospinal fibers to arm and leg are intermingled at subcortical levels. A cortical vascular lesion (thrombosis or embolus) is the most common cause of monoplegia, but a discrete traumatic lesion, tumor, or abscess may have the same effect. Multiple sclerosis and spinal cord tumor, early in their course, may cause isolated weakness of one extremity, usually the leg. Weakness due to damage of upper motor neurons is usually accompanied by spasticity, increased reflexes, and an extensor plantar reflex (Babinski's sign). In acute diseases affecting the lower motor neurons, such as poliomyelitis, the tendon reflexes are always reduced or abolished, but atrophy may not appear for several weeks. Hence one must take into account the mode of onset and the duration of the disease in evaluating the tendon reflexes, muscle tone, and degree of atrophy before reaching an anatomic diagnosis.

PARALYSIS WITH MUSCULAR ATROPHY   Atrophy of muscles in a paralyzed limb usually indicates a lesion of some portion of the motor unit (spinal cord, spinal roots, peripheral nerve, or muscle). Disease of the neuromuscular junction (e.g., myasthenia gravis) is not associated with muscular atrophy. In addition to the paralysis, reduced or abolished tendon reflexes, and decreased tone, there may be visible fasciculations. The EMG shows decreased numbers of motor units (often of large size), fasciculations at rest, and fibrillations. The location of the lesion can usually be decided by the distribution of the palsied muscles (whether the pattern is one of muscles, nerve, spinal root, or spinal cord involvement), by the associated neurologic symptoms and signs, and by special tests (CSF examination, CT or magnetic resonance imaging scans of the spine, myelogram, serum muscle enzymes, EMG, sensory evoked responses, and biopsy). A clinical approach to the signs and symptoms that assist the clinician in arriving at an anatomic diagnosis of diseases of the motor unit (spinal cord, spinal motor nerves, neuromuscular junction, or muscle) are described in more detail in Chaps. 382 and 383.

The anatomic pattern of paralysis with atrophy may suggest the clinical diagnosis. Atrophic monoplegia affecting the arm should suggest brachial plexus trauma in an infant; poliomyelitis in a child; and poliomyelitis, syringomyelia, amyotrophic lateral sclerosis, or neuritis of the brachial plexus in an adult. Crural monoplegia (affecting the leg) is more frequent than brachial monoplegia and may be caused by any lesion of thoracic or lumber cord, including trauma, tumor, myelitis, or multiple sclerosis. Multiple sclerosis almost never causes atrophy, and ruptured intervertebral disk and the many varieties of neuritis rarely paralyze all or most of the muscles of a limb. Muscular dystrophy may begin in one limb, but by the time the patient is seen, the typical pattern of symmetric proximal limb and trunk involvement is usually evident. A unilateral retroperitoneal tumor may paralyze the leg by implicating the lumbosacral plexus. Prolonged disuse of a limb may lead to atrophy, but this is usually not so marked as in diseases that denervate muscles. In disuse atrophy, the tendon reflexes are normal, and the responses of the muscles to electric stimulation and on EMG are unaltered.

Hemiplegia   Loss of strength in the arm, leg, and sometimes face on one side of the body is the most frequent distribution of paralysis. With rare exceptions (a few unusual cases of poliomyelitis or motor system disease), this pattern of paralysis is due to involvement of the descending motor tracts. The site or level of the lesion that produced hemiplegia can usually be deduced from the associated neurologic findings. Diseases localized in the cerebral cortex, cerebral white matter (corona radiata), and internal capsule usually produce weakness or paralysis of the face, arm, and leg on the side of the body contralateral to the brain lesion. The occurrence of convulsive seizures or the presence of a defect in speech (aphasia), a cortical type of sensory loss (astereognosis and loss of two-point discrimination), anosognosia, or defects in the visual fields suggest a cortical or subcortical rather than a capsular location. A pure, isolated motor hemiplegia affecting simultaneously the face, arm, and leg indicates a small, discrete lesion in the posterior limb of the internal capsule, cerebral peduncle, pons, or medullary pyramids. Damage to the corticospinal and corticobulbar tracts in the upper portion of the brainstem will cause paralysis of the face, arm, and leg in the side opposite the lesion, plus deficits in cranial nerve function on the same side as the lesion. These "crossed paralyses" that are so characteristic of brainstem diseases are described in Chap. 368.

Hemiplegia that spares cranial musculature may be caused by a lesion in the lateral column of the cervical spinal cord. At this level, however, the pathologic process often induces bilateral signs, with resulting quadriparesis or quadriplegia. Homolateral paralysis, if combined with a loss of vibratory and position sense on the same

side and contralateral loss of pain and temperature (Brown-Séquard syndrome), signifies disease of the spinal cord (Chap. 381).

Muscle atrophy of minor degree is often associated with hemiplegia but never reaches the proportions seen in diseases of the lower motor neurons. Atrophy secondary to upper motor neuron damage is largely due to disuse. There is an important exception to this rule: When the motor cortex and adjacent parts of the parietal lobe are damaged in infancy or childhood, the normal development of the muscles and the skeletal system in the affected limbs is retarded, and the palsied limbs and even the trunk on one side are small. Developmental atrophy does not occur, however, if the paralysis begins after puberty, when the greater part of skeletal growth has been attained. In hemiplegia due to spinal cord injury, muscles at the level of the lesion may undergo atrophy if there is associated damage to anterior horn cells or ventral roots.

Vascular diseases of the cerebral hemispheres and brainstem are the most common causes of hemiplegia. Trauma (brain contusion, epidural and subdural hemorrhage) ranks second, followed by other diseases such as brain tumor, demyelinative disease, brain abcess, and encephalitis. Complications of meningitis, tuberculosis, and syphilis were common causes of hemiplegia in the past but are much less evident in current practice.

Paraplegia   Paraplegia denotes a condition of weakness or paralysis of both lower extremities with sparing of the upper extremities. Paraplegia most commonly occurs in diseases of the spinal cord, spinal roots, or peripheral nerves. Among cerebral causes, parasagittal tumors and hydrocephalus cause leg weakness. If the onset is acute, it may be difficult to distinguish spinal from peripheral nerve or root causes of paralysis because sudden damage to either may result in flaccidity and abolition of reflexes. As a rule, in acute spinal cord diseases the paralysis affects all muscles below a given level; often, if the white matter is extensively damaged, sensory loss below a particular level (loss of pain and temperature sense from lateral spinothalamic tracts involvement and loss of vibratory and position sense from posterior columns damage) is conjoined. Also, in bilateral disease of the spinal cord the bladder and bowel sphincters are paralyzed. Alterations of CSF (dynamic block and increases in protein or cells) are frequent. In peripheral nerve diseases both sensory loss and motor loss tend to involve the distal muscles of the legs more than the proximal ones (an exception is acute idiopathic polyneuritis), and the sphincters are spared or only briefly deranged in function. Sensory loss, if present, is more likely to consist of distal impairment of touch, vibration, and position sense, with pain and temperature sense spared in many instances. The CSF protein level may be normal or elevated. Studies of nerve conduction through spinal roots (F waves) are always abnormal.

Acute paraplegia most commonly occurs after trauma or in association with metastatic neoplasia. Uncommon causes of acute paraplegia include a medial pontine lesion affecting the leg fibers which are near the midline (as in pontine infarction or central pontine myelinolysis), spontaneous hematomyelia with bleeding from a vascular malformation (angioma, telangiectasis), thrombosis of a spinal artery with infarction (myelomalacia), and dissecting aortic aneurysm or atherosclerotic occlusion of nutrient spinal arteries arising from the aorta with resulting infarction (myelomalacia). Postinfectious or postvaccinal myelitis, acute demyelinative myelitis (Devic's disease if the optic nerves are affected), necrotizing myelitis, and epidural abscess or hemorrhage with spinal cord compression tend to develop somewhat more slowly over a period of hours or days, but they may have an acute onset. Poliomyelitis, in those countries where immunization is incomplete, presents as a purely motor disorder with meningitis and must be distinguished from the other acute myelopathies.

Subacute or chronic paraplegia in adults results from such common diseases as cervical spondylosis and multiple sclerosis. Other causes are subacute combined degeneration, spinal cord tumor, ruptured cervical disk, syphilitic meningomyelitis, chronic epidural infections (fungus and other granulomatous diseases), motor system disease, and syringomyelia. Familial spastic paraparesis is a rare cause of paraplegia in which there is symmetric demyelination of the dorsolateral corticospinal tract. (See Chap. 381 for discussion of these spinal cord diseases.) The several varieties of polyneuritis, including Guillain-Barré syndrome and polymyositis, must be considered in the differential diagnosis of paraparesis. Friedreich's ataxia and familial spastic paraplegia, progressive muscular dystrophy, and the chronic varieties of polyneuritis tend to appear during late childhood and adolescence and are slowly progressive.

Paraplegia (or paraparesis) may be due to a lesion of the leg areas of the motor cortex. Arterial (anterior cerebral arteries) or venous (superior sagittal sinus and tributary cerebral veins) distribution cerebral infarctions are causes of acute paraplegia; parasagittal meningioma is a cause of asymmetric chronic paraplegia. Usually other signs such as confusion, stupor, or seizures indicate the cerebral localization, and differential diagnosis is not a problem.

Quadriplegia   All that has been written about the common causes of paraplegia applies to quadriplegia except that the lesion is in the cervical rather than the thoracic or lumbar segments of the spinal cord. If it is situated in the low cervical segments and involves the anterior half of the spinal cord, as in occlusion of the anterior spinal artery, the arm paralysis may be flaccid and areflexic and the leg paralysis spastic (anterior spinal syndrome). There are only a few points of difference between the common paraplegic and quadriplegic syndromes. One of the most common causes of subacute quadriplegia is the Guillain-Barré syndrome due to inflammatory demyelination of motor neuron axons in the anterior roots. Repeated cerebral vascular accidents may lead to bilateral hemiplegia, usually accompanied by pseudobulbar palsy. An unusual cause of quadriplegia is bilateral infarctions of the medullary pyramids.

Isolated paralysis   Paralysis of isolated muscle groups usually indicates a lesion of one or more peripheral nerves. The basis for diagnosing a lesion of an individual peripheral nerve is the presence of weakness or paralysis of the muscle or group of muscles and impairment or loss of sensation in the distribution of the nerve in question (Chap. 383). Complete transection or severe injury to a peripheral nerve is usually followed by atrophy of the muscles it innervates and by loss of their tendon reflexes. Trophic changes in the skin, nails, and subcutaneous tissue also may occur. It is of considerable importance to decide whether the lesion is only a temporary one (conduction block) or there has been a dissolution of axonal continuity, requiring nerve regeneration for recovery.

THE BASAL GANGLIA

The basal ganglia subserve motor functions that are distinct from those attributed to the pyramidal (corticospinal) tract. The term *extrapyramidal* underscores this distinction and calls attention to a set of neurologic illnesses caused by lesions that affect the basal ganglia.

ANATOMIC CONNECTIONS AND NEURONAL TRANSMITTERS IN THE BASAL GANGLIA   The basal ganglia are paired subcortical masses of gray matter that form anatomically distinct nuclear groups. The major nuclei are the caudate and the putamen (which together are called the *striatum*), the internal and external segments of the globus pallidus, the subthalamic nucleus, and the substantia nigra (Fig. 21-1). In contrast to the pyramidal system, the basal ganglia do not project directly to the spinal cord. The basal ganglia receive cortical input and project back to the frontal cortex through the thalamus. Together with parallel circuits originating in the cerebellum, the basal ganglia–thalamocortical circuit modulates activity in the corticospinal (pyramidal) motor system.

The striatum receives somatotopic cortical input from the frontal, sensory, motor, and parietotemporal-occipital association areas (see Fig. 21-1). Corticostriatal afferents release the excitatory amino acid glutamate. Another major afferent input to the striatum is from neurons in the substantia nigra pars compacta (SNc) which synthesize

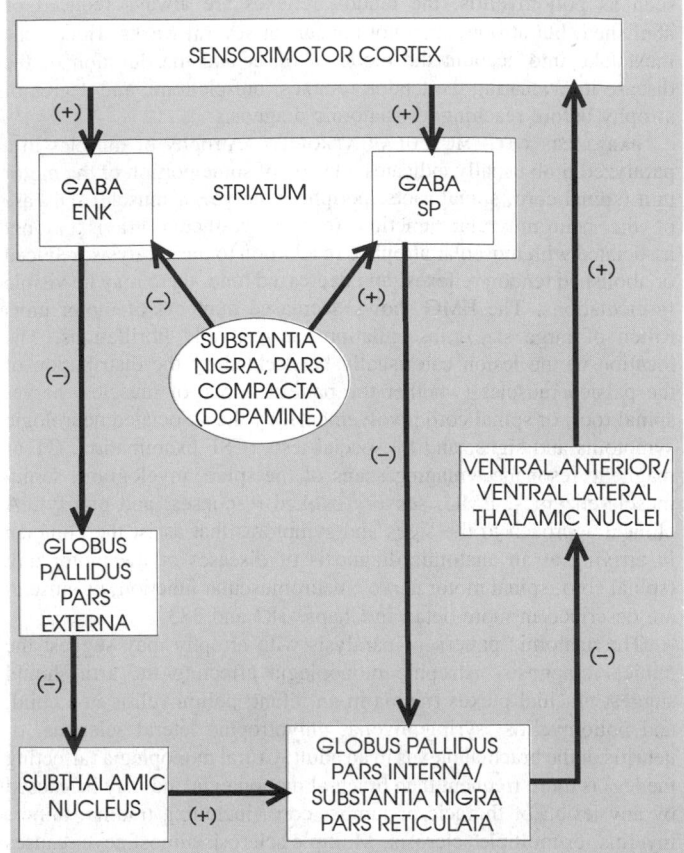

FIGURE 21-1   Diagram of the major functional connections of the basal ganglia. The striatum receives afferents (glutamatergic) from the sensorimotor cortex; the other major afferent arises from the substantia nigra pars compacta and contains dopamine. The major output of the striatum flows through the internal globus pallidus and substantia nigra pars reticulata to ventral anterior and ventral lateral nuclei of the thalamus. Abbreviations: GABA = gamma-aminobutyric acid; ENK = enkephalin; SP = substance P; (+) = excitatory pathway; (-) = inhibitory pathway. (*Diagram courtesy of Dr. Douglas G. Cole.*)

and release dopamine (DA). Additional afferents to the striatum arise from the intralaminar thalamic nuclei and the brainstem raphe (containing serotonin). The striatum contains two distinct classes of cells: local circuit neurons, whose axons do not project beyond the confines of the nucleus, and other neurons, whose axons project to the globus pallidus and substantia nigra. Many neurotransmitters are present in striatal local circuit neurons, but their role in basal ganglia function are not well understood. The one exception is acetylcholine, which is present in large local circuit striatal neurons and appears to act in a manner which is functionally antagonistic to DA. The major output nuclei of the basal ganglia, the internal segment of the globus pallidus (GPi) and the substantia nigra reticulata (SNr), send GABA-containing inhibitory projections to the ventral anterior, ventral lateral, and intralaminar thalamic nuclei, including the centromedian nucleus (see Fig. 21-1). The influence of the basal ganglia circuits on the cortical motor areas is completed by means of the excitatory pathway from the thalamus to precentral cortex (see Fig. 21-1).

Basal ganglia output nuclei (GPi and SNr) are inhibitory to thalamic nuclei and are differentially modulated by two GABA-containing efferent projections from the striatum. A *direct pathway* consists of inhibitory striatal (putaminal) efferents containing substance P which projects to the SNr (see Fig. 21-1). A parallel *indirect pathway*, containing enkephalin, projects to the GPi by way of the external globus pallidus (GPe) and subthalamic nucleus (STN). The two striatal efferent systems appear to exert opposing effects on the basal ganglia output nuclei and, in turn, on the thalamic target nuclei. Activation of the direct pathway results in net excitation of the thalamocortical circuits and facilitation of cortically initiated movements. Activation of the indirect pathway increases excitatory drive to the STN and the basal ganglia output nuclei, resulting in inhibition of the thalamocortical circuit. The influence of DA-containing nigrostriatal afferents is to enhance transmission through the direct pathway and suppress transmission through the indirect pathway. The net effect of DA, then, is to enhance positive feedback to the cortical motor areas and facilitate volitional movements.

Alterations in the balance between the indirect and direct pathways' influence on thalamocortical activity may result in hypokinetic and hyperkinetic movements seen in disorders of the extrapyramidal system. Increases in transmission through the direct pathway decrease thalamic inhibition and produce hyperkinetic disorders, and enhanced transmission through the indirect pathway increases thalamic inhibition and results in hypokinetic disorders. Deficiency of DA, as occurs in Parkinson's disease, increases transmission through the indirect pathway and decreases transmission through the direct pathway; the net effect is to increase the output through the STN and GPi/SNr, thereby inhibiting the facilitatory thalamocortical influences on motor function and producing hypokinesia. Consistent with this model, lesions of the STN have been reported to ameliorate motor impairments in experimental parkinsonism. This model also provides an explanation for hyperkinetic movement disorders. Damage to the STN, for example, is the usual cause of hemiballismus. In early Huntington's disease, when chorea is prominent, there is a selective loss of striatal GABA/enkephalin neurons that give rise to the indirect pathway.

Like the basal ganglia, the cerebellum receives cortical inputs and modulates pyramidal tract function through the thalamus. The major cerebellar output, which exits the cerebellum through the superior cerebellar peduncle, terminates with the pallidothalamic fibers in the ventral anterior and ventral lateral thalamic nuclei. This region of the thalamus, therefore, forms an essential link in the ascending fiber systems from both the basal ganglia and the cerebellum to the motor cortex. Although parallel, the basal ganglia and cerebellar circuits influence cortically initiated motor activity through segregated thalamic and cortical regions. Despite the apparently crucial nature of these structures, lesions placed stereotaxically in the ventral thalamus can abolish essential-familial tremor or the rigidity and tremor in Parkinson's disease without producing functional deficits.

PHYSIOLOGY OF THE BASAL GANGLIA Recordings from neurons in the globus pallidus and substantia nigra in awake, performing primates confirm the main motor function of the basal ganglia. Cells within these regions clearly participate in the initiation of movement, because they increase their firing rates before movement is observed clinically or detected by EMG. Discharges in the basal ganglia are related principally to contralateral rather than ipsilateral limb movements. Many neurons increase their firing rates during slow (ramp) movements, but some others discharge during more rapid (ballistic) movements. There is somatotopic localization of leg, arm, and face within the internal segment of the globus pallidus and pars reticulata of the substantia nigra. This observation provides a possible explanation for the occurrence of restricted dyskinesias: Focal dystonia and buccal-lingual-masticatory tardive dyskinesia may result from localized pallidal or nigral lesions that affect only regions with hand or face representation.

Although the basal ganglia are motor nuclei, it is not possible to identify a specific type of basal ganglia movement. Hypotheses about the function of the basal ganglia in human beings derive from correlations between clinical signs and sites of pathologic lesions in patients with extrapyramidal diseases. The basal ganglia are a constellation of nuclei centered around the globus pallidus, through which impulses are channeled to the thalamus and onward to the cerebral cortex (see Fig. 21-1). Neurons in each satellite nucleus contribute excitatory and inhibitory impulses, and the sum of these influences on the main pathway from basal ganglia to thalamus and cerebral cortex, modified by the cerebellum, determines smooth motor

function as expressed through the corticospinal and other descending cortical tracts. If one or more of the supporting nuclei are damaged, the sum of the impulses to the globus pallidus changes, and disordered mobility can occur. Hemiballismus is the most dramatic of these; damage to the subthalamic nucleus results in violent, involuntary, rotatory flinging movements of the contralateral arm and leg. Similarly, dysfunction of the caudate nucleus often results in chorea, whereas the opposite phenomenon, akinesia, typically occurs when dopamine-producing cells in the substantia nigra degenerate. Lesions restricted to the globus pallidus often cause flexion dystonia and impaired postural reflexes.

CLINICAL MANIFESTATIONS OF LESIONS OF THE BASAL GANGLIA Akinesia When extrapyramidal diseases are analyzed into primary functional deficits (negative symptoms due to loss of connectivity) and secondary release effects (positive symptoms of excessive activity), akinesia stands as a principal negative or deficit symptom. *Akinesia* refers to the inability to initiate changes in activity and to perform ordinary volitional movements rapidly and easily. The terms *bradykinesia* and *hypokinesia* are employed to describe lesser degrees of impairment. In contrast to paralysis, which is the negative symptom of corticospinal tract lesions, strength is preserved, although there is a delay in achieving peak power. Akinesia is the most disabling feature of Parkinson's disease. Akinetic patients display severe immobility and underactivity. They sit motionless for long periods of time without shifting postures and take more than the time normally required to eat, dress, and bathe. There is general poverty of movement, including loss of automatic associated motions, such as eye blinks and freely swinging arms when walking. Akinesia probably accounts for such common symptoms in Parkinson's disease as facial immobility, vocal hypophonia, micrographia, and difficulty in arising from a chair and beginning to walk. Akinesia can affect the mind as well; slowed speed of thought is called *bradyphrenia*. Although pathophysiologic details remain uncertain, clinical analysis of akinesia supports the hypothesis that the basal ganglia are mainly responsible for initiation and automatic execution of learned motor plans. Neuropharmacologic evidence suggests that akinesia itself results from DA deficiency.

Rigidity Muscle tone is defined as the amount of resistance encountered when a relaxed limb is moved passively. In rigidity, the muscles are in continuous contraction, and resistance to passive movement is constant. Rigidity secondary to extrapyramidal disorders may superficially resemble spasticity due to corticospinal tract lesions in that both produce increases in muscular tone. A few clinical guidelines provide help in distinguishing these conditions at the bedside (Table 21-2). The distribution of increased tone often differs in rigidity and spasticity. Although rigidity is present in both flexor and extensor muscle groups, it tends to be more prominent in those which maintain a flexed posture. Rigidity is easy to detect in large muscle groups, but smaller muscles of the face, tongue, and larynx are also often affected. In contrast to rigidity, spasticity usually produces increased tone in the extensor muscles of the legs and the flexor musculature of the arms. The quality of hypertonus also can be used to distinguish the two conditions. Resistance to passive

TABLE 21-2   Clinical characteristics of altered muscle tone

	Hypertonia		Hypotonia
	Spasticity	Rigidity	
Resistance to stretch	Increased "clasp knife"	Increased; "lead pipe"	Decreased
Associated findings	Increased DTRs, Babinski's sign	Bradykinesia, resting tremor	Decreased DTRs, muscle atrophy, ataxia, intention tremor
Clinical conditions	Upper motor neuron lesions	Extrapyramidal syndromes	Lower motor neuron lesions, cerebellar syndromes

movements is constant and independent of movement speed in rigidity, accounting for terms such as "lead pipe" and "plastic" resistance. In spasticity, increased tone is velocity-dependent; there may be a free interval followed classically by the clasp-knife phenomenon; muscles do not contract until they are stretched a bit, and later, during stretch, the augmentation in muscle tone quickly subsides. Deep tendon reflexes are normal in rigidity but increased in spastic states. Spasticity results from hyperactivity of the stretch reflex arc due to central changes but without increased sensitivity of the muscle spindle; spasticity can be abolished by sectioning posterior spinal roots. Rigidity has less relationship with hyperactivity of segmental reflex arcs and depends more on heightened discharge of alpha motor neurons. A special type of rigidity is the cogwheel phenomenon, which is commonly associated with tremor in Parkinson's disease. When the hypertonic muscle is passively stretched, the resistance may be rhythmically jerky, as though the resistance of the limb were controlled by a ratchet.

Chorea Derived from the Greek word meaning "dance," chorea refers to widespread arrhythmic movements of a forcible, rapid, jerky, restless type. Choreic movements are noted for their irregularity and variability; they are generally continuous, may be simple or quite elaborate, and affect any part of the body. They may resemble voluntary movement in complexity, but they are never combined into a coordinated act unless the patient incorporates them into a deliberate movement in order to make them less noticeable. Normal volitional movements are possible because there is no paralysis, but they may be excessively quick, poorly sustained, and deformed by choreic movements. Chorea may be generalized or limited to one side of the body. Generalized chorea is the predominant involuntary movement in Huntington's disease and in rheumatic (Sydenham's) chorea and usually involves the face, trunk, and limbs; it is often seen with levodopa toxicity in patients with Parkinson's disease. Another common choreiform disorder, tardive dyskinesia, occurs in association with chronic neuroleptic administration. Choreic movements in this disorder are generally restricted to the buccal, lingual, and mandibular musculature, although trunk and limbs may be involved in severe cases. Chorea may also occur in medical illnesses (e.g., systemic lupus erythematosus), cerebrovascular diseases, drug intoxications, and after infections (e.g., Sydenham's chorea). When alleviating the underlying disorder is not possible, benzodiazepines, reserpine, and neuroleptics may be moderately effective in suppressing chorea.

Athetosis This term is from a Greek word meaning "unfixed" or "changeable." Athetosis is characterized by an inability to sustain the muscles of the fingers, toes, tongue, or any other muscle group in one position. The maintained posture is interrupted by continuous, slow, sinuous writhing movements. These are most pronounced in the digits and hands and consist of extension, pronation, flexion, and supination of the arm with alternating flexion and extension of the fingers. Athetotic movements are slower than those associated with chorea, but gradations are commonly seen and termed *choreoathetosis* when it is impossible to distinguish between the two. Generalized athetosis may be seen in children with static encephalopathy (cerebral palsy); it also can occur in Wilson's disease, in torsion dystonia, and following cerebral anoxia. Posthemiplegic athetosis is unilateral and occurs especially in children who have suffered a stroke. Patients whose athetosis is due to cerebral palsy or cerebral anoxia have variable degrees of additional motor deficit due to associated corticospinal tract disease. Discrete individual movements of the tongue, lips, and hands are often impossible, and attempts to perform such voluntary movements result in contraction of all the muscles in the limb and other parts of the body. Variable degrees of rigidity are generally associated with all forms of athetosis and may account for the slower quality of movement in this disorder in contrast to chorea. Treatment of athetosis is generally unsatisfactory, although some patients improve with the drugs used to suppress chorea and dystonia.

The dystonias Dystonia refers to increased muscular tone that causes fixed abnormal postures. Some patients with dystonia also have shifting postures resulting from irregular, forceful twisting

movements that affect trunk and extremities and produce bizarre, grotesque movements and positions of the body. The mobile spasms of dystonia are similar to those of athetosis but are generally slower. Dystonic movements increase during volitional motor activity, nervousness, and emotional stress; they diminish during relaxation and, like most extrapyramidal movement disorders, disappear completely during sleep.

Dystonias may be classified in two ways: by etiology or by the pattern of affected body parts. *Primary idiopathic torsion dystonia*, formerly known as dystonia musculorum deformans, is frequently inherited as an autosomal dominant characteristic due to an abnormal gene on chromosome 9. Spontaneous cases without family histories of dystonia are also common. Manifestations of dystonia usually begin in the first two decades of life, but adult forms are recognized. Torsion dystonia is classified as an extrapyramidal disease even though no pathologic lesions have been observed in the basal ganglia or elsewhere in the brain. *Secondary dystonias* are those which result from a known illness. Examples include Wilson's disease, posthemiplegic dystonia, perinatal brain injury, kernicterus, and sequelae of neuroleptic drugs (e.g., acute dystonic reactions and tardive dystonia).

Focal dystonias are more common than generalized dystonias and include such disorders as spasmodic torticollis, writer's cramp, blepharospasm, and spastic dysphonia. In the focal dystonias, a single area of the body is affected. Focal dystonias occur more frequently in adults than in children, remain stable, and rarely spread to involve other body parts. Spasmodic torticollis is the most common focal dystonia. There are intermittent or continuous spasms of the sternocleidomastoid, trapezius, and other neck muscles, usually more prominent on one side than on the other, that cause turning or tipping of the head. Torticollis is involuntary and cannot be inhibited and thereby differs from habit spasm or tic. Torticollis is worse when the patient sits, stands, or walks; placing a finger to the chin or side of the jaw often alleviates the muscle imbalance. Women are affected twice as often as men; the average age of onset is 40 years old. *Segmental dystonia* indicates involvement of two or more continuous body parts. Meige syndrome (oromandibular dystonia and blepharospasm) is a segmental cranial dystonia. In *generalized dystonia*, most body parts, including the legs, are involved. *Hemidystonia* involves an arm and leg on the same side of the body.

Development of rational pharmacologic therapy for dystonia is limited by the lack of information regarding neuroanatomic and neurochemical abnormalities. For generalized and segmental dystonias, symptomatic relief is sometimes achieved with high doses of anticholinergic drugs, benzodiazepines, baclofen, carbamazepine, and reserpine; levodopa has been helpful in some types of dystonia. Focal dystonias, such as blepharospasm, have been treated successfully by injecting a dilute solution of botulinum toxin into the affected musculature. When spasmodic torticollis is severe, surgical denervation of the affected muscles (C1–C3 bilaterally and C4 on one side) has given favorable results in most patients.

Myoclonus This is a descriptive term for very brief, involuntary, random muscular contractions. Myoclonus can occur spontaneously at rest, in response to sensory stimuli, or with voluntary movements. Myoclonus may involve a single motor unit and simulate a fasciculation, or it may simultaneously involve groups of muscles that displace the limb or distort its voluntary movement. Myoclonus is a symptom that occurs in a wide variety of generalized metabolic and neurologic disorders collectively called the myoclonias. Posthypoxic intention myoclonus is a special myoclonic syndrome that occurs as a sequel to transient cerebral anoxia such as might occur, for example, during a brief cardiorespiratory arrest. Cognitive abilities are usually preserved; however, there are signs of cerebellar dysfunction, and voluntary movements are marred by action myoclonus involving the extremities, facial muscles, and even the voice. Action myoclonus deforms all movements and severely limits the patient's ability to eat, talk, write, or even walk. Myoclonus also may result from lipid storage disease, encephalitis, Creutzfeldt-Jakob disease, or metabolic

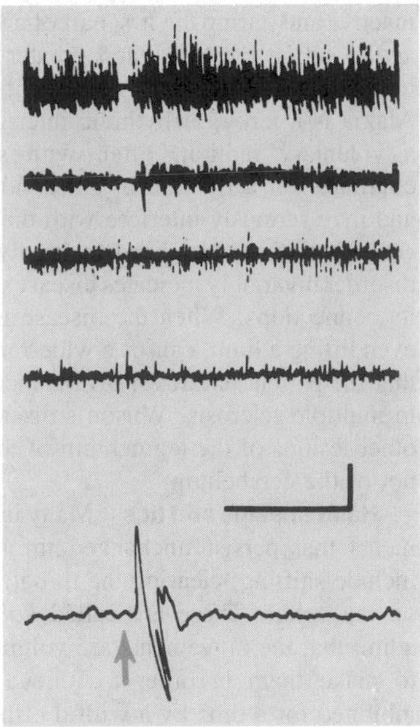

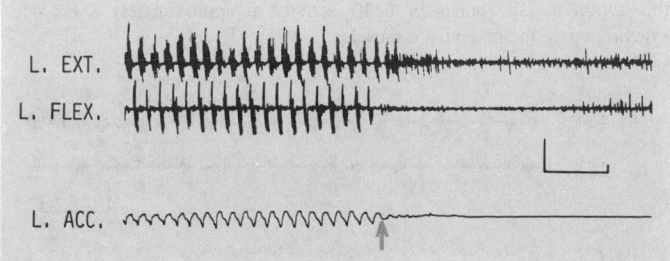

FIGURE 21-2 Asterixis recorded from the outstretched left arm of a patient with metrizamide-induced encephalopathy. The bottom trace is from an accelerometer on the dorsum of the hand. Calibration is 1 s. Note the continuous voluntary EMG interrupted at the arrow by a brief involuntary silent period in all four muscles. This silent period is followed by a lapse of posture and its jerky restitution, which is recorded by the accelerometer.

encephalopathies due to respiratory failure, chronic renal failure, hepatic failure, or electrolyte imbalance. Therapies for myoclonus include baclofen, clonazepam, and valproic acid.

Asterixis Quick arrhythmic movements that occur due to brief interruptions in background tonic muscular contractions are called *asterixis*; in a sense, asterixis may be considered as negative myoclonus. Asterixis may be observed in any voluntary muscle during contraction but is usually demonstrated clinically as a brief lapse of posture with prompt restoration during voluntary extension of the limb with dorsiflexion of the wrist or ankle. Asterixis is characterized by 50- to 200-ms silent periods in ongoing EMG activity in all muscle groups in one limb (Fig. 21-2). This results in a downward movement of the wrist or ankle due to gravity before muscular activity resumes and restores the limb to its original position. Asterixis is commonly observed bilaterally in metabolic encephalopathies, and its description in hepatic failure accounted for the original term "liver flap." Asterixis may be caused by drugs, including all anticonvulsants and the radiographic contrast agent metrizamide. Unilateral asterixis can occur after brain lesions in the distributions of the anterior or posterior cerebral arteries. The smallest brain lesion that can cause unilateral asterixis involves structures that are destroyed during stereotactic ventrolateral thalamotomy.

Hemiballismus Hemiballismus is a hyperkinetic movement disorder characterized by violent flinging motions in the arm contralateral to a lesion (usually vascular) in or near the subthalamic nucleus. The movements in ballism also have a rotary component at the shoulder and hip; there may be concomitant flexion and extension movements in the hand and foot as well. The involuntary motions persist throughout the day but generally attenuate during sleep. Strength and muscle tone may be slightly decreased in the affected extremities, and accurate movements are impaired, but patients with hemiballismus are not paralyzed. Both experimental and clinical observations indicate that the subthalamic nucleus probably exerts a controlling influence on the internal segment of the globus pallidus (see Fig. 21-1). Damage to the subthalamic nucleus destroys the excitatory input to the globus pallidus and thereby disinhibits thalamic facilitatory influences on motor cortex.

Tremor This common symptom consists of a rhythmic oscillation of a part of the body around a fixed point. Tremors usually involve the distal parts of limbs; the head, tongue, or jaw; and rarely the trunk. There are several different types of tremor, and each has its own clinical setting, pathophysiology, and therapeutic requirements. Often several different tremors exist in the same patient and must be treated individually. In a general hospital, most patients who appear

tremulous actually have asterixis as a manifestation of a metabolic encephalopathy. Tremors may be subdivided clinically according to their distribution, amplitude, and relationship to volitional movement.

Tremor at rest is a coarse tremor with an average rate of four to five beats per second. It is most often localized in one or both hands and, occasionally, in the jaw or tongue. It is frequently a feature of Parkinson's disease. It characteristically occurs with postural (tonic) contraction of axial and limb girdle musculature when the limb is in an attitude of repose; willed movement temporarily suppresses it (Fig. 21-3). If the proximal muscles are completely relaxed, the tremor usually disappears, but the average patient rarely achieves this state. In some cases the tremor is constant; in others it varies from time to time and may extend from one group of muscles to another as the disease progresses. In some patients with Parkinson's disease there is no tremor; in others the tremor tends to be rather gentle and more or less limited to the distal muscles, whereas in a minority of parkinsonian patients and in patients with Wilson's disease, tremor has a large amplitude and involves proximal muscles. In many cases there is a variable degree of plastic rigidity in the tremulous limb or elsewhere. Although it is a source of great embarrassment and often is deemed responsible for all of a patient's motor difficulties, rest tremor interferes with voluntary movements surprisingly little: It is not uncommon to see a patient who has been trembling violently raise a full glass of water to the lips and drain the contents without spilling a drop. It is the combination of tremor at rest, slowness of movement, rigidity, flexed postures without true paralysis, and postural instability that constitutes Parkinson's syndrome. Often patients with Parkinson's disease also suffer from the tremor of stage fright (one of the enhanced physiologic tremors—see below) or from essential-familial tremor. Both may be exaggerated by increased levels of catecholamines in the bloodstream and may be suppressed by drugs, such as propranolol, that block beta-adrenergic receptors.

Tremor at rest almost always reflects idiopathic Parkinson's disease. Other conditions in which rest tremor may occur include Wilson's disease and severe essential tremor. Patients with titubation and a proximal tremor at rest (rubral tremor) as a symptom of cerebellar system dysfunction can be differentiated by the presence of ataxia and dysmetria from those with Parkinson's disease.

Action tremor refers to tremors present when the limbs are active, either when maintained in a certain position, as when outstretched, or throughout voluntary movement. Tremor amplitude may increase slightly as the action of the limbs becomes more precise, but it never approaches the degree of augmentation seen with cerebellar ataxia/dysmetria. In contrast to tremor at rest, action tremors disappear when the limbs are relaxed. Some of the action tremors are an exaggeration of normal *physiologic tremor;* such enhanced physiologic tremors are extremely common. They are experienced occasionally by all normal persons as well as by patients with essential-familial tremor or Parkinson's disease. They involve the outstretched hand as well as

FIGURE 21-3 Tremor at rest in a patient with Parkinson's disease. The upper two traces are surface EMG recordings from extensors and flexors of the left wrist; the lower trace is from an accelerometer attached to the left hand. The horizontal calibration denotes 1 s. Note the tremor at rest results from alternating contractions of antagonistic muscles at approximately 5 Hz. At the arrow, the patient is asked to dorsiflex the left wrist, and the tremor at rest disappears.

TABLE 21-3 Conditions that enhance physiologic tremors

HYPERADRENERGIC STATES

Anxiety
Bronchodilators and other beta agonists
Excitement
Hypoglycemia
Hyperthyroidism
Pheochromocytoma
Peripheral metabolites of levodopa
Stage fright

POSSIBLE HYPERADRENERGIC STATES

Amphetamines
Antidepressants
Withdrawal from alcohol or opiates
Xanthines in tea and coffee

STATES OF UNCERTAIN ETIOLOGY

Glucocorticoid therapy
Exercise
Fatigue
Lithium therapy

head, lips, and tongue. In general, they are due to a hyperadrenergic state and sometimes are iatrogenic (Table 21-3). Activation of $beta_2$ receptors in muscle alters the mechanical properties of muscle, eliciting action tremor. These alterations are reflected in discharges of muscle spindle afferents which modify the timing of activity around the stretch reflex arc and serve to augment the amplitude of preexisting physiologic tremor. Only patients without functional stretch reflex arcs are immune to these tremors. Peripherally active drugs that block $beta_2$-adrenergic receptors diminish enhanced physiologic tremors. This type of tremor is seen in numerous medical, neurologic, and psychiatric diseases and is therefore more difficult to interpret than tremor at rest.

Essential-familial tremor (Fig. 21-4) is a somewhat slower action tremor which may occur as the only neurologic abnormality either sporadically or in several members of a family. It may begin in childhood but usually comes on later and persists throughout adult life. It becomes a source of embarrassment because it suggests to the onlooker that the patient is nervous. A curious fact about this tremor is that one or two drinks of an alcoholic beverage may abolish it, but it will become worse after the effects of the alcohol have worn off. Essential-familial tremors are suppressed by primidone or CNS-active beta-adrenergic blocking agents such as propranolol.

Intention tremor is an ambiguous term: The abnormal movements are certainly not intentional, and the abnormality is best described as an oscillatory ataxia generated proximally rather than as tremor. True tremors tend to affect distal musculature, and the movements are more rhythmic and tend to be in one plane. Cerebellar ataxia, in which the direction of abnormal movement varies from second to second, requires for its full expression the performance of an exacting, precise, willed movement. Ataxia is absent when the limbs are

FIGURE 21-4 Action tremor in a patient with essential-familial tremor. Recordings from the right upper extremity are with the hand actively dorsiflexed. The horizontal calibration denotes 500 ms. Note that during this action tremor, bursts of EMG activity at approximately 8 Hz occur synchronously in antagonistic muscles.

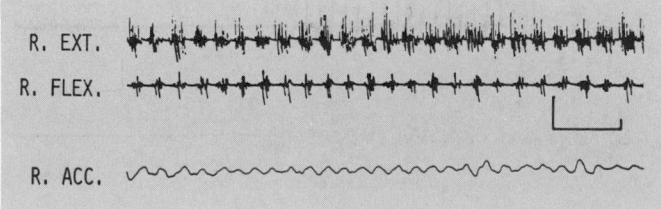

inactive and during the first part of a voluntary movement but develops as the action continues and greater precision is demanded (e.g., in touching a target such as the patient's nose or the examiner's finger). Ataxia is a jerky, arrhythmic interruption of forward progression in a voluntary motion, often with side-to-side oscillations. Ataxia continues for a fraction of a second or so after the act is completed and may seriously interfere with the patient's performance of skilled acts. Sometimes the head is involved (titubation). This movement disorder invariably indicates disease of the cerebellar system, including its connections. When the disease is very severe, every movement, even lifting a limb, causes a wide-ranging oscillation of such violence that the patient is thrown off balance. This state is occasionally seen in multiple sclerosis, Wilson's disease, and vascular, traumatic, and other lesions of the tegmentum of the midbrain and subthalamus but not of the cerebellum.

Habit spasms and tics   Many individuals develop habitual movements that persist unchanged throughout life. Common examples include sniffing, clearing the throat, protruding the chin, and pulling on the collar. These are called *habit spasms*. Affected individuals admit that the movements are voluntary but that they feel compelled to make them in order to relieve tension. Habit spasms can be inhibited for a time by a willful effort but reappear when attention is diverted. In certain cases they become so ingrained that the person is unaware of them and unable to control them. Children between 5 and 10 years of age are especially likely to have habit spasms.

Tics are characterized by stereotyped, purposeless, and irregularly repetitive movements. Gilles de la Tourette syndrome is the most common and severe form of multiple tic disorder. This syndrome is a neuropsychiatric disorder with motor and behavior abnormalities; it usually begins in the first two decades of life and affects boys four times more frequently than girls. Motor symptoms include multiple brief muscular spasms, known as *convulsive tics*, in the face, neck, and shoulders. Vocal tics, including grunts and barking sounds, are also common. Behavioral abnormalities include coprolalia (swearing and repeating other vile utterances) and repeating the words of others (echolalia). The cause of Tourette's syndrome is unknown, and its pathophysiology remains obscure. Treatment with neuroleptic drugs will decrease the severity and frequency of tics in 75 to 90 percent of patients with Tourette's syndrome, regardless of disease severity. The noradrenergic agonist clonidine also has been reported to suppress symptoms.

EXAMINATION OF EXTRAPYRAMIDAL SYNDROMES   In broad terms, all the extrapyramidal disorders should be viewed in terms of primary deficit (negative symptoms) and of the new phenomena (abnormal postures and involuntary movements) that have appeared. The positive symptoms are ascribed to release from inhibition or disequilibrium of undamaged motor parts of the nervous system. The physician must cultivate the habit of accurately observing and describing abnormalities of movement and must not be content merely to give the condition a name or to force it into some superficial category. The fully developed extrapyramidal motor syndromes can be recognized without difficulty once the physician has become familiar with the typical pictures. A mental picture of Parkinson's disease, with its slowness of movement, poverty of facial expression, tremor at rest, and muscular rigidity, should be fixed in mind. Similarly, the gross distortions of posture found in dystonia, whether widespread in trunk muscles or involving only neck muscles as in spasmodic torticollis, should be easily recognized. Athetosis, with its instability of postures, ceaseless movements of finger and hands, and intention spasm; chorea, with its rapid and complicated movements; and myoclonus, with its abrupt movements that flit over the body, are other standard syndromes. There tends to be a mild defect in the voluntary use of the affected parts in all extrapyramidal syndromes.

Early or mild forms of these conditions, like all medical diseases, may offer special difficulties in diagnosis. Cases of Parkinson's disease seen before the appearance of tremor are often overlooked. Uncertainty of balance and short gait (*marche à petit pas*) in the elderly is often incorrectly attributed to loss of confidence and fear of falling. Patients may complain of being nervous and restless and describe a stiffness and aching in parts of the body. Because there is no weakness or change in reflexes, the disorder may then be considered rheumatic or even psychogenic. Parkinson's disease often begins in a hemiplegic distribution, and for this reason, the illness may be misdiagnosed as cerebral thrombosis or tumor. Facial immobility, a suggestion of a limp, mild rigidity, failure of an arm to swing naturally in walking, or loss of certain movements of cooperation will help in diagnosis at this time. Every patient presenting with atypical extrapyramidal symptoms should be surveyed for Wilson's disease in order to avoid missing a treatable illness. Mild or early chorea is often mistaken for simple nervousness. Observing the patient at rest as well as in action is critical to the diagnosis. There are instances, nonetheless, in which it is impossible to distinguish simple fidgets from early chorea, especially in children, and there are no laboratory tests to aid in the diagnosis. The first postural manifestations of dystonia may suggest hysteria, and it is only with repeated examinations that an accurate diagnosis is reached.

Motor disorders seldom appear in pure form, and extrapyramidal syndromes often coexist with lesions in the corticospinal tract or cerebellar systems. For example, syndromes such as progressive supranuclear palsy, olivopontocerebellar atrophy, and the Shy-Drager syndrome have many elements of Parkinson's disease but also have paralysis of voluntary eye movements, ataxia, apraxia, postural hypotension, or spasticity with bilateral Babinski's signs. Wilson's disease usually displays tremor at rest, rigidity, slowness of movement, and flexion dystonia of the trunk, but exceptionally there are athetosis, dystonia, and intention tremor. Emotional or cognitive abnormalities may be the presenting signs in Wilson's disease. Hallervorden-Spatz disease may take the form of universal rigidity and flexion dystonia, but choreoathetosis is sometimes observed. In some forms of Huntington's disease, particularly with juvenile onset, rigidity replaces choreoathetosis. Corticospinal and various extrapyramidal disorders may be associated in patients with cerebral diplegia. Some of the neurodegenerative diseases in which corticospinal tract and basal ganglia lesions coexist are described in Chap. 371.

REFERENCES

ALBIN RL et al: The functional anatomy of basal ganglia disorders. Trends Neurosci 12:366, 1989

ALEXANDER GE, CRUTCHER MD: Functional architecture of basal ganglia circuits: Neural substrates of parallel processing. Trends Neurosci 13:266, 1990

BERGMAN H et al: Renewal of experimental parkinsonism by lesions of the subthalamic nucleus. Science 249:1436, 1990

DUM RP, STRICK PL: Premotor areas: Nodal points for parallel efferent systems involved in the central control of movement, in *Motor Control: Concepts and Issues: Dahlem Konferenzen*, DR Humphrey, HJ Freund (eds). Chichester, Wiley, 1991, pp 383–411

FAHN S et al: Classification and investigation of dystonia, in *Movement Disorders 2*, CD Marsden, S Fahn (eds). London, Butterworths, 1987, pp 332–358

FREUND HJ, HEFTER H: The role of basal ganglia in rhythmic movement. Adv Neurol 60:88, 1993

GROWDON JH et al: L-Threonine in the treatment of spasticity. Clin Neuropharmacol 14:403, 1991

HALLET M: Classification and treatment of tremor. JAMA 266:1115, 1991

JAGIELLA WM, SUNG JH: Bilateral infarction of the medullary pyramids in humans. Neurology 39:21, 1989

JANKOVIC J, BRIN MF: Therapeutic uses of botulinum toxin. N Engl J Med 325:1186, 1991

JANKOVIC J, SCHWARTZ KS: Longitudinal experience with botulinum toxin injections for treatment of blepharospasm and cervical dystonia. Neurology 43:834, 1993

KUYPERS HGJM: Anatomy of the descending pathways, in *Handbook of Physiology*, sec 1: *The Nervous System*, vol 2: *Motor Control*, part 1, VB Brooks (ed). Bethesda, American Physiological Society, 1981, pp 597–666

OHYE C: Dynamic aspects of striatothalamic connection studies in cases with movement disorder. Adv Neurol 60:78, 1993

OZELIUS L et al: Human gene for torsion dystonia located on chromosome 9q32–q34. Neuron 2:1427, 1989

PAPAGNO C et al: Ideomotor apraxia without aphasia and aphasia without apraxia: The anatomical support for a double dissociation. J Neurol Neurosurg Psychiatry 56:286, 1993

PARENT A, HAZRATI LN: Anatomical aspects of information processing in primate basal ganglia. Trends Neurosci 16:111, 1993

POLO JM et al: Hereditary "pure" spastic paraplegia: A study of nine families. J Neurol Neurosurg Psychiatry 56:175, 1993

22   ATAXIA AND DISORDERS OF BALANCE AND GAIT

SID GILMAN

In the assessment of patients with neurologic disorders, it is important when taking the history to inquire about posture and gait and to examine these functions routinely as part of the neurologic examination. Abnormalities of posture and gait can result from disorders affecting several levels of the nervous system, and the type of abnormality observed clinically often indicates the site affected.

NEURAL STRUCTURES REQUIRED FOR STANDING AND WALKING   The structures in the central nervous system that control standing and walking are the basal ganglia, a "locomotor region" in the mesencephalon, the cerebellum, and the spinal cord. The cerebral cortex doubtless is important in many aspects of standing and walking, but in experimental animals, complete removal of the cerebral cortex during the neonatal period, preserving the basal ganglia, thalamus, and lower structures, leaves stance and locomotion essentially normal. In the adult animal, if the cerebral cortex, basal ganglia, and thalamus are removed, leaving the mesencephalon and lower brainstem intact, standing and walking are still possible. Electrical stimulation in a region of the mesencephalon termed the *locomotor region* evokes walking motions, and the speed and form of locomotion can be modified from a slow walk to a trot or gallop with changes in stimulation strength. This region receives projections from the basal ganglia, including the subthalamic and endopeduncular nuclei and the substantia nigra.

The spinal cord contains neural circuitry that coordinates the muscles for locomotion. After transection of the spinal cord in the midthoracic region in experimental animals, the hindlimbs maintain the capacity to perform coordinated walking movements when placed on a moving treadmill. With increased treadmill speed, walking movements can switch to simultaneous movements of the hindlimbs, as in a gallop. After a high spinal transection, both the forelimbs and the hindlimbs can generate alternating movements, and the sets of limbs remain coordinated. Thus neural circuitry in the spinal cord can coordinate movements among all four limbs. The cerebellum controls many of the movements required for walking. Ablation of the cerebellum in animals results in severe disorders of standing and walking.

In summary, walking is the result of integrated activity of the basal ganglia, mesencephalon, cerebellum, and spinal cord. Sensory inputs from movements of joints and muscle afferents provide important components for the control of walking. Without appropriate sensory feedback information, the pattern of walking is severely disrupted.

THE CEREBELLUM   The cerebellum functions in concert with the motor cortex, basal ganglia, and many brainstem structures in executing a variety of movements. The cerebellum is needed to maintain proper posture and balance for walking and running; to perform fine voluntary movements such as those needed for writing, dressing, and eating; to carry out rapidly alternating and repetitive movements such as in playing a musical instrument or working with a computer; and to coordinate smooth tracking movements of the eyes. The cerebellum controls certain properties of movements, including trajectory, velocity, and acceleration. Voluntary movements can be performed in the absence of cerebellar function, but the movements are clumsy and disorganized. The disturbances of movement from cerebellar dysfunction are termed *dyssynergia* (also *asynergia* or *ataxia*).

The cerebellum consists of a midline vermal region and two hemispheres, which are attached to the medulla, pons, and midbrain by three peduncles on each side. A layer of gray matter, the cerebellar cortex, covers the cerebellar surface and encloses an internal core of white matter. Three pairs of deep cerebellar nuclei are buried within the cerebellum. From medial to lateral these consist of the fastigial, interposed (globose and emboliform), and dentate nuclei.

The cerebellum consists of three lobes. The *flocculonodular lobe*, which is the oldest part of the cerebellum phylogenetically (archicerebellum), consists of the paired flocculi and the nodulus. This lobe receives input principally from the vestibular nuclei. The *anterior lobe*, the second oldest part (paleocerebellum), consists of vermal and paravermal structures in the anterosuperior portion of the cerebellum. The anterior lobe receives input chiefly from the spinal cord. The *posterior lobe* is the largest and phylogenetically newest part of the cerebellum (neocerebellum) and is located between the other two lobes. The posterior lobe receives projections from the cerebral hemispheres via the pontine nuclei.

The cerebellar cortex contains three layers: an outermost *molecular layer*, a middle *Purkinje cell layer*, and an inner *granular layer*. The afferent fibers reaching the cerebellar cortex send collateral projections to the deep cerebellar nuclei and terminate either in the granule cell layer as *mossy fibers* or on the dendrites of Purkinje cells as *climbing fibers*. Mossy fiber afferents are derived from the spinal cord, pontine nuclei, vestibular receptors and nuclei, trigeminal nuclei, reticular nuclei, and deep cerebellar nuclei. Climbing fiber afferents are derived exclusively from the inferior olive. Both mossy fiber and climbing fiber inputs are excitatory to the deep cerebellar nuclei and the cerebellar cortex. Purkinje cells provide the only route for all information exiting from the cerebellar cortex and are inhibitory to the deep cerebellar and vestibular nuclei.

Projections to the cerebellum also originate in the locus coeruleus and the raphe nuclei of the brainstem. The afferents to the cerebellum from the locus coeruleus are noradrenergic; those from the raphe nuclei are serotonergic; and both sets of afferents are inhibitory. Several amino acids have been identified as putative neurotransmitters in the cerebellum. These include glutamate, which is used by mossy fibers and the axons of granule cells (parallel fibers); aspartate, which is used by climbing fibers; and γ-aminobutyric acid, which is used by the axons of Purkinje cells, Golgi cells, and basket cells.

The *inferior cerebellar peduncle* (*restiform body*) consists chiefly of afferent fibers. The peduncle contains a single efferent tract, the fastigiobulbar tract, which projects from the fastigial nuclei to the vestibular nuclei and completes a vestibular circuit through the cerebellum. Afferent fibers enter the inferior cerebellar peduncle from at least six sources (Fig. 22-1): (1) fibers from the vestibular nerve and nuclei, (2) olivocerebellar fibers from the inferior olivary nuclei, (3) the dorsal spinocerebellar tract, (4) some of the fibers from the ventral spinocerebellar tract, (5) the cuneocerebellar tract from the accessory cuneate nuclei in the medulla, and (6) reticulocerebellar fibers. The *middle cerebellar peduncle* (*brachium pontis*) consists almost entirely of crossed afferent fibers from the pontine nuclei in the gray substance of the basal part of the pons (pontocerebellar or transverse pontine fibers) (Fig. 22-2). The major projections to the pontine nuclei originate within the cerebral cortex. The *superior cerebellar peduncle* (*brachium conjunctivum*) consists principally of efferent projections from the cerebellum. Fibers arising in the dentate and interposed nuclei project to the reticular formation, red nucleus, and thalamus. Some fibers of the fastigiobulbar tract also run with the superior peduncle for a short distance before entering the inferior cerebellar peduncle. The superior cerebellar peduncle contains afferent projections from the ventral spinocerebellar tract, a portion of the dorsal spinocerebellar tract, and trigeminocerebellar projections.

Except for direct projections of Purkinje cells onto vestibular nuclei, the efferent pathways of the cerebellum begin with the deep nuclei. The fastigial nucleus sends fibers to the reticular and vestibular nuclei of the brainstem. These nuclei project into the spinal cord and are concerned with posture and balance. The interposed nuclei of each side of the cerebellum project axons through the superior cerebellar peduncle to the red nucleus of the contralateral side. The red nucleus sends fibers into the rubrospinal tract (see Fig. 22-2), and this tract crosses the midline before descending into the spinal cord. The origin of this pathway in the interposed nuclei and the terminal

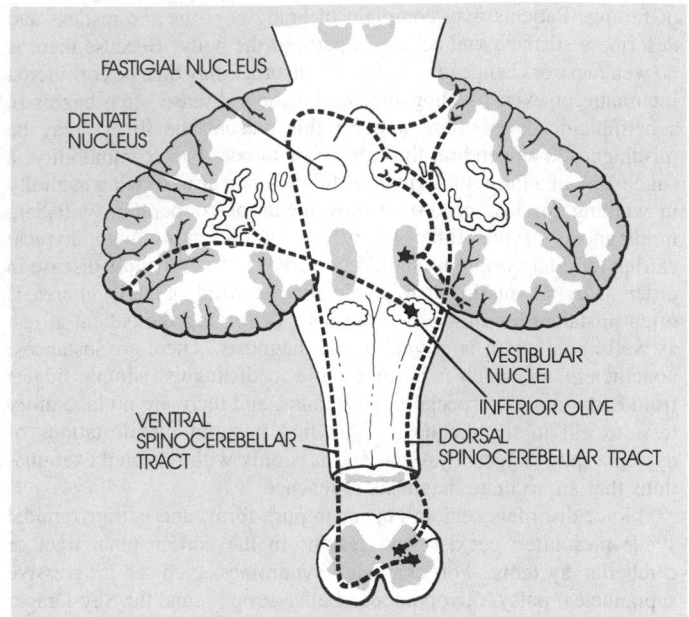

FIGURE 22-1 The central nervous system connections of the dorsal and ventral spinocerebellar tracts, the fastigial nuclei, and the vestibular nuclei. (*Adapted from S Gilman and S Winans Newman, Manter & Gatz's Essentials of Clinical Neuroanatomy and Neurophysiology, 8th ed, Philadelphia, Davis, 1992.*)

portion in the spinal cord are on the same side of the body. Both the dentate and the interposed nuclei send fibers through the superior cerebellar peduncle to the contralateral ventrolateral nucleus of the thalamus. The ventrolateral nucleus relays fibers to the motor regions of the ipsilateral frontal lobe. The thalamic endings in the cerebral cortex make connection with corticospinal neurons whose efferent fibers pass through the pyramidal tract and cross to the contralateral side of the spinal cord. Thus the origin of the cerebellothalamocortical

FIGURE 22-2 The central nervous system connections of the dentate nucleus and interposed (emboliform and globose) nuclei. (*Adapted from S Gilman and S Winans Newman, Manter & Gatz's Essentials of Clinical Neuroanatomy and Neurophysiology, 8th ed, Philadelphia, Davis, 1992.*)

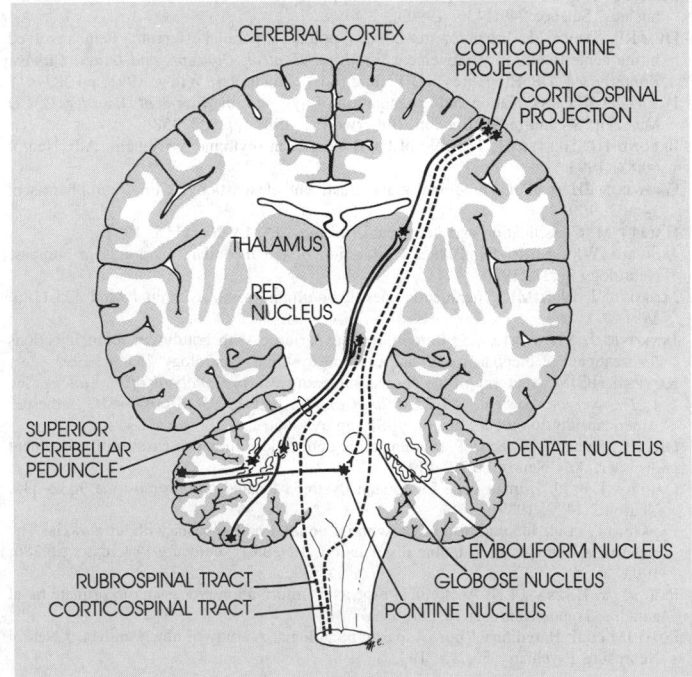

pathway in the dentate and interposed nuclei and its termination in the spinal cord are on the same side of the body (see Fig. 22-2).

For clinical purposes, a useful method of describing the cerebellum is based on the existence of longitudinal sagittal zones. Each half of the cerebellum is subdivided into three longitudinal strips arranged from medial to lateral, including the cerebellar cortex, underlying white matter, and deep cerebellar nuclei: (1) a midline zone consisting of the vermal region with the fastigial nucleus, (2) an intermediate zone, the paravermal region, with the interposed nuclei, and (3) a lateral zone consisting of the cerebellar hemisphere with the dentate nucleus. Lesions of the midline zone cause disorders of stance and gait, truncal ataxia and titubation, and rotated or tilted postures of the head. Lesions of the lateral zone lead to disturbances in coordinated limb movement (ataxia), dysarthria, hypotonia, nystagmus, and kinetic tremor. Lesions of the intermediate zone cause symptoms characteristic of involvement of both the midline and lateral zones.

Ataxia is the result of dysmetria and decomposition of movement. *Dysmetria* is a disturbance of the trajectory or placement of a limb during active movement in which the limb falls short of its target (*hypometria*) or extends beyond its target (*hypermetria*). *Decomposition of movement* refers to errors in the sequence and speed of the component parts of a movement. The result is a lack of speed and skill in acts requiring the smoothly coordinated activity of several muscles. Movements previously fluid and accurate become halting and imprecise. *Ataxia* appears clinically as a disturbance in the rate and extent of an individual movement and commonly occurs from lesions of the cerebellum or of the sensory systems. Ataxia of gait consists of irregularities in the rate, length, and consistency of walking movements, with veering to one side or the other.

PHYSIOLOGIC RESPONSES IMPORTANT IN STANDING AND WALKING Maintenance of the upright posture results from the actions of a number of postural reflex responses: (1) local static reactions acting on individual limbs, (2) segmental static reactions linking the extremities together, and (3) general static reactions resulting from the position of the head in space. *Local static reactions* include the stretch reflex and the positive supporting reaction. The simplest *stretch reflex* is illustrated by the muscle stretch response (deep tendon reflex), a brief muscle twitch evoked by rapid stretch of the muscle's tendon. Maintenance of muscle extension results in sustained contraction of that muscle through the stretch reflex. The *positive supporting reaction*, as elucidated in animal studies, results from a light cutaneous contact of the skin of the foot and also by proprioceptive stimulation owing to stretch of the interosseous muscles. The result of these stimuli is an extensor thrust by the limb.

The *segmental static reactions* include the crossed extension reflex and interlimb coordination. In the crossed extension reflex, application of noxious stimulation to an extremity results in flexion of that limb and simultaneous extension of the contralateral limb. With stronger stimulation, the crossed extension reflex triggered from a hindlimb can induce flexion in the contralateral forelimb and extension in the ipsilateral forelimb. Thus the whole body moves along a diagonal path through the extended contralateral hindlimb and ipsilateral forelimb, thereby removing the stimulated limb from the source of noxious stimulation. This diagonal pattern of interlimb coordination also provides postural adjustments in various situations.

The *general static reactions* consist of two general types. The first, the *tonic neck* and *labyrinthine reflexes*, function together to adjust body posture when the head moves relative to the trunk in space. The second, the *righting reflex*, is triggered by vestibular, neck proprioceptive, and visual stimuli and helps the animal to regain an upright position after a fall. The *grasp reflex* is a component of the righting reflex. Other forms of general static reactions include the placing and hopping reactions, as well as adjustment of body postures during limb movements.

CLINICAL APPROACH TO DISORDERS OF EQUILIBRIUM AND GAIT When evaluating a disorder of gait, the physician should inquire whether the disturbance occurs more in the dark than in the light; whether vertigo, giddiness, or lightheadedness accompanies the

disorder; and whether there is pain, numbness, or tingling of the limbs. Inquiry should search for weakness, bowel and bladder dysfunction, and limb stiffness or rigidity. The physician should ask whether there is difficulty in the initiation or termination of walking and whether walking up or down stairs or on uneven surfaces worsens the disturbance in walking.

Examination of stance and gait is performed best in a setting in which the physician can observe the patient walk from the front, back, and sides. The patient should rise quickly from a chair, walk normally at a slow pace, then more rapidly, and then turn around. The patient should walk on the heels, on the toes, and in tandem, placing the heel of one foot directly in front of the toes of the opposite foot, attempting to progress in a straight line. The patient should stand erect with the feet together and the head straight, first with the eyes open and then with the eyes closed to determine whether balance can be maintained (Romberg's sign). It is often helpful to observe the gait initially as the patient comes into the examining room when the patient is unaware that gait and stance are being examined.

With normal walking the body should be held erect, the head should be straight, and the arms should hang loosely at the sides, each moving in rhythm with movement of the opposite leg. The shoulders and hips should be level, and the arms should swing equally. The steps should be straight and equal in length. The head should not be tilted, and there should be no appreciable scoliosis or lordosis. With each step the hip and knee should flex smoothly, the ankle should dorsiflex, and the foot should clear the ground easily. The heel should strike the ground first, and the weight of the body should be transferred successively onto the sole of the foot and then onto the toes. The head and body should rotate slightly with each step without lurching or falling movements. Each person walks in a characteristic fashion that is often familial. Some people walk with the toes turned inward, others with the toes turned outward. Some people stride with large steps, and others shuffle, making small steps. A person's gait is often a reflection of personality traits and can reflect shyness and timidity or aggressiveness and self-confidence.

Hemiparesis The patient with weakness of the limbs on one side of the body from a lesion of the corticospinal tract usually develops a characteristic gait disorder. The severity of the disorder depends on the degree of weakness and stiffness of the affected limbs. The severely hemiparetic subject will stand and walk with the affected arm adducted at the shoulder and flexed at the elbow, wrist, and fingers and the affected leg stiffly extended at the hip, knee, and ankle. There is difficulty in flexing the hip and knee and dorsiflexing the ankle. Thus the paretic leg swings outward at the hip so that the foot does not scrape the floor. The leg is held stiffly and rotates in a semicircle, first away from and then toward the trunk in a circumduction movement. Often the upper body tilts slightly to the opposite side during the leg movement. The arm on the hemiparetic side usually swings little during walking. The loss of arm swing can be an early sign of a progressive hemiparesis. A person with a mild hemiparesis may show a gait disorder similar to that of the severely hemiparetic individual, but with a lesser degree of abnormality. In this case, a decrease in arm swing may be associated with subtle circumduction of the leg, without clear stiffness or weakness of the affected limbs.

Paraparesis Diseases of the spinal cord that affect the function of both legs produce a characteristic gait resulting from a combination of spasticity and weakness of the lower extremities. Walking requires considerable effort and consists of slow, stiff movements at the hips and knees. The legs are usually maintained extended or slightly flexed at the hips and knees and adducted at the hips. In some people with paraparesis the legs may cross with each step, producing a scissoring motion. The steps usually are regular and short, and the patient may move the trunk from side to side, attempting to compensate for the stiff movements of the legs. The legs circumduct at the hips, and the feet scrape along the floor so that the soles of the shoes become worn at the toes.

Parkinsonism Parkinson's disease produces a characteristic posture and gait. The severely affected individual stands in a posture of flexion, with the thoracic spine bent forward, the head bent downward, the arms moderately flexed at the elbows, and the legs slightly flexed at the hips and knees. The patient sits or stands with striking immobility, showing a fixed facial expression with infrequent blinking and making few automatic movements of the limbs. The patient seldom crosses the legs or adjusts body posture when seated in a chair. Although the arms are held immobile, often a tremor involves the fingers and wrists at four to five cycles per second. In some people the tremor also occurs at the elbows and even at the shoulders. In advanced cases there may be drooling and a rhythmic tremor of the jaw. The patient usually gets up slowly to walk, and with walking, the trunk bends even farther forward and the arms remain immobile at the sides of the body or become further flexed and are carried a bit ahead of the body. The arms fail to swing. As forward progression begins, the legs remain bent at the hips, knees, and ankles. Characteristically, the steps are short so that the feet barely clear the ground and the soles of the feet shuffle and scrape the floor. With forward locomotion the steps become successively more rapid, and the patient may fall unless assisted (*festination*). If the patient is pushed forward or backward, compensatory flexion or extension movements of the trunk fail to occur, and the patient is forced to make a series of propulsive or retropulsive steps.

Patients with Parkinson's disease often have great difficulty in rising from a chair or walking after standing still. The individual may initiate walking with several small steps before taking longer strides. Walking may stop involuntarily with attempts to pass through a doorway or into an elevator. Parkinsonian patients at times can walk with surprising speed and dexterity for brief intervals. In times of acute emergency, as in a fire, a person previously immobile can walk rapidly or even run briefly.

Cerebellar disease Disease of the cerebellum causes difficulty in standing without support and in walking. The disorder may result from lesions intrinsic to the cerebellum or from lesions in the connecting pathways to and from the cerebellum. The difficulty is worsened by attempts to walk with a narrow base. The affected person usually stands with the legs apart, and standing may provoke *titubation*, a coarse forward and backward tremor of the trunk. Attempting to stand with the feet together provokes swaying or falling. The instability is the same whether the eyes are open or closed. The patient walks cautiously, taking steps of varying lengths, and lurches from side to side. The patient complains of difficulty with balance, is fearful of walking without support, and may insist on holding onto objects such as a bed or chair, moving cautiously between these objects. Frequently the individual does not need to be supported; simply touching a wall or an object in the room makes it possible to walk with a greater sense of security. When a mild gait disorder is present, walking may deteriorate with attempts to walk in tandem in a straight line. This causes the patient to lose balance and, in response, to place one foot to the side to avoid falling. With unilateral lesions of the cerebellum, balance is lost toward the side of the lesion.

When disease is restricted to the midline (vermal) portions of the cerebellum, as occurs in alcoholic cerebellar degeneration, disorders of stance and gait may develop without other signs of cerebellar dysfunction such as limb ataxia or nystagmus. In contrast, disease of the cerebellar hemispheres, either unilaterally or bilaterally, often causes marked limb ataxia and nystagmus in association with a gait disorder. With a lesion confined to one cerebellar hemisphere, ipsilateral disturbances of posture and movement commonly accompany the gait disorder. The patient usually stands with the shoulder on the side of the lesion lower than the other, and there may be an accompanying scoliosis. The limbs on the side of the cerebellar lesion show diminished resistance to passive manipulation (hypotonia). On walking the patient staggers and deviates toward the affected side. This can be demonstrated by asking the patient to walk around a chair. Rotation toward the affected side results in a fall into the chair,

and rotation toward the normal side causes movement away from the chair in a spiral. The affected arm and leg show marked ataxia in tests of coordinated movement such as successively touching the patient's nose and then the examiner's finger (the "finger-nose-finger test") or running the heel of the affected leg down the shin of the opposite leg (the "heel-knee-shin test").

Sensory ataxia A characteristic gait disorder results from loss of sensation in the lower extremities due to disease processes in the peripheral nerves, dorsal roots, dorsal columns of the spinal cord, or medial lemnisci. The most disabling component of the sensory disorder is the loss of joint position sense, but loss of input from muscle spindle receptors, vibration detectors, and cutaneous receptors also contributes to the disability. People with sensory ataxia are unaware of the position of the lower extremities and consequently have difficulty in both standing and walking. The patient usually stands with the legs spread widely apart. The patient remains stable if asked to stand with the feet together and the eyes open but sways and often falls (positive Romberg's sign) when the eyes are closed. The test for Romberg's sign cannot be performed if the subject is unsteady when standing with the feet together and the eyes open, as may occur with cerebellar disease.

The patient with sensory ataxia walks with the legs spread widely apart, watching the ground carefully. The legs are lifted higher than necessary at the hips and are flung forward and outward in abrupt motions. The steps vary in length, and the feet make characteristic slapping sounds as they contact the floor. The patient usually holds the body somewhat flexed at the hips, often using a cane for support. If vision is impaired or the patient attempts to walk in the dark, the gait disturbance worsens. The patient becomes unsteady and often falls when attempting to wash the face because of the temporary loss of visual compensation occurring with closure of the eyes.

Cerebral palsy This term encompasses a number of different motor abnormalities, most of them resulting from hypoxic-ischemic injury to the central nervous system in the perinatal period. The severity of the gait disturbance varies with the nature and extent of the lesion. Mild limited lesions can lead to increased deep tendon reflexes and extensor plantar responses with a slight degree of talipes equinovarus, without a clear gait disorder. More severe and extensive lesions commonly lead to bilateral hemiparesis. The patient stands and walks with a paraparetic posture and gait. The arms are adducted at the shoulders and flexed at the elbows and wrists.

Movement disorders commonly alter the gait in people with cerebral palsy. Athetosis occurs frequently and consists of slow or moderately rapid serpentine movements of the arms and legs, with postures alternating between the extremes of flexion with supination and extension with pronation. On walking, people with athetotic cerebral palsy show involuntary limb movements that are accompanied by rotary movements of the neck and frequent facial grimacing. The arms are usually flexed and the legs are extended, but asymmetric limb postures can occur with ambulation. For example, one arm may flex and supinate, and the other may extend and pronate. Asymmetric limb postures commonly occur as the head rotates from side to side. Usually when the chin turns to one side, the arm on that side extends and the opposite arm flexes.

Chorea Individuals with choreic movements often develop a characteristic gait disorder. Chorea occurs most frequently in children with Sydenham's chorea, in adults with Huntington's disease, and occasionally in adults with Parkinson's disease treated with excessive amounts of dopamine agonist medications. Choreic movements consist of intermittent rapid movements of the face, trunk, neck, and limbs. Flexion, extension, and rotary movements of the neck occur along with grimacing movements of the face, twisting movements of the trunk and limbs, and rapid piano-playing movements of the digits. Frequently, in early chorea, flexion and extension movements of the hips occur so that the individual constantly seems to be crossing and uncrossing the legs. The patient may scowl, frown, and smile involuntarily. Walking usually accentuates the choreic movements. Sudden forward or sideward thrusting movements of the pelvis and rapid twisting movements of the trunk and limbs result in a gait that resembles a series of dance steps. The steps are usually irregular in size, and the patient has difficulty walking in a straight line. The rate of progression varies from slow to rapid owing to variability in the rate and amplitude of each step.

Dystonia   This is an involuntary postural and movement disorder affecting children (dystonia musculorum deformans or torsion dystonia) and adults (dystonia of adult onset). The condition may occur sporadically without known cause, as a genetic disorder, or as part of another process such as Wilson's disease. In dystonia musculorum deformans, which commonly begins in childhood, the first symptom often consists of an abnormal gait. Characteristically, the patient will walk with one foot inverted at the ankle, placing weight on the lateral side of the foot; as the disease progresses, this problem worsens, and other postural abnormalities develop. These include elevation of one shoulder, elevation of a hip, twisted postures of the trunk, and excessive flexion of the wrist and fingers of one upper limb. Intermittent spasms of the trunk and limbs may interfere with walking. Eventually, torticollis, tortipelvis, lordosis, and scoliosis may supervene. In extreme cases, the patient becomes unable to walk. Adult-onset dystonia often results in a similar progression of movement disorders.

Muscular dystrophy   Marked weakness of the muscles of the trunk and proximal portions of the legs causes a characteristic stance and gait. In attempting to rise from a seated position, the affected person bends forward, flexing the trunk at the hips, places the hands on the knees, and pushes the trunk upward by working the hands up the thighs. Standing occurs with exaggerated lumbar lordosis and a protuberant abdomen owing to weakness of the abdominal and paravertebral muscles. The patient walks with the legs spread widely apart and develops a waddling motion of the pelvis because of weakness of the gluteal muscles. The shoulders often slope forward, and winging of the scapulae may be seen with walking.

Frontal lobe disease   Bilateral frontal lobe disease causes a characteristic gait disorder that is usually associated with dementia and frontal lobe release signs, including grasp, suck, and snout reflexes. The patient characteristically stands with the feet spread widely apart and takes a first step only after a long delay. This hesitancy is followed by very small shuffling steps and then by a few steps of moderate amplitude, after which time the patient freezes, unable to continue walking. The cycle then is repeated. Affected individuals usually do not show muscular weakness, abnormalities of the deep tendon reflexes, sensory changes, or extensor plantar reflex responses. Usually the patient can perform the individual limb movements required for walking if asked to mimic walking movements while lying supine. The gait disorder with frontal lobe disease is a form of apraxia, i.e., a disturbance in the performance of a motor function in the absence of weakness of the muscles required for the function.

Normal-pressure hydrocephalus   Normal-pressure hydrocephalus (NPH) is a disorder characterized by dementia, gait apraxia, and urinary incontinence. Computed tomography reveals large cerebral ventricles, widening of the callosal angle, and lack of filling with cerebrospinal fluid of the subarachnoid space over the cerebral hemispheres. Injection of radioactive isotope into the lumbar subarachnoid space demonstrates pathologic reflux of the isotope into the ventricular system and inadequate penetration into the cortical subarachnoid spaces.

The gait in NPH resembles that seen in apraxia from frontal lobe disease, consisting of a series of small, shuffling steps, making it appear that the feet are glued to the floor. Initiation of walking is impaired, and slow and small angular displacements of the hip, knee, and ankle joints occur along with low clearance of the foot from the floor so that the patient appears to be sliding the feet along the floor. There is continuous contraction of the antigravity muscles of the legs but low muscle activity in the calf muscles. The gait disorder in NPH is thought to result from impaired function of the frontal lobes. In about half the patients with NPH the gait is improved by surgical shunting of cerebrospinal fluid from the cerebral ventricles into the venous system.

Aging   Changes in gait and difficulties with balance occur with aging. Elderly men develop forward flexion of the upper portion of the trunk with flexion of the arms and knees, decreased arm swing, and shortening of step length. Elderly women develop a waddling gait with shortening of step length. Abnormalities of gait and balance predispose the elderly to falls. About half the falls in the aged result from environmental factors, including poor illumination, stairs, and uneven or slippery surfaces. Other causes of falls include drop attacks, orthostatic hypotension, turning movements of the head, and vertigo.

Lower motor neuron disorders   Diseases of the lower motor neurons or peripheral nerves characteristically cause distal limb weakness. Foot drop is a common manifestation. In the case of lower motor neuron disease, the limb weakness occurs in association with fasciculations and muscle atrophy. The patient usually cannot dorsiflex the foot and compensates by raising the knees higher than usual, thereby walking with a "steppage gait." If proximal muscles are affected, the gait also can take on a waddling quality.

Hysterical gait disorders   Hysterical disorders of gait commonly appear in association with hysterical paralysis of one or more limbs. Usually the gait is bizarre, easily recognized as hysterical, and unlike any disorder of gait evoked by organic disease. In other instances, however, hysterical gait disorders may resemble organic gait disorders and can be difficult to identify. Hysterical gait disorders can occur in men or women and can appear in youth, young adulthood, and middle age.

In hysterical hemiplegia, the patient drags the affected leg along the ground behind the body and does not circumduct the leg or use it effectively to support the body weight. At times the hemiplegic leg may be pushed ahead of the patient and used mainly for support. The arm on the affected side often remains limp, hanging uselessly beside the body, and does not develop the flexed posture commonly seen in hemiplegia from organic causes. The patient with hysterical hemiplegia usually shows "give way" weakness. This is tested by asking the patient to make a maximum contraction of a set of muscles in an affected limb. Initially, a strong contraction may occur, but as the examiner attempts to oppose the contracting muscles, the contraction suddenly gives way. Hysterical patients also commonly contract their muscles very slowly upon request, displaying great concentration and effort to evoke the contraction. Objective signs of neurologic disease are absent; the affected limbs show normal resistance to passive manipulation, the deep tendon reflexes are equal on the two sides of the body, and the plantar responses are downgoing.

In hysterical paraplegia, the patient usually walks with one or two crutches or lies in bed with the legs maintained either completely limp or stiffly extended. The term *astasia-abasia* refers to patients who cannot stand or walk but who can carry out natural movements of the limbs when lying in bed. Some patients with hysterical paraparesis walk with seeming difficulty but show normal power and coordination when lying in bed. On walking, the hysterical person clings to the bed or the furnishings of the room. If asked to walk without support, the patient may lurch forward dramatically, veering from side to side at regular intervals. The patient can manage feats of extraordinary balance to avoid falling and may assume a variety of postures, walking with the legs in stiff extension, as if the legs are granite pillars, or walking with the legs in flexion and teetering from side to side. The hysterical patient may fall with walking, but only when a nearby physician or family member can catch the patient or when soft objects are available to cushion the fall. The gait disturbance is usually dramatic when an audience is present, and the patient can display remarkable agility in the rapid postural adjustments that occur.

REFERENCES

COLES SK et al: The mesencephalic centre controlling locomotion in the rat. Neuroscience 28:149, 1989

GILMAN S: Cerebellar deficit, in *Diseases of the Nervous System*, vol. 1: *Clinical Neurobiology*, 2d ed, AK Asbury et al (eds). Philadelphia, Saunders, 1992

——— et al: *Disorders of the Cerebellum*. Philadelphia, Davis, 1981

HORE J et al: Cerebellar dysmetria at the elbow, wrist, and fingers. J Neurophysiol 65:563, 1991

ITO M: Structural-functional relationships in cerebellar and vestibular systems. Arch Ital Biol 129:53, 1991

LEMPERT T et al: How to identify psychogenic disorders of stance and gait. J Neurol 238:140, 1991

MAZZIOTTA J, GILMAN S (eds): *Clinical Brain Imaging: Principles and Applications*. Philadelphia, Davis, 1992

ROSS CA et al: Messenger molecules in the cerebellum. Trends Neurosci 13:216, 1990

SANES JN et al: Motor learning in patients with cerebellar dysfunction. Brain 113:103, 1990

23 MUSCLE SPASMS, CRAMPS, AND EPISODIC WEAKNESS

ROBERT C. GRIGGS

Spontaneous or exercise-related discomfort from muscles or joints is usually benign and does not signal neuromuscular disease. Such symptoms may, however, provide clues to disabling disorders that too often evade diagnosis. The terms *pain*, *spasm*, and *cramp* are often used interchangeably by patients to describe symptoms referable to muscles. Other terms, including *aching*, *heaviness*, *stiffness*, and *rheumatism*, are also used and usually connote less certainty about the source or localization of the discomfort. In clinical terminology, *spasm* refers to a brief, unsustained contraction of a single or multiple muscles. *Cramp* is a paroxysmal, spontaneous, prolonged, and painful contraction of one or more muscles. Muscle pain may be associated with fatigue (asthenia) or weakness. This chapter discusses both fatigue and episodic weakness. The usual causes of weakness are considered in Chaps. 21 and 22.

SPASMS　Abnormal movements of muscle may arise from abnormal electrical activity of the central nervous system (CNS) mediated via the motor neuron or occur within the motor neuron or muscle fiber itself. It may be difficult on clinical grounds alone to determine the precise site of origin of the abnormal motor activity. In general, movements originating in the CNS affect the entire side of the body, an entire limb, or a group of muscles. Central disorders may be rhythmic or intermittent; those arising in the periphery are usually random. The electroencephalogram (EEG) may provide evidence for altered cortical activity in some conditions with a CNS etiology. The electromyogram (EMG) is less helpful because it reflects motor activity from any cause. EMG evidence of an underlying nerve or muscle disease may, however, be helpful in diagnosis (see Chaps. 366 and 382).

Intermittent, nonrhythmic movements of an entire limb, of the trunk, or of a portion of the face may result from cerebral seizure activity (Chap. 366) or from myoclonus (Chap. 21). Flexor and extensor spasms of an entire side or of the lower limbs result from a loss of motor inhibition within the CNS (Chap. 21). *Segmental myoclonus* results from focal disease within the brainstem or spinal cord that causes an abnormal discharge of groups of motor neurons. Localized vascular disease, tumor, or another lesion may be implicated.

Abnormal facial movements　*Hemifacial spasm* results from paroxysmal facial nerve activity, sometimes triggered by pressure from a tortuous blood vessel adjacent to the facial nerve as it leaves the brainstem. Hemifacial spasm commonly occurs in muscles about the eye but also may involve or spread to the entire side of the face. Symptoms are often intermittent and intensified when patients are using facial muscles in activities such as speaking. Hemifacial spasm is painless but embarrassing, especially to individuals dealing with the public. Since it is often intensified and more severe when the patient is in stressful situations, an erroneous diagnosis of tic (habit spasm) is often made. Cerebellopontine angle lesions can occasionally produce a similar disorder. Neuroradiologic investigation is indicated in patients with hemifacial spasm. Injection of botulinum toxin into involved muscles alleviated spasm for up to 3 months; surgical exploration and shielding of the facial nerve from the adjacent vessel is often curative (Chap. 380).

Facial *tics* (habit spasms) are stereotyped movements of the face such as eye blinking, head turning, or grimacing that are under voluntary control but may be suppressed only by effort and anxiety on the part of the subject (see Chap. 21). Some tics are so frequently encountered as to be considered mannerisms, analogous to excessive clearing of the throat. The repetitious elevation of the eyebrows by frontalis muscle contraction is an example. Certain hereditary movement disorders such as Gilles de la Tourette syndrome are characterized by multiple tics. Tics usually can be controlled by neuroleptic agents (Chap. 21).

Synkinesias of the face result from aberrant regeneration of the facial nerve following facial paralysis from Bell's palsy or other facial nerve lesions. Nearly 50 percent of patients who recover from Bell's palsy display such movements; an example is *jaw winking*, where voluntary movements of the lower face elicit contraction of the orbicularis oculi muscle with eye closure (see Chap. 380).

Trigeminal neuralgia (tic douloureux) is characterized by brief, paroxysmal, lancinating pain in one side of the face (see Chap. 380). Although the portion of the nerve involved is almost exclusively sensory, the severity of the pain causes involuntary contraction of facial muscles; hence the name *tic*. Abnormal movements do not occur in the absence of pain.

Facial myokymia refers to a nearly continuous, fine or coarse rippling and fascicular twitching of facial muscles. Although often benign, it may result from lesions of the pons such as a neoplasm or multiple sclerosis. Similar movements occur in motor neuron diseases such as amyotrophic lateral sclerosis or occasionally as an isolated, hereditary condition.

Abnormal limb movements　No movement should be visible in totally relaxed muscles. Diseases of motor neurons or their proximal axons are often associated with *fasciculations*, the spontaneous firing of an entire motor unit. Fasciculations are visible on inspection of muscle or perceived by the patient as a pulsation or quivering within muscle. Fasciculations occur at times in most normal individuals, and unless weakness is present, they are seldom of any significance. Fasciculations are normal if observed in incompletely relaxed muscles. *Myokymia*, consisting of numerous, repetitive fasciculations, also may occur in limb muscles, giving a writhing appearance. Myokymia disappears with neuromuscular blockade, proving that the activity originates in anterior horn cells or in peripheral nerve. In patients with long-standing muscle denervation and reinnervation, motor unit size enlarges and fasciculations may be so large as to produce movement of the limbs, particularly of the fingers, a condition termed *minipolymyoclonus*.

Certain conditions are characterized by a compulsion to move the extremities. *Akathisia*, or motor restlessness, occurs in Parkinson's disease and other disorders of the basal ganglia, including drug-induced movement disorders. The *restless legs syndrome* describes an uncomfortable sensation in muscles, usually in the legs and thighs, which occurs most commonly in middle-aged women. Patients feel they need to move their legs to relieve the abnormal sensation. The restless leg syndrome is frequent in uremia and may occur in other neuropathies, suggesting that the sensation is caused by an underlying neuropathy. It also may be familial, and detailed study of such patients has failed to demonstrate any evidence of neuropathy. The restless sensation may be accompanied by myoclonic jerks of muscle. These myoclonic jerks are similar to the myoclonus observed in normal individuals entering REM sleep (see Chap. 29).

These forms of muscle spasm and myoclonus are somewhat similar to a group of unusual *startle* syndromes or *hyperexplexias* characterized by sudden jerking of limbs or occasionally of trunk muscles. Sudden noise or touch may cause a patient to jump or to fling an extremity. Hyperexplexias may result from an abnormality of gamma-aminobutyric acid (GABA) receptors.

SUSTAINED MUSCLE CONTRACTIONS Distinguishing central from peripheral causes of sustained muscle contraction is often difficult. Abnormal muscle contractions with increased muscle tone usually result from CNS disease. Thus loss or disturbance of CNS inhibition may lead to abnormal muscle contraction characteristic of spasticity, rigidity, or "paratonic" rigidity. In most instances there is other evidence of CNS disorder (Chap. 21). Diseases of the basal ganglia, presumably resulting from altered neurotransmitter release, may lead to dystonia (see Chaps. 21 and 22).

Abnormal muscle contractions also may arise from repetitive depolarization of the component portions of the motor unit: the motor neuron, the peripheral axon of the neuron, the neuromuscular junction, or muscle fibers. Electrically inactive contractions may arise from disorders of the muscle contractile system.

Motor neuron disorders *Cramp* is a term often used by patients to refer to a painful, involuntary contraction of a single muscle or a muscle group. Muscle cramps can arise from spontaneous firing of groups of anterior horn cells followed by contraction of many motor units. EMG recordings indicate that motor units fire at a rate of up to 300 per second, much higher than occurs with voluntary contraction. Cramps occur frequently in the legs in elderly patients and, when severe, are followed by residual tenderness and evidence of muscle fiber necrosis, including elevation of serum creatine kinase. Cramps in the calf muscles are so common as to be considered normal, but more generalized cramps may be a sign of chronic disease of the motor neuron, such as amyotrophic lateral sclerosis. They may be particularly troublesome during pregnancy, in patients with electrolyte disturbances (hyponatremia), and in patients on hemodialysis. When recurrent and localized to one muscle group, they suggest nerve root disease. In many instances, however, it is impossible to determine the cause of cramps. Benign cramps, occurring commonly at night, may be relieved by quinine sulfate. Other causes of contractions arising from the motor neuron include *tetanus* (Chap. 106) and the *stiff-man syndrome*. In both disorders, a loss of inhibitory neuronal input to anterior horn cells may result in repeated firing of motor neurons, producing severe, painful muscle contraction. Antibodies to glutamic acid decarboxylase are present in the stiff-man syndrome, and the disorder may respond to plasma exchange. A similar clinical picture may occur acutely with *strychnine poisoning*. Diazepam improves these spasms but may cause respiratory depression in doses sufficient to alleviate muscle contraction.

Peripheral nerve *Tetany* is characterized by contractions of predominantly distal muscles, particularly in the hand (carpal spasm) and feet (pedal spasm). Laryngospasm also may occur. Tetany results from increased excitability of peripheral nerves. The muscle contractions are initially painless, but if sustained, they may cause muscle damage with pain. Severe tetany may involve spine musculature to produce opisthotonus. Tetany is usually caused by hypocalcemia, but it may occur with hypomagnesemia or severe respiratory alkalosis (see Chap. 357). Idiopathic normocalcemic tetany, *spasmophilia*, occurs in both hereditary and acquired forms. The acquired disorder is similar to Isaac's syndrome (neuromyotonia), in which hyperexcitability of peripheral nerve leads to muscle cramps and twitching. Such patients have responded to plasma exchange and it may be mediated by IgG autoantibodies to nerve membrane ion channels.

Muscle MYOTONIA Repetitive depolarization of muscle cells can cause muscle contraction resulting in muscle stiffness and impaired relaxation. Myotonia is usually painless, but it may disable patients by interfering with fine hand movements or by slowing ambulation. Myotonic dystrophy is the most common disorder associated with myotonia, although other manifestations of the disease such as cataracts and muscle weakness are usually more symptomatic (see Chap. 385). Myotonia congenita and paramyotonia congenita are less

common but more troublesome in terms of severity of myotonia. Myotonia is often worsened by cold and characteristically is attenuated by repeated muscle activity. *Myotonia congenita* has both autosomal dominant and recessive variants; myotonia results from defects in chloride channel function. *Paradoxical myotonia* worsens with repeated activity and is characteristic of paramyotonia congenita; these patients also suffer from episodic and cold-induced weakness (see Chap. 387). Myotonia can often be alleviated by quinine, phenytoin, or mexilitine. Impaired muscle relaxation that is electrically inactive is characteristic of the delayed relaxation of myxedema. This delay produces the characteristic "hung-up" ankle reflexes but is essentially asymptomatic.

CONTRACTURE Muscle contracture is a painful shortening of a muscle unassociated with muscle membrane depolarization. It occurs in disorders where a metabolic defect such as myophosphorylase deficiency limits the production of high-energy phosphates. Contractures are precipitated by exercise, are usually intensely painful, and result in muscle damage; widespread muscle contractures may cause sufficient myoglobinuria to precipitate renal failure. This use of the term *contracture* is confusing because the same word is used to describe the unrelated limitation of joint movement by shortening of muscle tendons seen in rheumatologic disorders, cerebral palsy, or chronic myopathies. Muscle rigidity from metabolic contracture can occur in the malignant hyperthermia syndrome, usually associated with general anesthesia (see Chap. 398). In the neuroleptic malignant syndrome, muscle rigidity arises from CNS overactivity, and intense electrical activity is present in muscle (see Chap. 398).

MUSCLE PAIN, ACHING, AND TENDERNESS Painful muscles do not always imply muscle disease. Joint and bone disease frequently produces complaints of muscle pain and may further confuse the anatomic localization of symptoms by resulting in disuse atrophy and moderate muscle weakness. Pain from disease of overlying subcutaneous tissue or fascia and of tendons also may be referred to muscle. Additionally, disease of major peripheral nerves or of their small intramuscular branches may produce both muscle pain and weakness. Muscle pain may be a major symptom in inflammatory, metabolic, endocrine, and toxic myopathies (see Chaps. 384 and 385).

Muscle trauma Vigorous activity, even in conditioned athletes, may be associated with muscle and tendon tears which lead to temporary acute muscle pain, swelling, and tenderness. Rupture of muscle tendons such as the biceps or gastrocnemius muscle may produce visible muscle shortening.

The almost-pleasurable ache and fatigue of muscles after strenuous activity is separable only by degree from more severe, but still normal pain following severe, unaccustomed activity. Such symptoms are often associated with laboratory evidence of profound muscle damage, including a rise in serum enzymes (creatine kinase), focal edema on MRI, and widespread muscle necrosis on biopsy. Myoglobinemia and myoglobinuria may occur. Particularly likely to produce muscle pain and necrosis are certain types of exercise: brief periods of contracting a muscle while it is lengthening (eccentric contractions) and prolonged exercise such as marathon running. The point at which such symptoms become abnormal is not clear. Many patients have pain with moderate activity. Such exertional muscle pain is also characteristic of metabolic disorders of muscle such as carnitine palmitoyl transferase deficiency and myoadenylate deaminase deficiency; patients with partial defects in *dystrophin* may have recurrent exercise-induced myalgias. Complete deficiency of this protein causes Duchenne muscular dystrophy (see Chap. 385). Deficiencies of enzymes of glycolysis are more commonly associated with contractures (see Chap. 385). The majority of patients with exertional and postexertional muscle pain do not have a definable abnormality.

Diffuse myalgias Muscle pain in the absence of muscle weakness can occur in acute infections caused by influenza virus and coxsackievirus. Fibrositis, fibromyalgia, and fibromyositis are synonyms for a disorder associated with pain and tenderness of muscle and adjacent connective tissue. Focal "trigger points" of tenderness can be identified, and systemic symptoms such as fatigue, insomnia, and depression are frequently present (see Chap. 384). Although patients often identify painful swellings, histologic evaluation discloses no abnormality of muscle or connective tissue. Symptoms may respond partially to amitriptyline or nonsteroidal anti-inflammatory agents, but the disorder tends to be chronic and unrelenting. A supportive program of physical reconditioning is sometimes helpful. Patients whose symptoms persist for months or years are often considered to have a psychiatric disorder, but its nature has not been defined.

Polymyalgia rheumatica occurs in patients over age 50 and is characterized by stiffness and pain in shoulder and hip musculature. Despite symptoms of pain localized to muscles, there is convincing evidence that the disease includes a proximal, inflammatory arthritis; joint effusions are often present in knees and other peripheral joints as well. Patients often develop profound disuse atrophy of muscles and complain of weakness, giving rise to a suspicion of polymyositis. However, creatine kinase levels are usually normal, and muscle biopsy shows atrophy without evidence of muscle necrosis or inflammation. The erythrocyte sedimentation rate is elevated in most patients, and temporal arteritis may be present (see Chap. 291). Treatment with nonsteroidal anti-inflammatory agents is advocated except in patients with temporal arteritis, for whom prednisone (40 to 60 mg daily) is recommended. Patients with polymyalgia rheumatica who fail to respond to nonsteroidal anti-inflammatory agents may require low-dose prednisone (10 to 20 mg daily). Myalgias are also frequent in other rheumatologic disorders, including rheumatoid arthritis, systemic lupus erythematosus, polyarteritis nodosa, scleroderma, and the mixed connective tissue syndrome. Patients with polymyositis and dermatomyositis may have myalgias, although in the majority muscle pain is lacking or minimal (see Chap. 384).

EPISODIC WEAKNESS   The term *weakness* is often used by a patient to describe a loss of stamina or decreased "energy." Even careful efforts at eliciting a history of true as opposed to subjective weakness may fail to distinguish the two conditions. The most helpful strategy is to ask the patient to identify whether a discrete loss of function has occurred and to elicit the circumstances in which symptoms are noted.

Weakness, whether true or perceived, may be due to disorders of the central or peripheral nervous system. Weakness from CNS disorders such as transient cerebral ischemia is usually associated with a change in level of consciousness or cognition, with increased muscle tone and muscle stretch reflexes, and often with alterations of sensation. Most neuromuscular causes of intermittent weakness are associated with normal mental function but diminished muscle tone and muscle stretch reflexes. The major causes of intermittent weakness are listed in Table 23-1. Central causes are considered in Chaps. 21 and 368.

EPISODIC ASTHENIA   Patients who describe intermittent "weakness" as *fatigue* and loss of *stamina* suffer from asthenia, which can be separated from true weakness by the fact that patients do not lack the ability to do a task but rather the ability to perform it repetitively. Asthenia is a major problem in many patients with serious renal, hepatic, cardiac, or pulmonary disease. Examination of such patients usually confirms their ability to do all functional activities at least once, such as rising from a knee bend, climbing stairs, or rising from a chair. Fatigue is also characteristic of relatively selective damage to CNS descending motor tracts, in which signs of neurologic abnormality may be minimal. Fatigue that is worsened by activity is characteristic of the *chronic fatigue syndrome* (see Chap. 388).

Intermittent weakness due to peripheral neuromuscular disease may result from abrupt changes in peripheral nerve function, intermittent destruction of muscle, alterations of electrophysiologic properties of muscle from abnormalities of blood electrolytes, and intermittent failure of neuromuscular transmission.

FAILURE OF PERIPHERAL NERVE CONDUCTION   A number of uncommon peripheral neuropathies are associated with recurrent weakness. *Hereditary liability to pressure palsies*, often termed *tomaculous* neuropathy because of the sausage-like appearance of

---

TABLE 23-1   Causes of episodic generalized weakness

Electrolyte disturbances
  Hypokalemia: Primary aldosteronism (Conn's syndrome); barium poisoning; renal tubular acidosis; juxtaglomerular apparatus hyperplasia (Bartter's syndrome); villous adenoma of colon; alcoholism; diuretics; licorice; para-aminosalicylic acid; glucocorticoids
  Hyperkalemia: Addison's disease; chronic renal failure; hyporeninemic hypoaldosteronism
  Hypercalcemia
  Hypocalcemic tetany
  Hyponatremia
  Hypophosphatemia
  Hypermagnesemia
Neuromuscular junction disorders
  Myasthenia gravis
  Lambert-Eaton syndrome
Muscle disorders
  Periodic paralyses
  Metabolic defects of muscle (impaired carbohydrate or fatty acid utilization)
Central nervous system causes
  Cataplexy and sleep paralysis associated with narcolepsy
  Multiple sclerosis
  Transient ischemic attacks
Disorders with only subjective weakness: Hyperventilation, hypoglycemia

---

myelin on nerve biopsy, is an autosomal dominant disorder characterized by abrupt paralysis following compression of a peripheral nerve. The paralysis is usually self-limited, lasting days to weeks. Other types of peripheral neuropathy also may predispose to the development of reversible, compressive neuropathies (see Chap. 383).

DISORDERED NEUROMUSCULAR JUNCTION TRANSMISSION   *Myasthenia gravis*, particularly in its initial manifestations, is characterized by transient weakness. Cranial muscles are usually affected first, causing double vision, ptosis, dysphagia, and dysarthria. Rarely, limb weakness may herald the onset of myasthenia gravis and in the absence of cranial muscle dysfunction may escape diagnosis for months. Diurnal variation in strength is typical, and reflexes are preserved. Other, less-common defects of the neuromuscular junction such as the Lambert-Eaton syndrome also may present with intermittent weakness (see Chap. 386).

INTERMITTENT ALTERATIONS IN ELECTROLYTES   Transient shifts in serum potassium are associated with profound alterations in muscle strength. Although the primary periodic paralyses (hypo- and hyperkalemic periodic paralysis) spring to mind in a patient with weakness and an abnormality in serum potassium, other causes of abnormal serum potassium are more frequently behind episodic weakness (see Chap. 387). Familial periodic paralysis seldom presents after age 30; other causes are usually present in older patients. Hypokalemic periodic paralysis may occur in patients with hyperthyroidism. Episodic weakness due to hypokalemia may occur with renal or gastrointestinal potassium loss (see Table 23-1).

Hyperkalemic weakness usually occurs in the setting of chronic renal or adrenal disease. Other electrolyte disturbances may produce intermittent weakness as the initial clinical manifestation of a severe metabolic abnormality (see Table 23-1). Correction of the metabolic derangement improves the weakness.

METABOLIC MUSCLE DISEASE   A number of uncommon defects in glycogen and lipid utilization are associated with impaired energy production by muscle and cause intermittent weakness, usually accompanied by muscle pain and evidence of muscle damage. Carnitine palmitoyl transferase deficiency is one such condition. Mitochondrial disorders such as cytochrome oxidase deficiency may produce severe exercise intolerance with fatigue and weakness associated with lactic acidosis. Muscle pain and destruction seldom occur. (See also Chap. 385.)

Recurrent attacks of a feeling of "weakness" often occur in patients with the *hyperventilation syndrome;* such patients are, however, of normal strength when tested. Similarly, *recurrent hypoglycemic episodes* are associated with subjective weakness, although hypoglycemia is uncommon as the cause of this symptom.

Central nervous system disorders may cause generalized weakness without an associated alteration of consciousness. *Drop attacks* resulting from impaired blood supply to the motor pathways of the brainstem cause sudden paraparesis or quadriparesis, usually lasting only a few seconds. Patients with narcolepsy may have sudden loss of muscle strength and tone during episodes of *cataplexy*. A disorder of the reticular activating system is responsible for these episodes as well as for *sleep paralysis* that occurs as narcoleptic patients are falling asleep or awakening (see Chap. 29).

REFERENCES

ARGOV Z: Phosphorus magnetic resonance spectroscopy (^{31}P MRS) in neuromuscular disorders. Ann Neurol 30:90, 1991

BARCHI RL, FURMAN RE: Pathophysiology of myotonia and periodic paralysis, in Diseases of the Nervous System, vol. 1: Clinical Neurobiology, AK Asbury et al (eds). Philadelphia, Saunders, 1992

BERTOLASI L et al: The influence of muscular lengthening on cramps. Ann Neurol 33:176, 1993

BROOKE MH: A Clinician's View of Neuromuscular Diseases. Baltimore, Williams & Wilkins, 1986

EDWARDS RHT et al: Muscle biochemistry and pathophysiology in postviral fatigue syndrome. Br Med Bull 47:826, 1991

FLECKENSTEIN JL et al: Magnetic resonance imaging of muscle injury and atrophy in glycolytic myopathies. Muscle Nerve 12:849, 1989

GEORGE AL et al: Molecular basis of Thomsen disease (autosomal dominant myotonia-congenita). Nature Genet 3:305, 1993

LAYZER RB: Muscle pain, cramps and fatigue, in Myology, AG Engel, BQ Banker (eds). New York, McGraw-Hill, 1986

24   NUMBNESS, TINGLING, AND SENSORY LOSS

ARTHUR K. ASBURY

Normal somatic sensation is a continuous process that commands considerable moment-to-moment nervous system activity. Little of the activity intrudes on consciousness or exacts notice. In contrast, disordered sensation, particularly pains and paresthesias, may be highly intrusive, alarming, and tenacious, and may dominate attention. Abnormalities of sensation tend to make patients seek medical attention quickly. When abnormal sensations are perceived as painful, medical advice is sought even more quickly. For a consideration of pain, see Chap. 11. The physician must have a framework of knowledge in order to assess abnormal sensations, estimate their likely site of origin, and recognize their implications.

POSITIVE AND NEGATIVE PHENOMENA It is useful to divide all abnormal sensory phenomena into two great categories, positive and negative. Positive phenomena include tingling, pins-and-needles, pricking, bandlike sensations, lightning-like shooting feelings (lancinations), aching, and knifelike, twisting, drawing, pulling, tightening, burning, searing, electrical, and raw sensations. These descriptors are frequently the actual words used by patients. Such sensations may or may not be experienced as painful. It is thought that the pathophysiologic basis of positive phenomena resides in the ectopic generation of volleys of impulses at some site of lowered neural threshold along the sensory pathways, either in peripheral or central sensory fibers. Such trains of ectopically generated afferent impulses arising from sites other than normal peripheral nerve receptors determine the quality of the abnormal sensation experienced, depending on the number, rate, and distribution of impulses and the type and function of nerve fibers in which they arise.

Positive phenomena represent heightened activity in sensory pathways; therefore, they are not necessarily associated with any demonstrable sensory deficit upon examination, an important point for the examiner to bear in mind.

Negative phenomena result from loss of sensory function and are characterized by numbness or diminution or absence of feeling in a particular distribution. Negative phenomena, in contrast to positive phenomena, are accompanied by abnormal findings on sensory examination. In disorders affecting peripheral sensation, it is estimated that at least half the afferent fibers innervating a given site must be lost or functionless in order for sensory deficit to be demonstrated. This estimate probably varies according to how rapidly sensory fibers have lost function. If the rate of loss is slow and chronic, lack of cutaneous feeling may be unnoticed by the patient and difficult to demonstrate on examination, even though few sensory fibers are functioning. Rapidly evolving sensory abnormality usually evokes positive phenomena of some type and is more readily recognized by patients than insidious deafferentation. Subclinical degrees of sensory dysfunction not demonstrable on clinical sensory examination may be revealed by sensory nerve conduction studies or somatosensory cerebral evoked potentials (see Chaps. 366 and 382).

Terminology Two general types of medical terms are used to characterize abnormal sensation, those referring to symptoms of which patients complain (both positive and negative phenomena) and those describing abnormalities found on examination (only negative phenomena). *Paresthesia* and *dysesthesia* are terms used to denote positive phenomena. Paresthesia carries the implication that the abnormal sensation is perceived without an apparent stimulus, whereas dysesthesia is a more general term used to describe all types of positive sensations whether a stimulus is evident or not. Abnormalities on examination are denoted by *hypesthesia* or *hypoesthesia* (reduction of cutaneous sensation to a specific type of testing such as pressure, light touch, and warm or cold stimuli), *anesthesia* (complete absence of skin sensation to the same stimuli plus pinprick), and *hypalgesia* (referring to loss of pain perception, i.e., nociception, such as the pricking quality elicited by a pin). *Hyperesthesia* connotes exaggerated perception of sensations in response to mild stimuli (light touch or stroking of the skin). Similarly, *allodynia* describes the situation in which an ordinarily nonpainful stimulus, once perceived, is experienced as painful, even excruciating. An example is elicitation of a painful sensation by application of a vibrating tuning fork. *Hyperalgesia* denotes an exaggerated response to a noxious stimulus, and *hyperpathia*, a broad term, encompasses all the phenomena described by hyperesthesia, allodynia, and hyperalgesia.

Disorders of deep sensation, arising from muscle spindles, tendons, and joints, deserve special comment. Normally these afferents subserve proprioception (position sense) and the moment-to-moment sense of the state of muscle contraction. If a significant number of these special nerve endings become denervated, the resulting manifestations include imbalance, particularly with eyes closed or in the dark, clumsiness of precision movements, and unsteadiness of gait, all of which is referred to as *sensory ataxia* (see Chap. 22). Other findings on examination include reduced or absent joint position and vibratory sensibility and absent deep tendon reflexes in the affected limbs. Romberg's sign is positive, which means that the patient sways or topples when asked to stand with feet close together and eyes closed.

In severe states of deafferentation involving deep sensation, the patient cannot walk or stand unaided or even sit unsupported. Continuous, sometimes wormlike involuntary movements, called *pseudoathetosis*, of the hands and arms occur, particularly with eyes closed. Such patients are severely disabled.

Normal sensation Cutaneous afferent innervation is subserved by a rich variety of receptors, both naked endings (nociceptors and thermoreceptors) and encapsulated terminals (mechanoreceptors). Each has its own set of sensitivities to specific stimuli, size and distinctness of receptive fields, and adaptational qualities. Much of the knowledge about these receptors has come from the development of techniques to study single intact nerve fibers intraneurally in alert unanesthetized human subjects. It is possible not only to record from single nerve fibers, large or small, but also to stimulate single fibers in isolation. A single impulse, whether elicited by a natural stimulus or evoked by electrical microstimulation, in a large myelinated afferent fiber may be both perceived and localized.

Afferent fibers in peripheral nerve trunks sort themselves into topographically coherent patterns as they approach the dorsal roots and enter the dorsal horn of the spinal cord. From there the polysynaptic projections of the smaller fibers (unmyelinated and small myelinated), which in general subserve nociception and temperature sensibility, cross and ascend in the contralateral spinothalamic tract through spinal cord, through brainstem, to the ventral posterolateral nucleus (VPL) of the thalamus, and ultimately project to the postcentral gyrus of the parietal cortex (see Chap. 11). This is the spinothalamic pathway. The larger fibers that subserve tactile and position sense and kinesthesia project rostrally in the ipsilateral posterior column of the spinal cord and finally make their first synapse in the gracile or cuneate nuclei of the lower medulla (see Fig. 24-1). The second-order neuron decussates and ascends in the medial lemniscus located medially in the medulla and in the tegmentum of the pons and midbrain and synapses in VPL. The third-order neuron projects to parietal cortex; this entire system is referred to as *lemniscal*.

Although the fiber types and functions that make up the spinothalamic and lemniscal systems are relatively well known, it has been found that many other fibers, particularly those associated with touch, pressure, and position sense, ascend in a diffusely distributed pattern both ipsilaterally and contralaterally in the anterolateral quadrants of the spinal cord. These anatomic facts explain why an individual with a known complete lesion of the posterior columns of the spinal cord may have little sensory deficit on examination.

EXAMINATION OF SENSATION   The initial step in examination of the somatosensory system is to do the tests of primary sensation, which by convention include the sense of pain, touch, vibration, joint position, and thermal sensation, both hot and cold. These tests have gradually become codified through tradition, but they do appear to assess, if crudely, the major afferent functions and pathways (see Table 24-1). Testing of both primary sensation and cortical sensory function can be carried out in the office or at the bedside with a minimum of special equipment.

Some general principles pertain to the sensory examination. First, it should be remembered that the examiner is depending on subjective patient response; therefore, discriminating responses depend on the level of alertness, motivation, and intelligence of the patient and also on the skill with which the examiner has made the task clear. In a stupefied or obtunded patient, the examiner is reduced to observing the briskness of withdrawal and the complexity of defensive movements of the patient in response to a pinch or other noxious stimulus. In the alert but uncooperative patient, it is often possible to get some idea of proprioceptive function by noting the patient's best performance in casually observed movements requiring balance and precision, but cutaneous sensation may be unexaminable.

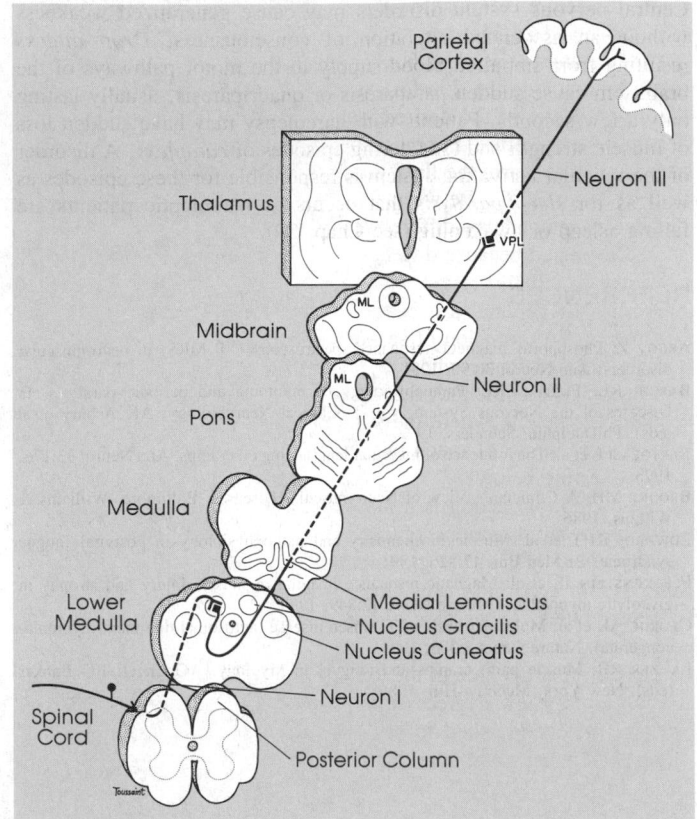

FIGURE 24-1   Schematic diagram of lemniscal system, which subserves proprioception and discriminative touch.

Second, sensory examination should not be pressed if the patient is fatigued. An abbreviated survey will suffice until a more extensive examination can be carried out when the patient has rested. Third, sensory examination in a patient who has no neurologic complaints should be quite abbreviated and may consist of pin, touch, and vibration testing in the hands and feet plus evaluation of station and gait, including Romberg's maneuver, which also tests the integrity of motor and cerebellar systems. Fourth, patients should be tested with their eyes closed or covered during both primary sensation and cortical sensory function examination.

Primary sensation (see Table 24-1)   The sense of pain is usually tested with a pin, asking the patient to focus on the pricking or unpleasant quality of the stimulus and not just the pressure or touch sensation elicited. Areas of hypalgesia should be mapped by

TABLE 24-1   Testing primary sensation

Sense	Test device	Endings activated	Fiber size mediating	Central pathway*
Pain	Pinprick	Cutaneous nociceptors	Small	SpTh, also D
Temperature, heat	Flask with warm water	Cutaneous thermoreceptors for hot	Small	SpTh
Temperature, cold	Flask with cold water	Cutaneous thermoreceptors for cold	Small	SpTh
Touch	Cotton wisp, fine brush	Cutaneous mechanoreceptors, also naked endings	Large and small	Lem, also D and SpTh
Vibration	Tuning fork, 128 Hz	Mechanoreceptors, especially pacinian corpuscles	Large	Lem, also D
Joint position	Passive movement of specific joints	Joint capsule and tendon endings, muscle spindles	Large	Lem, also D

*D = diffuse ascending projections in ipsilateral and contralateral anterolateral columns; SpTh = spinothalamic projection, contralateral; Lem = posterior column and lemniscal projection, ipsilateral.

proceeding from the most hypalgesic zones to less affected ones (see Figs. 24-2 and 24-3).

Temperature sensation, both to hot and to cold, is probably best tested by touching the skin for a couple of seconds with a water flask filled with water of the desired temperature, using a thermometer to verify the temperature. For most purposes, it is satisfactory if a patient can identify as warm the flask that is 35 or 36°C and as cool the one that is 28 to 32°C. Between 28 and 32°C, most individuals can distinguish temperature differences in 1°C steps. Both cold and warm should be tested because different receptors respond to each.

Touch is usually tested with a wisp of cotton or a fine camel's hair brush. In general, it is better to avoid testing touch on hairy skin because of the profusion of sensory endings that surround each hair follicle. The patients, whose eyes are covered, should be asked to say "now" each time they feel the stimulus. They also may be asked to point to the site where the stimulus was felt, although this tests not only the sense of touch but also touch localization (see cortical sensory testing below).

Joint position testing is a measure of proprioception, one of the most important functions of the sensory system. Joint position is usually tested first in the great toe and then in the fingers. Patients are asked to keep their eyes closed and to relax completely the part to be examined. In the case of the great toe, one starts with the toe in a neutral position and grasps it lightly between the thumb and the forefinger on either side of the toe (not top and bottom), and then the toe is moved a few degrees either in a dorsal or a plantar direction, and the patient is asked to say whether the movement was up or down. One must make sure that the patient understands that it is the

FIGURE 24-2 Anterior view of dermatomes (*left*) and cutaneous areas supplied by individual peripheral nerves (*right*). (*Modified from MB Carpenter and J Sutin, in Human Neuroanatomy, 8th ed, Baltimore, Williams & Wilkins, 1983.*)

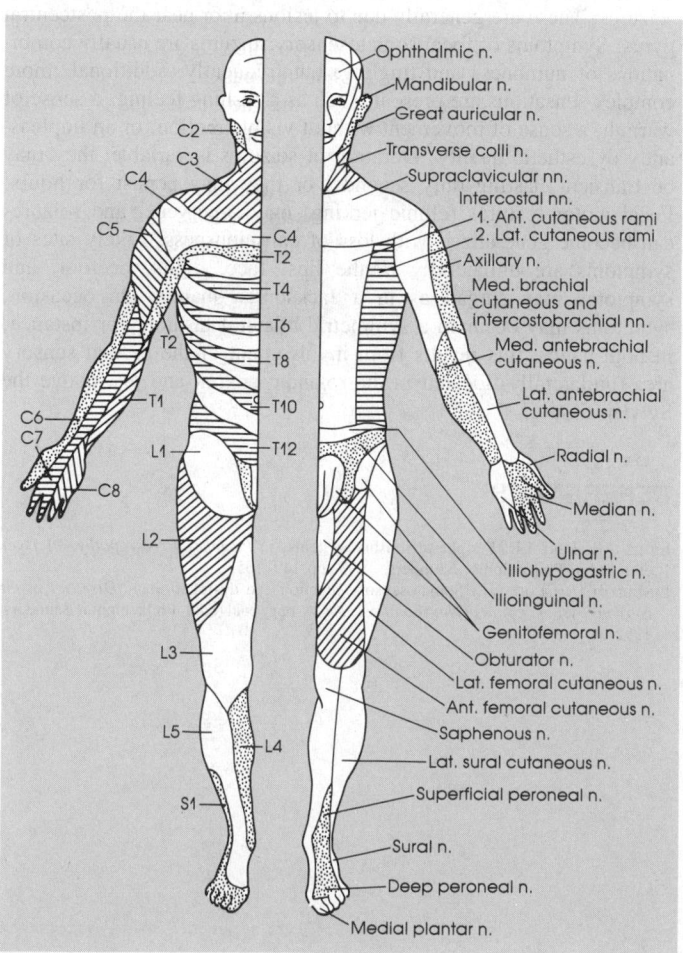

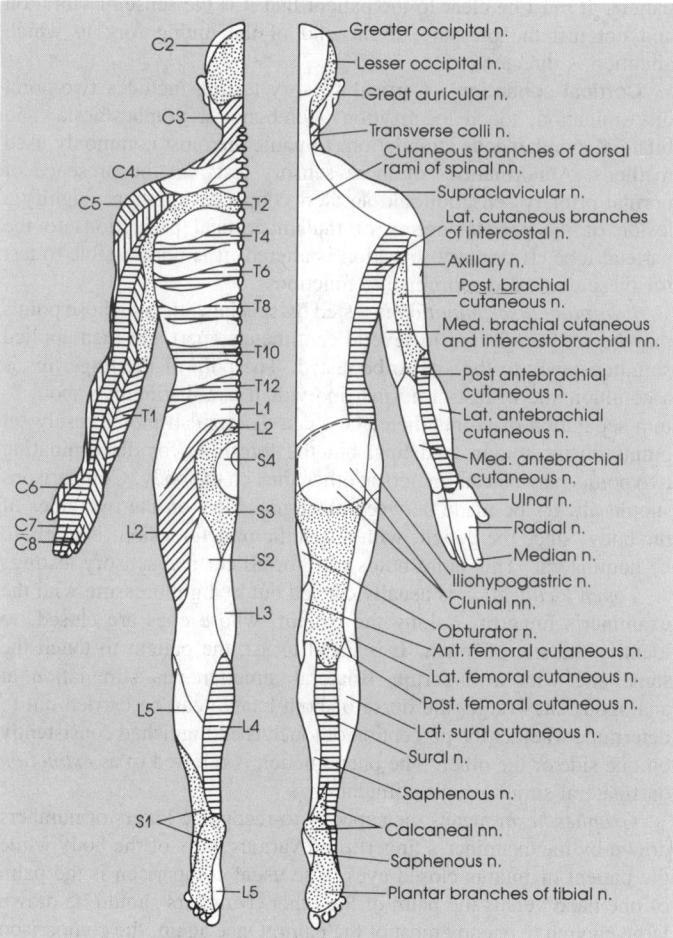

FIGURE 24-3 Posterior view of dermatomes (*left*) and cutaneous areas supplied by individual peripheral nerves (*right*). (*Modified from MB Carpenter and J Sutin, in Human Neuroanatomy, 8th ed, Baltimore, Williams & Wilkins, 1983.*)

direction of movement which is being tested and not the direction the toe is pointing when it stops. A patient with absence of position sense in the part being tested will have a 50 percent error rate because only two choices are available. Answers that are consistently greater than 50 percent in error should be viewed with skepticism. If errors are made in recognizing the direction of passive movements of the toe, then passive movements of the ankle or even of the knee should be undertaken in the same way. Similarly, position sense at the proximal interphalangeal joint of the index finger may be tested, and if abnormal, other finger joints and the wrist and elbow joints also should be tested. A test of proximal joint position sense, primarily at the shoulder, can be carried out by asking the patient to bring the two index fingers together with the arms extended and the eyes closed. Normal individuals should be able to do this quite accurately with errors of a centimeter or less.

The sense of vibration is tested with a tuning fork, preferably a large one that vibrates at 128 Hz. The decay of vibration using this fork is slow enough to be of quantitative use because it requires between 15 and 20 s to decay below the threshold of perceptibility. Vibration is usually tested at bony prominences, specifically the malleoli at the ankles, the patella, the anterior iliac spine, the spinous processes of the vertebral bodies, the metacarpal-phalangeal joints (knuckles), the styloid process of the ulna, the elbow, and the acromion of the shoulder. Control sites at which to test vibration are the sternum and the forehead. The examiner can compare the threshold at a given site in both patient and self. A crude approximation of degree of vibratory sense loss can be made by counting the seconds that the examiner can feel the sense of vibration longer than the patient. It must be clear to the patient that it is the sense of vibration and not just the pressure of the end of the tuning fork to which attention is directed.

Cortical sensation   Cortical sensory testing includes two-point discrimination, touch localization, stereognosis, graphesthesia, and bilateral simultaneous stimulation, to name the most commonly used methods. Abnormalities of these sensory tests, in the presence of normal primary sensation and an alert cooperative patient, signify a lesion of the parietal cortex or thalamocortical projections to the parietal lobe. If primary sensation is altered, it is not possible to test for these cortical discriminative functions.

Two-point discrimination is tested by special calipers whose points may be set from 2 mm to several centimeters apart and then applied simultaneously to the site to be tested. The pulp of the fingertips is a common site to test; a normal individual can distinguish about 3-mm separation of points there. One can distinguish more closely set points on the tongue and lips, but the threshold for discriminating two points may be centimeters at other sites on the body. Comparisons should always be made between analogous sites on the two sides of the body, since the deficit, with a specific parietal lesion, is likely to be hemilateral. This point holds true for all cortical sensory testing.

Touch localization is usually carried out by light pressure with the examiner's fingertip, asking the patient, whose eyes are closed, to identify the site of touch. It is usual to ask the patient to touch the same site with a fingertip. Bilateral simultaneous stimulation at analogous sites (e.g., the dorsa of both hands) can be carried out to determine whether the perception of touch is extinguished consistently on one side or the other. The phenomenon is referred to as *extinction* on bilateral simultaneous stimulation.

Graphesthesia means the capacity to recognize letters or numbers drawn by the examiner's fingertip on various parts of the body while the patient maintains closed eyes. The usual comparison is the palm of one hand versus the palm of the other. Numbers should be drawn large enough to occupy most of the palm. Once again, the comparison of one side with the other is of prime importance. Failure to recognize numbers or letters is termed *agraphesthesia*.

Stereognosis refers to the ability to identify common objects by palpation, recognizing their shape, texture, and size. Common standard objects are the best test objects, such as a marble, a paper clip, a small rubber ball, or coins. Patients with normal stereognosis should be able to distinguish a dime from a penny and certainly a nickel from a quarter. Patients should only be allowed to feel the object with one hand at time. If they are unable to identify it in one hand, it should be placed in the other for comparison. Individuals unable to identify common objects and coins in one hand who can do so in the other are said to have *astereognosis* of the abnormal hand. Note that the major comparison is one side of the body with the other.

Localization of sensory abnormalities   Peripheral neuropathies are generally graded, distal, and symmetric in their distribution of deficit. Although most peripheral neuropathies are pansensory and affect all modalities of sensation, selective sensory dysfunction according to nerve fiber size may occur. In small fiber neuropathies, the hallmark is burning, painful dysesthesias with reduced pinprick and thermal sensation but with sparing of proprioception, motor function, and even deep tendon jerks. Touch is variably involved, but when spared, the sensory pattern is referred to as *sensory dissociation* (see below). In contrast to small fiber neuropathies, large-fiber neuropathies are characterized by position sense deficit, imbalance, absent tendon jerks, variable motor dysfunction, but preservation of most cutaneous sensation and few or no dysesthesias.

Paresthesias and dysesthesias may be of either peripheral nerve or spinal cord origin and probably can arise in the brainstem, but in every instance they are thought to represent abnormal showers of impulses generated from an ectopic focus or foci. By themselves, paresthesias may not be localizable, but when accompanied by other signs of neuropathy or of myelopathy, the correct site of origin may be deduced.

Dissociated sensory deficit patterns, in which pinprick and thermal sensation are lost but touch is spared, are usually a sign of spinothalamic tract involvement in the spinal cord, especially if the deficit is unilateral and has an upper level on the torso. Bilateral spinothalamic tract involvement occurs with lesions affecting the center of the spinal cord, such as happens with expansion of the central canal in hydromyelia or syringomyelia. Sensory dissociation also may occur in peripheral neuropathies in which afferent cutaneous nerve fibers of small diameter are preferentially affected. Neuropathies in which sensory dissociation may occur include leprous neuritis, hereditary sensory neuropathy, and certain cases of amyloid and diabetic polyneuropathy (see Chap. 383).

Hemisensory disturbance with tingling numbness from head to foot is usually thalamic in origin. If abrupt in onset, the thalamic lesion is likely to be due to a small stroke (lacunar infarction). Occasionally, with lesions affecting the posterolateral thalamus (VPL) or adjacent white matter, a syndrome of thalamic pain, also called *Déjerine-Roussy syndrome*, may ensue. This is a persistent unrelenting hemipainful state often described in dramatic terms such as "like the flesh is being torn from my limbs" or "as though that side is bathed in acid" (see Chap. 11). Harlequin patterns of sensory disturbance, in which one side of the face and the opposite side of the body are affected, localize to the lateral medulla, where a small lesion may damage both the ipsilateral descending trigeminal tract and ascending spinothalamic fibers (lateral lemniscus) subserving the opposite arm, leg, and hemitorso (see "Lateral Medulla Syndrome" in Chap. 368).

With lesions of the parietal lobe, either of the cortex or of subjacent white matter, the most prominent symptoms are contralateral hemineglect, hemi-inattention, and a tendency not to use the contralateral hand and arm. Tests of primary sensation are usually normal or minimally altered, but tests of cortical sensation are often severely abnormal (see Chap. 27). Dysesthesias, or even a sense of numbness, are unusual except in the special circumstance of focal sensory seizures. These are generally due to lesions in or near the postcentral gyrus. Symptoms of focal somatosensory seizures are usually combinations of numbness and tingling, but frequently, additional, more complex sensations are present, such as a rushing feeling, a sense of warmth, a sense of movement without visible motion, or an unpleasantly dysesthetic quality. Duration of seizures is variable; they may be transient, lasting only seconds, or they may persist for hours. Focal motor features (clonic jerking) may supervene, and seizures can become generalized with loss of consciousness. Likely sites of symptoms are unilaterally in the lips, face, digits, or foot, and symptoms may spread as in a Jacksonian march. On occasion, symptoms may occur in a symmetric bilateral fashion, for instance, in both hands; this results from involvement of the second sensory area (unilaterally) located in the rolandic area at and just above the Sylvian fissure.

REFERENCES

LIGHT AR, PERL ER: Peripheral sensory systems, in *Peripheral Neuropathy*, PJ Dyck et al (eds). Philadelphia, Saunders, 1993, pp 149–165

LINDBLOM U, OCHOA JL: Somatosensory function and dysfunction, in *Diseases of the Nervous System: Clinical Neurobiology*, AK Asbury et al (eds). Philadelphia, Saunders, 1992

25 ACUTE CONFUSIONAL STATES, AMNESIA, AND DEMENTIA

MARTIN M. BROWN / VLADIMIR C. HACHINSKI

The complexity and vulnerability of neuronal function allow cognitive function to be easily disturbed. Many systemic and neurologic illnesses come to notice because of disruption of cognitive function, often without other symptoms or signs. Recognizing the patterns of the resulting syndromes avoids mistaken psychiatric diagnoses and allows early and appropriate management. Testing of individual cognitive functions allows identification of specific areas of abnormality and helps in establishing the cause of the disorder.

SYNDROME DEFINITION

CONFUSION Any disorder of cognitive function may cause confusion, i.e., a lack of clarity and coherence of thought, perception, understanding, or action. Confusion is often the first feature of cognitive impairment noticed by relatives or the examiner. Confusion also may appear to be the presenting complaint in isolated focal disorders of cognitive function such as aphasia or visuospatial agnosia (see Chap. 27), but careful examination will show that the confusion is related to a single deficit.

The acute confusional state is a common syndrome, consisting of global impairment of cognitive function accompanied by deficits in attention and consciousness. The impairment of cognition usually includes disorientation, abnormal perception, disordered reasoning, and poor memory. A wide variety of causes may be responsible.

DELIRIUM The term *delirium* is synonymous with the acute confusional state, although, strictly speaking, it describes a clinically distinct variety of acute confusional state characterized by periods of agitation, heightened mental activity, increased wakefulness, marked readiness to respond to certain stimuli (such as sudden noises), intrusive visual hallucinations, motor hyperactivity, and autonomic stimulation. Impairment of attention, essential to the acute confusional state, is present despite the apparent arousal (see ''Consciousness,'' below). The agitation of delirium characteristically fluctuates and may alternate with or progress to a subdued confusional state. The clinical picture is exemplified by the excited hallucinatory state of *delirium tremens* which follows alcohol withdrawal. However, delirium may be seen in acute confusional states from any cause.

DEMENTIA This is a syndrome of acquired global or multifocal impairment of cognitive function involving decline in intellect, memory, and personality in the presence of normal consciousness. Relatively normal alertness and attention distinguish dementia from the acute confusional state (see Table 25-1). The decline usually involves all intellectual functions, but the diagnosis may be established by impairment of any three of the following spheres: language, memory, visuospatial skills, emotion, personality, or cognition. Loss of a single intellectual function such as speech or memory, however devastating, is not sufficient. Dementia is not necessarily progressive, and in some instances it can be reversed or halted by appropriate treatment. It is therefore important to recognize dementia as a syndrome with many causes.

AMNESIA This term describes an isolated disorder of memory characterized by inability to remember past events and to learn new information despite normal consciousness and attention. Amnesia has a variety of possible causes.

OBSERVABLE COMPONENTS OF COGNITION

Despite the complexity of mental activity, certain aspects can be assessed reliably at the bedside as part of the neurologic examination.

TABLE 25-1 Clinical features of the acute confusional state and dementia compared

	Acute confusional state	Dementia
Onset	Acute	Usually insidious
Duration	Transient (hours to weeks)	Persistent (months to years)
Course	Fluctuating over hours; diurnal variation common	Stable over days
Sleep-wake cycle	Disrupted	Normal
Consciousness level	Depressed	Normal
Attention	Impaired	Normal
Orientation	Impaired	Impaired
Language	Incoherent	Aphasia common
Memory		
Digit span	Shortened	Normal
Long-term memory	Impaired	Impaired
Perception	Impaired (illusions, delusions, hallucinations)	Normal early, agnosia later
Mood	Agitation or fear common	Apathy or disinhibition common
Autonomic changes	Common	Unusual
Psychomotor changes (depressed motor activity or restlessness)	Common	Uncommon
Involuntary movements	Common	Uncommon
EEG	Diffuse slow-wave activity	Mild slowing

CONSCIOUSNESS Consciousness is the state of awareness of self and the environment and has various facets (see also Chap. 26). The *content* of consciousness represents the sum of cognitive and affective mental functions and can be assessed only by inference. *Arousal* is closely allied to the appearance of *alertness*, i.e., the readiness to respond to stimulation. *Attention* includes the capacity to attend selectively to relevant stimuli and to manipulate abstract ideas. Consciousness also includes the concepts of *insight* and recognition of self. *Clouding of consciousness* is an essential feature of acute confusional states and describes the mildest impairment of consciousness on the continuum from full consciousness to deep coma. In most instances, clouding of consciousness involves all facets of consciousness. In delirium the patient may appear aroused and excited, but the content of consciousness, awareness of the surroundings and self, and the capacity to attend selectively to relevant stimuli are all impaired.

PERCEPTION Perception involves conscious awareness, selection, and identification of a stimulus from the environment. Even under normal conditions the perception of a stimulus depends on numerous factors, both physiologic (such as lighting) and psychological (such as mood and expectation). With clouding of consciousness, attention falters, and perception becomes more subject to these influences. For example, poor vision or deafness may make the elderly more prone to misperception, and the advent of darkness often contributes to delirium. Coherent perception requires intact visuospatial and language function. Disturbances of perception are frequent in acute confusional states and include *illusions* (misperceptions of actual sensory stimuli) and *hallucinations* (perceptions experienced without apparent sensory stimulation). In dementia, misperception commonly results from focal impairments of visuospatial or language function such as agnosia or aphasia.

MEMORY Three classes of memory can be distinguished at the bedside depending on the length of recall. The *immediate memory* system holds information close to consciousness for a few seconds while it is used for mental activity. It can be tested by the reproduction of a string of numerals and has a finite capacity for information at around seven digits, which are retained for only seconds or minutes unless the information is rehearsed by internal repetition. Normal attention is required for immediate memory function, and impairment of immediate memory and a shortened digit span are diagnostic features of the acute confusional syndrome. Immediate memory is relatively normal in dementia and amnesic syndromes. Immediate memory appears to be mediated by a separate system that does not necessarily lead to longer-term storage. *Recent memory*, the recall of information presented within minutes, hours, or days, is distinguished from *remote memory*, the recall of events months or years earlier. Recall of information after a delay of a few minutes requires a process of consolidation or learning and is mediated by the *long-term*, or *secondary memory* system, with almost limitless capacity and durability. In contrast to immediate memory, recall of information from long-term memory is often selected by its relevance to the individual and usually incorporates the meaning of the information rather than exact words or pictures. Recent and remote memory probably both involve the same long-term memory system, but access to remote memories is less sensitive to interference (e.g., from the effect of head injury) than recent memory. Impaired recent memory is usual in dementia and acute confusional states and is the defining feature of amnesic syndromes.

MOOD AND PERSONALITY *Mood* refers to the prevailing emotional state, while *affect* is the emotional experience evoked by a particular stimulus. Individual reactions to any situation are closely related to underlying personality, previous experience, expectations, and degree of insight. The prevailing mood may have a profound influence on all aspects of cognition, especially at the extremes of the continuum of mood. Hypomania may be accompanied by illusions, flight of ideas, and extreme motor and verbal output sometimes mimicking delirium. In contrast, depression may exhibit slowing of thought, speech, and activity (psychomotor retardation) which, if severe, may be mistaken for dementia. Extreme anxiety also may interfere with the organization and coherence of thought and speech. Many diseases of the brain alter mood and affect. Frontal lobe lesions, in particular, may cause either lack of drive and initiative (abulia) with indifference to outcome or sometimes fatuous euphoria with social and sexual disinhibition.

PROBLEM SOLVING Thought is intangible and elusive. However, the processes of reasoning, logic, and the ability to solve problems using language or mathematics can be assessed more easily using tests of words or numbers. Disorder of these processes is an essential feature of the acute confusional states and dementia, but in contrast, reasoning is intact in the amnesic syndrome, except when recent memory is required. One manifestation of defective reasoning seen in acute confusional states and sometimes in dementia is the occurrence of delusions (false beliefs maintained in spite of convincing contradictory evidence). Delusions in psychiatric illnesses such as schizophrenia tend to be more organized and persistent than in acute confusional states.

APPROACH TO THE PATIENT WITH DISORDERS OF COGNITION

HISTORY A careful history taken from close relatives or friends is essential and may provide important clues about the underlying pathology. Questioning should establish the first appearance of intellectual impairment and the subsequent tempo of the disease. Was the onset over hours or days, suggesting an acute confusional state, or over months or years, making dementia a more likely diagnosis? Was there an organic precipitating event such as a head injury, or did the confusion follow an emotional crisis, suggesting a psychiatric cause or a drug overdose? Questioning should include inquiries about impairment of memory, personality and mood change, and how the patient copes with work, driving, and the activities of daily life. The history should include questioning about symptoms which suggest raised intracranial pressure (headaches, nausea, vomiting, and ataxia), strokelike events, or seizures. Attention to past medical and family history, drugs, alcohol, and toxic exposure is important (see also Chap. 363). The handedness of the patient should be determined to assess the likelihood that the left hemisphere is dominant for speech.

EXAMINATION OF COGNITIVE FUNCTION Careful examination of cognitive function is an important component of the neurologic examination. Cognitive impairment is frequently missed, especially in the elderly, because this part of the examination has been neglected. The main focus is to establish the level of consciousness and to determine whether the patient's deficit involves one aspect of intellectual function, suggesting a focal lesion at a single site, or more than one aspect, suggesting more global pathology. An initial step is to determine the patient's premorbid level of intellect. A rough indicator can be obtained from the patient's profession or occupation and the amount of schooling completed.

Examination of cognitive function needs to be adjusted according to the previous and current intellectual state, but it is useful to have a sequence of questions that the examiner has applied regularly to intellectually intact patients so as to have a good understanding of the normal range of replies. The Mini-Mental State Questionnaire provides an example of such a sequence that can be used to screen for cognitive impairment. However, the Mini-Mental State does not cover all aspects of intellectual function and does not always reveal mild or focal deficits, especially in younger or highly intelligent patients. It should therefore be supplemented by a fuller examination of cognitive function, as described below, if cognitive impairment is suspected. The patient's answers to questioning should be carefully recorded so that deterioration or improvement can be easily confirmed at a later evaluation. A number of pitfalls may cause the patient's intellectual function to be underestimated. Perseveration, usually a sign of frontal lobe disease, may cause the patient to repeat replies and have difficulty switching attention to a new task. Aphasia, with difficulty understanding commands or expressing the correct answer in response to questions, may cloud interpretation of the examination. The incoherence or mutism resulting from isolated expressive aphasia is commonly misinterpreted as a confusional state or dementia.

Orientation Orientation to person, place, and time (including date, time of day, month, and year) should be tested first. Usually, the more severe the impairment of memory, the more inaccurate is the date. If the patient cannot name the place accurately, ask the patient to identify the type of place (e.g., hospital or home).

Consciousness The normally alert individual engages in conversation or some other diversional activity, while the patient with impairment of consciousness remains quiet or engages in purposeless repetitive activities. Obtunded patients may drift into sleep when undisturbed but awaken promptly when questioned or examined. The demented patient may lack spontaneous activity or conversation but shows normal alertness and responsiveness to questioning.

Attention Attention is assessed during history taking. Does the patient pay attention to questions, or is the patient easily distracted? The capacity for sustained attention and concentration can be tested by asking for sequential subtraction of 7 from 100 down to zero, but the response should be interpreted with caution, since immediate memory and mathematical ability are also required. Forward and reverse digit spans are also specific tests of attention as well as of immediate memory (see below).

Abnormalities of perception Abnormalities of perception should be sought by specific questioning about perception of the environment. The presence of hallucinations may be betrayed by the patient brushing or picking nonexistent objects off the bed covers or turning to answer an imaginary question.

Language Aphasia results in nonfluency of speech, hesitation, circumlocution, neologisms, or jargon and is usually appreciated during routine conversation and history taking (see Chap. 28). It is also useful to ask the patient to name common and uncommon objects to assess for nominal aphasia and to give a complex command to test for minor degrees of receptive dysphasia. (For example, "If I take my pen out of my pocket, please touch your left ear with your right index finger.") Agraphia should be sought by asking the patient to write his or her name and a short spontaneous sentence. Reading should be assessed using a standard text or newspaper article, asking for an explanation of its meaning by the patient. Simple sums are given to assess mathematical skills.

Visuospatial function   The most useful test of visuospatial function is to ask the patient to copy a drawing, starting with a simple object such as a five-pointed star and progressing to a more difficult object such as a three-dimensional box. Constructional apraxia, or visuospatial agnosia, results in difficulty in drawing the lines required in the correct spatial orientation or position. Perseveration or visual neglect also may be revealed by this test. The visual recognition of common objects will have been tested when examining for nominal aphasia, but bedside testing for difficulty in recognition of faces (prosopagnosia) requires a newspaper or magazine containing photographs of famous people, unless individuals who should be well known to the patient can be presented without other clues such as voice to aid recognition.

Memory   *Immediate memory* and attention are tested by determining *digit span*. The patient is asked to repeat a string of numerals after the examiner starting with a short string and working up to the normal digit span of six or seven consecutive numbers presented at about half-second intervals. A shorter string of numerals or a short word can be given to repeat or spell backwards. This test requires sustained attention as well as immediate memory. *Recent memory* should be assessed by asking the patient to learn the names of three common objects or a simple address. After confirming that the patient has registered the information, recall is tested after 2 and 5 min, depending on the degree of anticipated amnesia. If the patient fails to recall the information, then the severity of the amnesia can be gauged by giving the patient a clue, and if this fails, recognition can be tested by asking the patient to identify the correct answer from a choice. Recent memory for events over the last few days or weeks is assessed by asking for a description of events of personal or world importance. A relative or friend may need to corroborate the appropriateness of the description. *Remote long-term memory* can be tested by asking for items of common general knowledge such as the dates of important past events, names of important political figures, or the locations of major cities.

Mood and personality   Judgments about personality, mood, affect, and insight should be made during history taking and examination. The appearance of the patient, content of conversation, and speed of movement provide the most useful clues to mood. Affect is signaled by language, facial expression, gestures, and posture, all of which should be studied closely. The presence of euphoria, disinhibition, or abulia should be noted.

Thought and problem solving   Incoherence of reasoning and logical thought will usually have been detected during history taking or testing of language skills and mathematics. More subtle disorder of thought is sometimes revealed by asking the patient to explain the meaning of well-known proverbs or sayings.

Cognitive scales   A number of scales (e.g., Blessed Dementia Scale; Mini-Mental State Examination) have been developed to make an approximate assessment of cognitive function. These are not true psychometric tests but questionnaires that can be completed fairly quickly by untrained staff to provide a score that roughly reflects the degree of intellectual and behavioral impairment. Another scale, the Ischemic Score, helps to distinguish multi-infarct from degenerative dementia. On the whole, these scales are less useful in diagnosis than a careful cognitive examination conducted in the manner described above.

ACUTE CONFUSIONAL STATES AND DELIRIUM

Acute confusional states occur in about 10 percent of all hospitalized patients and in 30 to 50 percent of hospitalized geriatric patients; patients with dementia are particularly vulnerable.

PATHOPHYSIOLOGY   *Neurologic diseases* cause confusional states in a variety of ways, including depression of consciousness. Consciousness is normally maintained by the ascending reticular activating system in the brainstem and thalamic regions (see Chap. 26). Focal diseases (such as a brain tumor or subdural hematoma) may depress consciousness by compression of the brainstem or thalamus or by producing hydrocephalus. Diffuse impairment of neuronal function (e.g., concussion or encephalitis) and multifocal disease (e.g., multiple metastases or multiple infarcts) also may present with confusion if the loci of disease cause several separate deficits of cognitive function with impaired attention. Usually lesions in both hemispheres are necessary, but occasionally a single right nondominant hemispheric lesion (usually a parietal infarct) presents with an acute confusional state because of impairment of attention, a predominant right hemisphere function.

Systemic diseases result in confusion from diffuse impairment of neuronal function. This may be due to inadequate supply of oxygen (hypoxia), glucose (hypoglycemia), or other factors required for metabolism, including vitamins and hormones. In metabolic encephalopathy, the mechanisms include acid-base disturbance, electrolyte imbalance, and circulating toxins (e.g., ammonia in liver failure). In systemic infections, there are several possible factors, including high fever, hypoxia, dehydration, and circulating bacterial toxins. Most drug-induced confusional states result from direct interference with synaptic transmission. In delirium following drug withdrawal, the excited state may result from the sudden exposure of neurotransmitter receptor sites.

In many cases of acute confusion, multiple mechanisms can be identified, particularly in the elderly. At any age, the brain may be made more vulnerable by preexisting brain damage, sleep or sensory deprivation, the effects of drugs, mild organ failure, or an unfamiliar environment.

CLINICAL FEATURES   Because most causes of the acute confusional state affect neuronal function diffusely, all aspects of intellectual function are impaired to a lesser or greater degree (see Table 25-1). The cardinal feature is *clouding of consciousness*, manifested by impaired alertness, awareness, and attention. This impairment is usually mild but can advance to coma if untreated. Depression of consciousness is distinguished from natural drowsiness by observing that the patient cannot be aroused easily. Reduced attentiveness can range from mild apathy and a failure to grasp complex details to reduced interaction with the examiner, lack of normal spontaneous comment or questions, and neglect of bodily needs. In delirium, arousal is evidenced by a readiness to respond to certain stimuli, insomnia, and excessive reactions to noise or bright lights. This is accompanied by a reduced ability to focus attention, distractibility, and inability to concentrate.

Variability in the level of arousal is a common feature of the acute confusional state. Reduced responsiveness may be interspersed with excited outbursts. Sleep-wake cycles are frequently disrupted or reversed, and confusion is often more marked during the night. The early symptoms of delirium often include insomnia and vivid, unpleasant dreams before a frank confusional state supervenes.

Impairment of memory with reduced digit span, poor recent memory, and defective recall for distant events is an important feature. One of the earliest signs of this impairment is disorientation for time and, later, disorientation for place. Knowledge of personal identity is usually retained if the patient can understand the question. The memory deficit is characteristically patchy so that distortions of memory (para-amnesia) and partially correct information may be incorporated into confabulatory answers or delusions. When the patient recovers, partial or total amnesia for the period of confusion is usual, although isolated events, especially vivid hallucinations, may be remembered in detail.

Impairment of cognitive function leads to difficulty performing tasks requiring logic, mathematics, or spatial organization. Thought processes are slowed, although the agitated delirious patient may have flight of ideas. Thinking is disorganized and disjointed. Speech is incoherent, rambling, and often inappropriate. Comprehension of complex material is impaired, and errors in the naming of objects or in writing may be elicited.

Impaired perception may compound confusion. The patient often misperceives surroundings and attendants as those more familiar to the patient. More concrete illusions and hallucinations are common, especially following drug withdrawal and in alcoholic delirium tremens. Hallucinations are most frequently visual but may involve any sensory modality.

Disturbances of emotion may include blunting of affect or emotional lability. Mood disturbances include dysphoria, depression, agitation, and fear, and these may be accompanied by appropriate autonomic responses. *Autonomic hyperactivity*, including tachycardia, diaphoresis, and anxiety, is marked in drug and alcohol withdrawal.

Psychomotor changes are common. In most patients, spontaneous motor activity is depressed, but hyperactivity and restlessness characterize delirium. Repetitive stereotyped motor behavior, such as plucking at the bed clothes or tossing from side to side, is frequent. *Involuntary movements*, including irregular tremor, asterixis, and myoclonus, are usually seen in drug withdrawal or metabolic encephalopathy. Rarely, patients show catatonic behavior.

DIFFERENTIAL DIAGNOSIS The first essential distinction to be made is whether the confusional state results from primary neurologic disease or as a complication of systemic illness (see Table 25-2). This distinction can often be made on examination but may require laboratory investigation.

Neurologic causes These can usually be recognized by the presence of focal neurologic signs in addition to disordered intellectual function. Examples include hemiparesis in *cerebral infarction*, neck stiffness in *meningitis* or *subarachnoid hemorrhage*, and gait disturbance in *hydrocephalus*. However, diffuse neurologic diseases such as *encephalitis, epileptic confusion*, or *small-vessel vasculitis* may cause no neurologic signs apart from the disorder of cognition. *Neoplasias* of the nervous system usually cause headache and focal signs, but midline tumors may present with a gradually evolving confusional state. Acute onset may be caused by brainstem compression or acute hydrocephalus.

Postictal confusion after a minor seizure lasts a few seconds and after a major seizure usually about an hour unless complicated by head injury, hypoxia, or status epilepticus. However, a persistent confusional state may occur with continuous or serial minor seizures *(minor epileptic status)* (see Chap. 367). Acute confusional states may accompany *encephalitis* or *brain abscess* without systemic signs of infection always being present.

Systemic causes Systemic causes are usually characterized by absence of focal neurologic signs apart from cognitive disorders, although minor signs such as reflex asymmetry or extensor plantar responses may be seen. An exception to this rule is occasionally seen in hypoglycemia, which may be accompanied in the elderly by hemiparesis. In *metabolic encephalopathy*, acidotic hyperventilation, tremor, asterixis, or myoclonus may suggest the diagnosis. *Wernicke's encephalopathy* (see Chaps. 377 and 390) should be considered in patients with a history of alcoholism or malnutrition. *Drugs* often cause confusion, especially in the elderly and those on multiple medications. *Endocrine dysfunction* (see Chaps. 331 and 334) rarely causes acute confusional state but should always be considered, particularly if there is hyponatremia. *Systemic infections*, especially *septicemia* and *subacute bacterial endocarditis*, can cause acute confusional states, particularly in the elderly, in whom fever may not always be evident, as can meningitis or brain abscess complicating the systemic infection.

Psychiatric causes In *anxiety*, extreme *grief*, or *depression*, orientation for person and place is usually preserved, and with encouragement, the patient can concentrate and improve cognitive performance. Hyperactivity, diminished need for sleep, pressure of speech, delusions, short attention span, and distractibility in *acute mania* may be confused with the hyperexcitability of delirium. Mania is characterized by a sustained elevation of mood and preservation of orientation. Hyperactivity persists throughout the manic episode in contrast to delirium, in which hyperactivity may be interspersed with somnolence. *Disassociative or hysterical disorders*, e.g., psychogenic

---

TABLE 25-2   Differential diagnosis of the acute confusional state

NEUROLOGIC (FOCAL SIGNS ARE COMMON)

Trauma
  Concussion
  Intracranial hematoma
  Subdural hematoma
Vascular disorders
  Multiple infarcts
  Right hemisphere or posterior circulation infarcts
  Hypertensive encephalopathy
  Vasculitis (e.g., systemic lupus erythematosus, polyarteritis nodosa, giant-cell arteritis)
  Air and fat embolism
  Subarachnoid hemorrhage
Neoplasia
  Multiple parenchymal metastases
  Meningeal carcinomatosis
  Midline brain tumors
  Brain tumors causing brainstem compression, edema, or hydrocephalus
  Paraneoplastic syndromes (limbic encephalitis)
Infections
  Meningitis and encephalitis (viral, bacterial, fungal, protozoal)
  Multiple abscesses
  Progressive multifocal leukoencephalopathy
Inflammations
  Acute disseminated encephalomyelitis
  Postinfectious encephalitis
Epilepsy
  Postictal state
  Temporal lobe status (complex partial status)

SYSTEMIC (FOCAL NEUROLOGIC SIGNS ARE UNCOMMON)

Substrate depletion
  Hypoglycemia
  Diffuse hypoxia
    Pulmonary
    Cardiac
    Carbon monoxide poisoning
Metabolic encephalopathy
  Diabetic ketoacidosis
  Renal failure
  Liver failure
  Electrolyte, fluid, and acid-base imbalance (especially Na^+, Ca^{2+}, Mg^{2+})
  Hereditary metabolic disease, e.g., porphyria, metachromatic leukodystrophy, mitochondrial cytopathy
Vitamin deficiency
  Thiamine (Wernicke's encephalopathy)
  Nicotinic acid (pellagra)
  B_{12} deficiency
Endocrine; over- or underactivity
  Thyroid
  Parathyroid
  Adrenal
Infection
  Septicemia
  Malaria
  Subacute bacterial endocarditis
  Focal infection, e.g., pneumonia
Thermal injuries
  Hypothermia
  Heat stroke
Hematologic disorders
  Hyperviscosity syndrome
  Severe anemia
Toxic causes
  Drug and alcohol intoxication (therapeutic, social, or illegal)
  Drug withdrawal, e.g., alcohol, barbiturates, narcotics
  Chemical toxins, e.g., heavy metals, organic toxins

PSYCHIATRIC

Acute mania
Depression or extreme anxiety
Schizophrenia
Hysterical fugue states

---

amnesia and fugue states, are usually distinguished from organic confusional states by the focal nature of the amnesia. *Acute schizophrenia* may simulate the acute confusional state, but consciousness, normal sleep-wake cycles, orientation, and attention are usually preserved (see Chap. 389).

INVESTIGATION Investigation is an urgent procedure. A *biochemical profile*, including blood sugar level, readily diagnoses the common metabolic disorders. A *blood count* detects hematologic disorders, and a neutrophilia suggests infection. If in doubt, a raised *erythrocyte sedimentation rate* supports the diagnosis of an organic disorder. *Arterial blood gas analysis* is a useful screen for hypoxia, respiratory failure, and acidosis. *Chest x-ray* and *blood and urine cultures* should be performed even if there is no fever. A complete infectious disease screen is indicated if there is a stronger suspicion of infection. *Endocrine tests* and *vitamin B$_{12}$* measurement may be indicated in individual patients. *Drug and toxicologic screens* are indicated for suspicion of drug overdose or toxic exposure. *Cerebrospinal fluid (CSF) examination* is mandatory in all patients with fever or neck stiffness so long as raised intracranial pressure or intracranial mass is not suspected and is also helpful in distinguishing metabolic from neurologic disease. The CSF white cell count is usually normal in metabolic disease, whereas leukocytosis implies neurologic disease, usually meningitis or encephalitis. The *electroencephalogram* (EEG) is useful if the presence of encephalopathy is uncertain; it is almost always abnormal in organic causes but does not necessarily distinguish between neurologic and systemic causes. Certain patterns may suggest metabolic disorders (particularly liver failure), encephalitis (especially herpes simplex), or epileptic status; and focal abnormalities may point to a stroke, abscess, or tumor. *Magnetic resonance imaging (MRI)* or *computed tomography (CT)* is not an emergency procedure unless examination or the EEG suggests a focal lesion but should be considered if no systemic cause is found after initial investigation.

MANAGEMENT The patient with acute confusional state is often agitated, and before the appropriate examination and investigations can be completed, the cooperation of the patient is required. Patients can frequently be calmed by a sympathetic and friendly physician. A relative or friend can often help and should be encouraged to stay with the patient. Nursing care should be given in a well-lit, relatively quiet environment with facilities for frequent observation. Sedation is seldom required. However, some agitated, violent, or paranoid patients may require a long-acting oral or intramuscular major tranquilizer such as chlorpromazine or haloperidol. For short-term sedation, such as during a CT or MRI scan, an intravenous benzodiazapine may be required. However, psychopharmaceutical agents may exacerbate an abnormal mental state or disguise the neurologic signs of deterioration.

Management begins with identification and correction of hypoxia, hypoglycemia, hyperthermia, or dehydration. Parenteral thiamine should be given to all patients suspected of Wernicke's encephalopathy. Later treatment depends on the underlying cause. If the confusional state does not resolve quickly, attention to hydration and nutrition is required to prevent perpetuation of the confusional state.

AMNESIA

PATHOPHYSIOLOGY The anatomic basis of memory is only partly understood, but it clearly involves the temporal lobes. Most lesions cause impairment of learning and recent memory loss without affecting immediate memory or attention. As a rule, significant amnesia occurs only after bilateral lesions of the medial temporal lobes. Unilateral lesions of the speech-dominant temporal lobe cause deficits of verbal memory, and unilateral lesions of the nondominant temporal lobe result in deficits in visual or nonverbal recall, but these deficits are rarely significant in the absence of preexisting contralateral temporal lobe pathology. The minimum lesion required to produce amnesia has not been established, but involvement of limbic structures appears crucial. Cholinergic neurons may play an important role. For example, anticholinergic drugs disrupt memory storage, and cholinergic drugs may on occasion improve memory.

CLINICAL FEATURES The classic example of amnesia is *Korsakoff's syndrome*, secondary to chronic alcoholism (see Chap. 377 and Chap. 390). The cardinal feature is an inability to recall new information despite a normal level of consciousness. Immediate memory, digit span, and attention are normal. Memory of knowledge acquired before the onset of illness is relatively intact, but memory for new events is severely impaired. Patients are disoriented in place and time and incapable of recalling information for more than the duration of immediate memory. They are thus condemned to be brief visitors to the present; their inner world consists only of memories of their remote past. On first encounter, they may seem relatively normal, taking part in ward routine and engaging in conversation. Because of intact immediate memory, they retain information briefly but forget as soon as they are distracted. In the pure syndrome, tests of intelligence not requiring long-term memory may be normal. Compensation is by confabulation, giving more or less plausible answers incorporating some relevant information and sometimes fantastic elaboration. Although characteristic, confabulation is not universal in Korsakoff's syndrome and may be seen in amnesia due to other causes as well as in acute confusional states. Amnesic subjects can slowly and laboriously learn some tasks, such as tactile or visual mazes, tunes on the piano, and the use of a computer. Despite evidence that the subjects acquire and·retain new skills, they do not recall learning and deny the new skills, demonstrating dramatically a disassociation between recollection and retention of information.

DIFFERENTIAL DIAGNOSIS The diagnosis of *Korsakoff's syndrome* is usually clear from its association with chronic alcoholism. It often follows an episode of Wernicke's encephalopathy, and the amnesic deficit becomes evident with recovery from the acute confusional state. Nonalcoholic causes of *thiamine deficiency* (see Chap. 377) may cause Korsakoff's syndrome. Similar clinical syndromes may occur after bilateral temporal lobe lesions resulting from *medial temporal lobectomy, head injury, herpes simplex encephalitis, strokes*, or *brain tumors. Alzheimer's disease* (see below) also may cause isolated amnesia before generalized dementia becomes evident.

Temporary amnesia is a common feature of *head injury* (see Chap. 376). The memory disturbance occurs both for events before *(retrograde amnesia)* and after *(posttraumatic amnesia)* the time of injury. *Anterograde amnesia* refers to impairment in learning new material, which accompanies posttraumatic amnesia. Almost invariably, retrograde amnesia causes permanent inability to recall the few minutes prior to the head injury, implying disruption of the immediate memory system and failure to register long-term memory. In severe head injuries, retrograde amnesia may extend back for hours or weeks. With recovery, the duration of retrograde amnesia shrinks and may resolve. During retrograde amnesia, remote memory is usually accessible. The length of posttraumatic amnesia generally corresponds to the length of postconcussive confusion and may continue despite normal immediate memory and digit span. The duration of posttraumatic amnesia indicates the severity of head injury, the ability to learn new material often being the last cognitive deficit to recover.

Transient global amnesia is a syndrome in which a previously well person suddenly becomes confused and amnesic. The attacks are usually spontaneous but occasionally follow immersion in cold or hot water, emotional stimuli, physical exertion, sexual intercourse, or travel in a motor vehicle. The patient appears bewildered and repeatedly asks questions about present and recent events. Orientation for person and sometimes place is preserved, but recent memory is impaired, and the patient cannot recall new information after a few minutes' delay. Behavior is otherwise normal and appropriate. Examination during an attack shows intact immediate memory but severe impairment of recall of recent and sometimes more distant events. General intellectual function is normal. By definition, no other neurologic signs are present. The attacks usually last 2 to 12 h. Headache, nausea, and vomiting may occur. Recovery is complete, and recurrence is unusual. The cause of transient global amnesia is a mystery. Similar symptoms may sometimes accompany migraine, temporal lobe ischemia or epilepsy. The disorder is usually benign; rarely, the attack is due to an underlying temporal lobe tumor.

Brief "blanks" in memory may cause difficulties in diagnosis. Occasionally, *complex partial seizures* may occur without the patient being conscious of any associated signs or loss of awareness, apart from the disruption of memory during the seizure. Amnesia also may rarely accompany *classical migraine*. A number of *drugs*, including alcohol and short-acting benzodiazepines, may impair memory and cause amnesia for events during the period of their use. *Electroconvulsive therapy* (ECT) causes temporary retrograde and anterograde amnesia.

Psychogenic amnesia for personally important memories is common, although whether this results from deliberate avoidance of unpleasant memories or from unconscious repression may be impossible to establish. This *event-specific amnesia* is particularly common after violent crimes such as homicide of a close relative or sexual abuse. It also may occur with severe drug or alcohol intoxication and sometimes with schizophrenia. More prolonged psychogenic amnesia occurs in *fugue states* that also commonly follow severe emotional stress. The patient with a fugue state suffers from a sudden loss of personal identity and may be found wandering far from home. In contrast to organic amnesia, fugue states are associated with amnesia for personal identity and events closely associated with the personal past. At the same time, memory for other recent events and the ability to learn and use new information are preserved. The episodes usually last hours or days and occasionally weeks or months while the patient takes on a new identity. On recovery, there is a residual amnesic gap for the period of the fugue.

MANAGEMENT The cause of temporary amnesia is usually evident from the history. In patients with transient global amnesia, investigations to exclude an underlying structural cause (MRI or CT), epilepsy (EEG), and vascular risk factors are appropriate. Unless the investigations are positive, reassurance is the only further measure required. The management of persistent amnesia is more demanding. Although Wernicke's encephalopathy responds to thiamine, established Korsakoff's syndrome does not, and the amnesia is usually permanent. Nevertheless, a course of thiamine should be given in newly diagnosed cases to prevent further deterioration.

DEMENTIA

Dementia is common, affecting about 4 million people in the United States alone. It is the major cause of long-term disability in old age. The prevalence of dementia increases rapidly with age, afflicting about 2 percent of the population between ages 65 and 70 and 20 percent of people above 80. With increasing longevity of the population and decreasing birth rates, the prevalence will continue to rise.

PATHOPHYSIOLOGY Some authorities separate dementia occurring before the age of 65 (presenile dementia) from that occurring after (senile dementia). This distinction was based on the assumption that the causes were different: rare neuronal degenerations in the young and vascular disease or senescence in the elderly. Although the expression of diseases may differ at different ages, the major findings in demented patients of all ages are similar, and the distinction is arbitrary.

Most diseases causing dementia are either widespread neuronal degenerations or multifocal disorders. The initial symptoms depend on where the dementing process starts, but the location and numbers of neurons lost that are required to cause dementia are difficult to establish. Aging results in a gradual loss of neurons and of brain mass, but this is not accompanied by significant intellectual decline in the absence of disease. Indeed, brain mass is a poor guide to intellectual function. Patients with a degenerative dementia in the sixth decade may have a greater brain mass than intellectually normal patients in their eighth decade. Consequently, documentation of generalized atrophy by CT scan is not a clear indication of dementia.

Dementia may result from cortical disease (e.g., Alzheimer's disease) or from disease of subcortical structures such as the basal ganglia, thalamus, and deep white matter (e.g., Huntington's disease or multiple sclerosis). Cortical dementia is characterized by loss of

cognitive functions such as language, perception, calculation; in contrast, subcortical dementia exhibits slowing of cognition and information processing (''bradyphrenia''), flattening of the affect, and disturbances of motivation, mood, and arousal. Memory is impaired in both types. The features of subcortical dementia also occur in cortical processes affecting the frontal lobes and probably reflect damaged projections to and from the frontal lobes.

In Alzheimer's disease, which is the most common cause of dementia, the dementia results from loss of cortical tissue especially in the temporal, parietal, and frontal lobes. This is accompanied in most cases by increased space between the gyri and enlargement of the ventricles. The histologic hallmark is the presence of numerous neurofibrillary tangles and senile plaques (see Chap. 370). Plaques and tangles are found in normal elderly brains but are increased in number in Alzheimer's disease, especially in the hippocampus and temporal lobes. The hippocampal involvement probably accounts for the memory disorder, which may be partially mediated by a reduction in cholinergic activity. The activities of other neurotransmitters, including norepinephrine, serotonin, dopamine, glutamate, and somatostatin, are also reduced. These changes are accompanied by reductions in cerebral blood flow and decreased metabolism of oxygen and glucose.

DIFFERENTIAL DIAGNOSIS The causes of dementia are numerous (Table 25-3). However, a small number of diseases account for most cases. In most of the western world, Alzheimer's disease is responsible for 50 to 90 percent and vascular disease for 5 to 10 percent of cases of dementia referred to hospital. In Japan and parts of Scandinavia, vascular disease appears to be more prevalent than Alzheimer's disease, at least in hospitalized patients. Cerebral infarction contributes to intellectual loss in a further 15 percent of patients with Alzheimer's disease documented at autopsy (*mixed dementia*). Dementia attributed to ethanol abuse may account for 5 to 10 percent of cases. Metabolic disturbances, cerebral neoplasms, subdural hematoma, and normal-pressure hydrocephalus account for around 10 percent of cases, and Huntington's chorea accounts for about 2 percent. The remainder of causes, including Creutzfeldt-Jakob disease, are rare, accounting for less than 1 percent of cases. In human immunodeficiency virus (HIV) infection, dementia occurs in 30 to 40 percent of patients and is an important cause in younger patients. Diffuse Lewy body disease increasingly is recognized as a cause of a degenerative dementia, although it remains unclear whether it is an entity or a variant of Alzheimer's disease (see Chap. 370).

The main aim of diagnosis is to identify treatable causes of dementia. The differential diagnosis depends primarily on a careful history and examination, supported by investigation. Illnesses that cause dementia can be divided into those in which dementia is the primary manifestation of the disease (other neurologic signs are absent), those in which dementia is secondary to other neurologic disorders (additional neurologic findings are usually present), and systemic diseases in which dementia is usually associated with signs outside the central nervous system.

In the elderly, dementia must be distinguished from the minor degree of forgetfulness that accompanies aging (*age-associated memory impairment* or *benign senescent forgetfulness*); the latter is often accompanied by slowing of physical and mental agility and rigidity of thinking. This is by no means universal with aging and may reflect an unidentified disease process. Benign senescent forgetfulness is not disabling in the activities of daily life and does not progress to more severe disability. Early on, dementias are often indistinguishable from benign senescence, and it is only the young age of the patient or progression of the symptoms that confirms the diagnosis of dementia.

Primary dementia The diagnosis of *Alzheimer's disease* is only certain at autopsy but is suggested by the characteristic history and signs, supported by negative investigations excluding other causes of dementia. Series of well-investigated patients with dementia attributed to Alzheimer's disease always include cases with an alternative diagnosis established at autopsy. The term *dementia of Alzheimer type* is sometimes used for patients with the characteristic clinical

TABLE 25-3 Differential diagnosis of dementia

Primary dementia with no other signs
   Alzheimer's disease
   Pick's disease
   Frontal lobe degeneration
Dementia with signs of vascular disease
   Multi-infarct dementia*
   Thalamic infarction
   "Binswanger's disease"* and lacunar state*
   Vasculitis,* e.g., systemic lupus erythematosus, polyarteritis nodosa,
      granulomatous angiitis of the central nervous system, Behçet's disease
Dementia with evidence of chronic infection†
   Human immunodeficiency virus
   Syphilis*
   Papovavirus (progressive multifocal leukoencephalopathy)
   Subacute sclerosing panencephalitis
   Creutzfeldt-Jakob disease (subacute spongiform encephalopathy)
   Tuberculosis,* fungal and protozoal infections*
   Sarcoidosis*
   Whipple's disease*
Secondary dementia with signs of the underlying neurologic condition
   Neoplasia and mass lesions
      Primary and secondary tumors*
      Carcinomatous meningitis
      Paraneoplastic encephalitis
      Chronic subdural hematoma*
      Hydrocephalus*
   Movement disorders
      Parkinson's disease
      Lewy body dementia
      Huntington's chorea
      Progressive supranuclear palsy (Steele-Richardson syndrome)
      Multisystem degeneration (Shy-Drager syndrome)
      Hereditary ataxias
   Motor neuron disease (amyotrophic lateral sclerosis)
   Multiple sclerosis
Dementia following diffuse brain damage‡
   Acute head injury
   Pugilistic dementia
   Anoxia
   Encephalitis
Endocrine disorders and vitamin deficiency
   Hypothyroidism*
   B_{12} deficiency*
   Thiamine deficiency*
   Nicotinic acid deficiency* (pellagra)
   Adrenal insufficiency* and Cushing's syndrome*
   Hypo-* and hyperparathyroidism*
   Chronic hypoglycemia*
Toxic disorders
   Drug and narcotic poisoning*
   Alcoholic dementia*
   Heavy metal intoxication*
   Organic toxins*
   Dialysis dementia*
Psychiatric
   Chronic schizophrenia
   Pseudodementia*
Additional conditions to consider in adolescents or young adults
   Movement disorders
      Wilson's disease*
      Hallervorden-Spatz disease
   Tuberous sclerosis
   Progressive myoclonic epilepsy*
   Metabolic diseases, e.g., leukodystrophies, mitochondrial cytopathy,
      storage diseases, Leigh's disease, homocystinuria

---

* Condition in which treatment may reverse or prevent progression of dementia.
† Systemic, hematologic or CSF findings suggest infection except in Creutzfeldt-Jakob
   disease.
‡ History of acute injury with depression of consciousness usual, except in pugilistic
   dementia.

picture and negative investigations in whom pathologic confirmation has not been obtained.

The mean duration from the onset of symptoms to death is 8 years, with a range of 2 to 15 years. The course may be more rapid in younger patients. The early features vary according to the initial brain site involved. The onset is insidious and subtle and can rarely be pinpointed. In most cases, insight is lost early, and intellectual failures are attributed to old age or oversight. Some patients have no spontaneous complaints but become disturbed when unable to answer simple questions. The history is almost invariably given by a relative. Early loss of spontaneity and initiative is frequent. The patient may give up hobbies and lose interest in social contacts or conversation. Lapses of memory, difficulty learning new information, and failure to remember names and appointments are noticed. At this stage, the memory deficit is more likely to involve recent events. In the early stages, social graces are usually preserved, and routine behavior and simple conversation are normal so that friends and relatives may be unaware that anything is wrong, unless the patient is tested by an unfamiliar situation or by a formal examination of cognitive function. As the disease progresses, inexplicable mistakes are made in the activities of everyday life, and dress, appearance, and personal hygiene are neglected. Spatial disorientation may become evident, especially in unfamiliar surroundings. The patient may oscillate between apathy and unprovoked irritability or aggression.

Examination in the early stage usually shows impairment of memory for recent events with varying degrees of other deficits. The patient often appears puzzled in response to questioning. Primitive reflexes such as palmomental response or suck reflex may be present.

As the disease advances, the impairments of memory, speech, and behavior become so marked that patients are unable to care for themselves, repeat questions over and over again, and fail to recognize friends and relatives. Restlessness is common, especially at night, and patients become lost if allowed to wander. Delusions, paranoia, and hallucinations may occur. On examination at this stage, the patient remains alert but is disoriented to time and place and has poor memory for recent and distant events. Digit span is usually preserved. Speech lacks spontaneity and fluency and exhibits minor aphasic errors, and there is difficulty understanding complex commands. Nonfluent aphasia, especially in younger patients, may be striking. Motor and constructional apraxia and agnosia may be present. Extrapyramidal signs, including stooped posture, slow shuffling gait, generalized bradykinesia, and rigidity, are common. The tendon reflexes may be brisk, but extensor plantar responses are rare. Grasp reflexes may be elicited. In the last stage, the patient is immobile, mute, and incontinent. The patient no longer recognizes relatives, and testing of cognitive function is not possible. Seizures and myoclonus may become prominent. Weight loss and a shrunken appearance may precede death, often from intercurrent infection.

Pick's disease is characterized by circumscribed cortical atrophy, usually confined to the frontal and temporal lobes, associated with a characteristic histologic appearance of degenerating neurons in the cortex, basal ganglia, and brainstem, which contain Pick's bodies (see Chap. 370). The age at onset and course are similar to Alzheimer's disease. Patients with Pick's disease suffer slowly progressive dementia and in the early stages may show frontal-temporal lobe features uncommon in Alzheimer's disease, including personality and emotional changes, disinhibition, lack of restraint, poor social and inappropriate sexual conduct, and lack of foresight. Later, patients may appear euphoric or retreat into increasing apathy and abulia in association with nonfluent aphasia, which progresses to mutism. Some cases of Pick's disease are indistinguishable clinically from Alzheimer's disease, and some cases of Alzheimer's disease show a frontal predominance so that the distinction may only be made at autopsy. A similar picture of *frontal lobe dementia* may occur in association with primary neuronal degeneration in the frontal and anterior temporal lobes without the neuropathologic findings of either Alzheimer's or Pick's disease.

Vascular dementia   Usually vascular dementia results from multiple areas of discrete infarction and not from chronic diffuse ischemia. The term *multi-infarct dementia* emphasizes this distinction. The diagnosis of vascular dementia is strongly suggested by an abrupt onset, especially if there is a history of previous stroke. The course characteristically fluctuates with periods of improvement and stepwise deterioration, in contrast to the steady progression of Alzheimer's disease. Hypertension is usual in vascular dementia but rare in Alzheimer's disease. Nocturnal confusion, relative preservation of personality, emotional lability, somatic complaints, and depression are more common in vascular dementia but not diagnostic. Focal neurologic signs (other than those of the cognitive deficits), including pseudobulbar palsy, visual-field deficits, hemiparesis, or extensor plantar responses, may suggest vascular dementia but also may be symptomatic of other neurologic causes such as a tumor.

Multi-infarct dementia can result from all types of cerebral vascular disease but is most likely to result from recurrent bilateral cerebral embolism from the heart or carotid arteries. It also can occur as a result of bilateral brain damage after a single episode of severe hypotension or cardiac arrest. Multi-infarct dementia may occur with widespread involvement of small vessels by vasculitis, from a few strategically placed large cortical infarcts, or from multiple small infarcts in subcortical structures, such as occurs in the *lacunar state* secondary to hypertensive small-vessel disease (see Chap. 368). Hypertensive or atherosclerotic disease with thickening of the perforating deep vessels and capillaries supplying the subcortical white matter also may cause *Binswanger's disease (subcortical arteriosclerotic encephalopathy)*, in which dementia is associated with diffuse loss of subcortical white matter and enlargement of the underlying ventricle. In contrast to multi-infarct dementia, major stroke is unusual in Binswanger's disease, and examination shows features of subcortical dementia (see above), a characteristic small-stepped, wide-based gait (*marche à petit pas*), pseudobulbar palsy, and corticospinal signs.

Chronic infections Chronic infections are important to consider, since the dementia may be treatable. Infections of the CNS are usually associated with systemic manifestations, meningeal involvement, abnormal CSF, and abnormalities on MRI or CT scan. Cerebral *syphilis* was a major cause and should still be excluded in all patients (see Chap. 133). *HIV* infection is an important cause of dementia in young people (see Chaps. 279 and 375) but should be considered in all patients at risk. The dementia may be the first manifestation of the infection. Dementia also may arise from "slow" virus infections. *Subacute sclerosing panencephalitis* causes dementia in children and occasionally in adolescents due to persistent replication of the measles virus in the brain many years after initial infection (see Chap. 375). *Creutzfeldt-Jakob disease (subacute spongiform encephalopathy)*, a rare dementia, has been transmitted by a novel agent, known as a *prion protein*, to animals and to humans by corneal transplantation, neurosurgical instrumentation, or injections of growth hormone extracted from human pituitaries. In most cases, the route of infection is unknown. After incubating for several years, the illness occurs in middle or late life and progresses to death within months. The dementia is often combined with ataxia, corticospinal signs, abnormal movements, cortical blindness, and myoclonus (see Chap. 375). Bizarre behavior and hallucinations are sometimes striking. In contrast to most other infections of the nervous system, signs of intracranial inflammation are absent and the CSF is normal, but characteristic EEG abnormalities (repetitive complexes) may be helpful in diagnosis. A rare genetic disorder, Gerstmann-Schenker-Straussler disease, is caused by a mutation in the prion protein.

Neoplasia and mass lesions *Primary or secondary brain tumors* may present with dementia, particularly slowly growing, deep, midline tumors of the corpus callosum or frontal lobe. Frontal meningiomas are the most important to consider in all patients because they are benign and the dementia is potentially curable. Other curable mass lesions include *chronic subdural hematoma*. The head trauma in such cases may have been remote, trivial, or forgotten, particularly in the elderly. Diffuse primary tumors and multiple secondary tumors also may cause dementia. Features of raised intracranial pressures (such as headaches or papilledema) and focal signs apart from the cognitive disorders may be absent, although minor signs such as a grasp reflex or extensor plantar response are often present. Most causes of dementia due to mass lesions or raised intracranial pressure are easily diagnosed from the MRI or CT scan.

Malignancy arising outside the nervous system also may cause dementia through *metastatic carcinomatous meningitis* or from a *nonmetastatic paraneoplastic encephalitis* (see Chaps. 328 and 369).

The latter condition usually begins insidiously and progresses slowly. Depression of consciousness is absent in the early stages, and psychiatric disturbances may be striking. The CSF is usually abnormal in these conditions.

Obstructive or communicating hydrocephalus in adults characteristically presents with subacute progressive dementia and is an important treatable cause. A history of headache may be obtained, and ataxia and gait disturbance are usual. Signs of raised intracranial pressure may be absent. The diagnosis is hampered in the elderly by the difficulty of distinguishing the scan appearances of hydrocephalus due to abnormal CSF dynamics from hydrocephalus ex vacuo secondary to atrophy. However, the combination of dementia, urinary incontinence, and gait disorder suggests the syndrome of *normal- or low-pressure hydrocephalus*. In this condition, routine measurements of CSF pressure at lumbar puncture or ventriculography are normal, but intermittent waves of increased CSF pressure may be detected if patients are monitored for several days. Such cases may respond to ventricular drainage.

Movement disorders A number of degenerative neurologic diseases other than the primary dementias also may cause dementia, usually as a late manifestation. Movement disorders provide the largest group, of which the most common is *idiopathic Parkinson's disease*, where dementia develops in the late stages of the disease in 15 to 30 percent (see Chap. 371). Another important cause is Huntington's chorea, partly because the diagnosis has genetic implications (see Chap. 370). In these conditions, the cause of the dementia is usually evident from the history or clinical signs of the underlying neurologic disease, but very occasionally the dementia may be the only feature.

Diffuse brain damage In dementia secondary to *head injury*, *anoxia, hypoglycemia*, or *encephalitis*, the cause is usually obvious from the history. The initial insult almost invariably causes loss of consciousness, and the dementia becomes evident when consciousness is regained after prolonged coma. If the patient recovers but then declines intellectually, the possibility of a secondary cause of dementia such as hydrocephalus should be considered. Repeated, less severe head trauma, such as occurs in boxers, may lead later in life to dementia associated with extrapyramidal signs, dysarthria, and ataxia (*dementia pugilistica*, or the "punch drunk" syndrome).

Endocrine disorders and vitamin deficiency Imbalances sufficient to affect neuronal function usually cause an acute confusional state with disturbance of attention and consciousness, but on occasion the presentation may be more chronic and mimic dementia. These conditions are treatable and cause reversible dementia, and they must be excluded in all patients. *Hypothyroidism* is the most common endocrine condition to present with dementia.

Toxic disorders Intoxications usually present with acute confusional state, often fluctuating according to the exposure. However, chronic intoxication may result in a reversible dementia. *Drugs* are an important cause, especially in the elderly, and the medication history should be carefully reviewed. The list of potential agents is large and includes drugs of abuse, psychotherapeutic agents (including barbiturates, sleeping tablets, tranquilizers, and antidepressants), drugs used in Parkinson's disease (levodopa and anticholinergics), and anticonvulsants. *Alcohol* is the most prevalent intoxicant implicated in dementia. Chronic inebriation results in reversible intellectual impairment but also may lead to a persistent deficit. In some cases, this is pure amnesia due to Korsakoff's psychosis, but in others it is a global dementia associated with cerebral atrophy. Factors accounting for dementia in alcoholics include vitamin deficiency, repeated head injury, anoxia or hypoglycemia during alcoholic stupor, chronic liver failure, or the rare complication of *Marchiafava-Bignami disease*, which causes widespread demyelination in the cerebral hemispheres.

Dementia in adolescents and young adults This requires consideration of a further group of conditions in addition to those already mentioned (Table 25-3). Late presentation of *Wilson's disease* is another important example of a treatable dementia and should be excluded in all patients under the age of 40. Metabolic diseases are the largest group. There is usually evidence of a systemic disorder such as a peripheral neuropathy, myopathy, retinopathy, or hepatosplenomegaly. Specific diagnosis relies on special investigation.

Pseudodementias Nonorganic causes of apparent intellectual decline are not rare, although it is probably more frequent for organic dementia to be misdiagnosed initially as a psychiatric illness. A mistaken diagnosis is particularly common in the elderly, in whom the behavioral changes of dementia may be attributed to depression. Conversely, the severely depressed patient may appear disoriented and perform poorly in all aspects of intellectual function. These deficits are caused by the psychomotor retardation, apathy, and loss of interest that accompanies depression. Such intellectual impairments may be due to reversible neurochemical changes that mimic the irreversible changes of degenerative dementias. The distinction may be difficult, but the correct diagnosis of depression is often suggested by a history of sudden onset, marked sleep disturbance, a previous history of psychiatric illness, or precipitation by an emotional event. In addition, depressed patients often complain to a greater extent about difficulties with mentation that seem justified from their performance on tests of intellectual function. In contrast, the patient with true dementia rarely complains appropriately about deficits that are obvious on examination. Dementia due to depression also may be suggested by inconsistency during the history; for example, patients may give a clear account of some topic of interest to them or recount the history and details of their personal lives reasonably well but then show inconsistent difficulties with specific questions, often failing even to attempt an answer. Variability in performance during testing, particularly improvement with encouragement, is characteristic. Negative neurologic investigation supports the diagnosis of pseudodementia but also may be found in organic dementia. The only way to confirm the diagnosis is to demonstrate improvement in intellectual functioning with appropriate psychiatric treatment (see Chap. 389).

Pseudodementias also may occur as a *hysterical phenomenon*, when amnesia is often striking. In one variety, Ganser syndrome, the answers to simple questions are often inaccurate, but the patient may retain a sense of the purpose of the question (''approximate'' answers), indicating that, despite the absurdity of the answer, the question is understood and the correct answer is known to the patient. In hysterical pseudodementia and Ganser syndrome, the apparent severe disturbance of intellect is not reflected in the patient's behavior. Frank simulation of dementia is rare, although the distinction between hysteria and malingering is not always clear. Intellectual impairment is a feature of *mania* and *schizophrenia;* the diagnosis is made from the accompanying thought disorder (see Chap. 389).

INVESTIGATION The age, history, and clinical findings will dictate the selection of screening tests. Investigations essential in all patients are aimed at excluding reversible causes of dementia. These include a full blood count, biochemical profile, thyroid function tests, serum vitamin B_{12}, and red cell folate. Syphilis and HIV serology also may be indicated. Ideally, every patient with dementia should have an *MRI* or *CT scan* to exclude treatable intracranial pathology, especially in the presence of focal clinical signs, a history of subacute illness, or a younger age of patient. Scanning is less likely to influence management if the patient is elderly and has a long history of degenerative dementia. In Alzheimer's disease, the scan may show progressive cortical atrophy and ventricular dilatation, but this is not invariable and also can be found in normal aging. The CT or MRI may show areas of low attenuation or abnormal signal in the deep white matter, particularly in the periventricular regions and centrum semiovale, referred to by the descriptive term *leukoaraiosis*. These findings are characteristic of Binswanger's disease but also can be seen in Alzheimer's disease, cerebrovascular disease, and in apparently normal subjects. The *EEG* may show features that support the diagnosis of Alzheimer's disease, subacute sclerosing panencephalitis, or Creutzfeldt-Jakob disease. *CSF examination* is normal in the primary degenerative dementias but may be useful if there is doubt about the diagnosis and is essential if there is a suspicion of intracranial infection. *Regional cerebral blood flow studies* (e.g., single-photon

or positron emission CT) may sometimes be useful in distinguishing between frontal lobe dementias and Alzheimer's disease or in demonstrating multifocal deficits in vascular dementia. *Cerebral angiography* is rarely helpful except for the investigation of suspected vascular dementia, vasculitis, or intracranial masses. *Neuropsychologic testing* (such as the Wechsler Adult Intelligence Scale) may help document intellectual decline or identify pseudodementia. *Meningeal and brain biopsy* may occasionally be justified when infection, vasculitis, or treatable tumor is suspected and occasionally in younger patients when etiology remains in doubt.

MANAGEMENT The initial management includes treatment of any reversible cause of dementia or superimposed confusional state. About 10 percent of patients with dementia have a treatable neurologic or systemic illness, 10 percent have pseudodementia due to treatable psychiatric illnesses, and 10 percent have a modifiable contributory cause such as alcoholism or hypertension. Unfortunately, the remainder have irreversible dementia so that management aims to support the patient and the family.

The mildly demented patient may continue relatively normal activities at home but rarely at work. As the dementia progresses, more supervision is required. As the disorder deepens, the patient requires increasing help with the activities of daily life. Some fairly severely impaired patients can live alone if they have support from the community, including daily visits from family or friends, regular visits by a community nurse, the provision of meals, and help from neighbors. Many mildly demented individuals become disoriented and confused when removed to unfamiliar surroundings such as a hospital.

In the early stages the patient may be helped by treatment of associated depression, anxiety, agitation, psychotic symptoms, or insomnia with appropriate psychotropic medication. However, psychotropic drugs may make demented patients more confused, requiring reduction or withdrawal of the medication. The demands on relatives caring for a severely demented patient are high, especially if the patient is restless at night and requires constant supervision to prevent wandering or personal harm. The fact that individuals may live for many years in such a state increases the burden. The situation often becomes intolerable when incontinence develops. Sleep deprivation and physical exhaustion aggravate the stress of caring for a demented relative, who may appear ungrateful, cantankerous, aggressive, or disinhibited. Sympathetic attention to the relatives of the demented is therefore important. It may help to obtain a ''baby sitter'' to allow the caregiver regular time off. If the caregiver can do so without undue feelings of guilt, an annual holiday while the patient is placed temporarily in a nursing home is invaluable.

Eventually, many demented patients require full-time nursing care in a residential home or hospital. Relatives should be encouraged to plan for this and should be counseled not to regard this outcome as a personal failure. In the later stages, management aims at preserving the patient's dignity and comfort.

REFERENCES

Brown MM, Hachinski VC: Vascular dementia. Curr Opinion Neurol Neurosurg 2:78, 1989

Cummings JL: Subcortical dementia: Neuropsychology, neuropsychiatry, and pathophysiology. Br J Psychiatry 149:682, 1989

Consensus Conference: Differential diagnosis of dementing diseases. JAMA 258:3411, 1987

Davies DC: Alzheimer's disease: Towards an understanding of the aetiology and pathogenesis, in *Current Problems in Neurology II*. London, Libbey, 1989

Dobkin BH, Hanlon R: Dopamine agonist treatment of antegrade amnesia from a mediobasal forebrain injury. Ann Neurol 33:313, 1993

Erickson KR: Amnestic disorders: Pathophysiology and patterns of memory dysfunction. West J Med 152:159, 1990

Fibiger HC: Cholinergic mechanisms in learning, memory and dementia: A review of recent evidence. Trends Neurosci 14:220, 1991

Gustafson L: Frontal lobe degeneration of non-Alzheimer type. Clinical picture and differential diagnosis. Arch Geront Geriat 6:209, 1987

Ho DD et al: The acquired immunodeficiency syndrome (AIDS) dementia complex (clinical conference). Ann Intern Med 111:400, 1989

HODGES JR, WARLOW CP: The aetiology of transient global amnesia: A case-control study of 114 cases with prospective follow-up. Brain 113:639, 1990

KOPELMAN MD: Amnesia: Organic and psychogenic. Br J Psychiatry 150:428, 1987

KRITCHEVSKY M, SQUIRE LR: Permanent global amnesia with unknown etiology. Neurology 43:326, 1993

LIPOWSKI ZJ: Delirium in the elderly patient. N Engl J Med 320:578, 1989

LISHMAN WA: Organic Psychiatry: The Psychological Consequences of Cerebral Disorder, 2d ed. Oxford, Blackwell, 1987

MALETTA GJ: Treatment considerations for Alzheimer's disease and related dementing illnesses. Clin Geriatr Med 4:699, 1988

ROMAN GC: Senile dementia of the Binswanger type: A vascular form of dementia in the elderly. JAMA 258:1782, 1987

ROTH M, IVERSEN LL (eds): Alzheimer's disease and related disorders. Br Med Bull 42:1, 1986

SCHOLTZ CL: Dementia in middle and late life. Curr Top Pathol 76:105, 1988

TATEMICHI TK et al: Clinical determinants of dementia related to stroke. Ann Neurol 33:568, 1993

WADE JPH, HACHINSKI VC: Multi-infarct dementia, in Dementia (Medicine in Old Age), BM Pitt (ed). London, Churchill Livingstone, 1987, pp 209–228

26 COMA AND OTHER DISORDERS OF CONSCIOUSNESS

ALLAN H. ROPPER / JOSEPH B. MARTIN

Coma is a common problem in general medicine; it is estimated that up to 3 percent of admissions to the emergency ward of large municipal hospitals are due to diseases that cause a disorder of consciousness. The importance of this class of neurologic disorders requires acquiring a systematic approach to their diagnosis and management.

The increased availability of computed tomography (CT) and magnetic resonance imaging (MRI) has focused attention on lesions that are radiologically detectable (e.g., hemorrhages, tumors, or hydrocephalus) in the diagnosis of coma. This approach, although at times expedient, is often imprudent because most coma is metabolic or toxic in origin. The physician confronted with an unresponsive patient should formulate a differential diagnosis based on the history and the clinical signs. The findings on general and neurologic examination allow the physician to narrow the possibilities responsible for the comatose state. A rational approach to defining the precise diagnosis and planning subsequent management can then be initiated and clinical changes anticipated. This chapter describes a practical approach to coma based on the anatomy and physiology of consciousness, the general and neurologic examination, and neuroimaging.

Coma is characterized by unresponsiveness and as such is easily recognized. A narrative description of the clinical state of the patient and of responses evoked by various stimuli, precisely as they are observed at the bedside, remains the optimal way to characterize coma and related disturbances of consciousness. Such a description is preferable to summary terms such as *semicoma* or *obtundation*, which are often ambiguous and commonly differ between observers. *Stupor*, as currently used, implies a state from which the patient can be aroused by vigorous stimuli, but verbal responses are slow or absent and the patient makes some effort to avoid uncomfortable stimuli; *coma* suggests a state from which the patient cannot be aroused by stimulation, and no purposeful attempt is made to avoid painful stimuli.

Although the definition of consciousness is a psychological and philosophical matter, the distinction between *level* of consciousness, or wakefulness, and *content* of consciousness, or awareness, has physiologic significance. Wakefulness or alertness is maintained by a diffuse system of upper brainstem and thalamic neurons, the reticular activating system (RAS), and its connections to the cerebral hemispheres. Therefore, depression of either hemispheral or RAS activity may cause reduced wakefulness. *Awareness* is dependent on integrated and organized material thoughts, subjective experience, emotions, and mental processes, each of which resides to some extent in anatomically defined regions of the brain. The inability to maintain a coherent sequence of thoughts, accompanied usually by inattention, is called *confusion* and is a disorder of content of consciousness (see Chap. 25). In special cases confusion is accompanied by illusions (misperceptions of environmental sight, sound, or touch) or hallucinations (spontaneous endogenous perceptions). The confused patient is usually subdued, not inclined to speak, and less active physically than usual. Psychiatrists use the term *delirium* for any confusion, but neurologists prefer to use delirium as a description for an agitated, hypersympathotonic, frequently hallucinatory state most often due to alcohol or drug withdrawal. Many processes that ultimately lead to coma begin with confusion or delirium, and diagnostic considerations should address the primary problem as an alteration in the level of consciousness. Focal cerebral lesions that cause deficits in language, orientation, or memory may make the patient appear to be confused (see Chap. 27).

ANATOMIC CORRELATES OF CONSCIOUSNESS A normal level of consciousness (wakefulness) depends on activation of the cerebral hemispheres by groups of neurons located in the brainstem RAS. All these components and the connections between them must be preserved for normal consciousness. The principal causes of coma are, therefore, (1) bilateral hemispheral damage or suppression by hypoxia, hypoglycemia, drugs, or toxins or (2) a brainstem lesion or metabolic derangement that damages or suppresses the RAS.

Reticular activating system The RAS is defined as a physiologic system, not an anatomic one. It is contained within the rostral reticular formation, which consists of loosely grouped neurons located bilaterally in the medial tegmental gray matter of the brainstem and extending from the medulla to the diencephalon. These neurons have been shown in neuroanatomic studies to span long rostrocaudal distances within the reticular formation. Animal experiments and human cliniconeuropathologic observations have established that the *neurons located in the region extending from the rostral pons to the caudal diencephalon are of primary importance for maintaining wakefulness.* Lesions here that produce coma also commonly affect adjacent brainstem structures concerned with control of pupillary constriction and eye movements (Fig. 26-1). *Abnormalities in these systems on physical examination provide signposts of brainstem damage.* Lesions confined to the cerebral hemispheres do not directly affect the brainstem RAS, although secondary dysfunction of the upper brainstem often results from compression by a mass in a cerebral hemisphere (see transtentorial herniation below).

Brainstem RAS neurons project rostrally to the cortex, primarily via "nonspecific" thalamic relay nuclei that exert a tonic influence on the activity of the cerebral cortex. Experimental work in primates suggests that the brainstem RAS indirectly affects the level of consciousness by suppressing the activity of the nonspecific nuclei. The basis of behavioral arousal by environmental stimuli (somesthetic, auditory, and visual) depends on the rich innervation of the RAS by each of these sensory systems.

The relay between the RAS and thalamic and cortical areas is accomplished by neurotransmitters. Of these, the influences of acetylcholine and biogenic amines on arousal have been studied most extensively. Cholinergic fibers connect the midbrain to other areas of the upper brainstem, thalamus, and cortex. These pathways are thought to mediate the clinical and EEG arousal observed after administration of cholinergic drugs such as physostigmine. Serotonin and norepinephrine also subserve important functions in the regulation of the sleep-wake cycle (see Chap. 29). Their roles in arousal and coma have not been clearly established, although the alerting effects of amphetamines are likely to be mediated by catecholamine release.

Cerebral hemispheres and consciousness The specialized functions of the cerebral cortex in language, control of movement, and perception are regionalized (see Chaps. 25, 27, and 28). In contrast, wakefulness is related in a semiquantitative way to the total mass of functioning cortex and is not focally represented in any region of the hemispheres, with the exception that large, purely unilateral

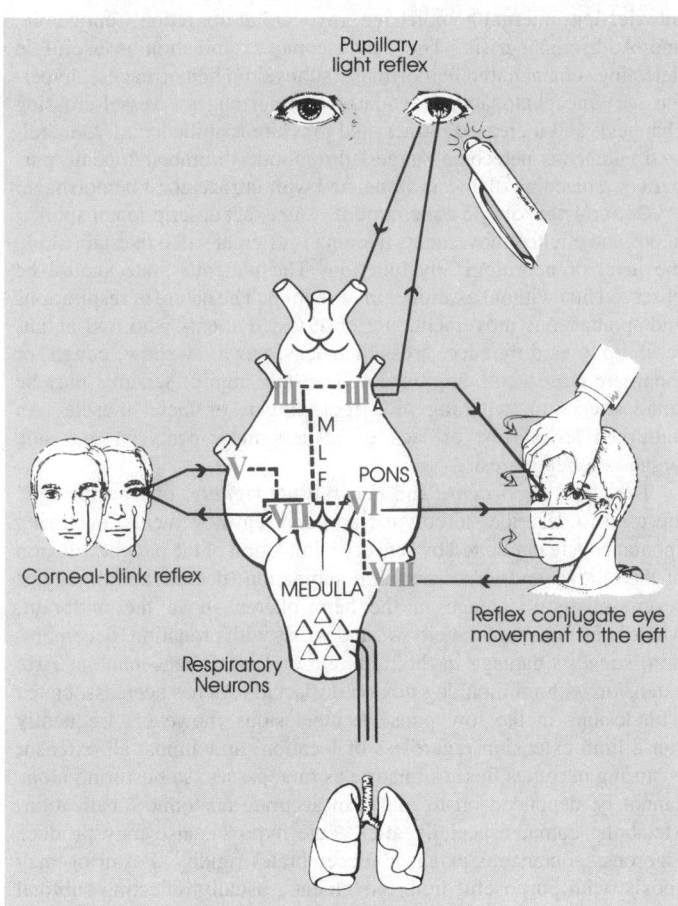

Pupillary
light reflex

Corneal-blink reflex

PONS

MEDULLA

Reflex conjugate eye
movement to the left

Respiratory
Neurons

FIGURE 26-1   Brainstem reflexes in the coma examination. Midbrain and third nerve function are tested by pupillary reaction to light, pontine function by spontaneous and reflex eye movements and corneal responses, and medullary function by respiratory and pharyngeal responses.

Reflex conjugate, horizontal eye movements are dependent on the medial longitudinal fasciculus (MLF) interconnecting the sixth and contralateral third nerve nuclei. Eye movements are elicited by head rotation (oculocephalic reflex) or caloric stimulation of the labyrinths (oculovestibular reflex). These reflex movements are suppressed in the awake patient by the cerebral hemispheres via their connections to the brainstem.

hemispheral lesions, particularly on the left, may cause transient drowsiness even in the absence of damage to the opposite hemisphere or RAS. Hemispheral lesions may cause coma in one of two ways: (1) most commonly, bilateral, generalized hemispheral lesions or metabolic derangements such as occur in encephalitis, hyperammonemia, hypoglycemia, generalized epilepsy, drug ingestion, global brain ischemia, and widespread traumatic damage interfere with awareness in a graded fashion and (2) large lesions in one or both hemispheres may compress the upper brainstem and diencephalic RAS causing coma indirectly. *The degree of decrease in alertness is related to the acuteness of onset of the cortical dysfunction or RAS compression.*

The concept of *transtentorial herniation* with progressive brainstem compression has been used to explain neurologic signs in coma caused by supratentorial mass lesions. *Herniation* refers to displacement of brain tissue away from a mass, past a less mobile structure such as dura, and into a space that it normally does not occupy. The common herniations seen at postmortem examinations are transfalcial (displacement of the cingulate gyrus under the falx in the anterior midline), transtentorial (medial temporal lobe displaced into the tentorial opening), and foraminal (the cerebellar tonsils forced into the foramen magnum). Uncal transtentorial herniation, or impaction of the uncal gyrus into the anterior portion of the tentorial opening, is thought to cause compression of the third nerve with pupillary

dilation. Subsequent coma is due to midbrain compression by the parahippocampal gyrus. Central transtentorial herniation denotes downward movement of the diencephalon (thalamic region) through the tentorial opening in the midline and is heralded by miotic pupils and drowsiness. These shifts in brain can cause an orderly progression of rostral to caudal compression of first the midbrain, then the pons, and finally the medulla leading to the sequential appearance of neurologic signs corresponding to the level damaged and to progressively diminished alertness. However, some patients with supratentorial masses do not follow these stereotypic patterns; for example, an orderly progression of signs from midbrain to medulla is rarely seen in catastrophic lesions, where all brainstem functions are lost almost simultaneously. Furthermore, drowsiness and stupor typically occur with moderate lateral shifts at the level of the diencephalon when there is only minimal vertical displacement of structures near the tentorial opening and before downward herniation is evident on CT or MRI scan.

PATHOPHYSIOLOGY OF COMA   The pathophysiologic basis of coma is either mechanical destruction of crucial areas of the brainstem or cerebral cortex (anatomic coma) or global disruption of brain metabolic processes (metabolic coma). Coma of metabolic origin may be produced by interruption of energy substrate delivery (hypoxia, ischemia, hypoglycemia) or by alteration of the neurophysiologic responses of neuronal membranes (drug or alcohol intoxication, toxic endogenous metabolites, or epilepsy).

The brain is dependent on continuous cerebral blood flow (CBF), oxygen, and glucose. CBF is approximately 75 mL per 100 g/min in gray matter and 30 mL per 100 g/min in white matter (mean = 55 mL per 100 g/min). Oxygen consumption is 3.5 mL per 100 g/min, and glucose consumption is 5 mg per 100 g/min. Brain stores of glucose provide energy for approximately 2 min after blood flow is interrupted, and consciousness is lost within 8 to 10 s. When hypoxia occurs simultaneously with ischemia, available glucose is exhausted more rapidly. When mean CBF is below 25 mL per 100 g/min, the EEG becomes diffusely slowed (typical of metabolic encephalopathies), and at 15 mL per 100 g/min brain electrical activity ceases. If all other conditions such as temperature and arterial oxygenation remain normal, CBF less than 10 mL per 100 g/min causes irreversible brain damage. The duration of ischemia is a major determinant of irreversible damage.

Coma due to hyponatremia, hyperosmolarity, hypercapnia, and the encephalopathies of hepatic and renal failure are associated with a variety of metabolic derangements of neurons and astrocytes. The toxic effects of these conditions on the brain are not well understood but may be multifactorial, producing impaired energy supplies, changes in resting membrane potentials, neurotransmitter abnormalities, and in some instances morphologic changes (see Chap. 377). For example, the high brain ammonia concentration associated with hepatic coma has been theorized to interfere with cerebral energy metabolism and the Na^+,K^+-ATPase pump, increase the number and size of astrocytes, result in increased concentrations of potentially toxic products of ammonia metabolism, and result in abnormalities of neurotransmitters, including possible "false" neurotransmitters, which may act competitively at receptor sites. Ammonia or other metabolites also may bind to benzodiazepine–γ-aminobutyric acid receptors to cause central nervous system (CNS) depression.

The exact cause of the encephalopathy of renal failure is also poorly understood. Unlike ammonia, urea itself does not produce CNS toxicity. A multifactorial cause is likely, including increased permeability of the blood-brain barrier to toxic substances such as organic acids and an increase in brain calcium or cerebrospinal fluid (CSF) phosphate content.

Abnormalities of osmolarity are involved in the coma and seizures caused by several systemic medical disorders, including diabetic ketoacidosis, the nonketotic hyperosmolar state, and hyponatremia. Brain water volume correlates best with level of consciousness in hyponatremic–hypoosmolar states, but other factors probably also play a role. Sodium levels below 115 mmol/L are associated with coma and convulsions, depending on the rapidity with which the hyponatremia develops. Serum osmolarity is generally above 350 mosmol/L in hyperosmolar coma.

Hypercapnia produces a diminished level of consciousness proportional to the P_{CO_2} tension in the blood and to acuteness of onset. A relationship between CSF acidosis and severity of symptoms has been established. The pathophysiologies of other metabolic encephalopathies such as hypercalcemia, hypothyroidism, vitamin B_{12} deficiency, and hypothermia are incompletely understood but probably reflect derangements of CNS biochemistry.

Central nervous system depressant drugs, anesthetics, and some endogenous toxins produce coma by suppression of both the RAS and cerebral cortex. For this reason, combinations of cortical and brainstem signs occur in drug overdose and other metabolic comas, which may lead to a specious diagnosis of structural brainstem damage.

Although all metabolic derangements alter neuronal electrophysiology, the disturbance of brain electrical activity most commonly encountered in clinical practice is epilepsy. Continuous, generalized electrical discharges of the cortex are associated with coma even in the absence of epileptic motor activity. Coma following seizures (postictal state) may be due to exhaustion of energy metabolites or be secondary to locally toxic molecules produced during the seizures. Recovery from postictal unresponsiveness occurs when neuronal metabolic balance is restored. The postictal state produces a pattern of continuous, generalized slowing of the background EEG activity similar to that of metabolic encephalopathy.

Endogenous "excitatoxins" such as glutamate released after injury have been found to cause secondary neuronal damage in experimental models of ischemia. These endogenous "neurotoxins" act to allow calcium influx into cells, a mechanism thought to lead to neuronal death. This mechanism may play a role in the genesis of coma, or at least in its neuropathologic changes, after global ischemia.

PRACTICAL APPROACH TO THE COMATOSE PATIENT   The diagnosis and acute management of coma depend on understanding the pitfalls of examining the comatose patient, an interpretation of brainstem reflexes, and the efficient use of diagnostic tests. Acute respiratory and cardiovascular problems should be attended to prior to neurologic diagnosis. The complete medical evaluation, except for the vital signs, funduscopy, and examination for nuchal rigidity, may be deferred until the neurologic evaluation has established the severity and nature of coma.

History   In many cases, the cause of coma is immediately evident (e.g., trauma, cardiac arrest, and known drug ingestion). In the remainder, historical information about the onset of coma is often sparse. The most useful historical points are (1) the circumstances and temporal profile of the onset of neurologic symptoms, (2) the precise details of preceding neurologic symptoms (weakness, headaches, seizures, dizziness, diplopia, or vomiting), (3) the use of drugs or alcohol, and (4) history of liver, kidney, lung, heart, or other medical disease. Telephone calls to family and observers on the scene are an important part of the initial evaluation.

Physical examination and general observations   The temperature, pulse, respiratory rate and pattern, and blood pressure should be measured. Fever suggests systemic infection, bacterial meningitis, or a brain lesion that has disturbed the temperature-regulating centers. High body temperature, 42 to 44°C, associated with dry skin should arouse the suspicion of heat stroke or anticholinergic drug intoxication. Hypothermia is observed with bodily exposure to lowered environmental temperature; alcoholic, barbiturate, or phenothiazine intoxication; hypoglycemia; peripheral circulatory failure; or hypothyroidism. Hypothermia causes coma only when the temperature is below 31°C. Aberrant respiratory patterns that may reflect brainstem disorders are discussed below. A change of pulse rate combined with hyperventilation and hypertension may signal an increase in intracranial pressure. Marked hypertension occurs in patients with hypertensive encephalopathy, cerebral hemorrhage, hydrocephalus, and acutely after head trauma. Hypotension occurs in the coma of alcohol or barbiturate

intoxication, internal hemorrhage, myocardial infarction, septicemia, and Addisonian crisis. The funduscopic examination is useful in detecting subarachnoid hemorrhage (subhyaloid hemorrhages), hypertensive encephalopathy (exudates, hemorrhages, vessel-crossing changes), and increased intracranial pressure (papilledema). Generalized cutaneous petechiae suggest thrombotic thrombocytopenic purpura or a bleeding diathesis associated with intracerebral hemorrhage.

General neurologic assessment   An exact description of spontaneous and elicited movements in coma is of great value in establishing the level of neurologic dysfunction. The patient's state should be observed first without examiner intervention. The nature of respirations and spontaneous movements are observed. Patients who toss about, reach up toward the face, cross their legs, yawn, swallow, cough, or moan are closest to being awake. The only sign of seizures may be small excursion twitching of a foot, finger, or facial muscle. An outturned leg at rest or lack of restless movements on one side suggests a hemiparesis.

The terms *decorticate* and *decerebrate rigidity*, or "posturing," are used to describe stereotyped arm and leg movements, occurring spontaneously or elicited by sensory stimulation of the patient. Flexion of the elbows and wrists and arm supination (decortication) suggest severe bilateral damage in the hemispheres above the midbrain, whereas extension of the elbows and wrists with pronation (decerebration) suggests damage in the midbrain or caudal diencephalon. Arm extension with minimal leg flexion or flaccid legs has been associated with lesions in the low pons. Acute lesions, however, frequently cause limb extension regardless of location, and almost all extensor posturing becomes flexor in nature as time passes, so posturing alone cannot be depended on to make an accurate anatomic localization. Metabolic coma, especially after acute hypoxia, also may produce vigorous spontaneous extensor (decerebrate) rigidity. Posturing may coexist with purposeful limb movements, usually reflecting subtotal damage to the motor system. Multifocal myoclonus is almost always an indication of metabolic disorder, particularly azotemia, anoxia, or drug ingestion. In an awake, confused patient, asterixis is a certain sign of metabolic encephalopathy or drug ingestion, particularly phenytoin.

Elicited movements and level of arousal   If the patient is not aroused by conversational voice, a sequence of increasingly intense stimuli is used to determine the patient's best level of arousal and the optimal motor response of each limb. Nasal tickle with a cotton wisp is a strong arousal stimulus. Pressure on the knuckles or bony prominences is the preferred and humane form of noxious stimulus. Pinching the skin over the face, chest, or limbs causes unsightly ecchymoses and is not necessary.

Responses to noxious stimuli should be appraised critically. Abduction avoidance movement of a limb is usually purposeful and denotes an intact corticospinal system to that limb. Stereotyped posturing following stimulation of a limb indicates severe dysfunction of the corticospinal system. Adduction and flexion of the stimulated limbs may be reflex movements and imply corticospinal system damage. Brief clonic or twitching limb movements frequently occur at the end of extensor posturing excursions and should not be mistaken for seizures.

Brainstem reflexes   Brainstem signs are a key to localization of the causative lesion in coma (see Fig. 26-1). As a rule, coma associated with normal brainstem function indicates widespread and bilateral hemispheral disease or dysfunction. The brainstem reflexes that are convenient to examine are pupillary light responses, eye movements, both spontaneous and elicited, and respiratory pattern. Pupillary reaction should be examined with a bright, diffuse light and, if the response is absent, confirmed with a magnifying lens. Light reaction in pupils smaller than 2 mm is often difficult to appreciate. Excessive room lighting mutes pupillary reactivity. Symmetrically reactive round pupils (2.5 to 5 mm in diameter) usually exclude midbrain damage as the cause of coma. An enlarged (greater than 5 mm) and unreactive or poorly reactive pupil results either from an intrinsic midbrain lesion (on the same side) or, far more commonly, is secondary to compression or stretching of the third nerve from transtentorial herniation or horizontal brainstem displacement. Unilateral pupillary enlargement usually denotes an ipsilateral mass but rarely occurs contralaterally, possibly by compression of the midbrain or third nerve against the opposite tentorial margin. Oval and slightly eccentric pupils often accompany early midbrain–third nerve compression. Bilaterally dilated and unreactive pupils indicate severe midbrain damage, usually from secondary compression by transtentorial herniation or from ingestion of drugs with anticholinergic activity. The use of mydriatic eye drops by a previous examiner, self-administration by the patient, or direct ocular trauma may cause misleading pupillary enlargement. Reactive and bilaterally small but not pinpoint pupils (1 to 2.5 mm) are most commonly seen in metabolic encephalopathy or after deep bilateral hemispheral lesions such as hydrocephalus or thalamic hemorrhage. This has been attributed to dysfunction of sympathetic nervous system efferents emerging from the posterior hypothalamus. Profound barbiturate-induced coma may produce similar-sized pupils. Very small but reactive pupils (less than 1 mm) denote narcotic overdose but also occur with acute, extensive bilateral pontine damage, usually from hemorrhage. The response to naloxone and the presence of reflex eye movements (see below) distinguish these. The unilaterally small pupil of a Horner's syndrome is detected by failure of the pupil to enlarge in the dark. It is rare in coma but may occur ipsilateral to a large cerebral hemorrhage that affects the thalamus. Lid tone, tested by lifting the eyelids, palpating resistance to opening, and speed of closure, is reduced progressively as coma deepens.

Eye movements are the second foundation of physical diagnosis in coma because their examination permits exploration of a large portion of the rostrocaudal extent of the brainstem. The eyes are first observed by elevating the lids and noting the resting position and spontaneous movements of the globes. Horizontal divergence of the eyes at rest is normally observed in drowsiness. As patients either awaken or coma deepens, the ocular axes become parallel again. An adducted eye at rest indicates lateral rectus paresis (weakness) due to a sixth nerve lesion, and when bilateral, it is often a sign of increased intracranial pressure. An abducted eye at rest, often accompanied by ipsilateral pupillary enlargement, indicates medial rectus paresis due to third nerve paresis. With few exceptions, vertical separation of the ocular axes, or *skew deviation*, results from pontine or cerebellar lesions.

Spontaneous eye movements in coma generally take the form of conjugate horizontal roving. This motion exonerates the midbrain and pons and has the same meaning as normal reflex eye movements (see below). Cyclic vertical downward movements are seen in specific circumstances. "Ocular bobbing" describes a brisk conjugate downward and slow upward movement of the globes associated with loss of horizontal eye movements and is diagnostic of bilateral pontine damage. "Ocular dipping" is a slow, arrhythmic downward movement followed by a faster upward movement in patients with normal reflex horizontal gaze and denotes diffuse anoxic damage to the cerebral cortex. The eyes may turn down and inward in thalamic and upper midbrain lesions.

"Doll's eye," or *oculocephalic*, responses are reflex movements tested by moving the head from side to side or vertically, first slowly then briskly; eye movements are evoked in the opposite direction to head movement (see Fig. 26-1). These responses are mediated by brainstem mechanisms originating in the labyrinths and cervical proprioceptors. They are normally suppressed by visual fixation mediated by the cerebral hemispheres in awake patients but appear as the hemispheres become suppressed or inactive. The neuronal pathways for reflex horizontal eye movements require integrity of the region surrounding the sixth nerve nucleus and are yoked to the contralateral third nerve via the medial longitudinal fasciculus (MLF) (see Fig. 26-1). Two pieces of information can be obtained from the reflex eye movements. *First*, in coma resulting from bihemispheral disease or metabolic or drug depression, the eyes move easily or "loosely" from side to side in a direction opposite to the direction of head turning. The ease with which the globes move toward the opposite side is a reflection of disinhibition of brainstem reflexes by damaged cerebral hemispheres. In drowsy patients, the first two or three head rotations cause opposite conjugate eye movements, following which the maneuver itself usually causes arousal and the reflex movements stop. *Second*, full conjugate oculocephalic movements demonstrate the integrity of brainstem pathways extending from the high cervical spinal cord and medulla, where vestibular and proprioceptive input from head turning originates, to the midbrain, at the level of the third nerve. Thus full and conjugate oculocephalic induced eye movements demonstrate the functional integrity of a large segment of brainstem and assist in excluding a lesion in the brainstem as the cause of coma. Incomplete adduction indicates an ipsilateral midbrain (third nerve) lesion or, alternatively, damage to the pathways mediating reflex eye movements in the MLF (i.e., internuclear ophthalmoplegia). Third nerve damage is usually associated with an enlarged pupil and horizontal ocular divergence at rest, whereas MLF destruction shows neither. Adduction of the globes is by nature more difficult to obtain with head turning than abduction, and subtle symmetric abnormalities in the "doll's eye" maneuver should be interpreted with caution.

Caloric stimulation of the vestibular apparatus (*oculovestibular* or *vestibuloocular response*) is a useful adjunct to the oculocephalic test and acts as a stronger stimulus to reflex eye movements. Irrigation of the external auditory canal with cold water causes convection currents in the endolymph of the labyrinths of the inner ear. With the head at approximately 30° elevation from the supine position, endolymph movement is induced primarily in the horizontal semicircular canals. An intact brainstem response is indicated, with variable latency, by tonic deviation of both eyes (lasting 30 to 120 s) to the side of cold-water irrigation. Bilateral conjugate eye movements have the same significance as full oculocephalic responses. If the cerebral hemispheres are intact, a rapid corrective conjugate movement is generated away from the side of tonic deviation. The absence of this saccadic, nystagmus-like quick phase signifies damage to the cerebral hemispheres.

Conjugate horizontal ocular deviation at rest or incomplete conjugate eye movements with head turning indicate damage in the pons on the side of the gaze paresis or frontal lobe damage on the opposite side. This phenomenon may be summarized by the aphorism "the eyes look toward a hemispheral lesion and away from a brainstem lesion." It is usually possible to overcome the ocular deviation associated with frontal lobe damage by oculocephalic testing. Seizures also may cause aversive (opposite) eye deviation with rhythmic, jerky movements to the side of gaze. On rare occasions, the eyes may turn paradoxically away from the side of a deep hemispheral lesion ("wrong-way eyes"). In hydrocephalus with dilatation of the third ventricle, the globes frequently rest below the horizontal meridian. Two types of rapid rhythmic eye movements may occur in stupor or coma. *Ocular myoclonus* is a rapid horizontal oscillatory nystagmus usually associated with a similar movement of the palate and due to damage to the central tegmental fasciculus, a longitudinal gray matter tract in the brainstem. *Opsoclonus* is an irregular, jerky, saccadic movement varying in direction that results from cerebellar lesions.

A major pitfall in coma diagnosis may occur when reflex eye movements are suppressed by drugs. The eyes then move with the head as it is turned as if locked in place, thus spuriously suggesting anatomic brainstem damage. Overdoses of phenytoin, tricyclic antidepressants, and barbiturates are commonly implicated as well as, on occasion, alcohol, phenothiazines, diazepam, and neuromuscular blockers such as pancuronium. The presence of normal pupillary size and light reaction will distinguish most drug-induced comas from brainstem damage (except for pontine infarction or hemorrhage, in which the pupils remain small). Small to midposition, 1- to 3-mm nonreactive pupils also may occur with very high serum levels of barbiturates or secondary to hydrocephalus (see below).

Although the *corneal reflexes* are rarely useful alone, they may corroborate eye movement abnormalities because they also depend on the integrity of pontine pathways. By touching the cornea with a wisp of cotton, a response consisting of brief bilateral lid closure may be observed. The corneal response may be lost if the reflex connections between the fifth and seventh cranial nerves within the pons are damaged. The normal efferent response is bilateral, with closure of both eyelids. CNS depressant drugs diminish or eliminate the corneal responses soon after the reflex eye movements become paralyzed but before the pupils become unreactive to light.

Respiration Respiratory patterns have received much attention in coma diagnosis but are of inconsistent localizing value. Shallow, slow, but well-timed regular breathing suggests metabolic or drug depression. Rapid, deep (Kussmaul) breathing usually implies metabolic acidosis but also may occur with pontomesencephalic lesions. Cheyne-Stokes respiration in its classic cyclic form, ending with a brief apneic period, signifies mild bihemispheral damage or metabolic suppression and commonly accompanies light coma. Agonal gasps reflect bilateral lower brainstem damage and are well known as the terminal respiratory pattern of severe brain damage. In brain-dead patients, shallow respiratory-like movements with irregular, nonrepetitive back arching may be produced by hypoxia and are probably generated by the surviving cervical spinal cord and lower medulla. Other cyclic breathing variations are not usually diagnostic of specific local lesions.

COMA-LIKE SYNDROMES AND RELATED STATES The simple observation of inability to arouse a patient characterizes most comatose states. Several syndromes, however, render patients unresponsive or insensate but are considered separately because of their unusual features. The *vegetative state*, an unfortunate term, describes patients who were earlier comatose but whose eyelids have subsequently opened giving the appearance of being awake. There may be yawning, grunting, and random limb and head movements but a complete inability to respond to commands or communicate. These are associated with signs of extensive damage to both cerebral hemispheres, i.e., Babinski signs, decerebrate or decorticate posturing, and absence of response to visual stimuli. Corrective nystagmus on oculovestibular testing fails to occur. Autonomic nervous system functions such as cardiovascular and thermoregulatory and neuroendocrine control are preserved and may be subject to periods of overactivity. The syndrome results from global damage to the cerebral cortex, most often in practice from global ischemia or head injury (see Chap. 376). *Akinetic mutism* refers to a partially or fully awake patient who is immobile and silent. The state may result from hydrocephalus, from masses in the region of the third ventricle, or from large bilateral lesions in the cingulate gyrus or other portions of both frontal lobes. *Abulia* is a mild form of akinetic mutism in which the patient is hypokinetic and slow to respond but generally gives correct answers. Lesions in the periaqueductal or low diencephalic regions may cause a similar state in which hypophonia is prominent. The *locked-in syndrome* (pseudocoma) describes patients who are awake but selectively deefferented, i.e., have no means of producing speech or limb, face, or pharyngeal movements. This results from infarction or hemorrhage of the ventral pons, which transects all descending corticospinal and corticobulbar pathways but spares the RAS arousal system, vertical eye movements, and lid elevation. Such eye movements can be used by the patient to signal to the examiner. A similar awake state simulating unresponsiveness may occur in severe cases of acute polyneuritis as a result of total paralysis of limb, ocular, or bulbar musculature. Unlike basilar artery stroke, vertical eye movements are not selectively spared.

Certain psychiatric states mimic coma by producing apparent unresponsiveness. *Catatonia* is a term for peculiar hypomobile syndrome associated with major psychosis. In the typical form, catatonic patients appear awake with eyes open but make no voluntary or responsive movements, although they blink spontaneously and may not appear distressed. There may be associated "waxy flexibility," in which limbs maintain their posture when lifted by the examiner. Upon recovery, such patients have some memory of events that occurred during their catatonic stupor. Patients with *pseudocoma conversion*

states have signs that indicate voluntary attempts to appear comatose. They may resist eyelid elevation, blink to threat when the lids are held open, and move the eyes concomitantly with head rotation, all signs belying brain damage.

LABORATORY EXAMINATION IN COMA Four laboratory tests are used most frequently in the diagnosis of coma: chemical-toxicologic analysis of blood and urine, CT or MRI, EEG, and CSF examination.

Chemical blood determinations are made routinely to investigate metabolic, toxic, or drug-induced encephalopathies. The major metabolic aberrations encountered in clinical practice are those of electrolytes, calcium, blood urea nitrogen (BUN), glucose, plasma osmolarity, and hepatic dysfunction. Toxicologic analysis is of great value in any case of coma where the diagnosis is not immediately clear. However, the presence of exogenous drugs or toxins, especially alcohol, does not ensure that other factors, particularly head trauma, may not also contribute to the clinical state.

The notion that a normal CT scan excludes anatomic lesions as the cause of coma is erroneous. Early bilateral hemisphere infarction, small brainstem lesions, encephalitis, mechanical shearing of axons as a result of closed head trauma, absent cerebral perfusion associated with brain death, sagittal sinus thrombosis, and subdural hematomas that are isodense to adjacent brain are some of the lesions that may be overlooked by CT. Nevertheless, in coma of unknown etiology, a CT scan should be obtained early in the evaluation. In those cases in which the etiology is clinically apparent, the CT provides verification and defines the extent of the lesion. With acute mass lesions, 3 to 5 mm of horizontal displacement of the pineal calcification from the midline generally corresponds to drowsiness, 5 to 8 mm corresponds to stupor, and greater than 8 mm corresponds to coma. As a supratentorial mass enlarges, the opposite perimesencephalic cistern is first compressed from lateral movement of the brainstem, the ipsilateral cistern is widened, and finally, both are compressed from the lateral mass effect. The lateral ventricle opposite the mass becomes enlarged as the third ventricle is compressed. These radiologic features of tissue shifts near the tentorial opening are helpful in correlating the clinical state with the progress of a mass lesion on scans (Fig. 26-2). They also suggest that transtentorial herniation is not necessary for upper midbrain compression and diminished consciousness. For technical reasons, MRI is difficult to perform in comatose patients, and it also does not demonstrate hemorrhages as well as CT (see Chap. 365). As MRI becomes more widely available and practical in comatose patients, some of the anatomic causes of coma that are not appreciated by CT scan, such as widespread white matter damage from trauma, will become better recognized.

The EEG is rarely diagnostic in coma, with the occasional exceptions of coma due to ongoing clinically unrecognized seizures, herpes virus encephalitis, and Creutzfeldt-Jakob disease. The EEG, however, may suggest metabolic encephalopathy and provide important information about the general state of the cortex. The amount of background slowing of the EEG is useful for gauging and following the severity of any diffuse encephalopathy. The EEG pattern of "alpha coma" is defined by widespread, invariant 8- to 12-Hz activity superficially resembling the normal alpha rhythm of waking but is unresponsive to environmental stimuli. Alpha coma results from either high pontine or diffuse cortical damage and is associated with a poor prognosis. Coma due to persistent epileptic discharges that are not clinically manifested may be revealed by EEG recordings. Normal alpha activity on the EEG also may alert the clinician to the locked-in syndrome. Computed on-line EEG analysis and evoked potential recordings (auditory and somatosensory) are currently under investigation as additional methods of coma diagnosis and monitoring.

Lumbar puncture is now used more judiciously than previously because the CT scan excludes intracerebral hemorrhages and most subarachnoid hemorrhages. The use of lumbar puncture in coma is limited to diagnosis of meningitis-encephalitis, occasional cases of subarachnoid hemorrhage, and cases with normal CT in which the

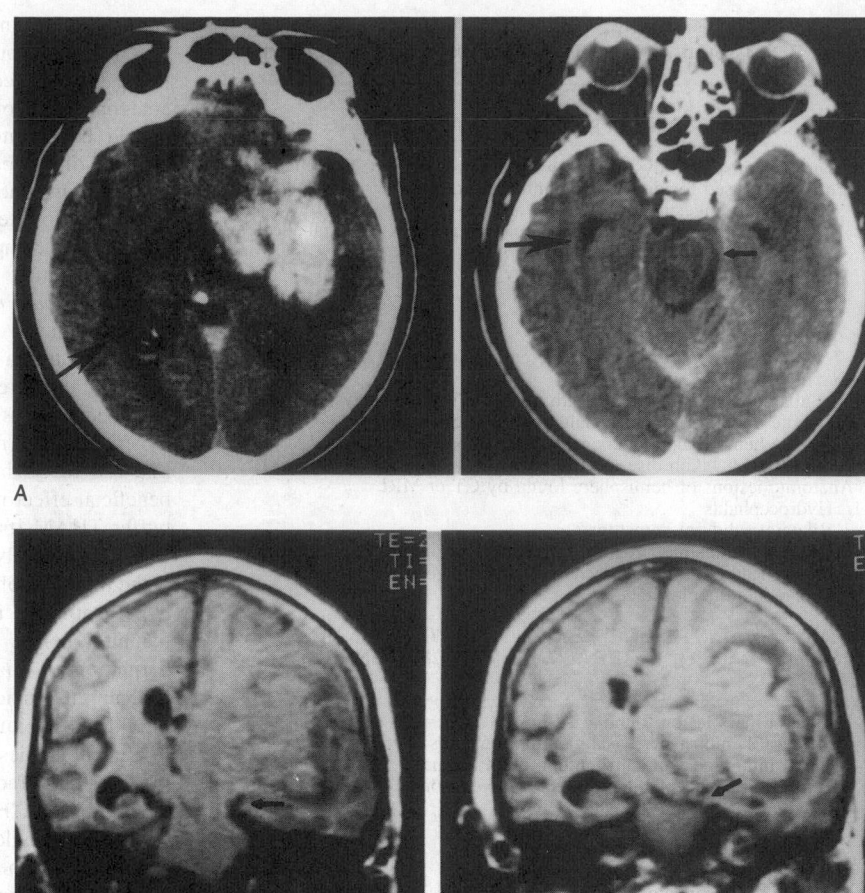

FIGURE 26-2 *A*. Axial CT scans from a comatose patient with a large cerebral hemorrhage showing the main radiologic signs of a unilateral intracranial mass. There is enlargement of the perimesencephalic cistern on the side of the mass (*small arrow*), compression contralaterally, and early enlargement of the lateral ventricle opposite the mass (*large arrow*). The pineal is shifted 8 mm from the midline. *B*. Coronal MRI scans from the same patient showing displacement of brain tissue across the midline, above the tentorium (*left, arrow*). The manner of horizontal displacement of the upper brainstem from a mass is appreciated, and the right scan shows a small uncal herniation (*arrow*).

origin of coma is obscure. If the CT is normal or unavailable and suspicion of meningeal infection or subarachnoid hemorrhage remains, then the CSF should be examined for white cells, microorganisms, and blood. In no case should lumbar puncture be deferred if meningitis is a strong clinical possibility. Xanthochromia is documented by spinning the CSF in a large tube and comparing the supernatant to water. Yellow coloration indicates preexisting blood in the CSF and permits exclusion of a traumatic puncture. In addition, initial and final tubes should be inspected for a decrement in the number of erythrocytes, indicating traumatic puncture.

DIFFERENTIAL DIAGNOSIS OF COMA In most instances, coma is part of an obvious medical problem such as known drug ingestion, hypoxia, stroke, trauma, or liver or kidney failure. Attention is then appropriately focused on the primary illness. A complete listing of all diseases that cause coma would serve little purpose, since it would not aid diagnosis. Some general rules, however, are helpful. Illnesses that cause sudden or acute coma are due to drug ingestion or to one of the catastrophic brain lesions—hemorrhage, trauma, hypoxia, or, rarely, acute basilar artery occlusion. Coma which appears subacutely is usually related to preceding medical or neurologic problems, including the secondary brain swelling that surrounds a preexisting lesion. Coma diagnosis, therefore, requires familiarity with the common intracerebral catastrophes. These are described in more detail in Chap. 368 but may be summarized as follows: (1) basal ganglia and thalamic hemorrhage (acute but not instantaneous onset, vomiting, headache, hemiplegia, and characteristic eye signs), (2) subarachnoid hemorrhage (instantaneous onset, severe headache, neck stiffness, vomiting, third or sixth nerve lesions, transient loss of consciousness, or sudden coma with vigorous extensor posturing), (3) pontine hemorrhage (sudden onset, pinpoint pupils, loss of reflex eye movements and corneal responses, ocular bobbing, posturing, hyperventilation, and sweating), (4) cerebellar hemorrhage (occipital headache,

vomiting, gaze paresis, and inability to stand), and (5) basilar artery thrombosis (neurologic prodrome or warning spells, diplopia, dysarthria, vomiting, eye movement and corneal response abnormalities, and asymmetric limb paresis). The most common stroke, namely, infarction in the territory of the middle cerebral artery, does not cause coma acutely. The syndrome of acute hydrocephalus causing coma may accompany many intracranial catastrophes, particularly subarachnoid hemorrhage. Acute symmetric enlargement of both lateral ventricles causes headache and vomiting followed by drowsiness that may progress quickly to coma, with extensor posturing of the limbs, bilateral Babinski signs, small nonreactive pupils, and impaired vertical oculocephalic movements.

If the history and examination are not typical for any neurologic diagnosis and metabolic or drug causes are excluded, then information obtained from CT may be used as outlined in Table 26-1. The neurologic examination remains preeminent because it allows localization of lesions to one or both hemispheres or to the brainstem (with the exceptions noted above). The CT scan is useful to focus the differential diagnosis, and because of its accuracy and general availability, the diagnoses which it facilitates are listed in the table. The majority of medical causes of coma are established without a CT or with the study being normal.

COMA AFTER HEAD TRAUMA Concussion is a common form of transient coma that probably results from torsion of the hemispheres about the midbrain-diencephalic junction with brief interruption of RAS function. Persistent coma after head trauma presents a more complex and serious problem (Chap. 376).

EMERGENCY TREATMENT OF THE COMATOSE PATIENT The immediate goal in acute coma is prevention of further CNS damage. Hypotension, hypoglycemia, hypoxia, hypercapnia, and hyperthermia should be corrected rapidly and assiduously. An oropharyngeal airway is adequate to keep the pharynx open in drowsy patients who are

TABLE 26-1 Approach to the differential diagnosis of coma

NORMAL BRAINSTEM REFLEXES, NO LATERALIZING SIGNS

A Bilateral hemispheral dysfunction without mass lesion (CT or MRI normal; primary test used for diagnosis is indicated in parentheses)
1 Drug-toxin ingestion (toxicologic analysis)
2 Endogenous metabolic encephalopathy (glucose, ammonia, calcium, osmolarity, P_{O_2}, P_{CO_2}, urea, sodium)
3 Shock, hypertensive encephalopathy
4 Meningitis (CSF analysis)
5 Nonherpetic viral encephalitis (CSF analysis)
6 Epilepsy (EEG)
7 Reye's syndrome (ammonia, increased intracranial pressure)
8 Fat embolism
9 Subarachnoid hemorrhage with normal CT (CSF analysis)
10 Acute disseminated encephalomyelitis (CSF analysis)
11 Acute hemorrhagic leukoencephalitis (repeat MRI)
12 Creutzfeldt-Jakob disease (EEG)
B Anatomic lesions of hemisphere found by CT or MRI
1 Hydrocephalus
2 Bilateral subdural hematomas
3 Bilateral contusions, edema, or axonal shearing of hemispheres due to closed head trauma, subarachnoid hemorrhage
4 Subarachoid hemorrhage

NORMAL BRAINSTEM REFLEXES (WITH/WITHOUT UNILATERAL 3D NERVE PALSY), LATERALIZING MOTOR SIGNS (CT OR MRI ABNORMAL)

A Unilateral mass lesion found
1 Cerebral hemorrhage (basal ganglia, thalamus)
2 Large infarction with surrounding brain edema
3 Herpes virus encephalitis (temporal lobe lesion)
4 Subdural or epidural hematoma
5 Tumor with edema
6 Brain abscess with edema
7 Vasculitis with multiple infarctions
8 Metabolic encephalopathy superimposed on preexisting focal lesions (i.e., stroke with hyperglycemia, hyponatremia, etc.)
9 Pituitary apoplexy
B Asymmetric signs accompanied by diffuse hemispheral dysfunction
1 Metabolic encephalopathies with asymmetric signs (blood chemical determinations)
2 Isodense subdural hematoma (MRI, CT with contrast)
3 Thrombotic thrombocytopenic purpura (blood smear, platelet count)
4 Epilepsy with focal seizures or postictal state (EEG)

MULTIPLE BRAINSTEM REFLEX ABNORMALITIES

A Anatomic lesions in brainstem
1 Pontine, midbrain hemorrhage
2 Cerebellar hemorrhage, tumor, abscess
3 Cerebellar infarction with brainstem compression
4 Mass in hemisphere causing advanced bilateral upper brainstem compression
5 Primary brainstem tumor, demyelination, or abscess
6 Traumatic brainstem contusion-hemorrhage
B Brainstem dysfunction without mass lesion
1 Basilar artery thrombosis causing brainstem infarction (clinical signs, angiogram)
2 Severe drug overdose (toxicologic analysis)
3 Brainstem encephalitis (CSF)
4 Basilar artery migraine

breathing normally. Tracheal intubation is indicated if there is apnea, upper airway obstruction, hypoventilation, or emesis, or if the patient is liable to aspirate. Mechanical ventilation is required if the patient is hypoventilating or if there is an intracranial mass and hypocapnia is therapeutically necessary. An intravenous access is established, and naloxone and dextrose are administered if narcotic overdose or hypoglycemia are even remote possibilities. Thiamine is generally administered with glucose in order to prevent an exacerbation of Wernicke's encephalopathy. The veins of intravenous drug abusers may be difficult to cannulate; in such cases, naloxone can be injected sublingually through a small-gauge needle. In cases of suspected basilar thrombosis with brainstem ischemia, intravenous heparin is administered after obtaining a CT scan, keeping in mind that cerebellar and pontine hemorrhages resemble the syndrome of basilar artery occlusion. Physostigmine, when used by experienced physicians with

careful monitoring, may awaken patients with anticholinergic-type drug overdose, but many physicians believe that this is justified only to treat associated cardiac arrhythmias. The use of benzodiazepine antagonists is promising for treatment of overdoses. Intravenous fluid should be monitored carefully in any serious acute CNS illness because of the potential for exacerbating brain swelling by excess water administration. Neck injuries must not be overlooked, particularly prior to attempting intubation or the oculocephalic maneuver. Headache accompanied by fever and meningismus indicates a need for examination of the CSF to diagnose meningitis, and *lumbar puncture should not be delayed while awaiting a CT scan.*

Enlargement of one pupil usually indicates secondary midbrain compression by a hemispheral mass and demands immediate reduction of intracranial pressure (ICP). Normal saline is the safest intravenous fluid because it is slightly hyperosmolar in most patients. Therapeutic hyperventilation may be used to achieve an arterial P_{CO_2} of 3.7 to 4.2 kPa (28 to 32 mmHg). This acts rapidly to reduce ICP, but the beneficial effect rarely lasts more than 1 to 2 h. The weak base and buffer THAM (tromethamine) may be a useful adjunct to keep the CSF alkalotic. Hyperosmolar therapy with mannitol or an equivalent is the mainstay of ICP reduction. It may be used simultaneously with hyperventilation in critical cases. It is generally best to administer mannitol before attempting to intubate a patient with impending herniation. A ventricular puncture is necessary to decompress hydrocephalus if medical measures fail to improve alertness. The use of high-dose barbiturates soon after cardiac arrest has not been shown in clinical studies to be beneficial, although they may still be useful in lowering intracranial pressure in other circumstances.

BRAIN DEATH Brain death results from total cessation of cerebral blood flow and global infarction of the brain at a time when respiration is preserved with artificial support and the heart continues to function. It is the only type of irrevocable loss of brain function currently recognized by law as death. Many sets of roughly equivalent criteria have been advanced for the diagnosis of brain death, and it is essential to adhere to those approved locally and recognized as standard practice. Ideal criteria are ones that are simple, conducted at the bedside, and which allow no chance of diagnostic error. Widespread cortical destruction is usually shown by unresponsiveness to the environment, midbrain damage by absent pupillary light reaction, pontine damage by absent oculovestibular and corneal reflexes, and medullary dysfunction by complete apnea. The pulse rate is invariant and unresponsive to atropine. Most patients have diabetes insipidus, but in some it develops after the clinical signs of brain death. The pupils need not be fully dilated but should not be constricted. The absence of spinal reflexes is not required because the spinal cord remains functional in many cases. Many centers use an isoelectric EEG as a confirmatory test for cortical death. The possibility of profound drug-induced or hypothermic CNS depression should always be excluded. Some period of observation, usually 6 to 24 h, is desirable during which this state is shown to be sustained. It is often advisable to delay clinical testing for up to 24 h if a cardiac arrest has caused brain death or if the inciting disease is not known.

The demonstration of apnea generally requires that the P_{CO_2} be high enough to stimulate respiration. This can be accomplished safely in most patients by removal of the respirator and use of diffusion oxygenation sustained by a tracheal cannula connected to an oxygen supply. In brain-dead patients, CO_2 tension increases approximately 0.3 to 0.4 kPa/min (2 to 3 mmHg/min) during apnea. At the end of an appropriate interval, arterial P_{CO_2} should be at least above 6.6 to 8.0 kPa (50 to 60 mmHg) for the test to be valid. Large posterior fossa lesions that compress the brainstem, CNS–depressant drugs, and profound hypothermia can simulate brain death, but adherence to recognized protocols for diagnosis will prevent these errors. Radionuclide brain scanning, cerebral angiography, or transcranial Doppler measurements also may be used to demonstrate the absence of cerebral blood flow in brain death. These techniques have the virtue of rapidity but, with the exception of Doppler, are cumbersome and have not been correlated extensively with pathologic material.

There is no implicit reason to make the diagnosis of brain death except when organ transplantation or difficult resource-allocation (intensive care) issues are involved. Although it is commonly accepted that the respirator can be disconnected from a brain-dead patient, most problems arise because of inadequate explanation and preparation of the family by the physician.

PROGNOSIS OF COMA   Interest in predicting the outcome of coma is oriented toward allocating medical resources and limiting the support of hopeless cases. To date, no collection of clinical signs except those of brain death assuredly predicts outcome of coma. Children and young adults may have ominous early clinical findings such as abnormal brainstem reflexes and yet recover. All schemes for prognosis should therefore be taken as only approximate indicators, and medical judgments must be tempered by other factors such as age, underlying disease, and general medical condition. In an attempt to collect prognostic information from large numbers of patients with head injury, a "Glasgow Coma Scale" has been devised that empirically has predictive value in cases of brain trauma (see Chap. 376). Major points include a 95 percent death rate in patients whose pupillary reaction or reflex eye movements are absent 6 h after onset of coma, and a 91 percent death rate if the pupils are unreactive at 24 h (although 4 percent make a good recovery).

Prognostication of nontraumatic coma is difficult because of the heterogeneity of contributing diseases. Unfavorable signs in the first hours after admission are the absence of any two of pupillary reaction, corneal reflex, or the oculovestibular response. One day after the onset of coma, the preceding signs, in addition to absence of eye opening and muscle tone, predict death or severe disability and the same signs at 3 days strengthen the prediction of a poor outcome. In many patients, precise combinations of predictive signs do not occur, and coma scales lose their value. The use of evoked potentials aids prognostication in head-injured and post–cardiac arrest patients. Bilateral absence of cortical somatosensory evoked potentials is associated with death or a vegetative state in most cases. Medical practitioners are becoming less reluctant to withdraw support from non-brain-dead but severely neurologically injured patients as predictions become more reliable and resources more limited.

REFERENCES

CELESIA GG et al: Persistent vegetative state—Report of the American Neurological Association Committee on Ethical Affairs. Ann Neurol 33:386, 1993
IVAN L, BRUCE D: *Coma.* Springfield, Ill., Charles C Thomas, 1982
JENNET B et al: Prognosis of patients with severe head injury. Neurosurgery 4:283, 1979
LEVY D et al: Prognosis in non-traumatic coma. Ann Intern Med 94:229, 1981
PLUM F, POSNER J: *The Diagnosis of Stupor and Coma,* 3d ed. Philadelphia, Davis, 1980
REICH JB et al: Magnetic resonance imaging measurements and clinical changes accompanying transtentorial and foramen magnum brain herniation. Ann Neurol 33:159, 1993
ROPPER AH: Lateral displacement of the brain and level of consciousness in patients with an acute hemispheral mass. N Engl J Med 314:953, 1986
———: Coma and acutely raised intracranial pressure, in *Diseases of the Nervous System,* 2d ed, A Asbury et al (eds). Philadelphia, Saunders, 1992
———: *Neurological and Neurosurgical Intensive Care,* 3d ed. New York, Raven, 1992

27   SYNDROMES DUE TO FOCAL CEREBRAL LESIONS

RAYMOND D. ADAMS / MAURICE VICTOR

In addition to the general syndromes described in Chap. 25, there are many others that relate to lesions of particular parts of the cerebrum. Recognition of the latter syndromes constitutes irrefutable evidence that all parts of the cerebrum are not functionally equivalent. Some of the symptoms and signs that make up these syndromes have the

same diagnostic value as a hemiplegia and, once identified, require the same type of clinical analysis as to cause and pathophysiologic mechanism.

These focal syndromes will be described in terms of the conventional anatomic divisions of the cerebrum, but it will be obvious that most diseases do not respect these boundaries. Furthermore, cerebral functions are not localized to discrete aggregates of cerebral cortical neurons but are organized in fairly widespread networks. A lesion in a particular part will cause a loss of function (negative symptoms), but the positive symptoms arising from the lesion are attributable to the now disinhibited functions of closely related intact parts of the cerebrum.

FRONTAL LOBES   In Fig. 27-1 it is seen that the frontal lobes lie anterior to the central (rolandic) sulcus and superior to the Sylvian fissure. They consist of several functionally different parts, which are conventionally designated in the neurologic literature by numbers (according to the scheme of Brodmann) or by letters (according to the scheme of von Economo and Koskinas).

The posterior parts, areas 4 and 6 of Brodmann, are specifically related to motor function. There is also a supplementary motor area, located in the posterior part of the superior frontal convolution and in close relationship to the anterior part of the cingulate gyrus. Voluntary movement in humans depends on the integrity of these

FIGURE 27-1   Diagram to show the cytoarchitectural zones of the human cerebral cortex (lateral surface) according to the scheme of Brodmann. Although the auditory association areas of Wernicke (areas 41 and 42) are shown on the lateral surface, they actually lie on the superior surface of the temporal lobe, deep within the sylvian fissure. *(From Adams and Victor.)*

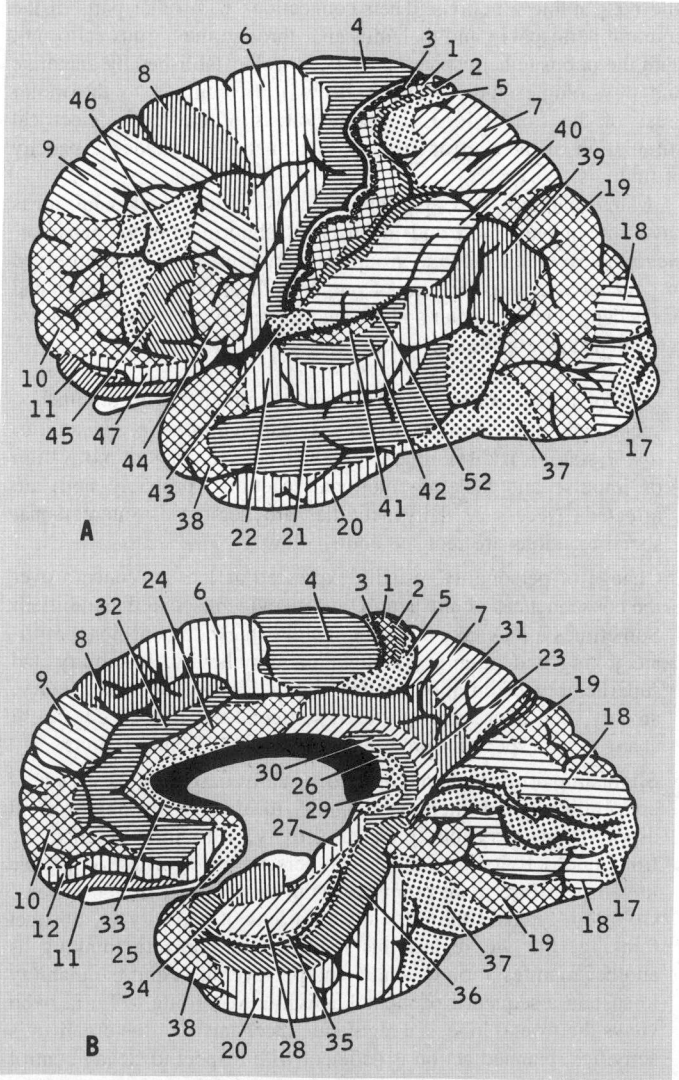

areas, and lesions in them produce a spastic paralysis of the contralateral face, arm, and leg. This is discussed in Chap. 21. A lesion limited more or less to the *premotor area* (area 6 and the supplementary motor area) is accompanied by less paralysis and more spasticity, as well as by a contralateral grasp reflex, and bilateral lesions of these parts are accompanied by a suck reflex. A lesion in area 8 of Brodmann interferes with the mechanism for turning the head and eyes contralaterally. In addition, a lesion of the left supplementary motor area can result in mutism at its onset; in time the condition resolves to a state of transcortical motor aphasia, with reduced language output but preserved capacity for repetition and naming. Ideomotor apraxia is another manifestation of area 6 lesions observed in some patients. A lesion in area 44 (Broca's area) of the dominant (usually the left) cerebral hemisphere and the parts of motor areas superior and posterior to it results in at least a temporary loss of verbal expression. As speech returns, it is characterized by loss of inflection (dysprosody), a phonetic-articulatory defect (cortical dysarthria), agrammatism, retention of "content words," and omission of articles, prepositions, and conjunctions. More extensive lesions, including adjacent insular and motor cortex, result in a more severe and persistent motor speech disorder, agraphia, and apraxia of the face, lips, and tongue (see Chap. 28). Lesions of the anterior cingulate gyrus, in the acute stages, may cause a speechless, aphonic state; with recovery, speech returns through whispering and hoarseness rather than dysarthria and aphasia, according to Brown. Lesions in the medial limbic or piriform cortex (areas 23 and 24), where the mechanisms controlling respiration, circulation, and micturition are organized bilaterally, have relatively unclear clinical effects.

The remaining parts of the frontal lobes (areas 9 to 12 of Brodmann), sometimes called the *prefrontal areas*, have less specific and measurable functions. Their connections with other parts of the cerebral hemisphere and thalamus and, through the corpus callosum, with the opposite hemisphere have been well established by anatomic and physiologic studies (Denny-Brown). In contrast to the motor areas of the frontal lobes and other areas of the brain, electrical stimulation of the prefrontal areas in humans has yielded a paucity of findings.

Many patients with gunshot wounds of the prefrontal areas have shown only mild and inconsistent abnormalities of behavior. Nevertheless, the following groups of symptoms have been observed in patients with large lesions of one or both of the frontal lobes and of the central white matter and the anterior part of the corpus callosum by which they are joined:

1 Lack of initiative and spontaneity in conjunction with diminished speech and motor activity—variously called *apathetic*, *akinetic*, or *abulic* state. It is difficult to distinguish between lack of motivation or impulse and lack of emotional reactions; probably both are affected. Necessary daily activities are neglected. Interpersonal social reactions are reduced and shallow.

2 Change of personality, usually expressed as lack of concern over the consequences of any action, and an evident social disinhibition. Sometimes it may take the form of childish excitement, inappropriate joking and punning, thoughtless impulsivity, instability and superficiality of emotion, or irritability. The capacity for worry, anxiety, and depression (tortured self-concern) is reduced. These changes are especially prominent with orbital frontal lesions.

3 Slight impairment of intelligence, usually described as a lack of concentration and attention, inability to analyze a problem in all aspects and carry out planned activity, difficulty in changing from one activity to another, or perseveration. These cognitive impairments are more prominent with dorsolateral frontal lesions. Goldstein reduced the difficulty to a loss of capacity for abstract thinking, but we regard this tendency to concrete thinking as another manifestation of abulia and perseveration and the inability to sustain a sequence of mental activity. According to Luria, who views the frontal lobe as a regulating mechanism of the organism's activities, planned action is deficient with respect to steady control

and goal orientation. Brown conceives of this difficulty as a manifest failure in one or more stages in an action sequence—a failure of activation, a faulty integration or final implementation. With left frontal lesions, intelligence is reduced more (10 points on the IQ scale) than with right frontal lesions, probably because of reduced verbal skills. There is also an impairment of memory, usually slight, probably because the mental strategies needed for memorization and recall are impaired. Only with extensive posterior orbital, preamygdaloid lesions has a severe memory defect been reported.

4 A decomposition of gait and upright stance, consisting of a wide-based gait, flexed posture, and small shuffling steps, culminating in an inability to stand (Bruns' frontal lobe ataxia or gait apraxia), reflex grasping or sucking, and incontinence of sphincters.

Some differences have been noted between the dominant (left) and right prefrontal lobes. In psychological tests, left-sided lesions impair verbal fluency and cause a greater degree of perseveration, and right-sided ones impair the learning of visual spatial patterns and cause impersistence (see Hecaen and Albert and Luria for details).

From all the foregoing comments it should be evident that the frontal lobes do not have a unitary function but comprise a number of interconnected functional components, each subserving a different aspect of motor function, speech, and behavior.

TEMPORAL LOBES   The boundaries of the temporal lobes are illustrated in Fig. 27-1. The Sylvian fissure separates the superior surface of each temporal lobe from the frontal lobe and anterior part of the parietal lobe. Posteriorly, there is no definite anatomic boundary between the temporal and the occipital and parietal lobes. The temporal lobe includes the superior, middle, and inferior temporal, fusiform, and hippocampal convolutions and the transverse convolutions of Heschl, which are the auditory receptive area on the superior surface, within the Sylvian fissure. The hippocampal convolution was once thought to be related to olfactory function, but lesions here do not cause anosmia. Only the medial and anterior parts of the temporal lobes (uncal regions) are related to smell. The lower fibers of the geniculocalcarine pathway (from the inferior retina) swing in a wide arc over the temporal horn of the ventricle into the white matter of the temporal lobe en route to the occipital lobes, and lesions that interrupt them characteristically produce a contralateral upper homonymous quadrantanopia. Hearing, localized in the superior surfaces of the temporal lobes (Heschl's gyri), is bilaterally represented, which accounts for the fact that both temporal lobes must be affected to cause deafness. Electrical stimulation (or a seizure discharge) of the superior surface of the temporal lobe, posterior to the auditory cortex, evokes vertigo. Disease in the superior convolution of the left temporal lobe and adjacent inferior parietal lobule in right-handed individuals results in Wernicke's aphasia. This syndrome, discussed in Chap. 28, consists of paraphasic speech or jargon aphasia and inability to read, write, repeat, or understand the meaning of spoken words.

Between the auditory and olfactory projection areas there is a large expanse of temporal lobe subserving three specific functional systems. In the inferolateral parts (areas 20, 21, and 37) are located some of the visual-associated projections from the striate and peristriate cortex of the occipital lobes. In the superolateral parts (areas 22, 41, and 42) are the primary and secondary areas for acoustic perception. In the mediobasal parts are the limbic structures (amygdaloid nuclei and hippocampi) containing the neural organizations for emotional and memory processes.

Bilateral lesions of the geniculocalcarine pathways result in cortical blindness; lesions of the visual cortex of the dominant temporal lobe result in a variety of agnosias, apparently based on a loss of visual memories: recognition of written words (alexia), visual naming (anomia), pattern discrimination, color recognition (achromatopsia), and object agnosia. Bilateral hippocampal/parahippocampal lesions produce a deficit in which the patient is unable to record events and information, i.e., has a loss of retentive memory (see Chap. 25). Also, the temporal lobes include a large part of the limbic system, which subserves the emotional and motivational aspects of behavior and vegetative functions ("visceral brain"). Lesions involving both the visual and limbic areas contribute to the Klüver-Bucy syndrome. This syndrome, first produced in monkeys by removal of both temporal lobes, has been observed only rarely in human beings, usually after an attack of herpes simplex encephalitis. It consists of apathy, impaired recognition of objects and persons, uncontrollable oral exploration, hypersexuality, amnesia, and bulimia. Usually the syndrome is incomplete.

Apart from aphasia, psychological studies have shown a difference between the effects of dominant and nondominant temporal lobe lesions. With dominant lesions there is impairment in learning auditorially presented verbal material; with nondominant lesions there is a failure in learning visually presented nonverbal material. In addition, about 20 percent of patients with either a right or left temporal lobectomy have shown an alteration of personality similar to that described after lesions in the prefrontal parts of the brain (see above).

The study of patients with uncinate seizures, with the characteristic dreamy state, olfactory or gustatory hallucinations, and masticatory movements, suggests that all these functions are organized through the temporal lobes. Stimulation of the posterior parts of the temporal lobes of fully conscious epileptic patients during surgical procedures arouses complex memories and visual and auditory images, some with strong emotional content. Stimulation of the amygdaloid nucleus, which is in the anteromedial part of the temporal lobe, may evoke symptoms like those of schizophrenia and mania. Complex emotional experiences may be revived. There are also autonomic effects: the blood pressure rises, pulse increases, respirations increase in frequency and depth, and the patient looks frightened. In temporal lobe epilepsy there may be an intensification of the patient's emotional reactions, vague preoccupation with moral and religious issues, a tendency to write excessively, and sometimes aggressiveness. Ablation of the amygdaloid nuclei has eliminated uncontrollable rage reactions in psychotic patients. Hippocampal and adjacent convolutions have been excised bilaterally, with a disastrous loss of ability to learn or to establish new memories (Korsakoff amnesic state).

The abnormalities consequent on lesions of the temporal lobes may be summarized as follows:

1 Effects of unilateral disease of the dominant temporal lobe:
   a Upper homonymous quadrantanopia
   b Wernicke's aphasia
   c Impairment in tests of verbal material presented through the auditory sense
   d Dysnomia or amnesic aphasia
   e Amusia (inability to name musical scores and to read and write music)
2 Effects of unilateral disease of nondominant temporal lobe:
   a Upper homonymous quadrantanopia
   b Inability to judge spatial relationships in rare cases
   c Impairment in tests of nonverbal visually presented material
   d Inability to recognize melodies and other nonlexical qualities of music
3 Effects of disease of either temporal lobe:
   a Auditory illusions and hallucinations
   b Psychotic behavior (aggressivity)
   c Upper homonymous quadrantanopia
4 Effects of bilateral disease:
   a Korsakoff amnesic defect
   b Apathy and placidity ⎫
   c Increased sexual activity ⎬ Klüver-Bucy syndrome
   d Sham rage ⎭
   e Cortical deafness
   f Loss of other unilateral functions

PARIETAL LOBES   This part of the brain lies between the fissure of Rolando and the parietooccipital notch. It includes Brodmann areas 1, 3, 5, 7, 31, 39, and 40.

The postcentral convolution is the terminus of somatic sensory pathways from the opposite half of the body. However, destructive lesions here do not abolish cutaneous sensation but cause mainly a defect in sensory discrimination with variable impairment of primary sensation. In other words, the perception of painful, tactile, thermal, and vibratory stimuli is affected little or not at all, whereas stereognosis (ability to recognize the size, shape, and texture of objects by touch), sense of position, distinction between single and double contacts (two-point threshold), and the localization of sensory stimuli are impaired or lost (atopognosia). There is also the phenomenon of extinction; i.e., if a stimulus (tactile, painful, visual) is delivered simultaneously to corresponding parts of the body or visual fields, only the stimulus on the normal side is perceived. This type of sensory disturbance, sometimes called *cortical sensory defect*, is really a disturbance of somatic sensory perception and is discussed in Chap. 24. Extensive lesions deep in the white matter of the parietal lobes produce an impairment of all forms of sensation contralaterally, and if these lesions encroach on the uppermost part of the temporal lobe, there may be a contralateral homonymous hemianopia, often incongruous and tending to be greater in the inferior quadrants. Lesions of the angular gyrus of the dominant hemisphere cause an inability to read (alexia).

In addition, the parietal lobes function in the perception of one's position in space, the interrelationships of objects in space, and the relationship of the various parts of the body to one another. Patients with large lesions of the minor parietal lobe are often unaware of their hemiplegia and hemianesthesia; Babinski called this condition *anosognosia*. Related psychological disorders are lack of recognition of the left arm and leg, neglect of the left side of the body (as in dressing) and of external space on the left side, and constructional apraxia (an inability to perceive and construct simple figures). While all these disorders may occur with left-sided lesions as well, they are observed less frequently, in part because the aphasia that occurs with lesions of the left hemisphere precludes adequate testing of other parietal lobe functions.

Another frequent constellation of symptoms, usually referred to as *Gerstmann's syndrome*, occurs only with lesions of the dominant parietal lobe. This consists of inability to write (agraphia), calculate (acalculia), distinguish right from left, and identify fingers (finger agnosia) and other parts of the body. This syndrome is a true *agnosia*, since it represents a defect in the formulation and use of symbolic concepts (including the significance of numbers and letters and the names of parts of the body) in which a unilateral (dominant) lesion evokes the defect bilaterally. An ideomotor apraxia may or may not be associated. *Apraxia* and *agnosia* are discussed in Chaps. 21 and 24.

The effects of disease of the parietal lobes may be summarized as follows:

1 Effects of unilateral disease of the parietal lobe, right or left:
   a Cortical sensory syndrome and sensory extinction (or total hemianesthesia with large acute lesions of white matter)
   b In children, mild contralateral hemiparesis and hemiatrophy
   c Visual inattention and sometimes anosognosia, constructional and dressing apraxias, and neglect of the opposite half of the body and extrapersonal space (all these defects are observed far more frequently with right than with left parietal lesions)
   d Abolition of optokinetic nystagmus to one side
2 Effects of unilateral disease of the dominant parietal lobe (left hemisphere in right-handed patients), additional phenomena:
   a Disorders of language (especially alexia)
   b Gerstmann's syndrome
   c Bimanual astereognosis (tactile agnosia)
   d Bilateral ideational or ideomotor apraxia

In all parietal lesions, if sufficiently extensive, there may be a bland mood, indifference to illness or neurologic defects, reduction in the capacity to think clearly, inattentiveness, and impaired memory.

OCCIPITAL LOBES   The occipital lobes, comprising Brodmann areas 17, 18, and 19, are the termini of the geniculocalcarine pathways and are essential for visual sensation and perception.

Destructive lesions in one occipital lobe result in a contralateral homonymous hemianopia, i.e., a loss of vision in part or all of the homonymous fields. Occasionally, patients complain of changes in the form and contour of visually perceived objects (metamorphopsia), as well as illusory displacement of images from one side of the visual field to another (visual allesthesia), or of abnormal persistence of the visual image after the object has been removed (palinopsia). Visual illusions and elementary (unformed) hallucinations also may occur. Bilateral lesions cause "cortical" blindness, a state of blindness without change in the optic fundi or pupillary reflexes.

Patients with lesions in Brodmann's areas 18 and 19 of the dominant hemisphere (see Fig. 27-1) are unable to recognize objects visually, even though by tests of visual acuity and perimetry they appear to see sufficiently well to do so—a state termed *visual object agnosia*; they are able to recognize objects by tactile or other nonvisual senses. In these terms, *alexia*, or inability to read, represents a visual verbal agnosia or "word blindness." Patients can see letters and words but do not know their meaning, although they can still recognize them through tactile or auditory senses. Several other types of agnosia are observed with bilateral occipital lesions: disorders of *spatial or topographic localization*, in which the patient cannot describe or find his or her way in familiar surroundings (usually due to bilateral occipitoparietal lesions); failure to identify a familiar face (*prosopagnosia*), often with achromatopsia (inferomesial occipitotemporal lesions); an inability to scan the peripheral field and to grasp an object under visual guidance, coupled with visual inattention (*Balint's syndrome*, due usually to bilateral occipitoparietal lesions); and a failure to perceive simultaneously all the elements of a scene (*simultanagnosia*). In actuality, these agnosias do not represent the effects of purely occipital lesions but of either occipitotemporal or occipitoparietal disconnections.

The details of these syndromes of the different lobes of the cerebrum can be found in the textbook of Adams and Victor and the monographs by Walsh and Mesulam.

CORPUS CALLOSUM AND THE DISCONNECTION SYNDROMES
Considerable attention has been devoted to the study of each of the two cerebral hemispheres in isolation. This is possible only when the corpus callosum, which forms a bridge between the two hemispheres, is absent (*agenesis*) or is surgically sectioned (for epilepsy) or destroyed by infarction or tumors. From these studies emerges the well-known fact that the left hemisphere is dominant in all language functions and auditory perception and the right hemisphere is superior in spatial and visual perception. Partial lesions of the corpus callosum or of the long tracts in the cerebral white matter are found to be associated with a number of interesting syndromes (commissural and intrahemispheric) described below.

When the corpus callosum is sectioned by a surgical procedure or destroyed by an anterior cerebral artery occlusion (anterior four-fifths), the language and perceptual areas of the left hemisphere are isolated from the sensory and motor areas of the right hemisphere. These patients, if blindfolded, are then unable to match an object held in one hand with an identical object in the other hand. Further, they cannot match an object seen in the right half of the visual field with one in the left half. If given verbal commands, they perform correctly with the right hand but not with the left. Without vision, objects placed in the right hand are named correctly, but not those in the left. In lesions confined to the posterior fifth of the corpus callosum (splenium), only the visual part of the disconnection syndrome occurs. Occlusion of the left posterior cerebral artery provides the best examples of the latter. Infarction of the left occipital lobe causes a right homonymous hemianopia, as a consequence of which all visual information needed for activating the speech areas of the left hemisphere must come from the right occipital lobe, across the splenium of the corpus callosum. If there is a lesion in the corpus callosum (or in other portions of the crossing fibers), the patient

cannot read or name colors because the visual information cannot reach the left angular gyrus. There is no difficulty in copying words, although the patient cannot read what he or she has written (alexia without agraphia); matching colors without naming them is done without error. Apparently the visual information for activating the left motor area crosses the corpus callosum more anteriorly. A lesion that is limited to the anterior third of the corpus callosum does not result in a left-sided apraxia (a failure of the left hand to obey commands, the right one performing perfectly). A section of the entire corpus callosum does result in such an apraxia, indicating that the fiber systems connecting the left to the right motor areas cross posterior to the genu (but anterior to the splenium).

There are also intrahemispheric disconnections, of which the most important are the following:

1 *Conduction aphasia* (also called *central aphasia*). The patient has fluent but paraphasic speech and writing with nearly perfect comprehension of spoken or written language. Repetition of what is heard or read is, however, severely impaired. The lesion is presumably in the arcuate fasciculus, which connects Wernicke's area with Broca's area.
2 *Pure word deafness*. Although the patient is able to hear and identify nonverbal sounds, there is a loss of ability to comprehend spoken language. The patient's speech remains normal. The defect has been attributed to a subcortical lesion undercutting Wernicke's area.

PATIENTS WITH FOCAL CEREBRAL LESIONS   Diagnosis and management involve the same principles described in Chap. 25. Special tests, mostly of the psychological type, are available for each of the focal cerebral syndromes. The investigation and care of individual patients also will be governed by the underlying disease, of course.

REFERENCES

ABSHER JR, BENSON DF: Disconnection syndromes—An overview of Geschwind's contributions. Neurology 43:862, 1993
ADAMS RD, VICTOR M: *Principles of Neurology*, 5th ed. New York, McGraw-Hill, 1993
BRODAL A: *Neurological Anatomy in Relation to Clinical Medicine*, 3d ed. New York, Oxford University Press, 1981
BROWN JW: Frontal lobe syndromes, in *Handbook of Clinical Neurology*, JAM Frederiks (ed). Amsterdam, Elsevier Science, 1985, vol 45, chap 3
DIMOND SJ: The disconnection syndromes, in *Modern Trends in Neurology*, D Williams (ed). London, Butterworth, 1975
GESCHWIND N: Disconnection syndromes in animals and man. Brain 88:237, 585, 1965
HECAEN H, ALBERT ML: Disorders of mental functioning related to the frontal lobes, in *Modern Trends in Neurology*, D Williams (ed). London, Butterworth, 1975
HEILMAN KM, VALENSTEIN E (eds): *Clinical Neuropsychology*, 2d ed. Oxford, Oxford University Press, 1985
LURIA AR: *The Working Brain: An Introduction to Neuropsychology*. New York, Basic Books (trans Penguin Books Ltd), 1973
MARLOWE WH et al: Complete Klüver-Bucy syndrome in man. Cortex 11:53, 1975
MESULAM M-M (ed): *Principles of Behavioral Neurology*. Philadelphia, Davis, 1985
WALSH KW: *Neuropsychology: A Clinical Approach*, 2d ed. London, Churchill Livingstone, 1987

28   DISORDERS OF SPEECH AND LANGUAGE

J. P. MOHR

Impairments of language and speech are among the most important consequences of brain disease because they affect the interaction between the victim and other people. The spectrum of impairment in communication ranges widely, from loss of all interpersonal communication at the most severe end of the spectrum to minor disturbances in intonation of normally selected words or minor flaws in selection at the other end. The more gross disturbances are easily recognized as signs of brain disease, whereas the minor disturbances may pass unnoticed by all but the most probing of examinations.

DEFINITIONS The site, size, and temporal proximity of a brain lesion influence speech and language in distinctively different ways. Disturbance in the comprehension or production of language in written or spoken forms is known broadly as *aphasia*. The disorder is usually incomplete and hence is often described as *dysphasia*. Because of its more common use, aphasia will be employed in this chapter. The term *language* has wide connotations and refers to the selection and serial ordering of words according to learned rules by which a person can use spoken or written modalities to communicate with others and to express cerebral activities involved with thinking and learning.

Brain lesions also may compromise the capacity to comprehend or produce the sights and sounds needed to convey language. Injuries to the main sensory and motor pathways can affect the skills involved in scanning visual displays and the selection of those shapes learned earlier to be letters, numbers, or marks of grammatical notation, such as apostrophes; listening to strings of sounds and selecting from among them the distinctive cluster that makes up the sounds of letters and syllables; and the execution of acquired motor skills for the pronunciation of these same items and marking down their graphic equivalents. A brain lesion also can disturb efforts of noting whether word strings seen or heard are given special emphasis or intonation, the intonation of strings of words to make questions or statements, the grouping of words into phrases, and the production of the speech "melody" that is distinctive for given languages and regional dialects. The needs of the patient can be exquisitely sensitive to such seemingly minor patterns of disturbance; e.g., a lesion that disturbs skills in vocal timing and emphasis could ruin the career of an actor but have no impact on that of a typist. While no general term has emerged to classify these disturbances in the sensory discrimination and motor production of the shapes and sounds of language, they are commonly referred to as *speech sensory* or *motor modalities*, as opposed to the language that they convey, and have a wide variety of terms that emphasize the focal nature of the disturbance. *Dysarthria*, a defect in articulation usually related to poor pronunciation of consonants, occurs with flaccid or spastic paralysis, rigidity, repetitive spasms (stuttering), or ataxia of the oropharynx and respiratory apparatus. *Dysphonia*, a defect in phonation (voice), is due to disease of the larynx or its innervation, causing inability to produce the basic vowel sounds. *Dysgraphia*, faulty writing skills, is due to disturbances of motor skills in writing. More complex disorders in understanding the meaning of words heard (word deafness) and seen (word blindness) are discussed below.

GENERAL PRINCIPLES As a general orientation, most lesions that lead to aphasia occur in the perisylvian regions (frontal, temporal, and parietal) of the dominant cerebral hemisphere, i.e., the left side in right-handed individuals. When the lesion is due to infarction as a result of arterial occlusion, hemorrhage, masses from various causes, or other focal conditions that cause gross changes in tissue characteristics, the anatomic site of the lesion can usually be demonstrated by computed tomography (CT scan) or magnetic resonance imaging (MRI). Focal dysfunction caused by cell death, atrophy, or impairment of cortical microvascular regulation may be evaluated by measurement of regional cerebral blood flow (rCBF) or by single-photon-emission tomography (SPECT) or positron-emission tomography (PET) (see Chap. 365).

Diseases of the cerebral surface gray matter produce a more significant deficit than those confined to the white matter; tumors, located largely in the white matter, usually reach a large size before causing a speech or language deficit. Small infarcts or traumatic lesions of a few centimeters in diameter are usually associated with an evanescent deficit that fades to functional insignificance within weeks or months. Improvements over weeks to months occur in all but the largest vascular lesions, whereas those due to tumors show progression. The site of the lesion determines the qualitative features

of the deficit, whereas size determines the severity of the syndrome. Furthermore, deficits in speech function predominate in smaller lesions, whereas major disturbances in language are superimposed on the speech disturbance with larger lesions.

The history of aphasiology has mirrored the notions of brain function popular at the time. Over a century ago, when sensory functions were thought to reside in the posterior half of the brain and motor in the anterior, it was popular to speak in broad terms of a sensory aphasia and a motor aphasia. When studies of the fiber pathways predominated, complex schemes were developed to show that aphasias could be cortical (brain surface, gray matter, centers), subcortical (affecting the pathways connecting the peripheral speech organs with the "cortical centers"), and transcortical (connecting various "cortical centers" with each other). PET studies have challenged these concepts. Most recently, awareness of the direct interactions between brain regions has led to the currently popular notion of neural networks. To date, however, the precise neural substrate of language continues to elude investigators, and it remains unknown what the brain does neurochemically and neurophysiologically when it is said to be thinking, comprehending words seen and heard, and formulating a reply. Even less is known about how improvements occur after lesions that destroy areas once thought essential for language function. It is not idle to speculate that the neurobiologic basis for language may prove as surprising and as clarifying as has research into the neural basis of vision.

CEREBRAL DOMINANCE: RELATION TO SPEECH AND HAND-EDNESS The side of the brain dominant for language is inferred to be the side opposite from the eye, hand, or foot preferentially used for intricate, complex acts. Over 90 percent of people are right-handed. The dominance is more complete in some persons than in others. Hereditary, anatomic, and developmental factors play a role, but there is considerable evidence of hemisphere specialization for certain types of tasks. In normal individuals, PET has shown the left hemisphere to be activated more for verbal tasks, whereas the right is more activated for spatial motor tasks. Left hemisphere dominance for language occurs in 95 percent of right-handed people and in 50 percent of those who are left-handed. Anatomic differences in size between the dominant and the nondominant cerebral hemispheres may explain the dominance: the planum temporale, adjacent to the auditory center of Heschl's transverse gyrus, is larger in the left hemisphere in right-handed individuals. Left-handedness may be hereditary or may result from disease of the left cerebral hemisphere in early life.

LESION LOCATION AND LANGUAGE DISTURBANCE Although language deficits are not always closely correlated with anatomic pathology, two large syndromic categories, recognized for over a century by the eponyms *Broca's* and *Wernicke's aphasia*, remain recognized by their distinctive clinical features. Large anterior lesions involving the bulk of the frontal operculum (that region that lies above the insula) and the insula itself result in Broca's aphasia, in which the main language disturbance is *agrammatism*. In its fully developed form, sentences have a sharply constricted structure, with absence of most small words and a preservation of words mainly serving predicative, interjectional, or substantive functions. The most severely affected patient may only be able to say *hi*, *no*, and *hello* or to use simple nouns, such as *ball*, *top*, and *key*.

Large posterior sylvian lesions cause Wernicke's aphasia, in which simple syllabic or word elements are missing or are replaced by substitutions so that the desired response is only approximated (*paraphasias*). These latter may consist of faulty pronunciations (*literal paraphasias*) or faulty word selections (*verbal paraphasias*). Verbal paraphasias may approximate the desired word with a similarity of sound or of spelling (formal verbal paraphasias), such as *stock* for *stop*, or by similarity of meaning (semantic verbal paraphasias), such as *slow* for *stop*. Disturbances in understanding language, both auditory and visual speech, occur in both types of major paraphasias and tend to be of the same type of disorder as that seen in language production.

LESION LOCATION AND DISTURBANCE IN SPEECH MODALITIES Focal left-sided sylvian lesions often disturb speech modalities. When small, the disturbance may occur with little or no accompanying aphasia, but when large, the aphasia often makes it difficult to determine the severity of the disturbances in speech. Anterior sylvian lesions, which lie close to the sensorimotor cortex for oropharyngeal movements, mainly disturb the act of speaking. These range from mutism through impaired articulation to disordered transitions from syllable to syllable to abnormalities in phrasing, intonation, and melody. Lesions just posterior to the lower rolandic region produce malpositioning of the tongue, lips, and other structures in the oropharynx, with anticipatory errors from some syllables occurring out of sequence. Lesions grouped around the posterior sylvian fissure, including the superior temporal lobe and its auditory gyri, are manifested by disordered understanding of spoken words, resulting in poor repetition of speech sounds. Those located more posteriorly over the left lateral parietal or occipital lobes interfere with reading.

Lesions well away from the sylvian region either fail to disturb human communicative skills or alter them only secondarily. A large lesion of the anterior frontal lobes, especially the medial and orbital parts, impairs all motor activities and often results in lack of attention and responsiveness (abulia), verging on the akinetic mute state (see Chap. 27). The speech is laconic, with long pauses between utterances, and there is an inability to sustain monologue and narrative, leaving an incorrect impression of aphasia. Extensive occipital lesions impair reading and reduce the utilization of all visual, lexical stimuli. Posterior thalamic and deep lesions in the adjacent temporal lobe impair alertness and cause fluctuating states of inattention and disorientation, thereby inducing fragmentation of words (*neologisms*) and phrases and protracted, uncontrollable talking (*logorrhea*). Strong stimulation to increase momentarily the level of awareness and alertness usually will show that such patients have intact language mechanisms. Lesions in the anterior thalamus, located beneath the genu of the internal capsule and the head of the caudate, may interrupt projection systems controlling rCBF over the convexity and produce short-lived reductions in the complexity and length of verbal responses. The deficit includes some elements of abulia but also disturbances in naming and in the proper use of grammatical forms. These syndromes usually improve within weeks or months, paralleling the improvement in rCBF. Recognition of these specific syndromes from isolated lesions separate from the more traditional aphasias has been increasing with improvements in brain imaging and may continue to proliferate.

The nondominant hemisphere provides the substratum for several types of behavior: motor responses of mimicry, social anticipation (smiling, handshaking, modesty reactions), and self-care (washing and feeding); avoidance behavior to noxious stimuli; and the capability of matching visually simple words with pictures.

APHASIA

TYPES OF APHASIA Disturbances of speech and language can result from several abnormalities. Classifications have been based on the predominant form, the presumed physiologic or psychological bases, and the anatomy of the underlying diseases. The classification utilized here has been formulated on the basis of the anatomic localization and the clinical presentation (see Table 28-1). The prognoses are helpful in management, particularly in the choice of therapy.

Aphasias also have been classified according to the severity of impediment to speech production and flow, the most obvious disturbance on brief personal contact with the patient. *Nonfluent aphasias* are characterized by slow, incorrectly articulated words and sentences; the lesion usually lies in the dominant frontal lobe. *Fluent aphasias* show runs of well-articulated speech, with basically normal rhythm and flow, although lacking in language meaning; the defect is usually a lesion in the dominant parietal or temporal lobe.

Total (global) aphasia The causative lesion is located in the left sylvian region, destroying a large part of the speech and language areas and leaving a severe aphasia with a poor prognosis for improvement. Most patients with total aphasia are initially mute or say few stereotyped words, such as *hi* and *yes*; they do not read or write even the simplest words, and they understand only a few words of the speech of others. Related signs include right hemiplegia, hemianesthesia, and homonymous hemianopsia. The alert patient may participate in common gestures of greeting, may show modesty and avoidance reactions, and is able to engage in self-help activities. Some improve months later with a persistent Broca's aphasia.

Infarction from occlusion of the left internal carotid or middle cerebral artery, a large hemorrhage, major tumor, or penetrating trauma is most often responsible for the deficit. In the rare instances of rapid improvement, the main cause is postconvulsive paralysis, posttraumatic edema, or transitory ischemia from a fragmenting embolus. Occasionally, hyperthermia, infection, or hyponatremia may cause temporary return of aphasia due to an old lesion.

Broca's aphasia (major motor aphasia) This term designates a complex syndrome with severely disturbed speech and writing, accompanied by simplified grammar skills (agrammatism) in speaking and writing and a less obvious impairment in language comprehension. It results from a large lesion involving cortex and subcortical structures in the anterior sylvian region and insula, including but usually extending beyond Broca's area (the inferior frontal convolution). The CT scan may underestimate the lesion because the angle of the imaged lesion may seem to merge with the sylvian fissure, but both coronal and true-axial MRI shows the real size. The lesion is smaller than that of total aphasia and usually involves the sensorimotor rolandic region, producing an accompanying persisting hemiparesis and hemisensory syndrome. Intitially, a transient ipsilateral deviation of the eyes is observed due to the frontal infarction.

In the acute phase, the entire language mechanism appears to be inactivated, and the helplessly mute, noncommunicative, and uncomprehending patient presents the syndrome of complete or global aphasia. Within weeks to years, the disorder of comprehension abates somewhat, and this improvement exceeds that found in speaking and writing, leaving the motor speech deficits that gave the syndrome its original name. For a time an apraxia of the lingual and oropharyngeal apparatus retards efforts to make purposeful movements. Imitation may be better performed than execution of acts on command. Certain stereotyped and simple phrases, such as *hi*, *good morning*, or curses are uttered more easily, and words of popular songs may be sung surprisingly well. The patient's efforts to speak and the facial expressions suggest an awareness of his or her ineptitudes and mistakes, and an accompanying exasperation and despair are common. Most patients with Broca's aphasia have a correspondingly severe impairment in communication by writing with either hand. However, communication by writing is superior to that of speaking, suggesting a certain independence between these two acts as vehicles of language.

As improvement occurs, words are enunciated slowly and laboriously, with greatly impaired melody of speech (prosody). Speech is sparse and consists mainly of nouns, transitive verbs, and important adjectives; many of the small words (articles, prepositions, conjunctions) are omitted, giving the speech an agrammatic and telegraphic character. The preservation of substantive words allows the patients to communicate despite the gross mechanical and agrammatic language difficulties. This hesitant, laconic speech has been termed *nonfluent aphasia*.

The syndrome is most often due to embolic occlusions of the upper division of the left middle cerebral artery; major putaminal hypertensive hemorrhage, huge frontal lobe tumor or abscess, metastatic lesions, subdural hematoma, and encephalitis are less common causes.

Minor motor aphasia More circumscribed focal lesions along the anterior and superior sylvian operculum and insula produce remarkably discrete effects on speech modalities which may resemble

TABLE 28-1	Classification of aphasic disorders			
	Clinical manifestations	Anatomic location	Etiology	Associated clinical symptoms
MAJOR SYNDROMES				
Global aphasia	Minimal speech; nonfluent aphasia; comprehension poor for spoken and written language	Large lesion of dominant frontal, parietal, and superior temporal lobe	Infarction in distribution of internal carotid or middle cerebral artery; trauma; tumor	Contralateral hemiplegia; hemisensory loss; hemianopsia
Broca's aphasia	Nonfluent aphasia; agrammatic sentences; poor articulation; dysprosody; may be mute	Cortical and subcortical lesion of prefrontal and frontal regions	Infarction in distribution of superior frontal branch middle cerebral artery; hemorrhage; tumor	Contralateral hemiparesis; minor or no sensory loss; no visual field disturbance; oral dyspraxia; cortical dysarthria; severe impairment in writing
Wernicke's aphasia (central or sensory aphasia)	Fluent speech; total incomprehension of spoken speech; inability to read or to repeat sounds or words; alexia, agraphia, paraphasia common	Posterior perisylvian structures of the parietal and temporal lobe	Infarction in distribution of lower division of middle cerebral artery; tumor; herpes simplex encephalitis	Parietal lobe sensory deficits; hemianopsia; no motor disturbance
MINOR CENTRAL APHASIA SYNDROMES				
Conduction aphasia	Paraphasia; difficulty in repetition of speech and in reading aloud; aware of deficit; adequate comprehension of written and spoken words	Upper bank of sylvian fissure; inferior parietal lobule	Embolic occlusion of posterior branches of middle cerebral artery	Contralateral hemihypesthesia or homonymous hemianopsia; abnormal optokinetic nystagmus
Mainly auditory (pure word deafness)	Impaired auditory comprehension; inability to repeat a sentence or write a dictation	Lesion in superior temporal gyrus	Infarction; tumor; abscess	Rarely deafness
Mainly visual (dyslexia with dysgraphia)	Visual language compromised more than auditory; cannot read or write	Parietooccipital lesion	Infarction; tumor, lobar hemorrhage	Hemianopsia
OTHER SYNDROMES				
Pure word blindness	Normal spoken language and writing, with inability to read	Left occipitostriate cortex, adjacent association cortex, and posterior corpus callosum (splenium)	Infarction in distribution of posterior cerebral artery; tumor, lobar hemorrhage	Hemianopsia
Isolation of speech areas	Parrot-like speech; echolalia	Ischemic infarction in border (watershed) zones between anterior, middle, and posterior cerebral artery distributions	Systemic hypotension or hypoxia; cardiac arrest	Decreased alertness and responsiveness; bilateral leg weakness
Amnesic-dysnomic aphasia	Inability to recall names of objects or parts of objects; difficulty with recent memory	Deep temporal lobe lesions, parahippocampal, hippocampal gyrus	Tumor; Alzheimer's disease; infarction in distribution posterior cerebral artery; herpes simplex encephalitis	Apraxia; dementia; no motor or sensory abnormalities; upper quadrantic visual field defect

major motor aphasia except for the satisfactory understanding of spoken and written words. The prognosis for nearly full recovery is excellent. Indeed, none of these focal lesions produces significant or lasting deficits in language usage.

Broca's area infarction affects the lower premotor cortex adjacent to the primary motor cortex controlling the oropharynx, larynx, and respiratory apparatus. The infarct interrupts skilled movements of these muscle groups, and the resultant dyspraxia in speech causes impaired transitions between syllables in words and disruption of the melodic intonation of phrases (dysprosody). Involvement of this region alone is insufficient to produce the major syndrome referred to as *Broca's aphasia*. *Rolandic infarction* involves the sensorimotor cortex itself; either the syndrome of dysprosody occurs or speech has poor articulation and lowered volume and pitch, while a nasal quality to the voice reveals the paresis of the nasopharyngeal musculature. *Postcentral, anterior parietal infarction* is associated with errors in the positioning of the oral cavity for individual sounds, syllables, and whole words; the acoustic features of the utterance are often distorted by these malpositions of the oral cavity and strike the ear as literal paraphasias.

Lesions in the more anterior parts of the dominant frontal lobe (sparing Broca's area) in the medial frontal lobe in the anterior cerebral artery territory, or in the head of the caudate and anterior

limb of the internal capsule also may cause an aphasic disorder. Usually, the speech output is reduced and nonfluent, and auditory comprehension is intact. Repetition of words spoken by the examiner is preserved. This condition has been called *transcortical motor aphasia* but is usually part of frontal lobe syndromes in which spontaneous speech is lacking (mutism) and all motor activity is reduced (akinesia).

Almost all these syndromes are due to stroke, usually infarction from embolism into a single branch. Other diseases rarely produce such circumscribed lesions. Exceptions supporting this view are the rare instances of highly focal penetrating head wounds from missile fragments. Deeper, larger lesions or larger emboli involving the stem of the upper division of the middle cerebral artery can cause several types of deficit in a single patient, making these individual distinctions less clear and blending with the major syndrome of Broca's aphasia. Facial, lingual, and sometimes brachial paresis and ideomotor dyspraxia of the face and left, nondominant limbs commonly accompany the speech disorder. Most of these syndromes recede within weeks or months (see Chap. 27).

Wernicke's aphasia (major central or sensory aphasia) This term encompasses syndromes that arise from lesions of the posterior perisylvian structures or the posterior temporal, parietal, and occipital regions supplied by the lower division of the middle cerebral artery.

When restricted to the temporal lobe, the main disturbance is in language tasks involving words heard; when more parietal and occipital, in words seen. Spoken and written communication, as well as auditory and visual comprehension, are affected, a combination that justifies the term *central aphasia*. Speech contains many language errors but is fluent, hence the term *fluent aphasia*.

In a severe or acute injury, the patient usually speaks easily in a series of incomprehensible syllables, makes illegible marks in attempts at writing, cannot repeat aloud or copy correctly, and treats the examiner's attempts at written and verbal communication as if they were in a wholly unfamiliar foreign language. Patients may seem puzzled that they are not communicating and may become angry and abusive. In less severe cases, the patient can repeat aloud and copy but echoes the words heard with faulty pronunciation or copies the words in a slavish manner, imitating even the examiner's handwriting style, as though the test words were unfamiliar. In the mildest cases, the deficits are manifested in errors in word comprehension and usage. The disturbance in language does not simply reflect a disturbance in hearing or vision. The patient may choose words that show approximation to the desired response, the words often belonging to the same functional class [i.e., *cow* for *pig*, but not *cow* for *yellow* (semantic verbal paraphasias)], or the words may be similar in sound or shape (formal verbal paraphasis) such as *flee* for *tree*; there may be errors in word structure, with improper tenses, prefixes, or suffixes (e.g., "beautifulling"), or other errors that resemble those of normal people unfamiliar with the language in question. Some patients pass for normal in brief or casual conversation. In its mildest form or later in the course of the illness, the speech resembles that of a person who is tired or distracted, and the abnormality is detected only on tests of complex language function.

Minor central aphasia syndromes   In time, Wernicke's aphasia improves, and a number of lesser syndromes appear. However, these latter syndromes may be present in comparatively pure form from the beginning when only a small, restricted lesion involves some part of the territory of the lower division of the middle cerebral artery. The posterior sylvian region, comprising posterosuperior temporal, opercular, supramarginal, and posterior insular gyri, appears to encompass a variety of language functions. Seemingly minor changes in size and locale of the lesion are associated with important variations in the elements of Wernicke's aphasia.

Depending on the location of the lesion, language behavior dependent on auditory function (hearing spoken words, echoing sounds and speech, relating the spoken to the written word, and finally, repeating and writing it) may be deranged partially or completely. The same is true of language behavior dependent on visual function when the left posterior parietal lobe is involved. These partial syndromes are termed *conduction aphasia*, *pure word deafness*, *dyslexia with dysgraphia*, *isolation of speech areas*, and *pure word blindness*.

CONDUCTION APHASIA   A clinical syndrome, which acquired its name for historical reasons not reflected in its pathoanatomy, conduction aphasia is characterized by disturbance in repeating words or sentences. This disturbance resembles that of Wernicke's aphasia; there is the same degree of paraphasia in self-initiated speech, in repeating what is heard, and in reading aloud. However, little or no difficulty is encountered in comprehending words that are heard or seen. Because the motor regions are unaffected, no element of dysarthria or dysprosody occurs. The patient is alert and fully aware of the deficit. The errors take the form of literal paraphasia, i.e., mispronunciations, many of which seem explained as errors in oropharyngeal positioning that produce detectably different sounds from those intended.

The lesion at autopsy is located in the cortex and subcortical white matter in the upper bank of the sylvian fissure, involving the supramarginal gyrus of the inferior parietal lobule. The posterior part of the superior temporal region is occasionally affected. The usual cause is an embolus in the ascending parietal or posterior temporal branch of the middle cerebral artery. Deeper, larger lesions that interrupt the arcuate fasciculus, once thought the explanation for the "disconnection" of the posterior and anterior language zones (hence the term *conduction aphasia*), rarely produce the syndrome.

PURE WORD DEAFNESS   This is considered to be the auditory form of Wernicke's aphasia. The most obvious findings are an impaired auditory comprehension and an inability to repeat what is said or to write to dictation. Spoken language is less impaired but rarely normal. Occasionally, the paraphasic speech leads to an initial diagnosis of Wernicke's aphasia. Little defect in hearing is found by audiometric testing. The patient frequently learns to use visual cues well enough to overcome much of the difficulty. Comprehension of visually presented material such as printed matter, although not normal, is better than auditory comprehension. When there is full preservation of reading skill, the traditional term *pure word deafness* can be applied. The syndrome is rare but has an excellent prognosis for functional recovery.

In most autopsy studies, the lesion has been focal and the result of embolism. The infarcts have been bilateral in the superior temporal gyrus in a position to damage the primary auditory cortex in the transverse gyrus of Heschl and to impair its relation to the associated areas of the superoposterior part of the temporal lobe. A unilateral infarct has rarely been found in this part of the major (dominant) temporal lobe, thought to encroach on those regions whose involvement precipitates the larger syndrome of Wernicke's aphasia.

DYSLEXIA WITH DYSGRAPHIA   This syndrome, often a late sequela of the larger syndrome of Wernicke's aphasia, is its visual form and thus is most evident in reading and writing. Errors occur in response to lexical stimuli. Auditory comprehension, while abnormal, is less impaired than visual comprehension. Since conversational testing is frequently the only type of clinical evaluation in such patients, satisfactory auditory comprehension, ability to repeat aloud, and mild paraphasic errors in spontaneous speech frequently lead to a misdiagnosis of mild Wernicke's aphasia. Detailed testing of reading aloud and reading for comprehension and tests of spontaneous writing and writing in response to dictated and visually presented material reveal a greater disturbance in these tasks.

The parietal and occipital regions are usually affected in the syndrome of dyslexia with dysgraphia. Although a discrete embolism is unusual, a small clot may pass through the more proximal territory and lodge distally. Tumors, abscess, and lobar hemorrhages usually disrupt other structures as well, and this syndrome is often a less conspicuous part of a larger clinical picture. Systemic hypotension and hypoxia may leave dyslexia with dysgraphia as a residual impairment, but more often they produce a more severe defect, described below under "Isolation of Speech Areas."

ISOLATION OF SPEECH AREAS   This rare syndrome is of importance to show that the act of repeating aloud can be accomplished without major portions of the parietal, temporal, and occipital lobes. Following prolonged hypoxia from cardiac arrest or other causes of hypotension, widespread cerebral ischemia can affect the vascular border zones linking the major cerebral arteries and their distal branches on the cerebral surfaces and can spread centripetally into their adjacent territories. The central fields of supply of these arteries are often spared. In the middle cerebral artery territory, this sparing leaves largely intact the sylvian region and its speech areas. Despite much of the rest of the brain that is inactive in patients who survive such episodes, spoken responses can be activated by words heard. The response is a parrot-like repetition of the sounds (*echolalia*) that is done well enough to indicate that the auditory-vocal loop is functional. Scant signs of comprehension or self-initiated conversation occur, reflecting the widespread injury outside the speech regions. The prognosis for full recovery is poor.

PURE WORD BLINDNESS   In the fully developed syndrome, victims lose the ability to read and usually to name colors. The patient is unable to name or point to a letter or word on command. However, understanding spoken language, repetition of what is heard, writing dictation, conversation, and writing are all intact. The condition is also sometimes termed *dyslexia without dysgraphia*. Because the victim may be unaware the deficit exists, the examiner is often required to test for its presence rather than simply assuming that the complaint will be volunteered. The errors may be minimal and the defect obscured if other visual cues are available, such as the bottle on which the words *Coca-Cola* appear. The naming of common colors presented singly and of objects is also impaired. When the syndrome is less severe, reading is impaired mainly in the affected visual field, producing a dyslexia for the letters on the affected side of the longer words (so-called hemidyslexia). Right homonymous hemianopsia, an amnesic defect, and a right hemisensory defect reflect respectively the involvement of the left occipial lobe and its callosal decussation, the left fornix, and the left thalamus. This combination nearly always signifies thrombosis or embolism of the left posterior cerebral artery, placing the origin of this syndrome rather remote from the main language zone supplied by the middle cerebral artery.

Autopsy usually demonstrates a lesion that destroys the left visual striate cortex (area 17) and visual association areas (18 and 19), as well as the connections of the right visual cortex and association areas with the temporoparietal region. This latter "disconnection" usually is due to interruption of the fibers passing through the posterior part (splenium) of the corpus callosum, which connect the visual association areas of the two hemispheres. Rarely, a lesion deep in the left parieto-occipital region prevents visual information from either occipital lobe from reaching the left language region. Right homonymous hemianopsia may be absent. Aside from infarction, the syndrome may occur from a primary or secondary tumor, multifocal leukoencephalopathy, or even multiple sclerosis.

In rare instances, the dyslexia has been found limited to the left side of space and to the initial letter or letters of a word. This partial left hemidyslexia has been explained by highly specific infarction or surgery done on the posterior end of the corpus callosum or fiber bundles passing through the callosum. The existence of such cases indicates the highly organized visual pathways serving reading.

Amnesic-dysnomic aphasia This may be a relatively early or isolated syndrome in patients with CNS disease. The patient has difficulty recalling names on demand, not only nouns, but also adjectives and other descriptive parts of speech. There are usually pauses in speech, groping for words, and substitution of another word or phrase that conveys the meaning (circumlocution). The function of an object may be described, but its name forgotten. The difficulty applies not only to common objects seen but also to the names of things heard or felt. By contrast, other verbal tasks, including recall of the names of the letters and digits, reading, writing, spelling, etc., are far better performed.

The causative lesion is usually deep in the temporal lobe, presumably interrupting connections of sensory speech areas with the hippocampal-parahippocampal regions concerned with learning and memory (see Chap. 27). Masses such as a tumor or abscess are the most frequent causes; as they enlarge, an upper contralateral quadrantic visual field defect or Wernicke's aphasia is added. Dysnomia may be part of the syndromes produced by occlusion of the temporal branches of the posterior cerebral artery. Alzheimer's or Pick's disease may begin with a dysnomic or amnesic type of aphasia; by the time the patient's difficulty is fully recognized, other disorders of speech and indifference, apathy, and abulia are conjoined. When Alzheimer's or Pick's disease is the cause, rCBF, SPECT, or PET studies may reveal reduced activity of the posterolateral parietal or occipital regions, even when the CT or MRI shows no major abnormalities. Dysnomia also may be present in confusional states caused by metabolic, infectious, intoxicative, or other acute medical illnesses, but then it has no particular localizing value.

The combination of dysnomia and major impairment of auditory comprehension, with a remarkable retention of the ability to repeat what is heard, is called *transcortical sensory aphasia*. The causative lesion spares the auditory cortex and Wernicke area and involves the inferior temporal cortices, particularly area 37.

DISORDERS OF ARTICULATION AND PHONATION

The highly coordinated act of speaking involves the larynx, pharynx, palate, tongue, lips, and respiratory musculature, which are innervated by the hypoglossal, vagal, facial, and phrenic nerves. Their nuclei are controlled through the corticobulbar tracts by both motor cortices and extrapyramidal influences from the cerebellum and basal ganglia.

In speaking, the current of air is produced by expiration and is finely regulated by the activity of the various muscles engaged in speech. Phonation, or the production of vocal sounds, is a function of the larynx. Changes in the size and shape of the glottis and in the length and tension of the vocal cords are controlled by the laryngeal muscles, which transmit their vibrations to the column of air passing over the vocal cords. Sounds thus formed are modified as they pass through the nasopharynx and mouth, which act as resonators. Articulation consists of contractions of the tongue, lips, pharynx, and palate that interrupt or alter the vocal sounds. Vowels are of laryngeal origin, as are some consonants, but the latter are formed for the most part during articulation. The consonants *m*, *b*, and *p* are labial; *l* and *t* are lingual; and *k* and *g* are nasoguttural.

Disorders of phonation (aphonia, dysphonia) prompt examination of the vocal cords, tongue, palate, and pharynx. Paresis of the respiratory movements, as in poliomyelitis and acute infectious polyneuritis, or incoordination as part of extrapyramidal disease may affect the voice because insufficient air is provided for phonation and speech. Reduced volume of speech due to limited excursion of the breathing muscles is common; the patient is unable to speak above a whisper or is unable to shout. Paresis of both vocal cords causes complete aphonia, with no voice, and the patient only able to speak in whispers. If one vocal cord is paralyzed, the voice becomes hoarse, low-pitched, and rasping. Involvement of one of the tenth cranial nerves by tumor, for example, also may cause a nasal voice because the posterior nares do not close during phonation. Consonants such as *b*, *p*, *n*, and *k* are followed by escape of air into the nasal passages. *Spastic dysphonia* is a poorly understood neurologic disorder similar to dystonia. Many patients who are middle-aged or elderly and otherwise healthy gradually lose the ability to speak quietly and fluently. Any effort to speak results in contraction of the speech musculature so that the voice is strained and phonation is labored. The condition differs from the stridor caused by spasm of the laryngeal muscles in tetany. It is nonprogressive but may be combined with restricted extrapyramidal disorders such as blepharospasm and spasmodic torticollis. Surgical section of the superior laryngeal nerve on one side has been found to at least partially diminish the rigidity.

Defects in articulation can be subdivided into paretic dysarthria, spastic and rigid dysarthria, and choreic, myoclonic, and ataxic dysarthria. *Paretic dysarthria* is due to a neural or bulbar (medullary) weakness or paralysis of the articulatory muscles (lower motor neuron paralysis). There is a special difficulty in the correct utterance of vibratives, such as *r*; the voice develops a nasal quality due to palatal weakness; and as the paralysis becomes more complete, lingual and labial consonants are not pronounced. In the advanced stages, the shriveled tongue lies inert on the floor of the mouth, and the lips are relaxed and tremulous. Bulbar palsy, peripheral neuropathies, and muscle diseases including myasthenia gravis are common causes. *Spastic and rigid dysarthria* is a supranuclear weakness of articulation from diseases that involve the corticobulbar or subcortical tracts, usually brainstem stroke. Unlike bulbar paralysis due to lower neuron involvement, this condition entails no atrophy or fasciculation of the paralyzed muscles, the jaw jerk and other facial reflexes are exaggerated, the palatal reflexes are retained, emotional control is poor (pathologic laughter and crying), and sometimes breathing is periodic (Cheyne-Stokes). When the frontal operculum alone is involved, the speech deficit may be a pure dysarthria but usually without the impairment in emotional control. In the beginning, the patient may be totally anarthric and aphonic, but when improvement occurs or when the patient has a milder version of the same condition, speech is notably slow, thick, and indistinct, much like that of a patient with partial bulbar paralysis. Choreic, myoclonic, and ataxic dysarthria may occur in Huntington's disease, cerebellar syndromes, and palatal myoclonus (see Chaps. 21 and 371). Speech is irregular, explosive, inarticulate, and unpredictable.

CLINICAL APPROACH TO LANGUAGE DISORDERS

DIAGNOSIS For aphasia, conversational testing permits quick assessment of the motor aspects of speech (praxis and prosody), apparent language formulation, and auditory comprehension. Disabilities in the purely motor aspects of speech suggest a motor aphasia. This possibility can be pursued by tests of repeating from dictation and tests of praxis of the oropharyngeal and respiratory apparatus. Disabilities in language formulation, such as literal paraphasias with impaired comprehension, are indicative of Wernicke's aphasia. Disorders confined to naming, generally without paraphasias, when other language functions (reading, writing, spelling, etc.) are adequate, are diagnostic of amnesic dysnomia.

Dyspraxia of limbs and speech musculature in response to spoken commands or to visual mimicry is generally associated with Broca's aphasia and sometimes with Wernicke's aphasia. Bilateral or unilateral homonymous hemianopsia without motor weakness is often linked with pure word blindness (alexia or dyslexia) or to amnesic-dysnomic aphasia. Bilateral hemiplegias due to extensive frontal lesions are accompanied occasionally by pure word muteness.

When conversation indicates virtually no disabilities, other tests may be revealing. Reading aloud single letters, words, and text may reveal pure word blindness, whereas tests of writing in this syndrome are normal. Literal and verbal paraphasic errors may appear in milder cases of Wernicke's aphasia as the patient reads aloud from text or from words in the examiner's handwriting. Similar errors occur more frequently when the patient is asked to explain the text, read aloud, or give explanations in writing. Adequacy of response channels is determined by presenting tasks that permit a response physically identical with the test stimulus, such as copying visual stimuli and repeating aloud from auditory stimuli. Inadequacy of speech modality functions such as vision, hearing, phonation/articulation, or body-part movements for writing precludes further analysis of language function via that channel. If reception and response channels are adequate in these initial tests, they may then be used in tests requiring all types of language function, such as writing from dictation, vocal naming of visual stimuli, and matching physically dissimilar stimuli having a name in common (e.g., the word *cow* and a picture of a cow). By using the same test material as in the earlier tests, direct comparison of performances in spoken naming, written naming, and matching can be made from visual, auditory, and palpated stimuli. A performance profile can be constructed separately for each type of stimulus material tested (objects, pictures, words, letters, numbers, colors, etc.). The resultant profile can then be used to determine whether the main deficits fall across one or more input or response channels. These data provide a baseline against which later changes may be compared.

Disturbances of articulation point to involvement of a different set of neural structures, such as the motor cortices, the corticobulbar pathways, the seventh, ninth, and tenth nuclei, the brainstem, and extrapyramidal nuclei and tracts. It may be necessary to use other neurologic findings to decide which of these areas is involved. There is no special treatment for the dysarthric disturbance of speech.

PROGNOSIS The outcome depends on the underlying disease and the magnitude of the lesion within the speech areas. Global aphasias lasting more than a week or two usually have had a bad long-term outcome. Seldom is there enough recovery of communicative speech to permit resumption of occupation or profession. Partial aphasias frequently improve, sometimes to a gratifying degree, if they are of vascular or encephalitic origin. Aphasias due to embolism, whether global or restricted, may disappear in hours to days or may persist. Most aphasias are due to vascular disease of the brain, and

some degree of spontaneous improvement usually occurs over days to months after the stroke. Sometimes recovery is complete within hours or days; at times, not more than a few words are regained after a year or two of assiduous speech training. Nevertheless, many experts in the field believe that speech training is worthwhile. Some of the methods used by specially trained therapists include melodic intonation therapy, which helps those with agrammatism; special programs to improve skills in syntax; and some programs to improve abilities to relate words heard to those seen and improve auditory comprehension at the level of sentences. Thus far, all such therapies have been based on insights into underlying brain mechanisms. When these insights become more firmly grounded, methods may improve, but the daunting problem facing all therapists is not simply to improve partially damaged functions, but to assist the brain in developing brand-new skills using tissues which may have had only marginal roles to play in speech and language before the brain injury.

REFERENCES

ALBERT ML et al: *Clinical Aspects of Dysphasia.* New York, Springer-Verlag, 1981

ALESANDER MP et al: Broca's area aphasias: Aphasia after lesions including the frontal operculum. Neurology 50:353, 1990

CHASE TN et al: Wechsler adult intelligence scale performance cortical localization by fluorodeoxyglucose F18-positron emission tomography. Arch Neurol 41:1244, 1984

COSTELLO AL, WARRINGTON EK: Dynamic aphasia: The selective impairment of verbal planning. Cortex 25:103, 1989

DAMASIO AR: Aphasia. N Engl J Med 325:531, 1992

———— (ed): Behavioral neurology. Sem Neurol 4:117, 1984

HART J, GORDON B: Delineation of single word semantic comprehension deficits in aphasia, with anatomical correlation. Ann Neurol 27:226, 1990

KARBE H et al: Profiles of language impairment in primary progressive aphasia. Arch Neurol 50:193, 1993

KEMPLER D et al: A metabolic investigation of a disconnection syndrome: Conduction aphasia. Ann Neurol 22:134, 1987

KERTESZ A: *Localization in Neuropsychology.* New York, Academic Press, 1983

LECOURS AR et al: *Aphasiology.* London, Bailliere Tindall, 1983

LUDLOW CL et al: Brain lesions associated with nonfluent aphasia fifteen years following penetrating head injury. Brain 109:55, 1986

METTER EJ et al: Brain behavior relationships in aphasia studied by positron emission tomography. Ann NY Acad Sci 620:153, 1991

MOHR JP et al: Broca aphasia: Pathologic and clinical aspects. Neurology 28:311, 1978

OJEMANN G et al: Cortical language localization in left, dominant hemisphere: An electrical stimulation mapping investigation in 117 patients. J Neurosurg 71:316, 1989

PETERSEN SE et al: Positron emission tomography studies of the cortical anatomy of single-word processing. Nature 331:585, 1988

POSNER MI et al: Localization of cognitive operations in the human brain. Science 240:1627, 1988

SHAYWITZ S et al: Evidence that dyslexia may represent the lower tail of a normal distribution of reading ability. N Engl J Med 326:145, 1992

VIGNOLO LA et al: Unexpected CT-scan findings in global aphasia. Cortex 22:55, 1986

29 DISORDERS OF SLEEP AND CIRCADIAN RHYTHMS

CHARLES A. CZEISLER / GARY S. RICHARDSON / JOSEPH B. MARTIN

Disturbed sleep is among the most frequent health complaints physicians encounter. One-third of adults in the United States experience occasional or persistent sleep disturbances. Sleep deprivation or disruption of the circadian timing system can lead to serious impairment of daytime functioning. Sleep disorders may either contribute to or result from related medical or psychiatric conditions. Twenty years ago, many such complaints were treated with hypnotic medications without further diagnostic evaluation. A distinct class of sleep and arousal disorders has now been identified, and the field of sleep disorders is now an established clinical discipline. Two principal neurobiologic systems govern the sleep-wake cycle: one that actively generates sleep and sleep-related processes and another that times sleep within the 24-h day. Either intrinsic abnormalities in these systems or extrinsic disturbances (environmental, drug- or illness-related) can lead to sleep or circadian rhythm disorders.

PHYSIOLOGY OF SLEEP AND WAKEFULNESS

Most adults sleep 7 to 8 h per night, although the timing, duration, and internal structure of sleep vary among apparently healthy individuals and as a function of age. At the extremes, infants and the elderly have frequent interruptions of sleep. In the United States, adults of intermediate age tend to have one consolidated sleep episode per day, although in some cultures sleep may be divided into a midafternoon nap and a shortened night sleep. While there is a wide range of normal sleep lengths, adults with habitual sleep durations of fewer than 4 h or greater than 9 have increased mortality rates as compared to those who sleep 7 to 8 h per night.

STATES AND STAGES OF SLEEP States and stages of human sleep are defined on the basis of characteristic patterns in the electroencephalogram (EEG), the electrooculogram (EOG—a measure of eye-movement activity), and the surface electromyogram (EMG). The continuous recording of this array of electrophysiologic parameters to define sleep and wakefulness is termed *polysomnography* (see Table 29-1).

Polysomnographic profiles define two states of sleep: (1) rapid-eye-movement (REM) sleep (also known as dreaming, paradoxical, desynchronized, or "D" sleep) and (2) non-rapid-eye-movement (NREM) sleep (also known as orthodox, synchronized, or "S" sleep). NREM sleep is in turn subdivided into four stages. NREM stage 1 is the transition from wakefulness and is characterized by disappearance of the regular alpha pattern and emergence of a low-amplitude, mixed-frequency pattern, predominantly in the theta range (2 to 7 Hz) (Fig. 29-1) and slow "rolling" eye movements. NREM stage 2 is defined by the occurrence of K complexes and sleep spindles superimposed upon a background activity similar to that of stage 1. K complexes are slow, high-amplitude, negative (upward) discharges followed immediately by a positive (downward) deflection. Sleep spindles are high-frequency (12 to 14 Hz) discharges lasting 0.5 to 2.0 s with a characteristic waxing-waning amplitude. Rapid-eye-movement activity is absent, and the EMG is similar to stage 1. NREM stage 3 is sleep with at least 20 percent but less than 50 percent high-amplitude ($\geq 75\ \mu$V) delta (0.5 to 2 Hz) activity. Sleep spindles may persist, eye-movement activity is absent, and EMG activity persists at a reduced level. In NREM stage 4, the high-voltage, slow EEG pattern of stage 3 comprises at least 50 percent of the record. NREM stages 3 and 4 are referred to, collectively, as "slow-wave," "delta," or "deep" sleep.

REM sleep is characterized by a low-amplitude, mixed-frequency EEG similar to that of NREM stage 1 (Fig. 29-1). Bursts of 3- to 5-Hz activity with sharp negative deflections are often superimposed on this pattern. The EOG shows bursts of REM similar to that seen

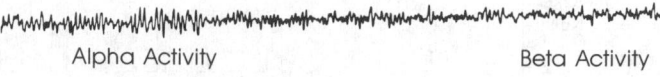

Awake

Alpha Activity   Beta Activity

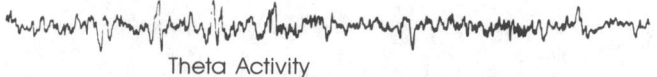

Stage 1 Sleep

Theta Activity

Stage 2 Sleep

K Complex

Spindle

Stage 3 Sleep

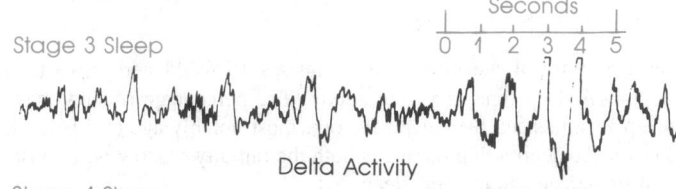

Seconds

Delta Activity

Stage 4 Sleep

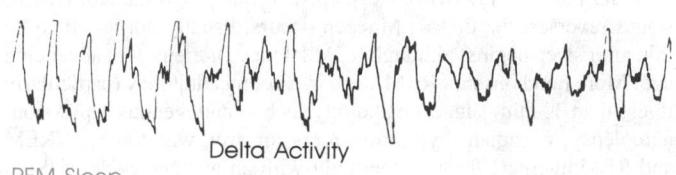

Delta Activity

REM Sleep

Theta Activity   Beta Activity

FIGURE 29-1 Electroencephalogram of human sleep stages. The first trace illustrates alpha activity seen in quiet wakefulness (eyes closed) and the beta activity of an alert subject. Stage 1 theta activity is seen in the second trace; stage 2 sleep (with associated sleep spindle and K complex) in the third. The fourth and fifth traces show slow-wave (stages 3 and 4) sleep, with prominent delta activity. This synchronous activity is absent in REM sleep (sixth trace), which resembles stage 1 EEG. However, REM sleep is accompanied by rapid eye movements and muscle paralysis. *(Reproduced from Horne.)*

during eyes-open wakefulness. EMG activity is absent, reflecting the complete brainstem-mediated muscle atonia that is characteristic of that state.

ORGANIZATION OF HUMAN SLEEP Normal nocturnal sleep in adults displays a consistent organization from night to night (Fig. 29-2). After sleep onset, sleep usually progresses through NREM stages 1 to 4 within 45 to 60 min. Slow-wave sleep predominates in

---

TABLE 29-1 Electrophysiologic correlates of human sleep states and stages

	Electroencephalogram	Electrooculogram	Electromyogram
Wake (eyes open)	Low amplitude, mixed, (high) frequency	Rapid	High, variable
Wake (eyes closed)	Low amplitude, alpha (8–13 Hz) dominates, particularly over occipital region	Absent, but slow "rolling" eye movements	Reduced
NREM stage 1	Low amplitude, mixed frequency (alpha absent)	Slow "rolling" eye movements	Reduced
NREM stage 2	Low amplitude with addition of characteristic EEG patterns (K complexes and sleep spindles)	Absent	Reduced
NREM stage 3	Increased amplitude, decreased frequency 20–50% of record dominated by delta (0.5–2.0 Hz)	Absent	Reduced
NREM stage 4	>50% of record dominated by delta EEG activity	Absent	Reduced
REM	Low amplitude, mixed frequency	Rapid, conjugate	Absent

SOURCE: Modified from: Rechtschaffen A, Kales A (eds): *A Manual of Standardized Terminology, Technique and Scoring System for Sleep Stages of Human Subjects.* Los Angeles, UCLA Brain Information Service/Brain Research Institute, 1968.

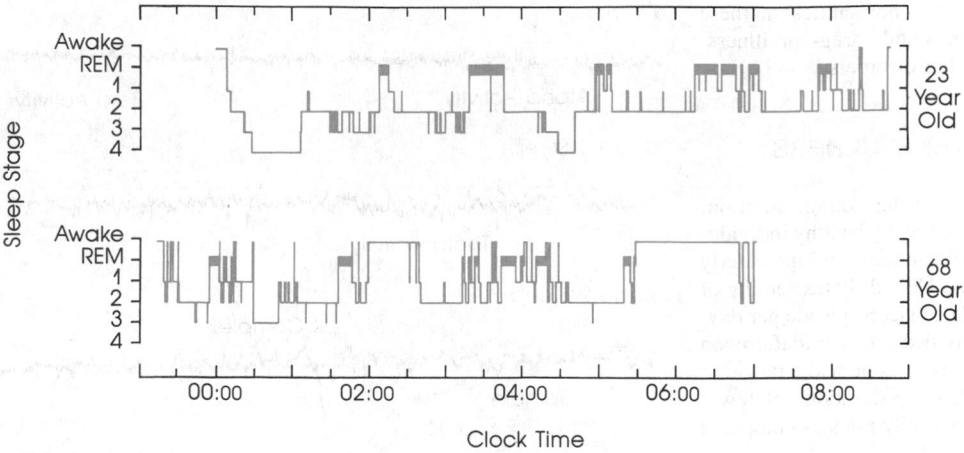

FIGURE 29-2 Plots of the stages of REM sleep (solid bars) and the four stages of NREM sleep over the course of the entire night for representative young (upper panel, age 23) and elderly (lower panel, age 68) adult men. The recording in the elderly subject illustrates the reduction of slow-wave sleep, frequent spontaneous awakenings, early sleep onset, and early morning awakening that are characteristic features of sleep in the aged, even in the absence of specific medical or psychiatric pathology. *(From the Center for Circadian and Sleep Disorders Medicine, Brigham and Women' Hospital.)*

the first third of the night and comprises 15 to 25 percent of total nocturnal sleep time in young adults. The percentage of slow-wave sleep is influenced by several factors, most notably age (see below). Prior sleep deprivation increases both the rapidity of slow-wave onset and its percentage of total sleep.

After the first slow-wave sleep episode, the progression of NREM stages reverses; the first REM sleep occurs, usually not less than 80 min after sleep begins, although REM latency shortens with advancing age. More rapid onset of REM sleep in a young adult may (particularly if less than 30 min) suggest pathology such as endogenous depression, narcolepsy, circadian rhythm disorders, or drug withdrawal. NREM and REM alternate through the night with an average cycle of 90 to 110 min (the "ultradian" cycle). As the sleep period lengthens, the portion of each cycle composed of slow-wave sleep decreases and that of REM sleep increases. Overall, REM sleep is 20 to 25 percent of total sleep, NREM stages (1 and 2) are 50 to 60 percent (increasing in elderly subjects).

BEHAVIORAL CORRELATES OF SLEEP STATES AND STAGES
Age has a large impact on sleep state organization (Fig. 29-2). Slow-wave sleep is most prominent during childhood, decreasing sharply at puberty and across the second and third decades of life. After age 30, there is a progressive, almost linear decline in the amount of slow-wave sleep, and the amplitude of delta EEG activity comprising slow-wave sleep is reduced. In the otherwise healthy elderly, slow-wave sleep may be completely absent, particularly in males.

A different age profile exists for REM sleep. In infancy, REM sleep may comprise 50 percent of total sleep time, and the percentage is inversely proportional to developmental age. The amount of REM sleep falls off sharply over the first postnatal year as a mature REM-NREM cycle develops. During the rest of life into extreme old age, REM occupies a more constant percentage of total sleep time than does slow-wave sleep.

Polysomnographic staging of sleep correlates with behavioral changes during specific states and stages. Sleep onset is associated with marked decrements in perception of both auditory and visual stimuli and lapses of consciousness. At stage 1 subjects may respond to faint auditory or visual signals without "awakening." Furthermore, although memory incorporation appears to be inhibited at the onset of NREM stage 1, subjects aroused from that stage frequently deny having been asleep. In contrast, subjective and objective assessments of sleep agree more closely for subjects awakened from NREM stage 2. This has led some investigators to define sleep onset as the occurrence of the first K complex or sleep spindle suggestive of NREM stage 2 and to define NREM stage 1 as a "transitional stage." The progression of subsequent NREM stages corresponds with increasing depth of sleep as measured by threshold for arousal with a variety of auditory stimuli.

Awakenings from REM sleep are associated with recall of vivid dream imagery more than 80 percent of the time. The reliability of dream recall increases with REM periods occurring later in the night.

Imagery may also be reported after NREM sleep interruptions, though these typically lack the detail and vividness of REM dreams. The incidence of NREM dream recall can be increased by selective REM sleep deprivation, suggesting that REM sleep and dreaming per se are not inexorably linked.

PHYSIOLOGIC CORRELATES OF SLEEP STATES AND STAGES
All major physiologic systems are influenced by sleep. In some cases, concomitant behavior changes such as supine posture or inactivity are the proximal causes of altered physiologic function, but in most cases the sleep state itself appears to be responsible. Changes in cardiovascular function include a decrease in blood pressure and heart rate during NREM and particularly during slow-wave sleep. During REM sleep, phasic activity (bursts of eye movements) is associated with variability in both blood pressure and heart rate mediated principally by the vagus. Cardiac dysrhythmias may occur selectively during REM sleep. Respiratory function also changes (see Chap. 229). Respiratory rate and minute ventilation decrease during NREM sleep and become variable during phasic REM sleep. The ventilatory response to carbon dioxide attenuates during NREM sleep, resulting in a higher P_{CO_2}. During REM sleep the ventilatory response to both hypercapnia and hypoxia shows marked variability. Respiratory musculature, including that responsible for upper airway patency, is hypotonic throughout sleep and more so during REM sleep, resulting in an increase in airway resistance. In addition, the cough reflex is attenuated or absent during sleep. These changes in respiratory function may be relevant to the pathogenesis of obstructive sleep apnea (OSA) and sudden infant death syndrome (SIDS) (see Chap. 229).

Endocrine function also varies with sleep. The most prominent changes are apparent in neuroendocrine parameters. Slow-wave sleep is associated with secretion of growth hormone in young men, while sleep in general is associated with augmented secretion of prolactin. Sleep has a complex effect on the secretion of luteinizing hormone (LH); during puberty sleep is associated with increased LH secretion, whereas sleep in the mature woman inhibits LH secretion in the early follicular phase of the menstrual cycle. Sleep onset (and probably slow-wave sleep) is associated with inhibition of thyroid-stimulating hormone (TSH) and of the adrenocorticotropic hormone (ACTH)–cortisol axis, an effect that is independent of the circadian rhythms in the two systems.

Sleep is also associated with alterations of thermoregulatory function. NREM sleep is associated with an attenuation of thermoregulatory responses to either heat or cold stress, and animal studies of thermosensitive neurons in the hypothalamus document a NREM-dependent reduction of the thermoregulatory set-point. REM sleep is associated with complete absence of thermoregulatory responsiveness, effectively resulting in poikilothermy. However, the potential adverse impact of this failure of thermoregulation is blunted by inhibition of REM sleep by extreme ambient temperatures.

Neuroanatomy of sleep Lesion studies in animals and neurologic diseases in humans have suggested distinct neuroanatomic sites in the generation of normal sleep and wakefulness. The studies of von Economo of patients with encephalitis lethargica suggested that the anterior hypothalamus contained a "sleep center" while the posterior hypothalamus contained a "wake center." Experimental studies in animals have variously implicated the medullary reticular formation, the thalamus, and the basal forebrain in the generation of sleep, while the brainstem reticular formation, the midbrain, the subthalamus, the thalamus, and the basal forebrain have all been suggested to play a role in the generation of wakefulness or EEG arousal (see also Chap. 26).

Despite many studies, there is little evidence for either a single, discrete "sleep center" or a single, discrete "wake center." Current hypotheses suggest that the capacity for sleep and wake generation is distributed along an axial "core" of neurons extending from the brainstem rostrally to the basal forebrain. Complex commingling of neuronal groups occurs at many points along this basal forebrain axis.

Nonetheless, the neuroanatomic correlates of REM sleep appear to be discretely localized. Specific regions in the pons are associated with each of the neurophysiologic correlates of REM sleep. Small lesions in the dorsal pons produce REM sleep without the descending muscle inhibition normally associated with that state; microinjections of carbachol into the same area produce atonia without other features of REM sleep. These experimental manipulations are mimicked by pathologic conditions in humans and animals. In narcolepsy, for example, abrupt, complete or partial paralysis (cataplexy) occurs in response to a variety of stimuli. In dogs with this condition, physostigmine, a central cholinesterase inhibitor, increases the frequency of cataplectic attacks while atropine decreases their frequency. Conversely, in REM sleep behavior disorder (see below), patients suffer from incomplete motor inhibition during REM sleep resulting in involuntary, occasionally violent movement during REM sleep.

Neurochemistry of sleep   Early experimental studies that focused on the raphe nuclei of the brainstem appeared to implicate serotonin as the primary sleep-promoting neurotransmitter, while catecholamines were considered to be responsible for wakefulness. Subsequent work has demonstrated that the raphe-serotonin system may facilitate sleep but is not necessary to its expression. The extensive pharmacology of sleep and wakefulness suggests roles for other neurotransmitters as well. The alerting influence of caffeine implicates adenosine, whereas the hypnotic effect of benzodiazepines and barbiturates suggests a role for endogenous ligands of the GABA-receptor complex.

A variety of sleep-promoting substances have been identified. These are principally peptides, and the hypnotic effect is commonly limited to NREM or slow-wave sleep, although peptides that increase REM sleep have also been reported. Many of these "sleep factors," including interleukin 1 and prostaglandin E_2, are immunologically active as well, suggesting a link between immune function and sleep-wake states.

PHYSIOLOGY OF CIRCADIAN RHYTHMICITY   The sleep-wake cycle is the most evident of the many 24-h rhythms in humans. Prominent daily variations also occur in endocrine, thermoregulatory, cardiac, pulmonary, renal, gastrointestinal, and cognitive functions. However, in evaluating a daily variation, it is important to distinguish between those rhythmic components passively evoked by periodic environmental or behavioral changes (e.g., the increase in blood pressure and heart rate upon assumption of the upright posture), and those actively driven by an endogenous oscillatory process (e.g., the circadian variation in plasma cortisol that persists under a variety of environmental and behavioral conditions).

The suprachiasmatic nuclei (SCN) of the hypothalamus act as the central neural pacemakers of the circadian timing system in mammals. Bilateral destruction of these nuclei results in a loss of endogenous circadian rhythmicity that can only be restored by transplantation of the same structure(s) from a donor animal. The period and phase of the endogenous neural oscillator are normally synchronized to the 24-h period of the environmental light-dark cycle. Entrainment of mammalian circadian rhythms by the light-dark cycle is mediated via the retinohypothalamic tract, a monosynaptic pathway that links the retina to the SCN.

The principal properties characterizing an endogenous circadian pacemaker are its *intrinsic period, phase, amplitude,* and *resetting capacity.* In human subjects living in controlled laboratory environments free of time cues *(free-running)*, the duration of the behavioral rest-activity cycle averages 25 h. However, the timing of the light-dark cycle has generally been uncontrolled in such free-running studies, with the subjects choosing to be exposed to light during their "subjective days" and to darkness during their "subjective nights." Recent work suggests that when the light-dark cycle is controlled, the observed period of the human circadian pacemaker is much closer to 24 h. Nonetheless, synchronization of the endogenous circadian pacemaker to the 24-h day requires that the pacemaker be reset each day, which is normally achieved by exposure to the environmental light-dark cycle.

Exposure to light can shift the phase of the endogenous circadian pacemaker, but both the magnitude and direction of the phase shifts induced by light depend on the timing and intensity of the light. Properly timed exposure to light of sufficient intensity can, within 2 to 3 days, reset the human circadian pacemaker (presumably the SCN) to any desired hour.

The timing and internal architecture of sleep are directly coupled to the output of the endogenous pacemaker. Spontaneous sleep duration, sleepiness, REM sleep propensity, and both the ability and the tendency to sleep vary with the circadian phase as marked by the endogenous circadian temperature cycle in humans. Sleep tendency, sleepiness, and REM sleep propensity all peak just after the nadir of the endogenous circadian temperature cycle (approximately 2 to 3 h before awakening). In addition, 85 percent of all spontaneous awakenings of subjects living in constant environmental conditions occur on the rising slope of the temperature cycle. Furthermore, there are certain times (wake maintenance zones) when it is very difficult to fall asleep, even for subjects who are sleep-deprived. Misalignment of the output of the endogenous circadian pacemaker with the desired sleep-wake cycle is thought to be responsible for certain types of insomnia, as well as for the decrements of alertness and performance in night-shift workers and after jet lag.

DISORDERS OF SLEEP AND WAKEFULNESS

An international classification of sleep disorders (Table 29-2) divides these conditions into three major groups: dyssomnias, parasomnias, and medical psychiatric sleep disorders. A detailed description of each of these disorders may be found in the publication of the American Sleep Disorders Association.

APPROACH TO THE PATIENT WITH A SLEEP COMPLAINT
Patients may seek help from a physician because of: (1) an acute or chronic inability to sleep adequately at night; (2) chronic fatigue, sleepiness, or tiredness during the day; or (3) a behavioral manifestation associated with sleep itself. Disruption or disturbance of nocturnal sleep is directly related to decreased alertness and impairment of daytime cognitive and psychomotor performance, which is often of serious concern to the patient.

Taking a careful history is critical in the evaluation of the patient with a sleep complaint. In particular, the duration, severity, and consistency of the complaint are important, along with the patient's estimate—in the case of an insomnia complaint—of the consequences of reported sleep loss on subsequent waking function. Information from a friend or family member can be an invaluable aid in assessing the severity of the complaint on daytime functioning, as some patients will underreport such potentially embarrassing symptoms as heavy snoring or falling asleep while driving.

Retrospective completion by the physician and patient of a day-by-day sleep-work-drug log in reverse chronologic order can help the physician better understand the nature of the complaint. Work times should be specified each day, as one in six working men and one in

TABLE 29-2   International classification of sleep disorders

DYSSOMNIAS

A Intrinsic sleep disorders
   1 Psychophysiologic insomnia
   2 Idiopathic insomnia
   3 Narcolepsy
   4 Recurrent or idiopathic hypersomnia
   5 Posttraumatic hypersomnia
   6 Sleep apnea syndromes
   7 Periodic limb movement disorder
   8 Restless legs syndrome
B Extrinsic sleep disorders
   1 Inadequate sleep hygiene
   2 Environmental sleep disorder
   3 Altitude insomnia
   4 Adjustment sleep disorder
   5 Sleep-onset association disorder
   6 Food allergy insomnia
   7 Nocturnal eating (drinking) syndrome
   8 Drug- or alcohol-dependent sleep disorders
C Circadian rhythm sleep disorders
   1 Time-zone change (jet-lag) syndrome
   2 Shift-work sleep disorder
   3 Delayed sleep phase syndrome
   4 Advanced sleep phase syndrome
   5 Non-24-h sleep-wake disorder

PARASOMNIAS

A Arousal disorders
   1 Confusional arousals
   2 Sleepwalking
   3 Sleep terrors
B Sleep-wake transition disorders
   1 Rhythmic movement disorder
   2 Sleep talking
   3 Nocturnal leg cramps
C Parasomnias usually associated with REM sleep
   1 Nightmares
   2 Sleep paralysis
   3 Impaired sleep-related penile erections
   4 Sleep-related painful erections
   5 REM sleep-related cardiac arrhythmias
   6 REM sleep behavior disorder
D Other parasomnias
   1 Sleep bruxism
   2 Sleep enuresis
   3 Nocturnal paroxysmal dystonia

SLEEP DISORDERS ASSOCIATED WITH MEDICAL/PSYCHIATRIC DISORDERS

A Associated with mental disorders
B Associated with neurologic disorders
   1 Cerebral degenerative disorders
   2 Parkinsonism
   3 Fatal familial insomnia
   4 Sleep-related epilepsy
   5 Sleep-related headaches
C Associated with other medical disorders
   1 Sleeping sickness
   2 Nocturnal cardiac ischemia
   3 Chronic obstructive pulmonary disease
   4 Sleep-related asthma
   5 Sleep-related gastroesophageal reflux
   6 Peptic ulcer disease
   7 Fibrositis syndrome

SOURCE: Modified from *International Classification of Sleep Disorders*, prepared by the Diagnostic Classification Steering Committee, Thorpy MJ, Chairman. Rochester, MN, American Sleep Disorders Association, 1990.

eight working women in the United States have an irregular work schedule that includes both day and night/evening work. Drug and alcohol use, including caffeine and hypnotics, should be noted each day. This log should be compared with a prospective sleep-work-drug log (including daytime naps and nocturnal awakenings) as recorded by the patient for at least 2 weeks. The resultant data should be plotted to facilitate recognition of circadian rhythm sleep disorders such as delayed sleep phase syndrome (see below). With the advent of objective measurements of sleep tendency (see below), quantifica-

tion of the impairment of daytime alertness is a valuable adjunct in the assessment of sleep problems. As a rule, the clinical approach to a patient with disrupted sleep but without impaired daytime alertness should be conservative. Chronic treatment of isolated insomnia with hypnotic medications is rarely justified.

Laboratory investigation   In addition to the three electrophysiologic variables used to define sleep states and stages (see above), the standard clinical polysomnogram includes measures of respiration (respiratory effort, air flow, and oxygen saturation), anterior tibialis EMG, and ECG. Evaluation of penile tumescence during nocturnal sleep also can be used to help determine whether the cause of erectile dysfunction in a patient is psychogenic or organic (see Chap. 47).

Assessment of daytime functioning as an index of the adequacy of sleep can be made with the multiple sleep latency test (MSLT), which involves repeated measurement of sleep latency (time to onset of sleep) under standardized conditions during a day following quantified nocturnal sleep. The average latency across four to six tests (administered every 2 h across the waking day) is taken as an objective measure of daytime sleep tendency. Disorders of sleep that result in pathologic, daytime somnolence can be reliably distinguished with the MSLT. In addition, the multiple measurements of sleep onset identify direct transitions from wakefulness to REM sleep that are indicative of specific pathologic conditions (e.g., narcolepsy).

INSOMNIA   Insomnia is the complaint of inadequate sleep; it is classified according to the nature of sleep disruption and the duration of the complaint. The nature of the sleep disruption provides important information about the possible etiology of the insomnia and is also central to the selection of specific and appropriate treatment. Insomnia is subdivided into difficulty falling asleep (*sleep onset insomnia*), frequent or sustained awakenings (*sleep maintenance insomnia*), or persistent sleepiness despite sleep of adequate duration (*nonrestorative sleep*). Similarly, the duration of the symptom is an important determinant of the nature of appropriate treatment. An insomnia complaint lasting one to several nights (within a single episode) is termed *transient insomnia*. Transient insomnia is typically the result of situational stress or a change in work schedule or environment (jet lag). *Short-term insomnia* lasts from a few days to 3 weeks. Disruption of this duration is usually associated with more protracted stress, such as recovery from surgery or short-term illness. *Long-term* or *chronic insomnia* lasts for months or years and commonly reflects the effects of psychiatric or other chronic medical conditions, medications, or a primary sleep disorder (see below). It is now clear that chronic insomnia may present as recurrent episodes of insomnia, not necessarily associated with parallel variation in the underlying cause. Although some clinicians refer to this as recurrent insomnia, others suggest that this may be the typical pattern of all chronic insomniacs.

While an occasional night of poor sleep, typically in the setting of stress or excitement about external events, is both common and without lasting consequences, persistent insomnia can have important adverse consequences in the form of impaired daytime function, mood disturbances, and increased risk of injury due to accidents. A complaint of persistent insomnia warrants specific investigation as to cause and intervention with appropriately designed treatment for either the underlying mechanism and/or the sleep disruption.

Psychophysiologic insomnia   Persistent psychophysiologic insomnia is a behavioral disorder in which patients are preoccupied with a perceived inability to sleep at night. The sleep disturbance is often triggered by an emotionally stressful event; however, the poor sleep habits acquired during the stressful period persist long after the initial incident. Such patients become hyperaroused by their own persistent efforts to sleep, and the insomnia is a conditioned or learned response. Patients with psychophysiologic insomnia fall asleep more easily at unscheduled times (when not trying) or outside the home environment. In these cases, polysomnographic recording reveals an objective sleep disturbance, often with an abnormally long sleep latency, frequent nocturnal awakenings, and an increased amount of stage 1 transitional sleep. Behavioral therapy is often beneficial; relaxation training can improve the sleep of patients in whom physical tension is prominent. Limited use of hypnotic medications, which can serve as a catalyst for successful behavioral therapy, may be appropriate. Extrinsic factors may contribute to this condition (see below). Rigorous attention should be paid to sleep hygiene (see below) and correction of counterproductive, arousing behaviors before bedtime.

Extrinsic insomnia A number of sleep disorders are the result of extrinsic factors that interfere with sleep. *Adjustment sleep disorder*, also called *transient situational insomnia*, can occur after a change in the sleeping environment (e.g., in an unfamiliar hotel or hospital bed) or before or after a significant life event, such as a change of occupation, loss of a loved one, illness, or anxiety over a deadline or examination. Increased sleep latency, frequent awakenings from sleep, and early morning awakening can all occur. Recovery generally occurs rapidly, certainly within 2 to 3 weeks. *Inadequate sleep hygiene* is characterized by a behavior pattern prior to sleep and/or a bedroom environment that is not conducive to sleep. On taking a careful history, physicians may learn that some insomniac patients are attempting to sleep with the television on throughout the night or are attempting to sleep just after coming home from work at midnight. Noise and/or light in the bedroom can interfere with sleep, as can a bed partner with periodic limb movements during sleep or one who snores loudly. Luminous clocks can arouse the patient, heightening anxiety about the time it has taken to fall asleep. Drugs that act on the central nervous system, large meals, vigorous exercise, or hot showers just before sleep may interfere with sleep onset. In preference to hypnotic medications, patients should be counseled to develop a soporific bedtime ritual and to prepare and reserve the bedroom environment for sleeping. Consistent, regular rising times should be charted daily; irregular naps should be avoided; total time in bed should be restricted to actual sleep time.

Altitude insomnia Sleep disturbance is a common consequence of exposure to high altitude. Periodic breathing of the Cheyne-Stokes type occurs during NREM sleep about half the time at altitude, with restoration of a regular breathing pattern during REM sleep. Central rather than obstructive sleep apnea appears to be responsible, characterized by regular respiratory pauses. Both hypoxia and hypocapnia are thought to be involved in the development of periodic breathing. Frequent awakenings and poor quality sleep characterize altitude insomnia, which is generally worst on the first few nights at high altitude but may persist. The duration of sleep is unchanged, but there are more arousals after sleep onset and less time in slow-wave (stages 3 and 4) sleep. Pretreatment with acetazolamide can decrease time spent in periodic breathing and substantially reduce hypoxia during sleep. Medroxyprogesterone acetate (MPA) also reduces periodic breathing but does not significantly reduce hypoxia during sleep at altitude.

Drug- or alcohol-dependent sleep disorders Disturbed sleep can result from ingestion of a wide variety of agents. Caffeine is perhaps the most common pharmacologic cause of insomnia in sensitive patients. It produces increased latency to sleep onset, more frequent arousals during sleep, and a reduction in total sleep time for up to 8 to 14 h after ingestion. Occasional patients are surprised to learn that their insomnia may be related to coffee consumption; a careful history will reveal that such patients may drink 15 to 20 cups per day. As few as 3 to 5 cups of coffee can significantly disturb sleep in some patients; therefore, a 1- to 2-month caffeine withdrawal period should be attempted in patients with these symptoms. Similarly, alcohol and nicotine can interfere with sleep, although many patients use them to relax and promote sleep. Although alcohol can increase drowsiness and shorten sleep latency, even moderate amounts of alcohol increase awakenings after sleep onset by interfering with the ability of the brain to maintain sleep. In addition, alcohol ingestion prior to sleep is contraindicated in patients with sleep apnea because of the inhibitory effects of alcohol on respiration. Acutely, amphetamines and cocaine suppress both REM sleep and total sleep time, which return to normal with chronic use. Withdrawal leads to a REM sleep rebound. Finally, rebound insomnia associated with the acute withdrawal of hypnotics can be severe, especially following the use of benzodiazepines with a short half-life. For this reason, hypnotics should rarely be prescribed for habitual use; doses should be low to moderate, the total duration of hypnotic therapy should be limited to 2 to 3 weeks, and drug dosage should be reduced prior to withdrawal.

NARCOLEPSY Excessive daytime sleepiness with involuntary daytime sleep episodes, disturbed nocturnal sleep, and cataplexy (sudden weakness or loss of muscle tone, often elicited by emotion) are the most common symptoms of narcolepsy. Some patients also experience muscular paralysis and/or hallucinations at sleep onset or upon awakening. The severity varies. Patients may have two to three cataplectic attacks per day or per decade, and the extent and duration of an attack may vary from a transient sagging of the jaw to flaccid paralysis of the entire voluntary musculature for up to 20 to 30 min, in rare cases.

Narcolepsy affects over 200,000 people in the United States and appears to have a genetic basis. Experiments in some canine models of narcolepsy suggest an autosomal recessive pattern of inheritance. First-degree relatives of narcoleptic patients commonly exhibit excessive daytime somnolence and have a much higher incidence of narcolepsy than the general population. In addition, nearly all narcoleptics are positive for the human leukocyte antigen DR2 (ordinarily found in 20 to 30 percent of the general population) (see Chap. 64).

Symptoms typically begin in the second decade, although the onset ranges from ages 5 to 50. An identifiable stress (e.g., sleep-wake cycle disruption, divorce, loss of a loved one) may precede symptom onset.

Diagnosis Classically, the diagnosis of narcolepsy required the presence of the "narcolepsy tetrad," consisting of (1) excessive daytime somnolence, (2) cataplexy, (3) hypnogogic hallucinations (the occurrence of vivid hallucinatory dream imagery at sleep onset), and (4) sleep paralysis (an awareness that voluntary musculature is paralyzed coincident with the onset of sleep). The last three symptoms of the tetrad are all manifestations of the abnormal REM sleep regulation inherent in the syndrome. All patients with narcolepsy have objectively verifiable daytime somnolence, but the other three symptoms are variably present. At least half have cataplexy of some degree and smaller percentages report hypnogogic hallucinations and/or sleep paralysis. Other associated symptoms are useful but not specific. A history of "automatic behavior" during wakefulness (a trancelike state during which simple motor behaviors persist) serves principally to corroborate the presence of daytime somnolence but is not specific for mechanism. Older patients with narcolepsy also commonly report severe disruption of nocturnal sleep.

A family history is important in the evaluation of the patient with excessive daytime somnolence. Careful observation of the children and siblings of known narcoleptics, particularly at the typical age of onset (second decade), can lead to early diagnosis. The diagnosis of narcolepsy in a patient with a suggestive history depends upon (1) objective verification of excessive daytime somnolence, typically using the MSLT after nocturnal sleep recording, and (2) documentation of abnormal REM sleep regulation as evidenced by REM sleep onset within 10 min of sleep onset, either during the nocturnal recording or on one or more of the MSLT determinations.

Treatment The treatment of narcolepsy is symptomatic. Somnolence is treated with stimulants. Methylphenidate is considered the drug of choice by most. Pemoline, a common second choice, has a longer half-life and is associated with fewer side effects but may not be as effective. Dextroamphetamine and methamphetamine are also frequently used, particularly when methylphenidate and pemoline are inadequate.

Treatment of cataplexy, hypnogogic hallucinations, and sleep paralysis requires antidepressants, which are effective, in part, because of potent REM-suppressive effects. Protriptyline is the most commonly used anti-cataplectic in the United States. Efficacy is limited largely by anticholinergic side effects. Compounds including viloxzine hydrochloride and fluoxetine are under evaluation for this condition.

Gamma-hydroxy-butyrate (GHB), a drug available in Europe and Canada but still under evaluation in the United States, appears to be particularly useful to reverse nocturnal sleep disruption.

SLEEP APNEA SYNDROMES   Respiratory dysfunction during sleep is a common, serious cause of excessive daytime somnolence as well as of disturbed nocturnal sleep. An estimated 2 to 5 million people in the United States stop breathing for 15 to 150 s, from a dozen to several hundred times every night during sleep. These cessations of breathing may be due to either an occlusion of the airway *(obstructive sleep apnea)*, absence of respiratory effort *(central sleep apnea)*, or a combination of these factors *(mixed sleep apnea)*. Failure to recognize and appropriately treat these conditions may lead to serious cardiovascular complications and increased mortality. This problem is particularly prevalent in overweight men and in the elderly and is often associated with hypertension. Occult sleep-related breathing disorders may result in significant impairment of daytime alertness and functioning in otherwise healthy elderly persons. Readers are referred to Chap. 229 for a comprehensive review of the diagnosis and treatment of patients with these conditions.

DYSSOMNIA ASSOCIATED WITH LIMB MOVEMENTS   Restless legs syndrome   Patients with dyssomnia associated with the restless legs syndrome report an irresistible urge to move their legs when awake and inactive, especially when lying in bed just prior to sleep. This interferes with the ability to fall asleep. They report a creeping or crawling sensation deep within the calves or thighs, or sometimes even in the upper limbs, that is only relieved briefly by movement, particularly walking. In contrast, paresthesia secondary to peripheral neuropathy persists with activity. The severity of this chronic, idiopathic disorder may wax and wane with time and can be exacerbated by caffeine, iron deficiency, anemia, renal failure, and pregnancy. Nearly all patients with restless legs also experience periodic limb movement disorder during sleep, although the reverse is not the case. Together, these conditions can be documented in one-eighth of patients with insomnia seen at sleep disorders centers, although they are often thought to be an incidental finding rather than the cause of disturbed sleep.

Periodic limb movement disorder   Periodic limb movement disorder, also known as *nocturnal myoclonus*, is the principal objective polysomnographic finding in 17 percent of patients with insomnia and 11 percent of those with excessive daytime somnolence. Stereotyped, rhythmic, 0.5- to 5.0-s extensions of the great toe and dorsiflexion of the foot recur every 20 to 40 s during NREM stages 1 and 2 sleep, in episodes lasting from minutes to hours. Most such episodes occur during the first half of the night. The disorder occurs in a wide variety of sleep disorders (including narcolepsy, sleep apnea, and various forms of insomnia) and is associated with frequent arousals and an increased number of sleep-stage transitions. However, it has not been demonstrated that these sleep disturbances lead to insomnia. In fact, periodic limb movement may be secondary to chronic sleep-wake disturbance rather than the cause of it. The incidence increases with age; 44 percent of healthy subjects over age 65 without a sleep complaint and almost all patients with the restless legs syndrome have periodic limb movements (see below). The pathophysiology is not well understood. Polysomnography with bilateral surface EMG recording of the anterior tibialis, extensor carpi radialis, triceps and/or biceps is used to establish the diagnosis. Treatment options are limited; some patients may respond to a combination of carbidopa and levodopa, clonazepam, or levodopa alone.

PARASOMNIAS   The term *parasomnia* refers to behavioral disorders during sleep that are associated with brief or partial arousals but not with marked sleep disruption or impaired daytime alertness. The presenting complaint is usually related to the behavior itself. Most are more common in children but may persist into adulthood when their occurrence may have more pathologic significance.

Sleepwalking (somnambulism)   Patients affected by this disorder carry out automatic motor activities that range from minor to complex. Individuals may leave the bed, walk, urinate inappropriately, or exit from the house while remaining unconscious or uncommunica-tive. Arousal is difficult, and untoward or even fatal activities can occur. Sleepwalking occurs in stage 3 or 4 NREM sleep. It is most common in children and adolescents. Episodes are usually isolated but may be recurrent in 1 to 6 percent of patients. The cause is unknown.

Sleep terrors   This disorder, also called *pavor nocturnus*, occurs primarily in young children during the first several hours after sleep onset, in stages 3 and 4 of NREM sleep. The child suddenly screams, exhibiting autonomic arousal with sweating, tachycardia, and hyperventilation. The individual may be difficult to arouse and rarely recalls the episode on awakening in the morning. Recurrent attacks are rare, and treatment is usually by way of reassurance of parents. Both sleep terrors and sleepwalking represent abnormalities of arousal. In contrast, *nightmares* (dream anxiety attacks) occur during REM sleep and cause full arousal, with memory for the dream-associated unpleasant episode.

REM sleep behavior disorder   This is a rare parasomnia arising from REM sleep instead of slow-wave sleep, as is characteristic of the other, more common parasomnias. It primarily afflicts men of middle age or older, many of whom have a history of prior neurologic disease (e.g., degenerative diseases, Guillain-Barré syndrome, dementia, subarachnoid hemorrhage, stroke). Presenting symptoms are of violent behavior during sleep, reported by a bed partner. In contrast to typical somnambulism, injury to patient or bystander is common, and, upon awakening, the patient reports vivid, often unpleasant dream imagery. The principal differential diagnosis is that of nocturnal seizures, which can be excluded with polysomnography. In REM sleep behavior disorder, seizure activity is absent, and the EEG/EOG REM sleep pattern exhibits a high-amplitude EMG. Complex, purposeful motor behavior occurs during REM sleep episodes. The pathogenesis is unclear, but the preexisting neurologic disease may have involved brainstem areas responsible for descending motor inhibition during REM sleep. In support of this hypothesis are the remarkable similarities between the REM sleep behavior disorder and the sleep of animals with bilateral lesions of the pontine tegmentum in areas controlling REM sleep motor inhibition. Treatment with clonazepam provides sustained improvement in almost all reported cases.

Sleep bruxism   Bruxism is an involuntary, forceful grinding of teeth during sleep that affects 10 to 20 percent of the population. The patient is usually unaware of the problem, and data on this parasomnia come from roommates and bed partners, alarmed by the loud grinding noise, and from dentists who see evidence of destruction of tooth enamel and dentum. The typical age of onset is 17 to 20 years, and spontaneous remission usually occurs by age 40. Sex distribution appears to be equal.

Hypotheses about the pathophysiology suggest contributory roles for dental abnormalities, e.g., malocclusion, and for central neural mechanisms. Psychological factors may also play a role in that stress exacerbates the disorder. Treatment is dictated by the risk of dental injury. In many cases, the diagnosis is made during dental examination, damage is minor, and no treatment is indicated. In more severe cases, treatment with a rubber tooth guard is necessary to prevent permanent and disfiguring tooth injury. Stress management or, in some cases, biofeedback can be useful when bruxism is a manifestation of severe stress. Useful pharmacologic therapy has not been described.

Sleep enuresis   Bedwetting, like sleepwalking and night terrors, is another parasomnia occurring during slow-wave sleep in the young. Before age 5 or 6, nocturnal enuresis should probably be considered a normal feature of development. The condition usually spontaneously improves at puberty, has a prevalence in late adolescence of 1 to 3 percent, and is rare in adulthood. The age threshold for initiation of treatment depends on parental and patient concern about the problem. Persistence of enuresis into adolescence or adulthood may reflect a variety of underlying conditions. In older patients with enuresis a distinction must be made between primary and secondary enuresis, the latter being defined as bedwetting in patients who have been fully continent for 6 to 12 months. Treatment of primary enuresis is reserved for patients of appropriate age (older than 5 or 6 years) and consists of bladder training exercises and behavioral therapy. Urologic abnormalities are more common in primary enuresis and must be assessed by urologic examination. Important causes of secondary enuresis include emotional disturbances, urinary tract infections, cauda equina lesions, epilepsy, sleep apnea, and urinary tract malformations. In the patient for whom enuresis may be a source of significant stress, symptomatic pharmacotherapy may be appropriate while attention is also paid to underlying causes. This is usually accomplished with oxybutynin chloride or imipramine. Intranasal desmopressin has been used in some patients.

Miscellaneous parasomnias Other clinical entities fulfill the definition of a parasomnia in that they occur selectively during sleep and are associated with some degree of sleep disruption. Examples include *jactatio capitis nocturna* (nocturnal headbanging), sleep talking, and nocturnal leg cramps.

SLEEP DISORDERS ASSOCIATED WITH MEDICAL/PSYCHIATRIC DISORDERS **Sleep disorders associated with mental disorders** Although some differences are present in sleep architecture and physiology in *schizophrenia* (such as a decreased amount of stage 4 sleep and a lack of augmentation of REM sleep following REM sleep deprivation), chronic schizophrenics usually sleep well. In contrast, patients with other psychiatric disorders (anxiety disorders, affective illness, obsessive-compulsive disorders, and chronic alcoholism) often sleep poorly. There is considerable heterogeneity, however, in the nature of the sleep disturbance both between conditions and among patients with the same condition.

Depression can be associated with sleep onset insomnia, sleep maintenance insomnia, and/or early morning wakefulness. However, hypersomnia occurs in some depressed patients, especially adolescents and those with either bipolar or seasonal (fall/winter) depression (see also Chap. 389). Indeed, sleep disturbance is an important vegetative sign of depression and may commence before any mood changes are perceived by the patient and then return to normal at the beginning of remission. Consistent polysomnographic findings in depression include decreased REM sleep latency, lengthened first REM sleep episode, and shortened first NREM sleep episode; however, these findings are not specific for depression and the extent of these changes varies with age and symptomatology.

In *mania* and *hypomania*, sleep latency is increased, and total sleep time can be reduced. Patients with *obsessive-compulsive disorders* have sleep disturbances similar to those of endogenously depressed patients. Finally, *chronic alcoholics* lack slow-wave sleep, have decreased amounts of REM sleep, and have frequent arousals throughout the night. This is associated with impaired daytime alertness. The sleep of chronic alcoholics remains disturbed for years after discontinuance of alcohol usage.

Sleep disorders associated with neurologic disorders A variety of neurologic diseases result in sleep disruption through both indirect, nonspecific mechanisms (e.g., pain in cervical spondylosis or low back pain) or by impairment of central neural structures involved in the generation and control of sleep itself.

For example, the dementias have long been associated with disturbances in the timing of the sleep-wake cycle, often characterized by nocturnal wandering and an exacerbation of symptomatology at night (so-called sundowning). Such clinical observations are consistent with the recent neuropathologic finding that 80 percent of the cells in the hypothalamic circadian pacemaker (the SCN) are lost in patients with senile dementia (Alzheimer's disease), though a causal association remains unproven.

Epilepsy may rarely present as a sleep complaint (see also Chap. 367). Often the history is of abnormal, occasionally violent activity during sleep, and the differential diagnosis includes REM sleep behavior disorder, sleep apnea syndrome, and periodic movements of sleep (see above). Diagnosis requires nocturnal EEG recording. Other neurologic diseases associated with abnormal movements, such as *Parkinson's disease*, *hemiballismus*, *Huntington's chorea*, and *Gilles de la Tourette syndrome*, are also associated with disrupted

sleep, presumably through secondary mechanisms. Headache syndromes may show sleep-associated exacerbations (*migraine* or *cluster headache*) (see also Chap. 14). The mechanism of association between sleep and headache is unknown.

Fatal familial insomnia is a rare hereditary disorder caused by bilateral degeneration of anterior and dorsomedial nuclei of the thalamus. Insomnia is a prominent early symptom. Progressively, the syndrome produces autonomic dysfunction, dysarthria, myoclonus, coma, and death. The pathogenesis of the thalamic destruction is unknown.

Sleep disorders associated with other medical disorders A number of medical conditions are associated with disruptions of sleep. The association may be nonspecific, for example, that between sleep disruption and chronic pain from rheumatologic disorders. Attention to this association is important in that sleep-associated symptoms are the presenting complaint of many such patients. In addition, sleep disruption may stem from the appropriate use of drugs such as steroids or from the symptoms of another illness.

Among the most prominent associations is that between sleep disruption and *asthma*. In many asthmatics there is a prominent daily variation in airway resistance, probably related to daily rhythms in catecholamine and histamine levels, which results in marked increases in asthmatic symptoms at night. In addition, treatment of asthma with theophylline-based compounds, adrenergic agonists, or glucocorticoids can independently disrupt sleep. When sleep disruption is a prominent side effect of asthma treatment, inhaled steroids (e.g., beclomethasone) that do not disrupt sleep may provide a useful alternative.

Cardiac ischemia may also be associated with sleep disruption. Variability in autonomic nervous system function during REM sleep may account for the association of sleep and angina, although this remains unproven. Patients may present with complaints of nightmares or vivid, disturbing dreams, with or without awareness of the more classical symptoms of angina. *Paroxysmal nocturnal dyspnea* can also occur as a consequence of sleep-associated cardiac ischemia that causes pulmonary congestion exacerbated by recumbent posture.

Chronic obstructive pulmonary disease is also associated with sleep disruption, the pathogenesis of which is presumed to be sleep-related exacerbation of hypoxia and hypercapnia secondary to alveolar hypoventilation. In addition, recumbent posture results in suboptimal ventilation-perfusion ratios. Other conditions associated with sleep disruption include *cystic fibrosis*, *menopause*, *hyperthyroidism*, *gastroesophageal reflux*, *chronic renal failure*, and *liver failure*.

CIRCADIAN RHYTHM SLEEP DISORDERS

A subset of patients presenting with either insomnia or hypersomnia may have a disorder of sleep *timing* rather than sleep *generation*. Disorders of sleep timing can either be organic (i.e., due to an intrinsic defect in the circadian pacemaker or its responsiveness to entraining stimuli) or environmental (i.e., due to a disruption of exposure to entraining stimuli from the environment). Regardless of etiology, the symptoms reflect the influence of the underlying circadian pacemaker on sleep-wake function. Thus, effective therapeutic approaches should aim to entrain the oscillator at an appropriate phase.

ENDOGENOUS CIRCADIAN PHASE ASSESSMENT Abnormal synchronization of the circadian pacemaker to the 24-h day can be assessed clinically by studying patients under standardized behavioral and environmental conditions. Exogenous factors (such as variations in light exposure, room temperature, activity level, posture, nutritional intake), which can evoke physiologic responses, must be held constant to assess the phase and amplitude of endogenous circadian rhythms. Patients are studied for 30 to 50 h of enforced semirecumbent wakefulness in constant indoor room light, with their daily nutritional and fluid intake equally divided into hourly snacks. During such a constant routine, the body temperature cycle serves as a reliable marker of the output of the endogenous circadian pacemaker. In normal young men, the endogenous component of the body temperature cycle under such conditions reaches its nadir about 2 to 3 h before the habitual waketime. The technique can be used to determine whether there is an organic basis consistent with a diagnosis of delayed sleep phase syndrome, non-24-h sleep-wake schedule, or advanced sleep phase syndrome.

RAPID TIME-ZONE CHANGE (JET LAG) SYNDROME More than 60 million people experience transmeridian air travel annually, which is often associated with excessive daytime sleepiness, sleep onset insomnia, and frequent arousals from sleep, particularly in the latter half of the night. Gastrointestinal discomfort is common. The syndrome is transient, typically lasting 2 to 14 days depending on the number of time zones crossed, the direction of travel, and the traveler's age and phase-shifting capacity. Travelers who spend more time outdoors reportedly adapt more quickly than those who remain in hotel rooms, presumably due to bright (outdoor) light exposure.

SHIFT-WORK SLEEP DISORDER About 7 million workers in the United States regularly work at night, either on a permanent or rotating schedule. Studies of shift workers indicate that the circadian timing system of the average night-shift worker fails to adapt successfully to such work schedules. This leads to a misalignment between the desired work-rest schedule and the output of the pacemaker and in disturbed daytime sleep. Consequent sleep deprivation and misalignment of circadian phase produce decreased alertness and performance and cause increased safety hazards among night-shift workers. In addition, shift workers are believed to have higher rates of cardiac, gastrointestinal, and reproductive disorders.

Treatment must be aimed at minimizing both circadian disruption and sleep deprivation. The work schedule should: (1) favor a phase delay (clockwise) direction of shift rotation; (2) minimize the frequency of shift rotation so that shifts do not rotate more than once every 2 to 3 weeks; and (3) reduce the number of consecutive days worked at night from 7 (which is typical) to 4 or 5. These steps can lead to marked improvements in employee health and performance and to reduced accident rates among shift workers. Future approaches may include strategic use of bright-light exposure to facilitate rapid adaptation to night shift work.

DELAYED SLEEP PHASE SYNDROME Delayed sleep phase syndrome is characterized by: (1) reported sleep onset and wake times intractably later than desired; (2) actual sleep times at nearly the same clock hours daily; and (3) essentially normal all-night polysomnography except for delayed sleep onset. Patients exhibit an abnormally delayed endogenous circadian phase, with the temperature minimum during the constant routine occurring later than normal. This delayed phase could be due to: (1) an abnormally long intrinsic period of the endogenous circadian pacemaker; (2) an abnormally reduced phase-advancing capacity of the pacemaker; or (3) an irregular prior sleep-wake schedule, characterized by frequent nights when the patient chooses to remain awake well past midnight (for social, school, or work reasons). In most cases, it is difficult to distinguish among these factors, since patients with an abnormally long intrinsic period are more likely to "choose" such late-night activities because they are unable to sleep at that time. Patients tend to be young adults. This self-perpetuating condition can persist for years and does not usually respond to attempts to reestablish normal bedtime hours.

Patients respond to a rescheduling regimen in which bedtimes are successively delayed by about 3 h per day until the desired (and earlier) bedtime is achieved. Treatment methods involving bright-light phototherapy during the morning hours also show promise in these patients.

ADVANCED SLEEP PHASE SYNDROME Advanced sleep phase syndrome is the converse of the delayed sleep phase syndrome and tends to occur in the elderly. Patients with this condition report excessive daytime sleepiness during the evening hours, when they have great difficulty remaining awake, even in social settings. The patients awaken from 3 to 5 A.M. each day, often several hours before their desired wake times. Although such patients have not been studied extensively, some of these patients may benefit from bright-

light phototherapy during the evening hours, designed to reset the circadian pacemaker to a later hour.

NON-24-H SLEEP-WAKE DISORDER This condition occurs when the maximal phase-advancing capacity of the circadian pacemaker is not adequate to accommodate the difference between the 24-h geophysical day and the intrinsic period of the pacemaker in the patient. Patients affected are not able to maintain a stable phase relationship between the output of the pacemaker and the 24-h day. Such patients typically present with an incremental pattern of successive delays in sleep onsets and wake times, progressing in and out of phase with local time. When the patient's endogenous rhythms are out of phase with the local environment, insomnia coexists with excessive daytime sleepiness. Conversely, when the endogenous rhythms are in phase with the local environment, symptoms remit. The intervals of alternation between symptomatic vs. asymptomatic intervals may last several weeks to several months. Blind subjects unable to perceive light are particularly susceptible to this disorder.

MEDICAL IMPLICATIONS OF CIRCADIAN RHYTHMICITY Understanding the role of circadian rhythmicity in the pathophysiology of illness may lead to improvements in diagnosis and treatment. For example, prominent circadian variations have been reported in the incidence of *acute myocardial infarction*, *sudden cardiac death*, and *stroke*, the leading causes of death in the United States. Platelet aggregability is increased after arising in the early morning hours, coincident with the peak incidence of these cardiovascular events. A better understanding of the possible role of circadian rhythmicity in the acute destabilization of a chronic condition such as atherosclerotic disease could improve the understanding of the pathophysiology.

Diagnostic and therapeutic procedures may also be affected by the time of day at which data are collected. Examples include blood pressure, body temperature, the dexamethasone suppression test, and plasma cortisol levels. The timing of chemotherapy administration has been reported to have an effect on the outcome of treatment. Few physicians realize the extent to which routine measures are affected by the time (or sleep/wake state) when the measurement is made.

In addition, both the toxicity and effectiveness of drugs can vary during the day. For example, more than a fivefold difference has been observed in mortality rates following administration of toxic agents to experimental animals at different times of day. Anesthetic agents are particularly sensitive to time-of-day effects.

Finally, it should be noted that the risk of errors and accidents due to inattention and/or sleepiness varies markedly with the time of day. Single-vehicle truck accidents, industrial errors and accidents, and lapses of attention all peak during a critical zone of vulnerability that typically occurs during the latter half of the night, coincident with maximal sleep drive within the brain. The physician must be increasingly aware of the public health risks associated with the ever-increasing demands made by the duty-rest-recreation schedules in our round-the-clock society.

REFERENCES

ALDRICH MS: Narcolepsy. Neurology 42 (Suppl 6):34, 1992

ANCH AM et al: *Sleep: A Scientific Perspective.* Englewood Cliffs, NJ, Prentice Hall, 1988

BLIWISE DL et al: Prevalence of self-reported poor sleep in a healthy population aged 50–65. Soc Sci Med 34:49, 1992

BRODEUR C et al: Treatment of restless legs syndrome and periodic movements during sleep with L-dopa: A double-blind controlled study. Neurology 38:1845, 1988

COLEMAN RM et al: Sleep-wake disorders based on a polysomnographic diagnosis: A national cooperative study. JAMA 247:997, 1982

CULEBRAS, A: Neuroanatomic and neurologic correlates of sleep disturbances. Neurology 42 (Suppl 6):19, 1992

CZEISLER, CA et al: Association of sleep-wake habits in older people with changes in output of circadian pacemaker. Lancet 340:933, 1992

——— et al: Exposure to bright light and darkness to treat physiologic maladaptation to night work. N Engl J Med 322:1253, 1990

DIAGNOSTIC CLASSIFICATION STEERING COMMITTEE, Thorpy MJ (chairman): *International Classification of Sleep Disorders: Diagnostic and Coding Manual.* Rochester, MN, American Sleep Disorders Association, 1990

DINGES DF, BROUGHTON RJ (eds): *Sleep and Alertness.* New York, Raven, 1989

FINDLEY LJ et al: Drivers with untreated sleep apnea. A cause of death and serious injury. Arch Intern Med 151:1451, 1991

HOFFSTEIN V et al: Treatment of obstructive sleep apnea with nasal continuous positive airway pressure, patient compliance, perception of benefits, and side effects. Am Rev Respir Dis 145:841, 1992

HORNE J: *Why We Sleep: The Functions of Sleep in Humans and Other Mammals.* Oxford, Oxford University Press, 1988

KLEIN DC et al (eds): *Suprachiasmatic Nucleus: The Mind's Clock.* New York, Oxford University Press, 1991

KRYGER MH et al (eds): *Principles and Practice of Sleep Medicine.* Philadelphia, Saunders, 1989

LEVINSON PD, MILLMAN RP: Causes and consequences of blood pressure alterations in obstructive sleep apnea. Arch Intern Med 151:455, 1991

LYDIC R, BIEBUYCK JF (eds): *Clinical Physiology of Sleep.* Bethesda, MD, American Physiological Society, 1988

MEDORI R et al: Fatal familial insomnia, a prion disease with a mutation at codon 178 of the prion protein gene. N Engl J Med 326:444, 1992

PRINZ PM et al: Geriatrics: Sleep disorders and aging. N Engl J Med 323:520, 1990

SCHENCK CH et al: Rapid eye movement sleep behavior disorder: A treatable parasomnia affecting older adults. JAMA 257:1786, 1987

SCHWARTZ WJ: A clinician's primer on the circadian clock: Its localization, function, and resetting. Adv Intern Med 38:81m, 1993

SOMERS VK et al: Sympathetic-nerve activity during sleep in normal subjects. N Engl J Med 328:303, 1993

VITIELLO MV et al: Sleep in Alzheimer's disease and the sundown syndrome. Neurology 42 (Suppl 6):83, 1992

WALSH JK et al: Insomnia, in *Sleep Disorders Medicine: A Comprehensive Textbook,* S Chokroverty (ed). Stoneham, MA, Butterworth, 1992

WARE JC, MOREWITZ J: Diagnosis and treatment of insomnia and depression. J Clin Psychiatry 52 (Suppl):55, 1991

WILLIAMS RL et al (eds): *Sleep Disorders: Diagnosis and Treatment,* 2d ed. New York, Wiley, 1988

section 4 # Alterations in circulatory and respiratory function

30 COUGH AND HEMOPTYSIS

EUGENE BRAUNWALD*

COUGH

Cough is an explosive expiration which provides a means of clearing the tracheobronchial tree of secretions and foreign bodies. It is one of the most frequent cardiorespiratory symptoms and one of the most common symptoms for which medical attention is sought. Reasons for the latter include exhaustion, insomnia, and concern for the cause of the cough, especially fear of cancer and AIDS.

MECHANISM Coughing may be initiated either voluntarily or reflexively. As a defensive reflex it has both afferent and efferent pathways. The *afferent limb* includes receptors within the sensory distribution of the trigeminal, glossopharyngeal, superior laryngeal, and vagus nerves. The *efferent limb* includes the recurrent laryngeal nerve (which causes glottic closure) and the spinal nerves (which cause contraction of the thoracic and abdominal musculature). The *sequence of a cough* includes an appropriate stimulus which initiates a deep inspiration. This is followed by glottic closure, relaxation of the diaphragm, and muscle contraction against a closed glottis so as to produce maximally positive intrathoracic and intraairway pressures. These positive intrathoracic pressures result in a narrowing of the trachea, produced by an infolding of its more compliant posterior membrane. Once the glottis opens, the combination of a large pressure differential between the airways and the atmosphere coupled with this tracheal narrowing produces flow rates through the trachea close to the speed of sound. The shearing forces which are developed aid in the elimination of mucus and foreign materials. A tracheostomy short-circuits and an endotracheal tube prevents glottic closure. Therefore, both decrease the effectiveness of the cough mechanism.

ETIOLOGY Cough is produced by inflammatory, mechanical, chemical, and thermal stimulation of the cough receptors. *Inflammatory* stimuli are initiated by edema and hyperemia of the respiratory mucous membranes, as in bacterial or viral bronchitis, the common cold, and excessive cigarette smoking. It also may be caused by irritation from exudative processes, such as postnasal drip and gastric reflux with aspiration. Such stimuli may arise either in the airways (as in laryngitis, tracheitis, bronchitis, and bronchiolitis) or in the alveoli (as in pneumonitis and lung abscess). *Mechanical* stimuli are produced by inhalation of particulate matter, such as dust particles, and by compression of the air passages and pressure or tension on these structures. Lesions associated with airway compression may be either extramural or intramural. The former include aortic aneurysms, granulomas, pulmonary neoplasms, and mediastinal tumors; intramural lesions include bronchogenic carcinoma, bronchial adenoma, foreign bodies, granulomatous endobronchial involvement, and contraction of airway smooth muscle (bronchial asthma). Pressure or tension on the air passages is usually produced by lesions associated with a decrease in pulmonary compliance. Examples of specific causes include acute and chronic interstitial fibrosis (Chap. 224), pulmonary edema, and atelectasis. *Chemical* stimuli may result from inhalation of irritant gases, including cigarette smoke and chemical fumes. Many other drugs can exert adverse effects on the respiratory system and thereby cause cough. However, cough *per se* is the major side effect of angiotensin converting enzyme inhibitors. Finally, *thermal* stimuli may be produced by inhalation of either very hot or cold air.

Cough is commonly associated with episodic wheezing secondary to bronchoconstriction in symptomatic patients with bronchial asthma (Chap. 217). Chronic, persistent cough may be the *sole* presenting manifestation of bronchial asthma ("cough asthma"). Such patients are characterized by (1) absence of a history of episodic wheezing and (2) no evidence of expiratory airflow obstruction by spirometry, but (3) hyperreactive airways (characteristic of asthma) when challenged with a cholinergic agent, methacholine.

DIAGNOSTIC EVALUATION The history is the most important aspect of the evaluation. It should address the following issues:

1 Is the cough acute or chronic?
2 Is it associated with fever? with wheezing?
3 Is it associated with sputum? If so, what is its character?
4 Is it seasonal?
5 Does the patient have important risk factors for disease? (e.g., homosexuality, cigarette smoking, intravenous drugs, immobilization, environmental exposures?)
6 What is the past medical history?

The physical examination, chest roentgenogram, sputum examination, and screening pulmonary function studies (static lung volumes and dynamic flow rates) may then indicate a specific cause. The *history* may indicate specific diagnoses. Acute episodes of cough may be associated with such viral infections as acute tracheobronchitis or pneumonitis or with bacterial bronchopneumonia. Cough associated with an acute febrile episode and associated with hoarseness is usually

---

* The late Gennaro M. Tisi was the senior author of this chapter in the eleventh and previous editions of this book, and this chapter represents a continuing revision of that work.

produced by viral laryngotracheobronchitis. Postnasal drip is also a common cause of chronic cough.

The character of the cough may suggest the anatomic site of involvement: The patient with a "barking" type of cough may have epiglottal involvement (i.e., "whooping cough" due to *Haemophilus pertussis* infection in young children), while the cough associated with tracheal or major airway involvement is often loud and "brassy." Cough associated with generalized wheezing may be produced by acute bronchospasm. The time of occurrence of a cough may indicate a specific cause: A cough which occurs selectively at night suggests congestive heart failure; one related to meals suggests gastrointestinal reflux into the tracheobronchial tree or a tracheoesophageal fistula, a hiatal hernia, or an esophageal diverticulum; a cough precipitated by a change in position suggests a lung abscess or a localized area of bronchiectasis. The description of sputum or secretions produced in conjunction with the cough should include color, consistency, odor, and volume. Purulent sputum and/or large amounts of sputum suggest lung abscess and bronchiectasis; bloody sputum, bleeding (see "Hemoptysis," below); frothy and pink-tinged sputum, pulmonary edema; mucoid and massive sputum, alveolar cell carcinoma.

The general *physical examination* may point to a nonpulmonary cause of cough, such as heart failure, primary nonpulmonary neoplasm, acquired immunodeficiency disease, etc. The character of the auscultatory findings may suggest the site of disease. Inspiratory stridor and wheezing may be present in laryngeal disease, inspiratory and expiratory rhonchi favor involvement of the trachea and major bronchi; coarse subcrepitant inspiratory rales may indicate interstitial fibrosis and/or edema; fine crepitant rales may indicate a process such as pneumonitis or pulmonary edema, which fills the alveoli with fluid. The *chest roentgenogram* may reveal the cause of the cough; it may show an intrapulmonary mass lesion (Chap. 227), an alveolar filling process which may be pneumonic or nonpneumonic, an area of honeycombing and cyst formation which may indicate an area of localized bronchiectasis, or bilateral hilar adenopathy which may indicate sarcoidosis or a lymphoma.

A careful *sputum examination* may be more enlightening than the patient's description of the character of the sputum. Examination shows whether the sputum is thin or viscid, purulent, foul-smelling, blood-tinged, or scant or copious. In pneumococcal pneumonia the sputum has a "rusty" color, while in *Klebsiella* pneumonia it may look like "currant jelly." Gram stain and culture of deep-cough specimens may reveal a specific bacterial, fungal, or mycoplasmal causation, while sputum cytology may result in a positive diagnosis of a pulmonary neoplasm.

Bronchoscopy may reveal the cause of otherwise unexplained chronic cough. *Pulmonary function* studies (Chap. 214) also may be helpful. Significant expiratory obstruction to airflow (as determined from a forced expiratory flow maneuver), coupled with a history of cough and significant sputum production, suggests that irrespective of other lesions the patient has significant bronchitis. Decreased lung volume (as determined from the static lung volumes) suggests that a restrictive type of lung disease (Chap. 224) is present. Perhaps more important than providing a specific diagnosis, pulmonary function studies are useful in quantifying the severity of disease, its progression over time, and the efficacy of an intervention.

Two features of cough should be highlighted: (1) A cough is often so common in the cigarette smoker as to be ignored or minimized. *Any change in the nature or character of a chronic cigarette cough should initiate immediate diagnostic evaluation, with particular attention directed to detection of bronchogenic carcinoma.* (2) Female patients are inclined to swallow sputum and not to expectorate as male patients do. This tendency may lead to the incorrect conclusion that a cough in a female patient is irritative and nonproductive.

COMPLICATIONS   Three complications may be produced by the coughing mechanism: Paroxysms of coughing may precipitate syncope (cough syncope, Chap. 17), and strenuous coughing may produce rupture of an emphysematous bleb, rib fractures, and costochondritis. A potential mechanism for cough syncope includes the development of markedly positive intrathoracic and alveolar pressures which decrease venous return, producing a decrease in cardiac output and resultant syncope. Although cough fractures of the ribs may occur in otherwise normal patients, their occurrence should at least raise the possibility of pathologic fractures, which are seen in multiple myeloma, osteoporosis, and osteolytic metastases.

THERAPY   Definitive treatment of cough depends on determining its precise cause and then initiating specific therapy for the underlying cause. When this is done, specific therapy is usually effective, as in smoking cessation, antibiotic therapy of a specific bacterial infection, or eliminating gastroesophageal reflux.

Symptomatic or nonspecific therapy of cough should be considered when (1) the cause of the cough is not known or specific treatment is not possible and (2) the cough performs no useful function or represents a potential hazard or causes marked discomfort. An irritative, nonproductive cough may be suppressed by an antitussive agent, which increases the latency or threshold of the cough center. Such agents include codeine (15 mg qid) or nonnarcotics such as dextromethorphan (15 mg qid). These drugs provide useful symptomatic therapy by interrupting prolonged, self-perpetuating paroxysms. However, a cough productive of significant quantities of sputum should usually not be suppressed, since retention of sputum in the tracheobronchial tree may interfere with the distribution of ventilation, alveolar aeration, and the ability of the lung to resist infection.

When secretions are tenacious and thick, adequate hydration, expectorants, and humidification of the air with an ultrasonic nebulizer with ipratroprium bromide, a class of bronchodilator with antimuscarinic actions given as two inhalations (36 µg qid), may be helpful. Iodinated glycerol (30 mg qid) may be especially useful in patients with cough asthma or chronic bronchitis and guaifenesin (100 mg tid) in acute or chronic bronchitis. Mucociliary clearance can be increased by beta-adrenergic agonists such as ephedrine (12.5 mg qid), especially in patients with cystic fibrosis, and theophylline (100 mg tid) in patients with chronic obstructive pulmonary disease.

Protussive (cough-enhancing) treatment is designed to increase the effectiveness of useful but inadequate cough. Hypertonic saline aerosol can increase the clearance of particles from the lower airways during coughing in patients with bronchitis, while amiloride aerosol has been shown to have a similar effect in patients with cystic fibrosis.

HEMOPTYSIS

Hemoptysis includes the expectoration from the respiratory tract of both blood-streaked sputum and gross blood. This symptom is often quite frightening to the patient. Any patient with gross hemoptysis should be given appropriate diagnostic tests so that a specific cause may be found. The patient with blood-streaked sputum also should be studied unless one can be certain that this type of hemoptysis is due to a benign condition. Recurrent episodes of hemoptysis should not be automatically ascribed to a previously established diagnosis, such as chronic bronchitis. Such an approach may result in missing a serious but potentially treatable lesion.

ETIOLOGY AND INCIDENCE   Prior to embarking on an extensive diagnostic workup of hemoptysis, it is essential to determine that the blood is in fact coming from the respiratory tract, not from the nasopharynx or gastrointestinal tract. Distinguishing hemoptysis from hematemesis is difficult at times. In hemoptysis, the prodrome is usually a tingling in the throat or a desire to cough, the blood is coughed up, is usually bright-red and *frothy*, and may be mixed with sputum; the pH is usually alkaline; and microscopic examination may show hemosiderin-laden macrophages. In hematemesis, the prodrome includes nausea and abdominal discomfort, the blood is vomited, and it is usually *dark red* in color. It may contain partially digested food, and the pH is usually acidic. Once this point is established, the diagnostic tests for hemoptysis may proceed. Although there are numerous single case reports of diseases which have been associated with hemoptysis, Table 30-1 presents the more common disorders.

The incidence of the diagnoses listed in Table 30-1 depends on the nature of the series reported and whether one includes both gross bleeding and blood streaking of the sputum. If both types of bleeding are included, then the major cause is chronic bronchitis. If the definition is restricted to gross bleeding (greater than several tablespoons), then the incidence depends on the type of series reported. Surgical series favor the incidence of mass lesions and operable lesions such as carcinoma. Those from centers with a large tuberculosis population obviously favor this condition. Combined medical-surgical series include a wider representation of those lesions which present with hemoptysis (carcinoma, bronchiectasis, bronchitis, other inflammatory lesions including tuberculosis, other lesions including the vascular, traumatic, and hemorrhagic etiologies listed in Table 30-1). Despite the most extensive of evaluations, 5 to 15 percent of cases entailing gross hemoptysis remain undiagnosed.

Two points should be highlighted with reference to diseases associated with hemoptysis: (1) hemoptysis is rare in metastatic carcinoma to the lung, and (2) although hemoptysis may occur at some time during the course of a viral or pneumococcal pneumonia, it is usually scanty and its occurrence should always raise the question of a more serious underlying process.

DIAGNOSIS   As is the case for cough, the *history* is of enormous value. Recurrent, chronic hemoptysis in a young, otherwise asymptomatic female favors the diagnosis of a bronchial adenoma; hemoptysis with chronic, marked sputum production [associated with ring shadows, tram lines (abnormal air bronchograms), and cyst formation on the roentgenogram, see below] suggests a diagnosis of bronchiectasis; putrid sputum production suggests lung abscess; weight loss and anorexia in a male smoker over age 40 raise the possibility of carcinoma of the lung; a recent history of blunt trauma to the chest suggests a lung contusion; and acute pleuritic chest pain raises the possibility of pulmonary embolism with infarction or some other pleurally based lesion (lung abscess, coccidioidomycosis cavity, and vasculitis). A history of a bleeding disorder or of anticoagulant drug administration should be sought.

Several findings on the *physical examination* of the patient with hemoptysis also may suggest a specific diagnosis: A pleural friction rub suggests those diagnoses just mentioned in connection with pleuritic pain; the findings of pulmonary hypertension raise the diagnostic possibilities of primary pulmonary hypertension, mitral stenosis, recurrent or chronic thromboembolism, and Eisenmenger's

TABLE 30-1   Major causes of hemoptysis

I **Inflammatory**
   A Bronchitis
   B Tuberculosis
   C Bronchiectasis
   D Cystic fibrosis
   E Lung abscess
   F Pneumonia, particularly *Kliebsiella*
   G Septic pulmonary embolism
   H Localized parenchymal disease caused by fungi and parasites
II **Neoplastic**
   A Lung cancer; squamous cell, adenocarcinoma, oat cell
   B Bronchial adenoma
III **Other**
   A Pulmonary thromboembolism
   B Mitral stenosis
   C Left ventricular failure
   D Tracheobronchial trauma, including foreign body and lung contusion
   E Bronchiolithiasis
   F Bronchovascular fistula
   G Primary pulmonary hypertension, arteriovenous malformation, Eisenmenger's syndrome
   H Idiopathic pulmonary hemosiderosis
   I Pulmonary vasculitis including Wegener's granulomatosis, Goodpasture's syndrome, connective tissue disorders
   J Hemorrhagic diathesis including anticoagulant therapy

syndrome; a localized wheeze over a major lobar airway suggests an intramural lesion such as a bronchogenic carcinoma or a foreign body; systemic arteriovenous communications or the presence of a murmur over the lung fields suggests the diagnosis of Osler-Rendu-Weber disease with pulmonary arteriovenous malformation; evidence of significant expiratory obstruction to airflow coupled with sputum production suggests that whatever other lesion may be present, the patient has significant bronchitis.

The *chest roentgenogram* is critical to identifying the cause of hemoptysis. The presence of ring shadows favors a diagnosis of bronchiectasis; an air-fluid level, the diagnosis of a lung abscess; enlargement of the left atrium, the diagnosis of mitral stenosis; and a mass lesion, the diagnosis of a central or peripheral pulmonary neoplasm. A mass lesion which may cause hemoptysis should be distinguished from an area of blood pneumonitis caused by aspiration of blood into contiguous areas. When the chest roentgenogram is normal, the airways are the usual site of bleeding.

A common challenging problem is the identification of the site of bleeding in a patient with normal findings on physical examination and a normal roentgenogram of the chest. A patient with hemoptysis tends to keep the bleeding side dependent and may report a burning or deep pain which may localize the side of bleeding; bronchoscopy may then be useful. This procedure generally is most helpful when the bleeding is scant and of least help when the bleeding is massive, since blood may be aspirated into contiguous airways. Such aspiration may produce alveolar filling (i.e., a "blood pneumonitis") that may obscure the etiology of the hemoptysis on the initial chest roentgenogram. Blood pneumonitis usually clears within a week, and once clearing has occurred, a repeat chest roentgenogram may disclose the origin of the hemoptysis.

Following the history and physical examination, the approach to a patient with hemoptysis includes whatever specialized studies and procedures are required to make a specific diagnosis. In patients who are not bleeding actively, the roentgenogram is followed by computed tomography and then bronchoscopy. In patients who are bleeding actively, bronchoscopy is carried out on an emergent or urgent basis. Rigid bronchoscopy permits visualization of the more central airways. It is of particular value when the source of bleeding is in this portion of the airway system, the degree of hemoptysis is massive, and selective endobronchial intubation is being considered. Fiberoptic bronchoscopy (Chap. 216) includes within the range of visualization airways as small as several millimeters in diameter. This endoscopic technique may provide definitive visual, biopsy, or cytologic information. Bronchography may be employed to (1) establish the presence of localized bronchiectasis (including a sequestered lobe) and (2) rule out the presence of more generalized bronchiectasis in a patient with localized disease who is regarded as a surgical candidate because of either repetitive hemoptysis or recurrent infections. The majority of patients with bronchiectasis have a normal chest roentgenogram, but the diagnosis can usually be established by computed tomography (Chaps. 215 and 216). A PPD and, if sputum is present, examination for acid-fast bacilli should be obtained. The laboratory evaluation also should rule out a bleeding disorder.

MANAGEMENT   Since hemoptysis is such an alarming symptom, there is a tendency to overtreat the patient. Usually hemoptysis is scant and will stop spontaneously without specific therapy. Following identification of the site and establishment of an etiologic diagnosis, the underlying disorder is treated. If the hemoptysis is substantial, the mainstays of therapy include keeping the patient calm, instituting complete bed rest, excluding unnecessary diagnostic procedures until the hemoptysis has begun to subside, and suppressing cough if it is present and an aggravating feature of the hemoptysis. Emergency care demands that intubation and suctioning equipment be at the bedside. Control of the airways must be obtained by endotracheal intubation in patients with massive hemoptysis (>500 mL/24h) to avoid asphyxiation. In patients in danger of asphyxiation by flooding of the lung contralateral to the side of hemorrhage, intubation by a technique which isolates the hemorrhaging lung and prevents contralateral aspiration of blood should be carried out. This can be accomplished by strategic location of a balloon catheter the introduction of which into the bronchus in question is facilitated by direct bronchoscopic visualization.

The management of massive, potentially lethal hemoptysis remains controversial. The choice between surgical and nonsurgical interventions hangs on the words *potentially lethal*. Massive hemoptysis is an alarming clinical situation in which asphyxiation due to aspiration of blood represents the principal threat to life. In many patients with massive hemoptysis, resectional surgery is ultimately carried out, but a strong effort is made to carry this out on an elective rather than emergent basis.

Since the source of massive hemoptysis is usually the bronchial arterial system, nonsurgical control includes bronchial arterial catheterization and embolization, a technique which is especially useful in patients with nonresectable lung cancer. Coagulation by means of a laser (neodymium:YAG—yttrium aluminum garnet) delivered through a bronchoscope and tamponading a proximal bleeding site with a balloon catheter or packing material applied through a rigid bronchoscope are also useful techniques.

The choice between surgical and nonsurgical management relates most often to the anatomic basis for the *massive* hemoptysis and its prognosis. In patients with cavitary tuberculosis, anaerobic lung abscess, and lung cancer, the risk of mortality is far greater than when the cause of the massive hemoptysis is bronchitis or bronchiectasis. Operation may occasionally be necessary in the former, but virtually never in the latter group. In either case the initial management should include the conservative measures suggested above. With such management, spontaneous cessation of bleeding usually occurs. Emergency surgical intervention should be considered in that small group of patients with a definable lesion on chest roentgenogram (i.e., cavitary disease, lung abscess, lung cancer) who have evidence of uncontrollable respiratory or hemodynamic compromise and who are considered to have pulmonary function that is sufficient to permit resection. If a patient is a surgical candidate, bronchoscopy should be performed to identify the specific site of bleeding. Otherwise, bronchoscopy should be deferred for several days because of the tendency of this procedure to aggravate cough and thereby perpetuate the hemoptysis.

REFERENCES

BENNETT WD et al: The acute effect of ipratropium bromide bronchodilator therapy on cough clearance in COPD. Chest 103:488, 1993

BUTCHER BL et al: High yield of chest radiography in walk-in clinic patients with chest symptoms. J Gen Intern Med 8:115, 1993

FITZGERALD JM et al: Chronic cough and gastroesophageal reflux. Can Med Assoc J 140:520, 1989

FREITAG L: Development of a new ballon catheter for management of hemoptysis with bronchofiberscopes. Chest 103:593, 1993

HENDELES L: Efficacy and safety of antihistamines and expectorants in nonprescription cough and cold preparations. Pharmacotherapy 13:154, 1993

IRWIN RS et al: Chronic cough: The spectrum and frequency of causes, key components of the diagnostic evaluation, and outcome of specific therapy. Am Rev Respir Dis 141:640, 1990

IRWIN RS, CURLEY FJ: The treatment of cough: A comprehensive review. Chest 99:1477, 1991

JONES DK, DAVIES R: Massive hemoptysis. Br Med J 300:299, 1990

KNOTT-CRAIG CJ et al: Management and prognosis of massive hemoptysis. Recent experience with 120 patients. J Thorac Cardiovasc Surg 105:394, 1993

PETTY TL: The National Mucolytic Study: Results of a randomized, double-blind, placebo-controlled study of iodinated glycerol in chronic obstructive bronchitis. Chest 97:75, 1990

POE RH et al: Chronic persistent cough: Experience in diagnosis and outcome using an anatomic diagnostic protocol. Chest 95:723, 1989

TAMURA S et al: Embolotherapy for persistent hemoptysis. Cardiovasc Intervent Radiol 16:85, 1993

THOMPSON AB et al: Pathogenesis, evaluation, and therapy for massive hemoptysis. Clin Chest Med 13:69, 1992

31   DYSPNEA AND PULMONARY EDEMA

ROLAND H. INGRAM, JR. / EUGENE BRAUNWALD

DYSPNEA

The breathing pattern is controlled by a series of higher central and peripheral mechanisms which can increase ventilation appropriate to increased metabolic demands during physical activity. It can also increase ventilation in excess of metabolic demands in conditions such as anxiety and fear. A normal resting person is unaware of the act of breathing, and while he or she may become conscious of breathing during mild to moderate exertion, no discomfort is experienced. However, during and following exhausting exertion, an individual may become unpleasantly aware of breathing yet feel reasonably assured that the sensation will be transitory and is appropriate to the level of exercise. Therefore, as a cardinal symptom of diseases affecting the cardiorespiratory system, *dyspnea* is defined as an *abnormally uncomfortable awareness of breathing*.

Although dyspnea is not painful in the usual sense of the word, it is, like pain, involved with both the perception of a sensation and the reaction to that perception. Patients experience a number of uncomfortable sensations related to breathing and use an even larger number of verbal expressions to describe these sensations, such as "cannot get enough air," "air does not go all the way down," "smothering feeling or tightness or tiredness in the chest," and a "choking sensation." It may be necessary, therefore, to review meticulously the patient's history in order to ascertain whether the more abstruse descriptions do, in fact, represent dyspnea. Once it is established that a patient does have dyspnea, it is of paramount importance to define the circumstances in which it occurs and to assess associated symptoms. There are situations in which breathing appears labored but in which dyspnea does not occur. For example, the hyperventilation associated with metabolic acidemia is rarely accompanied by dyspnea. On the other hand, patients with apparently normal breathing patterns may complain of shortness of breath.

QUANTITATION OF DYSPNEA   The gradation of dyspnea may usefully be based on the amount of physical exertion required to produce the sensation. In actual practice, the major functional classifications of patients with heart or lung disease are based largely on dyspnea in relation to degree of exertion. However, in assessing the severity of dyspnea, it is important to obtain a clear understanding of the patient's general physical condition, work history, and recreational habits. For example, the development of dyspnea in a trained runner upon running 2 mi may signify a much more serious disturbance than a similar degree of breathlessness in a sedentary person upon running a fraction of this distance. Another variable to consider in assessing the degree of dyspnea as an index of the severity of underlying heart or lung disease is the interindividual variation in perception. Some patients with extremely severe disease may complain of only mild dyspnea; others with mild disease may experience more severe shortness of breath. Thus, rather like variations in pain thresholds, patients have different degrees of subjective tolerance to cardiopulmonary dysfunction. There is some evidence that persons with relatively blunted ventilatory drives tolerate their disease with less dyspnea than those who have a heightened level of ventilatory responsiveness. Some patients with lung or heart disease may have such reduced capabilities due to other disease (e.g., peripheral vascular insufficiency or severe osteoarthritis of the hips or knees) that exertional dyspnea is precluded despite serious impairment of pulmonary or cardiac function.

Some patterns of dyspnea are not directly related to physical exertion. Sudden and unexpected dyspneic episodes at rest can be associated with pulmonary emboli, spontaneous pneumothorax, hypercapnea secondary to breath holding, or anxiety. Nocturnal episodes of severe paroxysmal dyspnea are characteristic of left ventricular failure. Dyspnea upon assuming the supine posture, *orthopnea* (see below), thought to be mainly characteristic of congestive heart failure, also may occur in some patients with asthma and chronic obstruction of the airways and is a regular finding in the rare occurrence of bilateral diaphragmatic paralysis. *Trepopnea* is used to describe the unusual circumstance in which dyspnea occurs only in the left or right lateral decubitus position, most often in patients with heart disease, while *platypnea* is dyspnea which occurs only in the upright position. Positional alterations in ventilation-perfusion relationships (see Chap. 214) have been invoked to explain these patterns. Platypnea can be seen with deficient abdominal musculature, a deficiency that results in loss of diaphragmatic support due to anterior protrusion of abdominal viscera in the upright posture. Upon lying down, the viscera resume support of the diaphragm, stretching it to its optimal operational length. This form of platypnea is alleviated by use of an abdominal binder.

MECHANISMS OF DYSPNEA Physicians usually relate the symptom of dyspnea to a process such as obstruction of the airways or congestive heart failure and generally proceed with further diagnostic and/or therapeutic attempts, having satisfied themselves that they understand the mechanism of the dyspnea. In fact, elucidation of the *actual* mechanism(s) of dyspnea has eluded clinical investigators.

Dyspnea occurs whenever the work of breathing is excessive. Increased force generation is required of the respiratory muscles to produce a given volume change if the chest wall or lungs are less compliant or if resistance to airflow is increased. Increased work of breathing also occurs when the ventilation is excessive for the level of activity. Although an individual is more apt to become dyspneic when the work of breathing is increased, the work theory does not account for the perceptual difference between a deep breath with a normal mechanical load and a normal-sized breath with an increased mechanical load. The work might be the same with both breaths, but the normal one with the increased load will be associated with discomfort. In fact, with respiratory loading, such as adding a resistance at the mouth, there is an increase in respiratory center output, as gauged by newer indexes, that is disproportionate to the increase in the work of breathing. It has been postulated that whenever the force that muscles actually generate during breathing approaches some fraction of their maximal force-generating ability, which may vary among individuals, dyspnea ensues due to transduction of mechanical to neural stimuli. Such a theory would still not explain why patients who are completely paralyzed, either by cord transections or neuromuscular blockade, experience dyspnea although aided by a mechanical ventilator. It is probable, in these circumstances, that signals from the lungs and/or airways travel via the vagus nerve to the central nervous system to account for the sensation.

In all likelihood, several different mechanisms operate to different degrees in the various clinical situations in which dyspnea occurs. There is a correlation between sensory descriptors of dyspnea and the method by which dyspnea is induced in normal subjects. In addition, there are correlations between certain clusters of sensory descriptions and the disease processes causing dyspnea. For example, patients with restrictive lung diseases may complain of rapid breathing, those with congestive heart failure may describe a need to sigh, and those with asthma may be most distressed by wheezing. Perhaps, in some circumstances, dyspnea is evoked by stimulation of receptors in the upper respiratory tract; in others it may originate from receptors in the lungs, airways, respiratory muscles, or some combination of these structures. In any event, dyspnea is characterized by an excessive or abnormal activation of the respiratory centers in the brainstem. This activation comes about from stimuli transmitted from or through a variety of structures and pathways, including (1) intrathoracic receptors via the vagi, (2) afferent somatic nerves, particularly from the respiratory muscles and chest wall, but also from other skeletal muscles and joints, (3) chemoreceptors in the brain, aortic and carotid bodies, and elsewhere in the circulation, (4) higher (cortical) centers, and perhaps (5) afferent fibers in the phrenic nerves. In general,

despite the interindividual variations described above, there is a reasonable correlation between the severity of dyspnea and the magnitude of disturbances of pulmonary or cardiac function which are responsible.

DIFFERENTIAL DIAGNOSIS   Obstructive disease of airways (See also Chaps. 217 and 223)   Obstruction to airflow can be present anywhere from the extrathoracic airways out to the small airways in the periphery of the lung. Large extrathoracic airway obstruction can occur acutely, as with aspiration of food or a foreign body or with angioedema of the glottis. Circumstantial evidence or testimony from witnesses should cause the physician to suspect aspiration, and an allergic history together with a few scattered hives should raise the possibility of glottic edema. The acute form of upper airway obstruction is a medical emergency. More chronic forms can occur with tumors or with fibrotic stenosis following tracheostomy or prolonged endotracheal intubation. Whether acute or chronic, the cardinal symptom is dyspnea, and the characteristic signs are stridor and retraction of the supraclavicular fossae with inspiration.

Obstruction of intrathoracic airways can occur acutely and intermittently or can be present chronically with worsening during respiratory infections. Acute intermittent obstruction with wheezing is typical of *asthma*. Chronic cough with expectoration is typical of *chronic bronchitis* and *bronchiectasis*. Most often there is a prolongation of expiration and coarse rhonchi which are generalized in chronic bronchitis and may be localized in the case of bronchiectasis. Intercurrent infection results in worsening of the cough, increased expectoration of purulent sputum, and more severe dyspnea. During such episodes, the patient may complain of nocturnal paroxysms of dyspnea with wheezing relieved by cough and expectoration of sputum. Despite the fact that severe limitation of expiratory flow and hyperinflation of the lung are characteristic of these diseases, the sensory experience is often that of an inability to take in a sufficiently deep breath rather than difficulty in exhaling.

The patient with predominant *emphysema* is characterized by many years of exertional dyspnea progressing to dyspnea at rest (Chap. 223). Although a parenchymal disease by definition, emphysema is invariably accompanied by obstruction of airways.

Diffuse parenchymal lung diseases (See also Chap. 224)   This category includes a large number of diseases ranging from acute pneumonia to chronic disorders such as sarcoidosis and the various forms of *pneumoconiosis*. History, physical findings, and radiographic abnormalities often provide clues to the diagnosis. The patients are often tachypneic with arterial P_{CO_2} and P_{O_2} values below normal. Exertion often further reduces the arterial P_{O_2}. Lung volumes are decreased, and the lungs are stiffer, i.e., less compliant than normal.

Pulmonary vascular occlusive diseases (See also Chap. 226)   Repeated episodes of dyspnea at rest often occur with recurrent pulmonary emboli. A source for emboli, such as phlebitis of a lower extremity or the pelvis, is quite helpful in leading the physician to suspect the diagnosis. Arterial blood gases are almost invariably abnormal, but lung volumes are frequently normal or only minimally abnormal.

Diseases of the chest wall or respiratory muscles (See also Chap. 229)   The physical examination establishes the presence of a chest wall disease such as severe kyphoscoliosis, pectus excavatum, or spondylitis. Although all three of these deformities may be associated with dyspnea, only severe kyphoscoliosis regularly interferes with ventilation sufficiently to produce chronic cor pulmonale and respiratory failure. Even though vital capacity, lung volumes, and airflow rates are normal with pectus excavatum, in the most severe cases cardiac compression from the posteriorly displaced sternum may interfere with diastolic filling of the ventricle during exercise. Hence a cardiogenic component to the dyspnea may be present in this condition.

Both weakness and paralysis of respiratory muscles can lead to respiratory failure and dyspnea (Chap. 229), but most often the signs and symptoms of the neurologic or muscular disorder are more prominently manifested in other systems.

Heart disease In patients with cardiac disease, exertional dyspnea occurs most commonly as a consequence of an elevated pulmonary capillary pressure; aside from uncommon causes such as congenital or acquired obstructive disease of the pulmonary veins (Chap. 199), pulmonary capillary hypertension is a consequence of left atrial hypertension, which in turn may be due to left ventricular dysfunction (Chaps. 194 and 195), reduced left ventricular compliance, and mitral stenosis. The elevation of hydrostatic pressure in the pulmonary vascular bed tends to upset the Starling equilibrium (see "Pulmonary Edema," below) with resulting transudation of liquid into the interstitial space, reducing the compliance of the lungs and stimulating J (juxtacapillary) receptors in the alveolar interstitial space. When prolonged, pulmonary venous hypertension results in thickening of the walls of small pulmonary vessels and an increase in perivascular cells and fibrous tissue, causing a further reduction in compliance. The competition for space between vessels, airways, and increased liquid within the interstitial space compromises the lumina of small airways, increasing the airways' resistance. Diminution in compliance and an increase in the airways' resistance increase the work of breathing, which, to some degree, is minimized by a reduction in tidal volume; the latter, in turn, is compensated for by an increase in frequency of respiration. In severe heart disease, usually involving elevation of both pulmonary and systemic venous pressures, hydrothorax may develop, interfering further with pulmonary function and intensifying dyspnea. In patients with heart failure and a severely diminished cardiac output, dyspnea also may be related to fatigue of the respiratory muscles as a consequence of their reduced perfusion. The metabolic acidosis characteristic of severe heart failure may play a contributory role. Dyspnea also may be associated with severe systemic and cerebral hypoxia, as occurs during exertion in patients with congenital heart disease and right-to-left shunts.

Cardiac dyspnea usually begins as breathlessness on strenuous exertion and, over the course of months or years, progresses until the patient is dyspneic at rest. Occasionally, a nonproductive cough developing in the recumbent position, particularly at night, may be the first complaint.

Orthopnea, i.e., dyspnea in the recumbent position, and *paroxysmal nocturnal dyspnea*, i.e., attacks of shortness of breath which usually occur at night and awaken the patient from sleep, are characteristic of more advanced forms of heart failure associated with elevations of pulmonary venous and capillary pressures and are discussed in Chap. 195. Orthopnea is the result of the alteration of gravitational forces when the recumbent position is assumed. This augmentation of intrathoracic blood volume elevates pulmonary venous and capillary pressures, which increases the pulmonary closing volume (Chap. 214) and reduces the vital capacity. An additional factor associated with recumbency is elevation of the diaphragm, which results in a lower end-expiratory lung volume. This combination of lower end-expiratory lung volume and increase in closing volume results in a significant alteration of alveolar-capillary gas exchange.

PAROXYSMAL (NOCTURNAL) DYSPNEA Also known as *cardiac asthma*, this condition is characterized by attacks of severe shortness of breath which generally occur at night and usually awaken the patient from sleep. The attack is precipitated by stimuli which aggravate the previously existing pulmonary congestion; frequently, the total blood volume is augmented at night because of the reabsorption of edema from dependent portions of the body during recumbency; the redistribution of blood volume which takes place results in an increase in intrathoracic blood volume and therefore produces pulmonary congestion. A sleeping patient can tolerate relatively severe pulmonary engorgement and may awaken only when actual pulmonary edema and bronchospasm have developed, with the feeling of suffocation and with wheezing respirations.

CHEYNE-STOKES RESPIRATION See Chap. 195.

DIAGNOSIS The diagnosis of cardiac dyspnea depends on the recognition of heart disease on the basis of the clinical examination supplemented by noninvasive testing. There may be a history of antecedent myocardial infarction, third and fourth heart sounds may be audible, and/or there may be evidence of left ventricular enlargement, jugular neck vein distention, and/or peripheral edema. Often there are radiographic signs of heart failure, with evidence of interstitial edema, pulmonary vascular redistribution, and accumulation of liquid in the septal planes and pleural cavity. Cardiomegaly is often present, but the overall heart size may be normal, particularly in patients with dyspnea due to acute myocardial infarction or mitral stenosis; an enlarged left atrium is usually evident in the latter condition. The electrocardiogram (Chap. 189) is rarely specific for heart disease and cannot specifically indicate whether a patient's dyspnea is caused by heart disease; however, it is rarely normal in patients with cardiac dyspnea. Echocardiography (Chap. 191) is particularly useful in establishing the diagnosis of structural heart disease, which can be responsible for dyspnea. Specifically, left atrial and/or left ventricular dilatation, left ventricular hypertrophy, a reduced left ventricular ejection fraction, and disorders of left ventricular wall motion may be clues to the presence of a cardiac etiology of otherwise unexplained dyspnea.

Differentiation between cardiac and pulmonary dyspnea In most patients with dyspnea there is obvious clinical evidence of disease of either the heart or lungs. The dyspnea of chronic obstructive lung disease tends to develop more gradually than that of heart disease; exceptions, of course, occur in patients with obstructive lung disease who develop an episode of infectious bronchitis, pneumonia, or pneumothorax or an exacerbation of asthma. Like patients with cardiac dyspnea, patients with chronic obstructive lung disease also may waken at night with dyspnea, but this is usually associated with sputum production; the dyspnea is relieved after these patients rid themselves of secretions.

The difficulty in the distinction between cardiac and pulmonary dyspnea may be compounded by the coexistence of diseases involving both organ systems. Patients with a history of chronic bronchitis or asthma who develop left ventricular failure tend to develop recurrences of bronchoconstriction and wheezing in association with bouts of paroxysmal nocturnal dyspnea and pulmonary edema. This condition, i.e., cardiac asthma, usually occurs in patients with overt clinical evidence of heart disease. Acute cardiac asthma is further differentiated from acute attacks of bronchial asthma by the presence of diaphoresis, more bubbly airway sounds, and the more common occurrence of cyanosis.

It is desirable to carry out pulmonary function testing in patients in whom the etiology of dyspnea is not clear, for these tests may be helpful in determining whether dyspnea is produced by heart disease, lung disease, abnormalities of the chest wall, or anxiety. In addition to the usual means of assessing patients for heart disease (Chap. 187), determination of the ejection fraction at rest and during exercise by echocardiography or radionuclide ventriculography (Chap. 191) is helpful in the differential diagnosis of dyspnea. The left ventricular ejection fraction is depressed in left ventricular failure, while the right ventricular ejection fraction may be low at rest or may decline during exercise in patients with severe lung disease. Both ejection fractions are normal at rest and during exercise in dyspnea due to anxiety or malingering. Careful observation during the performance of an exercise treadmill test will often help in the identification of the patient who is malingering or whose dyspnea is secondary to anxiety. Under these circumstances, the patient usually complains of severe shortness of breath but appears to be breathing either effortlessly or totally irregularly. In less than obvious cases, measurements of P_{O_2}, pH, and P_{CO_2} in arterial blood and CO_2 and O_2 levels in mixed expired gas may be helpful in establishing either that gas exchange is normal or that a significant abnormality that is not detectable at rest exists during exercise.

Anxiety neurosis Dyspnea experienced by someone with an anxiety neurosis is a difficult symptom to evaluate. The signs and symptoms of acute and chronic hyperventilation do not serve to distinguish between anxiety neurosis and other processes, such as recurrent pulmonary emboli. Another potentially confusing situation is seen when chest pain and electrocardiographic changes accompany the hyperventilation syndrome. When present and attributable to this condition, often referred to as *neurocirculatory asthenia* (Chap. 12), the chest pain is often sharp, fleeting, and in various loci, and the electrocardiographic changes are most often seen during repolarization; yet occasional ventricular ectopic activity can be seen as well. A rather extensive series of pulmonary and cardiac function tests, carried out both at rest and during exercise, may be needed to be certain that anxiety is, in fact, the cause of the dyspnea. Certain clues are helpful in leading one to suspect a psychogenic origin. Frequent sighing respirations and an irregular breathing pattern are helpful. Often the breathing pattern returns to normal during sleep.

PULMONARY EDEMA (See Table 31-1)

CARDIOGENIC PULMONARY EDEMA (see Table 31-1, IA)   An increase in pulmonary venous pressure, which results initially in engorgement of the pulmonary vasculature, is common in most instances of dyspnea in association with congestive heart failure. The lungs become less compliant, the resistance of small airways increases, and there is an increase in lymphatic flow which apparently serves to maintain a constant pulmonary extravascular liquid volume. At this early stage there is usually mild tachypnea, and if arterial blood gases are measured, the arterial P_{O_2} and P_{CO_2} are both lowered modestly

---

TABLE 31-1   Classification of pulmonary edema based on initiating mechanism

I IMBALANCE OF STARLING FORCES

A Increased pulmonary capillary pressure
  1 Increased pulmonary venous pressure without left ventricular failure (e.g., mitral stenosis)
  2 increased pulmonary venous pressure secondary to left ventricular failure
  3 Increased pulmonary capillary pressure secondary to increased pulmonary arterial pressure (so-called overperfusion pulmonary edema)
B Decreased plasma oncotic pressure
  1 Hypoalbuminemia
C Increased negativity of interstitial pressure
  1 Rapid removal of pneumothorax with large applied negative pressures (unilateral)
  2 Large negative pleural pressures due to acute airway obstruction alone with increased end-expiratory volumes (asthma)

II ALTERED ALVEOLAR-CAPILLARY MEMBRANE PERMEABILITY (ADULT RESPIRATORY DISTRESS SYNDROME)

A Infectious pneumonia—bacterial, viral, parasitic
B Inhaled toxins (e.g., phosgene, ozone, chlorine, Teflon fumes, nitrogen dioxide, smoke)
C Circulating foreign substances (e.g., snake venom, bacterial endotoxins)
D Aspiration of acidic gastric contents
E Acute radiation pneumonitis
F Endogenous vasoactive substances (e.g., histamine, kinins)
G Disseminated intravascular coagulation
H Immunologic—hypersensitivity pneumonitis, drugs (nitrofurantoin), leukoagglutinins
I Shock lung in association with nonthoracic trauma
J Acute hemorrhagic pancreatitis

III LYMPHATIC INSUFFICIENCY

A After lung tranplant
B Lymphangitic carcinomatosis
C Fibrosing lymphangitis (e.g., silicosis)

IV UNKNOWN OR INCOMPLETELY UNDERSTOOD

A High-altitude pulmonary edema
B Neurogenic pulmonary edema
C Narcotic overdose
D Pulmonary embolism
E Eclampsia
F After cardioversion
G After anesthesia
H After cardiopulmonary bypass

SOURCE: Reproduced with permission from Ingram and Braunwald.

---

with an increase in the alveolar-to-arterial oxygen difference. Tachypnea itself, which might result from stimulation of receptors in the pulmonary interstitium, apparently increases lymphatic flow by augmenting ventilatory pumping of lymphatic vessels. The changes described are seen well in advance of auscultatory findings or radiographic signs pointing to congestive heart failure. If sufficient both in magnitude and duration, the increase in intravascular pressure results in a net gain of liquid in the extravascular space despite further increases in lymphatic flow. It is at this point that symptoms worsen, tachypnea increases, gas exchange deteriorates further, and radiographic changes, such as Kerley B lines and loss of distinct vascular margins, are seen. It has been shown, even at this intermediate stage, that the capillary endothelial intercellular junctions have widened and allow passage of macromolecules into the interstices. Up to and including this stage, the edema is purely *interstitial*.

Further elevations in intravascular pressure result in disruption of the tighter junctions between alveolar lining cells, and alveolar edema ensues with outpouring of liquid which contains both red blood cells and macromolecules. At this point *alveolar edema* is present. Although at one time considered an early and subtle radiographic sign of interstitial edema, current evidence suggests that an antigravity redistribution of pulmonary blood flow (from the lung bases to the apices) occurs only after the onset of alveolar edema. With yet more severe disruption of the alveolar-capillary membrane, edematous liquid floods the alveoli and airways. At this point, full-blown clinical pulmonary edema with bilateral wet rales and rhonchi will occur, and the chest radiograph may show diffuse haziness of the lung fields with greater density in the more proximal hilar regions. Typically, the patient is anxious and perspires freely, and the sputum is frothy and blood-tinged. Gas exchange is more severely compromised with worsening hypoxia. Without effective treatment (Chap. 195), progressive acidemia, hypercapnia, and respiratory arrest ensue.

The earlier sequence of liquid accumulation described above follows the Starling law of capillary–interstitial fluid exchange:

$$\text{Liquid accumulation} = K[(P_c - P_{IF}) - \sigma(\pi_{pl} - \pi_{IF})] - Q_{\text{lymph}}$$

where K = hydraulic conductance (directly proportional to membrane surface area and inversely proportional to membrane thickness)
  P_c = mean intracapillary pressure
  π_{IF} = oncotic pressure of interstitial liquid
  σ = reflection coefficient of macromolecules
  P_{IF} = mean interstitial liquid pressure
  π_{pl} = oncotic pressure of the plasma
Q_{lymph} = lymphatic flow

The pressures tending to move liquid out of the vessel are $\dot{P}_c$ and π_{IF}, which are normally more than offset by pressures tending to move liquid back into the vasculature, i.e., the algebraic sum of P_{IF} and π_{pl}. Implicit in the preceding equation is that lymphatic flow can increase in the case of imbalance of forces and result in no net accumulation of interstitial liquid. Further elevations in P_c not only increase the outward movement of liquid in each capillary region but also recruit more of the capillary bed, which increases K. These two effects lead to liquid filtration that exceeds clearance capability by the lymphatics, and liquid accumulates in the loose interstitial spaces of the lung. Even greater increases in P_c open first the loose endothelial intercellular junctions and later the tight alveolar intercellular junctions with an increase in permeability to macromolecules. This secondary disruption of both the function and structure of the alveolar-capillary membrane leads to alveolar flooding.

NONCARDIOGENIC PULMONARY EDEMA (See Table 31-1, IB, IC, II, III, and IV)   Several clinical conditions are associated with pulmonary edema based on an imbalance of Starling forces other than through primary elevations of pulmonary capillary pressure. Although diminished plasma oncotic pressure in hypoalbuminemic states (e.g., severe liver disease, nephrotic syndrome, protein-losing enteropathy) might be expected to lead to pulmonary edema, the balance of forces normally so strongly favors resorption that even in these conditions some elevation of capillary pressure is necessary before interstitial edema develops. Increased negativity of interstitial pressure has been implicated in the genesis of unilateral pulmonary edema following rapid evacuation of a large pneumothorax. In this situation, the findings may be apparent only by radiography, but occasionally the patient experiences dyspnea with physical findings localized to the edematous lung. It has been proposed that large negative intrapleural pressures during acute severe asthma may be associated with the development of interstitial edema. If this proposal can be supported by sufficient clinical data, then asthma would represent an additional example of edema due to increased negativity of interstitial pressure. Lymphatic blockade secondary to fibrotic and inflammatory diseases or lymphangitic carcinomatosis may lead to interstitial edema. In such instances, both clinical and radiographic manifestations are dominated by the underlying disease process.

There are other conditions characterized by increases in the interstitial liquid content of the lungs which begin neither with an imbalance between intravascular and interstitial forces nor with alterations in lymphatics, but rather appear to be associated primarily with disruption of the alveolar-capillary membranes. Any number of spontaneously occurring or environmental toxic insults, including diffuse pulmonary infections, aspiration, and shock (particularly due to gram-negative septicemia and hemorrhagic pancreatitis and following cardiopulmonary bypass), are associated with diffuse pulmonary edema which clearly does not have a hemodynamic origin. These conditions, which may lead to the adult respiratory distress syndrome, are discussed in Chap. 230.

Other forms of pulmonary edema   There are three forms of pulmonary edema which have not been clearly related to increased permeability, inadequate lymphatic flow, or an imbalance of Starling forces; hence their precise mechanism remains unexplained. *Narcotic overdose* is a well-recognized antecedent to pulmonary edema. Although illicit use of parenteral heroin is the most frequent cause, parenteral and oral overdoses of legitimate preparations of morphine, methadone, and dextropropoxyphene also have been associated with pulmonary edema. Thus the earlier idea that injected impurities lead to the disorder is untenable. Available evidence suggests that there are alterations in the permeability of alveolar and capillary membranes rather than an elevation of pulmonary capillary pressure.

Exposure to high altitude in association with severe physical exertion is a well-recognized setting for pulmonary edema in unacclimatized, yet otherwise healthy persons. Recent data show that acclimatized high-altitude natives also develop this syndrome upon return to high altitude after a relatively brief sojourn at low altitudes. The syndrome is far more common in persons under the age of 25 years. The mechanism for high-altitude pulmonary edema remains obscure, and studies have been conflicting, some suggesting pulmonary venous constriction and others indicating pulmonary arteriolar constriction as the prime mechanisms. A role for hypoxia at altitude is suggested by the fact that patients respond to the administration of oxygen and/or return to lower altitudes. Hypoxia per se does not alter permeability of the alveolar-capillary membrane. Hence increased cardiac output and pulmonary arterial pressures with exercise combined with hypoxic pulmonary arteriolar constriction, which is more prominent in young persons, may combine to make this an example of prearteriolar, high-pressure pulmonary edema.

Neurogenic pulmonary edema has been suspected in patients with central nervous system disorders and without apparent preexisting left ventricular dysfunction. Although most experimental equivalents have implicated sympathetic nervous system activity, the mechanism whereby sympathetic efferent activity leads to pulmonary edema is a matter of speculation. It is known that a massive adrenergic discharge leads to peripheral vasoconstriction with elevation of blood pressure and shifts of blood to the central circulation. In addition, it is probable that a reduction in left ventricular compliance also occurs, and both factors serve to increase left atrial pressures sufficiently to induce pulmonary edema on a hemodynamic basis. Some experimental evidence suggests that stimulation of adrenergic receptors increases capillary permeability directly, but this effect is relatively minor as compared with the imbalance of Starling forces.

TREATMENT OF PULMONARY EDEMA   See Chap. 195.

REFERENCES

COLICE GL: Detecting the presence and cause of pulmonary edema. Postgrad Med 93:161, 169, 1993

CRAPO JD: New concepts in the formation of pulmonary edema. Am Rev Respir Dis 147:790, 1993

DePaso WJ et al: Chronic dyspnea unexplained by history, physical examination, chest roentgenogram and spirometry. Chest 100:1293, 1991

ELLIOTT MW et al: The language of breathlessness: Use of verbal descriptors by patients with cardiopulmonary diseases. Am Rev Respir Dis 144:826, 1991

INGRAM RH JR, BRAUNWALD E: Pulmonary edema: Cardiogenic and noncardiogenic, in *Heart Disease*, 4th ed, E Braunwald (ed). Philadelphia, Saunders, 1992, p 551

MAHLER DA et al: Measurement of breathlessness during exercise in asthmatics. Am Rev Respir Dis 144:39, 1991

SCHWARTZSTEIN RM et al: Dyspnea: A sensory experience. Lung 169:543, 1991

WASSERMAN K, CASABURI R: Dyspnea: Physiological and pathophysiological mechanisms. Annu Rev Med 39:503, 1988

32   HYPOXIA, POLYCYTHEMIA, AND CYANOSIS

EUGENE BRAUNWALD

HYPOXIA

The fundamental purpose of the cardiorespiratory system is to deliver oxygen (and substrates) to the cells and to remove carbon dioxide (and other metabolic products) from them. Proper maintenance of this function depends on intact cardiovascular and respiratory systems and a supply of inspired gas containing adequate oxygen. Changes in oxygen and in carbon dioxide tension as well as changes in the intraerythrocytic concentration of certain *organic phosphate compounds*, especially 2,3-biphosphoglyceric acid (2,3-BPG), cause shifts in the oxygen dissociation curve. These are discussed in detail in Chap. 302 and are illustrated in Fig. 302-4. When hypoxia results as a consequence of respiratory failure, Pa_{CO_2} usually rises (Chap. 214), and the oxygen dissociation curve is displaced to the right. Under these conditions, the percentage saturation of the hemoglobin in the arterial blood at a given level of alveolar oxygen tension (Pa_{O_2}) declines. Thus arterial hypoxia and cyanosis are likely to be more marked in proportion to the degree of depression of Pa_{O_2} when such depression results from pulmonary disease than when the depression occurs as the result of a decline in the partial pressure of oxygen in the inspired air, in which case Pa_{CO_2} falls and the oxygen dissociation curve is displaced to the left.

DIFFERENTIAL DIAGNOSIS   Anemic hypoxia   Any decrease in hemoglobin concentration is attended by a corresponding decline in the oxygen-carrying capacity of the blood. The Pa_{O_2} remains normal, but the absolute amount of oxygen transported per unit volume of blood is diminished. As the anemic blood passes through the capillaries and the usual amount of oxygen is removed from it, the P_{O_2} in the venous blood declines to a greater degree than would normally be the case.

Carbon monoxide intoxication (Chap. 395)   This condition is analogous to anemic hypoxia in that the hemoglobin which is combined with the carbon monoxide (carboxyhemoglobin) is unavailable for oxygen transport. In addition, the presence of carboxyhemoglobin shifts the dissociation curve of hemoglobin to the left so that the oxygen can be unloaded only at lower tensions. By such formation of carboxyhemoglobin, a given degree of reduction in oxygen-carrying power produces a far greater degree of tissue hypoxia than the equivalent reduction in hemoglobin due to simple anemia.

Respiratory hypoxia Arterial unsaturation is a common finding in advanced pulmonary disease. As discussed in Chap. 214, it may be caused by hypoventilation when it is associated with an elevation of Pa_{CO_2}. A second cause is shunting of blood from right to left by perfusion of nonventilated portions of the lung, as in pulmonary atelectasis or through vascular abnormalities of the lung with arteriovenous connections. The low Pa_{O_2} is not correctable by inspiring 100% O_2. The most common cause of respiratory hypoxia is ventilation-perfusion mismatch, which results from perfusion of poorly ventilated alveoli. The low Pa_{O_2} is usually readily correctable by inspiring 100% O_2.

Hypoxia secondary to right-to-left extrapulmonary shunting This cause of hypoxia resembles physiologically intrapulmonary right-to-left shunting but is caused by congenital cardiac malformations such as tetralogy of Fallot, transposition of the great arteries, and Eisenmenger's complex (Chap. 199). As in pulmonary right-to-left shunting, the Pa_{O_2} cannot be brought to normal with inspiration of 100% O_2.

Circulatory hypoxia As in anemic hypoxia, Pa_{O_2} is normal, but venous and tissue P_{O_2} values are reduced as a consequence of reduced tissue perfusion in the face of normal tissue oxygen consumption. Generalized circulatory hypoxia occurs in heart failure (Chap. 195) and in most forms of shock (Chap. 34).

Specific organ hypoxia Decreased circulation to a specific organ resulting in localized circulatory hypoxia may be due to organic arterial obstruction or may occur as a consequence of vasoconstriction. The latter is seen in the upper extremities in Raynaud's phenomenon. Reduced circulation may occur in all limbs in patients with heart failure or hypovolemic shock in an attempt to maintain adequate perfusion to more vital organs. Ischemic hypoxia with accompanying pallor occurs in organic arterial obliterative disease. Localized hypoxia also may result from venous obstruction and the resultant congestion and reduced arterial inflow. Edema, which increases the distance through which oxygen diffuses before it reaches the cells, also can cause localized hypoxia.

Increased oxygen requirements If the oxygen consumption of the tissues is elevated without a corresponding increase in volume flow per unit of time, the P_{O_2} in venous blood (and hence capillary and tissue P_{O_2}) may be reduced. This will occur even if oxygen diffusion into blood perfusing the pulmonary capillary bed is normal and the hemoglobin is qualitatively and quantitatively normal. Such a situation may be encountered when fever or thyrotoxicosis occurs in patients in whom the cardiac output is fixed and cannot rise normally. Under these conditions, the circulation may be considered deficient relative to the metabolic requirements.

Ordinarily, the clinical picture of patients with hypoxia due to an elevated metabolic rate is quite different from that in other types of hypoxia; the skin is warm and flushed, owing to increased cutaneous blood flow which dissipates the excessive heat produced, and cyanosis is usually absent.

Exercise is a classic example of increased tissue oxygen requirements. These increased demands are normally met by several mechanisms: (1) increasing the cardiac output and ventilation and thus oxygen delivery to the tissues, (2) preferentially directing the blood to the exercising muscles and away from resting muscles, skin, and viscera (by changing vascular resistances in various circulatory beds, directly and/or reflexly), (3) increasing oxygen extraction from the delivered blood and widening the arteriovenous oxygen differences, and (4) reducing the pH of the tissues and capillary blood, thereby unloading more oxygen from hemoglobin. If the capacity of these mechanisms is exceeded, then hypoxia, especially of the exercising muscles, will result.

Improper oxygen utilization Cyanide (Chap. 395) and several other similarly acting poisons cause a paradoxic state in which the tissues are unable to utilize oxygen, and as a consequence, the venous blood tends to have a high oxygen tension. This condition has been termed *histotoxic hypoxia*. Cyanide produces cellular hypoxia by paralyzing the electron-transfer function of cytochrome oxidase so that it cannot pass electrons to oxygen, whereas diphtheria toxin is believed to inhibit the synthesis of one of the cytochromes and thus interfere with oxygen consumption and energy production by the cells involved.

EFFECTS OF HYPOXIA Changes in the central nervous system, particularly the higher centers, are especially important. Acute hypoxia produces impaired judgment, motor incoordination, and a clinical picture closely resembling that of acute alcoholism. When hypoxia is long-standing, fatigue, drowsiness, apathy, inattentiveness, delayed reaction time, and reduced work capacity occur. As hypoxia becomes more severe, the centers of the brainstem are affected, and death usually results from respiratory failure. With reduction of Pa_{O_2}, cerebrovascular resistance decreases and cerebral blood flow increases, which tends to reduce the cerebral hypoxia. On the other hand, when the reduction of Pa_{O_2} is accompanied by hyperventilation and diminution of Pa_{CO_2}, cerebrovascular resistance rises, blood flow falls, and hypoxia is enhanced. Compared with the brain, the phylogenetically older spinal cord and peripheral nerves are relatively insensitive to hypoxia. Hypoxia also causes pulmonary arterial constriction, which serves the useful function of shunting blood away from poorly ventilated areas toward better-ventilated portions of the lung. However, it has the disadvantage of causing increased pulmonary vascular resistance and increased right ventricular afterload.

A complex disturbance of cellular functions results from the metabolic effects of severe acute hypoxia. In liver and muscles, the metabolism of the primary foodstuff, carbohydrate, normally proceeds anaerobically (i.e., without oxidation) to the stage of formation of pyruvic acid. The breakdown of pyruvate requires oxygen, and when this is deficient, increasing proportions of pyruvate are reduced to lactic acid, which cannot be broken down further (Chap. 46). Hence there is an increase in the blood lactate, with decrease in bicarbonate and a corresponding metabolic acidosis. Under these circumstances, the total energy obtained from foodstuff breakdown is greatly reduced, and the amount of energy available for continuing resynthesis of energy-rich phosphate compounds becomes inadequate, leading to a complex disturbance of cellular function.

Most of the useful respiratory response to hypoxia originates in special chemosensitive cells in the carotid and aortic bodies, although the respiratory center in the brainstem is also stimulated directly by oxygen lack. The resultant increase in ventilation, with loss of carbon dioxide, leads to respiratory alkalosis. On the other hand, the diffusion of additional quantities of lactic acid from the tissues into the blood tends to produce metabolic acidosis. In either case, the total amount of bicarbonate, and hence the carbon dioxide–combining power, tends to be diminished (Chap. 46).

Diminished oxygen tension in any tissue results in local vasodilatation, and the diffuse vasodilatation which occurs in generalized hypoxia causes an elevation of total cardiac output (Fig. 302-5). In patients with preexisting heart disease, the development of hypoxia and the requirements of the peripheral tissues for an increase of cardiac output may precipitate congestive heart failure. In patients with ischemic heart disease, a reduced Pa_{O_2} may intensify ischemia and further impair left ventricular function. Prolonged or severe hypoxia also may impair hepatic and renal function.

One of the important mechanisms of compensation for prolonged hypoxia is an increase in the hemoglobin concentration. This is due not to direct stimulation of the bone marrow but to the effect of erythropoietin (Chap. 302). Assayable levels of erythropoietin are increased by hypoxia, and its production has been found to be regulated by the balance between tissue oxygen supply and demand.

POLYCYTHEMIA (See also Chap. 309)

The term *polycythemia* signifies an increase above normal in the number of red blood cells in the circulating blood. This elevation is usually, although not always, accompanied by a corresponding increase in the quantity of hemoglobin and in the hematocrit. The

TABLE 32-1 Differential diagnosis of erythrocytosis

ABSOLUTE (↑ RED CELL MASS)

I **Autonomous erythroid proliferation** (↓ EP*); polycythemia vera
II **Secondary erythroid proliferation**
   A Autonomous or inappropriate increase in EP
      1 Neoplasm
      2 Renal lesions
      3 Familial erythrocytosis (autosomal recessive inheritance)
   B Secondary increase in EP
      1 Hypoxia (↓ arterial P_{O_2})
        a High altitude
        b Alveolar hypoventilation
        c Pulmonary disease
        d Cardiac right-to-left shunt
      2 Abnormal hemoglobin function (normal arterial P_{O_2})
        a High-affinity variants (autosomal dominant inheritance)
        b Congenital methemoglobinemia
        c Carboxyhemoglobin (smokers' polycythemia)
   C Hormonal stimulus to erythropoiesis
      1 Cushing's syndrome
      2 Androgen or corticosteroid administration

RELATIVE (REDUCED PLASMA VOLUME, NORMAL RED CELL MASS)

I **Dehydration**
II **Stress erythrocytosis**

* Erythropoietin.
SOURCE: Adapted from HF Bunn et al, *Human Hemoglobins*, Philadelphia, Saunders, 1988.

increase may or may not be associated with an elevation in the total quantity of red blood cells in the body. It is important to distinguish between *absolute* polycythemia (an increase in the total red cell mass) and *relative* polycythemia, which occurs when, through loss of blood plasma, the *concentration* of the red cells in the circulating blood becomes greater than normal. This may be the consequence of abnormally lowered fluid intake, of the loss of plasma into the interstitial fluid, or of the marked loss of body fluids, such as occurs in persistent vomiting, severe diarrhea, copious sweating, or acidosis.

Because the term *polycythemia* is used loosely to refer to all varieties of increase in the number of red corpuscles, the terms *erythrocytosis* and *erythremia* are preferred in referring to two forms of *absolute* polycythemia. *Erythrocytosis* denotes absolute polycythemia which occurs in response to some known stimulus, most commonly hypoxemia (secondary polycythemia); *erythremia* (polycythemia vera) refers to the disease of unknown etiology. Erythrocytosis develops as a consequence of a variety of factors and represents a physiologic response to conditions of hypoxia. An approach to the differential diagnosis of erythrocytosis should begin with a consideration of its mechanisms (Table 32-1).

SECONDARY POLYCYTHEMIA Sojourn at high altitudes leads to defective saturation of arterial blood with oxygen and stimulates the production of more red cells. The oxygen saturation, rather than oxygen tension, appears to be the more important determinant of the erythropoietic response to chronic hypoxia (Fig. 32-1). A condition known as *chronic mountain sickness* or *soroche* (Monge's disease) may set in insidiously after several years of continued residence at high altitude. This condition appears to be caused by the development of alveolar hypoventilation superimposed on a lowered inspired O_2 concentration. Prominent manifestations are a florid color which turns to cyanosis on mild exertion, impaired mental acuity, fatigue, and headache. Those affected are usually in the fourth to sixth decades. Return to sea level promptly relieves the symptoms. Living at high altitudes also evokes a number of compensatory reactions which act to increase oxygen delivery to the tissues. These include hyperventilation, which reduces the oxygen gradient between inspired and alveolar air, erythrocytosis, an augmentation of pulmonary capillary blood volume, an increase of diffusing capacity, and an increase in cardiac output.

Any pulmonary disease which produces chronic hypoxia may lead to erythrocytosis. The increased blood viscosity secondary to the polycythemia elevates pulmonary arterial pressure and, combined with the elevation of pulmonary vascular resistance resulting from hypoxia, further elevates right ventricular pressure, contributing to the development or intensification of cor pulmonale (Chap. 204). The *abnormal ventilatory conditions* present in very obese individuals may cause alveolar hypoventilation and result in arterial unsaturation, erythrocytosis, hypercapnia, and somnolence (the Pickwickian syndrome; Chap. 229). This syndrome is also observed in nonobese persons (sleep-apnea syndrome) in whom decreased sensitivity of the respiratory center to CO_2 may play a role (Chap. 229).

The partial shunting of blood from the pulmonary circuit (right-to-left shunts), such as occurs in *congenital heart disease*, causes the most striking erythrocytosis resulting from abnormalities in the heart or lungs (Chap. 199). Erythrocyte counts as high as 12×10^6 per microliter, which are possible only when the red corpuscles are smaller than normal, have been observed in such patients, with a hematocrit as high as 86 percent. As the polycythemia develops, there is a progressive elevation of blood viscosity, which begins to rise logarithmically when the volume of packed red blood cells exceeds 55 percent. The most common defects producing such polycythemia in the adult are tetralogy of Fallot and Eisenmenger syndrome. Other congenital cardiac malformations commonly responsible for polycythemia, but occurring more commonly in neonates, include transposition of the great arteries, tricuspid atresia, and persistent truncus arteriosus.

Rarely, patients with hepatic cirrhosis will be hypoxemic secondary to intrapulmonary shunts, or right-to-left shunts from the portal to the pulmonary veins. The polycythemia of cyanotic congenital heart disease may lead to spontaneous thrombosis at any site, including the central nervous system.

The increase in hematocrit and the sharp increase in viscosity which occur when these patients become dehydrated are particularly hazardous. Symptoms due to increased blood viscosity include reduced mentation, headache, fatigue, visual disturbance, and dizziness. This condition also may be accompanied by a variety of blood coagulation defects, including reduced fibrinogen and prothrombin concentrations, as well as thrombocytopenia. Reduction in red blood cell volume (phlebotomy with reinfusion of the plasma) is sometimes performed

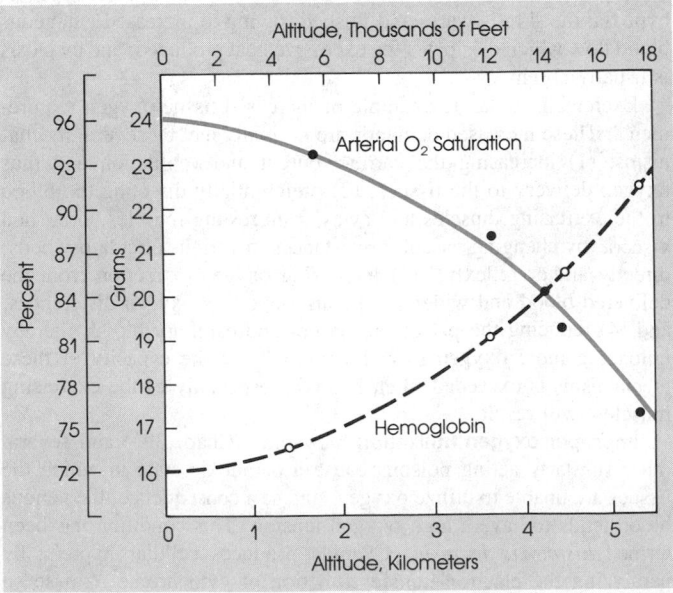

FIGURE 32-1 Relationship between mean arterial oxygen saturation (percent) and the mean hemoglobin content (grams per deciliter) in healthy male residents at various altitudes. *(From Hurtado, by permission of Annals of Internal Medicine.)*

in severely symptomatic patients with extremely high hematocrit levels, usually exceeding 65 percent, but it must be carried out slowly, with caution, and with the realization that the polycythemia is, in fact, an important compensatory mechanism. However, reduction of red blood cell volume may result in a reduction of the elevated blood viscosity which improves blood flow.

The excessive use of coal-tar derivatives and other forms of chronic poisoning, by producing abnormal hemoglobin pigments such as *methemoglobin* and *sulfhemoglobin* (Chap. 306), also may cause erythrocytosis. Patients with abnormal hemoglobins which displace the oxygen dissociation curve to the left and interfere with oxygen unloading in the tissues stimulate the production of erythropoietin and a secondary erythrocytosis *unassociated* with leukocytosis or thrombocytosis (Chap. 306).

Mild erythrocytosis is sometimes found in *Cushing's syndrome* and can be produced by the administration of large amounts of adrenocortical steroids and androgens. Especially intriguing are the instances of erythrocytosis observed in association with various *tumors* which produce erythropoietin or an erythropoietin-like substance. These include vascular tumors (hemangioblastomas) in the posterior fossa, renal tumors (renal cell carcinoma, adenoma, and sarcoma), uterine myoma, hepatic carcinoma, and pheochromocytoma. Erythrocytosis also occurs occasionally in patients with solitary and polycystic disease of the kidneys, hydronephrosis, and renal artery stenosis. Plasma erythropoietin levels have been found to be elevated in a number of these patients with tumors and indeed all forms of secondary polycythemia. Erythropoietin-like activity has been demonstrated in tumor extracts and in renal cyst fluid, and erythrocytosis has disappeared after the associated tumor was removed.

Stress erythrocytosis This term has been applied to the polycythemia seen occasionally in active, hard-working, middle-aged white males who are typically hypertensive, overweight, and in a state of anxiety and who appear florid but have none of the other characteristic signs of polycythemia vera, i.e., no splenomegaly or leukocytosis with immature white blood cells. In such persons, the total red blood cell mass is normal, and the plasma volume is below normal. Thus they have a moderately elevated hematocrit, usually 50 to 60 percent, and *relative* polycythemia. *Smokers' polycythemia* is a closely related condition, but the high carboxyhemoglobin concentration may cause a small absolute increase in red cell mass which is often associated with a reduced plasma volume. Smoking should be discontinued.

CLINICAL FEATURES AND DIFFERENTIAL DIAGNOSIS Patients with polycythemia present with (in addition to the symptoms of the underlying condition) a characteristic "ruddy" cyanosis, dizziness, headache, epistaxes, and an increased incidence of thrombotic complications.

The *differential diagnosis* of absolute polycythemia is discussed in Chap. 309. In polycythemia vera, erythropoietin levels are usually absent or below normal, leukocyte alkaline phosphatase, vitamin B_{12} binding capacity, and vitamin B_{12} levels and platelet and total white blood cells are usually elevated, and splenomegaly is common. Serum uric acid and lactate dehydrogenase (LDH) levels may be increased. The bone marrow shows hyperplasia of all elements. In secondary polycythemia with hypoxia, Pa_{CO_2} is usually reduced, erythropoietin levels are elevated, while levels of leukocyte alkaline phosphatase, serum vitamin B_{12}, platelet, total white blood cell, and differential counts are all normal. The liver and spleen are not enlarged, and the bone marrow shows only erythroid hyperplasia. In the absence of features of either polycythemia vera or polycythemia secondary to hypoxia or to a tumor, a hemoglobin with a high affinity for oxygen should be sought.

Workup of patients with polycythemia should include a chest roentgenogram, electrocardiogram, and arterial oxygen saturation determination to search for disease of the heart and lungs. In addition, imaging of the spleen should be carried out to assess its size and of the kidney to look for an erythropoietin-producing lesion. In patients who do not appear to have polycythemia vera or hypoxemia, the oxygen affinity of the patient's hemoglobin, i.e., the P_{O_2} at which 50

percent of the hemoglobin is deoxygenated (P_{50}) should be measured to detect hemoglobins which fail to release oxygen normally.

CYANOSIS

Cyanosis refers to a bluish color of the skin and mucous membranes resulting from an increased amount of reduced hemoglobin, or of hemoglobin derivatives, in the small blood vessels of those areas. It is usually most marked in the lips, nail beds, ears, and malar eminences. The florid skin characteristic of polycythemia vera (Chap. 309) must be distinguished from the true cyanosis discussed here. A cherry-colored flush, rather than cyanosis, is caused by carboxyhemoglobin (Chap. 395). The degree of cyanosis is modified by the quality of cutaneous pigment and the thickness of the skin, as well as by the state of the cutaneous capillaries. The accurate clinical detection of the presence and degree of cyanosis is difficult, as proved by oximetric studies. In some instances, central cyanosis can be detected reliably when the arterial saturation has fallen to 85 percent; in others, particularly in dark-skinned persons, it may not be detected until the saturation has declined to 75 percent.

The increase in the quantity of reduced hemoglobin in the cutaneous vessels which produces cyanosis may be brought about either by an increase in the quantity of venous blood in the skin as the result of dilatation of the venules and venous ends of the capillaries or by a reduction in the oxygen saturation in the capillary blood. In general, cyanosis becomes apparent when the mean capillary concentration of reduced hemoglobin exceeds 5 g/dL. It is the *absolute* rather than the *relative* quantity of reduced hemoglobin which is important in producing cyanosis. Thus, in a patient with severe anemia, the relative amount of reduced hemoglobin in the venous blood may be very large when considered in relation to the total amount of hemoglobin. However, since the concentration of the latter is markedly reduced, the *absolute* quantity of reduced hemoglobin may still be small, and therefore patients with severe anemia and even *marked* arterial desaturation do not display cyanosis. Conversely, the higher the total hemoglobin content, the greater is the tendency toward cyanosis; thus patients with marked polycythemia tend to be cyanotic at higher levels of arterial oxygen saturation than patients with normal hematocrit values. Likewise, local passive congestion, which causes an increase in the total amount of reduced hemoglobin in the vessels in a given area, may cause cyanosis. Cyanosis also is observed when nonfunctional hemoglobin such as methemoglobin or sulfhemoglobin (Chap. 306) is present in blood.

Cyanosis may be subdivided into *central* and *peripheral* types. In the *central* type, there is arterial blood unsaturation or an abnormal hemoglobin derivative, and the mucous membranes and skin are both affected. *Peripheral* cyanosis is due to a slowing of blood flow to an area and abnormally great extraction of oxygen from normally saturated arterial blood. It results from vasoconstriction and diminished peripheral blood flow, such as occurs in cold exposure, shock, congestive failure, and peripheral vascular disease. Often in these conditions the mucous membranes of the oral cavity or those beneath the tongue may be spared. Clinical differentiation between central and peripheral cyanosis may not always be simple, and in conditions such as cardiogenic shock with pulmonary edema there may be a mixture of both types.

DIFFERENTIAL DIAGNOSIS (See Table 32-2) **Central cyanosis** Decreased arterial oxygen saturation results from a marked reduction in the oxygen tension in the arterial blood. This may be brought about by a decline in the tension of oxygen in the inspired air without sufficient compensatory alveolar hyperventilation to maintain alveolar oxygen tension. Cyanosis does not occur to a significant degree in an ascent to an altitude of 2500 m (8000 ft) but is marked in a further ascent to 5000 m (16,000 ft). The reason for this becomes clear on studying the *S* shape of the oxygen dissociation curve (Fig. 302-4). At 2500 m (8000 ft) the tension of oxygen in the inspired air is about 120 mmHg, the alveolar tension is approximately 80 mmHg, and the

---

TABLE 32-2   Causes of cyanosis

CENTRAL CYANOSIS

A Decreased arterial oxygen saturation
  1 Decreased atmospheric pressure—high altitude
  2 Impaired pulmonary function
    a Alveolar hypoventilation
    b Uneven relationships between pulmonary ventilation and perfusion
      (perfusion of hypoventilated alveoli)
    c Impaired oxygen diffusion
  3 Anatomic shunts
    a Certain types of congenital heart disease
    b Pulmonary arteriovenous fistulas
    c Multiple small intrapulmonary shunts
  4 Hemoglobin with low affinity for oxygen
B Hemoglobin abnormalities
  1 Methemoglobinemia—hereditary, acquired
  2 Sulfhemoglobinema—acquired
  3 Carboxyhemoglobinemia (not true cyanosis)

PERIPHERAL CYANOSIS

A Reduced cardiac output
B Cold exposure
C Redistribution of blood flow from extremities
D Arterial obstruction
E Venous obstruction

---

hemoglobin is nearly completely saturated. However, at 5000 m (16,000 ft) the oxygen tensions in atmospheric air and alveolar air are about 85 and 50 mmHg, respectively, and the oxygen dissociation curve shows that the arterial blood is only about 75 percent saturated. This leaves 25 percent of the hemoglobin in the reduced form, an amount likely to be associated with cyanosis in the absence of anemia. Similarly, a mutant hemoglobin with a low affinity for oxygen (e.g., Hb Kansas) causes lowered arterial oxygen saturation and resultant central cyanosis (Chap. 306).

Seriously *impaired pulmonary function*, through alveolar hypoventilation or perfusion of unventilated or poorly ventilated areas of the lung, is a common cause of central cyanosis (Chap. 214). This may occur acutely, as in extensive pneumonia or pulmonary edema, or with chronic pulmonary diseases (e.g., emphysema). In the last situation polycythemia is generally present, and clubbing of the fingers may occur. However, in many types of chronic pulmonary disease with fibrosis and obliteration of the capillary vascular bed, cyanosis does not occur because there is relatively little perfusion of underventilated areas.

Another cause of decreased arterial oxygen saturation is *shunting of systemic venous blood into the arterial circuit*. Certain forms of congenital heart disease are associated with cyanosis (Chap. 199). Since blood flows from a higher-pressure to a lower-pressure region, in order for a cardiac defect to result in a right-to-left shunt, it must ordinarily be combined with an obstructive lesion distal to the defect or with elevated pulmonary vascular resistance. The most common congenital cardiac lesion associated with cyanosis in the adult is the combination of ventricular septal defect and pulmonary outflow tract obstruction (tetralogy of Fallot). The more severe the obstruction, the greater the degree of right-to-left shunting and resultant cyanosis. The mechanisms for the elevated pulmonary vascular resistance which may produce cyanosis in the presence of intra- and extracardiac communications without pulmonic stenosis (Eisenmenger syndrome) are discussed elsewhere (Chap. 199). In patients with patent ductus arteriosus, pulmonary hypertension, and right-to-left shunt, *differential cyanosis* results; i.e., cyanosis occurs in the lower but not in the upper extremities.

Pulmonary arteriovenous fistulas may be congenital or acquired, solitary or multiple, microscopic or massive. The degree of cyanosis produced by these fistulas depends on their size and number. They occur with some frequency in hereditary hemorrhagic telangiectasia. Arterial oxygen unsaturation also occurs in some patients with

cirrhosis, presumably as a consequence of pulmonary arteriovenous fistulas or portal vein–pulmonary vein anastomoses.

In patients with cardiac or pulmonary right-to-left shunts, the presence and severity of cyanosis depend on the size of the shunt relative to the systemic flow as well as on the oxyhemoglobin saturation of the venous blood. In patients with central cyanosis due to arterial oxygen unsaturation, the severity of cyanosis increases with exercise. With increased extraction of oxygen from the blood by the exercising muscles, the venous blood returning to the right side of the heart is more unsaturated than at rest, and shunting of this blood or its passage through lungs incapable of normal oxygenation intensifies the cyanosis. Also, since the systemic vascular resistance normally decreases with exercise, the right-to-left shunt is augmented by exercise in patients with congenital heart disease and communications between the two sides of the heart. Secondary polycythemia occurs frequently in patients with arterial unsaturation and contributes to the cyanosis.

Cyanosis can be caused by small amounts of circulating methemoglobin and by even smaller amounts of sulfhemoglobin (Chap. 306). Although they are uncommon causes of cyanosis, these abnormal hemoglobin pigments should be sought by spectroscopy when cyanosis is not readily explained by malfunction of the circulatory or respiratory systems. Generally, clubbing does not occur with them. The diagnosis of methemoglobinemia can be suspected, if, on mixing the patient's blood in a test tube and exposing it to air, it remains brown.

Peripheral cyanosis   Probably the most common cause of peripheral cyanosis is generalized vasoconstriction resulting from exposure to cold air or water. This is a normal response. When cardiac output is low, as in severe congestive heart failure or shock, cutaneous vasoconstriction occurs as a compensatory mechanism, so blood is diverted from the skin to more vital areas such as the central nervous system and heart (Chap. 195), and intense cyanosis associated with cool extremities may result. Even though the arterial blood is normally saturated, the reduced volume flow through the skin and the reduced oxygen tension at the venous end of the capillary result in cyanosis.

Arterial obstruction to an extremity, as with an embolus, or arteriolar constriction, as in cold-induced vasospasm (Raynaud's phenomenon; Chap. 211), generally results in pallor and coldness, but there may be associated cyanosis. If there is venous obstruction and the extremity is congested, as with stagnation of blood flow, cyanosis is also present. Venous hypertension, which may be local (as in thrombophlebitis) or generalized (as in tricuspid valve disease or constrictive pericarditis), dilates the subpapillary venous plexuses and thereby intensifies cyanosis.

APPROACH TO THE PATIENT WITH CYANOSIS   Certain features are important in arriving at the proper cause of cyanosis:

1 The history, particularly the duration (cyanosis present since birth is usually due to congenital heart disease), and possible exposure to drugs or chemicals which may produce abnormal types of hemoglobin.
2 Clinical differentiation of central as opposed to peripheral cyanosis. Objective evidence by physical or radiographic examination of disorders of the respiratory or cardiovascular systems. Massage or gentle warming of a cyanotic extremity will increase peripheral blood flow and abolish peripheral but not central cyanosis.
3 The presence or absence of clubbing of the fingers (see below). Clubbing without cyanosis is frequent in patients with infective endocarditis and in association with ulcerative colitis; it may occasionally occur in healthy persons, and in some instances it may be occupational, e.g., in jackhammer operators. Slight cyanosis of the lips and cheeks, without clubbing of the fingers, is common in patients with mitral stenosis and is probably due to minimal arterial hypoxia resulting from fibrotic changes in the lungs secondary to long-standing congestion combined with reduction of cardiac output (Chap. 201). The combination of cyanosis and clubbing is frequent in patients with certain types of congenital cardiac disease and is seen occasionally in persons with pulmonary

disease such as lung abscess or pulmonary arteriovenous shunts. On the other hand, peripheral cyanosis or acutely developing central cyanosis is not associated with clubbed fingers.

4 Determination of arterial blood oxygen tension or oxygen saturation, spectroscopic and other examinations of the blood for abnormal types of hemoglobin.

CLUBBING The selective bullous enlargement of the distal segments of the fingers and toes due to proliferation of connective tissue, particularly on the dorsal surface, is termed *clubbing*; an increase occurs in the sponginess of the soft tissue at the base of the nail. Clubbing may be hereditary, idiopathic, or acquired and associated with a variety of disorders, including cyanotic congenital heart disease, infective endocarditis, and a variety of pulmonary conditions (among them primary and metastatic lung cancer, bronchiectasis, lung abscess, cystic fibrosis, and mesothelioma), as well as with some gastrointestinal diseases (including regional enteritis, chronic ulcerative colitis, and hepatic cirrhosis). Clubbing in patients with primary and metastatic lung cancer, mesothelioma, bronchiectasis, and hepatic cirrhosis may be associated with *hypertrophic osteoarthropathy*. In this condition, the subperiosteal formation of new bone in the distal diaphyses of the long bones of the extremities causes pain and symmetric arthritis-like changes in the shoulders, knees, ankles, wrists, and elbows. The diagnosis of hypertrophic osteoarthropathy may be confirmed by bone radiographs and scans. Although the mechanism of clubbing is unclear, it appears to be secondary to a (presumably humoral) substance which causes dilation of the vessels of the fingertip.

REFERENCES

DOLL DC, GREENBERG BR: Cerebral thrombosis in smokers' polycythemia. Ann Intern Med 102:786, 1985

ERSLEV AJ: Erythrocytosis (Chaps 73–75), in *Hematology*, 4th ed, WJ Williams et al (eds). New York, McGraw-Hill, 1990, p 705

HANSEN-FLASCHEN J, NORDBERG J: Clubbing and hypertrophic osteoarthropathy. Clin Chest Med 8:287, 1987

HURTADO A: Some clinical aspects of life at high altitudes. Ann Intern Med 53:247, 1960

MURPHY S: Polycythemia vera. Dis Mon 38:165, 1992

SCHWARCZ TH et al: Thromboembolic complications of polycythemia: Polycythemia vera vs. smokers' polycythemia. J Vasc Surg 17:518, 1993

SMITH JR, LANDAW SA: Smokers' polycythemia. N Engl J Med 298:6, 1978

SZIDON JP, FISHMAN AP: Cyanosis and clubbing, in *Pulmonary Diseases and Disorders*, 2d ed, A Fishman (ed). Philadelphia, Saunders, 1988, p 351

TERRITO MC, ROSOVE MH: Cyanotic congenital heart disease: Hematologic management. J Am Coll Cardiol 18:320, 1991

33 EDEMA

EUGENE BRAUNWALD

Edema is defined as an increase in the interstitial fluid volume, which may expand by several liters before the abnormality is apparent clinically. Therefore, a weight gain of several kilograms usually precedes overt manifestations of edema, and a similar weight loss from diuresis can be induced in a slightly edematous patient before "dry weight" is achieved. *Ascites* (Chap. 43) and *hydrothorax* refer to accumulation of excess fluid in the peritoneal and pleural cavities, respectively, and are considered to be special forms of edema. *Anasarca* refers to gross, generalized edema.

Depending on its cause and mechanism, edema may be localized or have a generalized distribution; it is recognized in its generalized form by puffiness of the face, which is most readily apparent in the periorbital areas, and by the persistence of an indentation of the skin following pressure; this is known as "pitting" edema. In its more subtle form, it may be detected by noting that after the stethoscope

is removed from the chest wall, the rim of the bell leaves an indentation on chest skin for a few minutes. When the ring on a finger fits more snugly than in the past or when a patient complains of difficulty in putting on shoes, particularly in the evening, edema may be present.

PATHOGENESIS (See also Chap. 45) About one-third of the total-body water is confined to the extracellular space. This compartment, in turn, is composed of the plasma volume and the interstitial space. Normally the plasma volume represents about 25 percent of the extracellular space, and the remainder is interstitial fluid. The forces that regulate the disposition of fluid between these two components of the extracellular compartment are frequently referred to as the Starling forces (see p. 177). The hydrostatic pressure within the vascular system and the colloid oncotic pressure in the interstitial fluid tend to promote movement of fluid from the vascular to the extravascular space. In contrast, the colloid oncotic pressure contributed by the plasma proteins and the hydrostatic pressure within the interstitial fluid, referred to as the *tissue tension*, promote the movement of fluid into the vascular compartment. Consequently there is a movement of water and diffusible solutes from the vascular space at the arteriolar end of the capillaries. Fluid is returned from the interstitial space into the vascular system at the venous end of the capillary and by way of the lymphatics, and unless these channels are obstructed, lymph flow tends to increase if there is net movement of fluid from the vascular compartment to the interstitium. These forces are usually balanced so that a steady state exists in the sizes of the intravascular and interstitial compartments, and yet a large exchange between them is permitted. However, should any one of the hydrostatic or oncotic forces be altered significantly, a net movement of fluid from one component of the extracellular space to the other will occur.

An increase in capillary pressure as a cause of edema may result from an elevation of venous pressure due to local obstruction in venous drainage. This increase may be generalized as occurs in congestive heart failure, or rarely it may result from the simple expansion of the vascular volume by the administration of large volumes of fluid at a rate in excess of the ability of the kidneys to excrete them. The colloid oncotic pressure of the plasma may be reduced, owing to any factor that may induce severe hypoalbuminemia, such as malnutrition, liver disease, loss of protein into the urine or into the gastrointestinal tract, or a severe catabolic state.

Edema may also result from damage to the capillary endothelium, which increases its permeability and permits the transfer of protein into the interstitial compartment. Injury to the capillary wall can result from chemical or bacterial agents as well as from thermal or mechanical trauma. Increased capillary permeability may also be a consequence of a hypersensitivity reaction and is characteristic of immune injury. Damage to the capillary endothelium is presumably responsible for inflammatory edema, which is usually nonpitting, localized, and accompanied by other signs of inflammation—redness, heat, and tenderness.

To formulate a hypothesis about the pathophysiology of an edematous state, it is important to discriminate between the *primary* events, such as venous or lymphatic obstruction, reduction of cardiac output, hypoalbuminemia, trapping of fluid in spaces such as the peritoneal cavity, or an increase in capillary permeability, and the predictable *secondary* consequences, which include the renal retention of salt and water in an attempt to restore the plasma volume. Both the primary event and the secondary consequences may contribute to the formation of edema.

The development of edema depends on one or more alterations in the Starling forces so that there is a net movement of fluid from the vascular system into the interstitium or into a "third space" or from the arterial compartment of the vascular space into the chambers of the heart or into the venous circulation itself. In many forms of edema the *effective arterial blood volume*, an as yet poorly defined parameter of the filling of the arterial tree, is reduced, and as a consequence a series of physiologic responses designed to restore it to normal are

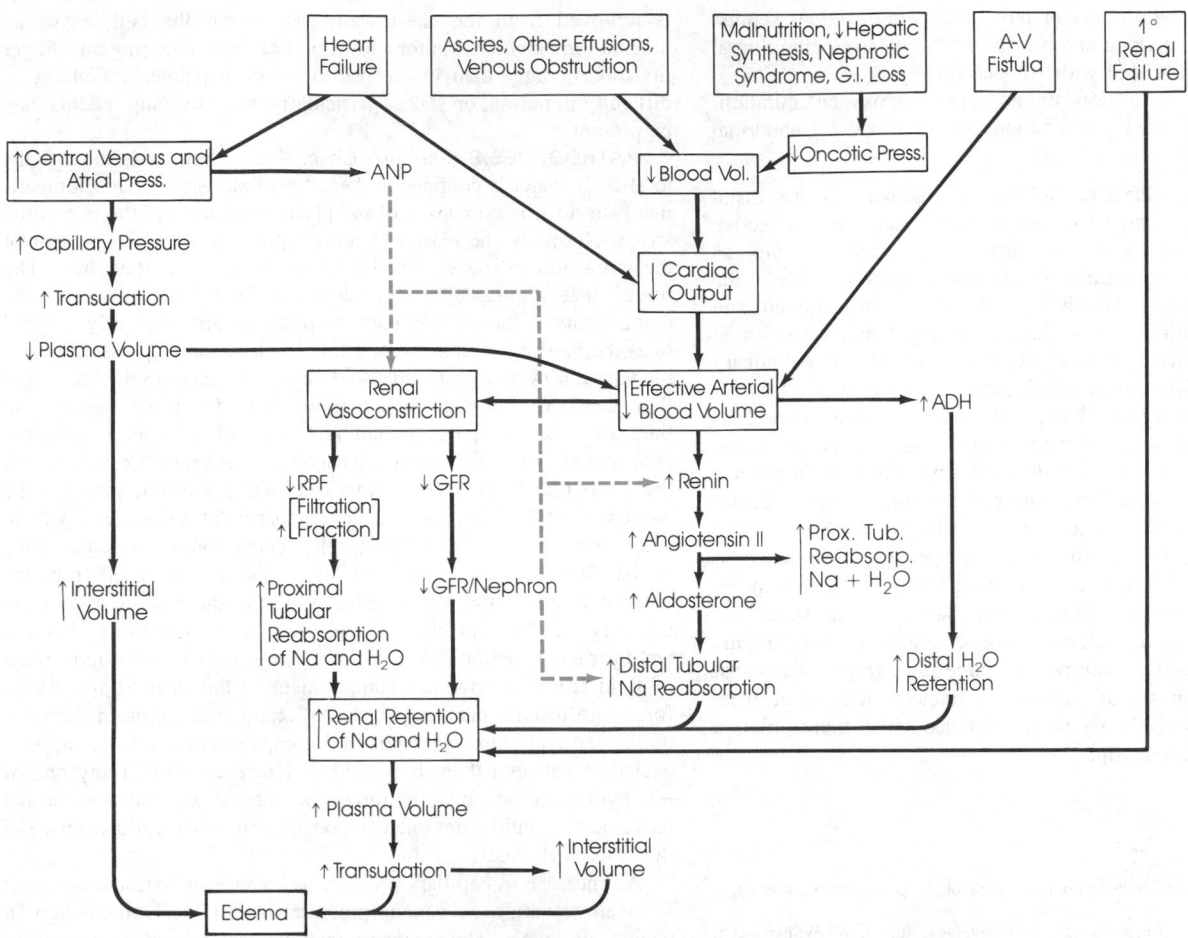

FIGURE 33-1 Sequence of events leading to the formation and retention of salt and water and the development of edema. ANP, atrial natriuretic peptide; RPF, renal plasma flow; GFR, glomerular filtration rate. Inhibitory influences are shown by colored dashed lines.

set into motion. A key element of these responses is the retention of an increment of salt and therefore of water, and in many instances this repairs the deficit of the effective arterial blood volume; often this occurs without the development of overt edema. If, however, the retention of salt and water is insufficient to restore and maintain the effective arterial blood volume, the stimuli are not dissipated, the retention of salt and water continues, and edema develops. This sequence of events is operative in dehydration and hemorrhage. Although in these conditions there is a reduction of effective arterial blood volume and activation of the entire sequence shown in the center of Fig. 33-1, including the diminished excretion of salt and water, edema does not occur because the net sodium and water balance is negative rather than positive. In most conditions that lead to edema the mechanisms responsible for maintaining a normal effective osmolality in the body fluids operate efficiently so that sodium retention promotes thirst and secretion of the antidiuretic hormone, which, in turn, lead to the ingestion and retention of approximately 1 L of water for each 140 mmol sodium retained. In edematous states, isotonic expansion of the extracellular fluid space may be massive, while the intracellular fluid volume is changed little or not at all.

Reduced cardiac output   A reduction of cardiac output, whatever the cause, is associated with a reduction of the effective arterial blood volume as well as of renal blood flow, constriction of the efferent renal arterioles, and an elevation of the filtration fraction, i.e., the ratio of glomerular filtration rate to renal plasma flow. In severe heart failure there is a reduction in the glomerular filtration rate. Activation of the sympathetic nervous system and of the renin-angiotensin systems are responsible for renal vasoconstriction. The finding that alpha-adrenergic blocking agents and/or angiotensin-converting enzyme inhibitors augment renal blood flow and induce diuresis

supports the role of these two systems in elevating renal vascular resistance and salt and water retention.

Renal factors   Reduced cardiac output lowers effective arterial blood volume. This increases the tubular reabsorption of glomerular filtrate which, in turn, plays a principal role in the salt and water retention of heart failure. There is evidence for both proximal and distal increases in sodium reabsorption in heart failure. Alterations in intrarenal hemodynamics appear to play a significant role. Heart failure, by augmenting renal arteriolar constriction, reduces the hydrostatic pressure and raises the colloid osmotic pressure in the peritubular capillaries, thus enhancing salt and water reabsorption in the proximal tubule. The reduction of renal perfusion pressure may be responsible for augmentation of sodium reabsorption in the ascending limb of the loop of Henle.

In addition, the diminished renal blood flow characteristic of states in which the effective arterial blood volume is reduced is translated by the renal juxtaglomerular cells into a signal for increased renin release (Chap. 335). The mechanisms responsible for this release include a baroreceptor response: reduced renal perfusion results in incomplete filling of the renal arterioles and diminished stretch of the juxtaglomerular cells, a signal that provides for the elaboration or release, or both, of renin. A second mechanism for renin release involves the macula densa; as a result of reduced glomerular filtration the sodium chloride load reaching the distal renal tubules is reduced. This is sensed by the macula densa, which in an undefined manner signals the neighboring juxtaglomerular cells to secrete renin. A third mechanism involves the sympathetic nervous system and circulating catecholamines. Activation of the beta-adrenergic receptors in the juxtaglomerular cells stimulates renin release. These three mechanisms generally act in concert.

The renin-angiotensin-aldosterone (RAA) system (See Chap. 335)   Renin, an enzyme with a molecular weight of about 40,000, acts on its substrate, angiotensinogen, an alpha$_2$ globulin synthesized by the liver, to release angiotensin I, a decapeptide, which is broken down to angiotensin II, an octapeptide. This has vasoconstrictor properties, especially on the efferent arterioles, and independently increases Na reabsorption in the proximal tubule. The intrarenal production of angiotensin II may also contribute to renal vasoconstriction and to the salt and water retention in heart failure. Angiotensin II also enters the circulation and stimulates the production of aldosterone by the zona glomerulosa of the adrenal cortex. In patients with heart failure, not only is aldosterone secretion elevated but the biologic half-life of aldosterone is prolonged, which further increases the plasma level of the hormone. A depression of hepatic blood flow, particularly during exercise, secondary to a reduction in cardiac output, is responsible for the reduced hepatic catabolism of aldosterone. The activation of the RAA system is most striking in the early phase of acute, severe heart failure and is less intense in patients with chronic, stable, compensated heart failure.

Although increased quantities of aldosterone are secreted in heart failure and in other edematous states and although blockade of the action of aldosterone by spironolactone often induces a moderate diuresis in edematous states, persistent augmented levels of aldosterone (or other mineralocorticoids) alone do not always promote accumulation of edema, as witnessed by the lack of striking fluid retention in most instances of primary aldosteronism (Chap. 335). Furthermore, although normal subjects retain some salt and water under the influence of a potent mineralocorticoid, such as deoxycorticosterone acetate or fludrocortisone, this accumulation is self-limiting, despite continued exposure to the steroid, a phenomenon known as mineralocorticoid escape. The failure of normal subjects receiving large doses of mineralocorticoids to accumulate large quantities of fluid and to develop edema is probably a consequence of an increase in glomerular filtration rate (pressure natriuresis) and through the action of natriuretic substance(s) (see below). The continued secretion of aldosterone may be more important in the accumulation of fluid in edematous states because patients with edema are generally unable to repair the deficit in effective arterial blood volume. As a consequence they do not develop pressure natriuresis nor do they elaborate normal quantities of atrial natriuretic peptide.

Blockade of the RAA system, by blocking angiotensin II receptors or inhibiting the angiotensin-converting enzyme (ACE) reduces efferent arterial resistance and increases renal blood flow. This action, combined with the rise in cardiac output secondary to afterload reduction as well as reduction in the secretion of aldosterone combine to cause diuresis. However, in patients with moderate or severe impairment of renal function interference with the RAA system can cause paradoxical sodium retention due to intensification of renal failure.

Atrial natriuretic peptide   Atrial distention and/or a sodium load cause release into the circulation of atrial natriuretic peptide (ANP), a polypeptide; a high-molecular-weight precursor of ANP is stored in secretory granules within atrial myocytes. Release of ANP causes (1) excretion of sodium and water by augmenting glomerular filtration rate, inhibiting sodium reabsorption in the proximal tubule, and inhibiting release of renin and aldosterone; and (2) arteriolar and venous dilatation. Thus, ANP has the capacity to oppose sodium retention and arterial pressure elevation in hypervolemic states.

There is also some evidence for the existence of a distinctly different natriuretic factor, a low-molecular-weight substance that is activated or released as a result of the expansion of the extracellular fluid and causes natriuresis by inhibiting renal sodium reabsorption through inhibiting ouabain-sensitive Na$^+$,K$^+$-ATPase. The roles of the latter factor and of ANP in normal and pathophysiologic conditions requires clarification. For example, it is not yet clear why patients with heart failure and hepatic cirrhosis have low rates of sodium excretion and edema despite often having high circulating levels of ANP, but it is likely that abnormal resistance of the end-organ, i.e.,

the renal tubule to ANP, plays a key role. This resistance to ANP in edematous states makes it unlikely that pharmacologic elevation of ANP will be very helpful in the management of edema.

Obstruction of venous (and lymphatic) drainage of a limb   In this condition the hydrostatic pressure in the capillary bed upstream to the obstruction increases so that more fluid than normal is transferred from the vascular to the interstitial space. Since the alternate route (i.e., the lymphatic channels) may also be obstructed, this event causes an increased volume of interstitial fluid in the limb, i.e., a trapping of fluid in the extremity, at the expense of the blood volume in the remainder of the body, thereby reducing effective arterial blood volume and leading to the consequences shown in Fig. 33-1.

As fluid accumulates in the interstitium of the limb in which venous and lymphatic drainage are obstructed, tissue tension rises until it counterbalances the primary alterations in the Starling forces, at which time no further fluid accumulates in that limb. When the additional accumulation of fluid has repaired the deficit in plasma volume the stimuli to retain more salt and water are dissipated. The net effect is a local increase in the volume of interstitial fluid, and the secondary responses repair the plasma volume deficit incurred by the primary event. This same sequence occurs in ascites and hydrothorax, in which fluid is trapped or accumulates in the cavitary space, depleting the intravascular volume and leading to secondary salt and fluid retention, as already described.

Congestive heart failure (See also Chap. 195)   In this disorder the defective systolic emptying of the chambers of the heart and/or the impairment of ventricular relaxation promotes an accumulation of blood in the heart and venous circulation at the expense of the arterial volume, and the aforementioned sequence of events (Fig. 33-1) is initiated. In mild heart failure, a small increment of total blood volume may repair the deficit of arterial volume and establish a new steady state because, through the operation of Starling's law of the heart, an increase in the volume of blood within the chambers of the heart promotes a more forceful contraction and may thereby increase the cardiac output (Fig. 195-1). However, if the cardiac disorder is more severe, retention of fluid cannot repair the deficit in effective arterial blood volume. The increment accumulates in the venous circulation, and the increase in capillary and lymphatic hydrostatic pressure promotes the formation of edema.

Incomplete ventricular emptying (systolic heart failure), and/or inadequate ventricular relaxation (diastolic heart failure), both lead to an elevation of ventricular diastolic pressure. If the impairment of cardiac function involves the right ventricle, pressures in the systemic veins and capillaries may rise, thereby augmenting the transudation of fluid into the interstitial space and enhancing the likelihood of peripheral edema. The elevated systemic venous pressure is transmitted to the thoracic duct with consequent reduction of lymph drainage, further increasing the accumulation of edema.

If the impairment of cardiac function (incomplete ventricular emptying and/or inadequate relaxation) involves the left ventricle, then pulmonary venous and capillary pressures rise [leading in some instances to pulmonary edema (Chap. 31)], as does pulmonary artery pressure; this in turn interferes with the systolic emptying of the right ventricle, leading to an elevation of right ventricular diastolic and of central and systemic venous pressures, enhancing the likelihood of formation of peripheral edema. Pulmonary edema impairs gas exchange and may induce hypoxia, which embarrasses cardiac function still further, sometimes causing a vicious cycle.

Nephrotic syndrome and other hypoalbuminic states (See also Chap. 240)   The primary alteration in this disorder is a diminished colloid oncotic pressure due to massive losses of protein into the urine. This promotes a net movement of fluid into the interstitium, causes hypovolemia, and initiates the edema-forming sequence of events described above, including activation of the RAA system. With severe hypoalbuminemia, the salt and water which are retained cannot be restrained within the vascular compartment, total and effective arterial blood volumes decline, and hence the stimuli to retain salt and water are not abated. A similar sequence of events occurs in other conditions which lead to *severe* hypoalbuminemia, including severe nutritional deficiency states, protein-losing enteropathy, congenital hypoalbuminemia, and severe, chronic liver disease. However, in the nephrotic syndrome, the impairment of renal function contributes to the retention of sodium.

Cirrhosis (See also Chaps. 43 and 268)   The *total* blood volume in hepatic cirrhosis is commonly increased when the disorder is accompanied by a system of dilated venous radicles and multiple small arteriovenous fistulas. On the other hand, tissue perfusion, the effective arterial blood volume, and the intrathoracic blood volume all are diminished, probably as a consequence of the passage of blood through these fistulas, as well as from the portal venous hypertension and the obstruction of the lymphatic drainage of the liver. Intrahepatic hypertension appears to be responsible for renal sodium retention. These alterations are frequently complicated by reduced serum albumin secondary to reduced hepatic synthesis, which reduces the effective arterial blood volume even further, leading to activation of the RAA system and other salt- and water-retaining mechanisms. The concentration of circulating aldosterone is elevated by the liver's failure to metabolize this hormone. Initially, the excess interstitial fluid is localized preferentially behind the congested portal venous system and obstructed hepatic lymphatics, i.e., in the peritoneal cavity. In later stages, particularly when there is severe hypoalbuminemia, peripheral edema may develop.

Idiopathic edema   This syndrome, which occurs almost exclusively in women, is characterized by periodic episodes of edema, frequently accompanied by abdominal distention. Fairly large, diurnal alterations in weight occur with orthostatic retention of sodium and water, so that the patient may weigh several pounds more after having been in the upright posture for several hours. Such large diurnal weight changes suggest an increase in capillary permeability which appears to fluctuate in severity and to be aggravated by hot weather. There is some evidence that a reduction in plasma volume occurs in this condition with secondary activation of the RAA system. Idiopathic edema should be distinguished from cyclical or premenstrual edema in which the sodium and water retention may be secondary to excessive estrogen stimulation. There are also some cases in which the edema appears to be "diuretic-induced." It has been postulated that in these patients, chronic diuretic administration leads to mild blood volume depletion which causes chronic hyperreninemia and juxtaglomerular hyperplasia. Salt-retaining mechanisms appear to overcompensate for the direct effects of the diuretics. *Acute* withdrawal of diuretics can then leave the sodium-retaining forces unopposed, leading to fluid retention and edema.

The treatment of idiopathic cyclic edema includes a reduction in salt intake, rest in the supine position for several hours each day, the wearing of elastic stockings which are put on before arising in the morning, and an attempt to understand any underlying emotional problems. A variety of pharmacologic agents including ACE inhibitors, progesterone, the dopamine receptor agonist bromocriptine, and the sympathomimetic amine dextroamphetamine have all been reported in observational studies to be useful when administered to patients who do not respond to simpler measures. Diuretics may be initially useful but may lose their effectiveness with continuous administration; accordingly, they should be employed sparingly, if at all. Persistent discontinuation of diuretics paradoxically leads to diuresis in "diuretic-induced" edema, described above.

DIFFERENTIAL DIAGNOSIS   As a rule, localized edema can be readily differentiated from generalized edema. The great majority of patients with generalized edema suffer from advanced cardiac, renal, hepatic, or nutritional disorders. Consequently, the differential diagnosis of generalized edema should be directed toward identifying or excluding these several conditions.

Localized edema (See also Chap. 211)   Edema originating from inflammation or hypersensitivity is usually readily identified. Localized edema due to venous or lymphatic obstruction may be caused by thrombophlebitis, chronic lymphangitis, resection of regional lymph nodes, filariasis, etc. Lymphedema is particularly intractable

because restriction of lymphatic flow results in increased protein concentration in the interstitial fluid, a circumstance which aggravates retention of fluid.

Edema of heart failure   Evidence of heart disease, as manifested by cardiac enlargement and gallop rhythm, together with evidence of cardiac failure, such as dyspnea, basilar rales, venous distention, and hepatomegaly, usually provides an indication on clinical examination that edema results from heart failure. Noninvasive tests such as echocardiography and radionuclide angiography may be helpful in establishing the diagnosis of heart failure (see also Chaps. 190 and 195).

Edema of the nephrotic syndrome   Marked proteinuria (>3.5 g/d), severe hypoalbuminemia (<2 g/dL), and in some instances hypercholesterolemia are present. This syndrome may occur during the course of a variety of kidney diseases, which include glomerulonephritis, diabetic glomerulosclerosis, and hypersensitivity reactions. A history of previous renal disease may or may not be elicited (see also Chap. 240).

Edema of acute glomerulonephritis and other forms of renal failure   The edema occurring during the acute phases of glomerulonephritis is characteristically associated with hematuria, proteinuria, and hypertension. Although some evidence supports the view that the fluid retention is due to increased capillary permeability, in most instances the edema in this disease results from primary retention of sodium and water by the kidneys owing to renal insufficiency. This state differs from congestive heart failure in that it is characterized by a normal or increased cardiac output and a normal arterial–mixed venous oxygen difference. Patients with edema due to renal failure commonly have evidence of pulmonary congestion on chest roentgenograms before cardiac enlargement is significant, but they usually do not develop orthopnea. Patients with chronic impairment of renal function (including some patients with the nephrotic syndrome *without* severe hypoalbuminemia) may also develop edema due to primary renal retention of sodium and water.

Edema of cirrhosis (Chap. 268)   Ascites and biochemical and clinical evidence of hepatic disease (collateral venous channels, jaundice, and spider angiomas) characterize edema of hepatic origin. The ascites is frequently refractory to treatment because it collects as a result of a combination of obstruction of hepatic lymphatic drainage, portal hypertension, and hypoalbuminemia. Edema may also occur in other parts of the body in these patients as a result of hypoalbuminemia. Furthermore, the sizable accumulation of ascitic fluid may increase intraabdominal pressure and impede venous return from the lower extremities; hence, it tends to promote accumulation of edema in this region as well.

Edema of nutritional origin   A grossly deficient diet over a prolonged period may produce hypoproteinemia and edema. The latter may be intensified by the development of beriberi heart disease, also of nutritional origin, in which multiple peripheral arteriovenous fistulas result in reduced effective systemic perfusion and effective arterial blood volume, thereby enhancing edema formation (Chap. 207). Edema may actually become intensified when these famished subjects are first provided with an adequate diet. The ingestion of more food may increase the quantity of salt ingested, which is then retained along with water. Refeeding edema may also be linked to increased release of insulin, which directly increases tubular sodium reabsorption. In addition to hypoalbuminemia, hypokalemia and caloric deficits may be involved in the edema of starvation.

Other causes of edema   These include hypothyroidism, in which the edema (myxedema) may be located typically in the pretibial region and which may also be associated with periorbital puffiness. Exogenous hyperadrenocortism, pregnancy, and administration of estrogens and vasodilators, particularly the calcium antagonist nifedipine, may also all cause edema.

Distribution   The distribution of edema is an important guide to the cause. Thus, edema of one leg or of one or both arms is usually the result of venous and/or lymphatic obstruction. Edema resulting from hypoproteinemia characteristically is generalized, but it is especially evident in the very soft tissues of the eyelids and face and tends to be most pronounced in the morning because of the recumbent posture assumed during the night. Less common causes of facial edema include trichinosis, allergic reactions, and myxedema. Edema associated with heart failure, on the other hand, tends to be more extensive in the legs and to be accentuated in the evening, a feature also determined largely by posture. When patients with heart failure have been confined to bed, edema may be most prominent in the presacral region. Unilateral edema occasionally results from lesions in the central nervous system affecting the vasomotor fibers on one side of the body; paralysis also reduces lymphatic and venous drainage on the affected side.

Additional factors in diagnosis The color, thickness, and sensitivity of the skin are significant. Local tenderness and increase in temperature suggest inflammation. Local cyanosis may signify a venous obstruction. In individuals who have had repeated episodes of prolonged edema, the skin over the involved areas may be thickened, indurated, and often red.

Measurement or estimation of the venous pressure is of importance in evaluating edema. Elevation in an isolated part of the body usually reflects localized venous obstruction. Generalized elevation of systemic venous pressure usually indicates the presence of congestive heart failure. Ordinarily, significant increase in venous pressure can be recognized by the level at which cervical veins collapse (Chap. 188); in doubtful cases and for accurate recording, the central venous pressure should be measured manometrically. In patients with obstruction of the superior vena cava, edema is confined to the face, neck, and upper extremities, where the venous pressure is elevated compared with that in the lower extremities. Measurement of venous pressure in the upper extremities is also useful in patients with massive edema of the lower extremities and ascites; it is elevated when the edema is on a cardiac basis (e.g., constrictive pericarditis or tricuspid stenosis) but is normal when it is secondary to cirrhosis. Severe heart failure may cause ascites that may be distinguished from the ascites caused by hepatic cirrhosis by the jugular venous pressure, which usually is elevated in heart failure and normal in cirrhosis.

Determination of the concentration of serum albumin aids importantly in identifying those patients in whom edema is due, at least in part, to diminished intravascular colloid oncotic pressure. The presence of proteinuria also affords useful clues. The total absence of protein in the urine is evidence against renal disease as a cause of edema. Slight to moderate proteinuria is the rule in patients with heart failure, whereas persistent massive proteinuria is characteristic of the nephrotic syndrome.

APPROACH TO THE PATIENT WITH EDEMA An important first question is whether the edema is localized or generalized. If it is localized, those phenomena that may be responsible should be concentrated upon. Localized edema includes hydrothorax, ascites, or both. Either may be a consequence of local venous or lymphatic obstruction, as in inflammatory disease or carcinoma.

If the edema is generalized, it should be determined, first, if there is hypoalbuminemia of significant degree, e.g., serum albumin concentration less than 2.5 g/dL. If there is, the history, physical examination, urinalysis, and other laboratory data will help evaluate the question of cirrhosis, severe malnutrition, protein-losing gastroenteropathy, or the nephrotic syndrome as the underlying disorder. If hypoalbuminemia is not present, it should be determined if there is evidence of congestive heart failure of a severity to promote generalized edema. Finally, it should be determined whether the patient has an adequate urine output, or if there is significant oliguria or even anuria. These abnormalities are discussed in Chaps. 44, 236, and 237.

REFERENCES

CODY RJ et al: Regulation of glomerular filtration rate in chronic congestive heart failure patients. Kidney Int 34:361, 1988

EDWARDS BS et al: Identification of atrial natriuretic factor within the tissue in hamsters and humans with congestive heart failure. J Clin Invest 81:82, 1988

GOLDEN MHN: Protein deficiency, energy deficiency, and the oedema of malnutrition. Lancet 1:1261, 1982

KELSCH RC, SEDMAN AB: Nephrotic syndrome. Pediatr Rev 14:30, 1993

MOE GW et al: Control of extracellular fluid volume and pathophysiology of edema formation, in *The Kidney*, 4th ed, BM Brenner, FC Rector Jr (eds). Philadelphia, Saunders, 1991, pp 623–676

MOORE J JR, CAROME MA: Proteinuria. Clin Lab Med 13:21, 1993

PACKER M: Neurohormonal interactions and adaptations in congestive heart failure. Circulation 77:721, 1988

ROSE BD: Edematous states, in *Clinical Physiology of Acid-Base and Electrolyte Disorders*. New York, McGraw-Hill, 1989, pp 416–463

SCHRIER RW: Pathogenesis of sodium and water retention in high-output and low-output cardiac failure, nephrotic syndrome, cirrhosis, and pregnancy. Part I. N Engl J Med 319:1065, 1988

STAUB NB, TAYLOR AE (eds): *Edema*. New York, Raven Press, 1984

STREETEN DHP: Idiopathic edema: Pathogenesis, clinical features, and treatment. Metabolism 27:353, 1978

34 SHOCK

JOSEPH E. PARRILLO

Shock may be defined as the state in which profound and widespread reduction in the effective delivery of oxygen and other nutrients to tissues leads first to reversible and then, if prolonged, to irreversible cellular injury.

CONTROL OF ARTERIAL BLOOD PRESSURE Maintenance of adequate perfusion of vital organs is critical for survival. Organ perfusion is dependent on an appropriate perfusion pressure, which, in turn, is determined by two variables, the cardiac output and the systemic vascular resistance. The latter is proportional to the vessel length and the viscosity of blood and inversely proportional to the fourth power of the vessel radius. Therefore, the cross-sectional area of a vessel is by far the most important determinant of the resistance to blood flow. Since vascular smooth-muscle tone regulates the cross-sectional area of the arteriolar bed (the major site of systemic resistance in the vascular tree), any variable that affects smooth-muscle tone has a profound effect on vascular resistance and, in turn, on perfusion pressure.

The second critical determinant of arterial pressure is the cardiac output, which itself is the product of stroke volume and heart rate. The stroke volume is a function of three major variables, as discussed in Chap. 194: (1) preload, generally reflected in the ventricular end-diastolic volume, (2) impedance to blood flow (afterload), which is related to the systemic vascular resistance, and (3) myocardial contractility.

Physiologic mechanisms can affect the arterial pressure by acting on one or more of the variables mentioned above. These mechanisms include the local release of vasodilator metabolites such as adenosine; the release from the endothelium of substances that relax (e.g., endothelium-derived relaxing factor, nitric oxide) or contract (e.g., endothelin) subjacent vascular smooth muscle; the activity of the autonomic (sympathetic and parasympathetic) nervous system and the modulation of this activity by baroreceptor reflexes and the vasomotor center in the brainstem, which, in turn, is acted on by higher centers in the nervous system; the release into the bloodstream of the catecholamines epinephrine or norepinephrine by the adrenal medulla and sympathetic nerve endings (Chap. 68); the activity of the renin-angiotensin system (Chap. 335); the release of vasopressin (Chap. 333); the release of vasodilators, including the kinins and prostaglandins; and alterations in intravascular volume via control of fluid and electrolyte balance (Chap. 33). All these mechanisms can affect the arterial pressure by altering the vascular resistance and/or cardiac output. Through the integrated operation of these several mechanisms, the mean arterial pressure (the average pressure throughout the cardiac

TABLE 34-1   Classification of forms of shock

CARDIOGENIC SHOCK

Myopathic (reduced systolic function)
   Acute myocardial infarction
   Dilated cardiomyopathy
   Myocardial depression in septic shock
Mechanical
   Mitral regurgitation
   Ventricular septal defect
   Ventricular aneurysm
   LV outflow obstruction (aortic stenosis, idiopathic hypertrophic subaortic
    stenosis)
Arrhythmic

EXTRACARDIAC OBSTRUCTIVE SHOCK

Pericardial tamponade
Constrictive pericarditis
Pulmonary embolism (massive)
Severe pulmonary hypertension (primary or Eisenmenger)
Coarctation of the aorta

OLIGEMIC SHOCK

Hemorrhage
Fluid depletion

DISTRIBUTIVE SHOCK

Septic shock
Toxic products, e.g., overdose
Anaphylaxis
Neurogenic shock
Endocrinologic shock

SOURCE: Adapted with permission from Parker and Parrillo.

cycle) in resting, young, healthy adults is maintained within a relatively narrow range of 90 to 100 mmHg.

CLASSIFICATION OF SHOCK   A classification of shock based on cause is shown in Table 34-1.

Oligemic or hypovolemic shock   Hemorrhage or a large loss of fluid secondary to vomiting, diarrhea, burns, or dehydration leads to inadequate ventricular filling, i.e., to severely decreased preload, reflected in decreased left and right ventricular end-diastolic volumes and pressures. These changes lead to shock by causing an inadequate stroke volume and inadequate cardiac output. This is probably the most frequent cause of shock and also the best studied, because all gradations of oligemic shock can be produced in animal models.

Cardiogenic shock (See Chap. 202)   This is due to a severe depression of systolic cardiac performance. Systolic arterial pressure is < 80 mmHg, the cardiac index is reduced below 1.8 L/min/m^2, and the left ventricular filling pressure is elevated, generally above 18 mmHg; pulmonary edema may or may not be evident. The patient is frequently obtunded, the urine output is less than 20 mL/h, and the extremities are cold and cyanotic. The most frequent cause is infarction involving 40 percent or more of the left ventricular myocardium, leading to a severe reduction in left ventricular contractility and failure of the left ventricular pump. Other causes include acute myocarditis and the depression of myocardial contractility following cardiac arrest and prolonged cardiac surgery.

Another form of cardiogenic shock is caused by mechanical abnormalities of the ventricle. Acute mitral or aortic regurgitation or acutely acquired ventricular septal defect or ventricular aneurysm, usually caused by acute myocardial infarction, can cause a severe reduction in *forward* cardiac output (blood flow throughout the aortic valve into the systemic arterial circulation) and thereby result in cardiogenic shock.

Extracardiac obstructive shock   This form of shock is best exemplified by pericardial tamponade (Chap. 206). Physiologically, the major abnormality is the inability of the ventricle to fill during diastole, markedly limiting the stroke volume and ultimately the

cardiac output. Another cause of extracardiac obstructive shock is massive pulmonary embolism (Chap. 226). Although the mechanism responsible for the reduced cardiac output in extracardiac obstructive shock differs from that in cardiogenic shock, the actual cause of shock, i.e., the severe reduction in tissue perfusion, is similar.

Distributive shock   Examples of this form of shock are septic shock (Chap. 83), neurogenic shock, and anaphylactic shock (Chap. 282), all of which usually cause a profound decrease in peripheral vascular resistance; the first is now the most common cause of death in intensive care units in the United States. The pathogenesis of septic shock involves abnormalities of both the peripheral vascular system and the heart. It is considered in detail below.

Patients may suffer from more than one form of shock simultaneously. Thus septic and oligemic shock sometimes coexist. These two forms of shock may produce dissimilar, even opposing cardiovascular effects, and treatment of one form may unmask the presence of the other.

PATHOGENESIS   Some characteristics of the pathogenesis of shock are the same regardless of the underlying cause. The final pathway of shock is cell death. Once large numbers of cells from vital organs have reached this stage, shock becomes irreversible, and death occurs despite correction of the underlying cause. This concept of irreversibility is useful because it emphasizes the need to prevent the progression of shock.

The pathogenetic mechanism leading to cell death is incompletely understood. One of the common denominators of the first three forms of shock listed in Table 34-1 is a low cardiac output (see Fig. 34-1). Patients with oligemic shock, cardiogenic shock, and extracardiac obstructive shock and a minority of patients with distributive shock develop a severe decrease in cardiac output and hence in perfusion of vital organs. Initially, compensatory mechanisms such as vasoconstriction may maintain arterial pressure at near-normal level. However, if the process causing shock continues, these compensatory mechanisms ultimately fail, leading to the clinical manifestations of the shock syndrome. If shock persists, cell death will ensue and result in irreversible shock.

Of the forms of shock with low cardiac output, *oligemic shock* has been studied the most carefully, both in humans and in animal models, and it provides lessons applicable to other forms of low-output shock. A healthy adult can compensate for the sudden loss of 10 percent of total blood volume using the mechanisms described previously, principally sympathetically mediated vasoconstriction. However, if 20 to 25 percent of the blood volume is lost rapidly, the compensatory mechanisms usually begin to fail, and the clinical shock syndrome ensues. The cardiac output declines, and there is hypotension despite generalized vasoconstriction. Regulation of local blood flow maintains perfusion of the heart and brain until late in the course, when these mechanisms also fail. Vasoconstriction, which begins as a compensatory mechanism in shock, may become excessive in some tissues and cause destructive lesions such as ischemic necrosis of the intestines or digits. A myocardial depressant factor has been identified in the dog with hemorrhagic shock, but this factor has not been clearly related to clinical myocardial dysfunction. Ultimately, if shock continues, end-organ damage occurs, precipitating the adult respiratory distress syndrome (Chap. 230), acute renal failure (Chap. 236), disseminated intravascular coagulation (Chap. 316), and multiorgan failure leading to death.

Distributive shock has a different and more complicated pathogenesis. Septic shock (Chap. 83) is characterized, at least initially, by a low systemic vascular resistance and an elevated cardiac output. As shown in Fig. 34-2, septic shock usually begins with a nidus of infection that releases microbes and/or one or more mediators into the bloodstream. Many mediators [e.g., histamine, kinins, most prostaglandins, lipid A (the toxic component of endotoxin), endorphins, tumor necrosis factor, interleukin 1, and interleukin 2] produce vascular dilatation, while others (e.g., some prostaglandins and leukotrienes) produce vasoconstriction. The peripheral vasodilatation results in a reduced systemic vascular resistance and a high cardiac

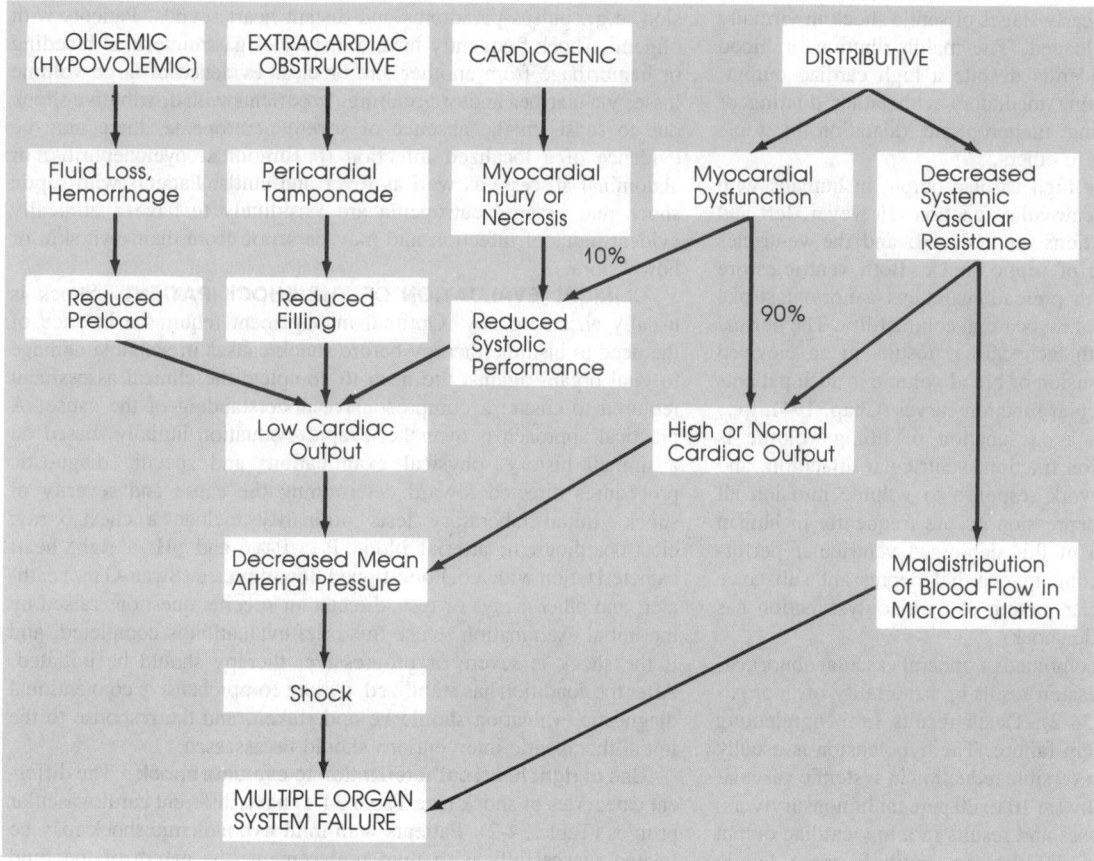

FIGURE 34-1 Pathogenesis of shock in humans. This schematic diagram depicts the present understanding of the pathogenetic relationships among the different types of shock and the cardiovascular abnormalities they usually produce.

FIGURE 34-2 Pathogenesis of human septic shock. This schematic diagram represents the present understanding of the interrelationships in the pathogenesis of septic shock in humans. (*From Parrillo et al, 1990.*)

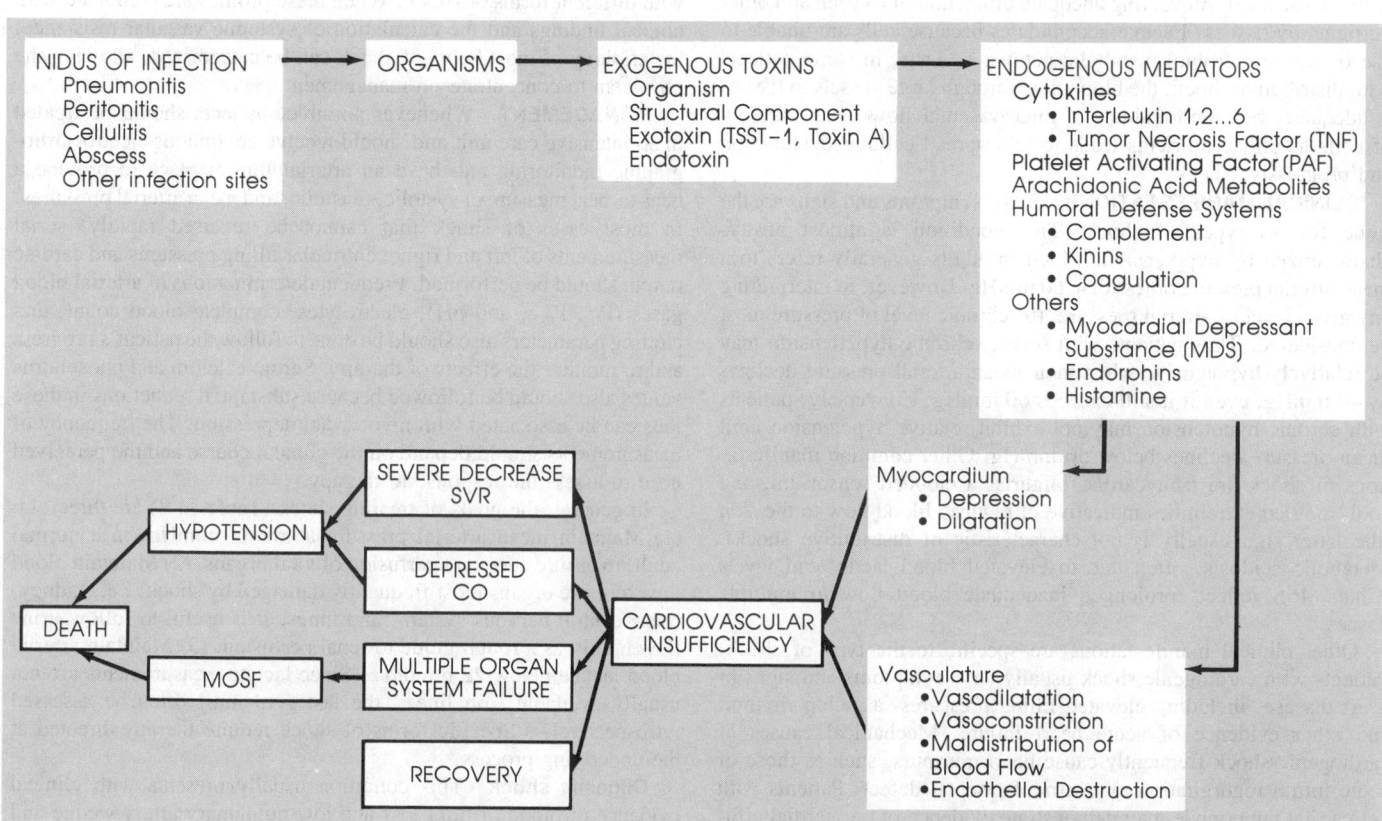

output; the latter occurs in the early stages of septic shock in virtually all patients who are volume-loaded. The maldistribution of blood flow, evidenced by lactic acidemia despite a high cardiac output, probably results from circulating mediators with either dilating or constricting properties, causing inappropriate dilatation in some vascular beds and constriction in others.

It has been argued that the high cardiac output in humans with septic shock indicates good ventricular function. However, left and right ventricular ejection fractions are reduced, and the ventricles dilate during the initial phase of septic shock. Both ventricles are usually dilated; the increase in preload maintains a normal stroke volume despite the depression of myocardial contractility. The normal stroke volume, combined with tachycardia, results in an elevated cardiac output. However, expansion of blood volume in such patients demonstrates depressed ventricular function curves (Chap. 194), i.e., the response of stroke work as a function of filling volume is subnormal. The reduced ejection fraction, ventricular dilatation, and decreased ventricular stroke work response to volume infusion all demonstrate that myocardial depression occurs frequently in human septic shock. The mechanism of this depressed ventricular performance is unknown; a circulating myocardial depressant substance probably plays a role. A similar pattern of cardiac dysfunction has been reported with anaphylactic shock.

If septic shock persists, the combined peripheral vascular abnormalities and the myocardial depression result in a mortality of approximately 50 percent (see Fig. 34-2). Death results from unrelenting hypotension and/or organ system failure. The hypotension is usually associated with a severe and irreversible reduction in systemic vascular resistance, although occasionally (in 10 to 20 percent of nonsurvivors) myocardial depression progresses and results in a low cardiac output that worsens the hypotension. Death from multiple-organ failure usually results from insufficiency of kidney, liver, brain, or lung function.

Other pathogenetic mechanisms in septic shock appear to relate to neutrophil aggregation, which produces microthrombi and endothelial cell injury; the latter, in turn, contribute to alterations in microvascular perfusion. In some forms of distributive shock, tissue blood flow appears adequate, but a mediator-induced "metabolic block" exists at the tissue level, preventing adequate utilization of oxygen and other nutrients by tissues. Lactate accumulates because cells are unable to use oxidative (aerobic) metabolic pathways. Thus, in some patients with distributive shock, the blood flow through large vessels to tissues is adequate, but abnormalities of microvascular flow or an inability of cells to utilize nutrients leads to widespread cellular dysfunction and progressive shock.

CLINICAL MANIFESTATIONS   Some symptoms and signs are the same for all types of shock. This condition is almost always characterized by hypotension, which in adults generally refers to a mean arterial pressure of less than 60 mmHg. However, in interpreting any given level of arterial pressure, the chronic level of pressure must be considered. Thus patients with severe, chronic hypertension may be relatively hypotensive when their mean arterial pressure declines by 40 mmHg, even if it still exceeds 60 mmHg. Conversely, patients with chronic hypotension may not exhibit relative hypotension until mean pressure declines below 50 mmHg. Other common manifestations of shock are tachycardia, oliguria, a clouded sensorium, and cool, mottled extremities indicative of reduced blood flow to the skin (the latter sign usually is not characteristic of distributive shock). Metabolic acidosis, often due to elevated blood lactic acid levels (Chap. 46), reflects prolonged inadequate blood flow to multiple tissues.

Other clinical manifestations are specific to the type of shock. Patients with cardiogenic shock usually have symptoms and signs of heart disease, including elevated filling pressures, a gallop rhythm, and other evidence of acute heart failure. Mechanical causes of cardiogenic shock frequently cause heart murmurs, such as those of acute mitral regurgitation or ventricular septal defect. Patients with pericardial tamponade may demonstrate evidence of pericardial effu-

sion, e.g., pulsus paradoxus and distant heart sounds. Patients with oligemic shock frequently have a history of gastrointestinal bleeding or hemorrhage from another site or clear evidence of large volume losses via diarrhea and/or vomiting. In patients with distributive shock due to sepsis in the absence of severe neutropenia, there may be evidence of a localized infection (pneumonitis, pyelonephritis, or abdominal abscess) as well as fever and chills. Patients with septic shock and severe neutropenia are less likely to have a clinically evident nidus of infection and may be septic from their own skin or bowel flora.

CLINICAL EVALUATION OF THE SHOCK PATIENT   Shock is usually an emergency. Optimal management requires a balance of the need to institute therapy before shock causes irreversible damage to vital organs against the need to complete the clinical assessment required to ensure a comprehensive understanding of the cause. A practical approach is to make a rapid evaluation initially, based on a limited history, physical examination, and specific diagnostic procedures directed toward determining the cause and severity of shock. Initial laboratory tests ordinarily include a chest x-ray; electrocardiogram; arterial blood P_{O_2}, P_{CO_2}, and pH; a right heart catheterization with a balloon-tipped flow-directed (Swan-Ganz) catheter; and other x-rays or tests directed at specific questions raised by the initial examination. Once this brief evaluation is completed, and if the shock is severe or progressive, therapy should be initiated. After the condition has stabilized, a more comprehensive conventional diagnostic evaluation should be undertaken, and the response to the initial therapeutic interventions should be assessed.

Use of right heart catheterization to evaluate shock   The different categories of shock (see Table 34-1) have different cardiovascular profiles (Table 34-2). Patients with mild hypovolemic shock may be treated successfully with fluid replacement, the nature of the fluid depending on the cause of the shock. However, in patients with moderate or severe shock, the flow-directed balloon-tipped pulmonary artery (Swan-Ganz) catheter is often useful for providing hemodynamic assessment and following the response to therapy, because clinical evaluation is frequently incorrect in estimating filling pressure and cardiac output.

Table 34-2 summarizes the usual hemodynamic profiles of patients with different forms of shock. When these profiles are combined with clinical findings and the calculation of systemic vascular resistance, the etiology of most bouts of shock can be categorized, allowing the physician to concentrate on management.

MANAGEMENT   Whenever possible, patients should be treated in an intensive care unit and should receive continuous electrocardiographic monitoring and have an arterial line in place to provide a beat-to-beat measure of systolic, diastolic, and mean arterial pressures. In most cases of shock that cannot be reversed rapidly, serial measurements of left and right ventricular filling pressures and cardiac output should be performed. Frequent determinations of arterial blood gases (P_{O_2}, P_{CO_2}, and pH), electrolytes, complete blood count, and clotting parameters also should be done to follow the patient's progress and to monitor the effects of therapy. Serum calcium and phosphorus values also should be followed because substantial reductions in these ions can be associated with myocardial depression. The frequency of measurements should depend on the clinical course and the perceived need to assess the response to therapy.

In general, the goals of treating shock (Table 34-3) are threefold: (1) Maintain mean arterial pressure above 60 mmHg (in a normal adult) to ensure adequate perfusion of vital organs. (2) Maintain blood flow to those organs most frequently damaged by shock, i.e., kidney, liver, central nervous system, and lungs. It is useful to follow urine flow hourly as a rough guide to renal perfusion. (3) Maintain arterial blood lactate below 22 mmol/L. (Since lactate measurements are not usually available "on line," the last goal must often be assessed retrospectively.) Specific forms of shock require therapy directed at the underlying process.

Oligemic shock   This condition usually presents with clinical evidence of blood or fluid loss and low pulmonary artery wedge and

---

TABLE 34-2   Use of right heart catheterization to diagnose the etiology of shock*

Diagnosis	Pulmonary capillary wedge pressure[†]	Cardiac output (CO)	Miscellaneous comments
Cardiogenic shock			
Cardiogenic shock due to myocardial dysfunction	↑ ↑	↓ ↓	Usually occurs with evidence of extensive myocardial infarction (>40% of left ventricular myocardium destroyed), severe cardiomyopathy, or myocarditis
Cardiogenic shock due to a mechanical defect			
Acute ventricular septal defect	↑ or nl	LVCO ↓ ↓ and RVCO > CO	If shunt is left to right, pulmonary blood flow is greater than systemic blood flow: oxygen saturation "step-up" occurs at right ventricular level
Acute mitral regurgitation	↑ ↑	Forward CO ↓ ↓	V waves in pulmonary capillary wedge pressure tracing
Right ventricular infarction	nl or ↓	↓ ↓	Elevated right atrial and right ventricular filling pressures with low or normal pulmonary capillary wedge pressures
Extracardiac obstructive forms of shock			
Pericardial tamponade	↑ ↑	↓ or ↓ ↓	Dip and plateau tracing in right and left ventricles. The right atrial mean, right ventricular end-diastolic, pulmonary artery end-diastolic, and pulmonary capillary wedge mean pressures are within 5 mmHg of one another
Massive pulmonary emboli	nl or ↓	↓ ↓	Usual finding is elevated heart pressure and with normal or low pulmonary capillary wedge
Oligemic shock (hypovolemia)	↓ ↓	↓ ↓	
Distributive forms of shock			
Septic shock	↓ or nl	↑ ↑ or nl, rarely ↓	
Anaphylactic shock	↓ or nl	↑ or nl	

* The hemodynamic profiles summarized in this table refer to patients with the diagnosis listed in the left column who are also in shock (MAP <60 mmHg).
† ↑ ↑ or ↓ ↓ designates a moderate-to-severe increase or decrease; ↑ or ↓ designates a mild-to-moderate increase or decrease; nl = normal; LV = left ventricular; RV = right ventricular.
NOTE: Systemic vascular resistance is increased, initially, in all forms of shock except distributive shock, in which it is usually reduced.
SOURCE: Modified from JE Parrillo, in *Major Issues in Critical Care Medicine*, JE Parrillo, SM Ayres (eds), Baltimore, William & Wilkins, 1984.

---

right atrial pressures. Rapid infusion of blood plasma or plasma expanders is the correct therapy while the source of blood or fluid loss is identified and corrected.

Cardiogenic shock   When it is due to myocardial infarction, after mechanical causes have been excluded (see Tables 34-1 and 34-2 and Chap. 202), therapy should be directed toward reducing ischemia and salvaging severely ischemic but reversibly damaged

---

TABLE 34-3   Guidelines for managing shock

Parameter	Therapeutic goal
Hemodynamic	
Mean arterial pressure	At least 60 mmHg
Pulmonary capillary wedge pressure	Between 14 and 18 mmHg
Oxygen delivery	
Hemoglobin	Above 10 g/dL
Oxygen saturation	Above 92%
Cardiac index	Nonseptic shock: above 2.2 L/min/m²
	Septic shock: above 4.0 L/min/m²
Organ system function	
Renal—blood urea nitrogen and creatinine levels, urinary output	Normalize values or otherwise reverse evidence of dysfunction
Hepatic—bilirubin level	
Pulmonary—alveolar-arterial gradient	
Cardiovascular—mean arterial pressure, cardiac index	
Central nervous system—mental status	
Blood lactate level	Normalization

SOURCE: Adapted from Dixon AC, Parrillo JE, in *The Principles and Practice of Medical Intensive Care*, Carlson RW, Geheb MA (eds), Philadelphia, Saunders, 1992.

---

myocardium at the infarct border. This may be accomplished by administration of oxygen and nitrates, institution of intraaortic balloon pumping to unload the ventricle mechanically and augment coronary perfusion, and, perhaps most important, attempts to restore myocardial perfusion to salvage nonirreversibly damaged myocardium. Depending on the specific situation, the latter may include the administration of thrombolytic agents, cardiac catheterization and coronary arteriography to define coronary anatomy, and early coronary angioplasty or coronary bypass surgery in patients with appropriate anatomy. This aggressive approach may reduce the mortality of cardiogenic shock from approximately 90 percent to around 60 percent. Prospective, randomized studies are needed to document the true efficacy of this approach. Cardiogenic shock also occurs after a prolonged period of induced cardiac arrest, often during reparative cardiac surgery. The impaired (stunned) myocardium may require hours or days to recover sufficiently to support the circulation. Treatment consists of the combination of intraaortic balloon counterpulsation and sympathomimetic amines such as dopamine or dobutamine (Table 34-4; see also Chap. 68). In cardiogenic shock due to mechanical abnormalities, such as acute mitral regurgitation or ventricular septal defect, surgical correction is usually necessary.

Pericardial tamponade   This is the prototype of extracardiac obstructive shock and may be recognized by clinical manifestations (hypotension, pulsus paradoxus, distended neck veins) and characteristic findings on electrocardiography (Chap. 206) or by echocardiography (Chap. 190). Although expansion of intravascular volume and the administration of inotropic agents, particularly sympathomimetic amines such as norepinephrine and/or dopamine, may temporarily improve hemodynamics and act as a "holding maneuver," pericardiocentesis or surgical pericardial drainage is the only effective treatment.

TABLE 34-4 Commonly used vasopressor agents (relative potency*)

Agent	Dose	Cardiac		Peripheral vasculature		
		Heart rate	Contractility	Vasoconstriction	Vasodilatation	Dopaminergic
Dopamine	1–4 (μg/kg)/min	2+	2+	0	2+	4+
	4–20 (μg/kg)/min	2+	2+	2–3+	0	0
Levarterenol (norepinephrine)	2–8 μg/min	2+	2+	4+	0	0
Dobutamine	1–10 (μg/kg)/min	1+	4+	1+	2+	0
Isoproterenol	1–4 μg/min	4+	4+	0	4+	0
Epinephrine	1–8 μg/min	4+	4+	4+	3+	0
Phenylephrine	20–200 μg/min	0	0	4+	0	0

* The 1 to 4+ scoring system represents an arbitrary quantitative scoring system to allow a judgment of comparative potency among these vasopressor agents.
SOURCE: Adapted from JE Parrillo, *Major Issues in Critical Care Medicine*, JE Parrillo, SM Ayres (eds), Baltimore, Williams & Wilkins, 1984.

Septic shock (See also Chap. 83)   This condition can be considered in three broad categories. First, the nidus of infection must be identified and eliminated, using surgical drainage, antimicrobial therapy, or both. Rapid institution of appropriate antimicrobial therapy has been associated with improved survival; however, the specific organisms causing septic shock are frequently not identified when patients present with this illness. Thus broad-spectrum antimicrobial therapy must be instituted that will be effective against all the likely causative microorganisms given a patient's clinical presentation and a hospital's organism-sensitivity profile. An antimicrobial regimen should be chosen that has a very high likelihood of covering the organisms subsequently isolated.

Second, using cardiovascular monitoring and support, adequate organ system perfusion and function must be maintained while antibiotics (and surgery, if necessary) eradicate the source of sepsis. Since antibiotics usually require 48 h or more to reverse a septic focus, maintenance of cardiovascular support (blood pressure and tissue oxygen delivery) is critical to a favorable outcome. Since oxygen delivery is the product of blood hemoglobin concentration, oxygen saturation, and cardiac output, maintenance of a blood hemoglobin level at greater than 10 g/dL, an oxygen saturation of higher than 92 percent, and a cardiac index of greater than 4.0 L/min/m² are important therapeutic guidelines.

Electrocardiographic, arterial, and pulmonary artery monitoring should be instituted. Specific hemodynamic goals of therapy (see Table 34-3) are similar to those for shock in general: maintenance of a mean arterial pressure of 60 mmHg or greater (in adults); maintenance of oxygen delivery; frequent monitoring and normalization of kidney, liver, respiratory, and cardiac function; and normalization of blood lactate. Initial cardiovascular therapy should be to optimize preload by administering volume to attain a pulmonary artery wedge mean pressure of 14 to 18 mmHg. In patients with a low hemoglobin (<10 g/dL), blood should be used as a volume expander. If the serum albumin level is low (<2 g/dL), concentrated albumin infusions may be used to increase intravascular plasma oncotic pressure. In other instances, crystalloid is the most convenient and inexpensive method to achieve optimal preload.

If volume fails to achieve adequate blood pressure and organ perfusion, inotropic and vasopressor therapy should be initiated (see Table 34-4). For the persistently hypotensive patient, dopamine will frequently raise blood pressure and maintain or enhance blood flow to the renal and splanchnic circulations. Patients who remain hypotensive despite the aforementioned measures, including dopamine administration, may be treated with norepinephrine. As mentioned above, myocardial function is frequently abnormal in septic shock patients. To optimize oxygen delivery to tissues, raising a low cardiac index to 3.0 L/min/m² or higher with inotropic therapy is a logical therapeutic endpoint. Dobutamine is a useful inotropic agent in this setting (see Table 34-4).

Refractory hypotension and multiple-organ failure are the two major causes of mortality in septic shock. Support of dysfunctional organ systems represents an important therapeutic goal. Patients with respiratory failure due to adult respiratory distress syndrome may require oxygen therapy, mechanical ventilation, and institution of positive end-expiratory pressure to ensure adequate oxygenation while lung injury heals (Chap. 230). Disseminated intravascular coagulation (DIC) should be treated with replacement of clotting factors and platelets. Renal failure may require dialysis. Several retrospective trials have documented that intensive care monitoring and organ system support directed by specialized critical-care personnel has been associated with a reduced mortality in septic shock patients.

A third general therapeutic goal is to interrupt the pathogenic sequence leading to septic shock. Several multicenter trials have documented that early corticosteroid administration fails to improve morbidity or mortality in septic shock. Patients with documented or suspected adrenal insufficiency should receive corticosteroids.

Inhibition of endorphin receptors with naloxone has been shown to cause a mild transient rise in blood pressure but no sustained benefit in septic shock patients. Inhibition of arachidonic acid metabolites has shown some promise in reversing septic adult respiratory distress syndrome.

A human monoclonal antibody directed against the lipid A (toxic) portion of endotoxin is under investigation (see Chap. 83). Inhibitors of other sepsis mediators (e.g., tumor necrosis factor and the interleukins) are presently undergoing clinical trials. Such inhibitors may allow interruption of the pathogenetic pathways of sepsis at multiple key steps and thereby reduce the high mortality associated with this disease.

REFERENCES

ALPERT JS, BECKER RC: Cardiogenic shock: Elements of etiology, diagnosis, and therapy. Clin Cardiol 16:182, 1993

BECKOW EC, ASTIZ ME: Mechanisms and management of septic shock. Crit Care Clin 9:219, 1993

BONE RC et al and the Methylprednisolone Severe Sepsis Study Group: A controlled clinical trial of high-dose methylprednisolone in the treatment of severe sepsis and septic shock. N Engl J Med 317:653, 1987

CONNORS AF et al: Evaluation of right-heart catheterization in the critically ill patient without acute myocardial infarction. N Engl J Med 308:263, 1983

GIROIR BP: Mediators of septic shock: New approaches for interrupting the endogenous inflammatory cascade. Crit Care Med 21L780, 1993

GUYTON AC: Cardiac output and circulatory shock, in *Human Physiology and Mechanisms of Disease*, 5th ed. Philadelphia, Saunders, 1991, pp 187–200

LEOR J et al: Cardiogenic shock complicating acute myocardial infarction in patients without heart failure on admission: Incidence, risk factors, and outcome. Am J Med 94:265, 1993

MORITZ A, WOLNER E: Circulatory support with shock due to acute myocardial infarction. Ann Thorac Surg 55:238, 1993

MOULOPOULOS SD: Effect of protracted dobutamine infusion on survival of patients in cardiogenic shock treated with intraaortic balloon pumping. Chest 103:248, 1993

NATANSON C et al: Gram-negative bacteremia produces both severe systolic and diastolic cardiac dysfunction in a canine model that simulates human septic shock. J Clin Invest 77:259, 1986

OGNIBENE FP et al: Depressed left ventricular performance in response to volume infusion in patients with sepsis and septic shock. Chest 93:903, 1988

PARKER MM, PARRILLO JE: Septic shock and other forms of distributive shock, in *Current Therapy in Critical Care Medicine*. Toronto, B. C. Decker, 1987, pp 44–55

PARRILLO JE: Septic shock in humans: Clinical evaluation, pathogenesis, and therapeutic approach, in *Textbook of Critical Care*, 2d ed, WC Shoemaker et al (eds). Philadelphia, Saunders, 1989, pp 1006–1023

———: Management of septic shock: Present and future. Ann Intern Med 115:491, 1991

———: Pathogenetic mechanisms of septic shock. N Engl J Med 328:1471, 1993

——— et al: A circulating myocardial depressant substance in humans with septic shock: Septic shock patients with a reduced ejection fraction have a circulating factor that depresses in vitro myocardial cell performance. J Clin Invest 76:1539, 1985

PINSKY MR et al: Serum cytokine levels in human septic shock. Relation to multiple-system organ failure and mortality. Chest 103:565, 1993

ROCK P et al: Efficacy and safety of naloxone in septic shock. Crit Care Med 13:28, 1985

ROUMEN RM et al: Intestinal permeability after severe trauma and hemorrhagic shock is increased without relation to septic complications. Arch Surg 128:453, 1993

SANDIN R: Kidney function in shock. Acta Anesthesiol Scand Suppl 98:14, 1993

35 CARDIOVASCULAR COLLAPSE, CARDIAC ARREST, AND SUDDEN DEATH

ROBERT J. MYERBURG / AGUSTIN CASTELLANOS

OVERVIEW AND DEFINITIONS

Cardiac disorders account for the vast majority of natural sudden deaths. The magnitude of the problem of *cardiac* causes is highlighted by estimates that more than 300,000 sudden cardiac deaths (SCD) occur each year in the United States and that as many as 50 percent of all cardiac deaths are sudden and unexpected. Since techniques and systems are now available to save patients who have out-of-hospital cardiac arrest, which was uniformly fatal in the past, understanding the SCD problem has practical importance.

SCD must be defined carefully. In the context of time, "sudden" was previously defined as death within 24 h of the onset of the clinical event which led to a fatal cardiac arrest; this was subsequently shortened for most clinical and epidemiologic purposes to 1 h or less between the onset of the terminal illness and death. However, because of community-based interventions, victims may remain biologically alive for days or weeks after a cardiac arrest that has resulted in irreversible central nervous system damage. Confusion in terms can be avoided by adhering strictly to definitions of death, cardiac arrest, and cardiovascular collapse, as outlined in Table 35-1. Death is biologically, legally, and literally an absolute and irreversible event. Death may be delayed in a survivor of cardiac arrest, but "survival

after sudden death" is contradictory. Currently, the accepted definition of SCD is *natural death* due to *cardiac* causes, heralded by abrupt loss of consciousness within *1 h* of the onset of acute symptoms, in an individual who may have known *preexisting* heart disease but in whom the *time* and *mode* of death are *unexpected*. When biologic death of the cardiac arrest victim is delayed because of interventions, the relevant pathophysiologic event remains the sudden and unexpected cardiac arrest which leads ultimately to death, even though delayed by artificial methods. Thus the terminology used should reflect the fact that the index event was a cardiac arrest and that death was due to its delayed consequences.

ETIOLOGY, INITIATING EVENTS, AND CLINICAL EPIDEMIOLOGY

Extensive epidemiologic studies have identified populations at high risk for SCD. In addition, a large body of pathologic data provides information on the underlying *structural abnormalities* in victims of SCD, and clinical/physiologic studies have begun to identify a group of *transient functional factors* which may convert a long-standing underlying structural abnormality from a stable to an unstable state (Table 35-2). This information is developing into an understanding of the causes and mechanisms of SCD.

Cardiac disorders constitute the most common causes of sudden *natural* death. After an initial peak incidence of sudden death between birth and 6 months of age (the sudden infant death syndrome), the incidence of sudden death falls abruptly and then increases to a second

---

TABLE 35-2 Cardiac arrest and sudden cardiac death

I STRUCTURAL CAUSES

A Coronary heart disease
   1 Coronary artery abnormalities
     a Chronic atherosclerotic lesions
     b Acute (active) lesions
       (plaque fissuring, platelet aggregation, acute thrombosis)
     c Anomalous coronary artery anatomy
   2 Myocardial infarction
     a Healed
     b Acute
B Myocardial hypertrophy
   1 Secondary
   2 Hypertrophic cardiomyopathy
     a Obstructive
     b Nonobstructive
C Cardiomyopathy—dilated or infiltrative
D Myocarditis
E Valvular heart disease
F Electrophysiologic abnormalities, structural
   1 Anomalous pathways in Wolff-Parkinson-White syndrome
   2 Conducting system disease

II FUNCTIONAL CONTRIBUTING FACTORS

A Transient ischemia and reperfusion
   1 Loss of energy substrates
   2 Generation of injurious substances (e.g., superoxide radicals)
   3 Disturbed membrane electrical properties (e.g., channels, pumps, receptors)
B Low cardiac output states
   1 Heart failure
     a Chronic
     b Acute decompensation
   2 Shock
C Systemic metabolic abnormalities
   1 Electrolyte imbalance (e.g., hypokalemia)
   2 Hypoxemia, acidosis
D Neurophysiologic disturbances
   1 Autonomic fluctuations—central, neural, humoral
   2 Receptor function
   3 Long QT syndrome, congenital
E Toxic responses
   1 Proarrhythmic drug effects
   2 Cardiac toxins (e.g., cocaine, digitalis intoxication)

TABLE 35-1 Distinction between death, cardiac arrest, and cardiovascular collapse

Term	Definition	Qualifiers or exceptions
Death	Irreversible cessation of all biologic functions	None
Cardiac arrest	Abrupt cessation of cardiac pump function which may be reversible by a prompt intervention but will lead to death in its absence	Rare spontaneous reversions; likelihood of successful interventions relates to mechanism of arrest and clinical setting
Cardiovascular collapse	A sudden loss of effective blood flow due to cardiac and/or peripheral vascular factors which may reverse spontaneously (e.g., vasodepressor syncope) or only with interventions (e.g., cardiac arrest)	Nonspecific term which includes cardiac arrest and its consequences and also events which characteristically revert spontaneously

peak in the age range of 45 to 75 years. Moreover, increasing age is a powerful risk factor for sudden *cardiac* death. It follows that the *proportion* of *cardiac* causes among all sudden *natural* deaths increases dramatically with advancing years. From 1 to 13 years of age, only one of five sudden *natural* deaths is due to cardiac causes. Between 14 and 21 years of age, the proportion increases to 30 percent, and then to 88 percent in the middle-aged and elderly.

Men and women have very different susceptibilities to SCD, and the gender differences decrease with advancing age. The overall male/female ratio is approximately 4:1, but in the 45- to 64-year-old age group, the male SCD excess is nearly 7:1. It falls to approximately 2:1 in the 65- to 74-year-old age group. The difference in risk for SCD parallels the risks for other manifestations of coronary heart disease in men and women. As the gap for other manifestations of coronary heart disease closes in the seventh and eighth decades of life, the excess risk of SCD narrows. Despite the lower incidence in women, the classic coronary risk factors still operate in the proportionately smaller subgroup of women—cigarette smoking, diabetes, hyperlipidemia, hypertension.

Hereditary factors contribute to the risk of SCD, but largely in a nonspecific manner: They represent expressions of the hereditary predisposition to coronary heart disease. Except for a few specific syndromes, such as the genetic hyperlipoproteinemias (Chap. 344) and congenital long QT interval syndromes (Chap. 198), there are no *specific* hereditary risk factors for SCD. Higher levels of life stress, lower levels of education, social isolation, changes in life-style after myocardial infarction, cigarette use, alcohol consumption, obesity, and absence of regular exercise all have been *suggested* as contributors to risk of SCD. Among women, those who are unmarried and those who have fewer children or have greater educational disparity with their spouses appear to be at higher risk.

The major categories of structural causes of, and functional factors contributing to, the SCD syndrome are listed in Table 35-2. Worldwide, and especially in western cultures, coronary atherosclerotic heart disease is the most common structural abnormality associated with SCD. Up to 80 percent of all SCDs in the United States are due to the consequences of coronary atherosclerosis. The cardiomyopathies (dilated and hypertrophic, collectively, Chap. 205) account for another 10 to 15 percent of SCDs, and all the remaining diverse etiologies cause only 5 to 10 percent of these events. The relative role of various factors contributing to the initiation of cardiac arrest has not been quantitated as well as the structural basis. Transient ischemia in the previously scarred or hypertrophied heart, hemodynamic and fluid and electrolyte disturbances, fluctuations in autonomic nervous system activity, and transient electrophysiologic changes caused by drugs or other chemicals (e.g., proarrhythmia) have all been implicated as mechanisms responsible for transition from electrophysiologic stability to instability. In addition, spontaneous reperfusion of ischemic myocardium, caused by vasomotor changes in the coronary vasculature and/or spontaneous thrombolysis, may cause transient electrophysiologic instability and arrhythmias.

PATHOLOGY   Data from necropsies of SCD victims parallel the clinical observations on the prevalence of coronary heart disease as the major structural etiologic factor. More than 80 percent of SCD victims have pathologic findings of coronary heart disease, and these commonly include ruptured atherosclerotic plaques and/or coronary thrombi. The most consistent *coronary artery* abnormality is extensive chronic coronary atherosclerosis. Seventy-five percent of the victims have two or more major vessels with ≥75 percent stenosis. In addition, in one study, atherosclerotic plaque fissuring, platelet aggregates, and/or acute thrombosis were observed in 95 of 100 individuals who had pathologic studies after SCD. Most of these acute changes were superimposed on preexisting chronic lesions. However, only 44 percent of the SCD victims had more than 50 percent luminal narrowing by recent coronary thrombi, raising issues about interactions between breakdown of preexisting noncritical lesions, local thrombus formation and spontaneous lysis, and acute coronary spasm with ischemia in the initiation of the terminal event.

The pathology of the *myocardium* in SCD reflects the extensive coronary heart disease which usually precedes the fatal event. As many as 70 to 75 percent of males who die suddenly have prior myocardial infarctions (MIs), and 20 to 30 percent have recent acute MIs. A high incidence of left ventricular (LV) hypertrophy coexists with prior MIs. Clinical, epidemiologic, and experimental data suggest that LV hypertrophy itself predisposes to SCD, and it is likely that coexistence with prior MI adds additional risk.

CLINICAL DEFINITION OF FORMS OF CARDIOVASCULAR COLLAPSE   The definitions of the terms listed in Table 35-1 have important clinical applications. *Cardiovascular collapse* is a general term connoting loss of effective blood flow due to acute dysfunction of the heart and/or peripheral vasculature. Cardiovascular collapse may be caused by vasodepressor syncope (vasovagal syncope, postural hypotension with syncope, neurocardiogenic syncope—see Chap. 17), a transient severe bradycardia, or cardiac arrest. The latter is distinguished from the transient forms of cardiovascular collapse in that it usually requires an intervention to achieve resuscitation. In contrast, vasodepressor syncope and many primary bradyarrhythmic syncopal events are transient, and the patient will regain consciousness spontaneously.

The most common electrical mechanism for true cardiac arrest is ventricular fibrillation (VF), which is responsible for 65 to 80 percent of cardiac arrests. Severe persistent bradyarrhythmias, asystole, and electromechanical dissociation (organized electrical activity is present but there is no mechanical response) cause another 20 to 30 percent. Sustained ventricular tachycardia (VT) with hypotension is a less common cause. Acute low cardiac output states, having precipitous onset, also may present clinically as a cardiac arrest. The causes include massive acute pulmonary emboli, internal blood loss from ruptured aortic aneurysm, intense anaphylaxis, cardiac rupture after myocardial infarction, and unexpected fatal arrhythmia due to electrolyte disturbances.

CLINICAL CHARACTERISTICS OF CARDIAC ARREST

PRODROME, ONSET, ARREST, DEATH   Long-term studies in both unselected and high-risk populations suggest that SCD may be presaged by days, weeks, or months of increasing angina, dyspnea, palpitations, easy fatigability, and other nonspecific complaints. However, these *prodromal complaints* are generally predictive of any major cardiac event; they are not specific for predicting SCD. In one study, nearly 50 percent of SCD victims saw a physician within the month prior to death, but the complaints generally appeared to be unrelated to the heart. Among survivors of out-of-hospital cardiac arrest, 28 percent retrospectively reported new onset of worsening angina pectoris or dyspnea prior to cardiac arrest. Prodromes are useful for identifying patients at risk for cardiovascular events but not for identifying the subgroup of SCD victims.

The *onset of the terminal event*, leading to cardiac arrest, is defined as an acute change in cardiovascular status preceding cardiac arrest by up to 1 h. When the onset is instantaneous or abrupt, the probability that the arrest is cardiac in origin and related to underlying coronary artery disease is >95 percent. Continuous ECG recordings, fortuitously obtained prior to a cardiac arrest, commonly demonstrate changes in cardiac electrical activity in the minutes or hours before the event. There is a tendency for the heart rate to increase and for advanced grades of premature ventricular contractions to evolve. Most cardiac arrests that occur by the mechanism of VF begin with a run of sustained or nonsustained VT which then degenerates into VF.

In the clinical classification proposed by Hinkle and Thaler, sudden unexpected loss of effective circulation was separated into "arrhythmic events" and "circulatory failure." Arrhythmic events are characterized by a high incidence of patients being awake and actively moving immediately prior to the event, are dominated by VF as the electrical mechanism, and have a short duration of terminal illness (<1 h). In contrast, circulatory failure deaths occur in patients who are inactive or comatose, have a higher incidence of asystole than VF, have a tendency to a longer duration of terminal illness, and are dominated by noncardiac events preceding the terminal illness.

The onset of cardiac arrest may be characterized by typical symptoms of an acute cardiac event, such as prolonged angina or the pain of onset of myocardial infarction, acute dyspnea or orthopnea, or the sudden onset of palpitations, sustained tachycardia, or light-headedness. However, in many patients, the onset is precipitous, without forewarning.

Cardiac arrest is, by definition, abrupt. Mentation may be impaired in patients with sustained VT during the onset of the terminal event. However, complete loss of consciousness is a *sine qua non* in cardiac arrest. Although rare spontaneous reversions occur, it is usual that cardiac arrest progresses to death within minutes (i.e., SCD has occurred) if active interventions are not undertaken promptly.

The ability to resuscitate the victim of cardiac arrest is related to the time from onset to institution of resuscitative efforts, the setting in which the event occurs, the mechanism (VF, VT, electromechanical dissociation, asystole), and the clinical status of the patient prior to the cardiac arrest. Those settings in which it is possible to institute prompt cardiopulmonary resuscitation (CPR) provide a better chance of a successful outcome. However, the outcome in intensive care units and other in-hospital environments is more heavily influenced by the patient's preceding clinical status. The immediate outcome is good for cardiac arrest occurring in the intensive care unit in the presence of an acute cardiac event or transient metabolic disturbance, but the outcome for patients with far-advanced chronic cardiac disease or advanced noncardiac diseases (e.g., renal failure, pneumonia, sepsis, diabetes, cancer) is no more successful in hospital than in the out-of-hospital environment.

The success rate for initial resuscitation and ultimate survival from an out-of-hospital cardiac arrest depends in part on the mechanism of the event. When the mechanism is VT, the outcome is best (67 percent); VF is the next most successful (25 percent), and asystole and electromechanical dissociation have dismal outcome statistics (Fig. 35-1). Advanced age also adversely influences the chances of successful resuscitation.

Progression to biologic death is a function of the mechanism of

cardiac arrest and the length of the delay before interventions. VF or asystole, without CPR within the first 4 to 6 min, has a poor outcome, and there are few survivors among patients who had no life-support activities for the first 8 min after onset. Outcome statistics are dramatically improved by lay bystander intervention (basic life support—see below) prior to definitive interventions (advanced life support—defibrillation) and by early defibrillation. The most common causes of death during hospitalization after resuscitated cardiac arrests are related to the severity of injury to the central nervous system. Anoxic encephalopathy and infections subsequent to prolonged respirator dependence account for 60 percent of the deaths. Another 30 percent occur as a consequence of low cardiac output states which fail to respond to interventions. Paradoxically, recurrent arrhythmias are the least common cause of death, accounting for only 10 percent of in-hospital deaths.

Outcome during hospitalization, particularly in patients with acute MI, is very different for patients with primary and secondary cardiac arrests. *Primary* cardiac arrests refer to those which occur in the absence of hemodynamic instability, and *secondary* cardiac arrests are those which occur in patients in whom abnormal hemodynamics dominate the clinical picture before cardiac arrest. The success rate for immediate resuscitation in primary cardiac arrest during acute MI should approach 100 percent. In contrast, as many as 70 percent of patients with secondary cardiac arrest succumb immediately or during the same hospitalization.

IDENTIFICATION OF PATIENTS AT RISK FOR SUDDEN CARDIAC DEATH Primary prevention of cardiac arrest depends on the ability to identify individual patients at high risk. One must view the problem in the context of the total number of events and the population pools from which they are derived. In Fig. 35-2A, the inverted triangle demonstrates that the annual incidence of SCD among an unselected adult population is 1 to 2 per 1000 population, largely reflecting the prevalence of those coronary heart disease patients among whom SCD is the first clinically recognized manifestation (20 to 25 percent of first coronary events are SCD). The incidence (percent per year) increases progressively with addition of identified coronary risk factors to populations free of prior coronary events. The most powerful factors are age, elevated blood pressure, LV hypertrophy, cigarette smoking, elevated serum cholesterol level, obesity, and nonspecific electrocardiographic abnormalities. These coronary risk factors are not specific for SCD but rather represent increasing risk for all coronary deaths. The proportion of coronary deaths that are sudden remains at approximately 50 percent in all risk categories. Despite the marked *relative* increased risk of SCD with addition of multiple risk factors (from 1 to 2 per 1000 population per year in an unselected population to as much as 50 to 60 per 1000 in the highest risk subgroups), the *absolute* incidence remains relatively low when viewed in terms of the relationship between the number of individuals who have a preventive intervention versus the number of events which can be prevented. Specifically, a 50 percent reduction in annual SCD risk would be a huge *relative* decrease but would require an intervention in up to 200 unselected individuals to prevent one sudden death. These figures highlight the importance of primary prevention of coronary heart disease. Control of coronary risk factors may be the only practical method to prevent SCD in major segments of the population, since the majority of events occur in the large unselected subgroups rather than in the specific high-risk subgroups (compare "Events/Year" with "Percent/Year" in Fig. 35-2A). In addition to population and clinical determinants of risk, there also appears to be time-dependent modulation of risk (Fig. 35-2B). Under most conditions of higher level of risk, particularly those related to a recent major cardiovascular event (e.g., myocardial infarction, recent onset of heart failure, survival after out-of-hospital cardiac arrest), the highest risk of sudden death occurs within the initial 6 to 18 months and then decreases toward baseline risk of the underlying disease. Accordingly, preventive interventions are most likely to be effective when initiated early.

For patients with acute or prior clinical manifestations of coronary

FIGURE 35-1 Initial electrophysiologic mechanisms recorded during out-of-hospital cardiac arrest. The figures highlighted by the boxes indicate the number of patients in each of three mechanism categories (ventricular fibrillation, ventricular tachycardia, and bradyarrhythmia/asystole). In each category, the data indicate the number of prehospital cardiac arrests (*top*), the number of patients successfully resuscitated in the field and transferred to the hospital alive (*middle*), and the number of patients who survived to be discharged from hospital (*bottom*). The percentages in parentheses indicate survivals between each level of care for each category. (*Modified from Myerburg RJ et al: Clinical, electrophysiologic, and hemodynamic profile of patients resuscitated from prehospital cardiac arrest. Am J Med 68:568, 1980, with permission*).

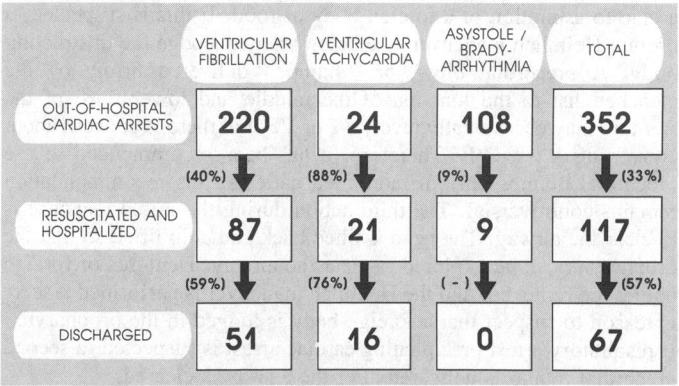

	VENTRICULAR FIBRILLATION	VENTRICULAR TACHYCARDIA	ASYSTOLE / BRADY-ARRHYTHMIA	TOTAL
OUT-OF-HOSPITAL CARDIAC ARRESTS	220	24	108	352
	(40%)	(88%)	(9%)	(33%)
RESUSCITATED AND HOSPITALIZED	87	21	9	117
	(59%)	(76%)	(–)	(57%)
DISCHARGED	51	16	0	67

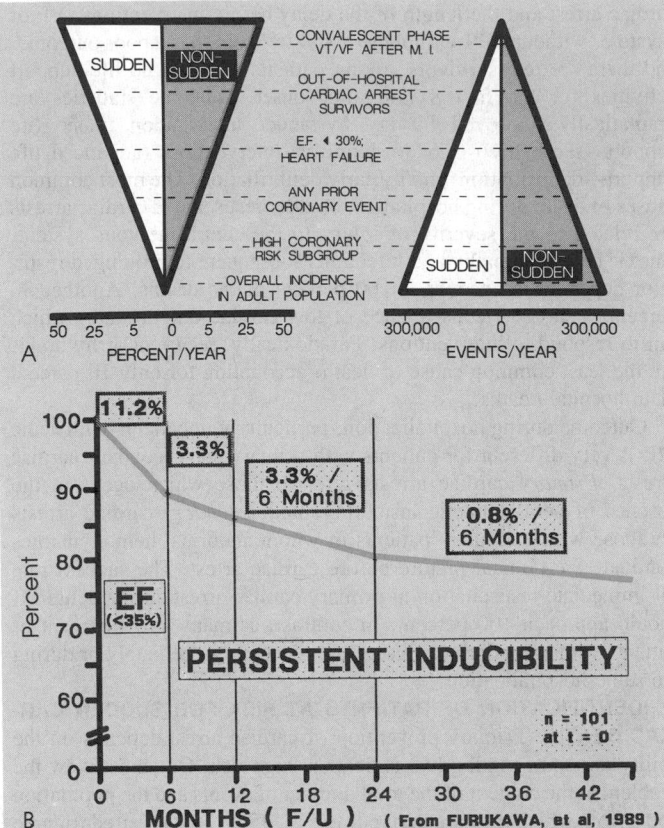

FIGURE 35-2 *A.* Incidence of sudden and nonsudden cardiac deaths in population subgroups, and the relation of total number of events per year to incidence figures. Approximations of subgroup incidence figures, and the related population pool from which they are derived, are presented. Approximately 50 percent of all cardiac deaths are sudden and unexpected. The incidence triangle on the left (''Percent/Year'') indicates the approximate percentage of sudden and nonsudden deaths in each of the population subgroups indicated, ranging from the lowest percentage in unselected adult populations (0.1 to 2 percent per year) to the highest percentage in patients with VT or VF during convalescence after an MI (approximately 50 percent per year). The triangle on the right indicates the total number of events per year in each of these groups, to reflect incidence in context with the size of the population subgroups. The highest risk categories identify the smallest number of total annual events, and the lowest incidence category accounts for the largest number of events per year. (EF = ejection fraction; VT = ventricular tachycardia; VF = ventricular fibrillation; MI = myocardial infarction.) *B.* Time dependence of risk among survivors of out-of-hospital cardiac arrest. Recurrence risk is highest in the first 6 months of the index event. Survival is expressed as a percentage. High risk is best predicted initially by an ejection fraction ≤ 35 percent during the first 6 months, and subsequently persistent inducibility of VT during electrophysiologic testing becomes an added major risk. *(Modified from Furukawa T et al, in Myerburg RJ et al. Reproduced with permission of the American Heart Association.)*

heart disease, high-risk subgroups having a much higher ratio of SCD risk to population base can be identified. The acute, convalescent, and chronic phases of MI provide large population subsets with more highly focused risk (Chap. 202). The potential risk of cardiac arrest from the onset through the first 72 h after acute MI (the acute phase) may be as high as 15 to 20 percent. The highest risk of SCD in relation to MI is found in the subgroup that has VT or VF during the convalescent phase (3 days to 8 weeks) after MI. A 50 to 80 percent mortality in 6 to 12 months has been observed among these patients, when managed with conventional therapy, and at least 50 percent of the deaths are sudden. Since the development of aggressive intervention techniques, the incidence has fallen dramatically to 15 to 20 percent in 18 months, or better.

Chronic premature ventricular complexes (PVCs) after the acute phase of MI identify a long-term risk for total cardiac mortality and SCD. Increasing *frequency* of PVCs, with a plateau above the range of 10 to 30 PVCs per hour on 24-h ambulatory monitor recordings, indicates increased risk, but advanced *forms* (salvos, nonsustained VT) are probably the more powerful predictor. PVCs interact strongly with the size of the MI, as reflected by decreased left ventricular ejection fraction (EF). The combination of frequent PVCs, salvos or nonsustained VT, and an EF ≤ 30 percent identifies patients who have an annual risk of 20 percent. The risk falls off sharply with decreasing PVC frequency and the absence of advanced forms, as well as with higher EF. Despite these risk implications of postinfarction PVCs, whether suppression of PVCs alters risk has not yet been determined. However, a large intervention trial, the Cardiac Arrhythmia Suppression Trial (CAST) demonstrated that, for the drugs studied, any potential benefit of suppression of PVCs was outweighed by a threefold increase in deaths among patients receiving the study drugs.

Beyond the specific problem of coronary heart disease, the general factors of extent of underlying disease due to any cause and a prior clinical expression of risk of SCD (i.e., survival after out-of-hospital cardiac arrest not associated with acute MI) identify very high risk patients. Survival after out-of-hospital cardiac arrest predicts a 30 percent 1-year recurrent cardiac arrest rate in the absence of specific interventions (see below) in this group of patients.

A general rule is that the risk of SCD is approximately one-half the total cardiovascular mortality rate. Thus the SCD risk is approximately 20 percent per year for patients with advanced coronary heart disease or dilated cardiomyopathy severe enough to result in a 40 percent 1-year total mortality rate. Figure 35-2A demonstrates a much more focused population fraction (''Percent/Year'') for identifying high-risk patients in the high-risk subgroups, but the impact on the overall population, indicated by the absolute number of preventable events (''Events/Year''), is considerably smaller.

MANAGEMENT OF CARDIAC ARREST

The individual who collapses suddenly is managed in five stages: (1) the initial response, (2) basic life support, (3) advanced life support, (4) postresuscitation care, and (5) long-term management. The initial response and basic life support can be carried out by physicians, nurses, paramedical personnel, and trained lay persons. There is a requirement for increasing skills as the patient moves through the stages of advanced life support, postresuscitation care, and long-term management.

INITIAL RESPONSE The initial response will confirm whether a sudden collapse is indeed due to a cardiac arrest. Observations for respiratory movements, skin color, and the presence or absence of pulses in the carotid or femoral arteries will immediately determine whether a life-threatening cardiac arrest has occurred. Agonal respiratory movements may persist for a short time after cardiac arrest, but it is important to observe for severe stridor with a persistent pulse as a clue to aspiration of a foreign body or food. If this is suspected, a prompt Heimlich maneuver (see below) may dislodge the obstructing body. A precordial blow, or ''thump,'' delivered firmly by the clenched fist to the junction of the middle and lower third of the sternum may occasionally revert VT or VF, but there is concern about converting VT *to* VF. Therefore, it has been recommended to use precordial thumps only in monitored patients; this recommendation remains controversial. The third action during the initial response is to clear the airway. The head is tilted back and chin lifted so that the oropharynx can be explored to clear the airway. Dentures or foreign bodies are removed, and the Heimlich maneuver is performed if there is reason to suspect that a foreign body is lodged in the oropharynx. If respiratory arrest precipitating cardiac arrest is suspected, a second precordial thump is delivered after the airway is cleared.

BASIC LIFE SUPPORT   More popularly known as cardiopulmonary resuscitation (CPR), basic life support is intended to maintain organ perfusion until definitive interventions can be instituted. The elements of CPR are the establishment and maintenance of ventilation of the lungs and compression of the chest. Mouth-to-mouth respiration may be used if no specific rescue equipment is immediately available (e.g., plastic oropharyngeal airways, esophageal obturators, masked Ambu bag). Conventional ventilation techniques during CPR require the lungs to be inflated once every 5 s when two persons are performing the resuscitation and twice in succession every 15 s when one person is carrying out both ventilation and chest wall compression.

Chest compression is based on the assumption that cardiac compression allows the heart to maintain a pump function by sequential filling and emptying of its chambers, with competent valves maintaining forward direction of flow. The technique is illustrated in Fig. 35-3. The palm of one hand is placed over the lower sternum, with the heel of the other resting on the dorsum of the lower hand. The sternum is depressed, with the arms remaining straight, at a rate of approximately 80 per minute. Sufficient force is applied to depress the sternum 3 to 5 cm, and relaxation is abrupt. This conventional technique for CPR is currently being compared with a new technique based on simultaneous compression and ventilation. While measurable carotid artery flow can be achieved with conventional CPR, experimen-

tal data and theoretical considerations suggest that flow may be optimized by a pumping action produced by pressure changes in the entire thoracic cavity, as is achieved by simultaneous compression and ventilation. However, it is not yet clear whether this technique causes an unacceptable impedance of coronary blood flow and whether the increased *carotid flow* produces equivalent increases in *cerebral perfusion*. Until these issues are clarified, conventional CPR remains the generally accepted technique.

ADVANCED LIFE SUPPORT   Advanced life support is intended to achieve adequate ventilation, control cardiac arrhythmias, stabilize the hemodynamic status (blood pressure and cardiac output), and restore organ perfusion. The activities carried out to achieve these goals include (1) intubation with an endotracheal tube, (2) defibrillation/cardioversion and/or pacing, and (3) insertion of an intravenous line. Ventilation with O_2 (room air if O_2 is not immediately available) may promptly reverse hypoxemia and acidosis. The speed with which defibrillation/cardioversion is carried out is an important element for successful resuscitation. When possible, immediate defibrillation should precede intubation and insertion of an intravenous line; CPR should be carried out while the defibrillator is being charged. As soon as a diagnosis of VT or VF is obtained, a 200-J shock should be delivered. Additional shocks at higher energies, up to a maximum of 360 J, are tried if the initial shock does not successfully abolish VT or VF. If the patient is less than fully conscious upon reversion, or if two or three attempts fail, prompt intubation, ventilation, and arterial blood gas analysis should be carried out. Intravenous $NaHCO_3$, which was formerly used in large quantities, is no longer considered routinely necessary and may be dangerous in larger quantities. However, the patient who is persistently acidotic after successful defibrillation and intubation should be given 1 mmol/kg $NaHCO_3$ initially and an additional 50 percent of the dose repeated every 10 to 15 min.

After initial defibrillation attempts, whether successful or not, a bolus of 1 mg/kg lidocaine is given intravenously (Chap. 202), and the dose is repeated in 2 min in those patients who have persistent ventricular arrhythmias or remain in VF. This is followed by a continuous infusion at a rate of 1 to 4 mg/min. If lidocaine fails to provide control, intravenous procainamide (loading infusion of 100 mg/5 min to a total dose of 500 to 800 mg, followed by continuous infusion at 2 to 5 mg/min) or bretylium tosylate (loading dose 5 to 10 mg/kg in 5 min; maintenance dose 0.5 to 2 mg/min) may be tried. For persistent VF, epinephrine (0.5 to 1.0 mg) may be given intravenously every 5 min during resuscitation with attempts to defibrillate between each dose. The drug may be given by an intracardiac route if intravenous access is not available. Intravenous calcium gluconate is no longer considered safe or necessary for routine administration. It is used only in patients in whom acute hyperkalemia is known to be the triggering event for resistant VF, in the presence of known hypocalcemia, or in patients who have received toxic doses of calcium channel antagonists.

Cardiac arrest secondary to bradyarrhythmias or asystole are managed differently. Once it is known that this type of rhythm is present, there is no role for external shock. The patient is promptly intubated, CPR is continued, and an attempt is made to control hypoxemia and acidosis. Epinephrine and/or atropine are given intravenously or by an intracardiac route. External pacing devices are now available to attempt to establish a regular rhythm, but the prognosis is generally very poor in this form of cardiac arrest. The one exception is bradyarrhythmic/asystolic cardiac arrest secondary to airway obstruction. This form of cardiac arrest may respond promptly to removal of foreign bodies by the Heimlich maneuver or, in hospitalized patients, by intubation and suctioning of obstructing secretions in the airway.

POSTRESUSCITATION CARE   This phase of management is determined by the clinical setting of the cardiac arrest. *Primary VF in acute MI* (Chap. 202) is generally very responsive to life-support techniques and easily controlled after the initial event. Patients are maintained on a lidocaine infusion at the rate of 2 to 4 mg/min for

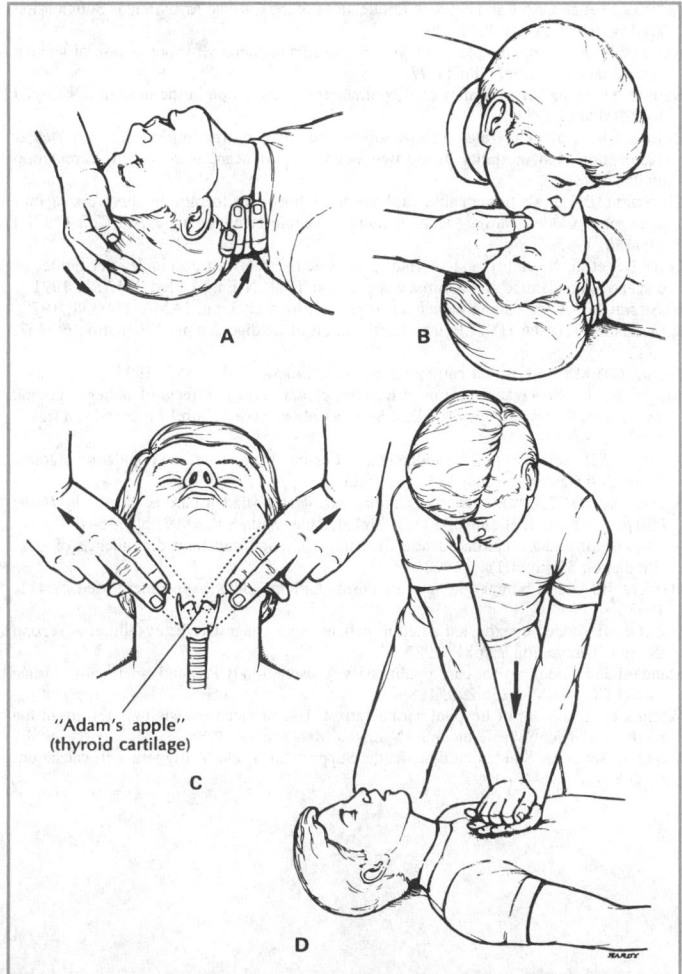

FIGURE 35-3 Major steps in cardiopulmonary resuscitation. *A.* Make certain the victim has an open airway. *B.* Start respiratory resuscitation immediately. *C.* Feel for the carotid pulse in the groove alongside the "Adam's apple" or thyroid cartilage. *D.* If pulse is absent, begin cardiac massage. Use 60 compressions a minute with one lung inflation after each group of 5 chest compressions. *(From J Henderson, Emergency Medical Guide, 4th ed, New York, McGraw-Hill, 1978.)*

"Adam's apple"
(thyroid cartilage)

24 to 72 h after the event. In the in-hospital setting, respirator support is usually not necessary or is needed for only a short time, and hemodynamics stabilize promptly after defibrillation or cardioversion. In *secondary VF in acute MI* (those events in which hemodynamic abnormalities predispose to the potentially fatal arrhythmia), resuscitative efforts are less often successful, and in those patients who are successfully resuscitated, the recurrence rate is high. The clinical picture is dominated by hemodynamic instability. In fact, the outcome is determined more by the ability to control hemodynamic dysfunction than by electrophysiologic abnormalities. Bradyarrhythmias, asystole, and electromechanical dissociation are commonly secondary events in hemodynamically unstable patients and are less responsive to interventions.

The outcome after in-hospital cardiac arrest associated with *noncardiac* diseases is poor, and in the few successfully resuscitated patients, the postresuscitation course is dominated by the nature of the underlying disease. Patients with cancer, renal failure, acute central nervous system disease, and uncontrolled infections, as a group, have a survival rate of less than 10 percent after in-hospital cardiac arrest. Some major exceptions to the poor outcome of cardiac arrest due to noncardiac causes are patients with transient airway obstruction, electrolyte disturbances, proarrhythmic effects of drugs, and severe metabolic abnormalities, most of whom may have an excellent chance of survival if they can be resuscitated promptly and maintained while the transient abnormalities are being corrected.

LONG-TERM MANAGEMENT AFTER SURVIVAL OF OUT-OF-HOSPITAL CARDIAC ARREST This form of care has evolved into a major area of specialized clinical activities since the development of community-based emergency rescue systems. Patients who do not suffer irreversible injury of the central nervous system and who achieve hemodynamic stability should have extensive diagnostic and therapeutic testing to guide long-term management. This aggressive approach is driven by the fact that statistics from the 1970s indicated survival after out-of-hospital cardiac arrest was followed by a 30 percent recurrent cardiac arrest rate at 1 year, 45 percent at 2 years, and a total mortality rate of almost 60 percent at 2 years. Historical comparisons suggest that these dismal statistics may be significantly improved by newer interventions, but the magnitude of the improvement is unknown because of the lack of concurrently controlled intervention studies.

Among those patients in whom a transmural, acute MI is the cause of out-of-hospital cardiac arrest, the management is the same as in any other patient who suffers cardiac arrest during the acute phase of a documented MI (see Chap. 202). For almost all other categories of patients, however, extensive diagnostic studies are carried out to determine etiology, functional impairment, and electrophysiologic instability as guides to future management. In general, patients who have out-of-hospital cardiac arrest due to chronic ischemic heart disease, without an acute MI, are evaluated to determine whether transient ischemia or chronic electrophysiologic instability was the more likely cause of the event. If there is reason to suspect an ischemic mechanism, anti-ischemic surgery or medical interventions (e.g., angioplasty, drugs) are used to reduce the ischemic burden. Electrophysiologic instability is best identified by the use of programmed electrical stimulation to determine whether sustained VT or VF can be induced in the patient (Chap. 198). If so, this information can be used as a baseline against which to evaluate drug efficacy for prevention of inducibility. It also can be used to determine suitability for map-guided antiarrhythmic surgery. Using this technique to establish drug therapy in patients with ejection fractions of 30 percent or more, the recurrent cardiac arrest rate is less than 10 percent during the first year of follow-up. The outcome is not as good for patients with ejection fractions under 30 percent but may be still better than the apparent natural history of survival after cardiac arrest. For patients for whom successful drug therapy cannot be identified by this technique, empiric treatment with amiodarone, insertion of an implantable cardioverter/defibrillator (ICD), or antiarrhythmic surgery (e.g., coronary bypass surgery, aneurysmectomy, cryoablation), can be considered options (Chap. 198). Primary surgical success, defined as surviving the procedure and reverting to a noninducible status without drug therapy, is better than 90 percent when patients are selected for ability to be mapped in the operating room. ICD therapy is also evolving into more sophisticated systems, including the ability to pace rather than shock out of some arrhythmias in selected patients. The array of interventions available for these patients, properly applied, is providing continuing improvement in long-term outcome.

PREVENTION OF SUDDEN CARDIAC DEATH

This remains a major unresolved challenge in modern medicine. Some progress appears to have been made in selected, very high risk subgroups. However, the majority of SCD cases, expressed in absolute numbers rather than relative risk, occur within those subgroups characterized by lesser degrees of risk (see Fig. 35-2). Major progress will therefore require effective measures for prevention of the underlying disease, plus the ability to identify and control transient initiating factors, and methods of identifying higher-risk clusters among the more general population groups.

REFERENCES

AKHTAR M et al: CAST and beyond: Implications of the Cardiac Arrhythmias Suppression Trial. Circulation 81:1123, 1990

AKHTAR M et al: Implantable cardioverter-defibrillator therapy for prevention of sudden cardiac death. Cardiol Clin 11:97, 1993

BEDELL SE et al: Survival after cardiopulmonary resuscitation in the hospital. N Engl J Med 309:569, 1983

BIGGER JT et al: The relationships among ventricular arrhythmias, left ventricular dysfunction, and mortality in the two years after myocardial infarction. Circulation 69:250, 1984

CRANDALL BG et al: Implantable cardioverter-defibrillator therapy in survivors of out-of-hospital sudden cardiac death without inducible arrhythmias. J Am Coll Cardiol 21:1186, 1993

ECHT DS et al: Mortality and morbidity in patients receiving encainide, flecainide, or placebo: The Cardiac Arrhythmia Suppression Trial. N Engl J Med 324:781, 1991

HEIMLICH HJ: A life-saving maneuver to prevent food choking. JAMA 234:398, 1975

HINKLE LA, THALER HT: Clinical classification of cardiac deaths. Circulation 65:457, 1982

JASTREMSKI MS: In-hospital cardiac arrest. Ann Emerg Med 22:113, 1993

JOSLYN ET AL: Survival from out-of-hospital cardiac arrest: Effects of patient age and presence of 911 Emergency Medical Services phone access. Am J Emerg Med 11:200, 1993

KANNEL WB, SCHATZKIN A: Sudden death: Lessons from subsets in population studies. J Am Coll Cardiol 5(suppl 6):141B, 1985

MYERBURG RJ, CASTELLANOS A: Cardiac arrest and sudden cardiac death, in *Heart Disease*, 4th ed, E Braunwald (ed). Philadelphia, Saunders, 1992, pp 756–789

——— et al: Sudden cardiac death: Structure, function and time dependence of risk. Circulation 85(suppl 1):2, 1992

ORNATO JP: Use of adrenergic agonists during CPR in adults. Ann Emerg Med 22:411, 1993

PACKER M: Sudden unexpected death in patients with congestive heart failure: A second frontier. Circulation 72:681, 1985

Standard and guidelines for cardiopulmonary resuscitation (CPR) and emergency cardiac care (ECC). JAMA 255:290, 1986

WILBER DJ et al: Out-of-hospital cardiac arrest: Use of electrophysiologic testing in the prediction of long-term outcome. N Engl J Med 318:19, 1988

WILLICH SN et al: Sudden cardiac death. Support for a role of triggering in causation. Circulation 87:1442, 1993

section 5   Alterations in gastrointestinal function

36   ORAL MANIFESTATIONS OF DISEASE

JOHN S. GREENSPAN*

A thorough oral examination, to include the oral and pharyngeal soft tissues as well as the teeth, is an important part of the physical examination. The common oral diseases are due to infection by bacteria, fungi, or viruses. The complex development of the orofacial structures leads to close interposition of a wide range of tissues, most of which are prone to developmental anomalies, growth disturbances, and neoplasia.

DISEASES OF THE TEETH

DENTAL CARIES, PULPAL AND PERIAPICAL DISEASE, AND COMPLICATIONS   Dental caries is a destructive disease of the hard tissues of the teeth due to infection with *Streptococcus mutans* and other bacteria. Formerly one of the most common human diseases, caries has shown marked changes in recent years. In the United States, fewer than half of those 17 years and younger now have carious lesions, although in many segments of the population and in developing countries this decrease has not occurred. Much of the decline is due to artificial fluoridation of drinking water to a level of 1 part per million, with additional effects due to fluoride-containing toothpastes and topical fluoride administration. Conversely, retention of teeth and the aging of the population have led to an increase in root caries. Increasing numbers of patients surviving with the consequences of cancer therapy and other special populations (diabetics and those with xerostomia due to Sjögren's syndrome or to medications) may experience severe caries unless appropriate topical fluoride prophylaxis is used. Treatment of caries involves removal of the softened and infected hard tissues, sealing of the exposed dentine, and restoration of the lost tooth structure with silver amalgam, composite plastic, gold, or porcelain.

If the carious lesion progresses, infection of the dental pulp may occur, causing *acute pulpitis*. The tooth may become sensitive to hot or cold, and then severe continuous throbbing pain ensues. At this stage, pulp damage is irreversible, and root canal therapy becomes necessary. The contents of the pulp chamber and root canals are removed, followed by thorough cleaning, antisepsis, and filling with an inert material. Alternatively, extraction of the tooth may be indicated.

If the pulpitis is not treated successfully, infection may spread beyond the tooth apex into the periodontal ligament. If the infection causes acute inflammation, pain on chewing or on percussion is present, and a *periapical abscess* may form, while chronic inflammation can produce a *periapical granuloma* within the alveolar bone. This may cause slight pain and tenderness or may be asymptomatic. Proliferation of epithelial cell rests may convert the granuloma into a *periapical cyst*. Both the granuloma and the cyst produce periapical radiolucencies, whereas the periapical abscess does not do so unless

it forms as a complication of one of the other two lesions. The pus in the periapical abscess may track through the alveolar bone into soft tissues, causing cellulitis and bacteremia, or may discharge into the oral cavity (*parulis* or *gumboil*), into the maxillary sinus, or through the skin of the face or submandibular area. A severe form of cellulitis, *Ludwig's angina*, originates from an infected mandibular molar, involves the submandibular space, and extends throughout the floor of the mouth, with elevation of the tongue, dysphagia, and difficulty in breathing. Glottal edema may occur, necessitating emergency tracheotomy.

EFFECT OF SYSTEMIC FACTORS ON TEETH   Systemic factors, occurring in utero or in infancy during the stages of crown formation, may influence the development and structure of the teeth. Enamel hypoplasia of the primary and/or permanent teeth, manifested by alterations ranging from white spots to gross defects in the surface structure of the crowns, may be caused by disturbances of calcium and phosphate metabolism such as are found in vitamin D–resistant rickets, hypoparathyroidism, gastroenteritis, and celiac disease. Premature birth or high fevers also may give rise to enamel hypoplasia. Tetracycline, when given during the second half of pregnancy, in infancy, and in childhood up to 8 years of age, causes both a permanent discoloration of the teeth and enamel hypoplasia. Daily ingestion of more than 1.5 mg fluoride can result in enamel discoloration (*mottling*). Prenatal factors appear to influence crown size. Larger teeth are associated with maternal diabetes, maternal hypothyroidism, and large birth size. Tooth size is reduced in Down syndrome. Premature loss of the deciduous dentition is frequently the first symptom in juvenile hypophosphatasia. Systemic disease may give rise to pain that simulates pulpal disease. Maxillary sinusitis is frequently manifested as pain in the maxillary teeth, including sensitivity to thermal changes and percussion. Cardiac disease with angina pectoris may result in pain referred to the lower jaw, probably through the vagus nerve.

PERIODONTAL DISEASES

In adults, chronic destructive periodontal disease becomes responsible for more loss of teeth than caries, particularly in the aged. However, the prevalence and incidence of periodontal disease also appears to be declining in the United States. The most common form of periodontal disease starts as inflammation of the marginal gingiva (*gingivitis*) which is painless, although the gingiva may bleed on brushing. The disease spreads to involve the periodontal ligament and alveolar bone. As the latter is slowly resorbed, there is loss of periodontal ligament attachment between tooth and bone. The soft tissue separates from the tooth surface, causing "pocket" formation with bleeding on probing and during chewing. Acute inflammation may become superimposed on this chronic process, with the production of pus and the formation of a *periodontal abscess*. Ultimately, extreme bone loss, tooth mobility, and recurrent abscess formation lead to tooth exfoliation or may mandate tooth extraction.

Gingivitis and periodontitis are infections associated with the accumulation of *bacterial plaque*, which may become mineralized (*calculus*) and which can be prevented by appropriate *oral hygiene* measures, including tooth brushing, flossing, antibacterial mouth rinses, and the removal of impacted food debris. Poorly fabricated or

* The author acknowledges the contribution of Dr. Paul Goldhaber in previous editions.

deteriorated restorations may contribute through overextended or inadequate margins, while the role of occlusal trauma is unclear. Therapy is directed at the causative microflora and consists of removal of plaque and calculus, debridement of the pocket lining and superficial infected cementum, and elimination of other contributing factors.

Periodontal disease appears to be a group of conditions, including *adult periodontitis*, associated with *Porphyromonas gingivalis*, *Prevotella intermedia*, and other gram-negative organisms. *Localized juvenile periodontitis* (LJP) causes rapid, severe pocketing and bone loss and is associated with *Actinobacillus actinomycetemcomitans* (*A.a*), *Capnocytophaga*, *Eikenella corrodens*, and other anaerobes. *Acute necrotizing ulcerative gingivitis* (ANUG) involves sudden inflammation of the gingivae with necrosis, tissue loss, pain, bleeding, and halitosis and is associated with *P. intermedia* and spirochetes. ANUG and an aggressive and rapid form of periodontitis (HIV-P) are seen in association with human immunodeficiency virus (HIV) infection. Some of these cases progress to a destructive gangrene-like lesion of oral soft tissues and bone (*necrotizing stomatitis*) resembling the *noma* formerly seen in severely malnourished populations. Therapy involves local antibacterial measures, debridement, and, in severe cases, systemic antibiotics effective against gram-negative anaerobes.

Host factors may be involved in the pathogenesis of periodontal disease in other populations as well. Thus familial defects in neutrophil chemotaxis are found in LJP, and these may predispose to tissue destruction caused by the toxins of *A.a.*, including leucotoxin, collagenase, endotoxin, and a factor further inhibiting neutrophil chemotaxis. Patients with IgA deficiency and agammaglobulinemia probably have less periodontal disease than matched healthy individuals, whereas in *Down syndrome* and *diabetes mellitus* severe periodon-tal disease may occur. During pregnancy there may be severe gingivitis and the formation of localized *pyogenic granulomas*. Certain drugs, notably the anticonvulsant *phenytoin* and the antiangina calcium channel blocker *nifedipine*, cause *fibrous hyperplasia* of the gingiva which may cover the teeth, interfere with eating, and be unsightly. Similar clinical appearances can be due to *idiopathic familial gingival fibromatosis*. Surgical management is used for both conditions, although a change in medication may be appropriate for the drug-induced form.

Periapical and periodontal bacterial infections can cause transient bacteremia after tooth extraction and even routine dental prophylaxis. These can lead to bacterial endocarditis in patients with a history of rheumatic fever, other valvular disease, valvular graft, or heart or joint prostheses. Antibiotic coverage is appropriate in such cases.

DISEASES OF THE ORAL MUCOSA

INFECTIONS   Most oral mucosal diseases involve microorganisms (see Table 36-1).

PIGMENTED LESIONS (See Table 36-2)

DERMATOLOGIC DISEASES (See Tables 36-1, -2, and -3 and Chaps. 50 to 55)

DISEASES OF THE TONGUE (See Table 36-4)

HALITOSIS (See Table 36-5)

HIV DISEASE AND AIDS (See Table 36-6 and Chaps. 151 and 279)   Immunosuppression induced by HIV infection predisposes to numerous oral infections, neoplasms, and autoimmune and idiopathic lesions. Some of these, such as *oral candidiasis* (Fig. A1-41) and *hairy leukoplakia* (Fig. A1-40) (a benign epithelial hyperplasia

---

TABLE 36-1   Vesicular, bullous, or ulcerative lesions of the oral mucosa

Condition	Usual location	Clinical features	Course
VIRAL DISEASES			
Primary acute herpetic gingivo-stomatitis (herpes simplex virus type 1, rarely type 2)	Lip and oral mucosa	Labial vesicles which rupture and crust, and intraoral vesicles which quickly ulcerate; extremely painful; acute gingivitis, fever, malaise, foul odor, and cervical lymphadenopathy; occurs primarily in infants, children, and young adults	Heals spontaneously in 10–14 days unless secondarily infected
Recurrent herpes labialis	Mucocutaneous junction of lip, perioral skin	Eruption of groups of vesicles which may coalesce, then rupture and crust; painful to pressure or spicy foods	Lasts about 1 week, but condition may be prolonged if secondary infection occurs
Recurrent intraoral herpes simplex	Palate and gingiva	Small vesicles which rupture and coalesce; painful	Heal spontaneously in about 1 week
Chickenpox (varicella-zoster virus)	Gingiva and oral mucosa	Skin lesions may be accompanied by small vesicles on oral mucosa that rupture to form shallow ulcers; may coalesce to form large bullous lesions that ulcerate; mucosa may have generalized erythema	Lesions heal spontaneously within 2 weeks
Herpes zoster (reactivation of varicella-zoster virus)	Cheek, tongue, gingiva, or palate	Unilateral vesicular eruption and ulceration in linear pattern following sensory distribution of trigeminal nerve or one of its branches	Gradual healing without scarring; postherpetic neuralgia is common
Infectious mononucleosis (Epstein-Barr virus)	Oral mucosa	Fatigue, sore throat, malaise, low-grade fever, and enlarged cervical lymph nodes; numerous small ulcers usually appear several days before lymphadenopathy; gingival bleeding and multiple petechiae at junction of hard and soft palates	Oral lesions disappear during convalescence
Warts (papillomavirus)	Anywhere on skin and oral mucosa	Single or multiple papillary lesions, with thick, white keratinized surfaces containing many pointed projections; cauliflower lesions covered with normal-colored mucosa or multiple pink or pale bumps (focal epithelial hyperplasia)	Lesions grow rapidly and spread

(Continued)

TABLE 36-1 Vesicular, bullous, or ulcerative lesions of the oral mucosa (continued)

Condition	Usual location	Clinical features	Course
VIRAL DISEASES			
Herpangina (coxsackievirus A; also possibly coxsackievirus B and echovirus)	Oral mucosa, pharynx, tongue	Sudden onset of fever, sore throat, and oropharyngeal vesicles, usually in children under 4 years, during summer months; diffuse pharyngeal congestion and vesicles (1–2 mm), grayish white surrounded by red areola; vesicles enlarge and ulcerate	Incubation period 2–9 days; fever for 1–4 days; recovery uneventful
Hand, foot, and mouth disease (type A coxsackieviruses)	Oral mucosa, pharynx, palms, and soles	Fever, malaise, headache with oropharyngeal vesicles which become painful, shallow ulcers	Incubation period 2–18 days; lesions heal spontaneously in 2–4 weeks
Primary HIV infection	Gingiva, palate, and pharynx	Acute gingivitis and oropharyngeal ulceration, associated with febrile illness resembling mononucleosis and including lymphadenopathy	Followed by HIV seroconversion, asymptomatic HIV infection and usually ultimately by HIV disease
BACTERIAL OR FUNGAL DISEASES			
Acute necrotizing ulcerative gingivitis ("trench mouth," Vincent's infection)	Gingiva	Painful, bleeding gingiva characterized by necrosis and ulceration of gingival papillae and margins plus lymphadenopathy and foul odor	Continued destruction of tissue followed by remission, but may recur
Prenatal (congenital) syphilis	Palate, jaws, tongue, and teeth	Gummatous involvement of palate, jaws, and facial bones; Hutchinson's incisors, mulberry molars, glossitis, mucous patches, and fissures of corners of mouth	Tooth deformities in permanent dentition irreversible
Primary syphilis (chancre)	Lesion appears where organism enters body; may occur on lips, tongue, or tonsillar area	Small papule developing rapidly into a large, painless ulcer with indurated border; unilateral lymphadenopathy; chancre and lymph nodes containing spirochetes; serologic tests positive by third to fourth weeks	Healing of chancre in 1–2 months, followed by secondary syphilis in 6–8 weeks
Secondary syphilis	Oral mucosa frequently involved with mucous patches, primarily on palate, also at commissures of mouth	Maculopapular lesions of oral mucosa, 5–10 mm in diameter with central ulceration covered by grayish membrane; eruptions occurring on various mucosal surfaces and skin accompanied by fever, malaise, and sore throat	Lesions may persist from several weeks to a year
Tertiary syphilis	Palate and tongue	Gummatous infiltration of palate or tongue followed by ulceration and fibrosis; atrophy of tongue papillae produces characteristic bald tongue and glossitis	Gumma may destroy palate, causing complete perforation
Gonorrhea	Lesions may occur in mouth at site of inoculation or secondarily by hematogenous spread from a primary focus elsewhere	Earliest symptoms are burning or itching sensation, dryness, or heat in mouth followed by acute pain on eating or speaking; tonsils and oropharynx most frequently involved; oral tissues may be diffusely inflamed or ulcerated; saliva develops increased viscosity and fetid odor; submaxillary lymphadenopathy with fever in severe cases	Lesions may resolve with appropriate antibiotic therapy
Tuberculosis	Tongue, tonsillar area, soft palate	A solitary, irregular ulcer covered by a persistent exudate; ulcer has an undermined, firm border	Lesions may persist
Cervicofacial actinomycosis	Swellings in region of face, neck, and floor of mouth	Infection may be associated with an extraction, jaw fracture, or eruption of molar tooth; in acute form resembles an acute pyogenic abscess, but contains yellow "sulfur granules" (gram-positive mycelia and their hyphae)	Acute form may last a few weeks; chronic form lasts months or years; prognosis excellent; actinomycetes respond to antibiotics (tetracyclines or penicillin) but not to antifungal drugs
Histoplasmosis	Any area in mouth, particularly tongue, gingiva, or palate	Numerous small nodules which may ulcerate; hoarseness and dysphagia may occur because of lesions in larynx, usually associated with fever and malaise	May be fatal
Candidiasis	Any area of oral mucosa	Pseudomembranous form has white patches which are easily wiped off leaving red, bleeding, sore surface; erythematous form is flat and red; rarely, candidal leukoplakia appears as white patch in tongue which does not rub off; angular cheilitis due to *Candida* involves sore cracks and redness at angle of mouth; *Candida* seen on KOH preparation in all forms	Responds to antifungals

(Continued)

TABLE 36-1   Vesicular, bullous, or ulcerative lesions of the oral mucosa *(continued)*

Condition	Usual location	Clinical features	Course
DERMATOLOGIC DISEASES			
Mucous membrane pemphigoid	Primarily mucous membranes of the oral cavity, but may also involve the eyes, urethra, vagina, and rectum	Painful, grayish white collapsed vesicles or bullae with peripheral erythematous zone; gingival lesions desquamate, leaving ulcerated area	Protracted course with remissions and exacerbations; involvement of different sites occurs slowly; glucocorticoids may temporarily reduce symptoms but do not control the disease
Erythema multiforme (Stevens-Johnson syndrome)	Primarily the oral mucosa and skin of hands and feet	Intraoral ruptured bullae surrounded by an inflammatory area; lips may show hemorrhagic crusts; the "iris," or "target" lesion, on the skin is pathognomonic; patient may have severe signs of toxicity	Onset very rapid; condition may last 1–2 weeks; may be fatal; acute episodes respond to steroids
Pemphigus vulgaris	Oral mucosa and skin	Ruptured bullae and ulcerated oral areas; mostly in older adults	With repeated recurrence of bullae, toxicity may lead to cachexia, infection, and death within 2 years; often controllable with steroids
Lichen planus	Oral mucosa and skin	White striae in mouth; purplish nodules on skin at sites of friction; occasionally causes oral mucosal ulcers and erosive gingivitis	Protracted course, may respond to topical steroids
NEOPLASTIC DISEASES			
Squamous cell carcinoma	Any areas in mouth, most commonly on lower lip, tongue, and floor of mouth	Ulcer with elevated, indurated border; failure to heal, pain not prominent; lesions tend to arise in areas of leukoplakia or in smooth or atrophic tongue	Invades and destroys underlying tissues and may metastasize to regional lymph nodes
Acute leukemia	Gingiva	Gingival swelling and superficial ulcerations followed by hyperplasia of gingiva with extensive necrosis and hemorrhage; deep ulcers may occur elsewhere on the mucosa complicated by secondary infection	Fatal if untreated
Lymphoma	Gingiva, palate, tongue, and tonsillar area	Elevated, ulcerated area which may proliferate rapidly, giving the appearance of a traumatic inflammatory lesion; swelling of regional lymph nodes	Fatal if untreated
Metastatic tumors	Deep in jaw bone, usually in premolar-molar area of mandible	May arise from carcinoma of distant organ such as breast, lung, or kidney; advanced lesion may expand and destroy bone, loosen and spread teeth, involve inferior alveolar nerve, cause pain and numbness of lower lip	Usually fatal
OTHER CONDITIONS			
Recurrent aphthous ulcers	Anywhere on nonkeratinized oral mucosa (lips, tongue, buccal mucosa, floor of mouth, soft palate, oropharynx)	Single or clusters of painful ulcers with surrounding erythematous border; lesions may be 1–2 mm in diameter in crops (herpetiform), 1–5 mm (minor), or 5–15 mm (major)	Lesions heal in 1–2 weeks but may recur monthly or several times a year; topical steroids give symptomatic relief; systemic glucocorticoids may be needed in severe cases; a tetracycline oral suspension may decrease severity of herpetiform ulcers
Behçet's syndrome	Oral mucosa, eyes, genitalia, gut, and CNS	Multiple aphthous ulcers in mouth; inflammatory ocular changes, ulcerative lesions on genitalia; inflammatory bowel disease and CNS disease	Ulcers may persist for several weeks and heal without scarring
Traumatic ulcers	Anywhere on oral mucosa; dentures frequently responsible for ulcers in vestibule	Localized, discrete ulcerated lesion with red border; produced by accidental biting of mucosa, penetration by a foreign object, or chronic irritation by a denture	Lesions usually heal in 7–10 days when irritant is removed, unless secondarily infected

associated with Epstein-Barr virus, or EBV), are common features of HIV disease and often precede or accompany full-blown AIDS. Some, such as oral Kaposi's sarcoma and lymphoma, are diagnostic of AIDS. Oral candidiasis is easily treated with topical or systemic antifungals. These include nystatin oral pastilles, clotrimazole oral troches, nystatin vaginal tablets used orally, fluconazole, and ketoconazole. While most oral lesions of HIV disease are also found in the general population, both hairy leukoplakia and HIV-P are strongly associated with HIV infection and are seen only very rarely in other

circumstances. Only small and variable amounts of HIV can be found in saliva, but blood, tissue fluid, and gingival crevicular exudate, found in the mouth as a result of lesions or of clinical manipulation, are certainly sources of other viruses, such as herpes simplex virus (HSV) and EBV, and the same may be true for HIV.

HEMATOLOGIC AND NUTRITIONAL DISEASE Gingival bleeding, necrotic ulcers, and enlargement due to malignant infiltrates are seen in all forms of leukemia, particularly *monocytic leukemia*. In *agranulocytosis* severe oral mucosal ulcers are seen, while in

TABLE 36-2 Pigmented lesions of the oral mucosa

Condition	Usual location	Clinical features	Course
Oral melanotic macule	Any area of the mouth	Discrete or diffuse localized, brown to black macule	Remains indefinitely
Diffuse melanin pigmentation	Any area of the mouth	Diffuse pale to dark-brown pigmentation; may be physiologic (''racial'') or due to smoking	Remains indefinitely
Nevi	Any area of the mouth	Discrete, localized, brown to black pigmentation	Remains indefinitely
Malignant melanoma	Any area of the mouth	Can be flat and diffuse, painless, brown to black, or can be raised and nodular	Expands and invades early; metastasis leads to death
Addison's disease	Any area in mouth but mostly on buccal mucosa	Blotches or spots of bluish-black to dark-brown pigmentation occurring early in the disease, accompanied by diffuse pigmentation of skin; other symptoms of adrenal insufficiency	Condition controlled by steroid therapy
Peutz-Jeghers syndrome	Any area in mouth	Dark-brown spots on lips, buccal mucosa, with characteristic distribution of pigment around lips, nose, eyes, and on hands; concomitant intestinal polyposis	Pigmented lesions remain indefinitely; polyps may become malignant
Drug ingestion (tranquilizers, oral contraceptives, antimalarials)	Any area in mouth	Brown, black, or gray areas of pigmentation	Disappears following cessation of drug
Amalgam tattoo	Gingiva and mucobuccal fold	Small blue-black pigmented areas associated with embedded amalgam particles in soft tissues; these may show up on radiographs as radiopaque particles in some cases	Remains indefinitely
Heavy metal pigmentation (bismuth, mercury, lead)	Gingival margin	Thin blue-black pigmented line along gingival margin; due to prior treatment for syphilis with bismuth or mercury or to accidental absorption of lead	Long-lasting
Black hairy tongue	Dorsum of tongue	Elongation of filiform papillae of tongue, which take on a brown to black coloration	Long-lasting but may disappear spontaneously
Fordyce's ''disease''	Buccal and labial mucosa	Aggregation of numerous small yellowish spots just beneath mucosal surface; no symptoms; due to hyperplasia of sebaceous glands	Remains without apparent change indefinitely

thrombocytopenia oral petechiae, ecchymoses, and gingival bleeding occur. In *Plummer-Vinson syndrome* (see Chaps. 302 and 303), atrophy of oral mucosa, particularly the tongue papillae, causes redness and soreness as well as dysphagia. This is associated with increased susceptibility to oral cancer. A smooth tongue also can be seen in *pernicious anemia* (Chap. 304). Severe oral mucositis with ulcers, candidiasis, bacterial infections, and xerostomia complicate local radiotherapy for head and neck malignancies as well as chemotherapy for both local and other malignancies. Although now rarely seen in the United States, oral features of vitamin deficiency include oral mucositis and ulcers, glossitis, and burning sensations in the tongue (*B group vitamins*) and petechiae, gingival swelling, bleeding, and ulceration as well as loosening of teeth (*scurvy* of vitamin C deficiency).

ORAL CANCER

Oral *squamous cell carcinoma* accounts for 2 to 4 percent of malignancies in the United States (when skin carcinomas are excluded) and in most western countries but represents up to 50 percent of malignancies in India. Globally, oral cancer is fourth in incidence for men and sixth for women. The disease is age-related, occurring in those over 40 years of age and increasing in incidence with age. The male/female ratio is 3:1, but the incidence of lip and mouth cancer is decreasing in white males and increasing in black males and in females. However, both the overall incidence and death rate are fairly static. *Lip cancer* has shown significant decreases in incidence in recent years, probably because of changes in pipe-smoking habits, while *tongue cancer* has become more common. The lip is still the most common oral site for cancer, followed by tongue, floor of

mouth, and other intraoral locations. The etiology involves *tobacco* smoked in pipes, cigars, and cigarettes or chewed or ''dipped.'' The role of pipe smoking in lip cancer also may include the effects of heat and other irritants. Other factors include *alcohol*, iron deficiency (Plummer-Vinson syndrome), and deficiencies of vitamins. Evidence linking oral *syphilitic* lesions and oral *candidiasis* with oral cancer is circumstantial, but a growing body of data indicates roles for *herpes simplex virus* and *human papillomavirus*. There are no data supporting the idea that irritation from sharp teeth or dental appliances causes oral cancer.

The most common precancerous lesion in the oral cavity presents as *leukoplakia*, a white patch on the mucosa that cannot be rubbed off. Histologically, such lesions show hyperkeratosis, acanthosis, and *atypia* (*dysplasia*). Leukoplakias include homogeneous and nonhomogeneous types. The nonhomogeneous nodular leukoplakias (white nodules on a red background) have a much higher potential for malignant transformation than homogeneous leukoplakia. Recent evidence suggests that the asymptomatic red velvety lesion (*erythroplasia*) of the floor of the mouth, ventrolateral aspect of the tongue, or soft palate–anterior pillar complex is more likely to be carcinoma in situ or invasive carcinoma than is the white lesion. All chronic ulcerative lesions that fail to heal within 1 to 2 weeks should be considered potentially malignant and must be biopsied in order to make a definitive diagnosis. It is noteworthy that in their early stages intraoral squamous cell carcinomas are rarely painful, in contrast to similar-appearing inflammatory lesions.

The prognosis for patients with carcinoma of the lip is usually good, since these malignant tumors are noted sooner and apparently metastasize later. Patients with carcinoma of the tongue have a poorer prognosis, particularly if the tumor occurs more posteriorly on the tongue. Intraoral carcinomas may spread by direct invasion to the

TABLE 36-3   White lesions of oral mucosa

Condition	Usual location	Clinical features	Course
Lichen planus	Buccal mucosa, tongue, gingiva, and lips; skin	Striae, white plaques, red areas, ulcers in mouth; purplish papules on skin; may be asymptomatic, sore, or painful; lichenoid drug reactions may look similar	Protracted; responds to topical steroids
White sponge nevus	Oral mucosa, vagina, anal mucosa	Painless white thickening of epithelium; adolescent/early adult onset; familial	Benign and permanent
Smoker's leukoplakia and smokeless tobacco lesions	Any area of oral mucosa, sometimes related to location of habit	White patch that may become firm, rough, or red-fissured and ulcerated; may become sore and painful but usually painless	Occasionally premalignant; may or may not resolve on cessation of habit
Nicotinic stomatitis	Palate in pipe smokers	White nodular elevations on hard palate with central red areas	Benign; usually resolves on cessation of pipe smoking
Frictional keratosis	Any area in mouth	Elevated white lesion due to hyperkeratosis and thickening of the oral epithelium secondary to chronic irritation	Removal of irritant leads to healing in 2–3 weeks
Candidiasis ("candidosis," "moniliasis")	Any area in mouth	*Pseudomembranous type* ("thrush"): creamy white curdlike patches that reveal a raw, bleeding surface when scraped; found in sick infants, debilitated elderly patients receiving high doses of glucocorticoids or broad spectrum antibiotics, or in patients with AIDS	Responds favorably to antifungal therapy and correction of predisposing causes where possible
		Erythematous type: flat, red, sometimes sore areas, same groups of patients	Course same as for pseudomembranous type
		Candidal leukoplakia: nonremovable white thickening of epithelium due to *Candida*	Responds to prolonged antifungals
		Angular cheilitis: sore fissures at corner of mouth	Responds to topical antifungals
Hairy leukoplakia	Usually lateral tongue, rarely elsewhere on oral mucosa	White areas ranging from small and flat to extensive and "hairy"; found in HIV carriers in all risk groups for AIDS; rarely causes discomfort	Due to EBV; many patients develop AIDS; responds to high dose acyclovir but recurs
Chemical burns	Any area in mouth	White slough due to necrosis of epithelium and underlying connective tissue caused by contact with agents (e.g., aspirin) applied locally or the use of undiluted sodium perborate or hydrogen peroxide as a mouthwash; removal of slough leaves a raw, painful surface	Lesion heals in several weeks if not secondarily infected

underlying bone. Depending on the site of origin of the intraoral carcinoma, metastases usually spread to the submaxillary or cervical lymph nodes. Death may result from recurrent or uncontrollable disease above the clavicles, metastatic disease beyond the neck, treatment complications, or a second primary cancer, usually in the oral cavity or the upper parts of the gastrointestinal or respiratory tract. Metastatic tumors to the jaw may occur from carcinomas of the lung, breast, kidney, or gastrointestinal tract.

DISEASES OF THE SALIVARY GLANDS

The major and minor salivary glands can be involved in mumps, sarcoidosis, tuberculosis, lymphoma, and Sjögren's syndrome (Chap. 288). The latter may cause dry eyes and dry mouth (xerostomia) and be associated with features of connective tissue diseases, including rheumatoid arthritis or systemic lupus erythematosus. Xerostomia also may be due to medications such as diuretics, antihistamines, or tricylic antidepressants as well as therapeutic irradiation for head and neck cancer. It may cause *cervical or incisal caries* and oral candidiasis. Management includes fluoride mouth rinses and topical applications, saliva substitutes, salivary stimulation with sugarless candies, and the avoidance of sugar-containing drinks or food. Candidiasis is treated with nystatin or other antifungals. Salivary stones (*sialolithiasis*), usually in the duct of a major salivary gland, cause *sialoadenitis* with pain and swelling, often on eating. Recurrent *parotitis* without apparent cause is seen in children.

The most common neoplasm of the salivary glands is the *pleomorphic adenoma*, which is benign but will recur unless fully enucleated; malignant tumors include *mucoepidermoid carcinoma*, *adenoid cystic carcinoma*, and *adenocarcinoma*. The pleomorphic adenoma causes a firm, slowly growing mass in the parotid, palate, or cheek, whereas malignant tumors grow faster and can cause ulceration and invade nerves, producing numbness or facial paralysis.

NEUROLOGIC DISTURBANCES AND OROFACIAL PAIN

The mouth and face may be the site of pain from a number of vascular, neurologic, muscle/connective tissue, or joint conditions. Interdisciplinary diagnosis and management programs involving neurologists, restorative dentists, oral surgeons, otorhinolaryngologists, and other specialists, together with new imaging techniques to diagnose or exclude organic lesions, have begun to clarify this complex field. *Temporal arteritis* causes pain in the face, jaws, and tongue and may mimic temporomandibular joint disease. Glucocorticoids may provide relief. *Myofascial pain* is a dull, constant ache with local tenderness in the muscles of the jaws and difficulty in opening the mouth. This may be related to clenching and grinding habits (*bruxism*). *Arthralgia* of the temporomandibular joint causes local pain which may extend to the face and head. Both myofascial pain and arthralgia can be relieved with heat, rest, and anti-inflammatory agents. Displacement of the meniscus or condyle may

TABLE 36-4 Alterations of the tongue

Type of change	Clinical features

SIZE OR MORPHOLOGY CHANGES

Macroglossia	Enlarged tongue that may be part of a syndrome found in developmental conditions such as Down syndrome; may be due to tumor (hemangioma or lymphangioma), metabolic disease (such as primary amyloidosis), or endocrine disturbance (such as acromegaly or cretinism)
Fissured ("scrotal") tongue	Dorsal surface and sides of tongue covered by painless shallow or deep fissures that may collect debris and become irritated
Median rhomboid glossitis	Congenital abnormality of tongue with ovoid, denuded area in median posterior portion of the tongue; may be associated with candidiasis and may respond to antifungals

COLOR CHANGES

"Geographic" tongue (benign migratory glossitis)	Asymptomatic inflammatory condition of the tongue, with rapid loss and regrowth of filiform papillae, leading to appearance of denuded red patches "wandering" across the surface of the tongue
Hairy tongue	Elongation of filiform papillae of the medial dorsal surface area due to failure of keratin layer of the papillae to desquamate normally; brownish-black coloration may be due to staining by tobacco, food, or chromogenic organisms
"Strawberry" and "raspberry" tongue	Appearance of tongue during scarlet fever due to the hypertrophy of fungiform papillae plus changes in the filiform papillae
"Bald" tongue	Atrophy may be associated with xerostomia, pernicious anemia, iron-deficiency anemia, pellagra, or syphilis; may be accompanied by painful burning sensation; may be an expression of erythmematous candidiasis and respond to antifungals

TABLE 36-5 Causes of halitosis

I **Upper respiratory infection**
   A Bronchiectasis
   B Lung abscess
II **Oral infection**
   A Acute primary herpetic gingivostomatitis
   B Acute necrotizing ulcerative gingivitis
   C Periodontal disease
   D Caries
III **Smoking**
IV **Hepatic failure (fishy odor)**
V **Azotemia (ammoniacal or urinary odor)**
VI **Diabetic ketoacidosis (sweet, fruity odor)**

TABLE 36-6 Oral lesions of HIV disease and AIDS

I **Fungal**
   A Candidiasis
      1 Pseudomembranous
      2 Erythematous
      3 Candidal leukoplakia
      4 Angular cheilitis
   B Histoplasmosis
   C Cryptococcosis
II **Bacterial**
   A Acute necrotizing ulcerative gingivitis
   B HIV-gingivitis
   C HIV-periodontitis
   D Necrotizing stomatitis
   E Mycobacterium avium intracellulare complex and tuberculosis
   F Stomatitis due to enteric organisms
III **Viral**
   A Herpes simplex
   B Herpes zoster
   C Hairy leukoplakia
   D Warts
IV **Neoplastic**
   A Kaposi's sarcoma
   B Lymphoma
V **Other**
   A Recurrent aphthous ulcers
   B Immune thrombocytopenic purpura
   C Xerostomia
   D Salivary gland enlargement

cause pain, clenching, or locking of the mandible in the open position. The joint may become involved in *osteoarthritis* with minimal symptoms, whereas *rheumatoid arthritis* causes pain and swelling in the joint, limitation of movement, and, in the *juvenile* form, severe malocclusion in children. *Ankylosis* may occur, necessitating condylectomy (see Chap. 285).

Trigeminal neuralgia (tic douloureux) causes sudden, severe, unilateral lancinating pain initiated by touching a "trigger zone" or occurring spontaneously. Confusion with pulpal or periapical pain is common, leading to inappropriate endodontic or surgical therapy. Many cases respond to carbamazepine and phenytoin, but for a few, surgical intervention to decompress the trigeminal nerve is indicated. Similar symptoms in the distribution of the ninth cranial nerve (tongue, pharynx, soft palate) are due to *glossopharyngeal neuralgia*, which may be triggered by swallowing and may produce referred pain in the temporomandibular joint. *Postherpetic neuralgia* may follow trigeminal herpes zoster (see Chap. 380) and cause burning, aching, and long-lasting pain. *Facial palsy* is usually unilateral and may be due to trauma, surgical intervention, tumor, or infection of the seventh cranial nerve. *Bell's palsy* is a form with acute onset and unknown cause, possibly viral infection such as herpes zoster. The corner of the mouth droops, and there may be difficulty in speech, eating, and in closing the eye. The symptoms usually disappear spontaneously, but residual facial immobility and lip drooping may persist. Abnormal or reduced *taste sensation* may be due to xerostomia, disturbances of the facial and glossopharyngeal nerves or their central connections, aging, or the wearing of dentures. Disease involving the hypoglossal nerve may cause atrophy of the tongue muscles with protrusion, if bilateral, or deviation toward the affected side, if unilateral.

REFERENCES

GENCO R et al: *Contemporary Periodontics.* St. Louis, Mosby, 1989
GREENSPAN D et al: *AIDS and the Mouth.* Chicago, Year Book, 1990
LYNCH MA et al: *Burket's Oral Medicine, Diagnosis and Treatment,* 8th ed. Philadelphia, Lippincott, 1983
NEWBRUN E: *Cariology,* 3d ed. Chicago, Quintessence, 1989
WRIGHT BA et al: *Oral Cancer: Clinical and Pathological Considerations.* Boca Raton, Fla, CRC Press, 1988

37   DYSPHAGIA

RAJ K. GOYAL

Dysphagia is defined as a sensation of "sticking" or obstruction of the passage of food through the mouth, pharynx, or the esophagus. It should be distinguished from other symptoms related to swallowing. *Aphagia* signifies complete esophageal obstruction, which is usually due to bolus impaction and represents a medical emergency. *Difficulty in initiating a swallow* occurs in disorders of the voluntary phase of swallowing. Once initiated, however, swallowing is completed normally. *Odynophagia* means painful swallowing. Frequently, odynophagia and dysphagia occur together. *Globus pharyngeous* is the sensation of a lump lodged in the throat. No difficulty, however, is encountered when actual swallowing is performed. *Misdirection of food*, resulting in nasal regurgitation and laryngeal and pulmonary aspiration of food during swallowing, is characteristic of oropharyngeal dysphagia. *Phagophobia*, meaning fear of swallowing, and *refusal to swallow* may occur in hysteria, rabies, tetanus, and pharyngeal paralysis due to fear of aspiration. Painful inflammatory lesions that cause odynophagia also may cause refusal to swallow. Some patients may feel the food as it goes down the esophagus. This esophageal sensitivity is not associated with sticking of the food or obstruction, however. Similarly, the *feeling of fullness in the epigastrium* that occurs after a meal or after swallowing air should not be confused with dysphagia.

PHYSIOLOGY OF SWALLOWING   The process of swallowing begins with a voluntary (oral) phase during which a bolus of food is pushed backward into the pharynx. The bolus activates oropharyngeal sensory receptors which initiate the involuntary (pharyngeal and esophageal) phase, or deglutition reflex. The deglutition reflex is a complex series of events which serves both to propel food through the pharynx and the esophagus and to prevent its entry into the airway. At the same time as the bolus is propelled backward by the tongue, the larynx moves forward and the upper esophageal sphincter opens. As the bolus moves into the pharynx, contraction of the superior pharyngeal constrictor against the contracted soft palate initiates a peristaltic contraction that proceeds rapidly downward to move the bolus through the pharynx and the esophagus. The lower esophageal sphincter opens as the food enters the esophagus and remains open until the peristaltic contraction has swept the bolus into the stomach. Peristaltic contraction in response to a swallow involves inhibition followed by sequential contraction of muscles along the entire swallowing passage and is called *primary peristalsis*. The inhibition that precedes the peristaltic contraction is called *deglutitive inhibition*. Local distention of the esophagus due to food activates intramural reflexes in the smooth muscle and results in *secondary peristalsis*, limited to the thoracic esophagus. *Tertiary contractions* are nonperistaltic as they occur simultaneously over a long segment of the esophagus. Tertiary contractions may occur in response to a swallow or esophageal distention, or they may occur spontaneously.

PATHOPHYSIOLOGY OF DYSPHAGIA   The normal transport of an ingested bolus through the swallowing passage depends on (1) the size of the ingested bolus, (2) the luminal diameter of the swallowing passage, (3) the peristaltic contraction, and (4) deglutitive inhibition, including normal relaxation of upper and lower esophageal sphincters during swallowing. Dysphagia caused by a large bolus or luminal narrowing is called *mechanical dysphagia*, whereas dysphagia due to incoordination or weakness of peristaltic contractions or to impaired deglutitive inhibition is called *motor dysphagia*.

Mechanical dysphagia   Mechanical dysphagia could be caused by a very large food bolus, intrinsic narrowing, or extrinsic compression of the lumen. In an adult, the esophageal lumen can distend up to a diameter of 4 cm because of the elasticity of the esophageal wall. When the esophagus cannot dilate beyond 2.5 cm in diameter, dysphagia can occur, but it is always present when it cannot distend beyond 1.3 cm. Circumferential lesions produce dysphagia more consistently than do lesions that involve only a portion of circumferences of the esophageal wall, as uninvolved segments retain their distensibility. The causes of mechanical dysphagia are listed in Table 37-1. Common causes include (1) carcinoma, (2) peptic and other benign strictures, and (3) lower esophageal ring.

Motor dysphagia   Motor dysphagia may result from difficulty in initiating a swallow or abnormalities in peristalsis and deglutitive inhibition due to diseases of the esophageal striated or smooth muscle.

Diseases of the striated muscle involve the pharynx, upper esophageal sphincter, and upper part of the esophagus. The striated muscle is innervated by a somatic component of the vagus with cell bodies of the lower motor neurons located in the nucleus ambiguus. These neurons are cholinergic and excitatory and are the sole determinant of the muscle activity. Peristalsis in the striated muscle segment is due to sequential central activation of neurons innervating muscles at different levels along the esophagus. Motor dysphagia of the pharynx results from neuromuscular disorders causing muscle paralysis, simultaneous nonperistaltic contraction, or loss of opening of the upper esophageal sphincter. Loss of opening of the upper sphincter is caused by paralysis of geniohyoid and other suprahyoid muscles or loss of deglutitive inhibition of the cricopharyngeus muscle. Because each side of the pharynx is innervated by ipsilateral nerves, a lesion of motor neurons occurring only on one side leads to unilateral pharyngeal paralysis. Although lesions of striated muscle also involve the cervical part of the esophagus, the clinical manifestations of pharyngeal dysfunction usually overshadow the manifestations due to esophageal involvement.

Diseases of the smooth muscle segment involve the thoracic part of the esophagus and the lower esophageal sphincter. The smooth muscle is innervated by the parasympathetic component of the vagal preganglionic fibers and postganglionic neurons in the myenteric ganglia. These nerves exert a predominantly inhibitory influence on the lower esophageal sphincter and cause inhibition followed by contraction in the esophageal body. Peristalsis in this segment is due to neuromuscular mechanisms in the wall of the esophagus itself. Dysphagia results when the peristaltic contractions are weak or nonperistaltic or when the lower sphincter fails to open normally. Loss of contractile power occurs due to muscle weakness, as in scleroderma, or to loss of myenteric neurons, as in achalasia. The cause of nonperistaltic contractions, typically seen in diffuse esophageal spasm, is not understood. Impairment of deglutitive inhibition of the lower esophageal sphincter is associated with a defect in inhibitory nerves to the sphincter and is the major cause of dysphagia in achalasia.

The causes of motor dysphagia are also listed in Table 37-1. The important causes are pharyngeal paralysis, cricopharyngeal achalasia, scleroderma of the esophagus, achalasia, diffuse esophageal spasm and related motor disorders.

APPROACH TO THE PATIENT WITH DYSPHAGIA   History   The history can provide a correct presumptive diagnosis in over 80 percent of patients. The type of food causing dysphagia provides useful information. Difficulty only with solids implies mechanical dysphagia with a lumen that is not severely narrowed. The impacted bolus may be forced through the narrowed area by drinking liquids. In advanced obstruction, dysphagia occurs with liquids as well as solids. In contrast, motor dysphagia due to achalasia and diffuse esophageal spasm is equally affected by solids and liquids from the very onset. Patients with scleroderma have dysphagia to solids that is unrelated to posture and to liquids in the recumbent but not in the upright posture. When peptic stricture develops in these patients, dysphagia becomes more persistent.

The duration and course of dysphagia are helpful in diagnosis. Transient dysphagia of short duration may be due to an inflammatory process. Progressive dysphagia of a few weeks' to a few months' duration is suggestive of carcinoma of the esophagus. Episodic dysphagia to solids of several years' duration indicates a benign disease and is characteristic of a lower esophageal ring.

TABLE 37-1 Causes of dysphagia

Mechanical dysphagia

I Luminal
  A Large bolus
  B Foreign body
II Intrinsic narrowing
  A Inflammatory condition causing edema and swelling
    1 Stomatitis
    2 Pharyngitis, epiglottitis
    3 Esophagitis
      a Viral (herpes simplex, varicella-zoster, cytomegalovirus)
      b Bacterial
      c Fungal (candidal)
      d Mucocutaneous bullous diseases
      e Caustic, chemical, thermal injury
  B Webs and rings
    1 Pharyngeal (Plummer-Vinson syndrome)
    2 Esophageal (congenital, inflammatory)
    3 Lower esophageal mucosal ring (Schatzki ring)
  C Benign strictures
    1 Peptic
    2 Caustic and pill-induced
    3 Inflammatory (Crohn's disease, candidal, mucocutaneous lesions)
    4 Ischemic
    5 Postoperative, postirradiation
    6 Congenital
  D Malignant tumors
    1 Primary carcinoma
      a Squamous cell carcinoma
      b Adenocarcinoma
      c Carcinosarcoma
      d Pseudosarcoma
      e Lymphoma
      f Melanoma
      g Kaposi's sarcoma
    2 Metastatic carcinoma
  E Benign tumors
    1 Leiomyoma
    2 Lipoma
    3 Angioma
    4 Inflammatory fibroid polyp
    5 Epithelial papilloma
III Extrinsic compression
  A Cervical spondylitis
  B Vertebral osteophytes
  C Retropharyngeal abscess and masses
  D Enlarged thyroid gland
  E Zenker's diverticulum
  F Vascular compression
    1 Aberrant right subclavian artery
    2 Right-sided aorta
    3 Left atrial enlargement
    4 Aortic aneurysm
  G Posterior mediastinal masses
  H Pancreatic tumor, pancreatitis
  I Postvagotomy hematoma and fibrosis

Motor (neuromuscular) dysphagia

I Difficulty in initiating swallowing reflex
  A Oral lesions and paralysis of tongue
  B Oropharyngeal anesthesia
  C Lack of saliva (e.g., Sjögren's syndrome)
  D Lesions of sensory components of vagus and glossopharyngeal nerves
  E Lesions of swallowing center
II Disorders of pharyngeal and esophageal striated muscle
  A Muscle weakness
    1 Lower motor neuron lesion (bulbar paralysis)
      a Cerebrovascular accident
      b Motor neuron disease
      c Poliomyelitis, postpolio syndrome
      d Polyneuritis
      e Amyotrophic lateral sclerosis
      f Familial dysautonomia
    2 Neuromuscular
      a Myasthenia gravis
    3 Muscle disorders
      a Polymyositis
      b Dermatomyositis
      c Myopathies (myotonic dystrophy, oculopharyngeal myopathy)
  B Simultaneous onset contractions or impaired deglutitive inhibition
    1 Pharynx and upper esophagus
      a Rabies
      b Tetanus
      c Extrapyramidal tract disease
      d Upper motor neuron lesions (pseudobulbar paralysis)
    2 Upper esophageal sphincter (UES)
      a Paralysis of suprahyoid muscles (causes same as paralysis of pharyngeal musculature)
      b Cricopharyngeal achalasia
III Disorders of esophageal smooth muscle
  A Paralysis of esophageal body causing weak contractions
    1 Scleroderma and related collagen vascular diseases
    2 Hollow visceral myopathy
    3 Myotonic dystrophy
    4 Metabolic neuromyopathy (amyloid, alcohol?, diabetes?)
    5 Achalasia (classical)
  B Simultaneous-onset contractions or impaired deglutitive inhibition
    1 Esophageal body
      a Diffuse esophageal spasm
      b Achalasia (vigorous)
      c Variants of diffuse esophageal spasm
    2 Lower esophageal sphincter
      a Disorders of achalasia
        (1) Primary
        (2) Secondary
          (a) Chagas' disease
          (b) Carcinoma
          (c) Lymphoma
          (d) Neuropathic intestinal pseudoobstruction syndrome
          (e) Toxins and drugs
      b Lower esophageal muscular (contractile) ring

The localization of the site of dysphagia by the patient is helpful in determining the site of esophageal obstruction; the lesion is at or below the perceived location.

Associated symptoms provide important diagnostic clues. Nasal regurgitation and tracheobronchial aspiration with swallowing are hallmarks of pharyngeal paralysis or a tracheoesophageal fistula. Tracheobronchial aspiration unrelated to swallowing may be secondary to achalasia, a Zenker's diverticulum, or gastroesophageal reflux. Severe weight loss out of proportion to the degree of dysphagia is highly suggestive of carcinoma. When hoarseness precedes dysphagia, the primary lesion is usually in the larynx. Hoarseness following dysphagia may suggest involvement of the recurrent laryngeal nerve by extension of esophageal carcinoma beyond the walls of the esophagus. Sometimes hoarseness may be due to laryngitis secondary to gastroesophageal reflux. Association of laryngeal symptoms and dysphagia also occurs in various neuromuscular disorders. Hiccups suggest a lesion in the distal portion of the esophagus. Unilateral wheezing with dysphagia indicates a mediastinal mass involving the esophagus and a large bronchus. Chest pain with dysphagia occurs in diffuse esophageal spasm and in related motor disorders. Chest pain resembling diffuse esophageal spasms also may occur in acute aphagia due to a large bolus. A prolonged history of heartburn and reflux preceding dysphagia indicates peptic stricture. Similarly, a history of prolonged nasogastric intubation, ingestion of caustic agents, ingestion of pills without water, previous radiation therapy, or associated mucocutaneous diseases may provide the cause of esophageal stricture. If odynophagia is present, candidal or herpes esophagitis should be suspected. In patients with AIDS or other immunodeficiency states, esophagitis due to opportunistic infections such as *Candida*, herpes simplex virus, cytomegalovirus, and tumors such as Kaposi's sarcoma and lymphoma should be suspected.

Physical examination Physical examination is important in motor dysphagia due to skeletal muscle, neurologic, and oropharyngeal diseases. Signs of bulbar or pseudobulbar palsy, including dysarthria, dysphonia, ptosis, tongue atrophy, and hyperactive jaw jerk, in addition to evidence of generalized neuromuscular disease, should be carefully searched for. The neck should be examined for thyromegaly or a spinal abnormality. A careful inspection of the mouth and pharynx should disclose lesions that may cause interference with passage of food from the mouth or esophagus because of pain or obstruction. Changes in the skin and extremities may suggest a diagnosis of scleroderma and other collagen-vascular diseases, or mucocutaneous diseases such as pemphigoid or epidermolysis bullosa which may involve the esophagus. Metastatic diseases to lymph nodes and liver may be evident. Pulmonary complications of acute aspiration pneumonia or chronic aspiration may be present.

Diagnostic procedures   Dysphagia is one of the major symptoms of esophageal disease, and a cause for this symptom can invariably be determined. Therefore, all patients with dysphagia must be thoroughly investigated until a specific cause is determined. This is particularly important because the treatment depends on the underlying cause of dysphagia. Barium swallow with cineradiography, esophago-gastroscopy with biopsy and exfoliative cytology, and esophageal motility study are the main diagnostic procedures (see Chap. 251). The treatment is dependent on the cause of dysphagia.

REFERENCES

CASTELL DO (ed): *The Esophagus.* Boston, Little, Brown, 1992

ENTERLINE H, THOMPSON J: *Pathology of the Esophagus.* New York, Springer-Verlag, 1984

GOYAL RK, PATERSON WG: Esophageal motility, in *Handbook of Physiology: Gastrointestinal System I.* Bethesda, MD, American Physiological Society, 1989, pp 865–908

KRESPI YP, BLITZER A (guest eds): Aspiration and swallowing disorders. Otolaryngol Clin North Am 21:595, 1988

OTT DJ: Radiologic evaluation of esophageal dysphagia. Curr Probl Diagn Radiol 17:1, 1975

SONIES B, DALAKAS M: Dysphagia in patients with the postpolio syndrome. N Engl J Med 324:1162, 1991

TYTGAT GNJ: Dilation therapy of benign esophageal stenoses. World J Surg 13:142, 1989

WEBB WA: Management of foreign bodies of the upper gastrointestinal tract. Gastroenterology 94:204, 1988

YAMATO S et al: Role of nitric oxide in lower esophageal sphincter relaxation to swallowing. Life Sci 50:1263, 1992

38   ANOREXIA, NAUSEA, VOMITING, AND INDIGESTION

LAWRENCE S. FRIEDMAN / KURT J. ISSELBACHER

ANOREXIA

Anorexia is a loss of appetite or lack of desire to eat. It must be differentiated from specific food intolerances and early satiety, a sense of fullness after the ingestion of a small amount of food. Anorexia is a prominent symptom in a wide variety of intestinal and extraintestinal disorders but as an isolated symptom is of little specific diagnostic value.

The mechanisms whereby hunger and appetite are modified in various disease states are poorly understood. Food intake is regulated by two hypothalamic centers—a lateral "feeding center" and a ventromedial "satiety center." The latter inhibits the feeding center following a meal, leading to the sensation of satiety. The brain-gut peptide cholecystokinin (CCK) appears to have a satiety effect and may be involved in the regulation of feeding behavior.

Anorexia is commonly seen in *diseases of the gastrointestinal tract and liver.* For example, it may precede the appearance of jaundice in acute hepatitis, or it may be a prominent symptom in gastric carcinoma. In the setting of intestinal disease, anorexia should be clearly differentiated from *sitophobia* (fear of eating because of subsequent abdominal discomfort). In such circumstances, appetite may persist, but the ingestion of food is curtailed nonetheless.

Sitophobia may occur, for example, in regional enteritis (especially with partial obstruction) or in chronic mesenteric vascular insufficiency ("abdominal angina").

Anorexia also may be a prominent feature of *extraintestinal diseases.* Chronic pain from any source may lead to loss of appetite. Anorexia may be profound in severe congestive heart failure and may be a major symptom in patients with uremia, respiratory failure, and various endocrinopathies (e.g., hyperparathyroidism, Addison's disease, and panhypopituitarism). In patients with cancer, anorexia may result from anxiety, depression, pain, a decreased sense of taste and smell, the effect of the tumor on the gastrointestinal tract (e.g., partial intestinal obstruction) or liver (metastases), chemotherapeutic agents, and, possibly, the release of an anorectic substance by the tumor (possibly tumor necrosis factor). Medications such as antihypertensives, diuretics, digitalis, and narcotic analgesics may cause anorexia. Finally, anorexia often accompanies psychogenic disturbances such as depression and may result from emotional upset, boredom, or exposure to unpleasant sights, odors, or thoughts. For a discussion of anorexia nervosa, see Chap. 74.

NAUSEA AND VOMITING

Nausea and vomiting may occur independently of each other but generally are closely allied and are presumed to be mediated by the same neural pathways, so they may be considered together. *Nausea* denotes the feeling of an imminent desire to vomit, usually referred to the throat or epigastrium. *Vomiting* (or *emesis*) refers to the forceful oral expulsion of gastric contents. *Retching* denotes the labored rhythmic contraction of respiratory and abdominal musculature that frequently precedes or accompanies vomiting.

Nausea often precedes or accompanies vomiting. It is usually associated with diminished functional activity of the stomach (e.g., hypotonicity, hypoperistalsis, and hyposecretion) and altered small-intestinal motility (e.g., hypertonicity and reversed peristalsis of the duodenum). Often accompanying severe nausea is evidence of altered autonomic (especially parasympathetic) activity, such as skin pallor, increased perspiration, hypersalivation, defecation, and, occasionally, hypotension and bradycardia (vasovagal syndrome); anorexia is also usually present.

Nausea, retching, and hypersalivation frequently precede the act of vomiting, which is a highly integrated sequence of involuntary visceral and somatic motor events. The stomach plays a relatively passive role in the vomiting process, the major ejection force being provided by the abdominal musculature. With relaxation of the gastric fundus and gastroesophageal sphincter, a sharp increase in intraabdominal pressure is brought about by forceful contraction of the diaphragm and abdominal wall muscles. This, together with concomitant annular contraction of the gastric pylorus, results in the expulsion of gastric contents into the esophagus. Increased intrathoracic pressure results in the further movement of esophageal contents into the mouth. Reversal of the normal direction of esophageal peristalsis may play a role in this process. Reflex elevation of the soft palate during the vomiting act prevents the entry of the expelled material into the nasopharynx, whereas reflex closure of the glottis and inhibition of respiration help to prevent pulmonary aspiration.

Repeated emesis may have deleterious effects in a number of ways. The process of vomiting, if forceful, may lead to pressure rupture of the esophagus (Boerhaave's syndrome) or to linear mucosal (Mallory-Weiss) tears in the region of the cardioesophageal junction with resulting hematemesis. Prolonged vomiting may lead to dehydration, the loss of gastric secretions (especially hydrochloric acid) resulting in metabolic alkalosis with hypokalemia, malnutrition with various deficiency states, and dental caries. In states of central nervous system depression (e.g., coma), gastric contents may be aspirated into the lungs, with a resulting aspiration pneumonitis.

VOMITING MECHANISM   The act of vomiting is under the control of two functionally distinct medullary centers: the *vomiting center* in the dorsal portion of the lateral reticular formation and the *chemoreceptor trigger zone* in the area postrema of the floor of the fourth ventricle. The vomiting center controls and integrates the actual act of emesis. It receives afferent stimuli from the gastrointestinal tract and other parts of the body, from higher brainstem and cortical centers, especially the labyrinthine apparatus, and from the chemoreceptor trigger zone. Persons vary considerably in the threshold of their vomiting centers to different stimuli. The important efferent pathways in vomiting are the phrenic nerves (to the diaphragm), the spinal nerves (to the intercostal and abdominal musculature), and visceral efferent fibers in the vagus nerve (to the larynx, pharynx, esophagus, and stomach). The vomiting center is located near other medullary centers regulating respiratory, vasomotor, and autonomic functions that may be involved in the act of vomiting.

The chemoreceptor trigger zone by itself is incapable of mediating the act of vomiting; rather activation of this zone results in efferent impulses to the medullary vomiting center, which in turn initiates emesis. The chemoreceptor trigger zone is an emetic chemoreceptor that can be activated by a variety of stimuli or drugs, including apomorphine and other opiates, levodopa (after decarboxylation to dopamine), digitalis, bacterial toxins, radiation, and metabolic abnormalities as occur with uremia and hypoxia.

CLINICAL CLASSIFICATION Nausea and vomiting are common manifestations of many organic and functional disorders. The precise mechanisms triggering vomiting in various clinical conditions are not well understood, making classification of mechanisms difficult.

Many *acute abdominal emergencies* which lead to the "surgical abdomen" are associated with nausea and vomiting. Vomiting may be seen with inflammation of a viscus, as in acute appendicitis or acute cholecystitis, intestinal obstruction, or acute peritonitis (see Chap. 260).

Other *disorders of the alimentary tract*, including those associated with chronic indigestion (see below), are frequently accompanied by nausea and vomiting. In peptic ulcer, emesis may be either spontaneous or self-induced and may lead to relief of symptoms, particularly if antral or pyloric edema has resulted in gastric outlet obstruction. Nausea and vomiting are also prominent in patients with disordered gastrointestinal motility, including postvagotomy, diabetic, or idiopathic gastroparesis (gastric atony), other gastric "dysrhythmias" resulting from abnormal myoelectric activity, and intestinal pseudo-obstruction due to abnormal intestinal myogenic or neurogenic function. Gastroparesis may be demonstrated by gastric scanning after a radiolabeled meal or by radiography after ingestion of indigestible radiopaque solid markers. Experimentally, some patients with otherwise unexplained nausea and vomiting have been demonstrated to have accelerated ("tachygastria") or irregular ("gastric tachyarrhythmia") gastric electrical activity as measured by electrodes implanted surgically on the serosa of the stomach or placed on the abdominal surface ("electrogastrogram"). Typically, intestinal obstruction of any cause (e.g., adhesions, malignancy, hernia, volvulus) leads to vomiting, as do other disorders of the liver, pancreas, and biliary tract. Nausea and vomiting may accompany the distention and pain seen in the aerophagic syndromes (see below).

Viral, bacterial, and parasitic *infections of the intestinal tract* are typically associated with severe nausea and vomiting, often with diarrhea. *Acute systemic infections* with fever, especially in young children, are also frequently accompanied by vomiting and often by severe diarrhea. The mechanism whereby infections remote from the gastrointestinal tract produce these manifestations may relate to stimulation of the medullary chemoreceptor trigger zone by toxins or abnormal metabolites.

Central nervous system disorders which lead to increased intracranial pressure (e.g., neoplasms, encephalitis, hydrocephalus) may be accompanied by vomiting, which is often *projectile* (intensely forceful). Vertigo due to disorders of the labyrinthine apparatus, such as acute labyrinthitis and Ménière's disease, may be accompanied by vomiting with nausea and retching. Similarly, motion sickness is typically associated with anorexia, nausea, and vomiting as well as

apathy, increased salivation, cold sweating, and headache. Additionally, migraine headaches, tabetic crises, acute meningitis, and the reactive phase of hypotension with syncope may be associated with nausea and vomiting.

Nausea and vomiting may be present in *acute myocardial infarction*, especially when posterior in location or transmural in extent, and in *congestive heart failure*, perhaps in relation to congestion of the liver. The possibility that these symptoms also may be due to drugs (e.g., opiates or digitalis) should always be borne in mind in patients with cardiac disease. Nausea and vomiting are common in cancer patients, especially those who are terminally ill.

Nausea and vomiting commonly accompany several *metabolic and endocrinologic disorders*, including uremia, diabetic ketoacidosis, hypo- and hyperparathyroidism, hyperthyroid crisis, and adrenal insufficiency, especially adrenal crisis. The morning sickness of early pregnancy is another instance of nausea and vomiting possibly related to hormonal changes; the term *hyperemesis gravidarum* is applied when fluid and electrolyte disturbances or nutritional deficiency results.

The *side effects of many drugs and chemicals* include nausea and vomiting. In some cases, drugs have central emetic effects, as with digitalis, morphine, histamine, and some chemotherapeutic agents. In other cases, drug-induced gastric irritation leads to stimulation of the medullary vomiting center, as with salicylates, aminophylline, and ipecac. The ingestion of a toxin (e.g., food poisoning) also may cause acute vomiting.

Psychogenic vomiting refers to chronic or recurrent vomiting which may result from an emotional or psychological disturbance. Often patients with emotional disorders and chronic vomiting maintain a relatively normal state of nutrition because only a relatively small amount of the ingested food is vomited. In some cases regurgitation rather than vomiting may predominate, and the degree of weight loss may be out of proportion to the patient's description of the frequency and severity of vomiting. As discussed in Chap. 74, anorexia nervosa and bulimia are emotional disturbances which may be associated with vomiting and weight loss.

DIFFERENTIAL DIAGNOSIS Vomiting should be distinguished from *regurgitation*, which refers to the expulsion of food in the absence of nausea and without the abdominal diaphragmatic muscular contraction associated with vomiting. Regurgitation of esophageal contents may occur with esophageal strictures or diverticula. Regurgitation of gastric contents is generally seen in gastroesophageal reflux disease due to gastroesophageal sphincter incompetence, in pyloric spasm or obstruction due to peptic ulcer, or in gastroparesis. *Hiccups* are a distinctive sound caused by contractions of the inspiratory muscles terminated abruptly by closure of the glottis. Brief episodes of hiccups may be caused by gastric distention, a sudden change in temperature, ingestion of alcohol, excess smoking, or excitement, whereas persistent hiccups may signify a serious underlying disease, such as a structural lesion or infection of the central nervous lesion, diaphragmatic irritation by a tumor or inflammatory process, metabolic derangement, vascular lesion, intraabdominal process, or systemic infection. In addition, a variety of drugs, including barbiturates and sedatives, general anesthesia, and psychogenic factors may lead to hiccups.

The temporal relationship of vomiting to eating may be of help diagnostically. Vomiting that occurs predominantly in the morning is often seen early in pregnancy and in uremia. Alcoholic gastritis is also commonly accompanied by early-morning retching and emesis, the so-called dry heaves. Vomiting that occurs during or shortly after eating may suggest psychogenic vomiting or peptic ulcer with pylorospasm. Vomiting that occurs 4 to 6 h or longer after eating and involves the elimination of large quantities of undigested food often indicates gastric retention (e.g., pyloric obstruction, gastroparesis) or certain esophageal disorders (achalasia, Zenker's diverticulum). Vomiting that is projectile or without antecedent nausea suggests the possibility of a central nervous system lesion.

Associated symptoms also may provide diagnostic clues. For

example, vertigo and tinnitus indicate the possibility of Ménière's disease. A long history of vomiting with little or no weight loss suggests psychogenic vomiting. Relief of abdominal pain with vomiting is typical of peptic ulcer. Early satiety is typical of gastroparesis.

The character of the vomitus also offers clues to the diagnosis. If the vomitus contains large amounts of free hydrochloric acid, gastric outlet obstruction due to an ulcer or a hypersecretory state such as Zollinger-Ellison syndrome should be considered. Absence of free hydrochloric acid is more compatible with gastric malignancy. A feculent or putrid odor reflects the results of bacterial action on the intestinal contents and may occur with distal intestinal obstruction, peritonitis, or gastrocolic fistula. Bile is commonly present in gastric contents whenever vomiting is prolonged; it has no significance unless constantly present in large quantities, when it may signify an obstructing lesion below the ampulla of Vater. The presence of blood in the gastric contents usually denotes bleeding from the esophagus, stomach, or duodenum.

TREATMENT Effective therapy of nausea and vomiting usually depends on correction of the underlying cause. *Antiemetic agents* vary in their usefulness depending on the cause of the symptoms, responsiveness of the patient, and occurrence of side effects. *Antihistamines* such as dimenhydrinate and promethazine hydrochloride are effective for the control of nausea and vomiting due to motion sickness and other inner ear disturbances and may be effective in pregnancy, uremia, and postoperative vomiting; they do not act on the chemoreceptor trigger zone and are of little value in other causes of vomiting. *Anticholinergics* such as scopolamine block central muscarinic receptors in afferent pathways of the vomiting reflex and are also effective in motion sickness. *Phenothiazine* derivatives such as prochlorperazine and the structurally related butyrophenone haloperidol inhibit cerebral dopamine receptors and act principally at the chemoreceptor trigger zone. They are often ineffective for severe nausea and vomiting and have the potential for causing sedation, hypotension, and Parkinson-like effects. *Metoclopramide* is the prototype of selective dopamine antagonists called *substituted benzamides*. Metoclopramide is useful in all types of vomiting except motion sickness and inner ear dysfunction. In contrast to the phenothiazines, which have anticholinergic effects, metoclopramide has powerful peripheral cholinergic effects that enhance gastric emptying. Metoclopramide may be superior to phenothiazines in the treatment of severe nausea and vomiting and is particularly useful in the treatment of gastroparesis. The usual oral dosage is 5 to 20 mg four times daily, but intravenous doses up to 1 to 3 mg/kg, which also inhibit 5-hydroxytryptamine$_3$ receptors, may be effective as prophylaxis prior to potent chemotherapeutic agents (e.g., cisplatin). Unfortunately, neurologic side effects are frequent, including drowsiness, dystonic reactions, anxiety, insomnia, depression, parkinsonism, confusion, and a rise in prolactin level. Experimental agents (not yet licensed for use in the United States) such as *domperidone* and *cisapride* exert peripheral antiemetic effects without the central nervous system side effects of metoclopramide. *Corticosteroids* are often combined with metoclopramide to control nausea and vomiting due to cancer chemotherapy; the mechanism of action may involve inhibition of prostaglandin formation. The sedative *lorazepam* may be added to this regimen. *Tetrahydrocannabinol*, the active ingredient of marijuana, is marketed as dronabinal for the prevention of nausea and vomiting after cancer chemotherapy; the mechanism of action is unknown. *Ondansetron*, a serotonin antagonist which binds to 5-hydroxytryptamine$_3$ receptors in the chemoreceptor trigger zone and gut, is particularly effective in preventing chemotherapy-induced nausea and vomiting. The recommended dose is 0.15 mg/kg intravenously infused over 15 min and given three times 4 h apart, beginning 30 min before the start of chemotherapy. The antibiotic *erythromycin*, which binds to motilin receptors in the gut, has been shown to enhance gastric emptying in patients with gastroparesis; however, stimulation of antral contractility by erythromycin leads to abdominal cramps, nausea, and bloating and may limit its usefulness.

INDIGESTION

Indigestion, or *dyspepsia*, is a term frequently used by patients to describe a variety of symptoms generally appreciated as upper abdominal distress and often associated with the intake of food. The term is nonspecific and may not have the same meaning for the patient and physician. Thus, in approaching the patient with indigestion, it is important for the physician first to elicit a precise description of this complaint. To some patients, indigestion refers to actual abdominal pain, pressure, or heartburn. Others may use the term to describe either a vague feeling that digestion has not proceeded naturally or intolerances to specific foods exist. Still others may use it to describe belching, a feeling of excessive gas, or flatulence.

After having ascertained the patient's definition of indigestion, it is important to determine (1) the location and duration of the discomfort, (2) the temporal relation of the symptoms to the ingestion of food, and (3) the possible relation of the symptoms to the ingestion of specific types of food (e.g., milk, fatty foods) or drugs.

Indigestion may occur in association with diseases of the gastrointestinal tract or pathologic states in other organ systems. As a result of a systematic clinical and laboratory investigation, a definable pathophysiologic process sometimes can be shown to be responsible for the symptoms in a given case of indigestion. Frequently, however, a clear etiologic explanation for the patient's complaint of indigestion cannot be established, and descriptive designations are applied. For example, the term *nonulcer dyspepsia* is often used to describe ulcer-like symptoms when no ulcer is found. The term *flatulent dyspepsia* is used when belching, abdominal distention, and early satiety are prominent symptoms; the term *dysmotility-like dyspepsia* has been applied to the same constellation of symptoms. Unfortunately, these terms do not imply that the symptoms described are attributable to a particular pathogenic process. The term *functional dyspepsia* also has been used when clinical evaluation fails to reveal an explanation for indigestion. In some cases of functional dyspepsia, sophisticated testing of gastrointestinal electrical activity and manometric studies may reveal disturbances of gastrointestinal motility, although the cause-and-effect relationship between such findings and the patient's symptoms may be difficult to prove. Indeed, some patients with functional indigestion also have features of the irritable bowel syndrome, suggesting a diffuse intestinal motility disturbance (see Chap. 256).

SYNDROMES COMMONLY DESCRIBED AS INDIGESTION
Pain A careful elucidation of the pattern of pain may provide important diagnostic information. Visceral abdominal pain is mediated by visceral afferent nerves which accompany the abdominal sympathetic pathways (see Chap. 13). Visceral pain is described as dull and aching in nature, with a diffuse midline localization, or as fullness or pressure. The location of the discomfort generally corresponds to the segmental level of neural innervation of the affected organ. Abdominal visceral pain, which can be produced experimentally by artificially increasing pressure in a hollow viscus, results from distention or exaggerated muscular contraction of the viscus. Inflammation generally lowers the threshold for pain from such stimuli.

The visceral pain of indigestion should be distinguished from the sharp, localized pain patterns of many acute abdominal processes involving the peritoneum. In contrast to visceral pain, this somatic pain is mediated by cerebrospinal afferent nerves.

In view of the diffuse nature of visceral abdominal pain, the main clue to the cause comes from the *location* of the pain and the corresponding segmental level of neural innervation; however, in any given segmental region there is no way of determining which of several viscera is the source of the pain (Table 38-1). The following rules, already described in Chap. 13, are useful: *Substernal pain* of gastrointestinal origin usually arises from disorders of the esophagus or cardia of the stomach. Because pain in this area can emanate from the heart, cardiac disease must be carefully considered and excluded. *Epigastric pain* is generally of gastric, duodenal, biliary, or pancreatic origin. (The epigastrium is also a frequent location for "functional"

TABLE 38-1 Distribution of visceral pain and examples of disorders frequently involving the specific organ

Organ	Common location of pain	Examples of disorders
Esophagus	Substernum, epigastrium	Peptic esophagitis, stricture, esophageal spasm, carcinoma
Stomach	Epigastrium	Gastritis, gastric ulcer, carcinoma
Duodenum (first and second portions)	Epigastrium	Duodenal ulcer
Small intestine (excluding first and second portions of duodenum)	Periumbilical region	Infectious gastroenteritis, regional enteritis, lymphoma, intestinal obstruction
Gallbladder	Epigastrium, right upper quadrant, right upper back	Cholelithiasis, cholecystitis
Pancreas	Epigastrium, left upper quadrant, left side of back	Pancreatitis, pancreatic carcinoma
Liver	Right upper quadrant	Hepatitis, cirrhosis, passive congestion
Colon	Below umbilicus	Infectious colitis, ulcerative colitis, carcinoma, partial obstruction

pain.) As pathologic processes in the biliary tract or pancreas become more intense, pain may lateralize and localize, e.g., biliary pain to the right upper quadrant and tip of the scapula and pancreatic pain to the left upper quadrant and back. *Periumbilical pain* is generally associated with disease involving the small intestine. *Pain below the umbilicus* is often of appendiceal, colonic, or pelvic origin.

The unraveling of the *temporal relationships* of the patient's symptoms often provides additional diagnostic clues. It is important to ascertain whether the symptoms are *constant* (continually present over extended periods of time), as may occur with an infiltrating gastric carcinoma, or *intermittent*, as in acute gastritis or biliary colic. The symptoms may have a *diurnal* pattern, as in reflux esophagitis in which pain often occurs nocturnally and with recumbency. Pain that awakens the patient from a sound sleep may occur with duodenal ulcer. Occasionally symptoms are *seasonal*, as in peptic ulcer disease, in which some patients experience more discomfort in the spring and autumn than at other times.

Another helpful diagnostic feature is the relation of pain to *food ingestion*. Early postprandial symptoms may reflect esophageal disease, acute gastritis, or gastric carcinoma. Late postprandial indigestion, i.e., occurring several hours after eating, may reflect failure of the stomach to empty adequately, as in gastric outlet obstruction, gastroparesis and other disorders of gastric motility, or duodenal ulcer, in which case pain results from exposure of ulcerated mucosa to acid secreted by the stomach and unbuffered by food. Conversely, the relief of pain following ingestion of food or antacids is characteristic of duodenal ulcer and is presumably due to the neutralization of acid. Late postprandial indigestion also may result from impaired digestive and absorptive processes, as in pancreatic insufficiency.

It is important to recognize that the pain patterns and relationships to the intake of food described above are generalizations, and many cases do not conform to classic "textbook" descriptions. For example, although pain limited to the right upper quadrant is often caused by gallbladder disease, about half of patients with this condition experience only epigastric pain. Similarly, there are some patients with peptic ulcer whose pain is not relieved by food or antacids; there are other patients with functional indigestion and even gastric carcinoma whose pain improves with food or antacids.

Nonulcer dyspepsia Nonulcer dyspepsia refers to symptoms that suggest a diagnosis of peptic ulcer despite the absence of an ulcer by endoscopy or barium x-ray studies and the absence of any other demonstrable organic disorder (e.g., biliary tract disease) or evidence of the irritable bowel syndrome to account for the symptoms. Nonulcer dyspepsia is twice as common as peptic ulcer and may affect up to 20 to 30 percent of the population. The pathogenesis is poorly understood; most patients with nonulcer dyspepsia have normal gastric acid secretion, and a relation between nonulcer dyspepsia and duodenitis or duodenal ulcer has not been demonstrated. Similarly, the role of *Helicobacter pylori* and associated chronic gastritis in causing dyspeptic symptoms in persons without peptic ulcer is uncertain (see Chap. 252). A role for disordered gastroduodenal and small-intestinal motility in nonulcer dyspepsia has been suggested but requires further investigation. In contrast to peptic ulcer, nonulcer dyspepsia improves inconsistently following antacids and other standard ulcer therapy.

Heartburn Heartburn, or pyrosis, is a sensation of warmth or burning located substernally or high in the epigastrium with radiation into the neck and occasionally to the arms. Occasional heartburn is common in normal persons, but frequent and severe heartburn is generally a manifestation of esophageal dysfunction. Heartburn may result from abnormal motor activity or distention of the esophagus, reflux of acid or bile into the esophagus, or direct esophageal mucosal irritation (esophagitis).

Heartburn is most often associated with gastroesophageal reflux (see Chap. 251). In this setting, heartburn typically occurs after a large meal, with stooping or bending, or when the patient is supine. It may be accompanied by the spontaneous appearance in the mouth of fluid which may be salty ("water brash"), sour (gastric contents), or bitter and green or yellow (bile). Heartburn may arise following the ingestion of certain foods (e.g., citrus fruit juices) or drugs (e.g., alcohol and aspirin). Characteristically, heartburn is alleviated promptly, even if only temporarily, by antacids.

Heartburn also may occur in the absence of a demonstrable anatomic or physiologic condition. In this setting, it is frequently accompanied by aerophagia, which may represent an attempt by the patient to relieve discomfort, and is often attributed to psychological factors for lack of other explanations.

Food intolerance In some persons, specific foods or types of foods appear to be related to indigestion. Careful documentation of this relationship is sometimes of great help in arriving at an etiologic diagnosis.

Some foods may be poorly tolerated because of their consistency. Patients with esophageal stricture or carcinoma may tolerate liquids well but may experience discomfort, especially substernal distress, after ingesting solids (see Chaps. 37 and 251). Citrus fruits, perhaps because of their relatively low pH, and spicy foods often provoke symptoms in patients with peptic ulcer disease or peptic esophagitis. Certain foods may be tolerated poorly because of impaired intestinal digestion or absorption, as with the ingestion of fatty foods in patients with pancreatic or biliary tract disease.

Patients may have a congenital or acquired *deficiency of a specific enzyme* required for intestinal absorption of a certain nutrient. One example is the deficiency of lactase, the intestinal mucosal enzyme which catalyzes the hydrolysis of lactose. In persons who are lactase-deficient, the ingestion of milk (which contains lactose) results in abdominal cramps, distention, diarrhea, and flatulence (Chap. 254). Sucrose may lead to similar symptoms in persons with hereditary sucrase-isomaltase deficiency. Certain nutrients may lead to profound systemic effects because of *biochemical defects* in the patient that render the substances particularly hazardous, as in galactose intolerance in persons with galactosemia (see Chap. 354).

Some foods or food additives may initiate *allergic reactions*, which should be suspected when symptoms occur after ingestion of a specific food, recur on challenge testing, and are associated with other features of an allergic reaction, such as lip swelling, urticaria, angioedema, asthma, or, rarely, anaphylactic shock. Acute IgE-mediated reactions are most commonly associated with cow's milk (in infants), shellfish, wheat, eggs, nuts, and chocolate and may be confirmed by the radioallergosorbent test (RAST) in some cases. Delayed hypersensitivity reactions also may occur; may be associated with less severe symptoms, including joint and muscle pain, fatigue, serous otitis, and altered spacial perception; and are more difficult to relate to specific foods. Some foods may exert *toxic effects* on the intestine in susceptible persons (e.g., gluten in patients with celiac sprue).

In many instances we do not understand the mechanism by which indigestion is associated with the ingestion of specific foods. Thus a history of fatty food intolerance or distress after eating spicy foods is commonly obtained from patients with indigestion; however, the mechanisms leading to these symptoms in these circumstances are often unclear.

Aerophagia Patients with a complaint of *chronic, repetitive eructation* (belching) can usually be observed to precede each belch with a swallow of air, most of which passes only partway down the esophagus and is then regurgitated. Thus excessive eructation results from *aerophagia*, or air swallowing, not from excessive gas production in the stomach or the intestine. A degree of aerophagia occurs in normal persons, but some individuals gulp air excessively because of chronic anxiety, rapid eating, drinking carbonated beverages or through a straw, gum chewing, sucking on hard candy, smoking cigarettes, postnasal drip, poorly fitting dentures, or esophageal speech. Because eructation which follows aerophagia may provide temporary relief to the patient, a vicious cycle of aerophagia and eructation may ensue.

About 20 to 60 percent of intestinal gas represents swallowed air. Because nitrogen and oxygen are the only gases present in the atmosphere in appreciable concentrations, and because they are not produced in the gastrointestinal tract, their detection on chromatographic analysis of intestinal gas indicates that swallowed air is the source. Swallowed air that is not eructated passes into the stomach and intestine. Accumulation of swallowed air in the stomach may lead to postprandial fullness and pressure and the finding by x-ray of a large amount of air in the gastric fundus. This symptom complex, referred to as the *magenblase* (i.e., gastric bubble) *syndrome*, may occur when a patient lies supine after a large meal, thereby permitting gastric air to be ''trapped'' below the gastroesophageal junction by overlying fluid and unable to be eructated. Inability to eructate is also thought to underlie the ''gas-bloat'' syndrome observed after surgical repair of a hiatal hernia. Acute gastric distention by swallowed air can sometimes produce sharp pains which may mimic angina pectoris. Swallowed air which successfully passes the stomach may either produce diffuse abdominal distention or become trapped in the splenic flexure of the colon. The latter condition, or *splenic flexure syndrome*, is characterized by a sensation of left upper quadrant fullness and pressure with radiation to the left side of the chest. Relief of pain often follows defecation or the expulsion of flatus. The diagnosis is suggested by the finding of increased tympany in the extreme left lateral portion of the upper abdomen on physical examination or of large amounts of air in the splenic flexure of the colon on a plain abdominal radiograph.

Gaseousness, bloating, and flatulence Despite the widely held belief that feelings of *diffuse abdominal pain and bloating* are often caused by excessive quantities of intestinal gas, studies employing an intestinal gas wash-out technique suggest that patients complaining of excessive gas have normal volumes of intestinal gas. The primary abnormality causing functional bloating and pain in such persons appears to be a motility disturbance that causes the patient to perceive pain with an intestinal gas volume that is well tolerated by normal subjects. Alternatively, intestinal motility may be normal in such persons, but they may be excessively responsive to normal impulses arising from the intestinal tract.

A major source of intestinal gas is the fermentative action of intestinal bacteria on carbohydrates and proteins within the lumen. Normally such bacteria are limited to the colon, and the principal gases produced are carbon dioxide and hydrogen (in addition to minute quantities of odoriferous gases—indoles, skatols, and sulfur-containing compounds—which give flatus its characteristic odor). In the upper small bowel carbon dioxide is also produced when hydrochloric acid from the stomach or ingested fatty acids are neutralized by bicarbonate. (This may explain, in part, indigestion associated with fatty foods.) About one-third of adults produce appreciable quantities of methane in the colon; this appears to be a familial trait and unrelated to food ingestion.

An increase in intraluminal gas production resulting in *abdominal distention, bloating, and flatulence* occurs following the ingestion of certain foods, such as legumes and some grains, which contain significant quantities of nonabsorbable complex carbohydrates that pass into the colon where they supply gas-forming substrates for colonic bacteria. The best-studied example of this is beans, which contain oligosaccharides (stachyose and raffinose) that cannot be split by intestinal mucosal enzymes but are metabolized by colonic bacteria. Less well appreciated is that fructose, a natural or added sweetener in fruit, fruit juices, soft drinks, figs, dates, prunes, and grapes and present in oligosaccharides in onions, asparagus, and wheat, may be incompletely absorbed in the small intestine and thereby contribute to abdominal distention, bloating, and flatulence. [In contrast, intestinal absorption of fructose is more likely to be complete when fructose is mixed with glucose or ingested as sucrose (glucose-fructose).] Intestinal malabsorption of sorbitol may underlie symptoms of abdominal distention, gaseousness, and diarrhea associated with certain fruits or when sorbitol is used as a sweetener in ''sugar-free'' gums and candies or as an ''inert'' ingredient in some medications. Increased intraluminal gas production also may result from abnormal bacterial colonization of the small intestine (bacterial overgrowth syndrome) or infection with *Giardia lamblia*.

Indigestion due to extraintestinal disease A number of extraintestinal diseases may lead to indigestion. Thus indigestion may be prominent in congestive heart failure, pulmonary tuberculosis, neoplastic disease, and uremia. Also, a variety of drugs such as aspirin, nonsteroidal anti-inflammatory agents, and glucocorticoids may cause indigestion because of their ulcerogenic properties.

DIAGNOSTIC APPROACH TO THE PATIENT WITH INDIGESTION
Indigestion represents a challenging and difficult diagnostic problem because of its nonspecific nature. It is essential to obtain a clear and detailed description of the specific symptoms, particularly the patient's definition of the term *indigestion*. The nature of the distress, its frequency and time of occurrence, its relationship to meals, and the special circumstances which lead to its exacerbation or relief should be elicited. Associated intestinal symptoms such as nausea and vomiting, abnormal bowel habits, diarrhea, steatorrhea, and melena should be sought, and an assessment of nutritional status, appetite, and changes in weight should be made. A careful history also should include an assessment of the patient's general health, including the possible presence of extraintestinal disorders which may produce indigestion. A careful dietary history is essential, and asking the patient to keep a diary of foods eaten may prove revealing. Similarly, the patient's medications should be reviewed, particularly for agents that may slow gut transit such as narcotics, anticholinergics, and calcium antagonists. Psychological factors may play an etiologic or contributory role, and the presence of anxiety, depressive symptoms, or hysteria should be noted.

Physical examination rarely establishes the specific diagnosis but may be useful in detecting diseases in other organ systems which can affect intestinal function (e.g., congestive heart failure). Stools should be examined for appearance and occult blood.

Whether further diagnostic studies are indicated depends on the specific nature of the patient's complaints and the patient's age (concern about the possibility of gastrointestinal malignancy being greater in older patients). Abdominal pain may be evaluated with radiologic and imaging studies of the esophagus, stomach, small intestine, colon, pancreas, and biliary tract. Esophagogastroscopy, endoscopic cholangiopancreatography, sigmoidoscopy, or colonoscopy may be considered depending on the specific symptoms. On the other hand, in patients under age 40 with epigastric pain typical of peptic ulcer, routine diagnostic studies are unlikely to disclose serious diseases (such as gastric carcinoma) and are often in fact negative; thus an empiric trial of antacids, H-2-receptor–blocking drugs, or sucralfate may be appropriate. Esophagogastroscopy may be reserved for patients with symptoms that persist despite therapy or that recur soon after therapy is discontinued. In patients with *H. pylori* on endoscopic antral biopsy and no other explanation for indigestion, eradication of *H. pylori*, which requires treatment with bismuth subsalicylate and two oral antibiotics, is cumbersome and of uncertain value but may be considered in selected cases. In individuals complaining of excessive eructation, the simple demonstration that aerophagia reproduces the symptoms may suffice to confirm the diagnosis and hopefully break the habit. Patients complaining of excessive gas, bloating, distention, and flatulence must be questioned carefully about dietary preferences and the relation of symptoms to ingestion of specific foods. In some cases, elimination of certain foods (e.g., milk, legumes) from the diet followed by rechallenge may be confirmatory. In other cases, a more detailed assessment, including stool examination for fat and muscle fibers and for parasites such as *G. lamblia*, breath tests to detect carbohydrate malabsorption or bacterial overgrowth, esophageal manometry and ambulatory pH monitoring, measurement of the rate of gastric emptying of a solid meal, and gastrointestinal motility studies, may be desirable. When no precise explanation for gaseousness can be identified, trials of activated charcoal to reduce gaseousness associated with carbohydrate malabsorption or simethicone to alter the elasticity of gas bubbles may be considered, although their value is uncertain.

In many cases of indigestion no clear explanation is obtained, even after careful diagnostic studies and therapeutic trials. Some cases represent nonulcer dyspepsia or intestinal motility disturbances, perhaps due to subtle physiologic derangements not detectable by currently available methods. In some such instances, an empiric trial of dopamine antagonists (e.g., metoclopramide) which augment gastrointestinal motility may be beneficial. Other cases represent early stages of actual disease processes which may only be diagnosed by conventional methods at a later date. Still others are psychogenic and may respond to appropriate psychiatric measures. The ultimate evaluation of indigestion requires, therefore, the utmost in sensitivity, diligence, and concern on the part of the examining physician.

REFERENCES

FELDMAN M: Nausea and vomiting, in *Gastrointestinal Disease*, 4th ed, MH Sleisenger, JS Fordtran (eds). Philadelphia, Saunders, 1989, pp 222–238

HANSON JS, MCCALLUM RW: The diagnosis and management of nausea and vomiting. Am J Gastroenterol 80:210, 1985

HEALTH AND PUBLIC POLICY COMMITTEE, AMERICAN COLLEGE OF PHYSICIANS: Endoscopy in the evaluation of dyspepsia. Ann Intern Med 102:266, 1985

LEVITT MD, BOND JH: Intestinal gas, in *Gastrointestinal Disease*, 4th ed, MH Sleisenger, JS Fordtran (eds). Philadelphia, Saunders, 1989, pp 257–263

MITCHELSON F: Pharmacologic agents affecting emesis: A review (part I). Drugs 43:295, 1992

OUYANG A: Approach to the patient with nausea and vomiting, in *Textbook of Gastroenterology*, T Yamada et al (eds). Philadelphia, Lippincott, 1991, pp 647–659

PERMAN JA, SALTZBERG DM: Approach to the patient with gas and bloating, in *Textbook of Gastroenterology*, T Yamada et al (eds). Philadelphia, Lippincott, 1991, pp 681–692

TALLEY NJ: Non-ulcer dyspepsia: Myths and realities. Aliment Pharmacol Ther 5(suppl 1):145, 1991

TYTGAT GNJ et al (eds): Towards understanding dyspepsia: An update and concensus from an International Working Party. Scand J Gastroenterol 26(suppl 182):1, 1991

39 DIARRHEA AND CONSTIPATION

LAWRENCE S. FRIEDMAN / KURT J. ISSELBACHER

NORMAL INTESTINAL FUNCTION

INTESTINAL FLUID ABSORPTION AND SECRETION On an average day, 9 L of fluid enters the gastrointestinal tract: 2 L by direct ingestion, 1 L as saliva, 2 L as gastric juice, and 4 L as biliary, pancreatic, and small intestine secretions. On passage through the small intestine, 4 to 5 L of fluid is reabsorbed in the jejunum and 3 to 4 L in the ileum. Therefore, approximately 1 L of residual enters the colon, where an additional 800 mL is reabsorbed before passage to the rectum and evacuation. Overall, the usual amount of fluid excreted in feces is approximately 200 mL/d.

In the intestine, water absorption follows active and passive sodium (Na^+) and nutrient absorption (Fig. 39-1). In the small intestine, Na^+ is cotransported with chloride (Cl^-) and nutrients such as glucose; in the terminal ileum, Na^+ is cotransported with bile salts; and in the colon, Na^+ is absorbed via Na^+ channels and by the electroneutral NaCl absorptive mechanism used in the small intestine. The cotransport mechanisms for Na^+ and nutrient absorption depend in part on Na^+ gradients across the apical membrane of intestinal epithelial cells created by the Na^+, K^+-ATPase pump of the basolateral membrane. The most important of these clinically is an Na^+-glucose cotransport carrier in the small intestine. Absorption of glucose by this mechanism results in accumulation of glucose in the epithelial cell, followed by its movement across the basolateral membrane by a facilitated transport mechanism, while Na^+ is actively pumped across the basolateral membrane by Na^+,K^+-ATPase. The absorption of Na^+ also promotes absorption of Cl^- through a paracellular pathway. Water absorption follows passively to maintain isoosmolality in the intercellular space. Because the Na^+-glucose cotransport mechanism remains unaffected by most diarrheal diseases, administration of a glucose-salt solution is useful clinically for the management of diarrhea and dehydration of most causes.

Other cotransport mechanisms exist. An Na^+-Cl^- cotransport mechanism is thought actually to be composed of an Na^+-H^+ exchange carrier and a Cl^--HCO_3^- exchange carrier. This mechanism permits entry of both Na^+ and Cl^- into a cell in exchange for H^+ and HCO_3^-. Additional transport mechanisms have been identified for potassium (K^+), which may be absorbed in exchange for H^+, and for calcium (Ca^{2+}), the absorption of which is regulated by vitamin D and 1,25-dihydroxyvitamin D_3, parathyroid hormone, calcitonin, and a number of calcium-binding proteins.

In addition to its absorptive function, the intestine has a secretory function. Cl^- can be secreted by intestinal crypt cells via an electrogenic mechanism, with Na^+, K^+, and water following passively through tight junctions. HCO_3^- is secreted in the duodenum, other parts of the small intestine, and into the bile and pancreatic ducts. Because of the large acid load from the stomach, secreted HCO_3^- is diluted and present in relatively low concentrations. However, in the distal gut, HCO_3^- gradually becomes the predominant anion, permitting conservation of Cl^- presumably via a Cl^--HCO_3^- exchange mechanism at the apical membrane of the epithelial cells. Intracellular cyclic nucleotides and ionized calcium (Ca^{2+}) initiate and regulate active Cl^- secretion (Fig. 39-2).

COLONIC FUNCTION As in the small intestine, an Na^+ absorptive mechanism exists in the colon. Na^+ absorption is predominantly electrogenic in that the absorbed Na^+ ion is unaccompanied by cation exchange or anion cotransport. Na^+ enters colonic epithelial cells through channels in the apical membrane and is pumped out across the basolateral membrane by Na^+, K^+-ATPase.

A variety of neural and nonneural mediators regulate colonic ion transport and motility, but the precise mechanisms are not well understood. The colon and rectum are innervated by nerve fibers that

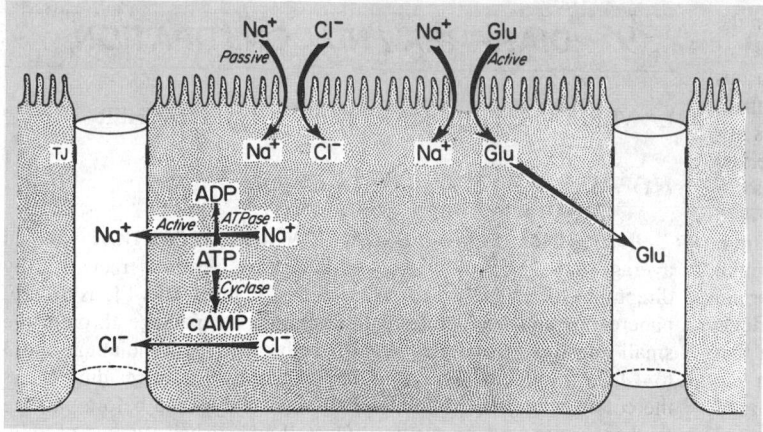

FIGURE 39-1   Sodium, chloride, and glucose transport by intestinal epithelial cells. Passive and active transport mechanisms for sodium (Na$^+$), chloride (Cl$^-$), and sodium-glucose coupled uptake are shown. Na$^+$ is pumped out at basolateral border by the active ATPase pump; Cl$^-$ in part accompanies Na$^+$ but also is actively extruded by cyclic AMP. TJ, tight junction.

release norepinephrine, acetylcholine, and other neurotransmitters. Parasympathetic nerves stimulate peristaltic contraction and electrolyte secretion, whereas adrenergic tone inhibits cholinergic stimulation and increases electrolyte absorption. Additional regulation is provided by local reflex arcs within the autonomous enteric nervous system and intrinsic contractile responses of the colonic smooth muscle.

Differences in basal motor activity of the various segments of the colon correlate with specific function. In the ascending colon, where most fluid absorption occurs, rhythmic retrograde contractions prolong fecal contact time. In the midcolon, segmental contractions continue the process of absorption, while feces is gradually advanced to the left colon. The distal colon, including the sigmoid colon and rectum, is under the greatest neurogenic control and propels feces caudally in preparation for defecation. Additionally, throughout the colon, massive peristalsis (mass movement) occurs several times a day.

DEFECATION   The defecatory reflex is initiated by acute distention of the rectum, which results in partial and transient relaxation of the internal anal sphincter via parasympathetic innervation. As sigmoid and rectal contractions increase the pressure within the rectum, the rectosigmoid angle created by tonic contraction of the puborectalis muscle, which forms a sling around the anorectal junction, is obliterated. Contraction of the external anal sphincter, which consists of at least three bundles of striated muscle surrounding the anal canal and innervated by the pudendal nerve, can delay defecation until a socially acceptable time. Concomitant relaxation of the internal and external anal sphincters then permits the evacuation of feces, which can be augmented by an increase in intraabdominal pressure created by the Valsalva maneuver.

DIARRHEA

DEFINITION   In developed countries, normal stool weight of an adult human is less than 200 g/d; stool water accounts for 60 to 85

percent of the weight. Normal bowel frequency ranges from three times a week to three times a day. Factors that influence stool weight, consistency, and frequency include the fiber content of the diet, gender (the average daily weight of stool in women is less than that of men), ingested medications, and possibly exercise and stress. *Diarrhea* is formally defined as an increase in daily stool weight above 200 g. Typically, the patient also may describe an abnormal increase in stool liquidity and frequency.

Diarrhea must be distinguished from *pseudodiarrhea* or *hyperdefecation*, which is an increased frequency of defecation without an increase in stool weight above normal, as occurs in patients with irritable bowel syndrome, proctitis, or hyperthyroidism. Diarrhea also must be distinguished from fecal *incontinence*, which is the involuntary release of rectal contents. Incontinence is more common when stool is liquid than solid and reflects abnormal function of the anorectum or pelvic muscles. Diarrhea is considered *acute* when lasting less than 7 to 14 days and *chronic* when lasting more than 2 to 3 weeks.

ACUTE DIARRHEA   The most common causes of acute diarrhea are infectious agents. Acute diarrhea also may be caused by ingested drugs or toxins, the administration of chemotherapy, resumption of enteral feeding following a prolonged fast, fecal impaction (overflow diarrhea), or particular situations, such as marathon running. Additionally, acute diarrhea may represent the onset of a chronic diarrheal illness.

Infectious diarrhea (see Chaps. 87, 102, 115, and 117 to 120) Worldwide, acute infectious diarrhea accounts for more than 4 million deaths each year in children less than age 5, especially in developing nations, where acute infectious diarrhea is a major cause of protein-calorie malnutrition and dehydration. Contributing factors include inadequate sewage disposal and water supplies, lack of refrigeration, overcrowding and lack of personal hygiene, poverty, lack of access to health care, and lack of education. Even in the United States, significant economic loss results from acute infectious diarrhea, which accounts for 250,000 hospital admissions and nearly 8 million office visits to physicians each year.

Most infectious diarrheas are acquired by fecal-oral transmission by way of water or food contaminated by human waste as a result of poor sewage systems or by wild or domestic animal feces in inadequately purified water. Beef, pork, or poultry may be the source of infection when improperly cooked. Food-preparing surfaces may be contaminated by organisms that are spread to uncooked food. Person-to-person transmission also may occur through aerosolization (Norwalk agent, rotavirus), contamination of hands (*Clostridium difficile*) or surfaces, or sexual activity.

In the United States, groups at particularly high risk of acute infectious diarrhea include travelers to or recently from developing nations, persons who ingest shellfish, male homosexuals (gay bowel syndrome), prostitutes, and intravenous drug users. Persons with AIDS in particular are at risk for a remarkable array of serious enteric infections (Table 39-1). Among children attending day-care centers, acute infectious diarrhea commonly results from person-to-person

FIGURE 39-2   Effect of increased mucosal cyclic AMP on stimulation of ion (chloride) secretion from intestinal crypt cells and inhibition of coupled Na$^+$ and Cl$^-$ absorption by intestinal villus cells.

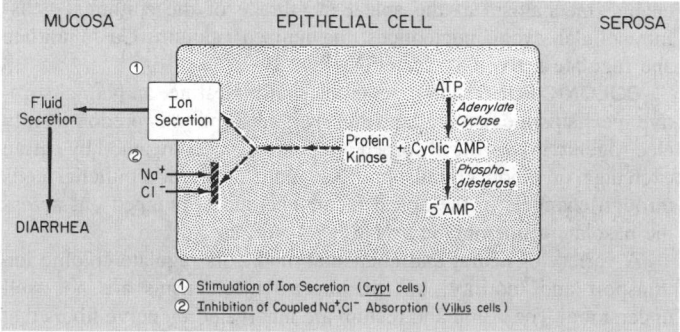

TABLE 39-1 Possible causes of diarrhea in patients with AIDS

Nonopportunistic pathogens
Shigella
Salmonella
Campylobacter
Entamoeba histolytica
Chlamydia
Neisseria gonorrhoeae
Treponema pallidum and other spirochetes
Giardia lamblia
Opportunistic infections
Protozoa
Cryptosporidium
Isospora belli
Microsporidia
Blastocystis hominis
Viruses
Cytomegalovirus
Herpes simplex
Adenovirus
Human immunodeficiency virus
Bacteria
Mycobacterium avium-intracellulare

transmission. The most common organisms involved in day-care outbreaks of diarrhea are *Shigella*, *Giardia lamblia*, and *Cryptosporidium*. Secondary attack rates ranging between 10 and 20 percent represent an important source of infection for parents and siblings. Additional high-risk institutions for outbreaks of acute infectious diarrhea include residential homes for the mentally and developmentally handicapped, nursing homes, and hospitals.

Clinical features Patients with acute infectious diarrhea typically present with nausea, vomiting, abdominal pain, fever, and diarrhea, which may be watery, malabsorptive, or bloody, depending on the cause. Patients ingesting *toxins* or those with *toxigenic infection* typically have nausea and vomiting as prominent symptoms but rarely a high fever. Abdominal pain is mild, diffuse, and crampy and results from the high volumes of secreted fluid that stimulate peristalsis and cause watery diarrhea. Vomiting that begins within several hours of ingesting a food should suggest food poisoning due to a preformed toxin. Parasites that do not invade the intestinal mucosa such as *Giardia lamblia* and *Cryptosporidium* usually cause only mild abdominal discomfort. *Giardia* also may be associated with mild steatorrhea, gaseousness, and bloating. *Invasive bacteria* such as *Campylobacter*, *Salmonella*, and *Shigella* and organisms that produce cytotoxins such as *C. difficile* and enterohemorrhagic *Escherichia coli* cause severe intestinal inflammation, abdominal pain, and often a high fever; occasionally, peritoneal signs may suggest a surgical abdomen. *Yersinia* often infects the terminal ileum and cecum and presents with right lower quadrant pain and tenderness suggestive of acute appendicitis. Watery diarrhea is typical of organisms that invade the intestinal epithelium with *minimal inflammation*, such as enteric viruses, or organisms that *adhere* to but do not destroy the epithelium, such as enteropathogenic or enteroadherent *E. coli*, protozoa, and helminths. Some organisms such as *Campylobacter*, *Aeromonas*, *Shigella*, and *Vibrio* species both produce enterotoxins and invade the intestinal mucosa, and patients therefore often present with watery diarrhea followed within hours or days by bloody diarrhea.

The presence of systemic symptoms may provide additional clues to the underlying cause of diarrhea. Both shigellosis and infection with enterohemorrhagic *E. coli* may be accompanied by the hemolytic-uremic syndrome, particularly in persons who are very young or very old. *Yersinia* infection and occasionally other enteric bacterial infections may be accompanied by Reiter's syndrome (arthritis, urethritis, and conjunctivitis), thyroiditis, pericarditis, or glomerulonephritis.

Differential diagnosis Virtually any *medication* can cause diarrhea, and a careful drug history should be obtained in any patient with acute diarrhea (Table 39-2). Other ingested toxins also must

be considered, including organophosphate insecticides, mushrooms, arsenic, and even caffeine. *Acute diverticulitis* may present with diarrhea accompanied by fever and abdominal pain. In patients with acute bloody diarrhea, diagnostic considerations may include *superior mesenteric arterial* or *venous thrombosis*, *ischemic* or *drug-induced colitis*, or *idiopathic inflammatory bowel disease* (ulcerative colitis or Crohn's disease). In the elderly patient with acute colitis, differentiating an ischemic cause from enterohemorrhagic *E. coli* may be difficult because both diseases may be associated with submucosal hemorrhage that presents as "thumbprinting" on a plain abdominal radiograph. While colonoscopic and radiographic findings may be indistinguishable in infectious colitis and idiopathic inflammatory bowel disease, histologic findings may be helpful in suggesting one diagnosis or the other, since the inflammatory infiltrate in acute infectious diarrhea consists mainly of polymorphonuclear leukocytes rather than the chronic inflammatory infiltrate with crypt distortion typical of idiopathic inflammatory bowel disease. The presence of pseudomembranes on colonoscopy points to *C. difficile* as the cause.

Laboratory diagnosis Acute infectious diarrhea is usually self-limited, often resolving by the time the patient seeks medical attention. Because of the expense of stool cultures and other diagnostic tests, considerable judgment is required in deciding which patients with acute diarrhea should be evaluated and treated with antibiotics. For the patient presenting without high fever, bloody diarrhea, or dehydration, symptomatic therapy with oral fluids in the absence of specific diagnostic testing may suffice. On the other hand, a high fever, systemic toxicity, bloody diarrhea, and dehydration favor diagnostic testing, as do a known outbreak of food poisoning, recent overseas travel, immunocomprise, male homosexuality, or recent antibiotic use. In these situations, freshly collected stool should be examined for *occult blood* and *white blood cells*. The finding of primarily polymorphonuclear leukocytes on a Wright's or methylene blue stain suggests *Salmonella*, *Shigella*, invasive *E. coli*, *Yersinia*, or *Entamoeba histolytica*. Although it is common practice to obtain a qualitative fecal fat determination in patients with acute diarrhea, the presence of a small amount of fat in the stool is not uncommon in patients with acute diarrhea of any cause and provides no particular diagnostic information. The cornerstone of diagnosis in patients with severe and especially bloody diarrhea or a suggestive epidemiologic history is *bacterial culture* and *microscopic examination* of the stool for ova and parasites. Most laboratories routinely examine stool specimens sent for culture for *Salmonella*, *Shigella*, *Yersinia*, and *Campylobacter*, but special requests must be made to identify other organisms, including *C. difficile* (culture and toxin) and enterohemorrhagic *E. coli*. Special cultivation or staining techniques also may be required to identify organisms that cause watery diarrhea, including *Aeromonas*, *Cryptosporidium*, and *Vibrio* species. Certain organisms

TABLE 39-2 Drugs that commonly cause diarrhea

Gastrointestinal drugs	**Hypolipidemic agents**
Magnesium-containing antacids	Clofibrate
Laxatives	Gemfibrozil
Misoprostol	Lovastatin
Olsalazine	Probucol
Cardiac drugs	**Neuropsychiatric drugs**
Digitalis	Lithium
Quinidine	Fluoxetine (Prozac)
Procainamide	Alprazolam (Xanax)
Hydralazine	Valproic acid
Beta blockers	Ethosuximide
Angiotensin-converting enzyme	L-Dopa
inhibitors	**Others**
Diuretics	Theophylline
Antibiotics	Thyroid hormones
Clindamycin	Colchicine
Ampicillin	Nonsteroidal anti-
Cephalosporins	inflammatory drugs
Erythromycin	
Chemotherapeutic agents	

such as *Giardia* and *Strongyloides* as well as *Cryptosporidium* and *Isospora belli* may be difficult to detect in stool and are better diagnosed by *duodenal aspiration* or intestinal biopsy. In patients with AIDS, electron microscopic examination of small intestinal biopsy specimens may facilitate detection of Microsporidia. *Sigmoidoscopy* and occasionally *colonoscopy* are generally reserved for patients with bloody diarrhea that does not improve within 10 days. As discussed above, mucosal changes may be nonspecific, although in some cases characteristic findings may be observed, such as pseudomembranes in *C. difficile*–induced colitis. *Barium radiographs* are also best deferred until the initial course of illness has been observed and appropriate stool specimens obtained. Even with the application of all available laboratory studies, between 20 and 40 percent of all acute infectious diarrheas remain undiagnosed.

Treatment   General and nonspecific treatment of acute infectious diarrhea includes rest and fluid replacement. Because death in most instances of acute diarrhea results from dehydration, careful attention must be paid to correction of fluid and electrolyte deficits. Intravenous fluid therapy may be necessary in severely dehydrated individuals, especially infants and the elderly. The use of oral sugar-electrolyte solutions, which has proved successful in the treatment of patients with cholera, also can be considered in patients with acute diarrhea due to other enterotoxin-producing bacteria. The use of antibiotic therapy in bacterial diarrheas is controversial and generally not necessary in patients with mild or resolving disease but should be considered in patients with shigellosis, traveler's diarrhea, pseudomembranous enterocolitis, cholera, and parasitic diseases. Regardless of the cause of infectious diarrhea, patients should be treated if they are immunocompromised, have a malignancy, have an abnormal heart valve or vascular or orthopedic prosthesis, have hemolytic anemia, or are extremely young or old. Anticholinergic drugs and opiates to control diarrhea should generally be avoided when an enteroinvasive organism is suspected because of the risk of prolonging colonization or causing an ileus. However, loperamide and bismuth subsalicylate have been shown to be safe in patients with traveler's diarrhea who have neither a high fever nor blood or pus in the stool.

CHRONIC DIARRHEA   Diarrhea that persists for weeks or months, whether constant or intermittent, requires evaluation. Although in the majority of cases the cause will prove to be irritable bowel syndrome, diarrhea may represent a manifestation of an underlying serious illness, and a careful search for organic disease must be undertaken. Chronic diarrhea can be categorized pathophysiologically as inflammatory diarrhea, osmotic diarrhea (malabsorption), secretory diarrhea, intestinal dysmotility, and factitious diarrhea (Table 39-3).

Inflammatory diarrhea   Inflammatory diarrheas are characterized generally by the presence of fever, abdominal tenderness, blood or leukocytes in the stool, and inflammatory lesions evident on intestinal mucosal biopsy. In some cases, hypoalbuminemia, hypoglobulinemia, and protein-losing enteropathy may be present. In addition to inflammation, the mechanism of diarrhea may include malabsorption or intestinal secretion.

In a patient who is not systemically ill, a liquid stool containing overt or occult blood raises the possibility of a *colonic neoplasm*. Patients with *ulcerative proctitis* also may present in this manner. In a patient who is systemically ill with chronic bloody diarrhea, the diagnosis of *inflammatory bowel disease* (either *ulcerative colitis* or *Crohn's disease*) is suggested. These diagnoses also should be suspected when chronic diarrhea is associated with prominent extraintestinal manifestations, including arthritis, skin lesions such as erythema nodosum or pyoderma gangrenosum, uveitis, or vasculitis. Diarrhea in inflammatory bowel disease may result from damage to absorptive surface epithelium as well as the release into the circulation of secretagogues such as leukotrienes, prostaglandins, histamine, and other cytokines which stimulate intestinal secretion or the enteric nervous system.

Inflammatory diarrhea is seen in patients with *chronic radiation enterocolitis* as a result of pelvic irradiation for malignancies of the

TABLE 39-3   Classification of chronic diarrhea

Mechanism	Clinical features	Examples
INFLAMMATORY		
Mucosal and submucosal inflammation Damaged epithelium In some cases impaired intestinal absorption and excessive secretion	Fever, abdominal pain, blood and/or leukocytes in stool	Ulcerative colitis Crohn's disease Radiation enterocolitis Eosinophilic gastroenteritis Infections associated with AIDS
OSMOTIC		
Nonabsorbed or nondigested intraluminal solute	Improvement of diarrhea with fasting Bulky, greasy, foul-smelling stools; weight loss Nutrient deficiencies Osmotic gap in fecal water	Pancreatic insufficiency Bacterial overgrowth Celiac disease Lactase deficiency Whipple's disease Abetalipoproteinemia Short bowel syndrome
SECRETORY		
Excessive secretion of electrolytes	Watery diarrhea, persists with fasting Dehydration Other systemic effects of hormones Absence of osmotic gap in fecal water	Carcinoid syndrome Zollinger-Ellison syndrome Vasoactive intestinal peptide-secreting pancreatic adenomas Medullary carcinoma of thyroid Villous adenoma of rectum Microscopic colitis Cholerrheic diarrhea
ALTERED INTESTINAL MOTILITY		
Rapid transit In some cases associated bacterial overgrowth	Alternating diarrhea and constipation Neurologic symptoms; bladder involvement	Irritable bowel syndrome Fecal impaction Neurologic diseases
FACTITIOUS		
Self-induced	Usually women Watery diarrhea with hypokalemia, weakness, edema	Laxative abuse

female urogenital tract or the male prostate. The segments usually involved are the terminal ileum, cecum, and rectosigmoid because they are fixed in the pelvis. The risk of radiation enterocolitis correlates with the radiation dose; the frequency is 1 to 5 percent with doses of 4500 to 5500 rad and 35 percent with higher doses. Chronic radiation injury is characterized by progressive swelling of the endothelial cells in small arterioles of the submucosa leading to obliterative endarteritis and vascular thrombosis and resulting in ischemia with fibrosis, bowel wall thickening, ulceration, and fissuring of the mucosa. Colonoscopy may show luminal narrowing, ulceration, diffuse inflammatory changes, and characteristic mucosal telangiectases which may bleed severely. Diarrhea also may result from bile acid malabsorption because of ileal inflammation or bacterial overgrowth resulting from intestinal strictures or stasis.

Eosinophilic gastroenteritis is characterized by infiltration of any portion of the gastrointestinal tract with eosinophils. In addition to diarrhea, patients present with abdominal pain, nausea, vomiting, weight loss, and, in 75 percent of cases, peripheral eosinophilia; some patients may develop steatorrhea and protein-losing enteropathy. Severe *protein-losing enteropathy* is manifested by peripheral edema, ascites, and occasionally anasarca. It may occur in a variety of disease states, including infections (viral gastroenteritis, bacterial overgrowth, parasitic infestation, *C. difficile* enterocolitis, or Whipple's disease), inflammatory bowel disease, lymphoma, or other conditions associated with lymphatic obstruction, such as congenital intestinal lymphangiectasia, Menetrier's disease, systemic lupus erythematosus, or milk allergy. Recently, an increasing number of infectious causes of chronic diarrhea have been associated with infection caused by the *human immunodeficiency virus* (HIV) or with AIDS (see Table 39-1). In many patients with AIDS and diarrhea, multiple potential pathogens may be present in the stool, although the exact cause of diarrhea may be uncertain because such pathogens may also be found in the stool of AIDS patients without diarrhea. HIV itself is also thought to cause diarrhea in some cases (AIDS enteropathy), but the mechanism is not understood.

Other miscellaneous diseases associated with inflammatory diarrhea include *Behçet's syndrome* and *graft-versus-host disease* following allogeneic bone marrow transplantation.

Osmotic diarrhea (see Chap. 254) Osmotic diarrhea occurs when an orally ingested solute is not fully absorbed in the small intestine and thereby exerts an osmotic force that draws fluid into the intestinal lumen. The increased luminal fluid volume overwhelms the capacity of the colon for reabsorption. The nonabsorbed solute can be a maldigested or malabsorbed nutrient or drug. Clinical symptoms are usually recognized because of the malabsorption of *fat (steatorrhea)* or *carbohydrates. Protein* or *amino acid* malabsorption (*azotorrhea*) is generally not recognized clinically unless it is severe enough to cause malnutrition or the consequences of a specific deficiency in an amino acid. The various disorders associated with malabsorption and maldigestion are discussed in more detail in other chapters, specifically, mucosal malabsorptive disorders in Chap. 254 and pancreatic exocrine deficiency and related disorders in Chap. 274.

Intraluminal maldigestion may result from *pancreatic exocrine insufficiency*, which occurs when at least 90 percent of the secretory capacity of the pancreas is lost in patients with *chronic pancreatitis* or occasionally *pancreatic ductal obstruction*. Maldigestion and weight loss occur despite preserved appetite. In children, *cystic fibrosis* may cause chronic pancreatic insufficiency. *Somatostatinoma* is a rare pancreatic islet tumor that leads to gallstones, diabetes, and steatorrhea thought to be caused by inhibition of pancreatic secretion. Intraluminal maldigestion also may result from *bile duct obstruction* as a result of cancer of the head of the pancreas or from severe liver disease with *cholestasis*. Deficiency of intraluminal bile salts usually results in only mild fat malabsorption. *Bacterial overgrowth* in a blind loop of intestine or a segment of stasis may result in steatorrhea due to deconjugation of the bile salts and impaired micelle formation; additional factors leading to diarrhea include brush border enzyme injury, mucosal inflammation, hydroxylation of fat causing fatty acid diarrhea, and altered intestinal motility.

Osmotic diarrhea may result from the chronic ingestion of certain fruits or candy, gum, dietetic foods, and medications sweetened with unabsorbed carbohydrates such as sorbitol or fructose. Congenital absence of specific brush border carbohydrate hydrolases and transport proteins also may lead to chronic diarrhea; the most common of these is lactase deficiency resulting in lactose intolerance.

The classic example of *mucosal malabsorption* is *celiac sprue*, or gluten-sensitive enteropathy (see Chap. 254). In addition to presenting with typical symptoms and signs of malabsorption, patients with celiac sprue may have atypical presentations, including failure to thrive, muscle wasting, abdominal distention, and irritability in young children, and unexplained iron deficiency anemia, growth retardation, and anorexia in adolescents or young adults. Later in life, patients may present with insidious nutritional deficiencies, infertility, and neuromuscular disease. Like celiac sprue, *tropical sprue* is characterized by malabsorption and histologic changes in the small bowel of villus atrophy, crypt hyperplasia, damaged surface epithelium, and a mononuclear infiltrate in the lamina propria. A disease affecting residents in certain tropical parts of the world, tropical sprue can occur even in visitors residing for as little as 1 to 3 months in an endemic area. The onset may be acute, suggesting an infectious etiology.

Intestinal malabsorption is typical of *Whipple's disease* due to *T. whippelii*, which usually affects middle-aged men but may present at any age and in patients of either sex. Additional manifestations include arthralgias, fever and chills, hypotension, lymphadenopathy, and involvement of the central nervous system (see Chap. 254). *Abetalipoproteinemia* is caused by the absence of Apo B resulting in defective chylomicron formation. Children with this disorder present with steatorrhea, acanthocytic red blood cells, ataxia, and retinitis pigmentosa (see Chap. 254). Steatorrhea also may result from infections with *Giardia, Isospora, Strongyloides*, and *Mycobacterium avium-intracellulare*. Ingestion of certain *drugs* may result in steatorrhea because of damage to enterocytes; examples include colchicine, neomycin, and *para*-aminosalicylic acid.

Intestinal lymphangiectasia (Chap. 254) causes protein-losing enteropathy with steatorrhea but preserved absorption of carbohydrates and is thus an example of *postmucosal obstruction of lymphatic channels*. The disease may be congenital or acquired as a result of trauma, lymphoma, carcinoma, or Whipple's disease.

Finally, extensive intestinal resection may result in the *short bowel syndrome*, in which steatorrhea results from an inadequate absorptive surface, decreased transit time, and a decreased bile salt pool. Other factors that may contribute to diarrhea in short bowel syndrome include the osmotic effect of nonabsorbed solutes, gastric hypersecretion, and in some cases bacterial overgrowth.

Secretory diarrhea Secretory diarrhea is characterized by a large volume of fecal output caused by abnormal fluid and electrolyte transport not necessarily related to the ingestion of food. Therefore, diarrhea usually persists with fasting. The term *watery diarrhea* is often used synonymously with secretory diarrhea. Because there is no malabsorbed solute, fecal osmolality in secretory diarrheas can be accounted for by normal ionic constituents with no fecal osmotic gap.

The classic examples of secretory diarrhea are those mediated by hormones (see Chaps. 252 and 276). Patients with metastatic *carcinoid tumors* of the gastrointestinal tract may have watery diarrhea as part of the carcinoid syndrome that includes episodic flushing, telangiectatic skin lesions, cyanosis, pellagra-like skin lesions, bronchospasm, and cardiac murmurs due to right-sided valvular lesions. The carcinoid syndrome results from secretion of a variety of vasoactive substances which are potent intestinal secretagogues, including serotonin, histamine, catecholamines, prostaglandin, and kinins. The *Zollinger-Ellison syndrome* is characterized by recurrent, refractory, and unusually located peptic ulcers due to a gastrinoma; diarrhea occurs in up to one-third of patients and may be the presenting symptom in 10 percent of cases. The diarrhea is not strictly secretory but is due in part to the high volumes of secreted hydrochloric acid in addition to maldigestion of fat caused by inactivation of pancreatic lipase and precipitation of bile acids at low pH. *Non-beta cell pancreatic adenomas* may secrete a variety of peptides, including vasoactive intestinal polypeptide (VIP), pancreatic polypeptide (PP), secretin, neurotensin, calcitonin, prostaglandins, and others. Those which secrete VIP may be associated with the *watery diarrhea hypokalemia achlorhydria* (WDHA) *syndrome*, characterized by often massive secretory diarrhea, achlorhydria, hypokalemia, hypomagnesemia, hypercalcemia without hyperparathyroidism, and in some cases flushing, myopathy, or nephropathy. Not all patients with WDHA syndrome have a *vipoma*, and in such cases, alternative mediators of intestinal secretion have been postulated. *Medullary carcinoma of the thyroid* (Chap. 343) may be sporadic or a feature of multiple endocrine neoplasia syndrome type IIa with pheochromocytomas and hyperparathyroidism. Watery diarrhea is thought to be mediated by calcitonin produced by the tumor, although in some cases other mediators may be found. The occurrence of diarrhea in medullary carcinoma of the thyroid is usually associated with metastases and a poor prognosis. *Systemic mastocytosis* (Chap. 254), which may be associated with the skin lesion urticaria pigmentosa, also may be associated with diarrhea that is secretory and mediated by histamine or malabsorptive and due to intestinal mucosal infiltration by mast cells.

Diarrhea associated with a *villous adenoma* (Chap. 257) of the rectum or rectosigmoid usually occurs with large tumors, often more than 3 to 4 cm in diameter. Hypokalemia due to potassium loss is common.

Microscopic or *lymphocytic colitis* and *collagenous colitis* (Chap. 255) may represent variants of the same disease. Their hallmarks are a characteristic histologic lesion despite a normal mucosal appearance on colonoscopy and diarrhea that is often secretory. In both disorders, histologic findings include infiltration of the lamina propria with inflammatory cells as well as intraepithelial lymphocytes, but only in collagenous colitis is there also a characteristic subepithelial collagen band.

Secretory diarrhea may result from *severe disease, resection, or bypass of the distal ileum* when less than 100 cm of the ileum is affected (Chap. 254). Presumably, diarrhea results from stimulation of colonic secretion by dihydroxy bile salts that escape absorption in the terminal ileum (cholerrheic diarrhea). By preventing gallbladder contraction and the delivery of large amounts of bile into the intestine, fasting eliminates this type of secretory diarrhea. When greater than 100 cm of terminal ileum is diseased or resected, hepatic synthesis cannot maintain an adequate intraluminal bile salt pool, and steatorrhea also ensues. Bile acid–induced diarrhea may occur following cholecystectomy because of the loss of the storage capacity of the gallbladder. Rarely, *primary (idiopathic) bile acid malabsorption* by the terminal ileum may account for otherwise unexplained secretory diarrhea. Rapid small intestinal transit resulting in increased delivery of bile acids to the colon also may account for *postvagotomy diarrhea*, which occurs in up to 30 percent of patients ungoing truncal vagotomy with a drainage procedure for peptic ulcer disease; diarrhea is much less common following selective or superselective vagotomy.

Altered intestinal motility Diarrhea may be associated with disorders that affect intestinal motility. The most common of these is *irritable bowel syndrome* (Chap. 256), in which typically diarrhea alternates with constipation and may be associated with abdominal pain, the passage of mucus, and a sense of incomplete evacuation. However, in some patients, constipation alone with lower abdominal cramps is the predominant clinical manifestation, while others present only with painless diarrhea presumably due to disordered intestinal motility. Diarrhea may occasionally occur paradoxically as a result of *fecal impaction* or an obstructing tumor with the overflow of liquid colonic contents around the impacted stool or obstruction. A variety of *neurologic diseases* also may be associated with diarrhea because of altered autonomic control of bowel function. Profuse watery diarrhea, often with incontinence, may be seen in young patients with *diabetes* and is often associated with severe neuropathy, nephropathy, and retinopathy. Additional contributing factors may include bacterial overgrowth secondary to intestinal dysmotility, pancreatic exocrine insufficiency, or, rarely, celiac disease. Diarrhea also may occur in patients with *traumatic neuropathy*, the *Shy-Drager syndrome*, or *lesions of the cauda equina*.

Factitious diarrhea Factitious diarrhea is self-induced by the patient and may result from intestinal infection, the addition of water or urine to the stool, or self-medication with laxatives. Patients are predominantly women with severe chronic watery diarrhea, abdominal pain, nausea and vomiting, weight loss, peripheral edema, and weakness resulting from hypokalemia. The diagnosis of factitious diarrhea should be suspected in a patient with a history of psychiatric disease or multiple previous negative evaluations for diarrhea. Additional diagnoses to consider in patients with chronic diarrhea of obscure origin are listed in Table 39-4.

History and physical examination A thorough history and physical examination are crucial initial steps in the evaluation of the patient with chronic diarrhea. The history in particular may direct the evaluation toward a general pathophysiologic mechanism or even a specific diagnosis and serves as a useful guide to the selection of a limited number of appropriate diagnostic studies.

Inflammatory diarrheas may be suggested by the presence of fever with abdominal pain, often localized to one of the lower quadrants.

TABLE 39-4   Causes of chronic diarrhea of obscure origin

Drugs (see Table 39-2)
Laxative abuse
Microscopic or collagenous colitis
Bacterial overgrowth
Carbohydrate malabsorption
Bile acid malabsorption (including after cholecystectomy and
 ileal resection)
Diabetic diarrhea
Chronic idiopathic secretory diarrhea
Fecal incontinence

Extraintestinal manifestations such as arthritis, skin lesions, or ocular symptoms suggest idiopathic inflammatory bowel disease. The presence of peripheral edema, ascites, or anasarca is compatible with protein-losing enteropathy. Intestinal malabsorption is suggested by bulky or greasy foul-smelling stools, flatulence, and weight loss. Malabsorption of specific essential nutrients may present as anemia, a bleeding tendency, osteopenia, amenorrhea, or infertility. Steatorrhea is typically more severe in pancreatic insufficiency than in intestinal mucosal disease, whereas flatulence and bloating are more typical of intestinal mucosal disease than pancreatic insufficiency because of associated carbohydrate malabsorption. Osmotic diarrhea of any cause often improves or resolves with fasting. In watery diarrheas, weight loss is unusual except in patients with advanced neuroendocrine tumors, which also may be suggested by characteristic systemic manifestations such as flushing. Symptoms of autonomic dysfunction such as postural hypotension, impotence, or disordered sweating are often found in patients with diabetic diarrhea. Diarrhea alternating with constipation is typical of the irritable bowel syndrome.

In addition to providing clues to the underlying cause of diarrhea, the physical examination is important in assessing the presence of volume depletion, as manifested by postural hypotension, tachycardia, absence of axillary sweat, decreased skin turgor, mental lethargy, and generalized weakness.

Evaluation Numerous laboratory studies may be employed in the evaluation of chronic diarrhea, but a "shotgun" approach should be avoided. The workup should be guided by the history and physical examination, and simpler investigations should be carried out before more complex diagnostic studies. In many patients it is helpful to start with routine blood studies such as a complete blood count and peripheral smear and serum electrolyte, calcium, phosphate, albumin, and quantitative immunoglobulin determinations.

Inflammatory diarrheas may be associated with leukocytosis, an elevated erythrocyte sedimentation rate, or hypoalbuminemia. The hallmark of inflammatory diarrheas is the presence of either *gross or occult blood and leukocytes* in the stool; leukocytes can be detected by a Wright's or methylene blue stain. Further evaluation usually involves *upper gastrointestinal endoscopy or colonoscopy* with diagnostic biopsies. An *upper gastrointestinal radiograph with a small bowel follow-through* also may be indicated to evaluate the small intestine. [111]*Indium-labeled white blood cell scans* may detect bowel inflammation not apparent on endoscopy or conventional barium radiography. In patients with AIDS and chronic diarrhea, multiple stool specimens for culture and examination for ova and parasites should be obtained prior to more invasive diagnostic testing.

A wide array of tests may be helpful in evaluating the patient with an osmotic diarrhea. Decreased levels of iron, folate, vitamin B_{12}, and vitamin D may suggest malabsorption. The prothrombin time may be prolonged due to vitamin K deficiency, and serum carotene, cholesterol, and albumin levels may be decreased. The cornerstone of testing for intestinal malabsorption is the measurement of *fecal fat*, which is described in detail in Chap. 254.

The capacity of the small intestine to absorb simple sugars can be assessed by the D-*xylose absorption test*, in which 25 g of this five-carbon sugar is administered orally and urine is collected for the subsequent 5 h; normally, at least 25 percent of the administered dose is excreted in the urine. The sensitivity of this test may be increased by obtaining a blood sample following the oral dose; a blood level of greater than 30 mg/dL at 2 h is normal (see Chap. 254).

The definitive test for malabsorption due to intestinal mucosal disease is the *small intestinal biopsy*, which may be performed via upper endoscopy with forceps biopsy of the distal duodenum or with a specialized small bowel biopsy instrument which reaches the jejunum. Small intestinal biopsy is generally diagnostic in diseases characterized by diffuse involvement of the small intestine such as Whipple's disease, *Mycobacterium avium-intracellulare* infection, or abetalipoproteinemia but may be falsely negative in diseases with a patchy distribution such as lymphoma, eosinophilic gastroenteritis, or amyloidosis. In celiac sprue, histologic findings may be suggestive, but the diagnosis can only be confirmed by demonstrating that the histologic lesion reverses following withdrawal of gluten from the diet.

Protein-losing enteropathy is best confirmed by assaying for α_1-*antitrypsin*, an endogenous protein, on an aliquot of lyophilized stool (Chap. 254). The most widely used test of *pancreatic function* is the *bentiromide test*, which depends on the ability of pancreatic chymotrypsin to cleave *para*-aminobenzoic acid (PABA) from the synthetic peptide *N*-benzoyl-L-tyrosyl *para*-aminobenzoic acid (bentiromide); the cleaved PABA is absorbed by the intestine, conjugated in the liver, and excreted in the urine. This and other tests of pancreatic function are discussed in Chap. 274.

The *Schilling test*, used in the evaluation of patients with suspected pernicious anemia, also can be used as a diagnostic test for pancreatic insufficiency, in which vitamin B_{12} absorption is impaired because gastric R-proteins are not cleaved from intrinsic factor as a result of diminished pancreatic proteolytic activity in the upper small intestine; vitamin B_{12} absorption improves when the test is repeated following oral administration of pancreatic enzymes.

Bacterial overgrowth may be detected by aspirating fluid from the upper small intestine through an endoscope or a small intestinal tube placed under fluoroscopic guidance and finding a *bacterial colony count* of greater than 10^5 per milliliter. Alternatively, the diagnosis of bacterial overgrowth is suggested by an increase in exhaled $^{14}CO_2$ within 60 minutes of the ingestion of 1 g ^{14}C-D-xylose (*^{14}C-xylose breath test*) or after the ingestion of ^{14}[C]cholylglycine (*bile acid breath test*) or the detection of increased breath H_2 within the first 2 h after ingestion of either glucose or rice flour (*breath hydrogen test*) (see Chap. 254).

Radiologic tests may play a diagnostic role in patients with suspected malabsorption. An abdominal radiograph may demonstrate pancreatic calcification in patients with chronic pancreatitis. *Abdominal ultrasonography*, *computed tomography*, or *endoscopic retrograde cholangiopancreatography* also may be useful in the evaluation of suspected pancreatic disease. Standard *barium radiographs* of the gastrointestinal tract may suggest thickening of the valvulae conniventes due to infiltrative disease such as Whipple's disease, lymphoma, or amyloidosis or dilatation of the small bowel with flocculation of the barium in celiac sprue. Additional relevant findings may include a gastrocolic fistula, blind loop, stricture, or multiple diverticula.

Fecal osmolality measurements may be helpful in distinguishing osmotic from secretory diarrhea when the diarrhea is watery. Measured osmolality can be compared with the calculated fecal osmolality, which is the sum of the measured Na^+ and K^+ concentrations multiplied by 2 (to account for anions). The osmotic gap is the measured fecal osmolality minus the calculated fecal osmolality and corresponds approximately to the concentration of poorly absorbed solutes in fecal water. Measured fecal osmolality should approximate plasma osmolality, which, in general, is 290 mosmol/kg H_2O. (In fact, a measured fecal osmolality greater than 300 mosmol/kg H_2O indicates bacterial degradation of nonabsorbed carbohydrate in the collection jar or the addition of urine to the jar.) A fecal osmotic gap greater than 50 mosmol/kg H_2O is significant and suggests osmotic diarrhea due to a poorly absorbed carbohydrate or excessive ingestion of magnesium-containing laxatives. If the fecal osmolality is much lower than that of the plasma (290 mosmol/kg H_2O), fluid has been added to the stool.

In patients with watery diarrhea, blood levels of *serotonin*, *gastrin*, *VIP*, *calcitonin*, and other potential secretagogues should be obtained, in addition to a *urinary 5-hydroxyindole acetic acid* (5-HIAA) level. *Flexible sigmoidoscopy* or *colonoscopy* should be considered to exclude villous adenoma of the rectum or sigmoid as well as microscopic or collagenous colitis. Colonoscopy also may reveal melanosis coli due to abuse of anthraquinone laxatives. Ingestion of phenolphthalein laxatives may be detected by *alkalinizing the stool* with either NaOH or KOH, which results in a pink or purple color. When the index of suspicion for laxative abuse is high, a cautious room search may be diagnostic.

In cases of suspected ileal bile salt malabsorption, a ^{75}*selenahomotaurocholic acid* (^{75}*SeHCAT*) test may be available in some centers. ^{75}SeHCAT acid is an analogue of taurocholic acid and is thus absorbed in the terminal ileum; scanning with a gamma camera can be used to quantitate ileal absorption and increased bile acid loss. Alternatively, a therapeutic trial of the bile salt–binding resin *cholestyramine* may be administered.

Antidiarrheal therapy While every effort should be made to identify and correct the specific cause of diarrhea, in many cases a cause that is specifically treatable may not be identifiable, and symptomatic therapy alone may be indicated. Psyllium and other hydrophilic agents absorb water and thereby enhance stool consistency. Most other available antidiarrheal agents act by altering intestinal motility; some also may have mild proabsorptive or antisecretory activity. *Opiate antidiarrheal agents* such as diphenoxylate and loperamide may be helpful in secretory diarrhea of mild to moderate severity. For patients with more severe symptoms, codeine or deodorized tincture of opium may be more successful. However, such antimotility agents may be contraindicated in diarrhea due to infectious agents because stasis may enhance tissue invasion by the organisms or delay their clearance from the bowel. In patients with severe inflammatory bowel disease, such drugs may contribute to the development of toxic megacolon and are contraindicated. *Octreotide*, a long-acting synthetic analogue of somatostatin, has a significant antisecretory effect in the carcinoid syndrome and other neuroendocrine tumors because of its specific inhibition of hormone secretion; it also may have some benefit in the short bowel syndrome. *Clonidine*, and alpha$_2$-adrenergic agonist, may be useful in the diarrhea of opiate withdrawal and diabetic diarrhea. H^+,K^+-*ATPase inhibitors*, such as omeprazole, and *H-2 receptor antagonists* are useful in the diarrhea that results from gastric hypersecretion in the Zollinger-Ellison syndrome. Other drugs that may have some benefit in the treatment of neuroendocrine tumors or unexplained secretory diarrheas include *phenothiazines* and *calcium antagonists*. *Indomethacin*, an inhibitor of prostaglandin synthesis and secretion, may have benefit in the diarrhea of medullary carcinoma of the thyroid and villous adenomas. A combination of H-1 and H-2 receptor antagonists may be helpful in treating the diarrhea of systemic mastocytosis. *Cholestyramine* is the drug of choice in diarrhea caused by ileal bile salt malabsorption.

CONSTIPATION

DEFINITION Constipation is a common complaint in clinical practice. Because of the wide range of normal bowel habits, constipation is difficult to define precisely. Most persons have at least three bowel movements per week, and *constipation* has been defined as a frequency of defecation of less than three times per week. However, stool frequency alone is not a sufficient criterion to use, because many constipated patients describe a normal frequency of defecation but subjective complaints of excessive straining, hard stools, lower abdominal fullness, and a sense of incomplete evacuation. Thus a combination of objective and subjective criteria must be used to define constipation.

CAUSES   Pathophysiologically, constipation generally results from *disordered colonic transit or anorectal function* as a result of a primary motility disturbance, certain drugs, or in association with a large number of systemic diseases that affect the gastrointestinal tract. Constipation of any cause may be exacerbated by chronic illnesses that lead to physical or mental impairment and result in inactivity or physical immobility. Additional contributing factors may include a lack of fiber in the diet, generalized muscle weakness, and possibly stress and anxiety.

In the patient presenting with the recent onset of constipation, an *obstructing lesion* of the colon should be sought. In addition to a *colonic neoplasm*, other causes of colonic obstruction include *strictures* due to colonic ischemia, diverticular disease, or inflammatory bowel disease; *foreign bodies*; or *anal strictures*. Anal sphincter spasm due to painful *hemorrhoids* or *fissures* also may inhibit the desire to evacuate.

In the absence of an obstructing lesion of the colon, *disturbed colonic motility* may mimic colonic obstruction. Disruption of parasympathetic innervation to the colon as a result of injury or lesions of the lumbosacral spine or sacral nerves may produce constipation with hypomotility, colonic dilatation, decreased rectal tone and sensation, and impaired defecation. In patients with *multiple sclerosis*, constipation may be associated with neurogenic dysfunction of other organs. Similarly, constipation may be associated with *lesions of the central nervous system* caused by parkinsonism or a cerebrovascular accident. In South America, the parasitic infection *Chagas disease* may result in constipation because of damage to myenteric plexus ganglion cells. *Hirschsprung's disease*, or aganglionosis, is characterized by absence of myenteric neurons in a segment of distal colon just proximal to the anal sphincter. This results in a segment of contracted bowel which produces obstruction and proximal dilatation. In addition, an absent rectosphincteric inhibitory reflex results in the failure of the internal anal sphincter to relax following rectal distention. Most patients with Hirschsprung's disease are diagnosed by 6 months of age, but in occasional cases symptoms are mild enough that the diagnosis may be delayed into adulthood.

Drugs that may lead to constipation include those with anticholinergic properties, such as antidepressants and antipsychotics, codeine and other narcotic analgesics, aluminum- or calcium-containing antacids, sucralfate, iron supplements, and calcium antagonists. In patients with certain endocrinopathies such as *hypothyroidism* and *diabetes mellitus*, constipation is generally mild and responsive to therapy. Rarely, life-threatening megacolon occurs in patients with myxedema. Constipation is common during *pregnancy*, presumably as a result of altered progesterone and estrogen levels which decrease intestinal transit. *Collagen vascular diseases* may be associated with constipation, which may be a particularly prominent feature of *progressive systemic sclerosis*, in which delayed intestinal transit results from atrophy and fibrosis of colonic smooth muscle.

In the large majority of patients with severe constipation, no obvious cause can be identified. In *idiopathic childhood constipation*, both psychological and physiologic factors are thought to play a role. Affected children often have slow colonic transit localized to the distal colon and rectum, and voluntary withholding behavior or abnormal anorectal function has been suggested to play a role in this disorder. Young to middle-aged women may present with severe constipation characterized by infrequent defecation, excessive straining when defecating, and unresponsiveness to fiber supplements or mild laxatives. In 70 percent of such cases, slow colonic transit (colonic inertia) may be demonstrated by the delayed passage of radiopaque markers through the proximal colon. In 30 percent of cases colonic transit is normal, and abnormalities of anorectal sensory and motor function may be demonstrated. The terms *outlet obstruction* and *anismus* have been used to describe this form of constipation, which appears to result from failed relaxation or inappropriate contraction of the puborectalis and external anal sphincter muscles. Because relaxation of these muscles involves cortical inhibition of the spinal reflex during defecation and may be modified by biofeedback, it

is speculated that such rectosphincteric dysfunction is an acquired or learned rather than an organic or neurogenic disease. Chronic straining at defecation itself may lead to descent of the perineal floor and stretching of the pudendal nerve, thus leading to an incompetent anal sphincter and fecal incontinence. Similarly, *rectal prolapse* may impair defecation as a result of rectal intussusception or chronic pudendal nerve injury. A *rectocele* is an anterior rectal herniation that may interfere with defecation by filling with feces preferentially during attempts at defecation.

Chronic idiopathic intestinal pseudo-obstruction is a rare disorder in which episodes of intestinal obstruction are unaccompanied by evidence of mechanical blockage (see Chap. 256). This disorder may be familial as a result of a neuropathy or myopathy involving the bowel and in some cases the bladder. *Idiopathic megacolon* or *megarectum* is characterized by a dilated colon or rectum, respectively, with constipation and defecatory difficulties attributed to neurogenic dysfunction.

In young to middle-aged adults, constipation is most commonly attributable to the *irritable bowel syndrome*. Unlike some of the idiopathic constipation syndromes described above, irritable bowel syndrome is typically accompanied by abdominal pain, especially in the lower abdomen, as well as by the passage of small, hard stools with a sense of incomplete evacuation and excessive straining. Patients also may complain of flatulence, abdominal bloating, heartburn, nausea, dysphagia, back pain, and genitourinary symptoms. Colonic transit is usually normal in such patients, and the precise pathophysiologic basis for the symptoms is uncertain (see Chap. 256).

HISTORY AND PHYSICAL EXAMINATION   A precise description of symptoms and their duration should be obtained. Constipation that is present from birth or early childhood is likely to be congenital in origin, whereas later onset suggests an acquired disease. A recent change in bowel habits in an adult always demands an evaluation for an obstructing neoplasm. A description of the frequency and nature of defecation should be obtained, including the presence of excessive straining, hard scybalous stools, or a sense of incomplete evacuation. The patient should be questioned about associated abdominal pain and bloating and upper gastrointestinal or genitourinary symptoms. It is especially important to obtain a history of prior laxative use and its duration. A gentle but careful assessment should be made for evidence of anxiety, emotional distress, or affective disorders and the use of mood-altering drugs.

Physical examination should be directed toward the detection of nongastrointestinal diseases that may contribute to constipation. Particular attention should be paid to the neurologic examination, including an assessment of autonomic function. The abdomen should be examined for evidence of prior surgery, bowel distention, or retained stool. A careful perineal and anorectal examination should be conducted for evidence of deformity, gluteal muscle atrophy, rectal prolapse, anal stenosis, anal fissure, rectal mass, or fecal impaction. The patient may be asked to strain to demonstrate evidence of a rectocele or rectal prolapse. The presence of an "anal wink" should be assessed by demonstrating reflex contraction of the anal canal following pinprick of the perineum. A variety of complications of constipation or its treatment also may be detected and may be the reason the patient seeks medical attention (Table 39-5).

EVALUATION   Studies of colorectal anatomy are important to exclude organic disease, although they provide little information

---

TABLE 39-5   Complications of constipation or its treatment

Hemorrhoids	Ischemic colitis
Anal fissure	Colonic volvulus
Rectal prolapse	Colonic perforation
Stercoral ulcer	Fecal incontinence
Melanosis coli	Urinary retention
Cathartic colon	Cardiac and cerebrovascular dysfunction
Fecal impaction	(e.g., syncope, arrhythmias, angina)

about colonic and anorectal function. *Flexible sigmoidoscopy or colonoscopy* may demonstrate melanosis coli as a brown-black discoloration of the bowel mucosa resulting from chronic use of anthraquinone laxatives. The absence of haustrations on endoscopy or barium enema suggests a "cathartic colon" due to laxative abuse. *Barium enema* also may demonstrate obstructing lesions of the colon, megacolon, or megarectum and in Hirschsprung's disease will show the characteristic denervated bowel segment with proximal dilatation of the colon. In such cases, rectal biopsies may be obtained to demonstrate the absence of neurons.

Studies of colonic and anorectal function should be reserved for patients with severe idiopathic constipation who fail to respond to simple therapeutic measures. In patients with a complaint of infrequent defecation, *colonic transit studies* may demonstrate colonic inertia. Radiopaque markers are ingested and their transit is monitored by serial abdominal radiographs until at least 80 percent have passed or a defined period of time has elapsed. The upper limit of normal for most adults is approximately 70 h. In patients with suspected outlet obstruction, *anorectal motility studies* provide information about rectal sensation, viscoelasticity, relaxation of the internal anal sphincter, and defecation of air-filled balloons of various sizes inserted into the rectum. For example, patients with constipation due to irritable bowel syndrome often have a low rectal compliance and tolerate rectal distention poorly, whereas those with megarectum have a very high rectal compliance. The absence of internal anal sphincter relaxation suggests Hirschsprung's disease. In some centers, anorectal manometry is supplemented by *electromyogram studies* to record external anal sphincter function and *defecography*, in which thickened barium approximating the consistency of stool is introduced into the rectum and its evacuation monitored by fluoroscopy while the patient sits on a commode.

TREATMENT   Treatment of constipation must be individualized, taking into account the duration and severity of constipation, potential contributing factors, the age of the patient, and the patient's expectations. Symptomatic therapy is quite empirical in that there is often little objective evidence to support a particular strategy. Initial therapy is usually dietary, with an emphasis on increasing dietary fiber intake. Although there is little evidence that constipated persons consume less dietary fiber than nonconstipated persons, many constipated persons do respond to increases in dietary fiber to between 20 and 30 g/d. Fiber supplementation may increase stool weight and the frequency of defecation and decrease gastrointestinal transit time. The bulking effect of fiber on stool may relate to both increased water retention and proliferation of colonic bacteria with the production of gases in the stool. Fiber supplementation is not appropriate for patients with obstructing lesions of the gastrointestinal tract or those with megacolon or megarectum.

Except for bulk laxatives, routine use of laxatives over long periods of time should be discouraged because of the risk of side effects such as lipid pneumonia due to mineral oil or damage to myenteric plexuses resulting in "cathartic colon" due to stimulant anthraquinone laxatives such as senna. *Bulk-forming laxatives* consist of natural (psyllium) or synthetic polysaccharides or cellulose derivatives that act in a manner similar to fiber. Fluid intake should be increased with the use of these preparations. *Emollient laxatives* include mineral oil, which when given orally or by enema penetrates and softens the stool, and docusate salts, which are anionic surfactants that lower the surface tension of stool to allow mixing of aqueous and fatty substances and thereby soften the stool. *Hyperosmolar agents* include mixed electrolyte solutions containing polyethylene glycol and nonabsorbable sugars such as lactulose and sorbitol, which act as osmotic agents and are used in bowel cleansing prior to colonoscopy. *Saline laxatives* contain nonabsorbable cations and anions that exert an osmotic effect to increase intraluminal water content. *Stimulant laxatives* include castor oil, anthraquinones such as senna, and diphenylmethanes such as phenolphthalein and bisacodyl. Castor oil is converted to ricinoleic acid, which stimulates intestinal secretion and increases intestinal motility. The anthraquinones increase

fluid and electrolyte accumulation in the distal ileum and colon. Phenolphthalein and bisacodyl stimulate colonic motor activity and inhibit glucose and sodium absorption. Recently, the experimental prokinetic agent cisapride has been shown to enhance intestinal transit through the proximal colon, but its role in the management of constipation is uncertain. A role for excessive endogenous opioids in constipation related to motility disorders has been hypothesized, and the benefit of opioid receptor antagonists in the treatment of constipation has been reported but requires further study. *Biofeedback* techniques have shown promise in the treatment of constipation resulting from inappropriate contraction of the pelvic floor muscles and external anal sphincter.

Surgical treatment for severe chronic constipation is generally controversial, except in Hirschsprung's disease, in which surgical resection of the aganglionic segment is the treatment of choice. In colonic inertia, subtotal colectomy with ileorectal anastomosis may be indicated in carefully selected patients in whom upper gastrointestinal motility is normal and anorectal dysmotility has been excluded. Surgery to reduce or resect a rectocele, intussusception, or prolapse should be undertaken with caution, because symptoms often are not alleviated.

REFERENCES

BERTOMEU A et al: Chronic diarrhea with normal stool and colonic examinations: Organic or functional? J Clin Gastroenterol 13:531, 1991

DANIELSSON A et al: Chronic diarrhoea after radiotherapy for gynaecological cancer: Occurrence and aetiology. Gut 32:1180, 1991

EHERER AJ, FORDTRAN JS: Fecal osmotic gap and pH in experimental diarrhea of various causes. Gastroenterology 103:545, 1992

FIELD M (ed): *Diarrheal Diseases*. New York: Elsevier, 1991

——— et al: Intestinal electrolyte transport and diarrheal disease. N Engl J Med 321:800, 1989

FINE KD, FORDTRAN JS: The effect of diarrhea on fecal fat excretion. Gastroenterology 102:1936, 1992

——— et al: Diarrhea, in *Gastrointestinal Disease: Pathophysiology, Diagnosis, Management*, MH Sleisenger, JS Fordtran (eds). Philadelphia, Saunders, 1989

GAZZARD BG: Diarrhea in human immunodeficiency virus antibody–positive patients. Semin Gastrointest Dis 2:3, 1991

GLEESON D: Acid-base transport systems in gastrointestinal epithelia. Gut 33:1134, 1992

HEATON KW et al: Defecation frequency and timing, and stool form in the general population: A prospective study. Gut 33:818, 1992

KAWIMBE BM et al: Outlet obstruction constipation (anismus) managed by biofeedback. Gut 32:1175, 1991

PEMBERTON JH et al: Evaluation and surgical treatment of severe chronic constipation. Ann Surg 214:403, 1991

POWELL DW: Approach to the patient with diarrhea, in *Textbook of Gastroenterology*, T Yamada et al (eds). Philadelphia, Lippincott, 1991

WALD A: Approach to the patient with constipation, in *Textbook of Gastroenterology*, T Yamada et al (eds). Philadelphia, Lippincott, 1991

WISTROM J et al: Empiric treatment of acute diarrheal disease with norfloxacin. Ann Intern Med 117:202, 1992

40   GAIN AND LOSS IN WEIGHT

DANIEL W. FOSTER

GENERAL PRINCIPLES   In normal persons weight is stable because food intake is matched to energy expenditure by the coordinated activity of "feeding" and "satiety" centers in the hypothalamus. The signals that regulate the interactions of these centers are multifactorial, and both short- and long-term controls are thought to be operative. Whatever the mechanisms, the system is normally efficient over periods of months to years.

Gain or loss in tissue mass is determined by the net balance between food intake and energy expenditure. Food intake is influenced by availability and attractiveness of food and by emotional and physical factors. The bulk of energy expenditure is due to basal metabolism and physical activity. The former is defined as the energy requirement when the body is in the supine position, motionless

TABLE 40-1 Percentage composition of mean daily weight loss in 13 young men during food restriction for 24 days

Days	Mean weight loss, kg/day	Water, %	Fat, %	Protein, %	Food equiv. of weight loss, kJ/kg (kcal/kg)
1–3	0.80	70	25	5	10,900 (2600)
11–13	0.23	19	69	12	29,500 (7000)
22–24	0.17	0	85	15	36,400 (8700)

SOURCE: After Brožek et al.

except for quiet respiration; it is the energy required to maintain structural and functional integrity of the body in the absence of physical activity. About half the total daily intake is normally consumed by basal processes. Nonsedentary persons spend about 40 percent of energy in physical activity; athletes may utilize 50 percent or more of ingested energy in exercise. Persons sedentary because of habit, illness, or obesity expend far less in activity. In nonobese, nonsedentary subjects 10 percent of ingested food is released as heat associated with the absorption of food, a process called *dietary thermogenesis*. This fraction, previously designated *specific dynamic action*, is usually considered a separate component of energy costs. Heat generated during and after exercise and heat released for maintenance of body temperature (*regulatory thermogenesis*) are components of the energy costs of physical activity and basal metabolism, respectively.

Change in body weight as a consequence of voluntary alteration in diet or exercise is usually not worrisome; change in weight that is not deliberately sought, on the other hand, is a frequent reason for consultation with the physician and often indicates the presence of disease. Changes in weight may reflect alteration in either tissue mass or body fluid content. Even when tissue mass is changing, fluid loss or gain plays a major role in the measured change in weight, particularly over the short run. This point is illustrated in Table 40-1, where the composition of weight loss was estimated during a 24-day period of semistarvation in 13 normal men [daily intake, 4200 kJ (1010 kcal)]. During the first 3 days 70 percent of the decrease in weight was due to water loss, while in subsequent stages weight loss was principally due to a diminution of body protein and fat. This varying contribution of fluid explains why a fixed formula cannot be used for predicting weight loss or gain. It is frequently stated that a net change of 32,000 kJ (7700 kcal) will be accompanied by a 1-kg change in body mass. While this estimate is reasonable for long-term changes in food intake, the apparent cost per kilogram of weight lost or gained varies with the accompanying fluid shifts. In the experiment summarized in Table 40-1, for example, a negative balance of only 10,900 kJ (2600 kcal) resulted in the loss of 1 kg of weight between days 1 and 3, while between days 22 and 24, loss of 1 kg of weight required a deficit of 36,400 kJ (8700 kcal). In general, if weight loss or gain occurs over a period of weeks or months, it is safe to assume that tissue mass has changed; weight loss or gain of short duration may be due to fluid shifts alone. Occasionally, true loss of tissue mass is obscured by fluid retention as in the patient with cirrhosis of the liver who develops ascites or the patient with anorexia nervosa who has edema.

WEIGHT GAIN

The diagnosis of obesity (see Chap. 73) is usually uncomplicated. Obese subjects often deny overeating, but the true situation can be assessed either by tabulating actual food intake and determining its caloric content from standard tables, by interviewing the patient's family and friends, or by estimating metabolic rates from indirect calorimetry.

Regardless of history, excess caloric intake is the usual cause of obesity. Pathologic causes are rare. In the adult, Cushing's syndrome can result in acquired obesity, but usually the diagnosis is suggested by the pattern of fat distribution and the clinical picture. Other endocrine diseases such as hypothyroidism, hypogonadism, and insulin-secreting tumors are frequently listed in the differential diagnosis of obesity but are not significant diagnostic problems. Congenital diseases that cause obesity such as the Prader-Willi, Laurence-Moon-Biedl, and Alström syndromes are also readily recognizable and appear early in life. Rarely, hypothalamic disease, such as craniopharyngioma, may cause acquired obesity. Extensive workup of the central nervous system is not indicated in obesity, however, in the absence of suspicious symptoms (headache, visual difficulties, vomiting, or endocrine changes).

WEIGHT LOSS

Weight loss in the absence of deliberate dieting is more serious than weight gain, because there is a high chance that organic disease is present. Sustained or continued weight loss in an obese person, even if dieting is in progress, should be a signal for concern, since sustained weight loss is rare in the obese. Mechanisms of pathologic weight loss include decreased food intake, accelerated metabolism, and loss of calories in urine or stool, acting singly or in combination. Almost any serious illness can cause weight loss either through direct effects or by inducing malaise and depression. The signals that cause decreased appetite and accelerated tissue loss are not known. The negative nitrogen balance that occurs following trauma, surgery, or stressful illness is likely mediated at least partially by glucagon and other catabolic hormones. Additional candidate molecules for disease-induced weight loss are cytokines such as tumor necrosis factor (cachectin) and adipsin, but proof of their involvement is lacking.

Several categories of disease need to be considered when weight loss is prominent:

DIABETES MELLITUS Initial weight loss with the onset of diabetes is largely fluid and is due to the osmotic diuresis induced by hyperglycemia. Subsequently, loss of tissue mass occurs in insulin-dependent diabetes as a result of caloric wastage (the consequence of glycosuria) and of the hormonal abnormalities that characterize the illness. Insulin deficiency and glucagon excess result in impaired synthesis of protein and fat and simultaneously cause accelerated proteolysis and lipolysis such that the net energy state is catabolic. Weight loss in diabetes is frequently associated with increased food intake.

ENDOCRINE DISEASE Hyperthyroidism usually causes weight loss. Increased appetite and food intake are the rule, and patients often consume a high-carbohydrate diet. Energy expenditure is enormous, primarily because of an increased metabolic rate and increased motor activity. The mechanism by which thyrotoxicosis causes weight loss is not settled. In rodents, thyroid hormone increases Na-K adenosine triphosphatase (ATPase) activity in many tissues resulting in a futile cycle of ATP synthesis and breakdown with energy lost as heat. This abnormality does not appear to operate in humans. Whatever the mechanism, metabolism is "uncoupled" in thyrotoxicosis, accounting for excess generation of heat and caloric wastage.

In "apathetic" hyperthyroidism, weight loss and weakness may predominate with little evidence of nervousness or other symptoms. Another endocrine cause of weight loss is pheochromocytoma, the inducing agent being catecholamine release. Panhypopituitarism and adrenal insufficiency can cause weight loss, largely as a consequence of diminished appetite secondary to cortisol deficiency.

GASTROINTESTINAL DISEASE Overt or occult steatorrhea due to sprue, chronic pancreatitis, or cystic fibrosis may produce wasting despite major increases in food intake. A variety of other diseases of the gastrointestinal tract cause weight loss: inflammatory bowel disease, parasites, esophageal strictures, obstruction secondary to chronic peptic ulcer, pernicious anemia, and cirrhosis of the liver. Mechanisms of weight loss include anorexia, obstruction with vomiting, malabsorption, and the effects of inflammation. Intraabdominal masses (e.g., massive splenomegaly) act by compressing the stomach, while weight loss in heart failure is due to visceral congestion.

INFECTION Hidden infection must always be sought in patients with unexplained weight loss. Tuberculosis, fungal disease, amebic abscess, and subacute bacterial endocarditis should be high on the list of suspects. Infection with human immunodeficiency virus must be considered, especially in high-risk groups (male homosexuals, intravenous drug users, recipients of multiple transfusions). Weight loss with infection is probably due to inflammatory cytokines.

MALIGNANCY Occult malignancy is probably the most common cause of weight loss in the absence of major signs and symptoms. In the search for malignancy, particular emphasis must be placed on the gastrointestinal tract, pancreas, and liver. Lymphoma and leukemia also should be considered. While silent (except for weight loss) malignancy can occur in any organ, the gastrointestinal tract is the most common site. Mechanisms of weight loss in cancer vary, and more than one factor is often operative. Anorexia is usually present, but increased metabolism also may play a role, particularly in lymphomas and leukemias. Tumor necrosis factor and other cytokines likely play a significant role in the weight loss of cancer.

PSYCHIATRIC DISEASE The classic psychiatric illness associated with profound weight loss is anorexia nervosa (Chap. 74). Conversion disorders, schizophrenia, and depression also may cause weight loss due to decreased food intake. In a study of weight loss in the elderly, depression was the cause as often as cancer.

RENAL DISEASE One of the earliest manifestations of uremia is anorexia. As a consequence, all patients with unexplained weight loss should be given screening renal function tests.

SUMMARY

Weight loss is more often a diagnostic problem than weight gain and more often a sign of serious organic illness. If the weight loss is associated with increased food intake, the diagnosis is likely diabetes, thyrotoxicosis, or malabsorption; less frequently, leukemias or lymphomas cause weight loss in the presence of increased food intake. If food intake is normal or decreased, malignancy, infection, renal disease, psychiatric disease, or endocrine deficiency is more likely.

REFERENCES

BEUTLER B, CERAMI A: Cachectin: More than a tumor necrosis factor. N Engl J Med 316:379, 1987

BROŽEK J et al: Changes in body weight and body dimensions in men performing work on a low calorie carbohydrate diet. J Appl Physiol 10:412, 1957

FOSTER DW: Eating disorders: Obesity and anorexia nervosa, in *Williams Textbook of Endocrinology*, 8th ed, JD Wilson, DW Foster (eds). Philadelphia, Saunders, 1992, p 1335

GARFINKEL PE et al: Differential diagnosis of emotional disorders that cause weight loss. Can Med Assoc J 129:939, 1983

MARTON KI et al: Involuntary weight loss: Diagnostic and prognostic significance. Ann Intern Med 95:568, 1981

MORLEY JE: Neuropeptide regulation of appetite and weight. Endocrine Rev 8:256, 1987

RAVUSSIN E et al: Determinants of 24-hour energy expenditure in man: Methods and results using a respiratory chamber. J Clin Inves 78:1568, 1986

ROMIJN JA, KLEIN S: One more reason for weight loss in patients with AIDS. Gastroenterology 101:861, 1991

THOMPSON MP, MORRIS LK: Unexplained weight loss in the ambulatory elderly. J Am Geriatr Soc 39:497, 1991

WILBER F: Neuropeptides, appetite regulation, and human obesity. JAMA 266:257, 1991

41 GASTROINTESTINAL BLEEDING

JAMES M. RICHTER / KURT J. ISSELBACHER

Hematemesis is defined as the vomiting of blood, and *melena* as the passage of stools rendered black and tarry by the presence of altered blood. These symptoms of gastrointestinal hemorrhage suggest a proximal source of bleeding. The color of vomited blood depends on the concentration of hydrochloric acid in the stomach and its mixture with the blood. Thus, if vomiting occurs shortly after the onset of bleeding, the vomitus appears red, and later the appearance will be dark red, brown, or black. Precipitated blood clots in the vomitus will produce a characteristic "coffee grounds" appearance. Hematemesis usually indicates bleeding proximal to the ligament of Treitz, because blood entering the gastrointestinal tract below the duodenum rarely enters the stomach.

While bleeding sufficient to produce hematemesis usually results in melena, less than half of patients with melena have hematemesis. *Melena* usually denotes bleeding from the esophagus, stomach, or duodenum, but lesions in the jejunum, ileum, and even ascending colon may cause melena provided the gastrointestinal transit time is sufficiently prolonged. Approximately 60 mL of blood is required to produce a single black stool; acute blood loss greater than this may produce melena for up to 7 days. After the stool color returns to normal, tests for occult blood may remain positive for over a week. The black color of melena results from contact of the blood with hydrochloric acid to produce hematin. Such stools are tarry ("sticky") and have a characteristic smell. This tarry consistency is in contrast to black or dark stools occurring after the ingestion of iron, bismuth, or licorice. Similarly, red stools may result from the ingestion of beets or intravenous administration of sulfobromophthalein. Gastrointestinal bleeding, even if detected only by positive tests for occult blood, indicates potentially serious disease and must be further investigated.

Hematochezia, the passage of red blood per rectum, generally signifies bleeding from a source distal to the ligament of Treitz. However, since blood must remain in the gut for approximately 8 h to produce melena, rapid hemorrhage into the esophagus, stomach, or duodenum also may result in hematochezia.

The clinical manifestations of gastrointestinal bleeding depend on the extent and rate of hemorrhage and the presence of coincidental diseases. Blood loss of less than 500 mL is rarely associated with systemic signs; exceptions include bleeding in the elderly or in the anemic patient in whom smaller amounts of blood loss may produce hemodynamic alterations. Rapid hemorrhage of greater volume results in decreased venous return to the heart, decreased cardiac output, and increased peripheral resistance due to reflex vasoconstriction (see Chap. 34). Orthostatic hypotension greater than 10 mmHg usually indicates a 20 percent or greater reduction in blood volume. Concomitant symptoms include syncope, lightheadedness, nausea, sweating, and thirst. When blood loss approaches 40 percent of blood volume, shock frequently ensues with pronounced tachycardia and hypotension. Pallor is prominent, and the skin is cool.

In the setting of rapid hemorrhage, the hematocrit may not accurately reflect the magnitude of blood loss, since equilibration with extravascular fluid and hemodilution require over 8 h. Common laboratory findings include mild leukocytosis and thrombocytosis which develop within 6 h after the onset of bleeding. The blood urea nitrogen may be elevated out of proportion to the creatinine, particularly in upper gastrointestinal bleeding, due to breakdown of blood proteins to urea by intestinal bacteria as well as from a mild reduction in the glomerular filtration rate.

Occult bleeding, detected by card test for hemoglobin peroxidase, is an important means of finding colorectal neoplasia at earlier, potentially curable stages. Testing is advocated for patients over age 40 as a part of the yearly checkup, and test kits are available for purchase by patients. The interpretation of the test is complicated by the need for examining multiple stools (usually two samples from three stools) and if positive, requires additional studies. A positive result can be due to physiologic blood loss, dietary peroxidases, or any cause of upper or lower gastrointestinal bleeding. Vitamin C ingestion over 500 mg daily may result in a false-negative test. To limit the confounding variables, patients should be tested on a high-fiber and low-meat diet with no ingestion of nonsteroidal anti-inflammatory agents or vitamin C. Quantitative and specific tests are being developed and advocated (Hemoquant) to improve the performance of fecal occult blood screening.

ETIOLOGY OF UPPER GASTROINTESTINAL BLEEDING   A careful history and physical examination of the oropharynx and nasal cavity should serve to exclude swallowed blood as a source of hematemesis or melena.

The four most common causes of upper gastrointestinal hemorrhage are (1) peptic ulceration, (2) erosive gastritis, (3) varices, and (4) esophagogastric mucosal tear. These entities account for up to 90 percent of all cases of upper gastrointestinal hemorrhage in which a definite lesion can be found.

Peptic ulcer   Peptic ulcer of the stomach or duodenum is the most common cause of upper gastrointestinal bleeding. Because hemorrhage may be the initial manifestation of a peptic ulcer, this lesion should be considered seriously even when a history characteristic of ulcer disease is not obtained.

Gastritis   Gastritis may be associated with recent alcohol ingestion or the use of anti-inflammatory drugs such as aspirin or ibuprofen (see Chap. 252). Gastric erosions also frequently develop in patients with major trauma, surgery, and severe systemic disease, particularly burn victims and patients with increased intracranial pressure. Because there are no characteristic physical findings, the diagnosis of gastritis must be suspected when the appropriate clinical setting is encountered.

Varices and portal hypertensive gastropathy   Variceal bleeding is characteristically abrupt and massive; chronic gastrointestinal blood loss is unusual. Bleeding from esophageal or gastric varices is usually the result of portal hypertension, secondary to cirrhosis. Although alcoholic cirrhosis is the most prevalent cause of esophageal varices in the United States, any condition producing portal hypertension may result in variceal bleeding. Further, while the presence of varices usually connotes long-standing portal hypertension, acute hepatitis or severe fatty infiltration of the liver may occasionally produce varices which disappear once the hepatic abnormality resolves. Although upper gastrointestinal bleeding in a patient with cirrhosis suggests a variceal source, approximately half those patients will be bleeding from peptic ulcer or portal hypertensive gastropathy. The latter results from gastric mucosal venous engorgement. Consequently, it is essential to determine the cause of bleeding so that the appropriate treatment can be instituted.

Esophagogastric mucosal tear (Mallory-Weiss syndrome)   With the advent of esophagogastroduodenoscopy, the Mallory-Weiss syndrome has been observed with increasing frequency as a cause of acute upper gastrointestinal hemorrhage (see also Chap. 38). Mucosal laceration occurs in the region of the esophagogastric junction and is often characterized historically by retching or nonbloody vomiting followed by hematemesis.

Other lesions   Less common bleeding esophageal lesions include esophagitis and carcinoma; these generally cause chronic blood loss and rarely produce massive bleeding.

Gastric carcinoma, lymphoma, polyps, and other tumors of the stomach and small bowel are uncommon and infrequently cause hemorrhage. Leiomyoma and leiomyosarcoma are likewise rare, but they can lead to massive hemorrhage. Bleeding from duodenal and jejunal diverticula is relatively unusual. Vascular insufficiency of the mesenteric vessels, including occlusive and nonocclusive disease, may lead to bloody diarrhea.

Rupture of arteriosclerotic aortic aneurysms into the small intestine is almost always fatal. Rupture usually occurs following arterial reconstructive surgery with fistula formation between synthetic graft and bowel lumen. A small or herald bleed may precede a sudden massive hemorrhage from an aortoenteric fistula. Sudden bleeding also may occur after trauma resulting in hepatic laceration; this may result in blood loss into the bile ducts (i.e., hemobilia).

Primary blood dyscrasias, vasculitis, and connective tissue disorders may result in significant gastrointestinal bleeding. Uremia may produce gastrointestinal blood loss; the most common presentation is chronic, occult bleeding from diffuse involvement of the mucosa of the stomach and small bowel.

ETIOLOGY OF LOWER GASTROINTESTINAL BLEEDING   Anal and rectal lesions   Small amounts of bright red blood on the surface of the stool and toilet tissue are often caused by hemorrhoids, anal fissures, or fistulas; such bleeding is generally precipitated by the strained passage of a hard stool. Proctitis is another source of rectal bleeding. It is often an idiopathic, limited variant of ulcerative colitis. In others, particularly male homosexuals or patients infected with HIV, proctitis may be due to CMV or gonorrheal or mycoplasmal infections. Rectal trauma is a cause of hematochezia, and the placement of foreign objects in the rectal vault may precipitate perforation as well as acute rectal hemorrhage. It must be emphasized that anal pathology does not preclude other sources of blood loss, and these must be sought and excluded.

Colonic lesions   Carcinoma of the colon, as well as colonic polyps, may produce chronic blood loss. Angiodysplasia, a mucosal telangiectasia usually involving the ascending colon, is a major source of acute or chronic bleeding in elderly patients. Frankly bloody diarrhea is common and may be the presenting symptom in patients with ulcerative colitis; it is less frequent in granulomatous colitis, but occult blood may be present in the stool. Bleeding also may accompany diarrhea due to infections with *Shigella*, amebae, *Campylobacter*, *C. difficile*, and rarely, *Salmonella*. In the elderly patient, ischemic colitis may be a cause of bloody diarrhea; this lesion also may be seen in younger women who use oral contraceptive agents.

Diverticula   Bleeding from colonic diverticula is a cause of massive lower gastrointestinal hemorrhage. The usual presentation of a diverticular hemorrhage is that of painless passage of a maroon-colored stool. Meckel's diverticulum, a congenital anomaly of the distal ileum, is present in about 2 percent of the population and is an important cause of acute hemorrhage in children and young adults. Although only about 15 percent of these diverticula contain gastric mucosa, half the lesions which cause acute bleeding contain gastric mucosa.

APPROACH TO THE PATIENT WITH GASTROINTESTINAL BLEEDING   The approach to the bleeding patient depends on the site, extent, and rate of bleeding. The primary consideration in the care of the bleeding patient is maintaining adequate intravascular volume and hemodynamic stability. Patients with hematemesis have usually bled greater amounts (often greater than 1000 mL) than those who have melena alone (usually 500 mL or less), and mortality with the former is about twice that of the latter. When first seen, the patient may be in shock. Prior to taking a history and performing a thorough physical examination, vital signs should be noted, blood sent for typing and cross-matching, and a large-bore intravenous line placed for infusion of saline or other plasma expanders.

History   A history or symptoms suggestive of ulcer disease may provide a useful clue. Similarly, recent heavy use of alcohol or anti-inflammatory drugs should make erosive gastritis suspect. If such alcohol use has been long-standing, esophageal varices may be a more likely source of hemorrhage. Prior history of gastrointestinal bleeding may be helpful, as may a family history of intestinal disease or hemorrhagic diathesis. Recent retching followed by hematemesis should suggest the possibility of the Mallory-Weiss syndrome. The acute onset of bloody diarrhea may indicate the presence of inflammatory bowel disease or an infectious colitis. Associated systemic illnesses, burns, or recent trauma may lead to erosive gastritis.

Physical examination   Following evaluation for orthostatic changes in pulse and blood pressure, clinical assessment of central venous pressure, and institution of volume repletion, the patient should be examined for clues to the underlying illness. A nonintestinal bleeding source should be excluded by careful examination of the oral cavity and nasopharynx. Dermatologic examination may disclose the characteristic telangiectasia of Osler-Weber-Rendu disease (although these will not be visible if severe anemia is present), the perioral pigmentation of Peutz-Jeghers syndrome, the dermal fibromas of neurofibromatosis, the sebaceous cysts and bony tumors of Gardner's syndrome, the palpable purpura frequently seen with vasculitis, or the diffuse pigmentation seen in hemochromatosis. Stigmata of chronic liver disease such as spider angiomata, gynecomastia, testicular atrophy, jaundice, ascites, and hepatosplenomegaly suggest portal hypertension resulting in bleeding from esophageal or gastric varices. Significant lymph node enlargement or abdominal masses may reflect underlying intraabdominal malignancy. Careful rectal examination is important to exclude local pathology as well as to observe the color of the stool.

Laboratory studies Initial studies should include the hematocrit, hemoglobin, careful assessment of red blood cell morphologic features (hypochromic, microcytic red blood cells suggest that blood loss is chronic), white blood cell count, differential, and platelet count. Prothrombin time, partial thromboplastin time, and other coagulation studies are needed to exclude primary or secondary clotting defects. Radiography of the abdomen is rarely helpful in establishing a diagnosis unless a perforated or ischemic viscus is suspected. Although the initial studies are valuable and essential, repeated evaluation of the laboratory data is important as one follows the clinical course of the bleeding.

Diagnostic and therapeutic approach The diagnostic approach to the patient with gastrointestinal hemorrhage must be individualized. When there is a history of melena or hematemesis or the suspicion of bleeding from the upper part of the gastrointestinal tract, the patient should have a nasogastric tube passed to empty the stomach and to determine whether the bleeding is proximal to the ligament of Treitz. If the initial nasogastric aspirate is clear, the tube should be left in place for several hours, since active duodenal bleeding may occur with an initially clear nasogastric aspirate. If the aspirate is negative for blood during a period of active bleeding, it is reasonable to conclude that active bleeding is not occurring in the gastroduodenal region, and the nasogastric tube can be removed. However, if there is no evidence of active bleeding at the time the nasogastric tube is placed, one cannot assume bleeding did not come from the stomach or duodenum, and endoscopy may be required.

If red blood or "coffee grounds" material is aspirated from the nasogastric tube, saline irrigation of the stomach should be initiated. Irrigation serves two purposes: It provides the clinician with an assessment of the rapidity of the bleeding, and it clears the stomach of old blood prior to possible endoscopy. Subsequent diagnostic maneuvers will depend on whether bleeding continues; this can be assessed by vital signs, transfusion requirements, and the number and consistency of stools.

If the bleeding has stopped and the patient is stable, one may proceed with esophagogastroduodenoscopy. Although studies have shown that emergency endoscopy and a vigorous diagnostic approach do not generally decrease patient morbidity or mortality, emergency endoscopy may be important in planning therapy in certain patients with previous gastric surgery, portal hypertension, or complex multisystem diseases. By identifying patients with visible vessels or varices, some patients may be treated endoscopically, and possible complications can be anticipated. Endoscopy is not required if the diagnosis and therapeutic approach are clear from clinical or other data.

Persistent upper gastrointestinal hemorrhage must be viewed differently, and most clinicians would proceed immediately to esophagogastroduodenoscopy (Fig. 41-1). Determination of the site and cause of bleeding is essential to plan for appropriate therapy. Anticipation of surgery, angiography, or the suspicion of bleeding varices are strong indications for esophagogastroduodenoscopy. Bleeding from an arteriole in a peptic ulcer may be controlled by endoscopic coagulation using Nd:YAG laser, heater probe, or electrocautery. However, esophagogastroduodenoscopy is more difficult in the evaluation of *massive* hemorrhage because large amounts of blood obscure visualization of mucosal pathology, and angiography may be required in addition to endoscopy.

Should bleeding continue and endoscopy fail to reveal the bleeding source, the site of hemorrhage may be beyond the ligament of Treitz. In this situation, angiography is frequently valuable in establishing a diagnosis. Angiographic demonstration of the bleeding site requires blood loss at a rate of at least 0.5 mL/min. Clinical correlates reflecting this degree of blood loss include postural hypotension and the necessity for blood transfusion to maintain stable vital signs. Emergency angiography may localize the site of bleeding; however, the cause of the bleeding may not be determined unless varices, vascular malformations, or aneurysms are present.

Therapeutic angiography is a helpful approach to the control of persistent hemorrhage. Continuous intraarterial infusion of vasoconstrictor agents, such as vasopressin, is often successful in controlling hemorrhage due to gastric ulcer or Mallory-Weiss tear. Additionally, embolic material may be injected directly into the artery perfusing the bleeding site.

If bleeding esophageal varices are identified on upper endoscopy, peripheral infusions of vasopressin may acutely control the bleeding. The response to such therapy depends on the general condition of the patient as assessed by clinical and laboratory parameters. It has been shown that intraarterial vasopressin is no more effective than intravenous administration in the control of variceal bleeding. Endoscopic sclerosis and banding of varices have emerged as effective

FIGURE 41-1 Endoscopic photographs from a patient with hematemesis. *A.* A gastric ulcer along the lesser curvature of the stomach is identified (*arrows*). *B.* The same ulcer is bleeding actively from a spurting artery (*arrows*).

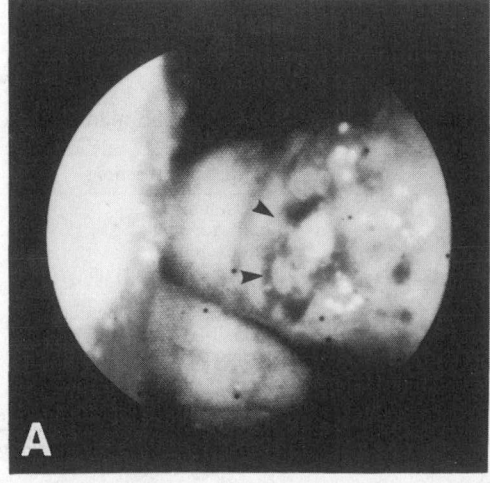
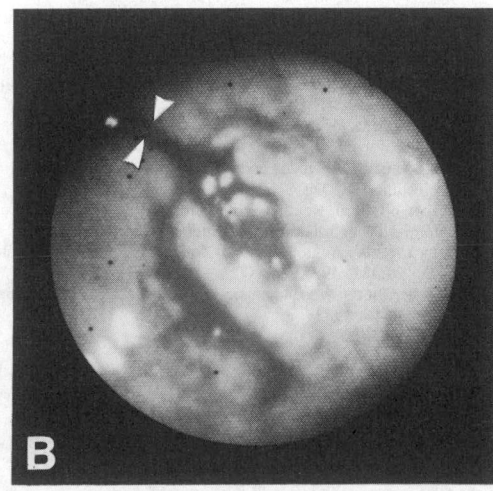

therapies for bleeding esophageal varices. Periodic endoscopic sclerotherapy and banding also appear to limit further bleeding in patients who have bled from varices but do not prolong life. Variceal bleeding also may be controlled by balloon tamponade with a Sengstaken-Blakemore tube. Like vasopressin, this technique is generally used as a stabilizing measure and should be followed by definitive therapy within 48 h whenever possible. Because of its morbidity, portosystemic shunting is reserved for the gravest circumstances. Liver transplantation may be an option for some patients with cirrhosis and bleeding varices.

In the evaluation of *lower gastrointestinal bleeding*, the most important procedures are the digital examination, anoscopy, and sigmoidoscopy. The last of these may identify a bleeding site or document bleeding coming from above the range of the instrument. In the latter case, preparation of the colon with saline lavage solutions permits a colonoscopic evaluation of the bowel within hours. Many colonic abnormalities can be detected and treated with polypectomy or electrocoagulation. If bleeding is brisk, arteriography may serve to localize the bleeding site and allow local infusion of vasoconstrictor agents to control bleeding. Because arteriography detects actively bleeding lesions only when blood loss exceeds 0.5 mL/min and gastrointestinal bleeding tends to be intermittent, arteriography is often nondiagnostic. Radiolabeled erythrocyte scanning is more sensitive than arteriography in detecting blood loss of 0.1 mL/min and may be used to investigate less severe bleeding. However, bleeding scans are less specific than arteriography, generally localizing the lesion but seldom making a discrete diagnosis. Bleeding scans are most helpful in detecting active, low-grade, or intermittent bleeding in order to better time arteriography and obtain the maximal diagnostic yield. Finally, a barium enema has a limited role in the evaluation of acute rectal bleeding. Although it may localize potential bleeding sources, it will not define the bleeding site. Furthermore, if brisk bleeding recurs, subsequent colonoscopy or angiography will be difficult to interpret due to retained contrast material. Therefore, it is advisable to withhold barium studies of both the upper and lower bowel for at least 48 h after the cessation of active bleeding.

Patients with positive tests for fecal occult blood are evaluated principally to exclude colorectal neoplasia. Any symptoms or history of disease should be investigated as well. If there are no symptoms, evaluation focusing on the colon with either a barium enema and sigmoidoscopy or colonoscopy is sufficient. Patients with anemia are unlikely to have a physiologic or trivial basis for their test result, and the evaluation should be pursued until a full explanation is obtained.

REFERENCES

AHLQUIST DA et al: Fecal blood levels in health and disease: A study using Hemoquant. N Engl J Med 312:1422, 1985

CELLO JP et al: Endoscopic sclerotherapy versus portacaval shunt in patients with severe cirrhosis and acute variceal hemorrhage; Long-term follow-up. N Engl J Med 316:11, 1987

CHOJKIER M et al: A controlled comparison of continuous intraarterial and intravenous infusions of vasopressin in hemorrhage from esophageal varices. Gastroenterology 77:540, 1979

LAINE L: Multipolar electrocoagulation in the treatment of active upper gastrointestinal tract hemorrhage. N Engl J Med 316:1613, 1987

LEVY M et al: Major upper gastrointestinal tract bleeding: Relation to the use of aspirin and other nonnarcotic analgesics. Arch Intern Med 148:281, 1988

LICHTENSTEIN JL: Accuracy and reliability of endoscopy and x-ray in upper gastrointestinal bleeding. Dig Dis Sci 26:70s, 1981

PETERSON WL et al: Routine early endoscopy in upper gastrointestinal tract bleeding: A randomized, controlled trial. N Engl J Med 304:925, 1981

RICHTER JM et al: Angiodysplasia: Clinical presentation and colonoscopic diagnosis. Dig Dis Sci 29:481, 1984

STEER ML, SILEN W: Diagnostic procedures in gastrointestinal hemorrhage. N Engl J Med 309:646, 1983

42 JAUNDICE

LEE M. KAPLAN / KURT J. ISSELBACHER

Accumulation of bilirubin in the bloodstream causes yellow pigmentation of the plasma, leading to discoloration of heavily perfused tissues. Serum bilirubin levels accumulate when its production from heme exceeds its metabolism and excretion. Imbalance between production and clearance may result either from excess release of bilirubin precursors into the bloodstream or from physiologic processes that impair the hepatic uptake, metabolism, or excretion of this metabolite (see Table 42-1). Clinically, hyperbilirubinemia appears as *jaundice* or *icterus*, yellow pigmentation of the skin and sclerae. Jaundice can usually be detected when the serum bilirubin level exceeds 34 to 43 μmol/L (2.0 to 2.5 mg/dL), or about twice the upper limit of the normal range, but may be detectable at lower bilirubin levels in patients with fair skin and profound anemia. Conversely, jaundice is frequently obscured in individuals with dark skin or edema. Scleral tissue is rich in elastin, which has a high affinity for bilirubin, so that scleral icterus is usually a more sensitive sign of hyperbilirubinemia than generalized jaundice. A similarly early sign of hyperbilirubinemia is darkening of the urine, which results from renal excretion of bilirubin in the form of bilirubin glucuronide. With pronounced jaundice, the skin may take on a greenish hue because of oxidation of some of the circulating bilirubin to biliverdin. This effect is seen more commonly in conditions with profound or long-standing *conjugated* hyperbilirubinemia such as cirrhosis (see below). Other causes of yellowed skin include *carotenemia*, usually developing as a result of ingestion and absorption of large amounts of β-carotene and related, pigmented compounds. In contrast to hyperbilirubinemia, however, carotenemia does not cause scleral icterus.

PRODUCTION AND METABOLISM OF BILIRUBIN **Sources and chemical characterization of serum bilirubin** Normal serum bilirubin concentrations range from 5 to 17 μmol/L (0.3 to 1.0 mg/dL). More than 90 percent of serum bilirubin in normal individuals is in the unconjugated form, a nonpolar molecule circulating as an albumin-bound complex. The remainder is conjugated to a polar group (primarily glucuronide), rendering it water-soluble and thus able to be filtered and excreted by the kidney. When measured by routine clinical assays, the conjugated, or direct, fraction is frequently overestimated, leading to reported normal values of 1.7 to 8.5 μmol/L (0.1 to 0.5 mg/dL).

Approximately 80 percent of circulating bilirubin is derived from senescent red blood cells. When circulating erythrocytes reach the end of their normal life span of approximately 120 days, they are destroyed by reticuloendothelial cells (Fig. 42-1). Oxidation of the heme moiety dissociated from the hemoglobin within these cells generates biliverdin, which is metabolized in turn to bilirubin. Approximately 15 to 20 percent of circulating bilirubin is derived

TABLE 42-1 Comparative properties of conjugated and unconjugated bilirubin

Properties and reactions	Unconjugated*	Conjugated
Water solubility	0	+
Affinity for lipids	+	0
Renal excretion	0	+
van den Bergh reaction	Indirect (total minus direct)	Direct
Binding to serum albumin (reversible)	+++	+
Formation of bilirubin-albumin complex (irreversible)	0	+[†]

* These properties apply to the naturally occurring bilirubin IXα. Other geometric and photoisomers behave like conjugated bilirubin. See text for details.
[†] Detectable in plasma under conditions of prolonged conjugated hyperbilirubinemia (see text).

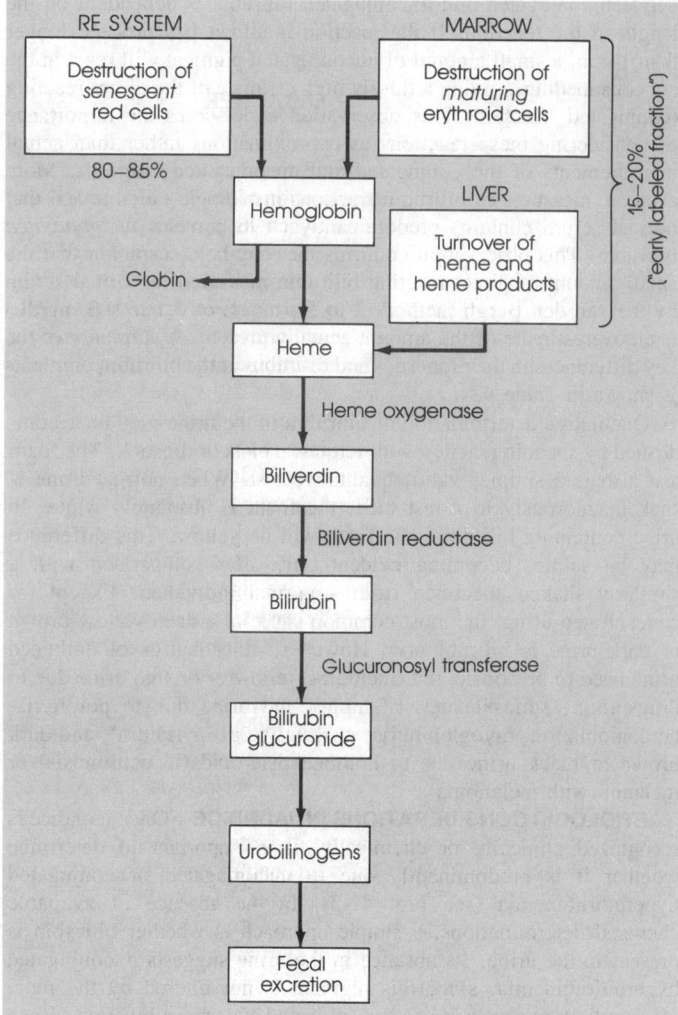

FIGURE 42-1 The sources and precursors of bilirubin and steps in its subsequent metabolism and excretion. RE, reticuloendothelial.

from sources other than senescent erythrocytes. The second major source of bilirubin is ineffective erythropoiesis resulting from destruction of maturing erythroid cells in the bone marrow. A smaller portion of circulating bilirubin derives from the metabolism of other heme-containing proteins, most notably hepatic cytochromes, muscle myoglobin, and widely distributed heme-containing enzymes.

Unconjugated bilirubin liberated into the plasma is bound tightly, but noncovalently to albumin. Certain organic anions, such as sulfonamides and salicylates, complete with bilirubin for binding sites on albumin, permitting the released pigment to enter tissues such as the central nervous system. This phenomenon may explain the neurotoxic effects of neonatal hyperbilirubinemia. Conjugated bilirubin is bound to albumin in two forms, reversible and irreversible. Reversible, noncovalent binding is similar to that of unconjugated bilirubin, although the complex is less stable. When present in serum for extended periods of time (e.g., with cholestasis, long-standing biliary obstruction, or chronic active hepatitis), conjugated bilirubin can form an irreversible, covalent complex with albumin (delta bilirubin or biliprotein). Because of the irreversibility of binding, this complex is not excreted by the kidney. This bilirubin-albumin conjugate has a serum half-life similar to that of albumin (15 to 20 days) and thus remains detectable in serum for up to several weeks after relief of biliary obstruction or during recovery from hepatocellular disease.

Bilirubin is present in body fluids (cerebrospinal fluid, joint effusions, ascites, pleural effusions, cysts, etc.) in proportion to their albumin content and is absent from true secretions such as tears,

saliva, and pancreatic juice. The appearance of jaundice is also influenced by blood flow and edema, with paralyzed extremities and edematous areas tending to remain uncolored.

Hepatic metabolism of bilirubin The liver has a central role in the metabolism of the bile pigments. This process can be divided into three distinct phases: (1) *hepatic uptake*, (2) *conjugation*, and (3) *excretion* into bile. Of these three phases, excretion appears to be the rate-limiting step and the one most susceptible to impairment when the liver cell is damaged.

UPTAKE Unconjugated bilirubin bound to albumin is presented to the liver cell, where the complex dissociates and the nonpolar bilirubin enters the hepatocyte by diffusion or transport across the plasma membrane. The uptake and subsequent hepatocyte storage of bilirubin involves binding of bilirubin to cytoplasmic anion-binding proteins, especially ligandin (glutathione-S-transferase B), that prevent efflux of bilirubin back into the plasma.

CONJUGATION Unconjugated bilirubin is water-insoluble unless complexed to an amphipathic molecule such as albumin. Since albumin is absent from bile, bilirubin must be converted to a water-soluble derivative before biliary excretion. This process is accomplished predominantly by conjugation of bilirubin to glucuronic acid, generating bilirubin glucuronide. The conjugation reaction occurs in the endoplasmic reticulum of hepatocytes and is catalyzed by bilirubin glucuronosyl transferase in a two-step reaction (see Fig. 42-2).

EXCRETION In normal circumstances, only conjugated bilirubin can be excreted into bile. Although the overall process is not well understood, bilirubin excretion appears to be an energy-dependent process limited to the canalicular membrane. Excretion is the rate-limiting step in the hepatic metabolism of this pigment. Impaired excretion leads to decreased bilirubin concentrations in the bile and concomitant "regurgitation" of *conjugated* bilirubin through the sinusoidal membrane of the hepatocyte into the bloodstream. The role of intracellular protein trafficking and membrane transport processes in normal and disordered bilirubin excretion are still poorly understood.

Intestinal phase of bilirubin metabolism After secretion into the bile, conjugated bilirubin is transported through the biliary ducts into the duodenum. Conjugated bilirubin is not reabsorbed by the intestinal mucosa. It is either excreted unchanged in the stool or metabolized by ileal and colonic bacteria to *urobilinogen* and related products. Urobilinogen can be reabsorbed from the small intestine and colon and enters the portal circulation. Some of the portal urobilinogen is taken up by the liver and reexcreted into the bile, and the remainder bypasses the liver and is excreted by the kidney. Under normal conditions, the daily urinary excretion of urobilinogen does not exceed 4 mg. When the hepatic uptake and excretion of urobilinogen is impaired (e.g., in hepatocellular disease) or the production of bilirubin is greatly increased (e.g., with hemolysis),

FIGURE 42-2 Scheme of bilirubin uptake, conjugation, and excretion by the liver cell. The conversion of BMG to BDG is catalyzed by glucuronosyl transferase of the endoplasmic reticulum. B, bilirubin; BMG, bilirubin monoglucuronide; BDG, bilirubin diglucuronide; UDP, uridine diphosphate.

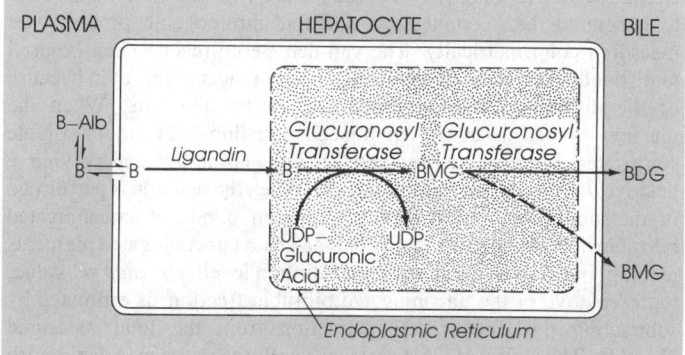

daily urinary urobilinogen excretion may increase significantly. In contrast, cholestasis or extrahepatic biliary obstruction interferes with the intestinal phase of bilirubin metabolism and leads to markedly decreased production and urinary excretion of urobilinogen. Measurement of urinary urobilinogen can thus be a useful tool in distinguishing possible causes of hyperbilirubinemia.

Renal excretion of bilirubin   The urine normally contains no detectable bilirubin by usual clinical assays, although traces may be detected by sensitive spectrophotometric procedures. Unconjugated bilirubin, being tightly bound into albumin, is not filtered by the renal glomeruli. Because there is no tubular secretory process for bilirubin, unconjugated bilirubin is not excreted in urine. In contrast, *conjugated* bilirubin is a polar molecule less tightly bound to albumin. A significant fraction circulates unbound, is filtered by the renal glomeruli, and appears in the urine. The presence of bilirubin in the urine is evidence of conjugated hyperbilirubinemia and can be a useful differentiating point early in the evaluation of jaundice. Bile salts enhance the glomerular filtration of conjugated bilirubin, and in conditions associated with increased circulating bile salts (e.g., cholestasis, extrahepatic biliary obstruction) renal bilirubin excretion is significantly enhanced. This phenomenon may explain the observation that serum conjugated bilirubin tends to plateau at levels below 510 to 680 μmol/L (30 to 40 mg/dL) in patients with *biliary tract obstruction*, while higher levels may occur in patients with severe hepatocellular injury.

For additional information about the production, metabolism, and excretion of bilirubin, please refer to Chap. 265.

PATHOPHYSIOLOGIC CONSEQUENCES OF HYPERBILIRUBI-NEMIA   In most cases, hyperbilirubinemia itself has little pathophysiologic effect. Unlike circulating bile salts, whose levels are also elevated in cholestasis and biliary obstruction, bilirubin does not become deposited in cutaneous tissues and does not produce pruritus. However, *unconjugated* plasma bilirubin that is not bound to albumin can cross the blood-brain barrier. In conditions such as neonatal jaundice or type I or II Crigler-Najjar syndrome (see below), extremely high concentrations (>340 μmol/L or >20 mg/dL) of unconjugated bilirubin can accumulate, and the resulting diffusion of bilirubin into the central nervous system can cause encephalopathy (kernicterus) and permanent impairment of nervous function. The risk of kernicterus is increased by conditions that favor elevated circulating levels of *unbound*, unconjugated bilirubin, such as hemolysis, hypoalbuminemia, acidosis, and increased levels of compounds that compete for albumin binding such as free fatty acids and drugs. Circulating concentrations of unconjugated bilirubin can be decreased by removing these contributory factors and by facilitating the biliary excretion of *unconjugated* bilirubin. Exposure to blue light causes conformational changes in unconjugated bilirubin, rendering it more polar and water soluble. These *photoisomers* are taken up and excreted by the liver and kidney, without need for normal conjugation. Intense treatment with blue light can provide sufficient isomerization of unconjugated bilirubin circulating through the skin to prevent kernicterus in patients with neonatal jaundice.

CHEMICAL TESTS FOR BILE PIGMENTS   The most widely employed chemical test for bile pigments in serum is the van den Bergh reaction. The bilirubin pigments are exposed to sulfanilic acid to generated diazo conjugates, and the chromogenic products are measured colorimetrically. The van den Bergh reaction can be used to distinguish between unconjugated and conjugated bilirubin because of the different solubility properties of the pigments. When the reaction is performed in an aqueous medium, the water-soluble conjugated bilirubin reacts directly with sulfanilic acid, giving a positive *direct* van den Bergh reaction. When the reaction is performed in methanol, the intramolecular hydrogen bonds of unconjugated bilirubin are broken; thus, both conjugated and unconjugated pigments react, giving a measure of the *total* bilirubin level. The *indirect* value, representative of the unconjugated bilirubin fraction, is estimated by subtracting the direct-reacting fraction from the total measured bilirubin. The ability of the *direct* van den Bergh reaction to distinguish

between conjugated and unconjugated bilirubin is dependent on the length of the reaction. If the reaction is allowed to proceed longer than 1 min, a small amount of unconjugated pigment will react in the aqueous medium, giving a falsely high estimate of the direct-reacting (conjugated) fraction. This observation underscores the importance of considering these reactions as approximations rather than actual measurements of the conjugated and unconjugated fractions. More accurate measures of bilirubin fractions in biologic fluids reveal that normal serum contains predominantly (>96 percent) *unconjugated* bilirubin. This observation confirms the long-held suspicion that the small amount of direct-reacting bilirubin measured in normal serum by the van den Bergh method (2 to 5 μmol/L or 0.1 to 0.3 mg/dL) is an overestimate of the amount actually present. A summary of the key differences in the properties and reactions of the bilirubin pigments is shown in Table 42-1.

Qualitative determination of bilirubin in the urine may be accomplished by specific reaction with Ictotest tablets or dipstick. The foam test also is a simple, valid, qualitative test. When normal urine is shaken vigorously in a test tube, the foam is absolutely white. In urine containing bilirubin, the foam will be yellow. This difference may be subtle, becoming evident only after comparison with a similarly shaken specimen from a normal individual. Except for concentrated urine, the most common cause of a deep yellow-brown or dark urine is bilirubinuria. However, other causes of darkened urine need to be considered, including yellow or orange urine due to drugs (e.g., sulfasalazine, rifampin), red urine due to porphyria, hemoglobinuria, myoglobinuria, or drugs (e.g., pyridium), and dark brown or black urine due to homogentisic acid (in ochronosis) or melanin (with melanoma).

ETIOLOGIC CONSIDERATIONS IN JAUNDICE   Once jaundice is recognized clinically or chemically, it is important to determine whether it is predominantly due to unconjugated or conjugated hyperbilirubinemia (see Fig. 42-3). In the absence of available chemical determinations, a simple approach is whether bilirubin is present in the urine. Its absence in the urine suggests unconjugated hyperbilirubinemia, since this pigment is not filtered by the renal glomeruli; its presence indicates conjugated hyperbilirubinemia. When chemical analysis (van den Bergh reaction) reveals 80 to 85 percent of the total serum bilirubin to be unconjugated, a patient is considered to have primarily *unconjugated hyperbilirubinemia*. A patient with more than 50 percent direct-reacting (conjugated) serum bilirubin is considered to have predominantly *conjugated hyperbilirubinemia*.

An approach to the classification of jaundice based on this important distinction is presented in Table 42-2. Derangements of bilirubin metabolism may occur through any of four mechanisms: (1) overproduction, (2) decreased hepatic uptake, (3) decreased hepatic conjugation, and (4) decreased excretion of bilirubin into bile (due either to intrahepatic dysfunction or extrahepatic mechanical obstruction). Jaundice may also be described on the basis of the pathogenic mechanisms or disease processes leading to increased bilirubin levels. Thus, the terms *hemolytic jaundice, hepatocellular jaundice,* and *obstructive* (or *cholestatic*) *jaundice* are often used. Though these classifications are helpful, in any one patient more than a single derangement in bilirubin metabolism may be operative, and more than a single "type" of jaundice may be present. For example, a patient with cirrhosis may have not only impaired liver cell function (and hence hepatocellular jaundice) but also hemolysis. Furthermore, as indicated above, obstructive jaundice or cholestasis may be due either to *mechanical* obstruction of the biliary radicles or to impaired *functional* hepatic excretion of bilirubin. This chapter presents a brief description of the major causes of jaundice. A more detailed discussion of individual diseases is found in Chap. 265.

Jaundice with predominantly unconjugated bilirubinemia   OVER-PRODUCTION OF BILIRUBIN   An increased amount of hemoglobin released from senescent or hemolyzed red blood cells leads to increased bilirubin production. Erythrocyte destruction leading to hyperbilirubinemia most commonly results from intravascular hemolysis (e.g., autoimmune, microangiopathic, or hemoglobinopathy-

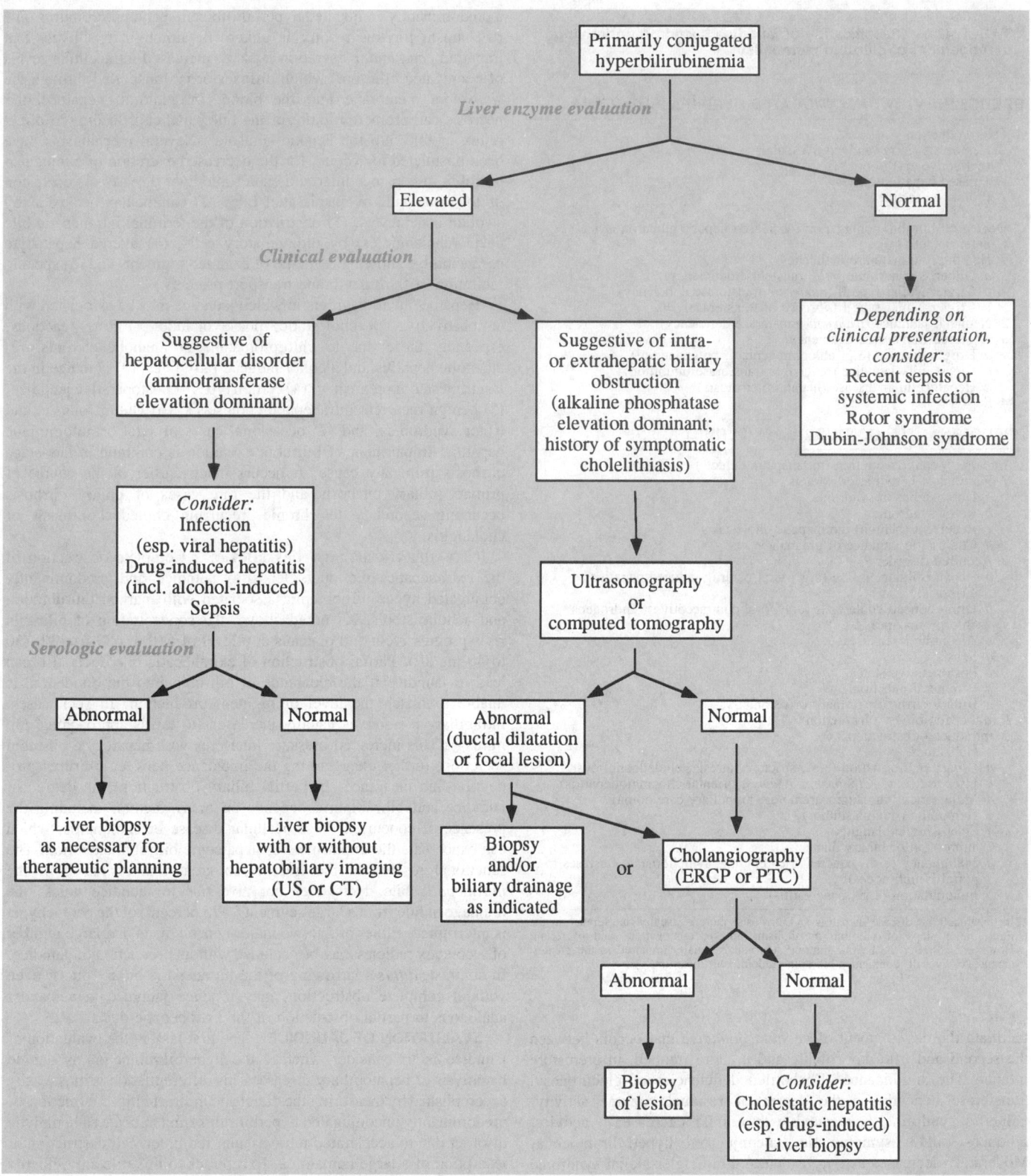

FIGURE 42-3 Algorithm for evaluation of conjugated hyperbilirubinemia. Abbreviations: CT, computed tomography, ERCP, endoscopic retrograde cholangiopancreatography; PTC, percutaneous transhepatic cholangiography; US, ultrasonography.

associated) or resorption of a large hematoma. Excess bilirubin production is reflected in increased serum bilirubin levels of up to 51 to 68 μmol/L (3 to 4 mg/dL), with a predominance of unconjugated bilirubin. For a more detailed discussion of the causes of increased bilirubin production, refer to Chap. 265.

IMPAIRED HEPATIC UPTAKE OF BILIRUBIN As indicated above, the uptake of bilirubin by hepatocytes requires dissociation of the nonpolar pigment molecule from albumin, transport across the cell membrane, and binding to ligandin. In rare cases of drug-induced jaundice (e.g., from flavaspidic acid) and possibly in some patients with Gilbert's syndrome, there may be a disruption of this phase of bilirubin handling.

IMPAIRED GLUCURONIDE CONJUGATION Deficiency in glucuronosyl transferase activity can occur as a result of both acquired and genetic defects. In the fetus and neonate, glucuronosyl transferase activity is normally low. This deficiency, although transient, can

TABLE 42-2 Classification of jaundice based on underlying derangement of bilirubin metabolism

PREDOMINANTLY *UNCONJUGATED* HYPERBILIRUBINEMIA

A Overproduction
   1 Hemolysis (intra- and extravascular)
   2 Ineffective erythropoiesis
B Decreased hepatic uptake
   1 Prolonged fasting
   2 Sepsis
C Decreased bilrubin conjugation (decreased hepatic glucuronosyl transferase activity)
   1 Hereditary transferase deficiency
     a Gilbert's syndrome (*mild* transferase deficiency)
     b Crigler-Najjar type II (*moderate* transferase deficiency)
     c Crigler-Najjar type I (*absence* of transferase)
   2 Neonatal jaundice (*transient* transferase deficiency)
   3 Acquired transferase deficiency
     a Drug inhibition (e.g. chloramphenicol, pregnanediol)
     b Breast milk jaundice (reversible transferase inhibition)
     c Hepatocellular disease (hepatitis, cirrhosis)*
   4 Sepsis

PREDOMINANTLY *CONJUGATED* HYPERBILIRUBINEMIA

A Impaired hepatic excretion (intrahepatic defects)
   1 Familial or hereditary disorders
     a Dubin-Johnson syndrome
     b Rotor syndrome
     c Recurrent (benign) intrahepatic cholestasis
     d Cholestatic jaundice of pregnancy
   2 Acquired disorders
     a Hepatocellular disease (e.g., viral or drug-induced hepatitis, cirrhosis)*
     b Drug-induced cholestasis (e.g., oral contraceptives, androgens, chlorpromazine)
     c Alcoholic liver disease
     d Sepsis
     e Postoperative state
     f Parenteral nutrition
     g Biliary cirrhosis (primary or secondary)
B Extrahepatic biliary obstruction
   1 Intraductal obstruction
     a Gallstones
     b Biliary malformation (e.g., stricture, atresia, choledochol cyst)
     c Infection (e.g., *Clonorchis, Ascaris,* oriental cholangiohepatitis)
     d Malignancy (cholangiocarcinoma, ampullary carcinoma)
     e Hemobilia (trauma, tumor)
     f Sclerosing cholangitis
   2 Compression of biliary ducts
     a Malignancy (e.g., pancreatic carcinoma, lymphoma, metastases to portal lymph nodes)
     b Inflammation (e.g., pancreatitis)

* In hepatocellular disease (hepatitis and cirrhosis) there is usually interference in the three major steps of bilirubin metabolism—uptake, conjugation, and excretion. However, excretion is the rate-limiting step and is usually impaired to the greatest extent. As a result, conjugated bilirubin predominates in serum.

facilitate the development of *neonatal jaundice* that occurs between the second and fifth days of life and is more frequent in premature infants. The significance of inherited deficiencies of glucuronosyl transferase depends on the degree of residual enzyme activity. Gilbert's syndrome, associated with a mild decrease in activity, produces mild, asymptomatic, unconjugated hyperbilirubinemia. Moderately decreased activity is detected in Crigler-Najjar syndrome type II, and this enzyme is total absent in Crigler-Najjar syndrome type I, an autosomal recessive disorder associated with kernicterus and childhood mortality from CNS dysfunction. Acquired defects in glucuronosyl transferase activity may be induced by drugs (i.e., direct enzyme inhibition) or be associated with liver disease generally. However, in most hepatocellular disorders, bilirubin excretion is impaired to a greater extent than bilirubin conjugation, leading to a primarily *conjugated* hyperbilirubinemia.

Jaundice with predominantly conjugated bilirubinemia
IMPAIRED BILIRUBIN EXCRETION BY HEPATOCYTES Interference with the biliary excretion of conjugated bilirubin by hepatocytes leads to "reentry" of this pigment into the systemic circulation, resulting in a predominantly conjugated hyperbilirubinemia and bilirubinuria. The mechanism for this reentry is unknown, although it is likely that impaired *canalicular* excretion leads to increased intracellular levels of conjugated bilirubin, which diffuses or is transported through the *sinusoidal* membrane into the blood. In addition, hepatocellular necrosis can promote rupture of the bile canaliculi, leading to direct reflux of bile into the hepatic sinusoids. Several mechanisms have been postulated to account for the decreased excretion of conjugated bilirubin in hepatocellular and cholestatic liver disease: (1) occlusion of the canaliculi by inspissated bile, (2) canalicular occlusion by swollen hepatocytes, (3) obstruction of the terminal intrahepatic bile ducts (cholangioles) by inflammatory cells, (4) altered hepatocyte permeability, allowing reuptake of excreted pigment, and (5) specific inhibition of transmembrane transport proteins.

Hepatocellular disorders in which jaundice may be associated with an obstructive, or cholestatic, phase include (1) drug reactions, especially those due to chlorpromazine or anabolic steroids, (2) alcoholic hepatitis and alcohol-induced fatty liver, (3) jaundice in the last trimester of pregnancy, (4) certain types of postoperative jaundice, (5) benign recurrent intrahepatic cholestasis, (6) Dubin-Johnson and Rotor syndromes, and (7) occasional cases of viral or autoimmune hepatitis. Impairment of bilirubin excretion is common in late-stage cirrhosis from any cause. It occurs much earlier in the course of primary biliary cirrhosis and the rare cases of biliary cirrhosis occurring secondary to chronic, recurring choledocholithiasis or cholangitis.

EXTRAHEPATIC BILIARY OBSTRUCTION Complete obstruction of the extrahepatic bile ducts leads to jaundice and predominantly conjugated hyperbilirubinemia associated with marked bilirubinuria and acholic stools. As noted above, the concentration of bilirubin rises progressively and plateaus at a level of 510 to 680 μmol/L (30 to 40 mg/dL). Partial obstruction of extrahepatic bile ducts also can lead to jaundice if the clearance of bilirubin into the duodenum is unable to match the level of pigment production. In such cases, intrabiliary pressure is usually increased (to levels approaching 250 mmHg). This increased pressure interferes with hepatocyte bilirubin secretion, further exaggerating the imbalance between bilirubin production and clearance. In partial biliary obstruction, the degree of jaundice and bilirubinuria depends on many factors, including the presence of concurrent hepatocellular disease or cholangitis, which can exacerbate the impairment of hepatocyte bilirubin excretion. The functional reserve of the liver is so great that occlusion of the *intrahepatic* bile ducts does not give rise to jaundice unless the drainage of bile from a large segment (>75 percent) of the parenchyma is interrupted. Either of the two major hepatic ducts or a large number of secondary radicles may be occluded without production of jaundice. In contrast, *diffuse* narrowing of the intrahepatic biliary ducts, even without complete obstruction, may produce jaundice in a manner analogous to partial obstruction of the extrahepatic ducts.

EVALUATION OF JAUNDICE The first task in the evaluation of jaundice is to consider whether the hyperbilirubinemia is due to hemolysis or hepatobiliary disease. This differentiation is most easily accomplished by measuring the direct and indirect bilirubin fraction. A predominantly unconjugated hyperbilirubinemia indicates a hemolytic disorder due to accelerated intravascular red blood cell destruction or resorption of a large hematoma. Exceptions to this rule are Gilbert's syndrome, the other, rare, hereditary disorders of glucuronosyl transferase, and end-stage hepatic failure. Further evaluation of the cause of hemolysis can then proceed as described in Chap. 304, Megaloblastic Anemias, Chap. 306, Disorders of Hemoglobin, and Chap. 307, Hemolytic Anemias.

Jaundice associated with a primarily (>50 percent) *conjugated* hyperbilirubinemia usually results from one of three groups of disorders, including hepatocellular disease, intrahepatic biliary obstruction ("cholestasis") and extrahepatic biliary obstruction. An early goal is the determination of which category of disease explains the patient's jaundice. Central to this determination is a careful *clinical* evaluation, including history, physical examination, basic tests of liver function, and a complete blood count. Using these simple tools, experienced clinicians can determine the overall nature of the jaundice in the majority of cases. Most importantly, however, the results of the clinical evaluation direct the physician to a logical progression of imaging studies, serological tests, and pathological evaluation. The initial clinical evaluation should focus on features of the patient's illness that distinguish between hepatocellular disease, intrahepatic cholestasis, and extrahepatic biliary obstruction. A general algorithm for the evaluation of jaundice due to conjugated hyperbilirubinemia is shown in Fig. 42-3.

History Historical evaluation should include determination of the length of symptoms, presence and character of abdominal pain, fever or other symptoms of active inflammation, changes in appetite, weight, and bowel habits. Specific attention should be directed to a history of blood transfusions, intravenous drug use, promiscuous sexual activity, and ethanol use. A history of medication use should be sought, particularly drugs known to cause either cholestasis, such as anabolic steroids and chlorpromazine, or hepatocellular necrosis, such as acetaminophen or isoniazid. A history of arthralgias may suggest acute viral hepatitis. Viral disease should also be considered in patients with a history of travel to developing countries endemic for enterally transmitted hepatitis E or East Asian countries, where the parenterally transmitted hepatitis B and C viruses are widespread. Pruritus is most commonly associated with chronic cholestasis, developing from either extrahepatic obstruction or cholestatic liver disease such as sclerosing cholangitis or primary biliary cirrhosis. In contrast, acholic stools develop more commonly in patients with extrahepatic biliary obstruction from tumor, choledocholithiasis, or secondary to a congenital biliary abnormality such as an inflamed choledochal cyst. The presence of acholic and heme-positive stool (silver stools) should suggest a tumor of the distal biliary tract such as ampullary, periampullary, or cholangiocarcinoma. This combination may also be seen in patients with pancreatic carcinoma eroding into the biliary tract or duodenum. Jaundice, in the setting of previous biliary surgery, may suggest retained or recurrent stone disease, a biliary stricture, or recurrent obstruction from an enlarging tumor. Finally, a preexisting or underlying condition predisposing to hepatobiliary disease should be solicited. For example, inflammatory bowel disease, particularly ulcerative colitis, may be associated with sclerosing cholangitis. Pregnancy predisposes to cholestasis, steatosis, and acute liver failure. Right heart failure may result in hepatic congestion and cholestasis, and sepsis can cause selective disruption of bilirubin transport or generalized intrahepatic cholestasis.

Physical examination The examination is also important for directing the subsequent evaluation. Excoriations suggest prolonged cholestasis or high grade biliary obstruction, and a greenish hue to the jaundice is associated with particular severe or long-standing liver disease, such as biliary cirrhosis, sclerosing cholangitis, severe, chronic hepatitis, or long-standing malignant obstruction. Fever and epigastric or right upper quadrant tenderness is frequently associated with choledocholithiasis and cholangitis or cholecystitis. In contrast, malignant biliary obstruction commonly presents as painless jaundice. An enlarged, tender liver suggests acute hepatic inflammation or a rapidly enlarging hepatic tumor, while a palpable gallbladder suggests distal biliary obstruction from a malignant tumor. The presence of splenomegaly may provide a clue to the presence of portal hypertension, from chronic active hepatitis, severe alcoholic or acute viral hepatitis, or cirrhosis. Cirrhosis is also associated with a hyperestrogenic state that may be reflected in gynecomastia, testicular atrophy, or spider angiomata. Testicular atrophy may be particularly prominent in cirrhosis due to alcoholic liver disease or hemochromatosis. Palmar erythema, facial telangiectasia, and Dupuytren's contractures are also associated with cirrhosis, particularly as a result of chronic ethanol ingestion. Wasting or lymphadenopathy suggests malignancy, and in the presence of splenomegaly, these signs may direct consideration to a pancreatic tumor obstructing the splenic vein or a widely metastatic lymphoma. In patients whose history or examination

suggests malignancy, particular attention should be directed toward physical findings suggestive of a primary tumor, including heme-positive stool, abdominal or breast masses, thyroid nodules, and supraclavicular lymphadenopathy. Physical findings associated with specific liver diseases include distended neck veins and hepatojugular reflux (right heart failure), xanthomata (primary biliary cirrhosis), and Kayser-Fleischer rings (Wilson's disease).

Laboratory tests Initial laboratory evaluation should focus on serum bilirubin fractionation. Predominantly *unconjugated* (indirect) hyperbilirubinemia should prompt consideration of a hemolytic disorder, such as an autoimmune or microangiopathic hemolytic anemia, ineffective erythropoiesis, or resorption of a large hematoma. The most common cause of mild elevations in the unconjugated fraction, however, is Gilbert's syndrome, an inherited condition resulting from a mild deficiency in hepatic glucuronosyl transferase. Individuals with Gilbert's syndrome experience variable elevations in circulating unconjugated bilirubin, especially in association with physical stress, fever, intercurrent infection or surgery, fasting, or heavy ethanol ingestion. This mild metabolic abnormality produces no symptoms other than jaundice, and is *not* associated with liver enzyme abnormalities or adverse long-term effects.

Conjugated (direct) hyperbilirubinemia usually results from hepatocellular or cholestatic liver disease, or extrahepatic biliary obstruction. Because hepatic glucuronosyl transferase activity is normally present in great abundance, adequate bilirubin glucuronide formation can occur even with severe liver disease. In patients with primarily conjugated hyperbilirubinemia, the presence and nature of liver enzyme abnormalities usually provide important clues about the nature of the underlying process. Conjugated hyperbilirubinemia without liver enzyme abnormalities is relatively uncommon, but can be seen in pregnancy, sepsis, or after recent surgery. Isolated conjugated hyperbilirubinemia is the primary manifestation of two heritable disorders, Rotor and Dubin-Johnson syndromes, and can also be seen in some patients with the syndrome of recurrent benign intrahepatic cholestasis. As described more fully in Chap. 263, elevation of the aminotransferases out of proportion to other liver enzymes suggests hepatocellular damage, most commonly seen in toxic, viral, or ischemic hepatitis, while prominent elevations of the alkaline phosphatase, 5'-nucleotidase and/or gamma-glutamyl transpeptidase are more suggestive of intrahepatic cholestasis or extrahepatic obstruction. Although these patterns are not invariably diagnostic, they are helpful in directing the ensuing evaluation.

Patients with a clinical evaluation and laboratory findings suggestive of hepatocellular disease should be evaluated for evidence of viral hepatitis, drug toxicity, hepatic congestion, such as that produced by right ventricular failure or acute obstruction of the hepatic veins, or ischemic hepatitis. In the appropriate clinical setting, serological studies are extremely helpful for diagnosing, or excluding the diagnosis of, hepatitis A, acute and chronic hepatitis B, and hepatitis C and D. Common causes of toxic hepatitis include acetaminophen, isoniazid, and halogenated anesthetic agents. Patients with alcoholic liver disease are particularly susceptible to acetaminophen toxicity, which may occur after therapeutic doses in these individuals. For patients with probable hepatocellular disease, liver biopsy can provide important diagnostic and prognostic information. The results of percutaneous, transjugular, or laparoscopic biopsy may also provide important information for optimal therapy. The role of hepatobiliary imaging in these patients is less clearly defined. In some cases, identification of focal lesions by computed tomography (CT), ultrasonography (US) or magnetic resonance imaging (MRI) can increase the diagnostic accuracy of liver biopsy. These imaging techniques can also aid in diagnosis by suggesting the presence of hepatic fat deposition, cirrhosis, or the excessive hepatic iron deposition of hemochromatosis. US is an exquisitely sensitive means of detecting ascites. Combined with Doppler flow analysis, it can also determine the patency and direction of flow in the portal and hepatic veins, frequently enabling noninvasive diagnosis of portal vein thrombosis and Budd-Chiari syndrome.

Hepatobiliary imaging   For patients whose clinical evaluation and liver chemistries suggest cholestasis or extrahepatic biliary obstruction, biliary imaging is an important early diagnostic tool to differentiate intrahepatic causes from extrahepatic obstruction. Both US and CT detect dilated extrahepatic biliary ducts with great sensitivity. In the absence of previous hepatobiliary surgery, the specificity of these tests for identifying dilated extrahepatic ducts is well above 90 percent. Both techniques are sensitive indicators of intrahepatic, portal, and pancreatic masses, and either can be effective in diagnosing biliary obstruction from tumors or impacted stones. In addition, US is an extremely effective means of detecting stones within the gallbladder and is somewhat more sensitive than CT. These imaging techniques are considerably less sensitive for detecting chole*docho*lithiasis. Both fail to detect approximately 40 percent of intraductal stones, although selected studies suggest that CT is somewhat better at detecting stones within *nondilated* ducts.

In patients with clinical and radiographic evidence of extrahepatic biliary obstruction, further evaluation should be directed at determining the cause of the obstruction and providing rapid relief. Masses identified by US, CT, or MRI, are usually accessible to radiographically directed percutaneous biopsy. Further definition and relief of extrahepatic biliary obstruction can frequently be accomplished by *percutaneous* or *endoscopic cholangiography*. In the hands of experienced practitioners, dilated biliary ducts can be accessed percutaneously in more than 90 percent of patients, nondilated ducts in up to 70 percent. Percutaneous transhepatic cholangiography (PTC) may be particularly useful for imaging and drainage of patients with biliary obstruction above the bifurcation of the common bile duct and in patients whose obstruction cannot be relieved during endoscopic cholangiography. Collection of bile for cytologic analysis may also allow identification of the obstructing lesion. *Endoscopic retrograde cholangiopancreatography* (ERCP) is frequently the preferred technique for diagnosing and treating distal biliary obstructions. In addition to cholangiography, ERCP provides the opportunity for inspection and biopsy of the ampulla of Vater and surrounding duodenum (common sites of tumors obstructing the bile ducts), visualization of the pancreatic ducts to detect evidence of pancreatic ductal stones or small pancreatic tumors, and direct biopsy of the bile duct epithelium and pancreatic head. Both PTC and ERCP can afford relief of malignant obstruction and dissolution or fragmenting of ductal stones. ERCP also provides the opportunity for long-term relief of stone disease via endoscopic papillotomy and is the preferred approach to intraductal stones remaining after surgical or laparoscopic cholecystectomy.

For patients with a clinical presentation of cholestasis who have ducts of *normal* caliber, attention should focus on intrahepatic cholestasis caused by primary biliary cirrhosis, drugs or toxins (including ethanol), and extrahepatic obstruction *without* ductal dilation, which can be caused by primary sclerosing cholangitis or intrahepatic arterial chemotherapy and is occasionally seen in patients with AIDS ("vanishing duct syndrome") and cholangiocarcinoma. If the clinical picture is more suggestive of cholestasis or biliary cirrhosis, liver biopsy may provide the most direct route to diagnosis. In contrast, cholangiography with cytologic analysis of the bile and/or biopsy of the ductal epithelium is indicated in patients whose presentation suggests extrahepatic obstruction, such as patients with jaundice and nondilated ducts in the setting of weight loss, lymphadenopathy, or inflammatory bowel disease.

REFERENCES

BERLIN N, BERK P: Quantitative aspects of bilirubin metabolism for hematologists. Blood 57:983, 1981

BLANKAERT N, FEVERY J: Physiology and pathophysiology of bilirubin metabolism, in *Hepatology*, 2d ed, D Zakim, T Boyer, eds. Philadelphia, Saunders, 1989, p 254

BORSCH G et al: Clinical evaluation, ultrasound, cholescintigraphy, and endoscopic retrograde cholangiography in cholestasis: A prospective clinical study. J Clin Gastroenterol 10:185, 1988

CRONIN JJ: Ultrasound diagnosis of choledocholithiasis: A reappraisal. Radiology 161:133, 1986

FRANK BB et al: Clinical evaluation of jaundice: A guideline of the patient care committee of the American Gastroenterological Association. JAMA 262:3031, 1989

FRANSON TR et al: Frequency and characteristics of hyperbilirubinemia associated with bacteremia. Rev Infect Dis 7:1, 1985

McDONAGH AF et al: Blue light and bilirubin excretion. Science 208:145, 1980

MURACA M et al: Analytic aspects and clinical interpretation of serum bilirubins. Semin Liver Dis 8:137, 1988

SCHARSCHMIDT BF et al: Approach to the patient with cholestatic jaundice. N Engl J Med 308:1515, 1983

SHERLOCK S, DOOLEY J (eds): *Diseases of the Liver and Biliary System,* 9th ed, Oxford, Blackwell, 1993, pp 199–213

VAN HOOTEGEM P et al: Serum bilirubins in hepatobiliary disease: Comparison with other liver function tests. Hepatology 5:112, 1985

WEISS JS et al: The clinical importance of a protein-bound fraction of serum bilirubin in patients with hyperbilirubinemia. N Engl J Med 309:147, 1983

43   ABDOMINAL SWELLING AND ASCITES

ROBERT M. GLICKMAN / KURT J. ISSELBACHER

ABDOMINAL SWELLING   Abdominal swelling or distention is a common problem in clinical medicine and may be the initial manifestation of a systemic disease or of otherwise unsuspected abdominal disease. *Subjective* abdominal enlargement, often described as a sensation of fullness or bloating, is usually transient and is often related to a functional gastrointestinal disorder when it is not accompanied by objective physical findings of increased abdominal girth or local swelling. *Obesity* and lumbar lordosis, which may be associated with prominence of the abdomen, may usually be distinguished from true increases in the volume of the peritoneal cavity by history and careful physical examination.

Clinical history   Abdominal swelling may first be noticed by the patient because of a progressive increase in belt or clothing size, the appearance of abdominal or inguinal hernias, or the development of a localized swelling. Often, considerable abdominal enlargement has gone unnoticed for weeks or months, either because of coexistent obesity or because the ascites formation has been insidious, without pain or localizing symptoms. Progressive abdominal distention may be associated with a sensation of "pulling" or "stretching" of the flanks or groins and vague low back pain. Localized *pain* usually results from involvement of an abdominal organ (e.g., a passively congested liver, large spleen, or colonic tumor). Pain is uncommon in cirrhosis with ascites, and when it is present, pancreatitis, hepatoma, or peritonitis should be considered. Tense ascites or abdominal tumors may produce increased intraabdominal pressure, resulting in *indigestion* and *heartburn* due to gastroesophageal reflux or *dyspnea, orthopnea,* and *tachypnea* from elevation of the diaphragm. A coexistent pleural effusion, more commonly on the right, presumably due to leakage of ascitic fluid through lymphatic channels in the diaphragm, also may contribute to respiratory embarrassment. The patient with diffuse abdominal swelling should be questioned about increased alcoholic intake, a prior episode of jaundice or hematuria, a change in bowel habits, or a past history of rheumatic heart disease. Such historical information may provide the clues that will lead one to suspect an occult cirrhosis, a colonic tumor with peritoneal seeding, congestive heart failure, or nephrosis.

Physical examination   A carefully executed *general physical examination* can yield valuable clues concerning the etiology of abdominal swelling. Thus palmar erythema and spider angiomas suggest an underlying cirrhosis, while supraclavicular adenopathy (Virchow's node) should raise the question of an underlying gastrointestinal malignancy. *Inspection* of the abdomen is an important but often cursorily performed aspect of the abdominal examination. By noting the abdominal contour, one may be able to distinguish localized from generalized swelling. The tensely distended abdomen with tightly stretched skin, bulging flanks, and everted umbilicus is characteristic of ascites. A prominent abdominal venous pattern with the direction of flow away from the umbilicus often is a reflection of portal hypertension; venous collaterals with flow from the lower part of the abdomen toward the umbilicus suggest obstruction of the inferior vena cava; flow downward toward the umbilicus suggests superior vena cava obstruction. "Doming" of the abdomen with visible ridges from underlying intestinal loops is usually due to intestinal obstruction or distention. An epigastric mass, with evident peristalsis proceeding from left to right, usually indicates underlying pyloric obstruction. A liver with metastatic deposits may be visible as a nodular right upper quadrant mass moving with respiration.

Auscultation may reveal the high-pitched, rushing sounds of early intestinal obstruction or a succussion sound due to increased fluid and gas in a dilated hollow viscus. Careful auscultation over an enlarged liver occasionally reveals the harsh bruit of a vascular tumor, especially a hepatoma, or the leathery friction rub of a surface nodule. A venous hum at the umbilicus may signify portal hypertension and an increased collateral blood flow around the liver. A fluid wave and flank dullness which shifts with change in position of the patient are important signs that indicate the presence of peritoneal fluid. In obese patients, small amounts of fluid may be difficult to demonstrate; on occasion, the fluid may be detected by abdominal percussion with patients on their hands and knees. Small amounts of ascites often can only be detected by ultrasound examination of the abdomen. Careful percussion should serve to distinguish generalized abdominal enlargement from localized swelling due to an enlarged uterus, ovarian cyst, or distended bladder. Percussion also can outline an abnormally small or large liver. Loss of normal liver dullness may result from massive hepatic necrosis; it also may be a clue to free gas in the peritoneal cavity, as from perforation of a hollow viscus.

Palpation is often difficult with massive ascites, and ballottement of overlying fluid may be the only method of palpating the liver or spleen. A slightly enlarged spleen in association with ascites may be the only evidence of an occult cirrhosis. When there is evidence of portal hypertension, a soft liver suggests that obstruction to portal flow is extrahepatic; a firm liver suggests cirrhosis as the likely cause of the portal hypertension. A very hard or nodular liver is a clue that the liver is infiltrated with tumor, and when accompanied by ascites, it suggests that the latter is due to peritoneal seeding. The presence of a hard periumbilical nodule (Sister Mary Joseph's nodule) suggests metastatic disease from a pelvic or gastrointestinal primary tumor. A pulsatile liver and ascites may be found in tricuspid insufficiency.

An attempt should be made to determine whether a mass is solid or cystic, smooth or irregular, and whether it moves with respiration. The liver, spleen, and gallbladder should descend with respiration unless they are fixed by adhesions or extension of tumor beyond the organ. A fixed mass not descending with respiration may indicate that it is retroperitoneal. Tenderness, especially if localized, may indicate an inflammatory process such as an abscess; it also may be due to stretching of the visceral peritoneum or tumor necrosis. Rectal and pelvic examinations are mandatory; they may reveal otherwise undetected masses due to tumor or infection.

Radiographic and laboratory examinations are essential for confirming or extending the impressions gained on physical examination. Upright and recumbent films of the abdomen may demonstrate the dilated loops of intestine with fluid levels characteristic of intestinal obstruction or the diffuse abdominal haziness and loss of psoas margins suggestive of ascites. Ultrasonography is often of value in detecting ascites, determining the presence of a mass, or evaluating the size of the liver and spleen. CT scanning provides similar information. CT scanning is often necessary to visualize the retroperitoneum, pancreas, and lymph nodes. A plain film of the abdomen may reveal the distended colon of otherwise unsuspected ulcerative colitis and give valuable information as to the size of the liver and spleen. An irregular and elevated right side of the diaphragm may be a clue to a liver abscess or hepatoma. Studies of the gastrointestinal

tract with barium or other contrast media are usually necessary in the search for a primary tumor.

ASCITES   The evaluation of a patient with ascites requires that the *cause* of the ascites be established. In most cases ascites will appear as a part of a well-recognized illness, i.e., cirrhosis, congestive heart failure, nephrosis, or disseminated carcinomatosis. In these situations, the physician should determine that the development of ascites is indeed a consequence of the basic underlying disease and not due to the presence of a separate or related disease process. This distinction is necessary even when the cause of ascites seems obvious. For example, when the patient with compensated cirrhosis and minimal ascites develops progressive ascites that is increasingly difficult to control with sodium restriction or diuretics, the obvious temptation is to attribute the worsening of the clinical picture to progressive liver disease. However, an occult hepatoma, portal vein thrombosis, spontaneous bacterial peritonitis, or even tuberculosis may be responsible for the decompensation. The disappointingly low success in diagnosing tuberculous peritonitis or hepatoma in the patient with cirrhosis and ascites reflects the too-low index of suspicion for the development of such superimposed conditions. Similarly, the patient with congestive heart failure may develop ascites from a disseminated carcinoma with peritoneal seeding. The thorough evaluation of each patient with ascites, even in the presence of an "obvious" cause, will help avoid these errors.

Diagnostic paracentesis (50 to 100 mL) should be part of the routine evaluation of the patient with ascites. The fluid should be examined for its gross appearance; and protein content, cell count, and differential cell count should be determined, and Gram's and acid-fast stains and culture performed. Cytologic and cell-block examination may disclose an otherwise unsuspected carcinoma. Table 43-1 presents some of the features of ascitic fluid typically found in various disease states. In some disorders, such as cirrhosis, the fluid has the characteristics of a transudate (<25 g protein per liter and a specific gravity of <1.016); in others, such as peritonitis, the features are those of an exudate. Rather than the total protein content of ascites, some authors prefer the use of a plasma-ascites albumin gradient to characterize ascites. If the difference between the plasma albumin and ascitic fluid albumin is greater than 1.1 g/dL, this is characteristic for uncomplicated cirrhotic ascites, while values less than 1.1 g/dL are seen in conditions characterized by exudative ascites. Although there is variability of the ascitic fluid in any given disease state, some features are sufficiently characteristic to suggest certain diagnostic possibilities. For example, blood-stained fluid with more than 25 g protein per liter is unusual in uncomplicated cirrhosis but is consistent with tuberculous peritonitis or neoplasm. Cloudy fluid with a predominance of polymorphonuclear cells and a positive Gram stain are characteristic of bacterial peritonitis; if most cells are lymphocytes, tuberculosis should be suspected. The complete examination of each fluid is most important, for occasionally only *one* finding may be abnormal. For example, if the fluid is a typical transudate but contains more than 250 white blood cells per microliter, the finding should be recognized as atypical for cirrhosis, nephrosis, or congestive heart failure and should warrant a search for tumor or infection. This is especially true in the evaluation of cirrhotic ascites where occult peritoneal infection may be present with only minor elevations in the white blood cell count of the peritoneal fluid (300 to 500 cells per microliter). Since Gram's stain of the fluid may be negative in a high proportion of such cases, careful culture of the peritoneal fluid is mandatory. Bedside innoculation of blood culture flasks with ascitic fluid results in a dramatically increased incidence of positive cultures when bacterial infection is present (90 versus 40 percent positivity with conventional cultures done by the laboratory). Direct visualization of the peritoneum (laparoscopy) may disclose peritoneal deposits of tumor, tuberculosis, or metastatic disease of the liver. Biopsies are taken under direct vision, often adding to the diagnostic accuracy of the procedure.

Chylous ascites refers to a turbid, milky, or creamy peritoneal fluid due to the presence of thoracic or intestinal lymph. Such a fluid

TABLE 43-1 Ascitic fluid characteristics in various disease states

Condition	Gross appearance	Specific gravity	Protein, g/dL	Cell count Red blood cells, >10,000/µL	White blood cells, per µL	Other tests
Cirrhosis	Straw-colored or bile-stained	<1.016 (95%)*	<25 (95%)	1%	<250 (90%);* predominantly mesothelial	
Neoplasm	Straw-colored, hemorrhagic, mucinous, or chylous	Variable, >1.016 (45%)	>25 (75%)	20%	>1000 (50%); variable cell types	Cytology, cell block, peritoneal biopsy
Tuberculous peritonitis	Clear, turbid, hemorrhagic, chylous	Variable, >1.016 (50%)	>25 (50%)	7%	>1000 (70%); usually >70% lymphocytes	Peritoneal biopsy, stain and culture for acid-fast bacilli
Pyogenic peritonitis	Turbid or purulent	If purulent, >1.016	If purulent, >2.5	Unusual	Predominantly polymorphonuclear leukocytes	+Gram's stain, culture
Congestive heart failure	Straw-colored	Variable, <1.016 (60%)	Variable, 15–53	10%	<1000 (90%); usually mesothelial, mononuclear	
Nephrosis	Straw-colored or chylous	<1.016	<25(100%)	Unusual	<250; mesothelial, mononuclear	If chylous, ether extraction, Sudan staining
Pancreatic ascites (pancreatitis, pseudocyst)	Turbid, hemorrhagic, or chylous	Variable, often >1.016	Variable, often >25	Variable, may be blood-stained	Variable	Increased amylase in ascitic fluid and serum

* Since the conditions of examining fluid and selecting patients were not identical in each series, the percentage figures (in the parentheses) should be taken as an indication of the order of magnitude rather than as the precise incidence of any abnormal finding.

shows Sudan-staining fat globules microscopically and an increased triglyceride content by chemical examination. Opaque milky fluid usually has a triglyceride concentration of more than 1000 mg/dL. A turbid fluid due to leukocytes or tumor cells may be confused with chylous fluid (pseudochylous), and it is often helpful to carry out alkalinization and ether extraction of the specimen. Alkali will tend to dissolve cellular proteins and thereby reduce turbidity; ether extraction will lead to clearing if the turbidity of the fluid is due to lipid. Chylous ascites is most often the result of lymphatic obstruction from trauma, tumor, tuberculosis, filariasis (see Chap. 182), or congenital abnormalities. It also may be seen in the nephrotic syndrome.

Rarely, ascitic fluid may be *mucinous* in character, suggesting either pseudomyxoma peritonei (Chap. 260) or rarely a colloid carcinoma of the stomach or colon with peritoneal implants.

On occasion, ascites may develop as a seemingly isolated finding in the absence of a clinically evident underlying disease. It is then that a careful analysis of ascitic fluid may indicate the direction the evaluation should take. A useful framework for the workup starts with an analysis of whether the fluid is an exudate or transudate. *Transudative ascites* of unclear etiology is most often due to occult cirrhosis, right-sided venous hypertension raising hepatic sinusoidal pressure, or hypoalbuminemic states such as nephrosis or protein-losing enteropathy. Cirrhosis with well-preserved liver function (normal albumin) resulting in ascites invariably is associated with significant portal hypertension (see Chap. 268). Evaluation should include liver function tests, liver-spleen scan, or other hepatic imaging procedure (i.e., CT or ultrasound) to detect nodular changes in the liver or a colloid shift of isotope to suggest portal hypertension. On occasion, a wedged hepatic venous pressure can be useful to document portal hypertension. Finally, if clinically indicated, a liver biopsy will confirm the diagnosis of cirrhosis and perhaps suggest its etiology. Other etiologies may result in hepatic venous congestion and resultant ascites. Right-sided cardiac valvular disease and particularly constrictive pericarditis should raise a high index of suspicion and may require cardiac imaging and cardiac catheterization for definitive diagnosis. Hepatic vein thrombosis is evaluated by visualizing the hepatic veins using imaging techniques (Doppler ultrasound, angiography, CT

scans, magnetic resonance imaging) to demonstrate obliteration, thrombosis, or obstruction by tumor. Uncommonly, transudative ascites may be associated with benign tumors of the ovary, particularly fibroma (Meigs's syndrome) with ascites and hydrothorax.

Exudative ascites should initiate an evaluation for primary peritoneal processes, most importantly infection and tumor. Routine bacteriologic culture of ascitic fluid often will yield a specific organism causing infectious peritonitis. Tuberculous peritonitis (see Table 43-1) is best diagnosed by peritoneal biopsy, either percutaneously or via laparoscopy. Histologic examination invariably shows granulomata that may contain acid-fast bacilli. Since cultures of peritoneal fluid and biopsies for tuberculosis may require 6 weeks, characteristic histology with appropriate stains allows antituberculosis therapy to be started promptly. Similarly, the diagnosis of peritoneal seeding by tumor can usually be made by cytologic analysis of peritoneal fluid or by peritoneal biopsy if cytology is negative. Appropriate diagnostic studies can then be undertaken to determine the nature and site of the primary tumor. Pancreatic ascites (see Table 43-1) is invariably associated with an extravasation of pancreatic fluid from the pancreatic ductal system, most commonly from a leaking pseudocyst. Ultrasound or CT examination of the pancreas followed by visualization of the pancreatic duct by direct cannulation (viz., endoscopic retrograde cholangiopancreatography, ERCP) will usually disclose the site of leakage and permit resective surgery to be carried out.

An analysis of the physiologic and metabolic factors involved in the production of ascites (see Chap. 268 for details), coupled with a complete evaluation of the nature of the ascitic fluid, will invariably disclose the etiology of the ascites and permit appropriate therapy to be instituted.

REFERENCES

EPSTEIN M: Treatment of refractory ascites. N Engl J Med 321:1675, 1989

GARCIA-TSAO G et al: The diagnosis of bacterial peritonitis. Hepatology 5:91, 1985

HOEFS JC: Globulin correction of the albumin gradient: Correlation with measured ascites colloid osmotic pressure gradients. Hepatology 16:396, 1992

PINTO PC et al: Large volume paracentesis in nonedematous patients with tense ascites: Its effect on intravascular volume. Hepatology 8:207, 1988

Rector WG Jr, Reynolds TB: Superiority of the serum: Ascites albumin difference over the ascites total protein concentration in separation of "transudative" and "exudative" ascites. Am J Med 77:83, 1988

Runyon BA: Ascitic fluid culture technique. Heptatology 8:893, 1988

————: Patients with deficient ascitic fluid opsonic activity are predisposed to spontaneous bacterial peritonitis. Hepatology 8:632, 1988

Runyon BA et al: The serum-ascites albumin gradient in the differential diagnosis of ascites. Ann Int Med 117:215, 1992

section 6 Alterations in urinary function and electrolytes

44 ALTERATIONS IN URINARY FUNCTION

FREDRIC L. COE

AZOTEMIA, OLIGURIA, AND ANURIA

AZOTEMIA Urea and creatinine concentrations in serum are often measured to assess the glomerular filtration rate (GFR). Both substances are produced at a reasonably constant rate, by the liver and muscles, respectively. As discussed in Chap. 235, they undergo complete glomerular filtration and are not reabsorbed extensively by the renal tubules; hence their clearances tend to reflect the GFR. An increase in their serum concentrations, termed *azotemia* (*azo*, "containing nitrogen"), occurs as the GFR falls. Creatinine is a more reliable index of GFR than urea because of the latter's lower back-diffusion from tubule lumen to peritubular blood. The GFR may be reduced by a fall in the filtration rates of individual functioning nephrons or by a reduction in the number of functioning nephrons. (See Table 44-1.)

Reduced single-nephron GFR TUBULAR FUNCTION NORMAL An important response of the normal kidney to a severe sodium-conserving stimulus, such as extracellular fluid volume depletion, is reduction of the single-nephron glomerular filtration rate (SNGFR) and subsequent reabsorption of an increased fraction of the reduced amounts of NaCl and water that enter the tubules. The resulting azotemia is called *prerenal azotemia*, in which urinary Na concentration falls below 20 (often below 1) mmol/L (see Table 44-1). The fractional excretion of Na can be calculated (see Chap. 236) and used as an additional index of prerenal azotemia. Secretion of vasopressin is stimulated by depletion of extracellular fluid volume, and as a consequence, the distal tubules and collecting ducts become fully permeable to water. The concentrating mechanisms in the inner medulla (Chap. 235) are efficient when flow rates through the loops of Henle and the collecting ducts are low. As a result, the filtrate that escapes reabsorption in the proximal tubule undergoes maximal osmotic concentration, the urine volume becomes small, and it has a high osmolality, above 500 mmol/kg of water. Most of the filtered creatinine escapes tubular reabsorption, and consequently, the ratio of the urine-to-plasma (U/P) creatinine concentrations is high, 40 or more. Because urea can back-diffuse more completely than creatinine, the blood urea nitrogen (BUN) level rises more than the serum creatinine concentration. Normally, the ratio of BUN to serum creatinine concentration is 10:1; with depletion of the extracellular fluid volume, this ratio rises. An elevated ratio also can be produced by unrelated factors such as tetracycline administration, glucocorticoid therapy, the presence of blood in the gastrointestinal tract, and increased protein turnover due to trauma or burn.

Prerenal azotemia can occur in any edema-forming condition during the phase in which NaCl and water accumulate. Typical examples include the nephrotic syndrome and hepatic cirrhosis with ascites (Chaps. 33 and 240). When a diuretic is administered to inhibit the tubular reabsorption of NaCl, urine volume and Na concentration may be normal or elevated, even though SNGFR falls in response to the combination of the underlying edema-forming stimulus and further extracellular fluid volume depletion from the drug. Oliguria may appear upon withdrawal of the drug as the renal tubules resume intense reabsorption of NaCl and water. Prerenal azotemia also may be seen when renal blood flow is reduced by systemic hypotension, partial renal arterial or venous occlusion, or other cause (Chap. 236). Acute incomplete obstruction of the ureter and acute glomerular injury also may reduce SNGFR and leave tubule function relatively intact; *postrenal azotemia* is a term often applied when acute obstruction lowers SNGFR and causes azotemia. Whenever chronic obstruction of any portion of the urinary tract or glomerulonephritis damages nephrons extensively, the high urinary osmolality, high U/P ratios for creatinine or urea, and low urinary Na concentrations disappear, and the kidneys behave as they do when nephron number is reduced.

TUBULE FUNCTION IMPAIRED Certain acute renal diseases that produce azotemia lower SNGFR and at the same time damage the tubules sufficiently to reduce or even abolish their reabsorptive function, producing *acute renal failure*. Acute tubular necrosis, nephrotoxic agents, and acute tubulointerstitial disease are excellent examples. Azotemia and oliguria appear, but the urinary Na concentration exceeds 20 mmol and usually 40 mmol/L; the U/P ratios for urea and creatinine are below 2 and 20, respectively; and urine osmolality is below 350 mmol/kg of water. The ratio of BUN to serum creatinine is not elevated (see Chap. 236).

Reduced nephron number INCREASED SNGFR If one kidney is removed, the other grows, its nephrons enlarge, and the SNGFR increases until the total GFR becomes nearly normal for two kidneys. The tubules are overperfused with filtrate, but they appear to cope with their increased reabsorptive burdens, perhaps in part because they are longer and wider and possess more cells. If more kidney tissue is removed, the remnant nephrons enlarge further, and their SNGFR rises. Extreme overperfusion of the tubules interferes with Na conservation. At the same time, total GFR comes to depend more and more on expansion of the extracellular fluid volume, largely because the increase in SNGFR is due not only to anatomic growth of the glomeruli but also to a relatively high rate of blood flow per glomerulus. Nephron adaptations to reduced nephron number are detailed in Chap. 235.

Azotemia ensues because the total GFR, i.e., the product of the elevated SNGFR and the markedly reduced nephron number, is low. Tubular conservation of filtered H_2O and Na conservation are poor, so fluid and salt intake must be liberal. Clinical states that produce this picture include surgical loss of renal substance secondary to trauma, neoplasm, stone, and destruction of kidneys by bacterial infection or tuberculosis, polycystic and medullary cystic renal diseases, and all the chronic tubulointerstitial nephropathies (Chaps. 242 and 244). In each of these disorders, the nephrons that remain viable are either fully intact or behave as though the SNGFR is better preserved than tubule function.

TABLE 44-1 Pathophysiologic mechanisms of azotemia

Mechanism of reduced GFR	Clinical examples	Laboratory findings					
		Oliguria	Urine osm, mosmol/kg	Urine [Na$^+$], mmol/L	$\left[\dfrac{U}{P}\right]_{creat}$	$\left[\dfrac{U}{P}\right]_{urea}$	$\dfrac{BUN}{Serum\ creat}$
REDUCED SNGFR							
Tubules normal (prerenal azotemia)	Severe dehydration, edema-forming states, diuretic agents, systemic hypotension, acute glomerular disease,* acute urinary obstruction, incomplete renal vascular obstruction	Nearly always present	>500	<20	>40	>8	>10
Tubules damaged (acute renal failure)	Acute tubular necrosis, nephrotoxic agents, glomerulonephritis with tubule injury	Common	<350	>40	<20	>2	10
REDUCED NEPHRON NUMBER							
Elevated SNGFR	Chronic tubulointerstitial-renal disease Surgical loss of renal tissue	Rare†	[290	>40	3–10	3–10]	10
Normal SNGFR	Diffuse chronic glomerulonephritis Diabetic nephropathy	Rare†	[100–350‡	10–100‡	>10	>3]	>10
Reduced SNGFR	Any of the factors that can reduce SNGFR (listed above) may lower SNGFR in a patient who has a reduced number of functioning nephrons	Common	290	>20	>10	<3	>10

* Acute obstruction causing reduced SNGFR is called *postrenal azotemia*.
† Occurs only when total GFR is below 5 percent normal; urine chemistry values are helpful only when oliguria is present and are therefore enclosed in brackets.
‡ Varies with diet and with the level of GFR. When GFR is below 20 percent normal, osmotic concentration of the urine is usually impossible.
NOTE: osm = osmolality; creat = creatinine concentration; U = urine; P = plasma.

SNGFR NORMAL The SNGFR does not appear to increase despite a reduction of nephron number in diseases such as glomerulonephritis and diabetic glomerulosclerosis, where the glomerulus is the primary site of damage. In these diseases, total GFR falls directly with nephron number and is not supported by elevated SNGFR. Since the tubules are not confronted with an excessive reabsorptive burden, sodium conservation is adequate. In these disorders, superimposed conditions that lower SNGFR, such as depletion of extracellular fluid volume, can cause oliguria with low urine sodium concentration and U/P ratios for creatinine and urea above 20 and 3, respectively. The serum urea-to-creatinine ratio will rise distinctly.

SNGFR REDUCED In patients with chronic renal disease in whom total GFR is sufficient to support life only because of a very high SNGFR, inadvertent dehydration or any other factor (Table 44-1 and Chaps. 235 and 236) that lowers the SNGFR can provoke oliguria and severe azotemia. Under these circumstances, urine Na concentration falls, but not below 20 mmol/L, as in the normal person, because SNGFR, though reduced from a previously high level, may still be above normal. The U/P ratios for creatinine and urea will be low, usually below 10 and 3, respectively, despite oliguria, and urine osmolality will not rise above the plasma level. The serum urea-to-creatinine ratio may rise, but not above 20. In less extreme situations, reduction of SNGFR worsens azotemia and alters urine chemistry in the same directions but to a lesser extent.

OLIGURIA AND ANURIA *Oliguria* refers to a urine volume insufficient to sustain life, usually less than 400 mL/d in an adult of average size. Daily urine volume is difficult to measure when flow rate is low, because small absolute errors of volume measurement, in the range of 50 to 100 mL/d of urine, or of timing of collection, may represent large percentage errors.

Anuria, which is the absence of urine flow, is caused usually by urinary obstruction, which must be excluded as a first step (Chap. 246), or by total renal arterial and venous occlusion. Severe renal diseases such as cortical necrosis and rapidly progressive glomerulonephritis produce anuria in the adult so rarely that anuria should never be ascribed to a primary renal disease until patency of the urinary tract and major renal blood vessels has been established.

Approach to the patient with azotemia or oliguria A critical issue is whether azotemia has been stable and long-standing (chronic renal failure; see Chap. 234) or is recent and increasing (acute renal failure; see Chap. 236; pre- and postrenal azotemia). If azotemia is recent and oliguria is present, the most discriminating additional measurements include serum urea and creatinine concentrations and the Na, urea, and creatinine concentrations and osmolality of a concurrent urine sample. Reduction of SNGFR with well-preserved tubule function is usually present when urine osmolality exceeds 500 mmol/kg of water, Na < 20 mmol/L, the U/P ratios for urea and creatinine > 8 and 40, respectively, the urinalysis is normal, and the BUN > 10 times the serum creatinine concentration. The prognosis for recovery of adequate GFR is good if the cause of reduced SNGFR can be reversed. When urine osmolality is below 350 mmol/kg of water, Na > 40 mmol, the U/P values for urea and creatinine < 2 and 20, respectively, and the BUN exceeds the serum creatinine by only tenfold, tubule function has been lost, and some form of acute or chronic renal failure is present.

ABNORMAL URINARY CONSTITUENTS

PROTEINURIA Normal adults may excrete up to 150 mg/d protein. Of this, only 5 to 15 mg is albumin; the rest is composed of over 30 different plasma proteins and of glycoproteins that derive from the renal cells. Tamm-Horsfall mucoprotein, the most prevalent urine protein that does not arise from plasma, is produced by the cells of the ascending limb of the loop of Henle and is excreted at the rate of 50 to 75 mg/d. Daily excretion of more than 150 mg protein is properly termed *pathologic proteinuria*, but in common usage the word *proteinuria* suffices. Protein excretion above 3.5 g/24 h is termed *massive* proteinuria and usually occurs when glomeruli have been damaged enough to allow plasma proteins, especially albumin, to enter the urine. Urinary albumin loss lowers serum albumin concentration, and the consequent fall in intracapillary oncotic pressure fosters the accumulation of tissue edema (Chap. 33); serum lipids rise, for reasons detailed in Chap. 240. The combination of *massive proteinuria, hypoalbuminemia, edema,* and *hyperlipidemia* is often called the *nephrotic syndrome,* but this term is also used for massive urinary protein loss alone. Massive proteinuria causes hypoalbuminemia, elevated blood lipids, and edema only when hepatic albumin synthesis, although normal or even increased, fails to compensate for urine albumin losses; these features are not a direct result of renal disease.

Detection of proteinuria   Proteinuria is usually detected by urine "dipsticks" that register a trace result in response to as little as 50 mg protein per liter and a distinct color change of the 1 + level at about 300 mg protein per liter. Since proteinuria can be missed if the urine is dilute, fasting morning samples that tend to be concentrated are usually studied. Dipsticks respond best to albumin, so a negative result can occur when large amounts of other protein, or protein fragments such as light chains, are excreted. Dipstick proteinuria requires additional documentation by the measurement of 24-h excretion rate. If total protein excretion is abnormal, it is helpful to characterize the proportions of albumin and globulins in the urine by cellulose acetate electrophoresis or other methods. Immunoelectrophoresis is required to identify immunoglobulin fragments, kappa or lambda light chains, when their presence is suggested by a monoclonal peak on routine urine electrophoresis.

Mechanisms of proteinuria   TUBULAR PROTEINURIA   Low-molecular-weight (<40,000) serum proteins, such as beta$_2$ microglobulin (11,600 mol wt), lysozyme (14,000 mol wt), or light chains (22,000 mol wt) are readily filtered by the glomeruli but are reabsorbed so efficiently that only trace amounts enter the urine. Diseases that selectively damage the tubules more than glomeruli (Chap. 242) cause excessive excretion of these small proteins with little or no increase in albumin excretion. The resulting proteinuria is usually between 1 and 3 g/24 h, and edema and lipid disorders do not occur because albumin losses are small. Bence Jones protein, which is probably a dimer of two light chains, light chains themselves, and myoglobin are examples of proteins whose plasma concentrations may increase as a consequence of disease. If the filtered load rises to exceed tubular reabsorptive capacity, "overflow" proteinuria may occur.

GLOMERULAR PROTEINURIA   Normal glomeruli filter little albumin or globulin. Glomerular capillary endothelial cells form a barrier penetrated by pores of about 100 nm diameter that holds back cells and other particles but offers no impediment to most proteins. The glomerular basement membrane traps molecules about 5 nm in effective radius, above 100,000 Da molecular mass. The *foot processes (podocytes)* of the visceral epithelial cells (Fig. 44-1) cover the urinary aspect of the glomerular basement membrane and produce a series of narrow channels through which molecules traverse the basement membrane. Anionic molecules, like albumin, are filtered less freely than are neutral or positively charged molecules of the same size, so little albumin enters the filtrate. This charge selectively appears to be due to anionic glycoproteins that cover the surfaces of the foot processes and contribute to the matrix structure of the basement membrane (Chap. 235). The glycoproteins are anionic due to their content of glutamate, aspartate, and sialic acid. At the pH of blood (7.4) or urine (4.5 to 7.5) carboxylic and sialic acid residues are dissociated and, therefore, have a negative charge; albumin also carries a negative charge. The negatively charged glycoproteins repel albumin and retard albumin filtration.

Glomerular disease can disrupt any of these filtration barriers. Injury limited to the polyanion glycoproteins tends to produce selective losses of anionic proteins, such as albumin, that would be filtered more completely by the normal glomerulus but for their charge. Extensive injury that involves the entire basement membrane, not only its polyanion components, may increase losses of very large proteins as well as albumin.

The selectivity of proteinuria varies with the extent of glomerular injury. However, the clinical value of measuring selectivity has not been fully defined. The basis of such measurements is to express the excretion rate of a protein as a fraction of its theoretical maximal filtered load, which is the product of its serum concentration and the

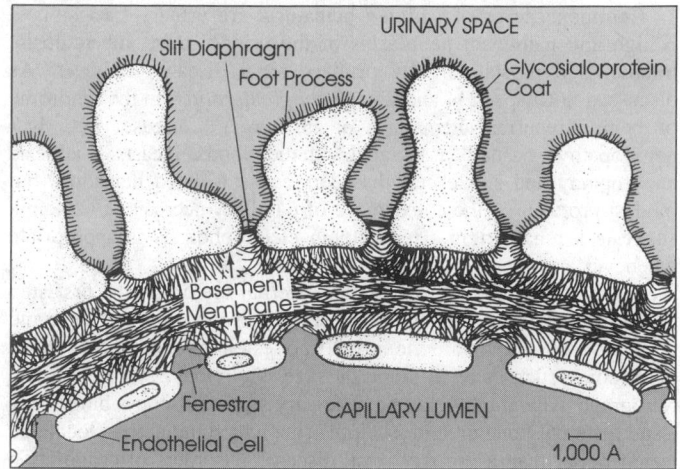

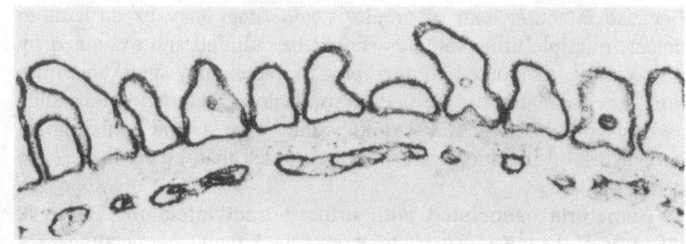

FIGURE 44-1   *(Top).* Diagram showing normal structures separating the capillary lumen and urinary space in the glomerulus. In the process of glomerular filtration, an ultrafiltrate of plasma traverses the glomerular capillary wall through endothelial fenestrae, basement membrane, and slit diaphragms. Macromolecules in the plasma are believed to be restricted from entry into glomerular urine by each of these wall structures. In addition, circulating polyanions (e.g., albumin) are thought to be retarded by negatively charged glycosialoproteins, which, as shown by the shaded area in the upper panel, are distributed throughout the glomerular wall. *(Bottom).* A corresponding electron micrograph of the same structures. *(Drawing by NL Gahan from BM Brenner, R Beeuwkes, Hosp Prac, vol 13, no 7, 1978. Reproduced with permission.)*

GFR. This fraction must reflect the relative filtration efficiency of the protein to that of a completely filtered GFR marker, usually inulin or creatinine, provided that tubular reabsorption and renal production or catabolism are negligible. The slope of a plot of the clearance ratio against molecular weight for a variety of serum proteins is one index of filtration selectivity. A more practical version of this test is based on the ratio of the clearance fractions of two proteins of different molecular weight, such as IgG and transferrin (Chap. 240).

Approach to the patient with proteinuria   If the dipstick proteinuria is 1 + or more, 24-h urine protein excretion should be measured. If it is above 150 mg, the proportions of albumin and other proteins should be determined by electrophoresis. Excretion mainly of albumin signifies a glomerular lesion. When the total daily protein excretion exceeds 3.5 g, by definition, the nephrotic syndrome is considered to be present; milder albuminuria is called an *asymptomatic urinary abnormality.* The initial steps in evaluating proteinuria are outlined in Chap. 234. Subsequent details of differential diagnosis are in Chaps. 240 and 241. Tubular proteinuria usually reflects a hereditary or acquired tubular disorder (Chap. 244) or tubulointerstitial nephropathy (Chap. 242). The presence of large amounts of Bence Jones protein suggests that multiple myeloma may be present (Chap. 280).

HEMATURIA AND CASTS   **Isolated hematuria**   Bleeding in the urinary tract from the urethra to the renal pelvis produces isolated hematuria, without significant proteinuria, cells, or urinary casts. Total hematuria, which occurs evenly throughout voiding, means that blood has had the opportunity to mix fully with the bladder urine. When bleeding occurs mainly at the beginning or end of micturition, a prostatic or urethral origin is more likely.

Common causes of *isolated* hematuria are urinary tract stones, benign and malignant neoplasms of the urinary tract, tuberculosis, trauma, and prostatitis; few primary renal diseases cause it. As discussed in Chaps. 234 and 240, *focal glomerulitis*, in the syndrome of benign recurrent hematuria or in Berger's disease, i.e., IgA nephropathy, is usually associated with red blood cell casts. Analgesic nephropathy and sickle cell disorders cause isolated hematuria but modest proteinuria; the coexistence of papillary necrosis or azotemia suggests a renal origin. Hemoglobin electrophoresis is appropriate whenever a sickle cell disorder is suspected.

Examination of the prostate and external urethra is the first step in the evaluation of isolated hematuria. Intravenous pyelography and renal ultrasonography are the next. If no lesion is found and no cause of bleeding such as renal stone passage is obvious, cystoscopy and retrograde pyelography may be necessary. At cystoscopy, blood may issue from only one ureter, a helpful clue which indicates a localized lesion rather than a primary renal disease. Disorders of coagulation and thrombocytopenia, as well as urinary infection, must be excluded. Because infection with tuberculosis and fungi may be difficult to detect, multiple urine samples should be cultured and examined by microscopy. Computed tomography of the kidney and sometimes renal arteriography may be needed to disclose anatomic lesions such as cysts or tumors. Urine cytology may give a clue to malignant neoplasms of the kidneys or urinary tract that otherwise escape detection.

Hematuria associated with urinary tract infection   Bacterial infection of the lower urinary tract or of the kidneys frequently causes hematuria. The presence of associated pyuria suggests the diagnosis, and the demonstration of pathogenic bacteria in concentrations above 10^5 colonies per milliliter of urine establishes it. Acute cystitis or urethritis in women is a common cause of gross hematuria; in such symptomatic patients, infection is established by documenting colony counts above 10^2 colonies per milliliter. Urinary tuberculosis can produce isolated hematuria, but pyuria often is present as well.

Hematuria with evidence of renal disease   NEPHRONAL HEMATURIA   Blood that enters the tubular fluid anywhere along the nephron can be trapped in a cylindrical mold of gelled Tamm-Horsfall protein to produce red blood cell casts. Tamm-Horsfall protein gels when concentrated at a low pH, as occurs during dehydration, or when exposed to myoglobin, hemoglobin, albumin, Bence Jones protein, or pyelographic contrast media. Degenerated red blood cells and clumps of hemoglobin can produce deeply pigmented casts that have the same significance—nephronal hematuria—as red blood cell casts.

Nephronal hematuria always connotes significant renal disease such as glomerulonephritis, tubulointerstitial injury, or a vasculitis that has damaged the circulation of the nephron. Glomerular or tubular proteinuria often accompanies renal bleeding, as a consequence of nephron injury. In general, nephronal hematuria and proteinuria alone arise from renal diseases that have a better prognosis than those in which proteinuria and hematuria occur in combination (Chap. 234).

Hematuria with proteinuria or casts   Frequently, hematuria is accompanied by proteinuria, but red blood cell and deeply pigmented granular casts are absent. The presumption is that bleeding is of nephronal origin, but a coincident independent lesion of the urinary tract must always be considered, because common renal diseases, such as diabetic glomerulosclerosis and arteriolar nephrosclerosis associated with hypertension, produce mainly proteinuria.

TYPES OF CASTS   Heavy albuminuria or dehydration can cause showers of transparent, refractile *hyaline* casts. During heavy proteinuria, tubule cells fill with cholesterol-rich lipid droplets that display a Maltese-cross appearance in polarized light. Casts that incorporate these cells are called *fatty casts* because the lipid droplets are prominent. The same lipid-rich cells free in urine are called *oval fat bodies*.

White blood cell and *epithelial cell casts* can occur in any inflammatory state that involves the nephrons. White blood cell casts are particularly common in pyelonephritis, in nephritis associated with systemic lupus erythematosus, and during transplant rejection.

When white blood or epithelial cells degenerate, they form granular nonpigmented casts that contain cellular debris and aggregated proteins. So-called *waxy* casts, with few granules and very distinct margins, arise when cell debris has broken down to a fine dispersion so that granules are no longer visible and are most common in chronic and progressive renal diseases.

Broad casts, of unusual width, are thought to arise in the dilated tubules of enlarged nephrons that have undergone compensatory hypertrophy in response to a reduction of functioning renal mass. A urine sample that contains a combination of broad and waxy casts as well as cellular or granular casts or red blood cells indicates a chronic smoldering process and has been termed a *telescoped* urine. This abnormality, first described in polyarteritis nodosa and systemic lupus erythematosus, also is found in many chronic forms of glomerulonephritis with active glomerulitis.

Approach to the patient with hematuria   Many urinalyses should be performed to determine whether the hematuria is isolated or associated with other features of primary renal disease, i.e., cells, casts, or proteinuria. The magnitude and type of associated proteinuria should be determined. Intravenous pyelography should be performed, if it can be done safely, even when the hematuria is of nephronal origin. Not only lesions of the urinary tract, but renal tumors or cysts, discrete areas of papillary necrosis, or signs of renal venous obstruction may be present. The source of isolated hematuria must always be ascertained, and this means a detailed examination of the urinary tract by cystoscopy, retrograde pyelography, and arteriography to disclose tumor, stone, cysts, or other cause. Renal ultrasonography and computed tomography are particularly helpful in detecting and evaluating renal cysts and tumors and should precede cystoscopy and arteriography. If all the studies disclose normal structures, a nephronal origin of hematuria is likely even if no red blood cell casts are present. The role of renal biopsy in such cases is detailed in Chaps. 240, 241, and 242. Hematuria with infection or overt renal disease usually requires no steps beyond intravenous pyelography. Evaluation of hematuria is detailed in Chap. 227.

POLYURIA AND NOCTURIA

POLYURIA   A reasonable definition of polyuria is a urine volume above 3 L/d, with the recognition that normal individuals who drink a large amount of fluid intake form large volumes of urine. Patients cannot always distinguish polyuria from urinary frequency, the frequent voiding of small volumes. Since voiding volumes may not be clear from the history, polyuria must be substantiated by 24-h urine collection before investigating the cause.

Causes   Polyuria can arise from inadequate secretion of vasopressin, failure of the renal tubules to respond to vasopressin, solute diuresis, or natriuresis (Table 44-2). It also may occur as a physiologic response to excessive water drinking. The physiology of urine formation and mechanisms for renal water conservation are discussed in Chap. 235.

DIABETES INSIPIDUS (See also Chap. 333)   The term *diabetes insipidus* is applied to situations in which inadequate renal water conservation causes polyuria and secondary thirst, either due to vasopressin insufficiency (central diabetes insipidus) or renal unresponsiveness to vasopressin (nephrogenic diabetes insipidus). In both, water reabsorption is reduced all along the distal nephron, because passive water movement from tubules into the hypertonic outer and inner medullary interstitium is slow. Even though the rate of water movement out of the collecting ducts is low for a given osmotic difference between the tubule lumen and interstitial fluid, however, the fluid that enters the collecting ducts is so dilute and copious in volume that more water reaches the inner medulla than normal and medullary solutes are washed into the vasa recta. Wash-out is incomplete; while vasopressin administration can lead to formation of a concentrated urine, the maximal urine osmolality attained is below normal.

TABLE 44-2 Causes of polyuria

INADEQUATE RENAL WATER CONSERVATION

A Diabetes insipidus
  1 Vasopressin-sensitive (posthypophysectomy; posttrauma; postpituitary ablation; idiopathic, supra- or intrasellar tumors or cysts; histiocystosis or granuloma; encroachment by aneurysm; Sheehan's syndrome, meningoencephalitis; Guillain-Barré syndrome; fat embolus; empty sella)
  2 Nephrogenic
    a Acquired tubulointerstitial renal disease (pyelonephritis, analgesic nephropathy, multiple myeloma, amyloidosis, obstructive uropathy, sarcoidosis, hypercalcemic or hypokalemic nephropathy, Sjögren's syndrome, sickle cell anemia, renal transplantation)
    b Drugs or toxins (lithium, demeclocycline, methoxyflurane, ethanol, diphenylhydantoin, propoxyphene, amphotericin)
    c Congenital (hereditary nephrogenic diabetes insipidus, polycystic or medullary cystic disease)
B Solute diuresis (glucosuria, high-protein tube feedings, urea or mannitol infusion, radiographic contrast media, chronic renal failure)
C Natriuretic syndromes (salt-losing nephritis, diuretic phase of acute tubular necrosis, diuretic agents)

PRIMARY POLYDIPSIA

A Psychogenic
B Hypothalamic disease
C Drugs (thioridazine, chlorpromazine, anticholinergic agents)

Vasopressin-sensitive (central) diabetes insipidus may be idiopathic or secondary to hypophysectomy or trauma or to neoplastic, inflammatory, vascular, or infectious causes (Table 44-2). Idiopathic diabetes insipidus can be inherited as an autosomal dominant trait; more commonly, it is sporadic and appears in childhood. In both forms there is selective destruction of the neurons that produce vasopressin in the supraoptic nucleus.

Rarely, nephrogenic diabetes insipidus is familial and congenital, but usually it is acquired (Table 44-2). Hypercalcemia and hypokalemic nephropathy are reversible causes of nephrogenic diabetes insipidus. Lithium carbonate, methoxyflurane anesthesia, and demeclocycline also can produce nephrogenic diabetes insipidus.

SOLUTE DIURESIS Excessive filtration of a poorly resorbed solute such as glucose, mannitol, or urea can depress reabsorption of NaCl and water in the proximal tubule and cause their loss in the urine, producing polyuria. Urine Na concentration is below that of blood, so more water than salt is lost from the body and the serum is hypertonic. Glucosuria in diabetes mellitus is a common cause of solute diuresis. Iatrogenic solute diuresis may arise from mannitol infusion, angiographic contrast media, and high-protein gavage feedings, which produce an excessive excretion of urea. Any solute diuresis can cause polyuria, so further evaluation of renal concentrating ability should be postponed until the solute diuresis is corrected.

NATRIURETIC SYNDROMES Excessive chronic Na loss may occur during the course of tubulointerstitial or cystic renal disease. Polyuria and polydipsia are accompanied by a large daily Na requirement. Examples include medullary cystic disease, Bartter's syndrome, and the diuretic phase of acute tubular necrosis, in which Na and water losses are large.

PRIMARY POLYDIPSIA Whether because of habit, predilection, psychiatric disorder, a specific lesion in the brain, or medication (Table 44-2), some people drink enough water every day to produce polyuria. The body and the kidneys rarely, if ever, are injured by chronic polydipsia, but the condition can be confused with diabetes insipidus, which it resembles closely. During deliberate polydipsia, extracellular fluid volume is normal or high, and vasopressin secretion is reduced to a basal level because serum osmolality tends to be near the lower limits of normal. Reabsorption of water from the distal convoluted tubule and collecting ducts is reduced so that all the surplus water can be excreted into the urine. The inner medulla loses its urea and NaCl gradients because of wash-out, as in diabetes insipidus. Wash-out may be more severe than in diabetes insipidus

because primary polydipsia tends to cause expansion of the extracellular fluid volume, whereas primary renal water loss does the opposite. Volume expansion raises total delivery of NaCl and water to the thick ascending limb of Henle and therefore to the inner medulla, all things being equal. It also raises renal blood flow, and increased flow through the vasa recta reduces their ability to trap solutes in the medulla.

Approach to the patient with polyuria Solute diuresis and natriuretic syndromes usually are apparent from the history, physical examination, urinalysis (glucosuria), clinical setting, blood count, blood glucose, and serum creatinine or BUN. Diagnostic problems occur mainly when stable, chronic polyuria and polydipsia of uncertain origin are present. Here one must try to distinguish between vasopressin-sensitive diabetes insipidus, nephrogenic diabetes insipidus, and primary polydipsia; the best way to make this distinction is by measuring the response of urine osmolality to water deprivation and the administration of vasopressin.

The subject should have free access to water and receive a normal diet that provides approximately 100 mmol NaCl per day for 3 days; then a total fast is instituted. During the fast, pulse and blood pressure should be measured every 30 min, and body weight should be measured every hour using an accurate balance. When 3 percent of the initial body weight has been lost or 14 h has elapsed, urine and serum osmolality are measured. In the normal subject urine volume will be below 0.5 mL/min, and urine osmolality will be above 700 mmol/kg of water. In complete diabetes insipidus, nephrogenic or vasopressin-sensitive, the urine osmolality will remain below 200 mmol/kg of water and urine flow above 0.5 mL/min, but some rise in osmolality and fall in flow occurs in incomplete diabetes insipidus. If urine osmolality is below 700 mmol/kg of water by the end of the fasting period, 5 mU/min aqueous arginine vasopressin or 1 μg desmopressin is administered by subcutaneous injection. Patients with complete or partial vasopressin-sensitive diabetes insipidus will raise their urine osmolality above the level achieved by fasting alone by more than 9 percent (see Chap. 333). No increase will occur in complete nephrogenic diabetes insipidus, although incomplete forms of nephrogenic diabetes insipidus will permit some response to vasopressin. Infusion of hypertonic saline (Chap. 333) is useful in defining defects of osmoregulator function.

Patients with primary polydipsia respond differently. During fluid restriction, the secretion of vasopressin increases, and at the completion of the test the flow rate and osmolality of the urine reflect a physiologic level of vasopressin acting on normal tubules that traverse a medullary interstitium whose urea and NaCl concentrations have been reduced by chronic wash-out. In other words, the wash-out sets the upper limit on urine osmolality, and patients with primary polydipsia thus demonstrate a submaximal concentrating ability despite intact vasopressin secretion. Exogenous vasopressin can increase urine osmolality very little (<9 percent) because medullary wash-out, not vasopressin insufficiency or insensitivity, is the main limiting factor. Usually the urine osmolality will be above 400 mmol/kg of water by the end of the fluid deprivation test, in contrast to the values of approximately 200 mmol/kg of water in patients with diabetes insipidus; in some cases it may be impossible to distinguish incomplete diabetes insipidus from primary polydipsia with the fluid deprivation test alone. Measurement of serum arginine vasopressin levels by radioimmunoassay is rarely of diagnostic help.

NOCTURIA Whether an individual sleeps through the night without urinating depends on a diurnal rhythm in which the volume of urine formed during sleep does not exceed bladder capacity, because of reduced renal osmotic concentration, high sodium excretion, solute diuresis, or low bladder capacity.

All polyuric states may cause nocturia. Urinary concentrating ability falls in most renal diseases (Chap. 235), often at an early stage. Even though overt polyuria may be absent, overnight urine volume frequently exceeds bladder capacity. Nocturia also occurs in edema-forming states. In congestive heart failure, nephrotic syndrome, and hepatic cirrhosis with ascites, fluid accumulates preferentially in dependent portions of the body during the day. At night, with recumbency, tissue capillary forces change, and some edema fluid is mobilized, producing the effect of an intravenous saline infusion. Venous insufficiency may produce dependent edema of the legs that is also mobilized at night, causing nocturia.

Reduced bladder capacity also causes nocturia. Infection, tumor, or stone can cause inflammation and increased bladder irritability. Chronic partial bladder outflow obstruction, from prostatic hyperplasia, urethral stricture, or benign or malignant neoplasm or stone, causes a stimulus to void and a thickening of the muscular wall that reduces its compliance. Frequent small voidings may be a clue to this cause of nocturia, but in its earlier phases bladder obstruction may cause only one nocturnal voiding of reasonable volume.

DYSURIA, FREQUENCY AND URGENCY, INCONTINENCE, AND ENURESIS

DYSURIA, FREQUENCY, AND URGENCY   *Dysuria* refers to pain or a burning sensation during urination. *Urinary frequency* means voiding at frequent intervals, due to a sense of bladder fullness that is due not to a full bladder but to an irritable bladder that feels full even when it is not. *Urgency* is an exaggerated sense of needing to urinate, due to an irritable or inflamed bladder.

Mechanisms of dysuria   REDUCED BLADDER COMPLIANCE When the ability of the bladder to expand is reduced, frequency, nocturia, and urgency result. When decreased expansion is due to inflammation of the mucosa (cystitis) from infection, radiation, chemicals, or foreign bodies (catheters, stones), a burning sensation usually is more intense than when it is due to infiltration of the muscle by tumors of the bladder or from adjacent organs (prostate, rectum, uterus).

INFECTION   Acute bacterial cystitis, which occurs more frequently in women, usually causes frequent urination day and night, a burning sensation on urination, and, not infrequently, gross hematuria. Prostatitis or prostatocystitis in men can cause a picture similar to acute cystitis in women. When only the prostate is involved, milder symptoms such as vague pain or discomfort in the lower abdomen, groin, perineum, rectum, testes, or penis occur. The symptoms may be associated with urination but usually is noticed at times other than during urination or ejaculation.

PSYCHOSOMATIC CYSTITIS   The *functional bladder syndrome* and *chronic glandular urethrotrigonitis* are synonyms for a very common but poorly understood affliction of middle-aged and older women, in which pain is usually vague, aching in nature, and in the lower abdomen or vagina. There is daytime frequency without nocturia; pyuria is absent. A complete urologic evaluation usually becomes necessary because symptoms are chronic and hard to eradicate. The functional bladder syndrome must be distinguished from the effects of a cystocele, which can be repaired surgically.

Approach to the patient with dysuria   The medical history should focus on past as well as present urinary problems. A pelvic examination in women and prostatic examination in men are necessary components of the physical examination. A two-glass urinary sediment in all patients and the prostatic fluid in men, obtained by prostatic massage, should be examined by microscopy. When the urethra is the principal site of inflammation or infection, the first 20 mL of a voiding, if collected separately, may contain a higher concentration of leukocytes and bacteria than the remainder of the voided urine. Normal prostatic fluid, not subjected to centrifugation, contains less than 10 leukocytes per high-power field; leukocytosis in the prostatic fluid is an important clue to prostatitis and may, when prostatitis is chronic, be the only detectable abnormality. Further diagnostic studies will depend on such features as a history of chronic or recurrent episodes or associated fever, which are rare in lower urinary tract infections except in acute prostatitis; an abnormality on physical examination, such as a pelvic or rectal mass or tenderness, hematuria, or pyuria; or increased excessive leukocytes and macrophages in the prostatic fluid.

Additional evaluation of dysuria, when the cause is not evident from clinical examination, may include cultures of urine and prostatic fluid for aerobic and anaerobic bacteria, tubercle bacilli, and mycoplasmas; excretory urography; and voiding cystourethrography. If these examinations do not reveal the diagnosis but symptoms are troublesome, urologic evaluations, including cystoscopy, urethroscopy, and endoscopic biopsies of visualized abnormalities, and dynamic urinary tract studies may be useful.

INCONTINENCE   *Incontinence*, the inability to retain urine in the bladder, results from neurologic or mechanical disorders of the system that controls normal micturition.

Normal bladder function   The detrusor muscle, which provides the propulsive force for emptying the bladder, consists of interlacing fibers of smooth muscle that are under parasympathetic autonomic control through the pelvic nerves from sacral spinal cord segments S2, S3, and S4. The smooth muscle of the trigonal portion of the bladder, between the ureteral orifices and the posterior area of the bladder outlet, is innervated by motor fibers from thoracolumbar segments (T11 to L2) of the sympathetic nervous system, in which alpha receptor sites predominate. This layer of muscle extends into the posterior urethra and acts as an involuntary internal sphincter that helps maintain urinary continence even in the absence of voluntary control. The external urethral sphincter and perineal muscles are under voluntary control via the pudendal nerves.

Sensory tracts of pain, temperature, and distention pass from the bladder via the pelvic nerves to sacral spinal levels S2, S3, and S4, creating a spinal voiding reflex between the bladder and the sacral spinal cord. The sensory tracts from the bladder further ascend through sacrobulbar pathways to the medulla of the brain and ultimately to cortical centers, from which impulses arise, pass back down the lateral and ventral reticulospinal tracts, and normally suppress the sacral spinal reflex arc controlling bladder emptying.

The normal adult bladder can accommodate approximately 400 mL fluid without a significant increase in intravesical pressure (<20 cmH_2O). Above this point, sensations of fullness are transmitted to the sacral cord. If not suppressed by cortical control, the sacral cord reflexly discharges motor impulses that cause powerful sustained detrusor contraction. Urination can be prevented by cortical suppression of the reflex arc or by voluntary contraction of the external sphincter and perineal muscles. Infants and adults with spinal cord damage above S2 urinate spontaneously when the bladder fills sufficiently.

Normal urination is initiated by voluntary suppression of cortical inhibition of the reflex arc and by relaxation of the muscles of the pelvic floor and the external sphincter. The base of the bladder falls; then the trigone contracts, an action that occludes the ureters as they pass through the bladder wall and helps to prevent vesicoureteral reflux of urine during voiding. Finally, the detrusor contracts, and voiding occurs.

Causes of incontinence   DETRUSOR INSTABILITY   In this condition, the bladder becomes prone to uncontrollable contractions—that cause incontinence—because inhibitory neural pathways are damaged. Among the elderly, detrusor instability causes as much as 70 percent of urinary incontinence and arises from diseases of the central nervous system such as cerebrovascular accidents, Alzheimer's disease, neoplasia, and, possibly, normal-pressure hydrocephalus. Any lesion that disrupts the lateral and ventral reticulospinal tracts can reduce or abolish descending inhibiting impulses to the sacral spinal reflex and result in detrusor instability. If the descending tracts are completely destroyed, the bladder will empty automatically. Bladder or pelvic infection or tumor, fecal impaction, uterine prolapse, and prostatic hypertrophy are other causes. Whatever the cause, the usual clinical picture is of unpredictable, involuntary voiding, usually >160 mL each time. Imipramine, 25 mg at bedtime, or calcium channel blockers (such as nifedipine) reduce detrusor contractions and improve continence. Local infection, tumors, or fecal impaction are treated conventionally.

STRESS INCONTINENCE   This condition is common in postmenopausal parous women. The structures of the female urethra atrophy when deprived of estrogen, and many women become unable to resist the passage of urine under the stress of increased intraabdominal pressure during coughing, sneezing, climbing stairs, and other physical activity, so small amounts of urine escape. Parturition may damage the pelvic support of the bladder so that the bladder and urethra can slip downward from their normal position above the pelvic diaphragm. As they do, the urethra shortens, and the normal urethrovesical angle, important in closing the urethral sphincter, is lost. In men, stress incontinence usually is secondary to prostatic surgery for benign prostatic hypertrophy or prostatic carcinoma. If the external sphincter is damaged during operation, total incontinence may result. Surgical elevation of the urethrovesical angle is helpful in women. Estrogen replacement therapy may prevent atrophy of the urethral mucosa.

MECHANICAL INCONTINENCE   Some congenital anomalies, extrophy of the bladder, patent urachus, and ectopic ureteral openings distal to the vesical neck cause mechanical incontinence. They are correctable only by surgery. Mechanical incontinence can follow transurethral resection of the prostate that damages both the internal and external sphincter mechanisms. Pelvic surgery or irradiation of the uterus or rectum may cause incontinence because of vesicovaginal, ureterovaginal, vesicoperineal, or ureteroperineal fistulas.

OVERFLOW OR PARADOXICAL INCONTINENCE   This form of incontinence arises from large residual volumes of urine secondary to obstruction at the bladder neck or the urethra (urethral stricture) or from neurologic damage. Benign prostatic hyperplasia afflicts upward of 75 percent of older men (see Chap. 323). It is manifested by nocturia, reduced size and force of the urinary stream, straining to urinate, and terminal dribbling, all due to outflow obstruction. Functional outflow obstruction can occur because of spinal cord disease; the detrusor and external sphincter contract dyssynergistically, i.e., at the same time. Hypotonic neurogenic bladders may occur in diseases that produce autonomic peripheral neuropathy, such as diabetes mellitus, uremia, hypothyroidism, chronic alcoholism, Guillain-Barré syndrome, collagen vascular diseases, and toxic neuropathies associated with some carcinomas (especially lung and kidney). It also may occur because of prolonged overdistention of the bladder. Hydronephrosis and impaired renal function can occur with chronic overflow incontinence. All causes produce a dilated, palpable bladder. Especially in diabetes, patients can control micturition but lose their sensory awareness of bladder filling. Their incontinence can be avoided by scheduled reminders. Outlet obstruction is treated surgically. If the bladder is adynamic because of prolonged overfilling, bethanechol chloride, 50 to 100 mg/d, may improve emptying.

PSYCHOGENIC AND FUNCTIONAL INCONTINENCE   Children and even some young adults draw attention to themselves by feigning incontinence and thereby derive some secondary emotional satisfaction. A complete diagnostic evaluation usually is necessary to rule out organic disease even when psychogenic incontinence is strongly suspected. In elderly people, especially those with a limited ability to walk or who are confused because of central nervous system disease or drugs, incontinence may be *functional*, i.e., due simply to an inability to reach a toilet in time. Treatment depends on correcting the individual problem in each case.

ENURESIS   *Enuresis* refers to the involuntary passage of urine at night or during sleep—hence the synonym *bed-wetting*. Some reserve the term enuresis for those bed-wetters who have no gross urologic abnormalities, but it is appropriate for bed-wetting in general.

The sacral spinal reflex arc alone controls urination in the infant; therefore, bed-wetting is normal under the age of 2 years. As the nervous system matures, development of cortical control over the spinal reflex arc results in the voluntary control over urination and defecation by the age of $2\frac{1}{2}$ years. Even so, enuresis beyond the age of 3 years occurs to some degree in approximately 10 percent of all otherwise normal children and probably is due to a delay in maturation of bladder control, which may be familial.

Although most bed-wetting ceases by the age of puberty, organic diseases, especially infections of the urinary tract, obstructive lesions

with overflow incontinence, neurovesical dysfunction, and polyuric conditions that overload the bladder must be suspected when enuresis persists beyond the age of 3 years. Patients with organic disease usually, but not always, are incontinent during the day as well as at night. For the majority, who have no overt lesions, imipramine (75 mg at bedtime) may be useful.

REFERENCES

Azotemia, oliguria, and anuria

ABUELO JG: Proteinuria: Diagnostic principles and procedures. Ann Intern Med 98:186, 1983

BRENNER BM, LAZARUS JM (eds): *Acute Renal Failure*, 2d ed. New York, Churchill-Livingstone, 1988

GLASSOCK RJ et al: Primary glomerular diseases, in *The Kidney*, 4th ed, BM Brenner, FC Rector Jr (eds). Philadelphia, Saunders, 1991, p 1182

HILBRANDS LB et al: Cimetidine improves the reliability of creatinine as a marker of glomerular filtration. Kidney Int 40:1171, 1991

KANWAR YS: Biophysiology of glomerular filtration and proteinuria. Lab Invest 51:7, 1984

KOHLER H et al: Acanthocytosis: A characteristic marker for glomerular bleeding. Kidney Int 40:115, 1991

LEVEY AS et al: Idiopathic nephrotic syndrome. Ann Intern Med 107:697, 1987

LOON N et al: Effect of angiotensin II infusion on the human glomerular filtration barrier. Am J Physiol 257:F608, 1989

MYERS BD et al: Mechanisms of proteinuria in human glomerulonephritis. J Clin Invest 70:732, 1982

PARDO V et al: Benign primary hematuria: Clinicopathologic study of 65 patients. Am J Med 67:817, 1979

Polyuria and nocturia

BERL T (ed): Disorders of water metabolism, in *Seminars in Nephrology*, vol 4. New York, Grune & Stratton, 1984, p 285

GOLDMAN MB et al: Mechanisms of altered water metabolism in psychotic patients with polydipsia and hyponatremia. N Engl J Med 318:397, 1988

ROBERTSON GL, BERL W: Pathophysiology of water metabolism, in *The Kidney*, 4th ed, BM Brenner, FC Rector Jr (eds). Philadelphia, Saunders, 1991, p 677

SCHRIER RW, BICHET DG: Osmotic and nonosmotic control of vasopressin release and the pathogenesis of impaired water excretion in adrenal, thyroid, and edematous disorders. J Lab Clin Med 98:1, 1981

Dysuria, frequency and urgency, incontinence, and enuresis

BRADLEY WE: Diagnosis of urinary bladder dysfunction in diabetes mellitus. Ann Intern Med 92:323, 1980

———, SCOTT FB: Physiology of the urinary bladder, in *Urology*, 4th ed, JH Harrison et al (eds). Philadelphia, Saunders, 1978, vol 1, p 87

DEGROAT WC, BOOTH AM: Physiology of the urinary bladder and urethra. Ann Intern Med 92:312, 1980

HINDMARSH HR, BYRNE PO: Adult enuresis: A symptomatic and urodynamic assessment. Br J Urol 52:88, 1980

JOHNSON JR, STAMM WE: Urinary tract infections in women: Diagnosis and treatment. Ann Intern Med 111:906, 1989

LIPSKY BA: Urinary tract infections in men. Ann Intern Med 110:138, 1989

MIKKELSEN EJ, RAPOPORT JL: Enuresis: Psychopathology, sleep stage, and drug response. Urol Clin North Am 7:361, 1980

PLATT R: Quantitative definition of bacteriuria. Infectious Diseases Symposium, July 28, 1983, p 44, Supplement to Am J Med

RESNICK NM et al: The pathophysiology of urinary incontinence among institutionalized elderly persons. N Engl J Med 320:1, 1989

TURNER-WARWICK R, WHITESIDE CG (eds): *Symposium on Clinical Urodynamics: The Urologic Clinics of North America*, vol 6. Philadelphia, Saunders, 1979

WILLIAMS ME, PANNELL FC: Urinary incontinence in the elderly. Ann Intern Med 97:895, 1982

45 FLUIDS AND ELECTROLYTES

NORMAN G. LEVINSKY

SODIUM AND WATER

PHYSIOLOGIC CONSIDERATIONS (See also Chap. 235)   Both physiologically and clinically, sodium and water metabolism are closely interrelated. The sodium content of the body depends on the balance between dietary intake and renal excretion of sodium. In health, extrarenal losses of sodium are negligible. Renal sodium excretion is closely regulated to match dietary content. Within 2 to 4 days after sodium intake stops, urinary excretion decreases to 5 mmol/d or less. If dietary sodium is abruptly increased, sodium excretion promptly rises and equals intake within a few days. Thus, in normal persons, the sodium content of the body remains quite constant despite wide variations in sodium intake; over the range of 0 to 400 mmol/d, total body sodium varies only by about 10 percent.

Renal sodium excretion   This is regulated by the interplay of multiple control mechanisms. Sodium loads or deficits tend to produce corresponding changes in the central blood volume. Receptors located in the atria, central arteries, and the juxtaglomerular apparatus in the kidney respond to changes in local pressure which signal the volume/capacity relation of the central circulation (*effective blood volume*). If the effective volume is depleted, salt retention is induced, whereas expansion triggers multiple factors that favor natriuresis. With volume (salt) depletion, renal blood flow falls, due to decreased cardiac output and increased renal sympathetic nerve activity, which causes afferent arteriolar vasoconstriction.

The renin-angiotensin system is activated by autonomic stimuli and by reduced pressure in the juxtaglomerular apparatus. Angiotensin II preferentially constricts efferent arterioles and causes glomerular mesangial cell contraction. Glomerular filtration tends to fall because of reduced renal blood flow, decreased glomerular capillary pressure caused by afferent arteriolar constriction, and reduced capillary filtration area caused by mesangial contraction. In moderate to severe volume depletion, these factors outweigh the effect of angiotensin-induced efferent arteriolar constriction, which tends to maintain glomerular filtration by enhancing capillary filtration pressure. The fall in glomerular filtration reduces filtered sodium. Tubular reabsorption of sodium is enhanced. Proximal reabsorption is stimulated by changes in Starling forces in the peritubular circulation. Hydraulic pressure in peritubular capillaries is decreased by arteriolar constriction. Oncotic pressure is enhanced by concentration of plasma proteins and by increased filtration fraction (glomerular filtration tends to fall less than renal blood flow). These changes in hydraulic and oncotic Starling forces promote proximal salt and water reabsorption. Proximal reabsorption also is stimulated by angiotensin II and by sympathetic nerves which innervate proximal segments directly. Distal tubular reabsorption is enhanced by aldosterone, which is secreted at an increased rate in response to stimulation of the adrenal gland by angiotensin.

Volume expansion leads to opposite changes in renal hemodynamics and in these various regulators of tubular transport. Moreover, one or more natriuretic hormones are released in response to increased extracellular volume. Natriuretic peptides are present in the atria, the brain, and probably the kidney itself. Such peptides can augment sodium excretion both by increasing glomerular filtration and by inhibiting sodium reabsorption in the collecting ducts. There is also evidence for a ouabain-like natriuretic hormone that reduces tubular salt transport by inhibiting Na^+,K^+-adenosine triphosphatase (N^+,K^+-ATPase). Prostaglandins and kinins secreted within the kidney reduce sodium reabsorption in distal nephron segments. The exact role of these natriuretic factors in the regulation of sodium excretion is uncertain.

Undoubtedly, other regulatory mechanisms remain to be defined.

The multiplicity of control mechanisms prevents abnormalities of any single mechanism from grossly distorting the regulation of sodium excretion. For example, increased aldosterone secretion leads only to limited and transient sodium retention, because the initial accumulation of sodium tends to increase glomerular filtration and stimulates opposing natriuretic factors which decrease tubular sodium reabsorption.

Distribution of sodium   All but 2 to 5 percent of the sodium in the body is located in the extracellular fluids. (Approximately 40 percent of total body sodium is in bone, but this fraction does not participate significantly in most physiologic processes and will not be considered further.) The electrolyte compositions of plasma and interstitial fluid differ slightly because of the Gibbs-Donnan effect of anionic plasma proteins, which increases cation and decreases anion concentrations by a few percent in plasma relative to interstitial fluid. For practical purposes, plasma composition can be considered representative of the entire extracellular compartment. Total extracellular volume approximates 20 percent of body weight. Of this, 5 percent represents plasma volume and 15 percent the volume of interstitial fluids. Thus, in a 70-kg individual with plasma sodium concentration of 140 mmol/L, extracellular sodium content will approximate 2000 mmol. The volume of intracellular fluid is approximately twice as great as that of extracellular fluid, i.e., about 40 percent of body weight. However, since intracellular sodium concentration is less than 5 mmol/L, total intracellular sodium content is only about 100 to 150 mmol. The asymmetric distribution of sodium across cell membranes is maintained by expenditure of a large fraction of the energy derived from cell metabolism, which is required constantly to pump sodium out of cells against its electrochemical gradient. All the principal electrolytes are asymmetrically distributed across cell membranes. The principal electrolytes of the extracellular fluids are sodium, chloride, and bicarbonate. The major electrolytes of the intracellular fluids are potassium, magnesium, calcium, and organic anions, including proteins.

Since sodium salts account for more than 90 percent of the total osmolality of the extracellular fluids, variations in plasma sodium concentration are almost always reflected in equivalent changes in plasma osmolality. Exceptions due to accumulation of other solutes in plasma are discussed later. Although the electrolyte compositions of intracellular and extracellular fluids differ markedly, they are always in osmotic equilibrium, since water moves rapidly across cellular membranes to dissipate osmotic gradients. Therefore, although sodium is largely confined to extracellular fluids, plasma sodium concentration is an index of not only the relative proportions of sodium and water in those fluids but also the relation between total body solute and total body water. An example is the effect of shift of sodium from extracellular to intracellular fluids without a change in total body solute. Movement of sodium into cells would not cause hyponatremia, since water would shift into cells with the sodium. On the other hand, a primary decrease in the concentration of osmotically active solute within cells would decrease total body solute; although there would be no change in total body sodium or water, hyponatremia would result from the shift of intracellular water into the extracellular compartment.

Role of antidiuretic hormone   A very effective mechanism involving the *hypothalamus*, the *neurohypophysis*, and the kidney regulates plasma osmolality. Changes of 2 percent or less in plasma osmolality can be detected by osmoreceptors in the hypothalamus. Small increases in osmolality stimulate the secretion of vasopressin (the antidiuretic hormone, ADH) from the neurohypophysis, while small decreases suppress secretion of the hormone. Normal plasma osmolality is approximately 280 to 300 mosmol/kg of water; the exact level is determined by the "set" of the hypothalamic osmoreceptors in a given individual. When ADH secretion is maximal, urine volume will be about 500 mL/d, and urine osmolality will be 800 to 1400 mosmol/kg. In the absence of ADH, minimal urine osmolality is 40 to 80 mosmol/kg, and maximum water diuresis can reach 15 to 20 L/d or more. The capacity of this receptor-effector system is sufficient to maintain plasma osmolality within narrow limits despite large variations in the volume and concentration of dietary fluids. ADH secretion is also regulated by changes in extracellular volume. A reduction of 10 percent or more may trigger ADH release even in the absence of changes in plasma osmolality. If volume contraction is sufficiently severe, volume-mediated stimulation of ADH may override osmotic signals and cause water retention despite progressive dilution of body fluids. Conversely, extracellular volume expansion tends to suppress ADH release even if the body fluids are hypertonic.

The total sodium *content* of the body is determined by the renal sodium regulatory mechanisms described earlier. However, the principal determinant of plasma sodium *concentration* is water metabolism rather than total body sodium content. If excess sodium were to be ingested and retained, hypernatremia would be only transient. Water intake would increase because of thirst, and the fluid ingested would be retained because hypernatremia (hyperosmolality) would stimulate ADH secretion. Expanded extracellular volume, not hypernatremia, would be the end result. Conversely, if the osmoregulatory system is functioning normally, loss of moderate amounts of sodium without water would not result in permanent reduction of plasma sodium concentration. The initial reduction would shut off secretion of ADH, and a water diuresis would ensue. The final outcome would be contraction of extracellular volume, while plasma sodium concentration would be restored to normal. It follows that changes in total sodium content tend to cause changes in extracellular volume. In this sense, the sodium content of the extracellular fluid determines extracellular volume. On the other hand, changes in plasma sodium concentration reflect altered regulation of water excretion, not changes in total body sodium content alone. Clinically, plasma sodium concentration per se gives no information about the amount of sodium present in the body. Total body sodium content is determined by the volume of extracellular fluids as well as by the concentration of sodium in these fluids. Extracellular volume is usually the dominant factor, since changes in volume tend to be proportionately greater than changes in sodium concentration. Plasma sodium concentration reflects the relative proportions of sodium and water (or, more exactly, of total body solute and water), not the absolute amount of sodium in the body. Either hyponatremia or hypernatremia may occur when total body sodium content is decreased, normal, or increased.

CLINICAL DISORDERS Deficits and excesses of sodium and water occur in a great variety of clinical circumstances. The manifestations of the underlying illness may overshadow the clinical features of the fluid and electrolyte disorder. Theoretically, disturbances of sodium and water metabolism can be classified into four categories, reflecting a primary excess or deficit of water or sodium. Practically, such isolated disturbances are uncommon. A primary excess of sodium leads to edema; it is not ordinarily considered as an electrolyte disorder but as a feature of underlying disease, such as congestive heart failure, hepatic cirrhosis, or nephrotic syndrome. Primary sodium deficits are nearly always accompanied by water depletion, leading to the clinical syndrome of extracellular volume depletion. Pure or disproportionate water excess leads to hyponatremia, relative or absolute water depletion to hypernatremia. A practical clinical classification of the principal disorders of sodium and water metabolism is given in Table 45-1.

VOLUME DEPLETION Combined sodium and water deficits are far more frequent than isolated deficits of either constituent. Although the term *dehydration* is often used for combined deficits, this usage is confusing. Dehydration should be used to describe relatively pure water depletion leading to hypernatremia; *volume depletion* or some similar term should be used for combined deficits.

Pathogenesis As noted earlier, elimination of sodium from the diet will not by itself lead to sodium depletion in the presence of normal renal function, since urinary sodium excretion will quickly fall to very low levels. Therefore, sodium depletion is always due either to extrarenal losses or to abnormal renal losses.

TABLE 45-1 Disorders of sodium and water metabolism*

I Combined sodium and water depletion (volume depletion)
  A Extrarenal losses
    1 Gastrointestinal (vomiting, diarrhea, gastrointestinal suction, fistulas)
    2 Abdominal sequestration (peritonitis, rapid reaccumulation of ascites)
    3 Skin (sweating, burns)
  B Renal losses
    1 Renal disease (diuretic phase of acute renal failure, postobstructive diuresis, chronic renal failure, salt-wasting tubular disease)
    2 Diuretic excess
    3 Osmotic diuresis (diabetic glycosuria)
    4 Mineralocorticoid deficiency (Addison's disease, hypoaldosteronism)
II Hyponatremia
  A Associated with extracellular volume depletion (see list of causes above)
  B Associated with extracellular volume excess and edema
  C Associated with normal or modestly expanded extracellular volume (no edema)
    1 Acute and chronic renal failure
    2 Temporary impairment of water diuresis (pain, drugs, emotion)
    3 Syndrome of inappropriate secretion of antidiuretic hormone (SIADH)
    4 Endocrine (glucocorticoid deficiency, hypothyroidism)
    5 Severe polydipsia
    6 Essential ("sick-cell syndrome")
  D Without plasma hyposmolality
    1 Osmotic (hyperglycemia, mannitol)
    2 Artifactual (hyperlipemia, hyperproteinemia, laboratory error)
III Hypernatremia
  A Due solely to water loss
    1 Extrarenal
      a Skin (insensible losses)
      b Lungs
    2 Renal
      a Diabetes insipidus (central, nephrogenic)
    3 Hypothalamic dysfunction
  B Due to water loss associated with sodium loss
    1 Extrarenal
      a Sweat
    2 Renal
      a Osmotic diuresis (glycosuria, urea)
  C Due to sodium gain
    1 Excessive sodium administration
    2 Adrenal hyperfunction (hyperaldosteronism, Cushing's syndrome)

* For differential diagnosis, see Fig. 45-1.

GASTROINTESTINAL The most common cause of volume depletion is loss of a significant fraction of the 8 to 10 L of gastrointestinal fluids secreted daily. As the sodium concentration of these fluids is high, their loss causes combined sodium and water deficits. Since the principal secretions contain potassium and hydrogen ion or bicarbonate in large amounts, volume depletion due to such losses is often combined with potassium depletion and acidosis or alkalosis.

Significant volume depletion may be caused by sequestration of secretions within an obstructed gastrointestinal tract or within the peritoneal cavity in peritonitis. Rapid reaccumulation of ascites after paracentesis may reduce the effective circulating blood volume.

SKIN The sodium concentration of sweat varies from 5 to 50 mmol/L; sodium concentration increases with higher rates of sweating and in adrenal insufficiency. Because sweat is always a hypotonic solution, sweating leads to water deficits out of proportion to sodium losses. In burns, capillary damage may lead to sequestration of large amounts of sodium and water in the injured skin.

RENAL Abnormal losses of sodium and water in the urine may occur in both acute and chronic renal diseases. Early in the recovery (diuretic) phase of *acute renal failure*, urinary sodium concentration tends to be high (50 to 100 mmol/L), and substantial deficits of both sodium and water may ensue. With rare exceptions, severe sodium and water wasting does not persist beyond the first few days. It is important to discriminate between increased excretion which eliminates excess retained during the oliguric period and true tubular sodium and water wasting which depletes normal extracellular volume. Only the latter requires replacement. Acute salt and water wasting due to tubular damage also may occur immediately after relief of prolonged *obstruction* of the urinary tract. Although such a postobstructive diuresis may be severe, it rarely persists for more than several days as a clinically important phenomenon.

Patients with *chronic renal failure* have limited ability to decrease sodium and water excretion in response to decreased intake. They will become progressively volume-depleted if their intake is restricted by the anorexia, nausea, and vomiting characteristic of uremia or because of their physician's instructions. Large deficits may develop insidiously over many days or weeks. A "self-perpetuating cycle" may result, in that volume depletion will tend further to compromise renal function. Severe sodium-wasting renal disease, i.e., negative sodium balance when dietary sodium is normal, is rare. It occurs in occasional patients with tubulointerstitial diseases of the kidney, especially medullary cystic disease.

Renal sodium wasting in the presence of normal intrinsic renal function occurs in three clinical circumstances. Perhaps the most common is sodium depletion due to continued administration of potent *diuretics* to patients after edema has been relieved or to patients whose edema is sequestered and cannot be mobilized. For example, attempted treatment of cirrhotics with ascites may result in depletion of extracellular volume rather than mobilization of ascitic fluid. An obligatory *osmotic diuresis* also may cause renal sodium and water wasting despite normal renal function. Marked glycosuria in uncontrolled diabetes mellitus is the most frequent clinical example. Volume depletion in patients receiving high-protein enteral or parenteral alimentation may be due to an osmotic diuresis of urea formed by protein metabolism. Administration of solutes such as mannitol, which act as osmotic diuretics, may cause volume depletion. Finally, renal sodium wasting despite normal intrinsic function occurs in Addison's disease and hypoaldosteronism due to a *deficiency of mineralocorticoids*.

Clinical features and diagnosis The cause of volume depletion can usually be suspected from a history of inadequate salt and water intake together with vomiting, diarrhea, or excessive sweating; the symptoms of poorly controlled diabetes mellitus or of renal or adrenal disease may be elicited. The key findings on physical examination are those of interstitial and plasma volume depletion. Decreased interstitial volume may be recognized from reduced skin turgor, which is usually present in patients with significant volume contraction but may be difficult to evaluate in the elderly. It can be estimated clinically by noting the slow rate of return of skin to its original position when it is raised between the examiner's fingers. An area of skin normally free of wrinkles and not subject to wide variations in the thickness of subcutaneous tissue, such as that over the sternum, should be selected for this maneuver. Oral mucous membranes may be dry and axillary sweating decreased; these are less reliable diagnostic features than decreased skin turgor. Plasma volume depletion is indicated by changes in blood pressure. With moderate volume depletion, blood pressure is usually normal when the patient is recumbent, although resting tachycardia may be present. Postural hypotension, i.e., a drop of at least 5 to 10 mmHg in the sitting or standing position, is often present. With greater degrees of volume depletion, even recumbent blood pressure is reduced, and frank shock may occur. The patient with moderate or severe degrees of volume contraction is often lethargic, weak, confused, or obtunded. Such patients are usually oliguric, even when recumbent blood pressure is normal. However, an osmotic diuresis, as occurs in hyperglycemia, tends to prevent oliguria despite volume contraction.

LABORATORY FINDINGS The hematocrit and plasma protein concentration are increased, but increases within the normal range are interpretable only if prior values are known. Plasma sodium concentration may be decreased, normal, or increased depending on the proportion between deficits of sodium and of water. Plasma creatinine and urea nitrogen are usually increased, since the glomerular filtration rate is decreased ("prerenal azotemia"). Blood urea nitrogen (BUN) tends to rise proportionately more than plasma creatinine. Urinary sodium concentration may be of value in differentiating extrarenal and renal sources of sodium loss if the probable cause is not clear from the history. With extrarenal losses, urinary sodium concentration is less than 10 mmol/L; the concentration will usually exceed 20 mmol/L if renal or adrenal disorders are at fault. However,

urinary sodium may ultimately fall below this level even in patients with renal salt wasting if sodium depletion becomes severe.

Treatment The principal clinical manifestations of extracellular volume depletion are due to reduction of plasma and interstitial fluid volume. Since there is no convenient clinical method for quantifying these volumes, the effect of treatment must be determined by following the changes in clinical features such as blood pressure, urine output, and skin turgor. Modest deficits of sodium and water often can be corrected by increased oral intake in patients not suffering from gastrointestinal disorders. Severe depletion requires therapy with intravenous solutions. Isotonic saline (0.85%) is the infusion of choice in patients whose serum sodium concentration is approximately normal. The amount to be infused can be estimated from the history of prior losses and from the severity of the physical findings of extracellular volume contraction. Patients with moderate volume contraction usually require replacement with 2 to 3 L of saline, while patients with severe depletion may require much larger volumes. The need for correction of other concurrent electrolyte abnormalities may alter the composition of the required infusion; e.g., some of the sodium may be given as bicarbonate to patients with volume contraction and metabolic acidosis, or potassium may be added in patients with concurrent potassium depletion. In estimating the total amount to be infused, allowance for ongoing losses must be included. Since the amount to be infused cannot be calculated precisely, patients should be monitored carefully to avoid fluid overload and congestive failure.

HYPONATREMIA Pathophysiology Hyponatremia indicates that the body fluids are diluted by an excess of water relative to total solute. Hyponatremia is not equivalent to sodium depletion, which is only one of the clinical states in which it may occur (see Table 45-1). Most types of hyponatremia result from defective urinary dilution. The normal response to dilution of body fluids is a water diuresis, which corrects the hyposmotic state. Normal water diuresis requires three factors: (1) secretion of ADH must be suppressed; (2) sufficient sodium and water must reach the diluting sites of the nephron, in the ascending limb of Henle's loop and the distal convoluted tubule; and (3) these nephron segments must function normally, reabsorbing sodium while remaining impermeable to water.

Correspondingly, three mechanisms may cause defective water diuresis in patients with hyponatremia: (1) Secretion of ADH may continue "inappropriately" despite hypotonicity of extracellular fluid, which normally shuts off secretion of the hormone. This may be due to unregulated release of ADH by neoplasms or to nonosmotic stimuli to ADH secretion. The latter include volume depletion, neural factors such as pain and emotion, and certain drugs. (2) Insufficient sodium may reach the diluting segments to permit the formation of an adequate amount of dilute urine. Inadequate delivery of tubular fluid to distal sites may be due to reduced glomerular filtration and/or enhanced proximal tubular reabsorption. Even in the absence of ADH, distal tubular segments are not absolutely impermeable to water; small amounts of water continue to leak from the hypotonic tubular fluid into the isotonic cortical and slightly hypertonic medullary interstitial fluid. The amount of water leaking back in this manner becomes an increasingly larger fraction of the volume of dilute urine formed, since the diluting process is progressively limited by decreasing delivery. Hence urine osmolality rises progressively. In some instances, this mechanism may even result in excretion of a urine hypertonic to plasma, despite the absence of ADH. (3) Sodium transport in the diluting segments may be defective, or water permeability may be excessive at these sites even in the absence of ADH. One of these three factors can account for most types of hyponatremia, as described below.

Types of hyponatremia (See Table 45-1) In patients with extracellular *volume depletion*, delivery of sodium and water to the diluting segments of the nephron is reduced because of decreased glomerular filtration, increased proximal tubular reabsorption, or both. ADH secretion is stimulated by the volume contraction. These changes in renal function and hormone secretion limit water diuresis during extracellular volume depletion. Hyponatremia per se is usually of little clinical significance in sodium (volume) depletion. The major features are those of extracellular volume contraction, described above. Reduction of plasma sodium concentration by more than 10 to 15 mmol/L is rare in the absence of obvious decreases in skin turgor, postural or recumbent hypotension, and some degree of azotemia. Treatment is directed to correction of the volume deficits. Restitution of extracellular volume will correct hyponatremia by reversing the pathophysiologic mechanisms which limit water diuresis. In the occasional symptomatic patient with sodium depletion whose plasma sodium concentration is less than 125 mmol/L, it may be desirable to administer some of the intravenous sodium replacement fluids as hypertonic saline (see "Treatment," below).

Multiple factors contribute to hyponatremia caused by *diuretics*. Salt loss may cause volume depletion, which limits water diuresis by mechanisms already described and stimulates thirst. Thiazides and loop diuretics (furosemide, bumetanide, and ethacrynic acid) inhibit salt reabsorption in the diluting segments of the nephron and thereby directly limit water diuresis. Thiazides are the diuretics most commonly associated with hyponatremia, because they interfere with elaboration of a hypotonic urine by inhibiting sodium reabsorption in the distal convoluted tubule but, unlike loop diuretics, do not limit urine concentration and water retention by interfering with salt transport in the loop of Henle. In addition, potassium depletion caused by many diuretics contributes to hyponatremia through uncertain mechanisms. Hyponatremia due to diuretic therapy of hypertension is frequent but usually minor in severity. However, moderate or severe hyponatremia may occur in patients who receive diuretics, usually thiazides, and who drink large quantities of water or other hypotonic fluids. Elderly women are especially prone to develop severe hyponatremia. Progressive hyponatremia is an important complication of diuretic therapy in edematous patients, in whom the underlying disease tends to cause hyponatremia (see below) and to whom large doses of diuretics may be given. The treatment of hyponatremia due to diuretics is water restriction and repletion of potassium deficits.

In *edematous states* such as congestive heart failure, cirrhosis, and the nephrotic syndrome, hyponatremia paradoxically appears to result from mechanisms similar to those which cause hyponatremia in patients with volume depletion. Although total extracellular volume is increased in edematous patients, it is believed that the "effective" volume is reduced by decreased cardiac output or sequestration of fluid outside the central circulation. The decrease in "effective" volume results in diminished delivery of sodium and water to nephron diluting segments because of reduced glomerular filtration, increased proximal tubular reabsorption, or both. Volume-mediated secretion of ADH is also triggered in these conditions. In some edematous patients, essential hyponatremia may be an additional mechanism (see below). In edematous states, the severity and frequency of hyponatremia correlate to some extent with the magnitude of the edema and the seriousness of the underlying condition. Hyponatremia is usually present in patients with advanced disease unless water intake is restricted. The hyponatremia itself is often of little clinical significance. The principal features are those of the underlying disease. However, symptomatic hyponatremia may occur, most often in connection with vigorous diuretic therapy or excessive oral or parenteral intake of dilute fluids.

Hyponatremia associated with edema responds to effective treatment of the underlying disease. Moderate nonprogressive hyponatremia in edematous patients usually does not cause symptoms. Attempts to correct such hyponatremia by restriction of fluid intake induce thirst and discomfort without improving the clinical picture or longevity. Patients with severe or progressive hyponatremia may require some restriction of water intake, especially during vigorous treatment with diuretics. However, moderate limitation to the range of 1 to 1.5 L/d will often suffice to avoid symptoms of progressive hyponatremia. More severe restriction should be instituted only if specific clinical or laboratory observations warrant. Since edematous

subjects have excess total extracellular sodium, hypertonic saline should not be administered except in rare instances in which clinical manifestations of extreme hyponatremia, such as coma or convulsions, justify emergency measures. Furosemide should be given concurrently in such cases to avoid further expansion of the extracellular space. Dialysis also can be used to correct severe hyponatremia without increasing volume in edematous patients.

Hyponatremia may result from *impaired water excretion* not associated with a substantial deficit or excess of salt. In this case, extracellular volume is only modestly expanded. Since excess water is distributed throughout both intracellular and extracellular fluids in proportion to their volumes, only one-third of a water excess will be retained in the extracellular compartment. *Oliguric* patients develop dilutional hyponatremia if the volume of oral and intravenous fluids is not restricted appropriately. The ability to excrete a normal volume of dilute urine is progressively limited in advancing *chronic renal failure*. Regulation of water intake by thirst usually prevents dilutional hyponatremia. However, hyponatremia may be precipitated by increased fluid intake (e.g., if the patient is instructed to force fluids). Since the ability to regulate salt excretion is also impaired in chronic renal failure, in many patients hyponatremia is associated with edema or salt depletion rather than normal extracellular volume. In patients with normal renal function, *water diuresis* may be *limited temporarily* by ADH secretion induced by various neural stimuli such as pain and narcotics. In the postoperative state, these factors, together with administration of large volumes of hypotonic fluids, may cause hyponatremia. The etiology of hyponatremia due to impaired water excretion is usually evident from the clinical setting and a careful review of fluid intake and output. This type of hyponatremia is treated by water restriction. Only if severe symptoms occur is hypertonic saline infusion required.

In the *syndrome* of *inappropriate antidiuretic hormone* (SIADH) secretion (see also Chap. 333), ADH is released "inappropriately" despite dilution of body fluids and increased extracellular volume. Hyponatremia in patients with SIADH is principally due to water retention, but urinary losses of sodium also may contribute to a mild negative sodium balance. Renal sodium wasting is due to water retention and consequent modest volume expansion, which increases sodium excretion by mechanisms discussed above. Clinically, SIADH is characterized by a number of features: (1) Urine osmolality is not maximally dilute even when marked hyponatremia is induced by water loading. In most cases, urine osmolality exceeds plasma osmolality. (2) Plasma creatinine and urea are normal or low, indicating that the glomerular filtration rate is normal or increased. (The elaboration of hypertonic urine is presumptive evidence of ADH secretion if the glomerular filtration rate is normal.) (3) During fluid loading (even if the fluid is saline), hyponatremia increases due to water retention and urinary sodium wasting. It should be noted that sodium wasting during volume expansion may be minimal or even absent in patients with extreme degrees of hyponatremia. (4) Since hyponatremia and salt wasting are not direct effects of vasopressin but are due to retention of ingested water, they are corrected by restriction of fluid intake. This response is helpful in occasional patients in whom it may be difficult to distinguish SIADH from mild volume depletion as the cause of hyponatremia. The plasma uric acid also may be of value in making this distinction. Since uric acid excretion tends to vary with "effective" extracellular volume, hyperuricemia is common in volume depletion, while hypouricemia is usual in SIADH.

SIADH occurs commonly in patients with oat cell carcinoma of the lung but also has been described in patients with a variety of other *neoplasms*. In some of these patients the tumor secretes ADH or a substance with analogous biologic activity (see also Chap. 333). The syndrome also has been reported in patients with various disorders of the *central nervous system*, including meningitis, encephalitis, tumors, trauma, and stroke, and in acute *porphyria*. It is assumed that ADH in these patients is secreted in response to direct stimulation of the hypothalamic osmoreceptors. *Pulmonary* diseases associated with

SIADH, in addition to tumors, include a wide variety of infections, asthma, and chronic obstructive lung disease.

Pharmacologic agents that induce SIADH include (1) the oral hypoglycemic agents chlorpropamide and tolbutamide, (2) the antineoplastic and immunosuppressive agents vincristine, vinblastine, and cyclophosphamide, and (3) psychoactive drugs such as haloperidol, thioridazine, carbamazepine, and amitriptyline. These agents exert their antidiuretic effect either by potentiating the tubular action of small amounts of ADH or by stimulating inappropriate secretion of ADH. The antipsychotic drugs also tend to stimulate fluid intake by their anticholinergic action, which dries mucous membranes.

Hyponatremia due to SIADH can be treated by limiting fluid intake; restriction to the range of 1 to 1.2 L/d is ordinarily adequate. Occasional patients who are symptomatic despite water restriction may be treated by enhancing water excretion. This can be accomplished either by increasing solute excretion (by taking a high-salt, high-protein diet or ingesting urea) or by antagonizing ADH with demeclocycline or lithium. Initial therapy with hypertonic saline infusions may be appropriate in a few symptomatic patients with marked hyponatremia. Concurrent administration of furosemide, which increases water excretion by limiting urinary concentration, may facilitate correction of hyponatremia in those patients who do not respond promptly to hypertonic saline alone.

Hyponatremia may occur in certain *endocrine* disorders, notably adrenal insufficiency and hypothyroidism. Multiple factors appear to play a role in limiting water diuresis in patients with *adrenal insufficiency*. Deficient secretion of mineralocorticoid hormones may lead to sodium depletion, with consequent reduction of glomerular filtration and enhancement of tubular sodium reabsorption. Moreover, glucocorticoid deficiency directly reduces filtration. Therefore, adrenal insufficiency will tend to decrease delivery of sodium to diluting sites. In addition, hormone deficiency prevents the maintenance of normal water impermeability in distal diluting segments of the nephron. This appears to be due in large part to inappropriate secretion of ADH, although there also may be direct effect of hormone deficiency on water permeability of distal tubular epithelium. Since patients with adrenal insufficiency may have the combination of defective dilution of the urine and sodium wasting, hyponatremia due to Addison's disease can occasionally be confused with SIADH. Usually, other clinical features of adrenal insufficiency such as hyperkalemia, pigmentation, and hypoglycemia suggest the correct diagnosis. However, specific tests of adrenal function are indicated whenever the diagnosis is in doubt. Hyponatremia due to adrenal insufficiency is corrected by appropriate hormonal therapy.

Hyponatremia may develop in moderate or severe *hypothyroidism*. Decreased delivery of tubular fluid to diluting segments and persistent release of ADH both limit water excretion in this condition. The diagnosis of this type of hyponatremia is made by recognizing the clinical features of hypothyroidism and from the response to treatment with thyroid hormone.

The normal kidney can excrete 15 to 20 L of dilute urine per day. Normal water intake, regulated by thirst and habit, is a small fraction of this maximum excretory capacity. Rarely, *psychogenic polydipsia* may be so severe that the rapid ingestion of huge quantities of fluids may overwhelm normal excretory capacity and produce symptomatic dilutional hyponatremia despite normal renal diluting mechanisms. Hyponatremia of this type is diagnosed from the history of massive fluid intake. The patients most often are women, usually with other evidence of psychiatric illness. Since water excretory capacity is normal, the urine is maximally dilute in this condition. Hyponatremia due to psychogenic polydipsia responds to water restriction. Rare patients who are symptomatic due to extreme degrees of hyponatremia may require intravenous infusion of hypertonic saline.

Low solute output will limit excretion of water. Since minimal urine osmolality is about 50 mosmol/kg, the kidney must excrete at least 50 mosmol of solute in order to excrete 1 L of water. In individuals consuming diets low in protein and electrolytes, urinary solute excretion may be reduced to less than half the usual 600 to 800 mosmol/d (mostly urea and electrolytes). Hyponatremia due to a diet which provides little urinary solute but large fluid intake has been described in beer drinkers who consume little else ("beer potomania").

Some patients may be hyponatremic in the absence of a defect in water diuresis. The terms *essential hyponatremia* and *"sick-cell" syndrome* have been applied to this category. Osmoreceptor cells in the hypothalamus are thought to be "reset" to maintain a decreased level of body fluid osmolality as though it were normal. Urine becomes dilute or concentrated, respectively, if plasma sodium falls or increases slightly from the new "normal" level for the particular patient. The genesis of such a syndrome is speculative. Changes in cellular metabolism may lead to a primary reduction in cellular osmolality. Another possibility is that essential hyponatremia is a variant of SIADH in which there is a nonosmotic stimulus to ADH secretion. When plasma osmolality is reduced sufficiently, osmotic suppression of ADH secretion overcomes the nonosmotic stimulus.

Essential hyponatremia may occur in a variety of chronic illnesses, such as pulmonary tuberculosis, congestive heart failure, and hepatic cirrhosis. This type of hyponatremia is asymptomatic; skin turgor, blood pressure, and renal function are normal, unless altered by the primary disease. Definitive diagnosis of essential hyponatremia requires the demonstration of normal urinary dilution in response to water loading, normal urinary concentration during dehydration, and normal renal sodium excretory responses to sodium loading and restriction. This type of hyponatremia does not require treatment.

Hyponatremia due to *accumulation of osmotically active solutes* in the plasma is the sole exception to the rule that hyponatremia means decreased plasma osmolality. In this type of hyponatremia, plasma osmolality is increased. Plasma sodium is diluted by movement of water out of cells along the osmotic gradient created by the addition of a solute such as glucose or mannitol. (High plasma urea levels in patients with renal failure do not cause hyponatremia because urea concentration is equal across cell membranes.) The diagnosis of hyponatremia due to increased plasma concentrations of osmotically active solutes is usually apparent from the history and clinical features of uncontrolled diabetes. Plasma sodium concentration will decrease by about 1.6 mmol/L with every elevation of 1 g/L in plasma glucose above normal. This type of hyponatremia also should be considered whenever there is a history of recent administration of mannitol, especially to oliguric patients unable to excrete it promptly. Since plasma osmolality is increased, clinical manifestations of hypotonicity are absent in this type of hyponatremia.

In patients with severe hyperlipemia or, very rarely, with extreme hyperproteinemia, *artifactual* hyponatremia may be reported by the laboratory. In severe hyperlipemia, part of any unit volume of plasma taken for analysis will be lipid, which is sodium-free. This type of hyponatremia rarely occurs unless the plasma is grossly milky. In patients with extreme hyperproteinemia, proteins occupy more than the normal 7 percent of plasma volume, thereby reducing the proportion of aqueous sodium-containing fluid per unit of plasma taken for analysis. In both cases, hyponatremia will be reported by the laboratory because the sodium concentration will be low in millimoles per liter of plasma. However, sodium concentration per liter of plasma water and plasma osmolality are normal; hence this type of hyponatremia has no clinical significance. Laboratories increasingly have adopted the sodium-selective electrode as the method for measuring plasma sodium. This technique eliminates artifactual hyponatremia because it gives accurate values regardless of plasma lipid or protein concentration.

Differential diagnosis Although the type of hyponatremia can be defined easily in most patients, precise diagnosis may be difficult in some. In Fig. 45-1 is a flowchart that outlines the major steps in determining the cause of hyponatremia. First, assess extracellular fluid (ECF) volume. The history and physical examination are usually sufficient to determine whether the hyponatremia is associated with a decreased, increased, or normal extracellular volume. In occasional patients, moderate volume depletion may not readily be separable from

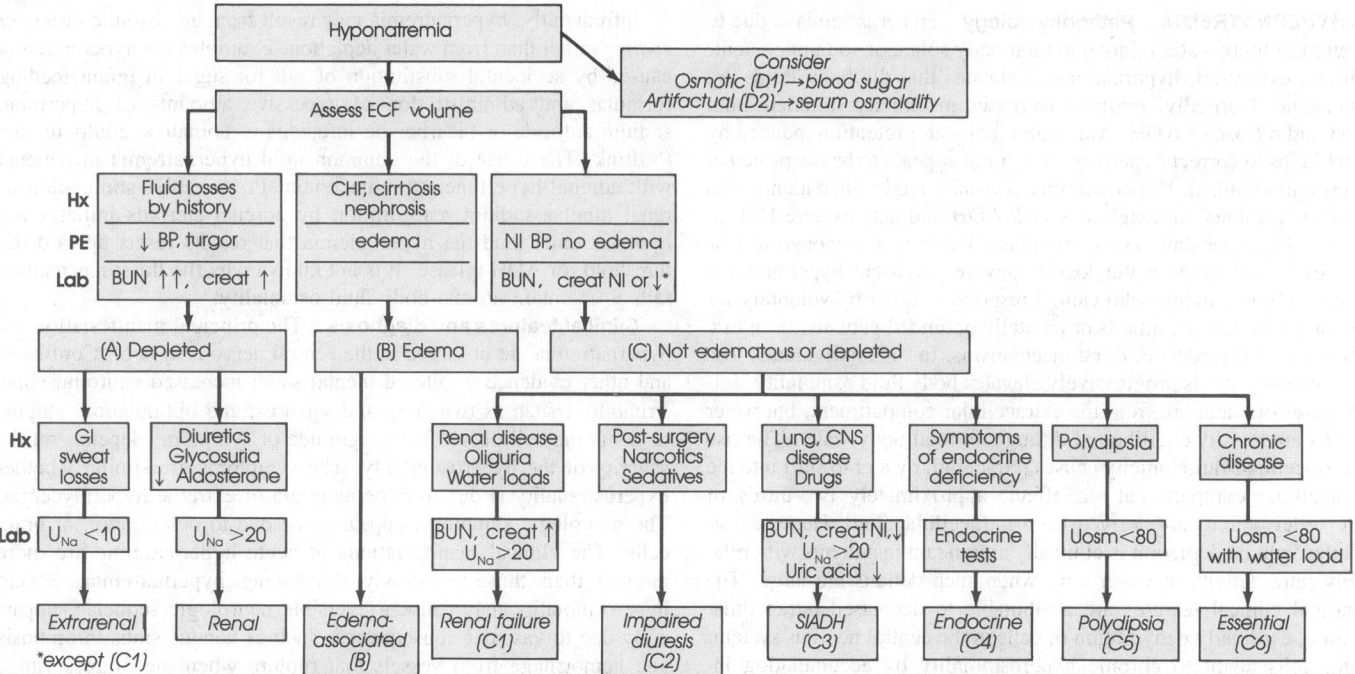

FIGURE 45-1 Flowchart for differential diagnosis of causes of hyponatremia. Categories (A, B, C, D) and types (C1–6) are keyed to Table 45-1, section II (Hyponatremia). Abbreviations: Nl = normal; ECF = extracellular fluid; creat = creatinine; CHF = congestive heart failure; BP = blood pressure; Uosm = urinary osmolality; U_{Na} = urinary Na, mmol/L; $\downarrow$ = decreased, $\uparrow$ = increased; Hx = history, PE = physical examination.

normovolemia by clinical examination. In that event, measurement of BUN and plasma creatinine may be helpful. The plasma creatinine and especially the BUN tend to be increased when hyponatremia is associated with volume depletion and normal or decreased when it is associated with a normal or expanded extracellular volume, as in SIADH. As noted above, plasma uric acid also may be helpful in making this distinction. The various types of normovolemic hyponatremia can frequently be recognized by a careful review of specific features of the history, such as associated diseases, drug therapy, and fluid intake. However, laboratory tests, such as measurement of serum cortisol, may be needed to confirm a diagnosis.

Measurements of urinary sodium concentration and osmolality are common in the workup. *Urinary sodium concentration* is low (under 10 mmol/L) if hyponatremia is associated with edema or with volume depletion due to extrarenal causes. Urine sodium concentration usually exceeds 20 mmol/L if hyponatremia is due to renal salt losses or to renal failure with water retention. In SIADH, urine sodium concentration usually exceeds 20 mmol/L unless fluid intake has been restricted. Since impaired water diuresis is the mechanism of most types of hyponatremia, measurement of *urinary osmolality* is not usually of value. A maximally dilute urine would be expected only in hyponatremia due to extreme polydipsia or during water loading in essential hyponatremia. With other causes, urinary osmolality exceeds 150 mosmol/kg of water; usually the urine is hypertonic to plasma.

Clinical manifestations Neurologic dysfunction is the principal clinical manifestation of hyponatremia. It is due to intracellular movement of water, leading to swelling of brain cells. The severity of symptoms is related both to the degree of hyponatremia and to the rapidity with which it develops. There is some evidence that women develop more severe manifestations than men. In chronic hyponatremia, the degree of brain swelling caused by any given reduction in body fluid osmolality is reduced by cellular volume regulatory mechanisms. These transport inorganic ions, such as potassium and chloride, and organic osmolytes, such as amino acids, out of swollen brain cells. Patients may be lethargic, confused, stuporous, or comatose. If hyponatremia develops rapidly, signs of hyperexcitability such as muscular twitches, irritability, and convulsions may occur. Hyponatremia rarely causes clinical symptoms when plasma sodium

is above 125 mmol/L, although symptoms may occur at higher levels if the decrease in concentration has been rapid.

Treatment Appropriate therapy for the various types of hyponatremia has been outlined. Hyponatremia itself is often of little significance and requires no specific treatment. If severe, symptomatic hyponatremia requires intravenous treatment; the amount of sodium required to increase plasma sodium concentration is calculated by multiplying the deficit in plasma sodium concentration (millimoles per liter) by the total body water (approximately 50 to 60 percent of body weight). Although the administered sodium will remain in the extracellular compartment, the osmotic effect of hypertonic saline will cause water to shift out of cells.

The appropriate rate and extent of initial correction of hyponatremia are controversial. Severe hyponatremia can cause major neurologic dysfunction. On the other hand, rapid correction of hyponatremia also can cause serious neurologic damage [osmotic demyelination, often prominent in the pons (central pontine myelinolysis)]. Both the rate and magnitude of initial correction of hyponatremia apparently influence the likelihood of this complication. The risk of neurologic damage appears to be very low in patients whose hyponatremia has developed rapidly, e.g., patients with psychogenic polydipsia. In patients with chronic hyponatremia, osmotic demyelination is more likely, although apparently still infrequent.

Although the issue of optimal treatment has not yet been resolved, the following regimen seems reasonable in the light of current information. Only patients with severe, symptomatic hyponatremia should be treated with hypertonic saline. If hyponatremia has developed over 24 h or less, 5% saline should be administered in an amount calculated to increase plasma sodium by no more than 1 to 2 mmol/L per hour. If hyponatremia is more chronic, plasma sodium should be raised by no more than 0.5 to 1 mmol/L per hour. In either case, plasma sodium should not be increased by more than 12 mmol/L over the first 24 h. The symptoms and clinical status, especially with respect to circulatory congestion, should be assessed carefully throughout the infusion. Furosemide may be given if fluid overload is present initially or develops during the infusion. Complete correction of hyponatremia, if indicated, is usually best carried out more slowly by water restriction or oral sodium supplementation if possible.

HYPERNATREMIA Pathophysiology Hypernatremia is due to a deficit of body water relative to total body solute or sodium content. Without exception, hypernatremia indicates that the body fluids are hypertonic. Normally, minimal increases in tonicity stimulate both thirst and release of ADH. Although renal water retention induced by ADH helps to correct hypernatremia, thirst appears to be the principal defense mechanism. Hypernatremia is usually modest in patients with diabetes insipidus, although they lack ADH and may excrete 15 L or more of urine per day. Thirst stimulates water intake enough to balance even such large water losses. Severe persistent hypernatremia occurs only in patients who cannot respond to thirst by voluntary ingestion of fluid, e.g., infants or mentally obtunded patients, or in rare patients with disorders of thirst mechanisms. In such individuals, loss of dilute body fluids progressively elevates body fluid osmolality. Initial losses of water are from the extracellular compartment, but water deficits are rapidly equilibrated throughout total body water. The rise in extracellular fluid tonicity causes intracellular water to shift into the extracellular compartment. In effect, approximately two-thirds of pure water deficits are derived from intracellular fluid. Hence extracellular volume depletion is clinically significant in patients with relatively pure deficits of water only when such deficits are large. The principal clinical features are attributable to decreased intracellular volume, especially dehydration of cells in the central nervous system. Brain cells adapt to chronic hyperosmolality by accumulating increased intracellular solute, principally potassium and amino acids. When hyperosmolality is rapidly corrected, the increase in total intracellular solute may promote brain swelling even at normal or slightly elevated plasma osmolality. These mechanisms may account for the fact that rapid correction of hypertonicity sometimes causes deterioration of central nervous function.

Pathogenesis (See Table 45-1) For clinical purposes it is useful to classify hypernatremia as due to water loss alone; to water deficits associated with, but proportionately in excess of, sodium deficits; or to retention of sodium. *Pure water deficits* may be due to extrarenal or renal water losses that are not replaced. Insensible losses of water from the skin or lungs may reach several liters per day, especially in patients with fever, increased respirations, or extensive burns. Renal losses may lead to hypernatremia in diabetes insipidus. Alert patients with diabetes insipidus ordinarily maintain normal or only slightly hypertonic body fluids despite massive renal water wasting by increasing fluid intake appropriately. However, diabetes insipidus may develop acutely after cerebral trauma or neurosurgical procedures. In such patients, careful attention to replacement of urinary losses is mandatory to avoid severe hypernatremia. Defective thirst and ADH regulation occurs in rare patients with hypothalamic disorders, which may be idiopathic ("essential hypernatremia") or due to specific causes such as tumors, granulomas, and cerebrovascular accidents.

Water losses leading to hypernatremia are often associated with sodium deficits. In such cases, the clinical features of extracellular volume depletion and hypernatremia may both be present, and either may predominate. Extrarenal losses of salt and water due to profuse sweating and renal losses due to osmotic diuresis are the major causes of hypernatremia in this category. Since sweat is hypotonic, hypernatremia will develop if profusely sweating patients cannot drink. In an osmotic diuresis, urinary sodium concentration is less than plasma concentration; therefore, hypernatremia tends to occur. Hypernatremia due to urea diuresis may develop when patients unable to complain of thirst are placed on high-protein feeding. Examples include patients with severe cerebrovascular accidents who are unable to swallow and postoperative neurosurgical patients. In the syndrome of hyperosmolar nonketotic diabetic coma, severe hyperosmolality of the body fluids is due to a combination of hyperglycemia and relative or absolute hypernatremia. The hypernatremia is a consequence of an intense glucose osmotic diuresis in patients who are unable to ingest fluids. Since hyperglycemia itself causes hyponatremia by inducing a shift of water from cells, the presence of hypernatremia in the face of extreme hyperglycemia indicates that total body water is severely depleted.

Infrequently, hypernatremia may result from an absolute *excess of sodium* rather than from water depletion. Examples are hypernatremia caused by accidental substitution of salt for sugar in infant feeding formulas and administration of excessive amounts of hypertonic sodium chloride or bicarbonate infusions to comatose adults unable to drink. The cause of the common mild hypernatremia in patients with adrenal hyperfunction is uncertain. Presumably, stimulation of renal tubular sodium reabsorption by adrenal steroids initiates the hypernatremia, and the hypervolemia that results resets upward the threshold for ADH release. It is not known why the thirst mechanism fails to maintain normal body fluid osmolality.

Clinical features and diagnosis The principal manifestations of hypernatremia are observed in the central nervous system. Confusion and other evidence of altered mental state; increased neuromuscular irritability, such as twitching and seizures; and obtundation, stupor, or coma may all occur. The magnitude of symptoms depends on the severity of the hyperosmolality. The symptoms are similar whether hyperosmolality is due to hypernatremia or extreme hyperglycemia. The neurologic symptoms appear to be due to dehydration of brain cells. The clinical manifestations of acute hypernatremia are more marked than those of slowly developing hypernatremia. Severe hyperosmolality may cause irreversible neurologic sequelae, apparently due to vascular consequences such as venous sinus thrombosis and hemorrhage from vessels that rupture when the brain shrinks. High mortality rates are associated with extreme hyperosmolality, especially in children and the elderly.

In patients with pure water deficits, manifestations of extracellular volume depletion are minimal because only one-third of the deficit is derived from extracellular fluid. As noted, combined deficits are common, especially in patients who sweat or experience an osmotic diuresis; in such individuals, the signs and symptoms of volume depletion may overshadow those of hypernatremia.

The cause of hypernatremia can usually be inferred from the history when it is due to extrarenal water loss, an osmotic diuresis, or sodium excess. In these cases, the urine is hypertonic to plasma. The differential diagnosis of pituitary and nephrogenic diabetes insipidus, in which urine concentrating ability is impaired, is discussed in Chap. 333.

Treatment Hypernatremia itself is corrected with water by mouth or by intravenous infusion of 5% dextrose in water. Calculation of water requirements must be based on total body water, since water deficits are drawn from both intracellular and extracellular fluid and both must be repleted. For example, suppose a 70-kg man has a plasma sodium of 160 mmol/L which is to be lowered to 140. Total body water is estimated as 60 percent of 70 kg, which is 42 L. To reduce plasma sodium, this volume must be increased to $(160/140) \times 42$ L, which equals 48 L. Thus a positive water balance of 6 L $(48 - 42)$ is required. Hypernatremia should be corrected slowly; no more than half the water deficit should be replaced in the first 12 to 24 h. As stated above, rapid correction of hypertonicity may cause central nervous function to deteriorate.

In patients with associated sodium deficits, saline solutions should be infused. If the predominant clinical feature is extracellular volume depletion with circulatory insufficiency, treatment should begin with 0.9% saline to replete extracellular volume promptly. If the neurologic effects of hypertonicity predominate, therapy can start with 0.45% saline. In patients with hyperosmolar diabetic coma, sodium deficits are usually large, due to prior glucose osmotic diuresis. Plasma hypertonicity is due to both hyperglycemia and hypernatremia. Treatment consists of isotonic saline (0.9%) to replete extracellular volume and insulin to lower plasma glucose and thereby partly correct hypertonicity. Later, hypotonic saline (0.45%) can replace the remaining water and salt deficits and return plasma sodium to normal.

POTASSIUM

PHYSIOLOGIC CONSIDERATIONS Potassium is the principal intracellular cation. Active transport mediated by Na^+,K^+–stimulated

ATPase in cell membranes maintains a cellular concentration of approximately 160 mmol/L, 40 times that in extracellular fluid. All but 2 percent of the 2500 to 3000 mmol potassium in the body is within cells. Since potassium is a large fraction of total cellular solute, it is a major determinant of the volume of the cell and the osmolality of the body fluids. Moreover, potassium is an important cofactor in a number of metabolic processes. Extracellular potassium, while a small fraction of the total, greatly influences neuromuscular function. The ratio of intracellular to extracellular potassium concentration is the principal determinant of membrane potential in excitable tissues. Since extracellular potassium concentration is low, small deviations in concentration produce large variations in this ratio; conversely, only large changes in intracellular potassium influence the ratio significantly. These relationships have practical consequences. For example, toxic effects of hyperkalemia can be mitigated by inducing movement of potassium from extracellular fluid into cells.

With the exception of changes in acid-base balance (see below), in most circumstances extracellular and intracellular potassium change in the same direction. Hence alterations in plasma potassium are a useful index of alterations in total body potassium. During potassium depletion, plasma potassium initially decreases about 1 mmol/L for each 100 to 200 mmol lost. However, plasma potassium falls more slowly after it reaches 2 mmol/L. Thus a plasma potassium in the range of 2 to 3.5 mmol/L is a reasonably accurate guide to the magnitude of depletion, but plasma potassium concentrations less than 2 mmol/L may reflect a wide range of deficits, from moderate to severe. Plasma concentration increases about 1 mmol/L after acute administration of 100 to 200 mmol potassium. Assuming an extracellular volume of 15 L, 150 mmol would be expected to raise plasma potassium by about 10 mmol/L. Thus the largest fraction of administered potassium rapidly enters cells. Renal excretion also increases promptly. Chronic exposure to high-potassium diets enhances both tissue uptake and renal excretion of the ion; the mechanism of these adaptations is uncertain. Sustained hyperkalemia rarely is caused by excess intake, because these mechanisms normally function so efficiently. Impaired renal excretion and cellular transfer are the usual causes of hyperkalemia.

The relation between plasma and cellular potassium is influenced by acid-base balance and by hormones. Acidosis tends to shift potassium out of cells, and alkalosis favors movement from extracellular fluid into cells. The relation between blood pH and plasma potassium is complex and is influenced by several factors, including the type of acidosis, the duration of the altered acid-base state, and the change in plasma bicarbonate per se. In general, plasma potassium changes less with respiratory acidosis than with metabolic acidosis and less with alkalosis than with acidosis. Metabolic acidosis due to organic acids such as lactic acid or ketoacids has little or no effect on plasma potassium, while mineral acids (e.g., hyperchloremic acidosis or renal failure acidosis) increase plasma potassium by about 0.5 to 1.0 mmol/L per 0.1-unit decrease in plasma pH. While the magnitude of the change in plasma potassium cannot be predicted from changes in blood pH alone, a patient with normal total body potassium tends to be hyperkalemic if acidotic and hypokalemic if alkalotic. Hormones appear to be important parts of the mechanism for moving potassium loads out of plasma. Insulin and beta-adrenergic catecholamines promote movement of potassium into cells. Conversely, alpha-adrenergic agonists impair potassium uptake into cells.

Of the usual potassium intake of 50 to 150 mmol/d, most is excreted in the urine. Normally, stool and sweat contain only about 5 mmol/d. As noted, the kidneys respond to acute and chronic changes in potassium intake by corresponding changes in excretion. Excess potassium is excreted promptly; about half of an acute load appears in the urine within 12 h. The renal response to potassium depletion is more sluggish. Excretion does not fall to minimal levels for 7 to 14 days. During this period, a deficit of 200 mmol or more may develop in an individual on a potassium-deficient diet. Renal excretory mechanisms for potassium are complex. Potassium in the urine is derived almost entirely from potassium secreted in the distal convoluted tubule and collecting duct; filtered potassium is nearly quantitatively reabsorbed in more proximal segments. Potassium secretion is influenced by the potassium concentration of tubular cells, aldosterone, distal tubular fluid flow rate, acid-base balance, and factors that alter distal tubular electronegativity. Aldosterone stimulates potassium secretion. Thus hyperkalemia increases potassium excretion by two mechanisms: It stimulates adrenal secretion of aldosterone, and it directly enhances renal secretion, presumably via increased tubular cell potassium. Potassium secretion in the distal tubule is flow-dependent; increased distal delivery of tubular fluid favors potassium excretion. For example, loop diuretics, which enhance distal volume delivery, increase potassium excretion, especially in patients with edema and secondary aldosteronism. Alkalosis enhances and acidosis depresses renal potassium secretion, probably by inducing corresponding changes in tubular cell potassium. If delivery to distal segments of sodium salts of unreabsorbable anions such as excess bicarbonate or carbenicillin is augmented, tubular electronegative potential will increase as sodium is reabsorbed. The enhanced electrical gradient will promote potassium excretion.

POTASSIUM DEPLETION AND HYPOKALEMIA Pathogenesis The principal causes of potassium depletion are listed in Table 45-2. As noted above, renal excretion of potassium falls slowly in persons on potassium-deficient diets. During the 10 to 14 days before balance is achieved, significant deficits may occur. Thus, in contrast to sodium, moderate potassium depletion may result from *poor intake* alone. Potassium deficiency is frequent in *gastrointestinal disorders* in which vomiting, diarrhea, or loss of gastrointestinal secretions is prominent. Diarrhea may cause large potassium deficits, since the potassium concentration of liquid stool is 40 to 60 mmol/L. *Loss of gastric secretions* through vomiting or nasogastric suction is also a common cause of potassium depletion. The potassium concentration of gastric fluid is only 5 to 10 mmol/L; direct losses contribute modestly to negative potassium balance. The potassium deficit is primarily due to increased renal excretion. Potassium excretion appears to be stimulated by three mechanisms. Loss of gastric acid leads to *metabolic alkalosis*, which increases tubular cell potassium concentration. The elevated plasma bicarbonate concentration also increases delivery of bicarbonate and fluid to the distal nephron. At that site, as noted above, excess bicarbonate acts as a nonreabsorbable anion to augment potassium excretion. Finally, secondary hyperaldosteronism due to associated extracellular volume contraction may play a role in maintaining potassium excretion at high levels despite potassium depletion.

TABLE 45-2 Causes of potassium depletion and hypokalemia

I Gastrointestinal
  A Deficient dietary intake
  B Gastrointestinal disorders (vomiting, diarrhea, villous adenoma, fistulas, ureterosigmoidostomy)

II Renal
  A Metabolic alkalosis
  B Diuretics, osmotic diuresis
  C Excessive mineralocorticoid effects
    1 Primary aldosteronism
    2 Secondary aldosteronism (including malignant hypertension, Bartter's syndrome, juxtaglomerular cell tumor)
    3 Licorice ingestion
    4 Glucocorticoid excess (Cushing's syndrome, exogenous steroids, ectopic ACTH production)
  D Renal tubular diseases
    1 Renal tubular acidosis (types I and II)
    2 Leukemia
    3 Liddle's syndrome
    4 Certain antibiotics
  E Magnesium depletion

III Hypokalemia due to shift into cells (no depletion)
  A Hypokalemic periodic paralysis
  B Insulin effect
  C Alkalosis
  D Increased beta-adrenergic activity

Diuretics are among the most frequent causes of hypokalemia and potassium depletion. Thiazides, loop diuretics, and carbonic anhydrase inhibitors all increase potassium excretion. These agents augment sodium and fluid delivery to the distal potassium secretory site by inhibiting reabsorption in more proximal nephron segments. Loop diuretics also inhibit potassium reabsorption by the Na^+-K^+-$2Cl^-$ transport mechanism in the ascending limb of Henle's loop. Carbonic anhydrase inhibitors such as acetazolamide, which inhibit proximal bicarbonate reabsorption, also enhance potassium excretion by increasing distal delivery of nonreabsorbable bicarbonate. Hypokalemia and potassium depletion are frequent when diuretics are used to treat edematous patients, in whom secondary aldosteronism is the rule. Although hypokalemia also occurs in patients receiving diuretics for treatment of hypertension, potassium depletion is modest if dietary potassium is normal. Surreptitious abuse of diuretics should be considered when hypokalemic patients have renal potassium wasting of uncertain cause.

Potassium excretion is increased during an *osmotic diuresis*. This mechanism leads to potassium depletion in patients with diabetic ketoacidosis, in whom the osmotic diuresis is due to glycosuria and to increased excretion of keto acid anions. However, despite potassium depletion plasma potassium may be normal or even high due to the shift of potassium out of tissues caused principally by insulin deficiency and renal insufficiency. Failure to recognize potassium depletion may lead to serious cardiotoxicity from sudden hypokalemia when the ketoacidosis is treated with insulin or alkali. A normal plasma potassium concentration in a patient with diabetic ketoacidosis strongly suggests potassium depletion.

Urinary potassium loss is often due to *excessive mineralocorticoid activity*. Hypokalemia is characteristic of *primary aldosteronism* (Chap. 335). It may be minimal in patients with restricted sodium intake because potassium excretion is limited by decreased distal salt and fluid delivery. *Secondary aldosteronism* causes renal potassium wasting and hypokalemia in patients with malignant hypertension, Bartter's syndrome, and renin-secreting renal tumors. However, patients with congestive heart failure, hepatic cirrhosis, and nephrotic syndrome usually are not hypokalemic despite secondary aldosteronism. The decrease in effective blood volume in such patients reduces distal delivery of salt and fluid, thereby limiting potassium excretion. As noted above, treatment with diuretics, which increase distal delivery, will often provoke hypokalemia in these patients. Patients who consume huge amounts of licorice may become hypokalemic. Glycyrrhizic acid in licorice inhibits 11-β-hydroxysteroid dehydrogenase, an enzyme which normally minimizes the mineralocorticoid activity of endogenous cortisol in the kidney by converting it to an inactive metabolite. Excessive levels of *glucocorticoids* stimulate secretion of renal potassium (and hydrogen), leading to hypokalemia and alkalosis in patients with *Cushing's syndrome* (Chap. 335) and some receiving *therapeutic steroids*.

Renal tubular potassium wasting is a feature of types I and II *renal tubular acidosis* (Chap. 244). Some patients with monocytic or myelomonocytic *leukemia* develop hypokalemia. The mechanism is uncertain. Renal potassium wasting in some patients appears to correlate with lysozymuria, and the enzyme may interfere with tubular function. In *Liddle's syndrome*, a rare familial disorder (Chap. 244), renal potassium wasting is an intrinsic tubular abnormality. Certain *antibiotics* may cause hypokalemia by increasing potassium excretion. Carbenicillin and rarely other penicillin derivatives given in large amounts promote distal tubular secretion by acting as unreabsorbed anions; amphotericin B alters distal tubular permeability. Gentamicin also has been reported to cause hypokalemia by unknown mechanisms.

Magnesium depletion can cause potassium depletion, apparently due to increased renal and possibly gastrointestinal losses. Increased aldosterone secretion may play a role in stimulating potassium excretion. Hypokalemia in this condition is associated with hypocalcemia.

Hypokalemia without potassium depletion occurs in a number of conditions in which *potassium shifts into cells*. Patients with *periodic paralysis* develop repeated episodes of muscle weakness, which may be severe or even life-threatening if respiratory muscles are involved. These are due to sudden movement of potassium into cells, which causes hypokalemia. *Insulin* promotes a shift of potassium into cells. Administration of large amounts of dextrose intravenously may cause mild hypokalemia by stimulating insulin secretion. This effect may be clinically significant if dextrose solutions are used to administer potassium to hypokalemic patients. Plasma *alkalosis* tends to decrease plasma potassium modestly (less than 0.5 mmol/L per 0.1-unit increase in pH) by promoting potassium movement into cells. Treatment of acidosis with bicarbonate infusions may have a greater effect on plasma potassium because potassium entry into cells is enhanced not only by increasing plasma pH but also by a direct effect of bicarbonate ion. As discussed above, hypokalemia in alkalotic patients also may reflect loss of potassium in the urine, e.g., with vomiting, diuretic use, or excessive mineralocorticoid effects. Exogenous or endogenous *beta-adrenergic catecholamines* may cause hypokalemia by stimulating potassium shifts into cells. This phenomenon may be one factor leading to cardiac arrhythmias during stress or during treatment of asthma with beta-adrenergic agonists.

Clinical features   The most prominent features of hypokalemia and potassium depletion are neuromuscular. Moderate degrees of depletion may be asymptomatic, especially if they develop slowly. Some patients, however, complain of muscle weakness, especially in the lower extremities. With more severe or acute degrees of hypokalemia and potassium deficiency, marked and generalized weakness of skeletal muscles is prominent. Very severe or abrupt development of hypokalemia may lead to virtually total paralysis, including the respiratory muscles. Rhabdomyolysis may occur. On physical examination, in addition to decreased motor power, the patient may demonstrate decreased or absent tendon reflexes. The smooth muscle of the gastrointestinal tract may be affected, resulting in paralytic ileus.

Abnormalities in the electrocardiogram are common. The characteristic changes include flattening and inversion of the T wave, increased prominence of the U wave, and sagging of the ST segment (Fig. 189-20A). These alterations are not well correlated with the severity of the disturbance in potassium metabolism and cannot be relied on as indexes of the clinical significance of a potassium deficit. Although moderate potassium depletion rarely affects cardiac action, severe or rapid reduction in serum potassium may cause cardiac arrest. Potassium deficiency enhances the cardiac toxicity of digitalis preparations. A variety of atrial and ventricular arrhythmias may occur in hypokalemia, especially in patients receiving digitalis.

Renal tubular function is markedly impaired by potassium depletion (Chap. 242). The most prominent abnormality is decreased concentrating ability, which may cause polyuria and polydipsia. Glomerular filtration rate is normal or slightly reduced; moderate reductions may occur with chronic potassium depletion nephropathy. Renal regulation of potassium excretion remains normal. The urinalysis is benign: Protein excretion is normal or minimally increased, and the urinary sediment is normal or demonstrates only a slight increase in hyaline or granular casts.

Diagnosis   The cause of hypokalemia and potassium depletion is usually evident from the history. However, patients whose potassium deficiency is caused by chronic abuse of laxatives; psychogenic, self-induced vomiting; or surreptitious use of diuretics rarely volunteer an accurate history. Patients with villous adenomas of the rectum sometimes report that their feces are formed; careful questioning will reveal the elimination of the characteristic mucous secretion of the tumor.

In Fig. 45-2 is a flowchart that outlines the steps in differential diagnosis of hypokalemia when the cause is not evident from the history. The presence of *hypertension*, which suggests hyperaldosteronism (except Bartter's syndrome) or glucocorticoid excess, may be a clue to diagnosis. Blood pressure is normal in patients whose potassium depletion is due to the other causes listed in Table 45-2. Evaluation of *urinary potassium excretion* may be helpful in

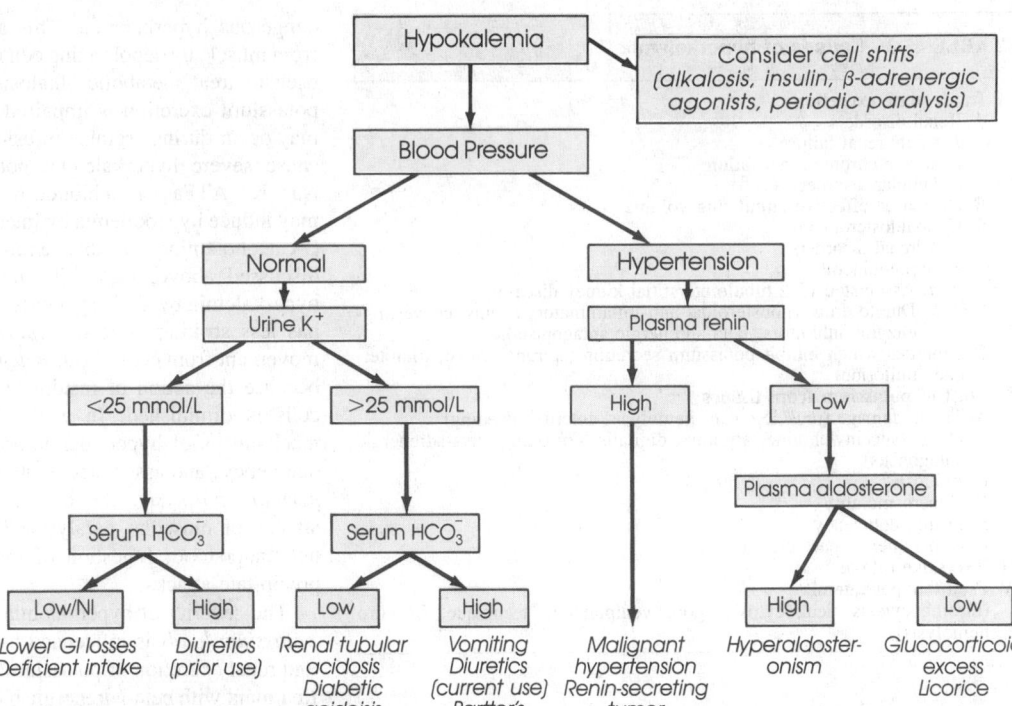

FIGURE 45-2 Flowchart for differential diagnosis of principal causes of hypokalemia. Nl = Normal.

determining the origin of the potassium deficit. If gastrointestinal losses have occurred, urinary excretion is usually less than 20 to 25 mmol/L or per day. Although renal conservation of potassium is slow, excretion falls to these levels by the time that clinically significant deficits of potassium have accumulated. On the other hand, when renal potassium wasting is the cause, urinary excretion usually exceeds 20 to 25 mmol/L or per day. However, lower concentrations and lower excretion rates may be found in severe depletion, in those patients with excessive mineralocorticoid activity while on low sodium intake, and in patients whose diuretics have been stopped at the time of examination. Evaluation of blood *acid-base status* may help in differential diagnosis. Hypokalemia is associated with metabolic acidosis in types I and II renal tubular acidosis, diarrhea, and diabetic ketoacidosis and in patients treated with carbonic anhydrase inhibitors. With other causes of hypokalemia, blood bicarbonate is normal or elevated due to associated metabolic alkalosis.

Treatment When possible, potassium depletion should be corrected by increased dietary intake or supplementation with potassium salts. Potassium chloride is the salt of choice, especially in alkalotic patients. It may be given in the form of an elixir or in tablets in which potassium chloride crystals are embedded in a wax. Enteric-coated potassium chloride tablets have been responsible for ulceration of the small bowel, due to release of high concentrations of potassium salts, and should be avoided. Organic salts such as gluconate or citrate are adequate in patients who are not severely alkalotic and often are used to treat hypokalemia due to renal tubular acidosis. In edematous patients treated with diuretics that cause hypokalemia, potassium deficits should be prevented or treated by increased dietary potassium intake, supplementation with potassium chloride, or addition of ‘‘potassium-sparing’’ diuretics such as spironolactone. More controversial is the need for routine dietary supplements in patients receiving diuretics for treatment of hypertension. Patients with adequate dietary potassium intake usually do not develop significant hypokalemia and probably do not require routine supplements to prevent potassium depletion. However, those who do develop hypokalemia despite adequate diets should probably receive potassium salts, since hypokalemia may be associated with an increased frequency of arrhythmias.

Intravenous treatment is required for patients with gastrointestinal disorders or when the potassium deficiency is severe. It must be emphasized that the potassium *concentration* in commonly available intravenous solutions of potassium chloride is 2000 mmol/L. Concentrations in intravenous infusions should not exceed 40 or at the most 60 mmol/L. The rate of infusion should not exceed 20 mmol/h or approximately 200 to 250 mmol/d, unless the need for more rapid infusion has been demonstrated in the individual patient by evidence of continuing losses large enough to justify more intensive therapy. The results of treatment are best monitored by repeated determinations of plasma potassium and evaluation of clinical symptoms such as muscular weakness or paralysis. Disappearance of electrocardiographic abnormalities correlates only roughly with improvement in total body potassium content. However, during rapid intravenous administration of potassium, the electrocardiogram should be monitored to avoid cardiac toxicity from inadvertent hyperkalemia.

Hypokalemia and hypocalcemia may occur together, e.g., in patients with malabsorption syndrome. The neuromuscular effect of each electrolyte abnormality is masked by the other. Treatment of either disorder alone may precipitate symptoms. Thus treatment of hypokalemia alone may precipitate tetany, and conversely, treatment of hypocalcemia without correcting the hypokalemia may exacerbate the manifestations of potassium deficiency.

HYPERKALEMIA Pathogenesis The causes of hyperkalemia are shown in Table 45-3. Inadequate renal excretion is a frequent cause (see also Chaps. 236 and 237). When oliguria or anuria is present, as in acute renal failure, progressive hyperkalemia is the rule. Plasma potassium rises by about 0.5 mmol/L per day if there are no abnormal loads. Chronic renal failure does not cause severe or progressive hyperkalemia unless oliguria supervenes. Adaptive changes increase potassium excretion per residual nephron as chronic renal failure progresses. However, patients with chronic renal failure function at the limits of their excretory capacity. Hence hyperkalemia may develop rapidly if the potassium load is increased or excretory capacity is limited, e.g., by administration of spironolactone. *Impaired tubular potassium secretion* has been described in a number of tubulointerstitial diseases. Causes include lupus erythematosus, sickle cell disease, rejection of a transplanted kidney, obstructive uropathy, and amyloidosis. Tubular H^+ secretion is often impaired as well, leading to the combination of hyperkalemia and hyperchloremic acidosis (type IV renal tubular acidosis). The defect in potassium secretion may result directly from a tubular disorder or may be due to hyporeninemic hypoaldosteronism (see below).

A *decrease in effective circulating volume* tends to impair potassium excretion. In conditions such as salt and water depletion or

TABLE 45-3 Causes of hyperkalemia

I Inadequate excretion
   A Renal disorders
      1 Acute renal failure
      2 Severe chronic renal failure
      3 Tubular disorders
   B Decreased effective circulating volume
   C Hypoaldosteronism
      1 Adrenal disorders
      2 Hyporeninemic
         a Associated with tubulointerstitial kidney disease
         b Due to drugs (nonsteroidal anti-inflammatory agents, converting-enzyme inhibitors, beta-adrenergic antagonists)
   D Diuretics which inhibit potassium secretion (spironolactone, triamterene, amiloride)
II Shift of potassium from tissues
   A Tissue damage (muscle crush, hemolysis, internal bleeding)
   B Drugs (succinylcholine, arginine, digitalis, poisoning, beta-adrenergic antagonists)
   C Acidosis
   D Hyperosmolality
   E Insulin deficiency
   F Hyperkalemic periodic paralysis
III Excessive intake
IV Pseudohyperkalemia
   (thrombocytosis, leukocytosis, poor venipuncture technique, in vitro hemolysis)

congestive heart failure, glomerular filtration rate is reduced and proximal fluid reabsorption is enhanced. This decreases delivery of fluid to the distal tubule, thereby limiting potassium secretion into the urine. Hyperkalemia may occur in some patients; it is usually modest and not progressive but may become severe if potassium loads are high.

Hyperkalemia is a cardinal feature of adrenal insufficiency (Addison's disease) and of certain congenital adrenal enzyme disorders, including selective *hypoaldosteronism*. Heparin inhibits aldosterone secretion; hyperkalemia may occur in patients treated with heparin who have other potentiating factors, such as volume depletion or renal insufficiency.

In adults, *hyporeninemic hypoaldosteronism* (see Chap. 335) is a frequent cause of hyperkalemia. In patients with this disorder, renin and aldosterone secretion are deficient. Hypoaldosteronism appears to be due both to the decrease in angiotensin, a major stimulus to aldosterone secretion, and to some secretory defect in the adrenal gland. Most patients have moderate renal insufficiency. In about half this is due to diabetic nephropathy, but a variety of chronic interstitial nephritides may cause this syndrome. Patients typically present with hyperkalemia, often associated with hyperchloremic acidosis (type IV renal tubular acidosis). Inhibition of the activity of the renin-angiotensin-aldosterone system by nonsteroidal anti-inflammatory drugs, converting enzyme inhibitors or beta-adrenergic blockers also may induce hyperkalemia due to hyporeninemic hypoaldosteronism. (Beta-adrenergic blockers also inhibit potassium entry into cells; see below.)

A kilogram of tissue such as muscle or erythrocytes contains about 80 mmol potassium, and damaged cells release potassium into the plasma. Hence hyperkalemia may be seen when there is muscle-crushing injury, hemolysis, or internal hemorrhage. Severe progressive hyperkalemia is not ordinarily a consequence of increased release of potassium from damaged or acidotic tissues alone. However, acidosis and tissue damage often occur together with acute renal insufficiency; under these circumstances, severe hyperkalemia may develop quickly. In contrast to the increase of 0.5 mmol/L per day typical of uncomplicated anuria, plasma potassium concentration in anuric patients with tissue damage may increase 2 to 4 mmol/L per day. Such rapidly progressive hyperkalemia may be an important cause of death in military casualties. Several *drugs* may cause hyperkalemia by altering tissue uptake of potassium. In patients with trauma, burns, or neuromuscular diseases such as paraplegia and multiple sclerosis, the muscle relaxant succinylcholine may cause

dangerous hyperkalemia. This agent apparently releases potassium from muscle by depolarizing cell membranes. Arginine hydrochloride, used to treat metabolic alkalosis, drives potassium out of cells. If potassium excretion is impaired, clinically significant hyperkalemia may occur during arginine infusions. Extreme digitalis poisoning may cause severe hyperkalemia; potassium leaks out of cells because Na^+,K^+-ATPase is inhibited by the drug. Beta-adrenergic blockers may induce hyperkalemia by interfering with the action of endogenous β-catecholamines to enhance movement of potassium into tissues. As discussed above, *metabolic acidosis* due to mineral acids causes hyperkalemia by shifting potassium out of cells. Respiratory acidosis has less striking effects. *Hyperosmolality* also enhances potassium movement from cells. *Insulin deficiency* is conducive to hyperkalemia because the action of insulin to promote potassium movement into cells is diminished. In acute diabetic ketoacidosis, the principal mechanisms of hyperkalemia appear to be hyperosmolality, insulin deficiency, and associated acute renal insufficiency. In *hyperkalemic periodic paralysis*, the hyperkalemia is associated with repeated attacks of muscular paralysis. The mechanism of this syndrome is not understood. Ingestion of increased amounts of potassium may precipitate attacks.

The severity of hyperkalemia caused by large oral or intravenous *potassium loads* is influenced by factors that modulate tissue uptake and renal excretion of potassium. For example, insulin deficiency and treatment with beta-adrenergic blockers tend to augment hyperkalemia by limiting tissue uptake. Volume depletion and administration of converting enzyme inhibitors or nonsteroidal anti-inflammatory agents enhance hyperkalemia by limiting the rate at which the kidney excretes such loads.

Patients with extreme thrombocytosis or, more rarely, extreme leukocytosis in leukemia may demonstrate the phenomenon of *pseudohyperkalemia*. Platelets or white blood cells release potassium during blood clotting in vitro. While serum potassium may be grossly abnormal, plasma potassium is not increased. Artifactual elevation of plasma potassium may occur if blood is drawn after repeated fist clenching to make veins more prominent during application of a tourniquet, due to leakage of potassium from exercising muscle. Improper technique during collection or processing of blood samples may cause hemolysis and hence hyperkalemia in vitro. Artifactual hyperkalemia may be suspected when electrocardiographic abnormalities are absent despite elevation of measured potassium levels.

Clinical features   The most important toxic effects of hyperkalemia are cardiac arrhythmias. The earliest manifestation is the development of high-peaked T waves, especially prominent in precordial leads. Hyperkalemia does not prolong the QT interval, unlike other disorders which induce peaking of the T waves. Later changes include prolongation of the PR interval, complete heart block, and atrial asystole. As plasma potassium rises further, ventricular complexes may deteriorate. The QRS complex becomes progressively prolonged and finally tends to merge with the T wave in a sinewave configuration. Terminally, ventricular fibrillation and standstill may occur.

Occasionally, moderate or severe hyperkalemia has striking effects on peripheral muscles. Ascending muscular weakness can occur, progressing to flaccid quadriplegia and respiratory paralysis. Cerebral and cranial nerve function are normal, as is sensation.

Diagnosis   Severe or progressive hyperkalemia is rare in the absence of renal insufficiency. Hence plasma creatinine and urine output should be determined promptly in hyperkalemic patients. Acute renal failure, especially if oliguric, will cause progressive hyperkalemia. Even in oliguric patients, an increase in plasma potassium of more than 0.5 mmol/L per day suggests the need to search for a source of potassium loads, e.g., from tissue breakdown in hematomas or muscle undergoing rhabdomyolysis. When hyperkalemia is detected in nonoliguric patients with chronic renal failure, the physician should look for sources of high dietary potassium intake or medications which interfere with potassium excretion. In the absence of such superimposed factors, hyperkalemia in these patients should suggest hyporeninemic hypoaldosteronism or a tubular disease which directly impairs tubular potassium secretion. This distinction is made by appropriate studies of renin and aldosterone levels (see Chap. 335), which are reduced in patients with hyporeninemic hypoaldosteronism but not in those with hyperkalemia due directly to tubular damage.

In all patients with hyperkalemia, the history should focus on medications that may cause elevated plasma potassium levels, such as converting enzyme inhibitors, nonsteroidal anti-inflammatory agents, beta-adrenergic blockers, and potassium-sparing diuretics. Sources of high potassium intake in the diet should be reviewed, e.g., potassium supplements or salt substitutes. Signs of extracellular volume depletion, Addison's disease, or edematous states with decreased effective extracellular volume should be sought on physical examination.

In addition to plasma creatinine, blood sugar and plasma bicarbonate levels should be determined to evaluate possible contributions of diabetes or acidosis to hyperkalemia. Urine potassium measurements are of little value in differential diagnosis. An electrocardiogram is important to evaluate the effects of hyperkalemia. In patients with no adequate explanation for hyperkalemia, especially if the electrocardiogram demonstrates no hyperkalemic features, the possibility of spurious hyperkalemia should be considered.

Treatment In considering therapy, it is helpful to classify hyperkalemia according to degree of severity. The seriousness of hyperkalemia is best estimated by considering both the plasma potassium concentration and the electrocardiogram. When the plasma potassium is less than 6 mmol/L and electrocardiographic changes are limited to peaking of T waves, hyperkalemia is mild. When the plasma potassium is 6 to 8 mmol/L and T-wave peaking is the only electrocardiographic abnormality, hyperkalemia is moderate. Severe hyperkalemia is present if the plasma potassium exceeds 8 mmol/L or if electrocardiographic abnormalities include absent P waves, widened QRS complexes, or ventricular arrhythmias.

Mild hyperkalemia can usually be treated by elimination of a cause, such as potassium-sparing diuretics, or by treatment of accompanying volume depletion or acidosis. Patients with Addison's disease require specific hormonal therapy (see Chap. 335). Those with renal tubular disorders can be treated with loop diuretics to increase potassium excretion. Patients with hyporeninemic hypoaldosteronism also respond to loop diuretics or may require mineralocorticoid therapy (see Chap. 335).

More severe or progressive hyperkalemia requires vigorous therapy. Severe cardiac toxicity responds most rapidly to infusion of calcium; 10 to 30 mL of 10% calcium gluconate may be infused intravenously within a period of 1 to 5 min under constant electrocardiographic monitoring. While calcium infusions do not alter plasma potassium, they counteract the adverse effects of potassium on neuromuscular membranes. The effect of calcium infusions, while almost immediate, is transient if the hyperkalemia is not treated directly.

In moderate or severe hyperkalemia, infusion of hypertonic glucose solutions decreases toxicity by provoking insulin release and shifting potassium into cells. In the first 30 min, 200 to 500 mL of 10% glucose may be given. An additional 500 to 1000 mL may be infused over the next several hours. Concurrently, 10 units of regular insulin is given intravenously or subcutaneously. This treatment may reduce serum potassium by 1 to 2 mmol/L within 30 to 60 min, and effects persist for a number of hours. The infusion of sodium bicarbonate also helps lower serum potassium rapidly by causing potassium to shift into cells; 50 to 150 mmol alkali (two to three ampuls) may be added to a liter of glucose. Although this agent is most valuable in acidotic patients, it also is effective in individuals with normal acid-base status. The effect occurs within 1 h and persists for a number of hours. The infusion of hypertonic sodium solutions also may be effective in reversing cardiac toxicity, especially in hyponatremic or volume-depleted patients. In part, the effect depends simply on dilution of plasma potassium, but there may be a direct effect of elevated plasma sodium to antagonize hyperkalemic neuromuscular

toxicity as well. Glucose, bicarbonate, and sodium may be combined in a "therapeutic cocktail," formulated by adding an ampul or two of sodium bicarbonate to a liter of 5% dextrose in 0.9% saline.

None of the measures just described removes potassium from the body. Cation-exchange resins such as sodium polystyrene sulfonate are useful to remove potassium in the treatment of moderate or severe hyperkalemia. Fifty grams of the resin is mixed with 100 mL of 35% sorbitol and given by retention enema. Enough potassium may be removed by a single enema to reduce potassium by 0.5 to 2 mmol/L within an hour, and repeated enemas can be given. These resins also can be given repeatedly by mouth to maintain low plasma potassium concentrations. Twenty grams is given three or four times a day together with 20 mL of a 70% sorbitol solution as required to ensure the passage of several loose stools daily. In patients with renal failure, hemodialysis and peritoneal dialysis effectively control hyperkalemia. However, they are relatively slow techniques, and patients with severe hyperkalemia should be treated first with one of the methods previously discussed.

REFERENCES

Sodium and water

DeVita MV, Michelis MF: Perturbations in sodium balance. Hyponatremia. Clin Lab Med 13:135, 1993

Kamel KS, Bear RA: Treatment of hyponatremia: A quantitative analysis. Am J Kidney Dis 21:439, 1993

Narins RG et al: Diagnostic strategies in disorders of fluid, electrolyte and acid-base homeostasis. Am J Med 72:496, 1982

Robertson GL: Thirst and vasopressin function in normal and disordered states of water balance. J Lab Clin Med 101:351, 1983

Sonnenblick, M et al: Diuretic-induced severe hyponatremia. Review and analysis of 129 reported patients. Chest 103:601, 1993

Strange K: Regulation of solute and water balance and cell volume in the central nervous system. J Am Soc Nephrol 3:12, 1992

Weisberg LS et al: Pseudohyponatremia: A reappraisal. Am J Med 86:315, 1989

Zerbe R et al: Vasopressin function in the syndrome of inappropriate diuresis. Ann Rev Med 31:315, 1980

Potassium

DeFronzo RA: Clinical disorders of hyperkalemia, in The Kidney: Physiology and Pathophysiology, 3d ed, DW Seldin, G Giebisch (eds). New York, Raven, 1992, p 2279

Knochel JP: The syndrome of hyporeninemic hypoaldosteronism. Ann Rev Med 30:145, 1979

————: Neuromuscular manifestations of electrolyte disorders. Am J Med 72:521, 1982

————: Hypokalemia. Adv Intern Med 30:317, 1984

Kupin WL, Narins RG: The hyperkalemia of renal failure: pathophysiology, diagnosis and therapy. Contrib Nephrol 102:1, 1993

Latta K et al: Perturbations in potassium balance. Clin Lab Med 13:149, 1993

Seldin DW, Giebisch G (eds): The Regulation of Sodium and Chloride Balance. New York, Raven, 1989

Sterns RH et al: Internal potassium balance and the control of the plasma potassium concentration. Medicine 60:339, 1981

Stokes JB: Potassium intoxication: Pathogenesis and Treatment, in The Regulation of Potassium Balance, DW Seldin, G Giebisch (eds). New York, Raven, 1989, p 269

Tannen RL: Diuretic-induced hypokalemia. Kidney Int 28:988, 1985

46 ACIDOSIS AND ALKALOSIS

NORMAN G. LEVINSKY

PHYSIOLOGIC CONSIDERATIONS Acids are produced continuously during normal metabolism. Despite the addition of some 20,000 mmol of carbonic acid and 80 mmol of nonvolatile acids to body fluids daily, the free hydrogen ion concentration of these fluids is fixed within a narrow range. The pH of extracellular fluids is normally between 7.35 and 7.45 (hydrogen ion, 45 to 35 nmol/L). The pH of intracellular fluids cannot be determined with precision, but most methods suggest a mean intracellular pH in the range of 6.9.

Intracellular hydrogen ion concentration is not uniform; it varies among intracellular organelles within individual cells. Although the free hydrogen ion concentration of body fluids is low, protons are so reactive that even minute changes in concentration influence enzymatic reactions and physiologic processes. Immediate defense against untoward changes in pH is provided by buffers that can take up or release protons instantaneously in response to changes in acidity of body fluids. Regulation of pH ultimately depends on the lungs and the kidneys.

Role of the lungs   The principal acid product of metabolism is carbon dioxide, equivalent to potential carbonic acid. The normal concentration of carbon dioxide in body fluids is fixed around 1.2 mmol/L [P_{CO_2} = 5.3 kPa (40 mmHg)] by the lungs; at this concentration, pulmonary excretion equals metabolic production. Although carbon dioxide reacts with water and body buffers during transport from cells to pulmonary alveoli, no net change in body fluid composition results, since the CO_2 excreted by the lungs is equal to the CO_2 produced by cells.

Nonvolatile acids   When a nonvolatile acid is produced by metabolism, the protons are removed instantaneously from body fluids by reaction with buffers. In extracellular fluid, bicarbonate is converted to water and carbon dioxide, which is excreted by the lungs. Although this mechanism minimizes changes in acidity, it destroys bicarbonate and uses up cell buffer capacity. The total buffer capacity of the body fluids is about 15 mmol/kg of body weight. The normal rate of production of nonvolatile acids would be sufficient to deplete the body buffers completely in 10 to 20 days, were it not for the ability of the kidney to eliminate protons from the body by secretion into the urine, thereby regenerating bicarbonate and cell buffer capacity.

The principal source of nonvolatile acid is metabolism of methionine and cystine in dietary proteins, which produces sulfuric acid. Additional sources include the incomplete combustion of carbohydrates and fats, which produces organic acids; the metabolism of nucleoproteins, which produces uric acid; and the metabolism of organic phosphorus compounds, which releases protons and inorganic phosphates. The diet does not normally contain significant amounts of preformed acid or alkali, but significant amounts of potential acid (e.g., an excess of cationic acids, such as lysine) or alkali (e.g., citrate) may be present.

Role of the kidney   The principal functions of the kidney in acid-base balance can be viewed as (1) retention of extracellular bicarbonate and (2) excretion of protons of nonvolatile acids produced by metabolic processes. Both functions are served by secretion of protons into tubular fluid, in proximal nephron segments via a sodium-proton exchanger and in distal segments by an H^+-ATPase pump. The protons secreted into tubular fluid are derived from carbon dioxide (carbonic acid); removal of protons generates bicarbonate in the tubular cell. This bicarbonate is reabsorbed with filtered sodium. When secreted protons are buffered by filtered bicarbonate, it is destroyed. The bicarbonate lost in this process is replaced by reabsorption of the bicarbonate generated in renal tubular cells, thereby conserving existing bicarbonate stores. When the secreted protons are buffered by urinary buffers other than bicarbonate, filtered bicarbonate is not destroyed; therefore, the new bicarbonate reabsorbed from tubular cells represents a net addition to extracellular bicarbonate. Normally, most protons are buffered by bicarbonate, thus reclaiming the approximately 4000 mmol/d of bicarbonate in glomerular filtrate. About 80 mmol/d is secreted onto nonbicarbonate buffers, thereby regenerating the buffer capacity used in buffering the daily production of nonvolatile acids. Of this amount, about one-third reacts with phosphate, converting HPO_4^{2-} to $H_2PO_4^-$; the remainder is titrated onto ammonia. The amount of free acid which can be excreted in the urine is negligible, even at the minimum urine pH of 4.8. However, acidification of the urine is essential for titration of protons onto phosphate and ammonia.

Changes in the pH of body fluids lead to regulatory responses by the kidney, mediated by parallel changes in renal tubular cell pH. Acidosis stimulates renal hydrogen ion secretion. Ammonia

production increases, and more protons can be excreted as ammonium, thus generating new extracellular bicarbonate. In extreme acidosis, ammonia production may increase tenfold or more above the normal rate of 40 to 50 mmol/d. Alkalosis inhibits renal proton secretion and thereby reduces reabsorption and generation of bicarbonate by renal tubules. Recent studies indicate that the kidney can secrete bicarbonate into distal tubular fluid via an HCO_3-Cl exchanger; alkalosis stimulates this process. If plasma bicarbonate rises, bicarbonate is excreted rapidly both because the increase in filtered load is not matched by a corresponding increase in tubular reabsorptive capacity and because bicarbonate is secreted. By these mechanisms, normal plasma bicarbonate is restored promptly. For example, chronic ingestion of even large amounts of sodium bicarbonate normally produces only minimal sustained elevation of plasma bicarbonate.

Renal acid-base regulatory mechanisms are influenced by a number of factors in addition to pH of body fluids, important among them the carbon dioxide tension and volume of the extracellular fluid, angiotensin, aldosterone, availability of chloride ion, and body potassium stores. Tubular bicarbonate reabsorption is directly related to the carbon dioxide concentration of body fluids, presumably because changes in CO_2 alter the pH of renal tubular acid-secreting cells. Hypercapnia, which induces intracellular acidosis, tends to stimulate renal bicarbonate reabsorption, while hypocapnia has the opposite effect. Effective extracellular volume also influences bicarbonate reabsorption. In volume-depleted states, proximal tubular bicarbonate reabsorption is increased. This effect appears to be mediated by angiotensin II, which stimulates proximal bicarbonate transport, and by a reduction in filtered load due to decreased glomerular filtration rate. Aldosterone increases proton secretion in distal tubular segments. This is due both to direct stimulation of the distal proton pump and to enhanced sodium reabsorption, which favors retention of protons in tubular fluid by increasing intraluminal electronegativity.

Chloride depletion tends to limit bicarbonate excretion. This may be due in part to reduced delivery of chloride to the collecting tubules, where it is needed for bicarbonate secretion via the HCO_3^--Cl exchanger. Moreover, sodium reabsorption is generally enhanced in chloride-depleted states owing to associated extracellular fluid volume depletion. When less chloride is available for reabsorption, a larger fraction of the sodium must be reabsorbed with bicarbonate (via increased proton secretion). In experimental animals, renal bicarbonate reabsorption is inversely related to body potassium stores. In humans, the relation is less clear, but severe potassium depletion has been associated with increased bicarbonate reabsorption and metabolic alkalosis. Hyperkalemia, on the contrary, may contribute to metabolic acidosis by suppressing renal ammonia production.

The respiratory response to changes in blood pH is almost instantaneous. Acidosis stimulates and alkalosis depresses ventilation. The respiratory center in the medulla appears to respond to a pH intermediate between those of blood and cerebrospinal fluid.

EVALUATION OF ACID-BASE BALANCE   In practice, classification of acid-base disorders is based on measurements of changes in the bicarbonate–carbonic acid system, the principal buffer of extracellular fluid. Because intracellular and extracellular buffers are functionally linked, measurement of the plasma bicarbonate system provides useful information about total body buffers. The relationship among the elements of the bicarbonate system is usually described in terms of the Henderson-Hasselbalch equation:

$$pH = pK + \log \frac{[HCO_3^-]}{[H_2CO_3]}$$

Acidosis is defined as a disturbance which tends to add acid or remove alkali from body fluids, whereas *alkalosis* is any disturbance which tends to remove acid or add base. Since compensatory processes may minimize or prevent a change in the hydrogen ion concentration of the plasma, some authors prefer to use the terms *acidemia* and *alkalemia* to indicate those situations in which the pH of the plasma is measurably altered. *Metabolic* disorders are those in which the primary disturbance is in the concentration of bicarbonate. Since bicarbonate appears in the numerator of the buffer salt/acid ratio in the Henderson-Hasselbalch equation, increased bicarbonate concentration causes increased pH (alkalemia), whereas a decrease in bicarbonate causes decreased pH (acidemia). *Respiratory* disorders are those in which the primary change is in the concentration of carbon dioxide (carbonic acid). As can be seen from the Henderson-Hasselbalch equation, a fall in carbon dioxide concentration causes alkalemia, whereas an increase in carbon dioxide concentration causes acidemia.

A major problem in the assessment of acid-base disorders results from the compensatory responses of the lungs and the kidneys. A primary change in carbon dioxide concentration induces a compensatory renal response which alters plasma bicarbonate in the same direction. Conversely, a primary alteration of plasma bicarbonate induces a compensatory respiratory response which changes plasma carbon dioxide in the same direction. Consider a patient with chronic respiratory insufficiency who has the following set of acid-base parameters: P_{CO_2} = 9.3 kPa (70 mmHg), [HCO_3^-] = 31 mmol/L, pH = 7.25. The clinician needs to know whether the elevation of plasma bicarbonate is merely the appropriate renal response to the primary hypercapnia or a metabolic acid-base disorder is superimposed. No calculations or a priori reasoning will provide the answer to this key question. Such information can be derived only from in vivo observations in which the usual compensatory response to a given degree of chronic hypercapnia is determined.

Clinical and experimental observations in humans (and animals) have been made in all common primary acid-base disturbances. They are most readily visualized and used for analysis of clinical acid-base disorders by the "confidence band" technique, as shown in Fig. 46-1. Each band represents the mean ± 2 SD, that is, 95 percent

FIGURE 46-1 Nomogram showing bands for uncomplicated respiratory or metabolic acid-base disturbances in intact subjects. Each "confidence" band represents the mean ± 2 SD for the compensatory response of normal subjects or patients to a given primary disorder. Ac = acute; chr = chronic, resp = respiratory; met = metabolic; acid = acidosis; alk = alkalosis. (*Modified from Arbus.*)

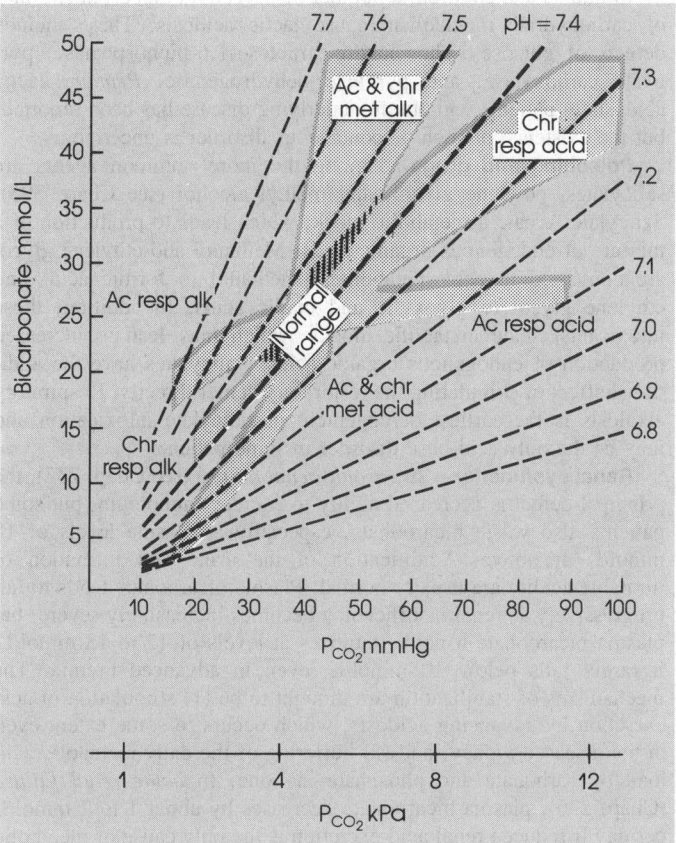

TABLE 46-1   **Approximate compensatory responses to primary acid-base disorders***

Metabolic acidosis
  P_{CO_2} ↓ ≈ 1.2 HCO_3^- ↓
Metabolic alkalosis
  P_{CO_2} ↑ ≈ 0.7 HCO_3^- ↑
Respiratory acidosis
  A Acute: HCO_3^- ↑ ≈ 0.1 P_{CO_2} ↑
  B Chronic: HCO_3^- ↑ ≈ 0.35 P_{CO_2} ↑
Respiratory alkalosis
  A Acute: HCO_3^- ↓ ≈ 0.2 P_{CO_2} ↓
  B Chronic: HCO_3^- ↓ ≈ 0.5 P_{CO_2} ↓

* P_{CO_2} measured in mmHg, HCO_3^- in mmol/L.

of observations, for the compensatory response to each primary disturbance. In the example under discussion, inspection of the confidence band marked *chronic respiratory acidosis* indicates that 95 percent of individuals with chronic elevation of P_{CO_2} to 9.3 kPa (70 mmHg) would have [HCO_3^-] between 34 and 44 mmol/L, due to renal compensation. Thus the [HCO_3^-] of 31 mmol/L in the example cannot be interpreted as the sole result of an appropriate compensatory response to chronic hypercapnia. A second acid-base disorder, presumably metabolic acidosis, must be superimposed to account for the fact that plasma bicarbonate, although increased in response to hypercapnia, is not as high as usually observed when P_{CO_2} is 9.3 kPa (70 mmHg). Obviously, the use of this figure is no panacea, nor does it obviate the need for commonsense clinical evaluation of alternative possibilities. For example, if the patient under discussion had only recently developed hypercapnia, the [HCO_3^-] of 31 mmol/L would be too high for a purely compensatory response to acute respiratory acidosis and would be interpreted as superimposed metabolic alkalosis. The difference between these two interpretations depends entirely on the clinical recognition of the chronicity of the primary respiratory disorder. The use of Fig. 46-1 in each type of acid-base disturbance is described in the appropriate sections of this chapter.* If the nomogram is unavailable, the "rules of thumb" in Table 46-1 are useful alternatives in interpreting acid-base data.

METABOLIC ACIDOSIS

PATHOPHYSIOLOGY Metabolic acidosis is caused by one of three mechanisms: (1) increased production of nonvolatile acids, (2) decreased acid excretion by the kidney, (3) loss of alkali. Extracellular bicarbonate is reduced by reaction with hydrogen ions or, in patients wasting alkali, by loss of bicarbonate in urine or stool. The decrease in pH stimulates respiration, and P_{CO_2} is lowered. Inspection of the confidence band for metabolic acidosis (Fig. 46-1) indicates that a decrease in P_{CO_2} of about 0.16 kPa (1.2 mmHg) can be expected for each decrement of 1 mmol/L in plasma bicarbonate. Complete respiratory compensation for primary metabolic acidosis does not occur. Respiratory compensation for acute acidosis tends to be somewhat greater than for chronic metabolic acidosis. The minimum level of P_{CO_2} that can be attained is approximately 1.3 kPa (10 mmHg); levels below 2 to 2.7 kPa (15 to 20 mmHg) are rarely maintained in chronic metabolic acidosis. When kidney function is normal, net acid excretion increases promptly in response to metabolic acidosis. Most of the initial rise is due to increased titration of urinary phosphate as urine pH falls below 5.2. Over several days, ammonia production by the kidney increases and becomes the most important mechanism for excreting excess protons. Net acid excretion may increase 5 to 10 times above normal, reaching a maximum of several hundred millimoles per day.

* Although the confidence band method does not permit automatic identification of simple or complicated acid-base disorders, it is preferable to techniques such as "buffer base" or "base excess-deficit" for reasons discussed in detail by Schwartz and Relman, N Engl J Med 268:1382, 1963. These terms are not used in this chapter.

TABLE 46-2   Causes of metabolic acidosis

INCREASED ANION GAP

I **Increased acid production**
  A Ketoacidosis
    1 Diabetic
    2 Alcoholic
    3 Starvation
  B Lactic acidosis
    1 Secondary to circulatory or respiratory failure
    2 Associated with various disorders (see text)
    3 Drugs and toxins
    4 Enzyme defects
  C Poisoning (salicylates, ethylene glycol, methanol)
II **Renal failure**

NORMAL ANION GAP (HYPERCHLOREMIC)

III **Renal tubular dysfunction**
  A Renal tubular acidosis
  B Hypoaldosteronism
  C "Potassium-sparing" diuretics
IV **Loss of alkali**
  A Diarrhea
  B Ureterosigmoidostomy
  C Carbonic anhydrase inhibitors
V **Production of HCl (ammonium chloride, cationic amino acids)**

TYPES OF ACIDOSIS The principal causes of metabolic acidosis are listed in Table 46-2.

Ketoacidosis In *diabetic ketoacidosis*, due to the hormonal abnormalities, acetoacetic and β-hydroxybutyric acids are produced more rapidly than they can be metabolized (see Chap. 337). Severe ketoacidosis may occur in *association* with *acute* and *chronic alcoholism*. Typically, patients give a history of prolonged abstention from food, protracted vomiting, and appreciable alcohol intake just before development of the ketoacidosis. β-Hydroxybutyrate, acetoacetate, and lactate accumulate in the plasma. The ketosis may be overlooked because the ratio of β-hydroxybutyrate to acetoacetate tends to be high; the nitroprusside test used for clinical detection of plasma ketones responds only to the latter. Blood sugar is usually normal or mildly elevated in these patients. *Starvation* may cause mild ketoacidosis; plasma bicarbonate usually falls no more than 3 to 4 mmol/L, although decreases of up to 10 mmol/L may occur with prolonged starvation. Reduced carbohydrate intake leads to low insulin and high glucagon levels in both starvation and alcoholic ketosis. These hormonal changes favor glycolysis and ketogenesis. In alcoholic ketosis, for uncertain reasons, fatty acid mobilization exceeds even that characteristic of starvation alone (see Chap. 337).

Lactic acidosis Metabolic production and consumption of lactate are normally in balance. Under basal conditions, the liver and kidney consume lactate produced by tissues such as erythrocytes, skin, intestine, and muscle. However, if oxygen delivery is inadequate to meet energy requirements, any tissue will generate lactate. Deficient oxygen impairs electron flow through the cytochrome transport chain; ATP formation is decreased, and cell redox pairs, such as NADH/NAD, are shifted toward the reduced state. Decreases in ATP and reciprocal increases in ADP and AMP concentrations activate phosphofructokinase, the key enzyme regulating glycolysis. Accelerated glycolysis leads to increased production of pyruvate, and the increase in NADH/NAD ratio decreases its oxidation. Pyruvate and lactate are in a near-equilibrium reaction catalyzed by lactic dehydrogenase, as follows:

$$\text{Pyruvate} + \text{NADH} + \text{H}^+ \rightleftharpoons \text{lactate} + \text{NAD}$$

Thus lactate will tend to increase when pyruvate concentration increases and when the ratio of NADH to NAD rises. Since both conditions occur when tissues are oxygen-deprived, lactate formation is increased. Lactate will accumulate because it can be consumed only by conversion back to pyruvate, which is blocked so long as pyruvate concentration and the NADH/NAD ratio are elevated. Since the overall process of glycolysis generates one H$^+$ for each lactate molecule produced, acid production increases proportionately with lactate production.

These mechanisms, probably compounded by decreased uptake or even production of lactate by the liver, account for the development of lactic acidosis in patients with *shock* due to any cause (e.g., sepsis, myocardial infarction, hemorrhage) or with respiratory arrest. Since severe acidosis depresses myocardial and arteriolar contractility, lactic acidosis may compound the underlying cause of shock. Less commonly, lactic acidosis may be caused by *pulmonary diseases* leading to extreme hypoxia or by diminished blood oxygen–carrying capacity in severe *anemia* and *carbon monoxide* poisoning. The mortality rate is high in patients with lactic acidosis secondary to shock and tissue hypoxia. During vigorous *exercise* or convulsions, local disproportion between oxygen supply and demand in contracting muscle may lead to transient, clinically benign lactic acidosis.

Lactic acidosis also is *associated* with disorders in which tissue hypoxia does not appear to be present. It has been reported in patients with leukemia, lymphoma, and solid tumors, with poorly controlled diabetes mellitus, and with severe hepatic failure. Mechanisms causing lactic acidosis in these disorders are poorly understood. Overproduction of lactate by neoplastic tissue probably is a factor in lactic acidosis associated with tumors. Insulin deficiency, which inhibits pyruvate oxidation, presumably is an important factor in patients with poorly controlled diabetes. Decreased hepatic lactate metabolism seems a likely mechanism in severe liver disease.

A variety of *drugs* and *toxins* have been associated with lactic acidosis. *Drugs* include fructose used in parenteral alimentation, sodium nitroprusside, epinephrine and norepinephrine infusions, and, before the drug was removed from general use, the biguanide hypoglycemic agent phenformin. Lactic acidosis may contribute to the severe acidosis in *poisoning* by salicylates, ethylene glycol, or methanol. Ethanol elevates serum lactate, but clinically significant lactic acidosis does not occur in alcohol intoxication unless there are associated disorders such as hepatic or circulatory failure.

In infants and children, a number of *congenital defects in enzymes* of carbohydrate metabolism cause lactic acidosis. These include defects of glucose-6-phosphatase, fructose-1,6-biphosphatase, pyruvate carboxylase, and pyruvate dehydrogenase. *Primary* lactic acidosis in patients without an underlying disease has been reported, but the existence of such a spontaneous disorder is uncertain.

Poisoning and drugs Among the more common agents are salicylates, ethylene glycol, and methyl alcohol (see Chap. 395). Salicylates create a metabolic block, which leads to production of a mixture of endogenous organic acids. Methanol and ethylene glycol are converted to acid metabolites, methanol to formic acid, and ethylene glycol to glyoxylic and oxalic acids. In addition, these intoxicants create metabolic blocks, which may lead to increased production of endogenous organic acids. Salicylates have the additional effect of stimulating the respiratory center directly. Respiratory alkalosis is the earliest derangement in salicylate intoxication and may be the only acid-base disorder in some patients.

Renal dysfunction In *chronic renal failure* (see Chap. 237), the principal defect is decreased ability to excrete ammonium, but some patients also waste bicarbonate, especially at plasma levels of 18 mmol/L or above. Acidification of the urine and formation of titratable acidity are usually normal. Plasma bicarbonate tends to fall progressively as renal insufficiency becomes increasingly severe, but plasma bicarbonate usually stabilizes at levels of 12 to 18 mmol/L; it rarely falls below 10 mmol/L, even in advanced uremia. The mechanisms of stabilization are thought to be (1) stimulation of acid excretion by advancing acidosis, which occurs to some extent even in the diseased kidney, and (2) buffering of the daily metabolic acid load by carbonate and phosphate in bone. In *acute renal failure* (Chap. 236), plasma bicarbonate decreases by about 1 to 2 mmol/L per day if reduced renal acid excretion is the only cause of metabolic acidosis. Greater rates of fall suggest the presence, in addition, of some cause of increased acid production.

Chronic metabolic acidosis is the hallmark of *renal tubular acidosis* (see Chap. 244), which may be an isolated disorder of tubular acid excretion; part of a Fanconi syndrome, in which other tubular functions are also abnormal; or associated with nonrenal primary disorders (see Chap. 352). The acidosis is due to defective renal tubular acidification mechanisms, which limit renal conservation and regeneration of bicarbonate.

Aldosterone stimulates distal tubular acid and potassium secretion. In *hypoaldosteronism*, loss of this effect leads to metabolic acidosis and hyperkalemia. The acidosis is due not only to loss of the direct effect of aldosterone on acid excretion but also to the hyperkalemia, which decreases renal ammonia production. The same factors account for metabolic acidosis caused by the diuretic spironolactone, which blocks the action of aldosterone, and other "potassium-sparing" diuretics such as triamterene and amiloride, which directly inhibit distal tubular secretion of acid and potassium.

Loss of alkali   Severe *diarrhea* or intestinal malabsorption usually causes mild to moderate acidosis due to the loss of bicarbonate in liquid stool, in which concentrations of 40 to 60 mmol/L may be present. *Ureterosigmoidostomy*, i.e., transplantation of the ureters into the sigmoid colon, leads to metabolic acidosis both because of exchange of chloride for bicarbonate by intestinal epithelium and because renal disease (obstructive uropathy and pyelonephritis) often develops. However, acidosis is not a problem with the more modern technique for urinary diversion, in which a bladder is formed from a small isolated loop of ileum. *Carbonic anhydrase inhibitors*, such as acetazolamide, cause mild to moderate acidosis by increasing bicarbonate loss in the urine.

Production of HCl   Acidosis can be caused by administration of ammonium chloride and lysine or arginine hydrochloride, which form HCl during metabolism. This type of acidosis also may occur during parenteral alimentation with amino acid infusates that contain an excess of the cationic amino acids arginine, lysine, and histidine.

CLINICAL FEATURES AND DIAGNOSIS   Acute metabolic acidosis is usually caused by overproduction of a nonvolatile acid (see Table 46-2, category I). Chronic metabolic acidosis is most frequently due to renal dysfunction. Diarrhea is a common cause of either acute or chronic acidosis.

There are few specific symptoms or signs of metabolic acidosis; diagnosis depends on recognition of the clinical setting and appropriate laboratory studies. In acute metabolic acidosis, hyperventilation is usual and may be intense (Kussmaul respiration). However, it is ordinarily impossible to detect increased respiration by physical examination in patients with chronic metabolic acidosis, despite substantial reduction of P_{CO_2}. Acute, severe acidosis produces a variety of nonspecific symptoms ranging from fatigue through confusion, stupor, and coma. Cardiovascular effects include decreased cardiac contractility and vasodilatation, which may lead to heart failure or hypotension. Chronic metabolic acidosis may produce no symptoms or may be associated with fatigue and anorexia, although it is usually difficult to determine whether these symptoms reflect the acidosis per se or are related to the underlying disease.

The characteristic laboratory features are reduction of plasma bicarbonate and blood pH, together with a compensatory reduction in P_{CO_2} (see Fig. 46-1). Hyperkalemia is often present, due to shift of potassium out of cells. This phenomenon may mask significant potassium depletion (see Chap. 45). Hypokalemia is a clue to conditions in which concomitant potassium depletion is severe, e.g., diarrhea or diabetic ketoacidosis, or in which renal potassium-regulating mechanisms are affected, e.g., renal tubular acidosis or administration of carbonic anhydrase inhibitors.

When the cause of metabolic acidosis is not evident from the history or clinical setting, calculation of unmeasured anions (anion gap) may help in differential diagnosis. Unmeasured anions are calculated by subtracting the sum of plasma bicarbonate and chloride concentrations from plasma sodium concentration; the normal value

is 8 to 16 mmol/L. The negative charges on plasma proteins, principally albumin, make up most of the anion gap. Phosphate, sulfate, and organic acid anions normally contribute to unmeasured anions to a lesser degree. When metabolic acidosis is due to increased acid production or renal insufficiency (categories I and II in Table 46-2), the anion gap is usually increased. In acidosis resulting from increased acid production, the increased anion gap is due to accumulation in plasma of the anions of the various acids such as acetoacetate or lactate, which are produced faster than they can be metabolized or excreted. In renal failure, the anion gap increases because sulfate, phosphate, and organic acid anions are not excreted efficiently.

The cause of acidosis with an increased anion gap usually is easily determined from the clinical setting and simple laboratory tests. *Ketoacidosis* should be considered when acidosis occurs in patients with uncontrolled diabetes mellitus (see Chap. 337), alcoholism, or starvation. Ketonemia can be detected by testing serum dilutions with nitroprusside (Acetest) reagent. In occasional patients this test, which reacts to acetoacetate but not β-hydroxybutyrate, may be misleading. If the clinical diagnosis is uncertain, a specific assay for β-hydroxybutyrate is available. The diagnosis of *lactic acidosis* is suspected in patients with severe circulatory insufficiency when other causes of acidosis can be ruled out. A specific assay for plasma lactate is available if the diagnosis is uncertain. Plasma salicylate concentration in the toxic range [>2.9 mmol/L (>40 mg/dL)] will confirm suspected *salicylate intoxication* (see Chap. 395). Acidosis due to *poisoning* with ethylene glycol or methanol (see Chap. 395) may be suspected if measured plasma osmolality exceeds calculated plasma osmolality [$(2 \times$ plasma Na$)$ + glucose/18 + BUN/2.8 (with plasma Na in mmol/L, glucose and BUN in mg/dL)]. This "osmolal gap" reflects the plasma level of methanol or ethylene glycol, small molecules that at toxic concentrations add significantly to plasma osmolality. (Since ethanol has a similar effect, it must be measured if alcohol intoxication is suspected.) Detection of a large "osmolal gap" in a patient with severe acidosis may permit prompt treatment to be instituted while awaiting confirmation of the diagnosis with specific tests for the toxins. However, for unknown reasons, moderately elevated "osmolal gaps" (up to 10 to 15 mosmol/kg) occur in some patients with lactic acidosis or alcoholic ketoacidosis. Hence an elevated "osmolal gap" is not a specific test for methanol or ethylene glycol poisoning; clinical judgment must be used in deciding on therapeutic strategy.

In all other types of metabolic acidosis (categories III, IV, and V in Table 46-2), the anion gap is normal because there is neither increased production nor decreased excretion of organic acids, sulfate, and phosphate. Plasma chloride concentration is increased approximately as much as plasma bicarbonate is decreased (hyperchloremic acidosis). In diabetic ketoacidosis, a variety of plasma acid-base patterns may develop, depending on the balance between production and renal excretion of ketoacid anions. In most patients there is renal dysfunction, and the anions are retained, leading to an anion-gap acidosis in which the elevation in plasma unmeasured anion is about equal to the reduction in bicarbonate concentration. Patients with normal renal function may present with a component of hyperchloremic acidosis due to renal excretion of ketone anions and retention of chloride. After therapy that repairs volume depletion and hence renal dysfunction, most patients develop some degree of hyperchloremia, due to the same mechanisms.

TREATMENT   The treatment of metabolic acidosis depends on its cause and severity. In *chronic renal failure*, mild or moderate metabolic acidosis does not require treatment. When plasma bicarbonate falls below 15 mmol/L, it is reasonable to treat patients with oral alkali, such as sodium bicarbonate or sodium citrate. The dose is gradually increased until plasma bicarbonate concentration rises to about 18 to 20 mmol/L. Some patients appear to benefit symptomatically from elevation of bicarbonate to this level, and fatigue, anorexia, and malaise tend to be alleviated. Caution must be exerted to avoid excessively rapid alkalination of the plasma, which may precipitate tetany; excess sodium given with alkali may aggravate hypertension or edema. Acidosis should be corrected as completely as possible in patients with type 1 (distal) *renal tubular acidosis;* this will avoid hypercalciuria, osteomalacia, nephrocalcinosis, and lithiasis. In type 2 (proximal) renal tubular acidosis, therapy is usually not required (see Chap. 244). Patients with *acute renal failure* also do not ordinarily require specific therapy for acidosis. Dialysis instituted for management of the renal failure should maintain an adequate plasma bicarbonate.

Diabetic *ketoacidosis* responds to insulin, and most patients do not require treatment with alkali (see Chap. 337). However, when acidosis is extreme (pH less than 7.1 or $[HCO_3^-]$ less than 6 to 8 mmol/L), intravenous bicarbonate therapy is justified. The ketoacidosis associated with alcoholism responds rapidly to infusions of glucose and saline. Insulin is not required, nor should alkali be given unless acidosis is extreme. The ketoacidosis of starvation is mild and requires no specific treatment.

In *lactic acidosis*, if the underlying disorder can be reversed, the acidosis will be corrected by metabolism of lactate, which generates bicarbonate. Since lactic acidosis is usually associated with severe circulatory or respiratory failure, the mortality rate is high. Because production of lactate and H^+ in lactic acidosis can be very rapid, it is usually resistant to treatment with alkali. Large amounts of bicarbonate may be required to raise or even to stabilize plasma bicarbonate. Some studies have suggested that alkali therapy in lactic acidosis may be counterproductive because correction of acidosis appears to increase lactate production. However, extreme acidosis may contribute to circulatory collapse (see above), thereby perpetuating the underlying cause of the lactic acidosis. Hence it seems reasonable to treat lactic acidosis with intravenous bicarbonate at a rate at least sufficient to maintain plasma bicarbonate at 8 to 10 mmol/L and pH above 7.10. If vigorous administration of sodium bicarbonate leads to circulatory overloading, diuretics should be given or dialysis with a bicarbonate-buffered fluid may be instituted. Dichloroacetate, an investigational agent that enhances pyruvate dehydrogenase activity, has shown promise for treating lactic acidosis in experimental and clinical studies.

The acidosis due to *diarrhea* or loss of alkaline upper intestinal secretions is usually associated with volume depletion and potassium deficiency. Treatment of such electrolyte disorders with intravenous infusions appropriate for the patient's specific abnormalities may be required.

Some general points about therapy with alkali deserve emphasis. Oral treatment with sodium bicarbonate usually should begin with 1 g three times daily and be increased to maintain the desired plasma bicarbonate level. Some patients find that sodium bicarbonate leads to upper gastrointestinal discomfort; a 10% sodium citrate solution may be more palatable. In the intravenous treatment of acute metabolic acidosis, sodium bicarbonate is the agent of choice. The amount of bicarbonate to be given depends on the severity of the acidosis and any associated disorders of serum sodium concentration. Typically, concentrations of bicarbonate between 50 and 150 mmol/L are achieved by adding one to three vials of sodium bicarbonate to a liter of dextrose in water. The concentration of bicarbonate in these vials is 1000 mmol/L (50 mmol in 50 mL); these bicarbonate solutions should never be given undiluted in the treatment of acidosis, since rapid infusion may induce serious or even fatal cardiac arrhythmias, especially if given as a bolus through a central venous catheter.

In metabolic acidosis, approximately equal amounts of acid appear to be buffered by extracellular bicarbonate and by intracellular buffers. (In severe acidosis, a greater fraction of the acid load may be buffered within cells.) Therefore, it is appropriate to calculate the amount of bicarbonate needed to raise plasma bicarbonate by assuming that approximately half will accept protons from intracellular buffers and be destroyed; the other half will elevate plasma bicarbonate concentration. Thus the calculation would be millimoles of bicarbonate required equals desired increment in plasma concentration (millimoles per liter) times 40 percent of body weight. The 40 percent figure represents twice the extracellular volume. It is rarely desirable to infuse enough alkali to elevate plasma bicarbonate to normal. Possible untoward effects include hypokalemic cardiac toxicity in patients who are substantially potassium-depleted, tetany in patients with renal failure or hypocalcemia, and congestive heart failure due to excess sodium. Moreover, alkalosis may supervene. Cerebrospinal fluid bicarbonate does not equilibrate rapidly with plasma. Hence the respiratory center, which responds to acidity both of blood and cerebrospinal fluid, maintains some degree of hyperventilation as plasma bicarbonate is increasing. This type of respiratory alkalosis may sometimes persist for several days after correction of metabolic acidosis. In acute acidosis due to overproduction of metabolic acids, successful treatment of the primary disorder will cause rapid metabolic conversion of lactate and ketone bodies to bicarbonate. Thus excessive administration of bicarbonate early in therapy also may lead to metabolic alkalosis at a later stage of treatment, when endogenous bicarbonate has been reconstituted by improvement in metabolism.

METABOLIC ALKALOSIS

PATHOPHYSIOLOGY   Metabolic alkalosis is usually initiated by increased loss of acid from the stomach or the kidney. However, excretion of bicarbonate at high plasma concentrations is normally so rapid that alkalosis will not be sustained unless bicarbonate reabsorption is enhanced or alkali is continuously generated at a great rate. Clinically, maintenance of metabolic alkalosis is most often due to stimulation of bicarbonate reabsorption by a volume (chloride) deficit. During volume depletion, renal conservation of sodium takes precedence over other homeostatic mechanisms, such as correction of alkalosis. Since in alkalosis a large fraction of plasma sodium is paired with bicarbonate, complete reabsorption of filtered sodium requires reabsorption of bicarbonate as well. Alkalosis is sustained until volume depletion is corrected by administration of sodium chloride. This diminishes tubular avidity for sodium and provides chloride as an alternative anion for reabsorption with sodium; excess bicarbonate can then be excreted with sodium. Chloride is required for bicarbonate secretion in the collecting duct via a bicarbonate-chloride exchanger. Provision of chloride probably also facilitates bicarbonate excretion by enhancing chloride delivery to this secretory site.

The other major mechanism which can maintain metabolic alkalosis is hypermineralocorticoidism. Mineralocorticoids stimulate renal hydrogen ion secretion. In patients with excess mineralocorticoid activity, elevation of plasma bicarbonate is initiated by increased urinary loss of protons as ammonium and titratable acidity. Stimulation of tubular acid secretion also enhances bicarbonate reabsorption, thereby sustaining the metabolic alkalosis. Patients with excess mineralocorticoid activity are not volume- or chloride-deficient. Hence this type of metabolic alkalosis does not respond to sodium chloride administration.

The relation between metabolic alkalosis and potassium is incompletely understood. Alkalosis and hypokalemia often occur together. Alkalosis may cause hypokalemia and potassium depletion through mechanisms discussed in Chap. 45. Conversely, potassium depletion may help to sustain metabolic alkalosis because tubular acid secretion, and hence bicarbonate reabsorption, is stimulated. This mechanism contributes to maintenance of alkalosis in hypermineralocorticoidism. Whether potassium depletion alone can generate metabolic alkalosis is uncertain; if so, severe potassium depletion is required.

Respiratory compensation for metabolic alkalosis is limited. Alveolar ventilation decreases, and P_{CO_2} is elevated. However, since this response is limited by hypoxia, P_{CO_2} rarely rises above 7.3 to 8 kPa (55 to 60 mmHg).

PATHOGENESIS   The principal causes of metabolic alkalosis are outlined in Table 46-3. *Vomiting* and *gastric drainage* usually induce only minimal or moderate alkalosis, but occasional patients, especially those with increased gastric acid secretion (e.g., with acid-peptic disease or the Zollinger-Ellison syndrome), may develop very severe

TABLE 46-3 Causes of metabolic alkalosis

I **Associated with volume (chloride) depletion**
  A Vomiting or gastric drainage
  B Diuretic therapy
  C Posthypercapnic alkalosis
II **Associated with hyperadrenocorticism**
  A Cushing's syndrome
  B Primary aldosteronism
  C Bartter's syndrome
III **Severe potassium depletion**
IV **Excessive alkali intake**
  A Acute
  B Milk-alkali syndrome

alkalosis. Loss of hydrochloric acid in the gastric fluid initiates the alkalosis. Water and sodium chloride are lost in the vomitus or gastric aspirate. Initially, sodium is lost in the urine as well, coupled with increased bicarbonate excretion (which results from elevation of plasma bicarbonate above the tubular reabsorptive threshold). These losses cause a volume (chloride) deficit, which stimulates tubular reabsorption of sodium and bicarbonate and presumably inhibits bicarbonate secretion. Thus the elevated plasma bicarbonate generated by gastric losses of hydrochloric acid is maintained.

Alkalosis may be present in patients treated with "loop" *diuretics* (furosemide, ethacrynic acid, bumetanide) or with thiazides. The diuretics cause extracellular volume contraction and inhibit sodium chloride reabsorption in the loop of Henle or distal convoluted tubule, which increases delivery of tubular fluid to more distal nephron segments. The volume deficit and consequent hyperaldosteronism, as well as concomitant hypokalemia, stimulate proton secretion in these segments, generating and maintaining the alkalosis. Alkalosis due to treatment with oral diuretics is usually mild. Acute administration of potent intravenous diuretics such as furosemide or ethacrynic acid to patients on low-sodium diets may induce more severe alkalosis due to rapid loss of sodium chloride in the urine. Sudden contraction of extracellular volume elevates plasma bicarbonate; renal excretion of excess bicarbonate is prevented by the mechanism discussed above. Diuretics that specifically inhibit bicarbonate reabsorption, such as acetazolamide, or inhibit distal cation secretion, such as spironolactone, amiloride, and triamterene, cause acidosis rather than alkalosis (see above).

Patients with chronic hypercapnia due to respiratory insufficiency maintain high plasma bicarbonate concentrations (see "Respiratory Acidosis," below). If respiration improves, P_{CO_2} falls promptly. However, urinary excretion of excess bicarbonate previously generated by renal compensatory mechanisms takes a number of days. In patients on low-salt diets or diuretics who have a volume (chloride) deficiency, *posthypercapnic* alkalosis of this type may persist indefinitely unless sodium or potassium chloride is added to the diet. The mechanism in this condition is the same as that which causes persistent alkalosis in vomiting, described earlier.

Alkalosis is variable in patients with excess mineralocorticoid activity. Minimal or moderate alkalosis is usually present in patients with *Cushing's syndrome* or *primary aldosteronism*. More marked alkalosis may be seen in patients with extreme adrenal hyperfunction associated with ACTH-secreting tumors, such as bronchogenic carcinoma. Moderate alkalosis is typical of patients with *Bartter's syndrome*.

Although alkalosis and *potassium depletion* are often associated, mild or moderate potassium depletion alone does not cause sustained metabolic alkalosis. However, extreme degrees of potassium depletion (serum potassium usually 2 mmol/L or less) may cause metabolic alkalosis. This type of alkalosis is not corrected by administration of sodium chloride but does respond to administration of potassium.

For reasons noted earlier, alkalosis due to administration of alkali cannot be sustained unless large amounts are given. When renal function is compromised, alkalosis may be sustained by small exogenous loads. This is apparently the mechanism of alkalosis in the milk-alkali syndrome, in which hypercalcemic nephropathy and alkalosis develop in response to excessive intake of absorbable alkali. The nephropathy limits bicarbonate excretion, thus maintaining the alkalosis.

CLINICAL FEATURES AND DIAGNOSIS There are no specific clinical signs or symptoms. Severe alkalosis may cause apathy, confusion, and stupor. If serum calcium is borderline or low, rapid development of alkalosis may lead to tetany. The diagnosis of metabolic alkalosis depends on recognition of the clinical setting and appropriate laboratory studies. Plasma bicarbonate is increased. P_{CO_2} increases by about 0.01 kPa (0.7 mmHg) for each mmol/L increase in bicarbonate. Elevation of P_{CO_2} is insufficient to prevent alkalemia (see Fig. 46-1). Plasma potassium concentration is often reduced, and the electrocardiogram may reveal changes in T and U waves typical of hypokalemia (Chap. 189). These changes may be due to alkalosis itself or to associated alterations in potassium metabolism. Despite elevation of plasma bicarbonate, the urine pH is usually less than 7 in patients with sustained metabolic alkalosis. This "paradoxical aciduria" reflects the fact that bicarbonate reabsorption must be increased if metabolic alkalosis is to be sustained.

Differential diagnosis is usually made from clinical features, such as a history of vomiting or the manifestations of Cushing's syndrome. If no cause is apparent, surreptitious vomiting or use of diuretics should be considered. The urinary chloride concentration may be a helpful clue if the cause of alkalosis is not evident. When the alkalosis is associated with volume contraction (category I in Table 46-3), urinary chloride is low, usually less than 10 mmol/L. When the alkalosis is caused by hyperadrenocorticism or severe potassium depletion (categories II and III), urinary chloride is higher, usually 20 mmol/L or more.

TREATMENT Mild or moderate metabolic alkalosis rarely requires specific treatment. In patients with gastric alkalosis, infusion of saline solutions is usually sufficient to enhance renal bicarbonate excretion and to correct alkalosis by mechanisms discussed above. Administration of potassium chloride is also helpful in treating or preventing alkalosis in these patients and those with diuretic-induced alkalosis. In patients with adrenal hyperfunction, alkalosis is corrected by specific treatment of the underlying disease. In Bartter's syndrome, hypokalemia, potassium wasting, and alkalosis may be partly corrected by treatment with prostaglandin synthetase inhibitors such as indomethacin. Whenever alkalosis and potassium depletion occur together, potassium depletion should be treated with potassium chloride.

Rarely, with prolonged gastric metabolic alkalosis, losses may be severe enough to require intravenous therapy with acidifying agents. Dilute hydrochloric acid or acidifying salts such as ammonium chloride or arginine hydrochloride may be given slowly under such circumstances. In most patients the use of acidifying agents can be avoided by appropriate treatment with saline and potassium chloride. In patients who are volume-expanded or in whom volume loading is inadvisable, therapy with acetazolamide, which enhances renal bicarbonate excretion, may be helpful.

RESPIRATORY ACIDOSIS

PATHOPHYSIOLOGY Failure of ventilation promptly increases P_{CO_2} (carbonic acid) because metabolic production of carbon dioxide is so rapid. Acute respiratory acidosis is modulated to a limited degree by tissue buffers. As can be seen from the curve labeled *acute respiratory acidosis* in Fig. 46-1, immediate tissue buffering elevates plasma bicarbonate only slightly, by about 1 mmol/L for each increase of 1.3 kPa (10 mmHg) in P_{CO_2}. If hypercapnia is sustained, renal acid excretion is enhanced, and bicarbonate reabsorption is stimulated. Over a period of several days, plasma bicarbonate rises approximately 3.5 mmol/L for each increase of 1.3 kPa (10 mmHg) in P_{CO_2}, thereby minimizing the degree of acidemia. The increment in plasma bicarbonate attributable to renal activity is represented by the difference between the curves marked *chronic respiratory acidosis* and *acute respiratory acidosis*.

PATHOGENESIS *Acute* respiratory acidosis occurs whenever there is a sudden failure of ventilation. Common causes include depression of the respiratory center by cerebral disease or drugs, neuromuscular disorders, and cardiopulmonary arrest. *Chronic* respiratory acidosis occurs in pulmonary diseases such as chronic emphysema and bronchitis, in which ventilation and perfusion are mismatched and effective alveolar ventilation is decreased. Chronic hypercapnia also may result from primary alveolar hypoventilation or from alveolar hypoventilation related to extreme obesity (Pickwickian syndrome). Acute and chronic diseases characterized principally by interference with alveolar gas exchange, such as chronic pulmonary fibrosis, pneumonia, and pulmonary edema, usually cause hypocapnia rather than hypercapnia. In these conditions, hypoxia stimulates increased ventilation; since carbon dioxide is much more diffusible than oxygen, excretion of carbon dioxide is enhanced despite the barrier to gas exchange. Hypercapnia occurs only with respiratory fatigue or extremely severe disease.

CLINICAL FEATURES AND DIAGNOSIS It is often difficult to separate the manifestations of respiratory acidosis from those of associated hypoxia. Moderate hypercapnia, especially if it develops slowly, probably has no specific clinical features. When P_{CO_2} exceeds 9.3 kPa (70 mmHg), patients become progressively confused and obtunded. Asterixis may be present. Papilledema may occur, apparently because intracranial pressure is increased by the cerebral vasodilation characteristic of hypercapnia. Dilatation of conjunctival and superficial facial blood vessels may be noted.

The diagnosis of acute respiratory acidosis is usually evident from the clinical situation, especially if respiration is obviously depressed. Proof requires laboratory confirmation that P_{CO_2} is elevated. Acidemia is always present in patients with *acute* hypercapnia. Acidosis in acute cardiopulmonary arrest is usually a combination of a metabolic lactic acidosis and acute respiratory acidosis. Patients with *chronic* hypercapnia are usually acidemic. However, some individuals with minimal or moderate chronic hypercapnia may have normal or even slightly elevated plasma pH, as may be seen from Fig. 46-1. The mechanism of full compensation or of "overcompensation" in such instances is unknown. However, significant elevation of pH in patients with chronic hypercapnia is almost always due to complicating metabolic alkalosis. Diuretics, low-sodium diets, and posthypercapnic alkalosis are frequent causes of this type of superimposed acid-base disorder.

Because of the differences between plasma bicarbonate in acute hypercapnia and in chronic hypercapnia, proper interpretation of acid-base parameters in respiratory acidosis depends on clinical information.

TREATMENT The only worthwhile approach to treatment of respiratory acidosis is correction of the underlying disorder. Rapid infusion of alkali is justified in cardiopulmonary arrest. In other circumstances, infusions of alkali have no role in practical management of respiratory acidosis.

RESPIRATORY ALKALOSIS

PATHOPHYSIOLOGY Acute reduction in carbon dioxide concentration releases hydrogen ion from tissue buffers, which minimize alkalemia by reducing plasma bicarbonate. Acute alkalosis also enhances glycolysis; increased production of lactic and pyruvic acids lowers serum bicarbonate and raises plasma concentrations of the corresponding anions by a millimole or two. In chronic hypocapnia, plasma bicarbonate is further reduced because the decreased P_{CO_2} inhibits tubular reabsorption and generation of bicarbonate. As in respiratory acidosis, compensation for the chronic state is much more complete than for the acute (see Fig. 46-1). In acute hypocapnia, plasma bicarbonate falls only about 2 mmol/L for each 1.3-kPa (10-mmHg) reduction in P_{CO_2}. In chronic hypocapnia, plasma bicarbonate

TABLE 46-4 Causes of respiratory alkalosis

I Hypoxia
   A Acute (e.g., pneumonia, asthma, pulmonary edema, hypotension)
   B Chronic (e.g., pulmonary fibrosis, cyanotic heart disease, high altitude, anemia)
II Respiratory center stimulation
   A Anxiety
   B Fever
   C Gram-negative sepsis
   D Salicylate intoxication
   E Cerebral disease (tumor, encephalitis, etc.)
   F Hepatic cirrhosis
   G Pregnancy
   H After correction of metabolic acidosis
III Excessive mechanical ventilation

is reduced by 4 to 5 mmol/L for each 1.3-kPa (10-mmHg) decrease in P_{CO_2}. The decrement in plasma bicarbonate attributable to renal compensatory activity is shown by the difference between the curves labeled *acute* and *chronic respiratory alkalosis* in Fig. 46-1.

PATHOGENESIS Respiratory alkalosis is due to acute or chronic hyperventilation, which lowers P_{CO_2}. The causes of respiratory alkalosis are shown in Table 46-4.

Hypoxia from any process which reduces arterial P_{O_2} to approximately 60 mmHg or less tends to cause hyperventilation and respiratory alkalosis. Hyperventilation in lung disorders appears to be caused not only by hypoxemia but also by activation of intrapulmonary receptors which stimulate the respiratory center via neural connections. Hyperventilation may occur in patients with hypotension or severe anemia, apparently due to decreased oxygen delivery to chemoreceptors in the great vessels.

A number of disease processes and medications directly stimulate the medullary respiratory center. Persistent acidosis of the cerebrospinal fluid may stimulate hyperventilation after correction of metabolic acidosis (see "Metabolic Acidosis," above).

CLINICAL FEATURES AND DIAGNOSIS Depending on its severity and acuteness, hyperventilation may or may not be clinically apparent. In acute respiratory alkalosis, the clinical picture is rather characteristic: Patients complain of paresthesias, numbness, and tingling; of light-headedness; and if alkalosis is sufficiently severe, of manifestations of tetany. Alkalosis directly enhances neuromuscular excitability; this effect, rather than the modest decrease in ionized plasma calcium induced by alkalosis, is probably the major cause of tetany. Severe respiratory alkalosis may cause confusion or loss of consciousness, perhaps due to cerebral vasospasm induced by hypocapnia.

The diagnosis may be suspected from the clinical setting but must be confirmed by analysis of the plasma bicarbonate system. Hypocapnia together with a variable degree of alkalemia is found; plasma bicarbonate is decreased but is rarely below 15 mmol/L.

TREATMENT The only successful treatment for respiratory alkalosis is elimination of the underlying disorder. In the acute hyperventilation syndrome, sedation, reassurance, and, if symptoms are sufficiently severe, rebreathing into a bag will usually terminate the attack.

MIXED DISORDERS

In some patients, acid-base disturbances are mixed; i.e., two or occasionally even three of the primary disorders described in preceding sections may coexist. Table 46-5 lists some common causes of mixed acid-base disorders.

Metabolic acidosis and respiratory acidosis This is the typical acid-base disorder in patients with acute *cardiopulmonary arrest* or severe *pulmonary edema*. The circulatory failure causes lactic acidosis, and the respiratory failure leads to hypercapnia. Patients, often elderly, who develop *salicylate toxicity* while under treatment for a chronic disorder such as arthritis also may be receiving sedatives or

TABLE 46-5   Some common causes of mixed acid-base disorders

I **Metabolic acidosis and respiratory acidosis**
   A Cardiopulmonary arrest
   B Severe pulmonary edema
   C Salicylate plus sedative overdose
   D Pulmonary disease with superimposed renal failure or sepsis
II **Metabolic acidosis and respiratory alkalosis**
   A Salicylate overdose
   B Sepsis
   C Combined hepatic and renal insufficiency
   D Recent alcohol binge
III **Metabolic alkalosis and respiratory acidosis**
   A Chronic pulmonary disease, with superimposed
     1 Diuretic therapy
     2 Steroid therapy
     3 Vomiting
     4 Reduction of hypercapnia by ventilator
IV **Metabolic alkalosis and respiratory alkalosis**
   A Pregnancy with vomiting
   B Chronic liver disease treated with diuretics
   C Cardiopulmonary arrest treated with bicarbonate and ventilator
V **Metabolic acidosis and alkalosis**
   A Vomiting superimposed on
     1 Renal failure
     2 Diabetic acidosis
     3 Alcoholic ketoacidosis

hypnotics. These medications can depress respiration, leading to respiratory acidosis and metabolic acidosis, rather than the respiratory alkalosis and metabolic acidosis typical of salicylate toxicity alone. Mixed metabolic and respiratory acidosis also may occur in patients with *pulmonary disease* who develop *renal failure* or *sepsis.*

The mixed acidosis may be suspected from the clinical setting. Definitive diagnosis requires interpretation of blood acid-base measurements. Acidemia usually is very severe. The acid-base measurements do not fit on the confidence band for either metabolic or respiratory acidosis. If analyzed as a respiratory acidosis, the bicarbonate concentration is found to be lower than appropriate for the P_{CO_2} level. If initially interpreted as a metabolic acidosis, the P_{CO_2} is inappropriately high for the measured bicarbonate. It should be emphasized that the P_{CO_2} need not be above 5.3 kPa (40 mmHg). Even a reduced P_{CO_2} may indicate a component of respiratory acidosis if it is higher than expected for the usual compensatory response to metabolic acidosis. For example, a P_{CO_2} of 3.9 kPa (30 mmHg) represents relative hypercapnia in a patient whose bicarbonate is 7 mmol/L (see Fig. 46-1). In most cases, the acid-base parameters will fall between the bands for metabolic acidosis and acute respiratory acidosis on the nomogram. However, in patients with chronic respiratory acidosis, superimposed metabolic acidosis may reduce bicarbonate only to the area between the acute and chronic respiratory acidosis bands or even to a position on the acute respiratory acidosis band (see Fig. 46-1). In such patients, correct diagnosis of the acid-base disorder depends on analysis of the clinical history and availability of prior acid-base measurements.

Metabolic acidosis and respiratory alkalosis   As discussed above, *salicylate toxicity* commonly causes this mixed (combined) disorder (see "Metabolic Acidosis," above). This mixed disorder occurs in *septic patients*; cardiovascular insufficiency causes lactic acidosis, whereas fever and endotoxemia stimulate the respiratory center and cause hypocapnia. Chronic respiratory alkalosis is often present in patients with *hepatic cirrhosis*. Acute renal failure, a frequent complication in these patients, will superimpose metabolic acidosis. Patients who recently binged on *alcohol* may develop ketoacidosis and also may hyperventilate due to delirium tremens. In patients who have vomited repeatedly, a component of metabolic alkalosis may be added, resulting in a triple disorder.

As the severity of the hypocapnia increases, acid-base values will shift to the left on the nomogram (Fig. 46-1). With mild hypocapnia, the patient's values will be in the area between the bands for metabolic acidosis and chronic respiratory alkalosis; in this case, the nature of

this disorder is relatively easily recognized. With more profound hypocapnia, the value may fall on the chronic respiratory alkalosis band or even on the area between chronic and acute respiratory alkalosis. In such patients, correct identification of the acid-base disorder depends on the clinical setting and history.

Metabolic alkalosis and respiratory acidosis   In patients with chronic respiratory acidosis due to *pulmonary disease,* metabolic alkalosis is often superimposed by treatment with *diuretics, steroids,* or *ventilators.* The pathogenesis of metabolic alkalosis with these forms of therapy is discussed in the section of this chapter on metabolic alkalosis.

This is an important disorder to recognize in patients with chronic lung disease because the metabolic alkalosis will reduce the acidemic stimulus to ventilation. In patients with this combined disorder, blood pH is usually close to normal. The diagnosis is suggested by the clinical history and confirmed by acid-base values that are to the left of the confidence band for chronic respiratory acidosis, typically falling between that band and the one for metabolic alkalosis. Appropriate therapy for the metabolic alkalosis may improve ventilation significantly.

Metabolic alkalosis and respiratory alkalosis   In *pregnant* patients, severe vomiting will superimpose metabolic alkalosis on the chronic hypocapnia characteristic of pregnancy. Diuretics or vomiting may produce a combined alkalosis in patients with the chronic respiratory alkalosis typical of *hepatic cirrhosis. Treatment of cardiopulmonary arrest* often leads to a combined alkalosis. Hypocapnia is caused by the ventilator setting. The blood bicarbonate level is elevated both by bicarbonate therapy and by metabolic conversion of lactate accumulated during the cardiac arrest to bicarbonate after the circulation is restored. A triple acid-base disorder also may occur during treatment of cardiopulmonary arrest. If the circulation is not adequately restored, lactic acidosis will persist, leading to the combination of metabolic acidosis (lactic acidosis), respiratory alkalosis (ventilator), and metabolic alkalosis (bicarbonate infusion).

It is important to recognize combined metabolic and respiratory alkalosis because the relatively normal blood bicarbonate concentration may conceal severe alkalemia. Most often analysis will show that acid-base parameters lie between the bands for each primary disorder on the nomogram (Fig. 46-1). During therapy of cardiac arrest, a triple disorder due to superimposed lactic acidosis is recognized from the clinical features and a persistent elevation of the anion gap (see below).

Metabolic acidosis and alkalosis   Most often this disorder results when metabolic alkalosis due to vomiting is superimposed on diabetic or alcoholic ketoacidosis or on the acidosis of chronic or acute renal failure. In some patients with diabetic ketoacidosis, ingestion of large amounts of absorbable antacids for self-treatment of accompanying symptoms of gastric discomfort may be an additional cause of metabolic alkalosis. As discussed above, during therapy of cardiopulmonary arrest, either this combined disorder or a triple disturbance including ventilator-induced respiratory alkalosis may occur.

Blood pH may be normal, acidemic, or alkalemic, depending on the relative magnitude of the primary disorders. The blood acid-base pattern is not diagnostic, since it can fall on the confidence band for either metabolic alkalosis or metabolic acidosis or be in the normal range if the two disorders balance each other. Recognition depends largely on the clinical setting and history. If the acidosis is of the high-anion-gap type (see Table 46-2), recognition of the increase in unmeasured anion concentration may be a clue to a hidden metabolic acidosis (see below). If the acidosis is characterized by a normal anion gap (see Table 46-2), diagnosis is essentially dependent on analysis of the clinical features.

Diagnosis   Diagnosis of combined acid-base disorders is principally dependent on evaluation of the clinical setting, especially the history, and on interpretation of blood acid-base patterns with the aid of the nomogram (Fig. 46-1). Values that do not fit on any confidence band strongly suggest a mixed disorder. However, values that do fit on the band for a single acid-base disorder do not eliminate the possibility of a mixed disorder. Even normal acid-base parameters may conceal mixed disorders.

Evaluation of the anion gap may help in interpreting complex acid-base disorders. An anion gap in excess of 25 mmol/L strongly suggests the presence of a component of metabolic acidosis even if plasma bicarbonate is normal or elevated. For example, consider a patient who has recently binged on alcohol and presents with these plasma values: [Na] = 134 mmol/L, [K] = 3.9 mmol/L, [Cl] = 81 mmol/L, [HCO_3^-] = 26 mmol/L. Although the [HCO_3^-] is normal, the anion gap is 27 mmol/L [134 − (81 + 26)]. In this clinical setting, the elevated anion gap suggests the possibility of alcoholic ketoacidosis, which can be confirmed by measurement of plasma ketones. History reveals that the patient has been vomiting. The normal [HCO_3^-] thus is probably the result of balancing metabolic alkalosis and ketoacidosis. Although helpful, an elevated anion gap is not unequivocal evidence of metabolic acidosis. It may be moderately increased and occasionally may even exceed 25 mmol/L in metabolic alkalosis.*

---

* The increase in unmeasured anions in metabolic alkalosis is due principally to increased albumin anions. Release of protons by albumin acting as a buffer increases the number of anions per molecule. Plasma albumin concentration may also be increased by associated

REFERENCES

ADROGUE HJ et al: Plasma acid-base patterns in diabetic ketoacidosis. N Engl J Med 307:1603, 1982

ARBUS GS: An in vivo acid-base nomogram for clinical use. Can Med Assoc J 109:291, 1973

EMMETT M, NARINS RG: Clinical use of the anion gap. Medicine 56:38, 1977

GENNARI FJ, MADDOX DA: Renal regulation of acid-base homeostasis: Integrated response, in The Kidney: Physiology and Pathophysiology, 3d ed, DW Seldin, G Giebisch (eds). New York, Raven, 1992, p 2695

HARRINGTON JT: Metabolic alkalosis. Kidney Int 26:88, 1984

KASSIRER JP, MADIAS NE: Respiratory acid-base disorders. Hosp Practice 15:57, 1980

MADIAS NE: Lactic acidosis. Kidney Int 29:752, 1986

NARINS RG, EMMETT M: Simple and mixed acid-base disorders: A practical approach. Medicine 59:161, 1980

PREUSS HG: Fundamentals of clinical acid-base evaluation. Clin Lab Med 13:103, 1993

ROCHER LL, TANNEN RL: The clinical spectrum of renal tubular acidosis. Ann Rev Med 37:319, 1986

STACPOOLE PW et al: Dichloroacetate in the treatment of lactic acidosis. Ann Intern Med 108:58, 1988

WRENN KD et al: The syndrome of alcoholic ketoacidosis. Am J Med 91:119, 1991

volume depletion. Small increases in plasma lactate contribute to the elevated anion gap in alkalosis.

section 7   Alterations in reproductive and sexual function

47   IMPOTENCE

JOHN D. MCCONNELL / JEAN D. WILSON

A variety of endocrine, vascular, neurologic, and psychiatric diseases disrupt normal sexual and reproductive function in men. Furthermore, sexual dysfunction may be the presenting symptom of systemic disease.

NORMAL SEXUAL FUNCTION   Penile erection is initiated by neuropsychological stimuli that ultimately produce vasodilation of the sinusoidal spaces and arteries within the paired corpora cavernosa. Erection is normally preceded by sexual desire (or libido), which is regulated in part by androgen-dependent psychic factors. Although nocturnal and diurnal spontaneous erections are suppressed in men with androgen deficiency, erections in response to erotic stimuli may continue. Thus continuing action of testicular androgens appears to be required for normal libido but not for the erectile mechanism itself.

The penis receives innervation from sympathetic, parasympathetic, and somatic fibers. Somatic fibers in the dorsal nerve of the penis form the afferent limb of the erectile reflex by transmitting sensory impulses from the penile skin and glans to the S2–S4 dorsal root ganglia via the pudendal nerve. Unlike the corpuscular-type endings in the penile shaft skin, the majority of afferent terminations in the glans are free nerve endings. The efferent limb begins with parasympathetic preganglionic fibers from S2–S4 which pass in the pelvic nerves to the pelvic plexus. Sympathetic fibers emerging from the intermediolateral gray areas of T11–L2 travel through the paravertebral sympathetic chain ganglia, superior hypogastric plexus, and hypogastric nerves to enter the pelvic plexus along with parasympathetic fibers. Somatic efferent fibers from S3–S4 traveling in the pudendal nerve to the ischiocavernosus and bulbocavernosus muscles and postganglionic sympathetic fibers innervating the smooth muscle of the epididymis, vas deferens, seminal vesicle, and internal sphincter of the bladder mediate rhythmic contraction of these structures at the time of ejaculation.

Autonomic nerve impulses, integrated in the pelvic plexus, project to the penis through the cavernous nerves which course along the posterolateral aspect of the prostate before penetrating the pelvic floor muscles immediately lateral to the urethra. Distal to the membranous urethra, some fibers enter the corpus spongiosum, while the remainder enter the corpora cavernosa along with the terminal branches of the pudendal artery and exiting cavernous veins. If disruption of the cavernous nerves occurs following pelvic trauma or surgery, erectile impotence may ensue.

The brain exerts an important modulatory influence over spinal reflex pathways that control penile function. A variety of visual, auditory, olfactory, and imaginative stimuli elicit erectile responses that involve cortical, thalamic, rhinencephalic, and limbic input to the medial preoptic–anterior hypothalamic area, which is an important integrating center. Other areas of the brain, such as the amygdaloid complex, may inhibit sexual function.

Although the parasympathetic nervous system is the primary effector of erection, the transformation of the penis to an erect organ is a vascular phenomenon. In the flaccid state the arteries, arterioles, and sinusoidal spaces within the corpora cavernosa are constricted due to active sympathetic-mediated contraction of smooth muscle in the walls of these structures. The venules between the sinusoids and the dense tunica albuginea surrounding the cavernosa open freely to the emissary veins. Erection begins when relaxation of the smooth muscles leads to dilation of the sinusoids and a decrease in peripheral resistance, causing a rapid increase in arterial blood flow through internal pudendal and cavernosa arteries. Blood is trapped in the expanding sinusoidal system, which compresses the venules against the tunica albuginea, resulting in venous occlusion. The increase in intracorporeal pressure leads to tumescence and rigidity. Full rigidity, however, may in addition require stimulation of somatic fibers in the pudendal nerve and contraction of the ischiocavernosus muscle.

Erection occurs when adrenergic-induced sinusoidal tone is antagonized by sacral parasympathetic stimulation. Sinusoidal relaxation is mediated primarily by nonadrenergic-noncholinergic (NANC) neurotransmitter(s) and by the acetylcholine-dependent release of an endothelium-derived relaxing factor (EDRF). In vitro electrical stimulation of isolated corpus cavernosum strips causes release of neurotransmitters within nerve terminals which produces smooth-muscle relaxation that is resistant to adrenergic and cholinergic blockers. Both EDRF and the NANC neurotransmitter—which acts independent of the endothelium—are nitric oxide–like factors. Inhibitors of nitric oxide synthesis and cyclic guanosine monophosphate (cGMP) synthesis, as well as nitric oxide scavengers, block sinusoidal relaxation. A variety of neuropeptides found in corporal tissues, including vasoactive intestinal peptide (VIP) and calcitonin gene–related peptide, produce tumescence when injected into the penis but have uncertain physiologic roles. Norepinephrine plays an important role in the adrenergic mechanism of detumescence.

Seminal emission and ejaculation are under control of the sympathetic nervous system. Emission results from alpha-adrenergic–mediated contraction of the epididymis, vas deferens, seminal vesicles, and prostate which causes seminal fluid to enter the prostatic urethra. Concomitant closure of the bladder neck prevents retrograde flow of semen into the bladder. Antegrade ejaculation results from contraction of the muscles of the pelvic floor including the bulbocavernosus and ischiocavernosus muscles.

Orgasm is a psychosensory phenomenon in which the rhythmic contraction of the pelvic muscles is perceived as pleasurable. Orgasm can occur without either erection or ejaculation and in the presence of retrograde ejaculation.

Detumescence after orgasm and ejaculation is incompletely understood. Presumably, active tone in the vessels of the sinusoidal spaces is restored by active (probably adrenergic-mediated) contraction of smooth muscles, which decreases the inflow of blood to the penis and promotes emptying of the erectile tissue. Following orgasm, there is a refractory period that varies with age, physical condition, and psychic factors during which erection and ejaculation are inhibited.

IMPOTENCE Simply defined, *impotence* is the failure to achieve erection, ejaculation, or both. Men with sexual dysfunction present with a variety of complaints, either singly or in combination: loss of libido, inability to initiate or maintain an erection, ejaculatory failure, premature ejaculation, or inability to achieve orgasm. Sexual dysfunction can be secondary to systemic disease processes or their treatment, to specific disorders of the urogenital or endocrine systems, or to psychological disturbance. Previously, it was felt that the cause of dysfunction in the majority of men with erectile impotency was psychogenic. It is now believed that the majority of impotent men have a component of underlying organic disease. Since the selection and success of subsequent therapy depends on the specific cause, it is essential to evaluate all aspects of the erectile mechanism.

Loss of desire A decrease in sexual desire, or libido, may be due to androgen deficiency (arising from either pituitary or testicular disease), psychological disturbance, or some types of prescribed or habitually abused drugs. The possibility of androgen deficiency can be tested by measurement of plasma testosterone and gonadotropin levels. The level of testosterone required for normal erectile function remains unknown. Hypogonadism also may result in the absence of emission secondary to decreased secretion of ejaculate by the seminal vesicles and prostate.

Failure of erection The organ causes of erectile impotence can be grouped into endocrine, drug, local, neurologic, and vascular causes (Table 47-1). Decreased plasma testosterone secondary to testicular failure is an uncommon but easily recognized and treated disorder. However, hyperprolactinemia may cause impotence in some men with pituitary tumors and may not be obvious on physical examination; hyperprolactinemia suppresses luteinizing hormone–releasing hormone (LHRH) production, resulting in plasma gonadotropin and testosterone values in the low or low-normal range. Bromocrip-

TABLE 47-1 **Some organic causes of erectile impotence in men**

ENDOCRINE CAUSES

A Testicular failure (primary or secondary)
B Hyperprolactinemia

DRUGS

A Antiandrogens
  1 Histamine—H-2 blockers (e.g., cimetidine)
  2 Spironolactone
  3 Ketoconazole
  4 Finasteride
B Antihypertensives
  1 Central acting sympatholytics (e.g., clonidine and methyldopa)
  2 Peripheral acting sympatholytics (e.g., guanadrel)
  3 Beta blockers
  4 Thiazides
C Anticholinergics
D Antidepressants
  1 Monoamine oxidase inhibitors
  2 Tricyclic antidepressants
E Antipsychotics
F Central nervous system depressants
  1 Sedatives (e.g., barbiturates)
  2 Antianxiety drugs (e.g., diazepam)
G Drugs of habituation or addiction
  1 Alcohol
  2 Methadone
  3 Heroin
  4 Tobacco

PENILE DISEASES

A Peyronie's disease
B Previous priapism
C Penile trauma

NEUROLOGIC DISEASES

A Anterior temporal lobe lesions
B Diseases of the spinal cord
C Loss of sensory input
  1 Tabes dorsalis
  2 Disease of dorsal root ganglia
D Disease of nervi erigentes
  1 Radical prostatectomy and cystectomy
  2 Rectosigmoid operations
E Diabetic autonomic neuropathy and various polyneuropathies

VASCULAR DISEASE

A Aortic occlusion (Leriche syndrome)
B Atherosclerotic occlusion or stenosis of the pudendal and/or cavernosa arteries
C Arterial damage from pelvic radiation
D Venous leak
E Disease of the sinusoidal spaces

tine, a dopamine agonist, may lower prolactin levels and reverse impotence in such patients.

Although many drugs are associated with impotence, antihypertensive agents, cimetidine, and monoamine oxidase inhibitors are more likely to lead to erectile dysfunction. Antihypertensive drugs with peripheral and central sympatholytic action or beta-adrenergic receptor blocking activity are the most frequently implicated. Angiotensin-converting enzyme inhibitors, calcium channel blockers, and peripheral vasodilators do not cause a significant incidence of sexual dysfunction. Histamine (H-2) receptor antagonists, such as cimetidine, have antiandrogenic properties in addition to increasing prolactin secretion. The 5α-reductase inhibitor finasteride, used commonly for the treatment of benign prostate hypertrophy, produces impotence or decreased libido in 3 to 4 percent of men. Monoamine oxidase inhibitors, antipsychotic drugs, and tricyclic depressants may impair sexual function via anticholinergic and sympatholytic actions.

Penile diseases, including previous priapism, penile trauma, and Peyronie's disease, can cause impotence due to fibrosis of the sinusoidal spaces of the corpora cavernosa, corporeal artery occlusion, or neurogenic mechanisms. Peyronie's disease is not rare; patients present with a painful plaque on the dorsum of the penis and may progress to development of penile curvature and decreased rigidity.

Many types of neurologic disorders cause impotence, including lesions in the anterior temporal lobe, spinal cord disorders, insufficiency of sensory input as in tabes dorsalis, or damage to parasympathetic nerves, e.g., following surgical procedures such as radical (total) prostatectomy or cystectomy. Furthermore, the nerve supply to the penis (the nervi erigentes) runs on the posterolateral surface of the prostate, and if the nerves are preserved during radical prostate and bladder surgery, potency can be preserved in many men. If spinal cord injury is above the sacral region, reflex erections may occur, whereas diffuse injury of the sacral spinal cord results in total impotence. As many as half of men with diabetes mellitus develop impotence within 6 years of the onset of diabetes, and impotence may be the first clinical manifestation of diabetic neuropathy. Several factors contribute to neuropathic impotence, including abnormalities in afferent sensory pathways, motor neuropathy in the cavernosa nerves (which carry the efferent pathways for vasodilation in the penis), and decreased level of cavernosa neurotransmitter. Although autonomic pathways in the penis can be tested by direct recording of electrical activity in the corporal smooth muscle, the test may not be necessary because most patients demonstrate other manifestations of autonomic neuropathy on careful examination. Many of the other polyneuropathies associated with impotence have similar effects.

Men with vasculogenic impotence may present with total erectile impotence, decreased penile rigidity, or loss of erection during intercourse. Vascular insufficiency may be due to aortic occlusion (Leriche syndrome) or to more distal atherosclerotic disease in the hypogastric, pudendal, and cavernosa arteries. Significant disease in the pudendal and cavernosa arteries can occur in the absence of other clinical manifestations of peripheral vascular disease. Impotence following pelvic radiation is probably due to vasculogenic causes. Together with neuropathy, vascular insufficiency contributes to the impotence in many men with diabetes mellitus.

Premature ejaculation This disorder seldom has an organic cause. It is usually related to anxiety in the sexual situation, unreasonable expectations about performance, or emotional disorder. A variety of successful therapeutic modalities have been described by Levine.

Absence of emission This symptom may be produced by (1) retrograde ejaculation, (2) sympathetic enervation, (3) androgen deficiency, or (4) drugs. Retrograde ejaculation may occur following surgery on the bladder neck or develop spontaneously in diabetic men. Demonstration of sperm in a postcoital urine specimen establishes the diagnosis. Following sympathectomy or occasionally after extensive retroperitoneal surgery, the autonomic innervation of the prostate and seminal vesicles is lost, resulting in absence of smooth-muscle contraction at the time of ejaculation. Androgen deficiency results in a decrease in secretions of the prostate and seminal vesicles and in a diminution of the volume of ejaculate. Finally, drugs such as guanethidine, phenoxybenzamine, and phentolamine primarily impair ejaculation rather than erection or libido.

Absence of orgasm If libido and erectile function are normal, the absence of orgasm is almost always due to a psychiatric disorder.

Failure of detumescence Priapism is a persistent painful erection, often unrelated to sexual activity. Priapism can be distinguished from a normal erection by the absence of tumescence of the glans penis. Priapism may be idiopathic but can be associated with sickle cell anemia, chronic granulocytic leukemia, spinal cord injury, or, rarely, injection of vasodilator agents (such as papaverine) into the penis. The disorder may be secondary to clotting of blood within the sinusoidal spaces of the penis or to abnormalities of the adrenergic-mediated mechanism for detumescence. Failure to treat priapism promptly usually results in fibrosis and subsequent loss of erectile function. In early phases, detumescence can sometimes be achieved by aspiration, irrigation of the corpora cavernosa, and injection of dilute vasoconstrictors. If this fails, surgical relief by shunting procedures may be necessary. In patients with priapism secondary to sickle cell anemia, conservative measures such as transfusion, oxygenation, and irrigation are generally preferred to shunting procedures.

EVALUATION OF IMPOTENCE The relative frequency of organic as opposed to psychogenic causes of erectile impotence is still debated. Nevertheless, anxiety and depressive states are common causes of impotence. Other psychological factors such as disinterest in the sexual partner, fear of sexual incompetence, martial discord, guilt about deviant sexual attitudes, worry, fatigue, and ill health often operate in various combinations to reduce sexual impulse. The central issue in the evaluation of impotence is to separate those instances due to psychological factors from those due to organic causes (see Table 47-1). Often, the separation can be made on the basis of history. With the exception of severe depression, men with psychogenic impotence usually have normal nocturnal and early morning erections. From early childhood through the eighth decade, erections occur during normal sleep. This phenomenon, termed *nocturnal penile tumescence* (NPT), occurs during rapid eye movement sleep, and the total time of NPT averages 100 min per night. Consequently, if the impotent man gives a history of rigid erections under any circumstances (often when awakening in the morning), the efferent neurologic and circulatory systems that mediate erection are intact, and dysfunction is probably due to a psychiatric disorder. In these patients the workup should be limited. (Occasional patients with early sensory neuropathy may have nocturnal erections.)

If the history of nocturnal erections is questionable, measurements of NPT can be made formally with the use of a strain gauge in a sleep laboratory or informally attached to a recorder by snap gauge or home monitor. Although false-negative and false-positive results are possible, this procedure helps to differentiate psychogenic and organic impotence. Patients with vasculogenic impotence may have some degree of penile tumescence without the development of adequate rigidity, which may result in a false-positive NPT test. An alternative to NPT testing is the visual sexual stimulation (VSS) test, which utilizes videotaped erotic material in a laboratory setting to monitor erection by strain gauge. Other features of organic impotence include a slow, insidious onset not associated with any particular psychiatric symptomatology, a previous uninterrupted period of normal erectile function, and persistent sexual desire.

Having deduced an organic cause, the fundamental problem is the differential diagnosis of the etiology (see Table 47-1). The history should be probed for diabetes mellitus, manifestations of peripheral neuropathy or bladder dysfunction, symptoms referable to the vascular system such as intermittent claudication, and symptoms of penile disease such as a history of priapism or penile curvature (Peyronie's disease). A thorough drug history should be obtained, and inquiry should be made concerning past surgery that may have produced neurologic damage. Smoking is a risk factor for atherosclerotic disease and may inhibit sinusoidal relaxation directly.

Physical examination should include a detailed genital examination to identify abnormalities of the penis, especially Peyronie's disease, which is usually easily felt as a fibrotic plaque on the dorsum of the penis. The testes should be palpated for size, symmetry, and abnormal masses; if the length is less than 3.5 cm, hypogonadism should be considered. Evidence of feminization such as gynecomastia and abnormal body hair distribution should be sought. All pulses should be palpated, and the presence of bruits should be sought. Often, the pulse in the dorsal penile artery can be felt. If there is an indication from either history or physical examination of a vascular cause, penile blood flow can be measured directly.

Pudendal arteriography provides the most accurate assessment of penile arterial disease, but it is expensive and invasive. Moreover, distal arterial lesions may not be identified unless the procedure is performed under conditions of chemical erection (e.g., papaverine injection). The penile/brachial index can be used to estimate penile blood flow by dividing the penile systolic blood pressure, as determined by Doppler technique, by the simultaneously determined supine brachial systolic pressure. An index of less than 0.6 is suggestive of vasculogenic impotence. However, the test evaluates flow only through the dorsal penile artery, which is not directly involved in the erectile process. Significant disease may be present in the cavernosa arteries despite normal flow through the dorsal artery. Pulsed Doppler analysis and high-resolution ultrasonography can be used in conjunction with intracorporeal papaverine to assess blood flow in the cavernosa arteries. Alternatively, dynamic infusion cavernosography, which measures pressure directly within the corpora, can be utilized to assess arterial inflow. Abnormalities in the venous occlusive mechanism of the penis can cause impotence due to venous leak and can be diagnosed with the use of dynamic infusion cavernosometry to demonstrate a rapid fall in corporal pressures, followed by cavernosography to document the anatomic site of leak. The incidence of venous leakage in men with normal erectile function is unknown. Moreover, venous leak is most commonly secondary to arterial inflow and sinusoidal disease. The failure rate of surgical or embolization procedures designed to obliterate the incompetent vein is high, suggesting that most patients have additional pathology.

The neurologic examination should measure anal sphincter tone, perineal sensation, and the bulbocavernosus reflex. This reflex is elicited by squeezing the glans penis and noting the degree of anal sphincter constriction. An examination for peripheral neuropathy, including assessment of distal muscle function, the tendon reflexes in the legs, and vibratory, position, tactile, and pain sensation also should be performed. In the presence of peripheral neuropathy, tests to evaluate penile neuropathy are seldom necessary. In cases with an uncertain neurogenic component, electromyographic sacral signal tracing of the bulbocavernosus reflex or direct electrical recording of the corpora cavernosa by needle or surface electrodes may be helpful. A specific test to document abnormalities in the penile autonomic efferent pathways is not available.

In the absence of hypogonadism or feminization, the serum testosterone level is usually normal. Hyperprolactinemia, however, may not be suspected on the basis of history and physical examination. Although the endocrine causes of erectile dysfunction are uncommon, serum prolactin and pooled serum testosterone and luteinizing hormone (see Chap. 339) should be measured, since abnormalities of these parameters are treatable.

TREATMENT OF IMPOTENCE Medical therapy with androgens offers little more than placebo benefit except in hypogonadal men, and empirical therapy may actually delay identification of organic causes. If a prolactin-secreting pituitary tumor is present, however, either surgical removal or treatment with bromocriptine usually results in return of potency. Yohimbine, an alpha$_2$-adrenergic antagonist, is widely prescribed but works only in psychogenic impotence by placebo effect. Surgical therapy may be useful in the treatment of decreased potency related to aortic obstruction; however, potency can be lost rather than improved after aortic surgery if the autonomic nerve supply to the penis is damaged. Penile revascularization is effective only in young men with traumatic arterial disease. Few men with venous leak impotency benefit from venous ligation.

A variety of vasoactive substances produce erection when injected into the corpora cavernosa. Self-injection with prostaglandin E and papaverine (with or without phentolamine) produces erection in patients with psychogenic, neurogenic, and mild vasculogenic impotency. Despite lack of FDA approval, occasional pain on injection, and the rare complications of priapism and penile fibrosis, use of this therapy is fairly widespread. Commercially available mechanical devices that utilize a vacuum to produce an erection and a rubber band to restrict venous return at the base of the penis provide a successful nonsurgical alternative in many patients, including some with diabetes mellitus.

Penile prostheses should only be implanted in impotent men refractory to other forms of therapy. Malleable Silastic rods inserted into the penis provide the simplest system and the lowest complication rates; however, the cosmetic and functional performance of the device is not uniformly satisfactory. Multicomponent, hydraulically operated prostheses offer the advantage of more physiologic erection and greater increase in penile diameter. However, these devices are subject to mechanical failure.

Even in patients with organic impotence, psychotherapy is often beneficial in alleviating concomitant psychogenic factors that limit the success of medical and surgical therapy.

REFERENCES

ABRAMOWICZ M et al: Drugs that cause sexual dysfunction. Med Lett 29:65, 1987

DEGROAT WC, STEERS WD: Neuroanatomy and neurophysiology of penile erection, in *Contemporary Management of Impotence and Infertility,* EA Tanagho et al (eds). Baltimore, Williams & Wilkins, 1988, pp 3–27

FISHMAN JF et al: Experience with inflatable penile prosthesis. Urology 23:86, 1984

GOLDSTEIN I: Overview of types and results of vascular procedures for impotence. Cardiovasc Intervert Radiol 11:240, 1988

———, KRANE RJ: Diagnosis and therapy of erectile dysfunction, in *Campbell's Urology,* PC Walsh et al (eds). Philadelphia, Saunders, 1992, pp 3033–3070

——— et al: Radiation-associated impotence: A clinical study of its mechanism. JAMA 251:903, 1984

KAISER FE, KORENMAN SG: Impotence in diabetic men. Am J Med 85(suppl 5A):147, 1988

KIM N et al: A nitric oxide–like factor mediates nonadrenergic-noncholinergic neurogenic relaxation of penile corpus cavernosum smooth muscle. J Clin Invest 88:112, 1991

KNISPEL HH: Penile venous surgery in impotence: Results in highly selected cases. Urol Int 47:144, 1991

KOLODNY RC et al: Sexual function in diabetic men. Diabetes 23:306, 1974

KORENMAN SG: Sexual dysfunction, in *Williams' Textbook of Endocrinology,* 7th ed, JD Wilson, DW Foster (eds). Philadelphia, Saunders, 1992, pp 1033–1048

KRANE RJ: Medical progress: Impotence. N Engl J Med 321:1648, 1989

KWAN M et al: The nature of androgen action on male sexuality: A combined laboratory–self-report study on hypogonadal men. J Clin Endocrinol Metab 57:557, 1983

LEE LM et al: Prostaglandin E, versus phentolamine/papaverine for the treatment of erectile impotence: A double-blind comparison. J Urol 141:549, 1989

LEVINE SB: Marital sexual dysfunction: Ejaculation disturbances. Ann Intern Med 84:575, 1976

LUE TF et al: Functional evaluation of penile veins by cavernosography in papaverine-induced erection. J Urol 135:479, 1986

——— et al: Vasculogenic impotence evaluated by high-resolution ultrasonography and pulsed Doppler spectrum analysis. Radiology 155:777, 1985

MEYER J: Disorders of sexual function, in *Textbook of Endocrinology,* vol 7, JD Wilson, DM Foster (eds). Philadelphia, Saunders, 1985, pp 476–491

MONTAGUE DK et al: Infusion pharmacocavernosometry and normal penile tumescence findings in men with erectile dysfunction. J Urol 145:768, 1991

RAJFER J: Nitric oxide as a mediator of relaxation in response to nonadrenergic, noncholinergic neurotransmission. N Engl J Med 326:90, 1992

SAENZ DE TEJADA I et al: Cholinergic neurotransmission in human corpus cavernosum: I. Responses of isolated tissue. Am J Physiol 254:H459, 1988

SAYPOL DC et al: Impotence: Are the newer diagnostic methods a necessity? J Urol 130:260, 1983

VIRAG R et al: Intracavernous self-injection of vasoactive drugs in the treatment of impotence: 8-year experience with 615 cases. J Urol 145:287, 1991

WABEK AJ: Bulbocavernosus reflex testing in 100 consecutive cases of erectile dysfunction. Urology 25:495, 1985

WALSH PC et al: Impotence following radical prostatectomy: Insight into etiology and prevention. J Urol 128:492, 1982

WINTER CC: Priapism. Urol Surv 28:163, 1978

WITHERINGTON R: Vacuum constriction device for management of erectile impotence. J Urol 141:320, 1989

ZORGNIOTTI AW: Autoinjection of the corpus cavernosum with a vasoactive drug combination for vasculogenic impotence. J Urol 133:39, 1985

48 DISTURBANCES OF MENSTRUATION AND SEXUAL FUNCTION IN WOMEN

BRUCE R. CARR / JEAN D. WILSON

Complaints related to the female reproductive tract can be categorized as disorders of menstruation, pelvic pain, disturbances in sexual function, or infertility. However, a single disorder, e.g., leiomyoma of the uterus, can present with symptoms referable to any one or more of these categories. Furthermore, sexual dysfunction can interdigitate with other complaints in several ways. On the one hand, in women with complaints related to other reproductive tract functions, the underlying problem may actually be severe sexual dysfunction or marital conflict. Alternatively, women with severe organic disorders of the pelvis, e.g., pelvic inflammatory disease, may present with sexual dysfunction such as dyspareunia which in fact is only a minor manifestation of the underlying disease.

Since normal reproductive function depends on the integrated action of the central nervous system, the endocrine glands, and the reproductive organs, menstrual cycle abnormalities, sexual dysfunction, and infertility may be the result of systemic and psychological disorders as well as of primary defects in the endocrine and reproductive organs. The endocrine and physiologic control—normal and abnormal—of puberty, reproductive life, and menopause are discussed in Chap. 340. The focus of this chapter is on the initial evaluation of women with disturbances of the reproductive tract.

DISTURBANCES IN MENSTRUATION   Disorders of menstruation can be divided into abnormal uterine bleeding and amenorrhea.

Abnormal uterine bleeding   The menstrual cycle is defined as the interval between the onset of one bleeding episode and the onset of the next. In normal women the cycle averages 28 ± 3 days, the mean duration of menstrual flow is 4 ± 2 days, and the average blood loss is 40 to 100 mL. Between menarche and menopause most women experience one or more episodes of abnormal uterine bleeding, here defined as any bleeding pattern outside the normal ranges of frequency, duration, and/or amount of blood loss. The decision to evaluate a patient with an abnormal bleeding pattern depends on the severity and frequency of the abnormal episodes.

When uterine bleeding is suspected, it is essential to establish first that the blood observed by the patient is derived from the uterine endometrium. Rectal, bladder, cervical, and vaginal sources of bleeding must be excluded. Once the bleeding is documented to be uterine in origin, a pregnancy-related disorder (such as threatened or incomplete abortion or ectopic pregnancy) must be excluded by physical examination and appropriate laboratory tests. Abnormal uterine bleeding also may be the initial or principal manifestation of a generalized bleeding diathesis. The remaining causes of abnormal uterine bleeding can be divided into those associated with ovulatory cycles and those associated with anovulatory cycles.

OVULATORY CYCLES   Menstrual bleeding with ovulatory cycles is spontaneous, regular in onset, predictable in duration and amount of flow, and frequently associated with discomfort. Uterine bleeding with ovulatory cycles is due to progesterone withdrawal at the end of the luteal (postovulatory) phase and requires prior estrogen priming of the endometrium during the follicular (preovulatory) phase of the cycle. When deviations from an established pattern of menstrual flow occur but the cycles are still regular, the usual cause is organic disease of the outflow tract. For example, regular, prolonged, excessive bleeding episodes unassociated with a bleeding diathesis can result from abnormalities of the uterus such as submucous leiomyomas, adenomyosis, or endometrial polyps. On the other hand, cyclic, predictable menstruation characterized by spotting or light bleeding suggests obstruction of the outflow tract as with uterine synechiae or scarring of the cervix. Intermittent bleeding between cyclic ovulatory menses is often due to cervical or endometrial lesions.

ANOVULATORY CYCLES   Uterine bleeding that is irregular in occurrence, unpredictable as to amount and duration of flow, and usually painless is called *dysfunctional uterine bleeding*. This type of bleeding is the result of a failure of normal follicular maturation with consequent anovulation and may be either transient or chronic. Transient disruption of the synchronous hypothalamic-pituitary-ovarian hormonal control necessary for ovulatory cycles occurs most often in the early menarcheal years, during the perimenopausal period, or as the consequence of a variety of stresses and intercurrent illnesses. Persistent dysfunctional uterine bleeding during the reproductive years can occur in several organic diseases that affect ovarian function and is most often due to estrogen breakthrough bleeding. Estrogen breakthrough bleeding occurs when prolonged continuous estrogen stimulation of the endometrium is not interrupted by cyclic progesterone withdrawal. For example, chronic acyclic estrogen production not associated with ovulation can occur in polycystic ovarian disease.

Amenorrhea   *Amenorrhea* is defined as failure of menarche by age 16, regardless of the presence or absence of secondary sexual characteristics, or the absence of menstruation for 6 months in a woman with previous periodic menses. Amenorrhea in a woman who has never menstruated is termed *primary*; cessation of menses is termed *secondary amenorrhea*. Because some disorders can cause both primary and secondary amenorrhea, we prefer a functional classification based on the nature of the underlying defect, namely, anatomic defects of the outflow tract (uterus, cervix, or vagina), ovarian failure, and chronic anovulation.

Anatomic defects of the outflow tract include congenital defects of the vagina, imperforate hymen, transverse vaginal septa, cervical stenosis, intrauterine adhesions (synechiae), absence of the vagina or uterus, and uterine maldevelopment. The diagnosis of an anatomic defect is usually made by physical examination and confirmed by demonstrating failure of bleeding following administration of estrogen plus a progestogen for 21 days. Pelvic ultrasonography, magnetic resonance imaging, hysterosalpingogram or hysteroscopy may be helpful in defining the defect.

Causes of *ovarian failure* include gonadal dysgenesis, deficiency of $P450_{17\alpha}$, resistant ovary syndrome, and premature ovarian failure. Ovarian failure encompasses disorders in which the ovary is deficient in germ cells and those in which the germ cells are resistant to FSH (follicle-stimulating hormone). The diagnosis of ovarian failure as the cause of amenorrhea is confirmed by a plasma FSH greater than 40 IU/L.

Women with *chronic anovulation* fail to ovulate spontaneously but have the capability of ovulating with appropriate therapy. In some women with chronic anovulation, estrogen production is adequate, but estrogen is not secreted in a cyclic fashion. In others, estrogen production is deficient.

Women who have adequate estrogen production and demonstrate withdrawal bleeding after progestogen challenge usually have polycystic ovarian disease (see Fig. 340-7). Other causes include hormone-secreting ovarian and adrenal tumors. Women with deficient or absent estrogen production, and therefore with absence of withdrawal bleeding after progestogen administration, usually have hypogonadotropic hypogonadism due to organic or functional disorders of the pituitary or central nervous system such as brain tumors, pituitary tumors (especially prolactin-secreting adenomas), primary hypopituitarism, or Sheehan's syndrome.

PELVIC PAIN   Pelvic pain may originate in the pelvis or be referred from another region of the body. A pelvic source is suggested by the history (e.g., dysmenorrhea and dyspareunia) and physical findings, but a high index of suspicion must be entertained for extrapelvic disorders that refer to the pelvis, such as appendicitis, cholecystitis, intestinal obstruction, and urinary tract infections (see Chap. 13).

"Physiologic" pelvic pain   PAIN ASSOCIATED WITH OVULATION ("MITTELSCHMERZ")   Many women experience low abdominal discomfort with ovulation, typically a dull aching pain at midcycle in one lower quadrant lasting from minutes to hours. It is rarely severe or incapacitating. The relationship of the pain to the process of ovulation is unknown. It may result from peritoneal irritation by follicular fluid released into the peritoneal cavity at ovulation. The onset at midcycle and short duration of pain are often diagnostic.

PREMENSTRUAL OR MENSTRUAL PAIN   In normal ovulatory women, somatic symptoms during the few days prior to menses may be insignificant or disabling. Such symptoms include edema, breast engorgement, and abdominal bloating or discomfort. A symptom complex of cyclic irritability, depression, and lethargy is known as the *premenstrual syndrome* (PMS). The cause of PMS is unknown, and there is no consensus about therapy.

Severe or incapacitating uterine cramping in women with ovulatory menses but no demonstrable disorders of the pelvis is termed *primary dysmenorrhea*. Primary dysmenorrhea is caused by prostaglandin-induced uterine ischemia and is treated with prostaglandin synthetase inhibitors or oral contraceptive agents.

Pelvic pain due to organic causes   Severe dysmenorrhea associated with disease of the pelvis is termed *secondary dysmenorrhea*. Organic causes of pelvic pain can be classified as (1) uterine, (2) adnexal, (3) vulvar or vaginal, and (4) pregnancy-associated.

UTERINE PAIN   Pain of uterine etiology is often chronic and continuous and increases in intensity during menstruation and intercourse. Causes include leiomyomas of the uterus (particularly submucous and degenerating leiomyomas), adenomyosis, and cervical stenosis. Infections of the uterus associated with intrauterine manipulation following dilatation and curettage or with intrauterine devices also can cause significant pelvic pain (see Chap. 340). Pelvic pain due to endometrial or cervical cancer is usually a late manifestation of disseminated disease (see Chap. 340).

ADNEXAL PAIN   The most common cause of pain in the adnexae (fallopian tubes and ovaries) is infection (see Chap. 89). Acute salpingo-oophoritis presents as low abdominal pain, fever, and chills; begins a few days after a menstrual period; and is usually due to chlamydia or gonococcal disease with or without a superimposed pyogenic infection. Chronic pelvic inflammatory disease results from either a single episode or multiple episodes of infection and may present as infertility associated with chronic pelvic pain that increases in intensity with menses and intercourse. On physical examination, the adnexae are tender, and adnexal thickening with or without masses may be present. Pelvic inflammatory disease may become a surgical emergency if peritonitis results from rupture of a tuboovarian abscess. Ovarian cysts or neoplasms may cause pelvic pain that becomes more severe with torsion or rupture of the mass, and ectopic pregnancy must be considered in the differential diagnosis (see below). Endometriosis involving fallopian tubes, ovaries, or peritoneum may cause both chronic low abdominal pain and infertility; the magnitude of tissue involvement does not always correlate with the severity of symptoms. Endometriosis pain typically increases with menstruation and, if the posterior ligaments of the uterus are involved, with intercourse.

VULVAR OR VAGINAL PAIN   Pain in these areas is most often due to infectious vaginitis caused by organisms such as *Monilia, Trichomonas*, or *Gardnerella* and is characteristically associated with vaginal discharge and pruritus. Herpetic vulvitis, condyloma acuminatum, and cysts or abscesses of Bartholin's glands also may cause vulvar pain.

PREGNANCY-ASSOCIATED DISORDERS   Pregnancy must be considered in the differential diagnosis of pelvic pain during the reproductive years. Threatened abortion or incomplete abortion often presents with uterine cramping, bleeding, or passage of tissue following a period of amenorrhea. Ectopic pregnancy may be insidious in presentation and result in severe intraperitoneal hemorrhage and maternal death.

Evaluation of pelvic pain   The evaluation of pelvic pain requires a careful history and pelvic examination. This often leads to the correct diagnosis and institution of appropriate treatment. If the pain is severe and the diagnosis is unclear, the workup should follow that outlined for the acute abdomen (Chap. 13). A culdocentesis is indicated if a ruptured ectopic pregnancy is suspected. If there is a question of an adnexal mass or if the patient is so obese as to preclude a thorough pelvic examination, sonography may be useful. Serial human chorionic gonadotropin (hCG) measurements may help in establishing a diagnosis of tubal pregnancy. Finally, diagnostic laparoscopy and laparotomy may be indicated with pain of undetermined etiology.

SEXUAL DYSFUNCTION   Some women with sexual dysfunction describe minor complaints related to the reproductive tract as a means of bringing sexual problems to the attention of the physician. Alternatively, sexual dysfunction may be thought to be the cause of low abdominal discomfort or dyspareunia when the actual etiology is organic. However, more and more women seek medical advice because of sexual problems that interface in provenance between medicine and sociology.

The normal sexual response begins with sexual arousal which causes genital vasocongestion that results in vaginal lubrication in preparation for intromission. The lubrication is due to the formation of a transudate in the vagina and in conjunction with genital congestion produces the so-called orgasmic platform prior to orgasm. Sexual stimuli (visual, tactile, auditory, and olfactory) as well as healthy vaginal tissue are prerequisites for genital vasocongestion and vaginal lubrication. During the second stage of the sexual response, involuntary contractions of the muscles of the pelvis result in a pleasurable cortical sensory phenomenon known as orgasm. Direct or indirect stimulation of the clitoris is important in the production of the female orgasm. In simple terms, sexual dysfunction can be due to interference with the arousal or orgasmic phases of the sexual response. Either disorder can be due to an organic or functional cause or both.

Illnesses that impair neurologic function such as diabetes mellitus or multiple sclerosis can prevent normal sexual arousal. Local pelvic diseases such as vaginitis, endometriosis, and salpingo-oophoritis may preclude normal sexual response because of resulting dyspareunia. Debilitating systemic diseases such as cancer and cardiovascular diseases may impair normal sexual response indirectly.

More commonly, failure of a normal sexual response is due to psychological factors that impair sexual arousal. Such problems include misinformation, e.g., the perception of sexual satisfaction as bad, or feelings of guilt about previous psychologically traumatic events such as incest, rape, or unwanted pregnancy. In addition, women who have had previous hysterectomy or mastectomy may perceive themselves as "incomplete." Stresses such as anxiety, depression, fatigue, and marital or interpersonal conflicts may lead to failure of the vasocongestive response and prevent normal vaginal lubrication. Women with such experiences may be unable to achieve normal sexual response unless they receive professional counseling by a family physician, psychiatrist, or sex therapist. Such problems are approached by attempting to identify and reduce the causative stresses.

Failure to achieve orgasm is a specific form of sexual dysfunction. In the absence of orgasm many women enjoy sexual encounters to variable degrees because of the pleasure derived from closeness in a cherished relationship, particularly with a loving partner. However, for other women sexual relations with rare or absent orgasms are frustrating and unsatisfying. In many instances, failure of orgasm is due to insufficient clitoral stimulation and may be rectified by appropriate counseling and patient education.

A specific entity, "vaginismus," painful, involuntary contractions of the musculature surrounding the entrance to the vagina, is a rare cause of dyspareunia. It is a conditioned response to a previous real or imagined frightening or traumatic sexual experience. Treatment is directed to elimination of the conditioned response by progressive vaginal dilation by the patient in conjunction with marital therapy.

REPRODUCTION   Problems of infertility are discussed in detail in Chap. 340. The approach to infertile couples always involves evaluation of both the man and woman. The history should elicit information as to the frequency of intercourse, the sexual responses of both, the use of contraceptives or lubricants, previous or past medical illnesses, and all medications taken.

Male-associated factors account for a third of infertility problems. Therefore, one of the first procedures in the workup of infertile couples should be a semen analysis (see Chap. 339). The initial evaluation of the woman includes documentation of normal ovulatory cycles. A history of regular, cyclic, predictable, spontaneous menses usually indicates ovulatory cycles, which may be confirmed by basal body temperature graphs, properly timed endometrial biopsies, or plasma progesterone measurements during the luteal phase of the cycle. Also, the diagnosis of luteal-phase dysfunction (low progesterone secretion during the luteal phase) can be established by these methods. If the woman is anovulatory, attempts to induce ovulation can be undertaken by a variety of methods including clomiphene, human menopausal gonadotropins, bromocriptine, luteinizing hormone–releasing hormone (LHRH) agonists, or wedge resection of the ovaries (Chap. 340).

The most common cause of infertility in women is tubal disease, usually due to infection (pelvic inflammatory disease) or endometriosis. Tubal disease can be evaluated by obtaining a hysterosalpingogram or by diagnostic laparoscopy. The treatment of tubal causes of infertility is primarily surgical.

A cervical factor as a cause of infertility is identified by a properly timed postcoital examination. During this examination, the sperm motility in cervical mucus is observed. Also, immunologic etiologies for infertility can be tested for by a variety of laboratory tests. The cause of infertility is unknown in 10 percent of couples. In many instances of infertility, it is now possible to use assisted reproductive technologies including in vitro fertilization and embryo transfer, gamete intrafallopian tube transfer, transfer of cryopreserved ova and embryos, and intrauterine insemination.

The desire for contraception is also a frequent cause for women to seek medical treatment or evaluation. The most widely used methods for fertility control include (1) rhythm and withdrawal techniques, (2) barrier methods, (3) intrauterine devices, (4) oral steroid contraceptives, (5) sterilization, and (6) abortion. These methods and their complications are discussed in Chap. 340.

REFERENCES

CUNNINGHAM FG et al: *Williams Obstetrics*, 18th ed. Norwalk, Appleton-Century-Crofts, 1989
HERBST AL et al: *Comprehensive Gynecology*, 2d ed. St. Louis, Mosby, 1992
FORDNEY DS: Dyspareunia and vaginismus. Clin Obstet Gynecol 21:205, 1978
HAMMOND DC: Screening for sexual dysfunction. Clin Obstet Gynecol 27:732, 1984
HATCHER RA et al: *Contraceptive Technology 1990–1992*. New York, Irvington, 1986
MASTERS W, JOHNSON V: *Human Sexual Response*. Boston, Little, Brown, 1966
——, ——: *Human Sexual Inadequacy*. Boston, Little, Brown, 1970
SPEROFF L et al: *Clinical Gynecologic Endocrinology and Infertility*, 4th ed. Baltimore, Williams & Wilkins, 1989

49   HIRSUTISM AND VIRILIZATION

WILLIAM J. KOVACS / JEAN D. WILSON

Hirsutism, male pattern hair growth in women, is a common and perplexing problem. The distribution and growth of hair in normal persons is under complex genetic and endocrine control so that there is considerable variability in hair growth among normal men and women. As a consequence, abnormal hair growth is difficult to define: Some patients may seek medical attention because of what the physician may consider an insignificant cosmetic defect. Others, because of personal or cultural differences, may be undisturbed by surprising degrees of hirsutism. The central issue in dealing with such patients is the separation of those infrequent instances in which hirsutism is a manifestation of a serious and remediable underlying disorder from the majority of hirsute women in whom excess hair is fundamentally a cosmetic problem.

CONTROL OF NORMAL HAIR GROWTH AND DISTRIBUTION
Endocrine control   Androgens are the major determinants of hair distribution in both sexes. There are three principal circulating androgens in women—dehydroepiandrosterone, derived from the adrenal; androstenedione, which is derived equally from adrenal and ovary; and testosterone, which is both secreted by the ovary and adrenal and formed in extraglandular tissue from circulating dehydroepiandrosterone and androstenedione. The production of adrenal androgen is regulated primarily by adrenocorticotropin while ovarian androgen secretion is regulated by luteinizing hormone (LH). These various androgens must be converted to testosterone (or dihydrotestos-

terone) before they can bind to the androgen receptor of target cells and induce an androgenic response. Thus, adrenal androgens virilize only in so far as they serve as precursors for testosterone and dihydrotestosterone.

Several types of relationships can be defined between hair growth and androgens in normal individuals. The growth of eyebrows, eyelashes, and vellus hair is not dependent on androgens, while axillary and lower pubic hair are sensitive to the small amounts of androgen secreted by the adrenal. Hair in these regions therefore grows to an approximately equal extent in men and women. Hair growth in some areas is more typical of males and appears to require the greater androgen levels normally produced by the testes; such areas include the face, upper pubic triangle, chest, and ears. Finally, scalp hair exhibits androgen-mediated regression. The reason different body regions respond differently to the same or similar androgen is unknown. Theoretically, the metabolism of androgens might differ in the various sites. The hair follicle, like some other androgen targets, requires conversion of testosterone to dihydrotestosterone for expression of androgen action, and hair follicles from all regions of the body perform this conversion. Moreover, the same receptor that is essential for androgen action in other cells (Chap. 339) mediates the effects of dihydrotestosterone in the hair follicle. Genetic disorders with normal testosterone production but absent androgen receptor have deficient or absent axillary, pubic, facial, truncal, and limb hair (Chap. 342). Regional differences in androgen responsiveness of hair in normal individuals may be the consequence of regional differences in the amount of androgen receptor in hair follicles.

Genetic factors   Despite similar hormone levels, the distribution of hair varies among individuals and among different racial groups. Dark-haired, darkly pigmented whites of either sex tend to be more hirsute than blond or fair-skinned persons. Orientals, American Indians, and blacks on average are less hirsute than whites. Orientals have scant facial and body hair except in the pubic and axillary regions, and American Indians, in addition, rarely develop baldness. Heterogeneity of hair patterns also exists within families. The inheritance of hair patterns is complex and probably polygenic in nature.

Other factors   Aging is a prerequisite for some types of hair development. For example, in men hair on the trunk and extremities frequently increases for several years after maximal levels of plasma androgens have been reached. Conversely, loss of androgen may not result in diminution of normal hair growth in men or complete reversal of hirsutism in women. The appearance of pubic hair is frequently the heralding event of puberty in females. Women in the first trimester of pregnancy commonly have increased hairiness of the face, extremities, and breasts. Menopause is often associated with the loss of hair in the pubic area, axillae, and extremities, whereas growth of hair on the face increases in postmenopausal women. These changes cannot be explained solely by changes in androgen levels.

PATHOLOGIC HAIR GROWTH AND DISTRIBUTION   A central consideration in the evaluation of women with hirsutism is whether evidence of virilization or defeminization is also present (Table 49-1) since such signs suggest androgen excess. In patients with overproduction of androgen, defeminizing signs, such as disturbances of menstruation, are more frequent than virilization. However, the

TABLE 49-1   Clinical signs of defeminization and virilization

Signs of defeminization	Signs of virilization
Amenorrhea	Frontal balding
Decrease in breast size	Increase in size of shoulder girdle
Loss of female body contours	muscles
	Clitoromegaly
	Coarsening of the voice
	Acne

After Karp L, Herrmann WL: Diagnosis and treatment of hirsutism in women. Obstet Gynecol 41:283, 1973.

presence or absence of overt virilization should be interpreted with caution for at least two reasons. First, signs of virilization (clitoromegaly, balding, coarsening of the hair, hirsutism) indicate androgen excess at some time in the patient's life but do not necessarily mean that active disease is present at the time of evaluation. It is necessary to measure plasma androgen levels and/or production rates to determine if androgen excess is ongoing. Second, severe overandrogenization may exist in the absence of marked virilization; i.e., at the same level of androgen production clitoromegaly may be present in one patient and not another.

Diagnostic considerations   DRUGS   Excessive hair growth can be caused by drugs that exert their effects independent of androgens and do not produce defeminization or virilization. Such drugs include phenytoin, minoxidil, diazoxide, cyclosporin, and hexachlorobenzene. Androgens produce hirsutism as well as virilization. Some synthetic progestogens have androgenic activity.

TUMORS   The rapid onset of hair growth with or without accompanying signs of frank virilization suggests a neoplastic source of androgen. Such tumors include adenomas and carcinomas of the adrenal and ovarian tumors such as arrhenoblastoma, which secrete androgens directly, and Krukenberg tumors of the ovary, which stimulate the surrounding ovarian stromal tissue to produce excess androgen.

POLYCYSTIC OVARIAN DISEASE   The most common cause of ovarian hyperandrogenism is polycystic ovarian disease. This disorder has a broad spectrum of manifestations that range from mild hirsutism to amenorrhea and virilization. The salient feature for the diagnosis is the pubertal onset of chronic anovulation and hirsutism; enlarged cystic ovaries, obesity, and amenorrhea (i.e., the Stein-Leventhal syndrome) are present in only half or fewer of women with this disorder and need not be present for the diagnosis (see Chap. 340). The fundamental abnormality in polycystic ovarian disease is not fully understood. Elevation of plasma LH causes enhanced androgen secretion by stromal and thecal cells of the ovary.

ATTENUATED FORMS OF ADRENAL HYPERPLASIA   The adrenal can be the source of excess androgen in the absence of tumor. Heritable defects in adrenal steroidogenesis (congenital adrenal hyperplasia) such as deficiencies of 21-hydroxylase ($P450_{C21}$), 11β-hydroxylase ($P450_{C11B}$), and 3β-hydroxysteroid dehydrogenase isomerase (3β-HSD) can produce virilization, and each can occur in a "late-onset" form in which hirsutism or virilization and menstrual irregularities appear at the time of expected puberty or in adulthood (see Chap. 342). The clinical presentation in these cases is usually indistinguishable from polycystic ovarian disease. Late-onset 21-hydroxylase deficiency is the most common of these attenuation forms of congenital adrenal hyperplasia and has been most extensively studied; its incidence in the general population of hirsute, oligomenorrheic women is probably on the order of one percent. The presence of elevated plasma levels of adrenal androgens (such as dehydroepiandrosterone sulfate) or of dexamethasone-suppressible hyperandrogenism does not necessarily imply that the overandrogenization is due to a specific adrenal steroidogenic defect, but these findings may be useful as a guide to therapy.

IDIOPATHIC HIRSUTISM   In many women with hirsutism a specific diagnosis cannot be made. The term *idiopathic hirsutism* applies to those women with evidence of androgen excess but with normal menses, normal-sized ovaries, no evidence of tumors of the adrenal or ovary, and normal adrenal function. Slight elevations of plasma androstenedione and testosterone are common in such women, and testosterone production rates are increased, although to a lesser degree than in patients with polycystic ovarian disease.

Experience outside the United States with the antiandrogen cyproterone acetate indicates that this form of hirsutism is androgen-mediated, since therapy results in improvement. Women with idiopathic hirsutism could constitute the extreme end of a normal continuum of androgen production or represent a true pathologic subset. Some women with the tentative diagnosis of idiopathic hirsutism actually have mild or early polycystic ovarian disease, but in most, hirsutism is not accompanied by or followed by signs of ovarian dysfunction. If such women are merely extremes of the normal range of androgen production, then their hirsutism is fundamentally a cosmetic defect.

DIAGNOSTIC EVALUATION   The decision as to when to undertake a complex diagnostic evaluation depends on several factors. Such evaluation is appropriate in all women with hirsutism accompanied by virilization; whether it should be performed in women with isolated hirsutism depends upon the severity, distribution, and rate of hair growth. An approach to the diagnostic evaluation of hirsute patients is shown in Fig. 49-1. The clinical history is taken with particular attention to drug ingestion and to the details of pubertal development and menstrual history and their relation to the onset of excessive hair growth. The physical examination is directed to the assessment of

FIGURE 49-1   Diagnostic approach to the hirsute patient. T = testosterone; DHEA-S = dehydroepiandrosterone sulfate.

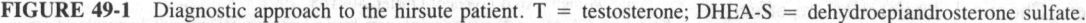
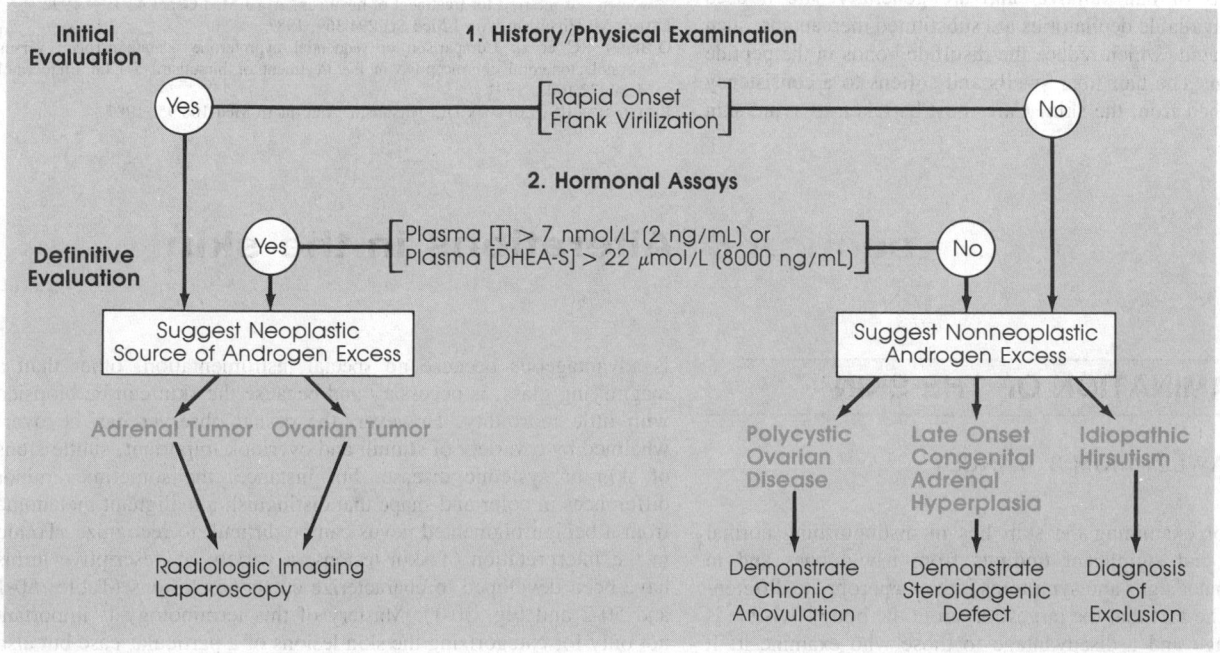

sites of growth of androgen-dependent hair (pubic, axillary, facial, truncal, and extremity) and evaluation for signs of virilization, which correlate with higher levels of androgen overproduction and raise the concern of androgen-producing neoplasms. Such signs include laryngeal enlargement (deepening of the voice), temporal balding, clitoromegaly, and increased muscle mass in the limb girdles. Signs of cortisol excess (plethora, centripetal obesity, striae, and dorsocervical and supraclavicular fat pads) should also be sought. Pelvic examination should include a search for palpable ovarian masses. Appropriate laboratory tests include measurement of serum androgens and, when appropriate, radiologic imaging of ovaries and adrenal glands. Basal measurements of dehydroepiandrosterone sulfate greater than 22 μmol/L (8000 ng/mL) or of serum testosterone over 7 nmol/L (2 ng/mL) suggest neoplastic sources of androgen excess; plasma testosterone levels in the normal range are more difficult to interpret because total levels in women do not necessarily reflect the free or unbound levels of hormone under conditions when testosterone-binding globulin levels are either increased or decreased. Suspected Cushing's syndrome should be evaluated with standard dexamethasone suppression testing if a screening test (such as urinary free cortisol excretion or overnight dexamethasone suppression test) is abnormal. The diagnosis of polycystic ovarian disease is made from the history and clinical features in a woman with chronic anovulation. Women may be screened for delayed-onset adrenal hyperplasia by the short ACTH stimulation test and measurement of plasma 17-hydroxy-progesterone (see Chap. 335).

MANAGEMENT In the case of drug-induced hirsutism and neoplastic disease of the ovary or adrenals treatment is straightforward; administration of the drugs should be stopped, or the tumor should be removed. Adrenal steroidogenic defects are treated with glucocorticoids to suppress excess ACTH and inhibit adrenal androgen secretion. In most instances (polycystic ovarian disease as well as idiopathic hirsutism) both cosmetic treatment and suppression of androgen production or antagonism of its action at the receptor level need to be employed.

Cosmetic therapy is directed at the concealment or removal of hair from exposed skin areas. Small amounts of hair can be bleached with hydrogen peroxide. Methods for removal of hair are classified as depilatory (removal of hair from the surface of the skin) or epilatory (removal of the intact hair with the root). Depilatory techniques include shaving and chemical methods. Shaving does not have an adverse effect on hair growth rate or coarseness (although the blunt ends may feel coarse), but shaving of areas other than axillae or legs is unacceptable to most women. Chemical depilatories are effective for limited areas of hair removal and are generally safe if used properly. Most available depilatories are substituted mercaptans, such as thioglycollic acid, which reduce the disulfide bonds in the peptide chains of keratin. The hair fiber swells and softens to a consistency that can be washed from the skin. Care must be taken to avoid skin irritation because of the alkalinity of these preparations. Temporary epilation can be achieved by plucking (useful only for isolated hairs) or wax treatment. The waxes are melted and applied to the skin. When the wax cools and sets, it is stripped off, removing hair with it. The procedure is uncomfortable, and best results can be obtained by salon treatments. Permanent epilation can be achieved only by electrolysis. The treatments are expensive and time-consuming, and success depends on the skill of the electrologist.

While cosmetic treatment is undertaken, attempts to suppress androgen overproduction may also be appropriate. Treatment with combination oral contraceptives suppresses ovarian androgen secretion when restoration of fertility is not an objective. To minimize side effects the lowest effective dosage of estrogen should be used. Women over 35 years of age, smokers, and those with hypertension, a history of thromboembolic disease, impaired liver function, or suspected estrogen-dependent neoplasm should not be treated with oral contraceptives. Suppression of adrenal androgen overproduction can be achieved with small doses of dexamethasone and is most useful in the treatment of women with late-onset 21-hydroxylase deficiency.

Antagonism of the effects of androgens at the hair follicle is the basis for the other main treatment modality, the antiandrogens. Cyproterone acetate has been used with success but is unavailable in the United States. Spironolactone has a dual action of blocking the androgen receptor and of inhibiting androgen production and is a useful alternative therapy. Cimetidine also binds to the androgen receptor and acts as an androgen antagonist but is not of general benefit in the treatment of hirsutism. The androgen antagonist flutamide has shown promise in some studies.

If pharmacologic therapy is undertaken, the patient should be prepared to make a commitment of 6 months for an adequate trial of efficacy. Even when treatment is long-term, dramatic reversal of established hair growth is unlikely to be achieved by interference with androgen synthesis or action. Such hormonal manipulations can arrest or slow the rate of hair growth, but established hair must be dealt with by use of cosmetic treatment.

REFERENCES

Cusan L et al: Treatment of hirsutism with the pure antiandrogen flutamide. J Am Acad Dermatol 23:462, 1990

Ehrman DA, Rosenfield RL: An endocrinologic approach to the patient with hirutism. J Clin Endocrinol Metab 71:1, 1990

Hassiokos DK et al: Late-onset congenital adrenal hyperplasia in a group of hyperandrogenic women. Arch Gynecol Obstet 249:165, 1991

Killeen AA et al: Prevalence of nonclassical congenital adrenal hyperplasia among women self-referred for treatment of hirsutism. Am J Med Genet 42:197, 1992

Leshin M: Hirsutism. Am J Med Sci 294:369, 1987

O'Brien RC et al: Comparison of sequential cyproterone acetate/estrogen versus spironolactone/oral contraceptive in the treatment of hirsutism. J Clin Endocrinol Metab 72:1008, 1991

Rittmaster RS, Loriaux DL: Hirsutism. Ann Intern Med 106:95, 1987

section 8 Alterations in the skin

50 EXAMINATION OF THE SKIN

THOMAS J. LAWLEY / KIM B. YANCEY

The challenge of examining the skin lies in distinguishing normal from abnormal and significant findings from trivial ones and in integrating pertinent signs and symptoms into an appropriate differential diagnosis. The fact that the largest organ in the body is visible is both an advantage and a disadvantage to those who examine it. It is advantageous because no special instrumentation, other than a magnifying glass, is necessary and because the skin can be biopsied with little morbidity. However, the casual observer can be overwhelmed by a variety of stimuli and overlook important, subtle signs of skin or systemic disease. For instance, the sometimes minor differences in color and shape that distinguish a malignant melanoma from a benign pigmented nevus can be difficult to recognize. To aid in the interpretation of skin lesions, a variety of descriptive terms have been developed to characterize cutaneous lesions (Tables 50-1 and 50-2 and Fig. 50-1). Mastery of this terminology is important not only for categorizing the skin lesions of a particular case but also

TABLE 50-1   Descriptions of primary skin lesions

1 **Macule:** A flat, colored lesion, <2 cm in diameter, not raised above the surface of the surrounding skin. A "freckle," or ephelid, is a prototype pigmented macule.
2 **Patch:** A large (>2 cm), flat lesion with a color different from the surrounding skin. This differs from a macule only in size.
3 **Papule:** A small, solid lesion, <1 cm in diameter, raised above the surface of the surrounding skin and hence palpable (e.g., a closed comedone, or whitehead, in acne).
4 **Nodule:** A larger (1–5 cm), firm lesion raised above the surface of the surrounding skin. This differs from a papule only in size (e.g., dermal nevus).
5 **Tumor:** A solid, raised growth >5 cm in diameter.
6 **Plaque:** A large (>1 cm), flat-topped, raised lesion; edges may either be distinct (e.g., in psoriasis) or gradually blend with surrounding skin (e.g., in eczematous dermatitis).
7 **Vesicle:** A small, fluid-filled lesion, <1 cm in diameter, raised above the plane of surrounding skin. Fluid is often visible, and the lesions are often translucent [e.g., vesicles in allergic contact dermatitis caused by *Rhus* (poison ivy)].
8 **Pustule:** A vesicle filled with leukocytes. Note: The presence of pustules does not necessarily signify the existence of an infection.
9 **Bulla:** A fluid-filled, raised, often translucent lesion >1 cm in diameter.
10 **Cyst:** A soft, raised, encapsulated lesion filled with semisolid or liquid contents.
11 **Wheal:** A raised, erythematous papule or plaque, usually representing short-lived dermal edema.
12 **Telangiectasia:** Dilated, superficial blood vessels.

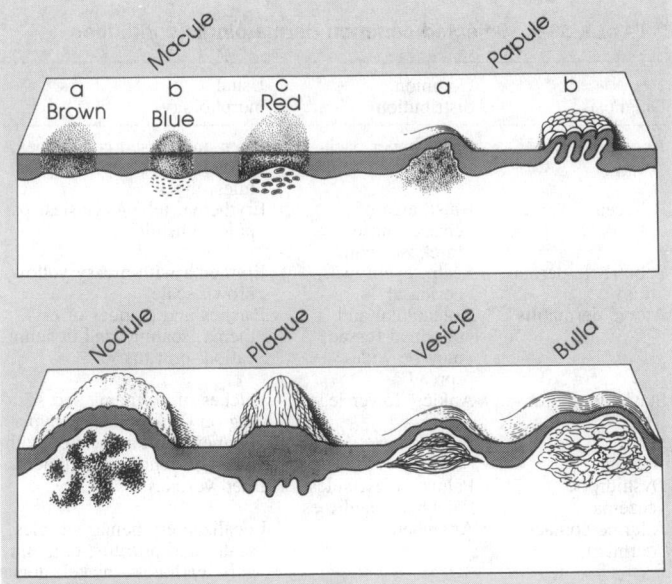

FIGURE 50-1   A schematic representation of several common primary skin lesions (see Table 50-1).

in formulating a differential diagnosis (Table 50-3). For instance, the finding of large numbers of scaling papules, usually indicative of a primary skin disease, places the patient in a different diagnostic category than would hemorrhagic papules, which may indicate vasculitis or sepsis. It is important to differentiate primary skin lesions from secondary skin changes. If the examiner focuses on linear erosions overlying an area of erythema and scaling, he or she may incorrectly assume that the erosion is the primary lesion and the redness and scale are secondary, while the correct interpretation would be that the patient has a pruritic eczematous dermatitis and the erosions have been caused by scratching.

AN APPROACH TO THE PATIENT   In examining the skin it is usually advisable to assess the patient before taking a history. This way, the entire cutaneous surface is sure to be evaluated, and objective findings can be integrated with relevant historical data. Four basic features of any cutaneous lesion must be noted and considered in the examination of skin: the distribution of the eruption, the type(s) of primary lesion, the shape of individual lesions, and the arrangement of the lesions. In the initial examination it is important that the patient be disrobed as completely as possible. This will minimize chances of missing important individual skin lesions and make it possible to assess accurately the distribution of the eruption. The patient should

first be viewed from a distance of about 1.5 to 2 m (4 to 6 ft) so that the general character of the skin and the distribution of lesions can be evaluated. Indeed, distribution of lesions often correlates highly with diagnosis (Fig. 50-2). For example, a hospitalized patient with a generalized erythematous exanthem is more likely to have a drug eruption than is a patient with a similar rash limited to the sun-exposed portions of the face. The presence or absence of lesions on mucosal surfaces also should be determined. Once the distribution of the lesions has been established, the nature of the primary lesion must be determined. Thus, when lesions are distributed on elbows, knees, and scalp, the most likely possibilities based solely on distribution are psoriasis or dermatitis herpetiformis. The primary lesion in psoriasis is a scaly papule that soon forms erythematous plaques covered with a white scale, whereas that of dermatitis herpetiformis is an urticarial papule that quickly becomes a small vesicle. In this manner, identification of the primary lesion directs the examiner toward the proper diagnosis. Secondary changes in skin also can be quite helpful. For example, scale represents excessive epidermis, while crust is the result of an inadequate or inconsistent epithelial cell layer. Palpation of skin lesions also can yield insight into the character of an eruption. Thus red papules on the lower extremities that blanch with pressure can be a manifestation of many different diseases, but hemorrhagic red papules that do not blanch with pressure indicate palpable purpura characteristic of necrotizing vasculitis.

The shape of lesions is also an important feature. Flat, round, erythematous papules and plaques are common in many cutaneous diseases. However, target-shaped lesions that consist in part of erythematous plaques are specific for erythema multiforme. In the same way, the arrangement of individual lesions is important. Erythematous papules and vesicles can occur in many conditions, but their arrangement in a specific linear array suggests an external etiology such as allergic contact or primary irritant dermatitis. In contrast, lesions with a generalized arrangement are common and suggest a systemic etiology.

As in other branches of medicine, a complete history should be obtained to emphasize the following features:

1 Evolution of lesions
   a Site of onset
   b Manner in which eruption progressed or spread
   c Duration
   d Periods of resolution or improvement in chronic eruptions

TABLE 50-2   Common dermatologic terms

1 **Lichenification:** A distinctive thickening of the skin that is characterized by accentuated skin-fold markings and that feels thick and firm on palpation.
2 **Crust:** Dried exudate of body fluids that may be either yellow (serous exudate) or red (hemorrhagic exudate).
3 **Milia:** Small, firm, white papules that are filled with keratin (and may in part resemble pustules).
4 **Erosion:** Epithelial deficit resulting in a superficial disruption of skin integrity.
5 **Ulcer:** Epithelial deficit resulting in a deep surface disruption.
6 **Excoriations:** Linear, angular erosions that may be covered by crust and are caused by scratching.
7 **Atrophy:** An acquired loss of substance. In the skin, this may appear as a depression with intact epidermis (i.e., loss of dermal or subcutaneous tissue) or as sites of shiny, delicate, wrinkled lesions (i.e., epidermal atrophy).
8 **Scar:** A change in the skin secondary to trauma or inflammation. Sites may be erythematous, hypopigmented, or hypertrophic depending on their age or character. Sites on hair-bearing areas may be characterized by destruction of hair follicles.

TABLE 50-3 Selected common dermatologic conditions

Diagnosis	Common distribution	Usual morphology	Diagnosis	Common distribution	Usual morphology
Acne vulgaris	Face, upper back	Open and closed comedones, erythematous papules, pustules, cysts	Seborrheic keratosis	Trunk, face	Brown plaques with adherent, greasy scale; "stuck on" appearance
Rosacea	Blush area of cheeks, nose, forehead, chin	Erythema, telangiectasias, papules, pustules	Folliculitis	Any hair-bearing area	Follicular pustules
Seborrheic dermatitis	Scalp, eyebrows, perinasal	Erythema with greasy yellow-brown scale	Impetigo	Anywhere	Papules, vesicles, pustules, often with honey-colored crusts
Atopic dermatitis	Antecubital and popliteal fossae; may be widespread	Patches and plaques of erythema, scaling, and lichenification; pruritus	Herpes simplex	Lips, genitalia	Grouped vesicles progressing to crusted erosions
			Herpes zoster	Dermatomal, usually trunk but may be anywhere	Vesicles limited to a dermatome (often painful)
Stasis dermatitis	Ankles, lower legs	Patches of erythema and scaling on background of hyperpigmentation associated with signs of venous insufficiency	Varicella	Face, trunk, relative sparing of extremities	Lesions arise in crops and quickly progress from erythematous macules to papules to vesicles to pustules to crusts
Dyshidrotic eczema	Palms, soles, sides of fingers and toes	Deep vesicles	Pityriasis rosea	Trunk (Christmas tree pattern) herald patch followed by multiple smaller lesions	Symmetric erythematous patches with a collarette of trailing scale
Allergic contact dermatitis	Anywhere	Localized erythema, vesicles, scale, and pruritus, e.g., fingers, earlobes—nickel; dorsal aspect of foot—shoe dermatitis; exposed surfaces—poison ivy dermatitis; etc.	Tinea versicolor	Chest, back, abdomen, proximal extremities	Scaly hyper- or hypopigmented macules
Psoriasis	Elbows, knees, scalp, lower back, fingernails (may be generalized)	Papules and plaques covered with silvery scale; nails have pits	Candidiasis	Groin, beneath breasts, vagina, oral cavity	Erythematous macerated areas with satellite pustules; white, friable patches on mucous membranes
Lichen planus	Wrists, ankles, mouth (may be widespread)	Violaceous flat-topped papules and plaques	Dermatophytosis	Feet, groin, beard, or scalp	Varies with site, e.g., tinea corporis—scaly annular patch
Keratosis pilaris	Extensor surfaces of arms and thighs, buttocks	Keratotic follicular papules with surrounding erythema	Scabies	Groin, axillae, between fingers and toes, beneath breasts	Excoriated papules, burrows, pruritus
Melasma	Forehead, cheeks, temples, upper lip	Tan to brown patches	Insect bites	Anywhere	Erythematous papules with central puncta
Vitiligo	Periorificial, trunk, extensor surfaces of extremities, flexor wrists, axillae	Chalk-white macules	Cherry angioma	Trunk	Red, blood-filled papules
			Keloid	Anywhere (site of previous injury)	Firm tumor, pink, purple, or brown
Actinic keratosis	Sun-exposed areas	Skin-colored or red-brown macule or papule with dry, rough, adherent scale	Dermatofibroma	Anywhere	Firm red to brown nodule that shows dimpling of overlying skin with lateral compression
Basal cell carcinoma	Face	Papule with pearly, telangiectatic border on sun-damaged skin	Acrochordons (skin tags)	Groin, axilla, neck	Fleshy papules
			Urticaria	Anywhere	Wheals, sometimes with surrounding flare, pruritus
Squamous cell carcinoma	Face, especially lower lip, ears	Indurated and possibly hyperkaratotic lesions often showing ulceration and/or crusting	Transient acantholytic dermatosis	Trunk, especially anterior chest	Erythematous papules
			Xerosis	Extensor extremities, especially legs	Dry, erythematous, scaling patches, pruritus

2 Symptoms associated with eruption
   a Itching, burning, pain, numbness
   b What, if anything, has relieved symptoms
   c Time of day when symptoms are most severe
3 Current or recent medications (prescribed as well as over-the-counter)
4 Associated systemic symptoms (e.g., malaise, fever, arthralgias)
5 Ongoing or previous illnesses
6 History of allergies
7 Presence of photosensitivity
8 Review of systems

DIAGNOSTIC TECHNIQUES Many skin diseases can be diagnosed on gross clinical appearance, but sometimes relatively simple diagnostic procedures can yield valuable information. In most instances, they can be performed at the bedside with a minimum of equipment.

Skin biopsy A skin biopsy is a straightforward minor surgical procedure; however, it is important to biopsy the anatomic site most likely to yield diagnostic findings. This decision may require expertise in skin diseases and knowledge of superficial anatomic structures in selected areas of the body. In this procedure, a small area of skin is anesthetized with 1% lidocaine with or without epinephrine. The skin lesion in question can be excised with a scalpel or removed by punch biopsy. In the latter technique, a punch is pressed against the surface of the skin and rotated with downward pressure until it penetrates to the subcutaneous tissue. The circular biopsy is then lifted with forceps, and the bottom is cut with iris scissors. Biopsy sites may or may not need suture closure depending on size and location.

KOH preparation A potassium hydroxide (KOH) preparation is performed on scaling skin lesions when a fungal etiology is suspected. The edge of such a lesion is scraped gently with a scalpel blade, and the removed scale is collected on a glass microscope slide and treated with 1 to 2 drops of a solution of 10 to 20% KOH. KOH dissolves keratin and allows easier visualization of fungal elements. Brief heating of the slide accelerates dissolution of keratin. When the preparation is viewed under the microscope, the refractile hyphae will be seen more easily when the light intensity is reduced. This technique can be utilized to identify hyphae in dermatophyte infections, pseudohyphae and budding yeast in *Candida* infections, and frag-

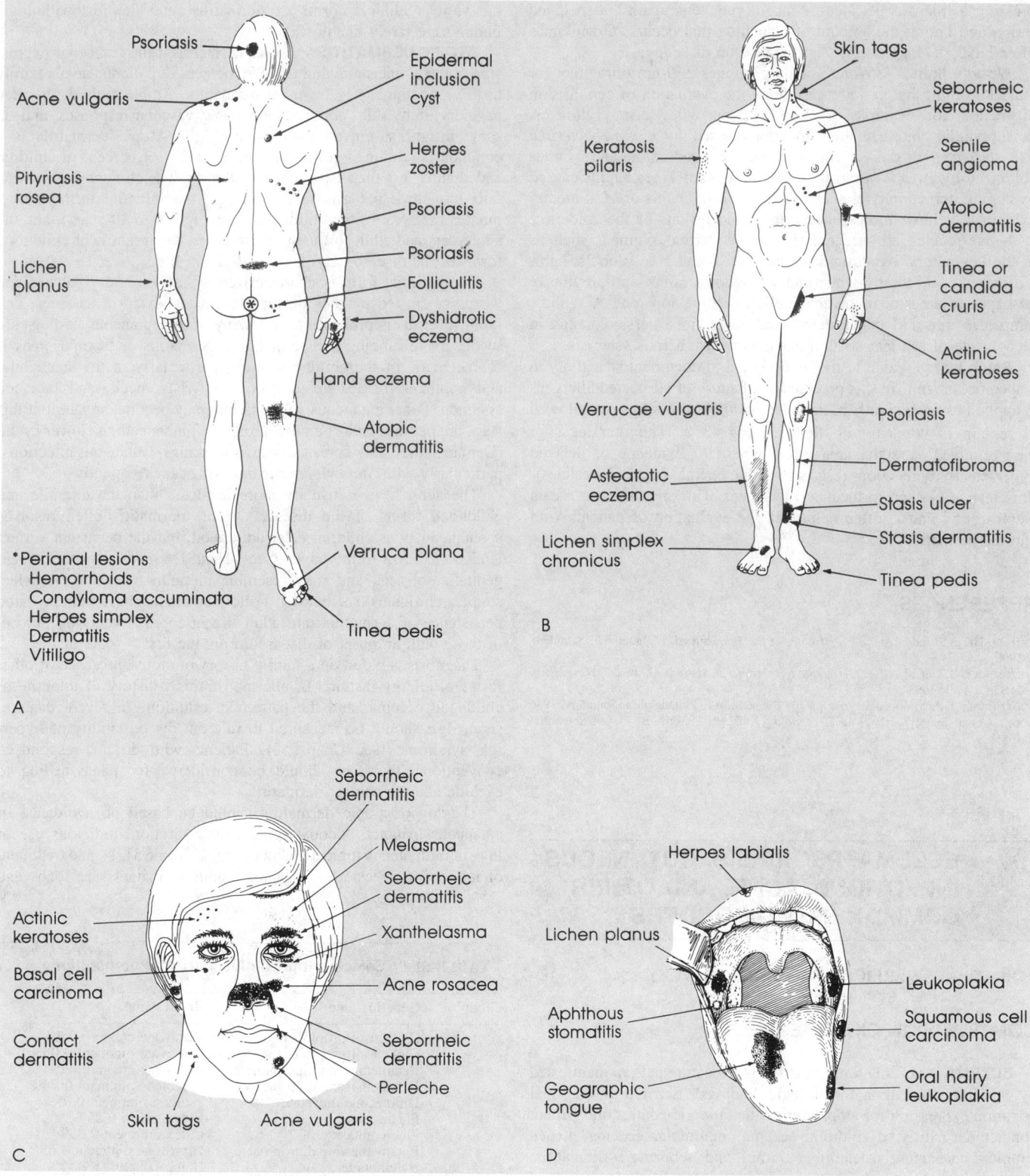

FIGURE 50-2 *A–D.* The distribution of some common dermatologic diseases and lesions.

mented hyphae and spores in tinea versicolor. The same sampling technique can be used to obtain scale for culture of selected pathogenic organisms.

Tzanck smear A Tzanck smear, named after Arnault Tzanck, is a cytologic technique most often used in the diagnosis of herpesvirus infections (simplex or varicella-zoster). An early vesicle, not a pustule or crusted lesion, is unroofed, and the base of the lesion is scraped gently with a scalpel blade. The material is then placed on a

glass slide, air-dried, and stained with Giemsa or Wright's stain. Multinucleated giant cells suggest the presence of herpes, but culture must be performed to identify the specific virus.

Diascopy Diascopy is designed to assess whether a skin lesion will blanch with pressure as, for example, in determining whether a red lesion is hemorrhagic or simply blood-filled. For instance, a hemangioma will blanch with pressure, whereas a purpuric lesion caused by necrotizing vasculitis will not. Diascopy is performed by pressing a microscope slide or magnifying lens against a specified lesion and noting the amount of blanching that occurs. Granulomas often have an "apple jelly" appearance on diascopy.

Wood's light   A Wood's lamp generates 360-nm ultraviolet (or "black") light that can be used to aid the evaluation of certain skin disorders. For example, a Wood's lamp will cause erythrasma (a superficial, intertriginous infection caused by *Corynebacterium minutissimum*) to show a characteristic coral red color, and wounds colonized by *Pseudomonas* to appear pale blue. Tinea capitis caused by certain dermatophytes such as *Microsporum canis* or *M. audouini* exhibits a yellow fluorescence. Pigmented lesions of the epidermis such as freckles are accentuated, while dermal pigment such as postinflammatory hyperpigmentation fades under a Wood's light. Vitiligo appears totally white under a Wood's lamp, and previously unsuspected areas of involvement often become apparent. A Wood's lamp also may aid in the demonstration of tinea versicolor and in recognition of ash leaf spots in patients with tuberous sclerosis.

Patch tests   Patch testing is designed to document sensitivity to a specific antigen. In this procedure, a battery of suspected allergens is applied to the patient's back under occlusive dressings and allowed to remain in contact with the skin for 48 h. The dressings are then removed, and the area is examined for evidence of delayed hypersensitivity reactions (e.g., erythema, edema, or papulovesicles). This test is best performed by physicians with special expertise in patch testing and is often helpful in the evaluation of patients with chronic dermatitis.

REFERENCES

ARNOLD HL et al (eds): *Andrew's Diseases of the Skin*, 8th ed. Philadelphia, Saunders, 1990

FITZPATRICK TB et al (eds): *Dermatology in General Medicine*, 4th ed. New York, McGraw-Hill, 1993

LOOKINGBILL DP, MARKS JG: *Principles of Dermatology*. Philadelphia, Saunders, 1986

ROOK A et al (eds): *Textbook of Dermatology*, 4th ed. Oxford, Blackwell Scientific, 1986

51   ECZEMA, PSORIASIS, CUTANEOUS INFECTIONS, ACNE, AND OTHER COMMON SKIN DISORDERS

ROBERT A. SWERLICK / THOMAS J. LAWLEY

COMMON SKIN DISORDERS

ECZEMA   Eczema, or dermatitis, is a reaction pattern manifested by variable clinical and histologic findings. Eczema is the final common expression for atopic dermatitis, allergic contact and irritant contact dermatitis, dyshidrotic eczema, nummular eczema, lichen simplex chronicus, asteatotic eczema, and seborrheic dermatitis. Primary lesions may include papules, erythematous macules, and vesicles, which can coalesce to form patches and plaques. In severe eczema, secondary lesions such as weeping and crusting may predominate. Long-standing dermatitis is often dry and is characterized by thickened, scaling skin (lichenification). The histologic changes correlate with the clinical findings. The histologic features of dermatitis have been divided into three patterns: acute, subacute, and chronic. Acute dermatitis shows a mixture of epidermal and dermal edema, epidermal vesiculation, and a mononuclear cell infiltrate. Chronic dermatitis demonstrates epidermal acanthosis, hyperkeratosis, upper dermal fibrosis, and a predominantly perivascular mononuclear cell infiltrate. Mixtures of these two histologic reaction patterns occur in subacute dermatitis. Any of these patterns may be associated with

the various clinical forms of dermatitis, and the histopathologic findings are rarely diagnostic.

ATOPIC DERMATITIS   Atopic dermatitis is the cutaneous expression of the atopic state, and up to 70 percent of patients have a family history of asthma, hay fever, or dermatitis. Atopic individuals often have dry, itchy skin, abnormal cutaneous vascular responses, and, in some instances, elevations in serum IgE. Atopic dermatitis is a common condition, with a prevalence of 2 to 3 percent in children and slightly less than 1 percent for all ages. The clinical presentation falls into three patterns related to age: the infantile form (ages 2 months to 2 years), the childhood form (ages 4 to 10 years), and the adolescent and adult form. In severe cases, the infantile or childhood forms of the disease may persist into adult life.

The infantile form is characterized by inflammatory patches and weeping, crusted plaques on the face, neck, extensor surfaces, and groin. Pruritus is prominent, and many of the cutaneous findings are secondary to rubbing and scratching. Dermatitis of flexural areas is characteristic of the childhood form, particularly in the antecubital and popliteal fossae. Lesions on the wrists, neck, and face are common. Other cutaneous stigmata that may become apparent at this stage are perioral pallor, an extra fold of skin beneath the lower eyelid (Dennie's line), and increased palmar markings. Cutaneous infections, particularly with *Staphylococcus aureus*, occur frequently.

The adult form is usually more localized than the infantile and childhood forms of the disease. Atopic dermatitis often resolves spontaneously as children enter adulthood, but the persistent variant tends to localize to the hands (see "Hand Dermatitis"), neck, face, genitalia, or legs and may resemble nummular eczema or lichen simplex chronicus (see below). Follow-up studies have demonstrated persistence of dermatitis into adult life in approximately 60 percent of those with an onset of disease during the first 5 years of life.

Diagnosis is based on a family history of atopy, presence of other forms of allergy (asthma or allergic rhinitis), history of infantile or childhood eczema, and the pattern of eruption. In severe disease, serum IgE should be measured to rule out the possibility of hyper-IgE syndrome (see Chap. 59). Patients who do not respond to conventional therapies should be considered for patch testing to exclude allergic contact dermatitis.

Therapy of atopic dermatitis should be based on avoidance of cutaneous irritants, adequate cutaneous hydration, judicious use of low- or midpotency topical glucocorticoids (Table 51-1), and treatment of infected skin lesions. The most common irritants are soaps and

TABLE 51-1   Selected topical glucocorticoid preparations*

Group[†]	Generic name	Brand name
1	Clobetasol propionate	Temovate cream 0.05%
	Clobetasol propionate	Temovate ointment 0.05%
	Betamethasone dipropionate	Diprolene cream 0.05%
	Betamethasone dipropionate	Diprolene ointment 0.05%
	Diflorasone diacetate	Psorcon ointment 0.05%
2	Flucinonide	Lidex cream 0.05%
	Flucinonide	Lidex ointment 0.05%
	Betamethasone dipropionate	Diprosone ointment 0.05%
	Halcinonide	Halog cream 0.1%
3	Betamethasone dipropionate	Diprosone cream 0.05%
	Betamethasone valerate	Valisone ointment 0.1%
	Diflorasone diacetate	Maxiflor cream 0.05%
4	Triamcinolone acetonide	Kenalog ointment 0.1%
	Triamcinolone acetonide	Aristocort ointment 0.1%
	Flurandrenolide	Cordran ointment 0.05%
5	Triamcinolone acetonide	Kenalog cream 0.1%
	Fluocinolone acetonide	Synalar cream 0.025%
	Hydrocortisone valerate	Westcort cream 0.2%
6	Desonide	Tridesilon cream 0.05%
	Desonide	DesOwen cream 0.05%
	Alclometasone dipropionate	Alcovate cream 0.05%
7	Hydrocortisone	Many

* List not meant to be comprehensive.
† Preparations grouped according to potency: Group 1 is most potent; group 7 is least potent.

hot water. Patients should bathe using warm, but not hot, water and should limit their use of soap, particularly on extremities. Immediately after bathing, the skin should be lubricated with a low- or midpotency topical glucocorticoid in a cream or ointment base. Crusted and weeping lesions should be treated with systemic antibiotics with activity against *S. aureus* and *Streptococcus pyogenes*, since secondary infection often exacerbates eczema. Antihistamines are useful to control the pruritus that accompanies eczema, but sedation may limit their usefulness.

The role of dietary allergens in atopic dermatitis is controversial, but there is little evidence that it plays any role except in infancy. A significant number of children under age 3 who do not respond to conventional therapy have food sensitivities. Unfortunately, parental histories of food intake do not correlate with actual food allergens, and identification of the offending agents is best done with double-blind food challenges.

Treatment with systemic glucocorticoids should be limited to severe exacerbations unresponsive to topical therapy. In the patient with chronic atopic eczema, therapy with systemic glucocorticoids will generally clear the skin only briefly, but cessation of the systemic therapy will invariably be accompanied by return, if not worsening, of the dermatitis. The side effects of daily doses of systemic glucocorticoids preclude chronic use in virtually all patients with atopic dermatitis, and the efficacy of alternate-day regimens in this disease is limited.

CONTACT DERMATITIS When dermatitis is induced by contact with an external agent, it is called *contact dermatitis*. When an external agent directly damages the skin, the ensuing eruption is referred to as an *irritant contact dermatitis* (ICD). This is different from *allergic contact dermatitis* (ACD), which is caused by an immunologic reaction to an allergen which comes into contact with the skin. The exact prevalence of contact dermatitis is not known, but previous surveys suggest that a significant proportion of occupation-related disease (almost 50 percent) is due to work-related skin injury, and the most commonly involved site is the hands (see Hand eczema). Contact dermatitis represents a significant economic problem. In 1975, a survey in California demonstrated that 95 percent of all occupation-related skin disease was contact dermatitis, which, in turn, represented almost half of all occupational claims that year. The most commonly recognized form of ACD is phytodermatitis or plant dermatitis. Members of the *Rhus* family, including poison ivy, poison oak, and poison sumac, cause an allergic reaction marked by erythema, vesiculation, and severe pruritus. The eruption is often linear, corresponding to areas where plants have touched the skin. Other allergens are much more difficult to identify, especially if the exposure is chronic and the skin becomes thickened and scaly.

If ACD is suspected and an offending agent is identified and removed, the eruption resolves. Usually, treatment with high-potency fluorinated topical glucocorticoids is enough to relieve symptoms while the ACD runs its course. Patients with particularly widespread disease, or disease involving the face or genitalia, may require treatment with oral glucocorticoids. Since the natural course of ACD is 2 to 3 weeks, therapy should be continued for that length of time. Treatment of ACD with short, rapidly tapered courses of oral glucocorticoids is usually followed by recurrence of skin lesions.

Identification of a contact allergen can be a difficult and time-consuming task. Patients with a dermatitis unresponsive to conventional therapy or with an unusual and patterned distribution should be suspected of having ACD. They should be questioned carefully regarding occupational exposures, topical medications, and oral medications. Common sensitizers include preservatives in topical preparations, nickel sulfate, potassium dichromate, neomycin sulfate, fragrances, formaldehyde, and rubber curing agents. Standard patch-test trays are helpful in identifying these agents but should not be used in patients with widespread active dermatitis or in those on systemic glucocorticoids.

HAND ECZEMA Hand eczema, a common chronic skin disorder, may be associated with other cutaneous disorders such as atopic dermatitis or psoriasis or may occur by itself. Like other forms of dermatitis, both exogenous and endogenous factors play important roles in the expression of hand dermatitis. Chronic, excessive exposure to water and detergents may initiate or aggravate this disorder. It may present with dryness and cracking of the skin of the hands, as well as with variable amounts of erythema and edema. Often the dermatitis begins under rings, where water and irritants are trapped. A variant of hand dermatitis, dyshidrotic eczema, presents with multiple, intensely pruritic, small papules and vesicles on the thenar and hypothenar eminences and the sides of the fingers. Lesions tend to occur in crops, slowly crust over, and are followed by another outbreak.

The overall prevalence of hand eczema has been estimated to be approximately 2 per 1000 persons. Its prevalence is highest in the 25- to 44-year-old age group where it is two- to threefold higher. The actual prevalence of hand eczema is probably much higher, since surveys that were used to estimate the prevalence of hand eczema and occupational contact dermatitis excluded homemakers and workers in industries which failed to report work-related skin injury.

Therapy of hand dermatitis is directed toward avoidance of irritants, identification of possible contact allergens, treatment of coexistent infection, and application of topical glucocorticoids. The most common hand irritants are soap and water. Health care professionals, housewives, and food handlers are prone to hand eczema. Use of mild soap, avoidance of hot water, and compulsive use of emollients can alleviate some symptoms. Whenever possible, the hands should be protected by gloves, preferably vinyl gloves, since many patients with hand eczema may become sensitive to curing agents in rubber gloves. Predominant involvement of the dorsal surfaces of the hands with sparing of the palmar surfaces should suggest a possible contact dermatitis. Most patients can be treated by application of cool, moist compresses (dressings) to dry and debride acute inflammatory lesions and to decrease swelling, followed by a midpotency topical glucocorticoid in a cream or ointment base. If allergic contact dermatitis is suspected, ointments are preferable. Chronic use of very high potency topical glucocorticoids can lead to cutaneous atrophy and is often accompanied by loss of effectiveness. As with atopic dermatitis, treatment of secondary infection with *Staphylococcus* or *Streptococcus* is essential. All patients with hand dermatitis should be examined for dermatophyte infection by KOH preparation and culture (see "Dermatophyte Infections").

NUMMULAR ECZEMA Nummular eczema is characterized by circular or oval "coinlike" lesions. Initially, this eruption consists of small edematous papules that become crusted and scaly. The most common locations are on the trunk or the extensor surfaces of the extremities, particularly on the pretibial areas or dorsum of the hands. It occurs most frequently in middle-aged men. The etiology is unknown but appears to be related to dryness of the skin and exogenous irritants. Unlike other forms of dermatitis, nummular eczema does not respond well to hydration, topical glucocorticoids, or antihistamines. Overt infection should be treated appropriately with antibiotics; however, even in instances where infection is not apparent, treatment with oral antibiotics, such as tetracycline or erythromycin, may be useful.

LICHEN SIMPLEX CHRONICUS Lichen simplex chronicus may represent the end stage of a variety of eczematous disorders. It consists of a well-circumscribed plaque or plaques with lichenified or thickened skin due to chronic scratching or rubbing. Common areas involved include the posterior nuchal region, dorsum of the feet, or ankles. Treatment of lichen simplex chronicus centers around breaking the cycle of chronic itching and scratching. High-potency topical glucocorticoids may be helpful in alleviating pruritus, but in recalcitrant cases, application of topical glucocorticoids under occlusion or intralesional injection of glucocorticoids may be required.

ASTEATOTIC ECZEMA Asteatotic eczema, also known as xerotic eczema or "winter itch," is a mildly inflammatory variant of eczematous dermatitis that develops most commonly on the lower legs of elderly individuals during dry times of year. Fine cracks, with or without erythema, resembling cracks seen in china or porcelain, characteristically develop on the anterior surfaces of the lower extremities. Pruritus is variable. Asteatotic eczema responds well to avoidance of excessive dryness, rehydration of the skin, and application of topical emollients, particularly those containing urea or alpha-hydroxy acids (lactic acid or glycolic acid).

STASIS DERMATITIS AND STASIS ULCERATION Stasis dermatitis develops on the lower extremities secondary to chronic edema and venous incompetence. The disorder usually begins as mild erythema and scaling associated with pruritus over the medial aspect of the ankle, often over a varicose vein. The dermatitis progresses to become pigmented as the result of extravasation of blood and hemosiderin deposition. Stasis dermatitis may become acutely inflamed, with crusting and exudation. Chronic stasis dermatitis is often associated with dermal fibrosis which results in brawny edema and may be complicated by the development of stasis ulcers.

Elevation of the legs, compression stockings, and topical emollients are the cornerstone of therapy. Patients should be instructed to elevate the affected extremity when sitting. Support stockings are a useful adjunct, particularly in individuals who stand for long periods of time. A graded compression stocking is more desirable than an antiembolism hose, which is designed for individuals confined to bed. The dermatitic component can be treated with cool dressings and the application of midpotency topical glucocorticoids. Glucocorticoids should not be applied to ulcerations, since they may retard healing. Secondarily infected lesions should be treated with appropriate oral antibiotics.

Stasis ulcerations are difficult to treat, and resolution of these lesions is slow even under the best of circumstances. The affected limb should be elevated as much as possible. External compression dressings such as an Unna boot are also helpful in aiding healing. The ulcer should be kept clear of necrotic material, and debridement may be facilitated by frequent soaks. The use of semipermeable and hydrocolloid dressings may be helpful. Some ulcerations may take months to heal and require skin grafting. Healed areas are prone to recurrent ulceration.

SEBORRHEIC DERMATITIS Seborrheic dermatitis is a common, chronic disorder usually affecting the central face and scalp and, on occasion, the groin, axilla, submammary folds, and gluteal cleft. Rarely, it may cause a widespread generalized dermatitis. Patients commonly complain of itching or burning. It is characterized by greasy scales overlying erythematous patches or plaques. In the scalp it may be recognized as severe dandruff. On the face it affects the eyebrows, eyelids, glabella, nasolabial fold, or ears. Scaling within the external ear is often mistaken for a chronic fungal infection (otomycosis), and postauricular dermatitis often becomes macerated and tender.

Seborrheic dermatitis may be evident in infancy in the scalp ("cradle cap"), face, or groin. It is not seen in children beyond infancy but becomes evident again during adult life. Although it is frequently seen in patients with Parkinson's disease, in those who have had cerebrovascular accidents, and in those with human immunodeficiency virus (HIV-1) infection, the overwhelming majority of individuals with seborrheic dermatitis have no underlying disorder.

Treatment with low- to midpotency topical glucocorticoids in conjunction with shampoos containing coal tar and/or salicylic acid is generally sufficient to control activity of this disorder. Selenium sulfide shampoos also may be effective. Fluorinated topical glucocorticoids should not be used on the face.

PAPULOSQUAMOUS DISORDERS

PSORIASIS Psoriasis is one of the most common dermatologic diseases, affecting 1 to 2 percent of people. It is a chronic inflammatory skin disorder characterized by erythematous, sharply demarcated papules and rounded plaques, covered by silvery micaceous scale. The lesions are variably pruritic. The most common areas of involvement are the elbows, knees, gluteal cleft, and scalp. Lesions tend to be symmetric. Traumatized areas are often involved (Koebner or isomorphic phenomenon). Most patients will have stable, slowly growing, infiltrated plaques, which remain unchanged for long periods. Eruptive psoriasis in children and young adults is notable for the development of many small lesions after upper respiratory tract infection with beta-hemolytic streptococci.

About half of patients have fingernail involvement, appearing as a punctate pitting, nail thickening, or subungual hyperkeratosis. About 5 to 10 percent of psoriatics have joint complaints, often when there is fingernail involvement. Although some have typical rheumatoid arthritis (see Chap. 285), many have joint disease specifically associated with psoriasis: (1) disease limited to a single or a few small joints (70 percent of cases), (2) a seronegative rheumatoid arthritis–like disease, (3) involvement of the distal interphalangeal joints, (4) severe destructive arthritis with the development of "arthritis mutilans," and (5) disease limited to the spine (see Chap. 298).

The histologic picture can be variable but is usually diagnostic in early lesions or at the advancing edge of a well-established plaque. The epidermis demonstrates elongation of the rete ridges, suprapapillary thinning, loss of the granular layer, parakeratotic keratin, and intraepidermal collections of neutrophils. Dilated capillaries and mononuclear cell infiltrates are common in the dermal papillae.

Treatment depends on the type, location, and extent of disease. All patients should be instructed to avoid excess drying or irritation of the skin and to maintain adequate cutaneous hydration. Most patients with localized plaque-type psoriasis can be managed with midpotency topical glucocorticoids, although their long-term use is often accompanied by loss of effectiveness. The effectiveness of topical glucocorticoids may be increased if used in conjunction with a keratolytic agent, such as salicylic acid, which removes surface scale and allows greater penetration. Crude coal tar (1 to 5% in an ointment base) is an old but useful method of treatment in conjunction with ultraviolet light therapy.

Ultraviolet light is useful for widespread psoriasis. The ultraviolet B (UV-B) spectrum is effective alone or may be combined with coal tar (Goeckerman regimen) or anthralin (Ingram regimen). Natural sunlight or an artificial light source can be used. The combination of the ultraviolet A (UV-A) spectrum and either oral or topical psoralens is also extremely effective for the treatment of psoriasis, but the photosensitizing potential of psoralens and unknown long-term toxicity may limit the use of this therapy.

Other agents can be used for widespread disease. Methotrexate is useful in patients with associated psoriatic arthritis. Long-term liver toxicity limits its use to patients with widespread disease not responsive to standard agents. The synthetic retinoid etretinate is effective in some patients with severe psoriasis, but it is a potent teratogen with an extremely long tissue half-life, thus precluding its use in women of childbearing age.

LICHEN PLANUS Lichen planus is a papulosquamous disorder in which the primary lesions are pruritic, polygonal, flat-topped, violaceous papules. Close examination of the surface of these papules will often reveal a network of grayish lines (Wickham's striae). The skin lesions have a predilection for the wrists, shins, lower back, and genitalia. Involvement of the scalp may lead to hair loss. Lichen planus commonly involves mucous membranes, particularly the buccal mucosa, where it can present as a netlike, whitish eruption. The etiology is unknown, but cutaneous eruptions clinically resembling lichen planus can occur after administration of numerous drugs, including thiazide diuretics, gold, antimalarials, and phenothiazines, and in patients with skin lesions of chronic graft-versus-host disease. Histologic examination of lesions of lichen planus will demonstrate hyperkeratosis, irregular acanthosis, a bandlike dermal infiltrate of lymphocytes adjacent to the epidermis, and damage to the epidermal basal cells. The course is variable, but most patients have spontaneous remissions 6 months to 2 years after the onset of disease. Topical glucocorticoids are the mainstay of therapy.

PITYRIASIS ROSEA Pityriasis rosea is a papulosquamous eruption of unknown etiology that occurs more commonly in the spring and fall. Its first manifestation is the development of a 2- to 6-cm annular lesion (the herald patch). This is followed in a few days to a few weeks by many smaller annular or papular lesions with a truncal predilection. The lesions are generally oval with their long axis parallel to the skin-fold lines. The individual lesions may be red to brown in color with an erythematous border and trailing scale. Many clinical features resemble the eruption of secondary syphilis, but palm and sole lesions are rare in pityriasis rosea. The eruption tends to be moderately pruritic and lasts 3 to 8 weeks. The histologic picture is often not diagnostic, because it can resemble an acute or subacute dermatitis. Treatment is generally directed at alleviating pruritus and consists of oral antihistamines, midpotency topical glucocorticoids, and, in some cases, the use of UV-B phototherapy.

CUTANEOUS INFECTIONS

IMPETIGO AND ECTHYMA Impetigo is a common superficial bacterial infection caused by group A beta-hemolytic streptococci or S. aureus. The primary lesion is a superficial pustule that ruptures and forms a characteristic yellow-brown "honey-colored" crust. Lesions caused by Staphylococcus may be tense, clear bullae, and this form of the disease is called bullous impetigo. Lesions may occur on normal skin or in areas already affected by another skin disease. Ecthyma is a variant of impetigo on the lower extremities and causes punched-out ulcerative lesions. In addition to improving hygiene, treatment of both ecthyma and impetigo involves gentle debridement of adherent crusts, which is facilitated by the use of soaks and topical antibiotics in conjunction with appropriate oral antibiotics.

ERYSIPELAS AND CELLULITIS See Chap. 103.

DERMATOPHYTOSIS Fungi that infect skin, hair, and nails include members of the species Trichophyton, Microsporum, and Epidermophyton. Infection of the foot is most common and is referred to as tinea pedis (athlete's foot). Tinea pedis is often chronic and is characterized by variable erythema and edema, scaling, pruritus, and occasionally vesiculation. Involvement may be widespread or localized, but almost invariably the web space between the fourth and fifth toes is affected. Infection of the nails (tinea unguium) is characterized by opacified, thickened nails and subungual debris. The groin is the next most commonly involved area, with men affected predominantly. It presents as a scaling erythematous eruption, which spares the scrotum. Microscopic examination of scale after digestion with potassium hydroxide (KOH preparation) of either untreated tinea pedis or tinea cruris usually demonstrates hyphae. However, even short courses of topical antifungal agents may make demonstration of hyphae difficult.

Dermatophyte infection of the scalp (tinea capitis) is quite common, particularly in inner-city clinics. The predominant organism, Trichophyton tonsurans, can produce a relatively noninflammatory infection that may present with either well-defined or irregular, diffuse areas of mild scaling and hair loss. Close examination of the scalp may reveal many broken off hairs appearing as small black dots. Unlike infections with Microsporum sp., which was previously the most common cause of tinea capitis, lesions caused by Trichophyton tonsurans are not fluorescent under a Wood's lamp. Tinea capitis caused by Microsporum audouini is characterized by a sharply delineated noninflammatory area in which hairs are broken off close to the surface. Hairs infected with M. audouini fluoresce bright bluish green when examined with a Wood's lamp. Tinea corporis, or widespread infection on non-hair-bearing skin, may have a variable appearance, depending on the extent of the associated inflammatory reaction. It may have the typical annular appearance of "ringworm" or appear as deep inflammatory nodules (on the scalp known as kerions) or granulomas. KOH examination of scale or hair from patients with tinea capitis or inflammatory tinea corporis often does not reveal hyphae, and diagnosis may require culture.

Both topical and systemic therapies may be used to treat dermatophyte infection. Topical imidazoles and triazoles, including miconazole, ketaconazole, and econazole, may be effective. Haloprogin, undecylic acid, ciclopirox olamine, and tolnaftate are also effective, but nystatin is not active against dermatophytes. Griseofulvin is the drug of choice for dermatophyte infections requiring systemic therapy. While older preparations of griseofulvin required the use of as much as 1 to 2 g of drug daily, newer microsized and ultramicrosized preparations are better absorbed and allow treatment with much lower doses of drug. Generally, a daily dose of 500 mg of microsized or 350 mg of ultramicrosized griseofulvin is adequate. Unresponsive infections may respond to doubling the dose. Griseofulvin is best absorbed if administered with a fatty meal. The most common side effects of griseofulvin are gastrointestinal distress and headache. It is also rarely associated with hematologic and liver function abnormalities, and patients on long-term therapy should be carefully monitored.

The choice of treatment depends on the site involved and the type of infection. For chronic noninflammatory tinea pedis, topical imidazoles or keratolytics are useful to limit pruritus and scaling but are rarely curative. Treatment with oral griseofulvin is effective but may require months of therapy for mycologic cure and, even then, is associated with a high relapse rate, particularly if the nails are involved. The therapy of tinea corporis depends on the extent of disease. Localized infection is best treated with topical imidazoles, but widespread disease, particularly in patients with decreased cellular immunity, requires systemic antifungal therapy.

Dermatophyte infection of hair-bearing areas (such as tinea capitis) requires systemic antifungal therapy, and treatment should be continued for 6 to 8 weeks. The adjunctive use of topical antifungals in addition to systemic therapy may be useful, but topical therapy alone is not adequate. Markedly inflammatory tinea capitis may result in scarring and hair loss, and systemic or topical glucocorticoids may prevent this sequela.

TINEA VERSICOLOR Tinea versicolor is caused by a nondermatophyte dimorphic fungus which is a normal inhabitant of the skin. As the yeast form (Pityrosporum orbiculare), it generally does not cause disease (except for folliculitis in certain individuals). However, in some individuals, it converts to the hyphal form and causes characteristic lesions. Infection is promoted by heat and humidity. The typical lesions consist of oval scaly macules, papules, and patches concentrated on the chest, shoulders, and back and rarely on the face or distal extremities. On dark skin they often appear as hypopigmented areas, while on light skin they are slightly hyperpigmented. In some darkly pigmented individuals, they may only appear as scaling patches. A KOH preparation from scaling lesions will demonstrate a confluence of short hyphae and round spores (so-called spaghetti and meatballs). There are many effective topical treatments for tinea versicolor. Solutions containing sulfur, salicylic acid, or selenium sulfide will clear the infection if used daily for a week and then intermittently thereafter. Topical imidazoles are also effective.

CANDIDIASIS Candidiasis is caused by a related group of yeasts, whose manifestations may be localized to the skin or may be systemic and life-threatening. The causative organism is usually Candida albicans but also may be C. tropicalis, C. parapsilosis, and C. krusei. These organisms are normal saprophytic inhabitants of the gastrointestinal tract but can overgrow (usually due to broad-spectrum antibiotic therapy) and cause disease at cutaneous sites. Other predisposing factors include diabetes mellitus, chronic intertrigo, and cellular immune deficiency. The oral cavity is commonly involved. Lesions may occur on the tongue or buccal mucosa (thrush) and appear as white plaques. Microscopic examination of scrapings demonstrates both pseudohyphae and yeast forms. Fissured, macerated lesions at the corners of the mouth (perleche) are often seen in individuals with poorly fitting dentures and also may be associated with candidal infection. Additionally, candidal infections have an affinity for sites that are chronically wet and macerated and may occur around nails (onycholysis and paronychia) and in intertriginous areas. Intertriginous lesions are characteristically edematous, erythematous, and scaly, with scattered "satellite pustules." In men there is often involvement of the penis and scrotum as well as the inner aspect of the thighs, and in women the introitus and vagina may be infected. Diagnosis is based on the clinical pattern and demonstration of yeast on KOH preparation or on culture. Treatment involves removing any predisposing factors such as antibiotic therapy or chronic wetness, the careful control of diabetes mellitus, if present, and the use of appropriate topical or systemic antifungal agents.

WARTS   Warts are cutaneous neoplasms caused by papillomaviruses. Over 50 different human papillomaviruses (HPV) have been described. Types 1, 2, 4, and 7 cause typical verrucae vulgaris. These lesions are sessile, dome-shaped, usually about a centimeter in diameter, and have a surface made up of many small filamentous projections. These papillomaviruses also cause typical plantar warts and filiform warts in intertriginous areas. Plantar warts are endophytic and are covered by thick keratin. Paring of the wart will generally demonstrate a central core of keratinized debris and punctuate bleeding points. Filiform warts are most common on the face, neck, and skin folds and present as papillomatous lesions on a narrow base. HPV types 3 and 10 are associated with flat warts or verrucae plana. These lesions are only slightly elevated and have a velvety, nonverrucous surface. They have a propensity for the face, arms, and legs and often are spread by shaving.

HPV types 6, 11, 16, 18, 31–35, 39, 48, and 51–54 cause genital tract lesions. Types 6 and 11 are associated with typical lesions of condyloma acuminata, which generally begin as small papillomas and may grow to form large, fungating lesions. In women, they may involve either the labia, perineum, or perianal skin. Additionally, the mucosa of the vagina, urethra, and anus can be involved, as well as the cervical epithelium. In men, the lesions often occur initially in the coronal sulcus, but they may be seen on the shaft of the penis, the scrotum, perianal skin, or in the urethra. They initially appear as soft, pink, filiform lesions, which may enlarge and coalesce to form large cauliflower-like aggregates. HPV types 6 and 11 also can cause juvenile laryngeal papillomas.

HPV also plays a role in the development of neoplasia of the uterine cervix and external genitalia. A high rate of coexistence of condyloma acuminata with cervical dysplasia or carcinoma was initially reported, and HPV DNA has been found in association both with cervical carcinoma and dyplasia and with cancerous and precancerous lesions of the external genitalia. HPV types 16 and 18 have been most intensely studied; other types are also implicated. In men, these lesions may initially appear as small, flat, hyperpigmented papules on the penis or perianal skin. The surface of the lesions is generally smooth and velvety, but it may be verrucous. The detection of subtle lesions may be improved by treatment with 5% acetic acid, which makes them appear white. In women, cutaneous lesions are generally multiple and often pigmented. They can be located on the labia majora and minora of the vulva and in the perianal region. Histologic examination of biopsies from affected sites may reveal changes associated with typical warts (hyperkeratosis, papillomatosis, and vacuolated cells) and/or features typical of intraepidermal carcinoma (Bowen's disease). Features in the latter include a disordered maturational sequence of dyskeratotic keratinocytes with hyperchromatic nuclei.

Squamous cell carcinomas are also associated with papillomavirus infections in extragenital skin. This has been seen in patients immunosuppressed after renal transplantation and in patients with the disorder epidermodysplasia verruciformis. Patients in both groups tend to develop multiple cutaneous squamous cell carcinomas on sun-exposed sites associated with several HPV types, including types 5, 8, and 14.

There are many ways to treat warts, but none is universally effective. Perhaps the most useful and convenient method is cryotherapy with liquid nitrogen. Equally effective, but requiring much more patient compliance is the use of keratolytic agents such as salicylic acid plasters or combinations of lactic acid and salicylic acid in flexible collodion. Keratolytic agents are of limited use on mucous membranes and genital lesions. For genital warts, podophyllin solution is moderately effective but may be associated with marked local reactions. Other topical agents used include trichloracetic acid or cantharidin. Electrodesiccation and curettage or carbon dioxide laser are also effective but require local anesthesia. Some caution should be exercised with electrodesiccation or carbon dioxide laser ablation because infectious viral particles may be in the vaporized tissue. Recurrence of warts appears to be common to all these modalities because viral genomic material is present in normal-appearing skin adjacent to the clinical lesions. Treatment should be tempered by recognition that most warts in normal individuals resolve spontaneously within 1 to 2 years. Also, only a fraction of warts are associated with neoplasia, and these are almost exclusively located on the genitalia or perianal skin.

HERPES SIMPLEX   See Chap. 143.
HERPES ZOSTER   See Chap. 144.

ACNE

ACNE VULGARIS   Acne vulgaris is usually a self-limited disorder of teenagers and young adults, although 10 to 20 percent of adults may experience some form of the disorder. The permissive factor for the expression of the disease is the increase in sebum release by sebaceous glands after puberty. Small cysts, called *comedones*, form in hair follicles due to blockage of the follicular orifice by retention of sebum and keratinous material. The action of lipophilic yeast *(Pityrosporum orbiculare)* and bacteria *(Proprionibacterium acnes)* within the comedones releases free fatty acids from sebum, causes inflammation within the cyst, and results in rupture of the cyst wall. An inflammatory reaction develops as a result of extrusion of oily and keratinous debris from the cyst.

The clinical hallmark of acne vulgaris is the comedo, which may be closed (whitehead) or open (blackhead). Closed comedones appear as 1- to 2-mm pebbly white papules that are accentuated when the skin is stretched. They are the precursors of inflammatory lesions, and the contents are not easily expressed. Open comedones, which rarely result in inflammatory acne lesions, have a large dilated follicular orifice and are filled with easily expressible oxidized, darkened, oily debris. Closed comedones are usually accompanied by inflammatory lesions: papules, pustules, or nodules.

The earliest lesions in adolescence are generally mildly inflamed or noninflammatory comedones on the forehead, followed by more typical inflammatory lesions on the cheeks, nose, and chin. The most common location for acne is the face, but the chest and back may be involved. Most diseases remain mild and do not lead to scarring; a subset of patients develop large inflammatory cysts and nodules, which may drain and result in significant scarring.

Exogenous and endogenous factors can alter the expression of acne vulgaris. Friction and trauma may rupture preexisting microcomedones and elicit inflammatory acne. This is commonly seen with headbands or chin straps of athletic helmets. Agents that predispose to comedone formation include topical agents in cosmetics or hair preparations such as lanolin, petrolatum, butylstearate, lauryl alcohol, and oleic acid and chronic topical exposure to certain industrial compounds that contain insoluble cutting oils (impure paraffin oil mixtures), halogenated hydrocarbons, and coal tar and its derivatives. Glucocorticoids, applied topically or administered systemically, also may elicit acne. Other systemic medications such as isoniazid, halogens, Dilantin, and phenobarbital may produce acneiform eruptions or aggravate preexisting acne.

Treatment is directed toward elimination of comedones, decreasing the population of lipophilic bacteria and yeast, and decreasing inflammation. Although areas affected with acne should be kept clean, removal of surface oils does not play an important role in therapy. Indeed, overly vigorous scrubbing may aggravate acne due to mechanical rupture of comedones. Oral tetracycline or erythromycin in doses of 250 to 1000 mg daily will decrease follicular colonization with some lipophilic organisms and may have an anti-inflammatory effect independent of antibacterial effects. Topical agents such as retinoic acid, benzoyl peroxide, or salicylic acid may alter the pattern of epidermal desquamation, prevent the formation of comedones, and aid in the resolution of preexisting cysts. Topical antibacterial agents such as benzoyl peroxide, topical erythromycin, clindamycin, or tetracycline are also useful adjuncts to therapy. Severe nodulocystic acne not responsive to oral antibiotics and topical therapy may be treated with the synthetic retinoid isotretinoin at doses of 0.5 to 1.0 mg/kg body weight per day for 15 to 20 weeks. The use of this drug is limited by its teratogenicity, and women must be screened for pregnancy prior to initiating therapy, maintain a fail-safe method of birth control during treatment, and be screened for pregnancy during treatment. Patients receiving this medication develop extremely dry skin and cheilitis and must be followed for development of hypertriglyceridemia. Patients treated with isotretinoin, particularly those on long-term therapy for disorders other than acne, are also at risk to develop calcifications of tendons and bony overgrowths of vertebrae.

ACNE ROSACEA Acne rosacea is an inflammatory disorder predominantly affecting the central face. It rarely affects patients under age 30. Rosacea is more common in women, but those most severely affected are men. It is characterized by erythema, telangiectasias, and superficial pustules and is not associated with comedones. Rosacea rarely involves the chest or back.

There is a relationship between the tendency for pronounced facial flushing and the subsequent development of acne rosacea. Initially, individuals with rosacea demonstrate a pronounced flushing reaction. This may be in response to heat, emotional stimuli, alcohol, hot drinks, or spicy foods. As the disease progresses, the flush persists longer and longer, eventually becoming permanent. Papules, pustules, and telangiectasias then become superimposed on the persistent flush.

Rosacea of long standing may lead to connective tissue overgrowth, particularly of the nose (rhinophyma), and may be complicated by inflammatory disorders of the eye, including keratitis, blepharitis, iritis, and recurrent chalazion. These ocular problems potentially threaten vision and warrant ophthalmologic evaluation.

Acne rosacea can generally be effectively treated with oral tetracycline in doses ranging from 250 to 1500 mg/d. Topical metronidazole is also effective, and low-potency, nonfluorinated topical glucocorticoids, particularly after cool soaks, may alleviate facial erythema. Fluorinated topical glucocorticoids should be avoided, since chronic use of these preparations may actually elicit rosacea. Topical therapy is not effective for ocular disease.

REFERENCES

FITZPATRICK TB et al (eds): *Dermatology in General Medicine*, 3d ed. New York, McGraw-Hill, 1987

KRANNING KK, ODLAND GF (eds): Analysis of research needs and priorities in dermatology. J Invest Dermatol 73 (Suppl 5):1, 1979

LEVER WP, LEVER GS: *Histopathology of the Skin*, 6th ed. Philadelphia, Lippincott, 1983

MOSCHELLA SL, HURLEY HH (eds): *Dermatology*, 2d ed. Philadelphia, Saunders, 1985

PETO R, ZUR HAUSEN H: *Viral Etiology of Cervical Cancer: Banbury Report*. Cold Spring Harbor, NY, Cold Spring Harbor Laboratory, 1986

PLEWIG G, KLIGMAN AM: *Acne: Morphogenesis and Treatment*. New York, Springer-Verlag, 1975

52 CUTANEOUS DRUG REACTIONS

BRUCE U. WINTROUB / ROBERT S. STERN

Cutaneous reactions are among the most frequent adverse reactions to drugs. Early in drug-induced illness, prompt therapeutic intervention may limit toxicity. This chapter focuses on adverse cutaneous reactions to drugs other than topical agents and reviews the incidence, patterns, and pathogenesis of cutaneous reactions to drugs and therapeutic agents.

USE OF PRESCRIPTION DRUGS IN THE UNITED STATES More than 1.5 billion prescriptions for 60,000 drug products, which include approximately 2000 different active agents, are dispensed each year in the United States. Hospital inpatients alone annually receive about 120 million courses of drug therapy, and half of adult Americans receive prescription drugs on a regular outpatient basis. As much as 15 percent of hospital days are devoted to treatment for drug toxicity.

INCIDENCE OF CUTANEOUS REACTIONS Although adverse drug reactions are common, it is difficult to ascertain their incidence, seriousness, and ultimate health effects. The fact that comprehensive information on these reactions is inadequate in part reflects the difficulty in establishing a system for postmarketing surveillance that is both economically feasible and capable of generating clinically useful data. Available information comes from evaluations of hospitalized patients, epidemiologic surveys, premarketing studies, and voluntary reporting.

In one study about 2 percent of medical inpatients had skin reactions consisting of rash, urticaria, or pruritus during hospitalization, and the overall reaction rate per course of drug therapy was 3:1000. Penicillins, sulfonamides, and blood products accounted for two-thirds of cutaneous reactions. Specific algorithmic estimates of drug-specific quantitative reaction rates for drugs commonly used in inpatients were calculated. Reaction rates for selected commonly used drugs are summarized in Table 52-1. This study showed that most cutaneous reactions occur within 1 week of exposure to the drug. Exceptions were semisynthetic penicillins and ampicillin; about half the reactions to these drugs occurred more than 1 week after initial administration. The risk of allergic reactions was not related to age, diagnosis, or blood level of urea nitrogen on admission. Skin reactions were more frequent among women.

The distribution of morphologic patterns of drug eruptions cared for within a Finnish hospital dermatology department with a special interest in fixed drug eruptions included exanthematous reactions (32 percent), urticaria and/or angioedema (20 percent), fixed drug eruptions (34 percent), erythema multiforme (2 percent), Stevens-Johnson syndrome (1 percent), exfoliative dermatitis (1 percent), and photosensitivity reactions (3 percent).

Documenting the risk of the most serious forms of drug eruptions associated with specific drugs remains an important challenge. Based on successful population-based retrospective case registries of toxic epidermal necrolysis and Stevens-Johnson syndrome in Germany and France, there are now prospective registries that serve as the basis

TABLE 52-1   Rates (per 1000 recipients) of skin reactions to selected medications

Drug	Reaction rate
Amoxicillin	51
Trimethoprim-sulfamethoxazole	34
Ampicillin	33
Other penicillins	20
Blood	21
Allopurinol	8
Centamycin	5
Barbiturates	4

SOURCE: Adapted from Bigby et al.

for case-control studies in these and other countries. These data, together with data from health-maintenance organizations and Medicaid, suggest that the risk of these reactions is from 1 to 10 per million person-years. The drugs most often associated with these reactions include the sulfonamide antibiotics, the aminopenicillins, phenytoin and structurally related antiseizure medications, and some nonsteroidal anti-inflammatory drugs.

PATHOGENESIS OF DRUG REACTIONS

Untoward cutaneous responses to drugs can arise as a result of immunologic or nonimmunologic mechanisms. Immunologic reactions require activation of host immunologic pathways and are designated *drug allergy*. Drug reactions occurring through nonimmunologic mechanisms may be due to activation of effector pathways, overdosage, cumulative toxicity, side effects, ecologic disturbance, interactions between drugs, metabolic alterations, exacerbation of preexisting dermatologic conditions, or inherited protein or enzyme deficiencies. Nonimmunologic cutaneous reactions to drugs are more common, and immunologic reactions are unpredictable when they do occur. It is often not possible to specify the responsible drug or pathogenic mechanism because the skin responds to a variety of stimuli through a limited number of reaction patterns. The mechanism of many drug reactions is unknown.

IMMUNOLOGIC DRUG REACTIONS   Drugs frequently elicit an immune response, but only a small number of individuals experience clinical hypersensitivity reactions. For example, most patients exposed to penicillin develop demonstrable antibodies to penicillin but do not manifest drug reactions when exposed to penicillin. Multiple factors determine the capacity of a drug to elicit an immune response, including the *molecular characteristics* of the drug and *host effects*.

Increases in *molecular* size and complexity are associated with increased immunogenicity, and macromolecular drugs such as protein or peptide hormones are highly antigenic. Most drugs are small organic molecules less than 1000 daltons in size, and the capacity of such small molecules to elicit an immune response depends on their ability to act as haptens, i.e., to form stable, usually covalent, bonds with tissue macromolecules. Fortunately, most drugs have little or no ability to form covalent bonds with tissue components, and clinical sensitization results from minor contaminants or conversion of the drugs themselves to reactive metabolic products.

Route of administration of a drug or simple chemical can influence the nature of the *host* immune response. For example, topical application of antigens tends to induce delayed hypersensitivity, and exposure to antigens via oral or nasal cavities stimulates production of secretory immunoglobins, IgA and IgE, and occasionally IgM. Some agents, such as pentadecacatechol, sensitize readily if applied to the skin but do so poorly if ingested orally or applied to a mucosal surface. Frequency of sensitization through intravenous administration of drugs varies, but anaphylaxis is a more likely clinical consequence with this route of exposure.

The degree of drug exposure and individual variability in absorption and metabolism of a given agent may alter immunogenic load. The variable degree of in vivo acetylation of hydralazine provides a clinical example of this phenomenon. Hydralazine produces a lupus-like syndrome associated with antinuclear antibody formation more frequently in patients who acetylate the drug slowly. Frequent high-dose and interrupted courses of therapy are also important risk factors for development of drug allergy.

Pathogenesis of allergic drug reactions   IgE-dependent drug reactions are usually manifest in the skin and gastrointestinal, respiratory, and cardiovascular systems (see Chap. 282). Primary symptoms and signs include pruritus, urticaria, nausea, vomiting, cramps, bronchospasm, and laryngeal edema and, on occasion, anaphylactic shock with hypotension and death. Immediate reactions may occur within minutes of drug exposure, and accelerated reactions occur hours or days after drug administration. Accelerated reactions are usually urticarial and may include laryngeal edema. IgE-dependent reactions are usually due to penicillins; manifestations are caused by release from sensitized tissue mast cells or circulating basophilic leukocytes of chemical mediators such as histamine, adenosine, leukotrienes, prostaglandins, platelet-activating factor, enzymes, and proteoglycans. Release is triggered when polyvalent drug protein conjugates cross-link IgE molecules fixed to sensitized cells. The clinical manifestations are determined by interaction of the released chemical mediator with its target organ, i.e., skin, respiratory, gastrointestinal, and/or cardiovascular systems. Certain routes of administration favor different clinical patterns (i.e., oral route: gastrointestinal effects; intravenous route: circulating effects).

Immune-complex–dependent reactions   Serum sickness is produced by circulating immune complexes and is characterized by fever, arthritis, nephritis, neuritis, edema, and an urticarial, papular, or pruritic rash (see Chap. 283). The syndrome requires an antigen that remains in the circulation for prolonged periods so that when antibody is synthesized, circulating antigen-antibody complexes are formed. Serum sickness was first described following administration of foreign sera, but drugs are now the usual cause. Drugs that produce serum sickness include the penicillins, sulfonamides, thiouracils, cholecystographic dyes, phenytoin, aminosalicylic acid, streptomycin, heparin, and antilymphocyte globulin. Symptoms develop 6 days or more after exposure to a drug, the latent period representing the time needed to synthesize antibody. The antibodies responsible for immune-complex–dependent drug reactions are largely of the IgG or IgM class.

Cytotoxic drug–induced reactions   Immunologic reactions to drugs may damage kidneys, heart, lungs, liver, muscle, peripheral nerves, or formed elements of the blood by at least three mechanisms. First, a drug may react with the tissue and introduce haptenic groups on a cell surface that renders the tissue susceptible to antibody- or lymphocyte-mediated cytotoxicity. Second, drug-antibody complexes formed in the fluid phase may bind to the cell surface and damage the cell as an "innocent bystander." Third, drugs may induce immune responses that involve formed blood elements such as platelets and erythrocytes but do not cause cutaneous allergic drug reactions.

Cell-mediated immune responses play a role in contact drug hypersensitivity and are suspected to participate in other allergic drug reactions (i.e., pulmonary infiltration).

NONIMMUNOLOGIC DRUG REACTIONS   Nonimmunologic mechanisms are responsible for the majority of drug reactions.

Nonimmunologic activation of effector pathways   Drug reactions may result from nonimmunologic activation of effector pathways by three mechanisms: First, drugs may release mediators directly from mast cells and basophils and present as anaphylaxis or as urticaria and/or angioedema. Urticarial anaphylactic reactions induced by opiates, polymyxin B, tubocurarine, radiocontrast media, and dextrans may occur by this mechanism. Second, drugs may activate complement in the absence of antibody. This is an additional mechanism through which radiocontrast media may act. Third, drugs such as aspirin and other nonsteroidal anti-inflammatory agents may alter pathways of arachidonic acid metabolism; such drugs inhibit the cyclooxygenase that catalyzes the generation of prostaglandins from arachidonic acid in vitro.

Overdosage   The manifestations of overdosage are predictable for most drugs; symptoms are an exaggeration of the drug's pharmacologic action. Overdosage can, at times, be observed in patients given the usual doses of a drug because of differing rates of absorption, metabolism, or excretion. An example is easy bruisability caused by warfarin overdose.

Phototoxicity   Phototoxic reactions may be drug-induced or may occur in metabolic disorders in which an appropriate photosensitizing chemical is overproduced. In each case the phototoxic reaction occurs when enough chromophore (drug or metabolic product) absorbs sufficient radiation in reactive tissue. Drug-induced phototoxic reactions can occur on first exposure, and the incidence of phototoxicity is a direct function of the concentration of sensitizer and amount of light. At least three distinct photochemical mechanisms have been described: First, the reaction between the excited state of a phototoxic molecule and a biologic target may cause formation of a covalent photoaddition product. Second, the phototoxic molecule may absorb protons to form stable photoproducts that are toxic to biologic substrates. Third, radiation of a phototoxic molecule may result in transfer of energy to oxygen molecules and cause formation of toxic oxygen species, such as singlet oxygen, superoxide anion, or hydroxyl radical. Interaction of these species with biologic targets produces photooxidized molecules. Serum protein–dependent systems and circulating effector cells play a role in acute in vivo phototoxic tissue damage due to exogenous agents; normal numbers of polymorphonuclear leukocytes and an intact complement system are required for the full development of demeclocycline-induced phototoxic lesions.

Cumulative toxicity The cumulative effects of drug deposition in skin may cause disturbance in skin color. In some instances, the drug is deposited in phagocytic cells of skin or mucous membranes, as occurs after prolonged administration of silver, bismuth, mercury, or gold. In other instances, the drug or its metabolic derivatives may bind to a component of the skin (e.g., melanin), as in patients taking high doses of chlorpromazine.

Secondary or side effects Secondary effects occur uniformly as part of the normal pharmacologic action of a drug but are not the primary therapeutic objective. Examples include alopecia, gastrointestinal disturbances, or hematopoietic depression during use of chemotherapeutic agents.

Ecologic disturbances These reactions result from drug-dependent alterations of normal flora of the skin, gut, or mucous membranes, permitting overgrowth of an organism (e.g., anogenital and oral candidiasis during administration of a broad-spectrum antibiotic).

Drug interactions Drugs may interact to cause adverse reactions. First, drugs may compete for the same plasma protein binding sites. For example, warfarin may be displaced from its binding site by phenylbutazone or aspirin and result in hemorrhage. Second, a drug may inhibit or stimulate metabolic enzymes important to its degradation or to that of another agent. Third, one drug may interfere with the excretion of another; for example, probenecid reduces penicillin excretion by the kidney.

Metabolic changes Drugs may sufficiently alter nutritional or metabolic status to induce cutaneous changes. For example, drugs, such as phenytoin, that interfere with folate absorption or metabolism increase the risk of aphthous stomatitis. In addition, drugs that alter lipid metabolism, such as isotretinoin, cause xanthomas by elevation of very low-density lipoproteins.

Exacerbation of preexisting diseases A variety of agents can exacerbate preexisting diseases. For example, lithium can exacerbate acne and psoriasis in a dose-dependent manner. Beta-blocking agents may induce a psoriasiform dermatitis, and withdrawal of glucocorticoids can exacerbate psoriasis or atopic dermatitis. Exacerbations of cutaneous lupus have been noted in association with cimetidine use. Vasodilators may exacerbate rosacea.

Inherited enzyme or protein deficiencies Drug reactions may also occur as the result of inherited enzyme deficiencies. For example, patients may be deficient in an enzyme required for metabolism of the drug or clearance of a toxic drug metabolite. The phenytoin hypersensitivity syndrome occurs in patients deficient in epoxide hydrolase, an enzyme required for metabolism of a toxic epoxide derived from phenytoin. Second, patients may be deficient in an enzyme required for normal function of a biochemical pathway, and further drug-induced lowering of the factor may cause pathologic manifestations. An example is warfarin sodium (Coumadin) necrosis of skin in patients with heterozygote deficiency of protein C, a proenzyme required for normal thrombolytic function. In contrast, heparin-induced cutaneous necrosis, which has some clinical similarity to warfarin necrosis, appears to be an immune-complex reaction.

Alterations of immunologic status Alterations in patients' immunologic status also may modify the risk of cutaneous reactions. Bone marrow transplant patients often experience cutaneous reactions to drugs. These reactions may be very difficult to differentiate from acute graft-versus-host reactions even when skin biopsy is obtained.

HIV-infected persons appear to be at very high risk of developing cutaneous eruptions, and this increased risk is not accounted for merely by the higher number of drugs utilized by these patients (see Chap. 279). The risk of these reactions increases as immunologic function deteriorates. Skin reactions to trimethoprim-sulfamethoxazole are seen in about a third of HIV-infected users of this drug. Dapsone, trimethoprim alone, and amoxicillin-clavulanate are also frequent causes of drug eruptions in these patients. Some drugs result in specific problems in HIV-infected persons. For example, foscarnet causes a painful penile ulcer in a substantial fraction of users. HIV-infected persons also appear to be at higher risk of the most serious types of reactions, including toxic epidermal necrolysis and Stevens-Johnson syndrome.

CHARACTERISTIC FEATURES OF CUTANEOUS DRUG REACTIONS

Cutaneous disorders induced by drugs by known mechanisms include urticaria, photosensitivity, disturbances of pigmentation, vasculitis, phenytoin hypersensitivity syndrome, and warfarin necrosis of skin. Reactions of uncertain mechanism include morbilliform reactions, erythema multiforme, fixed drug reactions, erythema nodosum, lichenoid reactions, bullous drug reaction, and toxic epidermal necrolysis.

REACTIONS OF KNOWN CAUSE **Urticaria** *Urticaria* is a skin reaction characterized by pruritic, red wheals. Lesions may vary from a small point to a large area. Individual lesions rarely last more than 24 h. When deep dermal and subcutaneous tissues are also swollen, this reaction is known as *angioedema*. Angioedema may involve mucous membranes and may be part of a life-threatening anaphylactic reaction. Urticarial lesions, along with pruritus and morbilliform (or maculopapular) eruptions, are among the most frequent types of cutaneous reactions to drugs.

Drug-induced urticaria may be caused by three mechanisms: an IgE-dependent mechanism, circulating immune complexes (serum sickness), and nonimmunologic activation of effector pathways. IgE-dependent urticarial reactions usually occur within 36 h but can occur within minutes. Reactions occurring within minutes to hours of drug exposure are termed *immediate reactions*, whereas those which occur 12 to 36 h after drug exposure are designated *accelerated reactions*. Immune-complex–induced urticaria associated with serum sickness may occur from 4 to 12 days after challenge. In this syndrome, the urticarial eruption may be accompanied by fever, hematuria, and arthralgias, hepatic dysfunction, and neurologic symptoms.

Certain drugs, such as nonsteroidal anti-inflammatory agents, the angiotensin-converting enzyme (ACE) inhibitors, and radiographic dyes, may induce urticarial reactions, angioedema, and anaphylaxis whose time course resembles that of immediate IgE-dependent reactions. Drug-specific antibody does not play a role in such reactions, and in some cases they are thought to be induced by the action of drug on cutaneous mast cells, complement, or arachidonic acid–dependent pathways. For the ACE inhibitors, inhibition of kinin may be responsible for these reactions, which can be life-threatening. Although aspirin, penicillin, and blood products are the most frequent causes of urticarial eruptions, urticaria has been observed in association with nearly all drugs.

Drugs also may cause chronic urticaria, which lasts more than 6 weeks. The mechanisms of chronic urticaria are unclear. Aspirin frequently exacerbates this problem.

Photosensitivity eruptions Photosensitivity eruptions are usually most marked in sun-exposed areas but may extend to sun-protected areas. Phototoxic reactions are more common than photoallergic reactions. Phototoxic reactions usually resemble sunburn, can occur with the first exposure to a drug, and are dose-related. The action spectrum for phototoxicity is similar to the ultraviolet absorption spectrum of the drug. No single test system seems to be a successful predictor of the photosensitivity potential for a given compound.

The mechanism for photoallergy to systemic medications is not well defined. Drug, immune response, and light are required to produce clinical photoallergy, and photoallergic reactions may be delayed hypersensitivity responses. Eruptions range from lichenoid papules to eczematous changes.

Orally administered drugs that cause photoallergic or phototoxic reactions include chlorpromazine, tetracycline, thiazides, nalidixic acid, and two nonsteroidal anti-inflammatory agents, the quinadone antibiotics benoxaprofen and piroxicam. Based on test systems, the majority of the common photosensitizers seem to have action spectrums in the long-wave ultraviolet (UV-A) range and are usually phototoxic. This is fortunate, since phototoxic reactions will abate with removal of either the drug or ultraviolet radiation, but some photoallergic reactions may persist after the drug is withdrawn. Because UV-A and visible light which trigger these reactions are not easily absorbed by nonopaque sunscreens, these reactions may be difficult to block.

Drugs also may induce photosensitivity diseases. For example, procainamide may induce systemic lupus erythematosus.

Pigmentation changes   Drugs may cause a variety of pigmentary changes in the skin. Some drugs stimulate melanocytic activity and increase pigmentation. Drug deposition also can lead to pigmentation; this phenomenon occurs with heavy metals. Phenothiazines may be deposited in the skin and cause a slate-gray color. Antimalarial drugs may cause a slate-gray or yellow pigmentation. Inorganic arsenic, once used to treat psoriasis, is associated with diffuse macular pigmentation. Other heavy metals that cause pigmentary changes include silver, gold, bismuth, and mercury. Long-term use of phenytoin can produce a chloasma-like pigmentation in women. Certain cytostatic agents also can cause pigmentary changes. Histologic examination is often diagnostic for drug deposition diseases.

Zidovudine (AZT) is a frequent cause of pigmentation, especially of the nails. Clofazimine, an aminophenazine dye used in the treatment of leprosy, causes a red skin color that is so marked that some patients discontinue therapy. Methysergide produces a red color in the skin and an orange-peel-like texture. Nicotinic acid in large doses may cause brown pigmentation. Oral contraceptives may produce chloasma, and adrenocorticotropin may cause a hypermelanosis similar to that of primary adrenal insufficiency. In addition, amiodarone may cause violaceous hyperpigmentation which is increased in sun-exposed skin. Drugs such as heavy metals, copper, antimalarial and arsenical agents, and ACTH also may discolor oral mucosa.

Vasculitis   Cutaneous necrotizing vasculitis often presents as palpable purpuric lesions that may be generalized or limited to the lower extremities or other dependent areas (see Chap. 291). Urticarial lesions, ulcers, and hemorrhagic blisters also occur. Vasculitis may involve other organs, including the liver, kidney, brain, and joints. Drugs are only one cause of vasculitis. Immune-complex–dependent mechanisms are probably responsible for drug-induced vasculitis and/or serum sickness. Propylthiouracil induces a cutaneous vasculitis that is accompanied by leukopenia and splenomegaly. Direct immunofluorescent changes in these lesions suggest immune-complex deposition. Drugs implicated in vasculitic eruptions include allopurinol, thiazides, penicillin, and phenytoin.

Phenytoin hypersensitivity reaction   The phenytoin hypersensitivity reaction, one of many phenytoin-induced cutaneous reactions, is an erythematous eruption that eventually becomes purpuric and is accompanied by fever, facial and periorbital edema, tender generalized lymphadenopathy, leukocytosis (often with atypical lymphocytes and eosinophils), hepatitis, and sometimes nephritis. The cutaneous reaction usually begins 1 to 3 weeks after phenytoin is begun and resolves rapidly with drug cessation and treatment with systemic glucocorticoids. The eruption recurs with rechallenge, and crossreactions with other anticonvulsants with similar structures, including carbamazepine and barbiturates, are frequent. This syndrome appar-

ently results from an inherited deficiency of epoxide hydrolase, an enzyme required for metabolism of a toxic intermediate arene oxide that is formed during metabolism of phenytoin by the cytochrome P450 system.

Warfarin necrosis of the skin   This rare reaction occurs usually between the third and tenth days of therapy with warfarin derivatives, usually in women. Lesions are sharply demarcated, erythematous, indurated, and purpuric and may resolve or progress to formation of large, irregular, hemorrhagic bullae with eventual necrosis and slow-healing eschar formation.

Development of the syndrome is unrelated to drug dose or underlying condition. Favored sites are breasts, thighs, and buttocks. The course is not altered by discontinuation of the drug after onset of the eruption. Similar reactions have been associated with heparin. Warfarin reactions are associated with protein C deficiency. Protein C is a vitamin K–dependent protein with a shorter half-life than other clotting proteins and is in part responsible for control of fibrinolysis. Since warfarin inhibits synthesis of vitamin K–dependent coagulation factors, warfarin anticoagulation in heterozygotes for protein C deficiency causes a precipitous fall in circulating levels of protein C, permitting hypercoagulability and thrombosis in the cutaneous microvasculature, with consequent areas of necrosis.

REACTIONS OF UNCERTAIN CAUSE   Morbilliform reactions   *Morbilliform* or *maculopapular eruptions* may be the most common of all drug-induced reactions, often start on the trunk or areas of pressure or trauma, and consist of erythematous macules and papules that are frequently symmetric and may become confluent. Involvement of mucous membranes, palms, and soles is variable; the eruption may be associated with moderate to severe pruritus and fever.

The pathogenesis is unclear. A hypersensitivity mechanism has been suggested, although these reactions do not always recur following drug rechallenge. Diagnosis is rarely assisted by laboratory tests; differentiation from viral exanthem is the principal differential diagnostic consideration. While these reactions usually require discontinuation of drug (dechallenge), eruptions occasionally may decrease or fade with continued use of the responsible drug.

Morbilliform reactions usually develop within 1 week of initiation of therapy and last 1 to 2 weeks; however, reactions to some drugs, especially penicillin, may begin more than 2 weeks after therapy has begun and last as long as 2 weeks after therapy has ceased. These eruptions are common in patients receiving ampicillin, amoxicillin, or allopurinol; trimethoprim-sulfamethoxazole causes frequent reactions in AIDS patients.

Erythema multiforme   *Erythema multiforme* is an acute, self-limited inflammatory disorder of skin and mucous membranes characterized by distinctive iris or target lesions, often associated with sore throat and malaise. Many drugs, including sulfonamides, penicillin, phenytoin, and phenylbutazone, can cause erythema multiforme; long-acting sulfonamides are the best-studied. Erythema multiforme resulting from sulfonamides typically begins after 1 to 2 weeks of drug therapy and is accompanied by fever and mucous membrane reaction (Stevens-Johnson syndrome). An immune-complex–induced, lymphocyte-mediated mechanism may be responsible.

Fixed drug reactions   These reactions are characterized by one or more sharply demarcated, erythematous lesions in which hyperpigmentation results after resolution of the acute inflammation; with rechallenge, the lesion recurs in the same (i.e., "fixed") location. Lesions often involve the face, genitalia, and oral mucosa and cause burning. Fixed drug eruptions have been associated with phenolphthalein, sulfonamides, tetracycline, phenylbutazone, and barbiturates. Although cross-sensitivity appears to occur between different tetracycline compounds, cross-sensitivity was not elicited when different sulfonamide compounds were administered to patients as part of provocation testing.

Documentation of a characteristic papillary-dermal mononuclear cell infiltrate in close approximation to the dermoepidermal junction may confirm the clinical diagnosis. Extensive basal cell degeneration can lead to formation of bullae and pigment dispersion. Even when lesions are completely healed, melanin-laden macrophages are present in the dermis.

Erythema nodosum *Erythema nodosum* is a panniculitis characterized by tender, subcutaneous, erythematous nodules, usually on the anterior portion of the legs. Drug hypersensitivity, frequently involving oral contraceptives, is one cause of this reaction. The mechanism is unknown.

Lichenoid drug eruptions A *lichenoid cutaneous reaction*, clinically and morphologically indistinguishable from lichen planus, is associated with a variety of drugs and chemicals. Eosinophils in lichen planus are more common when the reaction is drug-induced. Gold and antimalarials are most often associated with this eruption. Antihypertensive agents, including beta blockers and captopril, also have been reported to cause a lichenoid reaction.

Bullous eruptions Blisters accompany a wide variety of cutaneous reactions, especially the severe morbilliform eruptions, and may be an integral part of erythema multiforme, toxic epidermal necrolysis, and fixed drug eruptions. Nalidixic acid and furosemide cause blistering eruptions indistinguishable from the primary bullous diseases. Other examples are a pemphigus foliaceus–like eruption seen with penicillamine and cicatricial pemphigoid that has been seen with clonidine.

Pustular eruptions Active *pustular exanthemic eruptions* also are associated with exposure to drugs, most notably antibiotics. These eruptions can be distinguished from pustular psoriasis by more rapid onset of fever and pustulation and their rapid spontaneous resolution with drug withdrawal.

Toxic epidermal necrolysis *Toxic epidermal necrolysis* is the most serious cutaneous drug reaction and may be fatal. Drugs are the most frequent cause in adults. Onset is generally acute and is characterized by epidermal necrosis with a minimal dermal inflammatory process. This reaction is often associated with sulfonamides, aminopenicillins, anticonvulsants, nonsteroidal anti-inflammatory agents, and allopurinol and has been reported with measles vaccine, fumigants, and phenytoin.

DRUGS OF SPECIAL INTEREST

PENICILLIN The incidence of reactions to penicillin is about 1 percent. Not all adverse reactions are immunologic, as illustrated by ampicillin-induced morbilliform eruptions and central nervous system reactions to procaine penicillin.

IgG, IgM, and IgE antibodies can be produced; IgG and IgM anti-penicillin antibodies play a role in the development of hemolytic anemia, whereas anaphylaxis and serum sickness appear to be due to IgE antibodies in serum.

Since penicillin reactions often occur in patients without a prior history of penicillin allergy, the utility of accurate and easily administered tests for sensitization is apparent. Current practice is to perform skin testing with a commercially available penicilloyl determinant preparation (Pre-pen, Kremers-Urban) and with fresh penicillin and, if possible, with another source of minor (nonpenicilloyl) determinants such as aged or base-treated penicillin. Antibodies to minor determinants are common in patients experiencing anaphylaxis. Testing with major determinants alone detects most patients at risk for anaphylaxis.

Twenty-seven percent (10 to 36 percent) of patients with a positive history of penicillin allergy also have a positive skin test, while 6 percent (3 to 10 percent) with a negative history demonstrate a positive skin response to penicillin. Administering penicillin to those patients with a positive skin test produces reactions in a high proportion (50 to 100 percent); conversely, only a few patients (about 0.5 percent) with negative skin tests react to the drug, and reactions tend to be mild and to occur late. Since a negative skin test may occur during or just after an acute reaction, testing should be performed either prospectively or several months after a suspected reaction. As many as 80 percent of patients lose anaphylactic sensitivity and IgE antibody after several years. Radioallergosorbent test (RAST) and other in vitro tests offer no advantage over properly performed skin testing.

Some cross-reactivity exists between penicillin and nonpenicillin β-lactam antibiotics (e.g., cephalosporins). About half of patients who react to penicillin skin testing also react to cephalosporin skin testing; anaphylaxis from cephalosporins has occurred in patients testing positive to penicillin. The benefit of skin testing with penicillin derivatives and cephalosporins in addition to penicillin is uncertain; in one study, none of 120 patients with negative results to penicillin skin tests reacted to semisynthetic penicillinase-resistant agents.

In the face of a positive clinical history of penicillin reaction, another drug should be chosen. If this is not feasible or prudent (e.g., in a pregnant patient with syphilis; with enterococcal endocarditis), skin testing with penicillin is warranted. If skin tests are negative, cautious administration of penicillin is acceptable, although some recommend desensitization of such patients. In those with positive skin tests, desensitization is mandatory if therapeutic use of β-lactam antibiotics is to be undertaken. Various protocols are available, including oral and parenteral approaches. Oral desensitization appears to carry a lesser risk of serious anaphylactic reactions during desensitization. However, desensitization carries the risk of anaphylaxis regardless of how it is performed. After desensitization, many patients experience non-life-threatening IgE-mediated untoward reactions to penicillin during their course of therapy. Desensitization is not effective in those with exfoliative dermatitis or morbilliform reactions due to penicillin.

NONSTEROIDAL ANTI-INFLAMMATORY DRUGS Nonsteroidal anti-inflammatory drugs (NSAIDs), including aspirin (but not salicylates in general) and indomethacin (indometacin), cause two broad categories of allergic-like symptoms in susceptible individuals: (1) approximately 1 percent of persons experience urticaria or angioedema, and (2) about half as many (0.5 percent) experience rhinosinusitis and asthma; however, about 10 percent of adult asthmatics and one-third of individuals with nasal polyposis and sinusitis may respond adversely to aspirin.

Urticaria/angioedema may be delayed up to 24 h and may occur at any age. The rhinosinusitis-asthma syndrome generally develops within 1 h of drug administration. In young people, the reaction pattern often begins as watery rhinorrhea, which can be complicated by nasal and sinus infection, and polyposis, bloody discharge, and nasal eosinophilia. In many individuals with this syndrome, asthma eventually ensues that can be life-threatening whenever NSAIDs are subsequently ingested, and symptoms may persist despite avoidance of these drugs. Proof of the association of symptoms and NSAID use requires either clear-cut history of symptoms following drug ingestion or an oral challenge. For the latter to be performed with relative safety, (1) asthma must be under good control, (2) the procedure must be conducted in a hospital setting by experienced personnel capable of recognizing and treating acute respiratory responses, and (3) the challenge should begin with very low doses (i.e., <30 mg) of aspirin and increase every 1 to 2 h in doubling doses as tolerated to 650 mg. In a study of 50 consecutive patients with a positive history of aspirin-induced bronchospasm, 84 percent developed pulmonary or naso-ocular symptoms with aspirin, but 16 percent did not react; moreover, when subjects who initially tested positive to a challenge were reexposed to aspirin, the clinical reaction pattern was identical in only 60 percent.

While cross-reactivity between NSAIDs is common, it is not immunologic, and patients who are sensitive to NSAIDs cannot be identified by assessment of IgE antibody to aspirin, lymphocyte sensitization, or in vitro immunologic testing. All cross-reacting drugs are cyclooxygenase inhibitors, although salicylates also inhibit cyclooxygenase but (except for aspirin) do not cause the response.

"Desensitization" to the adverse effects of NSAIDs can be accomplished by the challenge procedure above, although repeated challenge at the initial provocation dose may be required. Desensitization works by unknown mechanisms, renders the subject tolerant to all NSAIDs yet studied, persists for at least 24 and up to 96 h, and is probably universal but does not have a positive effect on the underlying disorder.

RADIOCONTRAST MEDIA   Large numbers of patients are exposed to radiocontrast agents, and 5 to 10 percent of patients receiving them develop some reaction: urticaria in 1 percent, dyspnea in 0.25 percent, and death in 0.01 percent. Reactions consisting of urticaria and angioedema, asthma, and hypotension mimicking anaphylaxis occur in less than 1 percent of radiocontrast procedures. About one-third of those with mild reactions to previous exposure reexact on reexposure.

There is no proof of an immunologic mechanism for radiocontrast media reactions. Elevations in plasma histamine occur in those with and without reaction and may be due to the hypertonicity of these media. In addition, complement activation by both classical and alternative pathways occurs in normal and reactive individuals. In short, the mechanism for these reactions is not understood, and no test identifies patients at risk for a radiocontrast medium reaction. Because repeat reactions are common, obtaining a thorough history is the best available technique for identifying those most likely to experience an adverse reaction. Several pretreatment regimens are claimed to decrease repeat reaction rate to about 10 percent. One such regimen consists of 50 mg prednisone at 13, 7, and 1 h before the procedure and 50 mg diphenhydramine 1 h before the procedure.

HYDANTOINS   Phenytoin and other hydantoins cause morbilliform eruptions, erythema multiforme, and toxic epidermal necrolysis, as well as a hypersensitivity reaction (described above) and the pseudolymphoma syndrome. In one study, 5 percent of children treated with phenytoin developed a mild dose-dependent, maculopapular eruption lasting 3 to 5 days and occurring within 2 weeks of starting treatment.

The pseudolymphoma syndrome, consisting of lymphadenopathy and histopathologic lymph node atypia, is a more chronic form of the phenytoin hypersensitivity syndrome, and the cutaneous changes are less marked in this syndrome.

Use of phenytoin is frequently associated with gingival hyperplasia and rarely with a syndrome similar to systemic lupus erythematosus, severe exfoliative dermatitis, and polyarteritis nodosa. Because many hydantoin side effects may be dose-related, drugs that interfere with its elimination (e.g., chloramphenicol) effectively prolong those effects. Sulfasalazine, other sulfonamides, and allopurinol cause reactions that are indistinguishable from the phenytoin hypersensitivity syndrome.

THIAZIDES AND SULFONAMIDES   Thiazides are among the most common causes of drug-induced urticaria and morbilliform eruptions; they also cause erythema multiforme, drug-induced cutaneous vasculitis, and lichenoid and photosensitivity eruptions. Because they are substituted sulfonamides, antibodies to these diuretics may cross-react with sulfonamide antibiotics and sulfonamide-based hypoglycemic agents. The combination of sulfamethoxazole and trimethoprim causes two distinct cutaneous reactions: (1) an urticarial eruption beginning in the first few days of treatment and (2) a morbilliform eruption often occurring more than 1 week after therapy has begun. The morbilliform reaction is frequent in patients with AIDS and is associated with pancytopenia in some patients. The eruption may have an intensely purpuric characacter, independent of the presence of vasculitis. One patient developed toxic epidermal necrolysis and pancytopenia following administration of sulfamethoxazale-trimethoprim.

AGENTS USED IN CANCER CHEMOTHERAPY   Since many agents used in cancer chemotherapy inhibit cell division, rapidly proliferating elements of the skin, including hair, mucous membranes, and appendages, are sensitive to their effects; as a result, stomatitis and alopecia are among the most frequent dose-dependent side effects of chemotherapy. Onychodystrophy (dystrophic changes in nails) is also seen with bleomycin, hydroxyurea (hydroxycarbamide), and 5-fluorouracil. Sterile cellulitis and phlebitis and ulceration of pressure areas occur with many of these agents. Urticaria, angioedema, exfoliative dermatitis, and erythema of the palms and soles also have been seen, as has local and diffuse hyperpigmentation. Diagnosis and treatment of these reactions are especially difficult because of the underlying malignancy.

TETRACYCLINES   While urticaria and morbilliform eruptions are unusual, tetracyclines sometimes cause other cutaneous side effects, including a photosensitivity reaction (as a result of drug-induced phototoxicity) and onycholysis (sometimes with no apparent cutaneous photosensitivity). These reactions occur with demeclocycline, doxycycline, minocycline, tetracycline, and oxytetracycline. Tetracyclines also cause fixed drug and lichenoid eruptions. An acnelike, gram-negative folliculitis with long-term use of tetracycline is due to overgrowth of resistant bacteria.

Several pigmentary abnormalities have been noted. If used during pregnancy or early childhood, tetracycline stains the teeth, sometimes permanently. Minocyline can cause hyperpigmentation in sun-exposed areas and in areas of previous inflammation. Histiocytes that contain iron are responsible for the pigmentary changes. Tetracycline also has been associated with a flulike syndrome (accompanied by headaches, malaise, and eosinophilia) that recurred with rechallenge. A serum sickness–like reaction to minocycline also has been reported.

GLUCOCORTICOIDS   Both systemic and topical glucocorticoids cause a variety of skin changes, including acneiform eruptions, atrophy, striae, and other stigmata of Cushing's syndrome, and in sufficiently high doses can retard wound healing. Patients using glucocorticoids are at higher risk for bacterial, yeast, and fungal skin infections that may be misinterpreted as drug eruptions but are in fact drug side effects instead.

ANTIMALARIAL AGENTS   Antimalarial agents are used as therapy for several skin diseases, including the skin manifestations of lupus and polymorphous light eruption, but they also can induce cutaneous reactions. In patients with asymptomatic porphyria cutanea tarda, chloroquine increases porphyrin levels and may exacerbate the disease.

Pigmentation disturbances, including black pigmentation of the face, mucous membranes, and pretibial and subungual areas, occur with antimalarials, and quinacrine (mepacrine) causes generalized, cutaneous yellow discoloration. Antimalarial agents may exacerbate psoriasis, and exfoliative dermatitis, fixed drug eruptions, lichenoid dermatitis, and erythema annulare centrifugum have all been reported with their use.

GOLD   Chrysotherapy has been associated with a variety of dose-related dermatologic reactions (including maculopapular eruptions) that can develop as long as 2 years after initiation of therapy and require months to resolve. Erythema nodosum, psoriasiform dermatitis, vaginal pruritus, eruptions similar to pityriasis rosea, hyperpigmentation, and lichenoid eruptions resembling those seen with antimalarial agents have been reported. After a cutaneous reaction, it is sometimes possible to reinstitute gold therapy at lower doses without recurrence of the dermatitis.

DIAGNOSIS OF DRUG REACTIONS

Possible causes of an adverse reaction can be assessed as definite, probable, possible, or unlikely based on six variables: (1) previous experience with the drug in the general population, (2) alternative etiologic candidates, (3) timing of events, (4) drug levels or evidence of overdose, (5) patient reaction to dechallenge, and (6) patient reaction to rechallenge.

PREVIOUS EXPERIENCE   Tables of relative reaction rates are available and are useful to assess the likelihood that a given drug is responsible for a given cutaneous reaction. The specific morphologic pattern of a drug reaction, however, may modify these reaction rates by increasing or decreasing the likelihood that a given drug is responsible for a given reaction. For example, since fixed eruptions due to drug are more often seen with barbiturates than with penicillin, a fixed drug reaction in a patient taking both types of agents is more likely to be due to the barbiturate, even though penicillins have a higher overall drug reaction rate.

ALTERNATIVE ETIOLOGIC CANDIDATES A cutaneous eruption may be due to exacerbation of preexisting disease or to development of new disease unrelated to drugs. For example, a patient with psoriasis may have a flare-up of disease coincidental with administration of penicillin for streptococcal infection; in this case, infection is a more likely cause for the flare-up than drug reaction.

TIMING OF EVENTS Since most drug reactions of the skin occur within 1 to 2 weeks of initiation of therapy, reactions beginning after 2 weeks are less likely to be due to drugs.

DRUG LEVELS Some cutaneous reactions are dependent on dosage or cumulative toxicity. For example, lichenoid dermatoses due to gold administration appear more often in patients taking high doses.

DECHALLENGE Most adverse cutaneous reactions to drugs remit with dechallenge (removal of the suspected agent). A reaction is unlikely to be drug-related if improvement occurs without dechallenge or if a patient fails to improve after dechallenge and appropriate therapy.

RECHALLENGE Rechallenge provides the most definitive information concerning adverse cutaneous reactions to drugs, since a reaction failing to recur on rechallenge with a drug is unlikely to be due to that agent. Rechallenge is frequently impractical, however, because the need to ensure patient safety and comfort outweighs the value of the possible information derived from rechallenge.

DIAGNOSIS OF DRUG ALLERGY

Tests for IgE responses include in vivo and in vitro methods, but such tests are available only for a limited number of drugs, including penicillins and cephalosporins, some peptide and protein drugs (insulin, xenogeneic sera), and some agents used for general anesthesia. In vivo testing is accomplished by prick puncture and/or by intradermal skin testing. A wheal-and-flare response 2×2 mm greater than that seen with a saline control within 20 min is considered indicative of IgE-mediated mast cell degranulation, provided (1) the patient is not dermographic, (2) the drug does not nonspecifically degranulate mast cells, (3) the drug concentration is not high enough to be irritating, and (4) the buffer itself does not cause wheal-and-flare responses.

Skin testing with major and minor determinants of penicillins or cephalosporins has proved useful for identifying patients at risk of anaphylactic reactions to these agents. However, skin tests themselves carry a small risk of anaphylaxis. Negative skin tests do not rule out IgE-mediated reactivity, and the risk of anaphylaxis in response to penicillin administration in patients with negative skin tests is about 1 percent; about two-thirds of patients with a positive skin test and history of a previous adverse reaction to penicillin experience an allergic response on rechallenge. Skin tests may be negative in allergic patients receiving antihistamines or in those whose allergy is to determinants not present in the test reagent. Although less well studied, similar techniques can identify patients who are sensitive to protein drugs and to agents such as gallamine and succinylcholine. Most other drugs are small molecules, and skin testing with them is unreliable.

In vitro testing for IgE may be done by assessing the ability of serum to bind to antigen and then to bind radiolabeled antibody to IgE (RAST test) or by assessing the ability of the drug to cause histamine release from basophils from drug-sensitive individuals. The RAST test is sensitive and specific but is not available for most drugs; even in the case of penicillin it is available for major determinants only. Similarly, basophil histamine release is a research technique that is not generally available.

There are no generally available and reliable tests for sensitivity to NSAIDs, to agents that directly degranulate mast cells, or to drugs that cause manifestations via immune-complex–mediated complement activation. Although it is possible to screen for the absence of IgA antibody, the utility of this maneuver in preventing transfusion-associated anaphylaxis in IgA-deficient individuals has not been documented.

REFERENCES

Alanko K et al: Cutaneous drug reactions: Clinical types and causative agents. Five-year survey of inpatients (1981–1985). Acta Derm Venereol (Stockh) 69:223, 1989

Baum C et al: Prescription drug use in 1984 and changes over time. Med Care 26:105, 1988

Bielory L et al: Human serum sickness: A prospective analysis of 35 inpatients treated with equine anti-thymocyte globulin for bone marrow failure. Medicine 67:40, 1988

Bigby M et al: Drug-induced cutaneous reactions: A report from the Boston Collaborative Drug Surveillance Program on 15,438 consecutive inpatients, 1975–1982. JAMA 256:3358, 1986

Chan HL et al: The incidence of erythema multiforme, Stevens-Johnson syndrome, and toxic epidermal necrolysis: A population-based study with particular reference to reactions caused by drugs among outpatients. Arch Dermatol 126:43, 1990

Coopman SA, Stern RS: Cutaneous drug reactions in human immunodeficiency virus infection (editorial). Arch Dermatol 127:714, 1991

Levenson DE et al: Cutaneous manifestations of adverse drug reactions. Immunol Allergy Clin North Am 11:493, 1991

Roujeau JC et al: Toxic epidermal necrolysis (Lyeel syndrome): Incidence and drug etiology in France, 1981–1985. Arch Dermatol 126:37, 1990

——— et al: Acute generalized exanthematous pustulosis: Analysis of 63 cases. Arch Dermatol 127:1333, 1991

Shear NH, Spielberg SP: Anticonvulsant hypersensitivity syndrome: In vitro assessment of risk. J Clin Invest 82:1826, 1988

53 IMMUNOLOGICALLY MEDIATED SKIN DISEASES

KIM B. YANCEY / THOMAS J. LAWLEY

A number of immunologically mediated skin diseases and the cutaneous manifestations of immunologically mediated systemic disorders are now recognized as distinct entities with relatively consistent clinical, histologic, and immunopathologic findings. Many of these disorders are due to autoimmune mechanisms. Clinically, they are characterized by morbidity (pain, pruritus, disfigurement) and in some instances by mortality (largely due to loss of epidermal barrier function and/or secondary infection). The major features of the more common immunologically mediated skin diseases are summarized in this chapter. See Table 53-1.

PEMPHIGUS VULGARIS Pemphigus vulgaris (PV) is a blistering skin disease seen predominantly in elderly patients. Patients with PV have an increased incidence of the HLA-DR4 and -DRw6 serologically defined haplotypes. This disorder is characterized by the loss of cohesion between epidermal cells (a process termed *acantholysis*) with the resultant formation of intraepidermal blisters. Clinical lesions of PV typically consist of flaccid blisters on either normal-appearing or erythematous skin. These blisters rupture easily, leaving denuded areas that may crust and enlarge peripherally. Substantial portions of the body surface may be denuded in severe cases. Manual pressure to the skin of these patients may elicit the separation of the epidermis (Nikolsky's sign). This finding, while characteristic of PV, is not specific to this disorder and is also seen in toxic epidermal necrolysis, Stevens-Johnson syndrome, and a few other skin diseases. Lesions in PV typically present on the scalp, face, neck, axilla, trunk, and oral cavity. In half or more of patients, lesions begin in the mouth; approximately 90 percent of patients have oromucosal involvement at some time during the course of their disease. Involvement of other mucosal surfaces (e.g., pharyngeal, laryngeal, esophageal, conjunctival, vulval, or rectal) can occur in severe disease. Pruritus

TABLE 53-1   Immunologically mediated blistering skin diseases

Disease	Clinical	Histology	Immunopathology
Pemphigus vulgaris	Flaccid blisters, denuded skin, oromucosal lesions	Blister formed in suprabasal layer of epidermis	Cell surface deposits of IgG on keratinocytes
Pemphigus foliaceus	Crusts and shallow erosions on scalp, central face, neck, upper chest, and back	Blister formed in superficial layers of epidermis	Cell surface deposits of IgG on keratinocytes
Bullous pemphigoid	Large tense blisters on flexor surfaces, oromucosal lesions	Blister formed in subepidermal region, usually eosinophil-rich	Linear band of IgG or C3 at BMZ*
Dermatitis herpetiformis	Extremely itchy small papules and vesicles on elbows, knees, buttocks, and posterior nuchal area	Subepidermal blister with neutrophils in dermal papillae	Granular deposits of IgA in dermal papillae
Linear IgA disease	Extremely itchy small papules and vesicles on extensor surfaces, occasionally larger arciform blisters	Subepidermal blister with neutrophils in dermal papillae	Linear band of IgA at BMZ
Epidermolysis bullosa acquisita	Blisters, scarring, and milia on dorsum of hands, elbows, knees; oromucosal lesions	Blister is subepidermal and can be inflammatory or not	Linear band of IgG or C3 at BMZ

* BMZ = basement membrane zone.

may be a feature of early pemphigus lesions; extensive denudation may be associated with severe pain. Lesions usually heal without scarring, except at sites complicated by secondary infection or mechanically induced dermal wounds. Nonetheless, postinflammatory hyperpigmentation is usually present at sites of healed lesions for some time.

Biopsies of early lesions demonstrate intraepidermal vesicle formation secondary to loss of cohesion between epidermal cells (i.e., acantholytic blisters). Blister cavities contain acantholytic epidermal cells which appear as round homogeneous cells containing hyperchromatic nuclei. Basal keratinocytes remain attached to the epidermal basement membrane, hence blister formation is within the suprabasal portion of the epidermis. Lesional skin may contain focal collections of intraepidermal eosinophils within blister cavities; dermal alterations are slight, usually limited to an eosinophil-predominant leukocytic infiltrate. Direct immunofluorescence microscopy of lesional or normal skin shows deposits of IgG on the surface of keratinocytes; in contrast, deposits of complement are typically found in lesional but not normal skin. Keratinocyte IgG deposits are derived from a circulating autoantibody directed against cell surface antigens. Circulating autoantibodies can be demonstrated in 80 to 90 percent of PV patients by indirect immunofluorescence microscopy; monkey esophagus is the optimal substrate for demonstration of these autoantibodies. In PV, autoantibodies are directed against a 130-kDa desmosomal cadherin molecule that forms a complex with plakoglobin, an 85-kDa constituent of desmosomal and adherens junctions. These autoantibodies are responsible for dysadhesion of epidermal cells. The titer of circulating autoantibody (determined by indirect immunofluorescence microscopy) correlates roughly with disease activity. These immunopathologic findings aid the diagnosis of PV and its differentiation from other blistering skin diseases.

PV can be life-threatening. Prior to the availability of glucocorticoids, the mortality ranged from 60 to 90 percent. The current mortality is approximately 5 to 15 percent. Common causes of morbidity and mortality are infection and complications of treatment with glucocorticoids. Bad prognostic factors include advanced age, widespread involvement, and the requirement for high doses of glucocorticoids (with or without other immunosuppressive agents) for control of disease. The course of PV in individual patients is variable and difficult to predict. Some patients achieve remission after variable periods of treatment (40 percent of patients in some series), but others may require long-term treatment or succumb to complications of their disease or its treatment. The mainstay of treatment is systemic glucocorticoids. Patients with moderate to severe disease are usually started on prednisone 60 to 80 mg/d. If new lesions continue to appear after 1 to 2 weeks of treatment, the dose should be increased. Many regimens have combined an immunosuppressive agent with systemic glucocorticoids for control of PV. The two most frequently used are either azathioprine (1 mg/kg per day) or cyclophosphamide (1 mg/kg per day). It is important to bring severe or progressive disease under control quickly to lessen the severity and/or duration of this disorder.

PEMPHIGUS FOLIACEUS   Pemphigus foliaceus (PF) is distinguished from PV by several features. In PF, acantholytic blisters are located high within the epidermis, usually just beneath the stratum corneum. Hence PF is a more superficial blistering disease than PV. The distribution of lesions in the two disorders is much the same, except that in PF mucous membrane lesions are rare. Patients with PF rarely demonstrate intact blisters but rather exhibit shallow erosions associated with erythema, scale, and crust formation. Mild cases of PF resemble severe seborrheic dermatitis; severe PF may cause extensive exfoliation. Sun exposure (ultraviolet irradiation) may be an aggravating factor. A blistering skin disease endemic to south central Brazil known as fogo selvagem or Brazilian pemphigus is clinically, histologically, and immunopathologically indistinguishable from PF.

Patients with PF have immunopathologic features in common with PV. Specifically, direct immunofluorescence microscopy of normal, perilesional skin demonstrates IgG on the surface of keratinocytes. As in PV, patients with PF frequently have circulating IgG autoantibodies against keratinocyte cell surface antigens. Guinea pig esophagus is the optimal substrate for indirect immunofluorescence microscopy studies of sera from patients with PF. In PF, autoantibodies are directed against desmoglein, a 160-kDa desmosomal core glycoprotein that (like PV antigen) is complexed to plakoglobin.

Although pemphigus has been associated with several autoimmune diseases, its association with thymoma and/or myasthenia gravis is particularly notable. To date, more than 30 cases of thymoma and/or myasthenia gravis have been reported in association with pemphigus, usually with PF. Patients also may develop pemphigus as a consequence of drug exposure. The most frequently implicated agent is penicillamine; other offenders include captopril, rifampin, piroxicam, penicillin, and phenobarbital. Drug-induced pemphigus usually resembles PF rather than PV; autoantibodies in these patients have the same antigenic specificity as they do in other pemphigus patients. In most patients, lesions resolve following discontinuation of the drug; however, some patients require treatment with systemic glucocorticoids and/or immunosuppressives.

PF is generally a far less severe disease than PV and carries a better prognosis. Localized disease can be treated conservatively with topical or intralesional glucocorticoids; more active cases can usually be controlled with systemic glucocorticoids.

PARANEOPLASTIC PEMPHIGUS   Paraneoplastic pemphigus is a recently described autoimmune acantholytic mucocutaneous disease associated with an occult or confirmed neoplasm. Patients with paraneoplastic pemphigus typically show painful mucosal erosive lesions in association with pruritic papulosquamous eruptions that often progress to blisters. Palm and sole involvement is common in these patients and raises the possibility that prior reports of neoplasia-associated erythema multiforme actually may have represented unrecognized cases of paraneoplastic pemphigus. Biopsies of lesional skin from these patients show varying combinations of acantholysis, keratinocyte necrosis, and vacuolar-interface dermatitis. Direct immunofluorescence microscopy of patient skin shows deposits of IgG and complement on the surface of keratinocytes as well as similar immunoreactants in the epidermal basement membrane zone. Patients with paraneoplastic pemphigus have IgG autoantibodies that react with the surface of tissues containing desmosomes (i.e., complex and simple epithelia as well as myocardium). These autoantibodies immunoprecipitate a unique complex of four polypeptides (250, 230, 210, and 190 kDa) from keratinocyte cell extracts. In sodium dodecyl sulfate–polyacrylamide gel electrophoresis, the 250-kDa antigen comigrates with the desmosomal plaque–associated protein desmoplakin I, whereas the 230-kDa antigen comigrates with bullous pemphigoid antigen (see below); the identities of the other antigens in this complex have not yet been determined. Interestingly, passive transfer of patient immunoglobulin to neonatal mice produces keratinocyte detachment, indicating that patient autoantibodies are pathogenic mediators of tissue damage. Paraneoplastic pemphigus is generally treatment-resistant, although patients may improve (or even remit) following resection of the underlying neoplasm.

BULLOUS PEMPHIGOID   Bullous pemphigoid (BP) is a subepidermal blistering skin disease usually seen in the elderly. Lesions typically consist of tense blisters on either normal-appearing or erythematous skin. The lesions are usually distributed over the lower abdomen, groin, and flexor surface of the extremities; oral mucosal lesions are found in 10 to 40 percent of patients. Pruritus may be nonexistent or severe. As lesions evolve, tense blisters tend to rupture and be replaced by flaccid lesions or erosions with or without surmounting crust. Nontraumatized blisters heal without scarring. There is no ethnic or HLA association. Despite isolated reports, several studies have shown that patients with BP do not have an increased incidence of malignancy in comparison with appropriately age- and sex-matched controls.

While biopsies of early lesional skin demonstrate subepidermal blisters, the histologic features depend on the character of the particular lesion. Lesions on normal-appearing skin generally show a sparse perivascular leukocytic infiltrate with some eosinophils. Biopsies of inflammatory lesions typically show an eosinophil-rich, leukocytic infiltrate within the papillary dermis at sites of vesicle formation and in perivascular areas. In addition to eosinophils, these cell-rich lesions also contain mononuclear cells and neutrophils. It is not always possible to distinguish BP from other subepidermal blistering skin diseases by routine histologic techniques.

Immunopathologic studies have broadened our understanding of this disease and aided its diagnosis. Direct immunofluorescence microscopy of normal-appearing perilesional skin shows linear deposits of IgG and/or C3 in the epidermal basement membrane. The sera of approximately 70 percent of these patients contain circulating IgG autoantibodies that bind the epidermal basement membrane of normal human skin in indirect immunofluorescence microscopy. No correlation exists between the titer of these autoantibodies and disease activity. In BP, autoantibodies recognize 230- and (in approximately 50 percent of BP patients) 180-kDa hemidesmosome-associated glycoproteins in basal keratinocytes. Autoantibodies are thought to develop against these antigens, deposit in situ, and activate complement that subsequently produces dermal mast cell degranulation and granulocyte-rich leukocytic infiltrates that cause tissue damage and blister formation.

BP is generally benign, but it may persist for months to years, with exacerbations or remissions. Although extensive involvement may result in widespread erosions and compromise cutaneous integrity, the mortality rate is low even in the absence of treatment. Nonetheless, deaths may occur in elderly and/or debilitated patients. The mainstay of treatment is systemic glucocorticoids. Patients with local or minimal disease can sometimes be controlled with topical glucocorticoids alone; patients with more extensive lesions generally respond to systemic glucocorticoids either alone or in combination with immunosuppressive agents. Patients will usually respond to prednisone 40 to 60 mg/d. In some instances, azathioprine (1 mg/kg per day) or cyclophosphamide (1 mg/kg per day) are necessary adjuncts.

HERPES GESTATIONIS   Herpes gestationis (HG) is a rare, nonviral, subepidermal blistering disease of pregnancy and the puerperium. HG may begin during any trimester of pregnancy or present shortly after delivery. Lesions are usually distributed over the abdomen, trunk, and extremities; mucous membrane lesions are rare. Skin lesions in these patients may be quite polymorphic and consist of erythematous urticarial papules and plaques, vesiculopapules, and/or frank bullae. Lesions are almost always very pruritic. Severe exacerbations of HG frequently occur after delivery, typically within 24 to 48 h. HG tends to recur in subsequent pregnancies, often beginning earlier during such gestations. Brief flare-ups of disease may occur with resumption of menses and may develop in patients later exposed to oral contraceptives. Occasionally, infants of affected mothers demonstrate transient skin lesions.

Biopsies of early lesional skin show teardrop-shaped subepidermal vesicles forming in dermal papillae in association with an eosinophil-rich leukocytic infiltrate. Differentiation of HG from other subepidermal bullous diseases by light microscopy is often difficult. However, direct immunofluorescence microscopy of normal perilesional skin from HG patients reveals the immunopathologic hallmark of this disorder—linear deposits of C3 in the epidermal basement membrane zone. These deposits develop as a consequence of complement activation produced by a low titer IgG anti-basement membrane zone autoantibody. Recent studies have shown that the majority of HG sera contain autoantibodies that recognize the same 180-kDa hemidesmosome-associated glycoprotein that is targeted by autoantibodies in roughly 50 percent of patients with BP—a subepidermal bullous disease that resembles HG morphologically, histologically, and immunopathologically.

The goals of therapy in patients with HG are to prevent the development of new lesions, relieve intense pruritus, and care for erosions at sites of blister formation. Most patients require treatment with moderate doses of daily glucocorticoids (i.e., 20 to 40 mg of prednisone) at some point in their course. Mild cases (or brief flare-ups) may be controlled by vigorous use of potent topical glucocorticoids. Although HG was once thought to be associated with an increased risk of fetal morbidity and mortality, the best evidence now suggests that these infants may only be at increased risk of being slightly premature or "small for dates." Current evidence suggests that there is no difference in the incidence of uncomplicated live births in HG patients treated with systemic glucocorticoids and in those managed more conservatively. If systemic glucocorticoids are administered, newborns are at risk for development of reversible adrenal insufficiency.

DERMATITIS HERPETIFORMIS   Dermatitis herpetiformis (DH) is an intensely pruritic, chronic papulovesicular skin disease characterized by lesions symmetrically distributed over extensor surfaces (i.e., elbows, knees, buttocks, back, scalp, and posterior neck). The primary lesion in this disorder is a papule, papulovesicle, or urticarial plaque. Because pruritus is prominent, patients may present with excoriations and crusted papules but no observable primary lesions. Patients sometimes report that their pruritus has a distinctive burning or stinging component; the onset of such local symptoms reliably heralds the development of distinct clinical lesions 12 to 24 h later. Almost all DH patients have an associated, usually subclinical, gluten-sensitive enteropathy (also see Chap. 254), and more than 90 percent express the HLA-B8/DRw3 and HLA-DQw2 haplotypes. DH may present at any age, including childhood; onset in the second to fourth decades is most common. The disease is typically chronic.

Biopsy of early lesional skin reveals neutrophil-rich infiltrates within dermal papillae. Neutrophils, fibrin, edema, and microvesicle formation at these sites are characteristic of early disease. Older lesions may demonstrate nonspecific features of a subepidermal bulla or an excoriated papule. Because the clinical and histologic features of this disease can be variable and resemble other subepidermal blistering disorders, the diagnosis can be confirmed by direct immuno-fluorescence microscopy of normal-appearing perilesional skin. Such studies demonstrate granular deposits of IgA (with or without complement components) in the papillary dermis and along the epidermal basement membrane zone. IgA deposits in the skin are unaffected by control of disease with medication; however, these immunoreactants may diminish in intensity or disappear in patients maintained for long periods on a strict gluten-free diet (see below). Patients with granular deposits of IgA in their epidermal basement membrane zone do not have circulating IgA autoantibodies and should be distinguished from individuals with linear IgA deposits at this site (see below).

Although most DH patients do not report overt gastrointestinal symptoms or laboratory evidence of malabsorption, biopsies of small bowel usually reveal blunting of intestinal villi and a lymphocytic infiltrate in the lamina propria. As is true for patients with celiac disease, this gastrointestinal abnormality can be reversed by a gluten-free diet. Moreover, if maintained, this diet alone may control the skin disease and eventuate in clearance of IgA deposits from these patients' epidermal basement membrane zone. Subsequent gluten exposure in the latter patients alters the morphology of their small bowel, elicits a flare-up of their skin disease, and is associated with the reappearance of IgA in their epidermal basement membrane zone. Patients with DH also have an increased incidence of thyroid abnormalities, achlorhydria, atrophic gastritis, and antigastric parietal cell antibodies. These associations likely relate to the high frequency of the HLA-B8/DRw3 haplotype in these patients, since this marker is commonly linked to autoimmune disorders. The mainstay of treatment of DH is dapsone. Patients respond rapidly (24 to 48 h) to dapsone but require careful pretreatment evaluation and close follow-up to ensure that complications are avoided or controlled. All patients on more than 100 mg/d dapsone will have some hemolysis and methemoglobinemia. These are expected pharmacologic side effects of dapsone. It is important to employ the lowest possible maintenance dose of dapsone to control symptoms and lesions. Gluten restriction can control DH and lessen dapsone requirements, but this diet must rigidly exclude gluten to be of benefit. Moreover, many months of dietary restriction may be necessary before a beneficial result is achieved. Good dietary counselling by a trained dietitian is essential.

LINEAR IgA DISEASE   Linear IgA disease, once considered a variant form of dermatitis herpetiformis, is actually a separate and distinct entity. Clinically, these patients may resemble typical cases of DH, bullous pemphigoid, or other subepidermal blistering skin diseases. Lesions typically consist of papulovesicles, bullae, and/or urticarial plaques, predominantly on extensor (as seen in "classic" DH), central, or flexural sites. Oral mucosal involvement does occur in selected patients. Severe pruritus resembles that in patients with DH. Patients with linear IgA disease do not have an increased frequency of the HLA-B8/DRw3 haplotype or an associated enteropathy and hence are not candidates for a gluten-free diet.

The histologic alterations in early lesions may be virtually indistinguishable from those in DH. However, direct immunofluorescence microscopy of normal-appearing perilesional skin reveals linear deposits of IgA (and often C3) in the epidermal basement membrane zone. Many patients with linear IgA disease demonstrate circulating IgA autoantibodies against a 97-kDa protein in normal epidermal basement membrane. As in DH, these patients respond promptly to treatment with dapsone, 50 to 200 mg/d.

EPIDERMOLYSIS BULLOSA ACQUISITA   EBA is a rare, noninherited, polymorphic, subepidermal blistering skin disease. (The inherited form is discussed in Chap. 351.) Since lesions generally occur in sites prone to minor trauma (e.g., dorsum of the hands, elbows, knees, etc.), EBA is regarded as a mechanobullous disease. Patients with classic or noninflammatory EBA have blisters on noninflamed skin, atrophic scars, milia, nail dystrophy, and oral lesions. Other patients with EBA have widespread inflammatory, scarring, bullous lesions and oromucosal involvement that resembles severe BP. Interestingly, some patients present with an inflammatory bullous skin disease that subsequently evolves into the classic noninflammatory form of this disorder. In general, EBA is chronic; associations with multiple myeloma, amyloidosis, inflammatory bowel disease, and diabetes mellitus have been reported. The HLA-DR2 haplotype is found with increased frequency in these patients.

The histology of lesional skin varies depending on the type or character of the lesion being studied. Noninflammatory bullae show subepidermal blisters with a sparse leukocytic infiltrate and resemble those in patients with porphyria cutanea tarda. Inflammatory vesiculobullous lesions consist of a subepidermal blister and neutrophil-rich leukocytic infiltrates in the superficial dermis. EBA patients have continuous deposits of IgG (and frequently C3 as well as other complement components) in a linear pattern within the epidermal basement membrane zone. Ultrastructurally, these immunoreactants are found in the sublamina densa region in association with anchoring fibrils. Approximately 25 to 50 percent of EBA patients have circulating IgG autoantibodies directed against type VII collagen—the collagen species found in anchoring fibrils.

Treatment of EBA is generally unsatisfactory. Some patients with inflammatory EBA may respond to systemic glucocorticoids, either alone or in combination with immunosuppressive agents. Other patients (especially those with neutrophil-rich inflammatory lesions) may respond to dapsone. The chronic, noninflammatory form of this disease is largely resistant to treatment.

AUTOIMMUNE SYSTEMIC DISEASES WITH PROMINENT CUTANEOUS FEATURES

DERMATOMYOSITIS   The cutaneous manifestations of dermatomyositis (see Chap. 384) are often distinctive but at times may resemble those of systemic lupus erythematosus (SLE), scleroderma, or other overlapping connective tissue diseases. The extent and severity of cutaneous disease may or may not correlate with the extent and severity of the myositis. Patients with severe muscle involvement may have relatively minor skin changes, whereas patients with marked skin involvement may have mild muscle disease. The cutaneous manifestations of dermatomyositis are similar whether the disease appears in childhood or old age, except that calcification of subcutaneous tissue is a common late sequela in childhood dermatomyositis.

The cutaneous signs of dermatomyositis may precede or follow the development of myositis by weeks to years. Cases lacking muscle involvement (i.e., dermatomyositis sine myositis) also have been reported. The most common manifestation is a purple-red discoloration of the upper eyelids, sometimes associated with scaling ("heliotrope" erythema) and periorbital edema. Erythema on the cheeks and nose in a "butterfly" distribution may resemble the eruption in SLE. Erythematous or violaceous scaling patches are common on the upper anterior chest and the extensor surfaces of the arms, legs, and hands. Erythema and scaling may be particularly prominent over the elbows, knees, and the dorsal interphalangeal joints. Approximately one-third of patients have violaceous, flat-topped papules over the dorsal interphalangeal joints that are pathognomonic of dermatomyositis (Gottron's sign or Gottron's papules). These lesions can be contrasted with the erythema and scaling on the dorsum of the fingers in some patients with SLE which spares the skin over the interphalangeal joints. Periungual telangiectasia may be prominent, and a lacy or reticulated erythema may be associated with fine scaling on the extensor surfaces of the thighs and upper arms. Other patients, particularly those with long-standing disease, develop areas of hypopigmentation, hyperpigmentation, mild atrophy, and telangiectasia known as *poikiloderma vasculare atrophicans*. Poikiloderma is rare in both SLE and scleroderma and thus can serve as a clinical sign that distinguishes dermatomyositis from these two diseases. However, cutaneous changes may be similar in scleroderma and dermatomyositis and may include thickening and binding down of the skin of the hands (sclerodactyly) as well as Raynaud's phenomenon. However, the presence of severe muscle disease, Gottron's papules, heliotrope erythema, and poikiloderma serve to distinguish these patients as having dermatomyositis. Skin biopsy of erythematous, scaling lesions of dermatomyositis may reveal only mild nonspecific inflammation but sometimes may show changes indistinguishable from those found in SLE, including epidermal atrophy, hydropic degeneration of basal keratinocytes, edema of the upper dermis, and a mild mononuclear cell infiltrate. Direct immunofluorescence microscopy of lesional skin is usually negative. Treatment should be directed at the systemic disease. In the few instances where adjunctive cutaneous therapy is desirable, topical glucocorticoids are sometimes useful. These patients should avoid exposure to ultraviolet irradiation and use photoprotective measures such as sunscreens.

LUPUS ERYTHEMATOSUS The cutaneous manifestations of lupus erythematosus (LE) (see Chap. 284) can be divided into acute, subacute, and chronic (i.e., discoid LE) types. Acute cutaneous LE is characterized by erythema of the nose and malar eminences in a "butterfly" distribution. The erythema is often sudden in onset, accompanied by edema and fine scale, and correlated with systemic involvement. Patients may have widespread involvement of the face as well as erythema and scaling of the extensor surfaces of the extremities and upper chest. These acute lesions, while sometimes evanescent, usually last for days and are often associated with exacerbations of systemic disease. Skin biopsy of acute lesions may show only a sparse dermal infiltrate of mononuclear cells and dermal edema. In some instances, cellular infiltrates around blood vessels and hair follicles are notable, as is hydropic degeneration of basal cells of the epidermis. Direct immunofluorescence microscopy of lesional skin frequently reveals deposits of immunoglobulin(s) and complement in the epidermal basement membrane zone. Treatment is aimed at control of systemic disease; photoprotection in this, as well as in other forms of LE, is very important.

Subacute cutaneous lupus erythematosus (SCLE) is characterized by a widespread photosensitive, nonscarring eruption. About half of these patients have SLE in which severe renal and CNS involvement is uncommon. SCLE may present as a papulosquamous eruption that resembles psoriasis or annular lesions that resemble those seen in erythema multiforme. In the papulosquamous form, discrete erythematous papules arise on the back, chest, shoulders, extensor surfaces of the arms, and the dorsum of the hands but are uncommon on the face, flexor surfaces of the arms, and below the waist. The slightly scaling papules tend to merge into large plaques, some with a reticulate appearance. The annular form involves the same areas and also begins as an erythematous papule but tends to develop oval, circular, or polycyclic lesions. The lesions of SCLE are more widespread but have less tendency for scarring than do lesions of discoid LE. Skin biopsy reveals a dense mononuclear cell infiltrate around hair follicles and blood vessels in the superficial dermis, combined with hydropic degeneration of basal cells in the epidermis. Direct immunofluorescence microscopy of lesional skin reveals deposits of immunoglobulin(s) in the epidermal basement membrane zone in about half these cases. Most SCLE patients have anti-Ro antibodies. Local therapy is usually unsuccessful, and most patients require treatment with aminoquinoline antimalarials. Low-dose therapy with oral glucocorticoids is sometimes necessary; photoprotective measures against both ultraviolet B and A wavelengths are very important.

Discoid lupus erythematosus (DLE) is characterized by discrete lesions, most often on the face, scalp, or external ears. The lesions are erythematous papules or plaques with a thick, adherent scale that occludes hair follicles (follicular plugging). When the scale is removed, its underside will show small excrescences that correlate with the openings of hair follicles and is termed a "carpet tack" appearance. This finding is relatively specific for discoid LE. Long-standing lesions develop central atrophy, scarring, and hypopigmentation but frequently have erythematous, sometimes raised borders at

the periphery. These lesions persist for years and tend to expand slowly. Only 5 to 10 percent of patients with DLE meet the American Rheumatism Association criteria for SLE. However, typical discoid lesions are frequently seen in patients with SLE. Biopsy of discoid LE shows hyperkeratosis, follicular plugging, and atrophy of the epidermis. The dermal-epidermal junction reveals hydropic degeneration of basal keratinocytes, and a mononuclear cell infiltrate surrounds hair follicles and blood vessels. Direct immunofluorescence microscopy demonstrates immunoglobulin(s) and complement deposits at the basement membrane zone in about 90 percent of cases. Treatment is focused on control of local cutaneous disease and consists mainly of photoprotection and topical or intralesional glucocorticoids. If local therapy is ineffective, use of aminoquinoline antimalarials may be indicated.

SCLERODERMA AND MORPHEA The skin changes of scleroderma (see Chap. 286) usually begin on the hands, feet, and face, with episodes of recurrent nonpitting edema. Sclerosis of the skin begins distally on the fingers (sclerodactyly) and spreads proximally, usually accompanied by resorption of bone of the fingertips, which may have punched out ulcers, stellate scars, or areas of hemorrhage. The fingers may actually shrink in size and become sausage-shaped, and since the fingernails are usually unaffected, the nails may curve over the end of the fingertips. Periungual telangiectasias are usually present, but periungual erythema is rare. In advanced cases, the extremities show contractures and calcinosis cutis. Face involvement includes a smooth, unwrinkled brow, taut skin over the nose, shrinkage of tissue around the mouth, and perioral radial furrowing. Matlike telangiectasias are often present, particularly on the face and hands. Involved skin feels indurated, smooth, and bound to underlying structures; hyperpigmentation and hypopigmentation are also often present. Raynaud's phenomenon, i.e., cold-induced blanching, cyanosis, and reactive hyperemia, is present in almost all patients with scleroderma and can precede development of scleroderma by many years. The combination of calcinosis cutis, Raynaud's phenomenon, esophageal dysmotility, sclerodactyly, and telangiectasia has been termed the *CREST syndrome*. Anticentromere antibodies have been reported in a very high percentage of patients with the CREST syndrome but in only a small minority of patients with scleroderma. Skin biopsy reveals thickening of the dermis and homogenization of collagen bundles. Direct immunofluorescence microscopy of lesional skin is usually negative.

Morphea, which has been called *localized scleroderma*, is characterized by localized thickening and sclerosis of skin, usually affecting young adults or children. Morphea begins as erythematous or flesh-colored plaques that become sclerotic, develop central hypopigmentation, and demonstrate an erythematous border. In most cases, patients have one or a few lesions, and the disease is termed *localized morphea*. In some patients, widespread cutaneous lesions may occur, without systemic involvement. This form is called *generalized morphea*. Most patients with morphea do not have autoantibodies. Skin biopsy of morphea is indistinguishable from that of scleroderma. Linear scleroderma is a limited form of disease which presents in a linear, bandlike distribution and tends to involve deep as well as superficial layers of skin. Scleroderma and morphea are usually quite resistant to therapy with medications. For this reason, physical therapy to prevent joint contractures and to maintain function is employed and is often helpful.

Diffuse fasciitis with eosinophilia is a clinical entity that can sometimes be confused with scleroderma. There is usually the sudden onset of swelling, induration, and erythema of the extremities frequently following significant physical exertion. The proximal portions of extremities (arms, forearms, thighs, legs) are more often involved than are the hands and feet. While the skin is indurated, it is usually not bound down as in scleroderma. These skin findings are accompanied by peripheral blood eosinophilia, increased erythrocyte sedimentation rate, and sometimes hypergammaglobulinemia. Deep biopsy of affected areas of skin reveals inflammation and thickening of the deep fascia overlying muscle. An inflammatory infiltrate composed of eosinophils and mononuclear cells is usually found. Patients with eosinophilic fasciitis appear to be at increased risk to develop bone marrow failure or other hematologic abnormalities. While the ultimate course of eosinophilic fasciitis is uncertain, many patients respond favorably to treatment with prednisone in doses ranging from 40 to 60 mg/d.

The *eosinophilia-myalgia syndrome*, a newly recognized disorder reported in epidemic numbers in 1989 and linked to ingestion of manufactured tryptophan, is a multisystem disorder characterized by debilitating myalgias and absolute eosinophilia in association with varying combinations of arthralgias, pulmonary symptoms, peripheral edema, and neuropathies (see Chap. 286). The precise cause of this syndrome, which may resemble other sclerotic skin conditions, is unknown. However, the clustering of cases suggests that an impurity or contaminant in a manufactured tryptophan preparation is likely.

REFERENCES

ANHALT GJ et al: Paraneoplastic pemphigus: An autoimmune mucocutaneous disease associated with neoplasia. N Engl J Med 323:1729, 1990

BRAVERMAN IM: Connective tissue diseases, in *Skin Signs of Systemic Disease*. Philadelphia, Saunders, 1981

GAMMON WR et al: Epidermolysis bullosa acquisita—A pemphigoid-like disease. J Am Acad Dermatol 11:820, 1984

HALL RP: The pathogenesis of dermatitis herpetiformis: Recent advances. J Am Acad Dermatol 16:1129, 1987

KATZ SI et al: Dermatitis herpetiformis: The skin and the gut. Ann Intern Med 93:857, 1980

KORMAN N: Pemphigus. J Am Acad Dermatol 18:1219, 1988

SHORNICK JK: Herpes gestationis. J Am Acad Dermatol 17:539, 1987

SHULMAN LE: Diffuse fasciitis with eosinophilia: A new syndrome. Arthritis Rheum 20(Suppl):205, 1977

STANLEY JR: Pemphigus and pemphigoid as paradigms of organ-specific, autoantibody-mediated diseases. J Clin Invest 83:1443, 1989

YANCEY KB, LAWLEY TJ: The immunology of the skin, in *Allergy: Principles and Practice*, 3d ed, E Middleton et al (eds). St. Louis, Mosby, 1988

54   SKIN MANIFESTATIONS OF INTERNAL DISEASE

JEAN BOLOGNIA / IRWIN M. BRAVERMAN

It is now a generally accepted concept in medicine that the skin can show signs of internal disease. Therefore, in textbooks of medicine one finds a chapter describing in detail the major systemic disorders that can be identified by cutaneous signs. The underlying assumption of such a chapter is that the clinician has been able to identify the disorder in the patient and needs only to read about it in the textbook. In reality, concise differential diagnoses and the identification of these disorders are actually difficult for the nondermatologist because he or she is not well versed in the recognition of cutaneous lesions or their spectrum of presentations. Therefore, the authors of this chapter have decided to cover this particular topic of cutaneous medicine not by discussing individual disorders but by describing and discussing the various presenting clinical signs and symptoms that indicate the presence of these disorders. Concise differential diagnoses will be generated in which the significant diseases will be briefly discussed and distinguished from the more common disorders that have no significance for internal diseases. The latter disorders are reviewed in table form and always need to be excluded when considering the former. For a detailed description of individual diseases, the reader should consult a dermatologic text. The categories of skin lesions that are discussed include papulosquamous lesions, erythroderma, alopecia, figurate lesions, acne, pustules, telangiectasias, hypopigmentation, hyperpigmentation, vesicles/bullae, exanthems, urticaria, papulonodular lesions, purpura, and ulcers. In an attempt to determine

the appropriate category for a particular lesion, it is important to carefully examine its surface qualities, shape, and color in addition to the location and distribution (see Chap. 50).

PAPULOSQUAMOUS SKIN LESIONS (Table 54-1) When an eruption is characterized by elevated lesions, papules (<1 cm) or plaques (>1 cm), in association with scale, it is referred to as *papulosquamous*. The most common papulosquamous diseases—*psoriasis*, *tinea*, *pityriasis rosea*, and *lichen planus*—are primary cutaneous disorders (Table 54-2). When psoriatic lesions are accompanied by arthritis, the possibility of psoriatic arthritis or *Reiter's disease* should be considered. A history of oral ulcers, conjunctivitis, uveitis, and/or urethritis points to the latter diagnosis. In *guttate psoriasis* there is an acute onset of small, widely scattered, uniform lesions, often in association with a streptococcal infection. Lithium, beta blockers, human immunodeficiency virus (HIV) infection, and a rapid taper of systemic glucocorticoids are also known to exacerbate psoriasis. Epidermal hyperproliferation and incomplete maturation are responsible for the plaque formation and scale that is characteristic of psoriasis.

Whenever the diagnosis of pityriasis rosea or lichen planus is made, it is important to review the patient's medications because the eruption can be treated by simply discontinuing the offending agent. Pityriasis rosea–like drug eruptions are seen most commonly with beta blockers, captopril, clonidine, gold, griseofulvin, isotretinoin, metronidazole, and penicillin, while the drugs that can produce a lichenoid eruption include gold, antimalarials, thiazides, quinidine, phenothiazines, sulfonylureas, furosemide, griseofulvin, beta blockers, and captopril. Lichen planus–like lesions are also observed in chronic graft-versus-host disease. *Bowen's disease* represents squamous cell carcinoma in situ, and it usually presents as a single lesion. The plaque is well demarcated, pink to red in color, and the amount of scale varies. Bowen's disease is found in both sun-exposed and sun-protected areas of the body; the possibility of arsenic exposure should be explored in these patients, and an examination of the palms and soles for arsenical keratoses should be performed.

Parapsoriasis is an intermediate disease, for it can remain solely as a primary cutaneous disease or it can progress to cutaneous T cell lymphoma (CTCL) after a latency period of as long as 40 years. There are several forms of *parapsoriasis*, including small plaque (0.5 to 5 cm), large plaque (>6 cm), and retiform. The lesions of both small plaque and large plaque parapsoriasis are thin and salmon-pink in color with fine white scale. In small plaque forms, the lesions are commonly on the trunk but can be widely scattered. In large plaque forms, the most common location is the "girdle" area, and fine wrinkling secondary to epidermal atrophy is often seen. Retiform parapsoriasis forms a netlike pattern, and the individual papules are red-brown and flat-topped. The latter two forms of parapsoriasis, large plaque and retiform, can progress to CTCL.

Cutaneous T cell lymphoma (CTCL), *secondary syphilis*, *lupus* (see "Papulonodular Skin Lesions" below), and *Bazex' syndrome* are less common papulosquamous disorders that are associated with systemic disease. A clue to the development of *CTCL* within lesions

---

TABLE 54-1   Causes of papulosquamous skin lesions

Primary cutaneous disorders
  A Psoriasis
  B Tinea
  C Pityriasis rosea
  D Lichen planus
  E Parapsoriasis
  F Bowen's disease
Drugs
Systemic diseases
  A Lupus erythematosus
  B Cutaneous T cell lymphoma
  C Secondary syphilis
  D Reiter's disease
  E Bazex' syndrome

TABLE 54-2   Papulosquamous skin diseases (primary cutaneous disorders)

	Characteristic lesion	Location	Other findings	Diagnostic aids
Psoriasis	Pink-red, silvery scale, sharply demarcated	Elbows, knees, scalp, presacral area	Nail dystrophy: pitting, onycholysis, yellow discoloration Arthritis: primarily small joints (hands and feet)	Skin biopsy
Tinea	Pink-red, central clearing common, active, scaling border	Inner thigh (tinea cruris), palms, soles, any area of body	Invasion of stratum corneum by dermatophytes	KOH and/or fungal culture of scale
Pityriasis rosea	Salmon-pink, oval shape, long axis follows lines of cleavage in the skin, peripheral collarette of scale	Trunk, proximal extremities	Herald patch: initial lesion and usually the largest in size Spontaneous resolution over 2–3 months	Skin biopsy, VDRL to exclude secondary syphilis
Lichen planus	Violet-colored, polygonal, flat-topped, traversed by thin white lines (Wickham's striae)	Flexor wrists, ankles, presacral area, glans penis	Oral mucosa: lacelike white plaques and/or erosions Pruritus Nail dystrophy: pterygium, longitudinal ridging	Skin biopsy

of large plaque or retiform parapsoriasis is an increase in the palpable component of the plaque (increased infiltration). In its early stages, CTCL may be confused with ezcema or psoriasis, but it often fails to respond to the appropriate therapy for those inflammatory diseases. The diagnosis of CTCL is established by skin biopsy in which collections of atypical T lymphocytes are found in the epidermis and dermis. As the disease progresses, cutaneous tumors and lymph node involvement may appear.

In *secondary syphilis* there are scattered red-brown papules with thin scale. The eruption often involves the palms and soles, and it can resemble pityriasis rosea. Associated findings are helpful in making the diagnosis, and they include annular plaques on the face, nonscarring alopecia, condyloma lata (broad-based and moist), and mucous patches, as well as lymphadenopathy, malaise, fever, headache, and myalgias. The interval between the primary chancre and the secondary stage is usually 4 to 8 weeks, and spontaneous resolution without appropriate therapy is seen. When psoriasiform lesions are seen on the nose, ears, fingers, and toes, *Bazex' syndrome* should be considered. It is a distinctive paraneoplastic eruption associated with squamous cell carcinomas of the oropharynx, tracheobronchial tree, and esophagus.

ERYTHRODERMA (Table 54-3) *Erythroderma* is the term used when the majority of the skin surface is erythematous (red in color). There may be associated scale, erosions, or pustules as well as shedding of the hair and nails. Potential systemic manifestations include fever, chills, hypothermia, reactive lymphadenopathy, peripheral edema, hypoalbuminemia, increased transepidermal water loss, and high-output cardiac failure. The major etiologies of erythroderma are (1) *cutaneous diseases* such as psoriasis and dermatitis (Table 54-4), (2) *drugs*, (3) *systemic diseases*, most commonly CTCL, and (4) *idiopathic*. In the first three groups, the location and description of the initial lesions, prior to the development of the erythroderma, aid in the diagnosis. For example, a history of red scaly plaques on the elbows and knees would point to psoriasis. It is also important to examine the skin carefully for a migration of the erythema and

TABLE 54-3   Causes of erythroderma

Primary cutaneous disorders
  A Psoriasis
  B Dermatitis (atopic, stasis, contact, seborrheic)
  C Pityriasis rubra pilaris
Drugs
Systemic diseases
  A Cutaneous T cell lymphoma
  B Lymphoma
  C Necrolytic migratory erythema
Idiopathic

associated secondary changes such as pustules or erosions. Migratory waves of erythema studded with superficial pustules are seen in *pustular psoriasis*, whereas erosive migratory erythema of the girdle area is seen in *necrolytic migratory erythema* (glucagonoma syndrome).

An erythroderma secondary to an underlying cutaneous disease is most commonly due to *psoriasis* or one of the various forms of *dermatitis* (eczema). Each type of dermatitis has its own distinguishing features, but they may be limited to the initial lesions. Uncontrolled dermatitis can evolve into an erythroderma through a process known as *autosensitization* (conditioned hyperirritability), where initially uninvolved skin becomes pruritic and eventually dermatitic.

Drug-induced erythroderma (exfoliative dermatitis) may begin as a morbilliform eruption, or it may arise as diffuse erythema. Fever and peripheral eosinophilia often accompany the eruption. There are a number of *drugs* that can produce an erythroderma, including penicillins, sulfonamides, barbiturates, phenytoin, gold, allopurinol, captopril, sulfonylureas, and furosemide. Reactions to allopurinol also may be accompanied by hepatitis and nephropathy, especially in patients with impaired renal function given full doses of allopurinol plus a diuretic.

The most common malignancy that is associated with erythroderma is *CTCL*; in some series, up to 25 percent of the cases of erythroderma were due to CTCL. The patient may progress from isolated plaques and tumors, but more commonly the erythroderma is present throughout the course of the disease (Sézary syndrome). In the Sézary syndrome, there are circulating atypical T lymphocytes, pruritus, and lymphadenopathy. Additional findings include keratoderma and leonine facies. In cases of erythroderma where there is no apparent cause (idiopathic), longitudinal follow-up is mandatory to monitor for the possible development of CTCL. Other types of *lymphoma* can be associated with erythroderma, including Hodgkin's and non-Hodgkin's lymphoma, the former being more common. There also have been isolated case reports of erythroderma secondary to some solid tumors—lung, liver, prostate, thyroid, and colon—but it is usually in a late stage of the disease.

ALOPECIA (Table 54-5) The two major forms of *alopecia* are scarring and nonscarring. In *scarring alopecia* there is associated fibrosis, inflammation, and loss of hair follicles. A smooth scalp with a decreased number of follicular openings is usually observed clinically, but in some cases the changes are seen only in biopsy specimens from the affected areas. In *nonscarring alopecia* the hair shafts are gone, but the hair follicles are preserved, explaining the reversible nature of nonscarring alopecia.

Primary cutaneous disorders are the most common causes of nonscarring alopecia and they include *telogen effluvium, androgenetic alopecia, alopecia areata, tinea capitis,* and *traumatic alopecia* (Table 54-6). In women with androgenetic alopecia, an elevation in

TABLE 54-4   Erythroderma (primary cutaneous disorders)

	Initial lesions	Location of initial lesions	Other findings	Diagnostic aids
Psoriasis	Pink-red, silvery scale, sharply demarcated	Elbows, knees, scalp, presacral area	Nail dystrophy, arthritis, pustules	Skin biopsy
Dermatitis:				
Atopic	Acute: Erythema, fine scale, crust, indistinct borders Chronic: Lichenification (increased skin markings)	Antecubital and popliteal fossae, neck, hands	Pruritus Family history of atopy, including asthma, allergic rhinitis or conjunctivitis, and atopic dermatitis Rule out secondary infection with *S. aureus* Rule out superimposed irritant contact dermatitis	Skin biopsy
Stasis	Erythema, crusting, excoriations	Lower extremities	Pruritus, lower extremity edema History of venous ulcers, thrombophlebitis, and/or cellulitis Rule out cellulitis Rule out superimposed contact dermatitis, e.g., topical neomycin	Skin biopsy
Contact (local)	Erythema, crusting, vesicles, and bullae	Depends on offending agent	Irritant—onset often within hours Allergic—delayed-type hypersensitivity; lag time of 48 h	Patch testing
Contact (systemic)	Erythema, fine scale, crust	Generalized	Patient has history of allergic contact dermatitis to topical agent and then receives systemic medication that is structurally related, e.g., ethylenediamine (topical) aminophylline (IV)	Patch testing
Seborrheic	Pink-red, greasy scale	Scalp, nasolabial folds, eyebrows, intertriginous zones	Flares with stress, HIV infection Associated with Parkinson's disease	Skin biopsy
Pityriasis rubra pilaris	Orange-red, perifollicular, papules	Generalized, but characteristic "skip" areas of normal skin	Wax-like keratoderma Rule out cutaneous T cell lymphoma	Skin biopsy

circulating levels of androgens may be seen as a result of ovarian or adrenal gland dysfunction. When there are signs of virilization, such as a deepened voice and enlarged clitoris, the possibility of an ovarian or adrenal gland tumor should be considered.

Exposure to various *drugs* also can cause diffuse hair loss, usually by inducing a telogen effluvium. An exception is the anagen effluvium observed with antimitotic agents such as daunorubicin. Alopecia is a side effect of the following drugs: warfarin, heparin, propylthiouracil, carbimazole, vitamin A, isotretinoin, etretinate, lithium, beta blockers, levodopa, amphetamines, and thallium. Fortunately, spontaneous regrowth usually follows discontinuation of the offending agent.

Less commonly, nonscarring alopecia is associated with *lupus erythematosus* and *secondary syphilis*. In systemic lupus there are two forms of alopecia—one is scarring secondary to discoid lesions (see below) and the other is nonscarring. The latter form may be diffuse and involve the entire scalp, or it may localized to the frontal

TABLE 54-5   Causes of alopecia

Nonscarring alopecia	Scarring alopecia
A Primary cutaneous disorders	A Primary cutaneous disorders
1 Telogen effluvium	*1* Cutaneous lupus
2 Androgenetic alopecia	*2* Lichen planus
3 Alopecia areata	*3* Folliculitis decalvans
4 Tinea capitis	*4* Pseudopelade
5 Traumatic alopecia	*5* Linear scleroderma (morphea)
B Drugs	
C Systemic diseases	B Systemic diseases
1 Lupus erythematosus	*1* Lupus erythematosus
2 Secondary syphilis	*2* Sarcoidosis
3 Hypothyroidism	*3* Cutaneous metastases
4 Hyperthyroidism	
5 Deficiencies of protein, iron, biotin, and zinc	
6 HIV infection	

scalp in the form of multiple short hairs ("lupus hairs"). Scattered, poorly circumscribed patches of alopecia with a "moth-eaten" appearance are a manifestation of the secondary stage of syphilis (see "Papulosquamous Skin Lesions"). Diffuse thinning of the hair is also associated with hypothyroidism, hyperthyroidism, hypopituitarism, HIV infection, and deficiencies of protein, iron, biotin, and zinc.

Scarring alopecia is more frequently the result of a primary cutaneous disorder such as *lichen planus*, *folliculitis decalvans*, *cutaneous lupus*, or *linear scleroderma (morphea)* than it is a sign of systemic disease. Although the scarring lesions of *discoid lupus* can be seen in patients with systemic lupus, in the majority of cases the disease process is limited to the skin. Less common causes of scarring alopecia include *sarcoidosis* (see "Papulonodular Skin Lesions"), cutaneous *metastases*, and *pseudopelade*. The latter disease may be idiopathic and arise de novo, or it can represent the inactive end-stage phase of a previous inflammatory process such as lichen planus, sarcoid, or discoid lupus. The irregularly shaped areas of alopecia lack inflammation and often arise at an acute angle from the midline.

In the early phases of discoid lupus, lichen planus, and folliculitis decalvans, there are circumscribed areas of alopecia. Fibrosis and subsequent loss of follicles are observed primarily in the center of the individual lesions, while the inflammatory process is most prominent at the periphery. The areas of active inflammation in *discoid lupus* are erythematous with scale, whereas the areas of previous inflammation are often hypopigmented with a rim of hyperpigmentation. In *lichen planus* the peripheral perifollicular papules are violet-colored, and postinflammatory hyperpigmentation is a characteristic finding. Complete examination of the skin and oral mucosa combined with a biopsy and direct immunofluorescence microscopy will aid in distinguishing these two entities. The peripheral active lesions in *folliculitis decalvans* are perifollicular pustules that

TABLE 54-6   Nonscarring alopecia (primary cutaneous disorders)

	Clinical characteristics	Pathogenesis
Telogen effluvium	Diffuse shedding of normal hairs Follows either major stress (high fever, severe infection) or change in hormones (post partum) Reversible without treatment	Stress causes the normally asynchronous growth cycles of individual hairs to become synchronous; therefore, large numbers of growing (anagen) hairs simultaneously enter the dying (telogen) phase
Androgenetic alopecia	Miniaturization of hairs along the midline of the scalp Recession of the anterior scalp line in men and some women	Increased sensitivity of affected hairs to the effects of testosterone Increased levels of circulating androgens (ovarian or adrenal source)
Alopecia areata	Well-circumscribed, circular areas of hair loss, 2–5 cm in diameter In extensive cases, coalescence of lesions and/or involvement of other hair-bearing surfaces of the body Pitting of the nails	The germinative zones of the hair follicles are surrounded by T lymphocytes Occasional associated diseases: hyperthyroidism, hypothyroidism, vitiligo, Down's syndrome
Tinea	Varies from scaling with minimal hair loss, to discrete patches with "black dots" (broken hairs), to boggy plaque with pustules (kerion)	Invasion of hairs by dermatophytes, most commonly *Trichophyton tonsurans*
Traumatic alopecia	Broken hairs Irregular outline	Traction with curlers, rubber bands, braiding Exposure to heat or chemicals Mechanical pulling (trichotillomania)

routinely grow *Staphylococcus aureus* or normal flora. These patients often have other forms of acne and folliculitis and can develop a reactive arthritis.

FIGURATE SKIN LESIONS (Table 54-7)   In *figurate* eruptions, the lesions form rings and arcs that are usually erythematous but can be flesh-colored to brown. Most commonly, they are due to primary cutaneous diseases such as *tinea*, *urticaria*, *erythema annulare centrifugum*, and *granuloma annulare* (Table 54-8). An underlying systemic illness is found in a second, less common group of migratory annular erythemas. It includes *erythema gyratum repens*, *erythema migrans*, and *erythema marginatum*.

In *erythema gyratum repens*, one sees hundreds of mobile concentric arcs and wavefronts that resemble the grain in wood. A search

TABLE 54-7   Causes of figurate skin lesions

Primary cutaneous disorders
  A Tinea
  B Urticaria
  C Erythema annulare centrifugum
  D Granuloma annulare
Systemic diseases
  A Migratory
    1 Erythema migrans
    2 Erythema gyratum repens
    3 Erythema marginatum
    4 Pustular psoriasis
    5 Necrolytic migratory erythema
  B Nonmigratory
    1 Sarcoidosis
    2 Subacute lupus erythematosus
    3 Secondary syphilis
    4 Cutaneous T cell lymphoma
    5 Elastosis perforans serpiginosa

for an underlying malignancy is mandatory in a patient with this eruption. *Erythema migrans* is the cutaneous manifestation of Lyme disease, which is caused by the spirochete *Borrelia burgdorferi*. In the initial stage (3 to 30 days after tick bite), a single annular lesion is usually seen, which can expand to ≥10 cm in diameter. Within several days, approximately half the patients develop multiple smaller erythematous lesions at sites distant from the bite. Associated symptoms include fever, headache, myalgias, photophobia, arthralgias, and malar rash. *Erythema marginatum* is seen in patients with rheumatic fever, primarily on the trunk. Lesions are pink-red in color, flat to mildly elevated, and transient. If pustules are noted within a figurate eruption, consider *pustular psoriasis*, and if erosions are seen, consider *necrolytic migratory erythema*.

There are additional cutaneous diseases that present as annular eruptions, but they lack an obvious migratory component. Examples include *CTCL*, annular cutaneous *lupus*, also referred to as *subacute lupus* (see "Papulonodular Skin Lesions"), secondary *syphilis*, and *sarcoidosis* (see "Papulonodular Skin Lesions"). The most common clinical setting for the annular form of secondary lues is the face of black patients; a clue to this diagnosis is the presence of central hyperpigmentation. If keratotic plugs are noted within the annular or arciform lesions, particularly if they are localized to the neck and antecubital fossae, consider *elastosis perforans serpiginosa* (EPS). EPS is seen as a side effect of D-penicillamine and in patients with Down's syndrome and disorders of elastin and collagen. The latter include Ehlers-Danlos type IV and Marfan's syndromes, pseudoxanthoma elasticum, and osteogenesis imperfecta.

ACNE (Table 54-9)   *Acne vulgaris* and *acne rosacea* are the two major forms of acne (Table 54-10). Estrogens decrease sebaceous gland activity, whereas androgens enhance sebum production. Therefore, acne vulgaris in an adult, especially if it is of recent onset, may be a reflection of increased levels of circulating *androgens*.

TABLE 54-8   Figurate eruptions (primary cutaneous disorders)

	Clinical characteristics	Pathogenesis
Tinea	Active, scaling erythematous border with central clearing Expands slowly	Invasion of stratum corneum by dermatophytes
Urticaria	Central wheal with erythematous flare Transient and/or migratory Pruritic	Release of histamine from mast cells via immunologic (IgE, type 1 hypersensitivity) or nonimmunologic mechanisms (e.g., morphine)
Erythema annulare centrifugum	Enlarges slowly Erythematous, flat or slightly raised "Trailing scale"—scale on inner aspect of expanding ring Buttock, upper thighs	Not known Usually idiopathic Sometimes associated with tinea pedis, drug hypersensitivity Rarely, paraneoplastic
Granuloma annulare	Border composed of flesh-colored to red-brown papules Extremities	Granulomatous process is limited to the skin Unknown etiology Disseminated form is associated with diabetes mellitus

---

TABLE 54-9   Causes of acneiform eruptions

Primary cutaneous disorders
  A Acne vulgaris
  B Acne rosacea
Drugs
Systemic diseases
  A Increased androgen production
    1 Adrenal origin, e.g., Cushing's disease, 21-hydroxylase deficiency
    2 Ovarian origin, e.g., polycystic ovary disease
  B Cryptococcosis, disseminated
  C Behçet's disease

TABLE 54-11   Causes of folliculitis

Infections
  A Bacterial
    1 *Propionibacterium acnes*
    2 *Staphylococcus aureus*
    3 Gram-negative rods, e.g., *Pseudomonas*
      a Face and neck—in the setting of long-term antibiotic use
      b Trunk—"hot tub" folliculitis
  B Fungal
    1 *Pityrosporum*
      a AIDS
    2 Dermatophytes
      a Legs of women—*Trichophyton rubrum*
      b Beard area of men—*Trichophyton verrucosum*
      c Scalp—*Trichophyton tonsurans*
    3 *Candida*
      a Occluded areas
      b Diabetics
Inflammatory
  A Eosinophilic folliculitis
    1 AIDS
Drugs

Dysfunction of the ovary or adrenal gland, e.g., polycystic ovary disease, Cushing's syndrome, or partial deficiency of the enzyme 21-hydroxylase, can lead to the hormonal imbalance. Examination of the patient for signs such as hirsutism, androgenetic alopecia, hypertension, and redistribution of subcutaneous fat will aid in the diagnosis. In patients with *acne conglobata*, a more severe form of acne characterized by multiple cysts and bridging scars, an associated inflammatory arthritis has been described.

Exposure to chlorinated aromatic hydrocarbons such as dioxin (TCDD) leads to a particular form of acne known as *chloracne*, which is characterized by open comedones and straw-colored cysts. Patients exposed to dioxin also can develop the signs and symptoms of porphyria cutanea tarda (see "Vesicles"). Exacerbations of acne vulgaris follow the ingestion of several *drugs*, such as iodides, bromides, glucocorticoids, and lithium, as well as the application of oil-containing compounds. Acne-like lesions can be seen in patients with Behçet's disease (see "Ulcers"), and in immunocompromised hosts, disseminated *cryptococcosis* may present as an acneiform eruption.

Patients with the carcinoid syndrome have episodes of flushing of the head, neck, and sometimes the trunk. Resultant skin changes of the face, in particular telangiectasias, mimic the clinical appearance of acne rosacea. Suffusion of the face, as is seen in polycythemia vera, also can be confused with acne rosacea.

PUSTULAR LESIONS   *Acneiform eruptions* (see "Acne") and *folliculitis* represent the most common pustular dermatoses. An important consideration in the evaluation of perifollicular pustules is a determination of the associated pathogen (Table 54-11). Noninfectious forms of folliculitis include eosinophilic folliculitis and folliculitis secondary to drugs such as glucocorticoids and lithium. Eosinophilic folliculitis can be seen in HIV-infected individuals, and it is characterized by multiple pruritic lesions on the face and trunk. Administration of high dose oral glucocorticoids can result in a widespread eruption of perifollicular pustules on the trunk, characterized by lesions in the same stage of development. With regard to underlying systemic diseases, pustules are a characteristic component of pustular psoriasis and can be seen in septic emboli of bacterial or fungal origin (see "Purpura"). For example, the cutaneous lesions of disseminated gonococcemia often have a halo of erythema surrounding a central pustule.

TELANGIECTASIAS (Table 54-12)   In order to distinguish the various types of telangiectasias, it is important to examine the shape and configuration of the dilated blood vessels. *Linear telangiectasias* are seen on the face of patients with *actinically damaged skin* and *acne rosacea* and are found on the legs of patients with *venous hypertension* and *essential telangiectasia* (Table 54-13). Patients with an unusual form of *mastocytosis* (telangiectasia macularis eruptiva perstans), the *carcinoid* syndrome (see "Acne"), and *ataxia-telangiectasia* also have linear telangiectasias. In ataxia-telangiectasia, linear telangiectasias appear on the bulbar conjunctiva during childhood. Eventually, there is involvement of the ears, eyelids, cheeks, and/or flexural areas such as the antecubital and popliteal fossae. Lastly, linear telangiectasias are found in areas of cutaneous inflammation. For example, lesions of discoid lupus frequently have telangiectasias within them.

TABLE 54-12   Causes of telangiectasias

Primary cutaneous disorders	Systemic diseases
A Linear	A Linear
1 Acne rosacea	1 Carcinoid
2 Actinically damaged skin	2 Ataxia-telangiectasia
3 Venous hypertension	3 Mastocytosis
4 Essential telangiectasia	B Poikiloderma
B Poikiloderma	1 Dermatomyositis
1 Ionizing radiation	2 Xeroderma pigmentosa
2 Poikiloderma vasculare	C Mat
atrophicans	1 Scleroderma
C Spider angioma	D Periungual
1 Idiopathic	1 Lupus erythematosus
2 Pregnancy	2 Scleroderma
	3 Dermatomyositis
	E Papular
	1 Hereditary hemorrhagic
	telangiectasia
	F Spider angioma
	1 Cirrhosis

TABLE 54-10   Acne (primary cutaneous disorders)

	Clinical characteristics	Pathogenesis
Acne vulgaris	Erythematous papules, pustules, open comedones (blackheads), closed comedones (whiteheads), and cysts	Epithelial hyperproliferation within the infundibulum of the hair follicle leads to comedone formation
	Areas that contain sebaceous glands: face, neck, upper trunk	Additional factors: sebum-derived free fatty acids, *Propionibacterium acnes*
Acne rosacea	Papules, pustules; central face	Unknown
	Telangiectasias of nose and cheeks	No increased reactivity of cutaneous blood vessels to vasodilators
	Facial erythema	Sebum production normal
	Flushing reaction to hot foods and alcohol	
	Ocular involvement: conjunctivitis, blepharitis, keratitis	

TABLE 54-13   Telangiectasias (primary cutaneous disorders)

Type	Associated disorder	Clinical characteristics	Pathogenesis
Linear: Simple red or blue line that disappears with diascopy (pressure)	Acne rosacea	Face Associated with flushing, erythema, papulopustules, and rhinophyma	Vasodilatation
	Actinically damaged skin	Face, arms, upper trunk Associated with hypopigmentation, hyperpigmentation, and keratoses	Damage to supportive connective tissue
	Essential telangiectasia	Netlike sheets Begins on lower extremities May be widespread More common in women	Unknown
Spider angioma: Central pulsating punctum with radiating legs	Idiopathic Pregnancy	Upper half of the body Halo of pallor secondary to local steal phenomenon	Proliferation of blood vessels in association with increased circulating estrogens

Poikiloderma is a term used to describe a patch of skin with (1) reticulated hypo- and hyperpigmentation, (2) wrinkling secondary to epidermal atrophy, and (3) telangiectasias. Poikiloderma does not imply a single disease entity—it is seen in skin damaged by *ionizing radiation*, in the disorders *poikiloderma vasculare atrophicans* (PVA) and *xeroderma pigmentosum*, as well as in patients with connective-tissue diseases, primarily *dermatomyositis*. PVA is a precursor lesion of CTCL, and the areas of poikiloderma usually begin in the flexural areas of the axillae and groin.

In *scleroderma*, the dilated blood vessels have a unique configuration and are known as *mat telangiectasias*. The lesions are broad macules that usually measure 2 to 7 mm in diameter; occasionally, they are larger in size. Mats have a polygonal or oval shape, and their erythematous color may be uniform or the result of delicate telangiectasias. The most common locations for mat telangiectasias are the face, oral mucosa, and hands—peripheral sites that are prone to intermittent ischemia. One theory is that the mats represent a form of neovascularization in these areas. In the CREST variant of scleroderma (see Chap. 286), which is associated with a chronic course and anticentromere antibodies, the *T* stands for telangiectasias. Mat telangiectasias are an important clue to the diagnosis of the CREST syndrome as well as systemic scleroderma, for they may be the only cutaneous finding. A minority of the patients with scleroderma will have telangiectasias indistinguishable from those found in hereditary hemorrhagic telangiectasia (see below).

Periungual telangiectasias are pathognomonic signs of the three major connective tissue diseases—*lupus erythematosus*, *scleroderma*, and *dermatomyositis* (DM). They are easily visualized by the naked eye, and they occur in at least two-thirds of these patients. In both DM and lupus, there is associated nailfold erythema, and in DM, the erythema is often accompanied by ''ragged'' cuticles and fingertip tenderness. Under $10\times$ magnification, the blood vessels in the nailfolds of lupus patients are tortuous and resemble ''glomeruli,'' whereas in scleroderma and DM there is a loss of capillary loops and those which remain are markedly dilated.

In *hereditary hemorrhagic telangiectasia* (Osler-Rendu-Weber disease), the lesions usually appear during adulthood and are most commonly seen on the mucous membranes, face, and distal extremities, including under the nails. They represent arteriovenous (AV) malformations of the dermal microvasculature, are dark red in color, and are usually slightly elevated. When the skin is stretched over an individual lesion, an eccentric punctum with radiating legs is seen. Although the degree of systemic involvement varies in this autosomal dominant disease, the major symptoms are recurrent epistaxis and gastrointestinal bleeding. The fact that these mucosal telangiectasias are actually AV communications helps to explain their tendency to bleed.

HYPOPIGMENTATION (Table 54-14)   Disorders of hypopigmentation are classified as either diffuse or localized. The classic example of *diffuse* hypopigmentation is *oculocutaneous albinism* (OCA). The two most common forms are tyrosinase-negative OCA and tyrosinase-positive OCA; the former is characterized by a lack of enzyme

TABLE 54-14   Causes of hypopigmentation

Primary cutaneous disorders	Systemic diseases
A Diffuse	A Diffuse
1 Generalized vitiligo	*1* Oculocutaneous albinism
B Localized	B Localized
1 Vitiligo	*1* Vogt-Koyanagi-Harada
2 Chemical leukoderma	*2* Scleroderma
3 Piebaldism	*3* Melanoma-associated leukoderma
4 Nevus depigmentosus	*4* Tuberous sclerosis
5 Postinflammatory	*5* Hypomelanosis of Ito
6 Tinea versicolor	*6* Sarcoidosis
	7 Tuberculoid leprosy
	8 Cutaneous T cell lymphoma

activity. At birth, both types of OCA appear similar—white hair, gray-blue eyes, and pink-white skin. The patients with tyrosinase-negative OCA maintain this phenotype, whereas those with tyrosinase-positive OCA will acquire some pigmentation of the eyes, hair, and skin as they age. The degree of pigment formation is a function of their racial background, but a pigmentary dilution is readily apparent when they are compared to their first-degree relatives.

The ocular findings in OCA correlate with the degree of hypopigmentation, and they include decreased visual acuity, nystagmus, photophobia, and monocular vision. Patients with OCA, particularly those who reside in the tropics, develop cutaneous squamous cell carcinomas in association with severe actinic damage. The diagnosis of tyrosinase-positive OCA in a patient from Puerto Rico (Arecibo region) or southern Holland raises the possibility of the Hermansky-Pudlak syndrome. In addition to the signs and symptoms of OCA, these patients have a bleeding diathesis secondary to a platelet storage pool defect and restrictive lung disease secondary to deposits of ceroidlike material. Patients with Chédiak-Higashi syndrome also have tyrosinase-positive OCA, but their giant lysosomal granules fail to eradicate common pathogens such as *Staphylococcus aureus*. Generalized vitiligo, phenylketonuria, and homocystinuria are other unusual causes of diffuse pigmentary dilution. In generalized vitiligo, melanocytes are not found in affected skin, whereas in OCA they are present but have decreased activity. Appropriate laboratory tests exclude the other disorders of metabolism.

The differential diagnosis of *localized* hypomelanosis includes the following primary cutaneous disorders: *vitiligo*, *chemical leukoderma*, *piebaldism*, *nevus depigmentosus* (see below), *postinflammatory hypomelanosis*, and *tinea versicolor* (Table 54-15). In this group of diseases, the areas of involvement are macules or patches with a decrease or absence of pigmentation, and in the first four disorders, secondary changes such as scale or crust are absent. Patients with vitiligo have an increased incidence of several autoimmune disorders, including hypothyroidism, Graves' disease, pernicious anemia, Addison's disease, uveitis, alopecia areata, chronic mucocutaneous candidiasis, and the polyglandular autoimmune syndromes (types I, II, and III). Diseases of the thyroid gland are the most frequently associated disorders, occurring in up to 30 percent of patients with vitiligo.

TABLE 54-15 Hypopigmentation (primary cutaneous disorders, localized)

	Clinical characteristics	Wood's lamp examination (UV-A: peak = 365 nm)	Skin biopsy	Pathogenesis
Vitiligo	Acquired; progressive Symmetric areas of complete pigment loss Periorifical—around mouth, nose, eyes, nipples, umbilicus, anus Other areas—flexor wrists, extensor distal extremities Segmental form is less common—unilateral, dermatomal-like	More apparent Chalk-white	Absence of melanocytes Minimal inflammation	Possible autoimmune phenomenon that results in destruction of melanocytes—humoral and/or cellular Alternative hypothesis is self-destruction of melanocytes and circulating antibodies against melanocytes as a secondary phenomenon
Chemical leukoderma	Similar appearance to vitiligo Often begins on hands Satellite lesions in areas not exposed to chemicals	More apparent Chalk-white	Decreased number or absence of melanocytes	Exposure to chemicals that selectively destroy melanocytes, in particular, phenols and catechols (germicides; rubber products) Release of cellular antigens and activation of circulating lymphocytes may explain satellite phenomenon
Piebaldism	Autosomal dominant Congenital, stable White forelock Areas of hypomelanosis contain normally pigmented and hyperpigmented macules of various sizes Symmetric involvement of central forehead, ventral trunk, and mid regions of upper and lower extremities	Enhancement of leukoderma and hyperpigmented macules	Hypomelanotic areas—few to no melanocytes	Defect in migration of melanoblasts from neural crest to ventral skin or failure of melanoblasts to survive or differentiate in these areas Mutations within the *c-kit* proto-oncogene that encodes the tyrosine kinase receptor for mast/stem cell growth factor
Postinflammatory	Hypopigmentation can develop within active lesions, as in subacute lupus, or after the lesion fades, as in dermatitis	Depends on particular disease Usually less enhancement than in vitiligo	Type of inflammatory infiltrate depends on specific disease	Block in transfer of melanin from melanocytes to keratinocytes could be secondary to edema or decrease in contact time Destruction of melanocytes if inflammatory cells attack basal layer
Tinea versicolor	Common disorder Upper trunk and neck Shawl-like distribution Young adults Macules have fine white scale when scratched	Golden fluorescence	Hyphae and spores in stratum corneum	Invasion of stratum corneum by the yeast *Pityrosporum* Yeast is lipophilic and produces C_9 and C_{11} dicarboxylic acids which in vitro inhibit tyrosinase

Circulating autoantibodies are often found, and the most common ones are antithyroglobulin, antimicrosomal, and antiparietal cell antibodies.

There are three systemic diseases that should be considered in a patient with skin findings suggestive of vitiligo—*Vogt-Koyanagi-Harada syndrome*, *scleroderma*, and *melanoma-associated leukoderma*. A history of aseptic meningitis, nontraumatic uveitis, tinnitus, hearing loss, and/or dysacusis points to the diagnosis of the Vogt-Koyanagi-Harada syndrome. In these patients, the face and scalp are the most common locations of pigment loss. The vitiligo-like leukoderma seen in patients with scleroderma has a clinical resemblance to idiopathic vitiligo that has begun to repigment as a result of treatment; that is, perifollicular macules of normal pigmentation are seen within areas of depigmentation. The basis of this leukoderma is unknown; there is no evidence of inflammation in areas of involvement, but it can resolve if the underlying connective-tissue disease becomes inactive. In contrast to idiopathic vitiligo, melanoma-associated leukoderma often begins on the trunk, and its appearance should prompt a search for metastatic disease. The possibility exists that the destruction of normal melanocytes is the result of an immune response against malignant melanocytes.

There are two systemic disorders that may have the cutaneous findings of piebaldism (partial albinism) (see Table 54-15). They are *Hirschsprung's disease* and *Waardenburg's syndrome*. A possible explanation for both disorders is an abnormal embryonic migration or survival of two neural crest–derived elements, one of them being

melanocytes and the other myenteric ganglion cells (Hirschsprung's disease) or auditory nerve cells (Waardenburg's syndrome). The latter syndrome is characterized by congenital sensorineural hearing loss, dystopia canthorum (lateral displacement of the inner canthi but normal interpupillary distance), heterochromic irises, and a broad nasal root, in addition to the piebaldism.

In *tuberous sclerosis*, the earliest cutaneous sign is the ash leaf spot. These lesions are often present at birth; however, detection may require Wood's lamp examination, especially in fair-skinned individuals. The pigment within them is reduced but not absent. The average size is 1 to 3 cm, and the common shapes are oval, polygonal, and lance-ovate, whereas the less common shapes are dermatomal and confettilike. The terms *lance-ovate* and *ash leaf* are used to describe lesions with a particular shape, that is, tapered at one end and round at the other. Examination of the patient for additional cutaneous signs such as adenoma sebaceum (multiple angiofibromas of the face), ungual and gingival fibromas, fibrous plaques of the forehead, and connective-tissue nevi (shagreen patches) is recommended. It is important to remember that an ash leaf spot on the scalp will result in *poliosis*, which is a circumscribed patch of gray-white hair. Internal manifestations include seizures, mental retardation, central nervous system (CNS) and retinal hamartomas, renal angiomyolipomas, and cardiac rhabdomyomas. The latter can be detected in up to 60 percent of children (<18 years) with tuberous sclerosis by echocardiography.

Nevus depigmentosus is a stable, well-circumscribed hypomelanosis that is present at birth. There is usually a single circular or rectangular lesion, but occasionally, the nevus has a dermatomal or whorled pattern. It is important to distinguish this lesion from an ash leaf spot or hypomelanosis of Ito, for it is rarely associated with CNS findings. *Hypomelanosis of Ito* (incontinentia pigmenti achromians) is a neurocutaneous disorder in which swirls and streaks of hypopigmentation run parallel to one another. The pattern resembles that of a marble cake. Associated abnormalities are found in the musculoskeletal system (asymmetry), the CNS (seizures and mental retardation), and the eyes (strabismus and hypertelorism). Chromosomal mosaicism and diploid/triploid mixoploidy have been reported in these patients; this lends support to the hypothesis that the pattern is the result of the migration of two clones of primordial melanocytes, each with a different pigment potential.

Localized areas of decreased pigmentation are commonly seen as a result of cutaneous inflammation (see Table 54-15) and have been observed in the skin overlying active lesions of *sarcoidosis* (see "Papulonodular Skin Lesions") as well as *CTLC*. Cutaneous infections also present as disorders of hypopigmentation, and in *tuberculoid leprosy* there are a few asymmetric patches of hypomelanosis that have associated anesthesia, anhidrosis, and alopecia. Biopsy specimens of the palpable border show dermal granulomas that lack *Mycobacterium leprae* organisms.

HYPERPIGMENTATION (Table 54-16) Disorders of hyperpigmentation are also divided into two groups—localized and diffuse. The *localized* forms are due to an epidermal alteration, a proliferation of melanocytes, or an increase in pigment production. Both *seborrheic keratoses* and *acanthosis nigricans* belong to the first group (Table

---

TABLE 54-16 Causes of hyperpigmentation

Primary cutaneous disorders
  A Localized
    1 Epidermal alteration
      a Seborrheic keratosis
      b Acanthosis nigricans (obesity)
      c Pigmented actinic keratosis
    2 Proliferation of melanocytes
      a Lentigo
      b Nevus
      c Melanoma
    3 Increased pigment production
      a Ephelides (freckles)
      b Café au lait spots
  B Localized and diffuse
    1 Drugs
Systemic diseases
  A Localized
    1 Epidermal alteration
      a Seborrheic keratoses (sign of Leser-Trélat)
      b Acanthosis nigricans (endocrine disorders, paraneoplastic)
    2 Proliferation of melanocytes
      a Lentigines (Peutz-Jeghers, LEOPARD syndromes)
      b Nevi (LAMB and NAME syndromes)
    3 Increased pigment production
      a Café au lait spots (neurofibromatosis, Albright's syndrome)
      b Urticaria pigmentosa (see "Papulonodular Skin Lesions")
    4 Dermal pigmentation
      a Incontinentia pigmenti
      b Dyskeratosis congenita
  B Diffuse
    1 Endocrinopathies
      a Addison's disease
      b Nelson's syndrome
      c Ectopic ACTH syndrome
    2 Metabolic
      a Porphyria cutanea tarda
      b Hemochromatosis
      c Vitamin B_{12}, folate deficiency
      d Pellagra
      e Malabsorption, Whipple's disease
    3 Melanosis secondary to metastatic melanoma
    4 Autoimmune
      a Biliary cirrhosis
      b Scleroderma
      c POEMS syndrome
    5 Drugs and metals

54-17). Seborrheic keratoses are common lesions, but in one clinical setting they are a sign of systemic disease, and that setting is the sudden appearance of multiple lesions, often in association with acrochordons (skin tags) and acanthosis nigricans. This is termed the *sign of Leser-Trélat*, and it signifies an internal malignancy. *Acanthosis nigricans* also can be a reflection of an internal malignancy, most commonly of the gastrointestinal tract, and it appears as velvety hyperpigmentation (see Table 54-17). In the majority of patients, acanthosis nigricans is associated with obesity, but it may be a reflection of an endocrinopathy such as acromegaly, Cushing's syndrome, the Stein-Leventhal syndrome, or insulin-resistant diabetes mellitus (type A, type B, and lipoatrophic forms).

A proliferation of melanocytes results in the following pigmented lesions: *lentigo, melanocytic nevus,* and *melanoma* (see Table 54-17). In an adult, the majority of lentigines are related to sun exposure, which explains their distribution. However, in the Peutz-Jeghers and LEOPARD syndromes, lentigines do serve as a clue to systemic disease. The lentigines in patients with *Peutz-Jeghers syndrome* are located primarily around the nose and mouth, on the hands and feet, and within the oral cavity. While the pigmented macules on the face may fade with age, the oral lesions persist. However, similar intraoral lesions are also seen in Addison's disease and as a normal finding in darkly pigmented individuals. Patients with this autosomal dominant syndrome have multiple benign polyps of the gastrointestinal tract, ovarian tumors, and an approximately 6 percent risk of developing a gastrointestinal malignancy when the polyps arise in the stomach, duodenum, or colon.

In the multiple lentigines or *LEOPARD syndrome,* hundreds of lentigines develop during childhood and are scattered over the entire surface of the body. The syndrome consists of *L,* lentigines; *E,* ECG abnormalities, primarily conduction defects; *O,* ocular hypertelorism; *P,* pulmonary stenosis and subaortic valvular stenosis; *A,* abnormal genitalia (cryptorchidism, hypospadias); *R,* retardation of growth; and *D,* deafness (sensorineural). Lentigines are also seen in association with cardiac myxomas and have been described under the mnemonics *LAMB syndrome* and *NAME syndrome.* The findings in these two syndromes overlap and include *L,* lentigines; *A,* atrial myxomas; *M,* mucocutaneous myxomas; and *B,* blue nevi versus *N,* nevus; *A,* atrial myxoma; *M,* myxoid neurofibroma, and *E,* ephelides (freckles). These patients also can have evidence of endocrine overactivity in the form of Cushing's syndrome, acromegaly, or sexual precocity.

The third type of localized hyperpigmentation is due to a local increase in pigment production, and it includes *ephelides* (see Table 54-17) and café au lait spots. The latter are most commonly associated with two disorders—neurofibromatosis (NF) and Albright's syndrome. *Café au lait* (CAL) *spots* are flat, uniformly light brown in color, and can vary in size from 0.5 to 12 cm. Approximately 80 percent of the patients with *type I NF* will have six or more CAL spots measuring 1.5 cm or greater in diameter. Additional findings are discussed in the section on neurofibromas (see "Papulonodular Skin Lesions"). In comparison with NF, the CAL spots in patients with *Albright's disease* (polyostotic fibrous dysplasia with precocious puberty in females) are usually larger, more irregular in outline, respect the midline, and rarely contain macromelanosomes. CAL spots also have been associated with pulmonary stenosis, temporal dysrhythmia, tuberous sclerosis, the LEOPARD syndrome, and ataxia telangiectasia, but a few such lesions can be found in normal individuals.

In incontinentia pigmenti, dyskeratosis congenita, and bleomycin pigmentation, the areas of localized hyperpigmentation form a pattern—swirled in the first, reticulated in the second, and flagellate in the third. Patients with the X-linked dominant disorder *incontinentia pigmenti* can have linear blisters and verrucous papules during infancy. During childhood, parallel swirls and streaks of hyperpigmentation appear on the trunk, and occasionally streaks of hypopigmentation appear on the extremities. Associated findings include seizures, mental retardation, strabismus, cataracts, and delayed or impaired dentition. Biopsy of the streaks will show pigment within dermal macrophages ("incontinent pigment"). In *dyskeratosis congenita,* atrophic reticu-

TABLE 54-17 Hyperpigmentation (primary cutaneous disorders, localized)

	Clinical characteristics	Histopathology
Seborrheic keratosis	Tan to black papule Warty and/or greasy surface "Stuck on" appearance Trunk	Epidermal hyperplasia
Acanthosis nigricans	Velvety surface Neck, axillae, groin Occasionally on dorsum of the hand, corners of mouth	Epidermal folds Increased pigment in basal layer

Pigmented actinic keratosis	Brown macule, 3–10 mm
	Rough scale
	Sun-exposed areas, in particular
	  face and dorsum of hand
		Dysplasia of keratinocytes in lower third
		  of epidermis
		Increased pigment in epidermis

Ephelides (freckles)	2–5-mm macule Tan color Sun-exposed surfaces Darkens following sun exposure	Increased pigment in epidermis
Lentigo	0.3–1.5-cm macule Tan to black Most commonly in sun-exposed areas Face, upper trunk, and extremities	Increased number of melanocytes in epidermis Increased pigment in epidermis
Nevus		
Junctional	Brown to black macule 2–6 mm	Nests of melanocytes at dermoepidermal junction
Compound	Tan to brown papule 2–6 mm	Nests of melanocytes in epidermis and dermis
Dermal	Flesh-colored Papule	Nests of melanocytes in dermis
Melanoma	Variation in color—brown, black, blue, red, white Irregular outline and surface >5 mm in diameter Asymmetric	Malignant neoplasm of melanocytes

lated hyperpigmentation is seen on the neck, thighs, and trunk, and it is accompanied by nail dystrophy, pancytopenia, and leukoplakia of the oral and anal mucosa. The latter often develops into squamous cell carcinoma. In addition to the flagellate pigmentation (linear streaks) on the trunk, patients receiving bleomycin often have hyperpigmentation on the elbows, knees, and small joints of the hand.

Localized hyperpigmentation is seen as a side effect of several other *systemic medications*, including those which produce fixed drug reactions (phenolphthalein, tetracyclines, sulfonamides, barbiturates, and analgesics) and those which can bind to melanin (antimalarials). Fixed drug eruptions recur in the same location as circular areas of erythema that can become bullous and then resolve as brown macules. The eruption usually appears within hours of administration of the offending agent, and common locations include the genitalia, extremities, and perioral region. Chloroquine and hydroxychloroquine produce gray-brown to blue-black discoloration of the shins, hard palate, and face, while blue macules are seen on the lower extremities and in sites of inflammation with prolonged minocycline administration. Estrogen in oral contraceptives can induce melasma—symmetric brown patches on the face, especially the cheeks, upper lip, and forehead. Similar changes are seen in pregnancy, in patients receiving hydantoin, and in the adult form of Gaucher's disease. In the latter group there is also hyperpigmentation of the distal lower extremities.

In the *diffuse* forms of hyperpigmentation, the darkening of the skin may be of equal intensity over the entire body, or it may be accentuated in sun-exposed areas. The causes of diffuse hyperpigmentation can be divided into four groups—endocrine, metabolic, autoimmune, and drugs. The endocrinopathies that frequently have associated hyperpigmentation include *Addison's disease*, *Nelson's syndrome*, and *ectopic ACTH syndrome*. In these diseases, the increased pigmentation is diffuse, but it is accentuated in the palmar creases, sites of friction, scars, and the oral mucosa. An overproduction of any or all of the pituitary hormones α-MSH (melanocyte-stimulating hormone), ACTH, and β-lipotropin can lead to an increase in melanocyte activity. All these peptides are products of the proopiomelanocortin gene, and therefore, they exhibit homology; e.g., α-MSH and ACTH share 13 amino acids. A minority of the patients with Cushing's disease or hyperthyroidism have generalized hyperpigmentation.

The metabolic causes of hyperpigmentation include *porphyria*

cutanea tarda (PCT), *hemochromatosis*, *vitamin B₁₂ deficiency*, *folic acid deficiency*, *pellagra*, *malabsorption*, and *Whipple's disease*. In patients with *PCT* (see "Vesicles/Bullae"), the skin darkening is seen in sun-exposed areas and is a reflection of the photoreactive properties of porphyrins. The increased level of iron in the skin of patients with *hemochromatosis* stimulates melanin pigment production and leads to the classic bronze color. Patients with *pellagra* have a brown discoloration of the skin, especially in sun-exposed areas, as a result of nicotinic acid (niacin) deficiency. In the areas of increased pigmentation, there is a thin varnishlike scale. These changes are also seen in patients who are vitamin B₆ deficient, have functioning carcinoid tumors (increased consumption of niacin), or take isoniazid. Approximately 50 percent of the patients with *Whipple's disease* have an associated generalized hyperpigmentation in association with diarrhea, weight loss, arthritis, and lymphadenopathy. A diffuse slate-blue color is seen in patients with melanosis secondary to *metastatic melanoma*. There is a debate as to whether the color is due to single-cell metastases in the dermis or to a widespread deposition of melanin resulting from the high concentration of circulating melanin precursors.

Of the autoimmune diseases associated with diffuse hyperpigmentation, *biliary cirrhosis* and *scleroderma* are the most common, and occasionally, both disorders are seen in the same patient. The skin is dark brown in color, especially in sun-exposed areas. In biliary cirrhosis the hyperpigmentation is accompanied by pruritus, jaundice, and xanthomas, whereas in scleroderma it is accompanied by sclerosis of the extremities, face, and, less commonly, the trunk. Additional clues to the diagnosis of scleroderma are telangiectasias, calcinosis cutis, Raynaud's phenomenon, and distal ulcerations (see "Telangiectasias"). The differential diagnosis of cutaneous sclerosis with hyperpigmentation includes the *POEMS syndrome*: *P*, polyneuropathy; *O*, organomegaly (liver, spleen, lymph nodes); *E*, endocrinopathies (impotence, gynecomastia); *M*, M-protein; and *S*, skin changes. The skin changes include hyperpigmentation, skin thickening, hypertrichosis, hyperhidrosis, and angiomas.

Diffuse hyperpigmentation that is due to *drugs* or *metals* can result from one of several mechanisms—induction of melanin pigment formation, complexing of the drug or its metabolites to melanin, and deposits of the drug in the dermis. Busulfan; cyclophosphamide;

long-term, high-dose ACTH; and inorganic arsenic induce pigment production. Complexes containing melanin or hemosiderin plus the drug or its metabolites are seen in patients receiving chlorpromazine and minocycline. The sun-exposed skin as well as the conjunctivae of patients on long-term, high-dose chlorpromazine can become blue-gray in color. Patients taking minocycline may develop a diffuse blue-gray, muddy appearance in sun-exposed areas in addition to pigmentation of the mucous membranes, teeth, nails, bones, and thyroid. Administration of amiodarone can result in both a phototoxic eruption (exaggerated sunburn) and/or a brown or blue-gray discoloration of sun-exposed skin. Biopsy specimens of the latter show yellow-brown granules in dermal macrophages, which represent intralysosomal accumulations of lipids, amiodarone, and its metabolites. Actual deposits of a particular drug or metal in the skin are seen with silver (argyria), where the skin appears blue-gray in color; gold (chrysiasis), where the skin has a brown to blue-gray color; and clofazimine, where the skin appears reddish brown. The associated hyperpigmentation is accentuated in sun-exposed areas, and discoloration of the eye is seen with gold (sclerae) and clofazimine (conjunctivae). Recently, an epidemic of the eosinophilia-myalgia syndrome has been described that is presumably due to contaminated L-tryptophan preparations. In addition to maculopapular eruptions and alopecia, large areas of sclerodermalike induration are observed with overlying hyperpigmentation.

VESICLES/BULLAE (Table 54-18) Depending on their size, cutaneous blisters are referred to as *vesicles* (<0.5 cm) or *bullae* (>0.5 cm). The primary blistering disorders include *pemphigus vulgaris*, *pemphigus foliaceus*, *pemphigus erythematosus*, *bullous pemphigoid*, *herpes gestationis*, *cicatricial pemphigoid*, *epidermolysis bullosa acquisita*, and *dermatitis herpetiformis* (see Chap. 53).

Vesicles and bullae are also seen in *contact dermatitis*, both allergic and irritant forms (see "Erythroderma"). When there is a linear arrangement of vesicular lesions, an exogenous cause should be suspected. Bullous disease secondary to the ingestion of drugs can take one of several forms, including phototoxic eruptions, isolated bullae, toxic epidermal necrolysis, and erythema multiforme. Clinically, phototoxic eruptions resemble an exaggerated sunburn with diffuse erythema and bullae in sun-exposed areas. The most commonly associated drugs are thiazides, tetracyclines, sulfonylureas, sulfonamides, phenothiazines, griseofulvin, and psoralens. The development of a phototoxic eruption is dependent on the doses of both the drug and UV-A irradiation.

There are several drugs, including penicillins, sulfonamides, phenobarbital, phenytoin, furosemide, and nonsteroidal anti-inflammatory agents, that cause isolated bland bullae to arise on normal skin. The characteristics of these blisters are such that they cannot

be assigned to a particular cutaneous disease. The most common location for these isolated bullae is the distal extremity. In contrast, *toxic epidermal necrolysis* (TEN) is characterized by bullae that arise on widespread areas of erythema and then slough. This results in large areas of denuded skin. The associated morbidity, such as sepsis, and mortality are relatively high, and they are a function of the extent of epidermal necrosis. In addition, these patients also may have involvement of the mucous membranes and intestinal tract. Drugs are the primary cause of TEN, and the most common offenders are phenytoin, barbiturates, sulfonamides, penicillins, allopurinol, and phenylbutazone. Severe acute graft-versus-host disease (grade 4) also can resemble TEN.

In *erythema multiforme* (EM), the primary lesions are pink-red macules and edematous papules, the centers of which may become vesicular. The clue to the diagnosis of EM rather than of a drug-induced morbilliform exanthem is the development of a "dusky" violet color or petechiae in the center of the lesions. Target or iris lesions are also characteristic of EM, and they arise as a result of active centers and borders in combination with centrifugal spread. However, iris lesions need not be present to make the diagnosis of EM. Preferred sites of involvement include the hands, extensor forearms, palms, soles, and mucous membranes (oral, nasal, ocular, and genital). Hemorrhagic crusts of the lips are characteristic of EM, as well as two other blistering disorders—pemphigus vulgaris and TEN. Fever, malaise, myalgias, sore throat, and cough may precede or accompany the eruption. The lesions of EM usually resolve over 3 to 6 weeks, but they may be recurrent.

Drugs can induce EM, in particular sulfonamides, phenytoin, barbiturates, penicillins, and carbamazepine, but they do not cause the majority of cases, especially in young adults. Infections with herpes simplex are the most common cause of EM in this age group, and the lesions appear 7 to 12 days after the viral eruption. Other infectious agents associated with EM include *Mycoplasma pneumoniae*, *Histoplasma capsulatum*, *Coccidioides immitis*, *Yersinia enterocolitica*, and several viruses (echovirus, coxsackievirus, Epstein-Barr, and influenza). EM also can follow vaccinations with BCG, poliomyelitis, or vaccinia viruses; radiation therapy; and exposure to environmental toxins; and it has been observed in a few patients with lupus erythematosus, Wegener's granulomatosis, and internal malignancy.

In addition to primary blistering disorders and hypersensitivity reactions, bacterial and viral infections can lead to vesicles and bullae. The most common infectious agents are herpes simplex (see Chap. 143), herpes varicella-zoster (see Chap. 144), and staphylococci (see Chap. 102).

Staphylococcal scalded-skin syndrome (SSSS) and *bullous impetigo* are two blistering disorders associated with staphylococcal (phage group II) infection. In SSSS, the initial findings are redness and tenderness of the central face, neck, trunk, and intertriginous zones. This is followed by short-lived flaccid bullae and a slough or exfoliation of the superficial epidermis. Crusted areas then develop, characteristically around the mouth. SSSS is distinguished from TEN by the following features: younger age group, more superficial site of blister formation, no oral lesions, shorter course, less morbidity and mortality, and an association with staphylococcal exfoliative toxin ("exfoliatin"), not drugs. A rapid diagnosis of SSSS versus TEN can be made by a frozen section of the blister roof or exfoliative cytology of the blister contents. In SSSS the site of staphylococcal infection is usually extracutaneous (conjunctivitis, rhinorrhea, otitis media, pharyngitis, tonsillitis), and the lesions are sterile, whereas in *bullous impetigo* the lesions are the site of infection. Impetigo is more localized than SSSS, and it usually presents with honey-colored crusts. Occasionally, superficial purulent blisters also form. *Cutaneous emboli* from gram-negative infections may present as isolated bullae, but the base of the lesion is purpuric or necrotic, and it may develop into an ulcer (see "Purpura").

Several metabolic disorders are associated with blister formation, including diabetes mellitus, renal failure, and porphyria. Local

---

TABLE 54-18 Causes of vesicles/bullae

Primary cutaneous diseases	Systemic diseases
A Primary blistering diseases	A Infections
1 Pemphigus*	*1* Cutaneous emboli[†]
2 Bullous pemphigoid[†]	B Metabolic
3 Herpes gestationis[†]	*1* Diabetic bullae*,[†]
4 Cicatricial pemphigoid[†]	*2* Porphyria cutanea tarda[†]
5 Dermatitis herpetiformis[†]	*3* Porphyria variegata[†]
6 Epidermolysis bullosa[†]	*4* Pseudoporphyria[†]
acquisita	*5* Bullous dermatosis of
B Secondary blistering diseases	hemodialysis[†]
1 Contact*	
2 Erythema multiforme*,[†]	
3 Toxic epidermal ne-	
crolysis*,[†]	
C Infections	
1 Varicella/zoster*,[‡]	
2 Herpes simplex*,[‡]	
3 Staphylococcal scalded-skin	
syndrome*	
4 Bullous impetigo*	

* Intraepidermal.   [†] Subepidermal.   [‡] Also systemic.

hypoxia secondary to decreased cutaneous blood flow also can produce blisters, which explains the presence of bullae over pressure points in comatose patients (coma bullae). In *diabetes mellitus*, tense bullae with clear viscous fluid arise on normal skin. The lesions can be as large as 6 cm in diameter, and they are located on the distal extremities. There are several types of porphyria, but the most common form with cutaneous findings is *porphyria cutanea tarda* (PCT). In sun-exposed areas (primarily the face and hands), the skin is very fragile, and trauma leads to erosions and tense vesicles. These lesions then heal with scarring and formation of milia; the latter are firm, 2- to 3-mm white or yellow papules that represent epidermoid inclusion cysts. Associated findings can include hypertrichosis of the lateral malar region (males) or face (females) and, in sun-exposed areas, hyperpigmentation and firm sclerotic plaques. An elevated level of urinary uroporphyrins confirms the diagnosis and is due to a decrease in uroporphyrinogen decarboxylase activity. Precipitating agents include alcohol, estrogen, iron, and chlorinated hydrocarbons.

The differential diagnosis of PCT includes (1) *porphyria varie-gata*—the skin signs of PCT plus the systemic findings of acute intermittent porphyria; it has a diagnostic plasma porphyrin fluorescence emission at 626 nm; (2) *drug-induced bullous photosensitivity* (pseudoporphyria)—the clinical and histologic findings are similar to PCT, but porphyrins are normal; etiologic agents are furosemide, tetracycline, nalidixic acid, dapsone, naproxen, and pyridoxine; (3) *bullous dermatosis of hemodialysis*—the same appearance as PCT, but porphyrins are usually normal or occasionally borderline elevated; patients have chronic renal failure and are on hemodialysis; (4) PCT associated with hepatomas, hepatic carcinomas, and hemodialysis; and (5) *epidermolysis bullosa acquisita* (see Chap. 53).

EXANTHEMS (Table 54-19)   Exanthems are characterized by an acute generalized eruption. The two most common presentations are erythematous macules and papules (morbilliform) and confluent blanching erythema (scarlatiniform). *Morbilliform* eruptions are usually due to either *drugs* or *viral infections*. For example, at least 5 percent of the patients receiving penicillins, sulfonamides, captopril, phenytoin, or gold will develop a maculopapular eruption. Accompanying signs may include pruritus, fever, eosinophilia, and transient lymphadenopathy. Similar maculopapular eruptions are seen in the classic childhood viral exanthems, including (1) *rubeola* (measles)— a prodrome of coryza, cough, conjunctivitis, and Koplik's spots on the buccal mucosa whose onset coincides with a second fever spike; the eruption begins behind the ears, at the hairline, and on the forehead and then spreads down the body, often becoming confluent; (2) *rubella*—it begins on the forehead and face and then spreads down the body; it resolves in the same order and is associated with retroauricular and suboccipital lymphadenopathy; and (3) *erythema infectiosum* (fifth disease)—erythema of the cheeks is followed by a reticulated pattern on extremities; it is secondary to a parvovirus infection, and an associated arthritis is seen in adults.

Both measles and rubella are seen in unvaccinated young adults, and an atypical form of measles is seen in adults immunized with either killed measles vaccine or killed vaccine followed in time by live vaccine. In contrast to classic measles, the eruption of atypical measles begins on the palms, soles, wrists, and knuckles, and the lesions may become purpuric. The patient with atypical measles can have pulmonary involvement and be quite ill. Rubelliform and roseoliform eruptions are also associated with *Epstein-Barr virus* (5 to 15 percent of patients), *echovirus, coxsackievirus,* and *adenovirus* infections. Detection of specific IgM antibodies allows the proper diagnosis. Occasionally, a maculopapular eruption is the result of a drug-viral interaction. For example, about 95 percent of the patients with infectious mononucleosis who are given ampicillin will develop a rash.

Of note, early in the course of infections with *Rickettsia* and *meningococcus*, prior to the development of purpura, the lesions may be erythematous macules and papules. This is also the case in chickenpox prior to the development of vesicles. Maculopapular eruptions are associated with early *HIV infection*, early secondary *syphilis, typhoid fever,* and *acute graft-versus-host* disease. In the last, lesions frequently begin on the palms and soles; the macular rose spots of typhoid fever involve primarily the anterior trunk.

The prototypic *scarlatiniform* eruption is seen in *scarlet fever* and is due to an erythrotoxin produced by group A beta-hemolytic streptococcal infections, most commonly pharyngitis. There are a diffuse erythema, which begins on the neck and upper trunk, and red perifollicular puncta. Additional findings include a white strawberry tongue (white coating with red papillae) followed by a red strawberry tongue (red tongue with red papillae), petechiae of the palate, a facial flush with circumoral pallor, linear petechiae in the antecubital fossae, and desquamation of the involved skin, palms, and soles 5 to 20 days after onset of the eruption. A similar desquamation of the palms and soles is seen in toxic shock syndrome, Kawasaki's disease, and after severe febrile illnesses. Certain strains of staphylococci also produce an erythrotoxin that leads to the same clinical findings as in streptococcal scarlet fever, except that the antistreptolysin O titers are not elevated.

In *toxic shock syndrome* (TSS), staphylococcal (phage group I) infections produce an exotoxin that causes the fever and rash, as well as an enterotoxin. Initially, the majority of cases were reported in menstruating women who were using tampons. However, other sites of infection, including wounds and vaginitis, may produce TSS. The diagnosis of TSS is based on clinical criteria, and three of these involve mucocutaneous sites. The clinical criteria are (1) fever, (2) diffuse erythema of the skin, (3) desquamation of the palms and soles 1 to 2 weeks after onset of illness, (4) hypotension, and (5) involvement of three or more organ systems, including the gastrointestinal tract, muscles, kidney, liver, CNS, hematologic (thrombocytopenia), and mucous membranes. The latter is characterized as hyperemia of the vagina, oropharynx, or conjunctivae.

Although the cutaneous eruption in *Kawasaki's disease* (mucocutaneous lymph node syndrome) is polymorphous, the two common types are morbilliform and scarlatiniform. The majority of cases are seen in children less than 5 years of age, but adult cases have been reported. The diagnosis is based on a fever lasting more than 5 days plus four of the five following criteria: (1) bilateral conjunctival injection, (2) exanthem, (3) cervical lymphadenopathy, usually unilateral, (4) erythema and edema of the hands and feet followed by desquamation, and (5) diffuse erythema of the oropharynx, red strawberry tongue, and erosions with crusting on the lips. This clinical picture can resemble TSS and scarlet fever, but clues to the diagnosis of Kawasaki's disease are the cervical lymphadenopathy, lip erosions, and increased platelets. The most serious associated systemic finding in this disease is coronary aneurysm secondary to arteritis. Aneurysms may lead to sudden death, primarily within the first 30 days of the illness. Scarlatiniform eruptions are also seen in the early phase of SSSS (see ''Vesicles/Bullae'') and as reactions to drugs.

TABLE 54-19   Causes of exanthems

Morbilliform
A Drugs
B Viral
  1 Rubeola (measles)
  2 Rubella
  3 Erythema infectiosum
  4 Epstein-Barr, echovirus, coxsackievirus, and adenovirus
  5 Early HIV
C Bacterial
  1 Typhoid fever
  2 Early secondary syphilis
  3 Early *Rickettsia*
  4 Early meningococcus
D Acute graft-versus-host disease
Scarlatiniform
A Scarlet fever
B Toxic shock syndrome
C Kawasaki's disease

TABLE 54-20 Causes of urticaria

Primary cutaneous disorders
  A Acute and chronic urticaria
  B Physical urticaria
    1 Dermatographism
    2 Solar urticaria*
    3 Cold urticaria*
    4 Cholinergic urticaria*
  C Angioedema (hereditary and acquired)*
Systemic diseases
  A Urticarial vasculitis
  B Hepatitis B infection
  C Serum sickness
  D Angioedema (acquired)

* Also systemic.

URTICARIA (Table 54-20) *Urticaria* (hives) are transient lesions that are composed of a central wheal surrounded by an erythematous halo. Individual lesions are round, oval, or figurate, and they are often pruritic. *Acute* and *chronic* urticaria have a wide variety of allergic etiologies. Less common systemic causes of urticaria are mastocytosis (urticaria pigmentosa), hyperthyroidism, malignancy, and juvenile rheumatoid arthritis (JRA). In JRA, the lesions coincide with the fever spike, and they are transient but not migratory as in erythema marginatum.

The common *physical urticarias* include *dermatographism, solar urticaria, cold urticaria,* and *cholinergic urticaria.* Patients with dermatographism exhibit linear wheals following minor pressure or scratching of the skin. It is a common disorder, affecting approximately 5 percent of the population. Solar urticaria characteristically occurs within minutes of sun exposure and is a skin sign of one systemic disease—erythropoietic protoporphyria. In addition to the urticaria, these patients have subtle pitted scarring of the nose and hands. Cold urticaria is precipitated by exposure to the cold, and therefore, exposed areas are usually affected. In some cases, the disease is associated with abnormal circulating proteins—more commonly cryoglobulins and cold hemolysins and less commonly cryofibrinogens and cold agglutinins. Additional systemic symptoms include wheezing and syncope, thus explaining the need for these patients to avoid swimming in cold water. Cholinergic urticaria is precipitated by heat, exercise, or emotion and is characterized by small wheals with relatively large flares. It is occasionally associated with wheezing.

Whereas urticaria is the result of dermal edema, subcutaneous edema leads to the clinical picture of *angioedema.* Sites of involvement include the eyelids, lips, tongue, larynx, and gastrointestinal tract as well as the subcutaneous tissue. Angioedema occurs alone or in combination with urticaria, including urticarial vasculitis and the physical urticarias. Both acquired and hereditary (autosomal dominant) forms of angioedema occur (see Chap. 282), and in the latter, urticaria is rarely seen.

Urticarial vasculitis is an immune complex disease that may be confused with simple urticaria. In contrast to simple urticaria, individual lesions tend to last longer than 24 h, and they usually develop central petechiae that can be observed even after the urticarial phase has resolved. The patient also may complain of burning rather than pruritus. On biopsy, there is a leukocytoclastic vasculitis of the small blood vessels. Although many cases of urticarial vasculitis are idiopathic in origin, it can be a reflection of an underlying systemic illness such as lupus erythematosus, Sjögren's syndrome, or hereditary complement deficiency. There is a spectrum of urticarial vasculitis that ranges from purely cutaneous to multisystem involvement. The most common systemic signs and symptoms are arthralgias and/or arthritis, nephritis, and crampy abdominal pain, with asthma and chronic obstructive lung disease seen less often. Hypocomplementemia occurs in one- to two-thirds of patients, even in the idiopathic cases. Similar cutaneous, joint, and renal findings can be seen in the prodrome of *hepatitis B infection, serum sickness,* and *serum sickness–like illnesses.*

PAPULONODULAR SKIN LESIONS (Table 54-21) In the *papulonodular diseases,* the lesions are elevated above the surface of the skin, and they may coalesce to form plaques. The location, consistency, and color of the lesions are the keys to their diagnosis. This section is organized on the basis of color, and the color groups are white, flesh, pink, yellow, red, red-brown, blue, violaceous, purple, and brown-black.

White lesions In *calcinosis cutis* there are firm white to white-yellow papules with an irregular surface. When the contents are discharged, a chalky white material is seen. *Dystrophic* calcification is seen at sites of previous inflammation or damage to the skin. It develops in acne scars as well as on the distal extremities of patients with scleroderma and in the subcutaneous tissue and intermuscular fascial planes in dermatomyositis. The latter is more extensive and is more commonly seen in children. An elevated calcium phosphate product, as in secondary hyperparathyroidism, can lead to nodules of *metastatic* calcinosis cutis, which tend to be subcutaneous and periarticular. This form is often accompanied by calcification of muscular arteries and subsequent ischemic necrosis.

Flesh-colored lesions There are several types of flesh-colored lesions, including epidermoid inclusion cysts, lipomas, rheumatoid nodules, neurofibromas, angiofibromas, neuromas, and adnexal tumors such as tricholemmomas. Both *epidermoid inclusion cysts* and *lipomas* are very common mobile subcutaneous nodules—the former are rubbery and compressible, and they drain cheeselike material (sebum and keratin) if incised. Lipomas are firm and somewhat lobulated on palpation. When extensive facial epidermoid inclusion cysts develop in childhood or there is a family history of such lesions, the patient should be examined for other signs of Gardner's syndrome, including osteomas and desmoid tumors (see Chap. 256). *Rheumatoid nodules* are firm, 0.5- to 4-cm nodules that tend to localize around

TABLE 54-21 Papulonodular skin lesions according to color groups

White
  A Calcinosis cutis
Flesh
  A Rheumatoid nodule
  B Neurofibromas
    (von Recklinghausen's disease)
  C Angiofibromas
    (tuberous sclerosis)
  D Neuromas
    (multiple endocrine neoplasia syndrome, type 2b)
  E Adnexal tumors
    1 Basal cell epitheliomas
      (basal cell nevus syndrome)
    2 Tricholemmomas
      (Cowden's disease)
  F Primary cutaneous disorders
    1 Epidermal inclusion cysts
    2 Lipomas
Pink/translucent
  A Amyloidosis
  B Papular mucinosis
Yellow
  A Xanthomas
  B Tophi
  C Necrobiosis lipoidica
  D Pseudoxanthoma elasticum
  E Sebaceous adenomas
    (Torre's syndrome)
Red
  A Papules
    1 Angiokeratomas
      (Fabry's disease)
    2 Bacillary angiomatosis (primarily in AIDS)
  B Papules/plaques
    1 Cutaneous lupus
    2 Lymphoma cutis
    3 Leukemia cutis

  C Nodules
    1 Panniculitis
    2 Cutaneous polyarteritis nodosa
    3 Systemic vasculitis
  D Primary cutaneous disorders
    1 Arthropod bites
    2 Cherry hemangiomas
    3 Infections, e.g., erysipelas, sporotrichosis
    4 Polymorphous light eruption
    5 Lymphocytoma cutis (pseudolymphoma)
Red-brown
  A Sarcoidosis
  B Sweet's syndrome
  C Urticaria pigmentosa
  D Erythema elevatum diutinum (chronic leukocytoclastic vasculitis)
  E Lupus vulgaris
Blue
  A Cavernous hemangiomas (blue rubber bleb syndrome)
  B Primary cutaneous disorders
    1 Venous lake
    2 Blue nevus
Violaceous
  A Lupus pernio (sarcoidosis)
  B Lymphoma cutis
  C Cutaneous lupus
Purple
  A Kaposi's sarcoma
  B Angiosarcoma
  C Palpable purpura
Brown-black
  See "Hyperpigmentation"
Any color
  A Metastases

pressure points, especially the elbows. They are seen in approximately 20 percent of patients with rheumatoid arthritis and 6 percent of patients with Still's disease. Biopsies of the nodules show palisading granulomas. Similar lesions that are smaller and shorter-lived are seen in rheumatic fever.

Neurofibromas (benign Schwann cell tumors) are soft papules or nodules that exhibit the "button-hole" sign, that is, they invaginate into the skin with pressure in a manner similar to a hernia. Single lesions are seen in normal individuals, but multiple neurofibromas, usually in combination with six or more café au lait spots measuring >1.5 cm (see "Hyperpigmentation") and multiple Lisch nodules, are seen in von Recklinghausen's disease (NF type I). Lisch nodules are 1-mm yellow-brown spots within the iris that are best observed with slit-lamp examination. Additional manifestations include axillary freckling and peripheral and CNS tumors (see Chap. 378). In some patients the neurofibromas are localized and unilateral, whereas in others they are limited to the CNS.

Angiofibromas are firm, pink to flesh-colored papules that measure from 3 mm to several centimeters in diameter. When they are located on the central cheeks (adenoma sebaceum) or fibromas are seen around the nails, the patient has tuberous sclerosis. It is an autosomal disorder, and the associated findings are discussed in the section on ash leaf spots (see "Hypopigmentation").

Neuromas (benign proliferation of nerve fibers) are also firm, flesh-colored papules. They are more commonly found at sites of amputation and as rudimentary supernumerary digits. However, when there are multiple neuromas on the eyelids, lips, distal tongue, and/or oral mucosa, the patient should be investigated for other signs of the multiple endocrine neoplasia syndrome, type 2b. Associated findings include marfanoid habitus, protuberant lips, intestinal ganglioneuromas, and medullary thyroid carcinoma (>75 percent of patients) (see Chap. 343).

Adnexal tumors are derived from pluripotential cells of the epidermis that can differentiate toward hair, sebaceous, apocrine, or eccrine glands or remain undifferentiated. *Basal cell epitheliomas* (BCEs) are examples of adnexal tumors that have little or no evidence of differentiation. Clinically, they are translucent papules with rolled borders, telangiectasias, and central erosion. BCEs commonly arise in sun-damaged skin of the head and neck. When a patient has multiple BCEs, especially prior to age 30, the possibility of the basal cell nevus syndrome should be raised. It is inherited as an autosomal dominant trait and is associated with jaw cysts, palmar and plantar pits, frontal bossing, rib anomalies, and calcification of the falx cerebri and diaphragma sellae. *Tricholemmomas* are also flesh-colored adnexal tumors, but they differentiate toward hair follicles and can have a wartlike appearance. The presence of multiple tricholemmomas on the face and oral mucosa points to the diagnosis of Cowden's disease (multiple hamartoma syndrome). The oral tricholemmomas are found primarily on the tongue and gingiva and give these areas a cobblestone appearance. Internal organ involvement (in decreasing order of frequency) includes fibrocystic disease and carcinoma of the breast, adenomas and carcinomas of the thyroid, and gastrointestinal polyposis. Keratoses of the palms, soles, and dorsa of the hands are also seen.

Pink lesions The cutaneous lesions associated with primary systemic *amyloidosis* are pink in color and translucent. Common locations are the face, especially the periorbital and perioral regions, and intertriginous areas. On biopsy, homogeneous deposits of amyloid are seen in the dermis and in the walls of blood vessels; the latter lead to an increase in vessel wall fragility. As a result, petechiae and purpura develop in clinically normal skin as well as in lesional skin following minor trauma, hence the term "pinch purpura." Amyloid deposits are also seen in the striated muscle of the tongue, and these result in macroglossia.

Even though specific mucocutaneous lesions are rarely seen in secondary amyloidosis and are present in only about 30 percent of the patients with primary amyloidosis, a rapid diagnosis of systemic amyloidosis can be made by an examination of abdominal subcutaneous fat. By special staining, deposits are seen around blood vessels or individual fat cells in 40 to 50 percent of patients. There are also three forms of amyloidosis that are limited to the skin and that should not be construed as cutaneous lesions of systemic amyloidosis. They are macular amyloid (upper back), lichenoid amyloidosis (usually lower extremities), and nodular amyloidosis. In macular and lichenoid amyloidosis, the deposits are composed of altered epidermal keratin. Recently, macular amyloidosis has been associated with multiple endocrine neoplasia syndrome, type 2a.

Patients with *multicentric reticulohistiocytosis* also have pink-colored papules and nodules on the face and mucous membranes as well as on the extensor surface of the hands and forearms. They have a polyarthritis that can mimic rheumatoid arthritis clinically. On histologic examination, the papules have characteristic giant cells that are not seen in biopsies of rheumatoid nodules. Pink to flesh-colored papules that are firm, 2 to 5 mm in diameter, and often in a linear arrangement are seen in patients with *papular mucinosis*. This disease is also referred to as *lichen myxedematosus* or *scleromyxedema*. The latter name comes from the brawny induration of the face and extremities that may accompany the papular eruption. Biopsy specimens of the papules show localized mucin deposition, and serum protein electrophoresis demonstrates a monoclonal spike of IgG, usually with a λ light chain.

Yellow lesions Several systemic disorders are characterized by yellow-colored cutaneous papules or plaques—hyperlipidemia (xanthomas), gout (tophi), diabetes (necrobiosis lipoidica), pseudoxanthoma elasticum, and Torre's syndrome (sebaceous tumors). Eruptive xanthomas are the most common form of *xanthomas*, and they are associated with hypertriglyceridemia (types I, III, IV, and V). Crops of yellow papules with erythematous halos occur primarily on the extensor surfaces of the extremities and the buttocks in association with elevations of the circulating triglycerides. They spontaneously involute with a fall in serum lipids. Increased β-lipoproteins (primarily types II and III) result in one or more of the following types of xanthoma: xanthelasma, tendon xanthomas, and plane xanthomas. Xanthelasma are found on the eyelids, whereas tendon xanthomas are frequently associated with the Achilles and extensor finger tendons; plane xanthomas are flat and favor the palmar creases, face, upper trunk, and scars. Tuberous xanthomas are frequently associated with hypertriglyceridemia, but they are also seen in patients with hypercholesterolemia (type II) and are found most frequently over the large joints or hand. Biopsy specimens of xanthomas show collections of lipid-containing macrophages (foam cells).

Patients with several disorders, including biliary cirrhosis, can have a secondary form of hyperlipidemia with associated tuberous and planar xanthomas. However, patients with myeloma have *normolipemic* flat xanthomas. This latter form of xanthoma may be ≥12 cm in diameter and is most frequently seen on the upper trunk or side of the neck. It is also important to note that the most common setting for eruptive xanthomas is uncontrolled diabetes mellitus. The least specific sign for hyperlipidemia is xanthelasma because at least 50 percent of the patients with this finding have normal lipid profiles.

In *tophaceous gout* there are deposits of monosodium urate in the skin around the joints, particularly those of the hands and feet. Additional sites of *tophi* formation include the helix of the ear and the olecranon and prepatellar bursae. The lesions are firm, yellow in color, and occasionally discharge a chalky material. Their size varies from 1 mm to 7 cm, and the diagnosis can be established by polarization of the aspirated contents of a lesion. Lesions of *necrobiosis lipoidica* are found primarily on the shins (90 percent), and the majority of patients have diabetes mellitus or develop it subsequently. Characteristic findings include a central yellow color, atrophy (transparency), telangiectasias, and an erythematous border. Ulcerations also can develop within the plaques. Biopsy specimens show necrobiosis of collagen, granulomatous inflammation, and obliterative endarteritis.

In *pseudoxanthoma elasticum* (PXE) there is an abnormal deposition of calcium on the elastic fibers of the skin, eye, and blood vessels. In the skin, the flexural areas such as the neck, axillae, antecubital fossae, and inguinal area are the primary sites of involvement. Yellow papules coalesce to form reticulated plaques that have an appearance similar to that of plucked chicken skin. In severely affected skin, hanging, redundant folds develop. Some patients have a more subtle macular form of the disease, and careful inspection is required. Biopsy specimens of involved skin show swollen and irregularly clumped elastic fibers with deposits of calcium. In the eye, the calcium deposits in Bruch's membrane lead to angioid streaks and choroiditis; in the arteries of the heart, kidney, gastrointestinal tract, and extremities, the deposits lead to angina, hypertension, gastrointestinal bleeding, and claudication, respectively. Four types of PXE have been described—two with autosomal dominant and two with autosomal recessive inheritance. The extent of vessel and skin involvement varies depending on the type. Long-term administration of D-penicillamine can lead to PXE-like skin changes as well as elastic fiber alterations in internal organs.

Adnexal tumors that have differentiated toward sebaceous glands include sebaceous adenoma, sebaceous epithelioma, sebaceous carcinoma, and sebaceous hyperplasia. Except for sebaceous hyperplasia, which is commonly seen on the face, these tumors are solitary and uncommon. Patients with Torre's syndrome have *sebaceous adenomas*, and in the majority of cases there are multiple such tumors. These patients also can have sebaceous carcinomas and sebaceous hyperplasia as well as keratoacanthomas. The internal manifestations of Torre's syndrome include *multiple* carcinomas of the gastrointestinal tract (primarily colon) as well as cancers of the larynx, genitourinary tract, ovary, and endometrium. Some patients also have a strong family history of cancer.

Red lesions Cutaneous lesions that are red in color have a wide variety of etiologies, and in an attempt to simplify their identification, they will be subdivided into papules, papules/plaques, and subcutaneous nodules. Common red papules include *arthropod bites* and *cherry hemangiomas*; the latter are small, bright-red, dome-shaped papules that represent benign proliferation of capillaries. In patients with AIDS, the development of multiple red hemangioma-like lesions points to bacillary angiomatosis, and biopsy specimens show clusters of bacilli that stain positive with the Warthin-Starry stain; the pathogen has been identified as *Rochalimaea henselae*. Disseminated visceral disease is seen primarily in immunocompromised hosts, but it can occur in immunocompetent individuals.

Multiple *angiokeratomas* are seen in Fabry's disease, an X-linked recessive lysosomal storage disease that is due to a deficiency of α-galactosidase A. The lesions are red to red-blue in color and can be quite small in size (1 to 3 mm), with the most common location being the lower trunk. Associated findings include chronic renal failure, peripheral neuropathy, and corneal opacities (cornea verticillata). Electron photomicrographs of angiokeratomas and clinically normal skin demonstrate lamellar lipid deposits in fibroblasts, pericytes, and endothelial cells that are diagnostic of this disease. Widespread acute eruptions of erythematous papules are discussed in the section on exanthems.

There are several infectious diseases that present as erythematous papules or nodules in a sporotrichoid pattern, that is, in a linear arrangement along the lymphatic channels. The two most common etiologies are *Sporothrix schenckii* (*sporotrichosis*) and *Mycobacterium marinum* (atypical mycobacteria). The organisms are introduced as a result of trauma, and a primary inoculation site is often seen in addition to the lymphatic nodules. Additional causes include *Nocardia*, *Leishmania*, and other dimorphic fungi; culture of lesional tissue will aid in the diagnosis.

The diseases that are characterized by erythematous plaques with scale are reviewed in the papulosquamous section, and the various forms of dermatitis are discussed in the section on erythroderma. Additional disorders in the differential diagnosis of red papules/ plaques include *erysipelas, polymorphous light eruption, lymphocytoma cutis, cutaneous lupus, lymphoma cutis,* and *leukemia cutis.*

The first three diseases represent primary cutaneous disorders. Polymorphous light eruption (PMLE) is characterized by erythematous papules and plaques in a primarily sun-exposed distribution—dorsum of the hand, extensor forearm, and face. Lesions follow exposure to both UV-B and UV-A, and in northern latitudes PMLE is most severe in the late spring and early summer. A process referred to as "hardening" occurs with continued UV exposure, and the eruption fades, but in temperate climates it will recur in the spring. PMLE must be differentiated from cutaneous lupus, and this is accomplished by histologic examination and direct immunofluorescence of the lesions. Lymphocytoma cutis (pseudolymphoma) is a *benign* proliferation of lymphocytes in the skin that presents as infiltrated pink-red to red-purple papules and plaques. It must be distinguished from cutaneous lupus and lymphoma cutis.

Several types of red plaques are seen in patients with systemic *lupus*, including (1) erythematous urticarial plaques across the cheeks and nose in the classic butterfly rash, (2) erythematous discoid lesions with fine or "carpet-tack" scale, telangiectasias, central hypopigmentation, peripheral hyperpigmentation, follicular plugging, and atrophy located on the face, scalp, external ears, arms, and upper trunk, and (3) psoriasiform or annular lesions of subacute lupus with hypopigmented centers located on the face, extensor arms, and upper trunk. Additional cutaneous findings include (1) a violaceous flush on the face and vee of the neck, (2) urticarial vasculitis (see "Urticaria"), (3) lupus panniculitis (see below), (4) diffuse alopecia, (5) alopecia secondary to discoid lesions, (6) periungual telangiectasias and erythema, (7) erythema multiforme–like lesions that may become bullous, and (8) distal ulcerations secondary to Raynaud's phenomenon, vasculitis, or livedoid vasculitis. Patients with only discoid lesions usually have the form of lupus that is limited to the skin. However, 2 to 10 percent of these patients eventually develop systemic lupus. Direct immunofluorescence of involved skin shows deposits of IgG and C3 in a granular distribution along the dermal-epidermal junction.

In *lymphoma cutis* there is a proliferation of malignant lymphocytes or histiocytes in the skin, and the clinical appearance resembles that of lymphocytoma cutis—infiltrated pink-red to red-purple papules and plaques. Lymphoma cutis can occur anywhere on the surface of the skin, whereas the sites of predilection for lymphocytomas are the malar ridge, tip of the nose, earlobes, forearms, and scrotum. Patients with non-Hodgkin's lymphomas have specific cutaneous lesions more often than those with Hodgkin's disease, and occasionally, the skin nodules precede the development of extracutaneous non-Hodgkin's lymphoma. Arcuate lesions are sometimes seen in lymphoma and lymphocytoma cutis as well as in CTLC. *Leukemia cutis* has the same appearance as lymphoma cutis, and specific lesions are seen more commonly in monocytic leukemias than in lymphocytic or granulocytic leukemias. Cutaneous chloromas (granulocytic sarcomas) may precede the appearance of circulating blasts in acute nonlymphocytic leukemia and, as such, represent a form of aleukemic leukemia cutis.

Common causes of erythematous subcutaneous nodules include inflamed epidermoid inclusion cysts, acne cysts, and furuncles. *Panniculitis*, an inflammation of the fat, also presents as subcutaneous nodules and is frequently a sign of systemic disease. There are several forms of panniculitis, including erythema nodosum, erythema induratum, lupus profundus, Weber-Christian disease, α$_1$-antitrypsin deficiency, facticial, and fat necrosis secondary to pancreatic disease. In all these disorders, except for erythema nodosum, the lesions may break down and ulcerate or heal with a scar. The shin is the most common location for the nodules of erythema nodosum, whereas the calf is the most common location for lesions of erythema induratum. In erythema nodosum the nodules are initially red, but then they develop a blue color as they resolve. Patients with erythema nodosum and no underlying systemic illness can still have fever, malaise, leukocytosis, arthralgias and/or arthritis, and unilateral or bilateral hilar adenopathy. However, the possibility of an underlying illness should be excluded, and the most common associations are streptococcal infections, upper respiratory infections, sarcoidosis, and inflammatory bowel disease. The less common associations include tuberculosis, histoplasmosis, coccidioidomycosis, psittacosis, drugs (oral contraceptives, sulfonamides, aspartame, bromides, iodides), cat-scratch fever, and infections with *Yersinia*, *Salmonella*, and *Chlamydia*.

In most patients, erythema induratum/nodular vasculitis is an idiopathic disease, while in a few it may be a reflection of extracutaneous tuberculosis. The lesions of lupus profundus are found primarily on the face, upper arms, and buttocks (sites of abundant fat), and they are seen in both the cutaneous and systemic forms of lupus. The overlying skin may be normal, erythematous, or have the changes of discoid lupus. The subcutaneous fat necrosis that is associated with pancreatic disease is presumably secondary to circulating lipases and is seen in patients with pancreatic carcinoma as well as in patients with acute and chronic pancreatitis. In this disorder and in Weber-Christian disease there may be an associated arthritis, fever, and inflammation of visceral fat. Histologic examination of deep incisional biopsy specimens will aid in the diagnosis of the particular type of panniculitis.

Subcutaneous erythematous nodules are also seen in *cutaneous polyarteritis nodosa* (PAN) and as a manifestation of *systemic vasculitis*, e.g., systemic PAN, allergic granulomatosis, or Wegener's granulomatosis. Cutaneous PAN presents with painful subcutaneous nodules and ulcers within a red-purple, netlike pattern of livedo reticularis. The latter is due to slowed blood flow through the superficial horizontal venous plexus. The majority of lesions are found on the lower extremity, and while arthralgias and myalgias may accompany cutaneous PAN, there is no evidence of systemic involvement. In both the cutaneous and systemic forms of vasculitis, skin biopsy specimens of the associated nodules will show the changes characteristic of a vasculitis; the size of the vessel involved will depend on the particular disease.

Red-brown lesions The cutaneous lesions in *sarcoidosis* are classically red to red-brown in color, and with diascopy (pressure with a glass slide) a yellow-brown residual color is observed that is secondary to the granulomatous infiltrate. The waxy papules and plaques may be found anywhere on the skin, but the face is the most common location. Usually there are no surface changes, but occasionally the lesions will have scale. Biopsy specimens of the papules show "naked" granulomas in the dermis, i.e., granulomas surrounded by a minimal number of lymphocytes. Other cutaneous findings in sarcoidosis include annular lesions with an atrophic or scaly center, papules within scars, hypopigmented macules and papules, alopecia, acquired ichthyosis, erythema nodosum, and lupus pernio (see below). Additional physical findings are peripheral lymphadenopathy and parotid and lacrimal gland enlargement. When there is cutaneous involvement of the hands, radiographs often will show lytic lesions in the underlying bone.

The differential diagnosis of sarcoidosis includes foreign-body granulomas produced by chemicals such as beryllium and zirconium, late secondary syphilis, and *lupus vulgaris*. Lupus vulgaris is a form of cutaneous tuberculosis that is seen in previously infected and sensitized individuals. There is often underlying active tuberculosis elsewhere, usually in the lungs or lymph nodes. At least 90 percent of the lesions occur in the head and neck area, and they are red-brown plaques with a yellow-brown color on diascopy. Secondary scarring and squamous cell carcinomas can develop within the plaques. Cultures of the lesions should be done because it is rare for the acid-fast stain to show bacilli within the dermal granulomas.

Sweet's syndrome is characterized by red-brown plaques and nodules that are frequently painful and occur primarily on the head, neck, and upper extremities. The patients also have fever, neutrophilia, and a dense dermal infiltrate of neutrophils in the lesions. In approximately 10 percent of the patients there is an associated malignancy, most commonly acute nonlymphocytic leukemia. Lymphoma, chronic leukemia, myeloma, myelodysplastic syndromes, and solid tumors (primarily of the genitourinary tract) also have been reported. Extracutaneous sites of involvement include joints, muscles,

eye, kidney (proteinuria, occasionally glomerulonephritis), and lung (neutrophilic infiltrates). The idiopathic form of Sweet's syndrome is seen more often in women, following a respiratory tract infection.

A generalized distribution of red-brown macules and papules is seen in the form of mastocytosis known as *urticaria pigmentosa* (see Chap. 282). Each lesion represents a collection of mast cells in the dermis, with hyperpigmentation of the overlying epidermis. Stimuli such as rubbing and heat cause these mast cells to degranulate, and this leads to the formation of localized urticaria (Darier's sign). Additional symptoms can result from mast cell degranulation, and these include headache, flushing, diarrhea, and pruritus. Mast cells also infiltrate various organs such as the liver, spleen, and gastrointestinal tract in up to 30 to 50 percent of patients with urticaria pigmentosa, and accumulations of mast cells in the bones may produce either osteosclerotic or osteolytic shadows on radiographs. In the majority of these patients, however, the internal involvement remains fairly static. A subtype of chronic leukocytoclastic vasculitis, *erythema elevatum diutinum* (EED), also presents with papules that are red-brown in color. The papules coalesce into plaques on the extensor surfaces of knees, elbows, and the small joints of the hand. Flares of EED have been associated with streptococcal infections.

Blue lesions Lesions that are blue in color are the result of either vascular ectasias and tumors or melanin pigment in the dermis. *Venous lakes* (ectasias) are compressible dark blue lesions that are found commonly in the head and neck region. *Cavernous hemangiomas* are also compressible blue papules and nodules that can occur anywhere on the body, including the oral mucosa. When they are multiple rather than single congenital lesions, the patient may have the blue rubber bleb syndrome or Mafucci's syndrome. Patients with the blue rubber bleb syndrome also have hemangiomas of the gastrointestinal tract that may bleed, whereas patients with Mafucci's syndrome have associated dyschondroplasia and osteochondromas. In the case of single cavernous hemangiomas that are relatively large in size, there can be associated platelet consumption (Kasabach-Merritt syndrome) or musculoskeletal defects. *Blue nevi* (moles) are seen when there are collections of pigment-producing nevus cells in the dermis. These benign papular lesions are dome-shaped, and they occur most commonly on the dorsum of the hand and arm.

Violaceous lesions Violaceous papules and plaques are seen in *lupus pernio*, *lymphoma cutis*, and *cutaneous lupus*. Lupus pernio is a particular type of sarcoidosis that involves the tip of the nose and the earlobes, with lesions that are violaceous in color rather than red-brown. This form of sarcoidosis is associated with involvement of the upper respiratory tract. The plaques of lymphoma cutis and cutaneous lupus may be red or violaceous in color and were discussed above.

Purple lesions Purple-colored papules and plaques are seen in vascular tumors, such as *Kaposi's sarcoma* (see Chap. 279) and *angiosarcoma*, and when there is extravasation of red blood cells into the skin in association with inflammation, as in *palpable purpura* (see "Purpura"). Patients with congenital or acquired arteriovenous fistulas can develop purple papules on the lower extremities that can resemble Kaposi's sarcoma clinically and histologically, and this condition is referred to as pseudo-Kaposi sarcoma (acral angiodermatitis). *Angiosarcoma* is found most commonly on the scalp and face of elderly patients or within areas of chronic lymphedema, and it presents as purple papules and plaques. In the head and neck region the tumor often extends beyond the clinically defined borders and may be accompanied by facial edema.

Brown- and black-colored papules are reviewed in the section on hyperpigmentation.

Cutaneous metastases are discussed last because they can have a wide range of colors. Most commonly they present as either firm, flesh-colored subcutaneous nodules or firm, red to red-brown papulo-nodules. The lesions of lymphoma cutis range from pink-red to plum in color, whereas metastatic melanoma can be pink, blue, or black in color. Cutaneous metastases develop from hematogenous or lymphatic spread and are most often due to the following primary carcinomas: in men, lung, colon, melanoma, and oral cavity; and in women, breast, colon, and lung. These metastatic lesions may be the initial presentation of the carcinoma, especially when the primary site is the lung, kidney, or ovary.

PURPURA (Table 54-22) *Purpura* are seen when there is an extravasation of red blood cells into the dermis, and as a result, the lesions do not blanch with pressure. This is in contrast to those erythematous or violet-colored lesions that are due to localized vasodilatation—they do blanch with pressure. Purpura (≥3 mm) and petechiae (≤2 mm) are divided into two major groups, palpable and nonpalpable. The most frequent causes of *nonpalpable* petechiae and purpura are primary cutaneous disorders such as *trauma, solar purpura*, and *capillaritis*. Less common causes are *steroid purpura* and *livedoid vasculitis* (see "Ulcers"). Solar purpura are seen primarily on the extensor forearm, while glucocorticoid purpura (secondary to potent topical steroids) or endogenous or exogenous Cushing's syndrome can be more widespread. In both cases there is alteration of the supporting connective tissue that surrounds the dermal blood vessels. In contrast, the petechiae that result from capillaritis are found primarily on the lower extremities. In capillaritis there is an extravasation of erythrocytes as a result of perivascular lymphocytic inflammation. The petechiae are bright red, 1 to 2 mm in size, and scattered within annular or coin-shaped yellow-brown macules. The yellow-brown color is caused by hemosiderin deposits within the dermis.

Systemic causes of nonpalpable purpura fall into several categories, and those secondary to clotting disturbances and vascular fragility will be discussed first. The former group includes *thrombocytopenia* (see Chap. 314), *abnormal platelet function* as is seen in uremia, and *clotting factor defects*. The initial site of presentation for thrombocytopenia-induced petechiae is the distal lower extremity. Capillary fragility leads to nonpalpable purpura in patients with systemic *amyloidosis* (see "Papulonodular Skin Lesions"), disorders of collagen production such as *Ehlers-Danlos syndrome*, and *scurvy*. In scurvy there are flattened corkscrew hairs with surrounding hemorrhage on the lower extremities, in addition to gingivitis. Vitamin C is a cofactor for lysyl hydroxylase, an enzyme involved in the posttranslational modification of procollagen that is necessary for cross-link formation.

In contrast to the previous group of disorders, in which either capillary fragility or a clotting abnormality is responsible for the nonpalpable purpura, the purpura seen in the following group of diseases are associated with thrombi formation within vessels. It is important to note that these thrombi are demonstrable in skin biopsy specimens. This group of disorders includes *disseminated intravascular coagulation, monoclonal cryoglobulinemia, thrombotic thrombocytopenic purpura*, and *reactions to warfarin*. Disseminated intravascular coagulation (DIC) is triggered by several types of infection (gram-negative, gram-positive, viral, and rickettsial) as well as by tissue injury and neoplasms. Widespread purpura and hemorrhagic infarcts of the distal extremities are seen. Similar lesions are found in purpura fulminans, which is a form of DIC associated with fever and hypotension that occurs more commonly in children following an infectious illness such as varicella, scarlet fever, or an upper respiratory tract infection. In both disorders, hemorrhagic bullae can develop in involved skin.

Monoclonal cryoglobulinemia is associated with multiple myeloma, Waldenström's macroglobulinemia, lymphocytic leukemia, and lymphoma. Purpura, primarily of the lower extremities, and hemorrhagic infarcts of the fingers and toes are seen in these patients. Exacerbations of disease activity can follow cold exposure or an increase in serum viscosity. Biopsy specimens show precipitates of the cryoglobulin within dermal vessels. Similar deposits have been found in the lung, brain, and renal glomeruli. Patients with *thrombotic thrombocytopenic purpura* also can have hemorrhagic infarcts as a result of intravascular thromboses. Additional signs include thrombocytopenic purpura, fever, and microangiopathic hemolytic anemia (see Chap. 307).

Administration of *warfarin* can result in painful areas of erythema that become purpuric and then necrotic with an adherent black eschar. This reaction is seen more often in women and in areas with abundant subcutaneous fat—breasts, abdomen, buttocks, thighs, and calves. The erythema and purpura develop between the third and tenth day of therapy, most likely as a result of a transient imbalance in the levels of anticoagulant and procoagulant vitamin K–dependent factors. Continued therapy does not exacerbate preexisting lesions, and patients with an inherited or acquired deficiency of protein C are at increased risk for this particular reaction as well as for purpura fulminans.

Purpura secondary to *cholesterol emboli* are usually seen on the lower extremities of patients with atherosclerotic vascular disease. They often follow anticoagulant therapy or an invasive vascular procedure such as an arteriogram, but they also occur spontaneously from disintegration of atheromatous plaques. Associated findings include livedo reticularis, gangrene, cyanosis, subcutaneous nodules, and ischemic ulcerations. Multiple step sections of the biopsy specimen may be necessary to demonstrate the cholesterol clefts with the vessels. Petechiae are also an important sign of *fat embolism*, and they occur primarily on the upper body 2 to 3 days after a major injury. By using special fixatives, the emboli can be demonstrated in biopsy specimens of the petechiae. Emboli of tumor or thrombus are seen in patients with atrial myxomas and marantic endocarditis.

In the *Gardner-Diamond syndrome* (autoerythrocyte sensitivity), female patients develop large ecchymoses within areas of painful, warm erythema. An episode of significant trauma frequently precedes the onset of this syndrome. Intradermal injections of autologous erythrocytes or phosphatidyl serine derived from the red cell membrane can reproduce the lesions in most patients; however, there are instances where a reaction is seen at an injection site of the forearm but not in the midback region. The latter has led some observers to view Gardner-Diamond syndrome as a cutaneous manifestation of severe emotional stress. *Waldenström's hypergammaglobulinemic purpura* is a chronic disorder characterized by petechiae on the lower extremities. There are circulating complexes of IgG–anti-IgG molecules, and exacerbations are associated with prolonged standing or walking.

Palpable purpura are further subdivided into vasculitic and embolic. In the group of vasculitic disorders, *leukocytoclastic vasculitis* (LCV), also known as *allergic vasculitis*, is the one most commonly associated with palpable purpura (see Chap. 291). *Henoch-Schönlein purpura* is a subtype of acute LCV that is seen primarily in children and adolescents following an upper respiratory infection. The majority

---

TABLE 54-22 Causes of purpura

Primary cutaneous disorders	*c* Thrombotic thrombocyto-
A Nonpalpable	penic purpura
1 Trauma	*d* Warfarin reaction
2 Solar purpura	*4* Emboli
3 Steroid purpura	*a* Cholesterol
4 Capillaritis	*b* Fat
5 Livedoid vasculitis	*5* Possible immune complex
Systemic diseases	*a* Gardner-Diamond syn-
A Nonpalpable	drome (autoerythrocyte
1 Clotting disturbances	sensitization)
a Thrombocytopenia (in-	*b* Waldenström's hypergam-
cluding ITP)	maglobulinemic purpura
b Abnormal platelet	*B* Palpable
function	*1* Vasculitis
c Clotting factor defects	*a* Leukocytoclastic vascu-
2 Vascular fragility	litis
a Amyloidosis	*b* Polyarteritis nodosa
b Ehlers-Danlos syndrome	*2* Emboli
c Scurvy	*a* Acute meningococcemia
3 Thrombi	*b* Disseminated gonococcal
a Disseminated intravascu-	infection
lar coagulation	*c* Rocky mountain spotted
b Monoclonal cryoglobuli-	fever
nemia	*d* Ecthyma gangrenosum

of lesions are found on the lower extremities and buttocks. Systemic manifestations include fever, arthralgias (primarily of the knees and ankles), abdominal pain, gastrointestinal bleeding, and nephritis. Direct immunofluorescence examination shows deposits of IgA within dermal blood vessel walls. In *polyarteritis nodosa*, specific cutaneous lesions result from a vasculitis of arterial vessels rather than postcapillary venules as in LCV. The arteritis leads to ischemia of the skin, and this explains the irregular outline of the purpura (see below).

Several types of infectious emboli can give rise to palpable purpura. These embolic lesions are usually *irregular* in outline as opposed to the lesions of leukocytoclastic vasculitis, which are *circular* in outline. The irregular outline is indicative of a cutaneous infarct, and the size corresponds to the area of skin that received its blood supply from that particular arteriole or artery. The palpable purpura in LCV are circular because the erythrocytes simply diffuse out evenly from the postcapillary venules as a result of inflammation. Infectious emboli are most commonly due to gram-negative cocci (meningococcus, gonococcus), gram-negative rods (Enterobacteriaceae), and gram-positive cocci (staphylococcus). Additional causes include *Rickettsia* and, in immunocompromised patients, *Candida* and *Aspergillus*.

The embolic lesions in *acute meningococcemia* are found primarily on the trunk, lower extremities, and sites of pressure, and a gunmetal-gray color often develops within them. Their size varies from 1 mm to several centimeters, and the organisms can be cultured from the lesions. Associated findings include a preceding upper respiratory tract infection, fever, meningitis, disseminated intravascular coagulation, and, in some patients, a deficiency of the terminal components of complement. In *disseminated gonococcal infection* (arthritis-dermatitis syndrome), a small number of papules and vesicopustules with central purpura or hemorrhagic necrosis are found over the joints of the distal extremities. Additional symptoms include arthralgias, tenosynovitis, and fever. To establish the diagnosis, a Gram stain of these lesions should be performed. *Rocky mountain spotted fever* is a tick-borne disease that is caused by *Rickettsia rickettsii*. A several-day history of fever, chills, severe headache, and photophobia precedes the onset of the cutaneous eruption. The initial lesions are erythematous macules and papules on the wrists, ankles, palms, and soles. With time, the lesions spread centripetally and become purpuric.

Lesions of *ecthyma gangrenosum* begin as edematous, erythematous papules or plaques and then develop central purpura and necrosis. Bullae formation also occurs in these lesions, and they are frequently found in the girdle region. The organism that is classically associated with ecthyma gangrenosum is *Pseudomonas aeruginosa*, but other gram-negative rods such as *Klebsiella*, *E. coli*, and *Serratia* can produce similar lesions. In immunocompromised hosts, the list of potential pathogens is expanded to include *Candida* and *Aspergillus*.

ULCERS (Table 54-23) As an approach to the patient with a cutaneous ulcer, the etiologies are divided into two major groups: (1) primary cutaneous disorders and (2) underlying systemic diseases. Within the group of *primary cutaneous disorders*, there are three categories: vascular, tumor-associated, and infectious. The *peripheral vascular* group is the first to be discussed because it contains the most common cause of lower extremity ulcers in adults, *venous hypertension*. Stasis ulcers are characteristically painless and contain adequate granulation tissue. They are often found on the medial malleoli against a background of varicosities, stasis dermatitis, edema, and hemosiderin deposition (yellow-brown discoloration of the skin).

In contrast, lower extremity ulcers due to *arteriosclerosis obliterans* are often painful and are associated with cool, hairless, atrophic skin and dystrophic nails—all a reflection of a decrease in blood flow. The majority of patients are men, and they frequently have evidence of atherosclerosis in other large- and medium-sized arteries. *Thromboangiitis obliterans* (Buerger's disease) and *Mönckeberg's arteriosclerosis* are two less common arterial diseases that can lead to ulcers of the distal upper extremity as well as the lower extremity. The latter is found in patients with primary or secondary hyperparathyroidism, and the calcification of the tunica media of involved muscular arteries

TABLE 54-23 Causes of cutaneous ulcers
Primary cutaneous disorders
A Peripheral vascular disease
1 Venous
2 Arterial
B Livedoid vasculitis
C Squamous cell carcinoma, e.g., within scars
D Infections, e.g., ecthyma
Systemic diseases
A Legs
1 Leukocytoclastic vasculitis
2 Hemoglobinopathies
3 Cryoglobulinemia
4 Cholesterol emboli
5 Necrobiosis lipoidica
B Hands and feet
1 Raynaud's phenomenon
C Generalized
1 Pyoderma gangrenosum
D Mucosal
1 Behçet's syndrome
2 Erythema multiforme
3 Primary blistering disorders

is seen radiographically as a diffuse pipestem calcification. Buerger's disease occurs primarily in young men (ages 25 to 40) who smoke or have been smokers.

Livedoid vasculitis (atrophie blanche) represents a combination of a vasculopathy with intravascular thrombosis. Purpuric lesions and livedo reticularis are found in association with painful ulcerations of the lower extremities. These ulcers are often slow to heal, but when they do, irregularly shaped white scars are formed. The majority of cases are idiopathic in origin, but possible underlying illnesses include systemic lupus, the antiphospholipid syndrome, scleroderma, cryoglobulinemia, and cryofibrinogenemia. Patients with the antiphospholipid syndrome have anticardiolipin antibodies, biologic false-positive tests for syphilis, and prolonged activated partial thromboplastin times; the latter are due to a circulating lupus anticoagulant. These antiphospholipid antibodies are seen most commonly in patients with systemic lupus, but they are also associated with other connective tissue diseases. In addition to the lesions of livedoid vasculitis, patients with the antiphospholipid syndrome have recurrent venous thrombosis, arterial thrombosis (including cerebrovascular accidents), spontaneous abortions, and thrombocytopenia.

Several *carcinomas* can present as cutaneous ulcers, e.g., basal cell carcinoma, squamous cell carcinoma, and, less often, melanoma. When an ulcer on the lower extremity does not heal, despite appropriate treatment, it should be biopsied to rule out carcinoma, primarily squamous cell carcinoma. The same holds true for ulcers that develop within scars. Bacterial and viral *infections* also lead to cutaneous ulceration, and one of the more commonly isolated organisms is *Streptococcus*. The term *ecthyma* is used to describe the often widespread ulcerative lesions that are caused by this bacteria. Ecthyma is a primary cutaneous disorder and should not be confused with ecthyma gangrenosum, which is secondary to blood-borne emboli (see "Purpura"). In Meleney's ulcer, a gradually expanding ulcer begins at a site of trauma or surgery. The clinical appearance is similar to that of pyoderma gangrenosum, but it is due to a synergistic infection that usually includes anaerobic streptococci.

For one group of patients with cutaneous ulcers due to an underlying systemic disease, the lower extremity is the primary location for the lesions. In a young patient, ischemic cutaneous ulcers on the leg should raise the possibility of a *hemoglobinopathy* or *hereditary spherocytosis*. Intravascular thrombosis is the presumed cause of these ulcers, as well as for the ulcers seen in patients with *monoclonal cryoglobulinemia* (see "Purpura"). Primary and secondary forms of *LCV* as well as *emboli of cholesterol* can result in cutaneous ulceration, again primarily on the lower extremities (see "Purpura"). For example, lower extremity ulcers in patients with rheumatoid arthritis are often due to vasculitis. In addition, the yellow atrophic plaques of *necrobiosis lipoidica* can break down centrally into an ulcer (see "Papulonodular Skin Lesions").

Vasospasm occurs in patients with *Raynaud's phenomenon* and can lead to ulcerations of the hands as well as the feet. Raynaud's phenomenon is defined as a triphasic reaction of pallor, cyanosis, and hyperemia in response to cold or emotional stress. Vasospasm is also seen in patients who receive systemic norepinephrine, vasopressin, ergot, and bleomycin. The patient with Raynaud's phenomenon and ulcerations on the tips of the digits should be examined carefully for periungual and mat telangiectasias, the subtle signs of scleroderma. Raynaud's phenomenon is also seen in patients with dermatomyositis, systemic lupus, cryoglobulinemia, cervical rib and scalenus anticus syndromes, pneumatic hammer disease, and occupational acro-osteolysis (associated with the manufacture of polyvinyl chloride).

In *pyoderma gangrenosum*, the border of the ulcers has a characteristic appearance of an undermined necrotic bluish edge and a peripheral erythematous halo. The ulcers often begin as pustules that then expand rather rapidly to a size as large as 20 cm. Although these lesions are most commonly found on the lower extremities, they can arise anywhere on the surface of the body, including sites of trauma (pathergy). An estimated 30 to 50 percent of cases are idiopathic, and the most common associated disorders are ulcerative colitis and Crohn's disease. Less commonly, it is associated with chronic active hepatitis, seropositive rheumatoid arthritis, acute and chronic granulocytic leukemia, polycythemia vera, and myeloma. Additional findings in these patients, even those with idiopathic disease, are cutaneous anergy and a benign monoclonal gammopathy. Because the histology of pyoderma gangrenosum is nonspecific, the diagnosis is made clinically by excluding less common causes of similar-appearing ulcers such as necrotizing vasculitis, Meleney's ulcer (see above), dimorphic fungi, cutaneous amebiasis, spider bites, and facticial. In the myeloproliferative disorders, the ulcers may be more superficial with a pustulobullous border, and these lesions provide a connection between classic pyoderma gangrenosum and acute febrile neutrophilic dermatosis (Sweet's syndrome).

The clinical diagnosis of *Behçet's disease* (see Chap. 290) requires the presence of recurrent oral ulceration (at least three times in a 12-month period) in addition to two of the four following criteria: (1) recurrent genital ulcers, primarily of the vulva and scrotum, (2) eye lesions, either uveitis or retinal vasculitis, (3) skin lesions, and (4) a positive pathergy test. The oral ulcers are usually painful and well-defined with an erythematous halo, whereas the genital ulcers tend to be deeper and heal with scarring. Erythema nodosum, "pseudofolliculitis," papulopustular lesions, *or* acneiform nodules in a postadolescent patient not on glucocorticoids are the entities included under the heading of skin lesions. The test for pathergy, which is defined as a reproduction of cutaneous lesions by trauma, is performed by injecting sterile saline into the dermis. Before the diagnosis of Behçet's disease can be made, the following disorders must be excluded: recurrent erythema multiforme (see "Vesicles/Bullae"), herpes simplex, inflammatory bowel disease, systemic lupus, and primary blistering disorders.

FEVER AND RASH The major considerations in a patient with a fever and a rash are inflammatory diseases versus infectious diseases. In the hospital setting, the most common scenario is a patient who has a drug rash plus a fever secondary to an underlying infection. However, it should be emphasized that a drug reaction can lead to both a cutaneous eruption and a fever ("drug fever"). Additional inflammatory diseases that are often associated with a fever include pustular psoriasis, erythroderma, and Sweet's syndrome. Lyme disease, secondary syphilis, and viral and bacterial exanthems (see "Exanthems") are examples of infectious diseases that produce a rash and a fever. Lastly, it is important to determine whether or not the cutaneous lesions represent septic emboli (see "Purpura"). Such lesions usually have evidence of ischemia in the form of purpura, necrosis, or impending necrosis (gunmetal-gray color). In the patient with thrombocytopenia, however, purpuric lesions can be seen in inflammatory reactions such as morbilliform drug eruptions and infectious lesions.

REFERENCES

BORK K: *Cutaneous Side Effects of Drugs*. Philadelphia, Saunders, 1988
BRAVERMAN IM: *Skin Signs of Systemic Disease*, 2d ed. Philadelphia, Saunders, 1981
CALLEN JP: *Dermatology Clinics*, vol 8, no 2: *Skin Signs of Internal Disease II*. Philadelphia, Saunders, 1990
———, JORIZZO JL: *Dermatology Clinics*, vol 7, no 3: *Skin Signs of Internal Disease*. Philadelphia, Saunders, 1989
DEVITA VT JR et al (eds): *Cancer—Principles and Practice of Oncology*, 3d ed. Philadelphia, Lippincott, 1989
JORRIZZO JL: *Dermatology Clinics*, vol 3, no 1: *Urticaria*. Philadelphia, Saunders, 1985
LEVER WF, SCHAUMBURG-LEVER G: *Histopathology of the Skin*, 7th ed. Philadelphia, Lippincott, 1990
ROOK A et al (eds): *Textbook of Dermatology*, 5th ed. Oxford, Blackwell Scientific, 1991

55 PHOTOSENSITIVITY AND OTHER REACTIONS TO LIGHT

DAVID R. BICKERS

SOLAR RADIATION Sunlight is the most visible and obvious source of comfort in the environment, and it is in the nature of humans to love light. This natural proclivity for the sun has the beneficial results of warmth and vitamin D synthesis but also can produce pathologic consequences. Few effects due to sun exposure beyond those on the skin have been identified, but cutaneous exposure to sunlight can evoke immunosuppressive responses that may be relevant to the pathogenesis of nonmelanoma skin cancer.

The sun's energy encompasses a broad range from ultrashort ionizing radiation (10^{-2} μm) to ultralong radiowaves of very low photon energy (10^7 μm). Thus the emission spectrum has a range of nine orders of magnitude, but that reaching the earth's surface is narrow and is limited to components of the ultraviolet, visible light, and portions of the infrared. The cutoff at the short end of the ultraviolet is at approximately 290 nm, because stratospheric ozone is formed by ionizing radiation of wavelengths less than 100 nm and ozone in turn absorbs solar energy between 120 and 310 nm. In effect, stratospheric ozone prevents penetration to the earth's surface of the shorter, more energetic, potentially more harmful wavelengths of solar radiation. Indeed, concern about destruction of the ozone layer by chlorofluorocarbons released into the atmosphere has led to international agreements to reduce production of these chemicals.

Measurements of solar flux indicate that there is a twentyfold regional variation in the amount of energy at 300 nm that reaches the surface of the earth. This variability is in part related to seasonal effects, the path of sunlight transmission through ozone and air, the altitude (4 percent increase for each 300 m of elevation), the latitude (increasing intensity with decreasing latitude), and the amount of cloud cover, fog, and pollution.

The major components of the photobiologic action spectrum include the ultraviolet and visible wavelengths between 290 and 700 nm. In addition, the wavelengths beyond 700 nm in the infrared primarily evoke heat, but warming of the skin may enhance the response to wavelengths in the ultraviolet and visible spectrum.

The ultraviolet (UV) spectrum is arbitrarily divided into three major segments: C, B, and A. This includes the wavelengths between 10 and 400 nm. UV-C consists of wavelengths between 10 and 290 nm and does not reach the earth because of its absorption by stratospheric ozone. These wavelengths are not a cause of photosensitivity except in occupational settings where artificial sources of this energy are employed, e.g., for germicidal effects. UV-B consists of wavelengths between 290 and 320 nm. This portion of the photobiologic action spectrum is the most efficient in producing redness or erythema in human skin, and hence it is sometimes known as the "sunburn spectrum." UV-A represents those wavelengths between 320 and 400 nm and is approximately a thousandfold less efficient in producing skin hyperemia than is UV-B.

The visible wavelengths between 400 and 700 nm include the familiar white light which when directed through a prism can be shown to consist of various colors including violet, indigo, blue, green, yellow, orange, and red. The energy possessed by photons in the visible spectrum usually is not capable of damaging human skin in the absence of a photosensitizing chemical. Photon energy levels are critical to photosensitivity, since the absorption process requires that sufficient energy be present. The absorption of a photon is an all-or-none phenomenon, and when absorbed, the photon ceases to exist. The absorption of energy is critical to the development of photosensitivity. Thus the *absorption spectrum* of a molecule is defined as the range of wavelengths absorbed by it, whereas the *action spectrum* for an effect of incident radiation is defined as the range of wavelengths that evoke the response.

Photosensitivity occurs when a photon-absorbing chemical (*chromophore*) present in the skin absorbs incident energy, becomes excited, and transfers the absorbed energy to various structures or to oxygen. The absorbed energy must subsequently be dissipated by processes including heat, fluorescence, and phosphorescence. It is important to emphasize that absorption spectra and action spectra need not be superimposable, but there must be overlap at some point to produce photosensitization.

STRUCTURE AND FUNCTION OF SKIN The skin is accessible to incident solar radiation and has a structural heterogeneity that permits the absorption of some wavelengths and the transmission of others. Essentially, human skin is a sandwich of two distinctive compartments, the epidermis and dermis, separated by a basement membrane. The outer epidermis is a stratified squamous epithelium comprising the surface stratum corneum (a protein- and lipid-rich compact membrane), the stratum granulosum, stratum Malphigii, and the basal cell layer. The basal cell layer contains a heterogeneous population of cells, some of which migrate upward in the process of terminal differentiation that results in the expression of keratin genes and the formation of the stratum corneum. Epidermal cells include resident keratinocytes and melanocytes and immigrant cells, including the immunologically active Langerhans cells, lymphocytes, polymorphonuclear leukocytes, monocytes, and macrophages. The epidermis is a major component of the immune system. Branches of sensory nerve endings also reach into this compartment.

The second major component of skin is the dermis, which is relatively large and less densely populated with cells that include fibroblasts, endothelial cells within dermal vessels, and mast cells. Tissue macrophages and sparsely distributed inflammatory cells are also present. All these cells exist within an extracellular matrix of collagen, elastin, and glycosaminoglycans. In contrast to the epidermis, rich vascularization of the dermis allows it to play an important role in temperature regulation.

UV RADIATION (UVR) AND SKIN The epidermis and the dermis contain several chromophores capable of interacting with incident solar energy. These interactions include reflection, refraction, absorption, and transmission. The stratum corneum is a major impediment to the transmission of UV-B, and less than 10 percent of incident wavelengths in this region penetrate the basement membrane. Approximately 3 percent of radiation below 300 nm, 20 percent of radiation below 360 nm, and 33 percent of short visible radiation reaches the basal cell layer in untanned human skin. Proteins and nucleic acids absorb intensely in the short UV-B. In contrast, UV-A penetrates the epidermis efficiently to reach the dermis, where it likely produces changes in structural and matrix proteins that contribute to the aged appearance of chronically sun-exposed skin, particularly in individuals of light complexion.

One of the consequences of UV-B absorption by DNA is the production of pyrimidine, particularly thymine dimers. These structural changes can be repaired by mechanisms that result in their recognition, excision, and the reestablishment of normal base sequences. The efficient repair of these structural aberrations is crucial, since individuals with defective DNA repair are at high risk for the development of cutaneous cancer. For example, patients with xeroderma pigmentosum, an autosomal recessive disorder, are characterized by variably decreased repair of UV-induced pyrimidine dimers and may develop the xerotic appearance of photoaging as well as basal cell and squamous cell carcinomas and melanoma in the first two decades of life.

Cutaneous optics and chromophores Chromophores are endogenous or exogenous chemical components that can absorb physical energy. Endogenous chromophores of skin are of two types: (1) chemicals that are normally present, including nucleic acids, proteins, lipids, and cholesterol derivatives such as the precursor of vitamin D, and (2) chemicals, such as porphyrins, synthesized elsewhere in the body that circulate in the bloodstream and diffuse into the skin, where they can absorb incident radiation and evoke cutaneous photosensitivity. Normally, only trace amounts of porphyrins are present in the skin, but in the porphyrias, increased amounts of porphyrins are released into the circulation and are transported to the skin, where they absorb incident energy both in the Soret band around 400 nm (short visible) and to a lesser extent in the red portion of the visible spectrum (580–660 nm). This results in structural damage to the skin that may be manifest as erythema, edema, urticaria, or blister formation (see Chap. 346).

Acute effects of sun exposure The immediate cutaneous consequences of sun exposure include sunburn and vitamin D synthesis.

SUNBURN   This very common affliction of human skin is caused by exposure to UV radiation. Generally speaking, the ability of an individual to tolerate sunlight is inversely proportional to melanin pigmentation. Melanin is a complex polymer of tyrosine that functions as an efficient neutral-density filter with broad absorbance within the UV portion of the solar spectrum. Melanin is synthesized in specialized epidermal dendritic cells termed *melanocytes* and is packaged into *melanosomes* that are transferred via dendritic processes into *keratinocytes*, where they provide photoprotection. A single melanocyte can provide melanin pigment for approximately 36 keratinocytes, and this group of cells is termed the *epidermal-melanin unit*. Tolerance of sun exposure is a function of the efficiency of the epidermal-melanin unit and can usually be ascertained by asking an individual two questions: (1) Do you burn after sun exposure? and (2) Do you tan after sun exposure? By the answers to these questions, it is usually possible to divide the population into six skin types varying from type I (always burn, never tan) to type VI (never burn, always tan) (see Table 55-1).

There are two general theories about the pathogenesis of the sunburn response. First, the lag phase in time between skin exposure and the development of visible redness (usually 4 to 12 h) suggests an epidermal chromophore that causes delayed production and/or release of vasoactive mediator(s) that diffuse to the dermal vasculature to evoke vasodilatation. Second, it is possible that the small amount of incident UV-B radiation (10 percent or less) that penetrates to the dermis can be absorbed by endothelial cells in the vasculature, thereby directly resulting in vasodilatation. The issue remains unresolved.

TABLE 55-1   Skin type and sunburn sensitivity

Type	Description
I	Always burn, never tan
II	Always burn, sometimes tan
III	Sometimes burn, sometimes tan
IV	Sometimes burn, always tan
V	Never burn, sometimes tan
VI	Never burn, always tan

The action spectrum for sunburn erythema includes the UV-B and the UV-A regions. Photons in the shorter UV-B are at least a thousandfold more efficient than photons in the longer UV-B and the UV-A in evoking the response. However, UV-A may contribute to sunburn erythema at midday when much more UV-A than UV-B is present.

The mechanism of injury remains poorly defined, but the action spectrum for UV-B erythema closely resembles the absorption spectrum for DNA after adjusting for the absorbance of incident energy by the stratum corneum. Damaged keratinocytes (so-called sunburn cells) are visible histologically within an hour of exposure and are maximal within 24 h. UV-A is less effective than UV-B in producing sunburn cells. Mast cells may release inflammatory mediators after exposure to UV-B and UV-A. For example, erythema doses of both UV-B and UV-A increase histamine levels in suction blisters of human skin that return to normal by 24 h (before visible erythema has subsided). Prostaglandin E_2 (PGE_2) increases to approximately 150 percent of control levels by 24 h and then diminishes. Since prostaglandins evoke both pain and redness when injected intradermally, their presence in suction blisters after UV-B exposure suggests a role in UV-B erythema. There may be an age-related decline in the amount of inflammatory mediators detectable in human skin after UV-B irradiation. UV-A erythema results in few epidermal sunburn cells, but vascular endothelial injury is greater than with UV-B. In addition, there are increased levels of arachidonic acid and of prostaglandins D_2, E_2, and I_2 that peak within 5 to 9 h and then subside before peak redness occurs. Despite the evidence for elevated prostaglandins in both UV-B– and UV-A–irradiated skin, administration of nonsteroidal anti-inflammatory drugs is more effective in reducing erythema evoked by UV-B than by UV-A.

VITAMIN D PHOTOCHEMISTRY Cutaneous exposure to UV-B causes photolysis of epidermal provitamin D_3 (7-dehydrocholesterol) to previtamin D_3, which then undergoes a temperature-dependent isomerization to form the stable hormone vitamin D_3. This compound then diffuses to the dermal vasculature and circulates to the liver and kidney, where it is converted to the functional hormone 1,25-dihydroxy vitamin D_3 [1,25($OH)_2D_3$] (see also Chap. 356). Aging substantially decreases the ability of human skin to produce vitamin D_3. This, coupled with the widespread recommended use of sunscreens that filter out UV-B, has led to concern that vitamin D deficiency may become a significant clinical problem in the elderly. Indeed, studies have shown that the use of sunscreens can prevent the production of vitamin D_3 in human skin.

Chronic effects of sun exposure: nonmalignant The clinical features of photodamaged sun-exposed skin consist of wrinkling, blotchiness, telangiectasia, and a roughened, irregular, "weather-beaten" appearance. Whether these changes, which some refer to as *photoaging* or *dermatoheliosis*, represent accelerated chronologic aging or a separate and distinct process is not clear.

Within chronically sun-exposed epidermis there is thickening (acanthosis) and morphologic heterogeneity within the basal cell layer. Higher but irregular melanosome content may be present in some keratinocytes, indicating prolonged residence of the cells in the basal cell layer. These structural changes may help to explain the leathery texture and the blotchy discoloration of sun-damaged skin.

The dermis is the major site for sun-associated chronic damage, manifest as a massive increase in thickened irregular masses of tangled elastic fibers containing uncharacterized electron-dense material. Collagen fibers are also abnormally clumped in the deeper dermis. Fibroblasts are increased in number and show morphologic signs suggesting enhanced metabolic activity. Degraded mast cells may be present in the dermis, the relevance of which remains unclear.

These morphologic changes, both gross and microscopic, are features of chronically sun-exposed skin. The chromophore(s), the action spectra, and the specific biochemical events that result in these changes are unknown.

Chronic effects of sun exposure: malignant One of the major known consequences of chronic skin exposure to sunlight is nonmela-

noma skin cancer. The two types of nonmelanoma skin cancer are basal cell and squamous cell carcinoma (see Chap. 324). There are three major steps for cancer induction: initiation, promotion, and progression. Chronic exposure of animal skin to artificial light sources that mimic solar UVR results in *initiation*, a step whereby structural (mutational) changes in DNA evoke an irreversible change in the target cell (keratinocyte) that begins the tumorigenic process. Exposure to a tumor initiator is believed to be a necessary but not sufficient step in the malignant process, since initiated skin cells not exposed to tumor promoters do not generally develop tumors. The second stage in tumor development is *promotion*, a multistep process whereby initiated cells are exposed to chemical and physical agents that evoke epigenetic changes that culminate in the clonal expansion of initiated cells and cause the development, over a period of weeks to months, of benign growths known as *papillomas*. UV-B is a *complete carcinogen*, meaning that it can function as both an initiator and a promoter, leading to tumor induction. *Incomplete carcinogens* can initiate tumorigenesis but require additional skin exposure to tumor promoters to cause the production of tumors. The prototype tumor promoter is the phorbol ester 12-*O*-tetradecanoyl phorbol-13-acetate (TPA). Tumor promotion usually requires multiple exposures over time to evoke a neoplasm.

The final step in the malignant process is the conversion of benign precursors into malignant lesions, a process thought to require additional genetic alterations in already transformed cells.

Sun exposure is believed to cause nonmelanoma and melanoma cancers of the skin, although the evidence is far more direct for its role in nonmelanoma (basal cell and squamous cell carcinoma) than in melanoma cancers. Approximately 80 percent of nonmelanoma skin cancers develop on exposed body areas, including the face, the neck, and the hands. Men of fair complexion who work outdoors are twice as likely as women to develop these types of cancers. Whites of darker complexions (e.g., Hispanics) have one-tenth the risk of developing such cancers as do light-skinned individuals. Blacks are at lowest risk for all forms of skin cancer. Between 400,000 and 500,000 individuals in the United States develop nonmelanoma skin cancer annually, and the lifetime risk for a white individual to develop such a neoplasm is estimated at approximately 15 percent. A consensus exists that the incidence of nonmelanoma skin cancer in the population is rising for reasons that are unclear.

The relationship of sun exposure to melanoma is less clear-cut, but suggestive evidence supports an association. Melanomas may develop by the teenage years, indicating that the latent period for tumor growth is less than that of nonmelanomas. Epidemiologic studies of immigrants of similar ethnic stock indicate that individuals born in one area or who migrated to the same locale before age 10 have higher age-specific melanoma rates than individuals arriving later. It is thus reasonable to conclude that life in a sunny climate from birth or early childhood increases the risk of melanoma. In general, risk does not correlate with cumulative sun exposure but may relate to sequelae of sun exposure in childhood. Thus a blistering sunburn is associated with a doubling of melanoma risk at the site of the reaction.

Immunologic effects Exposure to solar radiation influences both local and systemic immune responses. UV-B appears to be most efficient in altering immune responses, likely related to the capacity of such energy to affect antigen presentation in skin by interacting with epidermal Langerhans cells. These bone marrow–derived dendritic cells possess surface markers characteristic of monocytes and macrophages. Following skin exposure to erythema doses of UV-B, Langerhans cells undergo both morphologic and functional changes that result in decreased contact allergic responses when haptens are applied to the radiated site. This diminished capacity for sensitization is due to the induction of antigen-specific suppressor T lymphocytes. Indeed, while the immunosuppressive effect of irradiation is limited to haptens applied to the irradiated site, the net result is systemic immune suppression to that antigen because of the induction of suppressor T cells that spread throughout the body.

Higher doses of radiation evoke diminished immunologic responses to antigens introduced either epicutaneously or intracutaneously at sites distant from the irradiated site. These suppressed responses are also associated with the induction of antigen-specific suppressor T lymphocytes and may be mediated by as yet undefined factors that are released from epidermal cells at the irradiated site. The implications of this generalized immune suppression in terms of altered susceptibility to cutaneous cancer or to infection remain to be defined.

It is known that UV-induced tumors in murine skin are antigenic and are rapidly rejected when transplanted into normal syngeneic animals. If the tumors are transplanted into animals previously exposed to subcarcinogenic doses of UVR, they are not rejected and instead grow progressively in the recipients. This failure of irradiated animals to reject the transplanted tumors is due to the development of T suppressor cells that prevent the rejection response. While the mechanism of suppression of tumor rejection is unknown, such a response might be a critical determinant of cancer risk in human skin.

PHOTOSENSITIVITY DISEASES   The diagnosis of photosensitivity requires a careful history to define the duration of the signs and symptoms, the length of time between exposure to sunlight and the development of subjective complaints, and visible changes in the skin. The age of onset also can be a helpful clue; for example, the acute photosensitivity of erythropoietic protoporphyria almost always begins in childhood, whereas the chronic photosensitivity of porphyria cutanea tarda typically begins in the fourth and fifth decades. A history of exposure to topical and systemic drugs and chemicals may provide important information. Many classes of drugs can cause photosensitivity on the basis of either phototoxicity or photoallergy. Fragrances such as musk ambrette contained in numerous cosmetic products are also potent photosensitizers.

Examination of the skin also may offer important clues. Anatomic areas that are naturally protected from direct sunlight such as the hairy scalp, the upper eyelids, the retroauricular areas, the infranasal, and the submental regions may be spared, whereas exposed areas show characteristic features of the pathologic process. These anatomic localization patterns are often helpful but not infallible in making the diagnosis. For example, airborne contact sensitizers that are blown onto the skin may produce dermatitis that can be difficult to distinguish from photosensitivity, despite the fact that such material may trigger skin reactivity in areas shielded from direct sunlight.

Many dermatologic conditions may be caused or aggravated by light (Table 55-2). The role of light in evoking these responses may be dependent on genetic abnormalities ranging from the well-described defect in DNA repair that occurs in xeroderma pigmentosum to the inherited abnormalities in heme synthesis that characterize the porphyrias. In certain photosensitivity diseases, the chromophore has been identified, whereas in the majority, the energy-absorbing agent is unknown.

Polymorphous light eruption   After sunburn, the most common type of photosensitivity disease is *polymorphous light eruption*, the mechanism of which is unknown. Many affected individuals never seek medical attention because the condition is often transient, becoming manifest each spring with initial sun exposure but then subsiding spontaneously with continuing exposure, a phenomenon known as "hardening." The major manifestations of polymorphous light eruption include pruritic (often intensely so) erythematous papules that may coalesce into plaques on exposed areas of the face and arms or other areas as well, making the distribution spotty and uneven.

The diagnosis can be confirmed by skin biopsy and by performing phototest procedures in which skin is exposed to multiple erythema doses of the UV-A and UV-B. The action spectrum for polymorphous light eruption is usually within these portions of the solar spectrum.

Treatment of this disease includes the induction of "hardening" by the cautious administration of light either alone or in combination with photosensitizers such as the psoralens (see below).

Phototoxicity and photoallergy   Another photosensitivity disorder is related to the topical or systemic administration of drugs and

TABLE 55-2 Classification of photosensitivity diseases	
Type	Disease
Genetic	Erythropoietic porphyria
	Erythropoietic protoporphyria
	Albinism
	Xeroderma pigmentosum
	Rothmund-Thompson disease
	Bloom's disease
	Cockayne's disease
	Familial porphyria cutanea tarda
	Phenylketonuria
	Hepatoerythropoietic porphyria
Metabolic	Sporadic porphyria cutanea tarda
	Variegate porphyria
	Hartnup disease
	Kwashiorkor
	Pellagra
	Carcinoid
	Pseudoporphyria
Phototoxic	
Internal	Drugs
External	Drugs, plants, food
Photoallergic	
Immediate	Solar urticaria
Delayed	Drug photoallergy
	Persistent light reaction
Neoplastic and degenerative	Photoaging
	Actinic keratoses
	Basal cell carcinoma
	Squamous cell carcinoma
	Melanoma
	Dysplastic nevus syndrome
	Bowen's disease
Idiopathic	Polymorphous light eruption
	Hydroa aestivale
	Actinic reticuloid
Photoaggravated	Lupus erythematosus
	Systemic
	Subacute cutaneous
	Dermatomyositis
	Pemphigus foliaceus
	Herpes simplex
	Lichen planus actinicus
	Acne vulgaris
	Atopic dermatitis
	Transient acantholytic dermatosis

other chemicals. Photosensitivity reactions are of two broad types, phototoxicity and photoallergy, both of which require the absorption of energy by a drug or chemical resulting in the production of an excited-state photosensitizer that can transfer its absorbed energy to a bystander molecule or to molecular oxygen, thereby generating tissue-destructive chemical species.

Phototoxicity is a nonimmunologic reaction caused by drugs and chemicals, a few of which are listed in Table 55-3. The usual clinical manifestations include erythema resembling a sunburn that quickly desquamates or "peels" within several days. In addition, edema, vesicles, and bullae may occur.

Photoallergy is distinct in that the immune system participates in the pathologic process. The excited-state photosensitizer may create highly unstable haptenic free radicals that bind covalently to macromolecules to form a functional antigen capable of evoking a delayed hypersensitivity response. Some of the drugs and chemicals that produce photoallergy are listed in Table 55-4. The clinical manifestations typically differ from those of phototoxicity in that an intensely pruritic eczematous dermatitis tends to be predominant and evolves into lichenified, thickened, "leathery" changes in sun-exposed areas. A small subset (perhaps 5 to 10 percent) of patients with photoallergy may develop a persistent exquisite hypersensitivity to light even when the offending drug or chemical is identified and eliminated. Known as *persistent light reaction*, this may be incapacitating for years.

Diagnostic confirmation of phototoxicity and photoallergy often can be obtained using phototest procedures. In patients with suspected phototoxicity, determination of the minimal erythema dose (MED) while the patient is exposed to a suspected agent and then repeating

TABLE 55-3 Phototoxic drugs and chemicals

	Topical	Systemic
Coal tar derivatives		
Acridine	+	
Anthracene	+	
Phenanthrene	+	
Drugs		
Amiodarone		+
Dacarbazine		+
5-Fluorouracil	+	+
Furosemide		+
Nalidixic acid		+
Phenothiazines		+
Psoralens	+	+
Retinoids	+	+
Sulfonamides		+
Sulfonylureas		+
Tetracyclines		+
Thiazides		+
Vinblastine		+
Dyes		
Anthraquinone		+
Eosin		+
Methylene blue		+
Rose bengal		+

the MED after discontinuation of the agent may provide a clue to the causative drug or chemical. Photopatch testing can be performed to confirm the diagnosis of photoallergy. This is a simple variant of ordinary patch testing in which a series of known photoallergens is applied to the skin in duplicate and one set is irradiated with a suberythema dose of UV-A. Development of eczematous changes at sites exposed to sensitizer and light is a positive result. The characteristic abnormality in patients with persistent light reaction is a diminished threshhold to erythema evoked by UV-B.

The management of drug photosensitivity is first and foremost to eliminate exposure to the chemical agents responsible for the reaction and to minimize sun exposure. The acute symptoms of phototoxicity may be ameliorated by cool, moist compresses, topical glucocorticoids, and systemically administered nonsteroidal anti-inflammatory agents. In severely affected individuals, a rapidly tapered course of systemic glucocorticoids may be useful. Judicious use of analgesics may be necessary.

TABLE 55-4 Photoallergenic drugs and chemicals

	Topical	Systemic
Antibiotics		
Sulfonamides		+
Antifungals		
Fenticlor	+	
Jadit	+	
Multifungin	+	
Diuretics		
Thiazides		+
Fragrances		
Musk ambrette	+	
6-Methylcoumarin	+	
Plant oleoresins	+	
Halogenated salicylanilides		
Bithionol	+	
Tetrachlorosalicylanilides	+	
Tribromosalicylanilide	+	
Nonsteroidal anti-inflammatory agents		
Piroxicam	+	
Phenothiazines		
Chlorpromazine	+	
Promethazine	+	
Sulfonylureas		+
Sunscreens		
p-Aminobenzoic acid and esters	+	
Whitening agents		
Stilbenes	+	

Photoallergic reactions require similar management techniques. Furthermore, individuals suffering from persistent light reactivity must be protected against light exposure. In selected patients in whom chronic systemic high-dose glucocorticoids pose unacceptable risks, it may be necessary to employ cytotoxic agents such as azathioprine or cyclophosphamide.

Porphyria   The porphyrias (see Chap. 346) are a group of diseases that have in common various derangements in the synthesis of heme. Heme is a nonchelated tetrapyrrole or porphyrin, and the porphyrins are potent photosensitizers that absorb light intensely in both the short (400–410 nm) and the long (580–650 nm) portions of the visible spectrum.

Heme cannot be reutilized and must be continuously synthesized, and the two body compartments with the largest requirement for its production are the bone marrow and the liver. Accordingly, the porphyrias originate in one or the other of these organs, with the end result of excessive endogenous production of potent photosensitizers. The porphyrins circulate in the bloodstream and diffuse into the skin, where they absorb solar energy, become photoexcited, and evoke cutaneous photosensitivity. The mechanism of porphyrin photosensitization is known to be a photodynamic or oxygen-dependent reaction that can be mediated by reactive oxygen species such as superoxide anions.

Two forms of human porphyria, porphyria cutanea tarda and erythropoietic protoporphyria, will be discussed briefly. *Porphyria cutanea tarda* is the most common type of human porphyria and is associated with decreased activity of the enzyme uroporphyrinogen decarboxylase. There are two basic types of porphyria cutanea tarda: the sporadic or acquired type, generally seen in individuals ingesting ethanol or receiving estrogens and associated with increased hepatic iron stores, and the inherited type, in which there is autosomal dominant transmission of deficient enzyme activity.

In both types of porphyria cutanea tarda, the predominant feature is a chronic photosensitivity characterized by increased fragility of sun-exposed skin, particularly areas subject to repeated trauma such as the dorsa of the hands, the forearms, the face, and the ears. The predominant skin lesions are vesicles and bullae that rupture, producing moist erosions often with a hemorrhagic base, and which heal slowly with crusting and purplish discoloration of the affected skin. Hypertrichosis, mottled pigmentary change, and scleroderma-like induration are associated features. Biochemical confirmation of the diagnosis can be obtained by measurement of urinary porphyrin excretion and by assay of uroporphyrinogen decarboxylase.

Treatment consists of repeated phlebotomies to diminish the excessive hepatic iron stores and/or intermittent low doses of the antimalarial drugs chloroquine and hydroxychloroquine. Long-term remission of the disease can be achieved if the patient eliminates exposure to porphyrinogenic agents.

Erythropoietic protoporphyria originates in the bone marrow and is due to a decrease in the enzyme ferrochelatase. The major clinical features include an acute photosensitivity characterized by subjective burning and stinging of exposed skin that often develops during or just after exposure. There may be associated skin swelling and, after repeated episodes, a waxlike scarring.

The diagnosis is confirmed by demonstration of elevated measurement of free erythrocyte protoporphyrin. Detection of increased plasma protoporphyrin helps to differentiate lead poisoning and iron-deficiency anemia, in both of which elevated erythrocyte protoporphyrin occurs in the absence of cutaneous photosensitivity and of elevated plasma protoporphyrin.

Treatment consists of reducing sun exposure and the oral administration of the carotenoid β-carotene, which is an effective scavenger of free radicals. Many affected individuals are able to tolerate sun exposure while ingesting this drug, but it has no effect on the metabolic defect in porphyrin-heme synthesis.

PHOTOPROTECTION   Since photosensitivity of the skin results from exposure to sunlight, it follows that avoidance of the sun would eliminate these disorders. Unfortunately, social pressures make this

TABLE 55-5 **Properties of selected sunscreens**

Ingredients	Trade names	SPF* (outdoors)	Substantivity[†]
p-Aminobenzoic acid (PABA) (5% in ethanol)	Pre-Sun-15	10–12	Excellent
p-Aminobenzoic acid esters (3.5% padimate A + 3.0% octyldimethyl PABA)	Original Eclipse	4–6	Fair
p-Aminobenzoic acid ester combinations (7.0% padimate 0 + 2.5% oxybenzone + 5.0% dioxybenzone)	Bain de Soleil	9	Excellent
Non-p-aminobenzoic acid (3% 2-hydroxy-4-methoxy benzophenone)	Ti-Screen-15	10–12	Excellent
Physical sunscreens (5% titanium dioxide + 5% methyl anthranilate)	A-Fil	4–6	Good

* SPF = sun protective factor.
† Substantivity = ability to remain on the skin.

an impractical alternative for most individuals, and this has led to a search for better approaches to photoprotection.

Natural photoprotection is provided by structural proteins in the epidermis, particularly keratin and melanin. The amount of melanin and its distribution in cells is genetically regulated, and individuals of darker complexion (skin types IV to VI) are at decreased risk for the development of cutaneous malignancy.

Other forms of photoprotection include clothing and sunscreens. Clothing constructed of tightly woven fabrics irrespective of color affords substantial protection. Wide-brimmed hats, long sleeves, and pants all reduce direct exposure. Sunscreens are of two major types—chemical and physical. Chemical sunscreening agents are chromophores that absorb energy in the UV-B and/or UV-A regions, thereby diminishing photon absorption by the skin (Table 55-5). Sunscreens are rated for their photoprotective effect by their *sun protective factor* (SPF). The SPF is simply a ratio of the time required to produce sunburn erythema with and without sunscreen application. SPF ratings of 15 or higher provide effective protection against UV-B and, to a lesser extent, UV-A. The major categories of chemical sunscreens include p-aminobenzoic acid and its esters, benzophenones, anthranilates, cinnamates, and salicylates. Physical sunscreens are light-opaque mixtures containing zinc oxide, talc, or titanium oxide that scatter light, thereby reducing absorption by the skin.

In addition to light absorption, a critical determinant of the photoprotective effect of sunscreens is their ability to remain on the skin, a property known as *substantivity*. In general, the PABA esters formulated in moisturizing vehicles provide the greatest substantivity.

Photoprotection also can be achieved by limiting the time of exposure during the day. Since as much as half an individual's total lifetime sun exposure may occur by the age of 18, it is important to educate parents and young children about the hazards of sunlight. Simply eliminating exposure at midday will achieve substantial reduction in UV-B exposure.

PHOTOTHERAPY AND PHOTOCHEMOTHERAPY While greatest attention has been paid to the damaging effects of sunlight in the skin, this same energy is employed in the management of selected dermatologic diseases. The administration of UV-B alone or in combination with topically applied compounds such as emollient ointments with or without crude coal tar induces remissions in psoriasis, an inflammatory disorder in which excessively rapid epidermal cell turnover is associated with thick scaling and redness of the skin.

Photochemotherapy in which UV-A radiation is administered in combination with topically applied or systemically administered psoralens (PUVA) is also effective in treating psoriasis and in the early stages of cutaneous T cell lymphoma and vitiligo. Psoralens are tricyclic furocoumarins which when intercalated into DNA and exposed to UV-A produce monofunctional adducts to pyrimidine bases and eventually form DNA cross-links. These structural changes are thought to decrease DNA synthesis and effect the improvement that occurs in psoriasis. The reason that PUVA photochemotherapy is effective in cutaneous T cell lymphoma is not clear.

In addition to its effects on DNA, PUVA photochemotherapy also stimulates melanin synthesis, and this provides the rationale for its use in the depigmenting disease vitiligo. Oral 8-methoxypsoralen and UV-A appear to be most effective in this regard, but as many as 100 treatments extending over 12 to 18 months may be required to promote satisfactory repigmentation.

The major side effects of phototherapy and PUVA photochemotherapy are due to the cumulative effects of photon absorption and include skin dryness, actinic keratoses, and an increased risk of nonmelanoma skin cancer. Despite these risks, the therapeutic index of these modalities is positive.

REFERENCES

FRAIN-BELL W: *Cutaneous Photobiology*. Oxford, Oxford University Press, 1985
HARBER LC, BICKERS DR: *Photosensitivity Diseases*, 2d ed. Toronto, Decker, 1989
HÖNIGSMANN H, STINGL G: *Therapeutic Photomedicine*. Basel, Karger, 1986
MAGNUS IA: *Dermatological Photobiology*. Oxford, Blackwell, 1976
MORISON WL et al: Photobiology. J Am Acad Dermatol 25:327, 1991
PATHAK MA et al: Preventive treatment of sunburn, dermatoheliosis, and skin cancer with sun-protective agents, in *Dermatology in General Medicine*, 4th ed, TB Fitzpatrick et al (eds). New York, McGraw-Hill, 1993

section 9 Hematologic alterations

56 ANEMIA

H. FRANKLIN BUNN

By definition, patients with anemia have a significant reduction in red cell mass and a corresponding decrease in the oxygen-carrying capacity of the blood. Normally, blood volume is maintained at a nearly constant level. Therefore, anemia entails a decrease in the concentration of red cells or hemoglobin in peripheral blood. Normal blood values for individuals of various ages are shown in the Appendix of this book. In women in the childbearing age group, these values are 10 percent lower than in men. At high altitudes, higher values are found, roughly in proportion to the elevation above sea level. Anemic patients have a reduction of more than 10 percent below the mean values for the sex. However, since the variations in normal hemoglobin values approach this limit, the documentation of mild anemia may be uncertain.

SIGNS AND SYMPTOMS OF ANEMIA The clinical presentation of the anemic patient depends on the underlying disease as well as on the severity and chronicity of the anemia. The manifestations of anemia per se can be explained by the pathophysiologic principles outlined in this chapter and in Chap. 302. Most of these signs and symptoms represent cardiovascular and ventilatory adjustments which compensate for the decrease in red blood cell mass.

The degree to which symptoms occur in an anemic patient depends on several contributing factors. If the anemia has developed rapidly, there may not be adequate time for compensatory adjustments to take place, and the patient may have more marked symptoms than if an anemia of equivalent severity had developed insidiously. Furthermore, the patient's complaints may depend on the presence of local vascular disease. For example, angina pectoris, intermittent claudication, or transient cerebral ischemia may be unmasked by the development of anemia.

Individuals with mild anemia are often asymptomatic. They may complain of fatigue as well as dyspnea and palpitation, particularly following exercise. Severely anemic patients will often be symptomatic at rest and unable to tolerate significant exertion. When the hemoglobin concentration falls below 75 g/L (7.5 g/dL), resting cardiac output rises significantly with an increase in both heart rate and stroke volume. The patient may be aware of this hyperdynamic state and complain of palpitation or a pounding pulse. Symptoms of cardiac failure may develop if the patient's myocardial reserve is reduced.

The symptoms of severe anemia extend to other organ systems. Patients often complain of dizziness and headache and may experience syncope, tinnitus, or vertigo. Many patients are irritable and have difficulty sleeping or concentrating. Because of decreased blood flow to the skin, patients may become hypersensitive to cold. Gastrointestinal symptoms such as anorexia, indigestion, and even nausea or bowel irregularity are attributable to shunting of blood away from the splanchnic bed. Females commonly develop abnormal menstruation, both amenorrhea and increased bleeding. Males may complain of impotence or loss of libido.

Physical findings *Pallor* is the physical finding most commonly associated with anemia. However, the usefulness of this sign is limited by other factors that affect the color of the skin. The thickness and texture of the skin vary widely among individuals. Furthermore, the blood flow to the skin can undergo wide fluctuations. The concentration of melanin in the epidermis is another important determinant of skin color. Individuals with a fair complexion may look pale even though they are not anemic. Conversely, pallor is difficult to detect in deeply pigmented individuals. Furthermore, acquired disorders of melanin pigmentation (e.g., Addison's disease, hemochromatosis) or jaundice may interfere with detection of pallor. Nevertheless, even in blacks, the presence of anemia may be suspected by the color of the palms or of noncutaneous tissues such as oral mucous membranes, nail beds, and palpebral conjunctivas. The color of the creases of the palm is a useful sign. When they are as pale as the surrounding skin, the patient usually has a hemoglobin of less than 70 g/L (7 g/dL).

Two factors contribute to the development of pallor in patients with anemia. There is, of course, a decrease in the hemoglobin concentration of blood perfusing the skin and mucous membranes. Also, blood is shunted away from the skin and other peripheral tissues, permitting enhanced blood flow to vital organs. Redistribution of blood flow is an important mode of compensation in anemia.

Other physical findings associated with anemia include tachycardia, wide pulse pressure, and a hyperdynamic precordium. A systolic ejection murmur is often heard over the precordium, particularly at the pulmonic area. In addition, a venous hum may be detected over the neck vessels. These cardiac findings disappear when the anemia is corrected. Patients with hemolytic anemia often have icterus and splenomegaly and occasionally develop superficial skin ulceration over the ankle bones.

APPROACH TO THE PATIENT WITH ANEMIA

In evaluating the anemic patient, the physician should proceed in an orderly fashion so that the correct diagnosis can be established with a minimum of laboratory tests and procedures. As in other clinical disciplines, a comprehensive history and meticulous physical examination are of paramount importance in the initial workup of the anemic patient. For example, a family history which reveals a dominant inheritance pattern provides strong support for the diagnosis of hereditary spherocytosis. The discovery of a heart murmur and splenomegaly raises the possibility that the anemic patient may have subacute bacterial endocarditis.

Under unusual circumstances, the blood values do not accurately reflect alterations in the red cell mass. For example, hemoglobin level and hematocrit are falsely elevated in patients who have sustained an acute reduction in plasma volume owing to hemorrhage, extensive burns, vigorous diuresis, or other types of severe dehydration. In contrast, the blood values may be falsely low in patients who have an expanded plasma volume, as in pregnancy or congestive heart failure.

The evaluation of the anemic patient should be based on a firm understanding of the pathophysiologic principles outlined in Chap. 302. As shown in Table 56-1, the clinician must first ask whether the anemia is due to a decreased production of red cells or to enhanced destruction. Moreover, the possibility of blood loss either as the sole cause or as a contributing factor must always be considered. The examination of the stool for occult blood is an indispensable part of the evaluation of all anemic patients.

RED CELL INDEXES Accurate measurements of the hematocrit, hemoglobin concentration, and red blood cell count enable the

TABLE 56-1   Initial evaluation of anemia

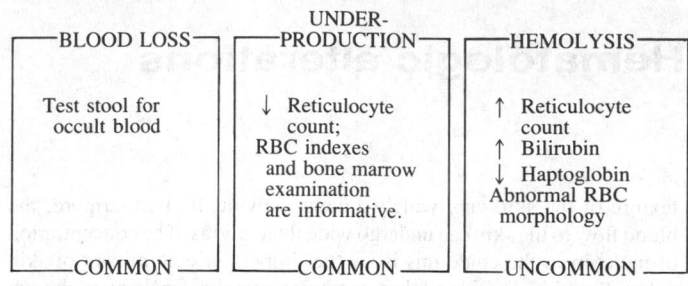

BLOOD LOSS	UNDER-PRODUCTION	HEMOLYSIS
Test stool for occult blood	↓ Reticulocyte count; RBC indexes and bone marrow examination are informative.	↑ Reticulocyte count ↑ Bilirubin ↓ Haptoglobin Abnormal RBC morphology
COMMON	COMMON	UNCOMMON

calculation of red cell indices which, as shown in Table 56-2, are very useful in the classification of anemias of underproduction. Measuring the hematocrit or PCV is the simplest and one of the most precise ways to ascertain the concentration of red cells in the blood. Generally, a small sample of anticoagulated blood is drawn into a capillary tube which is sealed at one end and centrifuged. The PCV is the ratio of the volume of packed red cells to the total volume. Alternatively, the concentration of hemoglobin can be determined spectrophotometrically from the absorbance of the cyanmethemoglobin form at a specific wavelength. With the advent of automated red blood cell counting technology, very precise measurements of red blood cell indexes are now readily available in nearly all hospitals and clinical laboratories. The electronic counter makes a direct measurement of the red cell count (RBC/μL) and the mean red cell volume (MCV):

$$MCV \ (fL) = \frac{PCV \ (L/L)}{(RBC/\mu L) \times 10^{-9}}$$

This instrument calculates the PCV from the direct measurement of MCV and RBC/μL. In addition, hemoglobin concentration is measured directly on a separate channel. The mean corpuscular hemoglobin concentration (MCHC) is then computed as follows:

$$MCHC \ (g/dL) = \frac{Hb \ (g/dL)}{PCV \ (L/L)}$$

TABLE 56-2   Anemias due to decreased red cell production

RBC Indexes	Marrow	Additional lab tests	Diagnosis
Hypochromic, microcytic (↓ MCV)	0 Iron	↓ Fe, ↑ TIBC	Iron deficiency
	+ Iron Ring sideroblasts	↑ Hb A₂ or ↑ Hb F ↓ Hb A₂	β Thalassemia Sideroblastic anemia
Macrocytic (↑ MCV)	Megaloblastic	↓ Serum B₁₂, achlorhydria	Vitamin B₁₂ deficiency, pernicious anemia
		↓ Serum folate	Folic acid deficiency
Normochromic, normocytic	Normal	↓ Fe, ↓ TIBC	Anemia of chronic inflammation
		↑ Creatinine	Anemia of uremia
		Abn LFT	Anemia of liver disease
		↓ T₄	Anemia of myxedema
	Aplastic	Pancytopenia	Aplastic anemia
Normoblasts, teardrops	Infiltrated: tumor, lymphoma, etc.	↑ LAP	Myelophthisic
	Fibrosis		Myeloid metaplasia

NOTE: Fe, iron; TIBC, total iron-binding capacity; Hb, hemoglobin; LAP, leukocyte alkaline phosphatase; LFT, liver function tests; Abn, abnormal; MCV, mean corpuscular volume.

A third red blood cell index, the mean corpuscular hemoglobin (MCH), is determined as follows:

$$MCH \ (pg) = \frac{Hb \ (g/dL)}{(RBC/\mu L) \times 10^{-7}}$$

Generally, an automated system provides a printout which includes hemoglobin concentration, red cell count, packed cell volume, and the three red cell indexes (MCV, MCHC, and MCH).

As Table 56-2 shows, the MCV is particularly useful in classifying the anemias due to decreased red cell production. Microcytic anemias have low MCV values. On microscopic examination, the red cells appear small and often pale. In contrast, in the macrocytic anemias the MCV is elevated, and large, oval cells (macroovalocytes) are seen on microscopic examination. Unlike the anemias of underproduction, nearly all the hemolytic anemias are normocytic or slightly macrocytic owing to the preponderance of young red cells which are somewhat large. Exceptions include the severe forms of thalassemia in which microcytic red cells are accompanied by brisk hemolysis.

RETICULOCYTE COUNT   This is the most useful laboratory test for distinguishing anemias secondary to underproduction of red blood cells from those caused by hemolysis. When an appropriate supravital stain is applied to a sample of peripheral blood, the 1- to 2-day-old red cells exhibit a network of purple strands which are aggregates of ribosomes. Reticulocytosis is a reflection of the release of an increased number of young cells from the bone marrow. The rate of red cell production can be assessed more quantitatively by determining the reticulocyte index, which uses the hematocrit or packed cell volume (PCV) and is calculated as follows:

$$Reticulocyte \ index = reticulocyte \ \% \times \frac{patient's \ PCV}{normal \ PCV}$$

This measure fails to consider the distribution of reticulocytes between the bone marrow and the peripheral blood. When the marrow is greatly stimulated, marrow reticulocytes enter the circulation prematurely. On a routinely prepared smear, these "shift reticulocytes" appear larger than average and have a lavender hue, so-called polychromatophilia. Since the circulation of "shift reticulocytes" in the peripheral blood is prolonged, the reticulocyte index should be divided by about 2. This factor varies from 1.5 to 3 depending on the severity of the anemia and the degree of erythropoietin stimulation. This correction should always be made if normoblasts are encountered in the peripheral blood, since this finding indicates the premature release of red cell precursors into the circulation.

A failure to produce red cells is reflected in an inappropriately low reticulocyte count. In contrast, a significant elevation of reticulocytes is suggestive of hemolysis. Exceptions include (1) the brisk reticulocyte response that is seen in a patient with hemorrhage, (2) reticulocytosis encountered in patients recovering from impaired erythropoiesis (e.g., an individual with pernicious anemia who received an injection of vitamin B₁₂ 1 week earlier), and (3) mild to moderate elevations in reticulocytes (3 to 7 percent) encountered in myelophthisic anemia in which the orderly release of cells is affected by alterations of the marrow stroma owing to tumor, fibrosis, or granulomata. These exceptions are often readily appreciated in the initial evaluation of the patient. Furthermore, a number of ancillary laboratory tests described below are useful in determining to what extent hemolysis is occurring. The measurement of unconjugated bilirubin in the serum is a particularly useful guide to the presence of accelerated red blood cell breakdown. Once this information is obtained, the workup can be directed toward the establishment of a specific etiology.

EXAMINATION OF THE BLOOD SMEAR   In the evaluation of a patient with anemia, the physician should take the time to examine a well-stained peripheral blood film. Figures A9-1 to A9-12 show examples of abnormalities in red cell morphology encountered in various types of anemia. Many subtleties escape the attention of the technologist whose primary purpose in examining the slide is to obtain a white cell differential count. Furthermore, the clinician can approach the specimen with a prepared mind and can scrutinize it for specific abnormalities. As suggested above, the examination can confirm the size and color of red cells as estimated by RBC indexes. Furthermore, while these indexes provide mean statistical values, the microscopic examination can reveal variation in red cell size (anisocytosis) or shape (poikilocytosis), changes which are helpful in the diagnosis of specific anemias. Examination of the blood smear is particularly important in evaluating a patient with hemolysis. Most hemolytic anemias have characteristic morphologic abnormalities. Finally, this practice may yield unexpected dividends. The finding of rouleaux suggests the presence of dysproteinemia, as occurs in multiple myeloma. The examination may provide the initial clue that the patient has significant thrombocytopenia.

BONE MARROW EXAMINATION A microscopic examination of the bone marrow is often useful and may be critical in the workup of any *unexplained* anemia. Study of the bone marrow is particularly informative in the anemias of underproduction. The more severe the anemia, the more likely it is that the procedure will be informative. An assessment of the quantity and quality of red cell precursors may determine whether there is a primary defect in cell production. A marrow biopsy is particularly useful in estimating overall cellularity. The normal differential of nucleated cells in the marrow is shown in the Appendix. The ratio of myeloid (M) to erythroid (E) precursors is normally about 2:1 but may be artifactually increased by the inclusion of circulating leukocytes. The ratio is increased in patients with infection, a leukemoid reaction, or neoplastic proliferation of myeloid cells. Rarely, a high M/E ratio is due to selective aplasia of the red cell precursors. A decreased M/E ratio indicates erythroid hyperplasia (seen in hemolysis or hemorrhage) or ineffective erythropoiesis (e.g., megaloblastic and sideroblastic anemias). The morphology of the precursors may reveal a maturation deficit such as megaloblastic anemia. The bone marrow examination is also important in demonstrating the presence of cellular infiltrates such as those found in leukemia, lymphoma, or multiple myeloma. The demonstration of tumor, fibrosis, or granulomata usually requires a biopsy. A portion of the marrow specimen should be stained with Prussian blue. In addition to providing an assessment of iron stores, this iron stain is required for the identification of sideroblasts.

VARIOUS FORMS OF ANEMIA

ANEMIA DUE TO BLOOD LOSS This form of anemia varies considerably in its clinical presentation depending on the site, severity, and rapidity of the hemorrhage. At opposite extremes are acute fulminant bleeding producing hypovolemic shock and chronic occult blood loss leading to iron-deficiency anemia.

Patients who have sustained an acute hemorrhage generally present with signs and symptoms secondary to hypoxia and hypovolemia. Depending on the severity of the process, the patient will have weakness, fatigue, lightheadedness, stupor, or coma and will often appear pale, diaphoretic, and irritable. Vital signs are a reflection of cardiovascular compensation for the acute blood loss (Chap. 34). The patient will have hypotension and tachycardia in proportion to the degree of hemorrhage. Elicitation of postural signs is useful in the initial evaluation of patients with acute blood loss. If the pulse rises 25 percent or more or the systolic blood pressure falls 20 mmHg or more upon going from a supine to sitting position, the patient is likely to have significant hypovolemia (blood loss >1000 mL) and requires prompt replacement. Acute blood loss in excess of 1500 mL usually leads to cardiovascular collapse.

If the blood loss has been acute and recent, the peripheral blood may not reveal a significant decrease in packed cell volume or hemoglobin, since the red cell mass and plasma volume are contracted in parallel. There often is a moderate leukocytosis and a "shift to the left" in the white cell differential count. Thrombocytosis may be encountered in both acute and chronic blood loss, particularly when the patient is iron-deficient. During the first few days following an acute hemorrhage there is usually an increase in reticulocytes. Occasionally, nucleated red cells may appear in the peripheral blood. Since young red cells are larger than old ones, the patient may develop slightly macrocytic red cell indexes (MCV = 95 to 105 fL). As mentioned above, sustained reticulocytosis will be seen if significant blood loss continues, or until iron stores have been exhausted. Internal bleeding may be accompanied by an increase in unconjugated bilirubin. This abnormality is a reflection of an increase in catabolism of heme from extravasated red cells. Patients with acute gastrointestinal blood loss will often have an elevation of blood urea nitrogen owing to impaired renal blood flow and perhaps to the absorption of digested blood protein.

It is of critical importance to assess these patients promptly and institute treatment without delay. A large-bore intravenous line should be placed. While blood is being typed and cross matched, saline, Ringer's lactate, or, preferably, a colloid such as 5% albumin should be infused to correct hypovolemia. Whole blood is then administered as soon as it is available. Monitoring of vital signs and central venous pressure is useful in determining the appropriate amount of volume replacement. During and following these emergency measures, diagnostic studies may reveal the site or sites of bleeding. If the bleeding is unexplained, an emergency coagulation profile should be obtained. Demonstration of bleeding from the gastrointestinal tract may require the insertion of a nasogastric tube. Appropriate radiologic studies may be indicated to determine sites of internal bleeding such as retroperitoneal hemorrhage.

Chronic blood loss is usually due to lesions in the gastrointestinal tract or the uterus. The testing of stool specimens for occult blood is an essential, though frequently overlooked, part of the evaluation of anemia. It may be necessary to examine serial specimens over a prolonged period of time, since gastrointestinal bleeding is often intermittent. The hematologic manifestations of chronic blood loss are those of iron-deficiency anemia, discussed in detail in Chap. 303.

ANEMIAS DUE TO DECREASED RBC PRODUCTION As shown in Table 56-2, red cell indexes are useful in classifying the anemias due to underproduction of red cells. They can be conveniently grouped into three major categories: microcytic, macrocytic, and normocytic.

The *microcytic* anemias include iron-deficiency anemia (Chap. 303), sideroblastic anemias (Chap. 303), and the thalassemias (Chap. 306). Collectively, they represent a decrease in the availability or synthesis of one of the three major constituents of the hemoglobin molecule: iron, porphyrin, and globin. Since hemoglobin makes up over 90 percent of the protein within the erythrocyte, it is not surprising that these defects in hemoglobin synthesis result in the formation of small, pale red cells. These disorders involve a variable degree of ineffective erythropoiesis (Chap. 302). In addition, the anemias of chronic inflammation and malignancy may be slightly microcytic (Chap. 305). This phenomenon is due to a defect in the availability of iron. However, these disorders are more often normocytic and have been so classified in Table 56-2. Measurement of serum iron and iron-binding capacity and evaluation of marrow iron stores are particularly useful in distinguishing between these anemias.

The *macrocytic* anemias generally are associated with megaloblastic morphology in the bone marrow. In most cases, a deficiency of either vitamin B_{12} or folic acid results in an impairment of the replication of DNA, particularly in cells having a high turnover rate. Because nuclear maturation lags behind cytoplasmic development, large red cells tend to be produced in the bone marrow. Megaloblastic anemias are discussed in detail in Chap. 304. Like the microcytic anemias, these disorders are maturation defects associated with ineffective erythropoiesis. Macrocytosis, generally of a lesser degree, also may be encountered in patients with liver disease, hypothyroidism, acute blood loss, hemolytic anemia, aplastic anemia, and alcoholism. However, in these conditions, the red cell precursors in the bone marrow do not appear megaloblastic. The macrocytes in liver disease and hypothyroidism may be related to an increased deposition of lipid in the red cell membrane.

The *normocytic* anemias of underproduction comprise a diverse group of disorders. As shown in Table 56-2, this group can be conveniently subdivided into two categories: those secondary to some other underlying disease and those due to intrinsic pathology within the bone marrow.

The primary disorders of the bone marrow, such as the leukemias, myelodysplasia, aplastic anemia, and myelophthisis, are best approached by microscopic examination of a marrow aspirate and biopsy. This group of anemias is often accompanied by leukopenia and thrombocytopenia. Pancytopenia, usually to a lesser degree, also can be seen in hypersplenism and in the megaloblastic anemias. Aplastic anemia, myelodysplasia, and the myelophthisic anemias are discussed in Chap. 308.

The diagnosis of anemia secondary to some underlying disease is usually quite straightforward. Conversely, the presence of an unexplained normocytic anemia should prompt the search for an underlying disorder such as chronic renal failure, infection, or myxedema. If the presence of such an illness is established, the physician is obliged to investigate whether other factors such as blood loss or a nutritional deficiency contribute to the patient's anemia. Generally, the anemias due to liver disease, chronic inflammation, or an endocrinopathy are of only moderate severity. Unlike the other "secondary" anemias, that due to chronic renal failure is often severe. All these anemias are discussed in more detail in Chap. 305.

HEMOLYTIC ANEMIAS   Hemolytic anemias (Table 56-3) are encountered much less frequently than the anemias due to decreased red cell production. Although they are a diverse group, the hemolytic anemias have a number of clinical features in common. Signs and symptoms of patients with hemolysis are briefly mentioned above.

A number of laboratory tests are available to establish the presence of accelerated breakdown of red cells. The reticulocyte count is the single most useful test. Patients with hemolysis nearly always have an elevated reticulocyte count. A variety of serum and urine tests are useful in confirming the presence of hemolysis and assessing its magnitude. Serum unconjugated bilirubin and haptoglobin are particularly useful (see Table 56-1). Others are described in detail in Chap. 307 and are summarized in Table 307-2.

Classification of hemolytic anemias   Once the presence of hemolysis is established, a large battery of laboratory tests is available for determining the specific diagnosis. Some of these tests are listed in Table 56-3. No other area of internal medicine is better suited to detailed and fruitful diagnostic probing. In the interest of time and

money, the clinician should use the available tests in an orderly fashion. This complex group of disorders is easier to approach diagnostically if a concise and workable classification is used. The hemolytic anemias can be grouped in several ways: congenital versus acquired, intracorpuscular versus extracorpuscular, or by anatomic site of the erythrocyte defect. The various kinds of hemolytic anemia are discussed in Chap. 307.

APPROACH TO THE TREATMENT OF ANEMIA

The effective treatment of anemia, like other disorders, is predicated on a thorough diagnostic evaluation. There is no reason to administer hematinics such as iron, vitamin B_{12}, or folic acid unless a specific deficiency of these substances has been demonstrated or is anticipated. Although the indiscriminate administration of vitamin B_{12} is not deleterious per se, it lulls both the patient and the physician into a sense of false security. In contrast, the inappropriate use of iron preparations over a prolonged period of time can be directly harmful, leading to a state of iron overload. Pyridoxine is indicated only in the treatment of sideroblastic anemias.

Many kinds of anemias can be corrected if a precipitating cause can be uncovered and reversed. If a drug or toxin can be incriminated, its withdrawal may allow full recovery. The outcome of the "secondary" anemias is dependent on whether the underlying condition can be corrected. Anemias due to an endocrinopathy or infection should respond favorably to appropriate treatment. Occasionally, the anemia of malignancy is corrected by removal of the primary tumor. One of the most dramatic sequelae of a successful renal transplant is the prompt correction of the "anemia of uremia." Moreover, the anemia associated with renal failure can be corrected by the administration of recombinant human erythropoietin. This agent also may prove to be effective in the treatment of anemia associated with other chronic disorders such as malignancies, rheumatoid arthritis, or AIDS.

Primary disorders of bone marrow such as aplastic anemia or myelophthisic anemia are often irreversible and are treated with supportive measures such as transfusions of red cells and platelets. *Androgens* are sometimes employed in this group of anemias, but their efficacy is marginal. The availability of recombinant hematopoietic growth factors may provide more specific and effective treatment. Because prognosis is so bleak in these disorders, a radical approach to treatment is justified. As described in Chaps. 308 and 313, bone marrow transplantation is a reasonable therapeutic alternative in selected cases of severe aplastic anemia and acute leukemia.

Several factors should be weighed in determining whether an anemic patient should be transfused. The risks and complications of the administration of blood products are discussed in Chap. 312. Patients with chronic or long-standing anemias are able to compensate in several ways, discussed earlier in this chapter. A considerable reduction in red cell mass can be surprisingly well tolerated, especially if the patient is young or sedentary. Transfusion is seldom indicated in a patient with a chronic anemia whose hemoglobin is 90 g/L (9 g/dL) or greater. Those who are expected to respond to the administration of a specific agent such as iron, folic acid, or vitamin B_{12} can usually be spared transfusions. If the anemia has precipitated an episode of congestive heart failure or myocardial ischemia, prompt but cautious administration of packed red cells is indicated. In general, whole blood should be given only if the patient is hypovolemic.

Glucocorticoids have only a limited role in the treatment of anemia. These agents are not effective in stimulating erythropoiesis. High doses of a glucocorticoid are indicated in the treatment of immunohemolytic anemia and pure red cell anemia. Otherwise, steroids should be prescribed sparingly unless some coexisting condition dictates their use.

Splenectomy is indicated in the treatment of certain hemolytic anemias. The efficacy of splenectomy correlates with the degree to which the abnormal or defective red cells are sequestered. Splenectomy

---

TABLE 56-3   Hemolytic anemias

Blood smear	Additional lab tests	Diagnosis
Schistocytes, helmet cells		Traumatic hemolytic anemia
Spherocytes	+ Coombs' test	Immunohemolytic anemia
	↑ Osmotic fragility	Hereditary spherocytosis
Spur cells	Abnormal LFT	Spur cell anemia
	+ Sucrose lysis	Paroxysmal nocturnal hemoglobinuria
Sickle cells	+ Sickle prep	Sickle cell syndromes
Target cells	Abn Hb electrophoresis	Hb C, D, etc.
Heinz bodies	Abn Hb electrophoresis	Congenital Heinz body hemolytic anemia
	↓ G6PD	G6PD deficiency

NOTE: Hb, hemoglobin; G6PD, glucose-6-phosphate dehydrogenase; LFT, liver function tests; Abn, abnormal.

is virtually curative in hereditary spherocytosis. The operation may be beneficial in selected patients with immunohemolytic anemia, congestive splenomegaly, spur cell anemia, and certain hemoglobinopathies and enzymopathies. The operative morbidity and mortality from elective splenectomy are very low. Occasional patients develop a left subphrenic abscess. Following splenectomy, young children are at risk of developing overwhelming septicemia. This complication is much rarer in adults. Thrombocytosis generally develops promptly following splenectomy. However, in most cases, it is transient. In patients with continued hemolysis or a myeloproliferative disorder (Chap. 309), the thrombocytosis usually persists and may occasionally be associated with thromboembolic phenomena.

REFERENCES

Babior BM, Stossel TP: *Hematology, A Pathophysiological Approach*, 2d ed. New York, Churchill Livingstone, 1990
Beck WS (ed): *Hematology*, 5th ed. Boston, MIT Press, 1991
Crosby WH: Red cell mass: Its precursors and perturbations. Hosp Prac 15:2, 71, 1980
Jandl JH: *Blood Pathophysiology*. Boston, Blackwell, 1991

57   BLEEDING AND THROMBOSIS

ROBERT I. HANDIN

Hemorrhage, intravascular thrombosis, and embolism are common clinical manifestations of many diseases. The normal hemostatic system limits blood loss by precisely regulated interactions between components of the vessel wall, circulating blood platelets, and plasma proteins. However, when disease or trauma damage large arteries and veins, excessive bleeding may occur, despite a normal hemostatic system. Less frequently, hemorrhage is caused by an inherited or acquired disorder of the hemostatic machinery itself. A large number of such bleeding disorders have now been identified.

In addition, unregulated activation of the hemostatic system may cause thrombosis and embolism, which can reduce blood flow to critical organs like the brain and myocardium. Although we understand less about the pathophysiology of thrombosis than of hemostatic failure, certain patient groups have been identified that are particularly prone to thrombosis and embolism. These include patients (1) immobilized after surgery, (2) with chronic congestive heart failure, (3) with atherosclerotic vascular disease, (4) with malignancy, or (5) who are pregnant. Most of these "thrombosis-prone" patients have no identifiable hemostatic disorder. However, there are certain patient groups who have inherited or acquired a "hypercoagulable" or "prethrombotic" state which predisposes them to recurrent thrombosis.

The cardinal manifestations of disordered hemostasis which cause bleeding or thrombosis are discussed below, along with the clinical approach to diagnosis and evaluation of these patients. Certain information in the patient's history, such as the mode of onset and sites of bleeding, a family bleeding tendency, and a record of drug ingestion help establish the correct diagnosis. Physical examination can identify bleeding in the skin or joint deformities due to previous hemarthroses. Ultimately, however, bleeding disorders are diagnosed by laboratory tests. General screening tests are utilized first, to document a systemic disorder, and are then supplemented by specific tests of coagulation protein or platelet function to arrive at an accurate diagnosis.

The hypercoagulable or prethrombotic patient can also be identified by a careful history. There are three important clues to this diagnosis: (1) repeated episodes of thromboembolism without an obvious predisposing condition; (2) a family history of thrombosis; and (3)

well-documented thromboembolism in adolescents and young adults. There are, as yet, no clinically useful screening tests for the prethrombotic state. However, several of the prethrombotic disorders can be diagnosed with specific immunologic and functional assays.

NORMAL HEMOSTASIS

Accurate diagnosis and treatment of patients with either bleeding or thrombosis requires some knowledge of the pathophysiology of hemostasis. The process can be divided into primary and secondary components and is initiated when trauma, surgery, or disease disrupt the vascular endothelial lining and blood is exposed to subendothelial connective tissue. *Primary hemostasis* is the name given to the process of platelet plug formation at sites of injury. It occurs within seconds of injury and is of prime importance in stopping blood loss from capillaries, small arterioles, and venules (see Fig. 57-1). *Secondary hemostasis* describes the reactions of the plasma coagulation system which result in fibrin formation. It requires several minutes for completion. The fibrin strands which are produced strengthen the primary hemostatic plug. This reaction is particularly important in larger vessels and prevents recurrent bleeding hours or days after the initial injury. Although presented here as separate events, primary and secondary hemostasis are closely linked. For example, activated platelets accelerate plasma coagulation, and products of the plasma coagulation reaction, such as thrombin, stimulate platelet aggregation.

Effective primary hemostasis requires three critical events—platelet adhesion, granule release, and platelet aggregation. Within a few seconds of injury, platelets adhere to collagen fibrils in vascular subendothelium via a specific platelet collagen receptor, glycoprotein Ia/IIa, which is a member of the integrin family. As shown in Fig. 57-2, this interaction is stabilized by the von Willebrand factor, an adhesive glycoprotein which allows platelets to remain attached to the vessel wall despite the high shear forces generated within the vascular lumen. The von Willebrand factor accomplishes this task by forming a link between a platelet receptor site on glycoprotein Ib/IX and subendothelial collagen fibrils. The adherent platelets then release preformed granule constituents and generate de novo mediators like those depicted in Fig. 57-1.

As in other cells, platelet activation and secretion are regulated by changes in the level of cyclic nucleotides, the influx of calcium,

FIGURE 57-1 Schematic presentation of the major events in primary hemostasis. The first event is platelet adhesion, the interaction of platelets with a nonplatelet surface such as vascular subendothelium. This is followed by platelet activation and secretion. Some of the products secreted by platelets are depicted. Abbreviations—ADP, adenosine diphosphate; PDGF, platelet-derived growth factor, vWF, von Willebrand's factor. The final event is the binding of activated platelets to the adherent monolayer in the process of platelet aggregation.

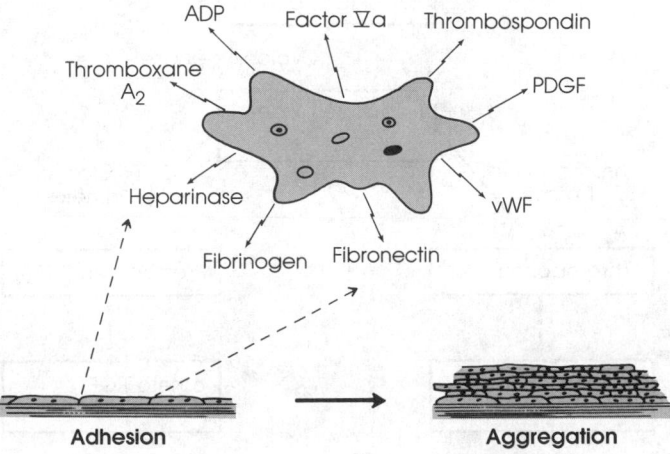

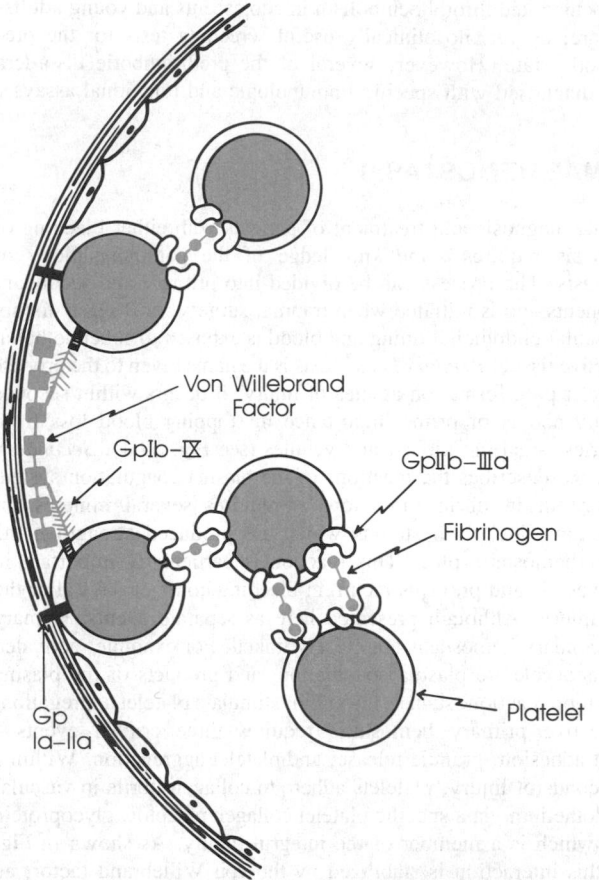

FIGURE 57-2 The molecular basis of platelet adhesion and aggregation. Adhesion of platelets to vascular subendothelium is facilitated by von Willebrand's factor, which forms a bridge between collagen fibrils in the vessel wall and receptors on platelet glycoprotein Ib/IX (GpIb–IX). In a similar manner, platelet aggregation is mediated by fibrinogen which links adjacent platelets via receptors on the platelet glycoprotein IIb and IIIa complex (GpIIb–IIIa).

hydrolysis of membrane phospholipids, and phosphorylation of critical intracellular proteins. The relevant pathways are depicted in Figs. 57-3 and 57-4. The binding of agonists such as epinephrine, collagen, or thrombin to platelet surface receptors activates two membrane enzymes—phospholipase C and phospholipase A₂. These enzymes catalyze the release of arachidonic acid from two of the major

FIGURE 57-3 Generation of thromboxane A₂ in platelets and prostacyclin (PGI₂) in endothelial cells.

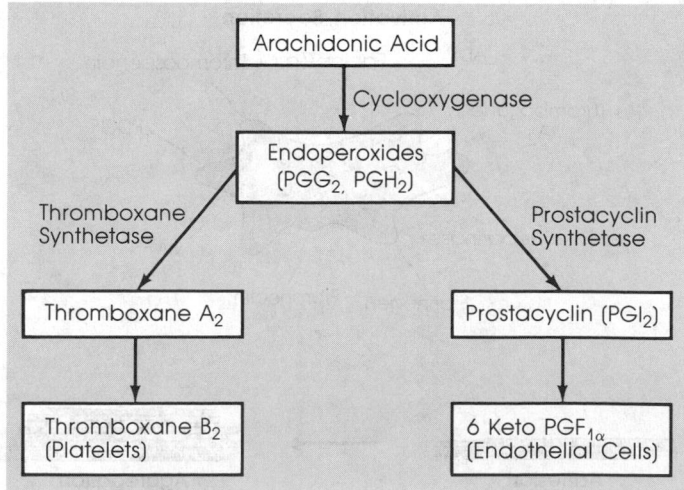

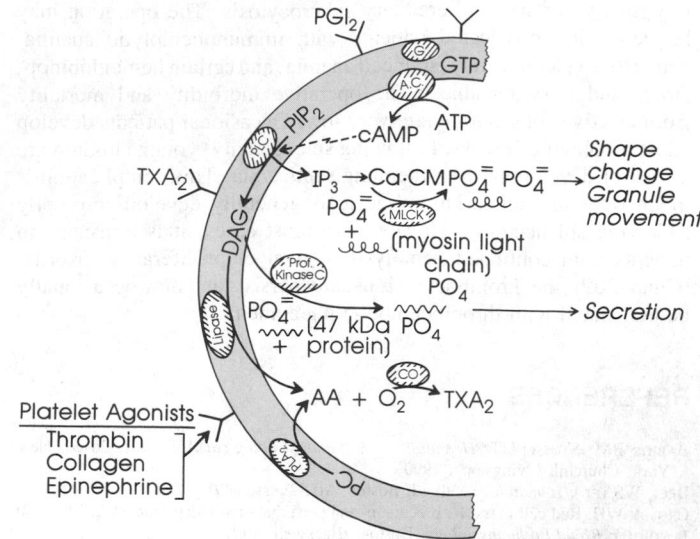

FIGURE 57-4 The biochemical basis of platelet activation and secretion. Binding of agonists such as thrombin, epinephrine, or collagen sets in motion a chain of events which hydrolyzes membrane phospholipids, inhibits adenylate cyclase, mobilizes intracellular calcium, and phosphorylates critical intracellular proteins. The net result is shape change, movement of granules to the canalicular system, generation of mediators like thromboxane A₂, and granule secretion. Abbreviations—A.C., adenylate cyclase; G, guanine nucleotide-binding protein; PIP₂, phosphatidylinositol-4,5-bisphosphate; PLC, phospholipase C; DAG, diacylglycerol; PLA₂, phospholipase A₂; PC, phosphatidylcholine; AA, arachidonic acid; CO, cyclooxygenase; O₂, oxygen; IP₃, inositol triphosphate; cAMP, cyclic AMP; Ca-CM, calcium calmodulin complex; MLCK, myosin light chain kinase.

membrane phospholipids, phosphatidylinositol and phosphatidylcholine. Initially, a small quantity of the released arachidonic acid is converted to thromboxane A₂ (TXA₂), which, in turn, can activate phospholipase C. The formation of TXA₂ from arachidonic acid is mediated by the enzyme cyclooxygenase (see Fig. 57-3). This enzyme is inhibited by aspirin and nonsteroidal anti-inflammatory drugs. Inhibition of TXA₂ synthesis is a cause of mild bleeding in some patients, as well as the basis for the action of some antithrombotic drugs.

Hydrolysis of the membrane phospholipid, phosphatidylinositol 4,5-bisphosphate (PIP₂), produces diacylglycerol (DAG) and inositol triphosphate (IP₃), both of which play critical roles in platelet metabolism. IP₃ mediates the movement of calcium into the platelet cytosol and stimulates the phosphorylation of myosin light chains. The latter interact with actin to facilitate granule movement and platelet shape change. DAG activates protein kinase C which, in turn, phosphorylates several substrates including myosin light chain kinase and a 47,000-Da protein (plekstrin). Phosphorylation of these or other proteins may regulate platelet granule secretion.

A finely balanced mechanism controls the rate and extent of platelet activation, which is illustrated in Fig. 57-3. TXA₂, a platelet product of arachidonic acid, stimulates platelet activation and secretion. In contrast, prostacyclin (PGI₂), an endothelial cell product of arachidonic acid, inhibits platelet activation by raising intraplatelet cyclic AMP levels. Similar pathways to regulate activation and secretion occur in other cells.

Following activation, platelets secrete their granule contents into plasma. Endoglycosidases and a heparin-cleaving enzyme are released from lysosomes; calcium, serotonin, and adenosine diphosphate (ADP) are released from the dense granules; and several proteins including the von Willebrand factor, fibronectin, thrombospondin, the platelet-derived growth factor (PDGF), and a heparin-neutralizing protein (platelet factor 4) are released from alpha granules. Released ADP binds to a specific purinergic receptor which, when activated, changes the conformation of the glycoprotein IIb/IIIa complex so that

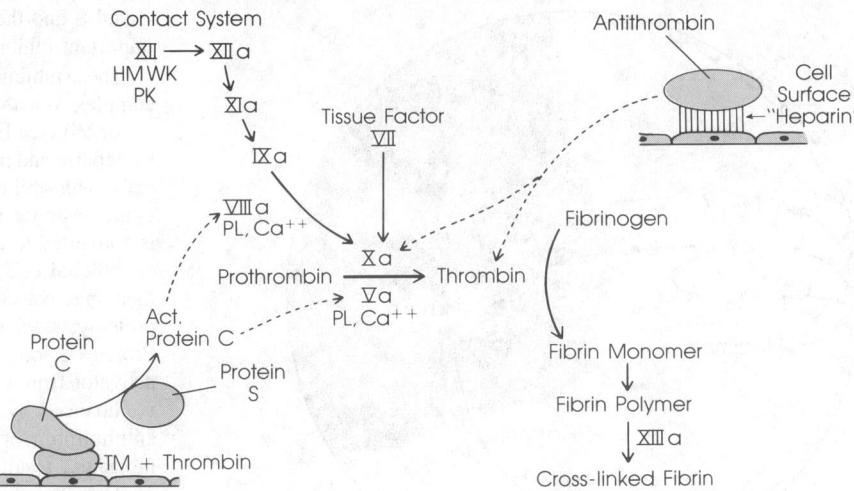

FIGURE 57-5 A schematic diagram of some of the clinically important coagulation reactions. The unactivated or precursor proteins are indicated by roman numerals, and the active form by the addition of a lowercase "a"—a standard convention. Other abbreviations are HMWK, high-molecular-weight kininogen; PK, prekallikrein; PL, phospholipid; TM, thrombomodulin; Ca^{2+}, calcium. There are two independent activation pathways, the contact system and the tissue factor–mediated or extrinsic system. They both merge at the point of factor X activation and lead to the generation of thrombin, which converts fibrinogen into fibrin. These reactions are regulated by antithrombin, which forms complexes with all of the coagulation protein serine proteases except factor VII, and the protein C–protein S system which inactivates factors V and VIII.

it binds fibrinogen, linking adjacent platelets into a hemostatic plug (Fig. 57-2). Released PDGF, stimulates the growth and migration of fibroblasts and smooth muscle cells within the vessel wall, which is an important part of the repair process.

As the primary hemostatic plug is being formed, plasma coagulation proteins are activated to initiate secondary hemostasis. An overall picture of the coagulation scheme, including the role of various inhibitors, is shown in Fig. 57-5. The coagulation pathway can be broken down into a series of reactions (outlined in Fig. 57-6) which culminate in the production of sufficient thrombin to convert a small portion of plasma fibrinogen to fibrin. Each of the reactions requires the formation of a surface-bound complex, the conversion of inactive precursor proteins into active proteases by limited proteolysis, and each is regulated by both plasma and cellular cofactors and calcium.

In *reaction 1*, the intrinsic or contact phase of coagulation, three plasma proteins, Hageman factor (factor XII), high-molecular-weight kininogen (HMWK), and prekallikrein (PK) form a complex on vascular subendothelial collagen. After binding to HMWK, factor XII is slowly converted to an active protease (XIIa), which then converts both PK to kallikrein and factor XI to its active form (XIa). Kallikrein (K) in turn accelerates XII conversion to XIIa, while XIa participates in subsequent coagulation reactions. Although these interactions are well-characterized in vitro, an alternative mechanism for the activation of factor XI may exist, as patients who are deficient in either factor XII, HMWK, or PK have apparently normal hemostasis and no clinical bleeding.

Reaction 2 provides a second pathway to initiate coagulation by converting factor VII to an active protease. In this extrinsic or tissue-factor-dependent pathway, a complex is formed between factor VII, calcium, and tissue factor, a ubiquitous lipoprotein present in cellular membranes which is exposed following cellular injury. There is increasing evidence that the tissue factor–VII pathway is continuously active and makes a major contribution to basal coagulation. Factor VII and three other coagulation proteins—factors II (prothrombin), IX, and X—require calcium and vitamin K for biologic activity. These proteins are synthesized in the liver, where a vitamin K–dependent carboxylase catalyzes a unique posttranslational modification which adds a second carboxyl group to certain glutamic acid residues. Pairs of these di-γ-carboxyglutamic acid (Gla) residues bind calcium, which anchors these proteins to negatively charged phospholipid surfaces and confers biologic activity. Inhibition of this posttranslational modification by vitamin K antagonists (e.g., warfarin) is the basis of one of the most common forms of anticoagulant therapy.

In *reaction 3*, factor X is activated by the proteases generated in the two previous reactions. In one reaction, a calcium- and lipid-dependent complex is formed between factors VIII, IX, and X. Within this complex, factor IX is first converted to IXa by factor XIa that was generated within the intrinsic pathway (reaction 1). Factor X is then activated by factor IXa in concert with factor VIII. Alternatively, both factors IX and X can be activated more directly by factor VIIa, which has been generated via the extrinsic pathway (reaction 2).

FIGURE 57-6 The major coagulation reactions are subdivided and depicted in schematic form to emphasize their similarity. They all rely on the formation of surface bound enzyme-cofactor complexes. Abbreviations are PK, prekallikrein; K, kallikrein; HMWK, high-molecular-weight kininogen; TF, tissue factor; Ca^{2+}, calcium; PT, prothrombin; Thr, thrombin. By convention other coagulation factors are indicated by roman numerals, with a lowercase "a" appended to indicate their active form. The ∧∧∧ is used to indicate the Gla (di-γ-carboxyglutamic acid)–containing domains of factors VII, IX, X, Xa, and PT which bind calcium and phospholipid. Hatching is used to indicate proteins that adhere to surfaces by hydrophobic interaction.

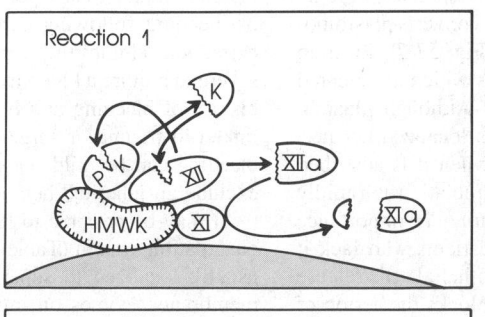

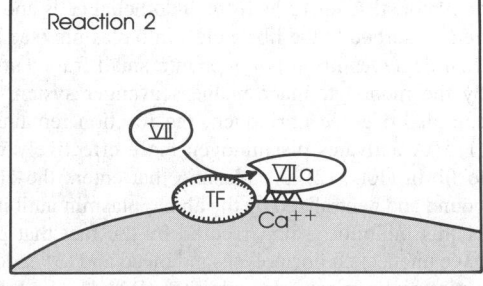

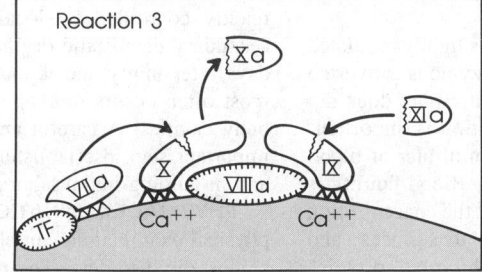

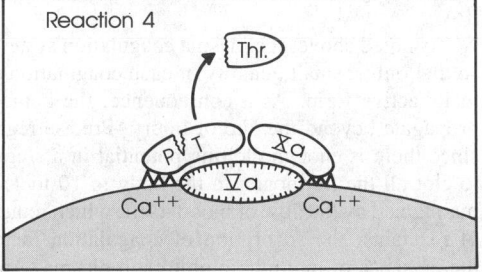

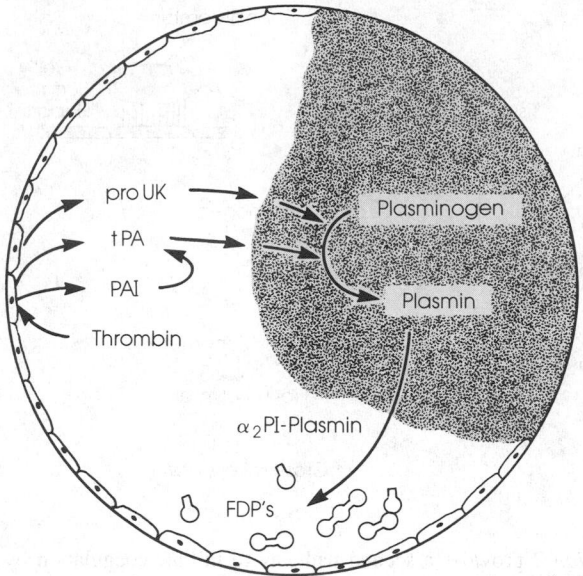

FIGURE 57-7   A schematic diagram of the fibrinolytic pathway. tPA (tissue plasminogen activator) is released from endothelial cells, enters the fibrin clot, and activates plasminogen to plasmin. Any free plasmin is complexed with α_2 PI (alpha$_2$ plasmin inhibitor). Fibrin is degraded to low-molecular-weight fragments, abbreviated as FDPs, fibrin degradation products.

Activation of factors IX and X provides an important link between the intrinsic and extrinsic coagulation pathways (see Fig. 57-5).

Reaction 4, the final step, converts prothrombin to thrombin in the presence of factor V, calcium, and phospholipid. Although prothrombin conversion can take place on various natural and artificial phospholipid-rich surfaces, it accelerates several-thousand-fold on the surface of activated platelets. Thrombin, the product of this reaction, has multiple functions in hemostasis. Although its principal role in hemostasis is the conversion of fibrinogen to fibrin, it also activates factors V, VIII, and XIII and stimulates platelet aggregation and secretion. Following the release of fibrinopeptides A and B from the alpha and beta chains of fibrinogen, the modified molecule, now called fibrin monomer, polymerizes into an insoluble gel. The fibrin polymer is then stabilized by the cross-linking of individual chains by factor XIIIa, a plasma transglutaminase (Fig. 57-5).

Clot lysis and vessel repair begin immediately after the formation of the definitive hemostatic plug. There are three major activators of the fibrinolytic system, Hageman factor fragments, urokinase (UK), and tissue plasminogen activator (tPA). The principal physiologic activator, tPA, diffuses from endothelial cells and converts plasminogen, adsorbed to the fibrin clot, into plasmin (see Fig. 57-7). Plasmin then degrades fibrin polymer into small fragments which are cleared by the monocyte-macrophage scavenger system. Although plasmin can also degrade fibrinogen, the reaction remains localized because (1) tPA activates plasminogen more effectively when it is adsorbed to fibrin clots, (2) any plasmin that enters the circulation is rapidly bound and neutralized by the alpha$_2$ plasmin inhibitor. The importance of this inhibitor is underscored by the fact that patients who lack it have unchecked fibrinolysis and bleed and (3) endothelial cells release a plasminogen activator inhibitor (PAI-1) which blocks the action of tPA.

As noted above, the plasma coagulation system is tightly regulated so that only a small quantity of each coagulation enzyme is converted to its active form. As a consequence, the hemostatic plug does not propagate beyond the site of injury. Precise regulation is important, since there is enough clotting potential in a single milliliter of blood to clot all the fibrinogen in the body in 10 to 15 s. Blood fluidity is maintained by the flow of blood itself, which reduces the concentration of reactants, the adsorption of coagulation factors to surfaces, and the presence of multiple inhibitors in plasma. Antithrombin, proteins

C and S and the tissue factor pathway inhibitor (TFPI) are the most important inhibitors which collectively maintain blood fluidity.

These inhibitors have distinct modes of action. Antithrombin forms complexes with all the serine protease coagulation factors except factor VII (see Fig. 57-5). Rates of complex formation are accelerated by heparin and heparin-like molecules on the surface of the endothelial cells. This ability of heparin to accelerate the activity of antithrombin is the basis for heparin's action as a potent anticoagulant. Protein C is converted to an active protease by thrombin after it is bound to an endothelial cell protein called thrombomodulin. Activated protein C then inactivates the two plasma cofactors V and VIII by limited proteolysis which slows down two critical coagulation reactions. Protein C may also stimulate the release of tissue plasminogen activator from endothelial cells. The inhibitory function of protein C is enhanced by protein S. As one might predict, reduced levels of antithrombin or proteins C and S, or dysfunctional forms of the molecule, result in a hypercoagulable or prethrombotic state.

The preceding description of blood coagulation implies that the process is uniform throughout the body. In fact, the process is not uniform and composition of the blood clot varies with the site of injury. Hemostatic plugs or thrombi that form in veins where blood flow is slow are richly endowed with fibrin and trapped red blood cells and contain relatively few platelets. They are often called red thrombi due to their appearance in surgical and pathologic specimens. The friable ends of these red thrombi, which often form in leg veins, can break off and embolize to the pulmonary circulation. Conversely, clots that form in arteries under conditions of high flow are predominantly composed of platelets and have little fibrin. These white thrombi may readily dislodge from the arterial wall and embolize to distant sites to cause temporary or permanent ischemia. This is particularly common in the cerebral and retinal circulation and may lead to transient neurologic dysfunction (transient ischemic attacks) including temporary monocular blindness (amaurosis fugax) or strokes. In addition, most episodes of myocardial infarction are due to thrombi which form after the rupture of atherosclerotic plaques within diseased coronary arteries. It is important to remember that there is little difference between hemostatic plugs, which are a physiologic response to injury, and pathologic thrombi. To underscore the similarity, thrombosis has been described as coagulation occurring in the wrong place or at the wrong time.

CLINICAL EVALUATION

HISTORY   Certain elements of the history are particularly useful in determining whether bleeding is caused by an underlying hemostatic disorder rather than a local anatomic defect. One clue is a history of bleeding following common hemostatic stresses such as dental extraction, childbirth, or minor surgery. Bleeding that is sufficiently severe to require a blood transfusion merits special attention. A family history of bleeding and bleeding from multiple sites that cannot be linked to trauma or surgery also suggest a systemic disorder. Since bleeding can be mild, lack of a family history of bleeding does not exclude an inherited hemostatic disorder.

It may be possible to localize the defect to the platelet or plasma coagulation system (Table 57-1). Bleeding from a platelet disorder is usually localized to superficial sites such as the skin and mucous membranes, comes on immediately after trauma or surgery, and is readily controlled by local measures. In contrast, bleeding from secondary hemostatic or plasma coagulation defects occurs hours or days after injury and is unaffected by local therapy. Such bleeding most often occurs in deep subcutaneous tissues, muscles, joints, or body cavities. A careful and thorough history is probably the most important step in establishing the presence of a hemostatic disorder and in guiding initial laboratory testing.

PHYSICAL EXAMINATION   In conjunction with a careful history, physical examination can also be of help in evaluating patients with hemostatic disorders. The most common site to observe bleeding is

TABLE 57-1 Differences in the clinical manifestations of disorders of primary and secondary hemostasis

	Primary hemostasis (platelet defect)	Secondary hemostasis (plasma proteins)
Onset of bleeding after trauma	Immediate	Delayed—hours or days
Sites of bleeding	Superficial—skin; mucous membranes; nose; gastrointestinal, genitourinary tracts	Deep—joints, muscle, retroperitoneum
Physical findings	Petechiae, ecchymoses	Hematomas, hemarthroses
Family history	Autosomal dominant	Autosomal or X-linked recessive
Response to therapy	Immediate; local measures effective	Requires sustained systemic therapy

TABLE 57-2 Causes of thrombocytopenia

Decreased marrow production of megakaryocytes
  A Marrow infiltration with tumor, fibrosis
  B Marrow failure—aplastic, hypoplastic anemias
Splenic sequestration of circulating platelets
  A Splenic hypertrophy—tumor, portal hypertension
Increased destruction of circulating platelets
  A Nonimmune destruction
    1 Vascular prostheses, cardiac valves
    2 Disseminated intravascular coagulation
    3 Sepsis
    4 Vasculitis
  B Immune destruction
    1 Autoantibodies to platelet antigens
    2 Drug-associated antibodies
    3 Circulating immune complexes—systemic lupus erythematosus, viral agents, bacterial sepsis

in the skin and mucous membranes. Collections of blood in the skin are called *purpura* and may be subdivided on the basis of the site of bleeding in the skin. Small pinpoint hemorrhages into the dermis due to the leakage of red cells through capillaries are called *petechiae* and are characteristic of platelet disorders—in particular, severe thrombocytopenia. Larger subcutaneous collections of blood due to leakage of blood from small arterioles and venules are *ecchymoses* (common bruises) or, if somewhat deeper and palpable, *hematomas*. They are also common in patients with platelet defects and result from minor trauma. There are other skin and mucous membrane lesions like dilated capillaries or *telangiectasia* that may cause bleeding without any hemostatic defect. In addition, the loss of connective tissue support for capillaries and small veins that accompanies aging increases the fragility of superficial vessels, such as those on the dorsum of the hand, leading to extravasation of blood into subcutaneous tissue—*senile purpura*. Menorrhagia is sometimes a serious problem in women with severe thrombocytopenia or platelet dysfunction. In addition, some patients with primary hemostatic defects, especially von Willebrand's disease, may have recurrent gastrointestinal hemorrhage.

As mentioned previously, bleeding into body cavities, retroperitoneum, or joints is a common manifestation of plasma coagulation defects. Repeated joint bleeding may cause synovial thickening, chronic inflammation, and fluid collections and may erode articular cartilage and lead to chronic joint deformity and limited mobility. Such deformities are particularly common in factors VIII and IX deficiency, the two sex-linked coagulation disorders referred to as the *hemophilias*. For unclear reasons, hemarthroses are much less common in other plasma coagulation defects. Blood collections in various body cavities or soft tissues can cause secondary necrosis of tissues or nerve compression. Retroperitoneal hematomas can cause femoral nerve compression, and large collections of poorly coagulated blood in soft tissues may occasionally mimic malignant growths—the pseudotumor syndrome. Two of the most life-threatening sites of bleeding are in the oropharynx, where bleeding can compromise the airway, and in the central nervous system. Intracerebral hemorrhage is one of the leading causes of death in patients with severe coagulation disorders.

LABORATORY TESTS The most important screening tests of the primary hemostatic system are (1) a *bleeding time* (a sensitive measure of platelet function) and (2) a *platelet count*. The latter is particularly useful as it is readily available and correlates well with the propensity to bleed. The normal platelet count is 150,000 to 450,000 platelets per cubic millimeter of blood. As long as the count is above 100,000 per cubic millimeter, however, patients are not symptomatic and the bleeding time remains normal. Platelet counts of 50,000 to 100,000 per cubic millimeter cause mild prolongation of the bleeding time so that bleeding occurs only after severe trauma or other stress. Patients with platelet counts less than 50,000 per cubic millimeter have easy bruising, which is manifested by skin purpura with minor trauma and bleeding after mucous membrane

surgery. Patients with a platelet count below 20,000 per cubic millimeter have an appreciable incidence of spontaneous bleeding, usually have petechiae, and may have intracranial or other spontaneous internal bleeding. The major causes of thrombocytopenia are outlined in Table 57-2.

Patients with qualitative platelet abnormalities have a normal platelet count and a prolonged bleeding time (Table 57-3). The bleeding time is ascertained by making a small, superficial skin incision and timing the duration of blood flow from the wounded area. Although this is a rather crude "bioassay," by careful standardization it has become a reliable and sensitive test of platelet function. The most widely used technique uses a template or an automated scalpel to control the length and depth of the incision (usually 1 mm deep by 9 mm long) and a sphygmomanometer inflated to 40 mmHg to distend the capillary bed of the forearm uniformly. In order to be useful the bleeding time must be performed by an experienced technician as small differences in techniques have a big effect on the outcome of the test. Although any patient with a bleeding time over 10 min has a slightly increased risk of bleeding, the risk does not become great until the bleeding time exceeds 15 or 20 min. As shown in Fig. 57-8, there is a roughly linear relationship between the platelet count and the bleeding time. When a defect in primary hemostasis is uncovered, specialized testing is needed to determine the cause of the platelet dysfunction (Table 57-3). A precise diagnosis is important since patients with bleeding due to a primary hemostatic disorder may need therapy with platelets, one of several hormones (desmopressin, estrogen, glucocorticoids), or plasma fractions, depending on the nature of the disorder. Occasional patients with a strong history of bleeding, particularly those with mild von Willebrand's disease, may have a normal bleeding time when initially tested due to cyclical variations in the level of the von Willebrand factor. They may need repeated testing to establish an accurate diagnosis.

Plasma coagulation function is readily assessed with a few simple

TABLE 57-3 Primary hemostatic (platelet) disorders

Platelet adhesion defects:
  Von Willebrand's disease
  Bernard-Soulier syndrome (absence, dysfunction of GpIb/IX)
Platelet aggregation defects
  Glanzmann's thrombasthenia (absence, dysfunction of GpIIb/IIIa)
Platelet release defects
  1 Decreased cyclooxygenase activity
    Drugs—aspirin, nonsteroidal anti-inflammatory agents
    Congenital
  2 Granule storage pool defects
    Congenital
    Acquired
  3 Uremia
  4 Platelet coating (e.g., penicillin or paraproteins)
Platelet coagulant defect
  Scott's syndrome

ABBREVIATION: Gp = glycoprotein.

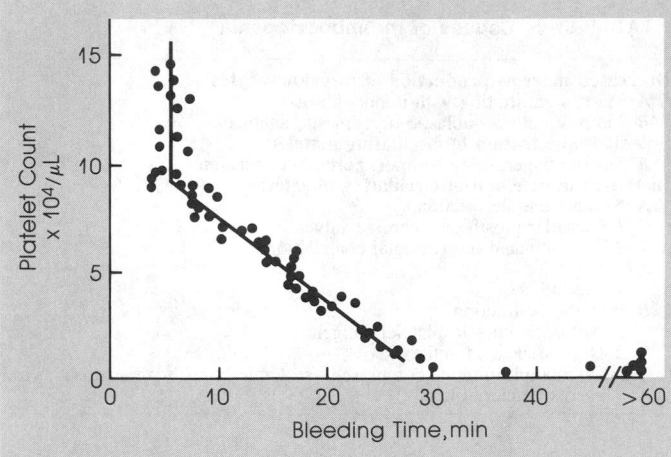

FIGURE 57-8 The relationship between the platelet count and the bleeding time. (*From Harker LA, Hemostasis Manual, 2d ed. Philadelphia, FA Davis Company, 1974.*)

laboratory tests—the partial thromboplastin time (PTT), prothrombin time (PT), thrombin time (TT), or a quantitative fibrinogen determination (Fig. 57-5, Table 57-4). The PTT screens the intrinsic limb of the coagulation system and tests for the adequacy of factors XII, HMWK, PK, XI, IX, and VIII. The PT screens the extrinsic or tissue factor–dependent pathway. Both tests also evaluate the common coagulation pathway involving all the reactions that occur after the activation of factor X. Prolongation of the PT and PTT that does not correct after the addition of normal plasma suggests a specific or nonspecific coagulation inhibitor. A specific test for fibrinogen conversion to fibrin is needed when both the PTT and PT are prolonged—either a TT or a clottable fibrinogen level can be employed. When abnormalities are noted in any of the screening tests, more specific coagulation factor assays can be ordered to determine the nature of the defect.

There are three rare coagulation abnormalities that may be missed as they do not perturb the screening tests just discussed. They are factor XIII deficiency, alpha₂ plasmin inhibitor deficiency, and Scott's syndrome, a platelet coagulant defect. A test for factor XIII–dependent fibrin cross-linking, such as clot solubility in 5 *M* urea, should be ordered when the PT and PTT are both normal but there is a strong

history of bleeding. The fibrinolytic system can be assessed by measuring the rate of clot lysis with the euglobulin lysis or whole blood clot lysis tests and by measuring the level of alpha₂ plasmin inhibitor. Scott's syndrome can be detected by ordering a serum prothrombin time, which assesses the amount of residual prothrombin.

There are no clinical tests to screen patients suspected of having hypercoagulable or prethrombotic disorders, although tests are being developed in research laboratories which measure small peptides or enzyme-inhibitor complexes generated during coagulation. For example, radioimmunoassays have been developed for fibrinopeptides A and B, for the thrombin-antithrombin complex, and for prothrombin cleavage fragments. Elevated levels of these products have been reported in patients with prethrombotic disorders and in patients with thromboembolism. At present, patients suspected of having a hypercoagulable state on the basis of clinical information, should have specific assays to screen for the small number of known defects. Currently available tests can identify 10 to 20 percent of the cases of familial thrombosis and represent only a small fraction of the many patients who present to physicians with thromboembolism.

Inhibitor syndromes or circulating anticoagulants are usually due to antibodies which impair coagulation factor activity. They are an infrequent cause of bleeding which require specialized diagnostic testing. Inhibitors are likely when screening test abnormalities cannot be reversed by adding normal plasma to patient plasma. Antibodies against specific coagulation factors may develop in (1) postpartum females; (2) patients with autoimmune disorders such as systemic lupus erythematosus; (3) patients taking drugs like penicillin and streptomycin; and (4) otherwise healthy elderly individuals. In addition, between 10 and 20 percent of patients with severe hemophilia who have received multiple plasma infusions develop inhibitor antibodies. Some patients, especially those with systemic lupus erythematosus, may also have a nonspecific form of anticoagulant antibody which interferes with phospholipid binding of coagulation factors and prolongs the PT and PTT but does not cause clinical bleeding. The presence of the lupus anticoagulant may increase the risk of thromboembolism and may cause placental infarction and recurrent midtrimester abortion. Occasionally, patients develop inhibitors that are not antibodies. For example, several patients with circulating mucopolysaccharides that have heparin-like activity have been described with clinical bleeding.

REFERENCES

BROZE GJ: The role of tissue factor pathway inhibitor in a revised coagulation cascade. Blood 29:159, 1992

COLMAN RW et al (eds): *Hemostasis and Thrombosis: Basic Principles and Clinical Practice*, 3d ed. Philadelphia, Lippincott, 1993

HANDIN RI et al (eds): *Blood: Principles and Practice of Hematology and Hematologic Oncology*, 4th ed. Philadelphia, Lippincott, 1993

HAWIGER J, HANDIN RI: Structure and function of platelets, in *Hematology of Infancy and Childhood*, 4th ed., DG Nathan et al (eds). Philadelphia, Saunders, 1992, pp 1512–1533

LIND SE: The bleeding time does not predict surgical bleeding. Blood 77: 2547, 1991

ROBERTS HR, LOZIER JN: New perspectives on the coagulation cascade. Hosp Prac Jan 1992, 97–112

ROSENBERG RD, SOFF G: Physiology of hemostasis: The fluid phase, in *Hematology of Infancy and Childhood*, 4th ed., DG Nathan et al (eds). Philadelphia, Saunders, 1992, pp 1534–1560

TABLE 57-4   Relationship between secondary hemostatic disorders and coagulation test abnormalities

Prolonged partial thromboplastin time (PTT)
No clinical bleeding—factors XII, HMWK, PK
Mild or rare bleeding—factor XI
Frequent, severe bleeding—factors VIII and IX
Prolonged prothrombin time (PT)
Factor VII deficiency
Vitamin K deficiency—early
Warfarin anticoagulant ingestion
Prolonged PTT and PT
Factor II, V, or X deficiency
Vitamin K deficiency—late
Warfarin anticoagulant ingestion
Prolonged thrombin time (TT)
Mild or rare bleeding—afibrinogenemia
Frequent, severe bleeding—dysfibrinogenemia
Heparin-like inhibitors or heparin administration
Prolonged PT and/or PTT not corrected with normal plasma
Specific or nonspecific inhibitor syndromes
Clot solubility in 5 *M* urea
Factor XIII deficiency
Inhibitors or defective cross-linking
Rapid clot lysis
Alpha₂ plasmin inhibitor

ABBREVIATIONS: HMWK = high-molecular-weight kininogen; PK = prekallikrein.

58 ENLARGEMENT OF LYMPH NODES AND SPLEEN

BARTON F. HAYNES

Lymph nodes and spleen constitute a major portion of the peripheral immune system and become enlarged in a wide spectrum of infectious, malignant, autoimmune, and metabolic diseases. Enlargements of lymph nodes (lymphadenopathy) and spleen (splenomegaly) are common clinical findings that can lead to a wide range of diagnostic and therapeutic procedures. The goal of this chapter is to serve as an introduction to these two components of the immune system and to highlight clinical features and diagnostic evaluation of some of the diseases in which lymphadenopathy and splenomegaly occur.

LYMPH NODES

LYMPH NODE STRUCTURE AND FUNCTION Lymph nodes are peripheral lymphoid organs that are connected to the circulation by afferent and efferent lymphatic vessels (Fig. 58-1) and by postcapillary high-endothelial venules. A number of cell types make up the lymph node supportive framework and stroma. Fibroblasts are the predominant cell type in the lymph node capsule and trabeculae. Fibroblast-derived reticular cells are supporting cells found frequently in the follicles and germinal centers, i.e., the B cell areas of lymph nodes. Tissue macrophages derived from circulating monocytes are present throughout the normal node. Within cortical areas are interdigitating reticular cells (also called *dendritic cells*) and Langerhans cells, both of which are specialized nonphagocytic, Ia-bearing cells of bone marrow origin that along with macrophages participate in antigen presentation to thymus-derived (T) and B cells (Chap. 277). The outer lymph node cortex contains lymphoid follicles with germinal centers that are the B cell areas of lymph node (see Fig. 58-1). Primary lymphoid follicles are aggregates of IgM- and IgD-bearing B cells and CD4 + helper/inducer T cells prior to antigenic challenge. Secondary lymphoid follicles are the result of antigen stimulation and contain an outer or mantle layer of IgM- and IgD-bearing B cells and an inner zone (germinal center) of activated B cells, macrophages, reticular cells, and scattered CD4 + helper T cells. Between primary and secondary follicle areas (interfollicular zones) and inner lymph node medullary regions are T cell (paracortical) areas. The majority of T cells in lymph nodes are CD4 + helper T cells (approximately 80 percent), while the minority are CD8 + suppressor/cytotoxic T cells (approximately 20 percent).

FIGURE 58-1 Schematic lymph node structure. Lymph flows into nodes via afferent lymphatics (A) and leaves nodes via efferent lymphatics (E). B cell areas are primary and secondary follicles in lymph node cortex while T cells are concentrated in paracortical areas.

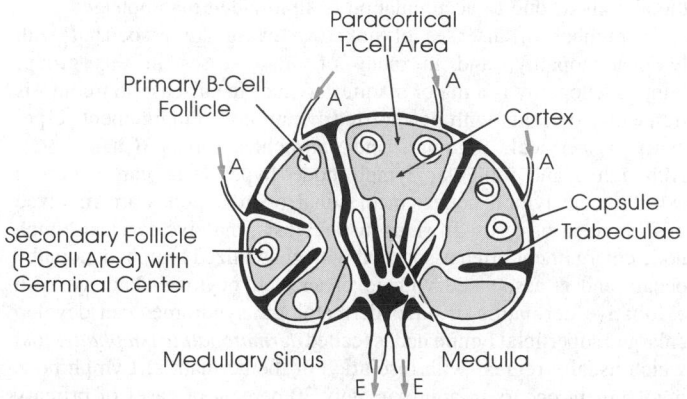

The two most important factors contributing to the composition and distribution of lymphoid cells within lymph node are (1) generation of memory B and T cells de novo from proliferation of antigen-stimulated precursors within lymph nodes and (2) selective recirculation to and homing of specific types of lymphoid cells to lymph nodes from the circulation. Traffic through lymph nodes is via two general routes (see Fig. 58-1). Afferent lymph, containing lymphocytes, macrophages, and antigens, enters the lymph node via the subcapsular space and drains through paracortical and medullary areas into medullary sinuses that converge to form efferent lymphatic vessels through which lymph exits. B cells from bone marrow and T cells from the thymus enter lymph nodes from the circulation by binding to specific receptors on cells of postcapillary high-endothelial venules. After activation by antigen and clonal expansion, sensitized T and B cells and antibody-secreting plasma cells leave the node in efferent lymph and rejoin the peripheral blood circulation via the thoracic duct.

Lymph nodes function as sites of antigen presenting cell, T cell, and B cell contact with antigen, with a specialized structure that gives rise to optimal T cell, B cell, and antigen presenting cell interactions. Under normal conditions, such interactions result in efficient recognition of antigen, activation of the cellular and humoral arms of the immune response, and ultimate elimination of antigen (see Chap. 277).

In normal immune responses, antigen stimulation of macrophages and lymphocytes in lymph nodes exerts profound influences on lymphocyte traffic. One of the earliest effects of antigen is to increase blood flow through the affected node, which during antigen stimulation may reach 10 to 25 times normal levels. Lymphocytes accumulate in antigen-stimulated nodes by increase in traffic through the node, decreased egress of lymphocytes from antigen-stimulated nodes, and proliferation of responding T and B cells. A lymph node may thus reach 15 times its normal size 5 to 10 days after antigenic stimulation.

DISEASES ASSOCIATED WITH LYMPHADENOPATHY Lymph node enlargement can be due to (1) an increase in the number of benign lymphocytes and macrophages during response to antigens, (2) infiltration by inflammatory cells in infections involving lymph nodes (lymphadenitis), (3) in situ proliferation of malignant lymphocytes or macrophages, (4) infiltration of nodes by metastatic malignant cells, or (5) infiltration of lymph nodes by metabolite-laden macrophages in lipid storage diseases. Under normal conditions in adults, the inguinal lymph nodes may be palpable and are generally 0.5 to 2 cm in size. Elsewhere in the body, smaller lymph nodes due to past infections may be present normally. Enlargement of lymph nodes requires investigation when there are one or more new nodes present equal to or greater than 1 cm in diameter and not known to arise from a previously recognized cause. However, this is not a rigid criterion, and under certain circumstances, new multiple or single smaller lymph nodes may warrant investigation as well. Important factors in assessing the significance of enlarged lymph nodes are (1) the patient's age, (2) the physical characteristics of the lymph node, (3) node locations, and (4) the clinical setting associated with lymphadenopathy. Lymphadenopathy reflects significant disease more often in adults than in children because children are more likely to respond to minor stimuli with lymphoid hyperplasia. Lymphadenopathy in patients under 30 years of age is due to benign causes in approximately 80 percent of cases, whereas in patients greater than 50 years of age lymphadenopathy is due to benign causes in only 40 percent of cases.

The physical characteristics of peripheral nodes are important. Nodes of lymphomas tend to be rubbery, firm, matted together, and nontender. Nodes involved with metastatic carcinomas are usually hard and fixed to underlying tissue. In acute infections, nodes are tender, asymmetrically enlarged, and matted together, and the overlying skin may be erythematous.

The clinical setting is important in assessing lymphadenopathy. In a young college student with fever and recent onset of lymph node enlargement, infectious mononucleosis syndromes are important to consider. In homosexuals, hemophiliacs, and intravenous drug users with systemic lymphadenopathy, AIDS an AIDS-related complex syndrome should be considered (see Chap. 279).

The location of enlarged lymph nodes may suggest important clues to the diagnosis. Enlarged posterior cervical nodes are frequently present in scalp infections, toxoplasmosis, and rubella, whereas anterior auricular nodes suggest infections of the eyelids and conjunctiva. Lymphomas commonly involve cervical lymph nodes and can occasionally involve posterior auricular and occipital nodes as well. Enlarged suppurative cervical nodes are seen in mycobacterial lymphadenitis (scrofula). Unilateral jugular or mandibular lymph node enlargement suggests lymphoma or nonlymphoid head and neck malignancy. Supraclavicular and scalene lymph node enlargement is always significant and frequently results from metastasis from intrathoracic or gastrointestinal malignancies or from lymphomas. Virchow's node is an enlarged left supraclavicular lymph node infiltrated with metastatic tumor usually from the gastrointestinal tract. Unilateral epitrochlear node enlargement is usually due to hand infections; bilateral epitrochlear node enlargement is seen in sarcoidosis, tularemia, and secondary syphilis.

Unilateral axillary adenopathy can be seen with breast carcinoma, lymphomas, infections of the upper extremities, cat-scratch disease, and brucellosis.

Bilateral inguinal adenopathy can be seen in a variety of venereal infections; however, lymphogranuloma venereum and syphilis are associated with unilateral inguinal adenopathy. Progressive inguinal lymph node enlargement without obvious infection suggests malignant disease. Femoral node involvement has been reported to occur in *Pasteurella pestis* infections and lymphomas.

Symptoms that should raise the suspicion of hilar or mediastinal node enlargement are cough or wheezing due to airway compression, recurrent laryngeal nerve compression with hoarseness, paralysis of the diaphragm, dysphagia with esophageal compression, and swelling of the neck, face, or arms due to superior vena cava or subclavian vein compression. Bilateral mediastinal adenopathy is frequently seen in lymphomas, especially the nodular sclerosing type of Hodgkin's disease. Unilateral hilar adenopathy indicates a high likelihood of metastatic carcinoma (usually lung), while bilateral hilar adenopathy is more often benign and is seen in sarcoidosis, tuberculosis, and systemic fungal infections. Bilateral hilar adenopathy in asymptomatic patients or in association with erythema nodosum or uveitis is almost always due to sarcoidosis (Chap. 292). The association of bilateral hilar adenopathy with an anterior mediastinal mass, pleural effusion, or pulmonary mass suggests neoplastic disease.

Enlarged retroperitoneal and intraabdominal nodes are not usually inflammatory in origin but are frequently due to lymphomas or other neoplastic diseases. Tuberculosis can cause mesenteric lymphadenitis with large matted and sometimes calcified nodes.

Some of the diseases associated with lymph node enlargement are listed in Table 58-1 and fall into six general categories: infectious diseases, immunologic diseases, malignant diseases, endocrine diseases, lipid storage diseases, and miscellaneous.

The manifestations of infectious diseases are protean and are best considered according to the type of infectious agent. The most common viral infection associated with systemic lymphadenopathy is Epstein-Barr (EB) virus–associated infectious mononucleosis (see Chap. 145). A variety of other viral diseases, including viral hepatitis, cytomegalovirus, rubella, and influenza, can cause clinical syndromes similar to those induced by the EB virus. AIDS is caused by a retrovirus, human immunodeficiency virus (HIV). In the HIV-associated lymphadenopathy syndrome, cervical, axillary, and occipital nodes are the most commonly involved (see Chap. 279).

Chronic bacterial infections as well as fungal infections may produce considerable lymph node enlargement without signs of local inflammation. Cat-scratch disease is a regional lymphadenitis occurring approximately 2 weeks following a cat scratch or bite. The nodes involved relate to lymph drainage of the wound site, with upper extremity adenopathy being the most common, occurring in 50 percent of cases. Fungi associated with primary pulmonary infections

TABLE 58-1   Diseases associated with lymph node enlargement

Infectious diseases
- A Viral infections: infectious hepatitis, infectious mononucleosis syndromes (cytomegalovirus, EB virus), AIDS, rubella, varicella–herpes zoster, vaccinia
- B Bacterial infections: streptococci, staphylococci, salmonella, brucella, Francisella tularensis, *Listeria monocytogenes, Pasteurella pestis, Haemophilus ducreyi*, cat-scratch disease, *Yersinia pseudotuberculosis, Y. enterocolitica*
- C Fungal infections: coccidioidomycosis, histoplasmosis
- D Chlamydial infections: Lymphogranuloma venereum, trachoma
- E Mycobacterial infections: tuberculosis, leprosy
- F Parasitic infections: trypanosomiasis, microfilariasis, toxoplasmosis
- G Spirochetal diseases: syphilis, yaws, endemic syphilis (bejel), leptospirosis

Immunologic diseases
- A Rheumatoid arthritis
- B Systemic lupus erythematosus
- C Dermatomyositis
- D Serum sickness
- E Drug reactions: phenytoin, hydralazine, allopurinol, silicone implants
- F Angioimmunoblastic lymphadenopathy
- G Sjögren's syndrome
- H Primary biliary cirrhosis and other forms of chronic hepatitis

Malignant diseases
- A Hematologic: Hodgkin's lymphoma, acute and chronic T, B, myeloid, and monocytoid cell leukemias and lymphomas, malignant histiocytosis
- B Metastatic tumors to lymph nodes: melanoma, Kaposi's sarcoma, neuroblastoma, seminoma, tumors of lung, breast, prostate, kidney, head and neck, gastrointestinal tract

Endocrine diseases: hyperthyroidism

Lipid storage diseases: Gaucher's and Niemann-Pick diseases

Miscellaneous diseases and diseases of unknown cause
- A Giant follicular lymph node hyperplasia (Castleman's disease)
- B Sinus histiocytosis
- C Dermatopathic lymphadenitis
- D Sarcoidosis
- E Amyloidosis
- F Mucocutaneous lymph node syndrome
- G Lymphomatoid granulomatosis
- H Multifocal Langerhans cell (eosinophilic) granulomatosis
- I Familial Mediterranean fever
- J Kikuchi's histiocytic necrotizing lymphadenitis

(coccidioidomycosis, histoplasmosis) can cause hilar adenopathy. Acute and chronic mycobacterial, parasitic, and spirochetal diseases against which there is a profound cellular and humoral immune response all can result in either systemic or regional enlarged lymph nodes depending on the clinical syndrome in question. Virtually any disease characterized by immune cell activation (systemic lupus erythematosus, rheumatoid arthritis, serum sickness, reactions due to drugs such as diphenylhydantoin, angioimmunoblastic lymphadenopathy) can be associated with regional or systemic adenopathy. Lymph node enlargement associated with malignant disease may be due to direct node involvement by tumor, lymphoid hyperplasia in response to tumor, or both. Generalized lymphoid hyperplasia may occur with hyperthyroidism. Patients with lipid storage diseases such as Gaucher's and Niemann-Pick can have enlarged lymph nodes, particularly in the abdomen, due to accumulation of lipid-laden macrophages.

A number of diseases of unknown cause are associated with lymphadenopathy, and in many of the diseases in this group, lymphadenopathy is a major manifestation of the disease. Sarcoidosis frequently presents with generalized lymph node enlargement, especially in cervical, inguinal, and epitrochlear areas (Chap. 292). Although giant follicular lymph node hyperplasia can occur in extrathoracic lymph nodes, mediastinal or hilar nodes are involved in 70 percent of cases. In sinus histiocytosis, massive cervical lymph node enlargement often associated with generalized lymphadenopathy occurs and is associated with fever and leukocytosis. Patients with exfoliative dermatitis or other dermatologic syndromes can develop enlarged superficial lymph nodes (called *dermatopathic lymphadenitis*) which usually regress with resolution of the dermatitis. Lymph node involvement occurs in approximately 30 percent of cases of primary and secondary amyloidosis; only rarely is amyloid lymphadenopathy the major or only organ involvement. The mechanism of node enlargement in amyloidosis is the accumulation of extracellular masses of amyloid fibrils that compress and eventually obliterate normal lymph node architecture (Chap. 281).

Mucocutaneous lymph node syndrome (Kawasaki's disease) is a systemic lymphadenopathy syndrome, the hallmarks of which are fever, conjunctivitis, erythema of the tongue with protrusion of papillae (strawberry tongue), a truncal exanthem with desquamation of palms and soles, and acute nonsuppurative enlargement of cervical lymph nodes (see Chap. 291).

Lymphomatoid granulomatosis is a disease characterized by infiltration of various organs (lungs, skin, central nervous system) with an angiocentric and angioinvasive polymorphic cellular infiltrate consisting of atypical lymphocytes and macrophages. The disease has characteristics of both an inflammatory granulomatous process and a lymphoproliferative disease, with progression to frank lymphoma in up to 50 percent of cases. Lymphadenopathy in the prelymphoma state of lymphomatoid granulomatosis occurs in 40 percent of cases affecting primarily intrathoracic nodes while peripheral adenopathy occurs only rarely (10 percent) (see Chap. 291).

Angioimmunoblastic lymphadenopathy is a disease characterized by fever, generalized lymphadenopathy, hepatosplenomegaly, polyclonal hypergammaglobulinemia, and Coombs-positive hemolytic anemia. Although it is not thought to be a malignant disease, it evolves into B cell lymphoma in 35 percent of patients (see Chap. 311).

Diseases characterized by benign and malignant proliferation of tissue macrophages (histiocytes) or of specialized bone marrow–derived cells called *Langerhans cells* have been termed *histiocytoses* or *histiocytosis X*. In the past, these terms encompassed a number of diseases, including unifocal and multifocal eosinophilic granuloma, Hand-Schüller-Christian syndrome, Letterer-Siwe disease, and frank neoplasms of undifferentiated histiocytes. However, the identification of the Langerhans cell as the predominant cell in forms of eosinophilic granuloma has prompted reevaluation of these syndromes.

One term currently in use for eosinophilic granuloma syndromes is *Langerhans cell (eosinophilic) granulomatosis*, and this term will be used here. The term *histiocytosis X* is an outmoded term that refers to a spectrum of diseases encompassing both the benign disorder of Langerhans cell (eosinophilic) granulomatosis and malignant lymphomatous disease.

The classic triad of the *Hand-Schüller-Christian syndrome* (exophthalmos, diabetes insipidus, and destructive bone lesions) occurs with 25 percent of cases of multifocal eosinophilic granuloma but also may occur in malignant lymphoma and carcinoma. *Letterer-Siwe disease* is an acute clinical syndrome of unknown cause in infants that consists of hepatosplenomegaly, lymphadenopathy, hemorrhagic diathesis, anemia, no familial occurrence, and generalized hyperplasia of tissue macrophages in a variety of organs. It is currently felt that Letterer-Siwe disease represents an unusual form of malignant lymphoma and is distinct from forms of eosinophilic granuloma.

Histologically, Langerhans cell granulomatosis consists of aggregates of mature eosinophils and Langerhans cells. Langerhans cells are bone marrow–derived cells normally found among epidermal cells of skin and rarely in B cell areas of lymph node and the medulla of thymus. Langerhans cells contain distinct cytoplasmic granules (Birbeck granules) and adenosine triphosphatase and alpha naphthyl acetate esterase. Surface markers of Langerhans cells include class II major histocompatibility complex antigens (Ia-like) and the CD1 antigen that is also expressed by the cortical (immature) thymocytes (see Chap. 277).

Unifocal Langerhans cell (eosinophilic) granulomatosis is a benign disease of children and young adults, predominantly in males. Occasionally, it occurs as late as 60 to 70 years of age and presents as a solitary osteolytic lesion in the femur, skull, vertebrae, ribs, or occasionally the pelvis. Since there are no consistent accompanying laboratory abnormalities, the diagnosis of unifocal Langerhans cell

granulomatosis requires biopsy of the lytic bone lesion. Treatment of choice of this condition is excision or curettage of the lesion. Rarely, lesions in inaccessible sites such as cervical vertebrae require moderate doses of irradiation [3 to 6 Gy (300 to 600 rad)]. After initial bone scan and radiographic survey to assess extent of disease, follow-up studies should be performed at 6-month intervals for 3 years. If no additional lesions are present 12 months after diagnosis, development of subsequent lesions is unlikely.

Multifocal Langerhans cell (eosinophilic) granulomatosis also usually presents in childhood and is characterized by the development of multiple bony lesions at virtually any site—though less commonly in the feet and hands.

Transient or permanent diabetes insipidus due to granulomatous involvement of the hypothalamus occurs in one-third of patients; 20 percent develop hepatomegaly, 30 percent splenomegaly, and 50 percent have focal or generalized lymph node involvement. Lesions also may involve the skin, vulva, gingiva, lung, and thymus. Laboratory studies are rarely helpful in the diagnosis of multifocal Langerhans cell granulomatosis, necessitating biopsy of lesions. While generally a benign disease, multifocal Langerhans cell granulomatosis is best treated with low to moderate doses of methotrexate, prednisone, or vinblastine, usually with regression of lesions.

Kikuchi's histiocytic necrotizing lymphadenitis was originally described in Japan in 1972 but also has been seen in the United States and Europe. This syndrome occurs most often in young adults and frequently presents with viral upper respiratory tract symptoms and fever. Lymphadenopathy occurs in most cases, with cervical adenopathy the most common site. Histologically, involved nodes show localized proliferation of histiocytes and immunoblasts associated with abundant nuclear debris and tissue necrosis. An increase in CD8 + TCRγδT cells has been reported in necrotizing lymphadenitis lymph nodes. Splenomegaly is also rarely seen in this condition. Although suspected to be caused by an infectious agent, no viral or bacterial etiologic agent has been identified.

EVALUATION OF THE PATIENT WITH LYMPHADENOPATHY

Good physical examination techniques for palpation and assessment of lymph nodes are essential for providing useful information on which diagnostic and therapeutic decisions can be based. For serial evaluation of nodes, the documentation of each node with regard to size, location, consistency, and mobility at each examination is critical. For cervical nodes, the examiner may stand behind or in front of the seated patient to palpate the neck and to examine in sequence the sites of various groups of nodes. Submental nodes are under the chin in the midline and on either side; submandibular nodes are under the jaw near its angle; jugular nodes are along the anterior border of the sternocleidomastoid muscle; supraclavicular nodes are found behind the midportion of the clavicle. Suboccipital nodes are found in the apex of the posterior cervical triangle, and pre- and postauricular nodes are found in front of and behind the ear pinnae, respectively. Central axillary nodes occur near the middle of the thoracic wall of the axilla; lateral axillary nodes are located near the upper part of the humerus along the axillary vein and are best felt by having the patient's arm elevated. Subscapular nodes can be felt under the anterior edge of the latissimus dorsi muscle, and pectoral nodes are beneath the lateral edge of the pectoralis major muscle. Infraclavicular nodes can be felt under the distal end of the clavicle. Epitrochlear nodes are located approximately 3 cm proximal to the medial humeral epicondyle. Palpation of epitrochlear nodes is best accomplished by palpation across the epitrochlear node area in an anterior to posterior direction. Enlarged abdominal lymph nodes can be difficult to palpate and may only be felt if the patient has a shallow abdominal cavity. Pelvic nodes are best evaluated with deep palpation of the lower abdomen by rolling the extended fingers over the pelvic brim.

The investigation of lymphadenopathy can be organized according to where nodes occur and the type of clinical symptoms present. Enlarged supraclavicular nodes most often result from lymphoma or gastrointestinal or intrathoracic tumors and should be biopsied. Acute onset of cervical adenopathy in young adults in the absence of head and neck infections suggests the diagnosis of infectious mononucleosis syndromes. If localized cervical node enlargement persists and serologic evaluation for EB virus, cytomegalovirus, and toxoplasmosis infections as well as chest x-ray and intermediate-strength PPD skin test are negative, then lymph node biopsy is indicated to seek lymphoma, sarcoidosis, carcinoma, and other diseases listed in Table 58-1.

Unilateral cervical adenopathy warrants a careful ear, nose, and throat examination for malignancy. In the asymptomatic patient with persistent new axillary and/or inguinal adenopathy, a biopsy specimen should be obtained. If fever and constitutional symptoms are present, the cause of infectious mononucleosis–like syndromes should be sought prior to node biopsy.

Generalized lymph node enlargement can be caused by systemic infections, drug reactions, malignancy, or one of the systemic lymphadenopathy syndromes (see Table 58-1). History and physical examination can yield clues regarding the possibility of these diagnoses and direct further evaluation (e.g., complete blood count, blood cultures, chest x-ray, serologies, skin tests). If systemic adenopathy persists without an obvious cause being identified, lymph node biopsy is warranted. Once the decision to perform lymph node biopsy has been made, tissue should be processed for culture of appropriate organisms, frozen in liquid nitrogen for lymphocyte typing or other special diagnostic studies for malignant cell types (such as Southern blot analysis of DNA for T cell receptor or immunoglobulin gene clonal rearrangements), and processed for routine pathologic evaluation. One can expect information that will lead to a diagnosis in 50 to 60 percent of lymph node biopsies. About 25 percent of patients with nondiagnostic lymph node biopsies will subsequently develop within a year a disease (usually a lymphoma) related to the indication for biopsy. Therefore, there should be little hesitation to repeat a nondiagnostic biopsy, especially if enlarged lymph nodes and symptoms persist.

The term *atypical hyperplasia of lymph nodes* refers to neither a clinical nor a pathologic entity but designates cases in which the pathologist expresses concern about neoplasia and is unable to unequivocally diagnose lymphoma. Since 30 percent of patients whose lymph node biopsies are read as atypical hyperplasia subsequently develop lymphoma, a repeat biopsy is recommended at a later date if node enlargement persists. Needle aspiration biopsy is a safe technique for initial evaluation of superficial adenopathy. While lymph node aspiration can aid in the diagnosis of metastatic tumor and infections, it is rarely helpful in the diagnosis of lymphomas and other hematologic malignancies.

SPLEEN

SPLEEN STRUCTURE AND FUNCTION   The spleen is a lymphoreticular organ that serves at least four major physiologic functions. First, it is an organ of the immune system and a major site of clearance of microorganisms and particulate antigens from the bloodstream and of generation of humoral or cellular responses to foreign antigens. Second, the spleen is instrumental in sequestration and removal of normal and abnormal blood cells. Third, the vasculature of the spleen plays a role in regulation of portal blood flow. Fourth, while hematopoiesis in the normal adult takes place primarily in the bone marrow, under pathologic conditions when the marrow is replaced or overstimulated to respond, the spleen may become a major site of extramedullary hematopoiesis.

The spleen is arranged into units of areas called *red* and *white pulp* (Fig. 58-2). Red pulp contains blood-filled sinuses and pulp cords lined by reticuloendothelial cells. White pulp contains centrally located arterioles, surrounded by densely packed small lymphocytes, which are primarily CD4 + helper T lymphocytes. Adjacent to the T cell periarteriolar lymphocyte sheath is the follicular zone of B lymphocytes which also contains germinal centers made up of B cells

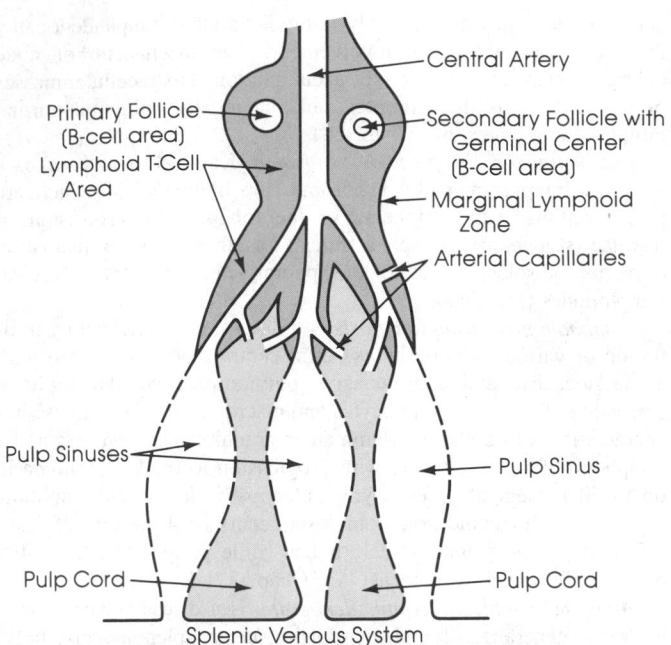

FIGURE 58-2   Schematic spleen structure. The spleen is made up of multiple units of red and white pulp centered around small branches of the splenic artery called central arteries. White pulp areas of spleen are lymphoid areas while red pulp areas include pulp sinuses and pulp cords. In white pulp, B cell areas are primary and secondary follicles and the marginal lymphoid zone, while T cell areas are lymphoid cells around follicles and arterial capillaries. (*Redrawn with permission from Videbaek et al.*)

and macrophages. The outermost portion of white pulp is another B cell layer called the *marginal zone* which blends into red pulp areas.

The blood supply and the route of blood flow are unique in the spleen, and splenic anatomy can best be defined in terms of route of blood flow (see Fig. 58-2). Blood enters the spleen by the splenic artery. The splenic artery divides into branches which penetrate into the spleen via connective tissue projections called *trabeculae* and from the trabeculae branch into smaller arteries called *central arteries*. From central arteries the bloodstream reaches the arterial capillaries. The periarteriolar lymphoid sheaths of T cells surrounding B cell follicles persist around the arterial vessels until they become small arterioles. Blood in central arterioles empties partly through arterial capillaries directly into splenic venules and then into splenic veins. The central arterioles also empty into macrophage-lined sinuses of red pulp and into the fibrous network of reticuloendothelial cells and tissue macrophages called *pulp cords*. Blood in red pulp sinuses and pulp cords empties directly into the splenic venous system. During red blood cell passage from central arteries to pulp cords, and finally to spleen sinuses, red cells are concentrated in the macrophage-rich pulp cords. Normally circulating red cells accumulate in pulp cords with subsequent passage through critical small openings of sinus endothelium into red pulp sinuses and on to the splenic venous system. Packing of red cells in pulp cords with subsequent passage through small slits into sinuses is termed *erythrocyte conditioning*. Upon senescence, red cells become less deformable and are unable to pass into sinuses; they are retained in pulp cords and phagocytosed by macrophages—a process termed *culling*. Erythrocyte particulate matter such as nuclear material (Howell-Jolly bodies), denatured hemoglobin (Heinz bodies), or malaria parasites can be pinched off during passage of red cells from pulp cords into sinuses and retained in the spleen while the rest of the red cell passes back into the circulation—a process termed *pitting*.

Many of the mechanisms of spleen enlargement are exaggerated forms of normal spleen function. While a wide variety of diseases are associated with enlargement of the spleen, there are six basic pathophysiologic mechanisms of splenic enlargement. (1) Splenic enlargement occurs from reticuloendothelial or immune system hyperplasia in infectious diseases such as bacterial endocarditis or in immune diseases such as Felty's syndrome. Reticuloendothelial hyperplasia also occurs in diseases associated with destruction of abnormal red blood cells such as hereditary spherocytosis, thalassemia, or early in the course of sickle cell disease. (2) Splenic enlargement occurs due to altered splenic blood flow in hepatic cirrhosis or splenic, hepatic, or portal vein thrombosis. (3) Malignant neoplasms can involve the spleen either primarily, as with lymphomas or angiosarcomas, or secondarily, as with leukemias or metastatic solid tumors. (4) Splenic enlargement can occur in situations leading to extramedullary hematopoiesis in the spleen, such as in myeloid metaplasia or other myelophthisic syndromes. (5) Infiltration of the spleen with abnormal material in amyloidosis and Gaucher's disease can result in splenomegaly. (6) Splenomegaly also can result from space-occupying lesions such as hemangiomas and cysts.

DISEASES ASSOCIATED WITH SPLENIC ENLARGEMENT A wide variety of diseases lead to an increase in cellularity and vascularity of the spleen (Table 58-2). Increase in cellularity in infections is due to lymphocyte and macrophage proliferation in both red and white pulp areas. Splenomegaly is often present in acute systemic bacterial infections. Infectious granulomas due to mycobacterial and fungal infections occur in both red and white pulp. In diseases associated with disordered immunoregulation such as rheumatoid arthritis and systemic lupus erythematosus, splenic enlargement is often due to lymphoid hyperplasia, with enlarged lymphoid follicles present in white pulp areas and increased numbers of plasma cells and macrophages around red pulp arterioles and pulp cords. Splenic enlargement associated with abnormal splenic blood flow is most commonly due to chronic passive congestion from increased portal vein pressure or from portal vein obstruction. *Banti's syndrome* is *congestive splenomegaly* with hypersplenism associated with cirrhosis and portal hypertension and is manifested histologically by red pulp congestion with accumulation and concentration of erythrocytes in widened pulp cords and sinuses. In congestive splenomegaly, reticuloendothelial hyperplasia occurs with proliferation of cells lining red pulp cords and sinuses. In splenic enlargement in conditions associated with abnormal erythrocytes such as hereditary spherocytosis, there is pooling of abnormal red cells in sinuses and pulp cords because of increased red cell rigidity and therefore decreased ability to traverse the red pulp sinusoidal endothelium.

Myelosclerosis with myeloid metaplasia is characterized by splenic intrasinusoidal extramedullary hematopoiesis involving all three myeloid cell lines associated with dilated and distended pulp sinuses. In cases of secondary extramedullary hematopoiesis such as in myelophthisic syndromes, extramedullary hematopoiesis may only involve one or two cell lineages, particularly red cells. Infiltrative malignant disease can cause focal or generalized increases in white pulp lymphoid cells, as in the case of Hodgkin's disease and lymphocytic lymphoma, or infiltration of red pulp areas with malignant cells, as in chronic granulocytic leukemia, acute leukemia syndromes, systemic mast cell disease, and metastatic carcinoma. Infiltrative diseases of the spleen such as Gaucher's and Niemann-Pick produce splenic enlargement by increasing the number of splenic red pulp histiocytes. Thyrotoxicosis can be associated with splenomegaly and is due to thyroid hormone–induced lymphoid hyperplasia. Sarcoidosis causes splenic enlargement by the development of areas of granulomatous inflammation in white pulp lymphoid tissue. A splenic artery aneurysm may cause unexplained splenomegaly, cramping, and left upper abdominal pain; a calcified ring in the splenic area may be seen on x-ray.

The degree of splenomegaly varies with the disease entity. Slight or mild enlargement occurs in chronic passive congestion of the liver due to congestive heart failure, acute malaria, typhoid fever, bacterial endocarditis, systemic lupus erythematosus, rheumatoid arthritis, and thalassemia minor. Moderate splenic enlargement occurs in hepatitis, cirrhosis, lymphomas, infectious mononucleosis, hemolytic anemias, splenic abscesses and infarcts, and amyloidosis. Massive enlargement of the spleen occurs in chronic myelocytic leukemia, agnogenic myeloid metaplasia with myelofibrosis, hairy cell leukemia, Gaucher's and Niemann-Pick diseases, sarcoidosis, thalassemia major, chronic malaria, congenital syphilis, leishmaniasis, and in some cases of portal vein obstruction.

DIAGNOSTIC EVALUATION OF THE PATIENT WITH SPLENIC ENLARGEMENT When normal in size and position, the spleen is generally inaccessible to abdominal palpation. A normal-sized spleen is about 12 cm long, 7 cm wide, and 250 cm^3. Because of the oblique orientation of the spleen to the abdominal cavity, its long axis lies behind and parallel to the tenth rib in the midaxillary line, with splenic width located between the ninth and eleventh ribs. Palpation of the left upper quadrant is performed with the patient supine or on the right side by the examiner's right hand; the examiner's left hand is placed under the lower thorax, grasping the lower ribs posteriorly. Palpation for spleen enlargement is performed with the patient taking deep breaths to permit the examiner to feel the inferior tip of an enlarged spleen. To avoid missing a massively enlarged spleen, palpation of the left upper quadrant should begin in the lower abdominal cavity with gradual movement up to the left upper quadrant.

Demonstration of mild to moderate splenic enlargement by physical examination may be difficult, particularly in obese patients. Other techniques for assessment of spleen size include ^{99}Tc-colloid liver-spleen scan, computed tomography, and ultrasound scanning of the left upper quadrant. These three techniques can be useful in defining

---

TABLE 58-2 Diseases associated with enlargement of the spleen

Infections
 A Infectious mononucleosis
 B Bacterial septicemias
 C Bacterial endocarditis
 D Tuberculosis
 E Malaria
 F Leishmaniasis
 G Trypanosomiasis
 H AIDS
 I Viral hepatitis
 J Congenital syphilis
 K Splenic abscess
 L Disseminated histoplasmosis

Diseases of disordered immunoregulation
 A Rheumatoid arthritis (Felty's syndrome)
 B Systemic lupus erythematosus
 C Immune hemolytic anemias
 D Angioimmunoblastic lymphadenopathy
 E Drug reactions with serum sickness syndromes
 F Immune thrombocytopenias and neutropenias

Diseases of disordered splenic blood flow
 A Laennec's and postnecrotic cirrhosis
 B Hepatic vein obstruction
 C Hepatic schistosomiasis
 D Portal vein obstruction or cavernous sinus transformation
 E Splenic vein obstruction
 F Chronic congestive heart failure
 G Splenic artery aneurysm

Diseases associated with abnormal erythrocytes
 A Spherocytosis
 B Sickle cell disease
 C Ovalocytosis
 D Thalassemia

Infiltrative diseases of the spleen
 A Benign—amyloidosis, Gaucher's disease, Niemann-Pick disease, Hurler's syndrome, Tangier disease, multifocal Langerhans cell (eosinophilic) granulomatosis, extramedullary hematopoiesis, hamartomas, fibromas, hemangiomas, lymphangiomas, splenic cysts
 B Malignant—leukemias, lymphomas, Hodgkin's lymphoma, primary splenic tumors, angiosarcomas, metastatic tumors, myeloproliferative syndromes

Miscellaneous diseases or diseases of unknown cause
 A Idiopathic splenomegaly
 B Thyrotoxicosis
 C Iron-deficiency anemia
 D Sarcoidosis
 E Berylliosis
 F Kikuchi's histiocytic necrotizing lymphadenitis

splenic defects such as cysts, infarct, or tumors or in defining accessory splenic tissue that may be due to congenital accessory spleens or residual foci of splenic tissue following splenic rupture (splenosis). One study has documented palpable spleens in 3 percent of entering college freshmen and no increased risk of any disease during the ensuing 6 years.

In evaluation of the patient with splenomegaly, it is helpful to consider splenomegaly with acute or subacute illnesses separately from splenomegaly with chronic illness. Acute left upper quadrant pain with an enlarged tender spleen suggests subcapsular hematoma, splenic rupture, or splenic infarcts. Rupture of the spleen with splenic hematoma most often follows direct or remote trauma but can occur as well in the setting of infectious diseases such as malaria, typhoid fever, and EB virus–induced infectious mononucleosis. Splenic infarcts due either to in situ red cell sickling (in sickle cell disease) or to emboli (from mural thrombus, atrial myxoma, or cardiac valve vegetation) can usually be detected by spleen scan or arteriogram. More unusual disorders presenting acutely are diffuse splenic metastatic disease and hemorrhage into a splenic cyst.

An acute febrile illness associated with splenomegaly may be due to bacterial endocarditis, infectious mononucleosis syndromes, tuberculosis, and histoplasmosis. Fever, peripheral adenopathy, and splenomegaly, with or without a rash or arthralgias, should suggest (in addition to infectious mononucleosis) sarcoidosis, Hodgkin's lymphoma, a collagen vascular disease such as systemic lupus erythematosus, or a serum sickness syndrome.

An acute illness with splenomegaly associated with the signs and symptoms of anemia, with or without bleeding, suggests autoimmune hemolytic anemia, myeloproliferative syndromes, or acute leukemia.

Splenomegaly with signs and symptoms of chronic illness suggests a wide range of disorders, many of which are listed in Table 58-2. Liver disease with portal hypertension is a common etiology of splenomegaly in this setting. Patients with congestive splenomegaly from liver disease or portal or splenic vein thrombosis are often asymptomatic. With clinical features of rheumatoid arthritis and leukopenia, Felty's syndrome should be considered. The presence of lymphadenopathy should suggest chronic lymphocytic leukemia or lymphoma. Plethora and an elevated hematocrit suggest polycythemia vera or chronic lung disease, with right-sided heart failure and congestive splenomegaly. Weight loss or other signs of chronic illness suggest leukemia or other myeloproliferative syndromes, as well as a variety of hemoglobinopathies. Bone marrow aspiration and biopsy can aid in the diagnosis of leukemia and lymphoma, lipid storage diseases, disseminated fungal or mycobacterial diseases, metastatic malignant diseases, and amyloidosis.

Occasionally, laparotomy and splenectomy are indicated in the evaluation of splenomegaly. The decision to perform diagnostic laparotomy in a patient with unexplained splenomegaly is difficult and must take into account the patient's age and clinical signs, symptoms, and laboratory abnormalities present. Palpation of moderately enlarged spleens (750 to 800 cm³) has been reported to miss up to 44 percent of spleens shown to be enlarged on radionuclide scan. In contrast, 97 percent of spleens are palpable when they reach three times normal size (900 cm³). In a study of older subjects (average age 49) who had undergone splenectomy for undiagnosed splenomegaly and had signs and symptoms of chronic illness, a diagnosis of an underlying disorder was obtained in the majority of patients by splenectomy.

HYPERSPLENISM   The term *hypersplenism* applies to any clinical situation in which the spleen removes excessive quantities of erythrocytes, granulocytes, or platelets from the circulation. General mechanisms of removal of formed blood elements include increased sequestration of cells due to hemodynamic abnormalities of splenic blood flow or production of anti–red cell, granulocyte, or platelet antibodies, making the cells vulnerable to clearance by splenic macrophages. Situations in which passive congestion of the spleen occurs produce abnormal sludging of blood in sinuses and red pulp cords. Under these conditions, there is plasma pooling, producing

marked intrasplenic hemoconcentration and hypoxia and making blood cells more vulnerable to the phagocytic action of pulp cord macrophages. Criteria for diagnosis of hypersplenism include (1) splenomegaly, (2) splenic destruction of one or more cell lines in the peripheral blood, (3) normal or hyperplastic cellularity of bone marrow with normal representation of the cell line deficient in the circulation, and (4) variably, evidence of increased cell turnover in the cell lines affected (i.e., reticulocytosis), increased band forms of neutrophils, or circulating immature platelet forms.

Therapy for hypersplenism relates in large part to the underlying disease or the underlying pathophysiologic process. If the underlying disorder responsible for hypersplenism cannot be corrected, splenectomy is an option for cases in which a severe deficit is present (see below for indications for splenectomy).

HYPOSPLENISM   The terms *hyposplenia* and *asplenia* are used to indicate diminished or absent splenic function, respectively. The usual causes of hyposplenism are splenectomy, congenital absence of the spleen, sickle cell anemia in patients older than 5 years (with autosplenectomy due to repeated infarcts), and splenic irradiation (Table 58-3). In sickle cell anemia, persistence of a palpable spleen after age 5 suggests coexisting α thalassemia. Findings in the peripheral blood that indicate diminished splenic function include the presence of nucleated red cells, erythrocyte Howell-Jolly bodies, erythrocyte Heinz bodies, basophilic stippling, as well as target and burr forms of red cells, and rarely, circulating nucleated red blood cells.

Splenectomized patients or patients with functional asplenia (such as in sickle cell disease) are prone to bacterial infections, which are frequently overwhelming and life-threatening, particularly with encapsulated organisms such as *Streptococcus pneumoniae*, *Neisseria meningitidis*, *Escherichia coli*, and *Haemophilus influenzae*. The overall risk of bacterial sepsis in splenectomized patients has been estimated to be approximately 7 percent over a 10-year period. In addition, patients with hyposplenia are susceptible to infections with the parasite *Babesia*, which causes the parasitic disease *babesiosis*. This is due to a reduction or absence of the filtration function of the spleen for clearance of antibody-coated bacteria as well as to decreased production of IgG and IgM antibodies (opsonins) needed to bind bacteria. Immunization with 23-valent pneumococcal vaccine is recommended in patients older than 2 years with hyposplenism and prior to elective splenectomy. The presence of peripheral blood manifestations of hyposplenism in a normal-sized or enlarged spleen suggests splenic infiltrative disease such as a primary splenic angiosarcoma.

TABLE 58-3   Causes of functional and anatomical hyposplenism

1 Congenital hyposplenism—Fanconi's syndrome
2 Surgical splenectomy
3 Hyposplenism of old age
4 Hyposplenism due to splenic congestion—sickle hemoglobinopathies, myeloproliferative disorders such as essential thrombocytosis and myelofibrosis
5 Hyposplenism due to impaired vascular supply to the spleen
6 Immunologic or autoimmune disorders—systemic lupus erythematosus, rheumatoid arthritis, systemic necrotizing vasculitis syndromes, sarcoidosis, bone marrow transplantation complicated by graft-versus-host disease, IgA deficiency, thyroiditis, and thyrotoxicosis
7 Gastrointestinal diseases—celiac disease, dermatitis herpetiformis, ulcerative colitis, regional enteritis, intestinal lymphangiectasia, chronic active hepatitis
8 Malignancies—Sézary syndrome, multiple myeloma, gastric carcinoma, breast carcinoma, primary splenic angiosarcoma, non-Hodgkins lymphoma, splenic irradiation, Thorotrast therapy
9 Miscellaneous—systemic amyloidosis, drug-induced (IV gamma globulin, methyldopa, glucocorticoids), nephrotic syndrome, splenosis following splenectomy or splenic trauma, malignant mastocytosis, disseminated varicella

SOURCE: *C Pochedly et al (eds)*.

INDICATIONS FOR SPLENECTOMY Splenic trauma, whether accidental blunt trauma or intraoperative iatrogenic injury, is the most common indication for splenectomy. En bloc removal of the spleen may be indicated either because of tumor involvement or for a splenorenal shunt. Staging laparotomy with splenectomy remains a major diagnostic procedure for many early stage Hodgkin's disease patients being considered for radiation therapy alone. Splenectomy for selected patients with idiopathic splenomegaly is often necessary when other investigations fail to produce a diagnosis; however, the spleen should not be removed simply because it is palpable. Hypersplenism in lymphomas can cause persistent cytopenias and in select cases responds to splenectomy. B cell hairy cell leukemia frequently presents with hypersplenism, and in those patients who fail medical treatments, splenectomy is beneficial.

Felty's syndrome (rheumatoid arthritis and hypersplenism) and Gaucher's disease both require splenectomy when splenomegaly leads to symptomatic neutropenia or other complications of hypersplenism. Immune thrombocytopenic purpura which persists after trials of medical therapy may benefit from splenectomy (see Chap. 314). Of the hemolytic anemias, hereditary spherocytosis, hereditary elliptocytosis, immune hemolytic anemia with warm-reacting IgG antibody, and pyruvate kinase deficiency have been improved by splenectomy. Splenectomy is usually necessary late in the course of thalassemia major when neutropenia or thrombocytopenia develops or when transfusion requirements double. Chronic lymphocytic leukemia (CLL), chronic granulocytic leukemia, and agnogenic myeloid metaplasia may be complicated by symptomatic hypersplenism or, in the case of CLL, immune hemolytic anemia and thrombocytopenia, often necessitating splenectomy (Chaps. 309 and 310.)

REFERENCES

Lymph node enlargement

BUTCHER E, WEISSMAN I: Lymphoid tissues and organs in *Fundamental Immunology*, WE Paul (ed). New York, Raven, 1984, pp 109–127

GREENFIELD S, JORDAN MC: The clinical investigation of lymphadenopathy, in primary care practice. JAMA 240:1388, 1978

IOACHIM HL: *Lymph Node Biopsy*. Philadelphia, Lippincott, 1982

LENNERT K, STEIN H: The germinal center, in *Morphology, Histochemistry, and Immunohistology in Lymphoproliferative Diseases of Skin*, M Goos, E Christopher (eds). Berlin, Heidelberg, New York, Springer-Verlag, 1982

LIEBERMAN PH et al: A reappraisal of eosinophilic granuloma of bone, Hand-Schüller-Christian syndrome, and Letterer-Siwe syndrome. Medicine 48:375, 1969

NATHWANI BN et al: Malignant lymphoma arising in angioimmunoblastic lymphadenopathy. Cancer 41:578, 1978

POPPEMA S et al: Distribution of T cell subsets in human lymph nodes. J Exp Med 153:30, 1981

SCHROER KR, FRANSSILA KO: Atypical hyperplasia of lymph nodes: A follow-up study. Cancer 44:1155, 1979

SINCLAIR S et al: Biopsy of enlarged, superficial lymph nodes. JAMA 228:602, 1974

THOMAS JA et al: Combined immunological and histochemical analysis of skin and lymph node lesions in histiocytosis X. J Clin Pathol 35:327, 1982

WINTERBAUER RH et al: A clinical interpretation of bilateral hilar adenopathy. Ann Intern Med 78:65, 1973

YEN-TSU N et al: Lymph node biopsy for diagnosis: A statistical study. J Surg Oncol 14:53, 1980

Splenic enlargement

BUTLER JJ: Pathology of the spleen in benign and malignant conditions. Histopathology 7:453, 1983

EICHNER ER, WHITFIELD CL: Splenomegaly: An algorithmic approach to diagnosis. JAMA 246:2858, 1981

ENRIQUEZ E, NEIMAN RS (eds): *The Pathology of the Spleen: A Functional Approach*. Chicago, American Society of Clinical Pathologists, 1976

HERMANN RE et al: Splenectomy for the diagnosis of splenomegaly. Ann Surg 168:896, 1964

LEWIS SM (ed): *Clinics in Haematology*, vol 12: *The Spleen*. London, Saunders, 1983, pp 361–608

McINTYRE OR, EBAUGH FG: Palpable spleens in college freshmen. Ann Intern Med 66:301, 1967

POCHEDLY C et al (eds): *Disorders of the Spleen: Pathophysiology and Management*. New York, Marcel Dekker, 1989

STEINBERG MH et al: Evidence of hyposplenism in the presence of splenomegaly. Scand J Haematol 31:437, 1983

VIDEBAEK A et al: *The Spleen in Health and Disease*. Chicago, Yearbook, 1982

ZHANGE B, LEWIS SM: A study of the reliability of clinical palpation of the spleen. Clin Lab Haematol 11:7, 1989

59 QUANTITATIVE AND QUALITATIVE DISORDERS OF PHAGOCYTES

JOHN I. GALLIN

Leukocytes are the major cellular components of inflammatory and immune responses and include neutrophils, T and B lymphocytes, monocytes, eosinophils, and basophils. These cells have been assigned specific functions, such as antibody production by B lymphocytes or destruction of bacteria by neutrophils, but in no single infectious disease is the exact role of each of the cell types completely established. Thus, whereas neutrophils are classically thought to be critical to host defense against bacteria, there is increasing evidence that neutrophils play important roles in viral infections.

The blood is the most readily obtainable source of leukocytes and serves as the vehicle for their delivery to the various tissues from the bone marrow, where they are produced. Normal blood leukocyte counts for adults are given in Table 59-1 and those for different ages in the Appendix. The various leukocytes are thought to derive from a common stem cell in the bone marrow. Three-fourths of the nucleated cells of bone marrow are committed to the production of leukocytes. Leukocyte maturation in the marrow is under the regulatory control of a number of different factors, known as colony stimulating factors and interleukins. Because an alteration in the number and type of leukocytes is a frequent association with disease processes, a total white blood count (WBC) (cells per microliter) and differential counts are obtained frequently. The lymphocytes and basophils are discussed elsewhere. This chapter focuses on the neutrophils, monocytes, and eosinophils.

NEUTROPHILS

MATURATION Important events in the neutrophil life are summarized in Fig. 59-1. In normal humans, neutrophils are only produced in the bone marrow. Best estimates indicate that the appropriate number of stem cells necessary to support hematopoiesis is between 400 and 500. There is convincing evidence that human blood monocytes and tissue macrophages produce colony stimulating factors, hormones required for the growth of monocytes and neutrophils in the bone marrow. The hematopoietic system not only produces enough neutrophils (approximately 1.3×10^{11} cells per 80-kg person per day) to carry out physiologic functions but also has a large reserve stored in the marrow which can be mobilized in response to inflammation or infection. An increase in the number of blood neutrophils is called *neutrophilia*, and the presence of immature cells is termed a "shift to the left." A diminution in the number of blood neutrophils is referred to as *neutropenia*.

Neutrophils evolve from pluripotent stem cells (Fig. 59-2). Proliferation of the earliest pluripotent stem cells appears to be augmented

TABLE 59-1 Normal values for concentration of blood leukocytes*

Cell type	Mean, cells per microliter	95% Confidence limits, cells per microliter
Neutrophil	3650	1830–7250
Lymphocyte	2500	1500–4000
Monocyte	430	200–950
Eosinophil	150	0–700
Basophil	30	0–150

* Total leukocyte counts from venous blood samples were done in a Coulter counter, and 200 leukocytes were differentiated on Wright-stained blood smears made on coverglass. (From DC Dale, in JD Wilson et al, eds, *Harrison's Principles of Internal Medicine*, 12th ed, Chap 64.)

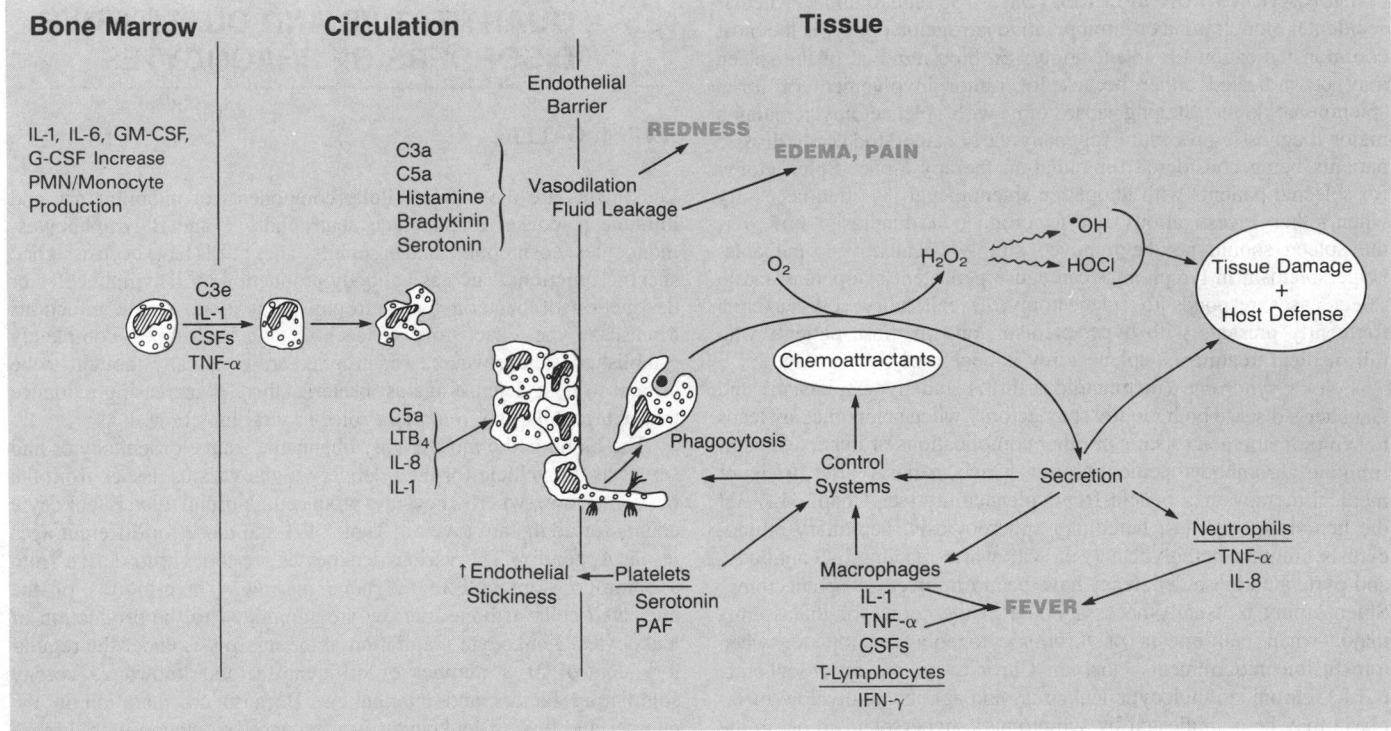

FIGURE 59-1 Events in inflammation. The four basic symptoms of inflammation are indicated by bold print.

by a multipotent growth factor (mgf). Interleukin 6 (IL-6) has no effect alone at this stage but synergistically augments the effect of mgf. As a consequence, the pluripotent stem cell is driven toward lymphocyte progenitors and toward granulocytes, erythrocytes, monocytes, megakaryocytes (GEMM), and mast cells. A multipotential colony stimulating factor known as interleukin 3 (IL-3) enhances proliferation toward erythrocytes, megakaryocytes, and mast cells, and interleukin 1 (IL-1) enhances proliferation at a later stage. Granulocyte-macrophage colony stimulating factor (GM-CSF) appears to act only on monomyeloid precursors. Granulocyte colony stimulating factor (G-CSF) is highly specific and influences neutrophil precursors only. By the myeloblast stage, cells under the influence of G-CSF enter the committed differentiation phase of development. The final stages of neutrophil development are characterized by the appearance of cells with distinct morphologic features. The myeloblast is the first recognizable precursor cell and is followed by the *promyelocyte* (see Fig. A9-15). The promyelocyte evolves when the classic lysosomal granules, called the *primary* or *azurophil granules*, are produced. The primary granules contain hydrolases, elastase, myeloperoxidase, cationic proteins, and bactericidal/permeability-increasing protein (BPI) important for killing gram-negative bacteria. Azurophil granules also contain *defensins*, a family of cystine-rich polypeptides with broad antimicrobial activity against bacteria, fungi, and certain enveloped viruses. The promyelocyte divides to produce the *myelocyte*, a cell responsible for the synthesis of the *specific* or *secondary granules* which contain unique (specific) constituents such as lactoferrin, vitamin B_{12}–binding proteins, membrane components of the NADPH oxidase required for hydrogen peroxide production, histaminase, and receptors for certain chemoattractants and adherence-promoting factors (CR3) as well as receptors for the connective tissue element laminin. The secondary granules do not contain acid hydrolases and therefore are not classic lysosomes. They are readily released extracellularly, and their mobilization is probably important in modulating inflammation. During the final stages of maturation there is no cell division, and the cell passes through the *metamyelocyte* stage and then to the *band* neutrophil with a sausage-shaped nucleus (see Fig. A9-17). As the band cell matures, the nucleus assumes a lobulated configuration. The nucleus of neutrophils normally contains

up to four segments. Excessive segmentation (greater than five nuclear lobes) may be a manifestation of folate or vitamin B_{12} deficiency. The Pelger-Hüet anomaly (see Fig. A9-19*B*), an infrequent dominant benign inherited trait, results in neutrophils with distinctive bilobed nuclei that must be distinguished from band forms. The physiologic role of the multilobed nucleus of neutrophils is unknown, but it may allow great deformation of neutrophils during migration into tissues at sites of inflammation.

In settings of severe acute bacterial infection, prominent neutrophil cytoplasmic granules called *toxic granulations* are occasionally seen (see Fig. A9-16). Toxic granulations are thought to be immature or abnormally staining azurophil granules. Cytoplasmic inclusions, also called *Doehle bodies* (see Fig. A9-17), can be seen during infection and probably represent fragments of ribosome-rich endoplasmic reticulum. Large neutrophil vacuoles are often present in acute bacterial infection and probably represent pinocytosed (internalized) membrane.

Neutrophils have long been thought to be a homogeneous population of cells. However, studies of neutrophil function have suggested that they are heterogeneous. Recently, monoclonal antibodies have been developed that recognize only a subset of mature neutrophils. The meaning of neutrophil heterogeneity is not known.

MARROW RELEASE AND CIRCULATING COMPARTMENTS
Specific signals, including interleukin 1, tumor necrosis factor-α, the colony stimulating factors, the complement fragment C3e, and perhaps other cytokines mobilize leukocytes from the bone marrow and deliver them to the blood in an unstimulated state. Under normal conditions, about 90 percent of the neutrophil pool is in the bone marrow, 2 to 3 percent in the circulation, and the remainder in the tissues. The blood pool exists as two compartments. The marginated pool is adherent to endothelial cells in capillary beds (especially in lung and spleen) and comprises about 50 percent of blood leukocytes. The freely flowing circulating pool makes up the remainder of blood leukocytes. In response to chemotactic stimuli from tissues (e.g., the complement product C5a, the arachidonic acid derivative leukotriene B_4, the cytokine interleukin 8, or the bacterial product *N*-formylmethionylleucylphenylalanine), neutrophil adhesiveness increases, and the circulating cells aggregate to each other and adhere to the endothelium.

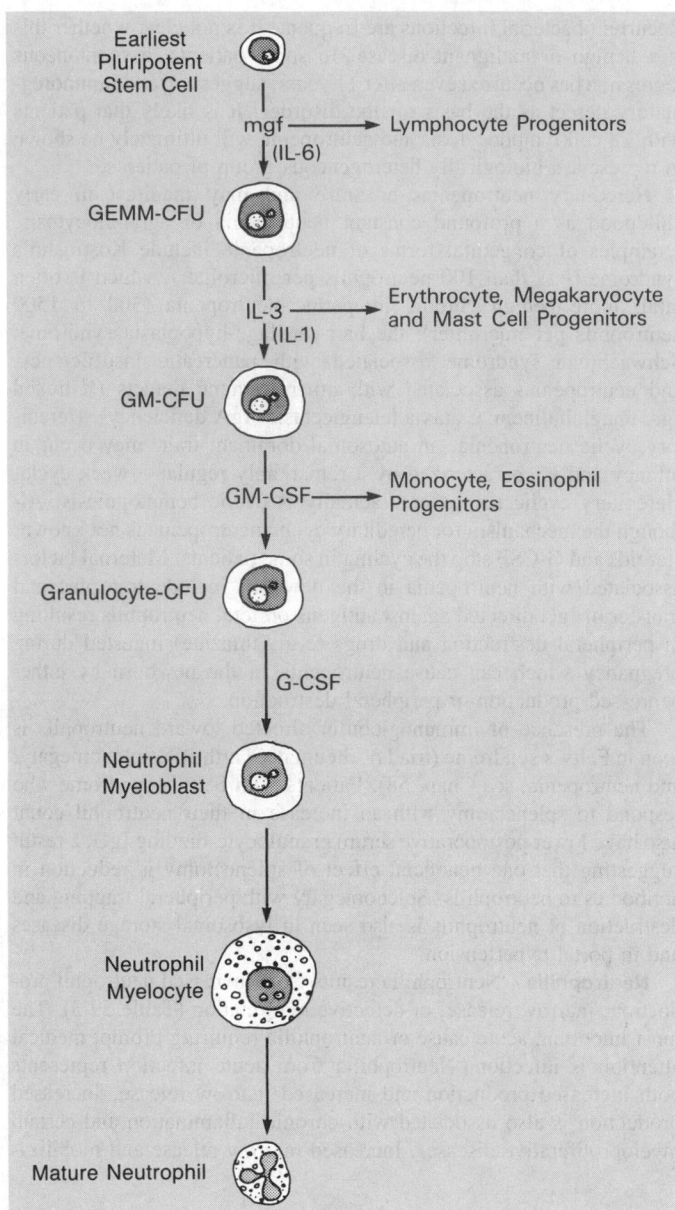

FIGURE 59-2   Regulation of myelopoiesis by growth factors (mgf, multipotent growth factor; IL, interleukin; GEMM, granulocyte, erythrocyte, monocyte, megakaryocyte; CFU, colony forming unit; CSF, colony stimulating factor; GM, granulocyte-macrophage; G, granulocyte).

An increased expression of the adhesion glycoprotein receptors called *integrins* [i.e., C3bi (also called CR3), LFA-1] on phagocytes is intimately involved with the increased adhesion. In addition, a novel family of adhesion molecules, called *selectins*, utilizes protein-carbohydrate interactions for specific cell-cell binding between leukocytes and endothelial cells. Receptors for chemoattractants and opsonins are also mobilized; the phagocytes orient toward the chemoattractant source in the extravascular space, increase their motile activity (chemokinesis), and migrate with direction (chemotaxis) into tissues. The biochemistry and cell biology of these processes are rapidly unfolding (see "References"). The process of migration into tissues is called *diapedesis* and involves the crawling of neutrophils between postcapillary endothelial cells which open junctions between adjacent cells to permit leukocyte passage. The endothelial responses (increased blood flow secondary to increased vasodilation and permeability) are mediated by anaphylatoxins (e.g., complement products C3a and C5a) as well as vasodilators such as histamine, bradykinin, serotonin, and prostaglandins E and I. In the healthy adult, most

neutrophils leave the body by migration through the mucous membrane of the gastrointestinal tract. Normally, neutrophils spend a relatively short time in the circulation, with a half-life of 6 to 7 h. Senescent neutrophils are cleared from the circulation by macrophages in the lung and spleen. Once in the tissues, neutrophils release enzymes such as collagenase and elastase, which may help establish abscess cavities. Neutrophils ingest (phagocytose) pathogenic materials that have been properly altered (opsonized) by substances such as immunoglobulin G (IgG) and the complement product C3b. Fibronectin and the tetrapeptide tuftsin facilitate the phagocytic process.

Concomitant with phagocytosis there is a burst of oxygen consumption and activation of the hexose-monophosphate shunt. A membrane-associated nicotinamide-adenine dinucleotide phosphate (NADPH) oxidase, consisting of membrane and cytosolic components, is assembled and catalyzes the reduction of oxygen to superoxide anion, which is then converted to hydrogen peroxide and other toxic oxygen products (e.g., hydrogen peroxide and hydroxyl radical). Hydrogen peroxide + chloride + neutrophil myeloperoxidase provide a particularly toxic system that generates hypochlorous acid, hypochlorite, and chlorine. These products oxidize and halogenate microorganisms and tumor cells and, when uncontrolled, can damage host tissue. Strongly cationic proteins and defensins also participate in microbial killing. Other enzymes, such as lysozyme and acid proteases, help digest microbial debris. After 1 to 4 days in tissues neutrophils die. Under certain conditions, such as in delayed-type hypersensitivity immunity, monocyte accumulation occurs within 6 to 12 h of initiation of inflammation. Neutrophils, monocytes, microorganisms in various states of digestion, and altered local tissue cells make up pus, which derives its characteristic green color from myeloperoxidase. Myeloperoxidase and other factors may be important in turning off the inflammatory process by inactivating chemoattractants and immobilizing phagocytic cells.

NEUTROPHIL DYSFUNCTION   A defect anywhere in the neutrophil life cycle (summarized in Fig. 59-1) can lead to dysfunction and compromised host defenses. Inflammation is often depressed, and the clinical result is often recurrent and severe bacterial and fungal infections creating novel and often difficult management problems. Diagnosis of phagocytic cell disorders is suggested by clinical evaluation. Aphthous ulcers of mucous membranes (gray ulcers without pus) and gingivitis and periodontal disease are common. Patients with congenital phagocyte defects can have infections within the first few days of life. Skin, ear, upper and lower respiratory tract, and bone infections are common. Sepsis and meningitis are rare. In some disorders the frequency of infection is variable, and patients can go for months or even years without major infection. In the past it was unusual for persons with congenital defects to live beyond the age of 30 years. However, aggressive management of these diseases has extended the life span of patients.

Neutropenia   The consequences of absent neutrophils are a dramatic demonstration of their importance in host defense. A large body of clinical data indicates that susceptibility to infectious diseases increases sharply when neutrophil levels fall below 1000 cells per microliter; when there are fewer than 200 cells per microliter, the inflammatory process is absent. The causes of neutropenia are multiple and are related to depressed production, peripheral destruction, and peripheral pooling. A falling neutrophil count or a significant decrease in neutrophils below steady state levels, together with a failure to increase neutrophil counts in the setting of infection or other challenge to the bone marrow reserve, requires investigation. Such acute neutropenia is more likely to be associated with increased risk of infection than neutropenia of long duration (months to years) that has a reversal in response to infection or carefully controlled administration of endotoxin (see "Laboratory Diagnosis," below).

Some causes of inherited and acquired neutropenia are listed in Table 59-2. The most common neutropenias are iatrogenic, resulting from the widespread use of cytotoxic or immunosuppressive therapies for malignancy or control of autoimmune disorders. These drugs cause neutropenia because they are toxic and result in decreased

TABLE 59-2 Causes of neutropenia

DECREASED PRODUCTION

Drug-induced—alkylating agents (nitrogen mustard, busulfan, chlorambucil, cyclophosphamide); antimetabolites (methotrexate, 6-mercaptopurine, 5-flurocytosine); noncytotoxic agents [antibiotics (chloramphenicol, penicillins, sulfonamides), phenothiazines, tranquilizers (meprobamate), certain diuretics, anti-inflammatory agents, antithyroid drugs, many others]
Hematologic diseases—idiopathic, cyclic neutropenia, Chédiak-Higashi syndrome, aplastic anemia, infantile genetic disorders (see text)
Tumor invasion, myelofibrosis
Nutritional deficiency—vitamin B$_{12}$, folate (especially alcoholics)
Infection—tuberculosis, typhoid fever, brucellosis, tularemia, measles, infectious mononucleosis, malaria, viral hepatitis, leishmaniasis, AIDS

PERIPHERAL DESTRUCTION

Antineutrophil antibodies and/or splenic or lung (alveolar macrophage) trapping
Autoimmune disorders—Felty's syndrome, rheumatoid arthritis, lupus erythematosus
Drugs as haptens—aminopyrine, α-methyl dopa, phenylbutazone, mercurial diuretics, some phenothiazines
Wegener's granulomatosis

PERIPHERAL POOLING (TRANSIENT NEUTROPENIA)

Overwhelming bacterial infection (acute endotoxemia)
Hemodialysis
Cardiopulmonary bypass

---

production of rapidly growing progenitor (stem) cells of the marrow. Cytotoxic chemotherapeutic agents fall into this category, but certain antibiotics such as chloramphenicol, trimethoprim-sulfamethoxazole, 5-flurocytosine, adenine arabinoside, and the antiretroviral drug zidovudine may cause neutropenia by inhibiting proliferation of myeloid precursors. The marrow suppression is generally dose-related and dependent on continued administration of the drug. Recombinant human G-CSF is an important drug for reversing this form of neutropenia and is particularly useful in cancer chemotherapy.

Another important mechanism for iatrogenically induced neutropenia is the effect of drugs that serve as immune haptens and sensitize neutrophils or neutrophil precursors to immune-mediated peripheral destruction. This form of drug-induced neutropenia can be seen within 7 days of exposure to the drug; with previous drug exposure, neutropenia may occur a few hours after administration of the drug. Although any drug can cause this form of neutropenia, the most frequent causes are commonly used antibiotics, such as sulfa-containing compounds, penicillins, and cephalosporins. Fever and eosinophilia also may be associated drug reactions, but often these signs are not present. Drug-induced neutropenia can be severe, but discontinuation of the sensitizing drug is sufficient for recovery, which is usually seen within 5 to 7 days and is complete by 10 days. Readministration of the sensitizing drug should be avoided, since abrupt neutropenia often will result. For this reason, diagnostic challenge, even with a brief exposure, should be avoided in most situations.

Autoimmune neutropenias caused by circulating antineutrophil antibodies are another form of acquired neutropenia that results in increased destruction of neutrophils. Acquired neutropenia also may be seen with viral infections, including those with the human immunodeficiency virus. Rarely, acquired neutropenia may be cyclic in nature, occurring at intervals of several weeks. Acquired cyclic neutropenia may be associated with increased natural killer (NK) cells and may be responsive to steroids.

Syndromes have been described in which clonal expansion of T8 cells is associated with neutropenia. T8 cells are granulated T lymphocytes, and patients with T8 cell lymphocytosis have moderate blood and bone marrow lymphocytosis, neutropenia, polyclonal hypergammaglobulinemia, splenomegaly, and absence of lymphadenopathy. Such patients have a chronic and relatively stable course.

Recurrent bacterial infections are frequent. It is not clear whether this is a benign or malignant disease. In some patients, a spontaneous regression has occurred even after 11 years, suggesting an immunoregulatory defect as the basis for the disorder. It is likely that patients with T8 cell lymphocytosis and neutropenia will ultimately be shown to represent a biologically heterogeneous group of patients.

Hereditary neutropenias are rare and may manifest in early childhood as a profound constant neutropenia or agranulocytosis. Examples of congenital forms of neutropenia include Kostmann's syndrome (less than 100 neutrophils per microliter), which is often fatal; more benign chronic idiopathic neutropenia (300 to 1500 neutrophils per microliter); the hair-cartilage-hypoplasia syndrome; Schwachman syndrome associated with pancreatic insufficiency; and neutropenias associated with other immune defects (X-linked agammaglobulinemia, ataxia telangiectasia, IgA deficiency). Hereditary cyclic neutropenia, an autosomal dominant trait, may occur in infancy and is characterized by a remarkably regular 3-week cycle. Hereditary cyclic neutropenia actually is cyclic hematopoiesis. Although the mechanism for hereditary cyclic neutropenia is not known, steroids and G-CSF stop the cycling in some patients. Maternal factors associated with neutropenia in the newborn include transplacental transfer of IgG directed against antigens on fetal neutrophils resulting in peripheral destruction and drugs (e.g., thiazide) ingested during pregnancy which can cause neutropenia in the newborn by either depressed production or peripheral destruction.

The presence of immunoglobulin directed toward neutrophils is seen in Felty's syndrome (triad of rheumatoid arthritis, splenomegaly, and neutropenia; see Chap. 58). Patients with Felty's syndrome who respond to splenectomy with an increase in their neutrophil count also have lower postoperative serum granulocyte-binding IgG, a result suggesting that one beneficial effect of splenectomy is reduction in antibodies to neutrophils. Splenomegaly with peripheral trapping and destruction of neutrophils is also seen in lysosomal storage diseases and in portal hypertension.

Neutrophilia   Neutrophilia results from increased neutrophil production, marrow release, or defective margination (Table 59-3). The most important acute cause of neutrophilia requiring prompt medical attention is infection. Neutrophilia from acute infection represents both increased production and increased marrow release. Increased production is also associated with chronic inflammation and certain myeloproliferative diseases. Increased marrow release and mobiliza-

---

TABLE 59-3 Causes of neutrophilia

INCREASED PRODUCTION

Idiopathic
Drug-induced—corticosteroids
Infection—bacterial, fungal, rarely viral
Inflammation—thermal injury, tissue necrosis, myocardial and pulmonary infarction, hypersensitivity states, collagen vascular diseases
Myeloproliferative diseases—myelocytic leukemia, myeloid metaplasia, polycythemia vera

INCREASED MARROW MOBILIZATION

Corticosteroids
Acute infection (endotoxin)
Inflammation—thermal injury

DEFECTIVE MARGINATION

Drugs—epinephrine, corticosteroids, nonsteroidal anti-inflammatory agents
Stress, excitement, vigorous exercise
Leukocyte adhesion protein [C3bi (CR3) receptor] deficiency

MISCELLANEOUS

Metabolic disorders—ketoacidosis, acute renal failure, eclampsia, acute poisoning
Drugs—lithium
Other—metastatic carcinoma, acute hemorrhage or hemolysis

tion of the marginated leukocyte pool are induced by corticosteroids. Release of epinephrine, as with vigorous exercise, excitement, or stress, will demarginate neutrophils in the spleen and lungs and double the neutrophil count. Administration of exogenous epinephrine is a useful test to distinguish neutrophilia due to decreased margination, as seen in leukocyte adhesion deficiency, from that due to increased marrow production or release. Leukocytosis with counts of 10,000 to 25,000 cells per microliter occurs in response to infection and other forms of acute inflammation and results from both release of the marginated pool and mobilization of marrow reserves. Persistent neutrophilia of 30,000 to 50,000 cells per microliter or greater is called a *leukemoid reaction*, a term often used to distinguish this degree of neutrophilia from leukemia. In a leukemoid reaction, the circulating neutrophils are usually mature.

ABNORMAL NEUTROPHIL FUNCTION The types of inherited and acquired abnormalities of phagocyte function are described in Table 59-4. The resulting diseases are best considered in terms of the functional defects of adherence, chemotaxis, and microbicidal activity. The distinguishing features of the important inherited disorders of phagocyte function are shown in Table 59-5, several of which are discussed below.

Patients with inherited (autosomal recessive) abnormal phagocyte adherence, *leukocyte adhesion protein deficiency*, lack the plasma membrane receptor for the fragment of the third complement component called C3bi (CR3 by other terminology). The mutation is in the gene of the beta subunit of the leukocyte adhesion molecules LFA-1, Mac-1, and gp150,95. The gene is located on the most distal portion of the long arm of chromosome 21. Variable expression of the defect determines the magnitude of clinical disease. Complete lack of expression of the leukocyte adhesion proteins by resting neutrophils results in the severe phenotype in which inflammatory cytokines do not increase the expression of leukocyte adhesion proteins on neutrophils or activated T and B cells. The functional abnormalities are predictable because of the role these molecules play in normal leukocyte function. Neutrophils (and monocytes) from patients with leukocyte adhesion protein deficiency adhere poorly to endothelial cells and protein-coated surfaces and exhibit defective spreading, aggregation, and chemotaxis. Patients with this syndrome have recurrent bacterial and fungal infections involving skin, oral and genital mucosa, and respiratory and intestinal tracts, persistent leukocytosis (15,000 to 20,000 neutrophils per microliter) because cells do not marginate, and usually a history of delayed separation of

the umbilical stump. Infections, especially of the skin, tend to become necrotic with progressively enlarging borders, slow healing, and the development of dysplastic scars. The most common bacteria are *Staphylococcus aureus* and enteric gram-negative bacteria.

Abnormal neutrophil and monocyte chemotaxis occurs in the *hyperimmunoglobulin E–recurrent infection (Job's) syndrome*. The molecular basis for the syndrome is not known. For many years the cold abscesses were thought to be a reflection of impaired chemotaxis with too few phagocytes arriving too late, perhaps secondary to a lymphocyte factor inhibiting chemotaxis. However, it is now clear that the chemotactic defect in these patients is variable and the fundamental basis for the impaired defenses is complex and inadequately delineated.

The most common neutrophil defect is *myeloperoxidase deficiency*, which is inherited as an autosomal recessive trait and may have an incidence as high as about 1 in 2000 persons. Isolated myeloperoxidase deficiency is not associated with severely compromised defenses, because other defense systems such as hydrogen peroxide generation are accelerated. Microbicidal activity of neutrophils is delayed but not absent. However, if another underlying defect in host defense, such as poorly controlled diabetes mellitus, accompanies myeloperoxidase deficiency, then host defenses are likely to be significantly compromised. An acquired form of myeloperoxidase deficiency occurs in myelomonocytic leukemia and acute myeloblastic leukemia (also referred to as *myelogenous leukemia*). Dapsone and sulfones also inhibit myeloperoxidase-mediated hypochlorous acid (bleach) production by neutrophils.

Chédiak-Higashi syndrome (CHS) is a rare disease with autosomal recessive inheritance. Neutrophils and all cells containing lysosomes from patients with CHS characteristically have large granules (see Fig. A9-19A). CHS patients have increased infections due to a multitude of infectious agents. CHS neutrophils and monocytes have impaired chemotaxis and abnormal rates of microbial killing due to slow rates of fusion of the lysosomal granules with phagosomes. Natural killer cell function is also impaired.

Chronic granulomatous disease (CGD) represents a group of patients with disorders of neutrophil and monocyte oxidative metabolism. Although CGD is rare, occurring about once in 1 million individuals, it is an important model of defective neutrophil oxidative metabolism. Most often CGD is inherited as an X-linked recessive pattern, although in 35 percent of patients the disease is inherited with an autosomal recessive pattern. Mutations of four genes corre-

---

TABLE 59-4 Types of phagocyte dysfunction

Function	Cause of indicated dysfunction		
	Drug-induced	Acquired	Inherited
Adherence-aggregation	Aspirin, colchicine, alcohol, glucocorticoids, ibuprofen, piroxicam	Neonatal state, hemodialysis	Leukoctye adhesion protein deficiency
Deformability		Leukemia, neonatal state, diabetes mellitus, immature neutrophils	
Chemokinesis-chemotaxis	Glucocorticoids (high dose), auranofin, colchicine (weak effect), phenylbutazone, naproxen, indomethacin, interleukin 2	Thermal injury, malignancy, malnutrition, periodontal disease, neonatal state, systemic lupus erythematosus, rheumatoid arthritis, diabetes mellitus, sepsis, influenza virus infection, herpes simplex virus infection, acrodermatitis enteropathica, Down syndrome, α-mannosidase deficiency, severe combined immunodeficiency, Wiskott-Aldrich syndrome, AIDS	Chédiak-Higashi syndrome, neutrophil specific granule deficiency, hyper IgE–recurrent infection (Job's) syndrome (in some patients)
Microbicidal activity	Colchicine, cyclophosphamide, glucocorticoids (high dose)	Leukemia, aplastic anemia, certain neutropenias, tuftsin deficiency, thermal injury, sepsis, neonatal state, diabetes mellitus, malnutrition, AIDS	Chédiak-Higashi syndrome, neutrophil specific granule deficiency, chronic granulomatous disease

TABLE 59-5   Inherited disorders of phagocyte function: Differential features

Clinical manifestations	Cellular or molecular defects	Diagnosis
CHRONIC GRANULOMATOUS DISEASES OF CHILDHOOD (60% X-LINKED, 30% AUTOSOMAL RECESSIVE)		
Severe infections of skin, ears, lungs, liver, and bone with catalase-positive microorganisms such as *S. aureus, Pseudomonas cepacia, Aspergillus* sp., *Chromobacterium violaceum*; often hard to culture organism; excessive inflammation with granulomas, frequent lymph node suppuration; granulomas can obstruct GI or GU tracts; gingivitis, aphthous ulcers, seborrheic dermatitis	Absent respiratory burst due to the lack of one of four NADPH oxidase subunits in neutrophils, monocytes, and eosinophils	NBT test; absent superoxide and H_2O_2 production by neutrophils
CHEDIAK-HIGASHI SYNDROME (AUTOSOMAL RECESSIVE)		
Recurrent pyogenic infections, especially with *S. aureus*; many patients get lymphomatous-like illness during adolescence; periodontal disease; partial oculocutaneous albinism, nystagmus, progressive peripheral neuropathy, mental retardation in some patients	Reduced chemotaxis and phagolysosome fusion, increased respiratory burst activity, defective egress from marrow, abnormal skin window	Clinical features, giant lysosomal granules in granule-bearing cells (Wright stain)
SPECIFIC GRANULE DEFICIENCY (AUTOSOMAL RECESSIVE?)		
Recurrent infections of skin, ears, and sinopulmonary tract; delayed wound healing; decreased inflammation; bleeding diathesis	Abnormal chemotaxis, impaired respiratory burst and bacterial killing, failure to upregulate chemotactic and adhesion receptors with stimulation, defect in transcription of granule proteins	Lack of Wright-stained secondary (specific) granules in neutrophils, absent neutrophil-specific granule contents (i.e. lactoferrin), and absent eosin-staining granulocytes due to abnormal eosinophil-specific granules, platelet alpha granule abnormality
MYELOPEROXIDASE DEFICIENCY (AUTOSOMAL RECESSIVE)		
Clinically normal except in patients with underlying disease such as diabetes mellitus; then candidiasis or other fungal infections	Absent myeloperoxidase due to pre- and posttranslational defects	Absent peroxidase in neutrophils
LEUKOCYTE ADHESION PROTEIN DEFICIENCY* (AUTOSOMAL RECESSIVE)		
Delayed separation of umbilical cord, sustained granulocytosis, recurrent infections of skin and mucosa, gingivitis, periodontal disease	Impaired phagocyte adherence, aggregation, spreading, chemotaxis, phagocytosis of iC3b coated particles; leukemoid reaction; defective production of beta subunit common to leukocyte adhesion proteins	Reduced phagocyte surface expression of leukocyte adhesion receptors using a monoclonal antibody against Mac-1
HYPER IgE–RECURRENT INFECTION SYNDROME† (NON-X-LINKED)		
Eczematoid or pruritic dermatitis, "cold" skin abscesses, recurrent pneumonias with *S. aureus* with bronchopleural fistulas and cyst formation, mild eosinophilia, mucocutaneous candidiasis, atopy, coarse facies, restrictive lung disease, scoliosis	Reduced chemotaxis in some patients, reduced suppressor T cell activity	Clinical features, serum IgE > 2000 IU/mL, high serum anti-*S. aureus* IgE, low or absent serum and salivary anti-*S. aureus* IgA

* C3bi (CR3) receptor, Mac-1,LFA-1, gp150,95 deficiency.
† Job's syndrome.

sponding to four proteins that assemble at the plasma membrane account for all patients with CGD. Two proteins (a 91-kDa protein, abnormal in X-linked CGD, and a 22-kDa protein, absent in autosomal recessive CGD) form the heterodimer cytochrome b-558 in the plasma membrane, and two other proteins (47 and 67 kDa, abnormal in autosomal recessive forms of CGD) are cytoplasmic in origin and interact with the cytochrome following cell activation to form NADPH oxidase, required for hydrogen peroxide production. Leukocytes from patients with CGD have severely diminished hydrogen peroxide production. The genes involved in each of the defects have been cloned and sequenced and the chromosome location identified. Patients with CGD characteristically have increased infection with catalase-positive microorganisms (organisms which destroy their own hydrogen peroxide). When patients with CGD become infected, they often have extensive inflammatory reactions, and lymph node suppuration is common despite the administration of appropriate antibiotics. Aphthous ulcers and chronic inflammation of the nares are usually present. Granulomas are frequent and can obstruct the gastrointestinal or genitourinary tracts. The excessive inflammatory reactions probably reflect abnormal turnoff of inflammation by failure to degrade chemoattractants and antigens which cause persistent neutrophil accumulation. Impaired killing of intracellular microorganisms by macrophages may lead to persistent cell-mediated immunity and granuloma formation.

MONONUCLEAR PHAGOCYTES

The mononuclear phagocyte system is defined as a continuum linking monoblasts, promonocytes, and monocytes with the structurally diverse tissue macrophages which make up what was previously referred to as the reticuloendothelial system. Macrophages are long-lived phagocytic cells capable of many of the functions of neutrophils. In addition, they are important secretory cells that, through their receptors and secretory products, participate in many complex immunologic and inflammatory processes not attributed to neutrophils. Monocytes leave the circulation by diapedesis more slowly than neutrophils and have a half-life in the blood of 12 to 24 h.

After blood monocytes arrive in the tissues, they differentiate into macrophages ("big eaters") with specialized functions suited for specific anatomic locations. Macrophages are particularly abundant in capillary walls of the lung, spleen, liver, and bone marrow, where they function to remove microorganisms and other noxious elements from the blood. Alveolar macrophages, liver Kupffer cells, splenic macrophages, peritoneal macrophages, bone marrow macrophages, lymphatic macrophages, brain microglial cells, and dendritic macrophages all have specialized functions. Macrophage-secreted products include lysozyme, neutral proteases, acid hydrolases, arginase, numerous complement components, enzyme inhibitors (plasmin, alpha₂ macroglobulin), binding proteins (transferrin, fibronectin, transcobalamin II), nucleosides, cachectin, and interleukin 1 (pyrogen). Interleukin 1 (see Chaps. 16 and 277) has many important functions, including stimulating the hypothalamus to initiate fever, mobilizing leukocytes from the bone marrow, as well as activating lymphocytes and neutrophils. Tumor necrosis factor (also called *cachectin*) is a pyrogen that duplicates many of the actions of interleukin 1 and plays an important role in the pathogenesis of gram-negative shock (see Chap. 83). It can stimulate vigorous production of hydrogen peroxide and related toxic oxygen species by macrophages and neutrophils. In addition, tumor necrosis factor induces catabolic responses of chronic inflammation which contribute to the profound wasting (cachexia) associated with many chronic diseases.

Other macrophage-secreted products include reactive oxygen metabolites, bioactive lipids (arachidonate metabolites and platelet-activating factors), a neutrophil chemoattractant, factors regulating synthesis of proteins by other cells, bone marrow colony stimulating factors, factors stimulating fibroblast and microvasculature proliferation, as well as factors inhibiting replication of lymphocytes, tumors, viruses, and certain bacteria (*Mycobacterium tuberculosis* and *Listeria monocytogenes*). Macrophages are key effector cells in the elimination of intracellular microorganisms. Their ability to fuse to form giant cells which coalesce into granulomas in response to some inflammatory stimuli is important in the elimination of intracellular microbes and may be under the control of interferon-γ.

Macrophages play an important role in the immune response (see Chap. 277). They process antigen for presentation to lymphocytes, their secreted products modulate lymphocyte function, and macrophages participate in autoimmune phenomena by removing immune complexes and other immunologically active substances from the circulation. Furthermore, they play a role in wound healing, in the disposal of senescent cells, and in the development of atheromas.

DISORDERS OF THE MONONUCLEAR PHAGOCYTE SYSTEM

Many disorders of neutrophils extend to mononuclear phagocytes. Thus drugs which suppress neutrophil production in the bone marrow usually lead to monocytopenia. Transient monocytopenia also can be seen after stress or glucocorticoid administration. Monocytosis is associated with certain infections such as tuberculosis, brucellosis, subacute bacterial endocarditis, Rocky Mountain spotted fever, and malaria. Monocytosis is also seen in kala azar, malignancies, leukemias, myeloproliferative syndromes, hemolytic anemias, chronic idiopathic neutropenias, granulomatous diseases such as sarcoidosis, regional enteritis, and some collagen vascular diseases. Patients with leukocyte adhesion protein deficiency, the hyperimmunoglobulin E–recurrent infection (Job's) syndrome, Chédiak-Higashi syndrome, and chronic granulomatous diseases all have defects in the mononuclear phagocyte system.

Certain viral infections impair mononuclear phagocyte function. For example, influenza virus infection is associated with abnormal monocyte chemotaxis. Mononuclear phagocytes can be infected by the human immunodeficiency virus (HIV), and abnormal monocyte chemotaxis and abnormal clearance of IgG-coated erythrocytes (discussed below) by macrophages is also seen in AIDS (see Chap. 279). It is likely that these defects of the monocyte-macrophage system in AIDS contribute to the disordered immunoregulation and increased susceptibility to opportunistic infection due to intracellular microorganisms such as *Pneumocystis carinii* and *Mycobacterium avium-intracellulare*. T lymphocytes produce interferon-γ, which induces Fc-receptor expression and phagocytosis and stimulates hydrogen

peroxide production by mononuclear phagocytes. In certain diseases, such as AIDS, interferon-γ production may be deficient, while in other diseases, such as T cell lymphomas, excessive release of interferon-γ is thought to cause erythrophagocytosis by splenic macrophages.

Specific defects of the mononuclear phagocytes have been described in certain autoimmune diseases. Removal of IgG-coated radiolabeled autologous erythrocytes, presumably via the Fc receptor of splenic macrophages, is profoundly abnormal in patients with active systemic lupus erythematosus. Patients with other autoimmune diseases characterized by tissue deposition of immune complexes, as seen in Sjögren's syndrome, mixed cryoglobulinemia, dermatitis herpetiformis, and chronic progressive multiple sclerosis, also have defects in Fc-receptor function as judged by clearance of IgG-coated erythrocytes (see Chap. 283). Clinically, normal subjects with genetic haplotypes commonly associated with autoimmune disease (i.e., HLA-B8/DRw3) also have an increased incidence of defective Fc-receptor–specific functional activity, suggesting that this defect may predispose individuals with this genetic profile to immune-complex disease.

Monocytopenia occurs with acute infections, with stress, and following administration of glucocorticoids. Monocytopenia also occurs in aplastic anemia and acute myelogenous leukemia and as a direct result of myelotoxic and immunosuppressive drugs.

EOSINOPHILS

Eosinophils and neutrophils share similar morphology, many lysosomal constituents, most chemotactic responses, phagocytic capacity, and oxidative metabolism. However, there are major differences between the two cell types, and little is known about the natural function of eosinophils. Eosinophils are much longer lived than neutrophils, and unlike neutrophils, tissue eosinophils can recirculate. During most infections, eosinophils do not appear to have any important function. However, in invasive parasite infections, such as hookworm, schistosomiasis, strongyloidiasis, toxocariasis, trichinosis, filariasis, echinococcosis, and cysticercosis, the eosinophil likely plays a central role in host defense. Eosinophils are also associated with bronchial asthma, cutaneous allergic reactions, and other hypersensitivity states.

The characteristic red-staining eosinophil granules (Wright's stain) contain a number of unique constituents. The distinctive feature of the eosinophil granule is its crystalline core consisting of an arginine-rich protein (major basic protein) with histaminase activity, which is probably important in host defense against parasites. Eosinophil granules also contain a unique eosinophil peroxidase which catalyzes the oxidation of many substances by hydrogen peroxide and may facilitate killing of microorganisms.

Eosinophil peroxidase, in the presence of hydrogen peroxide and halide, initiates mast cell secretion in vitro and thereby may contribute to inflammation. Other substances found in eosinophils include cationic proteins, some of which bind to heparin and reduce its anticoagulant activity. Eosinophil cytoplasm contains Charcot-Leyden crystal protein, a hexagonal bipyramidal crystal first described in leukemia and then in sputum from asthma patients, which is lysophospholipase and may function to restrict the toxicity of certain lysophospholipids. Eosinophils also contain a powerful neurotoxin. Because patients with hypereosinophilic syndrome and cerebral spinal fluid eosinophilia exhibit varied neurologic abnormalities, eosinophil-derived neurotoxin may play an important role in central nervous system disease.

Several factors enhance the eosinophil's function in host defense. For example, T cell–derived eosinophil stimulation promoter enhances the ability of eosinophils to kill parasites. Mast cell–derived eosinophil chemotactic factor of anaphylaxis (ECFa) increases the number of eosinophil complement receptors and enhances eosinophil killing of parasites. In addition, eosinophil colony stimulating factors produced by macrophages may not only increase eosinophil production in the bone marrow but also may activate eosinophils to kill parasites.

EOSINOPHILIA   Eosinophilia is the presence of more than 500 eosinophils per microliter of blood and is common in many settings besides parasite infection. Significant tissue eosinophilia can occur without an elevated blood count. The most common cause of eosinophilia is probably allergic reactions to drugs such as iodides, aspirin, sulfonamides, nitrofurantoin, penicillins, and cephalosporins. Allergies such as hay fever, asthma, eczema, serum sickness, allergic vasculitis, and pemphigus commonly are associated with eosinophilia. Eosinophilia is also seen in collagen vascular diseases (e.g., rheumatoid arthritis, eosinophilic fasciitis, allergic angiitis, periarteritis nodosa, and granulomatosis) and malignancies (e.g., Hodgkin's disease, mycosis fungoides, chronic myelogenous leukemia, and cancer of the lung stomach, pancreas, ovary, or uterus), as well as rare diseases such as Job's syndrome and the chronic granulomatous diseases; the mechanisms for the eosinophilia in these diseases are not known. Eosinophilia is commonly seen in helminthic infections, such as hookworm, strongyloidiasis, toxocariasis, trichuriasis, trichinosis, filariasis, schistosomiasis, echinococcosis, and cysticercosis. The most dramatic increases in eosinophils occur in hypereosinophilic syndromes, including Loeffler's syndrome, Loeffler's endocarditis, eosinophilic leukemia, and idiopathic hypereosinophilic syndrome (with counts as high as 50,000 to 100,000 per microliter).

The idiopathic hypereosinophilic syndrome represents a heterogeneous group of disorders with the common feature of prolonged eosinophilia of unknown cause and associated organ system dysfunction, including the heart, central nervous system, kidneys, lungs, gastrointestinal tract, and skin. The bone marrow is involved in all subjects, but the most severe complications involve the heart and central nervous system. Eosinophils are found in the involved tissues and are thought to cause tissue damage by local deposition of toxic eosinophil proteins such as eosinophil cationic protein and eosinophil major basic protein. In the heart, the pathologic changes lead to thrombosis, which may result in endocardial fibrosis and restrictive endomyocardiopathy. Similar pathologic changes are thought to contribute to the damage of tissues in other organ systems. Although the mechanism for the hypereosinophilia is not known, it has been shown that chemotherapy with glucocorticoids usually induces remission. In patients unresponsive to glucocorticoids, a cytotoxic agent such as hydroxyurea has been used successfully to lower the peripheral blood eosinophil counts and to improve markedly the prognosis. Aggressive medical and surgical approaches are also employed for management of patients with cardiovascular complications.

The *eosinophilia-myalgia syndrome* is a multisystem disease with prominent cutaneous, hematologic, and visceral manifestations that frequently evolves into a chronic course and can occasionally be fatal. The syndrome is characterized by blood eosinophilia (greater than 10^9 eosinophils per liter) and generalized disabling myalgias without other recognized causes. Eosinophil fasciitis, pneumonitis and myocarditis, neuropathy culminating in respiratory failure, and encephalopathy have been described. The association of the disease with ingestion of L-tryptophan–containing products originating from a single source has led to the identification and characterization of a putative etiologic agent present as a contaminant in these preparations. Although the accumulation of eosinophils, lymphocytes, macrophages, and fibroblasts in the affected tissues suggests that these cells play important roles in the pathogenesis of the eosinophilia-myalgia syndrome, the precise mechanism of their involvement has not been established. Several studies have demonstrated the activation of eosinophils and the deposition of eosinophil-derived toxic proteins in affected tissues. Fibroblast activation and increased expression of genes coding for various connective tissue macromolecules have been demonstrated with use of in situ hybridization with complementary DNAs. Furthermore, interleukin 5 and transforming growth factor-β have been implicated as potential mediators. Treatment has included withdrawal of L-tryptophan–containing products and the administration of corticosteroids. Most patients recover fully, remain stable, or show slow recovery, but in some patients (up to 5 percent) the disease can be fatal. This disease emphasizes the importance of chemical and environmental factors in the development of systemic disorders characterized by chronic inflammation and fibrosis.

EOSINOPENIA   This occurs with stress, such as acute bacterial infection, and following administration of glucocorticoids. The mechanism of eosinopenia of acute bacterial infection is unknown but is independent of endogenous glucocorticoids, since it occurs in animals following total adrenalectomy. There is no known adverse effect of eosinopenia.

LABORATORY DIAGNOSIS AND MANAGEMENT OF PHAGOCYTE DYSFUNCTION

Initial studies of white blood count and differential and often a bone marrow examination are followed by assessment of bone marrow reserves (steroid challenge test), marginated circulating pool of cells (epinephrine challenge test), and marginating ability (endotoxin challenge test). In vivo assessment of inflammation is possible with a Rebuck skin window test or an in vivo blister assay, which measures the ability of leukocytes and inflammatory mediators to accumulate locally within the skin. In vivo clearance of IgG-coated erythrocytes provides a useful way to monitor the mononuclear phagocyte system. In vitro tests of phagocyte aggregation, adherence, chemotaxis, phagocytosis, degranulation, and microbicidal activity (for *Staphylococcus aureus*) help pinpoint cellular or humoral lesions which can then be further characterized at the molecular level. Deficiencies of oxidative metabolism are screened with the nitroblue tetrazolium dye (NBT) test, which is based on the ability of products of oxidative metabolism to reduce yellow, soluble NBT to blue-black formazan, an insoluble material which precipitates intracellularly and can be seen microscopically. Further aspects of neutrophil oxidative metabolism are defined by studies of superoxide and hydrogen peroxide production.

The most important aspect of patient management is to appreciate that patients with leukopenias or leukocyte dysfunction often have delayed inflammatory responses. Therefore, clinical manifestations may be minimal despite overwhelming infection, and unusual infections must always be suspected in some patients. Early signs of infection demand prompt, aggressive culturing for microorganisms and use of antibiotics and surgical drainage of abscesses. Prolonged antibiotics are often required, and in life-threatening infections, daily white blood cell transfusions (enriched for neutrophils) are probably beneficial, although their use is still controversial. In patients with the chronic granulomatous diseases of childhood (CGD), prophylactic antibiotics (trimethoprim-sulfamethoxazole) probably diminish the frequency of life-threatening infections. Surgery is required for thorough drainage of abscesses in lung, liver, and bones. Short courses of glucocorticoids have had dramatic effects in the management of the granulomas of CGD. For example, obstruction of the gastrointestinal or genitourinary tract in CGD can be diminished with a short course of steroids followed by a long one of a nonsteroidal anti-inflammatory agent. Recent studies indicate that recombinant human interferon-γ, which nonspecifically stimulates phagocytic cell function, reduces the frequency of infections in CGD patients by 70 percent and reduces the severity of infection (hospital days for infection) as well. This effect of interferon-γ in CGD is additive to the effect of prophylactic antibiotics. Interferon-γ has been approved by the U.S. Food and Drug Administration for use in CGD at a recommended dose of 50 μg/m² of body surface area.

Rigorous oral hygiene reduces but does not eliminate the discomfort of gingivitis, periodontal disease, and aphthous ulcers; chlorhexidine mouth wash and tooth brushing with a hydrogen peroxide–sodium bicarbonate paste helps many patients. Ketoconazole has caused dramatic improvement of mucocutaneous candidiasis in patients with Job's syndrome. Treatment to restore myelopoiesis in patients with neutropenia due to impaired production has included use of androgens, glucocorticoids, lithium, and immunosuppressive therapy. Recombinant G-CSF is useful in the management of certain forms of neutropenia due to depressed production, especially that related to chemotherapy for cancer. Patients with chronic neutropenia with evidence of a good bone marrow reserve should not receive prophylactic antibiotics.

Patients with constant or cyclic neutrophil counts below 500 cells per microliter may benefit from prophylactic antibiotics. Oral trimethoprim-sulfamethoxazole (160/800 mg) twice daily is commonly used to prevent infection, although concerns about its predisposing to fungal infections have been raised. Increased fungal infection is not seen in CGD patients on this regimen. Oral quinolones such as norfloxacin and ciprofloxacin have been suggested alternatives.

In the setting of cytotoxic chemotherapy with severe, persistent neutropenia, the proven effectiveness of trimethoprim-sulfamethoxazole in preventing *Pneumocystis carinii* pneumonia may offer another incentive to use this form of prophylaxis. These patients, and patients with phagocytic cell dysfunction, should avoid heavy exposure to airborne soil, dust, or decaying matter (mulch, manure) which could be rich in spores of *Aspergillus* or other fungi. Restriction of activities or social contact probably makes little difference in risk of infection.

Cure of some congenital phagocyte defects is theoretically possible by bone marrow transplantation (see Chap. 313). However, complications of bone marrow transplantation are still great, and with rigorous medical care many patients with phagocytic disorders can go for years without a life-threatening infection. The identification of specific gene defects in patients with leukocyte adhesion protein deficiency and chronic granulomatous disease of childhood and the successful correction of B cells from these patients by gene transfection make gene therapy a likely and exciting future possibility.

REFERENCES

ANDERSON DC, SPRINGER TA: Leukocyte adhesion deficiency: An inherited defect in the Mac-1, LFA-1, and p150,95 glycoproteins. Annu Rev Med 38:175, 1987

BEUTLER B (ed): Tumor necrosis factors, in *The Molecules and Their Emerging Role in Medicine*. New York, Raven Press, 1992

CURNUTTE JT (ed): Phagocyte defects: Abnormalities outside the respiratory burst. Hematol Clin North Am 2, 1988

GALLIN JI: Interferon-γ in the management of chronic granulomatous disease. Rev Infect Dis 13:1973, 1991

—— et al: Delineation of the phagocyte NADPH oxidase through studies of chronic granulomatous diseases of childhood. Curr Opin Immunol 4:53, 1991

—— et al (eds): *Inflammation: Basic Principles and Clinical Correlates*, 2d ed. New York, Raven Press, 1992

GEHA RS, LEUNG DY: Hyper-immunoglobulin-E syndrome. Immunodefic Rev 1:155, 1989

GLEICH GJ, ADOLPHSON C: The eosinophil leukocyte: Structure and function. Adv Immunol 39:177, 1986

JOHNSTON RB: Monocytes and macrophages. N Engl J Med 318:747, 1988

KLEMPNER MS, MALECH HL: Phagocytes: Normal and abnormal neutrophil host defenses, in *Infectious Diseases*, SL Gorbach et al (eds). Philadelphia, Saunders, 1992

KUHNS DB et al: Dynamics of the cellular and humoral components of the inflammatory response elicited in skin blisters in humans. J Clin Invest 89:1734, 1992

LAWRENCE MB, SPRINGER TA: Leukocytes roll on a selectin at physiologic flow rates: Distinction from and a prerequisite for adhesion through integrins. Cell 65:859, 1991

LIESCHKE GJ, BURGESS AW: Granulocyte colony-stimulating factor and granulocyte-macrophage colony-stimulating factor. N Engl J Med 327:28, 99, 1992

LOMAX KJ et al: The molecular biology of selected phagocyte defects. Blood Rev 3:94, 1989

MALECH HL, GALLIN JI: Neutrophils in human diseases. N Engl J Med 317:687, 1987

METCALFE DM: Control of granulocytes and macrophages: Molecular, cellular and clinical aspects. Science 254:529, 1991

MOORE MAS: The clinical use of colony stimulating factors. Annu Rev Immunol 9:159, 1991

NAUSEEF WM: Myeloperoxidase deficiency. Hematol Pathol 4:165, 1990

SAMTER M (ed): *Immunological Diseases*, 4th ed. Boston, Little, Brown, 1988

VARGA J et al: The cause and pathogenesis of the eosinophil-myalgia syndrome. Ann Intern Med 116:140, 1992

WEISS SJ: Tissue destruction by neutrophils. N Engl J Med 320:365, 1989

60　GENETIC ASPECTS OF DISEASE

JOSEPH L. GOLDSTEIN / MICHAEL S. BROWN

GENETIC PRINCIPLES

More than one-fifth of the proteins (and hence genes) in each human being exist in a form that differs from the one present in the majority of the population. This remarkable genetic variability, or polymorphism, among "normal" people accounts for much of the normal variation in body traits such as height, intelligence, and blood pressure. These genetic differences also determine the ability of each individual to meet environmental challenges, including those which produce disease. All human diseases can be considered to result from an interaction between an individual's unique genetic makeup and the environment. In certain diseases, the genetic component is so overwhelming that it expresses itself in a predictable manner without a requirement for extraordinary environmental challenges. Such diseases are termed *genetic disorders*.

MOLECULAR BASIS OF GENE EXPRESSION　All hereditary information is transmitted from parent to offspring through the inheritance of deoxyribonucleic acid (DNA). DNA is a linear polymer composed of purine and pyrimidine bases whose sequence ultimately determines the sequence of amino acids in every protein made by the body. The four types of bases in DNA are arranged in groups of three, each triplet forming a code word, or codon, that signifies a particular amino acid. A *gene* represents the total sequence of bases in DNA that specifies the amino acid sequence of a single polypeptide chain of a protein molecule.

Genetic information encoded in the DNA of the chromosomes is first transcribed into a *ribonucleic acid* (RNA) copy. During transcription, the ribose nucleotides align themselves along the DNA according to base-pairing rules. Thus adenine of DNA pairs with uridine of RNA, cytosine pairs with guanine, thymine pairs with adenine, and guanine pairs with cytosine. The ribose bases are joined together by RNA polymerase. The resulting *RNA transcript* forms the template for translation into the amino acid sequence of a protein. The DNA and mRNA code words for each of the amino acids in protein are shown in Fig. 60-1.

A schematic diagram of the genetic control of protein synthesis in higher organisms is illustrated in Fig. 60-2. The DNA of most genes is fragmented into discrete coding regions (exons) separated by noncoding regions (introns or intervening sequences). The *coding regions* contain the bases that specify the sequence of amino acids in the polypeptide chain. The *intervening sequences* are composed of bases that act as spacers between the coding regions; they are not translated into protein. The transcription of DNA produces a faithful copy of the entire gene sequence; thus the RNA transcript contains alternating coding and intervening sequences. The RNA transcript is edited in the nucleus before it passes into the cytoplasm. In the editing process, the intervening sequences are excised, and the coding regions are spliced together to form one continuous RNA (Fig. 60-2).

FIGURE 60-1　The genetic code.

Second nucleotide

First nucleotide	A or U		G or C		T or A		C or G		Third nucleotide
A or *U*	**AAA** *UUU*⎫ Phe		**AGA** *UCU*⎫		**ATA** *UAU*⎫ Tyr		**ACA** *UGU*⎫ Cys		**A** or *U*
	AAG *UUC*⎭		**AGG** *UCC*⎬ Ser		**ATG** *UAC*⎭		**ACG** *UGC*⎭		**G** or *C*
	AAT *UUA*⎫ Leu		**AGT** *UCA*		**ATT** *UAA*⎫ Stop		**ACT** *UGA* Stop		**T** or *A*
	AAC *UUG*⎭		**AGC** *UCG*		**ATC** *UAG*⎭		**ACC** *UGG* Trp		**C** or *G*
G or *C*	**GAA** *CUU*⎫		**GGA** *CCU*⎫		**GTA** *CAU*⎫ His		**GCA** *CGU*⎫		**A** or *U*
	GAG *CUC*⎬ Leu		**GGG** *CCC*⎬ Pro		**GTG** *CAC*⎭		**GCG** *CGC*⎬ Arg		**G** or *C*
	GAT *CUA*		**GGT** *CCA*		**GTT** *CAA*⎫ Gln		**GCT** *CGA*		**T** or *A*
	GAC *CUG*⎭		**GGC** *CCG*		**GTC** *CAG*⎭		**GCC** *CGG*⎭		**C** or *G*
T or *A*	**TAA** *AUU*⎫		**TGA** *ACU*⎫		**TTA** *AAU*⎫ Asn		**TCA** *AGU*⎫ Ser		**A** or *U*
	TAG *AUC*⎬ Ile		**TGG** *ACC*⎬ Thr		**TTG** *AAC*⎭		**TCG** *AGC*⎭		**G** or *C*
	TAT *AUA*		**TGT** *ACA*		**TTT** *AAA*⎫ Lys		**TCT** *AGA*⎫ Arg		**T** or *A*
	TAC *AUG* Met		**TGC** *ACG*⎭		**TTC** *AAG*⎭		**TCC** *AGG*⎭		**C** or *G*
C or *G*	**CAA** *GUU*⎫		**CGA** *GCU*⎫		**CTA** *GAU*⎫ Asp		**CCA** *GGU*⎫		**A** or *U*
	CAG *GUC*⎬ Val		**CGG** *GCC*⎬ Ala		**CTG** *GAC*⎭		**CCG** *GGC*⎬ Gly		**G** or *C*
	CAT *GUA*		**CGT** *GCA*		**CTT** *GAA*⎫ Glu		**CCT** *GGA*		**T** or *A*
	CAC *GUG*⎭		**CGC** *GCG*⎭		**CTC** *GAG*⎭		**CCC** *GGG*⎭		**C** or *G*

Note: The DNA codons appear in boldface type; the complementary RNA codons are in italics. A = adenine, C = cytosine, G = guanine, T = thymine, U = uridine (replaces thymine in RNA). In RNA, adenine is complementary to thymine of DNA; uridine is complementary to adenine of DNA; cytosine is complementary to guanine, and vice versa. "Stop" = termination. The amino acids are abbreviated as follows:

Ala = alanine	Cys = cysteine	His = histidine	Met = methionine	Thr = threonine
Arg = arginine	Gln = glutamine	Ile = isoleucine	Phe = phenylalanine	Trp = tryptophan
Asn = asparagine	Glu = glutamic acid	Leu = leucine	Pro = proline	Tyr = tyrosine
Asp = aspartic acid	Gly = glycine	Lys = lysine	Ser = serine	Val = valine

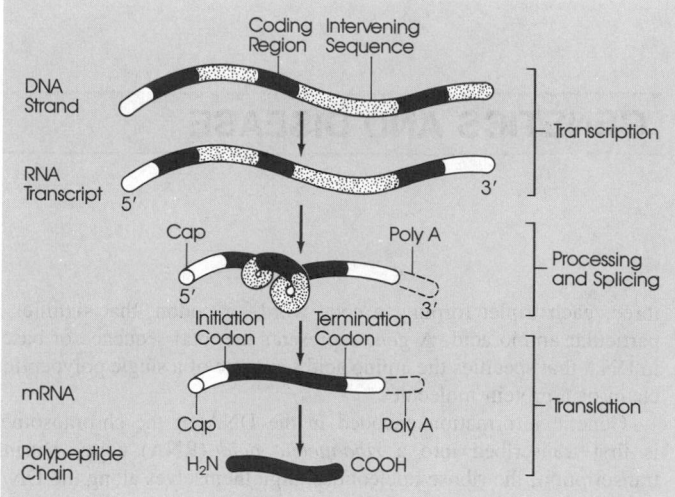

FIGURE 60-2 A schematic diagram of the genetic control of protein synthesis, illustrating the flow of genetic information from the base sequence of DNA to the RNA transcript (transcription) to mRNA (processing) to the polypeptide chain of a protein molecule (translation). Although DNA exists in a double-stranded form, only one of the two strands is used as a template for transcribing the RNA transcript. Solid sections represent coding regions in DNA, RNA transcript, mRNA, and amino acid sequence in polypeptide chain; dotted sections represent intervening sequences in DNA and RNA transcript.

After processing, the edited RNA, called *messenger RNA* (mRNA), leaves the nucleus and enters the cytoplasm, where it becomes associated with *ribosomes* and thereby serves as a template for the ribosomal synthesis of proteins. Each of the 20 amino acids is attached in the cell cytoplasm to a specific molecule called *transfer RNA* (tRNA). Each tRNA contains a triplet sequence of purine and pyrimidine bases that is "complementary" to a specific codon in the mRNA. These tRNA molecules with their attached amino acids line up along the mRNA molecule in the precise order dictated by the genetic code. Under the action of cytoplasmic enzymes (initiation factors, elongation factors, and termination factors), peptide bonds are formed between the various amino acids, and the completed protein is released from the ribosome. For a more detailed account of the molecular basis of gene expression, see Chap. 61.

MAINTENANCE OF GENETIC DIVERSITY THROUGH TRANSMISSION AND SEGREGATION OF GENES The amount of DNA in the nucleus of each human cell is sufficient to code for more than 50,000 genes and hence to specify more than 50,000 polypeptide chains. The genes are arranged in a linear sequence of DNA that together with certain histone proteins form rod-shaped bodies called *chromosomes*. Each somatic cell contains 46 chromosomes, arranged in 23 pairs, one of each pair derived from each parent. Thus each individual inherits two copies of each chromosome and hence two copies of each gene. The chromosomal location of the two copies of each gene is termed the *genetic locus*. When a gene occupying a genetic locus exists in two or more different forms, these alternate forms of the gene are referred to as *alleles*.

In humans, a given gene always resides at a specified genetic locus on one particular chromosome. For example, the genetic locus for the Rh blood group is on the short arm of chromosome 1; at this site there are two Rh genes, one on chromosome 1 derived from the mother and the other on chromosome 1 derived from the father. When two genes at the same genetic locus are identical, the individual is a *homozygote*. When the two genes differ (i.e., two different alleles are present at the locus), the individual is a *heterozygote*. Each normal human is heterozygous at approximately 20 percent of genetic loci and homozygous at 80 percent. A map of human chromosome 1,

shown in Fig. 60-3, illustrates the location of a representative sample of genes that have been assigned loci on this chromosome.

The genetic information carried on chromosomes is transmitted to daughter cells under two different sets of circumstances. One of these occurs whenever a somatic cell (i.e., a nongerm cell) divides. This process, called *mitosis*, transmits identical copies of each gene to each daughter cell, thus maintaining a uniform genetic makeup in all cells of a single individual. The other set of circumstances prevails when genetic information must be transmitted from one individual to an offspring. This process, called *meiosis*, produces germ cells (i.e., ova or spermatozoa) that possess only one copy of each parental chromosome, thus allowing for new combinations of chromosomes to occur when ovum and sperm cell fuse during fertilization.

During meiosis, the 46 chromosomes of an immature germ cell arrange themselves in 23 pairs at the center of the nucleus, each pair being composed of one chromosome derived from the mother and its homologous chromosome derived from the father. At a specified point in the meiotic process, the two partner chromosomes separate, only one of each pair going into each daughter cell, or gamete. Thus meiosis produces gametes with a reduction in the number of chromosomes from 46 to 23, each gamete having received one chromosome from each of the 23 pairs. The assortment of the chromosomes within each pair is random so that each germ cell receives a different combination of maternal and paternal chromosomes. During the process of fertilization, the fusion of ovum and sperm cell, each of which has 23 chromosomes, produces an individual with 46 chromosomes.

The independent assortment of chromosomes into gametes during meiosis produces an enormous diversity among the possible genotypes

FIGURE 60-3 Gene map of human chromosome 1, illustrating a representative sample of the more than 250 genes that have been localized to this chromosome. The black bands represent those genetic regions of the chromosome which stain brightly by a fluorescent dye such as quinacrine; the white bands are the negatively staining regions; the hatched area is a variable region that stains differently (i.e., either brightly or negatively) in the chromosomes of different individuals. Each gene is listed opposite its genetic locus on the right. (*Data provided by VA McKusick.*)

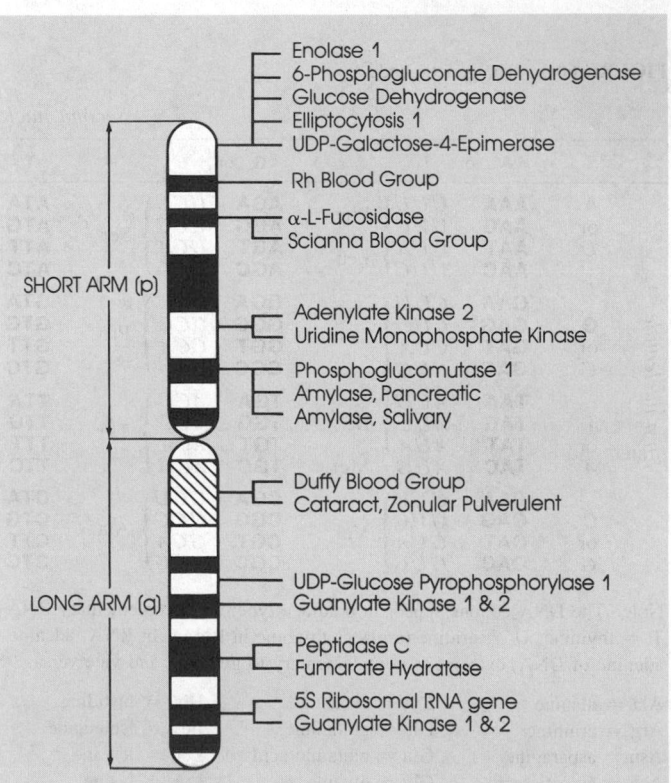

of the progeny. For each 23 pairs of chromosomes, there are 2^{23} different combinations of chromosomes that could occur in a gamete, and the likelihood that one set of parents will produce two offspring with the identical complement of chromosomes is 1 in 2^{23} or 1 in 8.4 million (assuming no monozygotic, or identical, twins).

RECOMBINATION Adding to the genetic diversity in humans is the phenomenon of *genetic recombination*. During meiosis, when homologous chromosomes are paired, bridges frequently form between corresponding regions of the chromosome pair. These bridges, or *chiasmata*, are regions in which the two chromosomes break at identical points along their length and subsequently rejoin, the distal segments having been switched from one homologous chromosome to another. This process is designated *crossing-over*. Although no net change in the amount of genetic material occurs during crossing-over, a recombination of genes does occur. For example, consider a chromosome with two loci, A and B, located at opposite ends of the same chromosome. On this particular chromosome, the A locus has a rare allele *x*, and the B locus also has a rare allele *y*. Without the phenomenon of recombination, every offspring that inherited the *x* allele at the A locus also would inherit the *y* allele at the B locus. However, if recombination occurs, the A locus with the *x* allele would then be on the opposite chromosome from the B locus with the *y* allele. In this case, any offspring that inherited the *x* allele at the A locus could not inherit the *y* allele at the B locus.

Crossing-over occurs with great frequency in every meiosis in humans, and the resultant recombination of genes may occur at any point on a chromosome. The farther apart two genes are on the same chromosome, the greater is the likelihood that a crossing-over will occur in the space between them. When two genes are on the opposite ends of a long chromosome, the probability of recombination is so great that their respective alleles are transmitted to offspring almost independently of one another, just as if the two gene loci were on different chromosomes. On the other hand, gene loci that are close together on the same chromosome are said to be *linked* so that there is a great likelihood that offspring will inherit the same combination of alleles that are present on the parental chromosome.

Several examples of *gene linkage* can be seen from the map of human chromosome 1 (Fig. 60-3). For example, the locus for the gene specifying the Rh blood group factor and the locus for the gene producing one form of the dominant trait·hereditary elliptocytosis occur in close proximity on this chromosome. Thus, if a subject with hereditary elliptocytosis transmits the disease to an offspring, the offspring will usually inherit the allele that is present at the Rh locus on this chromosome. If the Rh allele happens to be a rare one in the population (such as *r'*), one can assume that whichever offspring inherits the *r'* allele at the Rh locus also will inherit the abnormal allele at the elliptocytosis locus. On the other hand, if an offspring does not exhibit the *r'* allele, he or she will not usually have elliptocytosis. The concept of linkage does not imply an association between any particular set of Rh alleles and the disease state elliptocytosis, rather between the two genetic loci. Thus in different families the abnormal elliptocytosis allele may be linked to the R^1, R^0, r_2, or any other allele at the Rh locus depending on the allele that happened to be at that locus when the elliptocytosis mutation occurred. Stated another way, the elliptocytosis locus is linked to the Rh locus in every family, but the particular Rh allele with which it is associated differs from family to family.

MUTATION Broadly defined, a *mutation* is a stable, heritable alteration in DNA. Although the causes of mutation in humans are largely unknown, a variety of environmental agents, such as radiation, viruses, and chemicals, are among the factors that are implicated.

Mutations can involve a visible alteration in the structure of a chromosome, such as a deletion or translocation of a portion of a chromosome, or they can involve a minute change in one of the purine or pyrimidine bases of a single gene. Most commonly, such "point" mutations consist of the substitution of one base for another, changing the meaning of the codon containing that base, hence their

designation as *missense mutations*. For example, in the gene coding for the β chain of hemoglobin, the sixth position normally contains the nucleotide triplet CTC, which codes for the amino acid glutamic acid (Fig. 60-1). The mutation that gives rise to hemoglobin C produces a change of the first base of this triplet from cytosine to thymine, changing the triplet to TTC, which codes for lysine. On the other hand, the mutation that gives rise to hemoglobin S produces a change in the second base of the same triplet (from thymine to adenine), producing CAC, which codes for valine. Thus, in the sixth position of the β chain of hemoglobin, the normally occurring glutamic acid may be replaced with either lysine (producing hemoglobin C) or valine (producing hemoglobin S). More than 100 such single-base mutations in the hemoglobin β chain have been identified, and many of these mutations produce distinct clinical syndromes. Of the mutations so far elucidated in humans, most involve such single-base changes.

Besides producing an amino acid substitution, a single-base substitution also can cause another abnormality in protein synthesis—premature chain termination. Three mRNA code words (UAA, UAG, and UGA) normally do not specify an amino acid but constitute the signal that the message has ended and that the protein chain should be released from the ribosome (Fig. 60-1). If a change occurs in DNA that produces one of these mRNA code words [e.g., a switch in an mRNA triplet from UAU (tyrosine) to UAA (termination)], the polypeptide chain would be terminated prematurely when translation had reached that point. Such mutations, called *non-sense mutations*, produce short fragments of proteins that have reduced function.

CELLULAR MECHANISM BY WHICH MUTANT GENES PRODUCE DISEASES Critical to the understanding of heredity is the concept that the only information transmitted from generation to generation is the sequence of bases in DNA and that these sequences in turn specify only the primary structure of RNA and protein molecules. All other chemical reactions—such as the synthesis of complex lipids and carbohydrates, the formation of membranes and other cellular organelles, and the accumulation and partitioning of inorganic ions—occur as a secondary consequence of the action of specific proteins. Many of these proteins are enzymes that catalyze the biochemical conversion of one molecule into another. Others are structural proteins such as collagen and elastin, and still others are regulatory proteins that dictate how much of each enzyme and each structural protein is made.

Since proteins are the cellular molecules whose structures are encoded by genes, mutations in genes exert their deleterious effects by altering the structure of enzymes, structural proteins, or regulatory proteins. For example, in a disease such as glycogen storage disease, type I (von Gierke's disease), massive accumulation of glycogen in the liver is due not to a primary structural abnormality in the polysaccharide glycogen but to a structural abnormality in a protein, glucose-6-phosphatase, an enzyme that is required to liberate glucose so as to permit glycogen breakdown. Other examples of the biochemical mechanisms by which mutant genes alter cellular metabolism are discussed below under "Simply Inherited Disorders."

GENETIC HETEROGENEITY When two or more mutations can produce a similar clinical syndrome, *genetic heterogeneity* is said to exist. Hemophilia is an example of a genetically heterogeneous syndrome. A clinically similar bleeding disorder can be caused by mutations at either of two loci on the X chromosome, one leading to a deficiency of factor VIII (classic hemophilia) and the other causing a deficiency of factor IX (Christmas disease). Most, if not all, hereditary diseases, when carefully analyzed, will probably prove to be genetically heterogeneous.

Genetic heterogeneity may result from the existence of a series of different mutations at a single genetic locus (allelic mutations) or from mutations at different genetic loci (nonallelic mutations). For example, drug-induced hemolysis of red blood cells can occur in patients with several different types of allelic mutations at the glucose-6-phosphate dehydrogenase locus. On the other hand, hemophilia is an example of a syndrome in which nonallelic mutations can produce a similar clinical picture (see above).

In some cases of heterogeneity, both the genetic locus and the mode of inheritance differ. Diseases such as spastic paraplegia, Charcot-Marie-Tooth peroneal muscular atrophy, and retinitis pigmentosa are inherited as autosomal dominant traits in some families, as autosomal recessives in others, and as X-linked recessives in still others. The identification of such genetic heterogeneity in these disorders is of obvious importance for correct genetic counseling.

TAKING THE FAMILY HISTORY

The investigation of a patient with a possible genetic disorder begins with the *family history*. The first step is to obtain certain information on the *proband* or *index case* (i.e., the clinically affected person who has brought the family to attention) and on each of the *first-degree relatives* (i.e., the parents, siblings, and offspring of the proband). This information includes the given name, surname, maiden name, birth date or current age, age at death, cause of death, and name or description of any disease or defect.

The second step is to ask questions designed to survey the family for the presence of disease or defect. (1) Has any relative an identical or similar trait? (2) Has any relative a trait that is absent in the proband but is known to occur in some patients with the same disease? This question requires that the physician have some knowledge about the manifestations of the disease in question. For example, when obtaining the family history from a proband with dissecting aneurysm caused possibly by Marfan's syndrome, one should ask about the occurrence of eye abnormalities, cardiac abnormalities, and skeletal abnormalities in the relatives. (3) Has any relative a trait that is recognized to be genetically determined? The purpose of this question is to ascertain the occurrence of hereditary disease in the family even though the particular patient may not be involved. (4) Has any relative an unusual disease, or has any relative died of a rare condition? The purpose of this question is to identify a condition that might be genetically determined though not recognized as such by the informant. In addition, this question may help to identify conditions in relatives that might be etiologically related to the patient's problem. For example, a patient with pheochromocytoma should be suspected of having von Recklinghausen's disease if he or she has a brother with scoliosis and mental retardation, both of which can be manifestations of the neurofibromatosis (von Recklinghausen's) gene. (5) Is there any consanguinity in the family? This inquiry should be made directly. In addition, one should ask whether common last names appear in the families of husband-wife pairs. Consanguineous marriage may be the source of a rare autosomal recessive syndrome, and sometimes its presence in the family may not be known by the proband. (6) What is the ethnic origin of the family? Persons of various ethnic origins, such as blacks, Jews, and Greeks, have increased chances of specific genetic diseases. Table 60-1 lists examples of simply inherited disorders that are found with increased frequency in various ethnic groups.

CATEGORIES OF GENETIC DISORDERS

Genetic diseases generally fall into one of three categories: (1) *Chromosomal disorders* involve the lack, excess, or abnormal arrangement of one or more chromosomes, producing excessive or deficient genetic material. (2) *Mendelian, or simply inherited, disorders* are determined primarily by a single mutant gene. These disorders display inheritance patterns which can be classified into autosomal dominant, autosomal recessive, or X-linked types. (3) *Multifactorial disorders* are caused by an interaction of multiple genes and multiple exogenous or environmental factors. Although many of these multifactorial disorders, such as essential hypertension and cleft lip and palate, are said to run in families, the inheritance pattern is complex and the risk

TABLE 60-1   Examples of simply inherited disorders that occur with increased frequency in specific ethnic groups

Ethnic group	Simply inherited disorder
African blacks	Hemoglobinopathies, especially Hb S, Hb C, persistent Hb F, α and β thalassemias Glucose-6-phosphate dehydrogenase deficiency
Armenians	Familial Mediterranean fever
Ashkenazi Jews	Abetalipoproteinemia Bloom's syndrome Dystonia musculorum deformans (recessive form) Factor XI (PTA) deficiency Familial dysautonomia (Riley-Day syndrome) Gaucher's disease (adult form) Neimann-Pick disease Pentosuria Tay-Sachs disease
Chinese	α Thalassemia Glucose-6-phosphate dehydrogenase deficiency Adult lactase deficiency
Eskimos	Pseudocholinesterase deficiency Adrenogenital syndrome
Finns	Congenital nephrosis Mulibrey nanism
French Canadians	Tyrosinemia Homozygous familial hypercholesterolemia
Japanese	Acatalasemia
Lebanese	Homozygous familial hypercholesterolemia
Mediterranean peoples (Italians, Greeks, Sephardic Jews)	β Thalassemia Glucose-6-phosphate dehydrogenase deficiency Familial Mediterranean fever Glycogen storage disease, type III
Northern Europeans	Cystic fibrosis
Scandinavians	Alpha$_1$-antitrypsin deficiency LCAT (lecithin:cholesterol acyltransferase) deficiency
South African whites	Porphyria variegata Homozygous familial hypercholesterolemia

to relatives is less than in the single-gene (mendelian) disorders. Each of these categories presents different problems with respect to causation, prevention, diagnosis, genetic counseling, and treatment.

CHROMOSOMAL DISORDERS   The karyotype of an individual (i.e., the number and structure of the chromosomes) can be ascertained from readily accessible body tissues, such as peripheral blood lymphocytes or skin, by growing them in tissue culture until active cell proliferation occurs and then preparing single cells for examination of chromosomes by microscopy. Each individual chromosome can be identified by special staining of DNA sequences, e.g., by the affinity of fluorescent dyes (such as quinacrine hydrochloride) for certain chromosomal segments that can be visualized by fluorescence microscopy or by treatment with special dyes (Giemsa) and proteolytic enzymes (trypsin). These techniques produce characteristic *banding patterns* for each chromosome (Fig. 60-4).

The number of chromosomes in normal individuals is 46, of which 44 are the 22 pairs of *autosomes* and the other 2 are the *sex chromosomes*. Women have two X chromosomes (XX), and men have one X chromosome and one Y chromosome (XY). Each of the 22 pairs of autosomes and the 2 sex chromosomes can be distinguished on the basis of size, location of the centromere (which divides the chromosome into arms of equal or unequal length), and the unique banding pattern (Fig. 60-4). The relative length of the arms and the position of the centromere are used as further criteria to divide the human chromosomes into seven groups (designated A to G) (Fig. 60-4).

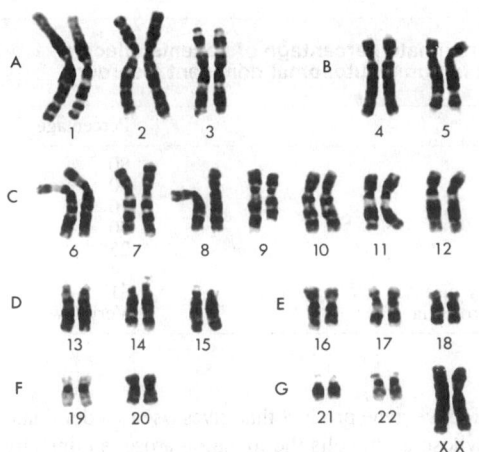

FIGURE 60-4 The karyotype of a normal woman showing the chromosomes of a single somatic cell in the metaphase stage of cell division. The photographic images of the chromosomes have been cut out and arranged according to descending length and varying arm ratio. The chromosomes have been stained by the Giemsa technique, which allows each chromosome pair to be identified by its unique banding pattern. Chromosomes 1 to 22 are the autosomes. The sex chromosomes in this normal female are both X. The normal male has an identical karyotype except for the absence of one X chromosome and the presence instead of one Y chromosome. (*Courtesy of David H. Ledbetter.*)

For a complete discussion of the etiology and clinical features of chromosomal abnormalities affecting humans, the reader is referred to Chap. 62.

SIMPLY INHERITED DISORDERS Disorders caused by the transmission of a single mutant gene show one of three simple (or mendelian) patterns of inheritance: (1) autosomal dominant, (2) autosomal recessive, or (3) X-linked. The distinction between "dominant" and "recessive" is one of convenience in pedigree analysis and does not imply a fundamental difference in genetic mechanism. The term *dominant* means that a mutation is clinically manifest when an individual has a single dose of this mutation (or is *heterozygous* for it), while *recessive* implies that a double dose (or *homozygosity*) is required for clinical detection. Genes are never dominant or recessive; their effects, however, produce clinical patterns that are classified as dominant or recessive. Despite their overall clinical "normality," individuals who are heterozygous for "recessive" genes often have biochemical abnormalities that are demonstrable in the laboratory; on the other hand, those who are homozygous for "dominant" genes are usually more severely affected than are the heterozygotes.

With few exceptions, each of the approximately 2500 mendelian diseases is rare. However, as a group, these disorders constitute an important cause of morbidity and death, accounting directly for more than 5 percent of all hospital admissions.

The genes for more than 450 simply inherited diseases have been assigned to specific chromosomes. Disease-producing genes assigned to the X chromosome outnumber those so far assigned to any single autosome. This is so because assignment to the X chromosome requires only pedigree studies showing X-linked inheritance (see below). Assignment to an autosome is more complicated, requiring sophisticated techniques of somatic cell hybridization or pedigree studies showing linkage between a disease-producing gene and a "marker" gene that is known to be on a certain chromosome.

Several hundred disease-producing genes have been cloned and analyzed at the molecular level. The vast majority of these genes, such as those responsible for the hemoglobinopathies, familial hypercholesterolemia, and glucose-6-phosphate dehydrogenase deficiency, have been identified after the protein product was characterized biochemically and functionally. In the past few years, a new strategy for cloning disease genes has emerged. This approach depends on first mapping the responsible gene to its correct chromosomal location

by means of linkage analysis or deletion mapping in affected patients. The relevant segment of DNA is then cloned, and the gene is identified by strategies designed to localize transcribed regions within the DNA segment. The sequence of the gene is thus obtained even before the protein has been identified. Inferences about the protein's function are drawn from the predicted protein sequence. This approach, originally referred to as *reverse genetics*, is more accurately called *positional cloning*. The first 13 disease genes that have been cloned and characterized by positional cloning are shown in Table 60-2.

The demonstration that a particular disease or syndrome shows one of the three mendelian patterns of inheritance implies that its pathogenesis, no matter how complex, is due to an abnormality in a single protein molecule. For example, in sickle cell anemia, the entire clinical syndrome, including such seemingly unrelated disturbances as anemia, pain crises, nephropathy, and predisposition to pneumococcal infections, is the consequence of having thymine instead of adenine at a specific site in the gene that codes for the β chain of hemoglobin, producing a substitution of a valine for a glutamic acid in the sixth amino acid position in the protein sequence.

In many mendelian disorders, especially in those with dominant inheritance, it is not possible to demonstrate directly the protein that is primarily altered by the mutation. In such cases (e.g., adult polycystic kidney disease and tuberous sclerosis), only the distal physiologic effects of the mutation are recognizable. Nevertheless, it is safe to assume that a single primary defect exists whenever a disease is transmitted by a single-gene mechanism and that the various manifestations of the disease all can be related to the mutational event by a more or less complicated "pedigree of causes." Table 60-3 lists the most commonly encountered mendelian disorders affecting adults.

Autosomal dominant disorders Dominant diseases are those manifest in the heterozygous state, i.e., when only one abnormal gene (*mutant allele*) is present and the corresponding partner allele on the homologous chromosome is normal. The gene responsible for an autosomal dominant disorder is located on one of the 22 autosomes, and both males and females can be affected. Since alleles segregate independently at meiosis, there is a 1 in 2 chance that the offspring of an affected heterozygote will inherit the mutant allele and, similarly, a 1 in 2 chance of the offspring inheriting the normal allele.

A typical pedigree involving an autosomal dominant trait is shown in Fig. 60-5. The following features are characteristic: (1) Each affected individual has an affected parent (unless the condition arose by a new mutation or is mildly expressed in the affected parent); (2) an affected individual will bear, on average, both normal and affected offspring in equal proportions; (3) normal children of an affected individual will have only normal offspring; (4) males and females are affected in equal proportions; (5) each sex is equally likely to transmit the condition to male and female offspring, with male-to-male transmission occurring; and (6) vertical transmission of the condition through successive generations occurs, especially when the trait does not impair reproductive capacity.

TABLE 60-2 Some disease genes identified by positional cloning

Disease locus	Chromosomal location	Date of identification
Chronic granulomatous disease	X	1986
Duchenne's muscular dystrophy	X	1986
Retinoblastoma	13	1986
Cystic fibrosis	7	1989
Wilm's tumor	11	1990
Sex determining gene	Y	1990
Choroideremia	X	1990
Fragile-X syndrome (mental retardation)	X	1991
Familial polyposis coli	5	1991
Kallman syndrome	X	1991
Aniridia	11	1991
Myotonic dystrophy	19	1991

TABLE 60-3   Some relatively frequent mendelian disorders affecting adults

AUTOSOMAL DOMINANT DISORDERS

Familial hypercholesterolemia
Hereditary hemorrhagic telangiectasia
Marfan's syndrome
Hereditary spherocytosis
Adult polycystic kidney disease
Huntington's chorea
Acute intermittent porphyria
Osteogenesis imperfecta tarda
von Willebrand's disease
Myotonic dystrophy
Idiopathic hypertrophic subaortic stenosis (IHSS)
Noonan's syndrome
Neurofibromatosis
Tuberous sclerosis

AUTOSOMAL RECESSIVE DISORDERS

Deafness
Albinism
Wilson's disease
Hemochromatosis
Sickle cell anemia
β Thalassemia
Cystic fibrosis
Hereditary emphysema (alpha$_1$-antitrypsin deficiency)
Homocystinuria
Familial Mediterranean fever
Friedreich's ataxia
Phenylketonuria

X-LINKED DISORDERS

Hemophilia A
Glucose-6-phosphate dehydrogenase deficiency
Fabry's disease
Ocular albinism
Testicular feminization
Chronic granulomatous disease
Hypophosphatemic rickets
Fragile-X syndrome (mental retardation)
Color blindness

TABLE 60-4   Approximate percentage of patients affected by new mutations in some autosomal dominant disorders

Disorder	Percentage
Achondroplasia	80
Tuberous sclerosis	80
Neurofibromatosis	40
Marfan's syndrome	30
Myotonic dystrophy	25
Huntington's chorea	4
Adult polycystic kidney disease	1
Familial hypercholesterolemia	Very low

however, cause a defective gene product that gives rise to a dominant trait. The parent in whose germ cells the mutation arose is clinically normal. Likewise, the siblings of the affected individual are normal, since the mutation affects only a single germ cell. However, the affected individual transmits the disease to half of his or her children.

The proportion of patients with dominant disorders who represent new mutations is inversely proportional to the effect of the disease in question on biologic fitness. The term *biologic fitness* refers to the ability of an affected individual to produce children who survive to adult life and reproduce. In the extreme case, if a dominant mutation produced absolute infertility, then all observed cases would, of necessity, represent new mutations, and it would be impossible to prove the genetic transmission of the trait. In less severe disorders, as in tuberous sclerosis, the severe mental retardation reduces biologic fitness to about 20 percent of normal, and the proportion of cases due to new mutations is about 80 percent. Other examples of the relation between biologic fitness and the proportion of new mutations in dominant disorders are shown in Table 60-4.

Many new mutations appear to occur in the germ cells of fathers who are of relatively advanced age. Such a "paternal age effect" is seen, for example, in Marfan's syndrome, in which the average age of fathers of sporadic or "new mutation" cases (37 years) is in excess of the mean age of fathers generally (30 years) and also in excess of the age of fathers who transmit Marfan's disease due to an inherited mutation (30 years).

Before one concludes that a dominant disorder in a given patient with unaffected parents is the result of a new mutation, it is important to consider two other possibilities: (1) that the gene may be carried by one parent in whom the disease is of low expressivity (discussed below) and (2) that extramarital paternity may have occurred. The latter is found in about 3 to 5 percent of randomly studied children in the United States.

Most autosomal dominant disorders show two characteristic features that are not usually seen in recessive syndromes: (1) *delayed age of onset* and (2) *variability in clinical expression*. Delayed age of onset is seen in disorders such as Huntington's chorea and adult polycystic kidney disease. These disorders do not manifest clinically until adult life, even though the mutant gene is present from the time of conception. Variability in clinical expression is illustrated dramatically by the multiple endocrine neoplasia syndrome. Patients in the same family inheriting the same abnormal gene may have hyperplasia or neoplasia of one or more endocrine glands (including the pancreas, parathyroid glands, and pituitary gland) as well as of adipose tissue. The resulting clinical manifestations are diverse; different members of the same family may develop peptic ulcers, hypoglycemia, kidney stones, multiple lipomas of the skin, or bitemporal hemianopsia. The recognition that each family member ṣuffers from the same genetic abnormality can be difficult, as ...ated by the family pedigree in Fig. 60-6.

Dominant mutations involve a type of gene product that produces clinical symptoms when only 50 percent of the gene product is defective. The defective genes usually do not encode enzymes, since a 50 percent deficiency of most enzymes produces no symptoms (see "Recessive Disorders" below). Rather, dominant diseases are likely

While half the offspring of an individual with an autosomal dominant condition will inherit the disease, it is not necessarily true that each affected person must have an affected parent. In every autosomal dominant disease a certain proportion of affected persons owe their disorder to a new mutation rather than to an inherited mutation. Since the estimated frequency of mutation is 5×10^{-6} mutations per gene per generation, and since a dominant trait, by definition, requires a mutation in only one of a pair of alleles, one would expect that about 1 in 100,000 newborn persons would possess a new mutation at any given genetic locus. Many of these mutations either do not impair the function of the gene product or involve a recessive function so that the mutation is clinically silent. Others,

FIGURE 60-5   Pedigree pattern of an autosomal dominant trait. Note the *vertical* pattern of inheritance.

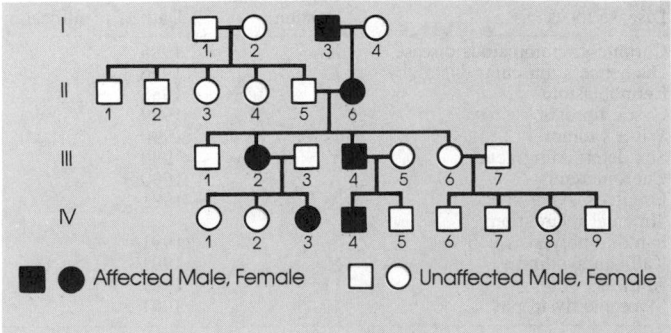

■ ● Affected Male, Female   □ ○ Unaffected Male, Female

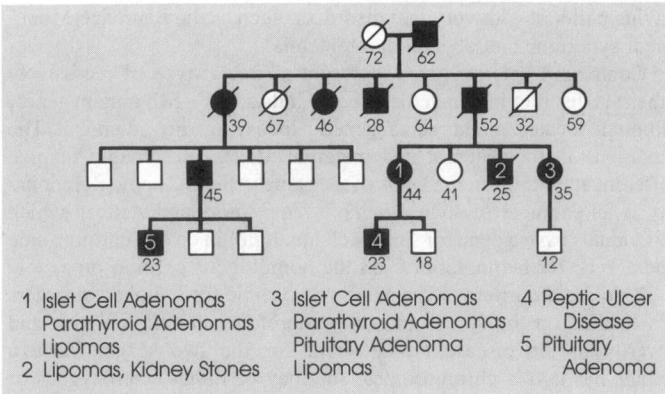

1 Islet Cell Adenomas
  Parathyroid Adenomas
  Lipomas
2 Lipomas, Kidney Stones

3 Islet Cell Adenomas
  Parathyroid Adenomas
  Pituitary Adenoma
  Lipomas

4 Peptic Ulcer
  Disease

5 Pituitary
  Adenoma

FIGURE 60-6 Pedigree of a family affected with the multiple endocrine neoplasia, type 1 (MEN-1) syndrome, a disorder inherited as an autosomal dominant trait. Circles denote females; squares, males. Open circles and squares denote unaffected relatives; closed circles and squares denote affected relatives. Deceased relatives are indicated by the oblique line. The age of each relative is indicated below his or her symbol. Note the marked variation in clinical expression among living affected heterozygotes.

to involve abnormalities in two classes of proteins: (1) those which regulate complex metabolic pathways, such as membrane receptors and rate-limiting enzymes in pathways under feedback control, and (2) key structural proteins, such as hemoglobin or collagen.

The basic biochemical defects have been identified in only a handful of the approximately 600 autosomal dominant disorders. These include familial hypercholesterolemia (abnormal cell surface receptor that binds plasma low-density lipoprotein and thereby regulates cholesterol metabolism); Marfan's syndrome (abnormal fibrillin molecule); osteogenesis imperfecta (abnormal collagen molecule); hereditary methemoglobinemia and several hemolytic anemias due to unstable forms of hemoglobin (abnormal hemoglobin molecule); hereditary angioedema (abnormal protein inhibitor of an enzyme involved in the serum complement system); acute intermittent porphyria (abnormal enzyme that catalyzes a rate-limiting step in the heme biosynthetic pathway); and pseudohypoparathyroidism, type 1 (abnormal guanine nucleotide-binding regulatory component or G-protein of the adenylate cyclase system).

Autosomal recessive disorders Autosomal recessive conditions are clinically apparent only in the homozygous state, i.e., when both alleles at a particular genetic locus are mutant. By definition, the gene responsible for an autosomal recessive disorder must be on one of the 22 autosomes; thus both males and females can be affected.

A pedigree in which an autosomal recessive trait is present in the family is shown in Fig. 60-7. The following features are characteristic: (1) The parents are clinically normal; (2) only siblings are affected and vertical transmission does not occur; and (3) males and females are affected in equal proportions.

FIGURE 60-7 Pedigree pattern of an autosomal recessive trait. Note the *horizontal* pattern of inheritance.

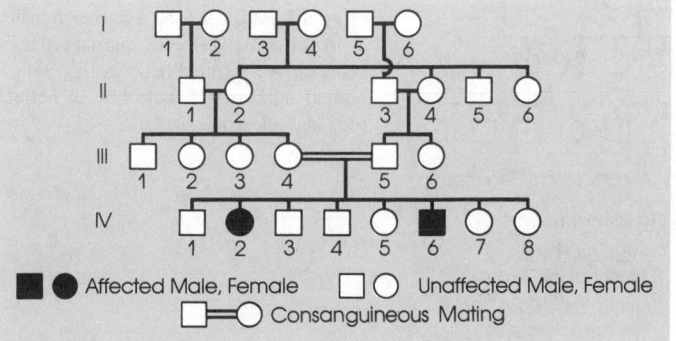

■● Affected Male, Female   □○ Unaffected Male, Female
□═○ Consanguineous Mating

The relative infrequency of recessive genes in the population and the requirement for two abnormal genes for clinical expression combine to create special conditions for autosomal recessive inheritance: (1) The more infrequent the mutant gene in the population, the stronger is the likelihood that affected individuals are the product of consanguineous matings (see below); (2) if a husband and a wife are both carriers for the same autosomal recessive gene, 25 percent of the children will be normal, 50 percent will be heterozygous carriers, and 25 percent will be homozygous and affected with the disease; (3) if an affected individual marries a heterozygote (as may occur with consanguineous marriage), half the children will be affected, and a pedigree simulating dominant inheritance will result; and (4) if two individuals with the same recessive disease marry, all their children will be affected.

The clinical picture in autosomal recessive disorders tends to be more uniform than that of dominant diseases, and the age of onset is often early in life. As a general rule, recessive disorders are more commonly diagnosed in children, while dominant diseases are more frequently encountered in adults.

Since with recessive inheritance only one of four children in a sibship is expected to be affected, multiple cases in a family may not occur. This is especially true in a society in which small families are common. Consider, for example, 16 families in which both parents are heterozygous for the same recessive disorder. If each family has two children, 9 of the families will have no affected children, 6 will have one affected and one normal child, and only 1 of the 16 families will have two affected children. In the United States, physicians usually see sporadic or isolated cases of a recessive disorder without an affected sibling to alert them to the possibility of a genetic disorder. Fortunately, because of the relatively uniform clinical picture of recessive disorders, and because most can be diagnosed directly by biochemical tests, the correct diagnosis usually can be made even when no other members of a family are clinically affected.

The basic biochemical lesions underlying many autosomal recessive disorders have been identified. Of the three types of proteins in which mutations could occur (i.e., enzymes, structural proteins, and regulatory proteins), the enzymes have been the easiest to study. A mutation that destroys the catalytic activity of an enzyme generally does not impair the health of a heterozygote (i.e., an individual who has one mutant allele specifying a functionless enzyme and one normal allele on the partner chromosome specifying a normal enzyme). In this situation, each cell in the body usually produces about 50 percent of the normal number of active enzyme molecules. However, normal regulatory mechanisms function to avert any clinical consequences of this 50 percent deficiency, and so heterozygotes·usually are clinically normal. On the other hand, when an individual inherits functionless alleles at both loci specifying an enzyme, the reduction in enzyme activity is too great for a compensatory mechanism to overcome, and a disease results. For example, heterozygotes for phenylketonuria have half the normal activity of phenylalanine hydroxylase, but they are clinically asymptomatic because the body compensates for the half-normal level of the enzyme by raising the substrate concentration approximately twofold. Under these conditions, a normal amount of phenylalanine can be metabolized with no symptoms. On the other hand, the homozygote for phenylketonuria has such a severe reduction in phenylalanine hydroxylase activity that enormous levels of phenylalanine and its derivatives accumulate, causing detrimental brain development. As in the case of phenylketonuria, the majority of enzyme deficiency states produce *simultaneously* both a simple accumulation of one or more metabolites preceding the enzymatic block and a deficient production of other metabolites distal to the block in the metabolic pathway.

Most of the genetic enzyme deficiencies that have been elucidated are not only inherited as recessive traits but also tend to involve enzymes that participate in catabolic pathways. Frequently these enzymes degrade organic molecules that are ingested in the diet, such as galactose (galactosemia), phenylalanine (phenylketonuria), and phytanic acid (Refsum's syndrome). A special class of such catabolic diseases is that in which the deficiency affects an acid hydrolase that occurs within lysosomes. In these *lysosomal storage disorders* the substrate, usually a complex lipid or polysaccharide, accumulates within swollen lysosomes in specific organs, giving the cells a foamy appearance. Examples of such lysosomal diseases include the mucopolysaccharidoses such as Hurler's syndrome (α-iduronidase deficiency) and the lipid storage diseases such as Gaucher's disease (glucocerebrosidase deficiency) (see Chap. 349).

In general, recessive diseases are rare because the reduced biologic fitness of homozygotes acts to remove the mutant gene from the population. However, a few recessive disorders, such as cystic fibrosis and sickle cell anemia, are common. To explain this paradox, it has been postulated that the biologic fitness of heterozygotes is greater than that of noncarriers for these genes. In such a case, the frequency of the gene in the population depends on the balance between the increased fitness of the relatively numerous heterozygotes and the reduced fitness of the less common homozygotes. A small selective advantage of the heterozygote over the normal results in a high gene frequency and hence a high birth frequency of homozygotes even when the disease is lethal. Thus about 1 in 22 Caucasians is a heterozygous carrier for the genetically lethal disease cystic fibrosis, and the disease occurs in about 1 in 2000 Caucasian births. To maintain such a high gene frequency, heterozygotes for cystic fibrosis must have a definite reproductive advantage over noncarriers, but the nature of this advantage is unknown. In sickle cell anemia, another recessive disorder with high frequency among certain populations, heterozygotes appear to have increased resistance to malaria.

Inasmuch as recessive diseases require the inheritance of a mutation at the same genetic locus from each parent, when the genes are rare, the likelihood of any two parents being carriers for the same defect becomes small. However, if the parents have a common ancestor and if that ancestor was a carrier for the recessive gene, then the likelihood that two of the descendants have inherited the gene becomes relatively great. The rarer the recessive gene, the stronger is the likelihood that an affected individual will have resulted from such a consanguineous mating. On the other hand, certain recessive genes are so common in the population that the likelihood of two random parents being carriers is great enough to eliminate the need for consanguinity. For common traits such as sickle cell anemia, phenylketonuria, cystic fibrosis, and Tay-Sachs disease, all of which have a high carrier frequency in certain populations, consanguinity in the parents is unusual.

In general, consanguinity is infrequent in families with recessive diseases in the United States. This is so because the rate of consanguinity in the general population is low. In most of the United States (as opposed to areas with relative geographic isolation such as northern Norway and Switzerland), a disorder must indeed be rare before it is associated with a high frequency of consanguinity. For example, consanguinity is expected in a large proportion of families having children with very rare disorders, such as the Laurence-Moon-Biedl syndrome and abetalipoproteinemia.

Compound heterozygotes represent a special type of recessively inherited disorder in which the affected individual's two mutant genes, although located at the same genetic locus, are not identical. The mutations in the paternal and maternal alleles presumably involve different alterations in the DNA of the same gene. SC hemoglobinopathy is an example of such a *heteroallelic* compound state in which individuals have a gene for sickle cell hemoglobin on one chromosome and a gene for hemoglobin C on the homologous chromosome.

X-linked disorders The genes responsible for X-linked disorders are located on the X chromosome; therefore, the clinical risk and severity of the disease are different for the two sexes. Since a female has two X chromosomes, she may be either heterozygous or homozygous for a mutant gene, and the trait may therefore demonstrate either recessive or dominant expression. Males, on the other hand, have only one X chromosome, so they can be expected to display the full syndrome whenever they inherit the gene regardless of whether the gene behaves as a recessive or as a dominant trait in the female. Thus the terms *X-linked dominant* or *X-linked recessive* refer only to the expression of the gene in women.

An important feature of all X-linked inheritance is the absence of male-to-male (i.e., father-to-son) transmission of the trait. This follows because a male must always contribute his Y chromosome to his sons; hence he can never contribute his X chromosome. On the other hand, a male contributes his one X chromosome to all his daughters.

The pedigree in Fig. 60-8 illustrates the characteristic features of X-linked recessive inheritance. (1) In contrast to the vertical transmission in dominant traits (parents and children affected) and the horizontal transmission in autosomal recessive traits (siblings affected), the pedigree pattern in X-linked recessive traits tends to be oblique because of the occurrence of the trait in the sons of normal carrier sisters of affected males (uncles and nephews affected) (Fig. 60-8A); (2) male offspring of carrier women have a 50 percent chance of being affected; (3) all female offspring of affected males are carriers, and affected males do not transmit the disease to their sons (Fig. 60-8C); (4) unaffected males do not transmit the trait to any offspring; and (5) affected homozygous females occur only when an affected male fathers the child of a carrier female (Fig. 60-8B).

Examples of X-linked recessive disorders in humans include hemophilia A, nephrogenic diabetes insipidus, the Lesch-Nyhan syndrome, Duchenne's muscular dystrophy, glucose-6-phosphate dehydrogenase deficiency, testicular feminization, and Fabry's disease. Color blindness is also inherited as an X-linked recessive trait, but it is so frequent (occurring in about 8 percent of white males) that the occurrence of homozygous color-blind females is no rarity.

X-linked dominant inheritance is illustrated by the pedigree in Fig. 60-9. Its characteristic features are as follows: (1) Females are

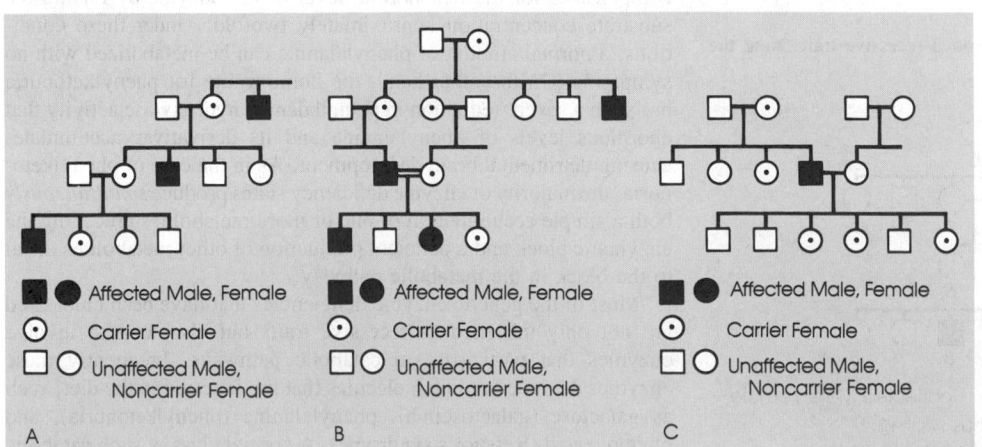

FIGURE 60-8 Pedigree patterns of an X-linked recessive trait. *A*. Note the oblique pattern of inheritance. *B*. An affected female can result from the mating of an affected male and a carrier female, as in the consanguineous marriage shown here. *C*. An affected male mating with a normal noncarrier female has all normal sons and all carrier daughters.

■ ● Affected Male, Female

⊙ Carrier Female

□ ○ Unaffected Male, Noncarrier Female

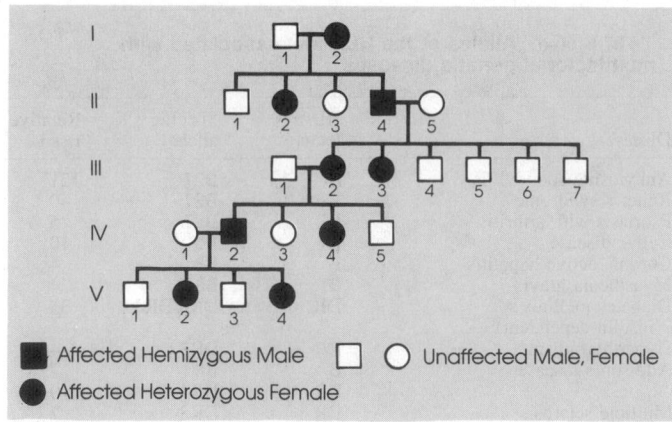

FIGURE 60-9   Pedigree pattern of an X-linked dominant trait.

affected about twice as often as males; (2) an affected female transmits the disorder to half her sons and half her daughters; (3) an affected male transmits the disorder to all his daughters and to none of his sons; and (4) the syndrome is more variable and less severe in heterozygous affected females than in hemizygous affected males. One common trait, the Xg(a+) blood group, is inherited as an X-linked dominant trait, as is hypophosphatemic rickets.

Some rare conditions may be inherited as X-linked dominant traits in which there is lethality in the hemizygous male. The characteristics of this form of inheritance are illustrated by the pedigree in Fig. 60-10: (1) The disorder occurs only in females who are heterozygous for the mutant gene; (2) an affected mother transmits the trait to half her daughters; and (3) an increased frequency of abortions occurs in affected women, the abortions representing affected male fetuses. Conditions that appear to be transmitted by this mode of inheritance include incontinentia pigmenti, focal dermal hypoplasia, orofaciodigital syndrome, and hyperammonemia due to ornithine transcarbamylase deficiency.

Expression of X-linked traits in females tends to be variable because of the phenomenon of X-chromosome inactivation. Early in embryonic development one of the two X chromosomes in each somatic cell of a female is inactivated. The inactivation process is random, so for each cell there is an equal probability that the paternally or maternally derived X chromosome will be inactivated. The inactivated X chromosome is rendered permanently nonfunctional, so all progeny of the initial cell inherit the same active and inactive X chromosomes. Thus each female is a mosaic; on average, half her cells express the X chromosome of the father, and half express the X chromosome of the mother. If a mutation in a gene is carried on one of the X chromosomes, about one-half of the cells in each tissue will be normal and the other half will manifest the mutant phenotype. However, chance or selection of one or the other set of clones of cells may disturb these proportions in any given individual. Depending on the proportions of mutant and normal X chromosomes in each tissue, a genetically heterozygous female may either be clinically

FIGURE 60-10   Pedigree pattern of an X-linked dominant trait lethal in the hemizygous male.

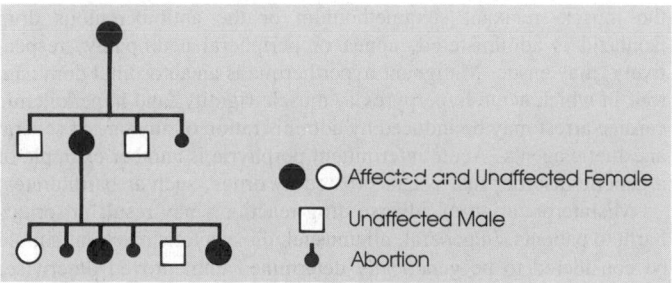

normal or have mild or severe manifestations of the disease. To illustrate, mothers of boys with the X-linked recessive Duchenne muscular dystrophy may occasionally show mild manifestations of the disease, such as limb girdle weakness or hypertrophied calves.

In each female cell the nonfunctional X chromosome can be visualized by several techniques. By ordinary staining, the inactivated X chromosome in metaphase appears heteropyknotic (condensed in appearance), and it replicates late in the mitotic cycle ("late-labeling" with tritiated thymidine). In nondividing cells the inactivated X chromosome can be observed as a clump of chromatin at the periphery of the nucleus—the so-called X chromatin or Barr body. In abnormal states with more than two X chromosomes such as 47,XXX, all but one of the X chromosomes are inactivated, so female cells may have multiple X chromatin bodies (see Chap. 62).

Since a single mutant allele is sufficient for the expression of X-linked recessive disorders, consanguinity does not increase the likelihood of expression in males, unlike the case in the rare autosomal recessive disorders. On the other hand, just as in the dominantly inherited disorders, new mutations can be a factor. In general, if an X-linked recessive condition reduces biologic fitness to zero, one-third of affected males will be a result of new mutations, and an additional one-third will be born to mothers who themselves are carriers as a result of a new mutation. Thus only one-third will come from a classic pedigree manifesting oblique transmission. An example of such a disease is Duchenne's muscular dystrophy in which affected hemizygous males are so severely disabled that they never reproduce. In hemophilia A, in which the biologic fitness is greater than zero, about 20 percent of affected males represent new mutations.

In families in which only one male is affected with an X-linked recessive disease and there is no other family history of the trait, it is essential for proper genetic counseling that the mother undergo biochemical tests or other relevant studies to determine whether she is a carrier. If she is a carrier, half her daughters will be carriers and half her sons will be affected. On the other hand, if her affected son represents a new mutation, only his daughters will inherit the gene. At present, biochemical tests can identify female carriers for several X-linked diseases, including the Lesch-Nyhan syndrome, Fabry's disease, Hunter's syndrome, hemophilia, testicular feminization, fragile X syndrome, and Duchenne's muscular dystrophy.

The distinction between X-linked inheritance and *sex-influenced autosomal dominant inheritance* is important. Baldness is probably inherited as an autosomal dominant trait, yet it is manifested mainly in men and rarely in women. Heterozygous females express the baldness gene only when a source of testosterone becomes available, as occurs with a virilizing tumor of the ovary.

MULTIFACTORIAL GENETIC DISEASES   The common chronic diseases of adults (such as essential hypertension, coronary heart disease, diabetes mellitus, peptic ulcer disease, and schizophrenia) as well as the common birth defects (such as cleft lip and palate, spina bifida, and congenital heart disease) have been long known to "run in families." They fit best into the category of *multifactorial genetic diseases*. The genetic element in these disorders rarely manifests itself in an all-or-none fashion as it does in the simply inherited (mendelian) disorders and in chromosomal aberrations. Instead, it is the interaction of multiple genes with multiple environmental factors that produces the familial aggregation.

In the multifactorial genetic diseases, there is a *polygenic component* consisting of a series of genes that interact in a cumulative fashion. An individual who inherits the right combination of these genes passes beyond a "threshold of risk," at which point an *environmental component* determines whether and to what extent that person is clinically affected. In order for another individual in the same family to express the same syndrome, the same or a similar combination of genes must be inherited. Since the first-degree relatives of an affected individual (i.e., parents, siblings, and offspring) each share half that person's genes, they are all at increased risk of exhibiting the same polygenic syndrome. Second-degree relatives (uncles, aunts, and grandparents) share, on average, one-fourth of an individual's genes, that is, $(\frac{1}{2})^2$, and third-degree relatives (cousins) share one-eighth, that is, $(\frac{1}{2})^3$. Thus, as the degree of relation becomes more distant, the likelihood of a relative inheriting the same combination of genes becomes less. Moreover, the chances of any relative inheriting the right combination of risk genes decrease as the number of genes required for the expression of a given trait increases.

Since the precise number of genes responsible for polygenic traits is unknown, the risk of inheritance for a relative of an affected individual is difficult to calculate, and the standard is based on empiric risk figures (i.e., a direct tally of the proportion of affected relatives in previously reported families). In contrast to the simply inherited disorders, in which 25 or 50 percent of the first-degree relatives of an affected proband are at genetic risk, multifactorial genetic disorders are generally observed empirically to affect no more than 5 to 10 percent of first-degree relatives. Moreover, in contrast to mendelian traits, the recurrence risk of multifactorial conditions varies from family to family, and its estimation is significantly influenced by two factors: (1) the number of affected persons already present in the family and (2) the severity of the disorder in the index case. The greater the number of affected relatives and the more severe their disease, the higher is the risk to other relatives. For example, the risk of cleft lip in the siblings of a child with unilateral cleft lip is about 2.5 percent, but if the lesion in the index case is bilateral, the risk in the siblings rises to 6 percent. Table 60-5 lists the empiric risk figures for the familial recurrence of a number of multifactorial genetic diseases.

The hypothesis of a polygenic component in the inheritance of multifactorial diseases has been given a sound basis by the demonstration that at least one-third of all gene loci harbor polymorphic alleles that vary among individuals. Such a large degree of variation in normal genes undoubtedly provides the substrate for variations in genetic predisposition with which environmental factors can interact. So far, the genetic loci most strikingly associated with predisposition to specific diseases are those which constitute the HLA system (also called the *major histocompatibility gene complex*) (see Chap. 64). The HLA gene complex is located on the short arm of chromosome 6. It consists of four closely linked but distinct loci (A, B, C, and D). The products of these genes are proteins that are found on the surfaces of body cells and that enable an individual's immune system to distinguish its own cells from those of someone else. Each HLA locus in the population consists of multiple alleles, each of which produces an immunologically distinct protein. For example, an individual may inherit any 2 of 20 alleles at the HLA-B locus.

An important observation of recent years has been the finding that certain alleles at the HLA loci predispose individuals to certain specific diseases. For example, if the B27 allele at the HLA-B locus is inherited by an individual, that person has a 121-fold greater chance of developing ankylosing spondylitis than an individual who lacks this allele (Table 60-6). Ankylosing spondylitis remains a multifactorial disease, however, because its development clearly requires one or

more other factors in addition to the B27 allele. Thus less than 15 percent of people who inherit this allele develop this disease. Table 60-6 lists some of the diseases associated with alleles at the HLA loci. Several of them are suspected to be of viral etiology, suggesting that the HLA loci may dictate the mode of expression of certain viral diseases. A more detailed discussion of the HLA system is presented in Chap. 64.

Multifactorial disorders are heterogeneous in the sense that the relative contribution of the polygenic factors ("risk genes") and environmental factors to the etiology vary greatly from patient to patient. However, it is important to remember that among common phenotypes which are largely multifactorial, often a small proportion will be created by major mutant genes. For example, although coronary heart disease is usually of multifactorial etiology, about 5 percent of subjects with premature myocardial infarctions are heterozygotes for familial hypercholesterolemia, a single-gene disorder that produces atherosclerosis in the absence of any other predisposing factor. Similarly, in a small proportion of patients with other common diseases such as peptic ulcer disease or "essential" hypertension, the condition is not multifactorial but determined by a single gene, as in the multiple endocrine adenoma–peptic ulcer syndrome or the medullary thyroid carcinoma–pheochromocytoma syndrome, respectively.

INTERACTION BETWEEN SINGLE GENETIC AND ENVIRONMENTAL FACTORS

Many diseases result from an interaction between a specific genotype and a specific environmental factor. In particular, inherited single-gene mutations may produce clinically significant and often life-threatening idiosyncratic responses to certain drugs.

Table 60-7 lists the most important of these *pharmacogenetic disorders*, which encompass all the mendelian modes of inheritance. Perhaps the most common is glucose-6-phosphate dehydrogenase deficiency, an X-linked recessive trait in which a variety of drugs may precipitate a hemolytic anemia. Plasma pseudocholinesterase deficiency and hepatic transacetylase deficiency are examples of autosomal recessive traits which alter drug catabolism so that when the muscle relaxant suxamethonium or the antituberculous drug isoniazid is administered, apnea or peripheral neuropathy, respectively, may ensue. Malignant hyperthermia is an autosomal dominant trait in which acute hyperpyrexia, muscle rigidity, and hyperkalemic cardiac arrest may be induced by administration of any one of several anesthetic agents. Acute intermittent porphyria is another example of a genetic disorder that is exacerbated by drugs, such as barbiturates.

Misinterpretation of adverse drug reactions may result in serious harm to patients. In general, all unusual idiosyncratic reactions should be considered to be genetically determined until proved otherwise. Fortunately, the pharmacogenetic disorders are a group of diseases

TABLE 60-6   Alleles at the HLA loci associated with multifactorial genetic diseases

Disease	HLA locus	Specific allele	Relative risk*
Ankylosing spondylitis	B	B27	121
Reiter's syndrome	B	B27	40
Psoriasis with arthritis	B	B27	5
Celiac disease	B	B8	10
Chronic active hepatitis	B	B8	4
Myasthenia gravis	B	B8	4
Diabetes mellitus (insulin-dependent)	DR	DR3/DR4	33
Hyperthyroidism	DR	DR3	4
Addison's disease	B	B8	7
	DR	DR4	10
Multiple sclerosis	DR	DR2	7

* *Relative risk* is the probability of the disease developing in an individual with the specific allele, divided by the probability of its development in an individual who does not possess this specific allele.

TABLE 60-5   Empiric risks for some common multifactorial genetic diseases affecting adults

Disorder in index case	Estimated absolute risk for first-degree relatives, %
Cleft lip and/or palate	3
Congenital heart disease	4
Coronary heart disease	8 for male relatives 3 for female relatives
Diabetes mellitus	5–10
Epilepsy	5–10
Hypertension	10
Manic-depressive psychosis	10–15
Psoriasis	10–15
Schizophrenia	15
Thyroid disease (autoimmune disorders including hyperthyroidism, thyroiditis, primary myxedema, simple goiter)	10

TABLE 60-7 Examples of inherited disorders involving an abnormal response to drugs

Disorder	Molecular abnormality	Mode of inheritance	Frequency	Clinical effect	Drugs producing abnormal response
Slow inactivation of isoniazid	Isoniazid acetylase in liver	Autosomal recessive	50% of U.S. population	Polyneuritis	Isoniazid, sulfamethazine, sulfamaprine, phenelzine, dapsone, hydralazine
Suxamethonium sensitivity	Pseudocholinesterase in plasma	Autosomal recessive	Several mutant alleles; most common affects 1 in 2500	Apnea	Suxamethonium, succinylcholine
Warfarin insensitivity	? Altered receptor or enzyme in liver with increased affinity for vitamin K	Autosomal dominant	Rare	Inability to achieve anticoagulation with usual doses of drug	Warfarin
Glaucoma	Unknown	? Autosomal dominant	Common	Increased intraocular pressure	Glucocorticoids
Malignant hyperthermia	Ryanodine receptor	Autosomal dominant	1 in 20,000 anesthetized patients	Severe hyperpyrexia, muscle rigidity, death	Such anesthetics as halothane, succinylcholine, methoxyflurane, ether, cyclopropane
Unstable hemoglobins: Hemoglobin Zurich	Arginine substitution for histidine at sixty-third position of β chain of hemoglobin	Autosomal dominant	Rare	Hemolysis	Sulfonamides
Hemoglobin H	Hemoglobin composed of four β chains	Autosomal dominant	Rare	Hemolysis	Sulfisoxazole
Glucose-6-phosphate dehydrogenase deficiency	Glucose-6-phosphate dehydrogenase in erythrocytes	X-linked recessive	$\sim 1 \times 10^8$ affected persons in world; common in persons of African, Mediterranean, Asiatic origin; multiple mutant alleles	Hemolysis	Analgesics, sulfonamides, antimalarials, nitrofurantoin, other drugs

SOURCE: Modified from ES Vesell, N Engl J Med 287:904, 1972.

for which therapy is straightforward: avoidance of the noxious drug by patient and relatives.

In addition to drugs, other factors in the environment may aggravate specific genetic traits. Cigarette smoke may have deleterious effects on persons homozygous and possibly heterozygous for alpha$_1$-antitrypsin deficiency, who are predisposed to the development of emphysema. Patients with xeroderma pigmentosa and anhydrotic ectodermal dysplasia are unusually sensitive to sunlight and high temperatures, respectively. Avoidance of milk at an early age prevents many of the complications ordinarily seen in persons with galactosemia.

Genetic-environmental interactions are particularly important in pregnancy. Women who are affected with phenylketonuria may develop high plasma phenylalanine levels during pregnancy, and thus their offspring may suffer from a variety of phenylalanine-induced birth defects even though the offspring may not themselves have phenylketonuria. Other examples of diseases resulting from an adverse genetic relation between the mother and fetus include erythroblastosis caused by Rh incompatibility and *diabetic embryopathy*, a term that refers to a series of major birth defects occurring in about 5 percent of the offspring of women who are clinically diabetic during pregnancy.

REFERENCES

GELEHRTER TD, COLLINS FS: *Principles of Medical Genetics*. Baltimore, Williams & Wilkins, 1990

LEWIN B: *Genes*, 4th ed. New York, Wiley, 1990

MCKUSICK VA: *Mendelian Inheritance in Man: Catalogs of Autosomal Dominant, Autosomal Recessive and X-Linked Phenotypes*, 11th ed. Baltimore, Johns Hopkins University Press, 1992

SCRIVER CR et al: *The Molecular and Metabolic Basis of Inherited Disease*, 7th ed. New York, McGraw-Hill, in press

THOMPSON MW et al: *Genetics in Medicine*, 5th ed. Philadelphia, Saunders, 1991

VOGEL F, MOTULSKY AG: *Human Genetics: Problems and Approaches*, 2d ed. Berlin, Springer-Verlag, 1986

WEATHERALL DJ: *The New Genetics and Clinical Practice*, 3d ed. Oxford, Oxford University Press, 1991

61 MOLECULAR GENETICS AND MEDICINE

ARTHUR L. BEAUDET / ANDREA BALLABIO

The haploid human genome is comprised of approximately 3×10^9 (3 billion) base pairs of DNA and is estimated to contain 30,000 to 100,000 genes encoding a large number of protein products. Each individual inherits one copy of the genome from each parent. In the cell, the genomic DNA is packaged as 23 pairs of chromosomes, each containing a single linear duplex DNA molecule. Most of the DNA sequences that encode proteins occur as unique (single copy) sequences in the genome. These protein coding genes are usually divided into coding exons and intervening introns in the genomic DNA. The messenger RNA (mRNA) is formed by splicing the RNA to link the exon and eliminate the introns. Many genes and their products show similarities in nucleotide and amino acid sequence and can be viewed as members of large gene families, e.g., the globin gene family, the immunoglobulin superfamily, or the serine protease family. Many proteins contain domains that are functionally distinct and show sequence homology to related domains in other proteins. Complex genes are believed to have commonly arisen by reassortment of preexisting protein domains through a protein of "exon shuffling." A large amount of DNA in the genome *appears* not to be functional, and hundreds, if not thousands, of repetitive DNA sequences of unknown function are present; some are dispersed, and some are clustered. The length of DNA frequently is quantitated in thousands of bases (kilobases, kb) or in millions of bases (megabases, Mb) so that the genome comprises 3 million kb or 3000 Mb.

If one were to print *one copy* of *one strand* of the haploid human genome, it would fill a text 170 times the size of *Harrison's*. The analogy of the human genome to a large text can be carried further. The text can be envisioned as being bound into 23 separate volumes of various sizes, each the equivalent of one chromosome. Individuals would inherit one paternal set of 23 volumes and one maternal set of 23 volumes. The mutation causing sickle cell anemia would be the equivalent of changing a single letter on one page of one volume, while deletion of the α-globin gene cluster in α-thalassemia might represent the equivalent of the loss of one or two pages of text in each set. The text can also be envisioned as having been copied over and over again for thousands of generations with frequent errors or alterations (mutations) being introduced and then passed to the progeny copies. Finally, to carry this analogy to the concept of crossing-over and linkage, one can envision a parent with two sets of 23 volumes needing to pass one set to an offspring. Each volume of each set will exchange parts with its corresponding partner at one to six sites per volume so that a unique 23 volume text comprised of mixed portions of the two available sets will be passed to the next generation. This results in the unique genotype that is the basis of genetic individuality.

The human genome is extraordinarily polymorphic so that the DNA of each individual (except identical twins) varies in millions of ways from the DNA of another. A polymorphic site or locus is any site in the genome that varies so much that more than 1 percent of the chromosomes have a sequence different from the most common sequence. Much of this variation involves single base substitutions (e.g., a C:G base pair versus a T:A base pair at a position). About 1 in 200 to 1 in 500 of the 3 billion base pairs in the genome is polymorphic, i.e., varies beyond the 1 percent criterion. Genetic variation or polymorphism includes the presence or absence of base pairs or longer segments. Genetic variation arises through single base mutation, deletion, insertion, unequal crossing-over, and other rearrangements of the DNA. This genetic variation gives rise to different alleles; an allele is defined as one of a series of possible alternative forms of a given gene, e.g., the sickle allele at the β-globin locus. The term allele is now commonly used to refer to differing DNA sequences for a DNA marker without regard to whether this occurs in a gene or not, as will be discussed below.

What are the phenotypic effects of this extensive variation in DNA? There is a tendency to think of the common variations in DNA and protein (i.e., the polymorphisms) as benign and without phenotypic effect, and this belief is justified to some extent. DNA sequence is more conserved in protein coding regions and more variable in introns and intergenic regions. The vast majority of variations in DNA presumably have little or no phenotypic effect, although they provide DNA markers of clinical utility as discussed below. Another class of genetic variation contributes to racial, ethnic, and individual differences but not in a way that affects health or susceptibility to disease. Of greater medical relevance are those genetic variations that affect disease susceptibility, often through the interaction of genes with nongenetic factors, giving rise to conditions of multifactorial etiology. This type of genetic variability contributes to the etiology and pathogenesis of most of the disease processes described in this textbook. Approximately 60 percent of individuals experience genetically influenced diseases during their lifetime, if multifactorial diseases of late onset are included. The separation between benign individuality and variation with subtle medical implications is often unclear, as exemplified by the variations in HLA loci and blood groups. Finally, in some instances a change (mutation) in the DNA of a single gene has a major phenotypic effect and causes a single gene defect or Mendelian disorder, since such disorders segregate in families according to simple Mendelian rules (see Chap. 60). Even for these "single gene" disorders, the phenotype is often influenced by genes at other loci and by nongenetic factors. Mutations causing single gene disorders can be common and exceed the 1 percent criterion for polymorphism (e.g., cystic fibrosis, sickle cell disease, and G6PD deficiency) so that polymorphism does not uniformly imply a benign circumstance. Although single gene disorders are the most obvious example of the role of genetic variation in disease processes, the genetic contribution to common multifactorial diseases is quantitatively more important, although more complex to unravel.

The molecular heterogeneity of individuals has an important implication for medical practice. Physicians should constantly be aware in their diagnostic and therapeutic activities that patients are as unique in biochemistry, physiology, pharmacologic responses, laboratory results, and disease processes as in their physiognomy and personality; everyone is different.

METHODS FOR ANALYSIS OF HUMAN DNA

Molecular analyses of clinical relevance rely on multiple features and strategies, including: (1) the ability to clone genes and DNA fragments using recombinant methods, (2) determination of the sequence of DNA fragments, (3) the specificity of nucleic acid hybridization, (4) the specificity of recognition sites of restriction endonucleases, and (5) the power of DNA amplification using the polymerase chain reaction. Various combinations of these capabilities are used for diverse diagnostic procedures.

MOLECULAR CLONING AND SEQUENCING The size, the complexity, and the variability of the human genome constitute barriers to the analysis of individual traits and genes. The feasibility for such analysis was greatly enhanced by the development of recombinant DNA technology, which allows for isolation of small DNA fragments and production of unlimited amounts of the cloned material. The methodology for gene cloning is now well established. Hundreds of human genes have been cloned, and progress in this regard has been extraordinary as the genes for cystic fibrosis, Marfan syndrome, polyposis of the colon, neurofibromatosis, myotonic dystrophy, fragile X mental retardation, Huntington's disease, and many other diseases have been cloned since the last edition of this text. Once cloned, the various genes and gene products can be utilized for studies of gene structure and function in normal and disease states with diagnostic, therapeutic, and research implications.

The cloning of DNA involves isolation of DNA fragments and their insertion into the nucleic acid from another biologic source (vector) for manipulation and propagation. The most widely used vectors are maintained in bacterial host cells and are based on bacterial plasmids or bacteriophage such as phage λ or M13, some variations of which (cosmids) can accommodate DNA fragments up to 45 kb in size. In addition, vectors designed to function as yeast artificial chromosomes are maintained in yeast host cells and can be utilized for cloning DNA fragments up to hundreds of kilobases in size. Space does not allow presentation of the various methods for DNA cloning, but these are well described in Watson et al.

Most genes encode proteins and are divided into coding exons and intervening introns in the genomic DNA. The messenger RNA (mRNA) from a gene is spliced to link the coding segments, and it is often useful to copy mRNA in vitro to synthesize cDNA (DNA complementary to mRNA) for analysis and cloning. Genomic DNA and cDNA clones have been isolated for hundreds of human genes. In addition, many hundreds of *anonymous* genomic DNA clones are in widespread use. These anonymous DNA clones are generally of interest because they represent a unique site in the genome and often are associated with polymorphic markers that map to that site, as will be discussed below. Radioactive, biotinylated, or otherwise modified copies of DNA can be prepared from any cloned fragment and can serve as specific molecular *probes*. Radioactive probes can be detected by autoradiography, and biotinylated probes can be detected with avidin and secondary detection methods. Sequencing of DNA is readily accomplished using manual or semiautomated methods. The amino acid sequence of a protein can be deduced from the cDNA sequence and frequently provides insight into the function of a gene. If a gene is cloned, it is relatively straightforward to analyze the DNA from a patient to determine if the sequence deviates from the normal. The availability of sequence data allows for the use of the polymerase chain reaction for DNA amplification. Thus, some of the fruits of molecular cloning are the availability of probes for analytical procedures, the availability of DNA sequence data both to deduce protein sequence and to allow for DNA amplification (see below), and the ability to analyze for disease mutations.

NUCLEIC ACID HYBRIDIZATION Many of the steps in recombinant DNA analysis take advantage of the complementary nature of nucleic acid interaction which is so essential for the synthesis of DNA and RNA (see Chap. 60). Linear pieces of double-stranded (native) DNA can be treated with heat or alkali to dissociate the two strands to yield single-stranded (denatured) DNA. When a strand is incubated under conditions that allow for nucleic acid hybridization, bases of the denatured DNA recognize complementary bases, and reformation of double-stranded molecules by base pairing takes place. Nucleic acid hybridization is so sensitive that a single-stranded DNA molecule can be hybridized specifically to a complementary strand of RNA or DNA present at about 1 part in 10,000. Many recombinant DNA studies involve the preparation of one radioactive or biotinylated strand of nucleic acid that is then used as a "probe" in the analysis. It is possible to identify and distinguish both fully homologous and partially homologous sequences. The specificity of nucleic acid hybridization, often in combination with fractionation or amplification procedures, allows detection of a single gene among tens of thousands or of a sequence from an infectious organism that may be present at a frequency of less than one copy per human cell.

A variation of nucleic acid hybridization involves the use of allele-specific oligonucleotides (ASO). The ASO probe is a synthetic, single-stranded oligonucleotide, usually 15 to 20 bases in length. Two probes are synthesized, usually differing at a mutation site by a single base, one perfectly matching the normal sequence and one perfectly matching the mutant sequence, with the variable nucleotide in the midportion of the oligonucleotide. Hybridization conditions are adjusted so that the oligonucleotide detects a perfectly matched sequence but fails to hybridize if there is a single base mismatch. Allele-specific oligonucleotides can be used in combination with Southern blotting or in combination with DNA amplification, as described below.

RESTRICTION ENDONUCLEASES The discovery in microorganisms of restriction endonucleases, commonly known as *restriction enzymes,* facilitated recombinant DNA manipulations. These enzymes recognize a specific short sequence in double-stranded DNA, typically 4 to 8 base pairs, and cleave the DNA at this site. Hundreds of enzymes are known, each recognizing a unique DNA sequence (Fig. 61-1). An example of an enzyme that recognizes sequences only four base pairs in length is *Hae*III, which cleaves the sequence 5′-GGCC-3′. By convention, only one strand of DNA is printed as the recognition site, but the enzymes recognize double-stranded DNA. The sequence specificity of restriction enzymes is a powerful tool in dissection of large genomes. When human DNA is digested with a particular restriction enzyme, hundreds of thousands of DNA fragments are generated with remarkable reproducibility. Such fragments can vary from a few base pairs to several thousand base pairs in length, depending on the enzyme used. Restriction enzymes that recognize a sequence only four base pairs long cleave the DNA into smaller fragments than enzymes that recognize longer sequences, since recognition sites of the former enzymes occur more often in a relatively random sequence. With the use of multiple restriction enzymes to analyze a particular segment of DNA, it is possible to construct a detailed map of restriction endonuclease cleavage sites for the region. Such a map can span a region of from hundreds to thousands of base pairs of DNA. Enzymes that cut DNA infrequently can be used to prepare DNA maps over megabase distances. As

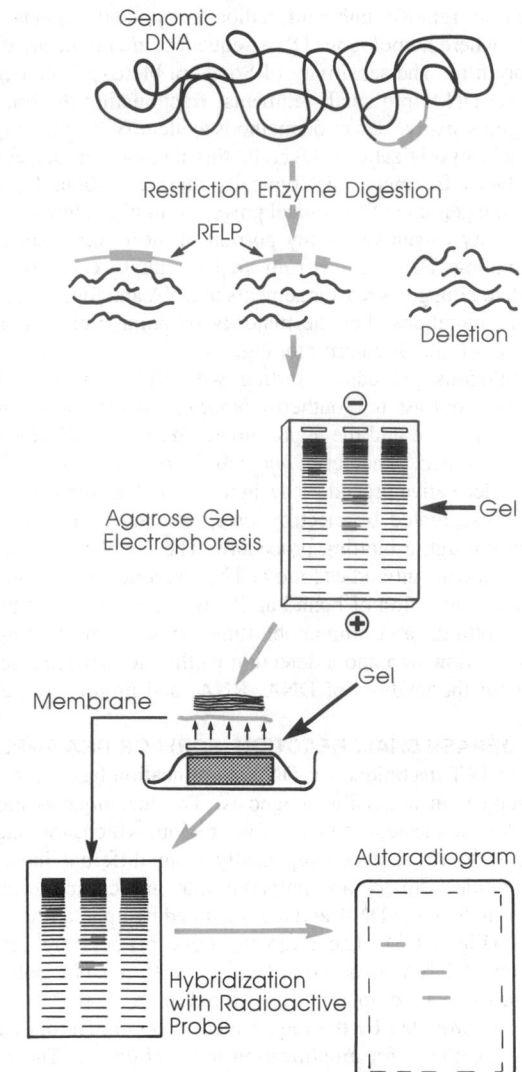

FIGURE 61-2 Southern blotting analysis of genomic DNA.

described below, variations in the sequences of cleavage sites can be analyzed as polymorphisms or mutations in the genome.

SOUTHERN BLOTTING Many analyses of the human genome utilize the blotting procedure developed by E. M. Southern, which involves hybridizing DNA in solution to DNA transferred to a membrane support. For clinical analysis, *Southern blotting* (Fig. 61-2) begins with the isolation of genomic DNA from any source but frequently from peripheral leukocytes or fetal cells. The high-molecular-weight genomic DNA is digested with a restriction enzyme to yield a series of reproducible fragments. These DNA fragments are separated by electrophoresis in agarose gels, and the DNA is transferred from the gel through the capillary action of a blotting procedure to a membrane that binds the DNA tightly. The membrane is treated to denature the DNA and is soaked in a solution containing a radioactive or otherwise labelled single-stranded nucleic acid probe. The probe will form a double-stranded nucleic acid complex at sites on the membrane where homologous DNA is present. The membrane

FIGURE 61-1 DNA sequence specificity and nuclease activity for three restriction endonucleases. Hae*III* leaves a blunt end while the other enzymes leave single-stranded ends.

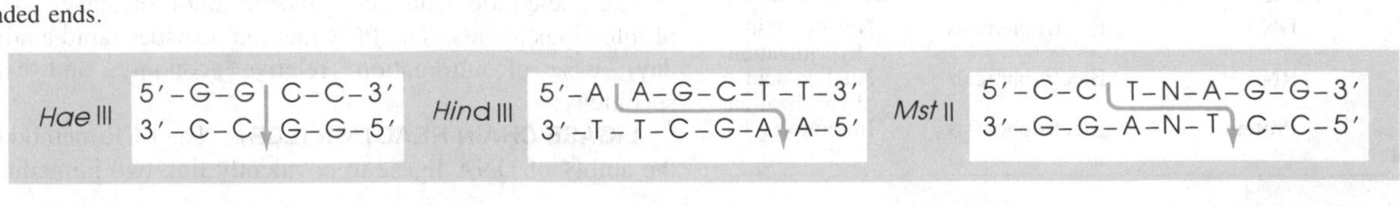

| *Hae* III | 5′–G–G C–C–3′
3′–C–C G–G–5′ | *Hind* III | 5′–A A–G–C–T–T–3′
3′–T–T–C–G–A A–5′ | *Mst* II | 5′–C–C T–N–A–G–G–3′
3′–G–G–A–N–T C–C–5′ |

is washed to remove unbound radioactivity, and regions on the membrane where homologous DNA sequences are bound are detected using x-ray film. The sensitivity of Southern blotting is enhanced by splitting the DNA into small segments, fractionating the fragments, and applying sensitive detection methods to identify specific fragments (nucleic acid hybridization). Overall, this method can detect unique genomic DNA fragments that typically represent about 1 part in 1 million in the genome. The clinical power of Southern blotting resides in the capacity to analyze a tiny portion of the primary structure of human genomic DNA taken from an individual. The procedure is ideal for detecting gross rearrangements in DNA and for distinguishing some point mutations, but the majority of point mutations are not detected by routine Southern blotting.

An analogous procedure starting with RNA has been termed *northern* (in contrast to Southern) *blotting*. In this procedure, the presence or absence and the approximate size of a particular mRNA can be determined. The term *immunoblotting* or *western blotting* describes a derivative procedure designed to analyze protein antigens. Proteins are separated by electrophoresis and transferred to a solid membrane through a blotting procedure. The membrane is analyzed by incubation with antibodies followed by a second step for enzymatic or radioactive detection of bound antibody. Thus, Southern blotting, northern blotting, and immunoblotting or western blotting each combines fractionation and a detection method to provide a sensitive technique for the analysis of DNA, RNA, and protein, respectively (Table 61-1).

POLYMERASE CHAIN REACTION (PCR) FOR DNA AMPLIFICATION   The PCR technique for DNA amplification has had a revolutionary impact on molecular diagnosis. The technique is based on knowing the nucleic acid sequence for a region, which, for diagnostic purposes, is to be analyzed repeatedly from different individuals. Oligonucleotide primers are prepared that are complementary to opposite strands of the DNA and are separated by up to a few hundred base pairs (Fig. 61-3). The oligonucleotide primers are incubated with the target DNA to be amplified and with a DNA polymerase that synthesizes a complementary strand in a 5'-to-3' direction. Specificity is provided by the requirement that primers must lead to convergent synthesis for amplification to be effective. The reaction is subjected to a sequence of temperature variations including a denaturing temperature where double-stranded DNA is dissociated to single-stranded DNA, an annealing temperature where oligonucleotide primers hybridize to target DNA, and a polymerization temperature for the synthetic step. The reaction is usually carried out using a thermostable polymerase so that the polymerase remains active during the temperature cycles (usually ranging from 50 to 95°C). After a number of such cycles, typically 20 to 30 or more, hundreds of thousands of copies of the original target sequence are synthesized as depicted in Fig. 61-3. The bulk of the product is a double-stranded DNA fragment of specific length. The technique is so sensitive that it can be used to amplify and analyze DNA from a single human sperm which contains one duplex target DNA molecule. PCR is easily performed with minimal preparation of crude and even degraded samples allowing analysis from whole blood, dried blood filters, mouthwash, old tissue sections, and other sources. Molecular diagnosis with PCR can include: (1) determining the presence or the absence of an amplified product, (2) digesting the amplified product with a

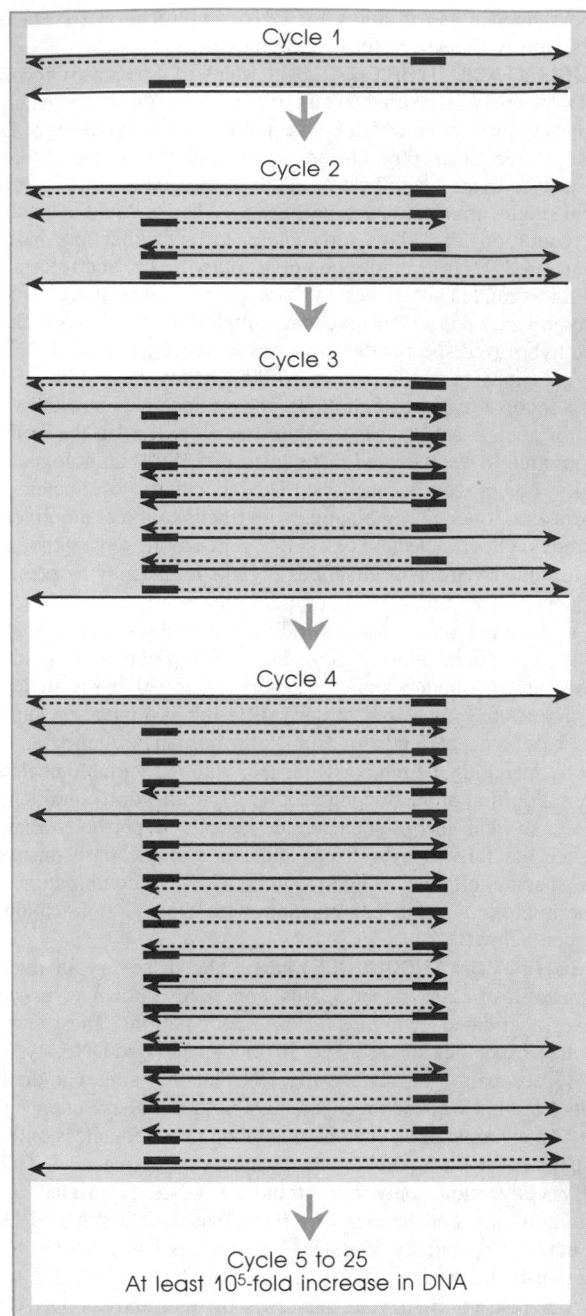

FIGURE 61-3 Polymerase chain reaction for amplification of DNA. The target DNA is shown as a solid line in cycle 1. Newly synthesized DNA is indicated by dotted lines in each cycle. Primer oligonucleotides are indicated by solid rectangles. Each DNA strand is marked with an arrow indicating 5'-to-3' orientation.

restriction enzyme, (3) hybridizing the PCR product with allele-specific oligonucleotides, and (4) direct sequencing of the PCR product. Many variations have been devised to take advantage of the PCR concept. These include synthesis of cDNA from mRNA using reverse transcriptase followed by amplification of the cDNA. Single-stranded DNA can be synthesized by altering the ratio of the oligonucleotide primers. Other applications include preparation of recombinant DNA constructs, mutagenesis of cloned DNA, detection of rare nucleotide sequences, and detection of nucleotide sequences of infectious agents. The PCR method provides rapid analysis (single day), ease of automation, relative economy, and extraordinary specificity.

LIGASE CHAIN REACTION (LCR)   The LCR method is based on the ability of DNA ligase to covalently link two immediate adjacent

TABLE 61-1 Analytical blotting procedures

Blot method	Material analyzed	Fractionation	Detection
Southern	DNA	Electrophoresis	Nucleic acid hybridization
Northern	RNA	Electrophoresis	Nucleic acid hybridization
Western or immunoblot	Protein	Electrophoresis	Immunologic

In the figure, the following labels appear:
Cycle 1
Cycle 2
Cycle 3
Cycle 4
Cycle 5 to 25
At least 10⁵-fold increase in DNA

oligonucleotides hybridized to a longer template that can bind both oligonucleotides. For example, if four 20-mer oligonucleotides forming two complementary, adjacent pairs are incubated with a heat stable ligase and the reaction is subjected to temperature cycles similar to PCR, oligonucleotides will be ligated to yield two longer complementary 40-mer oligonucleotides dependent on the presence or absence of a longer DNA template in the reaction. One useful feature of LCR is the ability to distinguish templates with single base differences at the ligation site. By placing six oligonucleotides in the reaction (two common and complementary on one side of a mutation, plus two matching the normal sequence and two matching the mutant sequence on the opposite side with the mutation site at the end adjacent to the common oligonucleotides to be ligated), a genotype analysis for a single base mutation is easily determined by the presence or absence of products that reflect the normal and/or mutant template. LCR has the potential advantage over most forms of PCR that the presence or absence of a distinct product is diagnostic, and the product does not need further characterization, although PCR offers greater versatility for many procedures. LCR is particularly useful in screening for known mutations in any given population.

ANALYZING THE HUMAN GENOME

The human genome map is the topographical description of human genomic DNA. Traditionally, the map is divided into regions corresponding to the chromosomal bands of the 24 chromosomes (22 autosomes and X and Y).

As of early 1993, over 2500 loci have been assigned to specific positions on the human genetic map. The main information contained in the map is the relative order and distance of genetic markers and their positions within a defined region. Two types of maps containing this kind of information have been developed, the genetic and the physical maps. There is a major conceptual difference between the two; the first is an indirect statistical analysis based on genetic recombination, whereas the second hinges on direct measurement of the length of DNA.

THE GENETIC MAP AND THE PRINCIPLE OF GENETIC LINKAGE
Genetic linkage is essential for preparation of the map of the human genome, and it is used routinely for molecular diagnosis in the clinical setting. Genetic distance, which is expressed in centimorgans (cM), is a measure of the likelihood of crossover between two loci. Two loci are 1 cM apart if there is a 1 percent probability of a crossover between them at meiosis. There are on average 30 to 35 crossovers per cell during meiosis in males and perhaps twice as many during meiosis in females. The frequency of meiotic crossing-over is not uniform along the length of the chromosomes.

One essential requirement for linkage analysis is the availability of DNA markers; the feasibility of human linkage analysis was revolutionized in 1978 when Kan and Dozy demonstrated genetic variation in the size of fragments generated after digestion of normal human DNA with restriction endonucleases. These restriction fragment length polymorphisms (RFLPs) are the consequence of the DNA sequence polymorphisms discussed above and are inherited according to Mendelian principles. Restriction enzyme digestion and Southern blotting made it possible to identify these polymorphisms and utilize them as genetic markers for sites within the genome. If one of the base pairs in the recognition sequence for a restriction enzyme is variable between individual copies of the genome or if there is a length variation in the DNA, there will be variation in the size of DNA fragments generated by the restriction enzyme digestion. The inheritance of an RFLP is depicted in Fig. 61-4.

A particularly informative subset of RFLPs occurs at variable number tandem repeat (VNTR) sites. These are sites of length variation in the genome in which a DNA sequence is tandemly repeated a different number of times on different chromosomes. The result is that there are many different sizes of DNA fragments, which can be regarded as different alleles at a VNTR site. The repeat unit

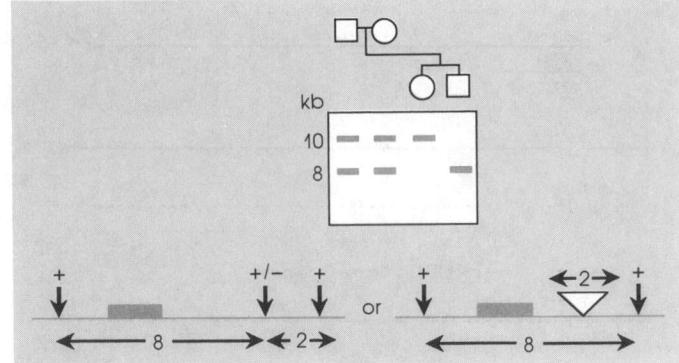

FIGURE 61-4 Example of restriction fragment length polymorphism (RFLP) in human DNA using Southern blotting. The solid blocks indicate segments of DNA used as probe. Parents are heterozygous and children are homozygous for the RFLP. Symbols above the arrows indicate cutting (+) or noncutting (−) by the restriction endonuclease. Numbers indicate DNA length in kilobases.

in VNTRs can be tens or hundreds of bases in length with variation arising through unequal crossing-over. In the case of the apolipoprotein for Lp(a), a VNTR repeat unit includes two exons giving rise to polymorphism in both the length of the gene and the protein. Another important group of polymorphic DNA markers is the short tandem repeats (STRs) which are repeats of tetra-, tri-, di-, and mononucleotides in the genome; variation arises through "slippage" of the DNA polymerase at replication to increase or decrease the number of repeat units on a chromosome. STRs are highly polymorphic, easily analyzed, and widely distributed in the genome. Dinucleotide repeats, of $(GT)_n$ on one strand and $(CA)_n$ on the other strand, with 10 to 40 repeat units, are the most common as depicted in Fig. 61-5. An

FIGURE 61-5 Depiction of a short tandem repeat (STR) polymorphism for a dinucleotide $(GT)_n$ repeat. Each repeat is separated by a vertical line. Sites for two primers for PCR are indicated by arrows. Four alleles of 24, 21, 18, and 15 GT repeats are indicated. Inheritance of the alleles in a family as detected by PCR is shown below.

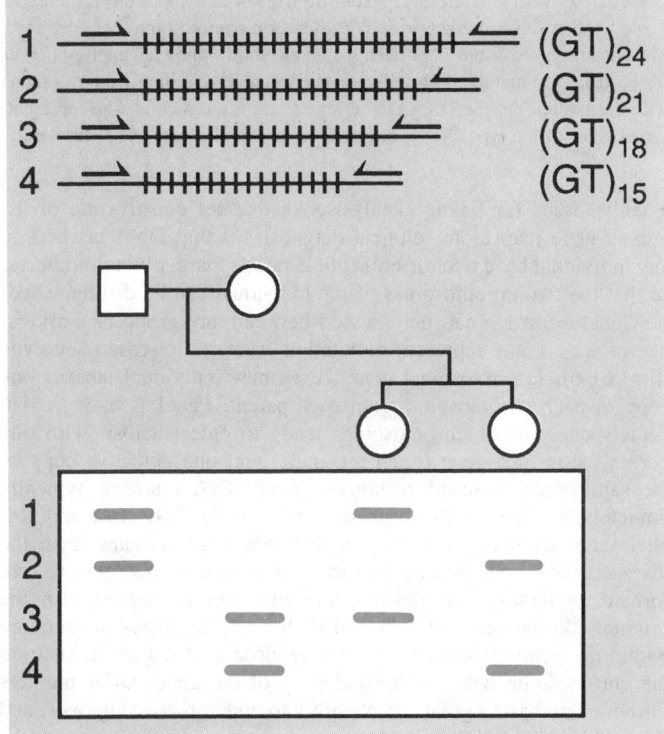

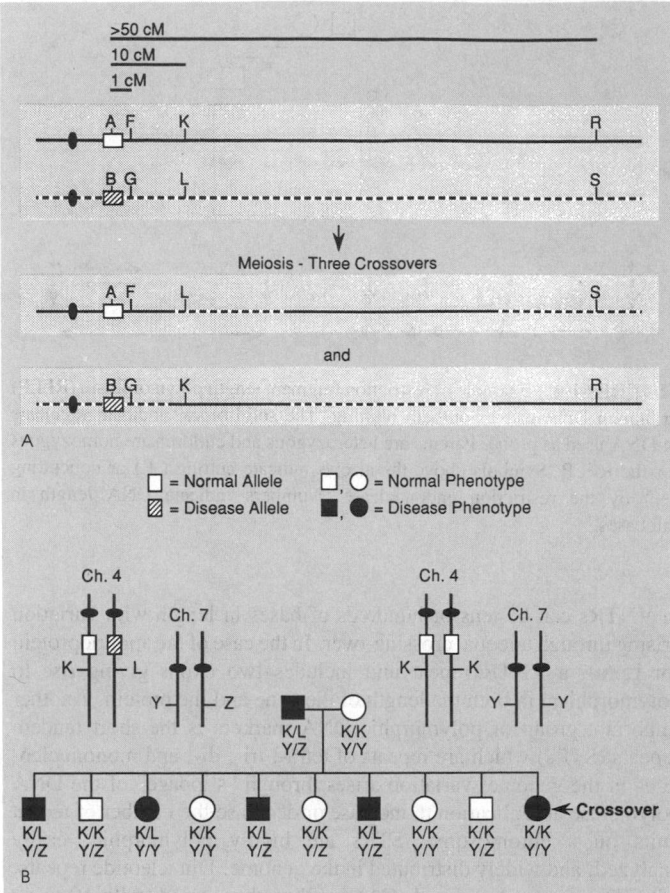

FIGURE 61-6 Depiction of meiotic crossing over and linkage analysis. Panel A shows two copies of one chromosome (one in solid line and one in dashed line) from an individual before (above) and after (below) meiotic crossing over. The individual is heterozygous for a disease locus with a normal allele (open rectangle) and a disease allele (hatched rectangle) and is heterozygous for four DNA markers with alleles A/B, F/G, K/L, and R/S at 0, 1, 10, and >50 centimorgans (cM) from the disease locus, respectively. Panel B depicts analysis in a family for an autosomal dominant disorder. The DNA marker with K/L alleles at 10 cM from the disease locus on chromosome 4 and another DNA marker with Y/Z alleles on chromosome 7 are depicted. The chromosomes 4 and 7 for each parent are shown and the genotypes given for each family member. The disease phenotype is inherited from the father with the L allele for the DNA marker except for the last child who represents a crossover of the type shown in the upper panel. See text for discussion.

essential issue for linkage analysis, whether for construction of the human gene map or for clinical diagnosis, is that DNA markers in any individual have two different alleles at the marker locus of interest so that the two chromosomes of the individual can be distinguished.

Genetic linkage can be assessed between any group of markers, one of which may represent a mutation causing a disease phenotype (Fig. 61-6). For autosomal genes, each new individual inherits one copy of each chromosome from each parent. Panel A of Fig. 61-6 depicts one pair of chromosomes ready to enter meiosis with one normal copy of a gene (open rectangle) and one defective copy of the same gene (hatched rectangle). Four DNA markers, typically dinucleotide repeat polymorphisms, with A/B, F/G, K/L, and R/S alleles are depicted at 0, 1, 10, and >50 centimorgans from the disease gene. After meiosis and three crossover events, gametes are formed containing one chromosome with various segments of the original chromosomes. The A and F alleles of the DNA markers are within the gene of interest (A) or very close to it (F) and remain on the chromosome with the normal copy of the gene. DNA markers further away have a greater probability to undergo crossing-over, and the L allele of one DNA marker is now on the chromosome with the

normal copy of the gene, although it was previously on the chromosome with the defective copy of the gene. The greater the distance between markers and genes, the greater the probability of crossovers. Alleles for a gene and a marker on different chromosomes are inherited independently.

Panel B of Fig. 61-6 depicts the analysis of DNA markers in a family with an autosomal dominant disease such as Huntington's chorea. Data are shown for the K/L DNA marker which is 10 cM from the disease gene and for a Y/Z DNA marker which resides on a different chromosome. A researcher trying to map a disease gene is likely to study many DNA markers like the Y/Z markers which show no correlation between which allele of the marker is inherited and whether or not the disease phenotype is inherited. Eventually a marker such as the K/L marker is discovered where there is significant linkage to the disease gene. Analysis of additional families can provide conclusive statistical evidence that a polymorphic DNA marker is near a disease gene. Identification of a genetic linkage allows for immediate application of the marker for predictive diagnosis within a family such as that shown in Fig. 61-6 (see "Diagnosis by Linkage Analysis," below) and opens the way for positional cloning of the disease gene (see "Cloning and Identifying Human Disease Genes," below). The frequency of crossovers as shown for the last offspring in Fig. 61-6 is a measure of the genetic distance between the DNA marker and the disease gene. Once a linked DNA marker is found, the gene is mapped to a specific site on a chromosome, and closer DNA markers can be identified rapidly.

With the availability of an unlimited number of polymorphic DNA markers, there is already a relatively detailed linkage map for the entire human genome. In one recent study, 814 polymorphic markers (dinucleotide repeats) were placed into 23 linkage groups corresponding to the 22 autosomes and the X chromosome and spanning 90 percent of the estimated length of the genome.

THE PHYSICAL MAP The physical map provides different information than the genetic map since it is based on direct DNA analysis and is not influenced by regional differences in recombination frequency. A physical map facilitates both the isolation of abundant DNA markers and the identification and cloning of all the genes in a region.

Four major strategies are used for physical mapping of the human genome: *in situ* hybridization, deletion mapping, long range restriction mapping, and isolation of yeast artificial chromosome clones. With *in situ* hybridization the direct hybridization of a DNA marker to a chromosome allows the assignment of the marker to a specific chromosomal band. With the advent of FISH (fluorescent *in situ* hybridization), the use of different colors for different probes makes it possible to map simultaneously more than one DNA marker. Hybridization to interphase nuclei allows determination of the order of markers within a particular chromosomal region. This technique is also useful for identification of chromosomal abnormalities, as described in Chap. 62.

Deletion mapping is based on the presence or absence of a particular region or locus in the DNA from patients with chromosomal abnormalities or from human/rodent somatic cell hybrids that retain known segments of the human chromosomes. Deletion mapping is particularly useful for mapping the X chromosome because of the large number of X chromosome abnormalities identified. Deletions of the X chromosome frequently result in a disease phenotype in males, and the deleted region can be identified without having to separate the abnormal chromosome from any normal homologue in somatic cell hybrids. Deletion mapping is also useful in establishing relative orders of sets of markers in the genome, although it does not provide precise information on the distance involved.

Information about physical distance is provided by long range restriction mapping. In this technique, high-molecular-weight DNA is cut into large fragments (from 100 kb up to 4 Mb) using restriction enzymes. These fragments are separated by pulsed field gel electrophoresis (PFGE) and then can be hybridized to DNA markers using conventional Southern blotting procedures. If two DNA probes hybridize, for example, to the same 200-kb restriction fragment, it can be concluded that the maximum distance between the two loci is 200 kb.

A particularly useful strategy in physical mapping utilizes yeast artificial chromosome (YAC) clones. The YAC cloning vectors are capable of carrying large-size fragments of genomic DNA (from 50 kb to 1 or 2 Mb). These vectors contain yeast telomeres and centromeres, and the clones are actually propagated as separate chromosomes in a yeast host. The human genome project will attempt the cloning of the entire human genome in overlapping YAC clones, and this has been accomplished for chromosomes 21 and Y. When this goal is achieved, physical mapping will be largely completed at one level of resolution, and further molecular analysis of the human genome will be facilitated because it will be possible to assign all genes and DNA markers to specific locations in the genome as defined by YAC clones.

THE HUMAN GENOME PROJECT   The human genome project is an international effort, started in the mid 1980s, aimed at the characterization of human genomic DNA. Specific goals of the human genome project are: (1) the development of detailed physical and genetic maps, (2) the cloning of the entire genome in overlapping YACs, (3) the identification and characterization of all genes, (4) the sequencing of all the 3×10^9 bp forming the haploid human genome, and finally (5) the biological interpretation of the information hidden in the nucleotide sequence. Although technology is now adequate to carry out the first two objectives and to identify a large fraction of all genes in a reasonable length of time (2 to 5 years), new methods of sequence determination and analysis will be needed for the last two goals. The human genome project will foster a tremendous advancement in basic biology and in medicine. In the latter field, the identification of genes involved in genetic predisposition to cancer and to common multifactorial disorders, such as hypertension and atherosclerosis, is among the most important goals.

CLONING AND IDENTIFYING HUMAN DISEASE GENES   Cloning of human disease genes can be categorized according to four general strategies: (1) knowledge and availability of the protein; (2) the ability to select for function of the gene; (3) knowledge of its genetic location (positional cloning); and (4) some combination of information regarding the phenotype, the genetic map location of the disease, and the genetic map location of biologically relevant genes (a regional candidate gene approach). Much of gene cloning relies on purification of a protein, determination of partial amino acid sequence, preparation of antibodies, and development of enzymatic or other assays. Using this information, cDNA clones can be isolated using approaches such as mRNA purification, hybridization screening with oligonucleotides based on available amino acid sequence, PCR amplification based on similar oligonucleotides, immunological screening of expression cDNA libraries, and other related approaches. In some instances, it has been possible to clone genes based on a functional property without knowing the protein or the genetic map location. For example, various genes involved in DNA repair disorders have been isolated using selection in tissue culture to identify clones that correct the cellular phenotype of defective DNA repair.

Positional cloning, often in the past, termed reverse genetics, is the isolation of a disease gene based on its location in the genome with no knowledge of its function. This strategy depends on the identification in samples from affected families of a DNA marker that is located close to the disease locus, as discussed above and depicted for an autosomal dominant disorder in Fig. 61-6B. Analogous efforts can be applied to autosomal recessive and X-linked diseases. Having localized the disease gene in a general way, it is possible to isolate the DNA of the relevant region in overlapping clones, identify genes in the region, and eventually prove which is the disease gene, often by identifying small mutations within one of the genes (Fig. 61-7). This strategy is facilitated if chromosomal translocations are available to assist in mapping and identifying the disease gene. This approach is labor intensive but has yielded landmark success in the case of genes for Duchenne's muscular dystrophy, cystic fibrosis, retinoblastoma, polyposis of the colon, neurofibromatosis, and Huntington's disease.

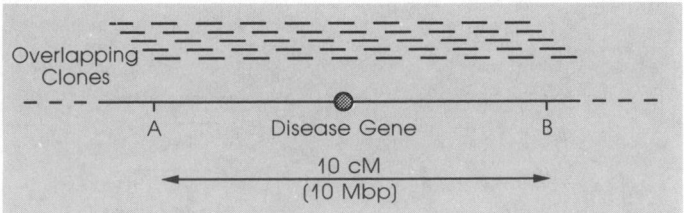

FIGURE 61-7   A positional cloning strategy. DNA markers at sites A and B are found to flank a disease gene. Overlapping DNA clones are isolated for the region, and the disease gene is identified within the region.

As human gene mapping becomes easier and as more genes are identified from human and other species, the regional candidate gene approach will be facilitated. A pure candidate gene strategy might involve simply guessing the disease gene from among known proteins based on the disease phenotype, but this is rarely possible. More often the candidate gene approach requires a limited amount of genetic mapping information for a disease, much less than would be adequate for a strictly positional cloning effort. Based on the limited mapping information, on information about relevant genes mapping to the general region, and perhaps taking into account information from other species such as the mouse, one can formulate and test the hypothesis that a particular gene is mutated in a specific genetic disease. Such testing is usually done by amplification and/or cloning of the gene in question from affected patients to search for mutations. A regional candidate gene approach led to the identification of mutations in the cardiac myosin heavy chain genes as the cause of familial hypertrophic cardiomyopathy. Use of information from the mouse led to the recognition that the *PAX3* gene is mutated in Waardenburg syndrome based on very limited mapping information and relevant information from the mouse. Many genes have been and will be cloned according to some combination of positional genetic information and candidate gene hypothesis, as exemplified by Marfan's syndrome, where mapping information and characterization of a candidate protein both contributed to the identification of the disease gene. One variation on the candidate gene approach would depend on the production of mice with targeted mutations and identification of candidate genes by phenotypes in humans that might resemble a phenotype observed in the mouse.

TRANSGENIC AND MUTANT MICE   Gene structure and function are usually similar in mouse and human, and studies in the mouse can provide insight into human disease. The germline DNA of mice can be manipulated in a variety of ways (Fig. 61-8). The creation of transgenic mice typically involves microinjection of cloned DNA sequences into the male pronucleus of fertilized mouse eggs. The injected DNA becomes integrated into the mouse chromosomal DNA in a fraction of the injected cells. The transgenic DNA can be expressed in the resulting animals and transmitted in the germ cells so that a series of transgenic descendant animals can be obtained. Each site of integration of foreign DNA behaves as a single Mendelian trait, and heterozygous and homozygous animals can be obtained.

Transgenic animals have been particularly useful for the evaluation of *cis*-acting regulatory DNA sequences that control tissue-specific and temporal aspects of gene expression. Putative regulatory sequences are linked to a reporter gene, which produces an easily detectable product. Using this strategy, short DNA sequences have been identified that provide exquisite tissue specificity for genes such as insulin and elastase, and more complex and distant regulatory sequences have been shown to control the expression of globin genes. The transgenic method has also been utilized to introduce viral or cellular oncogenes that induce tumors in animals, opening new approaches for the study of tumor biology. A tissue-specific regulatory sequence can be linked to the SV40 T antigen to produce tumors in specific cell types. Another transgenic mouse strategy involves linking of regulatory sequences to a toxin that will selectively kill cells that express the sequence. As an example, linking of insulin regulatory

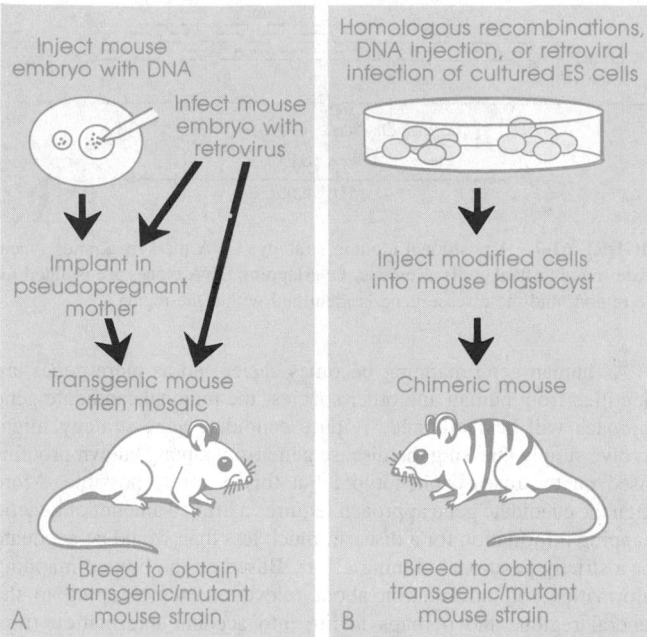

FIGURE 61-8 Various strategies for producing transgenic and mutant mice. DNA can be injected into the male pronucleus of fertilized mouse eggs followed by implantation in pseudopregnant mothers. Mouse embryos can be infected with retroviruses in vivo or in vitro. Transgenic mice may be mosaic, but the transgene can be recovered in nonmosaic form in the offspring of these mice. These strategies are depicted on the left. On the right, cultured embryonic stem (ES) cells can be modified by homologous or nonhomologous recombination or by retroviral infection. The modified cells can be selected and injected into a mouse blastocyst to produce a chimeric mouse with subsequent recovery of the mutation in the germline of the offspring of the chimeric mouse.

sequences to diphtheria toxin can generate mice with selective absence of pancreatic β cells. In yet another application, larger transgenic animals can be used for production of pharmaceuticals to be harvested from milk or blood.

Since integration of transgenic DNA is relatively random, it results in interruption of normal mouse genes in a certain percentage of cases. Retroviruses can also be used to infect mouse embryonic cells with the goal of relatively random insertional mutagenesis in the mouse. Mutant phenotypes can then be sought in the resulting heterozygous or homozygous offspring, including the identification of defects that are benign in heterozygotes but lethal in the homozygous state. Because the cloned DNA inserts at the site of the affected gene, it is possible to clone the gene associated with the mutant phenotype. Thus, it is possible to identify many new mutations and to clone the relevant genes.

The ability to carry out homologous recombination with mouse embryonic stem (ES) cells provides additional exciting opportunities. ES cells are totipotent cells that can be manipulated in culture and then reintroduced into mouse embryos. Using homologous recombination in ES cells, it is possible to target one specific gene for inactivation ("knockout") or subtle mutation. The injection of altered ES cells into recipient blastocysts results in chimeric animals composed partially of mutant cells derived from the ES cell culture. The genetically altered cells are often represented in the germ cells of the resulting chimeric animals, and mutant mice can be obtained and bred to study heterozygotes and homozygotes. The technique has allowed for the production of mouse models of many human genetic diseases including retinoblastoma, p53 oncogene deficiency (Li Fraumeni familial cancer syndrome), cystic fibrosis, Lesch-Nyhan syndrome, Gaucher's disease, apolipoprotein E deficiency, and others. In some instances there are major phenotypic differences for the same mutation in mouse and human, and delineation of the basis of these

differences will provide major insights into pathophysiology. In other cases, the phenotypes in mice and humans are similar, and the animals will be valuable for therapeutic trials. It is likely that mutant mice of these types will be particularly useful for unraveling the genetic factors in multifactorial disease processes such as atherosclerosis and for analysis of complex neurological functions. The ability to obtain mouse mutants for virtually any cloned gene provides an opportunity to analyze the function of cloned genes whose biologic roles are not delineated.

MOLECULAR DIAGNOSIS OF GENETIC DISEASE

NATURE AND ORIGIN OF MUTATIONS Typical genes which encode proteins are composed of promoters, exons, introns, and polyadenylation signals (see Fig. 60-2) and are subject to a wide variety of mutations. These include deletions, expanding triplet repeats, other gross rearrangements, and smaller mutations which can be characterized as missense, nonsense, frameshift, splicing, promoter, or other type. Some mutations are ancient in origin, and individuals in the population will carry the same mutation which originated from a rare event (a founder effect) as in the case of the common mutations for cystic fibrosis, sickle cell anemia, thalassemias, α_1-antitrypsin deficiency, Tay-Sachs disease, and other disorders. In the case of mutations that impair reproductive fitness and are eliminated from the population relatively quickly, disease mutations are more recent and tend to be different in each family, as in the case of X-linked lethal disorders and many dominant disorders including neurofibromatosis, Marfan's syndrome, and others. This consideration impacts on whether it is practical to search for known common mutations or to anticipate the need to search for an unpredictable mutation that is unique to a given family. In any consideration of molecular diagnosis, it is necessary to distinguish when one is dealing with the disease causing mutation as opposed to a variation in a DNA marker which is within or near the disease gene but is not the cause of the disease. Failure to distinguish the disease-causing mutation from variation in a DNA marker is a frequent source of misunderstanding in mutation analysis and linkage analysis.

Some mutations occur in stepwise fashion, progressing from premutation to mild mutation to severe mutation as exemplified by expanding triplet repeats in genes (see Caskey et al.). In addition, some genes are imprinted, in that only the paternal or maternal copy is expressed. This complicates the pattern of transmission of the phenotype within the family, since the appearance of the disease depends both on whether the disease gene was inherited or not and also on whether it was inherited from the mother or the father (see Hall). Imprinting is exemplified by the Prader-Willi syndrome where only the paternal copy of the gene appears to be active and the Angelman syndrome where only the maternal copy of the gene seems functional. The genes for Prader-Willi and Angelman syndromes appear to be distinct but close to each other on chromosome 15.

STRATEGIES FOR DIAGNOSIS OF MENDELIAN DISORDERS As for all clinical diagnosis, a detailed workup including family history and clinical examination, is the appropriate starting point. In some cases, the phenotype may be characteristic of a specific genetic disease, and the diagnostic information may be supplemented by family history or by specific biochemical laboratory tests. A general scheme for utilization of molecular methods for clinical diagnosis is depicted in Fig. 61-9.

Definite clinical and/or biochemical genetic diagnosis In many cases, a definite clinical genetic diagnosis is established before undertaking DNA analysis. The goals in such cases may include genotype/phenotype correlation, i.e., predicting the severity of the disease based on the mutations present. For example, some mutations cause nonneuronopathic Gaucher's disease, and others cause neuronopathic disease. Analysis may further confirm a diagnosis that is already considered to be established. Genotype/phenotype correlation and confirmation of diagnosis rely on mutation analysis and generally

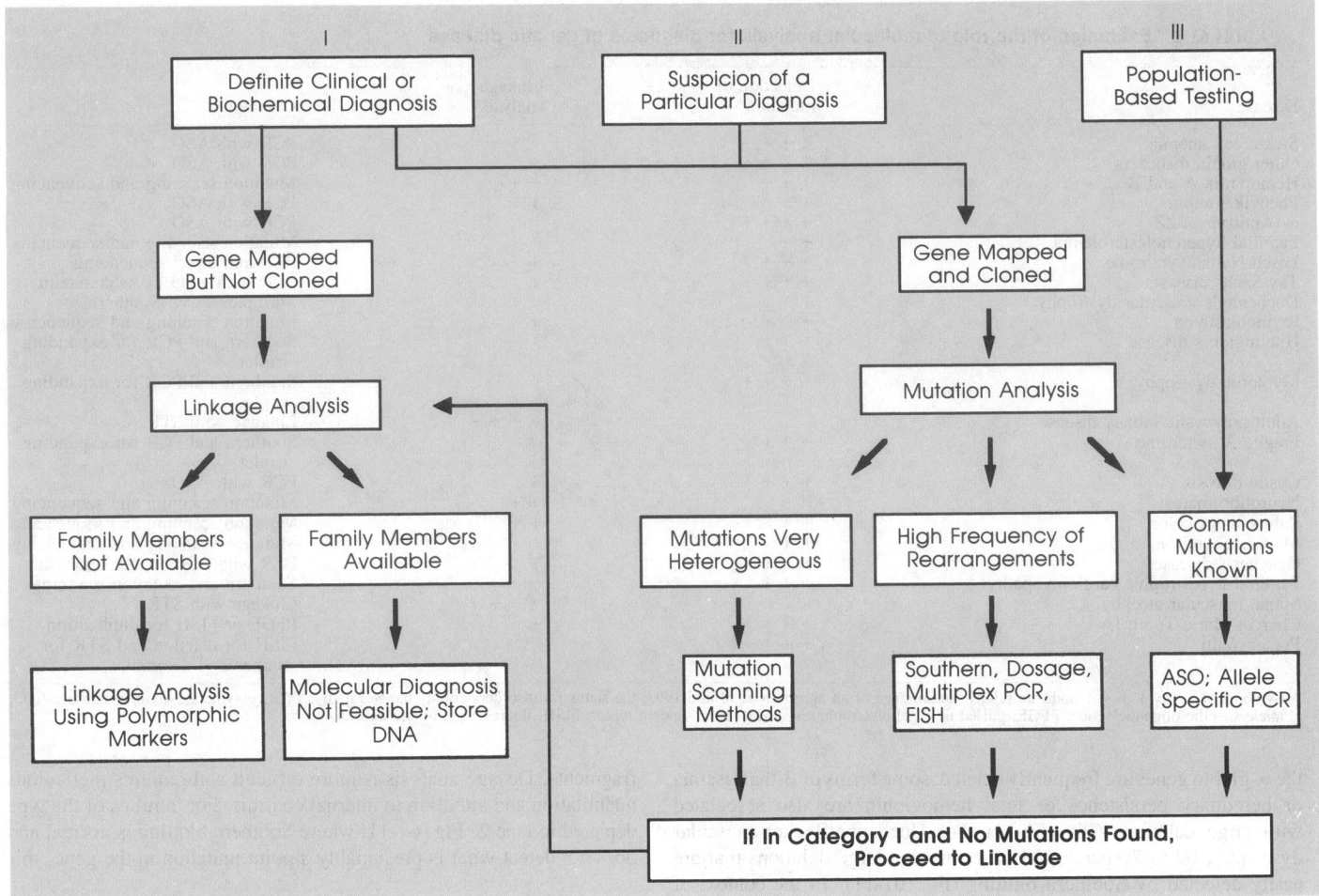

FIGURE 61-9 A scheme for utilization of DNA analysis for genetic diagnosis.

cannot be based on linkage analysis. Another application is studies of various family members for purposes of heterozygote detection, presymptomatic diagnosis, or prenatal diagnosis. Family studies should be performed using mutation analysis if possible and linkage analysis, where necessary, if suitable family members are available.

Clarification of a possible genetic diagnosis In some cases, there may be a suspicion of a particular genetic disease, but the findings may be inconclusive, the patient may be early in the clinical course, or the case may be atypical. This frequently occurs in a circumstance where it is possible to detect some fraction of the disease mutations but not to search the entire coding and flanking regions to exclude an undetected mutation. In the case of dominant disorders or X-linked diseases in males, a diagnosis may be established by demonstration of a single copy of a definitive deleterious change in the DNA such as a deletion, frameshift, or nonsense mutation. Failure to find a mutation usually does not rule out the diagnosis but in some diseases makes it less likely. For autosomal recessive disorders, the situation is more complex: Identification of pathologic mutations in both copies of the gene establishes a diagnosis; identification of one pathologic mutation increases the probability that the suspect phenotype is related to mutation at this locus but does not prove a diagnosis; and failure to identify any pathologic mutations lessens the likelihood that the disease is related to mutation at this locus, but does not eliminate that possibility. For example, failure to detect a mutation may mean that the mutation is outside the region analyzed or that the patient has a separate but similar disease. Linkage analysis is usually not a practical way of resolving diagnostic problems of this type.

Population based DNA testing Utilization of DNA testing for population-based screening offers the potential for many applications, similar to nonmolecular methods of population screening such as newborn screening; cholesterol measurements; mammography; measurement of prostate specific antigen; carrier screening for Tay-Sachs, sickle-cell, or thalassemia; and maternal serum α-fetoprotein screening. DNA testing may be useful for (1) presymptomatic detection of disease susceptibility with plans for intervention, (2) carrier screening and reproductive counseling, or (3) prenatal testing. Many forms of genotypic analysis based on protein methods (e.g., sickle cell, α₁-antitrypsin and Tay-Sachs testing) might be more specific and more economic using DNA methods. The question of whether DNA testing for carrier detection for cystic fibrosis should be offered routinely has been controversial but is likely to become widespread in time. With DNA variation of known or likely disease significance occurring in the genes for apolipoprotein E, apolipoprotein Lp(a), angiotensinogen, angiotensin-converting enzyme, α₁-antitrypsin, and many others, it is likely that population-based DNA testing might become a powerful preventive approach with pharmacologic and lifestyle interventions for individuals with high-risk genotypes. Such strategies might well apply to familial cancer risks, such as breast cancer. Novel technologies such as ASO analysis using DNA fixed on electronic chips to allow multiple determinations at very low cost offers the promise of both economical and preventive strategies.

EXAMPLES OF MUTATION DETECTION As indicated in Fig. 61-9, different methods of analysis are employed for molecular diagnosis depending on the most common type of mutation for a particular disorder, whether the mutations are usually large rearrangements or point mutations, and whether the mutations are usually of predictable type from ancient origins or are more heterogeneous and recent in origin. Examples of common genetic disorders are listed in Table 61-2 with the type of analysis that is most applicable for a disorder.

Examples of large defects in genes include α-thalassemia, where

TABLE 61-2   **Examples of the role of molecular analysis for diagnosis of genetic disease**

Disease	Detection of mutation*	Linkage analysis*	Comments
Sickle cell anemia	+ + + +		PCR with ASO
Other globin disorders	+ + + +	+	PCR with ASO
Hemophilia A and B	+ + +	+ +	Mutation scanning and sequencing
Phenylketonuria	+ +	+ +	PCR with ASO
α_1-Antitrypsin ZZ	+ + + +		PCR with ASO
Familial hypercholesterolemia	+ +	+ +	Mutation scanning and sequencing
Lesch-Nyhan syndrome	+ + + +	+	PCR and direct sequencing
Tay-Sachs disease	+ + +	+	PCR with ASO in Ashkenazim
Duchenne's muscular dystrophy	+ + +	+ +	Multiplex PCR, Southern
Retinoblastoma	+ + +	+	Mutation scanning and sequencing
Huntington's disease	+ + +		Southern and PCR for expanding triplet
Myotonic dystrophy	+ + + +		Southern and PCR for expanding triplet
Adult polycystic kidney disease		+ + + +	Linkage with STR
Fragile X syndrome	+ + + +		Southern and PCR for expanding triplet
Cystic fibrosis	+ + +	+	PCR with ASOs
Neurofibromatosis I	+ +	+ +	Mutation scanning and sequencing
Polyposis of colon	+ +	+ +	Mutation scanning and sequencing
Marfan's syndrome	+ +	+ +	Mutation scanning and sequencing
Gaucher's disease	+ + + +	+	PCR with ASO in Ashkenazim
Familial hypertrophic cardiomyopathy	+ + +	+	Southern and mutation scanning
Spinal muscular atrophy		+ + + +	Linkage with STR
Charcot-Marie-Tooth IA	+ + + +	+	PFGE or FISH for duplication
Prader-Willi	+ + + +		FISH for deletion and STR for uniparental disomy

* Symbols of + to + + + + indicate relative importance of an approach as of mid 1993; the status for disorders could change rapidly. PCR, polymerase chain reactions; ASO, allele specific oligonucleotide; PFGE, pulsed field gel electrophoresis; STR, short tandem repeat; FISH, fluorescence in situ hybridization.

the α-globin genes are frequently deleted; some forms of β-thalassemia or hereditary persistence of fetal hemoglobin are also associated with large deletions (Fig. 61-10). For Duchenne/Becker muscular dystrophy, 60 to 70 percent of cases involve large deletions that are easily detected by Southern blotting (Fig. 61-11). In the context of carrier detection for family members, a case such as lane 1 in Fig. 61-11 with a novel, junctional DNA fragment is optimal since the presence of this fragment will be absolutely diagnostic for carrier status for females in this family. For cases such as lane 3, heterozygote detection would depend on dosage analysis with one copy of the deleted fragments in carrier females, and two copies of the nondeleted

fragments. Dosage analysis is more difficult and requires meticulous quantitation and attention to internal controls. For families of the type depicted in lane 2, Fig. 61-11, where Southern blotting is normal and does not detect what is presumably a point mutation in the gene, this

FIGURE 61-11 Detection of deletions in the DNA isolated from Duchenne's muscular dystrophy patients using a dystrophin cDNA probe. Southern blot analysis detects deletions (absence of fragments) in five of eight patients (arrows). A junction fragment is clearly demonstrated in patients 1 and 6. *(From M Koenig et al, Cell 50:509, 1987.)*

FIGURE 61-10 Depiction of Southern blot analysis of human globin genes. Above, DNA was isolated from a normal individual and from patients with homozygous hereditary persistence of fetal hemoglobin (HPFH) or homozygous α-thalassemia. DNA was digested with the enzyme *Eco*RI. A mixed DNA probe was prepared by reverse transcription of reticulocyte globin mRNA. Below, arrows indicate *Eco*RI cut sites in the α- and β-globin regions, and numbers indicate DNA fragment sizes in kilobases. *(Adapted from YW Kan, AM Dozy, Proc Natl Acad Sci USA 75:5631, 1978.)*

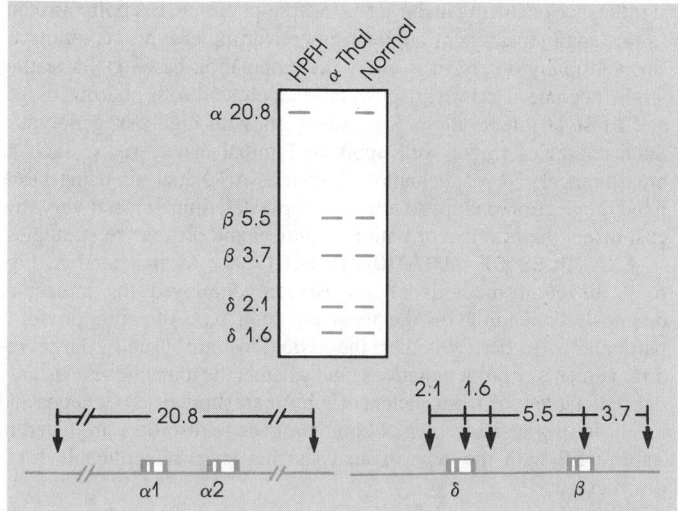

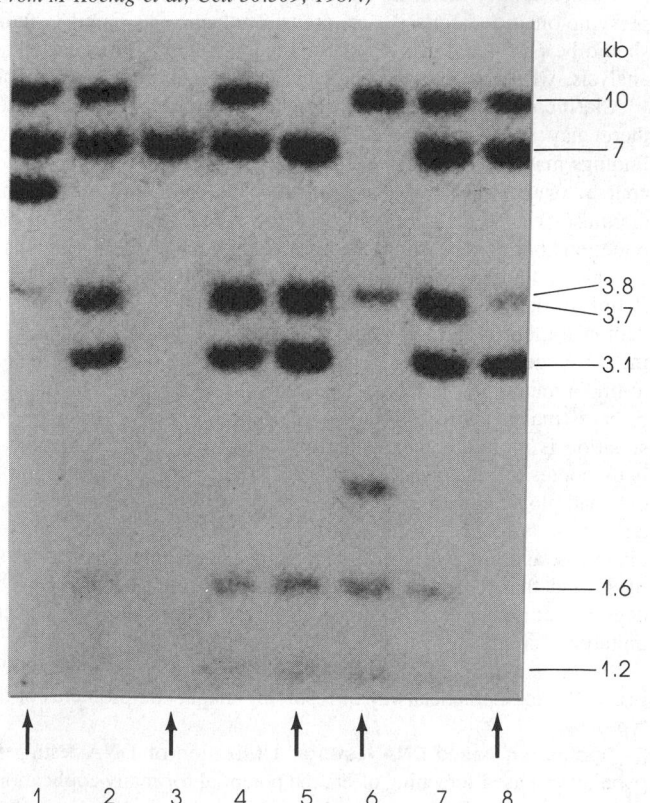

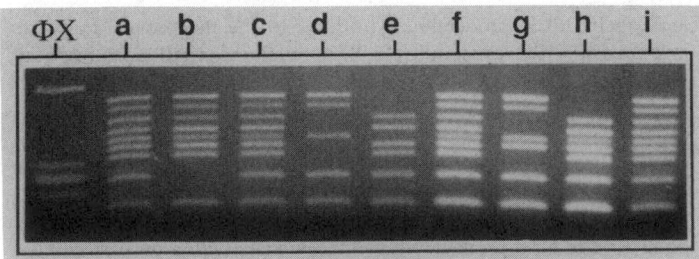

FIGURE 61-12 Multiple amplification of DNA using PCR to detect deletions in the dystrophin gene. Nine amplifications detecting fragments of nine different exons are performed in a single tube and analyzed on an agarose gel. Deletions can be seen as missing fragments for the Duchenne dystrophy patients shown in lanes b, d, e, g, and h, while no deletion is detected in lanes a, c, f, and i. φX indicates DNA markers. *(Used by permission, Multicenter Study Group: JAMA 267:2609, 1992.)*

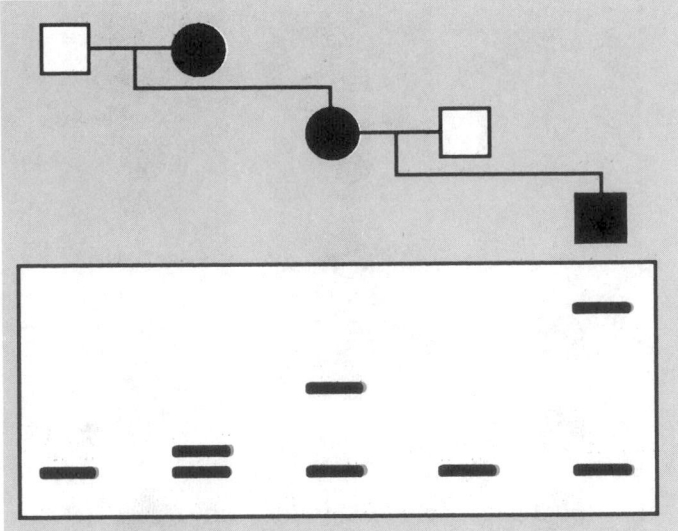

FIGURE 61-13 Diagramatic representation of Southern blot analysis revealing an expanding triplet mutation in a myotonic dystrophy family. A grandmother and mother with the adult form of the disease and a child with the infantile form of the disease are shown. The normal size genomic DNA fragment (lowest band) is present in homozygous form in the unaffected individuals and in heterozygous form in the affected family members. The larger mutant fragment is present in all affected individuals with increasing size from grandmother, to mother, to child.

analysis would not be useful for carrier detection. Deletions such as those seen in Duchenne/Becker dystrophy can also be detected using PCR to test for the presence or absence of various sites in the gene (Fig. 61-12). Deleted segments are identified by the absence of particular PCR products in a multiplex reaction testing for the presence of various sites along the length of the gene.

Expanding triplet repeat mutations have been described as the cause of myotonic dystrophy, fragile X mental retardation, Huntington's and Kennedy's syndrome, a form of spinomuscular atrophy associated with this type of mutation in the androgen receptor. In the case of fragile X mental retardation and myotonic dystrophy, there is increasing severity of the disease as permutation progresses to mild mutation and mild mutation progresses to severe mutation, a genetic phenomenon called anticipation (see Caskey et al). Depending on the size of the expanding triple repeat, these mutations can be detected by Southern blotting and/or PCR analysis. An example of an expanding triplet repeat mutation with anticipation and more severe disease in later generations is depicted in Fig. 61-13.

For many disorders, including all autosomal recessive disorders and autosomal dominant or X-linked disorders with minimal effect on reproduction, known mutations of ancient origin may be present in thousands or even millions of people in the population. Despite the fact that there may be ancient common mutations, there may still be extensive molecular heterogeneity as is depicted for β-thalassemia in Fig. 61-14. The situation is similar for cystic fibrosis where the

common mutation (designated ΔF508 for deletion of phenylalanine, F at position 508) accounts for about 70 percent of all mutations in most populations, but over 200 different mutations have been identified among the remaining 30 percent of mutant chromosomes. Common mutations of this type are usually best tested using some allele-specific method such as hybridization with ASOs. Typically, ASO analysis for a single disease may require testing for only a few alleles as in α_1-antitrypsin deficiency or for 10, 20, or more mutations as in the case of β-thalassemia or cystic fibrosis. A simple example of a traditional or "forward" ASO analysis is shown in Fig. 61-15 for S and C hemoglobin. In this case, PCR product is fixed on a filter, and the filter is hybridized to labeled oligonucleotide probes. In the reverse ASO or dot blot procedure, oligonucleotides are fixed on a membrane,

FIGURE 61-14 Point mutations in β-globin gene is shown with numbered hatched areas representing the coding regions of exons. Boxed open areas between the exons are introns, and boxed open areas at the 5' and 3' ends of

the gene are untranslated regions that appear in the messenger RNA. The various types of mutations are depicted by different symbols. *(From HH Kazazian, Jr., CD Boehm, Blood 72:1107, 1988.)*

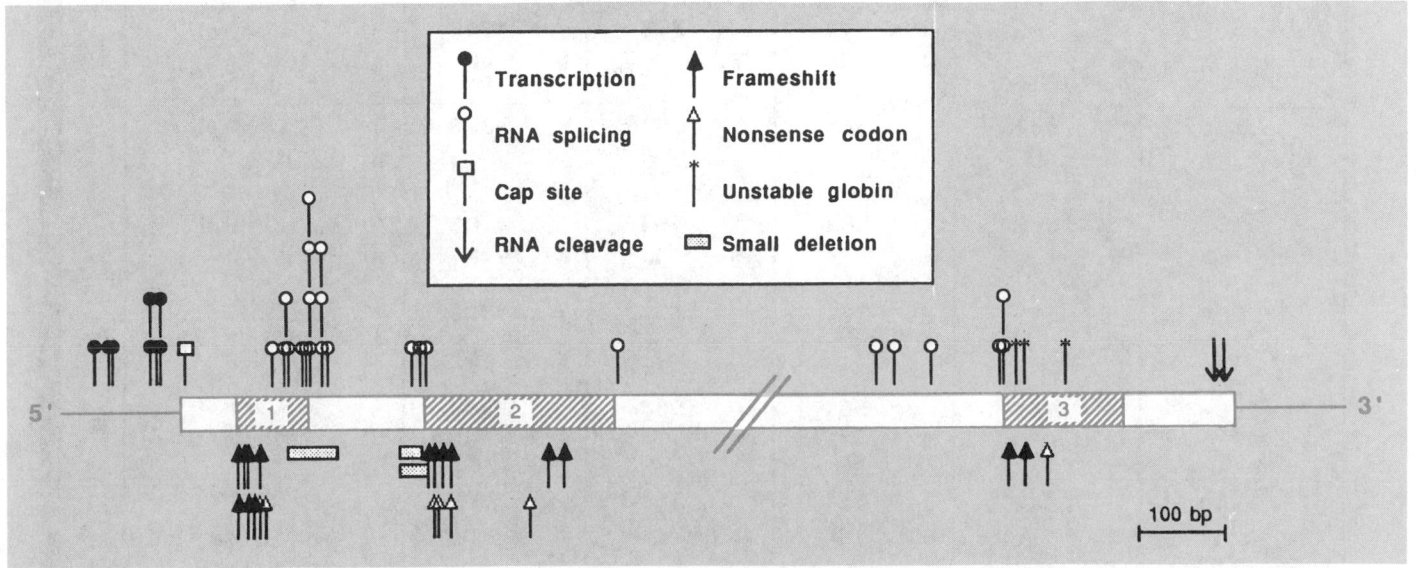

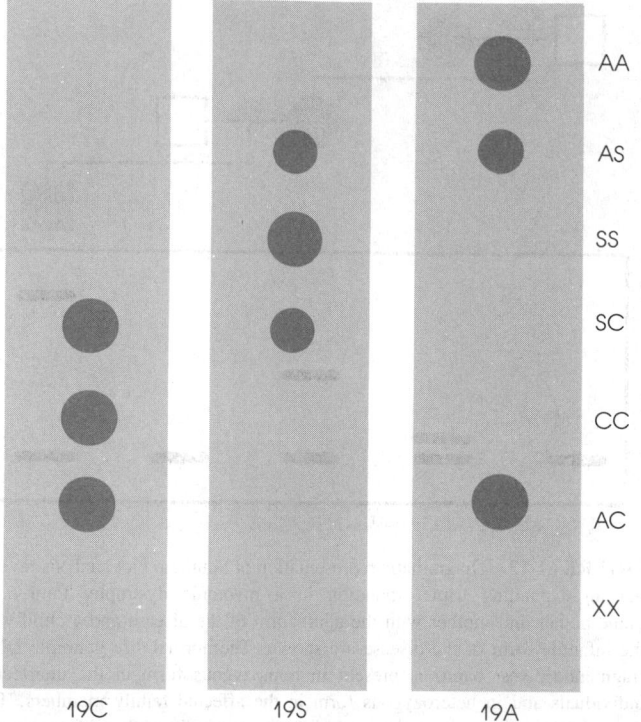

19C   19S   19A

AA
AS
SS
SC
CC
AC
XX

FIGURE 61-15 Genotype analysis of PCR amplified genomic DNA using allele-specific oligonucleotides (ASO) probes. DNA was extracted from the blood of individuals of β-globin genotypes AA, AS, SS, SC, CC, and AC and homozygous deletion (XX). The DNA was applied to replicate filters for hybridization with ASO as follows: β^A probe (19A), β^S probe (19S) or β^C probe (19C). *(From K Mullis et al, Cold Spring Harbor Symp Quant Biol 51:263, 1986.)*

FIGURE 61-16 Reverse dot ASO analysis for various point mutations causing cystic fibrosis. For each mutation, the PCR product is hybridized to an ASO dot on the left for the normal allele and on the right for the mutant allele. The positions for each ASO are indicated as follows: F and Δ for the ΔF508 mutation, G and X for the G542X mutation, G and D for the G551D mutation, R and X for the R553X mutation, N and K for the N1303K mutation, and 10 or 11 or 21 under control for the ASO to detect the amplification of exons of those numbers. Mutations are designated by single letter amino acid

and labeled PCR product is hybridized to the membrane. Forward and reverse ASO procedures yield similar information and are in widespread use today. An example of a reverse ASO analysis for cystic fibrosis mutations is shown in Fig. 61-16.

The data from mutation analysis is generally relatively straightforward to interpret, although it is important to determine which mutations are present in affected family members in some cases as depicted in Fig. 61-17. It is currently recommended that carrier testing be offered to all reproductive aged individuals with a positive family history of cystic fibrosis. In the case shown in Fig. 61-17, two uncles and an aunt undergo testing. Consider first the circumstance where the mutation analysis is not available on the index case and his parents, i.e., missing the shaded information in Fig. 61-17. One uncle is found to have the ΔF508 mutation and is a definite carrier without regard to other family information. The other uncle and the aunt have negative mutation studies, and the probability that they are carriers is substantially reduced from the approximate prior risk of 1 chance in 2, particularly for the male, since the ΔF508 mutation is present on his side of the family. Once DNA analysis is performed on the propositus and his parents, and it is determined that the father carries the common ΔF508 mutation and the mother carries an unidentified mutation, the carrier risk for the uncle with negative mutation studies remains at a very low level while that for the aunt rises substantially to the original 1 in 2 risk. This example demonstrates the importance of obtaining mutation analysis on appropriate family members and the significant impact of such information on risk calculations.

In some cases, mutation analysis is quite difficult because the majority of patients carry point mutations, and the point mutations are heterogeneous. This typically includes autosomal dominant disorders with some impairment of reproductive capacity and X-linked disorders that limit reproduction in males. The factors influencing the proportion of cases of autosomal dominant disorders due to new mutation are discussed in Chap. 60. In these cases of heterogeneous mutations,

code (X = non-sense) with the normal amino acid followed by the position number followed by the substituted amino acid. Thus G551D is substitution of aspartic acid (D) for glycine (G) at position 551. ΔF508 is described in the text. Letters at the right margin identify individuals of the following genotypes: A = no mutation, B = ΔF508/G542X compound heterozygote, C = ΔF508/R553X compound heterozygote; D = G542X heterozygote, E = G551D heterozygote, F = R553X heterozygote, and G = N1303K heterozygote. *(Modified from H. Erlich, Cetus Corporation.)*

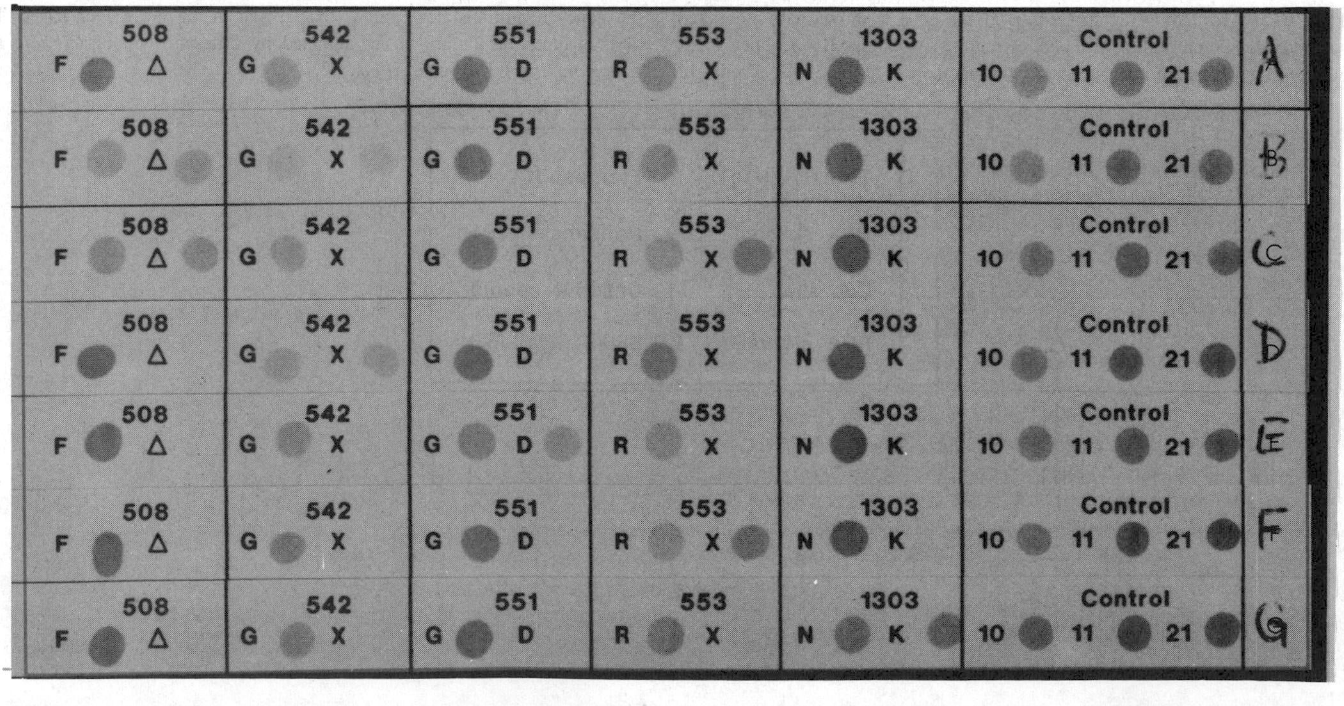

508	542	551	553	1303	Control	
F ● Δ	G ● X	G ● D	R ● X	N ● K	10 ● 11 ● 21 ●	A
F ● Δ ●	G ● X	G ● D	R ● X	N ● K	10 ● 11 ● 21 ●	B
F ● Δ	G ● X	G ● D	R ● X	N ● K	10 ● 11 ● 21 ●	C
F ● Δ	G ● X	G ● D	R ● X	N ● K	10 ● 11 ● 21 ●	D
F ● Δ	G ● X	G ● D	R ● X	N ● K	10 ● 11 ● 21 ●	E
F ● Δ	G ● X	G ● D	R ● X	N ● K	10 ● 11 ● 21 ●	F
F ● Δ	G ● X	G ● D	R ● X	N ● K	10 ● 11 ● 21 ●	G

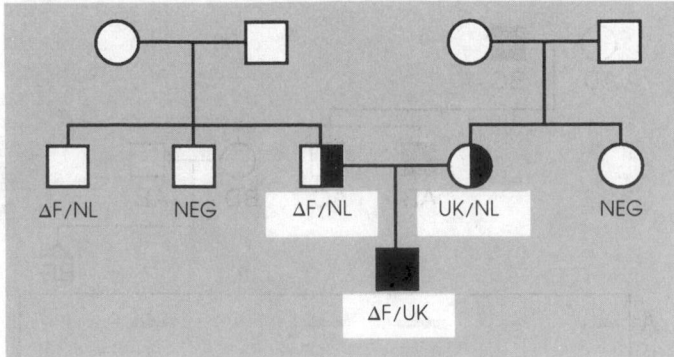

FIGURE 61-17 Mutational analysis in a cystic fibrosis family. Designations are as follows: ΔF = ΔF508 mutation, UK = unknown mutation, NL = normal allele, and NEG = negative mutation studies. See text for discussion.

some method of analyzing the entire gene is needed. Sequencing all of the exons of a gene is feasible in a few cases if the coding region of the gene is small, and this has been utilized for Lesch-Nyhan syndrome and to some extent for hemophilias A and B. However, this is impractical using current technology in most cases, and identification of mutations depends on a variety of procedures designed to detect single base differences in DNA sequences. In many cases, this remains an activity for research laboratories and is beyond the level of routine clinical service, although it would be extremely desirable to develop more powerful methods for detection of disease mutations in all families of this type.

DIAGNOSIS BY LINKAGE ANALYSIS If it is not possible to identify the mutation or mutations in the disease gene in a given family, then molecular diagnosis must be based on linkage analysis. In other cases, the disease gene may not be cloned but DNA markers

so close as to show negligible recombination with the disease phenotype may be available. In these cases, linkage diagnosis can be performed with a negligible possibility of crossovers. The general concepts for genetic recombination and linkage are discussed earlier in this chapter and in Chap. 60. For clinical linkage analysis, some genetic marker near the disease locus (or near the mutation if the locus is very large) must be *informative*. The genetic marker is informative if an individual has two different alleles at the marker locus. Linkage analysis often is appropriate when an individual carries one mutant gene and one normal gene and the goal is to determine which has been transmitted to the next generation. Most analyses can be made informative since highly polymorphic dinucleotide repeat polymorphisms are easily identified within and near genes causing diseases.

A second requirement for linkage analysis is that of *phase* information between the marker locus and the disease locus for genetic analysis. If an individual is heterozygous for a marker (genotype 1/2) that is tightly linked to a mutation, it must be determined whether allele 1 for the marker is on the chromosome with the disease allele or on the homologous chromosome with the normal allele, assuming that allele 2 for the marker would be on the chromosome with the alternate allele. When the genetic marker is informative and the phase is known, genetic diagnosis can be made for purposes of heterozygote detection, presymptomatic diagnosis, detection of failure of penetrance, and prenatal diagnosis. When the DNA probe or marker is within the gene that is mutated, crossing-over between the genetic marker and the disease-causing mutation is usually negligible. Duchenne's muscular dystrophy is an exception because it is an extremely large gene within which crossing-over occurs at a detectable frequency.

Examples of molecular diagnosis by linkage, when recombination between the loci is negligible, are presented in Fig. 61-18. Genetic marker data are presented as letters that might represent simple marker alleles or haplotypes of markers. A *haplotype* is a cluster of tightly

FIGURE 61-18 Examples of molecular diagnosis by genetic linkage with negligible recombination between the DNA probe and the disease locus. Letters below pedigree symbols indicate alleles for a DNA marker. Families A and B depict autosomal recessive disorders; C through E depict autosomal dominant disorders; and F through I depict X-linked disorders. Complete penetrance is assumed. See text for discussion.

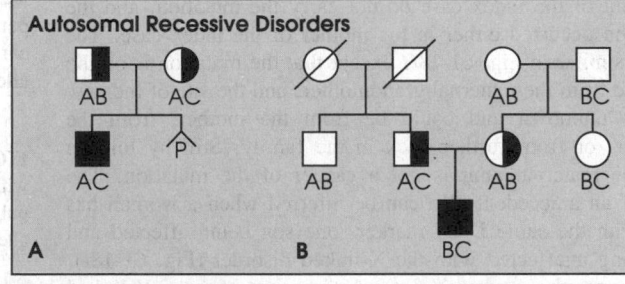

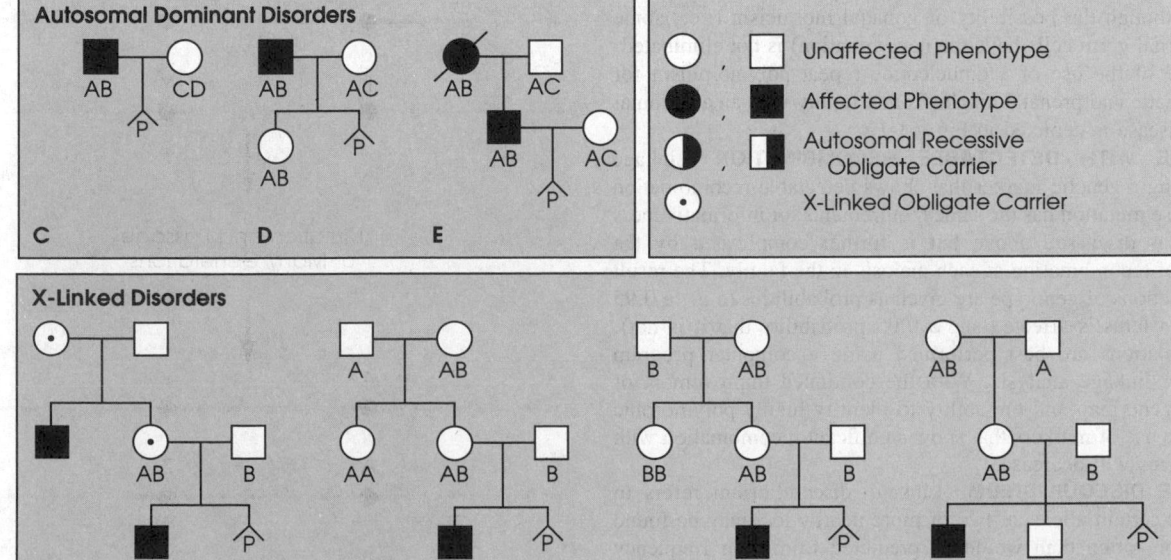

linked specific alleles on a chromosome. Phase can usually be determined from a single index case for autosomal recessive disorders (Fig. 61-18A). Fetuses of AC genotype are predicted to be affected in Fig. 61-18A while fetuses of AA or BC genotype are predicted to be carriers and those of AB genotype to be noncarriers. In Fig. 61-18B, carrier detection is sought for the aunt and uncle of the affected. The data on the maternal side require analysis of the grandparents and predict that the aunt is a noncarrier. Although the paternal grandparents are deceased, it is still possible to conclude that the uncle is a noncarrier since he does not inherit the C haplotype which is linked to disease allele on the paternal side. For autosomal dominant disorders, linkage phase usually cannot be determined from a single affected individual (Fig. 61-18C). Exceptions include retinoblastoma, when analysis of tumor DNA may distinguish the allele on the abnormal chromosome (often retained in the tumor) from the allele on the normal chromosome (often lost in the tumor). Linkage phase for autosomal dominant disorders can be determined from two appropriate individuals; it is not essential that both be affected if penetrance is complete (Fig. 61-18D and E). Fetuses of AA or AC genotype in Fig. 61-18D and fetuses of AB or BC genotype in Fig. 61-18E are predicted to be affected. For X-linked disorders, phase information is most readily obtained from a single affected male (Fig. 61-18F). In general, linkage information can be used to determine the genotype in children of individuals of known genotype. Linkage information generally cannot be used consistently to determine the genotype of antecedents because of the possibility of new mutation from one generation to the next. This is exemplified by an X-linked disorder, where linkage information will not clarify whether the mother of an isolated affected male is a heterozygote or whether there is a new mutation in the propositus (Fig. 61-18G). This represents an important difference between direct detection of a mutation and linkage analysis. Occasionally, linkage analysis can suggest the genotype of an antecedent. Note in Fig. 61-18G that the mutation arose on the chromosome that was inherited from the unaffected maternal grandfather; the maternal grandmother and the maternal aunt of the index case do not carry the mutation, and the new mutation occurred either in the mother or the index case. The situation is similar in Fig. 61-18H except that the mutation is on the chromosome from the maternal grandmother, and the site of the new mutation is unknown and could be from the mother, from the grandmother, or from further back in the family. Still by linkage analysis, the maternal aunt is not a carrier of the mutation. The genotype of an antecedent also can be inferred when a woman has two sons with the same DNA marker, one son being affected and one son being unaffected with the X-linked disorder (Fig. 61-18I). In this instance, the mother is not a heterozygote for the X-linked disorder, although the possibility of gonadal mosaicism (i.e., some of the maternal germ cells have the new mutation) is not eliminated. An example of the use of a dinucleotide repeat polymorphism for presymptomatic and prenatal diagnosis in a family with an autosomal dominant disease is depicted in Fig. 61-19.

LINKAGE WITH DETECTABLE RECOMBINATION Linkage analysis using a genetic marker that shows detectable recombination with a disease mutation has the same requirements for informativeness and phase as discussed above but is further complicated by the possibility of recombination at each meiosis in the family. The result is that predictions of genotype are given as probabilities (e.g., a 0.95 probability a fetus is affected and a 0.05 probability that it is not). These calculations are best performed using a computer program designed for linkage analysis. With the continued improvement of the human gene map and the ability to identify highly polymorphic markers, the use of markers that show significant recombination with a disease locus will decrease.

LINKAGE DISEQUILIBRIUM Linkage disequilibrium refers to the fact that certain alleles at two or more nearby loci may be found together more often than would be predicted from their frequency in the general population. Although linkage disequilibrium occurs routinely between multiple polymorphic sites, for purposes of genetic

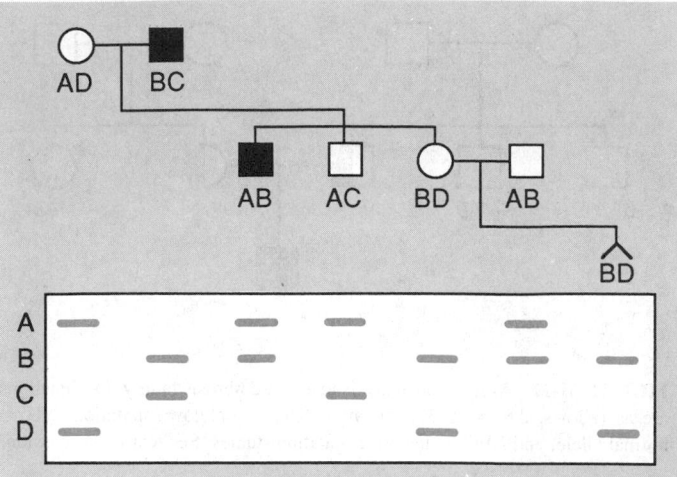

FIGURE 61-19 Linkage analysis in an autosomal dominant disorder with variable age of onset or incomplete penetrance. A dinucleotide repeat polymorphism is analyzed by PCR to detect alleles A–D. Solid symbols are affected and open symbols are asymptomatic. The brother of the affected in the second generation is predicted to carry the normal allele while the pregnant sister has received the disease allele. The fetus received the normal allele (with the D marker) from the mother. Thus presymptomatic diagnosis indicates an affected genotype for the pregnant sister and an unaffected genotype for the brother and fetus.

diagnosis this is most readily discussed in terms of a genetic marker and a disease mutation. In Fig. 61-20 is depicted the occurrence of a disease susceptibility mutation (Z) at a locus where the normal allele is represented as Y. The mutation arises on a chromosome carrying the A allele for a nearby polymorphic DNA marker. With the passage of time, chromosomes carrying the A allele for the DNA marker and the Z allele for the disease locus grow to represent 10 percent of the chromosomes in the population. Not all chromosomes carrying the A form of the marker carry the disease susceptibility allele, but the disease allele is carried only on chromosomes bearing

FIGURE 61-20 Depiction of the development of linkage disequilibrium within a population of chromosomes. A and B indicate alleles for a DNA polymorphism. Y represents a normal allele and Z a disease susceptibility allele at a locus. See text for discussion.

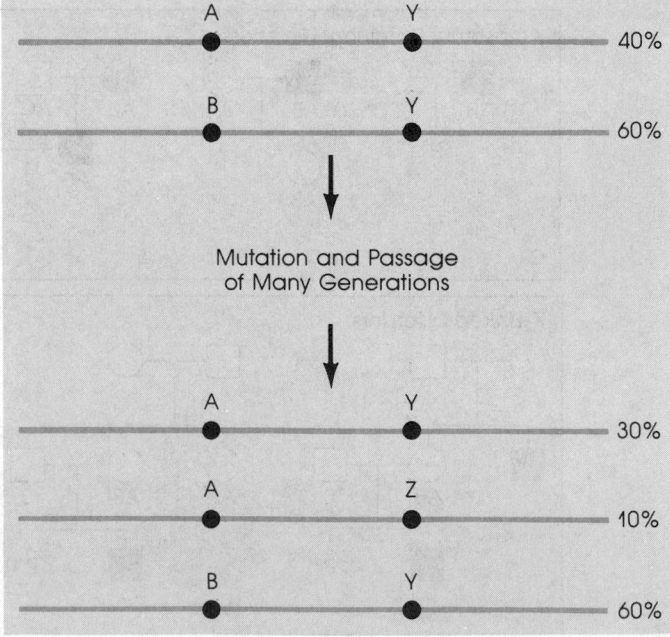

the A form of the marker. This model also implies that it might be possible at a future date to identify and detect directly the Z mutation to provide a more accurate prediction of disease susceptibility. For linkage disequilibrium to be present, the two genetic markers must be tightly linked. In addition there must be one or only a few origins for the disease mutations, or the mutations will be found randomly with different alleles for the marker site. Linkage disequilibrium can often be found using a group of close genetic markers to form a haplotype.

Linkage disequilibrium is extensive within the HLA complex, and numerous diseases are found in association with various HLA haplotypes (see Chap. 60 in this text and Chap. 9 in Scriver et al.). For example, insulin-dependent diabetes mellitus is associated with HLA-DR3 and HLA-DR4, and susceptibility to this disease may be attributable to the presence of an aspartic acid residue in position 57 of the HLA-DQβ locus. The genotype at this position can be directly determined using PCR and allele-specific oligonucleotides. By comparison to Fig. 6-20, the HLA-DR data for diabetes could be equivalent to the A/B marker, while the aspartic acid residue could be the equivalent of the Z mutation. By analogy, DNA polymorphisms near any gene might detect linkage disequilibrium with a disease susceptibility. Using this rationale, attempts have been made to determine if certain DNA markers adjacent to the apolipoprotein genes are associated with increased risk of atherosclerosis. If such associations are proven, they would imply that some genetic variation in the coding or regulatory portions of an apolipoprotein gene itself is responsible for the altered disease susceptibility. Ultimately these genetic variations could be used directly for assessment of disease risks.

MOLECULAR CYTOGENETICS Recombinant DNA techniques provide a bridge between single-gene disorders and cytogenetics (see Chap. 62 in this text and Chaps. 16 to 20 in Scriver et al.). Genetic alterations range in size from single-base changes to gain or loss of an entire chromosome. As an example, some patients with Duchenne's muscular dystrophy have gross cytogenetic abnormalities, some patients have large deletions of DNA detectable by molecular but not by conventional cytogenetic analysis, and presumably others have single-base changes. In some cases, large deletions may involve multiple adjacent disease genes giving rise to complex phenotypes (contiguous gene syndromes). Samples from patients with detectable constitutional cytogenetic abnormalities or with acquired abnormalities in tumors have facilitated the cloning of numerous X-linked and autosomal genes. Reciprocally, molecular probes have been used to define cytogenetic translocations, deletions, and insertions. DNA probes are used to detect Y chromosome–specific sequences including the testes-determining factor in 46,XX males and to demonstrate the absence of regions of the Y chromosome in 46,XY females.

The technique of FISH (fluorescence in situ hybridization) is a major breakthrough in diagnostic molecular genetics and cytogenetics (Chap. 62). In addition to its use in disorders traditionally considered as cytogenetic conditions, FISH makes possible diagnosis of deletions in Prader-Willi syndrome, DiGeorge's syndrome, and other conditions and detection of the typical duplications of chromosome 17 that cause Charcot-Marie-Tooth disease.

MOLECULAR ONCOLOGY Just as these diagnostic techniques can be used to detect mutations in the constitutional DNA of all cells, they can also detect somatic mutations in malignant cells. Southern blotting and/or PCR can be used to detect alterations affecting both dominant and recessive oncogenes. Single-base changes in dominant oncogenes such as substitutions in codon 12 of H-*ras*, have been demonstrated in human colon and pancreatic cancer among others. Oncogenes can be shown to be amplified in numerous human tumors. Loss of heterozygosity at loci for recessive oncogenes can be demonstrated, using polymorphisms linked to these loci, e.g., loss of heterozygosity on chromosomes 5, 17, and 18 in human colon cancer. Chromosomal translocations such as those between immunoglobin loci and oncogenes can be demonstrated by Southern blotting. Molecular techniques are invaluable in the analysis of the basic

alterations in tumor cells, in the classification and staging of tumors, and in the monitoring of therapeutic strategies (see Chap. 63 in this text and Chaps. 10 to 15 in Scriver et al.).

DIAGNOSTIC VIROLOGY AND MICROBIOLOGY Virtually all microorganisms have DNA or RNA sequences that can be detected by nucleic acid hybridization techniques. As discussed above, nucleic acid hybridization is sensitive and specific and can be combined with PCR to detect a low abundance of foreign nucleic acid sequences. Other diagnostic procedures such as detection of infectious antigens with monoclonal antibodies and detection of human immune responses with immunoblotting can also provide rapid, sensitive, and specific diagnostic procedures. Each strategy offers special advantages. Some advantages of the detection of foreign nucleic acid sequences are as follows: (1) sequences can be detected without the delay required for the host to mount immune responses, (2) sequences can be detected without regard to passive acquisition of antibody whether by maternal transfer or by transfusion, (3) sequences can be detected even if the host fails to mount an immune response, (4) sequences can be detected even if no foreign proteins are being synthesized, and (5) the extraordinary ability of PCR to detect even a single molecule in a sample may make it the most sensitive technique in many circumstances. These techniques have been used for a broad range of viral diagnoses including cytomegalovirus, rotavirus, Epstein-Barr virus, and others. PCR has been used to detect hepatitis B sequences in serum and to detect HIV-1 sequences in peripheral blood mononuclear cells. In one study using PCR, HIV-1 sequences were detected in all specimens from seropositive, virus culture-positive subjects and in 64 percent of specimens from seropositive, virus culture-negative subjects. DNA amplification required 3 days rather than the 3 to 4 weeks required for virus isolation. PCR can also be used to detect nucleic acids from infectious organisms.

IDENTITY TESTING Analysis for only a few highly polymorphic tandem repeat sites, often tetra-, tri-, or dinucleotide repeats, provides the ability to distinguish the genotype of virtually all individuals except identical twins. This powerful method of identification is useful in paternity testing, in settling immigration disputes, in criminal investigations, and in monitoring bone marrow transplantation. The use of PCR for analysis of short tandem repeats is particularly powerful for forensic analysis, since identification can be made from minuscule samples of semen, blood, hair root, skin, or other tissue. Tissue typing at the HLA loci is also feasible using molecular analysis of polymorphisms.

PROSPECTS FOR SOMATIC GENE THERAPY (See also Chap. 65)

The general visions regarding both the significance of the role for somatic gene therapy and mechanisms for implementation have evolved dramatically. One change involves the breadth of disorders which might be considered amenable to therapy. Thinking has expanded from treatment of single-gene disorders to include treatment of cancer, AIDS, and atherosclerosis; in addition, a recombinant protein therapy (e.g., insulin, erythropoietin, clotting factor) could be converted to in vivo production via somatic gene therapy. The repertoire of delivery systems has expanded from retroviral vectors to include vectors based on adenovirus, herpes virus, vaccinia, and other viruses. Nonviral systems such as liposomes, DNA-protein conjugates, and DNA-protein–defective virus conjugates are also promising. Emphasis has shifted from ex vivo modification of cells to in vivo delivery, although ex vivo manipulation of bone marrow cells, tumor cells, and cultured fibroblasts and epithelium remains attractive. In general, retroviral vectors provide integration of the foreign DNA and permanent alteration of the recipient cell, but they require dividing cells as a target and allow only low titers of virus to be generated and are therefore relatively impractical for most in vivo approaches. Adenoviral vectors, in contrast, offer high titer and easier ability to infect large numbers of cells in vivo, but there is concern about toxic effects on infected cells and about the transient nature of their expression. Vaccinia vectors and nonviral systems also cause only transient expression, since they are not integrated into DNA. There is little information as yet as to whether repeated administration of agents that provide transient expression is feasible. Transient expression may be acceptable for applications such as eliciting an altered immune response to malignant cells or treatment of acute disease. There is need for new delivery systems or vectors that can be delivered efficiently in vivo preferably by intravenous injection, targeted to specific cell types, alter resting or dividing cells, and persist indefinitely whether by integration into the chromosome or by an extrachromosomal (episomal) mechanism.

At least three strategies may be useful for integration of the expressed DNA for somatic gene therapy. In one, a cDNA might be inserted under the control of a foreign promoter so that the product is synthesized without proper regulation. In a second strategy, genomic DNA could include the sequences necessary for proper regulation of the level and tissue specificity of expression. Artificial "minigene" constructions that link genomic regulatory regions with cDNA may provide constructions that are of manageable size and that show proper regulation. These strategies would typically involve random insertion of DNA sequences into the chromosome, although expression of extrachromosomal sequences is also a possibility. A third strategy would utilize site-specific recombination so that the mutant region would be replaced by normal DNA sequence. This approach is theoretically optimal and, although challenging, is more feasible since homologous recombination has been achieved in various cultured cells. In the case of enzyme or other protein deficiencies, any of these three approaches might suffice. For hemoglobin disorders, the relative accessibility of bone marrow stem cells and the advantages of maintaining all the normal regulatory mechanisms make homologous recombination a desirable goal.

Retroviral vectors provide viral particles that encode foreign nucleic acid and contain mechanisms for chromosomal integration. One current strategy (Fig. 61-21) involves insertion of cDNA or minigene DNA constructions between two viral long terminal repeats (LTRs) in a plasmid vector. These constructions can be introduced into cultured cell lines that provide the viral proteins necessary to package pseudovirus particles that include the gene sequence of interest. For example, bone marrow cells could be removed from a patient with a specific defect, purified bone marrow stem cells could be infected with these viral particles, and the patient's bone marrow could be repopulated with the altered cells. Retroviral infection of hepatocytes ex vivo has also been tried for homozygous familial hypercholesterolemia, but in vivo alteration of hepatocytes is likely to be more useful.

Adenovirus vectors typically are deleted for an essential viral gene and are then produced in cultured cells which complement this defect to yield a vector that can infect target cells but not produce further virus. Human trials to deliver adenovirus encoding the cystic fibrosis cDNA to the airway of patients are being initiated, and adenoviral delivery to hepatocytes is feasible, although expression is expected to be transient in these cases. Various in vivo strategies for gene therapy are being explored (Fig. 61-21).

Several single-gene disorders are candidates for gene therapy, and many protocols are being developed (Table 61-3). Life-threatening, recessive diseases involving bone marrow–derived cells would be excellent choices (e.g., adenosine deaminase deficiency, chronic granulomatous disease, and leukocyte adhesion deficiency), as are disorders in which extracellular products such as hormones or clotting factors might be produced in altered bone marrow cells. Dominant, neurologic disorders such as Huntington's disease appear to be the least approachable. If proper regulation of globin genes could be achieved, sickle cell anemia and thalassemia would constitute important opportunities because of the accessibility of bone marrow for in vitro treatment.

FIGURE 61-21 Comparison of ex vivo and in vivo strategies for somatic gene therapy. A procedure for ex vivo retroviral infection of bone marrow stem cells is shown on the left. On the right, this is compared to delivery by inhalation of aerosol for a disease such as cystic fibrosis or parenteral injection for targeting to organs such as liver or muscle using a variety of vectors or delivery systems.

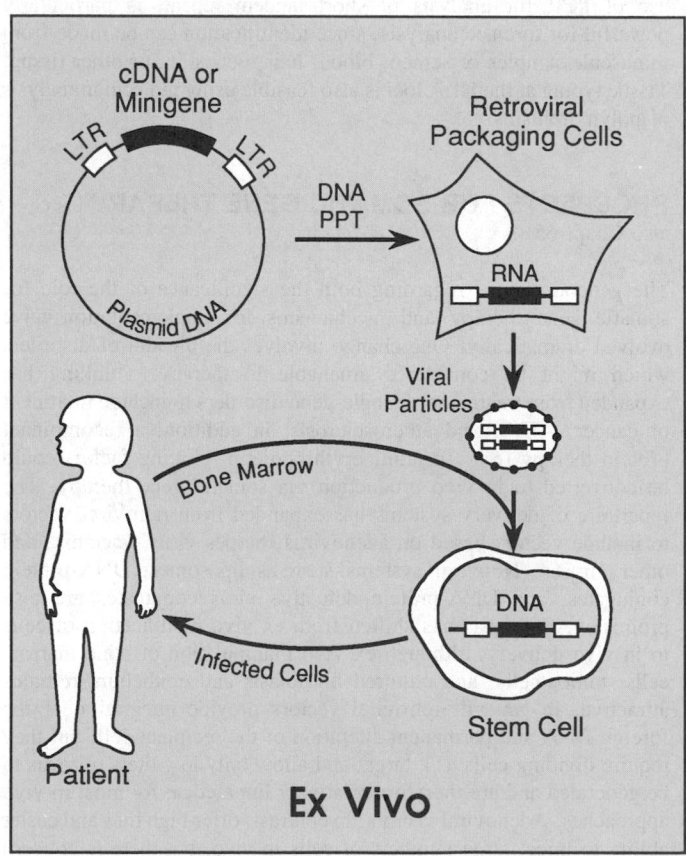

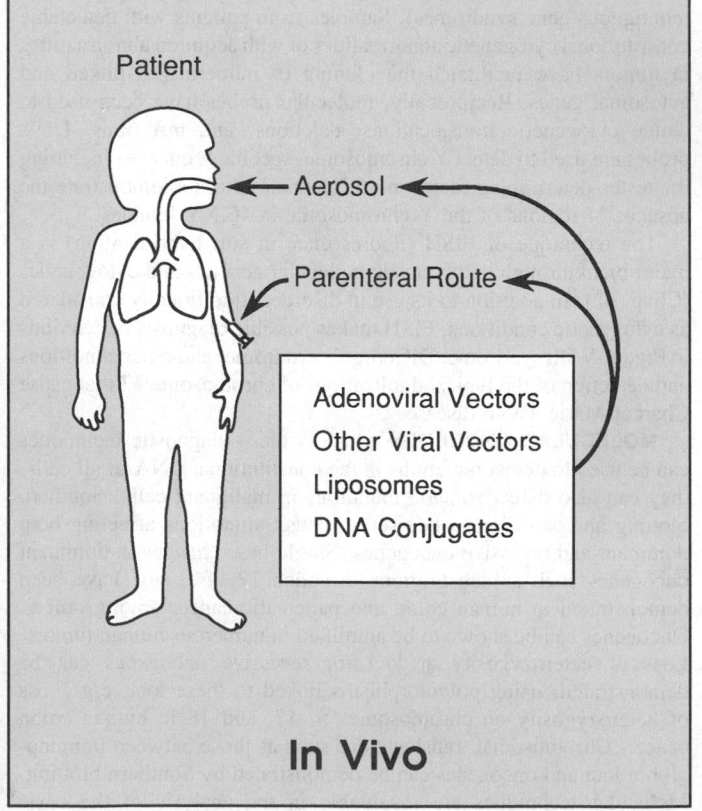

TABLE 61-3 Human diseases as candidates for gene replacement therapy*

Disorder	Burden of disease	Alternative treatment	Disease frequency	Requirement for tissue specificity	Regulation	Relative feasibility[†]
Hemoglobinopathies	Great	Transfusion, fair to poor	1 in 600 in ethnic groups	Erythroid	Required	+ + +
Lesch-Nyhan syndrome	Great	Poor	Rare	Brain, ?other	?Not essential	+ +
Adenosine deaminase and nucleoside phosphorylase deficiency	Great	Transplant, enzyme replacement, fair to good	Very rare	Bone marrow	?Not essential	+ + +
Leukocyte adhesion deficiency	Great	Transplant, fair to poor	Very rare	Bone marrow	?Not essential	+ + + +
Phenylketonuria	Small to moderate	Diet, good	1 in 11,000	Liver, ?other	?Not essential	+ +
Urea cycle disorders	Moderate to great	Diet, drug, good to poor	1 in 30,000 for all types	Liver, ?other	?Not essential	+ + +
α_1-Antitrypsin	Moderate	Poor, ?recombinant drug	1 in 3500	Liver, ?other	?Not essential	+ + +
Hemophilia A and B	Moderate to great	Replacement, fair	1 in 10,000 males	?Any organ,	?Not essential	+ + + +
Lysosomal storage diseases	Great	Poor	1 in 1500 for all types	Brain for many	?Not essential	+ +
Familial hypercholesterolemia	Great	Diet, drug, fair	1 in 500 heterozygotes	Liver, ?other	Some importance	+ +
Cystic fibrosis	Great	Supportive, fair/poor	1 in 2500 whites	Lung	?	+ + +
Duchenne's muscular dystrophy	Great	Poor	1 in 10,000 males	Muscle	?	+ +
Huntington's disease	Great	Poor	1 in 20,000	?Brain	?	?Poor
Various cancers	Great	Often poor	Very high	?Tumor cells	?	+ +
AIDS	Great	Poor	High	?Bone marrow	?	+ +
Atherosclerosis	Great	Fair	Very high	?Intravascular	?	+ +

* See Anderson for clinical protocols as of 1992.
† Attempts to take into account requirements for regulation, accessibility of target organs, alternative treatment, and risk vs benefit.

GENE THERAPY FOR CANCER, AIDS, ATHEROSCLEROSIS, AND PHARMACOTHERAPY The concept of somatic gene therapy has expanded beyond replacement strategies for genetic deficiencies (see Anderson). Many protocols for treatment of cancer are under evaluation, particularly for otherwise untreatable conditions. Strategies include (1) alteration of cancer cells or other host cells to produce cytokines or other molecules to alter the host response to the malignancy, (2) expression of antigens (e.g., allogeneic HLA proteins) on cancer cells to induce a host immune response, (3) insertion of tumor suppressor gene sequences or other sequences to slow cell growth, and (4) introduction of drug resistance genes into normal cells (e.g., bone marrow) to facilitate more aggressive chemotherapy. The first two "immunomodulatory" approaches are the basis of numerous research protocols.

A variety of strategies for gene therapy of bone marrow stem cells to introduce resistance to HIV or otherwise blunt expression of its effects are being proposed. In transgenic mice overexpression of apolipoprotein A-I can protect against atherosclerosis, and various strategies are being proposed for prevention and reversal of atherosclerosis whether of single-gene or multifactorial origin. As mentioned above, recombinant proteins could be produced in vivo rather than ex vivo with repeated injection. Transient and rapid expression of therapeutic proteins after injection of a viral or nonviral vector could greatly expand current therapeutic avenues.

ETHICAL CONSIDERATIONS Molecular genetic diagnosis provides an increasing capacity for presymptomatic and prenatal diagnosis of disease and disease susceptibility. It is possible to diagnose a newborn infant with familial polyposis of the colon, Huntington's disease, or dominant polycystic kidney disease decades before the onset of symptoms. What might be the impact of such diagnosis on the psychological development, career opportunities, and insurability of such individuals? Diagnosis of major increased susceptibility to coronary disease, diabetes mellitus, colon cancer, breast cancer, and other disorders is also likely to bring both the potential for therapeutic intervention and the risk of anxiety and discrimination. Prenatal diagnosis is now possible for diseases with a wide range of burden, such as α_1-antitrypsin deficiency, phenylketonuria, sickle cell anemia, muscular dystrophy, and familial hypercholesterolemia. Societies and individuals are divided regarding the option of abortion under such circumstances. Development of somatic gene therapy and other means

of treating presently untreatable genetic diseases may ultimately result in a reduced utilization of abortion.

Gene therapy raises other ethical considerations. Somatic gene replacement therapy requires conventional risk-benefit analyses for individual patients. So long as there is no modification of the germline DNA, few people have serious ethical concerns other than the question of whether such treatment is in the best interest of an individual patient. Experience with cancer chemotherapy suggests that some low level of damage to germline DNA might be an acceptable risk of such therapy if the patient received great benefit. In the future, it is conceivable that methods for site-specific recombination would allow replacement of mutant DNA in the germline with normal material. If one could permanently correct the cystic fibrosis mutation, the Huntington's disease mutation, or the sickle cell mutation in the germline of an individual and if such treatment were safe and effective, would society consider such therapeutic intervention? If introduction of an extra copy of a tumor suppressor gene into the germline of mice greatly protected against carcinogen-induced tumors without harmful effects, would this be relevant to humans?

REFERENCES

ANDERSON WF: Human gene therapy. Science 256:808, 1992

CASKEY CT et al: Triplet repeat mutations in human disease. Science 256:784, 1992

COOPER DN, SCHMIDTKE J: Diagnosis of genetic disease using recombinant DNA. Third edition. Hum Genet 87:519, 1991

ERLICH H et al (eds): *Polymerase Chain Reaction.* Cold Spring Harbor, Cold Spring Harbor Laboratory, 1989

HALL JG: Genomic imprinting: Review and relevance to human diseases. Am J Hum Genet 46:857, 1990

MULTICENTER STUDY GROUP: Diagnosis of Duchenne and Becker muscular dystrophies by polymerase chain reaction. JAMA 267:2609, 1992

PALMITER RD, BRINSTER RL: Germ-line transformation of mice. Annu Rev Genet 20:465, 1986

SAMBROOK J et al: *Molecular Cloning, A Laboratory Manual,* 2d ed. Cold Spring Harbor, Cold Spring Harbor Laboratory, 1989

SCRIVER CR et al (eds): *The Molecular and Metabolic Basis of Inherited Disease,* 7th ed. New York, McGraw-Hill, in press

WATSON JD et al: *Recombinant DNA,* 2d ed. New York, Scientific American Books, distributed by Freeman, 1992

WEISSENBACH J et al: A second-generation linkage map of the human genome. Nature 359:794, 1992

62   CYTOGENETIC ASPECTS OF HUMAN DISEASE

JAMES GERMAN

The chromosome complement is guarded carefully against change; most chromosome mutations, either structural or numerical, are deleterious. Only rarely is a structural rearrangement introduced into the population and transmitted from generation to generation, i.e., a chromosome mutation, that results in neither deficiency nor duplication of significant chromosome segments. As a rule an abnormal number of autosomes results in early death, except for trisomy of the shortest chromosome. In contrast, an abnormal number of sex chromosomes is often tolerated reasonably well although infertility or subfertility usually is present. Nevertheless, among human embryos abnormalities in chromosome structure and number are the major known cause of embryonic and early fetal wastage. However, not every fetus with an abnormal chromosome complement is aborted, and those that survive become the material of medical cytogenetics. Chromosome imbalance causes varying features including abnormal anatomic development, mental deficiency, behavioral disorders, and disturbances in growth and sexual development. Sometimes persons with abnormal chromosome complements whose own general development is normal present with infertility, repeated abortion, or the birth of malformed children.

The disorders just referred to are due to chromosome imbalance that affects tissues throughout the body. In addition, change can occur in the chromosome complement in a single cell of some somatic tissue. Such a mutant cell may have a proliferative advantage over normal cells if the mutation affects certain growth-controlling loci and is of a specific type, in which case a clone bearing the abnormal chromosome complement can develop among otherwise normal cells. Although such mutant clones are in many cases clinically insignificant, some are of importance in the etiology of cancer and possibly in other conditions that can be referred to as somatic mutational disease.

This chapter is addressed to those aspects of normal chromosome structure and function that constitute the basis for understanding the important chromosome alterations that have been or will be discovered. A selected number of those alterations and their consequences are mentioned as examples.

CHROMOSOME STRUCTURE AND FUNCTION   The human autosomes are numbered 1 through 22, and the sex chromosomes are denoted X and Y. (The normal human chromosome complement is shown in Fig. 62-1. In the legend of the figure several terms used in human cytogenetics are defined.) Only seven of the chromosomes can be identified microscopically by their relative lengths and centromere positions, but unique staining characteristics—banding patterns—make possible the identification of all.

A mammalian chromosome consists of one double-stranded helix of DNA that extends from one end through the centromere to the other end. The paternally and the maternally derived autosomes that compose a pair and the pair of X chromosomes in females are genetically homologous, their differences being qualitative, i.e., dependent on the alleles received from each parent at polymorphic loci. In contrast, the X and Y chromosomes in males are almost completely different with the exception of their *pseudoautosomal regions*, short homologous segments at the ends of the short arms. The two homologues of each autosomal pair synapse and exchange chromatid segments at meiosis, as do the pseudoautosomal regions, which in effect constitute a 24th autosomal pair. With respect to the sex chromosomes, in germ line cells in the ovary, the two Xs pair at meiosis and undergo *recombination* just as the autosomes do; in the male, pairing and recombination of the X and Y chromosomes normally is limited to the pseudoautosomal regions. In somatic cells of the female, except in early embryonic life, one X is extensively inactivated, thereby giving the male and female approximately equivalent numbers of active X-linked genes. Inactivation of an X

originates at a single active locus, *XIST*, on the long arm (band Xq13) of the inactivated X and affects most loci on that X, excluding the pseudoautosomal region. Similarly, one locus on the Y, *SRY* (Sex-determining Region on the Y chromosome), is pivotal in testis determination.

Cell-division cycle   Chromosomes must duplicate before cell division can occur. This duplication occurs prior to the onset of mitosis or meiosis in a phase of the cell cycle termed S, for synthesis of DNA (Fig. 62-2). Thus, from the completion of S to the completion of metaphase, each chromosome contains two identical double-stranded helices of DNA, and the nucleus contains four times as much DNA as a spermatozoon or ovum. During mitosis chromosomes are condensed, and the two sister chromatids can be visualized by late prophase or early metaphase (Fig. 62-1). (Metaphase is the stage in the cell-division cycle ordinarily employed for cytogenetic analysis.)

At the onset of anaphase the centromeric regions of each chromosome separate, and the two chromatids move quickly to opposite poles of the mitotic spindle. When the poles receive their full complements of chromatids (now called chromosomes), nuclear membranes assemble about each cluster to form the nuclei of the two sister cells that will emerge from mitosis. (The nuclear membrane had been disassembled late in prophase.) The sister cells emerge in what is called the G_1 phase of the cell cycle where they remain unreplicated unless another division is to be prepared for, in which case they enter S. Cells engaged in some differentiated function ordinarily remain unreplicated.

Most normal cells in the human body are diploid; i.e., they have twice the haploid number of chromosomes, the number in a gamete (haploid = 23, diploid = 46). In the germ line, the lineage of cells devoted to gamete formation, cells destined eventually to differentiate into spermatozoa or ova, undergo mitotic cell cycling until they enter *meiosis*, two specialized divisions unique to this lineage. In meiosis, pairing of homologous chromosomes takes place (the paternally derived chromosome 1 with the maternally derived chromosome 1, the paternal 2 with the maternal 2, and so on), and genetic recombination occurs by a process called *crossing-over*, an exchange of entire segments between paternal and maternal chromosomes whereby the genetic constitution of each is altered qualitatively (see Chap. 60). At the first meiotic division homologous chromosomes are segregated, and the diploid chromosome number is reduced to the haploid; i.e., each cell then contains one of each of the 22 (duplicated) autosomes plus one (duplicated) sex chromosome. No S phase takes place between the first and second meiotic divisions (depicted in Fig. 62-2, right), so that at the second division, in which sister chromatids separate, emerging cells maintain the haploid number of chromosomes but are reduced in their content of DNA to half the amount of diploid G_1 cells of somatic tissues. With fertilization, both the chromosome constitution and the DNA content of the zygote are restored to that of a G_1 somatic cell. An S period in the zygote then permits reinstitution of regular cell-division cycles characteristic of somatic cells.

Chromosome differentiation   A chromosome is differentiated along its length, and some aspects of this differentiation are resolvable microscopically. The DNA is complexed with a number of proteins in a highly specific way. The DNA-protein complex together with some associated RNA is referred to as *chromatin*. The fine structure, the manner in which the DNA is compacted and interacts with proteins, and the organization of chromatin in the interphase nucleus are thought to pertain to the control of RNA production and DNA replication and perhaps to cellular differentiation as well.

The sequences of nucleotide bases in DNA that constitute the genes and that can be transcribed into messenger RNA are distributed throughout the length of the various chromosomes. (These sequences are too short to be resolved microscopically.) Over 1500 genes have been assigned to specific chromosomes, in many cases to specific bands of a chromosome, where the order in which they are *linked* also has been determined.

Certain visible segments of at least 12 chromosomes vary in

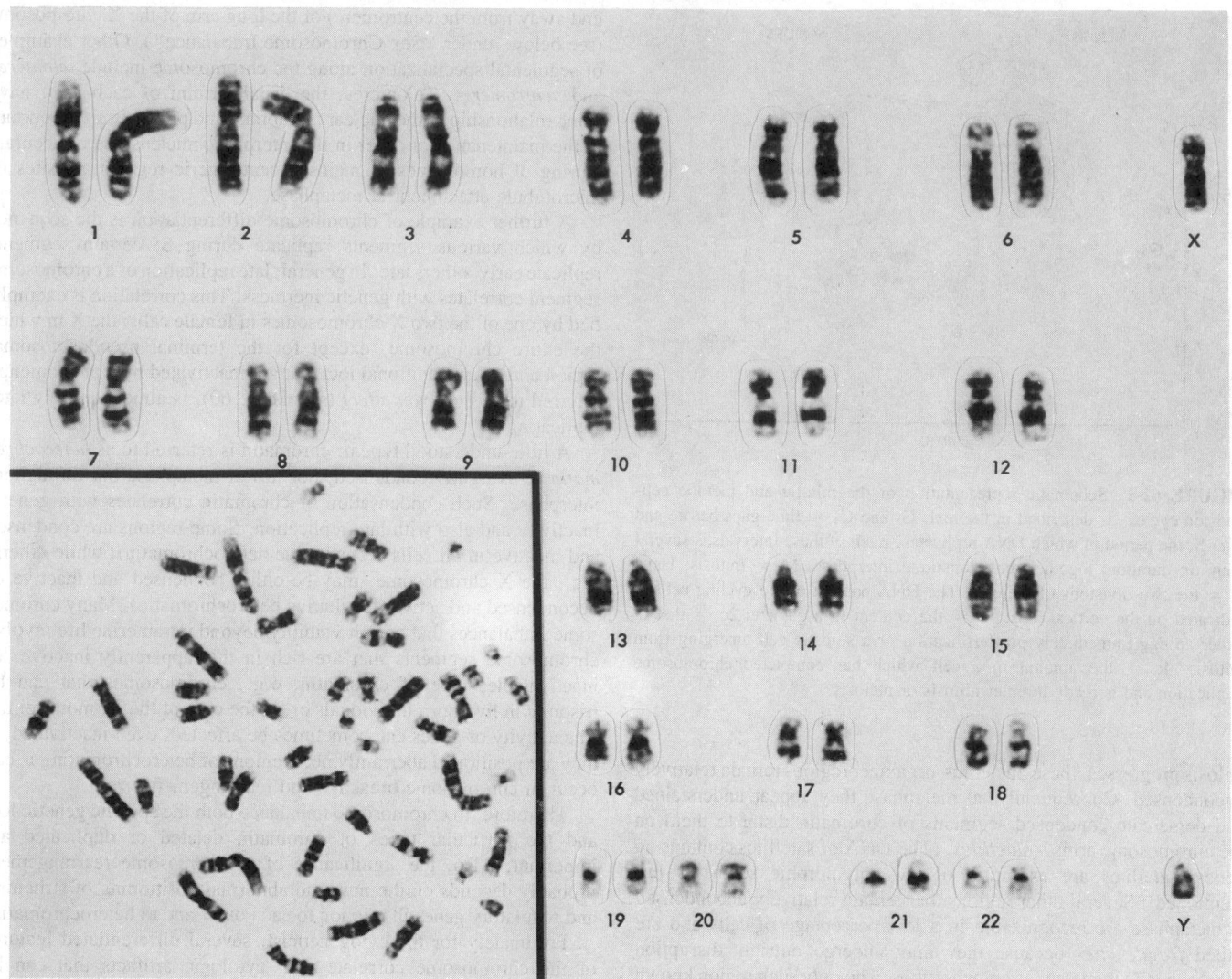

FIGURE 62-1   Normal human lymphocyte chromosomes arrested in metaphase and stained for G bands (G standing for Giemsa). The inset shows the arrangement of chromosomes in an intact cell, and the remainder of the figure shows their ordered arrangement into a karyotype. By the time mitosis begins, each chromosome consists of two identical parts called sister chromatids and is identified by its relative length, the location of its centromere, and a distinctive sequence of bands of varying lengths and depth of staining. The number of bands visible microscopically varies from cell to cell, depending on the degree of chromosome condensation. The 300 to 400 bands seen in this particular cell can be increased to several times that number if cells with longer chromosomes are chosen for analysis, i.e., many of the bands seen here will resolve into subbands. Normally, the band patterns of the two chromosomes of a pair are alike, with the exception of certain polymorphic regions, examples of which are shown in Fig. 62-3.

The centromere of a chromosome divides it into a short arm (p) and a long arm (q). Numbers 13 to 15, 21, 22, and Y are called acrocentric because of the nearly terminal positions of their centromeres; the minute p of each acrocentric autosome bears a nucleolus-organizing region which often causes a secondary constriction in the metaphase chromosome (the constriction at the centromere being the primary constriction).

By standard nomenclature, this karyotype is described as 46,XY, indicating that its chromosome number is 46, its sex chromosomes are an X and a Y, and the autosomes (those besides the X and Y) number 44. The following examples show the general use of this nomenclature: A normal female karyotype is described as 46,XX. A female cell with an extra chromosome 18 (trisomic for 18) would be described as 47,XX,+18. A cell with only one sex chromosome, an X, and with deletion in the short arm of chromosome 5 would be described as 45,X,5p−. A male cell with a translocation between chromosomes 2 and 3, with breakpoints in band 13 of 2p and band 22 of 3p, would be described as 46,XY,t(2;3)(p13;p22). (See also Table 62-2 footnote.)

length among individuals. These can be delineated by their staining characteristics (e.g., Fig. 62-3). The variable segments consist of nontranscribed, highly repetitive nucleotide sequences of DNA and are transmitted from parent to child in a straightforward mendelian fashion. The techniques of molecular genetics make possible the identification and molecular definition of innumerable heritable polymorphic segments of DNA, segments that, like genes themselves, are submicroscopic. These noncoding segments are referred to as *restriction fragment length polymorphisms* (RFLPs) or *variable number of tandem repeats* (VNTRs). Variations in both microscopically visible and invisible segments are usually unassociated with detectable phenotypic effect. However, they serve as useful genetic markers in prenatal diagnosis when they are tightly linked to disease-associated loci (e.g., in Duchenne's muscular dystrophy) and in the determination of zygosity of twins, paternity, and survival of transplants. Also, these DNA markers, especially those VNTRs composed of short oligonucleotide repeats that are highly polymorphic and are widely dispersed throughout the genome, are invaluable in the effort to map the human genome. In this undertaking, loci of importance in normal development and differentiated cell function, including those that when mutant result in human disease, are being assigned their correct order and relationship to one another along each of the chromosomes.

Microscopically recognizable segments in the short arms of the acrocentric autosomes (mentioned in the legend to Fig. 62-1) are devoted to the production of ribosomal RNA and nucleoli. As

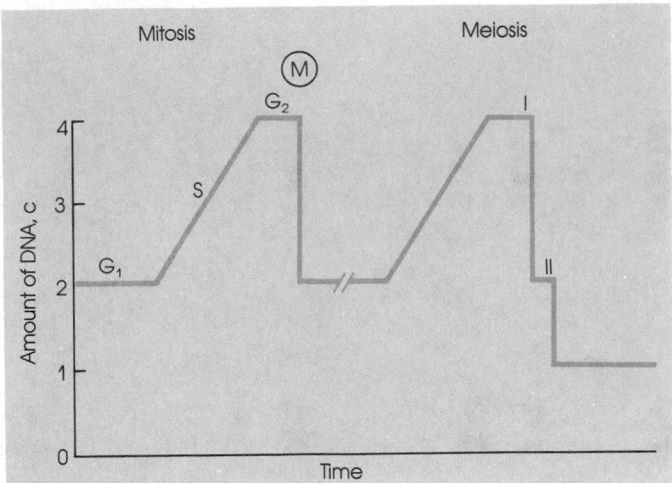

FIGURE 62-2 Schematic representation of the mitotic and meiotic cell-division cycles, as described in the text. G_1 and G_2 = time gaps before and after S, the period in which DNA replicates. Each of these intervals is several hours in duration; together they constitute interphase. M = mitosis; I and II = the two divisions of meiosis. The DNA content of the cycling cells is indicated on the vertical axis: 1c = the content in a gamete; 2c = that in either an egg immediately postfertilization or a somatic cell emerging from mitosis; 4c = the amount in a cell which has completed chromosome duplication and is ready to enter mitosis or meiosis.

mitosis progresses, these nucleolus-organizer regions remain relatively uncondensed. Consequently, at metaphase they appear understained and demarcate condensed segments of chromatin distal to them on the chromosome arms—*satellites*. (The DNA of satellites contains no genes; satellites are examples of the polymorphic segments just mentioned.) Several other regions that remain relatively uncondensed at metaphase are recognizable in a low percentage of cells and are called *fragile sites* because they may undergo outright disruption ("breakage") in metaphase preparations. The only such region known to be of significance in relation to a human trait, the clinical condition called the *fragile-X syndrome*, is one located near the distal end (the

FIGURE 62-3 Metaphase chromosomes stained for C bands (C standing for centromeric or constitutive heterochromatin), showing inherited variation in lengths of C bands in chromosome 1 (arrows).

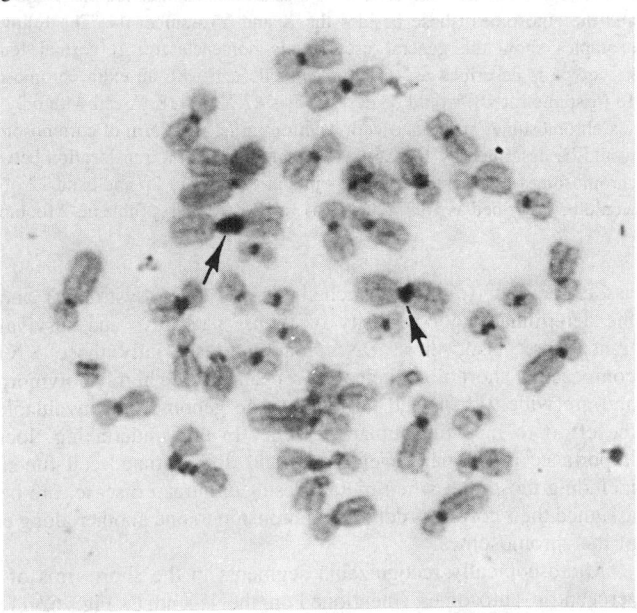

end away from the centromere) of the long arm of the X chromosome (see below, under "Sex Chromosome Imbalance"). Other examples of segmental specialization along the chromosome include *telomeres* and *centromeres*. Telomeres, the distal termini of each arm, have some relationship to the nuclear membrane and probably are important in the maintenance of order in the interphase nucleus and of accurate pairing of homologues in meiosis; centromeric regions are sites of microtubule attachment at metaphase.

A further example of chromosome differentiation is the sequence by which various segments replicate during S; certain segments replicate early, others late. In general, late replication of a chromosome segment correlates with genetic inertness. This correlation is exemplified by one of the two X chromosomes in female cells; the X in which the entire chromosome, except for the terminal pseudoautosomal region and a few additional loci that are inactivated by a phenomenon referred to as the *Lyon effect* (see Chap. 60), is almost entirely late-replicating.

A little-understood type of chromatin is referred to as *heterochromatin*. It is tightly condensed, not just at metaphase but throughout interphase. Such condensation of chromatin correlates with genetic inactivity and also with late replication. Some regions are condensed and inactive in all cells (constitutive heterochromatin), while others, e.g., the X chromosome, may be either condensed and inactive or decondensed and active (facultative heterochromatin). Many chromosome imbalances that permit viability beyond intrauterine life involve chromosome segments that are rich in this apparently inactive, or inactivatable, type of chromatin, e.g., chromosomes that can be trisomic in live-born individuals or, in the case of the X, monosomic. The activity of genes can sometimes be affected, even inactivated, if they are positioned aberrantly near regions of heterochromatin, as can occur in chromosome breakage and rearrangement.

Therefore, in chromosome imbalance both the specific genetic loci and the particular types of chromatin deleted or duplicated are important. Also, the significance of a chromosome rearrangement probably depends on the new and abnormal positioning of structural and regulatory genes in relation to each other and to heterochromatin.

Fortunately for the cytogeneticist, several differentiated features of the chromosome correlate with cytologic artifacts that can be produced and visualized in the laboratory. A number of techniques are now in use to display the constant pattern of bands of various lengths and staining characteristics already mentioned (Figs. 62-1 and 62-3). These patterns are identical in each chromosome 1, each chromosome 2, etc., varying only in the inert polymorphic regions mentioned above, so that they can be used in clinical cytogenetics to identify chromosomes and to detect and define structural rearrangements.

Sources of error   A large number of genetic loci must be active to produce the enzymes and structural proteins required to initiate and complete a cell-division cycle. Remarkable precision and accuracy are demanded over and over in matters such as the passage of a cell from G_1 into S, orderly progression of replication, assembly of the mitotic spindle, and the spindle action that segregates chromatids at mitosis. In the germ line additional loci are activated to permit a cell of the germ line to pass successfully through meiotic prophase including pairing of homologous chromosomes, genetic recombination, and then disjoining of recombined homologous chromosomes at anaphase of the first division. These mechanisms and processes are subject to errors, some spontaneous, others promoted by unfavorable environmental influences (e.g., Fig. 62-4) or the consequence of inherited or new mutations that affect one of the many steps in the cell cycle. Furthermore, the genetic material itself is subject to damage, and certain types of unrepaired or erroneously repaired lesions in DNA predispose to mutation, including chromosome rearrangement. Errors at many of these steps or errors introduced during the repair of damaged DNA lie behind chromosome imbalance. Mutations that arise in germ cells, during fertilization, or in early postfertilization divisions are important causes of embryonic maldevel-

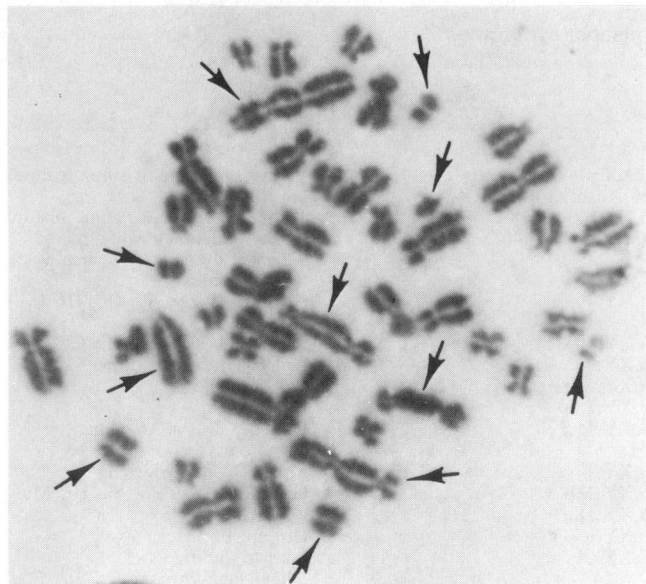

FIGURE 62-4 Breaks and rearrangements (arrows) in metaphase chromosomes of a blood lymphocyte that received ionizing irradiation before being stimulated by phytohemagglutinin to enter S and divide.

opment and infertility; mutations in somatic cells are important in causes of somatic mutational disease, particularly neoplasia.

CHROMOSOME ABNORMALITIES Mutations of a single base in a gene and deletions and duplications of chromosome segments involving even hundreds of base pairs are not visible microscopically. In fact, for the normal chromosome banding pattern to be detectably disturbed, a lengthy segment of DNA must be deleted, duplicated, or transposed. This means that a chromosome mutation that is microscopically detectable must involve large amounts of DNA. However, the same environmental agents that produce point mutations (mutagens in the usual sense) are also chromosome-breaking agents, and vice versa. Thus, it seems safe to assume the existence of a spectrum extending all the way from mutations visible to the cytogeneticist to those that must be defined by nucleotide sequencing. Visible mutations ordinarily exert a more widespread effect on development than do point mutations; ordinary genes—often many of them—as well as other specialized types of chromatin whose function or significance is unknown are involved in cytologically visible mutations.

If an entire chromosome is affected in an imbalance, the genome is said to be either *trisomic* or *monosomic* for the chromosome (thus, trisomy 13, monosomy X). Genes and chromatin carried on the affected chromosome then are present in triple or single dose, respectively, rather than the normal double—*disomic*—dose. Abnormal dosage affecting less than an entire chromosome, the result of chromosome breakage and rearrangement, is often termed *partial trisomy* or *partial monosomy*, to indicate that segments rather than entire chromosomes are involved (thus, partial trisomy 13q, partial monosomy 4p). Some of the recurring chromosome imbalances, both numerical and structural, are listed in Table 62-1.

Uniparental disomy refers to the situation in which both chromosomes of a pair, or perhaps just a segment of both, are erroneously inherited from a single parent. In such cases the presence of a homozygous chromosome segment can have unfavorable effects on development, presumably because of homozygosity of some recessive gene or genes that by chance were carried on that segment in the (heterozygous and therefore healthy) parent from whom the segment was inherited in double dose or possibly from an inappropriate balance of imprintable genes (see discussion of genomic imprinting under "Structural Abnormalities" below).

Incidence The frequency with which chromosome imbalance is detectable depends on the population investigated. It is estimated that a minimum of 1 in 10 human conceptions has a chromosome abnormality. In spontaneously aborted human embryos and fetuses, the incidence of chromosome imbalance is higher the earlier in pregnancy the sampling is made. The contribution of imbalance to late abortion and stillbirth, though not well studied, probably also is significant. From surveys of more than 65,000 live-born babies examined in different laboratories, approximately 1 in 200 has a significant chromosome abnormality, either numerical or structural. In such studies, at least 1 in 700 newborns is trisomic for one of the autosomes 21, 18, or 13; about 1 in 350 newborn males has the complement 47,XXY or 47,XYY. One in every several thousand newborns has monosomy X. One in 500 has some structural rearrangement, most of which are genetically balanced. Samplings of the general adult population reveal an occasional inherited balanced structural rearrangement as well as the expected number of XXY, XYY, and XXX complements; the inherited, apparently innocuous segmental polymorphisms (e.g., Fig. 62-3) and minor structural rearrangements demonstrable by banding techniques are found in abundance.

In individuals with mental deficiency, 10 to 15 percent have a significant chromosome abnormality, the proportion being greater if anatomic malformations are also present. In some groups of men with behavioral disorders or infertility, an increased incidence of individuals with an extra X or Y chromosome is found. Infertile women also include many individuals with extra or missing sex chromosomes and an appreciable number with structural chromosome rearrangement; approximately one-fourth of women with primary amenorrhea have some abnormality of the X chromosome. Among infertile men and women, individuals may have inherited mutations that interfere with meiosis, so-called meiotic mutants.

Numerical abnormalities Trisomy (47 chromosomes) is the most common chromosome imbalance in early spontaneous abortuses, followed by monosomy (45 chromosomes) and triploidy (69 chromosomes). The extra or missing chromosomes can be either paternal or maternal in origin, and the error in segregation of chromosomes can occur in the germ line, fertilized egg (zygote), or early embryo. Trisomy of every chromosome except the no. 1 has been observed in spontaneous abortions, trisomy 16 being the most frequent.

Sex chromosome trisomy (XXY, XYY, and XXX) is compatible with intrauterine survival; in contrast, autosomal trisomy rarely permits survival to term. However, a small proportion of autosomal trisomics are born alive. For practical purposes these are trisomy 21, 18, or 13, in decreasing frequency. Trisomies 18 and 13 cause death during infancy. Therefore, trisomies of significance in adults are only trisomy 21, XXY, XXX, and XYY. A few other autosomal trisomies, such as trisomy 8, occur rarely, usually in mosaicism with a normal cellular component. (*Mosaicism* is the coexistence in one individual of multiple, genetically different populations of cells, all derived originally, however, from a single zygote.)

Autosomal monosomy is rare even in abortion material. In contrast, monosomy X (45,X) occurs in approximately 1.5 percent of recognized conceptions. It is common among spontaneously aborted human embryos (approximately 10 percent) and is present in one in every several thousand live-born babies. The reason for the failure of 45,X embryos and fetuses to survive is unknown, although anatomic abnormalities probably contribute; cardiovascular and renal anomalies are common in the few that do survive. The genetic basis for the lethality may be hemizygosity for some vital locus or loci in the portions of the Y and in the portions of the second X in 46,XX individuals that fail to be inactivated by the Lyon effect, including the pseudoautosomal region. A possible explanation for the survival of an occasional 45,X individual is occult mosaicism, the nonmonosomic cells, perhaps limited just to a few tissues, going undetected. In monosomy X, the missing sex chromosome can have been either a Y or an X and either paternal or maternal in origin. Often the second

TABLE 62-1 Some recurring chromosome imbalances that result in distinct syndromes*

Class of imbalance	Chromosome affected	Karyotypes[†]	Clinical features[‡]
Monosomy	X	45,X	Turner syndrome
Segmental deficiency "partial monosomy"	X	46,XX,p−; 46,XX,q−; 46,X,r(X); 46,X,iso(Xp); 46,X,iso(Xq)	Turner syndrome or some features of it
	Y	46,XY,p−; 46,XY,q−; 46,X,r(Y); 46,X,iso(Yp); 46,X,iso(Yq)	Turner syndrome, or some features of it, sometimes with "mixed gonadal dysgenesis" when a 45,X cell line coexists
	4	46,XY,4p−	Gr, Cf, Mi, Ey, Sk, Ge, Ht, Co, Me
	5	46,XY,5p−	5p− syndrome: Cr, Mi, Cf, Me
	8	46,XY,8q−	Langer-Gideon syndrome
	11	46,XY,11p−	WT, Ge, Me
	13	46,XY,13q−	RB, Cf, Me
	15	46,XY,15q−	Prader-Willi (or Angelman) syndrome
	17	46,XY,17p−	Miller-Dieker syndrome
	18	46,XY,18p−	Gr, Cf, Ea, Te, Po, Sk, Ht, Me
	18	46,XY,18q−	Cf, Hy, Sk, Ey
	21	46,XY,r(21)	Cf, Hp, Ea, Me
Trisomy	X	47,XXX	Se, Me (mild), Ps
	X	47,XXY	Klinefelter syndrome
	Y	47,XYY	Ta, Ac, Su, B; but often normal
	8	46,XY/47,XY,+8	Cf, Sk, Me (moderate)
	13	47,XY,+13	Trisomy 13 syndrome: Cp, Ey, Pd, Po, Ht, D, V, Sc, F, Ar, Me
	18	47,XY,+18	Trisomy 18 syndrome: Cf, Ea, V, F, Gr, D, He, Me
	21	47,XY,+21	Trisomy 21 (Down syndrome)
Segmental duplication "partial trisomy"	Y	46,X,t(X;Y)[§]	XX male
	9	9p+[†]	Cf
	21	21q+(distal q)	Trisomy 21 syndrome
	22	22q+[¶]	Gr, Cf, Ea, Cp, Hy, Co
Chimerism	Entire complement	46,XY/46,XX	Pseudo- or true hermaphroditism; dimorphism of blood-cell-surface antigens
Triploidy	Entire complement	69,XXY	Hc, Me, Sy, Ht, Ge, D

* For complete listing, consult DeGrouchy and Turleau.
[†] The sex chromosome constitution might be either XY or XX, but in the example karyotypes given, XY arbitrarily is used in most.
[‡] The clinical features given include only some of the more constant ones. Deficiency of one segment often is accompanied by duplication of another, and the phenotypic effect is the consequence of the combined imbalance. Abbreviations are defined below.
[§] Translocation onto an X of a segment of the Y bearing the locus responsible for testicular differentiation.
[¶] Brought about through any of several rearrangements.
Abbreviations: Ac, acne; Ar, arrhinencephaly; B, behavior disorder; Cr, characteristically abnormal cry; Cf, characteristic craniofacial dysmorphism; Co, convulsions; Cp, cleft lip–palate; D, early death; Ea, characteristically abnormal ears; Ey, eye anomaly; F, characteristically flared, overlapping fingers; Ge, abnormality of external genitalia; Gr, severe growth deficiency; Hc, hydrocephaly; Hp, hypertonia; Ht, cardiac malformation; Hy, infantile hypotonia; Me, intellectual deficit; Mi, microcephaly; Om, omphalocele; Po, characteristically abnormal posture; Pd, polydactyly; Ps, psychotic predisposition; RB, retinoblastoma; Sc, scalp defect; Se, secondary amenorrhea; Sk, skeletal anomalies; Su, subfertility; Sy, syndactyly; Ta, tallness; Te, characteristically abnormal teeth; V, visceral anomalies; WT, Wilms's tumor with aniridia.

sex chromosome is not completely absent but is replaced by a structurally rearranged Y or X. Mosaicism is often demonstrable in live-borns with monosomy X; here, tissues are populated not only by cells with a 45,X complement but by other cells, perhaps with a normal complement, 46,XY or 46,XX, or with a complement in which the second sex chromosome is rearranged in some way.

The phenotypic effects of the autosomal trisomies, of 47,XXY, and of monosomy X (45,X) are characteristic and well defined so that their diagnosis usually is not difficult (see Chap. 342). The effects of the 47,XYY and 47,XXX constitutions are less striking, and therefore these complements are underdiagnosed. In mosaicism with coexistence of abnormal and normal populations of cells, the phenotype may approach the normal.

The mechanisms responsible for the numerical abnormalities are undefined and may be multiple. In trisomy 21 the extra chromosome is maternal in 95 percent of cases, and it usually results from nonsegregation of the no. 21 chromosomes at the first meiotic division. A maternal age effect exists in trisomies 21, 18, 13, XXY, and XXX. Over a third of babies with trisomy 21 are born to women over 35, whereas only about a tenth of all births occur in this group. The frequency of trisomy 21 rises from 0.5 to 0.7 per 1000 live births between ages 21 and 23 to 3 per 1000 at age 35, 10 per 1000 at age

40, and 34 per 1000 at age 45. After a child with trisomy 21 is born, the risk of recurrence in future pregnancies is approximately 1 percent. As to the cause of monosomy X, the frequent association of the 45,X complement in mosaicism with normal complements and with structural rearrangements of the X and Y suggests that the zygote or the preimplantation embryo is often the target of a chromosome-breaking event, rather than a nondisjunctional event during meiosis as in the trisomies.

Structural abnormalities Some structural chromosome rearrangements are inherited, and others represent new mutations. The cause of the new rearrangements is unknown, although they are assumed to be partly spontaneous and partly the effect of environmental agents such as mutagenic chemicals or ionizing radiation (Fig. 62-4) acting on the germ line, zygote, or early embryo. The majority of de novo rearrangements are in paternally derived chromosomes.

Many chromosome rearrangements have been detected only once or a few times. Others are detected repeatedly, the same one recurring in unrelated individuals and families. For example, the commonest translocation, one that can occur either as result of de novo mutation or by inheritance, affects one chromosome 13 and one 14 at or near their centromeres. In this translocation only inert chromatin or functional chromatin that is represented elsewhere in the genome—

the nucleolus-organizing regions and satellites referred to earlier—is lost from the tiny short arms. A similar recurring translocation affects chromosomes 14 and 21.

Chromosome complements bearing rearrangements can be genetically balanced or effectively so, thus imparting no unfavorable effect to their bearers; about two-thirds of rearrangements detected during surveys of live-born babies are balanced. Or, the complement can be unbalanced and impair development, the usual case when re-arrangements are detected during surveys of spontaneous abortuses or of individuals with multiple anomalies and mental deficiency.

A phenomenon that can influence the developmental consequence of chromosome abnormalities is *genomic imprinting*. Certain genetic loci are subject to functional modulation, presumably during passage through the germ line. The modulation differs, depending on whether the genome passed through spermatogenesis or oogenesis. The parental source of a chromosome mutation that affects an imprintable locus/loci can determine whether a developmental defect will arise and the nature of the defect. An example of imprinting concerns deletion of chromosome band 15q11 (fifteen-q-one-one): If the affected (deleted) chromosome 15 is the one inherited from the father, the Prader-Willi syndrome is the consequence; if from the mother, the Angelman syndrome (Table 62-1).

Some balanced chromosome rearrangements are transmitted from generation to generation without producing clinical effects. In other cases, they are responsible for the conception of embryos with unbalanced genomes. For example, inherited translocations involving chromosome 21 predispose to the trisomy 21 syndrome. Approximately 5 percent of live-borns with that syndrome have a translocation, and in about a fifth of those it is detectable in one of the parents. Because most babies with the trisomy 21 syndrome due to translocation are born to women under 30, a search for a translocation can be important when a child with this clinical syndrome is born to young parents. Different translocations bestow on their carriers different risks of having offspring with unbalanced rearrangements, i.e., partial trisomies or partial monosomies. These risks frequently cannot be predicted on theoretical grounds. Useful empiric risk figures have been accumulated for the common translocations; e.g., the 14;21 translocation bestows a 2 percent risk on a balanced male carrier and more than a 10 percent risk on a female carrier of having a child with the trisomy 21 syndrome. In contrast, the balanced carrier of a 21;21 translocation can expect unbalanced offspring almost exclusively. Information of this type is indispensable for counseling in relation to chromosome disorders.

DISEASE ASSOCIATIONS Various combinations of abnormalities in malformed and mentally defective individuals correlate with variations in the chromosome complement. (Many of the conditions are of little significance in adult medicine because of their lethality in infancy or early childhood.)

Autosome imbalance Of the three autosomal trisomies found in live-born babies, only trisomy 21 is compatible with survival past infancy. The phenotype produced by an extra chromosome 21, formerly known as *mongolism* but now called the *Down syndrome* or *trisomy 21 syndrome*, is characteristic and easily diagnosed. Cardiac malformations lead to death in infancy in a third of individuals with trisomy 21, and other malformations and infections may also cause early death. However, subjects who survive infancy often reach adulthood, and some old age. Affected females occasionally become pregnant, and, as expected, approximately half their children have trisomy 21.

Mosaicism of trisomy 21 with normal cells (46/47, +21) may occur in individuals with modified features of the trisomy 21 syndrome, or even in normal persons. The risk that a person with such mosaicism will have trisomic children is increased, but unfortunately the abnormal cell population usually is detected only after the birth of an affected child.

Partial trisomy, partial monosomy, or a combination of the two affecting any of many chromosomal segments throughout the genome explains many instances of multiple developmental defects combined with mental deficiency. Sometimes a balanced autosomal translocation is detected in normally developed adults who have repeated spontaneous abortion or subnormal fertility, with or without abnormal live-born children.

Although the phenotypic effects of many segmental chromosome imbalances are varied and nonspecific, the anomalies sometimes compose recognizable clinical syndromes. Two examples are the following: (1) If a rearrangement causes partial trisomy of just the distal band of 21q, the long arm of chromosome 21, the clinical features of the full Down syndrome associated with an extra entire 21 develop. (A triple dose of other segments of the long arm of chromosome 21 also produces adverse effects but not the Down syndrome.) (2) Partial monosomy of a short segment within the short arm of chromosome 5 causes mental deficiency, a characteristic facies, and a characteristic cry during infancy. This group of signs is known as the *5p−* (five-p-minus), or cri-du-chat, syndrome.

Additional recognizable syndromes produced by imbalance of many different chromosome segments now are known (Table 62-1), e.g., the 4p−, 9p partial trisomy, 13q−, and 18q− syndromes, to name a few. Furthermore, the application of high-resolution banding techniques and fluorescence in situ hybridization (FISH) (described below under "Technical Considerations") make possible identification of the exact band(s) deficient or duplicated. Rearrangements not previously described and their corresponding clinical syndromes still are being recognized. These syndromes may appear as the result either of de novo chromosome rearrangement or through formation of a genetically unbalanced gamete in a person carrying in balanced state a rearrangement affecting the segment involved.

In many individuals with chromosome imbalance, regardless of which segments are affected a degree of phenotypic similarity is present. These recurring and nonspecific features include mental deficiency, growth deficiency, dysmorphic ears, nose, and mouth, cardiac malformations of standard types, abnormalities of dermal ridges and creases, and dysmorphic digits. (As a rule, autosomal imbalance need not be considered in the etiology of anatomic defects unaccompanied by mental deficiency.) Why similar abnormalities occur with so many different segmental imbalances is unknown, but when several such features are observed in a single individual, they can be a valuable clinical indication for cytogenetic analysis. Imbalance affecting certain segments also causes specific phenotypic changes, examples being the 5p− syndrome, retinoblastoma [mutation of a particular band of chromosome 13 (band 13q14.2)], the WAGR syndrome (Wilms's tumor, aniridia, genital anomalies, and mental deficiency) caused by deletion of band 11p13, and the Prader-Willi syndrome, which is often the consequence of deletion of a specific band near the centromere of chromosome 15 (band 15q11). Whereas the nonspecific changes serve to call attention to the possibility of some chromosome imbalance, the specific features or constellation of features can suggest the exact segment of the genome affected. These conditions are sometimes referred to as contiguous gene-deletion syndromes, the case, for example, in the WAGR syndrome (above) and in deletions of segments of Xp that may result in loss of contiguous loci that individually are responsible for Duchenne's muscular dystrophy, chronic granulomatous disease, retinitis pigmentosa, and the MacLeod phenotype.

Sex chromosome imbalance (See also Chap. 342) In contrast to autosome imbalance, sex chromosome imbalance causes relatively mild phenotypic effects. This is because X chromosomes beyond one in the complement of somatic cells are usually almost totally inactivated, because the pseudoautosomal region is much shorter than any of the autosomes, and because the strictly sex-linked portions of the Y bears few genes. X-linked loci (in contrast to autosomal loci) function normally in single dose: the female is functionally hemizygous for most loci on the X through the Lyon effect; the male, with only one X chromosome, is hemizygous for X-linked genes with the exception of loci clustered in the pseudoautosomal segment and a few scattered in the proximal Yp and Yq. The addition of an extra sex chromosome has a phenotypic effect but insufficient to interfere with intrauterine survival. Since major anatomic defects are usually absent, men with the complements 47,XXY and 47,YYY and 47,XXX females often go unrecognized.

The *Klinefelter syndrome* (Chap. 342), which in classic form consists of small testes, infertility, gynecomastia, and variable degrees of underandrogenization, sometimes with mild mental deficiency, antisocial behavior, or both, is the consequence of the addition of an extra X to the male complement: 47,XXY. The extra X interferes with the survival of germ cells, and atrophy of the spermatogenic tubules and azoospermia are the consequence. Sometimes the phenotypic effects are mild, the testicular atrophy being the only noteworthy feature in otherwise healthy and socially well-adjusted men. The mosaicism 46,XY/47,XXY sometimes occurs and may ameliorate the phenotypic effect of the extra X. More extreme phenotypic effects and mental deficiency result when more than one extra X chromosome is added to the normal male complement: 48,XXXY or 49,XXXXY.

The phenotypic effect of 47,XYY is less well defined; although increased height, behavioral difficulties, and infertility are common, the extra Y is sometimes found in otherwise normal men. The rare complement 48,XXYY results in infertility. The phenotype associated with 47,XXX is also poorly defined; although women with mild mental deficiency, psychosis, and menstrual abnormalities sometimes have this complement, it is also detected in normal, healthy women. Further clarification is needed concerning the effects on personality and behavior of all three of the complements 47,XXY, 47,XYY, and 47,XXX.

Loss of the Y or of the second X has drastic effects on development. If it does not cause abortion (as already discussed), it may or may not be recognizable at birth. Loose nuchal skin folds and edema of the hands and feet in a newborn girl, with or without renal or cardiovascular anomalies, may point to the diagnosis of the 45,X complement. The *Turner syndrome* is the manifestation in subsequent life (Chap. 342): short stature, infantilism of otherwise normal female external and internal genitalia, germ-cell-free gonads referred to as gonadal streaks, and variable renal, cardiovascular, skeletal, and ectodermal anomalies.

The Turner syndrome may be the developmental consequence of several chromosome constitutions besides 45,X. Mosaicism as well as structural abnormalities affecting certain segments of a second sex chromosome, either a Y or an X, cause a spectrum of disorders at both the clinical and cytogenetic levels. A normal male or normal female cellular component may be present along with the 45,X cellular component, or one component may bear a structurally abnormal chromosome. Common abnormalities of the Y and X are isochromosome formation (one arm deleted and the other duplicated) or deletion of part or all of one arm. In some affected individuals all cells have 46 chromosomes, with one normal X plus an abnormal Y or X, for example, 46,XXp −, deletion of a segment of the short arm of one of the X chromosomes. In others a second or third cellular component may be present as well, for example, 45,X/46,XX/ 46,XXp −. Typical Turner syndrome may be found in association with various combinations of these karyotypes if one of them is either monosomic or partially monosomic for X. However, when Y-bearing cells coexist with the 45,X cells, for example, 45,X/46,XY, genital ambiguity often develops, and gonadal morphology ranges from streaks to functional testes (the syndrome of *mixed gonadal dysgenesis*); in mosaicism that includes 45,X cells and other cells with a Y the risk of gonadal neoplasia is significant. When 46,XX cells coexist with 45,X, varying degrees of ovarian function may be maintained, including ovulation. Although the phenotype may approach that of a normal male or female when normal and abnormal cells coexist, the effects of mosaicism are unpredictable. Thus, the phenotype associated with monosomy X and structurally abnormal Ys or Xs ranges from male through the Turner syndrome to female.

Two other rare disturbances of sexual development deserve mention here—*true hermaphroditism* and the *46,XX male* (see also Chap. 342). True hermaphroditism is present when testicular and ovarian tissue coexist in the same individual. In most cases the chromosome complement is 46,XX, and it appears normal by banding. Exceptionally, true hermaphrodites have the complement 46,XY, and sometimes *chimerism* 46,XY/46,XX is demonstrable, the two cellular components having been derived from different zygotes. Second, males occasionally have complement that appears by banding to be 46,XX. As in 47,XXY men, the second X interferes with meiosis and azoospermia results. In both the 46,XX true hermaphrodite and the 46,XX male, the rule that a Y is required for testicular differentiation appears to break down. The explanation in some XX males is that the testis-determining locus actually is present, having been erroneously translocated from Yp to Xp, demonstrable not by microscopy but by molecular cytogenetics.

In the general population more males than females are mentally deficient, and familial mental deficiency affects males preferentially. In some such kindreds, mental deficiency segregates as an X-linked trait, and several such syndromes are now recognized.

The commonest of these, the *fragile-X syndrome*, is characterized by mental retardation, a characteristic facies, and macroorchia. The condition can be recognized by cytogenetic techniques. In a variable but usually small proportion of metaphases from affected persons and in an even smaller number from the mothers, the abnormal X chromosome exhibits a so-called fragile site near the distal end of Xq. This site is responsible for the decondensed appearance of the region at metaphase, and its fragility is due to excess amplification of the trinucleotide sequence CGG. This base sequence is normally repeated 2 to 50 times at the fragile-X locus, whereas in the fragile-X syndrome the number of repeats expands to more than 160. This amplification is believed to affect the normal functioning of neighboring genetic determinants and thereby to cause the abnormal phenotype. Other examples of this mode of inheritance, heritable selective amplification of an oligonucleotide, are known, e.g., amplification of the trinucleotide CTG within a specific locus on chromosome 19 can cause familial myotonic dystrophy, though in this instance unassociated with a microscopically visible chromosome lesion.

Chromosome change in cancer The theory that chromosomal abnormalities may cause cancer was advanced many years ago, and with improved cytogenetic techniques and the advent of recombinant DNA technology firm evidence supporting the theory has become available. Indeed, most human cancers have chromosome complements that are altered in a microscopically detectable way.

Table 62-2 lists some of those found with regularity. In the leukemias, lymphomas, and certain myeloproliferative disorders the alterations are less extensive than in solid tumors and, therefore, easier to define. As examples, chromosome 14 is often found to have undergone structural rearrangement in certain lymphomas, with the breakpoint near or in the immunoglobulin heavy chain locus; the rearrangement translocates the *myc* locus from its normal position on chromosome 8 to chromosome 14. Also, in over 95 percent of cases of chronic granulocytic leukemia a translocation affecting chromosomes 9 and 22 (already mentioned) is detected, resulting in the Philadelphia, or Ph, chromosome, an abnormally short no. 22. (The abnormality in chromosome 9 is difficult to detect microscopically.) If the leukemia progresses into a "blastic" phase, the already mutated karyotype evolves; certain new chromosome changes are added stepwise in a nonrandom sequence. In this and certain other leukemias, the chromosome changes, demonstrable either by conventional cytogenetics techniques and microscopy or by microscopy supplemented by molecular techniques, may have diagnostic utility as well as some value in prognosis and choice of therapy. Common carcinomas such as of the lung, breast, and colon, although more difficult to study by conventional cytogenetics techniques, also have specific chromosome mutations, often analyzed more readily by molecular techniques.

The microscopically visible chromosome mutations that are found with regularity in human neoplasms often affect loci that play growth regulatory roles in normal cells. In some cases the chromosome breakpoints affect already known cellular oncogenes, but analysis of

TABLE 62-2 Some recurring chromosome abnormalities encountered in human neoplasms*

Neoplasm	Aberration	Chromosome region affected
Leukemia		
Chronic granulocytic	Translocation	9q34 and 22q11
Acute nonlymphocytic		
M1	Translocation	9q34 and 22q11
M2	Translocation	8q22 and 21q22
M3	Translocation	15q22 and 17q11
Chronic lymphocytic	Trisomy	12
Acute lymphocytic		
L1–L2	Translocation	9q34 and 22q11
L3	Translocation	4q21 and 11q23
	Translocation	8q24 and 14q32
Lymphoma		
Burkitt's	Translocation	8q24 and 14q32
Follicular	Translocation	14q32 and 18q21
Solid tumors		
Benign		
Meningioma	Deletion or monosomy	22q
Leiomyoma, uterus	Translocation	2q13–15 and 14q23–24
Adenomas, salivary gland	Translocation	3p25 and 8q12
Malignant		
Ewing's sarcoma	Translocation	11q24 and 22q12
Rhabdomyosarcoma, alveolar	Translocation	2q35–37 and 13q14
Germ cell tumors, testis	Isochromosome	12p
Lung, small cell carcinoma	Deletion	3p13–23
Liposarcoma, myxoid	Translocation	12q13 and 16p11
Sarcoma, synovial	Translocation	Xp11 and 18q11
Neuroblastoma	Deletion	1p31 to 3p36
Ovary, cystadenocarcinoma	Translocation	6q21 and 14q24
Retinoblastoma	Deletion	13q14
Wilms's tumor	Deletion	11p13

* For more complete listing see Solomon.

NOTE: The FAB (French-American-British) classification of leukemias is employed above. The chromosome breakpoint and band nomenclature is that of the Paris Conference (Birth Defects: Original Articles Series VIII (7):1–46, 1971). The chromosome and chromosome-arm designation (e.g., 9q means the long arm of chromosome no. 9) appears first and is followed by the chromosome region and band on that arm (e.g., 9q34 means the fourth band in the third region of the long arm of chromosome no. 9).

the breakpoints in the acute leukemias has resulted in identification of previously unrecognized genetic determinants in basic cell biology, e.g., transcription regulatory factors and loci concerned with the regulation of normal development. In the lymphoma examples given, *myc* in its new position on chromosome 14 is abnormally regulated, brought now under the influence of the activating elements of the transcribing immunoglobulin locus in cells differentiated to synthesize antibodies. In the Ph chromosome, the cellular-oncogene *abl* is translocated from its normal position on chromosome 9 into a specific region called *bcr* on chromosome 22, thereby creating what is referred to as a *fusion gene*; in myeloid cells, this mutant locus is transcribed, and the mRNA is translated into a novel protein that presumably plays a causative role in the autonomous growth of the neoplastic cell lineage that is recognized clinically as chronic granulocytic leukemia.

Another process that appears to be important in progression of some tumors is *gene amplification*. One particular chromosome segment is replicated selectively, sometimes to such a degree that the normal banding pattern at the chromosome region affected is visibly disturbed, a *homogeneously staining region* (HSR) being the result. Sometimes the region amplified rather than producing an HSR is released from the chromosome, and multiple tiny centromereless bodies of DNA, known as *double minutes* (DMs), accumulate in the nucleus and can be seen at metaphase. Presumably, in both HSRs and DMs, amplification of the DNA of some particular locus is of selective value to the neoplastic cell, thus enhancing the neoplastic clone's progression or perhaps resistance to chemotherapeutic agents.

Another chromosome mechanism in human neoplasia is *somatic crossing-over*. Through somatic crossing-over, a recessive mutation at a genetic locus concerned with growth regulation—a mutation that

preexisted in a cell but that had remained occult because of the presence of a normal locus on the homologous chromosome—can become homozygous. The recessive mutation may either have been inherited or arisen de novo in somatic cells. The consequence then of homozygosity at such a mutant locus is loss of normal growth control, i.e., acquisition of autonomous growth by the affected cell and its progeny. Such mutations were first recognized in the rare neoplasms retinoblastoma and Wilms's tumor, where the loci affected were on chromosomes 13 and 11, respectively. In some cases of retinoblastoma the original (recessive) mutation consisted of outright deletion of the locus; then, when somatic crossing-over occurred, homozygosity of the affected chromosome arm distal to the point of exchange was the consequence, and a cell and its progeny became *nullisomic* for the retinoblastoma locus. Transmission through the germ line of such occult recessive mutations at growth- or tumor-suppressor loci explains familial instances of those neoplasms.

Thus, chromosome mutations of at least four types constitute crucial steps in the initiation and progression of malignant neoplasia: (1) translocations that disturb the regulation of loci concerned with growth or that produce novel genes that affect growth; (2) deletion-mutation of recessive growth-controlling loci (e.g., the retinoblastoma locus just referred to), mutations that can either be inherited through the germ line or occur de novo in a somatic cell; (3) recombination yielding homozygosity for preexisting mutations affecting this last-mentioned type of locus; and (4) amplification of some locus that facilitates expansion of the neoplastic population. These mutations and their oncogenic consequences are the subject of intense investigation, both basic and clinical. In turn, the breakpoints in neoplasms are helping identify genetic determinants that together orchestrate normal cellular proliferation and tissue growth; thus the cytogenetics of human cancer is contributing not only to clinical medicine but also to the understanding of normal cell biology.

The cytogenetic findings in leukemias and solid tumors were some of the first evidence of the clonal nature of human cancer.

TECHNICAL CONSIDERATIONS Human metaphase chromosomes can be examined by light microscopy in any tissue in which sufficient cells are cycling. Preparations can therefore be made directly from almost any embryonic tissue and from adult bone marrow, lymphoid tissue, and selected malignant tissues. In searches for mosaicism and chimerism, the study of multiple tissues is often required. Some tissues unlikely to contain cells in metaphase can be placed in culture, and chromosome preparations can be made from cells that reach mitosis in vitro. Blood T lymphocytes stimulated to enter cell-division cycles by phytohemagglutinin are the standard material for diagnosing constitutional chromosome imbalance. In some myeloproliferative disorders and leukemias, unstimulated circulating blood cells will divide spontaneously after a few hours in culture. Long-term cultures of fibroblasts can be derived from minute skin biopsies or from fragments of many other types of tissue, although more elaborate laboratory facilities and a longer period of time are required before cytogenetic preparations can be made. Amniotic fluid is among the sources of cells suitable for culture, and the cells, which are fetal in origin, are widely used in the prenatal diagnosis of chromosome imbalance. Metaphase preparations also can be made from chorionic villi biopsied in the first trimester of pregnancy or from aborted fetal tissue.

Meiotic chromosome preparations from testicular biopsies are sometimes useful in obscure cases of infertility. Translocations and genetically determined disturbances of meiotic pairing may be identified there.

The combination of conventional techniques with those of recombinant DNA technology and fluorescence microscopy makes it possible to detect promptly abnormalities such as trisomy, translocation, and segmental duplication or deficiency and to characterize the abnormalities in some detail. The availability of molecular probes for many specific loci whose map position is known and that blanket the genome makes it possible to identify rearrangements not detectable by banding techniques alone. By FISH, molecular probes specific for each chromosome can be used to "paint" a chromosome differentially throughout its length, determining, for example, whether part of one chromosome might be translocated aberrantly to another, or whether some specific chromosome or chromosome segment might be trisomic. FISH also permits the exact chromosome localization of known DNA sequences including specific genes, even determining their order. For answering certain questions, study of interphase nuclei using either painting (chromosome-specific) probes or cloned gene sequences obviates the ordinary requirement of bringing cells into metaphase for identification of numerical or structural mutation. Often the use of FISH along with microscopy, Southern blotting, and polymerase chain reaction can provide minute definition of chromosome rearrangements, both constitutional ones and those in clones of neoplastic cell lineages.

Sometimes, metaphase or anaphase chromosomes are analyzed to determine whether damage to the genetic material has been induced by some environmental agent (radiation, chemical, virus), or whether constitutional genomic instability is present. Cells that have proliferated in vivo and then been incubated only briefly in vitro may be used in search of microscopically visible evidence of damage to the genetic material of a given person or of a population (e.g., Fig. 62-4). The number of chromatid gaps, breaks, and rearrangements can be estimated directly in cells reaching their first mitosis in vitro.

REFERENCES

CHAGANTI RSK, GERMAN J (eds): *Genetics in Clinical Oncology*. New York, Oxford, 1985

DE GROUCHY J, TURLEAU C: *Clinical Atlas of Human Chromosomes*, 2d ed. New York, Wiley, 1984

GERMAN JL: Studying human chromosomes today. Am Sci 58:182, 1970

GRUMBACH MM, CONTE FA: Disorders of sex differentiation, in *Williams Textbook of Endocrinology*, 8th ed, JD Wilson, DW Foster (eds). Philadelphia, Saunders, 1992, pp 853–951

SCHINZEL A: *Catalogue of Unbalanced Chromosome Aberrations*. Berlin and New York, W de Gruyter, 1983

SOLOMON E et al: Chromosome aberrations and cancer. Science 254:1153, 1991

63   GENES AND NEOPLASIA

STANLEY J. KORSMEYER

The past decade has witnessed enormous progress in understanding the genetic basis of human cancer. Cancer is nearly always of clonal origin, having originated from a single cell. Multiple genetic mutations are required for such a cell to result in a malignant tumor. Mutations that result in cancer can either be inherited in the germ line or acquired in somatic tissues. Cellular proto-oncogenes have emerged as the common targets for endogenous or exogenous events. Not infrequently, the same genes that are altered by carcinogens, radiation, or viruses also may be deregulated by translocation, amplification, or deletion.

Distinct aberrations of oncogenes are being defined for specific tumors at a rapid pace. This chapter will not attempt to provide a complete catalogue of mutations associated with human cancers. Instead, it will illustrate examples of genetic mechanisms to provide a framework for understanding developments in this field.

RNA TUMOR VIRUSES REVEAL ONCOGENES   Many malignancies of animals are transmissible. Extracts from chicken sarcomas were able to transmit the neoplasia to healthy recipients. The agent was proven to be the Rous sarcoma virus. A number of animal leukemias and carcinomas are induced within a matter of weeks by such acute transforming retroviruses. Retroviruses possess a single-stranded RNA genome. They are novel among viruses in that they

convert to a double-stranded DNA copy during their life cycle. After entry into the host cell via a cell surface receptor, the RNA template is copied into DNA by an RNA-dependent DNA polymerase known as *reverse transcriptase*. This viral DNA is efficiently integrated into the host cell's chromosomal DNA via specialized ends known as *long terminal repeats* (LTRs). LTRs are multifunctional, possessing promoter and enhancer elements as well as providing a signal for polyadenylation. The integrated DNA form of the virus is known as the *provirus*. The retroviral genome possesses genes which encode the core proteins of the viral capsid (gag), the reverse transcriptase (pol), and the viral envelope glycoproteins (env) (Fig. 63-1).

Retroviruses possessing only the gag, pol, and env genes may induce tumors but only after a long latency period. This results from *insertional activation*, whereby the integrated provirus activates a neighboring cellular gene which promotes transformation. In contrast the acute transforming retroviruses all carry a viral oncogene (v-*onc*). Often the v-*onc* gene interrupts one of the viral genes, necessitating a coinfection with a "helper virus" to provide the missing replicative machinery.

Insight into cancer pathogenesis was revolutionized by the discovery that v-*onc* genes represented copies of genes obtained from mammalian cells. The transforming element in Rous sarcoma virus, v-*src*, was shown to have originated from a normal cellular homologue in the chicken, c-*src*. v-*onc* genes lack introns, arguably because they were generated through an RNA intermediate. Moreover v-*onc* genes have been altered compared with their normal cellular counterparts in order to become transforming. They are often truncated, fused with viral proteins, or mutated. In contrast, the cellular homologues, c-*onc* genes, are correctly regulated in normal cells, where they frequently play pivotal roles in the control of cell growth and differentiation. However, it is these same c-*onc* genes that are often the sites of genetic alteration within human tumors.

THE SEARCH FOR HUMAN RETROVIRUSES   The observation that retroviruses were responsible for a number of malignancies in animals prompted an extensive search for retroviral counterparts in humans. However, only rarely have retroviruses been implicated in human tumorigenesis. The most notable exception is human T cell lymphotropic virus type I (HTLV-I), which causes adult T cell lymphoma/leukemia (ATL), an aggressive malignancy. ATL is characterized by leukemia, skin involvement, bone marrow infiltration, and hypercalcemia. A related virus, HTLV-II, was isolated from a patient with hairy cell leukemia. While the HTLVs do not possess a classic oncogene, an additional region, pX, was noted between env and the 3' LTR. This region encodes the 40-kDa tax protein that serves as a transcription factor capable of upregulating the IL-2 and IL-2 receptor genes. This may establish an autocrine loop important in the early stages of leukemogenesis. HTLV is endemic in southern Japan and the Caribbean, where the disease is more prevalent.

DNA TUMOR VIRUSES   Many DNA viruses can transform cells in culture or induce tumors in animal models. It has been more difficult to prove a causative role in humans because tumors arise during latent or persistent infection. Simian virus 40 (SV40) is a highly oncogenic virus isolated from monkeys that has proven highly instructive. SV40 encodes a transforming "early" gene product, large T antigen. Importantly large T antigen has been shown to bind to both the p53 and *Rb* tumor suppressor gene products of cellular origin. This finding has influenced the thinking concerning the pathogenic mechanism of DNA viruses implicated in human malignancies.

Epidemiologic studies have implicated papilloma virus, Epstein-Barr virus, and hepatitis B virus in human tumors. Human papilloma virus (HPV) induces condylomas and papillomas. Moreover, HPV has been implicated in cervical carcinoma in which invasive cervical cancers often contain HPV16 and 18. The *E6/E7* early genes of HPV have been mapped as the region responsible for transformation. Of interest, *E7* has been shown to interact with *Rb*, while E6 binds to p53.

Epstein-Barr virus (EBV) is a herpesvirus consistently detected in

FIGURE 63-1 Structure of a retrovirus as it would be integrated into genomic DNA as a provirus. LTR, long terminal repeats containing R, U5, U3 regulatory regions; gag, viral capsid; pol, reverse transcriptase; and env, envelope glycoproteins.

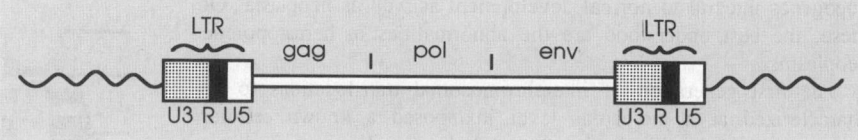

endemic Burkitt's lymphoma of Africa but in only 10 percent of sporadic cases. EBV infects B cells and is the etiologic agent of infectious mononucleosis. The virus has the ability to immortalize normal B cells in culture. EBV genome is also found in nasopharyngeal carcinomas, which are common in Southeast Asia.

Hepatitis B virus (HBV) has clearly been implicated in hepatocellular carcinoma. The acquisition of chronic infection by HBV in the Orient results in a several hundred–fold increased risk of hepatocellular carcinoma. Recent transgenic mouse models have indicated that overexpression of HBsAg results in progression to hepatocellular carcinoma.

TRANSFECTION OF TUMOR DNA IDENTIFIES ACTIVATED PROTO-ONCOGENES A valuable approach to detect activated oncogenes utilizes tumor DNA in a DNA-mediated gene transfer. Nonmalignant NIH3T3 mouse fibroblasts will take up exogenous DNA and incorporate portions into their own genome. DNA from chemically induced sarcomas was shown to transform NIH3T3 cells. Moreover, DNA from many human tumors also was capable of transforming these fibroblasts. Serial transfection of DNA from transformed foci enabled the isolation of a single human gene responsible for transformation. The transforming gene was often a member of the *ras* gene family. This includes the cellular homologues of viral Harvey ras (c-H-*ras*) and Kirsten ras (c-K-*ras*) as well as c-N-*ras*, which has no viral counterpart. Comparison of the DNA sequence of the transforming *ras* genes from tumors with their normal counterparts revealed an additional mechanism of tumorigenesis, somatic point mutations. Remarkably, single-base changes were noted to cluster in codons 12, 13, 59, or 61, resulting in amino acid substitutions responsible for the activation. The *ras* genes encode highly related p21^{ras} proteins that bind guanine nucleotides (GTP and GDP) and possess intrinsic GTPase activity (Fig. 63-2). Mutations which replaced gly^{12} with val^{12} or asp^{12} still retain the capacity to bind GTP but demonstrate less GTPase activity. The intrinsic GTPase activity of p21 is markedly accelerated by a GTPase-activating protein (GAP) which catalyzes the conversion of p21-GTP to p21-GDP. Oncogenic p21 molecules with mutations at position 12, 59, or 61 are resistant

to the effects of GAP. This locks the mutated ras protein in the GTP-ras activated form. While the precise role of mammalian ras proteins is under intensive scrutiny, it is known that they are located on the inner surface of the cell membrane and are similar to G proteins. This argues that ras proteins, which have been noted in some receptor complexes, may be intimately involved in the early phase of signal transduction. A wide variety of hematologic and solid tumors possess *ras* gene mutations. Mutated K-*ras* and H-*ras* are more common in cancers of epithelial origin, whereas N-*ras* mutations are noted in neural and hematologic malignancies. Mutations of *ras* genes are not a universal prerequisite for tumorigenesis. However, when present, the same alteration is found in all cells of the tumor, indicating a selective advantage. Moreover, activated *ras* genes have been noted in premalignant diseases, including myelodysplastic syndromes and adenomas of the colon, indicating that they can be an early event. In addition, the gene responsible for neurofibromatosis type 1 (NF-1) has substantial homology to the catalytic domains of GAP, suggesting an expanded role for this family in tumorigenesis.

GENE AMPLIFICATIONS IDENTIFY ONCOGENIC EVENTS Karyotypic analysis of neuroblastomas often reveals extrachromosomal double minute chromosomes or homogeneous staining regions (HSRs) within chromosomes. These regions were initially examined to determine if they bore genes involved in drug resistance. However, a survey of oncogenes indicated that the N-*myc* gene from chromosome 2 was uniformly amplified in these HSRs and double minutes. The sequence of events in amplification is felt to be an excision of a small chromosomal piece containing N-*myc* which is propagated as an extrachromosomal double minute. Later this can be randomly integrated into chromosomes resulting in HSRs.

Studies of primary tumors have indicated an important clinical correlation. Benign ganglioneuromas never have N-*myc* amplification. Low-stage neuroblastomas, generally associated with a good prognosis, have a low incidence of N-*myc* amplification (5 to 10 percent). However, those cases identified with N-*myc* amplification were destined to have rapid tumor progression similar to advanced-stage patients. *Over 30 percent of advanced-stage tumors have N-myc amplification* (Table 63-1). N-*myc* amplification appears to be an intrinsic biologic property of certain neuroblastomas, generally being present at the time of diagnosis rather than demonstrating acquisition over time.

CHROMOSOMAL TRANSLOCATIONS REVEAL NOVEL PROTO-ONCOGENES At the beginning of this century, it was proposed that chromosomal abnormalities would be the basis for malignant transformation. Since then, careful observations by cancer cytogeneticists have revealed over 125 recurrent cytogenetic abnormalities in a wide range of neoplasms. Specific interchromosomal translocations are found repeatedly within distinct types of malignancies but not their normal cellular counterparts. These sites of chromosomal breakage have proven an extremely rich source of novel proto-

FIGURE 63-2 Schematic of *ras* activation pathway and abnormalities induced by *ras* point mutation. GAP, GTPase-activating protein.

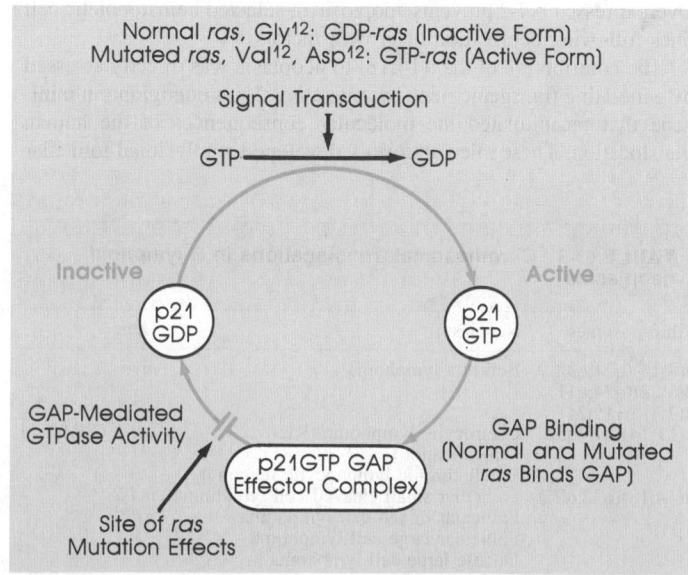

TABLE 63-1 N-*myc* copy number and stage in neuroblastoma

Stage at diagnosis	Frequency of N-*myc* amplification, %
Benign ganglioneuromas	0
Low stages (A, B; I, II)	3
Stage D-S or IVS	7
Advanced stages (C, D; II, IV)	31

SOURCE: Modified from Brodeur GM, Fong CT: Cancer Genet Cytogenet 41:153, 1989.

oncogenes integral to normal development as well as neoplasia. Of these, the best understood are the abnormalities in hematopoietic neoplasms.

The first generation of interchromosomal translocations to be characterized at a molecular level juxtaposed a known cellular oncogene, c-*myc*, with the immunoglobulin (Ig) locus in Burkitt's lymphoma (Table 63-2). A second generation of interchromosomal translocations introduces new putative proto-oncogenes into known loci. In B cell tumors this was often the immunoglobulin loci and in T cell malignancies the T cell receptor genes. The t(9;22), which generated the Philadelphia chromosome found in chronic myelogenous leukemia, serves as a prototype (see Table 63-2). This breakpoint revealed the *bcr* gene from chromosome segment 22q11 juxtaposed with the known c-*abl* gene on 9q34. Most translocations and deletions represent a third generation, and that presents the greatest challenge. The majority of chromosomal aberrations possess no certain candidate genes at either chromosomal site. Conquering these abnormalities requires new strategies that bridge the resolution gap between cytogenetics (≈5000 to 10,000 kb per band) and cosmid clones (50 kb). Yeast artificial chromosome (YAC) libraries of the human genome have permitted the isolation of large fragments containing over 1000 kb of human DNA. YACs have allowed the isolation of candidate oncogenes from the t(4;11) abnormality found in extremely aggressive mixed-lineage leukemias. Thus the technology now exists to address all these signatures of human cancer cells.

BURKITT'S LYMPHOMA JUXTAPOSES C-*MYC* WITH IMMUNO-GLOBULIN HEAVY OR LIGHT CHAIN LOCI The most common chromosomal aberration in the B cell lymphoma of childhood, Burkitt's lymphoma, is a t(8;14) reciprocal translocation that introduces the c-*myc* proto-oncogene from 8q24 into the immunoglobulin heavy chain locus at 14q32 (Fig. 63-3). This correlation between Burkitt's translocations and immunoglobulin gene loci was substantially strengthened when variant forms of Burkitt's translocations were shown to involve the home of the κ gene locus at 2p11 or the λ genes at 22q11 (see Table 63-3).

*The repositioning of c-*myc* next to an immunoglobulin gene markedly altered its regulatory control.* Immunoglobulin genes are actively transcribed at this stage of differentiation, and the c-*myc* gene may be influenced by mechanisms that augment antibody expression.

THE t(14;18) OF FOLLICULAR LYMPHOMA REVEALS THE *bcl*-2 PROTO-ONCOGENE The t(14;18) (q32;q21) is the most common translocation in hematologic malignancies (Table 63-3). Approximately 85 percent of follicular and 20 percent of diffuse B cell lymphomas possess this translocation. Molecular cloning of the

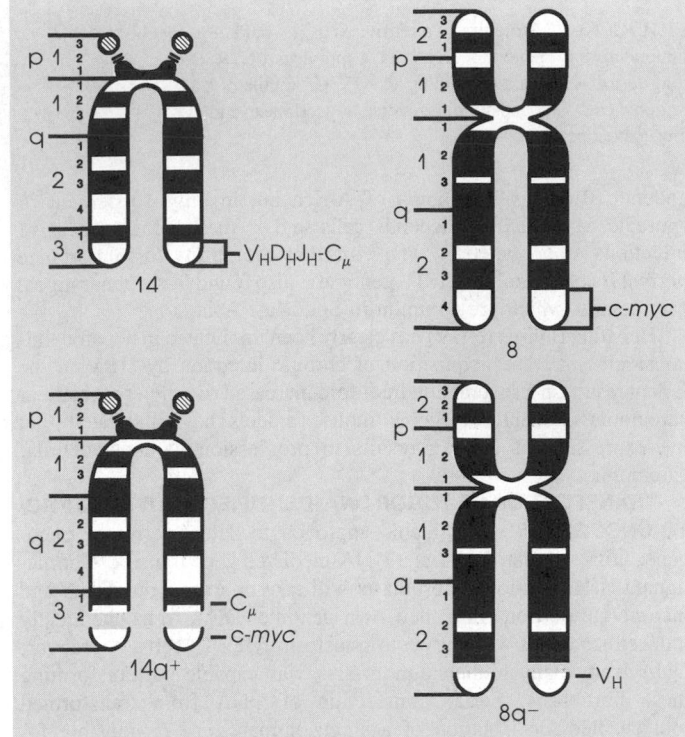

FIGURE 63-3 A schematic representation of the normal and reciprocally translocated chromosomes in Burkitt's lymphoma t(8;14). A normal chromosome 14 possesses an effective $V_H D_H J_H$ and $C\mu$ responsible for the IgM produced. The normal chromosome 8 retains a nonexpressed copy of c-*myc*. The 14q+ chromosome has received a portion of chromosome 8 bearing the c-*myc* gene. The 8q− chromosome breaks at 8q24 and receives part of chromosome 14, often including some V_H genes.

t(14;18) breakpoint revealed a putative proto-oncogene, *bcl*-2, at 18q21. Despite the mature B cell phenotype of lymphomas bearing t(14;18), the translocation appears to occur earlier in development at a pre-B cell stage. Immunoglobulin recombinase initiates the first attempt at rearrangement in pre-B development by cleaving at a D and J immunoglobulin segment (Fig. 63-4). Instead of completing that recombination, however, progenitor cells of follicular lymphoma introduce a broken *bcl*-2 gene from 18q21 into these sites.

The cloning of this second-generation breakpoint provided a new gene, *bcl*-2, which demonstrates the novel function of blocking programmed cell death (apoptosis) rather than promoting proliferation. Overexpressed *bcl*-2 prevents apoptosis in selected hematopoietic cell lines following deprivation of growth factors.

The contribution of the t(14;18) to neoplasia was directly assessed by generating transgenic mice bearing a *bcl*-2–immunoglobulin mini-gene that recapitulated the molecular consequences of the human translocation. These mice uniformly developed a polyclonal follicular

---

TABLE 63-2　Chromosomal translocations in lymphomas and leukemias

Candidate genes on both sides of breakpoint

	14q32	8q24
Burkitt's lymphoma t(8;14)	Ig H chain	c-*myc*

Candidate gene on one side, new gene on the other

	14q32	18q21
Follicular lymphoma t(14;18)	Ig H chain	*bcl*-2
	14q11	11p15, 11p13, 10q24
T acute lymphoblastic leukemia	α/δTCR	*ttg*-1, *ttg*-2, *Hox11*
Chronic myelogenous leukemia	9q34	22q11
Ph acute lymphoblastic leukemia	c-*abl*	*bcr*

No certain candidate gene on either side of breakpoint

	11q23	4q21
Mixed lineage leukemia t(4;11)	MLL	AF4

TABLE 63-3　Chromosomal translocations in B lymphoid neoplasms

Chromosomes	Neoplasm	Gene
t(8;14)(q24;q32) t(8;22)(q24;q11) t(2;8)(p11;q24)	Burkitt's lymphoma	*myc*
t(11;14)(q13;q32)	Centrocytic lymphoma (Kiel classification) B cell chronic lymphocytic leukemia	*bcl*-1 (*PRAD*-1)
t(14;18)(q32;q21)	Follicular small cleaved cell lymphoma Follicular mixed cell lymphoma Follicular large cell lymphoma Diffuse large cell lymphoma	*bcl*-2

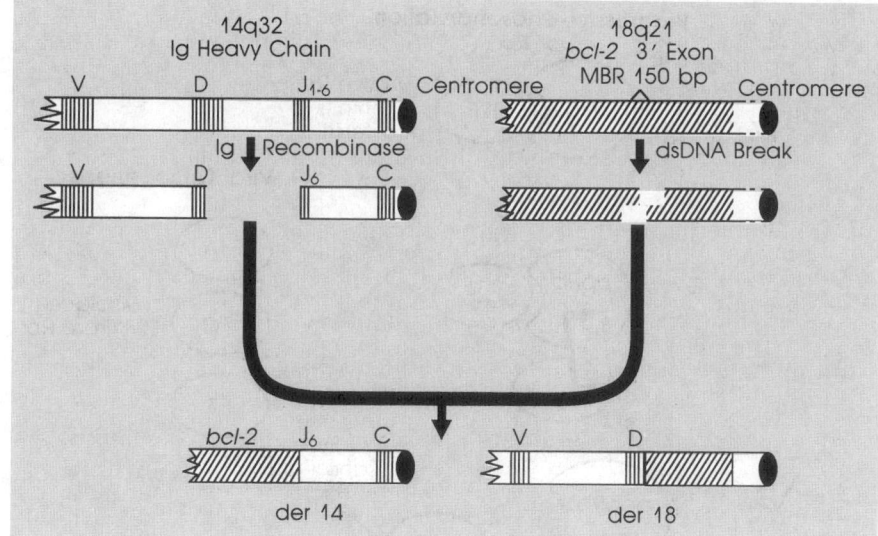

FIGURE 63-4 Mechanisms of the t(14;18) recombination. Der(14) chromosomes have breakpoints at J segments, while der(18) breakpoints involve D segments. This indicates that the translocation occurs at a pre-B cell stage following endonucleolytic cleavage at a D and J segment by immunoglobulin recombinase. Such ends illegitimately recombine with a double-stranded DNA break in the major breakpoint region (MBR) of *bcl*-2 exon III at 18q21.

lymphoproliferation that selectively expanded small resting B cells. These recirculating B cells accumulate as a result of extended survival rather than increased proliferation. Like patients with follicular lymphoma, these mice progress from indolent follicular hyperplasia to diffuse large cell lymphoma. This satisfies a molecular Koch's postulate for the t(14;18) in B cell lymphoma. Moreover, they also indicate that prolonged cell survival is oncogenic. Thus *bcl*-2 represents the first member of a new category of oncogenes, regulators of programmed cell death. Extended cell survival may prove to be a key event in carcinogenesis that enables the acquisition of further genetic changes (Fig. 63-5).

CLL, CENTROCYTIC LYMPHOMA, AND THE *bcl*-1 GENE, CYCLIN D1. One of the first interchromosomal breakpoints to be cloned was t(11;14) (q13;q32), first noted in a handful of B cell type chronic lymphocytic leukemias (CLLs). Once again, the immunoglobulin locus at 14q32 had recombined with a region on chromosome segment 11q13 entitled the *bcl*-1 locus. However certain intermediate-grade lymphomas, especially the centrocytic B cell lymphomas of the Kiel classification, have a much higher incidence (30 to 50 percent) of *bcl*-1 rearrangement. In parallel, a number of parathyroid adenomas bear clonal rearrangements of their phenotypic landmark gene, parathyroid hormone (PTH). This proved to be a translocation with 11q13 that overexpressed a newly identified gene located there, *PRAD*-1 (parathyroid adenomatosis). *PRAD*-1 encodes a novel cyclin that is expressed in the G_1 phase of the cell cycle and has been named *cyclin D1*. Cyclins regulate cell cycle transitions, and D cyclins appear to interact with a kinase protein (cdk) as well as Rb, the retinoblastoma gene product (Fig. 63-6). Cyclin D1 appears to be the *bcl*-1 gene, since it is also deregulated in B cell tumors t(11;14). This

FIGURE 63-5 Alternative pathways to neoplasia. Normal tissue homeostasis represents a balanced equation between input (cell proliferation) and output (cell death). Considerable evidence indicates that an increase in proliferation can lead to neoplasia. Studies of *bcl*-2 indicate that a decrease in the rate of cell death is also tumorigenic.

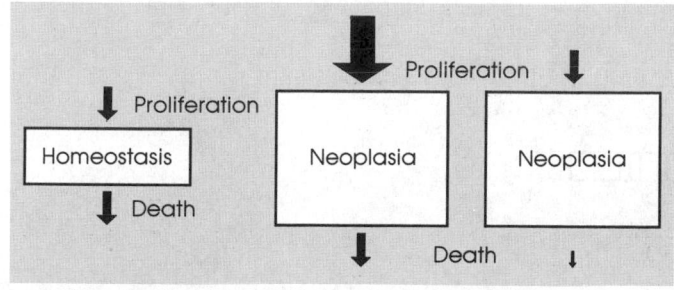

gene provides an avenue to determine how a cyclin which appears to act at the G_1–S boundary influences cell growth and neoplasia.

TWO MOLECULAR FORMS OF THE PHILADELPHIA CHROMOSOME IN CML AND ALL (See also Chaps. 309 and 310) The description in 1960 of the Philadelphia chromosome in chronic but not acute myelogenous leukemia initiated the field of cancer cytogenetics. The Philadelphia chromosome, Ph, is present in virtually all patients with chronic myelogenous leukemia (CML) and in approximately 25 percent of adults and 5 percent of children with acute lymphoblastic leukemia (ALL). CML is a disease of a multipotential hematopoietic stem cell in which multiple lineages including myeloid, erythroid, lymphoid, and megakaryocytic are affected. ALLs with Ph are of pre-B cell type. The t(9;22) (q34;q11) was found to involve c-*abl* on 9q34 and a limited region on 22q11 designated the *breakpoint cluster region* (bcr). Later this was shown to be part of a gene that spans over 90 kilobases. The molecular consequence of the t(9;22) is to generate a fusion gene between 5' *bcr* sequences and 3' *abl* sequences on the Ph chromosome. This results in a chimeric peptide that is part *bcr* and part *abl* (Fig. 63-7).

The breakpoints within the *bcr* gene at 22q11 are focused in two areas. The original breakpoint cluster region is within the heart of the *bcr* gene. This is where nearly all cases of CML break and results in a 8.5-kb *bcr-abl* fusion RNA and a fusion protein of p210 (210 kDa) size. In contrast, many ALLs break far upstream within the first intron of the *bcr* gene. This creates a smaller 7.0-kb fusion RNA and p190 fusion protein. Clinical studies indicate that Ph-positive ALL has a much worse prognosis than the Ph-negative ALL. Moreover, Ph-positive adult ALL can possess either the p210 form ($\approx$40 percent of cases) or the p190 form ($\approx$60 percent). The capacity of the p210 and p190 forms of the hybrid *bcr-abl* proteins to transform cells correlates with their augmented tyrosine kinase activity. Moreover, animal models bearing the p210 or p190 forms of *bcr-abl* develop leukemia. As the human disease first suggested, the molecular forms of *bcr-abl* may predetermine the type of disease. While it is not absolute, the p190 form appears to favor acute pre-B cell leukemia, whereas the p210 form favors a chronic stem cell leukemia.

T CELL TRANSLOCATIONS REDIRECT TRANSCRIPTION FACTORS The most frequent interchromosomal translocations within T cell neoplasms also involve their antigen receptor genes. Chromosome segment 14q11, the home of the α/δ TCR, is most frequently involved, but translocations into the β TCR locus at 7q34 are also noted. Analysis of transcripts from the other participating chromosome has proven rewarding. While TCR loci are involved on one side, a large number of different chromosomal partners participate on the far side. Characterization of six separate proto-oncogene candidates indicates that they belong to classic transcription factor families principally intended for lineages other than T cells. This includes *ttg*-1, *ttg*-2,

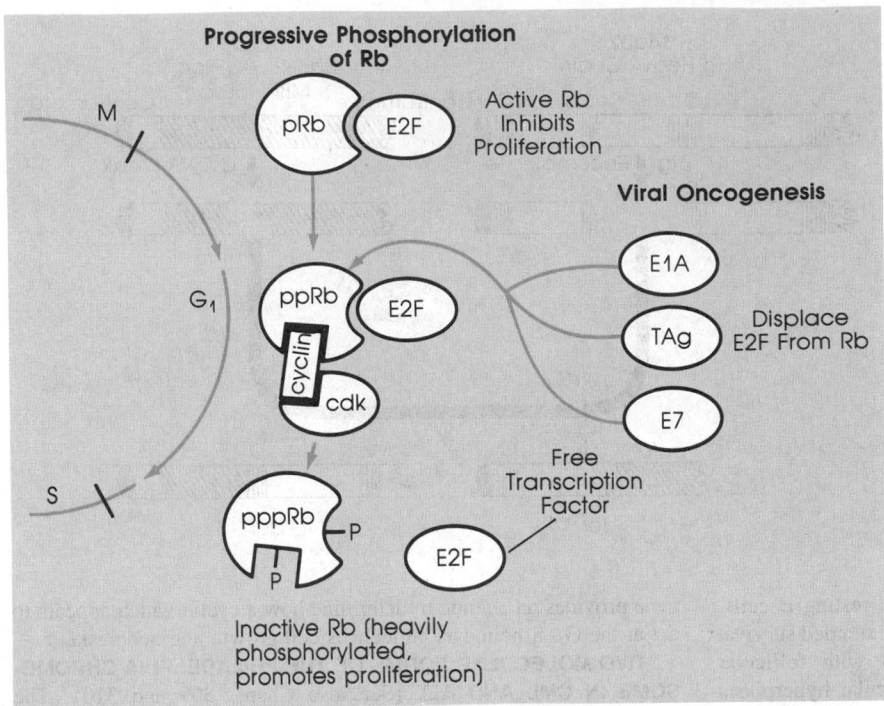

FIGURE 63-6 Schematic presentation of the role of the retinoblastoma protein Rb in the regulation of cell cycle. Rb is progressively phosphorylated during cell cycle progression. Underphosphorylated Rb is active in inhibiting proliferation and interacts with the E2F transcription factor, which is displaced by the viral oncogene products E1A, T antigen (TAg), and E7. Rb also may complex with the highly regulated cyclin proteins and cyclin-dependent kinases (cdks). Inactive Rb is hyperphosphorylated, which appears to displace a number of these interacting proteins.

scl, *tal-2*, and *lyl*-1. *HOX11* completes this group. Redirected expression of these transcription factors to the thymus results in T cell lymphoblastic lymphoma/leukemia. These aberrantly expressed products may substitute for homologues in T cells or inappropriately activate a gene program intended for another cell type.

EWING'S SARCOMA: SOLID TUMORS ALSO POSSESS RECIPROCAL TRANSLOCATIONS Highly recurrent interchromosomal translocations are not restricted to hematopoietic neoplasms. Ewing's sarcoma and related subsets of primitive neuroectodermal tumors bear a reciprocal translocation t(11;22) (q24;q12). Molecular cloning of the breakpoint has revealed the generation of a chimeric protein with the *fli*-1 proto-oncogene, a member of the *ets* family of oncogenes, located at 11q24.

TUMOR SUPPRESSOR GENES: THE RETINOBLASTOMA MODEL A class of cancer-related genes exists which suppresses tumorigenesis and contributes to neoplasia in a recessive manner. It has been noted that transfer of a single normal chromosome into certain tumor cells can suppress their tumorigenicity. For example,

a normal chromosome 11 will suppress the malignant behavior of a Wilms' tumor cell. These observations prompted the thesis that the absence or functional loss of such chromosomes would result in unchecked growth. Definitive data that indicated the existence of tumor suppressor genes were provided by several inherited forms of cancer, retinoblastoma and Wilms' tumor. Knudson advanced the "two hit" hypothesis to explain such pediatric tumors that occurred in families. In familial retinoblastoma he proposed that one mutation is present in the germ line while the second allele is altered in somatic development. In sporadic cases of retinoblastoma, both mutational events would occur in the retinal lineage cells. This accounts for the fact that familial retinoblastoma occurs at an earlier age and is typically bilateral.

Evidence for a recessive mechanism in retinoblastoma was first provided by cytogenetics in which deletions of the long arm of chromosome 13, 13q14, were noted in normal as well as tumor cells of some patients. This prompted the use of polymorphic genetic markers mapped to 13q14 to search for more refined losses in other

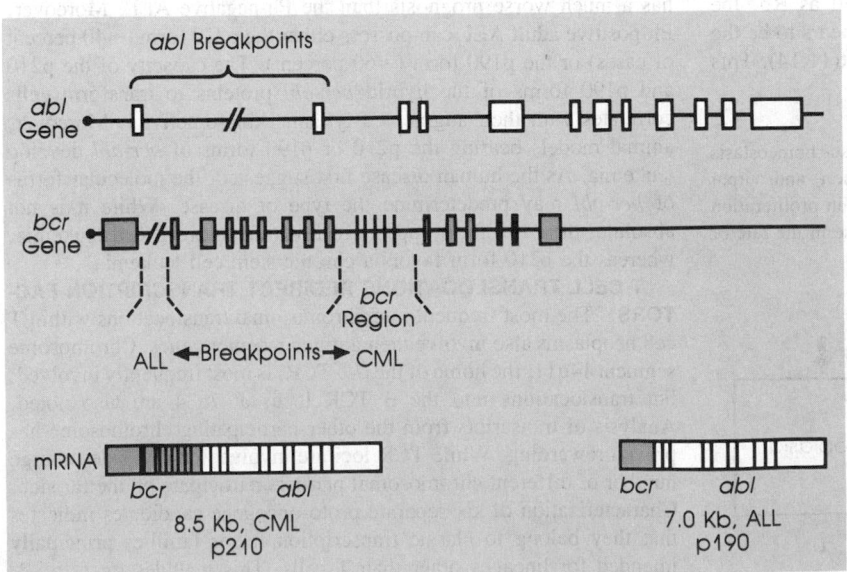

FIGURE 63-7 c-*abl* and *bcr* genes in CML and ALL. Normal genomic c-*abl* gene at 9q24; sites of breakpoints noted. Normal genomic *bcr* gene at 22q11; sites of ALL versus CML breakpoints noted. Two species of fusion RNAs, CML (8.5 kb) versus ALL (7.0 kb).

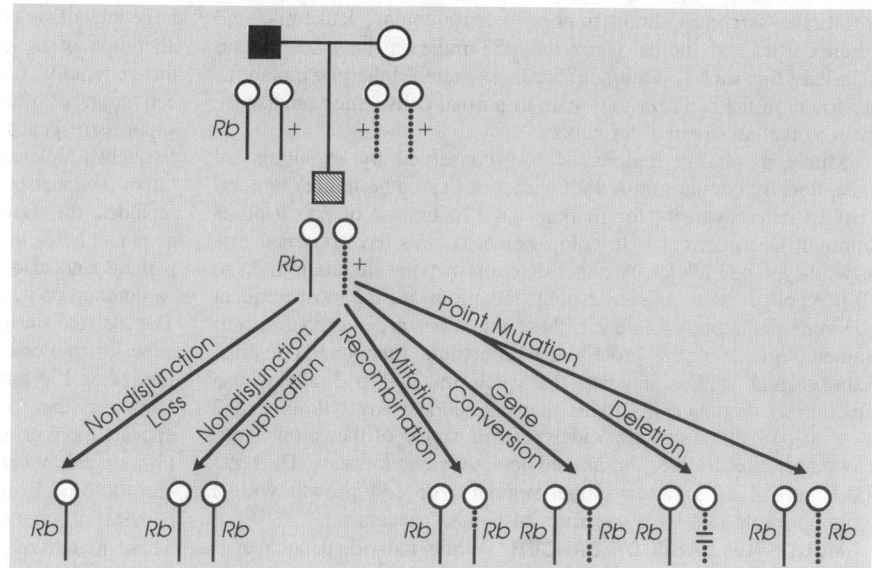

FIGURE 63-8 Schematic of the genetic mechanisms observed for the loss of heterozygosity in the *Rb* gene in familial retinoblastoma. *(Adapted from Cavenee et al, Nature 305, 780, 1983.)*

cases. These studies revealed a loss of heterozygosity for polymorphic DNA markers at 13q14 in tumor cells versus normal cells of patients. Loss of heterozygosity can occur by a number of genetic mechanisms (Fig. 63-8). While the second allele may be altered by a spontaneous mutation, other events are more common, including chromosomal nondisjunction, nondisjunction with duplication, mitotic recombination, and gene conversion. The loss of heterozygosity for a genetic marker has become the hallmark of a potential tumor suppressor gene.

The mapping of the locus to 13q24 soon led to the isolation of the retinoblastoma (*Rb*) gene. *Rb* encodes a 105-kDa nuclear phosphoprotein that has protein-protein interaction properties (see Fig. 63-6). The underphosphorylated form of *Rb* predominates in the G_1 phase of the cell cycle, whereas *Rb* is progressively phosphorylated toward the S phase. The underphosphorylated active form of Rb complexes with the E2F transcription factor, whereas the heavy phosphorylated inactive form of Rb releases E2F. Of note, the DNA viral oncoproteins T antigen of SV40, E1A of adenovirus, and E7 of the human papilloma virus all bind Rb and displace E2F. The loss of *Rb* protein results in neoplastic transformation and unregulated cell growth. Proof that the *Rb* gene was the responsible tumor suppressor gene was obtained when normal *Rb* was reintroduced into tumor cells and cell growth was arrested at the G_1 stage of the cell cycle.

WILMS' TUMOR AND THE INACTIVATION OF TUMOR SUPPRESSOR GENES Wilms' tumor is an embryonal malignancy of the kidney that represents the most common abdominal malignancy of childhood. Documented familial transmission is rare (≈ 10 percent), but 10 percent of Wilms' tumors present with bilateral disease. The mapping of genes involved in Wilms' tumor was advanced by the analysis of patients with associated congenital anomalies. Children with the WAGR syndrome (Wilms' tumor, aniridia, genitourinary abnormalities, and mental retardation) had overlapping deletions of chromosome segment 11p13. Molecular dissection of this common region of deletion yielded the *WT1* gene. *WT1* is a zinc finger containing transcription factor that interacts with a specific DNA motif. This DNA sequence is also recognized by other transcription factors involved in early growth response. This observation suggests how *WT1* might compete for target genes and function as a tumor suppressor. Initial studies had shown loss of heterozygosity for polymorphic DNA markers on 11p in sporadic cases of Wilms' tumor. Mutations have been documented for the *WT1* gene within sporadic Wilms' tumor. Moreover, germ-line mutations have been noted in cases with bilateral tumors.

The genetics of Wilms' tumor is complex, and loci beyond *WT1* are also implicated. The Beckwith-Wiedeman syndrome is characterized by congenital anomalies of macroglossia, hemihypertro-

phy, organomegaly, and an increased incidence of Wilms' tumor, adrenocortical carcinoma, and hepatoblastoma. Genetic linkage and cytogenetics have mapped the Beckwith-Wiedeman locus to 11p15. Moreover, some sporadic cases of Wilms' tumor demonstrate loss of heterozygosity of 11p15. In addition, evidence exists for differential imprinting of the parental genes at 11p15 in both Beckwith-Wiedeman syndrome and Wilms' tumor. It is believed that only the maternal or paternal copy is expressed, a phenomenon known as *parental imprinting*. Studies of Wilms' tumors suggest that mutations may be selective for the paternal chromosome, while the maternal allele may be prone to loss. Details of this differential regulation await the isolation of a putative *WT* gene at 11p15.

Familial cases of Wilms' tumor further emphasize the genetic complexity of this single disease. Genetic linkage analysis of several large pedigrees with multiple cases of Wilms' tumor excluded 11p13 and 11p15 as the sites of inherited susceptibility. Thus evidence exists that at least three genes can participate in the genesis of Wilms' tumor.

LI-FRAUMENI SYNDROME AND THE p53 GENE IN CANCER Mutation or loss of the p53 gene is the most common genetic alteration found in human cancer. p53 was first noted as a cellular origin protein that associated with T antigen in SV40-transformed cells. Reminiscent of the *Rb* tumor suppressor gene, p53 is also inactivated by the E1B product of adenovirus and the E6 oncoprotein of human papilloma virus. Indeed p53 was often found at much higher levels in tumor cells. This was demonstrated to reflect a marked prolongation of its normally short protein half-life. In fact, p53 was initially classified as a dominant-acting oncogene since an isolated p53 cDNA would cooperate with other oncogenes to transform cells. However, the transforming clones of p53 proved to be mutants. Subsequently, the wild-type form of p53 has been shown to suppress the transformation of cells. Reintroduction of wild-type p53 into tumor cells that had lost the gene arrested their growth by blocking the cell cycle at the G_1–S transition. p53 also had been shown to interact with other endogenous cellular proteins and to bind DNA. Those proteins include the heat shock protein Hsc70 as well as *mdm*2, a probable oncogene that is amplified in certain tumors. Thus p53 has emerged as a most important DNA-binding protein that regulates cell cycle progression at the G_1–S boundary.

Perhaps 5 to 10 percent of common cancers, including breast, ovarian, and colon cancer, cluster in families, reflecting an underlying genetic susceptibility. One of the best detailed familial cancer syndromes is the rare autosomal dominant Li-Fraumeni syndrome (LFS). Affected families have a high incidence of very diverse childhood and adult tumors. The spectrum includes breast carcinoma, soft tissue sarcomas, brain tumors, osteosarcomas, leukemia, and adrenocortical carcinoma. Germ-line p53 mutations have been found in at least five such Li-Fraumeni families studied. Inherited mutations are found in the heterozygous state in normal cells which predispose them to the development of cancer.

Mutations in the regions of p53 conserved by evolution are exceptionally common in a wide variety of sporadic human tumors. Loss of heterozygosity for markers on 17p or loss of p53 itself is common in cancer cells. In colon cancer studies have revealed loss of wild-type p53 alleles by either deletion or point mutation in 75 to 80 percent of cases. Missense point mutations are the most frequent p53 gene mutation. Of interest, these mutations are clustered in four limited regions of the protein that constitute functional domains. Experimental studies indicate that such mutated p53 alleles can function as dominant negatives that outcompete any wild-type p53 protein. p53 alterations are widespread in cancer of the colon, lung, esophagus, breast, liver, brain, and hematopoietic lineages. Thus p53 has emerged as a rather global regulator of cell growth with a prominent role in a wide spectrum of human cancers.

MULTISTEP BASIS OF CANCER While individual oncogenes have distinct effects on tumorigenesis, multiple events are usually required before a single cell is fully transformed. Transformation of embryonic fibroblasts requires the cooperation of two oncogenes. Epidemiologic studies of human cancer indicate an age-dependent tumor incidence that argues for multiple independent steps. Cytogenetic data indicate that many tumors acquire further chromosomal alterations with progression of the disease. This reflects a clonal evolution in which the most malignant cells are selected.

Detailed analysis of the molecular aberrations in colorectal carcinoma has provided the clearest evidence for the multistep progression of human cancer. Colon tumorigenesis represents a progression from benign adenomas to highly metastatic carcinoma (see Chap. 257). Approximately 10 percent of small adenomas and roughly half of

large adenomas possess a mutated *ras* gene, usually K-*ras*. Overall, alteration of at least four to five genes may often be required for the generation of malignant colon tumor. These reflect mutational activation of oncogenes together with the inactivation of tumor suppressor genes (Fig. 63-9). The chromosomes that are most frequently deleted include 5q, 17p, and 18q. Proven or candidate tumor suppressor genes have been isolated from each site. This includes the familial adenomatous polyposis (FAP) gene at 5q responsible for the hyperproliferative epithelium in these predisposed patients and also noted to be altered in sporadic examples of colon carcinoma. p53 appears to be the principal gene participating on 17p. The deleted in colon carcinoma (DCC) gene that resembles an adhesion molecule is the candidate recessive oncogene from 18q. Losses of 17p and 18q often occur in later stages of tumorigenesis. However, there is no strict order, and the accumulation of defects appears more critical than the order of events. Recently, a predisposition to colon cancer has been shown to be linked to a gene on chromosome 2. Most familial (nonpolyposis) colon cancers and 13 percent of sporadic colon cancers have mutations in this gene. These mutations are associated with widespread alterations in short (dinucleotide) repeat sequences throughout the genome, suggesting that numerous replication errors occurred during tumor development. Thus these cancers develop by a mechanism of genetic instability rather than by classic tumor suppressor genes.

The enormous progress in defining the sequential genetic events in carcinogenesis holds great promise and challenge for the future. Understanding changes that are inherited or acquired may enable the identification of environmental contributions and lead to preventive steps. Pinpointing the precise biochemical effect of each of these genetic changes should ultimately refine therapeutic approaches as well.

REFERENCES

BISHOP JM: Viral oncogenes. Cell 42:23, 1985
FEARON ER, VOGELSTEIN B: A genetic model for colorectal tumorigenesis. Cell 61:759, 1990
LEVINE AJ et al: The p53 tumour suppressor gene. Nature 351:453, 1991
MCCORMICK F: GTPase-activating protein: Signal transmitter and signal terminator. Cell 56:5, 1989
MITELMAN F: *Cancer Cytogenetics*. New York, Liss, 1987
RABBITTS TH: Translocations, master genes, and differences between the origins of acute and chronic leukemias. Cell 67:644, 1991
ROWLEY JD: Identification of the constant chromosome regions involved in human hematologic malignant disease. Science 216:749, 1982
WEINBERG RA: Tumor suppressor genes. Science 254:1138, 1991

FIGURE 63-9 Genetic changes depicted for stages of progression in colorectal tumorigenesis. Not shown are gene mutations on chromosome 2 that lead to colon cancer by causing replication errors throughout the genome. (*After Fearon and Vogelstein.*)

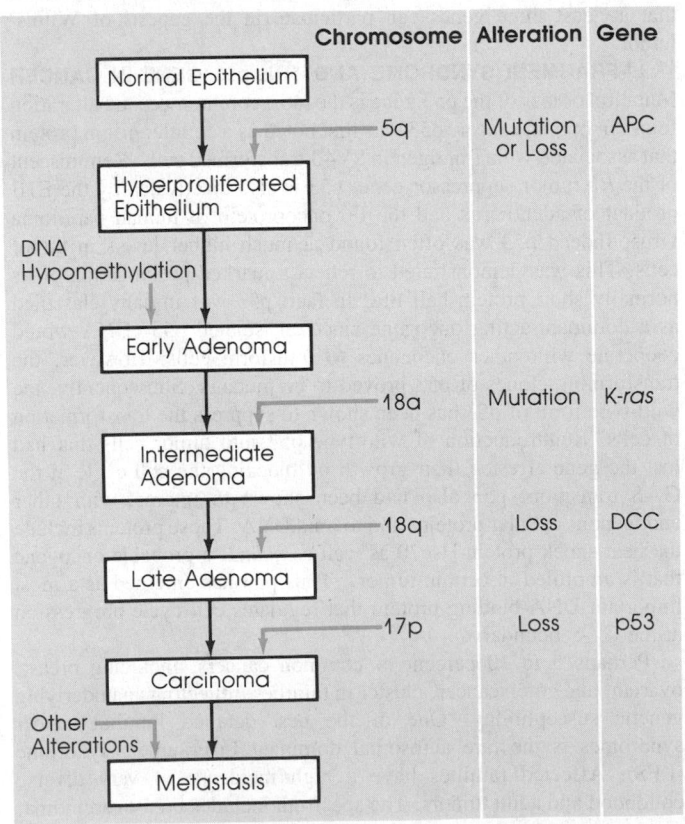

	Chromosome	Alteration	Gene
Normal Epithelium			
	5q	Mutation or Loss	APC
Hyperproliferated Epithelium			
DNA Hypomethylation			
Early Adenoma			
	18a	Mutation	K-*ras*
Intermediate Adenoma			
	18q	Loss	DCC
Late Adenoma			
	17p	Loss	p53
Carcinoma			
Other Alterations			
Metastasis			

64 THE MAJOR HISTOCOMPATIBILITY GENE COMPLEX

CHARLES B. CARPENTER

Antigenic differences between members of a species are called *alloantigens*, and when these play a determining role in the rejection of allogeneic tissue grafts, they are called *histocompatibility antigens*. Evolution has conserved a single closely linked region of histocompatibility genes, the products of which are prominently displayed on cell surfaces and provide a strong barrier to allotransplantation. The terms *major histocompatibility antigens* and *major histocompatibility gene complex* (MHC) refer to the gene products and genes of this chromosomal region. Their principal function is to bind peptide fragments so that they are optimally presented to T lymphocytes for recognition. Many minor histocompatibility antigens, in contrast, are encoded throughout the genome. They represent weaker allotypic differences on molecules that serve a variety of functions. Structures

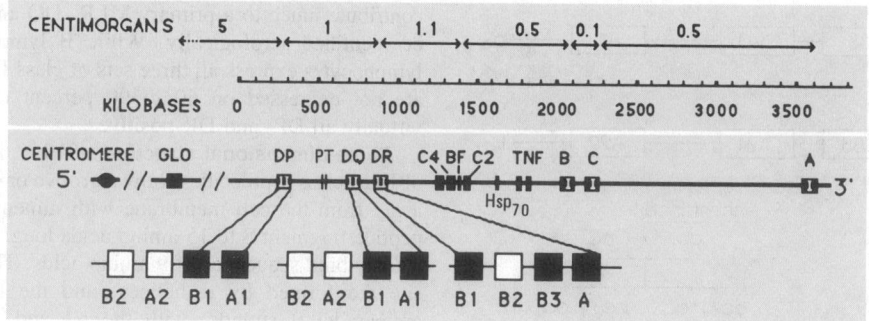

FIGURE 64-1 Schematic representation of human chromosome 6 showing the location of the HLA region in the 21 region of the short arm. The HLA-A, HLA-B, and HLA-C loci encode class I heavy chains (44,000 Da), while the beta$_2$-microglobulin light chain (11,500 Da) of the class I molecule is encoded by genes of chromosome 15. HLA-D region (class II) is centromeric to the A, B, and C loci, with genes for closely linked complement components C4A, C4B, Bf, and C2 in the B–D region. Two genes for tumor necrosis factor (TNFα,β) also lie between HLA-B and the complement genes. The order of the complement genes is uncertain. Additional loci shown are P for the proteosome (LMP) and T for the peptide transporter (TAP) genes and the Hsp$_{70}$ heat-shock protein gene. Each D region class II molecule is made up of an α and β chain (their genes are written as A and B). They appear on the cell surface in distinct heterodimers, DP, DQ, and DR. The numbers following A or B indicate that there are different genes for the chains of a given set; e.g., for DR, there are 9 β-chain genes (three are shown). The expressed molecule may be β1α(B1A) or β3α(B3A), for example. The β2 gene is not expressed (pseudogene). The antigens DR51, DR52, and DR53 are on the expressed B5, B3, and B4 chains, respectively, while the other DR antigens are on B1. DRA is not polymorphic, while the molecules bearing the DQ antigens have polymorphism in both A1 and B1 chains. DQA2 and DQB2 are pseudogenes. Polymorphism in DP is greater for B1 than for A1. The overall length of the HLA region is about 3 cM (3400 kilobases).

bearing MHC antigens play a major role in immunity and in self-recognition in the differentiation of cells and tissues. Much of the evidence for MHC control of the immune response comes from work in animal models in which immune-response genes have been mapped within the mouse (H-2), rat (RT1), and guinea pig (GPLA) MHC. In humans, the MHC is called *HLA*. The individual letters of HLA have various meanings, and by international agreement HLA is the logo for the human MHC.

Several generalizations can be made about the MHCs. *First*, three classes of gene products are encoded within the 4-kilobase region of the MHC. Class I molecules, expressed on virtually all cell surfaces, consist of one heavy and one light polypeptide chain and are the products of three reduplicated loci: HLA-A, HLA-B, and HLA-C. Class II molecules, restricted in expression to B lymphocytes, some monocytes, and activated T lymphocytes, consist of two polypeptide chains (α and β) of unequal length and are the products of several closely linked genes, collectively termed the HLA-D region. Class III molecules are the C4, C2, and Bf components of complement. *Second*, class I and class II molecules form complexes with immunogenic peptides (e.g., from bacteria or viruses), and they are conjointly recognized by T lymphocytes having appropriate antigen receptors. Selection of the T cell receptor repertoire occurs during development in the thymus, where various self-peptide + MHC combinations promote survival or elimination of T cell clones. Self versus nonself discrimination in the initiation and effector phase of the immune response is thereby intimately directed by class I and II molecules. *Third*, genes for enzyme systems having no apparent relationship to immunity are located in the region of the MHC, as are genes of importance in skeletal growth and development. *Fourth*, genes for tumor necrosis factors TNFα and TNFβ, heat-shock protein (Hsp$_{70}$), and peptide processing and transport lie also within the MHC. Loci of the HLA region on the short arm of chromosome 6 are shown in Fig. 64-1.

LOCI OF THE HLA SYSTEM   Class I antigens   HLA antigens of the class I type are defined serologically by human sera, principally from multiparous females, and to a limited extent by monoclonal antibodies. They are present in varying densities in most body tissues, including B cells, T cells, and platelets, but not in mature red blood cells. The number of serologically defined specificities is large, and the HLA system is the most polymorphic genetic system known in humans. Three clearly defined loci are recognized within the HLA complex for class I, serologically defined (SD), HLA antigens. Each class I antigen consists of an 11,500-Da beta$_2$-microglobulin subunit and a 44,000-Da heavy chain that carries the antigenic specificities

(Fig. 64-2). There are over 80 clearly defined A and B specificities, and 10 C-locus specificities are known. Antigens of the major complex are prefixed by HLA, but this may be omitted when the context is clear. The number following the locus designation is the name of the antigen. HLA antigens of African, Asian, and Oceanic peoples include many of the antigens commonly found in people of western European ancestry. However, the distribution of HLA antigens is distinctive for certain racial groups and can serve as anthropologic markers in the study of migration patterns and diseases.

Since chromosomes are paired, each individual has six serologically defined HLA-A, HLA-B, and HLA-C antigens, three from each parent. Each of these chromosomal sets is termed a *haplotype*, and

FIGURE 64-2 Schematic representation of class I and class II molecules on the cell surface. Class I molecules are composed of two polypeptide chains. The 44,000-Da heavy chain passes through the plasma membrane. Its external portion consists of three domains (α$_1$, α$_2$, α$_3$) formed by disulfide bonding. The beta$_2$-microglobulin (β$_{2μ}$) light chain (11,500 Da) encoded by chromosome 15 is noncovalently bound to the heavy chain. Amino acid sequence homology among class I molecules is 80 to 85 percent, falling to 50 percent or less in portions of α$_1$ and α$_2$ which represent the sites of alloantigenic polymorphism. Class II molecules consist of two noncovalently associated polypeptide chains, a 34,000-Da α and a 29,000-Da β. Each chain has two domains formed by disulfide bridging (the α$_1$ domain lacks a sulfide bridge). (*From Carpenter and Strom.*)

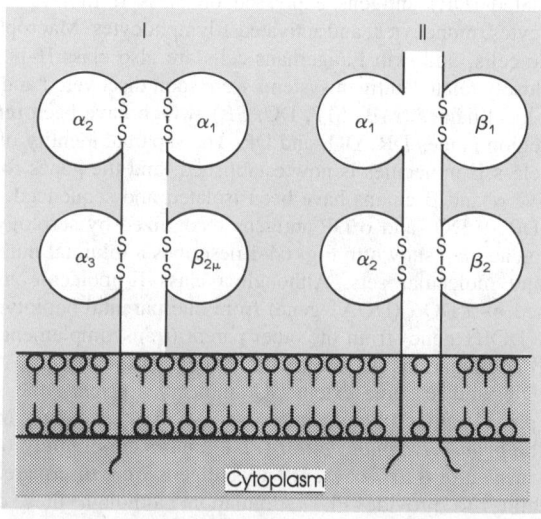

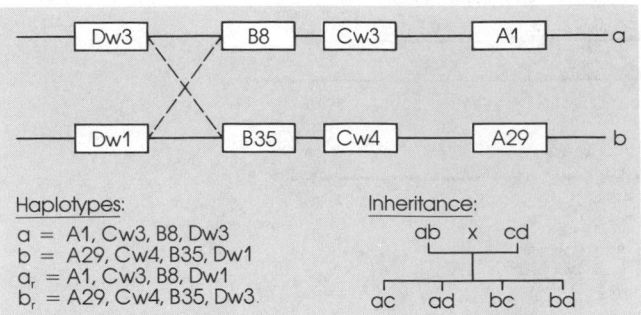

FIGURE 64-3 HLA region, chromosome 6: inheritance of HLA haplotypes. Each chromosomal segment of linked genes is termed a *haplotype*, and each individual inherits one haplotype from each parent. The A, B, C, and D antigens of haplotypes a and b are shown for this hypothetical individual in chromosomal order on the diagram and also below as they would be written in text. If individual ab were to marry cd, their offspring would be of four types only, as far as HLA is concerned. Occasionally (*dashed cross*) recombination occurs in the germ line (meiosis) of a parent, resulting in an altered haplotype. The frequency of recombinant children is a measure of the map distance (1 percent recombination frequency = 1 cM; see Fig. 64-1). (*From CB Carpenter, Kidney Int, 14:283, 1978.*)

by simple Mendelian inheritance, one-fourth of siblings have identical haplotypes, one-half share a haplotype, and the remaining one-fourth are completely incompatible (Fig. 64-3). Evidence that this gene complex plays the major role in the transplantation response comes from the fact that haplotype-matched sibling donor-recipient combinations show excellent results in kidney transplantation, in the vicinity of 85 to 90 percent long-term survival (see Chap. 238).

Class II antigens The HLA-D region is separated from the class I loci on the short arm of chromosome 6 by 1000 kilobases (see Fig. 64-1). This region encodes a series of class II molecules, each consisting of a 29,000-Da β chain and a 34,000-Da α chain (see Fig. 64-2). Incompatibility for this region, particularly concerning the DR antigens, determines the in vitro proliferative response of lymphocytes to mismatched haplotypes. This mixed lymphocyte response (MLR) is assessed by the degree of proliferation of a *mixed lymphocyte culture* (MLC) and is positive even when HLA-A, HLA-B, and HLA-C antigens are identical (see Fig. 64-3). When parental recombination has occurred between HLA-B and -DR, for example, a new haplotype appears in the child, who will be identical for class I but different for class II (a versus a_r in Fig. 64-3). HLA-D antigens are defined by reference-stimulating lymphocytes that are homozygous for HLA-D and are inactivated by x-irradiation or mitomycin C to make the reaction unidirectional. There are 26 such antigens recognized by homozygous typing cells.

Attempts to define HLA-D by serology first established a series of D-related (DR) antigens expressed on class II molecules of B lymphocytes, monocytes, and activated T lymphocytes. Macrophages, dendritic cells, and skin Langerhans cells are also class II–positive. Other closely related antigen systems were soon discovered and given various local names (MB, MT, DC, SB), which have been replaced by subregion names DR, DQ, and DP. The separate identity of these sets of class II molecules is now established, and the genes for their respective α and β chains have been isolated and sequenced. There are 24 DR, 9 DQ, and 6 DP antigens recognized by serology. The class II gene map shown in Fig. 64-1 describes a minimal number of genes and molecular sets. Although a class II molecule may be composed of a DQα (DQA1 gene) from one parental haplotype and a DQβ (DQB1 gene) from the other parent (transcomplementation), α and β combinations outside each DP, DQ, DR set rarely, if ever, occur. DR, and to some extent DQ, molecules provide the stimuli for the primary mixed lymphocyte response. The secondary MLR is called the *primed lymphocyte test* (PLT) and occurs rapidly over 24 to 36 h instead of 6 to 7 days. DP alloantigens were discovered from their ability to provide PLT stimulation, although they do not

contribute much to a primary MLR. DQ and DP molecules also can be identified serologically. While B lymphocytes and activated T lymphocytes express all three sets of class II molecules, DQ antigens are not expressed on 60 to 90 percent of monocytes, which are virtually all DP- and DR-positive.

Three-dimensional structure of HLA X-ray diffraction studies of HLA class I molecules show a groove or cleft on the surface facing away from the cell membrane with dimensions sufficient to bind a peptide fragment 8 to 15 amino acids long. In fact, class I molecules usually bind sequences of 9 amino acids. The margins of the binding site are formed by α helices, and the base is floored by eight antiparallel β strands, with the α1 and α2 domains contributing equally to each side of the structure (Fig. 64-4). The HLA variable regions which are recognized by alloantibodies or cytotoxic T cells lie along the α helices that form the margins of the groove. When the bound materials released by acidification of redissolved HLA class I crystals were analyzed by HPLC, hundreds of different peptides were found. Of those analyzed further, a 9 amino acid length and a binding consensus motif at positions 2 and 9 were characteristic. Although class II molecules have yet to be studied to the same resolution, preliminary results suggest a similar groove formed by the α1 and β1 domains, and the known sequence polymorphisms also lie along the presumed location of the groove. It is likely that virtually all MHC molecules come to the surface of the cell with a peptide in place. In the case of class I, the pathway is primarily one of selection of peptides endogenous to the cell (e.g., from intracellular viral infection), and for class II, the pathway is primarily an exogenous one which processes endocytosed or pinocytosed polypeptides. The latter function is classically performed by macrophages, but any cell which expresses class II MHC (e.g., B lymphocytes, epithelial cells) can serve as an antigen-presenting cell (APC). The phenomenon of MHC restriction, which requires the T cell to recognize both self-MHC and antigen, can now be viewed as the function of a single T cell receptor that binds to the surface formed by both α-helical sides of the HLA groove and peptide lying within it. Some of the MHC polymorphisms, those on the inner surfaces of the helices and on the floor of the groove, are not accessible in the presence of bound peptide; hence the polymorphisms serve to bind the peptide fragments having a certain sequence motif.

Molecular genetics Each polypeptide chain of class I and class II molecules bears several polymorphic sites in addition to the "private" antigen defined by alloantisera. In the *cell-mediated lympholysis* (CML) test, the specificity of killer T cells (T_c), which arise during the proliferative events in MLR, is determined by testing on target cells from donors other than those providing the MLR stimulus. Antigen systems defined by this method show a close but imperfect correlation with class I private antigens. Cloning of cytotoxic cells has revealed the presence of a variety of polymorphic target determinants on HLA molecules, some of which are identifiable by alloantisera or monoclonal antibodies derived from immunization of mice with human cells. Some of these reagents can be used to identify private determinants of HLA, while others are directed to more "public" (sometimes called *supertypic*) determinants. One such system of public HLA-B antigens has two alleles, Bw4 and Bw6. Most HLA-B private antigens are associated with either Bw4 or Bw6. Other systems are restricted to subsets of HLA antigen groups. For example, HLA-B–bearing heavy chains carry additional sites that are common to B7, B27, B22, and B40 or to B5, B15, B18, and B35. Other types of shared antigenic determinants exist, as exemplified by a monoclonal antibody which reacts with a site shared between HLA-A and HLA-B heavy chains.

The amino acid sequence and peptide maps of several HLA molecules show that the class I hypervariable regions are clustered in the peptide-binding region of the outer α_1 domain (see Fig. 64-2) and the adjacent portion of α_2. Variability in the sequences of class II molecules also differs in a similar manner. Remarkably, the class I α_3 domain, the class II α_2 and β_2 domains, and the portions of the CD8 (T8, Leu 2) cell surface molecule that function in T cell

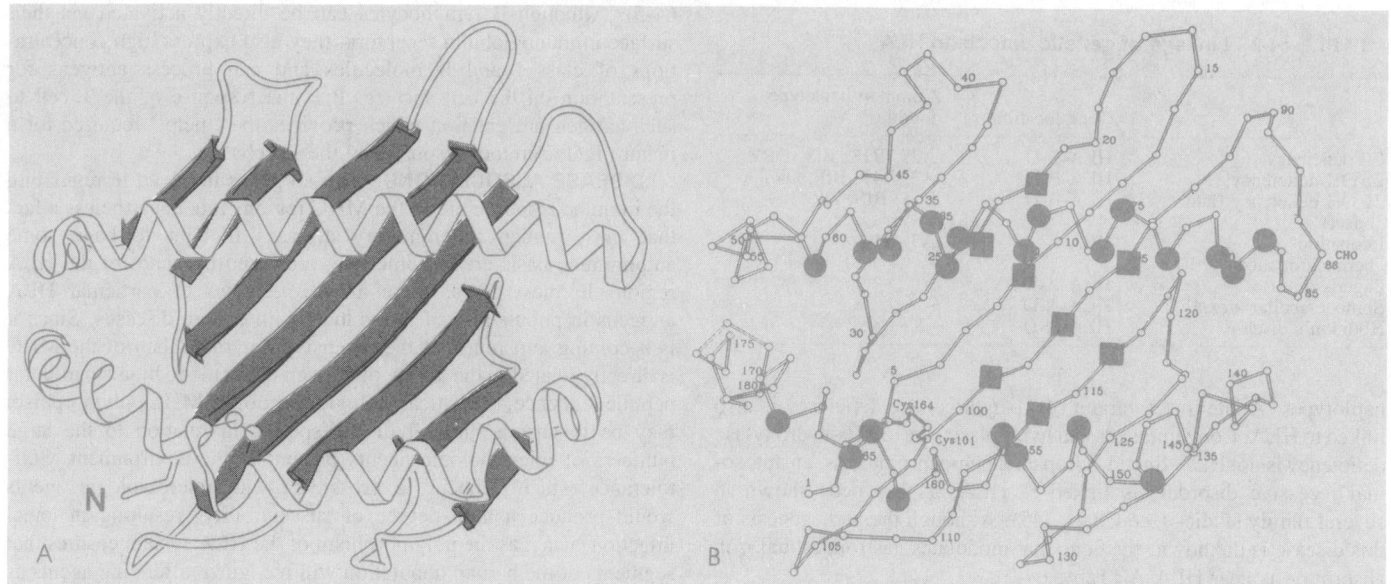

FIGURE 64-4 Structure of the HLA class I molecule as determined by x-ray crystallography. *A*. Shown is the face of the HLA-A2 molecule that points away from the cell surface. This ribbon diagram shows the groove that is formed by two α helices and is supported by a floor of eight β strands. N is the amino terminal of the α₁ domain; the two small circles represent a disulfide bond. (*From PA Bjorkman et al.*) *B*. Composite display of polymorphic sites from several human and mouse class I alleles using the HLA-A2 structure as the model. The symbols show a composite of the polymorphisms along the groove. Localization of variable amino acids and/or sites for alloantibody and/or cytotoxic T cell recognition is shown to be along the α helices (*circles*). Polymorphic sites exist also in the β strands (*squares*). The numbers indicate the amino acid sequence. (*After PA Bjorkman et al.*)

interactions, as well as the T cell receptor (TCR) itself, are all considered members of the immunoglobulin supergene family because of significant amino acid sequence homologies with immunoglobulin constant regions (see Chap. 277). These findings suggest evolutionary elaboration within a family of gene products that have immune recognition functions. When genomic DNA for HLA is examined, typical exon-intron sequences of DNA have been found for class I and class II, exons having been identified for signal peptides (5′), each of the domains, a transmembrane hydrophobic segment, and a cytoplasmic segment (3′). cDNA probes are available for most of the HLA chains, and enzymatic digests have been used to study patterns of *restriction fragment length polymorphisms* (RFLP), many of which correlate with class II serologic and MLR patterns. There are 20 to 30 class I genes, however, making assessment of polymorphism by RFLP difficult. Many of these genes are not expressed (pseudogenes), while some could represent additional class I loci that are expressed only on activated T cells and are of uncertain function. Tissue typing by the detection of variable nucleotide sequences begins with the polymerase chain reaction (PCR) technique to amplify specific segments of DNA, as defined by oligonucleotide primers, from genomic DNA obtained from a small sample of blood or tissue. The primers are usually locus-specific (e.g., the β1 chain of HLA-DR) or may be allele-specific (e.g., amplifying only genes having a particular polymorphic sequence. The products are then analyzed by hybridization with sequence-specific labeled probes or by RFLP analysis of the amplified DNA. The technique has already demonstrated ability to identify sequences in the human population in a more accurate fashion than with the established serologic technique. The official HLA nomenclature has been changed to reflect the definition of distinct sequences and to document the presence of polymorphisms not clearly understood from the definitions of classical serology (e.g., an HLA-DQ molecule is made up of both α and β chains, each of which is polymorphic). To illustrate, HLA-DR1 is written as DRB1*0101. DRB1 indicates the β chain of the DR locus, and *0101 indicates that it is antigen 1, first variant. In similar fashion, DQA1*0302 indicates the α chain of the DQ locus, antigen 3, variant 2. Many recent observations of disease associations wih HLA antigens use this more precise nomenclature in order to define the molecular

basis for peptide binding, as well as to provide better genetic markers for ethnic and population diversity.

Complement (class III) Structural genes for three complement components, C4, C2, and Bf (factor B), are present in the HLA-BD region (see Fig. 64-1). There are two loci for C4, coding for C4A and C4B, formerly recognized as the Rodgers and Chido red blood cell antigens, respectively. These antigens are, in fact, adsorbed plasma C4 molecules. Other complement components are not closely linked to HLA. No crossovers have been found between the C2, Bf, and C4 loci. They are all encoded within a 100-kilobase segment between HLA-B and HLA-DR. There are two alleles of C2, four of Bf, seven of C4A, and three of C4B, plus blanks (null genes) for each locus (QO). The extensive polymorphism of complement types (complotypes) makes them useful for genetic studies. The four most common extended haplotypes found in people of western European ancestry are shown in Table 64-1. MLRs between unrelated individuals who are matched for these extended haplotypes are nonreactive, whereas reactivity is common if unrelated individuals are matched for only HLA-DR and -DQ. Such identical extended haplotypes may be conserved from a common ancestor.

Other sixth-chromosome genes Deficiency of steroid 21-hydroxylase, an autosomal recessive trait, results in the syndrome of congenital adrenal hyperplasia (see Chaps. 335 and 342). The genes for the enzyme are also localized in the HLA-B-D region. The 21-hydroxylase gene adjacent to C4A is deleted in affected individuals along with C4A (C4AQO), and the HLA-B locus gene may have been altered to convert B13 to the rare B47 found only in affected

TABLE 64-1 Comnmon extended HLA haplotypes

HLA-B	HLA-DR	Bf	C2	C4A	C4B
8	3	S	C	QO	1
7	2	S	C	3	1
57	7	S	C	6	1
44	7	F	C	3	1

TABLE 64-2 Linkage of genetic defects to HLA

	Gene location	Common haplotype found
C2 deficiency	HLA-B-D	A25, B18, BfS, DR2
21-OH deficiency	HLA-B-D	A3, B47, BfF, DR7
21-OH deficiency (late onset)	HLA-B-D	B14, BfS, DR1
Idiopathic hemochromatosis	HLA-A	A3, B14
Paget's disease	HLA-A-D	
Spinocerebellar ataxia	HLA-A-D	
Hodgkin's disease	HLA-A-D	

haplotypes. A late-onset variant of 21-hydroxylase deficiency is also linked to HLA. Congenital adrenal hyperplasia due to 11β-hydroxylase deficiency is not HLA-linked. Idiopathic hemochromatosis, an autosomal recessive disorder, is linked to HLA, as has been shown in several family studies (see Chap. 345). Although the pathogenesis of this disease is unknown, the gene that modulates gastrointestinal iron absorption is near HLA-A (Table 64-2).

Immune-response genes As originally defined in the guinea pig and the mouse, high and low immune responsiveness to haptens or synthetic peptide motifs was shown to be determined by genes in the region of the MHC. It is now clear that these genes encode the class II molecules and that the ability to bind the relevant antigen is the major determinant of a strong T cell–dependent response initiated by CD4 + T cells. Class I genes are also important in the effector phases of a response, especially with regard to recognition by CD8 + T cells of foreign peptide bound to class I molecules. For example, human cell lines infected with the influenza virus are lysed by immune cytotoxic T cells (T_c) only if a class I (HLA-A or HLA-B) antigen is shared between the attacking and target cells. Class I and II molecules are said to be the *restriction elements* in immune responsiveness because they must be able to bind and present peptide fragments properly to T cells. In the allogeneic response, there is evidence that recognition may be of either the amino acid differences on the external face of the intact MHC molecule or of an MHC peptide fragment presented by a responder strain MHC molecule. In this special case, instead of restricting the response, the MHC antigenic differences become the stimulus. In transplantation, the induction and effector phases of a rejection response follow the general rules of CD4 + T_H and CD8 + T_c interacting with MHC class II and I, respectively (Fig.

64-5). Although B lymphocytes can be directly activated via their surface immunoglobulin receptors, they also express high concentrations of class I and II molecules and can process antigens for presentation on the cell surface. It is the response of the T cell to such antigen presentation which provides the "help" required for a mature IgG secretory response by the B cells.

DISEASE ASSOCIATIONS Not all genes involved in regulating the immune response are in the MHC region. It is nevertheless a fact that most human inflammatory diseases thought to have some autoimmune basis are in some way promoted by genes of the HLA region. In most cases, these are *associations* of particular HLA antigens in populations of individuals with certain diseases. Since it is becoming apparent that the extensive polymorphism of the MHC is directly related to the ability of a given molecule to bind a particular peptide sequence, the critical biologic function of MHC polymorphism may be to ensure survival of the species in relation to the large numbers of microbiologic agents present in the environment. Self-tolerance which happens to crossreact with microbiologic agents would produce a high degree of susceptibility, resulting in lethal infection, whereas the polymorphism of the HLA system ensures that segments of the human population will recognize offending agents as foreign and initiate the appropriate response. The importance of the MHC for species survival could be of the highest order, since there is need for local mechanisms, not entirely understood, to prevent allorecognition in the special case of pregnancy. The extent to which the MHC plays a role in immune surveillance against neoplasia and whether such a role contributes to survival in an evolutionary sense are not established.

Table 64-3 summarizes the most significant HLA and disease associations. It should be noted that such associations do not in themselves prove that variations in antigen presentation to T cells is necessarily at the root of autoimmunity. It also can be that HLA genes are markers for haplotypes in which mutations have occurred in other linked genes.

Most striking is the increased frequency of HLA-B27 in certain rheumatic diseases, particularly ankylosing spondylitis, a condition with a strong familial tendency. B27 is present in about 7 percent of people of western European ancestry, while it appears in 80 to 90 percent of patients with ankylosing spondylitis. Expressed as a relative risk, the antigen B27 confers a susceptibility to the development of ankylosing spondylitis that is 87 times that in the general population. Similarly, acute anterior uveitis, Reiter's syndrome, and reactive arthritis to at least three bacterial infections (*Yersinia, Salmonella,*

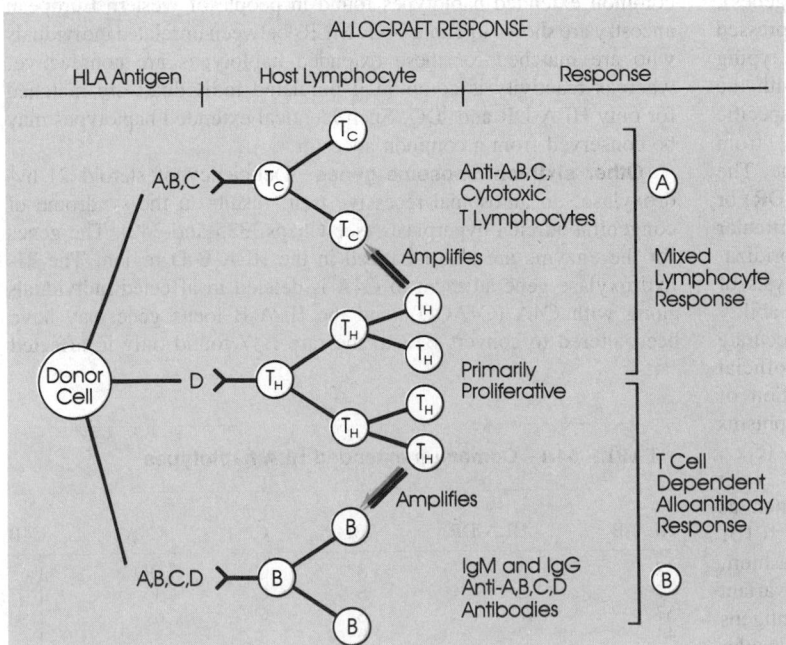

FIGURE 64-5 Schema of the relative roles of HLA-A, HLA-B, HLA-C, and HLA-D antigens in initiation of the alloimmune response and in the development of effector cells and antibodies. Two main classes of T lymphocytes recognize antigens: T_c, the precursors to the cytotoxic "killer" cells, and T_H, the helper cells for amplification of the cytotoxic response. T_H also provide help to B lymphocytes for production of a fully mature IgG response. Note that T_c generally recognize class I antigens, while the T_H signal is provided by antigens of the HLA-D region (class II). (*From CB Carpenter, Kidney Int, 14:283, 1978.*)

TABLE 64-3   HLA antigens and disease, showing the most highly associated antigens

Disease	Antigen	Relative risk*	Disease	Antigen	Relative risk*
RHEUMATIC			**ENDOCRINE**		
Ankylosing spondylitis	B27	69.1	Type 1 diabetes mellitus	DR4	3.6
Reiter's syndrome	B27	37.0		DR3	4.8
Acute anterior uveitis	B27	8.2		DR2	0.2
Reactive arthritis (*Yersinia, Salmonella,* gonococcus)	B27	18.0		BfF1	15.0
Psoriatic arthritis, central	B27	10.7	Hyperthyroidism (Graves')	B8	2.5
	B38	9.1		DR3	3.7
Psoriatic arthritis, peripheral	B27	2.0	Hyperthyroidism (Japanese)	B35	4.4
	B38	6.5		A2	2.2
Juvenile rheumatoid arthritis	B27	3.9		DP5	4.4
	DR8	3.6		A2 + DP5	10.5
Juvenile arthritis, pauciarticular	DR5	3.3	Adrenal insufficiency	Dw3	10.5
Rheumatoid arthritis	Dw4/DR4	3.8	Subacute thyroiditis (de Quervain)	B35	13.7
Sjögren's syndrome	Dw3	5.7	Hashimoto's thyroiditis	DR5	3.2
Systemic lupus erythematosus			Congenital adrenal hyperplasia	B47	15.4
Causasian	DR3	2.6			
Japanese	DR2	5.3	**NEUROLOGIC**		
Chinese	DQ3	11.5	Myasthenia gravis	B8	2.7
Systemic lupus erythematosus (hydralazine)	DR4	5.6		DR3	2.5
			Multiple sclerosis	DR2	6.0
GASTROINTESTINAL			Manic-depressive disorder	B16	2.3
Gluten-sensitive enteropathy	DR3	11.6	Narcolepsy	DR2	130.0
Chronic active hepatitis	DR3	6.8	Schizophrenia	A28	2.3
Ulcerative colitis	B5	3.8			
			RENAL		
HEMATOLOGIC			Idiopathic membranous glomerulonephritis	DR3	5.7
Idiopathic hemochromatosis	A3	6.7	Goodpasture's syndrome (anti-GBM)	DR2	15.9
	B14	26.7	Minimal change disease (steroid response)	B12	4.2
	A3, B14	90.0	Polycystic kidney disease	B5	2.6
Pernicious anemia	DR5	5.4	IgA nephropathy (Caucasians)	DR2	0.6
Hodgkin's disease			Gold nephropathy	DR3	14.0
Caucasian	DP3	2.0		DR4	0.3
Japanese	DP4	0.2			
			INFECTIOUS		
SKIN			Tuberculoid leprosy (Asians)	B8	6.8
Dermatitis herpetiformis	Dw3	17.3	Paralytic polio	B16	4.3
Psoriasis vulgaris	Cw6	7.5	Low vs. high response to vaccinia virus	Cw3	12.7
Psoriasis vulgaris (Japanese)	Cw6	8.5			
Pemphigus vulgaris (Jews)	DR4	14.6	**IMMUNODEFICIENCY**		
	A10	4.8	IgA deficiency (blood donors)	DR3	13.0
Behçet's disease					
Caucasian	B5	3.8			
Japanese	B51	12.4			
Chinese	B51	5.5			

* Relative risk = $\dfrac{(\% \text{ antigen-positive patients})(\% \text{ antigen-negative controls})}{(\% \text{ antigen-negative patients})(\% \text{ antigen-positive controls})}$

and gonococcus) show a high degree of association with B27. Although the ordinary form of juvenile rheumatoid arthritis (JRA) also shows a similar association with B27, the pauciarticular form of JRA with iritis is DR5-associated. The increased incidence of B27 in psoriatic arthritis is also significant for the central type (axial skeleton) of the disorder, while B38 is associated with both the central and peripheral types. Psoriasis is associated with Cw6. Patients with degenerative arthritis or gout show no alteration in antigen frequencies.

Most other disease associations are with HLA-D region antigens. The rheumatoid arthritis associations with DR4 involve 3 of the 12 DR4 variants (DRB1*0401, *0404, and *0405), as well as DRB1*0101 and DRB1*1402 in some ethnic groups. Narcolepsy is virtually 100 percent associated with DR2 in both Japanese and Caucasians. Affected individuals need inherit only a single gene dose of DR2. Although there is no apparent autoimmune component to this condition, there is speculation that an abnormality in a neurotransmitter or its receptor may be influenced by the DR2 gene or another closely linked gene. Gluten-sensitive enteropathy (celiac disease, nontropical sprue) in children and adults is associated with DR3 (relative risk = 12). Recent DNA typing shows a higher relative risk of 52 with DQA1*0501 and DQB1*0201. The actual percentage of such patients having DR3 ranges from 63 to 96 percent compared with 22 to 27 percent of controls. The same antigen is also present

in increased frequency in patients with chronic active hepatitis and in patients with dermatitis herpetiformis who also have gluten-sensitive enteropathy. Juvenile-onset insulin-dependent diabetes mellitus (type I) is associated with DR4 and DR3 and is negatively associated with DR2. Resistance to type I diabetes is strongly associated with the inheritance of aspartate at position 57 of the β chain of HLA-DQ, in linkage disequilibrium with HLA-DR2. Other amino acids at position 57, especially when HLA-DR3 or -DR4 are on the same haplotype, are associated with an increased risk of disease. Recent studies show that having nonaspartate at position 57 of DQB1 of both haplotypes confers a relative risk for type 1 diabetes of 7.4, whereas a single or double dose of aspartate at position 57, as with DQB1*0601 or *0602, provides protection (relative risk of 0.2). Maturity-onset diabetes is not HLA-associated. A rare allele of Bf (F1) is also found in 17 to 25 percent of patients with type I diabetes. Hyperthyroidism in Caucasians is associated with B8,DR3, while in Japanese populations the association is with B35, A2, and DP5. This is an example of a disease in which racial differences display different HLA associations in contrast with rheumatoid arthritis and type I diabetes, in which the DR4 associations are more universal. Sometimes an HLA marker is clearly associated only with a subgroup within a syndrome. For example, myasthenia gravis without thymoma is more strongly B8,DR3-associated, and the association of DR2 with multiple sclerosis is stronger in patients with rapidly progressive deterioration. The common DR2 and DQ haplotype found in normal individuals (DRB1*1501, DQA1*0102, DQB1*0602) is also most commonly increased in multiple sclerosis. Renal diseases strongly HLA-DR–associated are Goodpasture's syndrome due to an autoantibody to glomerular basement membrane (DR2), idiopathic membranous glomerulonephritis (DR3 in Caucasians, DR2 in Japanese) which may be an autoimmune process involving antibodies to an antigen of the glomerulus, and gold-induced nephritis (DR3). Studies of HLA associations with AIDS suggest that HLA-B35 is a risk factor for more rapid progression of the disease (see Chap. 279).

LINKAGE DISEQUILIBRIUM Although the distribution of HLA alleles varies in racial and ethnic populations, the most salient feature of population genetics of HLA antigens is the presence of linkage disequilibria among certain antigens of the A and B, B and C, and B, D, and complement loci. *Linkage disequilibrium* means that antigens of closely linked loci appear together more frequently than predicted by random association. The classic example is the linkage disequilibrium present between the A-locus antigen HLA-A1 and the B-locus antigen HLA-B8 in people of western European ancestry. The coincidence of A1 and B8 should be the product of their individual gene frequencies ($0.17 \times 0.11 \cong 0.02$). The observed frequency of A1 and B8 is 0.08, four times that expected, an increase of 0.06. The latter value is termed Δ (delta) and is a measure of the disequilibrium. Other A- and B-locus haplotype disequilibria have been recognized and include (A3, B7), (A2, B12), (A29, B12), and (A11, B35). Furthermore, some D-region determinants are in linkage disequilibrium with B-locus antigens (e.g., DR3 and B8), as are some B- and C-locus antigens. Serologically defined HLA antigens can serve as markers for the genes of an entire haplotype within a family and as markers for specific genes within a population, but only where a linkage disequilibrium exists.

Linkage disequilibrium is of importance because such gene associations may have some bearing on their function. For example, selective pressures during the course of evolution may have been the major factor in the survival of certain gene combinations in a haplotype. Such a theory suggests, for example, that A1 and B8, along with certain D-region and other determinants, conferred a selective advantage in the face of epidemics such as the plague or smallpox. It also would follow that the descendants of the survivors may display susceptibility to certain diseases because their unique gene complex happens to confer an abnormal response to other environmental agents. The major difficulty with this hypothesis is the assumption that selection must work on several genes simultaneously to account for the observed Δ's; however, the need for complex interactions among the products of the several loci of the major histocompatibility complex is only beginning to be appreciated, and selection might force multiple linkage disequilibria. The conservation of certain extended haplotypes, mentioned above, supports this view.

On the other hand, the selection hypothesis is not necessary to explain linkage disequilibrium. When a population lacking certain antigens is crossed with one in which a high frequency of antigens is in equilibrium, a Δ can develop within a few generations. For example, the increasing Δ value for A1,B8 found in populations from east to west, from India to western Europe, can be explained on the basis of migration and fusion. In smaller groups, consanguinity, founder effects, and gene drift may account for disequilibria. Finally, certain linkage disequilibria could occur as a result of nonrandom crossing over during gametic meiosis because of chromosomal segments which are either more or less likely to break. Unless there are selective pressures or restrictions in crossing over, linkage disequilibria disappear over a period of several generations. A large number of nonrandom associations occur throughout the HLA gene complex, and elucidation of the reasons for their existence may provide insight into the mechanism underlying certain disease susceptibilities.

LINKAGE AND ASSOCIATION The diseases listed in Table 64-2 are examples of HLA linkage wherein the inherited conditions are marked within families by the relevant HLA haplotypes. For C2

deficiency, 21-hydroxylase deficiency, and idiopathic hemochromatosis, the mode of inheritance is recessive, with heterozygotes showing partial deficiencies. These genetic defects are also HLA-associated, with an excess of certain HLA alleles in affected unrelated individuals. Also, C2 deficiency is commonly linked to the HLA-A25, B18, BfS, Dw/DR2 haplotype, and idiopathic hemochromatosis exhibits both linkage and strong association with HLA-A3 and -B14. The high degree of linkage disequilibria in these HLA-linked diseases may result from mutations in a single founder, and a sufficient period of time may not have passed to bring the gene pool back into equilibrium. In this view, the HLA antigens are simple markers for the linked gene. Alternatively, expression of the defect may require interaction with specific HLA alleles. This latter hypothesis would require a higher mutation rate, with defective gene expression occurring only when linked with certain HLA genes.

Paget's disease and spinocerebellar ataxia are HLA-linked autosomal dominant traits in families having multiple affected members, and Hodgkin's disease shows an HLA-linked recessive pattern of inheritance. Except for a weak association of HLA-DP3 with Hodgkin's disease, no HLA associations have been discerned for these disorders, suggesting that there were multiple founders with mutations of as yet undefined genes in linkage with different HLA alleles.

HLA linkage is readily recognized when recessive or dominant inheritance patterns are clear-cut, i.e., when expressivity is high and the process is mostly, if not entirely, determined by a single gene defect. In most of the associations, HLA markers represent risk factors involving the operation and modulation of the immune response under the influence of multiple genes. An example of a polygenic immunologic disease is atopic allergy, in which the association to HLA may be evident only in individuals whose genetically controlled (non-HLA) levels of IgE production are low. Another is IgA deficiency (see Table 64-3), which is HLA-DR3–associated.

CLINICAL APPLICATIONS The clinical value of HLA typing for diagnosis of disease is limited to B27 and ankylosing spondylitis, where nevertheless there are 10 percent false-positive and false-negative rates. HLA studies are also of value in genetic counseling and early recognition of disease in families with idiopathic hemochromatosis or congenital adrenal hyperplasia due to steroid 21-hydroxylase deficiency, particularly since HLA typing can be performed on cells obtained by amniocentesis. The high degree of polymorphism of the HLA system also makes it a powerful tool for paternity testing and other medicolegal applications. The implications for diseases such as type I diabetes mellitus and the other diseases showing HLA associations require further study of the components of the HLA system and their role in the pathogenesis of disease. Matching for HLA antigens in allogeneic transplantation is reviewed in Chap. 238.

REFERENCES

BJORKMAN PA et al: Structure of the human class I histocompatibility antigen, HLA-A2. Nature 329:506, 1987

——— et al: The foreign antigen binding site and T cell recognition regions of class I histocompatibility antigens. Nature 329:512, 1987

BODMER JG et al: Nomenclature for factors of the HLA system, 1991. Tissue Antigens, 39:161, 1992

BROWN MG et al: Structural and serological similarity of MHC-linked LMP and proteosome (multicatalytic proteinase) complexes. Nature 353:355, 1991

CARPENTER CB, STROM TB: Immunobiology of renal transplantation, in *Contemporary Issues in Nephrology*, vol 19: *Renal Transplantation*, EL Milford et al (eds). New York, Churchill Livingstone, 1989

DUQUESNOY RJ, TRUCCO M: Genetic basis of cell surface polymorphism encoded by the major histocompatibility complex in humans. CRC Crit Rev Immunol 8:103, 1988

EHRLICH HA, GYLLENSTEN UB: Shared epitopes among HLA class II alleles: Gene conversion, common ancestry and balancing selection. Immunol Today 12:411, 1991

GLYNNE R et al: A proteosome-related gene between the two ABC transporter loci in the class II region of the human MHC. Nature 353:357, 1991

ITESCU S et al: HLA-B35 is associated with accelerated progression to AIDS. J Acquired Immune Deficiency Syndrome 5:37, 1992

NELSON JL, HANSEN JA: Autoimmune disease and HLA. CRC Crit Rev Immunol 10:307, 1990

ROTZSCHE O, FALK K: Naturally occurring peptide antigens derived from the MHC class I–restricted processing pathway. Immunol Today 12:447, 1991

TROWSDALE J et al: Map of the human MHC, Immunol Today 12:443, 1991

65   TREATMENT AND PREVENTION OF GENETIC DISEASE

DAVID VALLE

Normal development and physiologic homeostasis depend on the coordinated interactions of the products of many genes working together in metabolic systems. These systems are adaptable within limits, allowing normal homeostasis to occur over a range of environmental conditions. For instance, the products of some 30 to 40 genes participate in blood glucose regulation; in concert they maintain a relatively constant blood glucose concentration despite intermittent and highly variable ingestion of glucose precursors. On a larger scale, developmental and homeostatic interactions of 10,000 or so gene products are believed to be necessary for normal development and function of the central nervous system. Mutations that reduce the adaptive capacity of these systems result in abnormalities that we recognize as genetic disease. The mutant gene may so compromise a particular developmental or homeostatic system that the system functions poorly or not at all under all circumstances, thereby producing a monogenic disorder. Alternatively, the mutant gene may have modest effects under ordinary conditions but in certain environments cause maldevelopment or dyshomeostasis that we recognize as a multifactorial disorder. Thus the role of the genes in health and disease is both central and complex. Consequently, treatment of genetic disease is both difficult and frequently less than completely effective.

TREATMENT

Effective treatment of genetic disorders requires accurate diagnosis, early intervention prior to development of irreversible tissue damage, and an understanding of the abnormal biochemistry or metabolic pathophysiology. Progress in delineating the molecular basis of genetic disease has improved our capability for accurate diagnosis of monogenic disorders. Understanding of the metabolic pathophysiology is increasing at a slower rate mainly because progress in this area often requires elucidation of integrative physiology by study of the intact organism. The development of noninvasive metabolic monitoring techniques such as positron emission tomography and topical magnetic resonance spectrometry, as well as new genetic technologies for the production of animal models of human genetic disease, offers promise for progress in this area.

Approaches to treatment of genetic disease can be organized proceeding from the clinical phenotype through the abnormal metabolites and dysfunctional protein to the level of the defective gene (Table 65-1).

TREATMENT OF THE CLINICAL PHENOTYPE Treatment of the clinical phenotype includes conventional medical practices such as patient education, pharmacologic interventions, and surgical procedures. It depends on a thorough understanding of the natural history of the particular disorder so that potential complications can be avoided or addressed early in the course to minimize the consequences. Although therapy at this level is not aimed at correcting the primary defect, it can markedly improve the quality of life. Examples include instruction to patients with albinism or xeroderma to limit sun exposure or to patients with glucose-6-phosphate dehydrogenase deficiency to avoid the offending drugs; administration of beta blockers to Marfan's syndrome patients to prevent or slow dilatation of the aortic root, anticonvulsants to patients with neurogenic disorders, or antihypertensive agents to patients with secondary hypertension; and a host of surgical interventions for patients with genetic malformations, skeletal dysplasias, and malignancies.

TREATMENT OF THE METABOLIC PHENOTYPE Treatment at the metabolite level involves nutritional or pharmacologic approaches

TABLE 65-1   Some treatments for monogenic disorders

Level of treatment and method	Disorder(s)
CLINICAL PHENOTYPE	
Patient education	
Avoidance of aggravating agents (high carbohydrate diet, exposure to cold)	Periodic paralysis syndromes
Avoidance of certain drugs	Pharmacogenetic disorders, acute intermittent porphyria
Avoidance of sun exposure	Xeroderma pigmentosa, albinism
Avoidance of certain physical activity	Chondrodystrophies
Notify physician for rapid increase in size of mass or tinnitus	Neurofibromatosis
Pharmacologic	
Beta blockers	Marfan's syndrome
Anticonvulsants	Neurodegenerative disorders
Surgical	
Orthopedic reconstruction	Chondrodystrophies
Colectomy	Familial polyposis coli
Plastic reconstruction of facial malformations	Treacher-Collins syndrome, several monogenic cleft lip and/or palate syndromes
METABOLIC PHENOTYPE	
Metabolite alteration	
Substrate restriction	
Phenylalanine	Phenylketonuria
Branch-chain amino acids	Maple syrup urine disease
Galactose	Galactosemia
Fructose	Hereditary fructose intolerance
Lactose	Lactase deficiency
Phytanic acid	Refsum's disease
Alternative pathway utilization	
Benzoate and phenylacetate	Urea cycle disorders
Glycine	Isovaleric acidemia
Carnitine	Organic acidosis
Cysteamine	Cystinosis
Penicillamine	Wilson's disease
Metabolic inhibition	
Allopurinol	Gout
Mevinolin	Familial hypercholesterolemia
Replacement of deficient products	
Glucose polymers (cornstarch)	Glycogen storage disease, types I and III
Uridine	Hereditary orotic aciduria
Glucocorticoids	Congenital adrenal hyperplasia
Thyroxine	Familial goiter
Biotin	Biotinidase deficiency
Protein alteration	
Activation of the mutant protein	
Pyridoxine (vitamin B_6)	Homocystinuria
Thiamine	Maple syrup urine disease
Hydroxycobalamin (vitamin B_{12})	Some forms of methylmalonic acidemia
Replacement of the mutant protein	
Growth hormone	Growth hormone deficiency
Factor VIII	Classic hemophilia
α_1-Antitrypsin	α_1-Antitrypsin deficiency
Polyethylene glycol-adenosine deaminase	Adenosine deaminase deficiency
Mannose-terminated glucocerebrosidase	Gaucher disease
Organ transplantation	
As a source for a specific protein	
Allogeneic bone marrow	Lysosomal storage diseases, β thalassemia
Liver	Glycogen storage disease, type I, familial hypercholesterolemia, ornithine transcarbamylase deficiency
As a protein source and replacement of damaged organ	
Liver	α_1-Antitrypsin deficiency, hepatorenal tyrosinemia
Kidney	Cystinosis

and is dependent on understanding the biochemical pathophysiology (Fig. 65-1). Deficient function of a mutant protein may result in a disease phenotype because a substrate accumulates to toxic levels (precursor toxicity), because the product of an alternative pathway is produced in excessive amounts (alternative pathway overflow), be-

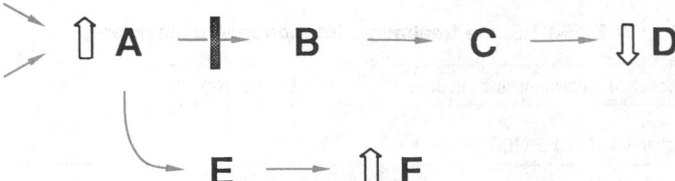

FIGURE 65-1 Pathophysiologic consequences of a genetic defect in a metabolic pathway. Substrate A is converted via a series of intermediates to a final product, D. The enzymes catalyzing these reactions are indicated by the horizontal arrows. A also is converted to F in an alternative pathway. Genetic deficiency of the enzyme converting A to B (indicated by the hatched rectangle) may have pathophysiologic consequences related to accumulation of A (precursor toxicity), overflow to F (alternative pathway overflow), reduced formation of D (product deficiency), or some combination of these possibilities.

cause of reduced formation of the reaction product or some downstream metabolite (product deficiency), or because of some combination of these possibilities. Although this paradigm is most easily visualized for enzymes in a metabolic pathway, it holds for virtually all proteins. The pathophysiology may be *local* within the cell or tissue normally expressing the mutant protein, or it may involve *distant* biochemical effects as a consequence of perturbations of metabolite concentrations in the extracellular fluid. For example, the neurologic phenotype of Tay Sachs disease results from destruction of neurons caused by deficiency of hexosaminidase A, whereas the mental retardation of untreated phenylketonuria due to deficiency of phenylalanine hydroxylase is mediated by the systemic accumulation of phenylalanine.

Precursor toxicity Correction of precursor toxicity frequently involves dietary restriction of a substrate whose major source is nutritional. Inborn errors of amino acid and carbohydrate metabolism are examples of this approach. A diet restricted in the branch-chain amino acids (leucine, isoleucine, valine) is effective in preventing the mental retardation associated with maple syrup urine disease caused by deficiency of branch-chain ketoacid decarboxylase (see Chap. 352). Such diets should be started soon after birth, continued for life, and monitored so that intake of these essential amino acids is just sufficient for normal growth. Illnesses that cause protein catabolism (e.g., those associated with intercurrent infections or trauma) periodically complicate this therapy by releasing large amounts of the offending amino acids from the breakdown of endogenous protein. These episodes may require hospitalization for administration of intravenous fluids or dialysis. Similarly, lifetime restriction of dietary galactose in patients with galactosemia due to deficiency of galactose-1-phosphate uridyl transferase corrects growth failure, prevents cataracts, and improves intellectual outcome (see Chap. 354).

Alternative pathway utilization For some disorders, alternative metabolic pathways may be utilized to remove toxic metabolites. The effectiveness of this approach is limited by the capacity of the alternative pathway and often must be combined with dietary restriction of the offending substrate. Administration of benzoate and phenylacetate to patients with inborn errors of urea metabolism is a good example of this approach. These compounds are conjugated with endogenous glycine and glutamine, forming hippurate and phenylacetylglutamine, respectively. When used in conjunction with restriction of dietary protein, this therapy reduces the accumulation of ammonia in patients with inborn errors of the urea cycle and organic acid metabolism. Similar approaches include the administration of carnitine, which conjugates with a variety of accumulated CoA esters, to patients with defects of organic acid metabolism; cysteamine, which helps to eliminate excess cystine in cystinosis; and penicillamine to reduce excessive stores of copper in Wilson's disease and iron in hemochromatosis.

Inhibition of an overactive pathway For other disorders, particularly those in which alternative pathway overflow produces a toxic

level of a particular metabolite, it may be possible to prevent the accumulation by inhibiting an enzyme in the affected pathway. This approach may lead to accumulation of upstream substrates that must be well tolerated if the treatment is to be successful. For instance, in gout and other disorders in which excessive purine degradation leads to uric acid accumulation, inhibition of xanthine oxidase by allopurinol reduces uric acid production and lowers the incidence of uric acid nephropathy and gouty arthritis. Xanthine, which accumulates as a consequence, has greater aqueous solubility than uric acid and usually is well tolerated. In a similar fashion, hypercholesterolemic patients heterozygous for mutations of the low-density lipoprotein receptor exhibit significant reductions in plasma cholesterol when treated with lovastatin, a drug that acts in part to inhibit hydroxymethylglutaryl coenzyme A reductase that catalyzes an early, rate-limiting step in the synthesis of cholesterol (see Chap. 344).

Product deficit For disorders in which the pathophysiology involves product deficit, nutritional or pharmacologic approaches to replenishing the product can be effective if the administered material reaches the appropriate physiologic compartment. For example, many of the inborn errors in hormone biosynthesis such as the various forms of congenital adrenal hyperplasia and hereditary defects in thyroid hormone biosynthesis respond well to pharmacologic replacement of the deficient hormones. By contrast, the administration of melanin to albinos would not correct the pigment deficit in melanocytes.

TREATMENT DIRECTED TO THE PROTEIN PHENOTYPE Therapy at the level of dysfunctional protein involves either activation or replacement of the mutant protein.

Activation of the mutant protein Activation may be possible if the protein requires a vitamin cofactor and the vitamin is one that is well tolerated in pharmacologic doses. Obviously, not all mutations of a gene encoding a vitamin-dependent protein will respond. Those that do are likely to be missense mutations that either decrease the affinity of an enzyme for its cofactor or destabilize a protein in a way that can be partially overcome by substantial increments in cofactor concentration. About one-third of the cases of homocystinuria due to deficiency of the pyridoxal phosphate–requiring enzyme cystathione-β-synthase exhibit a significant increment in the activity when treated with pharmacologic doses (50 to 500 mg/d) of pyridoxine (vitamin B_6). The actual increase in enzyme activity may be small, but it suffices to improve metabolic flux in the impaired pathway. Since activation of residual activity both reduces precursor accumulation and increases product formation, knowledge of the pathophysiologic mechanism is less critical for this form of treatment.

Protein replacement therapies An alternative approach involves replacement with an exogenous supply of the protein. To be efficacious, the protein must be administered directly into or reach the appropriate physiologic compartment. Thus blood proteins or proteins that traverse the vascular compartment (e.g., peptide hormones) are candidates for this approach. Other considerations include the availability, stability, and immunogenicity of the protein. In some instances, the administered protein may be modified to enhance stability and/or targeting to the appropriate cell or tissue. For example, linkage of adenosine deaminase to polyethylene glycol increases stability, and partial deglycolsylation of glucocerebrosidase exposes mannose residues on the surface of the protein that target it to macrophages via the mannose receptor. Recombinant DNA technology can sometimes be utilized to supply sufficient amounts of the pure protein (e.g., human growth hormone and α_1-antitrypsin). Other proteins (e.g., clotting factor VIII) are available from natural sources but may eventually be produced by recombinant technology. This advance ensures an adequate supply and avoids the risk of transmission of pathologic viruses contaminating the protein purified from natural sources.

ORGAN TRANSPLANTATION Organ transplantation is on the borderline between therapy at the level of the dysfunctional protein and gene therapy. On the one hand, a transplanted organ supplies a deficient protein; on the other, the transplant tissue also brings new genetic information which, in contrast to standard models of gene therapy, is not integrated into the recipient's genome. Kidney, liver, and bone marrow transplantation are utilized for a variety of genetic diseases. The development of more effective and specific immunosuppressants (cyclosporine and FK5061) and the inadequacy of many less invasive therapies account, in part, for the increased utilization of this form of treatment. In some instances, the goal of transplantation is to supply a tissue that can replace a mutant protein (e.g., liver transplant for deficiency of low-density lipoprotein receptor or one of the urea cycle enzymes). For other disorders (e.g., α_1-antitrypsin deficiency or hepatorenal tyrosinemia), the transplant both provides the protein and replaces a damaged organ. The pathophysiologic mechanism of the disease is relevant; the physician must consider if the newly supplied protein will only be used locally or, if not, will gain access to the involved tissue(s). The long-term efficacy and consequences of organ transplantation as treatment for genetic disorders remain to be determined.

PROSPECTS FOR GENE THERAPY Several methods are now available to introduce new genetic material into mammalian cells. These methods allow consideration of a more direct approach to treatment of genetic disease, namely, gene therapy or introduction of a functional gene to replace or supplement the activity of a resident defective gene. Typically, two strategies have been considered, germline and somatic cell gene therapy, which differ in the nature of the recipient cells. In the germline model, foreign DNA is introduced into the zygote or early embryo with the expectation that the newly introduced material will contribute to the germline of the recipient, i.e., be passed on to the next generation. By contrast, in somatic gene therapy models, genetic material is introduced only into somatic cells and is not transmitted to the germ cells. A third approach to gene therapy involves activation of endogenous genes to augment or circumvent a defective gene.

Much of the technology for germline gene therapy has been developed in transgenic mice. Fertilized mouse eggs are harvested from a superovulated female, microinjected with DNA molecules, and reimplanted in a pseudopregnant female. Several murine genetic diseases, including deficiency of growth hormone, myelin basic protein, and β-globin, have been "treated" in this fashion with the general result that the disease phenotype is markedly ameliorated. These experiments have provided considerable information on the regulation of gene expression and the pathogenesis of genetic disease. However, the method is inefficient: Only 15 to 20 percent of injected eggs produce transgenic animals, and of these, only 20 to 30 percent actually express the introduced gene. Furthermore, there are appreciable risks, including damage to a resident gene by the random insertion of the foreign DNA (insertional mutagenesis). For human disorders, availability of the molecular reagents for this approach makes prenatal diagnosis possible. The certainty of having an unaffected child as established by prenatal diagnosis is preferable to the uncertainty and risks of the transgenic approach. Thus germline gene therapy is not applicable to human genetic disease.

Conversely, somatic gene therapy experiments for human genetic disease are beginning (Fig. 65-2). The methods for introducing the genetic material and the recipient cells vary, depending, in part, on the disease to be treated. Currently, modified retroviral vectors that allow high-efficiency introduction of foreign DNA into dividing cells are favored. Other viral vectors that do not require the recipient cell to be dividing (e.g., replication-deficient recombinant adenovirus vectors) may also be useful. Bone marrow stem cells, hepatocytes, endothelial cells, fibroblasts, myoblasts, and epithelial cells are all candidates for recipient cells. Difficulties with long-term, high-level expression of the introduced gene and with reintroduction of the recipient cells into the organism are obstacles to progress in this area. Developments in directing the introduced gene to its normal location in the genome (homologous recombination) offer promise for achieving normal regulation of the introduced gene and elimination of possible detrimental effects of the endogenous mutant gene. The lessons learned from conventional therapies will apply to somatic gene therapy. The importance of early intervention, consideration of

pathophysiologic mechanism(s), and the need for regulated interactions of the product of the introduced gene with other members of the involved homeostatic system are all relevant. Each disorder will have its own therapeutic requirements and problems. These considerations suggest that many genetic disease will remain resistant to treatment despite advances in the ability to perform somatic gene therapy.

Activation of the expression of endogenous genes is another form of therapy that is being attempted for human genetic disease. Interferon γ, a potent transcriptional regulator of several genes, including those involved in X-linked chronic granulomatous disease (X-CGD), improves neutrophil function in that subset of X-CGD patients with mutations that impair a cytochrome involved in superoxide metabolism. Likewise, hydroxyurea increases the expression of the fetal globin genes in some patients with sickle cell disease, providing an alternative, nonsickling hemoglobin. The long-term efficacy and the possible detrimental effects of administering agents that affect the expression of many genes are unknown.

EVALUATION OF THERAPY FOR GENETIC DISEASE

Two general questions should be posed in an evaluation of therapy for a genetic disease. First, does the treatment provide therapeutic benefit? Second, does the treatment restore the patient to normality? These questions can be asked of any disease treatment but have special significance for genetic disorders that are predictable and preventable. Studies by Costa, Scriver, and Childs evaluated the effectiveness of therapy of 351 representative monogenic disorders on three basic variables: life span, reproductive capability, and social adaptation; in their study, available therapies returned life span to normal in 15 percent, allowed reproductive capability in 11 percent, and improved social adaptation in 6 percent of the disorders. Only slightly better outcomes were found with a subset of 65 diseases in which the basic defect is known. Because severe diseases are more quickly recognized, this sample may be skewed toward diseases most difficult to treat. Nevertheless, the results of therapy are worse than

FIGURE 65-2 One model for somatic gene therapy involving retroviral-mediated gene transfer into hepatocytes.

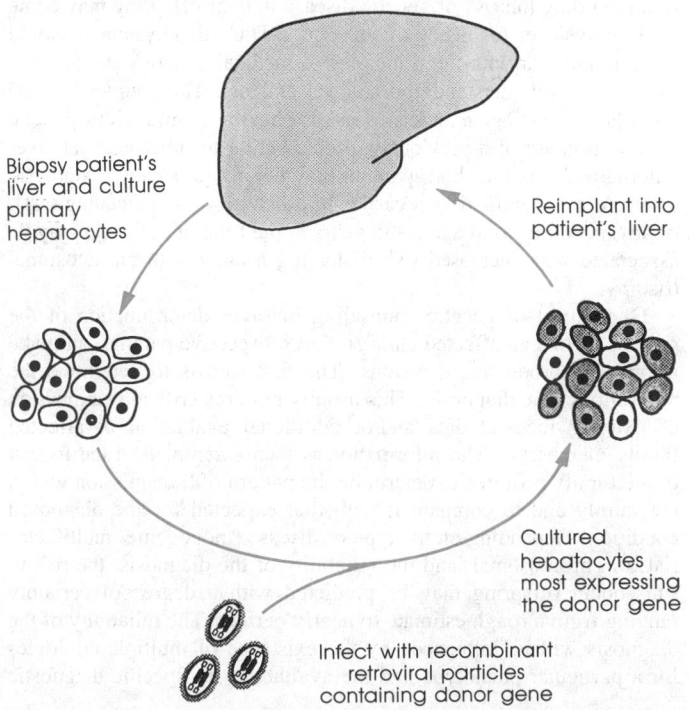

Biopsy patient's liver and culture primary hepatocytes

Reimplant into patient's liver

Cultured hepatocytes most expressing the donor gene

Infect with recombinant retroviral particles containing donor gene

expected, emphasize the difficulty in developing effective therapies for genetic diseases, and highlight the need for continued work in this area. The results also underscore the value of preventive measures as therapy for genetic disease.

PREVENTION OF GENETIC DISEASE

Recognition of the limitation of therapy in genetic disease plus the predictability of the pattern of transmission of genes from one generation to the next has focused attention on prevention as the most reliable and effective means of dealing with hereditary disorders. The preventive approach includes genetic screening, counseling, and prenatal diagnosis.

GENETIC SCREENING   There are two types of genetic screening programs for autosomal recessive disorders: Homozygote screening programs search for individuals who have the disorder; by contrast, heterozygote screening programs search for individuals who are carriers of a mutant gene and thus are at risk of having offspring with a particular disorder. Successful homozygote screening programs require an inexpensive and reliable test, the recognition of some benefit (treatment, counseling) of early diagnosis, and education of the individuals and/or families screened so that they understand the significance of the results. The best example of such programs are the newborn screening programs. The diseases screened vary from state to state but include phenylketonuria, homocystinuria, maple syrup urine disease, galactosemia, cystic fibrosis, hypothyroidism, and sickle cell disease. In each instance, the screening test allows early detection and the opportunity to initiate appropriate therapy prior to the onset of irreversible damage. Also, the parents of an affected individual are made aware of the risk to future offspring and have the option of prenatal diagnosis. Heterozygote screening programs are best exemplified by the program to detect carriers of Tay Sachs disease, a fatal autosomal recessive lysosomal storage disease for which there is no effective treatment. Heterozygote screening of defined subpopulations with an increased carrier frequency (e.g., Ashkenazi Jews, in whom the carrier frequency is approximately 1/25 as compared with approximately 1/300 in Anglo Saxons) identifies couples at risk in which both potential parents are carriers with a 25 percent chance of having an affected child. Prenatal diagnosis is possible, and the procedure provides a means for the couple to have unaffected children.

GENETIC COUNSELING   Prospective parents who seek information regarding the risk of genetic disease in their offspring may come to the physician for genetic counseling. Thus all physicians should become familiar with the principles of medical genetics and use this knowledge to understand and counsel patients. The couples may be identified as having an increased risk for having a child with a genetic disease because of a previously affected child or other near relative. Alternatively, one or both parents may belong to a known high-risk group (e.g., identified as a carrier in a heterozygote screening test), or advanced maternal age (>35 years at the time of delivery) may be associated with increased risk of having a baby with an autosomal trisomy.

One aspect of genetic counseling involves determination of the risk for having an affected child so that prospective parents can make informed reproductive decisions. The first step is to determine the reliability of the diagnosis. This usually requires critical examination of existing medical data and/or additional evaluation of affected family member(s). The information is then assembled in the format of the family pedigree to determine the pattern of transmission within the family and to compare it with that expected for the diagnosed condition. Depending on the type of disease (monogenic, multifactorial, or chromosomal) and the reliability of the diagnosis, the risk to subsequent offspring may be predicted with a degree of certainty ranging from a rough estimate to nearly perfect. The reliability of the diagnosis will be influenced by the existence of multiple etiologies for a particular phenotype and the availability of specific diagnostic tests. Molecular tests that directly and unambiguously determine the parental genotype are sometimes available and allow precise prediction of the risk of recurrence and prenatal diagnosis for some monogenic disorders (see Chap. 62). For autosomal recessive and X-linked disorders in which a primary biochemical defect is known, reliable diagnosis is possible by a functional test of the gene product (e.g., assay of enzyme activity). For most autosomal dominant disorders, the primary biochemical defect is not known, and identification of parental genotype is subject to error resulting from heterogeneity of manifestations. Availability of linked molecular markers, e.g., RFLPs, and identification of the involved genes will greatly improve the reliability and precision of counseling for some of these conditions.

Counseling for many common multifactorial disorders (e.g., diabetes mellitus, hypertension, atherosclerosis, congenital malformations, and psychiatric disorders) is imperfect and will be so until we have a better understanding of the interactions of the various genes and environmental factors that produce these diseases. In some families the etiology may involve a major contribution of a single gene, and in others a mix of multiple genes and environmental factors is the cause. In the former the risk may be predicted by a monogenic model, while in the latter no simple model suffices. In these instances, the physician must resort to empiric risk estimates derived from retrospectively assembled data based on the average outcome in many different families.

In addition to determining risk, other information should be obtained prior to counseling. The prognosis and treatment of the disorder should be reviewed, and the availability of prenatal diagnosis and carrier testing should be determined. Finally, the counselor must be sensitive to the emotional impact this information may have on those counseled.

During the counseling session, effective communication of the information depends on expressing the essentials in language understandable to those being counseled. Written notes and diagrams frequently are helpful and can be given to them at the end of the session. Finally, review at subsequent visits helps correct misconceptions and increase retention of the information. In this regard, the physician who has an established relationship with the family may have an advantage over a trained counselor who meets with the subjects on only one or two occasions.

PRENATAL DIAGNOSIS   Following genetic counseling, the couple at risk for having a child with a genetic disease has several options depending, in part, on the type of disorder. They may be reassured and proceed despite the risk without any subsequent monitoring. Or they may view the risks as too high and choose to have no additional children or to adopt. Alternatively, when both parents are heterozygous for an autosomal recessive disorder, they may choose to reduce the risk by utilizing artificial insemination by donor. The magnitude of the decrease in the risk provided by this option will depend on the carrier frequency for the particular disorder in the general population. For a couple with a 1 in 4, or 25 percent, chance of having a child with phenylketonuria, the risk with donor insemination will drop to 1 in 130 ($\frac{1}{2} \times \frac{1}{65}$), or less than 1 percent, because the carrier frequency in the general population is 1 in 65. When mutant alleles for the gene in question are preferentially associated with particular linked markers (linkage dysequilibrium), it may be possible to reduce the risk further by avoiding donors with the mutant-associated markers.

Finally, if the disorder can be detected antenatally, the couple may decide to proceed with reproduction and utilize prenatal diagnosis with elective abortion of affected fetuses. Because the risk of having an affected fetus ranges from a maximum of 50 percent for heterozygotes with autosomal dominant disorders to less than 10 percent for nearly all chromosomal and multifactorial disorders, the majority of pregnancies monitored by prenatal diagnosis have an unaffected fetus. This relatively low frequency of affected fetuses, together with an increase in reproductive activity which often results from the reassurance provided by the availability of prenatal diagnosis, leads to significant increases in the family size of at-risk couples. Thus, in contrast to some public misconceptions, availability of

TABLE 65-2   Major indications for prenatal diagnosis

Indication	Risk for affected fetus, %	Method of detection
CHROMOSOMAL DISORDERS		
Advanced maternal age (>35 y)	1–10 depending on maternal age	
Parent with a balanced trans-location	3–20 depending on the translo-cation	Chromosomal analysis of cells obtained by CVS* or amniocentesis
Previous child with chromosomal abnormality	~1	
MONOGENIC DISORDERS		
Couple at risk for having a child with an autosomal recessive inborn error of metabolism	25	Biochemical and/or molecular analysis of cells obtained by CVS or amniocentesis
Couple at risk for having a child with a monogenic disorder for which molecular markers are available	25–50	Molecular analysis of DNA obtained from cells obtained by CVS or by amniocentesis
Couple at risk for having a child with a monogenic malformation syndrome without biochemical or molecular markers	25–50	Fetal imaging by ultrasound
MALFORMATION DISORDERS		
Couples at risk for having a child with a neural tube defect (anencephaly or meningomyelocele) or other multifactorial malformation syndrome	1–10	Fetal imaging by ultrasound and, for neural tube defects, measurement of alpha fetoprotein and other fetal markers in amniotic fluid obtained by amniocentesis

* CVS, chorionic villus sampling

prenatal diagnosis actually results in increased numbers of offspring. The indications for prenatal diagnosis are based on a comparison of the risk of the procedures with the risk of having an affected child (Table 65-2).

Several methods for prenatal diagnosis are available (Table 65-3). Choice of a method depends on the disorder in question and on family preferences. Measurement of alpha fetoprotein (AFP) and other fetal proteins in maternal serum is noninvasive and can be used to screen for pregnancies at risk for neural tube defects (increased maternal serum AFP) and for fetal aneuploidies (decreased maternal serum AFP). It is possible by ultrasonography to visualize many fetal malformations and growth abnormalities and to monitor more invasive fetal sampling techniques with attendant reductions in the risks of the procedures. Although second-trimester (15 to 16 weeks of gestation) fetal sampling by amniocentesis is widely used for obtaining fetal cells, the techniques of transcervical and transabdominal chorionic villus sampling (CVS) also provide fetal cells and can be performed at 9 to 12 weeks of gestation. CVS has the advantage of allowing the diagnosis to be made earlier, and if an abortion is chosen, it will take place at a stage of pregnancy when maternal-fetal bonding is less. Finally, elective abortion at 12 weeks of gestation is a 2- to 3-h outpatient procedure, whereas a second-trimester elective abortion requires a 1- to 3-day hospitalization. The risks of CVS in experienced hands appear to compare well with those of amniocentesis. The tissue obtained at CVS is fetal trophoblastic tissue, expresses nearly all enzymes found in amniocytes, and provides an excellent source of fetal DNA.

REFERENCES

ANDERSON WF: Human gene therapy. Science 256:808, 1992

COSTA T, SCRIVER CR, CHILDS B: The effect of mendelian disease on human health: A measurement. Am J Med Genet 21:231, 1985

HARRISON MR et al: *The Unborn Patient: Prenatal Diagnosis and Treatment*, 2d ed. Philadelphia, Saunders, 1991

SCRIVER CR et al (eds): *The Molecular and Metabolic Basis of Inherited Disease*, 7th ed. New York, McGraw Hill, in press

TABLE 65-3   Methods of prenatal diagnosis

Method	Stage of gestation, weeks	Sample	Fetal disorders	Risks
Maternal serum sampling	15–18	Alpha fetoprotein and other fetal proteins	Neural tube defects, aneuploidies	Negligible
Fetal ultrasonography	6–40	Image	Fetal dating, morphologic abnormalities, skeletal dysplasis	Negligible
Fetal sampling				
Chorionic villus sampling	9–12	Fetal trophoblastic tissue	Cytogenetic, biochemical, molecular	1–2% fetal loss
Amniocentesis	15–18	Amniotic fluid and cells	Cytogenetic, biochemical, molecular, neural tube defects	0.2–0.5% fetal loss
Fetal biopsy	18–20	Fetal skin	Dermatologic	~2% fetal loss
		Fetal liver	Liver-specific, enzyme deficiencies	2–5% fetal loss
		Umbilical cord, blood	Blood disorders	~2% fetal loss

PART FOUR

66 PRINCIPLES OF DRUG THERAPY

JOHN A. OATES / GRANT R. WILKINSON

QUANTITATIVE DETERMINANTS OF DRUG ACTION

Safe and effective therapy with drugs requires their delivery to target tissues in concentrations within the narrow range that yields efficacy without toxicity. Optimal precision in achieving concentrations of drug within this therapeutic "window" can be achieved with regimens that are based on the kinetics of the drug's availability to target sites. This chapter deals with the principles of drug elimination and distribution that form the basis for loading and maintenance regimens for the average patient and considers instances in which elimination of the drug is impaired (e.g., renal failure). The basis for optimal utilization of plasma level data is also discussed.

PLASMA LEVELS AFTER A SINGLE DOSE The levels of lidocaine in plasma following intravenous administration decline in two phases, as illustrated in Fig. 66-1; such a biphasic decline is typical for many drugs. Immediately following rapid injection, essentially all of the drug is in the plasma compartment, and the high initial plasma level reflects its confinement to this small volume. Subsequently, the drug is transferred into the extravascular compartment, and the period of time during which this occurs is referred to as the *distribution phase*. For lidocaine the distribution phase is virtually complete within 30 min; then a slower rate of fall ensues, referred to as the *equilibrium phase* or *elimination phase*. During this latter phase, the drug levels in plasma and those in the tissues change in parallel.

Distribution phase Pharmacologic events during the distribution phase depend on whether the level of drug at the receptor site is similar to that in the plasma. If this is the case, the pharmacologic effects, whether favorable or adverse, may be inordinately great during this period because of the high initial levels in plasma. For example, following a small bolus dose (50 mg) of lidocaine, antiarrhythmic effects may be evident during the early distribution phase but disappear as levels fall below those which are minimally effective and even before equilibrium between plasma and tissue is reached. Thus larger single doses or multiple small doses must be administered to achieve an effect that is sustained into the equilibrium phase. Toxicity resulting from high levels of some drugs during the distribution phase precludes administration of a single intravenous loading dose that will achieve therapeutic levels during the equilibrium phase. For example, the administration of a loading dose of phenytoin as a single intravenous bolus can cause cardiovascular collapse due to the high levels during the distribution phase. If a loading dose of phenytoin is administered intravenously, it must be given in fractions at intervals sufficient to permit substantial distribution of the prior dose before the next is given (e.g., 100 mg every 3 to 5 min). For similar reasons, the loading dose of many potent drugs that rapidly equilibrate with their receptors is divided into fractional doses for intravenous administration.

After an oral dose that delivers an equivalent amount of drug into the systemic circulation, plasma levels during the initial period after administration are not as high as after an intravenous bolus dose.

Because the drug is not absorbed instantly after oral administration and is delivered into the systemic circulation more slowly, much of the drug is distributed by the time absorption is complete. Thus procainamide, which is almost totally absorbed after oral administration, can be given as a single 750-mg loading dose with little risk of hypotension; in contrast, loading of the drug by the intravenous route is more safely accomplished by giving the dose in fractions of about 100 mg at 5-min intervals to avoid the hypotension that might ensue during the distribution phase if the entire loading dose were given as a single bolus.

In contrast, other drugs are distributed slowly to their sites of action during the distribution phase. For example, levels of digoxin at the receptor site (and its pharmacologic effect) do not reflect plasma levels during the distribution phase. Digoxin is transported (or bound) to its cardiac receptors more slowly by a process that proceeds throughout distribution. Thus plasma levels fall during a distribution phase of several hours, while levels at the site of action and pharmacologic effect increase. Only at the end of the distribution phase, when the drug has reached equilibrium with the receptor, does the concentration of digoxin in plasma reflect pharmacologic effect. For this reason, there should be a 6- to 8-h wait after administration before plasma levels of digoxin are obtained for a guide to therapy.

Equilibrium phase After distribution has proceeded to the point where the concentration of drug in plasma is in dynamic equilibrium with that in the tissues outside the vascular compartment, the levels in plasma and tissues fall in parallel as the drug is eliminated from the body. Thus the *equilibrium phase* is sometimes also referred to as the *elimination phase*. Measurement of drug concentration in plasma provides the best reflection of drug level in tissues during this phase.

Most drugs are eliminated as a first-order process. During the equilibrium phase, a characteristic of the first-order process is that the time required for the level of drug in plasma to fall to one-half the original value (the half-life, $t_{1/2}$) is the same regardless of which

FIGURE 66-1 Concentrations of lidocaine in plasma following the administration of 50 mg intravenously. The half-life of 108 min is computed as the time required for levels to fall from any given value during the equilibrium phase ($Cp_{initial}$) to one-half that level. Cp_0 is the hypothetical concentration of lidocaine in plasma at time zero if equilibrium had been achieved instantly.

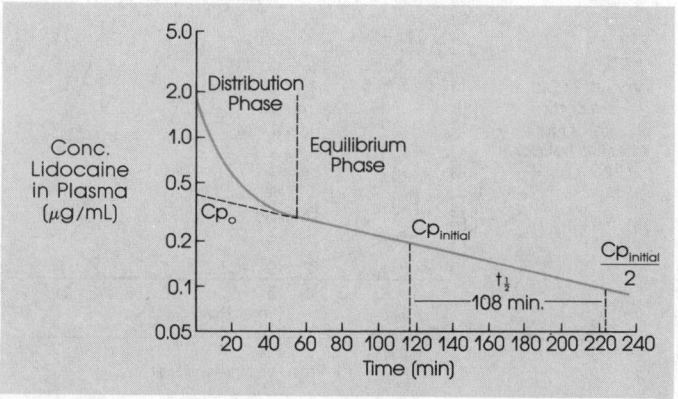

point on the plasma level curve is chosen as a starting point for the measurement. Another characteristic of the first-order process is that a semilogarithmic plot of the concentrations in plasma versus time during the equilibrium phase is linear. From such a plot (Fig. 66-1) it can be seen that the half-life of lidocaine is 108 min.

One can calculate what amount of the administered dose remains in the body at any multiple of the half-life interval following administration:

Number of half-lives	Amount of dose remaining in the body, %	Amount of dose eliminated, %
1	50	50
2	25	75
3	12.5	87.5
4	6.25	93.75
5	3.125	96.875

In principle, the elimination process never reaches completion. From a clinical standpoint, however, elimination is essentially complete when it has reached 90 percent. Therefore, for practical purposes, *a first-order elimination process reaches completion after 3 to 4 half-lives.*

DRUG ACCUMULATION—LOADING AND MAINTENANCE DOSES With repeated administration of a drug, the amount in the body accumulates if the elimination of the first dose is incomplete when the second dose is given, and both the amount of drug in the body and its pharmacologic effect increase with continuing administration until they reach a plateau. The accumulation of digoxin administered in repeated maintenance doses (without a loading dose) is illustrated in Fig. 66-2. Since digoxin's half-life is about 1.6 days in a patient with normal renal function, 65 percent of digoxin remains in the body at the end of 1 day. Thus the second dose will raise the amount of digoxin in the body (and average plasma level) to 165 percent of that following the first dose. Each subsequent dose will result in greater amounts in the body until a *steady state* is achieved. At this point, drug intake per unit of time is the same as the rate of elimination, with the fluctuation between peak and trough plasma levels remaining constant. If the rate of drug delivery is subsequently altered, a different and new steady state will be attained. Continuing infusion of a drug at constant rate also will result in progressive accumulation to a predictable steady state (Fig. 66-3). In this case, a constant plasma level (Cp_{ss}) is achieved which is between the peak and trough values attained when the same rate of drug delivery is administered in an intermittent fashion. For *all* drugs with first-order kinetics, the time required to achieve steady state levels can be predicted from the half-life because accumulation also is a first-order process with a half-life identical to that for elimination. Hence

FIGURE 66-2 The time course of digoxin accumulation when a single daily maintenance dose is given without a loading dose. Note that accumulation is more than 90 percent complete by the end of 4 half-lives.

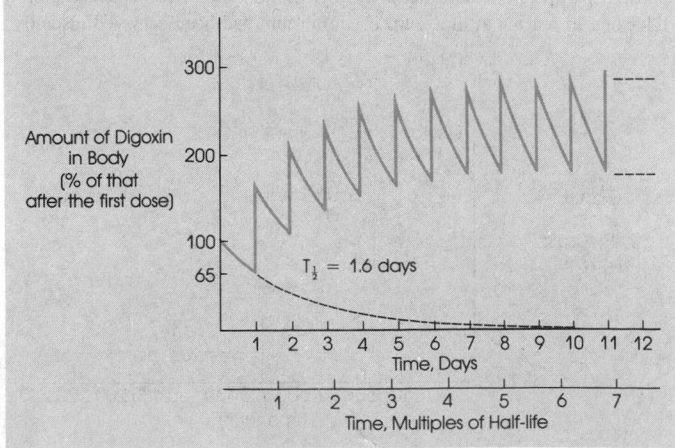

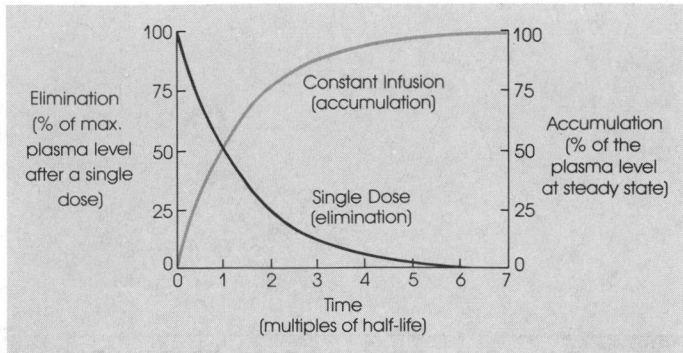

FIGURE 66-3 The time course of plasma levels of a drug following a single intravenous dose compared with those during a constant intravenous infusion. This relationship applies to all drugs that rapidly achieve equilibrium between plasma and tissues.

accumulation reaches 90 percent of steady state levels at the end of 3 to 4 half-lives. For digoxin, with a half-life of 1.6 days (with normal renal function), accumulation will be practically complete in 5 days. Continuous infusion of a drug at a constant rate also will result in progressive accumulation to a steady state with a time course predictable from the elimination curve for that drug (Fig. 66-3).

When the time required to reach steady state is longer than one wishes to wait, desired plasma levels may be achieved more rapidly by the administration of a *loading dose*. Loading entails the administration of an amount that will bring the concentration in plasma (at equilibrium) to the level present during steady state. If the desired plasma level (Cp_{ss}) is known, the loading dose can be estimated with knowledge of the extent of the drug's extravascular distribution at equilibrium, the apparent volume of distribution, or V_d:

$$\text{Loading dose} = \text{desired plasma level} \times \text{volume of distribution at steady state}$$

$$= Cp_{ss} \times V_d$$

Loading may be accomplished by the administration of the loading amount as a single dose, or in the case of drugs for which there is risk of toxicity if all the drug is introduced into the plasma compartment rapidly, the loading amount is administered in a series of fractions of the total loading amount. Since the accumulation of procainamide to 90 percent of steady state by infusion would require approximately 10 h (the $t_{1/2}$ is 3 h), a loading regimen is almost always desirable. The load required to suppress an arrhythmia, however, varies among individuals from 300 to 1000 mg, and rapid intravenous administration of the *average loading dose* causes hypotension during the distribution phase in some patients. Therefore, the intravenous loading dose of procainamide is given in fractions (e.g., 100 mg every 5 min) until the arrhythmia is controlled or adverse effects such as hypotension indicate that no further drug should be given. Dividing the loading dose into fractions is appropriate for most drugs that have a low therapeutic index (the *therapeutic index* is the ratio of toxic dose to the therapeutic dose). This permits better individualization of the loading amount and minimizes adverse effects.

The size of the loading dose required to achieve the plasma levels at steady state also can be determined from the fraction of drug eliminated during the dosage interval and the maintenance dose (in the case of intermittent drug administration). For example, if the fraction of digoxin eliminated daily is 35 percent and the planned maintenance dose is to be 0.25 mg daily, then the loading dose to achieve steady state levels should be 100/35 times the maintenance dose, or approximately 0.75 mg. Thus

$$\frac{\text{Loading}}{\text{dose}} = \frac{100}{\% \text{ of drug eliminated per dosage interval}} \times \text{maintenance dose}$$

The fraction of drug eliminated during any dosage interval can be determined from a semilogarithmic graph in which the total amount in the body at time zero is set at 100 percent and the fraction remaining at the end of one half-life is 50 percent.[1] Conversely, if the loading dose is known, the maintenance dose can be similarly calculated.

To calculate a loading dose designed to achieve the plasma concentration of a known infusion rate at steady state,

$$\text{Loading dose} = \frac{\text{infusion rate}}{k}$$

where k is the fractional elimination constant that describes the rate of drug elimination.[1]

Regardless of the size of the loading dose, *after maintenance therapy has been given for 3 to 4 half-lives, the amount of drug in the body is determined by the maintenance dose*. The independence of the plasma levels at steady state from the load is illustrated in Fig. 66-3, which indicates that the elimination of the loading dose would be practically complete after three to four half-lives.

DETERMINANTS OF PLASMA LEVELS DURING THE EQUILIBRIUM PHASE   An important determinant of the level of drug in plasma during the equilibrium phase after a single dose is the extent to which the drug is distributed outside the plasma compartment. For example, if the distribution of a 3-mg dose of a large macromolecule is confined to a plasma volume of 3 L, then the concentration in plasma will be 1 mg/L. However, if a different drug is distributed so that 90 percent of it leaves the plasma compartment, then only 0.3 mg will remain in the 3-L plasma volume and the concentration in plasma will be only 0.1 mg/L. The *apparent volume of distribution*, or V_d, expresses the relationship between the amount of drug in the body and the plasma concentration at equilibrium:

$$V_d = \frac{\text{amount of drug in body}}{\text{plasma concentration}}$$

The amount of drug in the body is expressed as mass (e.g., milligrams), and the plasma concentration is expressed as mass per volume (e.g., milligrams per liter). Thus V_d is a hypothetical volume into which a quantity of drug would distribute if its concentration in the entire volume were the same as that in plasma. Although it is not a real volume, it is an important concept because it determines the fraction of total drug in the plasma and therefore the fraction available to the organs of elimination. An approximation of V_d in the equilibrium phase can be obtained by estimating the concentration of drug in plasma at time zero (Cp_0) by back-extrapolation of the equilibrium-phase plot to zero time, as illustrated in Fig. 66-1. Then, after intravenous administration when the amount in the body at time zero is the dose, we have

$$V_d = \frac{\text{dose}}{Cp_0}$$

For the administration of the large macromolecule mentioned above, the measured Cp_0 of 1 mg/L after a 3-mg dose indicates a V_d that is a real volume, the plasma volume. This is the exception, however, for the V_d of most drugs is larger than plasma volume; many drugs are so extensively taken up by cells that tissue levels exceed those in plasma. For such drugs, the hypothetical V_d is large, even greater than the volume of body water. For example, Fig. 66-1 indicates that the Cp_0 obtained by extrapolation after administration of 50 mg lidocaine is 0.42 mg/L, yielding a V_d of 119 L.

Since elimination is performed largely by the kidneys and liver, it is useful to consider the elimination of drugs according to the *clearance* concept. For example, in the kidney, regardless of the

extent to which removal of drug is determined by filtration, secretion, or reabsorption, the net result is a reduction of the concentration of drug in plasma as it passes through the organ. The extent to which the concentration is reduced is expressed as the *extraction ratio*, or E, which is constant as long as first-order elimination occurs.

$$E = \frac{C_a - C_v}{C_a}$$

where C_a = arterial plasma concentration
C_v = venous plasma concentration

If the extraction is complete, $E = 1$. If the total plasma flow to the kidneys is Q (mL/min), the total volume of plasma from which drug is completely removed in a unit time (clearance from the body, Cl) is determined as

$$\text{Cl}_{renal} = QE$$

If the renal extraction ratio of penicillin is 0.5 and renal plasma flow is 680 mL/min, then penicillin's renal clearance is 340 mL/min. If the extraction ratio is high, as is the case for renal extraction of aminohippurate or hepatic extraction of propranolol, then clearance is a function of organ blood flow.[2]

Clearance from the body is the sum of clearance from all organs of elimination and is the best measure of the efficiency of the elimination processes. If a drug is removed by both the kidney and liver, then

$$\text{Cl} = \text{Cl}_{renal} + \text{Cl}_{hepatic}$$

Thus, if penicillin is eliminated by both renal clearance (340 mL/min) and hepatic clearance (36 mL/min) in a normal individual, total clearance is 376 mL/min. If renal clearance is reduced to half, total clearance is $170 + 36$ or 206 mL/min. In anuria, total clearance equals hepatic clearance.

Only the drug in the vascular compartment can be cleared during each passage through an organ. To ascertain the effect of a given plasma clearance by one or more organs on the rate of removal of drug from the body, the clearance must be related to the volume of "plasma equivalents" to be cleared, that is, the volume of distribution. If the volume of distribution is 10 L and clearance is 1 L/min, then one-tenth of the drug in the body is eliminated per minute. This fraction, Cl/V_d, is known as a *fractional elimination constant* and is designated as k:

$$k = \frac{\text{Cl}}{V_d}$$

If the fraction k is multiplied by the total amount of drug in the body, the actual rate of elimination at any given time can be determined:

$$\text{Rate of elimination} = k \times \text{amount in body} = \text{Cl}Cp$$

This is the general equation for all first-order processes and expresses the fact that rate is proportional to the declining quantity in a first-order process.

Since half-life is a temporal expression of the exponential first-order process, half-life ($t_{1/2}$) can be related to k as follows:

$$t_{1/2} = \frac{0.693}{k}$$

Because
$$k = \frac{\text{Cl}}{V_d}$$

then
$$t_{1/2} = \frac{0.693 V_d}{\text{Cl}}$$

As shown in the section on drug dosage in renal failure, the linear relationship of k to creatinine clearance makes k a useful parameter

---

[1] Alternatively, the fraction of drug lost from the body during a dosage interval can be determined nongraphically from this equation:

$$\text{Fraction of drug lost from body} = 1 - e^{-kt}$$

Values for e^{-kt} can be obtained from a table of natural exponential functions or by a calculator, where $k = (0.693/t_{1/2})$ is the fractional elimination constant (described in the next section) and t is the time interval after drug administration.

[2] When drug is present in the formed elements of blood, then calculation of extraction and clearance from blood is more physiologically meaningful than from the plasma.

upon which to estimate changes in drug elimination with reduction in creatinine clearance in renal insufficiency. Half-life is not linearly related to clearance.

The important relationship

$$t_{1/2} = \frac{0.693 V_d}{\text{Cl}}$$

indicates clearly the dependency of half-life, a measure of rate of elimination, on the two physiologically independent variables of volume of distribution and clearance, which expresses the efficiency of elimination. Thus half-life is shortened when phenobarbital induces the enzymes responsible for hepatic clearance of a drug, and half-life is lengthened when a drug's renal clearance is attenuated in renal failure. Also, the half-life of some drugs is shortened when their volume of distribution is reduced. If, as in the case of cardiac failure, the volume of distribution is reduced at the same time that clearance is reduced, there may be little change in drug half-life to reflect the impaired clearance, but steady state plasma levels will be increased, as is the case with lidocaine. In treating patients after an overdose, the effects of hemodialysis on a drug's elimination are dependent on its volume of distribution. When the volume of distribution is large, as with tricyclic antidepressants (V_d of desipramine equals more than 2000 L), the removal of drug, even with a high-clearance dialyzer, proceeds slowly.

The extent to which a drug is bound to plasma protein also determines the fraction extracted by the organ(s) of elimination. Altered binding changes the extraction ratio significantly, however, only when elimination is limited to the unbound (free) drug in plasma. The extent to which binding influences elimination depends on the relative affinity of the plasma binding versus the affinity of the drug for the extraction process. The high affinity of the renal tubular anion transport system for many drugs leads to extraction of bound and unbound drug, and the efficient process by which the liver removes propranolol extracts most of this highly bound drug from blood. However, in the case of drugs with low organ extraction ratios, only unbound drug is available for elimination.

STEADY STATE With a constant infusion of drug, the infusion rate equals elimination rate at steady state. Therefore,

Infusion rate	=	Cp_{ss}	×	Cl
(amt/unit time)		(amt/vol)		(vol/unit time)

when the units for amount, volume, and time are consistent.

Thus, if clearance (Cl) is known, the infusion rate to achieve a given steady state plasma level can be calculated. Estimation of drug clearance is discussed in the section on renal disease.

When the dose is given intermittently instead of by infusion, the above relationship between plasma concentration and the dose administered at each dosage interval can be expressed as

$$\text{Dose} = Cp_{av} \times \text{Cl} \times \text{dosage interval}$$

The average plasma concentration (Cp_{av}) implies, as seen in Fig. 66-2, that levels can be higher and lower than the average during the dosage interval.

When a drug is given orally, the fraction (F) of the administered dose that reaches the systemic circulation is an expression of the drug's *bioavailability*. A reduction in bioavailability may reflect a poorly formulated dosage form that fails to disintegrate or dissolve in the gastrointestinal fluids. Regulatory standards have reduced the extent of this problem. Drug interactions also can impair absorption after oral dosing. Bioavailability also may be reduced due to drug metabolism in the gastrointestinal tract and/or the liver during the absorption process, the *first-pass effect*. This is a particular problem for drugs that are extensively extracted by these organs, and considerable interpatient variability often exists in bioavailability. Lidocaine for the control of arrhythmias is not administered orally because of the first-pass effect. Drugs that are injected intramuscularly also may have low bioavailability, e.g., phenytoin. An unexpected drug

response should lead to consideration of bioavailability as a possible factor. Calculation of a dosage regimen should be corrected for bioavailability:

$$\text{Oral dose} = \frac{Cp_{av} \times \text{Cl} \times \text{dosage interval}}{F}$$

DRUG ELIMINATION THAT IS NOT FIRST-ORDER The elimination of some drugs such as phenytoin, salicylate, and theophylline does not follow first-order kinetics when amounts of drug in the body are in the therapeutic range. For these drugs, the clearance changes as levels in the body fall during elimination or after alterations in dose. This pattern of elimination is said to be *dose-dependent*. Accordingly, the time for the concentration to fall to one-half becomes less as plasma levels fall; this halving time is not truly a half-life, because the term *half-life* applies to first-order kinetics and is a constant. The elimination of phenytoin is dose-dependent, and when very high levels are present (in the toxic range), the halving time may be longer than 72 h, whereas as the concentration in plasma declines, the clearance increases and the concentration in plasma will halve in 20 to 30 h. When a drug is eliminated by first-order kinetics, the plasma level at steady state is directly related to the amount of the maintenance dose, and a doubling of the dose should lead to doubling of the steady state plasma level. However, for drugs with dose-dependent kinetics, increases in the dose may be accompanied by disproportionate increases in plasma level. Thus, if the daily dose of phenytoin is increased from 300 to 400 mg, plasma levels rise by more than 33 percent. The extent of increase is not predictable because of the interpatient variability in the extent to which clearance deviates from first order. Theophylline and salicylates also are eliminated by dose-dependent kinetics, and in children particular caution must be taken with the administration of salicylates in high doses. Changes in dosage regimens for such drugs should always be accompanied by surveillance for adverse effects and by measurement of the concentration of the drug in plasma after sufficient time to establish a new steady state. Ethanol metabolism also is dose-dependent, with obvious implications. The mechanisms involved in dose-dependent kinetics may include the saturation of the rate-limiting step in metabolism or a feedback inhibition of the rate-limiting enzyme by a product of the reaction.

INDIVIDUALIZATION OF DRUG THERAPY

Optimal drug therapy requires administration of just the right amount of drug for the particular patient—too little and efficacy is not likely, whereas too large a dose increases the risk of undesirable effects. When the desired response is a readily determined clinical effect, such as altered blood pressure or coagulation time, then an optimal dosage requirement can be achieved in an empirical fashion. Dosage alterations should, however, involve modest changes in amount (50 percent) and no more frequently than every two to three half-lives. In most cases, however, drug therapy must be guided by the concept of a "therapeutic window" within which drug concentrations must be achieved and maintained. If this therapeutic window is large, i.e., little dose-related toxicity, then maximal efficacy, should this be desired and achievable, may be obtained by administering a supraeffective dose. Such a strategy is often used for penicillins and many beta-adrenoceptor blocking agents. It is also possible under these circumstances to usefully extend the duration of action of the drug, especially when it is rapidly eliminated from the body. Thus 75 mg of captopril will result in reduced blood presure for up to 12 h, even though the elimination half-life of the ACE-inhibitor is about 2 h. The therapeutic window for most drugs, however, is much narrower, and in certain instances (see Table 66-4), as little as a twofold difference distinguishes the dose (concentration) of drug producing the desired response from that eliciting an adverse effect. In these cases, the application of pharmacokinetic principles is critical to achieving the defined therapeutic objective.

During long-term therapy, the most important pharmacokinetic factor is the drug's clearance, since this determines the steady state plasma concentration. Thus, after an oral dose, and assuming that clearance is constant regardless of the dose,

$$Cp_{av} = \frac{\text{dosage rate}}{\text{clearance}} = \frac{F \times \text{oral dose}}{Cl \times \text{dosage interval}}$$

Accordingly, steady state drug levels and, therefore, the intensity of response can be adjusted by changing the dosing rate. In most cases this is best achieved by changing the drug dose and maintaining the same dosage interval, e.g., 250 mg every 8 h versus 200 mg every 8 h—drug levels will change in a proportional fashion, but the relative fluctuation between the maximum and minimum values will remain the same. On the other hand, the steady state level may be changed by altering the frequency of intermittent dosing while maintaining the amount of administered drug the same. This strategy, however, will result in changes in the relative fluctuations around the average steady state concentration. If a drug is administered every half-life, the trough concentration at the end of the dosing interval will be about one-half that of the peak level, assuming that absorption is rapid. At shorter intervals the fluctuations will be smaller, with the ultimate smooth curve when the drug is continuously given by infusion. By contrast, reaching a given steady state using a longer dosage interval and a proportionally large dose leads to wider fluctuations between the maximum and minimum levels (Fig. 66-4). Only if very high concentrations are nontoxic and it is acceptable that drug concentrations are below the minimum effective concentration for a considerable period of time during the longer dosage interval can larger doses be given to achieve a desired average steady state level.

With drugs that have a long elimination half-life and in which, therefore, steady state is only achieved after a considerable period of time, the previously described loading-dose strategy may be appropriate. Also, knowledge of a drug's rate of elimination is important in predicting when the full effects of any dosage change made to alter a steady state will be expected, since this takes three to four times the elimination half-life.

RENAL DISEASE Where urinary excretion is an important route of elimination, renal failure results in decreased drug clearance and therefore slower removal of the drug from the body, so administration of the usual dosage leads to greater accumulation and an increased likelihood of toxicity. The goal in such cases is to modify the dosage schedule so that a similar drug concentration–time profile is achieved in the plasma of the patient with renal insufficiency and the steady

state is reached after a similar time interval as in the patient with normal renal function. This is particularly appropriate for drugs with long half-lives and narrow therapeutic indexes (e.g., digoxin). Since

$$Cp_{av} = \frac{\text{dose}}{\text{dose interval}} \times \frac{F}{Cl}$$

$$= \frac{\text{dose}}{\text{dose interval}} \times \frac{F}{k\,V_d}$$

the Cp_{av} achieved with normal renal function can be obtained in patients with renal impairment, i.e., decreased Cl, by either decreasing the dose while maintaining the normal dosing interval, administering the usual dose but less frequently, or a combination of the two. Moreover, the modification factor for the dosage regimen is dependent on the ratio of the drug's clearance or rate of elimination in renal failure to that in uncompromised patients. Although such pharmacokinetic strategies in renal failure result in the same Cp_{av} during the dosage interval, the peak-to-trough fluctuations differ considerably from those seen in patients with normal renal function. Selection of the most appropriate modifications, therefore, depends on the levels associated with efficacy or toxicity, e.g., peak, Cp_{av}, or trough, and the drug's therapeutic index.

One approach is to calculate the *fraction of the normal dose* that is to be given at the usual dosage interval. This fraction can be determined from either drug clearance (Cl) or the fractional rate constant (k) based on the fact that both renal clearance and k are proportional to creatinine clearance (Cl_{cr}). Creatinine clearance is best determined directly. However, serum creatinine (C_{cr}) may be used to estimate the value by the following equation which is applicable to men:

$$Cl_{cr} = \frac{(140 - \text{age}) \times \text{weight (kg)}}{72 \times C_{cr}\,(\text{mg/dL})} \,(\text{mL/min})$$

For women, the value should be reduced to 85 percent of that estimated by this equation. This approach to estimation of Cl_{cr} is invalid in severe renal insufficiency ($C_{cr} > 5$ mg/dL) or with rapidly changing renal function.

The clearance approach Calculation of drug dosage is most accurately based on the clearance of a drug. From data on the clearance of a drug, the dose in renal insufficiency ($Dose_{ri}$) may be calculated as follows:

$$Dose_{ri} = \text{dose} \times \frac{Cl_{ri}}{Cl}$$

where ri = renal insufficiency

    Cl = clearance from the whole body with normal renal function

    Cl_{ri} = clearance from the whole body with renal insufficiency

    Dose = maintenance dose with normal renal function ($Cl_{cr} \approx$ 100 mL/min)

The normal clearance and that in renal impairment can be obtained by employing the data in Table 66-1 in the following equations:

$$Cl = Cl_{renal} + Cl_{nonrenal}$$

$$Cl_{ri} = Cl_{renal} \times \frac{\text{measured } Cl_{cr}}{100 \text{ mL/min}} + Cl_{nonrenal}$$

The Cl_{renal} values in Table 66-1 are those found with $Cl_{cr} = 100$ mL/min, and the renal clearance of drug in renal insufficiency is obtained by multiplying Cl_{renal} by the ratio of measured Cl_{cr} (in milliliters per minute) to 100 mL/min.

For gentamicin, with a normal Cl_{renal} of 78 mL/min and $Cl_{nonrenal}$ of 3 mL/min, Cl = 81 mL/min. Therefore, with a Cl_{cr} of 12 mL/min, $Cl_{ri} = 78 \times (12/100) + 3 = 12.4$ mL/min. If the dose of gentamicin for a given infection should be 1.5 mg/kg per 8 h in the presence of normal renal function, then

$$Dose_{ri} = \frac{1.5 \text{ mg/kg}}{8 \text{ h}} \times \frac{12.4 \text{ mL/min}}{81 \text{ mL/min}} = \frac{0.23 \text{ mg/kg}}{8 \text{ h}}$$

FIGURE 66-4 Plasma concentrations of a drug with an elimination half-life of 12 h during chronic therapy using different dosage regimens for a period sufficient to reach steady state. Proportionally reducing or increasing both the size of the maintenance dose and the interval between dosage changes the magnitude of the fluctuations in plasma levels but has no effect on the average steady state (Cp_{av}) value, since this depends on the ratio between D and τ.

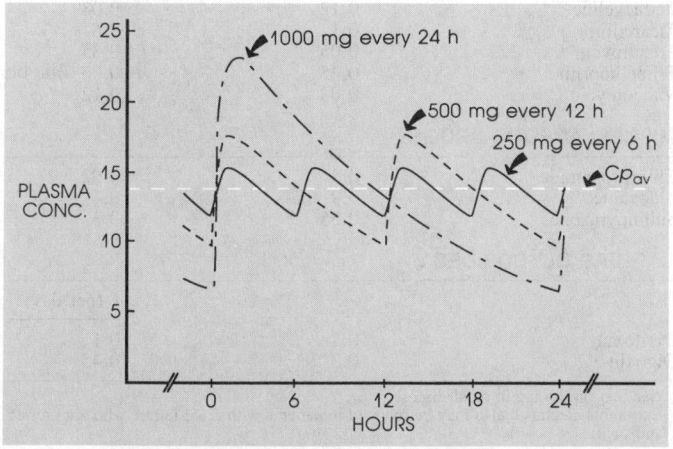

TABLE 66-1   Clearance of drugs

Drug	Renal clearance,* mL/min	Nonrenal clearance, mL/min
Ampicillin[†]	340	12
Carbenicillin	68	10
Digoxin[†]	110	36
Gentamicin	78	3
Kanamycin	60	0
Penicillin G[‡]	340	36

* The "normal" renal clearances are those associated with a clearance of creatinine of 100 mL/min.
† The fraction of digoxin absorbed after an oral dose (F) is approximately 0.75, and F for ampicillin is 0.5.
‡ One microgram of penicillin G = 1.6 units.

In the patient with renal insufficiency, this computation provides an average plasma level during a dosage interval that is the same as the average plasma level during the dosage interval with normal renal function; the fluctuations between peaks and troughs, however, will be less pronounced, but the peak value could be below the therapeutic level. Alternatively, the normal (1.5 mg/kg) dose of gentamicin could be administered but the dosage interval prolonged by the modification factor based on the change in clearance

$$8 \text{ h} \times \frac{81 \text{ mL/min}}{12.4 \text{ mL/min}} = 52 \text{ h}$$

In this case, the plasma levels may be subtherapeutic for a deleterious length of time during the dosage interval.

In some instances it may be desirable to calculate a dose that will yield a certain plasma level at steady state. This approach is most appropriate for constant intravenous infusions where 100 percent of the dose is delivered to the systemic circulation. When clearance of a drug in a patient with renal insufficiency is calculated as above, then

$$\underset{\text{(amt/unit time)}}{\text{Dose}_{ri}} = \underset{\text{(vol/unit time)}}{\text{Cl}_{ri}} \times \underset{\text{(amt/vol)}}{Cp}$$

where the time, amount, and volume terms are uniform.

If a plasma concentration of carbenicillin of 100 μg/mL is the therapeutic objective in a patient with a creatinine clearance of 25 mL/min, the infusion rate is calculated as follows. Carbenicillin clearance is

$$\text{Cl}_{ri} = \left(68 \times \frac{25}{100}\right) + 10 = 27 \text{ mL/min}$$

Therefore, carbenicillin should be infused at a rate of 2700 μg/min.

Should the method of calculating dose based on the desired plasma level be applied to intermittent-dose therapy, particular attention should be given to the fact that the calculation is based on an *average* plasma level and that peak plasma levels will be higher. In addition, if an oral drug is not completely absorbed, the computed dose must be divided by the fraction (F) that reaches the systemic circulation (see "Steady State" above).

The fractional rate constant (k) approach   For many drugs, clearance data in renal failure are not available. In these cases, the fraction of the normal dose that is required in a patient with renal failure can be approximated from the ratio of the fractional rate constant for elimination from the body in renal failure (k_{ri}) to that with normal renal function (k). This approach requires the assumption that the distribution of the drug (V_d) is not affected by renal disease. The approach is the same as that employed with clearance data:

$$\text{Dose}_{ri} = \text{dose} \times \frac{k_{ri}}{k}$$

Since the ratio k_{ri}/k is the fraction of the usual dose employed in a given degree of renal insufficiency, it is termed the *dose fraction* and

may be estimated from the information in Table 66-2 and the nomogram (Fig. 66-5). Table 66-2 gives the fraction of the usual dose of a drug required at a creatinine clearance of zero (dose fraction$_0$). The nomogram presents the dose fraction as a linear function of creatinine clearance.

To calculate the dose fraction$_{ri}$, the dose fraction$_0$ is obtained from Table 66-2, plotted on the left ordinate of the nomogram, and connected by a straight line to the upper right-hand corner of the nomogram. This line describes the dose fraction over a range of creatinine clearances from 0 to 100 mL/min. The point of intersection between the measured creatinine clearance (on the lower abscissa) and this dose-fraction line is a coordinate with the dose fraction (on the left ordinate) corresponding to that particular creatinine clearance. For example, if a patient with a creatinine clearance of 20 mL/min

TABLE 66-2   Estimated fraction of usual dose of drug required for a patient with a creatinine clearance of zero (dose fraction$_0$) and average overall fractional elimination rate constant for a patient with normal renal function (k)

Drug	Dose fraction$_0$	k (per hour)
ANTIBIOTICS		
Amikacin	0.05	0.4
Amoxicillin	0.15	0.7
Ampicillin	0.1	0.6
Aztreonam	0.25	0.4
Carbenicillin	0.1	0.6
Cefazolin	0.06	0.35
Cefotaxime*	0.3	0.7
Cefoxitin	0.1	0.8
Ceftazidime	0.1	0.4
Ceftriaxone[†]	0.5	0.09
Cephalexin	0.04	0.7
Cephalothin	0.02	1.4
Chloramphenicol	0.8	0.3
Ciprofloxacin	0.33	0.2
Clindamycin	0.8	0.2
Cloxacillin	0.25	1.2
Dicloxacillin	0.5	1.2
Doxycycline	0.8	0.03
Erythromycin	0.7	0.5
Gentamicin	0.05	0.3
Imipenem	0.25	0.7
Isoniazid:		
Fast inactivators	0.8	0.5
Slow inactivators	0.5	0.25
Methicillin	0.12	1.4
Minocycline	0.9	0.06
Nafcillin	0.4	1.2
Norfloxacin	0.5	0.2
Oxacillin	0.25	1.4
Penicillin G	0.1	1.4
Piperacillin	0.33	0.5
Rifampin	1.0	0.25
Streptomycin	0.05	0.25
Sulfadiazine	0.45	0.7
Sulfamethoxazole	0.85	0.07
Tetracycline	0.12	0.08
Ticarcillin	0.1	0.6
Tobramycin	0.05	0.35
Trimethoprim	0.45	0.06
Vancomycin	0.03	0.12
MISCELLANEOUS DRUGS		
Chlorpropamide	0.4	0.02
Lidocaine	0.9	0.4
Sulfinpyrazone	0.55	0.3
CARDIAC GLYCOSIDES		k (per day)
Digitoxin	0.7	0.1
Digoxin	0.3	0.45

* See text on dosage in renal disease.
† Extrarenal clearance also may be reduced in patients with renal failure who are uremic and/or ill.

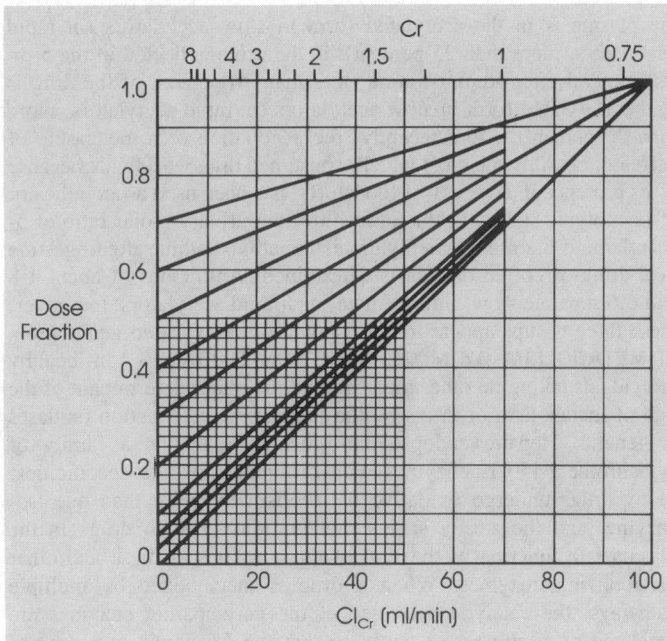

FIGURE 66-5 Nomogram for estimation of the dose fraction in patients with renal insufficiency. Cr = creatinine; Cl$_{cr}$ = creatinine clearance. (*From Dettli L, Clin Pharmacokin 1:126, 1976.*).

requires penicillin G for an infection that would be treated with 10 million units daily in patients with normal renal function, then an appropriate dose would be 2.8 million units daily. This dose is estimated by plotting the dose fraction$_0$ for penicillin G (0.1) on the left-hand ordinate and connecting it to the top right-hand corner of the nomogram (Fig. 66-5). On this dose-fraction line for penicillin G, the coordinate for a creatinine clearance of 20 mL/min corresponds on the left ordinate to a dose fraction of 0.28. Hence the dose is 0.28 × 10 million units daily.

The loading dose In addition to adjusting the maintenance dose in renal failure, consideration also must be given to the loading dose. Since this dose is designed to bring the plasma concentration, or more particularly, the amount of drug in the body, rapidly to the level at steady state, there is no need to modify the usual loading dose if one is normally used. The elimination of many drugs is sufficiently rapid in patients with normal renal function that the time required to reach steady state is not significant, and no loading dose is usually used. On the other hand, in renal failure, where the half-life may be significantly prolonged, this accumulation period may become unacceptably long. In such a case, a loading dose may be indicated; it would be the same amount of drug administered with normal renal function as described in "Drug Accumulation" above.

General considerations for determining dosage in renal insufficiency Because of the differences in volumes of distribution and rates of metabolism, calculations of drug dose in renal failure must be viewed as valuable approximations which prevent the use of doses that are grossly excessive or inadequate for most patients. However, *maintenance dosages are most accurate when plasma-level data are employed to enable adjustment of the dose where necessary.*

In all the above calculations, it is assumed that the nonrenal clearance and nonrenal k are constant in renal failure. In fact, when cardiac failure accompanies renal failure, metabolic clearance for many drugs is reduced. Accordingly, when a drug with a narrow therapeutic index, such as digoxin, is used in cardiac failure, an appropriate precaution would be to reduce the value for nonrenal clearance (or k) to about one-half.

Active or toxic metabolites of drugs also may accumulate in renal failure. Meperidine, for example, is cleared largely by metabolism, and its concentration in plasma is little altered by renal insufficiency.

However, the plasma concentration of one of its metabolites, normeperidine, is increased when its renal elimination is impaired. Since normeperidine has more convulsant activity than meperidine, its accumulation in patients with renal failure probably accounts for the signs of central nervous system excitation such as irritability, twitching, and seizures that result from the administration of multiple doses of meperidine to patients in renal insufficiency.

The metabolite of procainamide, *N*-acetylprocainamide, also has cardiac effects. Since *N*-acetylprocainamide is eliminated almost entirely by the kidney, its concentration in plasma is increased by renal failure. Thus the potential of procainamide to produce toxicity in renal insufficiency cannot be assessed by measuring the plasma concentration of procainamide alone. Cefotaxime is metabolized predominately to desacetylcefotaxime, which also has antimicrobial activity. Desacetylcefotaxime accumulates in renal failure to an even greater degree than does the parent drug, but no adverse effects are known to accrue to the accumulation of this metabolite.

LIVER DISEASE In contrast to the predictable decline in renal clearance of drugs when glomerular filtration is reduced, it is not possible to make a general prediction of the effect of liver disease on hepatic biotransformation of drugs (Chap. 261). Rather, in hepatitis and cirrhosis, changes may range from impaired to increased drug clearance. Even in advanced hepatocellular disease, the magnitude of impairment in drug clearance usually is only about two- to fivefold. The extent of such changes, however, cannot be predicted by the common tests of liver function. Consequently, even when it is suspected that drug elimination is altered in liver disease, there is no quantitative base on which to adjust the dosage regimen other than assessment of clinical response and concentration of drug in plasma.

Portacaval shunting creates a special condition because the effective hepatic blood flow is reduced. This situation has its greatest effect on drugs that normally have a high hepatic extraction ratio so that their clearance is largely a function of blood flow; thus the clearance of such drugs (e.g., propranolol and lidocaine) is remarkably reduced by portacaval shunting. In addition, the fraction of an administered oral dose reaching the systemic circulation is increased, because drug that is shunted around the liver during the absorption process escapes the first-pass metabolism by this organ (e.g., meperidine, pentazocine).

CIRCULATORY INSUFFICIENCY—CARDIAC FAILURE AND SHOCK Under conditions of decreased tissue perfusion, redistribution of the cardiac output occurs to preserve blood flow to the heart and brain at the expense of other tissues (Chap. 34). As a result, the drug is distributed into a smaller volume of distribution, higher drug concentrations are present in the plasma, and the tissues that are best perfused are exposed to these higher concentrations. If either the brain or heart is sensitive to the drug, an alteration in response will occur.

Furthermore, the decreased perfusion of the kidney and liver may impair drug clearance by these organs directly or indirectly. Thus, in severe congestive heart failure, in hemorrhagic shock, and in cardiogenic shock, the response to the usual dose of drug may be excessive, and dosage modification may be necessary. For example, the clearance of lidocaine is reduced by about 50 percent in cardiac failure, and therapeutic plasma levels are achieved at infusion rates of only about half those usually required. In cardiac failure there also is a significant reduction in lidocaine's volume of distribution, which results in the requirement of a smaller loading dose. Similar situations are thought to exist for procainamide, theophylline, and possibly quinidine. Unfortunately, predictors of these types of pharmacokinetic alterations are unavailable. Therefore, loading doses should be conservative, and continued therapy should be monitored closely, following clinical indicators of toxicity and plasma levels.

DISEASE-INDUCED CHANGES IN PLASMA BINDING Many drugs circulate in the plasma partly bound to the plasma proteins. Since only the unbound or free drug can distribute to the site of pharmacologic action, the therapeutic response should be related to the free rather than the total circulating plasma drug concentration.

In most cases the degree of binding is fairly constant across the therapeutic concentration range so that significant error is not caused by individualizing therapy on the basis of total drug levels in plasma. However, states such as hypoalbuminemia, liver disease, and renal disease can decrease the extent of drug binding, particularly of acidic and neutral drugs, so that at any total plasma level there is a greater concentration of free drug and a risk of increased response and toxicity. Other conditions, e.g., myocardial infarction, surgery, neoplastic disease, rheumatoid arthritis, and burns, that lead to an increased plasma concentration of the acute-phase reactant alpha₁-acid glycoprotein have the opposite effect on the basic drugs that are bound to this macromolecule. The drugs for which changes in binding are important are those which are normally highly bound in the plasma (>90 percent) because a small alteration in the extent of binding produces a large change in the amount of drug in the unbound form.

The consequences of these binding changes, particularly with respect to total drug levels, depend on whether the clearance and distribution are dependent on the unbound or total drug. For many drugs, elimination and distribution are largely restricted to the unbound fraction, and therefore, a decrease in binding leads to an increase in the clearance and distribution of the drug. The relative magnitudes of these changes are such that the net effect is to shorten the half-life. The appropriate modification of the dosage regimen in conditions with reduced drug binding, as is the case of phenytoin in renal failure, is simply to administer the usual daily dose of the drug but in divided doses at more frequent intervals. Individualization of therapy can then be based on either the clinical response or the plasma concentration of unbound drug. It is critical that the patient not be titrated into the usual therapeutic range for concentration of *total* drug in plasma, since this will lead to excessive response and toxicity.

In the case of drugs bound to alpha₁-acid glycoprotein, the disease-induced increase in binding has the opposite effects of reducing the clearance and distribution of total drug. Accordingly, constant rate infusion of lidocaine to control arrhythmias after myocardial infarction leads to an accumulation of total drug. However, the clearance of unbound and pharmacologically active drug remains essentially unchanged. Again, it is critical that the patient not be dosed on the basis of total drug concentrations in the plasma, since this will be associated with subtherapeutic levels of unbound drug.

VARIABLE ACTIONS OF DRUGS CAUSED BY GENETIC DIFFERENCES IN THEIR METABOLISM

ACETYLATION Isoniazid, hydralazine, procainamide, and a number of other drugs are metabolized by acetylation of a hydrazino or amino group. This reaction is catalyzed by N-acetyl transferase-2, an enzyme in the liver cytosol that transfers an acetyl group from acetyl coenzyme A to the drug. Individuals differ markedly in the rate at which drugs are acetylated, and there is a bimodal distribution of the population into "rapid acetylators" and "slow acetylators." The rate of acetylation is under genetic control; slow acetylation is an autosomal recessive trait.

Responses to hydralazine therapy are dependent on the acetylation phenotype. The hypotensive effect of hydralazine is greater in patients who acetylate the drug slowly, and the lupus erythematosus–like syndrome produced by hydralazine occurs almost exclusively in those with slow acetylation. Thus it may be of value to know the acetylation phenotype as a predictor of which patients with hypertension might benefit from an increase in the dose of hydralazine above the 200 mg daily that can be safely employed in the population at large.

Acetylation phenotype can be determined by measuring the ratio of acetylated to nonacetylated dapsone or sulfamethazine in plasma or urine following administration of a test dose of these acetylation substrates. The ratio of monoacetyldapsone to dapsone in plasma at 6 h after dapsone administration is less than 0.30 for slow acetylators and greater than 0.35 for rapid acetylators. At 6 h following the administration of sulfamethazine, less than 25 percent of the drug in the plasma is in the acetylated form in slow acetylators (in rapid acetylators, more than 25 percent); in the urine collected in the 5- to 6-h interval after administration, less than 70 percent of the drug is in the acetylated form in slow acetylators (in rapid acetylators, more than 70 percent). More recently, the acetylation of a metabolite of caffeine, possibly the most widely consumed drug worldwide because of its presence in a variety of foodstuffs, has been used as an indicator of phenotypic status. In this procedure, the urinary molar ratio of 5-acetylamino-6-amino-3-methyluracil to methylxanthine after ingestion of a drink of coffee or cola is determined. Antimodes of about 1.8 and 6.6 separate slow, intermediate, and rapid acetylators; moreover, these three groups appear to correspond to the expected genotypes.

METABOLISM BY MIXED-FUNCTION OXIDASES In healthy individuals taking no other medications, the major determinant of the rate of metabolism of drugs by the hepatic mixed-function oxidases is genetic. Hepatic endoplasmic reticulum contains a family of cytochrome P450 isoenzymes with different substrate specificities. Many drugs undergo oxidative metabolism by more than one isoenzyme, and the steady state concentrations of such drugs in the plasma is a function of the sum of the activities of these and other metabolizing enzymes. When a drug is metabolized by multiple pathways, the catalytic activities of the participating enzymes are regulated by a number of genes so that the frequency of clearance rates and steady state concentrations of the drug tend to distribute unimodally within the population. The range of activity may differ markedly (tenfold or more) between different individuals, as is the case for chlorpromazine, and there is no way to make a prior prediction of the rate.

For certain metabolic pathways, bimodally distributed activity suggests control by a single gene, and several polymorphisms have been identified. As a result, two phenotypic populations are usually present analogous to the situation with N-acetylation (see above). A majority of the population are extensive metabolizers (EM), and a smaller group of individuals of the poor metabolizer (PM) phenotype have an impaired, if not an absent, ability to metabolize the drug. For example, about 8 to 10 percent of whites are unable to form the 4-hydroxy metabolite of the test drug debrisoquin, and this trait is inherited in an autosomal recessive fashion. Importantly, the putatively involved cytochrome P450 isoenzyme 2D6 is also at work in the biotransformation of other drugs whose metabolic fate, therefore, cosegregates with the debrisoquin trait. These other drugs include antiarrhythmic agents (propafenone, flecainide), beta-adrenoceptor blockers (alprenolol, metoprolol, timolol), tricylic antidepressants (nortriptyline, desipramine, imipramine, clomipramine), neuroleptic drugs (perphenazine, thioridazine, and possibly fluoxetine), and certain opiates such as codeine. Thus a much reduced analgesic effect of codeine is obtained in PM patients because of impaired production of the active metabolite morphine. A similar situation occurs with the oxidative polymorphism that involves the metabolism of mephenytoin. The situation is further complicated by interethnic differences in the frequency of the polymorphisms. For example, impaired hydroxylation of mephenytoin is present in only 3 to 5 percent of whites, but the incidence is about 20 percent in individuals of Japanese descent; likewise, the frequency of the PM phenotype for debrisoquin hydroxylation appears to decrease as one moves from western (8 to 10 percent) to eastern (0 to 1 percent) population groups.

Polymorphisms in drug-metabolizing ability may be associated with large differences in the disposition of the drug among individuals, especially when the involved pathway is a major contribution to the overall elimination of the drug. For example, the oral clearance of mephenytoin differs 100- to 200-fold between individuals of the EM and PM phenotypes. As a result, peak plasma concentrations and bioavailability after oral administration may be profoundly increased and the rate of drug elimination decreased in PM individuals. This in turn results in drug accumulation and exaggerated pharmacologic responses, including toxicity, when usual drug dosages are administered to patients with the PM phenotype. Drug interactions between compounds that are metabolized by cytochrome P450 2D6 or which inhibit its activity noncompetitively, e.g., quinidine, may be of considerable clinical importance in patients with the EM phenotype, since such concomitant administration often leads to impaired drug handling similar to that in the PM phenotype. Effective individualization of drug therapy is even more critical when using drugs exhibiting polymorphic drug metabolism.

DRUG USE IN THE ELDERLY (See also Chap. 8)

The elderly (>65 years) constitute about 12 percent of the U.S. population, and will increase to about 20 percent, or 50 to 60 million individuals, over the next 20 years. These patients use a disproportionate amount of prescription medications (30 percent), and in addition, 70 percent of the elderly regularly use over-the-counter drugs, compared with only 10 percent in the general adult population. Aging results in changes in organ function, especially in those organs involved in drug disposition, as well as alterations in body size and composition. Not surprisingly, therefore, pharmacokinetic differences are often present in elderly individuals compared with younger cohorts. Unfortunately, few generalizations appear to exist with respect to the type, magnitude, or clinical importance of any age-related changes or their extent in an individual patient. Multiple diseases are also common in geriatric patients, and it is not unusual, therefore, that a large number of drugs are required, which may result in drug interactions that, along with increased vulnerability to morbidity and mortality, contribute to the higher incidence of adverse drug reactions in elderly patients. Increased sensitivity of target organs and impaired physiologic control systems, such as those involved in the regulation of the circulation, also may be a factor. Accordingly, optimization of drug therapy in the elderly, particularly frail patients, is often difficult, since a variety of factors that are frequently poorly defined accentuate the usual interindividual variability in drug response.

Although many individuals preserve good renal function into old age, as a group, elderly patients have an increased and predictable likelihood of impaired renal excretion of drugs. Even in the absence of kidney disease, renal clearance is generally reduced by about 35 to 50 percent in elderly patients. Dosage adjustments analogous to those in patients with kidney dysfunction (see above) are therefore necessary for drugs that are predominantly eliminated from the body by the renal route, e.g., digoxin, aminoglycosides, lithium, and other drugs listed in Table 66-2. In this regard, it is important to recognize that the reduced muscle mass present in older individuals results in a reduction in the rate of creatinine production; thus a normal serum creatinine concentration can be present even though creatinine clearance is impaired.

Aging also results in a decrease in liver size and blood flow, and possibly reduced activity of hepatic drug-metabolizing enzymes; accordingly, the hepatic clearance of some drugs is impaired in the elderly. Unfortunately, no consistent pattern of clinical application appears to be present. Moreover, changes that may exist are often modest relative to the interindividual variability within the patient population. However, even small reductions in hepatic extraction may result in a significant increase in oral bioavailability of drugs with a high first-pass effect, such as propranolol and labetalol.

As a consequence of impaired clearance and/or increased distribution, the elimination half-lives of drugs may increase with aging. Thus, if a dosage modification in an elderly patient is required, it is often possible to accomplish this by decreasing the frequency of drug administration, possibly along with a reduction in dose.

Even if the pharmacokinetics of a drug are not altered, elderly patients may require a smaller drug dosage because of an increase in pharmacodynamic sensitivity. Examples include increased analgesic effects of opioids, increased sedation from benzodiazepines and other central nervous system depressants, and increased risk of bleeding while receiving anticoagulant therapy, even when clotting parameters are well controlled. Exaggerated responses to cardiovascular drugs are also common because of the impaired responsiveness of normal homeostatic mechanisms. Such age-related changes require close monitoring of the patient's clinical response and appropriate dosage titration.

In general, drug therapy for the elderly should be attended by increased alertness to the possibility of moderate reductions in the clearance of drugs and instances of exaggerated pharmacodynamic responsiveness.

INTERACTIONS BETWEEN DRUGS

The effect of some drugs can be altered markedly by the administration of other agents. Such interactions can sabotage therapeutic intent by producing excessive drug action (with adverse effects) or decreasing the action of a drug, rendering it ineffective. Drug interactions must be considered in the differential diagnosis of unexpected responses to drugs, recognizing that patients often come to the physician with a legacy of drugs acquired during previous medical experiences. A meticulous drug history will minimize the unknown elements in the therapeutic milieu; it should include examination of the patient's medications and calls to the pharmacist to identify prescriptions, if necessary.

There are two principal types of interactions between drugs. *Pharmacokinetic interactions* result from alteration in the delivery of drugs to their sites of action. *Pharmacodynamic interactions* are those in which the responsiveness of the target organ or system is modified by other agents.

An index of the drug interactions discussed in this chapter is provided in Table 66-3. Included are interactions which have verified significance in patients and a few of such potential danger that cognizance should be taken of experimental data or case reports suggesting their likely occurrence.

I PHARMACOKINETIC INTERACTIONS CAUSING DIMINISHED DRUG DELIVERY

A Impaired gastrointestinal absorption Cholestyramine, an ionic exchange resin, binds thyroxine, triiodothyronine, and the cardiac glycosides with sufficiently high affinity to impair their absorption from the gastrointestinal tract. This resin probably also interferes with the absorption of other drugs, and it is safest not to give it within 2 h of their administration. Aluminum ions, present in antacids, form insoluble chelates with the tetracyclines, thereby preventing absorption of these drugs. Ferrous ions similarly block tetracycline absorption. Kaolin-pectin suspensions bind digoxin, and when the drugs are administered together, digoxin absorption is reduced by about one-half. However, when kaolin-pectin is administered 2 h after digoxin, there is no effect on absorption of digoxin.

Ketoconazole is a weak base that dissolves well only at acidic pH. Thus histamine-2 antagonists such as cimetidine, by neutralizing gastric pH, impair the dissolution and subsequent absorption of ketoconazole. By contrast, absorption of fluconazole is not impaired by increasing gastric pH. Oral administration of aminosalicylate interferes with the absorption of rifampin by an unknown mechanism.

Impaired absorption results in reduction in the total amount of drug absorbed, i.e., decreased bioavailability, F, with reduced area under the plasma level curve, reduced peak plasma levels, and lower steady state concentrations of the drug involved.

B Induction of hepatic drug-metabolizing enzymes When the elimination of the drug is largely by metabolism, an increase in the rate of metabolism reduces its availability to sites of action. The metabolism of most drugs occurs largely in the liver because of its mass, high blood flow, and concentration of enzymes that metabolize drugs. The initial step in metabolism of many drugs is mediated by a group of mixed-function oxidase isoenzymes in the endoplasmic reticulum. These enzyme systems containing cytochrome P450 oxidize drug molecules by a variety of reactions including aromatic hydroxylations, N-demethylations, O-demethylations, and sulfoxidations. The

TABLE 66-3   Drug interaction index

Drug	Section of chapter describing interaction
Acetohexamide	IIB
Allopurinol	IIA
p-Aminosalicylate	IA
Amiodarone	IIA, IIC
Amphetamine	IC
Antidepressants, tricyclic (desipramine, nortriptyline, imipramine, doxepin, protriptyline, amitriptyline)	IC
Aspirin	IIB, III
Azathioprine	IIA
Barbiturates (class)	IB
Bethanidine	IC
Carbamazepine	IB, IIA
Chlorpromazine	IC, IIA
Cholestyramine	IA
Cimetidine	IA, IIA, IIB
Clofibrate	IIA
Clonidine	IC
Codeine	IIA
Cyclosporin A	IB, IIA
Dexamethasone	IB
Digitoxin	IA, IB, IIC
Digoxin	IA, IIC
Diltiazem	IIA
Diuretics	III
Erythromycin	IIA
Ephedrine	IC
Ethanol	IIA
Famotidine	IIA
Guanadrel	IC
Guanethidine	IC
Haloperidol	IIA
Indomethacin	III
Isoniazid	IIA
Kaolin-pectin	IA
Ketoconazole	IA, IB, IIA
Lidocaine	IIA
Lovastatin	IIA
6-Mercaptopurine	IIA
Methadone	IB
Methotrexate	IIB
Methylprednisolone	IB, IIA
Metronidazole	IB, IIA
Metyrapone	IB
Mexiletine	IB
Nicardipine	IIA
Nifedipine	IIA
Nonsteroidal anti-inflammatory drugs	III
Oral contraceptive steroids	IB
Phenobarbital	IB
Phenylbutazone	IIA, IIB
Phenytoin (diphenylhydantoin)	IB, IIA
Piroxicam	III
Potassium	III
Prednisone	IB
Probenicid	IIB
Procainamide	IIB
Propranolol	III
Quinidine	IB, IIA, IIC, III
Ranitidine	IA, IIA
Rifampin	IA, IB
Salicylate	IIB
Spironolactone	III
Terfenadine	IIA
Tetracycline	IA
Theophylline	IIA
Thiazide diuretics	III
Tolbutamide	IIA
Triamterene	III
Triazolam	IIA
Verapamil	IB, IIA, IIC
Warfarin	IB, IIA, III

products of these reactions are usually more polar (and more readily excreted by the kidney).

The biosynthesis of some of the mixed-function oxidase isoenzymes is under regulatory control, and their content in the liver can be induced by a number of drugs. Phenobarbital is the prototype of these inducers, and all barbiturates in clinical use increase mixed-function oxidase isoenzymes. Induction with phenobarbital can occur with doses of as little as 60 mg daily. Mixed-function oxidases also are induced by rifampin, carbamazepine, phenytoin, and glutethimide, by smoking and exposure to chlorinated insecticides such as DDT, and by chronic alcohol ingestion.

Phenobarbital, rifampin, and other inducers lower plasma levels of many drugs, including warfarin, digitoxin, quinidine, mexiletine, verapamil, ketoconazole, cyclosporin A, dexamethasone, methylprednisolone, prednisolone (the active metabolite of prednisone), oral contraceptive steroids, methadone, metronidazole, and metyrapone. These interactions all have obvious clinical significance. With the coumarin anticoagulants, the patient is placed at major risk when an appropriate level of anticoagulation is achieved while the coumarin drug is coadministered with an inducing agent. Should the inducer then be discontinued, e.g., following discharge from the hospital, plasma levels of the coumarin anticoagulant will rise as the induction effect wears off, leading to excessive anticoagulation.

There is considerable variation among individuals in the extent to which drug metabolism can be induced. In some patients, phenobarbital leads to marked acceleration in the rate of drug metabolism, whereas little induction is seen in others.

In addition to inducing certain of the mixed-function oxidase isoenzymes, phenobarbital has other effects on hepatic function. It increases liver blood flow, bile flow, and the hepatocellular transport of organic anions. The conjugation of drugs and bilirubin also may be enhanced by inducing agents.

C Inhibition of cellular uptake or binding The guanidinium antihypertensives guanethidine, guanadrel, and bethanidine are transported to their site of action in adrenergic neurons by an energy-requiring membrane transport system for biogenic monoamines. Although the physiologic function of the transport system is reuptake of the adrenergic neurotransmitter, it also transports a variety of ring-substituted bases, including guanethidine and related guanidiniums, into the adrenergic neuron against a concentration gradient. Inhibitors of norepinephrine uptake prevent the uptake of the guanidinium antihypertensives into adrenergic neurons and thereby block their pharmacologic effects. The tricyclic antidepressants are potent inhibitors of norepinephrine uptake. Consequently, concomitant administration of clinical doses of tricyclic antidepressants, including desipramine, protriptyline, nortriptyline, and amitriptyline, almost totally abolishes the antihypertensive effects of guanethidine, guanadrel, and bethanidine. Although they are less potent inhibitors of norepinephrine uptake, doxepin and chlorpromazine produce dose-related antagonism of the action of the guanidinium antihypertensives. Ephedrine, a component of many drug combinations used in asthma, also antagonizes the effect of guanethidine. In patients with severe hypertension, the loss of control of blood pressure from these drug interactions can lead to stroke and malignant hypertension.

The antihypertensive effect of clonidine is partially antagonized by tricyclic antidepressants. Clonidine lowers arterial pressure by reducing sympathetic outflow from the blood pressure–regulating centers in the hindbrain (Chap. 209). This central hypotensive action is antagonized by the tricyclic antidepressants.

II PHARMACOKINETIC INTERACTIONS CAUSING INCREASED DRUG DELIVERY

A Inhibition of drug metabolism If the active form of a drug is eliminated largely by biotransformation, inhibition of its metabolism leads to a reduced clearance, prolonged half-life, and accumulation of the drug during maintenance therapy. Excessive accumulation due to inhibited metabolism can lead to adverse effects.

Cimetidine is a potent inhibitor of the oxidative metabolism of many drugs, including warfarin, quinidine, nifedipine, lidocaine, theophylline and phenytoin. Adverse reactions, many of them severe, have resulted from the administration of these drugs in conjunction with cimetidine. Cimetidine is a more potent inhibitor of mixed-function oxidases than ranitidine, whereas ranitidine is more potent as a histamine-2 antagonist. Thus ranitidine, when administered in doses of 150 mg twice daily, does not inhibit the oxidative metabolism of most drugs; where reduced drug elimination has been observed, the effects of ranitidine have been less than those of cimetidine and devoid of appreciable pharmacodynamic consequence. Doses of ranitidine higher than 150 mg, however, may produce greater inhibition of drug oxidation. Famotidine and nizatidine are not known to produce clinically appreciable inhibition of drug metabolism.

Knowledge of the P450 isoenzyme that catalyzes the predominant pathway of metabolism of a drug provides a basis for predicting and understanding drug interactions. For example, the P450 3A family of isoenzymes catalyzes the metabolism of many drugs that produce toxicity when their metabolism is blocked. Drugs that depend on P450 3A as a major route of metabolism include cyclosporin A, quinidine, lovastatin, warfarin, nifedipine, lidocaine, terfenadine, erythromycin, methylprednisolone, carbamazepine, midazolam, and triazolam.

Erythromycin and ketoconazole are potent inhibitors of enzymes in the P450 3A family. Some of the calcium antagonists, diltiazem, nicardipine, and verapamil also can inhibit P450 3A, as can some of its other substrates such as cyclosporin A. Thus serious toxicity from cyclosporin A can result from inhibition of its metabolism by erythromycin, ketoconazole, diltiazem, nicardipine, and verapamil. Lovastatin causes severe myopathy with rhabdomyolysis when administered together with erythromycin or cyclosporin A, and it is highly probable that other of the known inhibitors of P450 3A also can inhibit the disposition of lovastatin. Terfenadine-induced polymorphic ventricular tachycardia can occur when the metabolism of this antihistamine is blocked by ketoconazole and erythromycin.

Whenever erythromycin or ketoconazole are administered to patients, there should be a high level of alert regarding the potential for serious interactions with drugs that are metabolized by P450 3A.

The P450 2D6 isoenzyme that catalyzes the polymorphic metabolism of debrisoquin is markedly inhibited by quinidine and also is blocked by a number of neuroleptic drugs such as chlorpromazine, fluoxetine, and haloperidol. The analgesic effect of codeine depends on its metabolism to morphine via P450 2D6 in individuals with the extensive metabolizer phenotype. Thus quinidine abrogates the analgesic efficacy of codeine in extensive metabolizers. Since desipramine is cleared largely by metabolism via P450 2D6 in extensive metabolizers, its levels are increased substantially by concurrent administration of quinidine or the neuroleptic drugs that block P450 2D6.

Some drugs are inactivated by mechanisms other than the hepatic drug-metabolizing enzymes. Azathioprine is converted in the body to an active metabolite, 6-mercaptopurine, which in turn is oxidized by xanthine oxidase to 6-thiouric acid. When allopurinol, a potent inhibitor of xanthine oxidase, is administered concurrently with standard doses of azathioprine or 6-mercaptopurine, life-threatening toxicity (bone marrow suppression) can result.

Other drugs that inhibit biotransformation of pharmacologic compounds (with examples of drugs that have their metabolism blocked by the inhibitor listed in parenthesis) include:

Amiodarone (warfarin, quinidine)
Clofibrate (phenytoin, tolbutamide)
Excessive ingestion of ethanol (warfarin)
Isoniazid (phenytoin)
Metronidazole (warfarin)
Phenylbutazone (warfarin, phenytoin, tolbutamide)

***B* Inhibition of renal elimination** A number of drugs are secreted by the renal tubular transport systems for organic anions. Inhibition of this tubular transport system can cause excessive accumulation of a drug. Phenylbutazone, probenecid, and salicylates competitively inhibit this transport system. Salicylate, for example, reduces the renal clearance of methotrexate, an interaction that may lead to methotrexate toxicity. Renal tubular secretion contributes substantially to the elimination of penicillin, which can be inhibited by probenecid.

Inhibition of the tubular cation transport system by cimetidine impedes the renal clearance of procainamide and its active metabolite *N*-acetylprocainamide.

***C* Inhibition of clearance by multiple mechanisms** The concentrations of digoxin and digitoxin in plasma are elevated by quinidine, due largely to inhibition of renal elimination and in part to inhibition of nonrenal clearance as well. An increase in cardiac arrhythmia may occur when quinidine is given in conjunction with a cardiac glycoside.

Amiodarone, cyclosporin A, and verapamil also inhibit the clearance of digoxin and increase the concentration of digoxin in plasma.

***III* PHARMACODYNAMIC AND OTHER INTERACTIONS BETWEEN DRUGS** Therapeutically useful interactions occur in which the combined effect of two drugs is greater than that of either drug alone. These favorable drug combinations are described in specific therapeutic sections in this text, and the following is directed toward those interactions which create unwanted effects. Two drugs may act on separate components of a common process and yield effects greater than either alone. For example, small doses of aspirin (less than 1 g daily) do not alter the prothrombin time appreciably in patients who are on warfarin therapy. However, the addition of aspirin to patients anticoagulated with warfarin increases the risk of bleeding because aspirin inhibits platelet aggregation. Thus the combination of impaired functions of platelets and the clotting system increases the potential for hemorrhagic complications in patients receiving warfarin therapy.

Indomethacin, piroxicam, and probably other nonsteroidal anti-inflammatory drugs antagonize the antihypertensive effects of beta-adrenergic receptor blockers, diuretics, converting enzyme inhibitors, and other drugs. The resultant elevation in blood pressure ranges from trivial to severe. Aspirin and sulindac, however, do not elevate the blood pressure in treated hypertensive patients.

Polymorphic ventricular tachycardia (torsades de pointes) during quinidine administration occurs much more frequently in patients receiving diuretics, probably as a consequence of potassium and/or magnesium depletion.

The administration of supplemental potassium leads to more frequent and more severe hyperkalemia when potassium elimination is reduced by concurrent treatment with angiotensin-converting enzyme inhibitors, spironolactone, or triamterene.

CONCENTRATION OF DRUGS IN PLASMA AS A GUIDE TO THERAPY

Optimal individualization of therapy is assisted by measuring the concentration of certain drugs in plasma. Genetic variation in elimination rates, interactions with other drugs, disease-induced alterations in elimination and distribution, and other factors combine to yield a wide range of plasma levels in patients given the same dose. Furthermore, the problem of noncompliance with prescribed regimens during continuing therapy is an endemic and elusive cause of therapeutic failure (see below). Clinical indicators assist the titration of some drugs into the desired range, and no chemical determination is a substitute for careful observations of the response to treatment. However, the therapeutic and adverse effects are not precisely quantifiable for all drugs, and in complex clinical situations, estimates of the action of a drug may be misleading. For example, previously existing neurologic disease may obscure the neurologic consequences of intoxication with phenytoin. Because clearance, half-life, accumulation, and steady state plasma levels are difficult to predict, the measurement of plasma levels is often useful as a guide to the optimal dose. This is particularly so when there is a narrow range between the plasma levels yielding therapeutic and adverse effects. For drugs having such characteristics, e.g., digoxin, theophylline, lidocaine, aminoglycosides, and anticonvulsants, dose optimization should involve modification of the standard dose based on the pharmacokinetic principles described above. In certain instances, predictive nomograms and algorithms have been developed to facilitate the necessary modifications. However, the most flexible and accurate method for individualizing drug dosage appears to be a feedback approach using a small number of previously obtained plasma levels and Bayesian forecasting. In controlled studies, this type of computer-assisted dosing has been shown to improve patient care. However, the overall cost/benefit ratio of such methods in routine management still remains to be conclusively demonstrated.

For those drugs with a narrow therapeutic window that exhibit first-order elimination, then, dosage adjustments may be made on the basis that the average, maximal, minimum steady state concentrations are linearly related to the dosing rate. Accordingly, the dose may be adjusted on the basis of the ratio between the desired and measured concentrations:

$$\frac{Cp_{SS} \text{ (desired)}}{Cp_{SS} \text{ (measured)}} = \frac{\text{dose (new)}}{\text{dose (previous)}}$$

In instances where dose-dependent kinetics are present (e.g., phenytoin and theophylline), plasma concentrations change disproportionately more than the alteration in the dosing rate. Not only should changes in dose be small to minimize the degree of unpredictability, but plasma concentration monitoring also is critical to ensure appropriateness of the modification.

The variability among individual responses to given plasma levels must be recognized. This is illustrated by a hypothetical population concentration-response curve (Fig. 66-6) and its relationship to the therapeutic range or therapeutic window of desired plasma levels. The defined therapeutic window should include the levels at which the majority of patients achieve the intended pharmacologic effect. However, a few people, sensitive to the therapeutic effects, respond to lower levels, whereas others are sufficiently refractory as to require levels that impose the likelihood of adverse effects as a price for therapeutic benefit. For example, a few patients with strong seizure foci require plasma levels of phenytoin exceeding 20 μg/mL to control seizures. Dosages to achieve this effect may be appropriate.

As also illustrated in Fig. 66-6, some patients are prone to adverse effects at levels that are tolerated by most of the population, and therefore, elevation of levels to those with a high probability of therapeutic effect may bring on unwanted actions in the exceptional patient. Table 66-4 presents the concentrations of a number of drugs

TABLE 66-4   Concentrations of drugs in plasma: Relation to efficacy and adverse effects

Drug	Efficacy*	Adverse effects†
Amikacin (peak)	20 μg/mL	40 μg/mL
Carbenicillin	100 μg/mL‡	300 μg/mL
Carbamazepine	3 μg/mL	10 μg/mL
Digitoxin	12 ng/mL	25–30 ng/mL
Digoxin	0.8 ng/mL	2.0 ng/mL
Ethosuximide	40 μg/mL	100 μg/mL
Gentamicin (peak)	5 μg/mL	10 μg/mL
Gentamicin (predose)		2.5 μg/mL
Lidocaine	1.5 μg/mL	5 μg/mL
Lithium	0.5 mEq/L	1.3 mEq/L
Penicillin G	1–25 μg/mL¶	
Phenytoin (diphenylhydantoin)	10 μg/mL	20 μg/mL
Procainamide	4 μg/mL	10 μg/mL
Quinidine	2.5 μg/mL	6 μg/mL
Theophylline	8 μg/mL	20 μg/mL

* The therapeutic effect is infrequent or slight at levels below these.
† The frequency of adverse effects increases sharply when these levels are exceeded.
‡ Minimal inhibitory concentration (MIC) for most strains of *Pseudomonas aeruginosa*. MIC for other, more sensitive, organisms is less.
¶ There is a wide range of MIC of penicillin for various organisms, and the MIC of all those for which penicillin is used is < 20. "Massive" penicillin therapy with 20 million units daily achieves levels of 20 to 25 μg/mL in patients with clearance of creatinine of 100 mL/min.

in plasma that are associated with adverse and therapeutic effects in most patients. Its use within the guidelines discussed should permit more effective and safer therapy for those patients who are not "average."

EFFECTIVE PARTICIPATION OF THE PATIENT IN THERAPEUTIC PROGRAMS   Measurement of the concentration of a drug in plasma is the most effective approach to determine when patients have failed to take the drug. Such "noncompliance" is a frequent problem in the long-term treatment of diseases such as hypertension and epilepsy, occurring in 25 percent or more of patients in therapeutic environments that lack special efforts to involve patients in the responsibility for their own health. Occasionally, noncompliance can be uncovered by sympathetic, nonincriminating questioning, but more often it is recognized only after determining that the concentration of drug in plasma is nil or is recurrently low. Because other factors can cause plasma levels to be lower than expected, comparison with levels obtained during inpatient treatment may be required to confirm that noncompliance did, in fact, occur. Once the physician is certain of noncompliance, a nonaccusatory discussion of the problem with the patient may elucidate a reason for the noncompliance and serve as a basis for more effective cooperation of the patient. Many approaches have been tried to enhance patients' exercise of responsibility for their own treatment, most based on improved communication regarding the nature of the disease and the expectations of treatment success and treatment failure. This communication includes an opportunity for the patient to relate problems associated with treatment, and it may be improved by involving nurses and other paramedical personnel in the process. Minimizing the complexity of the regimen is helpful in terms of both the number of drugs and the frequency of administration. Educating patients to assume the principal role in their own health care requires a blend of the art and science of medicine.

FIGURE 66-6   The cumulative percentage of patients responding to increasing levels of drug in plasma with both therapeutic and adverse effects. The therapeutic window defines the range of concentrations of drug that will achieve therapeutic effects in most patients with adverse effects in only a small percentage.

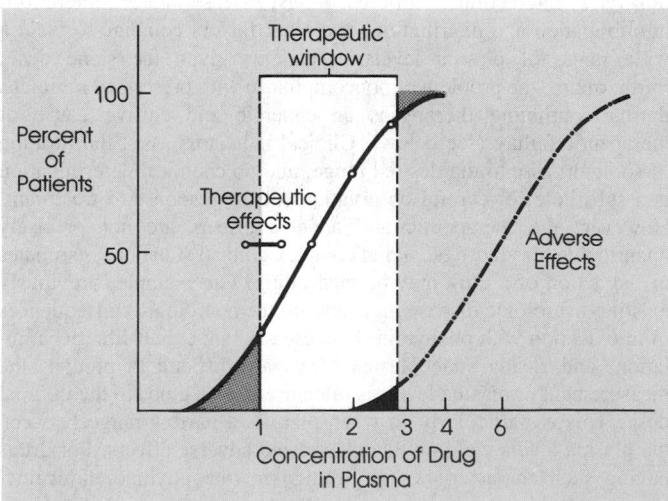

REFERENCES

BENET LZ, WILLIAMS RL: Design and optimization of dosage regimens: Pharmacokinetic data, in *Goodman and Gilman's The Pharmacological Basis of Therapeutics*, 8th ed, AG Gilman et al (eds). New York, Macmillan, 1990, p 1650, Appendix II

BENNETT WM et al: *Drug Prescribing in Renal Failure: Dosing Guidelines for Adults.* Philadelphia, American College of Physicians, 1987

BROWN GR et al: Drug concentration monitoring. An approach to rational use. Clin Pharmacokinet 24:187, 1993

MEYER UA: Drugs in special patient groups: Clinical importance of genetics in drug effects, in *Clinical Pharmacology: Basic Principles in Therapeutics*, 3rd ed, KL Melmon et al (eds). New York, McGraw-Hill, 1992, p 875

NEBERT DW et al: The P450 superfamily: Update on new sequences, gene mapping and recommended nomenclature. DNA Cell Biol 10:1, 1992

REYNOLDS DJ, ARONSON JK: ABCs of monitoring drug therapy. Making the most of plasma drug concentration measurements. BMJ 306:48, 1993

TUKEY RH, JOHNSON EF: Molecular aspects of regulation and structure of drug metabolizing enzymes, in *Principles of Drug Action: The Basis of Pharmacology*, 3d ed, WB Pratt, P Taylor (eds). New York, Churchill Livingstone, 1990, p 423

67   ADVERSE REACTIONS TO DRUGS

ALASTAIR J. J. WOOD*

The beneficial effects of drugs are coupled with the inescapable risk of untoward effects. The morbidity and mortality from these untoward effects often present diagnostic problems because they can involve every organ and system of the body and are frequently mistaken for signs of underlying disease.

Major advances in the investigation, development, and regulation of drugs ensure in most instances their uniformity, effectiveness, and relative safety, as well as identify their recognized hazards. However, the large number and variety of drugs available over the counter (OTC) or by prescription make it impossible for patient or physician to obtain or retain the knowledge necessary to use all drugs well. It is understandable, therefore, that many OTC drugs are used unwisely by the public and that restricted drugs may be prescribed incorrectly by physicians.

Most physicians use no more than 50 drug products in their practice, gaining familiarity with their effectiveness and safety. Most patients probably use only a limited number of OTC drugs. Nevertheless, many patients receive care and drug prescriptions from more than one physician, and in any 30-day period many patients consume more than three different OTC drug products containing nine or more different chemical agents.

Twenty-five to fifty percent of patients may make errors in self-administration of prescribed medicines, and this can be responsible for adverse drug effects. Elderly patients are most likely to commit such errors, perhaps reflecting their consumption of increased numbers of medicines. One-third or more of patients also may not take their prescribed medications. Similarly, patients commit errors in taking OTC drugs by not reading or following the directions for use of the medicines on the containers. Physicians must recognize that providing directions with prescriptions does not always guarantee compliance.

Every drug can produce untoward consequences, even when used according to standard or recommended methods of administration. When used incorrectly, the effectiveness may be reduced, and adverse reactions can be expected to occur more frequently. The administration of several drugs during the same period of time also may result in adverse interactions between drugs (see Chap. 66).

In the hospital, all drugs a patient is given should be under the control of a physician, and patient compliance is, in general, ensured. Errors may occur nevertheless, in that the wrong drug or dose may be given or the drug may be given to the wrong patient, although improved drug distribution and administration systems have reduced this problem. On the other hand, there are no means for controlling how ambulatory patients take prescription or OTC drugs.

EPIDEMIOLOGY   Epidemiologic studies of adverse drug reactions have been helpful in evaluating the magnitude of the overall problem, in calculating the rate of reactions to individual drugs, and in characterizing some of the determinants of adverse drug effects.

Patients receive, on average, 10 different drugs during each hospitalization. The sicker the patient, the more drugs are given, and there is a corresponding increase in the likelihood of adverse drug reactions. When fewer than 6 different drugs are given to hospitalized

patients, the probability of an adverse reaction is about 5 percent, but if more than 15 drugs are given, the probability is over 40 percent. Retrospective analyses of ambulatory patients have revealed adverse drug effects in 20 percent.

Thus the magnitude of drug-induced disease is large. Two to five percent of patients are admitted to the medical and pediatric services of general hospitals because of illnesses attributed to drugs. The case/fatality ratio from drug-induced disease in hospitalized patients varies from 2 to 12 percent. Furthermore, some fetal or neonatal abnormalities are due to medicines taken by the mother during pregnancy or parturition.

A small group of widely used drugs accounts for a disproportionate number of reactions; aspirin, digoxin, anticoagulants, diuretics, antimicrobials, steroids, antineoplastics, and hypoglycemic agents account for 90 percent of reactions.

ADVERSE DRUG REACTIONS IN THE ELDERLY   (See also Chap. 8)   The elderly as a group have a greater burden of disease and receive a greater number of medications. Thus it is not surprising that adverse drug reactions occur frequently in elderly patients. The issue of whether an elderly individual is more likely to develop an adverse drug reaction than a young person with a similar number of concurrent diseases and other therapy has not been unequivocally demonstrated. Although it is widely believed that the elderly are more sensitive to drugs than the young, this is not true for all drugs. For example, a consistent decrease in sensitivity to drugs acting at the beta-adrenergic receptor has been demonstrated in the elderly. The consequences of adverse drug effects may differ in the elderly because of their greater likelihood of other disease. For example, long half-life benzodiazepine use is linked to the occurrence of hip fractures in elderly patients, perhaps reflecting both a risk of falls from these drugs and the increased incidence of osteoporosis in elderly patients. Even when a drug impairs function similarly in different age groups the poorer baseline function in the elderly may put them at greater risk for an adverse drug reaction. When prescribing for an individual elderly patient the possibility that drug excretion, either by hepatic metabolism or renal excretion, may be impaired should be taken into account by the prescribing physician. Adverse drug effects in the elderly may be subtle and, as in all populations, the physician must be alert to the possibility that a patient's signs and symptoms may reflect an adverse effect of medication.

ETIOLOGY   Most adverse reactions can be classified into two groups. The most frequent result from the exaggerated but predicted pharmacologic action of the drug. Other adverse reactions ensue from toxic effects unrelated to the intended pharmacologic actions. These therefore are often unpredictable, are frequently severe, and result from recognized as well as undiscovered mechanisms. Some mechanisms of extrapharmacologic toxicity include direct cytotoxicity, initiation of abnormal immune responses, and perturbation of metabolic processes in individuals with genetic enzymatic defects.

EXAGGERATION OF THE INTENDED PHARMACOLOGIC EFFECT   By prior consideration of the known factors that modify drug action, these adverse reactions often are preventable.

Abnormally high drug concentration at the receptor site (site of action) due to the pharmacokinetic variability is the usual cause (see Chap. 66). For example, reduction in the volume of distribution, in the rate of metabolism, or in the rate of excretion all result in higher than expected concentration of drug at the receptor site with consequent increase in pharmacologic effect.

Recently, the specific cytochrome P450s involved in drug metabolism have been identified. Recognition of the polymorphic distribution of some of these enzyme activities within the population provides both an explanation for the interindividual variability in drug clearance and the expectation that as simple tests are developed to characterize an individual's specific cytochrome P450 activity it will be possible to identify, in advance, individuals at particular risk for concentration-related adverse effects. For enzymes whose activity is polymorphically distributed, a proportion of the population has low or absent enzyme activity. In these individuals, the concentration of drugs achieved will

* John A. Oates was coauthor in the 12th edition and this chapter represents a revision of that work.

be higher than normal and may produce toxicity. Conversely, where toxicity or efficacy is produced by a metabolite, the inability of poor metabolizers to produce that metabolite will limit toxicity or efficacy in such individuals. The polymorphic distribution of drug-metabolizing enzymes may explain some adverse drug effects previously labeled as idiosyncratic.

Alteration in the dose-response curve due to increased receptor sensitivity results in an increase in drug effect at the same concentration. An example of this is seen in the excessive response to the anticoagulant warfarin at normal or lower than normal blood levels in the elderly.

The shape of the dose-response curve itself also determines the likelihood of the development of adverse drug reactions. Drugs with a steep dose-response curve are more likely to be associated with dose-related toxicity because of the small increase in dose required to produce a large change in pharmacologic effect. An increase in the dose of drugs which exhibit nonlinear kinetics, such as phenytoin (see Chap. 66), may produce a proportionately greater increase in the blood level, resulting in toxicity.

Concomitant drug therapy may affect the pharmacokinetics or pharmacodynamics of other drugs. Pharmacokinetics may be affected by alterations in bioavailability, protein binding, or the rate of metabolism or excretion. Pharmacodynamics may be altered by competition for receptor sites, by preventing the drug from reaching its site of action, or by antagonism or enhancement of the drug's pharmacologic effect. Inhibition of the metabolism of one drug by another may occur when both drugs bind to the same cytochrome P450. Therefore, with increased identification of the specific cytochrome P450 responsible for metabolism of individual drugs, prediction of drug interactions is now on a more rational scientific basis (see Chap. 66).

TOXICITY UNRELATED TO A DRUG'S PRIMARY PHARMACO-LOGIC ACTIVITY Cytotoxic reactions The understanding of so-called idiosyncratic reactions has greatly improved with the recognition that many of these reactions are due to irreversible binding of drug or metabolites to tissue macromolecules by shared electron (covalent) bonds. Some chemical carcinogens such as the alkylating agents combine directly with DNA. Usually, it is only after metabolic activation to reactive metabolites that covalent binding occurs. This activation usually occurs in the microsomal mixed-function oxidase system, the hepatic enzyme system responsible for the metabolism of many drugs (Chap. 66). During the course of drug metabolism, reactive metabolites may covalently bind to tissue macromolecules, causing tissue damage. Because of the reactive nature of these metabolites, covalent binding often occurs close to the site of production, such as the liver, but the mixed-function oxidase system is found in other tissues as well.

An example of this type of adverse drug reaction is the hepatotoxicity associated with isoniazid, which is metabolized principally by acetylation to acetylisoniazid, which is then hydrolyzed to acetylhydrazine. The further metabolism of acetylhydrazine by the mixed-function oxidase system liberates reactive metabolites that covalently bind to hepatic macromolecules, causing hepatic necrosis. The administration of drugs known to increase the activity of the mixed-function oxidase system, such as phenobarbital or rifampin, together with isoniazid is associated with the production of increased amounts of reactive metabolites, increased covalent binding, and hepatic damage.

The hepatic necrosis produced by overdosage of acetaminophen is also caused by reactive metabolites. Normally these metabolites are detoxified by combining with hepatic glutathione. When glutathione becomes exhausted, the metabolites bind instead to hepatic protein, with resultant hepatocyte damage. The hepatic necrosis produced by the ingestion of acetaminophen can be prevented, or at least attenuated, by the administration of substances such as *N*-acetylcysteine, which reduce the binding of electrophilic metabolites to hepatic proteins. The risks of hepatic necrosis are increased in patients receiving drugs such as phenobarbital that increase the rate of drug metabolism and rate of production of toxic metabolite(s).

It is likely, though as yet not proven, that other idiosyncratic reactions are caused by the covalent binding of reactive metabolites to tissue macromolecules, with either direct cytotoxicity or via the initiation of an immunologic response.

Immunologic mechanisms Most pharmacologic agents are poor immunogens because they consist of small molecules with molecular weights less than 2000. Stimulation of antibody synthesis or sensitization of lymphocytes by a drug or one of its metabolites usually requires in vivo activation and covalent linkage to protein, carbohydrate, or nucleic acid.

Drug stimulation of antibody production may mediate tissue injury by one of several mechanisms. The antibody may attack the drug affixed to a cell by covalent linkage and thereby destroy the cell, as occurs in penicillin-induced hemolytic anemia. Complexes of antibody-drug-antigen may be passively adsorbed by a bystander cell which is destroyed by activation of complement; this occurs in quinine- and quinidine-induced thrombocytopenia. Drugs or their reactive metabolites may alter host tissue, rendering it antigenic, and stimulate autoantibodies; for example, hydralazine and procainamide can chemically alter nuclear material, stimulate formation of antinuclear antibodies, and occasionally cause lupus erythematosus. Autoantibodies may be stimulated by drugs which neither interact with the host antigen nor have any chemical similarity to the host tissue; e.g., alpha methyldopa frequently stimulates formation of antibodies to host erythrocytes, yet the drug does not itself attach to the erythrocyte or share any chemical similarities with the antigenic determinants on the erythrocyte.

Drug-induced *pure red cell aplasia* (Chap. 308) is due to an immunologic-based drug reaction. Red cell formation in bone marrow cultures can be inhibited by phenytoin and purified IgG obtained from a patient with pure red cell aplasia associated with phenytoin.

Serum sickness (Chap. 282) results from deposition of circulating drug-antibody complexes on endothelial surfaces. Complement activation occurs, chemotactic factors are generated locally, and an inflammatory response appears at the site of complex entrapment. Arthralgias, urticaria, lymphadenopathy, glomerulonephritis, or cerebritis may result. Penicillin is the most common cause of serum sickness today. Many drugs, particularly the antimicrobial agents, induce production of IgE, which affixes to mast cell membranes. Contact with a drug antigen initiates a series of biochemical events within the mast cell and results in the release of mediators that may produce urticaria, wheezing, flushing, rhinorrhea, and occasionally hypotension characteristic of anaphylaxis.

Drugs also may excite cell-mediated immune responses. Topically administered substances may interact with sulfhydryl or amino groups in the skin and react with sensitized lymphocytes to produce the rash characteristic of contact dermatitis. Other types of rashes also may appear from the interaction of serum factors, drugs, and sensitized lymphocytes. The role of drug-activated lymphocytes in the immune mechanisms governing destruction of visceral tissue is unknown.

Toxicity associated with genetically determined enzymatic defects In the porphyrias, drugs that increase the activity of enzymes proximal to the deficient enzyme in the biosynthetic pathway of porphyrins can increase the quantity of porphyrin precursors that accumulate proximal to the deficient enzyme (Chap. 346). These drugs are listed in Table 67-1.

Patients with a deficiency of glucose-6-phosphate dehydrogenase (G6PD) develop hemolytic anemia on primaquine and a number of other drugs (Table 67-1) that do not cause hemolysis in patients with adequate quantities of this enzyme (Chap. 307).

Diagnosis The manifestations of drug-induced diseases frequently resemble those of other diseases and may be produced by different and dissimilar drugs. Recognition of the role of a drug or drugs responsible for illness is dependent on appreciation of the possible adverse reactions to drugs in any disease, identification of a temporal relationship between drug administration and development of illness, and familiarity with the manifestations most often caused by particular drugs. Although specific reactions have been described

TABLE 67-1   Clinical manifestations of adverse reactions to drugs

I MULTISYSTEM MANIFESTATIONS

Anaphylaxis	Angioedema	Drug-induced lupus	Fever
ACE inhibitors and dialysis	ACE inhibitors	erythematosus	Aminosalicylic acid
Cephalosporins		Acebutolol	Amphotericin B
Demeclocycline		Asparaginase	Antihistamines
Dextran		Barbiturates	Novobiocin
Insulin		Bleomycin	Penicillins
Iodinated drugs or contrast		Cephalosporins	Hyperpyrexia
media		Hydralazine	Antipsychotics
Iron dextran		Iodides	Serum sickness
Lidocaine		Isoniazid	Aspirin
Penicillins		Methyldopa	Penicillins
Procaine		Phenolphthalein	Propylthiouracil
Streptomycin		Phenytoin	Streptomycin
Sulfobromophthalein		Procainamide	Sulfonamides
		Quinidine	
		Sulfonamides	
		Thiouracil	

II ENDOCRINE MANIFESTATIONS

Addisonian-like syndrome	Sexual dysfunction	Thyroid function tests,	Vaginal carcinoma
Busulfan	Impaired ejaculation:	disorders of	Diethylstilbestrol (given to
Etomidate	Bethanidine	Acetazolamide	mother)
Ketoconazole	Debrisoquin	Amiodarone	
Galactorrhea (may also	Guanethidine	Bromsulfophthalein	
cause amenorrhea)	Thioridazine	Chlorpropamide	
Methyldopa	Decreased libido and impotence:	Clofibrate	
Phenothiazines	Beta blockers	Colestipol and	
Reserpine	Clonidine	nicotinic acid	
Tricyclic antidepressants	Diuretics	Dimercaprol	
Gynecomastia	Lithium	Gold salts	
Calcium channel	Major tranquilizers	Iodides	
antagonists	Methyldopa	Lithium	
Digitalis	Oral contraceptives	Oral contraceptives	
Estrogens	Sedatives	Phenindione	
Ethionamide	Impairment of spermatogenesis	Phenothiazines (long-term)	
Griseofulvin	or oogenesis:	Phenylbutazone	
Isoniazid	Cytotoxics	Phenytoin	
Methyldopa	Priapism:	Sulfonamides	
Phenytoin	Trazodone	Tolbutamide	
Reserpine			
Spironolactone			
Testosterone			

III METABOLIC MANIFESTATIONS

Hyperbilirubinemia	Hyperkalemia	Hyperuricemia	Metabolic acidosis
Novobiocin	ACE inhibitors	Aspirin	Acetazolamide
Rifampin	Amiloride	Chlorthalidone	Paraldehyde (degraded)
Hypercalcemia	Cytotoxics	Cytotoxics	Phenformin
Antacids with absorbable	Digitalis overdose	Ethacrynic acid	Salicylates
alkali	Heparin	Fructose (IV)	Spironolactone
Thiazides	Lithium	Furosemide	Porphyria exacerbation
Vitamin D	Pentamidine	Hyperalimentation	Barbiturates
Hyperglycemia	Potassium preparations	Thiazides	Chlordiazepoxide
Chlorthalidone	including salt substitute	Hyponatremia	Chlorpropamide
Diazoxide	Potassium salts of drugs	Dilutional:	Estrogens
Encainide	Spironolactone	Antipsychotics	Glutethimide
Ethacrynic acid	Succinylcholine	Carbamazepine	Griseofulvin
Furosemide	Triamterene	Chlorpropamide	Meprobamate
Glucocorticoids	Hypokalemia	Cyclophosphamide	Oral contraceptives
Growth hormone	Alkali-induced alkalosis	Desmopressin	Phenytoin
Oral contraceptives	Amphotericin B	Diuretics	Rifampin
Thiazides	Carbenoxolone	Octreotide	Sulfonamides
Hypoglycemia	Corticosteroids	Vincristine	
Insulin	Diuretics	Salt wasting:	
Octreotide	Gentamicin	Diuretics	
Oral hypoglycemics	Insulin	Enemas	
Pentamidine	Laxative abuse	Mannitol	
Quinine	Mineralocorticoids,		
	some glucocorticoids		
	Osmotic diuretics		
	Sympathomimetics		
	Tetracycline (degraded)		
	Theophylline		
	Vitamin B_{12}		

(continued)

TABLE 67-1   Clinical manifestations of adverse reactions to drugs (continued)

IV DERMATOLOGIC MANIFESTATIONS

Acne
  Anabolic and androgenic
    steroids
  Bromides
  Glucocorticoids
  Iodides
  Isoniazid
  Oral contraceptives
  Troxidone
Alopecia
  Beta blockers
  Cytotoxics
  Ethionamide
  Heparin
  Oral contraceptives (withdrawal)
Eczema
  Captopril
  Cream and lotion
    preservatives
  Lanolin
  Topical antihistamines
  Topical antimicrobials
  Topical local anesthetics

Erythema multiforme or
    Steven-Johnson
    syndrome
  Barbiturates
  Chlorpropamide
  Codeine
  Ethosuximide
  Penicillins
  Phenylbutazone
  Phenytoin
  Salicylates
  Sulfonamides
  Sulfones
  Tetracyclines
  Thiazides
  Tocainide
Erythema nodosum
  Oral contraceptives
  Penicillins
  Sulfonamides
Exfoliative dermatitis
  Barbiturates
  Gold salts
  Penicillins
  Phenylbutazone
  Phenytoin
  Quinidine
  Sulfonamides
Fixed drug eruptions
  Barbiturates
  Captopril
  Foscarnet (penile ulceration)
  Phenolphthalein
  Phenylbutazone
  Quinine
  Salicylates
  Sulfonamides

Hyperpigmentation
  Bleomycin
  Busulfan
  Chloroquine and other
    antimalarials
  Corticotropin
  Cyclophosphamide
  Gold salts
  Hypervitaminosis A
  Oral contraceptives
  Phenothiazines
Lichenoid eruptions
  Aminosalicylic acid
  Antimalarials
  Chlorpropamide
  Gold salts
  Methyldopa
  Phenothiazines
Photodermatitis
  Captopril
  Chlordiazepoxide
  Furosemide
  Griseofulvin
  Nalidixic acid
  Oral contraceptives
  Phenothiazines
  Sulfonamides
  Sulfonylureas
  Tetracyclines, particularly
    demeclocycline
  Thiazides

Purpura (see also
    thrombocytopenia)
  Aspirin
  Glucocorticoids
  Rashes (nonspecific)
  Allopurinol
  Ampicillin
  Barbiturates
  Indapamide
  Methyldopa
  Phenytoin
Skin necrosis
  Warfarin
Toxic epidermal necrolysis
    (bullous)
  Allopurinol
  Barbiturates
  Bromides
  Iodides
  Nalidixic acid
  Penicillins
  Phenolphthalein
  Phenylbutazone
  Phenytoin
  Sulfonamides
Urticaria
  Aspirin
  Barbiturates
  Captopril
  Enalapril
  Penicillins
  Sulfonamides

V HEMATOLOGIC MANIFESTATIONS

Agranulocytosis (see also
    pancytopenia)
  Aprindine
  Captopril
  Carbimazole
  Chloramphenicol
  Cotrimoxazole
  Cytotoxics
  Gold salts
  Indomethacin
  Methimazole
  Oxyphenbutazone
  Phenothiazines
  Phenylbutazone
  Propylthiouracil
  Sulfonamides
  Tolbutamide
  Tricyclic antidepressants
Clotting abnormalities/
    Hypothrombinemia
  Cefamandole
  Cefoperazone
  Moxalactam
  Valproic acid
Eosinophilia
  Aminosalicylic acid
  Chlorpropamide
  Erythromycin estolate
  Imipramine
  L-Tryptophan
  Methotrexate
  Nitrofurantoin
  Procarbazine
  Sulfonamides

Hemolytic anemia
  Aminosalicylic acid
  Cephalosporins
  Chlorpromazine
  Dapsone
  Insulin
  Isoniazid
  Levodopa
  Mefenamic acid
  Melphalan
  Methyldopa
  Penicillins
  Phenacetin
  Procainamide
  Quinidine
  Rifampin
  Sulfonamides
Hemolytic anemia (in G6PD
    deficiency)
  Aminosalicylic acid
  Antimalarials, e.g.,
    primaquine
  Aspirin
  Chloramphenicol
  Cotrimoxazole
  Dapsone
  Nalidixic acid
  Nitrofurantoin
  Phenacetin
  Probenecid
  Procainamide
  Quinidine
  Sulfonamides
  Vitamin C
  Vitamin K

Leukocytosis
  Glucocorticoids
  Lithium
Lymphadenopathy
  Phenytoin
  Primidone
Megaloblastic anemia
  Cotrimoxazole
  Folate antagonists
  Nitrous oxide (repeated or
    prolonged exposure)
  Oral contraceptives
  Phenobarbital
  Phenytoin
  Primidone
  Triamterene
  Trimethoprim
Pancytopenia (aplastic anemia)
  Carbamazepine
  Chloramphenicol
  Cytotoxics
  Gold salts
  Mepacrine
  Mephenytoin
  Oxyphenbutazone
  Phenylbutazone
  Phenytoin
  Potassium perchlorate
  Quinacrine
  Sulfonamides
  Trimethadione
  Zidovudine (AZT)

Pure red cell aplasia
  Azathioprine
  Chlorpropamide
  Isoniazid
  Phenytoin
Thrombocytopenia
    (see also pancytopenia)
  Acetazolamine
  Aspirin
  Carbamazepine
  Carbenicillin
  Chlorpropamide
  Chlorthalidone
  Cotrimoxazole
  Digitoxin
  Furosemide
  Gold salts
  Heparin
  Indomethacin
  Isoniazid
  Methyldopa
  Moxalactam
  Novobiocin
  Oxyphenbutazone
  Phenylbutazone
  Phenytoin and other
    hydantoins
  Quinidine
  Quinine
  Thiazides
  Ticarcillin

(continued)

TABLE 67-1 Clinical manifestations of adverse reactions to drugs *(continued)*

VI CARDIOVASCULAR MANIFESTATIONS

Acute chest pain (nonischemic)	Arrhythmias	Fluid retention/congestive heart failure/edema	Hypertension
Bleomycin	Adriamycin	Beta blockers	Clonidine withdrawal
Angina exacerbation	Antiarrhythmic drugs	Calcium blockers	Corticotropin
Alpha blockers	Astemizole	Carbenoxolone	Cyclosporine
Beta-blocker withdrawal	Atropine	Diazoxide	Glucocorticoids
Ergotamine	Anticholinesterases	Estrogens	Monoamine oxidase inhibitors with sympathomimetics
Excessive thyroxine	Beta blockers	Indomethacin	
Hydralazine	Daunorubicin	Mannitol	NSAIDs (some)
Methysergide	Digitalis	Minoxidil	Oral contraceptives
Minoxidil	Emetine	Phenylbutazone	Sympathomimetics
Nifedipine	Erythromycin	Steroids	Tricyclic antidepressants with sympathomimetics
Oxytocin	Guanethidine	Verapamil	
Vasopressin	Lithium	Hypotension (see also arrhythmias)	Pericarditis
	Papaverine	Amiodarone (perioperative)	Emetine
	Phenothiazines, particularly thioridazine	Calcium channel blockers, e.g., nifedipine	Hydralazine
			Methysergide
	Sympathomimetics	Citrated blood	Procainamide
	Terfenadine	Diuretics	Pericardial effusion
	Theophylline	Interleukin 2	Minoxidil
	Thyroid hormone	Levodopa	Thromboembolism
	Tricyclic antidepressants	Morphine	Oral contraceptives
	Verapamil	Nitroglycerin	
	AV block	Phenothiazines	
	Clonidine	Protamine	
	Methyldopa	Quinidine	
	Verapamil		
	Cardiomyopathy		
	Adriamycin		
	Daunorubicin		
	Emetine		
	Lithium		
	Phenothiazines		
	Sulfonamides		
	Sympathomimetics		

VII RESPIRATORY MANIFESTATIONS

Airway obstruction (bronchospasm, asthma; see also anaphylaxis)	Cough	Pulmonary infiltrates	Respiratory depression
	ACE inhibitors	Acyclovir	Aminoglycosides
Beta blockers	Nasal congestion	Amiodarone	Hypnotics
Cephalosporins	Decongestant abuse	Azothioprine	Opiates
Cholinergic drugs	Guanethidine	Bleomycin	Polymyxins
NSAIDs, e.g., aspirin, indomethacin	Isoproterenol	Busulfan	Sedatives
	Oral contraceptives	Carmustine (BCNU)	Trimethaphan
	Reserpine	Chlorambucil	
Penicillins	Pulmonary edema	Cyclophosphamide	
Pentazocine	Contrast media	Melphalan	
Streptomycin	Heroin	Methotrexate	
Tartrazine (drugs with yellow dye)	Hydrochlorthiazide	Methysergide	
	Interleukin 2	Mitomycin C	
	Methadone	Nitrofurantoin	
	Propoxyphene	Procarbazine	
		Sulfonamides	

(continued)

as resulting from the use of particular drugs, there is always a "first," and any drug should be suspected of causing an adverse effect if the clinical setting is appropriate.

Illness related to a drug's pharmacologic action may be more easily recognized than illness attributable to immunologic or other mechanisms. For example, side effects such as cardiac arrhythmias in patients receiving digitalis, hypoglycemia in patients given insulin, and bleeding in patients receiving anticoagulants are more easily related to the drug than are symptoms such as fever or rash, which may be caused by many drugs or by other factors.

Once an adverse reaction is suspected, discontinuance of the suspected drug followed by disappearance of the reaction is presumptive evidence of a drug-induced illness. Reappearance of the reaction upon cautious readministration of the drug may provide confirmatory evidence of the relationship if such confirmation adds useful information to the future management of the patient without entailing undue risk. With concentration-dependent adverse reactions, lowering the dosage also may be followed by disappearance of the reaction, and

increasing the dose may cause it to reappear. When the reaction is thought to be allergic, however, readministration of the drug may be hazardous, since anaphylactic shock may develop. Readministration is unwise under these conditions unless alternative drugs are not available and treatment is mandatory.

If the patient is receiving many different drugs when an adverse reaction is suspected, the drugs most likely to be incriminated can usually be identified. All drugs may be discontinued at once, or if this is not practical, then drugs should be discontinued one at a time, starting with the drug under greatest suspicion, and the patient observed for signs of improvement. The time needed for a concentration-dependent adverse effect to disappear depends on the time required for the concentration to fall below the range associated with the adverse effect, and this, in turn, depends on the initial blood level and on the rate of elimination or metabolism of the drug. Adverse effects of drugs with long half-lives, such as phenobarbital, take a considerable time to disappear.

Drugs recognized as producing a number of reactions are listed in

TABLE 67-1 Clinical manifestations of adverse reactions to drugs (continued)

VIII GASTROINTESTINAL MANIFESTATIONS

Cholestatic hepatitis
- Acetohexamide
- Anabolic steroids
- Androgens
- Chlorpropamide
- Clavulanic acid/amoxicillin
- Cyclosporine
- Erythromycin estolate
- Flucloxacillin
- Gold salts
- Methimazole
- Nitrofurantoin
- Oral contraceptives
- Phenothiazines

Constipation or ileus
- Aluminum hydroxide
- Barium sulfate
- Calcium carbonate
- Ferrous sulfate
- Ganglionic blockers
- Ion exchange resins
- Opiates
- Phenothiazines
- Tricyclic antidepressants
- Verapamil

Diarrhea or colitis
- Antibiotics (broad-spectrum)
- Clindamycin
- Colchicine
- Digitalis
- Guanethidine
- Lactose excipients
- Lincomycin
- Magnesium in antacids
- Methyldopa
- Purgatives
- Reserpine
- Ticlopidine

Diffuse hepatocellular damage
- Acetaminophen (paracetamol)
- Acebutolol
- Allopurinol
- Aminosalicylic acid
- Amiodarone
- Aprindine
- Cyclophosphamide
- Dapsone
- Diclofenac
- Erythromycin estolate
- Ethionamide
- Glyburide
- Halothane
- Isoniazid
- Ketoconazole
- Labetalol
- Lovastatin
- Methimazole
- Methotrexate
- Methoxyflurane
- Methyldopa
- Monoamine oxidase inhibitors
- Niacin
- Nifedipine
- Nitrofurantoin
- Oxyphenisatin
- Phenytoin and other hydantoins
- Propoxyphene
- Propylthiouracil
- Pyridium
- Rifampin
- Salicylates
- Sodium valproate
- Sulfonamides
- Tetracyclines
- Verapamil
- Zidovudine (AZT)

Gallstones/biliary pseudolithiasis
- Ceftriaxone

Intestinal ulceration
- Solid KCl preparations

Malabsorption
- Aminosalicylic acid
- Antibiotics (broad spectrum)
- Cholestyramine
- Colchicine
- Colestipol
- Cytotoxics
- Neomycin
- Phenobarbital
- Phenytoin
- Primidone

Nausea or vomiting
- Digitalis
- Estrogens
- Ferrous sulfate
- Levodopa
- Opiates
- Potassium chloride
- Tetracyclines
- Theophylline

Oral conditions
- Dental discoloration:
  - Tetracycline
- Dry mouth:
  - Anticholinergics
  - Clonidine
  - Levodopa
  - Methyldopa
  - Tricyclic antidepressants
- Gingival hyperplasia:
  - Calcium antagonists
  - Cyclosporine
  - Phenytoin

Salivary gland swelling:
- Bethanidine
- Bretylium
- Clonidine
- Guanethidine
- Iodides
- Phenylbutazone

Taste disturbances:
- Acetazolamide
- Biguanides
- Captopril
- Griseofulvin
- Lithium
- Metronidazole
- Penicillamine
- Rifampin

Ulceration:
- Aspirin
- Cytotoxics
- Gentian violet
- Isoproterenol (sublingual)
- Pancreatin

Pancreatitis
- Azathioprine
- Ethacrynic acid
- Furosemide
- Glucocorticoids
- Opiates
- Oral contraceptives
- Sulfonamides
- Thiazides

Peptic ulceration or hemorrhage
- Aspirin
- Ethacrynic acid
- Glucocorticoids
- NSAIDs
- Reserpine (large doses)

IX RENAL MANIFESTATIONS

Bladder dysfunction
- Anticholinergics
- Disopyramide
- Monoamine oxidase inhibitors
- Tricyclic antidepressants

Calculi
- Acetazolamide
- Vitamin D

Concentrating defect with polyuria (or nephrogenic diabetes insipidus)
- Demeclocycline
- Lithium
- Methoxyflurane
- Vitamin D

Hemorrhage cystitis
- Cyclophosphamide

Interstitial nephritis
- Ciprofloxacin
- Allopurinol
- Furosemide
- NSAIDs
- Penicillins, esp. methicillin
- Phenindione
- Sulfonamides
- Thiazides

Nephropathies
- Due to analgesics (e.g., phenacetin)

Nephrotic syndrome
- Captopril
- Gold salts
- Penicillamine
- Phenindione
- Probenecid

Obstructive uropathy
- Extrarenal: methysergide
- Intrarenal: cytotoxics

Renal dysfunction
- Cyclosporin
- NSAIDs
- Pentamidine
- Triamterene

Renal tubular acidosis
- Acetazolamide
- Amphotericin B
- Degraded tetracycline

Tubular necrosis
- Aminoglycosides
- Amphotericin B
- Cephaloridine
- Colistin
- Cyclosporin
- Methoxyflurane
- Polymyxins
- Radioiodinated contrast medium
- Sulfonamides
- Tetracyclines

(continued)

Table 67-1. This table includes well-documented and some less well-documented reactions that are sufficiently devastating as to require consideration. It should be used to suggest the likely causative drug, but the absence of a drug from the table does not mean that it is not responsible for the reaction.

Serum antibody has been demonstrated in some persons with drug allergy involving cellular blood elements, as in agranulocytosis, hemolytic anemia, and thrombocytopenia. For example, both quinine and quinidine can produce platelet agglutination in vitro in the presence of complement and the serum from a patient who has developed thrombocytopenia following this drug.

Eliciting a drug history from patients is important for diagnosis.

Attention must be directed to nonprescription, or OTC, as well as to prescription drugs. Each type can be responsible for adverse drug effects, and adverse interactions may occur between OTC drugs and prescribed drugs. In addition, it is common for patients to be cared for by several physicians, and duplicative, additive, counteractive, or synergistic drugs may therefore be taken if the physicians are not aware of the patients' drug histories. Every physician should determine what drugs a patient has been taking, at least during the preceding 30 days, before prescribing any medications. A frequently overlooked source of additional drug exposure is topical therapy; for example, the patient complaining of bronchospasm who is using an ophthalmic beta blocker may not volunteer such drug use to the physician unless

TABLE 67-1   Clinical manifestations of adverse reactions to drugs (continued)

X NEUROLOGIC MANIFESTATIONS

Exacerbation of myasthenia
  Aminoglycosides
  Polymyxins
Extrapyramidal effects
  Butyrophenones,
    e.g., haloperidol
  Levodopa
  Methyldopa
  Metoclopramide
  Oral contraceptives
  Phenothiazines
  Reserpine
  Tricyclic antidepressants
Headache
  Bromides
  Ergotamine (withdrawal)
  Glyceryl trinitrate
  Hydralazine
  Indomethacin

Peripheral neuropathy
  Amiodarone
  Chloramphenicol
  Chloroquine
  Chlorpropamide
  Cisplatin
  Clioquinol
  Clofibrate
  Demeclocycline
  Disopyramide
  Ethambutol
  Ethionamide
  Glutethimide
  Hydralazine
  Isoniazid
  Methysergide
  Metronidazole
  Mustine
  Nalidixic acid
  Nitrofurantoin

  Perhexiline
  Phenelzine
  Phenytoin
  Polymyxin, colistin
  Procarbazine
  Streptomycin
  Tolbutamide
  Tricyclic antidepressants
  Vincristine
Pseudotumor cerebri (or
    intracranial hypertension)
  Amiodarone
  Glucocorticoids,
    mineralocorticoids
  Hypervitaminosis A
  Oral contraceptives
  Tetracyclines

Seizures
  Amphetamines
  Analeptics
  Imipenem
  Isoniazid
  Lidocaine
  Lithium
  Nalidixic acid
  Penicillins
  Phenothiazines
  Physostigmine
  Theophylline
  Tricyclic antidepressants
  Vincristine
Sleep disorders
  Lovastatin
Stroke
  Oral contraceptives
Tremor
  Beta-adrenergic agonists

XI OCULAR MANIFESTATIONS

Cataracts
  Busulfan
  Chlorambucil
  Glucocorticoids
  Phenothiazines
Color vision alteration
  Barbiturates
  Digitalis
  Methaqualone
  Streptomycin
  Sulfonamides
  Thiazides
  Troxidone

Corneal edema
  Oral contraceptives
Corneal opacities
  Chloroquine
  Indomethacin
  Mepacrine
  Vitamin D
Eye pain
  Nifedipine
Glaucoma
  Ipratropium bromide
  Mydriatics
  Sympathomimetics

Optic neuritis
  Aminosalicylic acid
  Chloramphenicol
  Clioquinol
  Ethambutol
  Isoniazid
  Penicillamine
  Phenothiazines
  Phenylbutazone
  Quinine
  Streptomycin

Retinopathy
  Chloroquine
  Phenothiazines

XII EAR MANIFESTATIONS

Deafness
  Aminoglycosides
  Aspirin
  Bleomycin
  Chloroquine
  Cisplatin
  Deferoxamine
  Erythromycin
  Ethacrynic acid
  Furosemide
  Mustine
  Nortriptyline
  Quinine

Vestibular disorders
  Aminoglycosides
  Mustine
  Quinine

XIII MUSCULOSKELETAL MANIFESTATIONS

Bone disorders
  Osteoporosis:
    Glucocorticoids
    Heparin
  Osteomalacia:
    Aluminum hydroxide
    Anticonvulsants
    Glutethimide

Myopathy or myalgia
  Amphotericin B
  Carbenoxolone
  Chloroquine
  Clofibrate
  Glucocorticoids
  Oral contraceptives
Rhabdomyolysis
  Gemfibrozil
  Lovastatin

XIV PSYCHIATRIC MANIFESTATIONS

Delirious or confusional states
  Amantadine
  Aminophylline
  Anticholinergics
  Antidepressants
  Bromides
  Cimetidine
  Digitalis
  Glucocorticoids
  Isoniazid
  Levodopa
  Methyldopa
  Penicillins
  Phenothiazines
  Sedatives and hypnotics

Depression
  Amphetamine withdrawal
  Beta blockers
  Centrally acting
    antihypertensives
    (reserpine, methyldopa,
    clonidine)
  Glucocorticoids
  Levodopa
Drowsiness
  Antihistamines
  Anxiolytic drugs
  Clonidine
  Major tranquilizers
  Methyldopa
  Reserpine
  Tricyclic antidepressants

Hallucinatory states
  Amantadine
  Beta blockers
  Levodopa
  Meperidine
  Narcotics
  Pentazocine
  Tricyclic antidepressants
Hypomania, mania, or excited
    reactions
  Glucocorticoids
  Levodopa
  MAO inhibitors
  Sympathomimetics
  Tricyclic antidepressants
Hypersexuality
  Antiparkinsonians

Schizophrenic-like or
    paranoid reactions
  Amphetamines
  Bromides
  Glucocorticoids
  Levodopa
  Lysergic acid
  Monoamine oxidase
    inhibitors
  Tricyclic antidepressants
Sleep disturbances
  Anorexiants
  Levodopa
  Monoamine oxidase
    inhibitors
  Sympathomimetics

specifically asked. A history of previous adverse drug effects in patients is common. Since these patients have a predisposition to other drug-induced illnesses, eliciting such a history should dictate added caution in prescribing drugs.

Patients with biochemical abnormalities such as erythrocyte G6PD deficiency can be identified; patients with the defect are usually blacks or of Mediterranean descent. Drug-induced hemolytic crisis can be avoided by testing for the enzyme defect before administering these drugs. Similarly, persons with an abnormal serum pseudocholinesterase may have abnormally prolonged apnea when given succinylcholine.

General comments   No drug is completely without side effects, and a side effect in one patient may be the desired pharmacologic effect in another. Current drug regulations allow physicians to prescribe drugs with considerable confidence in their purity, bioavailability, and effectiveness. However, physicians have to weigh the potential toxicity against the possible benefits. Thus toxicity that would be acceptable for an effective antineoplastic agent would not be permitted in an oral contraceptive. Because of the necessarily small number of patients treated in premarketing studies, rare adverse reactions cannot be identified, so the first responsibility for identifying and reporting these effects must rest with the practicing clinician through the use of the various national adverse reaction reporting systems, such as those operated by the Food and Drug Administration in the United States and the Committee on Safety of Medicines in Great Britain. The publication of a newly recognized adverse reaction can in a short time stimulate many similar such reports of reactions that previously had gone unrecognized.

The prevention of adverse drug reactions first involves a high index of suspicion that the development of a new symptom or sign may be drug-related. Reduction of the dose or discontinuation of the suspected agent usually clarifies the position in concentration-dependent toxic reactions. Physicians should be familiar with the common adverse effects of the drugs they use and, if they are in doubt, should consult the literature.

REFERENCES

BRENNAN TA et al: Incidence of adverse events and negligence in hospitalized patients: Results of the Harvard Medical Practice Study I. N Engl J Med 324:370, 1991

DAVIES DM: *Textbook of Adverse Drug Reactions*, 4th ed. New York, Oxford University Press, 1991

FELDMANN U: Design and analysis of drug safety studies, with special reference to sporadic drug use and acute adverse reactions. J Clin Epidemiol 46:237, 1993

HOIGNÉ R et al: Risk factors for adverse drug reactions: Epidemiological approaches. Eur J Clin Pharmacol 39:321, 1990

LEAPE LL et al: The nature of adverse events in hospitalized patients. Results of the Harvard Medical Practice Study II. N Engl J Med 324:377, 1991

Reactions Annual 89. Auckland, New Zealand, Adis Press, 1989

Reactions Annual 90. Auckland, New Zealand, Adis Press, 1990

RIEDER MJ: Immunopharmacology and adverse drug reactions. J Clin Pharmacol 33:316, 1993

STOUKIDES CA et al: Adverse drug reaction surveillance in an emergency room. Am J Hosp Pharm 50:712, 1993

WALLER PC: Measuring the frequency of adverse drug reactions. Br J Clin Pharmacol 33:249, 1992

68   PHYSIOLOGY AND PHARMACOLOGY OF THE AUTONOMIC NERVOUS SYSTEM

LEWIS LANDSBERG / JAMES B. YOUNG

FUNCTIONAL ORGANIZATION OF THE AUTONOMIC NERVOUS SYSTEM

The autonomic nervous system innervates vascular and visceral smooth muscle, exocrine and endocrine glands, and parenchymal cells throughout the various organ systems. Functioning below the conscious level, the autonomic nervous system responds rapidly and continuously to perturbations that threaten the constancy of the internal environment. The many functions governed by this system include the distribution of blood flow and the maintenance of tissue perfusion, the regulation of blood pressure, the regulation of the volume and composition of the extracellular fluid, the expenditure of metabolic

energy and supply of substrate, and the control of visceral smooth muscle and glands.

Autonomic responses, like those of the somatic nervous system, are induced promptly and dissipated quickly, in contrast to the slower, more prolonged effects of circulating hormones. The autonomic nervous system, like the endocrine system, regulates the rate of processes that have intrinsic activities of their own, while the somatic nervous system initiates responses de novo. Although certain autonomic responses are discriminating, many are generalized and influence a variety of effectors in different organs. The interface between the autonomic nervous system and the endocrine system is exemplified by the adrenal medulla. This gland, homologous in many respects with the postganglionic sympathetic neuron, secretes a hormone (epinephrine) into the circulation to interact with adrenergic receptors throughout the body.

ANATOMIC ORGANIZATION   The autonomic neurons, located in ganglia outside the central nervous system, give rise to the postganglionic autonomic nerves that innervate organs and tissues throughout the body (Fig. 68-1). The activity of autonomic nerves is regulated by central neurons responsive to diverse afferent inputs. After central integration of afferent information, autonomic outflow

FIGURE 68-1   Schematic representation of the autonomic nervous system. (*From Moskowitz M: Diseases of the autonomic nervous system. Clin Endocrinol Metab 6:77, 1977.*)

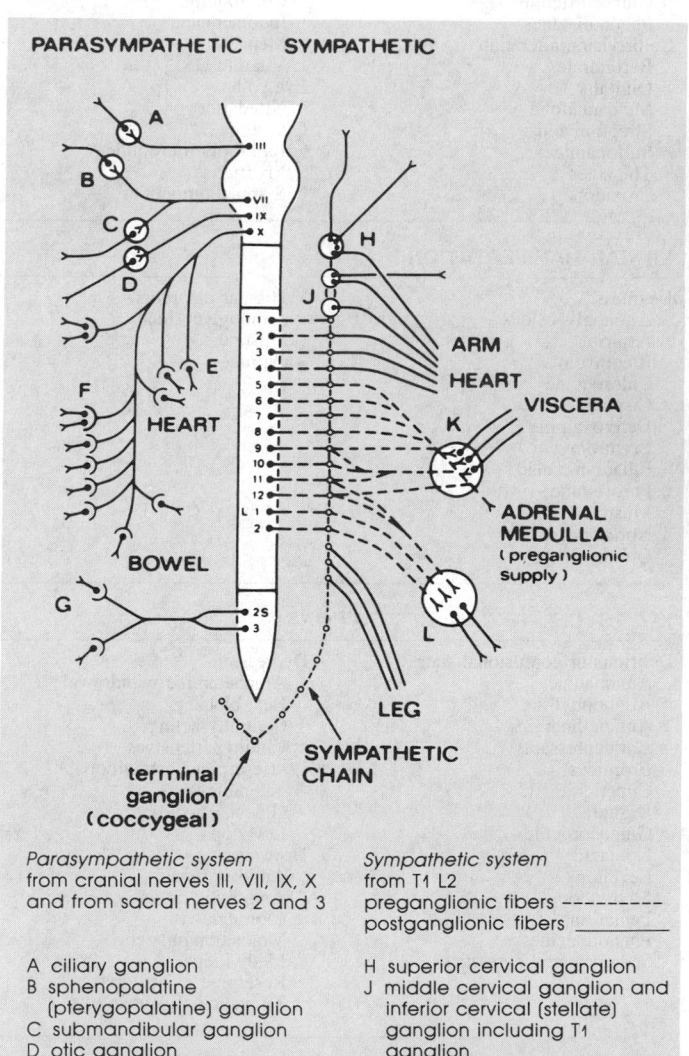

Parasympathetic system from cranial nerves III, VII, IX, X and from sacral nerves 2 and 3

Sympathetic system from T1 L2
preganglionic fibers ---------
postganglionic fibers _____

A ciliary ganglion
B sphenopalatine (pterygopalatine) ganglion
C submandibular ganglion
D otic ganglion
E vagal ganglion cells in heart wall
F vagal ganglion cells in bowel wall
G pelvic ganglia

H superior cervical ganglion
J middle cervical ganglion and inferior cervical (stellate) ganglion including T1 ganglion
K coeliac and other abdominal ganglia
L lower abdominal sympathetic ganglia

is adjusted to permit the functioning of the major organ systems in accordance with the needs of the organism as a whole. Connections between the cerebral cortex and the autonomic centers in the brainstem coordinate autonomic outflow with higher mental functions.

The sympathetic and parasympathetic divisions   The preganglionic neurons of the parasympathetic nervous system leave the central nervous system in the third, seventh, ninth, and tenth cranial nerves and in the second and third sacral nerves, while the preganglionic neurons of the sympathetic nervous system exit the spinal cord between the first thoracic and the second lumbar segments (Fig. 68-1). Responses to sympathetic and parasympathetic stimulation are frequently antagonistic, as exemplified by their opposing effects on heart rate and gut motility. This antagonism reflects highly coordinated interactions within the central nervous system; the resultant changes in parasympathetic and sympathetic activity, often reciprocal, provide more precise control of autonomic responses than could be achieved by the modulation of a single system.

Neurotransmitters   *Acetylcholine* (ACh) is the preganglionic neurotransmitter for both divisions of the autonomic nervous system, as well as the postganglionic neurotransmitter of the parasympathetic neurons. Nerves that release ACh are said to be cholinergic. *Norepinephrine* (NE) is the neurotransmitter of the postganglionic sympathetic neurons; these nerves are said to be adrenergic. Within the sympathetic outflow, postganglionic neurons innervating the eccrine sweat glands (and perhaps some blood vessels supplying skeletal muscle) are of the cholinergic type.

THE SYMPATHETIC NERVOUS SYSTEM AND THE ADRENAL MEDULLA

CATECHOLAMINES   All three of the naturally occurring catecholamines, NE, *epinephrine* (E), and *dopamine*, function as neurotransmitters within the central nervous system. NE, the neurotransmitter of postganglionic sympathetic nerve endings, exerts its effects locally, in the immediate vicinity of its release. E, the circulating hormone of the adrenal medulla, influences processes throughout the body. A peripheral dopaminergic system also exists but has not been characterized in detail.

Biosynthesis (Fig. 68-2)   Catecholamines are synthesized from the amino acid tyrosine, which is sequentially hydroxylated to form dihydroxyphenylalanine (dopa), decarboxylated to form dopamine, and hydroxylated on the beta position of the side chain to form NE. The initial step, the hydroxylation of tyrosine, is rate-limiting and is regulated so that synthesis of dopa is coupled to norepinephrine release. This regulation is achieved by alterations in both the activity and the amount of tyrosine hydroxylase. In the adrenal medulla and in those central neurons utilizing E as neurotransmitter, NE is *N*-methylated to E by the enzyme phenylethanolamine-*N*-methyltransferase (PNMT).

Catecholamine metabolism (Fig. 68-2)   The major metabolic transformations of catecholamines involve *O*-methylation at the meta-hydroxyl group and oxidative deamination. *O*-Methylation is catalyzed by the enzyme catechol-*O*-methyltransferase (COMT), and oxidative deamination is promoted by monoamine oxidase (MAO). COMT in liver and kidney is important in the metabolism of circulating catecholamines. MAO, a mitochondrial enzyme present in most tissues, including nerve endings, has a lesser role in the metabolism of circulating catecholamines but is important in regulating the catecholamine stores within the peripheral sympathetic nerve endings. The metanephrines and 4-hydroxy-3-methoxymandelic acid (VMA) are the major end products of N and NE metabolism. Homovanillic acid (HVA) is the end product of dopamine metabolism.

STORAGE AND RELEASE OF CATECHOLAMINES   In both the adrenal medulla and sympathetic nerve endings catecholamines are stored in subcellular granules and released by exocytosis. The large stores of catecholamines in these tissues provide an important physiologic reserve that maintains an adequate supply of catechol-

amines in the face of intense stimulation. A variety of substances may be stored along with catecholamines in sympathetic nerve endings and adrenal medulla and released with catecholamines during exocytosis. These substances, which may function as cotransmitters or neuromodulators, include peptides such as neuropeptide Y, substance P, and enkephalins; purines such as ATP and adenosine; and other amines such as serotonin. At the neuroeffector junction, coreleased neuromodulators modify the response to NE, while cotransmitters exert physiologic effects independent of those induced by NE.

Adrenal medulla   The adrenal medullary chromaffin tissue in a pair of normal human adrenal glands weighs about 1 g and contains approximately 6 mg catecholamines, 85 percent of which is E. Catecholamines are maintained in high concentration within the storage (chromaffin) granule by several complex processes including (1) an inwardly directed H^+-transporting ATPase in the chromaffin granule membrane which maintains a steep hydrogen ion concentration and an acidic (pH 5.5) internal milieu, (2) an amine carrier that is saturable, stereospecific, favors the naturally occurring substrate (dopamine), and is inhibited by the reserpine class of agents, and (3) an intragranular storage complex that involves ATP and acidic glycoproteins called *chromagranins*. The high internal H^+ concentration tends to trap catecholamines in their protonated form and provides the driving force for the amine pump; H^+ egress down its electrochemical gradient is coupled to carrier-mediated amine uptake from the cytoplasm. These mechanisms permit very high concentrations of catecholamines to be stored within the granules. Both the inwardly directed H^+-ATPase and chromagranins have a widespread distribution in the neurosecretory granules of other parts of the endocrine system, including the anterior pituitary, pancreatic islets, and parathyroids.

Catecholamine secretion, stimulated by ACh from the preganglionic sympathetic nerves, occurs after calcium influx triggers fusion of the chromaffin granule membrane and cell membrane; obliteration of the cell membrane at the point of fusion and extrusion of the entire soluble contents of the granule into the extracellular space complete the process of exocytosis (Fig. 68-2). Although the molecular mechanisms involved in the exocytotic process are only partially understood, evidence has accumulated that a specific calcium-binding protein is involved. Once bound, calcium induces a conformational change in this protein which forms a hydrophobic rod that penetrates chromaffin granule membranes favoring fusion of granules and docking of granules at the cell membrane. Approximately 2 to 10 percent of the total adrenal medullary catecholamine store is turned over each day.

Peripheral sympathetic nerve endings   The peripheral sympathetic nerve endings form a reticulum or ground plexus that brings the terminal fibers into close contact with effector cells. All the NE in peripheral tissues is in the sympathetic nerve endings, and heavily innervated tissues contain as much as 1 to 2 μg/g of tissue. NE stored in the nerve endings is in discrete subcellular particles analogous to the adrenal medullary chromaffin granules. MAO in the mitochondria of the nerve endings plays an important role in regulating the local concentration of NE (Fig. 68-2). Amines in storage vesicles are protected from oxidative deamination; amines within the cytoplasm, however, are deaminated to inactive metabolites. Release from the nerve ending occurs in response to action potentials propagated in terminal sympathetic fibers (Fig. 68-2).

THE PERIPHERAL ADRENERGIC NEUROEFFECTOR JUNCTION   Neuronal uptake   The peripheral sympathetic nerve endings possess an amine transport system that actively takes up amines from the extracellular fluid. A variety of synthetic and naturally occurring amines are substrates for this process. Neuronal uptake or recapture of locally released NE terminates the action of the transmitter and contributes to the constancy of the NE stores (Fig. 68-2). An NE transporter from human cells has been cloned and the amino acid sequence deduced. The structure of the protein inferred from the nucleotide sequence is remarkably similar to the transporter for gamma aminobutyric acid (GABA) as well as to recently cloned transporters

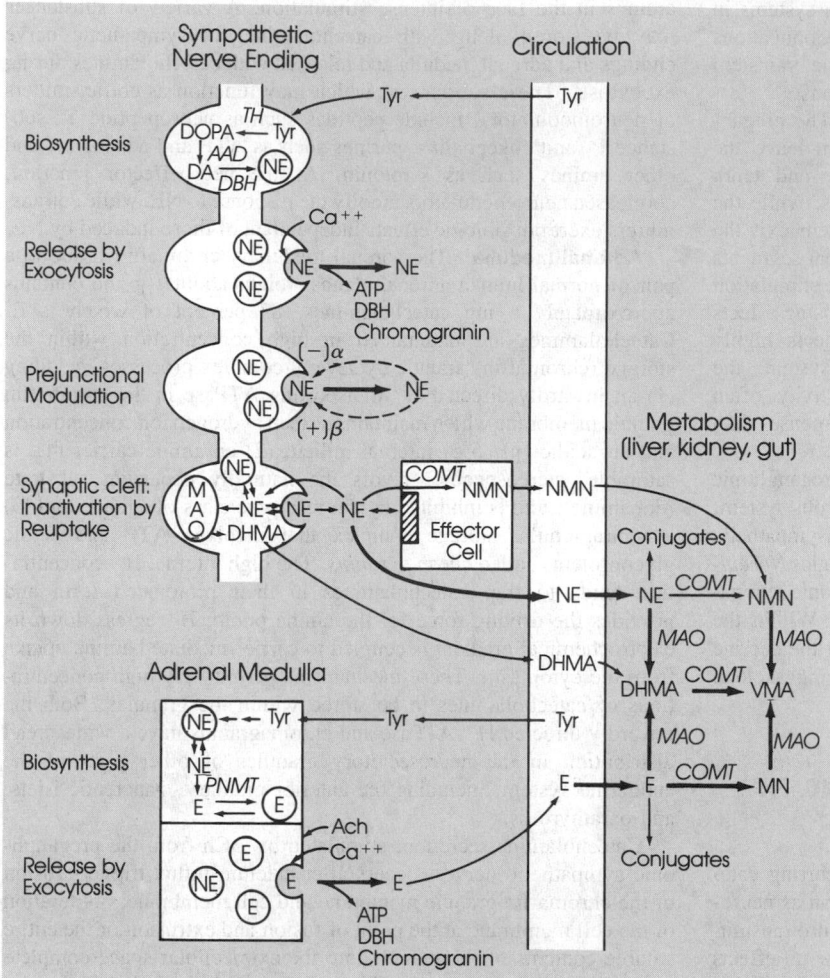

FIGURE 68-2 Catecholamine biosynthesis, release, and metabolism. Schematic representation of a peripheral sympathetic nerve ending is shown at the top; the bulbous areas on the terminal fiber represent varicosities identified by histochemical fluorescence techniques as areas of high neurotransmitter concentration. The processes of biosynthesis, release, modulation, and reuptake are shown sequentially for demonstration purposes only; in vivo they proceed concurrently. Adrenal medullary chromaffin cells are shown at the bottom of the diagram. (TH = tyrosine hydroxylase, AAD = aromatic-l-amino acid decarboxylase, DA = dopamine, DBH = dopamine-β-hydroxylase, NE = norepinephrine, PNMT = phenylethanolamine-N-methyltransferase, E = epinephrine, COMT = catechol-O-methyltransferase, NMN = normetanephrine, MAO = monoamine oxidase, DHMA = 3,4-dihydroxymandelic acid, VMA = 3-methoxy-4-hydroxymandelic acid.)

for dopamine and serotonin, suggesting the existence of a superfamily of neurotransmitter transporter genes.

Prejunctional modulation A variety of factors alter the relationship between neuronal impulse traffic and NE release. Diminished temperature and acidosis, for example, both decrease the amount of NE released in response to sympathetic impulses. Several chemical mediators operate at the peripheral sympathetic nerve ending (referred to as prejunctional or presynaptic sites) to modify sympathetic neurotransmission by influencing the amount of NE released in response to nerve impulses. Prejunctional modulation may be either inhibitory or facilitatory. Certain modulators, such as catecholamines and ACh, may either inhibit or facilitate NE release, antagonistic effects that are mediated by different adrenergic or cholinergic receptors, respectively. Those compounds exerting an *inhibitory* effect on NE release at the prejunctional nerve ending include the following: catecholamines (alpha$_2$ receptor), ACh (muscarinic receptor), dopamine (D-2 receptor), histamine (H-2 receptor), serotonin, adenosine, enkephalins, and prostaglandins. *Facilitatory* prejunctional modulators include catecholamines (beta$_2$ receptor), ACh (nicotinic receptor), and angiotensin II. The overall significance of prejunctional modulation, as well as the relative importance of the various mediators, has yet to be established, although increasing evidence indicates that many of these compounds exert a significant modulatory role in vivo. Antagonizing the facilitatory actions of angiotensin II at the neuroeffector junction may contribute to the antiadrenergic effects of angiotensin-converting enzyme inhibitors.

PREJUNCTIONAL ADRENERGIC RECEPTORS Catecholamines reduce NE release via prejunctional alpha receptors in a classic negative feedback system. Feedback regulation is complicated by the fact that beta-receptor activation facilitates NE release. This may be explained by the finding that prejunctional beta receptors (beta$_2$, see below) are

more sensitive to E than NE; this differential sensitivity could result in facilitation of NE release by circulating E. Infused E in fact augments NE release in humans. Release of E from sympathetic nerve endings (under conditions of intense adrenal medullary stimulation) also has been demonstrated, implying that E taken up in sympathetic nerve endings from the circulation and released as a cotransmitter may influence NE release as well.

PREJUNCTIONAL CHOLINERGIC RECEPTORS Though both inhibitory and facilitatory effects of ACh on NE release have been described, the inhibitory effect of ACh, mediated by the muscarinic cholinergic receptor, occurs at lower ACh concentrations and is probably of greater physiologic significance. This peripheral inhibitory effect of ACh on adrenergic neurotransmission may reinforce the reciprocal changes in central parasympathetic and sympathetic outflow that occur in the regulation of numerous physiologic responses.

CENTRAL REGULATION OF SYMPATHOADRENAL OUTFLOW

Brainstem sympathetic centers Sympathetic outflow is initiated from the reticular formation of the medulla oblongata and pons and from centers in the hypothalamus. The rostral ventral portion of the medulla, particularly the area designated the rostral ventrolateral medulla (RVLM), appears to contain especially important sympathoexcitatory areas. Descending fibers originating from these centers synapse in the intermediolateral cell column of the spinal cord with the preganglionic sympathetic neurons. The brainstem sympathetic centers, which have an intrinsic activity of their own, are regulated by many stimuli, including impulses from more rostral areas of the central nervous system (cortex, limbic lobe, hypothalamus), neural afferents that interact at the level of the brainstem centers and at the higher centers, and changes in the physical and chemical properties of the extracellular fluid, including the circulating levels of hormones and substrates. The area postrema, in the floor of the fourth ventricle, lies outside the blood-brain barrier and may play an important role in this regard. The higher centers, which have connections with the brainstem, coordinate sympathetic outflow with higher mental functions, emotional reactions, and the homeostatic needs of the internal environment. Although the hallmark of intense sympatho-adrenal stimulation is a global response (the fight-or-flight reaction of Cannon), discrete changes in sympathetic outflow to different organ systems continuously regulate many autonomic functions.

RELATIONSHIP BETWEEN THE SYMPATHETIC NERVOUS SYSTEM AND THE ADRENAL MEDULLA Sympathetic nervous system activity and adrenal medullary secretion are coordinated but not always congruent. During periods of intense sympathetic stimulation, such as cold exposure and exhaustive exercise, the adrenal medulla is progressively recruited, and circulating E reinforces the physiologic effects of sympathetic stimulation. In other situations, the sympathetic nervous system and the adrenal medulla are stimulated independently. The response to upright posture, for example, involves predominantly the sympathetic nervous system, while hypoglycemia stimulates only the adrenal medulla. An important role for the adrenal medulla may be to provide circulating catecholamines to support vital functions when the sympathetic nervous system is suppressed.

Sympathetic regulation of the cardiovascular system Stretch receptors in the systemic and pulmonary arteries and veins continuously monitor intravascular pressures; the resulting afferent impulses, after relay and integration in the brainstem, alter sympathetic activity in defense of blood pressure and blood flow to critical areas (Fig. 68-3).

ARTERIAL BARORECEPTORS An increase in blood pressure stimulates receptors in the carotid sinus and aortic arch. The ensuing afferent impulses, after relay within the nucleus of the solitary tract (NTS) in the brainstem, suppress the brainstem sympathetic centers (Fig. 68-3). This baroreceptor reflex arc forms a negative-feedback loop in which a rise in arterial pressure results in the inhibition of central sympathetic outflow. A brainstem noradrenergic pathway interacts with the NTS to participate in suppression of sympathetic outflow. This noradrenergic inhibitory pathway is stimulated by centrally acting alpha-adrenergic agonists and may be involved in the action of certain antihypertensive drugs, such as clonidine, that

potentiate the baroreceptor-mediated vasodepressor response (Chap. 209). In the opposite manner, when the blood pressure falls, decreased afferent impulses diminish central inhibition, resulting in an increase in sympathetic outflow and a rise in arterial pressure.

CENTRAL VENOUS PRESSURE Receptors in the walls of the great veins and within the atria are also involved in the regulation of sympathetic outflow. Stimulation of these receptors by high venous pressure suppresses the brainstem sympathetic centers; when central venous pressure is low, sympathetic outflow increases. The central connections are poorly understood, but the afferent impulses are carried in the vagus (Fig. 68-3).

ASSESSMENT OF SYMPATHOADRENAL ACTIVITY The clinical assessment of sympathoadrenal activity involves the measurement of catecholamines in plasma and of catecholamines and catecholamine metabolites in urine. Quantitation of urinary catecholamines and metabolites is useful in the diagnosis of pheochromocytoma (Chap. 336).

Plasma catecholamines Catecholamines in human plasma may be measured by radioenzymatic isotope derivative techniques or by high-performance liquid chromatography in conjunction with electrochemical detection. Plasma catecholamine measurements provide an index of sympathetic nervous system and adrenal medullary activity and have been widely used to assess sympathoadrenal activity in clinical investigation in human subjects. The usefulness of plasma catecholamine measurements is, however, compromised by factors that alter the relationship between the plasma concentration of catecholamines and the functional state of the sympathoadrenal system, and also by important regional differences in sympathetic outflow. Techniques utilizing tracer infusions of tritiated NE, which correct for changes in NE clearance when applied across a particular anatomic region, estimate regional sympathetic outflow with some precision and have helped to define differentiated sympathetic nervous system activity in the investigational setting. The clinical usefulness of plasma catecholamine levels remains limited to the evaluation of patients with autonomic insufficiency and, on occasion, patients with suspected pheochromocytoma (Chap. 336).

Basal plasma NE concentrations are in the range of 0.09 to 1.8 nmol/L (150 to 350 pg/mL); basal E levels are about 135 to 270 pmol/L (25 to 50 pg/mL). The half-time of disappearance of NE from the circulation is approximately 2 min. The plasma NE level is markedly affected by a variety of factors, including posture; accordingly, the conditions under which blood is obtained for assay must be controlled. By convention, basal plasma NE levels are those obtained through an indwelling intravenous line after the patient has rested supine in a relaxed environment for 30 min.

PLASMA NE RESPONSE TO UPRIGHT POSTURE The predictable increase in circulating NE concentration during upright posture provides a convenient test of sympathetic nervous system function. Five minutes of quiet standing results in a two- to threefold increase in plasma NE level. A normal response requires an intact afferent system, appropriate central nervous system relays, and an intact peripheral sympathetic nervous system; a defect of any of these components reduces the increment in circulating NE.

Plasma E levels are also dependent on the physical and mental state of the subject. Change in plasma E with upright posture is usually small. Hypoglycemia, strenuous exercise, and various types of mental stress, however, can cause large increments in the plasma E level.

PERIPHERAL DOPAMINERGIC SYSTEM

In addition to its role as neurotransmitter in the central nervous system, dopamine functions as an inhibitory transmitter in the carotid body and the sympathetic ganglia. A distinct peripheral dopaminergic system is also believed to exist. Dopamine elicits a variety of responses not attributable to stimulation of classic adrenergic receptors; it relaxes the lower esophageal sphincter, delays gastric emptying,

FIGURE 68-3 Symptomatic regulation of the circulation. Receptors in the venous and arterial circulations are stimulated by stretch, caused by an increase in pressure; afferent impulses from these receptors are carried to the central nervous system by the ninth (*IX*) and tenth (*X*) cranial nerves. The net result of these afferent impulses, after relay in the brainstem, is to inhibit central sympathetic outflow. The arterial baroreceptor reflex involves a relay in the nucleus of the tractus solitarius. (+ = stimulation; − = inhibition.)

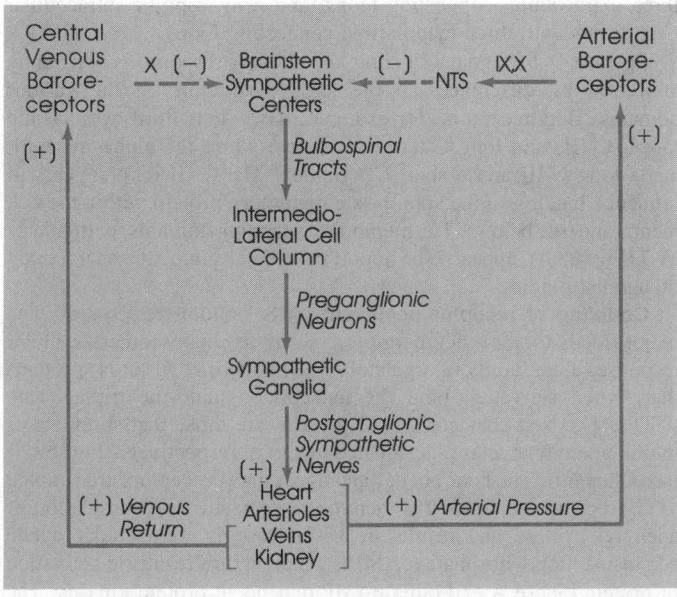

causes vasodilation in the renal and mesenteric arterial circulation, suppresses aldosterone secretion, directly stimulates renal sodium excretion, and suppresses NE release at sympathetic nerve terminals by a presynaptic inhibitory mechanism. The mediation of these dopaminergic effects in vivo is poorly understood. Dopamine does not appear to be a circulating hormone. Unequivocal evidence of peripheral autonomic dopaminergic nerves has not been produced, although such nerves may be present in the kidney. The kidney, furthermore, produces much of the dopamine in the urine, since the amount excreted each day (approximately 200 μg per 24 h) cannot be accounted for by clearance of plasma dopamine. Decarboxylation of circulating dopa, which is present in high concentration in the plasma [9 nmol/L (1500 pg/mL)] may contribute to urinary dopamine production. Dopamine generated from the decarboxylation of circulating dopa also might be involved in the mediation of dopaminergic effects in the kidney and other sites. Thus the nature of the peripheral dopaminergic system is obscure, but the existence of a dopaminergic system in those tissues that respond uniquely to dopamine seems likely.

ADRENERGIC RECEPTORS

Catecholamines influence effector cells by interacting with specific *receptors* on the cell surface. When stimulated by catecholamines, the adrenergic receptor initiates a series of membrane changes followed by a cascade of intracellular events that culminates in a measurable response. Compounds that elicit the response are referred to as *agonists;* those that block the interaction of the agonist with the receptor are referred to as *adrenergic receptor blocking agents* or *antagonists.*

Two major categories of response to catecholamines reflect the activation of two populations of adrenergic receptors, designated *alpha* and *beta*. Selective agonists and antagonists are available, enabling pharmacologic stimulation or blockade of the physiologic effects mediated by one receptor without influencing those mediated by the other. Both alpha and beta receptors have been further divided into subtypes that serve different functions and are susceptible to differential stimulation and blockade.

ALPHA-ADRENERGIC RECEPTORS   The alpha-adrenergic receptor mediates vasoconstriction, intestinal relaxation, and pupillary dilatation. E and NE are approximately equipotent as alpha-receptor agonists. Distinct alpha$_1$- and alpha$_2$-receptor subtypes are also recognized. Originally the postsynaptic or postjunctional alpha-adrenergic receptors on effector cells were designated alpha$_1$, while the prejunctional alpha-adrenergic receptors on the sympathetic nerve endings were designated alpha$_2$. It is now recognized that nonneuronal (postsynaptic) processes are mediated by the alpha$_2$ receptor as well. The alpha$_1$ receptor mediates the classic alpha effects, including vasoconstriction; phenylephrine and methoxamine are selective alpha$_1$ agonists, and prazosin is a selective alpha$_1$ antagonist. The alpha$_2$ receptor mediates presynaptic inhibition of NE release from adrenergic nerves and other responses, including inhibition of ACh release from cholinergic nerves, inhibition of lipolysis in adipocytes, inhibition of insulin secretion, stimulation of platelet aggregation, and vasoconstriction in some vascular beds. Specific alpha$_2$ agonists include clonidine and α-methylnorepinephrine; these agents, the latter derived from α-methyldopa in vivo, exert an antihypertensive effect by interacting with alpha$_2$ receptors within the brainstem sympathetic centers that regulate blood pressure. Yohimbine is a specific alpha$_2$ antagonist. Molecular biologic techniques support the further subdivision of both the alpha$_1$ and alpha$_2$ receptors into more or less distinct subtypes, suggesting the eventual potential for differential stimulation and blockade.

BETA-ADRENERGIC RECEPTORS   Physiologic events associated with beta-adrenergic receptor responses include stimulation of heart rate and contractility, vasodilation, bronchodilation, and lipolysis. Beta-receptor responses also can be divided into two types.

The beta$_1$ receptor responds equally to E and NE and mediates cardiac stimulation and lipolysis. The beta$_2$ receptor is more responsive to E than to NE and mediates responses such as vasodilation and bronchodilation. Isoproterenol stimulates and propranolol blocks both beta$_1$ and beta$_2$ receptors. Other agonists and antagonists that have partial selectivity for the beta$_1$ or beta$_2$ receptors have been used therapeutically where the desired response involves predominantly one of the two subtypes. Both pharmacologic and molecular genetic studies have suggested the possibility of an additional distinct beta$_3$-adrenergic receptor that subserves so-called atypical beta-adrenergic responses. Stimulation of heat production in brown adipose tissue has been suggested as a potentially important process mediated by this receptor. The full significance of this receptor remains to be elucidated.

DOPAMINERGIC RECEPTORS   Specific dopaminergic receptors, distinct from the classic alpha- and beta-adrenergic receptors, are present in the central and peripheral nervous system and in several nonneural tissues. Two types of dopaminergic receptors serve different functions and have different second messengers. Dopamine is a potent agonist of both types of receptors; the action of dopamine is antagonized by phenothiazines and thioxanthenes. The dopamine 1 receptor mediates vasodilation in the renal, mesenteric, coronary, and cerebral vascular beds. Fenoldopam is an investigational agonist selective for the dopamine 1 receptor. The dopamine 2 receptor inhibits transmission in the sympathetic ganglia, inhibits NE release from sympathetic nerve endings by an effect on the presynaptic membrane (Fig. 68-2), inhibits prolactin release from the pituitary, and causes vomiting. Selective agonists of the dopamine 2 receptor include bromocriptine, lergotrile, and apomorphine, while butyrophenones such as haloperidol (active within the central nervous system), domperidone (does not cross blood-brain barrier readily), and the benzamide sulpiride are relatively selective dopamine 2 antagonists.

STRUCTURE AND FUNCTION OF ADRENERGIC RECEPTORS
The utilization of recombinant DNA technology has substantially increased current understanding of the structure and function of adrenergic receptors. cDNAs of the four major adrenergic receptor subtypes have been cloned and their primary amino acid sequences deduced. It is clear from these studies that the adrenergic receptors belong to a superfamily of related membrane proteins that includes the visual protein rhodopsin and the muscarinic acetylcholine receptors. These proteins share significant sequence homologies and, as deduced from the properties of the constituent amino acids, a similar topographic structure in the cell membrane. The postulated structure of this family of receptor proteins is shown schematically in Fig. 68-4. The characteristic features include seven membrane-spanning hydrophobic domains containing 20 to 28 amino acids each (possibly arranged as alpha helices), a hydrophilic extracellular *N* terminus and three extracellular connecting loops, and a hydrophilic intracellular *C* terminus with three cytoplasmic connecting loops.

Specificity for agonist binding and effector response is apparently conferred by differences in the tertiary structure of the various domains. Beta receptors, for example, have short third cytoplasmic loops (C-III) and long *C*-terminal chains, while the alpha$_2$ receptor has a long C-III and a short *C* terminus. The C-III loop appears to influence binding to the appropriate regulatory protein within the cell membrane (see below). The membrane-spanning domains, particularly M-7 (Fig. 68-4), appear to be important in determining the characteristic agonist binding.

Coupling of receptor occupancy with cellular response   The major mediators of adrenergic (as well as many other) cellular responses are a family of regulatory proteins termed G (or N) proteins that, when activated, bind the nucleotide guanosine triphosphate (GTP). The best-characterized G proteins are those that stimulate or inhibit adenylyl cyclase, designated G$_s$ or G$_i$, respectively (Fig. 68-5) (see Chap 69). The beta$_1$, beta$_2$, and dopamine 1 receptors are coupled to G$_s$; receptor occupancy is therefore associated with stimulation of adenylyl cyclase and results in an increase in intracellular cyclic adenosine monophosphate (cAMP), which in turn results in activation of protein kinase A and other cAMP-dependent protein kinases. The

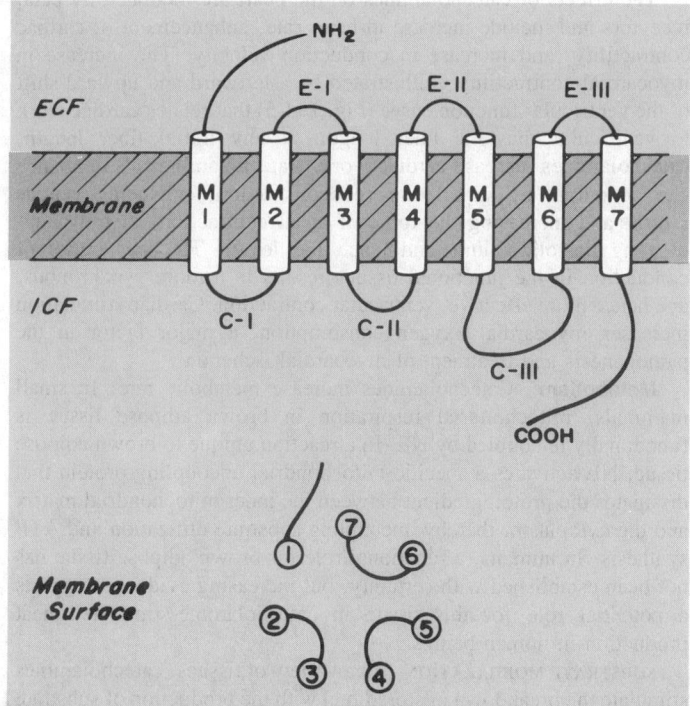

FIGURE 68-4 Proposed structure of adrenergic receptors as deduced from primary amino acid sequences. The single protein chain contains a hydrophilic N terminus (extracellular) and C terminus (intracellular) connected by seven lipophilic membrane-spanning regions (M-1 to M-7) which are interconnected by three extracellular loops (E-I to E-III) and three cytoplasmic loops (C-I to C-III). The beta$_1$, beta$_2$, alpha$_1$, and alpha$_2$ adrenergic receptors have appreciable sequence homologies and are believed to fit the general structural model represented. Specificity of agonist binding may be conferred by the tertiary structure of several of the membrane-spanning domains while specificity of intracellular response may be related to the length and tertiary structure of the cytoplasmic loops and C terminus. The top portion of the figure is a longitudinal representation of the receptor protein in the cell membrane; shown below is a hypothetical, more compact arrangement seen from the membrane surface. ECF = extracellular fluid; ICF = intracellular fluid. (*From Landsberg and JB Young, 1992.*)

resultant protein phosphorylation alters the activity of enzymes and the function of other proteins, culminating in a cellular response that is characteristic of the tissue being stimulated. The alpha$_2$, M-2 subtype of the muscarinic acetylcholine receptor and the dopamine 2 receptor are coupled to G$_i$, resulting in diminished adenylyl cyclase activity and a fall in cAMP. The subsequent alterations in enzyme activity and function of other proteins produce an alternate, frequently opposite, series of cellular responses. Although many alpha$_2$ responses can be explained by inhibition of adenylyl cyclase, other mechanisms may be involved as well.

The alpha$_1$-adrenergic receptor (as well as the M-1 subtype of the acetylcholine receptor) appears to be coupled to a different G protein that activates phospholipase C; this G protein has not been well characterized but is sometimes tentatively designated G$_p$. Receptor occupancy in this system stimulates phospholipase C, which catalyzes the breakdown of membrane-bound phospholipids, particularly phosphatidylinositol-4,5-bisphosphate (PIP$_2$) with the production of inositol-1,4,5-trisphosphate (IP$_3$) and 1,2-diacylglycerol (DAG), both of which act as second messengers (Fig. 68-5). IP$_3$ rapidly mobilizes calcium from intracellular stores within the endoplasmic reticulum, producing an increase in free cytoplasmic calcium which by itself and via calcium-calmodulin–dependent protein kinases influences cellular processes appropriate to the stimulated cell. The transient rise in calcium induced by IP$_3$ from the intracellular stores is reinforced in the presence of continued agonist stimulation by alterations in membrane calcium flux that result eventually in net calcium uptake from the extracellular fluid by mechanisms that have been incompletely defined.

DAG, the other second messenger produced by the action of phospholipase C on PIP$_2$ (as well as other membrane phospholipids), remains associated with the cell membrane and activates protein kinase C, which has different substrates than the calcium-calmodulin kinases stimulated by IP$_3$. Protein phosphorylation stimulated by protein kinase C contributes to the tissue-specific response in ways that remain poorly understood. Increases in intracellular calcium also potentiate the activation of protein kinase C (Fig. 68-5).

REGULATION OF ADRENERGIC RECEPTORS Radiolabeled adrenergic-receptor agonists and antagonists have been utilized as ligands to study adrenergic receptors. In combination with studies of peripheral tissue sensitivity, these studies demonstrated that changes

FIGURE 68-5 Interaction of autonomic agonists with membrane-bound regulatory proteins and cellular effectors systems. The designations α and β refer to adrenergic receptors, DA refers to dopaminergic receptors, and M, to muscarinic receptors. G designates the GTP-associated regulatory protein which may have a stimulatory (s) or inhibitory (i) effect on adenylyl cyclase or may stimulate phospholipase C (p). (+) designates stimulation; (−) designates inhibition. PIP$_2$ = phosphatidylinositol-4,5-bisphosphate; DAG = 1,2-diacylglycerol; IP$_3$ = inositol-1,4,5-trisphosphate. See text for details.

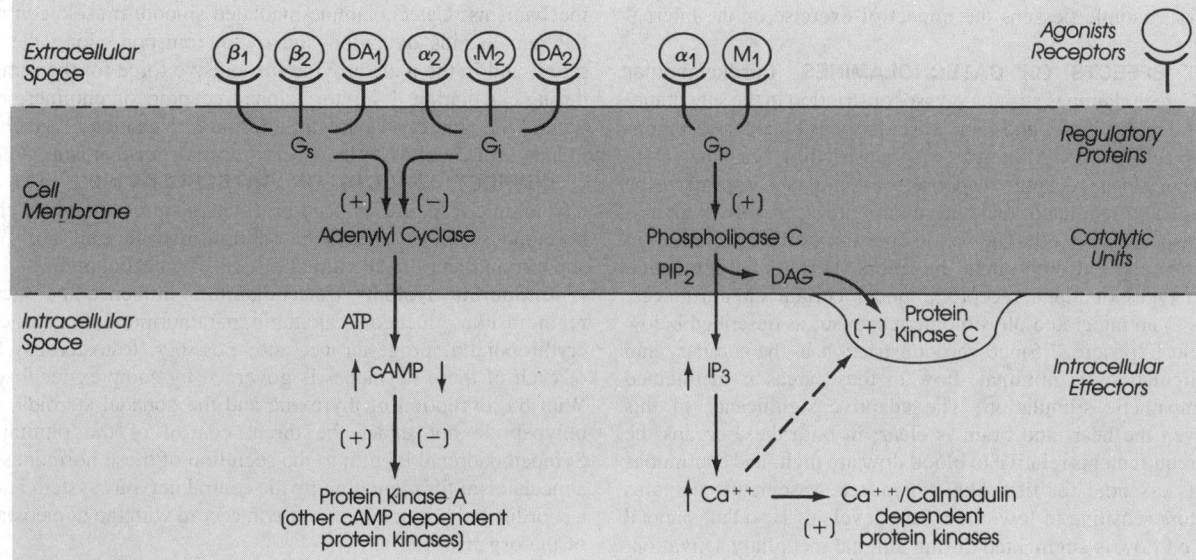

in adrenergic receptors occur under a variety of physiologic conditions. Prolonged exposure to alpha- or beta-adrenergic agonists decreases the number of corresponding adrenergic receptors on effector cells. Although the biochemical mechanisms involved are obscure, internalization of the beta-adrenergic receptor within the cell occurs during agonist exposure in some systems, suggesting that internal translocation contributes to the decrease in receptor number under these circumstances.

Alteration in agonist concentration also may affect the affinity of the receptor for the agonist. Adrenergic receptors that utilize adenylyl cyclase for the second messenger (beta receptors, alpha$_2$ receptors) exist in high and low affinity states; exposure to agonist diminishes the proportion of receptors in the high-affinity state. Such alterations in adrenergic receptors induced by adrenergic agonists are termed *homologous regulation*. Agonist-induced alterations in adrenergic-receptor density and affinity are believed to contribute to the diminished physiologic response that occurs after prolonged exposure of an effector tissue to adrenergic agonist, a phenomenon known as *tachyphylaxis* or *desensitization*. Recent evidence suggests that phosphorylation of the beta receptor by a specific beta-receptor kinase is involved in the desensitization phenomenon.

Adrenergic receptors are also influenced by factors other than adrenergic agonists, so-called *heterologous regulation*. Enhanced alpha-adrenergic-receptor affinity, for example, may underlie the potentiation of alpha-adrenergic responses that occur in response to lowered environmental temperatures. Thyroid hormones potentiate beta-receptor responses by alterations in beta-receptor number and in the efficiency of coupling receptor occupancy with physiologic response. Estrogen and progesterone alter the sensitivity of the myometrium to catecholamines by effects on alpha-adrenergic receptors. Glucocorticoids may influence adrenergic function by antagonizing agonist-induced decreases in adrenergic receptors, thereby counteracting tachyphylaxis in response to intense adrenergic stimulation. Some forms of heterologous desensitization may involve modifications in the membrane regulatory proteins or in adenylyl cyclase itself.

Alterations in sensitivity to catecholamines also occur as a consequence of postreceptor changes, although the latter remain poorly characterized.

PHYSIOLOGY OF THE SYMPATHOADRENAL SYSTEM

Catecholamines influence all the major organ systems. The effects take place in seconds as compared with the minutes, hours, or days that characterize the actions of the endocrine system and most other control systems that regulate bodily processes. The sympathoadrenal system, moreover, may respond in anticipation of physiologic requirement. An increase in sympathoadrenal activity prior to strenuous exercise, for example, lessens the impact of exercise on the internal environment.

DIRECT EFFECTS OF CATECHOLAMINES   Cardiovascular system   Catecholamines stimulate vasoconstriction in the subcutaneous, mucosal, splanchnic, and renal vascular beds by alpha-receptor–mediated mechanisms. Although vasoconstriction was originally considered an alpha$_1$-receptor response, vascular tone appears to be more complexly regulated and, in many areas, involves alpha$_2$-mediated responses as well. The venous portion of the circulation, in particular, is endowed with alpha$_2$ receptors. Differential regulation of the two types of alpha receptors, under certain circumstances, contributes to an integrated physiologic response, as described below under "Cold Exposure." Since vasoconstriction in the coronary and cerebral circulations is minimal, flow to these areas is maintained during sympathetic stimulation. The adaptive significance of this priority given the heart and brain is clear; in both these organs the metabolic requirements relative to blood flow are high, and continuous perfusion is essential for life. Skeletal muscle vasculature contains beta receptors sensitive to low circulating levels of E so that skeletal muscle blood flow is augmented during adrenal medullary activation.

The effects of catecholamines on the heart are mediated by beta$_1$ receptors and include increase in heart rate, enhancement of cardiac contractility, and increase in conduction velocity. The increase in myocardial contractility is illustrated by a leftward and upward shift of the ventricular function curve (Fig. 194-5) that relates cardiac work to ventricular diastolic fiber length; at any initial fiber length, catecholamines increase cardiac work. Catecholamines also enhance cardiac output by stimulating venoconstriction, enhancing venous return, and increasing the force of atrial contraction, thereby augmenting diastolic volume and hence fiber length. The acceleration of conduction in the junctional tissues results in a more synchronous, and hence more effective, ventricular contraction. Cardiac stimulation increases myocardial oxygen consumption, a major factor in the pathogenesis and treatment of myocardial ischemia.

Metabolism   Catecholamines increase metabolic rate. In small mammals, mitochondrial respiration in brown adipose tissue is functionally uncoupled by NE. In a reaction unique to brown adipose tissue, NE activates a specific mitochondrial uncoupling protein that dissipates the proton gradient between the inner mitochondrial matrix and the cytoplasm, thereby uncoupling substrate utilization and ATP synthesis. In humans, a functional role for brown adipose tissue has not been established with certainty, but increasing evidence suggests a potential role for this tissue in catecholamine-stimulated heat production in human beings.

SUBSTRATE MOBILIZATION   In a variety of tissues, catecholamines stimulate the breakdown of stored fuel with the production of substrate for local consumption; glycogenolysis in the heart, for example, provides substrate for immediate metabolism by the myocardium. Catecholamines also accelerate fuel mobilization in liver, adipose tissue, and skeletal muscle, liberating substrates (glucose, free fatty acids, lactate) into the circulation for use throughout the body. Activation of enzymes involved in fuel breakdown occurs by a beta-receptor (beta$_1$) mechanism for adipose tissue lipolysis and by alpha- and beta-receptor (beta$_2$) mechanisms for hepatic glycogenolysis and gluconeogenesis. In skeletal muscle, catecholamines stimulate glycogenolysis (beta receptor), thereby increasing lactate efflux.

Fluids and electrolytes   Catecholamines contribute to regulation of the volume and composition of extracellular fluid. By a direct action on the renal tubule, NE stimulates sodium reabsorption, thereby defending extracellular fluid volume. Dopamine, in contrast, promotes sodium excretion. NE and E also promote cellular uptake of potassium, thereby defending against the development of hyperkalemia. Effects of catecholamines on calcium, magnesium, and phosphate metabolism are complex and depend on a variety of factors.

Viscera   Catecholamines affect visceral function by actions on smooth muscle and glandular epithelium. Urinary bladder and intestinal smooth muscle are relaxed while the corresponding sphincters are stimulated. Gallbladder emptying also involves sympathetic mechanisms. Catecholamine-mediated smooth-muscle contraction in the female aids ovulation and ovum transport along the fallopian tubes, and in the male provides propulsive force for the seminal fluid during ejaculation. Inhibitory alpha$_2$ receptors on cholinergic neurons within the gut contribute to intestinal relaxation. Catecholamines induce bronchodilation by a beta$_2$-receptor mechanism.

INDIRECT EFFECTS OF CATECHOLAMINES   The ultimate physiologic response induced by catecholamines involves changes in hormone secretion and in blood flow distribution, both of which support and amplify the direct effects of catecholamines.

Endocrine system   Catecholamines influence the secretion of renin, insulin, glucagon, calcitonin, parathormone, thyroxine, gastrin, erythropoietin, progesterone, and, possibly, testosterone. Secretion of each of these hormones is governed by complex feedback loops. With the exception of thyroxine and the gonadal steroids, each is a polypeptide not under the direct control of the pituitary gland. Sympathoadrenal input into the secretion of these hormones provides a mechanism for regulation by the central nervous system and ensures a coordinated hormonal response in accord with the homeostatic needs of the organism.

RENIN (See also Chap. 209)   The juxtaglomerular apparatus of the kidney is heavily innervated. Sympathetic stimulation increases renin release by a direct beta-receptor effect independent of vascular changes within the kidney. The renin response to volume depletion is sympathetically mediated and is initiated by a fall in central venous pressure. Since renin secretion activates the angiotensin-aldosterone system, angiotensin-induced vasoconstriction supports the direct effects of catecholamines on blood vessels, while aldosterone-mediated sodium reabsorption complements the direct increase in sodium reabsorption induced by sympathetic stimulation. Beta-receptor blocking agents suppress renin secretion.

INSULIN AND GLUCAGON   The pancreatic islets also receive an extensive sympathetic innervation. Stimulation of pancreatic sympathetic nerves or an elevation in circulating catecholamines suppresses insulin and increases glucagon release. Inhibition of insulin secretion is mediated by the alpha$_2$ receptor, and stimulation of glucagon is mediated by the beta receptor. This combination of effects supports substrate mobilization, reinforcing the direct effects of catecholamines on hepatic glucose output and lipolysis. Although alpha-receptor–mediated suppression of insulin release usually predominates, a beta-receptor mechanism may augment insulin secretion under some circumstances.

SYMPATHOADRENAL FUNCTION IN SELECTED PHYSIOLOGIC AND PATHOPHYSIOLOGIC STATES   Support of the circulation

The sympathetic nervous system functions to maintain an adequate circulation. During upright posture and volume depletion, reduction of afferent venous and arterial baroreceptor impulse traffic diminishes an inhibitory input to the vasomotor center, thereby increasing sympathetic activity (Fig. 68-3) and reducing efferent vagal tone. As a result, heart rate is increased, and cardiac output is diverted from the skin, subcutaneous tissues, mucosa, and viscera. Sympathetic stimulation of the kidney increases sodium reabsorption, and sympathetically mediated venoconstriction enhances venous return. With pronounced hypotension, the adrenal medulla is recruited and E reinforces the effects of the sympathetic nervous system. A similar pattern of sympathetic activation occurs in the postprandial state when blood and extracellular fluid are sequestered in the splanchnic circulation and in the lumen of the gut, respectively.

The intense sympathoadrenal stimulation that accompanies severe volume depletion may contribute to the development of ketoacidosis in alcoholics as well as to the ketoacidosis sometimes seen in association with hyperemesis gravidarum. Under these circumstances, catecholamine-mediated suppression of insulin and stimulation of glucagon markedly potentiate ketogenesis. Volume resuscitation and provision of adequate glucose promptly reverse the ketoacidosis in most cases.

CONGESTIVE HEART FAILURE   The sympathetic nervous system also provides circulatory support during congestive heart failure (Chap. 195). Venoconstriction and sympathetic stimulation of the heart increase cardiac output while peripheral vasoconstriction directs blood flow to the heart and brain. The afferent signals are less clear than in simple volume depletion because the venous pressure is usually elevated. In severe heart failure, depletion of cardiac NE may impair the effectiveness of sympathetic circulatory support.

TRAUMA AND SHOCK   In acute traumatic injury or shock, adrenal catecholamines support the circulation and mobilize substrates. It is presumed, but unproved, that the sympathetic nervous system is activated as well, although some evidence suggests that suppression of the sympathetic nervous system may contribute to the hypotension that occurs in association with trauma. In the chronic, reparative phase following injury, catecholamines contribute to substrate mobilization and to the elevation in metabolic rate.

EXERCISE   Sympathetic activation during exercise increases cardiac output, maintains blood flow, and ensures sufficient substrate to meet the increased needs. Central neural factors, such as anticipation, and circulatory factors, such as fall in venous pressure, trigger the sympathetic response. Mild degrees of exercise stimulate the sympathetic nervous system alone; during more severe exertion the

adrenal medulla is activated as well. Conditioning is associated with a decrease in sympathetic nervous system activity both at rest and during exercise, in comparison with the untrained state.

Hypoglycemia (See also Chap. 338)   Hypoglycemia causes a marked increase in adrenal medullary E secretion. When glucose concentrations fall below overnight fasting levels, regulatory glucose-sensitive neurons in the central nervous system initiate a prompt increase in adrenal medullary secretion. The increase is especially intense at plasma glucose levels below 2.8 mmol/L (50 mg/dL), when plasma E levels increase 25 to 50 times above baseline, thereby increasing hepatic glucose output, providing alternative substrate in the form of free fatty acids, suppressing endogenous insulin release, and inhibiting insulin-mediated glucose utilization in muscle. Many clinical manifestations of hypoglycemia, such as tachycardia, palpitations, nervousness, tremor, and widened pulse pressure, are secondary to increased E secretion. These manifestations of E secretion constitute an "early warning" system in insulin-requiring diabetics. In patients with long-standing diabetes mellitus, however, the E response to hypoglycemia may be diminished or absent, leaving affected patients at greater risk to develop severe hypoglycemia.

Cold exposure   The sympathetic nervous system plays a critical role in the maintenance of normal body temperature during exposure to a cold environment. Receptors in the skin and central nervous system respond to a fall in temperature by activating hypothalamic and brainstem centers that increase sympathetic activity. Sympathetic stimulation leads to vasoconstriction in the superficial vascular beds, thereby diminishing heat loss. The sympathetic response involves a complex interaction between lowered environmental temperatures and alpha$_2$-adrenergic receptors. The superficial veins of the extremities are prominently endowed with alpha$_2$ receptors. Cold directly increases the vasoconstrictor response mediated by the alpha$_2$ receptor. The deep venous system, in contrast, is endowed with alpha$_1$ receptors which, in nonspecific fashion, diminish the constrictor response during environmental cooling. The net result is a shunting of blood from the superficial to the deep venous system. Since the deep veins run in close proximity to the major arteries supplying the limb, heat is efficiently returned to the central venous pool by a countercurrent exchange mechanism. Heat production is simultaneously increased by shivering, generation of metabolic heat, and substrate mobilization. Acclimatization during chronic cold exposure increases the capacity for metabolic heat production in response to sympathetic stimulation.

Dietary intake   Fasting suppresses and overfeeding stimulates the sympathetic nervous system. The reduction in sympathetic activity during fasting or starvation contributes to the decrease in metabolic rate, bradycardia, and hypotension in these states. Enhanced sympathetic activity during periods of increased caloric intake contributes to the elevation in metabolic rate associated with a chronic increase in dietary intake.

Hypoxia   Chronic hypoxia is associated with stimulation of the sympathoadrenal system, and some of the cardiovascular changes attendant to hypoxia are dependent on catecholamines.

THE SYMPATHETIC NERVOUS SYSTEM IN PATHOGENESIS OF SELECTED DISEASE STATES

HYPERTENSION (See also Chap. 209)   As shown in Fig. 68-6, regulation of arterial pressure by the sympathetic nervous system involves blood vessels, the heart, and the kidneys. The sympathetic nervous system increases peripheral resistance by direct stimulation of the resistance vessels and by activation of the renin-angiotensin system. Increased cardiac output is the result of enhanced cardiac contractility and augmented venous return, the latter a result of venoconstriction and increased renal sodium reabsorption. Stimulation of sodium retention alters the pressure natriuresis relationship, thereby diminishing the capacity of the kidney to compensate for the increase in blood pressure. Antiadrenergic agents lower blood pressure by interacting at many of the sites shown in Fig. 68-6.

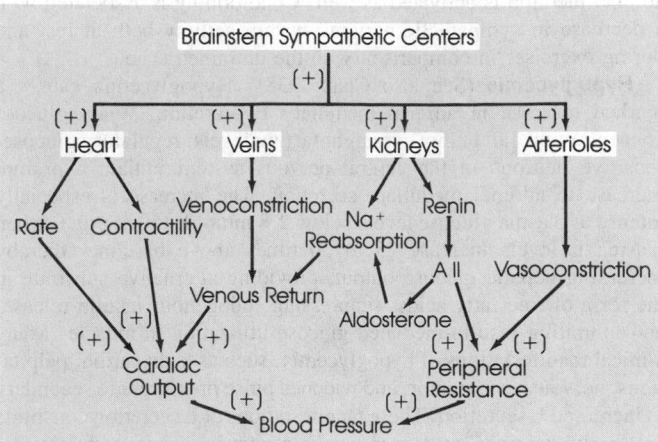

FIGURE 68-6 Sympathetic nervous system effects on blood pressure. Sympathetic stimulation (+) increases blood pressure by effects on the heart, the veins, the kidneys, and the arterioles. The net result of sympathetic stimulation is an increase in both cardiac output and peripheral resistance. AII = angiotensin II. *[From JB Young, L Landsberg, in P Sleight et al (eds), Scientific Foundations of Cardiology, London, Heinemann, 1981.]*

Whether primary sympathetic overactivity plays a role in the pathogenesis of essential hypertension is uncertain owing to the insensitivity of currently available methods of assessing regional sympathetic activity in humans. It is well established, however, that the sympathetic nervous system plays at least a permissive role in hypertension. Despite the elevated blood pressure, sympathetic nervous system activity is not suppressed in hypertensive patients, and reflex control of the circulation is retained, due in part to upward resetting of the baroreceptors. In addition, peripheral sensitivity of the vasculature to NE is either normal or enhanced. The maintenance of sympathetic nervous system activity in patients with hypertension accounts for the hypotensive effects of antiadrenergic agents.

During antihypertensive treatment with vasodilators or diuretics, the sympathetic nervous system may be activated in response to decreased pressure in either the venous or arterial circulation (Fig. 68-3). The heightened sympathetic activity that results, in addition to causing tachycardia, may oppose the antihypertensive therapy by activating the various effector systems shown in Fig. 68-6. Agents with antiadrenergic effects, therefore, have a fundamental role in the therapy of most hypertensive patients.

ANGINA PECTORIS (See also Chap. 203) Sympathetic stimulation of the cardiovascular system increases myocardial oxygen consumption as a consequence of elevated heart rate, enhanced myocardial contractility, and increased myocardial wall tension. Attacks of angina, therefore, are often precipitated by situations associated with sympathetic activation such as exercise, eating, and cold exposure. Beta blockade is beneficial in the treatment of angina because of reduction in sympathetic stimulation of the heart. Alpha-adrenergically mediated coronary vasoconstriction also may contribute to coronary spasm.

HYPERTHYROIDISM (See also Chap. 334) Many of the peripheral manifestations of hyperthyroidism suggest a hyperadrenergic state. Enhancement of beta-receptor responses in hyperthyroidism is due in part to effects on the beta receptor. Thyroid hormone, in some tissues and in some species, increases receptor number; in other tissues, even when beta-receptor number is not increased, coupling of receptor occupancy to the adenylate cyclase cyclic-AMP system is augmented to amplify catecholamine-induced responses. Since thyroid hormone excess does not suppress sympathetic nervous system activity (plasma NE levels are normal in thyrotoxic patients), a "normal" level of sympathetic activity may evoke an exaggerated physiologic response. Many of the adrenergic manifestations of hyperthyroidism are diminished by treatment with beta-receptor blocking agents.

ORTHOSTATIC HYPOTENSION The maintenance of arterial pressure during upright posture depends on an adequate blood volume, an unimpaired venous return, and an intact sympathetic nervous system. Significant postural hypotension, therefore, often reflects extracellular fluid volume depletion or dysfunction of the circulatory reflexes. Diseases of the nervous system, such as tabes dorsalis, syringomyelia, or diabetes mellitus, may disrupt these sympathetic reflexes with resultant orthostatic hypotension. Although any antiadrenergic agent may impair the postural sympathetic response, orthostatic hypotension is most prominent with drugs that block neurotransmission within the ganglia or adrenergic neurons.

The term *idiopathic orthostatic hypotension* refers to a group of degenerative diseases involving either the pre- or postganglionic sympathetic neurons. Involvement of the postganglionic sympathetic nervous system is characterized by low basal NE levels, while involvement at the level of the central nervous system or preganglionic sympathetic neurons is associated with normal basal plasma NE levels. In both cases, the plasma NE response to upright posture is deficient. Orthostatic hypotension caused by disruption of the preganglionic autonomic neurons within the intermediolateral cell column of the spinal cord often occurs in association with degenerative changes of basal ganglia and other portions of the central nervous system. In the latter situation, known as *multiple-systems atrophy*, or the *Shy-Drager syndrome*, orthostatic hypotension occurs along with a variety of neurologic disturbances, including Parkinson's disease.

Treatment of orthostatic hypotension is usually unsatisfactory except in the mildest cases. There is no way of reestablishing the normal relationship between fall in venous return and sympathetic neuronal activation. Volume expansion with fludrocortisone and a liberal salt diet in conjunction with fitted stockings to the waist, as well as elevation of the head of the bed to avoid recumbency, will maintain plasma volume and venous return and frequently provide symptomatic improvement. Rarely a beneficial response may be obtained from treatment with sympathomimetic amines (including clonidine).

PHARMACOLOGY OF THE SYMPATHOADRENAL SYSTEM

A variety of therapeutic agents affect sympathetic nervous system function or interact with adrenergic receptors, making it possible to stimulate or suppress effects mediated by catecholamines with some degree of specificity (Table 68-1).

SYMPATHOMIMETIC AMINES Sympathomimetic amines may directly activate adrenergic receptors (direct acting) or release NE from the sympathetic nerve endings (indirect acting). Many agents have both direct and indirect effects.

Epinephrine and norepinephrine The naturally occurring catecholamines act predominantly by the direct stimulation of adrenergic receptors. NE is employed to support the circulation and elevate the blood pressure in hypotensive states (Chap. 34). Peripheral vasoconstriction is the major effect, although cardiac stimulation occurs as well. E, also employed as a pressor, has special usefulness in the treatment of allergic reactions, especially those associated with anaphylaxis. E antagonizes the effects of histamine and other mediators on vascular and visceral smooth muscle and is useful in the treatment of bronchospasm.

Dopamine *Dopamine* is used in treating hypotension, shock (Chap. 34), and certain forms of heart failure (Chap. 195). At low infusion rates it exerts a positive inotropic effect both by a direct action on the cardiac beta$_1$ receptors and by the indirect release of NE from sympathetic nerve endings in the heart. At low doses direct stimulation of dopaminergic receptors in the renal and mesenteric vasculature also results in vasodilation in the gut and kidney and facilitates sodium excretion. At higher infusion rates interaction with alpha-adrenergic receptors results in vasoconstriction, an increase in peripheral resistance, and an elevation of blood pressure.

Beta-receptor agonists *Isoproterenol*, a direct-acting beta-receptor agonist, stimulates the heart, decreases peripheral resistance, and relaxes bronchial smooth muscle. It raises the cardiac output and accelerates atrioventricular conduction while increasing the automaticity of ventricular pacemakers. Isoproterenol is used in the treatment of heart block and bronchoconstriction. *Dobutamine*, a congener of dopamine with relative selectivity for the beta$_1$ receptor and with a greater effect on myocardial contractility than on heart rate, is also used in the treatment of congestive heart failure, often in combination with vasodilators (Chap. 195). In conjunction with radionuclide imaging or echocardiographic assessment of wall motion, dobutamine, as well as other investigational congeners that have a relatively greater effect on heart rate, is used in the diagnosis of demand-induced myocardial ischemia.

SELECTIVE BETA$_2$-RECEPTOR AGONISTS The cardiac stimulation caused by nonselective beta agonists, such as isoproterenol or epinephrine, is occasionally dangerous when these agents are used in the treatment of bronchoconstriction (see Chap. 217). Selective beta$_2$ agonists (*metaproterenol, albuterol, terbutaline, pirbuterol*, and *isoetharine*) improve the therapeutic ratio by achieving bronchial dilatation with less activation of the cardiovascular system (see Chaps. 217 and 223); selectivity is relative, and cardiac stimulation does occur with these agents, particularly at the higher dose levels. *Ritodrine*, another selective beta$_2$ agonist, is used as a tocolytic agent (as is *terbutaline*) to relax the uterus and antagonize premature labor.

Alpha-adrenergic agonists *Phenylephrine* and *methoxamine* are direct-acting alpha agonists that elevate blood pressure by increasing peripheral vasoconstriction. They are used primarily in the treatment of hypotension and paroxysmal supraventricular tachycardia (Chap. 198), in the latter case by increasing cardiac vagal tone through reflex baroreceptor stimulation. Phenylephrine and a related proprietary compound, *phenylpropanolamine*, are common constituents of decongestant medications (often combined with antihistamines) for the treatment of allergic rhinitis and upper respiratory infections.

Miscellaneous sympathomimetic amines with mixed actions *Ephedrine* has both direct beta-receptor agonist properties and an indirect effect on sympathetic nerve endings, from which it releases NE, and is used primarily as a bronchodilator. *Sudephedrine*, a congener of ephedrine, is less potent at dilating bronchi and serves as a nasal decongestant. *Metaraminol* has both direct and indirect effects on sympathetic nerve endings and is employed in the treatment of hypotensive states.

Dopaminergic agonists The dopamine 2–receptor agonist *bromocriptine* is used to suppress prolactin secretion (Chap. 331). *Apomorphine*, another dopamine 2–receptor agonist, is used to induce emesis.

ANTIADRENERGIC OR SYMPATHOLYTIC AGENTS (See also Chap. 209) **Agents inhibiting central sympathetic outflow** The antihypertensive agents *methyldopa, clonidine, guanabenz*, and *guanfacine* diminish central sympathetic outflow by stimulating a central alpha-adrenergic pathway (alpha$_2$ receptor) that diminishes vasomotor outflow. Central nervous system side effects such as sedation are common. When administration of clonidine is stopped abruptly, a withdrawal syndrome characterized by rebound hyperactivity of the sympathetic nervous system can produce a state resembling the crises of patients with pheochromocytoma. *Opiates* also may exert a central sympatholytic effect; the sympathetic excitation of morphine withdrawal responds to clonidine and vice versa. *Propranolol* and *reserpine* may exert some sympatholytic effects at the level of the central nervous system.

Ganglionic blocking agents Ganglionic transmission may be antagonized by drugs that block the (nicotinic) cholinergic synapse between the preganglionic and postganglionic autonomic nerves. These agents inhibit the parasympathetic as well as the sympathetic nervous system. Only *trimethaphan* is in general clinical use; its major application is in the treatment of hypertensive crises, particularly aortic dissection, when controlled hypotension and decreased myocardial contractility are desirable (Chap. 210).

Agents acting at the peripheral sympathetic nerve endings Adrenergic neuron-blocking agents depress the function of the peripheral sympathetic nerves by decreasing the amount of neurotransmitter released. *Guanethidine*, the prototype of this class of drugs, is concentrated in the sympathetic nerve endings by the amine-uptake mechanism. Within the terminal it blocks the release of NE in response to nerve impulses and eventually depletes the nerve of NE by displacing it from the intraneuronal storage granules. The drug is occasionally useful in the management of severe hypertension, although orthostatic hypotension is a limiting side effect. *Bretylium*, an agent whose effects are similar to those of guanethidine, is employed in the treatment of ventricular fibrillation (Chap. 198). Both guanethidine and bretylium are antagonized by agents that affect the amine-uptake transport process such as sympathomimetic amines, tricyclic antidepressants, phenoxybenzamine, and phenothiazines. The antihypertensive action of guanethidine may be rapidly reversed by these drugs.

Reserpine depletes catecholamines from the peripheral sympathetic nerve endings, the brain, and the adrenal medulla. Its antihypertensive effect in humans is usually attributed to depletion of peripheral NE stores within sympathetic nerve endings. The sedation and occasionally morbid depression attending its use result from NE depletion within the central nervous system.

Adrenergic-receptor blocking agents Adrenergic blocking agents antagonize the effects of catecholamines at the level of the peripheral tissue.

ALPHA-ADRENERGIC-RECEPTOR BLOCKING AGENTS *Phenoxybenzamine* and *phentolamine* are utilized principally in treating pheochromocytoma (Chap. 336). Phenoxybenzamine produces prolonged, noncompetitive alpha blockade, while phentolamine leads to reversible, competitive blockade. Because of its rapid action and short duration, phentolamine is commonly used in the treatment of acute hypertensive paroxysms secondary to catecholamine excess, such as occur with pheochromocytoma, with pressor reactions in patients receiving monoamine oxidase inhibitors, and in clonidine withdrawal. Both phentolamine and phenoxybenzamine antagonize alpha$_1$ and alpha$_2$ receptors, although phenoxybenzamine is more potent at the alpha$_1$ receptor site. *Prazosin*, an alpha-adrenergic blocking agent with selectivity for the alpha$_1$ receptor, possesses properties that resemble those of primary vasodilators and is used in the treatment of essential hypertension and as an afterload-reducing agent in congestive heart failure. Doxazosin and terazosin, long-acting selective alpha$_1$ blockers, are used in the treatment of essential hypertension. Selective alpha$_1$ blockers are potentially useful in the symptomatic treatment of urinary outflow track obstruction because they antagonize contraction of the sphincter at the bladder trigone.

BETA-ADRENERGIC-RECEPTOR BLOCKING AGENTS These drugs antagonize the cardiovascular effects of catecholamines in angina pectoris, hypertension, and cardiac arrhythmias. The benefit of beta blockade in angina derives from the decrease in myocardial oxygen consumption following reduction in heart rate and myocardial contractility (Chap. 203). The hypotensive effect of beta blockade is not clearly understood (Chap. 209). Diminished cardiac output, decreased NE release at postganglionic sympathetic nerve endings, reduced renin secretion, and suppressed central sympathetic outflow are possible mechanisms. The efficacy of beta blocking agents in the treatment of arrhythmias depends on reduction of the rate of spontaneous depolarization of pacemaker cells in the sinus node and junctional pacemakers and on slowing conduction within the atria and atrioventricular node. Beta blockade is also effective in the symptomatic management of hyperthyroidism and the control of tachycardia and arrhythmias in patients with pheochromocytoma. Beta-adrenergic blocking agents are also useful in the treatment of migraine, essential tremor, idiopathic hypertrophic subaortic stenosis, and aortic dissection. Several trials have demonstrated that beta-receptor blocking agents, administered long-term, diminish mortality following acute myocardial infarction. The mechanism of this cardioprotective effect may involve antiarrhythmic action, prevention of reinfarction, and reduction in infarct size (Chap. 202).

TABLE 68-1 Some commonly used autonomic drugs[a,b,c]

Agent	Indication	Dose and Route	Comment
ADRENERGIC AGONISTS[d]			
Epinephrine	Anaphylaxis	100–500 μg SC or IM (0.1–0.5 mL of 1/1000 solution of hydrochloride salt); 25–50 μg IV (slowly) every 5–15 min; titrate as needed	Nonselective alpha and beta agonist; increases BP, heart rate Bronchodilation
Norepinephrine	Shock Hypotension	2–4 μg of NE base/min IV; titrate as needed	Alpha and beta$_1$ agonist Vasoconstriction predominates Extravasation causes tissue necrosis; infuse through IV cannula
Isoproterenol	Cardiogenic shock Bradyarrhythmias AV block Asthma	0.5–5.0 μg/min IV; titrate as needed Inhalation	Nonselective beta agonist Increases cardiac rate and contractility (beta$_1$) Tachycardia limits usefulness Dilates bronchi (beta$_2$); cardiac stimulation also occurs
Dobutamine	Refractory CHF Cardiogenic shock	2.5–25 (μg/kg)/min IV	Selective beta$_1$ agonist with greater effect on contractility than heart rate; a congener of dopamine but not a dopaminergic agonist
Phenylephrine	Hypotension	40–180 μg/min IV	Selective alpha$_1$ agonist; useful in antagonizing hypotension of spinal anesthesia
	Supraventricular tachycardia	150–800 μg slow IV push	Pressor effect induces vagotonic response; do not exceed 160 mmH systolic BP
Terbutaline	Asthma	2.5–5.0 mg PO tid; 0.25–0.5 mg SC; inhalation every 4–5 h	Selective beta$_2$ agonist; beta$_1$ (cardiac) effects at higher doses
Albuterol	Asthma	2.0–4.0 mg PO tid or qid; inhalation every 4–6 h	Selective beta$_2$ agonist; beta$_1$ effects (cardiac) at higher doses
Isoetharine	Asthma	Inhalation every 2–4 h	Selective beta$_2$ agonist; some beta$_1$ effects
Metaproterenol	Asthma	10–20 mg PO tid or qid; inhalation every 3–4 h	Selective beta$_2$ agonist; some beta$_1$ effects
Pirbuteral	Asthma	Inhalation every 4–6 h	Selective beta$_2$ agonist; some beta$_1$ effects
Ritodrine	Premature labor	100–350 μg/min IV; 10–20 mg every 4–6 h PO	Selective beta$_2$ agonist; hypokalemia. hyperglycemia, hypotension, cardiac stimulation may occur Neonatal hypoglycemia, hypocalcemia reported
DOPAMINERGIC AGONISTS			
Dopamine	Shock	2–5 (μg/kg)/min IV (dopaminergic range) 5–10 (μg/kg)/min IV (dopaminergic and beta range) 10–20 (μg/kg)/min IV (beta range) 20–50 (μg/kg)/min IV (alpha range)	Pharmacologic effects are dose dependent: renal and mesenteric vasodilation predominate at lower doses; cardiac stimulation and vasoconstriction develop as the dose is increased
Bromocriptine	Amenorrhea-galactorrhea	2.5 mg PO bid or tid	Selective agonist of dopamine-2 receptor; inhibits prolactin secretion
	Acromegaly	5–15 mg PO tid or qid	Lowers growth hormone in a minority of patients with acromegaly
INHIBITORS OF CENTRAL SYMPATHETIC OUTFLOW			
Clonidine	Hypertension	0.1–0.6 mg PO bid	Selective alpha$_2$ agonist; potentiates central baroreceptor depressor reflex Abrupt discontinuation may result in withdrawal syndrome with rebound hypertension
Methyldopa	Hypertension	250–500 mg PO every 6–8 h	Metabolized by decarboxylation and beta hydroxylation to α-methyl-norepinephrine, a centrally active selective alpha$_2$ agonist
ADRENERGIC NEURON BLOCKING AGENTS			
Guanethidine	Hypertension	10–100 mg PO qd	Concentrated in sympathetic nerve endings; blocks release of NE in response to nerve impulses and depletes NE stores; prominent orthostatic hypotension
Bretylium	Ventricular fibrillation and tachycardia	5 mg/kg IV	In addition to blocking NE release, has direct effect on electrical properties of cardiac muscle
BETA BLOCKING AGENTS[e]			
Propranolol	Hypertension	40–160 mg PO bid (or higher)	Lipophilic, nonselective Dosage highly variable
	Angina	10–40 mg PO tid or qid	
	Myocardial infarction	60–80 mg PO tid	Prolongs survival post MI
	Arrhythmias	10–30 mg PO tid or qid; 1–3 mg IV	
	Hypertrophic cardiomyopathy	20–40 mg PO tid or qid	
	Pheochromocytoma	10–20 mg PO tid or qid; 0.5–2.0 mg IV	After alpha blockade initiated
	Essential tremor	20–80 mg PO tid	
	Migraine	20–80 mg PO bid or tid	
	Hyperthyroidism	10–60 mg PO tid or qid	
Metoprolol	Hypertension	50–200 mg PO bid	Selective beta$_1$ (cardiac), lipophilic
	Myocardial infarction	100 mg PO bid	Prolongs survival post MI

TABLE 68-1 Some commonly used autonomic drugs[a,b,c] (continued)

Agent	Indication	Dose and Route	Comment

BETA BLOCKING AGENTS[e] (continued)

Agent	Indication	Dose and Route	Comment
Nadolol	Hypertension Angina	80–320 mg PO qd 80–240 mg PO qd	Hydrophilic, nonselective; lengthen dosage interval with renal failure
Timolol	Hypertension Myocardial infarction	10–30 mg PO bid 10 mg PO bid	Lipophilic, nonselective Prolongs survival post MI
Atenolol	Hypertension	50–100 mg PO qd	Selective beta$_1$, hydrophilic; lengthen dosage interval with renal failure
Pindolol	Hypertension Angina	5–30 mg PO bid 10 mg PO qid	Nonselective, lipophilic with partial agonist activity
Acebutolol	Hypertension Arrhythmias	200–800 mg qid 200–600 mg bid	Selective beta$_1$, hydrophilic, partial agonist activity
Penbutolol	Hypertension	20–40 mg PO qd	Nonselective
Betaxolol	Hypertension	15–20 mg PO qd	Selective β_1, hydrophilic
Carteolol	Hypertension	2.5–10 mg PO qd	Nonselective, partial agonist activity, hydrophilic; lengthen dosage interval with renal failure
Esmolol	Supraventricular tachycardia	50–200 (µg/kg)/min IV after loading dose of 500 µg/kg/min for 1 min	Selective beta$_1$, very short duration of action

ALPHA BLOCKING AGENTS

Agent	Indication	Dose and Route	Comment
Phenoxybenzamine	Pheochromocytoma	10–60 mg PO bid; titrate as needed	Noncompetitive, nonselective alpha blockade
Phentolamine	Pheochromocytoma	5 mg IV (after test dose of 0.5 mg)	Competitive, nonselective alpha blockade
Prazosin	Hypertension CHF	1–5 mg PO bid or tid 2–7 mg PO qid	Competitive, selective alpha$_1$ blockade
Doxazosin	Hypertension	1–16 mg PO qd	Competitive selective alpha$_1$ blockade, long duration of action
Terazosin	Hypertension	1–5 mg PO qd	Competitive, selective alpha$_1$ blockade, long duration of action

COMBINED ALPHA-BETA BLOCKING AGENT

Agent	Indication	Dose and Route	Comment
Labetalol	Hypertension	100–1200 mg PO bid; titrate slowly as needed; 20–80 mg IV (by increments up to 300 mg); 2 mg/min by IV infusion	Competitive alpha and beta antagonist with relatively more activity against beta receptors

DOPAMINERGIC ANTAGONIST[f]

Agent	Indication	Dose and Route	Comment
Metoclopramide	Diabetic gastroparesis	10 mg PO qid	Competitive dopaminergic antagonist with prominent cholinergic agonist activity
	Gastroesophageal reflex Antiemetic (cancer chemotherapy)	10–15 mg PO qid 10 mg IV	

GANGLIONIC BLOCKING AGENT

Agent	Indication	Dose and Route	Comment
Trimethaphan	Hypertensive crisis (aortic dissection)	1–3 mg/min IV	Competitive ganglionic blocker; some direct vasodilating effects; inhibits parasympathetic as well as sympathetic nervous system

CHOLINERGIC AGENT

Agent	Indication	Dose and Route	Comment
Bethanechol	Urinary retention (nonobstructive)	10–100 mg PO tid or qid; 5 mg SC	M-2 receptor agonist

ANTICHOLINESTERASE AGENTS[g]

Agent	Indication	Dose and Route	Comment
Physostigmine	Central cholinergic blockade	1–2 mg IV (slow)	Tertiary amine; penetrates CNS well; may cause seizures; used to reverse central anticholinergic effects produced by overdose of atropine or tricyclic antidepressants
Edrophonium	Paroxysmal supraventricular tachycardia	5 mg IV (after 1.0-mg test dose)	Induces vagotonic response; rapid onset, short duration of action; effects reversed by atropine

CHOLINERGIC BLOCKING AGENTS[h]

Agent	Indication	Dose and Route	Comment
Atropine	Bradycardia and hypotension	0.4–1.0 mg IV every 1–2 h	Competitive inhibition of M-1 and M-2 receptor; blocks hemodynamic changes associated with increased vagal tone

[a] Consult complete prescribing information. [b] Doses for children are not given. [c] Only the more common indications and routes of administration are listed.
[d] Dopaminergic agonists are listed separately although dopamine, at high doses, is an adrenergic agonist as well.
[e] Clinical efficacy of most beta blockers appears similar for major indications. Not all beta blockers are FDA approved for all indications listed in the table. When beta blocking agents are discontinued, gradual dosage reduction is recommended. Both beta$_1$ selective and nonselective agents have cardioprotective effects after myocardial infarction.
[f] Neuroleptic and antipsychotic agents are also dopaminergic antagonists; these are not included in the table.
[g] A major use of cholinesterase inhibitors is in myasthenia gravis (Chap 386). These agents, quaternary amines that do not penetrate the CNS, are not included here.
[h] A wide variety of synthetic atropine derivatives are available for the purpose of (1) diminishing GI tract motility and secretion and (2) increasing urinary bladder capacity. Their usefulness is limited by anticholinergic side effects. Some may be useful as adjuncts in the treatment of peptic ulcer disease.

PHARMACOLOGIC PROPERTIES OF BETA-RECEPTOR BLOCKING AGENTS   Eleven beta blocking agents (atenolol, acebutolol, betaxolol, carteolol, esmolol, metoprolol, nadolol, pindolol, penbutolol, propranolol, and timolol) are available for use in the United States. Other agents (alprenolol, bevantolol, oxprenolol, sotalol, etc.) are in use in other countries and investigational within the United States. The utility of these agents is derived predominantly from blockade of beta-adrenergic receptors. In general, the various agents have similar clinical efficacy.

Although much has been written about other pharmacologic properties, including cardioselectivity, membrane stabilizing (local anesthetic) effects, intrinsic sympathomimetic (partial-agonist) activity, and lipid solubility, the clinical significance of these additional properties is small. Local anesthetic properties are most prominent with propranolol; however, membrane stabilization probably does not contribute substantially to the clinical utility. The various beta blockers do differ in their water and lipid solubility. The lipophilic agents (propranolol, metoprolol, oxprenolol) are readily absorbed from the gastrointestinal tract, metabolized by the liver, have large volumes of distribution, and penetrate the central nervous system well; the hydrophilic agents (acebutolol, atenolol, betaxolol, carteolol, nadolol, sotalol) are less readily absorbed, not extensively metabolized, and have relatively long plasma half-lives. As a consequence, the hydrophilic agents may be administered once per day. Hepatic failure may prolong the plasma half-life of the lipophilic agents, whereas renal failure may prolong the action of the hydrophilic group. The degree of lipid solubility, therefore, provides a basis for choice of a particular agent in patients with hepatic or renal insufficiency. Although the hydrophilic agents penetrate the central nervous system less well, central nervous system side effects (sedation, depression, hallucinations) are well described with the hydrophilic as well as with the lipophilic agents.

Some beta-adrenergic blocking agents possess beta-agonist activity. This has been referred to as "intrinsic sympathomimetic activity" (or ISA). Agents with partial agonist activity (pindolol, alprenolol, acebutolol, carteolol, oxprenolol) cause little or no depression of resting heart rate (partial agonist effect) while blocking the increase in heart rate that occurs in response to exercise or the administration of a beta agonist such as isoproterenol. The presence of partial agonist activity may be useful when bradycardia limits treatment in patients with slow resting heart rates. Although theoretically attractive in patients with depressed left ventricular function and reactive airways, no decisive advantage of these agents over beta blockers without partial agonist activity has been demonstrated under these circumstances. Pindolol also produces mild vasodilation, perhaps in part related to peripheral beta$_2$ stimulation. Agents with partial agonist activity appear to cause less change in blood lipid levels than agents without agonist properties. On theoretical grounds, intrinsic sympathomimetic activity would be undesirable in the treatment of thyrotoxicosis, idiopathic hypertrophic subaortic stenosis, aortic dissection, and tachyarrhythmias.

CARDIOSELECTIVE (BETA$_1$) ADRENERGIC RECEPTOR BLOCKING AGENTS   Propranolol, the prototype of the nonselective beta-adrenergic blocking agent, induces a competitive blockade of both beta$_1$ and beta$_2$ receptors. Other nonselective beta blocking agents include alprenolol, carteolol, nadolol, oxprenolol, penbutolol, pindolol, sotalol, and timolol. Metoprolol, acebutolol, atenolol, and betaxolol possess relative selectivity for the beta$_1$ receptor. Although beta$_1$-selective agents have the theoretical advantage of producing less bronchoconstriction and less peripheral vasoconstriction, a clear-cut clinical advantage of the cardioselective agents has not been demonstrated, since the beta$_1$ selectivity is only relative. Bronchoconstriction may occur when beta$_1$-selective agents are administered in full therapeutic doses.

ADVERSE EFFECTS OF BETA-RECEPTOR BLOCKING AGENTS   Aside from the effects on the central nervous system, most adverse reactions to beta blocking agents are consequences of beta-adrenergic blockade. These include the precipitation of heart failure in patients in whom cardiac compensation depends on enhanced sympathetic drive; the aggravation of bronchospasm in patients with asthma; predisposition to the development of hypoglycemia in insulin-requiring diabetics (blockade of catecholamine-mediated counterregulation and antagonism of the adrenergic warning signs of hypoglycemia); the development of hyperkalemia in diabetic or uremic patients with impaired potassium tolerance; the enhancement of coronary or peripheral arterial vasospasm; and elevation in triglycerides and depression of high-density lipoprotein (HDL) levels. The lipid effects are less (or absent) in agents with partial agonist activity.

MISCELLANEOUS ADRENERGIC BLOCKING AGENTS   Labetalol, approved for use in the United States as an antihypertensive agent, is a competitive antagonist of both alpha- and beta-adrenergic receptors. Although labetalol induces relatively more beta- than alpha-receptor blockade, fall in peripheral resistance may be marked following acute administration of the drug. Vasodilation may be mediated in part by a partial agonist effect on the beta$_2$-adrenergic receptor; labetalol does not possess partial agonist activity for the beta$_1$ (cardiac) receptor.

Metoclopramide is a dopaminergic antagonist with cholinergic agonist properties. It enhances gastric emptying, increases the tone of the lower esophageal sphincter, increases prolactin and aldosterone secretion, and antagonizes emesis induced by apomorphine. It is useful clinically in enhancing gastric emptying (in the absence of organic obstruction such as in diabetic gastroparesis), in antagonizing gastroesophageal reflux, and as an antiemetic during cancer chemotherapy.

THE PARASYMPATHETIC NERVOUS SYSTEM

ACETYLCHOLINE   Acetylcholine (ACh) serves as the neurotransmitter at all autonomic ganglia, at the postganglionic parasympathetic nerve endings, at the postganglionic sympathetic nerve endings innervating the eccrine sweat glands, and at the skeletal muscle end plate (neuromuscular junction). The enzyme choline acetyltransferase catalyzes the synthesis of ACh from acetyl CoA produced within the nerve ending and from choline, actively taken up from the extracellular fluid. Within the cholinergic nerve endings ACh is stored in discrete synaptic vesicles and released in response to nerve impulses that depolarize the nerve terminals and increase calcium influx.

Cholinergic receptors   Different receptors for ACh exist on the postganglionic neurons within the autonomic ganglia and at the postjunctional autonomic effector sites. Those within the autonomic ganglia and adrenal medulla are stimulated predominantly by nicotine (nicotinic receptors) and those on autonomic effector cells by the alkaloid muscarine (muscarinic receptors). Ganglionic blocking agents antagonize the nicotinic receptors, while atropine blocks the muscarinic receptors. The muscarinic (M) receptor, furthermore, has been recently subdivided into additional types. The M-1 receptor is localized to the central nervous system and perhaps parasympathetic ganglia; the M-2 receptor is the nonneuronal muscarinic receptor on smooth muscle, cardiac muscle, and glandular epithelium. Bethanechol is a selective agonist of the M-2 receptor; pirenzepine, an investigational agent, is a selective antagonist of the M-1 receptor. This agent markedly reduces gastric acid secretion. The M-2 receptor inhibits adenylyl cyclase and utilizes the regulatory G_i protein; the M-1 receptor interacts with G_p and stimulates phospholipase C (Fig. 68-5). The M-3 receptor, present on smooth muscle and secretory glands, is antagonized by atropine and utilizes phospholipase C, IP_3, and DAG as second messengers. Other subtypes have been identified by molecular biologic techniques but have not yet been fully characterized.

Acetylcholinesterase   Hydrolysis of ACh by acetylcholinesterase inactivates the neurotransmitter at cholinergic synapses. This enzyme (also known as specific or true cholinesterase) is present within neurons and is distinct from butyrocholinesterase (serum cholinesterase or pseudocholinesterase). The latter enzyme is present in plasma and nonneuronal tissues and is not primarily involved in the termination of the effects of ACh at autonomic effector sites. The pharmacologic effects of anticholinesterase agents are due to inhibition of neuronal (true) acetylcholinesterase.

PHYSIOLOGY OF THE PARASYMPATHETIC NERVOUS SYSTEM

The parasympathetic nervous system participates in the regulation of the cardiovascular system, the gastrointestinal tract, and the genitourinary system. Tissues such as liver, kidney, pancreas, and thyroid also receive parasympathetic innervation, suggesting a role for the parasympathetic nervous system in metabolic regulation as well, although cholinergic effects on metabolism are not well characterized.

Cardiovascular system Parasympathetic effects on the heart are mediated by the vagus nerve. ACh reduces the rate of spontaneous depolarization of the sinoatrial node and decreases heart rate. The heart rate in different physiologic states is the result of coordinated interaction between sympathetic stimulation, parasympathetic inhibition, and the intrinsic activity of the sinoatrial pacemaker. ACh also delays impulse conduction within the atrial musculature while shortening the effective refractory period, a combination of factors which may initiate or perpetuate atrial arrhythmias. At the atrioventricular node, ACh reduces conduction velocity, increases the effective refractory period, and thus diminishes the ventricular response during atrial flutter or fibrillation (Chap. 198). The decrease in inotropy induced by ACh is related to a prejunctional inhibitory effect on sympathetic nerve endings as well as to a direct inhibitory effect on the atrial myocardium. The ventricular myocardium is not much affected since innervation by cholinergic fibers is minimal. A direct cholinergic contribution to the regulation of peripheral resistance appears unlikely since parasympathetic innervation of the vasculature is not extensive. The parasympathetic nervous system, however, may influence peripheral resistance indirectly by inhibiting NE release from sympathetic nerves.

Gastrointestinal tract Parasympathetic innervation of the gut is via the vagus nerve and the pelvic sacral nerves. The parasympathetic nervous system increases the tone of gastrointestinal smooth muscle, enhances peristaltic activity, and relaxes the gastrointestinal sphincters. ACh stimulates exocrine secretion from the glandular epithelium and enhances the secretion of gastrin, secretin, and insulin.

Genitourinary and respiratory systems Sacral parasympathetic nerves supply the urinary bladder and genitalia. ACh increases ureteral peristalsis, contracts the urinary detrusor muscle, and relaxes the trigone and sphincter, thereby playing a critical role in the coordination of urination. The respiratory tract is innervated with parasympathetic fibers derived from the vagus nerve. ACh increases tracheobronchial secretions and stimulates bronchial constriction.

PHARMACOLOGY OF THE PARASYMPATHETIC NERVOUS SYSTEM

Cholinergic agonists ACh itself has no therapeutic role because of its widespread effects and short duration of action. Congeners of ACh are less susceptible to hydrolysis by cholinesterase and have a narrower range of physiologic effects. Bethanechol, the only systemic cholinergic agonist in general use, stimulates gastrointestinal and genitourinary smooth muscle with minimal effect on the cardiovascular system. It is used in the treatment of urinary retention in the absence of outflow tract obstruction and, less commonly, in gastrointestinal disorders such as postvagotomy gastric atony. Pilocarpine and carbachol are topical cholinergic agonists used in the treatment of glaucoma.

Acetylcholinesterase inhibitors Cholinesterase inhibitors enhance the effects of parasympathetic stimulation by diminishing the inactivation of ACh. The therapeutic application of reversible cholinesterase inhibitors depends on the role of ACh as neurotransmitter at the skeletal muscle neuroeffector junction and within the central nervous system and includes the treatment of myasthenia gravis (Chap. 386), the termination of neuromuscular blockade following general anesthesia, and the reversal of intoxication by agents with a central anticholinergic action. Physostigmine, a tertiary amine, penetrates the central nervous system well, while related quaternary amines (neostigmine, pyridostigmine, ambenonium, and edropho-

nium) do not. Organophosphorous cholinesterase inhibitors produce irreversible cholinesterase blockade; these agents are used principally as insecticides and are primarily of toxicologic interest. With regard to the autonomic nervous system, cholinesterase inhibitors are of limited use in the treatment of intestinal and bladder smooth-muscle dysfunction such as occurs in paralytic ileus and atonic urinary bladder. Cholinesterase inhibitors induce a vagotonic response in the heart and may be useful in terminating attacks of paroxysmal supraventricular tachycardia (Chap. 198).

Cholinergic-receptor blocking agents *Atropine* blocks muscarinic cholinergic receptors, with little effect on cholinergic transmission at the autonomic ganglia and the neuromuscular junctions. Many of the central nervous system actions of atropine and atropine-like drugs are attributable to blockade of central muscarinic synapses. The related alkaloid, *scopolamine*, is similar to atropine but causes drowsiness, euphoria, and amnesia, effects that make it suitable as a preanesthetic medication.

Atropine increases heart rate and enhances atrioventricular conduction, actions that may be useful in combating the bradycardia or heart block associated with heightened vagal tone. In addition, atropine reverses cholinergically mediated bronchoconstriction and diminishes respiratory tract secretions. These effects contribute to its utility as a preanesthetic medication.

Atropine also decreases gastrointestinal tract motility and secretion. Although various derivatives and congeners of atropine (such as *propantheline, isopropamide*, and *glycopyrrolate*) have been advocated in patients with peptic ulcer or with diarrheal syndromes, the chronic use of such agents is limited by other manifestations of parasympathetic inhibition such as dry mouth and urinary retention. The investigational selective M-1 inhibitor pirenzepine inhibits gastric secretion at doses that have minimal anticholinergic effects at other sites; this agent may be useful in the treatment of peptic ulcer. Atropine and its congener *ipratropium*, when given by inhalation, cause bronchodilation and have been used experimentally in the treatment of asthma.

REFERENCES

CARON MG, LEFKOWITZ RJ: Catecholamine receptors: Structure, function and regulation. Recent Prog Horm Res 48:277, 1993

CHALMERS J, PILOWSKY P: Brainstem and bulbospinal neurotransmitter systems in the control of blood pressure. J Hypertens 9:675, 1991

ESLER M et al: Overflow of catecholamine neurotransmitters to the circulation: Source, fate, and functions. Physiol Rev 70:963, 1990

HADCOCK JR, MALBON CC: Agonist regulation of gene expression of adrenergic receptors and G proteins. J Neurochem 60:1, 1993

HOLLENBERG MD: Structure-activity relationships for transmembrane signaling: The receptor's turn. FASEB J 5:178, 1991

KUPFERMANN I: Functional studies of cotransmission. Physiol Rev 71(3):683, 1991

LANDSBERG L, YOUNG JB: Catecholamines and the adrenal medulla, in *Williams' Textbook of Endocrinology*, 8th ed, DW Foster, JD Wilson (eds). Philadelphia, Saunders, 1992, p 621

————, ————: The influence of diet on the sympathetic nervous system, in *Neuroendocrine Perspective*, vol 4, EE Muller et al (eds). Amsterdam, Elsevier, 1985, p 191

LOKHANDWALA MF, AMENTA F: Anatomical distribution and function of dopamine receptors in the kidney. FASEB J 5:3023, 1991

LOW PA: Autonomic nervous system function. J Clin Neurophysiol 10:14, 1993

MEISTER B, APERIA A: Molecular mechanisms involved in catecholamine regulation of sodium transport. Semin Nephrol 13:41, 1993

PACHOLCZYK T et al: Expression cloning of a cocaine- and antidepressant-sensitive human noradrenaline transporter. Nature 350:350, 1991

RUFFOLO RR et al: Structure and function of α-adrenoceptors. *Pharmacol Rev* 43:475, 1991

SCHONDORF R: New investigations of autonomic nervous system function. J Clin Neurophysiol 10:28, 1993

WILLIAMS JL et al: Area postrema: A unique regulator of cardiovascular function. NIPS 7:30, 1992

69   G PROTEINS AND THE REGULATION OF SECOND MESSENGER SYSTEMS

MICHAEL FREISSMUTH / ALFRED G. GILMAN

Hormones, neurotransmitters, growth factors, and autacoids (local regulators such as histamine and adenosine) interact with specific receptors to produce biologic effects. These receptors are classified into distinct categories, based on structural homologies and on similarities in their mechanism of action. For example, the receptors for insulin and certain growth factors (e.g., platelet-derived growth factor) are membrane-bound tyrosine protein kinases, and this enzymatic activity is essential for their function (see Chap. 337). The binding site for ANF (atrial natriuretic factor; see Chap. 187) is in the extracellular domain of a guanylate cyclase that spans the plasma membrane; the intracellular portion of this protein synthesizes a second messenger, guanosine-3',5'-monophosphate (cyclic GMP). Steroid hormones and triiodothyronine form hormone-receptor complexes that act as regulators of gene transcription (see Chap. 329). Yet another class of receptors, exemplified by the nicotinic cholinergic receptor, acts as ligand-gated ion channels. Lastly, a large family of plasma membrane–bound receptors (the known number exceeds 100) activates heterotrimeric guanosine triphosphate–binding (GTP-binding) regulatory proteins, or *G proteins*, in the plasma membranes of cells. Each G protein, in turn, controls the activity of one or more membrane-bound effectors, such as adenylate cyclase, ion channels, and phospholipases (Table 69-1).

G PROTEIN–LINKED RECEPTORS   A diverse group of ligands interacts with G protein–linked receptors. These include peptide hormones (e.g., glucagon, ACTH), lipids (prostaglandins), nucleosides and nucleotides (adenosine, ATP), and amines (epinephrine, histamine). Nevertheless, almost all such receptors possess common structural features—including the topology of the proteins with respect to the plasma membrane (Fig. 69-1). The amino terminus of each receptor is outside the cell and is modified with N-linked oligosaccharides. The carboxyl terminus is intracellular and contains sites that can be phosphorylated and that play a crucial role in desensitization to hormone actions. The central portion of the receptor molecule is believed to fold into seven α helices that span the membrane bilayer and form the hydrophobic core of the receptor. The ligand-binding site lies within this hydrophobic core and is formed by reactive side chains that are contributed by more than one transmembrane helix. Portions of the intracellular loops that connect the individual membrane-spanning α helices form the sites of interaction between the ligand-bound receptor and the appropriate G protein.

G PROTEINS AND THEIR EFFECTORS   G proteins are composed of three different subunits designated α, β, and γ in order of decreasing mass. A few of the distinctive properties of individual G protein subunits are summarized in Table 69-1.

G protein α subunit   G proteins are classified on the basis of the α subunit. The hormone-sensitive adenylate cyclase system and the retinal cyclic GMP phosphodiesterase that participates in vision have served as models for the elucidation of the mechanisms of G protein–mediated transmembrane signaling. In both cases, the α subunit of the G protein interacts with and regulates the effector. The α subunits bind Mg^{2+} and guanine nucleotide (GTP or GDP) with high affinity and also possess GTPase activity that is essential for deactivation of the pathway. In addition, many G protein α subunits are substrates for bacterial toxins that catalyze the incorporation of an ADP-ribosyl moiety into the polypeptide at specific amino acid residues. G_s (the G protein that activates adenylate cyclase) and G_t (the major retinal G protein that activates the cyclic GMP phosphodiesterase) are substrates for cholera toxin; G_s in intestinal cells is the natural target for the toxin, since cholera is an intraluminal infection. The

incorporation of ADP-ribose into G_s causes its persistent activation, and this is the crucial reaction in the pathogenesis of cholera. The various isoforms of G_i, G_o, and G_t are ADP-ribosylated by pertussis toxin, and this modification blocks the ability of the G protein to interact with receptors. The precise role of ADP-ribosylation in the pathogenesis of whooping cough is not clear.

G_s ALPHA SUBUNIT   Apparently all molecular species of $G_{s\alpha}$ can activate each of the several isoforms of adenylate cyclase. $G_{s\alpha}$ also activates dihydropyridine-sensitive (L-type) Ca^{2+} channels in skeletal and cardiac muscle and inhibits cardiac NA^+ channels. The fact that a single G protein α subunit can interact with more than one effector is an important general point. Not only can G proteins integrate the input from several receptors, they also represent a branch point for regulation of multiple effectors in response to a single signal. In the olfactory neuroepithelium, G_{olf}, a specialized form of G_s, couples receptors for odorants to activation of adenylate cyclase.

G_i AND G_o ALPHA SUBUNITS   The G_i family consists of oligomers with at least three closely related α subunits, designated $G_{i\alpha1}$, $G_{i\alpha2}$, and $G_{i\alpha3}$; they are products of distinct genes and are broadly expressed in many cell types. Two splice variants of $G_{o\alpha}$ are closely related to the $G_{i\alpha}$ proteins and are expressed in neurons and neuroendocrine cells. The G_i proteins were discovered as mediators of hormonal inhibition of adenylate cyclase, although the mechanism of this effect is still not clear (see "Mechanism," below). The G_i proteins can

TABLE 69-1   Properties of G protein subunits

Families of subunits	Subunit	Toxin	Role
$G_{s\alpha}$ ($M_r \approx 45,000$)	α_s ($\times 4$)	Cholera toxin	Activates adenylate cyclase and L-type calcium channels; inhibit cardiac Na^+ channels
	$\alpha_{s,olf}$	Cholera toxin	Activates olfactory adenylate cyclase
$G_{i\alpha}/G_{o\alpha}$ ($M_r \approx 40,000$)	α_i ($\times 3$)	Pertussis toxin	Inhibit adenylate cyclase (indirectly?); stimulate K^+ channels; inhibit neuronal CA^{2+} channels
	α_o ($\times 2$)	Pertussis toxin	Regulates neuronal Ca^{2+} and K^+ channels; implicated in pertussis toxin–sensitive activation of phospholipase C
	α_z	None known	Unknown; structurally related to $G_{i\alpha}/G_{o\alpha}$
Transducins ($G_{t\alpha}$'s) ($M_r \approx 40,000$)	$\alpha_{t,r}$	Pertussis toxin, cholera toxin	Activate cyclic GMP phosphodiesterase in retinal rods
	$\alpha_{t,c}$	Pertussis toxin, cholera toxin	Activate cyclic GMP phosphodiesterase in retinal cones
	α_g	Pertussis toxin (?), cholera toxin (?)	Hypothesized to activate cyclic AMP phosphodiesterase in taste buds (gustducin)
$G_{q\alpha}$ ($M_r \approx 42,000$)	α_q, α_{11}	None known	Activate phospholipase C
	α_{14}, α_{15}, α_{16}	None known	
$G_{\alpha12}$ ($M_r \approx 42,000$)	α_{12}, α_{13}	None known	Unknown
βγ-complex (β: $M_r \approx 37,000$; γ: $M_r \approx 8000$–10,000):	β ($\times 5$) γ ($> \times 7$?)	— —	βγ required for interaction with receptor; direct regulation of effectors; modulation of effector response to G_α

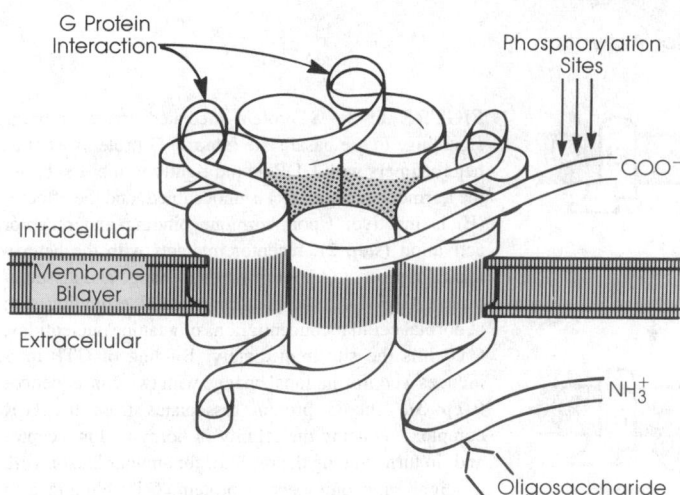

FIGURE 69-1 Schematic representation of the topology of a G protein–coupled receptor. The barrels represent membrane-spanning α helices. The ligand-binding site of the receptor is located within the core formed by these membrane-spanning segments.

activate K^+ channels in atrial myocardial cells. Stimulation of this pathway by muscarinic cholinergic agonists hyperpolarizes the cell and results in both negative chronotropic and inotropic responses. In the central nervous system, G_o and the G_i family apparently couple a variety of receptors to Ca^{2+} channels; G_o also can modulate K^+ currents in brain cells. The resulting ion fluxes mediate the actions of myriad neurotransmitters. Regulation of ion channels by G proteins results largely from direct interaction between the G protein α subunit and the channel-forming protein(s). Thus the structure of adenylate cyclase resembles that of an ion channel, and some adenylate cyclases serve a dual role, as both channel and enzyme.

G_t AND G_g ALPHA SUBUNITS   The retinal G proteins, G_t's or *transducins*, play a pivotal role in vision. The photon receptor, *rhodopsin*, is localized in membranous disks in the outer segments of retinal rod cells; analogous color receptors are present in the cones. These molecules resemble the other G protein–linked receptors. Upon activation by light, rhodopsin interacts with and activates G_t; G_t in turn activates a cyclic GMP–specific phosphodiesterase. Intracellular concentrations of cyclic GMP fall rapidly, resulting in the closing of Na^+ channels and hyperpolarization of the rod cells. This represents the initial electrical signal that is eventually transmitted to the visual cortex. Retinal rods and cones differ not only in their individual photon receptors; they also have distinct G_t molecules ($G_{t,r}$ and $G_{t,c}$) and distinct cyclic GMP phosphodiesterases.

G_g, or *gusducin*, the gustatory homologue of the transducins, is expressed exclusively in taste buds. Because of its close structural relationship to the transducins, it too is presumed to regulate a cyclic nucleotide phosphodiesterase.

G_q ALPHA SUBUNIT   The G_q α subunit and its homologues (α_{11}, α_{14}, α_{15}, and α_{16}) constitute a related group of proteins that are not substrates for pertussis toxin and are candidates for regulation of signaling pathways that cannot be disrupted by this toxin. In most cells, agonist-mediated, GTP-dependent activation of phospholipase C is not blocked by pertussis toxin, and, indeed, G_q and at least some of its homologues interact with and activate the β1-isoform of phospholipase C.

G protein βγ-subunit complex   The β and γ subunits form a tightly associated complex, and the proteins have not been resolved in their active forms. The βγ-subunit complex contributes to the receptor recognition site on the G protein oligomer and facilitates the attachment of the oligomer to the inner face of the plasma membrane (with the help of a lipid modification—a C-20 prenyl group—attached to γ). The βγ complex is believed to deactivate the α subunit by

formation of the intact G protein. In addition, free βγ also can interact with and regulate the activity of effectors such as adenylate cyclase or phospholipase C, either by itself or in concert with regulators such as G protein α subunits or calmodulin.

At least five genes encode closely related but distinct β subunits, while the number of different forms of γ is at least seven. The functional implications of this heterogeneity are discussed below.

MECHANISM OF G PROTEIN–MEDIATED SIGNAL TRANSDUCTION   A widely accepted model of the mechanism of G protein–mediated signal transduction is shown schematically in Fig. 69-2. The central thesis is that the G protein α subunit cycles between an inactive, GDP-liganded oligomeric form and an active, GTP-liganded monomeric state. *These two forms of the α subunit represent the "off" and "on" positions of a molecular switch.* The dissociation of GDP from α is the rate-limiting step. That is, the slow rate of spontaneous dissociation of GDP from α holds the switch in the off position. Interaction of the G protein with an agonist-receptor complex (H·R) facilitates dissociation of GDP. Binding of GTP to this ternary complex of hormone, receptor, and G protein has two consequences. First, the affinity of the receptor for the agonist is lowered, resulting in dissociation of the ternary complex. The receptor is thus free to recycle and activate additional G protein molecules, as long as agonist is present. As a result, considerable amplification occurs at this step. Second, the α subunit is activated by its dissociation from the βγ complex. The switch is now on, and the activated α subunit interacts with the appropriate effector and modulates its activity. The G protein switch is programmed to turn itself off automatically, since deactivation results from hydrolysis of bound GTP by the α subunit. However, the lifetime of the activated α subunit is relatively long (several seconds), since the intrinsic rate of hydrolysis of GTP is slow; this kinetic feature permits additional signal amplification. To complete the cycle, the GDP-bound α subunit associates with βγ, and the system relaxes to its basal state. As mentioned above, the free βγ subunit may itself regulate effectors directly.

Inhibition of adenylate cyclase may be due in part to the capacity of the βγ subunit, released on activation of G_i, to interact with and deactivate G_s; βγ can thus inhibit adenylate cyclase indirectly. This subunit exchange hypothesis predicts that the activation of one pathway can cause inhibition of effectors that are controlled by other G protein α subunits if the concentration of appropriate forms of βγ in the membrane is raised sufficiently.

Molecular heterogeneity   As the number of identified G protein subunits increases, the task of unraveling the complexity of the G protein–regulated cellular switchboard also expands. The known number of α, β, and γ subunits indicates roughly 1000 possible combinations; this number may get much larger. Furthermore, an individual cell must sort through a vast number of choices to complete its own customized G protein–controlled regulatory network. Additional complexity at each step in the signal transduction cascade compounds the problem. There is divergence and convergence of protein-protein interactions at both the receptor G protein level and the G protein effector level, and α and βγ subunits presumably interact to dictate the specificities of these choices and to control, synergistically or in opposition, the activities of effectors. Thus activation of a given receptor in different cells can produce a varied constellation of activated G proteins and effectors, and cellular responses will change with development or with exposure to regulatory signals. Such enormous "combinatorial power" endows cells and organisms with extraordinary capacity for fine-tuning both the magnitude and the nature of their responses to the environment.

SECOND MESSENGER SYSTEMS UNDER THE CONTROL OF G PROTEINS (Fig. 69-3)   **Cyclic AMP**   The conversion of ATP to cyclic AMP is accomplished by various isoforms of the enzyme adenylate cyclase. These membrane-bound proteins are believed to span the plasma membrane several times; their topology resembles that usually found in transporters and channels.

Cyclic AMP acts as a second messenger for a number of hormones. The primary mechanism of action of the cyclic nucleotide is to cause

1. Basal State

2. Receptor Activation

5. GTPase

3. Subunit Dissociation

4. Effector Activation

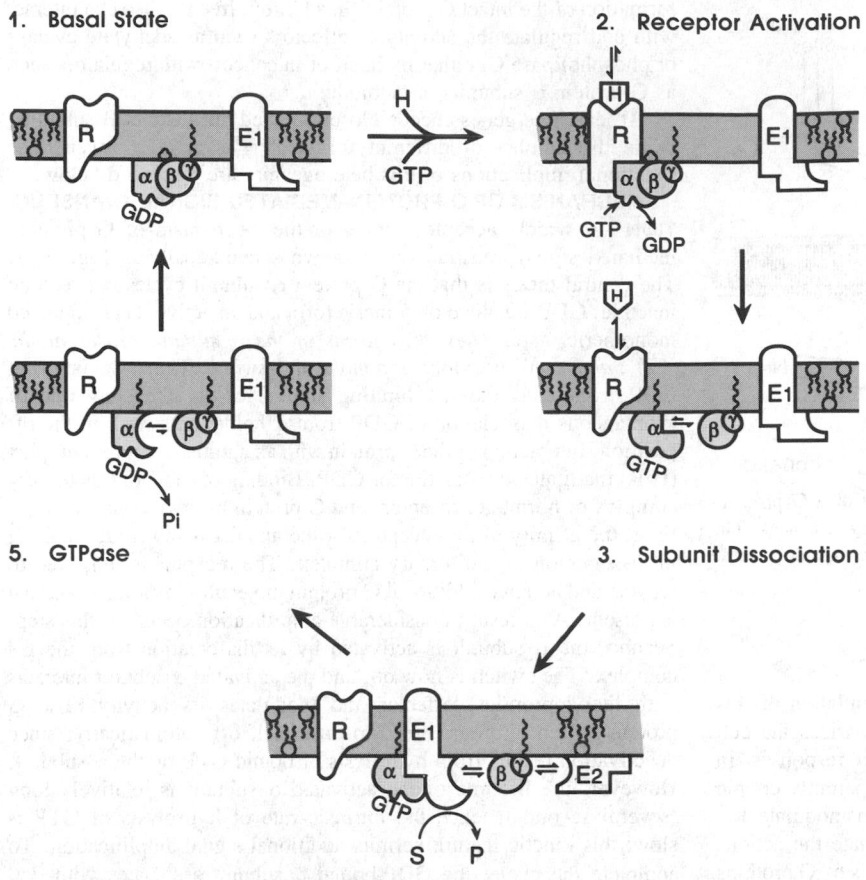

FIGURE 69-2 G protein–mediated transmembrane signaling. In the basal state (**step 1**),G proteins exist as heterotrimers with GDP bound tightly to the α subunit; the hormone receptor (R) is unoccupied, and the effector (E) is inactive. Upon hormone binding and receptor activation (**step 2**), receptor interacts with the heterotrimer to promote a conformational change and dissociation of GDP from the guanine nucleotide binding site; at normal cellular concentrations of guanine nucleotides, GTP fills the site immediately. Binding of GTP to α induces a conformational change with two consequences (**step 3**). The G protein dissociates from the H·R complex, reducing the affinity of hormone for receptor and, in turn, freeing the receptor for another liaison with a neighboring quiescent G protein. GTP binding also reduces the affinity of α for $\beta\gamma$, and subunit dissociation occurs. This frees α·GTP to fulfill its primary role as a regulator of effectors (**step 4**). At least in some systems, the free $\beta\gamma$ subunit complex may also interact directly with an effector (E$_1$) and modulate the activity of the active complex, or it may act independently at a distinct effector (E$_2$). α subunits possess an intrinsic GTPase activity (**step 5**). The rate of this GTPase determines the lifetime of the active species and the associated physiologic response. α-catalyzed hydrolysis of GTP leaves GDP in the binding site and causes dissociation and deactivation of the active complex. The GTPase activity of α is, in essence, an internal clock that controls an on/off switch. The GDP bound form of α has high affinity for $\beta\gamma$; subsequent reassociation of α·GDP with $\beta\gamma$ returns the system to the basal state (**step 1**).

dissociation of a dimer of cyclic AMP–binding regulatory subunits from the catalytic subunits of a protein kinase. The free catalytic subunits of the protein kinase are enzymatically active, and they transfer the γ phosphate from ATP to serine and threonine residues in target proteins. Such phosphorylation can either increase the activity (e.g., glycogen phosphorylase kinase, triacylglycerol lipase, protein phosphatase inhibitor 1) or decrease the activity (e.g., glycogen synthase, myosin light chain kinase) of the various substrates.

Termination of cyclic AMP action is accomplished by several mechanisms that are themselves subject to regulation by cyclic AMP and Ca^{2+}-calmodulin, a molecule with related second messenger functions (see below). Cyclic AMP is degraded to 5'-AMP by cyclic nucleotide phosphodiesterases. Some of these isoenzymes are activated by Ca^{2+}-calmodulin; they are inhibited by several drugs, including the methylxanthines (caffeine and theophylline) and milrinone. In addition, most cells possess a mechanism for the facilitated extrusion of cyclic AMP.

The regulatory effects of protein kinases are reversed by phosphoprotein phosphatases, which hydrolytically cleave the phosphate ester bond. These enzymes differ in their substrate specificities and in their regulation. For example, in the presence of elevated concentrations of cyclic AMP, protein phosphatase inhibitor 1 is phosphorylated by the cyclic AMP–dependent protein kinases; in this phosphorylated form, the inhibitor suppresses the activity of protein phosphatase 1. By contrast, protein phosphatase 2B is activated by Ca^{2+}-calmodulin. This network of stimulatory and inhibitory mechanisms integrates input from additional second messenger systems, which is necessary for efficient fine-tuning of cellular activities. All intracellular effects of cyclic AMP were initially believed to result from activation of protein phosphorylation, but ionic (Na$^+$) channels in olfactory neuroepithelial cells can be regulated (gated) directly by cyclic AMP.

Inositol trisphosphate, diacylglycerol, and calcium Inositol-1,4,5-trisphosphate (IP$_3$) and diacylglycerol are second messengers generated by activation of a family of phosphoinositidases, commonly termed *phospholipase C*. These enzymes use phosphatidylinositol-4,5-bisphosphate, a minor phospholipid component of the plasma membrane, as substrate. A large number of hormones and related molecules are known to activate phospholipase. Whereas the γ-isoform of phospholipase C is phosphorylated and activated by receptors belonging to the tyrosine kinase family, the β1-isoform is stimulated by G$_q$ and related G protein α subunits in most cells. However, in certain cells (e.g., granulocytes and mast cells) agonist-mediated, GTP-dependent activation of phospholipase C is blocked by pertussis toxin, presumably indicating a role for G$_i$ or G$_o$ (either their α or $\beta\gamma$ subunits.

Inositol trisphosphate releases Ca^{2+} from intracellular stores (endoplasmic/sarcoplasmic reticulum) and promotes Ca^{2+} influx from the extracellular fluid. Additional mechanisms for entry of Ca^{2+} into the cytosolic compartment include voltage-gated Ca^{2+} channels and exchange mechanisms activated by other ions. G proteins regulate the activity of some of these channels and exchangers.

Ca^{2+} both regulates the activity of target enzymes directly and, more important, exerts its second messenger functions by interactions with Ca^{2+}-binding proteins such as troponin C and calmodulin. Calmodulin is a ubiquitous intracellular protein that binds four molecules of Ca^{2+}. This Ca^{2+}-calmodulin complex regulates several enzymes of the cyclic AMP system, including at least one type of adenylate cyclase, certain cyclic nucleotide phosphodiesterases, and protein phosphatase 2B (calcineurin). Several protein kinases are also activated by Ca^{2+}-calmodulin; the resulting effect can be either synergistic with (e.g., activation of phosphorylase kinase) or antagonistic to (e.g., activation of myosin light chain kinase) the cyclic AMP–mediated action. The effects of Ca^{2+}-calmodulin on its target enzymes can be blocked by certain phenothiazine drugs. The relationship between this effect and the therapeutic efficacy or toxicity of these drugs is unknown.

Deactivation of the pathway is achieved by active transport of Ca^{2+} into intracellular compartments and extrusion of the ion by

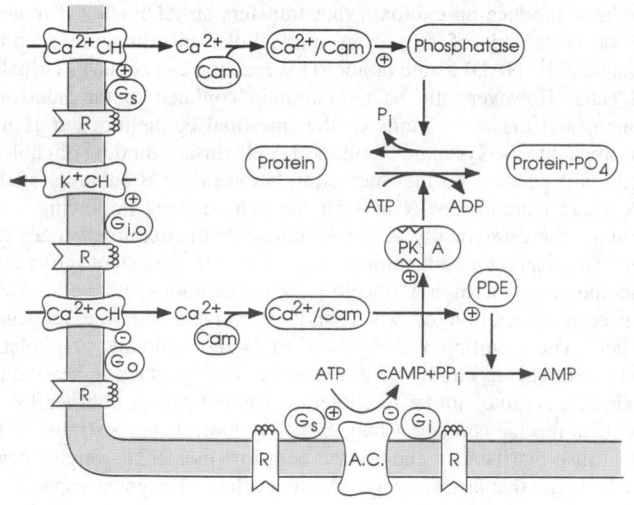

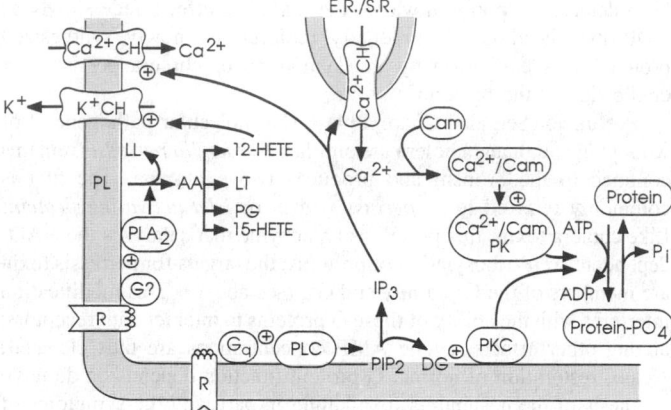

FIGURE 69-3   The role of G proteins in transmembrane signaling. The top panel shows G protein–regulated channels and adenylate cyclase. The bottom panel depicts pathways that involve activation of phospholipases.

AA = arachidonic acid
AC = adenylate cyclase
Ca^{2+}/Cam PKC = calcium-calmodulin-dependent protein kinase
Cam = calmodulin
CH = channel
DG = diacylglycerol
E.R./S.R. = endoplasmic/sarcoplasmic reticulum
G = G protein
12-HETE = 12-hydroxyeicosatetraenoic acid
15-HETE = 15-hydroxyeicosatetraenoic acid
IP_3 = inositol trisphosphate
LL = lysophospholipid
LT = leukotriene
PDE = cyclic nucleotide phosphodiesterase
PG = prostaglandin
PIP_2 = phosphatidylinositol trisphosphate
PLC = phospholipase C
PKA = cyclic AMP–dependent protein kinase
PKC = protein kinase C
R = receptor for hormone or agonist

plasma membrane–bound Ca^{2+}-pumping ATPases. Inositol trisphosphate is degraded by sequential dephosphorylation. The phosphatase that catalyzes the removal of phosphate from inositol-1-phosphate is inhibited by Li^+. This effect of Li^+ may be related to its efficacy in psychiatric disorders.

The second product of the phospholipase C reaction is diacylglycerol, which acts as a second messenger by activating a family of isoenzymes referred to as *protein kinase C*. Upon binding of diacylglycerol, the requirement of these enzymes for Ca^{2+} decreases into the range of free Ca^{2+} concentrations found in cytosol. Activated

protein kinase C phosphorylates many intracellular proteins, including some substrates of cyclic AMP–dependent protein kinase. The phorbol esters, which act as tumor promoters, are structurally related to diacylglycerol and also bind to and activate protein kinase C. This action is believed to explain their carcinogenicity.

The effect of diacylglycerol is terminated by enzymatic recycling to form phosphatidylinositol. Alternatively, diacylglycerol is broken down by a diacylglycerol lipase. Of interest, one of the fatty acids in the diacylglycerol molecule is usually arachidonate, the precursor of prostaglandins, leukotrienes, and other eicosanoids.

Stimulation of phospholipase A_2 and release of arachidonic acid
Release of arachidonate from membrane phospholipids is the rate-limiting step in the biosynthesis of prostaglandins, leukotrienes, and other eicosanoids (see Chap. 70). Free arachidonate can arise by two distinct mechanisms. First, a family of enzymes, termed *phospholipase A_2*, cleaves the ester bond at the 2 position of the glycerol moiety of membrane phospholipids, giving rise to equimolar amounts of arachidonate and lysophospholipids. The enzymes require Ca^{2+} for activity. Second, as mentioned above, free arachidonate can be produced by the sequential action of phospholipase C and diacylglycerol lipase. Thus hormones that stimulate the hydrolysis of phosphatidylinositol-4,5-bisphosphate also cause the release of arachidonate and the subsequent synthesis of eicosanoids. In addition, these hormones increase intracellular concentrations of free Ca^{2+} and stimulate protein kinase C through inositol trisphosphate and diacylglycerol, respectively. Both these effects also may contribute to the generation of free arachidonate via activation of phospholipase A_2. Phospholipase A_2 is activated by Ca^{2+}, and direct stimulation of protein kinase C by phorbol esters promotes release of arachidonate.

In view of the interdigitation of the regulatory mechanisms that control these pathways, it is not surprising that the regulation of phospholipase A_2 by G proteins is poorly understood. However, phospholipase A_2 can be activated independently of concomitant stimulation of phospholipase C.

Most eicosanoids are not second messengers as defined originally, since they produce their biologic effects by interacting with specific cell surface receptors coupled to G proteins. However, some metabolites of the 12-lipoxygenase pathway, in particular HEPETE (8-hydroxy-11,12-epoxy-5,9,14-icosotrienoic acid), may affect neuronal K^+ channels through a direct intracellular mechanism and thus act as typical second messengers.

Stimulation of phospholipase D   Phospholipase D utilizes phosphatidylcholine, another phospholipid component of the plasma membrane, as its preferred substrate and generates choline and phosphatidic acid. Phosphatidic acid may function directly as a second messenger or serve as an alternative source of diacylglycerol. This signaling pathway appears to be under the direct control of unidentified G proteins, both pertussis toxin–insensitive and –sensitive. Phospholipase D is also stimulated by Ca^{2+} and protein kinase C.

REGULATION OF RECEPTOR-EFFECTOR COUPLING   Desensitization   Prolonged exposure of cells to a hormonal stimulus leads to a gradual attenuation of the biologic response, despite the continuing presence of the stimulus; this phenomenon is termed *desensitization*, *refractoriness*, or *tolerance*. Such adaptation is a general biologic mechanism, as exemplified by pharmacodynamic tolerance to massive concentrations of opioids. Desensitization is traditionally divided into two categories. *Homologous* or *receptor-specific desensitization* refers to the refractoriness that develops only to agonists that act on the same receptor as the desensitizing stimulus. In addition, stimulation of a particular receptor by an agonist can lead to the subsequent attenuation of the response to multiple hormones that influence the same pathway through distinct receptors. This phenomenon is termed *heterologous desensitization*.

Beta-adrenergic-receptor–mediated stimulation of adenylate cyclase has served as a model system for elucidation of the molecular events that underlie desensitization, and both homologous and heterologous desensitization appear to result from phosphorylation of the receptor on its carboxyl-terminal domain.

Desensitization is a multistep process which can be considered in three phases: uncoupling (seconds to minutes), sequestration (minutes), and down-regulation (hours). Initially, receptors are uncoupled from G_s, as judged in part by their inability to stimulate adenylate cyclase. This process is reversible upon removal of agonist. Homologous desensitization is mediated by a novel protein kinase termed *beta-adrenergic-receptor kinase* (βARK), which specifically phosphorylates the agonist-bound receptor. Unliganded and antagonist-bound receptors do not serve as substrates. However, βARK also phosphorylates other agonist-bound receptors, including those that mediate inhibition of adenylate cyclase, such as the alpha$_2$-adrenergic and M$_2$-muscarinic receptors.

Heterologous desensitization of receptors that stimulate adenylate cyclase is probably mediated predominantly by a classic negative feedback loop. Activation of cyclic AMP–dependent protein kinase leads to phosphorylation of the receptors in a largely agonist-independent manner, and this modification also interferes with their ability to interact with G_s.

An analogous mechanism of desensitization is observed with receptors that mediate stimulation of phospholipase C (e.g., the alpha$_1$-adrenergic receptor). As a result of release of diacylglycerol, protein kinase C phosphorylates the receptors near the carboxyl terminus and is thereby presumed to interfere with the receptor–G protein interaction.

The mechanisms responsible for sequestration of beta-adrenergic receptors (the rapid removal of receptor into an ill-defined cellular compartment) are not well understood. The sequestered receptors may return to the functionally active pool upon hydrolytic cleavage of the incorporated phosphate by a phosphatase. Long-term exposure of cells to agonists leads to a decline in the number of receptors in the plasma membrane. This down-regulation is not readily reversible, and protein synthesis is required to replenish the receptors on the surface. Down-regulation results from both degradation of phosphorylated receptors and a cyclic AMP–dependent reduction in the steady state level of the mRNA that encodes the protein.

Additional forms of regulation   The steady state concentration of receptors in the plasma membrane represents the balance between synthesis and insertion into the bilayer versus internalization and degradation. As mentioned, the continuous presence of agonist tilts this balance in favor of degradation. Conversely, removal of agonist by pharmacologic blockade of the receptor, denervation of tissue, or extirpation of the source of the agonist favors accumulation of receptors on the cell surface and sensitization of target tissues to the appropriate agonist. Such sensitization may underlie the clinical syndrome associated with abrupt withdrawal of beta-adrenergic blocking agents.

Several other regulatory mechanisms influence signal transduction and thus the sensitivity of target cells to agonists. Since these events are not promoted by the receptor agonist, they are referred to as *heterologous regulation*. The most remarkable examples of heterologous regulation at the clinical level are the alterations in adrenergic receptor-effector coupling produced by thyroid and steroid hormones. Both triiodothyronine and glucocorticoids appear to be necessary to maintain normal coupling between beta-adrenergic receptors and G_s. In addition, thyroid hormones and glucocorticoids can increase transcription of mRNA for beta-adrenergic receptors. As one example, symptoms of increased sympathetic activity in the absence of elevated concentrations of plasma catecholamines are characteristic of hyperthyroidism. Similarly, heterologous regulation may underlie the permissive role of glucocorticoids in neurohormonal control of blood pressure.

ROLE OF G PROTEIN SYSTEMS IN DISEASE   The pivotal role of G proteins in regulatory biology is understood in considerable detail. Comparatively little is known about the degree to which perturbations of these pathways participate in pathophysiology. However, a link to alterations in a G protein–regulated second messenger system has been established in several entities.

Cholera (See also Chap. 120)   Pathogenic strains of *Vibrio cholerae* produce an exotoxin that transfers an ADP-ribosyl moiety to the α subunit of G_s, using intracellular nicotinamide adenine dinucleotide (NAD) as the donor. This reaction can occur in virtually all cells. However, the bacteria remain confined to the intestinal lumen, and the toxin binds to the intestinal epithelium but is not absorbed into the systemic circulation. Cell-surface binding of cholera toxin is dependent on the interaction between the B subunits of the toxin and gangliosides (GM$_1$) on the cell surface. Following such binding, the catalytically active A subunit of the toxin penetrates the cell. The ensuing modification of $G_{s\alpha}$ leads to its persistent activation, and the resultant high intracellular concentrations of cyclic AMP trigger the secretion of water and electrolytes into the intestinal lumen. The resulting watery diarrhea is the hallmark of cholera. Enteropathogenic strains of *Escherichia coli* produce a heat-labile toxin that is quite similar to cholera toxin and causes diarrhea by an identical mechanism (see Chap. 87). By contrast, other strains of *E. coli* cause diarrhea by elaboration of a low-molecular-weight, heat-stable toxin that activates guanylate cyclase. Enzymes capable of removing mono-ADP-ribosyl moieties from cellular proteins have not been detected. Upon removal of the toxin, its effects fade slowly as ADP-ribosylated $G_{s\alpha}$ is gradually replaced by newly synthesized protein. This explains why the symptoms of cholera persist after eradication of the bacteria.

Pertussis (See also Chap. 114)   The molecular pathogenesis of whooping cough and cholera are similar. *Bordetella pertussis* remains confined to the bronchi and produces two exotoxins. The first is commonly referred to as *pertussis toxin* or *islet-activating protein*. Like cholera toxin, this protein is an enzyme that catalyzes the NAD-dependent ADP-ribosylation of proteins; the targets for pertussis toxin are members of the $G_{i\alpha}$ family and $G_{o\alpha}$ (see above). This modification interferes with the ability of these G proteins to interact with receptors; among other effects, cyclic AMP concentrations are thus elevated. Again, restoration of normal G protein function depends on de novo synthesis of the α subunits, explaining in part why the symptoms of pertussis can persist for weeks after eradication of the microorganisms. In contrast to cholera, the sequence of events that links ADP-ribosylation of G protein α subunits to clinical symptoms is not understood. However, *B. pertussis* also interferes with cellular regulation of cyclic AMP concentrations by another mechanism, since the second exotoxin is itself an invasive calmodulin-dependent adenylate cyclase. Elevated concentrations of cyclic AMP in neutrophils impair their ability to kill ingested bacteria. In addition, ADP-ribosylation of G protein α_i subunits (presumably $G_{i\alpha1}$ and $G_{i\alpha2}$) uncouples the neutrophil chemotactic receptor from the pathway that controls superoxide generation and bactericidal activity. This may contribute to the increased susceptibility to pulmonary infection by other pathogens—a frequent complication of whooping cough.

Anthrax (See also Chap. 104)   Cutaneous infection with *Bacillus anthracis* produces a lesion characterized by central necrosis and prominent subcutaneous edema. The edema is due to the presence of a bacterial exotoxin, referred to as *edema factor*. Edema factor is an adenylate cyclase that shares many characteristics with the *B. pertussis* enzyme, including host cell penetration and dependence on calmodulin. Rare patients who ingest *Bacillus* organisms can develop a watery diarrhea indistinguishable from cholera. This syndrome may result from penetration of edema factor into cells of the intestinal mucosa.

Pseudohypoparathyroidism/Albright's hereditary osteodystrophy (See also Chap. 357)   Pseudohypoparathyroidism type I is an inherited disorder characterized by target-organ resistance to parathyroid hormone. In addition, many patients exhibit partial resistance to other hormones that act by stimulation of adenylate cyclase (e.g., thyroid-stimulating hormone, vasopressin, glucagon). In one variant of the disorder (termed *pseudohypoparathyroidism type Ia*), the molecular defect results in reduced cellular concentrations of $G_{s\alpha}$, and this partial deficiency is apparently due to lower cellular levels of the mRNAs that encode the polypeptide. The underlying genetic defect is heterogeneous. Several point mutations in one allele of the $G_{s\alpha}$ gene have been identified in affected kindreds. These result in aberrant splicing of the pre-mRNA, frame shifts, or loss of the codon for the initiating methionine residue. Pseudohypoparathyroidism type Ib is a similar syndrome in which cellular concentrations of $G_{s\alpha}$ are normal.

G proteins as products of oncogenes G proteins control pathways that are linked to cellular proliferation. Cyclic AMP is a trophic stimulus for endocrine target tissues (pituitary, thyroid, adrenals, gonads); stimulation of G_i-coupled receptors is mitogenic for many cells; tumor-promoting phorbol esters are believed to act via persistent stimulation of protein kinase C, and ectopic expression of receptors coupled to G_q and phospholipase C results in tumor formation. Certain point mutations within the genes that encode G protein α subunits interfere with the GTPase activity of the proteins. Such mutations cause constitutive activation of the pathways that they regulate and act in a dominant fashion. Activating point mutations have been identified in the genes encoding $G_{s\alpha}$ and $G_{i\alpha2}$. About 50 percent of growth hormone–producing pituitary adenomas contain a mutated $G_{s\alpha}$ allele (see Chap. 331); these mutations also occur in thyroid carcinomas and in the neoplastic lesions found in the McCune-Albright syndrome (see Chap. 362). A mutation in the $G_{i\alpha2}$ gene has been found in tumors derived from the adrenal cortex and the ovary. In addition, constitutively active mutant alpha$_2$-adrenergic (G_i-coupled) and alpha$_1$-adrenergic (G_q-coupled) receptors can be produced experimentally; expression of these mutated receptors causes transformation of the transfected cells. Thus alterations at any of several levels of the transmembrane signaling cascade that abolish the abnormal regulatory cycle of activation and deactivation may participate in carcinogenesis.

REFERENCES

DOHLMAN HG et al: Model systems for the study of seven-transmembrane-segment receptors. Annu Rev Biochem 60:653, 1991
GILMAN AG: G proteins and regulation of adenylyl cyclase. JAMA 262:1819, 1989
LYONS J et al: Two G protein oncogenes in human endocrine tumours. Science 249:655, 1990
PATTEN JL et al: Mutations in the gene encoding the stimulatory G protein of adenylate cyclase in Albright's hereditary osteodystrophy. N Engl J Med 322:1412, 1990
SIMON MI et al: Diversity of G proteins in signal transduction. Science 252:802, 1991
WATSON S, ABBOTT A: TIPS receptor nomenclature supplement. Trends Pharmacol Sci 12:S1, 1991
WEINSTEIN LS et al: Activating point mutations of the stimulatory G protein in the McCune-Albright syndrome. N Engl J Med 325:1688, 1991

70 EICOSANOIDS AND HUMAN DISEASE

R. PAUL ROBERTSON

This chapter focuses on the formation and mechanism of action of the physiologically active metabolites of arachidonic acid and on the biologic phenomena in which these compounds may be involved.

FORMATION OF THE EICOSANOIDS Prostaglandins, the first arachidonic acid metabolites to be recognized, were so named because they were originally identified in seminal fluid and thought to be secreted by the prostate. Subsequently, two major pathways relevant to human disease—the cyclooxygenase and the lipoxygenase pathways— were characterized. These synthetic pathways are summarized schematically in Fig. 70-1, and structures of representative metabolites are shown in Fig. 70-2. All products of both the cyclooxygenase and the lipoxygenase pathways are called *eicosanoids*. The products of the cyclooxygenase pathway—the prostaglandins and the thromboxanes—are termed *prostanoids*.

The initial synthetic step for both pathways involves the cleavage of arachidonic acid from phospholipid in the plasma membrane of

cells. Phospholipase A_2 cleaves arachidonic acid from phospholipid. A phospholipase-activating protein termed *PLAP* is present in some cells. Free arachidonic acid also can be derived by phospholipase C cleavage of diacylglycerol from phospholipids and subsequent cleavage of arachidonic acid from diacylglycerol. Free arachidonic acid can then be oxygenated by the cyclooxygenase or lipoxygenase pathway. The first product of the cyclooxygenase pathway is the cyclic endoperoxide prostaglandin G_2 (PGG_2), which is converted to prostaglandin H_2 (PGH_2). PGG_2 and PGH_2 are the key intermediates in the formation of physiologically active prostaglandins (PGD_2, PGE_2, $PGF_{2\alpha}$, and PGI_2) and thromboxane A_2 (TXA_2). Several lipoxygenase pathways, including 5-lipoxygenase and 12-lipoxygenase, are important to human physiology. The first product of the 5-lipoxygenase pathway is 5-hydroperoxyeicosatetraenoic acid (5-HPETE), which is an intermediate in the formation of 5-hydroxyeicosatetraenoic acid (5-HETE), and the leukotrienes (LTA_4, LTB_4, LTC_4, LTD_4, and LTE_4). 5-Lipoxygenase is activated by a membrane protein termed *FLAP*. The subscripts designate the number of double bonds between carbon atoms in the side chains. Arachidonic acid forms prostaglandin products with subscript 2 and leukotrienes with subscript 4. Two fatty acids other than arachidonic acid [3,11,14-eicosatrienoic acid (dihomo-γ-linolenic acid) and 5,8,11,14,17-eicosapentaenoic acid] can be converted to metabolites closely related to these eicosanoids. Prostanoid products of the former substrate carry the subscript 1; the leukotriene subscript is 3. Prostanoid products of the latter substrate have the subscript 3 while leukotrienes have the subscript 5. Omega-3 fatty acids found in fish oils can decrease production of some arachidonate metabolites and increase levels of prostanoids with the subscript 3. Feeding of these fatty acids has been used as a therapeutic strategy to diminish platelet aggregation by decreasing TXA_2 and increasing TXA_3 synthesis by platelets.

Virtually all cells have the necessary substrates and enzymes to form some of the metabolites of arachidonic acid, but tissues differ in enzyme profile and consequently in the products they form. Eicosanoids are synthesized in response to immediate need and are not stored in significant amounts for later release.

The cyclooxygenase products Prostaglandins D_2, E_2, $F_{2\alpha}$, and I_2 are formed from the cyclic endoperoxides PGG_2 and PGH_2. Of these, PGE_2 and PGI_2 exert the broadest physiologic effects. PGE_2 is synthesized by many tissues. PGI_2 (also called *prostacyclin*) is a dominant product in the endothelial and smooth muscle cells of vessel walls and in some nonvascular tissues. PGI_2 is a vasodilator, a bronchodilator, and an inhibitor of platelet aggregation. PGD_2 is also believed to play a role in platelet aggregation and brain function. $PGF_{2\alpha}$ plays a role in uterine and ovarian function. Both PGD_2 and $PGF_{2\alpha}$ are bronchoconstrictors.

Thromboxane synthetase catalyzes the incorporation of an oxygen atom into the ring of the endoperoxide PGH_2 to form the thromboxanes. TXA_2, which is synthesized by platelets, enhances platelet aggregation, and causes vasoconstriction and bronchodilation.

The lipoxygenase products The leukotrienes and HETE are the end products of the lipoxygenase pathway. The leukotrienes have histamine-like actions, including enhancement of vascular permeability and induction of bronchospasm, and appear to have mediator activities for leukocytes. On a molar basis, leukotrienes are more potent brochoconstrictors than histamine. LTC_4, LTD_4, and LTE_4 together have been identified as slow-reacting substance of anaphylaxis (SRS-A). (The pathophysiology of the leukotrienes is discussed in detail in Chap. 217.)

EFFECTS OF DRUGS ON THE SYNTHESIS OF EICOSANOIDS Many drugs block the synthesis of eicosanoids by inhibiting one or more enzymes in the biosynthetic pathways. Glucocorticoids and antimalarial drugs such as mepacrine interfere with the cleavage of arachidonic acid from phospholipids in some cells (Fig. 70-1). Cyclooxygenase is directly inhibited by nonsteroidal anti-inflammatory drugs including salicylates, indomethacin, and ibuprofen. Drugs under development inhibit more distal steps in the cyclooxygenase and lipoxygenase pathways. However, the fact that a drug inhibits

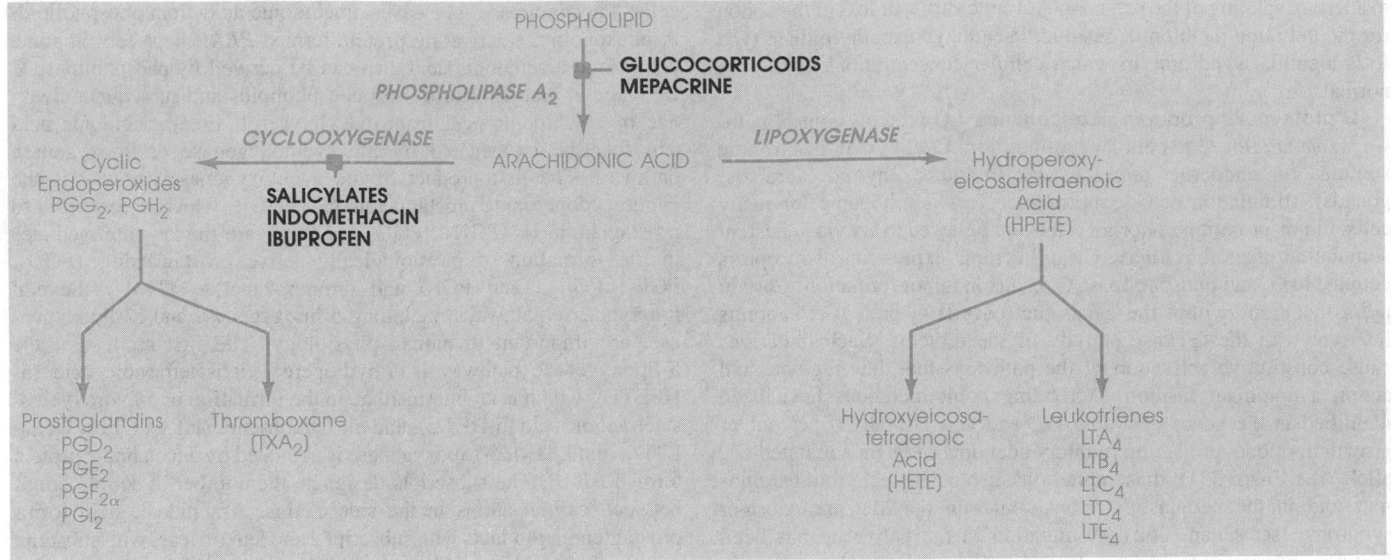

FIGURE 70-1 The overall scheme of arachidonic acid metabolism. The various drugs act at the various enzymatic steps to inhibit the reactions. The major pathways are the cyclooxygenase and the lipoxygenase pathways. PLAP and FLAP are proteins that activate, respectively, cyclooxygenase and 5- lipoxygenase. Phospholipase A_2 is inhibited by glucocorticoids and mepacrine, and cyclooxygenase is inhibited by certain salicylates, indomethacin, and ibuprofen. 5-Lipoxygenase is inhibited by zileuton.

the synthesis of a certain eicosanoid does not necessarily mean that a given effect of the drug is the direct result of a deficiency of that eicosanoid. Most currently available drugs inhibit early reactions in the synthetic pathways and therefore block the formation of more than one product. Additionally, some of the drugs have other effects. For example, indomethacin not only inhibits formation of cyclic endoperoxides by cyclooxygenase but also disrupts calcium flux across membranes, inhibits cyclic adenosine monophosphate (cyclic AMP)–dependent protein kinase and phosphodiesterase, and inhibits one of the enzymes responsible for degradation of PGE_2.

Truly specific synthesis inhibitors and receptor antagonists for individual arachidonic acid metabolites are needed for human use. The lack of such drugs has been a major barrier to elucidating the pathophysiologic roles of these metabolites.

METABOLISM AND ASSAY OF EICOSANOIDS Arachidonic acid metabolites are catabolized rapidly in vivo. Prostaglandins of the E and F series, although chemically stable, are almost completely degraded during a single passage through the liver or the lung. Thus essentially all nonmetabolized PGE_2 measurable in urine is derived

from renal and seminal vesicle secretion, whereas PGE_2 metabolites in urine represent total-body PGE_2 synthesis. PGI_2 and TXA_2 are both chemically unstable and also rapidly catabolized. Because PGE_2, PGI_2, and TXA_2 are short-lived in vivo, measurement of their inactive metabolites is commonly used as an index of the rates of their formation. As examples, PGE_2 is converted to 15-keto-13,14,-dihydro-PGE_2, PGI_2 is converted to 6-keto-$PGF_{1\alpha}$, and TXA_2 is converted to TXB_2, and these metabolites can be reliably measured. Six methods are generally available to measure arachidonic acid metabolites in physiologic fluids: bioassay, radioimmunoassay, enzyme immunoassay (ELISA), chromatography, receptor assay, and mass spectrometry. Bioassay provides direct physiologic data but is not very sensitive. Radioimmunoassay is the most convenient and sensitive but, as with bioassay and receptor assay, should be preceded by extraction and chromatography of samples to ensure specificity. ELISA is sensitive and eliminates the need for radioisotopes. Mass spectrometry preceded by chromatography is accurate but laborious. With each method precautions must be taken in handling samples because prostaglandin synthesis may be enhanced during the collection of biologic samples. For example, if blood is allowed to clot or if platelets are not carefully separated from plasma, the generation of large amounts of PGE_2 and TXA_2 during processing can lead to erroneous results. Use of an inhibitor of prostaglandin synthesis in the collection tube diminishes this problem.

PHYSIOLOGY Prostaglandins and leukotrienes have specific receptor sites on the plasma membranes of cells such as liver, corpus luteum, adrenal gland, adipocytes, thymocytes, uterus, pancreatic islets, platelets, and red blood cells. Most of the binding sites exhibit specificity for eicosanoids of a given type. For example, the liver plasma membrane PGE receptor binds PGE_1 and PGE_2 with high affinity but not prostaglandins of the A, F, and I configurations. The postreceptor mechanisms by which the binding of the prostaglandins alters cell function are poorly understood. Some involve modulation of cyclic AMP production through interactions with two G proteins, the stimulatory (G_s) and inhibitory (G_i) subunits of adenylate cyclase (see Chap. 69). The physiologic actions of eicosanoids are not mediated as circulating hormones. Instead, eicosanoids act as local, intercellular, and/or intracellular modulators of biochemical activity in the tissues in which they are formed (e.g., a paracrine function). They are autacoids, not hormones. Most are short-lived in the circulation because of chemical instability and/or rapid degradation.

FIGURE 70-2 Structures of representative biologically active eicosanoids.

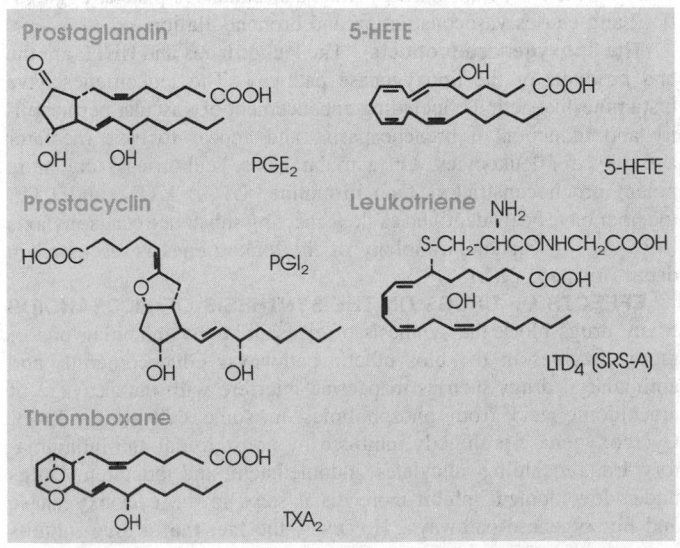

Lipolysis PGE_2 and PGI_2 are synthesized by adipose tissue and are potent endogenous regulators of lipolysis. Since the formation of cyclic AMP is necessary in the action of hormones that stimulate lipolysis, the interactions between PGE and adenylate cyclase have been examined in considerable detail. PGE inhibits lipolysis by decreasing the formation of cyclic AMP in response to epinephrine, adrenocorticotropic hormone (ACTH), glucagon, and thyroid-stimulating hormone (TSH). Thus PGE may act as an endogenous antilipolytic substance by interfering with the stimulation of cyclic AMP formation by hormones. During catecholamine-induced lipolysis, coordinate modulation is provided by the antilipolytic action of PGE_2 and the lipolytic action of PGI_2.

Insulin and PGE may act independently during their antilipolytic actions on the adipocyte. For example, insulin but not PGE inhibits the stimulation of lipolysis by exogenous cyclic AMP in isolated adipocytes, but both agents inhibit hormone-stimulated generation of cyclic AMP. This suggests a site of action of insulin distal to the stimulation of adenylate cyclase. In some animals, PGE inhibits glucagon-induced lipolysis whereas insulin does not.

Sodium and water balance The renin-angiotensin-aldosterone system is a major regulator of sodium homeostasis, and vasopressin exerts the principal control over water balance. Arachidonic acid metabolites influence both systems. PGE_2 and PGI_2 stimulate renin secretion, and inhibitors of prostaglandin synthesis have the opposite effect. PGI_2 and PGE_2 decrease renal vascular resistance and increase blood flow. Conversely, inhibitors of prostaglandin synthesis, such as indomethacin and meclofenamate, decrease total renal blood flow, which can lead to acute renal venoconstriction and decreased renal function in circumstances such as volume depletion and edematous states. PGE_2 is natriuretic, whereas cyclooxygenase inhibitors cause sodium and water retention.

Indomethacin also increases sensitivity to exogenous vasopressin in dogs. Conversely, PGE_2 decreases vasopressin-stimulated water transport. Since this effect of PGE_2 is circumvented by the administration of dibutyryl–cyclic AMP, PGE_2 most likely interferes with the stimulation of adenylate cyclase by vasopressin.

Platelet aggregation Platelets synthesize PGE_2 and PGD_2, but TXA_2 is the dominant eicosanoid produced. TXA_2 is a potent stimulator of platelet aggregation; in contrast PGI_2, formed by the endothelial cells of blood vessel walls, is an antagonist of platelet aggregation. TXA_2 and PGI_2 may exert their opposing effects by decreasing and increasing, respectively, platelet generation of cyclic AMP.

Inhibitors of endogenous prostaglandin synthesis interfere with platelet aggregation. For example, a single dose of aspirin can suppress normal platelet aggregation for 48 h and longer, presumably by suppressing cyclooxygenase-mediated TXA_2 synthesis. Cyclooxygenase inhibition by a single dose of aspirin is of longer duration in platelets than in other tissues, because the platelet, in contrast to nucleated cells that can synthesize new proteins, does not have the machinery to form new enzyme. Consequently, the effect of aspirin persists until newly formed platelets are released. Endothelial cells, on the other hand, rapidly recover cyclooxygenase activity following discontinuation of aspirin, and PGI_2 production is thus restored. This is one reason that aspirin therapy does not predispose to formation of excessive platelet thrombi. In addition, the platelet is more sensitive than the endothelial cell to aspirin.

Endothelial damage may lead to platelet aggregation along the blood vessel wall by causing a local decrease in PGI_2 synthesis, thereby allowing unbridled platelet aggregation at the site of vessel wall damage.

Vascular effects The vasoactive properties of arachidonic acid metabolites are among their most impressive actions. PGE_2 and PGI_2 are vasodilators, whereas $PGF_{2\alpha}$, TXA_2, and LTC_4-LTD_4-LTE_4 are vasoconstrictors in most vascular beds. These effects appear to be the result of direct action on the smooth muscle of the vessel wall. Provided that systemic blood pressure is maintained, the vasodilatory arachidonic acid metabolites act to increase blood flow. If blood pressure falls, however, blood flow decreases because with systemic hypotension catecholamine-induced vasoconstriction offsets the vasodilatory effect of the prostaglandins. Thus significant alterations in systemic blood pressure must be excluded when evaluating the effects of arachidonic acid metabolites on organ blood flow.

Gastrointestinal effects Prostaglandins of the E series influence gastrointestinal function. Infusion of either PGI_2 or PGE_2 into the gastric artery of dogs causes increases in blood flow and inhibition of acid output, and several PGE analogues both inhibit gastric acid output and directly protect the gastrointestinal mucosa when taken orally. In in vitro experiments prostaglandins stimulate gastrointestinal smooth muscle and thereby increase motility, but it is not clear whether these actions are physiologically important. Therapeutically, PGE analogues prevent damage to the stomach and duodenum by aspirin and other NSAIDs.

Neurotransmission PGE inhibits egress of norepinephrine from sympathetic nerve terminals. The effect of PGE on norepinephrine secretion appears to be prejunctional, i.e., at a site on the nerve terminal proximal to the synaptic cleft, and can be reversed by increases in calcium concentration in the perfusing medium. Therefore, PGE_2 may inhibit norepinephrine release by blocking calcium influx.

Catecholamines can release PGE_2 from a variety of tissues, probably by an alpha-adrenergic–mediated mechanism. For example, in innervated tissues such as the spleen, nerve stimulation or injection of norepinephrine causes release of PGE_2. This release is blocked after denervation or administration of alpha-adrenergic blockers. Thus a stimulus that activates the nerve causes release of norepinephrine, which in turn stimulates synthesis and release of PGE_2; PGE_2 then feeds back at the prejunctional level of the nerve terminal to decrease the amount of norepinephrine released.

Pancreatic endocrine function PGE_2 has primarily inhibitory effects on insulin secretion by the pancreatic beta cell in vitro and on insulin response to intravenous glucose. This effect is mediated by G proteins, since it is associated with decreased production of cyclic AMP and is preventable by pertussis toxin, an agent that inhibits G_i and G_o activity. This inhibitory effect appears to be specific for glucose because the insulin responses to other secretagogues are not influenced by PGE_2. Studies with inhibitors of prostaglandin synthesis support the concept that endogenous PGE_2 acts in vivo to inhibit insulin secretion. In general, such drugs augment insulin secretion and improve carbohydrate tolerance. An exception is indomethacin, which inhibits glucose-induced insulin secretion and can cause hyperglycemia. The discordant results with indomethacin are likely due to some action other than inhibition of cyclooxygenase. Aracidonic acid stimulates insulin secretion in vitro, and the lipoxygenase pathway appears to play a role in potentiating insulin secretion by participating in stimulus-secretion coupling. In this case a likely active arachidonic acid product may be 12-HPETE.

Luteolysis In the sheep, hysterectomy during the luteal phase of the ovarian cycle results in maintenance of the corpus luteum, suggesting that the uterus normally produces a luteolytic substance. A candidate for this substance is $PGF_{2\alpha}$, since it can cause luteal regression.

PATHOPHYSIOLOGY Most postulated roles for arachidonic acid metabolites in disease involve excessive production, but a few disorders may be the result of decreased production. The latter could result from dietary deficiency of arachidonic acid (an essential fatty acid), from damage to a tissue where prostaglandin synthesis takes place, or from therapy with drugs that inhibit enzymes in the synthetic pathway.

Bone resorption: Hypercalcemia of malignancy (See also Chaps. 327 and 357) Hypercalcemia occurs in association with nonparathyroid malignancies of many different types. Parathyroid hormone excess, as the result either of autonomous production by parathyroid tissue or ectopic formation by the tumor itself, is a rare cause. Most patients with hypercalcemia of malignancy do not have elevated plasma levels of parathyroid hormone, and secretion of parathyroid hormone–related peptide by tumors is the usual cause (see Chap. 357).

Prostaglandin E$_2$ is a potent inducer of bone resorption and of calcium release from bone, and PGE$_2$ production is elevated in certain hypercalcemic animals with transplantable tumors. Treatment of these animals with inhibitors of PGE$_2$ synthesis causes reduction of PGE$_2$ levels and a concomitant decrease in hypercalcemia. Likewise, rare patients with hypercalcemia and malignancy have excessive amounts of PGE$_2$ metabolites in urine. Drugs that inhibit prostaglandin synthesis may decrease circulating calcium levels in such patients. Thus a subset of approximately 5 percent of patients with hypercalcemia of malignancy have elevated PGE production and can be treated with drugs that inhibit prostaglandin synthesis.

The source of the excess PGE$_2$ in these patients has not been identified. Increased liver and lung degradation of PGE would be expected to compensate if large amounts of PGE were present in the circulation. It is possible, of course, that such large amounts of PGE$_2$ are released by a tumor into the circulation that liver and lung degradation cannot handle the load. Alternatively, if lung metastases are present, the venous drainage from the tumors could be delivered into the systemic circulation without passing through lung tissue. A third possible mechanism involves metastatic seeding of bone. Tumor cells synthesize PGE in culture, and metastatic tumor cells in bone could synthesize PGE that acts locally to cause bone resorption. Part of this hypothetical mechanism may involve PGE$_2$ production by circulating white cells which congregate at metastatic sites. Bone-resorbing effects of cytokines (particularly IL-1 and TNF) are mediated in part by local prostaglandin production in bone. Hypercalcemia of malignancy can occur in the absence of demonstrable bone metastases, but the clinical tools for excluding such metastases, such as radioisotope scans and computed tomography, may not be sensitive enough to detect many small lesions.

Bone resorption: Rheumatoid arthritis and dental cysts (See Chap. 285) Overproduction of PGE$_2$ has been postulated as a cause of the juxtaarticular osteoporosis and bony erosions in some patients with rheumatoid arthritis. Rheumatoid synovia synthesize PGE$_2$ in tissue culture, and media from these cultures promote bone resorption; moreover, the inclusion of indomethacin in the culture medium blocks this resorptive capacity.

Cells from benign dental cysts also cause bone resorption and synthesize PGE$_2$ in tissue culture. Again, bone resorption caused by the culture medium from such cells is decreased if indomethacin is added prior to the incubation. A related problem is that of alveolar bone resorption in patients with periodontal disease, a common inflammatory disease of the gums. PGE$_2$ levels in inflamed gingiva are greater than in healthy gingival tissue. Thus it is possible that alveolar resorption might be due, in part at least, to local overproduction of these metabolites.

Bartter's syndrome (See Chap. 244) Bartter's syndrome is characterized by elevated levels of plasma renin, aldosterone, and bradykinin; resistance to the pressor effect of angiotensin; hypokalemic alkalosis; and renal potassium wasting in the presence of normal blood pressure. A role for prostaglandins has been postulated since PGE$_2$ and PGI$_2$ stimulate the release of renin and since the pressor response to infused angiotensin is blunted by the vasodilator effects of PGE$_2$ and PGI$_2$. The increase in renin release leads to increased aldosterone secretion, which in turn can increase urinary kallikrein activity.

In keeping with this postulate, elevated levels of PGE$_2$ and 6-keto-PGF$_{1\alpha}$ are present in urine. Hyperplasia of renal medullary interstitial cells (which synthesize PGE in culture) also occurs. These findings led to therapeutic trials of inhibitors of prostaglandin synthesis in the disorder. Indomethacin (and other inhibitors) reverse virtually all the abnormalities except hypokalemia. Thus a prostaglandin, probably PGE$_2$ and/or PGI$_2$, probably mediates some of the manifestations of Bartter's syndrome.

Diabetes mellitus (See Chap. 337) Intravenous administration of glucose to normal individuals causes a sudden (first-phase) increase in secretion of insulin into plasma followed by a slower, more prolonged response termed *second-phase insulin secretion*. Patients with type II (non-insulin-dependent, adult-onset) diabetes mellitus have absent first-phase insulin release in response to glucose and a variable decrease in second-phase insulin secretion. Insulin response to other secretagogues, such as arginine, isoproterenol, glucagon, and secretin, is preserved. Thus diabetics appear to have a specific defect that interferes with normal recognition of glucose signals. Since PGE$_2$ inhibits glucose-induced insulin secretion in normal individuals, inhibitors of endogenous prostaglandin synthesis have been given to patients with type II diabetes to ascertain whether insulin secretion can be improved. Both sodium salicylate and aspirin elevate basal plasma insulin levels, partially restore the first-phase insulin response, increase second-phase insulin secretion, and improve glucose tolerance. This suggests that the defect in glucose-induced insulin secretion in patients with type II diabetes mellitus may be associated with excessive local production of, or hypersensitivity to, endogenous PGE$_2$.

Patients with diabetic ketoacidosis have elevated levels of PGE$_2$ metabolites, and diabetic animals have elevated levels of PGI$_2$ metabolites. PGE$_2$ production may be increased to inhibit lipolysis, and both PGE$_2$ and PGI$_2$ may play roles in the decreased vascular resistance and hypotension in diabetic ketoacidosis.

Patent ductus arteriosus (See Chap. 199) The ductus arteriosus in sheep is sensitive to the vasodilatory properties of PGE$_2$, and PGE-like material is present in the ductal wall. Thus enhanced endogenous PGE$_2$ might maintain prenatal patency of the ductus. Since inhibitors of prostaglandin synthesis cause constriction of the ductus of fetal lambs, trials with indomethacin were undertaken in premature human infants with isolated patent ductus arteriosus. Such treatment for several days is followed by closure of the vessel in the majority, although some require a second course of therapy, and a minority require surgical ligation. Infants under 35 weeks of gestational age are most likely to respond.

Patients with certain types of congenital heart disease require a patent ductus arteriosus to survive. Ductus-dependent pulmonary blood flow is essential under circumstances in which the ductus is the major channel by which nonoxygenated blood reaches the lungs from the aortic arch, e.g., in pulmonary atresia and tricuspid atresia. Since PGE relaxes the smooth muscle in the lamb ductus arteriosus, intravenous PGE has been administered to such patients to attempt to maintain patency of the ductus. Short-term PGE infusions cause a temporary increase in blood flow to the lungs and improve arterial oxygen saturation until the necessary corrective heart surgery can be performed. The large right-to-left shunt in these cardiac malformations allows the intravenously infused PGE$_2$ to escape pulmonary degradation before arriving at the ductus. In this instance, the disease process itself facilitates delivery of the therapeutic agent.

Peptic ulcer disease (See Chap. 252) Gastric acid secretion in patients with peptic ulcer disease is increased. Various analogues of PGE$_2$ inhibit gastric acid secretion and are also inherently cytoprotective. These agents are more effective than placebo in relieving pain and decreasing gastric acid secretion in patients with ulcer disease. Moreover, the healing of ulcer craters as assessed by endoscopic criteria is accelerated in patients receiving PGE analogues.

Dysmenorrhea (See Chap. 340) Dysmenorrhea is usually associated with increased uterine contractions. The fact that some analgesics used to treat this disorder also inhibit prostaglandin synthesis suggests that arachidonic acid metabolites may play a role in the pathogenesis of dysmenorrhea. Prostaglandins of the E and F series are present in human endometrium. Intravenous infusion of either produces uterine contractions, and PGF and PGE levels in menstrual blood are decreased by administration of prostaglandin synthesis inhibitors. Controlled trials in women with dysmenorrhea suggest that symptomatic improvement is greater following therapy with inhibitors of prostaglandin synthesis.

Asthma (See Chap. 217)

Inflammatory response and immune response (See Chaps. 277 and 282) Drugs such as aspirin have antipyretic, anti-inflammatory, and analgesic effects. Several arguments support a relation between inflammation and the arachidonic acid metabolites: (1) Inflammatory stimuli such as histamine and bradykinin release endogenous prostaglandins in parallel. (2) Leukotriene C_4-D_4-E_4 is more potent than histamine in causing bronchoconstriction. (3) Several arachidonic acid metabolites cause vasodilatation and hyperalgesia. (4) PGE_2 and LTB_4 are present in areas of inflammation. Polymorphonuclear cells release these products during phagocytosis, and they are chemotactic for leukocytes. (5) Some eicosanoids (PGD_2, PGE_2, LTC_4, LTD_4, LTE_4) cause increased vascular permeability, a feature of the inflammatory response that gives rise to local edema. (6) Vasodilation induced by PGE is not abolished by atropine, propranolol, methysergide, or antihistamines, known antagonists of other possible mediators of the inflammatory response. Thus PGE may have a direct inflammatory effect, and some mediators of inflammation may act by influencing PGE release. (7) Some arachidonic acid metabolites can cause pain in animal models and hyperalgesia or an increased sensitivity to pain in humans. (8) PGE can cause fever after injection into the cerebral ventricles or into the hypothalamus of animals. (9) Pyrogens cause increased concentrations of prostaglandins in cerebrospinal fluid, whereas prostaglandin synthesis inhibitors decrease fever and decrease release of prostaglandins into cerebrospinal fluid.

PGD_2 is believed to play a major role in the manifestations of systemic mastocytosis and other disorders of mast cell activation. These symptoms include flushing, tachycardia, hypotension, abdominal cramping, diarrhea, chest pain, headache, dyspnea, and pruritus. NSAIDs in combination with antihistamines are effective therapy, but a subset of patients have attacks provoked by aspirin.

Arachidonic acid metabolites also may play a role in the immune response. Small amounts of PGE_2 can suppress stimulation of human lymphocytes by mitogens such as phytohemagglutinin, and the inflammatory response is associated with the local release of arachidonic acid metabolites; thus these substances may act as negative modulators of lymphocyte function. The release of PGE by mitogen-stimulated mononuclear cells may play a role in the negative feedback control mechanism by which lymphocyte activity is regulated. Sensitivity of lymphocytes to the inhibiting effects of PGE_2 increases with age, and indomethacin augments lymphocyte responsiveness to mitogens to a greater degree in the elderly. Mononuclear cells from patients with Hodgkin's disease release more PGE_2 after the addition of phytohemagglutinin, and lymphocyte responsiveness is enhanced by indomethacin. When suppressor T cells are removed from the cultures, the amount of PGE_2 synthesized is diminished, and the responsiveness of the lymphocytes from the Hodgkin's patients and controls is no longer different. Depressed cellular immunity in patients with Hodgkin's disease may be the result of PGE inhibition of lymphocyte function.

REFERENCES

ADVANCES IN PROSTAGLANDINS AND GASTROENTEROLOGY. Symposium. Am J Med 83(1A): 1, 1987

HENDERSON WR: Eicosanoids and platelet-activating factor in allergic respiratory diseases. Am Rev Respir Dis 143:S86, 1991

HEYMAN MA: Prostaglandins and leukotrienes in the perinatal period. Clin Perinatol 14:857, 1987

NEEDLEMAN P et al: Arachidonic acid metabolism. Annu Rev Biochem 55:69, 1986

OATES JA et al: Clinical implications of prostaglandin and thromboxane A_2 formation. N Engl J Med 319(11):689, 1988 and 319(12):761, 1988

ROBERTSON RP (ed): Symposium on prostaglandins in health and disease. Med Clin North Am 65:711, 1981

———: Eicosanoids as pluripotential modulators of pancreatic islet function. Diabetes 37:367, 1988

SCHARSCHMIDT L et al: Glomerular prostaglandins, angiotensin II, and nonsteroidal anti-inflammatory drugs. Am J Med 81(2B):30, 1986

PART FIVE

71 NUTRITION AND NUTRITIONAL REQUIREMENTS

IRWIN H. ROSENBERG

Maintenance of nutrition is essential for both the management and the prevention of disease. Many complications can be prevented or modified by attention to nutritional status and prevention of nutritional deficits. The effective management of the sick patient, therefore, requires detailed evaluation of diet and nutritional status and a projection of the interaction of diet and nutritional status on the clinical course. Only then can proper goals and techniques of nutritional management be selected and nutritional guidance be provided for disease prevention and health promotion.

The purpose of this section is to summarize some of the basic considerations for the estimation of nutritional needs and the setting of goals for treatment. Determination of the nutritional needs of the individual patient must take into account both the physiologic responses to normal dietary intake and the nutritional impairments induced by disease.

EATING BEHAVIOR AND NUTRITIONAL NEEDS Eating behavior is by nature intermittent, yet energy needs are continuous. This feature of mammalian biology has resulted in the evolution of metabolic controls that promote the ebb and flow of nutrients after feeding and during the postabsorptive period and, in addition, provide for the maintenance of near-normal function during fasting.

In a nutritional perspective, the mechanisms that control appetite and eating behavior are directed to maintain energy intake adequate for the needs of the healthy adult, for growth in the child, and for the requirements of pregnancy and lactation. Under conditions of disease or trauma, the increased requirements must be met through appropriate modifications in eating behavior or caloric supplementation.

The usual remarkable stability of body weight and body composition requires that energy intake and expenditure be balanced over time. The nature of the internal signals that relay the information that caloric intake is appropriate for energy needs during the preceding days is not known. Such signals do not adjust eating behavior on a meal-to-meal time scale. With an individual meal, volume and chemoreceptors in the stomach and small bowel initiate neural and hormonal responses that contribute to satiety. The nutrient density of the food eaten, in terms of the protein or calorie content per unit volume, is not sensitively perceived, and therefore total energy or protein intake can fluctuate substantially over the short run. The neurophysiologic mechanisms that control eating behavior recognize calorie deficiencies on roughly a 24-h time scale and make compensatory changes in the volume of food eaten over periods of 1 to 2 days. That these controls work is attested to by the stability of body weight and general nutritional health of most people who have access to adequate food intake. Aberrations in these control factors can produce serious and even life-threatening imbalance, as evidenced by obesity and syndromes of anorexia and depletion.

METABOLIC RESPONSES TO CALORIC INTAKE When dietary or energy intake is adequate, several metabolic controls act to maintain essential body functions. One essential function is the maintenance of a steady fuel supply to the brain. Under the usual conditions the brain uses glucose for energy at a rate of about 5 g/h during both the fasted and fed states. The brain is also capable of utilizing ketones as an energy source and will do so in preference to glucose if the ketones are present in high concentration. In contrast to tissues such as skeletal muscle, the brain uses energy at a fairly constant rate, whether awake, sleeping, thinking, or dreaming.

During the influx of nutrients into blood after feeding and absorption, the energy and amino acid needs of the body are readily met by the supply entering from the gastrointestinal tract. When this flow of nutrients subsides, however, the body's needs are met by release of energy from stores. In the period immediately after feeding, these stores are generated under hormonal control, particularly insulin. The excess amino acids, fatty acids, and glucose not required immediately for energy are stored as proteins, triglycerides, and glycogen. This storage process also serves to mitigate the large extracellular osmotic shifts that might occur between the fed and the fasting states by depositing excess nutrients in intracellular depots.

NUTRITIONAL REQUIREMENTS To formulate a plan for nutritional management, one must consider the nutritional requirements of the patient and the impact of disease on these requirements. Energy balance means energy intake that maintains a steady body weight. Energy insufficiency is reflected in weight loss, and energy overabundance causes weight gain. Conditions that can modify nutritional requirements include infection, trauma, surgery, alcohol abuse, and malabsorption.

ESTIMATION OF ENERGY REQUIREMENT Although malnutrition, literally abnormal nutrition, could result from either excessive or inadequate energy balance, in general the term refers to undernutrition. Undernutrition can be due to inadequate intake or absorption or to increased metabolic requirements imposed by disease, including excessive loss of nutrients and drug-nutrient antagonisms.

The components of energy requirements in humans are summarized in Table 71-1. Total daily energy requirement consists of basal metabolic rate plus energy of activity and the thermic effect of food. Basal metabolic rate (BMR) or, more appropriately, resting metabolic rate (RMR) is a measure of the amount of energy expended at rest and without food; energy of activity is a measure of the energy

---

TABLE 71-1 Example of estimation of daily energy requirement

The information presented above can be utilized as in the following example: A 45-year-old, 70-kg male office worker presents with rheumatoid arthritis of mild severity. Calorie intake is good, but recent activity has been limited.

Resting energy expenditure*	7500 kJ (1800 kcal)
Activity-related expenditure	1700 kJ (400 kcal)
Illness-related expenditure	
(10 percent of 1800 kcal)	750 kJ (180 kcal)
Diet-induced thermogenesis	
(10 percent of 2380 kcal)	955 kJ (238 kcal)
Total	10,945 kJ (2618 kcal)

* Resting energy expenditure (RMR) is calculated as in Table 71-2.

TABLE 71-2   Estimation of resting metabolic rate (RMR)

Age (years)	Male		Female	
	kJ (a)	kcal (b)	kJ (a)	kcal (b)
3–10	Wt* × 95 + 2110	Wt* × 22.7 + 505	Wt* × 85 + 2033	Wt* × 20.3 + 486
10–18	Wt × 74 + 2754	Wt × 17.7 + 659	Wt × 56 + 2898	Wt × 13.4 + 693
18–30	Wt × 63 + 2896	Wt × 15.1 + 693	Wt × 62 + 2036	Wt × 14.8 + 487
30–60	Wt × 48 + 4653	Wt × 11.5 + 1113	Wt × 34 + 3538	Wt × 8.1 + 846
>60	Wt × 59 + 2459	Wt × 11.7 + 588	Wt × 38 + 2755	Wt × 9.1 + 659

*Body weight in kilograms
(a) To convert the RMR from kJ to kcal multiply kJ by 0.239.
(b) To convert the RMR from kcal to kJ multiply the kcal by 4.186.
SOURCE: Modified from WN Schofield.

expended to support a variety of physical activities; diet-induced thermogenesis (DIT) (also called *thermic effect of food* and previously termed *specific dynamic action*) is the increase in energy expenditure above basal values associated with consuming food. RMR accounts for about two-thirds of the total energy requirements and is affected by body size (height and weight), age, sex, and habitus (Table 71-2). Several methods are available for estimating resting energy expenditure. The most accurate technique for measuring total energy expenditure is the doubly labeled water technique, which utilizes the different distribution of ^{18}O and deuterium in CO_2 and body H_2O.

Estimation of resting metabolic rate (RMR) Most methods are based on calorimetry, a measurement of oxygen consumption under carefully controlled conditions, e.g., during fasting, in the morning, and for one hour. A more meaningful metabolic rate would reflect the rate at which energy is consumed in a normal life situation at rest throughout the day, including the period of food assimilation. Clinical estimates of RMR, based on indirect assessments rather than true measurements, are frequently very useful.

The estimations of Harris and Benedict for calculating BMR (in kcal/d) are as follows:

$$BMR_{women} = 655 + (9.5 \times W) + (1.8 \times H) - (4.7 \times A)$$
$$BMR_{men} = 66 + (13.7 \times W) + (5 \times H) - (6.8 \times A)$$

where W is actual or usual weight (kg), H is height (cm), and A is age (years).

The equations for RMR are simpler and are based on more comprehensive data. Because people of the same weight but of different heights have similar RMRs, the formulas are based only on weight, age, and sex (Table 71-2). It should be remembered that predicted RMR (or BMR) may over- or underestimate the measured values by 20 or even 30 percent for any individual.

Diet-induced thermogenesis (DIT) The ingestion of nutrients in food causes heat or energy production in excess of basal metabolic rates. A mixed diet causes approximately a 6 to 10 percent increase above basal in calories expended as heat. DIT can be divided into two components, *obligatory thermogenesis* and *facultative thermogenesis*. The former is the component of DIT that is expended in digestion, transport, and processing of food. The remainder is energy that may dissipate surplus energy and thus participate in weight maintenance and prevention of obesity. The thermogenic effect of protein is greatest, that of carbohydrate is next, and fat is least effective. The calorigenic effect of food seems to be closely related to the energy required for ATP formation, in which protein (via amino acid breakdown) is the oxidative substrate. Most of the effect is generated in the muscle and liver and occurs whether intake is enteral or parenteral. In hypermetabolic patients, diet-induced thermogenesis is less marked because heat production is already elevated. In calculating additional energy requirements for hypermetabolic patients, the DIT should be estimated at no more than 5 percent of total energy requirements.

Estimates of energy for activity The energy expenditure of physical activity accounts for about one-third of total energy expenditures under most conditions and can vary from 6 to 36 kJ (1.5 to 8.5

kcal) per kilogram body weight per hour (Table 71-3). This factor is obviously more important in calculating energy requirements for active, ambulatory patients. Some types of work (e.g., gardening) can cause fatigue without using a large number of calories. Usually, exercise that results in lifting the body from the ground (e.g., running) uses the most calories. Although precise measurements can be made for a wide range of activities, it is easiest to use an approximation when estimating energy needs.

Additional energy requirements of illness Heat production increases with fever and inflammation. However, as oxygen consumption increases, DIT decreases, and the energy of activity often declines owing to immobility. For these reasons, the daily energy requirement in ill persons is usually only slightly greater than the requirement when well. Indeed, the energy requirement for most patients, even during severe illness, rarely exceeds 12,500 kJ (3000 kcal) per day. (The earlier estimates of massively increased calorie requirements in patients with sepsis have not been substantiated.) Approximately 20 percent should be added to resting energy estimates for a patient confined to bed, and 30 percent should be added for ambulatory patients. Severe illness requires additional caloric supplementation, namely, addition of 10 percent of estimated RMR for mild illness, 25 percent for moderate illness, and 50 percent for severe illness.

Malabsorption is a special cause of increased energy requirement. The most accurate but impractical way to assess calorie loss would be calorimetry of the feces. However, fat excretion (in g/d) (as determined in a 72-h fecal fat assay) × 38 kJ (9 kcal) per gram equals the daily energy loss due to fat malabsorption. To estimate total fecal energy loss from all sources, the fecal energy loss from fat (in kJ or kcal) is multiplied by 2.5. This estimate assumes an average dietary composition and equivalent malabsorption of fat, carbohydrate, and protein.

ESTIMATION OF PROTEIN REQUIREMENT Protein balance, like energy balance, is a function of intake relative to utilization and loss. Normally, nitrogen derived from amino acids is lost in urine and feces and from skin. Unlike the energy stored in triglycerides and glycogen, no proteins (or amino acids) are stored in the body solely for subsequent utilization. Every protein serves either a structural or metabolic function; when excess protein is ingested the amino acids are transaminated, and the nonnitrogenous portion of the

TABLE 71-3   Estimation of additional energy expenditure by activity

Type of work	Calories added to BMR	
	kJ/d	kcal/d
Sedentary	1670–3350	400–800
Light: office, professional and clerical	3350–5000	800–1200
Moderate: walking, lifting	5000–7500	1200–1800
Heavy: construction, athletic	7500–19,000	1800–4500

SOURCE: Modified from DW Wilmore, *The Metabolic Management of the Critically Ill.* New York, Plenum Press, 1977.

molecule serves as a source of calories for storage as glycogen and/or fat.

Obligatory nitrogen losses Urea accounts for over 80 percent of urinary nitrogen. The remaining nitrogen is excreted as creatinine, porphyrins, and other nitrogen-containing compounds. Thus total urine loss of nitrogen = urinary urea nitrogen (mg/dL) × daily volume (dL) ÷ 0.8. Urinary nitrogen is related to the RMR. The larger the body muscle mass, the more transamination of amino acids occurs to fulfill energy needs. Each kilocalorie needed for basal metabolism leads to the excretion of 1 to 1.3 mg of urinary nitrogen. For the same reason, nitrogen excretion increases during exercise and heavy work.

Fecal and skin losses account for a large proportion of nitrogen loss from the body (about 40 percent) in normal circumstances, but the magnitude of these losses varies in disease states. Thus, measurement of urinary nitrogen often provides a useful index of daily nitrogen requirement.

Minimal nitrogen loss (in g/d) from a 70-kg person on a diet that is nitrogen free but energy adequate approximates 1.9 to 3.1 in urine, 0.7 to 2.5 in stool, and 0.3 from skin for a mean total loss of 4.4 g/d. Equivalent protein loss can be calculated by multiplying nitrogen loss by 6.25 so that total loss by metabolism of protein is 4.4 × 6.25 or 27.5 g/d or about 0.4 g/kg body weight for a 70-kg person. The recommended protein allowance for adults varies from 0.6 to 0.9 g/kg to allow for a margin of safety. Vigorous exercise may increase protein requirements to 1 g/kg body weight or higher.

Protein requirements are highest during the growth spurts of infancy and adolescence. During infancy, total body protein reserve is lowest, and obligatory losses are greatest. Thus, protein deficiency is most likely to occur during infancy. Protein requirements decline slightly during childhood and again increase with adolescence. Minimal requirements for these stages of life are about 1.5 g/kg body weight per day. The recommended allowance (2 g/kg body weight per day) allows a margin of safety for children who have increased needs or who ingest proteins of low biologic value. Low-quality proteins include certain vegetable proteins that do not support growth as well as protein from milk, eggs, or meat. The differences in the nutritional value of protein are largely due to the higher content of essential amino acids in animal proteins and to differences in digestibility. Protein (and energy) requirements also increase during pregnancy and lactation.

CALORIC REQUIREMENTS FOR PROTEIN UTILIZATION Amino acids ingested without other energy sources are not efficiently incorporated into protein partly because of the energy lost during amino acid metabolism. Moreover, incorporation of each amino acid molecule into peptides requires three high-energy phosphate bonds. Consequently, excess of dietary energy over basal needs improves the efficiency of nitrogen utilization. During the period of intense growth in children, about 300 kJ (76 kcal) of nonprotein energy are required for each gram of protein. In ambulatory adults about 200 kJ (50 kcal) from nonprotein sources are needed per gram of protein. This high ratio usually cannot be achieved with parenteral feeding, since energy intake is limited by the volume needed to be infused. Acceptable figures for parenteral nutrition are about 100 to 125 kJ (25 to 30 kcal) from nonprotein sources per gram of protein or 600 to 750 kJ (150 to 180 kcal) per gram of nitrogen.

RECOMMENDED DIETARY ALLOWANCES OF PROTEIN AND MICRONUTRIENTS Guidelines of nutritional requirements in health have been formulated in the reports, updated periodically, of the Food and Nutrition Board of the National Research Council of the United States. These Recommended Dietary Allowances, expressed for age and sex and modified for such conditions as pregnancy and lactation, are designed to cover the requirements of virtually all healthy individuals. With the exception of energy, the allowances are not average requirements but rather a recommended intake sufficient to meet the needs of all healthy individuals.

The recommended allowances for protein (nitrogen), iron, and calcium are based upon experiments in which normal requirement is

TABLE 71-4 Recommended dietary allowances for healthy adults

	Range of allowance	
	Men	Women
Protein, g	45–63	44–50
Vitamin A, μg retinol equivalents	1000	800
Vitamin D, μg	5–10	5–10
Vitamin E, mg α-tocopherol equivalents	10	8
Vitamin K, μg	45–80	45–65
Vitamin C, mg	50–60	50–60
Thiamine, mg	1.2–1.5	1–1.1
Riboflavin, mg	1.4–1.8	1.2–1.3
Niacin, mg niacin equivalents	15–20	13–15
Vitamin B$_6$, mg	1.4–2.0	1.4–1.6
Folate, μg	150–200	150–180[†]
Vitamin B$_{12}$, μg	2.0	2.0
Biotin, μg*	30–100	50–100
Pantothenic Acid, mg*	4–10	4–7
Calcium, mg	800–1200	800–1200
Phosphorus, mg	800–1200	800–1200
Magnesium, mg	270–400	280–300
Iron, mg	10–12	10–15
Zinc, mg	15	12
Iodine, μg	150	150
Selenium, μg	40–70	45–55
Copper, mg*	1.5–3	1.5–3
Manganese, mg*	2–5	2–5
Fluoride, mg*	1.5–4	1.5–4
Chromium, μg*	50–200	50–200
Molybdenum, μg*	75–250	75–250

* Estimated safe and adequate daily dietary intakes. From the National Research Council: *Recommended Dietary Allowances*, 10th ed. Washington, D.C., National Academy of Sciences, 1989.
† The allowance increases to 400–800 in women of childbearing age and for pregnancy.

defined as the intake necessary to achieve zero balance between intake versus output. For most vitamins the recommended allowance is the daily intake required to maintain full function and safe levels of body stores. Most estimates assume normal digestion and absorption and normal metabolism. In some cases, estimates of daily turnover are used to determine the amount of nutrient required to maintain body stores. It follows, therefore, that diseases that influence efficiency of absorption or that change the metabolism or nutritional requirements will change the safe allowance for that individual. It further follows that the recommended dietary allowances are at best a rough guide for requirements for enteral nutrient intake by any individual. Such allowances may be an overestimation of parenteral requirements, particularly in the case of micronutrients, since in that case no allowance need be made for the inefficiency of extraction from food and absorption. A listing of these essential nutrients and an estimation of the ranges of required intake for healthy adults are presented in Table 71-4.

The 1989 Recommended Dietary Allowances make little provision for changes in nutrient requirements for the elderly. Energy requirements decline progressively beyond age 50 or 60 as the lean (muscle) mass declines and as resting metabolic energy expenditure decreases. Energy needs for activity also decline as aging often leads to more sedentary lifestyle. At present, it is prudent to recommend full adult levels of protein, vitamins, and minerals even in the face of declining energy intake. For many elderly people, especially women, this may require careful dietary planning and dietary supplements. Increased physical activity at all ages promotes the retention of lean muscle mass and increases appetite and food intake.

REFERENCES

ALPERS DH et al: *Manual of Nutritional Therapeutics*. Boston, Little, Brown, 1987, chap 3

HAVEL RJ: Caloric homeostasis and disorders of fuel transport. N Engl J Med 1987:1186, 1972

KISSILEFF HR, VAN ITALLIE TB: Physiology of the control of food intake. Ann Rev Nutr 2:271, 1982

NATIONAL RESEARCH COUNCIL: *Recommended Dietary Allowances*, 10th ed. Washington, DC, National Academy of Sciences, 1989

SCHOFIELD WN: Predicting basal metabolic rate, new standards and review of previous work. Human Nutr Clin Nutr 39C(Suppl 1), 1985

WOO R et al: Regulation of energy balance. Ann Rev Nutr 5:411, 1985

72 PROTEIN-ENERGY MALNUTRITION

JOEL B. MASON / IRWIN H. ROSENBERG

Protein-energy malnutrition (PEM), also called protein-calorie malnutrition (PCM), is present when insufficient energy or protein is available to meet metabolic demands, thereby leading to impairments in normal physiologic processes. Inadequate dietary intake is only one of several mechanisms by which this may occur. Increased metabolic demands due to disease and increased nutrient losses are two other common mechanisms by which the body's protein and energy economy may become disrupted enough to cause PEM. Protein deficiency may also arise in the face of adequate protein intake if the dietary protein is of poor quality (i.e., the content of one or more essential amino acids is inadequate and thus becomes the limiting factor in protein utilization); such is the case when the entire protein intake is derived from a single vegetable source. Protein nutrition is also influenced by the intake of energy relative to the intake of protein because the efficient utilization of dietary protein requires energy from nonprotein calories.

Adaptive responses function over the short term when protein and energy sources are limited. As a consequence, the pathologic effects of undernutrition require a sustained inadequacy of protein or energy sources. The adaptive mechanisms that respond to protein and calorie deprivation are finite, particularly because protein has no storage form in the body.

The rapidity with which PEM develops and its severity depend on a number of factors, including the nutritional state when the nutritional deprivation begins, the underlying illness, and the developmental stage. Some of these factors are outlined in Table 72-1.

PROTEIN-ENERGY MALNUTRITION AS A GLOBAL PROBLEM Recognition of PEM emerged from studies in the tropics that were focused primarily on the problem in children. Preschool children, particularly those between the ages of 1 and 2 are more susceptible to PEM. They are dependent on others for determining the quantity and quality of food intake; their protein and energy requirements are substantially higher per unit weight; and unhygienic habits and immaturity of the immune system heighten susceptibility to infections.

Gastrointestinal infections, in particular, constitute a major precipitant of PEM in infants and children because such illnesses result in altered feeding habits, vomiting, decreased intestinal absorption, increased metabolic needs, and increased metabolic losses. The magnitude of the problem is immense; the World Health Organization estimated in 1983 that 300 million children have growth retardation secondary to malnutrition. Increased mortality and impaired cognitive, social, and economic development are additional features but are difficult to quantitate.

PROTEIN-ENERGY MALNUTRITION IN DEVELOPED NATIONS PEM is confined neither to children nor to the less-developed countries. Although the overall prevalence of PEM is low, specific sectors of the U.S. population, such as the institutionalized elderly and children of the poor, have a significant prevalence. For example, the Ten State Survey, which focused on low income areas in the United States, found that 22 to 35 percent of the children aged 2, 4, and 6 were below the 15th percentile for weight. In this survey income level and minority status were predictors of growth retardation among children. In a 1987 survey 11 percent of low income children had height for age below the 5th percentile standard. Moreover, in large urban teaching hospitals as well as smaller community hospitals 30 to 70 percent of general medical and surgical patients have anthropometric and/or biochemical evidence of PEM. Similar statistics have been noted in surveys of pediatric inpatients. It is perhaps more disturbing that the nutritional status of the majority of hospitalized patients *declines* during the course of hospitalization. Positive associations between the degree of PEM and the incidence of postoperative infections, impaired healing of surgical wounds, and prolongation of hospitalization indicate that more attention needs to be paid to the maintenance of adequate nutrition in individual patients. There are tangible benefits from such nutritional diligence. For example, aggressive preoperative nutritional restitution of malnourished patients can decrease perioperative morbidity such as infection.

Most modern-day hospital malnutrition is compounded by insufficient attention by medical personnel to nutrition (Table 72-2). Indeed, most factors contributing to the high prevalence of malnutrition in hospitalized patients are reversible or preventable.

PROTEIN-ENERGY METABOLISM DURING STRESS Physiological adaptation to starvation During periods of protein and/or energy deficit, compensatory mechanisms serve to lessen the pathologic impact of these deficiencies. To understand how malnutrition develops, it is important to understand the responses to such inadequate intake. During the first 24 h of fasting, circulating glucose, fatty acids, and triglycerides and liver and muscle glycogen are used as fuel sources. However, the sum of these stores in a 70-kg man is only about 5000 kJ (1200 kcal) and provides less fuel than is needed for basal metabolism for a single day. Triglycerides, derived primarily from adipose tissue, can be catabolized to fatty acids and ketone

---

TABLE 72-1 Factors that condition the response to inadequate nutrient intake

A Nutritional factors
 1 Underlying adequacy of reserves/depot of that nutrient
 2 Severity of the inadequate intake; duration of deprivation
 3 Concurrent deficiencies of other nutrients
B Underlying illnesses
 1 Fever, infection, trauma, and other conditions associated with increased requirements and catabolic losses
 2 Malabsorptive, maldigestive states
 3 Illnesses associated with excessive loss of nutrients (e.g., protein-losing enteropathy, nephrotic syndrome, enteric fistulas)
 4 Conditions associated with altered metabolism of nutrients (e.g., diabetes mellitus, hyperthyroidism)
C Physiologic states in which increased requirements are present
 1 Pregnancy, lactation
 2 Growth and development during infancy, childhood, and adolescence

---

TABLE 72-2 Undesirable practices that affect the nutritional health of hospital patients

1 Failure to record height and weight in the hospital chart
2 Diffusion of responsibility for patient care
3 Prolonged use of glucose and saline intravenous feedings
4 Failure to observe and record patients' dietary intake
5 Withholding meals because of diagnostic tests
6 Use of enteral or parenteral feedings of uncertain composition and in inadequate amounts
7 Ignorance of the composition of nutritional products
8 Failure to recognize increased nutritional needs due to injury or illness
9 Lack of communication and interaction between physician, nurse, and dietician
10 Delay of nutritional support until the patient is in a state of severe depletion
11 Limited availability of laboratory tests to assess nutritional status; failure to use those that are available
12 Limited emphasis on nutrition education in medical schools

SOURCE: Butterworth CE: The skeleton in the hospital closet. Nutr Today 9:4, 1974

bodies by most tissues. However, over the short run tissues such as the brain can only use glycolytic pathways to obtain energy. Since fatty acids are not converted to carbohydrate, these glycolytic tissues must utilize either glucose or substrates that can be converted to glucose. Amino acids derived primarily from skeletal muscle constitute the major endogenous substrate for glucose production for this purpose. Since there is no storage form of protein in the body, a fasting individual sustains a daily loss of functionally significant protein.

The provision of adequate fuel substrate to critical tissues, particularly the brain, has homeostatic priority during protein/energy deprivation. Brief starvation leads to acute adaptive responses that sustain the supply of glucose to tissues that require it and minimize the amount of protein breakdown to meet this need. To accomplish this end, certain tissues, such as the heart, kidney, and skeletal muscle, change their primary fuel substrate from glucose to fatty acids and ketone bodies. Other tissues, such as the bone marrow, renal medulla, and peripheral nerves, switch from the full oxidation of glucose to anaerobic glycolysis, resulting in the production of lactate and pyruvate. These compounds can be converted to glucose in the liver with energy derived from fat oxidation and then released for systemic consumption. This shuttle, the Cori cycle, enables energy stored as fat to be utilized for glucose synthesis and thus conserves protein energy that would otherwise be necessary for the de novo synthesis of glucose.

With more extended starvation other adaptations appear. A decrease in physical exertion decreases energy consumption, and the resting metabolic rate generally declines by about 10 percent. The brain, which ordinarily obtains energy only by glucose oxidation, acquires the ability to use keto acids for its fuel requirements, and this contributes further to protein conservation. Animal studies and, less definitively, human studies suggest that protein that is consumed during relative protein starvation is utilized more efficiently. Moreover, chronic protein deprivation leads to a reduced rate of protein turnover, and amino acids are reutilized more efficiently for the synthesis of new proteins, contributing to savings in both energy and amino acid requirements.

During relative or total caloric starvation, such adaptations allow the body to provide the energy necessary for metabolism and to minimize the obligatory loss of protein, which appears primarily as nitrogen-containing compounds in the urine. After several weeks of starvation, nitrogen loss in the urine may decrease by more than 65 percent. However, these homeostatic mechanisms do not compensate entirely for the imposed deficits, and eventually the negative caloric and/or protein balance lead to pathologic consequences.

Effects of physical stress Infection, trauma, and other physical stress cause inflammatory responses. In such situations, protein and energy metabolism change in ways that increase both energy demands and nitrogen losses and thereby predispose to the development of PEM.

Resting metabolic rate (RMR) increases dramatically during critical illness in a fashion that is roughly proportional to the severity of the stress. Patients with burns over more than 40 percent of the body have a RMR approximately twice normal, patients with sepsis have a RMR that is about one and a half times normal, and patients with a single bone fracture or a localized infection have RMRs that are about 1.3 times normal. Factors that contribute to the increased energy consumption include increases in circulating catecholamines, the increase in energy expenditure required for gluconeogenesis, and the hypermetabolism associated with fever.

Nitrogen loss during critical illness is also increased proportional to the severity of the stress, but the magnitude of the increase is generally larger than the increase in energy consumption. A healthy adult loses approximately 12 g of nitrogen in urine per day in the fasting state; sepsis and trauma commonly increase that value by 50 to 100 percent. Since 1 g of urinary nitrogen represents approximately 30 g of lean body mass, critical illness induces a daily loss of 0.6 kg of lean body mass. Most of this loss comes from the skeletal muscle,

and the efflux of amino acids from skeletal muscle increases two- to sixfold in critically ill patients. Increased efflux from skeletal muscle is probably due to increased protein catabolism rather than decreased protein synthesis.

The mobilization of amino acids from skeletal muscle is an adaptive response. The liberated amino acids are in part used as fuel. They are also taken up by the liver and other visceral organs (the ''visceral protein compartment''). The proteolysis of muscle under physical stress thus enables the body to shift protein substrate from skeletal muscle (the ''somatic protein compartment'') to visceral organs whose function is more critical for immediate survival. Hormonal factors play a significant role in this shift; circulating levels of cortisol, glucagon, epinephrine, and growth hormone are increased in physically stressed individuals. Increased local or circulating levels of interleukin 1 and tumor necrosis factor alpha (TNF-α) in patients with a systemic inflammatory process probably play a major role in sparing the visceral protein compartment at the expense of the skeletal muscle. Eventually, continued deficits in protein and energy, particularly when superimposed on sustained physical stress, lead to a contraction of the visceral protein compartment and its associated functions.

CLASSIFICATION AND ASSESSMENT OF PROTEIN-ENERGY MALNUTRITION Protein-energy malnutrition may be *primary*, due to an inadequate intake of protein and/or energy source, or *secondary*, due to illness that impairs intake or utilization of nutrients or that increases nutrient requirements or metabolic losses. Malignancy, intestinal malabsorption, inflammatory bowel disease, AIDS, and chronic renal failure are a few of the illnesses commonly associated with secondary PEM.

There are no universally accepted criteria for defining the severity of PEM although it is often categorized as mild, moderate, or severe. An effective nutritional assessment requires the synthesis of information provided by a dietary history, physical examination, biochemical data, and functional and/or anthropometric measurements of nutritional status. No single piece of evidence is sufficient to indicate the nutritional status. A corollary is that each parameter used to assess nutritional status can be, and often is, influenced by factors that have little to do with the nutritional state.

In adults, the most commonly used indication of caloric status is body weight. Standard tables of desirable or ideal body weight are available, but individual variation is so great that comparison with the pre-morbid weight of the individual is more informative. It therefore follows that an obese individual who has ongoing deficits in protein or caloric balance, although considerably above ideal body weight, can have PEM with its associated pathologic consequences.

The degree of unintentional weight loss in an ill individual correlates with the extent of total body protein depletion, the integrity of many physiologic functions, and clinical endpoints such as the rate of in-hospital infections and the duration of hospitalization. Consequently, an unintentional decrease of more than 20 percent of the usual body weight, which is almost always associated with a 25 to 35 percent decrease in lean body mass, significant impairment in many physiologic functions, a higher rate of in-hospital morbidity, and extended hospitalization, is the most accessible indicator of *severe* PEM. Patients whose weight loss is >10 and ≤20 percent (*moderate* PEM) have significant losses of body protein, impairments in physiologic functions, increased rates of in-hospital morbidity, and hospitalization stays that are intermediate between individuals with severe PEM and individuals whose weight loss is less than or equal to 10 percent. Unintentional weight loss of ≤10 percent is not associated with physiologic impairments or increased morbidity.

Fat stores are the major energy reserve in the body and, as such, also can be used to assess energy status. The reduction in subcutaneous fat is often evident by inspecting the extremities or face, although a significant reduction in fat mass is frequently overlooked unless more objective criteria than visual inspection are used. Skin-fold measurements or more sophisticated indicators of body consumption can be used to quantify the reduction in body mass that is composed

TABLE 72-3   Normative values for triceps skin-fold thickness

Age group, years	Mean, mm	Percentile						
		5	10	25	50	75	90	95
MEN								
18–74	12.0	4.5	6.0	8.0	11.0	15.0	20.0	23.0
18–24	11.2	4.0	5.0	7.0	9.5	14.0	20.0	23.0
25–34	12.6	4.5	5.5	8.0	12.0	16.0	21.5	24.0
35–44	12.4	5.0	6.0	8.5	12.0	15.5	20.0	23.0
45–54	12.4	5.0	6.0	8.0	11.0	15.0	20.0	25.0
55–64	11.6	5.0	6.0	8.0	11.0	14.0	18.0	21.5
65–74	11.8	4.5	5.5	8.0	11.0	15.0	19.0	22.0
WOMEN								
18–74	23.0	11.0	13.0	17.0	22.0	28.0	34.0	37.5
18–24	19.4	9.4	11.0	14.0	18.0	24.0	30.0	34.0
25–34	21.9	10.5	12.0	16.0	21.0	26.5	33.5	37.0
35–44	24.0	12.0	14.0	18.0	23.0	29.5	35.5	39.0
45–54	25.4	13.0	15.0	20.0	25.0	30.0	36.0	40.0
55–65	24.9	11.0	14.0	19.0	25.0	30.5	35.0	39.0
65–74	23.3	11.5	14.0	18.0	23.0	28.0	33.0	36.0

SOURCE: Heymsfield and Williams.

of fat. The triceps fat fold, when compared to standard values, provides an indication of the adequacy of body fat since more than half of total body fat is subcutaneous (Table 72-3). A triceps fat fold measurement that is less than the 10th percentile is indicative of a substantial deficit of fat stores.

Protein status can be assessed in several different ways. Separate assessments of the somatic and visceral protein compartments are useful and physiologically meaningful since these two protein depots are handled differently by the body. The somatic protein compartment can be objectively assessed by determining the mid-arm muscle area and comparing it to normative values such as in Table 72-4. Estimation of the creatinine-height index performs a similar function (Table 72-5). Physical examination also can provide evidence of decreased

muscle mass but tends to be an insensitive means of assessment. The visceral protein compartment can be estimated by several methods. The total lymphocyte count in the peripheral blood and the presence of delayed cutaneous hypersensitivity are effective in this respect. A total lymphocyte count less than 1500 cells per microliter or the absence of cutaneous hypersensitivity to common antigens suggests a deficit in the visceral protein compartment. The concentrations of certain serum proteins, albumin being the most common, are also useful parameters. However, the accuracy of serum albumin to reflect the status of the visceral protein compartment or the general state of nutrition is poor in the setting of acute or critical illness: the long half-life of albumin (20 days), the fact that it is distributed extensively in the extravascular and intravascular compartments, and the fact that its synthesis is influenced by circulating inflammatory mediators and by liver disease all contribute to its inaccuracy as a measure of nutrition. Other serum proteins with shorter half-lives such as transferrin, transthyretin (prealbumin) and retinol-binding protein are better in this regard (Table 72-6).

Alterations in body habitus and composition frequently occur in

TABLE 72-4   Normative values for midarm muscle area*

Age group	Arm muscle area percentiles, mm²						
	5	10	25	50	75	90	95
MEN							
16–16.9	3625	4044	4352	4951	5753	6576	6980
17–17.9	3998	4252	4777	5286	5950	6886	7726
18–18.9	4070	4481	5066	5552	6374	7067	8355
19–24.9	4508	4777	5274	5913	6660	7606	8200
25–34.9	4694	4963	5541	6214	7067	7847	8436
35–44.9	4844	5181	5740	6490	7265	8034	8488
45–54.9	4546	4946	5589	6297	7142	7918	8458
55–64.9	4422	4783	5381	6144	6919	7670	8149
65–74.9	3973	4411	5031	5716	6432	7074	7453
WOMEN							
16–16.9	2308	2567	2865	3248	3718	4353	4946
17–17.9	2442	2674	2996	3336	3883	4552	5251
18–18.9	2398	2538	2917	3243	3694	4461	4767
19–24.9	2538	2728	3026	3406	3877	4439	4940
25–34.9	2661	2826	3148	3573	4138	4806	5541
35–44.9	2750	2948	3359	3783	4428	5240	5877
45–54.9	2784	2956	3378	3858	4520	5375	5964
55–64.9	2784	3063	3477	4045	4750	5632	6247
65–74.9	2737	3018	3444	4019	4739	5566	6214

* Estimates based on data from the U.S. Health and Nutrition Examination Survey, 1971–1974 (HANES I). Mid-arm muscle area (MAMA) =

$$\frac{[\text{mid-arm circumference} - \pi(\text{triceps skin fold, mm})]^2}{4(\pi)}$$

SOURCE: AJ Frisancho, Am J Clin Nutr 34:2540, 1981.

TABLE 72-5   Normative values for creatinine excretion based on height

Men*		Women†	
Height, cm	Ideal creatinine, mg	Height, cm	Ideal creatinine, mg
157.5	1288	147.3	830
160.0	1325	149.9	851
162.6	1359	152.4	875
165.1	1386	154.9	900
167.6	1426	157.5	925
170.2	1467	160.0	949
172.7	1513	162.6	977
175.3	1555	165.1	1006
177.8	1596	167.6	1044
180.3	1642	170.2	1076
182.9	1691	172.7	1109
185.4	1739	175.3	1141
188.0	1785	177.8	1174
190.5	1831	180.3	1206
193.0	1891	182.9	1240

* Creatinine coefficient (men) = 23 mg/kg of ideal body weight.
† Creatinine coefficient (women) = 18 mg/kg of ideal body weight.

$$\text{Creatinine-Height Index} = \frac{\text{Actual 24-h urinary creatinine excretion}}{\text{normative value for height and sex}}$$

SOURCE: GL Blackburn et al., J Parent Ent Nutr 1:11, 1977.

TABLE 72-6   Serum proteins used in nutritional assessment

Serum protein	Approximate molecular mass, Da	Biosynthetic site	Normal value $\bar{X} \pm$ SD or (range)*	Half-life, days	Function	Comment[†]
Albumin	66,000	Hepatocyte	45 (35–50)	14–20	Maintain plasma oncotic pressure; carrier for small molecules	Serum levels are determined by many different processes
Transferrin	77,000	Hepatocyte	2.3 (2.0–3.2)	8–9	Binds Fe^{2+} in plasma and transports to bone	Iron nutriture influences plasma level; increased during pregnancy, estrogen therapy, and acute hepatitis; reduced in protein-losing enteropathy and nephropathy, chronic infections, uremia, and acute catabolic states; often measured indirectly as total iron-binding capacity
Transthyretin (Prealbumin)	61,000	Hepatocyte	0.30 (0.2–0.5)	2–3	Binds T_3 and to a lesser extent T_4. Carrier for retinol-binding protein	Increased in patients with chronic renal failure on dialysis; reduced in acute catabolic states, after surgery, in hyperthyroidism; serum level determined by overall energy and nitrogen balance
Retinol-binding protein (RBP)	21,000	Hepatocyte	0.0372 ± 0.0073[‡]	0.5	Transports vitamin A in plasma; binds noncovalently to prealbumin	Catabolized in renal proximal tubular cell; with renal disease RBP increases and $t_{1/2}$ is prolonged; low in vitamin A deficiency, acute catabolic states, after surgery, and in hyperthyroidism

* Units are g/L. Normal range varies between centers; check local values.
[†] All of the listed proteins are influenced by hydration and the presence of hepatocellular dysfunction.
[‡] Normal values are age- and sex-dependent. Table value is for pooled subjects.
SOURCE: Heymsfield and Williams.

acute illness: fluid retention, for example, may dilute the apparent concentration of serum proteins, alter anthropometric measurements of edematous body structures, and increase body weight. Because all the traditional measures of protein-energy status may fall prey to such artifacts in acutely ill individuals there is increasing reliance on functional measures of protein-calorie status. Measures of skeletal muscle strength correlate very highly with more conventional measures of somatic and visceral protein status, with total body protein, and with clinical outcomes. A handgrip dynamometer is a simple and highly effective tool in this regard (Fig. 72-1). Table 72-7 outlines parameters to classify an individual as either moderately or severely malnourished.

CLINICAL FEATURES   Weight loss and a reduction in subcutaneous fat are the most consistent physical features of mild to moderate PEM in adults. Children with PEM exhibit additional features related to retarded physical development such as a stunted (low height for

age) or wasted (low weight for height) body habitus and delayed puberty. PEM also causes retardation of cognitive and psychosocial development in children.

Mild to moderate PEM   The reduction in lean body mass in mild to moderate PEM is usually not as great as the reduction in fat but can be identified by measurement of the mid-arm muscle area or the creatinine-height index. The decrease in urinary urea nitrogen, in contrast, is more a reflection of the physiologic adjustments made by the body in response to inadequate protein and/or calories. A contraction of the visceral protein compartment may be reflected in decreased levels of serum albumin, transferrin, retinol-binding protein, and thyroxine-binding prealbumin, a reduction in the total lymphocyte count, or a loss of delayed cutaneous hypersensitivity. Functionally, there may be a decrease in handgrip strength; impairments in work capacity are usually evident only in individuals whose daily activities are particularly high in energy demands. Pregnant women with mild

FIGURE 72-1 Handgrip strength, expressed as percent predicted (*A*) correlates with visceral protein status (*B* and *C*), somatic protein status (data not shown), and total body protein (data not shown). Protein index = measured total body protein/predicted total body protein. Physiologic impairments are common when the protein index is <0.8. (*From Hill.*)

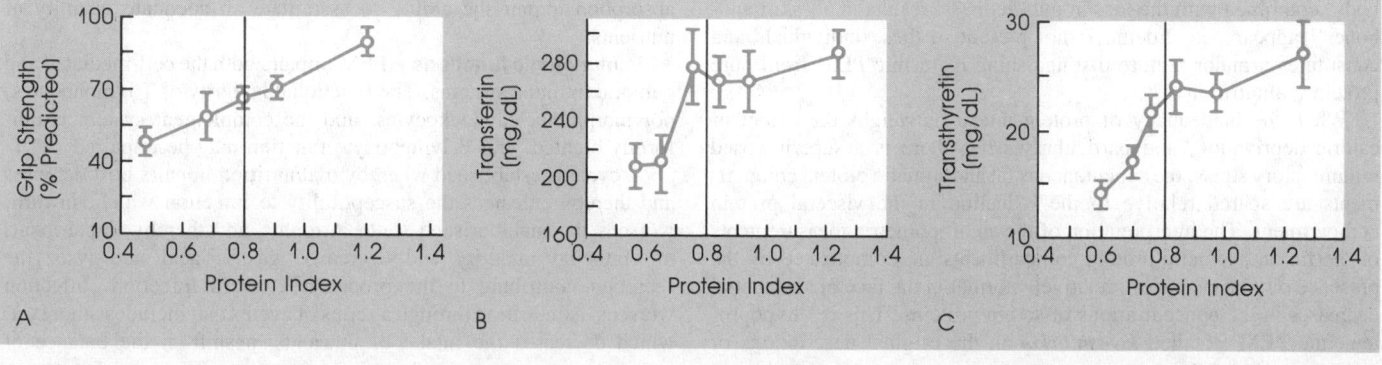

TABLE 72-7   Assessment of protein-energy status

Method of assessment	Moderate PEM	Severe PEM
Percent of premorbid weight	80–90	<80
Percent of ideal weight	60–80	<60
Creatinine-height index (see Table 72-5)	60–80	<60
Grip strength, % predicted	60–70	<60
Serum albumin, g/L	21–30	<21
Serum transferrin, g/L	1.0–1.5	<1
Total lymphocyte count, μL	800–1200	<800
Delayed hypersensitivity index*	1	0
Prognostic Nutritional Index, %[†]	40–50	>50

* Delayed hypersensitivity Index quantitates the amount of induration elicited by skin testing with a common antigen such as *Candida*, trichophyton, or mumps. Grading: 0 = <0.5 cm induration, 1 = 0.5 cm, 2 = 1.0 cm

[†] Prognostic Nutritional Index is a weighted combination of four measures (see Table 72-8): PNI % = 158 − [1.66 × albumin (g/L)] − [0.78 × triceps skin fold (mm)] − [2.0 × transferrin (g/L)] − [5.8 × delayed hypersensitivity index].

to moderate PEM are at risk of delivering an infant with low weight or length for gestational age. The volume of breast milk in such women is decreased as is its fat and energy content.

Severe PEM   More severe PEM is characterized by more severe alterations in the body habitus and in laboratory parameters. Deficiency states of specific micronutrients are common in conjunction with severe PEM although the latter usually has the most impact on health. There is further loss of subcutaneous fat and decrease in the somatic protein compartment as evidenced by muscle wasting in the extremities. The decrease in muscle mass can be identified by examining for atrophy of the interosseous muscles in the hand or the temporalis muscle on the sides of the head or by estimating the mid-arm muscle area. The loss of subcutaneous fat and muscle mass, in conjunction with a decrease in the elasticity of the skin, results in loose fitting, wrinkled skin with reduplicated folds. Skin lesions are common in advanced PEM, particularly over edematous areas. They may appear as shiny, erythematous, atrophic areas or as hyperkeratotic, hyperpigmented regions ("flaky paint" dermatitis). Decubitus ulcers are also common. The hair becomes sparse and dry, loses its usual sheen, and can be pulled out with little effort. The color of the hair may change to reddish or dull brown, and alternating periods of nutritional depletion and repletion may give rise to bands of color changes in the hair.

Lethargy is common. Alterations in gastrointestinal function include constipation and difficulty ingesting normal-sized meals due to early satiety and vomiting. The heart rate, blood pressure, and core body temperature may be subnormal. Infections may not be accompanied by appropriate hyperthermic and tachycardic responses.

When severe PEM arises from an inadequate intake of both protein and calories the diminution in the somatic protein compartment is disproportionately large compared to the decrease in the visceral protein compartment (*marasmic* PEM). Individuals with this form of PEM demonstrate marked muscle wasting in the extremities and trunk while maintaining relative normality of the visceral protein compartment. Weakness accompanies the loss in muscle mass and can be profound. The decrease in subcutaneous fat throughout the body, combined with the loss in muscle mass, results in a "skin-and-bones" appearance. Edema is not present in these individuals and constitutes a major feature distinguishing marasmic PEM from pure protein malnutrition.

When the inadequacy of protein intake outweighs the extent of caloric deprivation, and particularly when there is a superimposed inflammatory stress, the subcutaneous fat and somatic protein compartments are spared relative to the reduction in the visceral protein compartment. The interpretation of the anthropometric measurements of the fat and somatic protein compartments are complicated by the presence of edemas but are relatively normal in the face of substantial decreases in the concentrations of serum proteins. This is "hypoproteinemic PEM" (called *kwashiorkor* in the original descriptions of

children in under-developed nations). It is rare in its pure form among malnourished hospitalized patients but may occur in a mixed form with features of both hypoproteinemic and marasmic PEM. Such individuals have subnormal fat and somatic protein compartments, as indicated by anthropometric measurements, as well as depressed levels of serum proteins and the accompanying edema. The edema in hypoproteinemic PEM is usually dependent but may extend more cephalad and even be generalized. Individuals with hypoproteinemic PEM are particularly misleading because they do not have the marked fat and muscle wasting characteristic of marasmic protein-energy malnutrition. This does not imply that this type of PEM is associated with less morbidity. Indeed, hospitalized patients with hypoproteinemic PEM may have a worse prognosis than those with marasmic PEM, and there is a greater susceptibility for development of superimposed infections.

In hypoproteinemic PEM the liver may be enlarged and tender to palpation as a result of fatty infiltration: fat droplets initially appear in the periportal hepatocytes and, with increasing severity, spread to the pericentral regions of the hepatic lobule. Fatty liver is thought to be due to the inadequate transport of lipids out of the hepatic parenchyma due to the decreased availability of lipoproteins. Serum concentrations of VLDL and LDL are subnormal in hypoproteinemic PEM, and the severity of the fatty infiltration correlates with the degree of depression of these lipoproteins.

Several factors determine whether a malnourished individual develops a hypoproteinemic, marasmic, or combined form of PEM including the relative degree of protein versus energy deprivation, the presence of superimposed inflammatory processes, and individual host responses to the same type of nutritional deprivation and inflammatory insult. Children with marasmic PEM have higher glucocorticoid levels than those with hypoproteinemic PEM, and this hormonal difference may be responsible for maintaining the visceral protein compartment at the expense of the skeletal muscle.

PHYSIOLOGIC IMPAIRMENTS ASSOCIATED WITH PROTEIN-ENERGY MALNUTRITION   PEM impairs the function of all organs. Most, if not all, of the impairments are reversible with nutritional restitution.

Gastrointestinal tract   Alterations in gastrointestinal structure and function with PEM arise partially from undernutrition and partially from decreased stimulation of the gut by ingested nutrients. The sustained absence of nutrients in the intestine of nutritionally replete, parenterally fed individuals results in structural and functional atrophy of the intestine. The changes have been best described in children and are presumed to occur also in adult PEM and include both histologic and functional abnormalities. Marked blunting, or total absence, of the intestinal villi is associated with decreased levels of disaccharidases and aminopeptidases in the mucosa. Gastric and pancreatic secretions are reduced in volume and contain decreased concentrations of acid and digestive enzymes. The volume of bile and the concentration of conjugated bile acids in bile are reduced. Substantial populations of facultative and strict anaerobic bacteria are frequently present in the upper small bowel, probably explaining the increase in free bile acids. Malabsorption of carbohydrates, fat- and water-soluble vitamins, and fat may occur, the degree of steatorrhea being proportional to the severity of PEM. These alterations in absorption impair the ability to assimilate an adequate quantity of nutrients.

Immunologic functions   PEM impairs both the cell-mediated and humoral immune systems. The functional integrity of T lymphocytes, polymorphonuclear leukocytes, and the complement system is uniformly blunted, and B lymphocyte function may be impaired.

A cycle is established whereby malnutrition impairs host defenses and thereby enhances the susceptibility to infection which, in turn, worsens the malnourished state. Atrophy, and thereby impairment, of epithelial integrity and decreased gastric acid and lysozyme secretion contribute to the propensity toward infection. Infection worsens malnutrition through a series of events that includes: anorexia, which decreases the intake of nutrients; a shift in the balance of protein metabolism to the catabolic state, thereby promoting loss of lean body mass; and enhancement of the metabolic rate which increases about 13 percent for every 1°C elevation of body temperature. Interleukin 1, interleukin 6, and TNF-α appear to play roles in these processes. Tumor necrosis factor (sometimes called cachectin) also inhibits several enzymes of lipid metabolism and therefore impairs utilization of fat stores as an energy source.

The total lymphocyte count, delayed skin hypersensitivity, and some nutritional indices that incorporate these parameters (see below) correlate with the visceral protein compartment and can be used to predict the risk of postoperative infections and, in some cases, postoperative mortality. Additional factors other than nutritional status also influence lymphocytes, and nutritional status is therefore not the sole determinant of the predictive utility of these tests.

Endocrine system Hormonal alterations are common in PEM; most appear to be physiologic adaptations to the undernourished state. The inadequate intake of food leads to a decrease in the availability of circulating glucose and amino acids, low circulating levels of insulin, and increased levels of growth hormone. These alterations, in conjunction with the decreased levels of somatomedins and increased levels of cortisol in PEM, promote muscle protein catabolism and at the same time enhance incorporation of the liberated amino acids into visceral organs. Urea synthesis is inhibited, decreasing nitrogen loss and enhancing the reutilization of amino acids. The enhancement of lipolysis and gluconeogenesis provides substrate for energy.

The serum levels of triiodothyronine (T_3) and thyroxine (T_4) are commonly decreased in association with increased concentrations of reverse T_3 (3,5,5'-triiodothyronine), resembling the pattern observed in the *euthyroid sick syndrome*. The decreased concentrations of T_3 may play a role in the decrease in metabolic rate and decrease in protein catabolism in PEM.

Primary gonadal dysfunction is common in adults with moderate to severe PEM, including decreased levels of circulating testosterone and estrogen and impairment in reproductive potential. Amenorrhea is common. Fertility is further reduced in women by an increased risk of resorption of an implanted embryo. Impaired secretion of the hypothalamic hormone luteinizing hormone releasing hormone (LH-RH) may also play a role in the impaired reproduction. In prepubertal children with PEM the basal level of FSH and the response of this gonadatropin to LHRH are variously reported to be low or normal. Delay of puberty appears to be due to a decrease below a critical lean body mass. These changes in the pituitary-gonadal axis can be viewed as an adaptation, since the availability of energy and protein substrate is more critical for immediate survival than is the need for sexual maturation in children or reproduction in adults.

Cardiovascular system Moderate to severe PEM produces both quantitative and qualitative alterations in the heart. Myocardial mass is decreased, although proportionally less than the loss in body weight. Microscopic analysis of the myocardium reveals myofibrillar atrophy, edema, and, less commonly, patchy necrosis and infiltration with chronic inflammatory cells. Involvement of the myocardial conduction system may explain the conduction abnormalities in the PEM associated with anorexia nervosa and total starvation.

These structural changes are associated with alterations in myocardial performance, most evident under conditions of increased demand, as a decrease in cardiac output, stroke volume, and maximal work capacity. The cardiac alterations associated with PEM are reversible: both left ventricular mass and cardiac output increase with several weeks of nutritional repletion.

Respiratory system All muscles, including the diaphragm and the other respiratory muscles, undergo structural and functional atrophy, causing decreases in the inspiratory and expiratory pressures and in the vital capacity. Decreased respiratory muscle strength and a blunted ventilatory drive impair the ability to sustain ventilation in the severely malnourished individual. In tracheostomy patients, adherence of bacteria to tracheal epithelial cells correlates with the degree of malnutrition. Thus the immunologic integrity of the respiratory tract, as previously discussed, appears to be compromised by malnutrition.

Nutritional repletion leads to improvements in impaired pulmonary physiology and in the probability of weaning from a ventilator.

Wound healing Well-nourished individuals lay down more collagen at the site of a surgical wound than do those individuals with even mild malnutrition. Repletion of the malnourished surgical patient before surgery leads to better wound healing than if nutritional needs are only addressed postoperatively. Nevertheless, the provision of adequate nutrition after surgery enhances the deposition of collagen at the wound. Furthermore, intestinal anastomoses in well-nourished animals have a higher bursting strength than those in malnourished animals, and collagen deposition, tensile strength, and resistance to complications at the site of intestinal anastomses are greater in nutritionally replete animals.

Influence of malnutrition on the hospital course Numerous studies have demonstrated a correlation between protein-energy status and the outcome of hospitalization. For example, a depressed serum albumin or transferrin level, recent unintentional weight loss of >10 percent, a moderately depressed grip strength, a decreased total lymphocyte count (<1200 per microliter), or an anergic skin response to foreign antigens are all predictive of an increased incidence of morbid events within the hospital. Moreover, several of these parameters are predictors of the duration of postoperative hospitalization, in-hospital mortality, and the risk of morbidity following discharge.

Several nutritional indices, each of which incorporates various combinations of these parameters, have been utilized to assess the nutritional status of hospitalized patients (Table 72-8). However, every parameter used for the clinical assessment of nutritional status

TABLE 72-8 Prognostic indices in hospitalized patients

Index	Incorporated parameters	Correlates with	Reference
Likelihood of malnutrition	Serum folate, serum vitamin C, serum albumin, lymphocyte count, hematocrit, triceps skinfold, arm muscle circumference, weight	Duration of hospitalization	Am J Clin Nutr 32:418, 1979
Prognostic nutritional index	Serum albumin, serum transferrin, delayed hypersensitivity, triceps skinfold	Incidence of postoperative complications and mortality	Cancer 47:2375, 1981
Instant nutritional index	Serum albumin, lymphocyte count	Incidence of postoperative infection	J Parent Ent Nutr 12:195, 1988
Hospital prognostic index	Serum albumin, delayed hypersensitivity, presence of sepsis or cancer	Hospital mortality	Am J Clin Nutr 34:2013, 1981

and the indices that integrate several parameters, are influenced by disease as well as by nutritional status. Such indices are more properly considered assessments of the severity of illness and the "likelihood" of malnutrition rather than as indicators of nutritional status alone. Nevertheless, aggressive attention to nutritional restitution can mitigate the morbidity associated with PEM, confirming both the predictive and practical value of these nutritional measures. Furthermore, the response to nutritional intervention emphasizes the importance of attending to both nutritional assessment and therapy in hospitalized patients.

REFERENCES

BARACOS V et al: Stimulation of degradation of muscle proteins during fever. A mechanism for the increased degradation of muscle proteins during fever. New Engl J Med 308:553, 1983

BECKER DJ: The endocrine responses to protein calorie malnutrition. Ann Rev Nutr 3:187, 1983

BEUTLER B, CERAMI A: Cachectin: more than a tumor necrosis factor. New Engl J Med 316:379, 1987

BISTRIAN BR et al: Protein status of general surgical patients. JAMA 230:858, 1974
——— et al: Prevalence of malnutrition in general medical patients. JAMA 235:1567, 1976

BISTRIAN BR et al: Cytokines, muscle proteolysis, and the catabolic response to infection and inflammation. Proc Soc Exp Biol Med 200:220, 1992

CAHILL GF: Starvation in man. New Engl J Med 282:668, 1970

HEYMSFIELD SB, WILLIAMS PJ: Nutritional assessment by clinical and biochemical methods, in Modern Nutrition in Health and Disease, 7th ed, ME Shils, VR Young (eds). Philadelphia, Lea & Febiger, 1988

HILL GL: Body composition research: Implications for the practice of clinical nutrition. J Parent Ent Nutr 16:197, 1992

KEUSCH GT, FARTHING MJG: Nutrition and infection. Ann Rev Nutr 6:131, 1986

LONG CL, LOWRY SF: Hormonal regulation of protein metabolism. J Parent Ent Nutr 14:555, 1990

ROSENBLATT S et al: Exchange of amino acids by muscle and liver in sepsis. Arch Surg 118:167, 1983

73 OBESITY

JERROLD M. OLEFSKY

The ability to store food energy as fat provides survival value when the food supply is scarce or sporadic. Unlike glycogen or protein, triglyceride does not require water or electrolytes for storage purposes and can be retained essentially as pure fat; 1 g adipose tissue yields close to the full theoretical equivalent of 38 kJ (9 kcal). Because of the efficient storage of energy in adipose tissue, an individual of normal weight can survive up to 2 months of total starvation. However, western society is generally not characterized by periodic or insufficient food supply but rather by constant and abundant food. As a consequence, the ability to store fat frequently is of negative survival value because of overconsumption and resulting obesity.

DEFINITION AND INCIDENCE Obesity can most easily be assessed in terms of height and weight. One way is to relate weight to an average range for height and age. This measure of *relative weight* can lead to an underestimation of the incidence of obesity, since in the United States the "average" individual is somewhat obese. Tables of *ideal* and *desirable* weight are based on actuarial estimates of what is consistent with longest life expectancy. Such tables are more useful if adjusted for differences in body build. An alternative method of estimating obesity is the *body mass index* or *BMI* [body weight (in kilograms) divided by height (in meters)]. For adults ages 20 to 29, the 85th percentile for BMI is 27.8 for males and 27.3 for females. Although relative weight and BMI correlate with the degree of adiposity, excess weight can be either lean or fat tissue. For example, heavily muscled individuals would be considered obese using these measurements. Nevertheless, such assessments correlate fairly well with the risk of adverse effects on health and longevity. More precise assessment of obesity can be made with measurements of body density or with isotopic dilution methods, but these are unsuitable for routine use. Alternatively, anthropometry can be utilized for assessing the degree of adiposity. Assessment of skin-fold thickness over various areas of the body together with height, weight, and age can be used to assess the degree of adiposity. Triceps and subscapular skin folds are most commonly employed (see Chap. 72). From a health standpoint, certain patterns of obesity may be less desirable than others. Fat deposition about the waist and flank, as evidenced by a high ratio of waist to hip circumference, is associated with a greater health risk than fat deposition at the hips.

The term *obesity* implies an excess of adipose tissue, but the meaning of *excess* is hard to define. Aesthetic considerations aside, obesity is best defined as any degree of excess adiposity that imparts a health risk. This cutoff between normal and obese can only be approximated, and the health risk imparted by obesity is probably a continuum with increasing adiposity. The Framingham Study demonstrated that a 20 percent excess over desirable weight clearly imparted a health risk. A National Institutes of Health consensus panel on obesity agreed with this definition and concluded that a 20 percent increase in relative weight or a BMI above the 85th percentile for young adults constitutes a health risk; by use of these criteria, 20 to 30 percent of adult men and 30 to 40 percent of adult women are obese, with the highest rates among the poor and minority groups. Significant health risks at lower levels of obesity can occur in the presence of diabetes mellitus, hypertension, heart disease, or other associated risk factors.

The Surgeon General's 1988 report on obesity notes that even mild obesity increases the risk for premature death, diabetes mellitus, hypertension, atherosclerosis, gallbladder disease, and certain types of cancer. In the United States the prevalence of obesity has increased in the past few decades. Because of the frequency of obesity and its health consequences, its prevention and treatment should be a high public health priority.

ETIOLOGY When energy intake exceeds expenditure, the excess calories are stored in adipose tissue, and if this net positive balance is prolonged, obesity results; i.e., there are two components to weight balance, and an abnormality on either side (intake or expenditure) can lead to obesity.

The regulation of eating behavior is incompletely understood. To some extent, appetite is controlled by discrete areas in the hypothalamus: a feeding center in the ventrolateral nucleus of the hypothalamus (VLH) and a satiety center in the ventromedial hypothalamus (VMH). The cerebral cortex receives positive signals from the feeding center that stimulate eating (Fig. 73-1), and the satiety center modulates this process by sending inhibitory impulses to the feeding center. In animals, destruction of the feeding center results in decreased food intake, and destruction of the satiety center leads to overeating and obesity. Several regulatory processes may influence these hypothalamic centers. The satiety center may be activated by the increases in plasma glucose and/or insulin that follow a meal. It is of interest in this regard that the VMH contains insulin receptors and is insulin-sensitive. Meal-induced gastric distention is another possible inhibitory factor. The total adipose tissue mass also may influence the activity of the hypothalamic centers; i.e., there is a relatively fixed "set point" for body adiposity. An elevated set point may account for the frequent recidivism in obese patients who have lost weight. How the "set point" is established and how the hypothalamus senses total fat stores are unknown. Glycerol release from fat cells, ascending neural impulses, and/or circulation of adipocyte-derived peptides such as adipsin may be signals of adipose tissue size. Additionally, the hypothalamic centers are sensitive to catecholamines, and beta-adrenergic stimulation inhibits eating behavior. This provides at least one rationale for the anorexiant effects of amphetamines.

Ultimately, the cerebral cortex controls eating behavior, and impulses from the feeding center to the cerebral cortex are only one

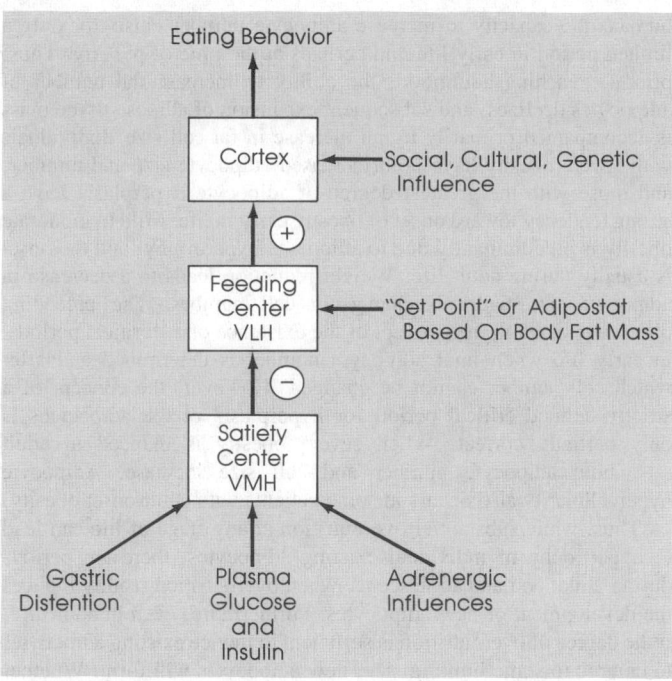

FIGURE 73-1 The regulation of eating. The ventromedial satiety center is considered to be inhibitory, and the ventrolateral feeding center stimulatory. See text for discussion.

input. Psychological, social, and genetic factors also influence food intake. In many obese subjects these influences are overriding; indeed, obese subjects usually respond to external signals such as time of day, social setting, and smell or taste of food to a greater extent than do persons of normal weight.

Although overeating is the usual cause of obesity, other factors may participate. Daily caloric needs normally range between 110 to 130 kJ (27 to 32 kcal) per kilogram of body weight; this figure is higher in active and lower in sedentary individuals. Physical activity clearly modulates overall caloric balance, and obese individuals tend to be less active. This can be a contributory factor in the maintenance of excess weight, but decreased physical activity is unlikely to be an important cause of major weight gain in most obese subjects. Rather, obesity leads to inactivity. The modest increase in weight that often accompanies the middle years may be related more directly to diminished physical activity. Injury or illness may lead to chronic restricted activity and predispose to weight gain unless caloric intake is appropriately curtailed. Perhaps the greatest factor tending to diminish energy output is simply a sedentary life-style.

Decreased caloric expenditure and a metabolic abnormality associated with overefficient caloric utilization also have been postulated as involved in the pathogenesis of obesity. With rare exceptions, major metabolic abnormalities have not been detected in obese individuals, although subtle defects may be undetected. There are three major components to overall energy expenditure: resting metabolic rate, exercise-induced thermogenesis, and the thermic response to food.

The resting metabolic rate accounts for 60 to 75 percent of daily energy expenditure and is measured in a thermoneutral environment while the subject is at rest following an overnight fast and several hours after any significant physical activity. An average resting metabolic rate in a 70-kg man is 6300 kJ (1500 kcal)/d. The resting metabolic rate should be expressed as a function of fat-free body weight (by subtracting the subject's total adipose mass from body weight), since triglyceride mass is metabolically inert in that negligible energy is expended to maintain triglyceride depots. When expressed in this way, the resting metabolic rate is normal in most obese subjects. However, a distinction must be made between static obesity

and the actual process of gaining weight. When normal subjects consume hypercaloric diets, less weight is gained than would be predicted on the basis of the excess calories ingested. This effect is most marked when carbohydrate is consumed and disappears when the excess calories consist of fat. Thus humans can apparently partially adapt to chronic excessive carbohydrate and protein intake, and this protective effect attenuates the weight gain. Part of this adaptive response is related to an increase in thermogenesis manifested as an increase in the resting metabolic rate. The mechanism of adaptive thermogenesis is unknown, but overeating of carbohydrate or mixed nutrients leads to increased plasma levels of triiodothyronine (T_3) and decreased levels of reverse T_3 (rT_3). A converse effect is seen in starvation, with decreased T_3 and increased rT_3 levels. The conversion of thyroxine to T_3 occurs largely in the liver; excess food may induce adaptive thermogenesis by increasing the concentration of T_3 relative to that of T_4 and rT_3. Increased central or peripheral sympathetic outflow leading to increased catecholamine-induced caloric utilization and increased heat production also may play a role in the thermogenic response to overnutrition. Adaptive thermogenesis can lead to a 10 to 15 percent increase in resting metabolic rate, and this effect is seen after a 2- to 3-week period of hypercaloric intake. The rate of onset and the degree of adaptive thermogenesis is the same in obese and nonobese individuals when expressed on the basis of fat-free body mass. Specifically, the increase in resting metabolic rate, changes in thyroid hormone metabolism, and thermic responses to infused catecholamines are similar in normal and obese subjects during periods of overnutrition.

Work performance, or energy expenditure per standard physical work load, can be normal or increased in obesity depending on the kind of work performed. The energy expenditure of exercise is increased in obese compared with lean subjects due to the extra effort involved in moving or supporting an increased body mass. When this effect of increased body mass is taken into account, work performance is normal in obesity. Clearly, normal or increased energy expenditure during physical work cannot contribute to the development of obesity. On the other hand, the total daily energy expenditure due to exercise is less in many sedentary obese subjects simply because they engage in less daily physical activity than their lean counterparts.

The third important aspect of caloric balance is the thermic response to food, so-called dietary thermogenesis. This consists of the heat, or energy, expended above the resting metabolic rate for several hours after the ingestion of a meal. About 75 percent of the thermic response to food is due to the energy cost of digestion, absorption, metabolism, and storage of foodstuffs; the remainder is probably due to activation of the sympathetic nervous system. The heat produced following nutrient ingestion is a form of caloric expenditure and is greater for protein and less for carbohydrate and fat. The thermic response to mixed meals can equal 10 to 15 percent of the calories ingested, and decreased thermic responses have been described in some studies of human obesity. This difference may be due to altered flux rates through different pathways of intermediary metabolism, with more energy-efficient pathways being favored in obesity. As an example, the higher the rate of glucose utilization, the greater the thermic response to carbohydrate-containing meals, and small decreases in the thermic response to food may be due to insulin resistance and decreased glucose disposal in obese subjects. It is clear that small differences in caloric utilization maintained over years can lead to a significant net positive caloric balance. However, while it is tempting to postulate that this decreased thermic response may contribute to obesity, most of the published comparisons have been made between normal persons and subjects who are already obese. Thus the obesity-associated changes in thermic response to food may be secondary to the obese state rather than a primary abnormality. More important, differences in the thermic response to meals between the obese and nonobese are at most in the range of 125 to 210 kJ (30 to 50 kcal) per day. Such minor differences can easily be counterbalanced by minor decreases in food intake and/or increases in exercise-induced thermogenesis. Since such compensation does not occur, it seems more probable that obesity is the result of impaired coupling between caloric intake and expenditure.

Another potential regulatory process in the control of adipose tissue mass involves adipose tissue lipoprotein lipase (ATLPL). This enzyme is synthesized within adipocytes, secreted into the extracellular space, and attaches to the luminal surface of nearby endothelial cells. At this location, ATLPL hydrolyzes fatty acids from the triglycerides of circulating triglyceride-rich lipoproteins. The released fatty acids are taken up by adipocytes, converted to triglycerides, and stored. Thus ATLPL participates in the storage of excess fat calories in adipose tissue. The *lipoprotein lipase hypothesis* holds that in some obese states excessive levels of this enzyme induce obesity by causing preferential deposition of fat calories in adipose tissue. In support of this hypothesis, ATLPL levels are increased in obese rodents and humans. More important, levels of this enzyme do not return to normal following weight reduction. This latter finding is of particular interest because it is one of the few characteristics of the obese state that is not corrected by weight reduction and could explain the propensity of obese patients to regain lost weight.

Environmental, cultural, and genetic influences all contribute to obesity, and in population studies it is impossible to quantitate the separate impact of these factors. Nevertheless, the role of genetics has been demonstrated in studies of twins and adopted siblings. The BMI of adopted individuals correlates better with that of the biologic rather than the adoptive parents. Among biologic and adoptive siblings, there is a genetic influence on the amount and distribution of fat, and similarities are not as close among adopted siblings. Most likely, both nature and nurture contribute to obesity.

SECONDARY OBESITY Hypothyroidism Obesity can result from hypothyroidism because of decreased caloric needs. However, only a minority of hypothyroid patients are truly obese, and an even smaller proportion of obese patients are hypothyroid. Indiscriminate use of thyroid hormone in the treatment of obesity is to be deplored and should never be instituted in the absence of decreased thyroid function.

Cushing's disease Cushing's disease is a rare cause of obesity. Hyperadrenocorticism elicits a typical pattern of obesity with predominantly centripetal fat stores, characteristic rounded or moon facies, and cervical or supraclavicular fat deposits.

Insulinoma Hyperinsulinemia, secondary to an insulinoma, can occasionally cause obesity, presumably because of increased caloric intake secondary to recurrent hypoglycemia. Most patients with islet cell tumors and hypoglycemia are not obese.

Hypothalamic disorders Froehlich's syndrome in boys is characterized by obesity and hypogonadotrophic hypogonadism with other variable features such as diabetes insipidus, visual impairment, and mental retardation. The anterior pituitary is usually normal, and the syndrome is thought to be the result of hypothalamic dysfunction. This syndrome likely includes a number of overlapping disorders having in common a hypothalamic lesion that leads to overeating and to hypogonadotrophism. Occasionally, pituitary tumors (as in Froehlich's original case) may physically impair the hypothalamus.

Other rare causes of obesity include the Laurence-Moon-Biedl syndrome, characterized by retinitis pigmentosa, mental retardation, skull deformities, polydactyly, and syndactyly and the Prader-Willi syndrome, which is associated with hypotonia, mental retardation, and a predilection for diabetes mellitus. In both these disorders obesity and hypogonadism are thought to be hypothalamic in origin.

PATHOLOGIC SEQUELAE Increased adipose tissue stores are deposited subcutaneously, around internal organs, throughout the omentum, and in the intramuscular spaces. Obese individuals also have an expansion of lean body mass, as evidenced by increased size of the kidneys, heart, liver, and skeletal muscle mass. Fatty livers are common in extreme obesity.

Adipocyte size and number Attempts have been made to classify obesity on the basis of the relative degree of adipocyte hypertrophy versus hyperplasia. This classification was generated as the result of experimental data indicating that in several rodent species and in humans the capacity to increase adipocyte number exists for only a limited period in early life and perhaps at the time of puberty. Thus, prior to reaching adulthood, the ability to increase the number of adipocytes declines, and subsequent expansion of adipose tissue mass is accompanied primarily by an increase in fat cell size. Individuals with severe obesity have both increased adipocyte size and number, and those with the greatest degree of adipocyte hyperplasia have a strong tendency toward onset of obesity early in life. Mild to moderate obesity is predominantly due to adipocyte hypertrophy, and the onset is usually during adult life. Weight reduction leads to a decrease in adipocyte size with no change in cell number. The preceding observations led to the concept of the existence of a "critical period" in early life when final adipocyte number is determined and after which cell number cannot be changed. However, the concept of a strictly defined critical period for hyperplasia of the adipocytes is only partially correct. When severe obesity is induced in adult rats, both adipocyte number and cell size increase. Adipocyte hypercellularity also occurs in some patients with adult-onset obesity.

Thus, while substantial overnutrition at any stage of life can lead to hypertrophy of individual existing adipocytes, there are periods during childhood and adolescence when overnutrition readily induces the development of new adipocytes. Furthermore, even in adult life, if the degree of overnutrition is sufficient to induce existing adipocytes to enlarge to some limiting size, new adipocytes will form. Whether this latter population of cells represents new cell formation or simply the filling with lipid of previously undetectable preadipocytes formed earlier in life is not known. Regardless of the cause or time of development of increased adiposity (adipocyte hypertrophy with or without hyperplasia), subsequent weight reduction only leads to a decrease in the size of existing adipocytes and not a decrease in adipocyte number. Thus, once a given complement of adipocytes is attained, this number is fixed and cannot be reduced.

METABOLIC SEQUELAE Obesity has a profound impact on diabetes mellitus and on various hyperlipoproteinemic states primarily through its influences on insulin secretion and insulin sensitivity.

Hyperinsulinemia: Insulin resistance Increased insulin secretion is a common feature of obesity. It occurs in the basal state and in response to a wide variety of insulinogenic agents. A correlation exists between the degree of obesity and the magnitude of the hyperinsulinemia—particularly the basal insulin levels. Some obese patients exhibit hyperglycemia or frank diabetes in the face of hyperinsulinemia. The combination of hyper- or euglycemia and hyperinsulinemia indicates an insulin-resistant state, and decreased hypoglycemic responses to insulin are common in obese humans and animals. Insulin resistance could be due to an abnormal beta cell product, circulating insulin antagonists, or tissue insulin insensitivity. Since abnormal islet secretory products or circulating antagonists have not been identified, it is thought that the insulin resistance of obesity is due primarily to tissue insensitivity. The initial step in insulin action involves binding to cell surface receptors in target tissues. Cells from obese animals and humans contain decreased numbers of insulin receptors, and this decrease doubtless plays a role in the insulin resistance. Binding of insulin to the receptor activates the tyrosine kinase activity of the cytoplasmic domain of the receptor, and this kinase activity is important for many, if not all, of insulin actions. While defects in insulin receptor tyrosine kinase activity have been found in several insulin-resistant states, including type II diabetes mellitus, receptor kinase activity is normal in obesity. Thus defects in insulin action distal to the insulin receptor participate in the insulin resistance of obesity. The enlarged adipocytes of obese rats have both a decrease in insulin receptors and an even greater defect in the capacity to metabolize glucose, suggesting a major biochemical abnormality downstream of the receptor mechanism. A similar postreceptor defect presumably exists in other insulin target tissues such as muscle and liver. In the obese human, insulin resistance is due to a combination of receptor and postreceptor defects in insulin action. In those obese patients with the mildest degree of hyperinsulinemia and insulin resistance, the decrease in insulin action is predominantly due to a decreased number of insulin receptors. As the insulin-resistant state worsens, a postreceptor defect emerges, and in obese subjects with the most severe degree of insulin resistance, the postreceptor defect is the predominant abnormality.

Diabetes mellitus (See also Chap. 337) Although only a minority of obese patients are diabetic, the converse is not the case. Non-insulin-dependent, or type II, diabetes comprises about 90 percent of the diabetic population in the United States, and 80 to 90 percent of type II diabetics are obese. Obesity is an important contributory factor to the diabetes in these patients, predominantly through its influences on insulin resistance. Obesity exacerbates the diabetic state, and in many cases diabetes can be ameliorated by weight reduction.

Hyperlipoproteinemia (See also Chap. 344) Most plasma cholesterol circulates in the low-density lipoprotein (LDL) fraction, and in the fasting state, very low density lipoproteins (VLDL) contain most of the circulating triglyceride. The association between obesity and elevated LDL levels is modest at best, especially when the relationship is corrected for factors such as age. Total-body cholesterol is increased in obesity, but this is mainly accounted for by adipose tissue cholesterol stores. Cholesterol turnover may be increased, leading to increased biliary excretion of cholesterol. This may contribute to the increased incidence of gallstone formation. Obesity has a more pronounced effect on VLDL metabolism. Hypertriglyceridemia is frequent, and the degree of obesity correlates with the level of hypertriglyceridemia. The increased triglyceride levels are due to increased hepatic VLDL production with no defect in the removal of VLDL from plasma. As discussed earlier, plasma insulin levels are elevated, particularly in the portal venous blood. Hyperinsulinemia can promote increased hepatic VLDL synthesis and secretion. In addition, increased plasma free fatty acid (FFA) turnover exists in obesity, and FFA extraction by the liver provides an important precursor for hepatic triglyceride synthesis. Thus the hypertriglyceridemia in obesity may be secondary to increased hepatic VLDL secretion due to hyperinsulinemia and augmented FFA availability.

MANIFESTATIONS AND COMPLICATIONS Gross obesity produces mechanical and physical stresses that aggravate or cause a number of disorders, including osteoarthritis (especially of the hips) and sciatica. Varicose veins, thromboembolism, ventral and hiatal hernias, and cholelithiasis are more common.

Hypertension In significantly obese persons, use of the standard size blood pressure cuff leads to erroneously high readings; an oversize cuff should always be used. A strong association between hypertension and obesity is observed even when accurate measurements are obtained. The mechanism by which obesity causes hypertension is uncertain, but peripheral vascular resistance is usually normal while blood volume is increased. Weight loss leads to reductions in systemic blood pressure independent of changes in sodium balance.

Hypoventilation syndrome (pickwickian syndrome) The obesity-hypoventilation syndrome is a heterogeneous group of disorders with differing clinical manifestations. The hypersomnolence that can occur in obesity is a manifestation of nighttime sleep apnea. In these individuals, once sleep begins, upper airway obstruction leads to hypoxemia and hypercapnia, causing arousal with return of normal respiration. Many such episodes occur each night, leading to chronic sleep deprivation and daytime somnolence. The combination of the obese habitus plus sleep-induced relaxation of the pharyngeal musculature is believed to be the cause of the intermittent upper airway obstruction. Occasionally, such episodes are life-threatening (causing serious cardiac arrhythmias) and require long-term tracheostomy. Chronic daytime hypoventilation is usually not as severe as that during sleep and may be due to abnormalities of the respiratory control centers. Patients with hypoventilation display blunted ventilatory responses to hypercapnia and hypoxia and often develop hypercapnia and hypoxemia due to decreased basal ventilation; in addition, ventilation-perfusion mismatch may result from mechanical factors. In severe cases, polycythemia, pulmonary hypertension, and cor pulmonale can result. Weight reduction will reverse these abnormalities if instituted before permanent cardiac damage develops. Some obese patients with sleep apnea and hypersomnolence do not have daytime hypoventilation and have normal ventilatory responses to hypoxia and hypercapnia. Progestational agents have been used therapeutically in the obesity-hypoventilation syndrome because they stimulate the ventilatory response to hypercapnia and hypoxia in normal subjects. Medroxyprogesterone increases ventilation and improves heart failure and erythrocytosis in these patients, although obstructive sleep apnea continues.

Adrenal function Although Cushing's disease can usually be distinguished from simple obesity on clinical grounds, laboratory testing is occasionally necessary. This can lead to confusion, since 24-h urinary 17-hydroxycorticoid excretion is often elevated in obesity. Less commonly, plasma cortisol levels are also increased. Glucocorticoid levels are usually suppressible with dexamethasone in obesity, but occasionally suppression is incomplete, rendering the diagnosis difficult (also see Chap. 335).

Growth hormone Secretory responses of growth hormone to a variety of stimuli such as hypoglycemia, exercise, and arginine infusion are reduced, and the starvation-induced rise in plasma growth hormone levels is attenuated.

Atherosclerosis Obesity is a risk factor for the development of coronary artery disease and stroke. Most of the risk is mediated through the associated hypertension, hyperlipoproteinemia, and diabetes. Nevertheless, even when these abnormalities are factored out, an additional, smaller risk can be ascribed to obesity per se.

TREATMENT Amelioration of hyperinsulinemia, insulin resistance, diabetes, hypertension, and hyperlipidemia can occur following weight loss. These changes are significant and enduring provided the weight loss is maintained. During weight loss, all adipose tissue depots diminish proportionately. Sometimes generalized loss does not produce the attractive cosmetic effects desired for those individuals wishing to achieve adipose tissue mass reduction in particular anatomic regions. Many techniques have been proposed to effect selective regional adipose tissue reduction, but none is effective.

Methods of weight reduction When obesity is secondary, the therapy is to treat the underlying disease. Most of the time, primary weight reduction must be undertaken.

Diet Caloric restriction is the cornerstone of weight reduction. For the patient and physician this is a frustrating and demanding undertaking. The basic principles are simple. If food intake is less than energy expenditure, stored calories, predominantly in the form of fat, will be consumed. In general, a deficit of 32,000 kJ (7700 kcal) leads to loss of about 1 kg fat. By estimating the patient's daily caloric needs [approximately 125 to 150 kJ (30 to 35 kcal) per kilogram of body weight], one can calculate the daily deficit necessary to achieve a given rate of weight loss.

Dietary restriction can range from total starvation to mild caloric deprivation, and these approaches will be discussed separately. Dietary recommendations are most effective when they are specific and geared to the patient's life-style. A dietitian or a similarly trained health professional should interview each patient and estimate average daily caloric intake, identify food preferences, and characterize the eating patterns. The amount of calories to be consumed on the restricted diet should be carefully explained in terms of amounts of specific foodstuffs. Frequently, the therapist must balance the degree of restriction against potential noncompliance. The more restrictive the diet, the more rapid is the weight loss, but this often leads to a greater rate of nonadherence. It is preferable to take the individual's needs and motivation into account and design a diet containing a degree of caloric restriction tailored to the patient's ability to comply. Such a diet should produce a consistent and relatively steady rate of weight loss.

Schemes for weight reduction have become a profitable business in the United States, and there are almost as many diets as there are therapists. Each proponent claims that the presence or absence of certain foodstuffs is desirable for more effective weight loss. However, little evidence exists that calorie for calorie one hypocaloric diet leads to greater weight loss than another. The relationship between the patient and the therapist, plus patient education and encouragement, is more important to success than the specific dietary constituents. The major virtue of "fad" diets is that patients are usually motivated to try them, at least initially, and patient cooperation is often better. Provided a particular diet is not harmful, the best course for the therapist is to maintain flexibility in the treatment program. Nevertheless, diets markedly deficient in any major class of foodstuff are to be avoided. For example, whole-food diets that are exceedingly low in carbohydrate are by nature high in fat and, depending on the type and quantity of fat ingested, may lead to hypercholesterolemia. The major virtue of a low-carbohydrate diet is the attendant ketosis (ketone bodies have a central anorexiant effect). This feature provided part of the rationale for the widely touted liquid or powdered protein diets that were previously popular. These diets have been dubbed "protein-sparing modified fasts" and were said to allow drastic long-term caloric restriction without inducing negative nitrogen balance. These claims have not been substantiated, nor has it been shown that the diets lead to a greater degree of true weight loss than mixed diets of equal caloric value. Basically, a calorie is a calorie whether it comes from protein, carbohydrate, or fat. Furthermore, deaths have been reported in otherwise healthy individuals participating in such long-term dietary programs, even under medical supervision. This has been attributed to the fact that some of these early diets contained mostly collagen-derived protein of low biologic value. The newer very low calorie diets involve formula preparations containing 500 to 800 kcal/d, with 50 to 80 g of high-quality protein. The remaining calories consist of carbohydrate and fat. Vitamin and micronutrient supplements are incorporated in the formula or provided as an added supplement. Such high-quality low-calorie diet formulas lead to relatively rapid weight loss but should not be taken continuously as the sole caloric source for more than 6 weeks. In the absence of coexisting diseases such as gout, renal insufficiency, cardiac arrhythmias, etc., such diets are safe when taken under medical supervision. As a general guideline, caloric intake below 800 kcal/d has been taken as the definition of a very low calorie diet (VLCD). Diets providing adequate high-quality protein and greater than 800 kcal/d are referred to as low-calorie diets (LCDs) and are safe in otherwise healthy obese individuals. While very low or low-calorie diets are often effective in achieving rapid and substantial amounts of weight loss, long-term maintenance of weight loss usually requires additive approaches (see below). There are several categories of subjects in whom VLCDs and LCDs are absolutely or relatively contraindicated; these include pregnant women, adolescents, growing children, and patients with significant liver, kidney, and cardiac diseases. In addition, there are conditions in which VLCDs and LCDs should only be used under medical supervision. Examples in this category are gout, diabetic patients taking insulin or oral hypoglycemic agents, preexisting gallbladder disease, and hypertensive patients on antihypertensive drugs.

Prior to therapy it is wise to warn patients that there is usually a marked initial weight loss when caloric restriction is started, in large part due to fluid loss, but such rapid rates of loss will not persist. Likewise, positive shifts in fluid balance can sometimes mask loss of adipose mass, a fact that can sometimes be demonstrated to the patient's satisfaction by recording skin-fold thickness at periodic intervals.

Total-starvation diets have been advocated for the treatment of obesity; provided gout, renal insufficiency, and ketosis-prone diabetes are not present, short-term (2- to 3-day) fasts are usually well tolerated. Ketonemia and hyperuricemia regularly develop during starvation but rarely lead to acidosis or gout. Because of these potential complications, total fasting should be carried out only under medical supervision. Probably the major usefulness of total fasting is as a motivational aid at the beginning of a dietary program or when weight loss has stopped. Even though much of the weight loss during short-term fasting represents fluid, this weight loss can be encouraging to frustrated patients and motivate them to improve compliance with the long-term weight reduction program.

The major problem in the treatment of obesity is not weight reduction but maintenance of the reduced weight. Provided the therapist works hard and long enough, most motivated patients can eventually lose weight. Unfortunately, only the rare patient maintains the weight loss permanently. Obesity is an eating disorder, and the underlying mechanisms are not reversed by limiting food intake.

Behavior modification   In recognition of the problems involved, the techniques of behavior modification have been applied to treat abnormal patterns of eating behavior. Many studies demonstrate that obese individuals respond less well than normal individuals to internal cues that regulate eating behavior such as gastric contractions, fear, and previous food ingestion. Conversely, obese subjects overrespond to external cues such as taste, smell, food attractiveness, food abundance, and the ease of obtaining food. Given the fact that the obese individual is unusually susceptible to external stimuli, food intake may be altered by changing the pattern and nature of these external cues, and this is the major premise underlying the behavior modification approach to weight reduction.

Behavior modification begins with a detailed individual history of the patient's eating patterns with respect to time of day, length of eating period, place of ingestion (restaurant, dining table, standing in front of open refrigerator), simultaneous activities (watching television, reading, idleness), emotional state, companions (relatives, friends, or alone), and finally the kinds and quantities of foods ingested. Once this detailed record is obtained, the therapist and patient can design specific behavioral changes aimed at disrupting or aborting recurring behavior patterns which initiate or prolong abnormal eating activity. As examples: if a patient eats in response to certain emotional states, then other activities can be substituted when the patient perceives such a state; if the patient snacks frequently from readily available food storage areas (refrigerators, cookie jars, etc.), then he or she is encouraged to eat only while sitting down at a table with a fixed place setting; if eating frequently occurs while watching television alone, then efforts to avoid this activity can be initiated. Results with behavior modification techniques indicate that many patients can maintain long-term weight reduction providing the new behavior patterns are truly "learned."

Exercise   Exercise has a place in any weight reduction program. However, the importance of exercise in terms of caloric balance must be clearly understood. Even moderate daily exercise would not lead to a large enough increase in energy expenditure to alter significantly the initial rate of weight reduction (Table 73-1). This does not mean that exercise is unimportant in weight reduction, since even modest increases in caloric expenditure can lead to large long-term differences in caloric balance, provided exercise is performed on a regular basis. For example, a daily increase in caloric expenditure of 1250 kJ (300 kcal) over a period of 4 months could lead to a 4.5-kg weight loss. More important, incorporation of regular exercise into the overall weight reduction program improves the chances that the weight loss will be maintained.

Drugs   Two classes of drugs are frequently used in the treatment of obesity: anorexiants and thyroid hormone. The addition of levothyroxine or liothyronine to a weight reduction program is ineffective in promoting adipose tissue loss and, if anything, accentuates lean tissue loss and causes negative nitrogen balance. Cardiotoxicity may occur. Thus, unless hypothyroidism is clear-cut, thyroid supplementation has no role in the treatment of obesity.

The major anorexiants are amphetamine-like agents that presumably exert their effect at the level of the hypothalamus. They probably have a modest effect in promoting short-term weight loss in some individuals. However, they are effective only for short periods, and problems of habituation, addiction, and drug abuse limit their usefulness. Two anorexiants, diethylpropion and fenfluramine, may be less addictive and, therefore, somewhat more useful. However, none of these agents treats the underlying eating disorder, and they are of little use in maintenance of weight reduction.

Injections of human chorionic gonadotropin (hCG) have been tried as an adjunct to weight reduction, but no evidence exists to indicate

TABLE 73-1 Energy equivalents of food calories expressed in minutes of activity

Food	Energy value, kJ (kcal)	Walking*	Riding bicycle[†]	Swimming[‡]	Running[§]	Reclining[¶]
			Activity			
Apple, large	422 (101)	19	12	9	5	78
Bacon, 2 strips	401 (96)	18	12	9	5	74
Beer, 1 glass	477 (114)	22	14	10	6	88
Bread and butter	326 (78)	15	10	7	4	60
Carbonated beverage, 1 glass	444 (106)	20	13	9	5	82
Carrot, raw	176 (42)	8	5	4	2	32
Cheese, cottage, 1 tbsp	113 (27)	5	3	2	1	21
Chicken, fried, ½ breast	971 (232)	45	28	21	12	178
Cookie, chocolate chip	213 (51)	10	6	5	3	39
Egg, fried	460 (110)	21	13	10	6	85
Ham, 2 slices	699 (167)	32	20	15	9	128
Ice cream, ⅛ qt	808 (193)	37	24	17	10	148
Mayonnaise, 1 tbsp	385 (92)	18	11	8	5	71
Milk, skim, 1 glass	339 (81)	16	10	7	4	62
Milk shake	1762 (421)	81	51	38	22	324
Orange, medium	285 (68)	13	8	6	4	52
Pancake with syrup	519 (124)	24	15	11	6	95
Peas, green, ½ cup	234 (56)	11	7	5	3	43
Pizza, cheese, ¼	753 (180)	35	22	16	9	138
Potato chips, 1 serving	462 (108)	21	13	10	6	83
Sandwiches:						
Hamburger	1456 (350)	67	43	31	18	269
Tuna fish salad	1163 (278)	53	34	25	14	214
Sherbet, ⅛ qt	741 (177)	34	22	16	9	136

* Energy cost of walking for 70-kg individual = 22 kJ (5.2 kcal)/min.
[†] Energy cost of riding bicycle = 34 kJ (8.2 kcal)/min.
[‡] Energy cost of swimming = 47 kJ (11.2 kcal)/min.
[§] Energy cost of running = 81 kJ (19.4 kcal)/min.
[¶] Energy cost of reclining = 5 kJ (1.3 kcal)/min.

a beneficial effect. The primary effectiveness of the hCG-diet program is due to the caloric restriction, frequent physician contact, and placebo effects. Comparable weight loss is achieved if saline injections are substituted for hCG, suggesting a placebo effect of parenteral injection.

Jejunoileal shunt Small-bowel bypass is an effective means of achieving weight reduction in morbidly obese patients. However, it is an experimental procedure and should be attempted only in institutions where a trained team is committed to regular, systematic, and long-term follow-up. Because of accompanying morbidity and mortality, most such institutions have abandoned this form of surgery in favor of the more benign and effective gastric plication or bypass approach described below.

The most common operative procedures for the jejunoileal bypass involve end-to-end or end-to-side anastomosis of about 38 cm of proximal jejunum to 10 cm of terminal ileum. Weight loss is initially rapid, reaching a plateau at 18 to 24 months. The mean weight loss is about 30 to 50 percent of initial excess weight, leaving patients still about 50 percent overweight once a steady state is reached. Although some malabsorption occurs, the major portion of the weight loss is due to decreased food intake.

Teams still performing this surgery select patients who are at least 50 kg overweight and in whom adequate attempts at medical management have failed repeatedly. Because of postoperative morbidity, older (>50 years) and psychologically unstable individuals are usually excluded.

The overall surgical mortality ranges from 0.5 to 7.8 percent, with an average of around 4 percent. Mortality is inversely related to the experience of the surgical team. The major postoperative morbidity is related to wound infection and thromboembolism. The common serious complications are cirrhosis and hepatic failure, nephrolithiasis, electrolyte imbalances, cholelithiasis, and arthritis (Table 73-2). Severe liver disease probably occurs in 5 percent of patients, and mild hepatic dysfunction is more common. The long-range implications of mild hepatic abnormalities are unknown. Possible causes of liver damage following small-bowel bypass include (1) protein and particularly essential amino acid deficiency, (2) accumula-

tion of hepatotoxic secondary bile salts, and (3) release of unknown toxic substances from the excluded bowel. Hypokalemia is likely secondary to diarrhea. Persistent deficiency of calcium and magnesium can result from malabsorption and must be treated with appropriate replacement. Transient depression of plasma 25-hydroxyvitamin D

TABLE 73-2 Complications of ileal bypass surgery

Complication	Percentage
EARLY	
Perioperative mortality	2–6
Thromboembolic disease	1–5
Wound infection	2–5
Renal failure	3
Severe nausea, vomiting	3
Wound dehiscence	1–3
LATE	
Urinary calculi	3–10
Severe electrolyte imbalance	5–8
Acute cholecystitis	0–5
Progressive liver disease	2–4
Intestinal obstruction	2
Peptic ulcer	1–2
Osteoporosis	?
Tuberculosis	1
MINOR	
Diarrhea	100
Weakness	80
Hypokalemia	80
Hypoproteinemia	50
Vomiting	50
Thirst	50
Hypocalcemia	30
Arthralgias	15
Incisional hernias	3
Hyperuricemia	<10
Anemias	<10

levels also may contribute to abnormal mineral metabolism. Nephrolithiasis occurs in up to 30 percent of patients and is due to hyperoxaluria secondary to calcium malabsorption. It can be treated by calcium supplements and a low oxalate intake. Migratory polyarthritis occurs in up to 6 percent of patients and may be due to circulating immune complexes. This operation is now rarely performed, in part due to the decision of many insurance companies not to pay for the procedure.

Gastric surgery Gastroplasty establishes a small upper gastric remnant connected to a larger lower gastric pouch by a narrow 1- to 1.5-cm channel. Gastric bypass excludes the lower 90 percent of the stomach pouch and maintains intestinal continuity of the upper 10 percent via a retrocolic gastrojejunostomy. Both these procedures cause patients to limit food intake by delaying gastric emptying and providing a small gastric reservoir so that fullness is experienced after a small meal. Weight loss with these procedures is comparable with that achieved with small-bowel bypass operations but without malabsorption, diarrhea, and hepatic dysfunction. The procedure can be reversed if a decision to restore normal anatomy is made at a later time. At institutions with a large experience with this procedure, operative mortality and morbidity are low, the efficacy is good, and weight loss is relatively long lasting. This surgical approach should only be considered in morbidly obese individuals who have failed repeated attempts at weight management through other means.

SUMMARY For most patients, obesity is an eating disorder, and a major hope for effective long-term treatment of this disease lies in understanding the causes of overeating. No single etiology explains all cases, and different causes exist for different individuals. At present, a variety of techniques are available to effect initial weight loss. Unfortunately, initial weight loss is not the real therapeutic goal. Rather, the problem is that most obese patients eventually regain their weight. Once obesity occurs, it is a lifelong, chronic illness requiring continuous treatment, even if successful weight loss has occurred. An effective means to sustain weight loss is the major challenge in the treatment of obesity today. The technique of behavioral modification, when professionally and rigorously applied and coupled with an appropriate exercise regimen, is the best tool for this task. As information develops concerning the hypothalamic "set point," or *adipostat*, and the factors that regulate it, other therapies may emerge that will effect long-term correction of abnormal eating patterns.

REFERENCES

BRAY GA: Obesity: An endocrine perspective, in *Endocrinology*, 2d ed, LJ DeGroot et al (eds). Philadelphia, Saunders, 1989, p 2303

——: Obesity: Basic aspects and clinical implications. Med Clin North Am 73:1, 1989

—— et al: Treatment of obesity: Diabetes Metab Rev 4:653, 1988

CARO JF: Clinical review 26: Insulin resistance in obese and nonobese man. J Clin Endocrinol Metab 73:691, 1991

FOSTER DW: Eating disorders: Obesity and anorexia nervosa, in *Williams' Textbook of Endocrinology*, 8th ed, JD Wilson, DW Foster (eds). Philadelphia, Saunders, 1992, p 1335

HENRY RR et al: Metabolic consequences of very low calorie diet therapy in obese non-insulin-dependent diabetic and non-diabetic subjects. Diabetes 35:155, 1986

HIRSCH J et al: Clinical review 28: A biological basis for human obesity. J Clin Endocrinol Metab 73:1153, 1991

KOLTERMAN OG et al: Mechanisms of insulin resistance in human obesity: Evidence for receptor and postreceptor defects. J Clin Invest 65:1272, 1980

NATIONAL INSTITUTES OF HEALTH CONSENSUS DEVELOPMENT PANEL: Gastrointestinal surgery for severe obesity. Ann Intern Med 115:956, 1991

NATIONAL INSTITUTES OF HEALTH CONSENSUS DEVELOPMENT PANEL: Health implications of obesity. Ann Intern Med 103:147, 1985

RAVUSSIN E et al: A brief overview of human energy metabolism and its relationship to essential obesity. Am J Clin Nutr 55:242S, 1992

STUNKARD AJ et al: An adoption study of human obesity. N Engl J Med 314:193, 1984

The Surgeon General's Report on Nutrition and Health, US Department of Health and Human Services Public Health Service (DHHS PHS) Publication 88-50210, 1988

WADDEN TA et al: Treatment of obesity by very low calorie diet, behavior therapy and their combination: A five-year perspective. Int J Obesity 13:39, 1989

WOO R et al: Regulation of energy balance, in *Annual Review of Nutrition*, vol. 5. Palo Alto, Calif., Annual Reviews, Inc, 1985, pp 411–433

74 ANOREXIA NERVOSA AND BULIMIA

DANIEL W. FOSTER

Anorexia nervosa and bulimia are eating disorders in young, previously healthy women who develop a paralyzing fear of becoming fat. The population at risk consists largely of white women from middle-class backgrounds. The disorders rarely occur in black or oriental women, in the poor, or in men. The driving force is the pursuit of thinness, all other aspects of life being secondary. In anorexia nervosa this aim is achieved primarily by radical restriction of caloric intake, the end result being emaciation. In bulimia massive binge eating is followed by vomiting and excessive use of laxatives. Weight loss in bulimic subjects is not great despite the obsession with food. Some authors consider anorexia nervosa and bulimia to be distinct illnesses, while others classify bulimia as a variant of anorexia nervosa. Overlap syndromes exist since emaciated patients fulfilling the criteria of true anorexia nervosa may exhibit bulimic behavior, subjects with bulimia often pass through a phase of anorexia. In this chapter it is assumed that the two disorders are different expressions of a psychologic obsession with body weight.

PREVALENCE Estimates of prevalence for anorexia nervosa range from 0.4 to 1.5 per 100,000 population. In adolescent white girls from middle- or upper-class families rates as high as 1 per 100 have been reported. Prevalence is believed to be increasing. Subclinical variants may occur in up to 5 percent of the group at highest risk. The incidence of bulimia is less certain. Vomiting after eating may occur in as many as 18 percent of women college students. The frequency of self-induced vomiting is probably 1 to 2 percent, but full-blown bulimia is less frequent.

DIAGNOSIS The diagnosis of both anorexia nervosa and bulimia is made on clinical grounds. No specific diagnostic tests exist. For many years the criteria of Feighner et al. were standard (Table 74-1). These criteria included both psychological and clinical/physical components. Revised criteria in the American Psychiatric Association's *Diagnostic and Statistical Manual of Mental Disorders, Third Edition, Revised* (DSM-IIIR) focus on the psychological components of the illnesses. "Softening" of the criteria allows inclusion of subjects that do not yet have a full blown eating disorder but who clearly have abnormal eating patterns.

In the revised criteria the weight loss required for diagnosis was decreased from 25 to 15 percent of expected or ideal weight. Three other features include intense fear of gaining weight or becoming fat even when underweight; disturbance in the way body weight, size, or shape is experienced such that the individual "feels fat"; and, in women, either primary amenorrhea or secondary amenorrhea for at least three consecutive periods. The Feighner criteria remain useful, although it seems reasonable to substitute the 15 percent figure for weight loss. Since the spectrum of restricted eating ranges from a mild disorder of little consequence to life-threatening starvation, neither set of criteria is definitive.

The diagnostic value of the disturbance in body image in patients with eating disorders has been questioned, and some authorities have recommended its omission on the grounds that many normal young women demonstrate the same perceptual distortion. In practice a presumptive diagnosis of anorexia nervosa is justified if the following elements are elicited: (1) a history of major weight loss; (2) absence of organic disease to account for weight loss; (3) absence of severe primary psychiatric illness that might account for failure to eat; (4) extreme restriction of food intake with or without intermittent induction of vomiting; (5) ritualized exercise; and (6) denial of hunger, fatigue, or emaciation. While there is an emphasis on the absence of organic disease to cause weight loss, anorexia nervosa may coexist with other disease that can cause loss of weight, for example, insulin-dependent diabetes mellitus. Late-onset disease is also now recognized although usually symptoms begin in the teen years or early adulthood.

TABLE 74-1 Diagnostic criteria for anorexia nervosa and bulimia nervosa

Anorexia nervosa		Bulimia nervosa
Feighner et al.	DSM-IIIR	DSM-IIIR

1 Onset prior to age 25.
2 Anorexia with weight loss of at least 25% of original body weight.
3 Distorted attitude toward eating, food, or weight that overrides hunger, admonitions, reassurances, and threats.
4 No known medical illness that could account for the weight loss.
5 No other known psychiatric disorder.
6 At least two of the following manifestations:
  a Amenorrhea
  b Lanugo hair
  c Bradycardia (persistent resting pulse of 60 beats per minute or less)
  d Periods of overactivity
  e Episodes of bulimia
  f Vomiting (may be self-induced)
	1 Refusal to maintain body weight over a minimal normal weight for age and height, e.g., weight loss leading to maintenance of body weight 15% below that expected; or failure to make expected weight gain during period of growth, leading to body weight 15% below that expected.
	2 Intense fear of gaining weight or becoming fat, even though underweight.
	3 Disturbance in the way in which one's body weight, size, or shape is experienced, e.g. the person claims to "feel fat" even when emaciated, believes that one area of the body is "too fat" even when obviously underweight.
	4 In women, absence of at least three consecutive menstrual cycles when otherwise expected to occur (primary or secondary amenorrhea). A woman is considered to have amenorrhea if periods occur only following hormone, e.g. estrogen, administration.
		1 Recurrent episodes of binge eating (rapid consumption of a large amount of food in a discrete period of time).
		2 A feeling of lack of control over eating behavior during the eating binges.
		3 The person regularly engages in either self-induced vomiting, use of laxatives or diuretics, strict dieting or fasting, or vigorous exercise to prevent weight gain.
		4 At least two binge-eating episodes a week for at least 3 months.
		5 Persistent overconcern with body shape and weight.

SOURCE: JP Feighner et al: American Psychiatric Association: Diagnostic and Statistical Manual of Mental Disorders, Third Edition, Revised. American Psychiatric Association, Washington D.C. 1987

The criteria for the diagnosis of bulimia in DSM-IIIR are also given in Table 74-1. The picture is that of a normal- or near-normal-weight subject whose life is dominated by gorging and regurgitation in the absence of profound weight loss.

ETIOLOGY The cause is unknown. Although primary dysfunction of the hypothalamus has been postulated, the associated hypothalamic abnormalities revert to normal with weight gain and thus are secondary rather than causal.

Most investigators favor a psychiatric etiology, but there is disagreement about its nature. One view holds that the disorders begin in response to inadequate or destructive interpersonal relationships in families that are goal-oriented and highly achieving. Despite an outward appearance of normality, interpersonal communication within the family tends to be inadequate, frequently following a pattern in which the father seeks success in his work while the mother turns to her children for fulfillment and in the process becomes overdirective. It is often stated that the families are "enmeshed," meaning that generational boundaries are blurred and that parents and children are constantly involved in each other's problems. Psychoanalytic interpretation tends to focus on anorexia as a mechanism whereby the patient reestablishes control of her own life independent of parental direction. It is not clear how this sequence might cause the intense fear of being fat that is the central feature of both anorexia and bulimia.

Although the absence of serious psychiatric disease is a common criterion for diagnosis (Table 74-1), it is now widely held that depression plays a significant role in the eating disorders, especially in bulimia. Abnormalities of neurotransmitter concentrations have been reported in blood and cerebrospinal fluid, but such changes are inconsistent and are likely secondary rather than primary.

Cultural issues are also important in anorexia nervosa. The quest for health and slimness is a powerful force in modern western society and may reinforce the fear of fatness in patients with established anorexia or tip the borderline case into full-blown disease. Occupation may play a role; dancers, for example, have a prevalence of anorexia nervosa 10 times that of the general population. Likewise athletes, particularly runners, often seek to decrease body fat to very low levels (5 to 7 percent). Thus far no genetic component has been identified.

Whatever the mechanism(s) involved, the behavioral response is obsessive and is difficult to treat.

CLINICAL PICTURE While anorexia nervosa and bulimia may coexist in the same patient, the clinical pictures are ordinarily distinct (Table 74-2).

Anorexia nervosa The anorexia nervosa syndrome usually begins before or shortly after puberty but may appear later (usually by the middle twenties). Many patients were overweight in childhood. Emaciation is equivalent to that seen in the concentration camp victims of World War II. Despite profound weight loss patients deny hunger, thinness, or fatigue. They are often physically active, and ritualized exercise is common. Frenzied calisthenics or running may follow food intake. There is a preoccupation with food, and elaborate meals may be prepared for others. If social circumstances require them to eat more than usual, vomiting is induced as soon as possible, often in a public restroom. As noted, episodic binge eating may occur and is also followed by emesis. Amenorrhea usually accompanies or follows weight loss but may appear prior to any physical change. Constipation and cold intolerance are common. The latter is presumably due to a defect in regulatory thermogenesis secondary to hypothalamic dysfunction.

In advanced cases bradycardia, hypothermia, and hypotension are present. Body fat is undetectable, and the bones protrude through the

TABLE 74-2 The eating disorders

	Anorexia nervosa	Bulimia
Predominant sex	Female	Female
Method of weight control	Restriction of intake	Vomiting
Binge eating	Uncommon	Invariant
Weight at diagnosis	Markedly decreased	Near normal
Ritualized exercise	Usual	Rare
Amenorrhea	100%	50%
Antisocial behavior	Rare	Frequent
Cardiovascular changes (bradycardia, hypotension)	Common	Uncommon
Skin changes (hirsutism, dryness, carotenemia)	Usual	Rare
Hypothermia	Usual	Rare
Edema	+/−	+/−
Medical complications	Hypokalemia, cardiac arrhythmias	Hypokalemia, cardiac arrhythmias, aspiration of gastric contents, esophageal or gastric rupture

NOTE: These features are characteristic of pure anorexia nervosa and pure bulimia. Overlap syndromes occur, and anorexia may evolve to bulimia (the bulimia → anorexia transformation is rare).

skin. Interestingly, breast tissue is often preserved. The skin may be dry and scaly and is often yellow due to carotenemia (particularly visible in the palms). Body hair is often increased; it is usually of fine, lanugo quality, but frank hirsutism may occur. Parotid glands may be enlarged as in other forms of starvation. Mitral valve prolapse is due to valve–ventricular volume mismatch secondary to starvation-induced decrease in left ventricular volume. Edema in the absence of hypoalbuminemia is thought to be due to failure of extracellular fluid volume to diminish proportionately with body mass during weight loss. Because of edema in the legs and parotid enlargement, which gives a fullness to the face, the true state of emaciation may be masked when the patient is fully dressed.

Laboratory abnormalities include anemia and leukopenia (with hypocellularity of the bone marrow), hypokalemia, and hypoalbuminemia. Serum β-carotene levels tend to be elevated. Prerenal azotemia may occur if vomiting or laxative use are prominent. The blood urea nitrogen may be as high as 21 to 25 mmol/L (60 to 70 mg/dL). Renal concentrating ability is impaired, possibly due to blunted responsiveness to vasopressin. Release of vasopressin in response to an osmotic stimulus is also abnormal. Plasma cholesterol is occasionally high, but triglyceride levels are not increased despite low activities of hepatic and lipoprotein lipases. Glucose tolerance is abnormal as in other forms of starvation.

Miscellaneous abnormalities include low levels of IgG, IgM, and a variety of complement proteins. Despite these findings immune function is generally preserved, and serious infections are rare. Plasma iron and ceruloplasmin are normal, but iron binding capacity is decreased. Serum zinc and copper are decreased, but concentrations of these metals are normal in hair. Serum amylase may be increased in the absence of pancreatitis.

Basal levels of luteinizing hormone (LH) and follicle-stimulating hormone (FSH) are low when weight loss is severe, and the LH response to luteinizing hormone–releasing hormone (LHRH) is impaired. FSH response to LHRH is normal, although time to peak increase may be delayed. Studies of the 24-h circadian pattern of LH secretion show regression of the mature stage to the pattern characteristic of prepubertal or early pubertal girls; i.e., episodic LH release is missing or occurs only during sleep. These findings presumably account, at least in part, for the amenorrhea. Menses return with weight gain, although the weight required for reinitiation of menstruation may be somewhat higher (about 10 percent) than that needed for the original induction of menarche. Ovulatory menses may be induced in subjects with anorexia nervosa by prolonged treatment with LHRH agonists, suggesting that pituitary gonadotropin release is impaired because of hypothalamic dysfunction. Prolactin levels are normal. Plasma estradiol levels are low, but plasma testosterone is in the normal female range. Testosterone levels are low in men with anorexia nervosa.

Growth hormone (GH) in the basal state may be normal or elevated. A rise in GH occurs after injection of thyrotropin-releasing hormone (TRH), as in other states with elevated basal levels of GH such as acromegaly, uremia, and protein-calorie malnutrition. Insulin-like growth factor I (somatomedin C) concentrations are low and may contribute to growth hormone elevation via diminished negative feedback. Plasma cortisol levels are high due to increased secretion of corticotropin-releasing hormone from the hypothalamus. The cortisol negative feedback mechanism in the hypothalamus is believed to be impaired. Dexamethasone suppression tests may be abnormal. Norepinephrine concentrations in plasma are depressed.

Thyroxine (T_4) levels are in the low-normal range; free T_4 is normal. Triiodothyronine (T_3) concentrations are reduced, while reverse T_3 (rT_3) levels are increased. Basal levels of thyroid-stimulating hormone (TSH) are usually normal, and TSH response to TRH is intact. The primary defect in thyroid hormone metabolism is decreased activity of the 5'-deiodinase that converts T_4 to T_3 and rT_3 to diiodothyronine in nonthyroidal tissues. These changes are characteristic of starvation and wasting diseases and are not specific for anorexia nervosa.

Bone density is decreased in women with anorexia nervosa. The mechanism is thought to be estrogen deficiency. Cortisol excess may contribute.

Bulimia Bulimia, which means "ox-hunger," refers to the episodic ingestion of large amounts of food in a compulsive fashion, coupled with awareness that the eating pattern is abnormal, a fear that eating cannot be stopped voluntarily, and feelings of depression at completion of the act. Bulimics have a morbid fear of becoming fat. While binge eating may occur in several types of emotional disorders, many patients give a history of overt or cryptic anorexia nervosa, suggesting that bulimia is a variant of anorexia nervosa. Episodes of binge eating are followed by induced vomiting, with or without the subsequent ingestion of laxatives. Initially vomiting is induced by placing a toothbrush or fingers in the throat, but eventually most patients learn to vomit reflexly.

Binge eating generally occurs daily in the active phase; in 40 patients the mean number of episodes per week was 12, ranging from 1 to 46. The duration of the eating period averaged 1.2 h but could last as long as 8 h. The amount of food ingested may be enormous, up to 200,000 kJ (50,000 kcal). High-carbohydrate foods are favored, and more than one food is usually eaten. The order of frequency in one report was: ice cream→bread→candy→doughnuts→soft drinks. The term "dietary chaos" describes the eating pattern. Because of the high sugar content of the diet, dental caries are frequent.

Other behavioral abnormalities are common. Secrecy about the eating-vomiting sequence is characteristic so that family and friends are often unaware. Stealing is common, and food is the item most often taken. There is a high rate of alcohol and drug abuse. Depression tends to be more severe than in anorexia nervosa, making suicide a definite risk. Hysterical behavior may occur. Families of patients with bulimia have a higher incidence of affective disorders, alcoholism, and illicit drug use than in families of patients with anorexia nervosa.

Despite the close relationship with anorexia nervosa, a number of differences are noted. While many patients with bulimia are thin, emaciation is not seen; generally weight is within 15 percent of the normal range as defined by life insurance tables of ideal weight. Fluctuating weight is common, with cyclical gains and losses. Some patients are modestly overweight. In contrast to anorexia nervosa, many patients continue to menstruate and may become pregnant. Persistent menstruation probably reflects the absence of extreme weight loss. Sexual activity is greater in bulimic subjects than in those with anorexia.

The physical findings are usually minimal, although more extensive weight loss may cause some of the changes seen with anorexia nervosa.

The most common laboratory abnormality is hypokalemia with metabolic alkalosis secondary to vomiting and laxative use. Endocrine abnormalities are similar to those in anorexia nervosa. One study suggested that LH response to LHRH is exaggerated in bulimic patients. It has been reported that peptide YY, a putative stimulant of feeding behavior in animals, is elevated in the cerebrospinal fluid of bulimic patients. Some also have deficient secretion of serotonin and cholecystokinin, thought to be satiety signals. The significance of these findings is not known. Dexamethasone suppression is frequently abnormal. Unlike patients with anorexia nervosa, some women with bulimia have low basal prolactin levels and an exaggerated prolactin response to TRH. Serum amylase may be elevated in the absence of pancreatitis in both anorexia and bulimia.

COMPLICATIONS Patients with anorexia nervosa are vulnerable to sudden death from ventricular tachyarrhythmias. Electrocardiograms show prolonged QT intervals. The risk of death becomes high when weight loss reaches 35 percent below ideal, probably because of protein deficiency. (Since there is no reserve store of protein, critical enzymes and cellular structures are affected by starvation-induced decreases in lean body mass; see Chap. 72.) Major complications include aspiration, esophageal or gastric rupture, pneumomediastinum, hypokalemia with cardiac arrhythmias, pancreatitis, and ipecac-induced myopathy and/or cardiomyopathy.

PROGNOSIS The course of anorexia nervosa is variable. In long-term follow-up about half of patients achieve normal weight, 20 percent improve but remain underweight, 20 percent continue anorexic, 5 percent become obese, and 6 percent die. Even when weight gain occurs, signs of persistent illness remain since intermittent dieting, binge eating, vomiting, and laxative use persist in up to two-thirds of patients. Death is usually due to starvation (cardiac arrhythmias primarily) or suicide. Poor prognostic signs include older age of onset, longer duration of illness, history of bulimia or vomiting, extreme weight loss, and presence of significant depression. Fewer reports of long-term follow-up are available for bulimia. Because the psychiatric disturbance tends to be more severe (suicide occurs at higher rates) and because the medical dangers of gorging are greater, prognosis is believed to be worse in bulimia than in anorexia. One report indicates that 40 percent of treated patients remained bulimic after 18 months of treatment and that relapse occurred in 65 percent after 1 year of recovery.

TREATMENT There is no specific treatment for anorexia nervosa or bulimia. The intense fear of becoming fat coupled with a perceptual disturbance that causes overestimation of body size results in powerful resistance to therapy. The benefits of psychiatric intervention are marginal. The same can be said of behavior modification techniques and for group and family therapy. Supportive care by an understanding physician may accomplish as much as formal psychotherapy. The patient should be seen regularly for a review of weight change, diet, and exercise patterns. It is often useful to establish a mutually agreeable explicit contract; e.g., if the patient weighs 65 pounds and ideal body weight determined from life insurance tables is 115 pounds, a goal of 90 pounds might be set as a first stage. At every visit the patient should be reassured by the physician that "we will not let you get fat." A calm but realistic review of the dangers of starvation, including sudden death, should be given, coupled with statements like "my job is to help you deal with this illness so that you can have a normal life expectancy with reasonable happiness." The physician must be perceived not as an enemy or a parental surrogate but an advisor and partner in the struggle.

A similar approach should also be used with bulimic patients. Even if the gorging-regurgitation cycle cannot be stopped, the lesser goal of limiting the load of food ingested (to minimize the chance of aspiration or gastric rupture) and decreasing the frequency of events may be achieved. Because depression and anti-social behavior are more common in bulimia, psychiatric therapy is usually required. Drug therapy appears to be of little use in anorexia nervosa although fluoxetine may help in preventing relapse in patients responding to behavior modification strategies. Antidepressant therapy appears to be superior to placebo in the treatment of bulemia nervosa. Potassium supplementation may be required for vomiters.

Hospitalization may be a lifesaving measure with severe anorexia nervosa. As noted above, sudden death may occur at weights more than 35 percent below ideal, particularly if weight loss has been rapid. Hypokalemia, hypotension, and prerenal azotemia due to volume depletion are other indications for hospitalization. A nasogastric tube may be required, but it is better to persuade the patient to eat. Supervision of every meal is initially required, ideally by the same person. During hospitalization the patient should never be allowed to eat alone. Total parenteral nutrition is rarely indicated. Instruction about nutrition, occupational therapy, group work with the family, and individual psychotherapy should be included in the treatment plan. The "safety" of eating and assurances that obesity will not result should be emphasized repetitively. Some specialists feel that all seriously affected anorexia patients benefit from initial hospitalization, but this is not a universal view. Hospitalization for bulimic subjects is normally only required for medical complications (e.g., aspiration).

Treatment of the anorexia-bulimia syndrome is a long-term proposition, rife with failure, and requires perseverance by the subject, family, and physician.

REFERENCES

FEIGHNER JP et al: Diagnostic criteria for use in psychiatric research. Arch Gen Psychiatry 26:57, 1972

FOSTER DW: Eating disorders: Obesity, anorexia nervosa and bulimia nervosa in *Williams Textbook of Endocrinology*, 8th ed, JD Wilson, DW Foster (eds). Philadelphia, Saunders, 1992, pp 1335–1365

HERZOG DB, COPELAND PM: Eating disorders. N Engl J Med 313:295, 1985

HERZOG DB et al: The course and outcome of bulimia nervosa. J Clin Psychiatry supp. 52:4, 1991

ISNER JM et al: Anorexia nervosa and sudden death. Ann Intern Med 102:49, 1985

KAYE WH, WELTZIN TE: Neurochemistry of bulimia nervosa. J Clin Psychiatry supp. 52:21, 1991

LEVY AB: Neuroendocrine profile in bulimia nervosa. Biol Psychiatry 25:98, 1989

—— et al: How are depression and bulimia related? Am J Psychiatry 146:162, 1989

LOVE L, GOLD PW: The hypothalamic-pituitary-adrenal axis in anorexia nervosa and bulimia nervosa: Pathophysiologic implications. Adv Pediatr 38:287, 1991

LUCAS AR et al: Anorexia nervosa in Rochester, Minnesota: A 45-year study. Mayo Clin Proc 63:433, 1988

MITCHELL JE et al: Medical complications and medical management of bulimia. Ann Intern Med 107:71, 1987

NEWMAN MM, HALMI KA: The endocrinology of anorexia nervosa and bulimia nervosa. Endocrin Metab Clin North Am 17:195, 1988

WALSH BT, DEVLIN MJ: The pharmacological treatment of eating disorders. Psychiatr Clin N Amer 15:149, 1992

75 DIET THERAPY

JOHANNA T. DWYER / JODI ROY

The primary aims of diet therapy are to prevent or treat malnutrition, control diet-related manifestations of disease, delay progression of chronic disease, and provide support for other medical or surgical treatments. Diet therapy also plays an important role in rehabilitation and in palliation, e.g., maintaining or enhancing the quality of life in the terminally ill. Dietary advice is useful for health promotion, disease prevention, nutritional support, and rehabilitation. Nutrition therapy may involve slight modifications of usual food intakes, use of special purpose oral supplements, or feeding by enteral or parenteral routes.

Four principles guide sound diet therapy. First a nutrition-related problem must be present for which an accepted dietary therapy exists. Second, the diet therapy must be based on a solid scientific rationale. Ideally, documentation of the effectiveness of the therapeutic diet in ameliorating symptoms, slowing progression, lessening secondary problems or offering other positive effects on function should be available. Anecdotal evidence alone is insufficient to warrant diet therapy. Third, the patient must be able and willing to eat and must have a functional gastrointestinal tract. (For patients who require parenteral or enteral nutrition therapy, see Chap. 76.) Finally, the patient must adhere to the diet. Little effort is required for a patient to consume a diet in the hospital since appropriate meals are served and no other food choice may be available, but a great deal of motivation is needed to prepare and eat therapeutic diets after discharge.

PLANNING DIET THERAPY

ASSESSMENT Dietary assessment attempts to discover what is eaten. It requires cataloguing what the individual usually eats and the nutritional quality and adequacy of that pattern. It also helps determine nutritional status, establishes or refines differential diagnoses, and furnishes the background information on food intakes and preferences that are needed for implementing diet therapy. Nutritional status assessment (Chap. 72) measures the interaction of diet, disease, and nutrition requirements by integrating information on food intake and clinical, biochemical and anthropometric measurements. Both dietary assessment and nutritional status assessment are needed to identify nutrition-related problems and plan therapeutic diets.

Dietary assessment can be performed at qualitative or quantitative levels. Qualitative assessment involves determining (1) whether the patient is currently eating and following a specific diet, and if so, the number of meals per day, any use of nutritional supplements (e.g., amounts and types of vitamin or mineral supplements), special dietary preferences or dietary practices (e.g., consumption of only one or a few foods), or medications that may influence nutritional status; (2) whether there has been recent weight loss or gain; (3) the physical state (e.g., chewing problems, dysphagia, diarrhea, ability to shop, cook and feed oneself); and (4) social circumstances that may influence intake (e.g., economic resources, social isolation, social support systems). If the qualitative assessment suggests that nutritional problems may exist, more quantitative approaches may be in order. For example, a complete record of all food intake (less uneaten food) and its ability to meet nutrient needs can be ordered if the patient is hospitalized. For outpatients, current dietary intake (e.g., the past day) can be catalogued using 24-h recalls. The patient is asked to describe what was consumed over the past 24 h, starting with the last meal eaten. Intake is then assessed by comparing it to a food grouping system or by calculating the nutrient contributions of each food from a table of food composition, and comparing the adequacy of nutrients with the Recommended Dietary Allowances or some other criteria of desirable food intake. Computer programs are now available for performing these analyses. This method is easy to administer, places little burden on the patient, and provides some estimate of intakes. However, one day may not be long enough to provide a truly representative intake, so habitual diet may not be assessed. If assessment of nutritional status is to be meaningful, dietary intake data must reflect a period of weeks or months. If changes in intake have occurred, it may also be helpful to probe previous intakes before the illness or other events that might have caused dietary alteration.

The habitual diet is assessed with either semiquantitative food frequency questionnaires, using a standardized list of foods and portion sizes, or the periodic collection of food records for several days at a time. Semiquantitative food frequency questionnaires can be analyzed on a computer. Food records are better for identifying the intake of unusual foods not included on food frequency questionnaires, but records are more difficult to obtain and analyze. Other methods for dietary assessment include the dietary history, in which the patient provides information on usual intakes in an interview with a dietitian. In skilled hands this can reveal dietary patterns quickly and is less burdensome to the patient than keeping food records, but training and time are required to interview in a reproducible manner.

PRESCRIPTION A diet prescription or diet order that specifies the dietary modifications needed for nutritional therapy is the first step in nutritional intervention. It is usually brief, stated in terms of the additional assessment needed, the disease to be treated, and the modifications to deal with the disease. The physician is also responsible for making appropriate changes in diet orders. Failure to make changes can result in such unfortunate events as keeping patients indefinitely on nutritionally inadequate "clear liquid" diets with resulting debilitation and/or delayed healing.

The rendering of nutrition care requires knowledge about food composition, dietary assessment, diet planning, and diet counseling techniques. In acute care and inpatient settings, the diet order is translated by dietitians into actual foods, menus, or eating plans acceptable to the patient. In outpatient settings, the physician may counsel patients directly, or they may be referred to dietitians.

CARE PLAN A nutrition care plan is then formulated for the implementation of the diet. The individual who undertakes diet therapy must record the nutritional care plan in the medical record and supervise its implementation. The care plan should include a summary of the needs uncovered during the assessment and an implementation plan for achieving nutritional objectives including additional resources needed, such as assistance in purchasing food, help with eating (if necessary) and any follow up plans for counseling

TABLE 75-1 Modifications in diet consistency

Consistency	Purpose	Use	Nutritional adequacy	Comments
Clear liquid: clear broth, gelatin, popsicles, ices; sugar, honey, hard candy; clear fruit juices; clear coffee, tea, and carbonated beverages (as tolerated); low-residue, high-protein, high-calorie clear oral supplements.	Short term (1–2 days preferably): to supply fluid and some energy [2500 kJ/d (600 kcal/d)] in a form that requires minimal digestion after surgery, trauma, or in acute illness.	Initial feeding after surgery or IV feeding to relieve thirst and hydrate, while minimizing the need to chew and GI-tract stimulation.	Falls seriously short of nutrient needs in energy, protein, vitamins, and minerals; if this diet is to continue beyond 3–5 days, nutritional support is necessary.	Produces few or no feces; greatly different from usual diets.
Full liquid: clear liquids plus: all milk and milk drinks, yogurt; vegetable and fruit juices; refined cooked cereals; butter, margarine; custard, ice cream, pudding; high-protein, high-calorie oral supplements.	Supply fluid and meet energy and other nutrient needs more completely with foods that are liquid at body temperature; usually higher in calories than clear liquid diet.	Transition between clear liquid and solid foods after surgery and in acute illness; in esophageal or stomach disorders with strictures or anatomical irregularity; and for inability to chew or swallow solid foods.	May be inadequate in niacin, folacin, and iron due to lack of meat, whole grain, and vegetable intake; adequacy may be improved using high-protein, high-calorie supplements or the addition of a multivitamin supplement.	More complete diet than clear liquid; beneficial as a transitional feeding for weak patients who cannot adequately chew food; greatly different from usual diets.
Soft	Provide foods that can be swallowed with little or no chewing.	For patients who are alert or acutely ill with difficulty in chewing/ swallowing, or who are too ill or weak to tolerate a usual diet; for head and neck surgical patients; those with esophageal strictures or poor dentition. Also useful for those with inflammatory ulceration, neurologic changes, or anatomic alterations.	Can be adequate in all nutrients based on menu selection. Oral nutritional supplements may be helpful as well.	Textures can range from pureed (blenderized, strained, or smooth foods) to ground, chopped, or soft solids.

and nutrition education. Special attention should be directed to easing the transition from special routes of feeding back to usual oral routes. Plans for review, follow-up, and evaluation of progress should also be specified.

IMPLEMENTING DIET THERAPY

USUAL INTAKE The starting point for planning therapeutic diets is the patient's usual intake. The fewer the changes from usual intake, the greater the likelihood that individual preferences will be met and that the new eating plan will be followed. If the usual intake is not nutritionally adequate, the therapeutic plan includes modifications to ensure nutritional sufficiency.

MODIFICATIONS Therapeutic diets can involve three basic alterations: modifications in food constituents, consistency, and route of feeding (see Chap. 76). The appropriate diet for a given condition depends on the stage or severity of disease, characteristics of the patient (age, sex, educational level, ethnicity), the treatment environment (e.g., inpatient, outpatient), and the social situation. For example, there are many diets for patients with diabetes mellitus, depending on individual needs such as whether the patient is on insulin, whether there is a need for weight reduction, and coexisting medical complications (such as hyperlipidemia, hypertension, or renal disease).

Additional considerations must be taken into account. The first is to meet the recommended dietary allowances (RDAs) for nutrients (see Table 71-4). The second is to deal with relevant medical concerns (such as ease of swallowing in a stroke patient or the timing of feeding in a patient with insulin-dependent diabetes mellitus), patient food preferences, and drug-nutrient interactions. Diet manuals in individual hospitals specify the diets available.

CONSISTENCY (See Table 75-1) Variations in consistency usually involve two factors. The first is liquidity; major categories are clear liquid, full liquid, and soft. The form and nature of the ingredients constitute the second factor. Options include common foods that have been chopped and blenderized, commercial nutritional supplements formulated with ingredients not usually available in the home, and "elemental diets" using nutrients in simple forms such as protein hydrolysates or amino acids. In general, the commercial products are more appetizing because they use stabilizers and other means to keep particles in suspension and because they are more palatable.

Nutritional adequacy and palatability must be considered in plans that alter consistency. Clear liquid diets are nutritionally inadequate and include only a few foods that most people eat regularly, but they may be necessary immediately after surgery or during severe medical emergencies. Full liquid diets include more foods and may be nutritionally adequate but are limited in choice compared to normal diets. Soft diets are also limited in terms of palatability. For these reasons, modifications in consistency should only be used when necessary and for as limited a time as feasible.

CONSTITUENTS (See Table 75-2) Modifications in the composition of diets may include energy level, type and amount of nutrients (e.g., lactose-free; low fat, low saturated fat), or type and amount of other constituents (e.g., 30-g soluble fiber, 300-mg cholesterol; low oxalate). Other therapeutic regimens are described in standard textbooks.

Several points need emphasis in planning alterations in dietary composition: First, the supporting evidence and documentation of

---

TABLE 75-2 Dietary modifications in various diseases

Therapeutic diet modification	Disease	Known benefit(s)	Possible benefit(s)
ENERGY			
Energy controlled	Diabetes mellitus	Increased glucose tolerance, decreased acute side effects	Decreased long-term complications (large vessel atherosclerosis, nephropathy, hypertension)
Low energy	Obesity	Weight loss	
	Hypertension	Decreased systolic and diastolic blood pressure	
	Non-insulin dependent diabetes mellitus	Increased glucose tolerance, decreased short-term symptoms	Decreased long-term complications
High energy	Anorexia, emaciation	Increased weight, lean body mass, and fat; promotes normal fat and lean tissue	
Small feedings	Gastroesophageal reflux	Decreased gastric volume, decreased likelihood of reflux (small feedings in an upright position)	
ENERGY-YIELDING NUTRIENTS			
Carbohydrate			
Low simple sugar	Postgastrectomy to prevent dumping syndrome (with low liquids) and to control symptoms due to lactose intolerance, sucrase or lactase deficiency, or other inborn errors of sugar absorption	Controls symptoms	
High carbohydrate (65–70% kcal)	When undertaken a week or so before event, increases muscle glycogen stores and energy reserves for endurance activities	May increase athletic performance by increasing energy reserves in muscle during long sustained activity in athletic events	
Protein			
Low protein	Chronic renal failure (end stage renal disease)	Control of blood urea nitrogen, electrolytes, and phosphorus levels (amino acid supplements are used)	
	Hepatic encephalopathy	Prevention of hepatic encephalopathy	
	Early chronic progressive renal insufficiency		Decreased decline in glomerular filtration rate
	Nephrotic syndrome		Decreased protein wasting

(continued)

TABLE 75-2 Dietary modifications in various diseases (continued)

Therapeutic diet modification	Disease	Known benefit(s)	Possible benefit(s)
ENERGY-YIELDING NUTRIENTS			
Fat			
Low fat	Steatorrhea, radiation enteritis, Gastroesophageal reflux	Decreased malabsorption Increased lower esophageal sphincter pressure	
	Acute hepatic, pancreatic, and gall bladder disease	Decreased need for bile salts	
	Crohn's disease	Decreased malabsorption in patients with functional lactase deficiency	
	Postgastrostomy dumping	Decreased malabsorption in patients with functional lactase deficiency	
	Colon, prostate, and breast cancers		Reduced risks in promotion stage via hormone actions
	Hyperlipidemia	Reduced serum lipids	
Low fat, low saturated fat, low cholesterol	Coronary heart disease	Reduced serum lipids	Some arterial plaques regress (if diet is extreme and long continued)
OTHER DIETARY ALTERATIONS			
Low sodium	Hypertension	Decreased blood-pressure in salt-sensitive persons	
	Congestive heart failure	Decreased sodium retention, reducing hypertension	
	Chronic renal failure	Decreased sodium retention, reducing hypertension	
	Ascites	Decreased sodium retention	
Low potassium	Hyperkalemia	Decreased serum potassium	
	Chronic renal failure	Decreased serum potassium	
High potassium	Hypokalemia	Increased serum potassium	
High calcium	Osteoporosis		Risk reduction in postmenopausal women
Low phosphorus	Hyperphosphatemia	Decreased serum phosphorus	
	Renal failure	Decreased serum phosphorus	
Low oxalate	Oxalate kidney stones	Decreased concentration of oxalate in the urine	
	Crohn's disease	Decreased malabsorption in patients with steatorrhea	
High fiber	Hyperlipidemia	Decreased serum cholesterol (if high water-soluble fiber or oat gum)	
Low fiber	Crohn's disease, inflammatory bowel disease, regional enteritis, ulcerative colitis (active phase)	Reduced diarrhea and pain	
	Crohn's disease (inactive phase)		Symptom control
Low fiber, low residue	Postoperative transition postostomy, diverticulitis, active inflammatory bowel disease, or other conditions with narrowed or stenosed colon	Symptom control and reduces total post-digestive luminal contents, decrease in fecal output	Unproved if diet improves gut healing
Sulfite restricted	Prevents adverse reactions such as asthma, hives, and anaphylaxis in sulfite sensitive persons	Decreases symptoms	
Phenylalanine restricted	Prevents adverse metabolic effects among persons with phenylketonuria or hyperphenylalaninemia	Decreases symptoms and reduces ill effects on mental function in children, and reduces fetal levels in utero of affected mothers	
Tyramine controlled	Prevents reactions from consumption of foods with tyramine and other amines while receiving monoamine oxidase inhibitor therapy	Reduces symptoms	
Purine restricted diet	Decreases elevated blood and urinary uric acid levels in patients with gout, urinary calculi, etc. when used in conjunction with other drug and diet therapy.	Other measures, such as drug therapy, weight reduction, limited alcohol intake, and control of hypertriglyceridemia also recommended if this is used	Not always required but may help to reduce drug doses
Gluten-free, gliadin free	Celiac disease	Decreased malabsorption and gut damage due to improved absorption	

benefits for therapeutic diets vary in their completeness (Table 75-2). For some diseases, such as the hyperlipidemias, the role of diet modification in decreasing serum cholesterol and risk of coronary artery disease is well documented. For other diseases, such as diabetes mellitus, diet can control acute and short-term complications, but the efficacy for long term sequelae, such as retinopathy and kidney disease, is not established. Patients need to be informed as to what can be expected from the diet instituted.

Second, changes both in consistency and in composition may be required. For example, simultaneous modifications in a number of constituents are mandatory in patients with diabetes mellitus and renal failure. Such a patient may require an eating plan that controls energy intake, type and amount of carbohydrate, timing of carbohydrate intake, amount of dietary fiber, and the content of fat, protein, and sodium. In some cases, there are so many constraints that priority ranking must be given to the important alterations. With other

TABLE 75-3 Recommendations of American Heart Association/National Cholesterol Education Program: step 1 (with PBR*) and step 2 diets for hypercholesterolemia

Indications
  LDL cholesterol >4.1 mmol/L (>160 mg/dL)
  LDL cholesterol >3.4 mmol/L (>130 mg/dL) with definite coronary disease or two other risk factors[†]

Minimal goals
  Without coronary disease or two risk factors: Lower LDL cholesterol below 4.1 mmol/L (150 mg/dL)
  With coronary disease or two risk factors: Lower LDL cholesterol below 3.4 mmol/L (130 mg/dL)

Recommended intake	% of total kilocalories	
	Step 1 diet and PBR* for persons of age >2 y	Step 2 diet (if serum lipid goal not reached)
Total fat	<30%	<25%
Saturated fatty acids	<10%	< 7%
Polyunsaturated fatty acids	<10%	<10%
Monounsaturated fatty acids	10–15%	10–15%
Carbohydrates	50–60%	50–60%
Protein	10–20%	10–20%
Cholesterol	<300 mg/d	<200 mg/d
Total energy intake	To achieve and maintain desirable weight	To achieve and maintain desirable weight

* Population Based Recommendations.
[†] Risk factors include male sex, family history of premature coronary distress, cigarette smoking, hypertension, low HDL cholesterol level, diabetes mellitus, history of definite cerebrovascular or occlusive peripheral vascular disease, severe obesity.
NOTE: LDL = low-density lipoprotein; HDL = high-density lipoprotein.
SOURCE: Adapted from National Cholesterol Education Program: Arch Intern Med 148:36, 1988; and National Cholesterol Education Program: *Report of the Expert Panel on Population Strategies for Blood Cholesterol Reduction*, U.S. Department of Health and Human Services, Public Health Service, National Institutes of Health, Bethesda MD, 1990.

TABLE 75-4 Nutritional goals for patients with diabetes mellitus

Energy intake: achieve and maintain a reasonable body weight
Carbohydrate: (1) up to 55–60% of total energy; (2) substitute unrefined complex carbohydrates high in fiber for highly refined carbohydrates; (3) modest amounts of sucrose and other refined sugars are acceptable depending on metabolic control; (4) individualization is important
Protein: no lower than the RDA for adults of 0.8 g/kg of ideal body weight, or approximately 12–20% of total calories, but further modifications and individualization may be needed for pregnancy, lactation, in aging, and in presence of renal complications.
Total fat: ideally <30% total calories from fat, with no more than 10% saturates, up to 10% polyunsaturated, and remainder from monounsaturated fatty acids
Dietary cholesterol: <300 mg/d
Fiber: up to 40 g/d recommended, with 25g/4200 kJ (100 kcal) calories if individual is on a low calorie diet
Sodium intake: <3000 mg/d, but may need further restrictions in presence of renal or other medical complications
Alcohol use: limit to 1–2 alcohol equivalents once or twice a week
Vitamins and minerals: at levels specified in Recommended Dietary Allowances
Alcohol: if at all, in moderation
Alternative sweeteners: nutritive and nonnutritive sweeteners both acceptable in moderation
Meal timing: in insulin-dependent diabetes, meal timing and size may need to be adjusted depending on type of insulin used, physical activity, sick days, and other factors
Other: presence of nephropathy, atherosclerosis, or high blood pressure may require further modifications

SOURCE: Modified and adapted from American Diabetes Association, Position statement: Nutritional recommendations and principles for individuals with diabetes mellitus. Diabetes Care 10:126, 1987; and Beebe CA: Kilocalorie and nutrient controlled diet for diabetes, in *Handbook of Clinical Dietetics*, 2d ed, American Dietetic Association 1992, pp 405–427.

modifications, less precision is acceptable. Otherwise, it may be impractical to implement diet therapy.

Third, modifications in nutrient composition may be necessary to meet physiologic needs (infancy, puberty, pregnancy, lactation, aging). Factors to be taken into account include inadequacies in recent intake, the timing of nutrient intake (as in insulin-dependent diabetes mellitus), and the presence of specific food allergies or intolerances (e.g., patients on monoamine oxidase inhibitors). Other problems, include inability to feed oneself, vegetarianism, religious beliefs that prohibit certain foods, alcoholism, and specific likes and dislikes.

Fourth, elaborate diet prescriptions place a burden on patients. Complicated diets may cause only minor problems in the hospitalized patients but create major compliance problems for outpatients. When

TABLE 75-5 Exchange list for meal planning for diabetics

Exchange list food group	Carbohydrate, grams	Protein, grams	Fat, grams	Energy intake, kilojoules (kilocalories)
Starch/bread	15	3	Trace	335 (80)
120 mL (½ cup) cereal, grain, or pasta				
30 g (1 oz) of a bread product				
Meat				
30 g (1 oz) cooked				
Lean	—	7	3	230 (55)
Medium-fat	—	7	5	315 (75)
High-fat	—	7	8	415 (100)
Vegetable	5	2	—	105 (25)
120 mL (½ cup) cooked or juice				
240 mL (1 cup) raw				
Fruit	15	—	—	250 (60)
120 mL (½ cup) fresh or juice				
60 mL (¼ cup) dried				
Milk				
240 mL (1 cup)				375 (90)
Skim	12	8	Trace	500 (120)
Low-fat	12	8	5	625 (150)
Whole	12	8	8	
Fat	—	—	5	190 (45)
5 mL butter, margarine, oil, mayonnaise (1 tsp.)				
15 mL salad dressing (1 Tbsp.)				

NOTE: Saturated fat, fiber and sodium intakes are controlled by choices within food groups
SOURCE: American Diabetes Association and the American Dietetic Association: *Exchange Lists for Meal Planning*, 1986.

the continuation of such diets is necessary, diet counseling prior to discharge should be supplemented by frequent outpatient visits.

Even within a given disease category, the role of dietary therapy may vary, and there may be no single "therapeutic diet" for a given disease. Rather, the appropriate dietary measures depend on symptoms and other manifestations of the disease.

Modifications for hypercholesterolemia The associations between diet and levels of serum cholesterol are well documented and, at least in men, predictable, and the association between lowering of serum cholesterol and decreases in the complications of coronary artery disease is clear-cut. Hence, diet therapy is the first step in the treatment of most hyperlipidemic states. Table 75-3 summarizes the current recommendations for diet therapy of those adults at high risk [(e.g., total serum cholesterol >6.2 mmol/L (<240 mg/dL)] jointly endorsed by the National Cholesterol Education Program (NCEP) and the American Heart Association and includes the indications for diet therapy in terms of the individual's serum lipid values (see also Chaps. 208 and 344).

The NCEP recommends a "step-care" approach in dealing with hyperlipidemia. Patients at risk are first placed on the step 1 diet (unless they are at very high risk), which is modified in total fat, saturated fat, cholesterol, and energy intake. After a period of 2 months the serum cholesterol is evaluated. Those who, despite adherence, do not achieve the goals of therapy on the step 1 diet are asked to continue the diet trial and are provided with additional assistance. Patients whose serum cholesterol is still not within acceptable levels are moved to the step 2 diet, which is even lower in saturated fat and cholesterol. If serum cholesterol levels are still not reduced sufficiently, drug therapy is added. Hyperlipidemic patients may also have hypertension, diabetes mellitus, chronic renal insufficiency, or other diseases that require additional dietary modifications.

Modifications for diabetes mellitus Table 75-4 outlines the nutritional recommendations for individuals with diabetes mellitus, and Table 75-5 summarizes a widely used tool—the exchange list. Exchange lists describe the serving size of various foods in groups that are similar in nutrient value. Exchange lists vary depending on the disease and the desired dietary modifications. Such lists provide an overall meal plan that allows selection of different foods and menus. However, the type and amount of dietary carbohydrate and fat and the energy intake ingested throughout the day need to be considered in planning the diet, drug administration schedule, and physical activity patterns. Diet therapy in diabetes is helpful in controlling the acute manifestations (excessive thirst, frequent urination, blurred vision, etc.) of hyperglycemia and may reduce the risk of accelerated atherosclerosis.

Alterations in dietary fiber Modifications in the type and amount of dietary fiber can sometimes ameliorate functional constipation or diarrhea. Increased dietary fiber intakes, particularly of water-insoluble fibers like wheat bran, also provide symptomatic relief in diverticulosis of the colon. Some water-soluble fibers in large doses may decrease serum cholesterol levels; these include fiber derived from oat bran, beans, and psyllium seeds.

Lactose-free diets Many adults, especially Orientals, blacks, and Ashkenazic Jews, have hereditary lactase deficiency. Lactose intolerance may also be secondary, either acquired or as a result of

TABLE 75-6 Rich food sources of vitamins

Vitamin	Alternative names	Richest sources
Vitamin A (plus carotenoids)	Retinol (vitamin A alcohol)	Liver, egg yolk, chicken meat; whole milk, butter; breakfast cereals and margarines fortified with vitamin A
Carotenoids	β-Carotene (most plentiful)	Dark-green leafy vegetables like spinach, chard; deep-yellow vegetables like carrots, squash; yellow fruits like mango, cantaloupe
Vitamin D	D_3 (cholecalciferol) D_2 (ergocalciferol)	Fatty fish like salmon and fish oils; eggs; butter; liver; milk fortified with vitamin D
Vitamin E	Alpha tocopherol	Oils from soybean, sunflower, corn, and cottonseed; germ of whole grains; fish liver oils; nuts
Thiamine	Vitamin B_1	Whole grains, dried legumes; pork muscle, liver; products made with enriched flour
Riboflavin	Vitamin B_2	Milk and milk products; eggs; whole- and enriched-grain products; lean meat, liver, poultry, fish; dark-green vegetables like spinach, asparagus
Niacin	Nicotinic Acid	Meats, poultry, fish; yeast; whole- and enriched-grain products; legumes; nuts; in addition, some of the tryptophan present in meats, poultry, fish, cheese, legumes, and seeds can be converted in the body to niacin
Vitamin B_6	Pyridoxine Pyridoxal Pyridoxamine	Meat, poultry, fish; bananas; yeast; bran; nuts
Vitamin B_{12}	Cobalamin	Only in foods of animal origin: liver, muscle meat, fish, eggs, and milk and milk products
Folacin	Folic Acid Folate	Liver; dark-green leafy vegetables like spinach, romaine lettuce; dried beans, peanuts, wheat germ, whole grains; yeast
Vitamin C	Ascorbic Acid	Citrus fruits like oranges, lemons, grapefruit; dark-green leafy vegetables like broccoli, asparagus

SOURCE: National Academy of Sciences Committee on Diet and Health: *Diet and Health: Recommendations to Reduce Chronic Disease Risk*, National Academy Press, Washington, 1989.

TABLE 75-7 Rich food sources of minerals

Mineral	Sources
Calcium	Milk, cheese, broccoli, dark-green leafy vegetables such as collard, turnip, and mustard greens
Phosphorus	Meat, milk products, grains, phosphate, food additives
Magnesium	Green vegetables, nuts, seeds, dried beans, whole grains, and meat
Iron	Liver, red meat, whole-grain and enriched-grain products, beans, nuts, and dark-green leafy vegetables
Zinc	Shellfish, meat, poultry, cheese, whole grains, dried beans, nuts
Copper	Crab meat, fresh vegetables and fruits, nuts, seeds, legumes
Sodium	Salt (sodium chloride); cured meats (ham, bacon, sausage, frankfurters, luncheon meats); cheeses; olives; pickles; condiment sauces; frozen and canned meat and fish entrees and dinners; canned and dried soups; commercial pasta, noodle, and potato dishes; salted snacks; commercial mixes for waffles, muffins, and cakes; canned vegetables with sauces; baking powder; baking soda; certain emulsifiers and other food additives; drinking water; drugs such as some antacids
Potassium	Milk, fruits (especially oranges, prunes, apples, pears, peaches, bananas, and grapefruit), vegetables (especially fresh broccoli, carrots, tomatoes, and potatoes), fish, shellfish, turkey, chicken, and cooked oatmeal

SOURCE: National Academy of Sciences Committee on Diet and Health: *Diet and Health: Recommendations to Reduce Chronic Disease Risk*, National Academy Press, Washington, 1989.

gastrointestinal disease. Elimination of lactose from the diet reduces the diarrhea due to the osmotic action of unabsorbed lactose in the gut lumen (see Chap. 254).

Gluten-free diets Gluten, a protein found primarily in wheat products, produces a toxic reaction causing villous atrophy in patients with sprue or celiac disease. Elimination of gluten from diet requires substitution of gluten-poor foods, e.g., rice or potato (Chap. 254).

Caffeine restriction Caffeine can cause untoward behavioral effects in large doses (e.g., 1000 mg or more, the equivalent of 10 cups of coffee a day, and in some individuals at lower doses). Some patients with reflux esophagitis, hypermotility syndrome, and peptic ulcer disease may also benefit from reducing or eliminating caffeine from the diet.

Questionable dietary remedies Many legitimate therapeutic diets exist in addition to those mentioned in Table 75-2. However, not all popular dietary remedies are documented to be useful. For example, there is no evidence that special diets have any role in alleviating or treating premenstrual syndrome, hyperactivity, fibrocystic disease of the breast, or acne; that a polyunsaturated fat diet is beneficial for multiple sclerosis; or that a macrobiotic diet is useful in patients with cancer.

HOW DIETARY CHANGES ARE ACHIEVED Dietary change is achieved by altering the amount and frequency of food consumption. Nutrients are not equally distributed throughout all foods. Tables 75-6 and 75-7 list food sources rich in selected vitamins and minerals.

Substitutions within food groups can alter diet composition. For example, using skimmed milk instead of whole milk lowers the amount of fat but does not alter its contribution of other nutrients (protein, calcium, and phosphorus). Lean cuts of meat, skinned chicken, and lean fish contain less fat than fried meats but have the same content of protein, vitamins, and minerals.

When many simultaneous reductions must be made in nutrient intakes, development of a reasonable eating plan can be time-consuming and difficult. Computerized menu planning systems or use of simplified exchanges' and menu-planning guides may be helpful in some circumstances. However, for most physicians the best first step is to consult a dietitian.

ORAL NUTRITIONAL SUPPLEMENTS WITH SPECIAL CHARACTERISTICS Diets to meet therapeutic needs may utilize readily available foods, but flexibility is enhanced by the use of specially formulated dietary products (Table 75-8). These products can be of great help in planning menus that are palatable and that permit some

TABLE 75-8 Nutrient composition of oral nutritional supplements

	Manufacturer	kJ/mL	kcal/mL	Protein	Fat	Carbohydrate	Comments
				Percent of energy			
CLEAR LIQUID FORMULAS							
Citrotein	Sandoz Nutrition	2.8	0.66	25	2	73	
Ross SLD (surgical liquid diet)	Ross	2.9	0.70	21	1	78	
FULL LIQUID FORMULAS							
Milk-based formulas							
Carnation Instant Breakfast	Carnation Company	4.4	1.06	21	27	52	
Meritene Liquid	Sandoz Nutrition	4.0	0.96	24	30	46	
Meritene Powder	Sandoz Nutrition	4.4	1.06	26	29	45	
Sustacal Nutritional Powder	Mead Johnson	5.4	1.30	23	23	54	
Sustagen	Mead Johnson	7.7	1.85	24	8	68	
Blenderized formulas							
Compleat Modified Formula	Sandoz Nutrition	4.5	1.07	16	31	53	Lactose-free; gluten-free
Compleat Regular Formula	Sandoz Nutrition	4.5	1.07	16	36	48	
Vitaneed	Sherwood Medical	4.2	1.00	16	35	49	Lactose-free
Formulas with fiber							
Enrich	Ross	4.6	1.10	14	29	57	Lactose-free; 14 g fiber per L
Sustacal with Fiber	Mead Johnson	4.4	1.06	17	29	54	Lactose-free; 5 g fiber per L
Jevity	Ross	4.4	1.06	16	30	54	Isotonic,* lactose-free; 14 g fiber per L
Nutren 1.0 with Fiber	Clinitec Nutrition Co.	4.2	1.0	16	33	51	Lactose free, 14 g fiber per L
Ultracal	Mead Johnson	4.2	1.06	17	37	46	Lactose free, 14 g fiber per L
Fibersource	Sandoz	4.4	1.20	14	30	56	Lactose free, 10 g fiber per L
Fibersource HN	Sandoz	5.0	1.20	18	30	52	Lactose free, 7 g fiber per L
Profiber	Sherwood	4.2	1.0	16	36	48	Lactose free, 12 g fiber per L
Newtrition Isofiber	OBrien/KMI	5.0	1.20	17	30	53	Lactose free, 14 g fiber per L
Lactose-free formulas							
Ensure	Ross	4.4	1.06	14	31	55	Low-residue*
Resource Plus Liquid	Sandoz Nutrition	6.2	1.50	15	32	53	Gluten-free; low-residue
Sustacal Liquid	Mead Johnson	4.2	1.01	24	20	56	Low-residue
Travasorb MCT Diet	Clinitec Nutrition Co.	6.7	1.60	20	30	50	
Resource Instant Crystals	Sandoz Nutrition	4.4	1.06	14	31	55	Low-residue
Resource Liquid	Sandoz Nutrition	4.4	1.06	14	31	55	Gluten-free; low-residue
Comply	Sherwood Medical	6.2	1.50	16	36	48	
Ensure Plus	Ross	6.2	1.50	15	32	53	Low-residue
Sustacal HC	Mead Johnson	6.4	1.52	16	34	50	Low-residue
Ensure Plus HN	Ross	6.2	1.50	17	30	53	Low-residue
Isocal HCN	Mead Johnson	8.4	2.00	15	45	40	
Magnacal	Sherwood Medical	8.4	2.00	14	36	50	Low-residue
Two Cal HN	Ross	8.4	2.00	17	40	43	

(continued)

TABLE 75-8   Nutrient composition of oral nutritional supplements (*continued*)

	Manufacturer	kJ/mL	kcal/mL	Percent of energy Protein	Fat	Carbohydrate	Comments
FULL LIQUID FORMULAS (*continued*)							
Isotonic formulas*							
Attain	Sherwood Medical	4.2	1.00	16	30	54	Lactose-free; low-residue
Osmolite	Ross	4.4	1.06	14	32	54	Lactose-free; low-residue
Precision Isotonic Diet	Sandoz Nutrition	4.0	0.96	12	28	60	Lactose-free; gluten-free
Isocal	Mead Johnson	4.4	1.06	13	37	50	Lactose-free; low-residue; gluten-free
Isosource	Sandoz Nutrition	5.2	1.20	14	30	56	Lactose-free; low-residue
Isotein HN	Sandoz Nutrition	5.0	1.20	23	25	52	Lactose-free; low-residue; gluten-free
Isosource HN	Sandoz Nutrition	5.4	1.20	18	30	52	High-nitrogen; isotonic; lactose-free; gluten-free; low-residue
Nutren 1.0	Clinitec Nutrition Co.	4.2	1.0	16	33	51	
Nutren 1.5	Clinitec Nutrition Co.	6.2	1.5	16	39	45	
Nutren 2.0	Clinitec Nutrition Co.	8.4	2.0	16	45	39	
Replete	Clinitec Nutrition Co.	4.2	1.0	25	30	45	
NEntrition	Clinitec Nutrition Co.	4.2	1.0	14	31	55	
Newtrition	O'Brien/KMI	4.4	1.06	15	32	54	
Osmolite HN	Ross	4.4	1.06	14	31	55	Lactose-free; low-residue
Specialized use formulas							
Amin-Aid Instant Drink	Kendall McGraw	8.2	1.90	4	21	75	Requires vitamin, mineral, and electrolyte supplementation
Attain L.S.	Kendall McGraw	8.2	1.90	16	36	48	Lactose-free; low-residue
Pre-Attain	Sherwood Medical	2.1	0.50	16	36	48	Lactose-free
Hepatic Aid II Instant Drink	Kendall McGraw	4.9	1.18				Requires vitamin, mineral, and electrolyte supplementation
Lonalac	Mead Johnson	4.2	1.00	21	49	30	
Portagen	Mead Johnson	4.2	1.01	14	40	46	Lactose-free
Precision High Nitrogen Diet	Sandoz Nutrition	4.4	1.05	9	1	90	Lactose-free; low-residue; gluten-free
Precision LR Diet	Sandoz Nutrition	4.2	1.10				Lactose-free; low-residue; gluten-free
Pulmocare	Ross	6.3	1.50	17	55	28	Lactose-free
Stresstein	Sandoz Nutrition	5.0	1.20	23	21	56	Lactose-free; no residue
Traum-Aid HBC	Kendall McGraw	4.2	1.00	24	6	70	Lactose-free; low-residue
TraumaCal	Mead Johnson	6.3	1.50	22	40	38	Lactose-free
Travasorb Hepatic	Clinitec Nutrition Co.	4.6	1.10	7	12	77	Low aromatic amino acids
Travasorb Renal	Clinitec Nutrition Co.	5.7	1.35	7	12	81	Requires vitamin, mineral, and electrolyte supplementation
Hydrolyzed protein-elemental formulas*							
Accept HPF	Sherwood Medical	4.2	1.0	16	76	9	Lactose-free
Carnation Peptamen Liquid, Isotonic, Complete, Elemental Diet	Clinitec Nutrition Co.	4.2	1.00	16	33	51	
Criticare HN	Mead Johnson	4.4	1.06	16	33	83	Lactose-free; low resid.
Pepti 2000	Sherwood Medical	4.2	1.00	18	12	70	Lactose-free; low-residue
Reabilan	Clinitec Nutrition Co.	4.2	1.0	13	35	54	
Tolerex	Norwich Eaton	4.2	1.0	15	3	73	
Travasorb HN	Clinitec Nutrition Co.	4.2	1.00	12	12	76	Lactose-free; low-residue
Travasorb STD	Clinitec Nutrition Co.	4.2	1.00	17	10	73	Lactose-free; low-residue
Vital High Nitrogen	Ross	4.2	1.00	17	1	82	Lactose-free; low-residue
Vivonex HN	Norwich Eaton	4.2	1.00	17	1	82	Lactose-free; no residue
Vivonex Standard	Norwich Eaton	4.2	1.00	9	1	90	Lactose-free; no residue
Vivonex T.E.N.	Norwich Eaton	4.2	1.00	15	3	82	Lactose-free; low-residue
HIGH CALORIE SOFT SUPPLEMENTS		kJ/g	kcal/g				
Puddings							
Ensure Pudding	Ross	7.5	1.8	11	35	54	Gluten-free
Sustacal Pudding	Mead Johnson	7.5	1.7	11	36	53	
Forta Pudding	Ross	7.5	1.6	11	35	54	Lactose-free

| TABLE 75-8 Nutrient composition of oral nutritional supplements (*continued*) | | | | | | | |

| | Manufacturer | kJ/mL | kcal/mL | Percent of energy | | | Comments |
				Protein	Fat	Carbohydrate	
MODULAR SYSTEMS (SINGLE NUTRIENT SOURCES)		kJ/g or /mL	kcal/g or /mL				
Protein modules							
Casec	Mead Johnson	15.5	3.7	96	4	<1	Powder
Nutrisource Amino Acids	Sandoz Nutrition	16.3	3.9	100	0	0	Powder
Nutrisource Amino Acids -High BCAA	Sandoz Nutrition	15.9	3.8	100	0	0	Powder
Nutrisource Protein	Sandoz Nutrition	16.7	4.0	75	10	6	Powder
Pro Mod	Ross	17.6	4.2	72	19	9	Powder
Propac	Sherwood Medical	16.7	4.0	77	18	5	Powder
RDP	Corpak, Inc.	15.1	3.6	84	10	6	Powder
Fat modules							
High Fat Supplement	Corpak, Inc.	25.5	6.12	3	70	27	Powder
MCT Oil	Mead Johnson	32.3	7.7	0	100	0	Liquid
Nutrisource Lipid—Long-Chain Triglycerides	Sandoz Nutrition	9.2	2.2	0	100	0	Liquid
Nutrisource Lipid—Medium-Chain Triglycerides	Sandoz Nutrition	8.4	2.0	0	100	0	Liquid
Microlipid	Sherwood Medical	18.8	4.5	0	100	0	Liquid
Carbohydrate modules							
Liquid Carbohydrate Supplement	Corpak, Inc.	10.5	2.5	0	0	100	Liquid
Moducal	Mead Johnson	15.9	3.8	0	0	100	Powder
Nutrisource Carbohydrate	Sandoz Nutrition	13.4	3.2	0	0	100	Liquid
Polycose Powder	Ross	15.9	3.8	0	0	100	Powder
Polycose Liquid	Ross	8.4	2.0	0	0	100	Liquid
Pure Carbohydrate Supplement	Corpak, Inc.	16.7	4.0	0	0	100	Powder
Sumacal	Sherwood Medical	15.9	3.8	0	0	100	Powder
LOW-PROTEIN PRODUCTS		kJ/20 g	kcal/20 g				
WelPlan low-protein pasta	Dietary Specialties Dist.	282	67	.006	2.4	97	Corn and potato starch
Aproten low-protein rusks	Dietary Specialties Dist.	353	84	.01	19	81	Melba toast-like product with wheat, rice, starch
WelPlan low protein brown bread	Dietary Specialties Dist.	180	43	.02	8.5	91	
Prono low protein gelled dessert	Dietary Specialties Dist.	328	78	.001	0	99	
DP low protein chocolate chip cookies	Dietary Specialties Dist.	420	100	.004	45	54	Wheat starch
Low Pro rice starch loaf	Med-Diet	265	63	.003	23	76	Rice starch
Poi Bread	Ener-G	282	67	.04	41	51	Gluten free rice flour and tapioca flour
Alterna Low Protein Milk Substitute	Ross	30.5	7.25	11	38	51	Comes in powder form (values are for prepared version, which compares to 2% milk)
Low protein cookies	Kingsmill	1046	250	<1	41	59	
FIBER SUPPLEMENTS		kJ/20 g	kcal/20 g				
Fiber Med	Purdue Frederick Co.	243	70	11	26	63	
Fiberall	Ciba-Geigy Corp.	331	79	5	46	49	
OTHER SPECIAL FORMULAS		kJ/g	kcal/mL				
Alitraq	Ross	4.2	1.0	21	13	66	Elemental nutrition with glutamine
Fibrael	Ross	29 kJ/9 g serving	5 kcal/9g serving				7 g dietary fiber per serving (9 g); concentrated dietary fiber supplement
Glucerna	Ross	4.2	1.0	17	50	33	Diabetic product
Impact	Sandoz	4.2	1.0	22	25	53	Critical care
Introlite	Ross	2.2	.53	17	30	54	Fortified .5 Calorie liquid nutrition
Lipisorb	Mead Johnson	4.2	1.0	14	40	46	MCT oil and corn oil mixture
Nepro	Ross	8.4	2.0	16	43	43	For dialysis patients
Replena	Ross	8.4	2.0	6	43	51	For predialysis patients

* Definitions: Low-residue = producing little or no stool; isotonic = having the tonicity of plasma (308 mosmol/L); hydrolyzed protein-elemental formula = nutrients partially or completely digested.
SOURCE: Modified from the American Dietetic Association: *Manual of Clinical Dietetics*, 1988.

latitude on the part of the patients. Some of the products are particularly useful for complex diets.

SPECIAL PROBLEMS IN DIET THERAPY

TRANSITIONS FROM ONE ROUTE OF FEEDING TO ANOTHER

Transitional feeding refers to the process of return to the usual feeding pattern after total parenteral nutrition, peripheral hyperalimentation, or enteral feeding by gastrotomy, jejunostomy, esophagostomy, or nasogastric tube. After extended periods of disuse, the gut may not function normally, and unless the transition process is carefully monitored, ad libitum oral intake and/or food absorption may be inadequate.

ADHERENCE TO DIET　Compliance with therapeutic dietary recommendations is relatively easy to monitor in the hospitalized patient. A menu that conforms to the diet orders is offered, and choices and made in line with the therapeutic prescription (and if choices are not appropriate, substitutions are made). However, the patient may refuse or be unable to eat or may miss meals because of diagnostic tests. Therefore, nutritional status and patient adherence should be monitored carefully even in the hospital.

To implement therapeutic diets in outpatients, the patient must be motivated and must understand the diet instructions and the changes in what is to be eaten. New food buying, food preparation, and eating habits may be required. Selections when dining out are also altered. These changes are difficult to make and even more difficult to sustain.

Psychological support; assistance in learning new food preparation, buying, and management skills; help with eating (in disabilities such as stroke); help in obtaining financial assistance to buy special foods; and general education about the importance of diet are as important as nutritional advice.

ASSURING THE CONTINUITY OF NUTRITIONAL CARE: THE TEAM CONCEPT

Nutrition is too important to be the sole responsibility of a single member of the health team. Nutritional counseling can and does change dietary habits, and each health-care provider has a critical role in assuring that nutrition is adequate. However, physicians rarely obtain thorough diet histories, address potential barriers to change in eating habits, or offer special guidance on food selection. The major role of physicians is to expand the content of the nutritional information they provide, to emphasize the health benefits of good nutrition to refer those requiring help to dietitians or other specialized providers.

REFERENCES

AMERICAN DIABETES ASSOCIATION, INC. AND THE AMERICAN DIETETIC ASSOCIATION: *Exchange Lists for Meal Planning,* Revised 1989. Alexandria, Va., American Diabetes Association, 1989

CHICAGO DIETETIC ASSOCIATION AND SOUTH SUBURBAN DIETETIC ASSOCIATION: *Manual of Clinical Dietetics,* 3rd ed. Chicago, The American Dietetic Association, 1992

COMMITTEE ON DIET AND HEALTH: *Diet and Health; Modifications to Reduce Chronic Disease Risk.* Washington, National Academy Press, 1993

Handbook of Clinical Dietetics, 2d ed. Chicago, American Dietetic Association, 1992

JOINT NATIONAL COMMITTEE V: *The Fifth Report of the Joint National Committee on Detection Evaluation and Treatment of High Blood Pressure* (JNCV), National High Blood Pressure Education Program. Bethesda, National Heart, Lung and Blood Institute, National Institutes of Health, 1992

NATIONAL RESEARCH COUNCIL: *Recommended Dietary Allowances,* 10th ed. Washington DC, National Academy of Sciences, 1989

Nutrition Interventions Manual for Professionals Caring for Older Americans. Washington DC, Nutrition Screening Initiative

Nutrition Screening Manual for Professionals Caring for Older Americans. Washington DC, Nutrition Screening Initiative

REPORT OF THE US PREVENTIVE SERVICES TASK FORCE: *Guide to Clinical Preventive Services: An Assessment of the Effectiveness of 169 Interventions.* Philadelphia, Williams & Wilkins, 1989

SHILS ME (ED): *Modern Nutrition in Health and Disease.* Philadelphia, Lea and Febiger, 1993

ZEMAN FJ: *Clinical Nutrition and Dietetics.* New York, Macmillan, 1983

76　PARENTERAL AND ENTERAL NUTRITION THERAPY

LYN HOWARD

Parenteral and enteral nutrition provide life-sustaining therapy for patients who cannot take adequate nutrition by mouth and who consequently are at risk for the debilitating effects of malnutrition. These effects include susceptibility to infection and the consequences of immobility, such as pulmonary embolism, aspiration pneumonia, and pressure sores, all of which delay recovery from illness and result in an increased mortality.

The term *enteral* refers to feeding via the gut and hence includes normal eating, but in the present context it implies the infusion of formulas via a tube inserted into the upper gastrointestinal tract. *Parenteral* refers to the infusion of nutrient solutions into the bloodstream. While these approaches to nutritional support are different, their goals are by and large the same. Where feasible, enteral nutrition is the preferred route because it sustains gastrointestinal function both from a digestive and an absorptive standpoint and as an immunologic barrier. Enteral feeding costs about one-tenth as much as parenteral feeding.

Enteral tube feeding initially involved large-bore rubber tubes placed via the nose or through an ostomy into the stomach or jejunum; these tubes have largely been replaced by small-bore pliable tubes that remain soft with exposure to digestive juices. Feeding tubes can now be placed directly (percutaneously) into the stomach or jejunum by endoscopic or radiologic techniques and seldom require surgical placement except when the gastrostomy is part of a larger operation. These advances have enhanced the acceptance of the technique by patients, and tube feedings are now used in medical conditions where malnutrition is due to impaired oral intake or defective nutrient assimilation as well as for swallowing or esophageal dysfunction.

Parenteral nutrition is more recent. After Gamble demonstrated in the 1940s that glucose (100 g/d) spares protein breakdown in fasting subjects, intravenous glucose infusions became routine therapy for hospitalized patients unable to eat. In the 1960s, Dudrick and colleagues showed that total nutrition (calories, amino acids, minerals, and vitamins) can be delivered on a long-term basis through infusion into a high-flow central vein. Such therapy results in positive nitrogen balance and promotes wound healing in adults and normal growth and development in children. Total parenteral nutrition is now available in all large hospitals and for certain patients at home. The development of high-energy, isotonic intravenous fat solutions also makes it possible to deliver adequate calories and other essential nutrients via a peripheral vein. However, peripheral veins usually cannot sustain nutrient infusions indefinitely, and long-term support requires central venous access.

THE DECISION PROCESS FOR USING PARENTERAL OR ENTERAL NUTRITION

The decision to use specialized nutrition support should be based on the likelihood that averting or redressing malnutrition will improve the quality of life or the ability to recover from a life-threatening condition. At least 15 to 20 percent of hospitalized patients have evidence of malnutrition. Some of these patients will benefit from specialized nutrition support, but for others wasting is an inevitable component of a terminal disease. Distinguishing between these possibilities requires critical clinical judgment: (1) knowledge of the potential benefits and risks of nutritional support, (2) the ability to communicate the benefits and risks to the patient and the family, and (3) awareness of the legal requirements pertinent to this issue. Figure 76-1 is a flow diagram of the steps involved in making this decision.

The first step requires the physician to formulate the nutritional implications of the disease process. Since it is easier to prevent than to treat malnutrition, this first step must be part of the initial workup. Clinicians can categorize a patient as severely, moderately, or

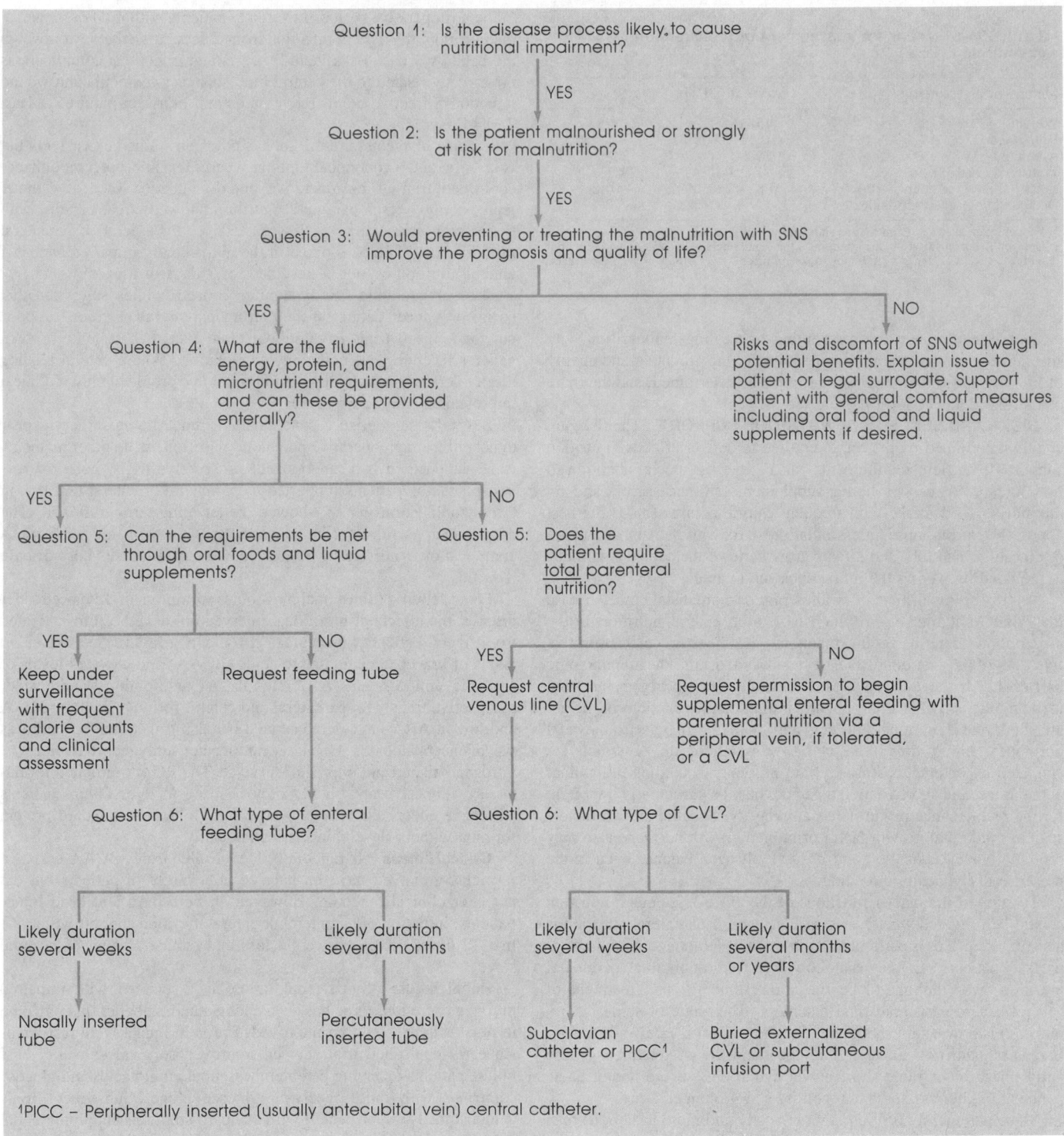

FIGURE 76-1 Should specialized nutrition support (SNS) be undertaken? An algorithm.

minimally malnourished by careful attention to the history and physical examination. The history must encompass recent weight change, the functional status of the patient, and the effects of the primary disease on food intake and assimilation. The physical examination must assess muscle wasting, fat stores, edema, anemia, and other signs of nutrient deficiencies (see Chap. 72). Table 76-1 summarizes some of the criteria for documenting protein-energy malnutrition. Except for delayed hypersensitivity testing, these criteria rely mainly on changes in body composition. In the future, more emphasis may be placed on functional tests of nutritional status, such as muscle strength, pulmonary reserve, and wound healing. Once it is recognized that the patient is at risk for or has developed

malnutrition, the question of whether artificially supplied nutrition is appropriate involves ethical and risk-versus-benefit considerations.

While the provision of food and water is a basic element of medical care, nutrition support delivered by enteral or parenteral means is associated with discomfort and should only be recommended if the benefits exceed the risks and only after obtaining the consent of the patient or the legal surrogate. In many situations the dividing line between comfort and medical therapy is not clear, especially in the incompetent patient. Physicians should advise all patients to address this issue by preparing advance directions such as a "living will" and designating a health care proxy. Without such preplanning, nutritional support may distressingly protract a terminal illness.

TABLE 76-1   Means for assessment of protein-energy malnutrition (PEM)

Method of assessment	Moderate PEM	Severe PEM
Weight loss, %	15–25	>25
Fat depletion*	<16 ± 6	<12 ± 5
Albumin, g/L	25–30	<25
Transferrin, g/L	1–2.0	<1
Total lymphocyte count, 10^6/L	0.8–1.2	<0.8
Delayed hypersensitivity index†	1	0

* Fat depletion assessed from triceps skin fold in millimeters.
† Delayed hypersensitivity index quantitates the centimeters of induration with common antigens such as *Candida*, trichophytin, or mumps: 0 = <0.5, 1 = 0.5, 2 = 1.0.

If it is determined that preventing or treating malnutrition with specialized nutrition support would improve the prognosis and quality of life, the nutritional requirements must be determined, and the route of nutrient delivery must be selected.

RISKS AND BENEFITS OF NUTRITION SUPPORT   The risks are chiefly determined by the route required to deliver effective nutrition support. If nutrient requirements can be met by special attention to oral intake, by use of liquid supplements (if necessary), and by monitoring food intake with frequent calorie counts, this is the best approach. Normal nutrient assimilation starts with the cephalic phase of digestion, and tube-fed infants grow better if the cephalic stimulus is provided by having the infant suck on a pacifier.

Anorexia, impairment of swallowing, or more distal bowel disease may limit oral intake, in which case tube enteral nutrition is the next option. Enteral feeding maintains the digestive and absorptive functions of the gastrointestinal tract and also sustains the immunologic barrier which the gut provides, preventing enteric organisms from invading the body. The nutrient and immunologic functions of the gut are supported by luminal nutrients and by the normal gastrointestinal hormones, blood flow, and neural stimulation, all of which are activated by enteral feeding. Certain nutrients, including glutamine, nucleotides, and short-chain fatty acids, may be particularly important for the maintenance of gut mucosal integrity. Specific growth factors such as epidermal growth factor or human growth hormone also may promote bowel adaptation and positive nitrogen balance even in the presence of hypocaloric feeding.

To support the barrier functions of the gut, some enteral nutrition should be provided whenever possible, even if parenteral nutrition is also required. This is particularly important in debilitated, immunosuppressed patients. In the past, bowel rest, through total parenteral nutrition, was thought to be the cornerstone for the treatment of several severe gastrointestinal disorders. The value of some enteral nutrition is now established, and strict bowel rest is rarely advocated. Parenteral nutrition alone is still the mainstay of treatment in the early phase of extreme short bowel syndrome, severe hemorrhagic pancreatitis, necrotizing enterocolitis, and prolonged ileus.

Since parenteral nutrition is more costly and more hazardous than enteral nutrition, most risk-versus-benefit studies to date have focused on parenteral nutrition. Increasingly, the end points required of such studies involve evidence that the therapy improves outcome, such as decreased mortality rates, a reduced incidence of major complications, or shorter duration of hospital stay. End points such as better nitrogen balance, increased levels of serum albumin, and improved delayed hypersensitivity are no longer acceptable.

Perioperative nutrition   While there is a clear-cut association between preoperative malnutrition and poor surgical outcome, it has been difficult to demonstrate a beneficial impact of preoperative parenteral nutrition on the outcome of surgery in malnourished patients. However, a meta-analysis of 18 small studies and a large cooperative Veterans Administration study suggests that preoperative parenteral nutrition does provide a net benefit for severely malnourished surgical patients. In treated patients, noninfectious complications (e.g., pulmonary emboli and delayed wound healing) were reduced

in the postoperative period. In surgical patients with mild or moderate malnutrition, the risks of infection from preoperative therapy outweigh the benefits. These risks include sepsis and infectious complications not directly related to the central line, such as pneumonia and wound infection. Effective preoperative parenteral nutrition requires at least 7 to 14 days.

Preoperative enteral nutrition has not been studied extensively but is a safe and economical option where feasible. A randomized, controlled trial of postoperative enteral nutrition (needle catheter jejunostomy) versus parenteral nutrition showed equal benefit, with the enteral approach being less expensive. Postoperative parenteral nutrition should be considered in the nutritionally impaired patient if enteral nutrition cannot be resumed for 7 days or longer.

Cancer cachexia   Early nonrandomized studies suggested that cachectic cancer patients benefit from parenteral nutrition support, but randomized trials have shown more risk than benefit for such patients receiving chemotherapy or radiation. Where enteral feeding is not tolerated, parenteral nutrition should be provided only if clinical improvement can be expected.

Severely malnourished cancer patients undergoing surgery appear to benefit from preoperative parenteral nutrition, as do other malnourished patients. In two randomized, prospective trials, bone marrow transplantation patients supported by parenteral or enteral nutrition in the cytoreduction phase showed better long-term survival. The nutrition support did not influence the frequency of initial infectious complications, nor was graft rejection or graft-versus-host disease reduced.

Liver failure   Since malnutrition is common in advanced liver disease, the effects of nutritional intervention have been investigated extensively. Patients with acute or chronic liver failure have decreased levels of branched chain amino acids (BCAA) and elevated levels of aromatic amino acids (AAA) in plasma and brain. Randomized, prospective trials with parenteral and enteral formulas high in BCAA and low in AAA have demonstrated better nitrogen balance and less risk of encephalopathy. One large multicenter study reported improved nitrogen balance and improved survival. The BCAA-enriched formulas are expensive and should only be used in liver failure patients who have encephalopathy or who cannot tolerate a standard protein formula without developing encephalopathy.

Critical illness   In randomized, controlled trials, BCAA-enriched formulas improved nitrogen balance in severely ill patients but did not alter clinical outcome. However, in both burn and head injury patients, initiation of parenteral or enteral nutrition support within the first 12 hours decreased weight loss and reduced length of hospital stay.

Renal failure   Since renal failure is associated with impaired nitrogen excretion, there has been a long-standing belief that outcome in renal failure would be improved if protein intake were restricted. An early controlled trial showed improved survival of acute renal failure patients receiving parenteral essential amino acids and glucose compared with those receiving glucose alone. Subsequent trials demonstrated similar benefit with standard solutions supplying equal amounts of essential and nonessential amino acids; thus the superiority of costly formulas rich in essential amino acids or their keto analogues is not established.

Pancreatitis   Parenteral nutrition does not improve the medical outcome of patients with mild or moderate pancreatitis. However, severe pancreatitis is associated with impaired nutrition, and survival decreases as malnutrition increases. These observations provide indirect evidence for the use of parenteral nutrition in severe pancreatitis. In the absence of severe hyperlipidemia or thrombocytopenia complicating pancreatitis, intravenous lipids are safe and are especially useful if glucose intolerance is present.

Inflammatory bowel disease (IBD)   Evidence of nutritional deficiencies such as weight loss, growth failure, anemia, and hypoalbuminia are common in IBD, more so in Crohn's disease than in ulcerative colitis (see Chap. 255). Nutrition support plays a role in redressing these nutritional deficiencies, particularly prior to elective surgery. Since IBD often improves with diversion of the fecal stream, the question has been raised as to whether bowel rest and parenteral nutrition might have a role as primary treatment. However, randomized, prospective studies have shown no special benefit from bowel rest. Elemental diets can be used in place of glucocorticoids for inducing remission in acute Crohn's disease, but relapse is common when a normal diet is resumed.

Because of the possibility that specific dietary fats may have a beneficial effect in several immune disorders, probably by altering prostaglandin pathways, diets high in omega 3 fatty acids are under investigation in IBD. While some studies suggest a benefit to IBD patients from high-fiber diets, this may cause problems in patients with strictures. In controlled studies, remissions may be longer in Crohn's disease if wheat and dairy products are eliminated.

Short bowel syndrome Before the advent of parenteral nutrition, patients with severe short bowel syndrome, as from mesenteric vascular infarction or surgical resection, seldom survived. Parenteral nutrition has allowed many patients with only a foot or two of small intestine to survive indefinitely. In some the short bowel eventually adapts so that only parenteral fluid and electrolyte support is required or they can graduate to enteral nutrition alone.

Acquired immunodeficiency syndrome Parenteral nutrition is frequently used in AIDS patients with severe gastrointestinal disease, weight loss, and intolerance for enteral feeding. There have been anecdotal reports of temporary clinical benefit, but there have been no randomized, controlled studies of parenteral support in these patients.

Pulmonary disease Weight loss in patients with advanced pulmonary disease is due to increased work of breathing and poor food intake. In cystic fibrosis, malnutrition may hasten pulmonary deterioration, and enteral feeding via gastrostomy tubes enhances growth and stabilizes or improves pulmonary function, particularly in young children. The criteria for selection of patients and the psychological costs of such treatment have not been defined. The use of a low-carbohydrate formula is beneficial in the weaning of patients from ventilators, but the superiority of such formulas in ambulatory patients with chronic lung disease is not established.

Pregnancy Severe hyperemesis gravidarum can make any oral or tube enteral nutrition impossible, and profound weight loss and ketosis may be harmful to the fetus. Hyperemesis is relieved by abortion or delivery, but the underlying mechanism is not understood. There are numerous reports of successful outcome of pregnancy following temporary support of the pregnant woman by parenteral nutrition, but nausea and vomiting tend to persist despite bowel rest.

THE DESIGN OF INDIVIDUAL REGIMENS Fluid requirements These can be estimated by adding the normal daily requirement (120 mL/kg of body weight for infants, 35 mL/kg of body weight for adults) to any abnormal loss. If the patient is on parenteral therapy, any enteral intake should be subtracted from the abnormal loss. For examples, see Table 76-2. Since abnormal loss of enteric fluid implies significant mineral losses, extra amounts of these nutrients (Table 76-3) also must be added to any standard parenteral or enteral formula.

Energy requirements These can be estimated as outlined in Chap. 71. Measurements of energy expenditure in ill patients have shown that the Harris-Benedict formula tends to overestimate expenditures. Direct measurements, using a bedside metabolic cart and calculation of energy requirements from gas exchange, are also difficult to interpret, since energy expenditure fluctuates throughout the day and calorimetry assessments are confounded by starvation or any ongoing nutritional support. A reasonable approach is to provide 100 kJ/kg (25 kcal/kg) per day for an unstressed patient and 125, 145, and 165 kJ/kg (30, 35, and 40 kcal/kg) per day, respectively, for mildly, moderately, and severely stressed patients.

The most desirable balance of carbohydrate to fat in parenteral and enteral solutions is unsettled. Wound healing, white blood cells, the brain, and the renal cortex depend on glucose metabolism. The majority of energy is usually supplied as glucose in parenteral solutions and as oligosaccharides and disaccharides in enteral solu-

tions. Parenteral lipid solutions are available as 10% or 20% emulsions of vegetable oils (soybean or safflower oils emulsified into artificial lipoproteins with egg phospholipid and made isotonic with glycerin). Parenteral lipids can be infused separately or as a "three in one" nutrient solution with amino acids and glucose. "Three in one" solutions are well tolerated and can obviate the need for an extra infusion pump for the separate solution. However, such solutions are not as stable as the more traditional glucose and amino acid mix, and destabilized fat particles have the potential of coalescing into larger droplets and becoming fat emboli. To be safe "three in one" solutions must be mixed by a pharmacist knowledgeable about the necessary mixing sequence of the separate ingredients and the amounts of divalent cations and trace elements that can be added. Patients who require parenteral iron or generous amounts of zinc must alternate between "three in one" and non-lipid-containing parenteral solutions.

Polyunsaturated vegetable oils are used in most enteral formulas because they are better absorbed by the compromised gastrointestinal tract. The fat in parenteral and enteral formulas must supply the

---

TABLE 76-2 Estimation of daily fluid requirements

NORMAL 70-KG MAN

Intake	Output
Normal requirement: 35 × 70 = ~2500 mL/d (derived from oral liquids of 1200 mL, or 5 glasses/cups per day, and solid food providing 1300 mL, 1000 mL from water in food, 300 mL from water generated by metabolism of foods)	Urine: 1600 mL/d Insensible loss: 800 mL/d Stool: 100 mL/d [sweat loss can be up to 2 L/d. Each degree of fever (C) = 200 mL/d]

TUBE ENTERAL PATIENT

A 58-kg woman recovering from total gastrectomy for gastric cancer and supported by jejunostomy feedings, taking nothing by mouth or intravenously, but experiencing 600 mL of diarrheal losses per day:
Normal requirement 35 × 58 = ~2000 mL/d
Abnormal loss (600 − 100) = 500 mL/d
Total requirement = 2500 mL/d

PARENTERAL PATIENT

A 66-kg man with a high jejunostomy following massive bowel resection for Crohn's disease with oral intake of 2000 mL/d and jejunostomy loss of 4000 mL/d:
Normal requirement 35 × 66 = 2300 mL/d
Abnormal loss (4000 − 100) minus oral intake (2000) = 1900 mL/d
Total requirement = 4200 mL/d

TABLE 76-3 Enteric fluid volumes and their sodium, potassium, chloride, and bicarbonate content*

	L/d†	Na mmol/L	K‡ mmol/L	Cl mmol/L	HCO₃§ mmol/L
Oral intake	2–3				
Enteric secretions					
Saliva	1–2	10	30	10	30
Gastric juice	2	60	9	90	0
Bile	2–3	150	10	90	70
Small bowel	1	100	5	100	20
Colon	Variable	40	100	15	60

* Enteric secretions are also rich in divalent cations (Ca, Mg, Zn, Cu), and their loss is increased by steatorrhea, a high bowel fistula, or prolonged suction.
† Of the 9 L/d of oral and enteric fluid presented to the upper small bowel, normally 50 percent is absorbed in the jejunum, 40 percent in the ileum, and 10 percent in the colon. In short bowel patients, the colon can absorb greater amounts, up to 3 L/d.
‡ Potassium losses are small except in secretions distal to the ileocecal valve. The colon ion exchange is partly controlled by aldosterone, and therefore, Na⁺ depletion increases K⁺ loss in the stool.
§ Bicarbonate losses must be replaced in parenteral solutions as acetate ingredients such as calcium by bicarbonate.

essential fatty acid requirement (1 to 2 percent of energy from linoleic and linolenic acid). The provision of 30 percent of energy as fat may reduce the problems that arise from providing excess carbohydrate calories (e.g., hepatic steatosis). Substitution of ordinary polyunsaturated vegetable fats by omega 3 polyunsaturated fish oils may reduce the inflammatory response to burn injury, trauma, and radiation by reducing the synthesis of prostaglandins that enhance gut mucosal permeability to enteric toxins.

Protein or amino acid requirements The recommended dietary protein allowance of 0.8 g/kg per day is adequate for nonstressed patients (e.g., a patient with a high-grade esophageal stricture or anorexia nervosa). Catabolic patients may require up to 1.5 g/kg per day of protein to induce positive nitrogen balance and reconstitute normal body mass. In a stable patient the adequacy of protein and energy support can be assessed by a balance study:

$$\text{Protein balance} = \text{protein intake} - \text{protein loss}$$

where protein loss = [24-h urine urea nitrogen (g) + 4] × 6.25, and by documenting wound healing, restoration of normal body composition, or resumption of longitudinal growth.

In states of disturbed protein utilization (e.g., renal and hepatic failure), azotemia and abnormal plasma amino acid patterns develop. The benefit of special enteral and parenteral solutions that correct these aberrations is not established.

Certain amino acids and peptides that are not essential nutrients (because they can be synthesized endogenously) may become essential in severely ill patients when endogenous production or salvage pathways are impaired. This is true of glutamine, arginine, and the products of methionine metabolism. Glutamine is an important fuel, particularly for the enterocyte. The oxidation of one molecule of glutamine produces 30 mmol ATP, which makes this amino acid almost as rich an energy source as glucose. The free amino acid pool of the enterocyte is glutamine-rich. Glutamine is fairly insoluble and is absent from many parenteral formulas and present only in low concentrations in most enteral formulas. Soluble glutamine-containing dipeptides are under investigation.

Parenteral amino acids are infused systemically rather than via the more physiologic portal route. Under these circumstances, methionine,

the only sulfur-containing amino acid in parenteral solutions, tends to be transaminated rather than transulfurated. As a result, downstream products such as carnitine, taurine, and glutathione become relatively deficient. Preliminary studies suggest the addition of *S*-adenosyl methionine to parenteral solutions results in less cholestasis.

Mineral and vitamin requirements (See Table 76-4) Parenteral requirements of some minerals and vitamins may be higher than the enteral requirements for several reasons: First, the micronutrients are delivered into the systemic rather than the portal circulation, thereby potentially bypassing the liver and being rapidly excreted into the urine. Second, many patients who require parenteral support have enteric losses that can result in sodium, potassium, chloride, and bicarbonate wasting (see Table 76-3) and in loss of divalent cations and vitamins that normally have an enterohepatic circulation, including folate, cobalamin, vitamin D, and other fat-soluble vitamins. The tubing and delivery bags and exposure to oxygen and light also can destroy vitamins (particularly vitamin A).

PARENTERAL NUTRITION Infusion technique and patient monitoring Partial and short-term parenteral nutrition can be provided via a peripheral vein if the majority of the energy intake is supplied by isotonic fat solutions, but long-term total parenteral support should be administered via a central vein catheter because the solutions contain hypertonic glucose that must be rapidly diluted in a high-flow system. The preferred sites for central vein access and the catheter choices available are summarized in Table 76-5, and typical nutrient content of a standard daily parenteral formula is given

---

TABLE 76-4 Daily enteral (EN) and parenteral (PN) requirements of essential fatty acids, minerals, and vitamins

Nutrient	Daily requirement, adult range	
	EN	PN
Essential fatty acids, % kcal	1–2	2–4
Calcium, g	0.8–1.2	0.4
Phosphorus, g	0.8–1.2	0.8
Potassium, g	2–5	3–4
Sodium, g	1–3	1–2
Chloride, g	2–5	2
Magnesium, g	0.3	0.3
Iron, mg	10	1–2
Zinc, mg	15	3–12
Copper, mg	2–3	0.3–0.5
Iodine, mg	0.15	0.15
Manganese, mg	2–5	2–5
Chromium, mg	0.05–0.2	0.015
Molybdenum, mg	0.15–0.3	0.01–0.5
Selenium, mg	0.05–0.02	0.05–0.1
Ascorbic acid, mg	60	100
Thiamine, mg	1.4	3.0
Riboflavin, mg	1–6	3.6
Niacin, mg	18	40
Biotin, μg	60	60
Pantothenic acid, mg	5	15
Pyridoxine, mg	2.0	4.0
Folic acid, μg	400	400
Cobalamin, μg	3.0	5
Vitamin A, μg	1000	1300
Vitamin D, μg	10	5
Vitamin E, mg	8–10	10–15
Vitamin K, μg	70–140	200

TABLE 76-5 Central vein parenteral nutrition catheters

SITES OF VENOUS ACCESS

A Distal tip of catheter best placed in midportion of superior vena cava
B Enters venous system via
　1 Percutaneous stick into the subclavian, external or internal jugular, or antecubital vein
　2 Cutdown site on external jugular (via common facial vein), femoral, axillary, or intercostal vein
C All catheters can be tunneled subcutaneously to a distal site, which
　1 May provide a barrier to skin organisms infecting the line
　2 Places exit site at convenient place for self-care in patients at home

TYPES OF CATHETERS

A Externalized
　1 Single, double, or triple lumen
　　a Second and third channels used for IV medications or drawing of blood
　　b Higher incidence of infectious complications with multiple-lumen catheters
　2 In home patients, avoids the need for a nightly needle stick but requires constant aseptic dressing
　3 Repair kits available if a leak or tear develops in the externalized portion
B Subcutaneous port
　1 Involves a small reservoir with an overlying rubber diaphragm that is self-sealing
　2 Port must be entered by a J-shaped needle
　3 Not all patients like the daily needle stick
　4 If line is not in use, the buried port makes taking showers and swimming less hazardous

CATHETER MATERIAL

A Polyvinylchloride, polyethylene, polyurethane, or polytetrafluoroethylene
　1 Advantage:
　　a Inherent stiffness may allow easy threading into the vein
　2 Disadvantages:
　　a Stiffness allows catheter to be in direct contact with vessel wall, causing phlebitis and thrombosis
　　b Stiffness increases with time, causing kinks or fractures
B Silicone rubber
　1 Advantages:
　　a Very pliable, less kinking
　　b Less traumatic to vessel wall
　　c Inert, inducing little reaction or adherence
　2 Disadvantages:
　　a Difficult to thread into vein
　　b Falls out more easily owing to nonadherence
　　c Potential for tearing

TABLE 76-6   Standard total parenteral nutrition solution (24 h) for a 70-kg adult

Fluid	3 L
Protein (amino acids)	0.2–0.3 g nitrogen/kg
Energy value*	100–165 kJ/kg (25–40 kcal/kg)
Essential fatty acids (lipids)	2% of total calories
Electrolytes	
Sodium	100 mmol
Potassium†	100 mmol
Chloride	130 mmol
Acetate/gluconate	90 mmol
Calcium	7.5 mmol
Magnesium	10 mmol
Phosphorous†	600 mg
Trace elements	
Zinc	5 mg
Copper	1.5 mg
Iodine	120 μg
Selenium	100 μg
Chromium	15 μg
Maganese	2 mg
Vitamins	
Ascorbic acid	100 mg
Thiamine	3 mg
Riboflavin	3.6 mg
Niacin	40 mg
Panthothenic acid	15 mg
Pyridoxine	4 mg
Biotin	60 μg
Folic acid	400 μg
Cobalamin	5 μg
Vitamin A	1300 μg
Vitamin D	10 μg
Vitamin E	15 mg
Vitamin K	200 μg

* Provided principally as dextrose.
† More potassium and phosphorus may be needed in the repletion phase after severe cachexia. Chronic starvation results in total-body potassium and phosphorus depletion.

in Table 76-6. The glucose content is increased gradually as the patient demonstrates tolerance of the high glucose load. Appropriate clinical and laboratory monitoring for patients on parenteral nutrition is summarized in Table 76-7.

Complications (See Table 76-8)   MECHANICAL   The insertion of a central venous catheter should only be done by trained personnel

TABLE 76-7   Monitoring the patient on total parenteral nutrition

CLINICAL DATA MONITORED DAILY

Sense of well-being: symptoms suggesting fluid overload, high or low blood glucose, electrolyte imbalance, etc.

Strength as judged by graded activity: getting out of bed, walking, stair climbing.

Vital signs: temperature, blood pressure, pulse rate and respiratory rate.

Fluid balance: weight; fluid input (intravenous +/− enteral) versus fluid output (urine, stool, gastric suction, etc.).

Delivery equipment for parenteral nutrition: composition of nutrient solution, tubing, pump, filter, catheter, dressing (skin checked for local infection at time of dressing change).

LABORATORY DATA

Plasma glucose	Four times daily until patient stable
Blood glucose Na^+, K^+, Cl^-, HCO_3^- Blood urea nitrogen	Daily until glucose infusion load and patient stable, then twice weekly
Serum albumin, transferrin (or TIBC) Liver function studies Serum creatinine Ca^{2+}, PO_4^{2-}, Mg^{2+} Hb/Hct, WBC	Baseline, then twice weekly
Prothrombin time, partial thromboplastin time Micronutrient tests as indicated	Baseline, then weekly

TABLE 76-8   Complications of total parenteral nutrition (TPN)

First 48 h	First 2 weeks	3 months onward
MECHANICAL		

Complications from catheter insertion:
  Cephalad displacement
  Pneumothorax
  Hemothorax
Detachment of line at catheter hub with blood loss or air embolism
	Catheter coming out of vein, more common if Silastic
	Detachment of line at catheter hub with blood loss or air embolism
		Detachment of line at catheter hub with blood loss or air embolism
		Fractures or tears in catheter

METABOLIC		
Fluid overload Hyperglycemia Hypophosphatemia Hypokalemia	Cardiopulmonary failure Hyperosmolar nonketotic hyperglycemic coma Acid-base imbalance Electrolyte imbalance	Essentially fatty acid deficiency Zinc, copper, chromium, selenium, molybdenum, deficiency Iron deficiency Vitamin deficiencies Refeeding edema TPN metabolic bone disease TPN liver disease
INFECTIOUS		
	Catheter-induced sepsis	Catheter-induced sepsis Tunnel infections

under stringent aseptic techniques. Major mechanical complications include pneumothorax, hemothorax from laceration of the subclavian artery or vein, brachial plexus injury, and malpositioning of the catheter in a cerebral vein, the azygos vein, or the right ventricle. The correct catheter position must be confirmed by x-ray before hypertonic nutrient solution is infused. Catheters can subsequently back out of the vein, develop leaks, or become detached from the hub and embolize into the heart or pulmonary artery. Catheter thrombosis may occur, especially if the catheter is used for withdrawing blood samples. Thrombosis of the catheter with involvement of the central vein is frequently coincident with infection. Thrombosed catheters can sometimes be unblocked by urokinase treatment. The addition of low-dose heparin (1000 units per liter) to limit thrombosis in parenteral catheters is controversial; no randomized, controlled studies demonstrate benefit, and heparin can contribute to loss of bone mineral, which is a particular problem in long-term parenteral nutrition.

METABOLIC   Fluid overload produces congestive heart failure especially in elderly and debilitated patients. Glucose overload can lead to osmotic diuresis and, via the stimulation of insulin, result in massive extracellular to intracellular shifts of phosphorous and potassium. Such shifts are most likely in cachectic patients with total-body phosphorus and potassium depletion; the reduction in plasma potassium and phosphorus levels can result in arrhythmias, cardiopulmonary dysfunction, and neurologic symptoms. To avoid these problems, parenteral nutrition should be started slowly and monitored carefully.

Late metabolic complications include cholestatic liver disease with bile sludging and gallstone formation. The exact cause of the liver disease is not understood, but defective sulfur amino acid metabolism may play a role. Cholestasis appears to be associated with the lack of enteral stimulation and is less likely to occur if some enteral feeding is maintained. Parenteral nutrition induces hypercalcuria, which can result in negative calcium balance and osteopenia. The hypercalcuria appears to be due to several factors, including effects of infused amino acid and the high fixed acid load of the bisulfite preservative. With earlier protein hydrolysate solutions aluminum contamination occurred which blocked bone mineralization; aluminum may still be a contaminant of some parenteral solution additives. Once patients on long-term parenteral nutrition move from catabolic breakdown to sustained anabolism, deficiencies of micronutrients such as essential fatty acids, trace minerals, and vitamins may develop unless they are provided in the parenteral nutrient solution (see Table 76-4).

INFECTIOUS   Infection of the access line rarely occurs in the first 72 h, and early fever is usually due to infection elsewhere or some other cause. Infection of the access line is likely if the patient defervesces when the infusion rate of the parenteral formula is tapered. Positive central line cultures suggest catheter sepsis, especially if no other infectious source is identified and if the organism is *Staphylococcus* or *Candida*. While removal of the central catheter may allow the patient to clear fungemia spontaneously, antibiotic therapy is usually necessary for bacterial infections. Catheter sepsis is less likely if central vein parenteral nutrition is provided via a single-lumen catheter; triple-lumen catheters, even if frequently replaced over a guidewire, are associated with a greater incidence of sepsis. Recurrent catheter sepsis may be avoided if small amounts of an antibiotic solution are left in the line along with a heparin lock.

ENTERAL NUTRITION   Tube placement and patient monitoring
The types, techniques of insertion, uses, and potential problems of enteral tubes are outlined in Table 76-9. Some of the available enteral formulas and their nutrient compositions are listed in Table 75-8 and in a more generic form in Table 76-10. Patients on enteral feeding are at risk for some of the same metabolic complications as parenterally fed patients and should receive the same clinical and laboratory monitoring (Table 76-10). Since small-bore tubes are easily displaced, tube position should be tested by aspirating and measuring the pH of the gut fluid (<4 in stomach, >6 in jejunum).

Complications   ASPIRATION   The debilitated patient with poor gastric emptying and an impaired swallow and cough mechanism is at risk for aspiration. In patients on respirators, effective tracheal suctioning induces coughing and provokes gastric regurgitation, and the cuff on the endotracheal tube or tracheostomy seldom provides adequate protection against aspiration. Under these circumstances, it may be safer to use a large-bore rubber feeding tube to allow for an accurate check of residual gastric contents and, if necessary, removal of gastric contents prior to tracheal suction.

Although normal gastric motility provides a churning and fragmenting activity with intermittent propulsion of liquid and small food fragments into the duodenum, constant gastric infusion of an enteral formula is better tolerated in sick patients than is intermittent bolus feeding. A continuous infusion is best achieved with an enteral feeding pump, especially with fine-bore feeding tubes that have a greater potential to clog. If long-term gastric feeding is anticipated, endoscopic, radiologic, or surgical placement of a gastric tube is

---

TABLE 76-9   Enteral feeding tubes

Placement technique	Clinical uses	Potential problems	Placement technique	Clinical uses	Potential problems
NASOGASTRIC TUBE			**GASTROSTOMY TUBE**		
External measurement: nostril, ear to xiphisternum; placed by professional or, with instruction, by family member or patient; tube stiffened by ice water or a stylet; position tested by injecting air and auscultating air bubble passing through fluid, by aspirating acid gastric contents, or by checking an x-ray.	Short-term clinical situations (a few weeks); placement can be intermittent; normal gastric emptying required; bolus feeds or continuous drip.	Aspiration pneumonia from regurgitated stomach contents; irritation of nasopharynx or esophagogastric junction with bleeding and/or stricture.	Tube placed through the abdominal wall into the stomach, either by a percutaneous radiologic or endoscopic technique using local anesthetic or surgically via an abdominal incision using a spinal or general anesthetic; can be converted to gastric "button" for long-term ambulatory patients.	Long-term access; once tract is established, tubes can be replaced; used when swallowing is impaired because of either mechanical obstruction or neurologic discoordination.	Irritation around tube site; aspiration of stomach contents; displacement of tube into peritoneal cavity or, if held in situ by balloon, migration and obstruction of the pylorus.
NASODUODENAL OR NASOJEJUNAL TUBE			**JEJUNOSTOMY TUBE**		
External measurement: nostril, ear to anterosuperior iliac spine in adults; to the medial malleolus in infants; weighted tube may pass spontaneously through pylorus if patient lies on right side; or tube is placed in jejunum with stiffening stylet under fluoroscopy; position tested by aspirating alkaline duodenal contents or by checking an x-ray.	Short-term clinical situations; used if gastric emptying is impaired or to infuse beyond a high bowel fistula such as an esophageal tear or gastric or duodenal fistula.	Passing tube through pylorus; preventing the spontaneous pulling back into stomach; continuous drip required and tends to cause diarrhea; tubes stiffen with time; can lacerate pylorus or gastroesophageal junction if pulled out rapidly.	Tube placed radiologically or surgically through abdominal wall into proximal loop of jejunum and tethered to anterior wall by suture; fine-bore tube inserted by diagonal tract into bowel lumen or large bore secured with an anchoring suture.	Long-term access; used for defective gastric emptying; fine-bore tube recommended as postoperative backup when prolonged gastric atony might occur.	Irritation at tube exit site, especially with large-bore tube; clogging or displacement of tube; continuous drip usually required; diarrhea
PHARYNGOSTOMY/ESOPHAGOSTOMY TUBE			**COMBINED GASTROJEJUNOSTOMY TUBE**		
Tube placed surgically through side of neck into pharynx.	Long-term access; no nasopharyngeal irritation; once tract is established, tubes can be replaced.	Aspiration; pharyngeal scarring causes distortion of normal anatomy.	Tube placed intragastrically with jejunal arm threaded beyond the pylorus.	Allows for simultaneous gastric suction and jejunal infusion; used in patient particularly at risk for aspiration of gastric contents.	Not yet widely available.

TABLE 76-10 Types of enteral feeding formulas

Description	Clinical indications	Delivery method	Comments on cost, amount needed to meet RDAs*
BLENDERIZED FORMULA			
Mixture of pureed meat, fruit, vegetables, sometimes added nonfat milk, fiber, vitamins, and minerals; highly viscous.	Normal digestion and absorption required; can be fed into esophagus, stomach, duodenum, or jejunum.	By sipping or via a large-bore tube (12–18 French); bolus or drip with pump.	Lowest cost; 2 L or more daily†
POLYMERIC FORMULA			
Mixture of whole proteins, polysaccharides, and triglycerides; seldom contain fiber; lower viscosity than blenderized formulas.	Normal digestion and absorption required; can be fed into esophagus, stomach, duodenum, or jejunum.	By sipping or via a small-bore tube (8–12 french); bolus or drip with pump.	2 L or more needed daily.
MONOMERIC FORMULA			
Mixture of predigested protein, carbohydrate (CHO), and a small amount of trigylceride; enough to provide essential fatty acids; contains no fiber; lowest viscosity of all formulas.	Used for inflammatory bowel disease, chronic pancreatitis, GI fistula, enteritis from radiation or chemotherapy, pan-malabsorption, or as a transition feeding from parenteral to enteral therapy.	Small-bore tube (5–8 French) drip with pump	Higher cost than polymeric formulas; 1.5–3 L needed daily.
DISEASE-RELATED FORMULA			
Devised to meet the nutritional needs of specific disease states; varying amounts of protein, amino acid ratios, CHO, electrolytes, and caloric density; low viscosity.	Used for fluid restricted, heart failure, renal failure, hepatic encephalopathy, high protein requirement, trauma, burn.	Small-bore tube (5–8 French) drip with pump	Highest cost; 1–2 L needed daily.
MODULAR FORMULA			
Made-to-order feedings of individual constituents; viscosity depends on quantities of protein, CHO, and fat.	Used for specific metabolic abnormalities, such as glycogen storage disease.	Varies, depending on viscosity.	Higher cost than monomeric formula; 1.5 L or more needed daily.

* RDA = recommended daily allowance of nutrient.
† Commercially made blenderized formulas are now available which can be delivered through small-bore tubes (8 French); relatively expensive.

preferred by most patients. For long-term ambulatory patients, a gastrostomy tube can be converted to a gastric "button," an access device that is flush with the skin.

A nasojejunal tube reduces the risk of aspirations. However, placement of such tubes through the pylorus is time-consuming, and such tubes frequently pull back into the stomach. Radiologic placement of a percutaneous gastric-jejunal tube is more reliable. If a debilitated patient with poor gastric emptying goes to surgery, it is appropriate to ask the surgeon to place a jejunostomy tube for feeding. This can involve a traditional (10 to 14 French) or a fine-bore (5 to 8 French) tube inserted through an oblique needle track that seals rapidly when the jejunostomy tube is removed.

DIARRHEA Enteral feeding often causes diarrhea, especially if absorption is compromised by bowel disease or drugs such as antibiotics. The diarrhea may be controlled by the use of continuous drip feeding or the addition of enteral bulking agents, such as psyllium hydrophilic mucilogs, or an anticholinergic medication, in the formula. Diarrhea, stimulated by enteral feeding, does not necessarily imply inadequate absorption of nutrients other than water and electrolytes. Furthermore, since luminal nutrients induce trophic effects on the gut mucosa and stimulate the enteric immunologic barrier, it may be appropriate to persist despite the diarrhea, even when this necessitates temporary supplemental parenteral fluid support.

THE COST OF NUTRITION SUPPORT Specialized nutrition support accounts for 1 percent of health care costs or approximately $6 billion per year in the United States. Most nutrition support is provided to hospitalized patients. Characteristically, such patients are among the most sick and have an above-average length of hospital stay, and many are high users of other life-sustaining therapies. Such patients are typically referred from smaller hospitals to tertiary-

care centers. With pressure mounting to contain health care costs, randomized, control trials such as those described above are important to determine the appropriate use of this treatment. The costs and complications of parenteral nutrition can be reduced if patient management is supervised by a nutrition support service. In one study, catheter sepsis decreased from 29 to 5 percent after such a service was instituted, and in another study, routine consultations with a nutrition support service resulted in a 20 percent reduction in average hospital stay and a 26 percent average reduction in costs per patient.

In patients with benign forms of extreme short bowel syndrome such as extensive surgical resection for Crohn's disease or mesenteric bowel infarction, home parenteral nutrition is associated with low morbidity and high rates of rehabilitation. Longitudinal data from a national registry for home parenteral nutrition patients show that 97 percent of Crohn's patients experience partial or complete rehabilitation. Home parenteral nutrition costs about half as much as in-hospital treatment. Enteral feeding is now common for many other debilitated patients both in nursing homes and at home. The clinical outcome for such patients has not been well studied.

REFERENCES

ALEXANDER WJ et al: The importance of lipid type in the diet after burn injury. Ann Surg 240:1, 1986
ALUN JONES V: Comparison of total parenteral nutrition and elemental diet in induction of remission of Crohn's disease. Dig Dis Sci 332:100S, 1987
ANDERSON GF, STEINBERG EP: DRGs and specialized nutritional support: The need for reform. J Parenter Enter Nutr 10:3, 1986
AMERICAN COLLEGE OF PHYSICIANS: Position paper: Parenteral nutrition in patients receiving cancer chemotherapy: A meta-analysis. Ann Intern Med 110:734, 1989

BOWER RH et al: Branched chain amino acid–enriched solutions in the septic patient: A randomized, prospective trial. Ann Surg 203:13, 1986

CERRA FB et al: Disease-specific amino acid infusion (FO80) in hepatic encephalopathy: A prospective, randomized, double blind, controlled trial. J Parenter Enter Nutr 9:288, 1985

CHIARELLI A et al: Very early nutrition supplementation in burned patients. Am J Clin Nutr 51:1035, 1990

DETSKY AS et al: Perioperative parenteral nutrition: A Meta-analysis. Ann Intern Med 107:195, 1987

Evaluating total parenteral nutrition: Assessment and practice guidelines forum, Georgetown University School of Medicine. Dig Dis Sci 34:489, 1989

FOX AD et al: Effect of glutamine-supplemented enteral diet on methotrexate-induced enterocolitis. J Parenter Enter Nutr 12:325, 1988

GIAFFER MH et al: Controlled trial of polymeric versus elemental diet in treatment of active Crohn's disease. Lancet 335:816, 1990

GREENBERG GR et al: Controlled trial of bowel rest and nutritional support in the management of Crohn's disease. Gut 29:1309, 1988

HILL A: Body composition research: Implications for the practice of clinical nutrition. J Parenter Enter Nutr 16:197, 1992

HOWARD L et al: Medical effectiveness of home parenteral nutrition support as judged by four years of North American Registry data. J Parenter Enter Nutr 15:384, 1991

KIRBY DF, CRAIG RM: The value of intensive nutritional support in pancreatitis. J Parenter Enter Nutr 9:353, 1985

——— et al: Intravenous nutritional support during pregnancy. J Parenter Enter Nutr 12:72, 1988

KOPPLE JD: Dietary considerations in patients with advance chronic renal failure, acute renal failure, and transplantation, in Diseases of the Kidney, vol 3, 4th ed, RW Schrier, CW Gohschalk (eds). Philadelphia, Saunders, 1988

LOCHS H et al: Comparison of enteral nutrition and drug treatment in active Crohn's disease. Gastroenterology 101:881, 1991

NAYLOR CD et al: Parenteral nutrition with branched-chain amino acids in heptic encephalopathy: A meta-analysis. Gastroenterology 97:1033, 1989

Perioperative total parenteral nutrition in surgical patients: Veterans Administration total parenteral nutrition cooperative study. N Engl J Med 325:525, 1991

RAPP RP et al: The favorable effect of early parenteral feeding on survival in head injured patients. J Neurosurg 58:90, 1983

RIGAUD D et al: Controlled trial comparing two types of enteral nutrition in treatment of active Crohn's disease: Elemental v. polymeric diet. Gut 32:1492, 1991

SAX HC et al: Early total parenteral nutrition in acute pancreatitis: Lack of beneficial effects. Am J Surg 153:117, 1987

SEIDMAN E: Nutritional management of inflammatory bowel disease. Gastroenterol Clin North Am 17:129, 1989

SITZMANN JV et al: Statement on guidelines for total parenteral nutrition. Dig Dis Sci 34:489, 1989

SZELUGA DJ et al: Nutritional support of bone marrow transplant recipients: A prospective, randomized clinical trial comparing total parenteral nutrition to an enteral feeding program. Cancer Res 47:3309, 1987

WEINSIER RL et al: Cost containment: A contribution of aggressive nutrition support in burn patients. J Burn Care Rehabil 6:436, 1985

WEISDORF S et al: Influence of prophylactic total parenteral nutrition on long-term outcome of bone marrow transplantation. Transplantation 43:833, 1987

77 VITAMIN DEFICIENCY AND EXCESS*

JEAN D. WILSON

Vitamins play several roles in human disease. Deficiencies of single vitamins are now rarely endemic, even in developing nations, and are more likely to occur either as a portion of states of general malnutrition, as a result of food faddism, as a complication of another disease such as malabsorption, as a consequence of complex therapy such as hemodialysis or total parenteral nutrition, or as the result of an inborn error of metabolism. Indeed, disorders of vitamin excess may now be more common than vitamin deficiency.

In considering the pathophysiology of vitamins, several points are worth emphasis: (1) The fact that organic compounds cannot be synthesized within the body and are required constituents of the diet is the result of mutations, and the provision of vitamins in the diet is a form of therapy for an inborn error of metabolism. In some instances, such as the limited ability to synthesize thiamine, the requirement is common to many, if not all, animals, and the mutation must have occurred early in evolution; in others, such as the single-gene defect that prevents ascorbic acid synthesis, humans share the defect with

* For vitamin D, see Chap. 358, and for the hematologic vitamins, see Chap. 304.

only a few species, such as the guinea pig. (2) The feature that separates vitamins from other necessary organic constituents in the diet is that small amounts are required in contrast to the relatively large amounts of essential amino acids and essential fatty acids. This is a consequence of the fact that vitamins function not as building blocks of tissue mass or as substrates for energy production but as prosthetic groups for quantitatively minor tissue constituents or as catalytic cofactors for biologic reactions; like most catalysts, they are required only in small amounts. (3) Deficiency of some vitamins (e.g., pantothenic acid) has never been described in humans, implying that these vitamins either are so ubiquitous in food sources or are conserved so efficiently by the body that deficiency can become manifest, if at all, only in the context of a mixed nutritional and vitamin deficiency. (4) Alcoholism is the background upon which many vitamin deficiencies develop. This is the consequence of several interlocking factors, including diminished intake, impairment of absorption and storage of vitamins, and, in some cases, predisposing genetic factors. (5) Biochemical means of proving vitamin deficiency, once suspected, are limited, and the role of vitamin deficiency in disease states is frequently not recognized because nonspecific vitamin therapy is a common part of standard supportive care. As a consequence, knowledge of the manifestations of vitamin deficiency and a high index of suspicion in the appropriate setting are essential for considering the diagnosis, and demonstration of a response to replacement therapy may be the most accurate way to confirm a diagnosis. (6) The consumption of excessive amounts of vitamins can occur either as the indirect consequence of dietary practice or, more commonly, as the result of deliberate ingestion. Syndromes of excess for the fat-soluble vitamins A and D are well characterized, whereas the toxicity syndromes produced by the water-soluble vitamins are inconsistent and less well understood.

DEFICIENCY STATES

NIACIN (PELLAGRA) **Biochemistry** *Niacin* is the generic term for nicotinic acid (pyridine-3-carboxylic acid) and derivatives that exhibit the nutritional activity of nicotinic acid (Fig. 77-1). In one sense, niacin is not a vitamin, since it can be formed from the essential amino acid tryptophan. In the human, an average of about 1 mg of niacin is formed from 60 mg of dietary tryptophan. Accordingly, estimates of the adequacy of dietary intake must take into account the tryptophan content of the diet as well as the content of niacin. Many foodstuffs, especially cereals, contain bound forms of niacin from which the vitamin is not nutritionally available.

The vitamin is absorbed rapidly from the intestine by both active and passive transport mechanisms. The capacity to absorb niacin is approximately 3 to 4 g/d in the human. Approximately one-fifth of the vitamin is decarboxylated to nicotinuric acid, and the remainder is excreted in the urine as methylated products, largely *N*-methylnicotinamide (NMN) and *N*-methyl-2-pyridone-5-carboxamide.

Mechanism of action Niacin is an essential component of nicotinamide adenine dinucleotide (NAD) and nicotinamide adenine dinucleotide phosphate (NADP), coenzymes for many oxidation-reduction reactions.

Requirements The requirements and recommended daily allowances for niacin and tryptophan are listed in Table 71-1. In contrast to most vitamins, the requirement for niacin does not appear to be increased during pregnancy. Requirement is determined primarily by the amino acid composition of the diet.

Experimental depletion After the institution of a diet deficient in niacin and tryptophan, the urinary excretion of niacin metabolites reaches minimal values (<1.5 mg/d) after 1 to 2 months. Clinical deficiency develops shortly thereafter and consists of dermatitis, glossitis, stomatitis, diarrhea, proctitis, mental depression, abdominal pain, vaginitis, dysphagia, and amenorrhea, findings similar to those in pellagra.

Vitamin	Active Derivative or Cofactor Form	Principal Function
Niacin 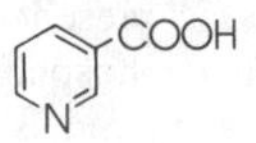	Nicotinamide Adenine Dinucleotide Phosphate (NADP) and Nicotine Adenine Dinucleotide (NAD)	Coenzymes for Oxidations and Reductions
Thiamine 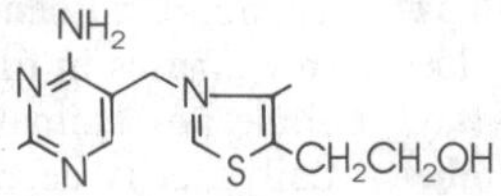	Thiamine Diphosphate	Coenzyme for Cleavage of Carbon-Carbon Bonds
Pyridoxine 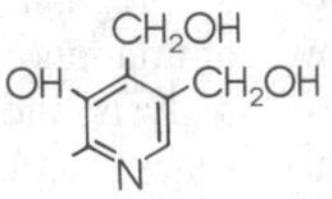	Pyridoxal Phosphate	Cofactor for Enzymes of Amino Acid Metabolism
Riboflavin 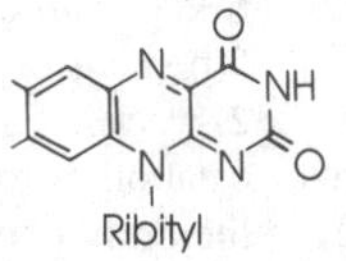	Flavin Mononucleotide (FMN) and Flavin Adenine Dinucleotide (FAD)	Cofactor for Oxidation-Reduction Reactions and Covalently Attached Prosthetic Groups for Some Enzymes
Ascorbic Acid 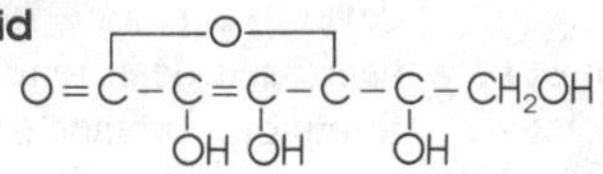	Ascorbic Acid and Dehydroascorbic Acid	Participation as a Redox Ion in Many Biological Oxidation Reactions
Biotin 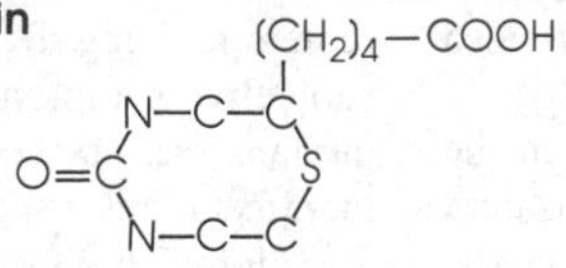	Biotin	Apoenzyme for Carboxylase Enzymes
Vitamin A 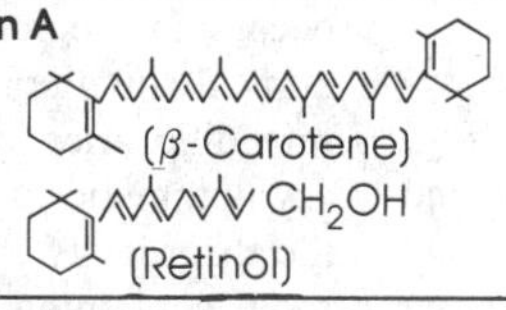	Retinol, Retinal, and Retinoic Acid	Formation of Carotenoid Proteins (Vision) and Glycoproteins (Epithelial Cell Function)
Vitamin E 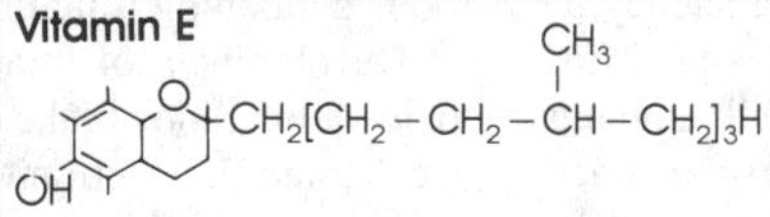	Tocopherol	Antioxidant
Vitamin K 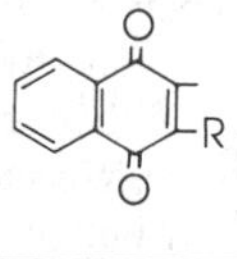	Menaquinone	Cofactor for Post-Translational Carboxylation of Many Proteins Including Essential Clotting Factors

FIGURE 77-1 The structure and principal functions of some of the vitamins associated with human disorders.

Clinical deficiency Pellagra was previously an endemic disease in the American South and in many other parts of the world. The endemic disease is usually associated with a high intake of maize (American corn) or of millet (sorghum, jowar) and can be cured by the administration of niacin; nevertheless, the fact that large populations of people exist on a diet in which maize is the major source of protein but are free of endemic pellagra implies that the relation between maize intake and the development of the disease is not straightforward. The niacin equivalent (available niacin and tryptophan) of maize, although low, is no lower than that of some cereals that are unassociated with endemic pellagra. As a consequence, the concept of the pathogenesis of pellagra has evolved from that of a pure vitamin deficiency or a mixed deficiency of tryptophan and available niacin in the diet to a more complicated etiology. The disorder may be due to an imbalance in dietary amino acids or to a complex deficiency

state. Alternatively, the milling of maize influences the bioavailability of the niacin in the cereal. Treatment of maize with alkali in the preparation of foods in Latin America may serve to hydrolyze bound nicotinic acid and inactivate toxins that accumulate in stored grain contaminated with molds. Alternatively, degermination of the cereal during the common milling process in the United States may inhibit the liberation of bound niacin. The effect of these treatments, respectively, would be to prevent or to predispose to the development of pellagra when maize is a major element of the diet.

Whatever the cause, endemic pellagra disappeared coincident with the improvement of nutritional education and the widespread supplementation of grain cereals with niacin. Pellagra is a rare manifestation of two disorders of tryptophan metabolism, the carcinoid syndrome, in which up to 60 percent of tryptophan is catabolized by what is ordinarily a minor pathway (see Chap. 276), and Hartnup disease (see Chap. 352), an inherited disorder in which several amino acids including tryptophan are absorbed poorly from the diet. In both conditions, pellagra is due to diminished availability of effective niacin equivalents and can be cured by the administration of large amounts of the vitamin.

Pellagra is a chronic wasting disease typically associated with dermatitis, dementia, and diarrhea. The dermatitis is bilateral, symmetric, and present in sites exposed to sunlight and is due to photosensitivity. The mental changes are less discrete; fatigue, insomnia, and apathy may precede the development of an encephalopathy characterized by confusion, disorientation, hallucination, loss of memory, and eventually, organic psychosis. Paresthesias and polyneuritis may be the result of coexisting deficiencies of other vitamins. Diarrhea, when present, results from widespread inflammation of the mucous surfaces; other mucosal abnormalities include achlorhydria, glossitis, stomatitis, and vaginitis. The skin lesions are characterized by hyperkeratosis, hyperpigmentation, and desquamation. The course is progressive over a several-year period, and death is usually due to secondary complications.

The relation between the coenzyme functions of NAD and NADP and the symptoms has not been defined. Levels of NAD and NADP in erythrocytes are low in patients with pellagra, but the coenzymes are essential to so many reactions in intermediary metabolism that profound deficiency of NAD and NADP is incompatible with life. The mental changes in pellagra may be due to diminished conversion of tryptophan to serotonin.

No biochemical test is of diagnostic value, and diagnosis must be based on suspicion and response to replacement therapy. As predicted, urinary excretion of the metabolites of nicotinic acid and tryptophan is low but not lower than in patients with generalized malnutrition. Plasma tryptophan and erythrocyte NAD and NADP levels are also low.

The administration of small amounts of niacin (10 mg/d) in the face of adequate amounts of dietary tryptophan is sufficient to cure endemic pellagra. Large amounts of niacin (40 to 200 mg/d) may be required in Hartnup disease and in the carcinoid syndrome.

THIAMINE (BERIBERI) **Biochemistry** Thiamine contains pyrimidine and thiazole moieties linked by a methylene bridge (see Fig. 77-1). The vitamin is synthesized by a variety of plants and microorganisms but not ordinarily by animals. However, rats and pigeons fed a thiamine-free diet can be protected from deficiency by large quantities of the pyrimidine and thiazole moieties, suggesting a small capacity to couple the subunits together. Small amounts may be synthesized by microorganisms in the gastrointestinal tract. Thiamine is absorbed both by an active-transport process and by passive diffusion. The capacity to absorb the vitamin in the human intestine is about 5 mg/d. Approximately 25 to 30 mg is stored in the body, 80 percent as thiamine diphosphate (pyrophosphate), 10 percent as thiamine triphosphate, and the remainder as thiamine monophosphate. Large amounts are present in skeletal muscles, heart, liver, kidneys, and brain. A number of thiaminase enzymes inactivate thiamine by splitting the vitamin into its two component parts. Several metabolites are excreted in the urine, principally thiamine itself (which is secreted by the renal tubules), an acetylated derivative, and derivatives of thiazole acetate and pyrimidine carboxylate.

Mechanism of action Thiamine diphosphate acts as a coenzyme for several reactions that cleave carbon-carbon bonds—the oxidative decarboxylation of α-keto acids (pyruvate and α-ketoglutarate) and keto analogues of leucine, isoleucine, and valine and the transketolase reaction in the pentose phosphate pathway. Many features of thiamine deficiency are the result of inhibition of these enzymatic reactions and/or the accumulation of the proximal metabolites. Thiamine also may have a specific role in neurons independent of its function in general metabolism; thiamine and its esters are present in axonal membranes, and electrical stimulation of nerves effects the hydrolysis and release of thiamine diphosphate and triphosphate.

Requirements The recommended daily allowances for thiamine are given in Table 71-1. The vitamin has a widespread distribution in food and is absent only from oils, fats, cassava, and refined sugar. In vegetable products, the vitamin is largely in the form of thiamine. The outer layers of cereal grains are especially rich in the vitamin; hence machine-milled rice is a poor source. In animal tissues, thiamine is present largely in the form of phosphate esters. The esters are dephosphorylated by phosphatases in the intestine, and only the free vitamin is absorbed. A substantial loss of the vitamin takes place during cooking above 100°C.

Several factors influence the absorption and metabolism of the vitamin (and hence alter daily requirements). One is the presence of thiaminases in foods such as fresh fish, clams, shrimp, mussels, and some raw animal tissues and in microorganisms in the colon. Two, daily needs decrease when fat forms a large part of the diet and increase as carbohydrate intake increases. Requirements are increased by pregnancy, lactation, thyrotoxicosis, and fever. Accelerated loss of thiamine may occur with diuretic therapy, hemodialysis, peritoneal dialysis, and diarrhea. Defective absorption can occur in malabsorption states, alcoholism, chronic malnutrition, and folate deficiency.

Experimental depletion Following the institution of a thiamine-free diet in control subjects, urinary thiamine excretion decreases to 5 percent of the control value after a week and is undetectable after 2 weeks. However, the excretion of the pyrimidine and thiazole catabolites remains unchanged for as long as a month, indicating that the body pool is slowly utilized when intake is low.

Within a week after the institution of a deficient diet, subjects develop a resting tachycardia, followed by the onset of weakness, decreased deep tendon reflexes, and (in some) sensory neuropathy. Symptoms include generalized malaise, headache, nausea, and aching of the muscles. Appearance of these symptoms is paralleled by a fall in red blood cell transketolase activity. Within a week of thiamine repletion (2 mg/d), all abnormal physical findings disappear, and the subjective symptoms clear after 2 weeks. (Experimental depletion in humans has not been carried to the point of development of severe manifestations.)

Clinical deficiency In developed nations, thiamine deficiency occurs in alcoholics or food faddists or in the context of special clinical situations, such as chronic peritoneal dialysis, hemodialysis, refeeding after starvation, or after the administration of glucose to asymptomatic but thiamine-depleted patients. In developing countries, the disorder is commonly due to the consumption of milled rice or foods containing thiaminases or (possibly) other antithiamine factors.

Development of thiamine deficiency in chronic alcoholics is due to low thiamine intake, impaired thiamine absorption and storage, accelerated destruction of thiamine diphosphate, and varying degrees of energy expenditure. However, clinical manifestations develop in only a fraction of alcoholics and other chronically malnourished persons. Genetic factors may be involved in susceptibility.

The two major manifestations of thiamine deficiency involve the cardiovascular (wet beriberi) and nervous systems (dry beriberi and the Wernicke-Korsakoff syndrome). The typical patient has mixed symptoms involving both the cardiovascular and nervous systems, but pure cardiovascular, neuropathic, and cerebral forms also occur. The relative preponderance of these manifestations is related in part to the duration and severity of deficiency, the degree of physical exertion, and the caloric intake. Severe physical exertion, high carbohydrate intake, and a moderate degree of chronic deficiency favor wet beriberi with little or no peripheral neuritis, whereas an equal deficiency with caloric restriction and relative inactivity favors the development of dry beriberi.

Beriberi heart disease comprises three major physiologic derangements: (1) peripheral vasodilatation leading to a high-output state, (2) retention of sodium and water leading to edema, and (3) biventricular myocardial failure. In the chronic form, peripheral vasodilatation leads to increased arteriovenous shunting of blood, rapid circulation time, tachycardia, increased cardiac output, and a venous congestive state characterized by elevated peripheral venous pressure, elevated right ventricular end-diastolic pressure, decreased arteriovenous extraction of oxygen, sodium retention, and edema. Decreased cerebral and renal blood flow and increased flow to muscles are common. Cardiac output increases so that notwithstanding the lowered peripheral vascular resistance, ventricular work, arterial blood pressure, and pulmonary wedge pressure tend to be elevated. Temporary appearance or worsening of hypertension may occur during thiamine repletion, presumably due to closing of arteriovenous shunts and temporary volume overload.

In acute fulminant cardiovascular (shoshin) beriberi, the myocardial lesion is the central feature of a course in which dyspnea, restlessness, and anxiety eventuate in acute cardiovascular collapse and death within hours to days. Physical findings include stocking-glove cyanosis, tachycardia, marked cardiomegaly, hepatomegaly, arterial bruits, and neck vein distention. The venous pressure is high, and the circulation time is rapid. Because of the fulminant course, edema may be minimal or absent. Administration of thiamine rapidly restores peripheral vascular resistance, but improvement in the myocardial abnormality may be delayed so that low-output failure supervenes during treatment.

Three types of nervous system involvement occur: peripheral neuropathy, Wernicke's encephalopathy (cerebral beriberi), and the Korsakoff syndrome. The neuropathy may or may not be painful and is characterized by a symmetric impairment of sensory, motor, and reflex function that affects predominately the distal segments of limbs. The histologic lesion is a noninflammatory degeneration of myelin sheaths. No meaningful distinction can be made between this disorder and so-called alcoholic neuropathy on the basis of clinical criteria.

Wernicke's encephalopathy ordinarily develops in an orderly sequence and consists of vomiting, nystagmus (horizontal more commonly than vertical), palsies of the rectus muscles leading to unilateral or bilateral ophthalmoplegia (and decrease in the nystagmus), fever, ataxia, and progressive mental deterioration that eventuates in a global confusional state and may progress to coma and death. Improvement occurs after thiamine replacement, although Korsakoff's syndrome may supervene. Thus the eye palsies are corrected, the nystagmus improves in one-half, the ataxia improves or disappears in two-thirds, and the global confusional state disappears to be replaced by Korsakoff's syndrome. The latter consists of retrograde amnesia, impaired ability to learn, and (usually) confabulation. The patient is typically alert and responsive and exhibits no serious defect in behavior. Recovery (complete or partial) from Korsakoff's syndrome occurs only in one-half.

In summary, Wernicke's encephalopathy and the amnesic psychosis of Korsakoff's syndrome are not separate clinical events; instead, the changing ocular and ataxic signs, the transformation of the global confusional state into the amnesic-confabulatory syndrome, and the development of a nonconfabulatory amnesic state are successive stages in the recovery from a single process. The clinical features, differential diagnosis, course, and pathology of cerebral beriberi are discussed in detail in Chap. 377.

Various biochemical tests to detect thiamine deficiency include the measurement of blood thiamine, pyruvate, α-ketoglutarate, lactate, and glyoxylate; measurement of the urinary excretion of thiamine and thiamine metabolites; the thiamine-loading test; and measurement of urinary methylglyoxal. The most reliable is the measurement of whole-blood or erythrocyte transketolase activity. Any enhancement in enzymatic activity resulting from added thiamine diphosphate (TPP) is referred to as the *TPP effect* (expressed in percent). If the activity of the enzyme is increased more than 15 percent by the added thiamine diphosphate, then a deficiency state is probably present. Due to variability in activity, measurement of isolated transketolase levels is not useful, but demonstration of an increase in activity after treatment coupled with a positive TPP test prior to treatment suggests thiamine deficiency.

Another criterion for the diagnosis is the assessment of clinical response to thiamine administration. Clinical improvement may be dramatic in cardiovascular beriberi, with an increase in blood pressure and a decrease in heart rate within 12 h after start of therapy and diuresis and reduction in heart size within 1 to 2 days.

Prompt administration of thiamine is indicated when beriberi is diagnosed or suspected. Fifty milligrams per day should be given intramuscularly for several days, after which 2.5 to 5 mg/d can be administered by mouth. Larger amounts are usually not absorbed. All patients also should receive other water-soluble vitamins in therapeutic quantities.

Thiamine-responsive inborn errors of metabolism   Thiamine-responsive inborn errors of metabolism, in which patients respond to pharmacologic doses of thiamine, include thiamine-responsive megaloblastic anemia, for which the mechanism is unknown; thiamine-responsive lactic acidosis, which is due to low activity of pyruvate carboxylase in liver; thiamine-responsive branched-chain ketoaciduria, which is due to low activity of a ketoacid dehydrogenase; and intermittent cerebellar ataxia, which may result from an abnormal pyruvate dehydrogenase. In addition, the autosomal recessive disorder subacute necrotizing encephalomyelopathy (Leigh's disease) may be related to a diminished amount of thiamine triphosphate in neural tissue; a factor has been isolated from the urine of such patients that inhibits the enzyme that synthesizes thiamine triphosphate. The response of patients with Leigh's disease to pharmacologic doses appears to be minor, however.

PYRIDOXINE (VITAMIN B$_6$)   Biochemistry   The biologic activity of the vitamin B$_6$ group is displayed by pyridoxine, pyridoxal, and pyridoxamine and their 5-phosphate esters (see Fig. 77-1). The coenzyme form is pyridoxal-5-phosphate, and the other compounds owe their activity to conversion to pyridoxal-5-phosphate. The vitamin is widely and uniformly distributed in all foods; muscle meats, liver, vegetables, and whole-grain cereals are among the best sources.

Mechanism of action   Pyridoxal phosphate acts as a cofactor for many enzymes involved in amino acid metabolism, including transaminases, synthetases, and hydroxylases. In humans, the vitamin is of particular importance in the metabolism of tryptophan, glycine, serine, glutamate, and the sulfur-containing amino acids. Pyridoxal phosphate is also required for the synthesis of the heme precursor δ-aminolevulinic acid. A large portion of body stores is in muscle phosphorylase, where it functions to stabilize the enzyme rather than as a catalyst. It also plays a poorly understood role in neuronal excitability, possibly as a result of its function in transsulfuration reactions or in γ-aminobutyric acid metabolism.

Requirements   The recommended daily allowances are given in Table 71-1. Even more than for most vitamins, the requirement is increased in pregnancy and by the administration of estrogens. Estrogens appear to inhibit the role of pyridoxal phosphate in tryptophan metabolism. Pyridoxine requirement also may be increased by high protein intake and by either chronic hemodialysis or peritoneal dialysis. The ethanol metabolite acetaldehyde displaces pyridoxal phosphate from proteins and thus enhances its degradation.

Experimental depletion   The feeding of pyridoxine-deficient diets leads to chemical evidence of deficiency (increased xanthurenic acid and decreased pyridoxine in urine) within a week. Electroencephalographic abnormalities occur within 3 weeks, and some subjects have grand mal seizures. Deficiency induced with the pyridoxine antagonist deoxypyridoxine causes, in addition, seborrheic dermatitis, cheilosis, glossitis, nausea, vomiting, weakness, and dizziness.

Clinical deficiency   The widespread occurrence of the vitamin in food is probably the reason that pure pyridoxine deficiency is rare except when the pyridoxine content of food is either destroyed or converted to less available protein-bound forms during processing, as has happened in some infant formulas. It is a paradox, therefore, that pyridoxine deficiency is now common because many drugs act as pyridoxine antagonists. Isoniazid, cycloserine, penicillamine, and carbonyl reagents in general form complexes with the aldehyde moiety of the vitamin and prevent normal function of the coenzyme. In each case abnormal tryptophan metabolism and convulsions can be prevented by supplementation with the vitamin.

Estimates of vitamin deficiency have been based on the correction of clinical signs of deficiency following administration of the vitamin, measurement of the excretion of tryptophan metabolites after tryptophan-loading tests, measurement of various amino acid transferase activities in blood, and measurement of the excretion of pyridoxine or its metabolites or of oxalate in urine. One index is the measurement of urinary tryptophan metabolites, particularly xanthurenic acid, following tryptophan loading. Alternatively, cystathionine can be assayed after administration of a methionine load. In vitro measurement of red blood cell glutamic pyruvic transaminase in the presence and absence of pyridoxal phosphate may be a better indicator of pyridoxine status than either loading test.

The appropriate management is prevention of deficiency. Supplementation of the diet with 30 mg pyridoxine returns tryptophan metabolism to normal in pregnancy, in users of oral contraceptives, and in patients taking isoniazid. Doses as high as 100 mg/d may be required in subjects taking penicillamine.

Pyridoxine-responsive diseases Several genetic disorders cause abnormalities in vitamin B_6 metabolism. In one group, infants develop convulsions and brain damage and die if not provided with large daily supplements of pyridoxine; these children have an apoenzyme for glutamic acid decarboxylase that has a decreased binding affinity for pyridoxal phosphate. Consequently, they do not form normal amounts of γ-aminobutyric acid, a physiologic inhibitor of neurotransmission. Another group has pyridoxine-responsive chronic anemia; pyridoxine supplementation results in prompt hematologic improvement but does not correct the morphologic abnormality in the erythrocytes.

The synthesis of cystathionine from homocystine and serine and its cleavage to cysteine and homoserine are catalyzed by two pyridoxal phosphate enzymes. The changes that occur with deficiency of these two enzymes and in xanthurenic aciduria due to kynureninase deficiency have been reviewed by Mudd. Some patients with vitamin B_6-responsive xanthurenic aciduria or cystathioninuria have a mutant apoenzyme that interacts abnormally with pyridoxal phosphate, a defect that can be largely corrected by elevated concentrations of the cofactor. In contrast, the vitamin B_6 response in patients with homocystinuria due to cystathionine synthetase deficiency results from enhancement of the activity of the residual amount of normal enzyme present rather than from a restoration of the affected enzyme levels to normal.

RIBOFLAVIN Riboflavin in the form of the coenzymes flavin mononucleotide (FMN) and flavin adenine dinucleotide (FAD) (see Fig. 77-1) participates in a variety of oxidation-reduction reactions. In addition, covalently attached flavins are essential to the structure of such enzymes as succinate dehydrogenase and monoamine oxidase. The vitamin is absorbed from the gastrointestinal tract either as free riboflavin or the 5′-phosphate by an active transport process. The recommended daily allowance is listed in Table 71-1. Covalently linked vitamin accounts for less than one-tenth of the tissue pool. The vitamin is excreted in urine predominantly in the free form, although a small fraction of the daily turnover is the result of catabolism by microorganisms in the gastrointestinal tract.

Riboflavin deficiency can be induced by feeding a riboflavin-deficient diet or by the administration of riboflavin antagonists such as galactoflavin. Deficiency is characterized by sore throat, hyperemia and edema of the oral mucous membranes, cheilosis, angular stomatitis, glossitis, seborrheic dermatitis, and normochromic, normocytic anemia due to red cell hypoplasia of the bone marrow. These features can be reversed by riboflavin administration. Thyroid hormones and adrenal steroids enhance FMN and FAD synthesis; phenothiazines and tricyclic antidepressants competitively inhibit flavin coenzyme biosynthesis, but these agents alone do not induce deficiency. Instead, riboflavin deficiency almost invariably occurs in combination with deficiencies of other water-soluble vitamins. Riboflavin requirements are increased in subjects on chronic hemodialysis or peritoneal dialysis.

VITAMIN C (SCURVY)   Biochemistry In most animals, ascorbic acid (vitamin C) can be synthesized from glucose. However, humans, other primates, and the guinea pig are unable to synthesize L-ascorbic acid and require vitamin C in the diet. These species can perform the various reactions required for the biosynthesis of the vitamin from D-glucose except for one step, the conversion of L-gluconogammalactone to L-abscorbic acid. The enzyme that catalyzes this reaction (L-gluconolactone oxidase) is missing because of a mutation; thus the need for vitamin C in the diet is the result of an inborn error in carbohydrate metabolism.

Mechanism of action L-Ascorbic acid readily undergoes reversible oxidation and reduction as follows:

$$\text{L-ascorbic acid} \rightleftharpoons \text{dehydro-L-ascorbic acid} + 2H^+ + 2e$$

This property of the vitamin is the key to understanding its role as a redox agent for biologic oxidation. However, ascorbic acid does not act as a conventional cofactor because its requirement can usually be replaced by other compounds with similar redox properties. The vitamin reduces the prosthetic metal ions in many enzymes to the required forms and performs other antioxidant functions by removing free radicals. The best understood function is in the synthesis of collagen; absence of the vitamin leads to impairment of peptidyl hydroxylation of procollagen and a reduction in collagen formation and secretion by connective tissue. Nonhydroxylated collagen cannot form the triple helix required for normal tissue structure. Many features of scurvy result from this defect in collagen synthesis, including the capillary fragility that underlies the hemorrhagic features, the poor healing of wounds, and (in part) the bony abnormalities of children. Collagens with the highest content of hydroxyproline are most severely affected, accounting for the early disruption of the adventitia, media, and basal laminae of blood vessels. Ascorbic acid also prevents oxidation of tetrahydrofolate and thus protects the active folic acid pool and regulates iron distribution and storage, probably by influencing the valence of stored iron and maintaining a normal ratio of ferritin to hemosiderin. Scorbutic patients excrete incompletely oxidized products of tyrosine metabolism, but the significance is not clear.

Requirements The recommended daily allowance for vitamin C is described in Table 71-1. The vitamin is present in milk and some meats (kidney, liver, fish) and is widely distributed in fruits and vegetables. A portion is lost after prolonged storage of unprocessed fruits and vegetables (e.g., potatoes), but it is partially preserved (half or greater) by most means of food processing (boiling, steaming, pressure cooking, preserving jams and jellies, freezing, dehydration, and canning). As a consequence, the recommended daily allowances can be met with even a modest intake of fruits and vegetables. Utilization of the vitamin is increased during pregnancy and lactation and in thyrotoxicosis, and absorption is decreased in diarrheal states and in achlorhydria.

Experimental depletion The total-body pool of vitamin C varies from 1.5 to 3 g. When a deficient diet is instituted, the pool is depleted at a rate that approximates 4 percent per day. In monkeys, the major catabolic pathway involves oxidation of the alcohol at carbon 6 to an aldehyde and then to an acid. Because of differences in initial pool size and rates of turnover, differences in the completeness of deficiency in various experimental diets, and variation among normal subjects at the cellular or enzymatic level, the time required for development of symptoms ranges from 1 to 3 months in different studies. Manifestations of deficiency correlate better with the total pool size than with plasma or blood levels. The first symptoms (petechial hemorrhages and ecchymoses) develop when the pool size is less than 0.5 g; with further depletion (pool size 0.1 to 0.5 g), manifestations include gum involvement, hyperkeratosis, congested hair follicles, arthralgias, Sjögren's syndrome, coiled hairs, and joint effusions. When depletion is extreme (pool size <0.1 g), dyspnea, edema, oliguria, and neuropathy supervene. Progress of the disease may then be rapid.

Symptoms do not improve until the pool is repleted, and the larger the therapeutic dose, the more rapid is the repletion. However, with doses as small as 6.5 mg/d the body pool eventually returns to normal, and amelioration of symptoms follows.

Clinical deficiency Scurvy now occurs for the most part in areas of urban poverty. An increased incidence occurs at 6 to 12 months of age in infants whose processed milk formulas are unsupplemented with citrus fruit or vegetables as a result of maternal error or neglect. Another peak occurs in middle and old age; edentulous men who live alone and cook for themselves are particularly prone. Clinical scurvy is more severe than the experimental disease, doubtlessly because affected individuals usually have deficiencies of other dietary constituents as well and because the groups at risk (infants and the elderly) are especially vulnerable.

In adults, the features include perifollicular hyperkeratotic papules in which hairs become fragmented and buried; perifollicular hemorrhages; purpura beginning on the backs of the lower extremities coalescing to become ecchymoses (Fig. 77-2); hemorrhage into the muscles of the arms and legs with secondary phlebothromboses; hemorrhages into joints; splinter hemorrhages in the nail beds; gum involvement (only in people with teeth) that includes swelling, friability, bleeding, secondary infection, and loosening of the teeth; poor wound healing and breakdown of recently healed wounds; petechial hemorrhages in the viscera; and emotional changes. Symptoms resembling those of Sjögren's syndrome may occur. Terminally, icterus, edema, and fever are common, and convulsions, hypotension, and death may occur abruptly.

In infancy and childhood, hemorrhage into the periosteum of long bones causes painful swellings and may result in epiphyseal separation. The sternum may sink inward, leaving a sharp elevation at the rib margins (scorbutic rosary). Purpura and ecchymoses may develop in the skin, and gum lesions occur if the teeth have erupted. Retrobulbar, subarachnoid, and intracerebral hemorrhages rapidly culminate in death if treatment is delayed.

FIGURE 77-2 Hemorrhages and ecchymoses in a patient with scurvy. *(Photograph courtesy of Leonard L. Madison.)*

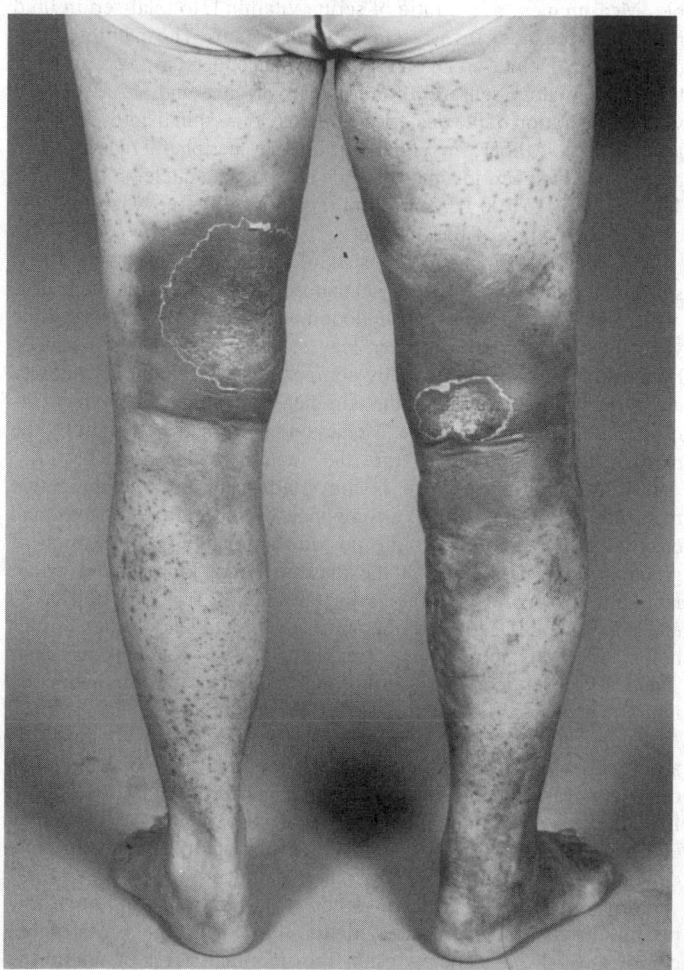

Normochromic, normocytic anemia is common and is due to bleeding into tissues. Anemia also may be macrocytic and/or megaloblastic (one-fifth of patients in one series). Many foods that contain vitamin C also contain folate, and diets that cause scurvy also may cause folate deficiency. However, ascorbic acid deficiency also results in an increased oxidation of formyl tetrahydrofolic acid to inactive folate metabolites and may cause a decrease in the active folate pool. Whether changes in iron distribution and storage are involved in the pathogenesis of the anemia is unclear. The anemia is corrected with replenishment of vitamin C and institution of a balanced diet.

In some hospitals, platelet ascorbic acid levels are useful in diagnosing scurvy and are usually less than one-fourth of the normal value. Plasma levels of the vitamin correlate less well with the clinical state. In infants, x-ray changes of the bones may be diagnostic. Bilirubin is frequently elevated. Capillary fragility is abnormal.

Scurvy is potentially fatal; if the diagnosis is suspected, blood should be obtained, and ascorbic acid therapy should be instituted promptly. The usual dose in adults is 100 mg three to five times a day by mouth until 4 g has been administered, then 100 mg/d. In infants and children, administration of 10 to 25 mg three times a day is adequate. A diet rich in vitamin C should be initiated simultaneously. Spontaneous bleeding usually ceases within 24 h, muscle and bone pains subside quickly, and the gums begin to heal within 2 to 3 days. Even large ecchymoses and hematomas resolve in 10 to 12 days, although pigmentary changes in areas of hemorrhage may persist for months. Serum bilirubin becomes normal within 3 to 5 days, and the anemia is ordinarily corrected within 2 to 4 weeks.

BIOTIN Biotin (see Fig. 77-1) functions as a cofactor in mammalian carboxylases. The vitamin is largely ingested in a form bound to protein, hydrolyzed by pancreatic biotinidase, and absorbed by what is probably an active transport process. The recommended daily allowance is given in Table 71-1. In cells, biotin is covalently attached to apocarboxylases to form four haloenzymes that catalyze the incorporation of biocarbonate into substrate, acetyl-CoA carboxylase, pyruvate carboxylase, methylcrotonyl CoA carboxylase, and propionyl CoA carboxylase. Biotin deficiency in the human occurs under at least three conditions: following the prolonged consumption of raw egg white (which binds biotin in the gut and prevents its absorption), after parenteral nutrition without biotin supplementation in patients with malabsorption, and in subjects with biotinidase deficiency. In all three conditions the common manifestations of biotin deficiency resemble those of essential fatty acid deficiency and include perioral dermatitis, conjunctivitis, alopecia, ataxia, and, in children, developmental delay. In addition, biotinidase deficiency may cause serious neurologic defects.

The diagnosis can be established by documenting reduced urinary excretion of biotin or by demonstrating resolution of the deficiency in response to supplementation with 100 μg/d.

VITAMIN A Biochemistry Vitamin A (retinol) can either be ingested or synthesized within the body from plant carotenes (see Fig. 77-1). The best sources of preformed vitamin A are liver, milk, and kidney, where it occurs largely in the form of fatty acid esters. The esters are hydrolyzed during digestion, absorbed in the free form, reesterified with fatty acids within the intestinal mucosa, and enter the circulation with lymph chylomicrons. The carotene substrates for synthesis of vitamin A, mainly β-carotenes, are widely distributed in plants. β-Carotene can either be absorbed intact or cleaved in the intestinal tract to form two molecules of retinaldehyde. Retinaldehyde is subsequently reduced by an aldehyde reductase to retinol. Retinol from whatever source is stored as retinyl esters in the liver. The normal body pool is 300 to 900 mg.

Prior to release from the liver, retinyl esters are hydrolyzed, and the free alcohol is bound to a specific transport protein, retinol-binding protein (RBP), for transport to peripheral tissues. In vitamin A deficiency, the release of RBP from the liver is inhibited, and the protein accumulates in liver; with repletion, RBP is rapidly released from preformed stores. Approximately equal amounts of retinol are excreted in the bile and urine.

Mechanism of action   The best-defined function of vitamin A is its role in vision; in the retina vitamin A constitutes the prosthetic group of carotenoid proteins that provide the molecular basis for visual excitation. In addition, vitamin A is required for growth, reproduction, and the maintenance of life. Retinol-phosphate-mannose glycolipid is present in a variety of cell membranes, and the vitamin plays a primary role in the synthesis of glycoproteins. The importance of glycoprotein to every cell implies that this is an equally important function of the vitamin. In all its functions, the vitamin is believed to act by binding to a transcription regulatory protein that controls gene expression (see Chap. 329).

Requirements   The recommended daily allowance for vitamin A is listed in Table 71-1. The assumed utilization efficiency for the conversion of β-carotene to vitamin A in the human is one-sixth (0.167). Other carotenoids with provitamin A activity have, on average, about half the activity of β-carotene. Pregnancy and disease states with impaired absorption or storage, excessive utilization, or increased excretion of vitamin A may lead to increased requirements.

Experimental depletion   When experimental subjects are fed a diet deficient in both retinol and carotene, plasma levels fall, and the body pool shrinks to less than half the control value. Deficiency is manifested by follicular hyperkeratosis, impaired dark adaptation, and abnormalities of the electroretinogram. These changes are corrected after supplementation with 150 μg retinol or 300 μg β-carotene per day.

Clinical deficiency   Endemic deficiency results from inadequate amounts of the vitamin and the provitamins in the diet and occurs in conjunction with deficiency of other nutrients or complicating diseases. In some developing countries, vitamin A deficiency is a major cause of blindness in the young as a consequence of failure to incorporate green leafy vegetables or other sources of the provitamin or vitamin into the diet. Such children appear to be particularly susceptible to the complications of measles. Vitamin A deficiency also may contribute to protein-calorie malnutrition, and here the deficiency is due in part to a defective release mechanism from the liver secondary to inadequate retinol-binding protein. In developed nations, vitamin A deficiency is usually due either to intestinal malabsorption (as in sprue or after intestinal bypass surgery), abnormal storage (liver disease), or enhanced destruction or excretion of the vitamin (proteinuria). Vitamin A deficiency also has occurred in patients receiving total parenteral nutrition because of loss of vitamin A after prolonged storage of intravenous fluid.

Night blindness is the earliest symptom of deficiency, followed by degenerative changes in the retina. The bulbar conjunctiva becomes dry (xerosis), and small gray plaques with foamy surfaces develop (Bitôt's spots). These early lesions are reversible with vitamin A. The more serious effects of deficiency are ulceration and necrosis of the cornea (keratomalacia), leading to perforation, endophthalmitis, and blindness. Dryness and hyperkeratosis of the skin may be present.

Vitamin A levels in plasma are not reliable for the assessment of stores in individual cases. Measurements of dark adaptation, rod scotometry, and electroretinography are useful indicators of vitamin A stores but require trained personnel and expensive equipment; consequently, the diagnosis is usually based on a high index of suspicion in malnourished children or in patients with predisposing factors for its development.

Night blindness and the milder conjunctival changes respond well to 30,000 IU vitamin A daily for a week. Corneal damage constitutes a therapeutic emergency, and the usual treatment is 20,000 IU/kg of body weight per day for 5 days. Children who are at risk for vitamin A deficiency and who develop measles should be given 200,000 IU orally each day for 2 days.

VITAMIN E   Biochemistry   Eight naturally occurring tocopherols possess vitamin E activity. The structure of alpha tocopherol, the most widely distributed and most active of the tocopherols, is shown in Fig. 77-1. The vitamin is absorbed from the gastrointestinal tract by a mechanism similar to that for other fat-soluble vitamins and enters the bloodstream via the lymph, associated first with chylomicrons and

then with plasma β-lipoproteins. Indeed, plasma levels correlate with plasma lipid levels. The vitamin is stored in all tissues, and the tissue stores can protect against vitamin deficiency for long periods. Approximately three-fourths of the vitamin is excreted in bile, and the balance is excreted as glucuronides in urine. Metabolites with quinone structures (including one similar to ubiquinone) are present in tissues.

Mechanism of action   The vitamin probably acts as an antioxidant rather than as a specific cofactor. In so acting it presumably inhibits oxidation of essential cellular constituents and prevents the formation of toxic oxidation products. Other antioxidants such as selenium, sulfur-containing amino acids, and the ubiquinone group can reverse the symptoms of vitamin E deficiency in animals.

Requirements   The recommended daily requirement is 10 to 30 mg/d (see Table 71-1). Diets containing large amounts of polyunsaturated fatty acids increase and diets containing antioxidants decrease the requirement. The vitamin is widely distributed in food, so a primary deficiency state has never been recognized in otherwise healthy children or adults. Newborn infants have plasma concentrations about one-fifth that of maternal levels, implying poor placental transfer, but human milk (in contrast to cow's milk) has sufficient levels to meet the requirements in infants.

Experimental depletion   In long-term studies, vitamin E concentrations in plasma declined significantly only after months on a deficient diet. No manifestations of the depletion were detected in normal volunteers, making it difficult to establish that tocopherol is a human vitamin.

Clinical deficiency   In the appropriate clinical setting, vitamin E deficiency is associated with a discrete syndrome. Rarely, deficiency is due to a selective malabsorption of the vitamin. More commonly, intestinal fat malabsorption can cause deficiency of all fat-soluble vitamins including vitamin E, and children with abetalipoproteinemia or chronic cholestatic liver disease appear to be particularly susceptible. Measurement of the ratio of serum vitamin E to total-serum lipid is the preferred index for assessing vitamin E status. The manifestations of deficiency include areflexia, gait disturbance, decreased proprioceptive and vibratory sensation, and paresis of gaze and are associated with degeneration of the posterior columns of the spinal cord, selective loss of large-caliber, myelinated axons in peripheral nerves, and appearance of spheroids in the gracile and cuneate nuclei of the brain. Treatment (50 to 100 IU/d by mouth) is most effective when initiated early in the course of the disease.

VITAMIN K   Vitamin K consists of a quinone ring attached to a side chain (labeled *R* in Fig. 77-1) that varies depending on the source of the vitamin. Vitamin K$_1$ (phylloquinone) is present in most edible vegetables, particularly in green leaves, and vitamin K$_2$ is produced by intestinal bacteria. The many compounds with vitamin K activity are structurally related to the simpler compound, 2-methyl-1,4-naphthoquinone (menadione). Menadione is formed in the gut by the removal of the side chain from the vitamin by intestinal bacteria. After absorption, menadione is converted in the body to the active menaquinone. The vitamin is a component of a specialized microsomal enzyme system that effects the posttranslational γ carboxylation of glutamic acid in proteins of the plasma, bone, kidney, and urine, including the precursor proteins for the clotting factors VII, IX, X, and possibly V. Death from hemorrhage in deficiency states ensues before deficiency of the other carboxylated proteins becomes manifest. The warfarin anticoagulant drugs induce hypoprothrombinemia by inhibiting the γ carboxylation of the precursor protein.

Under ordinary circumstances, about 80 percent of vitamin K is absorbed from the small bowel into the intestinal lymph. Deficiency can occur in association with diseases that interfere with fat absorption. In addition, long-term treatment with oral antibiotics may temporarily eliminate intestinal bacteria as a source for vitamin K and promote deficiency when the diet is marginal or deficient.

Newborn infants tend to be deficient in vitamin K and have low plasma levels of several coagulation factors in the prothrombin complex. Such deficiencies result from minimal stores of vitamin K at birth, lack of an established intestinal flora, and a limited dietary intake of the vitamin.

Routine determination of prothrombin should be performed prior to surgical procedures or delivery. Subjects with levels below 70 percent of normal should receive therapy with vitamin K. Vitamin K deficiency can be separated from hypoprothrombinemia of liver disease by demonstration of the noncarboxylated prothrombin precursor that accumulates in plasma in the vitamin deficiency.

VITAMIN EXCESS

According to the National Health Interview Survey, more than 50 percent of adults in the United States use vitamin and/or mineral supplements, and in many instances ingestion is within a potentially toxic range. Multivitamins are the most common type ingested by children, whereas single vitamins are consumed commonly among adults. Supplement use is higher with the level of education and income and in those whose health is good.

Fat-soluble vitamins are stored to a variable extent in the body and hence are more likely to cause adverse effects when taken in excess; excess states for vitamins D (see Chap. 358) and A are well characterized. Water-soluble vitamins are readily excreted in the urine and stored only to a limited extent. Consequently, toxicity states for these vitamins only occur when large amounts are taken for prolonged periods.

VITAMIN A AND CAROTENES Carotenemia Carotenemia results from excessive intake of vitamin A precursors in foods, principally carrots. Excess carotene is not injurious apart from the cosmetic effect; the fact that carotenemia does not cause hypervitaminosis A indicates that the conversion of carotene to vitamin A must be regulated. Carotenemia is manifested by yellowing of the skin with greatest intensity on the palms and soles and by a corresponding yellowness of serum. The yellowing of the skin differs from jaundice in that the sclerae remain white. Hypothyroid patients are particularly susceptible. The omission of carrots from the diet leads to the rapid disappearance of the pigmentation. Discoloration of the skin also can result from the consumption of large amounts of other colored fruits and vegetables.

Vitamin A toxicity Hypervitaminosis A can result from accidental overingestion by hunters or explorers (polar bear liver), as the result of food faddism (usually caused by overly solicitous parents), or as a side effect of inappropriate therapy. Acute toxicity from a single massive dose consists of abdominal pain, nausea, vomiting, headache, dizziness, sluggishness, papilledema, and in infants a bulging fontanel followed within a few days by generalized desquamation of the skin and recovery. Chronic toxicity occurs after ingestion of 25,000 units or more daily for protracted periods and is characterized by bone and joint pain, hyperostoses, hair loss, dryness and fissures of the lips, anorexia, benign intracranial hypertension, low-grade fever, pruritus, weight loss, and hepatosplenomegaly. The only diagnostic laboratory finding is elevation of the vitamin in serum, chiefly in the form of retinyl esters. The concentration of retinol-binding protein is normal, and the excess vitamin A circulates in association with lipoprotein. Relief is prompt on discontinuation of the vitamin.

VITAMIN E Relatively large doses of vitamin E have been taken by some for extended periods without apparent harm. In others, malaise, gastrointestinal complaint, headaches, and possibly hypertension have occurred. However, true toxicity appears to occur in two situations—in subjects receiving oral anticoagulants and in premature infants. In large amounts, vitamin E can antagonize vitamin K and prolong the prothrombin time; this phenomenon results in a potentiation of oral anticoagulants. Premature infants given parenteral vitamin E have developed ascites associated with hepatosplenomegaly, cholestatic jaundice, azotemia, and thrombocytopenia.

VITAMIN K Large amounts of vitamin K can block the effects of oral anticoagulants and when given to pregnant women can cause jaundice in the newborn.

PYRIDOXINE Most adults can consume up to 10 times the recommended daily allowance of 2 mg pyridoxine per day without adverse effects. However, severe peripheral neuropathies have developed after ingestion of several grams per day for prolonged periods; symptoms include ataxia, perioral numbness, and clumsiness of the hands and feet, and the findings include loss of position and vibration sense without impairment of reflexes or sensory function. Recovery is slow after ingestion ceases. Lower doses (25 mg/d) can antagonize the effects of levodopa in Parkinson's disease and decrease the anticonvulsant effects of phenytoin and barbiturates.

VITAMIN C Vitamin C is consumed by 85 percent of all vitamin users because of the claim that large amounts of the vitamin (a gram or greater per day) prevent or minimize the symptoms of the common cold. However, in controlled studies, no significant differences in occurrence, severity, or duration of colds have been demonstrated in subjects treated with the vitamin. Use of the vitamin in this way is unwarranted and probably unwise. The long-term use of ascorbic acid in these doses can interfere with the absorption of vitamin B_{12}, enhance blood levels of estrogens in women on exogenous estrogens, cause uricosuria, and predispose to formation of oxalate kidney stones. In addition, large doses enhance the development of metabolizing enzymes in the fetus and may cause rebound scurvy in the offspring of mothers who have ingested large amounts of the vitamin during pregnancy. However, pharmacologic doses (200 mg daily) may correct leukocyte abnormalities in patients with the Chédiak-Higashi syndrome (see Chap. 59).

NIACIN Large doses of niacin are used for treatment of hypercholesterolemia and occasionally for other purposes. The vitamin causes release of histamine, which in turn can cause severe flushing, pruritus, and gastrointestinal disturbances and may aggravate asthma. Acanthosis nigricans may occur. In doses of 3 g/d niacin can cause elevation of serum uric acid and of fasting glucose. Large doses can also cause hepatic toxicity including cholestatic jaundice.

In women who consume vitamin supplements, the median dose of pyridoxine approaches the level of 120 mg/d found to cause paresthesia and muscle weakness in all 103 volunteers who consumed the vitamin for 6 months or greater.

REFERENCES

General

BROWN ML: *Present Knowledge in Nutrition*. Washington, International Life Science Institute, 1990
COMBS GF JR: *The Vitamins*. San Diego, Academic, 1992
ELSAS LJ, McCORMICK DB: Genetic defects in vitamin utilization. Part I: General aspects and fat-soluble vitamins. Vitam Horm 43:103, 1986
GOODHART RS, SHILS ME (eds): *Modern Nutrition in Health and Disease*, 6th ed. Philadelphia, Lea & Febiger, 1980
HOYUMPA AM: Mechanisms of vitamin deficiencies in alcoholism. Alcoholism (NY) 10:573, 1986
LINDEN MC: *Nutritional Biochemistry and Metabolism*. New York, Elsevier, 1991
MUDD SH: Inborn errors of metabolism. Vitamin-responsive genetic disease. J Clin Pathol 27(Suppl) 8:38, 1974
RUDMAN D, WILLIAMS PJ: Nutrient deficiencies during total parenteral nutrition. Nutr Rev 43:1, 1984

Niacin deficiency

CARPENTER KJ: The relationship of pellagra to corn and the low availability of niacin in cereals. Experientia(Suppl) 44:197, 1983
———, LEWIN WJ: A reexamination of the composition of diets associated with pellagra. J Nutr 115:543, 1985
CASTIELLO RJ, LYNCH PJ: Pellagra and the carcinoid syndrome. Arch Dermatol 105:574, 1972
FU CS et al: Biochemical markers for assessment of niacin status in young men. J Nutr 119:1949, 1989
GOLDSMITH GA: Experimental niacin deficiency. J Am Dietetic Assoc 32:312, 1956
HENDERSON LM: Niacin. Ann Rev Nutr 3:289, 1983
JUKES TH et al: The conquest of pellagra. Fed Proc 40:1519, 1980
LEVY HL: Hartnup disorder, in *The Metabolic Basis of Inherited Disease*, 6th ed, CR Scriver et al (eds). New York, McGraw-Hill, 1989, p 2515

Thiamine deficiency

BROWN GM: Biogenesis and metabolism of thiamine, in *Metabolic Pathways*, 3d ed, DM Greenberg (ed). New York, Academic, 1970, p 369

DURAN M, WADMAN SK: Thiamine-responsive inborn errors of metabolism. J Inherited Metab Dis 8(Suppl 1):70, 1985

DYCKNER T et al: Aggravation of thiamine deficiency by magnesium depletion. Acta Med Scand 218:129, 1985

HAAS RH: Thiamin and the brain. Annu Rev Nutr 8:483, 1988

HARPER CG et al: Clinical signs in the Wernicke-Korsakoff complex: A retrospective analysis of 131 cases diagnosed at necropsy. J Neurol Neurosurg Psychiatry 49:341, 1986

HOYUMPA AM: Mechanisms of thiamine deficiency in chronic alcoholism. Am J Clin Nutr 33:2750, 1980

KAWAI C et al: Reappearance of beriberi heart disease in Japan. Am J Med 69:383, 1980

KOZAM RL et al: Cardiovascular beriberi. Am J Cardiol 30:418, 1972

KURIYAMA M et al: Blood vitamin B₁, transketolase, and thiamine pyrophosphate (TPP) effect in beriberi patients. Clin Chim Acta 108:159, 1980

VICTOR M et al: *The Wernicke-Korsakoff Syndrome.* Philadelphia, Davis, 1971

ZIPORIN ZZ et al: Excretion of thiamine and its metabolites in the urine of young adult males receiving restricted intakes of the vitamin. J Nutr 85:287, 1965

Pyridoxine deficiency

BASSIER KH: Megavitamin therapy with pyridoxine. Int J Vitam Nutr Res 58:105, 1988

BHAGAVAN HN, BRIN M: Drug–vitamin B₆ interaction. Curr Concepts Nutr 12:1, 1983

GERSHOFF SN: Vitamin B₆, in *Nutrition Reviews' Present Knowledge in Nutrition*, 4th ed, DM Hegsted et al (eds). Washington, The Nutrition Foundation, 1976, p 149

HARRIS JW, HORRIGAN DL: Pyridoxine-responsive anemia-prototype and variations on the theme, in *Vitamins and Hormones*, vol 22, RS Harris et al (eds). New York, Academic, 1964, p 721

LUHBY AL et al: Vitamin B₆ metabolism in users of oral contraceptive agents: I. Abnormal urinary xanthurenic acid excretion and its correction by pyridoxine. Am J Clin Nutr 24:684, 1971

ROSS EA et al: Vitamin B₆ requirements of patients on chronic peritoneal dialysis. Kidney Int 36:702, 1989

SAUBERLICH HE et al: Biochemical assessment of the nutritional status of vitamin B₆ in the human. Am J Clin Nutr 25:629, 1972

YOUNG RC, BASS JP: Iatrogenic nutritional deficiencies. Annu Rev Nutr 2:201, 1982

Riboflavin deficiency

BATES CJ: Human riboflavin requirements, and metabolic consequences of deficiency in man and animals. World Rev Nutr Diet 50:215, 1987

MERRILL AH JR et al: Formation and mode of action of flavoproteins. Annu Rev Nutr 1:281, 1981

PINTO JT, RIVLIN RS: Drugs that promote renal excretion of riboflavin. Drug Nutr Interact 5:143, 1987

——— et al: Mechanisms underlying the differential effects of ethanol on the bioavailability of riboflavin and flavin adenine dinucleotide. J Clin Invest 79:1343, 1987

Ascorbic acid deficiency

BARNESS LA: Nutritional aspects of vegetarianism, health foods, and fad diets. Nutr Rev 59:153, 1977

BOXER LA et al: Correction of leucocyte function in Chédiak-Higashi syndrome by ascorbate. N Engl J Med 295:1041, 1971

BURNS JJ et al: Third conference on vitamin C. Ann NY Acad Sci 498, 1987

ENGLAND S, SEIFTER S: The biochemical functions of ascorbic acid. Annu Rev Nutr 6:365, 1986

FRANCESCHI RT: The role of ascorbic acid in mesenchymal differentiation. Nutr Rev 50:65, 1992

HODGES RE et al: Clinical manifestations of ascorbic acid deficiency in man. Am J Clin Nutr 24:432, 1971

LEVINE M: New concepts in the biology and biochemistry of ascorbic acid. N Engl J Med 314:892, 1986

PADH H: Vitamin C: Newer insights into its biochemical functions. Nutr Rev 49:65, 1991

REID GM: Scurvy: Old disease—New insight. Med Hypotheses 12:167, 1983

REULER JB et al: Adult scurvy. JAMA 253:805, 1985

SATO P, UNDENFRIEND S: Studies on ascorbic acid related to the genetic basis of scurvy, in *Vitamins and Hormones*, vol 36, P Munson et al (eds). New York, Academic, 1978, p 33

TOLBERT BM et al: New information on synthesis and metabolism of ascorbic acid. Nutr Rev 35:22, 1977

VILTER RW: Effects of ascorbic acid deficiency in man, in *The Vitamins*, WH Sebrell Jr et al (eds). New York, Academic, 1967, vol 1, p 457

WALLERSTEIN RO, WALLERSTEIN RO JR: Scurvy. Sem Hematol 13:211, 1976

Biotin

MARSHALL MM: The nutritional importance of biotin—An update. Nutr Today 22:26, 1987

MOCK DM et al: Effects of biotin deficiency on serum fatty acid composition: Evidence for abnormalities in humans. J Nutr 188:342, 1988

SWEETMAN L, NYHAN WL: Inheritable biotin-treatable disorders and associated phenomena. Annu Rev Nutr 6:317, 1986

WOLF B et al: Biotinidase deficiency: Initial clinical features and rapid diagnosis. Ann Neurol 18:614, 1985

Vitamin A deficiency

BARCLAY AJG et al: Vitamin A supplements and mortality related to measles: A randomised clinical trial. Br Med J 294:294, 1987

DELUCA LM: The direct involvement of vitamin A in glycosyl transfer reactions of mammalian membranes, in *Vitamins and Hormones*, vol 35, PL Munson et al (eds). New York, Academic, 1977, p 1

GIGUERE V et al: Identification of a receptor for the morphogen retinoic acid. Nature 330:624, 1987

GOODMAN DS: Vitamin A and retinoids in health and disease. N Engl J Med 310:1023, 1984

HOWARD L et al: Vitamin A deficiency from long-term parenteral nutrition. Ann Intern Med 93:576, 1980

SAUBERLICH HE et al: Vitamin A metabolism and requirements in the human studied with the use of labeled retinol, in *Vitamins and Hormones*, vol 32, RS Harris et al (eds). New York, Academic, 1974

SMITH FR, GOODMAN DS: Vitamin A transport in human vitamin A toxicity. N Engl J Med 294:805, 1976

SOMMER A: New imperatives for an old vitamin (A). J Nutr 119:96, 1989

TIELSCH JM, SOMMER A: The epidemiology of vitamin A deficiency and xerophthalmia. Annu Rev Nutr 4:183, 1974

VAHLQUIST A: Clinical use of vitamin A and its derivatives—Physiological and pharmacological aspects. Clin Exp Dermatol 10:133, 1985

Vitamin A for measles. Lancet 1:1067, 1987

WALD G: Molecular basis of visual excitation. Science 162:230, 1968

Vitamin E deficiency

BIERI JG et al: Medical uses of vitamin E. N Engl J Med 308:1063, 1983

HORWITT MK: Interrelations between vitamin E and polyunsaturated fatty acids in adult men, in *Vitamins and Hormones*, vol 20, GF Marrian, KV Thimann (eds). New York, Academic, 1962, p 541

LLOYD JK: The importance of vitamin E in human nutrition. Acta Paediatr Scand 79:6, 1990

PERLMUTTER DH et al: Intramuscular vitamin E repletion in children with chronic cholestasis. Am J Dis Child 141:170, 1987

SITRIN MD et al: Vitamin E deficiency and neurologic disease in adults with cystic fibrosis. Ann Intern Med 107:51, 1987

SOKOL RJ et al: Vitamin E deficiency with normal serum vitamin E concentrations in children with chronic cholestasis. N Engl J Med 310:1209, 1984

——— et al: Isolated vitamin E deficiency in the absence of fat malabsorption—familial and sporadic cases: Characterization and investigation of causes. J Lab Clin Med 111:548, 1988

——— et al: Intestinal malabsorption of vitamin E in primary biliary cirrhosis. Gastroenterology 96:479, 1989

TRABER MG et al: Lack of tocopherol in peripheral nerves of vitamin E–deficient patients with peripheral neuropathy. N Engl J Med 317:262, 1987

Vitamin K deficiency

BERTINA RM et al: New method for the rapid detection of vitamin K deficiency. Clin Chim Acta 105:93, 1980

DOISY EA JR, MATSCHINER JT: Biochemistry of vitamin K, in *Fat-Soluble Vitamins*, vol 9, RA Morton (ed). Elmsford, NY, Pergamon, 1970, p 293

IBER FL et al: Vitamin K deficiency in chronic alcoholic males. Alcoholism (NY) 10:679, 1986

OLSON RE, SUTTIE JW: Vitamin K and α-carboxyglutamate biosynthesis, in *Vitamins and Hormones*, vol 35, PL Munson et al (eds). New York, Academic, 1977, p 59

SHEARER MJ et al: Studies on the absorption and metabolism of phylloquinone (vitamin K) in man, in *Vitamins and Hormones*, vol 32, RS Harris et al (eds). New York, Academic, 1974, p 513

SUTTIE JW: *Vitamin K Metabolism and Vitamin K-Dependent Proteins.* Baltimore, University Park Press, 1988

SUTTIE JW et al: Vitamin K deficiency from dietary vitamin K restriction in humans. Am J Clin Nutr 47:475, 1988

Vitamin excess

ALHADEFF L: Toxic effects of water-soluble vitamins. Nutr Rev 42:33, 1984

CHALMERS TC: Effects of ascorbic acid on the common cold. Am J Med 58:532, 1975

CORRIGAN JJ JR: The effect of vitamin E on warfarin-induced vitamin K deficiency. Ann NY Acad Sci 82:361, 1982

DALTON K, DALTON MJT: Characteristics of pyridoxine overdose neuropathy syndrome. Acta Neurol Scand 76:8, 1987

LEMONS JA, MAISELS MJ: Vitamin E—How much is too much? Pediatrics 76:625, 1985

LOMBAERT A, CARTON H: Benign intracranial hypertension due to A-hypervitaminosis in adults and adolescents. Eur Neurol 14:340, 1976

LORCH V et al: Unusual syndrome with fatalities among premature infants: Association with a new intravenous vitamin E product. Morb Mort Week Rep 33:198, 1984

MOSS AJ et al: Use of vitamin and mineral supplements in the United States. Advance Data No. 174. Hyattsville, Md: National Center for Health Statistics, 1989

SCHAUMBURG H et al: Sensory neuropathy from pyridoxine abuse: A new megavitamin syndrome. N Engl J Med 309:445, 1983

SHIN HB et al: Ascorbic acid–induced uricosuria: A consequence of megavitamin therapy. Ann Intern Med 84:385, 1976

Toxic effects of vitamin overdosage. Med Lett Drugs Ther 26:73, 1984

WOOLLISCROFT JO: Megavitamins: Fact and fancy. Dis-A-Month 24:1, 1983

78 DISTURBANCES IN TRACE ELEMENT METABOLISM

KENNETH H. FALCHUK

CLASSIFICATION AND FUNCTIONS The "trace elements" comprise metals in biologic fluids at concentrations <1 µg/g wet weight. Most are essential nutrients for humans (Table 78-1). Others (As, Ni, Sn, V, Si) are essential for some species and may be required by humans. The functions of trace elements and of more abundant metals (Na, K, Ca, Mg) are determined, in part, by their charges, mobilities, and binding constants to biologic ligands. Elements in one group (Na, K) bind weakly to negatively charged ligands and can cross cellular membranes without major impediment. They are used by living systems as charge carriers to conduct electric impulses along nerves, etc. Those in a second group (Mg, Ca) form moderately stable complexes with enzymes, nucleic acids, and other ligands. They act as biochemical "triggers," altering and/or controlling the functions of these molecules, e.g., Ca affects muscle contraction and relaxation (Chap. 385). Those in a third group (Fe, Zn, Cu, and others) form strong, static complexes with and become integral functional components of enzymes (Table 78-1).

METAL DEFICIENCY OR TOXICITY Metals can cause disease through deficiency, imbalance, or toxicity. Deficiency usually results when dietary intake is inadequate or when intake is adequate but other conditioning factors come into play. Deficiencies can be caused by metal malabsorption in chronic diarrheal diseases, surgical resection of the small intestine, or formation of metal complexes with dietary components that are not readily absorbed, e.g., between phytates and Zn. Deficiency states also can result from increased losses through urine, pancreatic juice, or other exocrine secretions or from metabolic imbalances produced by antagonistic or synergistic interactions between metals. Large amounts of Ca, for example, decrease the absorption and induce deficiency of Zn. Zinc supplements in excess of 10 times the recommended daily allowance cause a conditioned deficiency of copper including anemia. Similarly, Mo and Cu compete with each other; excessive Mo in cattle leads to Cu deficiency characterized by diarrhea and wasting. Trace element deficiencies in humans, except for iron, were previously thought to be rare but have been recognized more frequently with the use of total parenteral nutrition (TPN) (Chap. 76). Criteria for the recognition of deficiency states include decreases in metal content of whole blood, serum, hair and/or other accessible fluids and tissues, changes in the activities of metalloenzymes, and characteristic signs and symptoms (Table 78-2).

Toxic effects are dependent on the chemical form, the amount ingested, the route of entry into the body, the biologic ligands bound by the metal, the tissue distribution, the concentration achieved, and the excretion rate. Mechanisms of toxicity include inhibition of enzyme activity by binding to essential amino acid residues, alterations in nucleic acid function and structure, impairment in protein synthesis, effects on membrane permeability, and inhibition of phosphorylation, among others. Metal toxicity in patients undergoing chronic renal dialysis is important because of the frequency and severity of the resulting problems and because of the number of metals involved, e.g., Al, Zn, Cu, Ni, and Sn (Chap. 238). For example, even when present only in trace amounts in dialysis fluids, Al is readily absorbed into blood and accumulates in brain, bone, and erythroid tissues, causing disabling neurologic, skeletal, and hematologic disorders. These include malaise, memory loss, asterixis, dementia, twitches, and other manifestations of metabolic encephalopathy, including seizures and death. Osteomalacia unresponsive to vitamin D, fractures, muscular pain, weakness, and anemia may occur. Documentation of increase in plasma Al concentration following deferoxamine administration is diagnostic.

DISORDERS OF METABOLISM OF SPECIFIC METALS **Zinc** Absorption of Zn in the small intestine is decreased by fibers, phytate, phosphate, Ca, and Cu and increased by amino acids, peptides, iodoquinol and other chelating agents. Excretion of Zn occurs principally through secretions of the pancreas and intestine. Nearly 99 percent of total-body Zn is inside cells, the remainder in plasma

TABLE 78-1 **Requirements and functions of trace elements in humans**

Element	Requirements, mg/d*	Amount[†] Total, g/70 kg body weight	Serum µmol/L	Serum µg/dL	Selected biochemical functions	Enzymes Class	Enzymes Examples
Fe	10–20	4.0	18	100	Oxygen transport	Oxidoreductases	Cytochrome oxidase
Zn	15–20	3.0	15	100	Nucleic acid and protein synthesis and degradation, alcohol metabolism	Transferases, hydrolases, lyases, isomerases, ligases, oxidoreductases, transcription factors	RNA polymerases, alcohol dehydrogenases, glucocorticoid receptor
Cu	2–6	0.25	16	100	Hemoglobin synthesis, connective tissue metabolism, bone development	Oxidoreductases	Superoxide dismutase, ferroxidase (ceruloplasmin)
Co	0.0001	1.1	0.0001	0.0007	Methionine metabolism	Transferases	Homocysteine methyltransferase
Mn	2–5	0.02	0.001	0.06	Oxidative phosphorylation; fatty acid, mucopolysaccharide, and cholesterol metabolism	Oxidoreductases, hydrolases, ligases	Diamine oxidase, pyruvate carboxylase
Mo	0.15–0.5	0.07	0.007	0.07	Xanthine metabolism	Oxidoreductases	Xanthine oxidase
Se	0.05–0.2	(−)	1.6	13	Antioxidant	Oxidoreductases, transferases	Glutathione peroxidase
Ni	(−)	(−)	0.02	0.01	?Stabilizing RNA structure	Oxidoreductases, hydrolases	Urease
Cr	0.005–0.2	0.0006	0.004	0.02	?Binding of insulin to cells, glucose metabolism		

* Requirements may differ for different age groups and physiologic states, e.g., pregnancy.
[†] Reported normal values vary owing to differences in sample preparation, analytical instruments, and small quantities present in biologic materials.
(−), Reported values variable or not available.

TABLE 78-2   Disorders of metal metabolism in humans

Element	Deficiency	Toxicity*
Fe	Anemia	Hepatic failure, diabetes, testicular atrophy, arthritis, cardiomyopathy, peripheral neuropathy, hyperpigmentation
Zn	Growth retardation, alopecia, dermatitis, diarrhea, immunologic dysfunction, failure to thrive, psychological disturbances, gonadal atrophy, impaired spermatogenesis, congenital malformations	Gastric ulcer, pancreatitis, lethargy, anemia, fever, nausea, vomiting, respiratory distress, pulmonary fibrosis
Cu	Anemia, growth retardation, defective keratinization and pigmentation of hair, hypothermia, degenerative changes in aortic elastin, mental deterioration, scurvy-like changes in skeleton	Hepatitis, cirrhosis, tremor, mental deterioration, Kayser-Fleischer rings, hemolytic anemia, renal dysfunction (Fanconi-like syndrome)
Mn	Bleeding disorder (increased prothrombin time)	Encephalitis-like syndrome, Parkinson-like syndrome, psychosis, pneumoconiosis
Co	Anemia (B_{12} deficiency)	Cardiomyopathy, goiter
Mo	?Esophageal cancer	?Hyperuricemia
Cr	? Impairment of glucose tolerance	Renal failure, dermatitis (occupational), pulmonary cancer
Se	Cardiomyopathy, congestive heart failure, striated muscle degeneration	Alopecia, abnormal nails, emotional lability, lassitude, garlic odor to breath
Ni	?	Dermatitis (occupational), lung and nasal carcinomas, liver necrosis, pulmonary inflammation
Si	? Impaired early bone development	Pulmonary inflammation, granuloma, fibrosis
F	? Impaired bone and dental structure	Mottled dental enamel, nausea, abdominal pain, vomiting, diarrhea, tetany, cardiovascular collapse

* Symptoms are dependent on route of entry and tissue distribution (see text).

and extracellular fluids. Serum Zn, approximately 70 percent of which is bound to albumin and other proteins, is the source of metal for cellular needs. Serum Zn content is fairly constant, but small diurnal variations may occur. It decreases when intake or absorption is reduced (e.g., in regional enteritis) or when urinary losses are increased (e.g., in nephrotic syndrome, in cirrhosis of the liver or other hypoalbuminemic states, during the administration of penicillamine or other chelating agents, in high catabolic states as after trauma, burns, or surgery, and in hemolytic anemias and sickle cell disease). Plasma Zn also decreases with acute myocardial infarction, infections, malignancies, hepatitis, and other diseases. The decreases may be due to redistribution from plasma to tissues and are probably mediated by ACTH, cortisol, and/or cytokines (interleukins 2 and 6). Clinical deficiency may follow these decreases in serum content. The Zn requirement of the developing fetus, pregnant woman, and growing child or adolescent is higher than that of adult men or nonpregnant women. Therefore, the former groups are more susceptible to Zn depletion. Zn deficiency in pregnant animals can lead to fetal Zn deficiency, manifested by high mortality rates or congenital malformations of nearly all organ systems. Zinc deficiency has not been described in pregnant women but has been reported in adolescents who eat dirt, in patients who receive TPN without supplemental Zn

(see Chap. 76), and in patients with the autosomal recessive defect acrodermatitis enteropathica. In the latter disease, Zn deficiency may be the consequence of a defect in Zn absorption. The onset of symptoms often occurs when an affected infant is weaned from human to cow's milk. Zn also may play a role in the maintenance of normal taste and in wound healing.

Tissues with a high cellular turnover, including skin, gastrointestinal mucosa, chondrocytes, spermatogonia, and thymocytes are characteristically affected (Table 78-2). The dermatologic manifestations (hyperkeratosis, parakeratosis, acrodermatitis, and alopecia) call attention to the possibility of Zn deficiency. The usual distribution of the keratotic lesions is in areas that are readily traumatized (elbows, knees), but the lesions can develop in other areas as well. The keratotic lesions can become pustular or crusting, red, scaly plaques. Immunologic defects of T cell function are typical. The ability to mount an immunologic response to parasites is reduced. Superinfections are common with either fungi or bacteria.

Toxicity follows inhalation of Zn fumes (by welders), oral ingestion, or intravenous administration. Inhalation of high concentrations of zinc oxide fumes leads to an acute illness called *metal-fume fever* or *brass chills*, manifested by fever, chills, excessive salivation, headaches, cough, and leukocytosis. Dialysis fluids can be contaminated with Zn from the adhesive plaster used on the dialysis coils or from galvanized pipes. The toxic syndrome associated with hemodialysis is characterized by anemia, fever, and central nervous system disturbances (Table 78-2). Toxic amounts of Zn decrease chemotaxis, phagocytosis, pinocytosis, and platelet aggregation.

Copper   The liver, kidney, heart, and brain contain the highest amounts of Cu. Over 90 percent of plasma Cu is associated with ceruloplasmin, and 60 percent of that in red blood cells is bound to superoxide dismutase. The major excretory pathway is through the bile. The serum Cu concentration is normally constant. Increases occur in patients with acute myocardial infarction, leukemia, solid tumors, infections, cirrhosis of the liver, hemochromatosis, thyrotoxicosis, and connective tissue disorders. The consequences of the increases are unknown. Decreases occur in the nephrotic syndrome, kwashiorkor, the hepatolenticular degeneration of Wilson's disease (see Chap. 348), severe diarrheal diseases with malabsorption, and other conditions associated with increased excretion or decreased synthesis of ceruloplasmin. Premature infants who are fed diets deficient in Cu develop decreased serum ceruloplasmin and Cu levels, anemia, osteopenia, skin and hair depigmentation, and psychomotor retardation. Cu deficiency in subjects receiving TPN causes anemia and neutropenia.

A more complex disorder of Cu metabolism occurs in Menkes' disease, an X-linked recessive disorder (see also Chap. 353). Intestinal Cu uptake is normal, and tissue Cu content varies; that of intestinal, kidney, and skin (fibroblast) cells is normal or high, while that of serum, liver, brain, and (likely) vascular cells is low. Ceruloplasmin content and the activities of some Cu enzymes (e.g., connective tissue amine oxidases) are decreased. The clinical picture is similar to that of Cu deficiency in animals except that anemia does not occur (Table 78-2). The patients have kinky hair, and decreased amounts of mature collagen and elastin cause dissecting aneurysms, sudden cardiac rupture, emphysema, and osteoporosis. Death usually occurs in the first 5 years of life.

Excessive oral intake of Cu or hemodialysis with water contaminated with Cu is toxic. The acute symptoms include hemolytic anemia, nausea, vomiting, and diarrhea. The renal and hepatic failure and the central nervous system disorders that eventually develop (Table 78-2) are typical of the Cu toxicity syndrome in Wilson's disease (see Chap. 348).

Cobalt   Co is a component of vitamin B_{12}, and deficiency syndromes are those associated with deficiency of the vitamin (see Chap. 304). Pharmacologic amounts of Co induce erythropoiesis. Chronic administration blocks iodine uptake by the thyroid, resulting in development of goiter.

Cardiomyopathy, congestive heart failure with pericardial effusions, polycythemia, thyroid enlargement, and neurologic abnormalities have been reported as manifestations of Co toxicity in drinkers of beer to which the metal had been added as a foam stabilizer. Co accumulates in the heart, forms a complex with lipoic acid, and interferes with decarboxylation reactions critical to both pyruvate and fatty acid metabolism.

Manganese Mn acts both as an activator of enzymes and as a component of metalloenzymes (Table 78-1). Defects of the skeletal, central nervous, and gonadal systems occur in Mn deficiency in animals. Humans obtain sufficient Mn from normal dietary intake so that a deficiency syndrome is rare. Increase in prothrombin time, unresponsive to vitamin K, has been noted. In serum, Mn is bound to transmanganin. Mn is excreted primarily in bile and pancreatic secretions.

Serum Mn increases following myocardial infarction and decreases in children with convulsive disorders. Miners who inhale large quantities of Mn dust over long periods of time develop asthenia, anorexia, apathy, headache, impotence, leg cramps, speech disturbances, and occasionally even more severe symptoms (Table 78-2).

Selenium As a component of glutathione peroxidase, Se plays a critical role in the control of oxygen metabolism, particularly in catalyzing the breakdown of H_2O_2. The metal is required for the growth of human fibroblasts and other cells in tissue culture. Furthermore, Se cures or prevents Keshan disease, a syndrome endemic to Keshan Province in China, where the soil may be deficient in the metal. Keshan disease is characterized by multifocal myocardial necrosis and reduced serum Se content. The clinical severity varies from severe arrhythmias and cardiogenic shock to a mild form with cardiac enlargement as the only significant finding. Peripheral myopathies may develop as a consequence of muscle degeneration (Table 78-2). Children and women of childbearing age are particularly susceptible. Se protects animals from a number of carcinogenic chemicals and viruses; a role in human cancer prevention is not established. Se binds Cd, Hg, and other metals and mitigates their toxic effects, even though tissue levels of the metals remain elevated. Se poisoning has been reported due to ingestion of water containing large amounts of the metal.

Other trace elements *Silicon* is present in bone and skin and may play a role in the cross-linkage of collagen. Deficiency in animals results in decreased growth, abnormal bone development, and decreased hexosamine content of epiphyses and epiphyseal plates. Deficiency in humans has not been described. Inhalation of fine particles of SiO_2 causes granuloma formation and fibrosis (silicosis) of the lungs (see Chap. 219).

Fluoride is a constituent of teeth and bone. It prevents dental caries, and its use in patients with osteoporosis may result in increased mineralized bone (see Chap. 362). Complications of long-term ingestion by such patients include calcification of bony ligaments and tendons. Chronic intake of fluorides also causes fluorosis, a syndrome characterized by weakness, weight loss, anemia, brittle bones, and mottling of teeth (if taken during stages of enamel formation). Acute ingestion of toxic amounts, as found in some insect poisons, causes severe abdominal pain, nausea, vomiting, diarrhea, and hypocalcemia. Eventually, tetany and cardiorespiratory arrest occur.

Deficiencies of *arsenic, nickel, tin,* or *vanadium* cause pathologic manifestations in plants and some vertebrates. Their roles in human health are undefined.

REFERENCES

FALCHUK KH: Effect of acute disease and ACTH on serum zinc proteins. N Engl J Med 296:1129, 1977

KARCIOULU ZA, SARPER RM: *Zinc and Copper in Medicine*, Springfield, Ill., Charles C Thomas, 1980

Metabolic and physiological consequences of trace element deficiency in animals and man. Philos Trans R Soc Lond [Biol] 294:1, 1981

MILLINER DS et al: Use of the deferoxamine infusion test in the diagnosis of aluminum-related osteodystrophy. Ann Intern Med 101:775, 1984

PRASAD AS: *Trace Elements in Human Health and Disease*, vol 2. New York, Academic, 1976

REINHOLD JG: Trace elements—A selective survey. Clin Chem 21:476, 1975

TING-KAI L, VALLEE BL: The biochemical and nutritional roles of other trace elements, in *Modern Nutrition in Health and Disease*, 6th ed, RS Goodhart and ME Shils (eds). Philadelphia, Lea and Febiger, 1980

UNDERWOOD EJ: *Trace Elements in Human and Animal Nutrition*, 3d ed. New York, Academic, 1971

WILLIAMS RJP: The Tilden lecture. Q Rev Chem Soc (Lond) 24:331, 1970

section 1 Basic considerations in infectious disease

79 INTRODUCTION TO INFECTIOUS DISEASE: HOST-PARASITE INTERACTION

LAWRENCE C. MADOFF / DENNIS L. KASPER

Despite decades of dramatic progress in their treatment and prevention, infectious diseases remain a major cause of death and debility and are responsible for worsening the living conditions of many millions of people around the world. Infections, which must be considered in the differential diagnosis of syndromes affecting every organ system, frequently challenge the physician's diagnostic skill by involving a multitude of organ systems.

With the advent of antimicrobial agents, many people believed that infectious diseases would be relegated to medical history. Indeed, the years since World War II have seen the development of hundreds of chemotherapeutic agents, many of which are potent, safe, and effective not only against bacteria but also against viruses, fungi, and parasites. Yet we now realize that as antimicrobial agents developed, so did the ability of the microbes to elude our best strategies and to counterattack with their own strategies for survival. Antibiotic resistance occurs at an alarming rate among all classes of mammalian pathogens. Diseases once thought to have been nearly eradicated from the developed world—tuberculosis and rheumatic fever, for example—have rebounded with a new ferocity. Recently discovered and emerging infectious agents—the Lyme disease spirochete, the AIDS retrovirus, the hepatitis C virus, and the rickettsia causing ehrlichiosis—humble us even as our understanding of pathogenesis at the most basic, molecular level deepens. The role of infectious agents in the etiology of diseases once believed to be noninfectious is being increasingly recognized. For example, *Helicobacter pylori* has recently been shown to play a role in the development of gastrointestinal ulcers and perhaps malignancy. The possibility certainly exists that other diseases of unknown cause, such as rheumatoid arthritis, sarcoidosis, or inflammatory bowel disease, may in fact be infectious.

Medical advances over infectious diseases have been hindered by changes in the patient population. Immunocompromised hosts now constitute a significant proportion of the population who are being treated for infectious diseases. Physicians immunosuppress their patients to prevent the rejection of transplants and to treat neoplastic and inflammatory diseases. Some infections, most notably that caused by human immunodeficiency virus (HIV), immunocompromise the host. Lesser degrees of immunosuppression are associated with other infections, such as influenza and syphilis. Aging of and malnutrition in the host tip the survival balance toward the infecting pathogen. Implantable devices such as heart valves, automatic defibrillators, pacemakers, prosthetic joints, indwelling intravenous catheters, and ventriculoperitoneal shunts all provide foci predisposed to infection; many infections associated with implantable devices are difficult or impossible to cure without removal of the foreign hardware. Infectious agents that coexist peacefully with the immunocompetent hosts wreak havoc in those who lack a complete immune system. AIDS has brought to prominence once-obscure organisms such as *Pneumocystis carinii*, *Cryptosporidium parvum*, and *Mycobacterium avium*. Thus the understanding of infectious diseases remains crucial and ever-changing.

For any infectious process to occur, the parasite and the host must first encounter each other. Factors such as geography, environment, and behavior thus influence the likelihood of infection. Some organisms can be harbored in the host for years before disease becomes clinically evident. A detailed history, including information on travel, behavioral factors, exposures to animals or potentially contaminated environments, and living and occupational conditions, must be elicited and considered in the evaluation of a patient in whom infection is suspected. For example, the likelihood of infection by *Plasmodium falciparum* can be significantly affected by altitude, climate, terrain, season, and even time of day. Certain antibiotic-resistant strains are localized to specific geographic regions, and a seemingly minor alteration in a travel itinerary can dramatically influence the likelihood of acquiring chloroquine-resistant malaria. If such important details in the history are overlooked, inappropriate treatment may result in the death of the patient. Likewise, the chance of acquiring a sexually transmitted disease can be dramatically affected by relatively minor variation in sexual practices, such as the method used for birth control. Knowledge of the relationship between specific risk factors and disease allows the physician to influence a patient's health even before the development of infection by modifying these factors and administering appropriate vaccines.

Many specific host factors influence the likelihood of acquiring an infectious disease. Age, immunization history, prior illnesses, level of nutrition, pregnancy status, coexisting illness, and perhaps emotional state all have some impact on the risk of infection after exposure to a potential pathogen. The importance of individual host defense mechanisms, either specific or nonspecific, becomes apparent in their absence, and our understanding of these immune mechanisms is enhanced by studies of clinical syndromes developing in immunodeficient patients. For example, the frequent occurrence of meningococcal disease in people with deficiencies in specific complement proteins of the "membrane attack complex" underscores the importance of an intact complement system for preventing meningococcal infection.

Medical care itself increases the risk of acquiring an infection in several ways: (1) through contact with pathogens during hospitalization; (2) through breaching the skin (with intravenous devices or surgical incisions) or mucosal surfaces (with endotracheal tubes or bladder catheters); (3) through introduction of foreign bodies; (4)

through alteration of the natural flora with antibiotics; and (5) through treatment with immunosuppressive drugs.

Infection involves complicated interactions of parasite and host, inevitably affecting both. In most cases, several steps in the pathogenic process are required for the development of infection. Since the competent host has a complex series of barricades in place to prevent infection, the successful parasite must utilize specific strategies at each of these steps. The specific strategies used by bacteria (see Chap. 99), viruses (see Chap. 141), and parasites (see Chap. 170) have some remarkable conceptual similarities, but the strategic details are unique for each organism.

SURFACE CONTACT   Most often, the first contact between host and parasite is at a mucosal or cutaneous surface. In order to prevent the initiation of the infectious process during such contact, the host has developed highly effective defense mechanisms operating at the body's interface with the outside world. Many of these initial mechanisms of host defense are not specifically directed at individual species of organisms. Mechanical barriers, for example, including the tough cornified epithelium of the skin and the flow of secretions from glands tend to prevent infection by any potential pathogen. Chemical barriers, such as the acidic environment of the stomach and urinary bladder, represent hostile environments for most microorganisms. The normal microflora, composed of nonpathogenic organisms that inhabit mucosal surfaces, make colonization by pathogens more difficult by competing for environmental resources. Behavioral and neurologic mechanisms, such as gagging and coughing, help prevent infection of the lower respiratory tract.

We recognize the importance of these mechanisms when we observe the diseases that arise when they are impaired. Patients with suppressed coughing (for example, due to pain associated with a fractured rib) are very susceptible to pneumonia. Achlorhydric individuals are particularly likely to develop salmonellosis after the ingestion of contaminated food or drink because a lower inoculum is required. The abnormal bronchial secretions in cystic fibrosis usually lead to chronic pulmonary infection with *Pseudomonas aeruginosa*. A break in the skin resulting from an animal or insect bite, a burn, a scratch, trauma, or surgery allows the entry of pathogenic or opportunistic agents. The eradication of the normal bowel flora by antibiotics may render organisms such as *Clostridium difficile* pathogenic.

The host has also evolved an organism-specific immune system that functions at mucosal surfaces. Specialized macrophages and lymphocytes, which play a role in the specific defense system, reside in the epithelium of the gut, in the nasal mucosa, and at other sites that interface with the environment. This mucosa-associated lymphoid tissue appears to play a role in trapping antigens and allowing them to be presented to lymphocytes at the mucosal barrier. In certain areas, these tissues become recognizable anatomically; examples include the oropharyngeal tonsils, and—in the gastrointestinal tract—Peyer's patches and the appendix. Central to this defense system is the elaboration of surface immunoglobulins, particularly secretory IgA, which prevents adherence and penetration of organisms.

Pathogens have evolved an array of methods for breaching this well-developed boundary between the host and the outside world. In order to invade, most pathogens must first attach. Many microorganisms have developed a highly specialized apparatus for binding to the surface of the host. For example, pili of uropathogenic *Escherichia coli* recognize certain host glycoproteins that serve as sites for attachment to epithelial cells. The binding of Epstein-Barr virus to a specific complement receptor (CR2) on B lymphocytes allows the subsequent internalization of the virus. HIV binds to the CD4 complex present in certain human T lymphocytes. Many bacterial pathogens produce enzymes or surface components that bind to or inactivate secretory IgA. Others impair ciliary motility thus hindering their own clearance by this mechanism.

Some potentially pathogenic organisms are capable of living symbiotically with the host, colonizing but not infecting for extended periods. It is important for the astute clinician to distinguish coloniza-

tion from infection. *E. coli* are normally present in large numbers in the colon. At this site, these organisms are certainly harmless and may even be beneficial to the normal healthy host, contributing to the synthesis of vitamin K and inducing natural immunity to other gram-negative bacteria. It is only when *E. coli* penetrate the normal mucosal barriers and enter another site that they become opportunists and cause disease. The penetration of *E. coli* into the peritoneum through a mechanical breach in the bowel wall, their entry into the urinary bladder, and their invasion of the bloodstream are events associated with infection and disease. Some virulent pathogens, such as group A streptococci and *Neisseria meningitidis,* are able to colonize most individuals for prolonged intervals without untoward effects. In these cases the colonized individuals may already have developed specific immunity to the organism, or invasion may be prevented by nonspecific host defenses while specific immunity is being stimulated. Certain viruses (e.g., herpesviruses) inhabit tissue for the life of the host, causing little harm as long as the host's immune system is intact but inducing severe symptomatic disease if the immune status is altered.

INVASION   Microorganisms attached to a mucosal surface use specific mechanisms to invade deeper host structures. Meningococci and gonococci penetrate the mucosal barrier after engulfment by mucosal epithelial cells. *Haemophilus influenzae* penetrate by squeezing through the junction between epithelial cells. Salmonellae induce the host's gastrointestinal macrophages (i.e., in Peyer's patches) to engulf and phagocytose them; these bacteria then resist killing by the phagolysosome of the unactivated macrophage and subsequently proliferate, spilling into the bloodstream. Schistosomal cercariae enter the epidermis of hosts exposed to contaminated fresh water; in the presence of a specific host, they are able to uncoat, mature, and enter the circulation. Other pathogens, including bacteria (e.g., *Rickettsia rickettsii* and *Yersinia pestis*), viruses (e.g., dengue and eastern equine encephalitis virus), and parasites (e.g., *Plasmodium* and *Trypanosoma*), may enlist the aid of an insect vector to breach the protective skin and enter the circulation.

Infection has a major impact on the microorganism as well as the host. It is increasingly recognized that the invading microbe senses and adapts to changes in its environment through complex regulatory mechanisms, "turning on" the virulence factors necessary for invasion and survival in the host. For example, *Yersinia* sp., *Shigella* sp., and *Bordetella pertussis* all express virulence factors in response to exposure to the 37°C temperature likely to be encountered at the time of infection. Other virulence determinants—the Shiga-like toxin of enterohemorrhagic *E. coli,* for example—are expressed in response to the low-free-iron conditions existing in the host, where iron is tightly bound by transferrin and other proteins. Many such bacterial virulence factors are controlled by two-component regulatory systems: one protein component senses environmental changes and signals (often by phosphorylation) a second protein which coordinately regulates the expression of a group of genes whose products facilitate survival in the host milieu.

Once in the bloodstream or a normally sterile body site, the microorganism faces the host's tightly integrated cellular and humoral immune systems. Cellular immunity (Chap. 277), comprising T lymphocytes, macrophages, and NK cells, primarily recognizes and combats pathogens that proliferate intracellularly. Cellular immune mechanisms are important in immunity to all classes of infectious agents, including most viruses and many bacteria (e.g., *Mycoplasma, Chlamydia, Listeria, Salmonella, Mycobacterium*), parasites (e.g., *Trypanosoma, Toxoplasma, Leishmania*), and fungi (e.g., *Histoplasma, Cryptococcus,* and *Coccidioides*). Usually, T lymphocytes are activated by macrophages and B lymphocytes, which present foreign antigens along with the host's own major histocompatibility complex antigen. Activated T cells may then act in several ways to fight infection. They may directly attack and lyse host cells that express foreign antigens. Some act as helper T cells to stimulate the proliferation of B cells and the production of immunoglobulins. They may elaborate cytokines (interferon, for example) which directly inhibit the growth of pathogens or stimulate killing by host macrophages and cytotoxic cells. Cytokines also augment host immunity by stimulating the inflammatory response (fever, the production of acute-phase serum components, and the proliferation of leukocytes). Cytokine stimulation does not always result in a favorable response in the host; septic shock (see Chap. 83) and toxic shock syndrome (see Chap. 102) are among the conditions that are mediated by these inflammatory substances.

Extracellular pathogens, including most encapsulated bacteria (e.g., streptococci, staphylococci, and pathogenic *E. coli*), are attacked by the humoral immune system, comprising primarily the complement cascade, antibodies, and phagocytic cells. Polymorphonuclear leukocytes (PMNs) are short-lived blood cells that engulf and kill invading microbes; these migratory cells are capable of finding sites of inflammation via chemotaxis and exiting the circulation into infected tissue. In order to efficiently localize at the site of inflammation, PMNs make use of cellular adhesion molecules elaborated by endothelial cells in response to inflammation. For example, endothelial cells respond to inflammatory cytokines by transiently expressing the selectin molecules CD62 and ELAM-1. The binding of these molecules to specific receptors on PMNs results in the adherence of the latter to the endothelium. Other adhesion molecules, such as ICAM-1, may then bind to β_2 integrins on the PMN and facilitate diapedesis into the extravascular compartment. Although PMNs are capable of killing microorganisms without help, they function much more efficiently when pathogens are first "opsonized" (from the Greek for "to prepare for eating") by components of the complement system and/or by antibodies.

Antibodies are complex glycoproteins, also called immunoglobulins (Ig), that are produced by mature B lymphocytes and circulate in body fluids. They specifically recognize and bind to foreign antigens. One of the most impressive features of the immune system is the ability to generate an incredible diversity of antibodies capable of recognizing virtually every foreign antigen yet not reacting with self. In addition to their antigen specificity, antibodies of different structural and functional classes exist: IgG predominates in the circulation and persists for many years after exposure; IgM is the earliest specific antibody to appear in response to infection; IgA is important in immunity at mucosal surfaces; and IgE is important in allergic and parasitic diseases. Antibodies may act by directly impeding the function of an invading organism, by neutralizing secreted toxins and enzymes, or by facilitating the removal of the parasite by phagocytic cells. Immunoglobulins participate in cell-mediated immunity by promoting antibody-dependent cellular cytotoxicity functions of certain T lymphocytes. Antibodies also promote the deposition of complement components on the surface of the invader.

The complement system consists of a group of serum proteins that function as a cooperative, self-regulating cascade of enzymes that adhere to—and in some cases disrupt—the surface of invading organisms. Some of these surface-adherent proteins (e.g., C3b) can then act as opsonins for destruction of microbes by phagocytes. The later, "terminal" components (C7, C8, and C9) can directly kill some bacterial invaders (notably, many of the neisseriae) by forming a "membrane attack complex" and spoiling the integrity of the bacterial membrane. Other complement components, such as C5a, act as chemoattractants for PMNs. Complement activation and deposition occurs by either or both of two pathways: the classic pathway is primarily activated by immune complexes (i.e., antibody bound to antigen), and the alternative pathway is activated by microbial components, frequently in the absence of antibody. PMNs have receptors for both antibody and C3b, and antibody and complement function together to aid in the clearance of infectious agents.

Microbes have developed a variety of strategies for overcoming host immunity. Many bacteria are encapsulated with polysaccharides that allow them to evade host defense mechanisms and proliferate freely until the host is able to generate capsule-specific antibodies. Group B *Streptococcus* and serogroups B and C meningococci have capsules containing the sugar sialic acid, whose presence on the bacterial surface gives the organism an advantage in evading nonspecific (nonantibody-dependent) clearance by the alternative pathway of complement. The sialic acid residue increases the affinity of binding of the complement regulatory protein factor H to C3b on the bacterial surface; C3b bound to factor H is susceptible to degradation by another complement regulatory protein, factor I. Therefore, surface sialic acid prevents the accumulation of quantities of C3b on the bacterial surface that are sufficient to initiate the killing of organisms in the absence of specific antibody. Several gram-positive bacteria possess surface proteins that bind immunoglobulins, perhaps interfering with immune recognition. Other organisms even employ the host immune response as a survival strategy. *Schistosoma mansoni* recognizes the host lymphokine tumor necrosis factor (TNF) and responds to it by depositing eggs.

TOXINS AND ENZYMES Some pathogenic organisms elaborate toxins and enzymes that facilitate invasion of the host and are often responsible for the disease state. Pathogenic strains of *Vibrio cholerae* elaborate a potent and well-characterized toxin that enters host enterocytes via a specific receptor (the monosialyl GM_1 ganglioside) and then enzymatically inactivates the host cell adenylate cyclase system. This event in turn leads to the copious electrolyte and fluid secretion by the enterocyte and the voluminous watery diarrhea that is characteristic of cholera. *Staphylococcus aureus* expresses a large number of extracellular proteins that contribute to the variety of disease states associated with this bacterium. Enterotoxins cause staphylococcal food poisoning even though viable organisms may never enter the host. Toxic shock syndrome toxin 1 is responsible for the many systemic effects of toxic shock syndrome even though host tissue barriers may remain intact. Damage to mucosal surfaces, mediated by toxins, may permit a pathogen to proliferate at a mucosal site whether or not the organism invades. Pertussis toxin impairs the ability of ciliated epithelium to clear the pathogen from the host bronchial tree. Enteropathogenic *E. coli* and *V. cholerae* are examples of toxin-producing bacteria that normally do not invade. In contrast, other toxins are clearly capable of promoting invasion and spread. The extracellular enzymes of *Streptococcus pyogenes*, such as hyaluronidase, facilitate movement through tissue planes, and streptolysins O and S disrupt leukocyte membranes and thus impair host defense.

Integral components of pathogens are often responsible for much of the disease process that results from infection. Lipopolysaccharides of gram-negative bacteria act as a potent endotoxin ("endo" in this case referring to the fact that they are part of the bacterial membrane, not a secreted product) that is the proximate cause of the syndrome of sepsis. The cell walls of gram-positive bacteria appear to elicit a similar host inflammatory response. The anaerobic pathogen *Bacteroides fragilis* possesses a capsular polysaccharide that promotes abscess formation by the host.

TROPISM In order to successfully infect a host, many pathogens occupy highly specific niches within the host and thus are tropic to a particular body site or cell type. This type of tropism has many implications for the life cycle of the pathogen, for the immune system of the host, and for the disease process. Malaria sporozoites, for example, are rapidly cleared from the blood into hepatocytes, where they undergo maturation and release into the circulation; trophozoites, in turn, can infect only the erythrocyte. The bacterial pathogen *Helicobacter pylori* produces the enzyme urease, which, by cleaving urea to form ammonium ion, may allow the organism to inhabit a neutral microenvironment within the highly acidic gastric epithelium. Many viruses are tropic for specific tissues; for example, the hepatitis viruses are tropic for hepatocytes, HIV for CD4-bearing T lymphocytes, herpesviruses for neural tissues, and rhinoviruses for the nasal epithelium.

The central nervous system is uniquely protected from perturbations in the environment by a blood-brain barrier—a system of tight junctions at capillaries within the CNS that resists the entry of inflammatory cells, pathogens, and even macromolecules into the subarachnoid space. Yet certain pathogens have devised highly specialized, and as yet poorly understood, mechanisms for breaching this barricade. One strategy employed by organisms such as rabies and herpes simplex viruses in humans and by reovirus in experimental animals is to travel within peripheral nerves into the CNS. Other organisms, such as certain highly encapsulated bacteria and fungi, enter from the bloodstream and possess surface components that allow them to traverse the capillary tight junctions. The degree of specialization required for this mechanism is demonstrated by the predilection of certain serotypes of organisms within a species to cause meningitis. The type III strains account for the vast majority of cases of meningitis caused by group B *Streptococcus,* even though other serotypes cause much of the invasive disease outside the CNS. This disparity appears to be due solely to the arrangement of the component sugars of the capsular polysaccharide: other serotypes of group B *Streptococcus* rarely cause meningitis even though their capsules possess the same four component sugars in different structural arrangements.

CLINICAL MANIFESTATIONS OF INFECTION The clinical manifestations of infectious diseases at presentation are myriad, varying from fulminant, life-threatening processes to brief and self-limited conditions to indolent, chronic maladies. The clinician must use all of the skills of medicine to diagnose and prescribe appropriate treatment. First, a careful history is essential and must include details on underlying chronic diseases, medications, occupation, travel, risk factors for exposure to certain types of pathogens, such as those associated with sexual contacts, illicit drug use, particular animals, or bites of insect vectors. Since infectious diseases may involve many organ systems, the review of systems may elicit important clues as to the disease process. The physical examination must be thorough, and attention must be paid to seemingly minor details: a soft heart murmur that might indicate bacterial endocarditis; an evanescent skin rash that suggests rheumatic fever; a retinal lesion that suggests disseminated candidiasis.

LABORATORY INVESTIGATIONS Laboratory studies must be carefully considered and directed toward establishing an etiologic diagnosis in the shortest possible time, at the lowest possible cost, and with the least possible discomfort to the patient. Cultures must be performed in a manner that minimizes the likelihood of contamination while maximizing the yield. A sputum sample is far more likely to be valuable when elicited with careful coaching by the clinician than when collected in a container simply left at the bedside with cursory instruction. Gram stains of specimens should be interpreted carefully and the quality of the specimen assessed. The findings on gram staining should correspond to the results of culture. A discrepancy may suggest diagnostic possibilities such as infection due to fastidious or anaerobic bacteria.

The microbiology laboratory must be an ally in the diagnostic endeavor (see Chap. 80). Astute laboratory personnel will suggest optimal culture and transport conditions or alternative tests to facilitate diagnosis. If informed about specific potential pathogens, an alert laboratory staff will allow sufficient time for these organisms to become evident in culture, even when present in small numbers or when slow-growing. The parasitology technician who is attuned to the specific diagnostic considerations relevant to a particular case may be able to detect the rare, otherwise-elusive egg or cyst in a stool specimen. In cases where a diagnosis appears difficult, serum should be stored during the early acute phase of the illness so that a diagnostic rise in titer of antibody to a specific pathogen can be detected later. Bacterial and fungal antigens can sometimes be detected in body fluids, even when cultures are negative or are rendered sterile by antibiotic therapy. Newer techniques such as the polymerase chain reaction allow the amplification of specific DNA sequences so that minute quantities of foreign nucleic acids can be recognized in host specimens.

THERAPY Optimal therapy for infectious diseases requires a broad knowledge of medicine and careful clinical judgment. Life-threatening infections such as bacterial meningitis or sepsis, viral encephalitis, or falciparum malaria must be treated immediately, often before a specific causative organism is identified. Antimicrobial agents must be chosen empirically and must be active against the range of potential infectious agents consistent with the clinical scenario. Good clinical judgment is necessary in making decisions to withhold antimicrobials in a self-limited process or until a specific diagnosis is made. The dictum *primum non nocere* should be adhered to, and it should be remembered that all antimicrobials carry a risk (and a cost) to the patient. Direct toxicity may be encountered, e.g., ototoxicity due to aminoglycosides, bone marrow toxicity of zidovudine, and hepatotoxicity of antituberculous agents such as isoniazid and rifampin. Allergic reactions are common and can be serious. Since superinfection may follow eradication of the normal flora and colonization by resistant organism, one invariant principle is that infectious disease therapy should be directed toward as narrow a spectrum of infectious agents as possible. Treatment specific for the pathogen should result in as little perturbation as possible of the host's microflora. With few exceptions, abscesses require surgical or percutaneous drainage for cure. Likewise, infected foreign bodies, including medical devices, must generally be removed in order to eliminate an infection of the device or adjacent tissue. Other infections, such as necrotizing fasciitis, peritonitis due to a perforated organ, gas gangrene, and chronic osteomyelitis, require surgery as their primary means of cure, with antibiotics serving only an adjunctive role.

Recently, the role of immunomodulators in the management of infectious diseases has received increasing attention. Glucocorticoids have been shown to be of benefit in the treatment of *H. influenzae* meningitis in children and in therapy for *P. carinii* pneumonia in patients with AIDS. Their use in other infectious processes remains less clear, and in some cases (in cerebral malaria and septic shock, for example) is detrimental. Other agents that modulate the immune response include prostaglandin inhibitors, specific lymphokines, and TNF inhibitors. Specific antibody therapy has been shown to play a role in the treatment and prevention of many diseases. Specific immunoglobulins have long been known to prevent the development of symptomatic rabies and tetanus. More recently, cytomegalovirus (CMV) immune globulin has been recognized as important not only in preventing transmission of CMV during organ transplantation but also in treating CMV pneumonia in the bone marrow transplant recipient. There is a strong need for well-designed clinical trials to evaluate each new interventional modality.

PERSPECTIVE The genetic simplicity of many infectious agents allows them to undergo rapid evolution and to develop selective advantages that result in constant variation in the clinical manifestations of infection. Moreover, changes in the environment and the host can predispose new populations to infection. An epidemic of lethal respiratory failure on a Navajo reservation in the southwestern United States in 1993, which caused nationwide alarm, exemplifies the fear that new plagues induce in the human psyche. In this outbreak, patients presented with fever, myalgias, headache, and cough, which were followed by the rapid development of respiratory failure with unexplained noncardiogenic pulmonary edema. Among the etiologic agents potentially responsible for the clinical syndrome were the hantaviruses, which had never been described as human pathogens in the Western Hemisphere. Although patients had respiratory involvement, they lacked the renal failure and hemorrhagic manifestations previously described with hantavirus infection. Nonetheless, most of these patients demonstrated rises in antibody titer to the hantaviruses. This cluster of fatal illness emphasizes the propensity of new infectious diseases to arise in new populations. The potential for infectious agents to emerge in novel and unexpected ways requires that physicians and public health officials be knowledgeable, vigilant, and open-minded in their approach to the consideration of unexplained illness.

There has existed a perception that infectious diseases no longer represented as serious a concern to world health as they once did. The progress that science, medicine, and society as a whole have made in combatting these maladies is impressive, and it is ironic that, as we stand on the threshold of understanding the most basic biology of the microbe, infectious diseases are posing renewed problems. We are threatened by new diseases such as AIDS, hepatitis C, and Lyme disease and by the reemergence of old foes like tuberculosis, cholera, and rheumatic fever. True students of infectious diseases were, perhaps, the least surprised by these developments. Those who know pathogens are aware of their incredible adaptability and diversity. As ingenious and successful as therapeutic approaches may be, our ability to develop methods to counter infectious agents so far has not matched the myriad strategies employed by the sea of microbes that surrounds us. Their sheer numbers and the rate at which they can evolve are daunting. Though new vaccines, new antibiotics, and new modalities for treating and preventing infection will be developed, pathogenic microbes will continue to develop new strategies of their own, presenting us with an unending and dynamic challenge.

REFERENCES

DiRita VJ, Mekalanos JJ: Genetic regulation of bacterial virulence. Annu Rev Genet 23:455, 1989

Fields BN: Pathogenesis of viral infections, in *Virology*, BN Fields (ed). New York, Raven, 1990, pp 191–239

Gorbach SL et al (eds): *Infectious Diseases*. Philadelphia, Saunders, 1992

Kasper DL: Introduction to bacterial diseases, in *Principles and Practice of Infectious Diseases*, 3d ed, GL Mandell et al (eds). New York, Wiley, 1990, pp 1484–1489

Mahmoud A: Parasitic protozoa and helminths. Science 246:1015, 1989

Quagliarello V, Scheld MW: Bacterial meningitis: Pathogenesis, pathophysiology, and progress. New Engl J Med 327:864, 1992

Report of the Task Force on Microbiology and Infectious Diseases. NIAID. NIH Publication No. 92-3320, April 1992

80 LABORATORY DIAGNOSIS OF INFECTIOUS DISEASES

ANDREW B. ONDERDONK

The laboratory diagnosis of infection requires the demonstration, either directly or indirectly, of viral, bacterial, mycotic, or parasitic agents in tissues, fluids, or excreta of the host. Clinical microbiology laboratories are responsible for processing these specimens and also for determining antibiotic susceptibility for bacterial pathogens. Traditionally, the detection of pathogenic agents largely relies on either the microscopic visualization of pathogens in clinical material or growth of microorganisms in the laboratory. Identification is generally based on phenotypic characteristics, such as fermentation profiles for bacteria, cytopathic effects produced by viral agents in tissue culture, and microscopic morphology for fungi and parasites. These techniques are reliable but are often time-consuming.

DETECTION METHODS   Reappraisal of the methods employed in the clinical microbiology laboratory has led to development of strategies for detecting pathogenic agents through nonvisual biologic signal-detection systems. Much of this methodology is based on computerization of detection systems with relatively inexpensive, but sophisticated, computers. In this chapter, both the methods currently available and those under development will be discussed. Detection of parasitic agents is the subject of a separate chapter.

Biologic signals   A *biologic signal* is a material that can be reproducibly differentiated from other substances present in the same physical environment. The issue for biologic (and electronic) signals is distinguishing the signal from background "noise" and translating the signal into meaningful information. Examples of biologic signals as applicable to clinical microbiology include structural components of bacteria, fungi, and viruses; specific antigens; metabolic end products; unique DNA or RNA base sequences; enzymes; toxins or other proteins; and surface polysaccharides.

Detection systems   A detector is used to sense (or detect) a signal to allow discrimination between the signal and background noise. Detection systems range from morphologic variations that are detected by the trained eyes of a technologist to sensitive electronic instruments, such as gas-liquid chromatographs coupled to computer systems for signal analysis. The sensitivity with which signals can be detected varies widely. It is essential to utilize a detection system that discerns small amounts of signal (sensitivity) even when biologic background noise is present (specificity). Some common detection systems used in microbiology are immunofluorescence, substrate utilization reactions or end-product formation detected as color changes, enzyme activity detected as change in light absorbance, flame ionization detection of short- or long-chain fatty acids, turbidity changes, cytopathic effects in cell lines, and agglutination of particles.

Amplification   Amplification of weak signals enhances the sensitivity with which signals can be detected. The most common microbiologic amplification technique is growth of a single bacterium into a discrete colony on an agar plate or into a suspension containing many identical organisms. The advantage of growth as an amplification method is that it does not require anything but an appropriate medium; the disadvantage is the amount of time required for amplification to occur. More rapid, specific amplification of biologic signals can be achieved with techniques such as polymerase (ligase) chain reactions (for DNA/RNA), enzyme immunoassays (for antigens and antibodies), electronic amplification (for gas-liquid-chromatography assays), antibody capture methods for concentration and/or separation, and selective filtration or centrifugation.

Although a variety of methods are available for the amplification and detection of biologic signals on a research basis, thorough testing is required before they are validated as diagnostic assays.

DIRECT DETECTION   Microscopy   The field of microbiology has been defined largely by the development and use of the microscope. The examination of specimens by microscopic methods often provides rapid and useful diagnostic information. Staining techniques permit organisms to be seen more clearly. Some examples of common microbiologic stains are listed in Table 80-1.

The simplest method for microscopic evaluation is the wet mount, which is used for the examination of samples such as cerebrospinal fluid (CSF) for the presence of *Cryptococcus neoformans,* with India ink as a background against which to visualize yeasts with large capsules. Wet mounts with dark-field illumination are also used to detect spirochetes from genital lesions. Skin scrapings and hair samples can be examined with use of either 10% KOH wet mount preparations or the calcofluor white method and ultraviolet (UV) illumination to detect fungal elements as fluorescing structures. Stained wet mounts, such as the lactophenol cotton blue stain for fungal elements, are often used for morphologic identification. These techniques enhance signal detection and decrease the background by making it easier to identify specific fungal structures.

Staining   GRAM'S STAIN   Without staining, bacteria are difficult to see at the magnification (400 to 1000 ×) required for their detection. Although simple, one-step stains can be used, differential stains are more common. Gram's stain differentiates between those organisms with thick peptidoglycan cell walls (gram-positive) and those in which outer membranes can be dissolved with alcohol or acetone (gram-negative).

Gram's stain is particularly useful for examining sputum for the presence of polymorphonuclear cells (PMNs) and bacteria. Sputum specimens with 25 or more PMNs and fewer than 10 epithelial cells per low-power field often provide clinically useful information. However, "sputum" samples with more than 10 epithelial cells per low-power field and multiple bacterial types suggest contamination with oral microflora. Despite the difficulty in discriminating between normal microflora and pathogens, Gram's stain may prove useful for specimens from areas with a large resident microflora if a useful biologic marker (signal) is available. Gram's stain of vaginal swab specimens is useful for detecting epithelial cells covered with gram-positive bacteria, which are regarded as a sign of bacterial vaginitis. Similarly, examination of stool specimens for the presence of leukocytes is useful as a screening procedure before testing for *Clostridium difficile* toxin or other enteric pathogens.

TABLE 80-1   Selected microbiologic stains

Stain	Use	Expected result
Acridine orange (uses UV light)	Visualization of bacteria, yeast, and leukocytes	Bacteria and yeast are red-orange, and leukocytes are pale green.
Auramine/rhodamine (uses UV light)	Visualization of Mycobacterium spp.	Yellow fluorescing bacteria indicate Mycobacterium.
Calcofluor white (uses UV light)	Visualization of fungal elements	Fungal elements appear as green fluorescing structures.
Gram's	Visualization and differentiation of bacteria into two groups	Gram-positive bacteria appear purple, and gram-negative bacteria are red.
Kinyoun acid-fast	Detection of Mycobacterium spp.	Acid-fast bacteria are pink against a blue background.
Modified acid-fast	Detection of weakly acid-fast organisms, such as Nocardia	Weakly acid-fast organisms are pink against a blue background
Giemsa	Varied, used for visualization of chlamydiae and malarial and other intracellular parasites	Varied, depending on agent.
Methenamine-silver	Detection of Pneumocystis carinii	Cell wall of P. carinii appears black against a light green background.
Spore	Visualization of spores and cellular location	Spores are light green against a pink/red background, and bacteria stain red.
Toluidine blue	Detection of P. carinii	P. carinii cysts appear light purple/lavender against a blue background.
Wet mount India ink	Detection of Cryptococcus neoformans	Cryptococcus mucoid capsules appear as clear halos around a yeast cell against a dark background.
Lactophenol cotton blue	Visualization of fungal structures	Fungal elements stain a more intense blue against a light blue background.

SOURCE: After Eisenberg et al.

The examination of CSF and joint, pleural, or peritoneal fluid using Gram's stain is useful for determining whether bacteria and/or PMNs are present. The sensitivity is such that $>10^4$ bacteria per liter should be detected. Centrifugation is often performed before staining to concentrate specimens suspected of containing low numbers of organisms. The pellet is then examined after staining. This simple method is particularly useful for examination of CSF for bacteria and white blood cells or sputum for acid-fast bacilli.

ACID-FAST STAIN   The acid-fast stain differentiates organisms capable of retaining carbol fuchsin dye after acid/organic solvent disruption (Mycobacterium spp.). Modifications of this procedure also allow differentiation between Actinomyces and Nocardia or other weakly acid-fast organisms. The acid-fast stain is employed for sputum, gastric aspirates, tissue samples, or other fluids when acid-fast bacilli (Mycobacterium spp.) are suspected. The identification of the pink/red acid-fast bacilli (AFB) against the blue background of the counterstain requires a trained eye, since few AFB may be detected in an entire smear, even when the signal is amplified by centrifugation. An alternative is the auramine-rhodamine combination fluorescent dye technique.

FLUOROCHROME STAINS   Fluorochrome stains, such as acridine orange, are used to identify white blood cells, yeast, and bacteria in body fluids.

Other specialized stains, such as Dappe's stain, may be used for detecting Mycoplasma in cell cultures designated for this purpose.

Capsular, flagellar, and spore stains are also used for identification or demonstration of characteristic structure.

IMMUNOFLUORESCENT STAINS   Direct immunofluorescence staining (DFA) uses antibody coupled to a fluorescing compound, such as fluorescein, directed at a specific antigenic target to visualize organisms or subcellular structures. When samples are examined under appropriate conditions, the fluorescing compound absorbs the UV light and reemits light at a higher (visible) wavelength that can be detected by the human eye. In the indirect immunofluorescent antibody (IFA) technique, an unlabeled (target) antibody binds a specific antigen. The specimen is then stained with labeled polyclonal antibody directed at the target antibody. Because each unlabeled target antibody attached to the appropriate antigen has multiple sites for attachment of the second antibody, the visual signal can be intensified (amplification). This form of staining is called indirect because a two-antibody system is used to generate the signal for detection of the antigen. Both direct and indirect fluorescence methods can be used to detect cultured cells infected with viruses such as cytomegalovirus and herpes simplex and many difficult-to-grow bacterial agents such as Legionella pneumophila.

Macroscopic antigen detection   Latex agglutination assays and enzyme immunoassays (EIAs) are rapid and inexpensive methods for identifying organisms or extracellular toxins and viral agents using protein and polysaccharide antigens. Such assays may be performed directly on clinical samples or after growth on agar plates or in viral cell cultures. The biologic signal in each case is the antigen to be detected; such methods utilize monoclonal or polyclonal antibodies.

Techniques such as direct agglutination of bacterial cells with specific antibody are simple but relatively insensitive, while latex agglutination procedures and enzyme immunoassays are more sensitive. Some cell-associated antigens, such as capsular polysaccharides, lipopolysaccharides, and other surface-expressed antigens, can be detected by agglutination of a suspension of bacterial cells when antibody is added, a method useful for typing the somatic antigens of Shigella and Salmonella. Systems such as EIA employ monoclonal antibodies coupled to an enzyme in which antigen is detected by development of a color when colorless substrate is converted to a colored product after an antigen-antibody reaction has occurred. Because the coupling of an enzyme to the monoclonal antibody can amplify a weak biologic signal, the sensitivity of such assays is often high. In each instance, the basis for detection is antigen-antibody binding, with the detection system changed to accommodate the biologic signal. Most such assays provide information as to whether antigen is present but do not quantify the amount.

DETECTION OF PATHOGENIC AGENTS BY CULTURE   Specimen collection and transport   To culture bacterial, mycotic, or viral pathogens, an appropriate sample must be placed into the proper medium for growth (amplification). The success or failure of identification of a specific microbial pathogen often relies on the collection and transport process. Table 80-2 lists procedures for collection and transport of commonly obtained specimens. Because there are many pathogen-specific paradigms for these procedures, it is important to seek advice from the microbiology laboratory when in doubt about a particular situation.

Isolation of bacterial pathogens   The isolation of the suspect pathogen(s) from clinical material relies on the use of artificial media designed to support the growth of bacteria in vitro. Such media are composed of agar, which is not metabolized by bacteria, and nutrients to support the growth of the microbial species of interest, often in combination with substances to inhibit the growth of other bacteria. Broth for growth (amplification) of organisms is employed for specimens with low numbers of bacteria, such as peritoneal dialysis fluids, CSF, or samples in which anaerobes may be present. Two basic strategies are used to isolate pathogenic bacteria. The first uses enriched media to allow the growth of any bacteria that may be present in a sample such as blood or CSF. Since bacteria are not present in such fluids under normal conditions, the finding of organisms is usually significant. Broths that allow for the growth of

TABLE 80-2 Culture collection and transport

Body fluids
Specimen: Aseptically aspirated body fluids
Minimum volume: 1 mL
Container: Sterile tubes with a tight-fitting cap. The specimen may be left in the syringe used for collection if the needle is removed and a rubber cap placed over the barrel of the syringe before transport to the laboratory.
Other considerations: For some body fluids, such as peritoneal lavage samples, increased volumes are helpful for isolation of low numbers of bacteria.

Bronchial aspirates
Specimen: Transtracheal aspirate (TTA) or bronchoscopy specimen
Minimum volume: 1 mL of aspirate or brush in transport medium
Container: Sterile TTA or bronchoscopy tube, bronchoscopy brush in other sterile container

Cerebrospinal fluid (CSF or lumbar puncture)
Specimen: Spinal fluid
Minimum volume: 1 mL for routine cultures, 5 mL or greater for detection of *Mycobacterium*
Container: Sterile tube with tight-fitting cap

Genital sites
Specimen: Vaginal or urethral secretions, cervical swabs, uterine fluid, prostatic fluid, etc.
Minimum volume: 1 swab or 0.5 mL of fluid
Container: Transwab containing Amies transport medium or similar system containing holding medium for *Neisseria gonorrhoeae*
Other considerations: Vaginal swab samples for "routine culture" should be discouraged whenever possible, unless the presence of a particular pathogen is suspected. If detection of multiple organisms, such as group B *Streptococcus, Trichomonas, Chlamydia,* or *Candida* species is being requested, one swab per test should be sent.

Miscellaneous sterile sites
Specimen: Tissue removed at surgery, bone, anticoagulated bone marrow, biopsy samples, or other specimens from areas that are normally sterile sites
Minimum volume: 1 mL of fluid or a 1-g piece of tissue
Container: Sterile "culturette" type swab or similar transport system containing a holding medium. A sterile bottle or jar should be used for tissue specimens.
Other considerations: Accurate identification of the specimen and source is important for processing purposes. Enough tissue should be collected for both microbiologic and histopathologic evaluations.

Nares
Specimen: Swab from the nares
Minimum volume: 1 swab
Container: Sterile "culturette" or similar transport system containing holding medium
Other considerations: Swabs made of calcium alginate may be used.

Wounds
Specimen: Purulent material or abscess contents obtained from a wound or abscess without contamination by normal microflora
Minimum volume: Two swabs or 0.5 mL of aspirated pus
Container: "Culturette" swab or similar transport system or a sterile tube with a tight-fitting screw cap. If anaerobic cultures are to be ordered at the same time, send specimen in anaerobic transport device or closed syringe.
Collection: Abscess contents or other fluids should be collected in a syringe (see above) when possible to provide adequate sample volume and an anaerobic environment.

Sputum
Specimen: Fresh sputum (not saliva)
Minimum volume: 2 mL
Container: Commercially available sputum collection system or similar sterile container with a screw top
Cause for rejection: Care must be taken to ensure that the specimen is sputum and not saliva. Results of Gram's stain noting the number of epithelial cells and PMNs can serve as an important part of the evaluation process.

Stool for enteric pathogens
Synonyms: Stool for routine culture, stool for *Salmonella, Shigella,* and *Campylobacter*
Specimen: Rectal swab or a fresh, randomly collected stool (preferable)
Minimum volume: At least 1 g of stool or two rectal swabs
Container: Plastic-coated cardboard cup or plastic cup with a tight-fitting lid. Other leak-proof containers are also acceptable.
Other considerations: If *Vibrio* species are suspected, the laboratory must be notified, and appropriate collection and transport methods must be used.

Stool for *Yersinia*
Specimen: A fresh, randomly collected stool
Minimum volume: At least 1 g of stool
Container: Plastic-coated cardboard cup or plastic cup with a tight-fitting lid
Limitations: Procedure requires enrichment techniques.

Stool for *Aeromonas* and *Plesiomonas*
Specimen: A fresh, randomly collected stool
Minimum volume: At least 1 g of stool
Container: Plastic-coated cardboard cup or plastic cup with a tight-fitting lid
Limitations: Stool should not be cultured for *Aeromonas* or *Plesiomonas* unless culture for other enteric pathogens is also performed.

Throat
Specimen: Swab of posterior pharynx, ulcerations, or areas of suspected purulence
Minimum volume: 1 swab
Container: Sterile "culturette" or other sterile swab specimen collection system containing holding medium
Note: Normal microflora includes alpha-hemolytic streptococci, saprophytic *Neisseria* spp., diphtheroids, and nonhemolytic *Staphylococcus* spp. Aerobic culture of a throat ("routine") includes screening for and identification of beta-hemolytic *Streptococcus* species and any potentially pathogenic organism. Although considered normal microflora, organisms such as *Staphylococcus aureus, Haemophilus influenzae, Haemophilus parainfluenzae,* and *Streptococcus pneumoniae* will be identified by most laboratories, if requested. When *N. gonorrhoeae* or *Corynebacterium diptheriae* is suspected, a special culture request is recommended.

Urine
Specimen: Clear voided urine specimen or urine collected by catheter
Minimum volume: 0.5 mL
Container: Sterile, leak-proof container with a screw cap
Limitations: Isolates should be identified under the following circumstances:
 1 Clear voided specimen, midvoid specimen, and Foley or indwelling catheter-specimens that yield 50,000 organisms per milliliter or more and from which no more than three species are isolated.
 2 Straight catheterized, bladder tap, and similar urine specimens should have complete workup (identification and susceptibility test) for all potentially pathogenic organisms, regardless of colony count.
 3 Certain clinical problems (e.g., acute dysuria in women) may warrant identification and susceptibility testing of isolates present at concentrations lower than 50,000 organisms per milliliter.

Blood culture, routine
Synonyms: Blood culture for aerobes, anaerobes, and yeast
Specimen: Whole blood
Minimum volume: 10 mL, in each of two bottles for adults and children; 5 mL, if possible, in each of two bottles for infants, less for neonates
Containers: For adults, two bottles (smaller sizes are available for pediatric patients), one with dextrose phosphate, tryptic soy, or other appropriate broth and the other with thioglycollate or other broth containing reducing agents appropriate for isolation of obligate anaerobes. For special situations, e.g., suspected fungal identification, culture-negative endocarditis, or mycobacteremia, different blood collection systems may be used (Isolator systems, see below).
Collection: An appropriate disinfecting technique should be used on both the bottle septum and the patient. Do not allow air bubbles to get into anaerobic broth bottles.
Special considerations: There is no more important clinical microbiology test than the detection of blood-borne pathogens. The rapid identification of bacterial and fungal agents is a major determinant of patient survival. Bacteria may be present either continuously in blood, as is the case for endocarditis, overwhelming sepsis, and the early stages of salmonellosis and brucellosis, or intermittently, as is the case for most other bacterial infections in which bacteria are shed into the blood on a sporadic basis. Most blood culture systems employ two separate bottles containing broth medium, one that is vented in the laboratory for the growth of facultative and aerobic organisms and a second bottle that is maintained under anaerobic conditions. For suspected continuous bacteremia/fungemia, two to three samples should be drawn before the start of therapy, with additional sets obtained if fastidious organisms are suspected. For intermittent bacteremia, two to three sets should be obtained at least 1 h apart during the first 24 h.

Blood culture, fungus/*Mycobacterium* species
Volume of specimen: 10 mL in each bottle, as with routine blood cultures, or alternatively, request Isolator tube from the laboratory
Container: See Blood culture, routine.
Special instruction: Be sure to specify "hold for extended incubation," since many fungal agents require 7 to 14 days to grow in standard blood culture bottles.

Blood culture, Isolator (lysis centrifugation)
Specimen: Blood
Container: Isolator tubes
Note: Used mainly for the isolation of fungi, *Mycobacterium,* or other fastidious aerobes and for elimination of antibiotics from cultured blood in which organisms are concentrated by centrifugation.

TABLE 80-2 Culture collection and transport *(continued)*

Cultures: Fungus
Specimen: Specimen types listed in the aerobic culture section may be cultured for fungi. When urine or sputum are to be cultured for fungi, a first morning specimen is usually preferred.
Minimum volume: 1 mL or as specified for aerobic cultures under individual listing of specimens
Container: A sterile, nonleaking container with a tight-fitting cap
Collection: The specimen should be transported to the microbiology laboratory within 1 h of collection. Contamination with normal flora from the skin, rectum, vaginal tract, or other body surfaces should be avoided as much as possible.

Cultures: *Mycobacterium*
Synonyms: AFB culture, culture for acid-fast bacilli
Specimen: Sputum, tissue, urine, body fluids
Minimum volume: 10 mL of fluids or small piece of tissue. Swabs should not be used.
Container: A sterile container with a tight-fitting cap
Other considerations: The detection of *Mycobacterium* spp. is improved by the use of concentration techniques. Smears and cultures of pleural, peritoneal, and pericardial fluids often have low yields. Multiple cultures from the same patient are encouraged.

Cultures: *Legionella*
Specimen: Pleural fluid, lung tissue (biopsy), bronchial lavage (BAL), bronchial biopsy, transbronchial biopsy. Rapid transport to the laboratory is required.
Minimum volume: 1 mL of fluids; any size piece of tissue, although it is preferable to submit a 0.5-g sample when possible.

Cultures: Anaerobes
Specimen: Aspirated specimens in capped syringes or other transport devices designed to limit oxygen exposure are suitable for the cultivation of obligate anaerobes. A variety of commercially available transport devices may be used. Contamination of specimens with normal microflora from the skin, rectum, vaginal vault, or other body site should be avoided. Specimens cultured for obligate anaerobes should be cultured for facultative bacterial species as well.
Minimum volume: At least 1 mL of aspirated fluid or two swabs and an appropriate anaerobic transport device are required. Collection containers for aerobic culture, such as dry swabs, and inappropriate specimens, such as refrigerated samples, expectorated sputum, stool, gastric aspirates, vaginal, and throat, nose, and rectal swabs, should be rejected as unsuitable for culture.

Cultures: Viral agents
Specimen: Respiratory secretions, wash aspirates from the respiratory tract, nasal swabs, blood samples (including buffy coats), vaginal and rectal swabs, and swab specimens from suspect skin lesions. Stool samples may be employed for detection of some agents. Laboratories generally employ diverse methods for detecting viral agents, and the specific requirements for each specimen should be checked before sending a sample. In general, fluid samples or stool in sterile containers or swab samples in viral "culturette" devices kept on ice, but not frozen, are suitable. Plasma specimens and buffy coats in sterile collection tubes are adequate but should be kept at 4 to 8°C. If specimens are to be shipped or kept for extended periods of time, freezing at -80°C usually preserves viable replicating units.
Minimum volume: 1 mL of fluid, one swab, or 1 g of stool in each appropriate transport medium
Other considerations: Most samples for culture are transported to the laboratory in a holding medium containing antibiotics to prevent bacterial overgrowth and to provide an environment in which viral particles will not be inactivated. Many specimens should be kept cool but not frozen. Procedures and transport media vary depending on viral agent to be cultured and the length of time for transport.

TABLE 80-3 Examples of primary plating media

Medium	Incubation	Purpose
Blood agar(s), 5% defibrinated sheep blood in an enrichment agar base, chocolate agar with additives	CO_2 or anaerobic	Growth and amplification of many medically significant bacteria, including obligate anaerobes
MacConkey agar, deoxycholate agar, eosin–methylene blue agar	O_2	Select for Enterobacteriaceae and other gram-negative rods; inhibits growth of most gram-positive organisms; differentiate Lac-positive and Lac-negative organisms
Phenylethyl alcohol agar, Columbia CNA agar	CO_2	Select for gram-positive species, particularly *Staphylococcus* and *Streptococcus*; inhibits many gram-negative organisms
Hektoen enteric agar, deoxycholate-citrate, *Salmonella-Shigella* agar	O_2	Select for enteric pathogens; characteristics vary, depending on medium
GN broth, selenite broth, tetrathionate broth	O_2	Selective amplification for certain enteric pathogens
Thayer-Martin agar, Martin-Lewis agar, New York City agar	CO_2	Selective amplification for *Neisseria* spp.
Brain-heart infusion, tryptic digest, thioglycollate, chopped-meat glucose	O_2, CO_2, anaerobic	General-purpose amplification broths

SOURCE: After Eisenburg et al.

small numbers of organisms may be subcultured to solid media when growth is detected. The second is to isolate (amplify) specific bacterial species from stool, genital tract secretions, or sputum, which contain large numbers of bacteria under normal conditions. For this purpose, antimicrobial agents or other inhibitory substances are incorporated into the agar medium to inhibit growth of all but the bacteria of interest. Following incubation, organisms that grow on such media are further characterized to determine whether they are pathogens. Selection for organisms that may be pathogens from normal microflora shortens the time required to make the diagnosis. Some of the more common types of primary plating media and their uses for specific specimen types are listed in Tables 80-3 and 80-4.

IDENTIFICATION METHODS Once organisms are isolated, traditional methods of phenotypic characterization are used for the identification of specific isolates. Phenotypic characteristics include readily detectable traits (colony size, color, hemolytic reactions, odor) after growth on agar media, use of specific substrates and carbon sources (such as carbohydrates), the formation of specific end products during growth, and the microscopic appearance of the organisms themselves. Broth tubes containing specific substrates are commonly employed for such characterization procedures.

Classical phenotyping Automated systems allow identification of bacterial pathogens on the basis of phenotypic characteristics within a matter of hours. Most such systems are based on biotyping techniques, in which isolates are grown in multiple substrates and the pattern of reactions is compared with known patterns for various bacterial species. This procedure is relatively fast, and commercially available systems include a coding system to simplify recording of results, probability calculations for likely identification, and miniaturized biotyping methods. By automating the biotyping approach and coupling the reading process to computer-based data analysis, rapidly growing organisms, such as the Enterobacteriaceae, can be identified within hours of detection on agar plates.

To speed identification, several systems use preformed enzymes for 2- to 3-h identification methods. Such systems do not rely on bacterial growth per se to determine whether a substrate has been used or not. They employ a heavy inoculum in which enzymes are present in sufficient quantity to convert substrate to product rapidly. In addition, some systems use fluorogenic substrate/end-product detection methods to increase sensitivity (through signal amplification).

Gas-liquid chromatography Gas-liquid chromatography (GLC) is used for the detection of metabolic end products of bacterial fermentations. A common application of this technique is identification of the short-chain fatty acid products produced by obligate anaerobes during the fermentation of glucose. Because the types of volatile acids and relative concentrations differ among the various genera and

TABLE 80-4 Examples of commonly employed media by specimen type

Specimen	Medium	Time required for isolation and identification
Abscess or pus, deep wounds	Blood, chocolate, and MacConkey agar; anaerobic agar(s); enrichment broth	24–48 h for facultative species; 72–96 h for most anaerobes
Body fluids (other than blood, CSF, and urine)	Blood, chocolate agar enrichment broth; anaerobic agar(s), or MacConkey as indicated by site	Same as above
Blood	Enrichment broth for facultative and aerobic organisms; second enrichment broth for anaerobes	6 h to 14 days depending on organism; most facultative and anaerobic species detected in 7 days or less
CSF	Blood, chocolate, anaerobic agar(s), and enrichment broth; fungal agar as necessary	24–48 h for facultative species and dimorphic fungi; 72–96 h for most anaerobes
Intestinal tract (feces, rectal swabs, and ileostomy or colostomy contents)	MacConkey, Hektoenenteric, and other selective agar for *Salmonella* and *Shigella*; special agar(s) for *Campylobacter*, *Yersinia*, and *Vibrio*	18–24 h for *Salmonella* and *Shigella*; longer for other agents
Respiratory tract (bronchial lavage, sputum, tracheal aspirates)	Blood, chocolate, and MacConkey agars; medium for *Legionella*; medium for *Mycobacterium* if indicated	24–48 h for most facultative species; up to 14 days for *Legionella*; up to 2 months for *Mycobacterium* cultures
Throat swab for group A *Streptococcus*	Blood agar	18–24 h
Tissue (biopsy or surgical)	Blood, chocolate, MacConkey, and anaerobic agar; selective agar for gram-positives; fungal agar as required	24–48 h for most facultative species; longer for obligate anaerobes and fungal agents
Urine (clean voided or catheterized)	Blood and MacConkey agar; quantitative culture required	24–48 h

species that make up this group of organisms, such information serves as a metabolic "fingerprint" for identification of a particular isolate.

GLC also can be coupled to a sophisticated signal-analysis computer software system for identification and quantitation of long-chain fatty acids (LCFA) in the outer membranes and cell walls of bacteria and fungi. For any given species, the types and relative concentrations of LCFA are different enough to allow identification of even closely related species. Definitive identification may be obtained within a few hours after growth of the organism on appropriate media. LCFA analysis is one of the most advanced procedures currently available for phenotypic characterization.

Nucleic acid probes Organisms can be identified with absolute specificity by analysis of the unique DNA or RNA base sequences for that species. Probes have been developed for identification of a wide variety of pathogens from Epstein-Barr virus to *Mycoplasma* and *Cryptococcus*, and some of these are available for use in the clinical laboratory. The routine use of this methodology for direct detection from clinical specimens is limited at present because the sensitivity of this method without amplification is often less than that of other techniques. The use of ribosomal RNA as the target for oligonucleotide probes helps increase sensitivity, since there are many more rRNA molecules in a single bacterial cell than DNA molecules. Readily available probe technology can be used for the direct detection of *Chlamydia*, *Neisseria gonorrhoeae*, *Gardnerella*, and *Trichomonas* from vaginal/cervical swabs and for identification of bacterial agents such as *Salmonella* and *Mycobacterium*. Much work remains to be done with regard to signal amplification to provide adequate sensitivity for direct detection of pathogens such as *Mycobacterium* spp. in clinical material. An important application for probe technology, either directly on clinical specimens or by in situ hybridization, is the detection of viral agents such as HIV, human papilloma virus, hepatitis A, B, and C, cytomegalovirus, parvovirus, varicella zoster, and herpes simplex virus. In some cases, these techniques are more sensitive for direct detection of viral agents than are conventional culture or serologic methods. Many viral probes are now available only for research purposes, but DNA/RNA probes will probably become the method of choice for identification of hard-to-detect viral agents in the future.

One unresolved issue with regard to use of probes on a routine basis is how best to amplify weak biologic signals. The polymerase chain reaction requires repeated heating of the DNA or RNA to separate the two complementary strands of the double helix, hybridization of a primer sequence to the appropriate base sequence, target amplification via complementary strand extension, and signal detection via a labeled probe. At the present time, the complexity of this procedure often makes other methods for detection, including growth of organisms, easier and less expensive. One of the interesting advantages of probe technology is that live organisms need not be present to detect a positive biologic signal. The impact of detecting dead organisms and the inability to perform susceptibility testing remain to be elucidated.

SUSCEPTIBILITY TESTING One of the principal responsibilities of the clinical laboratory is to determine which antimicrobial agents are inhibitory for a specific bacterial isolate. Two approaches are useful for this purpose. The first is to use a qualitative assessment of susceptibility to categorize responses as susceptible, resistant, or intermediate. This qualitative approach can be accomplished either by placing paper disks containing antibiotics onto an agar surface inoculated with the bacterial strain to be tested (Kirby-Bauer or disk/agar-diffusion method) or by using broth tubes containing a set concentration of antibiotic (breakpoint method). These methods have been carefully calibrated against quantitative methods and clinical experience with each antibiotic.

The second is to inoculate the test strain of bacteria in a series of broth tubes (or agar plates) with increasing concentrations of antibiotic. The lowest concentration of antibiotic that inhibits microbial growth in this test system is known as the *minimum inhibitory concentration* (MIC). If tubes in which no growth occurs are subcultured, the minimum concentration of antibiotic required to kill the starting inoculum also can be determined. This measurement is called the *minimum bactericidal concentration* (MBC). A miniaturized version of the macrobroth dilution technique in microwell plates is called the *microbroth dilution method*. Quantitative susceptibility testing using the microbroth dilution technique lends itself to automation and is used commonly in larger clinical laboratories.

A novel version of the disk/agar-diffusion method employing a quantitative diffusion gradient uses an absorbent strip with a known gradient of antibiotic concentrations along its length. When the strip is placed on the surface of an agar plate seeded with a bacterial strain to be tested, antibiotic diffuses into the medium, and bacterial growth is inhibited. Quantitative measures of the MIC are estimated by determining the lowest point on the gradient strip that inhibits microbial growth.

AUTOMATION OF MICROBIAL DETECTION IN BLOOD The detection of microbial growth in blood is difficult because the numbers of organisms present in the sample are often low and because the integrity of the organisms and their ability to replicate may be damaged by humoral defense mechanisms or antimicrobial agents. Over the years, automated systems that relied on the detection of CO_2

produced by the organisms present in blood culture bottles have allowed for the automation of this procedure. The most common system involves inserting a sampling device into each bottle at periodic intervals and drawing off the head-space gas of the bottle. An infrared monitor is used to determine the CO_2 level. The system interprets levels exceeding a set concentration as indicative of microbial growth. Such methods are not any more sensitive than the human eye in detecting a positive culture, but because the bottles in an automated system are generally monitored more frequently, a positive culture is often detected more rapidly than by manual techniques, and consequently, important information, including Gram's stain and preliminary susceptibility assays, can be obtained sooner.

One technique for automated blood culture monitoring uses reflectance optics consisting of a photodiode and a light-emitting diode to monitor the amount of CO_2 produced in each blood culture bottle every 10 min through a self-contained sensor that is part of each bottle. Each reflectance measurement is then stored in computer memory, and when an appropriate change in reflectance occurs, the system alerts the clinical laboratory to the presence of a positive culture via audible and visible alarms. The continuous scanning of bottles used in this system provides shortened detection times with the concomitant advantage of early reporting for positive cultures, and the noninvasive monitoring procedure decreases the likelihood of laboratory contamination.

Automated systems also have been applied for detection of microbial growth from specimens other than blood, such as peritoneal and other normally sterile fluids. *Mycobacterium* spp. also can be detected in certain automated systems if appropriate media are used for culture.

DETECTION OF VIRAL AGENTS   Serologic methods   Measurement of antibodies provides an indirect marker for past or current infection with a specific viral agent. The biologic signal is usually either IgM or IgG antibody directed at viral antigen(s). The detection systems include those used for bacterial antigens (agglutination reactions, immunofluorescence, and EIA) and unique detection systems such as hemolysis inhibition and complement fixation. Serologic methods generally fall into two categories: tests to determine protective antibody levels or measurements of changing antibody titers as a method for detecting current infection. Documentation of an antibody response as a measure of current immunity is important for viral agents such as rubella or varicella zoster; assays for this purpose normally use one or two dilutions of serum for a qualitative determination of protective antibody levels. Quantitative serologic assays to detect increases in antibody titers most often employ paired serum samples obtained 10 to 14 days apart (acute and convalescent phase). Since the incubation period before symptoms are noted may be long enough for an antibody response to occur, the demonstration of acute phase antibody alone is often not enough to establish the diagnosis of active infection as opposed to past exposure. In such circumstances, the finding of IgM may be useful as a measure of an early, acute antibody response. A fourfold increase in total antibody titer or in EIA activity between the acute and convalescent samples is also regarded as evidence for active infection.

For certain viral agents, such as Epstein-Barr virus, the antibodies produced may be directed at different antigens during different phases of the infection. For this reason, most laboratories test for antibody directed at both viral capsid antigens and antigens associated with recently infected host cells to determine the stage of infection.

Culture methods   Pathogenic viral agents are often cultured when the presence of antibody is not a criterion of active infection or when an increase in serum antibody may not be detected during infection. The biologic signal, virus, is thus amplified to a level at which detection can occur. Although a number of techniques are available, the essential elements include a monolayer of cultured mammalian cells sensitive to infection with the suspect viral pathogen. These cells serve as the amplification system by allowing for the proliferation of viral particles. Virus may be detected by direct observation of the cultured cells for cytopathic effects or by immuno-

fluorescent detection of viral antigens following incubation. Culture methods are particularly useful for detection of rapidly propagated agents, such as cytomegalovirus or herpes simplex virus.

REFERENCES

EISENBERG HD et al: Specimen collection and handling, in *Manual of Clinical Microbiology,* 5th ed, A Ballows et al (eds). Washington, American Society for Microbiology, 1991

FUCCILLO DA et al: Rapid viral diagnosis, in *Manual of Clinical Laboratory Immunology,* 3d ed, Rose, NR et al (eds). Washington, American Society for Microbiology, 1986

HOPKIN JM et al: DNA hybridization for the diagnosis of microbial disease. Q J Med 75:415, 1990

LENNETTE DA: Preparation of specimens for virological examination, in *Manual of Clinical Microbiology,* 5th ed, A Ballows et al (eds). Washington, American Society for Microbiology, 1991

MURRAY PR: Comparison of the lysis-centrifugation and agitated biphasic blood culture systems for detection of fungemia. J Clin Microbiol 29:96, 1991

NOWINSKI RC et al: Monoclonal antibodies for diagnosis of infectious diseases in humans. Science 219:637, 1983

SCHOCHETMAN G et al: Polymerase chain reaction. J Infect Dis 158:1154, 1988

YOLKEN RH: Enzyme immunoassays for the detection of infectious antigens in body fluids: Current limitations and future prospects. Rev Infect Dis 4:35, 1982

81   INFECTIONS IN PATIENTS WITH INFLAMMATORY AND IMMUNOLOGIC DEFECTS

HENRY MASUR / ANTHONY S. FAUCI

DEFINITION   Qualitative or quantitative defects in inflammatory or immunologic host defenses are caused by a wide variety of processes, including primary congenital syndromes, cancer, trauma, malnutrition, retroviral infection, and drug therapy. When these defects—or those in other host protective mechanisms—are diminished significantly, patients develop increased susceptibility to infection and are considered "compromised hosts." Microbial processes are increasingly important causes of morbidity and mortality in compromised hosts because progressively more potent suppressive regimens are being used to manage conditions such as cancer and organ transplants and because patients are living longer as a result of improvements in the management of noninfectious complications.

HOST DEFENSE MECHANISMS

Antimicrobial defense mechanisms (Table 81-1) consist of complex, interacting systems that protect the host from endogenous and exogenous microbes (Chap. 79). The degree to which a patient becomes abnormally susceptible to infection by these microbes depends on the mechanism(s) compromised, the severity of the derangements, and their interactions. For instance, as isolated abnormalities, total absence of serum IgA or complement component C9 would probably have minor, if any, impact on host susceptibility to infection. In contrast, isolated abnormalities such as total absence of circulating neutrophils, serum IgG, or complement component C3 would lead to recurrent and life-threatening infections. Simultaneous damage to multiple host defenses may lead to especially ominous vulnerability. For instance, a combination of absent neutrophils and extensive disruption of the skin or mucous membranes would together constitute a particularly dangerous compromise that would likely be much worse than the sum of the risks posed by the individual abnormalities.

Recognition of which specific and nonspecific host defenses are compromised is important in order to develop effective clinical

TABLE 81-1 Mechanisms of host defense

Physical and chemical barriers
   Morphologic integrity of skin, mucous membranes
   Sphincters
   Epiglottis
   Normal secretory and excretory flow
   Endogenous microbial flora
   Gastric acidity
Inflammatory response
   Circulating phagocytes
   Complement
   Other humoral mediators (bradykinins, fibrinolytic systems, arachidonic
     acid cascade)
Reticuloendothelial system
   Tissue phagocytes
Immune response
   T lymphocytes and their soluble products
   B lymphocytes and immunoglobulins

strategies for predicting the probable timing of onset of infection and the most likely causative organisms, for formulating the appropriate diagnostic approach, and for developing the optimal therapeutic and preventive plan. However, based on an understanding of the mechanisms of host defenses, such an approach must be supplemented by clinical experience with specific patient populations. Because there are complexities of various host defense mechanisms that are not easily measured or fully understood, it cannot be assumed that all patient populations with the same measured deficiency in antimicrobial defense (as assessed by current laboratory techniques) will behave identically. For example, certain patients with AIDS and certain patients with hematologic malignancies will have neutrophil counts below 500 cells per microliter, but only the latter will have greatly increased frequency of infections due to gram-positive and gram-negative bacteria.

PHYSICAL AND CHEMICAL BARRIERS Physical and chemical barriers (Table 81-1) are part of a complex and interacting system of nonspecific host defense mechanisms that are essential for preventing the introduction and spread of endogenous and exogenous microbial organisms, including both those which normally colonize various anatomic sites and those which are highly pathogenic and whose presence is abnormal. These barriers utilize a wide variety of properties to protect the host, including the morphologic and functional integrity of skin or mucous membranes, the epiglottis, or sphincters; chemical processes (e.g., gastric acidity, pancreatic enzymes, cutaneous fatty acids or lysozyme); physical removal of organisms (e.g., peristalsis, sloughing of squamous cells, urine flow); and competition from less virulent flora. Interference with any of these mechanisms, e.g., by tumors, procedures, devices, infarcts, or drugs, can increase the host's susceptibility to infection. Common causes of disruption of physical and chemical barriers include intravenous catheters, which breach the skin; antacids, which remove the gastric barrier; and cytotoxic chemotherapy, which disrupts the gastrointestinal mucosa.

INFLAMMATORY RESPONSES Circulating phagocytes (neutrophils, monocytes, eosinophils, and basophils) arise from the bone marrow and upon appropriate signals enter the peripheral circulation and are distributed to local tissues, where they form the cornerstone of the inflammatory response. Recruitment of phagocytes from the bloodstream is a complicated process which involves the phagocytes' aggregation, adherence to the vascular endothelium, passage through endothelial spaces, and migration to local tissue sites (Chap. 59). An effective inflammatory response depends on the ability of the phagocyte to adhere, deform, have random locomotion, and respond to a chemical signal with directed movement. Humoral mediators influence local structures in ways that affect the phagocyte's ability to reach various loci; an example is the influence the complement cascade (especially C3a and C5a) has on the potential spaces between endothelial cells. Humoral mediators, including the complement system, the arachidonic acid cascade, kinin-generating systems, and cellular products such as interleukin 1 and tumor necrosis factor,

microbial peptides, or endotoxins, also promote directed locomotion of the phagocytes. Once the phagocyte arrives at a focus of infection, it may be able to adhere to the microorganism, ingest it, and digest it, particularly if the organism has been opsonized by antibodies or complement products. A wide variety of bacteria as well as fungi are killed by neutrophils in this manner.

RETICULOENDOTHELIAL SYSTEM Circulating microorganisms are cleared from the bloodstream by tissue phagocytes that are derived from circulating monocytes. These phagocytes include macrophages in the liver (Kupffer cells), spleen, lymph nodes, lung (alveolar macrophages), kidney (mesangial cells), and brain (microglial cells). The antimicrobial activities of these monocytes and macrophages are strongly influenced by opsonins such as IgG or C3b, which enhance the rate of particle ingestion, and by a large variety of soluble mediators produced primarily by mononuclear leukocytes (see Chap. 59). The efficacy of the reticuloendothelial system is also influenced by characteristics of specific organisms which allow the microbes to resist phagocytosis, lysosome-phagosome fusion (*Toxoplasma*), or intraphagosomal inactivation (*Leishmania*).

Immune response The major cellular components of the immune response are T lymphocytes and B lymphocytes (Chap. 277). These cells are distributed throughout the body in the bloodstream and at tissue sites. They interact in a highly complex fashion among themselves and with monocytes, macrophages, immunoglobulins, and the complement cascade. T lymphocytes are major components of the cell-mediated immune system. They secrete a multitude of cytokines which influence the functional status of other T lymphocytes, B lymphocytes, monocytes, and macrophages to eradicate infection and participate directly in cytotoxic reactions against tumor cells, HLA-incompatible cells, and certain virus-infected host cells. B lymphocytes and plasma cells secrete specific antibodies which have important roles in eradicating certain infections. The ability of the monocytes and macrophages to ingest and kill a wide variety of bacteria, fungi, and protozoa is augmented by lymphokines released by T lymphocytes, in particular, γ-interferon. Production of opsonizing, neutralizing, or microbicidal antibodies can also be profoundly influenced by the regulatory effect of T lymphocytes on B lymphocytes (Chap. 277).

ETIOLOGY AND PATHOGENESIS OF INFECTION

In compromised hosts, the development of infections reflects the interaction of impaired immunologic and nonimmunologic host defense mechanisms with the host's endogenous and exogenous microbial environment. Factors which change the microbial flora have an important impact on the organisms that are likely to cause disease. Such factors include antimicrobial therapy, invasive procedures or trauma, ingestion or inhalation of infected material, and hospitalization itself. The type of infections which develop are usually the consequence of specific alterations in host defenses, however.

Numerous processes can predispose to serious infection by compromising the anatomic and physical barriers of host defense. For example, the skin and mucous membranes can be breached by tumor invasion, tumor necrosis, or vascular insufficiency induced by arteritis or atherosclerosis; by injuries such as burns, pressure, or trauma; by radiation or cytotoxic chemotherapy; by a drug-induced cutaneous slough; and by procedures such as venipuncture or surgery. The respiratory tract can become the site of infection when its anatomic barriers are disrupted: the epiglottis may fail to protect the lower tract when the patient's consciousness is impaired or during intubation or bronchoscopy. The patient's ability to expel organisms may be adversely affected by infection, tumors, or drugs that alter the state of consciousness or prevent coughing; by disruption of mucociliary transport by a congenital disorder of ciliary subunits (such as Kartagener's syndrome) or by smoke or other inhaled toxins, anesthetic agents, or cytotoxic therapy; or by airway obstruction as a result of tumor, a foreign body, or lymph node enlargement.

The gastrointestinal tract can become a less effective barrier against entry of organisms if gastric acidity is abolished by a surgical procedure or antacid therapy (infections with *Salmonella* and other gram-negative rods are a typical consequence) or if its mucosa is eroded by tumor or cytotoxic therapy, especially in neutropenic patients. Obstruction of the intestinal or biliary tract by tumor, a stricture, or a stone allows endogenous or introduced flora to gain access to the involved tissues and often the bloodstream.

The genitourinary tract can become a portal of entry for infections if its mucosa is eroded by tumor, irradiation, or cytotoxic therapy or there is urinary obstruction. Renal failure associated with oliguria or anuria deprives the genitourinary system of the ability to flush out microorganisms and obviates the antimicrobial effects of urine itself. The insertion of foreign bodies into the urethra during catheterization or cystoscopy allows exogenous organisms to be introduced into the urinary tract.

Any locus in the body can become the site of infection if devitalized tissue or foreign bodies are seeded by bacteria or become infected by direct penetration. Hematomas, necrotic tissue, infarcts, calcified heart valves, and prosthetic devices (joints, heart valves, or central nervous system appliances) are particularly prone to bacterial infection.

Defects in inflammatory and immune function may permit infections that would normally be promptly eradicated to progress and cause clinically important disease. These quantitative or qualitative defects may be due to a congenital disorder, an underlying acquired disease, or drug therapy. Several specific types of defects are associated with particularly frequent or severe infectious complications.

LEUKOCYTE DISORDERS   The clinical consequences of leukocyte disorders depend on which subpopulations of leukocytes are numerically or functionally affected and the duration of the dysfunction (Table 81-2) (Chap. 59). Neutropenia (less than 1800 neutrophils per microliter) is the most commonly encountered defect in inflammatory host defense mechanisms (Chap. 59). When the neutrophil count falls below 1000 cells per microliter, there is a progressive increase in susceptibility to bacterial and fungal infections and a progressive decrease in the localizing signs and symptoms of inflammation. Susceptibility to infection increases dramatically when the peripheral neutrophil count falls below 500 cells per microliter, particularly when the count falls below 100 cells per microliter. The rate of decline and the duration of neutropenia are also important parameters which influence the development of infection. Neutropenia can occur because of bone marrow failure, peripheral destruction, or pooling or sequestration of cells. The most common causes of neutropenia are cytotoxic chemotherapy, neoplastic invasion of the bone marrow, aplastic anemia, and idiosyncratic drug reactions.

Neutrophil dysfunction also can result in a substantial predisposition to serious infection. Dysfunction may be a manifestation of a congenital disorder such as chronic granulomatous disease or Chédiak-Higashi syndrome (Chap. 59). Glucocorticoids and some multiple-drug chemotherapeutic regimens may alter both the number and the function of circulating neutrophils.

Lymphopenia in adults is defined as less than 1000 lymphocytes per microliter. The clinical consequences of lymphopenia depend on the subset(s) affected. Regardless of the total lymphocyte count, severe infections may occur if profound deficiencies of either B lymphocytes or T lymphocytes are present. Substantial reductions in helper T lymphocytes (CD4-positive lymphocytes) (<200 per microliter) can have particularly important infectious consequences, especially when caused by human immunodeficiency virus (HIV). The most common causes of lymphopenia are hematologic malignancies, glucocorticoid therapy, antilymphocyte globulins, cytotoxic drugs, and infection with certain viruses such as cytomegalovirus (Chap. 146) and HIV (Chap. 279). Congenital lymphopenias also can have severe consequences (Chap. 278).

Lymphocyte dysfunction can predispose to life-threatening infection even if the lymphocyte number is normal. Lymphocyte dysfunc-

tion is most often a consequence of therapy with glucocorticoids or cytotoxic drugs.

IMMUNOGLOBULIN DISORDERS   Decreased production of functional immunoglobulins, particularly IgG, can cause a marked increase in susceptibility to microbial disease (Chap. 278). Patients with significant reductions in IgG (usually less than 200 to 300 mg/dL) characteristically have recurrent infections due to encapsulated bacteria, particularly *Streptococcus pneumoniae*, *Haemophilus influenzae*, and *Neisseria meningitidis*, and to other organisms (*Pneumocystis carinii* and *Giardia lamblia*). Selective IgA deficiency can lead to respiratory or systemic bacterial infections (particularly when accompanied by IgG_2 deficiency) as well as intestinal giardiasis or severe viral hepatitis. The few documented cases of selective IgM deficiency also have been associated with severe infections, in particular with gram-negative organisms such as *Neisseria meningitidis*. Clinically important causes of immunoglobulin deficiency or dysfunction include congenital and acquired disorders, such as malignancies (multiple myeloma, chronic lymphocytic leukemia), sickle cell disease, and splenectomy (Table 81-2) (Chap. 278).

COMPLEMENT DISORDERS   The consequences of total absence of functional complement proteins depend on which of the specific components are deficient (Table 81-2) (Chap. 277). Deficiencies of C1 or C3 have been associated with pneumococcal infections, while deficiencies of C5, C6, C7, or C8 may lead to relapsing *Neisseria meningitidis* or *Neisseria gonorrhoeae* infections. Most severe deficiencies are due to inherited disorders, although there are reports of significant deficiencies in patients with systemic lupus erythematosus, cirrhosis, or splenectomy.

SPLENECTOMY   The spleen contains large numbers of B lymphocytes, monocytes, and macrophages and is a major site for T cell–independent immune responses such as the production of antibodies to polysaccharide antigens. The spleen has an important role in the phagocytosis of circulating opsonized organisms. Following splenectomy, young children are at high risk for fulminant infections due to *Streptococcus pneumoniae*, *Haemophilus influenzae*, *Neisseria meningitidis*, and the fastidious gram-negative bacterium DF-2. Adults who undergo splenectomy are also at increased risk for these infections, especially during the first 3 years after surgery. Splenectomized patients may develop fulminant infection with intraerythrocytic protozoa such as *Plasmodium malariae* and *Babesia*.

DIAGNOSIS

Clinicians managing compromised patients must recognize that the diagnosis of infectious processes requires special attention, persistence, and expertise. Compromised patients often present initially with manifestations that may be subtle or atypical. All infections can become life-threatening in extremely short time periods in many of these patients, so the diagnostic evaluation needs to begin promptly when the first signs or symptoms or laboratory abnormalities become apparent. These evaluations should proceed in rapid sequence, with use of tests that have the shortest feasible processing times. A thorough approach is necessary to make certain that the true etiologic agent is being treated and to minimize the likelihood that unnecessary drugs with toxic effects will be employed. The spectrum of potential etiologic agents is usually wide, so the diagnostic tests must often be broad-gauged as well. On the basis of a knowledge of the factors that render the patient compromised, the organisms associated with particular defects in host defense, and the patient's individual history and presentation, the clinician in concert with the laboratory must consider whether special testing should be done for unusual bacteria, fungi, viruses, helminths, protozoa, or other microorganisms. It is usually desirable to have a standard protocol for evaluating common clinical syndromes (e.g., pneumonia, fever, meningitis) in compromised patients, with modifications being made in the protocol as warranted by the individual patient's circumstances. For instance, when an HIV-infected patient has a helper T lymphocyte (T4-positive

TABLE 81-2 Infections associated with common defects in inflammatory or immunologic response

Host defect	Examples of diseases or therapies associated with defects	Common etiologic agents of infections
INFLAMMATORY RESPONSE		
Neutropenia	Hematologic malignancies, cytotoxic chemotherapy, aplastic anemia	Gram-negative enteric bacilli, *Pseudomonas* species, *Staphylococcus* species, *Candida* species, *Aspergillus* species
Chemotaxis	Chédiak-Higashi syndrome	*Staphylococcus aureus, Streptococcus pyogenes*
	Job's syndrome, protein-calorie malnutrition	*Staphylococcus aureus, Haemophilus influenzae*, gram-negative bacilli
Phagocytosis (cellular)	Systemic lupus erythematosus, chronic myelogenous leukemia, megaloblastic anemia	*Streptococcus pneumoniae, Haemophilus influenzae*
Splenectomy		*Haemophilus influenzae, Streptococcus pneumoniae*, other streptococci, DF-2, *Babesia microti, Salmonella* species
Microbicidal defect	Chronic granulomatous disease	Catalase-positive bacteria and fungi: staphylococci, *Escherichia coli, Klebsiella* species, *Pseudomonas aeruginosa, Aspergillus* species, *Nocardia* species
	Chédiak-Higashi syndrome	*Staphylococcus aureus, Streptococcus pyogenes*
COMPLEMENT SYSTEM		
C3	Congenital liver disease, systemic lupus erythematosus	*Staphylococcus aureus, Streptococcus pneumoniae, Pseudomonas* species, *Proteus* species
C5	Congenital	*Neisseria* species, gram-negative rods
C6, C7, C8	Congenital, systemic lupus erythematosus	*Neisseria meningitidis, Neisseria gonorrhoeae*
Alternate pathway	Sickle cell disease	*Streptococcus pneumoniae, Salmonella* species
IMMUNE RESPONSE		
T lymphocyte deficiency/dysfunction	Thymic aplasia, thymic hypoplasia, Hodgkin's disease, sarcoidosis, lepromatous leprosy	*Listeria monocytogenes, Mycobacterium* species, *Candida* species, *Aspergillus* species, *Cryptococcus neoformans*, herpes simplex virus, varicella-zoster virus
	Acquired immunodeficiency syndrome	*Pneumocystis carinii*, cytomegalovirus, herpes simplex, *Mycobacterium avium-intracellulare, Cryptococcus neoformans, Candida* species
	Mucocutaneous candidiasis	*Candida* species
	Purine nucleoside phosphorylase deficiency	Fungi, viruses
B cell deficiency/dysfunction	Bruton's X-linked agammaglobulinemia, agammaglobulinemia, chronic lymphocytic leukemia, multiple myeloma, dysglobulinemia	*Streptococcus pneumoniae*, other streptococci, *Haemophilus influenzae, Neisseria meningitidis, Staphylococcus aureus, Klebsiella pneumoniae, Escherichia coli, Giardia lamblia, Pneumocystis carinii*, enteroviruses
	Selective IgM deficiency	*Streptococcus pneumoniae, Haemophilus influenzae, Escherichia coli*
	Selective IgA deficiency	*Giardia lamblia*, hepatitis virus, *Streptococcus pneumoniae, Haemophilus influenzae*
Mixed T and B cell deficiency/dysfunction	Common variable hypogammaglobulinemia	*Pneumocystis carinii*, cytomegalovirus, *Streptococcus pneumoniae, Haemophilus influenzae*, various other bacteria
	Ataxia-telangiectasia	*Streptococcus pneumoniae, Haemophilus influenzae, Staphylococcus aureus*, rubella virus, *Giardia lamblia*
	Severe combined immunodeficiency	*Staphylococcus aureus, Streptococcus pneumoniae, Haemophilus influenzae, Candida albicans, Pneumocystis carinii*, varicella-zoster virus, rubella virus, cytomegalovirus
	Wiskott-Aldrich	Agents of infections seen in T and B cell abnormalities

or CD4-positive) count below 200 to 300 per microliter, and especially when the count falls below 100 per microliter, mild cough with fever must be evaluated promptly and aggressively because pneumocystis or cytomegalovirus pneumonia are much more likely than in HIV-positive patients with normal T4 counts. Kidney transplant recipients are known to be at very high risk for bacterial wound and urinary tract infections during the first postoperative month, while opportunistic viral, fungal, and protozoan diseases are more common during the second through sixth months. The development of fever during the first postoperative month should prompt an evaluation that focuses initially on the wound and urinary tract, while similar symptoms occurring several months after surgery should direct studies for protozoan, fungal, or viral infections.

Patients with leukemias and lymphomas need particular scrutiny for complicating bacterial or fungal infections when their neutrophil counts fall below 100 cells per microliter (a time that is usually predictable from the pharmacokinetics of the chemotherapeutic regimen).

THERAPY

In compromised patients the therapy of infectious complications should include drainage of localized collections of infected material, specific antimicrobials, and, if possible, reconstitution of deficient antimicrobial defenses. Examples of the last include the infusion of fresh frozen plasma to augment complement components, the administration of immune serum globulin to restore IgG levels, and the tapering of immunosuppressive drugs (such as glucocorticoids or cytotoxic agents) to restore cell-mediated immune mechanisms or neutrophil production. In certain neutropenic patients, augmentation or restoration of neutrophils can be achieved by the use of colony-stimulating factors (see Chap. 59) or white blood cell transfusions or permanently by bone marrow transplantation. Patients must be carefully selected for which of these procedures is likely to be effective.

Empiric antimicrobial therapy is clearly appropriate for some patient populations. For example, newly developing fever in severely neutropenic patients is frequently due to infection with bacteria, and therapy with a broad-spectrum regimen directed against potential major gram-positive and gram-negative pathogens before culture results are available can be lifesaving. The use of antibiotic combinations that are synergistic against infecting bacteria has been more successful in reducing morbidity and mortality from bacterial infection in neutropenic patients than single agents or nonsynergistic combinations. Examples of such combinations are vancomycin, ticarcillin, and amikacin or ceftazidime and amikacin (see Chap. 100). Empiric use of amphotericin B in the febrile neutropenic patient unresponsive after several days of antibacterial treatment is a common practice and may reduce morbidity from fungal superinfection.

PREVENTION OF INFECTION

In compromised patients, certain types of infections can be prevented by avoiding damage to physical barriers, bolstering host defenses, reducing acquisition of new potential pathogens, and suppressing colonizing flora. The use of invasive procedures, including repeated venipuncture, indwelling peripheral venous catheterization, and urinary catheterization, should be minimized or avoided completely. Surgical procedures should be chosen only when absolutely essential and should be performed with meticulous care. Bolstering host defenses can be accomplished directly in some patient groups. For example, immune serum globulin can be given prophylactically to hypogammaglobulinemic patients (see Chap. 278); hyperimmune varicella-zoster immunoglobulin can prevent or reduce the severity of varicella-zoster virus disease after acute exposure; immunization with vaccines against pneumococci, *Haemophilus*, and meningococci may be helpful for patients with conditions of particular susceptibility, such as those needing splenectomy (see Chap. 59).

Maintaining an optimal nutritional status will improve cellular immune mechanisms and aid wound repair. Most other methods to enhance depressed cell-mediated immunity have been clinically ineffective. Colony-stimulating factors offer promise in restoring neutrophil numbers and preventing infection in neutropenic subjects but require further investigation (see Chap. 59). Reducing the acquisition of potential pathogens can be facilitated by simple techniques, such as having hospital personnel wash their hands before patient contact, and by appropriate isolation from specific potentially contagious organisms, such as varicella-zoster virus, *Mycobacterium tuberculosis*, or multiply antibiotic-resistant gram-negative bacilli (see Chap. 98). More stringent measures, such as laminar flow isolation or control of sterility of food and water, have not proved to be useful or cost-effective for ultimate survival, although these measures will decrease the rate of infection for patients with prolonged and profound granulocytopenia. Selective or total suppression of endogenous bacteria or fungi is an important concept, since they cause more than 80 percent of infections in neutropenic cancer patients. Gut sterilization or prophylactic systemic antibiotics may have proved useful as temporary measures in certain neutropenic patients but cannot be practically sustained for more than a few weeks. Prolonged antimicrobial prophylaxis of certain specific infections that have exceedingly high attack rates in certain defined populations can be quite effective. The impressive protection provided by trimethoprim-sulfamethoxazole or aerosolized pentamidine against *Pneumocystis carinii* pneumonia in certain patients with AIDS or acute lymphocytic leukemia is a striking example.

REFERENCES

Bodey GP et al: Quantitative relationships between circulating leukocytes and infection in patients with acute leukemia. Ann Intern Med 64:328, 1966

Buckley RH, Schiff RI: The use of intravenous immune globulin in immunodeficiency diseases. N Engl J Med 325:110, 1991

Dwyer JM: Manipulating the immune system with immune globulin. N Engl J Med 326:107, 1992

Figueroa JE, Densen P: Infectious diseases associated with complement deficiencies. Clin Microbiol Rev 4:359, 1991

Hughes WT et al: Successful chemoprophylaxis for *Pneumocystis carinii* pneumonitis. N Engl J Med 297:1419, 1977

——— et al: Guidelines for the use of antimicrobial agents in neutropenic patients with unexplained fever. J Infect Dis 161:381, 1990

International Chronic Granulomatous Disease Cooperative Study Group: A controlled trial of interferon gamma to prevent infection in chronic granulomatous disease. N Engl J Med 324:509, 1991

Masur H et al: CD4 counts as predictors of pneumonias in human immunodeficiency virus–infected individuals. Ann Intern Med 111:223, 1989

Sande MA, Volberding PA: *The Medical Management of AIDS*, 2d ed. Philadelphia, Saunders, 1990

Shelhamer J et al (eds): *Respiratory Disease in the Immunosuppressed Host*. Philadelphia, Lippincott, 1991

Winston DJ et al: Beta-lactam antibiotic therapy in febrile granulocytopenic patients. Ann Intern Med 115:849, 1991

82 IMMUNIZATION PRINCIPLES AND VACCINE USE

GERALD T. KEUSCH / KENNETH J. BART

Most humans live their lives ignoring the certainty of their own mortality. Perhaps this explains why the adage "an ounce of prevention is worth a pound of cure" weighs so little in our everyday behavior. This is certainly true among adults, but even when it comes to acting to protect their young, humans are capable of either ignoring the potential mortality of their children in the developed world or accepting the certainty of childhood deaths in the developing world. In both settings, they all too often fail to seek out and demand the best preventive measures available. Unless mandated by the law in the former or provided by benevolent organizations or governments in the latter setting, universal immunization will invariably fall far short of the goal. Compulsion and benevolence, it seems, are two essential components of public health.

However, the integration of immunization practices (a major component of primary disease prevention) into routine health care services has provided caregivers with control over a substantial proportion of the disease and mortality that plagued the United States during the first half of the twentieth century (Table 82-1). For society today, immunization represents one of the most cost-effective means of preventing serious infectious disease. Presently, more than 50 biologic products are licensed in the United States and 11 antigens are used for routine immunization in the young, including diphtheria-tetanus-pertussis (DTP), trivalent polio, measles-mumps-rubella (MMR), *Haemophilus influenzae* type b (Hib), and hepatitis B vaccines. Five vaccines are designed for routine use in adults, including adult tetanus-diphtheria (Td) toxoids, hepatitis B virus, influenza virus, and polyvalent pneumococcal polysaccharides. The epidemiologically appropriate use of vaccines has resulted in the global eradication of smallpox, the virtual eradication of poliomyelitis in the Americas, and the near elimination of congenital rubella syndrome, tetanus, and diphtheria and a dramatic reduction in pertussis, rubella, measles, and mumps in the United States. Figure 82-1 shows the effect of vaccines on the incidence of *H. influenzae* type b meningitis. The Hib conjugate vaccines in particular have exerted a remarkable influence on invasive *Haemophilus* infections, presumably because they reduce nasopharyngeal carriage of *H.*

TABLE 82-1   Changes in vaccine-preventable disease incidence in the United States

		Cases reported	
	Peak year		1992*	Decreases, %
Diphtheria	1921	206,939	4	99.99
Measles	1941	894,134	2200	99.75
Mumps	1968	152,209	2460	98.38
Pertussis	1934	265,269	3359	98.73
Poliomyelitis (paralytic)	1952	21,269	0†	100.00
Rubella	1969	57,686	148	99.74
Congenital rubella syndrome	1964–5	20,000	9	99.96
Tetanus	1923	1,560	42	97.31

* Provisional.
† Projected to be 5 to 10 vaccine-associated cases.
SOURCE: Centers for Disease Control and Prevention, National Program for Immunization.

influenzae and induce protection before the period of greatest vulnerability in infancy.

Vaccine development depends on the systematic application of a four-phase strategy: (1) identify a protective antigen, (2) determine how to effectively present it to the immune system, (3) define the safety of the preparation, and (4) evaluate its efficacy in the target population. Each of these steps is simple in concept but difficult in execution, not the least so for the clinical trials necessary to assess safety and efficacy; failure at any level stops the development process. Progress in immunology has taught us much about the organization and function of the immune system (see Chap. 277); it also has taught us that the immune system is complicated and that details of antigen composition and presentation are critical for stimulating desired immune responses.

The development of vaccines goes beyond the technology and proof of principle to issues of development costs, manufacturers' liability and indemnity, perceived public health needs, and the likelihood of the product being used or sold. Given the complex science required, the costs of vaccine development are high and success is uncertain, adding risk to the development decision. It is unfortunate that the one certain implication of uncertainty in vaccine development is increased cost. In addition, a rational assignment of costs between public and private sectors in the United States has never been achieved. Under the National Vaccine Injury Compensation Program, the potential of associated or attributed adverse reactions following the use of vaccines adds to the risk and capitalization needs for vaccine development.

DEFINITIONS   *Vaccination* and *immunization* are often used as interchangeable terms; however, the former denotes only the administration of a vaccine or toxoid, whereas the latter describes the process of inducing or providing immunity by any means, whether by active or passive measures. Thus vaccination does not guarantee

FIGURE 82-1   *H. influenzae* vaccine doses sold or distributed and meningitis incidence in children more than 5 years old. *(From Centers for Disease Control and Prevention.)*

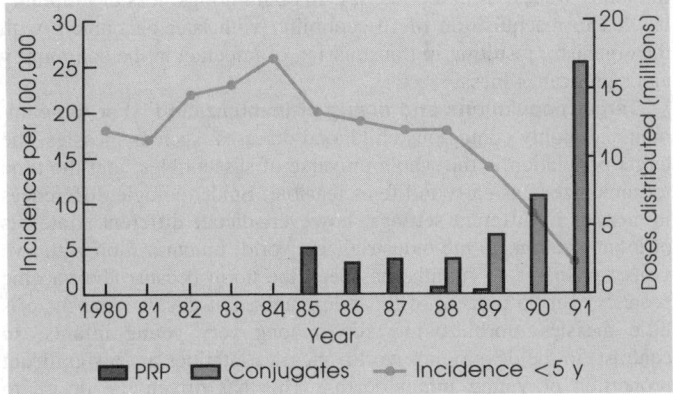

immunization. *Active immunization* refers to the induction of immune defenses by the administration of vaccines or toxoids, whereas *passive immunization* involves the provision of temporary protection by administration of exogenously produced immune substances. Immunizing agents thus include vaccines, toxoids, and antibody-containing immunoglobulin (Ig) preparations from human or animal donors (Table 82-2) and in the future may include immunocompetent cells, whether derived from the host himself or herself or from cell lines maintained in vitro or even DNA designed to express specific antigens which in turn induce protective antibodies or cell-mediated immunity.

PRINCIPLES OF IMMUNIZATION   Artificial induction of immunity closely follows two well-tested principles of nature. The first, active immunization, can be traced at least as far back as Thucydides, who noted that people surviving epidemics of plague in Athens were spared during later outbreaks of the same disease. Having symptomatic disease is an uncomfortable way of acquiring immunity, however, and some diseases do not provide subsequent resistance. The second, passive immunization, is a natural process as well, e.g., transplacental transmission of maternal antibodies to the fetus, which provides protection against several diseases during the first months of life. When practiced by clinicians, the two measures are complementary and only rarely mutually exclusive. Depending on whether there are multiple species or serotypes of an organism and whether there are common, cross-reactive, protective antigens, a specific vaccine may induce protection against all representative forms of an infectious agent or just the immunizing strain.

However, because the immune response to specific antigens is controlled genetically, individuals cannot be expected to respond equally to the same vaccine. One of the intrinsic virtues of whole-organism vaccines is that they potentially might contain all protective antigens of the organism. This is also an inherent problem of such vaccines: the possibility of adverse reactions to unnecessary materials present in the mix.

Approaches to active immunization   The principal approaches to active immunization are (1) the use of live, generally attenuated infectious agents (e.g., measles) and (2) the use of inactivated agents, detoxified extracts or toxins from them, or specific antigens obtained

TABLE 82-2   Definitions

Vaccine: A suspension of attenuated live or killed microorganisms or antigenic portions of these agents presented to a potential host to induce immunity and prevent disease.
Toxoid: A modified bacterial toxin that has been made nontoxic but retains the capacity to stimulate the formation of antitoxin.
Immune globulin: An antibody-containing solution derived from human blood obtained by cold ethanol fractionation of large pools of plasma and used primarily for the maintenance of immunity of immunodeficient persons or for passive immunization. Intramuscular and intravenous preparations are available.
Antitoxin: An antibody derived from the serum of animals after stimulation with specific antigens used to provide passive immunity.

by genetic recombination (e.g., hepatitis B virus). For many diseases (e.g., poliomyelitis, influenza), both approaches have been employed. Live, attenuated vaccines are believed to induce an immunologic response more nearly like that resulting from natural infection than the response induced by killed vaccines. Currently available inactivated or killed vaccines and those being developed consist of inactivated whole organisms (e.g., standard pertussis vaccine), detoxified protein exotoxins (e.g., tetanus toxoid), recombinant protein antigens (e.g., hepatitis B vaccine), fusion proteins with other antigens or carrier peptides or as conjugates with lipopolysaccharides, or in the case of carbohydrate antigens either as soluble purified capsular material (e.g., *Streptococcus pneumoniae* polysaccharides) or conjugated to a protein carrier (e.g., *H. influenzae* type b or group B streptococcal polysaccharides conjugated to diphtheria or tetanus toxoids).

Since the organisms in live vaccines multiply in the recipient host, antigen production generally increases logarithmically until checked by the onset of the immune response it is intended to induce. In those who respond, live, attenuated virus vaccines (e.g., measles, rubella, mumps) are believed to confer lifelong protection with one dose, although it is already clear that in some individuals immunity wanes and requires subsequent boosting for long-term protection. By contrast, except for purified polysaccharide antigens, killed vaccines generally do not induce permanent immunity with one dose, making both a series of multiple initial inoculations and subsequent periodic boosters necessary to develop and maintain high levels of antibody (e.g., diphtheria, rabies). Although the amount of antigen initially introduced is greater with inactivated vaccines, the multiplication of organisms in the host given live vaccines results in a cumulatively greater antigenic input.

Approaches to passive immunization Passive immunization is generally used to provide temporary immunity in an unimmunized subject exposed to an infectious disease when active immunization is either unavailable (e.g., hepatitis A) or has not been given prior to exposure (e.g., rabies). Passive immunization is used in the treatment of certain disorders associated with toxins (e.g., diphtheria), in certain bites (e.g., snake and spider), and as a specific [e.g., Rho(D) immune globulin] or nonspecific (e.g., antilymphocyte globulin) immunosuppressant.

Three types of preparations are used in passive immunization: (1) standard human immune serum globulin for general use (e.g., gamma globulin) and for intramuscular or intravenous administration, (2) special immune serum globulins with a known antibody content for specific agents (e.g., hepatitis B or varicella-zoster immune globulin), and (3) animal serums and antitoxins.

Determinants of the immune response The nature and extent of the response to vaccines or toxoids are determined by the chemical and physical states of the antigen, the mode of administration, the rate of antigen degradation, the genetic characteristics of the recipient, and various other host factors, some known and many unknown. The relationship between antigen dose and peak response describes a dose-response curve with a threshold at the low end and a plateau at the high end.

Route of administration The route of administration in part determines the rapidity and nature of the immune responses to vaccines. Parenterally administered vaccine may not induce mucosal secretory IgA, and mucosal immunization may or may not induce good systemic responses.

Age The age of the individual influences the response to vaccines, and therefore, recommended schedules for immunization are based on age-dependent responses and empirical data from clinical trials. The presence of high levels of maternal antibody and/or the immaturity of the immune system in the early months of life impairs the initial immune response to some antigens. In the elderly, vaccine responses may be diminished because of natural waning of the immune system. Hence larger amounts of an antigen may be required to produce the desired response (e.g., influenza).

Adjuvant potentiation The immune response to some antigens is potentiated by the addition of adjuvants such as aluminum salts or, in the case of polysaccharides (e.g., the polyribose phosphate polysaccharide of *H. influenzae* type b), by covalent conjugation to a peptide. Adjuvants, nonspecific boosters of immune responses, are used with inactivated products such as diphtheria and tetanus toxoids, acellular pertussis (aP), and hepatitis B vaccines. The mechanism for adjuvant enhancement of antigenicity is not well defined but may relate to the rendering of soluble antigens into a particulate form, the ability to mobilize phagocytes to the site of antigen deposition, and slower release of antigens, which prolongs stimulation of the immune response. Although many constituents of infectious microorganisms and their products, such as exotoxins, are or can be made to be antigenic, only a limited number stimulate a protective immune response.

Mucosal immunity Many pathogens replicate only at musocal surfaces (e.g., *Vibrio cholerae*), while other pathogens replicate at the mucosa before host invasion (e.g., poliovirus, rubella, or influenza). At the mucosal site, these organisms induce secretory IgA. Induction of secretory IgA by vaccines may be an efficient way to block the essential steps in pathogenesis, whether the organism is restricted to mucosal surfaces or systemically invades the host across mucosal surfaces.

Measurement of the immune response Immune responses to vaccines are often gauged by the concentration of specific antibody in serum. While seroconversion serves as a dependable indicator of an immune response, it measures only one immunologic parameter and does not necessarily indicate protection. The development of circulating antibodies after immunization often correlates directly with clinical protection (e.g., measles or rubella). Some responses may not in themselves reflect immunity but may be sufficiently associated with protection that they remain useful proxy measures (e.g., vibriocidal serum antibodies in cholera). At the same time, the absence of measurable antibody in a previously immunized individual does not mean that he or she is unprotected if a secondary protective IgG antibody response occurs rapidly enough after challenge. In some instances, the titer of antibody is critical, and for certain vaccines (e.g., tetanus), protection is predictable by the level of circulating antitoxin antibody.

Herd immunity It is not necessary to immunize every person to stop transmission of an infectious agent through a population. For those organisms dependent on person-to-person transmission, there may be a definable prevalence of immunity in the population above which it becomes difficult for the organism to circulate and reach new susceptibles. This prevalence is called *herd immunity,* and it permits the goals of immunization to be converted from the need to immunize every person in the community to a population goal, in which the target is to immunize a specified minimum percentage of the persons at risk. Herd immunity may be lost when individuals refuse to be immunized (as happened with pertussis in the United Kingdom in the 1970s because of the concerns about severe vaccine reactions, which exceeded the fear of the disease itself) or when immunity wanes (as in diphtheria). In both settings, loss of immunity has led to reacquisition of susceptibility with later encounters with the organism, resulting in transmission of infection in the community and significant illness.

Target populations and timing of immunization For the common and highly contagious childhood diseases, such as measles, the target population is the whole universe of susceptibles, and the time to immunize is as early in life as feasible. Epidemiologic differences in measles in different settings, however, dictate different strategies of immunization. In the industrialized world, immunization with live virus vaccine at 15 months has been the norm because the vaccine protects over 95 percent of those immunized at this age and there is little measles morbidity/mortality among very young infants. In contrast, in the developing world, measles fatalities are a significant proportion of young infant deaths. This has driven the desire to immunize in the first few months of life in order to close the window of vulnerability between the rapid decline of maternal antibody after 4 to 6 months and the subsequent vaccine-induced active immunity.

Problems have cropped up in measles immunization programs in both the developed and the developing world. In the United States, recent outbreaks of measles have occurred among unvaccinated infants younger than 15 months and preschoolers from underserved inner-city populations, as well as among previously vaccinated college students. These outbreaks represent both vaccine failure and program failure. Among the former, most are *primary* failures, i.e., no initial response to the vaccine. However, some are due to secondary loss of immunity with time after immunization, especially after the unstabilized pre-1980 vaccines, or when vaccines were given along with gamma globulin. Program failures represent an inability to reach and immunize the target population, often because no systematic program of immunization exists.

H. influenzae type b causes severe invasive disease and is the leading cause of meningitis, epiglotitis, and pneumonia in early childhood. Similar to measles, the majority of severe disease occurs in early childhood, rising sharply after the disappearance of maternally derived antibody. In contrast to measles vaccine, however, primary failure of Hib vaccine during infancy is due more to the age-related inability to respond to polysaccharide antigens. To overcome this innate deficit, the protective polysaccharide has been coupled with protein to convert it to a T cell–dependent antigen to which young infants respond.

In some diseases, such as rubella, infection is primarily a threat to the fetus, since young infants and children are not at risk of serious illness. While it is not clinically necessary to immunize early in life, the goal is to ensure immunity before females enter the reproductive age group. Theoretically, immunization of all reproductive-age women prior to pregnancy would be an ideal strategy. Because of the difficulties in systematically reaching all adolescents and young females and in ensuring the protection of as many women as possible, it was recognized that universal childhood immunization both to reach susceptibles and to interrupt transmission was necessary.

Some vaccines are now used primarily for adults, e.g., influenza virus and polyvalent pneumococcal polysaccharide vaccines to prevent pneumonia deaths in the elderly. They are, unfortunately, underused in large part because physicians and patients in the target group ignore the indication in otherwise healthy older adults and partly because there is a tendency to think about prevention with vaccines as a strategy for children. In addition, pneumococcal polysaccharide vaccine is recommended for children over 2 years who are at risk of severe, life-threatening pneumococcal infection, such as those with sickle cell disease, asplenia (whether functional or anatomic), renal failure and nephrotic syndrome, cerebrospinal fluid leak, and human immunodeficiency virus (HIV) infection or other immunosuppressive disease states. Because infection with *S. pneumoniae* is a major cause of otitis media, lung, and central nervous system infections in young children, however, the vaccine (which is immunogenic in infancy) may at some future time be considered for routine use in all children.

Biologic impediments Each of the vaccines mentioned below illustrates major technical problems to be overcome in vaccine development. Thus influenza virus, characterized biologically by its antigenic drift, periodically emerges in a new antigenic version capable of causing a global pandemic for which a new vaccine must be rapidly devised, produced, and distributed. In contrast to the circulation of one major antigenic type of influenza A at any one time, many prevalent pneumococcal polysaccharide serotypes are in circulation at all times. Because immunity is serotype-specific, however, an individual is susceptible to all serotypes for which he or she lacks antibody. The reality of serotype-specific protection is one reason why it was more difficult to develop an effective pneumococcal vaccine than it was to develop a vaccine for *H. influenzae,* where almost all severe disease is related to one capsular serotype, type b. To overcome this problem, pneumococcal vaccine includes 23

polysaccharides which represent approximately 80 percent of the commonly encountered virulent serotypes. Unfortunately, some serotype polysaccharides are poorly immunogenic, and immunized individuals will remain susceptible to the serotypes excluded from the vaccine. Improved immunization awaits either a safe, effective conjugate vaccine to break the polysaccharide-response barrier in early childhood or the development of a common protective protein antigen vaccine that protects against all pneumococcal serotypes.

The use of hepatitis B virus (HBV) vaccine illustrates another technical issue. Because hepatitis B is of low endemicity in the general population in the United States, the high cost of the original serum-derived vaccine led to its being targeted to populations at high risk of acquiring HBV infection and its sequelae, chronic active hepatitis, including medical personnel handling blood and blood products, injection drug users, and homosexuals. In contrast, the most important sequela of HBV in Africa and Asia is neither acute nor chronic hepatitis but rather the long-term effect of chronic infection acquired in infancy on the later induction of liver cancer in young adults. The need for immunization in the developing world was therefore different from in the United States, first to prevent liver cancer in adult life and only second to prevent acute and chronic hepatitis. To accomplish the first goal, it would be necessary to immunize as close to birth as possible. The advent of recombinant HBV vaccines and reductions in cost have permitted a change in strategy. HBV vaccine is now recommended for universal use in infants in the United States as well as in unimmunized older children and adults at high risk of infection, including household members exposed to HBV surface (HBVs) antigen–positive adopted or foster immigrant children from HBV-endemic countries. Universal immunization at birth has been adopted in a few African and Asian countries, but proof of its efficacy to prevent liver cancer will require decades of surveillance, and ambitious studies are now in progress.

Testing of vaccines In the development of vaccines, initial studies are typically carried out in animal models, if available, to demonstrate the production of immune responses, their ability to protect the host, and their relative safety. Ultimately, vaccines for humans must be tested in humans. There are three questions to be answered: (1) Is the vaccine immunogenic and safe? (2) Is the vaccine efficacious under controlled conditions? And (3) is the vaccine effective in reducing disease prevalence in a population? Thus, when initial in vitro and animal data look promising, graded doses of vaccine are given to small numbers of humans to assess immune responses and safety. Human clinical trials are then performed in larger numbers to demonstrate vaccine efficacy often by challenge of a group of informed volunteers with a virulent strain. After clinical trials in the community, typically involving 1000 to 10,000 vaccinees, licensure may be sought. Because of their limited size, however, these trials cannot be expected to detect rare but serious adverse effects. Thus licensing does not guarantee that a new vaccine is completely safe, and postlicensing monitoring of safety and efficacy is needed to ensure effectiveness and determine the occurrence of adverse effects of low frequency.

Vaccine formulations The development of the science of immunology has led to the understanding that living and dead antigens do not necessarily induce the same immune responses and that the requirements for protective immunity differ with the organism. These insights, together with the refinement of epidemiologic concepts surrounding immunization, have changed the strategy of vaccine development. Now the goal is not only to select the correct antigens but also to ensure that the vaccines will result in the type of immune response needed for protection, whether T cell–mediated macrophage activation or generation of cytotoxic T cells or B cell–mediated secretory IgA or a particular IgG subtype response to a specific polysaccharide epitope.

Living vaccines are selected or genetically altered to be avirulent or dramatically attenuated yet still remain immunogenic. In effect, these agents are expected to cause a subclinical illness that mimics natural infection except for the lack of clinical disease. They have the advantage of replication in vivo, which increases the antigenic load presented to the host immune system; they present a diversity of antigens to overcome immunogenetic restrictions in some hosts; they may reach the local sites most appropriate for inducing protective immunity; and they also may produce important protective antigens in vivo that are not efficiently expressed in vitro.

In contrast, with nonviable vaccines, in essence, what you give is what you get vis-à-vis antigen load and the specific antigenic determinants presented. In addition, these preparations often fail to elicit mucosal IgA-mediated immunity, since they lack a delivery system to the local antigen-processing cells as effective as a living organism, and, except for pure polysaccharide antigens, they almost always require multiple exposures to induce effective responses. However, killed vaccines can be extremely effective. For example, for hepatitis A, a nonviable vaccine formulation close to being licensed appears to be nearly 100 percent effective in inducing protective immunity.

Despite these characteristics, living vaccines are not always the preferred type. For example, there are populations in whom live oral polio vaccine (OPV) is less than ideally effective. Thus, in India, it requires up to 9 to 10 doses of Sabin vaccine to fully immunize the majority of subjects, whereas the usual series of the highly immunogenic enhanced-potency inactivated polio vaccine (IPV-e) will protect nearly all. There is a tradeoff, however, since the new killed vaccine does not immunize the gut and can neither reduce the circulation of wild-type poliovirus nor immunize contacts of vaccine recipients. There is also no risk of vaccine-strain poliomyelitis occurring. In some settings, a combination schedule of killed and living polio vaccine may make the most sense, and this strategy is currently being evaluated.

To create a deliverable vaccine, constituents other than the antigens are required (Table 82-3). These constituents can affect immunogenicity, efficacy, and safety of a vaccine, and they determine the success of one formulation over another.

Production of vaccines As products to be given to healthy individuals to prevent disease, there is a special requirement for vaccines to be not only efficacious but also without the capacity to cause harm. In the United States, this quality assurance is the responsibility of the manufacturers. Standards of manufacture of biologicals (quality control) are regulated and supervised by the Food and Drug Administration. Proof of both safety and efficacy is required, and sterility and purity of products are monitored. On rare occasions, either good manufacturing practice or quality assurance have broken down, e.g., the release of incompletely killed Salk polio vaccine in 1955, which caused an outbreak of poliomyelitis in nearly 200 vaccine recipients and their contacts. Unregulated and uncontrolled manufacture of vaccines in developing countries has sometimes led to the release and use of inactive products that fail to provide the expected protective immunity. These episodes are ordinarily not detected and their clinical consequences remain unmeasured.

Another problem in production of vaccines has cropped up unexpectedly in the past decade in violation of the basic law of supply and demand. For multiple reasons, including the high costs of vaccine development and testing, liability of pharmaceutical companies to claims of vaccine-related injury, and the prospect of much higher profitability from investing in other products, the number of vaccine manufacturers in the United States has declined and the costs of some basic childhood vaccines have increased. There is, therefore, legitimate concern about the future availability of these essential biologicals for national use. In addition, pricing decisions made within the private-sector pharmaceutical industry can have a major impact on vaccine use. This has stimulated an initiative toward increasing public oversight and price negotiations with industry. The recent increase in the UNICEF contract price of polio vaccine from 4 to 8 cents per dose has had no effect on the use of this vaccine in the United States but has severely stressed the ability of UNICEF to meet its vaccine procurement obligations for immunization in developing countries.

Administration of vaccines The number of vaccines that can be given at one time without interfering with response or increasing side effects—and the cost of buying and administering them—affect the ability to deliver vaccines. There is clearly as much art to the programming of vaccine administration as there is to the development and testing of protective antigens. Wherever effective primary health care systems ensure access to medical services for the majority and the population is educated about the need for and efficacy of vaccines, high coverage rates for basic immunization should be achieved, regardless of the route of administration of a vaccine or the number of doses necessary. However, without attention to the infrastructure needed for follow-up on multiple-dose vaccine schedules, coverage rates for second, third, and booster doses of vaccines may drop off significantly. The simple act of providing "road to health" cards to mothers in developing countries on which immunizations, growth, and major illnesses are recorded has increased the rates of complete basic immunization of infants because the mothers can more effectively participate in the process.

VACCINE USE Recommendations for vaccine use in the United States are developed by several different groups, including the Advisory Committee on Immunization Practices (ACIP) of the Centers for Disease Control and Prevention (CDC), the Committee on Infectious Diseases of the American Academy of Pediatrics (AAP, The Red Book), the American College of Physicians (ACP), the American Academy of Family Practice (AAFP), and the American College of Obstetrics and Gynecology (ACOG).

Vaccines recommended in 1993 for routine use for infants, children, and adults and vaccines for special use are shown in Tables 82-4 and 82-5, respectively. Intervals between doses longer than those recommended do not diminish the ultimate protective response but merely delay it. It is not necessary to restart an interrupted schedule from the beginning or to add an extra dose. In contrast, giving vaccines at shorter than recommended intervals may result in poor responses.

Recording and reporting requirements Certain aspects of vaccine use are directed by the National Childhood Vaccine Injury Act (NCVIA) of 1986. The act requires that all mandated childhood vaccinations be recorded by health care providers in the child's permanent medical record, including date of administration, the manufacturer and lot number, and the name of the provider administering the vaccine. Parents also should keep an up-to-date immunization record on their children. The act also requires that the benefits to the child and possible reactions be explained to parents. Educational materials providing the required information are available from the CDC or the AAP.

VACCINES FOR ROUTINE USE **Infants and children** Recommended schedules for administration of vaccines to infants and children are shown in Table 82-6. It is current practice that all children in the United States should receive DTP, polio, measles, mumps, rubella, *H. influenzae* type b, and HBV vaccines unless contraindicated (Table 82-7). Four doses of DTP and three doses of OPV constitute the primary series. A fifth dose of DTP is given at 4 to 6 years of age. Adult formulation tetanus-diphtheria (Td) boosters are recommended every 10 years thereafter. A fourth dose of OPV is also recommended

---

TABLE 82-3 Constituents of vaccines

Preservatives, stabilizers, antibiotics
Used to inhibit or prevent bacterial growth or to stabilize the antigen. Materials such as mercurials or antibiotics are used. Allergic reactions to any of the additives may occur.

Adjuvants
An aluminum salt is used in some vaccines to enhance the immune response (e.g., toxoids, hepatitis B).

Suspending fluid
Sterile water, saline, buffer, or more complex fluids derived from the growth medium or biologic system in which the agent is produced (e.g., egg antigens, cell culture ingredients, serum proteins).

TABLE 82-4 Routinely recommended vaccines for infants, children, and adults

Vaccine	Type of immunizing agent	Recommended route of administration	Efficacy	Adverse events
Diphtheria and tetanus toxoids and pertussis vaccine	Toxoids and inactivated whole bacteria	IM	D = 95% P = 80% T = 95%	Frequent local reactions; seizures, hypotonic hyporesponsive episodes, acute encephalopathy (DTP) Arthus-like reaction in persons who have received multiple boosters (Td)
Diphtheria and tetanus toxoids, pediatric				
Tetanus, diphtheria toxoids, adult				
Acellular pertussis	Inactivated bacterial antigen	IM	?	Reduce local reactions; no serious reactions reported
Haemophilus influenzae type b	Bacterial polysaccharide conjugated to protein	IM	90%	Local reactions, 10%; no serious reactions
Hepatitis B	Inactivated viral antigen	IM	80–95%	Mild local reaction; Guillain-Barré syndrome, rare
Influenza	Inactivated virus or viral components	IM	40–70%	Mild local reaction; Guillain-Barré syndrome with swine flu; rare allergic reaction in those allergic to eggs
Measles, mumps, rubella virus vaccine combined	Live viruses	SQ	M = 95% Mu = 95% R = 95%	Acute encephalopathy (measles) Parotitis and orchitis reported rarely (mumps) Arthralgia (40%); arthritis (<2%); rare arthropathy; 5–15% fever 5–21 days after vaccinations; 5% rash
Pneumococcal polysaccharide	Bacterial polysaccharide of 23 types	IM or SQ	60–80%	Local reactions—50% (pain); rare anaphylaxis; arthus-like reaction with booster doses
Poliomyelitis Oral polio virus	Live virus of three serotypes	Oral	95%	Vaccine-associated poliomyelitis, rare
Inactivated polio virus–enhanced (IPV-e)	Inactivated virus of three serotypes	SQ	95%	None significant

SOURCE: Recommendations of the Advisory Committee on Immunization Practices, the American Academy of Pediatrics, and the American College of Physicians.

TABLE 82-5 Special-use vaccines

Vaccine	Year licensed	Type of immunizing agent	Route of administration	Indications	Efficacy	Adverse events
Adenovirus types 4 and 7	1980	Unattenuated live viruses	Oral	Used solely for military recruits	>90%	Essentially non-existent
Anthrax	1970	Inactivated avirulent bacteria	SQ (6 doses primary; annual booster)	For high risk of exposure, i.e., persons in contact with or manufacture of animal hides, furs, bone meal, wool, goat hair	90% antibody response but efficacy uncertain	No serious adverse effects are known
Tuberculosis (BCG)	1950	Living bacteria	ID	PPD-negative individuals in prolonged contact with active TB patient	Controversial, reduces disseminated disease in children	Regional adenitis, disseminated BCG, osteitis
Cholera	1914	Inactivated bacteria	SC or ID	Not recommended for public health use	50% (short-lived)	Frequent fever, local pain, swelling
Meningococcal A, C, Y, W135	1981	Bacterial polysaccharide of four serotypes	SC	Military; principally travelers to epidemic areas	90% for 2–3-year-olds Annually for <4-year-olds	Rare
Plague	1911	Inactivated bacteria	IM	Laboratory workers; foresters in endemic areas; travelers	90% antibody response but efficacy uncertain	10% local reactions; rare sterile abscesses and hypersensitivity
Rabies (human diploid)	1980	Inactivated virus	IM or ID	Travelers; laboratory workers; veterinarians	Virtually 100%	25% local reactions; 6% arthropathy, arthritis, angioedema
Yellow fever	1953	Live virus	SC	Laboratory workers; travelers	High	Encephalitis; encephalopathy
Japanese encephalitis	1993	Inactivated virus	SC	Travelers	80–90%	Anaphylactic/severe delayed allergic reactions common; observe for 10 days
Typhoid				Not routinely recommended in United States		
Phenol and heat killed	1952	Killed whole bacteria	IM	Travelers, contact with carrier	50–70% (short-lived)	Frequent fever, local swelling, pain
Ty$_{21a}$	1992	Live mutant bacteria	Oral	Travelers, contact with carrier	50–70%	None

SOURCE: Recommendations of the Advisory Committee on Immunization Practices, the American Academy of Pediatrics, and the American College of Physicians.

TABLE 82-6 Recommended schedule of vaccinations for all children

Vaccine	2 Months	4 Months	6 Months	12 Months	15 Months	4–6 Years (before school entry)
DTP	√	√	√		√*	√
Polio	√	√			√*	√
MMR					√†	√‡
Hib						
Option 1§	√	√	√		√	
Option 2§	√	√		√		

	Birth	1–2 Months		6–18 Months
HBV				
Option 1	√	√¶		√¶
Option 2		√¶	√¶	√¶

NOTE: DTP: diphtheria, tetanus, and pertussis vaccine (combined); polio: live oral polio drops (OPV) or killed (inactivated) polio vaccine shots (IPV); MMR: measles, mumps, and rubella vaccine (combined); Hib: *Haemophilus* b conjugate vaccine; HBV: hepatitis B vaccine.
* Many experts recommend these vaccines at 18 months.
† In some areas this dose of MMR vaccine may be given at 12 months.
‡ Many experts recommend this dose of MMR vaccine be given at entry to middle school or junior high school.
§ HIB vaccine is given in either a four-dose schedule (1) or a three-dose schedule (2) depending on the type of vaccine used.
¶ Hepatitis B vaccine can be given simultaneously with DTP, polio, MMR, and *Haemophilus* b conjugate vaccine at the same visit.
SOURCE: ACIP: General recommendations on immunization. Morb Mort Week Rep 38:205, 1989.

TABLE 82-7 Vaccination contraindications and precautions[1]

Vaccine	Valid	Invalid
General for all vaccines (DTP/DTaP, OPV, IPV, MMR, Hib, HBV)	Anaphylactic reaction to a vaccine contraindicates further doses of that vaccine Anaphylactic reaction to a vaccine constituent contraindicates the use of vaccines containing that substance Moderate or severe illnesses with or without a fever	Mild to moderate local reaction (soreness, redness, swelling) following a dose of an injectable antigen Mild acute illness with or without low-grade fever Current antimicrobial therapy Convalescent phase of illnesses Prematurity (use same dosage and indications as for normal, full-term infants) Recent exposure to an infectious disease History of penicillin or other nonspecific allergies or fact that relatives have such allergies
DTP/DTaP	Encephalopathy within 7 days of administration of previous dose of DTP Fever of ≥40.5°C (105°F) within 48 h after vaccination with a prior dose of DTP[2] Collapse or shocklike state (hypotonic-hyporesponsive episode) within 48 h of receiving a prior dose of DTP[2] Seizures within 3 days of receiving a prior dose of DTP (see note 3 regarding management of children with a personal history of seizures at any time)[2] Persistent, inconsolable crying lasting ≥3 h within 48 h of receiving a prior dose of DTP[2]	Temperature of >40.5°C (105°F) following a previous dose of DTP Family history of convulsions[3] Family history of an adverse event following DTP administration Family history of sudden infant death syndrome
OPV[4]	Infection with HIV or a household contact with HIV Known immunodeficiency (hematologic and solid tumors; congenital immunodeficiency syndrome; and long term immunosuppressive therapy) Immunodeficient household contact Pregnancy[2]	Breast feeding Current antimicrobial therapy Diarrhea
IPV	Anaphylactic reactions to neomycin or streptomycin Pregnancy[2]	
MMR[4]	Anaphylactic reactions to eggs or to neomycin[5] Pregnancy Known immunodeficiency (hematologic and solid tumors; congenital immunodeficiency syndrome; and long term immunosuppressive therapy) Recent (within 3 months) IG administration[2]	Tuberculosis or positive PPD Simultaneous TB skin testing[6] Breast feeding Pregnancy of mother of recipient Immunodeficient family member or household contact Infection with HIV Nonanaphylactic reactions to eggs or neomycin
Hib	None identified	
HBV		Pregnancy
Influenza	Avoid during 1st trimester of pregnancy on theoretical grounds Anaphylactic reactions to eggs	
Pneumococcus	Has not been evaluated in pregnancy	

[1] Based on the recommendations of the Advisory Committee on Immunization Practices (ACIP) and those of the Committee on the Infectious Diseases (Red Book Committee) of the American Academy of Pediatrics (AAP) as of October 1992. Sometimes these recommendations vary from those contained in the manufacturers' package inserts. For more detailed information, providers should consult the current published recommendations of the ACIP, the AAP, the AAFP, and the manufacturers' package inserts.
[2] The events or conditions listed as precautions, although not contraindications, should be carefully reviewed. The benefits and risks of administering a specific vaccine to an individual under the circumstances should be considered. If the risks are believed to outweigh the benefits, the immunization should be withheld; if the benefits are believed to outweigh the risks (e.g., during an outbreak or foreign travel), the immunization should be given. Whether and when to administer DTP to children with proven or suspected underlying neurologic disorders should be decided on an individual basis. It is prudent on theoretical grounds to avoid vaccinating pregnant women. However, if immediate protection against poliomyelitis is needed, OPV, not IPV, is recommended.
[3] Acetaminophen given prior to administering DTP and thereafter every 4 h for 24 h should be considered for children with a personal or with a family history of convulsions in siblings or parents.
[4] There is a theoretical risk that the administration of multiple live virus vaccines (OPV and MMR) within 30 days of one another if not given on the same day will result in a suboptimal immune response. There are no data to substantiate this.
[5] Persons with a history of anaphylactic reactions following egg ingestion should be vaccinated only with extreme caution. Protocols have been developed for vaccinating such persons and should be consulted (J Pediatr 1983; 102:196–9, J Pediatr 1988; 113:504–6).
[6] Measles vaccination may temporarily suppress tuberculin reactivity. If testing can not be done the day of MMR vaccination, the test should be postponed for 4–6 weeks.
SOURCES: Standards for Pediatric Immunization Practices, Centers for Disease Control and Prevention; ACIP: Pneumococcal polysaccharide vaccine. Morb Mort Week Rep 38:64, 1989; ACIP: Prevention and control of influenza. Morb Mort Week Rep 40:73, 1991.

at 4 to 6 years of age. One dose of a combined measles, mumps, and rubella vaccine is recommended at 15 months and again at school entry or in middle school. DTP, MMR, OPV, and Hib vaccines may be given simultaneously at 15 months of age without increasing adverse reaction rates or impairing the immune response.

Adults All adults should be immune to diphtheria and tetanus. If not previously immunized, adults require a primary immunizing course of three doses of Td, with the second dose 4 to 8 weeks after the first and the third dose at 12 months, plus boosters administered every 10 years thereafter. Many individuals remain immune to tetanus into adulthood because they have received tetanus toxoid rather than Td after injuries, but they are commonly at risk of diphtheria. Routine immunization against polio is not recommended for adults unless they are at particular risk of exposure, as with travel to endemic regions of the world (see "Travel," below). Adults should be protected from measles, mumps, and rubella and should be vaccinated unless they are known to have either received vaccine on or after their first birthday or had physician-diagnosed disease. Rubella vaccine should be given to all women of childbearing age unless they have documentary proof of immunization after their first birthday or laboratory evidence of immunity. A history of prior rubella disease is unreliable and should not be accepted.

Current recommendations also include influenza vaccine for routine annual administration to adults 65 years of age and older and to individuals at any age with chronic illness. Polyvalent pneumococcal polysaccharide vaccine is similarly recommended for the elderly or chronically ill. Hepatitis B is recommended for individuals at high risk of exposure, including health care workers exposed to potentially infected blood, homosexuals, injection drug users, individuals living and working in institutions for the mentally retarded, and household contacts of known carriers of hepatitis B surface antigen.

Adverse events following vaccination Modern vaccines, while safe and effective, are associated with adverse effects which range from the very mild to the life-threatening. Because no vaccine can

be expected to be 100 percent effective, some persons who have received a full course of vaccine or toxoid may develop disease upon exposure. The decision to use a vaccine involves assessment of the risks of disease, the benefits of vaccination, and the risks associated with vaccination. These factors may change over time, and consequently, continued assessment of vaccines is essential. Table 82-7 presents a guide to contraindications to immunization and appropriate precautions in the use of specific vaccines.

All detected adverse events temporally related to vaccination are expected to be reported to both the local health department and the vaccine manufacturer. The NCVIA requires health care providers to report certain suspected adverse events after a mandated vaccine to the FDA's Vaccine Adverse Events Reporting System (VAERS) (Table 82-8). Although a temporal relationship does not establish cause and effect, surveillance is essential to collect data needed to form conclusions and make decisions.

Vaccine components, including the protective antigens, animal proteins introduced during vaccine production, and antibiotics or other preservatives or stabilizers, can cause allergic reactions in some recipients. These may be local or systemic, including serious anaphylaxis and urticaria. The most common extraneous allergen is egg protein introduced when vaccines are prepared in embryonated eggs, such as occurs with measles, mumps, influenza, and yellow fever vaccines. Local or systemic reactions can result from the too frequent administration of some vaccines, such as Td, DT, or rabies, and are probably due to antigen-antibody complexes.

In addition, live virus vaccines can interfere with tuberculin test responses. When a tuberculin skin test is indicated, it may be done either on the day of immunization or 6 weeks later.

USE OF VACCINES IN SPECIAL CIRCUMSTANCES Pregnancy Because of theoretical risks to the fetus and the risk of litigation to the practitioner, immunization of pregnant women is usually avoided. Notwithstanding, it is essential to ensure that pregnant women are immune to tetanus, since transfer of maternal antitoxin antibodies is

TABLE 82-8 Reportable events following vaccination, as required by the National Vaccine Injury Act of 1986

Vaccine/toxoid	Event	Interval from vaccination
DTP; P; DTP/polio combined	Anaphylaxis or anaphylactic shock	24 h
	Encephalopathy (or encephalitis)*	3 days
	Shock-collapse or hypotonic-hyporesponsive collapse*	3 days
	Residual seizure disorder*	(See Aids to Interpretation)
	Any acute complication or sequela (including death) of above events	No limit
	Events in vaccinees described in manufacturer's package insert as contraindications to additional doses of vaccine† (such as convulsions)	(See package insert)
Measles, mumps, and rubella, DT, Td, tetanus toxoid (TT)	Anaphylaxis or anaphylactic shock	24 h
	Encephalopathy (or encephalitis)*	15 days for measles, mumps and rubella; 3 days for DT, Td, TT
	Residual seizure disorder*	(See Aids to Interpretation)
	Any acute complication or sequela (including death) of above events	No limit
	Events in vaccinees described in manufacturer's package insert as contraindications to additional doses of vaccine†	(See package insert)
Oral polio vaccine (OPV)	Paralytic polio in a nonimmunodeficient recipient	30 days
	Paralytic polio in an immunodeficient recipient or vaccine-associated community case	6 months
	Any acute complication or sequela (including death) of the above	No limit
	Events in vaccinees described in manufacturer's package insert as contraindications to additional doses of vaccine†	(See package insert)
Inactivated polio vaccine–enhanced (IPV-e)	Anaphylaxis or anaphylactic shock	24 h
	Any acute complication or sequela (including death) of above events	No limit
	Events in vaccines described in manufacturer's package insert as contraindications to additional doses of vaccine†	(See package insert)

* Aids to Interpretation: Shock-collapse or hypotonic-hyporesponsive collapse may be evidenced by signs or symptoms such as decrease in or loss of muscle tone, paralysis (partial or complete), hemiplegia, hemiparesis, loss of color or turning pale white or blue, unresponsiveness to environmental stimuli, depression of or loss of consciousness, prolonged sleeping with difficult arousing, or cardiovascular or respiratory arrest. Residual seizure disorder may be considered to have occurred if no other seizure or convulsion unaccompanied by fevers or accompanied by a fever of less than 102°F occurred before the first seizure or convulsion after the administration of the vaccine involved; if in the case of measles, mumps, or rubella-containing vaccines, the first seizure or convulsion occurred within 15 days after vaccination; or in the case of any other vaccine, the first seizure or convulsion occurred within three days after vaccination, and, if two or more seizures or convulsions unaccompanied by fever or accompanied by a fever of less than 102°F occurred within 1 year after vaccination. The terms *seizure* and *convulsion* include grand mal, petit mal, absence, myoclonia, tonic-clonic, and focal motor seizures and signs. *Encephalopathy* means any significant acquired abnormality of, injury to, or impairment of function of the brain. Among the frequent manifestations of encephalopathy are focal and diffuse neurologic signs, increased intracranial pressure, or changes in level of consciousness lasting at least 6 h with or without convulsions. The neurologic signs and symptoms of encephalopathy may be temporary with complete recovery, or they may result in various degrees of permanent impairment. Signs and symptoms such as high-pitched and unusual screaming, persistent inconsolable crying, and bulging fontanel are compatible with an encephalopathy, but in and of themselves are not conclusive evidence of encephalopathy. Encephalopathy usually can be documented by slow wave activity on an electroencephalogram.
† The health-care provider must refer to contraindication section of the manufacturer's package insert for each vaccine.
SOURCE: National Childhood Vaccine Injury Act of 1986.

an important means of prevention of neonatal tetanus and pregnant women can safely receive tetanus as well as diphtheria toxoids. Although live virus vaccines, in general, should be withheld during pregnancy, polio and yellow fever vaccines are exceptions and may be administered if the risk of exposure to disease is great. If indicated, some inactivated virus vaccines, e.g., influenza, are safe to give to pregnant women.

Breast feeding Breast-fed infants can be immunized on a normal schedule. Breast feeding does not adversely affect the immune response and is not a contraindication for any vaccine. Breast-feeding women also may be vaccinated without problem. Although live vaccines multiply within the mother's body, most are not excreted in breast milk. Mothers may therefore receive oral polio or yellow fever vaccines without interrupting breast feeding.

Occupational exposure Immunization recommendations for most occupational groups remain to be developed. Specific requirements for immunization of health care workers against hepatitis B in the United States are now mandated by the Occupational Safety and Health Administration (OSHA). Those at particular risk of exposure to hepatitis B, such as health workers dealing with blood products or surgeons, must be immunized. Many medical institutions now give HBV vaccine to all health care workers and medical, dental, and nursing students. Transmission of rubella in medical facilities to and from health care workers, particularly in pediatrics, occurs as well. Health care workers who might transmit rubella to pregnant patients should therefore be immune to rubella, and it is prudent to screen them for antibodies to rubella and immunize susceptibles. Health care workers are also at greater risk from measles than the general public, and those likely to come in contact with measles patients should be immune. Health care workers caring for patients with chronic diseases can transmit influenza; such workers should be vaccinated annually. Unfortunately, these recommendations often are not fully implemented, even in academic institutions.

HIV infection and other immunocompromised states Limited studies in HIV-infected individuals have not shown an increased risk of adverse events from live or inactivated vaccines. However, immune responses in immunocompromised individuals may not be as vigorous as in subjects with a normal immune system. Except for polio, persons known to be HIV infected should be immunized with recommended vaccines as early in the course of their disease as possible in the same manner as individuals without immunocompromise, before significant impairment in immune function occurs. This includes the use of live, attenuated MMR vaccine (Table 82-9), although IPV-e should be used when vaccination against polio is indicated because the risk of vaccine-associated poliomyelitis is too great. Care should be taken to ensure that household contacts to be immunized against polio receive IPV-e and not OPV. However, it is not necessary to test for HIV before making immunization decisions for asymptomatic individuals from known HIV risk groups.

Live, attenuated vaccines are normally contraindicated in other immunocompromised patients such as the congenital immunodeficiency syndromes and in patients receiving immunosuppressive therapy. Passive immunization with immunoglobulin preparations or antitoxins can be considered in individual cases, either as postexposure prophylaxis or as part of the therapy of established infection.

Postexposure immunization For certain infections, active or passive immunization soon after exposure prevents or attenuates disease expression. The immune globulins and antitoxins currently available in the United States are listed in Table 82-10, and the recommended postexposure immunization regimens are compiled in Table 82-11. Measles immune globulins given within 6 days of exposure may prevent or modify infection, and administration of measles vaccine within the first few days after exposure may prevent symptomatic infection. Although clinical manifestations of rubella are minimized by postexposure passive immunization, this may not prevent viremia, fetal infection, and congenital rubella syndrome. Therefore, the administration of immune globulin is recommended only for women developing rubella during pregnancy who will not consider abortion under any circumstances. Tetanus immune globulin can be used in patients with tetanus; however, survivors with no history of tetanus immunization should receive a primary series of toxoid. Administration of rabies immune globulin plus rabies vaccine in the immediate postexposure period is highly effective in preventing disease. Similarly, the use of immune globulin within 2 weeks of exposure to hepatitis A is likely to prevent clinical illness. There are also good data indicating the efficacy of special human HBV immune globulin in preventing disease after exposure. While there is no high-titer preparation for postexposure protection against non-A, non-B hepatitis, standard human immune serum globulin is efficacious.

Simultaneous administration of vaccines The simultaneous administration of the most widely used live and inactivated vaccines has not resulted in impaired antibody responses or increased rates of adverse reactions. Simultaneous administration of vaccines is important to increase the probability that a child will ultimately be fully immunized and when there is imminent exposure to multiple infectious diseases in any age group in preparation for travel to endemic countries. Inactivated vaccines often can be given in a single injection or at separate sites at the same time. Vaccines that result in frequent local or systemic side effects, such as killed typhoid or plague vaccines, may result in accentuated reactions when given together.

Prior or simultaneous DTP or DT may be necessary to elicit an optimal response to certain *H. influenzae* conjugate vaccines (i.e., tetanus or diphtheria toxoid conjugates) but not others (conjugates with meningococcal outer membrane proteins). Administration of the

---

TABLE 82-9 Recommendations for routine immunization of HIV-infected persons in the United States

Vaccine	HIV clinical status		Comments
	Asymptomatic	Symptomatic	
DTP/Td	Yes	Yes	No change in usual immunization schedule
OPV	NO	NO	Increased risk of vaccine virus proliferation and paralytic polio IPV-e should be used for household contacts of HIV-infected persons
IPV-e	Yes	Yes	Antibody response may be impaired in symptomatic patients
MMR	Yes	Yes	No change in usual immunization schedule If high risk of exposure to measles, immunize at 6–11 months of age, with second dose at >12 months of age; with documented infection, measles immune globulin may be administered (see Table 82-10)
HIB conjugate	Yes	Yes	No change in usual immunization schedule
HBV	Yes	Yes	Antibody response may be impaired; a higher-dose vaccine is available, but there are no data addressing the optimal dose; it may be wise to check the antibody titer after immunization and give additional doses if inadequate
Pneumococcus	Yes	Yes	Should be given to all 2 years and older
Influenza	Yes	Yes	Antibody response may be impaired in symptomatic patients

SOURCE: Recommendations of the Advisory Committee on Immunization Practices (ACIP): Use of vaccines and immunoglobulins in persons with altered immunocompetence. Morb Mort Week Rep 42(No.RR-4):1, 1993.

TABLE 82-10 Preparations available for passive immunity*

Immunobiological	Indication(s)
STANDARD HUMAN IMMUNE GLOBULIN	
Intravenous immune globulin (IVIG)	Replacement therapy for antibody deficiency disorders; immune thrombocytopenic purpura (ITP); hypogammaglobulinemia in chronic lymphocytic leukemia; Kawasaki disease
Intramuscular immune globulin (IMIG)	Antibody immunodeficiency; hepatitis A pre- and postexposure prophylaxis; hepatitis B prophylaxis; hepatitis non-A, non-B prophylaxis; measles postexposure prophylaxis; chickenpox postexposure prophylaxis
SPECIAL HUMAN IMMUNE SERUM GLOBULIN	
Hepatitis B immune globulin (HBIG)	Perinatally exposed newborn infants; hepatitis B postexposure prophylaxis
Varicella-zoster immune globulin (VZIG)	Postexposure prophylaxis of susceptible immunocompromised persons, certain susceptible pregnant women, and perinatally exposed newborn infants
Rabies immune globulin† (RIG)	Rabies postexposure management of persons not previously immunized with HDCV
Tetanus immune globulin (TIG)	Tetanus treatment; postexposure prophylaxis of persons not adequately immunized with tetanus toxoid
Cytomegalovirus immune globulin, intravenous (CMV-IGIV)	Prophylaxis for bone marrow and kidney transplant recipients
Rho(D) immune globulin	Prevention of Rh hemolytic disease of the newborn
ANIMAL SERUM AND GLOBULINS	
Diphtheria antitoxin (equine)	Prevention or treatment of respiratory diphtheria
Botulinum antitoxin (equine)	Treatment of botulism

* Immune globulins and antitoxins are administered intramuscularly unless indicated otherwise.
† Rabies immune globulin is administered around wound in addition to the intramuscular injection.
SOURCE: Center for Biologics Evaluation and Research, Food and Drug Administration.

TABLE 82-11 Recommended postexposure immunization with immunoglobulin preparations in the United States

Disease	Indicated	Comments.
Measles	Yes	Standard human immune globulin recommended for exposed infants and adults with normal immunocompetence but contraindication to measles vaccine and for immunocompromised patients exposed to measles regardless of immunization status Patients should be immunized 3–6 months after immunoglobulin Recommended dose 0.25–0.5 mL/kg IM; maximum 15 mL
Rubella	No	Efficacy unreliable; therefore, standard human immune globulin is recommended for use only for antibody-negative pregnant women in the first trimester with a documented rubella exposure and who will not consider terminating pregnancy Recommended dose 0.55 mL/kg IM
Tetanus	Yes	Special human tetanus immune globulin (TIG) has replaced equine tetanus antitoxin because of the risk of serum sickness with equine serum Recommended dose for postexposure prophylaxis 250–500 units of TIG Recommended dose for treatment of tetanus 500–3000 units of TIG
Rabies	Yes	Special human rabies immune globulin (RIG) is preferred over equine rabies antiserum because of the risk of serum sickness, but RIG is not always available RIG or antiserum is recommended in nonimmunized individuals for all animal bites in which rabies cannot be ruled out and for other exposures to rabid animals Recommended dose of RIG 20 IU/kg; recommended dose of antiserum 40 IU/kg Rabies vaccine is given as well at 0, 3, 7, 14, and 28 days
Hepatitis A	Yes	Standard immune serum globulin is given in a single dose of 0.02–0.04 mL/kg or up to 0.06 mL/kg every 5 months for continuous exposure
Hepatitis B	Yes	Standard immune serum globulin is not reliably effective; special human hepatitis B immune globulin (HBIG) is useful and recommended for neonates born to an infected mother and after mucous membrane or parenteral contact with infected persons or infected blood or serum Recommended dose for neonates 0.5 mL IM within 12 h of birth; recommended dose for percutaneous or mucosal exposure is 0.06–0.12 mL/kg IM
Non-A, non-B hepatitis	Yes	Standard immune serum globulin may be valuable Recommended dose 0.12 mL/kg up to 10 mL

SOURCES: Recommendations of the Advisory Committee on Immunization Practices (ACIP): Use of vaccines and immunoglobulins in persons with altered immunocompetence. Morb Mort Week Rep 42(RR-4):1, 1993; Update on adult immunization: recommendations of the Immunization Practices Advisory Committee (ACIP). Morb Mort Week Rep 40(RR-12):1, 1991; Rabies prevention—United States, 1991: Recommendations of the Immunization Practices Advisory Committee (ACIP). Morb Mort Week Rep 40(RR-3):1, 1991; Hepatitis B virus: A comprehensive strategy for eliminating transmission in the United States through universal childhood immunization: Recommendations of the Immunization Practices Advisory Committee (ACIP). Morb Mort Week Rep 40(RR-13):1, 1991; Rubella prevention: Recommendations of the Immunization Practices Advisory Committee (ACIP). Morb Mort Week Rep 39(RR-15):1, 1990.

combined measles, mumps, and rubella vaccine (MMR) yields results comparable with administration of the individual vaccines given at different sites and has greatly increased the ease of achieving effective immunization for the three infections at little increase in cost. Although recent OPV is not a contraindication to use of MMR, in general, other live virus vaccines not given together on the same day should be given at least 30 days apart.

Neither OPV nor yellow fever vaccine responses are altered by administration of immune globulins. High doses of immune globulin may inhibit the efficacy of measles and rubella vaccines, and an interval of at least 3 months following administration of immune globulin is recommended. Postpartum vaccination of rubella-susceptible women should not be delayed because of the administration of anti-Rho(D) immune globulin or any other blood product during the last trimester or at delivery. If administration of an immune globulin preparation becomes necessary after vaccination, it should be postponed if possible for at least 14 days to allow time for vaccine virus replication and development of immunity to occur. In general, there is little interaction between immune globulin and inactivated vaccines, and postexposure passive prophylaxis can be given together with HBV vaccine or tetanus toxoid, resulting in both immediate and long-standing protection.

Travel The International Sanitary Regulations allow countries to impose requirements for yellow fever and cholera vaccines as a condition for admission, even though the currently available killed parenteral cholera vaccine is not an effective public health tool. Travelers should know whether these vaccines are required for entry into the countries on their itinerary to avoid being turned back or,

perhaps worse, immunized on the spot. Infants, children, and adults should be up to date with all routine immunizations before traveling, with particular attention to polio, measles, and DTP or Td. Pooled human gamma globulin for hepatitis A, at least until the vaccine is widely available, may be advisable for travelers to some locales. Use of rabies, meningococcal A and C polysaccharide, typhoid (oral live or Vi polysaccharide when available), Japanese encephalitis, and plague vaccines should be considered for those individuals who expect to go beyond the usual tourist routes or to spend extended time in rural areas in disease-endemic regions. In most U.S. cities, there are one or more travel clinics which maintain up-to-date epidemiologic monitoring, have supplies of the more uncommon vaccines available, and are prepared to provide general health information, including precautions for travelers' diarrhea and malaria prophylaxis.

DELIVERY OF VACCINES Over the past 20 years, considerable progress has been made to ensure that every child in the United States is fully immunized by the time of school entry. All 50 states now require immunization for school entry, and most have laws addressing attendance at preschool and day-care centers. As a result, up to 98 percent* of all children are immunized against nine vaccine-preventable diseases by the time they enter school. The impact of immunization, and other improvements in the health of the American population, on the incidence of vaccine-preventable illness is shown in Table 82-1 and Fig. 82-1.

Despite these successes, large numbers of preschool children are not fully immunized by 15 months of age. Only 37 to 56 percent of preschoolers in the United States have been completely immunized,† and this rate is as low as 10 percent in some communities. The failure to vaccinate preschool children was largely responsible for the resurgence of measles between 1989 and 1991, which included 55,467 cases and over 11,200 admissions to the hospital, with more than 44,100 hospital days and over 130 measles-related deaths. Congenital rubella syndrome also increased from 6 cases in 1988 to 47 in 1991. Outbreaks of pertussis and mumps have been on the rise for the same reason—low immunization rates among preschool children.

Standards for immunization practices National standards for immunization for pediatric and adult practice have been established which define common policies and practices for public health clinics and in physicians private offices (Table 82-12). These guidelines highlight the need to distinguish between true contraindications and conditions which often, but needlessly, preclude immunization. Among the true contraindications applicable to all vaccines are a history of anaphylaxis or allergic reaction to a vaccine or vaccine component and the presence of a moderate or severe illness with or without fever. Diarrhea, minor respiratory illness with or without fever, mild to moderate local reactions to a previous dose of vaccine, the concurrent or recent use of antimicrobials, mild to moderate malnutrition, and the convalescent phase of an acute illness are not valid contraindications to routine immunization. Failure to vaccinate children with these conditions is increasingly being viewed as a missed opportunity for immunization. Infants who develop an encephalopathy within 7 days of a dose of DTP should not receive further doses of DTP. Because of theoretical risks to the fetus, pregnant women should not receive MMR vaccine.

Access to immunization There are four major barriers to successful infant and childhood immunization within the health care system: (1) low public awareness and lack of public demand for immunization, (2) inadequate access to immunization services, (3) missed opportunities to administer vaccines, and (4) inadequate resources for public health and preventive programs. These problems are current public concerns and are a priority for national health policy in the United States.

In contrast, there has been little progress and virtually no publicity about the goals for adult immunization in the United States promulgated under *Healthy People 2000*, a set of national health promotion and disease prevention objectives for the year 2000 (Table 82-13). These objectives were established by the U.S. Department of Health and Human Services in consultation with the Institute of Medicine, the National Academy of Sciences, and after extensive public review and comment. Adult immunization goals are important, for as many as 60,000 adults are estimated to die each year from vaccine-

---

* These data do not include HBV vaccine and *H. influenzae* type b conjugate vaccine.
† By the second birthday, a fully immunized child will have received four doses of diphtheria and tetanus toxoids combined with pertussis vaccine (DTP), three doses of oral polio vaccine (OPV), one dose of measles, mumps, and rubella (MMR) vaccine, three doses of HBV vaccine, and three to four doses of a suitable *H. influenzae* type b conjugate vaccine (HibCV).

TABLE 82-12 Standards for immunization practices

PEDIATRIC PRACTICE

Standard 1: Immunization services are *readily available*.
Standard 2: There are *no barriers* or *unnecessary prerequisites* to the receipt of vaccines.
Standard 3: Immunization services are available *free* or for a *minimal fee*.
Standard 4: Providers utilize all clinical encounters to *screen* and, when indicated, *immunize* children.
Standard 5: Providers *educate* parents and guardians about immunization in general terms.
Standard 6: Providers *question* parents or guardians about *contraindications* and, before immunizing a child, *inform* them in specific terms about the risks and benefits of the immunizations their child is to receive.
Standard 7: Providers follow only true *contraindications*.
Standard 8: Providers administer *simultaneously* all vaccine doses for which a child is eligible at the time of each visit.
Standard 9: Providers use accurate and complete *recording procedures*.
Standard 10: Providers *co-schedule* immunization appointments in conjunction with appointments for other child health services.
Standard 11: Providers *report adverse events* following immunization promptly, accurately, and completely.
Standard 12: Providers operate a *tracking system*.
Standard 13: Providers adhere to appropriate procedures for *vaccine management*.
Standard 14: Providers conduct semiannual *audits* to assess immunization coverage levels and to review immunization records in the patient populations they serve.
Standard 15: Providers maintain up-to-date, easily retrievable *medical protocols* at all locations where vaccines are administered.
Standard 16: Providers operate with *patient-oriented* and *community-based* approaches.
Standard 17: Vaccines are administered by *properly trained individuals*.
Standard 18: Providers receive *ongoing education* and *training* on current immunization recommendations.

ADULT PRACTICE

Standard 1: Promote appropriate vaccine use through information campaigns for health-care practitioners and trainees, employers, and the public about the benefits of immunizations
Standard 2: Providers are completely immunized to protect themselves and prevent transmission to patients
Standard 3: Providers routinely determine the immunization status of their adult patients, offer vaccines for those for whom they are indicated, and maintain complete immunization records
Standard 4: Providers identify high-risk patients in need of influenze vaccine and develop a system to recall them for annual immunization
Standard 5: Providers and institutions identify high-risk adult patients in hospitals and other treatment centers and assure that appropriate vaccination is considered either prior to discharge or as part of discharge planning
Standard 6: Licensing/accreditation agencies support the development by health-care institutions of comprehensive immunization programs for staff, trainees, volunteer workers, inpatients, and outpatients
Standard 7: States establish preenrollment immunization requirements for colleges and other institutions of higher education
Standard 8: Institutions that train health-care professions, deliver health care, or provide laboratory or other medical support services require appropriate immunizations for persons at risk of contracting or transmitting vaccine-preventable illnesses
Standard 9: Health-care benefit programs, third part payers and government healt-care programs provide coverage for adult immunization services
Standard 10: Adopt a standard personal and institutional immunization record as a means of verifying the immunization status of patients and staff

SOURCE: Ad Hoc Working Group for the Development of Standards for Pediatric Immunization Practices. JAMA 269:1817, 1993
The National Coalition for Adult Immunization

---

preventable diseases for which effective vaccines are not being optimally used. As few as 40 percent of persons aged 65 and older receive influenza vaccine each year, and less than 15 percent have ever received pneumococcal vaccine (Table 82-14). Health care providers as often miss opportunities to vaccinate adults as they do infants and children. Between 60 and 90 percent of adults hospitalized for, or dying of, influenza-associated respiratory disease received medical care during the previous year during which they *could have* been immunized.

Financing immunization Many private health insurance policies do not provide adequate coverage for immunization, and physicians and other health care providers pass these costs directly on to patients.

TABLE 82-13 Vaccine-preventable disease targets

Vaccine-preventable diseases	1987 baseline	2000 target
Diphtheria among people aged 25 and younger	1	0
Tetanus among people aged 25 and younger	3	0
Polio (wild-type virus)	0	0
Measles	3058	0
Rubella	225	0
Congenital rubella syndrome	6	0
Mumps	4866	<500
Pertussis	3450	<1000

SOURCE: *Healthy People 2000: National Health Promotion and Disease Prevention Objectives*. Washington, U.S. Department of Health and Human Services, Public Health Service, 1990.

A major impediment to the delivery of vaccines under public-sector programs is the low reimbursement rates to providers of these services, which in 1990 served 5.3 million children under age 6 under Medicaid. Since states may reimburse Medicaid providers at less than the cost of the vaccines, let alone the cost of administration, there is little incentive for private providers to offer and promote immunizations for Medicaid-enrolled children. The result is that all too often children are referred to overburdened public clinics, thereby contributing to fragmentation of care and lower coverage rates against vaccine-preventable diseases. At the same time, 40 to 91 percent of unvaccinated preschool children who developed measles during the epidemic of 1989–1990 were enrolled in one or more public assistance programs which *could have* served as a referral source for children in need of immunization.

Similar gaps for immunization of adults exist under Medicare. While Medicare coverage includes the cost of influenza and pneumococcal vaccines and their administration to all enrolled individuals and HBV vaccine for those at high risk of exposure (i.e., renal dialysis patients), reimbursement is not adequate to encourage vaccine use among providers, and the program does not cover inexpensive vaccines such as tetanus-diphtheria toxoid (Td).

The role of industry With the exception of the states of Michigan and Massachusetts, which manufacture certain vaccines and immune globulin preparations, the American public is entirely dependent on the willingness of the commercial sector to make and market vaccines. This willingness has been in decline over the last two decades, and many manufacturers no longer produce vaccines. There are currently just one or two United States–based commercial sources for most childhood vaccines.

The National Vaccine Injury Compensation Program The use of mandated vaccines benefits society as a whole by reducing morbidity and the cost of care for preventable diseases and by reducing childhood mortality. For these reasons, and because the vaccines are sometimes associated with severe adverse reactions or sequelae, in the United States, society has assumed the obligation to care for those injured by the administration of mandated vaccines. The National

Childhood Vaccine Injury Compensation Act of 1986 is the instrument in use to ensure fairness to injured persons and protection for federal, state, and local immunization programs, private immunization providers, and vaccine manufacturers. The act was designed to carry out two vital public policies: (1) to provide prompt and fair compensation to the families of children who have died or have been injured as a result of routine mandated immunization and (2) to reduce the adverse impact of the tort system on vaccine supply, cost, and innovation and development. The intent is to encourage predictable, speedy, and equitable compensation for persons injured by vaccines. The success of immunization programs in the United States depends on the continued viability of the NVICP.

CONTROL OF VACCINE-PREVENTABLE DISEASE A continuing task of public health practice is to maintain individual and herd immunity. The job is not over once a population is fully vaccinated, since it is imperative to immunize each subsequent generation as long as the threat of the disease persists. Ongoing surveillance and prompt reporting of disease to local or state health departments are essential to this goal by ensuring a continuing awareness of the possibility of vaccine-preventable illness. Nearly all vaccine-preventable diseases are now notifiable and individual case data are routinely forwarded to the CDC. These data are used to detect outbreaks or other unusual events in need of investigation and to evaluate prevention and control policies, practices, and strategies.

A similar informations system for immunization coverage levels needs to be developed to determine if infants, children, and adults are actually receiving vaccines according to recommended schedules. This information could be used to ensure complete immunization of individuals, as well as to assess vaccine effectiveness and adverse events, to evaluate the performance of immunization programs, and to promote the efficient use of scarce resources.

Influencing acceptance of vaccines As a direct consequence of the success of immunization, vaccine-preventable disease has become less visible, and parents and health care providers can become complacent about immunization of children. Even among the affluent and educated, low levels of immunization may prevail, reflecting a gross misunderstanding of the continuing threat of disease with which parents and health care providers have limited experience and/or an inappropriately greater fear of vaccine adverse reactions than with the illness and death caused by vaccine-preventable diseases. Health care workers play an essential role in influencing the attitudes of patients regarding appropriate immunization, and therefore, it is essential for health care workers to continually update their own knowledge about vaccines and the epidemiology of vaccine-preventable illnesses.

VACCINE AND IMMUNIZATION RESEARCH To accomplish the preventive goals of *Healthy People 2000*, current immunization recommendations in the United States call for every child to receive nine different vaccines (many in combination and all requiring more than one dose) between birth and entry into kindergarten. This requires at least five visits to a health care provider by age 2, with an additional visit before starting school. This is a formidable task, particularly for those with limited access to health care, and compliance can be expected to become more difficult as new vaccines are licensed.

The Children's Vaccine Initiative The potential to eradicate selected diseases and build sustainable immunization programs that reach every child is not being achieved with existing vaccines and delivery technology. New vaccines or new formulations are required that will not only improve protective responses but also will simplify the immunization schedule. The Children's Vaccine Initiative (CVI) is an international effort to accomplish this goal. The ultimate ideal is to develop vaccines which may be administered orally early in life, provide lifelong protection to multiple infections, require one or a few doses, and be less reactive and more heat stable than current vaccines. Reaching these ambitious goals may take years or decades, but rapid progress is being made right now in developing new combinations of current vaccines to increase the feasibility of complete immunization. Thus DTP plus inactivated polio vaccine, Hib-conju-

TABLE 82-14 Estimates of vaccine coverage or immunity among adults, 1993

Vaccine	Percent
Influenza (age 65 +)	40
Pneumococcal (age 65 +)	14
Hepatitis B (age 65 +)	1–60*
Tetanus	16–59†
Diphtheria	34–51†
Measles	85–95†
Rubella	80–90†

* Varies by risk group.
† Varies by study.
SOURCE: Centers for Disease Control and Prevention: National Program on Immunization.

TABLE 82-15   Examples of directed scientific research to improve the immunization delivery system

Delivery system change desired	Scientific input	Products in process
Decrease number of visits required for full immunization	Developing new combination vaccines	MMRV, DTP-HIB-HBV, DTP-HIB
	Research on recombinant live multiantigen vaccines	Canarypox-measles, Canarypox-RSV, *Vaccinia*-rabies, *Vaccinia*-influenza, *Salmonella*, BCG
Decrease number of doses	Development of time-release products	Microencapsulated tetanus toxoid Microencapsulated hepatitis B Microencapsulated pertussis Microencapsulated influenza
Decrease number of injections	Reseach on oral vaccines	Pertussis
	Understanding mucosal immunity	Cholera
	Research in antigen presentation	Influenza
Immunization as early in life as possible	Research on maternal immunization	*Haemophilus* type B; *Meningococcus*
	Research on neonatal immunity	Group B streptococcus, *Pneumococcus*, influenza
Decrease in adverse events	Research on the mechanisms of adverse events	Acellular pertussis OPV neurovirulence, genetic determinants
Increase protection	Research on more immunogenic antigens	Group B streptococcus
	Development of conjugated vaccines	*Meningococcus*, *Pneumococcus*, influenza group B streptococcus
	Research on adjuvants	Typhoid
Increase thermal stability	Research on stabilizers	Polio, chemical stabilizer, freeze drying

SOURCE: National Vaccine Program Office, Office of the Assistant Secretary for Health, Department of Health and Human Services.

gate plus DTP, and HBV plus DTP vaccines are being evaluated, and a six-valent vaccine is a likely next step. Strategies of directed scientific research to improve vaccine delivery are listed in Table 82-15. The results will be applicable to both developed and developing country immunization programs.

Reemergence of controlled disease and emergence of new disease   The emergence of new pathogens is fostered by the genetic potential of microbes to evolve as well as by rapid changes in demographics and human behavior and in global ecology that create new or more hospitable hosts. The emergence of new infectious diseases such as HIV, Lyme borreliosis, and hepatitis C and the increase in global incidence and in drug resistance of familiar diseases such as tuberculosis and malaria, once considered under control, are proof of the need for continuing vaccine research. In addition, some common illnesses without a known etiology, such as peptic ulcer disease and cervical and nasopharyngeal cancer, are now epidemiologically linked to specific infection and thus may be vaccine-preventable.

Development of new vaccines   Many serious, life-threatening infectious diseases cannot be controlled because there are no effective vaccines. Many new vaccines are in development (Table 82-16); however, the task is proving to be very complex. Priority efforts for the United States are currently targeted toward HIV, acellular pertussis vaccine, group B streptococcus, respiratory syncytial virus, rotavirus, varicella, tuberculosis, hepatitis C, and two virus-associated tumors, human papilloma virus (cervical cancer) and Epstein-Barr virus (nasopharyngeal cancer).

INTERNATIONAL CONSIDERATIONS   Since the establishment of the World Health Organization's Expanded Programme on Immunization (EPI), immunization levels for the six basic children's vaccines have risen from 5 percent in the early 1980s to approximately 80 percent worldwide today. Each year, at least 2.7 million deaths from measles, neonatal tetanus, and pertussis and 200,000 cases of paralysis due to polio are prevented. Despite the successes of the EPI, many vaccine-preventable diseases remain prevalent in the developing world. Measles, for example, continues to kill an estimated 1.5 million children each year, and cases of diphtheria, whooping cough, polio, and neonatal tetanus still occur at unacceptably high levels. It is estimated that between 20 and 35 percent of all deaths in children under age 5 are associated with vaccine-preventable diseases.

Global targets   Eight antigens are recommended for routine use in the developing world by the EPI, including BCG, DTP, trivalent polio, and measles vaccines for children and tetanus toxoid for pregnant women. Others (Hib, Japanese B encephalitis, yellow fever, HBV, group A meningococcus, mumps, and rubella) are used

regionally, depending on disease epidemiology and resources. Polio has been targeted for eradication by the year 2000, and great progress has been achieved in the Americas by the Pan American Health Organization.

Because infectious diseases know no geographic or political boundaries, uncontrolled disease anywhere in the world poses a threat to the United States. Vaccines offer the opportunity to control and even eradicate some diseases, and successful eradication means that vaccines are no longer needed. The experience with smallpox has shown that the eradication of disease is a remarkably good economic investment. The entire sum that the United States spent for the global smallpox eradication campaign has been recouped, in 1968 dollars, every $2\frac{1}{2}$ months since 1971. A similar achievement with polio would save the United States over $300 million a year in vaccine and associated delivery costs, and the goal is feasible.

TABLE 82-16   Vaccines in human trial, 1993

Bacterial
Vibrio cholerae
Mycobacterium leprae
Salmonella typhi
Bordetella pertussis
Neisseria meningitidis
Streptococcus pneumoniae
Group B streptococcus
Shigella spp.
Enterotoxigenic *E. coli*
Lyme disease
Fungal
Cryptococcus neoformans
Parasitic
Plasmodium spp.
Viral
Hepatitis A
Dengue
Rotavirus
Japanese B encephalitis
Influenza A and B
Varicella
Measles
Cytomegalovirus
Rabies
Junin
Chikungunya
Rift Valley fever
Respiratory syncytial virus
Parainfluenza virus

SOURCE: National Vaccine Program Office, Office of the Assistant Secretary for Health, Department of Health and Human Services.

REFERENCES

AMERICAN ACADEMY OF PEDIATRICS: *Report of the Committee on Infectious Diseases* ("Red Book"), 22d ed, G. Peter et al (eds). Elk Grove Village, Ill., 1991

AMERICAN COLLEGE OF PHYSICIANS: *Guide for Adult Immunization*, 2d ed. Philadephia, American College of Physicians, 1990

AMERICAN PUBLIC HEALTH ASSOCIATION: *Control of Communicable Diseases in Man*, 15th ed, AS Benenson (ed). Washington, D.C., American Public Health Association, 1990

CENTERS FOR DISEASE CONTROL AND PREVENTION: Recommendations of the Advisory Committee on Immunization Practices (ACIP): Use of vaccines and immune globulins in persons with altered immunocompetence. Morb Mort Week Rep 42(RR-4):1, 1993

————: Standards for pediatric immunization practices. Morb Mort Week Rep 42(RR-5):1, 1993

————: Update on adult immunization. Recommendations of the Immunization Practices Advisory Committee (ACIP). Morb Mort Week Rep 40(RR-12):1, 1991

———— : *Health Information for International Travel* (published yearly) and *Advisory Memoranda on Travel* (published periodically)

section 2 Clinical syndromes—community acquired

83 SEPSIS AND SEPTIC SHOCK

ROBERT S. MUNFORD

DEFINITIONS The host reaction to invading microbes involves a rapidly amplifying polyphony of signals and responses that may spread beyond the invaded tissue. Fever or hypothermia, chills, tachypnea, and tachycardia often herald the onset of the systemic inflammatory response to microbial invasion, also called *sepsis*. Sepsis is usually limited by counterregulatory mechanisms. When these mechanisms are overwhelmed, often as the microbe moves from a local site to invade the bloodstream, homeostasis may fail, and dysfunction of major organs can supervene *(severe sepsis)*. Further failure of counterregulatory control leads to *septic shock,* characterized by hypotension as well as organ dysfunction. As sepsis progresses to septic shock, the risk of dying increases substantially. Early sepsis is usually reversible, whereas many patients with septic shock succumb despite aggressive therapy.

ETIOLOGY Sepsis can be a response to infection caused by any class of microorganism. Although gram-negative and gram-positive bacteria account for most cases, sepsis may occur with diseases caused by fungi, mycobacteria, rickettsiae, viruses, or protozoans. Microbial bloodstream invasion, with positive blood cultures, is not essential to the development of sepsis, since systemic spread of microbial signal molecules or toxins also can elicit the response. Approximately 30 to 60 percent of patients with sepsis and 60 to 80 percent of patients with septic shock have blood cultures that yield bacteria or fungi, and gram-negative bacteria account for approximately two-thirds of these isolates. The remaining cases are caused by gram-positive cocci (10 to 20 percent) or fungi (2 to 5 percent) or a mixture of microorganisms. In patients whose blood cultures are negative, the etiologic agent may often be established by culture or microscopical examination of infected material from a local site. Occasional patients with established bacteremia do not mount a septic response.

EPIDEMIOLOGY Sepsis now contributes to more than 100,000 deaths per year in the United States. The incidence is probably between 300,000 and 500,000 cases per year. Approximately two-thirds of the cases occur in hospitalized patients. Factors that predispose to gram-negative rod bacteremia include diabetes mellitus, lymphoproliferative diseases, cirrhosis of the liver, burns, invasive procedures or devices, and drugs that cause neutropenia. Major risk factors for gram-positive bacteremia include vascular catheters, indwelling mechanical devices, burns, and intravenous drug injection. Fungemia occurs most often in immunosuppressed patients with neutropenia, often after broad-spectrum antimicrobial therapy. The increasing incidence of sepsis in the United States is attributable to the aging of the population, the increasing longevity of patients with chronic diseases, and the relatively high frequency of sepsis in AIDS. The widespread use of antimicrobial agents, glucocorticoids, indwelling catheters and mechanical devices, and mechanical ventilation also contributes.

PATHOPHYSIOLOGY The septic response is usually triggered when commensal microorganisms spread from the gastrointestinal tract or skin into contiguous tissues. Localized infection in the genitourinary tract, biliary tract, lungs, or gastrointestinal tract may then lead to bloodstream infection. Microorganisms also may be introduced directly into the bloodstream (e.g., via intravenous catheters). In a minority of cases, no primary site of infection is apparent.

Microbial signals Animals recognize certain microbial molecules as signals that microorganisms have invaded. Lipopolysaccharide (LPS, also called *endotoxin*) is the most potent and best-studied gram-negative bacterial signal molecule. LPS binds to CD14 (and perhaps to other receptors) on monocytes, macrophages, and neutrophils. Plasma proteins, such as LPS-binding protein, facilitate the binding of LPS to CD14, thereby augmenting and accelerating the LPS-cell interaction. Cellular responses to LPS include the production and release of mediators that amplify and transmit the microbial signal to other cells and tissues. The peptidoglycan and lipoteichoic acids of gram-positive bacteria, certain polysaccharides, extracellular enzymes, and toxins elicit responses in animals that are similar to those induced by LPS. The molecular basis for the stimulatory potency of these molecules is less well understood than that for LPS.

Host responses Sepsis results from complex interactions among microbial signal molecules, leukocytes, humoral factors, and the vascular endothelium.

CYTOKINES The inflammatory cytokines may have endocrine, paracrine, and autocrine actions (see Chap. 277). Tumor necrosis factor alpha (TNFα) stimulates leukocytes and vascular endothelial cells to release other cytokines (as well as additional TNFα), to express cell-surface adhesion molecules, and to increase arachidonic acid turnover. Blood levels of TNFα are high in most patients with severe sepsis; in patients with fulminant meningococcemia, TNFα levels correlate with levels of circulating endotoxin and with clinical outcome. Moreover, intravenous infusion of TNFα can elicit many of the characteristic abnormalities of sepsis, including fever, tachycardia, tachypnea, leukocytosis, myalgias, and somnolence. In animals, larger doses of TNFα induce shock, disseminated intravascular coagulation (DIC), and death. Monoclonal antibodies to TNFα can abrogate the septic response and prevent the deaths of experimental animals from endotoxin challenge.

Although TNFα is a central mediator of sepsis, it is only one of many cytokines that contribute to the septic response. Interleukin 1β (IL-1β) is also present in the blood of patients with septic shock; this cytokine can elicit many of the same responses as TNFα when injected intravenously. Recombinant IL-1 receptor antagonist and monoclonal antibodies to IL-1β can protect animals from endotoxic death. Antibodies to IL-6 also may be protective. TNFα, IL-1β, IL-6, interferon-γ, and other cytokines probably interact synergistically with each other and with additional mediators. In addition, some mediators (such as IL-1 and TNFα) may enhance their own rates of synthesis by positive feedback. In animal models, the septic response can be interrupted by interventions that neutralize one or another of its many mediators; this observation testifies to the importance of mediator interactions for the overall result.

PHOSPHOLIPID-DERIVED MEDIATORS Arachidonic acid, released from membrane phospholipids by phospholipase A_2, is converted by the cyclooxygenase pathway into prostaglandins and thromboxanes. Prostaglandin E_2 and prostacyclin cause peripheral vasodilatation, whereas thromboxane is a vasoconstrictor and promotes platelet aggregation. Leukotrienes, products of the lipoxygenase pathway of arachidonate metabolism, are potent mediators of ischemia and shock; the principal arachidonate metabolite in human neutrophils is leukotriene B_4, which promotes leukocyte activation and may contribute to local vascular injury and thrombosis.

Another important phospholipid-derived mediator is platelet-activating factor (PAF), 1-O-alkyl-2-acetyl-sn-glycero-3-phosphocholine. Its precursor, lyso-PAF, is produced by the degradation of membrane choline phosphoglycerides by phospholipase A_2. PAF is a potent stimulus for neutrophil aggregation and degranulation, promotes platelet aggregation, and may contribute to tissue injury.

COAGULATION FACTORS   Intravascular deposition of fibrin, thrombosis, and DIC are important features of the septic response. Although LPS can activate the intrinsic clotting cascade in vitro, and although factor XII levels are low in patients with severe sepsis, LPS and TNFα probably promote intravascular coagulation initially by inducing blood monocytes to express tissue factor, by increasing the release of plasminogen activator inhibitor 1 (PAI-1), and by inhibiting the expression of thrombomodulin and plasminogen activator by vascular endothelial cells. Tissue factor is the high-affinity receptor and cofactor for factor VIIa. When tissue factor is expressed on monocytes, it complexes with factor VIIa to form an active complex that can convert factors X and IX to enzymatically active forms. The result is the activation of both extrinsic and intrinsic clotting pathways, culminating in the generation of thrombin. Decreased levels of antithrombin III and tissue plasminogen activator and increased concentrations of PAI-1 also promote clotting. Contact system activation may occur with severe sepsis, when denuded vascular basement membrane provides an appropriate activating surface.

COMPLEMENT   C5a and other products of complement activation may promote neutrophil chemotaxis, leukotriene synthesis, aggregation, degranulation, and oxygen radical production. When administered to animals, C5a induces hypotension, pulmonary vasoconstriction, neutropenia, and vascular leakiness due, in part, to endothelial damage. C5a-induced hypotension can be blocked by cyclooxygenase inhibitors.

ACTIVATION OF THE VASCULAR ENDOTHELIUM   Many tissues may be damaged by sepsis. The probable underlying mechanism is widespread vascular endothelial injury, with fluid extravasation and microthrombosis that decrease oxygen and substrate utilization by the affected tissues. Leukocyte-derived mediators and platelet-leukocyte-fibrin thrombi contribute to this injury, but the vascular endothelium itself also plays an active role. Stimuli such as LPS and TNFα induce vascular endothelial cells to produce and release cytokines, procoagulant molecules, PAF, endothelium-derived relaxation factor (nitric oxide), and other mediators. In addition, regulated cell adhesion molecules promote the adherence of neutrophils to endothelial cells. While these responses may attract phagocytes to infected sites and activate their antimicrobial arsenals, endothelial cell activation also can promote increased vascular permeability, microvascular thrombosis, DIC, and hypotension. Moreover, vascular integrity may be damaged by neutrophil enzymes (such as elastase) and toxic oxygen metabolites so that local hemorrhage ensues. Blocking the adhesion of leukocytes to endothelial cell surfaces, as with monoclonal antibodies to ICAM-1, can prevent tissue necrosis in response to endotoxin administration in animals.

SEPTIC SHOCK   The actual mediators of septic shock are not known. TNFα and IL-1β probably cause hypotension by triggering the release of additional mediators. Among the prominent hypotensive agents are β-endorphin, bradykinin, PAF, endothelium-derived relaxation factor (nitric oxide), leukotrienes, and prostacyclin. Agents that inhibit the synthesis or action of each of these mediators can prevent or reverse endotoxic shock in animals.

The sepsis cascade: Clues to the early events   Septic shock is associated with derangements of the proteolytic cascades that control clotting, kinin metabolism, and complement activation. Activation of the intrinsic (contact) clotting pathway, activation of kallikrein,

proteolytic inactivation of C1 inhibitor, and generation of C5a and other active complement components have been reported. In contrast, useful clues to the early changes during sepsis have come from studies of the effects of the intravenous administration of endotoxin. After injection of an endotoxin bolus, blood levels of TNFα, IL-6, and IL-8 increase (Fig. 83-1). Concentrations of TNFα typically increase by 30 min and peak at 90 min, whereas levels of IL-6 and IL-8 increase more slowly and peak around 2 to 4 h after infusion. Blood levels of tissue plasminogen activator and plasmin also increase transiently, and these rises are followed by a longer-lasting increase in PAI-1. An early fibrinolytic phase is thus followed by a period of hypercoagulability. Similar changes occur after infusion of TNFα. Activation of complement or of the intrinsic clotting pathway has not been detected in these studies; these derangements may occur only with more severe sepsis and may not be induced directly by endotoxin.

Ibuprofen, a cyclooxygenase inhibitor, blocks many of the responses to endotoxin infusion, including most symptoms (fever, myalgia, nausea, headache) and endotoxin-induced increases in adrenocorticotropin (ACTH), cortisol, epinephrine, and norepinephrine. On the other hand, ibuprofen does not prevent endotoxin-induced leukocytosis or hypoferremia, and blood levels of TNFα and IL-8 are actually higher after administration of ibuprofen and endotoxin than after endotoxin infusion alone. Prostanoids therefore mediate many of the effects of TNFα and IL-1β; some prostaglandins, such as prostaglandin E_2, appear to mediate certain cytokine actions (such as the production of fever and muscle proteolysis), yet they inhibit the production of TNFα and IL-8. They thus may provide an autoregulatory mechanism for limiting the inflammatory response.

Control mechanisms   Elaborate counterregulatory mechanisms limit the inflammatory response. Elevated plasma concentrations of ACTH occur within 1 h of intravenous endotoxin administration, and plasma cortisol levels peak shortly thereafter. Glucocorticoids inhibit cytokine synthesis by monocytes in vitro, and when administered with or shortly after the inflammatory stimulus, they may protect animals from septic shock. Presumably, endogenous glucocorticoids play a similar role in damping inflammatory responses. Certain cytokine antagonists also may dampen or control the septic response.

FIGURE 83-1   Typical time course and levels (relative to baseline) of cytokines (TNFα, IL-6, IL-8), tissue plasminogen activator (tPA), and plasminogen activator inhibitor-1 (PAI-1) in the plasma of volunteers receiving a bolus infusion of endotoxin. Data are taken from articles by Martich, van Deventer, and Suffredini. In patients with sepsis, multiple microbial signal molecules are probably produced and released intermittently at various tissue sites and in different doses. The host response is therefore much more complex than is shown here.

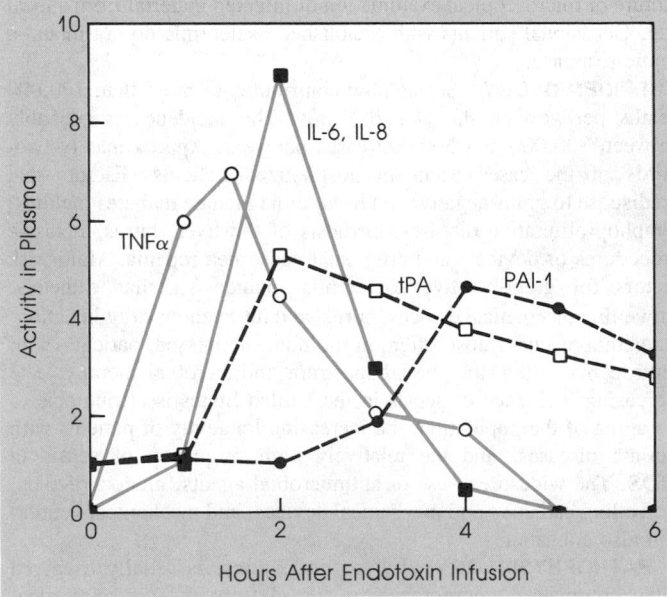

After endotoxin infusion into human subjects, for example, IL-1β rapidly appears in the blood, yet blood levels of IL-1 receptor antagonist rapidly exceed those of circulating IL-1β and may inhibit IL-1β binding to its receptors. IL-4, IL-6, IL-8, and IL-10 also can inhibit LPS-induced responses by human monocytes in vitro. Along with prostaglandin E₂, α-melanocyte-stimulating hormone, IL-1 receptor antagonist, and soluble TNF receptors, these molecules probably act to prevent the progression of most instances of sepsis to death. Much less is known about these control processes than about the activation arm of the septic response, however.

CLINICAL MANIFESTATIONS Sepsis is easily suspected in the patient with localized infection who abruptly develops fever, chills, tachycardia, tachypnea, altered mental status, and hypotension. However, the septic response may develop more slowly and have more subtle manifestations. For example, some septic patients have normal temperature or may even be hypothermic; the absence of fever is most common in neonates, in elderly patients, and in persons with uremia or alcoholism.

Hyperventilation is often a useful clue to the diagnosis, although its cause is poorly understood. Disorientation, confusion, and other manifestations of encephalopathy also may be early signs, particularly in the elderly and in individuals with preexisting neurologic impairment. Focal neurologic signs are uncommon, although preexisting focal deficits may become more prominent.

Hypotension and DIC predispose to acrocyanosis and ischemic necrosis of peripheral tissues, most commonly the digits. Cellulitis, pustules, bullae, or hemorrhagic lesions may develop when bacteria or fungi seed the skin or underlying soft tissues by hematogenous spread. Bacterial toxins also may be distributed hematogenously to elicit diffuse cutaneous reactions. On occasion, skin lesions may suggest specific pathogens. When sepsis is accompanied by cutaneous petechiae or purpura, infection with *Neisseria meningitidis* (or, less commonly, *Haemophilus influenzae*) should be suspected; in a patient who has been bitten by a tick while in an endemic area, petechial lesions also should suggest Rocky Mountain spotted fever. A cutaneous lesion seen almost exclusively in neutropenic patients is ecthyma gangrenosum, usually caused by *Pseudomonas aeruginosa* or *Aeromonas hydrophila*; a bullous lesion, surrounded by edema, undergoes central hemorrhage and necrosis. Histopathologic examination shows bacteria in and around the wall of a small vessel, with little or no neutrophilic response. Hemorrhagic or bullous lesions in a septic patient who has recently eaten raw oysters should suggest *Vibrio vulnificus* bacteremia, while in a patient who has recently suffered a dog bite, such lesions may indicate bacteremia due to *Capnocytophaga canimorsus* or *C. cynodegmi* (DF2). Generalized erythroderma in a septic patient should suggest the toxic shock syndrome due to *Staphylococcus aureus* or *Streptococcus pyogenes*.

Gastrointestinal manifestations such as nausea, vomiting, diarrhea, and ileus may suggest acute gastroenteritis. Stress ulceration can lead to upper gastrointestinal bleeding. Cholestatic jaundice, with elevated levels of serum bilirubin (mostly conjugated) and alkaline phosphatase, may precede other signs of sepsis. Hepatocellular or canicular dysfunction appears to underlie most cases, and hepatic function tests return to normal with resolution of the infection. Prolonged or severe hypotension may induce acute hepatic injury or ischemic bowel necrosis.

Blood lactate levels rise early, in part because of increased glycolysis in peripheral tissues with incomplete hepatic clearance of the resulting lactate and pyruvate. As hypoperfusion develops, tissue hypoxia generates more lactic acid, worsening the metabolic acidosis. The blood glucose concentration often increases, particularly in diabetics, although impaired gluconeogenesis and excessive insulin release may on occasion produce hypoglycemia. Hypertriglyceridemia reflects, at least in part, the inhibitory action of TNFα on lipoprotein lipase. The cytokine (IL-6, IL-1β, TNFα)–mediated acute-phase response inhibits albumin synthesis while enhancing the production of C-reactive protein, fibrinogen, complement components, and transferrin.

COMPLICATIONS Cardiopulmonary complications Ventilation-perfusion mismatching produces a fall in arterial P_{O_2} early in the course. Increasing alveolar capillary permeability results in increased lung water, which decreases pulmonary compliance and interferes with oxygen exchange. Progressive, diffuse pulmonary infiltrates, decreasing compliance, and arterial hypoxemia (often refractory to supplemental oxygen therapy, indicating right-to-left shunting) indicate development of the acute respiratory distress syndrome (ARDS). ARDS (or "shock lung") develops in 20 to 50 percent of patients with sepsis, and sepsis is the leading cause of ARDS. Leukocyte-induced pulmonary microvascular injury, with damage to pulmonary capillary endothelial cells, contributes to its pathogenesis. Respiratory muscle failure can worsen hypoxemia and hypercapnia. An elevated pulmonary capillary wedge pressure (>18 mmHg) suggests fluid volume overload or cardiac failure rather than ARDS. Pneumonia due to viruses or severe *Pneumocystis carinii* infection may be clinically indistinguishable from ARDS.

Septic shock usually results from a severe decrease in systemic vascular resistance, a generalized maldistribution of blood flow, and functional hypovolemia that is due, at least in part, to diffuse capillary leakage of intravascular constituents. Cardiac output is initially normal or elevated. Indeed, the normal or increased cardiac output and decreased systemic vascular resistance distinguish septic shock from cardiogenic, extracardiac obstructive, and hypovolemic shock; other processes that can produce this combination include anaphylaxis, beriberi, cirrhosis of the liver, and overdoses of nitroprusside or narcotics.

Depression of myocardial function, manifested as increased end-diastolic and systolic ventricular volumes with decreased ejection fraction, occurs within 24 h in most patients with severe sepsis. Cardiac output is maintained despite the low ejection fraction because ventricular dilatation permits a normal stroke volume. In survivors, myocardial function returns to normal over several days. While myocardial dysfunction may contribute to hypotension, refractory hypotension is usually due to a low systemic vascular resistance, and death results from refractory shock or the failure of multiple organs rather than from cardiac dysfunction per se.

Renal complications Oliguria, azotemia, proteinuria, and nonspecific urinary casts are frequent. Most renal failure is due to acute tubular necrosis induced by hypotension or capillary injury, although some patients also have glomerulonephritis, renal cortical necrosis, or interstitial nephritis. Drug-induced renal damage also may complicate therapy, particularly when hypotensive patients are given aminoglycoside antibiotics.

Coagulation abnormalities Although thrombocytopenia occurs in 10 to 30 percent of patients, the underlying mechanism(s) are not understood. Very low platelet counts (below 50,000 per microliter) are usually found in patients with DIC, typically reflecting diffuse endothelial injury (see Chap. 315).

Multiple organ dysfunction syndrome Dysfunction or failure of multiple organs, usually reflecting widespread vascular endothelial injury, is associated with high fatality rates. The severity of the insult and the risk of dying correlate with the number of organs affected.

LABORATORY FINDINGS In early sepsis, abnormalities often include leukocytosis with a left shift, thrombocytopenia, hyperbilirubinemia, and proteinuria. Leukopenia may occur. The neutrophils may contain toxic granulations, Döhle bodies, or cytoplasmic vacuoles. As the septic response becomes more severe, thrombocytopenia worsens (often with prolongation of the thrombin time, decreased fibrinogen, and the presence of D-dimers, suggesting DIC), azotemia and hyperbilirubinemia become more prominent, and levels of aminotransferases become elevated. Active hemolysis suggests clostridial bacteremia, malaria, a drug reaction, or DIC; in the case of DIC, microangiopathic changes may be seen on blood smear.

During early sepsis, hyperventilation induces respiratory alkalosis. With respiratory muscle fatigue and the accumulation of lactate, metabolic acidosis (with increased anion gap) typically supervenes. Arterial blood gases also reveal hypoxemia, initially correctable with supplemental oxygen but later refractory to 100% oxygen inhalation, indicating right-to-left shunting. The chest radiograph may be normal or may show an underlying pneumonia, volume overload, or diffuse infiltrates of ARDS. The electrocardiogram may show only sinus tachycardia or nonspecific ST-T wave abnormalities.

Most diabetics with sepsis develop hyperglycemia. Severe infection may precipitate diabetic ketoacidosis, which may worsen hypotension (see Chap. 337). Hypoglycemia occurs rarely. The serum albumin level, initially within the normal range, declines as sepsis continues. Serum lipid concentrations are often elevated. Hypocalcemia is rare.

DIAGNOSIS There is no reliable laboratory test. Suggestive findings include tachypnea, tachycardia, altered mental status, leukocytosis or leukopenia, and thrombocytopenia. The septic response can be quite variable, however. In one study, 36 percent of patients with sepsis had a normal temperature, 44 percent had a normal mental status, 60 percent had a normal respiratory rate, 10 percent had a normal pulse rate, and 78 percent had normal platelet counts. The typical symptoms and signs of sepsis are also not specific, since similar systemic responses (recently named the *systemic inflammatory response syndrome,* or SIRS) may occur in uninfected patients with other conditions. Strictly speaking, the diagnosis of *sepsis* requires confirmation that SIRS has a microbial cause. Conditions that may mimic sepsis include pancreatitis, burns, trauma, adrenal insufficiency, pulmonary embolism, dissecting or ruptured aortic aneurysm, myocardial infarction, occult hemorrhage, cardiac tamponade, anaphylaxis, and drug overdose.

Definitive diagnosis requires isolation of the microorganism from blood or a local site of infection. At least two blood samples (10 mL each) should be obtained, from different venipuncture sites, for culture. Gram-negative bacteremia is typically low grade (fewer than 10 organisms per milliliter of blood), so multiple blood cultures or prolonged culture incubation may be necessary for the diagnosis; *S. aureus* grows more readily, and most blood cultures will be positive within 48 h. In approximately one-third of cases, blood cultures are negative; this result can reflect prior antibiotic administration, the presence of slowly growing or fastidious organisms, or the absence of microbial invasion of the bloodstream. In these cases, Gram's stain and culture of the primary site of infection—or of infected cutaneous lesions—are necessary to establish the microbial cause. The skin and mucosae should be examined carefully and repeatedly for lesions that might yield diagnostic information. In patients with the staphylococcal toxic shock syndrome, for example, the clinical diagnosis is often supported by isolating *S. aureus* from a cutaneous lesion or mucosal site. With overwhelming bacteremia (e.g., pneumococcal sepsis in splenectomized individuals, fulminant meningococcemia), microorganisms are sometimes seen on buffy coat smears of peripheral blood.

TREATMENT Sepsis can kill quickly. Successful management requires urgent measures to treat the local site of infection, to provide hemodynamic and respiratory support, and to eliminate the offending microorganism. The outcome is also influenced by the patient's underlying disease, which should be aggressively treated.

Antimicrobial agents Antimicrobial chemotherapy should be initiated as soon as samples of blood and other relevant sites have been cultured. The choice of initial therapy can be based on knowledge of the likely pathogens at specific sites of local infection. Available information about antimicrobial susceptibility patterns in bacterial isolates from the community, the hospital, and the patient also should be taken into account. It is also important to recall that the signs and symptoms of sepsis can be elicited by many different microorganisms. Consequently, pending culture results, empirical antimicrobial therapy usually should be effective against both gram-positive and gram-negative bacteria. Maximal recommended doses of antimicrobial drugs should be given intravenously, with adjustment for impaired renal function when necessary. Cefotaxime (3 g IV every 6 h) or ceftazidime (2 g IV every 8 h) plus gentamicin or tobramycin (1.5 mg/kg every 8 h) is an appropriate initial empirical regimen in patients with no apparent site of primary infection. (If infection with *P. aeruginosa* is suspected, ceftazidime and tobramycin should be used.)

Nafcillin (3 g IV every 6 h) or vancomycin (15 mg/kg IV every 12 h) should be added if the patient has injected drugs intravenously or has an indwelling vascular catheter, and clindamycin (600 mg IV every 6 h) or metronidazole (500 mg IV every 6 h) should be added if an intraabdominal source is suspected. When culture results become known, the regimen often can be simplified, since a single antimicrobial agent is frequently adequate for the treatment of infection with a known pathogen. On the other hand, a combination of bactericidal antimicrobial agents (typically a β-lactam and an aminoglycoside) may be indicated for definitive treatment of sepsis in neutropenic patients and for the treatment of sepsis due to bacteria such as *P. aeruginosa* and enterococci, against which antimicrobial synergy has been documented.

Removal of the source of infection Removal or drainage of a focal source of sepsis is essential. Sites of occult infection should be sought carefully. Indwelling intravenous catheters should be removed, the tip should be rolled over a blood agar plate for quantitative culture, and a new catheter should be inserted at a different site. Foley and drainage catheters should be replaced if obstructed. Paranasal sinusitis (often caused by hospital-acquired gram-negative bacteria) should be considered in any patient who has undergone nasal intubation. In the neutropenic patient, cutaneous sites of tenderness and erythema should be sought, particularly in the perianal region. The possibility of pelvic or other soft tissue pus collections should be excluded (with use of computed tomography, if necessary) in patients with sacral or ischial decubitus ulcers. Ureteral obstruction, perinephric abscess, and renal abscess should be excluded by sonography or computed tomography in patients with urosepsis.

Hemodynamic support Here, the goal is to restore adequate oxygen and substrate delivery to the tissues. Effective intravascular volume depletion is common in septic patients, and initial management of the hypotensive septic patient should include the administration of intravenous fluids, typically 1 to 2 L of normal saline over 1 to 2 h. Larger volumes may be needed. Monitoring of the pulmonary capillary wedge pressure or central venous pressure is essential in patients with refractory shock or underlying cardiac or renal disease. To avoid pulmonary edema, the pulmonary capillary wedge pressure should be maintained between 12 and 15 mmHg or the central venous pressure between 10 and 12 cmH$_2$O. The urine output should be kept above 30 mL/h by continuing fluid administration; a diuretic such as furosemide may be used if needed. In about one-third of patients, hypotension responds to fluid resuscitation; a reasonable goal is to maintain a mean arterial blood pressure of >60 mmHg (systolic pressure > 90 mmHg). Dopamine is the most widely used pressor agent. When given in low doses [5 to 10 (μg/kg)/min] it has beta$_1$-adrenergic effects, increasing cardiac output and dilating tissue arterioles by stimulating dopaminergic receptors. Caution is necessary, however, since higher doses [>20 (μg/kg)/min] stimulate alpha-adrenergic receptors and can cause peripheral vasoconstriction, with ischemia and gangrene. Because of its alpha$_1$ stimulatory effect, norepinephrine should be carefully titrated to achieve a mean blood pressure of at least 60 mmHg; this agent is often reserved for patients who remain hypotensive despite dopamine therapy. Low-dose dopamine [1 to 4 (μg/kg)/min] may be combined with norepinephrine to maintain adequate renal and intestinal perfusion and achieve maximal pressor support.

Adrenal insufficiency, an uncommon complication of sepsis, should be considered in septic patients with refractory hypotension, fulminant *N. meningitidis* bacteremia, prior glucocorticoid use, disseminated tuberculosis, or AIDS. The cosyntropin (α$^{1-24}$-ACTH) stimulation test (see Chap. 335) may suggest absolute or partial adrenal insufficiency. Supplemental hydrocortisone (50 mg IV every 6 h) may be given while awaiting the results of the cosyntropin test.

Ventilator therapy is indicated for progressive hypoxemia, hypercapnia, neurologic deterioration, or respiratory muscle failure. Intubation is often undertaken to ensure adequate oxygenation, divert blood from the muscles of respiration, and reduce the cardiac afterload.

Blood or erythrocyte transfusion is indicated if oxygen delivery is compromised by a low hemoglobin concentration.

Therapy of acidosis and DIC Bicarbonate is sometimes administered for severe metabolic acidosis (arterial pH <7.2); efficacy is not established. DIC, if complicated by major bleeding, should be treated with transfusion of fresh frozen plasma and platelets. Successful treatment of the underlying infection is essential to reverse both acidosis and DIC.

Other measures Despite early diagnosis, surgical drainage of infected sites, prompt administration of appropriate antimicrobial therapy, and careful fluid and pressor resuscitation, many patients with sepsis die. Two kinds of agents are under investigation to prevent these deaths: drugs that neutralize bacterial endotoxin, thereby benefiting patients with gram-negative bacterial sepsis, and drugs that interfere with one or more mediators of the inflammatory response, thereby potentially benefiting patients with sepsis of all etiologies.

ANTIENDOTOXIN AGENTS The toxic moiety of endotoxin, called *lipid A*, is structurally conserved in the LPS of pathogenic gram-negative bacteria. Much effort has been devoted to developing antibodies to lipid A—or to a conserved core oligosaccharide moiety—that would neutralize endotoxin in vivo and protect patients from endotoxic shock. Studies with polyclonal antisera to endotoxin core structures seemed very promising, but in placebo-controlled trials, two monoclonal antibodies to lipid A did not prevent death among patients with gram-negative bacterial sepsis. These and other antibodies to endotoxin are being evaluated further. Other investigational agents include a human neutrophil protein that neutralizes endotoxin (bactericidal permeability-increasing protein) and nontoxic lipid A analogues that inhibit host responses to endotoxins.

ANTIMEDIATOR AGENTS Other adjunctive therapies for sepsis are designed to control the inflammatory response, regardless of the microbial stimulus. Of these agents, glucocorticoids have received most attention. However, two large-scale, randomized clinical trials of high-dose methylprednisolone therapy in patients with sepsis indicated that the regimens used did not prevent death or reverse septic shock. High-dose glucocorticoid therapy therefore is not currently recommended. Agents that directly interfere with cytokine actions, including recombinant IL-1 receptor antagonist, genetically engineered soluble receptors for TNFα, and monoclonal antibodies to TNFα, are now under evaluation. Since TNFα and IL-1β probably play some beneficial role in the host response to microbial invasion, anticytokine drugs could have both beneficial and detrimental consequences in patients with sepsis. Other investigational compounds include PAF antagonists, nitric oxide synthase inhibitors, pentoxifylline, soluble complement receptors (CR1), and anticoagulants such as recombinant α_1-antitrypsin Pittsburgh, antithrombin III, and protein C.

PROGNOSIS Overall, more than 25 percent of septic patients die. Although one-third of the deaths occur within the first 48 h after the onset of symptoms, mortality can occur 14 or more days later. Late deaths are often due to poorly controlled infection, complications of intensive care, or failure of multiple organs.

The risk of dying is influenced by the prior clinical condition of the patient and the rate at which complications develop. Patients with rapidly fatal diseases such as leukemia have higher case-fatality rates from sepsis than do patients with less severe underlying diseases. Analyses using prognostic stratification systems (such as the APACHE scoring system) indicate that factoring in the patient's age and certain physiologic variables results in more accurate estimates of the risk of dying. Variables associated with high case-fatality rates include ARDS, DIC, renal insufficiency, severe acidosis, hypothermia, altered mental status, and multiple organ dysfunction. Microbial variables are less important than host- and treatment-related factors, although high case-fatality rates have been observed for patients with sepsis due to *P. aeruginosa* and for patients with polymicrobial infection.

PREVENTION Prevention offers the best opportunity to reduce morbidity and mortality from sepsis. Most episodes of severe sepsis and septic shock are nosocomial complications; these cases might be prevented by reducing the number of invasive procedures, by limiting the use (and duration) of indwelling vascular and bladder catheters, by reducing the incidence and duration of profound neutropenia (<500 neutrophils per microliter), and by more aggressive treatment of localized nosocomial infections. Indiscriminate use of antimicrobial agents and glucocorticoids should be avoided, and optimal infection control measures (see Chap. 98) should be used. In addition, prompt and aggressive management of patients with early sepsis is imperative. Investigational approaches to preventing or damping the septic response include active and passive immunization to enhance antibody titers to key bacterial cell wall molecules, including endotoxin.

REFERENCES

AMERICAN COLLEGE OF CHEST PHYSICIANS/SOCIETY OF CRITICAL CARE MEDICINE CONSENSUS CONFERENCE COMMITTEE: Definitions for sepsis and organ failure and guidelines for the use of innovative therapies in sepsis. Crit Care Med 20:864, 1992

DANNER RL et al: Endotoxemia in human septic shock. Chest 99:169, 1991

GRANOWITZ EV et al: Production of interleukin-1-receptor antagonist during experimental endotoxaemia. Lancet 338:1423, 1991

HARRIS RL et al: Manifestations of sepsis. Arch Intern Med 147:1895, 1987

Increase in national hospital discharge survey rates for septicemia, United States, 1979–1987. Morb Mort Week Rep 39:31, 1990

KNAUS WA et al: The APACHE III prognostic system: Risk prediction of hospital mortality for critically ill hospitalized adults. Chest 100:1619, 1991

KREGER BE et al: Gram-negative bacteremia: IV. Re-evaluation of clinical features and treatment in 612 patients. Am J Med 68:344, 1980

MARTICH GD et al: Detection of interleukin 8 and tumor necrosis factor in normal humans after intravenous endotoxin: The effect of antiinflammatory agents. J Exp Med 173:1021, 1991

MARTIN MA et al: Gram-negative sepsis and the adult respiratory distress syndrome. Clin Infect Dis 14:1213, 1992

PARILLO JE: Septic shock in humans: Advances in the understanding of pathogenesis, cardiovascular dysfunction, and therapy. Ann Intern Med 113:227, 1990

SPRUNG CL et al: Impact of encephalopathy on mortality in the sepsis syndrome. Crit Care Med 18:801, 1990

SUFFREDINI AF et al: Promotion and subsequent inhibition of plasminogen activation after administration of intravenous endotoxin to normal subjects. N Engl J Med 320:1165, 1989

VAN DEVENTER SJH et al: Experimental endotoxemia in humans: Analysis of cytokine release and coagulation, fibrinolytic, and complement pathways. Blood 76:2520, 1990

VETERANS ADMINISTRATION SYSTEMIC SEPSIS COOPERATIVE STUDY GROUP: Effect of high-dose glucocorticoid therapy on mortality in patients with clinical signs of systemic sepsis. N Engl J Med 317:659, 1987

84 INFECTIOUS DISEASES OF THE UPPER RESPIRATORY TRACT

ROBERT LEBOVICS / ANN SULLIVAN BAKER

The head and neck form an anatomically complex region that includes the nose, paranasal sinuses, ears and mastoids, oral cavity, pharynx, and larynx. The functions of this region include the exchange and filtering of air, the intake and separation of food and liquids from the air stream entering the tracheobronchial tree, the expression of speech, and the senses of taste, smell, and hearing. Respiratory ciliated epithelium lines those portions involved in air exchange and filtration; squamous cells line the oral cavity, tongue, and oropharynx. The senses are controlled by a complex neural network, and local immunity is provided by a collection of lymphoid tissues. The proximity of these structures to the brain and mediastinum and the potential for airway obstruction require prompt recognition and treatment of head and neck infections.

NOSE AND FACE

EXTERNAL DISORDERS Any bacterial skin infection can affect the nose and face. Furunculosis commonly occurs around the nasal vestibule, in the region of the hair follicles. *Staphylococcus aureus* is the most commonly isolated pathogen. Infection in the nasal vestibule can spread to the cavernous sinus via facial veins that communicate with the central nervous system. Treatment of furunculosis should be prompt and consist of local heat and oral antibiotics with antistaphylococcal activity (see Chap. 102). Marked local edema, fever, or signs of generalized sepsis necessitate hospitalization and parenteral antibiotic therapy with careful evaluation for sinus or intracranial extension. Diabetic and immunocompromised patients are at especially high risk for rapid spread of infection. Incision and drainage of large lesions are usually necessary.

Staphylococcus aureus and group A beta-hemolytic *Streptococcus* (*e.g.*, *S. pyogenes*) are the foremost agents of impetigo and erysipelas of the nose and face. Impetigo features skin pustules overlaid with yellow crusts. Erysipelas is a form of cellulitis, commonly in a malar distribution, with an advancing border raised above the surrounding skin. The area is red-hot, erythematous, and tender. Intravenous antibiotics with coverage of gram-positive pathogens are required (see Chaps. 102, and 103).

Lupus vulgaris is a form of tuberculosis involving the external nose and adjacent facial structures. The lesions appear as brown gelatinous nodules. Confirmatory histology and positive mycobacterial cultures are usually required for diagnosis; the therapy is the same as for tuberculosis (see Chap. 130). Syphilis (see Chap. 133) of the nose and face is rare and usually presents with a painless ulcerative lesion or chancre at the mucocutaneous junction of the nose or within the nasal septum several weeks after infection. Widespread secondary lesions, which usually progress as the primary lesion disappears, appear as erythematous papulosquamous eruptions, annular lesions, or condylomata. Tertiary syphilis presents with a nasal gumma and circumscribed swellings covering the inflamed mucosa; the nasal septum is usually involved, and destruction of the septal cartilage may ultimately lead to a cosmetic deformity known as "saddle-nose."

INTERNAL NASAL INFECTIONS Infection with *Mycobacterium tuberculosis* (see Chap. 130) in the nasal cavity is uncommon in the United States. Symptoms may include pain, nasal obstruction, rhinorrhea, and epistaxis. The septum and inferior turbinate are most commonly affected. Septal perforations are common, and the gross appearance of the lesion varies from ulceration to a papillomatous growth. Diagnosis is made by smear, culture, and deep submucosal biopsies that demonstrate tissue invasion by mycobacteria. *M. leprae* (see Chap. 131), the pathogen of leprosy, causes a chronic granulomatous inflammation of the superficial tissues of the nose and may extend to the face to involve either skin or peripheral nerves. Symptoms include epistaxis, nasal obstruction, crusting, and generalized signs of atrophic rhinitis. Nasal septal perforations and saddle-nose deformity are common.

Pseudomonas mallei causes glanders, which is a nasal infection transmitted to humans from horses (see Chap. 116). It produces an extensive ulcerative granulomatous disease of the nasal mucosa that causes pain, with mucopurulent discharge. Diagnosis is confirmed by both culture and histology, and treatment is with appropriate antibiotics. Rhinoscleroma is a granulomatous infection caused by *Klebsiella rhinoscleromatis* (see Chap. 115), prevalent mainly in Central America, Central Europe, and the Middle East. Clinical presentation includes atrophic rhinitis with foul-smelling rhinorrhea and crusting. The granulomatous inflammation progresses to severe fibrosis and stenosis of the nasal cavity. Culture of *K. rhinoscleromatis* from infected tissue is diagnostic, and histologically the McKulicz cell (or foamy histiocyte) is characteristic. Tetracycline is the drug of choice. Rhinosporidiosis is caused by *Rhinosporidium seeberi*, a fungus-like organism. The lesion usually presents with either sessile or pedunculated nasal growths; epistaxis, foul odor, and nasal obstruction are common. Surgical excision is followed by administration of dapsone.

Mucormycosis (see Chap. 168) is a life-threatening illness that classically presents in patients with diabetic ketoacidosis or severe neutropenia. Rapid diagnosis and treatment are essential as the infection quickly spreads to the paranasal sinuses, orbits, and central nervous system. Black crusts overlying necrotic tissues within the nasal cavity should heighten suspicion of mucormycosis. Histologic sections of deep tissue biopsies are required to confirm the diagnosis.

Actinomyces israelii (see Chap. 127) can cause a purulent abscess in the nasal cavity. Sulfur granules are a distinguishing histologic feature, and long-term parenteral penicillin treatment is indicated.

Histoplasmosis (see Chap. 162) usually involves the lungs, larynx, and tongue. Nodules and ulcers are frequently visualized; a classic epithelioid or histiocytic granuloma is seen in addition to the organisms within the granuloma.

Cryptococcus neoformans (see Chap. 165) frequently infects the central nervous system but can be localized in the nasal cavity. *Cryptococcus* classically produces granulomatous lesions without acute inflammation. *Blastomyces hominis* (see Chap. 164) also causes granulomatous and suppurative inflammation that involves the respiratory tract and extends from the nose to the face and paranasal sinuses.

PARANASAL SINUSES

ANATOMY AND DEVELOPMENT The paranasal sinuses are cavities within the facial skeleton that are lined by ciliated respiratory epithelium and drain into the nose. The maxillary and ethmoid sinuses are present at birth; the ethmoid labyrinth grows and expands with age, so that the anterior ethmoid cells usually project above the orbital rim to develop into the frontal sinuses. Unilateral agenesis of the frontal sinuses is common. The anterior table of the frontal sinus is composed of marrow-containing bone. The sphenoid sinuses are the last to develop and often do not mature until individuals reach their early twenties. The cavernous sinus lies laterally and proximal to the sphenoid sinus and is traversed by cranial nerves II, III, IV, V_1, and VI.

SINUSITIS In the immunocompetent host acute sinusitis is usually a bacterial infection that often follows a viral infection of the upper respiratory tract. Rhinovirus, adenovirus, and influenza and parainfluenza viruses may be recovered along with bacteria in about one-fifth of cases. It is estimated that 1 to 3 percent of upper respiratory infections are complicated by sinusitis. Adults have approximately two to three episodes of upper respiratory infection and children six to eight per year.

The major factor leading to sinusitis is obstruction of the ostia of the anterior ethmoid and middle meatal complex. The ethmoid ostia are very small, ranging from 1 to 2 mm in size. A viral upper respiratory infection leads to retained secretions secondary to mucosal edema, with obstruction of the sinus ostia and impaired drainage and precipitation of acute purulent sinusitis. Obstruction may also be due to allergy with swelling of the mucosa or secondary to polyps. The maxillary sinuses are the most common site of infections, followed by the ethmoids, frontal, and sphenoid sinuses.

Sinusitis has been recognized as a frequent nosocomial infection in the intensive care unit. The single greatest risk factor for the development of nosocomial sinusitis is prolonged (more than 48 h) intubation with a nasal tracheal or nasal gastric tube. In one study, purulent sinusitis occurred in one (1.9 percent) of 53 patients with oral tracheal tubes and in 25 (43 percent) of 58 patients with nasal tracheal tubes.

Barotrauma from deep sea diving and airplane travel are recognized precipitating factors for sinusitis. Other predisposing conditions include quantitative and qualitative ciliary transport abnormalities (e.g., ciliary syndromes, cystic fibrosis, Young's syndrome), excessive production of secretions, chronic granulomatous disease (e.g., Wegener's granulomatosis, sarcoid), and midline granuloma. Chemical irritants such as chlorine may impair secretion clearance and foster microbial proliferation.

Symptoms of acute sinusitis depend on the site of involvement. Patients with maxillary sinusitis have pain over the malar area and upper teeth. The infraorbital nerve runs through the maxillary route and the first and second molars often project into the sinus floor. Patients with anterior ethmoid sinusitis may complain of headache in the temporal or retroorbital area or the upper nose. Patients with posterior ethmoid sinusitis present with pain over the distribution of the trigeminal nerve, particularly around the mastoid area. With sphenoid sinusitis, the patient may complain of pain in the frontal, retroorbital, or facial area. Facial complaints are found in one-third of the patients. Nasal congestion and discharge frequently occur.

Evaluation of acute sinusitis requires good clinical judgment. Radiographs are not necessarily required for the first episode of sinusitis. If one chooses to evaluate the patient by radiograph, sinus films that include a lateral view are optimal. CT scanning is useful for evaluating the orbital areas, the sphenoid sinus, and the possibility of osteomyelitis. MRI should be limited to evaluation for fungal concretions or tumor. The bacteriology in acute sinusitis has been incompletely defined. The most common organisms include *S. pneumoniae*, *Haemophilus influenzae*, streptococci, and *Moraxella*, and in the intensive care unit, gram-negative organisms. *Staphylococcus aureus* is more common in sphenoid sinusitis. Rhinovirus, adenovirus, and influenza and parainfluenza viruses may be recovered in one-fifth of cases.

Symptoms of chronic sinusitis include nasal congestion and discharge. Pain may be intermittent; fever is uncommon. Patients may have a chronic cough due to a postnasal drip. CT scan is most useful for revealing bony erosion, mucopyoceles, or sclerosis. In addition to the organisms isolated in acute sinusitis, anaerobic bacteria and *S. aureus* are frequently found in chronic sinusitis. Patients with chronic sinusitis should be evaluated for granulomatous disease, ciliary dysfunction, and hypogammaglobulinemia.

Therapy of sinusitis   Treatment must be directed at promoting adequate drainage. Patients should be instructed to decrease nasal swelling with vasoconstricting local agents such as oxymetazolin nasal spray. In addition to obstruction, the quality of mucus secretions is important. In patients with cystic fibrosis, for example, adequate hydration is often implemented to decrease mucus viscosity. Patients with sinusitis should inhale steam from a basin or hot shower to loosen secretions. Oral antihistamines thicken rather than liquify the material trapped within the sinuses and are not useful.

Antibiotic therapy is indicated in the setting of purulent discharge, fever, and leukocytosis. Amoxicillin-clavulanic acid, trimethoprim-sulfamethoxazole, or a second generation cephalosporin (such as cefuroxime-axetil) for 2 to 4 weeks are reasonable agents, assuming resolution of symptoms. Acute sinusitis that fails to clear completely after this time should be reevaluated and referred to the otolaryngologist for further medical and surgical attention.

Sinusitis is treated in the intensive care unit with removal of all nasal tubes and administration of appropriate antibiotics, including either oxacillin or vancomycin along with a third-generation cephalosporin or sulbactam-ampicillin. Sinus puncture by the otolaryngologist may be useful for obtaining aerobic and anaerobic material. Pus from the ostium is suboptimal culture material as the nasopharynx is colonized. Patients with sinusitis that has not resolved may be evaluated by endoscopy to investigate possible anatomic cause and obtain adequate specimens for culture. If symptoms persist in chronic sinusitis, endoscopic sinus surgery may be required to obtain a histologic diagnosis, remove polyps, and establish proper ventilation of the infected sinuses.

Complications of sinusitis   Infection of the frontal sinus mucosal wall may spread to the bone directly or by thrombophlebitis of the veins from sinus mucosa to diploic veins of the frontal bone. The infection may spread externally to the outer table and result in cortical breakthrough and periosteal abscess (Potts' puffy tumor). Inferior extension results in involvement of upper ethmoid cells and the roof of the orbit or in a periosteal abscess; posterior extension results in epidural abscess. Clinical presentation of frontal bone osteomyelitis includes a local soft doughy swelling. Evaluation should be by CT or MRI. Bacterial pathogens include *S. aureus*, streptococci,

anaerobes, and gram-negative organisms. Antibiotic therapy should be given intravenously for 4 weeks with a combination of agents such as (1) oxacillin, metronidazole, and a second- or third-generation cephalosporin or (2) ampicillin-sulbactam. Surgical drainage of the infected sinus is necessary should medical therapy fail.

Intracranial complications of sinusitis include cerebral epidural abscess, subdural empyema, cerebral abscess, and thrombosis of the large dural sinuses (cortical thrombophlebitis) (see Chap. 374). The most common intracranial complications of sphenoid sinusitis are meningitis and cavernous vein thrombophlebitis. The wall of the cavernous sinus surrounds the sphenoid sinus, thereby allowing easy access to the cavernous sinus and central nervous system. The patient with cavernous sinus thrombophlebitis presents with evidence of nerve palsies in cranial nerves III, IV, V_1, and VI. Patients should be evaluated with CT or MRI. Intravenous antibiotics are required, and drainage of the sphenoid sinus is important if the patient does not improve on antibiotics alone.

The most frequent extracranial complication is spread of infection to the orbit from an infected ethmoid sinus. The medial border of the orbit is also the lateral border of the ethmoid labyrinth. Acute ethmoid sinusitis can result in infection traversing the thin plate separating the bone to cause an orbital cellulitis. Orbital cellulitis is accompanied by pain, lid edema, and conjunctival chemosis (erythema, swelling). Orbital cellulitis requires hospitalization, broad spectrum intravenous antibiotics, and drainage of the sinus if no improvement is seen in 48 h.

FUNGAL SINUSITIS   This condition may be divided into (1) allergic, e.g., secondary to *Aspergillus* (see Chap. 167) or *Dreschlera* infection; (2) invasive sinusitis caused by organisms such as *Aspergillus*, *Curvularia*, and *Alternaria*; (3) rhinocerebral phycomycosis caused by genera of the class Zygomycetes. The patient with allergic fungal sinusitis may be treated symptomatically and may benefit from glucocorticoid therapy. Some patients may also have accompanying bronchopulmonary aspergillosis and a hypersensitivity type of allergic infection in the sinuses. Bronchospasm occurs, and Charcot-Leyden crystals (proteins originating in the cytoplasm of eosinophils) may be found in the discharge. Consultation with an allergist is advisable to coordinate possible glucocorticoid therapy. Patients with chronic invasive sinusitis should be treated with intravenous amphotericin or another antifungal agent appropriate for the specific organism (see Chap. 161). Patients with phycomycosis are often diabetic, leukemic, or otherwise immunocompromised. These patients need rapid, wide debridement of the infected area and intravenous amphotericin.

Candidiasis also can present as chronic sinusitis (see Chap. 166).

EAR

ACUTE OTITIS MEDIA   Viral upper respiratory tract infection is most commonly associated with acute otitis media. The hallmark of middle ear infection is pain. A sense of fullness, purulent otorrhea, hearing loss, vertigo or tinnitus, fever, and leukocytosis may be present. Otoscopic examination will confirm the diagnosis of acute otitis media by demonstrating a red, dull, and bulging or perforated tympanic membrane. *S. pneumoniae* (approximately 35 percent) and *H. influenzae* (approximately 20 percent) are the bacteria most frequently isolated from middle ear effusions in acute otitis media. The majority of *H. influenzae* isolates are nontypable strains. In children, infection by *H. influenzae* type b can cause severe systemic toxicity and may be associated with meningitis. Other commonly isolated bacteria include *Branhamella catarrhalis*, group A, *Streptococcus*, and *S. aureus*. Mixed anaerobic bacteria can occasionally cause acute otitis media. Respiratory viruses such as respiratory syncytial and influenza viruses are implicated in the pathogenesis but are rarely cultured.

Treatment of acute otitis media includes the use of antibiotics such as amoxicillin-clavulanic acid, trimethoprim-sulfamethoxazole, and cefuroxime-axetil. Antihistamines have not proven effective. Occasionally, in refractory cases, tympanocentesis is required for bacteriologic diagnosis. In persistent infection, a myringotomy with or without the insertion of a ventilating tube may be necessary. Severe pain, infection in immunologically compromised patients, and failure of antibiotic therapy are indications for surgical drainage of the middle ear space. Bullous myringitis may be associated with mycoplasma infection, while multiple perforations of the tympanic membrane suggest tuberculosis.

SEROUS OTITIS MEDIA   Serous otitis media with chronic effusion is a leading cause of hearing loss in children and occasionally in adults. Otoscopic examination will show a retracted tympanic membrane associated with fluid in the middle ear cavity. Pure tone audiometry and tympanometry can reveal a conductive hearing loss and a flat tympanogram consistent with restrictive disease in the middle ear space.

Therapy can be divided into conservative and surgical approaches. Decongestants, antihistamines, and glucocorticoids have been advocated in the treatment of serous effusions, although their usefulness is unproven. Antibiotics have been used as well as mechanical insufflation via the eustachian tube (politerization). Control of predisposing factors may include the treatment of allergy, nasal infection, or chronic sinus infection. Occasionally the use of ventilating tubes is required for management of a chronic effusion in the middle ear with or without infection. This provides drainage for an infected middle ear and will improve a conductive hearing loss caused by the accumulation of serous fluid in the middle ear. Unilateral serous otitis media in an adult should raise suspicion of a noninfectious process, e.g., tumor.

Mastoiditis   The mastoid air cells are patent with the middle ear unless blocked by an intervening mass. Because of the direct communication between the two cavities, every case of otitis media is in the truest sense a mastoiditis. The organisms causing mastoid infections are generally those that cause acute middle ear infections. Radiographs of the mastoid air cells frequently demonstrate fluid or mucosal thickening within the honeycomb labyrinth of the mastoid suggesting chronic infection. Treatment is similar to that of acute otitis media.

Intravenous antibiotics and emergency mastoidectomy are indicated when there are high fever and leukocytosis with radiographic evidence of destruction of trabeculae and the honeycombing of the mastoid air cells. Signs of acute otitis media are usually evident. A subperiosteal abscess may be present, in which case examination will reveal an ear that is displaced inferiorly and laterally, with a red fluctuant mass behind the pinna. When abscess is suspected clinically, CT scanning will usually confirm the diagnosis.

Chronic otitis media with otorrhea is defined as a chronic draining ear resulting from untreated acute or recurrent otitis media. The bacterial flora are variable. *Pseudomonas aeruginosa* and *S. aureus* are the most commonly isolated aerobic organisms, followed by *Escherichia coli* and *Proteus* species. Chronic, foul-smelling otorrhea may indicate anaerobic infection (one-third of patients). Chronic suppuration of the middle ear is associated with perforation of the tympanic membrane and may be associated with cholesteatoma (involuted squamous epithelium and keratin debris) formation. Imaging by conventional radiography or CT will show mucosal thickening in the middle ear space as well as in the mastoid cavity. Cholesteatoma may erode the temporal bone and rarely enters the cranial cavity. Treatment is directed at eradicating infection with a combination of local care, antibacterial ear drops, and systemic antibiotics selected according to antibiotic sensitivities defined by cultures. Cholesteatomas must be excised.

COMPLICATIONS OF OTITIS MEDIA AND MASTOIDITIS   Extracranial complications of otitis media and mastoiditis include conductive, sensorineural, and mixed hearing loss. Other complications include labyrinthitis manifested by vertigo as well as weakness or complete paralysis of the ipsilateral facial nerve. Gradenigo's syndrome consists of otalgia, a draining middle ear, and paralysis of the ipsilateral sixth cranial nerve, reflecting infection of the petrous

apex of the temporal bone. Cultures of draining material should be obtained. Therapy requires antibiotics directed at organisms that cause otitis media and they should be adjusted based on culture results. Surgical intervention should be reserved for refractory cases. Intracranial complications of otitis media include meningitis, brain abscess, epidural abscess, lateral sinus thrombophlebitis, and otitic hydrocephalus.

EXTERNAL OTITIS   The external auditory canals are lined by skin and are subject to the same diseases of skin as the rest of the body. Psoriasis may be the cause of an external otitis. Glands within the external auditory canal secrete cerumen, which acidifies the external auditory canal and minimizes the overgrowth of bacteria. Otitis externa ("swimmer's ear") is most common in the summer months and is thought to arise from a change in the milieu of the external auditory canal by increased alkalinization, which leads to the overgrowth of bacteria, most commonly *Staphylococcus, Streptococcus,* and *Pseudomonas* species. Treatment includes topical antibacterial ear drops, although occasionally systemic antibiotics (choice based on antibiotic sensitivities) are required. Mycotic infections causing otitis externa are diagnosed by smears and culture and are treated with topical antifungal ear drops. *Herpes zoster* in the external auditory canal can cause an associated loss of the sensory and motor functions of the facial nerve (Ramsay-Hunt syndrome); acyclovir is helpful in treating severe otalgia.

Necrotizing (malignant) otitis externa   This progressive necrotizing infection results in osteomyelitis of the temporal bone and is almost always caused by *P. aeruginosa.* The soft tissues and cartilage of the pinna may also be involved. The disorder occurs most commonly in patients with insulin-dependent diabetes mellitus. The diagnosis should be suspected in patients with swelling of the external canal and severe pain. Physical examination will often reveal granulation tissue in the posterior ear canal wall that is eroding into the temporal bone. The auricle and surrounding scalp may be swollen, tender, and necrotic. CT and bone scans are useful for making the diagnosis. Treatment consists of local care including debridement and antibacterial ear drops combined with intravenous antibiotics directed against *P. aeruginosa* (see Chap. 116). Good control of coexisting diabetes mellitus may hasten recovery. Occasionally radical surgical debridement of the temporal bone is required. Gallium scanning is helpful in monitoring recovery.

Perichondritis   Perichondritis is an infection or inflammation of the cartilage of the pinna usually arising after trauma. The most common organism isolated in infectious perichondritis is *P. aeruginosa.* The lobule is spared infection because it contains no cartilage. Relapsing polychondritis is an inflammatory disease of the external ear that initially may mimic infection and needs to be distinguished from perichondritis.

PHARYNX

ORAL CAVITY   The oral cavity begins at the vermilion border of the lips and extends posteriorly to the circumvallate papillae of the tongue. *Gingivitis* is inflammation of the gums covering the maxilla and mandible. Anaerobic bacteria are the usual cause of gingivitis. Poor oral and dental hygiene, tobacco use, and excessive alcohol are the main predisposing factors. Vincent's angina (also known as trench mouth or acute necrotizing ulcerative gingivitis) is usually caused by *Borrelia vincenti,* a fusiform bacillus. Patients will present with malodorous breath, excessive salivation, and frequent perigingival bleeding. Treatment is a combination of oral penicillin and hygiene.

Herpes viruses (see Chap. 143) infect the lip, causing common cold sores and lesions on the buccal mucosa, tongue, and pharyngeal wall. Patients complain of severe pain and odynophagia. Characteristic pustular eruptions are visible over the mucosa. Diagnosis is confirmed by viral culture or immunofluorescence staining. Herpes zoster can present similarly, and the treatment is a combination of local care, acyclovir, and analgesia. Herpangina, caused by group A coxsackievirus, can present with pain, dysphagia, odynophagia, and fever. Thrush, caused by *Candida albicans,* usually affects immunocompromised patients. Oral antifungals will control the overgrowth. Cancrum oris may occur in severely debilitated patients. Noma is a mixed bacterial infection of the oral cavity caused by fusospirochetal bacteria and/or streptococci. In developing countries with poor sanitation and hygiene, noma is associated with high rates of mortality. Treatment requires a combination of debridement, local care, and parenteral antibiotics directed at oral bacteria (see Chap. 128).

Ludwig's angina (see Chap. 128) is a rapidly progressing life-threatening infection that frequently follows a lower molar tooth infection with spread to the submandibular or sublingual space. Patients present with pain, dysphagia, drooling, fever, and leukocytosis. The floor of the mouth is red, inflamed, and swollen. The tongue is pushed posteriorly and superiorly and ultimately causes airway obstruction. Prompt hospitalization to control the airway, followed by possible incision and drainage and parenteral antibiotics (directed at oral bacteria) is the treatment of choice. The bacteriology is mixed, with anaerobic streptococci predominating.

OROPHARYNX The cause of acute pharyngitis is almost always infection, although pharyngeal inflammation and ulceration may be caused by agranulocytosis, trauma, or injury by chemicals or radiation. The major symptom of acute pharyngitis regardless of etiology is sore throat, with or without associated dysphagia. Examination may reveal exudate, erythema, and mucosal congestion with hypertrophy of the lymphoid tissue, particularly the palatine tonsils. The presence of exudate suggests bacterial infection, particularly by group A beta-hemolytic streptococci (see Chap. 103). *Neisseria gonorrhoeae* (see Chap. 110) can cause pharyngeal exudate but special culture technique is required to confirm its presence. *Corynebacterium diphtheriae* (see Chap. 104) pharyngitis can become life-threatening. A pseudomembrane over the mucosa can enlarge to the point of airway obstruction. Examination reveals a dark gray mucosa. *Mycoplasma pneumoniae* (see Chap. 139) and the TWAR strains of *Chlamydia* (see Chap. 140) can cause exudative pharyngitis. Exudate may be seen with a variety of viral infections, in particular those caused by Epstein-Barr virus, herpes simplex virus, or adenovirus. Infection with respiratory syncytial, parainfluenza, and influenza viruses may also cause pharyngitis without exudate; in rhinovirus infections a "scratchy" throat may be a prominent feature.

Pus that accumulates between the middle pharyngeal constrictor and the tonsillar capsule constitutes a peritonsillar abscess. Patients complain of fever, pain, dysphagia, and odynophagia and speak with a "hot potato" voice. Physical examination reveals trismus, unilateral swelling, and deviation of the uvula. Incision and drainage provides prompt relief.

LARYNX

SIGNS AND SYMPTOMS OF LARYNGEAL DISEASE Persistent, unexplained change in the voice, e.g., hoarseness or weakness, is pathognomonic of laryngeal disorders. Other symptoms include cough that may be dry or associated with the production of clear, purulent, or blood-streaked sputum; pain that may refer to other branches of the vagus nerve, manifested by otalgia; and upper respiratory obstruction causing stridor. Dysphagia and odynophagia may develop with either infectious or neoplastic lesions of the larynx. Besides evaluation of the neck, oropharynx, and gag and swallowing reflexes, physical examination should include an indirect mirror examination and, if available, flexible fiberoptic endoscopy. Vocal cord dysfunction, mass lesions, mucosal ulceration, infection of the larynx, structural abnormalities, and occasionally subglottic lesions will be evident on these inspections. Definitive diagnosis requires biopsy, usually under anesthesia, and culture, if possible.

LARYNGEAL INFECTIONS Acute epiglottitis (supraglottitis) This is a rapidly progressive cellulitis of the epiglottis and surrounding tissues in the supraglottic airway. It can cause acute airway obstruction. In infants and children the causative agent is most commonly *H. influenzae* type b, and bacteremia is frequent.

In adolescents and adults with acute bacterial epiglottitis, the clinical presentation may be less fulminant and other organisms have been implicated in some cases *(S. pneumoniae, S. aureus).* Frequently, the patient complains of dysphagia, odynophagia, and fever that has progressed over 1 to 2 days. Depending on the degree of respiratory obstruction, stridor may or may not be present, but hoarseness and loss of voice power are almost universal findings. As in children, the adult with epiglottitis usually leans forward, drooling oral secretions. Because the caliber of the airway is larger in the adult, intubation or tracheotomy may not be necessary, but the possibility of complete airway obstruction dictates management. Edematous, cherry-red epiglottis and surrounding pharyngeal mucosa are characteristic findings on fiberoptic examination, which in adults is the best way to confirm the diagnosis (see below). In infants and children this approach is contraindicated because of the threat of acute airway obstruction. A lateral radiograph of the neck may reveal an enlarged epiglottis—the so-called "thumb sign."

Until the possibility of airway obstruction has passed, the patient is best managed by admission to an intensive care unit where adequate monitoring is available. In adults, fiberoptic examination with a nasopharyngoscope should be performed only after preparations have been made to secure the airway by endotracheal intubation or, if necessary, tracheotomy. After blood is obtained for culture, appropriate intravenous antibiotic treatment is initiated with cefuroxime or a third-generation cephalosporin such as cefotaxime. Oxygen should be administered as dictated by O_2 saturations on pulse oximetry or arterial blood gas determination. Humidified air by face tent is advisable. If respiratory obstruction worsens, endotracheal intubation is required. Glucocorticoids have been administered as part of the treatment but with unproven benefit. Resolution of clinical manifestations usually occurs over 36 to 48 h. A child should not be extubated nor a patient removed from an intensive care setting unless the acute cellulitis has resolved, as confirmed by endoscopy.

Croup (laryngotracheobronchitis) Croup is a syndrome produced by acute infection of the lower air passages and is most commonly seen in children below age 3. The most common pathogen is the parainfluenza virus, but a variety of respiratory viruses and *Mycoplasma pneumoniae* can produce acute laryngotracheobronchitis and the croup syndrome. The pathophysiology is primarily one of circumferential mucosal inflammation in the subglottic larynx and trachea, with variable involvement and spasm of the vocal cords; the epiglottis is not involved. The clinical hallmark is a barking or brassy cough with or without stridor and hoarseness. Croup can be readily distinguished from epiglottitis by lateral films of the neck, which show no epiglottal edema, or by careful direct examination. Management of severe croup requires hospitalization, close observation, humidification, oxygenation as dictated by pulse oximetry, and rarely intubation. Glucocorticoid administration has been advocated by some, but the benefits are questionable.

Tuberculous laryngitis Tuberculous laryngitis is usually associated with active pulmonary tuberculosis. Characteristic manifestations include hoarseness, cough, and blood-tinged sputum; because of the large number of organisms in the sputum, it is usually highly contagious. The most common site of laryngeal disease is the interarytenoid fold (in the posterior portion of the larynx). Because granulomas tend to be subepithelial, deep submucosal biopsies may be essential for diagnosis. Treatment is the same as for pulmonary tuberculosis (see Chap. 130), and symptomatic measures include voice rest and analgesics for pain. Occasionally tracheostomy is needed to protect the airway.

Fungal infections The most commonly found fungal infections, usually in immunocompromised patients, are histoplasmosis (Chap. 162); candidiasis (Chap. 166); and blastomycosis (Chap. 164). Symptoms can include hoarseness, cough, dyspnea, dysphagia, and odynophagia. Examination may reveal oral and esophageal thrush (candidiasis) or nodules on the vocal cords with or without ulceration (histoplasmosis or blastomycosis). With the latter, diagnosis is confirmed by biopsy showing microabscesses in an epithelium infiltrated with giant cells, mononuclear cells, and yeast. Treatment with systemic antifungal agents is necessary.

Other laryngeal infections   These include tertiary syphilis, lepromatous leprosy, diphtheria, glanders, and actinomycosis. Biopsy is usually required for the diagnosis of syphilis and leprosy, both of which may produce infiltrating nodular lesions.

PERICHONDRITIS   Perichondritis in the larynx due to pyogenic bacterial infection or an inflammatory process may be difficult to distinguish from traumatic injury, certain neoplasms, or injury induced by radiation. The thyroid cartilage is the most common cartilage affected, and an abscess may form beneath the mucoperichondrium. Symptoms and signs include pain, tenderness, and swelling that are usually slowly progressive but occasionally acute. Hoarseness, airway compromise, dysphagia, and odynophagia require prompt radiographic evaluation to exclude the possibility of a foreign body. The airway should then be secured in the operating room. Treatment may require antibiotics directed at the causative agent or glucocorticoids and debridement of laryngeal granulations.

DEEP NECK INFECTIONS

Deep neck infections are often difficult to diagnose clinically, and the potential for rapid spread and death should not be underestimated. Detailed knowledge of neck spaces and fascial planes facilitates the understanding of etiology, symptoms, complications, and treatment of these infections. Infections of the submandibular, lateral pharyngeal (parapharyngeal), and retropharyngeal spaces are particularly onerous, because pus in these locations can cause airway obstruction or spread contiguously to such structures as the mediastinum or carotid sheath.

The lateral pharyngeal space (also called the parapharyngeal or pharyngomaxillary space) can become infected from a variety of sources, including the palatine tonsils, pharynx, parotid gland, and infected lymph nodes that drain the pharynx and nose. Dental infections, particularly those originating from the third mandibular molar can spread to either the submandibular or the lateral pharyngeal spaces. Diabetics are particularly susceptible to such infections. The mode of spread includes direct dissection through the fascial spaces or direct extension from other communicating spaces within the neck. Lymphatic spread or septic thrombosis of peritonsillar veins can also precede lateral pharyngeal space infection. Clinical manifestations include fever, leukocytosis, and deep neck pain. Dysphagia and/or odynophagia may be present. On physical examination, one may see edema over the parotid gland; on intraoral examination, there may be medial bulging and displacement of the pharyngeal wall. Trismus may also be present. CT scanning with contrast can help to define the location of infection. Treatment consists of securing the airway, following external drainage in the operating room. The most common complication is a septic thrombosis of the internal jugular vein; clinical features include shaking chills with fever spikes, and tenderness at the mandibular angle. The diagnosis is confirmed by MRI. Intravenous antibiotic treatment should be directed against *Fusobacterium, Peptostreptococcus, Porphyromonas,* and *Prevotella* (see Chap. 128) for several weeks. Surgical removal of the thrombosed vein is reserved for special circumstances. Anticoagulation therapy is controversial. Complications of the thrombosed internal jugular vein include septic pulmonary emboli, lateral sinus thrombosis, cavernous sinus thrombosis, and brain abscess. Carotid artery "blowouts" are a rare but possibly fatal complication of lateral pharyngeal space infections. Clinical features include sentinel bleeding from the nose, mouth, or ear. Ipsilateral Horner's syndrome and cranial neuropathy (IX to XII) can be associated with an impending blowout. Sentinel bleeding is an acute surgical emergency that necessitates major vessel ligation. Inferior spread of infection along the carotid sheath may progress into the chest causing mediastinitis. Mortality rates approach 50 percent when mediastinitis is present.

SUBMANDIBULAR SPACE INFECTIONS   See Ludwig's angina above under "Oral Cavity."

RETROPHARYNGEAL SPACE INFECTION   The retropharyngeal space extends from the base of the skull superiorly to the level of the tracheal bifurcation inferiorly. It contains lymph nodes and connective tissue. The source of infection is usually located cephalad from the nose, sinuses, adenoids, and nasopharynx. Infection may extend from the lateral pharyngeal space to the retropharyngeal space directly or secondary to lymphatic spread. The greatest number of retropharyngeal lymph nodes are found in children under the age of 5 years, which accounts for the greater incidence of retropharyngeal space abscesses in this age group. These lymph nodes, including the adenoidal lymphoid pad, involute over time and are thus less likely to cause infection in older children.

Retropharyngeal space infections in young children are primarily complications of acute upper respiratory tract infections. Dysphagia and odynophagia are common and, in advanced cases, drooling is present. There is cervical rigidity and a hot-potato voice. Advanced infections present with dyspnea and/or stridor. Treatment includes securing of an airway, emergency surgical drainage, and intravenous antibiotics. In some cases, intraoral drainage may be accomplished; advanced cases, however, may require an external approach. Complications include intraoral rupture of the abscess, with secondary aspiration and pneumonia. Mediastinitis and airway obstruction are potentially life-threatening complications.

The microbiology of the various deep neck infections is similar. The most common organisms are *Streptococcus pyogenes, Peptostreptococcus, Prevotella, Porphyramonas,* and *Fusobacterium.* Many deep neck infections have mixed flora, with the majority of bacteria sensitive to a combination of penicillin G and metrinidazole or ampicillin-sulbactam.

REFERENCES

ALLAN BP et al: Orbital abscess of odontogenic origin. Case report and review of the literature. Int J Oral Maxillofac Surg 20:268, 1991
BROOK I: Diagnosis and management of anaerobic infections of the head and neck. Ann Otol Rhinol Laryngol Suppl 155:9, 1992
CHOW AW: Life threatening infections of the head and neck. Clin Infect Dis 14:991, 1992
DE FOER et al: Sinus aspergillosis. J Craniomaxillofac Surg 18:33, 1990
DUDLEY JP: *Branhamella catarrhalis* and croup: Toxicity in the upper respiratory tract. Am J Otolaryngol 12:113, 1991
ENGLISH GM (ed): *Otolaryngology,* revised edition. New York, Harper & Row, 1993
EVANS et al: Sinusitis of the maxillary antrum. N Engl J Med 293:735, 1975
GOYCOOLES MV et al: Otitis media. Otolaryngol Clin Am 24:757, 1991
LEW D et al: Sphenoid sinusitis: A review of 30 cases. N Engl J Med 309:1149, 1983
PARADISE JL: Etiology and management of pharyngitis and pharyngotonsillitis in children: A current review. Ann Otol Rhinol Laryngol Suppl 155:51, 1992
RANDALL DA et al: Indications for tonsillectomy and adenoidectomy. Am Fam Physician 44:1639, 1991
RUBEN RJ et al: Recent advances in otitis media. Complications and sequelae. Ann Otol Rhinol Laryngol Suppl 139:46, 1989
SALORD E et al: Nosocomial maxillary sinusitis during mechanical ventilation: A prospective comparison of orotracheal versus the nasotracheal route for intubation. Intens Care Med 16:390, 1990
SINAVE CP et al: The Lemierre syndrome: Suppurative thrombophlebitis of the internal jugular vein secondary to oropharyngeal infection. Medicine 68:85, 1989

85   INFECTIVE ENDOCARDITIS

DONALD KAYE

DEFINITION   Infective endocarditis is an infection which produces vegetations on the endocardium. It is virtually always fatal if untreated. A heart valve is usually involved, but infection may be on a septal defect or mural endocardium. Infection of an arteriovenous shunt or coarctation of the aorta is more properly called *endarteritis* and produces a similar clinical syndrome. The subsequent discussion of endocarditis also applies to endarteritis.

CLASSIFICATION

Endocarditis can be divided into native valve endocarditis, endocarditis in intravenous drug abusers, and prosthetic valve endocarditis, each with different infecting microorganisms and courses. Endocarditis also can be classified as acute or subacute. Acute endocarditis most frequently is caused by *Staphylococcus aureus*, occurs on a normal heart valve, is rapidly destructive, produces metastatic foci, and, if untreated, is fatal in less than 6 weeks. Subacute endocarditis usually is caused by viridans streptococci, occurs on damaged valves, does not produce metastatic foci, and, if untreated, takes more than 6 weeks or even a year to be fatal. Correlations between organism and course are not perfect. Viridans streptococci can be associated with an acute course and *S. aureus* with a subacute course. Most important is classification by infecting organisms (e.g., *S. aureus* endocarditis), because the organism has implications for therapy as well as course.

NATIVE VALVE ENDOCARDITIS Etiology Although almost any bacteria can produce endocarditis, streptococci, enterococci, and staphylococci account for the vast majority of cases.

STREPTOCOCCI Streptococci cause about 55 percent of cases of native valve endocarditis in patients who do not abuse intravenous drugs. Viridans streptococci (most commonly *S. sanguis, S. mutans,* or *S. milleri*) account for about 75 percent of these; *S. bovis* and other streptococci cause 20 and 5 percent, respectively. Viridans streptococci are normal inhabitants of the oropharynx and generally are highly susceptible to penicillin. Two group D streptococci, *S. bovis* and *S. equinus,* are also highly susceptible to penicillin G. *S. bovis* endocarditis occurs in elderly individuals; 80 percent of cases are in persons over 60 years of age. More than a third of these individuals have a malignant or premalignant gastrointestinal lesion, most often colonic cancer or a villous adenoma or polyp of the colon.

Group A beta-hemolytic streptococci attack normal or damaged heart valves and may cause their rapid destruction. Group B streptococci, which have been reported as an increasing cause of endocarditis in recent years, also attack normal valves and result in large friable vegetations and large emboli. Other streptococci are much more likely to infect damaged valves and rarely cause rapid valve destruction. *S. milleri* can cause metastatic abscesses, which are uncommon with other streptococci.

ENTEROCOCCI Enterococci cause about 6 percent of cases of native valve endocarditis. Enterococci are alpha-, beta-, or gamma-hemolytic and are normal inhabitants of the gastrointestinal tract, the anterior urethra, and occasionally the mouth. All enterococci are in Lancefield's group D and may be distinguished from streptococci by biochemical tests. They are relatively resistant to penicillin G, and an aminoglycoside must be added to achieve a bactericidal effect. Enterococcal endocarditis is most common in males, who develop infection at an average age of 60, while the average age of women with enterococcal endocarditis is under 40. Many patients give a recent history of genitourinary tract manipulation, trauma, or disease (e.g., cystoscopy, urethral catheterization, prostatectomy, abortion, pregnancy, or cesarean section), which occur mainly in older men and younger women.

STAPHYLOCOCCI Staphylococci cause about 30 percent of cases of native valve endocarditis (with *S. aureus* 5 to 10 times more frequent than *S. epidermidis*). *S. aureus* attacks normal or damaged heart valves, often causing rapid destruction. The course is often fulminant, with death from bacteremia within days or heart failure within weeks. Abscesses are common at multiple sites (e.g., kidneys, lungs, and brain). *S. epidermidis* infects abnormal valves without causing rapid destruction.

HACEK ORGANISMS The HACEK group of bacteria (*Haemophilus, Actinobacillus, Cardiobacterium, Eikenella,* and *Kingella*) are part of the oropharyngeal flora. They produce endocarditis with a subacute presentation and very large vegetations. They are difficult to isolate from blood.

OTHER BACTERIA Almost all species of bacteria are occasional causes of endocarditis, including *Strep. pneumoniae, Neisseria gonorrhoeae,* enteric gram-negative bacilli, *Pseudomonas, Salmonella, Streptobacillus, Serratia marcescens, Bacteroides, Brucella, Mycobacterium, N. meningitidis, Listeria, Legionella,* and diphtheroids, and can result in an acute or chronic course.

FUNGI Fungi rarely cause native valve endocarditis in persons who do not abuse intravenous drugs. However, *Candida* and *Aspergillus* endocarditis can occur in patients with intravascular catheters who frequently have received glucocorticoids, broad-spectrum antimicrobial drugs, or cytotoxic agents. The course is usually subacute. Large friable vegetations are common and give rise to large emboli, often to the lower extremities. The prognosis is grave, partly because of the relatively poor activity of available antifungal agents.

OTHER MICROORGANISMS Spirochetes (e.g., *Spirillum minor*), cell wall–deficient bacteria, rickettsiae (*Coxiella burnetii*), and chlamydiae (*C. psittaci, C. pneumoniae,* and *C. trachomatis*) are rare causes of endocarditis.

Epidemiology In native valve endocarditis, the proportion of males is higher than females, and most patients are over age 50. Endocarditis is uncommon in children.

Between 60 and 80 percent of patients have an identifiable predisposing cardiac lesion. *Rheumatic valvular disease* accounts for about 30 percent of cases. The mitral valve is most commonly involved, followed by the aortic. Right-sided endocarditis usually affects the tricuspid valve but is rare on rheumatic valves.

Congenital heart disease other than mitral valve prolapse is the underlying lesion in about 10 to 20 percent of patients with endocarditis. Predisposing lesions include patent ductus arteriosus, ventricular septal defect, tetralogy of Fallot, coarctation of the aorta, pulmonary stenosis, and bicuspid aortic valve but not uncomplicated atrial septal defect. *Mitral valve prolapse* is the underlying lesion in about 10 to 33 percent of cases.

Degenerative heart disease predisposes to endocarditis. *Calcific aortic stenosis* (from degenerative disease or bicuspid valve) is an important lesion in the elderly. Other predisposing but unusual lesions are *asymmetric septal hypertrophy, Marfan's syndrome,* and *syphilitic aortic valve.* Arterioarterial or *arteriovenous fistulas* also can be underlying lesions. In 20 to 40 percent of patients with infective endocarditis, *no underlying heart disease* can be recognized.

ENDOCARDITIS IN INTRAVENOUS DRUG ABUSERS Drug abusers with endocarditis are frequently young males. The skin is the most frequent source of microorganisms responsible for endocarditis; contamination of drugs is less common. *S. aureus* causes over 50 percent of cases, streptococci and enterococci about 15 percent, and fungi (mainly *Candida*) and gram-negative bacilli (usually *Pseudomonas* species) about 10 percent each. Infection with multiple organisms is common. The onset is usually acute. Only about 20 percent of addicts with their first episode of endocarditis have previously damaged heart valves. The tricuspid valve is infected in over 50 percent of cases, the aortic in 25 percent, and the mitral in about 20 percent. Over 75 percent with *S. aureus* infection and a much lower percent with other organisms have tricuspid valve endocarditis. Pulmonary emboli or pneumonia consequent to septic pulmonary emboli is common in tricuspid valve endocarditis, and murmurs are frequently absent.

PROSTHETIC VALVE ENDOCARDITIS Any intravascular prosthesis predisposes to endocarditis and makes cure difficult. Infections of prosthetic valves now account for 10 to 20 percent of cases of endocarditis. Intravascular sutures, pacemaker wires, and Teflon-Silastic tubes also can be foci of infection. Patients with prosthetic valve endocarditis are mainly males over age 60. Endocarditis occurs in 1 to 2 percent of these patients during the first year after operation and in 1 percent per year thereafter. Aortic valve prostheses are much more likely to be involved than mitral valve prostheses. The infection is usually on the suture line.

Early-onset endocarditis (onset of symptoms within 60 days of surgery) is usually a consequence of valve contamination during the procedure or bacteremia perioperatively. *Late-onset endocarditis* (onset of symptoms after 60 days) may have the same pathogenesis as early endocarditis (especially during the first year) but with a long incubation period or may result from transient bacteremia.

About half the episodes of early and one-third of late endocarditis are caused by staphylococci, and *S. epidermidis* is more frequent than *S. aureus*. Gram-negative bacilli cause up to 15 percent and fungi (most commonly *Candida*) up to 10 percent of early cases and are less common in late endocarditis. A prosthetic valve may malfunction because of large vegetations (often fungal). Streptococci are the most frequent single cause of late endocarditis (about 40 percent of cases) but are uncommon in early endocarditis.

Early prosthetic valve endocarditis is often associated with valve dysfunction or dehiscence and a fulminant course. Although late endocarditis may be similarly fulminant, the course is commonly indistinguishable from that of patients without prosthetic valves, especially when the organism is a streptococcus.

PATHOGENESIS AND PATHOLOGY

The characteristic lesions of infective endocarditis are vegetations on valves or elsewhere on endocardium. The disease usually arises secondary to localization of microorganisms on sterile vegetations composed of platelets and fibrin. Sterile vegetations, termed *nonbacterial thrombotic endocarditis*, form over areas of trauma to the endothelium (e.g., from intracardiac foreign bodies), in areas of turbulence (as on deformed valves), over scars, or in patients with wasting disease, particularly malignancy (marantic endocarditis).

Infection of a sterile vegetation is most likely when bacteremia occurs with bacteria that adhere well to platelets, fibrin, and fibronectin. The vegetation of infective endocarditis then results from deposition of platelets and fibrin over the bacteria, forming a "protected site" into which phagocytic cells penetrate poorly.

Endocarditis tends to occur in high-pressure areas (left side of heart) and downstream from where blood flows through a narrow orifice at a high velocity from a high- to low-pressure chamber (e.g., distal to the constriction in coarctation of the aorta). Endocarditis is unusual in sites with a small pressure gradient, as in atrial septal defects. Endocarditis occurs more frequently in valvular incompetence than in pure stenosis and is characteristically on the atrial side of the regurgitant mitral valve and the ventricular surface of the regurgitant aortic valve. A high-velocity stream of blood can produce satellite-infected lesions at distant points of impact.

Microorganisms that possess little pathogenicity in other situations, e.g., viridans streptococci, usually implant only on deformed heart valves with nonbacterial thrombotic endocarditis, but more virulent microorganisms, e.g., *S. aureus* and *Strep. pneumoniae*, can infect apparently normal valves.

Transient bacteremia is common in various infections and during traumatic procedures involving epithelial surfaces that are colonized by a bacterial flora (oropharynx, genitourinary and gastrointestinal tracts, and skin). For example, after trauma to tissues of the mouth, viridans streptococci are the most common bacteria isolated from blood, alone or more often mixed with other bacteria. The frequency and magnitude of bacteremia are related to the severity of periodontal disease and the severity of trauma. The portal of entry for the initiating episode of bacteremia is usually not apparent in viridans streptococcal endocarditis. Dental procedures, the most common apparent portals of entry, precede viridans streptococcal endocarditis in only 15 to 20 percent of cases.

Bacteremia also is common with prostatic surgery, cystoscopy, urethral dilation or catheterization, and procedures on the female reproductive tract. The organisms are usually enterococci and gram-negative bacilli. About 50 percent of patients with enterococcal endocarditis have had a recent operation or instrumentation on the genitourinary or gastrointestinal tract. About 35 percent with staphylococcal endocarditis have had a preceding staphylococcal infection at a remote site.

The clinical features of endocarditis result from the vegetations and an immune reaction to the infection. Extensive vegetations, especially in fungal endocarditis, may occlude the valve orifice. Rapid destruction with consequent valvular regurgitation may occur, especially with *S. aureus*. Healing may cause scar formation with subsequent valvular stenosis or regurgitation. Infection may extend into the myocardium, producing burrowing abscesses. Conduction abnormalities, fistulas (between chambers of the heart and the pericardium or major vessels), or rupture of the chordae, a papillary muscle, or the ventricular septum may result.

Pieces of vegetation break off and embolize to the heart, brain, kidney, spleen, liver, extremities, and lung (in right-sided endocarditis). Infarcts and occasionally abscesses result. Septic embolization to the vasa vasorum or direct bacterial invasion of the arterial wall may result in formation of mycotic aneurysms, which may rupture. Mycotic aneurysms most often develop in the cerebral arteries, aorta, sinuses of Valsalva, ligated ductus arteriosus, and the superior mesenteric, splenic, coronary, and pulmonary arteries.

Patients with endocarditis usually have high antibody titers against the infecting microorganism. This contributes to formation of circulating immune complexes that may result in glomerulonephritis (focal, membranoproliferative, or diffuse), arthritis, or various mucocutaneous manifestations of vasculitis.

Myocarditis may be due to small coronary artery emboli, myocardial abscesses, or immune complex vasculitis.

MANIFESTATIONS

Symptoms of endocarditis generally start within 2 weeks of the precipitating event. With organisms of low pathogenicity (e.g., viridans streptococci), the *onset* is usually gradual, with mild fever and malaise. With organisms of high pathogenicity (e.g., *S. aureus*), the onset is often acute with high fever. *Fever* is present in almost all patients with endocarditis (except occasionally in the elderly or those with renal failure, congestive heart failure, or severe debility). The fever is usually low grade (less than 39.4°C) except with acute disease. Arthralgias are common, and arthritis occurs occasionally.

Cardiac murmurs are almost always present except early in acute endocarditis or in intravenous drug abusers with tricuspid valve infection. True changes in murmurs or the appearance of a new murmur is uncommon except in acute endocarditis, where a new murmur (particularly aortic regurgitation) is frequent. Changes in intensities of murmurs are often due to changes in heart rate and/or cardiac output (e.g., from anemia) and not necessarily to progressive valvular damage.

Splenomegaly and *petechiae* each tend to occur in about 30 percent of cases, mainly in disease of long duration. Petechiae are most frequently found on the conjunctivae, palate, buccal mucosa, and upper extremities. *Splinter hemorrhages* are subungual, linear, dark-red streaks that may appear in endocarditis but also commonly result from trauma. *Roth spots* (oval, retinal hemorrhages with a clear pale center) are seen in less than 5 percent of patients and also may occur in connective tissue disease and severe anemia. *Osler nodes* (small tender nodules, usually on the finger or toe pads, which persist for hours to days) occur in 10 to 25 percent of patients but also in other diseases. *Janeway lesions* are small hemorrhages with a slightly nodular character on the palms and soles and are most commonly seen in acute endocarditis. *Clubbing* of the fingers is present in some patients with long-standing disease. *Embolic episodes* are recognized in about one-third of patients and may occur during or after therapy. Emboli to large arteries (e.g., femoral arteries) are often the result of fungal endocarditis with its large friable vegetations. Pulmonary emboli are common in drug abusers with right-sided endocarditis and may be seen in left-sided endocarditis with left-to-right cardiac shunts.

Mycotic aneurysms occur in about 10 percent of patients. Symptoms are usually lacking but may be those of an expanding mass. The aneurysms can rupture during or even years after therapy. *Neurologic manifestations* are present in about one-third of patients with endocarditis and are more common with left-sided endocarditis than with right-sided disease and with *S. aureus* infection than with viridans streptococcal infection. Clinically apparent cerebral emboli occur in about 20 percent of patients, encephalopathy (from microemboli with or without microabscess formation) in 10 percent, leakage from mycotic aneurysm in less than 5 percent, and meningitis or macroscopic brain abscess in less than 5 percent. Major cerebral emboli as well as mycotic aneurysms usually involve the middle cerebral artery system. The majority of patients with brain abscess or purulent meningitis have *S. aureus* endocarditis. *Heart failure* may occur during the course of the disease or long after cure. Contributing factors are valve destruction, myocarditis, coronary artery emboli with infarction, and myocardial abscesses. *Myocardial abscess* most commonly occurs with acute endocarditis (most commonly *S. aureus*) or with a prosthesis. Conduction defects may result from ventricular septal invasion secondary to extension from a valve (most frequently the aortic valve). A valve ring abscess or less commonly a myocardial abscess may extend into the epicardium and cause pericarditis. Echocardiography may be helpful in the diagnosis of myocardial abscess, and surgery is often indicated, especially with a prosthesis. *Renal disease* is present in most patients with endocarditis and is due to renal emboli or glomerulonephritis. Renal insufficiency may result.

LABORATORY FEATURES

A normocytic normochromic anemia is usual in infective endocarditis. The white blood cell and differential counts are often normal. However, in acute disease, leukocytosis without anemia may be present. Proteinuria and/or microscopic hematuria is found in most patients, and the serum creatinine level may be elevated. The erythrocyte sedimentation rate is almost always elevated except when heart failure is present.

About 50 percent of patients with endocarditis of at least 6 weeks' duration have a positive serum test for rheumatoid factor, and virtually all have circulating immune complexes. These tend to disappear with cure. The serum complement level may be decreased, especially with diffuse glomerulonephritis. Bacteria can be seen inside leukocytes in buffy coat preparations of blood in about 50 percent of patients with endocarditis.

The critical diagnostic finding in endocarditis is bacteremia or fungemia. Blood cultures are positive in over 95 percent of patients. The bacteremia is continuous; if any cultures are positive, all are likely to be positive. There is no advantage to obtaining cultures at any particular time or body temperature. Arterial blood or bone marrow offers no advantage over antecubital vein blood.

In subacute disease, in the absence of previous therapy, three cultures should be obtained over 3 to 6 h and therapy initiated. With previous therapy, treatment may be expeditiously delayed in an attempt to obtain positive blood cultures. In general, in acute disease, therapy should not be delayed for more than 2 to 3 h while obtaining cultures. Only one culture should be obtained from each venipuncture; anaerobic as well as aerobic techniques should be used. Cultures should be spaced at least 30 to 60 min apart to demonstrate continuous bacteremia. The rate of positive cultures is increased by observing them over 3 weeks with periodic sampling for Gram stain and subculture even in the absence of turbidity. Addition of pyridoxal hydrochloride to the media will improve the chances of isolating nutritionally deficient variant streptococci.

Blood cultures may be negative in infections with fastidious organisms such as *Haemophilus parainfluenzae*. Fifty percent of patients with *Candida* endocarditis and almost all with *Aspergillus, Histoplasma*, and *Coxiella burnetii* endocarditis have negative blood cultures. With fungi, large peripheral emboli are common, necessitat-

ing embolectomy. Histologic examination and culture of the embolus may be diagnostic. Serologic tests for *C. burnetii* and *C. psittaci* are positive in endocarditis caused by these organisms.

Although not diagnostic, transthoracic echocardiograms will demonstrate the vegetation in 50 to 80 percent of patients with native valve endocarditis. Transesophageal echocardiograms are much more sensitive (positive in over 90 percent of cases) and are much more likely to demonstrate intracardiac abscesses. Serial phonocardiography and cineradiography are useful in evaluating infection on prosthetic valves. Disappearance of an opening click or sound produced by a closing valve suggests the presence of a vegetation. With dehiscence, cineradiography of the valve will show abnormal motion.

DIAGNOSIS

Endocarditis should be suspected either when a heart murmur and unexplained fever are present for at least 1 week or in febrile intravenous drug abusers, even in the absence of a murmur. However, a definitive clinical diagnosis requires positive blood cultures.

Atrial myxoma, nonbacterial thrombotic endocarditis, acute rheumatic fever, lupus erythematosus, and sickle cell disease can duplicate the syndrome of infective endocarditis. Any patient with an existing heart murmur can develop fever related to another occult illness or to drugs. Therefore, in the absence of positive blood cultures, a search must be made for other causes of fever.

Following cardiac surgery, fever may be related to infection at other sites, to the postcardiotomy syndrome, or to a "postpump syndrome" (e.g., cytomegalovirus infection).

TREATMENT

PRINCIPLES OF THERAPY Cure of endocarditis requires eradication of all microorganisms from the vegetation. Therefore, microbicidal drug regimens must be used in high enough concentrations and for a long enough duration to sterilize the vegetation. Regimens including penicillins, cephalosporins, and vancomycin give far better results than when these drugs cannot be used because of resistant organisms or drug reactions.

The minimal inhibitory and bactericidal concentrations (MIC and MBC) should be determined. To follow efficacy of therapy for a drug regimen, it may be useful to measure the bactericidal activity of the patient's serum against his or her isolate. A bactericidal titer of $\geq 1:8$ in serum drawn 30 min after drug infusion probably indicates adequate therapy. While this determination is not necessary in most cases, it may be useful when infection is caused by organisms other than gram-positive cocci, treatment has failed, or regimens do not include penicillins, cephalosporins, or vancomycin. Except for unusual circumstances, antibiotic administration should be parenteral to guarantee adequate absorption of drugs. The infecting microorganism should be saved for future testing (e.g., serum antibacterial activity, evaluation of different antibiotics, or comparison with a relapse strain).

SPECIFIC ANTIMICROBIAL REGIMENS Therapy before culture results are known The treatment of subacute infective endocarditis on a native valve while awaiting culture results should be for enterococci, which are more resistant to antibiotics than streptococci.

With an acute course, therapy should be directed against *S. aureus*. In intravenous drug abusers, initial therapy should be directed against *S. aureus*, and gentamicin should be included for the possibility of gram-negative bacilli. In many cities, most *S. aureus* isolated from drug abusers are methicillin-resistant, and vancomycin must be used. With prosthetic valves, vancomycin plus gentamicin should be used because of the high incidence of methicillin-resistant *S. epidermidis* and the need to cover enterococci.

Once the organism is isolated, the regimen should be altered appropriately. If cultures remain sterile and culture-negative endocarditis is likely, treatment is continued provided that the response is adequate.

Streptococci with MIC of ≤0.1 μg/mL penicillin G   Most streptococci are inhibited by serum concentrations of 0.1 μg/mL penicillin G. Three regimens including penicillin G (Table 85-1) can be used for these highly penicillin-susceptible strains. Penicillin G alone for 4 weeks (regimen A) gives cure rates of 99 percent. Addition of gentamicin or streptomycin (regimen B) results in a more rapid bactericidal effect and gives equivalent cure rates in 2 weeks. Regimen B should be standard for uncomplicated infection, but regimen A is preferred in patients likely to have side effects with aminoglycosides (i.e., those with renal insufficiency or eighth nerve disease or older than 65 years). Penicillin for 4 weeks with an aminoglycoside for the first 2 weeks (regimen C) is used for nutritionally deficient variant strains, a relapse, or complications (e.g., metastatic abscesses). Regimen D can be substituted with a history of a delayed rash to penicillin. Regimen E should be used with a history of anaphylaxis to penicillin.

Streptococci with MIC of > 0.1 μg/mL but < 0.5 μg/mL penicil­lin G   Endocarditis caused by streptococci with MIC of >0.1 but <0.5 μg/mL penicillin G is managed with regimen F, a compromise between the regimens for highly susceptible (MIC ≤ 0.1 μg/mL) and relatively resistant (MIC ≥ 0.5 μg/mL) streptococci.

Enterococci or streptococci with MIC of ≥ 0.5 μg/mL penicillin G   Penicillin, ampicillin, and vancomycin are not bactericidal for most enterococci. With the addition of an aminoglycoside, a synergistic bactericidal effect occurs. Enterococcal endocarditis requires penicillin, ampicillin, or vancomycin plus an aminoglycoside for cure of most patients (regimens G and H, with H used for hypersensitivity to penicillin G). An alternative to regimen H consists of skin testing with major and minor determinants of penicillin, followed by attempts at desensitization to penicillin. This process involves a scratch test through a drop of penicillin G (100 units per mL), followed in 30 min by graded amounts of penicillin intradermally, begun at 0.01

unit in 0.1 mL of saline solution and continued in tenfold increments every 30 min; with increasing amounts, administration is changed to the subcutaneous, intramuscular, and finally intravenous route. Epinephrine and diphenhydramine should be on hand for emergency use during the procedure in case of anaphylaxis, and preferably the procedure should be carried out in an intensive care unit. If a reaction occurs, alternative therapy should be initiated.

Therapy is usually given for 4 weeks but is prolonged to 6 weeks when symptoms have been present for longer than 3 months or the course is complicated. Cephalosporins cannot be used in enterococcal endocarditis because the organisms are highly resistant.

A synergistic bactericidal effect against enterococci occurs with penicillin and aminoglycosides only when growth is inhibited by 2000 μg/mL of the aminoglycoside. Synergism is most likely with gentamicin. However, enterococci resistant to 2000 μg/mL of gentamicin are now common. Some of these gentamicin-resistant strains are inhibited by 2000 μg/mL of streptomycin, but most are resistant to 2000 μg/mL of all aminoglycosides. With aminoglycoside-resistant strains, it may be best to exclude aminoglycosides from the regimen and treat for 6 to 8 weeks. However, relapses may occur. Isolates of enterococci have been observed that are highly resistant to penicillin (either by production of penicillinase or other mechanisms) or vancomycin. Therefore, in vitro susceptibility testing of enterococci is required to choose appropriate therapy.

Endocarditis caused by streptococci with MIC ≥ 0.5 μg/mL is managed in the same way as enterococcal endocarditis.

Staphylococci   Methicillin-susceptible *S. aureus* and *S. epidermidis* are treated with regimen I or J. Methicillin-resistant staphylococci are resistant to all penicillins and cephalosporins. In these cases, or in patients who cannot tolerate penicillins or cephalosporins, vancomycin as in regimens K and L must be used. Some experts advocate addition of gentamicin for the first 3 to 5 days because of

---

TABLE 85-1   Therapy of infective endocarditis caused by gram-positive cocci*

STREPTOCOCCI† WITH MIC ≤ 0.1 μg/mL PENICILLIN G

Regimen A	Penicillin G, 10–20 million units/d IV in divided doses every 4 h × 4 weeks *or*
Regimen B	Penicillin as in regimen A plus streptomycin, 7.5 mg/kg IM every 12 h or gentamicin, 1 mg/kg IV every 8 h, both × 2 weeks *or*
Regimen C	Penicillin plus streptomycin or gentamicin × 2 weeks as in regimen B with penicillin continued 2 weeks longer *or*
Regimen D	Cefazolin, 1–2 g IV or IM every 6–8 h × 4 weeks *or*
Regimen E	Vancomycin, 15 mg/kg IV every 12 h × 4 weeks

STREPTOCOCCI WITH MIC > 0.1 BUT < 0.5 μg/mL PENICILLIN G

Regimen F	Use regimen C *or* regimen E if penicillin allergic

ENTEROCOCCI OR STREPTOCOCCI WITH MIC ≥ 0.5 μg/mL PENICILLIN G

Regimen G	Penicillin G, 20–30 million units/d or ampicillin, 12 g/d IV in divided doses every 4 h plus gentamicin, 1 mg/kg IV every 8 h or streptomycin, 7.5 mg/kg IM every 12 h, both × 4–6 weeks *or*
Regimen H	Vancomycin, 15 mg/kg IV every 12 h plus gentamicin or streptomycin as in regimen G, both × 4–6 weeks

METHICILLIN-SUSCEPTIBLE *S. AUREUS* OR *S. EPIDERMIDIS*

Regimen I	Nafcillin, 2 g IV every 4 h × 4–6 weeks with or without gentamicin, 1 mg/kg IV every 8 h × the first 3–5 d *or*
Regimen J	Cefazolin, 2 g IV every 6 h × 4–6 weeks with or without gentamicin as in regimen I *or*
Regimen K	Vancomycin, 15 mg/kg IV every 12 h × 4–6 weeks with or without gentamicin as in regimen I

METHICILLIN-RESISTANT STAPHYLOCOCCI OR *CORYNEBACTERIUM SP.*

Regimen L	Vancomycin with or without gentamicin as in regimen K

ENDOCARDITIS CAUSED BY THE ABOVE ORGANISMS ON A PROSTHETIC VALVE

Regimen C but with 20 million units of penicillin each day and a longer duration of penicillin (a total of 6 weeks)
Regimen D × 6 weeks with gentamicin or streptomycin × the first 2 weeks
Regimen E × 6 weeks with gentamicin or streptomycin × the first 2 weeks
Regimen F, but continue penicillin × 6 weeks
Regimen G or H × 6 weeks
Regimen I, J, or K × 6–8 weeks with gentamicin × the first 2 weeks
Regimen L × 6–8 weeks with gentamicin × the first 2 weeks
In the presence of *S. epidermidis* also add rifampin, 300 mg orally every 8 h × 6–8 weeks. The use of rifampin with *S. aureus* is controversial.

* Peak serum concentrations of gentamicin should be about 3 μg/mL. Streptomycin peaks should be about 20 μg/mL. The maximum dose of vancomycin is 1 g every 12 h.
† For Group A streptococci or *S. pneumoniae* use regimen A.
NOTE: MIC = minimal inhibitory concentration.

and routine use of the drug is not recommended. Four weeks' therapy is standard, but with metastatic or intracardiac abscess (or other complications) therapy should be extended to 6 weeks or even longer.

Streptococci, enterococci, and staphylococci in prosthetic valve endocarditis Therapy should be prolonged (Table 85-1), and combinations with an aminoglycoside are usual. When a methicillin-resistant *S. epidermidis* is involved, addition of rifampin improves outcomes.

In vitro testing with added rifampin has shown a synergistic bactericidal effect with some staphylococci and an antagonistic one with others. Except for the case of *S. epidermidis*, addition of rifampin is controversial and therefore should be based on poor clinical response and in vitro evidence of synergism.

HACEK organisms Therapy for the HACEK group consists of ampicillin (2 g every 4 h IV) or a third-generation cephalosporin (e.g., ceftriaxone 1 g every 12 h IV or IM) plus gentamicin (1.7 mg/kg every 8 h IV) for 4 weeks.

Other organisms In endocarditis caused by other organisms, bactericidal antibiotics, preferably a penicillin, cephalosporin, or vancomycin with or without an aminoglycoside, should be given and therapy continued for 4 to 6 weeks. With gram-negative bacilli, the penicillin or cephalosporin which has the greatest potency against the infecting bacteria in vitro should be administered in large doses intravenously along with an aminoglycoside to which the bacterium is susceptible (e.g., ampicillin, 2 g every 4 h; piperacillin, 3 g every 4 h; cefotaxime, 2 g every 4 to 6 h; or ceftazidime, 2 g every 8 h; plus gentamicin, 1.7 mg/kg every 8 h). A quinolone such as ciprofloxacin alone, which is bactericidal for gram-negative bacilli, also should be useful.

With *Corynebacterium* species, which are often resistant to all penicillins and cephalosporins, regimen L in Table 85-1 is most likely to be effective.

When the organisms are resistant to penicillins, cephalosporins, quinolones, and vancomycin, therapy will probably be unsuccessful. Under these circumstances, treatment should be with the bactericidal drug grouping that demonstrates the best activity in vitro. If the response is poor or relapse occurs, antimicrobial therapy plus valve replacement will probably be necessary.

HOME THERAPY Home therapy is very cost effective and has been used successfully with stable, non-IV drug users who are highly motivated, able to administer the therapy, and living with someone else. Ceftriaxone, 2 g IV once daily, for streptococcal endocarditis, and vancomycin, 1 g IV every 12 h, for streptococcal and staphylococcal endocarditis, have been used most frequently.

SURGERY IN THE MANAGEMENT OF ENDOCARDITIS When appropriate microbicidal therapy is not available (as in fungal endocarditis) or positive blood cultures persist on therapy or relapse occurs after appropriate therapy, replacement of the valve should be considered. Ideally, surgery should be performed after several days of the best available antimicrobial therapy. With organisms that tend to produce metastatic foci, therapy should then be continued long enough to eradicate these foci. Persistence of infection with the same organism following valve replacement has been uncommon. Immediate replacement (even after only hours of therapy) is essential in patients developing heart failure secondary to severe valvular regurgitation. Surgery is necessary to drain myocardial or valve ring abscesses and should be considered with recurrent emboli despite adequate antimicrobial therapy. It also should be considered in patients with aortic valve endocarditis who develop first- and second-degree atrioventricular block. In some centers, the presence of a large vegetation on echocardiography may be an indication for surgery.

Replacement of a prosthesis is often necessary for infections with organisms other than streptococci, for valve dysfunction or dehiscence, or for myocardial invasion. Myocardial invasion is common with prosthetic valves and is suggested by continued fever after 10 days of therapy, a new regurgitant murmur, and/or atrioventricular conduction disturbance.

COURSE

Defervescence usually occurs after 3 to 7 days of antimicrobial therapy. Blood cultures should be obtained periodically during treatment and generally become negative after several days of therapy. Lack of response of fever and bacteremia may be associated with myocardial or metastatic abscess formation (especially associated with *S. aureus*).

The most common cause of persistent or recurrent fever during therapy is a drug reaction; less commonly, emboli are responsible. If a rash develops, therapy can be continued and antihistamines or even glucocorticoids given to suppress the reaction. If the rash is severe, therapy should be altered.

Weight gain and a rise in hemoglobin may not be seen until weeks after therapy has been completed. Petechiae, Osler nodes, and emboli may occur during and for weeks after successful antimicrobial therapy. Mycotic aneurysms may regress on drug therapy or may rupture weeks to years later. Heart failure may occur during or after therapy and is the principal cause of death.

Anticoagulants should be used only with a pressing indication (such as certain prosthetic valves, but not including infected emboli) because of increased risk of hemorrhage (especially intracranial). Warfarin is preferable to heparin. Blood cultures 2 and 4 weeks after discontinuation of the therapy detect the vast majority of relapses.

PROGNOSIS

Factors that predispose to a poor prognosis are (1) nonstreptococcal disease, (2) development of heart failure, (3) aortic valve involvement, (4) infection on a prosthetic valve, (5) older age, and (6) valve ring or myocardial abscess. The cure rate in streptococcal endocarditis is about 90 percent. Failures are not due to uncontrolled infection but to death from heart failure, embolus, rupture of mycotic aneurysm, or renal failure. The mortality rate in nonaddicts with *S. aureus* endocarditis is at least 40 percent, and most deaths are due to overwhelming infection or heart failure. In drug addicts with *S. aureus* infection on the tricuspid valve, cure rates are over 90 percent, and in the absence of infected emboli, therapy has been successful with 2 weeks of nafcillin plus an aminoglycoside. Results are poor in endocarditis caused by fungi and gram-negative bacilli resistant to penicillins and cephalosporins. The presence of large vegetations on echocardiogram may indicate a poorer prognosis than small or absent vegetations. About 10 percent of patients will have additional episodes of endocarditis, months or years later. The prognosis in early prosthetic valve endocarditis is much worse than in late disease, with mortality rates of 40 to 80 percent versus 20 to 40 percent.

ANTIMICROBIAL PROPHYLAXIS OF ENDOCARDITIS

Although the risk of endocarditis is small and there is no proof of efficacy, prophylaxis is recommended for patients with predisposing cardiac lesions undergoing procedures known to cause bacteremia. The conditions for which prophylaxis is recommended are valvular or congenital heart disease (except uncomplicated atrial septal defect), intracardiac prostheses, asymmetric septal hypertrophy, and previous episode of endocarditis. Mitral valve prolapse increases the risk of endocarditis to a low to moderate extent. However, it is so common that it is neither risk- nor cost-effective to give prophylaxis to all patients with prolapse for all procedures. It is, however, reasonable to use prophylaxis in individuals with mitral valve prolapse who have holosystolic murmurs and who presumably are at greatest risk. The finding of thickened redundant mitral valve leaflets on echocardiography apparently also selects a subset of patients at greater risk.

Oral hygiene should be optimal in patients with cardiac lesions that predispose to endocarditis, especially those who are to have prosthetic cardiac valves implanted.

For dental and other procedures in the mouth, nose, or throat likely to cause bleeding or significant trauma, prophylaxis is aimed at viridans streptococci. The regimen recommended by the American Heart Association is amoxicillin, 3 g orally 1 h before the procedure followed by 1.5 g 6 h later. With penicillin allergy, the recommendation is 800 mg oral erythromycin ethylsuccinate or 1.0 g erythromycin stearate 2 h before the procedure or 300 mg oral clindamycin 1 h before, in each case followed by half the dose 6 h later. In high-risk patients (e.g., those with prosthetic valves), an alternative but optional more stringent regimen is ampicillin, 2 g intramuscularly or intravenously, plus gentamicin, 1.5 mg/kg intramuscularly or intravenously, both 30 min before the procedure, and amoxicillin, 1.5 g orally, 6 h later or, with penicillin allergy, vancomycin, 1 g intravenously over 1 h starting 1 h before the procedure.

For genitourinary and gastrointestinal tract procedures likely to cause significant trauma (e.g., cystoscopy, prostatic surgery, and colonic or gallbladder surgery), prophylaxis is directed against enterococci. The regimen is ampicillin plus gentamicin as above. With penicillin allergy, the vancomycin regimen above is given, but 1.5 mg/kg gentamicin, given intravenously or intramuscularly, is added 1 h before the procedure. For low-risk patients, amoxicillin may be used, 3 g orally 1 h before the procedure, followed by 1.5 g 6 h later. Fiberoptic endoscopy, even with biopsy, is so low risk for endocarditis that prophylaxis is difficult to justify. If used, it should be only in high-risk patients.

Prophylaxis for cardiac surgery with placement of intracardiac prostheses, patches, or sutures is directed against staphylococci and has usually consisted of 2 g cefazolin intravenously plus 1.5 mg/kg gentamicin intravenously starting immediately preoperatively, followed by repeated doses 8 and 16 h later. However, since strains of *S. epidermidis* may be methicillin-resistant, substitution of vancomycin for cefazolin in a dose of 15 mg/kg intravenously over 1 h starting 1 h before the procedure, 10 mg/kg after completion of bypass, and then 7.5 mg/kg every 6 h for 3 doses is reasonable. Vancomycin also can be used when patients have hypersensitivity to penicillins and cephalosporins.

Patients with coronary artery bypass grafts or transvenous pacemakers in place do not require prophylaxis for endocarditis, nor is it indicated for patients undergoing cardiac catheterization.

REFERENCES

ABRUTYN E, KAYE D: Prevention of bacterial endocarditis: 1991. Ann Intern Med 114:803, 1991

BISNO AL et al: Antimicrobial treatment of infective endocarditis due to viridans streptococci, enterococci and staphylococci. JAMA 261(10):1471, 1989

CHAMBERS HF et al: Right-sided *Staphylococcus aureus* endocarditis in intravenous drug abusers: Two-week combination therapy. Ann Intern Med 109:619, 1988

DAJANI AS et al: Prevention of bacterial endocarditis: Recommendation by the American Heart Association. JAMA 264:2919, 1990

DANIEL WG et al: Improvement in diagnosis of abscesses associated with endocarditis by transesophageal echocardiography. N Engl J Med 324:795, 1991

DURACK D: Prophylaxis of infective endocarditis, in *Principles and Practice of Infectious Diseases*, 3d ed, GL Mandell et al (eds). New York, Churchill Livingstone, 1990

KANTER MC, HART RG: Neurologic complications of infective endocarditis. Neurology 41:1015, 1991

KAYE D (ed): *Infective Endocarditis*, 2d ed. New York, Raven Press, 1992

KORZENIOWSKI O, KAYE D: Infective endocarditis, in *Heart Disease*, 4th ed, E Braunwald (ed). Philadelphia, Saunders, 1992

MARKS AR et al: Identification of high-risk and low-risk subgroups of patients with mitral-valve prolapse. N Engl J Med 320:1031, 1989

SCHELD M, SANDE M: Endocarditis and intravascular infections, in *Principles and Practice of Infectious Diseases*, 3d ed, GL Mandell et al (eds). New York, Churchill Livingstone, 1990

SHIVELY BK et al: Diagnostic value of transesophageal compared with transthoracic echocardiography in infective endocarditis. J Am Coll Cardiol 18:391, 1991

STECKELBERG JM et al: Emboli in infective endocarditis: The prognostic value of echocardiography. Ann Intern Med 114:635, 1991

THRELKELD M, COBBS G: Infections of prosthetic valves and intravascular devices, in *Principles and Practice of Infectious Diseases*, 3d ed, GL Mandell et al (eds). New York, Churchill-Livingstone, 1990

86 INTRAABDOMINAL INFECTIONS AND ABSCESSES

DORI F. ZALEZNIK / DENNIS L. KASPER

Intraperitoneal infections generally arise because a normal anatomic barrier is disrupted. This disruption may occur when the appendix, a diverticulum, or an ulcer ruptures; when the bowel wall is weakened by ischemia, tumor, or inflammation (e.g., in inflammatory bowel disease); or with adjacent inflammatory processes, such as pancreatitis or pelvic inflammatory disease, in which enzymes (in the former case) or organisms (in the latter) may leak into the peritoneal cavity. Whatever the inciting event, once inflammation develops and organisms usually contained within the bowel or another organ enter the normally sterile peritoneal space, a predictable series of events takes place. Intraabdominal infections occur in two stages: peritonitis and—if it goes untreated—abscess formation. The types of microorganisms predominating in each stage of infection are responsible for the pathogenesis of disease.

PERITONITIS

The peritoneal cavity is large but divided into compartments. The upper and lower peritoneal cavities are divided by the transverse mesocolon; the greater omentum extends from the transverse mesocolon and from the lower pole of the stomach to line the lower peritoneal cavity. The pancreas, duodenum, and ascending and descending colons are located in the anterior retroperitoneal space; the kidneys, ureters, and adrenals are found in the posterior retroperitoneal space. The other organs, including liver, stomach, gallbladder, spleen, jejunum, ileum, transverse and sigmoid colon, cecum, and appendix, are found within the peritoneal cavity itself. Normally the cavity is lined with a serous membrane that can serve as a conduit for fluids— a property utilized in peritoneal dialysis. A small amount of fluid sufficient to allow movement of organs is normally present in the peritoneal space. This fluid is serous, with a protein content (consisting mainly of albumin) of <30 g/L and fewer than 300 white blood cells (WBCs, generally mononuclear cells) per microliter. Certain of the compartments in the peritoneal cavity more commonly than others collect fluid or pus in the presence of infection. These include the pelvis (the most dependent portion), the subphrenic spaces on both the right and left, and Morrison's pouch, which is a posterior, superior extension of the subhepatic spaces and is the most dependent area of the paravertebral groove when a patient is recumbent. The falciform ligament separating the right and left subphrenic spaces appears to act as a barrier to the spread of infection; consequently, it is unusual to find bilateral subphrenic collections.

SPONTANEOUS BACTERIAL PERITONITIS Peritonitis is either primary (without apparent inciting event) or secondary. The types of organisms found and the clinical presentation of these two processes are different. In adults primary or spontaneous bacterial peritonitis (SBP) occurs most commonly in conjunction with cirrhosis of the liver (frequently the result of alcoholism). It virtually always develops in patients with ascites. Nevertheless, it is not a common event, occurring in no more than 10 percent of cirrhotic patients. The cause of SBP has not been established definitively but is believed to involve hematogenous spread of organisms with the diseased liver and altered portal circulation resulting in a defect in the usual filtration function. Organisms are able to multiply in ascites, a good medium for growth. The proteins of the complement cascade have been found in peritoneal fluid, with lower levels in cirrhotic patients than in patients with other causes of ascites. The opsonic and phagocytic properties of neutrophils are also decreased in patients with advanced liver disease.

The presentation of SBP differs from that of secondary peritonitis. The most common manifestation is fever, which is documented in as many as 80 percent of patients. Ascites is found but virtually always predates infection. Abdominal pain, an acute onset of symptoms, and peritoneal irritation detected during physical examination can be helpful diagnostically, but the absence of any of these findings does not exclude this often subtle diagnosis. It is vital to sample the peritoneal fluid of any cirrhotic patient with ascites and fever. The finding of more than 300 polymorphonuclear leukocytes (PMNs) per microliter is diagnostic for SBP, according to Conn. The microbiology of SBP also is distinctive. While enteric gram-negative bacilli such as *Escherichia coli* are the most common organisms encountered, gram-positive organisms such as streptococci, enterococci, or even pneumococci are sometimes found. The characteristic microbiologic features of SBP are that generally only a single organism is recovered and anaerobes are rarely found. This microbiologic picture contrasts with that of secondary peritonitis, in which a mixed flora, including anaerobes, is the rule. In fact, if SBP is suspected and multiple organisms, including anaerobes, are recovered from the peritoneal fluid, the diagnosis must be reconsidered and a source of secondary peritonitis sought.

The diagnosis of SBP is not easy. The level of suspicion needs to be high. It may be difficult to recover organisms from cultures of peritoneal fluid, presumably because the burden of organisms is low. The yield can be improved if 10 mL of peritoneal fluid is placed directly into a blood culture bottle. Bacteremia may accompany SBP; therefore, blood should be cultured simultaneously. No specific radiographic studies are helpful in the diagnosis of SBP. A plain film of the abdomen would be expected to show ascites. Chest and abdominal radiography should be performed in cases with abdominal pain to exclude free air, which signals a perforation. Treatment for SBP is directed at the isolate from blood or peritoneal fluid. Until culture results become available, empirical therapy should cover gram-negative aerobic bacilli and gram-positive cocci. Empirical coverage for anaerobes is not necessary.

SECONDARY PERITONITIS Secondary peritonitis develops when bacteria contaminate the peritoneum as a result of spillage from an intraabdominal process. The organisms found almost always constitute a mixed flora in which aerobic gram-negative bacilli and anaerobes predominate, especially when the source is colonic. Early in the course of infection, free-flowing exudate with PMNs is found. Early mortality is attributable to gram-negative bacillary sepsis and potent endotoxins circulating in the bloodstream (see Chap. 83). Gram-negative bacilli, particularly *E. coli*, are common bloodstream isolates, but *Bacteroides fragilis* bacteremia is common as well. The severity of abdominal pain and the clinical course depend on the inciting process. The types of organisms isolated from the peritoneum also vary with the initial process and the normal flora present. There also are differences in peritonitis that primarily results from chemical irritation and that resulting primarily from bacterial contamination. For example, as long as the patient is not achlorhydric, a ruptured gastric ulcer will release low pH gastric contents that will serve as a chemical irritant. The normal flora of the stomach comprises the same organisms found in the oropharynx (see Chap. 128) but in numbers at least two logs lower. The surfaces of teeth contain approximately 10^7 aerobic and 10^7 anaerobic organisms per milliliter of saliva; the normally acidic stomach contains an equal ratio of aerobic and anaerobic species, but in concentrations more in the range of 10^5 per milliliter. After meals, when gastric acidity is highest, this number may fall to 10^3. The bacterial burden, then, in a ruptured gastric ulcer—or even duodenal ulcer—is negligible compared with that in a ruptured appendix. The normal flora of the colon below the ligament of Treitz contains about 10^{11} anaerobic organisms per gram of feces but only 10^8 aerobes per gram; therefore, anaerobic species account for 99 percent of the bacteria. There is not a significant chemical peritonitis from leakage of colonic contents (pH 7 to 8), but infection from the heavy bacterial load is severe.

Depending on the inciting event, local symptoms may initially be found in secondary peritonitis—for example, epigastric pain from a ruptured gastric ulcer. In appendicitis the initial presenting symptoms often are vague, with periumbilical discomfort and nausea followed in a number of hours by pain more localized to the right lower quadrant. Variable locations of the appendix (including a retrocecal position) can complicate this presentation further. Once infection has spread to the peritoneal cavity, however, pain increases, particularly with infection involving the parietal peritoneum, which is innervated extensively. Patients usually lie motionless, often with knees drawn up to avoid stretching the nerve fibers of the peritoneal cavity. Coughing and sneezing, which increase pressure within the peritoneal cavity, are associated with sharp pain. There may or may not be pain localized to the infected or diseased organ from which secondary peritonitis has arisen. Patients with secondary peritonitis generally have abnormal abdominal examinations with marked voluntary and involuntary guarding of anterior abdominal musculature. Later findings include tenderness, especially rebound tenderness. In addition, there may be localized findings in the area of the inciting event. In general, patients are febrile, with marked leukocytosis and a left shift of the WBCs to earlier granulocyte forms.

While recovery of organisms from peritoneal fluid is easier in secondary than in primary peritonitis, a tap of the abdomen is rarely the procedure of choice in secondary peritonitis. An exception is in cases involving trauma, where the possibility of a hemoperitoneum may need to be excluded early. Treatment for secondary peritonitis includes administration of early antibiotics targeted particularly at aerobic gram-negative bacilli and anaerobes as well as etiologic studies. Most secondary peritonitis requires both surgical intervention to address the inciting process and antibiotic administration to treat early bacteremia, to decrease the incidence of abscess formation and wound infection, and to avoid more distant spread of infection. In SBP in adults, surgery is rarely indicated. In secondary peritonitis, surgery may be life-saving.

INTRAPERITONEAL ABSCESSES

Abscess formation is common in untreated peritonitis if overt gram-negative sepsis either does not occur or does occur but is not fatal. In experimental models of abscess formation, mixed aerobic and anaerobic organisms have been implanted intraperitoneally. Without therapy directed at anaerobes, animals develop intraabdominal abscesses. As in patients, these experimental abscesses may stud the peritoneal cavity, lie within the omentum or mesentery, or even develop on the surface of or within viscera such as the liver.

ROLE OF BACTERIAL VIRULENCE FACTORS *B. fragilis*, although accounting for only 0.5 percent of the normal colonic contents, is found in 65 percent of intraabdominal infections and is the most common anaerobic bloodstream isolate. Therefore, it appears to be uniquely virulent on clinical grounds. Moreover, *B. fragilis* causes abscesses in the animal model of intraabdominal infection, whereas most other *Bacteroides* species must be implanted with a facultative organism in order for abscesses to form.

Several virulence factors have been identified in *B. fragilis* and some are critical to abscess formation. The most important virulence factor is the capsular polysaccharide complex (CP) found on the surface of this organism. Two distinct surface polysaccharides comprise the CP of most, if not all, *B. fragilis* strains. The CP by itself can provoke abscesses. Structural analysis of each polysaccharide in the CP shows unusual features thought to be responsible for abscess formation. In addition, immunization of animals with CP leads to immunity from abscess formation. Other virulence properties of *B. fragilis* CP include the ability to adhere to peritoneal mesothelial cells and antiphagocytic activity.

B. fragilis also contains a surface lipopolysaccharide that lacks the potency of the endotoxins produced by aerobic gram-negative bacilli. In addition, *B. fragilis* elaborates an important enzyme, superoxide dismutase, which facilitates bacterial survival in the presence of oxygen by counteracting the toxic effects of superoxide radicals. One reason that anaerobic species thrive in intraabdominal infections is the reduced oxidation-reduction potential associated with necrotic tissue. The oxidation-reduction potential in the center of an abscess also is low, but, before an abscess becomes established, some oxygen is present. Anaerobic species such as *B. fragilis,* which display a degree of oxygen tolerance, have an enhanced ability to survive.

PATHOGENESIS AND IMMUNITY   There is often disagreement about whether an abscess represents a disease state or a host response. In a sense, it represents both: while an abscess is an infection in which viable organisms and PMNs are contained within a fibrous capsule, it is also a process by which the host confines microbes to a limited space, thereby preventing further spread of infection. Experimental work has helped to define both the host cells involved in abscess formation and the bacterial virulence factors responsible— most notably those of the most common gram-negative anaerobic isolate, *B. fragilis.* Several host factors have been found experimentally to participate in abscess formation, including the alternative pathway of complement and fibrinogen. T cells also are important; nude mice can form small abscesses, but animals depleted of CD4 + / CD8 + T cells cannot. Although most organisms involved in abscess induction are extracellular pathogens and would be expected to elicit an immune response that is primarily humoral, in intraabdominal abscess the immune response to *B. fragilis* is T cell dependent and directed to the CP. Two different CD8 +, non-H$_2$–restricted T cells are responsible for immunity to experimental intraabdominal abscesses. While antibodies to CP are not critical in immunity to abscesses, they enhance bloodstream clearance of *B. fragilis.*

CLINICAL PRESENTATION   Most intraperitoneal abscesses result from secondary bacterial peritonitis due to fecal spillage from a colonic source, such as an inflamed appendix. Seventy-four percent of intraabdominal abscesses are intraperitoneal or retroperitoneal and are not associated with a specific organ. Abscesses arise from a number of different processes as well. They usually form within weeks of the development of peritonitis and may be found in a variety of locations from omentum to mesentery, pelvis to psoas muscles, and subphrenic space to the surface of (or deeper in) viscera such as the liver. Infections of the female genital tract and pancreatitis are among the more common causative events. When abscesses occur in the female genital tract—either as a primary infection (e.g., tuboovarian abscess) or as an infection extending into the pelvic cavity or peritoneum—*B. fragilis* figures prominently among the organisms isolated. *B. fragilis* is not found in large numbers in the normal vaginal flora. It is encountered less commonly in pelvic inflammatory disease and endometritis, for example, without an associated abscess. In pancreatitis with leakage of damaging pancreatic enzymes, inflammation is prominent. Therefore, clinical findings such as fever, leukocytosis, and even abdominal pain do not distinguish pancreatitis itself from complications such as pancreatic pseudocyst, pancreatic abscess, or intraabdominal collections of pus. Some authors have advocated early needle aspiration of pancreatic collections under computed tomographic (CT) guidance as a means of distinguishing pseudocyst from abscess, but this procedure is associated with some hazard, and the recovery of organisms is not of clear significance.

The psoas muscle of the anterior back is another location in which abscesses are encountered. These abscesses may arise from a presumed hematogenous source, from contiguous spread from an intraabdominal or pelvic process, or from contiguous spread from nearby bony structures such as vertebral bodies. Associated osteomyelitis due to spread from bone to muscle or from muscle to bone is common in psoas abscess. When Pott's disease was common, *Mycobacterium tuberculosis* was a frequent cause of psoas abscess. Currently in the United States, the usual isolates from psoas abscesses are either *Staphylococcus aureus* or a mixture of enteric organisms including aerobic gram-negative bacilli. *S. aureus* is most likely to be isolated when a psoas abscess arises from hematogenous spread or a contiguous focus of osteomyelitis; a mixed enteric flora is most likely when the abscess has an intraabdominal or pelvic source.

DIAGNOSIS   A variety of scanning procedures have facilitated considerably the diagnosis of intraabdominal abscesses. Abdominal CT scans probably have the highest yield, although ultrasonography is particularly useful for the right upper quadrant, kidneys, and pelvis. Both gallium- and indium-labeled WBCs tend to localize in abscesses and may be useful in finding a collection. Since gallium is taken up in the bowel, indium-labeled WBCs may have a slightly greater yield for abscesses near the bowel. Neither gallium- nor indium-labeled WBC scans serve as a basis for a definitive diagnosis, however; both need to be followed by other, more specific studies, such as CT, if an area of possible abnormality is identified. Abscesses contiguous with or contained within outpouchings of bowel are particularly difficult to diagnose with scanning procedures. Occasionally, a barium enema may detect a diverticular abscess not diagnosed by other procedures, although barium should not be injected if a free perforation is suspected. If one study is negative, a second study sometimes reveals a collection. On occasion, exploratory laparotomy still must be undertaken if an abscess is strongly suspected on clinical grounds, although this procedure has been less commonly used since the advent of CT.

TREATMENT   The treatment of intraabdominal infections involves the establishment of the initial focus of infection, the administration of broad-spectrum antibiotics targeted at organisms involved in the associated infection, and the performance of a drainage procedure if one or more definitive abscesses have formed already. It cannot be overemphasized that antimicrobial therapy, in general, is adjunctive to drainage and/or surgical correction of an underlying lesion or process in intraabdominal abscesses. Unlike the intraabdominal abscesses precipitated by most infections, for which drainage of some kind generally is required, abscesses associated with diverticulitis usually wall off locally after rupture of a diverticulum, so that surgical intervention is not routinely required.

A number of antimicrobial agents exhibit excellent activity against aerobic gram-negative bacilli. Since mortality in intraabdominal sepsis is linked to gram-negative bacteremia and endotoxin release, empirical therapy for intraabdominal infection always needs to include adequate coverage of these organisms. Aminoglycosides and second- and third-generation cephalosporins are the agents most widely tested and used in intraabdominal processes. Newer antibiotics such as aztreonam, imipenem, ticarcillin/clavulanic acid, and quinolones (e.g., ciprofloxacin) cover these organisms as well, although at a higher cost. Second-generation cephalosporins such as cefoxitin or cefotetan are not as uniformly active as the other agents against all of the aerobic gram-negative species. Aztreonam, ciprofloxacin, aminoglycosides, and most of the third-generation cephalosporins are not active against anaerobes and therefore need to be used in combination with another antibiotic. There are conflicting studies in the literature about the anaerobic activity of ceftizoxime, a third-generation cephalosporin. There may be a discrepancy between in vitro sensitivities and in vivo activity. Since a number of antibiotics highly effective against anaerobes are available, third-generation cephalosporins should generally not be considered for treatment of anaerobes.

The most active and cost-effective antibiotic for anaerobic coverage currently is metronidazole. Although rare isolates of *B. fragilis* have been reported to be resistant to this drug, the clinical significance of resistance in anaerobic species is not known. Other first-line agents include cefoxitin and clindamycin. Neither metronidazole nor clindamycin covers aerobic gram-negative bacilli; thus these drugs must be combined with other agents. Cefotetan has a spectrum of activity similar to that of cefoxitin and including *B. fragilis,* but its lesser activity against other *Bacteroides* species limits its utility. The rate of resistance to cefoxitin or clindamycin among *B. fragilis* isolates has ranged from 6 to 30 percent in certain areas, although, again, the clinical significance of this finding is unclear. Among newer agents, imipenem, ticarcillin/clavulanic acid, and ampicillin/sulbactam are highly active against anaerobes. Chloramphenicol, which exhibits strong activity against *B. fragilis* in vitro, nevertheless should probably not be considered a first-line drug for anaerobes since failures of treatment have been documented in both experimental and clinical intraabdominal infections. The emerging surgical literature on scoring systems and stratification by diagnosis, severity of disease, and outcome measures should permit more accurate clinical trials of antibiotic regimens for the treatment of intraabdominal infections.

VISCERAL ABSCESSES Liver abscesses The liver is the organ most commonly subject to the development of abscesses. Altemeier and associates studied 540 intraabdominal abscesses over a 12-year period. Visceral abscesses accounted for 26 percent of these abscesses; moreover, liver abscesses made up 13 percent of the total number, or 48 percent of all visceral abscesses. Liver abscesses may be solitary or multiple; they may arise from hematogenous spread of bacteria or from local spread from contiguous infections within the peritoneal cavity. In the past, appendicitis with rupture and subsequent spread of infection was the most common route for the development of a liver abscess. Currently, associated disease of the biliary tract is the most common etiology. Suppurative pylephlebitis, usually arising from infection in the pelvis but also from infection elsewhere in the peritoneal cavity, is another common source for bacterial seeding of the liver.

Fever is the most common presenting sign of liver abscess. Some patients, particularly those with active associated disease of the biliary tract, have symptoms and signs localized to the right upper quadrant, including pain, guarding, punch tenderness, and even rebound tenderness. Nonspecific symptoms such as chills, anorexia, weight loss, nausea, and vomiting also may develop. Only 50 percent of patients with liver abscesses, however, have hepatomegaly, right upper quadrant tenderness, or jaundice; thus half of patients have no symptoms or signs that would direct attention to the liver. Fever of unknown origin (FUO) may be the only presenting manifestation of liver abscess, especially in the elderly. Diagnostic studies of the abdomen, especially the right upper quadrant, should be a part of any FUO workup. The single most reliable laboratory finding is an elevated serum concentration of alkaline phosphatase, which is documented in 90 percent of patients with liver abscesses. Other tests of liver function may yield normal results, but 50 percent of patients have elevated serum levels of bilirubin and 48 percent have elevated concentrations of aspartate aminotransferase. Other associated laboratory findings include leukocytosis in 77 percent of patients, anemia (usually normochromic, normocytic) in 50 percent, and hypoalbuminemia in 33 percent. Concomitant bacteremia is found in one-third of patients. A liver abscess is sometimes suggested by chest radiography, especially if a new elevation of the right hemidiaphragm is seen; other suggestive findings include a right basilar infiltrate and a right pleural effusion.

Imaging studies are the most reliable methods for diagnosing liver abscesses. These studies include ultrasonography, CT scan, gallium- or indium-labeled WBC scans, and even magnetic resonance imaging. In an occasional case, more than one such study may be required. Organisms recovered from liver abscesses vary with the etiology. In liver infection arising from the biliary tree, enteric gram-negative aerobic bacilli and enterococci are common isolates. Unless previous surgery has been performed, anaerobes are not generally involved in liver abscesses arising from biliary infections. In contrast, in liver abscesses arising from pelvic and other intraperitoneal sources, a mixed flora including aerobic and anaerobic species (especially *B. fragilis*) is common. With hematogenous spread of infection, usually only a single organism is encountered; this species may be *S. aureus* or a streptococcal species such as *Streptococcus milleri*.

Liver abscesses also may be caused by *Candida* species; such abscesses usually follow fungemia in patients receiving chemotherapy for cancer and often present as a return of neutrophils after a period of neutropenia. Treatment of candidal liver abscesses usually entails lengthy administration of amphotericin B, although recent reports have described successful maintenance therapy with fluconazole after an initial course of amphotericin (see Chaps. 96 and 166).

Amebic liver abscesses are not an uncommon problem (see Chap. 173). Amebic serology gives positive results in more than 95 percent of cases; thus a negative result assists in excluding this diagnosis.

While drainage—either percutaneous with a pigtail catheter kept in place or surgical—remains the mainstay of therapy for intraabdominal abscesses (including liver abscesses), there is growing interest in medical management alone for pyogenic liver abscesses. Cases treated without definitive drainage generally require longer courses of antibiotic therapy. When percutaneous drainage was compared with open surgical drainage, the average length of hospital stay for the former was almost double that for the latter, although both the time required for fever to resolve and mortality were the same for the two procedures. Mortality was appreciable despite treatment, averaging 15 percent. Several factors may predict the failure of percutaneous drainage and therefore may favor primary surgical intervention. These include the presence of multiple, sizable abscesses; viscous abscess contents which tend to plug the catheter; associated disease (e.g., of the biliary tract) that requires surgery; or the lack of a clinical response to percutaneous drainage in 4 to 7 days.

Splenic abscesses Splenic abscesses are much less common than liver abscesses. In fact, no splenic abscesses were observed in Altemeier's series of 540 intraabdominal abscesses. The incidence of splenic abscesses has ranged from 0.7 to 0.22 percent in various autopsy series. The clinical setting and the organisms isolated usually differ from the corresponding findings for liver abscesses. The degree of clinical suspicion for splenic abscess needs to be high as this condition frequently is fatal if left untreated. Even in the most recently published series, diagnosis was made only at autopsy in 37 percent of cases. While splenic abscesses may arise occasionally from contiguous spread of infection or from direct trauma to the spleen, hematogenous spread of infection is the usual mode of development. Bacterial endocarditis is the most common associated infection. Splenic abscesses also are seen in patients who have received extensive immunosuppressive therapy (particularly those who have malignancy involving the spleen) and in patients with hemoglobinopathies or other hematologic disorders (especially sickle cell anemia).

While approximately 50 percent of patients with splenic abscesses have abdominal pain, the pain is localized to the left upper quadrant in only half of these cases. Splenomegaly is found in approximately 50 percent of patients. Fever and leukocytosis generally are present; the development of fever preceded diagnosis by an average of 20 days in a recent series. Left-sided chest findings may include abnormalities to auscultation, and chest radiographic findings may include an infiltrate or a left-sided pleural effusion. When splenic abscesses are being considered in a differential diagnosis, CT scan of the abdomen has been the most sensitive diagnostic tool. Ultrasonography can yield the diagnosis, but cases have been missed with this modality. Liver-spleen scan or gallium scan also may be useful. Streptococcal species are the most common bacterial isolates from splenic abscesses and *S. aureus* is the next most common organism; presumably these prevalences reflect the bacterial cause of the associated endocarditis. An increase in the frequency of isolation of gram-negative aerobic organisms from splenic abscesses has been reported; these organisms often derive from a urinary tract focus, with associated bacteremia, or another intraabdominal source. *Salmonella* species are seen fairly commonly, especially in patients with sickle cell hemoglobinopathy. Anaerobic species accounted for only 5 percent of isolates in the largest collected series, but the reporting of a number of "sterile abscesses" may indicate that optimal techniques for the isolation of anaerobes were not employed. Because of the high mortality figures reported for splenic abscesses, the treatment of choice is splenectomy with adjunctive antibiotics. However, percutaneous drainage was recently successful in one group of patients. The most important factor in successful treatment of splenic abscesses is early consideration of the diagnosis.

Perinephric and renal abscesses Perinephric and renal abscesses are not common: the former accounted for only about 0.02

percent of hospital admissions and the latter for about 0.2 percent in Altemeier's series of 540 intraabdominal abscesses. While liver abscesses generally arise from contiguous foci of infection or track from other intraabdominal sources and splenic abscesses usually arise from hematogenous spread (e.g., bacterial endocarditis), perinephric and renal abscesses have a different pathogenesis. Before antibiotics became available, the majority of renal and perinephric abscesses were hematogenous in origin, with *S. aureus* most commonly recovered. In contrast, at the present time, more than 75 percent of perinephric and renal abscesses arise from an initial urinary tract infection. Infection ascends from the bladder to the kidney, with pyelonephritis occurring first. Bacteria may directly invade the renal parenchyma from medulla to cortex. Local vascular channels within the kidney may also facilitate the transport of organisms. Areas of abscess developing within the parenchyma may rupture into the perinephric space. The kidneys and adrenal glands are surrounded by a layer of perirenal fat that, in turn, is surrounded by Gerota's fascia, which extends superiorly to the diaphragm and inferiorly to the pelvic fat. When abscesses extend into the perinephric space, tracking may occur through Gerota's fascia into the psoas or transversalis muscles, into the anterior peritoneal cavity, superiorly to the subdiaphragmatic space, or inferiorly to the pelvis. Of the several risk factors that have been associated with the development of perinephric abscesses, the most important is the presence of concomitant nephrolithiasis producing local obstruction to urinary flow. Twenty to sixty percent of patients with perinephric abscess have renal stones. In addition, other structural abnormalities of the urinary tract, a prior history of urologic surgery, trauma, and diabetes mellitus all have been identified as risk factors.

The organisms most frequently encountered in perinephric and renal abscesses are *E. coli*, *Proteus* sp., and *Klebsiella* sp. *E. coli*, the aerobic species most commonly found in colonic flora, seems to have unique virulence properties in the urinary tract, including factors promoting adherence to uroepithelial cells. The urease of *Proteus* sp. splits urea, thereby creating a more alkaline and hospitable environment for bacterial proliferation. *Proteus* sp. frequently are found in association with large struvite stones caused by the precipitation of magnesium ammonium sulfate in an alkaline environment. These stones serve as a nidus for recurrent urinary tract infection. While a single bacterial species usually is recovered from a perinephric or renal abscess, multiple species also may be found. If a urine culture is not contaminated with periurethral flora and is found to contain more than one organism, a perinephric abscess or renal abscess should be considered in the differential diagnosis. Urine cultures also may be polymicrobial in cases of bladder diverticulum.

Candida sp. is another organism to consider in the etiology of renal abscesses. This fungus may spread to the kidney via the hematogenous route or by ascension from the bladder. The hallmark of the latter route of infection is ureteral obstruction with large fungal balls.

The presentation of perinephric and renal abscesses is quite nonspecific. Flank pain and abdominal pain are common. At least 50 percent of patients are febrile. Pain may be referred to the groin or leg, particularly with extension of infection. The diagnosis of perinephric abscess, like that of splenic abscess, is frequently delayed, and mortality in some series is appreciable although lower than in the past. Perinephric or renal abscess should be most seriously considered when a patient presents with symptoms and signs of pyelonephritis and remains febrile after 4 or 5 days, by which time the fever should have resolved. Moreover, when a urine culture yields a polymicrobial flora, when a patient has known renal stone disease, or when fever and pyuria coexist with a sterile urine culture, the diagnosis of perinephric or renal abscess should be entertained.

Renal ultrasonography and abdominal CT scan are the most useful diagnostic modalities. If a renal abscess or perinephric abscess is diagnosed, nephrolithiasis should be excluded, especially when a high urinary pH suggests the presence of a urea-splitting organism. Treatment for perinephric or renal abscesses, like that for other

intraabdominal abscesses, includes drainage of pus and antibiotic therapy directed at the organism(s) recovered. For perinephric abscesses, percutaneous drainage usually is successful.

REFERENCES

Altemeier WA et al: Intra-abdominal abscesses. Am J Surg 125:70, 1973

Chun CH et al: Splenic abscess. Medicine 59:50, 1980

Hutchison FN, Kaysen GA: Perinephric abscess: The missed diagnosis. Med Clin North Am 72:993, 1988

Levison ME, Bush LM: Peritonitis and other intra-abdominal infections, in *Principles and Practice of Infectious Diseases*, 3d ed, GL Mandell et al (eds). New York, Churchill Livingstone, 1990

Maher JA et al: Successful medical treatment of pyogenic liver abscess. Gastroenterology 77:618, 1979

Nystrom P-O et al: Proposed definitions for diagnosis, severity scoring, stratification, and outcome for trials on intraabdominal infection. World J Surg 14:148, 1990

Tzianabos AO et al: The capsular polysaccharide of *Bacteroides fragilis* comprises two ionically linked polysaccharides. J Biol Chem 267:18230, 1992

Zaleznik DF, Kasper DL: *Bacteroides* species, in *Principles and Practice of Infectious Diseases*, 3d ed, GL Mandell et al (eds). New York, Churchill Livingstone, 1990

87   ACUTE INFECTIOUS DIARRHEAL DISEASES AND BACTERIAL FOOD POISONING

JOAN R. BUTTERTON / STEPHEN B. CALDERWOOD

Ranging from mild annoyances during vacations to devastating dehydrating illnesses that can kill within hours, acute gastrointestinal illnesses rank second only to acute upper respiratory illnesses as the most common diseases worldwide. In children less than 5 years old, attack rates range from 2 to 3 illnesses per child per year in developed countries to as high as 10 to 18 illnesses per child per year in developing countries. In Asia, Africa, and Latin America, acute diarrheal illnesses are not only a leading cause of morbidity in children—producing an estimated 1 billion cases per year—but also the major cause of mortality, being responsible for 4 to 6 million deaths per year, or a sobering total of 12,600 deaths per day. In some areas, more than 50 percent of deaths of children are directly attributable to acute diarrheal illnesses. In addition, by contributing to malnutrition and thereby reducing resistance to other infectious agents, gastrointestinal illnesses may be indirect factors in a far greater burden of disease.

The wide range of clinical manifestations observed in acute gastrointestinal illnesses is matched by the wide variety of infectious agents, which include viruses, bacteria, and parasitic pathogens, that can cause these diseases (Table 87-1). This chapter will discuss factors that enable gastrointestinal pathogens to cause disease, review host defense mechanisms, and present an approach to the evaluation and treatment of patients presenting with acute diarrhea. Detailed discussions of individual organisms are presented in subsequent chapters.

PATHOGENIC MECHANISMS   Enteric pathogens have developed a variety of tactics to overcome host defenses and ultimately cause disease by a number of mechanisms. Understanding the virulence factors employed by these organisms is important in the diagnosis and treatment of clinical disease.

Inoculum size   The number of microorganisms that must be ingested to cause disease varies considerably from species to species. For *Escherichia coli*, *Salmonella*, and *Vibrio cholerae*, for example, 10^5 to 10^8 organisms must be ingested orally to cause disease, whereas for *Shigella*, *Giardia lamblia*, and *Entamoeba* as few as 10 to 100 bacteria or cysts can produce infection. The ability of organisms to overcome host defenses has important implications for transmission;

TABLE 87-1 Gastrointestinal pathogens causing acute diarrhea

Mechanism	Location	Illness	Stool findings	Examples of pathogens involved
Noninflammatory (enterotoxin)	Proximal small bowel	Watery diarrhea	No fecal leukocytes	*Vibrio cholerae* Enterotoxigenic *Escherichia coli* (LT and/or ST) *Clostridium perfringens* *Bacillus cereus* *Staphylococcus aureus* *Aeromonas hydrophila* *Plesiomonas shigelloides* Rotavirus Norwalk-like viruses Enteric adenoviruses *Giardia lamblia* *Cryptosporidium*
Inflammatory (invasion or cytotoxin)	Colon	Dysentery	Fecal polymorphonuclear leukocytes	*Shigella* sp. *Salmonella enteritidis* *Campylobacter jejuni* Enterohemorrhagic *Escherichia coli* Enteroinvasive *E. coli* *Vibrio parahemolyticus* *Clostridium difficile* ?*Aeromonas hydrophila* ?*Plesiomonas shigelloides* *Entamoeba histolytica*
Penetrating	Distal small bowel	Enteric fever	Fecal mononuclear leukocytes	*Salmonella typhi* *Yersinia enterocolitica*

SOURCE: After Guerrant, in Mandell et al.

Shigella, *Entamoeba*, and *Giardia* can spread by person-to-person contact, whereas bacteria such as *Salmonella* may have to grow in food for several hours before reaching an effective infectious dose.

Adherence Many organisms must adhere to the gastrointestinal mucosa as an initial step in the pathogenic process; thus organisms that can compete with the normal bowel flora and colonize the mucosa have an important advantage in causing disease. Specific cell-surface proteins involved in attachment of bacteria to intestinal cells are important virulence determinants. *V. cholerae*, for example, adheres to the brush border of small intestinal enterocytes via specific surface adhesins, including the toxin-coregulated pilus (Tcp) and other accessory colonization factors. Enterotoxigenic *E. coli* produces an adherence protein, called *colonization factor antigen* (CFA), that is necessary for colonization of the upper small intestine by the organism prior to its production of enterotoxin. Enteropathogenic strains of *E. coli* produce virulence determinants that allow these organisms to attach to and efface the brush border of the intestinal epithelium, while enterohemorrhagic strains of *E. coli* produce fimbriae that mediate attachment of bacteria to cells in culture.

Toxin production The production of one or more exotoxins is important in the pathogenesis of numerous enteric organisms. Such toxins include *enterotoxins,* which cause watery diarrhea by acting directly on secretory mechanisms in the intestinal mucosa; *cytotoxins*, which cause destruction of mucosal cells and associated inflammatory diarrhea; and *neurotoxins*, which act directly on the central or peripheral nervous system. Some exotoxins act by more than one mechanism; *S. dysenteriae* type 1, for example, produces an exotoxin that has neurotoxic, enterotoxic, and cytotoxic activities.

The prototypical enterotoxin is cholera toxin, a heterodimeric protein composed of one A and five B subunits. The A subunit contains the enzymatic activity of the toxin, while the B subunit pentamer binds holotoxin to the enterocyte surface receptor, the ganglioside G_{M1}. After the binding of holotoxin, a fragment of the A subunit is translocated across the eukaryotic cell membrane into the cytoplasm, where it catalyzes the ADP-ribosylation of a GTP-binding protein and causes persistent activation of adenylate cyclase. The end result is an increase of cAMP in the intestinal mucosa, which increases Cl^- secretion and decreases Na^+ absorption, leading to loss of fluid and the production of diarrhea.

Enterotoxigenic strains of *E. coli* may produce a protein, called *heat-labile enterotoxin* (LT), that is similar to cholera toxin and causes secretory diarrhea by the same mechanism. Alternatively, enterotoxigenic strains of *E. coli* may produce *heat-stable enterotoxin* (ST), which causes diarrhea by activation of guanylate cyclase and elevation of intracellular cGMP. Some enterotoxigenic *E. coli* produce both LT and ST.

Bacterial cytotoxins, in contrast, destroy intestinal mucosal cells and produce the syndrome of dysentery, with bloody stools containing inflammatory cells. Enteric pathogens that produce such cytotoxins include *S. dysenteriae*, *V. parahemolyticus*, and *Clostridium difficile*. Enterohemorrhagic strains of *E. coli*, most commonly serotype 0157:H7, also produce potent cytotoxins that are highly related to Shiga toxin from *S. dysenteriae* and have been termed *Shiga-like toxins* (SLTs). Such strains of *E. coli* have been associated with outbreaks of hemorrhagic colitis and hemolytic-uremic syndrome.

Neurotoxins usually are produced by the responsible organism outside the host and therefore produce symptoms soon after ingestion. These include the staphylococcal and *Bacillus cereus* toxins, which act on the central nervous system to produce vomiting.

Invasion Dysentery may result not only from the production of cytotoxins but also from bacterial invasion and destruction of intestinal mucosal cells. Infections due to *Shigella* and enteroinvasive *E. coli*, for example, are characterized by invasion of mucosal epithelial cells, intraepithelial multiplication, and subsequent spread to adjacent cells. *Salmonella*, on the other hand, causes inflammatory diarrhea by invasion of the bowel mucosa but is generally not associated with destruction of enterocytes or the full clinical syndrome of dysentery. *S. typhi* and *Yersinia enterocolitica* can penetrate intact intestinal mucosa, multiply intracellularly in Peyer's patches and intestinal lymph nodes, and then disseminate through the bloodstream to cause enteric fever, a syndrome characterized by fever, headache, relative bradycardia, abdominal pain, splenomegaly, and leukopenia.

HOST DEFENSES Given the enormous number of microorganisms ingested with every meal, it is evident that the normal host must possess effective defense mechanisms to combat a constant influx of potential enteric pathogens. Observations of infections in patients with alterations in these defenses has led to a greater understanding of the variety of ways in which the normal host can protect itself against disease.

Normal flora The large numbers of bacteria that normally inhabit the intestine act as an important host defense by preventing colonization by potential enteric pathogens. Persons with fewer intestinal bacteria, such as infants who have not yet developed normal enteric colonization or patients receiving antibiotics, are at significantly greater risk of developing infections with enteric pathogens. The composition of the intestinal flora is as important as the number of organisms present. More than 99 percent of the normal colonic flora is anaerobic bacteria, and the acidic pH and volatile fatty acids produced by these organisms appear to be critical elements in the colonization resistance offered by the normal enteric flora.

Gastric acid The acidic pH of the stomach is an important barrier to enteric pathogens, and an increased frequency of *Salmonella*, *Shigella*, *G. lamblia*, and a variety of helminthic infections has been observed in patients who have undergone gastric surgery or are otherwise achlorhydric. Neutralization of gastric acid with antacids or with H-2 blockers, as commonly occurs in hospitalized patients, similarly increases the risk of enteric colonization. Some microorganisms, however, can survive the extreme acidity of the gastric environment; rotavirus, for example, is highly stable to acid.

Intestinal motility Normal peristalsis is the major mechanism for clearance of bacteria from the proximal small intestine, although gastric acidity and secreted immunoglobulins also play a role in limiting the number of organisms present. When intestinal motility is impaired, as by treatment with opiates or other antimotility drugs, anatomic abnormalities (diverticulas, fistulas, or afferent-loop stasis following surgery), or hypomotility states (as in diabetes mellitus or scleroderma), the frequency of bacterial overgrowth and infection of the small bowel with enteric pathogens is much increased. Some patients with *Shigella* infection treated with diphenoxylate hydrochloride with atropine (Lomotil) demonstrate prolonged fever and shedding of organisms, while patients treated with opiates for mild *Salmonella* gastroenteritis have a higher frequency of bacteremia.

Immunity Both cellular immune responses and antibody production play important roles in protecting susceptible hosts from enteric infections. The wide spectrum of gastrointestinal viral, bacterial, parasitic, and fungal infections in patients with AIDS highlights the importance of cell-mediated immunity in protecting the normal host from these pathogens. Humoral intestinal immunity is also important and consists both of systemic IgG and IgM and secretory IgA. Growing evidence supports the concept of a common mucosal immune system for secretory IgA in which binding of bacterial antigens to the luminal surface of M cells in the distal small bowel and subsequent presentation to subepithelial lymphoid tissue leads to the proliferation of sensitized lymphocytes that circulate and populate all of the mucosal tissues of the body as IgA-secreting plasma cells.

CLINICAL EVALUATION History The answers to questions with high discriminating value can quickly narrow the potential cause of diarrhea and help determine if treatment is needed: (1) What is the *duration* of symptoms? Is the diarrhea acute or chronic? Diarrhea lasting more than 2 weeks generally is defined as chronic; in such cases, many of the causes of acute diarrhea are much less likely, and a new spectrum of causes needs to be considered. (2) Is there *fever*? Fever often implies invasive disease, although fever and diarrhea also may result from infection outside the gastrointestinal tract, as with malaria and a variety of febrile illnesses in children. (3) What is the *appearance of the stool*? Stools that contain blood or mucus indicate ulceration of the large bowel. Bulky, white stools suggest a small-intestinal process that is causing malabsorption. Profuse, "rice-water" stools suggest cholera or a similar toxigenic process. (4) What is the *frequency* of bowel movements? The number of stools over a given period can be the first warning of impending dehydration. (5) Does the patient have *abdominal pain*? Abdominal pain may be most severe in inflammatory processes, such as with *Shigella*, *Campylobacter*, and necrotizing toxins. Painful abdominal muscle cramps, caused by electrolyte loss, can be seen in severe cases of cholera. Bloating is common in giardiasis. (6) Is there *tenesmus* (cramps in the rectum felt after a bowel movement)? Tenesmus may be present when there is inflammation of the rectum, as is seen with shigellosis. (7) Has the patient been *vomiting*? Vomiting implies an acute infection, such as with a toxin-mediated illness or food

poisoning, but also can be prominent in a variety of systemic illnesses (e.g., malaria) and in intestinal obstruction. (8) Is there evidence of a *common source* of infection? Asking patients if anyone else is sick is a more efficient means of identifying a common source than is constructing a list of recently eaten foods. If a common source seems likely, specific foods can then be investigated.

Epidemiology TRAVEL HISTORY Of the 12 to 20 million people who travel from temperate industrialized countries to tropical regions of Asia, Africa, and Central and South America each year, 20 to 50 percent will experience a sudden onset of abdominal cramps, anorexia, and watery diarrhea, making *traveler's diarrhea* the most common travel-related illness. The onset is usually 3 days to 2 weeks after the traveler's arrival in a tropical area, with most cases beginning within the first 3 to 5 days. The illness is generally self-limited, lasting 1 to 5 days. The high rate of diarrhea in travelers to underdeveloped areas is related to the ingestion of contaminated food or water.

The organisms that cause traveler's diarrhea vary considerably with location. In all areas, enterotoxigenic *E. coli* is the organism most commonly isolated in cases of the classical secretory traveler's diarrhea syndrome, ranging from a high of approximately 50 percent in Latin America to a low of 15 percent in Asia. *Shigella*, *Salmonella*, and *Campylobacter* spp. are classically considered to cause more invasive, dysenteric disease than enterotoxigenic *E. coli*, but clinical differentiation can be difficult. *Shigella*, *Salmonella*, and *Campylobacter* are isolated in 1 to 15 percent of cases, with different organisms being more common in different locations. *Vibrio* species are most common in Asia, although *V. cholerae* disease reached epidemic proportions in parts of Central and South America in 1991 and has become a significant concern to travelers to these regions. Less common bacteria are *Aeromonas hydrophila* and *Plesiomonas shigelloides*, which have been isolated in travelers to Thailand. Parasitic causes of traveler's diarrhea include *Entamoeba histolytica*, which is responsible for up to 5 percent of cases in Mexico and Thailand, and *G. lamblia*, which has been associated with contaminated freshwater supplies in many areas of the world. *Giardia* is found in association with zoonotic reservoirs in the northern United States and poses a risk for hikers and campers who drink from freshwater streams. A striking association also has been noted with contaminated water supplies in St. Petersburg. *Cryptosporidium* has been recognized as a problem in travelers to the Commonwealth of Independent States, Mexico, and Africa. Viruses, such as rotavirus and Norwalk-like viruses, have been isolated in up to 12 percent of visitors to Latin America, Asia, and Africa.

LOCATION Day-care centers are sites of particularly high attack rates of enteric infections. Rotavirus is most common in children less than 2 years old, with attack rates of 75 to 100 percent among those exposed. *G. lamblia* is more common in older children, with somewhat lower attack rates. Other common organisms, often spread by fecal-oral contact, are *Shigella*, *C. jejuni*, and *Cryptosporidium*. A characteristic feature of infection in day-care centers is the high rate of secondary cases among family members.

Similarly, hospitals are sites for concentrations of enteric infections. In medical intensive-care units and pediatric wards, diarrhea is among the most common nosocomial infections. *C. difficile* and *Salmonella* species are predominant causes of nosocomial diarrhea in the United States; viral pathogens, especially rotavirus, can spread rapidly in pediatric wards. Enteropathogenic *E. coli* has been associated with outbreaks of diarrhea in newborn nurseries. One-third of elderly patients in chronic-care institutions develop a significant diarrheal illness each year. Surveillance stool cultures suggest that 25 percent of these residents harbor cytotoxin-producing *C. difficile*, which causes more than one-half the cases of diarrhea in this population. Antimicrobial therapy can predispose to pseudomembranous colitis by altering normal colonic flora and allowing multiplication of *C. difficile*.

AGE The majority of the morbidity and mortality from enteric pathogens is in children less than 5 years of age. Breast-fed infants are protected from contaminated food and water and derive some protection from maternal antibodies, but their risk of infection rises dramatically when they begin to eat solid foods. Infants and younger children are more likely than adults to develop rotaviral disease, while older children and adults are more commonly infected with Norwalk-like viruses. Other organisms that produce disease with higher attack rates in children than in adults include enterotoxigenic and enteropathogenic *E. coli*, *C. jejuni*, and *G. lamblia*. In children, the incidence of *Salmonella* infections is highest in infants under 1 year of age, while the attack rate for *Shigella* infections is greatest in children aged 6 months to 4 years.

Physical examination   The examination of patients for signs of dehydration provides essential information about the severity of the diarrheal illness and the need for rapid therapy. Mild dehydration is indicated by thirst, dry mouth, decreased axillary sweat, decreased urine output, and slight weight loss. Signs of moderate dehydration include an orthostatic fall in blood pressure, skin tenting, and sunken eyes or, in infants, a sunken fontanelle. Signs of severe dehydration range from hypotension and tachycardia to confusion and frank shock.

Diagnostic approach   The most important distinction that the clinician must make is between *inflammatory* and *noninflammatory* disease. By using the history and epidemiology as guides to this distinction, the clinician can rapidly assess the need for further efforts to define a specific etiology and the need for therapeutic intervention. Examination of a stool sample is an important addition to the narrative history. Grossly bloody or mucoid stool suggests an inflammatory process, but all stools should be examined for fecal leukocytes by making a thin smear of the stool on a glass slide, adding a drop of methylene blue, and examining the wet mount. Causes of acute infectious diarrhea, divided into inflammatory and noninflammatory etiologies, are listed in Table 87-1.

BACTERIAL FOOD POISONING   If the history and stool examination indicate a noninflammatory etiology of diarrhea and there is evidence of a common-source outbreak, questions concerning the ingestion of specific foods and the time of onset of the diarrhea after a meal can provide clues to the bacterial cause of the illness. Potential etiologies of bacterial food poisoning are shown in Table 87-2. Bacteria that cause disease by an enterotoxin elaborated outside the host, such as *Staphylococcus aureus* and *Bacillus cereus*, have the shortest incubation periods, averaging 1 to 6 h, and illness generally lasts less than 12 h. The majority of cases of staphylococcal food poisoning are

caused by contamination from infected human carriers. Staphylococci can multiply at a wide range of temperatures, so if food is left to cool slowly and remains at room temperature after cooking, the organisms will have the opportunity to form enterotoxin. Outbreaks following picnics where potato salad, mayonnaise, and cream pastries were served are classic examples of staphylococcal food poisoning. Diarrhea, nausea, vomiting, and abdominal cramping are common, while fever is less so. *B. cereus* produces both a syndrome with a short incubation period, the *emetic* form, mediated by a staphylococcal type of enterotoxin, and one with a longer incubation period (8 to 16 h), the *diarrheal* form, caused by an *E. coli* LT type of enterotoxin in which diarrhea and abdominal cramps are characteristic but vomiting is uncommon. The emetic form of *B. cereus* food poisoning is associated with contaminated fried rice; the organism is common in uncooked rice, and its heat-resistant spores survive boiling. If cooked rice is not refrigerated, the spores can germinate and produce toxin. Frying before serving may not destroy the preformed, heat-stable toxin. Food poisoning due to *C. perfringens* also has a slightly longer incubation period (8 to 14 h) and results from the survival of heat-resistant spores in inadequately cooked meat, poultry, or legumes. Toxin is produced after ingestion in the intestinal tract, causing moderately severe abdominal cramps and diarrhea; vomiting is rare, as is fever. The illness is self-limited, rarely lasting for more than 24 h.

Not all food poisoning has a bacterial cause; diagnostic confusion can result from diarrhea caused by nonbacterial causes of short-incubation food poisoning. These include the chemical effects of capsaicin, which is found in hot peppers, and of a variety of toxins found in fish and shellfish.

LABORATORY EVALUATION   Many cases of noninflammatory diarrhea are self-limited or can be treated empirically, and for these, the clinician may not need to determine a specific etiology. Potentially pathogenic *E. coli* cannot be distinguished from normal fecal flora by routine culture. Special tests to detect LT and ST are not available in most clinical laboratories. In situations in which cholera is a concern, stool should be cultured on thiosulfate citrate bile salt sucrose agar (TCBS). A latex agglutination test has made the rapid detection of rotavirus in stool practical for many laboratories, but electron microscopy or measurement of serologic response with a radioimmunoassay is still necessary for identification of Norwalk-like viruses. At least three stool specimens should be examined for *Giardia* cysts or stained for *Cryptosporidium* if clinical suspicion for these organisms is high.

All patients with fever and evidence of inflammatory disease should have stool cultured for *Salmonella*, *Shigella*, and *Campylobacter*. *Salmonella* and *Shigella* can be selected on MacConkey's agar as non-lactose-fermenting (colorless) colonies or grown on *Salmonella-Shigella* agar or in selenite enrichment broth, both of which inhibit most organisms except these pathogens. Isolation of *Campylobacter* requires inoculation of fresh stool on selective growth media and incubation at 42°C in a microaerophilic atmosphere. Enterohemorrhagic *E. coli* strains of serotype 0157:H7 can be identified in specialized laboratories by serotyping but also can be identified presumptively as lactose-fermenting, indole-positive colonies that are nonsorbitol fermenters (white colonies) on sorbitol MacConkey plates. Fresh stools should be examined for amebic cysts and trophozoites. Pathogenic strains of *C. difficile* generally produce two toxins, A and B. Toxin B can be detected with a cytotoxin assay; if the toxin is present, a monolayer culture of fibroblasts will show cytopathic effects within 6 to 24 h. Rapid enzyme immunoassays and latex agglutination tests for both toxin A and toxin B are a recent development.

TREATMENT   In many cases, a specific diagnosis is not necessary or available to guide treatment; the clinician can proceed with the information available from the history, stool examination, and evaluation of the severity of dehydration of the patient.

Nonspecific therapy   Most causes of noninflammatory diarrhea can be treated effectively with nonspecific therapy. The mainstay of

TABLE 87-2   Bacterial food poisoning

Organisms	Symptoms	Common food sources
1 TO 6 H INCUBATION		
Staphylococcus aureus	Nausea, vomiting, diarrhea	Ham, poultry, potato and egg salad, mayonnaise, cream pastries
Bacillis cereus	Nausea, vomiting, diarrhea	Fried rice
8 TO 16 H INCUBATION		
Clostridium perfringens	Abdominal cramps, diarrhea (vomiting rare)	Beef, poultry, legumes, gravies
Bacillus cereus	Abdominal cramps, diarrhea (vomiting rare)	Meats, vegetables, dried beans, cereals
>16 H INCUBATION		
Vibrio cholerae	Watery diarrhea	Shellfish
Enterotoxigenic *Escherichia coli*	Watery diarrhea	Salads, cheese, meats, water
Salmonella sp.	Inflammatory diarrhea	Beef, poultry, eggs, dairy products
Shigella sp.	Dysentery	Potato and egg salad, lettuce, raw vegetables
Vibrio parahemolyticus	Dysentery	Mollusks, crustaceans

treatment is adequate rehydration. The treatment of cholera and other dehydrating diarrheal diseases was revolutionized by the promotion of oral rehydration solutions, which depend on the fact that glucose-facilitated sodium and water absorption in the small intestine remains intact in the presence of cholera toxin. The availability of oral rehydration solutions has reduced the mortality from cholera from greater than 50 percent in untreated cases to less than 1 percent. The World Health Organization recommends a solution containing 3.5 g sodium chloride, 2.5 g sodium bicarbonate, 1.5 g potassium chloride, and 20 g glucose (or 40 g sucrose) per liter of water. Patients who are severely dehydrated or in whom vomiting precludes the use of oral therapy should be treated with intravenous solutions such as Ringer's lactate.

Bismuth subsalicylate, marketed in the United States as Pepto-Bismol since 1918, is hydrolyzed in the stomach to salicylic acid and insoluble bismuth salts. It has been demonstrated to be an active antimicrobial compound in vitro and to have antisecretory and anti-inflammatory properties, yet it does not significantly affect normal bowel flora. It effectively treats traveler's diarrhea when given at a dosage of 2 tablets (525 mg) every 30 to 60 min for up to 8 doses following the onset of symptoms. It should not be taken with other salicylate-containing drugs.

Antiperistaltic agents such as codeine, diphenoxylate hydrochloride with atropine (Lomotil), or loperamide (Imodium) also can reduce the frequency of stools and hasten the relief of symptoms in traveler's diarrhea. Loperamide, at a dose of 4 mg at the onset of symptoms followed by 2 mg after each loose stool (not to exceed 16 mg/d), is effective more rapidly than bismuth subsalicylate. Antiperistaltic agents should be avoided in patients with inflammatory disease, since they may prolong diarrhea in patients with infection due to *Shigella* and other invasive organisms.

Antibiotics Although most secretory forms of traveler's diarrhea, most commonly due to enterotoxigenic *E. coli,* can be treated effectively with nonspecific therapy, antimicrobial agents can shorten the duration of illness from 3 to 4 days to 24 to 36 h. Trimethoprim-sulfamethoxazole, doxycycline, and ciprofloxacin, each given in a 3-day course, have all been found to be effective. Patients with dysenteric disease should receive empirical therapy tailored to the most likely infectious agent. Ampicillin, trimethoprim-sulfamethoxazole, and ciprofloxacin are effective in treating shigellosis, depending on the local antimicrobial resistance pattern of the organism. *C. jejuni* infections can be treated with erythromycin (see Chap. 119). Treatment of *Salmonella* gastroenteritis (see Chap. 117) with ciprofloxacin may reduce fecal shedding and the duration of illness, but other oral antibiotics have not been shown to be efficacious and may prolong fecal shedding of bacteria. Therapy should be directed toward other organisms if they are likely on epidemiologic grounds. *V. cholerae* infections (see Chap. 120.), for example, can be shortened by treatment with tetracycline or a fluoroquinolone. *C. difficile* colitis (see Chap. 108) may be treated by discontinuing any implicated antibiotics and, if necessary, with oral metronidazole or vancomycin.

Prophylaxis Improvements in hygiene to reduce fecal-oral spread of enteric pathogens will be necessary before significant reductions in the prevalence of diarrheal diseases will be seen in developing countries. Travelers can reduce their risk of diarrhea by eating only hot, freshly cooked food; by avoiding raw vegetables, salads, and unpeeled fruit; and by drinking only boiled or treated water and avoiding ice.

Bismuth subsalicylate is an inexpensive method of prophylaxis against traveler's diarrhea, when taken at a dosage of 2 tablets (525 mg) four times a day. Treatment appears to be effective and safe for up to 3 weeks. Prophylactic antimicrobial agents, although effective, are not generally recommended for the prevention of traveler's diarrhea. The risk of side effects from antibiotic therapy and the possibility of developing an infection with a drug-resistant organism or with more serious, invasive bacteria make a short course of therapy once symptoms have developed a more reasonable therapeutic approach.

The possibility of exerting a major impact on the worldwide morbidity and mortality of diarrheal diseases has led to intense research activity in the development of effective vaccines against the common bacterial and viral enteric pathogens. The currently available vaccines for cholera and typhoid fever are not highly effective. Recent research has shown promising advances in the development of vaccines against these organisms as well as against rotavirus, *Shigella*, and enterotoxigenic *E. coli.*

REFERENCES

BELL DR: *Lecture Notes on Tropical Medicine,* 2d ed. Oxford, Blackwell, 1987, chap. 15

BLACK RE: Epidemiology of travelers' diarrhea and relative importance of various pathogens. Rev Infect Dis 12(suppl 1):S73, 1990

GUERRANT RL: Principles and syndromes of enteric infection, in *Principles and Practice of Infectious Diseases,* 3d ed, GL Mandell et al (eds). New York, Churchill Livingstone, 1990, chap 81

—— et al: Diarrhea in developed and developing countries: Magnitude, special settings, and etiologies. Rev Infect Dis 12(suppl 1):S41, 1990

LEVINE MM: *Escherichia coli* that cause diarrhea: Enterotoxigenic, enteropathogenic, enteroinvasive, enterohemorrhagic, and enteroadherent. J Infect Dis 155:377, 1987

LUND BM: Foodborne disease due to *Bacillus* and *Clostridium* species. Lancet 336:982, 1990

PETRUCCELLI BP: Treatment of traveler's diarrhea with ciprofloxacin and loperamide. J Infect Dis 165:557, 1992

TRANTER HS: Foodborne staphylococcal illness. Lancet 336:1044, 1990

88 SEXUALLY TRANSMITTED DISEASES

KING K. HOLMES / H. HUNTER HANDSFIELD

In all societies, sexually transmitted diseases (STDs) are among the most common of all infections. In the developing countries, three bacterial STDs—gonorrhea, chlamydial infections, and syphilis—rank among the top 10 to 20 diseases causing the loss of years of healthy, productive life due to major complications such as salpingitis, infertility, ectopic pregnancy, and perinatal morbidity. Among the viral STDs, infection with human immunodeficiency virus (HIV) has become the leading cause of death in some developing countries within the past decade, while two of the most common sexually transmitted viruses—human papillomavirus (HPV) and hepatitis B virus (HBV)—are important causes of cervical carcinoma and hepatocellular carcinoma. There is also a growing awareness of the sexual transmission of human T lymphotropic virus type I (HTLV-I) in many developing countries of Latin America, Africa, and the Caribbean. Although the bacterial STDs remain extremely common in all parts of the world, their incidence is rapidly declining in virtually all the industrialized countries except some parts of the United States. The Centers for Disease Control and Prevention in Atlanta estimates that at least 12 million U.S. residents acquire an STD each year, and some authorities estimate that half or more of all Americans acquire an STD by age 35. In industrialized countries, the unexpectedly high prevalence of certain incurable viral STDs [e.g., HPV infection, genital herpes, and cytomegalovirus (CMV) infection] is being increasingly recognized. The marked enhancement of the efficiency of transmission of HIV by both the genital ulcerative and the genital mucosal STDs adds to the urgency of STD prevention and control.

CLASSIFICATION OF AND GENERAL APPROACH

STDs can be classified on the basis of either cause or clinical manifestations. Table 88-1 summarizes the etiologic classification of STDs. Several of the pathogens listed are also transmitted nonsexually,

TABLE 88-1 Sexually transmitted pathogens

Bacteria	Viruses	Other*
TRANSMITTED IN ADULTS PREDOMINANTLY BY SEXUAL INTERCOURSE		
Neisseria gonorrhoeae	Human immunodeficiency viruses (HIV-1 and -2)	*Trichomonas vaginalis*
Chlamydia trachomatis	Human T lymphotropic virus type I (HTLV-I)	*Phthirus pubis*
Treponema pallidum	Herpes simplex virus type 2 (HSV-2)	
Calymmatobacterium	Human papillomavirus (multiple types)	
granulomatis	Hepatitis B virus†	
Ureaplasma urealyticum	Cytomegalovirus	
	Molluscum contagiosum virus	
SEXUAL TRANSMISSION REPEATEDLY DESCRIBED BUT NOT WELL DEFINED OR NOT THE PREDOMINANT MODE		
Mycoplasma hominis	Human T lymphotrophic virus type II (HTLV-II)	*Candida albicans*
Gardnerella vaginalis and	(?) Hepatitis C, D viruses	*Sarcoptes scabiei*
other vaginal bacteria	Herpes simplex virus type 1 (HSV-1)	
Group B streptococcus	(?) Epstein-Barr virus (EBV)	
TRANSMITTED BY SEXUAL CONTACT INVOLVING ORAL-FECAL EXPOSURE; OF DECLINING IMPORTANCE IN HOMOSEXUAL MEN		
Shigella spp.	Hepatitis A virus	*Giardia lamblia*
Campylobacter spp.		*Entamoeba histolytica*

* Includes protozoa, ectoparasites, and fungi.
† Among U.S. patients for whom a risk factor can be ascertained, most hepatitis B virus infections are sexually transmitted.

but in each instance sexual transmission is clinically and epidemiologically important.

No single STD can be regarded as an isolated problem because multiple infections are common and because the presence of one STD denotes high-risk sexual behavior that is often associated with other, more serious infections. STDs are not endogenous, and rarely if ever are they transmitted by fomites, food, flies, or casual contact. *At least one sexual partner is always infected*; the apparent exceptions usually can be attributed to prolonged subclinical infection in one or both partners. The elicitation of a sexual history and the management of sexual partners are therefore of paramount importance. The failure to identify and to examine or refer the infected partner represents a failure in management, both at the community level (since sources of spread of infection are not identified) and at the individual patient level (since reinfection is not prevented).

Most persons with overt genital discharge, lesions, or pain cease sexual activity and seek medical care. Accordingly, those who transmit infection usually are among the minority who are infected but asymptomatic or who do not understand the implications of their symptoms and thus do not seek medical attention spontaneously. Physicians must see that such partners are examined and treated or referred. In the United States, local health departments will usually help to identify and treat contacts of patients with some of the curable diseases [e.g., syphilis, gonococcal pelvic inflammatory disease (PID)] and will help notify partners of persons with HIV infection, but for most STDs this responsibility is shared by the patient and the clinician.

In general, persons with a new-onset STD have a *source contact* from whom it was acquired; in addition, they may have a *secondary contact* (also known as a *spread contact* or *exposed contact*). The identification and treatment of both types of contacts are important but generally for different reasons. Identification and treatment of the source contract (often a casual contact who, by definition, is spreading infection) are of greatest importance from the public health/community standpoint, since these measures will prevent further transmission. Identification and treatment of the recently exposed secondary contact (more often a spouse or steady sexual partner) will help prevent the development of serious complications, such as PID.

The increasing importance of the viral STDs, most of which are incurable and lifelong, underscores the central role of primary prevention. Whereas early detection and treatment can curtail the spread of the bacterial STDs, control of the viral STDs depends entirely on the avoidance of unprotected exposure to infected persons; the sole exception is vaccination against HBV infection.

Because STDs disproportionately affect women and newborn children, the prevention of these diseases is an important women's health issue. Many STDs are transmitted more efficiently from men to women than from women to men. Early in the course of infection, women are more likely than men to have subclinical infections or minor, nonspecific symptoms—a situation than can result in delayed diagnosis. The lesser specificity of clinical findings and the lesser sensitivity of several microbiologic tests make the diagnosis of STDs more difficult in women than in men. Most important, women and newborn children are at far greater risk than are men for long-lasting or permanent sequelae.

STDs are propagated most efficiently in populations with frequent changes of sexual partners and with poor access to or low motivation in obtaining early treatment. In most of the United States, these groups consist predominantly of young individuals of low socioeconomic status. These individuals often reside within circumscribed, deteriorating, crowded urban neighborhoods, although rates of STDs are also high in rural areas (in the southeastern United States, for example). The treatable bacterial STDs, such as syphilis, gonorrhea, and chancroid, are increasingly concentrated in "core populations" and increasingly involve prostitutes and their sexual partners and persons involved in the use of illicit drugs, particularly "crack" cocaine in the United States. Members of these core populations have been difficult to reach for the purposes of education and contact tracing and may continue to be sexually active despite STD symptoms. Other STDs are more evenly distributed in society. For example, chlamydial infection and the incurable viral STDs persist (often asymptomatically) and are propagated widely in populations that do not share the characteristics of STD core groups.

Various STDs differ in the extent to which their spread and persistence in the population depend on high rates of sexual partner change. In general, the initial rate of spread of an STD pathogen within a population depends on the product of three factors: the average rate of partner change in the population, the average duration of infectiousness of the pathogen, and the average efficiency of transmission per exposure of a susceptible person to an infected person. For diseases with a high efficiency of transmission and/or a long duration of infectiousness, rates of partner change need not be very high to sustain an epidemic. For STDs with a low efficiency of transmission (e.g., HIV infection) or a short duration of infectiousness (e.g., chancroid), high rates of partner change may be necessary to sustain an epidemic. Efforts to prevent and control STDs involve attempts to decrease the duration of infectiousness (through early diagnosis and treatment), to decrease the efficiency of transmission (through promotion of condom use), and to decrease the rate of partner change (through provision of information, health education, and counseling and efforts to change the norms of sexual behavior).

MANAGEMENT OF COMMON STD SYNDROMES

Table 88-2 lists some of the most common clinical STD syndromes and their associated complications. Strategies for the management of some of the common STD syndromes are outlined below. AIDS is discussed in Chap. 279.

An overall approach to the management of a patient with an STD begins with risk assessment (of sexual behaviors, specific exposures, and sociodemographic and other markers for high risk) and clinical assessment (elicitation of specific symptoms and signs of STDs). In light of the results of these assessments, confirmatory diagnostic tests or screening tests (e.g., culture, antigen detection test, most serologic tests) may be ordered. In developing countries and in office practices in most industrialized countries, treatment is usually given on a syndromic basis (i.e., it is selected to cover the most likely causes) while the results of confirmatory tests are pending. For certain syndromes in industrialized countries, rapid tests may be used to narrow the spectrum of this initial therapy (e.g., wet mount for women with vaginal discharge, Gram's stain for men with urethral discharge). After the institution of syndromic treatment (or of specific treatment when rapid tests have been diagnostic), it is essential to complete the first phase of STD management with what has been termed "the three C's": contact notification and treatment; condom promotion, where appropriate; and counseling regarding the reduction of future risk.

The following approach to the management of common STD syndromes is geared toward clinicians in industrialized countries, where rapid tests and confirmatory tests are widely available but less widely used then they should be.

URETHRITIS IN MEN   Urethritis is the most commonly recognized STD syndrome in men. During the past decade, the incidence of gonococcal urethritis has fallen precipitously in nearly all industrialized countries, while that of nongonococcal urethritis (NGU) remains high—a pattern suggesting that current measures for control of NGU are relatively ineffective. In general, gonorrhea and NGU occur with similar frequencies among men seen in STD clinics in the United States, whereas NGU is several times more common than gonorrhea among men seen by physicians in most other settings.

About 30 to 40 percent of NGU cases are caused by *Chlamydia trachomatis*, although the proportion may have declined in populations where chlamydial control programs have been implemented. Herpes simplex virus (HSV) and *Trichomonas vaginalis* each cause a small proportion of NGU cases in the United States. However, most cases cannot be attributed to any of these three pathogens. *Ureaplasma urealyticum* has been implicated in case-control studies as a probable cause of many of the *Chlamydia*-negative cases. A few cases are caused by coliform bacteria in men who are the insertive partners in unprotected anal intercourse. The diagnosis of male urethritis usually does not include specific tests for pathogens aside from *Neisseria gonorrhoeae* and *C. trachomatis*. However, diagnostic testing for *C. trachomatis* is now widely available; the agent can be isolated from tissue cell culture, or its antigens or genetic material can be detected. The following steps should be taken in evaluating sexually active men with symptoms of urethral discharge and/or dysuria.

1 Establish the presence of urethritis. The first step is examination for purulent or mucopurulent urethral discharge. Sometimes the urethra must be milked after the patient has not voided for several hours, preferably overnight. Whether or not an abnormal discharge is evident, inflammation should be evaluated by examination of a Gram-stained smear after passage of a small swab 2 to 3 cm into the urethra; the presence of 5 or more neutrophils per $1000\times$ field in areas containing cells suggests urethritis. Alternatively, the centrifuged sediment of the first 20 to 30 mL of voided urine can be examined for inflammatory cells, either by microscopy or by the leukocyte esterase test. Patients with symptoms who lack objective evidence of urethritis on two occasions 1 week apart may have functional rather than organic problems and generally do not benefit from repeated courses of antibiotics.

2 Evaluate for complications or alternative diagnoses. Epididymitis and systemic complications, such as the gonococcal arthritis-dermatitis syndrome and Reiter's syndrome, should be excluded by a brief history and examination. Bacterial prostatitis and cystitis should be excluded by appropriate testing of men with dysuria who lack evidence of urethritis and of sexually inactive men with urethritis. Digital examination of the prostate gland is seldom informative in the evaluation of sexually active young men with urethritis.

3 Evaluate for gonococcal and chlamydial infection. Gonorrhea is diagnosed by the demonstration of typical gram-negative diplococci within neutrophils, and a preliminary diagnosis of NGU is warranted if gram-negative diplococci are not found. Confirmation of gonococcal urethritis by culture is optional if the Gram's stain is interpreted by an experienced reader as positive; culture is recommended if the Gram's stain is equivocal. Diagnostic testing for *C. trachomatis* is also recommended, even if empirical treatment for chlamydial infection is planned, because the results predict the patient's prognosis and guide the counseling given to the patient and the management of the patient's sexual partner(s).

TABLE 88-2   Common STD syndromes and etiologic agents

Syndrome	Primary sexually transmitted (ST) agents
Urethritis: males	*N. gonorrhoeae, C. trachomatis, U. urealyticum,* HSV
Epididymitis	*C. trachomatis, N. gonorrhoeae;* **non-ST agents:** urinary tract pathogens
Lower genital tract infections: females	
Cystitis/urethritis	*C. trachomatis, N. gonorrhoeae,* HSV; **non-ST agents:** urinary tract pathogens
Mucopurulent cervicitis	*C. trachomatis, N. gonorrhoeae*
Vulvovaginitis	*C. albicans, T. vaginalis;* **non-ST agents:** chemical irritants, allergens
Bacterial vaginosis (BV)	BV-associated bacteria (see text)
Acute pelvic inflammatory disease	*N. gonorrhoeae, C. trachomatis,* BV-associated bacteria; **non-ST agents:** coliform bacteria
Ulcerative lesions of the genitalia	HSV-1, *T. pallidum, H. ducreyi, C. trachomatis* (LGV strains), *C. granulomatis;* **non-ST agents:** *C. albicans,* pyogenic bacteria
Proctitis	*C. trachomatis, N. gonorrhoeae,* HSV, *T. pallidum*
Enteritis, enterocolitis, proctocolitis	*G. lamblia, Campylobacter* spp., *Shigella* spp., *E. histolytica,* other enteric pathogens
Acute arthritis	*N. gonorrhoeae* (e.g., DGI), *C. trachomatis* (e.g., Reiter's syndrome), HBV, HIV
Genital and anal warts	Human papillomavirus (genital types)
AIDS	HIV-1, HIV-2; also many opportunistic pathogens
Mononucleosis syndrome	Cytomegalovirus, HIV, EBV
Viral hepatitis	HBV; **non-ST agents:** HAV, HCV, HDV
Neoplasias	
Squamous cell cancer of the cervix, anus, vulva, or penis	Human papillomavirus (especially types 16, 18, 31)
Kaposi's sarcoma	HIV; other (?)
Lymphoid neoplasia	HIV, HTLV-I
Hepatocellular carcinoma	HBV
Tropical spastic paraparesis	HTLV-I
Scabies	*S. scabiei*
Pubic lice	*P. pubis*

Abbreviations: HSV = herpes simplex virus; DGI = disseminated gonococcal infection; EBV = Epstein-Barr virus; HAV, HBV, HCV, HDV = hepatitis A, B, C viruses and "delta" agent.

4 Treat the urethritis. In practice, urethritis is treated with a regimen effective for NGU if gonorrhea is excluded by Gram's stain; for example, doxycycline (100 mg orally, twice daily) or tetracycline (500 mg orally, four times daily) for 7 days may be administered. If gonococci are demonstrated by Gram's stain or if no diagnostic tests are performed, treatment should include one of the single-dose regimens for gonorrhea (see Chap. 110) plus a 7-day course of doxycycline or tetracycline for possible chlamydial infection. Sexual partners should be tested for gonorrhea and chlamydial infection and should receive the regimen given to the male index case.

EPIDIDYMITIS Acute epididymitis is almost always unilateral and must be differentiated from testicular torsion, tumor, and trauma. Torsion, a surgical emergency, usually occurs in the second or third decade of life and is suggested by sudden onset of pain, elevation of the testicle within the scrotal sac, rotation of the epididymis from a posterior to an anterior position, and absence of blood flow on Doppler examination or ^{99m}Tc scan. Testicular tumor is suggested by persistence of symptoms after a course of therapy. In sexually active men under age 35, acute epididymitis is caused most frequently by *C. trachomatis* and less commonly by *N. gonorrhoeae* and is usually associated with overt or subclinical urethritis. Antimicrobial agents are the mainstays of therapy; the optimal syndromic treatment for epididymitis due to *C. trachomatis* or *N. gonorrhoeae* is ceftriaxone (250 mg intramuscularly) followed by doxycycline (100 mg orally, twice daily for 10 days). Alternatively, ofloxacin (300 mg orally, twice daily for 10 days) is effective against both *N. gonorrhoeae* and *C. trachomatis* as well as against Enterobacteriaceae.

Acute epididymitis in older men or following urinary tract instrumentation is usually caused by gram-negative bacilli or other urinary pathogens. Similarly, epididymitis in young homosexual men is often caused by Enterobacteriaceae. Urethritis is usually absent in these cases, but bacteriuria is present.

LOWER GU TRACT INFECTION IN WOMEN Infections of the female lower urinary tract, cervix, vulva, and vagina produce various combinations of dysuria, vulvar irritation, dyspareunia, and increased or altered vaginal discharge. Diagnostic confusion may be attributable to the nonspecific symptomatology, to the tendency of specific pathogens to produce inflammation and symptoms at multiple contiguous sites (e.g., genital herpes can cause dysuria, vulvar pain, and vaginal discharge), and to the lack of consistent application of available laboratory tests. Two steps are required in the evaluation of symptoms of the lower genitourinary tract in women: (1) differentiation among cystitis, urethritis, vulvovaginitis, and cervicitis and (2) exclusion of associated upper tract disease (e.g., pyelonephritis, salpingitis).

Urethritis and the urethral syndrome *C. trachomatis, N. gonorrhoeae*, and occasionally HSV are causes of symptomatic urethritis— with or without cervicitis— in women. Sexually acquired urethritis in women often presents as the *urethral syndrome*, characterized by "internal" dysuria (usually without urinary urgency or frequency) and pyuria, with $\geq 10^2$ *Escherichia coli* or other uropathogens per milliliter of urine. The urethral syndrome in the absence of pyuria usually is idiopathic, associated with neither uropathogens nor STD pathogens. Although dysuria occurs more frequently in bacterial urinary tract infection (UTI) or urethral syndrome than in vulvar or vaginal infection, this symptom is often attributable to vulvovaginitis because in many settings the latter are more common than UTI. The dysuria associated with vulvar herpes or vulvovaginal candidiasis (and perhaps with trichomoniasis) is often described as "external," being caused by painful contact of urine with the inflamed labia or introitus.

Among women with acute dysuria and frequency, the first step in diagnosis is to exclude the possiblity of acute pyelonephritis (e.g., costovertebral pain and tenderness and fever). The management of bacterial UTI is discussed in Chap. 90. The next step in diagnosing cases in sexually active women is the differentiation of cystitis from urethritis or vaginal infection. Among women without signs of vulvovaginitis, bacterial UTI must then be differentiated from the urethral syndrome by assessment of risks, evaluation of the pattern of symptoms and signs, and specific microbiologic testing. An STD etiology is suggested by young age, more than one current sexual partner or a new partner within the past month, or coexisting mucopurulent cervicitis (see below). Bacterial cystitis is suggested by acute onset, hematuria, or suprapubic bladder tenderness. The finding of a single conventional urinary pathogen, such as *E. coli* or *Staphylococcus saprophyticus*, in a concentratoin of $\geq 10^2$ per milliliter in a properly collected specimen of midstream urine from a symptomatic woman with pyuria indicates probable bacterial UTI, whereas pyuria with $< 10^2$ conventional uropathogens per milliliter of urine ("sterile" pyuria) suggests acute urethral syndrome due to *C. trachomatis* or *N. gonorrhoeae*. Gonorrhea should be evaluated by Gram's staining and culture of specimens from the cervix and urethra. Chlamydial infection should be evaluated by culture or other specific tests for chlamydial antigen in urethral and cervical specimens. Treatment with a tetracycline (e.g., doxycycline, 100 mg twice daily for 7 days) alleviates dysuria in women with sterile pyuria but not in women without pyuria or isolation of a uropathogen.

Vulvovaginal infections Vulvovaginal symptoms are among the most common reasons for visits to physicians by young women. Further, vulvovaginal infections may have serious sequelae and may increase sexual transmission of HIV; rarely, vulvovaginal symptoms may represent serious upper genital tract or systemic disease. A recent multicenter study (sponsored by the National Institutes of Health) of vaginal infections in pregnancy found that vaginal trichomoniasis and bacterial vaginosis early in pregnancy were independent predictors of premature onset of labor. Bacterial vaginosis also appears to be a risk factor for PID and may be involved in the pathogenesis of anaerobic bacterial infection of the upper genital tract. Trichomoniasis has been associated with about a twofold increase in the risk of acquiring HIV infection in one study of prostitutes in Zaire. Vaginitis may be an early and prominent feature of toxic shock syndrome, and recurrent or chronic vulvovaginal candidiasis develops with increased frequency among women with systemic illnesses, such as diabetes mellitus or HIV infection with impaired immunity (although only a very small proportion of women with recurrent vulvovaginal candidiasis in the United States actually have a serious predisposing illness). Vaginal discharge may be the presenting manifestation of mucopurulent cervicitis caused by gonorrhea or chlamydial infection and may reflect the presence of PID.

Thus vulvovaginal symptoms or signs warrant careful evaluation and appropriate therapy that is specific for the anatomic site and type of infection. A careful pelvic examination is, in fact, within the purview of general medicine and should usually precede more invasive or expensive tests in the evaluation of women with vulvovaginal, pelvic, or abdominal symptoms—and even in the evaluation of some systemic illnesses.

Bacterial vaginosis is the most common cause of vulvovaginal symptoms in most clinical settings; next most common are candidiasis, then trichomoniasis. Vaginal infection may be characterized by one or more of the following: increased volume of discharge; abnormal yellow color of discharge caused by increased concentration of polymorphonuclear leukocytes; vulvar pruritus, irritation, or burning, often with external dysuria; vulvar dyspareunia; and vaginal malodor. An important component of the clinical evaluation of vaginal discharge is ascertaining by speculum examination whether this discharge emanates from the vagina or the cervix and whether it is, in fact, abnormal. Occasionally, increased discharge or other vaginal signs and symptoms are not associated with objective signs of vaginitis or cervicitis. The diagnosis and treatment of the three types of vaginal infection are summarized in Table 88-3.

VAGINAL TRICHOMONIASIS (See also Chap. 179) Sexual transmission of *T. vaginalis* is well documented. Routine culture indicates that many infected women and most infected men are asymptomatic. However, treatment of asymptomatic as well as symptomatic cases

TABLE 88-3 Diagnostic features and management of vaginal infection

Feature	Normal vaginal examination	Vulvovaginal candidasis	Trichomonal vaginitis	Bacterial vaginosis (BV)
Etiology	Uninfected; *Lactobacillus* predominant	*Candida albicans* and yeasts	*Trichomonas vaginalis*	Associated with *G. vaginalis*, various anaerobic bacteria, and mycoplasmas
Typical symptoms	None	Vulvar itching and/or irritation, increased discharge	Profuse purulent discharge; vulvar itching	Malodorous, slightly increased discharge
Discharge				
Amount	Variable; usually scant	Scant to moderate	Profuse	Scant to moderate
Color*	Clear or white	White	Yellow	White or gray
Consistency	Nonhomogeneous, floccular	Clumped; adherent plaques	Homogeneous	Homogeneous, low viscosity; uniformly coats vaginal walls
Inflammation of vulvar or vaginal epithelium	None	Erythema of vaginal epithelium, introitus; vulvar dermatitis common	Erythema of vaginal and vulvar epithelium; colpitis macularis	None
pH of vaginal fluid[†]	Usually ≤4.5	Usually ≤4.5	Usually ≥5.0	Usually >4.5
Amine ("fishy") odor with 10% KOH	None	None	May be present	Present
Microscopy[‡]	Normal epithelial cells; lactobacilli predominant	Leukocytes, epithelial cells; yeast, mycelia, or pseudomycelia in up to 80%	Leukocytes; motile trichomonads seen in 80% to 90% of symptomatic patients, less often in the absence of symptoms	Clue cells; few leukocytes; lactobacilli outnumbered by profuse mixed flora, nearly always including *G. vaginalis* plus anaerobic species on Gram's stain
Usual treatment	None	Miconazole or clotrimazole intravaginally, each 100 mg nightly for 3 to 7 nights	Metronidazole, 2 g orally (single dose)	Clindamycin, 2% vaginal cream, twice daily for 7 days Metronidazole, 0.75% vaginal gel, twice daily for 5 days Metronidazole, 500 mg orally, twice daily for 7 days
		Fluconazole, 150 mg orally (single dose)	Metronidazole, 500 mg orally, twice daily for 7 days	
Usual management of sexual partner	None	None; topical treatment if candidal dermatitis of penis is present	Examination for STD; treatment with metronidazole, 2 g orally (single dose)	Examination for STD; no treatment if normal

* Color of discharge is best determined by examination against the white background of a swab.
[†] pH determination is not useful if blood is present.
[‡] To detect fungal elements, vaginal fluid is digested with 10% KOH prior to microscopic examination; to examine for other features, fluid is mixed (1:1) with physiologic saline. Gram's stain is also excellent for detecting yeasts and pseudomycelia and for distinguishing normal flora from the mixed flora seen in bacterial vaginosis, but it is less sensitive than the saline preparation for detection of *T. vaginalis*.
SOURCE: From KK Holmes et al.

is recommended to reduce the reservoir of infection and the risk of transmission and to prevent the later development of symptoms.

Symptomatic trichomoniasis characteristically produces a profuse, yellow, purulent, homogeneous vaginal discharge and vulvar itching. The vaginal and vulvar epithelium are often visibly inflamed, and petechial lesions are seen by colposcopy on the cervix ("strawberry cervix") in about 50 percent of cases. The pH of vaginal fluid is usually 5.0 or greater. In women with typical symptoms and signs of trichomoniasis, the diagnosis usually can be confirmed by the demonstration of motile trichomonads and polymorphonuclear leukocytes in vaginal secretions mixed with normal saline and promptly examined microscopically. In such cases, wet-mount examination is at least 80 percent as sensitive as culture. However, in women without symptoms or signs, culture is often required for detection of the organism. The diagnosis of *T. vaginalis* infection in men is more difficult and requires culture of early-morning first-voided urine sediment or of a urethral swab specimen obtained before voiding. New methods of identifying *T. vaginalis* by immunofluorescence or by use of oligonucleotide probes are under investigation and may prove diagnostically helpful for cases in both men and women.

Nitroimidazoles are the only drugs that are consistently effective for the treatment of trichomoniasis. Several studies show that a single 2.0-g oral dose of metronidazole is at least 90 percent as effective as more prolonged dosage schedules. Other nitroimidazoles such as tinidazole and ornidazole have longer half-lives than metronidazole but have not been shown clearly to give better results in trichomoniasis. Routine treatment of sexual partners is recommended to reduce both the risk of reinfection and the reservoir of infection. Vaginal treatment with 0.75% metronidazole gel, although effective for bacterial

vaginosis (see below), is not highly effective for vaginal trichomoniasis. Metronidazole is not recommended during the first trimester of pregnancy. Alcohol must be avoided for 24 h after its use because of occasional disulfiram-like effects. When practical, the partners of patients with trichomoniasis (or with any sexually transmitted infection, for that matter) should be seen in person rather than treated without examination and counseling.

BACTERIAL VAGINOSIS Vaginal discharge not associated with *T. vaginalis*, yeast, or cervical infection is usually due to bacterial vaginosis. This syndrome (formerly termed *nonspecific vaginitis*, *anaerobic vaginitis*, or *Gardnerella-associated vaginal discharge*) is characterized by vaginal malodor and a slightly to moderately increased white discharge that is homogeneous, low in viscosity, and smoothly coats the vaginal mucosa. It is unclear whether bacterial vaginosis is a sexually transmitted infection. The syndrome is associated with STD risk factors, such as multiple sexual partners and recent intercourse with a new partner, but no single sexually transmitted pathogen has been clearly implicated as the cause. Antibiotic treatment of male partners does not seem to influence the rate of recurrence among affected women. Formerly considered a benign condition, bacterial vaginosis has been implicated as a risk factor for acute salpingitis, premature labor, and related neonatal and perinatal complications.

The increased prevalence and concentrations of *G. vaginalis*, *Mycoplasma hominis*, and several anaerobic bacteria [e.g., *Mobiluncus* spp., *Prevotella* spp. (formerly *Bacteroides* spp.), and some *Peptostreptococcus* spp.] in vaginal fluid of women with bacterial vaginosis probably contribute to its pathogenesis. Of the various microorganisms associated with bacterial vaginosis, *Prevotella* spp.

and *M. hominis* have been most strongly correlated with premature delivery. However, none of these organisms is found only among women with this syndrome, and *G. vaginalis* has been isolated from the vagina of up to 50 percent of healthy women. The hydrogen peroxide–producing *Lactobacillus* spp., which constitute most of the normal vaginal flora (with *L. acidophilus* and *L. jensenii* most commonly found), are usually absent from the vagina in bacterial vaginosis. Hydrogen peroxide–producing lactobacilli may protect against a variety of vaginal and cervical pathogens, and it has been hypothesized that selective depletion of these organisms facilitates the overgrowth of the vagina by anaerobic bacteria, *M. hominis*, and *G. vaginalis*.

In a patient with symptoms of abnormal vaginal discharge and malodor or with objective signs of increased white homogeneous vaginal discharge, bacterial vaginosis can be diagnosed with reasonable certainty by the following:

1 *Exclusion of candidal and trichomonal vaginitis and mucopurulent cervicitis.* This process must include the collection of endocervical specimens to be tested for *C. trachomatis* and *N. gonorrhoeae.*

2 *Liberation of a distinct fishy odor immediately after mixing of vaginal secretions with a 10% solution of KOH.* This odor is attributable to volatile amines (e.g., trimethylamine, putrescine, and cadaverine) in the vaginal fluid, presumably resulting from anaerobic bacterial metabolism.

3 *Demonstration of a pH of vaginal secretions of > 4.5.* The elevated pH may be partly due to the presence of amines as well as to decreased production of lactate.

4 *Microscopic demonstration of "clue cells" and characteristic alterations of the vaginal microflora.* Clue cells are vaginal epithelial cells coated with coccobacillary organisms. On wet mount, prepared by mixing of vaginal secretions with normal saline in a ratio of approximately 1:1, clue cells have a granular appearance and indistinct borders (Fig. 88-1). Clue cells also can be detected on a Gram-stained smear. The Gram-stained smear permits assessment of the vaginal flora; the normally predominant lactobacilli (large, gram-positive rods) are mostly or completely replaced by a profusion of bacterial morphotypes consistent with *G. vaginalis* and anaerobic organisms. The demonstration of many clue cells by wet mount microscopy and the documentation of characteristically altered vaginal flora by Gram's stain represent the most sensitive, specific, and objective criteria for the diagnosis of bacterial vaginosis in women with symptoms and/or signs of this condition.

Attempts to isolate *G. vaginalis*, genital mycoplasmas, or anaerobic bacteria are of little utility in the diagnosis of bacterial vaginosis because these organisms are components of the vaginal flora in many women without the syndrome. However, semiquantitative techniques that detect high concentrations of *G. vaginalis* (equivalent to $\geq 10^6$ organisms per milliliter) are being evaluated.

The standard regimen for bacterial vaginosis has been metronidazole (500 mg orally, twice daily for 7 days). Clindamycin (300 mg orally, twice daily for 7 days) is also effective. Recent data suggest that intravaginal treatment with 2% clindamycin cream (5 g each night for 7 nights) or 0.75% metronidazole gel (5 g twice daily for 5 days) is comparable to oral therapy in efficacy but produces fewer adverse reactions. Intravaginal clindamycin cream is likely to become the treatment of choice for pregnant women with bacterial vaginosis. Oral amoxicillin formerly was considered a therapeutic option, but is much less effective than metronidazole or clindamycin (perhaps because it is active against *Lactobacillus* spp., preventing reestablishment of a protective *Lactobacillus* flora) and is no longer recommended. Sulfonamide-containing vaginal creams are usually ineffective, probably because sulfonamides are inactive against both *G. vaginalis* and many vaginal anaerobes, and there is no rationale for their use. Tetracycline therapy also is ineffective. No controlled data support the use of vaginal or oral preparations of *Lactobacillus* spp. in the treatment of bacterial vaginosis. However, few if any of the commercial preparations of lactobacilli used so far have contained

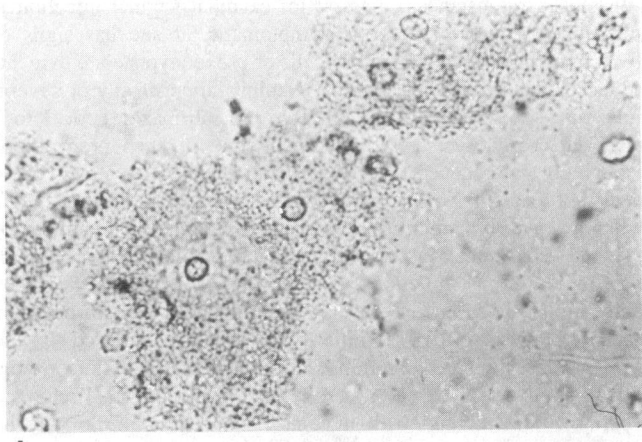

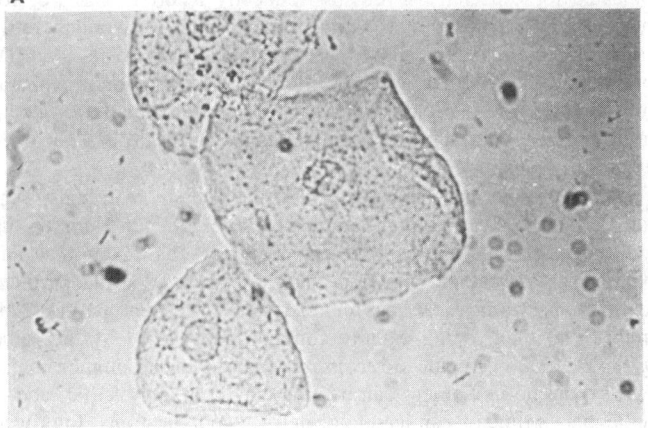

FIGURE 88-1 *A.* Vaginal epithelial "clue cells." Note granular appearance due to adherent *G. vaginalis* and indistinct cell margins (400×). *B.* Normal vaginal epithelial cells. The cell margins are distinct and lack granularity.

hydrogen peroxide–producing vaginal strains, and studies with such isolates will be of interest.

Treatment of male partners of women with bacterial vaginosis does not seem to prevent recurrence in these women and therefore is not indicated.

VULVOVAGINAL CANDIDIASIS The predominant symptom in vulvovaginal candidiasis is vulvar pruritus. There is usually no distinct odor. Vulvar erythema is common. The vaginal discharge typically is white and scanty and sometimes takes the form of thrushlike plaques or cottage cheese–like curds adhering loosely to the vaginal mucosa. *Candida albicans* accounts for about 80 percent of yeasts isolated from the vagina, while *Torulopsis glabrata* and other less commonly encountered *Candida* spp. are found in the remainder. Most cases of vulvovaginal candidiasis probably result from increased growth of yeasts that previously colonized the vagina or the intestinal tract. However, occasional cases of recurrent vulvovaginal candidiasis may be due to sexual transmission from a colonized male, and some men whose partners have vulvovaginal candidiasis develop symptomatic yeast dermatitis of the penis.

The diagnosis of vulvovaginal candidiasis involves the demonstration of fungi by microscopic examination of vaginal fluid in saline or 10% KOH or by Gram's stain. Demonstration of pseudohyphae strengthens the diagnosis of vaginitis due to *C. albicans*. Polymorphonuclear leukocytes often are present. Microscopic examination is less sensitive than culture, but correlates better with symptoms. Culture commonly detects coincidental colonization in women who may not require therapy. The pH of vaginal secretions is usually less than 4.5, and no amine odor is produced when vaginal secretions are mixed with 10% KOH. Vulvitis often accompanies vaginitis and may result in superficial erosions or fissures that must be differentiated from genital herpes and other causes of genital ulcer.

In most circumstances, therapy for candidal vaginal infection is indicated only if the patient is symptomatic, if she has signs of vulvovaginitis, or if inflammatory cells or pseudohyphae are evident. The usual treatment is intravaginal administration of any of several imidazole antibiotics (e.g., miconazole or clotrimazole) for 3 to 7 days. The recent over-the-counter marketing of such preparations undoubtedly has reduced the cost of care and made treatment more convenient for many women with yeast vulvovaginitis. However, the symptoms of vulvovaginitis are nonspecific, and self-treatment of presumed yeast infections may delay the detection and treatment of other, more serious infections. Therefore, self-treatment should be strictly limited to women with classic symptoms in whom previous episodes of yeast vulvovaginitis have been documented by an experienced clinician. Single-dose oral treatment with fluconazole (150 mg) is also effective and is preferred by many patients. Prolonged or periodic oral therapy with fluconazole or ketoconazole may be indicated for especially severe or frequently recurrent cases or for those which do not respond to intravaginal or single-dose oral therapy. Such patients probably should be evaluated for diabetes or HIV infection, although such systemic illnesses are uncommon explanations for recurrent vulvovaginal candidiasis. Treatment of sexual partners is not routinely indicated, although its value has not been studied rigorously.

Mucopurulent cervicitis *Mucopurulent cervicitis* refers to inflammation of the columnar epithelium and subepithelium of the endocervix and of any contiguous columnar epithelium that lies exposed in an ectopic position on the exocervix. Mucopurulent cervicitis in women can be regarded as the "silent partner" of urethritis in men, being equally common and caused by the same agents but more difficult to recognize. It is the most common major STD syndrome in women, can be a harbinger or sign of PID, and—in pregnant women—can lead to obstetrical complications. Improved recognition and treatment of this syndrome would greatly facilitate the control of STDs. Mucopurulent cervicitis is caused most commonly by *C. trachomatis* and sometimes by *N. gonorrhoeae*; the relative proportions of cases due to these two organisms depend on their prevalence in the community. However, up to one-half of cases are associated with neither of these organisms and currently must be considered idiopathic. The syndrome usually can be differentiated clinically from cervicitis caused by HSV, which produces lesions on the stratified squamous epithelium of the exocervix as well as on the columnar epithelium.

The diagnosis is made by the demonstration of mucopurulent discharge from the cervical os or of increased numbers of polymorphonuclear leukocytes in Gram-stained or Papanicolaou smears of endocervical mucus. Edematous cervical ectopy (see below) and endocervical bleeding induced by gentle swabbing are common signs of mucopurulent cervicitis due to *C. trachomatis*. The color of cervical mucus on a white swab removed from the endocervix should be noted; a yellow color indicates the presence of polymorphonuclear leukocytes. The mucus should be rolled *thinly* on a slide for Gram's staining. An area of the slide should be identified that contains strands of cervical mucus not contaminated by vaginal squamous epithelial cells or vaginal bacteria. The presence of 30 or more polymorphonuclear cells per $1000\times$ microscopic field within strands of cervical mucus suggests cervicitis. A characteristic pattern of inflammatory cells on endocervical Papanicolaou smears is sometimes considered by cytopathologists to suggest chlamydial infection. However, such findings are not sufficiently specific to warrant a diagnosis of chlamydial infection; they signify only a need for specific confirmatory testing.

Mucopurulent cervicitis requires antimicrobial therapy. An etiologic diagnosis should always be established to guide the management of sexual partners, but therapy for these men should be initiated against the most likely causes of this syndrome while results of diagnostic tests are pending.

In settings where both gonorrhea and chlamydial infection are common, therapy should include a single-dose regimen effective for gonorrhea, such as ceftriaxone (125 mg intramuscularly), followed by doxycycline (100 mg orally, twice daily for 1 week). When doxycycline is contraindicated, erythromycin base or stearate (500 mg four times daily for 7 days) can be substituted. Ofloxacin (300 mg orally, twice daily for 7 days) is an alternative regimen that is effective for both gonorrhea and chlamydial infection. In settings where gonorrhea is much less common than chlamydial infection, initial therapy for mucopurulent cervicitis may be designed to cover chlamydial infection only (e.g., a regimen of doxycycline, erythromycin or azithromycin). Azithromycin in a single dose of 1.0 g orally can be substituted for a 7-day course of doxycycline or erythromycin but is not reliable for the treatment of gonorrhea. The sexual partner(s) of a woman with mucopurulent cervicitis should be examined and given a regimen similar to that chosen for the woman unless results of tests for gonorrhea or chlamydial infection in either partner warrant a change in therapy. Gonococcal cervicitis is diagnosed by culture of an endocervical specimen. When carefully collected endocervical specimens are examined by experienced personnel, Gram's stain is an insensitive but fairly specific test, and the observation of intracellular gram-negative diplococci indicates gonococcal infection even if the culture is negative. The sensitivity of a single endocervical culture for *N. gonorrhoeae* is 80 to 90 percent (see Chap. 110). Chlamydial infection of the cervix can be confirmed by culture, antigen detection, or DNA probe or DNA amplification tests (see Chap. 140).

Cervical ectopy Cervicitis must be differentiated from *cervical ectopy*, which is often mislabeled "cervical erosion." Ectopy represents the presence of the one-cell-thick columnar epithelium extending from the endocervix out onto the visible ectocervix. In ectopy, the cervical os may contain clear or slightly cloudy mucus but usually does not include yellow mucopus. Colposcopy shows that the epithelium is intact and not ulcerated. Ectopy is normally found during early adolescence and gradually recedes as squamous metaplasia replaces the ectopic columnar epithelium. Oral contraceptive use favors the persistence or reappearance of ectopy. Cauterization for the elimination of ectopy is not warranted. Ectopy may make the cervix more susceptible to infection with *N. gonorrhoeae* or *C. trachomatis* by exposing a larger area of susceptible columnar epithelium. Moreover, ectopy may increase susceptibility to HIV infection. If mucopurulent cervicitis supervenes, the area of ectopy may become edematous and fragile, with bleeding induced by gentle swabbing. In addition, edema of the cervix may result in eversion of the os, with enlargement of the apparent area of ectopy.

PELVIC INFLAMMATORY DISEASE PID is a syndrome that comprises various combinations of endometritis, salpingitis, and pelvic peritonitis resulting from ascending genital infection, which usually arises from gonococcal or chlamydial mucopurulent cervicitis and/or from bacterial vaginosis (see Chap. 89). PID and its sequelae predominantly affect sexually active adolescents and young women, in whom at least 90 percent of cases are sexually acquired. Although sometimes clinically severe, with tuboovarian abscess or overt peritonitis, most cases of acute PID are relatively mild or even subclinical; however, such cases can nevertheless result in significant tubal damage, as evidenced by the frequent lack of history of PID or pelvic pain in *Chlamydia*-seropositive women with tubal scarring and infertility or ectopic pregnancy. Accordingly, the clinician must have a low threshold for considering PID in the differential diagnosis of mild or even trivial abdominal pain in young women. The approach represents a shift in thinking from the days when PID was considered likely only in women with severe adnexal tenderness plus an elevation in temperature, white blood cell count, or erythrocyte sedimentation rate.

The proportion of cases caused by *N. gonorrhoeae* recently has declined in most industrialized countries, a trend reflecting the declining incidence of gonococcal infections in general. *C. trachomatis* remains a common cause of PID in many countries. Numerous other pathogens contribute to PID, including *M. hominis* and various anaerobic members of the vaginal flora found in bacterial vaginosis.

Recent data also suggest that vaginal douching is an important risk factor for ascending pelvic infection. PID is discussed in detail in Chap. 89.

ULCERATIVE LESIONS OF THE GENITALIA The incidence and etiology of ulcerative lesions of the genitalia vary greatly in different areas of the world (Table 88-4). In Asia and Africa, genital ulcers are seen as frequently as gonorrhea in some STD clinics; chancroid is the most common cause, while genital herpes is relatively uncommon. In the industrialized western countries, genital ulcers are considerably less common than urethritis, mucopurulent cervicitis, and vaginitis; genital herpes is the most common cause, and chancroid is relatively uncommon. Syphilis is the second most common form of genital ulcer in almost all areas of the world, and the possiblity of its presence must always be excluded. Lymphogranuloma venereum (LGV) and donovanosis (granuloma inguinale) are very rare in North America and Europe. Other causes of genital ulcer include candidiasis and traumatized genital warts, both of which are usually readily recognized, and various non-sexually transmitted dermatoses.

Trauma is an uncommon cause of genital ulcer unless there is clear history of definite injury accompanied by bleeding. Chancroid, syphilis, genital herpes, and probably all causes of genital ulcer enhance the efficiency of sexual transmission and acquisition of HIV. Moreover, genital ulcers, especially chancroid and syphilis, are most common in inner-city populations with low socioeconomic status and high rates of prostitution and illicit drug use—independent risk factors for HIV infection. In the late 1980s in the United States, chancroid and syphilis spread at epidemic rates in such populations, although these rates began to decline in the early 1990s.

In industrialized countries, the differential diagnosis of genital ulceration usually includes genital herpes, syphilis, and chancroid. The clinical findings are occasionally definitive (e.g., the presence of herpetic vesicles), and clinical findings plus epidemiologic considerations can usually guide initial therapy pending the results of further studies. Nevertheless, most genital ulcerations cannot be diagnosed confidently on clinical grounds. It is axiomatic to exclude syphilis by appropriate serologic studies in all cases. All lesions except those highly characteristic of infection with HSV should be subjected to dark-field examination or a direct immunofluorescence test for *Treponema pallidum*. Selective enrichment media are available for isolation of *Haemophilus ducreyi*.

The following general guidelines are recommended for management of ulcerative genital lesions:

Lesions typical of genital herpes In industrialized countries, where the probability of prior herpes is high, a clinical diagnosis of genital herpes is warranted if typical vesicles or pustules are evident or if there is a cluster of painful ulcers that was preceded by vesiculopustular lesions. These clinical presentations are sufficiently typical that confirmation of the diagnosis by isolation of HSV, immunochemical detection of the virus, or type-specific serology is optional. A serologic test for syphilis should be performed not primarily for diagnostic purposes, but because screening is indicated in all patients with a newly diagnosed STD.

All other acute genital ulcers The appearance of genital herpetic lesions is highly variable, and—except in the relatively clear-cut cases described above—a specific test for HSV is indicated whenever feasible. Isolation of HSV by culture or immunochemical identification of HSV antigens or genetic material should be attempted. Type-specific serologic tests may be useful in some cases, but commercially available serologic tests do not distinguish between antibodies to the two types of HSV and are of little use (see Chap. 143). Cytologic methods (Tzanck preparation with Wright-Giemsa or Papanicolaou staining) for the detection of HSV-infected multinucleated cells are very insensitive except in the presence of intact vesicles and are seldom useful in diagnosing genital ulcer disease. An attempt should be made to isolate *H. ducreyi* if the genital ulcer is painful and inguinal lymphadenopathy with fluctuance or overlying erythema is noted; if chancroid is prevalent in the community; if the patient is at high risk for chancroid (e.g., through the use of injection drugs or "crack" cocaine or through prostitution); or if the patient has recently had a sexual exposure in a chancroid-endemic area (e.g., a developing country or certain North American cities). Enlarged, fluctuant lymph nodes should be aspirated for culture and Gram's staining to detect *H. ducreyi* and pyogenic bacteria. Syphilis should be excluded by dark-field examination and serologic testing, and the latter should be repeated 1 to 2 weeks later if the results are initially negative and if another diagnosis cannot be established.

Lesions typical of syphilis If lesions are at all suggestive of syphilis (e.g., painless, nontender, indurated) or there are epidemiologic reasons to suspect syphilis (e.g., recent exposure), dark-field examination and a rapid serologic test for syphilis should be performed. If the results are negative and the patient is reliable in terms of follow-up and sexual abstinence, there should be two more dark-field examinations on successive days before treatment is attempted, and the serologic test should be repeated 1, 2, and 6 weeks later. Direct immunofluorescence staining of *T. pallidum* is quite reliable and should be used if dark-field examination by experienced examiners is impossible.

Chronic genital ulceration When genital ulcers persist beyond the usual course of herpes (2 to 3 weeks) or chancroid or syphilis (up to 6 weeks) and do not resolve with syndromic antimicrobial therapy, then—in addition to the usual tests for herpes, syphilis, and chancroid—biopsy is indicated to exclude donovanosis, carcinoma, and other nonvenereal dermatoses. A test for HIV infection should be done, since chronic, persistent genital herpes is common in HIV infection with reduced concentrations of CD4 cells.

Ideally, treatment for genital ulceration should be withheld until the diagnosis is secure. However, immediate syndromic treatment for acute genital ulcerations (after collection of all necessary diagnostic specimens) is sometimes necessary, e.g., when it is believed that a patient may not return for follow-up. Initial treatment in such cases should generally include 2.4 million units of benzathine penicillin G for possible primary syphilis. Immediate empirical therapy for chancroid also is indicated if the patient has been exposed in an area where chancroid is endemic and especially if regional lymph node suppuration is evident or appears imminent (see Chap. 112). Prompt systemic therapy with acyclovir is indicated for patients with initial episodes of genital or anorectal herpes (see Chap. 143). Finally, empirical antimicrobial therapy may be indicated if ulcers persist and the diagnosis remains unclear after 1 to 2 weeks of observation and repeated attempts to diagnose herpes, syphilis, and chancroid.

PROCTITIS, PROCTOCOLITIS, ENTEROCOLITIS, AND ENTERITIS Sexually acquired proctitis, or inflammation limited to the rectal mucosa, results from direct rectal inoculation of typical STD pathogens. In contrast, inflammation that extends from the rectum to the colon (proctocolitis), that involves both the small and the large bowel (enterocolitis), or that involves the small bowel alone (enteritis) can result from ingestion of typical intestinal pathogens through sexual contact involving oral-fecal exposure. Anorectal pain and

TABLE 88-4 Etiologies of genital ulcer disease in industrialized and tropical developing countries

Diagnosis	Percent of cases	
	Industrialized countries	Tropical developing countries
Genital herpes	50–70	0–10*
Syphilis	10–20	10–20
Chancroid	0–10†	50–60
Donovanosis	<1	<1‡
Other/unknown	10–20	10–30

* The proportion of genital ulcers caused by HSV appears to be increasing as the prevalence of HIV infection increases in developing countries.
† Highly variable; may account for >25% of cases in selected U.S. cities during chancroid outbreaks.
‡ Donovanosis accounts for higher proportions of cases in some geographic areas (e.g., southern Africa, western Australia, Papua New Guinea, and the Indian subcontinent).

mucopurulent or bloody rectal discharge suggest proctitis or proctocolitis. Proctitis is commonly associated with tenesmus (causing frequent attempts to defecate, but not true diarrhea) and constipation, whereas proctocolitis and enterocolitis are more often associated with true diarrhea. In all three conditions anoscopy usually shows the presence of mucosal inflammation with exudate and easily induced mucosal bleeding (i.e., a positive "wipe test"). Petechiae or mucosal ulcers also may be observed. Exudate should be sampled for microbiologic studies and Gram's staining. Sigmoidoscopy or colonoscopy—which should be performed, if possible, without an enema—shows inflammation limited to the rectum (in proctitis) or disease extending at least into the sigmoid colon (in proctocolitis).

Most cases of sexually transmitted intestinal infection in the past have involved homosexual men. During the AIDS era, there has been an extraordinary shift in the clinical and etiologic spectrum of intestinal infections among homosexual men. The number of opportunistic intestinal infections (see Chap. 279) has risen rapidly among persons with AIDS. At the same time, the number of sexually transmitted intestinal infections (as described below) has fallen rapidly as high-risk sexual behaviors have become less common in this group.

Most cases of infectious proctitis are due to *N. gonorrhoeae*, HSV, or *C. trachomatis;* these are acquired via receptive anorectal intercourse. Primary and secondary syphilis also can produce anal or anorectal lesions, with or without symptoms. Proctitis due to *N. gonorrhoeae* or to common strains of *C. trachomatis* typically involves the most distal rectal mucosa and the anal crypts and is clinically mild, without systemic manifestations. In contrast, primary proctitis due to HSV and proctocolitis due to the strains of *C. trachomatis* that cause LGV usually produce severe anorectal pain and often cause fever. Perianal ulcers and inguinal lymphadenopathy, most commonly due to HSV, also can occur in LGV or syphilis. Sacral nerve root radiculopathies, usually presenting as urinary retention, laxity of the anal sphincter, or constipation, are common in primary herpetic proctitis. Sigmoidoscopy most commonly shows ulcerative proctitis in either herpes or LGV but may reveal intact vesicopustular lesions in anorectal herpes. In herpes, biopsy of the rectal mucosa shows microulcerations and may show intranuclear inclusions or perivascular lymphocytic cuffing. In LGV, biopsy typically shows crypt abscesses, granulomas, and giant cells—findings that may be indistinguishable from those of Crohn's disease. Syphilis also can produce rectal granulomas, usually in association with infiltration by plasma cells or other mononuclear cells.

The occurrence of diarrhea and abdominal bloating or cramping pain without anorectal symptoms and in association with normal anoscopy and sigmoidoscopy is consistent with inflammation of the small intestine (enteritis) or with proximal colitis. In homosexual men without HIV infection, enteritis limited to the small intestine is often attributable to *G. lamblia*. Sexually acquired proctocolitis is most often due to *Campylobacter* spp., *Shigella* spp., or *E. histolytica*.

HUMAN PAPILLOMAVIRUS INFECTION AND GENITAL WARTS
Genital warts and infection with HPV were long considered inconvenient but benign conditions. However, evolving evidence indicates that some strains of HPV—e.g., types 16, 18, and 31—are closely linked with (and probably a direct cause of) moderate to severe squamous dysplasia and overt cancer of the cervix, anus, vulva, vagina, and penis; thus infection with this virus is now recognized as one of the most important STDs. The number of visits to clinicians because of genital warts has been estimated at more than 1.2 million each year in the United States. However, most HPV infections are subclinical, and increasingly sensitive tools for the detection of HPV (e.g., the polymerase chain reaction) show that most sexually active young men and women seen at STD clinics have genital HPV infection, usually without visible clinical abnormalities. Treatment of HPV infection yields largely unsatisfactory results; destruction of visible condylomata with cryotherapy, other chemical or physical cytotoxic agents, or surgery does not cure subclinical infection of adjacent tissues. Accordingly, the primary goal of treatment of genital warts is cosmetic, and therapy should be conservative. Although genital warts are no more predictive than other STDs of severe cervical dysplasia (since the types of HPV that commonly cause genital warts are not the types that cause severe dysplasia or invasive cancer), women with any STD should undergo routine cervical cytologic screening. These conditions are addressed in detail in Chap. 149.

ACUTE ARTHRITIS The gonococcal arthritis-dermatitis syndrome and Reiter's syndrome are among the most common forms of acute arthritis in sexually active young adults. These two syndromes must be differentiated from each other, from other forms of infective arthritis, from various diseases associated with immune-complex deposition, from crystal-induced arthritis, from acute rheumatoid arthritis, and from other, less common rheumatic disorders, such as systemic lupus erythematosus. Meningococcemia, infection with *Yersinia*, sarcoidosis, and syphilis are other occasional causes of acute arthritis in young adults.

Demonstration of *N. gonorrhoeae* by culture or by a specific immunochemical method in synovial fluid, blood, skin lesions, or cerebrospinal fluid is diagnostic of disseminated gonococcal infection (DGI). Gonococcal arthritis is highly probable if such tests fail to detect the organism, if it is recovered from a mucosal site of infection or from the patient's sexual partner, and if there are typical pustular or hemorrhagic skin lesions distributed primarily on the extremities. Suspected and confirmed cases of DGI should be treated promptly with an antibiotic effective against antibiotic-sensitive and antibiotic-resistant gonococci, such as ceftriaxone (see Chap. 110).

Reiter's syndrome occurs in a sporadic (apparently sexually transmitted) form that usually follows chlamydial infection and in a postdysenteric form that usually follows infection with *Yersinia*, *Campylobacter*, or *Shigella* spp. Discrete epidemics of the latter form are sometimes documented (see Chap. 289).

HEPATITIS B VIRUS, CYTOMEGALOVIRUS, AND HUMAN T LYMPHOTROPIC VIRUSES HBV and CMV are carried in the blood, are shed in genital secretions, and can be transmitted through sexual and perinatal exposure as well as through contact with blood. Sexual transmission and perinatal transmission predominate with HTLV-I, whereas transmission by injection drug users predominates with HTLV-II. HTLV-II also is endemic among some Native American tribes. All these agents cause primary infections that usually are asymptomatic, with subsequent chronic or latent infection and a potential for complications or transmission for many years—perhaps indefinitely.

Sexually transmitted HBV infection was an extremely common problem among homosexual and bisexual men until the mid-1980s, and sexual contact among men continues to account for 5 to 10 percent of adult HBV infections in the United States. About 25 percent of cases of hepatitis B in adults currently are attributed to heterosexual transmission and 30 percent to sharing of injection equipment by illicit drug users. The route of acquisition is unknown in 35 to 40 percent of cases, many of which are probably acquired sexually. Hepatitis B is the only STD for which an effective vaccine is available, and current recommendations in the United States include universal vaccination of infants and targeted vaccination of adolescents in high-risk communities, people with multiple sexual partners or other STDs, sexual partners of individuals with acute hepatitis B, and seronegative sexual partners of chronic carriers of the hepatitis B surface antigen.

Sexual contact is the most important mode of transmission of CMV in some settings. Among initially seronegative women attending STD clinics, the annual incidence of seroconversion is 8 to 30 percent. CMV is among the most common causes of congenital neurodevelopmental abnormalities and of life-threatening morbidity in patients with advanced cellular immunodeficiency due to HIV, malignancy, or chemotherapy. Until an effective vaccine is developed, the prevention of sexually transmitted CMV infection will be problematic.

HTLV-I is endemic as a sexually transmitted virus in parts of the Caribbean, Latin America, Asia, and Africa and is associated with

T cell leukemia and tropical spastic paresis (HTLV-I–associated myelopathy). HTLV-II is found in up to 15 to 20 percent of injection drug users in the United States. The clinical consequences of infection with this virus have yet to be defined.

PREVENTION AND CONTROL OF STDs

The control of bacterial STDs has traditionally depended on early diagnosis and treatment. The emergence of the incurable viral STDs has required increasing emphasis on health education and health promotion as a means of discouraging casual sex and high-risk sexual practices and encouraging the use of condoms. Medical students and physicians require training in eliciting a sexual history, determining the extent to which their patients (especially adolescents and young adults) are at risk for STDs, and counseling these patients appropriately. Public education and personal counseling should begin in early adolescence and should emphasize responsible sexual behavior (abstinence, maintenance of monogamous relationships); the use of condoms for nonmonogamous sexual encounters; the avoidance of traumatic sexual practices, such as anal intercourse; the recognition of early symptoms and signs of STDs; and the importance of early health care for such symptoms and signs.

Maintenance of clinical skills in the recognition, diagnosis, and treatment of STDs is essential to the prevention of STD transmission and STD complications. Screening tests for gonorrhea, chlamydial infection, syphilis, and HIV infection as well as cervical cytology should be made widely available and should be used by physicians serving populations at risk. In region X (the Northwest) of the United States, a federally funded program for selective chlamydial diagnostic screening in more than 150 family planning clinics was associated with a decline in chlamydial prevalence from 10 to 5 percent during a 5-year period from 1987 to 1992. It is appalling that, as of early 1993, other regions still had not implemented similar programs for this preventable STD. Health departments should provide high-quality STD clinical services and screening for high-risk populations; these departments are also responsible for STD surveillance and for the coordination of targeted control measures—efforts that require the cooperation of physicians in reporting cases. Notification of the sexual partners of infected persons is the joint responsibility of the patient and the physician. In most communities, the local health department will assist in this effort for cases of syphilis, for some cases of gonorrhea, and increasingly, for cases of HIV infection.

REFERENCES

General

ADIMORA A et al: *Sexually Transmitted Diseases, 2d ed, Companion Handbook.* New York, McGraw-Hill, 1993
ARAL SO, HOLMES KK: Sexually transmitted diseases in the AIDS era. Sci Am 264:62, 1991
BRANDT AM: *No Magic Bullet: A Social History of Venereal Disease in the United States Since 1890,* 2d ed. New York, Oxford Univ Press, 1989
CENTERS FOR DISEASE CONTROL: 1989 sexually transmitted diseases treatment guideline. Morb Mort Week Rep 38(suppl 8):1, 1989
HOLMES KK et al (eds): *Sexually Transmitted Diseases,* 2d ed. New York, McGraw-Hill, 1990
HANDSFIELD HH: *Color Atlas and Synopsis of Sexually Transmitted Diseases.* New York, McGraw-Hill, 1992

Urethritis in males

BOWIE WR: Urethritis in males, in *Sexually Transmitted Diseases,* 2d ed, KK Holmes et al (eds). New York, McGraw-Hill, 1990, chap 52
——— et al: Etiology of nongonococcal urethritis: Evidence for *Chlamydia trachomatis* and *Ureaplasma urealyticum.* J Clin Invest 59:735, 1977
KREIGER J et al: Clinical manifestations of trichomoniasis in men. Ann Intern Med 118:844, 1993
SHAFER MD et al: Urinary leukocyte esterase screening test for asymptomatic chlamydial and gonococcal infection in males. JAMA 262:2562, 1989

Epididymitis

BERGER RE et al: Etiology and manifestations of epididymitis in young men: Correlation with sexual orientation. J Infect Dis 155:1341, 1987

Urethral syndrome

STAMM WE et al: Urinary tract infection: From pathogenesis to treatment. J Infect Dis 159:400, 1989

Vaginal infections

ESCHENBACH DA et al: Diagnosis and clinical manifestations of bacterial vaginosis. Am J Obstet Gynecol 158:819, 1988
HILLIER SL et al: The relationship of hydrogen peroxide–producing lactobacilli to bacterial vaginosis and genital microflora in pregnant women. Obstet Gynecol 79:369, 1992
SOBEL J: Genital candidiasis, in *Sexually Transmitted Diseases,* 2d ed, KK Holmes et al (eds). New York, McGraw-Hill, 1990
WØLNER-HANSSEN P et al: Clinical manifestations of vaginal trichomoniasis. JAMA 261:571, 1989

Mucopurulent cervicitis

BRUNHAM RC et al: Mucopurulent cervicitis—The ignored counterpart in women of urethritis in men. N Engl J Med 311:1, 1984

Genital ulcers

KOUTSKY LA et al: Underdiagnosis of genital herpes by current clinical and viral isolation procedures. N Engl J Med 326:1533, 1992
SIMONSEN JN et al: Human immunodeficiency virus infection among men with sexually transmitted diseases. N Engl J Med 319:274, 1988

Proctitis, proctocolitis, enterocolitis, and enteritis

QUINN TC et al: The polymicrobial etiology of intestinal infections in homosexual men. N Engl J Med 309:576, 1983

Arthritis

HANDSFIELD HH, POLLOCK PS: Arthropathies associated with sexually transmitted diseases, in *Sexually Transmitted Diseases,* 2d ed, KK Holmes et al (eds). New York, McGraw-Hill, 1990

Pelvic inflammatory disease

SOPER DE: Diagnosis and laparoscopic grading of acute salpingitis. Am J Obstet Gynecol 164:1370, 1991
WØLNER-HANSSEN P et al: Association between vaginal douching and acute pelvic inflammatory disease. JAMA 263:1936, 1990

HPV/warts

KOUTSKY LA et al: A cohort study of the risk of cervical intraepithelial neoplasia grade 2 or 3 in relation to papillomavirus infection. N Engl J Med 327:1272, 1992

HBV, CMV, HTLV-I, and HTLV-II

ALTER MJ et al: The changing epidemiology of hepatitis B in the United States: Need for alternative vaccination strategies. JAMA 263:1218, 1990
COLLIER AC et al: Cytomegalovirus infection in women attending a sexually transmitted disease clinic. J Infect Dis 162:46, 1990

89 PELVIC INFLAMMATORY DISEASE

KING K. HOLMES

DEFINITION The term *pelvic inflammatory disease* (PID) usually refers to ascending infection of the endometrium and/or fallopian tubes. Intrauterine infection can be primary (spontaneously occurring and usually sexually transmitted) or secondary to invasive intrauterine surgical procedures (e.g., dilatation and curettage, termination of pregnancy, insertion of an intrauterine device, or hysterosalpingography) or to parturition. Endometritis or endomyometritis is particularly common following delivery by cesarean section.

PID is uncommon during pregnancy itself. The uterotubal junction is closed as early as the seventh week of pregnancy, and the chorioamnion becomes approximated to the endocervical os, sealing off the intrauterine cavity, at the twelfth to fifteenth week of gestation. As a consequence, ascending intrauterine infection prior to the twelfth week of gestation may be associated (as either cause or effect) with endometritis and spontaneous abortion, while ascending infection after the twelfth week may be associated with chorioamnionitis. Rarely, infection may extend secondarily to the pelvic organs from adjacent foci of inflammation, such as appendicitis, regional ileitis, or diverticulitis; as a result of hematogenous dissemination, such as tuberculosis; or as a rare complication of certain tropical diseases, such as schistosomiasis.

Spontaneously occurring PID can be divided into chronic and acute types. Chronic PID due to tuberculosis has become uncommon in industrialized countries. However, subacute or chronic PID caused by chronic infection with *Chlamydia trachomatis* is thought to be common.

PID is the term most often used today to refer to cases of acute spontaneously occurring infection ascending from the cervix or vagina. The clinical diagnosis of PID is imprecise. Use of endometrial biopsy together with laparoscopy provides evidence of a continuum, progressing from cervicitis alone to endometritis, to salpingitis, to pelvic peritonitis, to generalized peritonitis, perihepatitis, or pelvic abscess. In this chapter, PID is used to refer to the clinical syndrome which includes each of these conditions, and the term *salpingitis* is restricted to patients with visually or histopathologically confirmed inflammation of the fallopian tubes. The distribution between endometritis and salpingitis may be important, because long-term sequelae are common after salpingitis. These sequelae include infertility due to bilateral tubal occlusion, peritubal adhesions, ectopic pregnancy due to tubal damage without occlusion, chronic pelvic pain, and recurrent PID.

ETIOLOGY   The etiology of PID has seemed to vary greatly in several studies for reasons related to patient selection as well as methodology. As is summarized in Table 89-1, the agents most often implicated in acute PID include those which are primary causes of cervicitis (*Neisseria gonorrhoeae* and *C. trachomatis*) and those which can be regarded as abnormal components of the vaginal flora.

In the United States, gonococci were isolated from 44 percent of women with acute PID in a multicity cooperative study during the 1970s. From 1980 through 1990 in Seattle, *N. gonorrhoeae* or *C. trachomatis* were found in 85 percent of patients with proven salpingitis and endometritis, with gonorrhea being nearly twice as common as chlamydial infection and dual infection being common. However, in Scandinavian countries, where gonococcal infection is under much better control, endocervical gonococcal infection has been found in a declining proportion of women with PID during the past decade, while chlamydial infection remains more common in this group. In general, PID is most often associated with gonorrhea where there is a high incidence of gonorrhea, e.g., in developing countries and in indigent, inner-city populations in developed countries. In several studies of women with PID, up to two-thirds with positive endocervical cultures for *N. gonorrhoeae* have had positive endometrial, peritoneal, or tubal cultures for this organism. Similarly, studies of women with proven PID have shown that *C. trachomatis* can be demonstrated by culture or immunofluorescent staining in the endometrium or tubes of the majority of those who have endocervical chlamydial infection.

Anaerobic and facultative anaerobic organisms (especially *Prevotella* spp., peptostreptococci, *Escherichia coli*, and group B streptococci) and genital mycoplasmas have been isolated from specimens obtained at laparoscopy from the peritoneal fluid or fallopian tubes in a varying proportion—typically one-fourth to one-third—of women with PID studied in the United States. These vaginal organisms can be found in association with chlamydial or gonococcal infection, as well as in women without them. The importance of vaginal organisms in salpingitis has probably been overestimated in studies based on culture of specimens obtained by culdocentesis or endometrial aspiration, procedures in which contamination of the aspirated specimen by vaginal flora could occur. However, specimens obtained by laparoscopy also have contained anaerobic and facultative species in some patients with PID. It is extremely difficult to determine the exact microbial etiology in the individual patient with PID because of the frequency of mixed infection, the difficulty in sampling the fallopian tube itself, and the complexity of microbiologic techniques required to detect the various fastidious pathogens involved.

In general, first episodes of acute PID are particularly likely to be caused by *N. gonorrhoeae* and/or *C. trachomatis*. These sexually transmitted pathogens are somewhat less often implicated in recurrent bouts of acute PID, episodes occurring in IUD users, and episodes precipitated by invasive intrauterine diagnostic or therapeutic procedures, which are often associated with ascending infection caused by certain components of the endogenous vaginal flora.

EPIDEMIOLOGY   It has been estimated that the annual incidence of PID in the United States during the mid-1970s was about 850,000 cases per year. PID is not a reportable disease in the United States; surveillance of physicians in private practice and of hospital discharges suggests that the incidence of PID increased from the mid-1960s through the mid-1970s and may then have decreased. Hospitalization for acute PID declined from 1982 through 1990, but visits to physicians' offices remained steady during that period. The 1988 National Survey of Family Growth indicated that 11 percent of women have been treated for PID.

Acute PID is almost exclusively a disease of sexually active women. The risk may be greater in sexually active teenagers than among older women. Important risk factors other than young age include a history of salpingitis, recent history of vaginal douching, and use of an intrauterine device, particularly the Dalkon shield. In most studies, the relative risk of PID among IUD users was higher in nulliparous than in parous women, and was greatest during the first few months after insertion. The increased risk of PID among IUD users appears mainly among those with multiple sex partners. On the other hand, women using oral contraceptives appear to be at decreased risk of PID. Barrier methods of contraception also prevent PID by reducing the risk of chlamydial and gonococcal infection. Tubal sterilization reduces (but does not completely eliminate) the risk of salpingitis by preventing intraluminal spread of infection into the tubes.

PATHOGENESIS   Factors cited as possibly contributing to intracanalicular upward spread of gonococci and *Chlamydia* from the endocervix to the endometrium and endosalpinx include estrogen-dominated (thin) cervical mucus, attachment to sperm which migrate upward into the tubes, use of an intrauterine device, vaginal douching, and menstruation. The onset of symptoms of gonorrhea-associated PID and of *Chlamydia*-associated PID often occurs during or soon after the menstrual period. In fallopian tube organ cultures in vitro, gonococci attach to the surface of the secretory columnar cells (but not the ciliated cells) of the endosalpinx. Gonococcal pili and perhaps other surface proteins are important in this attachment. Gonococci then are taken into the secretory cells by endocytosis. They pass through the cells, and perhaps between cells, and are extruded through the base of the cell into the submucosal connective tissue. Ciliary motion ceases, and then ciliated cells, although not directly invaded by gonococci, are sloughed from the mucosa during this process—a factor which may render the tubes more susceptible to superinfection by other organisms. It is uncertain whether this loss of ciliated cells is irreversible in vivo. Gonococcal endotoxin and peptidoglycan and certain cytokines appear responsible for these cytotoxic effects.

TABLE 89-1   Cervical and vaginal organisms most often implicated in acute PID

Cervical pathogens	Vaginal flora
N. gonorrhoeae	**Anaerobic bacteria**
C. trachomatis	*Prevotella* spp., Peptostreptococci, *Mobiluncus* spp., *Actinomyces* spp.
	Facultative bacteria
	Enterobacteriaceae, *H. influenzae*, *G. vaginalis*, Group B, streptococcus
	Mycoplasmas
	M. hominis,
	U. urealyticum

Gonococci associated with PID have been significantly more resistant to penicillin and less likely to belong to the Arg-Hyx-Ura auxotype than are strains causing uncomplicated gonorrhea.

C. trachomatis also infects the columnar cells of the fallopian tube but produces little damage in tubal organ cultures, perhaps because the host response is more important than directly toxic effects of bacterial products in the pathogenesis of chlamydial salpingitis. In chlamydial mucopurulent cervicitis (MPC), cervical biopsies show inclusions containing *Chlamydia* within columnar cells; columnar epithelial infiltration by neutrophils; submucosal and stromal infiltration by plasma cells, lymphocytes, histiocytes, and neutrophils; and lymphoid aggregates containing transformed lymphocytes. Routine endometrial biopsies from consecutive women with chlamydial MPC show endometritis in approximately one-half. Although endometritis detected in this way is sometimes associated with uterine tenderness, abnormal menstrual bleeding, and leukocytosis, symptoms of abdominal pain and fever, as well as signs of adnexal tenderness, are usually lacking, underscoring the subclinical nature of many cases of upper genital tract chlamydial infection. It is not known what proportion of those with endometritis also have salpingitis, since laparoscopy has not been performed in the absence of more suggestive symptoms and signs of salpingitis. However, among women with chlamydial MPC who do have such symptoms and signs, the great majority who undergo endometrial biopsy and laparoscopy have both endometritis and salpingitis. Chlamydial inclusions are demonstrable by direct immunofluorescence in columnar epithelial cells of the endometrium and endosalpinx. The endometrial biopsies usually show neutrophils infiltrating the epithelium and plasma cells infiltrating the stroma, findings also seen in gonococcal endometritis but not in the uninfected endometrium. Other inflammatory changes analogous to those seen in the cervix are also found in the endometrium with chlamydial infection. Experimental inoculation of the fallopian tubes of lower primates produces mild acute salpingitis and ciliary sloughing, which is transient and reversible. However, if experimental tubal inoculation is preceded by repeated inoculation of the fallopian tubes or cervix, a more intense salpingitis results and progresses to peritubular scarring. This suggests that in the female genital tract, as in the eye, repeated exposure to *C. trachomatis* leads to the greatest degree of tissue inflammation and damage.

The pathogenesis of PID attributable to mycoplasmas or other vaginal anaerobic or facultative organisms is less well studied. It is possible that other vaginal organisms implicated in PID often cause tubal infection in women whose tubes have already been damaged by a primary sexually transmitted pathogen (i.e., *N. gonorrhoeae* or *C. trachomatis*). The organisms and mycoplasmas implicated in PID are found in the vagina most often and in greatest concentration in bacterial vaginosis (nonspecific vaginitis), and there is epidemiologic evidence that bacterial vaginosis itself is a predisposing factor for PID (just as poor oral hygiene is a risk factor in aspiration pneumonia).

Certain other iatrogenic factors, such as dilatation and curettage or cesarean section, are known to increase the risk of PID in women with endocervical gonococcal or chlamydial infection. Recent evidence indicates that among women undergoing cesarean section, the presence of bacterial vaginosis increases the risk of postpartum endometritis.

CLINICAL MANIFESTATIONS Tuberculous salpingitis Unlike nontuberculous salpingitis, genital tuberculosis often occurs in older women, about half of whom are postmenopausal. In a large review of cases in Sweden, 38 percent had had previously diagnosed tuberculosis. The most common presenting symptoms were abnormal vaginal bleeding, pain (including dysmenorrhea), and infertility. Most had normal bimanual pelvic examinations, though about one-quarter had adnexal masses. The most common method of diagnosis was endometrial biopsy, showing tuberculous granulomas, often associated with a positive culture.

Nontuberculous salpingitis The evolution of symptoms classically proceeds from a mucopurulent vaginal discharge caused by

cervicitis—possibly associated with dysuria and frequency due to urethritis or with anorectal pain, tenesmus, rectal discharge, and bleeding due to proctitis—to midline abdominal pain and abnormal vaginal bleeding caused by endometritis, followed by bilateral lower abdominal and pelvic pain caused by salpingitis, with nausea and vomiting and increased abdominal tenderness caused by peritonitis. Some patients have diffuse abdominal pain caused by generalized peritonitis or pleuritic right upper quadrant pain caused by perihepatitis. The pattern in which symptoms evolve varies from patient to patient and is also related to the etiology of the PID.

The onset of IUD-associated PID is typically gradual and may be preceded by typical malodorous vaginal discharge characteristic of bacterial vaginosis. The onset of gonococcal PID has been more acute than that of chlamydial PID in some, but not all studies, and both are often associated with menses.

The abdominal pain is usually described as dull or aching. In some cases, pain is lacking or is atypical, and active inflammatory changes can be found in the course of an unrelated evaluation or procedure such as a tubal ligation or laparoscopic evaluation for infertility. Abnormal uterine bleeding precedes or coincides with the onset of pain in about 40 percent of women with PID, symptoms of urethritis occur in 20 percent, and symptoms of proctitis occasionally are seen in those with gonococcal or chlamydial infection.

Speculum examination shows evidence of mucopurulent cervicitis in the majority of women with gonococcal or chlamydial PID. Cervical motion tenderness is produced by stretching of the adnexal attachments on the side toward which the cervix is pushed. Bimanual examination reveals uterine fundal tenderness due to endometritis and abnormal adnexal tenderness due to salpingitis which is usually, but not necessarily, bilateral. Adnexal swelling is palpable in about one-half of women with acute salpingitis, but evaluation of the adnexae in a patient with marked tenderness is not reliable, even by an experienced examiner. An initial temperature >38°C is found in only about one-third of patients with acute salpingitis, and fever is not required for the diagnosis.

Laboratory findings include elevation of the erythrocyte sedimentation rate (ESR) in 75 percent and elevation of the peripheral white blood cell count in up to 60 percent of patients with acute salpingitis. Microscopic examination of a saline wet-mount preparation of vaginal fluid has revealed more than one polymorphonuclear leukocyte per vaginal epithelial cell, or findings consistent with bacterial vaginosis, in nearly all patients with laparoscopically confirmed salpingitis in Swedish studies. However, exceptions have not been uncommon in U.S. studies.

Certain clinical manifestations of acute PID have been correlated with etiologic findings. For example, the onset of salpingitis is related to menses in women with gonorrhea or chlamydial infection. Women with gonorrhea or *Chlamydia*-associated salpingitis are significantly younger than women with other forms of salpingitis. In a Swedish study, women with *Chlamydia*-associated salpingitis had a more indolent disease with mild symptoms of significantly longer duration and with less fever than women who had gonorrhea-associated salpingitis. It is suspected that for all recognized cases of symptomatic *Chlamydia* salpingitis, there is a comparable number of unrecognized cases of indolent subclinical *Chlamydia* salpingitis, and that subclinical chronic or recurrent *Chlamydia* salpingitis may be a major cause of infertility in women.

IUD-associated PID has been much less common since withdrawal of the Dalkon shield from the market. It tends to be indolent and is associated less often with fever, but more often with adnexal masses, than is PID not associated with IUD use.

Perihepatitis and periappendicitis Symptoms of perihepatitis, including pleuritic upper abdominal pain and tenderness, usually localized to the right upper quadrant, occur in 3 to 10 percent of women with acute PID. The onset of symptoms of perihepatitis occurs during or after onset of symptoms of PID and may overshadow the lower abdominal symptoms, leading to a mistaken diagnosis of cholecystitis. In perhaps 5 percent of cases of acute salpingitis, laparoscopy performed early reveals inflammation ranging from edema and erythema of the liver capsule to exudate with fibrinous adhesions between the visceral and parietal peritoneum. When treatment is delayed and laparoscopy is performed late, dense "violin-string" adhesions are seen over the liver; these cause chronic exertional or positional right upper quadrant pain when traction is placed on the adhesions. Although perihepatitis, also known as the *Fitz-Hugh–Curtis syndrome*, was for many years attributed to gonococcal PID, in recent studies most cases of perihepatitis have been associated with chlamydial salpingitis. In patients with chlamydial salpingitis, serum microimmunofluorescent antibody titers against *C. trachomatis* are typically much higher when perihepatitis is present than when it is absent, and it has been suggested that repeated chlamydial infections are responsible for perihepatitis.

Physical findings include right upper quadrant tenderness and usually include adnexal tenderness and cervicitis, even in patients whose symptoms are not suggestive of salpingitis.

Liver function tests are nearly always normal, since inflammation is largely limited to the liver capsule, usually sparing the parenchyma. Oral cholecystogram may show nonfunction of the gallbladder, but ultrasonography of the right upper quadrant is normal. The presence of mucopurulent cervicitis and pelvic tenderness in a young woman with subacute pleuritic right upper quadrant pain with normal ultrasonography of the gallbladder points to a diagnosis of perihepatitis.

Periappendicitis (appendiceal serositis without involvement of the intestinal mucosa) has been found in approximately 5 percent of patients undergoing appendectomy for suspected appendicitis and can occur as a complication of gonococcal or chlamydial salpingitis.

DIAGNOSIS Early diagnosis and initiation of therapy are essential to minimize tubal scarring. Appropriate treatment must not be withheld from patients who have an equivocal diagnosis. Since delay in therapy may lead to progression of tubal scarring, it is better to err on the side of overdiagnosis and overtreatment. On the other hand, it is essential to differentiate between salpingitis and other pelvic pathology, particularly surgical emergencies such as appendicitis and ectopic pregnancy.

No clinical or laboratory finding short of laparoscopy is pathognomonic for salpingitis, and there is reluctance to perform laparoscopy in all cases of suspected salpingitis. Most patients with acute PID have lower abdominal pain of less than 3 weeks' duration, pelvic tenderness on bimanual pelvic examination, and evidence of lower genital tract infection (e.g., white blood cells outnumber all other cells in the vaginal fluid). Approximately 60 percent of such patients have salpingitis at laparoscopy. Among the patients with these findings, a rectal temperature above 38°C, a palpable adnexal mass, and elevation of the ESR over 15 mm/h also raise the probability of salpingitis, which has been found at laparoscopy in 68 percent of patients with one of these additional findings, 90 percent of patients with two or more, and 96 percent of patients with three or more additional findings. However, only 17 percent of all patients with laparoscopy-confirmed salpingitis had all three additional findings.

Mucopurulent cervicitis is probably responsible for the presence of neutrophils in vaginal fluid in PID. In a woman with pelvic pain and tenderness, demonstration of an increased number of neutrophils (≥30 per 1000× microscopic field in strands of cervical mucus) increases the predictive value of a clinical diagnosis of acute PID.

Several clinical features other than the presence of cervicitis also favor the diagnosis of acute PID. These include onset with menses, history of recent mentrual bleeding, presence of an IUD, history of previous salpingitis, and exposure to a male with urethritis. Detection of polymorphonuclear leukocytes in fluid aspirated by culdocentesis supports a diagnosis of suspected salpingitis. Urethritis or proctitis may occur in chlamydial or gonococcal infection but also may represent a urinary tract infection or an intestinal source for the patient's symptoms. Early onset of nausea and vomiting favors appendicitis or other disorders of the gut. A missed menstrual period dictates evaluation for ectopic pregnancy. The more sensitive assays

for human beta-chorionic gonadotropin are usually positive. Ultrasonography is sometimes useful to identify tuboovarian abscess or pelvic abscess, and intravaginal ultrasound assessment of the tubes has recently been reported to show increased tubal diameter, intratubal fluid, or tubal wall thickening in salpingitis (confirmatory experience is needed).

Laparoscopy is the most specific method for diagnosis of acute salpingitis. Although laparoscopy may be normal if inflammation is limited to the endosalpinx or endometrium, patients with suspected PID who have normal laparoscopy have a better prognosis, with few, if any, sequelae, than patients who have abnormal laparoscopic findings. The primary and uncontested value of laparoscopy in women with lower abdominal pain is exclusion of other surgical problems. Table 89-2 clearly shows that the most common and serious problems that may be confused with salpingitis are usually unilateral. Unilateral pain or pelvic mass, though not incompatible with PID, is a strong indication for laparoscopy unless the clinical picture warrants laparotomy instead. Atypical clinical findings such as the absence of lower genital tract infection, a missed menstrual period, or failure to respond to appropriate therapy are other frequent indications for laparoscopy.

Laparoscopic criteria used for the diagnosis of salpingitis include (1) erythema of the fallopian tube, (2) edema of the fallopian tube, and (3) seropurulent exudate or fresh, easily lysed adhesions at the fimbriated end or on the serosal surface of a fallopian tube.

Endometrial biopsy is relatively sensitive and specific for the diagnosis of endometritis when the endometrial changes described above are found, and the presence of endometritis correlates well with the presence of salpingitis. Endometritis is found in at least three-fourths of women with laparoscopically confirmed salpingitis and is absent in women without PID.

The etiologic diagnosis of PID can be further studied by cultures or other tests on specimens obtained by endocervical swab, endometrial aspiration, or culdocentesis or by laparoscopy or laparotomy. Endocervical swab specimens should be examined by Gram's stain for neutrophils and gram-negative diplococci and by culture for *N. gonorrhoeae*. The sensitivity of Gram's stain is about 60 percent, and specificity is more than 95 percent, compared with culture. The endocervical swab specimen also should be tested for *C. trachomatis* by culture, immunofluorescence, or assays for chlamydial DNA or RNA. Although isolation of either *N. gonorrhoeae* or *C. trachomatis* from the cervix does not prove that either agent is also present in the upper genital tract, this finding strongly supports the diagnosis of PID. The clinical diagnosis of PID made by expert gynecologists is confirmed by laparoscopy or endometrial biopsy in only about 60 percent of all consecutive patients but in about 90 percent of those who also have positive cultures for *N. gonorrhoeae* or *C. trachomatis*. There is no evidence that isolation of anaerobes or facultative aerobes from the cervix or vagina correlates with the presence of these organisms in the upper genital tract in acute PID, but this has not been well studied. The value of culture of culdocentesis and endometrial aspirate specimens is disputed because of the risk of contamination

TABLE 89-2 Laparoscopic findings in patients with false-positive or false-negative clinical diagnoses of acute PID

False-positive clinical diagnosis		False-negative clinical diagnosis, unexpected PID at laparoscopy	
Laparoscopic diagnosis	Percent	Clinical diagnosis	Percent
Acute appendicitis	24	Ovarian tumor	20
Endometriosis	16	Acute appendicitis	18
Corpus luteum bleeding	12	Ectopic pregnancy	16
Ectopic pregnancy	11	Chronic salpingitis	6
Pelvic adhesions only	7	Acute peritonitis	6
Benign ovarian tumor	7	Endometriosis	5
Chronic salpingitis	6	Uterine myoma	5
Miscellaneous	15	Atypical pelvic pain	6
		Miscellaneous	6

SOURCE: L Jacobsen and L Weström, Am J Obstet Gynecol 105:1088, 1969.

of the specimen with vaginal flora. When laparoscopy is performed, material can be obtained directly from the cul-de-sac or the fimbriated opening of the tube or by tubal aspiration if pyosalpinx is present. Such specimens should be cultured for anaeorbic and facultative pathogens, as well as for *N. gonorrhoeae* and *C. trachomatis*.

TREATMENT Hospitalization should be considered in all women with PID and is strongly recommended when (1) the diagnosis is uncertain, (2) surgical emergencies such as appendicitis and ectopic pregnancy must be excluded, (3) a pelvic abscess is suspected, (4) severe illness precludes outpatient management, (5) the patient is pregnant, (6) the patient is an adolescent (among adolescents, compliance is less predictable), (7) the patient is assessed as unable to follow or tolerate an outpatient regimen, (8) the patient has failed to respond to outpatient therapy, or (9) clinical follow-up after 48 to 72 h of instituting antibiotic treatment cannot be arranged. Treatment should cover *N. gonorrhoeae*, *C. trachomatis*, gram-negative facultative bacteria (especially *E. coli*), vaginal anaerobes, and group B streptococcus. No single agent is active against the entire spectrum of pathogens (Table 89-3). Several antimicrobial combinations do provide a broad spectrum of activity against the major pathogens in vitro, but many have not been adequately evaluated for clinical efficacy in PID.

A recent survey showed that physician antibiotic prescribing for PID improved from 1979 (when only 32 percent of patients received an antichlamydial drug) to 1989 (when 74 percent received such treatment). However, in 1989, only 21 percent of patients received a two-drug regimen that included an antichlamydial agent.

Examples of combination regimens with broad activity against major pathogens in PID Clinicians have had extensive experience with the following two inpatient regimens:

1 Doxycycline 100 mg, twice a day, IV, plus cefoxitin 2.0 g, four times a day, IV, or cefotetan 2.0 g, every 12 h, IV. These drugs should be continued IV for at least 48 h after the patient improves. Doxycycline should be continued in a dose of 100 mg by mouth, twice a day, after discharge from the hospital to complete 14 days of therapy. This regimen provides excellent coverage for *N. gonorrhoeae*, including penicillinase-producing *N. gonorrhoeae* (PPNG), and *C. trachomatis*.

2 Clindamycin 900 mg, every 8 h, IV, plus gentamicin 2.0 mg/kg, IV, followed by 1.5 mg/kg, every 8 h, IV, in patients with normal renal function. These drugs should be continued for at least 48 h after the patient improves. After discharge from the hospital, doxycycline 100 mg orally, twice a day, should be given to complete 14 days of therapy. This regimen provides good activity against anaerobes and facultative gram-negative rods and is active against *C. trachomatis* and *N. gonorrhoeae*. Doxycycline provides definitive therapy for chlamydial infection.

Patients who are not hospitalized also should receive a combined regimen with broad activity, such as ceftriaxone 250 mg, IM, followed by doxycycline, 100 mg, by mouth, twice a day for 14 days. Cefoxitin, 2.0 g, IM, given concurrently with probenecid 1.0 g, orally, can be used in place of ceftriaxone. Tetracycline also can be used in a dose of 500 mg, four times·a day, in place of doxycycline but requires more frequent dosing, which is a major drawback in the treatment of PID. An alternative outpatient regimen, which requires more evaluation but which provides good coverage of the major pathogens, is ofloxacin, 400 mg, twice daily, plus either metronidazole, 500 mg, twice daily, or clindamycin, 450 mg, four times daily, for 14 days.

Management of sexual partners All persons who are sexual partners of patients with PID should be examined for STD and promptly treated with a regimen effective against uncomplicated gonococcal and chlamydial infection. Treatment of PID should be considered inadequate until sexual partners have been properly evaluated and treated.

Follow-up All patients who are treated as outpatients should be clinically reevaluated in 48 to 72 h. Those not responding favorably should be hospitalized. A culture for *N. gonorrhoeae* or *C. trachomatis* to test whether cure has been achieved should be performed as needed.

Removal of an intrauterine device Although possible benefit of IUD removal on the response of acute salpingitis to antimicrobial therapy and on the risk of recurrent salpingitis has not been proven, removal of the IUD soon after antimicrobial therapy has been initiated seems reasonable. When an IUD is removed, contraceptive counseling is necessary.

Surgery Surgery is necessary only rarely for treatment of salpingitis, except in the face of life-threatening infection such as rupture or threatened rupture of a tuboovarian abscess or for drainage of an abscess. Ultrasonography is useful for diagnosing and following pelvic abscesses. When surgery is performed, conservative procedures are usually sufficient. Pelvic abscesses often can be drained by posterior colpotomy, and peritoneal lavage can be used if there is generalized peritonitis.

PROGNOSIS In a cooperative trial in the United States, nearly 20 percent of women treated for PID on an ambulatory basis with IM penicillin followed by a 10-day course of ampicillin or with a 10-day course of tetracycline alone were judged to be clinical failures.

Among 900 women who underwent long-term follow-up for a mean period of 8 years after successful treatment of the acute episode with various regimens in Sweden, late sequelae included infertility due to bilateral tubal occlusion, ectopic pregnancy due to tubal scarring without occlusion, chronic pelvic pain, and recurrent salpingitis. Chronic pain lasting longer than 6 months was seen in 18 percent of patients and infertility due to tubal occlusion in 17 percent; 4 percent of pregnancies that did occur were ectopic, representing approximately a sixfold increase over the expected rate of ectopic pregnancies. The rate of infertility after salpingitis was found to be related to age of the patient, duration of symptoms when treatment was started, severity of salpingitis by laparoscopy at the time of

TABLE 89-3 Relative activities of the antimicrobial agents most commonly used to treat PID

| | | | Vaginal anaerobes | | Facultative | |
	N. gonorrhoeae	C. trachomatis	GPC*	GNR†	GNR	M. hominis
Ampicillin/amoxicillin	2+	2+	4+	2+	2+	0
Tetracycline HCl	2+	4+	4+	2+	2+	2+
Doxycycline	2+	4+	4+	3+	2+	2+
Cefoxitin, cefotetan	3+	0	4+	3+	4+	0
Ceftriaxone	4+	0	3+	2+	4+	0
Gentamicin/tobramycin	2+	0	1+	0	4+	2+?
Ofloxacin	4+	3+	1+	1+	4+	1+
Clindamycin	1+	3+	4+	4+	0	3+
Metronidazole	0	0	4+	4+	0	0

* GPC = Gram-positive cocci (peptostreptococci).
† GNR = Gram-negative rods (anaerobic GNR include *Prevotella*; facultative GNR include Enterobacteriaceae, *H. influenzae*).
NOTE: No single antimicrobial agent offers optimal activity against all of these pathogens, but certain combinations (e.g., cefoxitin plus doxycycline, gentamicin plus clindamycin) or ofloxacin plus metronidazole have complementary activity. Relative activity is indicated on a 0→4+ scale.

diagnosis, and number of episodes of salpingitis. The rate of infertility due to tubal occlusion among women exposed to a chance of pregnancy was 14 percent for women 15 to 24 years of age and 26 percent for women 25 to 34 years of age; the risk for women of all ages combined was 11 percent after one episode of salpingitis, 23 percent after two episodes, and 54 percent after three or more episodes. The risk of infertility after gonococcal salpingitis was comparable with the risk after chlamydial salpingitis in one small prospective study. A study of outcomes of PID at the University of Washington found a sevenfold increase in risk of ectopic pregnancy and an eightfold increase in hysterectomies after PID.

A striking relationship also has been shown in several countries between infertility due to tubal occlusion and the prevalence and titer of antibody to *C. trachomatis*. Recurrent salpingitis has been seen in approximately 15 to 25 percent of women treated for salpingitis in various studies.

PREVENTION   Prevention of PID depends first on the effective control of gonococcal and chlamydial infection. Effective methods include promotion of changes in sexual behavior and use of barrier contraceptives while providing ready access to modern methods of diagnosis and effective treatment of sex partners to control further spread. The decline in popularity of the intrauterine device, particularly in nulliparous women, has undoubtedly helped to reduce the incidence of PID. It is also possible, but not proven, that use of oral contraceptives and avoidance of vaginal douching may reduce the risk of PID.

The complications of salpingitis can be minimized by early diagnosis and prompt treatment. It seems logical, but is unproven, that broad-spectrum therapy effective against all of the common causes of PID would offer the best outcome. Similarly, hospitalization to ensure rest and adequate compliance may improve the rather dismal long-term prognosis for tubal function. One placebo-controlled study showed that concurrent anti-inflammatory therapy with prednisolone hastened the reduction of acute inflammatory changes but did not improve the end results as measured by fertility, hysterosalpingographic findings, or chronic pain. However, the potential value of anti-inflammatory therapy remains to be evaluated adequately.

REFERENCES

CATES WJ et al: Worldwide patterns of infertility: Is Africa different? Lancet 2:596, 1985

CENTERS FOR DISEASE CONTROL: Policy guidelines for the prevention and management of pelvic inflammatory disease. Morb Mort Week Rep 40RR-5:1, 1992

ESCHENBACH DA et al: Polymicrobial etiology of acute pelvic inflammatory disease. N. Engl J Med 293:166, 1975

FALK V et al: Genital tuberculosis in women. Am J Obstet Gynecol 138:974, 1980

GERMAINE A et al: *Reproductive Tract Infections: Global Impact and Priorities for Women's Reproductive Health*. New York, Plenum, 1992

KIVIAT N et al: Endometrial histopathology in patients with culture-proven upper genital tract infection and laparoscopically diagnosed acute salpingitis. Am J Surg Pathol 14:167, 1990

LANDERS DV et al: Combination antimicrobial therapy in the treatment of acute pelvic inflammatory disease. Am J Obstet Gynecol 164:849, 1991

MÅRDH PA et al: *Chlamydia trachomatis* infection in patients with acute salpingitis. N Engl J Med 296:1377, 1977

PLUMMER FA et al: Postpartum upper genital tract infections in Nairobi, Kenya: Epidemiology, etiology, and risk factors. J Infect Dis 156:92, 1987

REED SD et al: Antibiotic treatment of tuboovarian abscess: Comparison of broad-spectrum beta-lactam agents versus clindamycin-containing regimens. Am J Obstet Gynecol 164:1556, 1991

SOPER DE et al: Microbial etiology of urban emergency department acute salpingitis: Treatment with ofloxacin. Am J Obstet Gynecol 167:653, 1992

ST JOHN RK, BROWN ST (eds): International symposium on pelvic inflammatory disease. Am J Obstet Gynecol 138:845, 1980

SVENSSON L et al: Differences in some clinical and laboratory parameters in acute salpingitis related to culture and serologic findings. Am J Obstet Gynecol 138:1017, 1980

——— et al: Infertility after acute salpingitis—With special reference to *Chlamydia trachomatis*–associated infections. Fertil Steril 40:322, 1983

WASHINGTON AE, KATZ P: Cost of and payment source for pelvic inflammatory disease: Trends and projections, 1983 through 2000. JAMA 266:2565, 1991

WASSERHEIT JN et al: Microbial causes of proven pelvic inflammatory disease and efficacy of clindamycin with tobramycin. Ann Intern Med 104:187, 1986

WØLNER-HANSSEN P et al: Atypical pelvic inflammatory disease: Subacute, chronic, or subclinical upper genital tract infections in women, in *Sexually Transmitted Diseases*, 2d ed, KK Holmes et al (eds). New York, McGraw-Hill 1990, pp 615–620

90   URINARY TRACT INFECTIONS AND PYELONEPHRITIS

WALTER E. STAMM

DEFINITIONS   Acute infections of the urinary tract can be subdivided into two general anatomic categories: lower tract infection (urethritis, cystitis, and prostatitis) and upper tract infection (acute pyelonephritis and intrarenal and perinephric abscesses). Infections at these various sites may occur together or independently and may be asymptomatic or present as the clinical syndromes outlined below. Infections of the urethra and bladder are often considered superficial (or mucosal) infections, while prostatitis, pyelonephritis, and renal suppuration signify tissue invasion.

Microbiologically, urinary tract infection exists when pathogenic microorganisms are detected in the urine, urethra, bladder, kidney, or prostate. In most instances, growth of more than 10^5 organisms per milliliter from a properly collected midstream "clean catch" urine sample indicates infection. However, significant bacteriuria may be absent in some circumstances when true urinary infection exists. Especially in symptomatic patients, a smaller number of bacteria (10^2 to 10^4 per milliliter of midstream urine) may accompany infection. In urine specimens obtained by suprapubic aspiration or "in and out" catheterization, or from a patient with an indwelling catheter, colony counts of 10^2 to 10^4 per milliliter generally indicate infection. Conversely, colony counts in excess of 10^5 per milliliter of midstream urine are occasionally due to specimen contamination, especially when multiple species are present.

Recurrent infections after antibiotic therapy can be due to persistence of the originally infecting strain, as judged by species identification, serotype, and antibiogram, or to reinfection with a new strain. "Same strain" recurrent infections that occur within 2 weeks of cessation of therapy can result from unresolved renal or prostatic infection (termed *relapse*) or from persistent vaginal colonization that leads to rapid reinfection of the bladder.

Symptoms of dysuria, urgency, and frequency unaccompanied by significant bacteriuria have been termed the *acute urethral syndrome*. Although widely used, this term lacks anatomic precision because many cases of urethral syndrome are actually bladder infections. Moreover, since the causative agent can usually be identified in these patients, the term *syndrome*, implying unknown causation, is inappropriate.

Chronic pyelonephritis refers to chronic interstitial nephritis believed to result from bacterial infection of the kidney (see Chap. 242). Many noninfectious diseases also cause an interstitial nephritis indistinguishable pathologically from chronic pyelonephritis.

ACUTE INFECTIONS OF THE URINARY TRACT: URETHRITIS, CYSTITIS, AND PYELONEPHRITIS

EPIDEMIOLOGY   Epidemiologically, urinary tract infections should be subdivided into catheter-associated (or nosocomial) infections and non-catheter-associated (or community-acquired) infections. In either category, infections may be symptomatic or asymptomatic. Acute infections in noncatheterized patients are very common, especially in women, and account for over 6 million office visits annually in the United States. These infections occur in 1 to 3 percent of schoolgirls and then increase markedly in incidence with the onset of sexual activity in adolescence. The vast majority of acute symptomatic infections occur in young women. Acute symptomatic urinary infections are unusual in men under the age of 50. The occurrence of asymptomatic bacteriuria parallels that of symptomatic infection and is rare in men under 50 but is common in women between the ages of 20 and 50. Asymptomatic bacteriuria is very common in elderly men and women, being identified in up to 40 to 50 percent of patients in some studies.

ETIOLOGY   Many different microorganisms can infect the urinary tract, but by far the most common agents are the gram-negative bacilli. *Escherichia coli* causes approximately 80 percent of acute infections in patients without catheters, urologic abnormalities, or calculi. Other gram-negative rods, especially *Proteus* and *Klebsiella* and occasionally *Enterobacter*, account for a smaller proportion of uncomplicated infections. These organisms, plus *Serratia* and *Pseudomonas*, assume increasing importance in recurrent infections and infections associated with urologic manipulation, calculi, or obstruction. They play a major role in nosocomial, catheter-associated infections (see below). *Proteus* species, by virtue of urease production, and *Klebsiella* species, through production of extracellular slime and polysaccharides, predispose to stone formation and are isolated more frequently from patients with calculi.

Gram-positive cocci play a lesser role in urinary tract infections. However, *Staphylococcus saprophyticus*, a novobiocin-resistant, co-agulase-negative staphylococcus, accounts for 10 to 15 percent of acute symptomatic urinary tract infections in young females. Enterococci and *Staphylococcus aureus* cause infections in patients with renal stones or previous instrumentation. Isolation of *S. aureus* from the urine should arouse suspicion of bacteremic infection of the kidney.

About one-third of women with dysuria and frequency have either a nonsignificant number of bacteria in midstream urine cultures or completely sterile cultures and have been previously defined as having the urethral syndrome. About three-quarters of these women have pyuria, while one-quarter have no pyuria and little objective evidence of infection. In the women with pyuria, two groups of pathogens account for the majority of infections. Low quantities (10^2 to 10^4 bacteria per milliliter) of typical bacterial uropathogens such as *E. coli*, *S. saprophyticus*, *Klebsiella*, or *Proteus* in midstream urine specimens are found in the majority of these women. They are probably the causative agents in these women because they can usually be isolated from a suprapubic aspirate, are associated with pyuria, and respond to appropriate antimicrobial therapy. In other women with acute urinary symptoms, pyuria, and sterile urine (even on suprapubic aspiration), sexually transmitted urethritis-producing agents such as *Chlamydia trachomatis*, *Neisseria gonorrhoeae*, and herpes simplex virus are important etiologic agents. These sexually transmitted agents are most frequently found in young, sexually active women with new sexual partners.

The causative role of nonbacterial pathogens in urinary tract infections remains poorly defined. *Ureaplasma urealyticum* has frequently been isolated from the urethra and urine of patients with acute dysuria and frequency but is also found in many patients without urinary symptoms. Thus ureaplasmas probably account for some cases of urethritis and cystitis. *U. urealyticum*, as well as *Mycoplasma hominis*, has also been isolated from prostatic and renal tissues in patients with acute prostatitis and pyelonephritis and probably accounts for some of these infections. Adenoviruses cause acute hemorrhagic cystitis in children and in some young adults, often in epidemics. Although many other viruses can be isolated from urine (cytomegalovirus, Jakob-Creutzfeldt virus, and others), they are not thought to cause urinary infection. *Candida* and other fungal species often colonize the urine of catheterized patients or diabetics and in some patients progress to symptomatic invasive infection (see Chap. 166). Mycobacterial infection of the genitourinary tract is discussed in Chap. 130.

PATHOGENESIS AND SOURCES OF INFECTION   The urinary tract should be viewed as a single anatomic unit connected by a continuous column of urine that extends from the urethra to the kidney. In the vast majority of infections, bacteria gain access to the bladder via the urethra. Ascent of bacteria from the bladder may then follow and is probably the usual pathway for most renal parenchymal infections.

The vaginal introitus and distal urethra are normally colonized with diphtheroids, streptococcal species, lactobacilli, and staphylococcal species but not with the enteric gram-negative bacilli that commonly cause urinary tract infections. In females prone to development of cystitis, however, enteric gram-negative organisms residing in the bowel colonize the introitus, the periurethral skin, and the distal urethra prior to and during episodes of bacteriuria. Factors predisposing to periurethral colonization with gram-negative bacilli remain poorly understood but probably involve alteration of the normal perineal flora by antibiotics, other genital infections, or contraceptives, especially diaphragms and spermicide. Small numbers of periurethral bacteria probably gain entry to the bladder frequently, facilitated in some women by urethral massage during intercourse. Whether bladder infection ensues then depends on interaction between the pathogenicity of the strain, the inoculum size, and local and systemic host defense mechanisms.

Under normal circumstances, bacteria placed in the bladder are rapidly cleared. This results partly from the flushing and dilutional effects of voiding but also from direct antibacterial properties of urine and the bladder mucosa. Due mostly to high urea concentration and high osmolarity, the bladder urine of many normal persons inhibits or kills bacteria. Prostatic secretions possess antibacterial properties as well. Polymorphonuclear leukocytes in the bladder wall also appear to play a role in clearing bacteriuria. The role of locally produced antibody remains unclear.

Hematogenous pyelonephritis occurs most often in debilitated patients who either have chronic illnesses or are receiving immunosuppressive therapy. Staphylococcal pyelonephritis may follow bacteremia from distant foci of infection in the bone, skin, endothelium, or elsewhere.

CONDITIONS AFFECTING PATHOGENESIS   **Gender and sexual activity**   The female urethra appears particularly prone to colonization with colonic gram-negative bacilli, owing to its proximity to the anus, its short length (about 4 cm), and its termination beneath the labia. Urethral massage, as occurs during sexual intercourse, causes introduction of bacteria into the bladder and appears to be important in the pathogenesis of urinary infections in younger women. (Voiding after intercourse has been shown to reduce the risk of cystitis, probably because it promotes eradication of bacteria introduced during intercourse.) In addition, diaphragm and spermicide use dramatically alter the normal introital bacterial flora and have been associated with a marked increase in vaginal colonization with *E. coli* and risk of urinary infection. In males, prostatitis or urethral obstruction due to prostatic hypertrophy are important factors predisposing to bacteriuria. Homosexuality also predisposes to an increased risk of cystitis, probably associated with rectal intercourse. HIV-infected men with CD-4-positive T cell counts less than 200 cells per microliter have recently been shown to have an increased risk of both bacteriuria and symptomatic urinary tract infection. Finally, lack of circumcision has been identified as a risk factor for urinary tract infection in both neonates and young men.

Pregnancy   Depending on socioeconomic status, urinary infections are detected in 2 to 8 percent of pregnant women. In particular, symptomatic upper tract infections occur more commonly during pregnancy; fully 20 to 30 percent of pregnant women with asymptomatic bacteriuria subsequently develop pyelonephritis. This predisposition to upper tract infection during pregnancy results from the decreased ureteral tone, decreased ureteral peristalsis, and temporary incompetence of the vesicoureteral valves seen in pregnancy. Bladder catheterization during or after delivery causes additional infections. Cystitis and pyelonephritis are no more common in women with toxemia of pregnancy than in other pregnant women. An increased prevalence of prematurity and newborn mortality may result from urinary infections during pregnancy, particularly those involving the upper urinary tract.

Obstruction   Any impediment to the free flow of urine—tumor, stricture, stone, or prostatic hypertrophy—results in hydronephrosis and a greatly increased frequency of urinary tract infection. Infection superimposed on urinary tract obstruction may lead to rapid destruction of renal tissue. It is of utmost importance, therefore, when infection is present, to repair obstructive lesions. On the other hand, with minor degrees of obstruction that are not progressive or associated with infection, great caution should be exercised in attempting surgical correction. The introduction of infection in such patients may be more damaging than uncorrected minor obstructions that do not significantly impair renal function.

Neurogenic bladder dysfunction   Interference with the nerve supply to the bladder, as in spinal cord injury, tabes dorsalis, multiple sclerosis, diabetes, or other diseases, may be associated with urinary tract infection. The infection may be initiated by the use of catheters for bladder drainage and is favored by the prolonged stasis of urine in the bladder. An additional factor often present in these patients is bone demineralization due to immobilization, which causes hypercalciuria, calculus formation, and obstructive uropathy.

Vesicoureteral reflux   This condition is defined as reflux of urine from the bladder cavity up into the ureters and sometimes into the renal pelvis. It occurs during voiding or with elevation of pressure in the bladder. In practice, vesicoureteral reflux exists when retrograde movement of radiopaque or radioactive material can be demonstrated during a voiding cystourethrogram. An anatomically impaired vesicoureteral junction facilitates reflux of bacteria and thus upper tract infection. However, since a fluid connection between the bladder and kidney always exists even in the normal urinary system, some retrograde movement of bacteria probably occurs during infection but is not detected by radiologic techniques.

Vesicoureteral reflux is common in children with anatomic abnormalities of the urinary tract and in children with anatomically normal but infected urinary tracts. In the latter group, reflux disappears with advancing age and probably results from causes other than urinary infection. Long-term follow-up of children with urinary tract infection who were found to have reflux establishes that renal damage correlates with marked reflux, not with infection.

The routine search for reflux would be aided by development of noninvasive tests applicable to young children, where the need is greatest. In the meantime, it appears reasonable to search for reflux in anyone with unexplained failure of renal growth or renal scarring, because urinary tract infection per se is an insufficient explanation for these abnormalities. On the other hand, it is doubtful that all children with recurrent urinary tract infections but normal urinary tracts on pyelography should be subjected to voiding cystoureterography merely to detect the rare patient with marked reflux that did not reveal itself on the intravenous pyelogram.

Bacterial virulence factors   Bacterial virulence factors influence the likelihood that a given strain, once introduced into the bladder, will cause urinary tract infection. Not all *E. coli* are equally able to infect the intact urinary tract. The majority of strains that cause symptomatic urinary tract infections in noncatheterized patients belong to a small number of specific O, K, and H serogroups, produce hemolysin, and share certain other "uropathogenic" properties. Adherence of bacteria to uroepithelial cells is a critical first step in the initiation of infection. For both *E. coli* and *Proteus*, fimbriae (hairlike surface proteinaceous appendages) mediate bacterial attachment to specific receptors on epithelial cells. Nearly all *E. coli* strains that cause pyelonephritis in patients with anatomically normal urinary tracts possess a particular pilus (the P pilus or gal-gal pilus) that mediates attachment to the digalactoside portion of glycosphingolipids present on uroepithelium. Strains that produce pyelonephritis are also usually hemolysin producers, have aerobactin (a siderophore for scavenging iron), and are resistant to the bactericidal action of human serum. Since most strains that produce acute pyelonephritis in the intact host possess all or nearly all these virulence factors, the concept has arisen that a small number of uropathogenic clones cause most such cases of infection. In patients with structural or functional abnormalities of the urinary tract, infections are frequently caused by bacterial strains that lack these uropathogenic properties, implying that these properties are not needed for infection of the compromised urinary tract.

Genetic factors   Increasing evidence suggests that host genetic factors influence susceptibility to urinary infection. The number and type of receptors on uroepithelial cells to which bacteria may attach are at least in part genetically determined. Many of these structures to which uropathogenic bacteria bind are components of blood group antigens and are present on erythrocytes and uroepithelial cells. For example, P fimbriae mediate attachment of *E. coli* to P-positive erythrocytes and are present on nearly all strains causing acute uncomplicated pyelonephritis. Conversely, P blood group–negative individuals, who lack these receptors, have a decreased likelihood of pyelonephritis. It also has been demonstrated that nonsecretors of blood group antigens may have an increased risk of recurrent urinary infection, which may relate to a different profile of genetically determined glycolipids that are present on the uroepithelial cells of nonsecretors.

LOCALIZATION OF INFECTION   Infections involving the upper urinary tract usually cause a significant rise in serum antibodies directed against the O antigen of the infecting strain. They also produce a temporary defect in renal concentrating ability in many patients and may be associated with formation of leukocyte casts. Lower tract infections rarely result in increased antibody titers, concentrating defects, or white cell casts. Unfortunately, these methods of distinguishing renal parenchymal infection from cystitis are neither reliable nor convenient enough for routine clinical use. More sensitive tests for distinguishing pyelonephritis from cystitis (bilateral ureteral catheterization and the bladder wash-out technique originated by Fairley) are inherently invasive and too complex for routine clinical practice. A simpler, noninvasive test to separate upper and lower tract infections based on antibody coating of bacteria in the urine does not have sufficient sensitivity and specificity to be of value in the routine clinical management of patients. An elevated C-reactive protein often accompanies acute pyelonephritis and rarely is seen in cystitis, but this acute-phase reactant is nonspecific and occurs in infections other than pyelonephritis as well.

CLINICAL PRESENTATION   Clinical signs and symptoms cannot be relied on to diagnose urinary tract infection accurately or to localize the site of infection. Many patients with significant bacteriuria (including some with upper tract infection) have no symptoms at all. Of those with significant bacteriuria and symptoms of cystitis, about two-thirds have lower tract infection and about one-third have clinically silent upper tract infection that is evident only upon performing localization studies. Clinical symptoms and signs of pyelonephritis, though usually suggestive, do not always indicate upper tract infection. Finally, among women presenting with acute dysuria and frequency, only 60 to 70 percent have significant bacteriuria, but the majority of those without significant bacteriuria also have urinary tract or urethral infections.

Enumeration of the number and type of bacteria in the urine is an extremely important diagnostic procedure. In symptomatic infections of the urinary tract, uropathogenic bacteria are usually demonstrable in the urine in large numbers. Quantitative estimation of the number of bacteria in voided urine specimens as a rule makes it possible to distinguish contaminants from true bacteriuria, and 10^5 or more bacteria per milliliter has been the criterion traditionally used for this purpose. However, in symptomatic women with pyuria, bacterial colony counts of 10^2 to 10^4 *E. coli*, *Klebsiella*, *Proteus*, or *S. saprophyticus* per milliliter of midstream urine usually indicate infection, not contamination, and should not be disregarded. In asymptomatic patients, two or three consecutive urine specimens should be examined bacteriologically before instituting therapy, and 10^5 or more per milliliter of a single species should be demonstrable in the repeated specimens. Since the large number of bacteria in the bladder urine is due in part to bacterial multiplication during residence in the bladder cavity, samples of urine from the ureters or renal pelvis may contain fewer than 10^5 bacteria per milliliter and yet indicate infection. Similarly, the presence of bacteriuria of any degree in suprapubic aspirates or of 10^2 or more bacteria per milliliter of urine obtained by catheterization usually indicates infection. In some circumstances (antibiotics, high urea concentration, high osmolarity, low pH), urine will inhibit bacterial multiplication, resulting in a lower number of bacteria in the presence of infection. For this reason, antiseptic solutions should not be used in washing the periurethral area prior to collection of the urine specimen. Water diuresis or recent voiding also reduces the bacterial counts in urine.

Rapid methods of detection of bacteriuria have been developed as alternatives to standard culture methods. They detect bacterial growth using photometry, bioluminescence, or other means and provide results rapidly, usually in 1 to 2 h. These methods generally achieve a sensitivity of 95 to 98 percent and >99 percent negative predictive value as compared with urine cultures when bacteriuria is defined as 10^5 colony forming units per milliliter. However, the sensitivity of these tests falls to 60 to 80 percent when bacteriuria of 10^2 to 10^4 colony forming units per milliliter is the standard of comparison.

Microscopy of urine from symptomatic patients can be of great diagnostic value. Microscopic bacteriuria, which is best assessed using Gram-stained, uncentrifuged urine, is found in over 90 percent of specimens from patients whose infections have colony counts of 10^5 per milliliter and is a very specific finding. However, bacteria cannot usually be detected microscopically in lower colony count infections (10^2 to 10^4 per milliliter). The presence of bacteria on urinary microscopy is firm evidence of infection, but its absence does not exclude the diagnosis. When carefully sought using a chamber count microscopy method, pyuria is a highly sensitive indicator of urinary tract infection in symptomatic patients. Pyuria is present in nearly all patients with acute bacterial urinary tract infection, and its absence should cause the diagnosis to be questioned. The leukocyte esterase "dipstick" method is less sensitive than microscopy in identifying pyuria but is a useful alternative where microscopy is not available.

Cystitis Patients with dysuria, frequency, urgency, and suprapubic pain usually have cystitis. The urine often becomes grossly cloudy, malodorous, and, in about 30 percent of cases, bloody. White cells and bacteria should be present on examination of the unspun urine in most patients. However, some women with cystitis have only 10^2 to 10^4 bacteria per milliliter of urine, which cannot be seen on a Gram stain of unspun urine. Physical examination generally reveals only a tender urethra or suprapubic tenderness. If a genital lesion or a vaginal discharge is present, especially with fewer than 10^5 bacteria per milliliter on culture, causes of urethritis, vaginitis, or cervicitis such as *C. trachomatis*, gonorrhea, *Trichomonas, Candida*, and herpes simplex virus should be considered. Prominent systemic manifestations such as temperature >38.3°C (101°F), nausea, vomiting, and costovertebral angle tenderness usually indicate concomitant renal infection. However, the absence of these findings does not ensure that infection is limited to the bladder and urethra.

Acute pyelonephritis Symptoms generally develop rapidly over a few hours or a day and include temperature ≥39.4°C (103°F), shaking chills, nausea, vomiting, and diarrhea. Symptoms of cystitis may or may not be present. Besides fever, tachycardia, and generalized muscle tenderness, physical examination reveals marked tenderness on deep pressure in one or both costovertebral areas or on deep abdominal palpation. In some patients, signs and symptoms of gram-negative sepsis predominate. Most patients have significant leukocytosis, pyuria with leukocyte casts in the urine, and bacteria on a Gram stain of unspun urine. Hematuria may be present during the acute phase of the disease, but if it persists after acute manifestations of infection have subsided, a stone, tumor, or tuberculosis should be considered.

Except in individuals with papillary necrosis or urinary obstruction, the manifestations of acute pyelonephritis usually subside within a few days, even without specific antibacterial therapy. However, despite the absence of symptoms, bacteriuria or pyuria may persist. With severe pyelonephritis, fever subsides more slowly and may not disappear for several days, even after appropriate antibiotic treatment has been instituted.

Urethritis Approximately 30 percent of women with acute dysuria, frequency, and pyuria have midstream urine cultures that show either no growth or nonsignificant bacterial growth. Clinically, these women cannot be readily distinguished from those with cystitis. In these women, distinction should be made between those with sexually transmitted pathogens such as *C. trachomatis, Neisseria gonorrhoeae*, or herpes simplex virus, and those with low-count *E. coli* or staphylococcal infection of the urethra and bladder. Women with a gradual onset of illness, no hematuria, no suprapubic pain, and a history of more than 7 days of symptoms should be suspected of having chlamydial or gonococcal infection. The additional history of a recent sex partner change, especially if the patient's partner has recently had chlamydial or gonococcal urethritis, should heighten the suspicion of a sexually transmitted infection, as would the finding of mucopurulent cervicitis. Gross hematuria, suprapubic pain, abrupt onset of illness, a duration of illness of less than 3 days, and a history of previous urinary tract infections favor *E. coli* or staphylococcal infection.

Catheter-associated urinary tract infections Bacteriuria occurs in at least 10 to 15 percent of hospitalized patients with indwelling urethral catheters. The risk of infection is about 3 to 5 percent per day of catheterization. *Proteus, Pseudomonas, Klebsiella*, and *Serratia*, in addition to *E. coli*, usually cause these infections. Many infecting strains show marked antimicrobial resistance compared with organisms that cause community-acquired urinary infections. Factors associated with an increased risk of infection include female sex, lengthy period of catheterization, severe underlying illness, disconnection of the catheter and drainage tube, other types of faulty catheter care, and absence of systemic antimicrobials.

Infection occurs when bacteria reach the bladder by one of two routes: by migrating through the column of urine in the catheter lumen (intraluminal route) or by moving up the mucous sheath outside the catheter (periurethral route). Hospital-acquired pathogens reach the patient's catheter or urine-collecting system on the hands of hospital personnel, in contaminated solutions or irrigants, and via contaminated instruments or disinfectants. Entry of bacteria into the catheter system usually occurs at the catheter–collecting tube junction or at the drainage bag portal. Bacteria then ascend intraluminally into the bladder within 24 to 72 h. Alternatively, the patient's own bowel flora colonize the perineal skin and periurethral area and reach the bladder via the external surface of the catheter. This route is particularly common in women. Recent studies have demonstrated the important role of attachment and growth of bacteria on the inner surface of the catheter in the pathogenesis of catheter-associated urinary tract infection. Such bacteria growing in biofilms on the inner surface of the catheter eventually produce encrustations consisting of bacteria, bacterial glycocalyxes, host urinary proteins, and urinary salts. Encrustations provide a refuge for bacteria and may protect them from antimicrobials and phagocytes.

Clinically, most catheter-associated infections cause minimal symptoms and no fever and often resolve after withdrawal of the catheter. The frequency of upper tract infection associated with catheter-induced bacteriuria is unknown. Gram-negative bacteremia, which follows 1 to 2 percent of cases of catheter-associated bacteriuria, is the most significant recognized complication of catheter-induced urinary infections. The catheterized urinary tract has repeatedly been demonstrated to be the most common source of gram-negative bacteremia in hospitalized patients. It also has been suggested that bacteriuria in hospitalized catheterized patients is associated with an adjusted increased relative risk of death of approximately threefold compared with similar patients without bacteriuria.

Catheter-associated urinary tract infections can be partially prevented in patients catheterized less than 2 weeks by use of a sterile closed collecting system, by attention to aseptic technique during insertion and care of the catheter, and by measures to minimize cross-infection. Other preventive approaches, including short courses of systemic antimicrobials, topically applied periurethral antimicrobial ointments, preconnected catheter–drainage tube units, and antimicrobials added to the drainage bag, have all been protective in one or more controlled trials but are not recommended for general use. Despite precautions, the majority of patients catheterized longer than

2 weeks eventually develop bacteriuria. The need for treatment and, if given, the optimal type and duration of treatment for such patients with asymptomatic bacteriuria have not been established. Removal of the catheter and a short course of antibiotics to which the organism is susceptible are probably the best course of action and nearly always eradicate the bacteriuria. Treatment of asymptomatic catheter-associated bacteriuria may be of greatest benefit in elderly women, who more often develop symptoms if left untreated. If the catheter cannot be removed, antibiotic therapy usually proves to be unsuccessful and may result in infection with a more resistant strain. In this situation, the bacteriuria should be ignored unless the patient develops symptoms or is at high risk of developing bacteremia. In these cases, systemic antibiotics or urinary bladder antiseptics may reduce the degree of bacteriuria and the likelihood of bacteremia. Because of spinal cord injury, incontinence, or other factors, some patients in hospitals or nursing homes require long-term or semipermanent bladder catheterization. Preventive measures have been largely unsuccessful, and essentially all such chronically catheterized patients develop bacteriuria. If feasible, intermittent catheterization by a nurse or by the patient appears to reduce the occurrence of bacteriuria and associated complications in such patients. Treatment should be provided when symptomatic infections arise, but treatment of asymptomatic bacteriuria in such patients has no apparent benefit.

DIAGNOSTIC TESTING   Although many authorities have recommended that urine culture and antimicrobial susceptibility testing be performed in any patient with a suspected urinary tract infection, it may be more practical and cost-effective to manage women who have symptoms and urinalysis findings characteristic of acute uncomplicated cystitis without an initial urine culture. Thus women with symptoms and signs of acute cystitis in whom no complicating factors are present can be managed with urinary microscopy (or alternatively, a leukocyte esterase test). If positive for pyuria, hematuria, and/or bacteriuria, these tests provide sufficient documentation of infection such that urine culture and susceptibility testing can be omitted and the patient treated empirically. Urine culture should be obtained, however, in women in whom symptoms and urine examination findings leave the diagnosis of cystitis in question. Pretherapy cultures and susceptibility testing are also essential in the management of all patients with suspected upper tract infections and those in whom complicating factors are present, since in these situations a variety of pathogens may be present and antibiotic therapy is best tailored to the individual organism.

TREATMENT   Several therapeutic principles should underlie treatment of urinary tract infections:

1 In most circumstances, a quantitative urine culture, a positive Gram stain, or an alternative rapid diagnostic test should be obtained to confirm infection before starting treatment. When cultures are obtained, antimicrobial sensitivity testing should be used to direct therapy.
2 Factors predisposing to infection, such as obstruction, neurogenic bladder, calculi, etc., should be identified and corrected if possible.
3 Relief of clinical symptoms does not always indicate bacteriologic cure.
4 After completion of therapy, each treatment episode should be classified as a failure (symptoms and/or bacteriuria not eradicated during therapy or in the immediate posttreatment culture) or a cure (resolution of symptoms and elimination of bacteriuria). Recurrent infections should be classified as same strain or different strain and early (within 2 weeks of stopping therapy) or late.
5 In general, uncomplicated infections confined to the lower urinary tract respond to low doses and short courses of therapy, while upper tract infections require longer periods of treatment. After therapy, early recurrences with the same strain may result from an unresolved upper tract focus of infection but often (especially after short-course therapy for cystitis) result from persistent vaginal colonization rather than from recurrent bladder infection. Recurrences more than 2 weeks after the cessation of therapy are nearly

always reinfections, even though some may be with the same strain.
6 Community-acquired infections, especially initial infections, are usually due to antibiotic-sensitive strains.
7 Patients with repeated infections, instrumentation, or recent hospitalization should be suspected of harboring resistant strains.

The anatomic location of a urinary tract infection greatly influences success or failure of a therapeutic agent. Bladder bacteriuria (cystitis) can usually be eliminated with nearly any antimicrobial to which the infecting strain is sensitive; in the past, it was demonstrated that as little as a single dose of 500 mg of intramuscular kanamycin eliminated bladder bacteriuria in most patients. Currently, a 7-day course of therapy with oral drugs appears more than adequate. With upper tract infections, however, single-dose therapy fails in the majority of cases, and even a 7-day course will be unsuccessful in many patients. Longer periods of treatment (2 to 6 weeks) aimed at eradicating a persistent focus of infection may be necessary in some cases.

In *acute uncomplicated cystitis*, more than 80 percent of infections are due to *E. coli*, and although resistance patterns vary geographically, most strains are sensitive to many antibiotics. Single doses of trimethoprim-sulfamethoxazole (4 single-strength tablets), trimethoprim (400 mg), sulfa alone (2.0 g), and most fluoroquinolones (norfloxacin, ciprofloxacin, ofloxacin) have been used successfully to treat acute uncomplicated episodes of cystitis. A single 3-g dose of amoxicillin (amoxicilline) appears to result in lower cure rates than these other agents, especially in women infected with amoxicillin-resistant strains. In most areas, about one-third of *E. coli* strains causing acute cystitis are amoxicillin-resistant. The advantages of single-dose therapy include less expense, ensured compliance, fewer side effects, and perhaps less intense selective pressure for emergence of resistant organisms in the gut or vaginal or perineal flora. However, several studies now suggest that more recurrences with the same strain occur shortly after single-dose therapy than after 3 to 7 days of treatment and that single-dose therapy does not effectively eradicate vaginal colonization with *E. coli*. Nevertheless, single-dose therapy does appear safe and efficacious for women presenting with *acute uncomplicated cystitis*. Single-dose therapy should be used only in reliable patients, in whom posttreatment follow-up can be ensured, and in patients in whom symptoms have been present for less than 7 days. Three days of therapy with trimethoprim-sulfamethoxazole, norfloxacin, ciprofloxacin, or ofloxacin appears to preserve the lower side-effects rate of single-dose therapy but improves efficacy. Neither single-dose nor 3-day therapy should be used in women with symptoms or signs of pyelonephritis, in women with urologic abnormalities or stones, or in women with previous infections due to antibiotic-resistant organisms. Males with urinary tract infection often have urologic abnormalities or prostatic involvement and hence are not candidates for single-dose or 3-day therapy.

Treatment of women with acute urethritis depends on the etiologic agent involved. In chlamydial infection, doxycycline (100 mg orally bid for 7 days) should be used. Women with acute dysuria and frequency, negative urine cultures, and no pyuria do not usually respond to antimicrobial agents.

Acute uncomplicated pyelonephritis in women without accompanying clinical evidence of calculi or urologic disease is due to *E. coli* in most cases. Although the optimal route and duration of therapy have not been established, a 14-day course of trimethoprim-sulfamethoxazole, trimethoprim alone, a fluoroquinolone, an aminoglycoside, or a cephalosporin usually provides adequate therapy. Ampicillin or amoxicillin should not be used as initial therapy because 20 to 30 percent of *E. coli* are now resistant in vitro. Intravenous antibiotics, at least for the first few days of treatment, should probably be given to most patients, but mildly symptomatic patients can be treated with 2 weeks of oral antibiotics (usually trimethoprim-sulfamethoxazole, ciprofloxacin, or ofloxacin). Patients who relapse following therapy should be investigated to determine whether unrecognized suppurative foci, calculi, or urologic disease is present. If not, treatment should be extended to 2 to 6 weeks to eliminate a presumed upper tract focus causing recurrent bacteriuria.

Complicated urinary tract infections (those arising in the setting of catheterization, instrumentation, urologic anatomic or functional abnormalities, stones, obstruction, immunosuppression, renal disease, or diabetes) are typically due to hospital-acquired bacteria, including *E. coli*, *Klebsiella*, *Proteus*, *Serratia*, *Pseudomonas*, enterococci, or staphylococci. Many of these strains are antibiotic-resistant. Thus initial empiric antibiotic therapy for complicated urinary tract infections ideally should provide broad-spectrum coverage against these pathogens. In patients with minimal symptoms, oral therapy with a fluoroquinolone such as ciprofloxacin or ofloxacin can be utilized until culture results and antibiotic sensitivities are known. In patients with more severe illness attributable to complicated urinary tract infection, including acute pyelonephritis or suspected urosepsis, hospitalization and parenteral therapy should be provided. Commonly used empiric regimens include imipenem alone, a penicillin or cephalosporin plus an aminoglycoside, ceftriaxone, and ceftazadime (when enterococci are unlikely). When the antimicrobial sensitivity pattern of the infecting strain becomes available, a more specific antimicrobial regimen can be selected. Therapy should generally be provided for 7 to 21 days, depending on the severity of the infection. Follow-up cultures 2 to 4 weeks after cessation of therapy should be obtained to demonstrate cure.

In *pregnancy*, acute cystitis can be managed with 3 to 7 days of amoxicillin, nitrofurantoin, or a cephalosporin. All pregnant women should be screened for asymptomatic bacteriuria during the first trimester, and if bacteriuric, they should be treated with one of the regimens just outlined. After treatment, a culture should be obtained to ensure cure and repeated monthly thereafter. Acute pyelonephritis in pregnancy should be managed with hospitalization and parenteral antibiotics, generally a cephalosporin or an extended-spectrum penicillin. Continuous low-dose prophylaxis with nitrofurantoin should be given to women who have recurrent infections during pregnancy.

Asymptomatic bacteriuria should be documented with at least two positive cultures before treatment is given. Seven days of an oral agent to which the organism is sensitive should be given initially. If bacteriuria persists, it can be followed without further treatment in most patients. High-risk patients with neutropenia, renal transplants, or other complicating conditions may require longer periods of treatment.

UROLOGIC EVALUATION Very few women with recurrent urinary tract infections have correctable lesions discovered at cystoscopy or upon intravenous pyelography, and these procedures should not be performed routinely in such patients. In selected women, namely those with relapsing infection, those with a history of childhood infections, those with stones or painless hematuria, and those with recurrent pyelonephritis, urologic evaluation should be performed. Most males with urinary infection should be considered to have complicated infection and thus be evaluated urologically. Exceptions may include young men who have sexually associated cystitis, are uncircumcised, or have AIDS. Men or women presenting with acute infection and signs or symptoms suggestive of an obstruction or stones should undergo urologic evaluation, generally by means of ultrasound.

PROGNOSIS In patients with uncomplicated cystitis or pyelonephritis, treatment ordinarily results in complete resolution of symptoms. In fact, symptoms usually remit even without specific therapy. Lower tract infections in adult women are of concern mainly because they cause discomfort, minor morbidity, and time lost from work. Cystitis also may result in upper tract infection or in bacteremia (especially during instrumentation), but there is little evidence to suggest that renal impairment follows. When repeated episodes of cystitis occur, they are nearly always reinfections, not relapses.

Uncomplicated acute pyelonephritis in adults rarely progresses to functional impairment and chronic renal disease. Repeated upper tract infections often indicate relapse rather than reinfection, and a vigorous search for renal calculi or an underlying urologic abnormality should be undertaken. If neither is found, 6 weeks of chemotherapy may be useful in eradicating an unresolved focus of infection.

Repeated symptomatic urinary tract infections in children, and in adults with obstructive uropathy, neurogenic bladder, structural renal disease, or diabetes, more often progress to chronic renal disease. Asymptomatic bacteriuria in these groups, as well as in adults without urologic disease or obstruction, predisposes to increased episodes of symptomatic infection but does not result in renal impairment in most instances.

PREVENTION Patients with frequent symptomatic infections may benefit from long-term low-dose antibiotics directed at preventing recurrences. A single dose of trimethoprim-sulfamethoxazole (80 mg trimethoprim and 400 mg sulfamethoxazole), trimethoprim alone (100 mg), or nitrofurantoin (50 mg) given daily or thrice weekly has been particularly effective. Prophylaxis should be initiated only after bacteriuria has been eradicated with a full-dose treatment regimen. Women having more than two infections every 6 months should be considered for such preventive antibiotics. These same regimens can be used after sexual intercourse to prevent episodes of symptomatic infections in women whose infectious episodes are temporally related to intercourse. Other patients for whom prophylaxis appears to have some merit include men with chronic prostatitis; patients undergoing prostatectomy, both during the operation and in the postoperative period; and pregnant women with asymptomatic bacteriuria. All pregnant women should be screened for bacteriuria in the first trimester and should be treated if bacteriuria is found.

PAPILLARY NECROSIS

When infection of the renal pyramids develops in association with vascular diseases of the kidney or with urinary tract obstruction, renal papillary necrosis is likely to result. Patients with diabetes, sickle cell disease, chronic alcoholism, and vascular disease seem peculiarly susceptible to this complication. Hematuria, pain in the flank or abdomen, and chills and fever are the most common presenting symptoms. Acute renal failure with oliguria or anuria sometimes occurs. Rarely, sloughing of a pyramid may take place without symptoms in a patient with chronic urinary infection, and the diagnosis is made when the necrotic tissue is passed in the urine or identified as a "ring shadow" on pyelography. If renal function deteriorates suddenly in a diabetic or a patient with chronic obstruction, the diagnosis of renal papillary necrosis should be entertained, even in the absence of fever or pain. Although renal papillary necrosis is often bilateral, when it is unilateral, nephrectomy may be lifesaving in the management of overwhelming infection.

RENAL AND PERINEPHRIC ABSCESS

See p. 529.

PROSTATITIS

The term *prostatitis* has been used for various inflammatory conditions affecting the prostate, including acute and chronic infections with specific bacteria and, more commonly, instances in which signs and symptoms of prostatic inflammation are present but no specific organisms can be detected. Patients with acute bacterial prostatitis can usually be identified on the basis of typical symptoms and signs, pyuria, and bacteriuria. To classify patients with suspected chronic prostatitis correctly, each patient should be evaluated using first-void and midstream urine specimens, a prostatic expressate, and a postmassage urine specimen. All specimens should be quantitatively cultured and evaluated for numbers of leukocytes. Based on the results of these studies, patients can be classified as having chronic bacterial prostatitis, chronic nonbacterial prostatitis, or prostatodynia. Patients with suspected chronic prostatitis usually have low back pain, perineal or testicular discomfort, mild dysuria, and lower urinary obstructive symptoms. Microscopic pyuria may be the only objective manifestation of prostatic disease.

ACUTE BACTERIAL PROSTATITIS This disease generally affects young male adults when it occurs spontaneously, but it also may be associated with an indwelling urethral catheter. It is characterized by fever, chills, dysuria, and a tense or boggy, extremely tender prostate on examination. Although prostatic massage usually produces purulent secretions with a large number of bacteria on culture, bacteremia may result from manipulation of the inflamed gland. For this reason, and because the etiologic agent can usually be identified on urine Gram stain and culture, vigorous prostatic massage should be avoided. In non-catheter-associated cases, the infection is generally due to common gram-negative urinary tract pathogens (*E. coli* or *Klebsiella*). Initially, intravenous trimethoprim-sulfamethoxazole, a cephalosporin, a fluoroquinolone, or an·aminoglycoside can be utilized if gram-negative rods are seen in the urine Gram stain, and a cephalosporin or nafcillin if gram-positive cocci are seen. Although many of these drugs do not readily diffuse into the noninflamed prostate gland, the response to antibiotics in acute bacterial prostatitis is usually prompt, perhaps because drugs penetrate more readily into the acutely inflamed prostate. In catheter-associated cases, a broader spectrum of etiologic agents is seen, including hospital-acquired gram-negative rods and enterococci. In such cases, an aminoglycoside, a fluoroquinolone, or a third-generation cephalosporin should be used for initial therapy until the organism has been isolated and susceptibilities determined. The long-term prognosis is good, although in some instances acute infection may result in abscess formation, epididymoorchitis, seminal vesiculitis, septicemia, and residual chronic bacterial prostatitis. Since the advent of antibiotics, the frequency of acute bacterial prostatitis has diminished markedly. Many so-called cases of acute prostatitis are probably posterior urethritis.

CHRONIC BACTERIAL PROSTATITIS This entity is now infrequent but should be considered in men with a history of recurrent bacteriuria. Symptoms are usually absent, and the prostate usually feels normal on palpation. Obstructive symptoms or perineal pain occurs in some patients. Intermittently, infection spreads to the bladder, producing frequency, urgency, and dysuria. A pattern of relapsing infection in a middle-aged man strongly suggests chronic bacterial prostatitis. Classically, the diagnosis is established by culturing *E. coli*, *Klebsiella*, *Proteus*, or other uropathogenic bacteria in higher quantities from the expressed prostatic secretion or postmassage urine than are found in first-void or midstream urine. Antibiotics promptly relieve the symptoms associated with acute exacerbations but have been less effective in eradicating the focus of chronic infection in the prostate. The relative ineffectiveness of antimicrobials, in terms of long-term cure, in part results from the poor penetration of most antibiotics into the prostate because the low pH which prevails in this organ precludes solubility of most drugs. Sulfonamide-trimethoprim, ciprofloxacin, and ofloxacin have been employed successfully in some cases, but they must be given for at least 12 weeks to be effective. Patients with frequent episodes of acute cystitis can be managed with prolonged courses of antimicrobials (usually sulfonamide, trimethoprim, or nitrofurantoin), with a view toward suppressing symptoms and keeping the bladder urine sterile. Total prostatectomy produces cure of chronic prostatitis but is associated with considerable morbidity. Transurethral prostatectomy is safer but cures only one-third of patients.

NONBACTERIAL PROSTATITIS Patients who present with symptoms and signs of prostatitis, increased leukocytes in their expressed prostatic secretions and postmassage urine, and no bacterial growth in cultures are classified as having nonbacterial prostatitis. In addition, such patients do not have a history of recurrent episodes of bacterial cystitis. Prostatic inflammation can be considered present when the expressed prostatic secretion and postmassage urine contain at least tenfold more leukocytes than the first-void and midstream specimens or when the expressed prostatic secretion contains ≥1000 leukocytes per microliter. The presumed infectious etiology of this condition remains unidentified. Evidence for the causative role of both *Ureaplasma urealyticum* and *Chlamydia trachomatis* has been presented but is not conclusive. Since most cases of nonbacterial prostatitis occur in young, sexually active men, and since many cases arise following an episode of nonspecific urethritis, the causative agent may well be sexually transmitted. The effectiveness of antimicrobial agents in this condition remains uncertain. Some patients benefit from a 4- to 6-week course of erythromycin, doxycycline, trimethoprim-sulfamethoxazole, or a fluoroquinolone, but controlled trials are lacking.

PROSTATODYNIA Patients who have symptoms and signs of prostatitis but no evidence of prostatic inflammation (normal leukocyte counts) and negative urine cultures are classified as having prostatodynia. Despite their symptoms, these patients most likely do not have prostatic infection and should not be given antimicrobial agents.

REFERENCES

HOOTON TM et al: *Escherichia coli* bacteriuria and contraceptive method. JAMA 265:64, 1991

——, STAMM WE: Management of acute uncomplicated urinary tract infection in adults. Med Clin North Am 75:339, 1991

JOHNSON JR, STAMM WE: Diagnosis and treatment of urinary tract infections. Infect Dis Clin North Am 1:773, 1987

KRIEGER JN: Complications and treatment of urinary tract infections during pregnancy. Urol Clin North Am 13:685, 1986

KUNIN CM: *Detection, Prevention and Management of Urinary Tract Infections*, 4th ed. Philadelphia, Lea & Febiger, 1987

LIPSKY BA: Urinary tract infections in men. Ann Intern Med 110:138, 1989

MEARES EM JR: Acute and chronic prostatitis: Diagnosis and treatment. Infect Dis Clin North Am 1:855, 1987

PEZZLO M: Detection of urinary tract infections by rapid methods. Clin Microbiol Rev 1:268, 1988

STAMM WE et al: Causes of the acute urethral syndrome in women. N Engl J Med 303:409, 1980

—— et al: Diagnosis of coliform infection in acutely dysuric women. N Engl J Med 307:463, 1982

—— et al: Urinary tract infections: From pathogenesis to treatment. J Infect Dis 159:400, 1989

——: Catheter-associated urinary tract infections: Epidemiology, pathogenesis, prevention. Am J Med 91(suppl 3B):B655, 1991

SVANBORG-EDEN C et al: Host-parasite relationship in urinary tract infection. J Infect Dis 157:421, 1988

WARREN JW: Catheter-associated urinary tract infections. Infect Dis Clin North Am 1:823, 1987

91 INFECTIOUS ARTHRITIS

DANIEL ROTROSEN

NONGONOCOCCAL SEPTIC ARTHRITIS Acute bacterial arthritis is a common medical problem affecting individuals of all ages. Prompt recognition and treatment are important to avoid permanent articular disability.

Etiology, pathogenesis, and predisposing factors Approximately 75 percent of nongonococcal pyoarthroses are due to gram-positive cocci, with *Staphylococcus aureus* isolated particularly often. Pneumococci and group A beta-hemolytic and viridans streptococci collectively account for fewer than half of isolates. Among immunocompromised individuals, group G streptococci are an infrequent cause of septic arthritis; among neonates, group B streptococci are an important cause of arthritis. *Staphylococcus epidermidis* is the leading cause of prosthetic joint infection.

Gram-negative bacilli account for approximately 20 percent of cases, typically in patients with obvious risk factors for gram-negative bacteremia. *Pseudomonas aeruginosa* is an important cause of septic arthritis in intravenous drug addicts and neonates. *Haemophilus influenzae* type b is a prominent cause of pyoarthrosis among children under age 5.

Septic arthritis usually results from direct hematogenous seeding of the synovium. Factors that predispose to septic arthritis include infancy, immunosuppressive therapy, alcoholism, drug abuse, some chronic systemic illnesses, hemoglobinopathies, complement and immunoglobulin deficiencies, phagocytic cell dysfunction, chronic arthritis, and previous joint damage. Infection may occur as a complication of arthroscopy, intraarticular glucocorticoid injection, or prosthetic joint surgery. A history of minor joint trauma is a common but often-overlooked feature in patients with suppurative arthritis. An extraarticular focus of infection (e.g., cutaneous abscesses) can be identified in about 25 percent of patients and can be helpful in establishing a cause and choosing antibiotics before results of joint fluid cultures become available.

The synovium is well vascularized and lacks a limiting basement membrane, allowing relatively free access of bloodborne microorganisms to the joint space once extravasation has occurred. In experimentally induced arthritis, microorganisms are found scattered throughout the synovium 1 to 2 h after inoculation. Within 1 to 2 days, vascular congestion, leukocyte infiltration, and hyperplasia of the synovial lining cells are prominent. The host response may be sufficient to eradicate infection, but early changes usually progress to purulent effusion and microabscess formation within the synovium and subchondral bone. Increased intraarticular pressure causes ischemia and impairs cartilage biomechanics and nutrition. The formation of granulation tissue and release of chondrolytic enzymes contribute to the destruction of articular cartilage, subchondral bone, and the joint capsule.

Clinical and experimental observations suggest that host immune mechanisms play a critical role in the development and maintenance of synovial inflammation. For example, sterile bacterial products, including endotoxins, exotoxins, and cell wall peptidoglycan, induce acute and chronic arthritis in laboratory animals. Deposition of immune complexes in the synovium and periarticular tissues may be followed by a sterile synovitis during the convalescent phase of certain bacterial and viral infections. In addition, individuals who develop postinfectious arthritis or Reiter's syndrome following *Shigella*, *Salmonella*, *Yersinia*, and *Campylobacter* infection of the gastrointestinal tract are more likely than matched controls to have the specific histocompatibility antigen HLA-B27.

Manifestations Nongonococcal septic arthritis presents as a monarticular synovitis with a predilection for large weight-bearing joints. The knee is the most frequently involved joint in children and adults, followed by the hip. The ankle, wrist, elbow, shoulder, sternoclavicular, and sacroiliac joints are involved less often. The interphalangeal joints are rarely affected in bacterial arthritis, except in patients with gonococccal synovitis or mycobacterial infection. Gram-positive coccal arthritis usually presents as an acute illness with severe constitutional symptoms accompanied by swelling, pain, warmth, and restricted motion of the involved joint. In septic arthritis of the hip, effusion may not be readily appreciated, and pain may be minimal or referred to the groin, buttock, lateral thigh, or anterior knee. Patients with suppurative arthritis usually seek medical attention within 3 to 4 days of the onset of symptoms. Signs of inflammation may be masked in patients taking glucocorticoids or other immunosuppressive medications and in those with chronic debilitating illnesses. Individuals with coexistent rheumatoid or gouty arthritis often attribute their symptoms to a flare-up of the underlying disease and consequently delay medical evaluation. In this setting a high degree of suspicion is warranted, and studies to exclude infection are important when articular symptoms fail to respond to anti-inflammatory agents.

If medical attention is sought early in the illness, a source of bacteremia is usually identified, and the responsible pathogen can be isolated from the blood in about 50 percent of cases. In contrast to the gram-positive arthritides, gram-negative bacillary arthritis follows a more indolent course with less prominent articular manifestations.

These differences contribute to the more prolonged time to diagnosis in gram-negative bacillary arthritis (typically 3 weeks from the onset of symptoms) and to the high incidence of coexistent osteomyelitis at the time of diagnosis.

Prosthetic joint infection is associated with mild symptoms and an indolent course resulting in a mean diagnostic delay of 2 to 8 months. *S. epidermidis* and *S. aureus* account for most of these infections, but polymicrobial infections or infections due to gram-negative bacilli or anaerobes are not uncommon. Infection occurs in 1 to 4 percent of prostheses followed for 10 years and is more frequent after revision of a previous total joint replacement. It invariably is accompanied by osteomyelitis at the site of implantation. Eradication of the infection usually requires removal of the prosthesis.

Certain pathogens are likely to cause infection at unusual sites. Spinal arthritis is often associated with osteomyelitis of adjacent vertebral bodies. It is usually due to *S. aureus*, but *Brucella*, *Salmonella*, and *Mycobacterium tuberculosis* also preferentially involve the spine. Among intravenous drug addicts, *P. aeruginosa* infection can occur in the sternoclavicular and sacroiliac joints.

Laboratory findings and diagnosis Analysis of synovial fluid is essential in the evaluation of suspected bacterial arthritis. Fluid sufficient for complete analysis usually can be obtained by percutaneous arthrocentesis. Care should be taken not to contaminate the joint space by inserting the needle through an area of overlying cellulitis or through an infected bursa. Fluoroscopic guidance may facilitate aspiration of the hip, shoulder, spinal, or sacroiliac joints. When joints are difficult to aspirate, arthrotomy may be required to obtain fluid or synovial tissue. Synovial fluid in septic arthritis is usually turbid or grossly purulent. The synovial fluid leukocyte count is greater than 100,000 per microliter (range < 10,000 to > 300,000 per microliter, usually > 90 percent polymorphonuclear neutrophils) in one-third to one-half of patients. In patients with unexpectedly low leukocyte counts on initial evaluation, repeat joint aspiration 12 to 24 h later almost always demonstrates leukocytosis. The synovial fluid leukocyte count and differential are of limited value in establishing an infectious cause because of overlap with other acute inflammatory arthritides. However, serial counts are important in monitoring response to therapy.

Gram's stain of synovial fluid is important in establishing the cause of septic arthritis. Stains are positive in 75 to 95 percent of gram-positive coccal and in approximately 50 percent of gram-negative bacillary infections. Regardless of the results of Gram's stain, synovial fluid should be cultured aerobically and anaerobically to identify specific pathogens and to provide data on antimicrobial sensitivity. Joint fluid cultures are positive in most patients with nongonococcal bacterial arthritis. If the patient has taken oral antibiotics prior to arthrocentesis, the microbiology laboratory should be notified, because growth of the organism may be delayed and cultures may require special handling. Blood cultures should be obtained, and a diligent search should be made for occult sources of bacteremia. Bacterial antigen detection by counterimmunoelectrophoresis has been advocated as a rapid diagnostic test for certain etiologic agents (e.g., *Streptococcus pneumoniae* and *H. influenzae*) but is not widely used.

In septic arthritis the synovial fluid glucose level may be low and lactate elevated compared with the corresponding levels in serum, but neither test is sufficiently sensitive or specific to be generally used. Elevated synovial fluid protein and poor mucin clot are nonspecific.

Unless arthritis arises by extension of adjacent osteomyelitis, distention of the joint capsule and periarticular soft tissue swelling are the only radiographic findings expected on initial evaluation. Nonetheless, early films are useful to establish a baseline. Destructive changes are rarely noted before the second to third week of untreated infection. At that time, periosteal elevation, juxtaarticular osteoporosis, bony erosions on the articular surface, and joint space narrowing may be apparent. In prosthetic joint infection radiographic evidence of implant loosening and osteomyelitis is usually seen.

In the setting of staphylococcal or gram-negative bacillary arthritis, computed tomography (CT) or magnetic resonance imaging (MRI) is helpful, particularly when the sternoclavicular joint or the hip is involved. These joints are poorly visualized by conventional techniques, and CT or MRI may reveal extensive bony involvement and parasynovial abscesses when conventional x-ray films are negative. Such findings have important implications for surgical intervention and for the duration of antimicrobial therapy. Radioisotope scans lack diagnostic specificity and may be positive in noninfectious inflammatory joint disease. However, scans are useful to identify inapparent foci of osteomyelitis and to substantiate suspicions of low-grade infection in the hip, shoulder, spine, and sacroiliac joints.

Other conditions to be considered in the differential diagnosis of oligoarticular arthritis include septic bursitis (usually olecranon or prepatellar), adult or juvenile rheumatoid arthritis, psoriatic arthritis, acute rheumatic fever, Reiter's syndrome, sarcoid arthropathy, trauma, villonodular synovitis, aseptic necrosis, and intermittent hydroarthrosis. Lyme disease and infections caused by mycobacteria and fungi typically present as oligoarticular arthritis.

Management and outcome Optimal management of suppurative arthritis includes parenteral antimicrobial therapy, drainage, and articular rest. Most antibiotics achieve therapeutic levels in the infected joint following parenteral administration. There is no rationale for intraarticular administration of antibiotics, and direct injection of antibiotics can induce chemical synovitis. The initial choice of antibiotics should be guided by Gram's stain of synovial fluid and revised as dictated by culture results. Antibiotic regimens for specific organisms are provided in the chapters dealing with these organisms and in Chap. 100. When no organisms are seen on Gram's stain, the antimicrobial regimen should be tailored to cover the likely pathogens based on the patient's age and the clinical setting. Infants under 1 month of age should be treated with a semisynthetic penicillin and an aminoglycoside to provide coverage against *S. aureus*, gram-negative bacilli, and group B streptococci. In children under 5 years of age, therapy should be targeted against *S. aureus* and ampicillin-resistant *H. influenzae*. Children over 5 years and adults should receive a semisynthetic penicillin and an aminoglycoside until culture results are available. Vancomycin is the drug of choice in patients with serious penicillin allergy, renal failure, or prosthetic joint infection. The results of single-drug therapy of gram-negative bacillary arthritis have been disappointing, despite in vitro sensitivity to the agents used. Because of the high rates of failure and relapse in this setting, combination chemotherapy is generally advised. After an initial clinical response, substitution of a newer β-lactam or quinolone antibiotic may avoid the toxicities of prolonged aminoglycoside therapy.

Most cases of streptococcal arthritis are cured by a 10- to 14-day course of antibiotics, whereas staphylococcal and gram-negative bacillary infections require longer treatment, usually 3 to 6 weeks. Drainage of purulent joint fluid is essential to relieve pain, to diminish the risk of loculation and pressure necrosis, and to remove chondrolytic products that promote destructive changes within the joint. Drainage of acidic, purulent fluid improves the bactericidal activity of neutrophils and certain antibiotics. Percutaneous needle aspiration and joint irrigation can be performed daily or twice daily for the first 5 to 7 days. The development of loculations, continued culture positivity, and persistence of a purulent effusion are indications that arthroscopy or open drainage may be required. When the hip is involved, surgical intervention is usually warranted from the outset, especially in children, because of the difficulty of repeated percutaneous aspiration and the risk of vascular compromise from elevated intracapsular pressure. Exploratory arthrotomy and open drainage have been beneficial in septic arthritis of the shoulder and sternoclavicular joints. Persistence of culture positivity despite adequate drainage is an indication for repeat studies to look for the emergence of antibiotic-resistant strains.

During the acute phase the joint should be immobilized in a position that minimizes capsular tension, usually midway between full extension and flexion. Passive range-of-motion exercises should be started as the synovitis improves, but weight bearing should be avoided until pain and signs of inflammation are gone.

Most cases of streptococcal arthritis resolve without sequelae, whereas in staphylococcal and gram-negative bacillary arthritis the response is generally less salutary. In this setting healing may be delayed by a sterile, postinfectious synovitis. Such patients may be left with limitation of motion and persistence of pain. Other major determinants of a poor outcome are failure to recognize and treat the infection within 7 days of onset and involvement of the hip joint. In children with hip or ankle arthritis, impaired ambulation and shortening of the extremity are not uncommon.

GONOCOCCAL ARTHRITIS (See Chap. 110) Gonococcal infection is the leading cause of bacterial arthritis in young adults and the most common form of infectious arthritis seen at urban medical centers. It may be a complication of sexual abuse in young children. In disseminated gonococcal infection, an early arthritis-dermatitis syndrome is typically followed by a joint-localization stage. The early phase is characterized by constitutional symptoms, migratory tenosynovitis and arthralgias, vesiculopustular skin lesions, and minimal joint effusion. The knee, shoulder, wrist, and interphalangeal joints of the hands are commonly involved. Cultures of blood and skin lesions may be positive at this stage of the illness, whereas culture and Gram's stain of synovial fluid are usually negative. A presumptive diagnosis can be made if the gonococcus is isolated from a silent primary focus (e.g., urogenital tract, pharynx, or rectum). Without treatment, constitutional symptoms and dermatitis usually abate, but joint involvement progresses to a purulent mon- or polyarticular arthritis. Synovial fluid cultures may be positive at this stage, whereas blood cultures are almost always negative. In 30 to 40 percent of patients a biphasic pattern of illness is not observed, and some patients present with a monarticular purulent arthritis and few systemic manifestations. Terminal complement component deficiencies, menstruation, and pregnancy predispose to gonococcal dissemination.

The differential diagnosis of disseminated gonococcal infection includes acute rheumatic fever, Reiter's syndrome, chronic meningococcemia, and *Streptobacillus moniliformis* infection. In Reiter's syndrome, constitutional toxicity is usually less pronounced, there is often a history of symptomatic urethritis and conjunctivitis, and distinct but subtle mucocutaneous lesions are usually present. Sacroiliitis and Achilles tendonitis are more common in Reiter's syndrome, and involvement of the upper extremity, especially the wrist, is unusual. A clinical response to antibiotics (in gonococcal disease) or to salicylates (in rheumatic fever) may help to differentiate among these syndromes.

In the United States most gonococcal isolates causing disseminated infection are penicillin-sensitive. However, penicillin resistance is increasingly common in some urban areas and in the Philippines, Southeast Asia, and Africa. Ceftriaxone or spectinomycin is effective. After an initial response, therapy can be continued with cefuroxime or amoxicillin plus clavulanic acid. Hospitalization and administration of parenteral antibiotics are warranted for unreliable patients and for those with purulent monarticular arthritis or uncertain diagnoses.

CHRONIC MONARTICULAR ARTHRITIS Certain mycobacteria and fungi cause chronic oligoarticular arthritis that is clinically and histologically distinct from other forms of septic arthritis.

Tuberculous arthritis (See Chap. 130) *Mycobacterium tuberculosis* causes a slowly progressive arthritis that is monarticular in up to 90 percent of cases. With the decline in primary tuberculosis in developed countries, spinal arthritis is rare, and involvement of the knee, hip, wrist, ankle, or small joints of the hand is more common. These sites become infected by reactivation of long-dormant lymphohematogenous foci. Rupture of such a focus (often in the epiphyseal region of long bones) into the joint space causes effusion and a progressive granulomatous reaction of synovial membranes, articular cartilage, and tendons. Localized pain may precede other signs of inflammation or x-ray changes by weeks or even months. The insidious nature of the infection usually delays diagnosis by weeks or months (the average time elapsed was 19 weeks from onset in one series). The granulomatous process eventually imparts a boggy, doughy feeling to the joint and periarticular structures. Cold abscesses and draining sinuses may develop. Constitutional symptoms are not prominent, and active pulmonary tuberculosis is unusual. Most patients are tuberculin-positive. Radiographs initially show subchondral osteoporosis and periarticular bone destruction with overlying periosteal thickening. Eventually, destructive changes are noted within the joint. The synovial fluid leukocyte count ranges from about 1000 to >100,000 per microliter (average about 15,000 per microliter), with a preponderance of polymorphonuclear neutrophils when counts are high, but frankly purulent fluid is uncommon. Acid-fast bacilli are not often seen on smears of synovial fluid (approximately 20 percent yield), but cultures of synovial fluid or tissue are positive in 80 to 90 percent of cases. Granulomatous changes in synovium are indications for antituberculous therapy while awaiting culture results. Infection due to atypical mycobacteria (e.g., *M. kansasii*, *M. marinum*, *M. avium-intracellulare*) may produce a chronic granulomatous arthritis with similar clinical and histopathologic features. These organisms are highly resistant to antimicrobial agents. The correct diagnosis and choice of an appropriate regimen depend on isolation of the organism (Chaps. 130 and 132). In spinal tuberculosis, surgery is usually reserved for drainage of abscesses or stabilization of the spine and is rarely required for treatment of other joints. Arthritis due to *Brucella* sp., *Nocardia asteroides*, and fungi may resemble mycobacterial infection.

Fungal arthritis Any of the invasive mycoses may involve bone and articular structures (see Chaps. 161–169). With the exception of acute arthritis due to *Candida* sp. or blastomycosis, the fungal arthritides tend to be slowly progressive and may elude accurate diagnosis for months or years. All show a predilection for involvement of large weight-bearing joints, especially the knee, and joint infection usually occurs without extraarticular dissemination. A history of serious underlying illness is common in blastomycotic arthritis but not in other fungal arthritides.

In acute pulmonary *coccidioidomycosis* (see Chap. 163), self-limited sterile synovitis is a component of the acute hypersensitivity syndrome known as "desert fever." Persistent coccidioidal synovitis may arise via direct hematogenous seeding of the synovium or via extension from an adjacent osteomyelitic focus. In the former case the disease tends to follow an indolent course with recurrent effusion, maintenance of joint space integrity, no evidence of osteomyelitis, and only late progression to a destructive villonodular arthritis with pannus formation. With extension from an adjacent bony focus, effusion is less prominent, and destructive changes tend to occur earlier. Diagnosis depends on culture and histology of synovial tissue; joint fluid cultures are positive in < 5 percent of cases.

Sporotrichotic arthritis (see Chap. 169) usually occurs in the absence of the more familiar lymphocutaneous syndrome. There is a predilection for involvement of the small joints of the hand and wrist in addition to the knee. Articular disability is uncommon until late in the disease. The etiologic agent, *Sporothrix schenckii*, is easily cultured from synovial fluid. As opposed to cutaneous sporotrichosis, articular disease is relatively refractory to iodide therapy, and response to amphotericin B may be slow.

Isolated articular involvement is unusual in *blastomycosis* (see Chap. 164), and patients usually present with a rapidly progressive "pulmonary-cutaneous-arthritic" syndrome. Involvement of multiple joints is the rule. In contrast to other granulomatous arthritides, articular blastomycosis is characterized by frankly purulent joint fluid, and the organism is easily visualized on wet-mount microscopy of synovial aspirates.

Candida arthritis usually follows direct hematogenous seeding of synovium in patients with risk factors for disseminated candidiasis (see Chap. 166). The acute articular infection may spread to adjacent bone.

In *histoplasmosis* (see Chap. 162), a migratory polyarthritis

accompanied by erythema nodosum may be analogous to the acute hypersensitivity syndrome of coccidioidomycosis; osseous and articular infection is exceedingly rare.

In disseminated *cryptococcal* infection, bone involvement is common, but synovitis is unusual.

Successful management of fungal arthritis usually requires prolonged administration of amphotericin B; surgical debridement is helpful in cases with extensive pannus formation.

VIRAL ARTHRITIS Self-limited polyarthritis is a common manifestation of rubella, type B hepatitis, human immunodeficiency virus infection, and arboviral diseases not found in the Western Hemisphere (chikungunya and O'nyong-nyong in Africa and Ross River arthritis in Australia). Synovitis is less common in mumps, varicella, adenoviral infection, and parvoviral infection. Destructive joint changes are uncommon in viral arthritis, even with recurrent disease.

Arthritis occurs in natural *rubella* infection and following immunization with live, attenuated rubella virus. Approximately 15 percent of postpubertal women develop frank arthritis in the course of natural rubella infection. Large and small joints may be involved; the small joints of the hand and wrist are most severely affected. Occasional involvement of the distal interphalangeal joints helps to differentiate this syndrome from the onset of rheumatoid arthritis. The onset of arthritis in rubella usually occurs at the same time as—or within a few days of—the rash in natural infection and within 2 to 10 weeks after immunization. Rubella arthritis usually abates spontaneously within 1 to 2 weeks; recalcitrant cases respond to salicylates. Joint symptoms may recur for a year or more in natural rubella, but rarely recur after rubella immunization.

The synovitis that accompanies *type B hepatitis* resembles serum sickness, with abrupt onset of fever and articular symptoms. Symmetric polyarthritis of the small joints of the hand may be associated with rheumatoid arthritis–like morning stiffness. The knee, shoulder, ankle, elbow, and wrist are also involved, but the joints of the feet are typically spared. Synovitis is usually accompanied by an urticarial rash, but the rash may be erythematous, maculopapular, or petechial. The possibility of hepatitis-associated arthritis is rarely entertained at the onset of the illness because synovitis usually occurs in the anicteric/prodromal phase. Over a third of patients never become jaundiced, but liver function tests show evidence of hepatitis. Immune complexes containing hepatitis B antigens are present in serum and synovium during the prodromal stage of hepatitis, lending support to the concept that this form of synovitis is immunologically mediated.

In contrast to that of rubella, the arthritis of *mumps* has a predilection for men. It usually occurs after parotitis has subsided, may be accompanied by high fever, and does not respond to salicylates. In children and adults, *coxsackieviral* and *adenoviral* infections have been associated with recurrent fever, polyarthritis, and a polyserositis resembling Still's disease. *Parvoviruses* cause a self-limited acute polyarthritis, predominately in women.

SPIROCHETAL ARTHRITIS Articular disease occurs in congenital, secondary, and tertiary *syphilis* (see Chap. 133). Congenital syphilis is associated with metaphyseal osteochondritis of the long bones that abates spontaneously after 6 months of age. Periostitis continues after that age, and at puberty a painless bilateral synovitis of the knees and elbows (Clutton's joints) may develop. Synovial fluid shows a lymphocytic pleocytosis. Arthralgias, arthritis, and tenosynovitis may accompany the classic signs of secondary syphilis. Gummatous synovitis of the large joints occurs in tertiary syphilis. Neurogenic joint degeneration (Charcot's joint) occurs in neurosyphilis. Articular manifestations also may occur in the nonvenereal treponematoses.

Lyme disease (see also Chap. 137) is a multisystem disorder caused by a spirochete, *Borrelia burgdorferi*, that is transmitted by the bite of *Ixodes dammini* or related ticks. The hallmark of the disease is a characteristic rash, erythema chronicum migrans, during the early phase of infection. Weeks to months later, neurologic and cardiac abnormalities occur, accompanied by polyarthralgias and tenosynovitis. Joint manifestations may evolve to frank arthritis, particularly of the large joints, and recur for years. Prompt oral therapy with tetracycline or amoxicillin eradicates the rash and generally prevents late manifestations, whereas erythromycin does not reliably prevent sequelae. Less than 5 percent of patients are seronegative but develop late manifestations, possibly related to a spirochetal ''persister'' state induced by suboptimal antibiotic therapy. Established late manifestations are cured by parenteral penicillin or ceftriaxone; response to therapy may take several months, and repeated treatment may be necessary.

REFERENCES

BAYER AS, GUZE LB: Fungal arthritis. II. Coccidioidal synovitis: Clinical, diagnostic, therapeutic, and prognostic considerations. Semin Arthritis Rheum 8:200, 1979

GOLDENBERG DL, REED JI: Bacterial arthritis. N Engl J Med 312:764, 1985

HOFFMAN GS: Mycobacterial and fungal infections of bones and joints, in *Textbook of Rheumatology*, 2d ed, WN Kelley, ED Harris, Jr, S Ruddy (eds). Philadelphia, Saunders, 1985

STEIGBIGEL NH: Diagnosis and management of septic arthritis, in *Current Clinical Topics in Infectious Diseases*, JS Remington, MN Swartz (eds). New York, McGraw-Hill, 1983, vol 4, pp 1–29

92　OSTEOMYELITIS AND INFECTIONS OF PROSTHETIC JOINTS

JAMES H. MAGUIRE

Osteomyelitis, an infection of bone, is caused most commonly by pyogenic bacteria and mycobacteria. Case classification on the basis of the causative agent and the route and duration of infection provides a useful framework for evaluating the patient and planning treatment.

PATHOGENESIS AND PATHOLOGY Microorganisms enter bone by the hematogenous route, by direct introduction from a contiguous focus of infection, or by a penetrating wound. Trauma, ischemia, and foreign bodies enhance the susceptibility of bone to microbial invasion. Phagocytes attempt to contain the infections and, in the process, release enzymes that lyse bone. Pus spreads into vascular channels, raising intraosseous pressure and impairing the flow of blood; as the untreated infection becomes chronic, ischemic necrosis of bone results in the separation of large devascularized fragments (*sequestra*). When pus breaks through the cortex, subperiosteal or soft tissue abscesses form, and the elevated periosteum deposits new bone (the *involucrum*) around the sequestrum. Bacteria escape host defenses by adhering tightly to damaged bone and by coating themselves and underlying surfaces with a protective biofilm.

Microorganisms, infiltrates of neutrophils, and congested or thrombosed blood vessels are the principal histologic findings of acute osteomyelitis. The distinguishing feature of chronic osteomyelitis is necrotic bone, which is recognized by the absence of living osteocytes. Mononuclear cells predominate in chronic infections, and granulation and fibrous tissues replace bone that has been resorbed by osteoclasts. In the chronic stage, organisms may be too few to be seen.

HEMATOGENOUS OSTEOMYELITIS Hematogenous infection accounts for approximately 20 percent of cases of osteomyelitis and primarily affects children, in whom the long bones are infected, and older adults and intravenous drug users, in whom the spine is the usual site of infection.

Acute hematogenous osteomyelitis Infection usually involves a single bone, most commonly the tibia, femur, or humerus. Bacteria settle in the well-perfused metaphysis, where functioning phagocytes are scarce and a network of venous sinusoids slows the flow of blood. Because of a different vascular anatomy in children and adults, hematogenous infection of long bones is uncommon during adulthood and, when it occurs, usually involves the diaphysis.

In children, the source of bacteremia is often inapparent, although there may have been recent blunt trauma to the extremity. On presentation, the child usually appears acutely ill, with high fever, chills, localized pain and tenderness, and leukocytosis. Cutaneous erythema and swelling indicate extension of pus through the cortex. During infancy and after puberty, infection may spread through the epiphysis into the joint space.

Plain radiographs initially show soft tissue swelling, but the first change in bone—a periosteal reaction—is not evident until at least 10 days after the onset of infection. Lytic changes can be detected after 2 to 6 weeks, when 50 to 75 percent of bone density has been lost. Rarely, a well-circumscribed lytic lesion, or *Brodie's abscess*, is seen in a child who has had pain for several months but no fever.

Chronic hematogenous osteomyelitis With prompt treatment, fewer than 5 percent of cases of acute hematogenous osteomyelitis progress to chronic osteomyelitis. On average, 10 days are required for the formation of necrotic bone, but plain radiographs are unable to detect sequestra or sclerotic new bone for many weeks.

A protracted clinical course, long periods of quiescence, and recurrent exacerbations are characteristic of chronic osteomyelitis. Sinus tracts between bone and skin may drain purulent material and occasionally pieces of necrotic bone. An increase in drainage, pain, or the erythrocyte sedimentation rate (ESR) signals an exacerbation. Fever is unusual except when obstruction of a sinus tract leads to soft tissue infection. Rare late complications include pathologic fractures, squamous cell carcinoma of the sinus tract, and amyloidosis.

Vertebral osteomyelitis Organisms reach the well-perfused vertebral body of adults via spinal arteries and quickly spread from the end plate into the disk space and then to the adjacent vertebral body. The infection may originate in the urinary tract and reach the spine via the prostatic venous (Baston's) plexus; such cases develop particularly often among elderly men. Other sources of the bacteremia include endocarditis, soft tissue infection, and a contaminated intravenous line; these sources usually are obvious. Penetrating injuries and surgical procedures to the vertebrae may cause nonhematogenous vertebral osteomyelitis.

Most patients with vertebral osteomyelitis complain of neck or back pain, although 15 percent describe atypical pain in the chest, abdomen, or an extremity that is due to irritation of nerve roots. Symptoms are localized to the lumbar spine (over 50 percent) more often than the thoracic (35 percent) or cervical spine in pyogenic infections, but the thoracic spine is involved most commonly in tuberculous spondylitis (Pott's disease). Percussion over the involved vertebra elicits tenderness, and physical examination may reveal spasm of the paraspinal muscles and a limitation of motion. Approximately 50 percent of patients experience a subacute illness in which a vague, dull pain gradually intensifies over the course of 2 to 3 months; fever is low grade or absent, and the white blood cell count is normal. An acute presentation with high fever and toxicity is less common and suggests an ongoing bacteremia.

Usually, by the time the patient seeks medical attention, the ESR is elevated, and plain radiographs show irregular erosions in the end plates of adjacent vertebral bodies and narrowing of the intervening disk space. This radiographic pattern is virtually diagnostic of bacterial infection because tumors and other diseases of the spine rarely cross the disk space. Computed tomography (CT) or magnetic resonance imaging (MRI) may demonstrate epidural, paraspinal, retropharyngeal, mediastinal, retroperitoneal, or psoas abscesses that originate in the spine. An epidural abscess may evolve suddenly or over the course of several weeks; irreversible paralysis may be the consequence of failure to recognize the classic clinical presentation of a spinal epidural abscess, consisting of spinal pain progressing to radicular pain and weakness.

Microbiology Over 95 percent of cases of hematogenous osteomyelitis are caused by a single organism. *Staphylococcus aureus* accounts for 50 percent of isolates. Vertebral osteomyelitis is due to *Escherichia coli* and other enteric bacilli in approximately 25 percent of cases. *Pseudomonas aeruginosa* and *Serratia* infections are associated with intravenous drug use in some parts of the United States and may involve the sacroiliac, sternoclavicular, or pubic joints as well as the spine. *Salmonella* spp. and *S. aureus* are the major causes of long bone osteomyelitis complicating sickle cell anemia and other hemoglobinopathies. Tuberculosis and brucellosis affect the spine more often than other bones.

Unusual causes of hematogenous osteomyelitis include disseminated histoplasmosis, coccidioidomycosis, and blastomycosis in endemic areas. Immunocompromised persons on rare occasions develop osteomyelitis due to species of *Candida, Cryptococcus, Aspergillus,* or *Pneumocystis.* Syphilis, yaws, varicella, and vaccinia may involve bone. The etiology of chronic relapsing multifocal osteomyelitis, an inflammatory condition of children characterized by recurrent episodes of painful lytic lesions in multiple bones, has not yet been identified.

OSTEOMYELITIS SECONDARY TO A CONTIGUOUS FOCUS OF INFECTION   Clinical features   This broad category includes infections introduced by penetrating injuries and surgical procedures and direct extension of infection from adjacent soft tissues. It accounts for the greatest number of cases of osteomyelitis and occurs most commonly in adults.

Frequently the diagnosis is not made until the infection has already become chronic. The pain, fever, and inflammatory signs due to acute osteomyelitis may be attributed to the original injury or soft tissue infection. An indolent infection may become apparent only weeks or months later when a sinus tract develops, a surgical wound breaks down, or a fracture fails to heal. It may be impossible to distinguish the radiographic abnormalities due to osteomyelitis from those due to the precipitating condition.

A special category of contiguous focus osteomyelitis occurs in the setting of peripheral vascular disease and nearly always involves the small bones of the feet of adult diabetics. Diabetic neuropathy exposes the foot to frequent trauma and pressure sores, and the patient may be unaware of infection as it spreads into bone. Poor tissue perfusion impairs normal inflammatory responses and wound healing and creates a milieu that is conducive to anaerobic infections. It is often during the evaluation of a nonhealing ulcer or acute cellulitis that a radiograph provides the first evidence of osteomyelitis.

Microbiology   *S. aureus* is a pathogen in more than half of cases, but in contrast to hematogenous osteomyelitis, these infections often are polymicrobial and more likely to involve gram-negative and anaerobic bacteria. Hence a mixture of staphylococci, streptococci, enteric organisms, and anaerobic bacteria may be isolated from a diabetic foot infection or pelvic osteomyelitis underlying a decubitus ulcer. Aerobic and anaerobic bacteria cause osteomyelitis following surgery or soft tissue infection of the oropharynx, paranasal sinuses, gastrointestinal tract, or female genital tract. *S. aureus* is the principal cause of postoperative infections; coagulase-negative staphylococci are common pathogens following implantation of orthopedic appliances; and these organisms as well as gram-negative enteric bacilli, atypical mycobacteria, and *Mycoplasma* may cause sternal osteomyelitis after cardiac surgery. Infection with *P. aeruginosa* is frequently associated with puncture wounds of the foot or thermal burns, and *Pasteurella multocida* infection commonly follows cat bites (see Chap. 95).

DIAGNOSIS   Early diagnosis of acute osteomyelitis is critical because prompt antibiotic therapy may prevent the necrosis of bone. The evaluation usually begins with plain radiographs because of their ready availability, although they frequently show no abnormalities during early infection. The ESR is elevated in most cases of active osteomyelitis, including those in which constitutional symptoms and leukocytosis are missing. It is not a specific test for osteomyelitis, however, and occasionally is normal in early infections. In 95 percent of cases the technetium radionuclide scan using ^{99m}Tc diphosphonate is positive within 24 h of onset of symptoms. Falsely negative scans usually indicate obstruction of blood flow to the bone. Because the uptake of technetium reflects osteoblastic activity and skeletal vascularity, the bone scan cannot differentiate osteomyelitis from fractures, tumors, infarction, or neuropathic osteopathy. ^{67}Ga citrate–

and ^{111}In-labeled leukocyte or immunoglobulin scans, which have greater specificity for inflammation, may help distinguish infectious from noninfectious processes and indicate inflammatory changes within bones that are already abnormal by radiography and the technetium scan for other reasons.

MRI is as sensitive as the bone scan for the diagnosis of acute osteomyelitis because it is able to demonstrate changes in the water content of marrow. MRI gives better anatomic resolution of epidural abscesses and other soft tissue processes than CT and is currently the imaging technique of choice for vertebral osteomyelitis.

The role of diagnostic imaging in chronic osteomyelitis is to determine the presence of active infection and delineate the extent of debridement necessary to remove necrotic bone and abnormal soft tissues. Although plain films accurately reflect chronic changes, the CT scan is more sensitive for detecting sequestra, sinus tracts, and soft tissue abscesses. Sequential technetium and gallium or indium scans may help determine whether infection is active and may distinguish infection from noninflammatory bone changes; they do not, however, provide good anatomic detail. MRI gives detailed information about the activity and the anatomic extent of infection but does not always distinguish osteomyelitis from healing fractures and tumors. MRI is particularly useful in distinguishing cellulitis from osteomyelitis in the diabetic foot; however, no imaging modality consistently distinguishes infection from neuropathic osteopathy.

Appropriate samples for microbiologic studies should be obtained in all cases of suspected osteomyelitis before initiation of antimicrobial therapy. Blood cultures are indicated in acute cases and are positive in over one-third of children with hematogenous osteomyelitis and 25 percent of adults with vertebral osteomyelitis. If the clinical picture demands immediate antibiotic therapy or if blood cultures are negative, samples from needle aspiration of pus in bone or soft tissues or a bone biopsy should be obtained for culture.

The results of culture of specimens obtained by swabbing a sinus tract or the base of an ulcer correlate poorly with the organisms infecting the bone. For this reason, in cases of chronic osteomyelitis and contiguous focus osteomyelitis, samples for aerobic and anaerobic culture should be obtained by percutaneous needle aspiration, percutaneous biopsy, or intraoperative biopsy at the time of debridement. Isolates of coagulase-negative staphylococci and other organisms of low virulence should not be automatically disregarded as contaminants, especially in the presence of prosthetic materials. Special culture media may be necessary to isolate mycobacteria, fungi, and other less common pathogens. In some cases, histopathologic examination of biopsy specimens may be the only way to make a diagnosis.

TREATMENT   Antiobiotic therapy   Antibiotics are administered only after appropriate specimens have been obtained for culture. The antibiotics selected should be bactericidal for the organism(s) isolated from bone or blood and in most cases should be given intravenously in the same high doses used to treat endocarditis. When necessary, empirical therapy is guided by the findings of a Gram-stained specimen from the bone or abscess or is chosen to cover the most likely pathogens. Empirical therapy in most cases should include an agent active against *S. aureus,* such as oxacillin, nafcillin, a cephalosporin, or vancomycin and, if gram-negative organisms are likely to be involved, a third-generation cephalosporin, an aminoglycoside, or a fluoroquinolone.

The duration of therapy is typically 4 to 6 weeks; in some cases, at-home intravenous administration of antibiotics or oral therapy is appropriate. Children with acute hematogenous osteomyelitis routinely receive oral antibiotics after 5 to 10 days of parenteral therapy if signs of active infection have resolved; such treatment has been as successful as the standard parenteral therapy. The doses of oral penicillins or cephalosporins required for treating osteomyelitis are several times higher than the doses of these drugs given for common infections. Adults do not tolerate these high doses as well as children, and except in case of the fluoroquinolones, there are few data to support the use of oral antibiotics by adults. Oral administration of an agent such as ciprofloxacin (750 mg every 12 h) has been as successful as the intravenous administration of β-lactam antibiotics. Caution should be exercised in the use of these agents as the sole treatment of infection due to *S. aureus* or *P. aeruginosa* because resistance may develop during therapy.

Serum minimal bactericidal concentrations (MBC) against isolates of the responsible pathogen should be measured to document compliance and adequate serum levels in patients who receive an oral antibiotic. Otherwise, there are few data to support the routine use of the MBC to monitor therapy of osteomyelitis.

Acute osteomyelitis Early treatment of acute hematogenous osteomyelitis of childhood with 4 to 6 weeks of an appropriate antibiotic is usually successful; treatment for less than 3 weeks has resulted in a 10-fold greater rate of failure. Surgical intervention in childhood cases is indicated for intraosseous or subperiosteal abscesses, concomitant septic arthritis, and failure of the acute signs of infection to improve in 24 to 48 h. Acute hematogenous osteomyelitis of bones other than the spine in adults often requires surgical debridement.

Four to 6 weeks of an appropriate antibiotic are usually sufficient to cure vertebral osteomyelitis. Failure of the ESR to drop to at least two-thirds of pretreatment levels is an indication for longer treatment. Surgery is seldom necessary, even in cases of many months' duration, except in the case of spinal instability, new or progressive neurologic deficits, large soft tissue abscesses, or a failure of medical treatment. Patients should maintain bed rest until back pain has declined to the point at which ambulation is possible. Body casts are no longer used.

Contiguous focus osteomyelitis usually requires surgery in addition to 4 to 6 weeks of appropriate antibiotics, even when diagnosed early, because of underlying soft tissue infection or damage to bone from an injury or surgery.

Chronic ostemyelitis The risks and benefits of aggressive therapy of chronic osteomyelitis should be weighed before any attempt to eradicate the infection is undertaken. Some patients with extensive disease prefer to live with their infections rather than undergo multiple surgical procedures, take prolonged courses of antimicrobial therapy, and face the risk of loss of an extremity. Such persons often benefit from intermittent courses of oral antibiotics to suppress acute exacerbations.

Once the decision has been made to treat chronic osteomyelitis aggressively, antibiotics should be started several days before surgery to reduce inflammation if the etiology of the infection is known preoperatively. If not, antibiotic therapy should be withheld until surgical debridement. An empirical antibiotic regimen is started intraoperatively after culture specimens are obtained. Four to 6 weeks of appropriate antibiotic therapy are given postoperatively on the basis of the susceptibility pattern of organisms isolated from the bone. The benefit of prolonged oral antibiotic therapy following 4 to 6 weeks of parenteral therapy remains unproven. There currently is insufficient information to recommend the routine use of hyperbaric oxygen to enhance the killing of microorganisms by phagocytes or instillation pumps and antibiotic-impregnated methacrylate beads to deliver high levels of antibiotics to the bone.

Success in treating chronic osteomyelitis rests largely on the complete surgical removal of necrotic bone and abnormal soft tissues. Modern imaging techniques allow accurate preoperative delineation of tissues to be debrided, but it remains difficult for the surgeon to determine intraoperatively whether all necrotic and infected tissue has been removed. In the past, the inability to restore large defects in bone and soft tissue limited the extent of debridement. Muscle flaps and skin grafts are now used routinely to cover large soft tissue defects and fill dead space, and bone grafts and vascularized bone transfer may restore a seriously compromised bone to a functional state.

In infections of recent fractures, internal fixators are often left in place, and the infection is controlled by limited debridement and suppressive antibiotic therapy. Definitive surgical antimicrobial ther-apies are delayed until after bony union of the fracture is achieved. If there is nonunion of the fracture or loosening of the fixator, the appliance should be removed and an external fixator applied.

Osteomyelitis of the small bones of the feet in persons with vascular disease also requries surgery for successful treatment. The effectiveness of the surgery is limited by the blood supply to the site and the patient's ability to heal the wound. Revascularization of the extremity is indicated if the vascular disease involves large arteries. In cases of decreased perfusion due to small-vessel disease, treatment is likely to fail, and the best option is suppressive therapy or amputation. The duration of antibiotic therapy depends on the surgical procedure performed. When the infected bone is removed entirely but residual infection of soft tissues remains, 2 weeks of antibiotics should be given; if amputation eliminates infected bone and soft tissue, standard surgical prophylaxis is given; otherwise 4 to 6 weeks of postoperative antibiotics are required.

INFECTIONS OF PROSTHETIC JOINTS Infection complicates 1 to 4 percent of total joint replacements. The majority of infections are acquired intraoperatively or in the immediate postoperative period due to wound breakdown or infection and, less commonly, at any time after joint replacement by the hematogenous route or by direct inoculation. The presentation may be acute with fever, pain, and local signs of inflammation, especially in infections due to *S. aureus*, pyogenic streptococci, and enteric bacilli, or infection may persist for months or years without causing constitutional symptoms when less virulent organisms such as coagulase-negative staphylococci or diphtheroids are involved. Such indolent infections are usually acquired during joint implantation and are discovered during evaluation of chronic unexplained pain or after a radiograph shows loosening of the prothesis; the ESR is usually elevated in such cases.

The diagnosis is best made by needle aspiration of the joint; accidental introduction of organisms during aspiration must be meticulously avoided. Synovial fluid pleocytosis with a predominance of polymorphonuclear leukocytes is highly suggestive of infection, since other inflammatory processes uncommonly affect prosthetic joints. Culture and Gram's stain usually yield the responsible pathogen. Special media for unusual pathogens such as fungi, atypical mycobacteria, and *Mycoplasma* may be necessary if routine and anaerobic cultures are negative.

Treatment includes surgery and high doses of parenteral antibiotics, which are given for 4 to 6 weeks because bone is usually involved. In most cases, the prosthesis must be replaced in order to cure the infection. Implantation of a new prothesis is best delayed for several weeks or months because relapses of infection occur most commonly within this time frame. In some cases, reimplantation is not possible, and the patient must manage without a joint, with a fused joint, or, at times, with amputation. Cure of infection without removal of the prosthesis occasionally is possible in cases of infection due to streptococci or pneumococci and without radiologic evidence of loosening of the prosthesis. In these cases, antibiotic therapy must begin within several days of the onset of infection, and the joint should be vigorously drained either by open arthrotomy or arthroscopically.

To avoid the disastrous consequences of infection, candidates for joint replacement should be selected with care. Rates of infection are particularly high in patients with rheumatoid arthritis, persons who have undergone previous surgery on the joint, and persons with medical conditions requiring immunosuppressive therapy. Perioperative antibiotic prophylaxis, usually cefazolin, and measures to decrease intraoperative contamination, such as laminar flow, have decreased the rates of perioperative infection to less than 1 percent in many centers. Following implantation, measures should be taken to prevent and rapidly treat extraarticular infections that might give rise to hematogenous spread of infection to the prosthesis. The effectiveness of prophylactic antibiotics for prevention of hematogenous infection following dental procedures has not been demonstrated, and in fact, viridans streptococci and other components of the oral flora are extremely unusual causes of prosthetic joint infection.

REFERENCES

Esolen LM et al: *Pneumocystis carinii* osteomyelitis in a patient with common variable immunodeficiency. N Engl J Med 326:999, 1992

Esterhai JL Jr (ed): Orthopedic infection. Orthop Clin North Am 22:363, 1991

Mader JT et al: Evaluation of new anti-infective drugs for the treatment of osteomyelitis in adults. Clin Infect Dis 15(suppl 1):S155, 1992

May JW Jr et al: Treatment of chronic traumatic bone wounds. Microvascular free tissue transfer: A 13-year experience in 96 patients. Ann Surg 214:241, 1991

Norden CW (ed): Osteomyelitis. Infect Dis Clin North Am 4:361, 1990

Waldvogel FA et al: Osteomyelitis: A review of clinical features, therapeutic considerations, and unusual aspects. N Engl J Med 282:198, 1970

93 INFECTIONS OF THE SKIN, MUSCLE, AND SOFT TISSUES

DENNIS L. STEVENS

ANATOMICAL RELATIONSHIPS: CLUES TO THE DIAGNOSIS OF SOFT TISSUE INFECTIONS Protection against infection of the epidermis is dependent upon the mechanical barrier afforded by the stratum corneum, since the epidermis itself is devoid of blood vessels (Fig. 93-1). Disruption of this layer by burns, bites, abrasion, or foreign body allows penetration of bacteria to the deeper structures. Similarly, the hair follicle can serve as a portal for either normal flora *(Staphylococcus)* or for extrinsic bacteria *(Pseudomonas—*hot tub folliculitis). Intracellular infection of the squamous epithelium with vesicle formation may arise from cutaneous inoculation with viruses such as herpes simplex 1, from the dermal capillary plexus with viruses associated with viremia (varicella), or from cutaneous nerve roots (herpes zoster). Bacteria infecting the epidermis such as *Streptococcus pyogenes* may be translocated laterally to deeper structures via lymphatics, thus resulting in the rapid superficial spread of erysipelas. Later, engorgement or obstruction of lymphatics causes flaccid edema of the epidermis, another characteristic of erysipelas.

The rich plexus of capillaries beneath the dermal papillae provides nutrition to the stratum germinativum, and physiologic responses of this plexus provide important clinical signs and symptoms. For example, infective vasculitis of the plexus results in petechiae, Osler's nodes, Janeway lesions, and palpable purpura, which are important clues for the existence of endocarditis (Chap. 85). In addition, metastatic infection within this plexus can also result in cutaneous manifestations of disseminated fungal infection (Chap. 166), gonococcal infection (Chap. 110), salmonella infections (Chap. 117), pseudomonas infection, i.e. ecthyma gangrenosa (Chap. 116), meningococcemia (Chap. 109), and staphylococcal infection (Chap. 102). This plexus also provides access for bacteria to the circulation, thereby facilitating local spread or bacteremia. Postcapillary venules of this plexus are a major site of polymorphonuclear leukocyte sequestration, diapedesis, and chemotaxis to the site of cutaneous infection. Exaggeration of these physiologic mechanisms by excessive cytokines or bacterial toxins causes leukostasis, venous occlusion, and pitting edema. Edema with purple bullae and ecchymosis suggests loss of vascular integrity and requires exploration of the deeper structures for evidence of necrotizing fasciitis or myonecrosis. To make an earlier diagnosis requires a high level of suspicion in patients with unexplained fever and pain and tenderness in the soft tissue, even in the absence of acute cutaneous inflammation.

INFECTIONS ASSOCIATED WITH VESICLES (Table 93-1) Vesicle formation due to infection is caused by viral proliferation within the epidermis. In variola, viremia precedes the onset of a diffuse centrifugal rash that progresses from macules to vesicles, then pustules, and finally scabs over the course of 1 to 2 weeks. Vesicles of varicella have a "dew drop" appearance and occur in crops randomly about the trunk, extremities, and face over the course of 3 to 4 days. Herpes zoster occurs in a single dermatome and is preceded by pain for several days before the appearance of vesicles. Zoster occurs predominately in elderly patients and AIDS victims, whereas most varicella occurs in young children. Vesicles due to herpes simplex (HSV) are found on or around the lips (HSV-1) or genitals (HSV-2) but may appear on the head and neck in young wrestlers (herpes gladitorum) or on the digits (herpetic whitlow) in health care workers. Coxsackie A-16 characteristically causes vesicles on the

FIGURE 93-1 Structural components of the skin and soft tissue are identified at the left. Superficial infections are depicted along the top of the figure and infections of the deeper structures of the soft tissue at the right edge. The rich capillary network beneath the dermal papillae plays a key role in localizing infection and in the development of the acute inflammatory reaction.

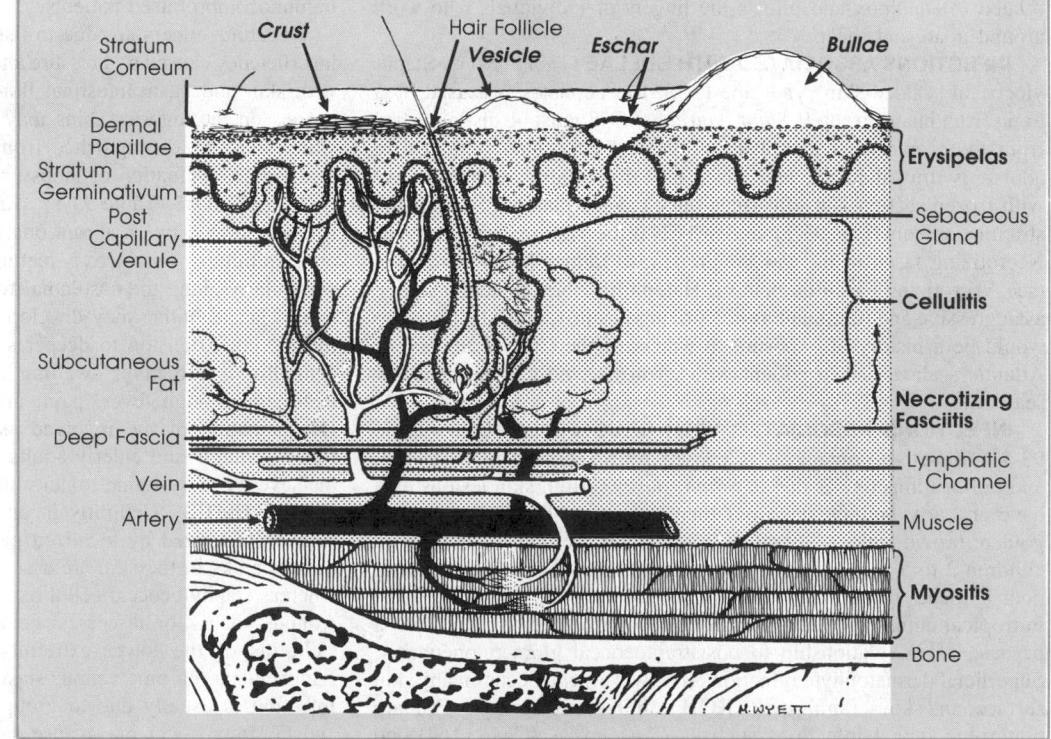

TABLE 93-1   Skin and soft-tissue infections

Lesion	Agent/ Clinical syndrome	Chapter Reference
Vesicles	Variola (smallpox)	147
	Varicella (chickenpox)	144
	Herpes zoster (shingles)	144
	Herpes simplex types I and II	143
	Coxsackie A-16 (hand, foot, and mouth disease)	154
	Orf	147
Bullae	Staphylococcal scalded-skin syndrome	102
	Necrotizing fasciitis	128
	Gas gangrene	108
	Halophilic vibrio	120
Crusted lesions	Impetigo	103
	Superficial dermatophytes	169
	Systemic dimorphic fungi	162
	Cutaneous leishmaniasis	175
	Mucocutaneous candidiasis	166
	Cutaneous tuberculosis	130
	Nocardiosis	126
Folliculitis	*Staphylococcus aureus*	102
	Pseudomonas aeruginosa (hot tub folliculitis)	116
	Schistosomiasis (swimmer's itch)	183
	Acne vulgaris	51
Ulcers with or without eschars	Anthrax	104
	Cutaneous diptheria	104
	Ulceroglandular tularemia	122
	Bubonic plague	123
	Mycobacterium ulcerans	132
	Mycobacterium leprae	131
	Mycobacterium tuberculosis	130
Erysipelas	*Streptococcus pyogenes*	103
Necrotizing fasciitis	*Streptococcus pyogenes*	103
	Mixed aerobic/anaerobic infection	128
Myositis	Pyomyositis	102
	Streptococcal necrotizing myositis	103
	Gas gangrene	108
	Nonclostridial (crepitant) myositis	128
	Synergistic nonclostridial anaerobic myonecrosis	128

hands, feet, and mouth in children. Orf is caused by a DNA virus related to smallpox and infects the fingers of individuals who work around goats and sheep.

INFECTIONS ASSOCIATED WITH BULLAE (Table 93-1)   Staphylococcal scalded-skin syndrome (SSSS) in neonates is caused by a toxin from phage group II *Staph. aureus*. SSSS must be distinguished from toxic epidermal necrolysis (TEN) which occurs primarily in adults, is drug induced, and has a higher mortality. Punch biopsy with frozen section is useful since the cleavage plane in SSSS is the stratum corneum (Fig. 93-1), and in TEN is the stratum germinativum. Necrotizing fasciitis and gas gangrene also induce bullae formation (see Necrotizing Fasciitis, below). Halophilic vibrio infection can be as aggressive and fulminant as necrotizing fasciitis, and a helpful clue would be a history of exposure to waters of the Gulf of Mexico or Atlantic seaboard, or a patient with cirrhosis who has ingested raw seafood.

INFECTIONS ASSOCIATED WITH CRUSTED LESIONS (Table 93-1)   Impetigo contagiosa is caused by *Streptococcus pyogenes*, and bullous impetigo is due to *Staph. aureus*. Both skin lesions may have an early bullous stage but then appear as thick crusts with a golden brown color. Streptococcal lesions are most common in children 2 to 5 years of age, and epidemics may occur in settings of poor hygiene, particularly in children of lower socioeconomic status in tropical climates. It is important to recognize impetigo contagiosa because of its relationship to poststreptococcal glomerulonephritis. Superficial dermatophyte infections (ringworm) can occur on any skin surface, and skin scrapings with KOH staining are diagnostic. Primary dimorphic fungal infections such as *Blastomyces* (Chap. 164) and

Sporothrix schenkii (Chap. 169) can initially present as crusted skin lesions resembling ringworm. Disseminated *Coccidioides immitis* (Chap. 163) also can involve skin, and biopsy and culture should be performed on crusted lesions in patients from endemic areas.

FOLLICULITIS (Table 93-1)   Hair follicles serve as a portal of entry for a number of bacteria, though *Staph. aureus* is the most common cause of localized folliculitis. Sebaceous glands empty into hair follicles and ducts, which if blocked (sebaceous cyst), may resemble staphylococcal abscess or may become secondarily infected. Infection of sweat glands (hidradenitis suppurativa) can also mimic infected hair follicles particularly in the axillae. Chronic folliculitis is uncommon except in acne vulgaris where normal flora, e.g., *Propionibacterium acnes,* may play a role.

Diffuse folliculitis occurs in two settings. "Hot-tub folliculitis" is caused by *Pseudomonas aeruginosa* in waters that are insufficiently chlorinated and maintained at temperatures between 37 and 40°C. Infection is usually self-limited, though bacteremia and shock have been reported. Swimmer's itch occurs when a skin surface is exposed to water infested with freshwater avian schistosomes. Warm water temperatures and alkaline pH are suitable for molluscs that serve as intermediate hosts between bird and human. Free-swimming schistosomal cercariae (see Chap. 183) readily penetrate human hair follicles or pores but quickly die and elicit a brisk allergic reaction causing intense itching and erythema.

ULCERS WITH OR WITHOUT ESCHARS (Table 93-1)   Cutaneous anthrax begins as a pruritic papule which develops within days to an ulcer with surrounding vesicles and edema and then to an enlarging ulcer with black eschar. Cutaneous diphtheria may cause chronic nonhealing ulcers with an overlying dirty-gray membrane, though lesions may also mimic psoriasis, eczema, or impetigo. Ulceroglandular tularemia may have associated ulcerated skin lesions with painful regional adenopathy. Although bubos are the major cutaneous manifestation of plague (see Chap. 123), cutaneous lesions in 25 percent of cases include ulcers with eschars, papules, or pustules.

Mycobacterium ulcerans typically causes chronic skin ulcers on the extremities of individuals living in the tropics. *M. leprae* may be associated with cutaneous ulcerations in patients with lepromatous leprosy associated with the Lucio phenomenon or during reversal reactions. *M. tuberculosis* may also cause ulcerations, papules, or erythematous macular lesions of the skin in both normal and immunocompromised patients.

Decubitus ulcers are due to tissue hypoxia secondary to vascular insufficiency caused by pressure and may become secondarily infected with skin and gastrointestinal flora including anaerobes. Ulcerative lesions on the anterior shins may be due to pyoderma gangrenosa, which must be distinguished from infectious etiology by means of histological evaluation of biopsy sites.

ERYSIPELAS (Table 93-1)   Erysipelas is due to *S. pyogenes* and is characterized by an abrupt onset of fiery, red swelling of the face or extremities. Distinctive features are its well-defined margins, particularly along the nasolabial fold, rapid progression, and intense pain. Flaccid bullae may develop during the second or third day of illness, but extension to deeper soft tissues is rare. Treatment with penicillin is effective; swelling may progress despite appropriate treatment, though fever, pain, and the intense red color diminish. Desquamation of the involved skin occurs 5 to 10 days into the illness. Infants and elderly adults are most commonly afflicted, and the severity of systemic toxicity may vary.

CELLULITIS   Cellulitis is an acute inflammatory condition of skin characterized by localized pain, erythema, swelling, and heat. Small breaks in the skin are associated with streptococcal infection, whereas staphylococcal cellulitis is commonly associated with larger wounds, ulcers, or abscesses. Fever suggests streptococcal infection. Cellulitis of the lower extremity is more common with chronic lymphedema, chronic venous stasis, and saphenous vein donor sites. Infection is usually due to group A streptococci, though group C and G streptococci may cause saphenous donor site infections. *S.*

agalactiae infection may occur in diabetes mellitus or peripheral vascular disease. *Haemophilus influenzae* causes periorbital cellulitis in children in association with sinusitis, otitis media, or epiglottitis.

Exogenous bacteria may be introduced into the skin by a variety of means: *Pasteurella multocida*—cat bites; *Staph. intermedius*—dog bites; *Aeromonas hydrophila*—cuts in fresh water; *P. aeruginosa*—sweaty tennis shoe syndrome; *Erysipelothrix rhusiopathiae*—fish monger's cellulitis; *Mycobacterium marinum*—fish tank exposure; and gram-negative rod cellulitis—compromised hosts.

Bacterial diagnosis is difficult in acute cellulitis, and needle aspiration or even punch biopsy yields positive cultures in only about 20 percent of cases. The low number of bacteria identified suggests that toxins or host response to infection may be largely responsible for the signs and symptoms of cellulitis.

NECROTIZING FASCIITIS (Table 93-1) Necrotizing fasciitis, formerly called streptococcal gangrene, may be associated with group A streptococcus, mixed aerobic-anaerobic bacteria, or as part of gas gangrene caused by *Clostridium perfringens*. Early diagnosis may be difficult when pain or unexplained fever are the only presenting symptoms and signs. Swelling then occurs and is followed by brawny edema and tenderness. With progression, dark red induration of the epidermis appears along with bullae filled with blue or purple fluid. Later skin becomes friable and takes on a bluish, maroon, or black color. By this stage, extensive thrombosis of blood vessels occur in the dermal papilla (see Fig. 93-1). Extension of infection to the level of the deep fascia causes a brownish-gray appearance. Rapid spreading occurs along fascial planes, through venous channels and lymphatics. Patients in the later stages are toxic and frequently manifest shock and multiorgan failure.

Necrotizing fasciitis caused by mixed aerobic-anaerobic bacteria begins with a breach in integrity of a mucous membrane barrier such as the mucosa of the gastrointestinal or genitourinary tract. The portal can be a malignancy, diverticulum, hemorrhoid, anal fissure, or urethral tear. Other predisposing factors include peripheral vascular disease, diabetes mellitus, surgery, or penetrating injury to the abdomen. Leakage into the perineal area results in a syndrome called *Fournier's gangrene,* characterized by massive swelling of the scrotum and penis with extension into the perineum, or abdominal wall, and legs.

Necrotizing fasciitis caused by *S. pyogenes* has increased in frequency and severity since 1985. It frequently begins deep at the site of nonpenetrating minor trauma such as a bruise or muscle strain. Seeding of the site by transient bacteremia is likely, though most patients deny antecedent streptococcal infection. Necrotizing fasciitis due to mixed aerobic-anaerobic bacteria may be associated with gas in the deep tissue, but gas is not usually present when the cause is *S. pyogenes.* Toxicity is severe, and renal impairment may precede the development of shock. In 20 to 40 percent of cases, myositis occurs concomitantly, and, as in gas gangrene (see below), serum creatinine phosphokinase values may be markedly elevated. Prompt surgical exploration down to the deep fascia and muscle is essential. Necrotic tissue must be surgically removed, and Gram's stain of material will be useful to establish whether group A streptococci, mixed aerobic-anaerobic bacteria, or *Clostridium* species are present. (See "Treatment," below.)

MYOSITIS (Table 93-1) Muscle involvement can occur with virus infection [influenza, dengue, coxsackievirus B (pleurodynia)]; or parasitic invasion [*Trichinella spiralis* (trichinosis), *Taenia solium* (cysticercosis), *Toxoplasma gondii* (toxoplasmosis)]. Although myalgia can occur in most of these infections, severe muscle pain is the hallmark of pleurodynia, trichinosis, and bacterial infection. Acute rhabdomyolysis predictably occurs with clostridial and streptococcal myositis but may also be associated with influenza, echovirus, coxsackievirus, Epstein-Barr virus, and *Legionella* infection.

Pyomyositis is usually due to *Staph. aureus,* is common in tropical areas, and commonly has no known portal of entry. Infection remains localized and unless organisms produce toxic shock syndrome toxin

1 or certain enterotoxins, shock does not occur. In contrast, *S. pyogenes* may induce a primary myositis referred to as *streptococcal necrotizing myositis,* which is associated with severe systemic toxicity. Such infections occur as part of the streptococcal toxic shock syndrome.

Gas gangrene usually occurs following severe penetrating injuries that result in interruption of blood supply and introduction of soil into wounds. Such cases of traumatic gangrene are usually caused by *C. perfringens, C. septicum,* or *C. histolyticum*. Rarely, latent or recurrent gangrene can occur years after penetrating trauma, most likely due to dormant spores that reside at the previous site of injury. Spontaneous nontraumatic gangrene among patients with neutropenia, gastrointestinal malignancy, diverticulosis, or recent radiation therapy to the abdomen is caused by *C. septicum*. Tolerance of this anaerobe to oxygen probably explains why *C. septicum* can initiate infection spontaneously in normal tissue anywhere in the body.

Synergistic nonclostridial anaerobic myonecrosis, also known as necrotizing cutaneous myositis and synergistic necrotizing cellulitis, is a variant of necrotizing fasciitis caused by mixed aerobic and anaerobic bacteria with the exclusion of clostridial organisms (see "Necrotizing Fasciitis," above).

TREATMENT OF DEEP-SEATED SOFT TISSUE INFECTIONS
Early and aggressive surgical exploration is essential in patients with suspected necrotizing fasciitis, myositis, or gangrene in order to (1) visualize the deep structures, (2) remove necrotic tissue, (3) reduce compartment pressure, and (4) obtain suitable material for Gram's stain and aerobic and anaerobic cultures. Appropriate empirical antibiotic treatment pending culture results could be either A or B below:

A 1 Clindamycin 600–800 mg IV every 8 h or metronidazole 750 mg every 6 h
plus
2 Ampicillin or ampicillin/sulbactam 2–3 grams IV every 6 h
plus
3 Gentamicin 1.0–1.5 mg/kg every 8 h
or
B Ampicillin/sulbactam or cefoxitin alone

For Group A streptococcal and clostridial infection of the fascia and/or muscle, mortality of 20 to 50 percent occurs with penicillin treatment. In experimental models of streptococcal and clostridial necrotizing fasciitis/myositis, clindamycin has superior efficacy, but no comparative trials have been performed in humans. Hyperbaric oxygen treatment may also be useful in gas gangrene due to clostridia species. Antibiotic treatment should be continued until all signs of systemic toxicity have resolved, all devitalized tissue has been removed, and granulation tissue has developed (Chaps. 103, 108, 128).

In summary, infections of the skin and soft tissues are diverse in presentation and severity and offer a great challenge to the clinician. This chapter is meant to provide an approach to diagnosis and understanding of the pathophysiologic mechanisms. More in-depth information may be found in individual chapters.

REFERENCES

HOOK EW et al: Microbiologic evaluation of cutaneous cellulitis in adults. Arch Intern Med 146:295, 1986
SIMMONS RL, AHRENHOLZ DH: Infections of the skin and soft tissue, in *Surgical Infectious Diseases*, 2d ed, RJ Howard, RL Simmons (eds). Norwalk, Appleton & Lange, 1988, pp 377–441
STEVENS DL: Invasive group A Streptococcus infections. Clin Infect Dis 14:2, 1992
STEVENS DL et al: Spontaneous, nontraumatic gangrene due to *Clostridium septicum*. Rev Infect Dis 12(2):286, 1990

94   INFECTIONS (EXCLUDING AIDS) IN INJECTION DRUG USERS

GERALD H. FRIEDLAND / PETER A. SELWYN

The injection of illicit drugs is a widespread practice whose prevalence has increased dramatically since the 1950s in association with successive epidemics of heroin and cocaine use. Injection drug users are a hidden population, engaging in an illegal and societally disapproved activity. It is impossible to determine their precise number and, therefore, the true incidence of infectious complications in this population. In the 1980s, the total number of heroin addicts in the United States was estimated yearly at 500,000, with heavy concentrations in urban areas, particularly but not exclusively in the Northeast. The number of injection drug users may be almost three times this figure when users of cocaine and occasional injection users are included. In addition, there are large numbers of injection drug users in Europe and increasing numbers in developing countries, often at sites of drug production and along routes of drug trade and distribution.

Markedly higher age-specific mortality among injection drug users than in the general population was documented even before the epidemic of infection with human immunodeficiency virus (HIV) and AIDS (see Chap. 279). For example, in New York City between 1965 and 1972, the death rate among young (20- to 54-year-old) adult heroin addicts not involved in drug treatment programs was estimated to be five times greater than that among age-matched, non-heroin-addicted adults (28.2 per 1000 versus 5.6 per 1000). A substantial portion of this excess mortality was the result of infectious complications of injection drug use. Data from the New York City Medical Examiner during the 1960s indicated that 27 percent of narcotic-related deaths were associated with infections. During this period, a wide array of infectious complications of injection drug use was described. More recently, as a consequence of the HIV epidemic, overall mortality and cause-specific mortality secondary to both AIDS and bacterial infections have dramatically increased in this population. Mortality rates of 3.41 per 100 person-years from AIDS and 1.08 per 100 person-years from bacterial infection preceding AIDS have been reported in HIV-infected injection drug users.

Most infectious complications in injection drug users reflect the events surrounding drug injection and associated life-style issues rather than the direct effects of the illicit drugs themselves. Drugs are purchased in powdered form and often contain adulterants such as quinine, talc, and dextrose. The drugs are dissolved in water (obtained from any available source) or occasionally in saliva in bottle caps or "cookers," filtered through cotton wool or gauze, aspirated into tuberculin or diabetic syringes, and injected intravenously or subcutaneously. Skin preparation is usually minimal and may consist of rubbing saliva on the injection site. A small amount of blood may remain in the needle and syringe after use and may be diluted by rinsing in tap water or bleach. Needles and syringes are often shared among injection drug users, either by a few friends or relatives or by larger numbers of users sequentially and anonymously in "shooting galleries." These clandestine locations where injection drug users gather to rent injection equipment and administer drugs are ideal sites for the transmission of bloodborne infectious agents.

Within this setting, the characteristics of injection drug users that increase the risk of infection are (1) increased rates of skin, mucous membrane, and nasopharyngeal carriage of pathogenic organisms, particularly staphylococci, (2) unsterile injection technique resulting in the introduction of components of the skin or nasopharyngeal flora into soft tissues or the bloodstream, (3) contamination of injection equipment or drugs with viral, bacterial, and parasitic microorganisms, which may be present in residual blood in shared injection equipment or in contaminated water used to dissolve drugs before injection or to rinse equipment afterward, (4) humoral, cell-mediated, and phagocytic defects induced by HIV infection and/or drug use (even before the HIV/AIDS epidemic, injection drug users were known to have abnormal immunologic parameters, including high levels of globulins, false-positive serologic reactions to multiple antigens, and abnormalities in phagocytosis, and these defects have been markedly exacerbated by HIV-induced B and T cell dysfunction), (5) poor dental hygiene and drug-induced impairment of gag and cough reflexes, (6) alteration of the normal microbial flora by intermittent antibiotic use, (7) low socioeconomic status, with increased prevalence of exposure to certain pathogens (notably *Mycobacterium tuberculosis*), (8) behaviors associated with injection drug use, such as cigarette smoking, alcohol use, or exchange of sex for drugs or money, and (9) decreased access to and/or lack of appropriate use of preventive and primary health care services, resulting in low levels of immunization and prophylaxis and delay in the diagnosis and treatment of minor infectious complications.

SPECIFIC INFECTIONS OCCURRING AMONG INJECTION DRUG USERS

SKIN AND SOFT TISSUE INFECTIONS (See also Chap. 93) Infections of the skin and soft tissues represent the most common bacterial infectious complication of injection drug use and, before the AIDS epidemic, were the most common cause of hospital admissions of injection drug users. The clinical spectrum of infection is broad, ranging from simple cellulitis and abscess to life-threatening necrotizing fasciitis and septic thrombophlebitis. The high frequency of skin and soft tissue infections is attributable to several factors: the practice of injecting drugs subcutaneously ("skin popping"), the extravasation of drugs into soft tissue during intravenous injection, the presence in injected material of adulterants that may cause tissue necrosis, and the increased skin carriage of pathogenic organisms.

Most skin and soft tissue infections occur on the upper and lower extremities, but occasionally atypical sites (e.g., the abdomen or back, groin, scrotum, and neck) may be involved as a result of injection into the jugular or femoral veins. Cellulitis may extend from a fresh injection site or may result from superinfection of an open wound sustained earlier. The clinical appearance is often atypical because of chronic damage to the skin and to venous and lymphatic systems in both the upper and the lower extremities, with resultant underlying lymphedema, hyperpigmentation, scarring, and regional lymphadenopathy. Nevertheless, careful examination often reveals characteristic redness, warmth, and tenderness, with tender inguinal or axillary lymph nodes. Fever is variable and bacteremia infrequent.

Uncomplicated cellulitis is most frequently due to group A streptococci, other streptococci, or *Staphylococcus aureus*. Unless an associated open, draining wound is present or bacteremia develops, the precise microbial etiology is difficult to determine. For localized abscesses presenting either as draining lesions or as fluctuant subcutaneous masses, Gram's staining and culture of pus or aspirated material are required. Although these abscesses are usually staphylococcal in etiology, they are sometimes due to a more complex mixture of anaerobic and aerobic bacteria. A foul odor and Gram's staining of pus suggest the presence of mixed organisms.

Treatment consists of hospitalization in most cases, incision and drainage in instances of abscess formation, and administration of intravenous antistaphylococcal β-lactam antibiotics such as oxacillin or nafcillin. Cefazolin may be an alternative choice. In areas where methicillin-resistant *S. aureus* is highly prevalent, vancomycin should be used empirically pending the results of susceptibility tests. The total duration of therapy should be 10 to 14 days; for the latter part of this course, oral agents may or may not be used, depending on the individual's clinical response. For injection drug users who have an established realtionship with a health care provider, mild infections may be treated with oral agents on an outpatient basis; therapy should be followed by frequent visits at which the response is assessed.

Indolent skin ulcers are common. These lesions are shallow and indurated and may become superinfected. Their etiology is unclear, but they are likely the result of foreign-body inflammatory changes, necrosis, and low-grade infection. They usually respond to local wound care and oral or topical antibiotic treatment. Occasionally, these ulcers are extensive enough to require skin grafting. When lesions heal, they leave depressed, hyperpigmented scars.

Necrotizing fasciitis and myositis and septic thrombophlebitis are life-threatening local complications of injection drug use. Although infrequent, they should always be considered when skin or soft tissue infection develops in injection drug users. The presence of fasciitis and myositis is associated with exquisite pain and tenderness at the injection site and with toxicity and hemodynamic instability out of proportion to the local lesion. Crepitus may be noted, and soft tissue radiographs may reveal gas in tissues. Immediate surgical exploration, with extensive drainage and debridement of infected and nonviable tissue, is required. These infections often have a polymicrobial etiology that includes S. aureus, aerobic and anaerobic streptococci, enteric gram-negative bacilli, and other anaerobes. Parenteral antibiotic therapy aimed at gram-positive and gram-negative organisms, with anaerobic coverage, is essential. Several regimens, including vancomyicin or nafcillin, plus metronidazole or clindamycin, plus an aminoglycoside, a third-generation cephalosporin, or an expanded-spectrum penicillin, are indicated.

Septic thrombophlebitis of extremity, jugular, or femoral veins often appears as septic pulmonary emboli. Bacteremia is invariably found, and pus may be expressed from injection sites of infected vessels. Parenteral antibiotic therapy as well as ligation and excision of infected thrombosed veins (if technically feasible) is advocated. The value of heparin remains unproved, and it is generally not recommended.

Other, infrequent complications of injection drug use under unsterile circumstances include wound botulism, tetanus, malaria, and disseminated candidiasis. The first two have been sporadically reported, usually in long-term users and often in "skin poppers," whereas outbreaks of malaria have resulted from the sharing of needles contaminated with infected blood. Botulism should be considered in patients with unusual, progressive cranial nerve palsies; wounds should be cultured for *Clostridium botulinum*. Tetanus should be suspected in drug users with seizures, muscle rigidity, and autonomic hyperactivity.

ENDOCARDITIS (See Chap. 85) Although bacterial endocarditis is less frequent than skin and pulmonary infections among injection drug users, its potential life-threatening complications and the usual need for prolonged intravenous antibiotic therapy in the hospital make it a disease of great consequence in this population. In several studies of consecutive hospital admissions of injection drug users before the AIDS epidemic, endocarditis accounted for 5 to 16 percent of admissions and for 2 to 8 percent of all deaths.

Microbiology The predominant organism causing endocarditis in injection drug users is *S. aureus*. In various published series, this organism has accounted for 60 percent to more than 90 percent of cases. In many geographic locations, a substantial and increasing proportion of *S. aureus* isolates are resistant to methicillin. Although this organism was originally believed to be a contaminant of drugs and injection paraphernalia, it is now clear that *S. aureus* is part of the patient's own flora, carried in the nares and oropharynx and on the skin and subsequently introduced into the bloodstream by unsterile injection. In the published studies, 60 to 100 percent of injection drug users with *S. aureus* endocarditis on admission to the hospital had an identical organism in the blood and at one or more of these sites, while cultures of heroin and injection equipment were negative for *S. aureus*.

Certain bacteria are encountered more frequently in right-sided rather than in left-sided endocarditis. Right-sided endocarditis is caused by *S. aureus* in more than 80 percent of cases, whereas the organisms isolated in aortic or mitral valve endocarditis are more similar to those found in other patients. Streptococci and enterococci, including α-hemolytic viridans streptococci and *Enterococcus fae-*

calis, are the second most common organisms but account for only 5 to 10 percent of cases of endocarditis in various series. Geographic and temporal clustering of more unusual infecting organisms has occasionally been reported. These organisms include *Pseudomonas aeruginosa*, which was isolated from injection drug users in Chicago and Detroit in the 1970s and early 1980s in relation to pentazocine and tripelennamine abuse; *Pseudomonas cepacia*, isolated in New York; *Serratia marcescens*, isolated in San Francisco; enterococci, isolated in Cleveland; and recently, methicillin-resistant *S. aureus*, isolated in Detroit. Infrequent cases of endocarditis due to *Candida* spp., *Bacillus* spp., diphtheroids, and fastidious gram-negative or anaerobic components of the oral flora have been described as well. *Bacillus* spp. have been the most frequent contaminants of drugs and injection paraphernalia. Polymicrobial endocarditis due to both gram-positive and gram-negative organisms has been documented.

Pathogenesis and clinical presentation Longer duration and increased frequency of the use of drugs are associated with a cumulative increase in the risk of endocarditis. Most cases of endocarditis in this populatoin involve the right side of the heart and the tricuspid valve. In one series, 76 percent of cases of endocarditis in injection drug users were right-sided, while the corresponding figure was only 9 percent among non-drug-using patients.

The frequency of involvement of the tricuspid valve may be a function of its proximity to the injection site and its consequent bombardment with injected particulate matter, including talc and cotton. Microscopic examination of uninfected tricuspid valve surfaces in injection drug users reveals pitting and disruption of the smooth endothelial lining—changes that may facilitate the attachment of pathogenic organisms. Left-sided endocarditis may occur with or without right-sided involvement and usually develops in the setting of underlying valvular heart disease.

The various characteristic clinical presentations depend on the site of valvular involvement. In tricuspid valve endocarditis, the predominant picture is one of an abrupt illness with persistent high fever, pulmonary involvement, and an absence of systemic embolic or microvascular phenomena. Approximately 50 percent of patients present with cough and pleuritic chest pain, and some exhibit hemoptysis; these signs and symptoms are the result of multiple septic pulmonary emboli and infarctions. The characteristic murmur of tricuspid regurgitation may be heard in 50 percent of patients: a midsystolic medium-ptiched murmur at the lower left sternal border that increases in intensity with inspiration.

Characteristically, the chest x-ray shows multiple patchy or nodular infiltrates which progress to cavitation during therapy and eventually resolve. Endocarditis involving the mitral and aortic valves also has an acute onset, with high fever, toxicity, and signs and symptoms resulting from multiple systemic emboli (including arterial emboli and septic infarcts of the skin, liver, spleen, kidneys, and central nervous system). Toxic encephalopathy, focal neurologic abnormalities (the result of mycotic aneurysm or brain abscess), and bacterial meningitis may ensue. Petechiae and splenomegaly occur in approximately 50 percent of patients, and aortic and mitral regurgitant murmurs are reported in almost all cases.

Diagnosis The diagnosis of endocarditis in injection drug users can be problematic, even in the emergency room setting, where most febrile drug users are evaluated and this diagnosis is often suspected. Right-sided endocarditis may be particularly difficult to diagnose because systemic emboli and a regurgitant murmur are usually absent. The diagnosis rests on a composite of clinical, microbiologic, radiologic, and imaging data.

The clinical criteria used include sustained bacteremia involving an organism likely to cause endocarditis and the presence of compatible pulmonary, systemic, or cardiac findings. A clinically useful case definition employed by Marantz et al. divides cases into definite (pathologic confirmation), probable (several positive blood cultures, new regurgitant murmur, or peripheral or pulmonary embolic phenomena), and presumed (several positive blood cultures and no other source found). However, the diagnostic accuracy of emergency room evaluation to predict endocarditis in febrile injection drug users was quite low. Of 87 consecutive febrile injection drug users, 13 percent ultimately met the case definition for definite or probable endocarditis. Only 4 of 12 suspected of having endocarditis in the emergency room proved to have this diagnosis, while 8 of 30 admitted with other diagnoses ultimately proved to have endocarditis. In this series, bacterial pneumonia and minor illnesses were more frequent. The authors conclude that the emergency room diagnostic accuracy is insufficient to distinguish between endocarditis and nonendocarditis and that febrile injection drug users in emergency rooms should be admitted for observation and/or therapy.

Injection drug users may self-medicate with oral antibiotics. Although, unfortunately, this behavior is not always disclosed when the patient's medical history is taken, it may be critically important in the evaluation of patients with suspected endocarditis because blood cultures may be falsely negative. In addition, a large-scale study from Detroit suggested that use of nonprescribed antibiotics before admission to the hospital was an important factor predicting endocarditis due to methicillin-resistant *S. aureus* among drug injectors.

As the above comments indicate, all febrile injection drug users should have a careful history taken, with an emphasis on the frequency and type of drug injection and on antibiotic use. The physical examination should focus attention on the presence of septic emboli in the skin and on mucosal surfaces and of regurgitant murmurs. Chest radiography should be used to detect the characteristic radiologic findings of septic emboli or focal infections that may result in bacteremia. Typically, the radiograph shows multiple patchy or nodular infiltrates that progress to cavitation during therapy and eventually resolve. Ideally, three sets of blood cultures—spaced over several hours, as clinical exigency permits—should be obtained. Gram's staining of peripheral lesions and buffy coat smear of blood may provide a more rapid diagnosis in some cases of bacterial infection. Cardiac imaging studies are a valuable adjunct to diagnosis, although they cannot usually be undertaken at the time of initial presentation and are of variable sensitivity and specificity; false-negative results are frequent in right-sided involvement, and false-positive results also have been documented. Echocardiography may be invaluable in following patients with potentially unstable lesions (i.e., valve incompetence or intramyocardial abscess).

Therapy　After blood cultures are obtained, empirical antibiotic therapy should be instituted if patients are acutely ill, if left-sided endocarditis is highly suspected, and/or if septic pulmonary emboli are seen on radiographs. However, it is not necessary to institute therapy for endocarditis in all injection drug users with fever. In fact, it is often reasonable to withhold antibiotics and to observe the patient carefully until the results of blood cultures are known. Some patients will be found to have a minor transient illness or a pyrogenic or hypersensitivity reaction to injected drugs and will defervesce within 24 h. In others, an alternative diagnosis will become apparent.

Appropriate empirical antibiotic therapy should be given parenterally and should always include an antistaphylococcal agent. Depending on local susceptibility patterns and the severity of the patient's illness, the agent selected is usually either a β-lactam antibiotic, such as oxacillin or nafcillin or—if infection with methicillin-resistant *S. aureus* is suspected—vancomycin. If local patterns warrant, gram-negative coverage with an added aminoglycoside may be appropriate. For endocarditis due to methicillin-susceptible staphylococci, conventional therapy consists of 4 weeks of oxacillin or nafcillin at a dose of 1.5 to 2 g every 4 hours. In severe endocarditis, some clinicians add an aminoglycoside, usually gentamicin (1.5 mg/kg every 8 h) for the first 2 weeks of therapy; this addition may result in more rapid resolution of bacteremia, although an improved outcome has never been shown. In cases of allergy to penicillin or infection with methicillin-resistant *S. aureus*, vancomycin (1 g every 12 h) is given. Therapy targeting other organisms should be selected on the basis of antimicrobial susceptibility patterns. There is no evidence that treatment for 6 weeks instead of 4 weeks improves outcome. A few

studies have reported successful treatment of uncomplicated right-sided endocarditis with a 2-week course of a β-lactam antibiotic plus an aminoglycoside. Given the difficulty of obtaining long-term secure intravenous access, this alternative regimen may prove valuable in selected cases. Its value in HIV-infected injection drug users with endocarditis remains to be determined. Most experts advocate parenteral therapy for the duration of the course, although this decision often necessitates the placement of an indwelling central line.

The prognosis of right-sided staphylococcal endocarditis in this population is excellent, with only rare deaths and infrequent lack of response to medical therapy. Endocarditis caused by other organisms and left-sided involvement carries a more serious prognosis with higher complication and fatality rates. These are largely determined by valve destruction and site and severity of peripheral arterial emboli. The role of surgery remains controversial in this as in other populations with endocarditis (see Chap. 85). The same criteria for surgical intervention should apply: intractable heart failure, undrained myocardial abscess, and failure of medical therapy, particularly in candidal or fungal endocarditis. The surgical approach varies with the cardiac valve(s) involved. Valve excision alone appears to be sufficient for severe tricuspid endocarditis. In mitral and aortic valve endocarditis, valve replacement is required and usually can be accomplished safely. Concerns about subsequent reinfection in the setting of continued injection drug use engender heated debates and require medical, surgical, and patient joint decisions.

PNEUMONIA　(See also Chap. 220)　Community-acquired bacterial pneumonia, most often caused by *Streptococcus pneumoniae* and *Haemophilus influenzae*, was commonly described among drug injectors in the 1960s and 1970s. Although population-based epidemiologic data were lacking, these infections were thought to be more frequent among drug users than among the general population. The putative risk factors in drug users included pulmonary aspiration resulting from intermittent overdose, deleterious effects of opiates on lung defenses and cough reflex, hypoventilation due to respiratory depression, and smoking. These factors have all been outweighed by HIV infection, which has dramatically increased the risk of bacterial pneumonia in drug injectors. Beginning in the mid-1980s, epidemiologic surveillance data from New York City showed rising mortality from bacterial pneumonia and other bacterial infections among drug injectors—a phenomenon linked to HIV infection. In some cases, HIV-infected drug users died from pyogenic bacterial infections even before the diagnosis of AIDS. Prospective studies demonstrated that even when they were not actively injecting drugs, HIV-infected drug users had a four- to fivefold greater risk of bacterial pneumonia and sepsis (up to 10 cases per 100 person-years) than their HIV-seronegative counterparts. Among febrile drug users presenting to an emergency room, pneumonia was the single largest diagnostic category, accounting for 38 percent of admissions. The 1993 Revised AIDS Case Definition of the Centers for Disease Control and Prevention includes recurrent bacterial pneumonia in persons with HIV infection as an AIDS-defining condition; the inclusion of this criterion is expected to increase the proportion of AIDS cases reported among injection drug users. The organisms involved in HIV-related pneumonia among drug injectors are predominantly those reported in the earlier literature on community-acquired pneumonia in this group, i.e., *S. pneumoniae* and *H. influenzae*.

The clinical presentation of bacterial pneumonia and the strategies for its diagnosis and therapy are similar in injection drug users and in other populations, despite an expanded array of differential diagnostic possibilities. The typical presentation includes fever, productive cough, pleuritic chest pain, and findings of consolidation and segmental or lobar infiltrate on chest radiography. Specific etiologic diagnosis requires cultures of sputum and/or blood. Therapy aimed at *S. pneumoniae* and/or *H. influenzae*, given parenterally for 10 days to 2 weeks, is recommended, with modifications based on Gram's stain and culture results and on clinical course.

Among other infectious entities to be considered in the differential diagnosis of pulmonary infiltrates in this population of patients are septic pulmonary emboli, tuberculosis, and *Pneumocystis carinii* pneumonia (in patients infected with HIV). Noninfectious pulmonary complications of injection drug use also should be considered. Heroin-induced pulmonary edema, the most common of these complications, occurs most often in drug-use neophytes but also develops in experienced users exposed to particularly potent opiates and results rapidly in death by asphyxiation unless treated promptly with a narcotic antagonist (e.g., naloxone) and respiratory support. Heroin users who relapse and return to drug injection after a period of abstinence appear to be at especially high risk for the complication. Other noninfectious pulmonary complications of drug injection include (1) pulmonary vascular or talc granulomatosis, which develops in fewer than 5 percent of injectors and is caused by repeated intravenous injection of crushed oral medications or by injection of cotton or other particulate material that may contaminate injected drugs (a syndrome characterized by a diffuse reticulonodular pattern on chest radiography and often by disabling symptoms of pulmonary hypertension), (2) bullous disease, which often involves the peripheral upper lobe areas and which is of uncertain etiology but may be another complication of particulate matter injection, (3) reactive airway disease, which may be exacerbated by heroin use or by "crack" cocaine inhalation, and (4) mechanical complications, such as pneumothorax resulting from attempted venous injection into the deep veins of the neck ("pocket shot") or (as has been described more recently in cocaine smokers) pulmonary barotrauma with pneumothorax or pneumomediastinum resulting from intense Valsalva's or other maneuvers used in the inhalation of drugs.

Finally, the virtual universality of heavy cigarette smoking among drug injectors may not only predispose them to the usual sequelae of this behavior but also complicate the differential diagnosis of pulmonary symptoms (e.g., cough, shortness of breath, sputum production).

TUBERCULOSIS (See also Chap. 130) The other important pulmonary infection described in drug injectors is tuberculosis. Infections due to *M. tuberculosis* were well documented in drug users before the AIDS epidemic, accounting for greater morbidity and mortality in this population than in the non-drug-using population. Although some authors attributed this greater impact to poverty, poor housing, and the social and demographic factors associated with both drug use and tuberculosis, others found an elevated risk of tuberculosis among drug users even after attempting to control for these other factors. AIDS has now overwhelmed all other potential risk factors and has resulted in a new epidemic of resurgent tuberculosis among HIV-infected drug users and their contacts (see Chaps. 130 and 279). Among persons with HIV infection, tuberculosis has disproportionately affected injection drug users. This observation may reflect higher levels of latent infection with *M. tuberculosis* in drug-using populations, associated environmental factors, or a combination of factors. In parts of the urban northeastern United States, where 20 percent of drug injectors have evidence of latent *M. tuberculosis* infection and 40 percent are infected with HIV, the overlap of these two endemic infections has resulted in an unprecedented increase in the incidence of tuberculosis since 1985. This finding highlights the importance of aggressive chemoprophylaxis with isoniazid in this population.

Pulmonary tuberculosis should always be suspected and included in the differential diagnosis in injection drug users with pneumonia. Particularly among those with HIV infection, extrapulmonary tuberculosis has greatly increased in frequency. The therapy administered to injection drug users is similar to that given to other populations, but special efforts must be made to ensure long-term adherence to the regimen.

SKELETAL INFECTIONS (See Chap. 92) Skeletal infections in injection drug users result both from hematogenous dissemination and, less commonly, from contiguous spread from chronically infected skin and soft tissue sites to underlying bone. In one series, skeletal infections represented 9 percent of admissions of injection drug users to a large urban hospital. Septic arthritis of large synovial joints may be seen during the course of staphylococcal endocarditis or of bacteremia arising from other infected sites and may appear as a complication of disseminated gonococcal disease. The joints most frequently involved are the knees, hips, shoulders, and elbows, but there is predilection for involvement of unusual joints as well—e.g., the vertebral column, the symphysis pubis, and the sternoclavicular, sternochondral, and sacroiliac joints. These infections are usually unilateral and subacute, with an indolent, progressive course characterized by pain, limitation of motion, and absence of fever. The diagnosis may be easily missed or overlooked. Point tenderness over the affected joint is usually elicited. Sternoarticular infections are often associated with soft tissue swelling of the chest wall and bacteremia. Vertebral osteomyelitis may be associated with paraspinal soft tissue masses and (in cases of posterior extension) with the formation of spinal epidural abscesses. Radiologic and imaging studies may suggest the diagnosis by findings which are most characteristic of vertebral osteomyelitis, where the disk space is lost, contiguous bone erosion and new bone formation are evident, and several vertebrae are involved. Infection of the sacroiliac joints and symphysis pubis results in joint space separation and erosion of the articular surfaces.

S. aureus is the pathogen most commonly isolated from sites of skeletal infection, but gram-negative organisms—notably *P. aeruginosa*, *Serratia marcescens*, and fungi—also have been well documented. *M. tuberculosis* should be included in the differential diagnosis, particularly in cases of vertebral osteomyelitis. Because etiologic agents and their antimicrobial susceptibilities vary, efforts should be made to obtain a specific microbiologic diagnosis. This process may involve diagnostic aspiration or closed or open biopsy, with fluid or material sent for staining and culture for bacterial, mycobacterial, and fungal pathogens.

Treatment consists of a combination of drainage of the synovial joints and the contiguous soft tissue collections and prolonged administration of appropriate antimicrobial agents.

CENTRAL NERVOUS SYSTEM COMPLICATIONS The nervous system, especially the CNS, is another important site for adverse sequelae of drug injection. Drug injectors are at increased risk for certain noninfectious complications, including intracerebral hemorrhage and other stroke syndromes (especially in cocaine and amphetamine users), particulate emboli to the brain and spinal cord, vasculitis, and the consequences of head trauma. Among the infectious complications, the most common is systemic embolization to the brain as a result of bacterial endocarditis or bacteremia, which frequently involves multiple small septic emboli, from either aortic or mitral valve vegetations or, even more commonly given the more frequent occurrence of right-sided endocarditis in drug users, from pulmonary arteriovenous shunting or bacteremic seeding of the meninges and brain. Patients may present with focal neurologic deficits, seizures, altered mental status, and/or meningismus. *S. aureus* and other bacteria that cause endocarditis in drug injectors are most commonly involved in these manifestations. Cerebral mycotic aneurysms and spinal and epidural abscesses also have been described as complications of endocarditis in this population. Less commonly, drug users have been reported to be at risk for focal brain abscesses, not related to endocarditis, caused by organisms such as *Aspergillus*, *Mucor*, other fungi, and *Nocardia*. There is also evidence that tuberculous meningitis and focal tuberculomas of the brain may be more common in drug users than in other patients with tuberculosis, with and without HIV infection. Finally, ocular infections, including episcleritis, chorioretinitis, and endophthalmitis have been well described in drug injectors, involving such organisms as *B. cereus*, *Aspergillus*, and *C. albicans* (the last often in conjunction with the syndrome of systemic candidiasis, described in several populations of European drug injectors in the early 1980s, associated with "brown" heroin and the use of lemon juice as a medium for dissolving the drug).

HEPATITIS (See also Chaps. 266 and 267) Injection drug users have long been known to be at high risk for hepatitis, primarily through parenteral transmission of bloodborne infectious agents. The incidence of hepatitis B has risen over the past decade in the United States, and the proportion of all cases occurring among injection drug users has increased from 15 percent to close to 30 percent since the mid-1980s. The acquisition of hepatitis B is a relatively early event for most drug injectors, occurring within the first several years of illicit drug use. Since the 1970s, seroprevalence studies in a wide range of drug-using populations have indicated that 75 to 90 percent of long-term drug injectors have serologic evidence of past exposure to hepatitis B. Approximately 5 to 10 percent of these individuals will remain chronic carriers of hepatitis B surface antigen; the remainder will develop immunity to hepatitis, producing antibody to hepatitis B core antigen and/or that to hepatitis B surface antigen. While most hepatitis B–infected drug users do not progress to chronic forms of clinically significant hepatitis or cirrhosis, at least 40 percent of most series of entrants in drug-treatment programs exhibit abnormalities of liver function. In addition to infectious causes, the toxic effects of adulterants used in the production of illicit drugs and the hepatotoxic effects of alcohol are responsible in part for these abnormalities. Indeed, while chronic active and chronic persistent hepatitis have been linked to infection with hepatitis B virus and ongoing injection of illicit drugs, hepatic cirrhosis in drug users is most often associated with coexisting alcohol abuse.

Another infectious agent commonly found in drug injectors is hepatitis D virus, previously referred to as the *delta agent*. This defective hepatotropic RNA virus depends on coexisting infection with hepatitis B virus for expression and replication. First detected in Italy in the mid-1970s, hepatitis D virus has since been documented in numerous seroprevalence studies among drug users in the United States, Europe, and Southeast Asia. In most such surveys, antibody to hepatitis D virus has been found in 10 to 15 percent of patients with antibody to hepatitis B surface or core antigen and in as many as 50 to 70 percent of patients with chronic carriage of hepatitis B surface antigen. Fulminant hepatitis B may show a characteristic biphasic pattern in the setting of hepatitis D coinfection. Moreover, hepatitis D has been associated among drug users with chronic active hepatitis and persistent abnormalities of liver function. Among persons with hepatitis B in the United States, coexisting hepatitis D infection has shown a greater predilection for injection drug users and hemophiliacs than for homosexual men; thus the parenteral route may be important in the transmission of hepatitis D virus.

The third significant bloodborne agent of hepatitis in injection drug users is hepatitis C virus. This virus, which has been identified in recent years as the cause of a large proportion of cases of what had previously been termed non-A, non-B hepatitis, is highly prevalent in many different populations of drug users. In seroprevalence studies in the United States and Europe, antibody to hepatitis C virus has been detected in up to 70 percent of drug injectors—a rate reflecting a level of infection comparable with that for hepatitis B. Like hepatitis B, hepatitis C appears to be acquired relatively soon after the start of illicit drug injection. While hepatitis C has been associated with chronic active hepatitis, persistent abnormalities of liver function, and cirrhosis, further studies must fully elucidate the natural history of this infection in drug users. Preliminary data suggest that interferon-α may be of benefit in patients with progressive hepatitis B or hepatitis C. This treatment has not yet been widely administered to drug users, however, and its requisite duration is unknown. Preliminiary follow-up studies suggest that disease quickly recrudesces after cessation of therapy.

Although not considered to be a bloodborne infection, hepatitis A has been associated with injection drug use. In 1970, 60 percent of more than 1000 entrants in a drug-treatment program at the Federal Addiction Treatment Center in Lexington, Kentucky, showed serologic evidence of exposure to hepatitis A. While the high rate of seropositivity in this study cannot be compared with the background rate in the general population at the time, several surveillance-based investigations since then have indicated that injection drug users may have up to a 50-fold higher risk of acquiring hepatitis A than noninjection drug users. In addition, recent outbreaks of hepatitis A have been linked to groups of injection drug users in both the United States and Europe. While the exact mechanism of spread has not been determined, investigation of these outbreaks has suggested that fecal-oral contamination, close personal contact, and poor hygiene are the most likely factors; viral contamination of drugs or injection equipment was considered less likely but could not be ruled out.

These observations suggest that in long-term drug injectors with known past exposure to hepatitis B and/or hepatitis C, hepatitis A (and—for chronic carriers of hepatitis B—hepatitis D) should be strongly considered in the differential diagnosis of new-onset acute hepatitis syndromes. The acquisition of bloodborne hepatitis soon after the start of illicit injection drug use suggests the importance of developing public health strategies for reaching adolescent and young-adult drug users with information about preventive interventions (such as hepatitis B vaccine) and risk-reducing behaviors.

HTLV-I/II Injection drug users are at relatively high risk not only for infection with HIV but also for that with human T lymphotropic retrovirus types I and II (see Chap. 151). In the United States, injection drug use has been the most important behavioral factor associated with the presence of antibody to HTLV-I/II in blood donors screened for retroviral infection. Seroprevalence studies in the United States have documented HTLV-I/II infection in more than 10 percent of certain populations of drug users; in some areas the rate of HTLV infection has exceeded that of HIV infection. HTLV infection has often been associated with black race, older age, and a history of heroin injection. Rates of infection have shown wide geographic variation. Molecular genetic techniques have recently indicated that more than three-fourths of the HTLV infections in drug injectors are due to HTLV-II; this observation may account for the relatively low rate of clinical disease reported to date in patients with such infections. Two studies have suggested, however, that coinfection with HTLV-I/II and HIV may be associated with more rapid progression of HIV infection and early mortality; if corroborated, this observation might make serologic testing for HTLV-I/II an important prognostic tool for HIV-infected drug users.

HARM REDUCTION FOR INJECTION DRUG USERS

The myriad infectious consequences of injection drug use mandate the development of preventive harm-reduction strategies which are based on the underlying principle that if people are going to inject drugs, they should do so in a way that minimizes harm to themselves and others. Prevention of the infectious complications of injection and education about more hygienic injection practices are primary goals. Needle- and syringe-exchange programs are the most obvious example of the harm-reduction approach. In addition to the distribution or exchange of injection equipment, these programs typically include AIDS education, condom distribution, and enrollment in a variety of medical and social services.

Provision of primary medical care services linked to drug-abuse treatment is a way to promote preventive regimens to enhance harm reduction. In this and all other clinical settings, injection drug users should be routinely screened for hepatitis B, latent *M. tuberculosis* infection, and syphilis and other sexually transmitted diseases. They should be offered pneumococcal, influenza, tetanus, and hepatitis B immunization and (when appropriate) prophylaxis for tuberculosis and complications of HIV disease.

Clearly, the ultimate goal of harm-reduction strategies should be the reduction or prevention of illicit drug use itself. A high priority must be assigned to the development of strategies that will minimize the serious medical consequences of drug abuse as well as to those that will eliminate drug abuse and its root causes.

REFERENCES

CHAMBERS HF et al: *Staphylococcus aureus* endocarditis: Clinical manifestations in addicts and non-addicts. Medicine 62:170, 1983
——— et al: Right-sided *Staphylococcus aureus* endocarditis in intravenous drug users: Two-week combination therapy. Ann Intern Med 109:619, 1988

CHANDRASEKAR PH, NARULA AP: Bone and joint infections in intravenous drug abusers. Rev Infect Dis 8:904, 1986

DONAHUE JG et al: Antibody to hepatitis C virus among cardiac surgery patients, homosexual men and intravenous drug users in Baltimore, Maryland. Am J Epidemiol 134:1206, 1991

FELTON CP: Pulmonary infections in the addict, in *Medical Aspects of Drug Abuse*, RW Richter (ed). Hagerstown, MD, Harper & Row, 1975

HAVERKOS HW, LANGE WR: Serious infections other than human immunodeficiency virus among intravenous drug users. J Infect Dis 161:894, 1990

HIND CRK: Pulmonary complications of intravenous drug users: I. Epidemiology and noninfective complications. Thorax 45:891, 1990; II. Infective and HIV-related complications. Thorax 45:957, 1990

KHABBAZ RA et al: Seroprevalence of HTLV-I and HTLV-II among intravenous drug users and persons in clinics for sexually transmitted diseases. N Engl J Med 326:375, 1992

LANGE WR et al: The Lexington addicts, 1971–72: Demographic characteristics, drug use patterns, and selected infectious disease experience. Int J Addict 24:609, 1989

LETTAU LA et al: Outbreak of severe hepatitis due to delta and hepatitis B viruses in parenteral drug abusers and their contacts. N Engl J Med 317:1256, 1987

LEVINE DP, SOBEL JD (eds): *Infections in Intravenous Drug Abusers*. New York, Oxford University Press, 1991

MARANTZ PR et al: Inability to predict diagnosis in febrile intravenous drug abusers. Ann Intern Med 106:823, 1987

NOVICK DM et al: Hepatitis D virus antibody in HBsAg-positive and HBsAg-negative substance abusers with chronic liver disease. J Med Virol 15:351, 1985

SANDE MA et al: Endocarditis in intravenous drug users, in *Infective Endocarditis*, 2d ed, D Kaye (ed). New York, Raven, 1992, pp 345–359

SELWYN PA et al: Clinical manifestations and predictors of disease progression in drug users with human immunodeficiency virus infection. N Engl J Med 327:1697, 1992

SHEAGREN JN: Endocarditis complicating parenteral drug abuse, in *Current Clinical Topics in Infectious Diseases*, 2d ed, JS Remington, MN Schwartz (eds). New York, McGraw-Hill, 1981, pp 211–233

STIMSON GV: Editorial review: Syringe exchange programs for injection drug users. AIDS 3:253, 1989

STONEBURNER RL et al: A larger spectrum of severe HIV-1 related disease in intravenous drug users in New York City. Science 242:916, 1988

VON HAASTRECHT HJA et al: The course of the HIV epidemic in Amsterdam, The Netherlands. Am J Public Health 81:59, 1991

95   INFECTIONS FROM BITES AND SCRATCHES, BURNS, AND ENVIRONMENTAL ORGANISMS

JAMES L. BREELING / LOUIS WEINSTEIN

ANIMAL BITES AND SCRATCHES

Infections following animal bites are caused by deep inoculation of bacteria into the skin or soft tissues. Early culture of the wound often discloses small numbers of organisms representative of a particular animal's oral flora; many bites never become overtly infected. Patients with infected wounds usually present 12 to 24 h after the injury with inflammation caused by invasion by common organisms.

EPIDEMIOLOGY   Most domestic animal bites are inflicted by pets. There are more than 100 million dogs and cats in the United States. Dogs inflict 80 to 90 percent of the bites and cats about 6 percent. (Other animals that inflict bites are monkeys, rodents, livestock, and reptiles.) However, 20 to 50 percent of the bites by cats and about 5 percent by dogs become infected. Most of the 2 to 4 million bite wounds each year result in minor injury: 10 percent may require suturing, and an estimated 1 to 2 percent require hospitalization. Children are bitten more often than adults. Occupational groups at high risk include animal breeders, veterinary surgeons, zookeepers, wild animal trainers, laboratory workers, and postal carriers. The hands and arms are the most common sites of bites. Wounds of the hands tend to become infected most often. Because of the structure of the hand and the ease with which infection spreads along tissue planes, every bite on the hand must be considered potentially serious.

ETIOLOGY   The oropharynx of an animal is the most important source of organisms involved in infections following a bite. However, the microflora of the skin, soil, and excreta also may be involved in the development of infection. The average dog or cat harbors a wide range of pathogens, such as *Pasteurella*, *Staphylococcus aureus*, streptococci, and mixed oral anaerobic organisms. The oral microfloras of other animal species have been less well studied. Infections caused by *Actinobacillus* may occur following bites by horses or sheep. Bites by dolphins may lead to infection by halophilic and waterborne organisms such as *Mycobacterium marinum*. An unidentified agent that responds to tetracycline is responsible for infection following a bite by a seal ("seal finger"). Bites by monkeys may lead to the development of fatal encephalomyelitis caused by herpesvirus simiae. Leptospirosis, brucellosis, and tularemia have been attributed to animal bites, although documentation of actual transmission has been scanty. Rabies is transmitted by the bite of some animals (see Chap. 158).

Bites by animals may lead to damage of soft tissues and loss of skin, acute cellulitis, chronic localized infection of deep tissues (septic arthritis, osteomyelitis), or septicemia with or without disseminated intravascular coagulation.

SPECIFIC ORGANISMS   *Pasteurella multocida*   *P. multocida* is a small gram-negative coccobacillus present in the naso-oropharynx and gastrointestinal tract of mammals and birds. Cats have the highest carriage rate (70 to 90 percent), but dogs, great cats (lions and tigers), swine, sheep, cattle, rabbits, and rats may harbor the organism. The most common human infection is cellulitis surrounding the wound, but localized abscess, osteomyelitis, septic arthritis, peritonitis, mycotic aneurysm, meningitis, acute epiglottis, pneumonia, and chorioamnionitis may occur. *P. multocida* infections may follow nonbite exposure to animals, including scratches and respiratory spread of droplets from carrier animals to the respiratory tract of patients with chronic pulmonary disease. Patients with cirrhosis who come into contact with animal saliva are at risk of developing primary bacteremia.

Pasteurella infections following animal bites are characterized by the rapid development in <24 h of intense inflammation and purulent drainage. Because bites are often small but penetrate deeply, the possibility of septic arthritis, tendon sheath involvement, or osteomyelitis is great, even when the puncture wounds are trivial.

The preferred oral treatment of wounds infected by *Pasteurella* is penicillin VK (500 mg orally every 6 h) or, in the penicillin-allergic patient, tetracycline (500 mg orally every 6 h). Erythromycin, cephalosporins, clindamycin, and dicloxacillin are ineffective and should not be used.

***Capnocytophaga canimorsus* (CDC group DF-2)**   Formerly an unclassified microorganism (CDC group DF-2 for dysgonic fermenter), *C. canimorsus* is a gram-negative rod associated with septicemia following dog bites, particularly in immunocompromised alcoholics or splenectomized subjects (see Chap. 112).

Fever is the most common presenting symptom. The illness is usually mild in patients with an intact spleen, but systemic meningitis and endocarditis can cause an overall mortality rate approaching 30 percent. In splenectomized patients, disseminated intravascular coagulation (DIC), gangrene of the extremities, adrenal hemorrhage, hemorrhagic pulmonary edema, and fulminant sepsis may occur. The organism can be seen on microscopic examination of the buffy coat (with use of Wright's or Gram's stain) in splenectomized patients. *Capnocytophaga* is generally sensitive to penicillin, tetracycline, clindamycin, and erythromycin.

CLINICAL MANIFESTATIONS   The likelihood of infection depends on the location and nature of the wound. Signs of infection almost always appear 1 to 3 days after injury; disease produced by *Pasteurella* usually presents in 12 to 24 h. Redness, swelling, and tenderness are accompanied by drainage that may be scant or purulent. Localization of infection in the hand usually occurs, but the process can spread through the tendon sheath to distant sites. In patients with systemic signs and symptoms out of proportion to the degree of local injury, sepsis with *Pasteurella* or *Capnocytophaga* should be suspected. Persistence of local inflammation after treatment of an infected wound warrants a search for deeper infection in joints, bones, or subcutaneous spaces.

DIAGNOSIS AND TREATMENT　After infection is established, Gram's stain and culture of a wound swab or exudate may be helpful in the evaluation of its etiology. However, interpretation of the frequently complex results of early culture (within 8 h of injury) may be misleading. Thorough cleansing of the lesion (high-pressure irrigation and careful debridement) followed by closure in low-risk injuries (e.g., dog bites, bites not involving the hand) is often sufficient for healing. For wounds first seen 24 h after injury and those clearly infected at presentation, specimens for culture should be labeled as "bite wound" to alert the microbiology laboratory to the possibility of anaerobes and unusual organisms. Primary closure of older wounds is rarely advisable; provision should be made for observation of such wounds over the next few days. Prophylaxis for tetanus (see Chap. 106) and rabies (see Chap. 158) and administration of antimicrobial prophylaxis should be considered (1) at the time of debridement and/or closure of wounds seen later than 24 h after injury, (2) for puncture wounds from cats, (3) for deep wounds (especially of the hand) involving tendons or bone, and (4) for facial wounds. In addition, splenectomized patients with dog bites are at extra risk of *C. canimorsus* sepsis and should receive penicillin prophylaxis. *Pasteurella* spp. are generally sensitive to penicillin, but most *S. aureus* strains require penicillinase-resistant penicillins. Treatment with penicillin VK and dicloxacillin, cephalexin, or amoxicillin/clavulanic acid offers coverage for most potential pathogens. Established wound infections are usually treated for 10 to 14 days. Prophylaxis for apparently noninfected but high-risk wounds should be given for 3 to 5 days. Tetracycline offers some degree of coverage for the penicillin-allergic patient. Erythromycin may be considered in the pregnant woman or the child with severe allergy. Response to treatment should be monitored carefully; surgical intervention and parenteral antibiotics may be required.

RAT-BITE FEVER　Fever and arthralgias following a rat bite may be caused by two microorganisms: *Streptobacillus moniliformis* and *Spirillum minus*. Infection becomes manifest after the wound heals, distinguishing rat-bite fever from the animal bites described above.

Both *S. moniliformis* and *S. minus* normally reside in the rodent oral cavity. Rat-bite fever may be transmitted by rats, laboratory animals, and domestic and wild rodents. Also, outbreaks of rat-bite fever have been associated with the ingestion of contaminated milk or drinking water (Haverhill fever).

S. moniliformis is a pleomorphic gram-negative rod. The incubation period is usually 3 to 10 days, sufficient time for the original rodent bite wound to heal. High-grade fever, rigors, headache, vomiting, and myalgias followed by regional lymphadenopathy, arthralgias, and arthritis constitute the clinical syndrome. A maculopapular rash on the palms and soles may progress to petechial hemorrhages. If the patient is not treated, fever persists, and the patient may die.

S. minus is a spirochete that causes febrile illness approximately 1 to 3 weeks after a bite. A healed initial wound may break down at the onset of systemic illness. High-grade fever, rigors, and myalgias develop, but joint involvement is rare. Unlike streptobacillary rat-bite fever, there is no rash. Transmission by contaminated food or water has not been reported, but other spirochetes present in animals (*Leptospira* spp. and *Anaerobiospirillum succiniciproducens*) may be transmitted in this fashion. Spirillar rat-bite fever is more common in Asia than in the United States and should be considered in travelers from Asia who develop cryptic fever.

The diagnosis of streptobacillary rat-bite fever is established by culture of the organism from blood or infected tissues, which may require the use of special media. The diagnosis of spirillar rat-bite fever is made only by dark-field examination of blood, examination of infected tissues, or animal inoculation. *S. minor* infection may cause the serologic test for syphilis to be falsely positive.

Treatment of either form of rat-bite fever with procaine penicillin G (600,000 units IM twice daily for 14 days) is curative. Alternative therapy for penicillin-allergic patients is tetracycline (500 mg orally four times daily for 14 days).

CAT-SCRATCH DISEASE　**Definition and etiology**　Tender regional lymphadenopathy persisting for 3 weeks or longer, frequently preceded by a primary skin lesion after contact with cats, has been called *benign inoculation lymphoreticulosis, nonbacterial regional lymphadenitis, cat-scratch fever,* and *cat-scratch disease.* Cat-scratch disease appears to be caused by a small, pleomorphic, gram-negative bacillus that has been identified in the excised lymph nodes of patients. This organism has been grown in vitro, and a new genus and species name, *Afipia felis,* has been assigned. The organism belongs to the alpha-2 subgroup of the class Proteobacteria. This class contains other pathogens such as *Bartonella, Brucella,* and *Rochalimaea* (see Chap. 124). Cats acquire the organisms from the soil and carry it orally and/or on their paws. Inoculation of a human occurs with a scratch or bite.

Epidemiology　Cat-scratch disease occurs throughout the world and most often in children. Exposure to an immature cat is the most common means of transmission, although older cats and dogs may transmit the disease. Scratches are the most common mode of infection, but transmission may occur by licks, bites, and handling of objects with which a cat has recently made contact or by inoculation of organisms into mucous membranes (e.g., conjunctiva). Most cases occur from July to October.

Clinical manifestations　Three to five days after a bite, scratch, or lick by a cat, the patient may develop a papule that progresses to a pustule which crusts over. Within 1 to 2 weeks, tender regional lymphadenopathy develops. Since the hands are most often involved, epitrochlear, axillary, pectoral, and cervical lymph node involvement is common. Mild generalized aching, malaise, and/or anorexia is rarely accompanied by fever unless secondary bacterial infection produces suppuration of the lymph node. Conjunctival inoculation may lead to Parinaud's oculoglandular syndrome with conjunctivitis and preauricular lymphadenopathy. The lymphadenopathy usually persists for 3 to 6 weeks but may be protracted. Other manifestations not limited to immunocompromised hosts include encephalitis, meningitis, transverse myelitis, granulomatous hepatitis, osteomyelitis, and disseminated infection. In patients with AIDS, two additional manifestations, bacillary (epithelioid) angiomatosis and bacillary peliosis hepatitis, have been described and appear to be more strongly related to another recently described organism, *Rochalimaea hensleae* (see Chap. 124). Lack of serologic cross-reactivity between the two organisms, despite their occurrence in similar types of disease, suggests that the exact cause of cat-scratch disease is still unclear.

Diagnosis　Cat-scratch disease should be suspected if the patient has lymphadenopathy, exposure to a cat, and a skin lesion at the site of inoculation. Other causes of regional or generalized lymphadenopathy should be excluded (see Chap. 58). The diagnosis may be confirmed by pathologic examination of the involved nodes. Concern about transmission of viral illness has lessened the utility of a skin test with cat-scratch antigen because the antigen is prepared from material aspirated from human lymph nodes. Typical pathology includes granulomas, central necrosis of the germinal centers, and infiltration by neutrophils.

Treatment　Cat-scratch disease is generally benign and self-limited and does not require treatment with antibiotics for resolution. Antipyretics and analgesics may be used as needed. Immunocompromised patients and those with severe or long-lasting illness have been treated with a variety of agents, including aminoglycosides, erythromycin, doxycycline, and ciprofloxacin. Since no comparative antibiotic trials have been carried out, firm recommendations for therapy cannot be made at this time.

HUMAN BITE INFECTIONS

Human bites may occur in adults during fights or child abuse, in hospital personnel bitten while caring for patients, in partners during sexual play, and in persons sustaining "clenched fist" injuries involving the metacarpophalangeal joint.

ETIOLOGY Human bites (occlusional and clenched-fist) are thought to be more prone to infection than animal bites because the human oropharyngeal flora contains a large number of species of microorganisms, including anaerobic bacteria (see Chap. 128). Anaerobes are present in 39 percent of animal bites, in 50 percent of human bites, and in 56 percent of clenched-fist injuries. Anaerobes, including the oral *Bacteroides* spp. (now called *Prevotella* and *Porphyromonas*), and aerobic organisms, such as *S. aureus, Eikenella corrodens,* and non-beta-hemolytic streptococci, are commonly involved.

Clenched-fist injuries inflicted by humans have a worse prognosis than other bites, perhaps because the injury occurs with the fingers flexed, and when the fingers are extended, bacteria are sealed beneath the skin. Infection of clenched-fist injuries also may appear to be more common because many patients report the injury only after infection has developed, usually 24 or 48 h later. The rates of infection following human bites of the face or lip are much lower, possibly because patients with these injuries are likely to seek more immediate medical attention.

CLINICAL MANIFESTATIONS Clenched-fist injuries are produced by piercing of the thin skin over the flexed metacarpophalangeal joint, the teeth often penetrating the joint. There is often delayed development of pain and a proximally spreading swelling of the hand, with or without discharge. Suppurative arthritis, ankylosis, and osteomyelitis may develop. Radiographs must be examined for the presence of foreign bodies, fractures, or air in the joints. Plain films may show early osteomyelitis.

Occlusional bites on any body surface may lead to the development of cellulitis, tenosynovitis, osteomyelitis, or septic arthritis. In addition to organisms of the normal oral flora that cause infection, hepatitis B, syphillis, and tuberculosis have been transmitted by human bite.

TREATMENT Clenched-fist injuries must be treated aggressively. Patients presenting more than 24 h after injury or those with obviously infected wounds should be considered for admission, surgical exploration, irrigation, and parenteral antibiotic therapy. Aerobic and anaerobic cultures are required. Empirical antimicrobial therapy must be effective against *Bacteroides, S. aureus,* and *E. corrodens.* Organisms expressing β-lactamases (*Bacteroides, S. aureus*) and pathogens usually resistant to clindamycin but sensitive to penicillin (*Eikenella*) make monotherapy difficult. Among the drugs thought to provide adequate coverage are clindamycin, amoxicillin and clavulanic acid in combination and cefoxitin or cefotetan alone. The duration of therapy is usually 10 to 14 days when the infection appears to be responding. When osteomyelitis is present, antibiotics should be given intravenously for 4 to 6 weeks. Some patients require a second surgical debridement and may suffer residual disability.

Although HIV-1 may be present in saliva, human bites have not been documented to transmit the virus. The issue of counseling victims of human bites to be tested for HIV is unclear, but testing is probably advisable.

BURN-WOUND INFECTION

Each year 130,000 persons in the United States are hospitalized for thermal burns. About 70,000 require intensive care. Infection is the major cause of death in nearly 10,000 patients. Thermal burns to the skin are often complicated by smoke injury to the lungs.

ETIOLOGY During the first or second week after thermal injury, host immunity becomes depressed: concentrations of immunoglobulins, complement, and fibronectin fall; clearance of particulates by the reticuloendothelial system is impeded; phagocytic function is depressed and there is a decline in cell-mediated immunity, as evidenced by the impairment of cutaneous hypersensitivity, rejection of skin allografts, decreased activity of natural killer cells, lessened

mitogen responses, and decreased numbers of helper T cells. Suppressor T cells become activated. The magnitude of burn-induced changes in humoral and cellular immunity is related to the extent of the burn. The relation between the magnitude of injury and the risk of infection is linear. Mortality due to infection increases when burns cover more than 40 percent of the body surface area.

The combination of destruction of the skin barrier to bacteria and immunodeficiency permits colonizing bacteria to multiply and invade adjacent viable tissue or even to enter the systemic circulation (burn-wound sepsis). Thermal injury, hypermetabolism, and the catabolic state caused by a burn and endotoxemia from infected wounds also appear to promote "translocation" of intestinal bacteria into the portal and systemic circulations by causing a breakdown in the mucosal barriers and immune defenses of the normal gut. Intensive resuscitation and surgical intervention, including intubation and mechanical ventilation (especially in patients with adult respiratory distress syndrome or smoke inhalation), predispose to pneumonia, the third major route of systemic infection in burn patients.

CLINICAL MANIFESTATIONS Burned skin is initially free of major bacterial contamination. However, because of the exudation of body fluid, necrosis of tissues, and contamination from environmental sources, the surface area of the burn wound rapidly becomes colonized with the microbial flora of the hospital unit. Early use of topical antimicrobial agents (sodium mafenide, silver sulfadiazine, nystatin) serves to delay but not prevent infection of a burn wound. If bacterial counts reach a level of 10^5 organisms per gram of tissue, invasion of viable subcutaneous tissue with bloodstream dissemination is likely. Gram-negative, gram-positive, fungal, and even viral (herpes simplex) pathogens may cause sepsis. Suppurative thrombophlebitis and suppurative chondritis may develop.

DIAGNOSIS Quantitative bacterial cultures of biopsy specimens of a burn wound at 48-h intervals provide adequate monitoring of the wound. High densities of organisms in the area of a burn increase the risk of sepsis and interfere with the ability of skin allografts to "take," thus delaying closure of open areas.

TREATMENT Current surgical approaches to early excision of a wound and closure with autografts or skin substitutes within the first week of a burn have improved survival. Removal of the necrotic eschar appears to reverse many of the immunologic defects that occur. Debridement also promotes drainage of seromas and hematomas and improves the delivery of host resistance factors and antibiotics to the sites of injury and inflammation. Topical and appropriate systemic antimicrobial therapy and early enteral nutrition also improve survival. Selective decontamination of the intestine with antibacterial and antifungal agents may be helpful.

Systemic antimicrobial therapy must be directed toward the microorganism responsible for clinical sepsis. Since no single agent or combination of agents destroys all organisms, and because multidrug therapy may promote development of resistance, parsimonious use of antibiotics administered long enough to reverse sepsis but not long enough to permit secondary infection must be the rule.

MISCELLANEOUS ENVIRONMENTAL ORGANISMS

AEROMONAS HYDROPHILA *A. hydrophila,* a gram-negative, facultative anaerobe of the family Vibrionaceae, may cause a variety of infections in persons who have had contact with flowing or stagnant fresh water, aquaria, tap water, or freshwater fish. If ingested, *A. hydrophila* may cause gastroenteritis. When inoculated into the skin via puncture or contamination of simple wounds, it may cause rapid-onset cellulitis and even septicemia in immunocompromised or cirrhotic individuals. The skin is characteristically necrotic; formation of bullae is common. Involvement of muscle may occur early, especially in cases of wounds contaminated by water. Metastatic complications include osteomyelitis, peritonitis, meningitis, and endocarditis. Inoculation into the eye may cause conjunctivitis. A closely related species, *Plesiomonas shigelloides,* may produce rapid-onset wound infections and sepsis after marine contact. Antibiotic sensitivity patterns suggest the use of trimethoprim-sulfamethoxazole, aminoglycosides, quinolones, or third-generation cephalosporins.

PSEUDOMONAS Many species of *Pseudomonas,* including *P. aeruginosa,* are present in fresh and salt water and may cause cutaneous infection via inoculation (see Chap. 116). *Pseudomonas* folliculitis is associated with contaminated heated indoor whirlpool hot tubs, and saunas. It is treated with topical agents such as chlorhexidine and povidone-iodine; antibiotics are reserved for patients with cellulitis. Otitis externa, "swimmer's ear," is produced by *Pseudomonas* as well as other aquatic species in individuals with exposure to pools for long periods of time during the summer months. Puncture wounds of the foot by nails may lead to the development of osteomyelitis, septic arthritis, and infection of soft tissues by soil or aquatic microorganisms. The risk is especially high for infection by *Pseudomonas,* perhaps because the organism can survive and proliferate in the moist, humid environment of the inside of a shoe. Treatment usually involves surgical debridement and long courses of antipseudomonal agents.

ERYSIPELOID (ERYSIPELOTHRIX RHUSIOPATHIAE) *E. rhusiopathiae* is a small, slender, gram-positive rod found in many mammals, birds, and fish. Human infection follows a scratch or a puncture of the skin, usually the fingers, while handling fish, shellfish, or organic matter containing the organism. The infection is an occupational hazard for fish handlers, farmers, and veterinarians. A purplish, painful pruritic area appears at the site of inoculation after 1 to 4 days and is followed by a slowly spreading erythematous rash, pruritic vesicles, and papules. Fever and regional lymphadenopathy are uncommon. Rare cases of disseminated infection or endocarditis have been reported. The disease may be self-limited and run a course of several weeks. Erysipeloid responds to treatment with penicillin or erythromycin. Persons at risk of inoculation are advised to wear puncture-proof gloves and wash their hands frequently.

REFERENCES

BRENNER DJ et al: Proposal of *Afipia* gen. nov., with *Afipia felis* sp. nov. (formerly the cat scratch disease bacillus), *Afipia clevelandensis* sp. nov. (formerly the Cleveland Clinic Foundation strain), *Afipia broomeae* sp. nov., and three unnamed genospecies. J Clin Microbiol 29:2450, 1991

GOLDSTEIN EJC: Bite wounds and infection. Clin Infect Dis 14:633, 1992
—— et al: Role of anaerobic bacteremia in bite-wound infections. Rev Infect Dis 6(suppl):S177, 1984

HICKLIN H et al: Dysgonic fermenter-2 septicemia. Rev Infect Dis 9:884, 1987

JACOBS RF et al: *Pseudomonas* osteochondritis complicating puncture wounds of the foot in children: A 10-year evaluation. J Infect Dis 160:657, 1989

KULLBERG BJ et al: Purpura fulminans and symmetrical peripheral gangrene caused by *Capnocytophaga canimorsus* (formerly DF-2) septicemia: A complication of dog bite. Medicine 70:287, 1991

MARGILETH AM et al: Systemic cat-scratch disease: Report of 23 patients with prolonged or recurrent severe bacterial infection. J Infect Dis 155:390, 1987

MCEVOY M et al: Outbreak of fever caused by *Streptobacillus moniliformis.* Lancet 2:1361, 1987

PITLIK S et al: Nonenteric infections acquired through contact with water. Rev Infect Dis 9:54, 1987

ROBERGE RJ: Cat-scratch disease. Emerg Med Clin North Am 9:327, 1991

SCHLOSSBERG D et al: Culture-proved disseminated cat-scratch disease in acquired immunodeficiency syndrome. Arch Intern Med 149:1437, 1989

SCHWARTSMAN WA: Infections due to Rochalimaea: The expanding clinical spectrum. Clin Infect Dis 15:893, 1992

WEBER DJ et al: *Pasteurella multocida* infections: Report of 34 cases and review of literature. Medicine 63:133, 1984

section 3   Clinical syndromes— nosocomial infections

96   INFECTIONS IN THE IMMUNOCOMPROMISED HOST

ROBERT FINBERG

In dealing with infections in immunocompromised patients, the type of defect and the anticipated infection should guide therapy (Tables 96-1 and 96-2). This chapter will discuss the approach to diagnosis and treatment of infections in patients who are immunocompromised by virtue of chemotherapy-induced granulocytopenia and immunosuppression related to organ or bone marrow transplantation. Many defects in host response are covered in other areas of this book.

INFECTIONS IN NEUTROPENIC PATIENTS

INITIAL MANAGEMENT The neutropenic patient is unusually susceptible to bacterial infection, so antibiotic therapy should be initiated promptly to cover likely pathogens if infection is suspected. Indeed, early initiation of antibacterial agents is mandatory to prevent fatal events. These patients are susceptible to common gram-positive and gram-negative organisms found on the skin and in the bowel (Table 96-3). Treatment with narrow-spectrum agents leads to infection with organisms not covered by the antibiotics used, and for this reason, the initial regimen should be designed to treat pathogens likely to be initial causes of bacterial infection in neutropenic hosts (see Table 96-3).

Selection of antibiotics Hundreds of antibiotic regimens have been tested for use in this setting. Many of these studies involved small populations in which the outcomes were generally good, and most did not have the statistical power to detect differences among the regimens studied. Each febrile neutropenic patient should be approached as a unique problem, with particular attention to previous infections and recent exposures to antibiotics. Several general guidelines are useful in the initial therapy of neutropenic patients with fever (Fig. 96-1):

1 It is necessary to treat with antibiotics active against both gram-negative and gram-positive pathogens (see Table 96-3) in the initial regimen.

2 An aminoglycoside or ciprofloxacin alone is not adequate therapy in this setting.

3 The agents used should reflect both the epidemiology and the antibiotic resistance pattern of the hospital [e.g., in hospitals where there is gentamicin resistance, amikacin-containing regimens should be considered, and in hospitals with frequent *Pseudomonas aeruginosa* infections, a regimen with the highest activity against this pathogen (such as tobramycin plus a semisynthetic penicillin) would be a reasonable initial regimen].

4 A single third-generation cephalosporin is an appropriate initial regimen for many hospitals (if the pattern of resistance justifies its use).

5 Most standard regimens are designed for patients who have not been treated previously with prophylactic antibiotics. The development of fever in a patient receiving antibiotics affects the choice of subsequent therapy (which should be tailored to treat resistant organisms or organisms known to cause infections in patients being treated with the antibiotics used at the time).

TABLE 96-1   Normal barriers to infections

Type of defense	Specific lesion	Cells involved	Organism	Disease
Physical barrier	Breaks in skin	Epithelial cells	Staphylococci, streptococci	Cellulitis, extensive skin infection
Phagocytosis	Splenectomy	Reticuloendothelial cells	S. pneumoniae, H. influenzae, N. meningitidis	Rapid overwhelming bacteremia
Phagocytosis	Lack of granulocytes	Granulocytes (neutrophils)	Staphylococci, streptococci, enteric organisms	Bacteremia
Humoral immunity	Lack of antibody	B cells	S. pneumoniae, H. influenzae, N. meningitidis	Infections with encapsulated organisms, sinusitis, pneumonia
Cellular immunity	Lack of T cells	T cells and macrophages	M. tuberculosis, Listeria, herpes viruses, fungi, other intracellular parasites	Infections with intracellular bacteria, fungi, parasites

The initial regimen should be refined on the basis of culture results (see Fig. 96-1). Blood cultures are the most relevant culture on which to base therapy; surface cultures of skin and mucous membranes may be misleading. In the case of bacteremia or other gram-positive infections, it is important that the antibiotic is optimal for the organism isolated. If the infection is caused by certain gram-negative pathogens (especially *P. aeruginosa*), a synergistic combination of antibiotics, usually a semisynthetic penicillin (such as mezlocillin) plus an aminoglycoside (such as tobramycin), may be appropriate. Although it is not desirable to leave the patient unprotected, adding more and more antimicrobials is not appropriate unless there is a clinical or microbiologic reason to do so. *Planned progressive therapy* (the serial, empirical addition of one drug after another without culture data) is not efficacious in most settings and may have unfortunate consequences. Cephalosporins can cause bone marrow suppression, and vancomycin is associated with neutropenia in some normal people. Furthermore, the addition of multiple cephalosporins may induce β-lactamase production in some organisms (cephalosporins and particularly double β-lactam combinations probably should be avoided altogether in the case of *Enterobacter* infections).

Antifungal therapy   Most clinicians add amphotericin B to antibiotic regimens after a patient has been febrile on antibacterial agents for 4 to 7 days. The rationale for the "empirical" addition of amphotericin B is based on the difficulty in culturing fungi prior to

their causing disseminated disease and the high fatality rate of disseminated fungal infections in granulocytopenic patients. The imidazoles (especially fluconazole) may have prophylactic efficacy in this regard, but the spectrum of the imidazoles is less broad than that of amphotericin B. Amphotericin B is the mainstay of therapy for disseminated *Candida* or *Aspergillus* infection in the neutropenic patient. The use of the combination of an imidazole and amphotericin B is controversial because of the theoretical antagonistic effects of these agents.

Other therapeutic modalities   Another way to address the problems of the febrile neutropenic patient is to replace the neutrophils. Although granulocyte transfusions may be efficacious in refractory gram-negative bacteremia, they do not have a documented role in prophylaxis. Because of the expense, the risk of leukoagglutinin reactions (although this risk is probably decreased because of improved cell separation procedures), and the risk of transmitting cytomegalovirus (CMV) in unscreened donors, granulocyte transfusion is reserved for patients unresponsive to antibiotics. This modality may be efficacious for documented gram-negative bacteremia refractory to antibiotics, particularly in situations where the granulocytes will be depressed for only a short period. A variety of cytokines, including granulocyte colony stimulating factor (G-CSF) and granulocyte macro-

TABLE 96-2   Infections and cancer

Cancer	Underlying immune abnormality	Organisms causing infection
Multiple myeloma	Hypogammaglobulinemia	S. pneumoniae, H. influenzae, N. meningitidis
CLL	Hypogammaglobulinemia	S. pneumoniae, H. influenzae, N. meningitidis
AML, ALL	Granulocytopenia, skin and mucous membrane lesions	Extracellular gram-positive and gram-negative organisms, fungi
Hodgkin's disease	Abnormal T cell function	Intracellular pathogens (M. tuberculosis, Listeria, Salmonella, Cryptococcus, M. avium-intracellulare)
Non-Hodgkin's lymphoma and ALL	Steroid chemotherapy, T and B cell dysfunction	P. carinii
Colon and rectal tumors	Local abnormalities*	S. bovis bacteremia
Hairy cell leukemia	Abnormal T cell function	Intracellular pathogens (M. tuberculosis, Listeria, Cryptococcus, M. avium-intracellulare)

* The reason for this association is not well defined.

TABLE 96-3   Organisms likely to cause infections in granulocytopenic patients

GRAM-POSITIVE COCCI

Staphylococcus epidermidis
Staphylococcus aureus
Streptococcus viridans
Streptococcus fecalis (enterococcus)
Streptococcus pneumoniae

GRAM-NEGATIVE RODS

E. coli
Klebsiella
Pseudomonas aeruginosa
Pseudomonas nonaeruginosa (often IV catheter-associated)
Enterobacter
Serratia
Acinetobacter (ofter IV catheter-associated)
Citrobacter

GRAM-POSITIVE RODS

Diphtheroids
JK bacillus (often associated with IV catheters)

FUNGI

Candida species
Aspergillus species

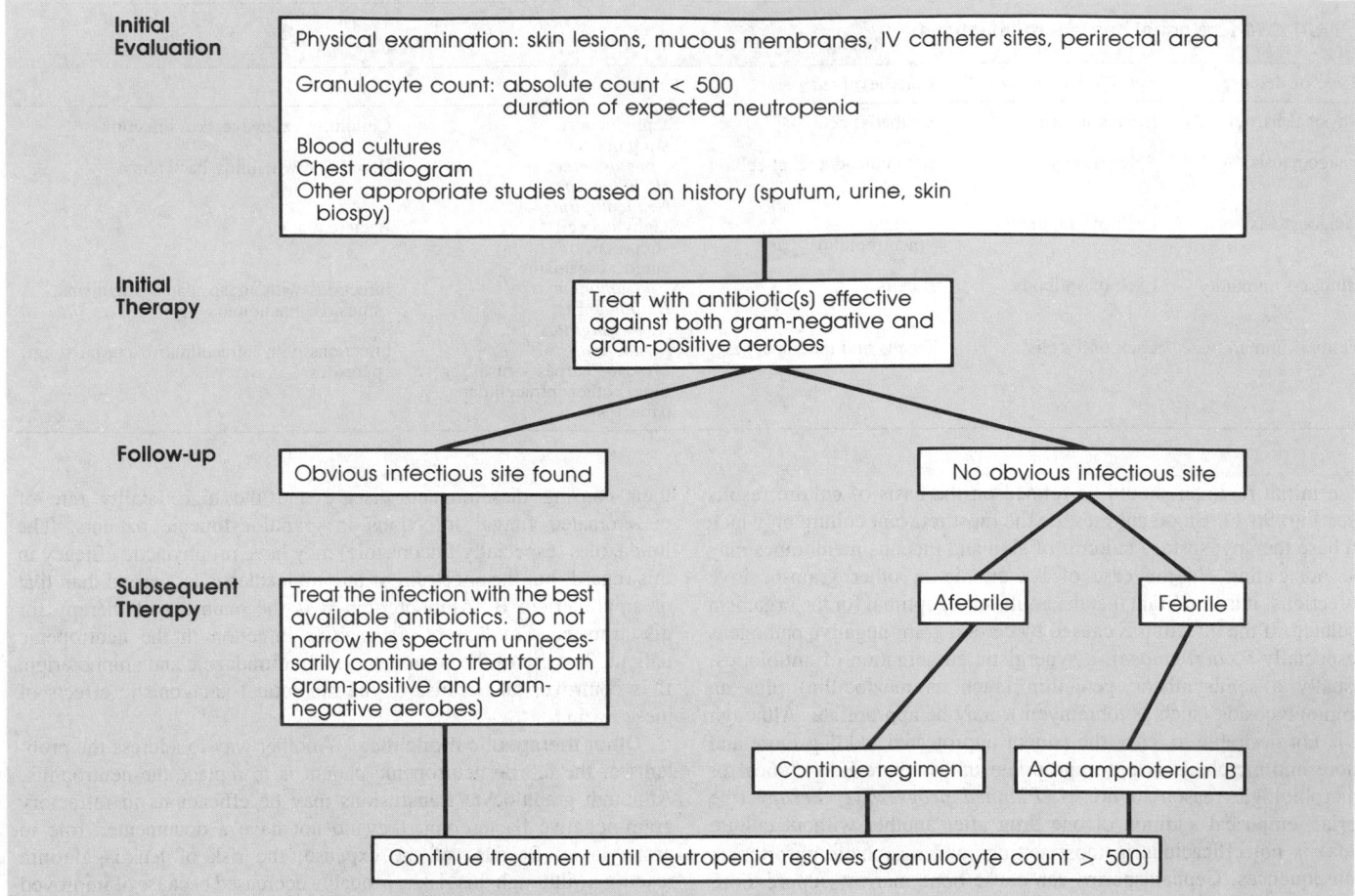

FIGURE 96-1   Diagnosis and treatment of febrile neutropenic patients: an algorithm.

phage colony stimulating factor (GM-CSF), enhance granulocyte recovery after chemotherapy and consequently shorten the period of maximal vulnerability to fatal infections. The role of other cytokines, such as macrophage colony stimulating factor (M-CSF) for monocytes or interferon (IFN-γ), in preventing or treating infections in granulocytopenic patients is under investigation.

Catheter infections   Infections of catheters in the neutropenic patient can be caused by both bacteria and fungi. The decision to remove the line should be based on the necessity of its remaining (it is always easier to treat the infection if the line can be removed). In general, an infection that involves the tunnel (the area where the catheter runs underneath the skin) mandates removal of the catheter. Infections at the exit site can be treated without removing the catheter with variable success depending on the organism causing the infection. Most coagulase-negative staphylococcal infections can be treated even with the line in place. Treatment of coagulase-positive staphylococcal or fungal infections has a high rate of failure and complication. Treatment of catheter infections due to JK bacilli or *Pseudomonas* species with antibiotics alone also is often associated with failure, and removal of the catheter may be required to achieve a cure.

Duration of therapy   In general, therapy should be continued until the granulocytopenia resolves in an infected (or febrile) neutropenic patient. If there is no evidence of focal infection and the fever resolves with resolution of granulocytopenia, antibiotics can be discontinued after the neutrophil count rises.

DISORDERS UNIQUE TO NEUTROPENIC HOSTS   **Skin lesions** The appearance of skin lesions in a neutropenic patient merits careful attention, since these lesions are often an important clue to serious infection. While most lesions (whether due to bacteria or fungi) begin as innocent-looking macules or papules, in the neutropenic host they may progress rapidly to ulceration with a necrotic center (ecthyma gangrenosum) (Fig. 96-2). Ecthyma gangrenosum, which is usually

painless, is often associated with *Pseudomonas* bacteremia but can be caused by other gram-negative rods (e.g., *Escherichia coli*) or fungi. The use of occlusive dressings is associated with the development of infection with *Rhizopus* and *Aspergillus* species. Biopsy should be considered when a skin nodule develops in a neutropenic patient, since histologic identification and positive bacterial or fungal cultures may precede the development of blood cultures positive for the infecting agent. Such lesions may evolve rapidly (even with the patient on appropriate antibiotics), and surgical debridement may be required (see Fig. 96-2*A–E*).

Sweet's syndrome   Sweet's syndrome, acute febrile neutrophilic dermatosis, usually presents as fever and multiple painful cutaneous plaques or tender nodules (and sometimes as pustules, vesicles, or bullae) on the face and upper extremities (see Fig. 96-2*F*) or at intravenous sites (Koebner phenomenon) and is characterized by a dermal infiltrate of neutrophils, often with edema, and elevated erythrocyte sedimentation rates. The syndrome was originally described in middle-aged women with elevated neutrophil counts unassociated with malignancy. In the last two decades it has been recognized increasingly as a cancer-associated syndrome [particularly associated with acute myelogenous leukemia (AML)] and, paradoxically, may occur in the setting of profound neutropenia. Cultures and stains of biopsy specimens for microorganisms are negative. Patients respond dramatically to prednisone, with lysis of fever within hours and resolution of skin lesion in days.

Typhlitis   Typhlitis (cecitis) is an inflammatory process of the cecum in granulocytopenic patients, particularly children with acute lymphocytic leukemia (ALL), that presents like appendicitis, with fever and right lower quadrant pain and tenderness. Pathologically, the involved bowel has ulcerations, necrotic tissue, and dilated blood vessels. Masses of organisms are often found, and the disease is associated with gram-negative bacteremia (particularly with *Pseudo-*

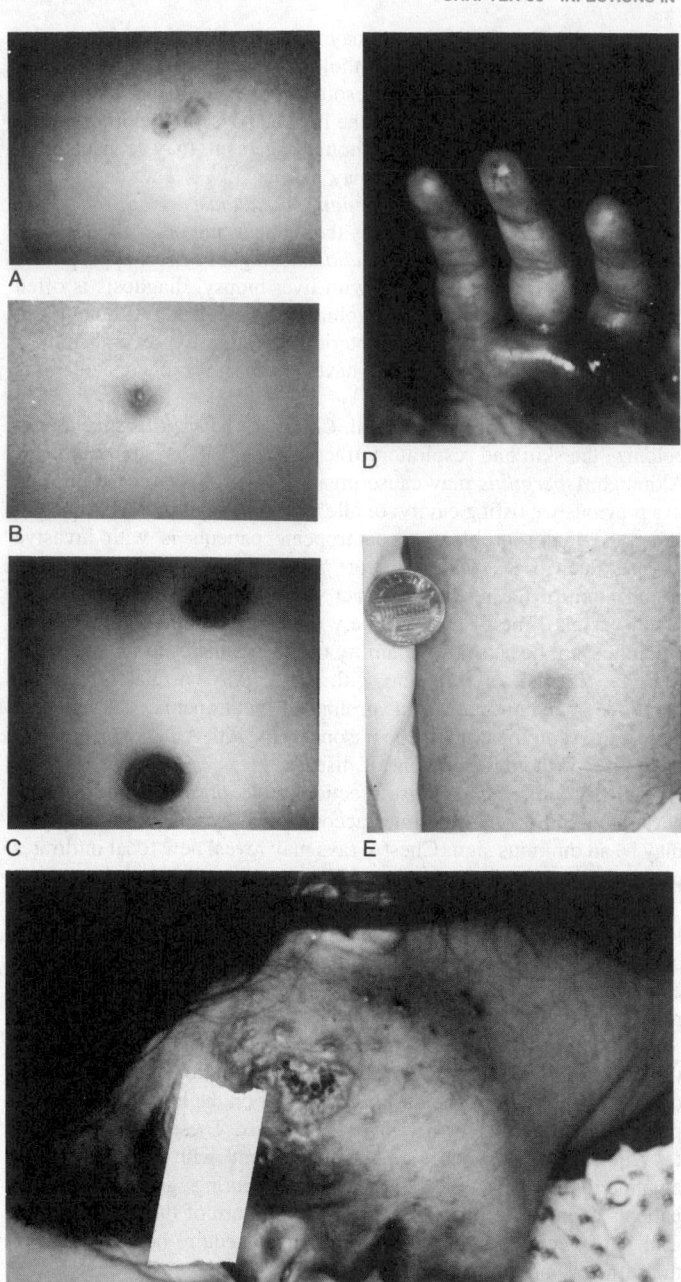

FIGURE 96-2 Skin lesions of neutropenic patients. *A.* Papules related to *E. coli* bacteremia in a neutropenic patient with acute lymphocytic leukemia. *B.* The same papule 2 h later. *C.* The same patient the following day. *D.* Ecthyma gangrenosum in a neutropenic patient with *P. aeruginosa* bacteremia. *E.* Papule in a neutropenic patient with *C. tropicalis* fungemia. *F.* Plaques of Sweet's syndrome in a patient with acute myelocytic leukemia.

Perirectal infections Leukemic patients (especially those with myelomonocytic leukemias) frequently develop perirectal infections. These infections, which like other infections in neutropenic patients often present with a minimum of physical findings, are usually caused by aerobic gram-negative organisms, and do not necessarily mandate the use of agents active against intestinal anaerobes such as *Bacteroides fragilis*. In the presence of deep infection or intestinal fistulas, antibiotics should be changed to include agents with activity against *B. fragilis* (e.g., metronidazole) (see Chap. 128).

***Clostridium difficile*–induced diarrhea** Neutropenic patients, because of exposure to multiple antibiotics, commonly develop *C. difficile*–induced diarrhea. While this diarrhea must be distinguished from chemotherapy-induced diarrhea, patients with *C. difficile* toxin–positive stools respond to therapy with oral vancomycin. The intravenous vancomycin preparation can be given as an elixir at low dose (125 mg PO qid). Therapy with metronidazole is an alternative (see Chap. 108).

Pneumonias in neutropenic patients Pneumonias in immunocompromised patients may be difficult to diagnose because conventional methods of diagnosis depend on the presence of neutrophils. Bacterial pneumonias in neutropenic patients may present without purulent sputum or without any sputum and may not produce physical findings suggestive of chest consolidation (rales or egophony).

Chest x-rays are needed in the situation of persistent or recurrent fever in granulocytopenic patients. The x-ray pattern may provide localizing information which is helpful in further defining which investigative tests and procedures and in narrowing therapeutic options (Table 96-4). The difficulties in management of pulmonary infiltrates relates in part to the difficulties in performing diagnostic procedures on these patients. When platelet counts can be increased to adequate levels with transfusion, microscopic and microbiologic evaluation of the fluid obtained by endoscopic bronchial lavage is often diagnostic. Lavage fluid should be cultured for *Mycoplasma, Chlamydia, Legionella, Nocardia,* fungi, and the usual bacterial pathogens. In addition, *Pneumocystis carinii* pneumonia should be considered, especially in ALL and lymphoma patients who have not had prophylactic trimethoprim-sulfamethoxazole. The characteristics of the infiltrate may be helpful in determining further diagnostic and therapeutic maneuvers. Nodular infiltrates suggest fungal pneumonia (e.g., *Aspergillus* or *Mucor*). Diffuse interstitial infiltrates suggest a viral or parasitic pneumonia. If the patient has a diffuse interstitial pattern on chest x-ray, it may be reasonable to treat empirically with trimethoprim-sulfamethoxazole (for *Pneumocystis*) and erythromycin (for *Chlamydia, Mycoplasma,* and *Legionella*) while considering invasive diagnostic procedures. Noninvasive procedures such as staining of sputum smears for *Pneumocystis* and serum *Cryptococcus* antigen tests may be helpful on occasion. In transplant recipients who are CMV-seropositive, culturing CMV from another site may be worthwhile.

While bleomycin is the most common cause of chemotherapy-induced lung disease, other causes include alkylating agents (such

monas). It is difficult to diagnose the disease without surgical intervention or postmortem examination. Surgery in neutropenic patients can be difficult, because healing is likely to be impaired and the risk of infectious complications is high. Therapy of typhlitis is controversial. Surgical resection has been successful in some patients. On the other hand, in many neutropenic patients, right lower quadrant pain and fever resolve with antibiotics alone, making it hard to define the role of surgery. In general, if the underlying problem can wait until the neutropenia has resolved, surgery is likely to be less complicated. If surgery is absolutely required during the neutropenic period, the patient should be treated with appropriate antibiotics and the necessary procedure should be performed, assuming adequate platelet support can be given.

TABLE 96-4 Differential diagnosis of chest infiltrates in immunocompromised patients

	Cause of pneumonia	
Infiltrate	Infectious	Noninfectious
Localized	Bacteria, *Legionella,* Mycobacteria	Local hemorrhage or embolism, tumor
Nodular	Fungi (e.g., *Aspergillus* or *Mucor*), *Nocardia*	Recurrent tumor
Diffuse	Viruses (especially CMV), *Chlamydia, P. carinii, T. gondii,* mycobacteria	Congestive heart failure, radiation pneumonitis, drug-induced lung injury, diffuse alveolar hemorrhage (described after BMT)

as cyclophosphamide, chlorambucil, and melphalan), nitrosoureas (BCNU, CCNU, methyl-CCNU), busulfan, procarbazine, methotrexate, procarbazine, and hydroxyurea. Both infectious and drug- and/or radiation-induced pneumonitis can cause fever and chest x-ray abnormalities, so the differential diagnosis of an infiltrate in a patient receiving chemotherapy is broad (see Table 96-4). Since the treatment of radiation pneumonitis (which may respond dramatically to glucocorticoid) or drug-induced pneumonitis is different than that of infectious pneumonia, a biopsy may be important in the diagnosis. Unfortunately, a definitive diagnosis is not made in approximately 30 percent of cases even after bronchoscopy.

Open lung biopsy is the standard of diagnostic techniques. Biopsy via a visualized thoracostomy may replace an open procedure in many cases. When a biopsy cannot be performed, empirical treatment may be undertaken with erythromycin and trimethoprim-sulfamethoxazole in the case of diffuse infiltrates or amphotericin B in the case of nodular infiltrates. The risks should be weighed carefully in these cases. Empirical treatment may result in drug toxicity from administration of inappropriate drugs or in a failure to administer appropriate therapy, either of which may be more harmful than biopsy.

FUNGAL INFECTIONS IN NEUTROPENIC PATIENTS　Neutropenic patients are predisposed to the development of invasive fungal infections, most commonly including *Candida* species and *Aspergillus* and, on occasion, *Fusarium, Trichosporon,* and *Dreschlera.* Cryptococcus infection, which is common in patients on immunosuppressive agents, is uncommon in neutropenic patients receiving chemotherapy for AML. Invasive candidal disease is usually caused by *C. albicans* or *C. tropicalis* but can be caused by *C. krusei, C. parapsilosis,* and *C. glabrata.*

Candida infections in other settings include superficial candidiasis, candidal sepsis, and hepatic (or hepatosplenic) candidiasis.

Superficial or mucous membrane infection with *Candida*　As with any patients who receive antibiotics for prolonged periods, superficial colonization with *Candida* is likely to occur in the skin, mouth, and anal and genital areas. Such colonization is usually unassociated with evidence of tissue invasion. Local care and treatment of the area may be all that is required. Prophylactic oral nystatin, as commonly employed to prevent these mucocutaneous "superinfections," is probably of little or no efficacy. Treatment with fluconazole is effective against *C. albicans* but may be associated with an increased risk of *C. kruseii* or *Aspergillus* infection. Colonization of mouth, skin, and stool with *C. tropicalis* but not with *C. albicans* may be predictive of invasive disease in neutropenic patients. *Candida* esophagitis, often a complication of antibiotic treatment, may respond to low doses of amphotericin or imidazole and may be accompanied by invasive disease.

Candida sepsis　Early in neutropenia, *Candida* may cause acute sepsis with fungemia, skin nodules, and hypotension—manifestations similar to those of gram-negative bacteremia. *Candida* may seed almost any organ; joint disease and thyroid disease have been reported, and the organism appears to have a predilection for the kidney and for retinal embolization. The presence of a maculopapular rash and subcutaneous nodules is suggestive of *C. tropicalis* infection. If the candidemia results from colonization of an indwelling catheter, the catheter should be removed as soon as possible. Although transient candidemia may not always require therapy in the noncompromised patient, documentation of candidemia in the neutropenic host should lead to immediate administration of amphotericin B.

Hepatic candidiasis　Hepatic candidiasis in neutropenic patients usually develops around the time of resolution of the neutropenia. The characteristic picture is that of persistent fever unresponsive to antibiotics, abdominal symptoms, and elevated serum alkaline phosphatase levels in a patient with hematologic malignancy who has recently recovered from neutropenia. The diagnosis of this disease (which may present in an indolent manner and persist for several months) is based on the finding of yeasts or pseudohyphae in granulomatous lesions. Hepatic ultrasound or computed tomographic (CT) scans may reveal bull's eye lesions. In some cases, magnetic

resonance imaging (MRI) scans may reveal small lesions not seen by other imaging modalities. The pathology (revealing a granulomatous response) and the timing (with resolution of neutropenia and higher granulocyte counts) suggest that the host response is important in the manifestations. In many cases, although organisms may be visualized, cultures of biopsied material may be negative. The designation *hepatosplenic candidiasis* or *hepatic candidiasis* is a misnomer because the disease often involves the kidneys and other tissues, and the term *chronic disseminated candidiasis* might be more appropriate. Because of the risk of bleeding with liver biopsy, diagnosis is often made on the basis of radiographic abnormalities. Although the traditional therapy is with amphotericin B (often for several months until all manifestations of disease have disappeared), fluconazole may be useful for outpatient therapy.

***Aspergillus* infection**　As with *Candida, Aspergillus* species can colonize the skin and respiratory tract or cause fatal systemic illness. Although *Aspergillus* may cause invasive aspergillosis, aspergilloma in a previously existing cavity, or allergic bronchopulmonary aspergillosis, the major problem of neutropenic patients is with invasive disease due to *A. fumigatus* or *flavus.* Entry is often through colonization of the respiratory tract with subsequent invasion of the blood vessels. The disease is likely to present with a thrombotic or embolic event because of the ability of the organisms to invade blood vessels. The risk of infection with *Aspergillus* correlates with the duration of neutropenia. In prolonged neutropenia, surveillance cultures for colonization of the nasopharynx with *Aspergillus* may be predictive of the development of disease.

Patients with *Aspergillus* infection often present with pleuritic chest pain and fever sometimes accompanied by cough. Hemoptysis may be an ominous sign. Chest x-rays may reveal new focal infiltrates or nodules (see Table 96-4). Chest CT scans may reveal a characteristic "halo" consisting of a masslike infiltrate surrounded by an area of low attenuation. The presence of a "crescent sign" on chest x-ray or chest CT, in which the mass progresses to central cavitation, is characteristic of invasive *Aspergillus* but may occur only with resolution of the lesions.

In addition to pulmonary presentations, *Aspergillus* may invade through the nose or palate, with deep sinus penetration. The appearance of a discolored area in the nasal passages or on the hard palate should prompt investigation for invasive *Aspergillus.* These cases are likely to require surgical debridement. Treatment with high doses of amphotericin B has been successful in curing granulocytopenic patients of invasive *Aspergillus* following return of the granulocytes. Catheter infections with *Aspergillus* usually require both removal of the catheter and antifungal therapy.

PREVENTION OF INFECTIONS IN NEUTROPENIC PATIENTS
Air handling　Outbreaks of fatal *Aspergillus* infections have been associated with construction and construction materials in several hospitals. The association between spore counts and risk of infection suggests the need for a high-efficiency air handling system in hospitals that care for large numbers of neutropenic patients. The use of laminar flow rooms and prophylactic antibiotics has decreased the number of infectious episodes in severely neutropenic patients. But because of the expense of such a program and the failure to show any dramatic effects on mortality, most centers do not routinely use laminar flow to care for neutropenic patients. Some centers use "reverse isolation," in which health care providers and visitors to a patient who is neutropenic are dressed in gowns and gloves. Since most of the infections the patients develop are due to organisms that colonize the patients' own skin and bowel, the validity of such schemes is dubious, and limited clinical data do not support their use. Hand washing may prevent spread of resistant organisms.

Food　The presence of large numbers of bacteria (particularly *P. aeruginosa*) in certain foods (particularly fresh vegetables) has led some to recommend a special low-bacteria diet. A diet consisting of cooked and canned food is satisfactory to most neutropenic patients and does not involve elaborate disinfection or sterilization protocols. Some spices (such as black pepper) are likely to be contaminated with fungal spores, and these, like fresh flowers and live plants, probably should be avoided during the period of severe neutropenia.

Antibiotic prophylaxis There is no consensus on the use of prophylactic antibiotics in neutropenic patients. The incidence of infection is decreased in patients treated prophylactically with broad-spectrum antibiotics, and trimethoprim-sulfamethoxazole appeared to prevent infections in some series. Because of a prolongation of neutropenia which may be associated with use of trimethoprim-sulfamethoxazole, some clinicians have used such broad-spectrum agents as the quinolones (e.g., ciprofloxacin). Either regimen can be given orally, and both have the theoretical advantage that the antibiotics are not active against anaerobic organisms and are thus less likely to disrupt the bowel flora and permit colonization with new aerobes or *Candida*. However, both have adverse effects and can lead to resistance in a hospital. For this reason, many clinicians reserve their use for patients with the longest periods of neutropenia (e.g., bone marrow transplant recipients; see below). The same issues exist concerning the use of antifungal agents; again, the administration of antifungals such as fluconazole may prevent infections with susceptible organisms (e.g., *C. albicans*) but cause a concomitant increase in infections due to resistant fungi (e.g., *C. krusei*). Thus the decision to use antifungal prophylaxis may vary depending on what fungi are endemic in a given hospital.

Treatment after resolution of the neutropenic episode Once neutropenia has resolved, the patient is not at high risk of infection. However, patients who continue on chemotherapeutic protocols, depending on what drugs they receive, continue to be at high risk for certain diseases. Any patient on more than a maintenance level of glucocorticoids (including many diffuse lymphoma treatment regimens) should have prophylactic trimethoprim-sulfamethoxazole because of the risk of *P. carinii* infection; those with ALL should be maintained on trimethoprim-sulfamethoxazole prophylaxis for as long as they are receiving chemotherapy.

INFECTIONS IN BONE MARROW TRANSPLANT (BMT) RECIPIENTS

Bone marrow transplantation for either immune deficiency or cancer results in a transient state of complete immune incompetence. Immediately following transplantation, both phagocytes and immune cells (T cells and B cells) are absent, and the host is susceptible to infection. The reconstitution that occurs following transplantation has been likened to maturation of the immune system in neonates. The analogy does not entirely predict infections seen in these patients, however, because the new marrow is usually expressed in an old host who has several latent infections already (Table 96-5).

TIMETABLE OF COMMON INFECTIONS (See also Fig. 96-3) In the first month after transplantation, infectious complications are similar to those in granulocytopenic patients receiving chemotherapy for AML or ALL (see above). Because of the anticipated 3- to 4-week duration of neutropenia in this population, many centers give prophylactic antibiotics to patients with the initiation of chemotherapy.

TABLE 96-5 Herpes group virus syndromes in transplant recipients

Virus	Reactivation disease
Herpes simplex type 1	Oral lesions, sometimes with spread (pneumonia described in BMT patients)
Herpes simplex type 2	Severe and/or persistent anogenital lesions
Varicella zoster	Zoster (dissemination may occur)
Cytomegalovirus	Associated with graft rejection, fever
Epstein-Barr virus	B cell lymphoproliferative disease
Human herpes virus 6	Fever, rash,* pneumonitis
Human herpes virus 7	Undefined

* A characteristic rash (seen in primary infection) has not been well defined.

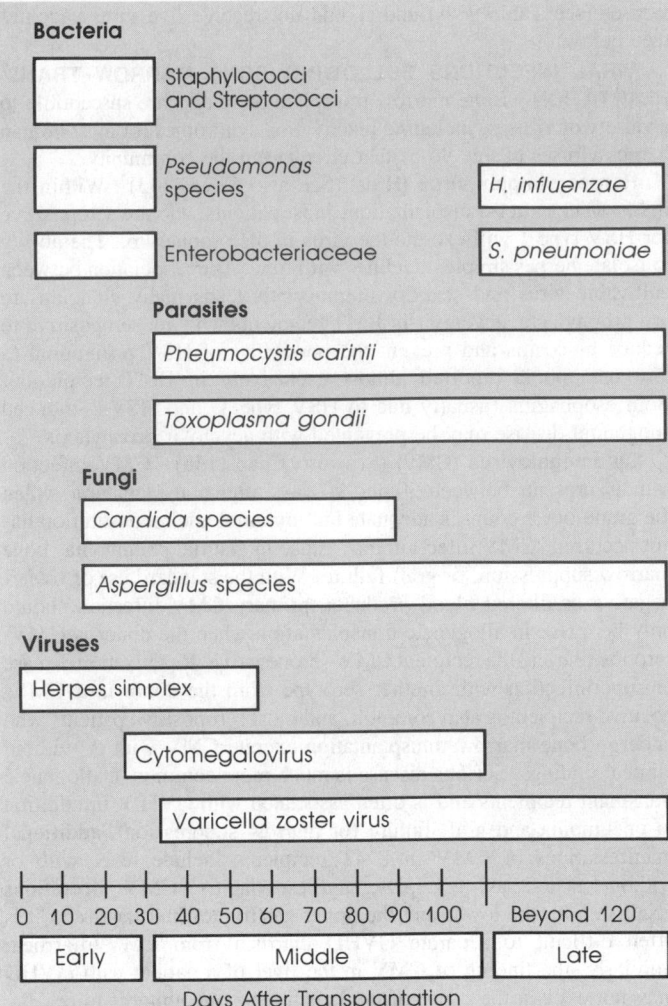

FIGURE 96-3 Infections after bone marrow transplantation.

Prophylactic trimethoprim-sulfamethoxazole or ciprofloxacin decreases the incidence of gram-negative bacteremia in these patients.

In the second month after transplantation, a major concern (particularly in allogeneic transplant recipients) is CMV disease. The diagnosis of pneumonia in these patients presents some special problems (see Table 96-4). Because they have been treated with multiple chemotherapeutic agents and radiation, the differential diagnosis of pneumonitis in this group should include CMV pneumonitis, diffuse alveolar hemorrhage (DAH), viral and fungal causes of pneumonia, and parasites. Because of the high risk of *P. carinii* pneumonia (especially in patients being treated for hematologic malignancies), most patients should be maintained on prophylactic doses of trimethoprim-sulfamethoxazole. Trimethoprim-sulfamethoxazole also may provide protection for patients seropositive for *Toxoplasma gondii,* which may cause a pneumonia in the early weeks after transplantation or central nervous system (CNS) lesions later.

The late posttransplantation period (6 months following bone marrow reconstitution) is marked by bacteremias due to encapsulated organisms and reactivation of varicella zoster virus (Fig. 96-3). The advantages of maintaining patients on trimethoprim-sulfamethoxazole for 1 year after transplantation include protection against late bacterial infections with pneumococci and *Haemophilus influenzae* which are a consequence of the inability of the immature bone marrow to respond to polysaccharide antigens (see Fig. 96-3). After recovery from transplantation and full restoration of immune function, patients should be revaccinated with all recommended vaccines (based on the age of the patient). Patients who continue to take immunosuppressive drugs for graft-versus-host disease (GVHD) are susceptible to intracellular pathogens such as *Listeria, Nocardia*, fungi, *Pneumocystis,* and viruses (see Table 96-1) and should not receive live virus vaccines (see below).

VIRAL INFECTIONS FOLLOWING BONE MARROW TRANSPLANTATION

Bone marrow transplant recipients are susceptible to a variety of viruses, including reactivation syndromes for most human herpes viruses (Table 96-5) that circulate in the community.

Herpes simplex virus (HSV) (See also Chap. 143) Within the first 6 weeks after transplantation, most patients who are seropositive for HSV type 1 will excrete the virus in the oropharynx. The ability to isolate herpes simplex declines with time. The association between cultivable virus and severity of mucositis leads many clinicians to use prophylactic acyclovir in BMT recipients who are seropositive to reduce mucositis and prevent the possibility of HSV pneumonia (a rare pneumonia reported almost exclusively in BMT recipients). Both esophagitis (usually due to HSV type 1) and HSV-2–induced anogenital disease may be prevented with acyclovir prophylaxis.

Cytomegalovirus (CMV) (See also Chap. 146) CMV infection usually presents between 30 and 90 days after transplantation, when the granulocyte count is adequate but immunologic reconstitution has not occurred. CMV infection may cause interstitial pneumonia, bone marrow suppression, or graft failure. With the standard use of CMV-negative or filtered blood products, primary CMV infection should only be a risk in allogeneic transplantation when the donor is CMV-seropositive and the recipient CMV-seronegative. Reactivation disease or superinfection with another serotype from the donor in a CMV-positive recipient is also common, and most seropositive patients who undergo bone marrow transplantation excrete CMV with or without clinical findings. Serious disease is much more common in allogeneic transplant recipients and is often associated with GVHD. In addition to pneumonia and graft failure (or marrow suppression), additional manifestations of CMV in BMT recipients include fever with or without arthralgias, myalgias, and esophagitis. CMV ulcerations occur in both the lower and the upper gastrointestinal tract, and it is often difficult to separate GVHD diarrhea from CMV diarrhea. Similarly, the finding of CMV in the liver of a patient with GVHD may not explain the cause of the hepatic enzyme abnormalities.

Because of the high fatality rate of CMV pneumonia in bone marrow transplantation and the difficulty in diagnosing infection early, prophylactic ganciclovir is given in some centers during the period of maximum vulnerability (from engraftment to day 120 after transplant). The major problem with its administration relates to adverse effects that include a dose-related neutrophil suppression. Because the frequency of CMV pneumonia is lower in autologous transplant recipients (2 to 7 percent versus 10 to 40 percent for allogeneics), prophylactic therapy in this group will not become the rule unless a less toxic antiviral agent is available. A common practice among many centers treating allogeneic transplant patients is to culture blood and urine (and bronchial secretions in some) and treat those patients who have positive CMV cultures with ganciclovir as prophylaxis against the development of CMV pneumonia. The development of improved antigen testing methods should make surveillance of those at high risk for CMV disease more reliable. Treatment of CMV pneumonia in BMT recipients requires both IVIG and ganciclovir, although ganciclovir alone is effective prophylactically.

Varicella zoster (VZV) (See also Chap. 144) Reactivation of herpes zoster may occur as early as 1 month but more commonly occurs several months after transplantation. Attack rates are approximately 40 percent for allogeneic and 25 percent for autologous transplant recipients. Localized zoster can spread in the face of immunosuppressives. Fortunately, disseminated disease usually can be controlled with high doses of acyclovir (Fig. 96-4; see also Chap. 142). Because of the high incidence of dissemination of herpes zoster in patients with skin lesions, acyclovir is given prophylactically in some centers to prevent severe disease. Low doses of acyclovir (400 mg PO tid) appear to be effective prophylaxis for preventing reactivation of varicella zoster virus. However, administration of acyclovir inhibits development of VZV-specific immunity. Thus, administration for only 6 months following transplantation does not prevent zoster

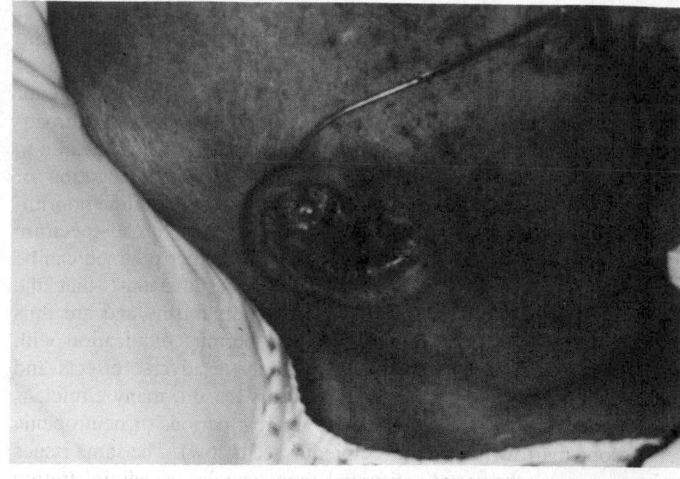

A

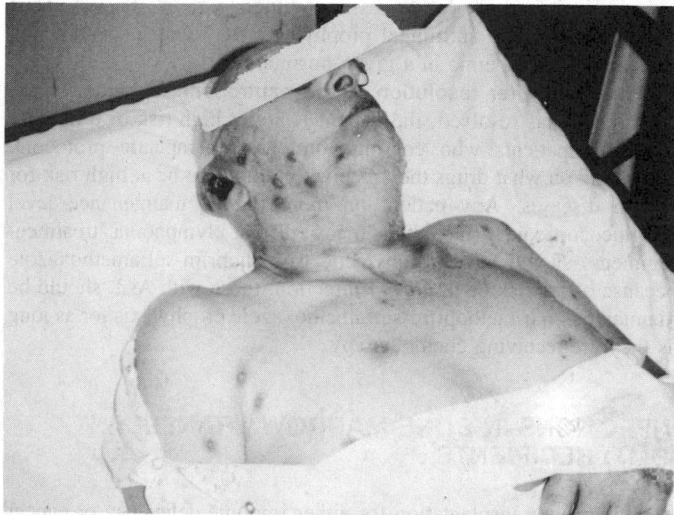

B

FIGURE 96-4   Spread of herpes zoster with chemotherapy. *A.* The patient complained of external ear pain. A vesicular rash on the concha and antihelix suggested Ramsey-Hunt syndrome. *B.* Following chemotherapy for prostate cancer, the patient developed disseminated zoster which was eventually controlled with acyclovir.

infection from occurring when acyclovir is stopped. Some data suggest that administration of low doses of acyclovir for an entire year following transplantation is effective and may eliminate most post-transplantation zoster.

Epstein-Barr virus (See also Chap. 145) Primary Epstein Barr virus (EBV) infection can be fatal in transplant recipients, and EBV reactivation can cause a B cell lymphoproliferative disease (EBV lymphoproliferative syndrome), which also may be fatal in patients taking immunosuppressive drugs. The localization of EBV to B cells leads to several interesting phenomena in marrow transplants. The marrow ablation that occurs as part of the bone marrow transplantation procedure eliminates latent EBV from the host. The disease can then be reacquired following transplantation when a susceptible pool of B cells is regenerated.

The EBV lymphoproliferative syndrome can develop in the recipient's B cells (if any should survive marrow ablation) but is more likely to be a consequence of reactivation in the donor cells. Reactivation of EBV is more likely during immunosuppression (e.g., it is associated with GVHD and the use of anti-T cell antibodies). Although less likely in the autologous transplant recipient, it can occur in the case of T cell–depleted autologous recipients (e.g., patients being treated for a T cell lymphoma with marrow depletion using anti-T cell antibodies). The EBV lymphoproliferative syndrome usually presents 1 to 3 months after engraftment and can cause high fevers and cervical adenopathy, similar to those in infectious mononucleosis, but more commonly resembles disseminated lymphoma. An incidence of 0.6 percent has been found among allogeneic bone marrow transplants recipients, in contrast to the figures of approximately 5 percent for renal transplant recipients and 20 percent after cardiac transplantation. In all cases, EBV lymphoproliferative syndrome is more likely to occur with continued immunosuppression (especially with the use of anti-T cell antibodies and cyclosporin).

Other (nonherpes) viruses Both respiratory syncytial virus (RSV) and parainfluenza virus type 3 can cause severe and sometimes fatal pneumonias in BMT recipients. Infections with both these agents can occur as disastrous nosocomial epidemics. Therapy with ribavirin has been reported to ameliorate disease. Influenza is also seen in BMT recipients and generally mirrors the presence of infection in the community. In addition, adenovirus can be isolated at rates varying from 5 to 18 percent of BMT recipients. Although hemorrhagic cystitis, pneumonia, and fatal disseminated infection have been reported, adenovirus infection, which usually occurs in the first or second month after transplantation (similar to CMV), is often asymptomatic. No treatment has proven efficacy. Infections with B19 parvovirus (presenting with anemia) and enteroviruses (with fatalities) can occur, rotaviruses are a common cause of gastroenteritis in BMT recipients, and BK and JC virus can be found in the urine of some transplant recipients.

VACCINATION OF BMT RECIPIENTS Because of their lack of immunologic memory, BMT recipients should be vaccinated against organisms they are likely to encounter. Vaccines against pneumococci and *H. influenzae* should be administered (see Table 96-9), particularly if the patient is splenectomized. In addition patients should be inoculated against poliovirus with an inactivated vaccine. Because of the risk of spread, household contacts of marrow transplant recipients (or patients immunosuppressed by virtue of chemotherapy) should receive the inactivated polio vaccine as well. It is safe to give live measles, mumps, and rubella vaccine to allogeneic transplant recipients 2 years after transplantation if they are free of overt GVHD. This vaccine also has a lower risk of spreading to a household contact than the polio vaccine. In patients who have active GVHD and/or are maintained on high doses of glucocorticoids, it may be prudent to avoid all live virus vaccines.

INFECTIONS IN SOLID ORGAN TRANSPLANT RECIPIENTS

The most important cause of death among early kidney transplant recipients was infection with organisms not susceptible to conventional antibiotic therapy. These infections occurred in patients requiring prolonged courses of glucocorticoids and other immunosuppressive drugs. Morbidity and mortality in solid organ transplantation have been reduced with the use of better antibiotics.

The organisms that cause infections in these patients are different from those in BMT recipients because solid organ recipients do not go through a period of neutropenia. On the other hand, since organ transplant patients are immunosuppressed for more prolonged periods (usually permanently), they are susceptible to the same organisms as cancer patients with impaired T cell immunity (see Table 96-1). In addition, since the transplantation procedure involves surgery, the recipients are subject to wound infections.

TIMETABLE OF INFECTIONS (See also Table 96-6) During the early period (less than 1 month after transplantation), infections are most often caused by extracellular bacteria (staphylococci, streptococci, *E. coli,* other gram-negative organisms) which often originate in surgical wound or anastomotic sites. Thus the infections are largely determined by the type of transplant.

In subsequent weeks, the consequences of the administration of agents that suppress cell-mediated immunity and of the acquisition (from the transplanted organ) or reactivation of parasites and viruses become apparent. CMV is often a problem at this time and may present as severe systemic disease or as an infection of the transplanted organ. CMV is associated not only with generalized immunosuppression but also (in some series) with organ-specific, rejection-related syndromes. CMV is associated with glomerulopathy in kidney transplant recipients, bronchiolitis obliterans in lung transplant recipients, premature atherosclerosis in heart transplant recipients, and the vanishing bile duct syndrome in liver transplant recipients. Whether these syndromes are actually caused by CMV, which itself is an opportunistic invader, or are merely associated has not been established. It is clear that the presence of CMV and CMV disease is associated with a poor outcome after transplantation. For this reason, considerable attention has focused on the diagnosis, treatment, and prophylaxis of CMV in organ transplant recipients.

During the period beyond 6 months after transplantation, infections characteristic of patients with defects in cell-mediated immunity develop. Thus infections with *Listeria monocytogenes, Nocardia,* various fungi, and other intracellular parasites may be a problem. Elimination of these late infections will not be possible until specific tolerance to the transplanted organ can be achieved without the administration of drugs that lead to generalized immunosuppression. Meanwhile vigilance, prophylaxis (when indicated), and rapid diagnosis and therapy of infections can be lifesaving in the solid organ transplant recipient who, unlike most BMT recipients, continues to be immunosuppressed.

Solid organ transplant recipients are susceptible to EBV lymphoproliferative disease from as early as 2 months to many years after transplantation. The prevalence of this complication is increased by potent immunosuppressive drugs and may be reversed (in some cases) by decreasing the immunosuppression. The proliferation of B cells, which is the pathologic problem in this disease, occurs with increased frequency in renal and liver transplantation. Among organ transplant

---

TABLE 96-6 Infections after renal transplantation

	Period after transplantation		
	Early (<1 month posttransplant)	Middle (1–4 months posttransplant)	Late (>6 months posttransplant)
Urinary tract	Bacteria (*E. coli, Klebsiella,* Enterobacteriaceae, *Pseudomonas,* enterococcus), associated with bacteremias and pyelonephritis, *Candida*	Cytomegalovirus (fever alone is common)	Bacteria, late UTIs usually not associated with bacteremia
Lungs	Bacteria (including *Legionella* in endemic settings)	CMV diffuse interstitial pneumonitis, *P. carinii, Aspergillis, Legionella*	*Nocardia, Aspergillis, Mucor*
CNS		*Listeria monocytogenes,* bacteremia and meningitis, CMV encephalitis, toxoplasmosis	CMV retinitis, listerial meningitis, cryptococcal meningitis, *Aspergillis, Nocardia*

patients, lung and heart transplants are most likely to present with EBV-induced B cell proliferation in the lungs. Whether the tendency of EBV lymphoproliferation to present in the transplanted organ relates to local factors (e.g., lack of access of host T cells to the transplanted organs because of disturbed lymphatics) or to the differences in major histocompatibility loci between the host T cells and the organ (which may lead to lack of cell migration or lack of effective T cell–macrophage cooperation) has not been established.

INFECTIOUS COMPLICATIONS OF KIDNEY TRANSPLANTATION **Early infections** Early infections following kidney transplantation are often caused by bacteria associated with skin or wound infections. Some data indicate a role for perioperative antibiotic prophylaxis, and many centers give cephalosporins or a penicillin with an aminoglycoside to decrease the risk of postoperative complications. Immediately after transplantation, urinary tract infections are usually related to anatomic alterations due to surgery (see Table 96-6). Such early infections may require prolonged treatment as for pyelonephritis (6 weeks of antibiotics). Urinary tract infections that occur more than 6 months after transplantation do not seem to be associated with the high rate of pyelonephritis or relapse seen with infections that occur in the first 3 months and may be treated for shorter time periods.

Prophylaxis with trimethoprim-sulfamethoxazole, i.e., 1 double-strength tablet (800 mg sulfamethoxazole and 160 mg trimethoprim) per day, for the first 4 months following transplantation decreases the incidence of early and middle period infections (see below and Table 96-7).

Middle-period infections Because of continuing immunosuppression, renal transplant recipients are predisposed to lung infections characteristic of patients with T cell deficiencies (i.e., *Listeria, Mycobacteria, Nocardia,* fungi, viruses, and parasites). The high mortality associated with *Legionella pneumophila* infection led to the closing of renal transplant units in hospitals with endemic *Legionella*. Fifty percent of all renal transplant recipients presenting with fever in the period 1 to 4 months after transplantation have evidence of CMV disease, and CMV itself accounts for over two-thirds of the fevers, making it the predominant pathogen during this period. CMV infection also may present as arthralgias or myalgias. CMV can cause primary disease (in the case of a seronegative recipient who receives a kidney from a seropositive donor) or may present as either reactivation disease or superinfection during this period. Patients may have an atypical lymphocytosis, but unlike nonimmunosuppressed patients, they often do not have lymphadenopathy or splenomegaly, thereby making clinical suspicion (and laboratory confirmation) necessary for diagnosis. The clinical syndrome may be accompanied by bone marrow suppression (particularly leukopenia). CMV is associated with an increased incidence of other opportunistic infections (e.g., fungal infections) and glomerulopathy. Because of the frequency and severity of CMV disease, a considerable effort has been addressed to its prevention and treatment in renal transplant recipients. Administration of an immune globulin preparation enriched for antibodies to cytomegalovirus (CMV-Ig) decreases the incidence in the group at highest risk for severe infections (seronegative recipients of seropositive kidneys). Ganciclovir is useful for the treatment of serious CMV disease.

The other herpes group viruses may present within 6 months of the transplant or later. Early after transplantation, herpes simplex may cause either oral or anogenital lesions that are usually responsive to acyclovir. Large ulcerating lesions in the anogenital area may lead to bladder and rectal dysfunction as well as predisposing to bacterial infection. VZV may cause a fatal disseminated infection in nonimmune renal transplant recipients, but immune patients usually do not have dissemination of reactivation zoster outside the dermatome; thus it is a less fearsome complication in renal than in bone marrow transplantation.

EBV reactivation disease is more serious; it often presents as a polyclonal proliferation of B cells that invade the CNS, nasopharynx, liver, small bowel, heart, and transplanted kidney. The disease is diagnosed by the finding of a proliferation of EBV-positive B cells. The incidence of the syndrome is higher in patients on high doses of cyclosporin. Fortunately, the B cells usually regress with withdrawal of immunosuppression with or without antiviral therapy (acyclovir). Human herpes virus type 6 infection and reactivation also occur after renal transplantation.

The papovaviruses BK and JC have been cultured from the urine of renal transplant recipients (as they have from BMT recipients). BK virus excretion is associated with ureteral strictures, and JC virus with progressive multifocal leukoencephalopathy. Adenoviruses also may persist in patients with continued immunosuppression.

Renal transplant recipients are also subject to infections with other intracellular organisms. These patients are likely to have pulmonary infections with *Nocardia, Aspergillus,* and *Mucor* and infections with other pathogens in which the T cell–macrophage axis plays an important role. In patients without intravenous catheters, *L. monocytogenes* is the most common cause of bacteremia 1 month or more after transplantation. Renal transplant recipients also may have *Salmonella* bacteremia, which can lead to endovascular infections and require prolonged therapy. Pulmonary infections with *P. carinii* are common unless the patient is maintained on trimethoprim-sulfamethoxazole prophylaxis. The addition of cyclosporine to azathioprine and prednisone is probably associated with an increased risk of *P. carinii* pneumonia. *Nocardia* infection may present in the skin, bones, lungs, or CNS (usually single or multiple brain abscesses). *Nocardia* infection usually occurs 1 month or more after transplantation and may follow treatment (increased immunosuppression) for an episode of rejection. Pulmonary findings are nonspecific; localized disease with or without cavities is most common, but the disease may disseminate. The diagnosis is made by culture of the organism from sputum or from the involved nodule. Most patients are now cured with prolonged sulfonamide therapy. Prophylaxis with trimethoprim-sulfamethoxazole also appears to be efficacious in the prevention of disease. *Nocardia* infections can occur more than 2 years after transplantation, suggesting that long-term prophylaxis is justified.

Toxoplasmosis occurs in seropositive patients, usually in the first few months after transplantation. In endemic areas, histoplasmosis, coccidioidomycosis, and blastomycosis may cause pulmonary infiltrates or disseminated disease.

Late infections Late infections (more than 6 months after transplantation) include CMV retinitis and a variety of CNS complica-

TABLE 96-7 Prophylaxis against infections in transplant recipients

Risk factors	Organism	Prophylactic antibiotics	Examinations
Travel or residency in area with known risk of fungal infection	Coccidiodomycosis, histoplasmosis, blastomycosis	? Imidazoles* or amphotericin B	Chest radiogram
Latent viruses	Herpes simplex, varicella zoster, EBV, CMV	Acyclovir after BMT for HSV and VZV; ganciclovir in some settings	Serology—test for HSV, VZV, CMV, EBV
Latent parasites	*P. carinii, T. gondii*	Trimethoprim-sulfamethoxazole or dapsone plus pyrimethamine	Serology for *Toxoplasma*
History of exposure to tuberculosis	*M. tuberculosis*	Isoniazid, if recent conversion for positive chest x-ray and no previous treatment	PPD and chest radiogram

* The use of imidazoles in this setting is under study.

tions. Patients (and particularly those in whom immunosuppression has been increased) are also at risk for subacute meningitis due to *Cryptococcus* as well as aspergillomas (usually originating from a lung source) and for cryptococcal disease, which may present in an insidious manner (sometimes as a skin infection before the development of clear CNS findings). *Listeria* meningitis may present acutely and requires prompt therapy to avoid a fatal outcome.

In addition, patients who remain on glucocorticoid therapy are predisposed to infection. "Transplant elbow" is a recurrent bacterial infection in and around the elbow that is said to result from a combination of poor tensile strength of the skin of steroid-treated patients and steroid-induced proximal myopathy that requires patients to push themselves up with their elbows to get out of chairs. Recurrent bouts of cellulitis (usually caused by *Staphylococcus aureus*) occur until patients are provided with elbow protection.

These patients are susceptible to other fungal infections with *Aspergillus* and *Rhizopus*, for example, which may present as superficial lesions before dissemination disease. Mycobacteria (particularly *M. marinum*) can be diagnosed by skin examination. *Prototheca wickerhamii* (an achlorophyllic alga) has been diagnosed by skin biopsy. Warts caused by human papillomaviruses are a late consequence of persistent immunosuppression. Local therapy is usually satisfactory treatment.

INFECTIONS IN HEART TRANSPLANT RECIPIENTS **Early infections** Mediastinitis is an early complication of heart transplantation. An indolent course is common, with fever or a mildly elevated white blood cell count preceding the development of site tenderness or drainage. Clinical suspicion based on evidence of sternal instability and failure to heal may lead to the diagnosis. Although common skin organisms such as *S. aureus* and *S. epidermidis* are common pathogens, mediastinitis in these patients also can be due to *Mycoplasma hominis*. Since these organisms require an anaerobic environment for growth and may be difficult to see on conventional medium, the laboratory should be alerted that *M. hominis* is suspected. *M. hominis* mediastinitis has been cured with a combination of surgical debridement (sometimes requiring muscle flap placement) and clindamycin and tetracycline. Other organisms, including *P. aeruginosa* and *Candida,* can cause mediastinitis. The organisms may be cultured from accompanying pericarditis fluid.

Middle-period infections *Toxoplasma gondii* may be transmitted to a seronegative recipient in the heart of a seropositive donor, thus making serologic screening for *T. gondii* infection important in the months after transplantation. The incidence of disease is so high in this setting that some centers have advocated prophylaxis with pyrimethamine. CMV and HIV also have been transmitted by heart transplantation. CNS infections can be due to *Toxoplasma, Nocardia,* and *Aspergillus,* and *L. monocytogenes* meningitis should be considered in heart transplant recipients with fever and headache.

CMV infection is associated with poor outcomes after heart transplantation. The virus is usually cultivable 1 to 2 months after transplantation, causes manifestations (usually fever and atypical lymphocytosis, often associated with leukopenia and thrombocytopenia) in 2 to 3 months, and develops into severe disease such as pneumonia 3 to 4 months after transplantation. Seropositive recipients usually develop cultivable virus faster than patients whose primary CMV infection is a consequence of the transplant. Between 40 and 70 percent of patients develop symptomatic CMV disease: (1) CMV pneumonia, the most likely to be fatal, (2) CMV esophagitis and gastritis, sometimes accompanied by abdominal pain with or without ulcerations and bleeding, and (3) the CMV syndrome, comprising CMV in the blood, fever, leukopenia, thrombocytopenia, and hepatic enzyme abnormalities. Ganciclovir is efficacious in the treatment of CMV infection; prophylaxis with ganciclovir may reduce the incidence of CMV-related disease.

Late infections EBV infection usually presents as a lymphoma-like proliferation of B cells as a late complication, particularly with increased immunosuppression. A subset of heart-lung transplant recipients may develop early (within 2 months of transplantation)

fulminant EBV lymphoproliferative disease, often in the transplanted lung. Prophylaxis against *P. carinii* infection is required for these patients (see below and Table 96-8).

LUNG TRANSPLANTATION **Early infections** It is not surprising that lung transplants are predisposed to the development of pneumonia. The combination of ischemia and the resulting mucosal damage together with accompanying denervation and lack of lymph drainage probably contribute to the high rate (66 percent in one series) of pneumonia. The prophylactic use of high doses of broad-spectrum antibiotics for the first 3 to 4 days after surgery decreases the incidence of pneumonia. Gram-negative pathogens (Enterobacteriaceae and *Pseudomonas* species) are troublesome in the first 2 weeks after surgery (the period of maximum vulnerability). Pneumonia also can be caused by *Candida* (possibly as result of colonization of the donor lung), *Aspergillus,* and *Cryptococcus.*

Mediastinitis Mediastinitis may occur at an even higher rate than in heart transplant recipients. *Staphylococcus, M. hominis,* and *C. albicans* are common causes of mediastinitis that occurs within 2 weeks of surgery. Mediastinitis due to CMV (which may be transmitted as a consequence of the transplant) usually presents between 2 weeks and 3 months after surgery, with primary disease occurring later than reactivation disease. The incidence of CMV infection, either reactivation or primary, is between 75 and 100 percent if either the donor or the recipient is seropositive for CMV. CMV-induced disease appears to be more severe in recipients of lung and heart-lung transplants. Whether this relates to the mismatch in lung antigen-presenting and host immune cells or occurs for other (nonimmune) reasons is not known. Over half of lung transplant recipients with symptomatic CMV disease have pneumonia, and it may be difficult to distinguish the radiographic picture of CMV from organ rejection, thereby further complicating therapy. CMV also can be associated with bronchiolitis obliterans in lung transplants. The development of pneumonitis related to herpes simplex has led to use of acyclovir for the prevention of herpes simplex pneumonia. Acyclovir prophylaxis also may affect CMV isolation. Ganciclovir is probably more efficacious than acyclovir in lung transplant recipients.

EBV lymphoproliferative syndrome As in other transplant recipients, infection with EBV may cause either a mononucleosis-like syndrome or lymphoproliferative disease. The tendency of the B cell blasts to present in the lung appears to be greater after lung than in other organ transplantation. Reduction of cyclosporine dosage causes remission in most cases, but lymph node compression can cause fatalities.

Late posttransplantation infections The incidence of *P. carinii* infection (which may present with a paucity of findings) is high in lung or heart-lung transplants. Some form of prophylaxis against *P. carinii* pneumonia (PCP) is indicated in all organ transplant situations (see Table 96-7 and Table 96-8). Trimethoprim-sulfamethoxazole prophylaxis for 12 months after transplantation may be sufficient to prevent disease in patients whose immunosuppression is not increased.

LIVER TRANSPLANTATION **Early complications** As in the case of other transplantation, early bacterial infections are a major problem following liver transplantation. Many centers administer systemic broad-spectrum antibiotics for the first 5 days following

TABLE 96-8 Prophylactic antibiotics or vaccination for immunocompromised patients

Underlying problem	Therapy
Splenectomy	Vaccination for pneumococci, *H. influenzae*, meningococci*
T cell defects (e.g., solid organ transplantation)	Prophylaxis for *P. carinii* while patient is immunosuppressed
Antibody defects (e.g., BMT, CLL, or multiple melanoma)	Vaccination for *Pneumococcus, H. influenzae, N. meningitidis*

* Patients should be advised of the importance of seeking immediate medical attention for suspected infections [it may be advisable for patients to have antibiotics (e.g., amoxicillin or amoxicillin/clavulanate) at home].

surgery, even in the absence of documented infection. However, despite prophylaxis, infectious complications are still common and are correlated with duration of surgical procedure and the type of biliary drainage. An operation of greater than 12 h is associated with an increased likelihood of infection. Patients with a choledochojejunostomy with drainage of the biliary duct to a roux en Y jejunal bowel loop have more fungal infections than those whose bile is drained via a choledochocholedochostomy (with anastomosis of the donor common bile duct to the recipient common bile duct).

Cholangitis The development of postoperative biliary stricture predisposes to cholangitis. These patients may lack the characteristic signs and symptoms of cholangitis: fever, abdominal pain, and jaundice. In fact, even if present, these findings may suggest graft rejection. The diagnosis of cholangitis in liver transplant recipients therefore requires documentation of bacteremia or demonstration of aggregated neutrophils in bile duct biopsy specimens. Unfortunately, invasive studies of the biliary tract (either T-tube cholangiograms or endoscopic retrograde cholangiopancreatography) may lead to cholangitis. For this reason, many clinicians recommend prophylactic antibiotics covering gram-negative organisms and anaerobes when these procedures are performed in liver transplant recipients.

Peritonitis Peritonitis and intraabdominal abscesses are common complications. Bacterial peritonitis may result from biliary leaks and primary or secondary infection following leakage of bile. Peritonitis in liver transplant recipients is often polymicrobial, commonly due to enterococci, aerobic gram-negative organisms, staphylococci, anaerobes, or *Candida*. Only one-third of patients with intraabdominal abscesses have bacteremia. Abscesses within the first postoperative month may occur not only over the liver but also in the spleen, pericolic area, and pelvis. Treatment includes antibiotics and drainage as necessary.

As is true of other transplant recipients, liver transplant patients have a high incidence of fungal infections, and the occurrence of fungal infection (often candidiasis) correlates with preoperative use of glucocorticoids, duration of treatment with antibacterial agents, and posttransplant use of immunosuppressive agents.

Viral infections Viral hepatitis is a common complication of liver transplantation (see Chap. 266). As in other transplant settings, reactivation disease with herpes group viruses is common (see Table 96-5). Herpes simplex, human herpes virus 6, and CMV can be transmitted in donor organs. Although CMV hepatitis occurs in about 4 percent of liver transplant recipients, it is usually not so severe as to require retransplantation. While CMV disease develops in the majority of seronegative recipients who receive organs from CMV-positive donors, fatality rates are lower than in lung or heart-lung transplant recipients. CMV disease is associated with the vanishing bile duct syndrome after liver transplantation. While patients respond

to treatment with ganciclovir, prophylaxis with CMV-Ig and acyclovir may modify disease. EBV lymphoproliferative disease after liver transplantation shows a propensity for involvement of the liver.

PANCREAS TRANSPLANTATION Transplantation of the pancreas is complicated by early abdominal infection in approximately 20 percent of cases. To prevent contamination of the allograft with enteric bacteria and yeasts, some surgeons, instead of draining the pancreas through the bowel, drain secretions into the urinary tract or bladder. A cuff of duodenum if often utilized in the anastomosis between the pancreas graft and the bladder. In addition to the attendant bicarbonate loss, this technique causes a high rate of urinary tract infections (30 to 40 percent), possibly related to the retention of the duodenum. An alternative method, the transplantation of only the islet cells, may eliminate the problems of wound and urinary tract sepsis which are characteristic of pancreas transplant recipients.

Issues related to the development of CMV infection, EBV lymphoproliferative disease, and infection with opportunistic pathogens are similar in patients receiving pancreas as in other solid organ transplant recipients.

VACCINATION OF TRANSPLANT RECIPIENTS

In addition to antibiotic prophylaxis (Table 96-8), transplant recipients should be vaccinated against likely pathogens (Table 96-9). In the case of BMT recipients, optimal responses cannot be achieved until after reconstitution; allogeneic transplant BMT recipients require reimmunization to be protected against pathogens, despite previous immunization of the donor and recipient. The situation is complex in the case of autologous transplants. T and B cells in the peripheral blood may reconstitute the response if they are transferred in adequate numbers. However, cancer patients (particularly those with Hodgkin's disease, in whom it has been extensively studied) on chemotherapy do not respond normally to immunization, and titers to infectious agents fall more rapidly than in normal hosts. Therefore, even immunosuppressed patients who have not had marrow transplants may need booster vaccine injections. If memory cells are specifically eliminated as part of a marrow "cleanup" procedure, it will be necessary to reimmunize the recipient with a new primary series. Optimal times for immunization for different transplant populations are currently being evaluated.

In the absence of compelling data as to the best time to immunize BMT recipients, it is reasonable to vaccinate both autologous and allogeneic transplant recipients with pneumococcal vaccine at 12 months after transplantation followed by another injection 12 months later (since the response to the initial vaccine is weak in the early posttransplantation period). The *H. influenzae* conjugate vaccine, *N. meningitidis* polysaccharide vaccine, and diphtheria, tetanus, and inactivated polio vaccines can all be given at these same intervals (12 and 24 months after transplantation). Some authorities recommend instead a new primary series for tetanus/diphtheria and inactivated polio vaccine (vaccination at 12, 14, and 16 months after transplantation). The live-virus measles/mumps/rubella vaccine can be given to autologous transplant recipients 24 months after transplantation and to most allogeneic bone transplant recipients if they are not maintained on immunosuppressive drugs and do not have ongoing GVHD.

In the case of solid organ transplant recipients, vaccination with all usual vaccines and the indicated booster shots should be given prior to immunosuppression, if possible, since responses will be improved. For patients on immunosuppressive agents, administration of the pneumococcal vaccine should be repeated every 6 years. No data are available for the meningococcal polysaccharide vaccine, but it is probably reasonable to administer it along with the pneumococcal vaccine. The *H. influenzae* conjugate vaccine is safe and should have efficacy in this population; therefore, administration is recommended prior to transplantation. Booster doses of this vaccine are not recommended in adults. Solid organ transplant recipients who remain on immunosuppressive drugs (glucocorticoids, cyclosporine) should

TABLE 96-9 Vaccination for bone marrow or solid organ transplant recipients

Vaccine	Bone marrow	Solid organ
Pneumococcus, H. influenzae, Meningococcus	After transplantation (optimal timing not established) preimmunization*	Immunize prior to transplant and every 6 years for Pneumovax (others not established)
Seasonal influenza	Yes	Before transplantation if possible
Poliomyelitis	Inactivated vaccine	Inactivated vaccine; live vaccine may be given prior to immunosuppression
Measles/ mumps/ rubella	Immunize 24 months after transplantation if no graft-versus-host disease	Prior to transplant
Tetanus, diptheria	Reimmunize after transplantation	Before transplantation; boosters at 10 years or as required; does not require new primary series

* Some studies suggest that it may be helpful to "immunize the graft" prior to transplant.

not receive live-virus vaccines. Thus a person in this group exposed to measles should be given immune globulin. Similarly, an immunocompromised patient who is seronegative for varicella and who comes in contact with a person who has chickenpox should be given varicella zoster immune globulin (VZIG) as soon as possible (and certainly within 96 h).

Immunocompromised patients who travel benefit from some but not all vaccines. If patients travel to areas where *N. meningitidis* meningitis or polio is common, they should be protected against these diseases. The current typhoid vaccines are not recommended for use in most immunocompromised patients because the inactivated preparation has too many adverse effects and the live vaccine is contraindicated. The yellow fever live vaccine also should not be administered. Phenol-inactivated cholera vaccine is probably of little use in this setting. On the other hand, immunization with the purified protein hepatitis B vaccine is reasonable if patients are likely to be exposed. The inactivated hepatitis A vaccine has not been licensed at this time but may have efficacy in this population as well. In the absence of an approved vaccine for hepatitis A, travelers should consider receiving passive protection with immune globulin (the dose depends on the length of travel in the high-risk area).

REFERENCES

ANAISSIE E et al: Fluconazole therapy for chronic disseminated candidiasis in patients with leukemia and prior amphotericin B therapy. Am J Med 91:142, 1991

DAUBER JH et al: Infectious complications in pulmonary allograft recipients. Clin Chest Med 11(2):291, 1990

DENNING DW, STEVENS DA: Antifungal and surgical treatment of invasive aspergillosis: Review of 2,121 published cases. Rev Infect Dis 12(6):1147, 1990

EMANUEL D et al: Cytomegalovirus pneumonia after bone marrow transplantation successfully treated with the combination of ganciclovir and intravenous immune globulin. Ann Intern Med 109:777, 1988

EORTC INTERNATIONAL ANTIMICROBIAL THERAPY COOPERATIVE GROUP: Empiric antifungal therapy in febrile granulocytopenic patients. Am J Med 86:668, 1989

ETTINGER NA, TRULOCK EP: Pulmonary considerations of organ transplantation (parts 1, 2, and 3). Am Rev Respir Dis 144:1386, 144:213, 144:433, 1991

GOODRICH JM et al: Early treatment with ganciclovir to prevent cytomegalovirus disease after allogeneic bone marrow transplantation. N Engl J Med 325:1601, 1991

HUGHES WT et al: Guidelines for use of antimicrobial agents in neutropenic patients with unexplained fever. J Infect Dis 161:381, 1990

KRAMER MR et al: Trimethoprim-sulfamethoxazole prophylaxis for *Pneumocystis carinii* infections in heart-lung and lung transplantation: How effective and for how long? Transplantation 53:586, 1992

KUSNE S et al: Infections after liver transplantation: An analysis of 101 consecutive cases. Medicine 67(2):132, 1988

RAAD II, BODEY GP: Infectious complications of indwelling vascular catheters. Clin Infect Dis 15:197, 1992

RUBIN RH, YOUNG LS (eds): *Clinical Approach to Infection in the Compromised Host.* New York, Plenum, 1988

——— et al: Infection in the renal transplant recipient. Am J Med 70:405, 1981

SHAH G et al: Incidence, prevalence and clinical course of hepatitis C following liver transplantation. Gastroenterology 103:323, 1992

SNYDMAN DR et al: Use of cytomegalovirus immune globulin to prevent cytomegalovirus disease in renal-transplant recipients. N Engl J Med 317:1049, 1987

STRATTA RJ et al: Successful prophylaxis of cytomegalovirus disease after primary CMV exposure in liver transplant recipients. Transplantation 51:90, 1991

THALER M et al: Hepatic candidiasis in cancer patients: The evolving picture of the syndrome. Ann Intern Med 108:88, 1988

TSEVAT J et al: Which renal transplant patients should receive cytomegalovirus immune globulin? Transplantation 52:259, 1991

WINGARD JR et al: Cytomegalovirus infection after autologous bone marrow transplantation with comparison to infection after allogeneic bone marrow transplantation. Blood 71:1432, 1988

WOLFSON JS et al: Dermatologic manifestations in immunocompromised patients. Medicine 64:115, 1985

WRIGHT TL et al: Recurrent and acquired hepatitis C viral infection in liver transplant recipients. Gastroenterology 103:317, 1992

ZUTTER MM et al: Epstein-Barr virus lymphoproliferation after bone marrow transplantation. Blood 72:520, 1988

97 EVALUATION AND MANAGEMENT OF PATIENTS WITH HOSPITAL-ACQUIRED INFECTIONS

DORI F. ZALEZNIK

Nosocomial infections are defined as infections acquired during or as a result of hospitalization. Generally, a patient who has been in the hospital for less than 48 h and develops an infection is considered to have been incubating the infection prior to hospital admission. Most infections manifested after 48 h are considered to be *nosocomial*. Patients may still develop a nosocomial infection after hospital discharge if the organism presumably was acquired in the hospital. Surgical wound infection developing in the weeks after hospital discharge is an example of nosocomial infection.

INCIDENCE AND COSTS Nosocomial infections contribute significantly to morbidity and even mortality, as well as to excess costs, for hospitalized patients. It is estimated that 3 to 5 percent of patients admitted to an acute care hospital in the United States acquire a new infection, which accounts for about 2 million nosocomial infections per year and an annual cost in excess of 2 billion dollars. Some estimate that the odds of death double in patients who develop a nosocomial infection, although clearly such factors as underlying disease and severity of illness also play an important role.

Although immunosuppressed hosts are especially vulnerable to infections acquired in a hospital, there are common nosocomial infections that occur even in normal hosts. The most common hospital-acquired infection is a urinary tract infection, accounting for about 40 to 45 percent of all nosocomial infections. Pneumonia accounts for 15 to 20 percent, surgical wound infection 25 to 30 percent, and bacteremia, mainly associated with intravascular devices, 5 to 7 percent.

The potential impact of nosocomial infections is considerable when assessed in terms of incidence, morbidity, mortality, and increased financial burden. These types of analyses examine nosocomial infections as medical and economic issues. The clinical problem for the physician is a patient in the hospital developing a new fever. In the evaluation of such a patient, information about the most common categories of infection may not be helpful. The clinician must use clinical clues from the patient's presentation and hospitalization as well as information about common hospital-acquired infections to diagnose a nosocomial infection.

The evaluation of a hospitalized patient with new fever should include a careful history. Particular attention should be paid to symptoms of headache, cough, abdominal pain, diarrhea, flank pain, dysuria, urinary frequency, and leg pain. Other features related to the hospitalization also are important, such as presence and type of intravenous devices, history or current use of a urinary catheter, surgical procedure if any was performed, and new medications administered, including those for surgical prophylaxis. The physical examination should be directed at possible sources of infection and should pay particular attention to the skin to look for rash or possible embolic lesions; lungs; abdomen, especially the right upper quadrant; costovertebral angles; surgical wounds, if present; and calves and current and old intravenous sites for signs of phlebitis. The laboratory evaluation of all hospitalized patients with new fever should include a complete blood count with differential, chest radiograph, and blood and urine cultures. Other diagnostic tests to consider, depending on the patient, include liver function tests, plain film or other study of the abdomen, routine aerobic cultures of sputum, stool, or other relevant body fluids, and testing of stool for *Clostridium difficile* toxin in cases of diarrhea.

CATEGORIES OF INFECTION Pneumonia Although the astute clinician will question the patient thoroughly and perform a rapid, comprehensive physical examination, one way to approach the development of fever in a hospitalized patient is to consider potential infectious sites which may be life-threatening. One important infection to consider is pneumonia. Patients most at risk for developing nosocomial pneumonia are those in an intensive care unit (ICU), especially intubated patients; patients with altered levels of consciousness, especially those with nasogastric tubes; elderly patients; patients with chronic lung disease; postoperative patients; and any of the above patients taking H-2 blockers or antacids. Nosocomial pneumonia in the National Nosocomial Infections Surveillance (NNIS) Registry is diagnosed 0.6 to 1.0 times per 100 hospitalizations and is common in postoperative patients. In patients on ventilators, the occurrence of pneumonia may be 10 to 20 times higher. Mortality figures for nosocomial pneumonia are as high as 33 percent.

Oropharyngeal and gastric colonization play a critical role in the pathogenesis of pneumonia in the hospitalized patient. The oropharynx of hospitalized patients can become colonized by many species of aerobic gram-negative organisms within 48 h of hospitalization. Aspiration occurs commonly during sleep and is increased by such factors as a nasogastric tube, altered consciousness, decreased gag reflex, or delayed gastric emptying. In recent years, the role of gastric colonization in nosocomial pneumonia has been recognized. Bacterial counts in the stomach rise in the presence of medications that raise gastric pH, such as H-2 blockers and antacids, as well as in malnourished, achlorhydric, or some elderly patients. The prevalence of pneumonia in intubated patients is reportedly two to three times higher in patients receiving H-2 blockers or antacids for stress ulcer prophylaxis than in those receiving sucralfate, a medication that heals ulcers without altering gastric pH.

Gastric colonization is believed to influence development of pneumonia by retrograde colonization of the oropharynx. Ventilated patients are also at risk of developing pneumonia by leakage of bacteria around the cuff of the endotracheal tube and by nebulized bacteria from nebulizers, condensate within ventilator circuits, and humidifiers.

In patients outside intensive care, pneumonia should be suspected when a patient develops a new cough, fever, leukocytosis, sputum production, and a new infiltrate on chest x-ray. Diagnosis can be complicated in patients with congestive heart failure, in whom concomitant chest x-ray abnormalities are present, or in patients with chronic sputum production. Some organisms, such as *Legionella* spp., may not be associated with peripheral leukocytosis.

The signs of pneumonia are more subtle, and therefore, diagnosis of pneumonia often is more complex in ICU patients, especially those who are intubated. In particular, chest x-ray films are much more difficult to interpret, since fluid overload, congestive heart failure, and adult respiratory distress syndrome (ARDS) are all common findings in intubated patients. Polymorphonuclear leukocytes (PMNs) often are present on Gram's stains of the purulent secretions common in intubated patients. An important clue to pneumonia is a change in output or character of these secretions. If increased quantity or thickness or change in color of secretions is noted, a sputum Gram's stain should be performed and pneumonia seriously considered in the differential diagnosis. Serial Gram's stains are useful, since the number of PMNs may increase substantially, and the type(s) of organisms may shift. For example, the baseline sputum from an intubated patient may contain about 25 PMNs per high-power field and have mixed gram-positive and gram-negative organisms of several morphologic types in moderate amounts. On the day of a new fever, the same patient may have copious amounts of more tenacious sputum with more PMNs and a predominance of enteric-appearing gram-negative rods. Even without distinct changes in chest x-ray, this patient would be considered to have developed pneumonia. Another subtle sign of pneumonia in the intubated patient is a requirement for change in ventilator settings in the absence of (1) fluid overload, (2) a mechanical alteration such as a shift in endotracheal tube placement, or (3) the presence of a pneumothorax.

The major organisms of concern in nosocomial pneumonia are gram-negative aerobic organisms. In the NNIS survey, *Pseudomonas*

aeruginosa was the leading pathogen causing nosocomial pneumonia in 1984, followed by *Staphylococcus aureus*, *Klebsiella pneumoniae*, and *Enterobacter* spp. While surveys of this kind are useful, it is essential to know which pathogens are common in a particular institution, since there are differences among hospitals in resident flora, particularly in ICUs. In some institutions, methicillin-resistant *S. aureus*, *Xanthomonas* spp., *Flavobacterium* spp., and even *Legionella* spp. may be of particular concern. Viruses such as respiratory syncytial virus and adenovirus as etiologic agents in nosocomial pneumonia in the adult and the pediatric population are receiving more attention. Viruses have been underrepresented as agents of nosocomial pneumonia because diagnosis is more difficult, and many microbiology laboratories do not have the capability to isolate viruses.

Antibiotic resistance is another important issue to address in the hospitalized patient. In addition to knowing the sensitivity patterns of the hospital flora, one must consider whether a patient has been on continuous or multiple courses of antibiotic therapy. To reduce the likelihood of altering the sensitivity patterns of the patient's flora, antibiotic courses for pneumonia should be kept as short as possible, with coverage as narrow as possible for the organism(s) involved.

Bacteremia Another potentially life-threatening nosocomial infection to consider in the evaluation of the patient with a new fever is bacteremia, which is usually related to the presence of an intravascular device. While many common nosocomial infections such as pneumonia or urinary tract infection can be accompanied by bacteremia, a primary bacteremia is defined by isolation of a recognized pathogen from the blood without an infection at another site. The NNIS survey from 1989 reported bloodstream infection rates at 1.3 to 6.5 per 1000 patient discharges, with large teaching hospitals having the highest rates. In one study, bacteremia led to 14-fold higher in-hospital mortality, with length of stay increased by at least 2 weeks.

One difficulty in assessing the significance of bacteremia is to distinguish true pathogens from contaminating skin flora. This problem is especially important in establishing an infection of an indwelling intravascular catheter because organisms that inhabit the skin, such as coagulase-negative staphylococci, also commonly cause infection. The most common entry site for infection related to intravascular devices is at the insertion site, with spread of infection along the outside of the device initially. Other sources of entry, however, include contaminated infusates and tubing, introduction of organisms through ports or leaking connections, and hematogenous seeding of a catheter during bacteremia. While gram-negative aerobic bacilli are probably the most feared nosocomial bloodstream pathogens, the NNIS survey from 1980–1989 showed that these organisms had not increased in frequency of isolation over the decade. The bacteremia-associated group of organisms that increased the most in frequency was the coagulase-negative staphylococci, followed by *Candida* spp. Other leading causes of line-related bacteremia were *S. aureus* and enterococci.

For practical purposes, establishing an infection of an intravascular device or primary bacteremia as the cause of fever in a hospitalized patient is a diagnosis of exclusion. If a patient has a fever and signs of cutaneous involvement (erythema, induration, tenderness, or purulent drainage) at the insertion site of a catheter, full cultures should be obtained, the vascular access line removed, and the catheter tip sent for quantitative culture. Studies have correlated growth of 15 colonies or more from a catheter tip with infection of the line. More commonly, the exit site does not show signs of infection, and there is considerable debate about the necessity of removing a line at that point in a febrile patient. Unless another site of infection is obvious, it is generally advisable to remove a line when a patient develops a new fever. While central line changes over a guidewire have been shown to be safe, it is not clear that maintaining the same insertion site with possible line infection is wise. In general, when a line is removed for possible infection, the site should be changed. If vascular access is a problem and one wishes to continue intravascular therapy despite the intravascular device infection, it is probably not necessary to change the line over a guidewire. Traditional teaching suggested automatic removal of an infected intravenous device. In current practice, however, especially with surgically implanted intravenous catheters, a decision may be made to attempt treatment with antibiotics leaving the catheter in place. This practice often is successful when the infecting organism is a coagulase-negative *Staphylococcus* and less so with other organisms, particularly *Candida* spp.

Another controversial management issue is whether to draw blood for culture through a line. While some studies document correlation of cultures drawn through vascular access lines in the 90 percent range with peripheral blood cultures, there are both false-positive and false-negative cultures of blood obtained through a line. If the culture is positive and no peripheral blood has been drawn, it is impossible to determine whether the patient has a true bacteremia or the culture merely reflects bacteria associated with the line. In turn, if multiple peripheral blood cultures are positive, it is reasonable to assume that the line is at least infected secondarily. Whether a bacteremia is high grade or sustained may influence duration of antibiotic therapy and cannot be determined from cultures of specimens obtained through a line.

Surgical wound infection   Evaluation of fever in the postoperative patient must include careful evaluation of the surgical wound. Although surgical wound infection accounts for 25 to 30 percent of nosocomial infections, the true incidence of postoperative wound infection is difficult to assess, particularly at a time when patients are hospitalized for shorter periods. In a number of studies, careful follow-up for the development of wound infections after discharge, especially observation of the wound by a trained observer such as a nurse, has shown the actual rates of wound infections in all categories of surgery to be greater than reported rates. Surgical procedures have long been classified as clean, clean-contaminated, contaminated, and dirty-infected. The risk of wound infection varies from 2.9 percent for clean procedures to 12.6 percent for already infected sites. In 1985, a more sophisticated system was proposed for assessing risk of wound infection. This index uses abdominal operation, surgery lasting >2 h, contaminated or dirty-infected surgery by the classic wound classification system, and the presence of three or more diagnoses in the patient and predicts wound infection rates between 1 and 27 percent.

Other risk factors for the development of postoperative wound infection include the presence of a drain; preoperative length of stay, with the rates doubling for each week of extra preoperative hospitalization; preoperative shaving of the field, especially 24 h or more before the procedure; length of surgery; presence of an untreated remote infection; and surgeon. Perioperative antibiotic prophylaxis has been shown to decrease wound infection rates in a number of careful studies, including those of clean surgical procedures. Antibiotic coverage after the surgical wound is closed has not been shown to provide additional benefit.

A surgical wound should be examined for erythema extending more than 2 cm beyond the margin of the wound, localized tenderness and induration, fluctuance, drainage of purulent material, or dehiscence of sutures. Mechanical factors, as well as infection, can cause wound dehiscence. Sternal wounds following cardiac surgery are of special concern, since the consequence of infection can be great. The surface of the wound may not present an obvious cause for concern, but in some patients ongoing fevers and especially development of rocking or instability of the sternum may be sufficient cause for surgical exploration of the wound. Mediastinitis or sternal osteomyelitis is a severe complication of cardiac surgery. Wounds associated with the placement of prosthetic devices such as mechanical joints also are of special concern. Infection of these wounds can lead to infection of the prosthesis, which generally requires surgical removal to clear the infection.

Urinary tract infection   Urinary tract infections (UTIs) are the most common nosocomial infection and generally the easiest to treat with the least severe sequelae. In a study that controlled for potential confounding factors such as severity of illness, length of hospitaliza-

tion, and duration of catheterization, the overall case-fatality rate was 2.8 times higher in bacteriuric patients than in patients without bacteriuria. A follow-up study of sealed catheter junctions showed a decrease in this mortality rate associated with a decrease in UTIs. Four principal risk factors have been associated repeatedly with the development of UTI in hospitalized patients: female sex, duration of urinary catheterization, absence of systemic antibiotics, and breach of appropriate catheter care. Administration of systemic antibiotics in patients with urinary catheters in place for 1 to 5 days has been associated with a decrease in rates of bacteriuria. For patients with catheters in place for 6 or more days, however, this benefit is no longer observed.

The pathogenesis of catheter-associated UTI appears to differ in men and women. In women, periurethral colonization with fecal flora, with tracking of organisms up the catheter to the bladder, resembles the pathogenesis of UTI in noncatheterized female patients, in whom bacteria track up the short female urethra. In contrast, periurethral colonization often cannot be demonstrated in men; the majority of infections seem to arise from intraluminal spread of organisms to the bladder. Some organisms such as *Proteus* and *Pseudomonas* spp. appear to facilitate growth of a biofilm along the inside of the urinary catheter which encrusts and obstructs the flow of urine.

Although UTI is an extremely common nosocomial infection, it is important to define infection precisely. Especially in evaluating a febrile hospitalized patient, it is crucial to think carefully about all possible sources of infection and not to assume UTI is the probable cause. In patients who have had urinary catheters in place for a number of days, fever, dysuria, frequency, leukocytosis, and especially flank pain or costovertebral angle tenderness are highly suggestive of bladder infection or pyelonephritis. In patients with fever but no other symptoms or signs referable to the urinary tract, one should look for ancillary findings suggestive of urinary tract involvement, such as white blood cells without epithelial cells in the urine sediment or leukocyte esterase or nitrite on urinalysis. A urine culture positive for a single organism should not be accepted as definitive evidence of UTI in an asymptomatic patient. While one might treat the febrile patient with a positive urine culture with antibiotics, it is prudent to repeat the culture before the institution of therapy. Inability to recover an organism or the same organism on repeat culture, particularly if the patient does not respond to antibiotics, should raise questions about the validity of the diagnosis of UTI. In addition, isolation of two or more bacteria in a single specimen is most likely due to contamination unless there is reason to suspect a bladder diverticulum or a perinephric abscess.

Other infectious sources of fever   Several other types of infections may cause fever in the hospitalized patient and should be considered in the differential diagnosis of new fever. In patients who have received antibiotics, even a single dose as surgical prophylaxis, antibiotic-associated diarrhea may develop. This is caused usually by the spore-forming organism *C. difficile*, which produces toxins that cause diarrhea. Some patients may appear quite toxic with this infection, with high fevers, leukocytosis, and profuse diarrhea. The organism is quite hardy and is difficult to eradicate from the hospital environment. The hands of hospital personnel have been implicated as a mode of transmission of this organism, as have electronic rectal thermometers despite use of individual covering sheaths for each patient. The colon may become colonized with *C. difficile* while the patient is in the hospital, but particularly for patients still on antibiotics when sent home, diarrhea may not present until after discharge. Other infections to consider in the hospitalized patient include decubitus ulcers, particularly in patients on chronic care wards or confined to bed rest for prolonged periods, and sinusitis, especially in patients with nasotracheal tubes.

NONINFECTIOUS SOURCES OF FEVER   Several common noninfectious causes of fever in hospitalized patients also are part of a thorough evaluation of new fever. Drugs are the major noninfectious cause of fever. Drug fever may occur with or without an accompanying rash or eosinophilia and can be caused by new medication or by medications the patient has been receiving for some time. Particular agents associated with drug fever include phenytoin, H-2 blockers, procainamide, and antibiotics, most notably sulfonamides. Fevers, even drug-associated, can be quite high in some patients and may take up to 5 days to resolve after removal of the offending agent. Other noninfectious causes of fever include phlebitis, often at the site of an old intravenous line and sometimes followed by suppurative thrombophlebitis with clots or septic emboli, and pulmonary emboli, especially in patients on prolonged bed rest, although prophylactic heparin or mechanical boots often are used to reduce the risk of pulmonary embolism in these patients.

The range of possibilities for the etiology of a new fever in a hospitalized patient is quite broad. Attention to detail, a careful history and physical examination and knowledge of infections and organisms likely to cause nosocomial problems usually lead to an accurate diagnosis.

REFERENCES

HALEY RW et al: Identifying patients at high risk of surgical wound infection: A simple multivariate index of patient susceptibility and wound contamination. Am J Epidemiol 121:206, 1985

HOLTZ TH, WENZEL RP: Postdischarge surveillance for nosocomial wound infection: A brief review and commentary. Am J Infect Control 20:206, 1992

MARTONE WJ, GARNER JS (eds): Proceedings of the Third Decennial International Conference on Nosocomial Infections. Am J Med 91(suppl 3B), 1991

PLATT R et al: Epidemiology of nosocomial infections, in Infectious Diseases, SL Gorbach et al (eds). Philadelphia, Saunders, 1992, p 96

—— et al: Mortality associated with nosocomial urinary tract infection. N Engl J Med 307:637, 1982

WEBER DJ et al: Relative frequency of nosocomial pathogens at a university hospital during the decade 1980 to 1989. Am J Infect Control 20:192, 1992

98   INFECTION CONTROL IN THE HOSPITAL

ROBERT A. WEINSTEIN

The costs of nosocomial (hospital-acquired) infections are great, whether measured in dollars or in morbidity and mortality (see Chap. 97). Although infection control and hospital epidemiology activities have been the subjects of increasing scientific study over the past 20 years, efforts to lower infection risks have been continually challenged by the growing numbers of immunocompromised patients, of antibiotic-resistant bacteria, of fungal and viral superinfections, and of new invasive devices and procedures. Three international decennial conferences on infection control, organized by the Centers for Disease Control and Prevention (CDC), have clearly documented these formidable trends. This chapter reviews the basic surveillance and prevention activities that have been developed to deal with these problems and that form the foundation for current hospital epidemiology programs.

ORGANIZATION AND RESPONSIBILITIES OF INFECTION-CONTROL PROGRAMS The standards of the Joint Commission on Accreditation of Healthcare Organizations require all accredited hospitals to have an active program for surveillance, prevention, and control of nosocomial infections and a multidisciplinary infection control committee that meets not less than quarterly to oversee the program. The agents of the committee are the chairperson, preferably an infectious disease physician, and the infection control practioner(s), who are usually trained in nursing or medical technology and in epidemiology and public health.

In the 1970s, the CDC's extensive Study on the Efficacy of Nosocomial Infection Control found that hospitals that established programs with organized surveillance and control activities, a trained, effectual infection-control physician, and 1 infection-control practitioner per 250 beds experienced a 32 percent reduction in nosocomial infection rates, while rates in hospitals without effective programs increased by 18 percent. Since that study, however, the responsibilities and roles of hospital epidemiology programs have expanded in several ways. Diagnosis-related reimbursement has led hospital administrators to place increased emphasis on cost containment and on documenting that infection control is cost-effective. The quality-improvement movements and the Joint Commission's Agenda for Change have redirected infection-control attention, in part, beyond just writing policies and procedures to improving the actual processes and optimizing the outcomes. In a few hospitals, epidemiology programs have even taken on additional pharmacoepidemiologic and antibiotic utilization review reponsibilities. Finally, all programs must now respond to increasing governmental regulation of hospital waste and to Occupational Safety and Health Administration (OSHA)–mandated standards for protecting health care workers from occupational exposure to bloodborne pathogens and tuberculosis.

SURVEILLANCE Traditionally, infection-control practitioners survey inpatients for the occurrence of nosocomial infections (defined as those neither present nor incubating at the time of admission). Surveillance involves review of microbiology laboratory results, "shoe leather" epidemiology on the nursing wards, standardized definitions of infection, ongoing dialogue with hospital workers, and common sense. Some innovative infection-control programs have taken advantage of the increased use of computerized pharmacy, microbiology, and other data bases in hospitals to create algorithm-driven surveillance activities.

Because total hospital surveillance leaves little time for data analysis and education, most hospitals now aim surveillance at infections that have high morbidity (e.g., ICU-related infections and nosocomial pneumonia), are costly (e.g., cardiac surgery wound infections) or difficult to treat (e.g., those due to antibiotic-resistant bacteria), present recurring epidemic problems (e.g., Clostridium difficile–related diarrhea), and are potentially preventable (e.g., vascular access–related infections). Quality assurance activities in infection control have led to increased surveillance of personnel compliance with policies (e.g., monitoring actual use of universal precautions).

The results of surveillance are expressed as rates; e.g., 5 to 10 percent of patients develop nosocomial infections. Although such overall statistics are often requested of hospitals by administrators or surveyors, they have little value unless qualified by site of infection, by patient population, and by exposure to risk factors. Meaningful denominators for infection rates include the number of patients exposed to a specific risk (e.g., rates of pneumonia in patients on mechanical ventilators) and the number of intervention days (e.g., pneumonias per patient-days on a ventilator).

Temporal trends in rates should be reviewed, and ideally, rates should be compared with regional and national norms. However, even comparison rates generated by the CDC's ongoing National Nosocomial Infection Surveillance (NNIS) system, which collects data from over 100 hospitals that use standardized definitions of nosocomial infections, have not been validated independently and represent a nonrandom sample of hospitals. Interhospital comparisons are easily confounded by the wide range in risk factors and severity of underlying illnesses—unless rates are adjusted for these factors, comparisons may be misleading. Unfortunately, systems for making such adjustments either are rudimentary or have not been well validated.

The ongoing analysis of an individual hospital's infection rates helps to determine whether ongoing control efforts are succeeding and where increased education and control measures should be focused. Knowledge of infection rates also helps in discussions with the hospital administration regarding areas to which additional resources should be directed.

PREVENTION AND CONTROL MEASURES **Epidemiologic basis and general measures** Nosocomial infections follow basic epidemiologic patterns that help to direct prevention and control measures. Nosocomial pathogens have reservoirs, follow predictable modes of transmission, and require susceptible hosts. Reservoirs and sources exist in the inanimate environment (e.g., tap water contaminated with *Legionella*) and in the animate environment (e.g., infected or colonized health care workers, patients, and visitors). The modes of transmission most often are either cross-infection (e.g., indirect spread of pathogens from one patient to another on the inadequately washed hands of hospital personnel) or autoinoculation (e.g., aspiration of oropharyngeal flora into the lung along an endotracheal tube). Occasionally, pathogens (e.g., group A streptococci and many respiratory viruses) are spread indirectly from person-to-person by infectious droplets released by coughing or sneezing. Much less common, but often devastating in epidemic risk, is true airborne spread of droplet nuclei (e.g., as in nosocomial chickenpox) or common-source spread by contaminated materials (e.g., iodophors contaminated with *Pseudomonas*). Factors that increase host susceptibility include underlying conditions discussed elsewhere in this text and the many medical-surgical interventions and procedures that bypass normal host defenses.

The hospital's infection-control committee, through its infection control program, must determine the general and specific measures used to control infections and must review and recommend the specific antiseptics and disinfectants for hospital use. Given the prominence of cross-infection, handwashing is the single most important preventive measure in hospitals. There have been many studies of the antimicrobial activity of a large variety of antiseptic-containing handwashing agents. Such agents are important for handwashing before invasive procedures and possibly in intensive care unit (ICU) settings; however, given the poor general compliance with handwashing recommendations, the importance of handwashing with any hand cleanser between patient contacts cannot be overemphasized.

The fact that 25 to 50 percent of nosocomial infections are due to the combined effect of the patient's own flora and invasive devices highlights the importance of improvements in use and design of devices. Intensive educational programs can be associated with at least temporary reduction in infection rates through improved asepsis in handling and earlier removal of invasive devices, but sustaining such gains is often difficult. Nevertheless, it is encouraging to note that epidemiologic studies have been used increasingly to assess the value of newer devices and site-specific control measures, which are discussed below, and to debunk some traditional yet ineffective and costly measures, such as routine culturing of the environment and personnel for "pathogens."

Urinary tract infections Although urinary tract infections (UTIs) cause 40 to 45 percent of nosocomial infections, they contribute only 10 to 15 percent to prolongation of hospital stay and to extra costs. Almost all nosocomial UTIs are associated with preceding instrumentation or indwelling bladder catheters, which increase the risk of UTI by about 7 percent per day. As discussed in Chap. 97, UTI is caused by pathogens that spread up the periurethral space from the patient's perineum or gastrointestinal tract and by cross-infection via caregivers who are irrigating catheters or emptying drainage bags. Occasionally, pathogens come from inadequately disinfected urologic equipment and rarely from contaminated supplies (e.g., dilute aqueous benzalkonium chloride, an ineffective disinfectant).

Attempts at prevention have included the use of topical meatal antimicrobials, drainage bag disinfectants, antimicrobial-coated catheters, and sealed catheter–drainage tube junctions to eliminate inadvertent breaks in the system. Because of conflicting study results, none of these measures is considered routine. Systemic antimicrobials given for other purposes decrease the risk of UTI during the first 4 days of catheterization, after which resistant bacteria or yeasts emerge

as pathogens. Selective decontamination of the gut also is associated with a reduced risk; however, neither approach is routine. Moreover, irrigation of catheters, with or without antimicrobials, may actually increase the risk of infection.

Pneumonia Pneumonia causes 15 to 20 percent of nosocomial infections but is responsible for 24 percent of extra hospital days and 39 percent of extra costs. Almost all bacterial nosocomial pneumonias are caused by aspiration of endogenous or hospital-acquired oropharyngeal and gastric flora (viral pneumonias, which are particularly important in pediatric and immunocompromised patients, are discussed in Chaps. 96 and 220). Nosocomial pneumonia is associated with mortality rates up to 50 percent in ICUs; however, prevention of pneumonia often does not reduce overall ICU mortality, thereby suggesting that this infection is a marker for patients with otherwise heightened mortality risk. Surveillance and accurate diagnosis of pneumonia are often problematic because many ICU patients have abnormal chest roentgenograms, fever, and leukocytosis attributable to multiple causes.

Control measures are aimed at remediable risk factors in general patient care (e.g., minimizing supine aspiration-prone positioning and possibly avoiding prophylactic gastric alkalization because of increased risk of colonization with gram-negative rods when gastric pH is over 4) and at meticulous aseptic care of respirator equipment (e.g., disinfecting or sterilizing all in-line reusable components such as nebulizers, replacing tubing circuits at ≥48-h intervals rather than more frequently to lessen the number of breaks into the system, and teaching aseptic technique for suctioning). Two additional, more controversial issues have been the infection-control benefits of sucralfate, which provides stress ulcer prophylaxis without altering gastric pH, and of selective decontamination of the oropharynx and gut with nonabsorbable antimicrobials. Each approach warrants further investigation.

Surgical wound infections Wound infections cause approximately 25 to 30 percent of nosocomial infections but contribute up to 57 percent of extra hospital days and 42 percent of extra costs. They are usually caused by the patient's endogenous or hospital-acquired skin and mucosal flora and occasionally by airborne spread of skin squames that may be shed into the wound from members of the operating room team. True airborne spread of infection due to droplet nuclei is rare in operating rooms unless there is a "disseminator" (e.g., of group A streptococci or of staphylococci) among the staff. Because the average wound infection incubation period is 5 to 7 days, which is now longer than many postoperative stays, and because many procedures now are performed on an outpatient basis, over 50 percent of wound infections may not be detected unless postdischarge surveillance is performed.

The most important risk factors are the surgeon's judgment and operative technique, the patient's general health (e.g., presence of diabetes), and the specific operative procedure and its duration. The most important control measures include use of antimicrobial prophylaxis at the start of high-risk procedures, attention to technical surgical issues and operating room asepsis (e.g., not shaving the preoperative site until surgery and avoiding open or prophylactic drains), and preoperative therapy of any active infection. Reporting of surveillance results to surgeons also has been associated with reductions in infection rates. Interest in reporting results to surgeons, and the growing review of infection rates by regulatory agencies and payor sources, emphasizes the importance of stratifying rates by patient risk factors and of developing meaningful systems for interhospital comparisons.

Infections related to vascular access and monitoring Infection rates for peripheral intravenous (IV) catheters are very low (approximately 0.2 to 0.5 percent), but infections of central venous and arterial catheters are at least 20-fold more frequent, depending primarily on duration of use. Control measures include moving peripheral or arterial catheters to a new site at specified intervals (e.g., every 72 h for peripheral IVs), which may be facilitated by use of an IV team; using disposable transducers and aseptic technique when accessing transducers or other vascular ports; and removing "idle" catheters. Unresolved issues include the frequency for rotating central venous catheter sites (guidewire-assisted catheter changes at the same site do not lessen infection risk); the best antiseptics for site preparation and for catheter dressing; the appropriate role for mupirocin ointment, a topical antibiotic with excellent antistaphylococcal activity, for site care; whether newer designs—tunneled, totally implanted, or peripherally inserted central catheters (PICC lines)— offer a lessened infection risk than percutaneous central catheters; and the role of other costly catheter innovations, such as impregnating catheters with antimicrobials or attaching subcutaneous cuffs that contain bactericidal silver. In several studies, the use of semitransparent polyurethane dressings has increased infection rates, although these dressings have potential nursing benefits (ease of bathing and site inspection and protection of site from secretions).

Isolation techniques   Written policies for isolation of infectious patients are a standard component of infection-control programs. The CDC recommends that hospitals use either category-specific (based on suspected infection) or disease-specific (based on likely mode of transmission) isolation. The category-specific system includes *strict* (e.g., for chickenpox), *contact* (e.g., for staphylococcal wound infections), *respiratory* (e.g., for untreated bacterial meningitis), *acid-fast bacillus*, or AFB (for *M. tuberculosis* infection, which has specific ventilation requirements, described below), *isolation and enteric* (e.g., for bacterial diarrhea), and *drainage/secretion* (e.g., for minor wound infections) precautions. Some hospitals also use blood and body fluid precautions, although universal precautions have largely supplanted them. For each of the six category-specific modes, a door sign lists the necessary protective measures (e.g., gown, gloves, and mask for strict isolation). In the disease-specific system, the caregiver checks off the appropriate measures on a generic isolation sign, on the basis of an understanding of the patient's infection and its specific mode(s) of transmission.

In body substance isolation, the preceding systems are abandoned in favor of instructing personnel to wear gloves for contact with any body substance or mucous membrane. Other barriers, such as gowns, are required if soiling or splashing is anticipated. For patients with airborne pathogens such as tuberculosis, additional isolation precautions are required (see below).

In addition to these three alternative systems, all hospitals are mandated by OSHA to provide annual in-service training in and to monitor compliance with universal precautions to protect health care workers from bloodborne pathogens, including HIV and hepatitis B and C viruses. In essence, these precautions are similar to body substance isolation and require gloves, gown, mask, and/or eye protection depending on the likelihood of contact or splash with *any* blood or potentially contaminated body fluids. Some hospitals use additional guidelines for handling infected mothers and their newborns and antibiotic resistance precautions for patients colonized or infected with problematic strains.

EPIDEMIC PROBLEMS   Outbreaks are always big news but probably account for less than 5 percent of nosocomial infections. The investigation and control of epidemics in hospitals require that infection-control personnel develop a case definition, confirm that an outbreak really exists (since many apparent epidemics are actually pseudo-outbreaks due to surveillance or laboratory artifacts), review aseptic practices and disinfectant use, determine the extent of the outbreak, perform an epidemiologic investigation to determine modes of transmission, work closely with microbiology personnel to culture for common sources or personnel carriers as appropriate and to type epidemiologically important isolates, and heighten surveillance to judge the effect of control measures. Control measures generally include early reinforcement of routine aseptic practices while seeking compliance problems that may have fostered the outbreak, ensuring appropriate isolation of cases (and instituting cohort isolation and nursing if needed), and implementing further controls on the basis of the findings of the investigation. Examples of some potential epidemic problems follow.

Chickenpox   When health care workers are exposed to chickenpox in the community or by patients with initially unrecognized infections or work during the 24 h before developing chickenpox, infection-control practitioners institute a varicella exposure investigation and control plan, which includes obtaining names of exposed workers and patients, reviewing medical histories and (if needed) obtaining serologic tests for immunity, notifying physicians of susceptible exposed patients, administering prophylactic varicella-zoster immune globulin and/or instituting early acyclovir treatment where appropriate, and furloughing susceptible exposed employees during the at-risk period for disease. The varicella vaccine, if approved by the FDA, could be used to decrease risk for susceptible employees.

Tuberculosis   The resurgence of pulmonary tuberculosis in the United States since 1987 and a series of nosocomial outbreaks of multiply drug-resistant strains primarily involving patients with AIDS and caregivers have led to a reevaluation of tuberculosis control. Important control measures include prompt recognition, isolation, and treatment of cases; recognition of atypical presentations (e.g., lower-lobe infiltrates without cavitation); use of negative pressure, 100 percent exhaust, private isolation rooms with closed doors, and six air changes per hour; use of particulate respirator face masks by caregivers entering isolation rooms; possible use of HEPA (high-efficiency particulate arrest) filter units and/or ultraviolet lights for disinfecting air when other engineering controls are not feasible or reliable; and follow-up skin-testing of susceptible personnel who have been exposed to infectious patients before isolation.

Group A streptococci   The potential for a group A streptococcal outbreak should be suspected when even a single nosocomial case occurs. Most outbreaks involve surgical wounds and are due to the presence of an asymptomatic carrier in the operating room. Investigation can be confounded by extrapharyngeal sites of carriage, such as the rectum and vagina. Carriers who have been linked to nosocomial transmission of group A streptococci are removed from patient care and are not returned until carriage has been eliminated by antimicrobial therapy.

Aspergillus   *Aspergillus* spores are common in the environment, particularly on dusty surfaces. When hospital ceiling tiles are removed for access to electrical wiring or plumbing or when dusty areas are disturbed during hospital renovation, the spores become airborne. Inhalation of spores by immunosuppressed, particularly neutropenic, patients creates a risk of pulmonary and/or paranasal sinus infection and disseminated aspergillosis. Routine surveillance among neutropenic patients for infections with filamentous fungi, such as *Aspergillus* and *Fusarium*, helps hospitals to determine whether they have undue environmental loads. To lower the risk, hospitals should inspect and clean air-handling equipment on a routine schedule, review all planned hospital renovations with infection-control personnel and construct appropriate barriers, remove immunosuppressed patients from renovation sites, and consider use of HEPA filters for air supplied to rooms housing immunosuppressed patients.

Legionella   Sporadic and epidemic cases of nosocomial *Legionella* pneumonia are most often due to contaminated potable water or to contamination of air-handling systems and predominantly affect immunosuppressed patients, particularly those receiving glucocorticoid medication. The nosocomial risk varies greatly by geographic region and within an area depending on the extent of hospital hot-water contamination, on the presence of high-risk patient populations, and on specific hospital practices (e.g., use of nonsterile water in respiratory therapy equipment.) Laboratory-based surveillance for nosocomial *Legionella* should be performed, and a diagnosis of legionellosis should probably be considered more often than it is. If cases are detected, environmental cultures (e.g., hot-water tank sediment, faucets, and showerheads) should be obtained. If cultures grow *Legionella* and typing of clinical and environmental isolates correlate, eradication measures should be pursued (see Chap. 113).

An alternative approach is to periodically culture water tanks and water on wards housing high-risk patients. If *Legionella* is found, a concerted effort should be made to culture for *Legionella* in all patients with nosocomial pneumonia.

Antibiotic-resistant bacteria   Outbreaks of antibiotic resistance reflect Darwinian selection of bacterial chromosomal mutations, spread of plasmid- and/or transposon-borne resistance among bacterial species, and/or (re)admission of patients chronically infected with resistant bacteria—all further complicated by clonal dissemination of resistant strains by cross-infections and occasionally by personnel carriers and/or environmental contamination. Outbreak control depends on close laboratory surveillance to allow early detection of problems, on reinforcing routine asepsis (e.g., handwashing), on barrier precautions for all colonized and/or infected patients, on use of patient surveillance culture surveys to more fully ascertain extent of patient colonization, on use of antibiotic control policies, and on timely epidemiologic investigation when rates increase. Colonized personnel who are implicated in nosocomial transmission and problematic patients may be decontaminated; e.g., methicillin-resistant *Staphylococcus aureus* colonization may be controlled by use of oral antibiotics, such as trimethoprim-sulfamethoxazole and rifampin, and topical agents, including hexachloraphene or chlorhexidine and mupirocin. In a few ICUs, selective decontamination has been used successfully as an emergency control measure for outbreaks of infection due to gram-negative bacilli.

EMPLOYEE HEALTH SERVICE ISSUES   Employee health services (EHSs) are a critical component of infection control. New employees should be processed through the EHS where a contagious disease history can be taken; evidence of immunity to a variety of diseases, such as hepatitis B, chickenpox, measles, and rubella can be determined; immunizations for hepatitis B, measles, and rubella can be given as needed and a reminder about need for yearly influenza immunization can be imparted; a baseline PPD skin test can be performed; and education about personal responsibility for infection control can begin. Evaluations of employees should be codified to meet the requirements of accrediting and regulatory agencies; e.g., the CDC recommends at least annual PPD skin testing of susceptible caregivers, and OSHA requires that employees who have potential exposure to blood or blood-containing fluids must receive free hepatitis B vaccination or sign a specific declination form.

The EHS must have protocols for dealing with employees who have been exposed to contagious diseases. The newest problem is counseling, treating, and following personnel after percutaneous or mucosal exposure to blood of HIV-infected patients. Protocols are also needed for dealing with caregivers who have common contagious diseases, such as chickenpox, group A streptococcal infections, respiratory infections, and infectious diarrheas, and for caregivers who have less common but very high visibility public health problems, such as chronic hepatitis B or HIV—for which exposure-control guidelines have been published recently by the CDC.

REFERENCES

BENNETT JV, BRACHMAN PS (eds): *Hospital Infections*, 3d ed. Boston, Little, Brown, 1992

CENTERS FOR DISEASE CONTROL: Report of the Nosocomial Infections Surveillance (NNIS) System: Nosocomial infection rates for interhospital comparison: Limitations and possible solutions. Infect Control Hosp Epidemiol 12:609, 1991

HALEY RW et al: The efficacy of infection surveillance and control programs in preventing nosocomial infections in U.S. hospitals. Am J Epidemiol 121:182, 1985

MARTONE WJ, GARNER JS (eds): Proceedings of the Third Decennial International Conference on Nosocomial Infections. Am J Med 91(suppl 3B):1S, 1991

section 4   Bacterial disease: general considerations

99   MOLECULAR MECHANISMS OF BACTERIAL PATHOGENESIS

GERALD B. PIER

The past decade has seen an explosion of information about the bacterial and host molecules that contribute to the infectious and disease processes, which are thought by many to consist of three stages: (1) bacterial entry and colonization of the host; (2) bacterial invasion and growth in host tissues along with elaboration of toxic substances; and (3) the host response. These three stages reflect the more traditional concepts of *infection* (presence of bacteria in a host) and *disease* (reaction to the infection)—terms that are often used interchangeably. Bacterial pathogenesis is the measure of an organism's capacity to cause disease and is a function of the myriad pathogenic or virulence factors elaborated by bacteria. These virulence factors may be classified in two groups: those that promote bacterial colonization and infection (usually surface molecules) and those that cause disease (often, but not exclusively, secreted toxins or toxic metabolites). In addition, the host's inflammatory response to infection can contribute greatly to the observed disease and its attendant clinical signs and symptoms. Knowledge of the molecular architecture of the bacterial surface (Fig. 99-1), its interaction with the host, and the host response are critical to an understanding of the basic process of infection and disease.

CELL WALL STRUCTURE OF GRAM-POSITIVE AND GRAM-NEGATIVE BACTERIA

GRAM-POSITIVE BACTERIA   Gram-positive bacteria have a typical lipid bilayer cytoplasmic membrane surrounded by a rigid cell wall that gives the organisms their characteristic shape, differentiates them from eukaryotic cells, and allows them to survive in osmotically unfavorable environments. The cell wall is composed mainly of peptidoglycan, a polymer of *N*-acetylglucosamine and its lactyl ether, *N*-acetylmuramic acid, with peptide side chains covalently bound to the lactyl group. The peptide chains consist of alternating D and L amino acids and are usually linked to each other by a pentaglycine bridge binding a terminal D-alanine on one peptide substituent to the penultimate L-lysine on a neighboring peptide. Variations in this basic structure have been described for a number of bacterial genera.

In addition, the cell walls of gram-positive bacteria contain teichoic acids, phosphate-linked polymers of ribitol or glycerol that can have additional compounds linked to available side groups. Lipid tails anchor these acids to the cytoplasmic membrane, giving rise to lipoteichoic acids. Some organisms have cell wall teichoic acids wherein the glycerol or ribitol phosphate polymer is directly linked to *N*-acetylmuramic acid in the peptidoglycan. The various substituents on teichoic acids are often responsible for the biologic and immunologic properties associated with disease due to pathogenic gram-positive bacteria.

Most pathogenic gram-positive bacteria have additional extracellular structures. These include surface polysaccharides (such as the

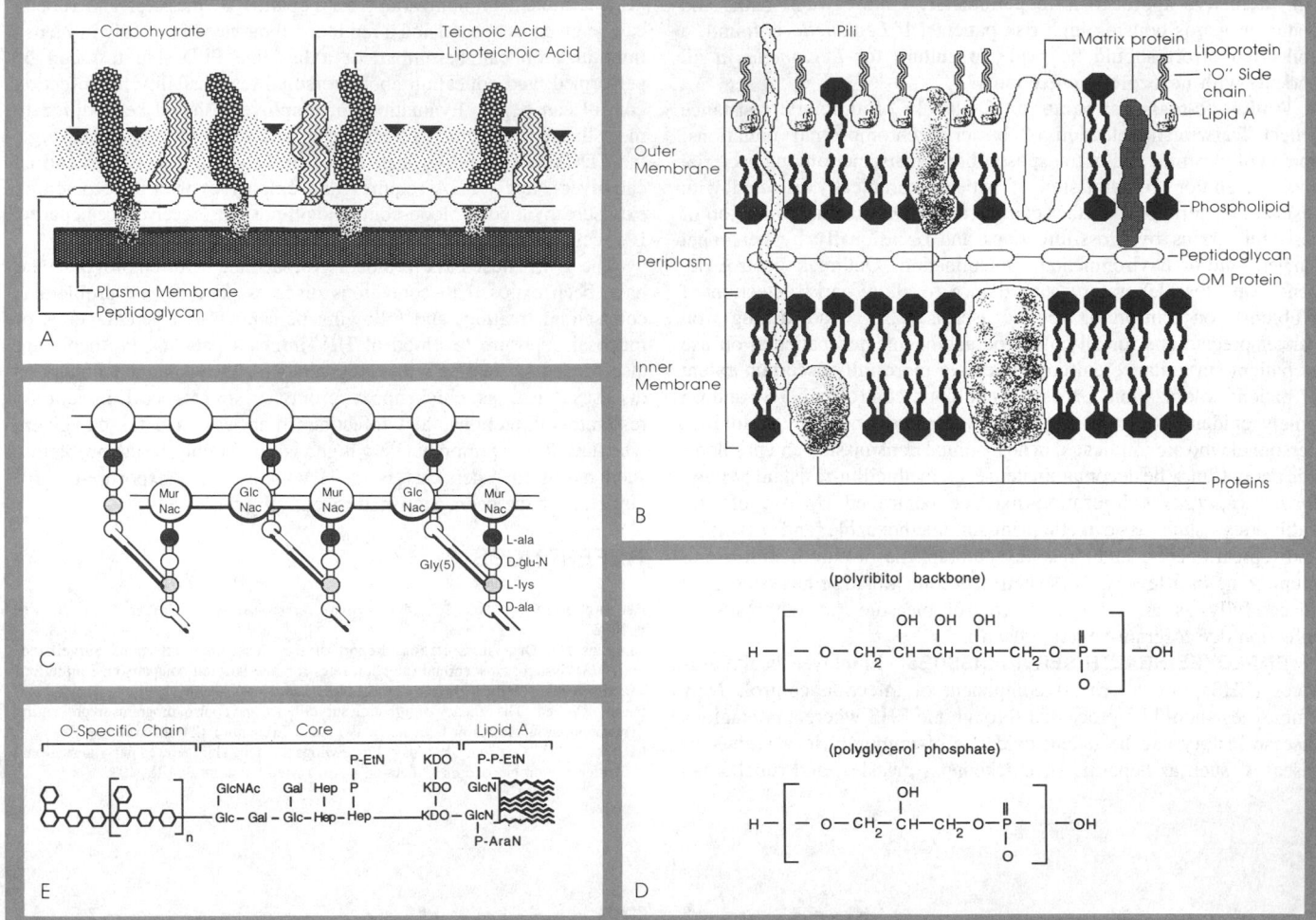

FIGURE 99-1 Schematic representations of bacterial surface structures. *A.* Cytoplasmic membrane and cell wall typical of gram-positive bacteria. *B.* Outer structure of a gram-negative organism (*OM* = outer membrane). *C.* Detailed structure of peptidoglycan showing backbone of *N*-acetylmuramic acid (*MurNac*) and *N*-acetylglucosamine (*GlcNac*); tetrapeptide bridges composed of L-alanine (L-*ala*), D-glutamate (D-*Glu-N*), L-lysine (L-*Lys*), and D-alanine (D-*ala*); and pentaglycine [*Gly(5)*] cross-bridges. *D.* Teichoic acid backbone. *E.* Detailed structure of lipopolysaccharide typical of *Salmonella* spp., including the lipid A sugars glucosamine (*GlcN*) and 4-amino arabinose (*AraN*) and the core sugars 2-keto-3-deoxyoctonate (*KDO*), heptose (*Hep*), glucose (*Glc*), galactose (*Gal*), and *N*-acetylglucosamine (*GlcNAc*). Hexagons depicting the O-specific chain represent variable monosaccharide residues that comprise this structure. (*Drawing courtesy of T.J. DiCesare.*)

group antigens of streptococci), capsular polysaccharides, and surface proteins and polypeptide capsules needed for survival in blood or useful for epidemiologic classification.

GRAM-NEGATIVE BACTERIA In addition to having a cytoplasmic membrane and a peptidoglycan layer similar to but reduced from that found in gram-positive organisms, gram-negative bacteria are characterized by an outer membrane that is covalently linked to the tetrapeptides of the peptidoglycan layer by a lipoprotein; this protein also contains a special lipid substituent on the terminal cysteine that embeds the lipoprotein in the outer membrane. The outer layer of the outer membrane contains the lipopolysaccharide (LPS) constituent, and embedded in this membrane are special proteins with important functions, including maintaining the outer membrane's integrity, acting as a selective barrier for diffusion of molecules into the cell, serving as receptors for bacteriophages, and binding siderophores that scavenge iron for transport into the bacterial cell.

Lipopolysaccharide The LPS is made up of a relatively conserved di-*N*-acetylglucosamine backbone linked β 1→6, containing phosphate groups on the reducing 1 and nonreducing 4′ carbons. The hydroxyl and amino groups on carbons 2, 3, 2′, and 3′ are esterified with 2-hydroxy fatty acids of varying length, and these fatty acids also can be derivatized on their 2-hydroxy residue with additional fatty acids. This structure is termed *lipid A* and likely possesses most

of the important biologic properties associated with LPS or endotoxin. Attached to carbon 6′ is the inner polysaccharide core, which is usually, but not always, composed of a di- or trisaccharide of 2-keto-3-deoxyoctonate (KDO). Some pathogens, such as *Vibrio cholerae*, do not use KDO here. Additional sugar substituents are linked to the inner core, forming a complete core that is somewhat conserved among related gram-negative pathogens. Attached to the complete core are the O polysaccharide side chains, which, when present, confer serologic variability on different strains within a species and provide protection for the cell against host proteins such as lytic complement components. O polysaccharides can be composed of a variety of monosaccharides, ranging from the common pentoses and hexoses to more complex and often unique structures such as pseudaminic acid (5,7- diamino-3,5,7,9-tetradeoxynonulosonic acid), which is found in LPS from some strains of *Pseudomonas aeruginosa* and *Shigella boydii* type 7. These sugars can be substituted by a variety of components, such as formyl, acetyl, and hydroxy-butyryl side chains; amino acids or peptides; and phosphate groups. This high level of chemical variability is thought to be key to bacterial pathogenesis in that it allows various strains of pathogenic organisms to avoid host defenses.

Pili Pili or fimbriae extend through the outer membrane into the external environment. They are seen in electron micrographs as hairlike projections that may be confined to either one of the organism (polar pili) or distributed more evenly over the surface, with up to several hundred per cell. An individual cell may make multiple pili with different functions. Most pili comprise a major pilin protein subunit with a molecular weight of 17,000 to 30,000 that polymerizes to form the pilus. Some pili, such as the gal-gal binding pili of *Escherichia coli*, have additional proteins located at their tips that are functionally critical. The major function attributed to pili to date is mediation of the binding of bacteria to host tissues.

Flagella   Flagella are long appendages attached to either one or both ends of the bacterial cell (polar flagella) or distributed over the entire cell surface (peritrichous flagella). Flagella, like pili, are composed of a polymerized or aggregated basic protein. In flagella, the protein subunits form a tight helical structure and show serologic variability among different species. Spirochetes such as *Treponema pallidum* and *Borrelia burgdorferi* have axial filaments similar to flagella running down the long axis of the center of the cell and swim by rotation around these filaments. Some bacteria can glide over a surface in the absence of obvious motility structures.

INITIAL STAGE OF BACTERIAL INFECTION: COLONIZATION OF HOST SURFACES

Most bacterial pathogens initially enter the host through a mucosal surface of the respiratory, ocular, gastrointestinal, or genitourinary tract. The skin can be an important site of bacterial colonization (particularly for staphylococci), and direct inoculation of pathogens into the host is always a risk factor for subsequent disease. Successful colonization usually requires bacterial adherence to the mucosal surface. The ability to adhere is most often attributed to the pili, capsular polysaccharides, and lipoteichoic acids exposed on the cell surface, although any surface structure is capable of mediating adherence to host tissues. Host targets for bacterial adherence are either the epithelial cells lining mucosal tracts or the mucous layer itself. In the latter case, the bacteria must circumvent the host's normal ability to clear mucus-embedded cells. Such circumvention is thought to occur in states like ciliary dyskinesia in the respiratory tract or chronic *P. aeruginosa* colonization of the respiratory tract of individuals with cystic fibrosis.

It now appears that an individual bacterial cell expresses multiple, often serologically variable adhesins and that the cell uses different adhesins during different stages of colonization. For example, most strains of *E. coli* express type 1 pili, whose binding to host tissues is inhibited by D-mannose. These pili appear to help these organisms bind to mucus. Strains of *E. coli* causing pyelonephritis express a different adhesin, the Pap or P pilus, that mediates binding to digalactose residues on globosides of the human P blood groups. Adherence here is due to minor components of the pilus proteins that are found only on the tip. *E. coli* cells causing diarrheal disease express receptors for enterocytes on the small bowel, along with other receptors termed *colonization factors*.

A common type of pilus found in *Neisseria* spp., *Moraxella* spp., *V. cholerae*, and *P. aeruginosa* appears to be involved in adherence of these organisms to target surfaces. These pili tend to have a relatively conserved amino-terminal region and a more variable carboxy-terminal region. For some species such as *N. gonorrhoeae* and *N. meningitidis*, the pili are critical for attachment to mucosal epithelial cells. For others, such as *P. aeruginosa*, the pili mediate only some of the epithelial cell adherence. *V. cholerae* cells appear to use two different types of pili for intestinal colonization. While interference with this stage of colonization would appear to be an effective antibacterial strategy, attempts to develop pilus-based vaccines for human diseases have not been highly successful to date. In some instances, diarrhea due to *E. coli* in pigs, calves, and lambs has been prevented by pilus immunization, but a recent trial of a gonococcal pilus vaccine in humans failed to demonstrate efficacy. The serologic variability among pili is one barrier to this approach.

Other bacterial structures involved in adherence to host tissues include specific proteins found among staphylococci that bind to human proteins such as fibrin, fibronectin, laminin, and collagen. These bacterial structures probably promote the normal colonization of the nares and skin. Fibronectin appears to be a commonly used receptor for various pathogens; a particular sequence, Arg-Gly-Asp or RGD, is critical to binding. Surface lipoteichoic acids promote adherence of streptococci to mucosal surfaces. The mucoid exopolysaccharide or alginate capsule of *P. aeruginosa* promotes binding of mucoid strains to respiratory mucins. Coagulase-negative staphylococci have emerged as important pathogens through their ability to colonize prosthetic devices and catheters commonly used in medical care; the surface capsular polysaccharide of these organisms promotes binding to the prosthetic material.

TISSUE INVASION AND TISSUE TROPISM

TISSUE INVASION   Bacteria may invade deeper layers of mucosal tissue via intracellular uptake by epithelial cells or via traversal of epithelial cell junctions. Among virulent *Shigella* strains and invasive *E. coli*, outer membrane proteins are critical to epithelial cell invasion and bacterial multiplication. *Neisseria* and *Haemophilus* penetrate mucosal cells by poorly understood mechanisms before dissemination into the bloodstream. Staphylococci and streptococci elaborate a variety of extracellular enzymes, such as hyaluronidase, lipases, nucleases, and hemolysins, that are probably important in breaking down cellular and matrix structures and allowing the bacteria access to deeper tissues and blood. Organisms that colonize the gastrointestinal tract can often translocate through the mucosa into the blood and, under circumstances in which host defenses are inadequate, cause bacteremia. *Yersinia enterocolitica* can invade the mucosa through the activity of the invasin protein. Some bacteria (e.g., *Brucella*) can be carried from a mucosal site to a disant site by phagocytic cells (e.g., polymorphonulcear leukocytes, or PMNs) that ingest but fail to kill the bacteria.

A number of major pathogens cause disease without further invasion of host tissues; these include *Bordetella pertussis*, *V. cholerae*, *Clostridium tetani*, *Clostridium botulinum*, *Corynebacterium diphtheriae*, *Mycobacterium tuberculosis*, and *Mycobacterium leprae*. Some pathogens can cause both local disease (such as pharyngitis and epiglottitis, skin ulcerations, or diarrhea) and disease due to tissue invasion. Some pathogens require a breach in host tissues to cause deeper infections; an example of this situation is peritonitis due to *Bacteroides fragilis* or other intestinal organisms after bursting of the appendix or intestinal trauma. In such cases, bacterial factors are not critical for invasion.

TISSUE TROPISM   The propensity of certain bacteria to cause disease by infecting specific tissues has been known since the early days of bacteriology, yet the molecular basis for this propensity is much less well understood than is viral tissue tropism. By analogy, receptor-ligand interactions may be expected to underlie bacterial tissue tropism, and some good evidence from studies of gastrointestinal infection supports this possibility. However, there is no well-accepted explanation of why *N. gonorrhoeae* colonizes and infects the human genital tract, while the closely related species *N. meningitidis* principally colonizes the human oropharynx. *N. meningitidis* expresses a capsular polysaccharide, while *N. gonorrhoeae* does not; however, there is no indication that this property plays a role in the different tissue tropisms displayed by these two bacterial species. *N. gonorrhoeae* can use the enzyme sialytransferase from host tissues to add *N*-acetyl neuraminic acid (sialic acid) to its LPS O side chain, and this alteration appears to make the organism resistant to host defenses. Whether this enzyme is present in a special form or amount in the genital tract of humans is not known. Bacteria with sialic acid sugars in their capsules, such as *N. meningitidis*, *E. coli* K1, and group B streptococci, have a propensity to cause meningitis, but this generalization has many exceptions. For example, all six recognized serotypes of group B streptococci contain sialic acid in their capsules, but only one of these serotypes (type III) is responsible for most cases of meningitis due to infection by these organisms. In addition, both *H. influenzae* and the pneumococcus can readily cause meningitis, and these organisms do not have sialic acid in their capsules.

DISEASE

Disease is a complex phenomenon resulting from bacterial colonization, invasion, toxin elaboration, and host response. Toxin elaboration is one of the best-characterized molecular mechanisms of bacterial pathogenesis, while host factors such as interleukin 1 (IL-1) and IL-6, tumor necrosis factor α (TNFα), kinins, inflammatory proteins and products of complement activation, and mediators derived from arachidonic acid metabolites (leukotrienes) and cellular degranulation (histamines) readily contribute to the severity of disease.

TOXINS Among the first diseases emanating from bacterial infection to be understood were those due to toxin-elaborating organisms. Diphtheria, botulism, and tetanus toxins are responsible for the disease associated with local infections due to *C. diphtheriae*, *C. botulinum*, and *C. tetani*, respectively. Enterotoxins produced by *E. coli*, *Salmonella*, *Shigella*, *Staphylococcus*, and *V. cholerae* contribute to diarrheal disease caused by these organisms. Staphylococci, streptococci, *P. aeruginosa*, and *Bordetella* elaborate a variety of toxins that cause or contribute to disease, including toxic shock syndrome toxin 1 (TSST-1), erythrogenic toxin, exotoxin A, and pertussis toxin. A number of these toxins (e.g., cholera toxin, diphtheria toxin, pertussis toxin, *E. coli* heat-labile toxin, and *P. aeruginosa* exotoxin) have adenosine diphosphate (ADP)–ribosyltransferase activity, wherein the toxins enzymatically catalyze the transfer of the ADP-ribosyl portion of nicotinamide adenine diphosphate to target proteins and inactivate them. The staphylococcal enterotoxins, TSST-1, and streptococcal pyogenic exotoxins have been shown recently to behave as "superantigens," stimulating certain T cells to proliferate without processing of the protein toxin by antigen-presenting cells. Part of this process involves stimulation of the antigen-presenting cells to produce IL-1 and TNFα, which have been implicated in many of the clinical features of diseases such as toxic shock syndrome and scarlet fever.

ENDOTOXIN The lipid A portion of gram-negative LPS has potent biologic activities that are thought to cause many of the clinical features seen in gram-negative bacterial sepsis. These include fever, muscle proteolysis, uncontrolled intravascular coagulation, and shock. This effect appears to be mediated by production from mononuclear cells of IL-1, TNFα, and perhaps IL-6. These molecules exhibit potent hypothermic activity via effects in the hypothalamus, increase vascular permeability, alter the activity of endothelial cells, and induce these cells to procoagulant activity. Numerous therapeutic strategies aimed at neutralizing the effects of endotoxin are under study, including the use of antibodies to lipid A and to TNF and the administration of the IL-1 receptor antagonist (IL-1RA), which blocks the binding of IL-1 to its cellular receptor. Unfortunately, the clinical trial of one human monoclonal antibody to endotoxin, HA-1A, was halted in January 1993 because of excess mortality in the treated group, and disappointing results with the IL-1RA clinical trial reported in February 1993 have raised some doubts about the efficacy of this drug. Whether future clinical trials of these reagents will show efficacy is unclear at this time.

BACTERIAL INVASION Some diseases are likely caused primarily by the presence of bacteria in tissue sites that are normally sterile. Invasion of the bloodstream by gram-negative rods gives rise to sepsis and bacteremia without obvious exotoxin involvement, although endotoxin is very important in this situation. Pneumococcal pneumonia is mostly attributed to the growth of *Streptococcus pneumoniae* in the lung and the attendant host inflammatory response; there is little evidence that bacterial toxins are important in this disease. Disease following bacteremia and invasion of the meninges by meningitis-producing bacteria such as *N. meningitidis*, *H. influenzae*, *E. coli*

K1, and group B streptococci appears to be due solely to the ability of these organisms to get into these tissues and multiply. Most of the tissue destruction here results from bacterial growth and host inflammation.

If organisms are to effectively invade host tissues (particularly the blood), they must avoid the major host defenses of complement and phagocytic cells. This avoidance is most often accomplished through the presence of cell surface polysaccharides—either capsular polysaccharides or long O side chain antigens characteristic of the smooth LPS of gram-negative bacteria. These molecules appear to function by preventing activation and/or deposition of complement opsonins or by limiting access of phagocytic cells with receptors for complement opsonins to these molecules when they are deposited on the bacterial surface below the capsular layer. Another potential mechanism of microbial virulence is the ability of some organisms to present the capsule as an apparent self-antigen via molecular mimicry. For example, the polysialic acid capsule of group B *N. meningitidis* is chemically identical to an oligosaccharide found on human brain cells. The M proteins of group A streptococci appear to convey resistance to phagocytic activity in blood. Some bacteria such as *Brucella*, *Yersinia*, *Listeria*, *Francisella*, and *Mycobacterium* resist destruction inside phagocytic cells. Even in the absence of an obvious bacteremic phase, such as that seen in shigellosis, production of a smooth LPS is critical for bacterial pathogenesis and disease.

Immunochemical studies of capsular polysaccharides have led to an appreciation of the tremendous chemical diversity that can result from the linking of a few monosaccharides. For example, three different hexoses can link up in more than 300 different, potentially serologically distinct ways, while three different amino acids have only six different possible peptide combinations. This immunochemical diversity may be the reason why many pathogenic bacteria use capsular polysaccharides to avoid host defenses. Capsular polysaccharides have been employed as effective vaccines against meningococcal meningitis as well as pneumococcal and *H. influenzae* infections and are currently under development as vaccines against infections due to group B streptococci, *P. aeruginosa*, *Klebsiella*, *S. aureus*, and *S. epidermidis*. In fact, capsular polysaccharides can function as a vaccine against any organism expressing a nontoxic, immunogenic capsular polysaccharide. In addition, most encapsulated pathogens become virtually avirulent when capsule production is interrupted via genetic manipulation; this observation emphasizes the importance of this structure in bacterial pathogenesis. Some encapsulated bacteria may alter their expression of capsular antigens during pathogenesis, producing a capsule when avoiding host defenses (such as during bloodstream dissemination) but not when adhering to and invading an epithelial cell during mucosal colonization.

HOST RESPONSE The inflammatory response of the host is critical for interruption and resolution of the infectious process but also is often responsible for the signs and symptoms of disease. Bacterial infection promotes a complex series of host responses involving the complement, kinin, and coagulation pathways. Most likely, the initial recognition of a foreign pathogen involves the activation of complement, and the generation of molecules such as C3a and C5a initiate inflammation. Consequently, changes take place in endothelial membranes; receptors for inflammatory cells are produced on the luminal side of the blood vessel, causing these cells to adhere to the endothelium and migrate through the vessel wall to the site of infection. The subsequent production of factors such as IL-1, IL-6, and TNF leads to fever, muscle proteolysis, and other effects noted above. An inability to kill or contain the microbe usually results in further damage due to the progression of inflammation and infection. For example, in many chronic infections, degranulation of host inflammatory cells can lead to release of host proteases, elastases, histamines, and other toxic substances that can degrade host tissues. Chronic inflammation in any tissue will eventually lead to the destruction of that tissue and to clinical disease associated with loss of organ function, such as sterility from pelvic inflammatory disease caused by chronic infection with *N. gonorrhoeae*.

The nature of the host response is often a critical factor in the type of pathology associated with a particular infection. Most bacterial pathogens provoke either local or systemic inflammation or the formation of a granuloma or an abscess. Local inflammation, as noted above, produces local tissue damage, while systemic inflammation, such as that seen during sepsis, can result in the signs and symptoms of septic shock. The latter can occur with either gram-negative or gram-positive infections, and its severity is associated with the degree of production of host effectors such as IL-1 and TNFα. Disease due to intracellular parasitism arising from infection with bacteria that cause tuberculosis, leprosy, or brucellosis results from the formation of granulomas, wherein the host attempts to wall off the parasite inside a fibrotic lesion surrounded by fused epithelial cells that make up so-called multinucleated giant cells. A number of pathogens, particularly anaerobic bacteria, staphylococci, and streptococci, provoke the formation of an abscess. It has been suggested that a network of T cells is involved in abscess formation following inoculation of *B. fragilis* into the peritoneum of experimental animals to mimic human peritonitis. IL-8 may play a role in recruiting and activating PMNs during abscess formation. The outcome of a bacterial infection will depend on the balance between an effective host response that eliminates a pathogen and an excessive inflammatory response that is associated with an inability to eliminate a pathogen and with the resultant tissue damage that leads to disease.

REFERENCES

BITTERSUERMANN D: Influence of bacterial polysialic capsules on host defense: Masquerade and mimicry, in *Polysialic Acid,* J Roth et al (eds). Basel, Birkhauser-Verlag, 1993, p 11

BOSLEGO JW et al: Efficacy trial of a parenteral gonococcal pilus vaccine in men. Vaccine 9:154, 1991

CRABB JH et al: T cell regulation of *Bacteroides fragilis*–induced intraabdominal abscesses. Rev Infect Dis 12:S178, 1990

DAVIS BD: Bacterial architecture, in *Microbiology,* BD Davis et al (eds). Philadelphia, Lippincott, 1990, p 21

DENICH K et al: Frequency and organization of *papA* homologous DNA sequences among uropathogenic digalactoside-binding *Escherichia coli* strains. Infect Immun 59:2089, 1991

DINARELLO CA, THOMPSON RC: Blocking IL-1: Interleukin-1 receptor antagonist in vivo and in vitro. Immunol Today 12:404, 1991

GREENMAN RL et al: A controlled clinical trial of E5 murine monoclonal IgM antibody to endotoxin in the treatment of gram negative sepsis. JAMA 266:1097, 1991

ISBERG RR: Discrimination between intracellular uptake and surface adhesion of bacterial pathogens. Science 252:934, 1991

MARRACK P, KAPPLER J: The staphylococcal enterotoxins and their relatives. Science 248:705, 1990

MEKALANOS JJ: Environmental signals controlling expression of virulence determinants in bacteria. J Bacteriol 174:1, 1992

PIER GB et al: Complement deposition by antibodies to *Pseudomonas aeruginosa* mucoid exopolysaccharide (MEP) and by non-MEP specific opsonins. J Immunol 147:1869, 1991

ZIEGLER EJ et al: Treatment of gram-negative bacteremia and septic shock with HA-1A human monoclonal antibody against endotoxin: A randomized, double-blind, placebo-controlled trial. N Engl J Med 324:429, 1991

100   TREATMENT AND PROPHYLAXIS OF BACTERIAL INFECTIONS

GORDON L. ARCHER / RONALD E. POLK

The discovery and development of drugs able to prevent and cure bacterial infections have represented one of this century's major contributions toward improving human longevity and quality of life. Antibacterial agents are among the most commonly prescribed drugs of any kind worldwide. Used properly and appropriately, these drugs are lifesaving. However, their indiscriminate use drives up the cost of health care, leads to a plethora of side effects and drug interactions, and fosters the emergence of bacterial resistance, rendering valuable

drugs useless. The rational use of antibacterial agents is dependent on an understanding of their mechanisms of action; their pharmacokinetics, toxicities, and interactions; bacterial strategies for resistance; and testing in vitro for susceptibility of bacteria to antibacterial activity. In addition, patient-associated parameters, such as the site of infection and both the immune and the excretory status of the host, are critically important to appropriate therapeutic decisions.

This chapter provides specific data required for making an informed choice of antibacterial agent. Throughout the chapter the term *antibacterial agent* is used to refer to all natural, synthetic, and semisynthetic compounds that kill bacteria or inhibit their growth. The term *antibiotic* is reserved for those compounds produced by living organisms.

MECHANISMS OF ACTION

Antibacterial agents, like all antimicrobial drugs, are directed against unique targets not present in mammalian cells. The goal is to limit toxicity to the host and maximize chemotherapeutic activity affecting invading microbes only. The mechanisms of action of the antibacterial agents to be discussed in this section are summarized in Table 100-1.

INHIBITION OF CELL WALL SYNTHESIS   One major difference between bacterial and mammalian cells is the presence in bacteria of a rigid wall external to the cell membrane. The wall protects bacterial cells from osmotic rupture because of the difference between the markedly hyperosmolar (up to 20 atm) cell interior and the usually isosmolar or hyposmolar host environment. The structure conferring cell wall rigidity and resistance to osmotic lysis in both gram-positive and gram-negative bacteria is peptidoglycan, a large, covalently linked sacculus that surrounds the bacterium. In gram-positive bacteria, peptidoglycan is the only layer external to the cell membrane and is large (20 to 80 nm); in gram-negative bacteria, there is an outer membrane external to a very thin (1-nm) peptidoglycan layer.

Chemotherapeutic agents directed at any stage of the synthesis, export, assembly, or cross-linking of peptidoglycan lead to inhibition of bacterial cell growth and, in most cases, to cell death. Peptidoglycan is composed of a backbone of two alternating sugars, *N*-acetylglucosamine and *N*-acetylmuramic acid; a chain of four amino acids that extend down from the backbone (stem peptides); and a peptide bridge that cross-links the peptide chains. Peptidoglycan is formed by the addition of subunits (a sugar with its five attached amino acids) that are assembled in the cytoplasm and transported through the cytoplasmic membrane to the cell surface. Subsequent cross-linking is driven by cleavage of the terminal stem peptide amino acid. Antibacterial agents act to inhibit cell wall synthesis in the following ways.

Bacitracin, a cyclic peptide antibiotic, inhibits the conversion to its active form of the lipid carrier that moves the water-soluble cytoplasmic peptidoglycan subunits through the cell membrane to the cell exterior. Cell wall subunits accumulate in the cytoplasm and cannot be added to the growing peptidoglycan chain.

Glycopeptides (vancomycin and teichoplanin) are high-molecular-weight antibiotics that bind to the terminal D-alanine–D-alanine component of the stem peptide when the subunits are external to the cell membrane and still linked to the lipid carrier. This binding sterically inhibits the addition of subunits to the peptidoglycan backbone.

β-Lactam antibiotics (penicillins, cephalosporins, carbapenems, and monobactams; see Table 100-2), characterized by a four-membered β-lactam ring, prevent the cross-linking reaction called *transpeptidation.* Energy for attaching a peptide cross-bridge from the stem peptide of one peptidoglycan subunit to another is derived from the cleavage of a terminal D-alanine residue from the subunit stem peptide. The cross-bridge amino acid is then attached to the penultimate D-alanine by transpeptidase enzymes. The β-lactam ring of the antibiotic forms an irreversible covalent acyl bond with the

TABLE 100-1 Mechanisms of action and resistance for major classes of antibacterial agents

Antibacterial agent*	Major cellular target	Mechanism of action	Major mechanisms of resistance
β-Lactams (penicillins and cephalosporins)	Cell wall	Inhibits cell wall cross-linking	1 Drug inactivation (β-lactamase) 2 Insensitive target (altered penicillin-binding protein) 3 Decreased permeability (altered gram-negative outer-membrane porins)
Vancomycin	Cell wall	Interferes with the addition of new cell wall subunits (muramyl pentapeptides)	Alteration of target (substitution of terminal amino acid of peptidoglycan subunit)
Bacitracin	Cell wall	Prevents addition of cell wall subunits by inhibiting recycling of membrane lipid carrier	Not defined
Macrolides (erythromycin)	Protein synthesis	Binds to 50 S ribosomal subunit	Alteration of target (ribosomal methylation)
Lincosamides (clindamycin)	Protein synthesis	Binds to 50 S ribosomal subunit	Alteration of target (ribosomal methylation)
Chloramphenicol	Protein synthesis	Binds to 50 S ribosomal subunit	Drug inactivation (chloramphenicol acetyltransferase)
Tetracycline	Protein synthesis	Binds to 30 S ribosomal subunit	1 Decreased intracellular drug accumulation (active efflux) 2 Insensitive target
Aminoglycosides (gentamicin)	Protein synthesis	Binds to 30 S ribosomal subunit	Drug inactivation (aminoglycoside-modifying enzyme)
Mupirocin	Protein synthesis	Inhibits isoleucine t-RNA synthetase	Insensitive target (mutation of target gene or acquisition of gene for new, insensitive enzyme)
Sulfonamides and trimethoprim	Cell metabolism	Competitively inhibits enzymes involved in two steps of folic acid biosynthesis	Production of insensitive targets [dihydropteroic acid (sulfonamides) and dihydrofolic acid (trimethoprim)] that bypass metabolic block
Rifampin	DNA synthesis	Inhibits DNA-dependent RNA polymerase	Insensitive target (mutation of polymerase gene)
Metronidazole	DNA synthesis	Intracellularly generates short-lived reactive intermediates by electron transfer system	Not defined
Quinolones (ciprofloxacin)	DNA synthesis	Inhibition of DNA gyrase (A subunit)	1 Insensitive target (mutation of gyrase genes) 2 Decreased intracellular accumulation (active efflux)
Novobiocin	DNA synthesis	Inhibition of DNA gyrase (B subunit)	Not defined
Polymixins (polymyxin B)	Cell membrane	Disrupts membrane permeability by charge alteration	Not defined
Gramicidin	Cell membrane	Forms pores	Not defined

* Compounds in parentheses are major representatives for the class.

transpeptidase enzyme (probably because of the antibiotic's steric similarity to the enzyme's D-alanine–D-alanine target), preventing the cross-linking reaction. Transpeptidases and similar enzymes involved in cross-linking are called *penicillin-binding proteins* (PBPs) because they all have active sites that bind β-lactam antibiotics.

Virtually all the antibiotics that inhibit bacterial cell wall synthesis are bactericidal. That is, they eventually result in the cell's death due to osmotic lysis. However, much of the loss of cell wall integrity following treatment with cell wall–active agents is due to the bacteria's own cell wall–remodeling enzymes (autolysins) that cleave peptidoglycan bonds in the normal course of cell growth. In the presence of antibacterial agents that inhibit cell wall growth, autolysis proceeds without normal cell wall repair; weakness and eventual cellular lysis occur.

TABLE 100-2 β-Lactam antibiotics

Class	Route of administration	
	Parenteral	Oral
Penicillins		
β-Lactamase susceptible		
Narrow spectrum	Penicillin G	Penicillin V
Enteric active	Ampicillin	Amoxicillin, ampicillin
Enteric active and antipseudomonal	Carbenicillin, ticarcillin, mezlocillin, azlocillin, piperacillin	Indanyl carbenicillin
β-Lactamase resistant		
Antistaphylococcal	Methicillin, oxacillin, nafcillin	Cloxacillin, dicloxacillin
Combinations with β-lactamase inhibitors	Ticarcillin plus clavulanic acid, ampicillin plus sulbactam	Amoxicillin plus clavulanic acid
Cephalosporins		
First generation	Cefazolin, cephalothin, cephapirin	Cephalexin, cephradine, cefadroxil
Second generation		
Haemophilus active	Cefamandole, cefuroxime, cefonicid, ceforanide	Cefaclor, cefuroxime axetil, cefixime,* cefprozil, cefpodoxime,* loracarbef
Bacteroides active	Cefoxitin, cefotetan, cefmetazole	None
Third-generation		
Extended-spectrum	Ceftriaxone, cefotaxime, ceftizoxime	None
Extended-spectrum and antipseudomonal	Ceftazidime, cefoperazone	
Carbapenems	Imipenem-cilastatin	None
Monobactams	Aztreonam	None

* Some sources classify cefixime and cefpodoxime as a third-generation oral agents because of a marginally broader spectrum.

INHIBITION OF PROTEIN SYNTHESIS Most of the antibacterial agents that inhibit protein synthesis interact with the bacterial ribosome. The difference between the composition of bacterial and mammalian ribosomes gives these compounds their selectivity.

Aminoglycosides (gentamicin, kanamycin, tobramycin, streptomycin, netilmicin, neomycin, and amikacin) are a group of structurally related compounds containing three linked hexose sugars. They exert a bactericidal effect by binding irreversibly to the 30 S subunit of the bacterial ribosome and blocking initiation of protein synthesis. The reason for the lethal effect of aminoglycosides—as opposed to the largely bacteriostatic effect of other protein synthesis–inhibiting antibacterial drugs (macrolides, lincosamides, chloramphenicol, and tetracycline)—is not completely understood. Uptake of aminoglycosides and their penetration through the cell membrane constitute an aerobic, energy-dependent process. Thus aminoglycoside activity is markedly reduced in an anaerobic environment. *Spectinomycin*, an aminocyclitol antibiotic, also acts on the 30 S ribosomal subunit but has a different mechanism of action from the aminoglycosides and is bacteriostatic rather than bactericidal.

Macrolides (erythromycin, clarithromycin, and azithromycin) are antibiotics that consist of a large lactone ring to which sugars are attached. They bind specifically to the 50 S portion of the bacterial ribosome. After attachment of mRNA to the initiation site of the 30 S ribosomal subunit (the process blocked by aminoglycosides), the 50 S subunit becomes bound to the 30 S component to form the 70 S ribosomal complex, and protein chain elongation proceeds. Binding of macrolides to the 50 S ribosomal subunit inhibits protein chain elongation.

Lincosamides (clindamycin and lincomycin), although structurally unrelated to macrolides, bind to a site on the 50 S ribosome nearly identical to the binding site for macrolides. Although the mechanism and site of action of macrolides and lincosamides are similar, the number and type of bacteria against which these two groups of agents are active differ.

Chloramphenicol, a small antibiotic with a single aromatic ring and short side chain, binds reversibly to the 50 S portion of the bacterial ribosome at a site close but not identical to the sites binding the macrolides and lincosamides. The ribosomal binding of chloramphenicol inhibits peptide bond formation.

Tetracyclines (tetracycline, doxycycline, and minocycline) consist of four aromatic rings with various substituent groups. They interact reversibly with the bacterial 30 S ribosomal subunit, blocking the binding of aminoacyl tRNA to the mRNA-ribosome complex. This mechanism is markedly different from that of the aminoglycosides, which also bind to the 30 S subunit. The specificity of tetracyclines for bacteria depends both on their selectivity for bacterial (as opposed to mammalian) ribosomes and on their requirement for active, energy-dependent transport into the bacterial cell by a system not found in mammalian cell membranes.

Mupirocin (pseudomonic acid) is produced by the bacterium *Pseudomonas fluorescens*. Its mechanism of action is unique in that it inhibits the enzyme isoleucine tRNA synthetase by competing with bacterial isoleucine for its binding site on the enzyme. Inhibition of this enzyme depletes cellular stores of isoleucine-charged tRNA and therefore leads to a cessation of protein synthesis. The antibiotic is selective for bacteria because of the lack of affinity of mammalian isoleucine tRNA synthetase for the compound.

INHIBITION OF BACTERIAL METABOLISM The antimetabolites are all synthetic compounds that interfere with bacterial synthesis of folic acid. Products of the folic acid synthesis pathway function as coenzymes for the one-carbon transfer reactions that are essential for the synthesis of thymidine, all purines, and several amino acids. Inhibition of folate synthesis leads to cessation of cell growth and, in some cases, to bacterial cell death. The principal antibacterial antimetabolites are sulfonamides (sulfisoxazole, sulfadiazine, and sulfamethoxazole) and trimethoprim.

Sulfonamides are structural analogues of *p*-aminobenzoic acid (PABA), one of the three structural components of folic acid (the other two being pteridine and glutamate). The first step in the synthesis of folic acid is the addition of PABA to pteridine by the enzyme dihydropteroic acid synthetase. Sulfonamides compete with PABA as substrates for the enzyme. The selective effect of sulfonamides is due to the fact that bacteria synthesize folic acid while mammalian cells cannot synthesize the cofactor and must have exogenous supplies. However, the activity of sulfonamides can be greatly reduced in the presence of excess PABA or by the exogenous addition of end products of one-carbon transfer reactions (e.g., thymidine and purines). High concentrations of the latter substances may be present in some infections as a result of tissue and white cell breakdown, compromising sulfonamide activity.

Trimethoprim is a diaminopyrimidine, a structural analogue of the pteridine moiety of folic acid. It is a competitive inhibitor of dihydrofolate reductase, the enzyme responsible for reduction of dihydrofolic acid to tetrahydrofolic acid, the essential final component in the folic acid synthesis pathway, necessary for all one-carbon transfer reactions. Like the sulfonamides, trimethoprim is bactericidal in the absence of thymine but is only bacteriostatic when this pyrimidine is present in high concentration. The selective antibacterial activity of trimethoprim is based on the extreme sensitivity of bacterial dihydrofolate reductase to inhibition by this drug in comparison with the mammalian enzyme. The bacterial enzyme is approximately 50,000 times more sensitive to such inhibition.

INHIBITION OF NUCLEIC ACID SYNTHESIS OR ACTIVITY Numerous antibacterial compounds have disparate effects on nucleic acids. The *quinolones*, including nalidixic acid and its fluorinated derivatives (norfloxacin, ciprofloxacin, ofloxacin, and lomefloxacin), are synthetic compounds that inhibit the activity of one of the subunits (the A subunit) of the bacterial enzyme DNA gyrase. DNA gyrase is responsible for negative supercoiling of DNA, an essential conformation for DNA replication in the intact cell. Inhibition of the activity of DNA gyrase is lethal to bacterial cells. The antibiotic *novobiocin* also interferes with the activity of DNA gyrase, but it interferes with the B subunit.

Rifampin, used primarily as an antituberculous agent, is an antibiotic that is also active against a variety of bacteria other than *Mycobacterium tuberculosis*. Rifampin binds tightly to bacterial DNA–dependent RNA polymerase, thus inhibiting transcription of DNA into RNA. Mammalian cell RNA polymerase is not sensitive to the compound.

Nitrofurantoin, a synthetic compound, causes DNA damage. The nitrofurans, compounds containing a single five-membered ring, are reduced by a bacterial enzyme to highly reactive, short-lived intermediates that are thought to cause DNA strand breakage, either directly or indirectly.

Metronidazole, a synthetic compound, is an imidazole that has activity against a wide range of anaerobic bacteria and protozoa. This activity is totally dependent on the organism's system for anaerobic energy production. In the presence of the anaerobic electron transport system, the nitro group of metronidazole is reduced to a series of transiently produced, reactive intermediates that are thought to cause DNA damage. Although the unique redox system of anaerobes accounts for the selective antibacterial activity of metronidazole, this compound is also a mutagen and a radiosensitizer of hypoxic mammalian cells.

ALTERATION OF CELL MEMBRANE PERMEABILITY The *polymyxins* (polymyxin B and colistin, or polymyxin E) are cyclic, basic polypeptides. They behave as cationic, surface-active compounds that disrupt the permeability of both the outer and the cytoplasmic membranes of gram-negative bacteria.

Gramicidin A is a polypeptide of 15 amino acids that acts as an ionophore, forming pores or channels in lipid bilayers.

MECHANISMS OF RESISTANCE

Some bacteria are *intrinsically resistant* to certain classes of antibacterial agents (e.g., obligate anaerobic bacteria to aminoglycosides and gram-negative bacteria to vancomycin). Clearly these agents can never be used alone in the treatment of infections caused by resistant bacteria. However, bacteria that are ordinarily susceptible to antibacterial agents can acquire resistance. *Acquired resistance* is one of the major limitations to effective antibacterial chemotherapy. Resistance can develop by mutation of resident genes or by acquisition of new genes. New genes mediating resistance are usually spread from cell to cell by way of mobile genetic elements such as plasmids, transposons, and bacteriophages. The resistant bacterial populations flourish in areas of high antimicrobial use, where they enjoy a selective advantage over susceptible populations.

The major mechanisms used by bacteria to resist the action of antimicrobial agents are destruction of the compound, alteration or overproduction of the antibacterial target, decreased permeability of the cell envelope to the agent, and active elimination of the compound from the interior of the cell. Specific mechanisms of bacterial resistance to the major antibacterial agents are outlined below and are summarized in Table 100-1.

β-LACTAMS Bacteria develop resistance to β-lactam antibiotics by a variety of mechanisms. Most common is the destruction of the drug by β-lactamases. These enzymes have a higher affinity for the antibiotic than the antibiotic has for its target. Binding results in hydrolysis of the β-lactam ring. Genes encoding β-lactamases have been found in both chromosomal and extrachromosomal locations and in both gram-positive and gram-negative bacteria; these genes are often on mobile genetic elements. One strategy that has been devised for circumventing resistance mediated by β-lactamases is to combine the susceptible β-lactam with an inhibitor that avidly binds the inactivating enzyme, preventing its attack on the antibiotic. Unfortunately, the inhibitors (e.g., clavulanic acid and sulbactam) do not bind all classes of β-lactamase and cannot be depended on to prevent the inactivation of β-lactam antibiotics by all β-lactamases. No β-lactam antibiotic or inhibitor has been produced that can resist all of the many β-lactamases that have been identified.

A second mechanism of bacterial resistance to β-lactam antibiotics is an alteration in PBP targets so that the PBPs have a markedly reduced affinity for the drug. While this alteration may occur by mutation of existing genes, the acquisition of new PBP genes (as in staphylococcal resistance to methicillin) or of new pieces of PBP genes (as in pneumococcal, gonococcal, and meningococcal resistance to penicillin) is more important.

A final resistance mechanism is the alteration by gram-negative bacteria of their outer membrane so that it is no longer permeable to the antibiotic. Mutations of genes encoding the outer membrane proteins called *porins* mediate this alteration in permeability. The resistance of Enterobacteriaceae to some cephalosporins and that of *Pseudomonas* spp. to ureidopenicillins are the best examples of this mechanism. More than one of these resistance mechanisms commonly coexist in the same bacterial cell.

VANCOMYCIN Clinically important resistance to vancomycin was first described among enterococci in France in 1988. Vancomycin-resistant enterococci have subsequently become disseminated worldwide. The genes encoding resistance are carried on plasmids that can transfer themselves from cell to cell. Resistance is mediated by enzymes that alter the terminal amino acid on the peptidoglycan stem peptide so that there is no longer an appropriate target for vancomycin binding. This alteration does not appear to affect cell wall integrity, however. Vancomycin resistance is so far confined to enterococci and one species of coagulase-negative staphylococci (*Staphylococcus haemolyticus*); *S. aureus* and *S. epidermidis* remain susceptible.

AMINOGLYCOSIDES The most common resistance mechanism is inactivation of the antibiotic. Aminoglycoside-modifying enzymes, usually encoded on plasmids, transfer phosphate, adenyl, or acetyl residues from intracellular molecules to hydroxyl or amino side groups on the antibiotic. The modified antibiotic is less active because of decreased transport across the cytoplasmic membrane and diminished binding to its ribosomal target. Modifying enzymes that can inactivate any of the available aminoglycosides have been found in both gram-positive and gram-negative bacteria.

A second resistance mechanism that is uncommon but has been identified in clinical isolates of *P. aeruginosa* is decreased antibiotic uptake, presumably due to alterations in the outer membrane.

MACROLIDES AND LINCOSAMIDES Resistance in gram-positive bacteria, the usual target organisms for macrolides and lincosamides, is due to the production of an enzyme—most commonly plasmid-encoded—that methylates ribosomal RNA, interfering with binding of the antibiotics to their target. Methylation mediates resistance to erythromycin, newer macrolides, and clindamycin. However, the enzyme usually needs to be induced by exposure to low concentrations of macrolides before resistance is fully expressed; clindamycin is a poor inducer. The need for induction can lead to false reports of susceptibility when bacterial isolates are tested in vitro.

CHLORAMPHENICOL Most bacteria resistant to this antibiotic produce a plasmid-encoded enzyme, chloramphenicol acetyltransferase, that inactivates the compound by acetylation. Occasionally, gram-negative bacteria acquire a mutation affecting the permeability of the outer membrane to this antibiotic.

TETRACYCLINE The most common mechanism of resistance in gram-negative bacteria is a plasmid-encoded active-efflux pump that is inserted into the cytoplasmic membrane and extrudes antibiotic from the cell. Resistance in gram-positive bacteria is due either to active efflux or to ribosomal alterations that diminish binding of the antibiotic to its target. Genes involved in ribosomal protection are found on mobile genetic elements.

MUPIROCIN Although this topical compound was only recently introduced into clinical use, resistance is already becoming widespread in some areas. The mechanisms appear to be mutation of the target isoleucine tRNA synthetase so that it is no longer inhibited by the antibiotic or plasmid-encoded production of a form of the target enzyme that binds mupirocin poorly.

TRIMETHOPRIM AND SULFONAMIDES The most prevalent resistance mechanism in both gram-positive and gram-negative bacteria is the acquisition of plasmid-encoded genes that produce a new, drug-insensitive target. Bacteria produce an insensitive dihydrofolate reductase for trimethoprim and an altered dihydropteroate synthetase for sulfonamides.

QUINOLONES Resistance to the newer fluoroquinolones emerged rapidly among *Staphylococcus* and *Pseudomonas* spp. after the introduction of these agents. The most common mechanism is the development of one or more mutations in the target DNA gyrase so that the antibacterial agent no longer interferes with the activity of the enzyme. Some gram-negative bacteria also acquire mutations in their outer-membrane porins so that cells are no longer permeable to the drugs; some gram-positive bacteria develop a mutation that allows them to actively pump the antibacterial agents from the cell.

RIFAMPIN Bacteria rapidly become resistant to rifampin by developing mutations in RNA polymerase that render the enzyme unable to bind the antibiotic. The rapid selection of resistant mutants is the major limitation to the use of this antibiotic against otherwise susceptible staphylococci and requires that it be used in combination with another antistaphylococcal agent.

MULTIPLE ANTIBIOTIC RESISTANCE Acquired resistance of one bacterium to multiple antibacterial agents is becoming increasingly common. The two major mechanisms are the acquisition of multiple unrelated resistance genes and the development of mutations in a single gene or gene complex that mediate resistance to a series of unrelated compounds. The construction of multiresistant strains by acquisition of multiple genes occurs by sequential steps of gene transfer and environmental selection in areas of high antimicrobial use. In contrast, mutations in a single gene can conceivably be selected in a single step. Bacteria that are multiresistant by virtue of the acquisition of new genes include hospital-associated gram-negative bacteria, enterococci and staphylococci, and community-acquired strains of salmonellae, gonococci, and pneumococci. Most of the latter bacterial isolates originated in other countries but have become established in some areas of the United States. Mutations that confer resistance to multiple unrelated antimicrobial agents occur in the outer-membrane proteins (porins) of gram-negative bacteria. These mutations affect the permeability of these bacteria to β-lactams, quinolones, tetracycline, chloramphenicol, and trimethoprim. Multi-resistant bacterial isolates pose increasing problems in U.S. hospitals; strains resistant to all available antibacterial chemotherapy have already been identified.

PHARMACOKINETICS

The *pharmacokinetic profile* of an antibacterial agent refers to concentrations in serum and tissue versus time after administration of the drug and reflects the processes of absorption, distribution, metabolism, and excretion. Important characteristics include peak and trough serum concentrations and mathematically derived parameters such as half-life, clearance, and distribution volume. Pharmacokinetic information is useful for estimating the appropriate antibacterial dose and frequency of administration, for adjusting dosages in patients with impaired excretory capacity, and for comparing one drug with another.

ABSORPTION Data on absorption can refer to oral, intramuscular (IM), or intravenous (IV) administration.

Oral administration Most patients with infection are treated with oral antibacterial agents in the outpatient setting. Advantages of oral therapy over parenteral therapy include lower costs, generally fewer adverse effects (including complications of indwelling lines), and greater acceptance by patients. The percentage of an orally administered antibacterial agent that is absorbed (i.e., the agent's *bioavailability*) ranges from as little as 10 to 20 percent (erythromycin and penicillin G) to nearly 100 percent (clindamycin, metronidazole, doxycycline, and trimethoprim-sulfamethoxazole). These differences in bioavailability are not clinically important as long as concentrations at the site of infection are sufficient to inhibit or kill the pathogen. However, therapeutic efficacy may be compromised when absorption is reduced as a result of physiologic or pathologic conditions (such as the presence of food for some drugs or the shunting of blood away from the gastrointestinal tract in the patient with hypotension), drug interactions (such as that of quinolones and metal cations), or noncompliance. The oral route is usually used for patients with relatively mild infections in whom absorption is not thought to be compromised by the preceding conditions.

Intramuscular administration Although the IM route of administration usually results in 100 percent bioavailability, it is not as widely used in the United States as the oral and IV routes, in part because of the pain often associated with IM injections and the relative ease of IV access in the hospitalized patient. Intramuscular injection may be suitable for specific indications requiring an "immediate" and reliable effect (e.g., with long-acting forms of penicillin, including benzathine and procaine, and with single doses of ceftriaxone for uncomplicated gonococcal infection).

Intravenous administration The IV route is appropriate when oral antibacterial agents are not effective against a particular pathogen, when bioavailability is uncertain, or when larger doses are required than are feasible with the oral route. After IV administration, bioavailability is 100 percent, and peak serum concentrations occur at the end of the infusion. For many patients requiring long-term therapy, outpatient IV administration using convenient portable pumps may be cost-effective and safe when oral therapy is not feasible. Alternatively, some newer oral antibacterial drugs are sufficiently active against some organisms to rival parenteral therapy; their use may allow the patient to return home earlier or to avoid hospitalization entirely.

DISTRIBUTION After absorption, the resulting serum concentrations of most antibacterial agents must exceed the minimum concentra-

tion required to inhibit bacterial growth (MIC; see Chap. 80) to be effective. Since most infections are extravascular, an antibiotic also must *distribute* to the site of infection. Concentrations of most antibacterials in interstitial fluid are similar to free drug concentrations in serum. However, when the infection is located in a "protected" site where penetration is poor, such as cerebrospinal fluid, the eye, the prostate, or infected cardiac vegetations, high parenteral doses or local administration for prolonged periods may be required for cure. In addition, even though an antibacterial agent may penetrate to the site of infection, its activity may be antagonized by local factors, such as an unfavorable pH or inactivation by cellular degradation products. For example, since the activity of aminoglycosides is reduced at acidic pH, the acidic environment in many infected tissues may be partly responsible for the relatively poor efficacy of aminoglycoside monotherapy. In addition, the abscess milieu reduces the activity of many antibacterial compounds so that surgical drainage is required for cure.

Most bacteria causing human infections are located extracellularly. Intracellular pathogens such as *Legionella, Chlamydia, Brucella,* and *Salmonella* may persist or cause relapse if the antibacterial agent does not enter the cell. In general, β-lactams, vancomycin, and aminoglycosides penetrate cells poorly, whereas macrolides, tetracyclines, metronidazole, chloramphenicol, rifampin, trimethoprim-sulfamethoxazole, and quinolones penetrate cells well.

METABOLISM AND ELIMINATION Like other drugs, antibacterial agents are disposed of by hepatic elimination (metabolism or biliary elimination), by renal excretion in unchanged or metabolized form, or by a combination of the two processes. For most antibacterial drugs, metabolism leads to loss of in vitro activity, although some agents such as cefotaxime, rifampin, and clarithromycin have bioactive metabolites that may contribute to their overall efficacy.

The most practical consequence of the mode of excretion of an antibacterial agent is the need to adjust the dosage when elimination capability is impaired. Direct, nonidiosyncratic toxicity from antibacterial drugs most often results from failure to reduce the dosage appropriately in a patient with impaired elimination. For agents that are primarily cleared intact by glomerular filtration, drug clearance is linearly correlated with creatinine clearance. Commonly used antibacterial drugs that require dosage adjustment in patients with renal impairment are listed in Table 100-3. Unfortunately, for drugs whose elimination is primarily hepatic, no simple marker (such as serum creatinine) is useful for dosage adjustment in subjects with liver disease. Even in patients with severe hepatic disease, residual metabolic capability is usually sufficient for the avoidance of accumulation and toxic adverse effects. However, for drugs that undergo hepatic metabolism and have a narrow therapeutic index (such as chloramphenicol), alternative therapy may be warranted in patients with liver disease, since the technology for the monitoring of serum levels is not widely available.

PRINCIPLES OF ANTIBACTERIAL CHEMOTHERAPY

The choice of an antibacterial compound for a particular patient and a specific infection involves more than just a knowledge of the agent's mechanism of action and pharmacokinetic profile. The basic tenets of chemotherapy, to be elaborated on below, include the following: First, whenever possible, material containing the infecting organism(s) should be obtained so that presumptive identification can be made by microscopic examination of stained specimens and the organism can be grown for definitive identification and susceptibility testing. Second, once the organism is identified and its susceptibility to antibacterial agents is determined, the regimen with the narrowest effective spectrum should be chosen. Third, the choice of antibacterial agent is guided by the pharmacokinetic and adverse-reaction profile of active compounds, the site of infection, the immune status of the host, and evidence of efficacy from well-performed clinical trials.

TABLE 100-3 Pharmacokinetics of selected antibacterial agents

Drug	Dose, route	Peak serum concentration, μg/mL	Breakpoint,* μg/mL	Half-life, h	Dose alteration in renal disease
Penicillin G	2×10^6 U, IV	60	0.1[†]	0.5	Yes
Ampicillin	1000 mg, IV	40	8[‡]	1	Yes
Dicloxacillin	500 mg, PO	15	2	1	No
Nafcillin	1000 mg, IV	40	2	1	No
Ticarcillin	3000 mg, IV	160	16[‡]	1	Yes
Cefazolin	1000 mg, IV	188	8	2	Yes
Cefaclor	500 mg, PO	15	8	1	Yes
Cephalexin	500 mg, PO	15	8	1	Yes
Cefoxitin	1000 mg, IV	110	8	1	Yes
Cefuroxime	1000 mg, IV	100	8	1.5	Yes
Ceftriaxone	1000 mg, IV	150	8	8	Yes
Ceftazidime	2000 mg, IV	170	8	2	Slight
Aztreonam	2000 mg, IV	200	8	2	Yes
Imipenem	500 mg, IV	43	4	1	Yes
Gentamicin	1.5 mg/kg, IV	8	4	2	Yes
Amikacin	7.5 mg/kg, IV	35	16	2	Yes
Doxycycline	100 mg, PO	2.5	4	18	Yes
Tetracycline	500 mg, PO	4	4	8	§
Erythromycin	500 mg, PO	1	0.5	0.5–2.0	No
Clindamycin	600 mg, IV	10	0.5	2.4	No
Metronidazole	500 mg, PO	10	NA¶	6	No
Vancomycin	1000 mg, IV	30	4	6	Yes
Trimethoprim-sulfamethoxazole	160/800 mg, PO	2/40	2/38	11/9	Yes
Ciprofloxacin	500 mg, PO	3	1	4	Yes
Ofloxacin	400 mg, PO	6	2	6	Yes

* For fully susceptible organisms.
† For most gram-positive organisms.
‡ For Enterobacteriaceae.
§ Contraindicated in renal impairment.
¶ NA = not applicable.

Finally, if all other factors are equal, the antibacterial regimen that is the least expensive should be chosen.

SUSCEPTIBILITY OF BACTERIA TO ANTIBACTERIAL DRUGS IN VITRO (See also Chap. 80) The determination of the susceptibility of the patient's infecting organism to a panel of appropriate antibacterial agents is an essential first step in devising a chemotherapeutic regimen. The details of susceptibility testing are discussed elsewhere (Chap. 80). However, susceptibility testing is designed to estimate the susceptibility of a bacterial isolate to an antibacterial drug under standardized conditions that favor rapidly growing aerobic or facultative organisms. Under certain circumstances, specialized testing is required. (1) Strict anaerobes require testing under anaerobic conditions. Problems with poor growth of the inoculum or unstable activity of some antibacterial agents (i.e., metronidazole) in testing media have led to significant interlaboratory variation. (2) Production of β-lactamase by such fastidious organisms as *Haemophilus influenzae* and *Neisseria gonorrhoeae* has a major effect on therapy. Therefore, production of this enzyme must be measured directly; β-lactam susceptibility testing cannot be relied on. (3) Resistance genes that require induction for expression may require longer incubation (e.g., erythromycin resistance in staphylococci) or detection of inducible enzymes (e.g., β-lactamase production by staphylococci). (4) Methicillin resistance in staphylococci requires specialized testing with larger inocula, longer incubation, and the addition of salt to the medium because of the variable expression of resistance under standardized testing conditions. (5) Resistance of enterococci to aminoglycosides needs to be assessed with use of very high levels of antibiotics in testing media because of intrinsic resistance. Resistance of enterococci to greater than 2000 μg/mL of an aminoglycoside such as gentamicin suggests that the isolate will be resistant to the bactericidal synergy of a β-lactam plus an aminoglycoside. (6) The minimum bactericidal concentration (MBC) of an antibacterial agent for a particular bacterial isolate may need to be determined rather than the minimal inhibitory concentration (MIC) that is the result of routine susceptibility testing. It must be performed manually by broth dilution with a carefully standardized protocol that defines the endpoint for growth after subculture to agar. It is generally only indicated for certain patients with endocarditis or osteomyelitis.

RELATIONSHIP OF PHARMACOKINETICS AND IN VITRO SUSCEPTIBILITY TO RESPONSE The relationship between the report of susceptibility in vitro and the clinical pharmacokinetics of the antibacterial agent helps predict clinical response. Bacteria are usually considered to be *susceptible* to a drug if the achievable peak serum concentration exceeds the MIC by at least fourfold. The *breakpoint* is the concentration of the antibiotic that separates susceptible from resistant bacteria. When a majority of the isolates of a given bacterial species are inhibited at concentrations below the breakpoint, the species is within the spectrum of the drug (see "Choice of Antibacterial Therapy," below). Antibacterial agents are frequently administered every 3 to 4 half-lives, since serum concentrations will by then be below the breakpoint and may be below the MIC for the organism. These relationships are illustrated in Fig. 100-1. *Pharmacodynamics* refers to the relationship between drug concentrations in serum and tissues, in vitro susceptibility, and microbial response at the site of infection. Pharmacodynamic parameters that appear to correlate with reduction in the number of bacteria at the site of infection include the ratio of the peak antibacterial concentration to the MIC (especially for aminoglycosides and quinolones), the length of time that concentrations exceed the MIC (especially for β-lactams), and the postantibiotic effect (or length of time that bacterial growth is inhibited after concentrations fall below the MIC). For some drugs, such as the aminoglycosides, it is not necessary to maintain serum concentrations above the MIC for the entire dose interval. Many microbiology laboratories report quantitative susceptibilities (MIC); Table 100-3 lists peak serum concentrations and breakpoints for some common antibacterial agents.

STATUS OF THE HOST Various host factors must be considered when devising antibacterial chemotherapy. The host's antibacterial *immune function* is of importance, particularly as it relates to opsonophagocytic function. Since the major host defense against acute, overwhelming bacterial infection is the polymorphonuclear leukocyte, patients with neutropenia must be treated aggressively and

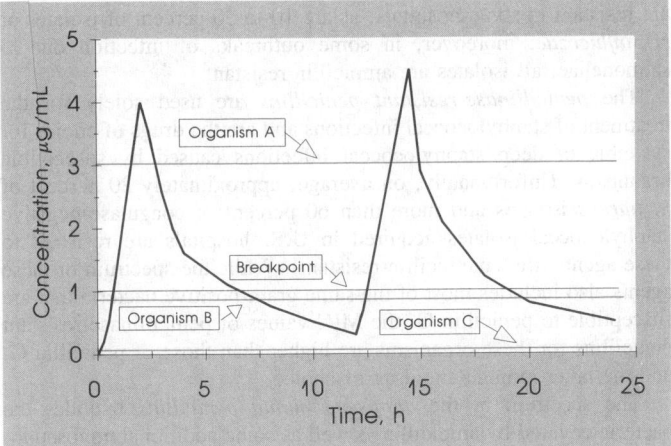

FIGURE 100-1 Relationship between pharmacokinetics of an antibiotic and susceptibility. Organism A is resistant, organism B is moderately susceptible, and organism C is very susceptible.

empirically with bactericidal drugs for suspected infection (see Chap. 96). Likewise, patients who have deficient humoral immunity (e.g., those with chronic lymphocytic leukemia and multiple myeloma) and individuals with surgical or functional asplenia (e.g., those with sickle cell disease) should be treated empirically for infections with encapsulated organisms, especially the pneumococcus.

Genetic factors may determine the type of infection, the pathogen, and susceptibility to antibacterial side effects. For example, in patients with chronic granulomatous disease, the survival of catalase-positive microorganisms (e.g., *S. aureus*) inside phagocytes is enhanced, and therapy not only must be directed against these bacteria but also must include agents that are taken up by phagocytes and are active intracellularly.

Pregnancy increases the risk of toxicity of certain antibacterial drugs for the mother (e.g., the hepatic toxicity of tetracycline), affects drug disposition and pharmacokinetics, and—because of the risk of fetal toxicity—severely limits the choice of agents for treating infections. Certain antibacterials are contraindicated in pregnancy either because safety has not been established or because of known toxicity. These include all fluoroquinolones, clarithromycin, erythromycin estolate (but not erythromycin base), and tetracyclines. Data on the safety of many other antibacterial drugs are limited, but they may be used cautiously when there is no suitable alternative and the perceived benefit outweighs the risk. These include aminoglycosides, azithromycin, clindamycin, imipenem, metronidazole, trimethoprim, and vancomycin. The following drugs are contraindicated in the third trimester but can be used cautiously in the first two trimesters: chloramphenicol, nitrofurantoin, and sulfonamides.

In patients with *concomitant viral infections*, the incidence of adverse reactions to antibacterial drugs may be unusually high. For example, persons with infectious mononucleosis and those infected with HIV may react more often to ampicillin and folic acid synthesis inhibitors, respectively.

In addition, the patient's age, sex, racial heritage, and excretory status all determine the incidence and type of side effects that can be expected with certain antibacterial agents.

SITE OF INFECTION The location of the infected site may play a major role in the choice and dose of antimicrobial drug. Patients with suspected *meningitis* should receive drugs that can cross the blood–cerebrospinal fluid (CSF) barrier; in addition, because of the relative paucity of phagocytes and opsonins at the site of infection, the agents should be bactericidal. Chloramphenicol, one of the standard drugs for therapy, is bactericidal for common organisms causing meningitis (i.e., meningococcus, pneumococcus, and *H. influenzae, not* enteric gram-negative bacilli), is highly lipid-soluble, and enters the CSF well. However, β-lactams, the mainstay of therapy for most of these infections, do not normally reach high levels in

CSF. Their efficacy is based on the increased permeability of the blood-brain and blood-CSF barriers to hydrophilic molecules during inflammation and the extreme susceptibility of most infectious organisms to even small amounts of β-lactam drug.

The vegetation that is the major site of infection in *bacterial endocarditis* is also a focus that is protected from normal host defense mechanisms. Antibacterial therapy needs to be bactericidal, administered at a dose that produces serum levels at least eight times higher than the MBC for the infecting organism, and given parenterally for a prolonged period. Likewise, *osteomyelitis* involves a site that is somewhat resistant to opsonophagocytic removal of infecting bacteria; furthermore, avascular bone (sequestrum) represents a foreign body that thwarts normal host defense mechanisms. *Chronic prostatitis* is exceedingly difficult to cure because most antibiotics do not penetrate nonfenestrated capillaries serving the prostate, especially when acute inflammation is absent. Drugs that are "ion trapped" after entering prostatic tissue, such as trimethoprim and fluoroquinolones, may be uniquely effective because of this mechanism. *Intraocular infections*, especially endophthalmitis, are difficult to treat because drug penetration into the vitreous from blood is hindered by retinal capillaries lacking fenestration. Inflammation does little to disrupt this barrier. Thus direct injection into the vitreous is necessary in many cases. *Abscesses* also represent infections where antibiotic penetration is usually poor. In addition, even when an antibiotic does penetrate into the abscess, local conditions, such as low pH or the presence of enzymes that hydrolyze the drug, may antagonize activity. In contrast, *urinary tract infections*, when confined to the bladder, are relatively easy infections to cure, in part because of the higher concentration of most antibiotics in the urine than in blood. Since blood is the usual reference fluid in defining susceptibility, even organisms found to be "resistant" to achievable serum concentrations may be susceptible to achievable urine concentrations. For drugs that are used only for the treatment of urinary tract infections, such as nitrofurantoin and methenamine salts, achievable urine concentrations are used to determine susceptibility.

COMBINATION CHEMOTHERAPY One of the tenets of antibacterial chemotherapy is that if the infecting bacterium has been identified, the most specific chemotherapy possible should be used. The use of a single agent with a narrow spectrum of activity against the pathogen diminishes the alteration of normal flora and thus limits overgrowth of resistant nosocomial organisms (e.g., *Candida albicans*, enterococci, *C. difficile*, or methicillin-resistant staphylococci), limits the potential toxicity of multiple drug regimens, and reduces cost. However, certain circumstances call for the use of more than one antibacterial agent. These are summarized below.

1 *Prevention of the emergence of resistant mutants.* Spontaneous mutations occur at a detectable frequency in certain genes encoding the target proteins for some antibacterial agents. The use of these agents can eliminate the susceptible population, select out resistant mutants at the site of infection, and result in the failure of chemotherapy. Resistant mutants are usually selected when the MIC of the antibacterial agent for the infecting bacterium is close to achievable levels in serum or tissues and/or when the site of infection limits the access or activity of the agent. The most common examples are rifampin for staphylococci, imipenem for *Pseudomonas*, and ciprofloxacin for staphylococci and *Pseudomonas*. Small-colony variants of staphylococci resistant to aminoglycosides also emerge during monotherapy with these antibiotics. A second antibacterial agent with a mechanism of action different from that of the first is added to prevent the emergence of these resistant mutants (e.g., imipenem plus an aminoglycoside for systemic *Pseudomonas* infections). However, since resistant mutants have emerged following combination chemotherapy, this approach is not uniformly successful.

2 *Synergistic or additive activity.* Against some bacteria, two antibacterial agents are clearly more active than one; whether or not this is the case is usually judged on the basis of testing in vitro.

Synergistic or *additive activity* is defined as a lowering of the MIC or MBC of *each* of two drugs tested in combination against a specific bacterium. Thus *each* agent is more active when combined with a second drug than it would be alone. The best examples of a synergistic or additive effect, confirmed both in vitro and by animal studies, are the enhanced bactericidal activities of certain β-lactam–aminoglycoside combinations against enterococci, viridans streptococci, and *P. aeruginosa*. The synergistic or additive activity of these combinations also has been demonstrated for selected isolates of enteric gram-negative bacteria and staphylococci. The combination of trimethoprim and sulfamethoxazole also has synergistic or additive activity against many enteric gram-negative bacteria. Most other antimicrobial combinations show indifferent activity (i.e., the combination is *no better* than the more active of the two agents alone), and some combinations (e.g., penicillin plus tetracycline against pneumococci) may be antagonistic (i.e., the combination is *worse* than either drug alone).

3 *Therapy directed against multiple potential pathogens.* For certain infections, either a mixture of pathogens is documented or the patient is desperately ill; in these situations, the most important infecting bacteria need to be covered by therapy until culture and susceptibility results become available. Examples of the former infections are intraabdominal or brain abscesses and infected limbs in diabetic patients with microvascular disease. The latter situations include fevers in neutropenic patients, acute pneumonia from aspiration of oral flora by hospitalized patients, and septic shock or sepsis syndrome. However, in circumstances where presumptive therapy with more than one agent is begun, monotherapy should always be given subsequently if a single infecting bacterium that can be treated effectively with one agent is identified.

CHOICE OF ANTIBACTERIAL THERAPY

The antibacterial spectrum of specific agents and the infections for which they represent the treatment of choice are detailed below. No attempt has been made to include all the potential situations in which antibacterial agents may be used. A more detailed discussion of specific bacteria and infections that they cause can be found elsewhere in this volume.

β-LACTAMS (See also Table 100-2) All *penicillins* (except for the semisynthetic, penicillinase-resistant, antistaphylococcal agents) are hydrolyzed by β-lactamases and are ineffective against isolates that produce these enzymes. Penicillin G has a spectrum that includes spirochetes (*Treponema pallidum, Borrelia*, and *Leptospira*), streptococci (groups A and B, viridans, and *Streptococcus pneumoniae*), enterococci, most *Neisseria* spp., a few staphylococci, many fastidious oral bacteria [*Bacteroides (Porphyromonas* and *Prevotella), streptococci, Actinomyces,* and *Fusobacterium*], *Clostridium* spp. (except *C. difficile*), *Pasteurella multocida, Erysipelothrix rhusiopathiae,* and *Streptobacillus moniliformis*. However, resistance is widespread among staphylococci, is increasing among gonococci and enterococci, and is emerging among pneumococci, oral strains of *Bacteroides (Porphyromonas* and *Prevotella*), and meningococci. Penicillin G is the drug of choice for syphilis, yaws, leptospirosis, group A and B streptococcal infections, pneumococcal infections (in the United States), actinomycosis, oral and periodontal infections, meningococcal meningitis and meningococcemia, viridans streptococcal endocarditis, clostridial myonecrosis, tetanus, anthrax, rat-bite fever, *P. multocida* infections, and erysipeloid (*E. rhusiopathiae*).

Ampicillin extends the spectrum of penicillin G to some gram-negative rods. It is active against some isolates of *Escherichia coli, Proteus mirabilis, Salmonella, Shigella,* and *H. influenzae* and is one of the drugs of choice for susceptible organisms causing urinary tract infections, salmonellosis, *H. influenzae* meningitis and epiglottitis, and *Listeria monocytogenes* meningitis. High rates of resistance have lessened its value as empirical therapy in some situations. For example, more than 80 percent of isolates of *E. coli* and *P. mirabilis*

are resistant in some hospitals, as are 10 to 30 percent of isolates of *H. influenzae*; moreover, in some outbreaks of infection due to salmonellae, all isolates are ampicillin-resistant.

The *penicillinase-resistant penicillins* are used solely for the treatment of staphylococcal infections and are the drugs of choice for systemic or deep staphylococcal infections caused by susceptible organisms. Unfortunately, on average, approximately 20 percent of *S. aureus* isolates and more than 60 percent of coagulase-negative staphylococcal isolates acquired in U.S. hospitals are resistant to these agents (i.e., methicillin-resistant). While the spectrum of these agents also includes most of the same gram-positive bacteria that are susceptible to penicillin G, the MIC values of penicillinase-resistant penicillins for these organisms are higher than those of penicillin G, and the latter remains the drug of choice.

The spectrum of the *antipseudomonal penicillins* includes the bacteria covered by ampicillin as well as some additional nonpseudomonal enteric gram-negative bacilli. For example, piperacillin is active against many indole-positive *Proteus, Enterobacter, Klebsiella, Providencia,* and *Serratia* spp. However, the susceptibility of these penicillins to β-lactamase markedly limits their utility as empirical therapy when infections caused by gram-negative enteric organisms are suspected. The major use of these compounds is in the treatment of proven or suspected infections with *P. aeruginosa* and *Acinetobacter*, for which they are among the drugs of choice. Their relative antipseudomonal activities can be ranked as follows: piperacillin > mezlocillin, ticarcillin > carbenicillin.

The addition of β-*lactamase inhibitors* (clavulanic acid or sulbactam) to ampicillin, amoxicillin, or ticarcillin extends the spectrum of these agents to include many organisms that are resistant by virtue of β-lactamase production. These species include *E. coli, Klebsiella,* all *Proteus* spp., *H. influenzae, Moraxella* (formerly *Branhamella*) *catarrhalis, Providencia,* and *B. fragilis*. Such combinations are also active against staphylococci that produce β-lactamase but are not methicillin-resistant. However, the efficacy of these combinations in serious staphylococcal infections has not been adequately proven. Furthermore, *Enterobacter, Pseudomonas, Acinetobacter,* and various enteric gram-negative isolates either produce β-lactamases not inhibited by these compounds or develop resistance attributable to non-β-lactamase-mediated mechanisms.

The *first-generation cephalosporins* have a spectrum that includes penicillinase-producing, methicillin-susceptible staphylococci and streptococci. While these drugs may be used when infections with gram-positive bacteria are suspected, they are *not* the drugs of choice for such infections. They have excellent activity against many isolates of *E. coli, K. pneumoniae,* and *P. mirabilis* and are among the drugs of choice in presumptive therapy for non-hospital-acquired urinary tract infections. They have no activity against *B. fragilis*, enterococci, methicillin-resistant staphylococci, *Pseudomonas, Acinetobacter, Enterobacter*, indole-positive *Proteus*, and *Serratia* and poor activity against *H. influenzae*.

The *parenteral second-generation cephalosporins* extend the gram-negative spectrum of first-generation compounds. The various second-generation agents have differing activities. Cefuroxime and cefamandole retain activity against gram-positive cocci and are also active against *H. influenzae, Neisseria*, some *Enterobacter* isolates, and indole-positive *Proteus* but exhibit poor activity against *B. fragilis*. Cefoxitin and cefotetan have reasonably good activity against *B. fragilis*, but cefotetan is less effective against some other *Bacteriodes* spp. (see Chaps. 86 and 128). However, they display poor activity against gram-positive cocci and *Enterobacter*. No second-generation cephalosporin is active against *Pseudomonas* or *Acinetobacter*.

Oral second-generation cephalosporins have fair activity against gram-positive cocci and *H. influenzae* and are widely used in outpatient therapy for otitis media, sinusitis, and lower respiratory tract infections, although cheaper agents that are equally effective are preferable. Cefixime is one of the drugs of choice for single-dose treatment of gonococcal urethritis.

Third-generation cephalosporins all have a broad spectrum of activity against enteric gram-negative rods and are especially useful for treating hospital-acquired infections caused by multiresistant organisms. In addition, ceftazidime has excellent antipseudomonal activity. Cefoperazone has modest antipseudomonal activity, and the other third-generation cephalosporins have poor antipseudomonal activity. Since resistance to third-generation cephalosporins is increasing among all nosocomial gram-negative rods, the use of these agents should be guided by susceptibility testing. The gram-positive spectrum of the third-generation cephalosporins is variable, the relative rank being cefotaxime, ceftizoxime, ceftriaxone > cefoperazone > ceftazidime. Because of its excellent gram-negative spectrum, its activity against *Haemophilus*, *S. pneumoniae*, and penicillin-resistant *Neisseria*, its long serum half-life, and its high serum and CSF levels, ceftriaxone has become one of the drugs of choice for presumptive therapy for bacterial meningitis (except that caused by *Listeria*), all gonococcal infections, salmonellosis, and typhoid fever and is one of the drugs of choice for nonpseudomonal, hospital-acquired pneumonia. Third-generation cephalosporins have poor activity against *B. fragilis* and no activity against methicillin-resistant staphylococci, *Enterococcus*, *Acinetobacter*, or *Xanthomonas*.

The only *carbapenem* currently available in the United States is imipenem, marketed in combination with the renal dipeptidase inhibitor cilastatin, which enables imipenem to escape renal inactivation, thus increasing urinary levels of the drug. Imipenem has a spectrum that provides excellent activity in vitro against virtually all bacterial pathogens except *Xanthomonas*, methicillin-resistant staphylococci, and *E. faecium*. Limitations to its use are its relatively low blood levels, short serum half-life, central nervous system side effects, and cost. Resistance to imipenem is a problem only among nosocomial isolates of *P. aeruginosa*, approximately 20 percent of which are resistant. Imipenem is *not* the drug of choice for any bacterial infection, but because of its broad spectrum, it can be used as presumptive therapy for serious nosocomial infections thought to be caused by multiple bacterial species or multiresistant organisms. This antibiotic is often held in reserve as therapy for nosocomial infections due to gram-negative pathogens resistant to third-generation cephalosporins.

The only *monobactam* currently available is aztreonam. This antibiotic has a spectrum limited to facultative, gram-negative enteric bacilli. It has no activity against any gram-positive or anaerobic bacterium. Its gram-negative spectrum is similar to that of ceftazidime, with equally good activity against *Pseudomonas*. Its primary advantages are its theoretical ability to preserve the normal gram-positive and anaerobic flora and the lack of cross-reactive immediate hypersensitivity reactions in patients with histories of these reactions to other β-lactam antibiotics.

VANCOMYCIN The spectrum of vancomycin is limited to gram-positive cocci, especially streptococci and staphylococci. It is second-line therapy for most gram-positive bacterial infections but is the drug of choice for infections caused by methicillin-resistant staphylococci or the JK group of *Corynebacterium* and for serious infections in penicillin-allergic patients. Given orally (a route by which it is not absorbed), it is one of the drugs of choice for antibiotic-associated pseudomembranous colitis caused by *C. difficile*.

AMINOGLYCOSIDES The aminoglycosides are rapidly bactericidal in vitro at low concentrations, with activity limited to facultative gram-negative bacteria and staphylococci. They have no activity against anaerobic bacteria and are not effective in environments that are acidic or have a low oxygen tension. However, their spectrum includes virtually all gram-negative bacteria that are not strict anaerobes, and they are among the drugs of choice for any suspected gram-negative bacteremic infection, particularly in neutropenic patients. Aminoglycosides are synergistically bactericidal in combination with a penicillin for treating staphylococcal, enterococcal, or viridans streptococcal endocarditis and are usually combined with a β-lactam antibiotic for treating gram-negative bacteremia. Aminoglycosides are also among the drugs of choice for severe infections of the upper urinary tract. The major limitations to aminoglycoside use are their

renal and otic toxicity, their diminished activity at certain sites of infection (e.g., abscesses and the central nervous system), the resistance of target bacteria, and the need to monitor serum levels to minimize the risk of toxicity and to ensure adequate concentrations. Among the available agents, gentamicin is generally preferred because of its low cost, but tobramycin has slightly greater activity against *P. aeruginosa*, and amikacin retains activity against many tobramycin- and gentamicin-resistant gram-negative bacteria because it is inactivated by fewer aminoglycoside-modifying enzymes. Streptomycin is still one of the drugs of choice in initial therapy for tularemia, plague, glanders, and brucellosis and is a second-line agent for treating tuberculosis.

MACROLIDES Erythromycin has broad spectrum activity against gram-positive bacteria, with additional activity against *Legionella*, *Mycoplasma, Campylobacter*, and some *Chlamydia* isolates. It is the drug of choice for infections due to *Legionella, Campylobacter*, and *Mycoplasma* and is one of the drugs of choice for pneumococcal pneumonia and pharyngitis and for skin and soft tissue infections due to group A streptococci in penicillin-allergic patients. However, resistance to erythromycin among group A streptococci and pneumococci is increasing in some countries. Erythromycin also appears to be one of the drugs of choice for infections caused in immunocompromised patients by the newly identified agent of bacillary angiomatosis (*Rochalimaea henselae*). The newer macrolides clarithromycin and azithromycin have an antibacterial spectrum similar to that of erythromycin in vitro. However, azithromycin has greater activity against *Chlamydia*. Both are active against nontuberculous mycobacteria, and both appear to have fewer gastrointestinal side effects than does erythromycin.

LINCOSAMIDES The only lincosamide used in the United States is clindamycin. It shares the gram-positive coccal spectrum of erythromycin but is more active, in some cases showing bactericidal activity, against susceptible staphylococci. However, resistance among staphylococci and many streptococci, mediated by the same genes responsible for macrolide resistance, limits clindamycin's usefulness against gram-positive cocci. In general, all gram-positive cocci resistant to erythromycin should be considered resistant to clindamycin regardless of the results of in vitro susceptibility testing. Clindamycin is one of the drugs of choice for anaerobic infections because of its broad spectrum of activity against both gram-positive and gram-negative strict anaerobes. In contrast, clindamycin, like erythromycin, has no clinically significant activity against facultative gram-negative enteric bacilli. Appropriate use is limited only by resistance or the development of pseudomembranous colitis, the major serious side effect of this drug.

CHLORAMPHENICOL Chloramphenicol has a broad spectrum of activity against gram-positive and gram-negative bacteria, although plasmid-mediated resistance has diminished its effective spectrum. However, this antibiotic is rarely used in adult infections because of the rare idiosyncratic side effect of irreversible bone marrow aplasia and the availability of other agents with similar activity. It remains one of the drugs of choice for typhoid fever and plague and is still useful for the treatment of brucellosis and both pneumococcal and meningococcal meningitis in penicillin-allergic patients.

TETRACYCLINES Tetracyclines have a broad spectrum of bacteriostatic activity against gram-positive and gram-negative bacteria and are widely used in a variety of non-hospital-acquired infections. These agents are among the drugs of choice for chronic bronchitis, granuloma inguinale, brucellosis (with streptomycin), tularemia, glanders, melioidosis, spirochetal infections caused by *Borrelia* (Lyme disease and relapsing fever; doxycycline), infections caused by *Vibrio vulnificus*, some *Aeromonas* infections, infections caused by *Xanthomonas* (minocycline), and plague. The tetracyclines are also used in penicillin-allergic patients for treating leptospirosis, syphilis, actinomycosis, and skin and soft tissue infections caused by gram-positive cocci. They are among the drugs of choice for infections due to chlamydiae (doxycycline) and rickettsiae and for granulomatous skin infection due to *M. marinum* (minocycline).

SULFONAMIDES AND TRIMETHOPRIM   The folic acid synthesis inhibitors have a broad spectrum of bacteriostatic activity individually; in combination, they can be bactericidal against facultative gram-negative bacteria and staphylococci. The fixed combination of sulfamethoxazole and trimethoprim, the major folic acid synthesis inhibitors used in therapy for bacterial infections, has only modest activity against some streptococci and no activity against strict anaerobes. The individual sulfonamides are rarely used in the treatment of bacterial infections but are among the drugs of choice for treating nocardial infections, leprosy (dapsone, a sulfone), and toxoplasmosis (sulfadiazine). Trimethoprim-sulfamethoxazole is the drug of choice for the treatment of uncomplicated urinary tract infections (except for those caused by enterococcci) and is widely used in the treatment of otitis media. It can be used in therapy for upper respiratory tract infections in which *H. influenzae* and *M. catarrhalis* are suspected, gonococcal and meningococcal infections, chancroid, and infections thought to be caused by *Aeromonas, Xanthomonas, P. cepacia, Acinetobacter*, and *Yersinia enterocolitica*. For nosocomial infections due to *Xanthomonas*, trimethoprim-sulfamethoxazole is the drug of choice.

FLUOROQUINOLONES   The fluoroquinolones have excellent activity against most facultative gram-negative rods, fair activity against staphylococci, variable to poor activity against streptococci, and no activity against obligate anaerobes. They are the oral agents with greatest activity against *P. aeruginosa*; ciprofloxacin is the most active against this species. All the quinolones have good to excellent oral absorption, while ciprofloxacin and ofloxacin are also administered as intravenous formulations. Treatment with norfloxacin can be used for urinary tract infections, and it has been recommended for infectious diarrhea. However, it should not be used for systemic gram-negative infections; the other quinolones should be used for this purpose. The quinolones are among the drugs of choice for complicated urinary tract infections, bacterial gastroenteritis, and enteric fever and may be useful in therapy for chronic infections caused by gram-negative organisms, such as osteomyelitis and chronic otitis externa in adults. The use of quinolones is limited by the development of resistance among staphylococci and *P. aeruginosa* and by interactions with other drugs.

RIFAMPIN   Rifampin has been used in combinations for the treatment of serious infections due to methicillin-resistant staphylococci (e.g., coagulase-negative staphylococcal foreign-body infections). Because the spontaneous selection of rifampin-resistant mutants occurs rapidly, rifampin should never be used alone in treating staphylococcal infections. Rifampin is also used in the chemoprophylaxis of persons at risk for developing meningococcal meningitis and in the therapy of *Legionella* pneumonia.

METRONIDAZOLE   Metronidazole has a spectrum limited to anaerobic bacteria. It is one of the drugs of choice for the treatment of any abscess in which the involvement of obligate anaerobes is suspected (e.g., lung, brain, or intraabdominal abscesses) because of its spectrum and its ability to penetrate into the area of infection. Other antibacterial agents should be used in combination with metronidazole if additional facultative and aerobic pathogens are suspected. Metronidazole is also one of the drugs of choice for treating bacterial vaginosis and antibiotic-associated pseudomembranous colitis.

URINARY TRACT ANTISEPTICS   Urinary tract antiseptics are active only in the lower urinary tract and cannot be used for treating upper urinary tract or systemic infections. Their activity is limited to susceptible gram-negative enteric bacteria. The available agents in this category include nitrofurantoin and methenamine salts.

TOPICAL ANTIBACTERIAL AGENTS   Mupirocin is available only as a topical preparation for use against staphylococci and streptococci. Its major applications are for impetigo and eradication of the staphylococcal carrier state. It is the drug of choice for the elimination of nasal carriage of both methicillin-susceptible and methicillin-resistant staphylococci. Unfortunately, the emergence of resistance is limiting its usefulness in some hospitals.

Although their efficacy has never been well documented, topical preparations that include sulfonamides, polymyxin B, neomycin, bacitracin, gramicidin, and novobiocin in a variety of combinations are widely used as eye drops, irrigation solutions, and ointments for superficial skin infections.

ADVERSE REACTIONS

Adverse drug reactions are frequently classified by mechanism as either dose-related ("toxic") effects or unpredictable reactions. Unpredictable reactions are further categorized as either idiosyncratic or allergic. Dose-related reactions include aminoglycoside nephrotoxicity, penicillin-induced seizures, and vancomycin anaphylactoid reactions. Many of these reactions can be avoided by reducing dosage, limiting the duration of therapy, or reducing the frequency or rate of administration. Adverse reactions to antibacterial agents are a common cause of morbidity, requiring alteration in therapy and additional expense, and they occasionally result in death. The elderly, often those with the more severe infections, may be especially prone to certain adverse reactions. These reactions to antibacterial agents are summarized below.

β-LACTAMS   The therapeutic index for β-lactam antibiotics is large, and dose-related adverse reactions are uncommon and largely preventable. The greatest concern is allergic reactions. All types can occur, including anaphylaxis (type 1, hypersensitivity reactions), nephritis and Coombs-positive hemolytic anemia (type 2, cytotoxic reactions), drug fever and serum sickness (type 3, immune-complex formation), contact dermatitis (type 4, cell-mediated effects), and maculopapular eruption (type 5, idiopathic reactions). Approximately 1 to 4 percent of treatment courses result in an allergic reaction, and approximately 0.004 to 0.015 percent of treatment courses result in anaphylaxis. Fewer than half the patients who claim an allergy to penicillin react to skin testing with the major and minor determinants (penicilloyl polylysine and benzylpenicillin degradation products, respectively); those with negative skin tests only rarely react adversely to subsequent therapeutic doses. However, a careful history for allergy is still required before any β-lactam is administered, since the consequences may be life-threatening. Generally, a suitable alternative to β-lactams is available for patients who have a severe allergy, and penicillin desensitization can be carefully undertaken if there is no suitable alternative. A small number of persons (<2 percent) who are allergic to penicillin react similarly when a cephalosporin is administered; thus the latter drugs are contraindicated in patients with a history of an immediate reaction to penicillin (although they are often used in patients with a history of mild reactions). The same precaution applies to imipenem, but aztreonam is antigenically distinct and can be administered safely to the penicillin-allergic patient.

Other reactions thought to have an allergic basis include nephritis (associated with methicillin), hepatitis (related to oxacillin), leukopenia (following high doses of most β-lactams administered for prolonged periods), and severe skin rashes (toxic epidermal necrolysis and Stevens-Johnson syndrome). These reactions are not IgE-mediated, and skin testing is not predictive of their occurrence. For unclear reasons, most patients who have infectious mononucleosis develop a rash when given ampicillin.

Miscellaneous reactions to β-lactams include gastrointestinal side effects ranging in severity from mild diarrhea (5 to 10 percent) to pseudomembranous colitis (<1 percent). Drugs excreted to a large extent through the bile, such as ampicillin, ceftriaxone, and cefoperazone, may be especially prone to cause diarrhea. The addition of clavulanic acid to amoxicillin further increases the frequencey of diarrhea. Ceftriaxone, because of extremely high concentrations in bile, can cause "sludging" in the gall bladder and occasionally cause symptoms compatible with acute cholecystitis.

In high doses—and most often in patients with renal impairment who receive an excessive dose—penicillins (especially carbenicillin, ticarcillin, and penicillin G) can cause bleeding from impaired platelet aggregation. In addition, bleeding also is occasionally associated with use of cephalosporins containing a methylthiotetrazole group at the 3′ position (most commonly, cefamandole and cefoperazone); this reaction may result from impairment of prothrombin formation. These same cephalosporins can cause a disulfiram-like reaction if ethanol is administered. Carbenicillin and ticarcillin are disodium salts and in high doses can cause hypokalemia and fluid overload.

Seizures are occasionally observed with β-lactams, especially penicillin G and imipenem. This reaction is most common when excessive doses relative to renal function are administered or in patients with a history of seizures.

VANCOMYCIN   When vancomycin was first used clinically in 1956, local intolerance at the infusion site was common, as were systemic reactions, including ototoxicity and nephrotoxicity. Current formulations are of higher purity and, with proper dosage guidelines, are very safe, although phlebitis can still be troublesome. The most common adverse reaction is called *red man syndrome* and is characterized by pruritus, flushing, and erythema of the head and upper torso. This anaphylactoid reaction usually follows the first dose, is dependent on dose and infusion time, and results from vancomycin-induced release of histamine. The reaction is usually mild in adult patients who receive 1 g over 60 min and diminishes with repeated doses. If vancomycin is mistakenly given as a bolus, severe hypotension may result. In unusually sensitive patients, extending the infusion time or administering H-1 receptor antagonists is usually effective in preventing this reaction or reducing its severity. Patients with this reaction must not be mislabeled as having an allergy to vancomycin, since vancomycin may be the only effective treatment for certain infections, such as those due to methicillin-resistant staphylococci.

Nephrotoxicity from vancomycin is mild and occurs in fewer than 5 percent of patients. Although some data suggest that aminoglycosides and vancomycin are synergistically nephrotoxic, this is difficult to prove, and the simultaneous use of these agents should not be avoided if clinically indicated, as in the treatment of enterococcal endocarditis in penicillin-allergic patients.

Ototoxicity from vancomycin is rare as long as doses are appropriately reduced in patients with renal insufficiency. Other uncommon adverse reactions include leukopenia, skin rashes, and true allergy.

AMINOGLYCOSIDES   Aminoglycoside antibiotics have a narrow therapeutic index. The two most common adverse reactions are nephrotoxicity and ototoxicity. Rarely, respiratory depression is observed. Nephrotoxicity results from accumulation of the aminoglycoside in the peritubular space, with damage to the proximal tubule and a corresponding reduction in the glomerular filtration rate. The incidence of nephrotoxicity, defined as a greater than 0.5 percent increase over baseline in serum creatinine, is approximately 5 to 10 percent among adult patients who receive a therapeutic course for 10 to 14 days. However, many cofactors also influence the frequency of toxicity, such as extremes of age (toxicity is uncommon among children, more common among the elderly), concomitant drug therapy, hydration status, and magnitude of serum concentrations. Toxicity is manifested clinically by a gradual rise in serum creatinine after a few days of therapy and is reversible if the dosage is reduced or discontinued. Serum creatinine levels should be monitored every 3 to 5 days or more often if changes are seen. There is not an important difference in the frequency of nephrotoxicity among the most useful agents (gentamicin, tobramycin, and amikacin); streptomycin is a rare cause of nephrotoxicity.

Ototoxicity from aminoglycoside therapy presents as either auditory or vestibular damage. Since the aminoglycosides can destroy hair cells within the inner ear, this ototoxicity may be permanent. The risk of ototoxicity increases with prolonged therapy, higher serum concentrations (especially in patients with renal impairment), hypovolemia, and concurrent treatment with other ototoxins, especially ethacrynic acid. Clinically apparent ototoxicity, manifested by diminished acuity or vestibular imbalance, is uncommon (probably occurring in <1 percent of cases) when serum concentrations are monitored and the duration of therapy is kept to a minimum. With

more sensitive monitoring, e.g., audiograms, asymptomatic high-tone hearing loss is more commonly noted. There are no clinically important differences in the overall frequency of ototoxicity among the aminoglycosides.

Neuromuscular depression from aminoglycosides is caused by reduced acetylcholine activity at postsynaptic membranes and can result in rare but severe respiratory depression. Risk factors include hypocalcemia, peritoneal administration, use of neuromuscular blockers, and preexisting respiratory depression. It is largely avoided by administering the aminoglycoside IV over 30 min or by IM injection; if respiratory depression occurs, it is antagonized by the administration of calcium.

Fear of toxicity should not prevent the use of aminoglycosides when there is a legitimate indication, since toxicity is usually mild and reversible. Serum concentrations are monitored both to minimize the risk of toxicity and to ensure that sufficient drug is administered to treat targeted infections.

MACROLIDES   Serious adverse reactions to the macrolide antibiotics are very rare. Gastrointestinal effects, such as burning, nausea, and vomiting, are the most common adverse reactions to the macrolides; depending on dosage, these reactions may occur in up to 50 percent of patients, occasionally requiring early discontinuation of therapy. The mechanism is thought to be the binding of erythromycin to motilin receptors, with a consequent increase in gastrointestinal motility. Gastrointestinal side effects appear equally common for all the oral formulations and also occur with IV administration. Clarithromycin and possibly azithromycin may be better tolerated than erythromycin, although gastrointestinal distress is still their most common adverse effect.

Less common reactions include hepatotoxicity and ototoxicity. Hepatotoxicity is a rare, nonfatal complication of treatment with erythromycin estolate and appears as an allergic cholestatic jaundice. Ototoxicity is rare after oral administration but may occur in a dose-dependent pattern in up to 20 percent of adults who receive IV erythromycin (4 g/d) and have audiograms performed. Ototoxicity is usually reversible and mild. Allergic cutaneous reactions are observed in rare cases.

LINCOSAMIDES   The most common adverse effect of clindamycin is gastrointestinal distress. Diarrhea has been reported in up to 20 percent of patients and pseudomembranous colitis in 0.01 to 10 percent. The mechanism of pseudomembranous colitis is production of a toxin by *C. difficile* (see Chap. 108). *C. difficile* colonizes the gastrointestinal tract, and may produce a toxin when normal flora is suppressed by clindamycin. This toxin causes mucosal damage that results in cramps, pain, and diarrhea that may be bloody. Pseudomembranous colitis may follow both IV and oral administration and may not become manifest until after completion of therapy. Oral metronidazole or vancomycin is effective in treating symptomatic patients with toxin-positive stools, but some spores may survive and relapse is frequent. Although diarrhea and pseudomembranous colitis can be caused by most antibacterial agents, the incidence in relation to the amount used appears to be highest for clindamycin. Allergic reactions (such as rashes and fever), hepatotoxicity, and neutropenia are observed only rarely.

CHLORAMPHENICOL   Chloramphenicol causes two types of bone marrow suppression; a dose-related, reversible suppression of all elements, which occurs commonly during therapy at the maximal recommended doses (4 g/d in adults), and an idiosyncratic, irreversible aplastic anemia, which occurs in approximately 1 in every 25,000 to 40,000 exposures. The irreversible form has been reported to follow all types of chloramphenicol treatment, including ocular administration, and often develops months after therapy is discontinued.

In premature neonates and infants, chloramphenicol can cause a dose-related "gray syndrome" characterized by cyanosis, hypotension, and death resulting from an inability of the newborn to metabolize chloramphenicol. These potentially serious toxicities and the availability of newer drugs have substantially reduced the indications for chloramphenicol.

TETRACYCLINES Gastrointestinal effects are the most common adverse reactions to the tetracyclines. These problems may be related to a direct irritant effect, since tetracyclines also can cause esophageal ulceration when they dissolve before reaching the stomach. Concurrent food intake may improve tolerance, but absorption of tetracycline HCl is impaired when it is taken with food.

Hepatotoxicity has been reported after administration of more than 2 g of tetracycline IV and at lower doses during pregnancy. There are currently no indications for IV tetracycline treatment in pregnancy. All tetracyclines can cause phototoxic skin reactions, although they are most common with doxycycline. Other dermal reactions, including rash, are uncommon. Tetracyclines are contraindicated in children less than 8 years of age because of mottling of the permanent teeth, although doxycycline may be less likely to cause this problem. Worsening of renal function in patients with preexisting renal dysfunction has been reported with use of tetracycline, although some of the increased azotemia may be due to amino acid catabolism. Doxycycline and perhaps minocycline appear to be free from these renal side effects. Alternative effective agents are nearly always available for use in such patients. Minocycline can cause vertigo in up to 70 percent of women receiving therapeutic doses, with a lower frequency in men.

SULFONAMIDES AND TRIMETHOPRIM The sulfonamides are generally safe, but the list of possible adverse reactions is very long. These compounds occasionally cause a number of allergic reactions, from relatively minor skin rashes (including maculopapular rashes and urticarial reactions typically appearing after a week of therapy) to severe, life-threatening reactions such as erythema multiforme, Stevens-Johnson syndrome, and toxic epidermal necrolysis. The severe hypersensitivity reactions have occurred most commonly after treatment with the "long-acting" sulfonamides, such as sulfamethoxypyridazine, which are no longer used. Fansidar (pyrimethamine plus sulfadoxine), used for malaria prophylaxis, may cause severe allergic reactions, including hepatic and hematologic toxicities, in addition to dermatologic toxicity. Photosensitivity reactions are also relatively common with sulfonamides.

For reasons that are not clear, many patients infected with human immunodeficiency virus (HIV) who receive trimethoprim-sulfamethoxazole have adverse dermatologic reactions. These are usually not life-threatening and appear to regress in many cases despite continuation of therapy.

Sulfonamides and trimethoprim also may cause severe hematologic complications, including agranulocytosis, hemolytic and megaloblastic anemia, and thrombocytopenia. These dose-related side effects may be greater in patients with renal insufficiency. Hemolytic anemia is most common in patients with glucose-6-phosphate dehydrogenase (G6PD) deficiency who take long-acting compounds; trimethoprim-sulfamethoxazole rarely causes hemolysis in such subjects. Granulocytopenia from trimethoprim-sulfamethoxazole is especially common in HIV-infected patients, occurring in 10 to 50 percent of subjects.

Renal insufficiency, caused by crystals of the relatively insoluble acetyl metabolite, is observed primarily with the long-acting sulfonamides. A number of cases of crystalluria in HIV-infected patients taking sulfadiazine for toxoplasmosis have been reported. A high level of fluid intake and urinary alkalization may prevent this complication.

It is recommended that sulfonamides not be administered to the newborn because of concerns that bilirubin may be displaced from protein binding sites, with subsequent jaundice and kernicterus.

In addition to the preceding problems, sulfonamides may occasionally cause drug fever with serum sickness, hepatic toxicity (including necrosis), systemic lupus erythematosus, and central nervous system symptoms such as drowsiness, fatigue, and insomnia.

FLUOROQUINOLONES Fluoroquinolones are relatively safe; adverse reactions rarely require discontinuation of therapy. The most common reactions include gastrointestinal distress, such as nausea or diarrhea (<5 percent), and central nervous system effects, including insomnia and dizziness (<5 percent). Rarely, hepatic and renal dysfunction and anaphylactoid and allergic reactions are observed. The use of these drugs is contraindicated in children less than 18 years of age because of evidence in animals of cartilage damage in developing joints. In carefully selected situations, in which the perceived benefits outweigh the risks, such as in adolescent patients with cystic fibrosis who have pulmonary exacerbations, fluoroquinolones may be useful for short-term therapy. They are contraindicated in pregnancy because of concern for the developing fetus. Temafloxacin was withdrawn after a few months on the world market because it occasionally caused hypoglycemia in the elderly and hemolysis with renal failure.

RIFAMPIN Rifampin is generally well tolerated but has several important side effects. Some patients have transient rises in hepatic transaminases, but these levels usually return to normal without discontinuation of the drug. Although hepatitis from rifampin itself develops only rarely, the drug is thought by some investigators to potentiate the hepatic toxicity of concomitantly administered isoniazid. Intermittent administration of rifampin, usually less than three times per week, has been associated with symptoms that seem to have an immunologic basis. These include flulike symptoms and (rarely) hemolysis, thrombocytopenia, shock, and renal failure. Minor gastrointestinal side effects, skin rashes, and interstitial nephritis also have been reported. Patients should be warned that rifampin and its metabolites cause secretions such as urine, tears, sweat, and saliva to turn orange and that contact lenses may be stained.

METRONIDAZOLE Serious adverse reactions to metronidazole are uncommon. Gastrointestinal side effects such as nausea are most frequent but rarely necessitate discontinuation of therapy. Pseudomembranous colitis in association with metronidazole has been reported but appears to be very rare. A metallic taste is relatively common, and stomatitis and glossitis are occasionally reported. Disulfiram-like reactions can occur if ethanol is administered. Peripheral neuropathy occurs in some patients, and seizures and encephalopathy have been reported after high doses or in patients with hepatic failure.

Concerns about mutagenicity and carcinogenicity from metronidazole have led to recommendations that it not be used in pregnancy (especially during the first trimester) when alternative agents are available. Although retrospective studies have found no association between metronidazole and carcinogenesis, long-term administration of high doses should be avoided when therapeutic alternatives are available.

DRUG INTERACTIONS

Historically, clinically important interactions involving antibacterial drugs were generally of little concern, since β-lactams were the most widely used agents and rarely interacted with other drugs in a manner that affected the patient adversely. However, fluoroquinolones, macrolides, and rifampin are more widely used, and interactions are of increasing concern. Table 100-4 lists the most common and best documented interactions and their clinical relevance. Coadministration of two of the drugs paired in Table 100-4 does not necessarily result in clinically important adverse consequences. The result also depends on timing of administration, dose and duration of therapy, baseline serum concentration of the non-antibacterial drug administered, the patient's susceptibility to the pharmacologic effect of the non-antibacterial drug, and other less well described cofactors. Recognition of the potential for an interaction before the administration of an antibacterial agent is crucial to the rational use of these drugs, since adverse consequences often can be prevented if the interaction is anticipated. Table 100-4 is intended only to heighten awareness of the potential for an interaction. Additional sources should be consulted to identify appropriate options.

MACROLIDES Erythromycin can inhibit the hepatic metabolism of many concurrently administered drugs, such as theophylline, carbamazepine, terfenadine, warfarin, and ergot alkaloids—an effect

TABLE 100-4 Interactions of antibacterial agents with other drugs

Antibacterial agent (A)	Drug (B)	Effect	Clinical relevance*
Erythromycin	Theophylline	Increased levels of B	1
	Carbamazepine	Increased levels of B	1
	Digoxin	Increased levels of B	3
	Triazolam	Increased levels of B	2
	Ergotamine	Increased levels of B	1
	Warfarin	Increased levels of B	2
	Cyclosporine	Increased levels of B	1
	Terfenadine/astemazole	Increased levels of B	1
	Valproate	Increased levels of B	2
Fluoroquinolones	Theophylline	Increased levels of B[†]	2
	Divalent/trivalent cations (Al, Fe, Mg, etc.)	Decreased levels of A	1
Tetracyclines	Divalent/trivalent cations	Decreased levels of A	1
	Digoxin	Increased levels of B	3
Sulfonamides	Oral hypoglycemic agent	Increased levels of B	2
	Phenytoin	Increased levels of B	2
	Warfarin	Increased levels of B	2
Metronidazole	Ethanol	Disulfiram-like reaction	2
	Warfarin	Increased levels of B	2
Rifampin	Warfarin	Decreased levels of B	1
	Oral contraceptive	Decreased levels of B	1
	Cyclosporine	Decreased levels of B	1
	Oral hypoglycemic	Decreased levels of B	1
	Glucocortoids	Decreased levels of B	1
	Methadone	Decreased levels of B	1
	Digoxin/digitoxin	Decreased levels of B	1
	Quinidine	Decreased levels of B	1
	Azole antifungal agent	Decreased levels of B	2
	Phenytoin	Decreased levels of B	2
	Zidovudine	Decreased levels of B	1
	Diltiazem	Decreased levels of B	1
	Verapamil	Decreased levels of B	1

* 1 = a well-documented interaction with clinically important consequences; 2 = an interaction of uncertain frequency but possible clinical importance; 3 = an unusual interaction of possible clinical importance in some patients.
† Enoxacin > ciprofloxacin > norfloxacin/ofloxacin > lomefloxacin.

leading to increased serum concentrations and toxicity. The magnitude of the theophylline interaction is highly variable and proportional to the dose and duration of erythromycin treatment. In contrast, cyclosporine levels predictably increase when erythromycin is administered, since erythromycin inhibits the specific enzyme responsible for cyclosporine metabolism. Decreased metabolism of terfenadine and probably astemazole has been reported to cause severe cardiac dysfunction. Clarithromycin appears to be similar to erythromycin in its inhibitory potential, although azithromycin may have little effect on the metabolism of other drugs. In approximately 10 percent of patients receiving digoxin, concentrations will increase when erythromycin is also given; the mechanism is increased absorption of digoxin because of the killing of digoxin-metabolizing bacteria by erythromycin.

TETRACYCLINES Drug interactions with tetracyclines are relatively uncommon. The most important interaction is the reduction in absorption when tetracyclines are coadministered with di- and trivalent cations, such as antacids, iron compounds, or dairy products. A similar interaction is seen with quinolones (see below). Food also adversely affects absorption of most tetracyclines. Inducers of hepatic isoenzymes, such as phenytoin and barbiturates, increase the clearance of doxycycline; although the clinical significance of this effect is unknown, use of an alternative antibiotic may be appropriate.

SULFONAMIDES Sulfonamides may increase the hypoprothrombinemic effect of warfarin by inhibition of metabolism of the more potent isomer of warfarin and possibly by protein-binding displacement. Sulfonamides also may potentiate the effects of oral hypoglycemic agents and phenytoin through reduction in metabolism or displacement from serum protein.

FLUOROQUINOLONES There are two clinically important drug interactions with fluoroquinolones. First, as with tetracyclines, divalent and trivalent cations chelate all fluoroquinolones and prevent most of the dose from being absorbed. Second, certain fluoroquinolones (enoxacin, ciprofloxacin, and, to a lesser extent, norfloxacin and

ofloxacin, but not lomefloxacin) can inhibit hepatic enzymes which metabolize theophylline, with resultant theophylline toxicity. The same mechanism accounts for increases in serum caffeine concentrations, but the clinical significance of this interaction is unknown. Scattered reports indicate that quinolones also can potentiate the nephrotoxicity of cyclosporine, exaggerate the effects of warfarin, and increase neurotoxicity when coadministered with nonsteroidal anti-inflammatory agents. However, these interactions have not been confirmed by controlled trials.

RIFAMPIN Rifampin is an excellent inducer of many cytochrome P450 enzymes and increases the hepatic clearance of a number of drugs, including the following (with the indicated predictable outcomes): oral contraceptives (pregnancy), warfarin (decreased prothrombin times), cyclosporine and prednisone (organ rejection or exacerbations of any underlying inflammatory condition), and verapamil and diltiazem (increased dosage requirements).

METRONIDAZOLE Metronidazole can cause a disulfiram-like syndrome when alcohol is ingested, and patients should be instructed to avoid alcohol. Inhibition of the metabolism of warfarin by metronidazole leads to significant rises in prothrombin times.

PROPHYLAXIS OF BACTERIAL INFECTIONS

INDICATIONS FOR PROPHYLAXIS Antibacterial agents are occasionally indicated for use in patients who have no evidence of infection but who have been or are expected to be exposed to bacterial pathogens under circumstances that constitute a major risk of infection. The basic tenets of antimicrobial prophylaxis are as follows: First, the risk or potential severity of infection should be greater than the risk of side effects from the antibacterial agent. Second, the antibacterial agent should be given for the shortest period necessary to prevent target infections. Third, the antibacterial agent should be given before the expected period of risk (e.g., surgical prophylaxis) or as soon as

TABLE 100-5   Prophylaxis of bacterial infections in adults

Condition	Antibacterial agent	Duration of prophylaxis
Nonsurgical		
Cardiac lesions susceptible to bacterial endocarditis	Amoxicillin*	Before and after procedures causing bacteremia
Recurrent *S. aureus* infections	Mupirocin	Intranasally for 5 days
Contact with patient with meningococcal meningitis	Rifampin	2 days
Bite wounds[†]	Penicillin V or amoxicillin–clavulanic acid	3–5 days
Recurrent cystitis	Trimethoprim-sulfamethoxazole	3 times per week for up to 1 year or after sexual intercourse
Surgical		
Clean (cardiac, vascular, neurologic, orthopedic)	Cefazolin (vancomycin)[‡]	Before and during procedure
Ocular	Topical combinations and subconjunctival cefazolin	During and at end of procedure
Clean-contaminated (head and neck, high-risk gastroduodenal, biliary tract, cesarean section, hysterectomy)	Cefazolin (or clindamycin for head and neck)	Before and during procedure
Clean-contaminated (colorectal, appendectomy)	Cefoxitin or cefotetan (add oral neomycin + erythromycin for colorectal)	Before and during procedure
Dirty[†] (ruptured viscus)	Cefoxitin or cefotetan ± gentamicin (clindamycin + gentamicin) or another appropriate regimen directed at anaerobes and gram-negative aerobes	Before and for 3–5 days after procedure
Dirty[†] (traumatic wound)	Cefazolin	Before and for 3–5 days after trauma

* Gentamicin should be added to amoxicillin for high-risk gastrointestinal and gentourinary procedures.
[†] In these cases, use of antibacterial agents is actually treatment of infection rather than prophylaxis.
[‡] Vancomycin is recommended only in those institutions which have a high incidence of infection with methicillin-resistant staphylococci.

possible after contact with an infected individual (e.g., prophylaxis for meningococcal meningitis).

Table 100-5 lists the major indications for antibacterial prophylaxis in adults. (The use of antibacterial agents in children to prevent rheumatic fever and otitis media under certain circumstances is also common practice.) The table includes only those indications which are widely accepted, supported by well-designed studies, or recommended by expert panels. Those conditions for which prophylaxis is also used but is less widely accepted include administration of antibacterials to prevent recurrent cellulitis in conjunction with lymphedema, recurrent pneumococcal meningitis in patients with deficiencies in humoral immunity or CSF leaks, traveller's diarrhea, gram-negative sepsis in neutropenic patients, and spontaneous bacterial peritonitis in patients with ascites.

The major use of antibacterial prophylaxis in the United States is for infections following surgical procedures. Antibacterial agents are administered just before and, for long operations, during the surgical procedure in order to ensure high levels in serum and tissues during surgery. The objective is to eradicate bacteria originating from the air of the operating suite, the skin of the surgical team, or the patient's own flora that may contaminate the wound. In all but colorectal surgical procedures, prophylaxis is predominantly directed against staphylococci. Prophylaxis is intended to prevent wound infection or infection of implanted devices, not all infections that may occur during the postoperative period (e.g., urinary tract infections or pneumonia). Prolonged prophylaxis merely alters normal flora and favors infections with organisms resistant to the antibacterial agents used.

ANTIBACTERIAL COSTS AND INAPPROPRIATE USE   Use of antibacterial agents in hospitals in the United States accounts for 20 to 50 percent of all drug costs and represents the largest expenditure for any pharmacologic class. In the outpatient setting, costs of antibacterial drugs are second only to those of cardiovascular agents. It is not unusual for the purchase cost (in 1993 dollars) of a newer parenteral antibiotic to be $1000 to $2000 for a 10- to 14-day course of treatment. Therapy with a new oral antibiotic can easily cost $50 to $60. Administration costs, monitoring costs, and pharmacy charges must be added to these figures. While some newer antibacterial agents

undeniably represent important advances in therapy, many newer drugs offer no advantage over older, less expensive agents.

Clinicians are understandably confused by the bewildering array of available drugs. Numerous surveys have reported that approximately 50 percent of antibiotic use is in some way "inappropriate." Aside from the monetary cost of unnecessary antibiotics, there are the costs of excess morbidity from adverse effects and drug interactions and the eventual costs of treating more resistant organisms. The following suggestions are intended to provide guidance through the antibiotic maze. First, objective evidence regarding the merits of newer drugs is available through publications such as *The Medical Letter*, including the annual update of *Drugs of Choice*. Second, clinicians should become comfortable using a few drugs recommended by independent experts and should resist the temptation to use a new drug unless the merits are clear. A new antibacterial agent with a "broader spectrum and greater potency" or a "longer half-life and higher tissue levels" does not necessarily mean greater clinical efficacy. Third, the clinician must become familiar with local bacterial susceptibility profiles. It may not be necessary to use a new drug with "improved activity against *P. aeruginosa*" if that pathogen is rarely encountered or if it retains full susceptibility to older drugs. Finally, with regard to inpatient use of antibacterial drugs, appropriate empirical treatment with one or more broad-spectrum agents may often be simplified with use of a narrower-spectrum agent or even an oral drug once the results of cultures and susceptibility tests become available. While there is an understandable temptation to not alter effective therapy, no data suggest that switching to a more specific agent, once the patient has improved clinically, alters efficacy. If these guidelines are followed, the care of patients will not be compromised, many unnecessary complications and expenses can be avoided, and the useful life of valuable drugs will be extended.

REFERENCES

Antimicrobial prophylaxis in surgery. Med Lett Drugs Ther 34:5, 1992
DONOWITZ GR, MANDELL GL: Beta-lactam antibiotics. N Engl J Med 319:419, 1988
EBERT SC, CRAIG WA: Pharmacodynamic properties of antibiotics: Application of drug monitoring and dosage regimen design. Infect Control Hosp Epidemiol 11:319, 1990

Handbook of Adverse Drug Interactions: New Rochelle, The Medical Letter, 1991

HOOPER DC, WOLFSON JS: Fluoroquinolone antimicrobial agents. N Engl J Med 324:384, 1991

JACOBY GA, ARCHER GL: Mechanisms of disease: New mechanisms of bacterial resistance to antimicrobial agents. N Engl J Med 324:601, 1991

KUNIN CM: Problems in antibiotic usage, in *Principles and Practice of Infectious Disease*, GL Mandell et al (eds). New York, Churchill Livingstone, 1990, pp 427–434

O'HANLEY P et al: Infectious disorders, in *Basic Principles in Therapeutics*, KL Melmon et al (eds). New York, McGraw-Hill, 1992, pp 642–720

PRATT WB, FEKETY R (eds): *The Antimicrobial Drugs.* New York. Oxford University Press, 1986

The choice of antibacterial drugs: Med Lett Drugs Ther 34:49, 1992

section 5 Diseases caused by gram-positive bacteria

101 PNEUMOCOCCAL INFECTIONS

ROBERT AUSTRIAN

ETIOLOGY The pneumococcus *(Streptococcus pneumoniae)* is a gram-positive encapsulated coccus that usually grows in pairs or short chains. In the diplococcal form, the adjacent margins are rounded and the opposite ends slightly pointed, giving the organisms a lancet shape. In stained preparations of exudate, gram-negative forms are sometimes present. Pneumococcal colonies are surrounded by greenish discoloration on or in blood agar and are confused at times with other alpha-hemolytic streptococci to which they are closely related. Their isolation from respiratory secretions may be facilitated by inclusion of 5 μg gentamicin per milliliter in the medium. Pneumococci can be distinguished by their bile solubility and mouse virulence or by serologic typing. Another method with approximately 90 percent specificity, utilizing inhibition of pneumococci by Optochin-impregnated paper disks, is less cumbersome.

The capsular substances are complex polysaccharides and are the basis for dividing pneumococci into serotypes. Organisms exposed to type-specific antiserum show a positive capsular precipitin reaction, the Neufeld quellung reaction; by this means, 84 serotypes have been identified. All are pathogenic for human beings, but types or groups 3, 4, 6, 7, 9, 12, 14, 18, 19, and 23 are encountered currently most often in clinical practice. Types or groups 6, 9, 14, 19, and 23 frequently cause pneumonia and otitis media in children.

Specific typing of pneumococci remains of great clinical importance if pneumococcus is to be identified with regularity, and recognition of pneumococcus has decreased significantly since the abandonment of capsular typing by most clinical laboratories. The detection of pneumococcal capsular polysaccharides in sputum and other body fluids by immunologic methods such as counter-immuno-electrophoresis (CIE) or latex agglutination provides an alternative to bacteriologic techniques for the presumptive diagnosis of pneumococcal infection. Because of cross reactions between the polysaccharides of pneumococci and of other bacterial species, immunologic diagnosis is less specific than bacteriologic diagnosis.

PATHOGENESIS The mechanism by which pneumococci damage the mammalian host is obscure, and no toxin elaborated by the organism has been shown to play a major pathogenic role in pneumococcal infection, although the teichoic acid component of the cell wall may cause inflammation. The capsular polysaccharides, although nontoxic, are known to be necessary factors in virulence and to offer some protection of the organism from phagocytosis.

Although "pneumococcal pharyngitis" is a doubtful clinical entity, invasion of nasopharyngeal tissue may occur in the infant and occasionally in the nonimmune adult and be followed by spread to the circulation via the cervical lymphatics. At times, secondary infection of serous cavities in the absence of demonstrable focal infection of the upper or lower respiratory tract may occur. The

organisms multiply readily in vivo and may produce acute inflammation of the lungs, serous cavities, and endocardium.

The normal human respiratory tract is provided with a variety of mechanisms which guard the lungs from infection. The lower respiratory tract is protected by the glottis and larynx, and material passing these barriers stimulates the expulsive cough reflex. Removal of small particles impinging on the walls of the trachea and bronchi is facilitated by their mucociliary lining (see Chap. 220), and growth of bacteria reaching normal alveoli is inhibited by their relative dryness and by the phagocytic activity of alveolar macrophages. Any anatomic or physiologic derangement of these coordinated defenses tends to augment the susceptibility of the lungs to infection. Anesthesia, alcoholic intoxication, convulsions, and disturbed innervation of the larynx depress the cough reflex and may permit aspiration of infected material. Alterations in the tracheobronchial tree leading to anatomic changes in the epithelial lining or to localized obstruction increase the vulnerability of the lungs to infection. Pulmonary edema, local or generalized, resulting from viral infection, inhalation of irritant gases, cardiac failure, or contusion of the chest wall provides a fluid menstruum in the alveoli for the growth of bacteria and their spread to adjacent areas of the lung. Viral infection of the respiratory epithelium with concomitant disruption of its component cells interferes significantly with the clearance of bacteria from the lungs, an observation in accord with the high incidence of pneumococcal pneumonia during epidemics of viral influenza and its frequent clinical association with sporadic viral respiratory infections.

Pneumonia usually begins in the right lower, right middle, or left lower lobe, those areas to which gravity is most likely to carry upper respiratory secretions aspirated during sleep. Bronchial embolization with infected mucinous secretions during the course of an upper respiratory infection appears to be the initiating factor in many cases of pneumococcal pneumonia. Protected initially from phagocytosis by mucinous material, the bacteria multiply and, in infected alveoli, evoke the outpouring of proteinaceous fluid which serves both as a nutrient and as a vehicle for spread to adjacent alveoli. Soon thereafter, polymorphonuclear leukocytes migrate from the pulmonary capillaries to phagocytize a part of the pneumococcal population before the appearance of detectable antibody. Delay in the polymorphonuclear leukocytic response occurs during alcoholic intoxication and certain forms of anesthesia, permitting spread of infection. Glucocorticoids also may interfere with leukocyte migration. Later, as the pneumonic lesion evolves, macrophages appear in the exudate and remove the debris of fibrin and cells. It is probable that antibody to the capsular polysaccharide of the invading pneumococcus makes its appearance locally in the lung before being detectable in the circulation. Such antibody increases the efficiency of phagocytosis approximately twofold and causes agglutination of the organisms and their adherence to alveolar walls, thereby slowing their dissemination in the lung. The outcome of infection depends, therefore, on the rate at which bacteria can multiply in the edema fluid and spread and on the host's ability to immobilize and destroy them by phagocytosis. Individuals with deficiencies of the early components of complement or hypogam-maglobulinemia and patients with multiple myeloma (see Chap. 81) incapable of producing anticapsular antibody are prone to recurrent attacks of pneumococcal pneumonia. Repeated infection with the same pneumococcal type should always prompt a search for dysgam-maglobulinemia.

The attack rates of bacterial pneumonia and of pneumococcal bacteremia are markedly increased in individuals infected with HIV both before and after the development of AIDS. Neither the clinical manifestations of pneumococcal infection nor the distribution of capsular types causing infection differ significantly from those of the general population.

Failure of local defense mechanisms in the lung results in lymphatic spread of pneumococci to the hilar lymph nodes. In the sinusoids of these organs, a sequence of events not unlike that in the lung ensues. If infection is not checked in this secondary line of defense, organisms find their way into the thoracic duct and then into the circulation. Although transient bacteremia may occur at the onset of many cases of pneumococcal pneumonia, it is detectable in only 20 to 30 percent of cases. Bacteremia, which reflects the body's inability to localize the pulmonary infection, is a poor prognostic sign and carries with it the danger of metastatic infection. The mortality of treated or untreated bacteremic pneumococcal pneumonia is four times that resulting from comparably managed nonbacteremic infections. Metastatic infection secondary to bacteremia may occur in the meninges, joints, or peritoneum or on the endocardium. Direct spread from the infected lung may give rise to empyema or to pericarditis.

Natural recovery from pneumococcal infection coincides usually, but not invariably, with the appearance of detectable type-specific antibody in the circulation and is often accompanied by a dramatic and abrupt fall in temperature, the so-called crisis. Antibody aids recovery by increasing the efficiency of phagocytosis and by limiting dissemination of the organisms. Bacteriostatic drugs, such as sulfon-amides, facilitate control of the infection by limiting the size of the pneumococcal population, but the host's defense mechanisms are still required for the elimination of the bacteria. Bactericidal agents, such as penicillin, cause the death of pneumococci in the lung and are effective when some of the host's defense mechanisms are compromised. With the arrest of infection, the alveolar exudate undergoes liquefaction, the inflammatory debris is removed by expectoration and via the lymphatic channels, and the lung is restored to its normal state. Necrosis of pulmonary tissue as a result of pneumococcal infection is distinctly uncommon. Primary pneumococ-cal lung abscess is a rare clinical entity, although the diagnosis is mistakenly made at times when pneumococcal infection complicates lung abscess of other origins.

In addition to causing pneumonia and its metastatic sequelae, pneumococcus can extend from the nasopharynx to its adjacent structures, giving rise to otitis media, mastoiditis, paranasal sinusitis, or conjunctivitis. Soft tissue abscesses are rare but may occur, notably in patients with systemic lupus erythematosus and complement deficiency.

PNEUMOCOCCAL PNEUMONIA

Pneumococcal pneumonia is a disease of considerable uniformity, in contrast to other infections such as typhoid fever and tuberculosis. The diseases produced by different pneumococcal serotypes show little variation in severity or in clinical manifestations. The prognosis in type 3 pneumococcal pneumonia is usually regarded as poor, probably because type 3 infections occur frequently in the aged and in patients with other debilitating diseases, such as diabetes and congestive heart failure. The usual lesion in adults is segmental or lobar in distribution, but in children and the aged, bronchopneumonia, characterized by patchy involvement, is frequent.

MANIFESTATIONS   Pneumonia is often preceded for a few days by coryza or some other form of common respiratory disease. The onset is frequently so abrupt that the patient can state the exact hour that illness began. There is a sudden *shaking chill* in more than 80 percent of the cases and a rapid rise in temperature, with corresponding tachycardia and an increase in respiratory rate (tachypnea). Most patients with pneumococcal pneumonia have a single rigor unless antipyretic drugs are administered, and repeated chills should suggest another etiologic agent.

About 75 percent of patients develop severe *pleuritic pain* and *cough*, productive of pinkish or "rusty" mucoid sputum, within a few hours. The chest pain is agonizing, and respirations become rapid, shallow, and grunting as the patient tries to splint the affected side. Many patients are mildly cyanotic as a result of hypoxia caused by $\dot{V}/\dot{Q}$ (ventilation-perfusion ratio) abnormality or shunt, which accompanies altered respiration, and show dilatation of the alae nasi when first seen. Patients appear acutely ill, but nausea, headache, and malaise are not prominent, and most individuals are alert. Pleuritic pain and dyspnea are the dominant complaints.

In the untreated disease, there are sustained fever of 39.2 to 40.5°C (103 to 105°F) and continued pleuritic pain, cough, and expectoration; and *abdominal distention* is frequent. *Herpes labialis* is a common complication. After 7 to 10 days, there are diaphoresis, abrupt defervescence, and dramatic improvement in well-being, the "crisis."

In cases which terminate fatally, there is usually extensive pulmonary involvement, and dyspnea, cyanosis, and tachycardia are prominent. Circulatory collapse or a picture resembling adult respiratory distress syndrome has been observed. Death in a few patients is associated with empyema or some other suppurative complication such as meningitis or endocarditis.

Physical examination reveals restricted motion of the affected hemithorax. Tactile fremitus may be decreased during the initial day of illness but is usually increased when consolidation is fully established. Deviation of the trachea away from the affected lung suggests pleural effusion or empyema. The percussion note is dull, and if the lesion is in an upper lobe, impaired motion of the diaphragm can be detected on the affected side. Very early in the course of infection, breath sounds are diminished, but as the lesion evolves, they become tubular or bronchial in quality, and bronchophony and whispered pectoriloquy can be elicited. These findings are accompanied by fine crepitant rales.

EFFECT OF SPECIFIC CHEMOTHERAPY   Pneumococcal pneu-monia usually improves promptly when an appropriate antimicrobial drug is given. Within 12 to 36 h after initiation of treatment with penicillin, temperature, pulse, and respiration begin to fall and may reach normal values, pleuritic pain subsides, and the spread of the inflammatory process is halted. The temperature of approximately half the patients, however, requires 4 days or longer to become normal, and failure of the patient's temperature to reach normal in 24 to 48 h should not prompt a change in antibacterial therapy in the absence of other indications.

COMPLICATIONS   The typical course of pneumococcal pneumo-nia can be modified by the development of one or more local or distant complications:

In the lung   ATELECTASIS   Atelectasis of all or part of a lobe may occur during the active stage of pneumonia or after treatment has been instituted. The patient may complain of sudden recurrence of pleuritic pain and show rapid respirations. Small areas of atelectasis are often detected by x-ray in the absence of symptoms. These areas usually clear with coughing and deep breathing, but bronchoscopic aspiration is occasionally necessary. If atelectasis is allowed to persist, the affected area becomes fibrotic and functionless.

DELAYED RESOLUTION   Return of physical findings in the lung to normal after pneumococcal pneumonia is usually complete within 2 to 4 weeks. X-ray evidence of residual pulmonary consolidation, however, may persist as long as 8 weeks, and other radiologic manifestations of the infection (volume loss, stranding, and pleural disease) may persist for up to 18 weeks. The process of resolution may require a longer time in those over 50 years of age and in those with chronic obstructive airway disease or alcoholism.

ABSCESS Lung abscess is a rare sequel to pneumococcal infection, although pneumococcal pneumonia is a not uncommon complication of lung abscess of other origins. It is manifested by continued fever and profuse expectoration of purulent sputum. X-ray shows one or more cavities. This complication is exceedingly rare in patients who receive penicillin therapy and is most likely to follow infection with pneumococcus type 3.

In adjacent structures PLEURAL EFFUSION Pleural effusion detectable in lateral decubitus x-rays of the chest occurs in approximately half of patients with pneumococcal pneumonia and is associated with delay in the initiation of therapy and with bacteremia. Usually the effusion is sterile and is absorbed spontaneously within a week or two. At times, however, the effusion is large and requires aspiration or drainage.

EMPYEMA Before the introduction of effective chemotherapy, empyema occurred in 5 to 8 percent of patients with pneumococcal pneumonia; it is now observed in less than 1 percent of treated cases. It is manifested by persistent fever or pleuritic pain, together with signs of pleural effusion. In the early stages, the gross appearance of infected fluid may not differ from that of a sterile pleural effusion; later, there is a profuse outpouring of polymorphonuclear leukocytes and fibrin, resulting in an exudate of thick greenish pus containing large clots of fibrin. The quantity of exudate may become large enough to displace mediastinal structures. In neglected cases, this process leads to extensive pleural scarring, with limitation of thoracic movement. Rupture and drainage through the chest wall (*empyema necessitatis*) occur but are rare. Metastatic *brain abscess* is an occasional complication of chronic empyema.

PERICARDITIS A particularly serious complication is spread of infection to the pericardial sac. This lesion is characterized by pain in the precordial region, a friction rub synchronous with the heartbeat, and distention of cervical veins, although one or all of these findings may be absent. The possibility of coexisting purulent pericarditis should be considered whenever a very ill patient with pneumonia develops empyema.

Metastatic infections *Arthritis* occurs more often in children than in adults. The affected joint is swollen, red, and painful, with a purulent effusion. It usually subsides promptly with systemic administration of penicillin, although aspiration and intraarticular injection of penicillin may be necessary in adults.

Acute bacterial endocarditis and *meningitis*, complications of pneumococcal pneumonia, are discussed subsequently.

Paralytic ileus Gaseous abdominal distention is commonly present and in severely ill patients may assume such serious proportions that the term *paralytic ileus* is justified. This complication further impairs respiratory movement by elevation of the diaphragm and constitutes a difficult problem in management. A rarer and more serious gastrointestinal complication is acute gastric dilatation.

Impaired liver function Alterations in hepatic function are common during the course of pneumococcal pneumonia, and mild jaundice is not at all rare. The pathogenesis of the jaundice is not entirely clear, although in some patients it appears to be related to glucose-6-phosphate dehydrogenase deficiency.

LABORATORY FINDINGS *Sputum* should be obtained in the physician's presence before the administration of antimicrobial drugs to ensure its quality. Although resort to transtracheal aspiration or lung puncture may be necessary on occasion to establish the cause of pneumonia, routine use of these invasive techniques is not recommended because of their attendant, albeit infrequent, complications. When stained by Gram's method, the sputum shows polymorphonuclear leukocytes and variable numbers of gram-positive cocci, singly and in pairs. These can be typed directly by the Neufeld quellung technique, and this procedure should be used to facilitate diagnosis whenever possible. The *blood culture* is positive for pneumococci during the first days of untreated illness in 20 to 30 percent of cases. The white blood cell count usually shows a polymorphonuclear *leukocytosis* ranging from 12×10^9 to 25×10^9 cells per liter (12,000 to 25,000 cells per microliter). A normal white count or leukopenia is sometimes observed in patients with overwhelming infection and bacteremia. Occasionally, pneumococci may be seen directly in granulocytes of patients with bacteremia by examining the buffy coat after staining with Wright's stain. These patients often have asplenia. *X-ray of the chest* usually reveals a homogeneous density in the affected area of the lung. In well-established cases, the density may occupy one or more entire lobes. Atypical patterns of consolidation may be seen in patients with underlying chronic pulmonary disease.

EXTRAPULMONARY PNEUMOCOCCAL INFECTION

PNEUMOCOCCAL MENINGITIS The pneumococcus is second only to the meningococcus as a cause of purulent meningitis in adults; in children, meningitis caused by *Haemophilus influenzae* is also more frequent than pneumococcal infection.

Pneumococcal meningitis can develop as a "primary" disease without preceding signs of infection elsewhere; as a complication of pneumococcal pneumonia; by extension from otitis, mastoiditis, or sinusitis; or following a skull fracture which creates an opening between the subarachnoid space and the nasal cavity or paranasal sinuses. Patients with pneumococcal endocarditis frequently develop meningeal infection. Patients with multiple myeloma and with sickle cell disease seem to be prone to pneumococcal infection of the meninges, just as they are to pneumonia.

The *manifestations* are those of any acute pyogenic meningitis (see Chap. 374) and include chills, fever, headache, nuchal rigidity, Kernig's and Brudzinski's signs, delirium, and cranial nerve palsies. Evidence of otitis, sinusitis, or pneumonia should be carefully sought by physical and roentgenographic examination in all patients.

The *spinal fluid* is under increased pressure, appears cloudy, often with a greenish tint, and shows a high protein and low glucose content. Stained smears usually reveal gram-positive diplococci and polymorphonuclear leukocytes; in some patients, the number of cells in the spinal fluid is surprisingly small, and much of the cloudiness is produced by the bacterial content. The diagnosis can be established rapidly by identification of pneumococci in the spinal fluid by Gram's stain or by the Neufeld quellung reaction. Immunologic tests (CIE or latex agglutination) are positive in approximately 80 percent of culture-positive cases and may provide a presumptive bacterial cause of infection in some patients from whose spinal fluid no organism is recovered.

With appropriate chemotherapy, recovery can be expected in 70 percent of cases; the prognosis is better in children than in infants or adults, and limited but inconclusive data suggest that anti-inflammatory therapy may be of benefit. Relapse may occur but is unusual if adequate treatment is carried out. Subarachnoid block, the result of accumulation of large amounts of thick exudate in the meningeal space and at the base of the brain, is an infrequent complication.

PNEUMOCOCCAL ENDOCARDITIS Endocarditis is a rare complication of pneumonia or meningitis. The clinical picture is that of acute bacterial endocarditis (see Chap. 85), with remittent fever, splenomegaly, and metastatic infection of the lungs, meninges, joints, eye, and other tissues. Petechiae are uncommon. The infection can attack normal valves and is particularly likely to occur on the aortic valve. The valvular infection is destructive, and loud murmurs and heart failure develop rapidly. Rupture or perforation of cusps or even rupture of the aorta may occur. The blood culture is consistently positive for the pneumococcus in the absence of treatment with antimicrobial drugs, yet at the same time antibodies to the infecting organism may be demonstrable in the blood, a combination of findings seldom observed except in endocarditis or brucellosis. Although the infection is relatively easy to cure with penicillin, damage to valve leaflets, especially to the cusps of the aortic valve, may be followed by rapidly progressive heart failure. Surgical repair or replacement of damaged valvular structures should be carried out early, before heart failure becomes intractable.

PNEUMOCOCCAL PERITONITIS   Pneumococcal peritonitis is a rare disease and is probably the sequel to transient pneumococcal bacteremia, although, because of its somewhat greater frequency in young girls, it has been hypothesized that the organism may gain entry to the peritoneum via the vagina and fallopian tubes. Peritonitis was formerly a common complication of the nephrotic syndrome, particularly in children, but it occurs now with a frequency of less than 2 percent. In adults, the disease is seen in association with cirrhosis or with carcinoma of the liver. The diagnosis is made by examination of the ascitic fluid; blood cultures are often positive, and a polymorphonuclear leukocytosis is the rule.

TREATMENT

SPECIFIC ANTIMICROBIAL THERAPY   Although resistance of pneumococci to antimicrobial drugs was long regarded as an insignificant problem, increasing numbers of strains from widely separated geographic areas throughout the world have been found in the last decade to be resistant to one or to all of the following agents: penicillins, cephalosporins, tetracyclines, chloramphenicol, erythromycin, clindamycin, cotrimoxazole, and aminoglycosides. For this reason, sensitivity of the infecting organism to the drug(s) to be used should be determined, particularly in treating extrapulmonary infection. In the absence of resistance or of hypersensitivity to it, penicillin G (benzylpenicillin) is the drug of choice for all manifestations of pneumococcal infection. Strains of pneumococcus manifesting increased resistance to penicillin are being recovered with increasing frequency from humans in a number of areas throughout the world. Although the level of such resistance rarely precludes treatment with this antibiotic when infection is confined to the lung, awareness of the phenomenon is necessary. A dose of 600,000 units daily provides a good margin of safety in treating adults with bacteremic or nonbacteremic infection in the absence of an extrapulmonary focus when caused by pneumococci lacking increased resistance to the drug, but the occurrence of pneumococci showing increased resistance to penicillin makes the initiation of therapy with larger amounts desirable. Treatment may be started with doses of 600,000 units of aqueous crystalline penicillin G or procaine penicillin administered at 6-h intervals to be continued until the patient has been afebrile for 48 to 72 h. Pneumococcal pneumonia can be treated with an oral penicillin, preferably one resistant to gastric acid (see Chap. 100), in dosage equivalent to 2.4 to 4.8 million units of penicillin G. *Peritonitis* caused by sensitive strains responds usually within 36 to 48 h to 2 to 4 million units of penicillin daily.

Pneumococcal meningitis in adults should be treated with 18 to 24 million units of penicillin G daily intravenously. Larger amounts should not be used, to avoid neurotoxicity from excessive dosage. Intrathecal administration of penicillin is unnecessary, and supplementation of penicillin with broad-spectrum bacteriostatic drugs such as tetracyclines may exert a deleterious effect. All pneumococcal isolates from cerebrospinal fluid should be tested promptly for their sensitivity to antibacterial drugs, including ceftriaxone, resistance to which has been demonstrated. Vancomycin is the drug of choice for treatment of meningitis caused by pneumococci resistant to multiple antimicrobial agents.

Moderate doses of penicillin G are used to treat pneumococcal endocarditis—8 to 12 million units daily by intravenous infusion. Rapidly developing heart failure as a result of valvular injury and a tendency to form myocardial abscess, however, often lead to a fatal outcome despite the use of antibiotics. Prompt surgical repair or replacement of damaged heart valves should be considered when cardiac failure develops.

Cephalosporins in parenteral doses of 1 to 2 g daily are effective in pneumococcal pneumonia but must be administered with caution to those hypersensitive to penicillin. Many members of this class of β-lactam drugs cannot be used to treat meningitis because of their poor ability to penetrate the blood–cerebrospinal fluid barrier. Several of the newer cephalosporins, including cefotaxime and ceftriaxone, show promise of efficacy in treating pneumococcal meningitis, although experience with each is limited. The tetracyclines in doses of 1 to 2 g daily, erythromycin in doses of 1.6 g daily, or clindamycin in doses of 1.2 g daily are effective treatment for pneumococcal pneumonia if it is caused by a sensitive strain, but they are recommended only for patients who have had untoward reactions to penicillins or cephalosporins. Despite its efficacy, chloramphenicol should not be used to treat pneumococcal infections other than meningitis in patients hypersensitive to penicillin who are infected with a drug-sensitive strain. For patients with illness caused by multiply drug-resistant pneumococci, vancomycin in doses of 2 g daily is the drug of choice. Sulfonamides have little place in the present-day treatment of pneumococcal pneumonia and are useless in endocarditis and meningitis. Aminoglycosides, such as gentamicin, tobramycin, and amikacin, should not be employed to treat pneumococcal infection.

Pneumococcal arthritis responds to systemic penicillin, but aspiration and intraarticular instillation of the drug may be necessary.

Empyema should be detected and treated as early as possible. When an effusion is found, fluid should be removed and examined for bacteria, leukocytes, glucose concentration, and pH. The presence of bacteria or pus, a pH below 7.0, and/or a pleural fluid glucose level below 2.2 mmol/L (40 mg/dL) are indications for institution of closed chest tube drainage. Failure to cure empyema early may be followed by pleural fibrosis and may necessitate subsequent surgical decortication of the lung to restore pulmonary function.

OTHER MEASURES   Oxygen administered through a face mask should be used to treat significant cyanosis, cardiac failure, and delirium. In the presence of adult respiratory distress syndrome, positive end-expiratory pressure may be indicated. Codeine, 32 to 64 mg every 4 h, will usually control pleuritic pain. When pain is severe, it may require intercostal nerve block with 1% to 2% procaine for relief.

PROGNOSIS AND PREVENTION

Although the mortality from pneumococcal pneumonia has diminished significantly since the advent of antimicrobial drugs, available evidence indicates that the incidence of the disease has changed little, if at all. The fatality rate in patients over the age of 12 years with bacteremic pneumococcal pneumonia treated with an antibiotic is 18 percent, and in patients over the age of 50 and in those with underlying systemic illness, it is significantly higher.

Signs of poor prognosis in pneumonia include leukopenia, bacteremia, multilobar involvement, any extrapulmonary focus of pneumococcal infection, presence of preexisting systemic disease, asplenia, circulatory collapse, and occurrence of the infection in the first year of life or after the age of 55. Infection with pneumococcus type 3 has a higher mortality rate than that caused by other pneumococcal types. Death is most likely to occur in individuals sustaining irreversible physiologic damage early in the course which is unaltered by antimicrobial therapy. Until the nature of the injury produced by pneumococcus is understood and ways are devised to repair it, vaccination will remain the principal means of protecting those at high risk of a fatal outcome.

A 23-valent vaccine containing the capsular polysaccharides of pneumococcal types 1, 2, 3, 4, 5, 6B, 7F, 8, 9N, 9V, 10A, 11A, 12F, 14, 15B, 17F, 18C, 19F, 19A, 20, 22F, 23F, and 33F, which include the serotypes or groups responsible for 90 percent of bacteremic infections in the United States, is recommended for prevention of pneumococcal infection caused by these serotypes in individuals at high risk of a fatal outcome. In immunocompetent subjects, the vaccine has an aggregate efficacy of 61 percent in preventing infection with any of the pneumococcal types represented in it. Those at higher-than-average risk are individuals over the age of 55 and patients with a variety of chronic systemic illnesses, including heart disease, chronic bronchopulmonary disease, hepatic disease, renal insufficiency, diabetes, and a variety of malignancies. Persons of all ages with sickle cell disease have an increased risk of developing pneumococcal infection, and the vaccine is recommended for those with this disorder over the age of 2 years. Since anatomic or functional asplenia is associated with fulminant overwhelming pneumococcal septicemia with disseminated intravascular coagulation, giving rise to a clinical picture resembling that of the Waterhouse-Friderichsen syndrome, such individuals also should be immunized. However, the vaccine does not contain the antigens of all pneumococcal types, and infection caused by nonincluded types may occur occasionally in immunized subjects. Reactions to the vaccine are usually absent or mild, although in the occasional individual they may resemble those following immunization with typhoid vaccine: local pain, erythema, and elevation of temperature. Recent evidence suggests gradual waning of immunity induced by pneumococcal vaccine over a period of several years, especially in individuals over age 65. Reimmunization of such individuals at intervals of 5 years may be beneficial, although evidence to support such a practice is lacking currently. The aggregate efficacy of vaccine in preventing bacteremic infection is 60 to 70 percent in immunocompetent adults. It may afford little, if any, protection, however, to those with agamma- or dysgammaglobulinemia or to patients who have been subjected recently to intensive antitumor chemotherapy and radiation. Although the efficacy of polyvalent pneumococcal vaccine in those infected with HIV has not been quantified, and although the immunologic responses of small numbers of infected individuals are less than those in their uninfected counterparts, administration of the vaccine to the former should be considered in view of the potential benefit it may confer to those at greatly increased risk and its lack of harmful side effects. In children, immunologic responsiveness to different capsular antigens develops at different times prior to puberty as a result of maturational characteristics of the human immune system and, in infancy, may be manifested only by antibodies of the IgM class. Currently, vaccines of capsular polysaccharide conjugated to proteins such as diphtheria toxoid, which are antigenic in infancy, are under development for pediatric populations. If circumstances dictate, pneumococcal vaccine may be administered concomitantly with influenza viral vaccine, provided each vaccine is injected from a separate syringe at a separate site.

REFERENCES

AUSTRIAN R: *Life with the Pneumococcus.* Philadelphia, University of Pennsylvania Press, 1985

————: Untreated pneumococcal bacteraemia of cryptic origin in the human adult with spontaneous recovery. S Afr Med J 70(suppl):46, 1986

BRADLEY JS, CONNOR JD: Ceftriaxone failure in meningitis caused by *Streptococcus pneumoniae* with reduced susceptibility to beta-lactam antibiotics. Pediatr Infect Dis J 10:871, 1991

DINUBILE MJ et al: Pneumococcal soft-tissue infections: Possible association with connective tissue diseases. J Infect Dis 163:897, 1991

FRUCHTMAN SM et al: Adult respiratory distress syndrome as a cause of death in pneumococcal pneumonia. Chest 83:598, 1983

HEFFRON R: *Pneumonia with Special Reference to Pneumococcus Lobar Pneumonia.* Cambridge, Mass, Harvard University Press, 1979

KLUGMAN KP: Pneumococcal resistance to antibiotics. Clin Microbiol Rev 3:171, 1990

LEE BL et al: Infectious complications with respiratory pathogens despite ciprofloxacin therapy. N Engl J Med 325:520, 1991

REDD SC et al: The role of human immunodeficiency virus infection in pneumococcal bacteremia in San Francisco residents. J Infect Dis 162:1012, 1990

RESEARCH COMMITTEE, BRITISH THORACIC SOCIETY: Community acquired pneumonia in adults in British hospitals in 1982–83: A study of aetiology, mortality, prognostic factors and outcome. Q J Med 62:195, 1987

ROSS JC, DENSEN P: Complement deficiency states and infection: Epidemiology, pathogenesis and consequences of neisserial and other infections in an immune deficiency. Medicine 63:243, 1984

SHAPIRO ED et al: The protective efficacy of polyvalent pneumococcal polysaccharide vaccine. N Engl J Med 325:1453, 1991

STEPHAN JJ et al: The radiographic resolution of *Streptococcus pneumoniae* pneumonia. N Engl J Med 293:798, 1975

TUOMANEN E et al: Induction of pulmonary inflammation by components of the pneumococcal cell surface. Am Rev Respir Dis 135:869, 1987

VILADRICH PF et al: Evaluation of vancomycin for therapy of adult pneumococcal meningitis. Antimicrob Agents Chemother 35:2467, 1991

102 STAPHYLOCOCCAL INFECTIONS

RICHARD M. LOCKSLEY

The staphylococci, of which *Staphylococcus aureus* is the most important human pathogen, are hardy, gram-positive bacteria that colonize the skin of most human beings. If the skin or mucous membranes are disrupted by surgery or trauma, staphylococci may gain access to and proliferate in the underlying tissues, giving rise to a typically localized, superficial abscess. Although these cutaneous infections are most commonly harmless and self-limited, the multiplying organisms may invade the lymphatics and the blood, leading to the potentially serious complications of staphylococcal bacteremia. These complications include septic shock, which may be indistinguishable from that caused by gram-negative bacteria, and serious metastatic infections, including endocarditis (see Chap. 85), arthritis (see Chap. 91), osteomyelitis (see Chap. 92), pneumonia (see Chap. 220), and abscesses (see Chap. 86) in virtually any organ. Certain strains of *S. aureus* produce toxins that cause skin rashes or that mediate multisystem dysfunction, as in toxic shock syndrome. Coagulase-negative staphylococci, particularly *S. epidermidis*, are important nosocomial pathogens, with a predilection for infecting vascular catheters and prosthetic devices. *S. saprophyticus* is a common cause of urinary tract infection.

ETIOLOGY AND MICROBIOLOGY Staphylococci are gram-positive, nonmotile, aerobic or facultatively anaerobic, catalase-positive cocci within the family Micrococcaceae. The name derives from the typical clustering of organisms (the Greek *staphyle*, "bunch of grapes") observed microscopically in stained specimens taken from colonies grown on solid media. Pathogenic staphylococci are distinguished from nonpathogenic micrococci by the ability of staphylococci to ferment glucose anaerobically and by their sensitivity to lysostaphin endopeptidase. *S. aureus*, the most important human pathogen in the genus, is named for the golden color of colonies grown aerobically on solid media. Staphylococcal strains producing coagulase are designated *S. aureus*. In contrast to coagulase-negative staphylococci, *S. aureus* ferments mannitol, produces DNase, and displays greater susceptibility to lysostaphin. *S. aureus* strains are generally hemolytic when cultured on blood agar and exhibit greater expression of biochemical activity (production of coagulase, toxins, hemolysis) than coagulase-negative staphylococci.

There are 21 recognized species of coagulase-negative staphylococci. Twelve are part of the normal human flora, of which *S. epidermidis* and *S. saprophyticus* are the most important clinically.

Differentiation among strains of *S. aureus* or *S. epidermidis* has been used to identify a common source during epidemics or intrahospital outbreaks of staphylococcal disease. Strains may be distinguished by antimicrobial susceptibility profiles, patterns of lysis by staphylococcal bacteriophages (phage typing), biochemical testing (biotyping), and molecular analysis of plasmids or of plasmid or chromosomal DNA. Of these tests, antibiotic susceptibility testing has the least, and molecular analysis the most, discriminatory ability.

EPIDEMIOLOGY The coagulase-negative staphylococci are part of the normal flora of the skin, mucous membranes, and lower bowel; *S. epidermidis* is the most common species isolated. *S. aureus* transiently colonizes the anterior nares in 70 to 90 percent of persons and may be recovered for relatively prolonged periods of time in 20 to 30 percent of them. Nasal carriage is often accompanied by secondary colonization of the skin. Independent colonization of the perineal area occurs in 5 to 20 percent of persons, and vaginal carriage has been demonstrated in 10 percent of menstruating females. Higher carriage rates of *S. aureus* have been documented in hospital employees (including physicians and nurses), hospitalized patients, persons with atopic dermatitis, and patients whose care requires frequent puncture of the skin, e.g., with insulin-dependent diabetes, dialysis-dependent renal failure, or frequent desensitization injections for allergies. Drug abusers who use needles also have enhanced *S. aureus* carriage rates. Presumably, disturbances in the local cutaneous barrier allow *S. aureus* to establish and maintain colonization successfully.

S. saprophyticus demonstrates greater adherence to urothelial cells than *S. epidermidis*. Approximately 5 percent of healthy males and females have low colony counts of *S. saprophyticus* in the urethral or periurethral areas (see Chap. 90).

Although staphylococci can survive in the environment for prolonged periods of time and airborne spread of organisms can be demonstrated, person-to-person transfer via contaminated hands is the most important mechanism for transmission of these organisms. Hospitalized patients with active staphylococcal infection or those who become heavily colonized, particularly at cutaneous sites (surgical wounds, burns, decubitus ulcers), constitute the greatest reservoir for nosocomially acquired infection. Such patients shed an enormous number of organisms, and the hands of hospital personnel caring for these patients are readily colonized. Failure to use aseptic technique and neglect of hand washing allow transmission of the organisms to the skin of other patients. Strains of both *S. aureus* and *S. epidermidis* may become endemic in areas of the hospital housing patients with large integumental defects, particularly when widespread antimicrobial use favors the acquisition of multiply resistant strains (burn units, intensive care units, bone marrow transplant units). Less frequently, otherwise healthy hospital employees who are nasal carriers have been implicated in nosocomial outbreaks. Upon careful examination, most of these carriers will have active dermatologic infections during the time that effective transmission of staphylococci is documented.

If infections arising from the urinary tract are excluded, *S. aureus* and *S. epidermidis* together have become the most common cause of nosocomial infection in U.S. hospitals. They are the most frequently isolated pathogens in both primary and secondary bacteremias and in cutaneous and surgical wound infections.

PATHOGENESIS   Infection by staphylococci usually results from a combination of bacterial virulence factors and diminution in host defense. Important microbial factors include the ability of the staphylococcus to survive under harsh conditions, its cell wall constituents, the production of enzymes and toxins that promote tissue invasion, its capacity to persist intracellularly in certain phagocytes, and its potential to acquire resistance to antimicrobials. Important host factors include an intact mucocutaneous barrier, an adequate number of functional neutrophils, and removal of foreign bodies or devitalized tissues.

Microbial factors   Cell wall components of *S. aureus* include a large peptidoglycan complex that confers rigidity on the organism and enables it to survive under unfavorable osmotic conditions, a unique teichoic acid linked to peptidoglycan, and protein A, found both attached to peptidoglycan over the outermost parts of the cell and released in soluble form. Most isolates of *S. aureus* are coated by serologically distinct, thin, polysaccharide capsules. Serotypes 5 and 8 are most prevalent. Both peptidoglycan and teichoic acid are capable of activating the complement cascade via the alternative pathway. Although important for opsonization of organisms for ingestion by phagocytes, complement activation also may play a role in the pathogenesis of shock and disseminated intravascular coagulation. Protein A binds in the Fc portion of certain classes of IgG as well as to the Fc receptor on phagocytes and may serve as a blocking factor preventing neutrophil ingestion of the organism. Specific receptors for laminin and fibronectin may mediate the widespread metastatic potential of *S. aureus*. Activation of tissue factor (procoagulant activity) occurs when endothelial cells and monocytes are incubated with *S. aureus*. The cell wall of certain strains of *S. epidermidis* is also capable of activating complement; shock and disseminated intravascular coagulation during infections by these organisms have been described, although less frequently than with *S. aureus*. The capacity of *S. epidermidis* to adhere to intravascular cannulas and prosthetic devices may explain the propensity of these organisms to cause foreign-body infections. These

organisms bind fibronectin and other matrix proteins that coat catheters and secrete an exopolysaccharide slime that forms a protective biofilm over the colonizing organisms.

Certain enzymes produced by *S. aureus* may play a role in virulence. Catalase degrades hydrogen peroxide and may protect the organism during phagocytosis, when it must withstand the phagocyte's respiratory burst. Coagulase is present in both soluble and cell-bound forms and causes plasma to clot by formation of thrombin-like material. The high correlation between coagulase production and virulence suggests that this substance is important in the pathogenesis of staphylococcal infections, but its precise role as a determinant of pathogenicity has not been determined. Many strains also produce hyaluronidase, an enzyme that degrades hyaluronic acid in the connective tissue matrix and that may promote spreading of infection. A trypsin-like protease from some strains enhances influenza virus infection by proteolytic cleavage of the viral precursor hemagglutinin into its active fragments and may contribute to the morbidity of such coinfections. *S. saprophyticus* produces urease, an enzyme capable of breaking down urea to ammonium, alkalinizing the urine and favoring the formation of struvite stones.

S. aureus may produce numerous extracellular toxins. The expression of multiple toxins, as in gram-negative bacilli, is coordinately regulated by an accessory gene regulator protein, presumably in response to physicochemical environmental stimuli. Toxins may be encoded by chromosomal or plasmid DNA. Four different red cell hemolysins—designated alpha, beta, gamma, and delta toxins—have been identified. Alpha toxin is also dermonecrotic when injected subcutaneously into animals. Delta toxin inhibits water absorption by elevating cyclic AMP in guinea pig ileum and may play a role in the acute watery diarrhea seen in some cases of staphylococcal infection. Leukocidin lyses granulocyte and macrophage membranes by producing membrane pores permeable to cations.

While the role of the above factors in virulence is incompletely understood, the exfoliatin toxins A and B, the staphylococcal enterotoxins, and the toxic shock syndrome toxin—TSST-1—have been implicated in disease. These exotoxins belong to the enlarging family of microbial superantigens. Superantigens bind to regions that lie outside of the normal peptide recognition domains on both MHC class II molecules and certain families of T cell antigen receptors, thus bridging antigen-presenting cells and T cells, resulting in activation. A number of cytokines are produced that subsequently mediate local or systemic effects depending on the amount of toxin formed, the immune status of the host, and the access of the toxin to the circulation.

The exfoliatin toxins mediate the dermatologic manifestations of the staphylococcal scalded-skin syndrome and bullous impetigo. These toxins cause intraepidermal cleavage of the skin at the stratum granulosum, leading to bullae formation and denudation. Antibodies to the toxins are protective in both humans and animals. Seven distinct enterotoxins (A, B, C1, C2, C3, D, and E) have been implicated in food poisoning due to *S. aureus*. The toxins enhance intestinal peristalsis and seem to induce vomiting by a direct effect on the central nervous system. Enterotoxins B and C1 also may mediate toxic shock syndrome (TSS), although this is more frequently due to TSST-1. TSST-1 is produced by over 90 percent of *S. aureus* recovered from women with menstrual TSS and over 60 percent of nonmenstrual cases. Most TSST-1–negative strains produce enterotoxin B and, rarely, enterotoxin C1. These superantigens activate large numbers of T cells and monocyte/macrophages, resulting in release of a number of cytokines, including tumor necrosis factor (TNF), that mediate most of the symptoms of TSS (see Chaps. 16 and 83). The *tst* gene encoding TSST-1 is present in 5 to 25 percent of clinical isolates of *S. aureus* as part of a large, mobile, transposon-like element. Similar elements encode the enterotoxin B and C genes.

Antimicrobial resistance by staphylococci favors their persistence in the hospital environment. Over 90 percent of both hospital and community strains of *S. aureus* causing infection are resistant to penicillin. Resistance is due to the production of β-lactamases; the genes for these enzymes are usually carried by plasmids. A subgroup of *S. aureus* hyperproduce β-lactamase in vitro and show borderline in vitro susceptibility to oxacillin that disappears when clavulanic acid (β-lactamase inhibitor) is added. Infections due to these organisms with "acquired resistance to oxacillin" can be treated safely with penicillinase-resistant β-lactam antimicrobial agents. The true penicillinase-resistant *S. aureus* organisms, called methicillin-resistant *S. aureus* (MRSA), are resistant to all the β-lactam antimicrobials, as well as to the cephalosporins, despite the fact that standard disk susceptibility testing may indicate sensitivity to cephalosporin drugs. Resistance of MRSA is chromosomally mediated and involves production of an altered penicillin-binding protein (PBP 2a or PBP 2′) with a low binding affinity for β-lactams. Not uncommonly, MRSA has acquired R plasmids mediating resistance to some combination of erythromycin, tetracycline, chloramphenicol, clindamycin, and aminoglycosides. MRSA has become increasingly common worldwide, particularly in tertiary-care referral hospitals. In the United States, approximately 5 percent of hospital isolates of *S. aureus* are MRSA; one-third of hospitals surveyed have experienced bacteremias due to MRSA. The isolation of these organisms has remained relatively constant since 1980. Outbreaks continue to occur periodically in the form of intrahospital epidemics. The community carriage rate of MRSA is low, although selected patient populations, such as parenteral drug abusers, may have MRSA at the time of admission to the hospital. These isolates remain susceptible to vancomycin.

Tolerance of staphylococci to β-lactams is an in vitro phenomenon characterized by resistance to the lethal action of normally cidal antimicrobials. It is characterized by a marked discrepancy between the minimal inhibitory and the minimal bactericidal concentrations of the drug. The mechanism may relate to a defect in the normal activation of autolytic enzymes of the bacteria by cell wall–active antimicrobials. Demonstration of the trait is influenced markedly by physicochemical conditions. Although tolerance has been reported to influence the outcome of severe staphylococcal infection adversely, it has been difficult to incriminate tolerance to β-lactams as a significant cause of antibiotic failure because of the in vitro observation that continued treatment with β-lactams will kill tolerant *S. aureus*, although killing proceeds more slowly.

Most cases of *S. epidermidis* infection are nosocomially acquired, and the infecting strains typically express greater variability and degrees of antimicrobial resistance than those of *S. aureus*. Virtually all isolates contain R plasmids that produce β-lactamase and are resistant to penicillin. Approximately one-third are resistant to aminoglycosides and two-thirds are resistant to tetracycline, erythromycin, clindamycin, and chloramphenicol. Hospital isolates of *S. epidermidis* containing multiple antimicrobial-resistant plasmids can serve as important reservoirs for the acquisition of resistance by *S. aureus* and *Enterococcus* species.

Methicillin resistance is common among *S. epidermidis* strains; over 80 percent of isolates from cases with prosthetic valve endocarditis in one study were methicillin-resistant. Conditions of temperature, pH, osmolality, and the presence of chelating agents and heavy metals all may influence the demonstration of resistance. Methicillin-resistant isolates may appear susceptible by routine susceptibility testing. The most reliable identification of these organisms is by their growth from a large inoculum (10^7 cells) spread on agar containing 6 μg/mL oxacillin. Cross-resistance to the other β-lactam antimicrobials and to the cephalosporins is always present, although, as with MRSA, these bacteria may appear susceptible to cephalosporins by conventional disk testing. As with *S. aureus*, *S. epidermidis* strains remain susceptible to vancomycin, although resistance has occurred in strains of *S. haemolyticus*. Although the quinolone antibiotics may be active against methicillin-resistant staphylococci, resistance is widespread due to rapid, single-step mutations in the DNA gyrase or expression of an active efflux transporter.

HOST FACTORS The importance of host factors in resisting staphylococcal infections is demonstrated by the observation that enormous numbers of bacteria are required to establish experimental infections in humans and animals. Areas where skin or mucosal continuity is broken provide portals of entry for staphylococci. More than 50 percent of serious staphylococcal infections of deep tissues arise from cutaneous foci; a smaller number originate from the respiratory, gastrointestinal, or less frequently, the genitourinary tract. Direct inoculation of organisms into the blood is an important route of infection in hospitalized patients with intravenous catheters and in drug abusers.

Staphylococci often invade the integument via plugged hair follicles and sebaceous glands or areas involved by burns, wounds, abrasions, insect bites, or dermatitis. Colonization and invasion of the lungs may occur when the normal mucociliary clearance mechanisms are either bypassed, as occurs with endotracheal intubation, or depressed, as occurs following viral infections of the lung (influenza) or in patients with cystic fibrosis. Mucosal damage to the gastrointestinal tract following cytotoxic chemotherapy or radiotherapy predisposes to invasion from that site.

Once the integument has been breached, local bacterial multiplication is accompanied by inflammation and tissue necrosis at the site of infection. Neutrophils rapidly enter the area and ingest large numbers of staphylococci. Thrombosis of surrounding capillaries occurs; fibrin is deposited about the periphery; later, fibroblasts create a relatively avascular wall about the area. The fully developed staphylococcal abscess consists of a central core of dead and dying leukocytes and bacteria which gradually liquefies to form characteristic thick, creamy pus, surrounded by a fibroblastic wall. When host mechanisms fail to contain the cutaneous or submucosal infection, staphylococci may enter the lymphatics and the bloodstream. Common sites of metastatic seeding include the diaphyseal ends of long bones in children and the lungs, kidneys, cardiac valves, myocardium, liver, spleen, and brain.

Polymorphonuclear leukocytes appear to be the major protective mechanism against staphylococcal disease. Persons with neutropenia or inherited or acquired defects of neutrophil chemotaxis, ingestion, or killing are particularly susceptible to staphylococcal infections. A low number of staphylococci are capable of surviving within phagocytes, which may account for the relatively slow response of staphylococcal infections to antimicrobials and the potential for relapse.

Although infections may occur in all age groups, serious staphylococcal infections most commonly afflict the young and old—particularly those with underlying debilitating disease. Primary staphylococcal pneumonia is common in infants but rare in adults. Superficial staphylococcal pyoderma is more frequent in infants, whereas actual abscess formation occurs more often in adults. While these examples suggest some role for immunity in resistance against staphylococci, there has been no satisfactory demonstration that human staphylococcal disease is followed by effective immunity or that infection can be modified significantly by vaccination. Virtually 100 percent of adults possess antistaphylococcal antibodies in their serum. Except for the efficacy of neutralizing antibodies to toxins in staphylococcal toxin–mediated diseases, the role of humoral immunity in modifying or protecting against staphylococcal infection is unclear.

The presence of a foreign body such as a suture or a prosthetic device markedly decreases the inoculum of staphylococci required to produce experimental infection. Once established, such infections are very difficult to cure without removal of the foreign body. Strains of *S. epidermidis* are capable of adhering firmly to and invading plastic catheters and of secreting a protective glycocalyx covering the adherent colonies. Neutrophil function is also altered in the presence of a foreign body; phagocytosis and killing of *S. aureus* are diminished.

DIAGNOSIS The diagnosis of all staphylococcal infections is made by Gram stain and culture of purulent material, either aspirated pus or involved tissue, or by culture of normally sterile body fluids. Typical clustering of organisms may not be seen in clinical specimens; individual cocci and even short chains of three or four organisms may be present. Bacteria in the static phase or within leukocytes may appear gram-negative. Abundant neutrophils, many containing intracellular organisms, are usually present, except in severely neutropenic patients.

SPECIFIC DISEASES **Superficial infections** Infection of hair follicles manifested as a collection of minute erythematous papules without involvement of the surrounding skin or deeper tissues is termed *folliculitis*. A more extensive and invasive follicular or sebaceous gland infection with some involvement of subcutaneous tissues is termed a *furuncle*, or *boil*. Itching and mild pain are followed by progressive local swelling and erythema, and the overlying skin becomes exquisitely painful on pressure or motion. Relief of pain occurs promptly after spontaneous or surgical drainage.

Furuncles occur most commonly in areas subject to maceration or friction and poor personal hygiene or involved by acne or dermatitis. The face, neck, axillae, buttocks, and thighs are common sites. Staphylococcal infection may involve the apocrine sweat glands in the axilla or groin (hidradenitis suppurativa). These infections may be deep-seated and slow to localize and drain and are prone to recurrence and scarring.

Staphylococcal infections within the thick, fibrous, inelastic skin of the back of the neck and upper part of the back lead to formation of a *carbuncle*. The relative thickness and impermeability of the overlying skin lead to lateral extension and loculation, and a large, indurated, painful lesion with multiple ineffective drainage sites results. Carbuncles produce fever, leukocytosis, extreme pain, and prostration. Bacteremia is common.

Staphylococci frequently colonize impetiginous lesions, but most impetigo is due to group A streptococci. However, staphylococcal impetigo does occur, and while it cannot be clearly differentiated on the basis of its clinical features from streptococcal impetigo, it tends to produce multiple superficial, localized lesions at different stages of development, has a grayish rather than golden-yellow crust, and less often produces high fever. Staphylococcal bullous lesions are caused by exfoliatin-producing strains.

Treatment of most superficial infections does not require the use of antibiotics. Local moist heat, attention to personal hygiene, and washing with germicidal soaps that leave an inhibitory residue on the skin (hexachlorophene, chlorhexidine, triclosan) are usually sufficient. For more severe or recurrent disease, oral antibiotic therapy with dicloxacillin or cloxacillin (2 g/d in four divided doses) for 7 to 10 days may be effective. Incision and drainage should be utilized selectively. Disease presenting with prominent constitutional symptoms or facial or periorbital infection should be treated with intravenous doses of appropriate antimicrobials as outlined in the section on bacteremic disease.

Toxin-mediated staphylococcal diseases STAPHYLOCOCCAL SCALDED-SKIN SYNDROME (SSSS) SSSS is a generalized exfoliative dermatitis complicating infection by toxin (exfoliatin)–producing strains of *S. aureus*. The disease typically occurs in newborns (Ritter's disease) and in children under the age of 5; it is rare in adults. Strains of *S. aureus* causing SSSS in the United States are frequently phage group II. The disease begins with a localized cutaneous infection often accompanied by a nonspecific virus-like prodrome. Fever and leukocytosis are mild. A scarlatiniform rash begins in the perioral area, becomes generalized over the trunk and extremities, and finally desquamates. The disease may consist of rash alone (staphylococcal scarlet fever), or large, flaccid bullae develop that may be localized (more common in adults) or generalized. The bullae burst, resulting in red, denuded skin resembling a burn. Friction applied to healthy areas of skin causes the epidermis to wrinkle and separate (Nikolsky's sign). *S. aureus* can usually be recovered from the skin and nasopharynx. Most adults with SSSS are immunosuppressed or have renal insufficiency. Blood cultures are frequently positive, and mortality is significant. Therapy includes antistaphylococcal antibiotics and local skin care. Recovery usually occurs in infants and children.

In adults, SSSS has been grouped with other severe scalding syndromes such as toxic epidermal necrolysis (Lyell's disease). Drug reactions are the most frequent cause of toxic epidermal necrolysis in adults, and the syndrome may be differentiated from SSSS by skin biopsy. Cleavage of the skin in drug-induced toxic epidermal necrolysis occurs at the basal cell layer, resulting in full-thickness denudation, with a greater potential for superinfection and significant fluid and electrolyte loss. In SSSS, cleavage occurs within the epidermis. Kawasaki's disease and toxic shock syndrome also should be considered in the differential diagnosis of SSSS.

TOXIC SHOCK SYNDROME Toxic shock syndrome (TSS) was described in 1978 as a multisystem disease presenting with high fever, a "sunburn" rash that subsequently desquamated, and hypotension in children who had group I *S. aureus* isolated from mucosal or sequestered sites. In 1980, TSS became epidemic among young, primarily white, women, with onset during menstruation. A strong correlation was found between TSS and recovery of *S. aureus* from vaginal or cervical cultures of affected patients. Subsequently, a marker toxin, TSST-1, that mediates most cases of this syndrome was identified. Staphylococcal enterotoxins B or C1 also may mediate TSS. The pathogenesis involves establishment of a toxin-producing strain in a nonimmune individual under conditions favoring toxin formation, i.e., an aerobic, nutrient environment favoring late log to stationary phase growth of the organism. The attack rate of TSS among the 10 percent of persons lacking sufficient levels of antitoxin antibodies approaches 25 percent in those infected with toxin-positive strains.

Epidemiologically, TSS was associated with the introduction of certain brands of hyperabsorbent tampons. Public education and removal of hyperabsorbent tampons from the market have resulted in a marked decrease in the number of reported cases of TSS. Although the majority of cases continue to occur among menstruating females, nonmenstrual TSS now accounts for up to 45 percent of TSS cases in the United States.

The diagnosis of TSS is based on clinical criteria that include high fever, a diffuse rash that desquamates on the palms and soles over the subsequent 1 to 2 weeks, hypotension that may be orthostatic, and evidence of involvement in three or more organ systems. Such involvement commonly includes gastrointestinal dysfunction (vomiting or diarrhea), renal or hepatic insufficiency, mucous membrane hyperemia, thrombocytopenia, myalgias with elevated creatine phosphokinase (CK) levels, and disorientation with a normal cerebrospinal fluid examination. Hypocalcemia is common. Milder forms of the syndrome have been reported.

The onset is acute and typically occurs around the start of menses in a young woman using tampons or barrier contraception methods. The vaginal mucosa is hyperemic, and *S. aureus* can be cultured from the vaginal discharge. Blood cultures are usually negative. Clinical findings are the same in nonmenstrual-associated TSS. Cutaneous infections, postpartum vaginal and cesarean section wound infections, focal tissue infections (abscesses, empyema, osteomyelitis), postinfluenza pneumonia, and rarely, primary staphylococcal bacteremia have been associated with TSS. Signs of infection may be minimal among patients with postoperative wound infections where the onset typically occurs on the second day after surgery. Nosocomial transmission has been described. The mortality rate of TSS is 3 percent and is most often due to refractory hypotension and the development of the adult respiratory distress syndrome (ARDS) with or without disseminated intravascular coagulation.

Treatment is directed at correcting shock and treating renal failure, pulmonary insufficiency, and disseminated intravascular coagulation when present. Antistaphylococcal antibiotics should be administered parenterally. Focal collections of *S. aureus* must be drained. Because neutralizing antibodies are widespread, the use of intravenous pooled gamma globulin is being investigated. Up to 30 percent of menstruating women with TSS may have recurrences with subsequent menses, although these are generally milder. The use of antistaphylococcal antibiotics to treat TSS and discontinuation of tampon use significantly decrease the likelihood of recurrences.

The differential diagnosis of TSS includes Rocky Mountain spotted fever, meningococcemia, streptococcal scarlet fever, toxic epidermal necrolysis, and Kawasaki's syndrome. A similar syndrome has been described following group A streptococcal infection.

Staphylococcal food poisoning See Chap. 87.

Invasive staphylococcal infections BACTEREMIA AND ENDOCARDITIS Bacteremia due to *S. aureus* may arise from any local infection, at either extravascular (cutaneous infections, burns, cellulitis, osteomyelitis, arthritis) or intravascular foci (intravenous catheters, dialysis access sites, intravenous drug abuse). Up to one-third of patients do not have an identifiable focus.

Rarely, patients with bacteremia die within 12 to 24 h with high fever, tachycardia, cyanosis, and vascular collapse. Disseminated intravascular coagulation may produce a disease mimicking meningococcemia. Commonly, the disease progresses more slowly, with hectic fever and metastatic abscess formation in the bones, kidneys, lungs, myocardium, spleen, brain, or other tissues.

A major complication of *S. aureus* bacteremia is endocarditis (see Chap. 85). *S. aureus* is the second most common cause of endocarditis and the most common cause among drug addicts. Among nonaddicts, normal valves are involved in 30 to 60 percent of cases, and older, frequently hospitalized, patients with underlying medical disease are most often infected. The mitral, aortic, or both valves may be involved. The disease typically pursues an acute course with high fever, progressive anemia, and frequent embolic and extracardiac septic complications. Progressive valvular insufficiency leads to significant murmurs in 90 percent of patients. Valve ring and myocardial abscesses are common. The mortality rate is 20 to 30 percent. Infection of the aortic valve, the development of uncontrolled congestive heart failure, or evidence of central nervous system involvement are poor prognostic signs; these patients frequently require surgical intervention.

Among addicts, *S. aureus* frequently involves the tricuspid valve. Evidence for septic pulmonary emboli (chest pain, hemoptysis, nodular infiltrates) is common. Audible murmurs and peripheral stigmata of endocarditis are less common than in nonaddicts. Myalgias and back pain may be the major presenting symptoms and obfuscate the diagnosis. The mortality rate is 2 to 10 percent.

Differentiation of bacteremia from endocarditis may be difficult. Patients with normal heart valves with an identifiable, easily managed or removable primary focus of infection, who receive and respond promptly to appropriate antibiotic therapy, and who do not develop evidence of metastatic complications during the subsequent 2 weeks on therapy usually can be treated for bacteremia alone. Patients with underlying valvular disorders, with murmurs of valvular regurgitation, with community-acquired disease and no obvious focus, with infection secondary to drug abuse, with evidence for embolic events, or with echocardiographic evidence for vegetations should be treated for endocarditis. The presence of antibodies to the teichoic acid cell wall component of *S. aureus* after 2 weeks of illness does not distinguish reliably between endocarditis or bacteremia with metastatic foci and uncomplicated bacteremia.

Three carefully collected blood cultures are adequate for the diagnosis in most instances; usually all are positive for *S. aureus*. More cultures may be required if the patient has previously received antibiotics. Purulent skin lesions and urine also should be cultured before instituting antibiotic therapy. The urine may be positive in up to a third of cases of staphylococcal bacteremia (with colony counts typically lower than 10^5 per milliliter); staphylococcal bacteriuria in this setting does not indicate metastatic renal infection.

Intravenous therapy should be initiated with a penicillinase-resistant agent. Nafcillin (1.5 g every 4 h) and oxacillin (2.0 g every 4 h) are preferred to methicillin because of the high incidence of interstitial nephritis with methicillin. Gentamicin (1 mg/kg every 8 h, adjusted for renal function) may be added for the first 48 to 72 h because of evidence for synergy with β-lactam antimicrobials against *S. aureus* and the tendency for patients treated with both drugs to

defervesce more rapidly and to achieve earlier sterilization of the bloodstream. Rare isolates that do not produce β-lactamase should be treated with intravenous penicillin G (4×10^6 units every 4 h). First-generation cephalosporins (cephalothin, cefazolin) also have been used successfully in infections with both penicillinase-positive and -negative strains of *S. aureus*. Patients with serious penicillin allergy or with infections due to methicillin-resistant *S. aureus* should be treated with vancomycin 30 mg/kg per day in two or three divided doses, adjusted for renal function.

Cases of uncomplicated *S. aureus* bacteremia can be treated for 2 weeks. These patients should be followed carefully; relapses should be treated as endocarditis. Uncomplicated right-sided endocarditis in drug addicts has been treated successfully with 2 weeks of intravenous nafcillin plus tobramycin or gentamicin. All other cases of endocarditis should receive 4 to 6 weeks of parenteral antimicrobials. Prosthetic valve endocarditis should be treated with an appropriate penicillin or vancomycin plus gentamicin, with or without rifampin, for 6 weeks. Most cases will require surgery as well.

The response to antimicrobials in staphylococcal endocarditis may be slow, particularly when MRSA is treated with vancomycin. The fever may not disappear until the second week of therapy. Persistent fever or signs of sepsis should prompt a search for metastatic abscesses that require drainage.

S. epidermidis is the most common isolate in primary nosocomial bacteremias and the most frequent organism infecting intravenous access devices. It has been recognized as a major cause of bacteremia among neutropenic cancer patients, arising either from long-term indwelling central catheters or from the gastrointestinal tract, and among high-risk neonates receiving intravenous lipid emulsions. Continued fever, progressive sepsis, multiple pulmonary abscesses, and death may result if this complication is left untreated.

Although an uncommon cause of native valve endocarditis, *S. epidermidis* is the most common cause of prosthetic valve endocarditis (40 percent of cases). Most cases are due to inoculation of organisms at the time of surgery but may not become clinically apparent until 1 year later. Infections frequently involve the valve ring and require surgical intervention. Over 50 percent of patients die.

Because coagulase-negative staphylococci are frequent blood culture contaminants, distinguishing infection from contamination can be difficult. Positive blood cultures demand careful inspection of catheter sites and repeat blood cultures, even in the absence of symptoms, in patients with indwelling catheters or with prosthetic heart valves or vascular grafts. Speciation of multiple isolates may be useful if isolates can be demonstrated to be the same; plasmid analysis may be required. Catheters should be removed and cultured, although antibiotic therapy alone has been successful for treatment of bacteremic catheter-related infections.

Hospital-acquired *S. epidermidis* infections are usually multiply antibiotic-resistant. Methicillin resistance is heterotypic and difficult to exclude. For these reasons, all serious *S. epidermidis* infections should be treated with vancomycin in doses used for *S. aureus*. Prosthetic valve endocarditis should be treated for 6 weeks with vancomycin plus gentamicin, with or without rifampin. Monitoring of renal function and ototoxicity is required.

OSTEOMYELITIS *S. aureus* is responsible for the majority of cases of acute osteomyelitis (see Chap. 92). Although most common in persons under the age of 20, adults over 50 make up an increasingly prevalent group, particularly with involvement of the spine. A primary portal of entry is frequently not identified. In children, the frequent localization in the diaphyseal end of the long bones is thought to be due to the endarterial circulation of the diaphysis. Many patients give a history of preceding trauma to the involved area. Clavicular osteomyelitis has complicated septic thrombosis of a catheterized subclavian vein.

Once established, infection spreads through the newly formed juxtaepiphyseal bone to the periosteum or along the marrow cavity. If the infection reaches the subperiosteal space, the periosteum is lifted, a subperiosteal abscess forms, and rupture with infection of the subcutaneous tissues may occur. Rarely, the joint capsule is penetrated, producing pyogenic arthritis. There is death of bone, producing a sequestrum, followed by new bone formation, the involucrum. Occasionally, indolent staphylococcal infections of bone may persist for years within dense granulation tissue about a central necrotic cavity, a so-called Brodie's abscess.

Osteomyelitis in children may present as an acute process beginning abruptly with chills, high fever, nausea, vomiting, and progressive pain at the site of bony involvement. Muscle spasm about the affected bone is a common early sign, and the child may refuse to move the affected limb. Leukocytosis is common. Blood cultures are positive for *S. aureus* in 50 to 60 percent of cases early in disease. The tissues overlying the involved bone become edematous and warm, and the skin becomes erythematous. Anemia develops during the course of untreated disease.

Staphylococcal vertebral osteomyelitis in the adult differs considerably from acute osteomyelitis in the child. The onset is less abrupt, and there is a greater tendency for bony fusion with obliteration of the disk space. The lumbar spine is most frequently affected.

Osteomyelitis should be suspected in any child with fever, limb pain, and leukocytosis. Similarly, back or neck pain in an adult, when accompanied by fever, should raise the possibility of vertebral osteomyelitis. A history of a preceding cutaneous infection, local tenderness over the bone, and culture of *S. aureus* from the blood are confirmatory. Roentgenograms are usually normal during the first week, but radionuclide and MRI scans are generally abnormal. Bony rarefaction, local periosteal elevation, and new bone formation can frequently be seen during the second week. Needle aspiration or bone biopsy should be performed if necessary to obtain a specific etiologic diagnosis prior to institution of chemotherapy. In chronic osteomyelitis, sinus tracts are often present, but cultures of the sinus tracts are not reliable in the diagnosis.

Therapy should be initiated parenterally using a penicillinase-resistant semisynthetic penicillin as outlined for bacteremia and endocarditis and continued for 4 to 6 weeks. Cephalosporins and clindamycin also have been used. Uncomplicated osteomyelitis in children has been managed with 2 weeks of intravenous therapy followed by 2 to 4 weeks of oral therapy. Vancomycin can be used in penicillin-allergic patients and in infections due to methicillin-resistant organisms. Surgery may be required to remove devitalized bone and to drain soft tissue and periosteal abscesses. Neurologic findings due to epidural abscess and cord compression complicating vertebral osteomyelitis demand early surgical intervention. Aggressive treatment of acute osteomyelitis has decreased the incidence of chronic osteomyelitis, with its penchant for recurrent flare-ups and sinus formation. The cure rate for acute staphylococcal osteomyelitis is approximately 90 percent, and death is rare.

PNEUMONIA   (See Chap. 207) *S. aureus* causes approximately 3 percent of community-acquired bacterial pneumonias. This disease occurs sporadically except during influenza outbreaks, when staphylococcal pneumonia is relatively more common, although still less frequent than pneumococcal pneumonia.

Primary staphylococcal pneumonia in infants and children frequently presents with high fever and cough. Multiple thin-walled abscesses, or pneumatoceles, are present on the chest roentgenogram. Empyema formation is common. Cough may be nonproductive, and blood cultures are usually negative, frequently necessitating empiric antistaphylococcal therapy. In older children and healthy adults, staphylococcal pneumonia is generally preceded by an influenza-like respiratory infection (influenza, measles, or other viruses). Onset of staphylococcal involvement is abrupt, with chills, high fever, progressive dyspnea, cyanosis, cough, and pleural pain. The sputum may be bloody or frankly purulent.

Staphylococci frequently colonize the bronchiectatic airways in children with cystic fibrosis and may cause recurrent episodes of bronchopneumonia. Nosocomial staphylococcal pneumonia typically occurs in intubated patients in intensive care units and in debilitated patients who are prone to aspiration. Residents of nursing homes may have an increased incidence of staphylococcal pneumonia. Infections distal to an obstructing bronchogenic carcinoma also may be caused by *S. aureus*. These infections can begin insidiously, with increasing fever, tachycardia, and tachypnea the only indications of infection. The disease also may be less abrupt when pulmonary involvement occurs during the course of staphylococcal bacteremia, as in patients with right-sided endocarditis or septic thrombophlebitis. Cavitation and pleural effusions are common, but empyema is unusual.

The course of staphylococcal pneumonia may be stormy despite adequate antimicrobial therapy. Gradual defervescence starting 48 to 72 h after the initiation of therapy is typical.

Staphylococcal pneumonia must be differentiated from other pneumonias. The preceding influenza-like illness, rapid onset of pleural pain, cyanosis, and prostration out of proportion to physical findings should suggest primary staphylococcal pneumonia. Sputum Gram stain showing masses of neutrophils and gram-positive intraleukocytic cocci provides supportive evidence. Leukocytosis is generally present. Blood cultures are positive in 20 to 30 percent of cases. When pneumonia develops suddenly or insidiously in debilitated hospital patients, staphylococci should be considered.

Parenteral therapy should be initiated with antistaphylococcal antimicrobials as outlined for serious bacteremia and endocarditis. Two weeks of intravenous therapy is usually adequate if complications do not develop. Empyema usually necessitates chest tube drainage and may be complicated by the formation of loculations or bronchopleural fistulas. Ultrasound or computed tomography (CT) scan may be required to identify loculated collections of pus for drainage.

CNS INFECTION   *S. aureus* causes 1 to 9 percent of cases of bacterial meningitis and 10 to 15 percent of brain abscesses. Most commonly, spread from a focus outside the CNS, typically from infective endocarditis or by extension from a paraspinal or parameningeal abscess, or nosocomial infection following neurosurgical procedures have been involved. Blood cultures are usually positive. Over 50 percent of epidural abscesses are due to *S. aureus*; up to half these cases may be associated with vertebral osteomyelitis. The thoracic spine and lumbar spine are most frequently involved. Patients present with either acute (<2 weeks) or chronic back pain, usually with low-grade fever and malaise. The onset of radicular pain is an ominous sign that portends progression to frank neurologic dysfunction and ultimate paralysis. The diagnosis is most reliably established using magnetic resonance imaging, although CT scanning and myelography have been useful. Surgical drainage, often with decompression laminectomy, and parenteral antibiotics are required. The duration of therapy is dependent on the adequacy of drainage and the presence or absence of coexisting osteomyelitis.

URINARY TRACT INFECTION   *S. saprophyticus* is, after *Escherichia coli*, the most common cause of primary, nonobstructive urinary tract infection in sexually active young women (see Chap. 90). It is responsible for 10 to 20 percent of infections in healthy outpatients. Symptoms of urgency, frequency, and burning are indistinguishable from urinary infections due to other agents. Fever is absent or low-grade. Although lower tract infection is most common, pyelonephritis has been reported.

The diagnosis is established by examination of the urinary sediment, which characteristically reveals pyuria, microscopic hematuria, and cocci in clumps. The organism may be identified by its resistance to novobiocin and nalidixic acid. *S. saprophyticus* grows readily on blood agar but less well on MacConkey agar and may be missed by currently available rapid diagnostic methods that depend on nitrate reduction or glucose utilization. The criterion for greater than 10^5 bacteria per milliliter developed for gram-negative urinary tract infection is unreliable.

The organism is susceptible to most antimicrobials used for urinary tract infection, including ampicillin, trimethoprim, sulfonamides, and nitrofurantoin. Relapses after appropriate therapy should raise the consideration of infected renal calculi, which may be formed because of the organism's capacity to produce urease.

Isolation of *S. aureus* from a well-collected urine specimen should prompt consideration of staphylococcal bacteremia, which may have been complicated by renal, perinephric, or prostatic abscesses.

Other infections Infection of the vascular access site with *S. aureus* is a major cause of morbidity and death among patients on hemodialysis. Chronic nasal carriage is the source of most infections. The use of 5-day courses of oral rifampin and topical bacitracin every 3 months significantly decreases the incidence of infection and should be considered in hemodialysis centers where such infections are endemic. *S. epidermidis* and *S. aureus* rank first and second among pathogens infecting prosthetic devices and intravascular grafts and are particularly problematic in AIDS patients with indwelling catheters. Acute *S. aureus* pyomyositis also may complicate the course of HIV infection. *S. epidermidis* infections tend to be more insidious and frequently pursue a prolonged course with high morbidity due in part to the temptation to regard positive cultures as contaminants. *S. epidermidis* is a common cause of endophthalmitis complicating ocular surgery. *S. aureus* is a frequent cause of mastitis among nursing mothers.

CONTROL OF HOSPITAL OUTBREAKS (See Chap. 98) Hospital outbreaks of staphylococcal disease may develop rapidly in burn units, intensive care units, or neonatal care units—areas housing debilitated patients under continuous antibiotic pressure. The index case is frequently a patient recently discharged or transferred from another hospital where the organism is endemic. The implicated strains of *S. aureus* are frequently methicillin-resistant (MRSA).

Control demands the rapid identification of the patient reservoir in the affected care units by cultures of wounds, nares, and perineum; urine cultures should be performed for patients with indwelling urinary catheters. Isolation of culture-positive patients together with reinforcement of the need for proper aseptic technique and hand washing by hospital personnel decreases transmission. Housekeeping antisepsis using phenolic cleaning agents should be carried out in the rooms of colonized patients. Early discharge of colonized patients should be encouraged. Charts should be labeled and the patient returned to strict isolation upon readmission to the hospital until shown to be culture-negative.

Although nasal carriers among hospital personnel may transmit the organism, efficient dissemination is by cutaneous diseases (eczema, atopic dermatitis) that have become colonized with *S. aureus*. Such personnel should be removed from clinical duties until they become culture-negative either spontaneously or following therapy.

Decolonization of the skin and nares in patients and personnel has been accomplished by whole-body washing with antiseptic soaps that leave an inhibitory residue on the skin—hexachlorophene, chlorhexidine, or triclosan. Topical antibiotics are generally ineffective. Although intranasal application of mupirocin has eradicated carriage, resistance can develop. Oral antibiotics may be required to abolish the carrier state. Rifampin (600 mg every day for 5 days) has been used successfully alone or, depending on the sensitivity of the staphylococcal isolate, combined with trimethoprim-sulfamethoxazole, doxycycline, or dicloxacillin to prevent the emergence of rifampin resistance.

REFERENCES

BOHACH GA et al: Staphylococcal and streptococcal pyrogenic toxins involved in toxic shock syndrome and related illnesses. Crit Rev Microbiol 17:251, 1990

BRUMFITT W, HAMILTON-MILLER J: Methicillin-resistant *Staphylococcus aureus*. N Engl J Med 320:1188, 1989

ESPERSEN F et al: Changing pattern of bone and joint infections due to *Staphylococcus aureus*: Study of cases of bacteremia in Denmark, 1959–1988. Rev Infect Dis 13:347, 1991

MARTIN MA et al: Coagulase-negative staphylococcal bacteremia: Mortality and hospital stay. Ann Intern Med 110:9, 1989

RAAD II, SABBAGH MF: Optimal duration of therapy for catheter-related *Staphylococcus aureus* bacteremia: A study of 55 cases and review. Clin Infect Dis 14:75, 1992

SCHWARTZMAN WA et al: Staphylococcal pyomyositis in patients infected by the human immunodeficiency virus. Am J Med 90:595, 1991

TRUCKIS M et al: Emerging resistance to fluoroquinolones in staphylococci: An alert. Ann Intern Med 114:424, 1991

103 STREPTOCOCCAL INFECTIONS

MICHAEL R. WESSELS

Many varieties of streptococci are found as part of the normal human flora colonizing the respiratory, gastrointestinal, and genitourinary tracts. Several species are important causes of human disease. Group A streptococcus, or *Streptococcus pyogenes,* is the organism responsible for streptococcal pharyngitis, one of the most common bacterial infections of school-age children, and for the postinfectious syndromes of acute rheumatic fever and poststreptococcal glomerulonephritis. Group B streptococcus, or *S. agalactiae,* is the leading cause of bacterial sepsis and meningitis in newborns and a major cause of endometritis and fever in parturient women. Enterococci are important causes of urinary tract infection, intraabdominal infections, and endocarditis. Viridans streptococci are the most common cause of bacterial endocarditis.

Streptococci are gram-positive bacteria of spherical to ovoid shape that characteristically form chains when grown in liquid media. Most streptococci that cause human infections are facultative anaerobes, although some are strict anaerobes. Streptococci are relatively fastidious organisms, requiring enriched media for growth in the laboratory. No single scheme for classification of streptococci is entirely satisfactory. Consequently, clinicians and clinical microbiologists commonly identify streptococci by any of several classification systems, including hemolytic pattern, Lancefield group, species name, or a common or trivial name. Many of the streptococci associated with human infection produce a zone of complete hemolysis around the bacterial colony when cultured on blood agar, a pattern known as *beta hemolysis.* The beta-hemolytic streptococci can be classified by the Lancefield system, a serologic grouping based on the reaction of specific antisera with cell wall carbohydrate antigens of the bacteria. With rare exceptions, organisms belonging to Lancefield groups A, B, C, and G are all beta-hemolytic streptococci, and each is associated with characteristic patterns of human infections. Other streptococci produce a zone of partial, or alpha, hemolysis, often imparting a greenish appearance to the agar. These alpha-hemolytic streptococci are further identified by biochemical testing and include *S. pneumoniae,* an important cause of pneumonia, meningitis, and other infections (discussed in Chap. 101), and several species of streptococci referred to collectively as the *viridans streptococci,* part of normal oral flora and important as agents of subacute bacterial endocarditis. Finally, some streptococci are nonhemolytic, a pattern sometimes called *gamma hemolysis.* Classification of the major groups of streptococci responsible for human infections is outlined in Table 103-1. Among the group D streptococci, the species previously designated as *S. faecalis* and *S. faecium* have recently been renamed *Enterococcus faecalis* and *E. faecium,* respectively, on the basis of DNA homology studies. Although, technically, these organisms now fall into a separate genus from true streptococci, they will be discussed in this chapter, since clinical syndromes associated with the enterococci are generally considered within the context of other streptococcal infections from which they must be distinguished.

GROUP A STREPTOCOCCUS

Lancefield's group A consists of a single species, *S. pyogenes.* As its species name implies, this organism is associated with a variety of suppurative infections. In addition, group A streptococci are unique among known bacterial pathogens in their capacity to trigger the postinfectious syndromes of acute rheumatic fever (see Chap. 200) and poststreptococcal glomerulonephritis (see Chap. 240).

Group A streptococci elaborate a number of cell surface components and extracellular products important both in the pathogenesis of infection and in the immune response of the human host. The cell

TABLE 103-1 Classification of streptococci

Lancefield group	Representative species	Hemolytic pattern	Typical infections
A	S. pyogenes	Beta	Pharyngitis, impetigo, cellulitis, scarlet fever
B	S. agalactiae	Beta	Neonatal sepsis and meningitis, puerperal infections, urinary tract infection, diabetic ulcer infection, endocarditis
C	S. equi	Beta	Cellulitis, bacteremia, endocarditis
D	Enterococci E. faecalis E. faecium	Usually nonhemolytic	Urinary tract infection, wound infection, endocarditis
	Nonenterococci S. bovis	Usually nonhemolytic	Bacteremia, endocarditis
G	S. canis	Beta	Cellulitis, bacteremia, endocarditis
Variable or nongroupable	Viridans streptococci S. mutans S. sanguis	Alpha	Endocarditis, dental abscess, brain abscess
	Intermedius or milleri group S. milleri	Beta	Brain abscess, visceral abscess
	Anaerobic streptococci Peptostreptococcus magnus	Usually nonhemolytic	Sinusitis, pneumonia, empyema, brain abscess, liver abscess

wall contains a carbohydrate antigen that may be released from the bacterial cells by treatment with acid. The reaction of such acid extracts with group A–specific antiserum is the basis for the definitive identification of a streptococcal strain as *S. pyogenes*. The major surface protein of group A streptococci is M protein, which occurs in more than 80 antigenically distinct types and is the basis for serotyping strains with specific antisera. The M protein molecules are fibrillar structures anchored in the cell wall of the organism and extending as hairlike projections away from the cell surface. The amino acid sequence of the distal or amino-terminal portion of the M protein molecule is quite variable, accounting for the antigenic variation of the different M types, while more proximal regions of the protein are relatively conserved. The presence of M protein correlates with the capacity of a strain to resist phagocytic killing in fresh human blood, a phenomenon that appears to be due, at least in part, to binding of plasma fibrinogen to M protein molecules on the streptococcal surface, thereby interfering with complement activation and deposition of opsonic complement fragments on the bacterial cell. This resistance to phagocytosis may be overcome by M protein–specific antibodies, accounting for the observation that individuals with antibodies to a given M type acquired as a result of prior infection are protected against subsequent infection with organisms of the same, but not different, M types. Group A streptococci also elaborate, to varying degrees, a polysaccharide capsule composed of hyaluronic acid. Certain strains produce large amounts of hyaluronic acid capsule, resulting in a characteristic mucoid appearance to the bacterial colonies. The capsular polysaccharide also plays an important role in protecting the organisms from ingestion and killing by phagocytes. In contrast to M protein, the hyaluronic acid capsule is a weak immunogen, and antihyaluronate antibodies have not been shown to be important in protective immunity, presumably because of the apparent structural identity between streptococcal hyaluronic acid and the hyaluronic acid of mammalian connective tissues.

Group A streptococci produce a large number of extracellular products that may be important in local and systemic toxicity and in facilitating the spread of infection through tissues. These products include streptolysins S and O, toxins that damage cell membranes and account for the hemolysis produced by the organisms; streptokinase; DNAses; protease; and pyrogenic exotoxins A, B, and C. The pyrogenic exotoxins, previously known as *erythrogenic toxins,* cause the rash of scarlet fever. More recently, exotoxin A–producing strains of group A streptococcus have been linked to unusually severe, invasive infections, including necrotizing fasciitis and a systemic syndrome termed the *streptococcal toxic shock–like syndrome.* Several extracellular products stimulate specific antibody responses useful in serodiagnosis of recent streptococcal infection. These antibody tests are used primarily as evidence of preceding streptococcal infection in cases of suspected acute rheumatic fever or poststreptococcal glomerulonephritis.

PHARYNGITIS Group A streptococcal pharyngitis is one of the most common bacterial infections of childhood, accounting for 20 to 40 percent of cases of exudative pharyngitis. Streptococcal pharyngitis is seen in patients of all ages; it is most common in children but is rare in children under the age of 3. Younger children may manifest streptococcal infection with a syndrome of fever, malaise, and lymphadenopathy without exudative pharyngitis. Infection is acquired through contact with another individual carrying the organism. Respiratory droplets are the usual mechanism of spread, although other routes are well described, including food-borne outbreaks.

Clinical features The incubation period is 1 to 4 days. Symptoms include sore throat, fever and chills, malaise, and sometimes abdominal complaints and vomiting, particularly in children. Both symptoms and signs are quite variable, ranging from mild throat discomfort with minimal physical findings to high fever and severe sore throat associated with intense erythema and swelling of the pharyngeal mucosa and the presence of purulent exudate over the posterior pharyngeal wall and tonsillar pillars. Enlarged, tender anterior cervical lymph nodes are commonly found accompanying exudative pharyngitis.

The differential diagnosis of streptococcal pharyngitis includes the many other bacterial and viral causes of pharyngitis. Other infections commonly producing exudative pharyngitis include infectious mononucleosis and adenovirus infection. Now rare in the United States, the pseudomembrane of diphtheria also may give a similar appearance. *Corynebacterium (Arcanobacterium) hemolyticum* may cause pharyngitis, often in association with a scarlet fever–like rash. Other causes of pharyngitis, usually without a purulent exudate, include coxsackievirus, influenza, *Mycoplasma, Neisseria gonorrhoeae,* and acute infection with HIV. Because of the range of clinical presentations of streptococcal pharyngitis and the large number of other agents that can produce the same clinical picture, diagnosis of streptococcal pharyngitis on clinical grounds alone is not reliable.

The throat culture remains the gold standard for diagnosis of streptococcal pharyngitis. When properly collected (a sterile swab rubbed vigorously over both tonsillar pillars) and processed, the throat culture is the most sensitive and specific means available to make a definitive diagnosis. Rapid diagnostic kits using latex agglutination or enzyme immunoassay of swab specimens are now widely available and can serve as a useful adjunct to the throat culture. While precise figures on sensitivity and specificity vary among studies, in general, the rapid diagnostic kits are highly specific (greater than 95 percent), so a positive result can be relied on for definitive diagnosis and precludes the need for a throat culture. However, the rapid diagnostic tests are less sensitive than throat culture, with a relative sensitivity ranging from 55 to 90 percent in comparative studies, so a negative rapid diagnostic test should be confirmed with a throat culture.

The usual course of uncomplicated streptococcal pharyngitis is resolution of symptoms after 3 to 5 days. The course is shortened little by treatment, which is given primarily to prevent suppurative complications and rheumatic fever. Prevention of rheumatic fever depends on eradication of the organism from the pharynx, not simply on resolution of symptoms, and requires 10 days of penicillin treatment, either as a single intramuscular dose of benzathine penicillin G or as a 10-day course of oral penicillin (Table 103-2). Erythromycin may be substituted for individuals allergic to penicillin. Follow-up culture after treatment is no longer routinely recommended, though it may be warranted in selected cases, such as patients or families with frequent streptococcal infections or situations in which the risk of rheumatic fever is thought to be high, e.g., when cases have occurred recently in the community.

Suppurative complications of streptococcal pharyngitis have become uncommon with the widespread use of antibiotics for most cases of symptomatic streptococcal infection. These complications arise as a result of spread of infection from the pharyngeal mucosa to deeper tissues, either by direct extension or via hematogenous or lymphatic spread, and may include cervical lymphadenitis, peritonsillar or retropharyngeal abscess, sinusitis, otitis media, meningitis, bacteremia, endocarditis, and pneumonia. Local complications such as abscess formation in the peritonsillar or parapharyngeal space should be considered in a patient with unusually severe or prolonged symptoms or localized pain associated with high fever and toxic appearance.

ASYMPTOMATIC CARRIER STATE Surveillance cultures have shown that up to 20 percent of individuals, in certain populations, may have asymptomatic pharyngeal colonization with group A streptococci. There are no definitive guidelines for management of these asymptomatic carriers or of asymptomatic individuals with a positive throat culture after a full course of treatment for symptomatic pharyngitis. A reasonable course of action is to give a single 10-day course of penicillin for symptomatic pharyngitis but not to retreat if positive cultures persist unless symptoms recur. Studies of the natural history of streptococcal carriage and infection have shown that the risk both of developing rheumatic fever and of transmitting infection to others is substantially less in asymptomatic carriers than in individuals with symptomatic pharyngitis, so overly aggressive attempts at eradicating carriage are probably not justified under most circumstances. An exception to this general statement is the situation in which an asymptomatic carrier is a source of infection to others. Outbreaks of food-borne infection and nosocomial puerperal infections have been traced to asymptomatic carriers who may harbor the organisms in the throat, on the skin, or in the vagina or anus. In cases in which a carrier is transmitting infection to others, attempts to eradicate carriage are warranted, although data are limited on the best regimen to clear the organism after penicillin alone has failed. The combination of penicillin and rifampin has been used to eliminate pharyngeal carriage, and addition of oral vancomycin has been successful in eradicating rectal colonization, although there is not extensive experience with any regimen.

TABLE 103-2 Treatment of group A streptococcal infections

Infection	Treatment
Pharyngitis	Benzathine penicillin G, 1.2 million units IM or penicillin V, 250 mg PO qid x 10 days (Children <27 kg: Benzathine penicillin G, 600,000 units IM or penicillin V, 125 mg PO qid x 10 days)
Impetigo	Same as pharyngitis
Erysipelas/cellulitis	Severe: Penicillin G, 1 to 2 million units IV q4h Mild to moderate: Procaine penicillin, 1.2 million units IM bid
Necrotizing fasciitis/ myositis	Surgical debridement plus penicillin G, 2 to 4 million units IV q4h
Pneumonia/empyema	Penicillin G, 2 to 4 million units IV q4h plus drainage of empyema

* Penicillin allergy: Erythromycin (10 mg/kg PO qid up to maximum of 250 mg per dose) may be substituted for oral penicillin. Alternative agents for parenteral therapy include first-generation cephalosporins if the nature of the allergy is not an immediate hypersensitivity reaction (anaphylaxis or urticaria) or other potentially life-threatening manifestation (e.g., severe rash and fever) or vancomycin.

SCARLET FEVER Scarlet fever is streptococcal infection, usually pharyngitis, accompanied by a characteristic rash. The rash arises from the effects of one of three toxins, currently designated streptococcal pyrogenic exotoxins A, B, and C and known previously as erythrogenic or scarlet fever toxins. Scarlet fever was thought to reflect infection of an individual lacking toxin-specific immunity with a toxin-producing strain of group A streptococcus. Susceptibility to scarlet fever was correlated with results of the Dick test: A small amount of erythrogenic toxin injected intradermally produced local erythema in susceptible individuals but no reaction in those with specific immunity. Subsequent studies have suggested that development of the scarlet fever rash may reflect a hypersensitivity reaction requiring prior exposure to the toxin. For reasons that are not clear, scarlet fever has become less common in recent years, although strains of group A streptococci that produce exotoxins B or C continue to be prevalent in the population. The symptoms of scarlet fever are the same as for pharyngitis alone. The rash typically begins on the first or second day of illness over the upper trunk, spreading to involve the extremities but sparing the palms and soles. The rash is made up of minute papules, giving a characteristic "sandpaper" feel to the skin. Associated findings include circumoral pallor, "strawberry tongue" (enlarged papillae on a coated tongue which may later become denuded), and accentuation of the rash in the skin folds (Pastia's lines). The rash subsides after 6 to 9 days and is followed after several days by desquamation of the palms and soles. The differential diagnosis of scarlet fever includes other causes of fever and generalized rash, such as measles and other viral exanthems, Kawasaki's disease, toxic shock syndrome, and systemic allergic reactions such as drug eruptions.

SKIN AND SOFT TISSUE INFECTIONS Group A streptococci, and occasionally other streptococcal species, cause a variety of infections involving the skin, subcutaneous tissues, muscles, and fascia. While several clinical syndromes, recognized according to the tissues involved, are a useful means for classification of skin and soft tissue infections, not all cases fit exactly into a single category. The classic syndromes should be considered as general guides to predicting the level of tissue involvement in a particular patient, the likely clinical course, and the likelihood that surgical intervention or aggressive life support will be required.

Impetigo (pyoderma) Impetigo is a superficial infection of the skin caused primarily by group A streptococci, occasionally by other streptococci or by *Staphylococcus aureus*. Impetigo is seen most often in young children, tends to occur during the warmer months, and is more common in semitropical or tropical climates than in cooler regions. Infection is more common among children living under conditions of poor hygiene. Prospective studies have shown that colonization of unbroken skin with group A streptococci precedes the development of clinical infection. Minor trauma, such as a scratch or insect bite, may then serve to inoculate organisms into the skin. Impetigo is best prevented, therefore, by attention to adequate hygiene. The usual sites of involvement are the face, particularly around the nose and mouth, and the legs, although lesions may occur at other locations. Individual lesions begin as red papules that evolve quickly to vesicular and then pustular lesions which break down and coalesce to form characteristic honey-like crusts. Lesions are generally not painful, and patients do not appear ill. Fever is not a feature of impetigo and, if present, should suggest infection extending to deeper tissues or another diagnosis.

The classic presentation of impetigo usually is not difficult to diagnose. Cultures of impetiginous lesions often show *S. aureus* as well as group A streptococci, but longitudinal studies have shown that, in almost all cases, streptococci can be isolated initially, with staphylococci appearing later, presumably as secondary colonizing flora. Penicillin is nearly always effective in these infections, although most staphylococcal strains are resistant, further supporting the primary role of streptococci in the infection. An exception to this general rule is bullous impetigo due to *S. aureus*, distinguished from streptococcal infection by the presence of more extensive, bullous lesions that break down and leave thin, paper-like crusts, in contrast to the thick, amber crusts of streptococcal impetigo. Other skin lesions which may be confused with impetigo include herpetic lesions, either of orolabial herpes simplex or of chicken pox or zoster. Herpetic lesions can generally be distinguished by their appearance as more discrete, grouped vesicles and by a positive Tzanck test. In difficult cases, cultures of vesicle fluid should yield group A streptococci in the case of impetigo and the responsible virus in herpesvirus infections.

Treatment of impetigo is the same as for streptococcal pharyngitis. Rheumatic fever is not a sequel to streptococcal skin infections, in contrast to pharyngitis, although poststreptococcal glomerulonephritis may follow either skin or throat infection. The reason for this difference is not known. One hypothesis is that the immune response necessary for development of rheumatic fever only occurs following infection of the pharyngeal mucosa. In addition, the strains of group A streptococci that cause pharyngitis are generally of different M-protein types from those associated with skin infections, suggesting that the strains that cause pharyngitis may have rheumatogenic potential, while the skin strains do not.

Cellulitis Inoculation of organisms into the skin may lead to infection involving the skin and subcutaneous tissues, or cellulitis. The portal of entry may be a traumatic or surgical wound, an insect bite, or any break in skin integrity. Often, no entry site is apparent.

A particular form of streptococcal cellulitis is known as *erysipelas*. Erysipelas is characterized by a bright red appearance of the involved skin which forms a plateau, sharply demarcated from surrounding normal skin. The lesion is warm to touch, may be tender, and appears shiny and swollen. The skin often has a *peau d'orange* texture, thought to reflect involvement of superficial lymphatics; superficial blebs or bullae may form, usually 2 or 3 days after onset. The lesion typically develops over a few hours and is associated with fever and chills. Erysipelas tends to occur in certain characteristic locations; the malar area of the face, often with extension over the bridge of the nose to the contralateral malar region, and the lower extremities are the usual sites. After one episode, recurrence at the same site, sometimes years later, is not uncommon.

Classic cases of erysipelas, with the typical features described above, are almost always due to group A streptococci. Often, however, the appearance of streptococcal cellulitis is not sufficiently distinctive to permit a specific diagnosis on clinical grounds; the area of involvement may be other than one of the typical sites for erysipelas, the lesion may be less intensely red and may fade into surrounding skin, and patients may appear only mildly ill. In such cases, it is prudent to broaden empirical antimicrobial therapy to include other potential pathogens, particularly *S. aureus*, that can produce cellulitis with the same appearance.

Streptococcal cellulitis tends to occur at anatomic sites in which the normal lymphatic drainage has been disrupted, such as sites of prior episodes of cellulitis, the arm ipsilateral to a mastectomy and axillary lymph node dissection, a lower extremity previously involved with deep venous thrombosis or chronic lymphedema, and the leg from which a saphenous vein has been harvested for coronary artery bypass grafting. The organism may enter via a breach in the dermal barrier at a location some distance from the eventual site of clinical cellulitis. For example, some patients with recurrent episodes of leg cellulitis following saphenous vein removal have stopped having recurrent episodes only after treatment of tinea pedis on the foot of the affected extremity, fissures in the skin presumably having served as a portal of entry for streptococci which then produced infection more proximally in the leg at the site of previous injury. Another setting in which streptococcal cellulitis may occur is recent surgical wounds. Group A streptococci are among the few bacterial pathogens that typically produce signs of wound infection and surrounding cellulitis within the first 24 h after surgery. These wound infections are usually associated with a thin exudate and may spread rapidly, either as cellulitis in the skin and subcutaneous tissue or as a deeper tissue infection (see below). Streptococcal wound infection or localized cellulitis also may be associated with *lymphangitis,* manifested by red streaks extending proximally along superficial lymphatics from the site of infection.

Deep soft tissue infections *Necrotizing fasciitis,* also referred to as *hemolytic streptococcal gangrene,* is an infection involving the superficial and/or deep fascia investing the muscles of an extremity or the trunk. The source of the infection is either organisms on the skin, introduced into the tissue as a result of trauma that may be trivial, or bowel flora released during abdominal surgery or from an occult enteric source such as a diverticular or appendiceal abscess. The site of inoculation in both forms of necrotizing fasciitis may be inapparent and often is some distance from the site of clinical involvement, e.g., minor trauma to the hand associated with clinical infection of the tissues overlying the shoulder or chest. In cases of necrotizing fasciitis associated with bowel flora, the infection is usually polymicrobial, involving a mixture of anaerobic bacteria, such as *Bacteroides fragilis* or anaerobic streptococci, and facultative organisms, usually gram-negative bacilli. Cases unrelated to contamination from bowel organisms are most commonly caused by group A streptococci, either alone or in combination with other organisms, most often *S. aureus*. Overall, group A streptococci are implicated in about 60 percent of cases of necrotizing fasciitis. The onset of symptoms is usually quite acute and is marked by severe pain at the site of involvement, malaise, fever, chills, and a toxic appearance. The physical findings, particularly early in the illness, may not be striking, with only minimal erythema of the overlying skin. Pain and tenderness are usually severe, in contrast to more superficial cellulitis in which the skin appearance is more abnormal, but pain and tenderness are only mild or moderate. As the infection progresses, often in a matter of several hours, the severity and extent of symptoms worsen, and skin changes become more apparent, with the appearance of dusky or mottled erythema and edema. The marked tenderness of the involved area may evolve to anesthesia, as the spreading inflammatory process produces infarction of cutaneous nerves. Once the diagnosis is suspected, early surgical exploration is indicated, both to confirm the diagnosis and for treatment. The findings at operation are necrosis and inflammatory fluid tracking along the fascial planes above and between muscle groups, without involvement of the muscles themselves. The process usually is found to extend beyond the area of clinical involvement, and extensive debridement is required. Drainage and debridement are central to the management of necrotizing fasciitis; antibiotic treatment is useful as adjunctive therapy (see Table 103-2), but surgery is lifesaving.

Group A streptococci may produce abscesses in skeletal muscles *(streptococcal myositis)* with little or no involvement of surrounding fascia or overlying skin. This syndrome is more commonly due to *S. aureus* infection but is occasionally caused by group A streptococci. Presentation is usually subacute, but a fulminant form of streptococcal myositis has been described, associated with severe systemic toxicity, bacteremia, and a high mortality. The fulminant form may reflect the same basic disease process as that seen in necrotizing fasciitis, but with extension of the necrotizing inflammatory process into the muscles themselves, rather than remaining limited to fascial layers. Treatment for streptococcal myositis is surgical drainage, usually by an open procedure, to evaluate the extent of the infection and ensure adequate debridement of involved tissues and high-dose penicillin (see Table 103-2).

PNEUMONIA AND EMPYEMA Group A streptococci are an occasional cause of pneumonia, generally in previously healthy individuals. Onset of symptoms may be abrupt or gradual. Pleuritic chest pain, fever, chills, and dyspnea are the usual symptoms. Cough is usually present but may not be prominent. Approximately one-half of patients with group A streptococcal pneumonia have an accompanying pleural effusion. In contrast to the sterile parapneumonic effusions typically seen with pneumococcal pneumonia, those complicating streptococcal pneumonia are almost always infected. The empyema fluid is usually visible by chest x-ray on initial presentation and may enlarge rapidly. These pleural collections should be drained early because they tend to become loculated rapidly, resulting in a chronic fibrotic reaction that may require thoracotomy for removal.

BACTEREMIA, PUERPERAL SEPSIS, AND STREPTOCOCCAL TOXIC SHOCK–LIKE SYNDROME Bacteremia with group A streptococcus is usually associated with an identifiable local infection. Bacteremia occurs rarely with otherwise uncomplicated pharyngitis, somewhat more frequently with cellulitis or pneumonia, and relatively frequently in patients with necrotizing fasciitis. Occasionally, there is no apparent source for the bacteremia. Bacteremia without an identified source should raise suspicion of endocarditis, an occult abscess, or osteomyelitis. A variety of focal infections may arise secondarily from streptococcal bacteremia, including endocarditis, meningitis, septic arthritis, osteomyelitis, peritonitis, and visceral abscesses.

Group A streptococci are occasionally implicated in infectious complications of childbirth, usually endometritis and associated bacteremia. In the preantibiotic era, puerperal sepsis was commonly caused by group A streptococci, but currently it is more often caused by group B streptococci. Several nosocomial outbreaks of puerperal infections due to group A streptococci have been traced to an asymptomatic carrier, usually an individual present at the time of delivery of the infant. The site of carriage may be the skin, throat, anus, or vagina.

In 1987, Cone and associates described a series of patients with group A streptococcal infections associated with shock and multisystem disease. Several subsequent reports have described the same syndrome, which has been called the *streptococcal toxic shock–like syndrome* because it shares certain features with staphylococcal toxic shock syndrome. While a formal case definition has not been established, the general features of the illness include fever, hypotension, renal impairment, and respiratory distress syndrome. Various types of rashes have been described, but rash is usually absent. Laboratory abnormalities include a marked shift to the left in the white blood cell differential, with many immature granulocytes, hypocalcemia, hypoalbuminemia, and thrombocytopenia, which usually becomes more pronounced on the second or third day of illness. In contrast to those with staphylococcal toxic shock, the majority of patients with the streptococcal syndrome are bacteremic. The most common associated infection is a soft tissue infection—necrotizing fasciitis, myositis, or cellulitis—although a variety of other local infections have been described in association with the syndrome, including pneumonia, peritonitis, osteomyelitis, and myometritis. Streptococcal toxic shock–like syndrome is associated with a 30 percent mortality, with most deaths secondary to shock and respiratory failure. Because of the rapidly progressive and lethal course of the illness, early recognition of the syndrome is essential. Patients should be given aggressive supportive care in the form of fluid resuscitation, pressors, and mechanical ventilation, in addition to antimicrobial therapy and, in cases associated with necrotizing fasciitis, surgical debridement. Exactly why certain patients develop this fulminant syndrome is not known; however, studies of the streptococcal strains isolated from patients with streptococcal toxic shock–like syndrome have shown a strong association with production of pyrogenic exotoxin A. While exotoxin A–producing strains currently are rare among clinical isolates from other types of infections, 80 to 90 percent of the strains associated with streptococcal toxic shock–like syndrome have been exotoxin A producers, suggesting that the toxin may play a role in pathogenesis of the syndrome. In light of the possible role of this or other streptococcal toxins in streptococcal toxic shock–like syndrome, treatment of these patients with clindamycin has been advocated by some authorities, who argue that, through its direct action on protein synthesis, clindamycin is more effective than penicillin, a cell wall agent, in rapidly terminating toxin production. Support for this view comes from studies of an experimental model of streptococcal myositis, in which mice treated with clindamycin

had improved survival over those that received penicillin. Comparable data for treatment of human infections are not available.

GROUP C AND G STREPTOCOCCAL INFECTIONS

Group C and group G streptococci are beta-hemolytic streptococci that occasionally cause infections in humans similar to those caused by group A streptococci, including pharyngitis, pneumonia, cellulitis and soft tissue infections, bacteremia, septic arthritis, and endocarditis. Bacteremia due to group C or G streptococci occurs most commonly in patients who are elderly or chronically ill and, in the absence of an obvious local infection, is likely to reflect endocarditis. Septic arthritis, sometimes involving multiple joints, may complicate endocarditis or occur in the absence of endocarditis. Response to treatment is slow, and patients with joint infections often require repeated aspiration or open drainage and debridement for cure. Penicillin is the drug of choice for therapy of infections due to group C or G streptococci; because of poor clinical response in some patients treated with penicillin alone, the addition of gentamicin (1 mg/kg every 8 h for patients with normal renal function) is recommended for treatment of endocarditis or septic arthritis.

GROUP B STREPTOCOCCUS

Identified first as a cause of mastitis in cows, streptococci belonging to Lancefield's group B have since been recognized as a major cause of sepsis and meningitis in human neonates. Group B streptococci are also a frequent cause of peripartum fever in women and an occasional cause of serious infection in nonpregnant adults. Lancefield group B consists of a single species, *S. agalactiae*. Definitive identification of the organism is made serologically using antiserum specific for the group B cell wall–associated carbohydrate antigen. Presumptive identification of a streptococcal isolate as belonging to group B may be made on the basis of biochemical testing, including hydrolysis of sodium hippurate (99 percent are positive), hydrolysis of bile esculin agar (99 to 100 percent are negative), bacitracin susceptibility (92 percent are resistant), and production of so-called CAMP factor (98 to 100 percent are positive). CAMP factor is a phospholipase produced by group B streptococci that results in synergistic hemolysis with β-lysin produced by certain strains of *S. aureus*. Its presence can be demonstrated by cross-streaking the test isolate and staphylococcal strain on a blood agar plate. Most group B streptococci causing human infections are encapsulated by one of six antigenically distinct polysaccharides. The capsular polysaccharide has been shown experimentally to be important in virulence of the organism. Antibodies to the capsular polysaccharide afford protection against group B streptococci of the same, but not of different, capsular type.

INFECTION IN NEONATES Two general types of infections in infants are defined by the age of the patient at presentation. Early-onset infections occur within the first week of life, with a median age at onset of illness of 20 h. Approximately half these infants have signs of group B streptococcal disease at birth. The infection is acquired during or shortly before birth from organisms colonizing the maternal genital tract. Surveillance studies have shown 5 to 40 percent of women are vaginal or rectal carriers of group B streptococci. Approximately 50 percent of infants vaginally delivered from carrier mothers become colonized, although only 1 to 2 percent of those colonized develop clinically evident infection. Prematurity and maternal risk factors of prolonged labor, obstetric complications, and maternal fever are often present. The presentation of early-onset infection is the same as that of other forms of neonatal sepsis. Typical findings include respiratory distress, lethargy, and hypotension. Essentially all infants with early-onset disease are bacteremic, one-third to one-half have pneumonia and/or respiratory distress syndrome, and one-third have meningitis. Late-onset infections occur in infants between 1 week and 3 months of age, with a mean age of 3 to 4 weeks. Acquisition of the infecting organism may occur during birth, as in early-onset cases, or later from contact with a colonized mother, nursery personnel, or other sources. Meningitis is the most common manifestation of late-onset infection and in 80 to 90 percent of cases is associated with infection by a strain of capsular type III. Infants present with fever, lethargy or irritability, poor feeding, and seizures. Poor prognostic signs include presentation with hypotension, coma, status epilepticus, and the presence of neutropenia. Up to 50 percent of survivors have some degree of long-term neurologic impairment ranging from mild language delay or hearing loss to profound mental retardation, blindness, and uncontrolled seizures. A variety of other types of late-onset infections occur, including bacteremia without an identified source, osteomyelitis, septic arthritis, and facial cellulitis associated with submandibular or preauricular adenitis.

Penicillin is the treatment of choice for all group B streptococcal infections. Neonates with suspected bacterial sepsis are generally begun on empirical broad-spectrum therapy with ampicillin and gentamicin until culture results are known. If cultures return positive for group B streptococci, many pediatricians will continue gentamicin, along with ampicillin or penicillin, for a few days, until clinical improvement is evident. The basis for this practice is in vitro studies showing synergistic killing of group B streptococci by the two agents in combination. Certainly for infants with group B streptococcal meningitis, combined therapy for the first few days is recommended, although rigorous clinical data to support this view are lacking. Therapy with penicillin alone should be continued for 10 days for bacteremia and local infections and for a minimum of 14 days for meningitis because of the risk of relapse in patients treated with shorter courses.

Because the usual source of the organism in infected neonates is the mother's birth canal, efforts have been made to prevent group B streptococcal infections by identification and treatment of high-risk carrier mothers with various forms of antibiotic or immunoprophylaxis. This approach has been hampered by the logistical difficulties of identifying colonized women before delivery, since vaginal cultures early in pregnancy are poor predictors of carrier status at the time of delivery. Rapid diagnostic tests are available, using latex agglutination or enzyme immunoassay, for testing vaginal swab specimens directly; however, these tests currently are less sensitive than cultures, with a false-negative rate of approximately 10 to 30 percent. The incidence of group B streptococcal infection is increased in infants of women with risk factors: preterm delivery, prolonged rupture of membranes (>24 h), prolonged labor, fever, or chorioamnionitis. While prophylactic administration of ampicillin to such patients during delivery has been shown to prevent infection of the newborn, it should be emphasized that indiscriminate antibiotic treatment of colonized women is likely to do more harm than good, since the risk of adverse reactions to the antibiotic outweighs the risk of infection in the absence of maternal risk factors. Prophylaxis should be reserved for women with vaginal or rectal colonization *and* one or more of the risk factors noted above or a history of having delivered an infant with group B streptococcal infection. Because transplacental passage of maternal antibodies produces protective levels in the newborn, efforts are underway to develop a vaccine against group B streptococci that could be given to childbearing women before or during pregnancy.

INFECTION IN ADULTS   The majority of group B streptococcal infections in adults are related to pregnancy and parturition. Peripartum fever is the most common manifestation, sometimes accompanied by symptoms and signs of endometritis or chorioamnionitis (abdominal distention and uterine or adnexal tenderness). Blood cultures are often positive, as are cultures of vaginal swabs. Bacteremia is usually transitory but occasionally results in meningitis or endocarditis. Infections in adults not associated with the peripartum period generally occur in individuals who are elderly or have some underlying chronic illness, particularly diabetes mellitus or a malignancy. Infections that occur with some frequency include cellulitis and soft tissue infections

(including infected diabetic skin ulcers), urinary tract infections, pneumonia, endocarditis, and septic arthritis. Other reported infections include meningitis, osteomyelitis, and intraabdominal or pelvic abscesses.

Group B streptococci are less sensitive to penicillin than group A, requiring 10- to 100-fold higher concentrations for inhibition of growth in vitro. Therefore, somewhat higher doses of penicillin are needed for treatment of group B infections. Adults with serious localized infections (pneumonia, pyelonephritis, abscess) should receive doses in the range of 12 million units of penicillin G daily, while patients with endocarditis or meningitis should receive 18 to 24 million units per day, in divided doses. Vancomycin is an acceptable alternative for patients allergic to penicillin.

GROUP D STREPTOCOCCAL INFECTIONS

Group D includes the enterococci, organisms now classified in a separate genus from other streptococci, and nonenterococcal group D streptococci. Enterococci are distinguished from nonenterococcal group D streptococci by their ability to grow in the presence of 6.5% sodium chloride and other biochemical tests. The enterococcal species that are significant pathogens for humans are *E. faecalis* and *E. faecium*. They tend to produce infection in patients who are elderly or debilitated or who have had disruption of mucosal or epithelial barriers or alterations in the balance of normal flora through antibiotic treatment. Urinary tract infections due to enterococci are quite common, particularly in patients who have had antibiotic treatment or instrumentation of the urinary tract. These organisms account for 10 to 20 percent of cases of bacterial endocarditis on both native and prosthetic valves. The presentation of enterococcal endocarditis is usually subacute but may be acute with rapidly progressive valve destruction. Enterococci are frequently cultured from bile and are commonly involved in infectious complications of biliary surgery and in liver abscesses. Enterococci are often isolated from mixed infections arising from bowel flora, such as intraabdominal abscesses. Similarly, enterococci are often found in polymicrobial infections arising from abdominal surgical wounds and in diabetic foot ulcers. While such mixed infections are often cured by antimicrobials not active against enterococci, specific therapy directed against enterococci is warranted in circumstances in which these organisms are the predominant species or in which enterococci are isolated from blood cultures.

Unlike other streptococci, enterococci are not reliably killed by penicillin or ampicillin alone at concentrations of antibiotic achieved clinically in the blood or tissues. Because in vitro testing has shown evidence of synergistic killing by the combination of penicillin or ampicillin with an aminoglycoside for most enterococcal strains, combined therapy is recommended for serious enterococcal infections. Ampicillin reaches sufficiently high urinary concentrations to be adequate as single-drug therapy for uncomplicated urinary tract infections. For other types of enterococcal infections, however, addition of gentamicin at moderate doses (e.g., 1 mg/kg every 8 h for patients with normal renal function) is recommended. Vancomycin, in combination with gentamicin, may be substituted for penicillin in allergic patients. Enterococci are resistant to all cephalosporins, and this class of antibiotics should not be used for treatment of enterococcal infections.

Antimicrobial susceptibility testing should be performed routinely on enterococcal isolates from patients with serious infections. Most enterococci are resistant to streptomycin, and this drug should not be used for treatment of enterococcal infection unless in vitro testing of the strain indicates susceptibility. Though less widespread than streptomycin resistance, high-level resistance to gentamicin (minimum inhibitory concentration greater than 2000 µg/mL) has become common. Gentamicin-resistant enterococci should be tested for susceptibility to other aminoglycosides. If the isolate is resistant to all aminoglycosides, treatment with penicillin or ampicillin alone may be successful. Prolonged (at least 6 weeks), high-dose (e.g., 12 g/d ampicillin) therapy is recommended for endocarditis due to these highly resistant enterococci. β-Lactamase production (mediating resistance to penicillin and ampicillin) has been reported but currently appears to be rare among clinical isolates. β-Lactamase–producing strains may be treated with vancomycin plus gentamicin or with ampicillin combined with a β-lactamase inhibitor such as sulbactam in combination with gentamicin.

The main nonenterococcal group D streptococcal species that causes human infections is *S. bovis*. *S. bovis* endocarditis is often associated with neoplasms of the gastrointestinal tract, most often a colon carcinoma or polyp, but is also reported in association with other bowel lesions. When occult gastrointestinal lesions are carefully sought, abnormalities have been found in 60 percent or more of patients with *S. bovis* endocarditis. In contrast to the enterococci, nonenterococcal group D streptococci such as *S. bovis* are reliably killed by penicillin as a single agent, and penicillin is the treatment of choice for *S. bovis* infections.

VIRIDANS AND OTHER STREPTOCOCCI

Consisting of multiple species of alpha-hemolytic streptococci, the viridans streptococci are a heterogeneous group of organisms important as agents of bacterial endocarditis. Several species of viridans streptococci, including *S. salivarius*, *S. mutans*, *S. sanguis*, and *S. mitis*, are part of the normal mouth flora, where they live in close association with the teeth and gingiva. Some contribute to development of dental caries. Transient bacteremia induced by eating, tooth brushing and flossing, and other minor trauma, together with the ability of these organisms to adhere to biologic surfaces, is thought to account for their predilection for causing endocarditis. Viridans streptococci are also isolated, often as part of a mixed infection, in sinusitis, brain abscess, and liver abscess. A group of organisms referred to variously as *S. milleri*, *S. intermedius*, and *S. anginosus* are often considered as viridans streptococci, although they differ somewhat from other viridans streptococci in both hemolytic pattern (usually beta-hemolytic) and disease syndromes. These organisms often cause suppurative infections, particularly abscesses of brain and abdominal viscera.

Most viridans streptococci are sensitive to penicillin. Occasional isolates from blood cultures of patients with endocarditis fail to grow when subcultured on solid media. These *nutritionally variant streptococci* require supplemental thiol compounds or active forms of vitamin B_6 (pyridoxal or pyridoxamine) for growth in the laboratory. Because treatment failure and relapse appear to be more common for cases of endocarditis due to nutritionally variant streptococci than for usual viridans streptococci, the addition of gentamicin (1 mg/kg every 8 h for patients with normal renal function) to penicillin is recommended for therapy of endocarditis due to these organisms.

S. suis is an important pathogen in swine and has been reported to cause meningitis in humans, usually in individuals with occupational exposure to pigs. Strains of *S. suis* associated with human infections have generally reacted with Lancefield group R typing serum and sometimes with group D as well. Isolates may be alpha- or beta-hemolytic and have been sensitive to penicillin. *Anaerobic streptococci* are part of the normal flora of the oral cavity, bowel, and vagina. They are involved, usually in mixed infections, in brain abscess, sinusitis, dental abscess, and other odontogenic infections (Ludwig's angina, abscesses of the retropharyngeal or lateral pharyngeal space); in aspiration pneumonia, lung abscess, and empyema; and in intraabdominal and pelvic abscesses. Anaerobic and microaerophilic streptococci, together with facultative bacteria, also may play a role in invasive soft tissue infections, generally related to trauma or surgical wounds. Management of these infections involves debridement of infected tissues and treatment with high-dose penicillin (12 to 18 million units per day for serious infections).

REFERENCES

BASILIERE JL et al: Streptococcal pneumonia. Am J Med 44:580, 1968

BISNO AL: Group A streptococcal infections and acute rheumatic fever. N Engl J Med 325:783, 1991

CONE LA et al: Clinical and bacteriologic observations of a toxic shock–like syndrome due to *Streptococcus pyogenes*. N Engl J Med 317:146, 1987

EDWARDS MS, BAKER CJ: *Streptococcus agalactiae* (group B streptococci), in *Principles and Practice of Infectious Diseases*, 3d ed, GL Mandell et al (eds). New York, Churchill Livingstone, 1990, p 1554

KLEIN RS et al: Association of *Streptococcus bovis* with carcinoma of the colon. N Engl J Med 297:800, 1977

LANCEFIELD RC: A serological differentiation of human and other groups of hemolytic streptococci. J Exp Med 57:571, 1933

MOELLERING RC JR.: Emergence of *Enterococcus* as a significant pathogen. Clin Infect Dis 14:1173, 1992

STEVENS DL et al: Severe group A streptococcal infections associated with a toxic shock–like syndrome and scarlet fever toxin A. N Engl J Med 321:1, 1989

VARTIAN C et al: Infections due to Lancefield group G streptococci. Medicine 6:75, 1985

VIGLIONESE A et al: Recurrent group A streptococcal carriage in a health care worker associated with widely separated nosocomial outbreaks. Am J Med 91(suppl 3B):329S, 1991

WANNAMAKER LW: Differences between streptococcal infections of the throat and of the skin. N Engl J Med 282:23, 78, 1970

WELLS VD et al: Infections due to beta-lactamase–producing, high-level gentamicin-resistant *Enterococcus faecalis*. Ann Intern Med 116:285, 1992

YODER EL et al: Spontaneous gangrenous myositis induced by *Streptococcus pyogenes*: Case report and review of the literature. Rev Infect Dis 9:382, 1987

104 DIPHTHERIA, OTHER CORYNEBACTERIAL INFECTIONS, AND ANTHRAX

RANDALL K. HOLMES

DIPHTHERIA

DEFINITION Diphtheria is a localized infection of mucous membranes or skin caused by *Corynebacterium diphtheriae*. A characteristic pseudomembrane may be present at the site of infection. Some strains of *C. diphtheriae* produce diphtheria toxin, a protein that can cause myocarditis, polyneuritis, and other systemic toxic effects. Respiratory diphtheria is usually caused by toxinogenic (tox$^+$) *C. diphtheriae*, but cutaneous diphtheria is frequently caused by nontoxinogenic (tox$^-$) strains.

ETIOLOGY *C. diphtheriae* is an aerobic, nonmotile, nonsporulating, irregularly staining, gram-positive rod. The bacteria are 2 to 6 μm long, 0.5 to 1 μm wide, club shaped, and often arranged in clusters (Chinese letters) or parallel arrays (palisades). *C. diphtheriae* forms gray to black colonies on selective media containing potassium tellurite. Three biotypes, designated *gravis*, *mitis*, and *intermedius*, are distinguished on the basis of colonial morphology, hemolytic activity, sugar fermentation reactions, and other biochemical tests. Both tox$^+$ and tox$^-$ strains cause infections, and tox$^+$ strains of all three biotypes can cause severe disease. Individual strains of *C. diphtheriae* within a biotype can be identified by phage typing, analysis of bacterial polypeptides or DNA restriction patterns, DNA hybridization tests or polymerase chain reactions with specific probes, ribotyping, or other methods.

The gene for diphtheria toxin is present in specific corynephages. Nontoxinogenic *C. diphtheriae* acquires the ability to produce diphtheria toxin by infection with tox$^+$ phages, a process termed *phage conversion*. Growth of *C. diphtheriae* under low-iron conditions mimicking the environment of host tissues induces the synthesis of diphtheria toxin and the expression of a siderophore-dependent, high-affinity iron uptake system.

IMMUNOLOGY Treatment of diphtheria toxin with formaldehyde converts it to a nontoxic product called *diphtheria toxoid*. Immunization with the toxoid elicits antibodies (antitoxin) that neutralize the toxin and prevent diphtheria. Antitoxin does not prevent colonization by *C. diphtheriae* or eradicate the carrier state. If most individuals in a population have antitoxic immunity, the carriage of tox$^+$ strains of *C. diphtheriae* decreases to a low level. Thus herd immunity reduces the risk that nonimmune individuals in the population will be exposed to tox$^+$ *C. diphtheriae*. Nonimmune individuals may contract diphtheria if they travel to regions where the disease is present or if tox$^+$ strains of *C. diphtheriae* are introduced into their community.

No specific amount of antitoxin provides absolute protection against diphtheria, but the attack rate and the mortality rate for diphtheria are much lower among individuals with more than 0.01 unit of antitoxin per milliliter. This antitoxin level is often used, therefore, as an index of immunity for epidemiologic studies. Antitoxic immunity is also demonstrated by the Schick test, in which standardized doses of diphtheria toxin and toxoid are injected intracutaneously at separate sites on the volar surface of the forearm. A tender, swollen, erythematous lesion reaching maximal intensity in 4 to 5 days at the site of the toxin injection only (a positive reaction) is caused by the direct action of diphtheria toxin and indicates that the individual is not immune. The absence of a lesion at either site (a negative reaction) indicates that the toxin has been neutralized by circulating antitoxin and that the individual is immune. Tuberculin-like reactions at both sites that reach a maximum in 2 to 3 days and then fade (pseudoreaction) indicate delayed hypersensitivity to toxin/toxoid in an immune individual. Delayed hypersensitivity reactions at both toxin administration sites combined with a subsequent positive reaction at the site of toxin administration only (a combined reaction) indicate delayed hypersensitivity in an individual who does not have a protective level of antitoxin.

EPIDEMIOLOGY AND IMMUNITY   Humans are the reservoir for *C. diphtheriae*. The organism is transmitted primarily by close contact of diphtheria patients or carriers with susceptible individuals, but the risk of transmission from patients appears to be substantially greater than that of transmission from asymptomatic carriers. Transmission involving fomites and indirect routes is less common, although *C. diphtheriae* can survive for weeks to months in the environment. The incubation period for respiratory diphtheria is typically 2 to 5 days and rarely up to 8 days. Cutaneous diphtheria is usually a secondary infection whose signs develop an average of 7 days (range 1 to >21 days) after the appearance of primary skin lesions.

In populations in temperate climates, diphtheria primarily involves the respiratory tract, occurs throughout the year with a peak incidence in colder months, and is usually caused by tox$^+$ *C. diphtheriae*. Before the introduction of active immunization, diphtheria was usually a disease of children, affected up to 10 percent of this group, and sometimes occurred in devastating epidemics. Most infants were immune because of transplacental transfer of maternal IgG antitoxin, but children became susceptible by 6 to 12 months of age. Approximately 75 percent of individuals became immune by age 10 as a result of clinical or subclinical infection with *C. diphtheriae*. Mortality rates of 30 to 40 percent were common in untreated disease and sometimes exceeded 50 percent in epidemics. Treatment with antitoxin reduced the case mortality rate to 5 to 10 percent.

Routine immunization of children in the United States resulted in a progressively decreasing incidence of diphtheria and a shift of cases to older age groups, but the case mortality rate remained at 5 to 10 percent. More than 206,000 cases of diphtheria occurred in 1921. Only 22 cases were reported in 1980–1987, and 5 cases were reported in 1991. Forty-eight percent of cases in 1971–1981 were in persons over 15 years of age. Rates of immunization by school entry are high (96 percent), but rates for younger children are substantially lower. Many older adults (25 to 50 percent) are susceptible to diphtheria.

Large local outbreaks of diphtheria occurred in San Antonio, Texas (1969–1970, 201 cases), and Seattle, Washington (1972–1982, 1100 cases). Alcoholism, low socioeconomic status, crowded living conditions, and Native American ethnic background were significant risk factors in these and other recent diphtheria outbreaks. A recent report from England documented pharyngeal infections by tox$^-$ *C. diphtheriae* developing predominantly among homosexual men, often causing symptomatic pharyngitis and sometimes resulting in a tonsillar exudate.

In the tropics, cutaneous diphtheria is more common than respiratory diphtheria, occurs throughout the year, and often develops as a secondary infection complicating other dermatoses. Isolates of *C. diphtheriae* from skin lesions are more often tox$^-$ than tox$^+$. A study in Rangoon, Burma, demonstrated *C. diphtheriae* (18.5 percent tox$^+$ strains) in more than 60 percent of bacterially infected skin lesions in patients under 12 years of age. Eighty percent of isolates were from impetiginous scabies, with most of the remainder from impetiginous eczema or impetigo. Cutaneous diphtheria also has been increasingly recognized in temperate climates during the past two decades and accounted for 86 percent of the 1100 cases in Seattle.

Molecular epidemiologic studies demonstrated that the Seattle epidemic actually consisted of three discrete but overlapping outbreaks involving intermedius, gravis, and mitis strains, respectively. The intermedius strains (433 tox$^+$ isolates in 1972–1977) and gravis strains (8 tox$^+$ and 8 tox$^-$ isolates in 1973–1976; 3 tox$^+$ and 173 tox$^-$ isolates in 1978–1982) were shown to be distinct clones of *C. diphtheriae*, with tox$^-$ variants of the gravis clone predominating late in the epidemic. The mitis strains isolated throughout the epidemic, all but 4 of which were tox$^-$, were heterogeneous and represented multiple clones. In Sweden, a recent outbreak (1984–1986) with high mortality (>20 percent) was found to be caused by a single tox$^+$ mitis strain that differed from *C. diphtheriae* strains isolated concurrently from carriers. These observations suggest that traits of *C. diphtheriae* in addition to toxinogenicity contribute to virulence. In England, evidence was found for the initiation of an epidemic by phage conversion of tox$^-$ to tox$^+$ strains in vivo in one individual, with subsequent dissemination to other susceptible subjects.

PATHOLOGY AND PATHOGENESIS   *C. diphtheriae* infects mucous membranes, most commonly in the respiratory tract, and also invades open skin lesions resulting from insect bites or trauma. In infections caused by tox$^+$ *C. diphtheriae*, initial edema and hyperemia are often followed by epithelial necrosis and acute inflammation. Coagulation of the dense fibrinopurulent exudate produces a pseudomembrane, and the inflammatory reaction accompanied by vascular congestion extends into the underlying tissues. The pseudomembrane contains large numbers of *C. diphtheriae* cells, but the bacteria are rarely isolated from the blood or internal organs.

Diphtheria toxin acts both locally and systemically. Very small amounts cause dermonecrosis (as in the Schick test), and toxin presumably contributes to pseudomembrane formation. The lethal dose of diphtheria toxin for nonimmune humans and highly susceptible animals is about 0.1 μg/kg of body weight. Absorbed toxin can cause myocarditis, neuritis, and focal necrosis in various organs, including the kidneys, liver, and adrenal glands. Early changes in diphtheritic myocarditis include cloudy swelling of muscle fibers and interstitial edema. These are followed within weeks by hyaline and granular degeneration of muscle fibers (sometimes with fatty degeneration of the myocardium) progressing to myolysis and finally to the replacement of lost muscle by fibrosis. Thus diphtheria can cause permanent cardiac damage. In diphtheritic polyneuritis, pathologic changes include patchy breakdown of myelin sheaths in peripheral and autonomic nerves, but recovery of damaged nerves is the rule if the patient survives.

Diphtheria toxin is produced by *C. diphtheriae* as an extracellular polypeptide. It is cleaved by proteases to form nicked toxin consisting of fragments A and B, which remain linked by a disulfide bond. Fragment B binds to a plasma membrane receptor (an integral membrane protein corresponding to the precursor of a heparin-binding growth factor resembling epidermal growth factor) on cells from humans or susceptible animals, and the bound toxin is internalized by receptor-mediated endocytosis. Fragment A is translocated across the endosomal membrane and released into the cytoplasm, where it catalyzes the transfer of the adenosine diphosphate ribose moiety from nicotinamide adenine dinucleotide (NAD) to a modified histidine residue (diphthamide) on elongation factor 2, thereby inactivating this factor and inhibiting protein synthesis. One molecule of fragment A in the cytoplasm can kill a cell. Other metabolic alterations in intoxicated cells are secondary to inhibition of protein synthesis. The depletion of carnitine noted in the intoxicated heart may contribute to the pathogenesis of diphtheritic myocarditis. Diphtheria toxin and exotoxin A of *Pseudomonas aeruginosa* have the same enzymatic activity, and their catalytic domains are structurally homologous. Nevertheless, their biologic effects differ because they bind to different cell-surface receptors and exhibit different cellular tropisms.

CLINICAL MANIFESTATIONS Patients with *C. diphtheriae* in the respiratory tract are classified as diphtheria cases if they have symptoms consistent with local infection and as diphtheria carriers if they are asymptomatic. Signs and symptoms vary with the site and severity of the local infection, the patient's age, and the presence or absence of preexisting nasopharyngeal disease or concomitant systemic disease. Onset is often gradual, but most patients seek medical care within a few days of becoming ill. Sore throat is the most common symptom, but children are less likely than adults to complain of sore throat and are more likely to have nausea and vomiting. Fever of 37.8 to 38.9°C (100 to 102°F) and dysphagia are documented in about half of patients, but cough, hoarseness, chills, and rhinorrhea are less common. Systemic manifestations are primarily due to the effects of diphtheria toxin. Patients without toxicity exhibit discomfort and malaise associated with local infection, whereas severely toxic patients may have listlessness, pallor, and tachycardia that can progress rapidly to vascular collapse.

Primary infection in the respiratory tract is most often tonsillopharyngeal (one-half to two-thirds of cases) but also may be (in decreasing order of frequency) laryngeal, nasal, and tracheobronchial. Multiple sites are frequently involved, and secondary spread of pharyngeal infection upward to the nasal mucosa or downward to the larynx and tracheobronchial tree is much more common than primary infection at those sites. Systemic toxicity is usually less severe in nasal diphtheria than in tonsillopharyngeal diphtheria and is most severe when extensive pseudomembrane extends from the tonsils and pharynx into contiguous regions. A small percentage of patients present with malignant, or "bull neck," diphtheria, with abrupt onset, extensive pseudomembrane formation, foul breath, massive swelling of the tonsils and uvula, thick speech, cervical lymphadenopathy, striking edematous swelling of the submandibular region and anterior neck, and severe toxicity.

In tonsillopharyngeal diphtheria, only erythema may be noted initially, but isolated spots of gray or white exudate are common. These often extend and coalesce within a day to form a confluent, sharply demarcated pseudomembrane that becomes progressively thicker, more tightly adherent to the underlying tissue, and darker gray. Unlike the exudate in streptococcal pharyngitis, the diphtheritic pseudomembrane often extends beyond the margin of the tonsils onto the tonsillar pillars, palate, or uvula. Dislodging the membrane is likely to cause bleeding. Estimates of the proportion of patients with pharyngeal diphtheria who develop typical pseudomembranes vary widely, from as few as one-third to almost all. The higher estimates may be biased by failure to consider and confirm the diagnosis of diphtheria in patients who do not develop pseudomembranes. Patients with nasal diphtheria often present with serosanguineous nasal discharge, which may be unilateral or bilateral, and may cause irritation of the nares or lip. Laryngeal diphtheria often presents with hoarseness and cough. Demonstration of laryngeal pseudomembrane by laryngoscopy is helpful for distinguishing diphtheria from other infectious forms of laryngitis. Primary or secondary diphtheritic infection occasionally involves other mucous membranes, including the conjunctiva and the membranes of the genitourinary and gastrointestinal tracts.

Cutaneous diphtheria usually presents as an infection by *C. diphtheriae* of preexisting dermatoses involving (in decreasing order of frequency) the lower extremities, upper extremities, head, or trunk.

The clinical features are similar to those of other secondary cutaneous bacterial infections. In the tropics, the presentation of cutaneous diphtheria occasionally includes morphologically distinct "punched-out" ulcers that are covered by necrotic slough or membrane and have well-demarcated edges.

COMPLICATIONS Obstruction of the respiratory tract, presenting as tachypnea, dyspnea, stridor, cyanosis, and use of accessory muscles of respiration, can be caused by extensive pseudomembrane formation and swelling during the first few days of the disease or by sloughed pseudomembrane that becomes lodged in the airways at a later stage. The risk of respiratory obstruction is greater when infection involves the larynx or the tracheobronchial tree and is higher in children because of the small size of the airways.

Myocarditis and polyneuritis are the most prominent toxic manifestations of diphtheria. The risk of developing these manifestations is proportional to the severity of local disease, and the two can occur together in the same patient. Myocarditis may present during the acute phase of illness, develop as local disease is resolving, or begin insidiously after several weeks. One-half to two-thirds of patients with typical diphtheria have subtle evidence of cardiac dysfunction, including electrocardiographic abnormalities, but clinically apparent myocarditis develops in 10 to 25 percent of patients and is usually more severe when the onset is early. Electrocardiographic abnormalities include ST-T-wave changes, varying degrees of heart block, and arrhythmias, including atrial fibrillation, ventricular premature beats, ventricular tachycardia, or ventricular fibrillation. Clinical signs include diminished heart sounds, gallop rhythm, systolic murmurs, and (less commonly) acute or insidiously progressive congestive heart failure. Serum levels of aspartate aminotransferase reflect the intensity of myocardial damage and can be used to monitor its course.

Polyneuritis is uncommon in mild diphtheria but occurs in approximately 10 percent of cases of average severity and in up to 75 percent of severe cases. Bulbar dysfunction typically develops during the first 2 weeks. Palatal and pharyngeal paralysis usually develops first. Swallowing is difficult, the voice sounds nasal, and ingested fluids may be regurgitated through the nose. With unilateral pharyngeal infection, ipsilateral palatal paralysis is more common than contralateral or bilateral paralysis. Additional bulbar signs may develop over several weeks, with oculomotor and ciliary paralysis occurring more often than facial or laryngeal paralysis. Peripheral polyneuritis typically begins from 1 to 3 months after the onset of diphtheria with proximal weakness of the extremities that spreads distally. The severity of the disease varies from mild weakness of the pelvic muscles with unsteady gait to total paralysis, including failure of respiration. Paresthesias may develop, most often in a glove-and-stocking distribution. Approximately one-half of patients with diphtheritic neuropathy have evidence of cardiac vagal denervation, and a smaller proportion of this group has abnormal baroreceptor function. Polyneuritis usually resolves completely, with the time needed for improvement approximately equal to that elapsing from exposure to the development of symptoms. Severe muscular weakness may develop 1 to 2 weeks before maximal abnormalities in the peripheral nerve conduction velocity are demonstrated, the result being a striking dissociation between clinical and electrophysiologic findings. Cerebrospinal fluid (CSF) most often contains moderately increased levels of albumin, occasionally with pleocytosis, but the abnormalities in CSF do not determine prognosis.

Pneumonia occurs in more than half of fatal cases of diphtheria. Less common complications include renal failure, encephalitis, cerebral infarction, pulmonary embolism, and bacteremia or endocarditis due to invasive infection by *C. diphtheriae*. Serum sickness may result from antitoxin therapy.

COURSE AND PROGNOSIS Most cases of diphtheria occur in nonimmunized patients. The attack rate, severity of disease, and risk of complications are much lower in immunized patients. The pseudomembrane may continue to increase in size during the first day after administration of antitoxin. During the next several days to a week, it becomes softer, less adherent, and nonconfluent and eventually disappears as the normal mucosa is regenerated. In the preantibiotic era, *C. diphtheriae* persisted in the throat for about 2 weeks in one-half of patients and for 1 month or more in about one-fifth. Mortality increases with the severity of local disease, the extent of pseudomembrane formation, and the delay between onset of local disease and administration of antitoxin. The death rate is highest during the first week of illness; among patients with "bull neck" diphtheria; among patients with myocarditis who develop ventricular tachycardia, atrial fibrillation, or complete heart block; among patients with laryngeal or tracheobronchial involvement; among infants and patients over 60 years of age; and among alcoholics. In cutaneous diphtheria both mortality and the risk of myocarditis or peripheral neuropathy are significantly lower than in respiratory diphtheria.

DIAGNOSIS   A characteristic pseudomembrane on the mucosa of the oropharynx, palate, nasopharynx, nose, or larynx suggests diphtheria but is not uniformly present. Diphtheritic pseudomembrane must be distinguished from other pharyngeal exudates, including those of group A beta-hemolytic streptococcal infections, infectious mononucleosis, viral pharyngitides, fusospirochetal infection, and candidiasis. Diphtheria should be considered in patients with sore throat, cervical adenopathy or swelling, and low-grade fever, especially when these manifestations are accompanied by systemic toxicity, hoarseness, stridor, palatal paralysis, and/or serosanguineous nasal discharge with or without demonstrable pseudomembrane. Treatment with diphtheria antitoxin should be begun as soon as the clinical diagnosis of diphtheria is made.

Definitive diagnosis of diphtheria depends on the isolation of *C. diphtheriae* from local lesions. The laboratory should be notified that diphtheria is suspected so that use of selective tellurite medium appropriate for the isolation of *C. diphtheriae* is ensured. All isolates of *C. diphtheriae* should be subjected to toxicity testing. Primary isolates can be rapidly screened for toxinogenicity by the polymerase chain reaction, although occasional strains of *C. diphtheriae* that carry an inactive toxin gene may give false-positive results. The biochemical tests needed to differentiate *C. diphtheriae* from corynebacteria of the normal flora (diphtheroids) require several days. Group A beta-hemolytic streptococci and *Staphylococcus aureus* are also isolated frequently from patients with diphtheria.

Although, as has been mentioned, cutaneous diphtheria may present as a characteristic "punched-out" ulcer with a membrane, it is more often indistinguishable from other inflammatory dermatoses. Diagnosis depends on a high degree of suspicion and on culture of cutaneous lesions on laboratory media appropriate for the isolation of *C. diphtheriae*. Throat samples from all patients with cutaneous diphtheria should be cultured for *C. diphtheriae*.

TREATMENT   The decision to administer diphtheria antitoxin must be based on the clinical diagnosis of diphtheria without definitive laboratory confirmation, since each day of delay is associated with increased mortality. Because diphtheria antitoxin is produced in horses, it is necessary to inquire about possible allergy to horse serum and to perform a conjunctival or intracutaneous test with diluted antitoxin for immediate hypersensitivity. Epinephrine must be available for immediate administration to patients with severe allergic reactions. Patients with immediate hypersensitivity should be desensitized before a full therapeutic dose of antitoxin is given. The dose of diphtheria antitoxin currently recommended by the Committee on Infectious Diseases of the American Academy of Pediatrics is based on the site of the primary infection and the duration and severity of disease: 20,000 to 40,000 units for disease present for 48 h or less and involving the pharynx or larynx, 40,000 to 60,000 units for nasopharyngeal infections, and 80,000 to 100,000 units for disease that is extensive, has been present for 3 or more days, or is accompanied by brawny anterior cervical edema. Antitoxin is administered intravenously by infusion in saline over 60 min to neutralize unbound toxin rapidly. The approximately 10 percent risk of serum sickness is acceptable because of the established therapeutic value of antitoxin in decreasing mortality from respiratory diphtheria. During the early phase of the Seattle epidemic, all patients with cutaneous

diphtheria received 20,000 units of antitoxin. Later, when most isolates were tox⁻, antitoxin was withheld initially and administered only to patients from whom tox⁺ strains of *C. diphtheriae* were isolated. The potential systemic complications of cutaneous diptheria must be weighed against the potential adverse effects of antitoxin treatment; authorities are not unanimous in recommending antitoxin therapy for cutaneous diphtheria.

Antibiotics have little demonstrated effect on healing of the local infection in diphtheria patients treated with antitoxin. The primary goal of antibiotic therapy for patients or carriers is therefore to eradicate *C. diphtheriae* and prevent its transmission from the patient to susceptible contacts. Erythromycin, penicillin G, rifampin, or clindamycin is recommended by most authorities. Commonly recommended regimens for the treatment of adults with respiratory diphtheria are erythromycin (500 mg four times daily, parenterally or orally) or intramuscular procaine penicillin G (600,000 units at 12-h intervals) for 14 days. Patients with cutaneous diphtheria and carriers can be treated orally with erythromycin (500 mg four times daily) or rifampin (600 mg once daily) for 7 days. If compliance is in question, a single dose of benzathine penicillin G (1.2 to 2.4 million units intramuscularly) can be administered. Eradication of *C. diphtheriae* should be documented by negative cultures of samples taken on two or three successive days, beginning at least 24 h after the completion of antibiotic therapy. Some authorities also recommend a repeat throat culture 2 weeks later. The small percentage of patients who continue to be infected with *C. diphtheriae* after treatment should receive an additional 10-day course of oral erythromycin or rifampin. Plasmid-mediated erythromycin resistance of the MLS type emerged transiently in *C. diphtheriae* during the Seattle epidemic, but its frequency declined dramatically after the routine use of erythromycin was discontinued.

Patients with respiratory or cutaneous diphtheria caused by tox⁺ *C. diphtheriae* or strains of unknown toxinogenicity should be hospitalized, kept in bed initially, handled with isolation procedures appropriate for the site of infection, and given supportive care as needed. Respiratory and cardiac function must be monitored closely. Early intubation or tracheostomy is recommended when the larynx is involved or signs of impending airway obstruction are present. Tracheobronchial membrane can sometimes be mechanically removed via the endotracheal tube or tracheostomy. Primary or secondary pneumonia should be diagnosed and treated promptly. Sedative or hypnotic drugs that may mask respiratory symptoms are contraindicated. Close electrocardiographic monitoring, treatment of arrhythmias, and electrical pacing for heart block are essential. Congestive heart failure should be treated as described in Chap. 195. Glucocorticoids do not reduce the risk of diphtheritic myocarditis or polyneuritis. Oral therapy with DL-carnitine (100 mg/kg per day, given in twice-daily doses for 4 days) may be beneficial in diphtheritic myocarditis, but such therapy should be considered experimental until additional data becomes available. Ulcerative or ecthymatous cutaneous lesions should be treated with Burow's solution applied on wet compresses after debridement of necrotic areas, and treatment for associated conditions such as pediculosis, scabies, or underlying dermatoses should be instituted.

PREVENTION   Vaccines available in the United States for immunization against diphtheria include diphtheria and tetanus toxoids and pertussis vaccine adsorbed (DTP), diphtheria and tetanus toxoids adsorbed (DT) (for pediatric use), and tetanus and diphtheria toxoids adsorbed (Td) (for adult use). Each vaccine contains one dose in 0.5 mL and is administered intramuscularly. The adsorbent is alum, which functions as an adjuvant and enhances immunogenicity of the vaccines. Td contains less diphtheria toxoid than DTP or DT and causes fewer adverse reactions in adults.

Initial immunization against diphtheria requires completion of a primary series. Booster doses are required periodically throughout life for the maintenance of immunity. The recommended primary series for immunization of children up to the seventh birthday consists of four doses of DTP: the first at 6 weeks of age or older, the second and third doses after successive intervals of 4 to 8 weeks, and the fourth 6 to 12 months after the third. DT is substituted for DTP if pertussis vaccine is contraindicated (see Chap. 114). If primary immunization is delayed until after the seventh birthday, the primary series consists of three doses of Td, with the second dose given 4 to 8 weeks after the first and the third dose given 6 to 12 months after the second. If primary immunization is interrupted, the series should simply be completed; there is no need to start a new series. Children who complete a primary series should receive a booster dose of DTP before entering kindergarten unless the final dose of the primary series was given after the fourth birthday. Adults with an uncertain history of immunization should receive a primary series. Patients with diphtheria should be actively immunized after recovery. Booster doses of Td should be given at intervals of 10 years throughout life, preferably at the middecade ages (15 years, 25 years, etc).

Close contacts of patients with diphtheria should be cultured for *C. diphtheriae*, kept under surveillance for 1 week, and treated with appropriate antibiotics if cultures are positive. Previously immunized close contacts should receive an appropriate booster containing diphtheria toxoid if their last booster was given more than 5 years earlier. If the immunization status is uncertain, close contacts should receive an antibiotic regimen appropriate for carriers and a primary immunization series appropriate for their age.

OTHER CORYNEBACTERIAL INFECTIONS

DEFINITION Medically important *coryneform bacteria* (formerly called *diphtheroids*) include members of the normal flora that cause opportunistic infections, human pathogens of relatively low virulence, and animal pathogens that cause occasional zoonotic infections. Reported infections caused by coryneform bacteria have increased substantially in number over the last two decades. Isolates of *C. jeikeium* and group D-2 coryneform bacteria are often resistant to multiple antibiotics.

ETIOLOGY AND LABORATORY FEATURES Because coryneform bacteria are potential pathogens, it is important not to dismiss them as constituents of the normal flora or contaminants when they are found in clinical specimens. Laboratory differentiation of coryneform bacteria is important when they are isolated repeatedly, when they are recovered in pure culture or in large numbers, or when they form pigmented or hemolytic colonies.

The coryneform bacteria are a large, taxonomically heterogeneous, poorly classified group of gram-positive, pleomorphic, irregularly staining bacilli or coccobacilli that superficially resemble *C. diphtheriae*. The scheme recommended by the Centers for Disease Control and Prevention (CDC) for the classification of coryneform bacteria assigns them to several genera, including *Actinomyces, Arcanobacterium, Corynebacterium, Oerskovia,* and *Rhodococcus,* as well as to several groups that have not yet been categorized at the genus and species level.

ECOLOGY AND EPIDEMIOLOGY Humans are the probable natural habitat for *C. xerosis, C. pseudodiphtheriticum* (formerly *C. hofmanii*), *C. striatum, C. minutissimum, C. jeikeium* (fomerly CDC group JK), *Arcanobacterium haemolyticum* (formerly *C. haemolyticum*), and members of CDC coryneform groups A-4, D-2, G, I, 1, and 2. Animals are the probable natural habitat for *Actinomyces pyogenes* (formerly *C. pyogenes;* cows, sheep, pigs), *C. ulcerans* (cows, horses), and *C. pseudotuberculosis* (sheep, goats, horses). The natural habitat for *Rhodococcus equi* (formerly *C. equi*) is soil. The ecologic niches for most other coryneform bacteria of medical importance are not well defined.

The coryneform bacteria found most frequently as components of the normal flora include *C. pseudodiphtheriticum* (pharynx, skin), *C. xerosis* (conjunctival sac, nasopharynx, skin), and *C. striatum* (anterior nares, skin). Those which often colonize the skin of hospitalized patients include *C. jeikeium* (axilla, groin, perineum) and CDC group D-2. *C. jeikeium* most frequently colonizes patients with malignancies

or severe immunodeficiency; it also can be isolated from environmental sources (surfaces, air) in hospitals and from the hands of ward staff. *C. ulcerans* infections are acquired by consumption of raw milk. *C. pseudotuberculosis* infections are acquired by contact with animals or animal products or by consumption of raw milk.

PATHOGENESIS AND CLINICAL MANIFESTATIONS *C. jeikeium* was recognized in 1976 as a cause of infections in immunocompromised hosts. It also causes infections in immunocompetent hosts, but severe infections continue to be most frequent in patients with hematologic malignancies and neutropenia. Colonization of the skin precedes clinical infection. Additional risk factors for nosocomial *C. jeikeium* sepsis include prolonged hospitalization, breaks in the integument, chronic intravascular catheterization, and prior treatment with broad-spectrum antibiotics. Other presentations of *C. jeikeium* infection include endocarditis, device-related infections, pulmonary infiltrates, cutaneous septic emboli, soft tissue infections, and skin rashes. Endocarditis due to *C. jeikeium* occurs primarily in patients with prosthetic heart valves. *C. jeikeium* is a rare cause of infections of the central nervous system in patients with ventricular shunts.

Group D-2 coryneform bacteria were identified in 1985 as a significant cause of nosocomial urinary tract infections, including acute and chronic cystitis and pyelonephritis. These organisms closely resemble *C. jeikeium* but differ by producing urease and failing to convert glucose to acidic metabolites. Hydrolysis of urea by urease causes alkalinization of the urine and formation of ammonium magnesium phosphate (struvite) stones. Group D-2 coryneform bacteria cause alkaline-encrusted cystitis in patients with preexisting bladder lesions that serve as foci for precipitation of struvite crystals. Risk factors associated with symptomatic urinary tract infections include preexisting immunosuppression, recent urologic procedures (including renal transplantation), underlying disorders of the genitourinary tract, and a history of urinary tract infections.

A. haemolyticum causes pharyngitis, with 90 percent of cases occurring in patients between 10 and 30 years old. In this age group, *A. haemolyticum* pharyngitis is 5 to 13 percent as frequent as *Streptococcus pyogenes* pharyngitis. An erythematous rash is present in 30 to 67 percent of cases. The rash is usually scarlatiniform and most pronounced on the extremities, but it sometimes resembles urticaria or erythema multiforme. Because rash is more common in *A. haemolyticum* infections than in *S. pyogenes* infections, older children and adults presenting with the scarlet fever syndrome are as likely to have *A. haemolyticum* as *S. pyogenes* infection. Infection due to *A. haemolyticum* also can present with extensive pharyngeal exudate and can mimic diphtheria. *A. haemolyticum* occasionally causes peritonsillar abscess, sepsis, endocarditis, or meningitis.

C. minutissimum is frequently isolated from the lesions of erythrasma, a common superficial skin infection characterized by the presence in intertriginous areas of reddish brown, scaly, pruritic, macular patches that exhibit coral-red fluorescence under a Wood's light. The etiology of erythrasma has not been definitively established; infection of the skin by *C. minutissimum* has been shown to develop after the onset of maceration and scaling. Deep infections caused by *C. minutissimum* are rare and include abscesses, bacteremia, and endocarditis.

Among coryneform bacteria that cause disease in animals and occasionally in humans, *R. equi* is emerging as a potentially important intracellular opportunistic pathogen in immunocompromised patients. Most reported cases are pulmonary infections that resemble tuberculosis in patients with severely defective cell-mediated immunity. Several cases of *R. equi* infection have recently been documented in patients with AIDS. *A. pyogenes* causes bovine mastitis, a disease transmitted by flies. Yearly epidemics of leg ulcers infected with *A. pyogenes* occurred among schoolchildren in Thailand between 1979 and 1984 and were postulated to have resulted from introduction of the organism into traumatic skin lesions by flies. Reported *A. pyogenes* infections among adults in Denmark have included abscesses, cystitis, intraabdominal infections, and mastoiditis with bacteremia. Infections due to *C. ulcerans* in humans usually present as pharyngitis and can mimic respiratory diphtheria, whereas infections caused by *C. pseudotuberculosis* typically present as suppurative granulomatous lymphadenitis. *C. ulcerans* and *C. pseudotuberculosis* can be lysogenized by tox⁺ phages and can produce diphtheria toxin. Human infections by tox⁺ strains of *C. ulcerans*—but not by tox⁺ strains of *C. pseudotuberculosis*—have been reported.

C. pseudodiphtheriticum, a commensal of low virulence, is an uncommon cause of pneumonia in men with AIDS and of endocarditis, necrotizing tracheitis, tracheobronchitis, and urinary tract infection in patients without known immune deficiencies. Likewise, *C. xerosis* and *C. striatum* occasionally cause infections in humans.

DIAGNOSIS The clinical features of *C. jeikeium* infections are not pathognomonic. Thus the diagnosis of *C. jeikeium* infections is based on a high index of suspicion, identification of the organism by culture from appropriate clinical specimens, and exclusion of other likely causes of infection.

Group D-2 coryneform bacteria often are not detected by routine urine cultures; rather, it is necessary to incubate the cultures for 24 to 48 h on blood agar or special media. Cultivation should be prolonged in selected cases—i.e., those involving patients (especially elderly men who have preexisting genitourinary abnormalities) with alkaline urine, ammonium magnesium phosphate stones, gram-positive bacilli in the urine, or negative standard urine cultures despite clinical evidence of bacteriuria. Other microbes that can cause urinary tract infections with alkaline urine include *Proteus*, *Ureaplasma*, and some *staphylococci* and *streptococci*. Alkaline-encrusted cystitis is an anatomic diagnosis made by cystoscopy.

The differential diagnosis of *A. haemolyticum* pharyngitis with rash includes scarlet fever; rubella; staphylococcal and streptococcal toxic shock syndromes; infections caused by Epstein-Barr virus, cytomegalovirus, and enteroviruses (especially coxsackieviruses); disseminated gonococcal infection; secondary syphilis; and drug allergy. Routine diagnostic methods of throat culture are not ideal for the detection of *A. haemolyticum*, nor is this organism detected by rapid tests for *S. pyogenes* that are sometimes substituted for throat cultures. Pharyngitis caused by *A. haemolyticum* in adolescents and adults is likely to be underdiagnosed until improved tests for the organism are used by diagnostic laboratories.

Erythrasma is diagnosed clinically. Because of uncertainty about the etiologic role of *C. minutissimum*, culture of erythrasma lesions is not currently recommended. Pharyngitis caused by tox⁺ strains of *C. ulcerans* may be clinically indistinguishable from diphtheria. The presentations of infections caused by other coryneform bacteria are not usually diagnostic; cultures are required for identification of the causal organisms.

TREATMENT AND PREVENTION Strains of *C. jeikeium* are typically resistant to most antibiotics except vancomycin, which is the drug of choice. Some recent isolates of *C. jeikeium* are susceptible or only moderately resistant to β-lactam antibiotics. Infections due to fully susceptible strains can be treated with β-lactam antibiotics alone, and those due to moderately resistant strains can be treated with β-lactam antibiotics plus an aminoglycoside. Quinolones, especially ciprofloxacin, exhibit excellent in vitro activity against *C. jeikeium*, but clinical data on their therapeutic effectiveness are not yet available. For device-related *C. jeikeium* infections, removal of the infected device is usually required in addition to appropriate antibiotic therapy.

Group D-2 coryneform bacteria are often resistant to the antibiotics used commonly for the treatment of urinary tract infections. Early isolates were uniformly susceptible to vancomycin and quinolones, but recent isolates have exhibited increasing resistance to norfloxacin and ciprofloxacin. Isolates are often susceptible to erythromycin, rifampin, novobiocin, and tetracyclines. Treatment of urinary tract infections due to group D-2 strains is often difficult; several courses of antibiotic may be necessary for bacteriologic cure. Patients with alkaline-encrusted cystitis require resection of the encrusted lesions in addition to antibiotic therapy.

Controlled trials of treatment for infections caused by *A. haemolyticum* have not been performed. In vitro tests have demonstrated susceptibility to erythromycin but tolerance or relative resistance to penicillin. Limited data suggest that the clinical course of *A. haemolyticum* pharyngitis may be shortened by treatment with erythromycin.

Infections caused by *C. ulcerans* that present like diphtheria or that are known to be caused by tox⁺ strains should be treated like diphtheria. Oral erythromycin is usually effective for the treatment of erythrasma. Initial treatment of infections caused by other coryneform bacteria should be based on the identity of the organism and on published data regarding antibiotic susceptibility. Therapy should be modified, when necessary, in light of the results of antibiotic susceptibility tests. All isolates of *Corynebacterium* and of coryneform bacteria reported to date have been susceptible to vancomycin.

ANTHRAX

DEFINITION Anthrax is an acute bacterial infection caused by *Bacillus anthracis* that occurs most frequently in herbivorous animals. Humans become infected when spores of *B. anthracis* are introduced into the body by contact with infected animals or contaminated animal products, insect bites, inhalation, or ingestion. In humans, the most common form is cutaneous anthrax, which is characterized by a localized skin lesion with a central eschar surrounded by marked nonpitting edema. Inhalation anthrax (woolsorters' disease) typically involves hemorrhagic mediastinitis, rapidly progressive systemic infection, and very high mortality. Gastrointestinal anthrax is rare and is associated with high mortality.

ETIOLOGY *B. anthracis* is a large (1 to 1.5 μm by 4 to 10 μm), nonmotile, encapsulated, chain-forming, aerobic, gram-positive rod that forms centrally located, oval spores. Oxygen is required for sporulation but not for germination of spores, and sporulation does not take place in living animals. The rectangular shape of the individual bacteria gives chains of *B. anthracis* a boxcar-like appearance. On blood agar, virulent *B. anthracis* usually forms nonhemolytic or weakly hemolytic, grayish white, rough colonies that have irregular, comma-shaped projections and are said to resemble a medusa's head; however, if the medium contains bicarbonate and incubation is carried out in the presence of excess CO_2, the colonies are smooth and mucoid. Virulent strains of *B. anthracis* are pathogenic for animals, including mice and guinea pigs. Known virulence factors include three proteins collectively called *anthrax toxin* (see below) and an antiphagocytic capsular polypeptide composed of D-glutamic acid residues linked by peptide bonds involving the gamma carboxyl group. The genes that determine the production of anthrax toxin and of capsular polypeptide are on separate plasmids of *B. anthracis*. Determination of susceptibility to bacillus phage gamma and demonstration of species-specific antigens by direct fluorescent antibody tests or by hemagglutination tests are helpful in laboratory identification of *B. anthracis*. Spores of *B. anthracis* can survive for years in dry earth but are destroyed by boiling for about 10 min, by treatment with oxidizing agents such as potassium permanganate or hydrogen peroxide, or by dilute formaldehyde. Most strains of *B. anthracis* are susceptible to penicillin.

EPIDEMIOLOGY The distribution of anthrax is worldwide. All animals are susceptible to varying degrees, but the disease is most prevalent among domestic herbivores (including cattle, sheep, horses, and goats) and wild herbivores.

Grazing animals become infected when they are foraging for food in areas contaminated with spores of *B. anthracis* under appropriate climatic conditions. Anthrax in herbivores tends to be severe, with high mortality. Terminally ill animals have overwhelming bacteremia and often bleed from the nose, mouth, and bowel, thereby contaminating soil or watering places with vegetative *B. anthracis* that can subsequently sporulate and persist in the environment. The carcasses of infected animals provide additional potential foci of contamination. Whether or not *B. anthracis* multiplies to any significant extent in the soil is controversial, and environmental factors affecting the probability that animals grazing in contaminated areas will become infected have not been fully defined. Epidemics among animals may spread from an initial focus to contiguous geographic areas in a pattern consistent with the movement of infected animals. Biting flies also have been implicated as vectors for the spread of anthrax, and vultures that feed on infected carcasses are believed to be involved in the occasional spread of anthrax from a contaminated area to noncontiguous areas, probably by contamination of surface water pools. A striking example of the impact of anthrax in animals is provided by an outbreak on a pig farm in northern Wales in 1989 that necessitated the slaughter and incineration of 4492 pigs; decontamination of excrement, farm buildings, equipment, paths, roadways, and farmland with formalin; and disposal of the decontaminated excrement as toxic waste–all at public expense.

The natural resistance of humans to anthrax is greater than that of herbivorous animals. It is difficult to determine the annual worldwide incidence of human anthrax because many cases do not receive medical attention and are not reported; estimates of 20,000 to 100,000 cases per year have been made. Human cases are classified as agricultural or industrial on the basis of the epidemiologic setting in which they occur. Agricultural cases result most often from contact with animals that have anthrax (during skinning, butchering, dissecting, etc.), from bites of contaminated or infected flies, and, in rare instances, from consumption of contaminated meat. Industrial cases are associated with exposure to contaminated hides, goat's hair, wool, or bones. Anthrax in animals has been a long-standing problem in Iran, Turkey, Pakistan, and Sudan, and the probability is high that animal products (especially goat's hair) originating from these areas will be contaminated with anthrax spores.

Only 4 cases of human anthrax were documented in the United States from 1984 through 1988, and gastrointestinal anthrax has never been documented in this country. Large epidemics of anthrax occurred in the former Soviet Union at Sverdlovsk in 1979 and in Zimbabwe between 1978 and the early 1980s. Initially, the cases in Sverdlovsk were reported to be cutaneous and gastrointestinal anthrax and were attributed to exposure to meat from infected animals. Intense international interest was stimulated by the suspicion that the release of *B. anthracis* from a nearby military facility was responsible for the outbreak. A recent analysis of 42 necropsies from the Sverdlovsk outbreak, including most of the fatal cases, describes the pathologic findings and documents that the disease was, in fact, inhalation anthrax. The outbreak in Zimbabwe involved more than 9700 cases of agricultural anthrax in humans. This massive outbreak occurred during wartime and was associated with disruption of the veterinary and medical infrastructure and cessation of veterinary anthrax vaccination programs (see below).

PATHOGENESIS   *B. anthracis* is an extracellular pathogen that can evade phagocytosis, invade the bloodstream, multiply rapidly to a high population density in vivo, and kill quickly. Capsular polypeptide and anthrax toxin are recognized as the principal virulence factors of *B. anthracis*. The capsule of *B. anthracis* consists of poly-D-glutamic acid and confers resistance to phagocytosis. Anthrax toxin consists of three proteins called *protective antigen* (PA), *edema factor* (EF), and *lethal factor* (LF). The toxin was discovered by the demonstration that the transfer of sterile blood from guinea pigs dying of anthrax to uninfected guinea pigs killed the recipients.

PA, EF, and LF have been purified and characterized and their structural genes cloned and sequenced. PA binds to plasma membranes of target cells and is cleaved by a cellular protease into two fragments. The larger fragment remains on the cell surface and displays a binding site for a domain that is present in both EF and LF, but the smaller fragment is released. The larger PA fragment on the cell surface serves as a specific receptor that mediates entry of either EF or LF into the target cells by receptor-mediated endocytosis. Recent studies have demonstrated that PA also can be cleaved in the blood of infected animals and that the larger PA fragment can interact with LF to form circulating complexes. EF is a calmodulin-dependent adenylate cyclase, and EF activity is expressed within human or animal cells that provide both the calmodulin activator and the ATP substrate for EF. The biologic effects of EF, which include formation of edema in anthrax lesions and inhibition of polymorphonuclear leukocyte functions, are mediated by the cyclic AMP that is formed intracellularly from ATP by the enzymatic action of EF. PA-mediated entry of LF into susceptible cells leads to cell death, but the mechanism of action of LF has not yet been determined.

Cutaneous anthrax is initiated by the introduction of spores of *B. anthracis* into the skin through cuts or abrasions or by biting flies. The spores germinate within hours, and the vegetative cells multiply and produce anthrax toxin. Histologically, the lesion in cutaneous anthrax is characterized by necrosis, vascular congestion, hemorrhage, and gelatinous edema. The number of leukocytes is disproportionately small in comparison with the amount of tissue damage. The clinical description of this lesion as a "malignant pustule" is not in concordance with the pathologic findings.

In inhalation anthrax, *B. anthracis* spores in airborne particles less than 5 μm in diameter are deposited directly into the alveoli or alveolar ducts. The spores are phagocytized by alveolar macrophages, and some are carried to and germinate in mediastinal nodes. Hemorrhagic necrosis of the nodes, in association with hemorrhagic mediastinitis and overwhelming *B. anthracis* bacteremia, may develop rapidly. Secondary pneumonia sometimes occurs.

Gastrointestinal anthrax usually results from ingestion of inadequately cooked meat from animals with anthrax. Primary infection can be initiated in the intestine by organisms that survive passage through the stomach, but an oropharyngeal form of the disease also has been described. Lesions in the throat or intestine are usually accompanied by hemorrhagic lymphadenitis.

B. anthracis bacteremia can develop in any form of anthrax and is documented in almost all fatal cases. Autopsies reveal large numbers of bacteria in blood vessels, lymph nodes, and many organs.

CLINICAL MANIFESTATIONS   Approximately 95 percent of human cases of anthrax are the cutaneous form and about 5 percent the inhalation form. Gastrointestinal anthrax is rare. Anthrax meningitis occurs in a small percentage of all cases and is a frequent complication of overwhelming *B. anthracis* bacteremia.

Cutaneous anthrax   The cutaneous lesion in anthrax is most often found on exposed areas of skin. In the Zimbabwe outbreak, lesions in children under 5 years old were significantly more likely to be on the head, neck, or face and less likely to be on the upper limbs than in adults. This distribution correlates with the fact that children have less contact than adults with carcasses of infected animals and are more likely to acquire infection through fly bites.

Within days after inoculation of *B. anthracis* spores into the skin, a small red macule appears. During the next week the lesion typically progresses through papular and vesicular or pustular stages to the formation of an ulcer with a blackened necrotic eschar surrounded by a highly characteristic, expanding zone of brawny edema. The early lesion may be pruritic, and the fully developed lesion is painless. Small satellite vesicles may surround the original lesion, and painful nonspecific regional lymphadenitis is common. Most patients are afebrile, with mild or no constitutional symptoms; in severe cases, however, edema may be extensive and associated with shock. Spontaneous healing occurs in 80 to 90 percent of untreated cases, but edema may persist for weeks. In the 10 to 20 percent of untreated patients who have progressive infection, bacteremia develops and is often associated with high fever and rapid death. The differential diagnosis includes staphylococcal skin infections, tularemia, plague, and orf. Cutaneous anthrax should be considered when patients have painless ulcers associated with vesicles and edema and have had contact with animals or animal products.

Inhalation anthrax   The frequent similarity of the presenting symptoms of inhalation anthrax (woolsorters' disease) to those of severe viral respiratory diseases makes early diagnosis difficult. After 1 to 3 days an acute phase supervenes, with increasing fever, dyspnea, stridor, hypoxia, and hypotension usually leading to death within 24 h. Occasionally, patients present with fulminant disease. A characteristic radiologic finding associated with hemorrhagic medi-astinitis is symmetrical mediastinal widening.

Gastrointestinal anthrax   Symptoms of gastrointestinal anthrax are variable and include fever, nausea and vomiting, abdominal pain, bloody diarrhea, and sometimes rapidly developing ascites. Diarrhea is occasionally massive, causing hemoconcentration and severe con-traction of intravascular volume. The major features of oropharyngeal anthrax are fever, sore throat, dysphagia, painful regional lymphade-nopathy, and toxemia; respiratory distress may be evident. The primary lesion is most often on the tonsils.

LABORATORY DIAGNOSIS   *B. anthracis* is present in large numbers in cutaneous lesions of anthrax and can be demonstrated by Gram's stain, direct fluorescent antibody staining, or culture unless the patient has been treated with antibiotics. A small proportion of patients with anthrax have bacteremia, but the disease may progress to death before blood cultures become positive. Patients with anthrax meningitis have bloody spinal fluid containing large numbers of *B. anthracis* cells demonstrable by staining or culture. The virulence of suspected isolates of *B. anthracis* can be demonstrated by the inoculation of guinea pigs; death results within 24 h with positive cultures of heart blood. Patients with mild disease usually have normal leukocyte counts, but patients with disseminated disease typically have polymorphonuclear leukocytosis. Tests for antibody to *B. anthracis* are useful in confirming the diagnosis of anthrax. A sensitive and specific polymerase chain reaction method developed for the detection of spores of *B. anthracis* may be useful for rapid testing of potentially contaminated animal or agricultural products.

TREATMENT   Viable *B. anthracis* disappears from the lesions of cutaneous anthrax within 5 h of the initiation of treatment with parenteral penicillin G. Recommended therapy for adults is 2 million units of penicillin G at intervals of 6 h until edema subsides, with the subsequent administration of oral penicillin to complete a 7- to 10-day course. For penicillin-sensitive adults, erythromycin or tetracycline (500 mg every 6 h) can be substituted. Chloramphenicol also has been used successfully. Antibiotics decrease local edema and systemic toxicity in patients with cutaneous anthrax but do not prevent eschar formation. Cutaneous lesions should be cleaned and covered, and used dressings should be decontaminated. For inhalation anthrax, high-dose penicillin therapy (2 million units at 2-h intervals) is recommended; for gastrointestinal anthrax or anthrax meningitis, the recommended regimen is similar. A rational case can be made for passive immunization with anthrax antitoxin in addition to antibiotic therapy in severely ill patients with anthrax, but an appropriate antitoxin is not commercially available.

PREVENTION   Inhalation anthrax was essentially eliminated in England before 1940 through the development of methods to decon-taminate wool and goat's hair and the improvement of working conditions for handlers of animal products.

Nonliving vaccines consisting of alum-precipitated or aluminum hydroxide–adsorbed extracellular components of unencapsulated *B. anthracis* are used in the United Kingdom and the United States for agricultural workers, veterinary personnel, and others at risk of exposure to anthrax. The major active component of these vaccines is PA. Live attenuated vaccines containing spores of *B. anthracis* are used in both developed and developing countries for the immunization of domestic herbivores; these preparations are also used for the immunization of humans in Russia but not in the United States. The probable basis for attenuation of the original Pasteur spore vaccine is partial loss of the plasmid that encodes anthrax toxin during prolonged incubation of *B. anthracis* cultures at 42°C. The basis for attenuation of the current Sterne spore vaccine is loss of the plasmid that encodes capsular polypeptide.

Improved anthrax vaccines for humans are needed because the current vaccines are impure and chemically complex, elicit only slow-onset protective immunity, provide incomplete protection, and cause significant adverse reactions. In addition to agricultural and industrial anthrax, the possible use of *B. anthracis* as an agent of biological warfare is stimulus to the development of an improved vaccine.

Current strategies for vaccine development include purification of candidate protective antigens, expression of protective antigens in recombinant microbial vaccines, and construction of improved live attenuated strains of *B. anthracis*. A mutant form of PA that lacks the protease-sensitive sequence and that cannot be processed to interact with EF or LF to mediate toxicity has been produced by genetic engineering as one candidate vaccine against anthrax.

Carcasses of animals that succumb to anthrax should be buried intact or cremated. Necropsies or butchering of infected animals should be avoided because sporulation of *B. anthracis* occurs only in the presence of oxygen.

PROGNOSIS   The mortality rate is 10 to 20 percent for untreated cutaneous anthrax but is very low with appropriate antibiotic therapy. In contrast, the mortality rate for inhalation anthrax approaches 100 percent, and therapy is usually unsuccessful. The mortality rate for treated gastrointestinal anthrax is approximately 50 percent. Meningitis as a complication of anthrax is usually fatal.

The opinions expressed herein are those of the author and do not necessarily represent the views of the Department of Defense or the Uniformed Services University of the Health Sciences.

REFERENCES

ABRAMOVA FA et al: Pathology of inhalational anthrax in 42 cases from the Sverdlovsk outbreak of 1979. Proc Natl Acad Sci USA 90:2291, 1993

AKSARAY N et al: Cutaneous anthrax. Trop Geogr Med 42:168, 1990

CENTERS FOR DISEASE CONTROL: Diphtheria, tetanus, and pertussis: Recommendations for vaccine use and other preventive measures: Recommendations of the Immunization Practices Advisory Committee (ACIP). Morb Mort Week Rep 40(No. RR-10):1, 1991

COHEN Y et al: *Corynebacterium pseudodiphtheriticum* pulmonary infection in AIDS patients. Lancet 340:114, 1992

COMMITTEE ON INFECTIOUS DISEASES: Diphtheria, in *Report of the Committee on Infectious Diseases*, 22d ed. Elk Grove Village, IL, American Academy of Pediatrics, 1991, p 91

COYLE MB et al: The molecular epidemiology of three biotypes of *Corynebacterium diphtheriae* in the Seattle outbreak from 1972–1982. J Infect Dis 159:670, 1989

COYLE MB, LIPSKY BA: Coryneform bacteria in infectious diseases: Clinical and laboratory aspects. Clin Microbiol Rev 3:227, 1990

FARIZO KM et al: Fatal respiratory disease due to *Corynebacterium diphtheriae:* Case report and review of guidelines for management, investigation, and control. Clin Infect Dis 16:59, 1993

HARNISH JP et al: Diphtheria among alcoholic urban adults. A decade of experience in Seattle. Ann Intern Med 111:71, 1989

HEDLUND KW: Anthrax toxin: History and recent advances and perspectives. J Toxicol Toxin Rev 11:41, 1992

HÖFLER W: Cutaneous diphtheria. Int J Dermatol 30:845, 1991

KAIN KC et al: *Arcanobacterium hemolyticum* infection: Confused with scarlet fever and diphtheria. J Emerg Med 9:33, 1991

LAFORCE FM: Bacillus anthracis (anthrax), in *Principles and Practice of Infectious Diseases*, 3d ed, GL Mandell et al (eds). New York, Churchill Livingstone, 1990, p 1593

MORRIS A, GUILD I: Endocarditis due to *Corynebacterium pseudodiphtheriticum:* Five case reports, review, and antibiotic susceptibilities of nine strains. Rev Infect Dis 13:887, 1991

RAPPUOLI R et al: Molecular epidemiology of the 1984–1986 outbreak of diphtheria in Sweden. N Engl J Med 318:12, 1988

ROZDZINSKI E et al: *Corynebacterium jeikeium* bacteremia at a tertiary care center. Infection 19:201, 1991

SORIANO F et al: Urinary tract infection caused by *Corynebacterium* group D2: Report of 82 cases and review. Rev Infect Dis 12:1019, 1990

TURNBULL PCB: Anthrax vaccines: Past, present and future. Vaccine 9:533, 1991

WILSON APR et al: Unusual nontoxigenic *Corynebacterium diphtheriae* in homosexual men. Lancet 339:998, 1992

105 INFECTIONS CAUSED BY *LISTERIA MONOCYTOGENES*

ANNE SCHUCHAT / CLAIRE V. BROOME

Listeria monocytogenes is a gram-positive rod which can be isolated from soil, vegetation, and many animal reservoirs. Human disease due to *L. monocytogenes* generally occurs in the setting of pregnancy or immunosuppression due to illness or medication. A substantial portion of human listeriosis occurs through food-borne transmission of *L. monocytogenes*. Unlike the majority of food-borne pathogens which primarily cause gastrointestinal illness, *L. monocytogenes* causes invasive syndromes such as meningitis, sepsis, chorioamnionitis, and stillbirth.

ETIOLOGY *Listeria* are aerobic or facultatively anaerobic nonsporulating bacilli that grow well at temperatures between 1 and 45°C and have a characteristic tumbling motility when cultured at 20 to 25°C. Characteristics which help distinguish *L. monocytogenes* from other *Listeria* species include formation of a narrow zone of beta hemolysis on sheep blood agar and production of acid from glucose, maltose, and rhamnose but not from xylose or mannitol. Determination of serotype of *L. monocytogenes* is based on somatic (O) and flagellar (H) antigens. Most cases of human disease are caused by serotypes 1/2a, 1/2b, and 4b. Molecular subtyping techniques, including multilocus enzyme electrophoresis, phage typing, and ribosomal DNA analysis, have improved the ability to discriminate among strains of *Listeria*, thus complementing efforts to link environmental or food isolates with clinical infections.

PATHOGENESIS *L. monocytogenes* is an intracellular pathogen with a predilection to cause illness in persons with deficient cell-mediated immunity. The organism is present in normal gastrointestinal flora in healthy individuals. Lack of gastric acidity and abnormal gastrointestinal function may increase the risk of invasive disease following exposure to the organism in the gastrointestinal tract. Invasion, intracellular multiplication, and cell-to-cell spread of the organism appear to be mediated through proteins such as internalin, the hemolysin listeriolysin O, and phospholipase C. Local immunosuppression at the maternal-fetal interface of the placenta may facilitate intrauterine infection following transient maternal bacteremia.

EPIDEMIOLOGY Long recognized as a veterinary pathogen, *L. monocytogenes* causes basilar meningitis ("circling disease") and stillbirth in sheep and cattle. The occurrence of listeriosis among humans has received increasing attention as a result of recognition of the role of contaminated foods in the pathogenesis of epidemic listeriosis and the increased reports of disease associated with the expanding immunosuppressed population.

Invasive listeriosis confirmed by culture of blood or cerebrospinal fluid occurs in approximately 7.4 per million population annually in the United States, or an estimated 1850 cases per year. Perinatal listeriosis complicates 16 of every 100,000 births. These are minimal estimates of the real disease burden, which includes milder or unrecognized illness. Recent multistate surveillance suggests that 23 percent of infections are fatal or result in stillbirth, although higher case-fatality rates have been observed during listeriosis epidemics and in earlier series. Although the majority of disease due to *L. monocytogenes* occurs sporadically, investigation of several listeriosis outbreaks during the 1980s demonstrated that common-source food-borne transmission caused human illness and that the incubation period for disease following consumption of contaminated food may be 2 to 6 weeks. The largest North American outbreak, in Los Angeles in 1985, involved over 100 cases and resulted in 48 deaths or stillbirths. Foods implicated in outbreaks include contaminated cole slaw, pasteurized milk, soft cheeses, paté, and pork tongue. Epidemiologic studies also have implicated consumption of undercooked chicken, uncooked hot dogs, soft cheeses, and food from store delicatessen counters as risk factors for sporadic listeriosis. *Listeria* contamination of foods is relatively common. Among foods contaminated with the organism, those which are ready-to-eat, contaminated with serotype 4b, and contaminated at a relatively high level may be the most likely to cause illness. The long incubation period associated with listeriosis contributes to the difficulty of implicating specific foods as the cause of both common-source outbreaks and sporadic cases.

Although food-borne transmission appears to be the major cause of epidemic and sporadic disease, several clusters of late-onset neonatal infection suggest that nosocomial transmission of *L. monocytogenes* can occur. Contaminated multiuse materials and equipment have been suggested as causes for some nosocomial clusters. Listeriosis has been reported in veterinarians and others with close contact with infected animals.

CLINICAL PRESENTATION *Pregnancy-associated listeriosis* may occur during any stage of pregnancy, although the majority of infections are detected during the third trimester, possibly because of failure to obtain bacterial cultures in abortions and stillbirths occurring earlier in gestation. One-half to two-thirds of pregnant women with perinatal listeriosis experience a mild illness characterized by fever, myalgias, malaise, and backache, sometimes accompanied by diarrhea, abdominal pain, nausea, and/or vomiting during the bacteremic phase of illness. Blood cultures should be used for diagnosis, since isolation of the organism from rectal or vaginal culture is not diagnostic. Transplacental spread of the organism results in intrauterine infection, which can lead to chorioamnionitis, premature labor, intrauterine fetal demise, or early-onset infection (<7 days of age) of the newborn. Women with listeriosis diagnosed during pregnancy have a favorable clinical outcome following antibiotic therapy or delivery. Although often included in the differential diagnosis of recurrent abortion, infection with *L. monocytogenes* appears to cause fewer than 2 percent of stillbirths.

Neonatal listeriosis can be classified by the same categories used in group B streptococcal infection (see Chap. 103), with early-onset infection evident during the first week of life and late-onset disease occurring thereafter. Infants may be symptomatic at birth; most infants with early-onset infection are symptomatic by the second day of life. Aspiration of infected amniotic fluid contributes to pathogenesis. Early-onset disease may include sepsis, respiratory distress, skin lesions, and the syndrome *granulomatosis infantisepticum*, which is characterized by disseminated abscesses involving the liver, spleen, adrenal glands, lung, and other sites. Infants with late-onset neonatal disease (≥7 days of age) are more likely than those with early-onset disease to develop meningitis. While early-onset disease often occurs in association with obstetrical complications such as premature delivery and chorioamnionitis, late-onset disease typically affects infants born at term by uncomplicated deliveries. Infants may acquire the organism during passage through the birth canal, but with the exception of several clusters of late-onset neonatal infection linked to nosocomial transmission, the pathogenesis of late-onset disease is not well understood.

Listeriosis not associated with pregnancy usually occurs in persons with immunosuppressive conditions, although invasive disease also can occur in immunocompetent adults, particularly the elderly. Data from a multistate study of listeriosis revealed that the most common underlying conditions seen in nonpregnant adults with listeriosis were the chronic use of glucocorticoid medications and the presence of solid or hematologic malignancies, diabetes mellitus, renal disease, liver disease, or AIDS. Although the incidence of listeriosis in AIDS patients is much higher than the incidence in the general population, listeriosis is a relatively uncommon opportunistic infection in AIDS. Bacteremic and central nervous system (CNS) disease are the most common presentations of listeriosis in nonpregnant adults.

Sepsis Recent clinical series have shown that bacteremic infection without evident focus is the most common clinical manifestation of listeriosis, followed by CNS infection. Listerial sepsis cannot be distinguished clinically from bacteremia due to other organisms. Patients are usually febrile, often appear extremely ill, and may have prodromal symptoms including myalgia, nausea, vomiting, and diarrhea. Immunocompromised patients with listeriosis are less likely than other adults to present with CNS infection. Immunocompromised patients may be more likely to have blood cultured during febrile episodes, while in other adults transient bacteremia due to *L. monocytogenes* may go unrecognized.

Central nervous system infection   The majority of CNS infections due to *L. monocytogenes* are meningitic. Meningitis due to *L. monocytogenes* is not distinguishable clinically from other types of bacterial meningitis, and presenting symptoms include fever, headache, and altered level of consciousness. Typically, examination of cerebrospinal fluid (CSF) reveals pleocytosis, increased protein, and normal glucose, although other patterns (including low CSF sugar) can occur. As is the case in other forms of bacterial meningitis, Gram's stain is often unrevealing; the diagnosis is made when *L. monocytogenes* is identified on culture. Despite its name, *L. monocytogenes* infection is rarely associated with monocytosis of either the CSF or blood. Other syndromes seen with CNS infection include encephalitis, cerebritis, and brainstem, spinal cord, or intracranial abscesses. Symptoms may include fever, ataxia, seizures, personality changes, and coma. Nuchal rigidity is rare. CSF cultures may be sterile, and blood cultures are usually diagnostic.

Endocarditis   Like most forms of bacterial endocarditis, endocarditis due to *L. monocytogenes* typically occurs in patients with prosthetic or previously damaged valves. The organism has a predilection for the left side of the heart, and endocarditis due to *L. monocytogenes* is often associated with systemic embolization.

Focal infections   Other focal infections that can occur following unrecognized bacteremia include endophthalmitis, peritonitis, osteomyelitis, visceral abscess, pleuropulmonary infection, and cholecystitis. Cutaneous lesions may occur without systemic involvement and have been reported in veterinarians and poultry workers.

Recurrent infection with *L. monocytogenes* has been reported but is rare. Many recurrences are due to the subtype responsible for the initial infection, suggesting that recurrences result either from insufficient treatment of a focus of primary infection or from repeated exposure to a persistently contaminated source.

DIAGNOSIS   Listeriosis is diagnosed when the organism is cultured from usually sterile sites such as blood, CSF, or amniotic fluid. The organism will grow readily within 36 h on routine culture media, but there are morphologic similarities between *Listeria* and both diphtheroids and streptococci; biochemical tests are needed to identify the species. Serologic assays have not been useful in diagnosing listeriosis, because exposure to the organism may be common and infected individuals may not show elevated antibody titers following infection. Culture of the organism from nonsterile sites such as vaginal and rectal specimens is not useful for diagnosis because the organism may be carried in approximately 5 percent of healthy individuals.

Differential diagnosis of prematurity, spontaneous abortion, or stillbirth includes infectious diseases such as group B streptococcal infection, congenital syphilis, and toxoplasmosis; pathogens such as group B streptococci and *Escherichia coli* are more common than *L. monocytogenes* as causes of meningitis and sepsis in the newborn period. Because *L. monocytogenes* is not sensitive to cephalosporins, these agents should not be used as a single agent in empirical therapy of neonatal sepsis and meningitis. Listerial infection should always be considered in the differential diagnosis of meningitis in immunosuppressed persons, particularly in transplant recipients and others receiving glucocorticoid treatment, as well as in patients with hematologic malignancy or HIV infection. Among healthy adults, meningitis is much more likely to be caused by *Neisseria meningitidis*, *Streptococcus pneumoniae*, or viral pathogens than by *L. monocytogenes*.

TREATMENT   The treatment of choice for listeriosis is intravenous therapy with either ampicillin or penicillin, often in combination with an aminoglycoside. Trimethoprim-sulfamethoxazole has been used successfully in patients with penicillin allergy, although clinical experience with this regimen is limited. *L. monocytogenes* is suscepti-

TABLE 105-1   Dietary recommendations for the prevention of food-borne listeriosis

Recommendations to all individuals
1. Thoroughly cook raw food from animal sources such as beef, pork, and poultry.
2. Wash raw vegetables thoroughly before eating.
3. Keep uncooked meats separate from vegetables and from cooked foods and ready-to-eat foods.
4. Avoid raw (unpasteurized) milk or foods made from raw milk.
5. Wash hands, knives, and cutting board after handling uncooked foods.

Additional recommendations to high-risk individuals*
1. Avoid soft cheeses such as Mexican-style, feta, Brie, Camembert, and blue-veined cheese. There is no need to avoid hard cheeses, cream cheese, cottage cheese, or yogurt.
2. Left-over foods or ready-to-eat foods such as hot dogs should be reheated until steaming hot before eating.
3. Although the risk of listeriosis associated with foods from delicatessen counters is relatively low and poorly characterized, pregnant women and immunosuppressed persons may choose to avoid these foods or to thoroughly reheat cold cuts before eating.

* Persons immunocompromised by illness or medications and pregnant women.

ble in vitro to penicillin G, ampicillin, erythromycin, trimethoprim-sulfamethoxazole, chloramphenicol, rifampin, tetracyclines, aminoglycosides, and imipenem. However, chloramphenicol and rifampin may antagonize the bactericidal effect of penicillins. Cephalosporins are not recommended.

Dosages and duration of therapy have not been subjected to controlled trials. For treatment of neonatal listeriosis and listeriosis in pregnancy, a 2-week course of either penicillin G (240,000 to 320,000 units per kilogram per day) or ampicillin (150 to 200 mg/kg per day) in six divided doses is recommended. Addition of an aminoglycoside (gentamicin, 6 mg/kg per day in four divided doses) should be considered for neonatal infection. Higher dosage may be appropriate for CNS disease (penicillin G, 320,000 to 480,000 units per kilogram per day, or ampicillin, 200 to 300 mg/kg per day, in six divided doses). Penicillin-allergic patients may be treated with trimethoprim-sulfamethoxazole, as 15/75 mg/kg per day, intravenously, in three equal doses every 8 h. Meningitis in a patient without immunosuppression may require 2 to 3 weeks of antibiotic therapy following defervescence. Bacteremia, endocarditis, and nonmeningitic listeriosis in immunosuppressed patients should be treated longer, probably 4 to 6 weeks.

PROGNOSIS   Treatment of maternal bacteremia during pregnancy can prevent neonatal infection. Antibiotic therapy for the newborn can limit sequelae, although the widely disseminated disease characteristic of granulomatosis infantisepticum is frequently fatal regardless of treatment. Early-onset disease carries a higher mortality rate than late-onset infection, and immunocompromised hosts have a worse prognosis than do otherwise healthy adults with listeriosis.

PREVENTION   *L. monocytogenes* is frequently isolated from foods; the U.S. Food and Drug Administration, U.S. Department of Agriculture, and manufacturers are actively pursuing further measures to reduce *L. monocytogenes* contamination of foods that have been subjected to listericidal processing. Prevention of listeriosis requires dietary counseling of persons at increased risk of disease (Table 105-1). There is no role for prophylaxis of contacts of patients with listeriosis. Clinicians are encouraged to report cases of listeriosis to local or state health departments to facilitate early recognition of listeriosis outbreaks and prevention of subsequent cases.

REFERENCES

NIEMAN RE, LORBER B: Listeriosis in adults: A changing pattern. Report of eight cases and review of the literature, 1968–1978. Rev Infect Dis 2:207, 1980

PINNER RW et al: Role of foods in sporadic listeriosis: II. Microbiologic and epidemiologic investigation. JAMA 267:2046, 1992

SCHLECH WF et al: Epidemic listeriosis—Evidence for transmission by food. N Engl J Med 308:203, 1983

SCHUCHAT A et al: Role of foods in sporadic listeriosis: I. Case-control study of dietary risk factors. JAMA 267:2041, 1992

——— et al: Epidemiology of human listeriosis. Clin Microbiol Rev 4:169, 1991

SEELIGER HPR: *Listeriosis*. Basel, Karger, 1961

106   TETANUS

ELIAS ABRUTYN

DEFINITION   Tetanus is a neurologic disorder, characterized by increased muscle tone and spasms, that is caused by tetanospasmin, a powerful protein toxin elaborated by *Clostridium tetani*. Tetanus occurs in several clinical forms, including generalized, neonatal, and localized disease.

MICROBIOLOGY   The organism is an anaerobic, motile gram-positive rod that forms an oval, colorless, terminal spore creating a shape that resembles a tennis racket or drumstick. It is found worldwide in soil, in the inanimate environment, in animal feces, and occasionally in human feces. Spores may survive for years in some environments and are resistant to various disinfectants and boiling for 20 min. Vegetative cells, however, are easily inactivated and are susceptible to several antibiotics (penicillin and others).

Tetanospasmin is formed in vegetative cells under plasmid control. It is a single-polypeptide chain. With autolysis, the single-chain toxin is released and cleaved to form a heterodimer consisting of a heavy chain (100,000 mol wt) and a light chain (50,000 mol wt) joined by a disulfide bond. The amino acid structures of the two most powerful toxins known, botulinum and tetanus toxin, are partially homologous.

EPIDEMIOLOGY   Tetanus occurs sporadically and almost always affects nonimmunized or partially immunized persons, or fully immunized individuals who fail to maintain adequate immunity with booster doses of vaccine. Although entirely preventable by immunization, worldwide the burden of disease is large. The disease is common where soil is cultivated, in rural areas, in warm climates, during summer months, and in males. In countries without a major immunization program, neonatal tetanus and tetanus in the young predominate; worldwide an estimated 800,000 neonates die each year. In the United States and other nations with successful immunization programs, neonatal tetanus rarely occurs, and the disease affects other age groups and those in groups inadequately reached by immunization such as nonwhites. The elderly, in particular, are prominently involved. Under 100 cases have been reported to the Centers for Disease Control annually: 94 percent of cases occurred in persons over 20 years of age and 68 percent in individuals over 50. The burden of illness, however, is greater because reporting is incomplete.

In the United States, most tetanus occurs after an acute injury, such as a puncture wound, laceration, or abrasion, and is often acquired indoors, during farming or gardening, or in other outdoor settings. The injury may be major but often is trivial, so medical attention is not sought. The disease may complicate chronic conditions such as skin ulcers, abscesses, and gangrene. Tetanus is also associated with burns, frostbite, ear infection, surgery, abortion, childbirth, and drug abuse, notably skin "popping." In some patients no portal of entry can be identified.

PATHOGENESIS   Contamination of wounds with spores is probably frequent. Germination and toxin production, however, only occur in wounds with low oxidation-reduction potential such as those containing devitalized tissue, foreign bodies, or active infection. *Clostridium tetani* does not itself evoke inflammation, and the portal of entry appears benign unless infection from other organisms is present.

Toxin released in the wound binds to peripheral alpha motor neuron terminals, enters the axon, and is transported to the nerve cell body in the brainstem and spinal cord by retrograde intraneuronal transport. Toxin then migrates across the synapse to presynaptic terminals, where it blocks release of the inhibitory neurotransmitters glycine and gamma-aminobutyric acid (GABA). With diminished inhibition, the resting firing rate of the alpha motor neuron increases, producing rigidity. With lessened activity of reflexes, which limits polysynaptic spread of impulses (a glycinergic activity), agonists and antagonists may be recruited rather than inhibited, thereby producing

spasms. Loss of inhibition also may affect preganglionic sympathetic neurons in the lateral gray matter of the spinal cord and produce sympathetic hyperactivity and high circulating catecholamine levels. Tetanospasmin, like botulinum toxin, also may block neurotransmitter release at the neuromuscular junction and produce weakness or paralysis; recovery requires sprouting of new nerve terminals.

In local tetanus, only the nerves supplying the affected muscles are involved. Generalized tetanus occurs when toxin released in the wound enters the bloodstream and is spread to other nerve terminals; the blood-brain barrier blocks direct entry into the central nervous sytem. Assuming equal intraneuronal transport times for all nerves, short nerves are affected before long nerves; this fact explains the sequential involvement of nerves of the head, trunk, and extremities in generalized tetanus.

CLINICAL MANIFESTATIONS   Generalized tetanus, the most common form, is characterized by increased muscle tone and generalized spasms. The median onset after injury is 7 days; 15 percent of cases occur within 3 days and 10 percent after 14 days.

Typically, the patient first notices increased tone in the masseter muscles (trismus or lockjaw). Dysphagia or stiffness or pain in the neck, shoulder, and back muscles occurs concurrently or appears soon thereafter. Then other muscles are involved, producing a rigid abdomen and stiff proximal limb muscles; the hands and feet are relatively spared. Sustained contraction of the facial muscles produces a grimace or sneer (risus sardonicus), and contraction of the back muscles produces an arched back (opisthotonos). Some patients develop paroxysmal, violent, painful, generalized muscle spasms that may cause cyanosis and threaten ventilation. They occur repetitively and may be spontaneous or provoked by even the slightest stimulation. A constant threat during generalized spasms is reduced ventilation or apnea or laryngospasm. The severity of illness may be mild (muscle rigidity and few or no spasms), moderate (trismus, dysphagia, rigidity, and spasms), or severe (frequent explosive paroxysms). The patient may be febrile, although many have no fever; mentation is unimpaired. Deep tendon reflexes may be increased. Dysphagia or ileus may preclude oral feeding.

Autonomic dysfunction commonly complicates severe cases and is characterized by labile or sustained hypertension, tachycardia, arrhythmias, hyperpyrexia, profuse sweating, peripheral vasoconstriction, and increased plasma and urinary catecholamine levels. Periods of bradycardia and hypotension also may occur and are usually easily reversed by physical stimulation such as suctioning; however, pacemaker insertion is occasionally required. Sudden cardiac arrest occurs, but the basis for it is unknown.

Complications include pneumonia, fractures, muscle rupture, deep vein thrombophlebitis, pulmonary emboli, decubitus ulcer, and rhabdomyolysis.

Neonatal tetanus usually occurs as generalized tetanus and untreated is usually fatal. It develops in children born to inadequately immunized mothers, frequently after unsterile treatment of the umbilical cord stump. The onset generally occurs during the first 2 weeks of life. Poor feeding, rigidity, and spasms occur.

Local tetanus is an uncommon form in which manifestations are restricted to muscles near the wound. The prognosis is excellent.

Cephalic tetanus, a rare form of local tetanus, follows head injury or ear infection. Trismus and dysfunction of one or more cranial nerves, often the seventh nerve, are found. The incubation period is a few days and the mortality is high.

DIAGNOSIS   The diagnosis of tetanus is made entirely on the basis of clinical findings. Tetanus is unlikely if a reliable history indicates completion of a primary vaccination series and receipt of appropriate booster doses. Wound cultures should be done. However, *C. tetani* can be isolated from wounds of patients without tetanus, and frequently the organism cannot be recovered from the wounds of those with tetanus. The leukocyte count may be elevated. The cerebrospinal fluid examination is normal. Electromyograms may show continuous discharge of motor units and shortening or absence of the silent interval normally seen after an action potential. Nonspecific changes may be seen on the electrocardiogram. Muscle enzyme levels may be raised. Serum antitoxin levels of 0.01 units/mL or higher are considered protective and would make tetanus unlikely.

The differential diagnosis includes local conditions also producing trismus such as alveolar abscess, strychnine poisoning, dystonic drug reactions (e.g., phenothiazines and metoclopramide), and hypocalcemic tetany. Other conditions possibly confused with tetanus include meningitis/encephalitis, rabies, and an acute intraabdominal process (because of the rigid abdomen). The marked increased tone in central muscles (face, neck, chest, back, and abdomen) with superimposed generalized spasms and relative sparing of the hands and feet strongly suggests tetanus.

TREATMENT   **General measures**   The goals of therapy are to eliminate the source of toxin, neutralize unbound toxin, prevent muscle spasms, and provide support, especially respiratory support, until recovery. Patients should be admitted to a quiet room in an intensive care unit where observation and cardiopulmonary monitoring can be maintained continuously, but stimulation can be minimized. Protection of the airway is vital. Wounds should be explored, carefully cleansed, and thoroughly debrided.

Antibiotic therapy   Although it is of questionable benefit, parenteral penicillin (10 to 12 million units daily for 10 days) is administered to eradicate vegetative cells, the source of the toxin. Clindamycin, erythromycin, or metronidazol may be given as a substitute to patients with penicillin allergy. Specific therapy should be given for active infection caused by other organisms.

Antitoxin   Given to neutralize circulating toxin and unbound toxin in the wound, antitoxin effectively lowers mortality; toxin already bound to neural tissue is unaffected. Tetanus immune globulin (human) (TIG) is the preparation of choice and should be given promptly. The dose is 3000 to 6000 units intramuscularly, usually in divided doses, because the volume is large. The optimal dose is not known, however, and results from one study indicated that 500 units was as effective as higher doses. It may be best to administer antitoxin before manipulating the wound; the value of injecting a dose proximal to the wound or infiltrating the wound is unclear. Additional doses are unnecessary because the half-life of the antitoxin is long. Antibody does not penetrate the blood-brain barrier. Intrathecal administration should be considered experimental. Equine tetanus antitoxin (TAT) is also available. It is cheaper, but the half-life is shorter and hypersensitivity and serum sickness are common; doses up to 100,000 units are given, part intramuscularly and part intravenously, but 10,000 units may suffice.

Control of muscle spasms   Many agents, alone and in combination, have been used to treat the muscle spasms, which are painful and can threaten ventilation by causing laryngospasm or sustained contraction of ventilatory muscles. Ideal therapy would abolish spasmodic activity without causing oversedation and hypoventilation. Diazepam, a benzodiazepine and GABA agonist, is in wide use. The dose is titrated, and large doses (250 mg/d or more) may be required. Lorazepam, with a longer duration of action, and midazolam, whose short half-life necessitates administration by continuous intravenous infusions, are other options. Barbiturates and chlorpromazine are also used. Neuromuscular blockade (with vecuronium or equivalent agent) with mechanical ventilation is highly effective for treating severe spasms unresponsive to medication or spasms that threaten ventilation. Dantrolene and baclofen are being investigated as treatment to shorten the period of therapeutic paralysis.

Respiratory care   Intubation or tracheostomy, with or without mechanical ventilation, may be required for hypoventilation from oversedation or laryngospasm or to avert aspiration in patients with trismus, disordered swallowing, or dysphagia. The need should be anticipated, and the procedure performed electively and early.

Autonomic dysfunction   The optimal therapy for sympathetic overactivity has not been defined. Considerations include labetalol (an alpha- and beta-adrenergic blocking agent that is recommended by some experts, but sudden death has been reported), esmolol by continuous infusion (a beta blocker whose short half-life may be

advantageous in the event of hypotension or bradycardia), clonidine (a centrally acting antiadrenergic drug), and morphine sulfate. Parenteral magnesium sulfate and continuous spinal anesthesia have been used but may be more difficult to administer and monitor. The relative efficacy of these modalities is yet to be determined.

Vaccine   Active immunization should be initiated because immunity is not induced by the small amount of toxin that produces disease.

Additional measures   These include hydration to control insensible and other fluid losses, which may be high; increased nutritional requirements, which can be met by enteral or parenteral means; physiotherapy to prevent contractures; and heparin to prevent pulmonary emboli. Bowel, bladder, and renal function must be monitored. Gastrointestinal bleeding and decubitus ulcers must be prevented, and intercurrent infection should be treated.

PREVENTION   **Active immunization**   All partially immunized and unimmunized adults should receive vaccine, as should those recovering from tetanus. The primary series for adults consists of three doses: the first and second doses are given 4 to 8 weeks apart, and the third dose is given 6 to 12 months after the second. A booster dose is required every 10 years and may be given at middecade ages, 35, 45, and so on. Combined tetanus and diphtheria toxoid adsorbed (for adult use) (Td) rather than single-antigen tetanus toxoid is preferred for persons over 7 years of age.

Wound management   Proper wound management requires consideration of the need for (1) passive immunization with TIG and (2) active immunization with vaccine, preferably Td in those over age 7. For clean, minor wounds, Td is administered to persons who have (1) unknown tetanus immunization histories, (2) received less than three doses of adsorbed tetanus toxoid, (3) received three or more doses of adsorbed vaccine but more than 10 years have elapsed since the last dose, and (4) received three doses of *fluid* (nonadsorbed) vaccine. The recommendations for contaminated or severe wounds are identical, except that vaccine should be given to those who received three or more doses of adsorbed tetanus toxoid if more than 5 years have elapsed since the last dose. TIG is not recommended for clean, minor wounds but is given for all other wounds if the vaccination history indicates unknown or partial immunization. The dose of TIG for passive immunization of wounds of average severity is 250 units intramuscularly, which produces a protective antibody level in the serum for at least 4 to 6 weeks; the dose of equine antitoxin is 3000 to 6000 units. Vaccine and tetanus antitoxin should be administered at separate sites in separate syringes.

Neonatal tetanus   Preventive efforts include maternal vaccination, even during pregnancy, measures to increase the number of in-hospital births, and training for nonmedical birth attendants.

PROGNOSIS   The application of methods to support respiration has markedly improved the prognosis in tetanus; mortality rates as low as 10 percent have been reported from units accustomed to handling such cases. In the United States, the overall mortality for the years 1987 to 1988 was 2 percent. The outcome is poor in neonatal tetanus and the elderly and in those with a short incubation period, a short interval from the onset of symptoms to admission, or a short period from onset of symptoms to the first spasm (period of onset).

The course of tetanus extends over 4 to 6 weeks, and patients may require ventilatory support for 3 weeks during this period. Increased tone and minor spasms can last for months, but recovery is usually complete.

REFERENCES

ABRUTYN E, BERLIN JA: Intrathecal therapy of tetanus: A meta-analysis. JAMA 266:2262, 1991

BLECK TP: Tetanus, in *Infections of the Central Nervous System*, WM Scheld et al (eds). New York, Raven, 1991

CENTERS FOR DISEASE CONTROL: Diphtheria, tetanus, and pertussis: Recommendations for vaccine use and other preventive measures. Recommendations of the Immunization Practices Advisory Committee. Morb Mort Week Rep 40(RR-10):1, 1991

———: Tetanus—United States, 1987 and 1988. Morb Mort Week Rep 39:37, 1990

KING WW, CAVE DR: Use of esmolol to control autonomic instability of tetanus. Am J Med 91:425, 1991

ROOS KL: Tetanus. Semin Neurol 11:206, 1991

SUTTON DN et al: Management of autonomic dysfunction in severe tetanus: The use of magnesium sulphate and clonidine. Intensive Care Med 16:75, 1990

TRAVERSON HP et al: A reassessment of risk factors for neonatal tetanus. Bull WHO 69:573, 1991

WRIGHT KD et al: Autonomic nervous system dysfunction in severe tetanus: Current perspectives. Crit Care Med 17:371, 1989

WESLEY AG, PATHER M: Tetanus in children: An 11-year review. Ann Trop Pediatr 7:32, 1987

107   BOTULISM

ELIAS ABRUTYN

DEFINITION   Botulism is a paralytic disease that begins with cranial nerve involvement and progresses caudally to involve the extremities. It is caused by potent protein neurotoxins elaborated by *Clostridium botulinum*. Cases may be classified as (1) *food-borne botulism*, from ingestion of preformed toxin in food contaminated with *C. botulinum*, (2) *wound botulism*, from toxin produced in wounds contaminated with the organism, (3) *infant botulism*, from ingestion of spores and production of toxin in the intestine of infants, (4) *adult infant botulism*, for older children and adults whose mechanism for disease resembles that found in infant botulism, or (5) *indeterminate*.

ETIOLOGY   *C. botulinum*, a heterogeneous group of anaerobic gram-positive organisms that form subterminal spores, is found in soil and marine environments throughout the world and elaborates the most potent bacterial toxin known. Types A through G have been distinguished by the antigenic specificities of their toxins. Rare strains of other clostridial species—*C. butyricum* and *C. baratii*— also have been found to produce toxin. Types of *C. botulinum* with proteolytic activity can digest food and produce a spoiled appearance; nonproteolytic types leave the appearance of food unchanged.

Eight distinct toxin types (A, B, C_1, C_2, D, E, F, and G) have been described. All are neurotoxins, except for C_2, which is a cytotoxin of unknown significance that has vascular permeability and lethal, but not paralytic, activities. Botulinum neurotoxin, whether ingested or produced in the intestine or a wound, enters the vascular system and is transported to peripheral cholinergic nerve terminals, including neuromuscular junctions, postganglionic parasympathetic nerve endings, and peripheral ganglia. The central nervous system is not involved. Active neurotoxin (150,000 Da) is composed of a heavy chain (100,000 Da) and a light chain (50,000 Da). The heavy chain attaches to a receptor and enables translocation of the light chain into the nerve cell. Once intracellular, the light chain irreversibly blocks release of the neurotransmitter acetylcholine by an undefined mechanism(s) that may involve depression of calcium-mediated release reactions. Cure follows sprouting of new nerve terminals. The toxin resists degradation by acid and proteolytic enzymes but is inactivated by heat at 100°C for 10 min, as during routine home cooking. Spores, in contrast, are highly heat resistant, requiring exposure to 120°C for inactivation, as in steam sterilizers or pressure cookers.

Toxin types A, B, E, and rarely F cause human disease; type G has been associated with sudden death in a few patients in Switzerland; and types C and D cause animal disease.

EPIDEMIOLOGY   Human botulism occurs worldwide. In the United States, the geographic distribution of cases by toxin type parallels the distribution of organism types found in the environment. Type A predominates west of the Rocky Mountains; type B is generally distributed but is more common in the East; and type E is found in the Pacific Northwest, Alaska, and the Great Lakes area. In the United States, food-borne botulism has been associated primarily with home-canned food, particularly vegetables, fruit, and condiments, and less commonly with meat and fish. Type E outbreaks are frequently associated with fish products. Commercial products occasionally cause outbreaks, but some of these have resulted from improper handling after purchase. Outbreaks in restaurants, schools, and private homes have been traced to uncommon sources (commercial pot pies, beef stew, turkey loaf, sauteed onions, baked potatoes, and chopped garlic in oil). Food-borne botulism can occur when (1) a food to be preserved is contaminated with spores, (2) preservation does not inactivate the spores but kills other putrefactive bacteria that might inhibit growth of *C. botulinum* and also provides anaerobic conditions at a pH and temperature that allow germination and toxin production, and (3) food is not heated to a temperature that destroys toxin before being eaten.

CLINICAL MANIFESTATIONS   Food-borne botulism   Following ingestion of food containing toxin, illness varies from a mild one for which no medical advice is sought to very severe disease which may result in death in 24 h. The incubation period is usually 18 to 36 h but depending on toxin dose ranges from a few hours to several days. A symmetric descending paralysis is characteristic and can lead to respiratory failure and death. Cranial nerve involvement, which almost always marks the onset of symptoms, usually produces diplopia, dysarthria, and/or dysphagia; weakness progresses, often rapidly, from the head to involve the neck, arms, thorax, and legs. Nausea, vomiting, and abdominal pain may occur before or after onset of paralysis. Dizziness, blurred vision, dry mouth, and very dry, occasionally sore throat are common. Occasionally, the weakness is asymmetric. Patients are generally alert and oriented, but they may be drowsy, agitated, and anxious. Typically, fever is absent. Ptosis is frequent; the pupillary reflexes may be depressed, and fixed or dilated pupils are seen in half the patients. The gag reflex may be suppressed, and deep tendon reflexes may be normal or decreased. Paralytic ileus, severe constipation, and urinary retention are common.

Wound botulism   When wounds are contaminated with *C. botulinum* spores, the spores may germinate to vegetative organisms that produce toxin. This rare condition resembles food-borne illness except that the incubation period is longer, averaging about 10 days, and gastrointestinal symptoms are absent. Wound botulism has been noted after traumatic wounds contaminated with soil, in chronic drug abusers, and after cesarean delivery. The illness has occurred even when antibiotics were given to prevent wound infection. When present, fever is probably from concurrent infection with other bacteria. The wound may appear benign.

Infant botulism   In infant botulism, the most common form of disease, toxin is produced in and absorbed from the intestine following germination of ingested spores. The severity ranges from mild illness with failure to thrive to fulminant, severe paralysis with respiratory failure and may be one cause of sudden infant death, but this is controversial. Ingestion of contaminated honey has been defined as one source of spores, leading to the recommendation that honey not be fed to children less than 12 months of age. Most cases cannot be attributed to a particular food source. The factors permitting intestinal colonization with *C. botulinum* are not fully defined, but cases usually occur in infants under 6 months of age; susceptibility may decrease as normal intestinal flora develop.

Adult infant botulism   Also called *adult enteric infectious botulism* or *adult infectious botulism of unknown source*, this disorder resembles infant botulism in that toxin is produced in the intestine of persons colonized with the organism. Toxin and organisms may be found in the stool over prolonged periods, and spores, but not toxin, may be found in the suspect food. Gastrointestinal disease or surgery may predispose to illness. Previously, such cases would have been classified as *indeterminate*.

DIAGNOSIS   Botulism must be considered in afebrile, mentally intact patients who have a symmetric descending paralysis without sensory findings. Conditions often confused with botulism include myasthenia gravis, which may be excluded by electromyography and appropriate antibody studies, and the Guillain-Barré syndrome, which is characterized by ascending paralysis, sensory abnormalities, and elevation in cerebrospinal fluid protein. The Miller-Fisher variant of Guillain-Barré—a descending paralysis—can be difficult to differentiate. Other conditions that may mimic botulism include poliomyelitis, tick paralysis, acute abdomen, pharyngitis, cerebrovascular accidents, and intoxications from mushrooms, medications, or chemicals.

The demonstration of toxin in serum by bioassay in mice is definitive, but the test may be negative, particularly in wound and infant botulism. It is only performed by specific laboratories, which can be identified by contacting regional public health authorities. The demonstration of toxin or the organism in vomitus, gastric fluid, or stool is strongly suggestive, because intestinal carriage is rare. Isolation of the organism from food without toxin is insufficient for diagnosis. Wound cultures showing the organism are suggestive. The edrophonium chloride (Tensilon) test for myasthenia gravis may be falsely positive in botulism but is usually less dramatic. Nerve conduction velocity is normal, but on routine electromyography, action potentials are decreased with a supramaximal stimulus and facilitation is found after repetitive stimulation at high frequency. Single-fiber electromyography may be helpful. The white blood cell count and sedimentation rate are normal.

TREATMENT Patients should be hospitalized and monitored closely both clinically and by spirometry, pulse oximetry, and measurement of arterial blood gases for incipient respiratory failure. Intubation and mechanical ventilation should be strongly considered when the vital capacity is less than 30 percent of predicted, especially when paralysis is progressing rapidly and hypoxemia with absolute or relative hypercarbia is present (see Chap. 231). Serial measurement of the maximal static inspiratory pressure may be useful in predicting respiratory failure.

In food-borne illness, trivalent (types A, B, and E) equine antitoxin should be administered as soon as possible after obtaining specimens for laboratory analysis. Laboratory confirmation, which may take days, is unnecessary before initiating treatment. After testing for hypersensitivity to horse serum, two vials are given, either both intravenously or one intravenously and one intramuscularly; the dose may be repeated in 2 to 4 h. Anaphylaxis and serum sickness are risks inherent in use of the equine product, and in allergic patients desensitization may be necessary. If there is no ileus, cathartics and enemas may be given to purge the gut of toxin; emetics or gastric lavage is used also if the time since ingestion is brief, e.g., only a few hours. Antibiotics to eliminate an intestinal source for possible continued toxin production and guanidine hydrochloride and other drugs used to reverse paralysis are of unproven value. In the United States, antitoxin and help in clinical management and laboratory confirmation are available at *any* time by calling the state health department or the Centers for Disease Control.

Treatment of infant botulism requires supportive care. Neither equine antitoxin nor antibiotics have been shown to be beneficial, and the value of human botulism immune globulin, an experimental preparation, is under evaluation. In wound botulism, equine antitoxin is administered. The wound should be thoroughly explored and debrided, and an antibiotic such as penicillin should be given to eradicate *C. botulinum* from the wound, although the benefit of this therapy is unproven; results of wound cultures should guide the use of other antibiotics.

PROGNOSIS Type A disease is generally more severe than type B, and mortality is higher above age 60. With improved respiratory and intensive care, the case-fatality rate in food-borne illness has fallen to about 7.5 percent and is low in infant botulism as well. Artificial respiratory support may be required for months in severe cases. Some patients experience residual weakness and autonomic dysfunction for as long as a year after disease onset.

BOTULINUM TOXIN THERAPY Botulinum toxin is being used as therapy for strabismus, blepharospasm, and other dystonias and appears safe and effective.

REFERENCES

ELSTON HR et al: Arm abscesses caused by *Clostridium botulinum*. J Clin Microbiol 29:2678, 1991

HAMBLETON P: *Clostridium botulinium* toxins: A general review of involvement in disease, structure, mode of action and preparation for clinical use. J Neurol 239:16, 1992

HATHEWAY CL: Toxigenic clostridia. Clin Microbiol Rev 3:66, 1990

JANKOVIC J, BRIN MF: Therapeutic uses of botulinum toxin. N Engl J Med 324:1186, 1991

MCCARTHY JD et al: Fever, dyspnea, and slurred speech following lower extremity trauma. Rev Infect Dis 13:172, 1991

MCCROSKEY LM, HATHEWAY CL: The large intestine as the site of *Clostridium botulinum* colonization in human infant botulism. J Clin Microbiol 26:1052, 1988

MORSE DL et al: Garlic-in-oil associated botulism: Episode leads to product modification. Am J Public Health 80:1372, 1990

SCHREINER MS et al: Infant botulism: A review of 12 years' experience at the Children's Hospital of Philadelphia. Pediatrics 87:159, 1991

SCHWARZ PJ, ARNON SS: Botulism immune globulin for infant botulism arrives—one year and a Gulf War later. West J Med 156:197, 1991

SMITH LDS, SUGIYAMA H: *Botulism: The Organism, Its Toxins, the Disease*, 2d ed. Springfield, Ill., Thomas, 1988

WILCOX PG et al: Recovery of the ventilatory and upper airway muscles and exercise performance after type A botulism. Chest 98:620, 1990

108 GAS GANGRENE AND OTHER CLOSTRIDIAL INFECTIONS

DENNIS L. KASPER / DORI F. ZALEZNIK

DEFINITION Bacteria of the genus *Clostridium* are gram-positive, spore-forming, obligate anaerobes that are ubiquitous in nature. There are over 60 recognized species of clostridia, many of which generally are considered saprophytic. Some of these species are pathogenic for humans and animals, particularly under conditions of lowered oxidation-reduction potential. Infections associated with these organisms range from localized wound contamination to overwhelming systemic disease. The four major disease categories for which clostridia are responsible include intestinal disorders, deep tissue suppurative infections, skin and soft tissue infections, and bacteremias (see Table 108-1). Toxins play a major role in some of these syndromes.

ETIOLOGY In humans, clostridia normally reside in the gastrointestinal tract and in the female genital tract, although they occasionally can be isolated from the skin or the mouth. As with other pathogenic anaerobic bacteria, clostridia are quite aerotolerant. Of the known species of the genus *Clostridium*, at least 30 have been isolated from human infections. Clostridia characteristically produce abundant gas

TABLE 108-1 Classification of diseases caused by other clostridia

Intestinal syndromes
 A Food poisoning
 B Enteritis necroticans
 C Antibiotic-associated colitis

Suppurative deep tissue infections
 A Mixed bacterial infections
 B Only microorganism isolated

Skin and soft tissue infections
 A Simple contamination
 B Local infection without systemic signs
 C Spreading cellulitis and fasciitis
 D Myonecrosis

Bacteremia
 A Transient bacteremia
 B Sepsis

in artificial media and form subterminal endospores. *C. perfringens*, one of the most important of the species, is encapsulated, nonmotile, and rarely sporulates in artificial media; the spores usually can be destroyed by boiling. *C. tetani* and *C. botulinum* are discussed in Chaps. 106 and 107, respectively.

Clostridia are present in the normal colonic flora in concentrations of 10^9 to 10^{10} per gram. Of the 30 or more species that normally colonize humans, *C. ramosum* is the most common, followed by *C. perfringens*. These organisms are universally present in soil in concentrations of up to 10^4 per gram. Clostridia are gram-positive organisms, but in clinical specimens or stationary phase cultures, many species may appear to be gram-negative. Therefore, Gram's stains of cultures or clinical material should be interpreted with great care.

C. perfringens is the most common of the clostridial species isolated from tissue infections and bacteremias, followed in frequency by *C. novyi* and *C. septicum*. In the category of enteric infections, *C. difficile* is an important cause of antibiotic-associated colitis, and *C. perfringens* is associated with food poisoning and enteritis necroticans.

PATHOGENESIS Despite the isolation of clostridial species in many severe, traumatic wounds, the incidence of severe infections due to these organisms is low. Essential to the development of severe disease appears to be the presence of tissue necrosis and a low oxidation-reduction potential. *C. perfringens* requires about 14 amino acids and 6 or 7 additional growth factors for optimal growth. These nutrients are not found in appreciable concentrations in normal body fluids but are present in necrotic tissue. When *C. perfringens* grows in necrotic tissue, a zone of tissue damage due to the toxins elaborated by the organism allows for progressive growth. In contrast, when only a few bacteria leak into the bloodstream from a small defect in the intestinal wall, the organisms do not have the opportunity to multiply rapidly because blood as medium for growth is relatively deficient in certain amino acids and growth factors. Therefore, in a patient without tissue necrosis, bacteremia is usually benign.

C. perfringens possesses 17 possible virulence factors, including 12 active tissue toxins and enterotoxins. *C. perfringens* has been divided into five types (A through E) on the basis of four major toxins: alpha, beta, epsilon, and iota. The alpha toxin is a phospholipase C (lecithinase) that splits lecithin into phosphorylcholine and diglyceride. This alpha toxin has been associated with gas gangrene and is known to be hemolytic, destroy platelets and polymorphonuclear leukocytes, and cause widespread capillary damage. When injected intravenously, it causes massive intravascular hemolysis and damages liver mitochondria. Alpha toxin may be important in the initiation of muscle infections that may progress to gas gangrene. Experimentally, the higher the concentration of alpha toxin present in the culture fluid, the smaller the infecting dose of *C. perfringens* required to produce infection. The protective effect of antiserum is directly proportional to its content of alpha antitoxin. Beta, epsilon, and iota toxins are also known to increase capillary permeability.

C. difficile produces two major toxins, designated A and B. Toxin B is a cytotoxin and is the toxin measured in the sensitive tissue culture assay system employed in many clinical laboratories as the gold standard for diagnosing antibiotic-associated diarrhea. Toxin A is an enterotoxin which is believed to play an important role in causing diarrhea but is not reliably measured in assays currently in widespread use. Diarrheal disease due to *C. difficile* is toxin-mediated. Teaching about pathogenesis of this disease has centered on overgrowth of *C. difficile* when antibiotics suppress normal bowel flora. The mechanism is probably more complex, since many of the antibiotics that cause this disease are active against *C. difficile* as well as other bowel flora, and many patients who become colonized with *C. difficile* do not develop diarrhea. Critical features in the pathogenesis of this disease include mechanisms of toxin production and the interaction of *C. difficile* with other bowel flora. Some antibiotics may actually trigger toxin production by the organism. In turn, other bowel flora may

suppress or inhibit toxin production. *C. sordellii*, for example, neutralizes cytotoxin B in vitro. In addition, when antibiotics eliminate more sensitive bowel flora, more resistant organisms may produce enzymes such as β-lactamases that can inactivate antibiotics and thereby facilitate growth of *C. difficile*.

CLINICAL MANIFESTATIONS **Intestinal disorders** FOOD POISONING *C. perfringens* is the second or third most common cause of food poisoning in the United States (see Chap. 87). Outbreaks generally have resulted from problems in the cooling and storage of foods cooked in bulk. The food sources primarily involved are meat, meat products, and poultry. Generally, the implicated meats have been cooked, allowed to cool, and then recooked the following day, often in a stew or hash. Strains of *C. perfringens* that contaminate meat manage to survive initial cooking. During reheating, the organisms sporulate and germinate. The disease is associated with an attack rate often as high as 70 percent. Symptoms of food poisoning from type A strains develop 8 to 24 h after ingestion of foods heavily contaminated with the organism. The primary symptoms include epigastric pain, nausea, and watery diarrhea lasting 12 to 24 h. Fever and vomiting are uncommon. Symptoms usually last less than 24 h. Diarrhea appears to be caused by a heat-labile protein enterotoxin. The enterotoxin inhibits glucose transport, damages the intestinal epithelium, and causes protein loss into the intestinal lumen.

ENTERITIS NECROTICANS Enteritis necroticans (*pigbel*), caused by type C strains of *C. perfringens*, has been the cause of necrotizing enteritis and death, occurring after a feast, in children and adults in New Guinea. A similar disease, *darmbrand*, was epidemic in Germany after World War II and also was reported from an evacuation site on the Thai-Kampuchean border. Clinical features include acute abdominal pain, bloody diarrhea, vomiting, shock, and peritonitis; death occurs in 40 percent of patients. Pathologically, there is an acute ulcerative process of the bowel restricted to the small intestine. The mucosa is lifted off the submucosa, forming large denuded areas. Pseudomembranes composed of sloughed epithelium are common, and gas may dissect into the submucosa. The source of the organisms may be the patient's own intestinal flora, because cultures of ingested pork have failed to yield the organism. Antitoxin against the beta toxin of *C. perfringens* has been of considerable benefit in changing the course of established disease, and in a large-scale trial, children immunized with *C. perfringens* beta toxoid were protected.

ANTIBIOTIC-ASSOCIATED COLITIS Strains of *C. difficile* that produce toxins detectable in the stool have been identified as the major cause of colitis in patients with antibiotic-associated diarrhea. In order to diagnose this type of colitis, there should be no other identifiable cause of diarrhea and the onset of symptoms must occur either during antimicrobial administration or within 4 weeks after the implicated agent has been discontinued. Essentially any antibiotic can cause this syndrome, and even metronidazole and vancomycin, which treat the disease, have been implicated as etiologic agents in some cases. On a per-use basis, clindamycin, which was the first antibiotic described to cause this entity, is the most commonly implicated antibiotic. But since other antibiotics are prescribed more often than clindamycin in the United States, currently cephalosporins are the antibiotics which most commonly cause *C. difficile* enterocolitis, followed by penicillins.

Antimicrobial-associated diarrhea can be divided into four categories based on the appearance of the colon: (1) normal colonic mucosa, (2) mild erythema with some edema, (3) granular, friable, or hemorrhagic mucosa, and (4) pseudomembrane formation. Most patients with antibiotic-associated diarrhea have a normal, minimally erythematous colonic mucosa with some edema. Occasionally, colitis is more severe and is characterized by granular, friable, or hemorrhagic mucosa. Stool examination in these patients may reveal large numbers of red blood cells and some leukocytes. Biopsy shows subepithelial edema with round cell infiltration of the lamina propria and focal extravasation of erythrocytes. *C. difficile* cytotoxin B has been found in 15 to 46 percent of stools from patients in these first three categories, suggesting that either toxin A or other factors exist in the pathogenesis of antibiotic-associated diarrhea. The most characteristic form of antibiotic-associated colitis caused by *C. difficile* is pseudomembranous colitis (PMC). More than 95 percent of patients with documented PMC have positive stool toxin assays. Close inspection of pseudomembranes reveals exudative, punctate, raised plaques with skip areas or edematous hyperemic mucosa. These plaques can enlarge and coalesce over large segments of intestine in the later stages of disease. The clinical spectrum of antibiotic-associated PMC is diverse. Diarrhea is the common feature and is usually watery, voluminous, and without gross blood or mucus. Most patients have abdominal cramps and tenderness, fever, and leukocytosis. However, the symptoms may vary considerably. At one end of the spectrum are patients with annoying diarrhea but no systemic signs or symptoms, while at the other end there is severe systemic toxicity, fever to 40 or 40.6°C (104 or 105°F), and peripheral white blood cell counts of up to 50,000 per microliter. Fecal examination frequently reveals leukocytes. Without specific therapy, the course is highly variable. Some patients have prompt resolution of symptoms with discontinuation of the drug, while others have protracted diarrhea with large stool volumes for up to 8 weeks, with resultant hypoalbuminemia and electrolyte imbalance. Severely ill patients with toxic megacolon and colonic perforation have been reported. In those who are severely ill, mortality rates may be as high as 30 percent, while most patients with minimal symptoms have resolution of disease with discontinuation of antibiotics alone. In the majority of patients, symptoms begin 4 to 10 days after antibiotic therapy is initiated. However, about 25 percent of patients do not have symptoms until the implicated antimicrobial has been discontinued, in some cases as long as 4 weeks afterward. Some cases have been reported within hours after initiation of antibiotic therapy or after a single dose of antibiotic administered for surgical prophylaxis.

Diagnostic evaluation of patients with PMC should include examination of the stool for the presence of *C. difficile* cytotoxin. Although several assays are available, the tissue culture assay is the most practical and sensitive. The assay is performed by incubating stool filtrates with tissue culture cells and monitoring for a cytopathic effect which can be neutralized by antitoxin to either *C. sordellii* (which is cross-reactive with *C. difficile* but does not cause PMC) or *C. difficile*. Endoscopy, although useful in establishing the presence of PMC, does not establish the etiology and should be reserved for more serious disease manifestations to exclude alternative diagnoses. Isolation of *C. difficile* from stool cultures is difficult, and *C. difficile* may be present as part of the "normal" flora in asymptomatic patients, particularly infants.

Suppurative deep tissue infection Clostridia are recovered frequently from various suppurative conditions in conjunction with other anaerobic and aerobic bacteria but also can be the only organisms isolated. These conditions exist with severe local inflammation but usually without systemic signs induced by clostridial toxins. These infections include intraabdominal sepsis, empyema, pelvic abscess, subcutaneous abscess, frostbite with gas gangrene, infected stumps in amputees, brain abscess, prostatic abscess, perianal abscess, conjunctivitis, infection of a renal cell carcinoma, and infected aortic grafts.

Clostridia are isolated in approximately two-thirds of patients with intraabdominal infections resulting from intestinal perforation. *C. ramosum*, *C. perfringens*, and *C. bifermentans* are the most commonly isolated species. The presence of clostridial species does not affect the clinical presentation or outcome of these infections (see Chap. 128).

An association has been made between malignancy and the isolation of *C. septicum* in the absence of grossly contaminated deep traumatic wounds. A major site for these malignancies is the gastrointestinal tract, particularly the colon. An association with leukemia or with other solid tumors also has been noted. Some of these patients present with *C. septicum* bacteremia and have a fulminant clinical course (discussed below). Others develop localized

suppurative infection in the abdomen or the abdominal wall without bacteremia. Presumably this infection arises from a silent perforation that leads to intraabdominal abscess formation.

Clostridia have been isolated from suppurative infections of the female genital tract, particularly tuboovarian and pelvic abscess. The major species involved has been *C. perfringens*. Most of these are mild suppurative infections without evidence of uterine gangrene. Isolation of *C. perfringens* has been reported in as many as 20 percent of diseased gallbladders at surgery. One clinical syndrome, emphysematous cholecystitis, is caused by clostridial species at least 50 percent of the time. In this syndrome there is gas formation in the biliary radicles and the wall of the gallbladder. It is seen most often in diabetic patients. Although the mortality rate in this entity is higher than in more common forms of cholecystitis, there is no evidence of myonecrosis.

Clostridia are among the many organisms found in empyema fluid or isolated by transtracheal aspiration from patients with lung abscesses. There is no clinical clue to the presence of clostridia (as opposed to other organisms) in these infections. *C. perfringens* has been reported as a cause of empyema arising from aspiration pneumonia, pulmonary emboli, and infarction. However, the majority of cases of clostridial empyema are secondary to trauma.

Skin and soft tissue infections Various categories of traumatic wound infections due to clostridia have been described: simple contamination, anaerobic cellulitis, fasciitis with or without systemic manifestations, and anaerobic myonecrosis.

SIMPLE CONTAMINATION Clostridia are cultured most often from wounds in the absence of clinical signs of sepsis. As many as 30 percent of battle wounds can be contaminated by clostridia without signs of suppuration, and 16 percent of penetrating abdominal wounds yield clostridia on culture despite treatment with cephalothin and kanamycin. In cases of trauma, clostridia are isolated with equal frequency from suppurative and well-healing wounds. Based on these findings, the diagnosis of clostridial infection should be clinical rather than bacteriologic.

LOCALIZED INFECTION OF THE SKIN AND SOFT TISSUE WITHOUT SYSTEMIC SIGNS This condition was originally referred to as *anaerobic cellulitis*. It is a localized infection involving the skin and soft tissue due to clostridia in pure or mixed culture. There are no systemic signs of toxicity, although the infection may invade locally, producing necrosis. These infections tend to be relatively indolent, spreading slowly to contiguous areas. Localized infections tend to be relatively free of pain and edema. Perhaps because of the lack of edema, gas that is limited to the wound and the immediately surrounding tissue may be more evident than in gas gangrene. In these localized infections, gas is never found intramuscularly. Cellulitis, perirectal abscesses, and diabetic foot ulcers are typical infections from which clostridial species can be isolated. If inadequately treated, these localized infections advance by extension through subcutaneous tissue and fascial planes into muscle and may produce severe systemic disease with signs of toxemia.

A localized form of suppurative myositis has been described in heroin addicts. These patients develop local pain and tenderness in discrete areas (particularly the thigh and forearm) with the subsequent appearance of fluctuance and crepitance that require surgical drainage. The unusual aspect of these infections is that they remain localized without systemic signs of toxicity. Moreover these local areas are not necessarily sites of trauma or heroin injection. Pathologically, there are subcutaneous abscesses, purulent myositis, and fasciitis from which clostridia are recovered in pure culture; on occasion, mixed infections involving aerobes and anaerobes are found.

SPREADING CELLULITIS AND FASCIITIS WITH SYSTEMIC TOXICITY This is diffuse spreading cellulitis and fasciitis, but myonecrosis is absent, and only mild inflammation is seen in muscle. These patients present with the abrupt onset of a syndrome which progresses rapidly through the fascial planes within hours. When suppuration and gas in soft tissues as well as overwhelming toxemia are present, the infection is rapidly fatal. On physical examination there is subcutaneous crepitance but little localized pain. Surgery is of no proven value because there are no discretely involved tissues amenable to resection, as may be the case in myonecrosis. However, incision of the affected area should be performed, because in rapidly advancing fasciitis, it is still the cornerstone of therapy. The initial local lesion may be quite innocuous and arises from an area involved by tumor or other infection and not from injury. The systemic toxic effects include hemolysis and injury of capillary membranes. Usually, this infection is uniformly fatal within 48 h, despite intensive therapy involving antitoxin and exchange transfusion. This syndrome is seen most commonly in patients with carcinoma, especially of the sigmoid or the cecum. Presumably, the tumor invades the fascia, and colonic contents leak into the abdominal wall. These patients present with extreme toxicity and occasionally with total-body crepitance. The syndrome differs from necrotizing fasciitis caused by other organisms in three respects: (1) rapid mortality, (2) rapid tissue invasion, and (3) the systemic effects of the toxin typified by massive hemolysis.

CLOSTRIDIAL MYONECROSIS (GAS GANGRENE) Clostridial myonecrosis occurs when bacteria invade healthy muscle from adjacent traumatized muscle or soft tissue. The infection originates in a wound contaminated with clostridia. Despite the fact that more than 30 percent of deep wounds are infected with clostridia, the incidence of clostridial myonecrosis is quite low. These infections occur in military or civilian settings. An essential factor in the genesis of gas gangrene appears to be trauma, particularly involving deep lacerated muscle wounds. The entity of clostridial myonecrosis is relatively uncommon after simple, through-and-through bullet wounds without shattering of bone and relatively common following shrapnel fragmentation wounds, particularly when deep muscle is involved. In civilian cases, gas gangrene can occur after trauma, surgery, or intramuscular injection. The trauma need not be severe; however, the wound must be deep, necrotic, and without communication to the surface.

The incubation period of gas gangrene is usually short: almost always less than 3 days and frequently less than 24 h. Eighty percent of cases are caused by *C. perfringens*, while *C. novyi*, *C. septicum*, and *C. histolyticum* cause most of the other cases. Typically, gas gangrene begins with the sudden appearance of pain in the region of the wound, which helps to differentiate it from spreading cellulitis. Once established, the pain increases steadily in severity but remains localized to the infected area and only spreads if the infection spreads. Soon after pain develops, local swelling and edema, accompanied by a thin, often hemorrhagic exudate, appear. These patients frequently develop marked tachycardia, but elevation in temperature may be only minimal. Gas usually is not obvious at this early stage and may be completely absent. Frothiness of the wound exudate may be noted. The skin is tense, white, often marbled with blue and cooler than normal. The symptoms progress rapidly; swelling, edema, and toxemia increase, and a profuse serous discharge, which may have a peculiar sweetish smell, appears. Gram's stain of the wound exudate shows many gram-positive rods with relatively few inflammatory cells.

At surgery, muscle may appear pale because of the amount of edema, but it does not contract when probed with a scalpel. When dissected, the muscle is beefy red and nonviable and can progress to become black, friable, and gangrenous. It is important to establish a diagnosis early, preferably by frozen section biopsy of muscle.

Despite hypotension, renal failure, and often body crepitance, patients with myonecrosis often have a heightened awareness of their surroundings until just before death, when they lapse into toxic delirium and coma. In untreated cases, as the local wounds progress, the skin becomes bronzed; bullae appear, become filled with dark red fluid, and are accompanied by dark patches of cutaneous gangrene. Gas appears in later phases but may not be as obvious as in anaerobic cellulitis. Jaundice is rarely seen in wound gas gangrene (in contrast to uterine infections) and, when it does appear, is almost invariably associated with hemoglobinuria, hemoglobinemia, and septicemia. There have been reports of cases of clostridial myonecrosis without a history of trauma. These patients have bullous lesions and crepitance

of the skin; they present with a rapidly worsening course which includes myonecrosis, especially of the extremities.

Bacteremia and clostridial septicemia The relatively common entity of transient bacteremia due to clostridia can arise in any hospitalized patient but is most common with a predisposing focus in the gastrointestinal tract, biliary tract, or uterus. Fever frequently resolves within 24 to 48 h without therapy. Despite the finding of clostridial bacteremia following septic abortions and the frequent isolation of clostridia from the lochia, most of these patients do not have evidence of septicemia. In one series of 60 patients with clostridial bacteremia, half the cases could be associated with an infected site, while the other half had a totally unrelated illness, such as tuberculous pneumonia, meningitis, or benign gastroenteritis. Frequently, by the time the blood culture reports return, the patients are completely well and sometimes have been discharged. Therefore, when a blood culture report is positive for clostridia, the patient must be assessed clinically rather than simply treated for the positive blood culture.

Clostridial septicemia is an uncommon but almost invariably fatal illness occurring after clostridial infection primarily of the uterus, colon, or biliary tract. This entity must be differentiated from transient clostridial bacteremia, which is much more common than septicemia. *C. perfringens* causes the majority of septicemic infections, as well as the majority of cases of transient bacteremia. *C. septicum*, *C. sordellii*, and *C. novyi* account for most of the remainder of cases. Clostridia account for 1 to 2.5 percent of all positive blood cultures in major hospital centers.

The majority of cases of clostridial septicemia originate from the female genital tract following septic abortion. Introduction of a foreign body is a common antecedent event. In the uterus there may be residual necrotic fetal and placental tissues and traumatized endometrium that allow the growth of clostridia. Only a small fraction of cases of septic abortion (1 percent) are followed by serious septicemic illness.

In these patients, sepsis, fever, and chills begin from 1 to 3 days after the attempted abortion. The initial signs are malaise, headache, severe myalgias, abdominal pain, nausea, vomiting, and occasionally diarrhea. Frequently a bloody or brown vaginal discharge is noted. Patients may rapidly develop oliguria, hypotension, jaundice, and hemoglobinuria. The hemolysis, which is secondary to *C. perfringens* alpha toxin, causes a characteristic bronzing of the skin. As in myonecrosis, the mental status of severely ill patients is characterized by increased alertness and apprehension. Local examination of the pelvis reveals foul cervical discharge, occasionally with gas. Frequently, laceration marks around the cervix or perforation of the cervical segment are evident. If the infection involves the myometrium or has spread to the adnexa, extreme tenderness, guarding, and an adnexal mass may be found.

Laboratory studies in septicemic patients reveal an elevated white count and may show pink, hemoglobin-tinged plasma. Anemia is proportional to the degree of hemolysis, and the hematocrit may be extremely low. Platelets may be reduced, and there is often evidence of disseminated intravascular coagulation. Oliguria or anuria, increasingly refractory hypotension, and hemorrhage and bruising may develop.

Clostridia may enter the bloodstream from the gastrointestinal or biliary tract. This occurrence is associated with ulcerative lesions or obstruction of the small or large intestine, necrotic or infiltrating malignancy, bowel surgery, or various abdominal catastrophes. The patient may present with an acute febrile illness with chills and fever but no other signs of localized infection. Intravascular hemolysis occurs in as many as half the cases. Biliary or gastrointestinal symptoms, if present, may be the only clue to the etiology. Positive blood cultures provide the definitive clue for the diagnosis.

Patients with malignant disease also can develop rapidly fatal clostridial sepsis, particularly from a gastrointestinal focus. The most common species in this setting is *C. septicum*. Characteristic signs and symptoms include fever, tachycardia, hypotension, abdominal pain or tenderness, nausea, vomiting, and, preterminally, coma. The tachycardia may be out of proportion to the fever. Only about 20 to 30 percent of patients develop hemolysis. A striking feature of this syndrome is the rapidity of death, which frequently occurs in less than 12 h.

DIAGNOSIS The diagnosis of clostridial disease must be based primarily on clinical findings. Because of the presence of clostridia in many wounds, their mere isolation from any site, including the blood, does not necessarily indicate severe disease. Smears of wound exudates, uterine scrapings, or cervical discharge may show abundant large gram-positive rods as well as other organisms. Cultures should be placed in selective media and incubated anaerobically for identification of clostridia.

The urine of patients with severe clostridial sepsis may contain protein and casts, and some patients may develop severe uremia. Profound alterations of circulating erythrocytes are seen in severely toxemic patients. Patients have a hemolytic anemia, which develops extremely rapidly, along with hemoglobinemia, hemoglobinuria, and elevated levels of serum bilirubin. Spherocytosis, increased osmotic and mechanical red blood cell fragility, erythrophagocytosis, and methemoglobinemia have been described. Disseminated intravascular coagulation may be seen in patients with severe infection. In patients with severe septicemia, a Wright's or Gram's stain smear of peripheral blood or buffy coat may demonstrate clostridia.

X-ray examination sometimes provides an important clue to the diagnosis by revealing gas in muscles, subcutaneous tissue, or the uterus. However, the finding of gas is not pathognomonic for clostridial infection. Other bacteria, particularly anaerobes, mixed with aerobic organisms may produce gas.

The diagnosis of clostridial myonecrosis can be established by frozen section biopsy of muscle. The diagnosis of C. difficile–associated colitis is made by the identification of C. difficile toxin in stool.

TREATMENT The treatment of choice for clostridial infection is penicillin G, 20 million units a day in adults. In cases of penicillin sensitivity or allergy, other antibiotics should be considered, but all should be tested for in vitro efficacy because of the occasional isolation of resistant strains. Chloramphenicol, 4 g/d, usually is an effective alternative. Clostridia are frequently, but not universally, susceptible in vitro to cefoxitin, carbenicillin, clindamycin, metronidazole, doxycycline, minocycline, tetracycline, third-generation cephalosporins, and vancomycin. For severe clostridial infections, sensitivity testing should be done before using an antimicrobial with unpredictable susceptibility. Simple contamination of a wound with clostridia should not be treated with antibiotics. Localized skin and soft tissue infection can be managed by debridement rather than with systemic antibiotics. Drugs are required when the process extends into adjacent tissue, or when fever and systemic signs of sepsis are present. Surgery is an important mainstay of therapy in clostridial myonecrosis or gas gangrene. Amputation may be required for rapidly spreading infection involving a limb. Hysterectomy is required for uterine myonecrosis. Repeated surgical debridement of all involved muscle is necessary for abdominal wall myonecrosis where ongoing myonecrosis usually occurs despite initial aggressive surgery and antibiotics.

Suppurative infections should be treated with antibiotics. Frequently, broad-spectrum antibiotics must be used because of mixed flora in these infections. Aminoglycosides can be used for the aerobic gram-negative bacteria in mixed infections.

The use of a polyvalent gas gangrene antitoxin is still recommended by some authorities. At present, the antitoxin is not produced in the United States, and most centers have discontinued its use in management of patients with suspected gas gangrene or clostridial postabortion sepsis because of questionable efficacy and the substantial risk of hypersensitivity to horse serum.

The use of hyperbaric oxygen in the treatment of gas gangrene is also controversial. Studies in humans are not well designed to answer questions on efficacy, but several knowledgeable authors believe that hyperbaric oxygen therapy has contributed to dramatic clinical improvement. It may, however, be associated with untoward effects due to oxygen toxicity and high atmospheric pressure. Some centers without hyperbaric chambers have reported acceptable mortality rates, indicating that expert surgical and medical management and control of complications are probably the most important factors in treating gas gangrene.

Treatment of C. difficile enterocolitis The treatment of C. difficile–associated colitis requires discontinuation of the offending antimicrobial agent. In some patients, symptoms will resolve over a period of 2 weeks. However, specific therapy shortens the duration of symptoms. The most widely used agent in the treatment of antibiotic-associated diarrhea ascribed to C. difficile is oral vancomycin. Most strains of C. difficile are susceptible to achievable concentrations of oral vancomycin. This antibiotic is poorly absorbed after oral administration and high levels appear in the stool. Dosing should begin with 125 mg orally four times a day for 7 to 10 days, but the dose may be increased to 500 mg orally four times a day. A randomized trial comparing vancomycin with metronidazole demonstrated equal efficacy between the two regimens. The dose of metronidazole used was 250 mg four times a day, although 500 mg three times a day should be equally effective. Relapse rates were 8 to 9 percent for both regimens. Because metronidazole is considerably less costly than vancomycin, initial treatment should begin with this agent. If diarrhea persists, therapy should be changed to vancomycin. In patients with refractory symptoms and fever unresponsive to either regimen, the addition of rifampin to vancomycin has helped in some cases. Since resistance can develop to rifampin, it should not be used alone. A number of patients who respond to initial therapy present with relapse of symptoms and a repeat positive toxin assay. A number of options are available. Some patients have been shown to acquire a different strain of C. difficile despite the appearance of relapsing disease. These patients respond to a second trial of the same agent used to treat the first episode. Alternatively, patients who receive vancomycin and relapse can be treated with metronidazole, and vice versa. Some authors report success with tapering regimens of vancomycin given daily or every other day for 2 weeks to avoid relapse. The resin cholestyramine binds the cytotoxin of C. difficile and has been used with some success to treat severe cases. Since cholestyramine also binds vancomycin, the two agents should not be used in combination. Efforts to repopulate the normal colonic flora also have been tried in relapsing disease. Ingestion of capsules of the yeast Saccharomyces boulardii showed some promise in one trial.

REFERENCES

BARTLETT JG: Antibiotic-associated diarrhea. Clin Infect Dis 15:573, 1992
———: Gas gangrene (other clostridium-associated diseases), in Principles and Practice of Infectious Diseases, 3d ed, GL Mandell et al (eds). New York, Churchill Livingstone, 1990
——— et al: Antibiotic-associated pseudomembranous colitis due to toxin-producing clostridia. N Engl J Med 298:531, 1978
BORNSTEIN DL: Clostridial myonecrosis, in Medical Microbiology and Infectious Diseases, A Braude (ed). Philadelphia, Saunders, 1981, chap 239
BUGGY BP et al: Therapy of relapsing Clostridium difficile–associated diarrhea and colitis with the combination of vancomycin and rifampin. J Clin Gastroenterol 9:155, 1987
FINEGOLD SM: Anaerobic Bacteria in Human Disease. New York, Academic, 1977
———: Anaerobic infections and Clostridium difficile colitis emerging during antibacterial therapy. Scand J Infect Dis (Suppl)49:160, 1986
GORBACH SL, THADEPALLI H: Isolation of Clostridium in human infections: Evaluation of 114 cases. J Infect Dis 131:S81, 1975
JENDRZEJEWSKI JW et al: Nontraumatic clostridial myonecrosis. Am J Med 65:542, 1978
JOHNSON S et al: Enteritis necroticans among Khmer children at an evacuation site in Thailand. Lancet 2:496, 1987
KORANSKY JR et al: Clostridium septicum bacteremia. Am J Med 66:63, 1979
PETERSON LR et al: Detection of Clostridium difficile toxin A (enterotoxin) and B (cytotoxin) in clinical specimens. Am J Clin Pathol 86:208, 1986
PRITCHARD JA, WHALLEY PJ: Abortion complicated by Clostridium perfringens infection. Am J Gynecol 111:484, 1971
SMITH LDS: Virulence factors of Clostridium perfringens. Rev Infect Dis 1:254, 1979
TEASLEY DG et al: Prospective, randomized trial of metronidazole versus vancomycin for Clostridium difficile–associated diarrhea and colitis. Lancet 2:1043, 1983

section 6 Diseases caused by gram-negative bacteria

109 MENINGOCOCCAL INFECTIONS

J. McLEOD GRIFFISS

DEFINITION *Neisseria meningitidis* is an ordinary commensal of the human oropharynx that can cause a variety of diseases, most notably bacteremia and meningitis. Its pathogenic potential can be expressed as epidemic disease or as sporadic cases and focal outbreaks.

ETIOLOGY Meningococci are gram-negative single cocci or diplococci with flattened adjacent sides. They grow well on media containing blood at temperatures between 35 and 37°C in a moist atmosphere reduced in oxygen and containing 5 to 10 percent CO_2. The organism is recovered readily when fresh specimens are inoculated on warm chocolate agar and incubated 18 to 24 h in a candle jar or other apparatus that provides a suitable environment.

Neisseria make cytochrome oxidase, which is responsible for the positive "oxidase" test; species are differentiated by their ability to use simple and compound sugars as sources of energy. Typically, meningococci use both glucose and maltose. Meningococci differ from other *Neisseria* in that they are surrounded by a polysaccharide "capsule."

Meningococci are divided into serologic groups on the basis of antigenic differences among their capsular polysaccharides. Groups A, B, C, W, and Y cause most serious disease; other groups frequently colonize the oropharynx but only very rarely disseminate. The serogroups are further divided into serotypes and subtypes based on independent antigenic differences among outer membrane protein and glycolipid constituents.

EPIDEMIOLOGY The natural habitat of meningococci is the human throat. Transmission from person to person is through inhalation of droplets of infected oropharyngeal secretions. Colonization only rarely proceeds to disease, because specific antibodies and complement lyse the organisms as they enter the bloodstream and thereby provide an effective barrier to dissemination. The incidence of disseminated infection varies cyclically, with peaks of increased frequency occurring every 10 to 15 years and lasting 4 to 6 years. Each cycle spreads slowly and is called a *hyperendemic wave* to distinguish it from the truly endemic disease that occurs between waves. Hyperendemic waves are often punctuated by focal outbreaks. Widespread epidemics have been rare in developed areas of the world since the end of World War II; hyperendemic waves continue to occur. The between-waves endemic incidence in temperate climates is a fairly constant 1 reported case per 100,000 population per year. The prevalence of meningococcal infection is also subject to seasonal influences; the lowest attack rate occurs in midsummer and the highest in winter and early spring.

Epidemic disease receives the greatest public attention. An epidemic begins as a focal outbreak in a demographically discrete population in which a strain of a single serotype, the *epidemic strain*, emerges from among the endemic strains. In less developed areas the outbreak quickly spreads, develops high attack rates, and involves large segments of the community. It remains either multicentric or evolves in the same pattern as a hyperendemic wave. Each focal outbreak in multicentric epidemics lasts 1 to 3 years, while the epidemic as a whole may last 5 or more years. In developed areas foci usually involve economically deprived segments of the population and do not spread or develop into generalized epidemics.

Group A strains caused most epidemics in the United States in the first half of this century; since World War II, groups B and C meningococci have caused outbreaks in both military and civilian populations. Hyperendemic waves are caused by group B, C, or W organisms that share a limited set of serotypes. Group A strains do not share serotypes with other groups and do not cause hyperendemic waves. Group W strains have been associated with endemic and hyperendemic disease only. Group Y organisms only cause sporadic disease in older children and teenagers. Endemic disease predominantly is caused by group B organisms of diverse serotypes.

The attack rate of endemic meningococcal disease is highest for children between 6 and 36 months of age. The age distribution of epidemic cases is always shifted to proportionately older individuals, and those of any age may be involved. The attack rate in household contacts of sporadic cases is up to 1000 times the overall endemic rate and may be as much as 15,000 times that of the general population in epidemic periods.

Carriers Between epidemics, 2 to 30 percent of individuals, depending on age, carry meningococci on their throats. When sporadic disease occurs, the carrier rate in close contacts may rise to 40 percent, and in closed populations or during epidemics, it may approach 100 percent. However, the prevalence of meningococcal disease cannot be attributed to the prevailing carrier rate. Only a small proportion of the meningococci carried on the throats of those who share a patient's environment are of the same clonotype as the patient's, and individual levels of immunity to it will vary. Case-to-case transmission of infection is rare; carriers, not patients, are the foci from which disease is spread. Although some individuals harbor meningococci for years, oropharyngeal infection is usually transient, and in 75 percent of carriers the organism disappears within a few weeks to a few months.

Immunity The occurrence of clinical disease is most dependent on the immunologic status of the host. Natural immunity is usually type-specific and develops in most individuals within the first two decades of life. Natural immunization may result from pharyngeal colonization during the first few years of life by a closely related bacterium, *Neisseria lactamica*. *N. lactamica* strains are genetically diverse but many share important outer-membrane protein and lipooligosaccharide antigens with virulent strains of *N. meningitidis*. They are not encapsulated and therefore do not survive in the bloodstream to cause disseminated disease. *N. lactamica* colonizes the throat earlier in life than does *N. meningitidis;* colonized infants develop bactericidal antibodies that initiate complement-mediated lysis of a broad range of potentially pathogenic meningococci.

Colonization with *N. meningitidis* gradually replaces that with *N. lactamica* as the child grows older, and *N. lactamica* carriage is only rarely encountered in teenagers, in whom meningococcal carrier rates of 15 to 25 percent are the rule, regardless of season. Meningococcal carriage induces antibodies to the infecting strain as well as to other strains, thereby reinforcing and broadening naturally acquired immunity. Many enteric bacteria make capsules that are chemically similar to those of meningococci. Asymptomatic colonization with them can induce group-specific antibody. Second episodes of meningococcal disease are encountered. Deficiency of properdin or one of the terminal complement components, C5, C6, C7, C8, or C9, is a risk factor for repeated episodes of bacteremia with pathogenic *Neisseria* and should always be sought in patients with second episodes.

PATHOGENESIS Meningococcal infection begins in the oropharynx. In most instances, this infection is subclinical, but occasionally mild symptoms develop. Dissemination from the pharynx is via the bloodstream and generally is followed by clinical manifestations. Purulent meningitis, the most common manifestation, may predominate, or it may be associated with signs and symptoms of meningococcemia. Rarely, extensive inflammation may cause an acute diffuse encephalitis.

There is a correlation between susceptibility to meningococcal disease and the absence of complement-mediated bactericidal activity in serum. The pathogenetic mechanisms that account for the different epidemiologic forms of meningococcal disease all interfere with the generation of bactericidal activity by the membrane attack complex of complement (C5–9) (see Chap. 277). Hypogammaglobulinemia, deficiencies of complement components, and interference by the organism's capsular polysaccharides with the effective deposition of the attack complex into its outer membrane account for endemic disease. Primary isolated IgM deficiency is a rare cause of susceptibility that is disproportionately reported. Deficiencies of complement components are seen more frequently in patients than in the general population. They may be either primary or secondary and should always be sought in patients infected with the less common W, X, Y, Z, and 29E serogroups or in those with recurrent disseminated meningococcal or gonococcal infections. Inheritance of properdin deficiency and ineffective alternative pathway complement activity is sex-linked. Males in these pedigrees are at extremely high risk of fulminant meningococcal disease. Several systemic diseases, notably systemic lupus erythematosus and membranoproliferative glomerulonephritis, can result in secondary deficiencies of complement components and sporadic meningococcal disease. People with functional asplenia are also at increased risk of sporadic meningococcal disease, although pneumococcal infection is a more common complication.

The generation of hyperendemic waves remains incompletely understood. An "out-of-phase" response to fluctuations in antibody levels in the population is a possible mechanism. Focal outbreaks during hyperendemic waves can be correlated with the presence of elevated levels of circulating strain-specific IgA which blocks initiation of complement-mediated lysis by IgM or IgG, but the precise contribution of IgA-mediated susceptibility to hyperendemic waves remains unclear. When a sufficiently large part of the population has developed blocking serum IgA, conditions are established for an epidemic to occur. The environmental events that cause IgA levels to be elevated within the epidemic focus are not known with certainty, but epidemic disease has been correlated with prevalent enteric colonization with cross-reacting organisms. The extent of induction of blocking IgA in the epidemic focus may explain the extent and intensity of the epidemic as well as the failure of focal outbreaks to develop into generalized ones. Asplenia and coincidental diseases that interfere with the normal hepatic clearance of IgA, such as alcoholism, biliary tract disease, hemoglobinopathies, and hemosiderosis, increase susceptibility within the epidemic focus.

The meningococcal outer membrane contains lipooligosaccharides (LOS) that are chemically and biologically similar to the lipopolysaccharide endotoxins of enteric bacilli. They induce tumor necrosis factor (TNF-α) and interleukins 1 (IL-1) and 6 (IL-6), which seem to be responsible for the hypotension and vascular collapse observed in fulminant meningococcemia, the purpura and visceral hemorrhages associated with meningococcal bacteremia, and the influx of leukocytes into the cerebrospinal fluid during meningitis. Release of cytokines is associated with a fatal outcome (see Chap. 83). The presence of LOS sialic acid and release of redundant outer-membrane blebs into the circulation have been correlated with "virulence" and a poor prognosis, respectively.

CLINICAL MANIFESTATIONS Of patients with meningococcal disease, 90 to 95 percent have meningococcemia and/or meningitis.

Meningococcemia Thirty to fifty percent of patients who develop overt disease have meningococcemia without meningitis. The onset of clinical illness may be abrupt, but patients usually have nonspecific prodromal symptoms of cough, headache, and sore throat followed by the sudden development of spiking fever, chills, arthralgias, and myalgias. Patients usually appear acutely ill with an inordinate degree of prostration. In addition to high fever, tachycardia, and tachypnea, mild hypotension may be present. However, clinical shock does not occur unless fulminant meningococcemia supervenes. In the course of meningococcal bacteremia, about three-fourths of the patients develop a characteristic petechial rash. Lesions are frequently sparse, and the axillae, flanks, wrists, and ankles are most commonly involved. Often petechiae are located in the center of lighter-colored macules, and they may become nodular as the disease progresses. The diagnosis of meningococcemia occasionally can be established by demonstrating gram-negative diplococci in scrapings from these nodular lesions. In severe cases, purpuric spots or large ecchymoses develop, and a widespread petechial or purpuric eruption suggests fulminating disease. However, the absence of rash does not necessarily indicate that the illness will be mild. The levels of circulating endotoxin, or of the cytokines it induces, are sensitive markers for the development of fulminant disease and a poor prognosis. Patients with terminal complement-component deficiencies have a more favorable prognosis; those with properdin deficiency usually do not survive.

Fulminant meningococcemia, or the Waterhouse-Friderichsen syndrome, is meningococcemia associated with vasomotor collapse and shock. It occurs in the 10 to 20 percent of patients in whom high levels of endotoxin circulate. The onset is abrupt, and profound prostration frequently occurs within a few hours. Petechiae and purpuric lesions enlarge rapidly, and hemorrhage into the skin may be extensive. Early in the preshock stage, there is generalized vasoconstriction; patients are alert and pale, with circumoral cyanosis and cold extremities. In the early shock stage, however, the cardiac output decreases, and the blood pressure falls; mentation decreases, and coma may develop. Despite appropriate therapy, 40 to 60 percent of patients die from cardiac and/or respiratory failure. Patients who recover may have extensive sloughing of skin lesions or loss of digits because of gangrene.

Occult meningococcemia is an uncommon form of meningococcal infection that affects children between the ages of 3 and 24 months. It is characterized by fever and bacteremia without an obvious source. Infection usually resolves without treatment but may lead to the development of meningitis or other metastatic infection.

Chronic meningococcemia is a very rare form of meningococcal infection that may be associated with terminal complement component deficiencies, lasts for weeks or months, and is characterized by fever, rash, and arthritis or arthralgia. Typically, the fever is intermittent, and during afebrile periods, which may last several days, patients appear remarkably well. The usual maculopapular or polymorphous rash waxes and wanes with the fever. Petechial and nodular lesions are occasionally seen. Joint involvement is present in two-thirds of the patients, and splenomegaly is detected in about 20 percent. If treatment is delayed, meningitis, carditis, or nephritis may occur.

Meningitis Meningitis is a common form of meningococcal disease that occurs primarily in children from 6 months to 10 years of age. Fever, vomiting, headache, and confusion or lethargy are the most common symptoms; in about one-fourth of patients, symptoms begin abruptly and rapidly increase in severity. The more typical patient, however, has symptoms of an upper respiratory tract infection followed by an illness that progresses over several days. Twenty to forty percent of patients have meningitis without clinical evidence of meningococcemia, and the diagnosis depends on bacteriologic examination of the cerebrospinal fluid. However, when meningitis occurs in association with a petechial or purpuric rash, a presumptive diagnosis of meningococcal disease is warranted because this pattern of illness is seen only rarely in other infections.

Rarer manifestations The meningococcus may cause purulent conjunctivitis or sinusitis. Primary pneumonia occurs rarely, but secondary pneumonia not infrequently follows viral respiratory infections, particularly influenza. Bacterial endocarditis, primary pericarditis, arthritis, and osteomyelitis also have been reported. Meningococci also can produce genital infections clinically indistinguishable from gonococcal disease, including urethritis and endometritis.

LABORATORY FINDINGS Aside from bacteriologic data, laboratory studies are of little value in establishing a specific diagnosis of meningococcal infection. Polymorphonuclear leukocyte counts usually are elevated but may be normal or low in meningococcemia; a left shift usually is present. Patients with hemorrhagic manifestations may have low platelet counts and decreased levels of circulating clotting factors as a result of disseminated intravascular coagulation (see Chap. 57). In meningitis, the cerebrospinal fluid (CSF) pressure is increased; the fluid usually contains from 1000 to 40,000 polymorphonuclear leukocytes per microliter; the protein content is increased, and the concentration of glucose is low (see Chap. 374).

Meningococci usually can be recovered from cultures of blood or spinal fluid and, on occasion, of material aspirated from skin lesions or joints. In addition, gram-negative diplococci may be seen in stains of nodular petechiae or the buffy coat of blood from patients with meningococcemia. In meningococcal meningitis, a smear of the spinal fluid is diagnostic in about half the patients but often shows only a few intracellular bacteria, which are located with difficulty, particularly early in the course of the infection, when organisms may be present in the absence of CSF abnormalities. The infecting organisms shed their capsular polysaccharide, which usually can be detected in CSF, joint fluid, serum, or urine with use of highly specific antibodies in counterimmunoelectrophoresis (CIE) or latex agglutination (LA) assays. The sensitivity of these assays is dependent on the antibodies used and is least for group B; LA is somewhat more sensitive and easier to perform. In general, the immunoassays are more sensitive than culture alone and in combination with Gram's stain will provide a diagnosis in over 98 percent of cases. They are particularly helpful early in infection and when the patient has been treated with antibiotics, causing negative cultures.

COMPLICATIONS Herpes labialis occurs in 5 to 20 percent of patients with meningococcal disease. Other complications, which result from neurologic damage or secondary foci of infection, are uncommon following appropriate treatment and are often transient. Seizures or deafness occur in 10 to 20 percent of patients during the acute stages of meningitis, but postmeningitic epilepsy is rare, and the frequency of permanent nerve damage is probably less than 5 percent. A number of patients complain of recurrent headache, emotional lability, insomnia, backache, memory loss, and difficulty in concentrating for months after an episode of meningitis. These symptoms usually disappear a year or two after the infection.

Septic arthritis is a not uncommon complication of meningococcemia that may accompany meningitis or occur as the only metastatic manifestation. The joint fluid usually contains many granulocytes (see Chap. 91), but meningococci are recovered infrequently. It can be diagnosed by Gram's stain, CIE, or LA or by recovery of the organism on culture. It is treated in the same way as meningitis; recovery without sequelae is to be expected.

Immune-complex arthritis occurs in about 10 percent of patients during convalescence. As a rule, multiple joints are involved, primarily the larger ones. Inflammation appears between days 7 and 15 of treatment when newly produced antibodies form insoluble complexes with the infecting organism's capsular polysaccharide. No specific therapy is indicated; permanent joint changes are rare.

Other pyogenic complications have become extremely uncommon since antibiotics have been used routinely. Bacterial endocarditis is quite rare, but a high proportion of patients who die of meningococcal infection have myocarditis. A pericardial friction rub or electrocardiographic changes of pericarditis are seen in about 5 percent of patients; rarely, purulent pericarditis may develop.

DIAGNOSIS The diagnosis of meningococcal disease depends on recovering *N. meningitidis* or detecting antigens in blood, spinal fluid, joint fluid, urine, or petechial scrapings from patients with a typical clinical picture. Capsular polysaccharides of serogroups A, B, C, Y, and W can be detected in fluids by LA or CIE. Recovery of meningococci from the pharynx does not establish the diagnosis of meningococcal disease; throat cultures are not indicated.

Few diseases need to be considered seriously in the differential diagnosis of meningococcal disease. If meningococcal meningitis is not accompanied by rash or other manifestations of bacteremia, it is indistinguishable from meningitis caused by other common pathogens (see Chap. 374). Occasionally, the common viral exanthems, *Mycoplasma* infection, Rocky Mountain spotted fever (see Chap. 138), and vascular purpuras (see Chaps. 53 and 291) may be confused with meningococcemia.

TREATMENT In the absence of fulminant meningococcemia, the treatment of meningococcal disease is not difficult, and the mortality rate should not exceed 5 percent. Therapy should be instituted as early as possible. Penicillin G remains the drug of choice, although low-level penicillin resistance has been reported in Europe, and should be administered intravenously. The usual dosage for treatment of meningitis in adults with normal renal function is 12 to 24 million units per day (2 to 4 million units intravenously every 4 h), and in the pediatric age group, 200,000 to 300,000 units per kilogram per day, intravenously every 4 h in divided doses. When treatment is continued for a minimum of 7 days, or 4 to 5 days after the patient becomes afebrile, relapse is extremely rare. Chloramphenicol is just as effective as penicillin and may be the drug of choice in less-developed countries. It should be used when a patient is allergic to penicillin in a dosage of 75 to 100 mg/kg per day or, in adults, 2.0 to 4.0 g/d in divided doses every 6 h given intravenously until the patient is able to take oral medication. Cefotaxime, ceftriaxone, and cefuroxime (see Chaps. 100 and 374), are also effective and are often used to initiate therapy when the etiology of meningitis is uncertain. A significant proportion of meningococci are resistant to sulfonamides, so these should not be used routinely unless the infecting organism is shown to be susceptible. Sulfadiazine (2 to 3 g initially followed by 1 g every 6 h thereafter given intravenously until the patient can take oral medication) or trimethoprim-sulfamethoxazole (160/800 mg intravenously every 6 h) is effective treatment for susceptible strains. The dosages must be reduced in renal failure and in children, depending on age (see Chap. 100).

Patients with meningococcal infections require supportive treatment as well as antimicrobial therapy. Maintenance of fluid and electrolyte balance and prevention of respiratory complications in comatose patients are of primary concern. When shock occurs, visceral perfusion must be improved. Vasoactive drugs should be employed according to the pathophysiologic derangement (see Chaps. 34 and 83). When disseminated intravascular coagulation is recognized, treatment with heparin, whole blood, or fibrinogen can be tried, but these are not certain to be effective.

PROGNOSIS Before the introduction of antibiotics, meningococcal meningitis and meningococcemia were almost invariably fatal. With prompt and appropriate chemotherapy, the mortality rate of meningitis without fulminant meningococcemia has dropped to less than 10 percent in the United States, and neurologic sequelae are rare. The mortality of fulminant infection remains high primarily because patients are often in irreversible shock when treatment is instituted. Most deaths occur within 24 to 48 h of admission, and the capacity of the meningococcus to kill a previously healthy individual within a few hours remains one of the most awesome characteristics of this disease.

PREVENTION The capsular polysaccharides from organisms of serogroups A, C, Y, and W induce group-specific bactericidal antibody responses after subcutaneous injection. A tetravalent vaccine containing these antigens is available for use to prevent or control outbreaks. Routine immunization of recruits has eliminated nearly all disease among military personnel, but in the United States, immunization is recommended routinely only for travelers to areas where epidemic disease is occurring and for individuals with complement deficiencies or splenic dysfunction. An effective group B vaccine has not been developed. Chemoprophylaxis should be administered to intimate household, day-care center, and nursery school contacts of sporadic cases. If the organism isolated from the patient is sensitive to sulfonamides, 2 days of prophylaxis with one of these drugs is recommended. When sensitivities are not known or the organism is resistant to sulfonamides, rifampin in a dosage of 10 mg/kg, up to 600 mg, every 12 h for 2 days for children and adults and 5 mg/kg every 12 h for infants can be expected to eradicate the carrier state temporarily and minimize spread of meningococci. Resistance to rifampin has been reported, however. Vaccination is over 99 percent effective in preventing secondary cases (as compared with approximately 89 percent effectiveness for rifampin chemoprophylaxis), and vaccination of household or other intimate contacts should be encouraged.

REFERENCES

COUNTS GW et al: Group A meningococcal disease in the U.S. Pacific Northwest: Epidemiology, clinical features, and effect of a vaccination control program. Rev Infect Dis 6:640, 1984

DENSEN P et al: Familial properdin deficiency and fatal meningococcemia: Correction of the bactericidal defect by vaccination. N Engl J Med 316:922, 1987

FIJEN CA et al: Complement deficiencies in patients over ten years old with meningococcal disease due to uncommon serogroups. Lancet 2:585, 1989

GRIFFISS J McL: Epidemic meningococcal disease: Synthesis of a hypothetical immunoepidemiologic model. Rev Infect Dis 4:159, 1982

JARVIS GA et al: Sialic acid of group B Neisseria meningitidis regulates alternative complement pathway activation. Infect Immun 55:174, 1987

KIM JJ et al: Neisseria lactamica and Neisseria meningitidis share lipooligosaccharide epitopes but lack common capsular and class 1, 2, and 3 protein epitopes. Infect Immun 57:602, 1989

MOORE PS et al: Intercontinental spread of an epidemic group A Neisseria meningitidis strain. Lancet 2:260, 1989

WAAGE A et al: The complex pattern of cytokines in serum from patients with meningococcal septic shock: Association between interleukin 6, interleukin 1, and fatal outcome. J Exp Med 169:333, 1989

WOLF RE, BIRBARA CA: Meningococcal infections at an army training center. Am J Med 44:243, 1968

110   GONOCOCCAL INFECTIONS

KING K. HOLMES / STEPHEN A. MORSE

DEFINITION Gonorrhea, an infection of columnar and transitional epithelium caused by *Neisseria gonorrhoeae*, is the most common reportable communicable disease in the United States. Anatomic sites which can be infected directly by the gonococcus include the urethra, rectum, conjunctivas, pharynx, and endocervix. Local complications include endometritis, salpingitis, peritonitis, and bartholinitis in the female and periurethral abscess and epididymitis in the male. Systemic manifestations of gonococcemia include arthritis, dermatitis, endocarditis, and meningitis as well as myoperi-carditis and hepatitis.

ETIOLOGY *Neisseria gonorrhoeae* is a gram-negative coccus usually found in pairs with flattened adjacent sides. It forms oxidase-positive colonies and is differentiated from other *Neisseria* by its ability to utilize glucose but not maltose, sucrose, or lactose; by nucleic acid probes; and by specific immunologic reactions.

Organisms present in colonies examined within 20 h of inoculation from clinical specimens are covered by fimbriae (pili). Pili mediate attachment to various epithelial cells and interfere with neutrophil phagocytosis. Each pilus is composed of repeating peptide subunits (pilin) which have a molecular weight of about 20,000. The pilin subunits consist of conserved and variable regions. Pili undergo both *antigenic* and *phase variation*. Chromosomal rearrangements, leading to expression of any one of a large number of incomplete (silent) pilin genes, lead to antigenic variation in pili. If the rearrangement involves a defective pilin gene, piliated gonococci (pil⁺) produce nonpiliated variants (pil⁻), a process known as *phase variation*. Piliated organisms cause infection and urethritis after inoculation into the urethras of male volunteers, whereas nonpiliated organisms do not. Antigenic variation of pilin may allow gonococci to attach to different types of epithelial surfaces and to evade the host's antibody response to pilin. Phase variation from pil⁺ to pil⁻ may permit detachment and facilitate spread.

The trilaminar outer membrane of the gonococcus contains several classes of proteins, including proteins I, II, and III, and lipopolysaccharide (Fig. 110-1). Like pili, protein II (now referred to as *opacity-associated outer membrane proteins*, or *OPAs*) also is thought to function as a ligand, mediating the attachment of gonococcus to various types of human cells. An individual gonococcus can possess about a dozen OPA genes and can express zero to three or more OPAs at a time. Gonococci possessing certain OPAs adhere to and are phagocytosed by human neutrophils in the absence of serum. Certain OPAs may be responsible for the clumping of gonococci that is so evident on Gram-stained smears of urethral exudate.

Opaque colonies contain organisms that express OPAs and predominate in isolates from the male urethra and in cervical isolates obtained from women in midcycle. Transparent colonies often lack OPAs and predominate in isolates from women during menses and in isolates from blood, synovial fluid, or fallopian tubes.

Protein I is quantitatively the major outer membrane protein; it exhibits intrastrain differences in molecular mass that vary between 34,600 and 37,700 Da. Protein I molecules associate in a trimeric structure, forming anion-selective transmembrane channels (porins) that permit the exchange of hydrophilic molecules through the outer membrane. Protein I also interacts with other outer membrane components, such as protein III and lipopolysaccharide (LPS), to form complex outer membrane structures. Protein I molecules have been shown to move rapidly from gonococcal outer membranes to the more fluid cytoplasmic membrane of human cells, where they form pores. This process may initiate endocytosis of the gonococcus, the first step in gonococcal invasion of the epithelium.

The LPS of the gonococcus contains lipid A and an oligosaccharide. Features that distinguish gonococcal LPS from enteric LPS are the highly branched oligosaccharide structure and the absence of repeating O-antigen subunits. For these reasons, gonococcal LPS is often referred to as *lipooligosaccharide (LOS)*. Gonococci produce several discrete LOS components. The type of LOS produced can be altered by a mechanism that is not well understood. Host-derived cytidine monophospho-*N*-acetylneuraminic acid can be used by gonococci to sialylate the oligosaccharide component of one of its LOSs. This sialylation results in the conversion of a serum-sensitive organism into one that is serum-resistant and markedly reduces nonopsonic interactions of OPA-expressing gonococci with human neutrophils. Gonococci observed in urethral exudate are sialylated, thereby indicating that sialylation occurs in vivo. Recent structural and immunochemical analyses of gonococcal LOS revealed that the antigenicity and immunogenicity of the LOS is complex due in part to the structural similarity of the oligosaccharide to host glycosphingo-lipids. No capsular polysaccharide has been isolated, but high-molecular-weight surface polyphosphates have been demonstrated that may have functions similar to those of capsular polysaccharides in other organisms.

Gonococcal typing Gonococcal strains can be typed on the basis of nutritional requirements (auxotyping) or antigenic differences of protein I (serotyping). Unlike pili and protein II, the protein I expressed by any single strain of gonococcus is antigenically stable, although there is considerable antigenic heterogeneity of protein I between strains. There are two structurally related forms of protein I, known as IA and IB, and individual strains contain either but not both. Protein IA and IB genes are alleles of the same gene. Monoclonal antibodies against different epitopes of protein IA and protein IB can be used to classify gonococci into a large number of serovariants, known as serovars IA1 to IA24 and IB1 to IB32.

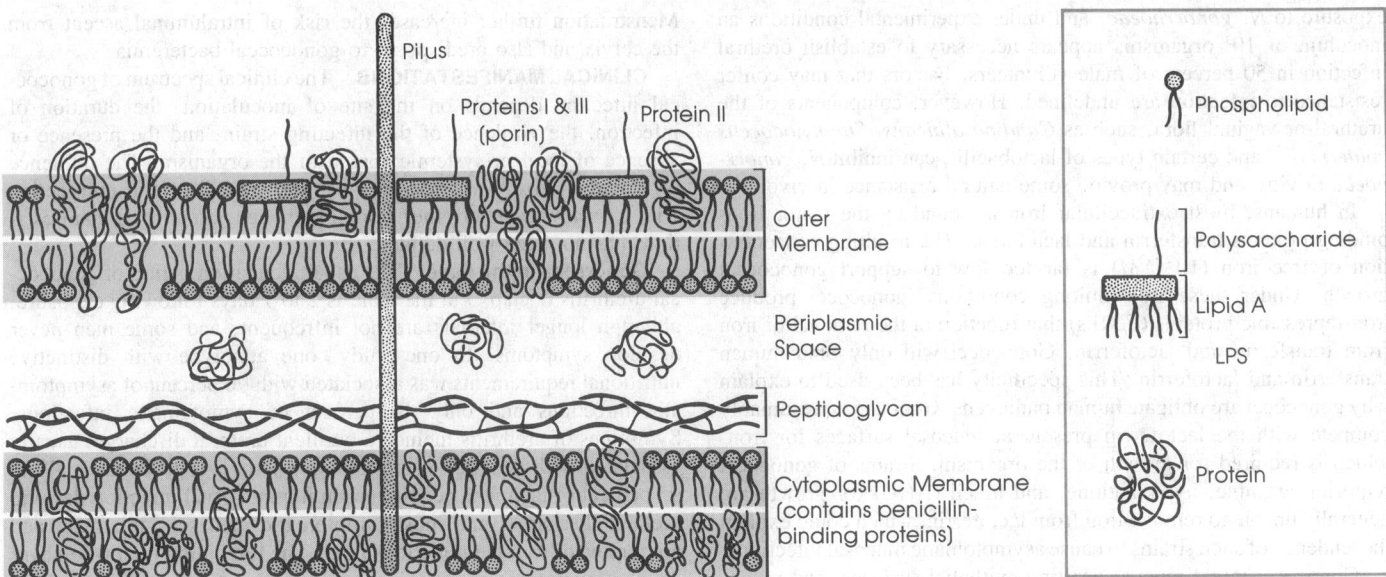

FIGURE 110-1 Diagram of the envelope of *N. gonorrhoeae*, showing structures thought to influence pathogenesis, antimicrobial susceptibility, and antigenicity.

EPIDEMIOLOGY The only natural hosts for *N. gonorrhoeae* are humans. In the United States, the annual age-specific incidence rates tripled from 1963 to 1975, when over 1 million cases were reported and an equal number probably went unreported. During this period of epidemic gonorrhea, the incidence increased fastest in young white females. The incidence of gonorrhea has decreased from a peak of 473 cases per 100,000 in 1975 to about 277 per 100,000 in 1990.

Gonorrhea incidence and prevalence rates are known to be related to age, sex, sex preference, race, socioeconomic status, marital status, urban residence, and level of education—risk factors which influence sexual behavior, illness behavior, and accessibility of health care. Among sexually active individuals, the highest rates occur in teenagers, in nonwhites, in the poor and poorly educated, in large cities, and in unmarried persons—particularly those who live alone. Such individuals comprise a "core group" of "efficient transmitters" who play a disproportionate role in the spread of gonorrhea. Since 1985, the incidence of gonorrhea has continued to fall among white and Hispanic men and women but has leveled off among black men and women. There is some evidence that the spread of gonorrhea, like that of syphilis and chancroid, is associated with the "crack" cocaine epidemic and with exchange of sex by women for illegal drugs such as cocaine. The incidence of gonorrhea is highest in men, while the prevalence is highest in women. The prevalence rate remains so high among women in the United States that routine endocervical cultures have been advocated for gonorrhea case detection in asymptomatic women age 30 or under who are considered to be at high risk because of sexual behavior or demographic factors cited above. However, greater reliance should be placed on partner notification (contact tracing), which is far more efficient for control of gonorrhea, than on routine endocervical culturing, which is expensive and does not focus on those most likely to transmit the infection. The single most important axiom about the epidemiology of this disease is that *gonorrhea is usually spread by carriers who have no symptoms or have ignored symptoms.* Symptomatic patients, male or female, have usually been recently infected by such carriers, who must in turn be traced and treated to prevent reinfection. *Men and women with symptomatic gonorrhea should always be interviewed to identify their recent sex contacts, who should be examined and treated if infected.* The growing association of gonorrhea, syphilis, and chancroid with the exchange of sex for drugs such as "crack" cocaine presents a new and unique challenge for sexually transmitted disease (STD) control and calls for intensified and innovative control efforts.

There are interesting regional differences in the antibiotic resistance of *N. gonorrhoeae*. In 1976, penicillinase-producing strains of *N. gonorrhoeae* (PPNG), completely resistant to penicillin and ampicillin, appeared almost simultaneously in two areas of the world: in England, where they had probably been imported from West Africa, and in the United States, where they had been imported from the Philippines. PPNG first became established and then spread in areas of the world where prostitution is exceptionally common and where access to subcurative antimicrobial therapy is unrestricted. PPNG now comprise 50 percent or more of all gonococci in many areas of Africa and Asia and have by now become well established in many regions of the United States and Europe. Plasmid-borne penicillin resistance results from the presence of a TEM-type β-lactamase gene on one of six small R factors which make up a very closely related family of plasmids. Plasmid-borne, tetracycline resistance (TRNG) resulted from introduction of the streptococcal resistance determinant *tetM* into *N. gonorrhoeae*, where it resides on a plasmid derived in part from a gonococcal conjugative plasmid. This new plasmid is self-transmissible and retains the capacity to mobilize some of the β-lactamase plasmids. TRNG are clinically resistant to tetracycline, minocycline, and doxycycline. Strains possessing both penicillin and tetracycline resistance plasmids are increasing in prevalence in some parts of the country, and one or the other type of plasmid was present in about one-fifth of gonococcal isolates in the United States by 1992. Of equal importance has been the spread of gonococci with chromosomally mediated resistance to penicillin and tetracycline. These strains are referred to as chromosomally mediated resistant *N. gonorrhoeae* (CMRNG). Auxotyping and monoclonal antibody serotyping have shown that in a midsized metropolitan city, as many as 60 to 100 different gonococcal strains are circulating, and new strains are being continuously introduced. Against this background, local outbreaks of PPNG, TRNG, or CMRNG belonging to a single auxotype-serovar class have been identified, and public health efforts have at times been successfully focused on the control of such strains.

Recent epidemiologic studies have shown interesting relationships between gonorrhea and HIV infection. Gonorrhea in female prostitutes has been associated with increased susceptibility to acquiring HIV infection; gonococcal urethritis has been associated with shedding of HIV in urethral exudate in HIV-seropositive men; and HIV infection in prostitutes has been associated with both increased risk of gonococcal reinfection and increased risk of clinical signs of salpingitis when gonococcal infection occurs.

IMMUNOLOGY AND PATHOGENESIS Epidemiologic data suggest that only about one-third of men become infected after a single exposure to *N. gonorrhoeae*, and under experimental conditions an inoculum of 10^3 organisms appears necessary to establish urethral infection in 50 percent of male volunteers. Factors that may confer resistance to infection are undefined. However, components of the urethral or vaginal flora, such as *Candida albicans, Staphylococcus epidermidis*, and certain types of lactobacilli, can inhibit *N. gonorrhoeae* in vitro and may provide some natural resistance in vivo.

In humans, most extracellular iron is bound by the major iron-binding proteins transferrin and lactoferrin. The resulting concentration of free iron ($10^{-18} M$) is far too low to support gonococcal growth. Under these iron-limiting conditions, gonococci produce iron-repressible proteins (FeRPs) that function in the removal of iron from transferrin and lactoferrin. Gonococci will only bind human transferrin and lactoferrin. This specificity has been used to explain why gonococci are obligate human pathogens. Gonococci presumably compete with the lactoferrin present at mucosal surfaces for iron, which is required for growth of the organism. Strains of gonococci requiring arginine, hypoxanthine, and uracil (AHU) for growth are generally unable to remove iron from lactoferrin, which could explain the tendency of such strains to cause asymptomatic mucosal infections.

Gonococci infect mucus-secreting epithelial surfaces, and mucus could be a physical barrier or competitive inhibitor. Attachment of gonococci to mucosal cells is mediated in part by pili and by protein II. Local antibody to pili or protein II can partially block attachment. Pili also impede phagocytosis of gonococci by neutrophils, and antibody to pili (as well as antibody to protein II) is opsonic. An enzyme produced by the pathogenic *Neisseria*, IgA1 protease, which inactivates sIgA1, may interfere with IgA-mediated antiadherence activity, resulting in increased attachment.

Following attachment to columnar or transitional epithelium, gonococci penetrate through or between cells to reach the subepithelial connective tissue. Transfer of gonococcal protein I into the host cell may initiate endocytosis by the epithelial cell. Gonococcal LOS produces mucosal damage in fallopian tube organ cultures. Recent evidence suggests that gonococcal LOS stimulates the production of tumor necrosis factor (TNF) in fallopian tube organ cultures; inhibition of TNF with specific antiserum prevents tissue damage. Peptidoglycan fragments are also toxic for fallopian tube mucosa and may contribute to the intense inflammatory reactions characteristic of gonococcal disease. Gonococci also produce several proteases, peptidases, and phospholipases which may play a role in pathogenesis. In subepithelial tissue, as well as in blood, gonococci presumably interact with serum antibody, including natural IgM antibody directed against LOS antigens, with generation of the chemotactic factor C5a and formation of the bactericidal C5b-C9 attack complex. Insertion of the attack complex into the outer membrane of serum-sensitive gonococci results in gonococcal cell lysis, making antibody to LOS (like antibody to protein I) bactericidal. Although an attack complex is also formed when serum interacts with gonococci characterized by stable serum resistance, insertion of the complex into the outer membrane of the organism has an abnormal configuration which does not result in rapid cell lysis. Furthermore, human serum also appears to contain complement-fixing IgG antibody directed against epitopes on protein III which blocks the bactericidal antibodies directed against other antigens. Protein III has extensive homology to the enterobacterial Omp A protein and the meningococcal class 4 protein. Since Enterobacteriaceae and *N. meningitidis* are both common commensal microorganisms, it is possible that the protein III–blocking antibodies result from prior exposure to cross-reacting proteins from other microbial species.

Oxygen-independent antimicrobial mechanisms contribute significantly to intraleukocytic killing of gonococci following their phagocytosis by neutrophils. Despite effective intraleukocytic killing of gonococci in in vitro assay systems, a small but reproducible number survive. Whether gonococci survive within neutrophils in vivo remains a subject of controversy.

Spread of gonococci from the cervix to the endometrium and salpinges may be enhanced in women using an intrauterine device.

Menstruation further increases the risk of intraluminal ascent from the cervix and also predisposes to gonococcal bacteremia.

CLINICAL MANIFESTATIONS The clinical spectrum of gonococcal infection depends on the site of inoculation, the duration of infection, the virulence of the infecting strain, and the presence or absence of local or systemic spread of the organism. The influence of inoculum size, variations in host susceptibility, and coinfection with *C. trachomatis* or other genital pathogens on clinical manifestations has not been well-defined.

Gonorrhea in the male The usual incubation period of gonococcal urethritis (''clap'') in the male is 2 to 7 days following exposure, although longer intervals are not infrequent, and some men never develop symptoms. In one study, one auxotype with distinctive nutritional requirements was associated with 96 percent of asymptomatic infections and only 40 percent of symptomatic infections. Symptoms of urethritis include a purulent urethral discharge, usually associated with dysuria, and meatal erythema. Approximately 90 to 95 percent of men who acquire urethral gonococcal infection develop urethral discharge, and most symptomatic men seek treatment and are removed from the infectious pool. The remaining men who never develop symptoms or who ignore their symptoms constitute about two-thirds of the infected men at any point in time, and they serve as the main source of spread of infection to women. Before antibiotic treatment became available, symptoms of urethritis persisted for an average of 8 weeks, and unilateral epididymitis occurred in 5 to 10 percent of untreated men. Epididymitis is now an uncommon complication (see below), and gonococcal prostatitis occurs rarely, if at all. Other local complications of gonococcal urethritis which are now unusual include inguinal lymphadenitis, edema of the penis due to dorsal lymphangitis or thrombophlebitis, submucous inflammatory ''soft'' infiltration of the urethral wall, periurethral abscess or fistula, unilateral inflammation or abscess of Cowper's gland (which lies between the thumb and forefinger when the forefinger is in the anal canal and the thumb is positioned anteriorly on the perineum), and, rarely, seminal vesiculitis.

In homosexual men, the frequency of gonococcal infection fell by 90 percent or more throughout the United States during the early AIDS era of the 1980s, but a disturbing resurgence of gonorrhea in young homosexual men has been seen in a few cities during the early 1990s. Gonococcal isolates from homosexual men tend to be more resistant to antimicrobials than are isolates from heterosexuals. This may be due to the fact that certain highly susceptible strains are rapidly killed by bile salts and fatty acids in feces and rarely occur in homosexual men, while gonococci possessing a gene for multidrug resistance (*mtr*) are more resistant to bile salts and fatty acids and occur with increased frequency in homosexual men. Rectal infection may be asymptomatic from the outset or may produce anorectal pain, pruritus, tenesmus, and a bloody, mucopurulent rectal discharge. Proctoscopy and appropriate laboratory studies are essential to exclude several other conditions which cause similar symptoms (see Chap. 88). These symptoms may subside without treatment, leaving a chronic asymptomatic carrier state. Pharyngeal gonococcal infection occurs in approximately 20 percent of homosexual men or heterosexual women who engage in fellatio with men who have urethral infection and in a smaller proportion of heterosexual men who engage in cunnilingus. Pharyngeal infection may produce exudative tonsillitis but frequently is asymptomatic; asymptomatic pharyngeal gonococcal infection usually clears spontaneously over several weeks, even without therapy.

Gonorrhea in the female Acute uncomplicated gonorrhea in the female often causes dysuria, increased vaginal discharge due to exudative endocervicitis, abnormal menstrual bleeding due to endometritis, and anorectal discomfort. While dysuria in young men arouses the suspicion of gonococcal urethritis, the same symptom in a young woman is often automatically attributed to ''cystitis.'' Actually, some of those without bacteriuria have gonococcal or chlamydial infection of the urethra. Young women with dysuria should have a thorough pelvic examination. Compression of the urethra through the anterior vaginal wall against the symphysis pubis may express urethral exudate which can be examined by Gram's stain and culture. Symptomatic young women with "sterile pyuria" (i.e., ≥ 10 neutrophils per $100 \times$ microscopic field in the centrifuged sediment of clean-catch midstream urine; no uropathogens isolated from the urine) should be evaluated for gonococcal and chlamydial infection. Acute symptoms of gonococcal urethritis in the female may subside spontaneously or following subcurative therapy with sulfonamides or urinary antiseptics. The proportion of women with gonorrhea who never develop symptoms is undefined.

Asymptomatic gonococcal infection in the female involves the endocervix, urethra, anal canal, and pharynx, in decreasing order of frequency. Extension of infection from the endocervix to the fallopian tubes occurs in at least 15 percent of women with gonorrhea. This tends to occur soon after acquisition of infection or during menstruation and results in acute endometritis, with abnormal menstrual bleeding and midline low abdominal pain and tenderness, followed by *acute salpingitis*, the major complication of gonorrhea. Coexisting *C. trachomatis* infection may increase the rate of pelvic inflammatory disease (PID). Extension of infection to the pelvis may produce signs of pelvic peritonitis, accompanied by nausea and vomiting, and may lead to pelvic abscess. Early antibiotic treatment, before development of adnexal masses, restores normal tubal function and fertility in nearly all cases of gonococcal salpingitis. However, if prominent adnexal swelling has occurred before treatment is begun, bilateral tubal damage occurs in 15 to 25 percent.

Spread of gonococci or chlamydiae into the upper abdomen may cause *perihepatitis* (Fitz-Hugh–Curtis syndrome), manifested by right upper quadrant or bilateral upper abdominal pain and tenderness and occasionally by a hepatic friction rub.

Acute inflammation of Bartholin's gland is usually unilateral and frequently is due to gonococcal infection. The acutely infected duct is surrounded by a red halo and exudes pus at the posterior third of the labium majus. Occlusion of the duct results in formation of a Bartholin's abscess. Chronic Bartholin cysts are rarely caused by active gonococcal infection.

There is evidence that peripartum endocervical gonococcal infection is associated with premature rupture of membranes, preterm delivery, and postpartum endometritis.

Gonorrhea in children   During childbirth, the gonococcus may infect the conjunctivas, pharynx, respiratory tract, or anal canal of the newborn. The risk of infection increases with prolonged rupture of membranes. Prevention of gonococcal ophthalmia by prophylactic use of 1% silver nitrate eyedrops or ophthalmic preparations containing erythromycin or tetracycline is a cost-effective measure in most areas of the world, including the United States. However, with the emergence of TRNG, it is not certain whether ophthalmic tetracycline prophylaxis is effective in preventing neonatal conjunctivitis caused by such strains of *N. gonorrhoeae*. Since neonates and young infants lack bactericidal IgM antibody against *N. gonorrhoeae*, they may be at increased risk for gonococcal bacteremia. During the first year of life, infection of the infant usually results from accidental contamination of the eye or vagina by an adult. Between 1 year of age and puberty, many cases of gonorrhea involve vulvovaginitis in females who have been molested, and medicolegal considerations necessitate a complete bacteriologic diagnosis and child welfare consultation. Auxotyping and serotyping of isolates from the sexual assault victim and accused assailant have been used as evidence in court.

Disseminated gonococcal infection   The incidence of disseminated gonococcal infection (DGI) varies with time and place in relation to the local incidence of infection with strains of gonococci that have a propensity to produce bacteremia. Approximately two-thirds of patients with DGI are women, and symptoms of bacteremia often begin during menses. The majority of men and women with gonococcemia do not have symptoms of urogenital, anorectal, or pharyngeal gonococcal infection.

Patients typically present either with symptoms and signs of gonococcemia or with purulent arthritis affecting one or two joints.

The onset of gonococcemia is characterized by fever, polyarthralgias, and papular, petechial, pustular, hemorrhagic, or necrotic skin lesions. Approximately 3 to 20 such lesions appear, usually on the distal extremities. Gonococci are demonstrable by immunofluorescent staining in about two-thirds of gonococcal skin lesions. The initial joint involvement is characteristically limited to tenosynovitis involving several joints asymmetrically. The wrists, fingers, knees, and ankles are most often involved. Circulating immune complexes have been demonstrated at this stage of infection in some studies. Serum complement levels are normal (except in those with complement deficiency), and the role of immune complexes, if any, is uncertain. Without treatment, the duration of gonococcemia is variable; the systemic manifestations of bacteremia may subside spontaneously within a week. Alternatively, septic arthritis ensues, often without prior symptoms of fever, polyarthralgias, or skin lesions. Pain and swelling then increase in one or, very occasionally, more joints, with accumulation of purulent synovial fluid, leading to progressive destruction of the joint if treatment is delayed.

IgM antibody to gonococcal LOS, present in normal human serum, is bactericidal for most strains of gonococci in the presence of complement. Gonococci isolated from patients with DGI have stable resistance to normal human serum. These strains usually contain outer membrane protein IA and are highly susceptible to penicillin. They often require arginine, hypoxanthine, and uracil for growth, and belong to the AHU auxotype. The decline in incidence of such strains in the United States during the past two decades has been associated with a sharp decline in incidences of DGI as well. Patients deficient in complement components C5, C6, C7, and C8 are uniquely susceptible to gonococcemia and meningococcemia because they cannot mount a serum bactericidal response to gonococci or meningococci. Although perhaps 5 percent of patients with a first episode of gonococcemia or meningococcemia are complement-deficient, the porportion is higher among those with recurrent gonococcemia or meningococcemia. Strains isolated from these patients may not be resistant to normal human serum. However, gonococci isolated from DGI patients without complement deficiency are resistant to pooled normal human serum. Isolates from patients with tenosynovitis and skin lesions are even more serum-resistant than are isolates from patients with purulent arthritis, suggesting that the two different DGI syndromes may be determined by characteristics of the causative organism.

The probability of positive blood cultures decreases after 48 h of illness, and the probability of recovery of gonococci from synovial fluid increases with increasing duration of illness. Gonococci are infrequently recovered from early effusions containing less than 20,000 leukocytes per microliter but are usually recovered from effusions containing more than 80,000 leukocytes per microliter. In the individual patient, gonococci are seldom recovered from blood and synovial fluid simultaneously.

Other common manifestations of disseminated gonococcal infection include mild myopericarditis and "toxic" hepatitis. Endocarditis and meningitis are infrequent but severe complications. Endocarditis is suggested by pathologic or changing heart murmurs, major embolic phenomena, severe myocarditis, deterioration of renal function, or an unusually large number of skin lesions.

DIFFERENTIAL DIAGNOSIS   Gonococcal infection produces several common clinical syndromes which have multiple etiologies or which mimic other conditions. In particular, the epidemiology and clinical manifestations of *Chlamydia trachomatis* infections closely resemble those of gonococcal infections. The differential diagnosis of urethritis, epididymitis, and proctitis in men; vaginitis and cervicitis in women; and acute arthritis in young adults is discussed in Chap. 88. The differential diagnosis of pelvic inflammatory disease is discussed in Chap. 89.

LABORATORY DIAGNOSIS   A presumptive diagnosis of gonorrhea may be made if intracellular gram-negative diplococci are observed in leukocytes on Gram-stained smears of urethral or endocervical exudate. A diagnosis is equivocal if only extracellular or atypical gram-negative diplococci are seen and is negative if no gram-negative diplococci are seen. When these criteria are employed by experienced microbiologists, the sensitivity and specificity of Gram's stain of the urethral exudate approach 100 percent. Presumptive diagnosis of gonorrhea cannot be made on the basis of gram-negative diplococci in pharyngeal smears because other *Neisseria* spp. are normal flora at this site. In areas where resistant gonococci are seen, culture should be performed to allow testing of isolates for antimicrobial resistance. The specificity of Gram's stain of purulent cervical exudate also is high, but the sensitivity is only about 50 percent. Selective media, i.e., Thayer-Martin (TM) medium, modified TM medium, and Martin-Lewis medium, which contain antibiotics to selectively inhibit most other organisms, are most useful for recovering the gonococcus from the urethra, endocervix, and pharynx. Rectal specimens are plated on modified TM medium or equivalent media containing trimethoprim lactate, which suppresses swarming organisms such as *Proteus* spp. The concentration of vancomycin in the selective medium should not exceed 3 μg/mL, and even this concentration may inhibit a small proportion of gonococci. After inoculation, the medium should be placed in a chamber with 70 percent humidity and an atmosphere containing 3 to 10 percent carbon dioxide to permit growth of the gonococcus. This can be accomplished in a candle jar, by generation of carbon dioxide chemically within packets that are sealed after inoculation, or within special CO_2 incubators. Inoculated media should be incubated at 35 to 37°C for 24 to 48 h, and putative gonococcal colonies should be confirmed by oxidase reaction, Gram's stain, and either sugar utilization tests, rapid enzyme tests, nucleic acid probes, or agglutination reactions using antibodies that are specific for *N. gonorrhoeae*. The last four tests are especially important for isolates from the pharynx and rectum, for cultures obtained from populations which have a low prevalence of gonorrhea, such as prenatal patients, and for isolates from victims of rape or sexual child abuse.

In men with incubating or chronic asymptomatic urethral infection without exudate or as a test of cure following treatment, a very thin swab should be inserted 2 cm into the anterior urethra and used to inoculate TM or other selective medium. Cultures of the pharynx and rectum should be obtained from homosexual men with suspected gonorrhea.

The most efficient test for gonorrhea in women is the endocervical culture, which is positive on a single examination in approximately 80 to 90 percent of those with gonorrhea. This diagnostic yield can be increased by performing a second endocervical culture and by performing cultures of the rectum, urethra, and pharynx.

Standard blood culture broth medium (tryptic soy, Columbia, brain-heart infusion) should be used in culturing blood and is also recommended for culturing synovial fluid. The broth should be vented and incubated under increased CO_2 tension. Synovial fluid also can be plated onto chocolate agar rather than a selective medium because it is not likely to be contaminated with commensal bacteria. In pus from skin lesions, *N. gonorrhoeae* is demonstrable by immunofluorescent staining, but this test is seldom performed. Techniques designed to detect gonococcal infection by testing of a single serum for antibody to *N. gonorrhoeae* have been limited by an inability to differentiate antibody due to past gonorrhea from antibody due to current infection and by false-positive tests caused by cross-reactive antibody to *N. meningitidis*. For these reasons, serologic tests for gonorrhea have had a very low predictive value and are not used in clinical practice.

Another diagnostic approach is the detection of gonococcal antigen in urethral or cervical secretion by enzyme-linked immunosorbent assay (ELISA). In men with urethritis, the Gram's stain is just as accurate, quicker, and cheaper. In women, such tests may be an acceptable alternative to culture for diagnosis of endocervical gonococcal infection in settings where culture is not feasible. However, the positive predictive value of antigen detection tests requires careful study, particularly in populations with a low prevalence of gonorrhea. Nucleic acid probes also have been used to detect gonococci in urethral and cervical specimens. However, additional evaluations are required. The medicolegal and psychosocial implications of a false-positive diagnosis of gonorrhea can be troublesome for both the physician and patient.

TREATMENT Until 1986, the preferred drugs for gonococcal infection were penicillin G, ampicillin or amoxicillin, tetracycline hydrochloride, and spectinomycin. Although long-acting forms of penicillin (such as benzathine penicillin G) are effective in syphilotherapy, they have *no place* in the treatment of gonorrhea. Penicillin V and the isoxazolyl penicillins are not recommended for the treatment of gonococcal infection. Similarly, first-generation cephalosporins are not used for gonorrhea. In 1986, the Centers for Disease Control published new guidelines for treatment of gonorrhea. These 1986 guidelines, which are presented in this chapter but modified by the authors to include newer, single-dose oral regimens which appear to be highly effective alternatives, are based on several observations: the importance of single-dose efficacy; the increasing proportion of infections due to antibiotic-resistant strains of *N. gonorrhoeae*, including PPNG, TRNG, and strains with chromosomally mediated resistance to multiple antimicrobials; the high frequency of coexisting chlamydial infections in persons with gonorrhea; the absence of a cheap, rapid test for chlamydial infection; and the severity of complications of gonococcal and chlamydial infections. The guidelines do not represent a comprehensive list of all possible treatment regimens. As is shown in Table 110-1, a regimen combining a single intramuscular 125-mg dose of ceftriaxone, together with a 7-day course of tetracycline or doxycycline, is recommended for uncomplicated urethral, endocervical, rectal, or pharyngeal gonococcal infections in heterosexual adults. This combination regimen can be expected to provide adequate therapy for gonorrhea at any site and

TABLE 110-1 Recommended treatment for gonococcal infection

Diagnosis	Treatment of choice
Uncomplicated urethral, endocervical, rectal, or pharyngeal infection	Ceftriaxone, 125 mg single IM dose *plus* Doxycycline, 100 mg PO twice daily for 7 days.
Treatment failure	True treatment failure with the above regimen has so far occurred rarely, if ever. Evaluate for reinfection, alternative diagnosis.
Alternative regimens (all given with 7 days of doxycycline)	Cefixime, 400 mg single oral dose Ofloxacin, 400 mg single oral dose Spectinomycin, 2 g single IM dose Ciprofloxacin, 500 mg single oral dose
Gonorrhea in pregnancy	Ceftriaxone, 125 mg single IM dose *plus* Erythromycin base 500 mg PO four times daily for 7 days. Equivalent dose of erythromycin stearate (500 mg) or ethylsuccinate (800 mg) can be used.
Disseminated gonococcal infection (DGI)	Hospitalization is recommended. Ceftriaxone, 1 g IM or IV every 24 h *or* Ceftizoxime, 1 g IV every 8 h *or* Cefotaxime, 1 g IV every 8 h (see text for duration of inpatient and subsequent ambulatory therapy).
Gonococcal PID	Hospitalization is recommended. See Chap. 89 for recommended therapy.
Gonococcal epididymitis	See Chap. 88.
Pediatric gonococcal infections Infants	Ceftriaxone, 25–50 mg/kg once daily *or* Cefotaxime, 25 mg/kg twice daily. Usual duration of therapy is 7 days (longer for meningitis or endocarditis).
Children	Children who weigh 100 lb (45 kg) should receive adult doses; for those weighing less, see text.

will eliminate coexisting *C. trachomatis* infections. Tetracycline hydrochloride, 500 mg orally four times daily, can be substituted for doxycycline. Pregnant women and those unable to tolerate doxycycline or tetracycline can instead be given erythromycin base or stearate, 500 mg by mouth four times daily for 7 days, or erythromycin ethylsuccinate, 800 mg by mouth four times daily for 7 days, to accompany the ceftriaxone. All tetracyclines are ineffective as single-dose therapy for gonorrhea, and even a 7-day course of tetracycline has been ineffective in a growing proportion of patients owing to the spread of TRNG and the high proportion of strains with chromosomal resistance to tetracycline. Ceftriaxone can be prepared in 1% lidocaine as diluent (for intramuscular injection only) to reduce discomfort due to the injection. Other intramuscular β-lactam antibiotics (cefotaxime, cefuroxime, ceftizoxime) are also very effective for resistant gonorrhea, but the long half-life of ceftriaxone, together with its in vitro activity, makes it the optimal drug for single-dose therapy of gonorrhea. For patients who cannot take ceftriaxone, the preferred alternative is spectinomycin, 2 g intramuscularly as a single dose. Although spectinomycin resistance has emerged where that drug was used commonly for gonorrhea (e.g., in England and Korea), it has been rare in the United States. Other convenient alternatives to ceftriaxone for uncomplicated urethral, endocervical, or rectal gonorrhea include cefixime, given as a single 400-mg oral dose, ofloxacin, as a 400-mg single oral dose, or ciprofloxacin, in a 500-mg single oral dose. Although the fluoroquinolones ofloxacin and ciprofloxacin remain highly effective for gonorrhea, lessened gonococcal susceptibility to these drugs has been seen in Asia and recently in England, Canada, and the United States.

All patients with gonorrhea should have a serologic test for syphilis at the time of diagnosis and should be offered confidential testing for human immunodeficiency virus (HIV). Patients with incubating seronegative syphilis, without clinical signs of syphilis, are likely to be cured of syphilis by the recommended ceftriaxone-doxycycline regimen. However, patients with gonorrhea who also have syphilis or who are established contacts of someone with syphilis should be given additional treatment appropriate to the stage of syphilis (see Chap. 133).

Follow-up and treatment failure Treatment failure following combined ceftriaxone-doxycycline therapy is exceedingly rare; therefore, a follow-up culture is not essential. Patients should be advised to return for reexamination if any symptoms persist or recur after completion of treatment. Persistent or recurrent symptoms or signs after treatment for gonorrhea should be evaluated by culture for *N. gonorrhoeae* and a specific test for chlamydial infection. Any gonococcal isolate should be tested for antibiotic susceptibility. Additional treatment for persistent or recurrent gonorrhea should be with ceftriaxone, 250 mg intramuscularly, or with spectinomycin, 2.0 g intramuscularly (except in areas where spectinomycin resistance is a problem). Recurrent gonococcal infections after treatment with the recommended schedule are almost certainly due to reinfection, and indicate a need for improved sex partner referral and patient education.

Postgonococcal urethritis (PGU) usually becomes apparent about 2 to 3 weeks after treatment of gonorrhea with a penicillin or a cephalosporin. PGU often is caused by *C. trachomatis* which may have been acquired at the same time as gonorrhea but did not become clinically apparent until later because of the longer incubation period of chlamydial infection. When PGU occurs, it can be managed, like nongonococcal urethritis, with doxycycline, 100 mg orally twice daily, or tetracycline, 0.5 g four times a day, for 7 days. Similarly, mucopurulent cervicitis in women which often persists or appears after treatment of gonorrhea with cephalosporin, penicillin, or spectinomycin is often caused by *C. trachomatis* and can be treated like PGU. Men and women exposed to gonorrhea should be examined, cultured, and treated with one of the recommended treatment schedules.

All pregnant women should be cultured for *N. gonorrhoeae* (and tested for *C. trachomatis* infection and syphilis) at the time of the first visit as an integral part of the prenatal care. A second culture late in the third trimester (as well as tests for chlamydial infection and syphilis) should be obtained from women at high risk of sexually transmitted disease.

The regimen of choice for gonorrhea in pregnancy is ceftriaxone, in a single 125-mg intramuscular dose, plus erythromycin for a possible coexisting chlamydial infection. Pregnant women allergic to β-lactams can be treated with a single dose of spectinomycin, 2.0 g intramuscularly, plus erythromycin. Doxycycline and tetracycline should not be used in pregnant women because of potential toxic effects for mother and fetus.

The management of pelvic inflammatory disease is discussed in Chap. 89.

Treatment of gonococcal arthritis can be accomplished satisfactorily with several regimens. Gonococci recovered from patients with gonococcal arthritis have been significantly less resistant to penicillin or tetracycline than isolates from patients with uncomplicated gonorrhea. However, several cases of DGI caused by PPNG have been reported. Because of the threat of endocarditis, meningitis, and joint sepsis, all patients with disseminated infection should be hospitalized and treated with ceftriaxone intravenously, 1 g once a day, or with the alternatives listed in Table 110-1. Reliable patients without endocarditis or meningitis can be discharged 24 to 48 h after symptoms resolve, to complete a total of 7 to 10 days' therapy with an oral regimen of cefixime, 400 mg twice a day. If the infecting gonococcus is shown to be penicillin-sensitive, treatment can be completed with oral amoxicillin, 500 mg three times a day, without clavulanic acid. Failure to improve with appropriate antimicrobial regimens as listed above strongly suggests a diagnosis other than disseminated gonococcal infection. Repeated joint aspiration or closed irrigation of the joint with sterile saline may be required to reduce inflammation in patients with high synovial fluid leukocyte counts. Open drainage is seldom, if ever, required for gonococcal arthritis, except in infants with hip infection. Temporary immobilization of the joint may reduce discomfort and may be useful during initial ambulation in patients with persistent effusions of the knee or ankle. Antibiotics should not be injected directly into the joint. Once the diagnosis of gonococcal arthritis is proven, then occasional patients may benefit from use of anti-inflammatory agents along with antimicrobial therapy. However, if the diagnosis is suspected, but not proven, then early use of anti-inflammatory drugs will prevent monitoring the response to antimicrobial therapy, which is usually rapid and often of diagnostic importance in gonococcal arthritis.

Meningitis and endocarditis caused by the gonococcus require high-dose intravenous therapy with an agent effective against the strain causing the disease: ceftriaxone, 1 g intravenously every 12 h, for 10 to 14 days for meningitis and for 1 month for endocarditis. Patients with gonococcal endocarditis or meningitis, and perhaps all patients with DGI, should be evaluated for complement deficiency.

Gonococcal conjunctivitis in the adult or in children over 20 kg should be managed as a medical emergency by irrigation of the conjunctiva with saline, together with ceftriaxone, 1 g in a single intramuscular dose. All patients must have careful ophthalmologic evaluation, including slit-lamp examination.

Pediatric gonococcal infection The infant born to a mother with gonorrhea is at high risk of infection and requires prophylactic treatment with a single injection of ceftriaxone, 50 mg/kg intravenously or intramuscularly, not to exceed 125 mg. Ceftriaxone should be given with caution to hyperbilirubinemic infants, especially premature babies. Topical prophylaxis for neonatal ophthalmia is not adequate treatment for infections at other sites. Infants with gonococcal infection at any site (e.g., eye) should be evaluated for DGI by examination and culture of blood and CSF. They should be treated for 7 days with ceftriaxone, 25 to 50 mg/kg in a single daily intravenous or intramuscular dose. Alternatively, cefotaxime can be used in a dose of 25 mg/kg twice daily intravenously. Limited data suggest that uncomplicated gonococcal ophthalmia in the infant can be cured with a single injection of ceftriaxone, 50 mg/kg, up to a dose of 125 mg. Irrigation of the eyes with saline or buffered ophthalmic solutions should be performed immediately and then repeated as often as necessary to eliminate discharge. Topical antibiotic preparations alone are not sufficient or required when appropriate systemic antibiotic therapy is given. Both the parents of a newborn with gonococcal ophthalmia must be treated for gonorrhea. The parents and infant also should be tested for chlamydial infection.

Children who weigh 45 kg or more should be treated with adult regimens. Children who weigh less than 45 kg should be treated as follows: For uncomplicated vulvovaginitis, cervicitis, urethritis, proctitis, and pharyngitis, the recommended treatment is ceftriaxone, a single 125-mg intramuscular dose. The alternative regimen is spectinomycin, a single 40-mg/kg intramuscular dose. Children 8 years of age or older can, in addition, be given doxycycline, 100 mg twice a day for 7 days. Children with gonorrhea should be evaluated for coexisting syphilis and chlamydial infection.

Topical and/or systemic estrogen therapy is of no benefit in gonococcal vulvovaginitis. All children should have follow-up cultures, and the source of infection should be identified, examined, and treated. Child abuse should be carefully considered and evaluated. For treatment of complicated disease, the alternative regimens recommended for adults may be used in appropriate pediatric dosages.

Treatment of gonorrhea in developing countries   The proportion of gonococcal infections caused by PPNG, TRNG, or CMRNG is highest in developing countries, which can least afford ceftriaxone, spectinomycin, or other new antimicrobials effective against these strains. Inexpensive alternatives to penicillin G and tetracycline, the traditional mainstays of gonorrhea therapy, have been disappointing. For example, a sulfonamide-trimethoprim combination which initially cured over 95 percent of cases of gonorrhea in African countries fell to less than 75 percent efficacy within 2 years after it became a popular regimen in Kenya. One approach has been the use of 4.8 million units of procaine penicillin G intramuscularly plus 1.0 g probenecid orally (a standard regimen for non-PPNG infections) together with 125 mg of clavulanic acid (in the form of one capsule of amoxicillin-clavulanate) to inhibit gonococcal β-lactamase. This inexpensive regimen has been effective in small trials in Kenya, even against PPNG infections. Gentamicin, in a single 280-mg intramuscular dose, also has been used effectively in this setting. Newer cephalosporins in lower than recommended doses, to reduce cost, should be discouraged. Norfloxacin, ciprofloxacin, and ofloxacin are increasingly prescribed or dispensed without prescription for urethritis in developing countries. None of these drugs is effective as a single-dose regimen for chlamydial urethritis, and the impact of increased fluoroquinolone use on gonococcal resistance to the quinolones remains to be assessed. There is a growing need for clinical trials with less expensive regimens and for ongoing surveillance of in vitro sensitivity of *N. gonorrhoeae*.

PREVENTION AND CONTROL   There is probably no more striking illustration than gonorrhea of the failure of a specific treatment alone to eradicate a communicable disease. Vaccination is not available. A field trial of a purified gonococcal pili vaccine in U.S. soldiers in Korea showed that the vaccine was not effective. Use of the condom can prevent transmission, and the extensive use of condoms for contraception may be responsible for the low rates of gonorrhea in some countries (e.g., Japan). Spermicidal preparations used with a diaphragm or cervical sponges impregnated with nonoxynol-9 probably offer some protection against gonorrhea and chlamydial infection. Prophylactic antibiotics (e.g., 200 mg minocycline or doxycycline taken soon after sexual exposure) reduce the risk of infection but are not recommended for general use or for individuals with known exposure to gonorrhea, who should receive one of the regimens recommended for established gonorrhea.

To contain the increasing spread of antimicrobial-resistant gonococci, several measures are important: (1) routine use of diagnosis by cultures and testing of isolates for antimicrobial resistance or β-lactamase production, (2) routine use of highly effective antibiotics, such as ceftriaxone, to prevent gonorrhea treatment failures, and (3)

rapid identification and treatment of sexual partners of patients with gonorrhea, particularly partners of those with recurrent infection and those known to be infected with resistant gonococci. One of the most effective public health measures now available for control of gonorrhea is treatment of sexual partners of infected patients. In addition, public health education and individual patient counseling are essential to promote fewer sexual partners, condom use during casual sexual encounters, and early health care for symptoms of urethritis or unusual vaginal discharge, with or without lower abdominal pain.

REFERENCES

BOSLEGO JW et al: Effect of spectinomycin use on the prevalence of spectinomycin resistant and of penicillinase-producing *Neisseria gonorrhoeae*. N Engl J Med 317:272, 1987

BRITIGAN BE, SPARLING PF: Gonococcal infection: A model of molecular pathogenesis. N Engl J Med 312:1683, 1985

CENTERS FOR DISEASE CONTROL: 1989 Sexually transmitted diseases treatment guidelines. Morb Mort Week Rep 38(Suppl 8):1, 1989

————: Policy guidelines for the detection, management, and control of antibiotic resistant strains of *Neisseria gonorrhoeae*. Morb Mort Week Rep 36(5S):1, 1987

COHEN MS, SPARLING PF: Mucosal infection with *Neisseria gonorrhoeae*. Bacterial adaptation and mucosal defenses. J Clin Invest 89:1699, 1992

HANDSFIELD HH et al: Localized outbreak of penicillinase-producing *Neisseria gonorrhoeae:* Paradigm for introduction and spread of gonorrhea in a community. JAMA 261:2357, 1989

———— et al: A comparison of single-dose cefixime with ceftriaxone as treatment for uncomplicated gonorrhea. N Engl J Med 325:1337, 1991

KNAPP JS et al: Serologic classification of *Neisseria gonorrhoeae* using monoclonal antibodies directed against outer membrane protein I. J Infect Dis 150:44, 1985

MANDRELL RE et al: In vitro and in vivo modification of *Neisseria gonorrhoeae* lipooligosaccharide epitope structure by sialylation. J Exp Med 171:1649, 1990

MORSE SA et al: High-level tetracycline resistance in *Neisseria gonorrhoeae* is result of acquisition of streptococcal *tetM* determinant. Antimicrob Agents Chemother 30:664, 1986

———— (eds): Perspectives on pathogenic *Neisseria* spp. Clin Microb Rev 2:1S, 1989

RICE PA et al: Immunoglobulin G antibodies directed against protein III block killing of serum-resistant *Neisseria gonorrhoeae* by immune serum. J Exp Med 164:1735, 1986

RICE R et al: Sociodemographic distribution of gonorrhea incidence: Implications for prevention and behavioral research. Am J Public Health, 81:1252, 1991

SCHWARCZ SK et al: National surveillance of antimicrobial resistance in *Neisseria gonorrhoeae*: The Gonococcal Isolate Surveillance Project. JAMA 264:1413, 1990

SPARLING PF: Biology of *Neisseria gonorrhoeae*, in *Sexually Transmitted Diseases*, 2d ed; KK Holmes et al (eds). New York, McGraw-Hill, 1990, pp 131–147

VAN PUTTEN JPM: Iron acquisition and the pathogenesis of meningococcal and gonococcal disease. Med Microbiol Immunol 179:289, 1990

111   MORAXELLA (BRANHAMELLA) CATARRHALIS, OTHER MORAXELLA SPECIES, AND KINGELLA

DANIEL M. MUSHER

MORAXELLA (BRANHAMELLA) CATARRHALIS

This gram-negative coccus has undergone three changes of name in as many decades. Originally called *Micrococcus catarrhalis*, it was renamed *Neisseria catarrhalis* in the 1960s because of its morphologic similarity to *Neisseria* species, and then, in 1970, it was given status as a distinct genus, *Branhamella*, on the basis of DNA homology. In 1979 this organism was placed into the genus *Moraxella*, although many authorities continue to call it *Moraxella (Branhamella) catarrhalis*. A component of normal bacterial flora of the upper airways, *M. catarrhalis* has been increasingly recognized as a cause of otitis media, sinusitis, and bronchopulmonary infection.

BACTERIOLOGY AND IMMUNITY   On Gram's stain, *M. catarrhalis* appears as large round cocci that tend to retain crystal violet during the decolorizing step and occasionally are confused with *Staphylococcus aureus*. Colonies grow well on blood or chocolate agar and are readily distinguishable from *Neisseria* species by biochemical tests.

Unlike many other pathogenic bacteria, *M. catarrhalis* shows a surprising degree of homogeneity of outer-membrane proteins. Antibody to certain of these proteins is generally present in serum of children over the age of 4 years; however, isolates that cause disease are generally serum resistant; i.e., they survive in serum despite this naturally present antibody and complement. Bactericidal antibody emerges following natural infection and may be directed against one or more conserved outer-membrane proteins, a property of potential value in vaccine development.

EPIDEMIOLOGY With use of selective media, *M. catarrhalis* can be isolated from the upper respiratory tract or saliva of 50 percent of healthy school children and from the nasopharynx of up to 7 percent of healthy adults. The rate of nasopharyngeal colonization increases to 86 percent in children who have otitis media. Investigators in both the Northern and Southern Hemispheres have reported a striking seasonal variation in the isolation of this organism from clinical specimens, with a peak in late winter/early spring and a nadir in late summer/early fall. Direct contact has not been shown to contribute to community-acquired infection, but nosocomial spread of infection has rarely been documented.

OTITIS MEDIA, SINUSITIS *M. catarrhalis* has repeatedly been shown to be the third most common bacterial isolate from middle ear fluid of children who have otitis media, following *Streptococcus penumoniae* and nontypable *Haemophilus influenzae*. Recent studies also show this organism to be a prominent isolate from sinus cavities in acute and chronic sinusitis.

PURULENT TRACHEOBRONCHITIS, PNEUMONIA *M. catarrhalis* causes acute exacerbations of chronic bronchitis (increased production and/or purulence of sputum), purulent tracheobronchitis (above, plus fever and leukocytosis), and pneumonia. The great majority of infected persons are greater than 50 years of age with a long history of cigarette smoking and underlying chronic obstructive pulmonary disease (COPD); lung cancer is often present as well. In one recent study, 76 percent of affected persons had COPD (often severe), together with lung cancer in one-third of cases; most patients also had clinical evidence of malnutrition. In one extensive series of cases, *Branhamella* pneumonia was not discovered in an otherwise healthy host.

Symptoms of patients with *M. catarrhalis* pneumonia have been regarded as modest in severity, perhaps due more to a diminished febrile response because of the advanced age of the affected individuals than to any lack of pathogenic capacity of this organism. Cough usually is increased, as are the amount and purulence of the sputum, but these symptoms may not be noticeably increased above baseline. Chills are present in one-quarter of patients, pleuritic pain in one-third, and malaise in 40 percent. The majority of patients have peak temperatures < 101°F (38.3°C), and peripheral white blood cell counts are < 10,000 per cubic millimeter in nearly one-quarter of cases. Microscopic examination of a good sputum specimen following Gram's stain regularly reveals profuse numbers of organisms (approximately 2×10^8 colony forming units per milliliter). A variable radiologic appearance is seen; in one study, 43 percent of subjects had segmental or lobar infiltrates, and the remainder had a mixed pattern of subsegmental, segmental, interstitial, and diffuse involvement. These clinical, laboratory, and radiographic findings do not differ from those of pneumococcal pneumonia in an older patient population. By comparison with pneumococcal infection, however, a far lesser degree of bloodstream invasion is apparent; in one series, none of 25 patients with *M. catarrhalis* pneumonia had bacteremia. Nevertheless, *Branhamella* pneumonia is a marker for severe underlying disease in that nearly one-half of patients die within 3 months of onset.

OTHER SYNDROMES Local extension causing empyema is very uncommon, and as might be inferred from the low rate of bacteremia,

metastatic complications of *Branhamella* pneumonia such as septic arthritis are exceedingly rare. As of 1990, 27 cases of bacteremic infection due to *M. catarrhalis* had been reported, mainly in children less than 10 years or adults more than 60 years of age; most occurred in immunocompromised patients. Syndromes have included bacteremia with no apparent focus, endocarditis, and meningitis. A petechial or purpuric rash, reminiscent of that observed in meningococcal sepsis and associated with disseminated intravascular coagulation, has been described in a few cases, nearly all in children.

TREATMENT Treatment of presumed *M. catarrhalis* infection with a penicillin–clavulanic acid combination seems highly appropriate. Penicillin resistance first appeared in *Branhamella* isolates in the mid-1970s but is now found in 85 percent of clinical isolates. Resistance is mediated by two closely related β-lactamases, BRO-1 and BRO-2 (acronyms derived from *Branhamella* and *Moraxella*) that are present in 90 and 10 percent, respectively, of resistant isolates. These enzymes are active against penicillin, ampicillin, and amoxicillin but less so against cephalosporins, especially third-generation cephalosporins, and they bind avidly to clavulanic acid and sulbactam.

Cephalosporins, especially of the second and third generations, are effective alternatives. A 5-day course of therapy has been shown to cure respiratory infection, although a slightly longer course may be required in sinusitis. Isolates in the United States are nearly uniformly susceptible to tetracycline, erythromycin, and chloramphenicol, although tetracycline resistance, perhaps due to Tet B determinants, is increasing in Europe and Asia and has been documented in two isolates in the United States. *M. catarrhalis* is also susceptible to trimethoprim-sulfamethoxazole and to quinolones.

After the identification of gram-negative cocci in a Gram-stained specimen and pending final identification by culture, the severity of the condition and the potential presence of other infecting organisms should dictate antibiotic selection. For example, an exacerbation of bronchitis caused by *Branhamella* might be treated with tetracycline or trimethoprim-sulfamethoxazole, but in a patient with pneumonia, the possibility that pneumococci resistant to these agents also might be present dictates the choice of ampicillin sulbactam, at least until results of culture are available.

MORAXELLA

Moraxella species cause a wide range of infections, including bronchitis, pneumonia, empyema, endocarditis, meningitis, conjunctivitis, urinary infection, septic arthritis, and wound infection. In a report of all *Moraxella* isolates submitted to the Centers for Disease Control (CDC) between 1953 to 1980, certain clinical associations were apparent (Table 111-1). *M. osloensis* and *M. nonliquefaciens* were the most commonly isolated species, emanating from a wide range of body sites including blood, cerebrospinal fluid, and joints. *M. osloensis* was the *Moraxella* species most commonly isolated from blood; *M. nonliquefaciens* tended to be isolated from the ears, nose, or throat (47 percent) or sputum (8 percent). *Moraxella* M-5 (an as yet unnamed group) had a striking association with infected wounds from dog bites (72 percent of all isolates), whereas *M. lacunata* was associated with conjunctivitis and keratitis (70 percent of isolates). *M. urethralis* was isolated most often from urine and the genital tract and is probably the *Moraxella* species that had previously been implicated in urethritis. More than one-half of isolates of *M. phenylpyruvica* and *M. atlantis* were obtained from normally sterile sites. The clinical features of such infections and the nature of the hosts in which they occur are not fully characterized.

KINGELLA

Kingella kingae was originally *Moraxella* new species 1 (M-1) and was subsequently named in honor of Dr. Elizabeth King of the CDC,

TABLE 111-1 *Moraxella* species and *Kingella*

Species	Number of isolates	Common sites/ clinical association	Number (percent) for each site
M. osloensis	199	Blood	44 (22)
		CSF	18 (9)
		Urine	17 (9)
		Respiratory tract	24 (12)
M. nonliquefaciens	356	Blood	27 (8)
		CSF	6 (2)
		Respiratory tract	196 (55)
M-5	74	Dog bite wound	53 (72)
M-6	47	Blood, bone	15 (32)
M. lacunata	33	Conjunctivitis, keratitis	23 (70)
M. urethralis	28	Urine	16 (57)
		Genital tract	3 (11)
M. phenylpyruvica	73	Blood	19 (26)
		CSF	8 (11)
		Urine	12 (16)
M. atlantis	44	Blood	20 (45)
		CSF	5 (11)
Kingella kingae	79	Blood	38 (48)
		Joint	10 (13)
		Bone	11 (14)

SOURCE: Taken from a summary of CDC experience (Graham et al, Rev Infect Dis 12:423, 1990).

who first described it. A fastidious organism, *K. kingae* has been found to cause endocarditis, arthritis, and osteomyelitis (see Table 111-1); isolated instances of other infections have been recorded. Most bone and joint infections occur in young children. The failure to implicate this organism more frequently as a cause of pneumonia may indicate true tissue tropism for heart valve, bones, and joints, or it may reflect the difficulty in separating *Kingella* from normal respiratory flora on sputum culture.

Most moraxellae and kingellae remain susceptible to penicillins, cephalosporins, tetracyclines, and chloramphenicol, but some strains of *Moraxella* produce BRO β-lactamases, and clinical specimens must be tested for lactamase production and antibiotic susceptibility. Initial therapy with a penicillin or cephalosporin is reasonable pending susceptibility testing.

REFERENCES

CATLIN BW: *Branhamella catarrhalis:* An organism gaining respect as a pathogen. Clin Microbiol Rev 3:293, 1990

DEGROOT R et al: Bone and joint infections caused by *Kingella kingae:* Six cases and review of the literature. Rev Infect Dis 10:998, 1988

GRAHAM D et al: Infections caused by *Moraxella, Moraxella urethralis, Moraxella*-like groups M-5 and M-6, and *Kingella kingae* in the United States, 1953–1980. Rev Infect Dis 12:423, 1990

HAGER H et al: *Branhamella catarrhalis* respiratory infections. Rev Infect Dis 9:1140, 1987

MORRISON VA, WAGNER KF: Clinical manifestations of *Kingella kingae* infections: Case report and review. Rev Infect Dis 11:776, 1989

NASH DR et al: Comparison of the activity of cefixime and activities of other oral antibiotics against adult clinical isolates of *Moraxella (Branhamella) catarrhalis* containing BRO-1 and BRO-2 and *Haemophilus influenzae.* Antimicrob Agents Chemother 35:192, 1991

VERGHESE A, BERK SL: *Moraxella (Branhamella) catarrhalis.* Infect Dis Clin North Am 5:523, 1991

WALLACE RJ JR et al: Antibiotic susceptibiolities and drug resistance in *Moraxella (Branhamella) catarrhalis.* Am J Med 88(suppl 5A), 1990

WRIGHT PW et al: A descriptive study of 42 cases of *Branhamella catarrhalis* pneumonia. Am J Med 88(suppl 5A):5A, 1990

112 INFECTIONS DUE TO *HAEMOPHILUS INFLUENZAE,* HACEK GROUP, *CAPNOCYTOPHAGA,* AND *H. DUCREYI*

MICHAEL A. APICELLA

***HAEMOPHILUS INFLUENZAE* INFECTIONS** The species *H. influenzae* encompasses a group of pleomorphic gram-negative human pathogens whose sole ecologic niche is the human environment. When visualized by Gram's stain directly from biologic specimens (CSF or sputum), these organisms can appear coccobacillary with deeply staining polar bodies that cause misidentification as gram-positive cocci. *H. influenzae* is not a fastidious species and can be recovered readily from clinical specimens. However, it has an absolute growth requirement for hemin (factor X) and/or nicotinamide adenine dinucleotide (factor V). These factors can be supplied by direct addition to the medium. Factor V is heat labile and must be added to the media after autoclaving. Hemin can be supplied from the autoclaved hemoglobin of lysed erythrocytes as in chocolate media. Factor V is produced by certain bacteria such as *Staphylococcus aureus. H. influenzae* will grow around a staphylococcal streak on routine blood agar. This is a useful means of identifying factor V–requiring *Haemophilus* organisms. Species of *Haemophilus* that do not require factor V are designated by the *para* prefix (*H. parainfluenzae*).

There are six capsular serotypes of *H. influenzae,* a to f. *H. influenzae* serotype b (Hib) is the capsular serotype most frequently involved in human disease. Encapsulation is best detected by counter-immunoelectrophoresis of extracts prepared from organisms. Alternatively, agglutination can be used to determine capsular type. Genetic analyses indicate that Hib strains are clonally related. Unencapsulated *H. influenzae* strains are termed *nontypable H. influenzae* (NTHi). Unlike Hib strains, NTHi strains have wide genetic and antigenic diversity.

Pathogenesis *H. influenzae* is part of the normal flora of the upper respiratory tract. The mechanism by which it invades the mucosal surface has been studied in human adenoidal organ culture models. Some mucosal pathogens such as *Neisseria gonorrhoeae, N. meningitidis,* and strains of *H. influenzae* biogroup *aegyptius* cross the mucosal barrier through nonciliated epithelial cells. In contrast, most *H. influenzae* move across by passing between rather than through cells.

The capsular polysaccharide of Hib strains, which is a polymer of ribosyl-ribitol phosphate, acts as an antiphagocytic barrier and is an important virulence factor. *H. influenzae* has a potent endotoxin (LPS) that can act systemically to induce CSF inflammation and signs associated with sepsis. Locally LPS can damage mucosal cells in the respiratory tract during middle ear infection and acute bronchitis. *H. influenzae* strains express pili which are probably important because of their ability to colonize the respiratory mucosal surface. The outer membrane proteins have been well defined, and antibodies to several (P2, P4, and P6) have been shown to be protective in experimental animals, suggesting that they may be useful as future human vaccines.

NTHi strains primarily cause disease by damaging the respiratory mucosal epithelial cell surface. The factors associated with invasiveness of *H. influenzae* biogroup *aegyptius* have not been identified. Its members are not encapsulated but contain LPS and outer membrane proteins similar to other NTHi strains.

Epidemiology Vaccines composed of Hib polyribosyl-ribitol phosphate (PRP) capsule, chemically conjugated to modified diphtheria toxoid, tetanus toxoid, or proteosomes, have greatly reduced the incidence of Hib infections in infants below the age of 6 months since their use in the United States beginning in 1991. Before introduction of these vaccines, approximately 10,000 cases of Hib meningitis occurred per year in the United States in children below the age of 2. In regions of the world where this vaccine is not being utilized, the yearly incidence of Hib meningitis still ranges between 20 and 50 cases per 100,000 children between 6 months and 2 years of age.

H. influenzae infections also cause morbidity and mortality in adults. In one study in Atlanta, invasive *H. influenzae* infections in adults had an annual incidence of 5.6 cases per 100,000 population. Over 75 percent of the patients (representing 70 percent of the cases) were women with bacteremic pneumonia and most of them had underlying conditions, such as chronic lung disease. Other risk factors include pregnancy, HIV infection, and malignancy. Overall the mortality in adults was 28 percent, and more than half of the pregnancy-related infections resulted in fetal death. Approximately one half of the strains isolated from invasive *H. influenzae* infections in adults were nontypable.

Clinical aspects PNEUMONIA AND TRACHEOBRONCHITIS *H. influenzae* is an important cause of community-acquired bacterial pneumonia in adults. NTHi strains account for over 80 percent of these infections. The patients are generally elderly and have chronic lung disease or a long smoking history. Patients with HIV infection are also susceptible to serious respiratory infection by Hib and NTHi and appear to have an increased incidence of bacteremia. The clinical features of pneumonia caused by *H. influenzae* are indistinguishable from those of other bacterial pneumonias; fever, cough, and purulent sputum, usually of several days' duration. Chest radiographs show either lobar or patchy infiltrate and are not specific.

NTHi may play a role in acute exacerbations of chronic bronchitis in patients with obstructive lung disease. However, the organism can be found in serial cultures of sputum in the majority of patients with chronic bronchitis during quiescent periods so that the mere presence of the organism does not imply a pathogenic role in this setting. Nevertheless, the isolation of NTHi from sputum during exacerbations, the development of serum antibodies to NTHi after exacerbations, and the response of patients to antibiotics suggest that NTHi is the etiologic agent in many acute exacerbations of chronic bronchitis.

MENINGITIS AND SEPSIS *H. influenzae* is the most common cause of meningitis in children between the ages of 2 months and 2 years, with 95 percent of these cases attributable to Hib. As mentioned above, the introduction of the PRP Hib capsule vaccine in 1991 has reduced the incidence of Hib meningitis. In adults, *H. influenzae* is a relatively uncommon cause of meningitis, and approximately 50 percent of the isolates are NTHi. In children, spread to the meninges is hematogenous after invasion of the organism across the nasopharyngeal barrier. In young children, Hib is the leading cause of septic arthritis which is frequently associated with sepsis. Hib cellulitis with sepsis is also a cause of serious morbidity and mortality in this age group. In adults, infection commonly spreads to the meninges from a contiguous site, an infected sinus, CNS trauma with a CSF leak, or a middle ear infection. Since the upper respiratory tract is frequently colonized, NTHi is the second most common cause (after *Pneumococcus*) of recurrent meningitis. The clinical presentation of meningitis due to Hib and NTHi is otherwise no different from that due to other bacterial pathogens.

H. influenzae biogroup *aegyptius* is the cause of Brazilian purpuric fever, a serious systemic illness of children that begins with purulent conjunctivitis and is characterized by fever, petechiae, purpura, and shock.

OTITIS MEDIA AND SINUSITIS NTHi strains are responsible for 20 to 40 percent of bacteriologically confirmed cases of otitis media in children. It is the most common illness during early childhood; some 60 to 70 percent of children experience one to three ear infections before the age of 2 years.

OBSTETRIC AND NEONATAL INFECTIONS Obstetric infections due to *H. influenzae* are a serious complication of pregnancy as both the mother and the child become infected and there appears to be maternal-fetal transmission of the organism. The isolates are almost invariably

NTHi. Symptoms in mother and child occur within 24 h of birth, and there is a high frequency of prematurity. Infant mortality is high.

ADULT EPIGLOTTITIS *H. influenzae* is an important cause of adult epiglottitis. In one large review, the incidence of acute epiglottitis in adults was 9.7 cases per million population. The average age was 44 years with an equal sex distribution. Patients presented with an elevated temperature, sore throat (90 percent), dysphagia (80 percent), respiratory difficulty (45 percent), and hoarseness or drooling. Visualization by indirect laryngoscopy of an inflamed epiglottis has proven to be more reliable in making the diagnosis (positive in 86 percent of cases) than by soft-tissue x-rays of the neck. Laryngoscopy can induce laryngospasm, particularly in children, and clinicians should be prepared to maintain the airway with tracheostomy when this procedure is performed. Mortality is 7 percent, with all deaths related to airway obstruction. It has been suggested that an airway should be established at the time of presentation rather than waiting for a worsening clinical picture. Antibiotic therapy of epiglottitis in adults is primarily directed against *H. influenzae*, group A streptococci, and pneumococci.

OTHER INFECTIONS Less common manifestations of *H. influenzae* infection in adults include empyema, pericarditis, osteomyelitis, endocarditis, cholecystitis, intraabdominal infections, urinary tract infections, mastoiditis, and aortic graft infection.

Management of *H. influenzae* infections Resistance has become more prevalent among isolates. It varies, but overall 10 to 20 percent of *H. influenzae* strains exhibit β-lactamase-mediated resistance and approximately 3 percent of strains exhibit nonenzymatic resistance secondary to modified penicillin-binding proteins or outer membrane proteins. Antibiotic resistance is approximately twice as frequent among Hib strains as among NTHi strains. Chloramphenicol resistance is a significant problem in less-developed countries and in the United States. Fortunately, there are a number of effective therapeutic choices. All isolates from seriously ill patients should be assumed resistant to ampicillin until proven otherwise, and initial therapy should be based on this assumption. Once the sensitivity of the organism is known, therapy should be adjusted to minimize cost and risk of superinfection. For serious systemic infection, combined therapy with ampicillin and chloramphenicol is recommended. In addition, several third-generation cephalosporins (including ceftriaxone and cefotaxime) penetrate the CSF to therapeutic levels and are effective in management of serious *H. influenzae* infection. The early administration of glucocorticoids may reduce the incidence of hearing loss in children with type b meningitis. Preschool contacts of children with the infection should receive prophylaxis with rifampin (20 mg/kg per day) for 4 days. This has been shown to reduce the risk of secondary cases significantly.

Less serious infections, such as otitis, sinusitis, and acute bronchitis due to ampicillin-sensitive strains, can be treated with ampicillin or amoxicillin. Infections due to ampicillin-resistant strains can be managed with ampicillin/β-lactamase inhibitors, trimethoprim-sulfamethoxazole, cefadroxil, or quinolones. Penicillin-allergic patients can be treated with trimethoprim-sulfamethoxazole, cefadroxil, or quinolones.

HACEK GROUP INFECTIONS The group of organisms including *Haemophilus aphrophilis*, *H. paraphrophilis*, *H. parainfluenzae*, *Actinobacillus actinomycetemcomitans*, *Cardiobacterium hominis*, *Eikenella corrodens*, and *Kingella kingae* is known as HACEK. Culture of these fastidious organisms requires incubation in an atmosphere containing carbon dioxide. They require longer incubation for isolation in blood than *H. influenzae* organisms. When HACEK organisms are suspected, blood cultures should be observed for at least 7 days. The improved ability to isolate these fastidious organisms may be the reason for the reported increased incidence. The pathogenicity of these species is lower than that of *H. influenzae*.

Haemophilus species cause about 5 percent of infective endocarditis. The course of the endocarditis is similar to that due to viridans streptococci. Underlying valvular disease, intravenous drug abuse, and prosthetic valves are predisposing factors. Vegetations tend to be large. Embolization, a frequent complication (up to 60 percent of cases), may be due in part to delay in diagnosis as a result of the difficulty in isolation of these species.

Therapy should ultimately be based on antibiotic sensitivity. Initial treatment with ampicillin and aminoglycosides, which are synergistic against some *Haemophilus* species, is recommended. Even in effectively managed cases, the mortality in *Haemophilus* endocarditis is between 10 and 15 percent.

Actinobacillus actinomycetemcomitans is part of the endogenous flora of the mouth. It is often recovered from the sites of lesions associated with juvenile periodontitis. It can cause endocarditis (especially on damaged or prosthetic valves) and has been isolated from infections of the meninges, bone, urinary tract, and pericardium. It is susceptible to the newer cephalosporins, rifampin, trimethoprim-sulfamethoxazole, quinolones, and chloramphenicol.

Cardiobacterium hominis is a small gram-negative rod. Almost all clinical isolates of *C. hominis* have been associated with endocarditis, usually of abnormal or prosthetic valves. The valvular infection tends to be insidious, and patients present with splenomegaly, anemia, and hematuria indicative of a long-standing infection before diagnosis. It is frequently difficult to determine antibiotic susceptibility because the organisms are slow-growing. *C. hominis* is usually susceptible to penicillin, chloramphenicol, and tetracycline. Penicillin alone or combined with aminoglycosides is the most common therapy. Complications caused by embolization, mycotic aneurysm, or heart failure have necessitated valvular replacement in a number of cases.

Eikenella corrodens is a gram-negative facultative anaerobic bacillus and a part of the normal oral and respiratory mucosal flora. The most common clinical types of infection are human bites, head and neck infections, and respiratory tract infections. Gynecologic infections may be associated with intrauterine devices. Other sites of *Eikenella* infection include synovial fluid, bone, and brain abscess. As with other organisms in the HACEK group, *Eikenella corrodens* has been associated with endocarditis. *Eikenella* species are resistant to clindamycin. Ampicillin, penicillin, second- and third-generation cephalosporins have been reported effective in management of such infections.

The *Kingella* genus contains three species, *K. kingae*, *K. indologenes*, and *K. denitrificans*. *Kingella* have been associated with mucous membrane, joint, bone, and valvular infections. *Kingella* infections have been treated successfully with β-lactam–aminoglycoside combinations.

Capnocytophaga infections *Capnocytophaga* are gram-negative facultative anaerobic bacilli that grow optimally under anaerobic conditions in the presence of 5 to 10 percent carbon dioxide on blood or chocolate media. *Capnocytophaga* are motile on agar but lack flagellae. They are commonly isolated from the gingival sulcus and can cause gingival ulcers in neutropenic patients. *Capnocytophaga* cause serious infections predominantly in immunocompromised patients, but bacteremia and endocarditis can occur in patients with normal immune function. *Capnocytophaga* species are sensitive to a wide range of antibiotics including penicillin, clindamycin, erythromycin, quinolones, third-generation cephalosporins, metronidazole, chloramphenicol, and imipenem.

HAEMOPHILUS DUCREYI INFECTIONS The etiologic agent associated with soft genital ulcers (the chancroid ulcer) is a short, compact, rodlike organism that initially could not be cultured. Its role in soft ulcer disease was established by documenting its ability to cause ulcers by autoinoculation. The chancroid bacillus was designated *Haemophilus ducreyi* because of the requirement for factors X and V, but genetic studies suggest that *H. ducreyi* does not belong within this genus. An enriched chocolate medium is necessary for reliable cultivation of the organisms from ulcers, and vancomycin can be added to the medium to reduce contamination with gram-positive bacteria. Samples for culture are usually taken from the base and sides of the ulcers. Aspiration of inguinal buboes is a less-common source of positive cultures.

Epidemiology of chancroid ulcer disease Genital ulcers from *H. ducreyi* occur on a world-wide basis but are more common in less-developed tropical countries. In Africa, chancroid ulcers are implicated as a cofactor in the transmission of HIV. In the United States before 1960 there were approximately 10,000 cases reported per year. This number dropped to an average of 1000 cases per year during the 1960s and 1970s and increased during the 1980s. In 1991, 3476 cases were reported to the Centers for Disease Control and Prevention. Outbreaks in several major cities occurred among heterosexual blacks and Hispanics, mostly men, a fact suggesting that a small number of females was infecting a large number of males. The failure to identify an asymptomatic carrier state for *H. ducreyi* suggests that female prostitution is the mechanism of transmission.

Pathogenesis and clinical features *H. ducreyi* invades via a break in the integrity of the epithelium and causes, over 4 to 7 days, an ingress of polymorphonuclear leukocytes, with edema and disruption of epithelial cells. A small papule surrounded by an erythematous halo ruptures within 2 to 4 days to form a sharply defined ulcer with ragged edges and minimal induration. The base of the ulcer contains grey or yellow friable granulomatous material and bleeds easily. While the papular stage may go unnoticed by the patient, chancroid ulcers are always painful. The most common sites of involvement in men are the distal prepuce, the mucosal surface of the prepuce on the frenulum, and the coronal sulcus. Local extension can occur to other regions in the genital area. In women most lesions are at the entrance to the vagina including the fourchette, labia, vestibule, and clitoris. Painful unilateral inguinal lymphadenopathy occurs in over half of patients. Buboes can form and rupture with the formation of inguinal ulcers. Despite the development of large ulcers, systemic invasion by *H. ducreyi* is rare.

Management Oral erythromycin (500 mg four times a day) for 7 days is effective therapy. Other drugs used include ceftriaxone as a single dose agent (250 mg intramuscularly) and trimethoprim-sulfamethoxazole for 5 to 7 days; considerably less clinical experience is available for the latter therapies.

REFERENCES

FARLEY MM et al: Invasive *Haemophilus influenzae* disease in adults: A prospective population based surveillance. Ann Intern Med 116:806, 1992

MAYOSMITH MF et al: Acute epiglottis in adults. An eight-year experience in the state of Rhode Island. N Engl J Med 314:1133, 1986

MEYER DJ, GERDING DN: Favorable prognosis of patients with prosthetic valve endocarditis caused by gram-negative bacilli of the HACEK group. Am J Med 85:104, 1988

MORSE FS: Chancroid and *Haemophilus ducreyi*. Clin Microbiol Rev 2:137, 1989

MURPHY TF, APICELLA MA: Nontypable *Haemophilus influenzae*: A review of clinical aspects, surface antigens and the human immune response to infection. Rev Infect Dis 9:1, 1987

PARKER SW et al: *Haemophilus* endocarditis in two patients with complications. Arch Intern Med 143:48, 1983

SCHLAMM HT, YANCOVITZ SR: *Haemophilus influenzae* pneumonia in young adults with AIDS, ARC or risk of AIDS. Am J Med 86:11, 1989

WESTERINK MAJ et al: Septicemia due to DF-2; cause of a false-positive cryptococcal latex agglutination test. Am J Med 83:155, 1987

---

113 LEGIONELLA INFECTIONS

MICHAEL S. BERNSTEIN / RICHARD M. LOCKSLEY

DEFINITION The family Legionellaceae consists of over 30 species of fastidious gram-negative, aerobic bacilli. The organisms are ubiquitous in the environment and cause disease when a sufficient environmental inoculum is aerosolized and inhaled by a human host. The course of the subsequent disease is determined both by virulence factors of the bacterium and by the immune competence of the host. The organism in humans behaves as a facultative intracellular bacterium. Legionnaires' disease, a fulminant pneumonia caused by *Legionella pneumophila*, is the prototypic illness caused by these organisms. Pontiac fever is a self-limited, flulike syndrome that occurs in immunocompetent individuals. The spectrum of disease caused by these organisms is designated *legionellosis*.

HISTORY *Legionnaires' disease* refers to an epidemic of pneumonia that affected 221 people and caused 34 deaths during the American Legion Convention at the Bellevue-Stratford Hotel in Philadelphia during July and August 1976. Initially referred to as the *Legionnaires' disease agent*, the organism was shown to be a new species of bacterium and subsequently designated *L. pneumophila*. Serotyping revealed that this organism had been responsible for previous epidemics of pneumonia, including 20 cases of severe pneumonia among attendees at a convention in Philadelphia at the same hotel in 1974. Furthermore, in July 1968, 144 employees and visitors in a health department building in Pontiac, Michigan, developed a self-limited illness consisting of fever, myalgias, headache, and malaise, subsequently termed *Pontiac fever*. Exposure of guinea pigs to aerosols of water from the building's air conditioning system led to isolation of the organism, eventually identified as *L. pneumophila*.

The discovery of *L. pneumophila* led rapidly to the isolation of related organisms within the family Legionellaceae (Table 113-1). There are more than 50 species (33 named) and over 60 distinct serogroups. Many isolates cause pneumonia indistinguishable from that caused by the initial strain, designated *Legionella pneumophila* serotype 1. This isolate accounts for 50 percent of human infection, followed in frequency by serotype 6 (10 percent). *L. micdadei* (Pittsburgh pneumonia agent) accounts for 7 percent of cases. The serologically unrelated, unnamed legionellae are designated *Legionella*-like organisms (LLOs).

ETIOLOGY The legionellae are classified in a single genus, *Legionella*, within the family Legionellaceae. The legionellae are gram-negative, aerobic, nonencapsulated bacilli measuring 0.3 to 0.9 μm in width and 2 to 5 μm in length. They are non-spore-forming, and most are motile due to polar or subpolar flagellae. Electron microscopy reveals multiple fimbriae (pili) extending from the surface. Legionellae have complex growth requirements and do not grow on standard bacteriologic media. All species require supplementation of growth media with L-cysteine and ferric salts and grow best at pH 6.8 to 7.0. Legionellae display an unusual dependence on amino acids, as opposed to carbohydrates, for energy and carbon sources. The fatty acids of legionellae contain an unusually high proportion of branched-chain acids, permitting identification by gas-liquid chromatography.

In most clinical laboratories, legionellae are recognized by their growth on selective media. Identification is confirmed by serologic reactivity with defined antisera. A commercially available slide agglutination test identifies 22 *Legionella* species and 33 serogroups. Further identification of a *Legionella* isolate may require analysis in a reference laboratory. Biochemical analysis, autofluorescence, immunofluorescence staining, and gas-liquid chromatography are used to characterize different species and strains. Less widely available techniques include restriction endonuclease analysis, alloenzyme typing, and plasmid DNA profiling.

ECOLOGY AND TRANSMISSION Legionellae are ubiquitous in aquatic environments. Diverse natural *reservoirs* harbor these organisms, including mud, frozen streams, hot springs, and stagnant lakes. Certain algae provide all the nutritional and growth requirements for *L. pneumophila*. Some amebas and ciliated protozoa ingest legionellae and support their intracellular multiplication, protecting the bacteria from disinfectants and other adverse conditions. Legionellaceae have no animal or human reservoir.

Amplifiers are man-made water supplies that favor the growth of legionellae. Growth is enhanced by elevated temperatures (36 to 70°C), a source of iron and simple nutrients, and low levels of other competing bacteria. Hot water systems and heat exchange units are frequently contaminated due to stagnation, infrequent decontamination, and the presence of sediment or decayed plumbing, all of which contribute to suboptimal levels of chlorine. Decomposing rubber gaskets and sealing washers are capable of supporting the growth of these organisms. Legionellae have been isolated from such diverse man-made aqueous environments as potable water systems, ice machines, hot tubs, and humidifiers.

Disseminators facilitate transmission to the human respiratory tract by generating infectious aerosols. Airborne transmission by environmentally generated aerosols was suggested by epidemiologic evidence and has been reproduced in experimental animals. Aerosolized *L. pneumophila* can survive for more than 2 h and have been isolated nearly 1 mile downwind of cooling towers. Infectious aerosol particles are less than 5 μm in diameter and can be inhaled directly into the alveoli. A variety of sources have been identified in outbreaks of Legionnaires' disease, including cooling towers, air-conditioning systems, humidifiers, whirlpool baths, respiratory nebulizers, showers, and vegetable misters used in grocery stores. Aerosolized legionellae have been traced to contaminated soil disturbed by excavation and to industrial lubricants used to cool machinery.

Other routes of transmission may exist. Microaspiration of drinking water may be a mechanism of infection, particularly in sporadic, community-acquired disease. Postoperative wound infections have developed following exposure to contaminated tap water and whirlpool baths. There is no evidence of person-to-person transmission.

EPIDEMIOLOGY *Legionella* infections account for up to 7 percent of community-acquired pneumonias and, in some studies, up to one-fourth of "atypical" community-acquired pneumonias. *L. pneumophila* may be responsible for 10 percent of nosocomial pneumonias and as much as 30 percent during endemic hospital outbreaks. About half of adults show evidence of prior exposure to at least one *Legionella* species.

Legionella infections occur in epidemic outbreaks, sporadic cases,

TABLE 113-1 Identified *Legionella*

Species (serogroups)	Pneumonia	Pontiac fever	DFA*
L. pneumophila (15)	X	1,6[†]	1–10
L. micdadei	X	X	X
L. bozemanii (2)	X		1
L. dumoffii	X	?	X
L. gormanii	X		X
L. longbeachae (2)	X		1,2
L. jordanis	X		X
L. oakridgensis	X		
L. wadsworthii	X		
L. feeleii (2)	X	X	
L. sainthelensi (2)	X	?	
L. anisa	X		
L. maceachernii	X		
L. jamestownensis			
L. rubrilucens			
L. erythra			
L. hackeliae (2)	X		
L. spiritensis		?	
L. parisiensis			
L. cherrii	X		
L. steigerwaltii			
L. santicrucis			
L. israelensis			
L. cincinnatiensis	X		
L. quinlivanii			
L. birminghamensis	X		
L. moravica			
L. brunensis			
L. tucsonensis	X		
L. gratiana			
L. fairfieldensis			
L. adelaidensis			
L. shakespearei			
L. lansingensis	X		

* Direct fluorescent antibody reagents available.
† Numbers refer to serogroups.

or highly endemic clusters related to sustained nosocomial outbreaks. Both pneumonic and nonpneumonic legionelloses exist in epidemic form but differ in their attack rates and incubation periods. *Legionella* pneumonia has an attack rate of 1 to 7 percent, whereas Pontiac fever affects 95 to 100 percent of those exposed. The incubation period for pneumonia is 2 to 12 days, while that for nonpneumonic outbreaks is 24 to 48 h. There is a higher incidence of legionellosis during summer, presumably due to warmer water temperatures and increased use of water-cooling systems that transmit the organism.

Pneumonic legionellosis affects men three times as often as women and is uncommon in children. Other risk factors for pneumonic disease include cigarette smoking, heavy alcohol use, advanced age, chronic illness, and use of immunosuppressive medication. Organ transplant patients appear to be at particular risk. *Legionella* infection remains uncommon among patients infected with HIV. Nonpneumonic legionellosis has no demonstrable risk factors.

PATHOGENESIS AND PATHOLOGY Direct alveolar deposition of infectious aerosols containing legionellae is the predominant form of inoculation in *Legionella* infections. The short incubation period and the association with environmental aerosols are consistent with this mechanism. The inoculum of aerosolized bacteria and variability in virulence among strains may be important in determining the outcome of infection. Common-source exposures can result in nonpneumonic illness or severe pneumonia in different individuals, depending on the extent of exposure to infectious aerosols.

Legionellae appear to be susceptible to clearance by the mucociliary apparatus. Asymptomatic colonization does not occur, and during disease, pathologic findings are limited to the lower respiratory tract. Alveolar deposition via aerosol and factors, such as smoking, that impair mucociliary clearance permit the organism to establish infection within resident alveolar macrophages. In the human host, legionellae are facultative intracellular pathogens of monocytes and macrophages. The organisms activate complement by the classic pathway but are resistant to lysis. Mononuclear phagocytes ingest *L. pneumophila* by a mechanism termed *coiling phagocytosis* that is mediated by complement receptors CR1 and CR3 following C3 deposition on the major outer membrane protein of the bacterium. A surface protein designated *macrophage infectivity potentiator*, or mip, has been shown to enhance infectivity and virulence in experimental systems. Proteins for mip-related proteins are present in all *Legionella* species. Interestingly, the sequence of mip reveals significant homology to mammalian isomerases that bind the immunosuppressive drug FK506. Ingested organisms inhibit fusion of the phagosome to primary and secondary lysosomes, blocking the transfer of microbicidal substances into the phagosome and interfering with acidification of the vacuole. The sequestered organisms divide by binary fission within unusual vacuoles studded by host ribosomes and surrounded by glycogen granules and mitochondria. Continued replication results in lysis of the mononuclear cell and spread to adjacent cells. Both neutrophils and monocytes are recruited to the developing inflammatory lesion but are unable to inhibit bacterial growth efficiently. Specific antibody is produced, but the organisms remain resistant to antibody-mediated complement lysis. Phagocytosis is enhanced by specific antibody, thus further targeting the bacteria to the intracellular environment.

From the initial site, infection spreads by endobronchial, hematogenous, and lymphatic routes or by contiguous invasion. Bacteremia occurs in as many as one-third of patients with legionellosis and is the most common source of extrapulmonary infection.

As with infections due to other intracellular pathogens, *Legionella* infection is contained as cell-mediated immunity appears. Sensitized T lymphocytes secrete macrophage activating factors, primarily interferon-γ, that enable the cell to inhibit intracellular replication. Interleukin 2–activated natural killer cells are also capable of destroying *Legionella*-infected monocytes in vitro. The importance of cell-mediated immunity is supported by the increased incidence and severity of legionellosis among immunosuppressed patients, particularly transplant recipients.

Macroscopically, bronchopneumonia ranges from a patchy lobular process to more extensive multilobar consolidation. Round, nodular lesions are sometimes present. Abscesses with central necrosis occur in 25 percent of fatal cases. Pleuritis and small serosanguinous pleural effusions are common, but empyema is rare. Microscopically, infection is characterized by intense alveolitis and bronchiolitis. Alveolar spaces are filled with polymorphonuclear leukocytes, macrophages, fibrin, and proteinaceous exudate. Many inflammatory cells have undergone leukocytoclasis, leaving only nuclear debris and fibrin. Organisms can be visualized using the Gimenez stain, Dieterle silver impregnation stain, or direct fluorescent antibody and are predominantly located within phagocytes. Alveolar septae and interstitial spaces are thickened by edema and inflammatory cells. More severe disease, including diffuse alveolar damage with hyaline membrane formation, occurs in immunocompromised patients. Pathologic changes do not extend proximal to terminal bronchioles, a finding consistent with inoculation by aerosol. Pathologic changes are usually limited to the lungs. Brain tissue is normal even in cases with neurologic abnormalities.

CLINICAL MANIFESTATIONS Legionnaires' disease and Pontiac fever are the two well-described syndromes. The complete spectrum of infection by Legionellaceae remains undefined, however, and probably includes asymptomatic seroconversion, mild self-resolving illness, and isolated extrapulmonary manifestations.

Pneumonic illness typically begins with an abrupt prodrome of malaise, headache, myalgia, and weakness. Fever and intermittent rigors appear 24 h later, with temperatures exceeding 40°C in more than half of patients. Nonproductive cough is common. About half of patients eventually produce thin or minimally purulent sputum, and one-third may have scant hemoptysis. Pleuritic chest pain and dyspnea can raise the suspicion of pulmonary embolism. Gastrointestinal symptoms include diarrhea, nausea, vomiting, and abdominal pain. Altered mental status suggesting toxic encephalopathy may include confusion, disorientation, lethargy, hallucinations, depression, delirium, obtundation, or coma. Seizures are rare, but cranial or peripheral neuropathy and cerebellar dysfunction are not uncommon. Physical examination usually shows a toxic appearance and high fever. Relative bradycardia is common. Lung examination reveals rales and consolidation, but the physical findings are mild when compared to radiographic findings. Complications and systemic manifestations include lung abscess, empyema, respiratory failure, hypotension, shock, rhabdomyolysis, disseminated intravascular coagulation (DIC), thrombotic thrombocytopenic purpura (TTP), and renal failure.

Pontiac fever is an acute, self-limited illness lasting 2 to 5 days. A prodrome of malaise, myalgia, and headache is followed rapidly by fever, chills, and, variably, cough, coryza, and sore throat. Diarrhea, nausea, and mild neurologic symptoms such as dizziness or photophobia may be present.

Legionellae also may cause extrapulmonary infections related to bacteremia at the time of pneumonia or local exposure to contaminated water. Pericarditis, myocarditis, pyelonephritis, pancreatitis, sinusitis, peritonitis, and hemodialysis fistula infections; abscesses in liver, skin, and the perirectal area; and postoperative wound infections have been reported. *L. pneumophila* and *L. dumoffii* can cause subacute and chronic prosthetic valve endocarditis with annular and myocardial abscesses. The organisms are nosocomially acquired during the perioperative period when the primary infection may cause a postpericardiotomy-like syndrome. Emboli are rare.

LABORATORY FINDINGS *Legionella* pneumonia is usually accompanied by leukocytosis with an increase in early granulocyte forms; the total leukocyte count exceeds 20,000 cells per microliter in 10 to 20 percent of cases. None of the laboratory abnormalities associated with pneumonic legionellosis is specific, although hyponatremia occurs in 50 to 70 percent, more commonly than in other forms of pneumonia. Other laboratory findings may include hypophosphatemia, azotemia, microhematuria, proteinuria, and abnormal tests of liver function. Hematologic findings are typically normal unless the illness is complicated by DIC or TTP. Cerebrospinal fluid examination is usually normal, although pleocytosis and elevated protein have been reported. Gram stain of the sputum may show inflammatory cells, but legionellae stain poorly or not at all in clinical specimens. *L. micdadei* is acid-fast by Kinyoun and modified Ziehl-Neelsen stains.

Early roentgenographic patterns include diffuse patchy infiltrates or ill-defined nodular densities. Pneumonia progresses to bilateral infiltrates in 50 percent of patients; a lobar-segmental pattern predominates. Small pleural effusions are present in 20 to 50 percent. Cavitation is uncommon but may occasionally be seen, particularly in immunosuppressed patients.

Leukocytosis is frequently the only laboratory abnormality in Pontiac fever.

DIAGNOSIS The diagnosis of *Legionella* infection may be made by culturing the organism, identifying its antigens or nucleic acids in tissue or secretions, or demonstrating a serologic response in the host (Table 113-2). A positive culture is diagnostic, since no carrier state occurs. Cultures are performed on buffered charcoal yeast extract agar with α-ketoglutarate (BCYE-α agar), but 2 to 5 days may be required to identify the organism. BCYE-α agar is not selective, and supplementation with antibiotics or acidification is required for sputum samples to inhibit the growth of other bacteria. Typical results of the culture of clinical specimens are listed in Table 113-2. Blood cultures must be subcultured on BCYE-α agar after 24 h of aerobic incubation.

Legionellae may be visualized in clinical specimens by direct fluorescent antibody (DFA) staining. Clinical specimens are treated with fluorescein-conjugated rabbit antibody and examined by fluorescence microscopy. The test requires only 2 to 4 h. Commercially available DFA reagents detect over 90 percent of strains responsible for clinical disease (see Table 113-1). However, the relatively low sensitivity (50 percent) and the need for an experienced technician are disadvantages. DFA may be less sensitive after a patient has received appropriate antibiotics.

Available tests for *Legionella* antigens in urine include an enzyme-linked immunosorbent assay, radioimmunoassay, and latex agglutination. The relative ease of specimen collection and assay performance may make urinary diagnosis an attractive rapid test. However, antigenuria may persist for months, obscuring the distinction between acute and past infection. A radiolabeled nucleic acid hybridization kit is moderately sensitive and detects all *Legionella* species, although false-positive results have been reported. The radioactive isotope limits the shelf life of the assay.

Serum antibody is most commonly measured by the indirect fluorescent antibody (IFA) assay. Routinely available reagents detect antibody directed only against *L. pneumophila* serogroup 1, believed to account for half of human disease. A diagnosis of legionellosis is made by a fourfold rise in titer between acute and convalescent sera to at least 1:128 or by a single titer of 1:256 or greater. Serum samples should be obtained acutely and after 3 weeks, although as many as one-fourth of patients may seroconvert within the first week of illness. Seroconversion develops in 80 percent of patients by 10 weeks.

While no clinical features of *Legionella* pneumonia are unique, the diagnosis should be suspected in a patient with severe pneumonia, high fever, nonproductive cough, hyponatremia, and altered mental status, particularly in the setting of immunosuppression. Each of the tests employed to diagnose legionellosis has its limitations. Combined approaches are recommended. No diagnostic test may be used to exclude the disease absolutely. Thus clinical judgment must often prevail in decisions regarding therapy.

The diagnosis of Pontiac fever requires a compatible clinical illness, evidence of serologic conversion, and, preferably, isolation of the organism from the environment. Viable legionellae have never been isolated from a case of Pontiac fever, raising the possibility that the pathogenesis involves hypersensitivity to bacterial antigens rather than true infection.

TREATMENT Erythromycin is the antibiotic of choice for pneumonic legionellosis. For serious infection, patients should receive 4 g/d intravenously. Dosage reduction may be necessary in renal or hepatic failure to avoid ototoxicity. Immunocompromised patients and those with severe disease should receive rifampin (rifampicin) concurrently in a dose of 600 mg twice daily. Immunosuppressive medications should be tapered when possible. Response to therapy occurs in 24 to 48 h, although fever may persist for up to a week. With improvement, erythromycin may be reduced to 2 g/d orally. Therapy should continue for 3 weeks; shorter courses have been associated with relapse. Doxycycline, trimethoprim-sulfamethoxazole, ciprofloxacin, and other quinolones are potential alternatives when erythromycin is not tolerated or in the rare patients failing to respond to erythromycin. Clarithromycin also has been effective in treating severe legionellosis. Effective antibiotics are those which diffuse readily into phagocytic cells, suggesting that their role may be to arrest intracellular multiplication until effective cellular immunity develops.

Legionella prosthetic valve endocarditis usually requires valve replacement and prolonged antibiotic therapy (3 to 12 months). Pontiac fever is a self-limited illness requiring no therapy.

PROGNOSIS AND IMMUNITY Overall case fatality rates for *Legionella* pneumonia are approximately 15 percent. Mortality is 80 percent among untreated immunosuppressed patients and is reduced to 25 percent with appropriate antibiotic treatment. Untreated immunocompetent hosts have a 25 percent mortality rate; with proper therapy, only 7 percent succumb.

Patients who survive usually have no permanent sequelae. Full recovery of pulmonary function is usual, although pulmonary fibrosis with respiratory disability has been reported. Immunocompetent individuals who recover from infection are immune to reinfection with the same strain. Reinfection with an identical serotype has been reported in an immunocompromised patient.

PREVENTION AND CONTROL Understanding the chain of transmission of legionellae from natural reservoirs to man-made amplifiers and disseminators is important in devising control strategies. Surveillance efforts should concentrate on documenting human infection, rather than routinely screening the environment. During epidemic or endemic outbreaks, sentinel cases occur among immunosuppressed patients. Once detected, a careful search for the environmental source should be conducted. Multiple legionellae may be recovered from environmental cultures, many of which are not associated with human disease. Therefore, clinical isolates should be characterized so that control measures can focus on the source of pathogenic strains. Legionellosis is a reportable infection, and local health departments can provide assistance in the isolation and characterization of environmental strains.

Sources of environmental aerosols (disseminators), such as shower heads and air-conditioning systems, must be identified so that transmission can be interrupted. Contaminated water systems (amplifiers) can be sterilized. Legionellae may be present in low titer in potable water systems and may thus require culture of large volumes on selective media or pretreatment with heat or acid to enhance recovery. Rusted plumbing and decayed rubber gaskets should be replaced. Sites of stagnation and sediment in water tanks may require elimination. Decontamination of potable water systems is accomplished by hyperchlorination (2 to 3 ppm) and/or intermittent

---

TABLE 113-2 Laboratory tests in Legionnaires' disease

Test	Sensitivity, %	Specificity, %
Culture		
Sputum	60	100
Transtracheal	80	100
Lung biopsy	90	100
Blood	38	100
DFA	50	95
Urine antigen*	80	99
DNA probe	70	99
Serology (IFA)*	80	99

* *L. pneumophila* serogroup 1 only.

heating to 60°C with flushing of distal outlets. During nosocomial outbreaks, prophylactic treatment of high-risk patients with oral erythromycin has been effective. Periodic monitoring of hospital water may be necessary to detect reemergence of the organism.

REFERENCES

CIANCIOTTO NP et al: A mutation in the *mip* gene results in attenuation of *Legionella pneumophila* virulence. J Infect Dis 162:121, 1990

FANG GD et al: Disease due to the Legionellaceae (other than *Legionella pneumophila*): Historical, microbiological, clinical, and epidemiologic review. Medicine 68:116, 1989

FRASER DW et al: Legionnaire's disease: Description of an epidemic of pneumonia. N Engl J Med 297:1189, 1977

LOWRY PW et al: A cluster of *Legionella* sternal-wound infections due to postoperative topical exposure to contaminated tap water. N Engl J Med 324:109, 1991

MASTRO TD et al: Nosocomial Legionnaires' disease and use of medication nebulizers. J Infect Dis 163:667, 1991

NGUYEN MH et al: Legionellosis. Infect Dis Clin North Am 5:561, 1991

SNYDER MB et al: Reduction in *Legionella pneumophila* through heat flushing followed by continuous supplemental chlorination of hospital hot water. J Infect Dis 162:127, 1990

STOUT JE et al: Potable water as a cause of sporadic cases of community-acquired Legionnaires' disease. N Engl J Med 326:151, 1992

114   PERTUSSIS

GEORGE R. SIBER / MATTHEW H. SAMORE

DEFINITION   Pertussis, or whooping cough, is an acute infection of the respiratory tract caused by *Bordetella pertussis*. The name *pertussis*, coined by Sydenham in 1679, means "violent cough" and describes the most characteristic feature of this disease. The Chinese call this illness "the cough of 100 days" because of its chronic nature. A dramatic inspiratory whoop following a paroxysmal cough is a hallmark of severe pertussis in children but is frequently absent, particularly in infants and adults. Thus the term *whooping cough* may mislead clinicians by implying that whoops are an essential feature of the disease.

The clinical features that should suggest pertussis are a chronic cough lasting 2 weeks or longer and coughing spells that are typically sudden in onset and paroxysmal in nature. The episodes may, in severe cases, be followed by a whoop or vomiting. Fever is absent or low, unless a superinfection has occurred. An absolute lymphocytosis may provide an additional clue to the diagnosis, particularly in unimmunized children.

MICROBIOLOGY   The etiologic agent of pertussis, *B. pertussis*, was first isolated by Bordet and Gengou in 1900 using the medium that bears their names. Humans are the only known host of *B. pertussis*. Other species in the genus include *B. parapertussis*, which is associated with a milder, less chronic respiratory illness in humans, and *B. bronchiseptica*, an animal pathogen that on rare occasions causes respiratory or opportunistic infections in humans.

B. pertussis is a small, nonmotile, gram-negative coccobacillus that is slow growing and fastidious in its growth requirements. After 3 to 6 days of growth at 36°C on special medium such as Bordet-Gengou agar, glistening pinpoint colonies with surrounding zones of hemolysis appear. Preliminary identification is accomplished by direct fluorescent antibody staining or by agglutination with antiserum to *B. pertussis*. *B. pertussis* is distinguished from *B. bronchiseptica* and *B. parapertussis* by further tests such as motility and nitrate reduction. *B. pertussis*, *B. parapertussis*, and *B. bronchiseptica* show extensive DNA homology and share many non-virulence-related enzymes and some virulence factors. However, only *B. pertussis* expresses pertussis toxin.

Like many other bacterial pathogens, *B. pertussis* possesses a precise mechanism for coordinated regulation of its virulence factors that is under control of a central genetic locus. This process is typically mediated by a two-component system consisting of a sensory protein and a regulatory protein which transmits specific environmental signals to regulatory genes. In *B. pertussis*, the central regulatory locus is called the *Bordetella* virulence gene (*bvg*). Reversible down-regulation of virulence factors (i.e., pertussis toxin, filamentous hemagglutinin, pertactin, fimbriae, adenyl cyclase, dermonecrotic toxin) and up-regulation of other proteins occur in response to environmental stimuli such as high sulfate, high nicotinic acid, or low temperature. This process, called *antigenic modulation*, is mediated by transmembrane sensory protein (BvgS) and a gene regulatory factor (BvgA). In addition, mutations in the *bvg* locus that occur at a frequency of 10^{-3} to 10^{-6} organisms may abolish expression of virulence factors. This process is called *phase variation*.

Both antigenic modulation and phase variation occur in vitro and in vivo. It is likely that these processes play a critical role in the ecology of the organism and its adaptation to the environment. It has been suggested that phase variation or antigenic modulation may facilitate expulsion of the organism from the respiratory tract by lowering adherence, enable it to survive hostile environmental conditions during transmission, or enable it to survive intracellularly in a quiescent state protected from attack by immune mechanisms directed toward its virulence factors.

PATHOGENESIS   *B. pertussis* initiates colonization of the respiratory tract by adhering to ciliated epithelial cells, grows to high numbers producing local mucosal damage, and induces the paroxysmal cough which enhances its expulsion and transmission to contacts. A number of virulence factors that enable the organism to produce this cycle of events have been described. Fimbriae or pili, hairlike appendages on the surface of the organism, may play a role in the initial stages of adherence to ciliated cells. The fimbriae induce serotype-specific agglutinating antibodies (agglutinins) and are therefore called *agglutinogens*. Filamentous hemagglutinin, a large 220-kDa rodlike surface protein, and pertactin, a 69-kDa protein residing in the outer membrane, enable the organism to adhere closely to ciliated and other mammalian cells. Both these adherence factors have arginine, glycine, aspartic acid repeat sequences (RGD) typical of eukaryotic adhesins that stick to the integrin family of mammalian cell surface proteins.

A variety of toxins then impair local defenses (tracheal cytotoxin by inducing ciliostasis and adenyl cyclase by inhibiting phagocytes) and cause local tissue damage (tracheal cytotoxin and dermonecrotic toxin), thereby enhancing the supply of nutrients and perhaps facilitating systemic absorption of pertussis toxin. Pertussis toxin conforms to the general A/B model of enzymatic bacterial exotoxins. It contains an enzymatic moiety, the A subunit, consisting of a single peptide (S1), and a binding moiety, the B-oligomer, consisting of four peptides (S2, S3, S4, and S5) in a molar ratio of 1:1:2:1. The B-oligomer adheres to mammalian cells and delivers the A subunit to its targets. The B-oligomer exerts some biologic functions directly (e.g., mitogenesis of T cells) and may contribute to adherence of the whole organism to mammalian cells. The A subunit transfers ADP-ribose from NAD to certain members of a family of guanine nucleotide–binding regulatory membrane proteins (G proteins) in target cells. By this mechanism pertussis toxin produces a variety of biologic effects, including the inhibition of normal lymphocyte migration, which results in lymphocytosis (lymphocytosis-promoting factor), the sensitization of mice to histamine and serotonin (histamine-sensitizing factor), the enhancement of insulin secretion in response to regulatory signals such as beta-adrenergic stimulation (islet-activating protein), and the enhancement of certain immune functions such as the production of IgG and IgE class antibodies.

The mechanisms whereby the organism produces the paroxysmal cough typical of pertussis have not been elucidated. The best evidence that pertussis toxin plays a critical role in producing the pertussis syndrome was provided by studies in which infants immunized only with pertussis toxoid had an 80 to 90 percent lower rate of severe pertussis than did controls.

EPIDEMIOLOGY Pertussis is a highly communicable disease, with attack rates of 90 to 100 percent in nonimmune household contacts. Transmission of the organism is mediated via exposure to respiratory droplets expelled in large numbers by symptomatic individuals.

Before the introduction of pertussis vaccine in the late 1940s, 115,000 to 270,000 cases of pertussis were reported annually in the United States (average incidence 150 per 100,000 population per year). Epidemics of pertussis recurred at 3- to 4-year intervals without significant seasonality. Incidence was highest in children aged 1 to 5 years and was 10 to 20 percent higher in females than in males. In infants, attack rates were lower than in older children, perhaps due to maternally derived antibodies. However, case fatality rates were highest in infants. During the years 1940–1948, pertussis caused more infant deaths than did diphtheria, polio, measles, meningitis, and scarlet fever combined. Most adults were immune due to long-lasting protection induced by natural disease and perhaps boosting by frequent reexposure.

The incidence of pertussis declined 100- to 150-fold after adoption of universal whole-cell pertussis vaccination. Discontinuation or curtailment of pertussis vaccine use was associated with a rapid resurgence of pertussis in countries such as Great Britain, Sweden, and Japan. In the United States, the incidence of pertussis has been increasing gradually after reaching a low point in the mid-1970s; an average of 2783 cases were reported per year from 1980 to 1989. The reported incidence of pertussis is highest in young infants and declines with age. Approximately two-thirds of children with pertussis in the United States have not received the appropriate number of immunizations for their age group. In developed countries, mortality from pertussis has declined markedly. In the United States, the case-fatality rate is 0.4 percent overall but 1.3 percent in infants less than 2 months of age. From 1980 to 1989, infants less than 1 year of age accounted for 50 percent of reported pertussis cases and 79 percent of pertussis deaths.

Epidemiologic studies suggest that the actual incidence of pertussis is much higher than estimates based on passively reported cases. Only one-third of patients hospitalized with pertussis and an even smaller proportion of patients with less severely symptomatic pertussis are reported to the Centers for Disease Control and Prevention. Furthermore, pertussis rates continue to peak cyclically at 3- to 4-year intervals, indicating that widespread transmission still occurs in the population despite childhood immunization.

Persons aged 15 years or older comprised 13 percent of pertussis cases reported from 1980 to 1989 in the United States. The proportion of all cases that were within this age group rose during this period. In some states with active surveillance and serologic investigation of outbreaks, the proportion of pertussis in adolescents and adults is much higher. Data from pertussis outbreaks indicate that vaccine-induced protective immunity wanes after about 12 years, in contrast to natural pertussis, which usually induces life-long immunity. Consequently, a progressively larger proportion of adolescents and adults are susceptible to pertussis. Large outbreaks of pertussis that have occurred in schools, nursing homes, hospitals, and residential facilities indicate the high transmissibility of this organism in susceptible adolescent and adult populations.

Careful studies of household contacts show that while 40 to 80 percent of family members have serologic evidence of infection, only one-third to one-half of them were ever clinically symptomatic. Symptomatic undiagnosed pertussis in adults is believed to be an important source of transmission to infants and children and a mechanism of perpetuating the disease in the population. There is no evidence that asymptomatic individuals transmit *B. pertussis* to others. Chronic carriers of pertussis have not been identified.

CLINICAL MANIFESTATIONS Pertussis is typically a prolonged illness, with an average duration of 6 to 8 weeks. The incubation period ranges from 5 to 14 days but is usually 7 to 10 days. The symptoms of pertussis generally evolve through three stages: the catarrhal, the paroxysmal, and the convalescent. The catarrhal stage lasts 1 to 2 weeks and is characterized by nonspecific symptoms of coryza, mild cough, lacrimation, malaise, and low-grade fever. The paroxysmal stage, which usually lasts 2 to 4 weeks, is characterized by the paroxysmal cough, defined as sudden, forceful, repetitive coughing. The number of coughs per spasm is variable, ranging from 10 to 30; the paroxysms of pertussis characteristically occur during a single exhalation, a feature useful in distinguishing it from the repetitive cough caused by other pathogens in which there are inspirations between coughs. In severe cases, the physical effort associated with each spasm may be extreme, and there may be neck vein distention, bulging of the eyes, and cyanosis. The distinctive whoop is heard in 40 to 60 percent of pediatric cases and is due to sudden inspiration against a closed glottis at the end of the paroxysm. The paroxysm, which often results in the expectoration of viscous respiratory secretions, may be triggered by external stimuli, such as loud noises or physical contact. Typically, 10 to 25 paroxysms occur per 24-h period, with disruption of nocturnal sleep. Posttussive vomiting is common and should be considered suggestive of pertussis. Fever is generally absent during the paroxysmal stage, unless there is bacterial superinfection. Most complications of pertussis occur during the paroxysmal stage. The convalescent stage is defined by the gradual waning in intensity of the cough. Complete resolution of the cough may require several months, and superimposed viral or bacterial respiratory infections may lead to severe clinical exacerbations with recurrence of paroxysmal coughing.

An absolute lymphocytosis is a characteristic but not universal laboratory finding in children with pertussis. Typically, the total white blood cell count ranges between 10,000 and 30,000 cells per microliter, with 50 to 75 percent lymphocytes. Lymphocytosis is much less common in teenagers and adults.

The most common presentation of pertussis in adolescents and adults is cough, with or without paroxysms, persisting for 2 weeks or more. Other useful clinical clues are shortness of breath during coughing spells, nocturnal cough, a tingling sensation in the back of the throat, posttussive vomiting, and a history of exposure to other patients with prolonged coughing illness. Whooping and lymphocytosis are infrequently present. Thus, as the pool of susceptible adults increases, this nonclassical presentation of pertussis has become more common than the classical presentation seen in preschool children.

B. pertussis has been isolated from human immunodeficiency virus–infected patients with chronic respiratory symptoms. It is not known whether the incidence of pertussis is increased in these patients.

COMPLICATIONS Minor complications of pertussis secondary to increased intrathoracic pressure include subconjunctival hemorrhage and upper torso petechiae. Episodes of cyanosis and apnea are common in infants and small children (prevalence 20 to 50 percent). Malnutrition and weight loss may occur because of inadequate caloric intake. The major respiratory complication of pertussis is pneumonia, usually a secondary infection due to encapsulated bacterial pathogens such as *Streptococcus pneumoniae* and *Haemophilus influenzae*. Pneumonia is more common in infants (incidence 21 percent) than in children aged 1 to 2 (12 percent) or in adults (3 percent). Nonimmune infants may develop a severe primary pneumonia due to *B. pertussis*. Neurologic complications are infrequent and include encephalopathy (0.7 percent) and seizures (2 percent). The mechanisms of pertussis-associated encephalopathy, though unknown, are postulated to include hypoxia, hypoglycemia due to pertussis toxin, hemorrhages secondary to increased venous pressure, effects of neurotoxins, and co-infection by neurotoxic viruses.

DIAGNOSIS Laboratory confirmation should be attempted in all cases of suspected pertussis. The standard diagnostic test is isolation of *B. pertussis* on nasopharyngeal swab culture. A calcium alginate swab is inserted into the nares and maintained in contact with the nasopharynx for 10 s to permit moistening. The swab should be placed immediately into transport medium (such as Regan-Lowe charcoal medium) or plated directly onto fresh Bordet-Gengou agar or other suitable agar. A nasopharyngeal aspirate collected with a syringe attached to a fine plastic catheter is a suitable alternative specimen and should be handled in the same fashion. Growth typically requires 3 to 5 days of incubation at 36°C. Suspicious colonies may be presumptively identified by direct fluorescent antibody staining or agglutination. The fluorescein-labeled antibody also may be used to detect organisms directly in nasopharyngeal secretions but with less sensitivity and specificity than culture. Nasopharyngeal cultures are positive in 70 to 80 percent of cases when obtained within 2 weeks of the onset of symptoms (during the catarrhal and early paroxysmal stage). The diagnostic yield declines rapidly thereafter. By 4 weeks, cultures are rarely positive. Newer diagnostic tests, such as detection of *B. pertussis*–specific DNA from nasopharyngeal swabs by polymerase chain reaction, promise to enhance the detection of this organism.

Serologic tests for pertussis have been used more frequently in outbreak and contact investigation than for routine clinical diagnosis. Typically, ELISA is used to measure IgG and IgA antibodies to filamentous hemagglutinin and to pertussis toxin in acute and convalescent sera. High titers of one or more of these antibodies on a single specimen (e.g., >3 SD above the mean of appropriately matched controls) or a significant rise in at least one of the antibody titers is considered diagnostic evidence of pertussis. However, antibody levels increase early in the disease course, particularly in previously immunized individuals, so that in practice the rise in titer is frequently missed. Serologic assays are particularly useful in evaluating adults in whom the disease was not suspected until more than 2 weeks after onset, when cultures are no longer sensitive. Adequately standardized serologic assays for pertussis are not yet available in most areas of the United States.

DIFFERENTIAL DIAGNOSIS A variety of respiratory pathogens may cause paroxysmal cough. However, the constellation of prolonged (>2 weeks) paroxysmal cough accompanied by whoops and lymphocytosis is highly specific for *B. pertussis*. *B. parapertussis* typically causes a milder respiratory illness. Although the organisms are distinct species, *B. parapertussis* and *B. pertussis* are occasionally associated epidemiologically. They have been isolated from the same patients simultaneously or sequentially.

Viruses such as respiratory syncytial virus and adenovirus have been isolated from patients with clinical pertussis (with or without isolation of *B. pertussis*). However, there is no convincing evidence that these viruses alone can cause the full pertussis syndrome with whooping and lymphocytosis.

TREATMENT **Antibiotics** The major aim of antibiotics is to eradicate *B. pertussis* from the respiratory tract. Erythromycin, preferably the estolate form, at a dose of 50 mg/kg per day (maximum 2 g/d) in two to four divided doses, reliably eradicates the organism from nasopharyngeal cultures within 5 days. Treatment should be continued for a full 14 days to prevent bacteriologic relapse. Patients unable to tolerate erythromycin may be treated with trimethoprim-sulfamethoxazole (8/40 mg/kg per day in two divided doses), but its efficacy is unproven.

Erythromycin ameliorates the clinical illness when begun during the catarrhal phase. According to classic teaching, antibiotics have little effect once paroxysmal cough occurs, but recent studies indicate some reduction in whooping when erythromycin is begun within 2 weeks of onset of paryoxysmal cough.

Supportive care Infants have the highest rates of complications and death due to pertussis. Accordingly, most infants and those older patients with severe pertussis should be hospitalized. Supportive care includes monitoring for apnea and cyanosis, gentle nasotracheal suctioning, oxygen, hydration, and nutritional support. Glucocorticoids and the beta-adrenergic stimulant salbutamol have been advocated but not proven to be effective. Cough suppressants are ineffective.

Isolation of hospitalized patients Patients should be placed on respiratory isolation for 5 days after initiation of erythromycin or for 3 weeks if unable to tolerate appropriate antimicrobial therapy.

PREVENTION **Management of contacts** All household and other close contacts, whether children or adults and irrespective of immunization status, should receive chemoprophylaxis with erythromycin (preferably the estolate) at 40 to 50 mg/kg per day in four divided doses (maximum 2 g/d) for 14 days. Prompt use of erythromycin is effective in limiting secondary transmission. Children younger than 7 years should have pertussis immunization initiated or continued according to the recommended schedule.

Vaccines The vaccine currently used for primary immunization of infants consists of killed whole-cell pertussis organisms combined with diphtheria and tetanus toxoids (DTP) adsorbed to aluminum phosphate adjuvant. The standard schedule involves three primary doses at 2-month intervals initiated at 6 to 8 weeks of age, followed by booster doses at 15 to 18 months and 4 to 6 years of age. The vaccine is not recommended for anyone above the age of 6 but has been used in special circumstances for control of nosocomial outbreaks.

The whole-cell vaccine is believed to be 80 to 95 percent efficacious in preventing pertussis during 3 years following immunization. Thereafter, protective immunity wanes, with attack rates reaching 95 percent in household contacts exposed more than 12 years after immunization. Fortunately, the disease in previously immunized individuals is usually mild.

Injection of DTP containing a whole-cell pertussis component is associated with a variety of adverse effects. Local reactions and fever occur after one-third to one-half of injections and are maximal during the first 24 h. Fever of 40.5°C (105°F) or greater occurs after 1 in 300 doses, persistent crying (>3 h) after 1 in 100 doses, and high-pitched, unusual crying after 1 in 1000 doses. More severe reactions include seizures, which are usually febrile (1 in 1750 doses), and collapse or shocklike state (1 in 1750 doses).

There appears to be an excess incidence of acute neurologic illness during the 7 days after DTP administration, but the rate is extremely low, and a causal relationship with the vaccine has not been shown. There is no evidence for a causal relation between DTP administration and chronic neurologic illnesses, infantile spasms, or sudden infant death syndrome. Anaphylaxis is estimated to occur 1 in 50,000 DTP doses.

Two acellular pertussis vaccines formulated with diphtheria and tetanus toxoids (DTaP) have been licensed in the United States for use as booster doses at 15 to 18 months and 4 to 6 years of age in children previously immunized with three primary doses of whole-cell DTP. Both DTaP vaccines contain acellular pertussis components developed and manufactured by Japanese manufacturers. The Biken-type vaccine contains purified formalin-treated pertussis toxin and filamentous hemagglutinin. The Takeda-type vaccine contains a mixture of formalinized antigens including filamentous hemagglutinin, the predominant component, as well as smaller amounts of pertussis toxin, pertactin, and agglutinogen 2. Both acellular pertussis vaccines have shown epidemiologic evidence of efficacy in children 2 years of age or older in Japan, and both induce booster antibody responses to their constituent antigens similar to those of whole-cell pertussis vaccine. Both DTaP vaccines produce significantly fewer local reactions, fever, and other systemic symptoms than does whole-cell DTP and are therefore preferred for booster immunization in children. Whether rare severe reactions are less frequent after DTaP administration is unknown.

Licensure of DTaP vaccines for primary immunization of infants awaits the outcome of clinical efficacy studies currently underway comparing DTaP vaccines containing from 1 to 5 purified pertussis antigens and whole-cell DTP vaccine.

Neither DTaP nor whole-cell DTP vaccine is currently approved for use in adults. Whole-cell DTP has been used rarely in the control of hospital outbreaks of pertussis but is associated with high rates of adverse reactions. Routine use of DTaP vaccines in adults may offer a means for reducing symptomatic pertussis in older children and adults, thereby enhancing herd immunity and reducing transmission to incompletely immunized infants and children. However, further studies are needed before this approach can be recommended routinely.

REFERENCES

ADDISS DG et al: A pertussis outbreak in a Wisconsin nursing home. J Infect Dis 164:704, 1991

AD HOC GROUP FOR THE STUDY OF PERTUSSIS VACCINES: Placebo-controlled trial of two acellular pertussis vaccines in Sweden: Protective efficacy and adverse events. Lancet 1:955, 1988

AOYAMA T et al: Pertussis in adults. Am J Dis Child 146:163, 1992

COOTE JG: Antigenic switching and pathogenicity: Enviromental effects on virulence gene expression in *Bordetella pertussis*. J Gen Microbiol 137:2493, 1991

FARIZO KM et al: Epidemiological features of pertussis in the United States, 1980–1989. Clin Infect Dis 14:708, 1992

HERWALDT LA: Pertussis in adults: What physicians need to know. Arch Intern Med 151:1510, 1991

KELLER MA et al: Etiology of pertussis syndrome. Pediatrics 66:50, 1980

LONG SS et al: Widespread silent transmission of pertussis in families: Antibody correlates of infection and symptomatology. J Infect Dis 161:480, 1990

MINK CAM et al: A search for *Bordetella pertussis* infection in university students. Clin Infect Dis 14:464, 1992

Pertussis outbreaks: Massachusetts and Maryland, 1992. Morb Mort Week Rep 11:197, 1993

OLSON LC: Pertussis. Medicine 54:427, 1975

PITTMAN M: The concept of pertussis as a toxin-mediated disease. Pediatr Infect Dis J 3:467, 1984

STEKETEE RW et al: Evidence for a high attack rate and efficacy of erythromycin prophylaxis in a pertussis outbreak in a facility for the developmentally disabled. J Infect Dis 157:434, 1988

SUTTER RW, COCHI SL: Pertussis hospitalizations and mortality in the United States, 1985–1988. JAMA 267:386, 1992

115 DISEASES CAUSED BY GRAM-NEGATIVE ENTERIC BACILLI
(*Escherichia coli, Klebsiella, Enterobacter, Serratia, Proteus, Morganella, Providencia,* and *Acinetobacter*)

BARRY I. EISENSTEIN

The gram-negative enteric bacilli frequently reside in the human colon without causing disease. They also normally colonize other environmental niches with which hospitalized patients come in contact. Because of their ubiquity within and outside the body, they often cause opportunistic infections, such as pneumonia, in debilitated patients. As a group, the enteric bacteria account for approximately one-third of the septicemia isolates, two-thirds of the bacterial gastroenteritis isolates, and three-quarters of the urinary tract isolates in all infected patients. One of the organisms, *Escherichia coli,* is also the most frequent cause of urinary tract infection and of bacterial gastroenteritis in otherwise healthy individuals.

GENERAL PROPERTIES

CLASSIFICATION AND PHYSIOLOGY These organisms belong to the family Enterobacteriaceae, which includes other pathogens (*Shigella, Edwardsiella, Salmonella, Citrobacter, Yersinia*) discussed elsewhere. Some characteristics of members of this family are the lack of spore formation, the ability to grow both aerobically and anaerobically (i.e., facultative anaerobes), the ability to ferment glucose to acid, lack of oxidase production, and variable motility (depending on the presence of flagella).

STRUCTURE Enterobacteriaceae share with all bacteria a peptidoglycan-containing cell wall, a single circular chromosome consisting of double-stranded DNA located throughout the cytoplasm, and prokaryote-type ribosomes (see Chap. 99). These structures are different enough from those of eukaryotes to make them ideal targets for antimicrobial chemotherapy (see Chap. 100). For example, β-lactam antibiotics, the most frequently used agents for these organisms, bind to the bacterial cytoplasmic membrane and inhibit the cross-linking of the peptidoglycan. Gram-negative bacteria possess a unique multilayered cell envelope consisting of the typical inner (cytoplasmic) membrane, a surrounding polymeric peptidoglycan, and a complex outer membrane. The outer layer contains lipopolysaccharide (LPS or endotoxin), porins (multimeric proteins that are important channels for the penetration of antimicrobials and nutrients), and the polysaccharide capsule, which generally serves an antiphagocytic function. Many bacterial strains with intrinsic or acquired drug resistance contain porins that are impermeable to at least some antimicrobial agents.

Three classes of surface antigens have been used for serotyping for the clonal identification of *E. coli* and *Salmonella* strains: (1) the O or somatic antigens, (2) the H or flagellar antigens, and (3) the K or capsular antigens. (At present, genetically based methods are the preferred way of identifying bacteria both for taxonomy and epidemiology.) All gram-negative bacteria have the core part of LPS, which includes the toxic moiety, lipid A, responsible for the endotoxic shock seen in many episodes of bacteremia. Most pathogenic strains (at least in *E. coli*) also contain O antigens, which are repeating polysaccharide side chains attached to the core LPS. The O antigenic types are widely shared among all the Enterobacteriaceae, but in some cases cross-reactivity is particularly pronounced, even extending to cell-surface antigens from mammalian tissue. These O antigens are found on "smooth" strains and distinguish them from "rough" strains (terms that refer to differences in colonial morphology) and, along with other surface factors, mediate bacterial resistance to the killing effect of normal serum. Serum-resistant isolates, by surviving longer in the bloodstream, typically cause more severe disease.

A number of the O, H, and K serogroupings of *E. coli* act as markers for strains capable of causing a particular infectious disease; these strains also possess additional virulence factors required for pathogenesis. Thus certain O serogroups possess adhesive/colonization factors needed for urinary tract infection, other O serogroups have colonization factors and toxins that cause gastroenteritis, and another O serogroup is associated with the hemolytic-uremic syndrome. H antigens, which are proteins found on bacterial flagella, are also linked to the hemolytic-uremic syndrome (i.e., serogroup O157:H7), and the K1 capsular antigen is associated with neonatal meningitis, bacteremia, and urinary tract infection.

THE HOST-PARASITE INTERACTION Many enteric bacteria, like relatively nonpathogenic strains of *E. coli*, colonize the gastrointestinal tract without causing symptoms. Significant disease requires either an exceptionally virulent organism, debilitated host (or one with broached defenses), or some combination of the two. A particularly pathogenic bacterium, such as *Shigella dysenteriae*, can produce dysentery even in normal hosts. A normally colonizing bacterium, such as a commensal strain of *E. coli*, can produce peritonitis or bacteremia in an otherwise healthy individual with a ruptured appendix or in a granulocytopenic individual receiving chemotherapy for cancer. A moderately pathogenic bacterium, such as K1-encapulated strains of *E. coli*, can cause meningitis in newborns, who are particularly susceptible to this illness.

Regardless of the initial state of the host defenses, disease due to enteric bacteria consists of several sequential stages, beginning with the entry into and colonization of the gastrointestinal tract, nasopharynx, or oropharynx. Those bacteria which colonize the gastrointestinal tract, whether they are pathogenic or merely commensal, must survive the acidity of the stomach, the alkalinity and high concentrations of detergent (bile salts) and digestive enzymes in the small intestine, the immune system, and phagocytic cells. The cell wall of the gram-negative organism is well suited for coping with these challenges. Moreover, these bacteria, to avoid dislodgment by the passing intestinal contents, must attach to epithelial cell receptors or to the cell-associated mucus. This attachment is a function of hairlike proteinaceous organelles, known as *fimbriae* or *pili*, which cover the entire surface of the bacterial cell and contain lectin-like molecules that bind to specific mucosal receptors. The fimbriae of strains of *E. coli* that cause gastroenteritis have binding specificities appropriate to the gastrointestinal tract, and strains of *E. coli* associated with urinary tract infections contain P fimbriae (so-called because of affinity for the P blood group antigen found on uroepithelial cells), also called *pyelonephritis-associated pili* (PAP).

Normal host defenses limit the majority of bacterial interactions to benign commensalism. Therefore, to produce disease in healthy hosts, these organisms need additional attributes, known as *virulence factors*. For localized diseases (e.g., diarrhea, dysentery), the bacteria use secretory and cytologic toxins and, occasionally, cellular invasive factors. For successful penetration into the bloodstream, capsules inhibit opsonization, and other factors (such as smooth LPS and outer-membrane proteins) inhibit the bactericidal effect of serum.

In contrast, infections in debilitated individuals can occur with relatively avirulent organisms (see Chap. 96). Such organisms are typically robust enough to survive in various hospital environments (e.g., water supplies, the hands of caregivers) and sufficiently drug resistant to be part of the flora of an antibiotic-treated host. A debilitated host recovering from surgery or trauma or suffering from organ failure or immunodeficiency can become ill merely from the inadvertent relocation of a commensal strain to a site either normally sterile or normally not colonized with enteric bacteria. Examples include colonization of the upper airways, which with aspiration can lead to gram-negative pneumonia, and contamination of surgical wounds or intravascular or urinary catheters. The resultant "opportunistic" infections can be particularly severe because of the inability of the host to mount a normal immune response. Moreover, because the setting is most often the antimicrobial-laden hospital environment, the bacteria, preselected for drug resistance, are particularly difficult to treat.

Whether the pathogen is a virulent invader or an opportunistic commensal, the host response and appropriate antimicrobial therapy are the major determinants of recovery. Some bacteria, by possessing such antiopsonic and anticomplementary shields as K1 capsule and smooth LPS, are able to withstand the immune response of the host and can produce severe and complicated infections. Paradoxically, the normal immune response also can potentiate the disease by eliciting inflammatory responses beyond those needed for bacterial containment. Complement activation, the liberation of cytokines (e.g., tumor necrosis factor, the numerous interleukins), leukocyte mobilization and degranulation, and platelet and coagulation pathway activation can mediate the lethal manifestations of endotoxemia, including excessive fluid extravasation and circulatory collapse, renal tubular necrosis, adult respiratory distress syndrome, and damage to the central nervous system in cases of meningitis. Therapy of severe gram-negative infection is directed not only toward eliminating the invading microbe but also toward attenuating the immune response.

DRUG RESISTANCE AND VIRULENCE FACTORS Successful therapy for bacterial infection depends on the use of antimicrobial agents to which the infecting microbe is susceptible. Unfortunately, bacteria have enormous ability to evade the effects of these drugs (see Chap. 100). Most drug resistance occurs from the acquisition of new genes, usually in the form of transposons. Transposons (a segment of DNA which can migrate between plasmids and between chromosomes) are more typically found on R-plasmids, which are self-replicating, nonchromosomal units of DNA that are frequently capable of being transferred from one bacterial cell to another, even of a different species, by conjugation.

The genetic organization of genes involved in drug resistance promotes their spread through the Enterobacteriaceae. Since R-plasmids move across bacterial populations readily, the presence of several antimicrobials in the environment readily selects those bacteria which contain multiple-drug-resistance elements. With time and the continued use of many drugs in the hospital and in agriculture, R-plasmids have become larger; each now consists of many different transposons strung together like pearls on a necklace. Many individual

virulence factors, including colonization factors, enterotoxins, and hemolysin, are found on plasmids, occasionally R-plasmids, which promote their spread. Also, some virulence factors can be carried together and need to be present together to cause disease, as is seen with genes for enterotoxin production and colonization factor antigens in some strains of enterotoxigenic *E. coli*.

ESCHERICHIA COLI INFECTIONS

ETIOLOGY, EPIDEMIOLOGY, AND MANIFESTATIONS *E. coli*, primarily a commensal in the gastrointestinal tract, can be associated with disease in a number of settings. Normal individuals, if exposed to certain pathogenic strains, will develop gastroenteritis or other enteric infections. Debilitated individuals can develop pneumonia, sepsis, or urinary tract infection from otherwise avirulent strains, particularly with the placement of foreign bodies (such as endotracheal, endovascular, or endovesicular catheters). Previously healthy individuals are subject to contiguous infection from normal contents of a ruptured intestine, as may occur with appendicitis or abdominal trauma. Some otherwise healthy individuals, particularly sexually active females, are subject to repeated urinary tract infections from contiguous spread of uropathogenic strains from the gastrointestinal tract.

Enteric infections First recognized as an agent of infantile diarrhea in the 1920s, *E. coli* is also the major cause of bacterial gastroenteritis in individuals traveling abroad. As discussed in Chap. 87, this organism comes in multiple pathogenic varieties. The most important are enterotoxigenic *E. coli* (ETEC), a cause of travelers' diarrhea; enteropathogenic (enteroadherent) *E. coli* (EPEC), a cause of childhood diarrhea; enteroinvasive *E. coli* (EIEC), which causes a dysentery-like disease; and enterohemorrhagic *E. coli* (EHEC), which causes hemorrhagic colitis and the hemolytic-uremic syndrome in children.

In industrialized countries, travelers' diarrhea typically occurs in otherwise healthy individuals visiting tropical or subtropical regions that lack advanced hygienic conditions. The organism is passed by the fecal-oral route, usually through contamination of unbottled water and salad vegetables. The inoculum of organisms must be high enough to resist the normal defensive barriers of the acid pH of the stomach. (Individuals with achlorhydria are more susceptible.) In most cases, the patient, within 1 to 2 days of exposure, develops symptoms of abdominal cramps and frequent explosive bowel movements lasting 3 to 4 days. The major manifestations are a consequence of the copious outpouring of fluid from the gastrointestinal tract due to the action of enterotoxin(s) on the gastrointestinal mucosa. The clinical presentation is similar whether the enterotoxin is of the heat-stable (ST) or heat-labile (LT) variety. Gastroenteritis in travelers also can be caused by other bacteria (e.g., *Shigella*, *Salmonella*, *Campylobacter*), viruses (e.g., rotavirus, Norwalk agent), and parasites (e.g., *Giardia*, *Entamoeba*). Cholera, which is caused by *Vibrio cholerae*, develops into a much more severe, life-theatening disease.

EPEC strains cause childhood diarrhea, especially in underdeveloped countries and in nursery outbreaks. These bacteria bind to the membranous cells of Peyer's patches and disrupt the overlying mucous gel of the host cell. In contrast to ETEC and EPEC, the EIEC strains, rare in the United States, invade the host cell and provoke a significant inflammatory response. Manifestations are those of bacterial dysentery with fever and bloody diarrheal stool containing polymorphonuclear leukocytes.

EHEC strains, which all belong to the serotype O157:H7, cause hemorrhagic colitis. These strains produce shiga-like toxins that kill certain cells in tissue culture. Although the typical patient is afebrile, the sequelae can be severe. In the elderly the disease is often confused with ischemic colitis and can lead to death. Children and occasionally adults with EHEC infection can develop the hemolytic-uremic syndrome (HUS), which also can lead to death. HUS is seen occasionally with bacteria other than O157:H7, including other *E. coli* serotypes and *Shigella*.

Urinary tract infections (See also Chap. 90) Unlike the gastrointestinal tract, the urinary tract is normally sterile. Most uncomplicated urinary tract infections (i.e., those lacking foreign bodies, anatomic defects, prior surgery, pregnancy, stones, or prostate or other obstructions) are due to *E. coli*. The typical acute infection occurs in a sexually active woman following bacterial colonization of the periurethral region and ascension up the urethra. Disease can include asymptomatic bacteriuria, urethritis, cystitis, and pyelonephritis. Patients with the predisposing problems listed above also become infected with other Enterobacteriaceae and strains of *Pseudomonas* and are more likely to develop chronic or relapsing infection.

Intraabdominal infections (See also Chap. 86) *E. coli* represents a small part of the normal bowel flora—over 99 percent of the bacteria are strict anaerobes—but is a significant pathogen in those infections resulting from spillage of normal bowel contents into previously sterile environments. Studies in animals indicate that the aerobic flora (including *E. coli*) of normal bowel contents are primarily responsible for the early septicemia associated with bowel spillage, whereas the anaerobic species are required for abscess formation. Thus *E. coli* is usually cultured from peritonitis resulting from a perforated appendix, diverticulum, or peptic ulcer and is often found in the bloodstream of patients with more severe cases. It is also associated with intraabdominal abscesses and cholecystitis and ascending cholangitis. Severe intraabdominal infections can occur with ischemia of the bowel or other organs, as frequently occurs in patients with diabetes mellitus and atherosclerotic vascular disease. Such individuals are at risk for developing acute emphysematous cholecystitis, characterized by gangrene and perforation, and septic thrombophlebitis of the portal vein (pylephlebitis), leading to liver abscesses. *E. coli* is a prominent pathogen in each of these processes.

Bacteremia (See also Chap. 83) Bloodstream invasion by *E. coli* is most likely to lead to severe sequelae including death. Septic shock, which can be caused by the bloodstream invasion of virtually any bacterial species, is mediated by the inflammatory response of the host to the invading pathogen or to circulating constituents of the pathogen (e.g., the lipopolysaccharide, or endotoxin, of gram-negative organisms). By definition, septic shock includes hypotension, which often occurs 12 to 16 h after bacteremia but may be present from the onset. Bacteremia also can give rise to a milder "sepsis syndrome" not associated with hypotension and characterized by the sudden onset of fever and chills, tachycardia, tachypnea, and mental confusion. (The sepsis syndrome also can occur with bacterial infection in the absence of demonstrated bacteremia.) Septic shock also can occur with only one or two signs predominating, so bacteremia should be considered in any patient with unexplained confusion or hypotension. Hypothermia, rather than fever, occurs in 5 to 10 percent of patients. Combinations of uremia, hepatic failure, respiratory failure [adult respiratory distress syndrome (ARDS)], stupor, and coma can develop. The most common antecedent diseases are urinary tract, biliary, and intraperitoneal infections, and the most typical patient is the elderly man with prostatic obstruction and a history of urethral instrumentation and catheterization. Patients with persistent bacteremia despite adequate therapy often have undrained abscesses, most typically intraabdominally. Some patients, especially those with poor filtering capacity in the liver (i.e., those with cirrhosis or portosystemic shunts), diminished reticuloendothelial function, or diminished numbers of circulating phagocytic cells, may have no obvious portal of entry. In most of these the gastrointestinal tract is the source.

Other manifestations *E. coli* can produce abscesses anywhere in the body as a consequence of bacteremia or contiguous spread. Individuals with vascular disease, especially common in diabetics, are prone to infections of the distal extremities and of surgical wounds, whereas those with diminished numbers of circulating phagocytes are prone to perirectal abscesses. Many of these subcutaneous infections are polymicrobial, with anaerobic as well as aerobic organisms, and, particularly in diabetics, gas may be demonstrable in the tissues by crepitation or by x-ray. *E. coli* may cause septic arthritis, perinephric

abscess, endophthalmitis, suppurative thyroiditis, brain abscess, endocarditis, osteomyelitis, sinusitis, pneumonia, and other infections. Neonates, most notably premature infants, are especially susceptible to bacteremia and meningitis with K1-encapsulated *E. coli*.

E. coli and other gram-negative bacteria are frequently cultured from endotracheal tubes and chronic indwelling Foley catheters, particularly in individuals on antimicrobial therapy. Whether such infestations reflect true infection requiring specific therapy or instead indicate mere colonization requires broader assessment of the patient's condition.

DIAGNOSIS The diagnosis of *E. coli* infection depends on the combination of clinical findings (e.g., signs and symptoms of urinary tract infection) and isolation of *E. coli* by the clinical microbiology laboratory. In general, infections by *E. coli* either are due to a single organism in a previously sterile (e.g., urinary tract infections, meningitis) or nonsterile background (e.g., gastroenteritis) or are part of a polymicrobial process (e.g., ruptured appendix, infected foot in a diabetic). These distinctions are important in the interpretation of laboratory results. Thus the genital tract flora in women will contaminate urine during culturing unless assiduous attempts at obtaining and processing a clean-catch specimen are made. Urine samples from which other microbes grow along with *E. coli* should be considered contaminated. Because of the normal presence of *E. coli* in the stool, diagnosis of *E. coli* gastroenteritis is problematic but can be attempted with techniques that screen for specific strains of *E. coli* (e.g., sorbitol positivity in EHEC). Recovery of *E. coli* from tracheal aspirates in intubated patients must be analyzed in the context of the patient's clinical state to distinguish between colonization and infection (either tracheitis or pneumonia). In contrast, any growth of *E. coli* in the normally sterile environs of the bloodstream, cerebrospinal fluid, biliary tract, pleural fluid, or peritoneal cavity (the latter often in the context of polymicrobial growth) should be assumed to be diagnostic of *E. coli* infection at the site of recovery of the organism.

Rapid identification of gram-negative organisms at the site of infection is possible with Gram's stain, but this technique is unable to distinguish well among the other gram-negative bacteria that often cause similar infectious diseases. Techniques that involve amplification of nucleic acid show promise in identifying virulence genes and drug-resistance genes associated with specific microbes. One great advantage of the culture method, although it is slow, is the opportunity for antimicrobial susceptibility testing, which is particularly important with the emergence of drug-resistant pathogens.

TREATMENT As for any infectious process, the mainstay of treatment is appropriate antimicrobial therapy and elimination of suppuration, necrotic tissue, and foreign bodies. Duration and breadth of antimicrobial therapy depend on the site and severity of the infection. For example, uncomplicated cystitis in otherwise healthy women often can be managed with a single dose of drug, whereas septicemia typically requires 2 weeks of therapy, and prostatitis or deep-seated renal infection requires as much as 6 weeks of treatment; a ruptured appendix requires coverage of anaerobic bacteria in addition. When a microorganism(s) can be recovered, antimicrobial susceptibility testing is indicated and should direct subsequent therapy of each of these conditions. Until test results are available, empirical therapy should be based on the severity and site of the infection, the status of the host, and the known drug resistance patterns in the treatment setting. For more detailed recommendations, the reader is referred to the chapters dealing with specific sites of infections.

KLEBSIELLA, ENTEROBACTER, AND SERRATIA INFECTIONS

The genera *Klebsiella*, *Enterobacter*, and *Serratia* belong to the tribe Klebsielleae and are typically differentiated only by certain amino acid decarboxylase tests and the fact that strains of *Klebsiella* are usually nonmotile and form large mucoid colonies on solid media. Like *E. coli*, all are colonizers of the human gastrointestinal tract and are rarely associated with disease in the normal host; however, they are a major cause of nosocomial and opportunistic infection. In many hospitals, strains of *Klebsiella* are among the most antimicrobial-resistant microbes isolated, with their ready acquisition of R-plasmids carrying aminoglycoside-inactivating enzymes, a wide variety of β-lactamases, and other drug resistance genes.

K. pneumoniae (the Friedlander bacillus) can cause community-acquired lobar pneumonia, found typically in alcoholic men over 40 with diabetes mellitus or chronic obstructive pulmonary disease. The disease is clinically indistinguishable from pneumococcal pneumonia, except for the greater tendency for disease due to *K. pneumoniae* to progress to lung abscess and empyema. Occasionally, this type of pneumonia causes the radiographic features of bulging fissures and loss of lung volume, findings that can be seen in any severe bacterial pneumonia. Gram's stain of the sputum reveals a predominance of short, plump, gram-negative bacilli, often surrounded by a capsule, which appears as a clear space. Because of the severity of the infection and to delay the emergence of resistance, acceptable antibiotic regimens should include a combination of a cephalosporin and an aminoglycoside, depending on susceptibility results.

In the hospital, *K. pneumoniae* and its tribal relatives are major causes of infections (in order of frequency) of the urinary tract, lower respiratory tract, biliary tract, and surgical wounds. Many of these infections are associated with bacteremia and life-threatening septic shock. Less common conditions caused by strains closely related to *K. pneumoniae* include rhinoscleroma, a chronic granulomatous disease involving the mucosa of the upper respiratory system leading occasionally to bony invasion and airway obstruction, associated with *K. rhinoscleromatis*, and ozena, a chronic severe rhinitis associated with turbinate atrophy and progressive anosmia, associated with *K. ozenae*. These strains actually belong to the species *K. pneumoniae*, and indole-positive strains of *K. pneumoniae* have been assigned to a new species, *K. oxytoca*.

The genus *Enterobacter* consists of *E. aerogenes*, *E. cloacae*, *E. agglomerans* (formerly called *erwinia*), and several other species. These organisms were originally lumped into the classification, *Klebsiella-Aerobacter*. *Enterobacter* strains are opportunistic pathogens clinically indistinguishable from *Klebsiella* but may produce cephalosporinases that inactivate even third-generation cephalosporins. *E. cloacae* accounts for the majority of hospital-acquired infections with this genus.

Like the genus *Enterobacter*, *Serratia* is an opportunist that has been recognized as a human pathogen only since the 1960s. Only *S. marcescens* and *S. liquifaciens* have been associated with human disease. The epidemiology of *S. marcescens* is somewhat different from that of other Enterobacteriaceae in that *S. marcescens* is less likely to colonize the gastrointestinal tract but more likely to colonize the respiratory and urinary tracts of hospitalized adults. Serious infections due either to *Enterobacter* or *Serratia* should be treated with a combination of antibiotics to which the organisms are susceptible. Two-drug combinations typically include an aminoglycoside and a cephalosporin (assuming susceptibility).

PROTEUS, MORGANELLA, AND PROVIDENCIA INFECTIONS

Proteeae are actively motile bacteria that do not ferment lactose. This tribe consists of at least three genera, *Proteus*, *Morganella*, and *Providencia*, and seven species, *Proteus vulgaris*, *Proteus mirabilis*, *Proteus myxofaciens*, *Morganella morganii* (previously *Proteus morganii*), *Providencia alcalifaciens*, *Providencia stuartii*, and *Providencia rettgeri* (previously *Proteus rettgeri*). Virtually all *P. mirabilis* strains, which cause the majority of *Proteus* infections, are indole-negative, whereas most strains in the tribe are indole-positive. *Proteus* strains are unique in their ability to swarm on moist agar media. These organisms are normally found in soil, water, and sewage

and are part of the normal fecal flora. Except for urinary tract infections, *Proteus* rarely causes primary disease in otherwise healthy individuals but is a common opportunistic invader in debilitated individuals on broad-spectrum antimicrobial therapy. Like other gram-negative bacteria, *Proteus* can contaminate burns, decubitus ulcers, and surgical wounds and is associated with destructive chronic infections of the middle ear and mastoid that occasionally lead to deafness or extension to the central nervous system with lateral sinus thrombosis, meningitis, brain abscess, and death. Although not as important as *Pseudomonas* in this regard, following trauma to the eye, *Proteus* can cause corneal ulcers, leading to panophthalmitis. *Proteus* is also an important cause of chronic urinary tract infections, in part by possession of the enzyme urease, which produces ammonium hydroxide by splitting urea and raises urinary pH to levels that promote struvite stone formation. These stones act as foreign bodies that obstruct urinary flow, serve as a nidus for persistence of infection, and promote destruction of renal parenchyma.

As with other gram-negative bacteria that cause focal infections, a serious complication of *Proteus* infection is bloodstream invasion. Clinical manifestations are typical of gram-negative sepsis, even including shock. The urinary tract serves as the portal of entry in the majority of cases, followed by the biliary tree, gastrointestinal tract, and other foci. A surgical procedure often precedes bloodstream invasion. Like *Proteus* infections, those due to *Providencia rettgeri* and *stuartii* may cause nosocomial urinary tract infections and are often resistant to multiple antimicrobials.

Treatment of these infections is similar to that of the other gram-negative bacteria, with two differences. Most strains of *P. mirabilis* are sensitive to most β-lactam and aminoglycoside antibiotics and are less difficult to treat. Nevertheless, the occurrence of struvite stones in these infections poses a challenge; by providing a nidus of bacterial persistence, untreated obstruction can lead to rapid renal destruction and sepsis. Contaminated stones often require surgical intervention for eradication of the infection.

ACINETOBACTER INFECTIONS

Acinetobacter organisms are ubiquitous water and soil saprophytes, which, along with the genera *Moraxella*, *Neisseria*, and *Kingella*, belong to the family Neisseriaceae. The two well-characterized pathogens are *Acinetobacter calcoaceticus* var. *lwoffi*, formerly called *Mima polymorpha*, and *Acinetobacter calcoaceticus* var. *anitratis*, formerly called *Herellea vaginicola*. Like other family members, they are gram-negative diplococci when grown on agar but differ by typically negative oxidase reactions, simple growth requirements, and bacillary appearance in broth. Unlike Enterobacteriaceae, they give a negative nitrate reaction.

The infections caused by members of this genus are similar in many respects to those of the Enterobacteriaceae, particularly nosocomial and community-acquired infections of the urinary tract, meninges, and lower respiratory tract. Likewise, *Acinetobacter* strains can cause bacteremia and both subacute and acute endocarditis. With their low innate virulence but high prevalence on the skin of normal individuals, these bacteria demonstrate a predilection for bloodstream invasion in individuals with intravenous catheters, surgical wounds, or burns. Occasionally, a bacteremic episode can be fulminant and suggestive of meningococcemia, with high fever, shock, and petechiae. Many of the bacteremias are polymicrobial.

Given the ubiquity of these organisms, disease due to *Acinetobacter* must be distinguished from mere colonization. True infection may be difficult to treat because it frequently occurs in debilitated patients and because these bacteria are frequently resistant to standard antimicrobials. Until susceptibility test results are available, the infection should be treated with the combination of an extended-spectrum β-lactam agent plus an aminoglycoside, any foreign body should be removed, and necrotic tissue, if present, should be debrided.

REFERENCES

Enterobacteriaceae: General

BONE RC: The pathogenesis of sepsis. Ann Intern Med 115:457, 1991

EISENSTEIN BI: Enterobacteriaceae, in *Principles and Practice of Infectious Diseases*, 3d ed, GL Mandell, RG Douglas, JE Bennett (eds). New York, Churchill Livingstone, 1990

————: New molecular techniques for microbial epidemiology and the diagnosis of infectious diseases. J Infect Dis 161:595, 1990

MURRAY BE: New aspects of antimicrobial resistance and the resulting therapeutic dilemmas. J Infect Dis 163:1184, 1991

SCHABERG DR et al: Major trends in the microbial etiology of nosocomial infection. Am J Med 91(suppl 3B):72S, 1991

Escherichia coli infections

GRANSDEN WR et al: Bacteremia due to *Escherichia coli:* A study of 861 episodes. Rev Infect Dis 12:1008, 1990

JOHNSON JR: Virulence factors in *Escherichia coli* urinary tract infection. Clin Microbiol Rev 4:80, 1991

OSTROFF SM et al: Infections with *Escherichia coli* O157:H7 in Washington State. JAMA 262:355, 1989

RUBINOFF MJ, FIELD M: Infectious diarrhea. Annu Rev Med 42:403, 1991

Klebsiella, Enterobacter, and Serratia infections

BODEY GP et al: Bacteremia caused by *Enterobacter:* 15 years of experience in a cancer hospital. Rev Infect Dis 13:550, 1991

CARPENTER JL: *Klebsiella* pulmonary infections: Occurrence at one medical center and review. Rev Infect Dis 12:672, 1990

CHOW JW et al: *Enterobacter* bacteremia: Clinical features and emergence of antibiotic resistance during therapy. Ann Intern Med 115:585, 1991

SCHWIMMBECK PL, OLDSTONE MB: Molecular mimicry between human leukocyte antigen B27 and *Klebsiella:* Consequences for spondyloarthropathies. Am J Med 85:51, 1988

Proteus infections

RAIMONDI A et al: Imipenem- and meropenem-resistant mutants of *Enterobacter cloacae* and *Proteus rettgeri* lack porins. Antimicrob Agents Chemother 35:1174, 1991

Acinetobacter infections

HARTSTEIN AI et al: Multiple intensive care unit outbreak of *Acinetobacter calcoaceticus* subspecies *antitratus* respiratory infection and colonization associated with contaminated, reusable ventilator circuits and resuscitation bags. Am J Med 85:624, 1988

116 PSEUDOMONAS INFECTIONS

MATTHEW POLLACK

Pseudomonas species are ubiquitous, free-living, opportunistic gram-negative pathogens. *P. aeruginosa*, the most common human pathogen among this group, is the primary subject of this chapter. Also discussed are *P. cepacia*, primarily an opportunistic pathogen; *Xanthomonas maltophilia*, which primarily infects hospitalized patients; *P. pseudomallei*, an organism that inhabits soil and water (primarily in the tropics) and that causes melioidosis—a systemic disease with acute or chronic manifestations—in nonimmunocompromised patients; and *P. mallei*, a pathogen of animal origin that occasionally produces glanders in humans.

P. AERUGINOSA INFECTIONS

P. aeruginosa is a small, aerobic gram-negative rod belonging to the family Pseudomonadaceae. It is motile by virtue of its single polar flagellum. More than half of clinical isolates produce the blue-green pigment pyocyanin; this pigment is helpful in the identification of the organism and accounts for the species name *aeruginosa*, which refers to the distinctive color of copper oxide. *P. aeruginosa* is readily identified in the clinical laboratory. It is a straight or slightly curved, nonsporulating, motile gram-negative rod that grows aerobically on most common media.

EPIDEMIOLOGY *P. aeruginosa* is widespread in nature, inhabiting soil, water, plants, and animals, including humans. It has a predilection for moist environments. This organism occasionally colonizes the skin, external ear, upper respiratory tract, or large bowel of healthy humans. Rates of carriage are relatively low, however, except in patients who have serious underlying disease, whose host defenses have been naturally or iatrogenically compromised, who have received prior antibiotic therapy, and/or who have been exposed to the hospital environment. Under these circumstances, colonization with *P. aeruginosa* frequently precedes infection, and factors that predispose to the former also increase the likelihood of the latter.

Most *P. aeruginosa* infections are hospital acquired. Many potential reservoirs of infection have been identified, including respiratory equipment, cleaning solutions, disinfectants, sinks, vegetables, flowers, endoscopes, and physiotherapy pools. Most reservoirs are associated with moisture. It is assumed that the organism is transmitted to patients via the hands of hospital personnel or via fomites.

While some infecting strains of *P. aeruginosa* appear to be endemic within the hospital environment, others are traced to a common source associated with a specific outbreak or epidemic. Epidemiologic investigation is facilitated by serotyping (immunotyping) of strains on the basis of differences in lipopolysaccharide structure or by the use of DNA probes.

PATHOGENESIS The pathogenesis of infections due to *P. aeruginosa* is complex, as is evidenced by the clinical diversity of the diseases related to this organism and by the multiplicity of virulence factors it produces. *P. aeruginosa* rarely causes disease in the healthy host. It may undergo a "malignant" transformation, however, when normal cutaneous or mucosal barriers have been breached or bypassed (e.g., by burn injury, penetrating trauma, surgery, endotracheal intubation, urinary bladder catheterization, or intravenous drug abuse); when immunologic defense mechanisms have been compromised (e.g., by chemotherapy-induced neutropenia, hypogammaglobulinemia, extremes of age, diabetes mellitus, cystic fibrosis, cancer, or AIDS); when the protective function of the normal bacterial flora has been disrupted by broad-spectrum antibiotic therapy; and/or when the patient has been exposed to reservoirs associated with a hospital environment. The ubiquity of the organism, its flexible nutritional and metabolic requirements, its environmental resiliency, and its relative resistance to antibiotics help account for the frequency and success with which it acts as an opportunistic pathogen.

Infections caused by *P. aeruginosa* usually begin with bacterial attachment and superficial colonization of cutaneous or mucosal surfaces and progress to localized bacterial invasion and damage to underlying tissues. This process may continue with bloodstream invasion, dissemination, sepsis syndrome, and ultimately death. Alternatively, the infection may remain anatomically localized or may spread by direct extension to contiguous structures. The organism and its products may cause tissue injury at primary and secondary sites of infection, while the release of systemically acting toxins may contribute directly or indirectly to the sepsis syndrome.

The initial attachment of *P. aeruginosa* to the respiratory epithelium and other epithelial surfaces appears to be mediated by bacterial organelles called *pili* or *fimbriae* and by the mucoid exopolysaccharide termed *alginate*, which is produced by mucoid strains. Receptors for these adhesins are found, for example, on tracheal epithelial cells and tracheobronchial mucin and are composed, at least in part, of *N*-acetylneuraminic acid (sialic acid) and *N*-acetylglucosamine, respectively.

Surface moieties of *P. aeruginosa*, including exopolysaccharide and lipopolysaccharide, may protect the organism from direct antibody- and complement-mediated bactericidal mechanisms and from opsonophagocytosis. Meanwhile, the organism produces a number of extracellular enzymes, including alkaline protease, elastase, phospholipase, cytotoxin, and exoenzymes (or exotoxins) A and S. The breakdown of host tissues by these extracellular bacterial products creates conditions conducive to enhanced bacterial proliferation, invasion, and tissue injury.

The preceding process is particularly likely to culminate in bloodstream invasion and dissemination in the face of immune compromise such as that resulting from profound neutropenia. Septicemia or sepsis syndrome due to *P. aeruginosa* shares many of the features of gram-negative sepsis caused by other bacteria, and the lipopolysaccharide or endotoxin produced by this organism, like that produced by other bacterial species, is thought to play a pivotal role in the pathogenesis of this syndrome.

In addition to lipopolysaccharide, which is a structural component of the bacterial outer membrane, the extracellular enzyme exotoxin A, diphtheria-like toxin, is produced by most clinical isolates of *P. aeruginosa*. Exotoxin A inhibits mammalian protein synthesis by transferring the adenosine diphosphate (ADP) ribose moiety of the nicotinamide adenine dinucleotide into covalent linkage with elongation factor 2, an enzyme that catalyzes the elongation step in polypeptide assembly but is inactivated by exotoxin-mediated ADP ribosylation. Exotoxin A appears to cause both local and systemic disease. It is cytotoxic in vitro and necrotizing in vivo and produces fatal shock in experimental animals, including nonhuman primates. Toxinogenic clinical isolates are more virulent than nontoxinogenic strains. Moreover, the rate of survival is higher among patients with *P. aeruginosa* bacteremia in the presence of adequate preexisting levels of exotoxin A–specific serum antibodies.

CLINICAL MANIFESTATIONS AND DIAGNOSIS Respiratory infections

Lower respiratory tract infections due to *P. aeruginosa* occur mainly in immunocompromised patients. Primary or nonbacteremic pneumonia results from aspiration of upper respiratory tract secretions, often develops in patients with chronic lung disease or congestive heart failure, and is most common in an intensive care setting. Bacteremic pneumonia, in contrast, complicates hematopoietic malignancies, especially after chemotherapy that induces severe neutropenia. Chronic infection of the lower respiratory tract with *P. aeruginosa* is prevalent among patients with cystic fibrosis. It occurs typically in older children or young adults and is caused almost exclusively by mucoid strains.

Primary or nonbacteremic pneumonia caused by *P. aeruginosa* may present as an acute, life-threatening infection characterized by fever, chills, severe dyspnea, cyanosis, productive cough, apprehension, confusion, and other signs of severe systemic toxicity. Chest roentgenograms typically show bilateral bronchopneumonia with nodular infiltrates and small areas of radiolucency; pleural effusions are common; empyema is rare; and lobar consolidation is occasionally seen. Pathologic lesions include alveolar necrosis, focal hemorrhages, and microabscesses.

Bacteremic pneumonia due to *P. aeruginosa*, typically associated with neutropenia, begins as a respiratory infection, but subsequent bloodstream invasion and resulting metastatic spread produce characteristic lesions in the lung and other viscera. Alveolar hemorrhage and necrosis are common. The signs and symptoms of this fulminant disease include those described for nonbacteremic pneumonia caused by this organism as well as those associated with gram-negative sepsis. Chest roentgenograms characteristically demonstrate a rapid progression from pulmonary vascular congestion to interstitial edema, to pulmonary edema, to diffuse necrotizing bronchopneumonia with cavity formation. The patient typically dies 3 to 4 days after initial presentation.

Mucoid strains of *P. aeruginosa* infect the lower respiratory tract of patients with cystic fibrosis, contributing to the acute exacerbations and chronic progression that characterize pulmonary disease in these individuals. Colonization with *P. aeruginosa* correlates with bronchial airway disease in cystic fibrosis patients. It is unclear whether mucus plugging precedes infection or vice versa. This uncertainty notwithstanding, airway obstruction appears to begin with bronchiolitis, which causes mucus plugging and predisposes to *P. aeruginosa* infection. The latter produces more mucus plugging, chronic suppuration, bronchiectasis, atelectasis, and ultimately fibrosis. This process progresses to pulmonary insufficiency, hypoxemia, and alterations in cardiopulmonary dynamics resulting in pulmonary hypertension and cor pulmonale.

Clinical manifestations of lower respiratory tract infections due to *P. aeruginosa* in cystic fibrosis vary with the severity and duration of underlying lung disease and with the frequency and intensity of acute episodes. Early in the disease, patients may experience recurrent upper respiratory symptoms followed by a lingering cough. Episodes of pneumonia develop later, with persistent cough between acute episodes. Eventually, patients exhibit a chronic productive cough, diminished appetite, weight loss, and decreased activity. Other symptoms may include wheezing, tachypnea, and irritability. Acute exacerbations are typically accompanied by low-grade fever and heightened respiratory symptoms. Physical signs include evidence of malnutrition, increase in anteroposterior diameter, intercostal retractions, cyanosis, inspiratory and expiratory wheezing, rhonchi, moist rales, abdominal distention, and clubbing of the fingers and toes. Laboratory abnormalities include leukocytosis with a left shift and hypoxemia with or without hypercarbia. Tests of pulmonary function demonstrate obstructive and restrictive defects. Chest roentgenograms reveal overaeration, patchy atelectasis, peribronchial fibrosis, and patchy infiltrates associated with pneumonia. In more advanced disease, there may be evidence of severe overaeration, depressed diaphragms, increased anteroposterior diameter, extensive peribronchial infiltration, generalized bronchiectasis, and cyst formation.

Bacteremia *P. aeruginosa* causes one of the most common and life-threatening forms of gram-negative bacteremia in immunocompromised patients. *P. aeruginosa* bacteremia is usually associated with nosocomial infections and is frequently iatrogenic. It is either primary (no identifiable source) or secondary to a discrete extravascular focus. *P. aeruginosa* bacteremia is associated with underlying abnormalities such as hematologic malignancies, neutropenia, immunoglobulin deficiencies, severe burns, dermatitis, diabetes mellitus, AIDS, and prematurity. Predisposing iatrogenic factors include cancer chemotherapy resulting in neutropenia or mucosal ulceration, genitourinary instrumentation or catheterization, placement of intravascular hardware, recent surgery, steroid therapy, and antibiotic administration.

The clinical features of *P. aeruginosa* bacteremia are similar to those of other forms of bacteremia. Common primary sites of infection include the urinary tract, gastrointestinal tract, lungs, intravascular foci, skin, and soft tissues. Fever, tachypnea, tachycardia, and prostration are common. Disorientation, confusion, or obtundation may be evident. Hypotension can progress to refractory shock. Renal failure, adult respiratory distress syndrome, or disseminated intravascular coagulation may occur as complications. Jaundice is seen more commonly in *P. aeruginosa* bacteremia than in other forms of gram-negative sepsis.

Pathognomonic skin lesions termed *ecthyma gangrenosum* develop in a relatively small minority of patients with *P. aeruginosa* bacteremia. The lesions begin as small, hemorrhagic vesicles surrounded by a rim of erythema and undergo central necrosis with subsequent ulceration. They occur singly or in small numbers on the perineum, buttocks, and extremities; in the axillae; or elsewhere. Ecthyma-like lesions are occasionally noted on the mucous membranes of the mouth or gingiva. Histologic study shows that these lesions contain numerous bacteria invading blood vessels but few inflammatory cells. Bacteria are readily visible on Gram's stain and may be cultured from aspirated material.

Endocarditis *P. aeruginosa* infects native heart valves in intravenous drug users as well as prosthetic heart valves. The source of *P. aeruginosa* strains infecting drug users appears to be standing water contaminating drug paraphernalia. Moreover, foreign materials that are mixed with heroin may cause injury to valve leaflets or mural endocardium leading to fibrosis. These factors, combined with the apparent high affinity of the organism for human endocardium, may explain the association between *P. aeruginosa* endocarditis and intravenous drug use. The particularly frequent exposure of the tricuspid valve to both trauma and bacteria apparently accounts for the high incidence of tricuspid involvement in association with intravenous drug use.

The pulmonic, mitral, or aortic valve or the mural endocardium of either atrium also may be affected in *P. aeruginosa* endocarditis. Multiple-valve infections are common. Tricuspid or right-sided involvement is often associated with septic pulmonary emboli. Right-sided *P. aeruginosa* endocarditis usually presents subacutely, while the appearance of left-sided disease is likely to be more acute or even fulminant. Fever is almost invariable, and murmurs are usually detectable at initial presentation or shortly thereafter. Septic pulmonary emboli associated with right-sided disease result in cough, pleuritic chest pain, sputum production, pulmonary infiltrates (with or without abscess formation), and pleural effusions. Left-sided infections may present as intractable heart failure or large systemic emboli. Mycotic aneurysms, cerebritis, or brain abscess may occur; septic infarcts are occasionally found in the spleen, but skin and soft tissue manifestations, including Janeway lesions, Osler's nodes, and ecthyma gangrenosum, are relatively uncommon.

The diagnosis of *P. aeruginosa* endocarditis is based on a positive blood culture in the absence of an extracardiac source; an indication of valvular dysfunction or vegetation on an echocardiogram; evidence of septic pulmonary lesions on a chest roentgenogram (in right-sided disease); and the actual demonstration of infected heart valves at the time of surgery.

Central nervous system infections   *P. aeruginosa* infections of the central nervous system include meningitis and brain abscess. These infections follow extension from a contiguous, parameningeal structure such as the ear, mastoid, or paranasal sinus; direct inoculation into the subarachnoid space or brain through head trauma, surgery, or diagnostic procedures; or bacteremic spread from a distant site such as the urinary tract, lung, or heart valve. Like *P. aeruginosa* infections at other anatomic sites, central nervous system infections are documented almost exclusively in patients with compromised local or systemic immune defense mechanisms. Predisposing factors include recent neurosurgical procedures, penetrating head trauma, lumbar puncture or spinal anesthesia, cancer of the head and neck, parameningeal infection, and *P. aeruginosa* infections occurring at distant sites and associated with bloodstream invasion.

The clinical signs of *P. aeruginosa* meningitis, like those of other forms of acute bacterial meningitis, include fever, headache, stiff neck, confusion, and obtundation. The onset of illness may be acute or even fulminant, particularly in bacteremic patients, with a precipitous downhill course, shock, coma, and early death. In nonbacteremic patients, *P. aeruginosa* meningitis or brain abscess may present more insidiously, with a paucity of systemic symptoms. This presentation is especially common in infections resulting from recent neurosurgery, cancer of the head and neck, or direct extension from a parameningeal focus of chronic infection. Occasionally, *P. aeruginosa* meningitis runs a subacute or relapsing course that is thought to be related to the intermittent release of bacteria from a loculated site of infection. Chronic or recurrent meningitis may result from altered cranial anatomy associated with central nervous system tumors, traumatic injury, neurosurgical procedures, indwelling hardware, or cerebrospinal fluid leaks.

Ear infections   *P. aeruginosa* is often found in the external auditory canal, particularly under moist conditions and in the presence of inflammation or maceration (as in "swimmer's ear"). Moreover, this organism is the predominant pathogen associated with external otitis, a usually benign inflammatory process affecting the external auditory canal. This self-limited condition provides a local environment conducive to the growth of *P. aeruginosa*, which, in turn, appears to contribute to the inflammatory process. The ear is painful or merely itchy, there is a purulent discharge, and pain is elicited by pulling on the pinna. The external canal appears edematous and is filled with detritus that often prevents visualization of the tympanic membrane.

P. aeruginosa occasionally penetrates the epithelium overlying the floor of the external auditory canal at the junction between bone and cartilage and invades underlying soft tissue. The ensuing invasive process, which involves soft tissue, cartilage, and cortical bone, is typically slow but destructive. Termed *malignant external otitis*, this condition occurs predominantly in elderly diabetics but is reported occasionally in young infants with other underlying diseases and rarely in elderly nondiabetic patients. Virtually all cases of malignant external otitis are caused by *P. aeruginosa*. From the external ear, the infection advances to the retromandibular area or parotid space and enters the mastoid air cells and temporal bone. Advancing osteomyelitis at the base of the skull often involves the seventh, ninth, tenth, and eleventh cranial nerves. The cavernous sinus can become involved, as can the contralateral petrous apex. The middle ear is commonly spared; meningitis and brain abscess are relatively rare complications.

Otalgia and otorrhea are common presenting symptoms of malignant external otitis. Facial nerve paralysis tends to occur early, while other cranial nerve palsies appear later. There may be a loss of hearing, the pinna of the ear is typically tender, and trismus indicates temporomandibular involvement. Constitutional symptoms such as fever and weight loss are relatively uncommon. Physical examination almost always reveals abnormalities of the external auditory canal, including swelling, erythema, purulent discharge, debris, and granulation tissue in the canal wall. The tympanic membrane is often hidden from view and is sometimes perforated. Inflammation may involve the pinna as well as the periauricular, retromandibular, and mastoid areas. Bilateral disease is unusual but does occur.

Peripheral leukocytosis is relatively infrequent in malignant external otitis, while the erythrocyte sedimentation rate usually is markedly elevated. Cerebrospinal fluid occasionally exhibits pleocytosis and an elevated protein level. Computed tomographic (CT) scans or polytomograms of the mastoid or temporal bone typically reveal bony erosions and new bone formation, while the floor of the skull may have soft tissue densities associated with areas of cellulitis. Magnetic resonance imaging (MRI) may delineate soft tissue involvement with greater sensitivity and accuracy than CT scans. Technetium 99m bone scans and gallium 67 scans also are frequently positive. Cultures of samples from the external auditory canal and surgical specimens are almost always positive for *P. aeruginosa*.

P. aeruginosa is commonly implicated in chronic suppurative otitis media in children and adults. It is either the sole bacterial isolate or among the organisms isolated from the middle or external ear in a majority of cases and is thought to play a central pathogenic role.

Eye infections   *P. aeruginosa* causes bacterial keratitis or corneal ulcer and endophthalmitis in the human eye. Keratitis due to *P. aeruginosa* may result from even minor corneal injury, which interrupts the integrity of the superficial epithelial surface and permits bacterial access to the underlying stroma. Corneal ulcer may complicate contact lens use, particularly when extended-wear soft contact lens are involved. Contact lens solutions or the lens themselves may be the source of the organism, which is probably inoculated into the eye at sites of minor lens-induced corneal damage. Patients who have sustained serious burns, have undergone ocular irradiation or tracheostomy, have been exposed to the intensive care environment, and/or are in a coma are also susceptible to *P. aeruginosa*–associated corneal ulcers. *P. aeruginosa* keratitis usually starts as a small central ulcer; spreads concentrically to involve a large portion of the cornea, sclera, and underlying stroma; and in some cases progresses to posterior corneal perforation.

The clinical manifestations of *P. aeruginosa* keratitis include a rapidly expanding, necrotic stromal infiltrate in the bed of an epithelial injury; surrounding epithelial edema; an anterior chamber reaction; and mucopurulent discharge adherent to the ulcer's surface. Corneal ulcer due to *P. aeruginosa* may advance rapidly to involve the entire cornea in 2 days or less or may evolve subacutely over several days. Systemic symptoms are uncommon. Complications include corneal perforation, anterior chamber involvement, and endophthalmitis.

P. aeruginosa endophthalmitis may complicate penetrating injuries of the eye, intraocular surgery, hematogenous spread from other sites of *Pseudomonas* infection, or posterior perforation of corneal ulcers. It is typically a rapidly progressive, sight-threatening condition that demands immediate therapeutic intervention. Clinical manifestations may include eye pain, conjunctival hyperemia, chemosis, lid edema, decreased visual acuity, hypopyon, severe anterior uveitis, and signs of possible vitreous involvement. Panophthalmitis may result from this intraocular infection.

Bone and joint infections Vertebral osteomyelitis due to *P. aeruginosa* is associated with complicated urinary tract infection, genitourinary instrumentation or surgery, and intravenous drug abuse. Vertebral infections associated with a urinary tract source most often develop in the elderly and usually affect the lumbosacral spine. Drug use–related infections typically occur in younger patients and may affect the cervical or lumbosacral spine. *P. aeruginosa* vertebral osteomyelitis is usually an indolent disease. Accordingly, the duration of symptoms before diagnosis may be weeks or even months. Back or neck pain is generally reported, while fever and systemic symptoms are relatively uncommon. Local tenderness and decreased range of motion of the affected spine are typical. Neurologic deficits are documented in a minority of patients. Leukocytosis may be noted, the erythrocyte sedimentation rate is almost always markedly elevated, and blood cultures are sometimes positive. Roentgenograms reveal loss of bone density, narrowed intervertebral space, destruction of vertebral end plates, lytic lesions of vertebral bodies, sclerosis, and possible osteophyte formation. CT or MRI may be the most sensitive means of defining the lesions. Technetium bone scans and gallium scans are usually positive, while myelograms are revealing only if granulation tissue impinges on the epidural space. An etiologic diagnosis requires culture of material obtained by needle aspiration or biopsy of the affected spine under fluoroscopic guidance, while open biopsy is occasionally needed.

Sternoclavicular pyarthrosis caused by *P. aeruginosa* is another complication of intravenous drug abuse; in some cases it is associated with *P. aeruginosa* endocarditis, but more often it is not. Joint involvement is usually monoarticular, with the sternoclavicular joint more often affected than sternochondral joints. Localized pain in the anterior chest wall is the usual presenting complaint, movement of the homolateral shoulder may be restricted by discomfort, associated fever is common, and symptoms typically last for months (although some cases do have more acute presentations). Physical examination reveals tenderness, erythema, and swelling over the affected joint. Leukocytosis is common, and an elevated erythrocyte sedimentation rate is almost invariable. Roentgenograms show soft tissue edema, bone demineralization, lytic lesions, and periosteal elevation of the clavicular head, rib, or sternum. Material obtained by arthrocentesis or synovial biopsy yields *P. aeruginosa* in culture.

P. aeruginosa infections of the symphysis pubis are associated with pelvic surgery and intravenous drug use. The symphysis pubis, like other fibrocartilaginous joints, exhibits a peculiar susceptibility to bloodborne infection with *P. aeruginosa*. Affected patients report pain in the groin, hip, thigh, and/or lower abdomen that is made worse by walking. Fever is variable, and the duration of symptoms before diagnosis ranges from days to months. As in other bone and joint infections caused by *P. aeruginosa*, leukocytosis is variable, while the erythrocyte sedimentation rate is markedly elevated. Roentgenograms show irregularities of the pubic margins, separation of the symphysis pubis, and osteomyelitic abnormalities of the pubic rami that may be extensive. Bone scans are usually positive. Needle aspiration or biopsy is necessary to obtain material for culture. A positive culture is particularly important for the discrimination of *P. aeruginosa* infections and other pyogenic infections from osteitis pubis, which is thought to be a noninfectious condition complicating pelvic surgery, childbirth, or trauma.

P. aeruginosa osteochondritis of the foot follows puncture wounds of the foot, primarily in children. The organism infects the small joints and bones of the foot, including the proximal phalanges, metatarsals, metatarsophalangeal joints, tarsal bones, and calcaneus. *P. aeruginosa* shows a particular predilection for cartilage. Systemic symptoms are usually lacking. On average, symptoms last for several weeks. There may be plantar cellulitis over the involved area or tenderness upon deep palpation. Roentgenograms and bone scans are

generally positive. Aspiration of the affected joint usually yields purulent material in which *P. aeruginosa* can be demonstrated by Gram's stain and by culture.

P. aeruginosa is one of the most common causative agents in a variety of other, less specific syndromes involving nonhematogenous infections of bones and joints and collectively referred to as *chronic contiguous osteomyelitis*. These infections may result, for example, from compound fractures, contamination associated with open reduction and fixation of closed fractures, sternotomy performed in conjunction with cardiac surgery, contiguous spread from infected ischemic ulcers related to peripheral vascular disease or diabetes mellitus, and cellulitis in general. The chronicity, indolence, and heterogeneity of these infections explain their varied clinical manifestations and the frequent need for complicated long-term management.

Gastrointestinal infections *P. aeruginosa* infections involving virtually every portion of the human gastrointestinal tract—from oropharynx to rectum—have been documented. *P. aeruginosa*–associated gastrointestinal disease is most common in young infants and in adults with hematologic malignancies and neutropenia. Moreover, asymptomatic large-bowel colonization resulting from prolonged exposure to the hospital environment and the selective pressure of antibiotics may be a silent source of organisms that subsequently invade the bloodstream during severe chemotherapy-induced neutropenia or other forms of immunosuppression.

P. aeruginosa causes necrotizing enterocolitis in young infants and a similar disease in neutropenic patients with cancer. The most common sites of involvement are the distal ileum, cecum, and colon. The pathologic lesions are hemorrhagic and necrotic ulcers that begin in the bowel mucosa and extend into the submucosa. Vascular invasion by bacteria may be documented in the submucosa, with associated bacteremia, local spread to the muscularis and serosa, and subsequent perforation leading to peritonitis. Necrotic ulcers are also documented occasionally in the oropharynx, esophagus, stomach, or proximal small bowel. Typhlitis, a disease developing most frequently in patients with leukemia, involves localized lesions of the cecum that are associated with necrosis and gangrene and sometimes result in perforation, bacterial peritonitis, and early death; *P. aeruginosa* is the agent most commonly identified in this condition. This organism is also among the pathogens most frequently isolated from rectal abscesses in neutropenic patients with cancer. These lesions, which may be associated with few signs and symptoms, must be carefully sought in susceptible patients because they may give rise to life-threatening sepsis if not surgically drained.

P. aeruginosa has been implicated in epidemics of moderate to severe diarrhea in children, a form of enteric fever sometimes referred to as *Shanghai fever*, and a cholera-like illness attributed to a putative but still-unidentified *Pseudomonas* enterotoxin.

Urinary tract infections *P. aeruginosa* is one of the most common causes of complicated and nosocomial infections of the urinary tract. These infections may result from urinary tract catheterization, instrumentation, surgery, or obstruction; they may arise from persistent foci (e.g., the prostate or stones) and may be chronic or recurrent. The urinary tract may be a target for bloodborne infection in patients with *P. aeruginosa* bacteremia but more often is the source of bacteremia. Chronic *P. aeruginosa* infections of the urinary tract are relatively common in patients with indwelling Foley catheters, altered urinary tract anatomy secondary to diversionary procedures, and paraplegia.

The clinical features of urinary tract infections due to *P. aeruginosa* are usually indistinguishable from those of other bacterial infections. However, *P. aeruginosa* infections exhibit a propensity for persistence, chronicity, resistance to antibiotic therapy, and recurrence. More unusual forms of urinary tract involvement peculiar to *P. aeruginosa* include ulcerative lesions of the renal pelvis, ureters, and bladder that cause sloughing of vesical membrane in the urine and bacterial invasion of renal blood vessels that produces ecthyma-like lesions in association with *Pseudomonas* sepsis.

Skin and soft tissue infections As indicated above, *P. aeruginosa* bacteremia may be associated with ecthyma gangrenosum. These disseminated skin lesions, which frequently begin as small vesicles, are characterized by hemorrhage, necrosis, surrounding erythema, and histologic evidence of blood vessel invasion by bacteria. *P. aeruginosa* can almost always be cultured from the lesions. Other, less common skin manifestations of *P. aeruginosa* sepsis include vesicular or pustular lesions, bullae, subcutaneous nodules, deep abscesses, and cellulitis. Metastatic lesions of the skin or mucous membranes complicate *Pseudomonas* sepsis and occasionally produce massive necrosis or gangrene of the extremities, perineum, face, or oropharynx.

Primary *P. aeruginosa* pyoderma occurs when the skin breaks down secondary to trauma, burn injury, dermatitis, or ulcers related to peripheral vascular disease or pressure sores. Moist conditions, such as those in the perineum or diaper area of infants, contribute to the development of *P. aeruginosa* pyoderma. Neutropenia also may predispose to this condition. The clinical appearance of primary *P. aeruginosa* pyoderma, which frequently includes hemorrhage and necrosis, resembles that of metastatic *P. aeruginosa* skin lesions. Histologic studies document vascular invasion by bacteria in both diseases. A rare distinguishing feature of *P. aeruginosa* pyoderma is its association with a blue-green exudate and a characteristic fruity odor.

P. aeruginosa wound sepsis complicating extensive third-degree burn injuries results from colonization of the burn site or burn eschar, invasion of the subeschar space and underlying dermis, vascular invasion, and systemic spread. The development and progression of *P. aeruginosa* burn wound sepsis are facilitated by the injury-associated breakdown of normal skin, antibiotic selection, and burn-related immune defects. Local manifestations include black, dark brown, or violaceous discoloration of the burn eschar; degeneration of underlying granulation tissue, hemorrhage, and premature eschar separation; edema, hemorrhage, and necrosis of skin adjacent to the burn site; erythematous nodular lesions in unburned skin; and formation of brown or black neoeschars. Systemic manifestations include fever or hypothermia, confusion or obtundation, oliguria, hypotension, ileus, and sometimes respiratory failure or pneumonia. The diagnosis of *P. aeruginosa* burn sepsis is based on these local and systemic clinical manifestations and a burn wound biopsy that reveals $> 10^5$ colony-forming units of *P. aeruginosa* per gram of tissue and histologic evidence of bacterial invasion of unburned tissue, vasculitis, or intense inflammation at the burn margin.

P. aeruginosa causes diffuse pruritic maculopapular and vesiculo-pustular rashes associated with exposure to contaminated hot tubs, spas, whirlpools, and swimming pools. Most cases of *P. aeruginosa* dermatitis have occurred as part of a common-source outbreak. At least two nosocomial common-source outbreaks—one related to a physiotherapy pool—have been reported. Skin rashes may be limited to areas covered by swimsuits or may be more diffuse, sparing only the head and neck. Associated symptoms may include dizziness, headache, earache, sore eyes, sore nose, sore throat, swollen breasts, or abdominal cramps. Low-grade fever is uncommon. The illness is usually self-limited, and the rash resolves without specific therapy after cessation of exposure. One nosocomial outbreak involving immunocompromised patients, however, resulted in *P. aeruginosa* folliculitis evolving into full-blown ecthyma gangrenosum.

TREATMENT AND PROGNOSIS Most types of *P. aeruginosa* disease are treated with one or more antibiotics to which the infecting organism is sensitive. Exceptions are external otitis (nonmalignant) and dermatitis associated with exposure to contaminated water. Both these infections are self-limited and usually require no specific antimicrobial therapy.

In general, the choice of antibiotics with antipseudomonal activity includes the aminoglycosides (e.g., gentamicin, tobramycin, netilmicin, amikacin), selected third-generation cephalosporins (e.g., ceftazidime, cefoperazone), selected extended-spectrum penicillins (e.g., carbenicillin, ticarcillin, ticarcillin/clavulanate, piperacillin, mezlocillin, azlocillin), carbapenem (imipenem), monobactams (e.g., aztreonam), and fluoroquinolones (e.g., ciprofloxacin, ofloxacin). All these agents are available in parenteral form; ciprofloxacin and ofloxacin are also available in oral form. Local patterns of antimicrobial susceptibility should influence the initial choice of antibiotic agents, while the susceptibility profile of the isolate from a particular case should dictate definitive antibiotic therapy.

In most severe or life-threatening infections due to *P. aeruginosa*, two antibiotics to which the infecting strain is (or is likely to be) sensitive should be administered together. The combination of an aminoglycoside and a β-lactam antibiotic is usually appropriate. The goals of combined therapy are to achieve additive or synergistic killing, to exploit the pharmacologic strengths and offset the pharmacologic limitations of each agent, and to prevent the emergence of antibiotic resistance. Particularly in acute or fulminant infections, antibiotics should be employed at the maximal doses consistent with safety. Likewise, when sites of infection are relatively inaccessible (e.g., the central nervous system or the heart), maximal or even supramaximal antibiotic doses may be required for the attainment of therapeutic concentrations in infected tissues.

The appropriate duration of antibiotic therapy for disease caused by *P. aeruginosa* depends on the type, location, and severity of infection. Precise, prospectively defined treatment guidelines are sometimes problematic; it may be more appropriate to tailor the duration of therapy to the specific cirumstances of a case, including the initial response to treatment. In general, chronic infections associated with extensive tissue injury, disruption of normal anatomy, foreign or prosthetic material, or suboptimal antibiotic accessibility require therapy for weeks or even months rather than days. More acute infections may be treated aggressively but for shorter periods.

Infections of the lower respiratory tract in patients with cystic fibrosis pose a special challenge because they represent long-standing, chronic conditions complicated by acute exacerbations and a downhill course. Antibiotic therapy for acute exacerbations clearly results in clinical improvement. A more aggressive approach featuring periodic, expectant courses of antimicrobial therapy may limit disease progression. Frequent pulmonary toilet is important in the management of this disease, while periodic bronchial lavage has been employed to good effect to relieve symptoms associated with mucus plugging. Aerosolized antibiotics also have been used successfully in some instances.

Optimal management of infections due to *P. aeruginosa* often requires surgical intervention as well as antimicrobial therapy. The presence of necrotic tissue or of prosthetic or foreign material necessitates surgical debridement (e.g., in malignant external otitis and some cases of chronic osteomyelitis or osteochondritis); loculated pus demands drainage (e.g., in sternoclavicular pyarthrosis, brain abscess, and endophthalmitis); left-sided endocarditis is an indication for early valve replacement; perforated bowel requires laparotomy and bowel resection (e.g., in necrotizing enterocolitis); and urinary tract obstruction may necessitate appropriate surgery.

All infections caused by *P. aeruginosa* are treatable and—with the possible exception of lung infections in patients with cystic fibrosis—potentially curable. The heterogeneity of these infections, however, accounts for major differences in short- and long-term prognosis. At one end of the spectrum are acute fulminant infections such as bacteremic pneumonia, septicemia, burn wound sepsis, and meningitis, which are associated with extremely high mortality despite appropriate therapy. At the other end of the spectrum are more chronic, indolent infections, including certain cases of chronic contiguous osteomyelitis, malignant external otitis, and lower respiratory tract infections in patients with cystic fibrosis. Although the latter infections may not be imminently life-threatening, they are often difficult to eradicate and (as in the case of cystic fibrosis lung disease) may end fatally in the longer term.

INFECTIONS CAUSED BY OTHER PSEUDOMONAS SPECIES

P. cepacia, like *P. aeruginosa*, is primarily an opportunistic pathogen that is implicated in both endemic infections and occasional nosocomial outbreaks. Hospital epidemics are most frequently associated with a liquid reservoir or a moist environmental surface. Under these circumstances, the organism may colonize various body sites, with the subsequent development of invasive disease. The distinction between colonization and true infection is often difficult and may hinge on the presence of clinical signs of infection as well as a positive culture. *P. cepacia* has been reported to cause pneumonia, urinary tract infections, meningitis, peritonitis, surgical and burn wound infections, bacteremia, and endocarditis related to injection drug use. In addition, *P. cepacia* has been implicated, either alone or together with *P. aeruginosa*, in chronic infections of the lower respiratory tract in patients with cystic fibrosis. In some of these patients, the appearance of *P. cepacia* has been associated with fulminant necrotizing pneumonia, bacteremia, and a rapid downhill course.

The treatment of *P. cepacia* infections is complicated by the resistance of the organism to aminoglycosides and many β-lactam agents. Although trimethoprim-sulfamethoxazole and chloramphenicol have been used successfully in the treatment of *P. cepacia* infections, resistance to these two antimicrobial agents has been reported. Third-generation cephalosporins and fluoroquinolones have variable activity against *P. cepacia*. However, ciprofloxacin and ampicillin-sulbactam may be considered as alternative agents for use against sensitive strains. While in vitro synergy has been demonstrated for certain antibiotic combinations, such as ciprofloxacin, imipenem, and rifampin, the clinical efficacy of such combinations has not been fully documented.

Xanthomonas (formerly *Pseudomonas*) *maltophilia* is a ubiquitous, free-living opportunistic pathogen that colonizes and occasionally infects hospitalized patients, particularly in an intensive care setting. This organism has been associated with pneumonia, urinary tract infection, wound infection, peritonitis, cholangitis, meningitis, bacteremia, and endocarditis. *X. maltophilia*, like other *Pseudomonas* species, has been implicated in pseudoinfections, particularly pseudobacteremia related to contaminated blood-drawing materials. It is thus essential to consider clinical signs and symptoms in distinguishing exogenous contamination or simple colonization from genuine infection. Urinary tract infection is usually associated with a chronic indwelling urinary catheter or with urinary tract instrumentation; line-related sepsis complicates intravenous therapy; peritonitis has occurred in patients undergoing chronic ambulatory peritoneal dialysis; native valve endocarditis has been described in intravenous drug users; and prosthetic valve endocarditis also has been reported. Acute *X. maltophilia* pneumonia is being seen increasingly often in debilitated patients on intensive care units; it can be a devastating disease and is frequently associated with bacteremia.

Antibiotic resistance in *X. maltophilia*, based on both low outer-membrane permeability and inducible β-lactamases, is at least partly responsible for the emergence of this organism as a nosocomial pathogen under the selective pressure of antibiotic treatment. Trimethoprim-sulfamethoxazole is often useful for the treatment of infections due to drug-resistant strains. Alternative agents include ticarcillin-clavulanate, ciprofloxacin, and minocycline or doxycycline. The third-generation cephalosporins cefoperazone and ceftazidime may be active against *X. maltophilia* in some instances, but in vitro susceptibilities should be tested in each case. The aminoglycosides and imipenem are usually inactive.

P. fluorescens occasionally causes human disease; it is implicated particularly often in infections related to the administration of contaminated (stored) blood products and other pseudoinfections. Additional *Pseudomonas* spp. that are associated only rarely with human infections include *P. putida*, *P. stutzeri*, *P. alcaligenes*, *P.*

pseudoalcaligenes, *P. pickettii*, *P. acidovorans*, *P. testosteroni*, *P. diminuta*, and *P. vesicularis*.

MELIOIDOSIS

Infections caused by *P. pseudomallei* constitute a broad spectrum of acute and chronic, local and systemic, clinical and subclinical disease processes collectively called *melioidosis*. *P. pseudomallei* and the infections it causes are found mainly in the tropics and are endemic in Southeast Asia and surrounding areas. *P. pseudomallei* is a free-living, small, motile, aerobic gram-negative rod belonging to rRNA homology group II of *Pseudomonas* and related species. The organism is a saprophyte that is normally found in soil, ponds, and rice paddies and on produce from endemic areas. It is occasionally a pathogen for animals. Humans contract the disease through soil contamination of abrasions, ingestion, nasal instillation, or inhalation. Person-to-person transmission is apparently rare.

Acute infections most often involve the lungs, although lesions sometimes develop in other organs. Pulmonary lesions tend to be more extensive and dissemination to other organs tends to be more widespread in subacute melioidosis. Acute abscesses exhibit necrosis, polymorphonuclear leukocyte infiltration, and surrounding hemorrhage; multinucleated histiocytes are observed in areas of necrosis. Subacute lesions, in contrast, are characterized by caseation necrosis, with mononuclear and plasma cell infiltration.

Melioidosis presents in different forms. High rates of seropositivity in endemic areas such as Vietnam, Thailand, and Malaysia suggest that many infections are clinically inapparent. The occasional diagnosis based solely on abnormal routine chest roentgenograms represents asymptomatic pulmonary infection. Acute, localized, suppurative skin infections associated with nodular lymphangitis and regional lymphadenitis result from direct inoculation at sites of minor skin trauma. Acute pulmonary infections may originate in the respiratory tract or result from hematogenous spread, their severity varying from mild bronchitis to extensive necrotizing pneumonia. Onset may be sudden or gradual. Fever, productive cough, and marked tachypnea are frequent. Chest roentgenograms typically reveal upper lobe consolidation or thin-walled cavities. Progressive upper lobe disease mimics tuberculosis.

Acute suppurative infections or pulmonary disease may give rise to hematogenous dissemination and the acute septicemic form of melioidosis. This progression is more likely in chronically debilitated patients, such as those with diabetes mellitus or alcoholism. Patients with pulmonary infections in particular may present with severe tachypnea, confusion, headache, pharyngitis, diarrhea, and pustular lesions of the head, trunk, and extremities. The skin may be flushed or cyanotic; signs of meningitis or arthritis may be apparent; the liver and spleen may be enlarged; and muscle tenderness may be striking. Chest roentgenograms show diffuse nodular densities that may expand, coalesce, and finally cavitate. The acute septicemic form of melioidosis usually follows a rapid downhill course ending in early death unless arrested by early and aggressive therapy.

Chronic suppurative melioidosis is characterized by acute or chronic abscesses of the skin and various organs. Recrudescent disease arising from inactive sites of infection and perhaps triggered by intercurrent illness or other events may present in any acute or chronic form.

The diagnosis of melioidosis should be entertained when a febrile patient who has been in an endemic area presents with an acute lower respiratory tract illness associated with tachypnea, exhibits unusual skin or subcutaneous lesions, or has a chest roentgenogram suggesting tuberculosis in the absence of sputum-associated tubercle bacilli. An etiologic diagnosis may be made by microscopic demonstration of small, irregularly staining, gram-negative rods in exudate material; by characteristic bipolar ("safety-pin") staining of organisms with methylene blue; and by a culture positive for *P. pseudomallei* and/or a fourfold or greater rise in the titer of serum antibody to the organism.

The mainstay of treatment for melioidosis is antibiotic administration combined with appropriate surgical drainage of abscesses and aggressive support for patients with septicemic forms of the disease. The guidelines for antibiotic therapy are somewhat imprecise. Subclinical infection or mere seropositivity does not usually require specific therapy. Ceftazidime may be the agent of choice for clinical disease, while trimethoprim-sulfamethoxazole, cefotaxime, imipenem, and amoxicillin/clavulanate are possible alternatives. Therapy with a combination such as ceftazidime plus trimethoprim-sulfamethoxazole is indicated in severe forms of melioidosis. However, the resistance of many strains of *P. pseudomallei* to trimethoprim-sulfamethoxazole, particularly in Southeast Asia, necessitates other antibiotic choices. Acute septicemic infections probably should be treated with combinations of multiple agents administered parenterally. Patients with acute pulmonary infections should receive antibiotics for 60 to 150 days, while chronic disease associated with persistently positive sputum cultures may require longer treatment. Extrapulmonary suppurative disease is appropriately treated for 6 months to 1 year. When initial therapy for acute infections involves a third-generation cephalosporin such as ceftazidime, a switch can often be made after 30 days to an oral agent such as trimethoprim-sulfamethoxazole or amoxicillin-clavulanate.

Most cases of melioidosis are curable if appropriately treated. However, septicemic infections are still associated with very high mortality despite optimal therapy, while all forms of melioidosis are subject to possible early or very late recrudescence.

GLANDERS

Glanders is primarily a systemic equine disease that is caused by *P. mallei* and is associated with pulmonary involvement, subcutaneous ulcerative lesions, and lymphangitis. Once widespread, glanders still occurs in Africa, Asia, and South America but not in the United States or western Europe. The infection may be communicated to humans during close contact with horses, mules, or donkeys, probably by cutaneous inoculation or nasal exposure to contaminated discharges. Glanders assumes the following forms in humans: acute localized suppurative infection, acute pulmonary infection, acute septicemic infection, and chronic suppurative infection. Inoculation of *P. mallei* into the skin usually produces a nodule with an area of lymphangitis. Fever, malaise, and prostration are common. Mucous membrane infection results in the production of a mucopurulent discharge from the eye, nose, or lips, with the subsequent development of granulomatous ulcers. Pulmonary infection secondary to inhalation of the organism is accompanied by typical local and systemic signs and symptoms of pneumonia. Lymphadenopathy and splenomegaly may be documented. Chest roentgenograms reveal circumscribed densities suggesting early lung abscesses; bronchopneumonia or lobar consolidation also may be evident. Chronic suppurative infection presents as multiple subcutaneous and intramuscular abscesses, particularly often involving the extremities; visceral lesions are documented in some patients. The acute septicemic form of glanders may be associated with a diffuse papular or pustular eruption, severe systemic symptoms, and early death.

The diagnosis of glanders may be suggested by the clinical setting (including a history of close contact with equines) and confirmed by culture of the causative agent from clinical material and by demonstration of *P. mallei*–specific seroconversion.

Optimal antimicrobial therapy for glanders has not been adequately defined. Sulfadiazine has proven effective historically both in animals and in humans. It has been suggested, however, that rational therapy consists of the same antibiotics recommended for the treatment of melioidosis, with the specific agent chosen on the basis of in vitro susceptibility testing. Antibiotics are administered for at least 30 days in uncomplicated infections and longer in complicated cases. Abscesses may require surgical drainage, and appropriate supportive measures are necessary in acute septicemic forms of the disease.

REFERENCES

Pseudomonas aeruginosa infections

BARKER LF: The clinical symptoms, bacteriologic findings and postmortem appearances in cases of infection of human beings with the *Bacillus pyocyaneus*. JAMA 29:213, 1897

BODEY GP et al: *Pseudomonas* bacteremia: Retrospective analysis of 410 episodes. Arch Intern Med 145:1621, 1985

FICK RB (ed): *Pseudomonas aeruginosa: The Opportunist, Pathogenesis and Disease.* Boca Raton, CRC, 1992

KORVICK JA, YU VL: Antimicrobial agent therapy for *Pseudomonas aeruginosa.* Antimicrob Agents Chemother 35:2167, 1991

MORRISON AF, WENZEL RP: Epidemiology of infections due to *Pseudomonas aeruginosa.* Rev Infect Dis 6(suppl):S267, 1984

POLLACK M: The virulence of *Pseudomonas aeruginosa.* Rev Infect Dis 6(suppl):S617, 1984

————: *Pseudomonas aeruginosa,* in *Principles and Practice of Infectious Diseases,* 3d ed, GL Mandell et al (eds). New York, Churchill Livingstone, 1990, pp 1673–1691

Infections caused by other *Pseudomonas* species

ELTING LS, BODEY GP: Septicemia due to *Xanthomonas* species and non-aeruginosa *Pseudomonas* species: Increasing incidence of catheter-related infections. Medicine 69:296, 1990

GOLDMANN DA, KLINGER JD: *Pseudomonas cepacia:* Biology, mechanisms of virulence, epidemiology. J Pediatr 108:806, 1986

MURRAY AE et al: Blood transfusion-associated *Pseudomonas fluorescens* septicemia: Is this an increasing problem? J Hosp Infect 9:243, 1987

POLLACK M: *Pseudomonas,* in *Infectious Diseases,* SL Gorbach et al (eds). Philadelphia, Saunders, 1992, pp 1502–1513

TOMASHEFSKI JF et al: *Pseudomonas cepacia*–associated pneumonia in cystic fibrosis. Arch Pathol Lab Med 112:166, 1988

Melioidosis

LEELARASAMEE A, BOVORNKITTI S: Melioidosis: Review and update. Rev Infect Dis 11:413, 1989

SANFORD JP: *Pseudomonas* species (including melioidosis and glanders), in *Principles and Practice of Infectious Diseases,* 3d ed, GL Mandell et al (eds). New York, Churchill Livingstone, 1990, pp 1692–1696

117 SALMONELLOSIS

GERALD T. KEUSCH

Organisms of the genus *Salmonella* are capable of causing a large variety of infections in humans, including typhoid (or enteric) fevers, focal systemic infections, septicemias, and gastroenteritis varying clinically from watery diarrhea to dysentery. *Nontyphoidal salmonellosis* usually refers to enteric disease caused by many members of the genus except *S. typhi.* Convalescent carriage of gastroenteritis strains is usually transient. A few subjects, generally young children under 5 years of age, may become long-term (longer than 1 year) asymptomatic carriers, although they are not important in the spread of infection. Patients with *S. typhi* are more likely to become long-term carriers, for years or possibly for life, and they serve as reservoirs for the spread of infection.

ETIOLOGY The salmonellae are nonencapsulated gram-negative bacilli, almost always motile by means of peritrichous flagella, expressing two or more forms of H antigens. They are generally lactose nonfermenters, and this property is used for initial selection in the clinical microbiology laboratory. The salmonellae ferment glucose, resulting in a typical acid butt and alkaline slant on triple sugar iron agar (TSI). They generally produce H_2S, which is detectable as a black reaction product and serves initially to distinguish isolates from *Shigella*, which also give an alkaline/acid TSI reaction. There are a very large number of *Salmonella* O and H antigens, allowing the separation of over 2200 different organisms on the basis of the patterns of the O and H antigens. Since these isolates have often been named after the place they were first detected, *Salmonella* classification more closely resembles geography. On the basis of major somatic antigens, a limited number of serogroups have been defined, and most human pathogens are members of groups A to D.

More rational classification schemes have been introduced that divide the genus into three species. One scheme includes *S. cholerasuis*, the prototype species; *S. typhi*, the major cause of typhoid (enteric) fever; and *S. enteritidis*, a catchall designation for all the remaining serotypes only some of which are pathogenic for humans. These serotypes do not have the taxonomic rank of species and should not be italicized, but for clinical and epidemiologic ease the convention is to use only the serotype name. Thus *S. enteritidis* serotype typhimurium becomes *S. typhimurium*, and *S. enteritidis* serotype enteritidis becomes *S. enteritidis*.

Some salmonellae are highly host-adapted to humans (e.g., *S. typhi*, *S. paratyphi A*, and *S. paratyphi B*), while most animal-adapted species cause no human disease. Others infect both humans and lower animals causing gastroenteritis or, less commonly, localized or septicemic infections.

TYPHOID FEVER

Typhoid fever is a distinctive acute systemic febrile infection of the mononuclear phagocytes and deserves separate consideration. Since it may be caused by several *species (S. typhi, S. paratyphi A* and *paratyphi B*, and occasionally *S. typhimurium)*, many clinicians prefer the term *enteric fever*. But because typhoid is fundamentally not an enteric disease, this term is also inappropriate. On balance, *typhoid fever* is still the best term, for it is understood by nearly all clinicians to describe a particular syndrome that is, in fact, due primarily to *S. typhi*.

EPIDEMIOLOGY Because the cause of clinical typhoid fever is almost always a human-adapted *Salmonella*, most cases can be traced to a human carrier. The proximate cause may be water (the most common route) or food contaminated by a human carrier. Chronic carriers are generally over 50 years old, are more commonly women, and often have gallstones. *S. typhi* reside in the bile, even within the interiors of stones, and intermittently reach the lumen of the bowel and are excreted in the stool, thereby contaminating water or food.

With improvements in environmental sanitation in the United States, the incidence of typhoid has gradually dropped. Compared with 1920 when almost 36,000 cases were detected, the annual number now is approximately 500. Over 80 percent of these are active typhoid cases, and the others are convalescent carriers. The median age of patients is around 24 years, while the median age of carriers is over 60 years. Data gathered by the Centers for Disease Control and Prevention (CDC) show that the incidence in the United States dropped fivefold from 1955 to 1966, from 1 per 100,000 to 0.2 per 100,000 population, and has remained steady since then. At the same time, the proportion of infections acquired abroad increased from 33 percent in the 1960s to over 60 percent in the 1980s and continues to increase. Mexico is the leading source for Americans, accounting for 39 percent of cases from 1975 to 1984, although the risk to travelers to Peru, Chile, India, and Pakistan is significantly greater. Students are most at risk. In England, the majority of cases are also acquired abroad, usually in India or Pakistan. Known hot spots for typhoid include Alexandria, Egypt; Jakarta, Indonesia; and Santiago, Chile.

Typhoid contracted in the United States is primarily due to association with known or newly diagnosed carriers (30 percent) or from food-borne outbreaks (28 percent). The highest rates occur in states bordering Mexico. Other than travelers, the groups most likely to be at risk are bacteriology laboratory workers and household contacts of known carriers. The number of patients in the United States is clearly underestimated, and an unknown proportion of patients escape detection because appropriate cultures are not done or the patients have already taken antibiotics.

In *S. typhi*–endemic regions, the rate of clinical typhoid is approximately 25-fold greater in HIV-positive than in HIV-negative individuals in the 15- to 35-year-old age group and as much as 60-fold greater than in the general population. Asymptomatic HIV-positive patients have a typical clinical presentation and response to therapy; AIDS patients can present with fulminant diarrhea and/or colitis and are far more likely to relapse. While this fact has little practical significance for AIDS patients in low-typhoid countries, it may become a problem for those who travel to highly endemic countries.

PATHOGENESIS Following ingestion of a suitable inoculum, *S. typhi* pass the gastric barrier to reach the small bowel. Experimental human infections with the Quailes strain have revealed that 10^3 organisms will not cause symptomatic disease but that 10^5 bacteria cause symptoms in 27 percent of volunteers. Higher doses result in more frequent illness, especially if the organisms produce the Vi capsular polysaccharide antigen. Animal studies suggest that *S. typhi* invade the host in the upper small bowel and produce a transient and asymptomatic bacteremia. The organisms are ingested by mononuclear phagocytes and must survive and multiply intracellularly to cause illness.

Persistent bacteremia initiates the clinical phase of infection. The ability of the inoculum to invade mononuclear cells and multiply intracellularly determines whether or not this secondary bacteremia occurs. The absence of bactericidal antibodies allows organisms to be phagocytized in a viable state. Intracellular survival is dependent on microbial factors that promote resistance to killing and on specific host T lymphocyte–activated cell-mediated immunity, which is under genetic control. Dose dependence of clinical disease appears to be governed by the balance between bacterial multiplication and acquired host extracellular and intracellular defenses. When the number of intracellular bacteria surpasses a critical threshold, secondary bacteremia occurs and results in the invasion of the gallbladder and Peyer's patches of the intestine. The sustained bacteremia is responsible for the persistent fever of clinical typhoid, while inflammatory responses to tissue invasion determine the pattern of clinical expression (cholecystitis, intestinal hemorrhage, or perforation). With invasion of the gallbladder and Peyer's patches, bacteria regain entry to the bowel lumen, and may be recovered in stool cultures beginning in the second week of clinical disease. Seeding of the kidney leads to positive urine cultures but in a much lower percentage of patients than those with positive blood cultures. The lipopolysaccharide endotoxin of *S. typhi* may contribute to causing fever, leukopenia, and other systemic symptoms, but the occurrence of such symptoms in subjects made tolerant to endotoxin supports a role for other factors, such as cytokines released from infected mononuclear phagocytes, that can mediate inflammation (see Chap. 16).

CLINICAL MANIFESTATIONS The incubation period is variable and depends on both the inoculum size and the state of host defenses. A range of 3 to 60 days has been reported. The disease classically presents with a steplike daily increase in temperature to 40 to 41°C, associated with headache, malaise, and chills. The hallmark of typhoid fever is prolonged, persistent fever (4 to 8 weeks in untreated patients). Mild and brief illness may occur, but in some patients acute, severe infection with disseminated intravascular coagulation and central nervous system involvement rapidly results in death. In other patients, necrotizing cholecystitis or intestinal bleeding and perforation can occur in the third or fourth week of illness, when the patient is otherwise improving. In most, the onset of these complications is dramatic and clinically obvious. Intestinal perforation appears to be less common in children under 5 years of age.

Early intestinal manifestations include constipation, especially in adults, or mild diarrhea in children, associated with abdominal tenderness. Mild hepatosplenomegaly is detectable in the majority of

COLOR ATLASES

Atlas of Dermatology

Atlas of Dermatology

Stephen F. Templeton
Thomas J. Lawley

1 Common Skin Diseases and Lesions

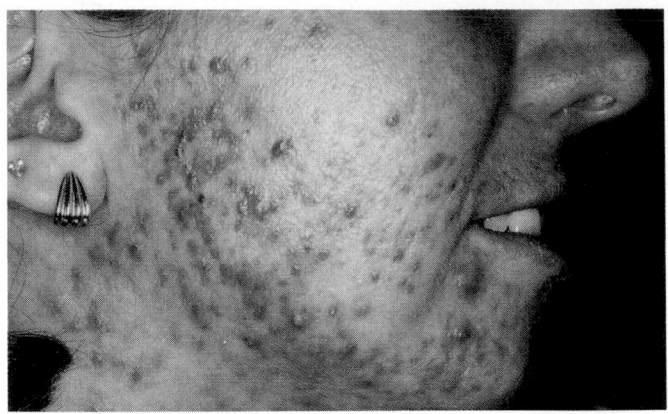

A1-1 **Acne vulgaris** with inflammatory papules, pustules, and comedones.

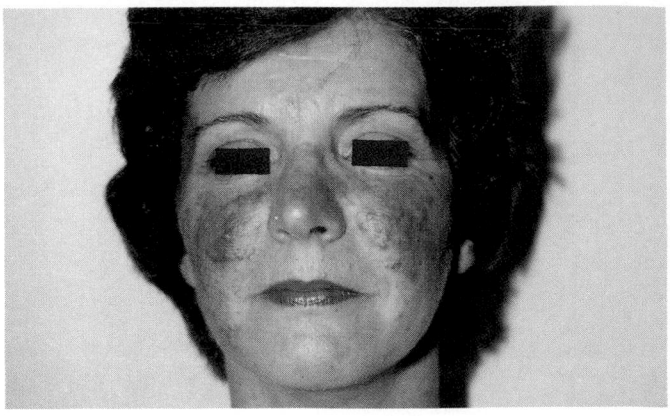

A1-2 **Acne rosacea** with prominent facial erythema, telangiectasias, scattered papules, and small pustules.

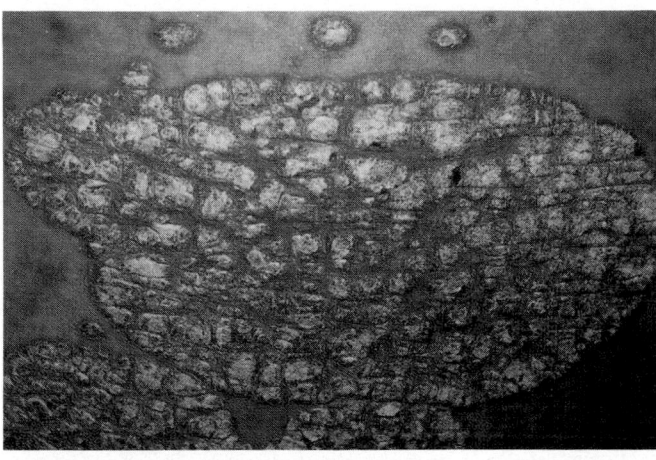

A1-3 **Psoriasis** is characterized by small and large erythematous plaques with adherent silvery scale.

A1-4 **Atopic dermatitis** with excoriated, lichenified plaques in the popliteal fossa.

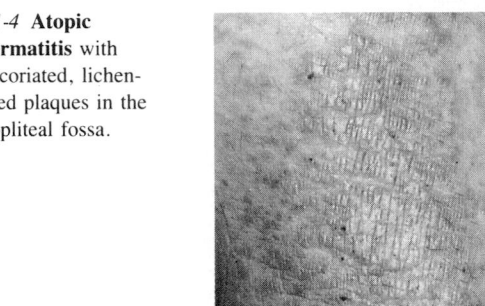

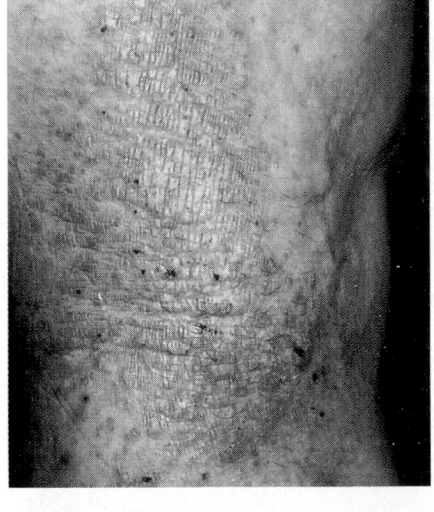

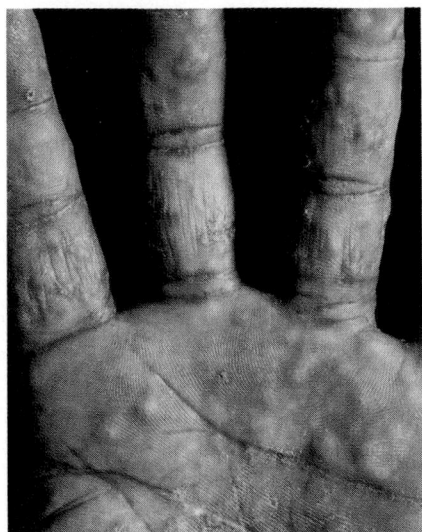

A1-5 **Dyshidrotic eczema,** characterized by deep-seated vesicles and scaling on palms and lateral fingers, is often associated with an atopic diathesis.

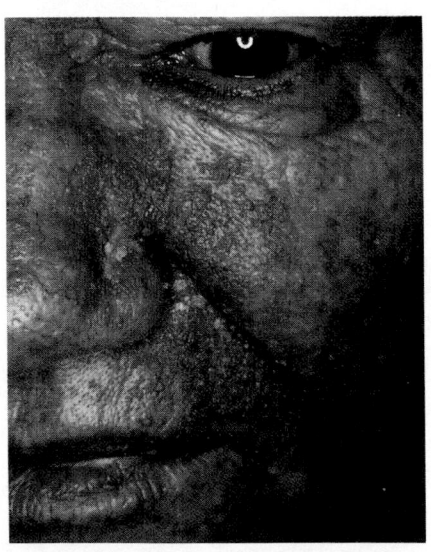

A1-6 **Seborrheic dermatitis** showing central facial erythema with overlying greasy, yellowish scale.

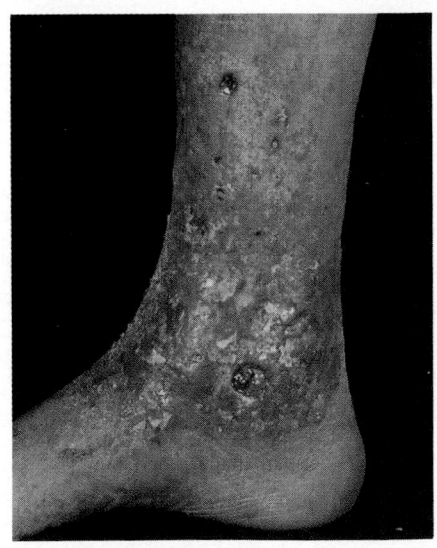

A1-7 **Stasis dermatitis** showing erythematous, scaly, and oozing patches over the lower leg. Several stasis ulcers are also seen in this patient.

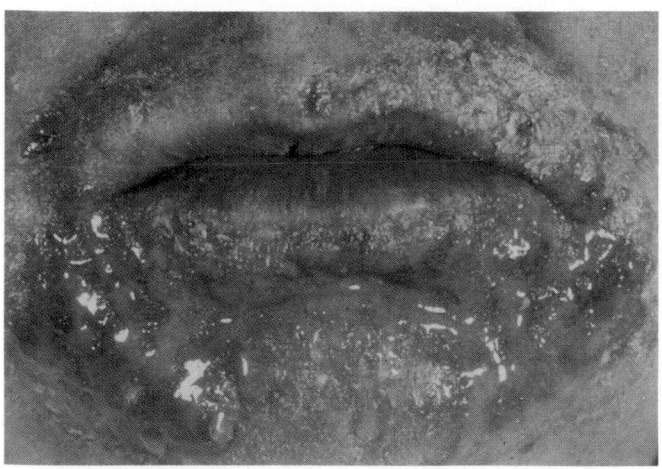

A1-8 **Allergic contact dermatitis,** acute phase, with sharply demarcated, weeping, eczematous plaques in a perioral distribution.

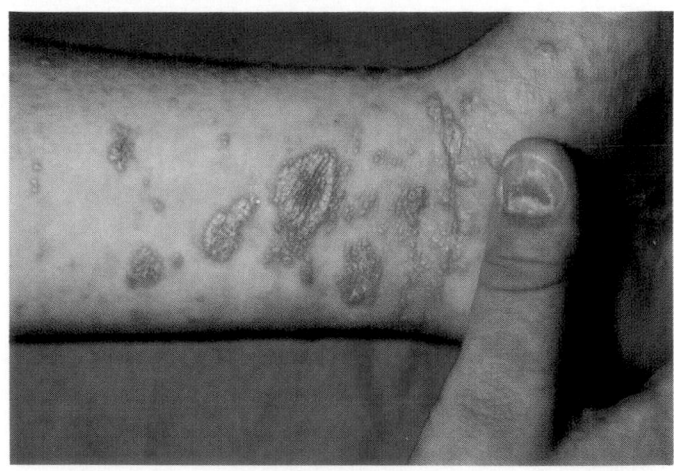

A1-9 **Lichen planus** showing multiple flat-topped, violaceous papules and plaques. Nail dystrophy as seen in this patient's thumbnail may also be a feature.

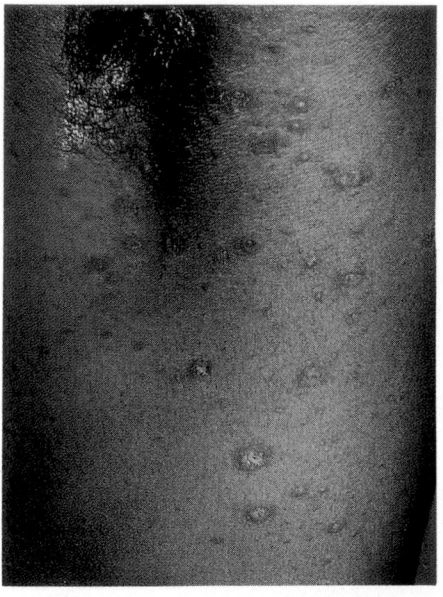

A1-10 **Pityriasis rosea.** Multiple round to oval erythematous patches with fine central scale are distributed along the skin tension lines on the trunk.

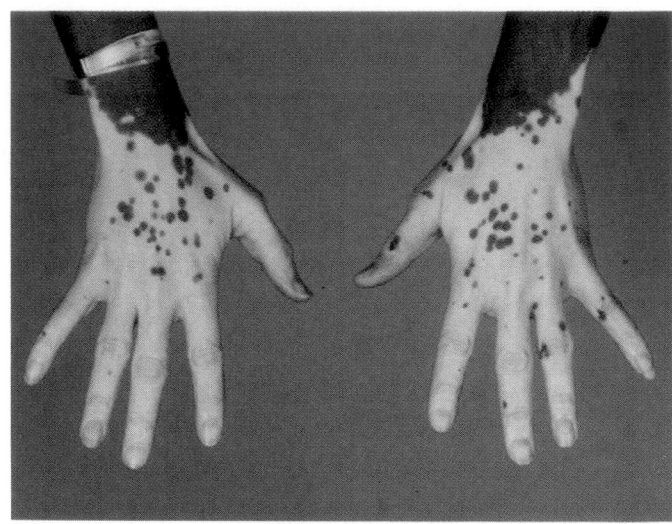

A1-11 **Vitiligo** in a typical acral distribution demonstrating striking cutaneous depigmentation, as a result of loss of melanocytes.

A1-13 **Urticaria** showing characteristic discrete and confluent, edematous, erythematous papules and plaques.

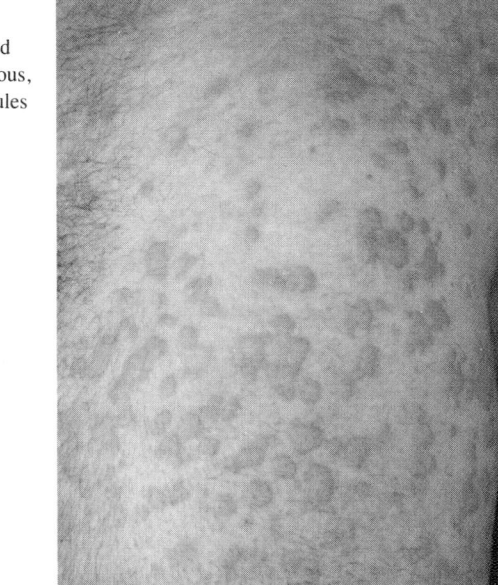

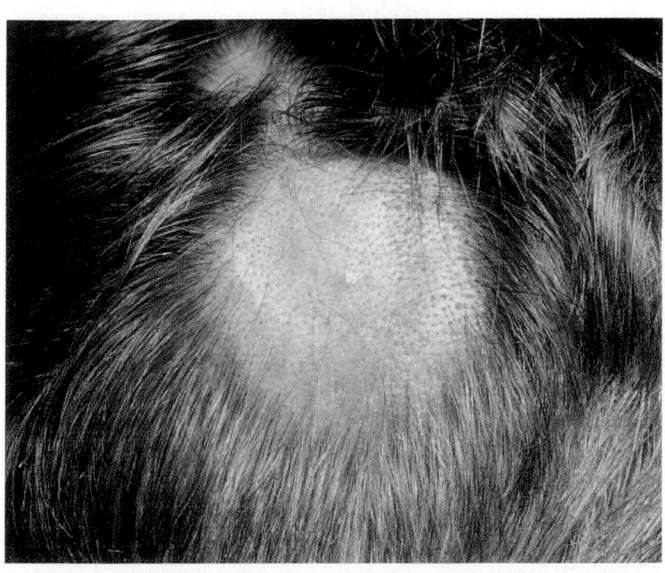

A1-12 **Alopecia areata** characterized by a sharply demarcated circular patch of scalp completely devoid of hairs. Follicular orifices are preserved, indicating a nonscarring alopecia.

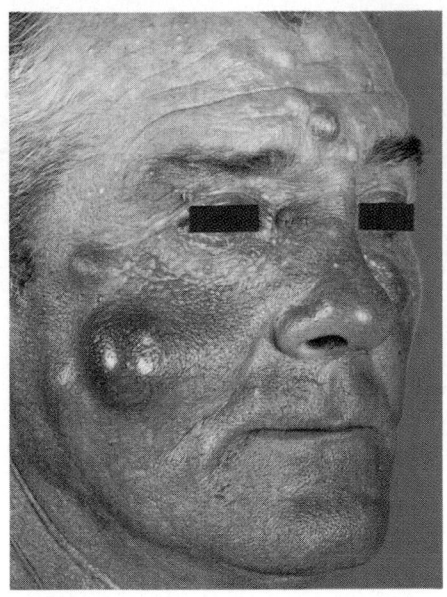

A1-14 **Epidermoid cysts.** Several inflamed and noninflamed firm, cystic nodules are seen in this patient. Often a patulous follicular punctum is observed on the overlying epidermal surface.

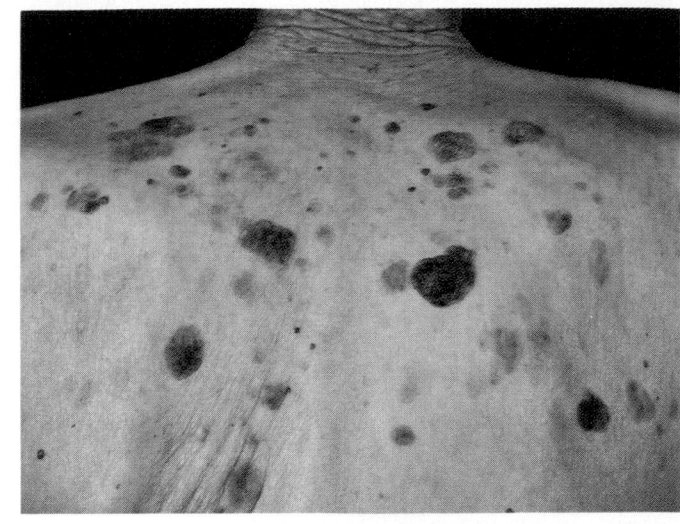

A1-15 **Seborrheic keratoses** are seen as "stuck on," waxy, verrucous papules and plaques with a variety of colors ranging from light tan to black.

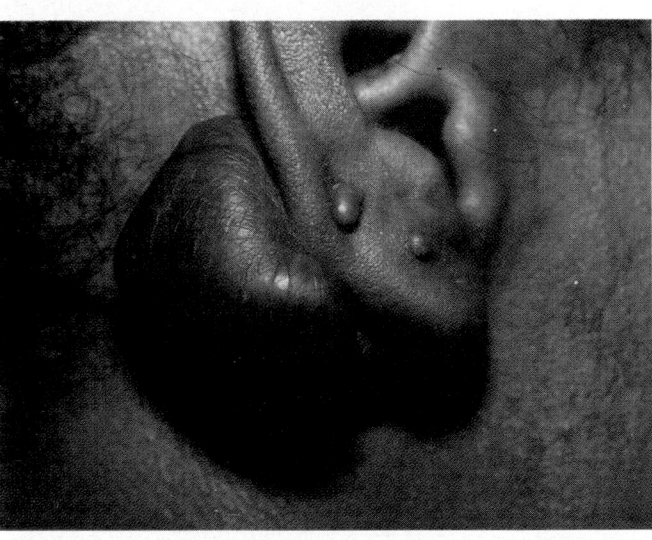

A1-16 **Keloids** resulting from ear piercing, with firm exophytic flesh-colored to erythematous nodules of scar tissue.

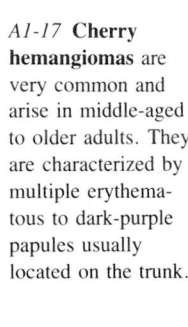

A1-17 **Cherry hemangiomas** are very common and arise in middle-aged to older adults. They are characterized by multiple erythematous to dark-purple papules usually located on the trunk.

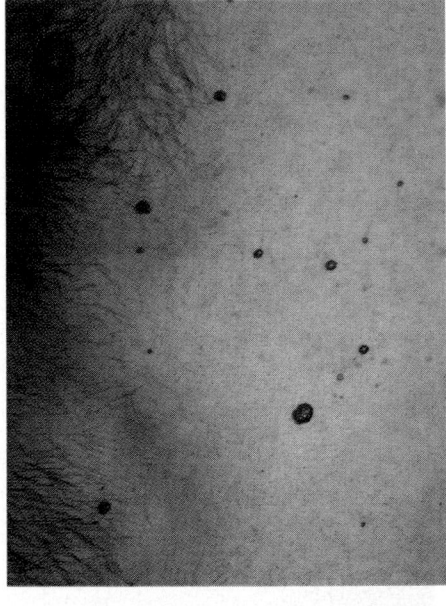

2 Cutaneous Neoplasms

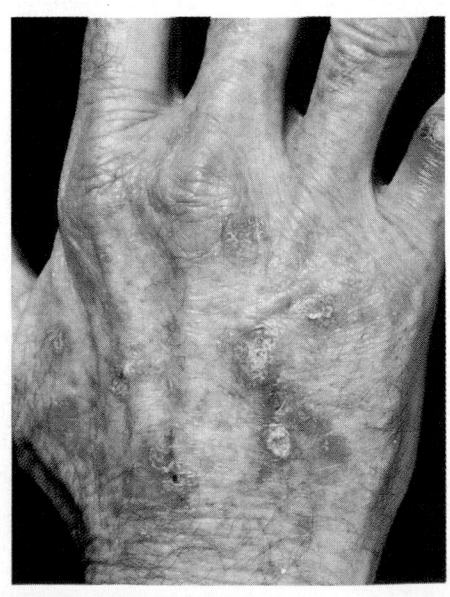

A2-18 **Actinic keratoses** consist of hyperkeratotic erythematous papules and patches on sun-exposed skin. They arise in middle-aged to older adults and have some potential for malignant transformation.

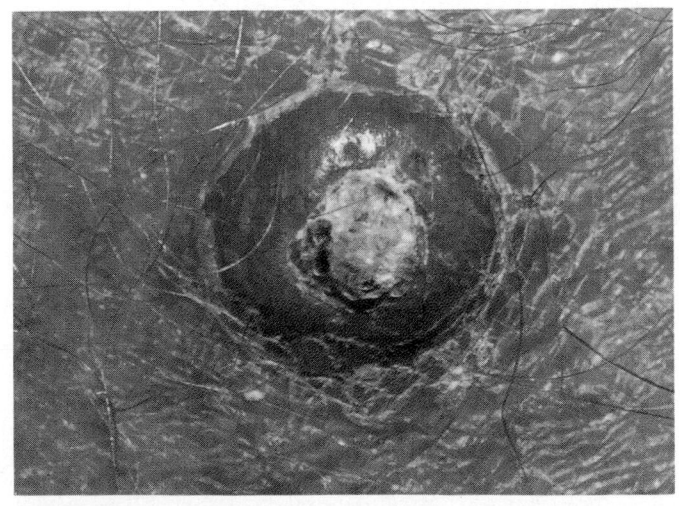

A2-19 **Keratoacanthoma** is a low-grade squamous neoplasm characterized by an exophytic nodule with central keratinous debris.

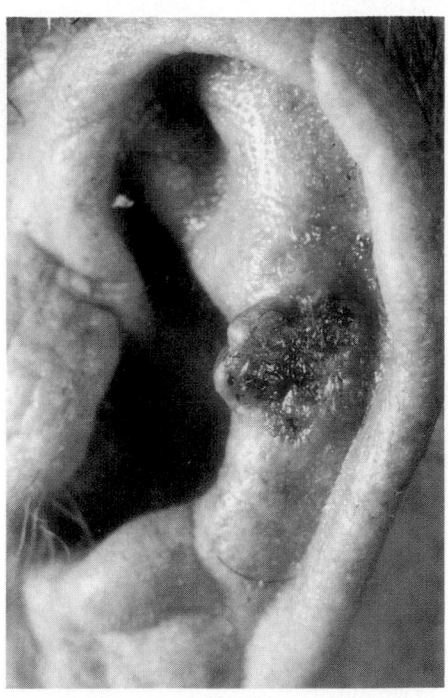

A2-20 **Basal cell carcinoma** showing central ulceration and a pearly, rolled, telangiectatic tumor border.

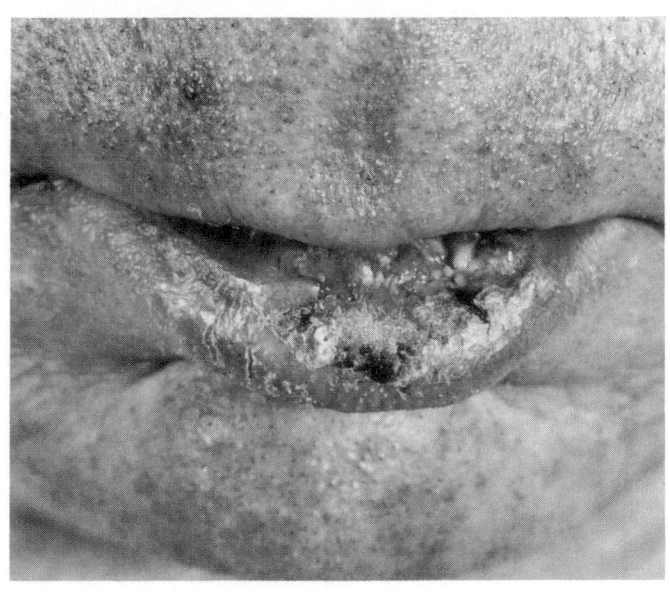

A2-21 **Squamous cell carcinoma** seen here as a hyperkeratotic crusted and somewhat eroded plaque on the lower lip. Sun-exposed skin such as the head, neck, hands, and arms are other typical sites of involvement.

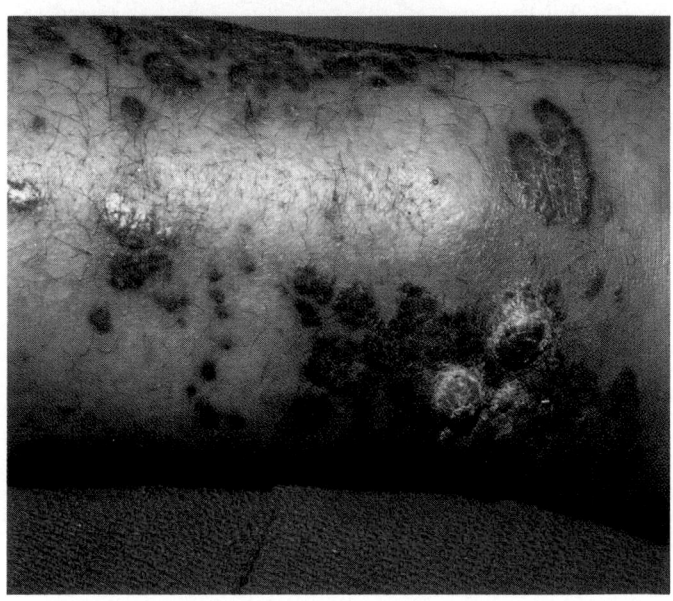

A2-22 **Kaposi's sarcoma** in a patient with AIDS demonstrating patch, plaque, and tumor stages.

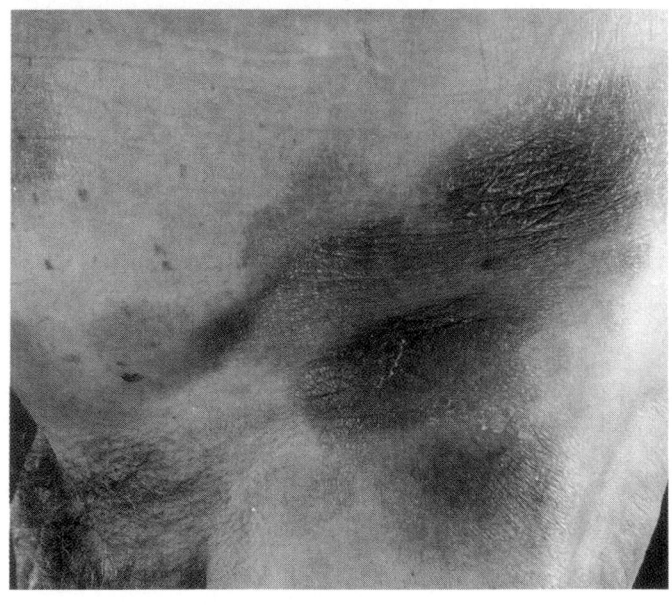

A2-23 **Mycosis fungoides** is a cutaneous T cell lymphoma, and plaque stage lesions are seen in this patient.

A2-25 **Metastatic carcinoma** to the skin is characterized by inflammatory, often ulcerated dermal nodules.

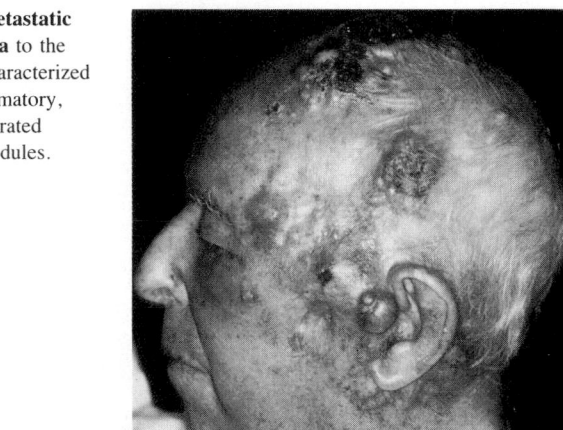

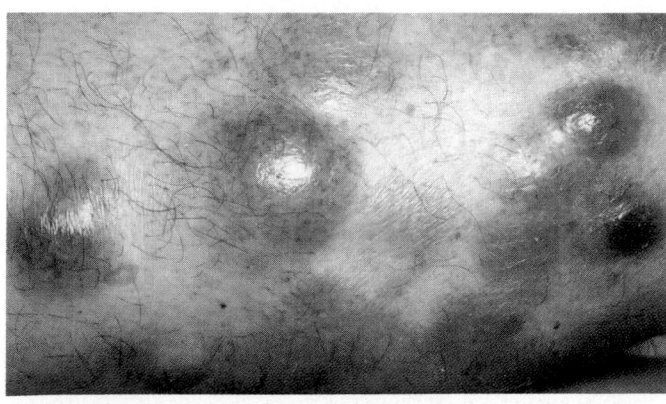

A2-24 **Non-Hodgkin's lymphoma** involving the skin with typical violaceous, "plum-colored" nodules.

3 Pigmented Lesions—Benign and Malignant

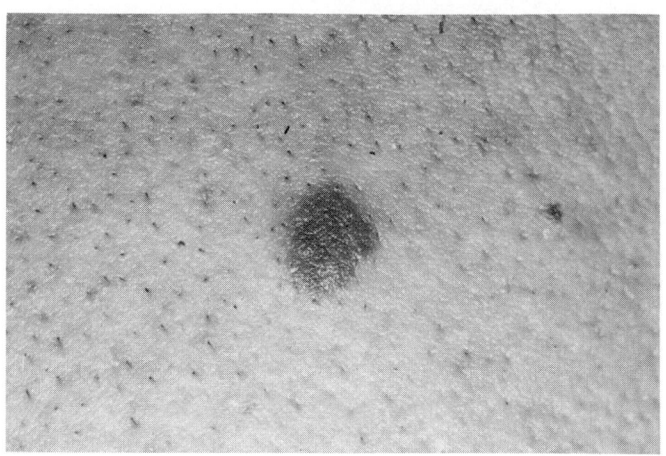

A3-26 **Nevus.** Nevi are benign proliferations of nevomelanocytes characterized by regularly shaped hyperpigmented macules or papules of a uniform color.

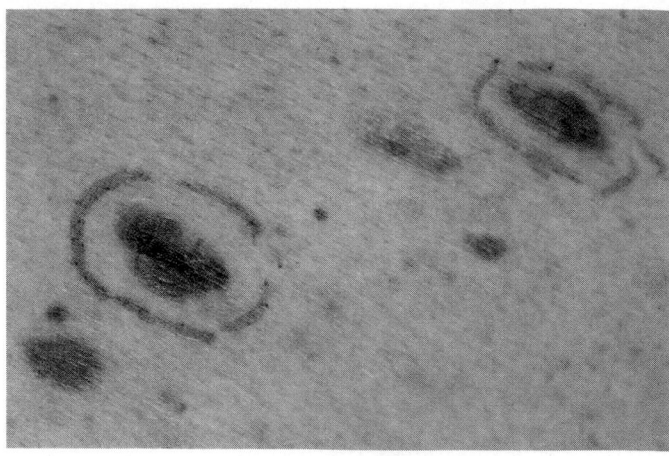

A3-27 **Dysplastic nevi** are irregularly pigmented and shaped nevomelanocytic lesions which may be associated with familial melanoma.

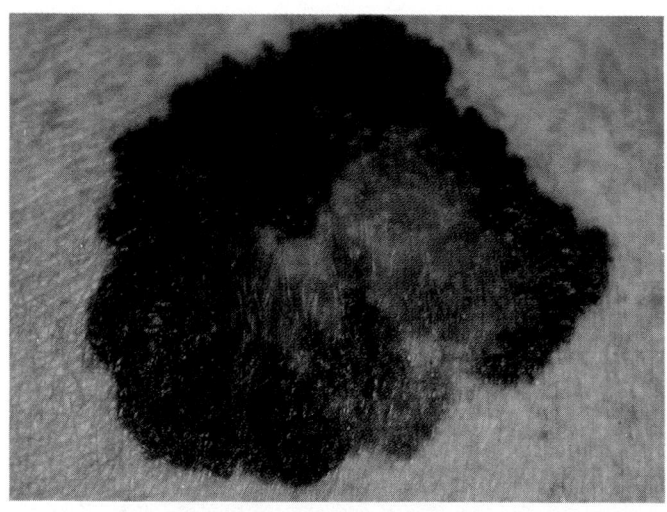

A3-28 **Superficial spreading melanoma** is the most common type of malignant melanoma and demonstrates color variegation (black, blue, brown, pink, and white) and irregular borders.

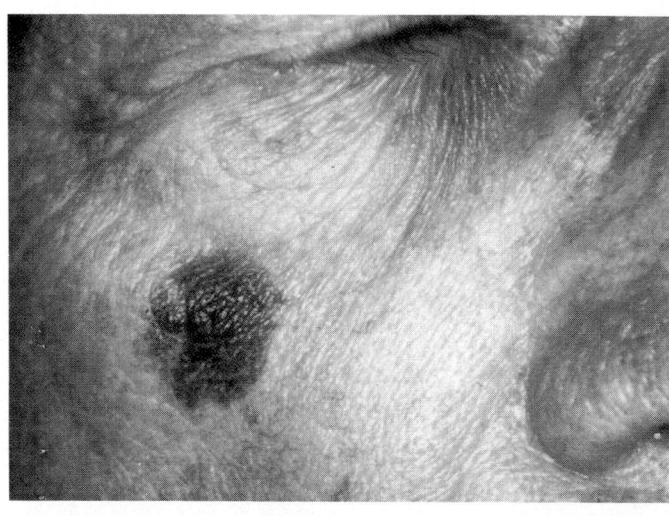

A3-29 **Lentigo maligna melanoma** occurs on sun-exposed skin as a large, hyperpigmented macule or plaque with irregular borders and variable pigmentation.

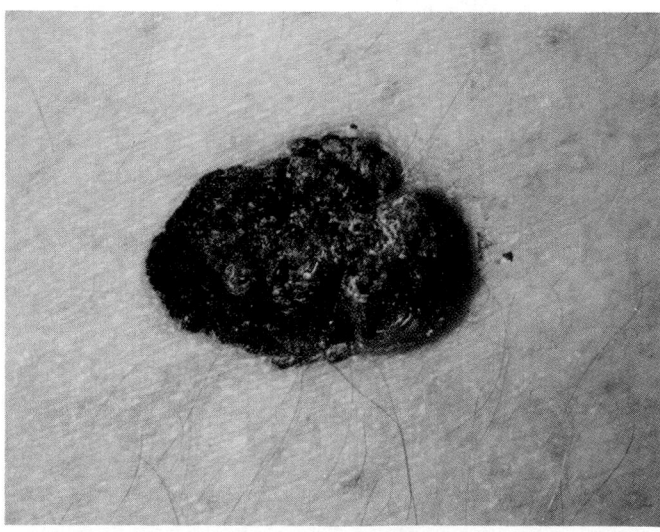

A3-30 **Nodular melanoma** most commonly manifests itself as a rapidly growing, often ulcerated or crusted black nodule.

A3-31 **Acral lentiginous melanoma** is more common in blacks, Orientals, and Hispanics and occurs as an enlarging hyperpigmented macule or plaque on the palms and soles. Lateral pigment diffusion is present.

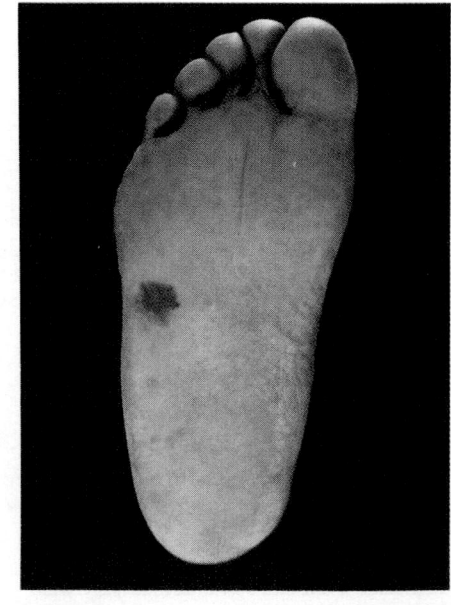

4 Infectious Disease and the Skin

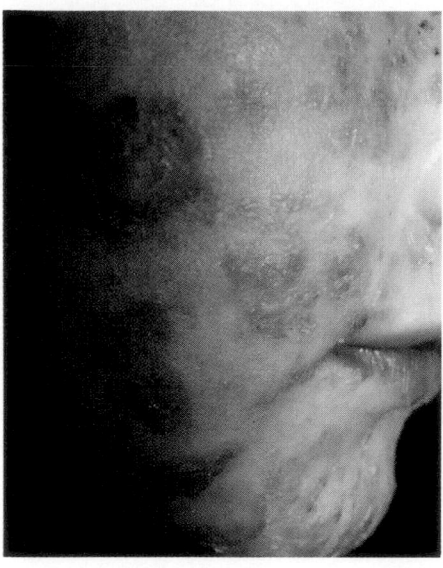

A4-32 **Impetigo contagiosa** is a superficial streptococcal or *Staph. aureus* infection consisting of honey-colored crusts and erythematous weeping erosions. Occasionally bullous lesions may be seen.

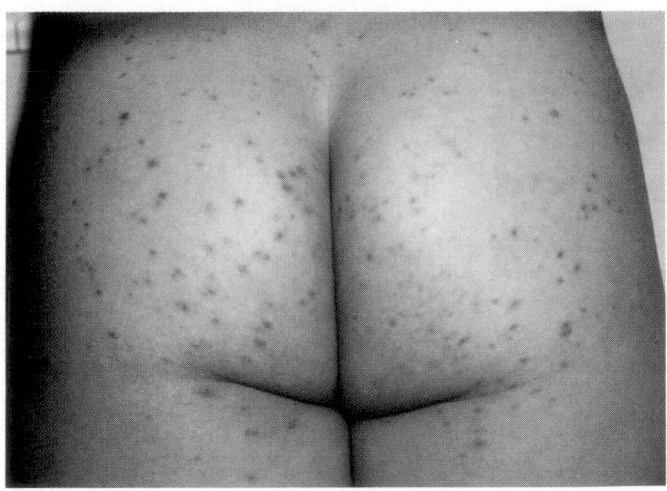

A4-33 **Folliculitis** is a bacterial infection of hair follicles and is seen as erythematous follicular papules and pustules.

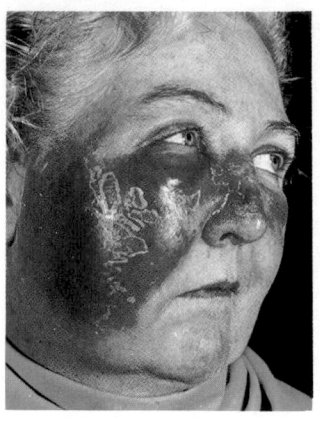

A4-34 **Erysipelas** is a streptococcal infection of the superficial dermis and consists of well-demarcated, erythematous, edematous, warm plaques.

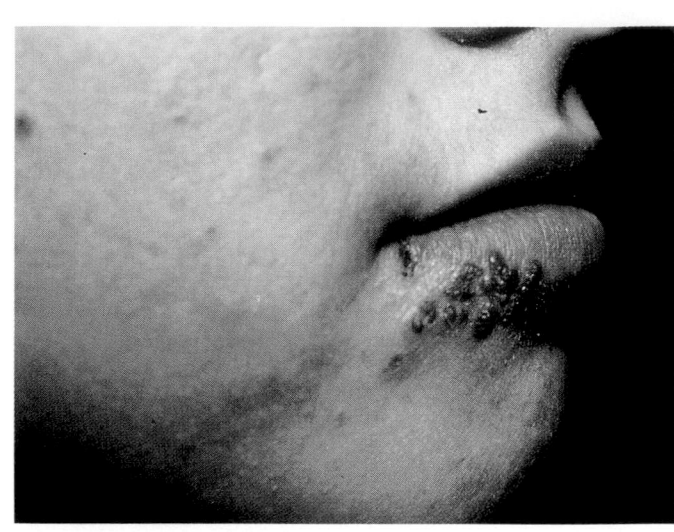

A4-35 **Herpes simplex.** Grouped vesiculopustules on an erythematous base characterize primary HSV infections.

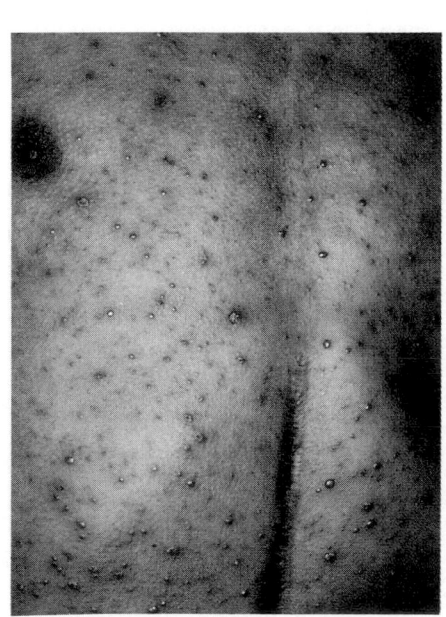

A4-36 **Varicella** showing numerous lesions in various stages of evolution: vesicles on an erythematous base, umbilicated vesicles, and crusts.

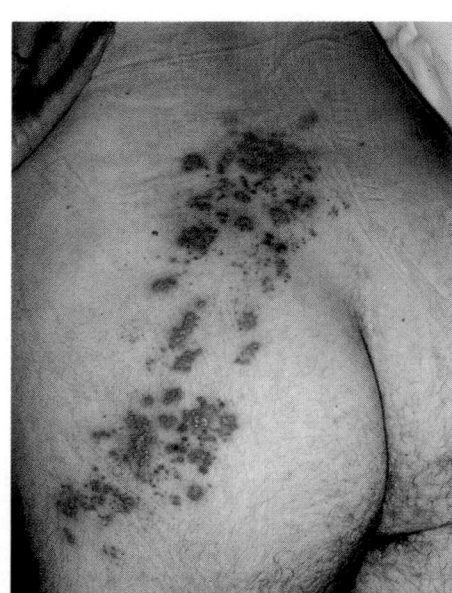

A4-37 **Herpes zoster** seen in this HIV-infected patient as hemorrhagic vesicles and pustules on an erythematous base grouped in a dermatomal distribution.

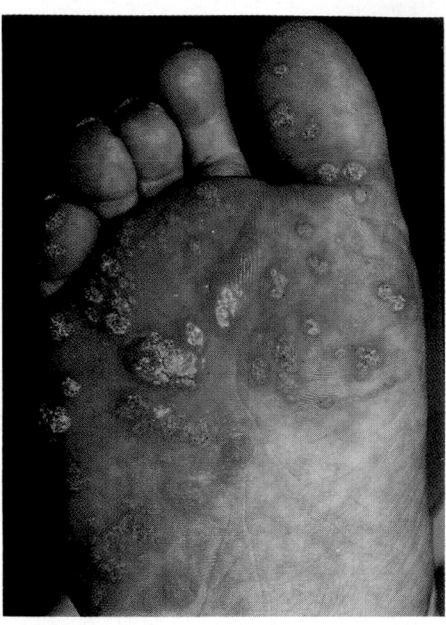

A4-38 **Verrucae** characterized as multiple hyperkeratotic, verrucous papules.

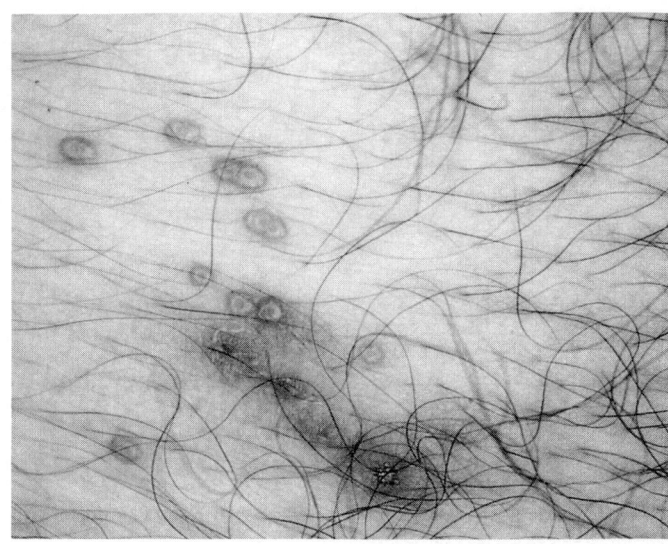

A4-39 **Molluscum contagiosum** is a cutaneous poxvirus infection characterized by multiple umbilicated flesh-colored or hypopigmented papules.

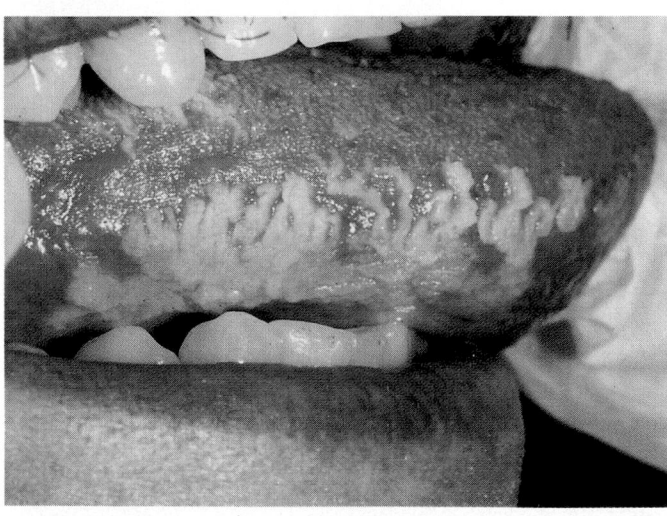

A4-40 **Oral hairy leukoplakia** often presents as white plaques on the lateral tongue and is associated with Epstein-Barr virus infection.

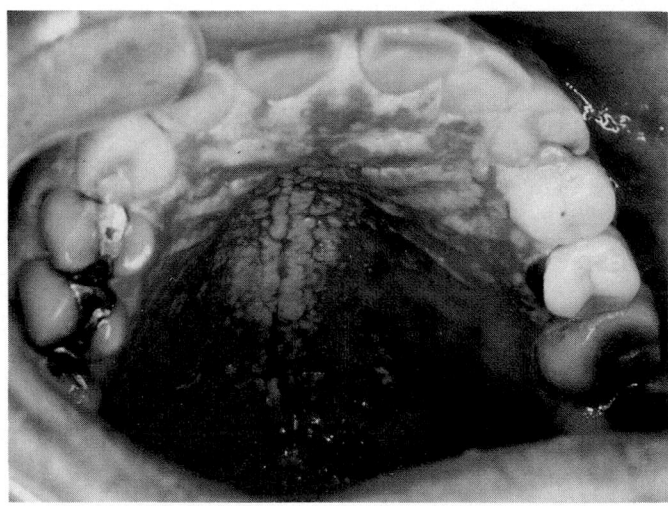

A4-41 **Pseudomembranous oral candidiasis.** Adherent white, mucoid plaques with an erythematous halo seen here on the palate often indicates an immunocompromised state.

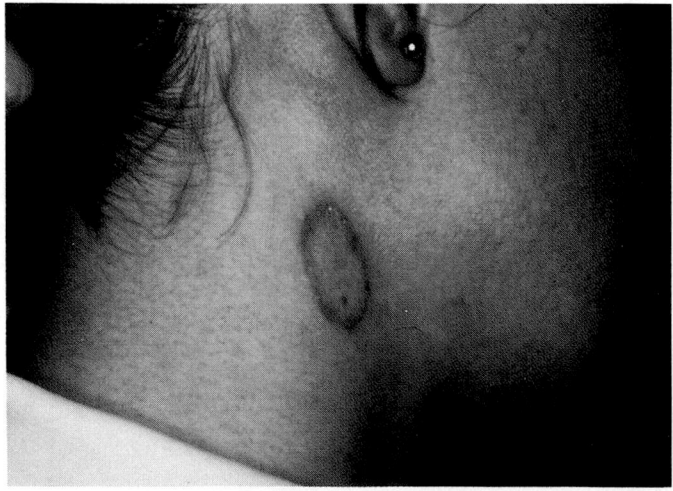

A4-42 **Tinea corporis** is a superficial fungal infection seen here as an erythematous annular scaly plaque with central clearing.

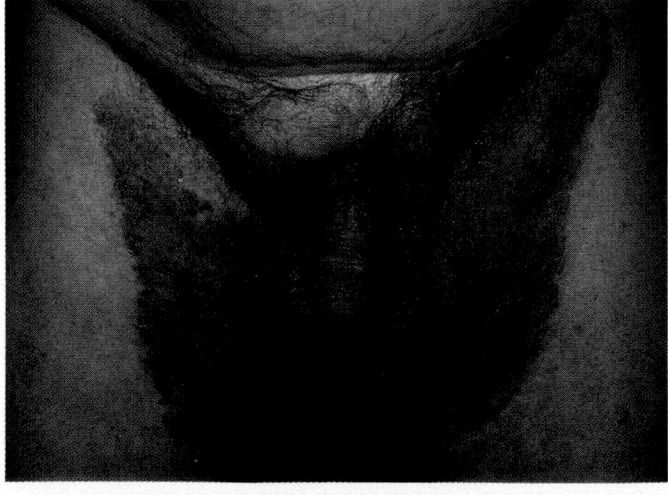

A4-43 **Tinea cruris** is a superficial dermatophyte infection with bilateral scaly, erythematous, annular plaques extending from the inguinal crease to the upper thighs.

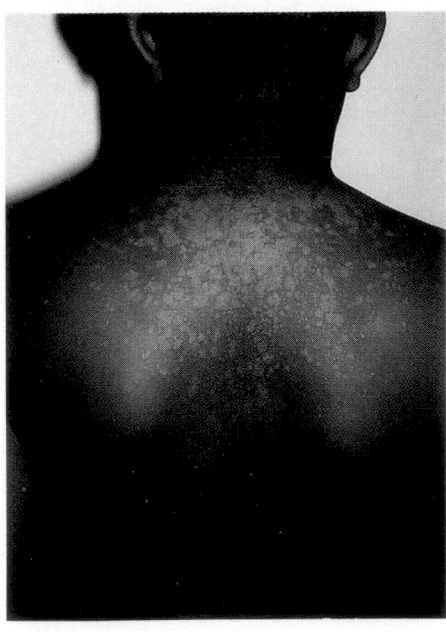

A4-44 **Tinea versicolor** is a superficial cutaneous fungal infection showing a wide variety of lesions. Finely scaling patches may be small or large, hyperpigmented or hypopigmented.

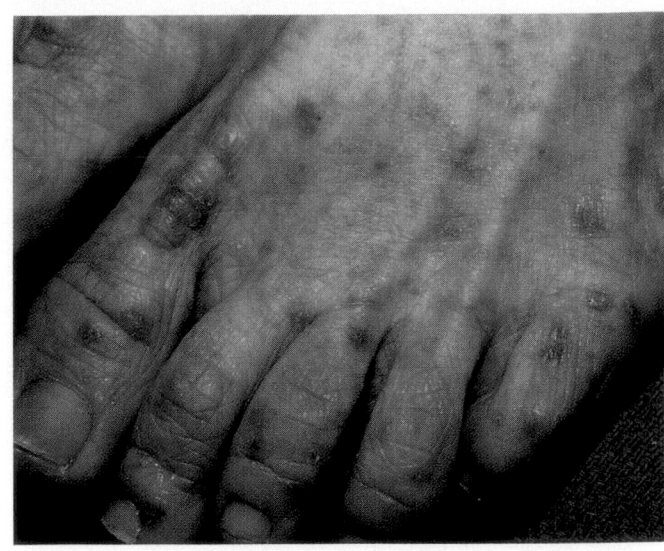

A4-45 **Scabies** showing typical scaling erythematous papules and few linear burrows.

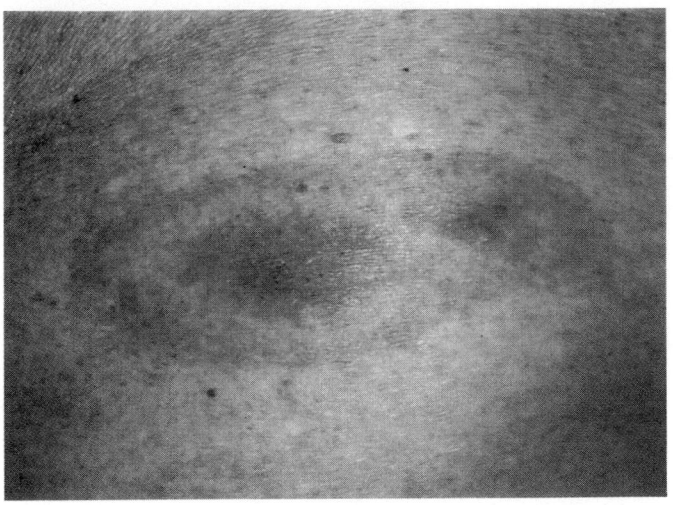

A4-46 **Erythema chronicum migrans** is the early cutaneous manifestation of Lyme disease and is characterized by erythematous annular patches, often with a central erythematous papule at the tick bite site.

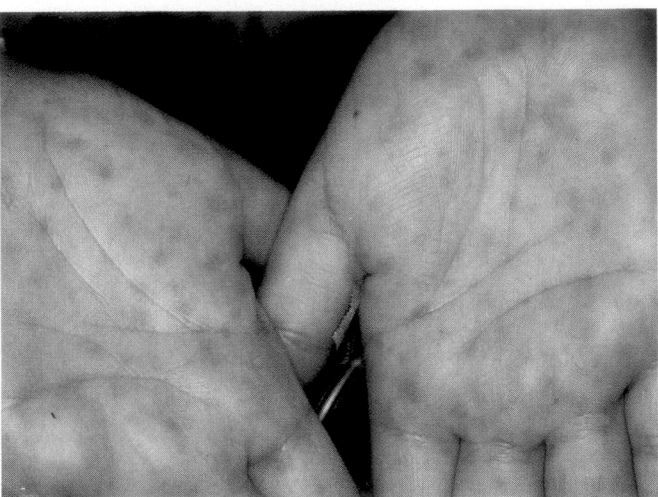

A4-47 **Rocky Mountain spotted fever** demonstrating faint erythematous palmar macules in the early phase of the disease. Lesions may become hemorrhagic (purpuric) as the disease progresses.

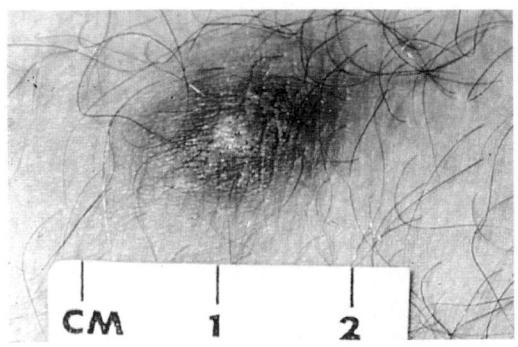

A4-48 **Disseminated gonococcemia** in the skin is seen as hemorrhagic papules and pustules with purpuric centers in an acral distribution.

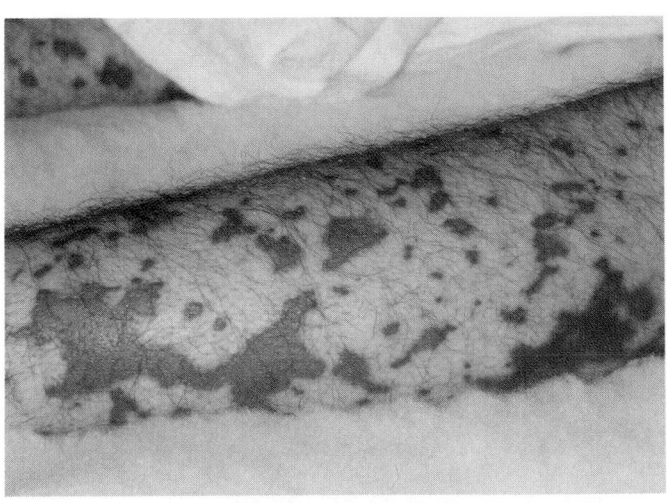

A4-49 **Fulminant meningococcemia** with extensive angular purpuric patches.

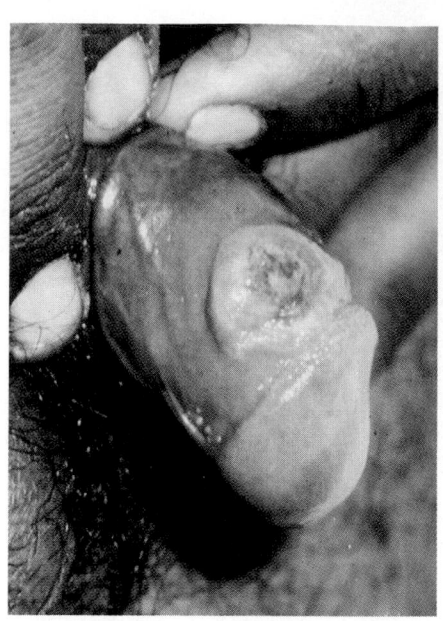

A4-50 **Primary syphilis** with a firm, nontender chancre.

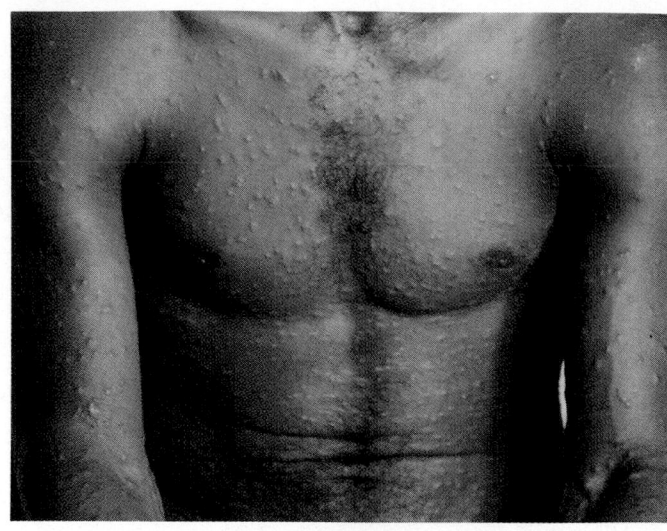

A4-51 **Secondary syphilis** demonstrating the papulosquamous truncal eruption.

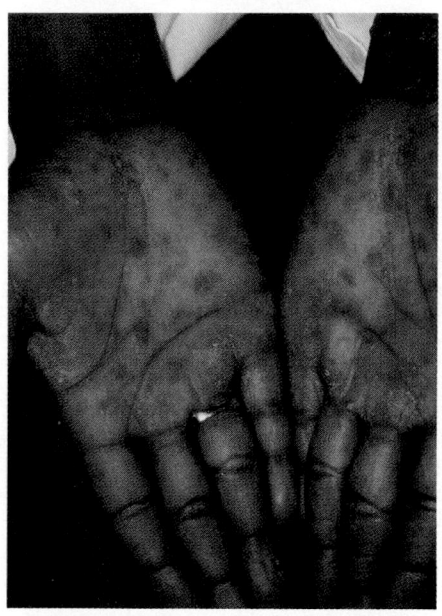

A4-52 **Secondary syphilis** commonly affects the palms and soles with scaling, firm, red-brown papules.

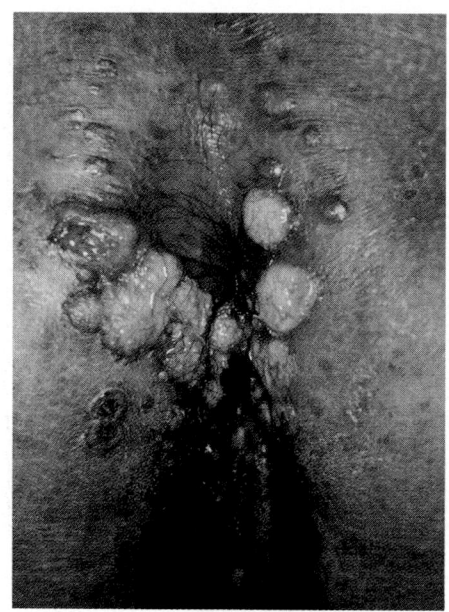

A4-53 **Condylomata lata** are moist somewhat verrucous intertriginous plaques seen in secondary syphilis.

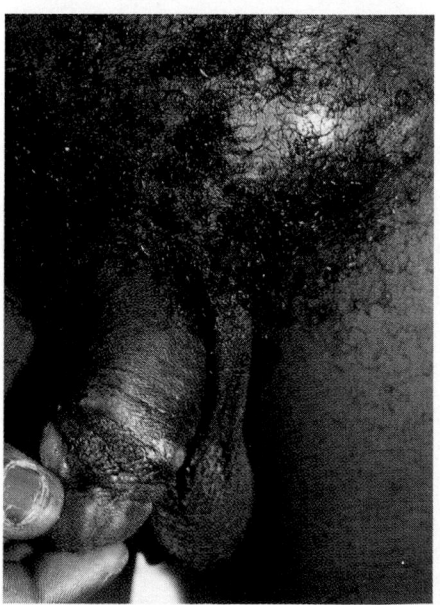

A4-54 **Chancroid** with characteristic penile ulcers and associated left inguinal adenitis (bubo).

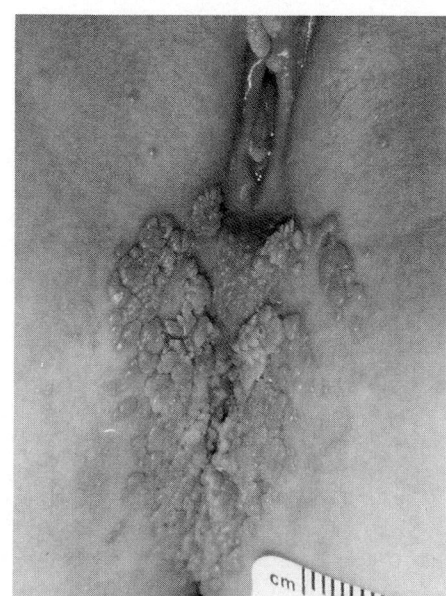

A4-55 **Condylomata acuminata** are lesions induced by human papillomavirus (HPV) and in this patient are seen as multiple verrucous papules coalescing into plaques.

5 Immunologically Mediated Skin Disease

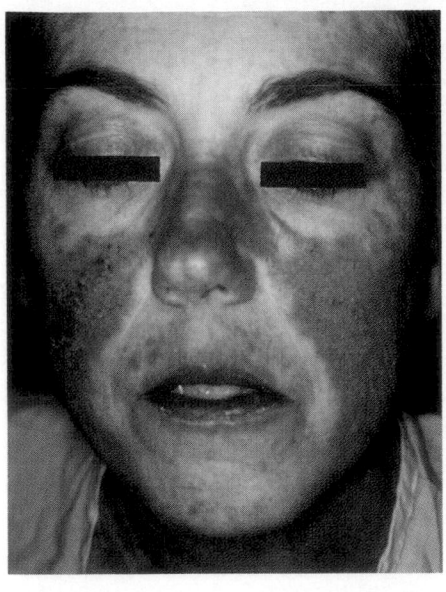

A5-56 **Systemic lupus erythematosus** showing prominent, scaly, malar erythema. Involvement of other sun-exposed sites is also common.

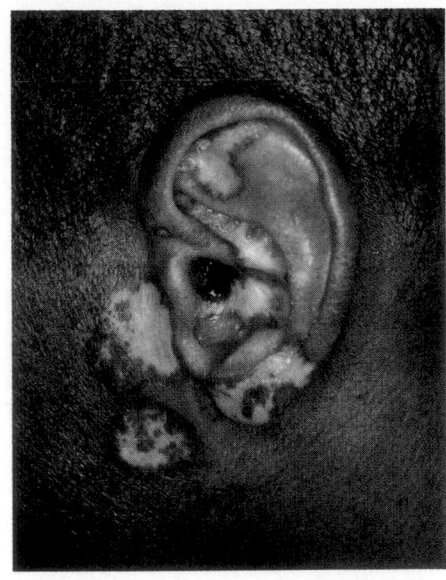

A5-57 **Discoid lupus erythematosus.** Violaceous, hyperpigmented, atrophic plaques, often with evidence of follicular plugging, which may result in scarring, are characteristic of this cutaneous form of lupus.

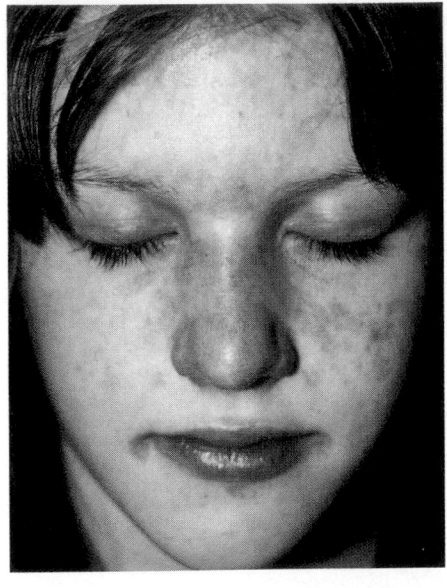

A5-58 **Dermatomyositis.** Periorbital violaceous erythema characterizes the classic heliotrope rash.

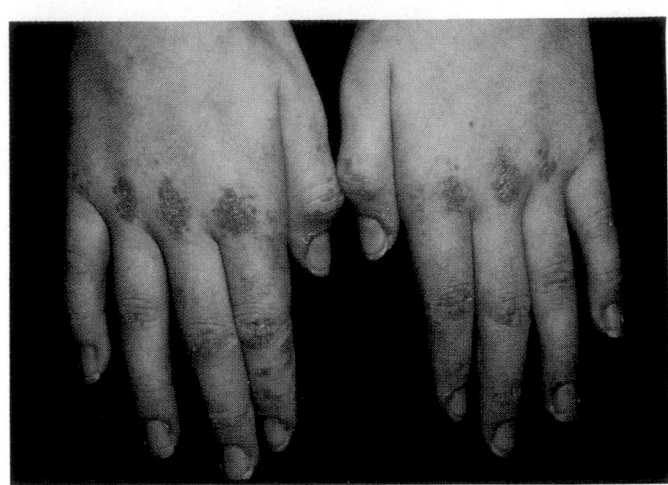

A5-59 **Dermatomyositis** often involves the hands as erythematous flat-topped papules over the knuckles (Gottron's sign) and periungual telangiectasias.

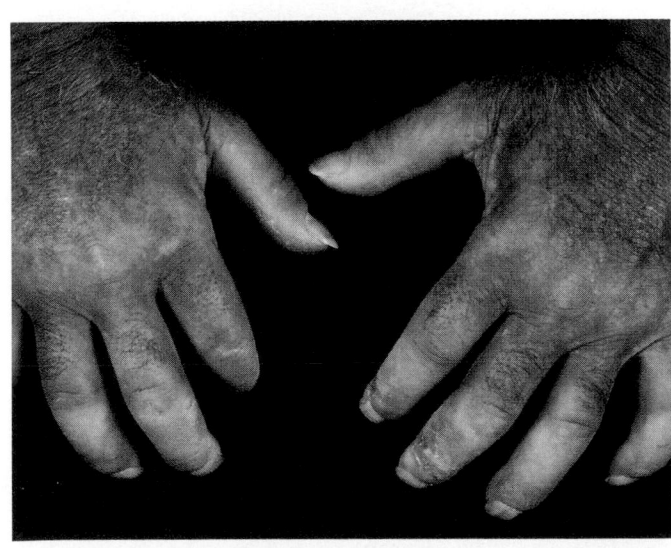

A5-60 **Scleroderma** showing acral sclerosis and focal digital ulcers.

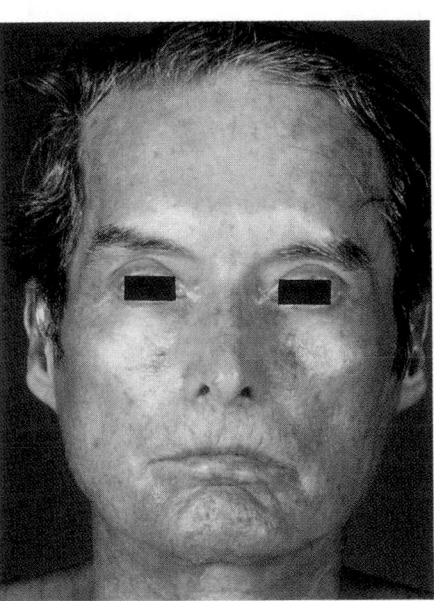

A5-61 **Scleroderma** characterized by typical expressionless, mask-like facies.

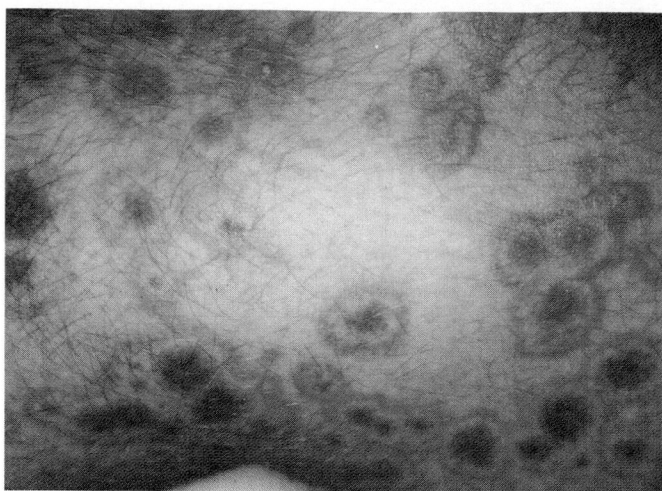

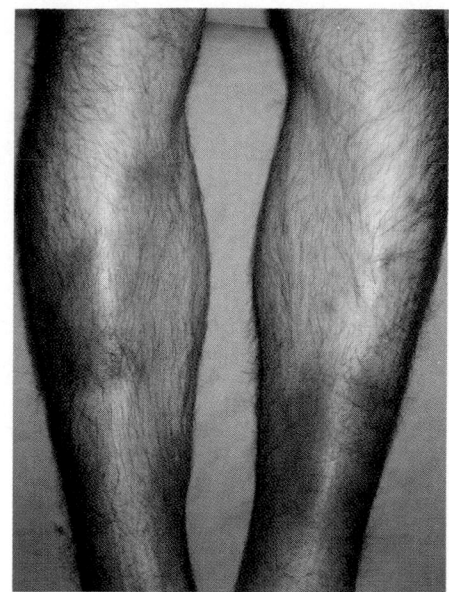

A5-63 **Erythema nodosum** is a panniculitis characterized by tender deep-seated nodules and plaques usually located on the lower extremities.

A5-62 **Erythema multiforme** is characterized by multiple erythematous plaques with a target or iris morphology and usually represents a hypersensitivity reaction to drugs or infections (especially herpes simplex virus).

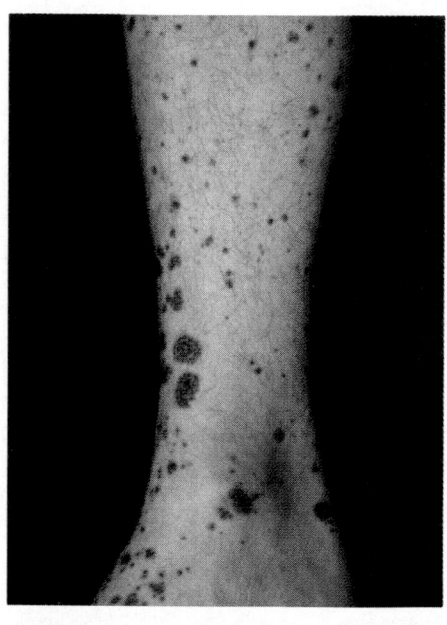

A5-64 **Vasculitis.** Palpable purpuric papules on the lower legs are seen in this patient with cutaneous small vessel vasculitis.

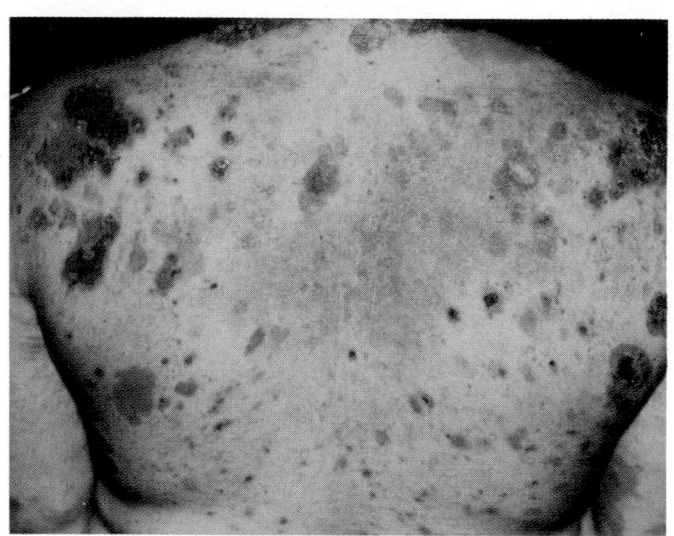

A5-65 **Pemphigus vulgaris** demonstrating flaccid bullae which are easily ruptured, resulting in multiple erosions and crusted plaques.

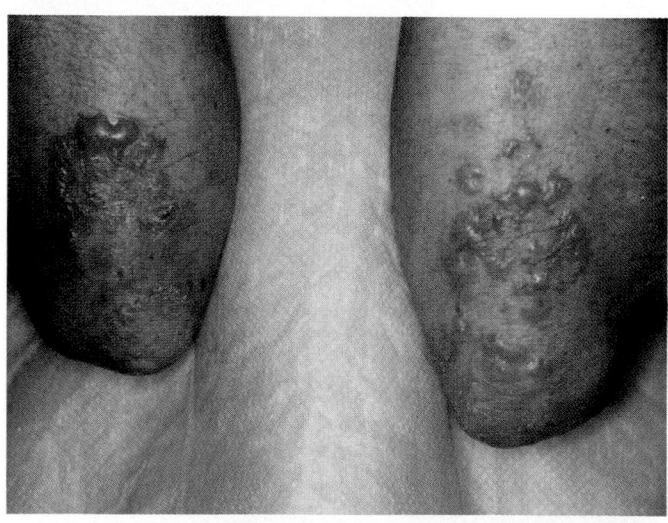

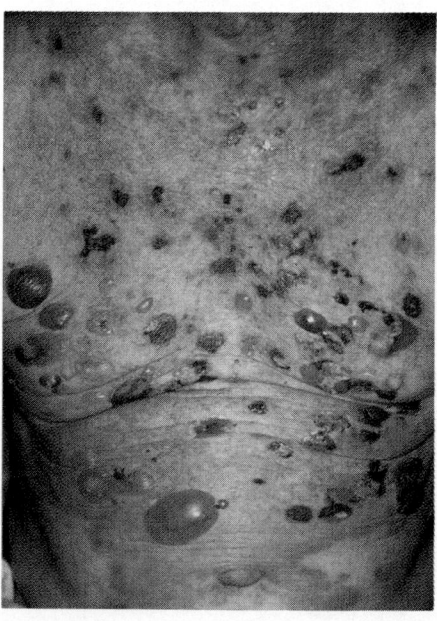

A5-67 **Bullous pemphigoid** with tense vesicles and bullae on an erythematous, urticarial base.

A5-66 **Dermatitis herpetiformis** manifested by pruritic, grouped vesicles in a typical location. The vesicles are often excoriated and may occur on knees, buttocks, and posterior scalp.

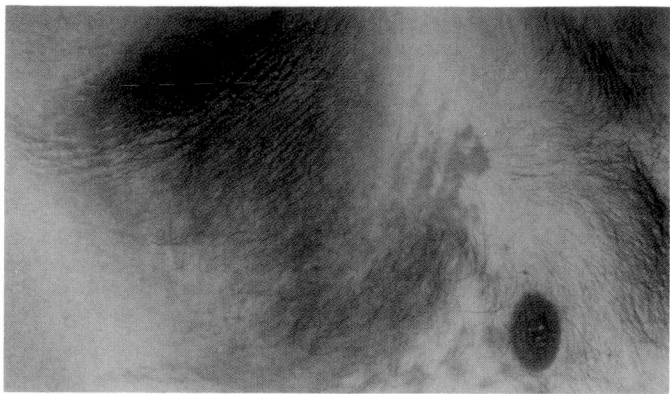

A6-68 **Acanthosis nigricans** demonstrating typical hyperpigmented axillary plaques with a velvet-like, verrucous surface.

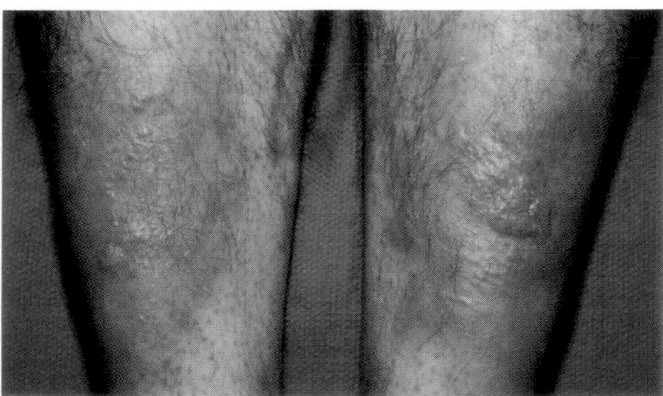

A6-69 **Pretibial myxedema** manifesting as waxy, infiltrated plaques in a patient with Graves' disease.

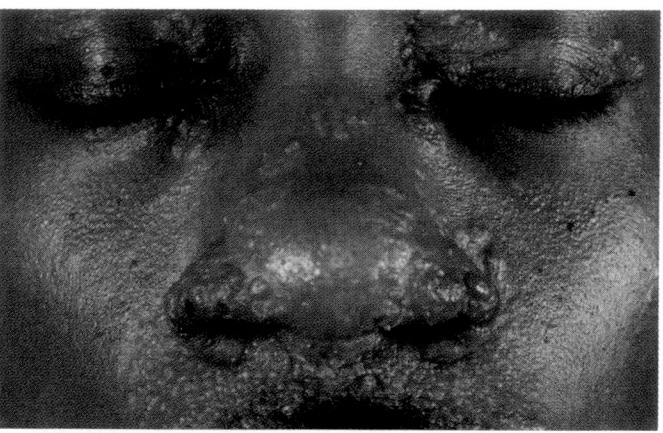

A6-70 **Sarcoid.** Infiltrated papules and plaques of variable color are seen in a typical paranasal and periorbital location.

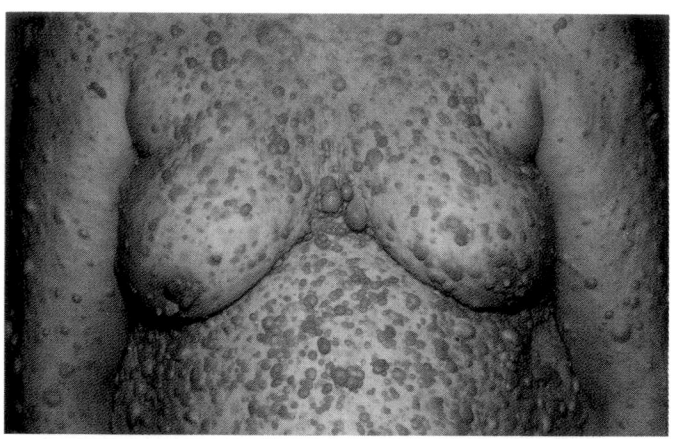

A6-71 **Neurofibromatosis** demonstrating numerous flesh-colored cutaneous neurofibromas.

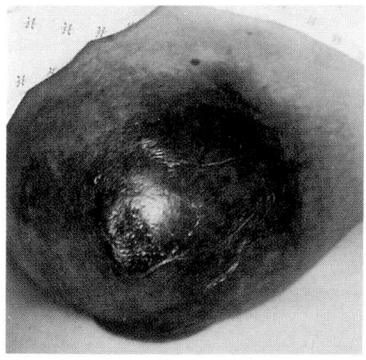

A6-72 **Coumarin necrosis** showing cutaneous and subcutaneous necrosis of a breast. Other fatty areas such as buttocks and thighs are also common sites of involvement.

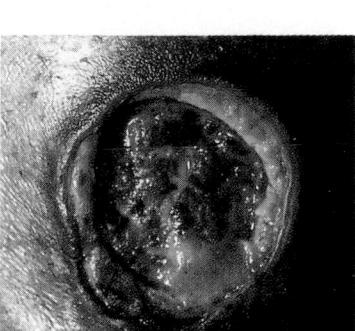

A6-73 **Pyoderma gangrenosum** showing a somewhat purulent ulcer with violaceous and undermined wound edges.

Sources of Photographs

Robert Swerlick, M.D. (*A1-2*) acne rosacea, (*A1-9*) lichen planus, (*A1-12*) alopecia areata, (*A4-33*) folliculitis, (*A5-63*) erythema nodosum, (*A5-64*) vasculitis

S. Wright Caughman, M.D. (*A3-30*) nodular melanoma, (*A4-35*) herpes simplex, (*A4-49*) fulminant meningococcemia, (*A4-55*) condylomata acuminatum

Alvin Solomon, M.D. (*A3-29*) lentigo maligna melanoma, (*A4-52*) secondary syphilis of the palms

Mary Spraker, M.D. (*A4-32*) impetigo contagiosa

Kim Yancey, M.D. (*A6-72*) coumarin necrosis

John Greenspan, Ph.D. (*A4-40*) oral hairy leukoplakia, (*A4-41*) pseudomembranous oral candidiasis

Gregory Cox, M.D. (*A4-50*) primary syphilis

Marilynne McKay, M.D. (*A5-57*) discoid lupus erythematosus

James Krell, M.D. (*A5-58*) dermatomyositis

Yale Resident's Slide Collection (*A4-39*) molluscum contagiosum, (*A4-47*) Rocky Mountain spotted fever, (*A5-67*) bullous pemphigoid, (*A4-46*) erythema chronicum migrans, (*A4-53*) condylomata lata, (*A5-62*) erythema multiforme

Kalman Watsky, M.D. (*A1-1*) acne vulgaris

Jean Bolognia, M.D. (*A1-6*) seborrheic dermatitis, (*A2-24*) non-Hodgkin's lymphoma

Robert Hartman, M.D. (*A4-36*) varicella

Irwin Braverman, M.D. (*A1-4*) atopic dermatitis

Harrison's Principles of Internal Medicine (*A4-34*) erysipelas, (*A4-48*) disseminated gonococcemia

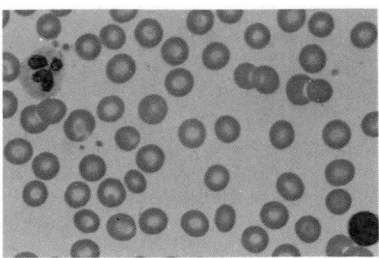

A9-1 **Normal blood smear.** Normal red blood cells are round, possess an area of central pallor, appear slightly smaller than the nucleus of a mature lymphocyte, and vary little in size (anisocytosis) or in shape (poikilocytosis).

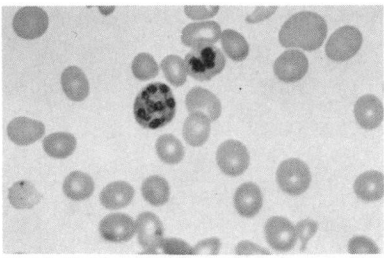

A9-2 **Megaloblastic anemia.** Oval macrocytes, well filled with hemoglobin, are admixed with lesser numbers of small teardrop-shaped red blood cells. Note also hypersegmented granulocyte.

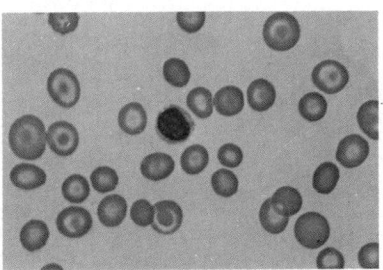

A9-3 **Liver disease.** Round macrocytes of rather uniform size are seen. Many of the macrocytes are also target cells.

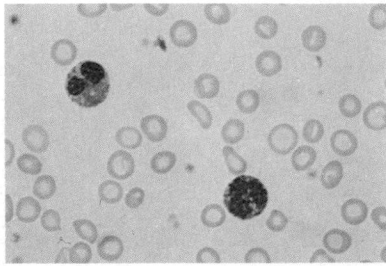

A9-4 **Iron-deficiency anemia.** In severe iron deficiency, the red blood cells are smaller than normal (microcytosis), and their central area of pallor is expanded (hypochromia) so that the cells appear to have only a thin rim of hemoglobin.

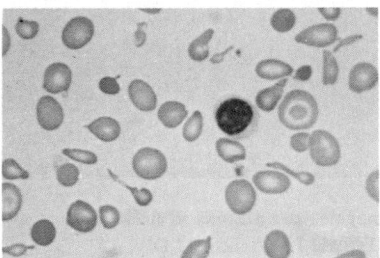

A9-5 **β Thalassemia intermedia.** Microcytic and hypochromic red blood cells are seen that resemble the red blood cells of severe iron deficiency anemia shown in Fig. A9-4. Many elliptical and teardrop-shaped red blood cells are noted.

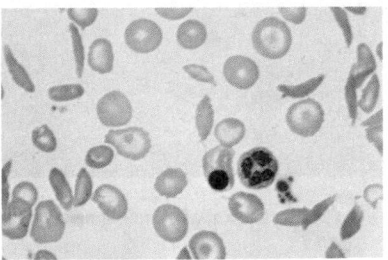

A9-6 **Sickle cell anemia.** The elongated and crescent-shaped red blood cells seen on this smear represent circulating irreversible sickled cells. Target cells and a nucleated red blood cell are also seen.

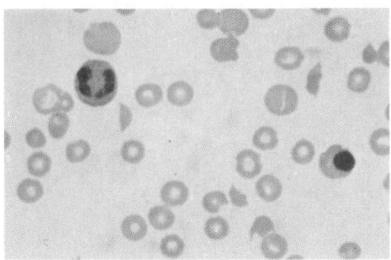

A9-7 **Traumatic hemolysis.** The helmet-shaped red blood cell and the small triangular-shaped red blood cells seen on this smear represent morphologic evidence of mechanical damage to red blood cells within the circulatory tree.

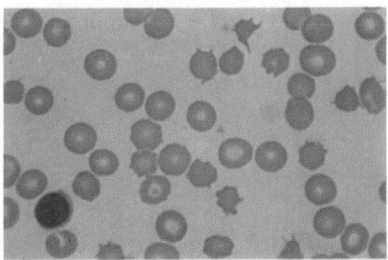

A9-8 **Spur cell anemia.** Spur cells are recognized as distorted red blood cells containing several irregularly distributed thornlike projections. Cells with this morphologic abnormality are also called acanthocytes.

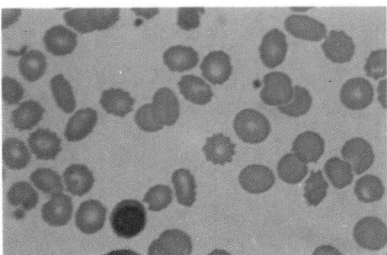

A9-9 **Uremia.** The red blood cells in uremia may acquire numerous, regularly spaced, small spiny projections. Such cells, called burr cells or echinocytes, are readily distinguishable from the irregularly spiculated acanthocytes shown in Fig. A9-8.

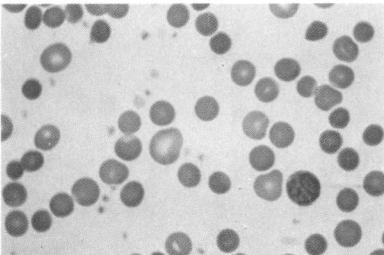

A9-10 **Hereditary spherocytosis.** Small, densely staining red blood cells are seen that have lost their central area of pallor (microspherocytes). Microspherocytes may also be found in other hemolytic disorders (Fig. A9-11).

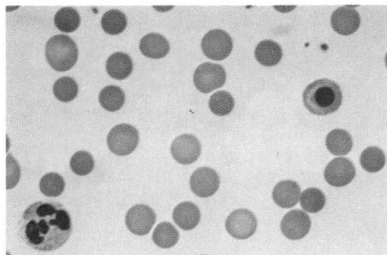

A9-11 **Immunohemolytic anemia.** Microspherocytes are seen on this blood smear along with several macrocytes with a slight purple tinge (polychromasia). The latter represent new red blood cells released early from the bone marrow. The microspherocytes seen in immunohemolytic anemia may be indistinguishable from the microspherocytes seen in hereditary spherocytosis (Fig. A9-10).

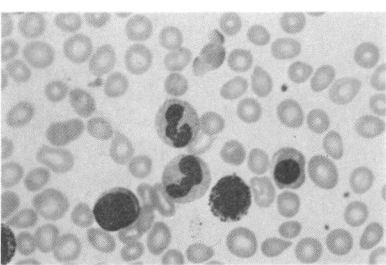

A9-12 **Myeloid metaplasia.** Teardrop-shaped red blood cells, a nucleated red blood cell, and immature myeloid cells are seen on this blood smear.

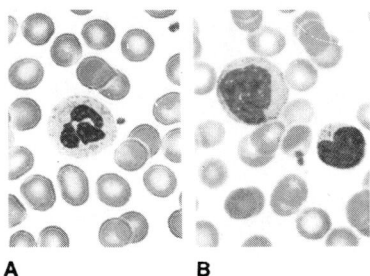

A   **B**

A9-13 A. **Normal granulocyte.** The normal
granulocyte has a segmented nucleus with
heavy, clumped chromatin; fine neutrophilic
granules are dispersed throughout its cytoplasm. *B.* **Normal monocyte and lymphocyte.** The normal monocyte is a large cell
with an indented or folded nucleus containing
loose, strandliké chromatin; the cytoplasm is
a blue-gray color and usually contains fine
azurophilic granules. The normal lymphocyte
is a smaller cell. Its nucleus is usually round
but may be indented, as in the cell shown in
this plate. The nuclear chromatin has a
smudgy appearance; the cytoplasm is a blue
color.

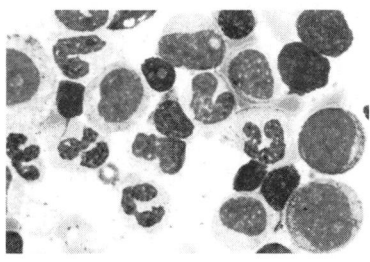

A9-15 **Normal granulocyte precursors in
marrow.** The earliest granulocytic precursor
(myeloblast) possesses a round nucleus with
fine, punctate chromatin and one or more
nucleoli; the cytoplasm is blue. As nuclear
differentiation proceeds, the nucleoli disappear, the chromatin coarsens, and the nucleus
becomes increasingly indented and finally
segmented. As cytoplasmic differentiation
proceeds, azurophilic granules appear and
the cytoplasm changes color from blue to the
yellow-pink-gray hue of the mature granulocyte, and as this occurs the azurophilic
granules become obscured by fine neutrophilic granules.

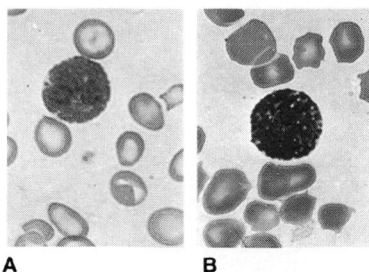

A   **B**

A9-14 A. **Normal eosinophil.** The eosinophil contains large, bright-orange granules;
the nucleus is bilobed. *B.* **Basophil.** The
basophil contains large purple-black granules
which fill the cell and obscure the nucleus.

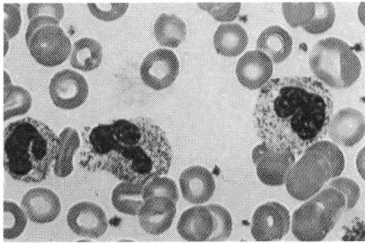

A9-16 **Neutrophils with toxic granulation.**
In infection and other toxic states, azurophilic
granules may become visible in mature granulocytes as coarse, dark-staining cytoplasmic
granules.

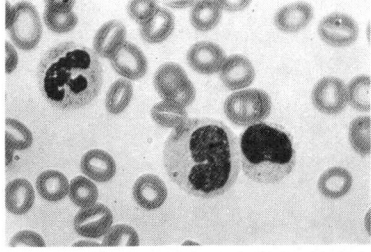

A9-17 **Band with Döhle body** (center).
Döhle bodies are discrete, blue-staining non-
granular areas found in the periphery of the
cytoplasm of the neutrophil in infections and
other toxic states. They represent aggregates
of rough endoplasmic reticulum.

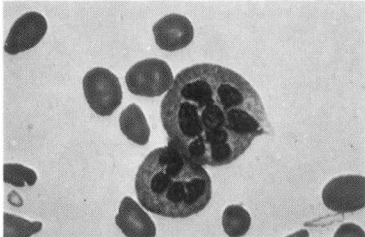

A9-18 **Hypersegmentation.** Frequent five-lobed granulocytes on a blood smear or granulocytes with more than five lobes are evidence of hypersegmentation, an important clue to the diagnosis of megaloblastic anemia.

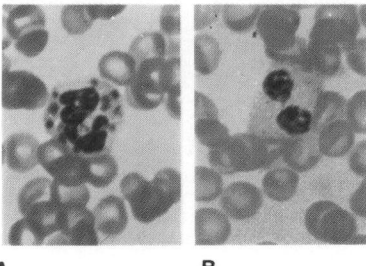

A   **B**

A9-19 A. **Chédiak-Higashi anomaly.** In this ultimately fatal disorder, the granulocytes contain huge cytoplasmic granules, formed from aggregation and fusion of azurophilic and specific granules. Large, abnormal granules are found in other granule-containing cells throughout the body. *B.* **Pelger-Hüet anomaly.** In this benign disorder, the majority of granulocytes are bilobed. The nucleus frequently has a spectacle-like or "pince-nez" configuration.

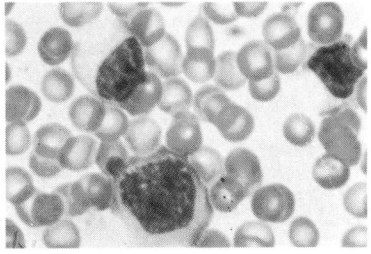

A9-20 **Reactive lymphocytes** (infectious mononucleosis). Reactive lymphocytes are usually large, cytoplasmic lymphocytes. The nucleus may be eccentrically placed and may have irregular borders and indentations (not seen on this plate). The cytoplasm contains areas that stain a darker blue due to their increased content of RNA. The cytoplasm may be indented where it abuts against a red blood cell.

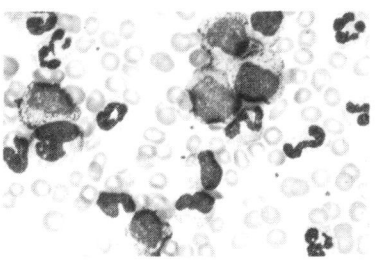

A9-21 **Chronic granulocytic leukemia.** The peripheral blood WBC count is high due to increased numbers of granulocytes and their precursors. The majority of the WBCs are segmented granulocytes or band forms, but as seen on this plate, myelocytes and promyeloblasts (not seen on this plate) may also be found on review of the blood smear.

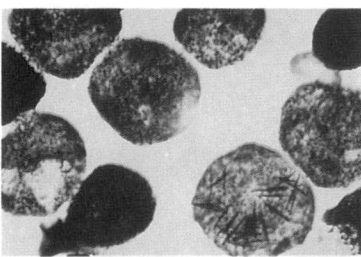

A9-22 **Leukemic cell in acute promyelocytic leukemia.** Note multiple Auer rods.

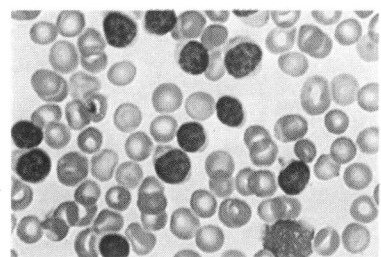

A9-23 **Chronic lymphocytic leukemia.** The peripheral blood WBC count is high due to increased numbers of small, well-differentiated lymphocytes. However, the leukemic lymphocytes are fragile, and substantial numbers of broken, smudged cells are usually also present on the blood smear.

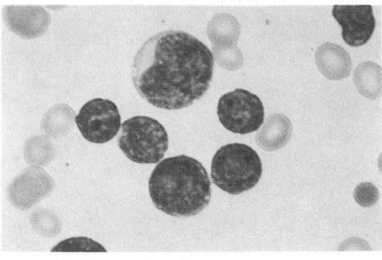

A9-24 **Leukemic cells in acute lympho-blastic leukemia** characterized by round or convoluted nuclei, high nuclear/cytoplasmic ratio and absence of cytoplasmic granules.

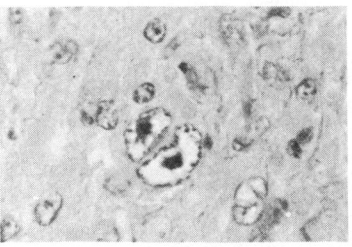

A9-25 **Hodgkin's disease:** Reed-Sternberg cell in marrow (center). The Reed-Sternberg cell is recognized by its bilobed, mirror-image nucleus, which contains in each lobe a giant, inclusion body-like nucleolus. The cytoplasmic borders of the cell cannot be identified on this plate.

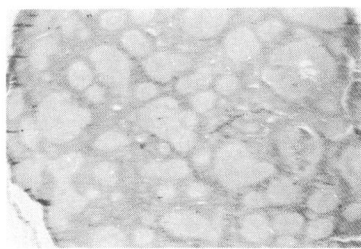

A9-26 **Non-Hodgkin's nodular lymphoma** (lymph node). This low-power view illustrates that a proliferative process has caused the normal architecture of the lymph node to be replaced by multiple nodules of varying size that extend throughout the entire lymph node.

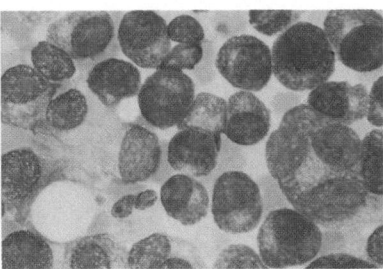

A9-27 **Multiple myeloma** (marrow). The cells bear the characteristic morphologic features of plasma cells, round or oval cells with an eccentric nucleus composed of coarsely clumped chromatin, a densely basophilic cytoplasm, and a perinuclear clear zone (hof) containing the Golgi apparatus. Binucleate and multinucleate malignant plasma cells also can be seen.

patients. Bradycardia relative to the height of the fever may be a clinical clue to typhoid but is present in a minority of patients. Epistaxis may occur in the early stages of illness. "Rose spots," appearing as small, pale red, blanching, slightly raised macules, are occasionally seen on the chest and abdomen during the first week. They also can evolve into nonblanching small hemorrhages that are difficult to see in dark-skinned patients. The major characteristics of untreated typhoid are persistent high fever, severe anorexia, weight loss, and changes in sensorium, but a variety of other complications may develop, including hepatitis, meningitis, nephritis, myocarditis, bronchitis, pneumonia, arthritis, osteomyelitis, parotitis, and orchitis. Excepting relapse, the frequency of all these complications, including hemorrhage and perforation, is reduced by prompt use of appropriate antibiotics.

Multidrug-resistant *S. typhi* is becoming more prevalent in many endemic countries. These patients present with more severe illness, they look "toxic," and they have a higher incidence of disseminated intravascular coagulation and hepatomegaly and a threefold increased mortality rate thought to be related to the longer duration of disease and prior ineffective oral antibiotic therapy.

Around 3 to 5 percent of patients become long-term asymptomatic carriers, some for life unless treated. Many carriers give no history of typhoid fever and probably had an undiagnosed mild infection.

LABORATORY FINDINGS In around 25 percent of patients, leukopenia and neutropenia are present. In most patients, the white blood cell count is normal, albeit low in relation to the degree of fever, which may be a clue to the diagnosis. Rarely, severe leukopenia (<2000 cells per microliter) can occur. In the event of intestinal perforation or pyogenic complications, secondary leukocytosis develops. The anemia of blood loss may be superimposed on the anemia of chronic infection.

Definitive diagnosis depends on isolation of the organism. The recovery of organisms from blood is highest in the first week of illness, when it approaches 90 percent. Bacteremia is detectable in 50 percent in the third week and at a progressively lower frequency later on. Early in the illness culture of bone marrow aspirates will yield the organism in the majority of patients with negative blood cultures, even after brief prior antimicrobial treatment. Stool cultures are frequently negative in the first week but become positive in 75 percent of patients during the third week. By the eighth week, stools are positive in only 10 percent of patients but in approximately 3 to 5 percent of patients will remain so for at least 1 year. The frequency of positive urine cultures parallels the yield from stools and may represent, in some patients, contamination with feces.

Serologic diagnosis is less reliable than culture. Most, but not all, patients will develop agglutinating antibodies to O, H, and Vi antigens (the Widal test). In the absence of recent immunization, a high titer of antibody to O antigen (>1:640) is suggestive but not specific because other serogroup D salmonellae share the antigen used in the Widal test, as do some organisms in groups A and B. H antibodies may be found in even higher titer but because of their broad cross-reactivity are difficult to interpret. A fourfold rise in antibody in paired samples is a good criterion but is of little use in the acutely ill patient and may be blunted by early effective antimicrobial therapy. The earlier the baseline sample is obtained, the more likely a significant rise will be detected. Vi antibodies typically rise later, after 3 to 4 weeks of illness, and are of less use in the early diagnosis of infection.

DIFFERENTIAL DIAGNOSIS When all the classic clinical manifestations are present, including rose spots, prolonged fever, relative bradycardia, and leukopenia, the diagnosis of typhoid will be strongly suggested. However, most cases do not fit this "typical" profile. Differential diagnosis includes infections associated with prolonged fever such as the rickettsioses, brucellosis, tularemia, leptospirosis, miliary tuberculosis, viral hepatitis, infectious mononucleosis, cytomegalovirus infections, and malaria, as well as noninfectious causes such as lymphoma (see Chap. 16). In the United States, typhoid should be considered in any patient with prolonged, unexplained fever, especially after recent travel to places with endemic typhoid fever.

TREATMENT Since its introduction, chloramphenicol has been the antimicrobial gold standard for treatment. No drug has been better in promoting a favorable clinical response, which usually becomes apparent within 24 to 48 h of the start of treatment in the appropriate dosages (3 to 4 g/d in adults or 50 to 75 mg/kg of body weight per day in young children). The drug is given orally for 2 weeks, and the dose may be reduced to 2 g/d or 30 mg/kg per day when the patient becomes afebrile, which usually is not before day 5 of treatment. However, because of the specter of aplastic anemia associated with chloramphenicol, the drug is little used in the United States. Other effective oral regimens include amoxicillin (4 to 6 g/d in four divided doses in adults or 100 mg/kg per day in children), trimethoprim-sulfamethoxazole (640 and 3200 mg, respectively, in two divided doses daily in adults or 185 mg/m^2 of body surface area per day of the trimethoprim component for children), or in those over 17 years of age a 4-fluoroquinolone such as ciprofloxacin or ofloxacin.

A variety of intravenous drugs are also effective, and both chloramphenicol and trimethoprim-sulfamethoxazole can be given intravenously in those unable to take oral medications. Other effective parenteral antimicrobials include high-dose ampicillin, cefotaxime, aztreonam, and the 4-fluoroquinolones. However, none has been as rapidly acting or as effective as ceftriaxone, which rivals or betters chloramphenicol in rapidity of defervescence. Initial recommendations for a 7-day course of ceftriaxone have since been pared down to 3 days of 3 to 4 g once daily in adults or 80 mg/kg once daily for 5 days in children without apparent loss of efficacy. In addition, compared with that associated with other drugs, the relapse rate appears lower in adults or children given ceftriaxone; however, the number of patients reported is still small.

Prevalence of multidrug resistance of *S. typhi* to first-line oral drugs has been rising in developing countries, sometimes strikingly, due to acquisition of plasmids encoding inactivating β-lactamase and chloramphenicol acetyl transferase enzymes. In regions where this multidrug resistance is a problem, ceftriaxone or a 4-fluoroquinolone should be used initially for adults over 17 years of age, with ceftriaxone as the best choice for children, at least until the new quinolones are proven safe for young children. The higher cost of ceftriaxone is somewhat offset by the efficacy of a short course and the economy of once-daily dosing.

Studies in Indonesia of patients with severe typhoid who present with central nervous system manifestations and/or evidence of disseminated intravenous coagulation suggest that intravenous dexamethasone, 3 mg/kg as a loading dose over 30 min followed by 1 mg/kg every 6 h for 24 to 48 h, in addition to parenteral antimicrobials, reduces mortality. Salicylates should be avoided to diminish the danger of intestinal hemorrhage. Prompt surgical management of bleeding and bowel perforation reduces mortality, which is associated primarily with peritonitis. Bowel perforations should be closed in two layers for best results. Antibiotics should be selected to treat not only *S. typhi* but also the facultative and anaerobic bowel flora. Selective angiography, radioisotopic scanning methods, or sometimes endoscopy (see Chap. 46) to localize the bleeding site can facilitate operative repair. In developing countries, however, patients often present late after perforation, they may be severely malnourished and poor surgical risks, and only limited surgical and postoperative care may be available. Supportive medical care and antibiotics alone have been recommended in this setting, although limited surgery to close the perforation site without bowel resection is increasingly favored. With the use of double-layer closure of the lesion and an inexpensive broad antibiotic regimen including chloramphenicol, gentamicin, and metronidazole, mortality rates have been reduced from 25 to 30 percent to well under 10 percent.

The early use of effective antimicrobials is associated with a relatively high rate of relapse; relapse rates of 20 percent can be expected, compared with 5 to 10 percent in untreated patients. This is presumably because prompt therapy inhibits the development of an adequate immune response. Relapses are usually milder than the initial attack and will respond to the same antimicrobial used initially.

Eradication of the chronic carrier state, especially in the presence of gallstones, is notoriously difficult. Traditional regimens have used 100 mg/kg per day of ampicillin or amoxicillin plus probenecid (30 mg/kg per day) or trimethoprim-sulfamethoxazole (160/800 mg) twice daily plus rifampin (600 mg) once daily for at least 6 weeks. Recent studies suggest that a 4-week course of a 4-fluoroquinolone is at least as good and probably much better because the organism is exquisitely sensitive in vitro and the drugs reach the gut lumen, liver, gallbladder, and bile in active form. The new quinolones provide the best chance of eradicating *S. typhi* in the presence of gallstones, and because of simplicity and safety, they should be the first choice in patients without stones as well. The optimal dose and duration of treatment have yet to be defined. These drugs would be the best choice for chronic suppression of typhoid relapse in AIDS patients as well.

PREVENTION AND CONTROL   Worldwide experience has shown that improvement of environmental sanitation, including sewage disposal and water supplies, will sharply reduce the incidence of typhoid fever. Where this approach is not yet possible, and for travelers, immunization has been used. The protective efficacy of multiple doses of traditional heat-killed phenol-extracted whole typhoid vaccine is, at best, 65 percent and lasts just a few months, at a cost of certain local pain and fever. It has been largely replaced in the United States by three doses of a first-generation live oral vaccine (Ty21a). While this strain is invasive, because it is also metabolically defective, it dies after a few cycles of replication and therefore is avirulent. Nonetheless, it provides protection equivalent to the killed vaccine and lasts for at least several years. In Europe, one dose of purified Vi polysaccharide vaccine has proven as effective and long lasting as multiple doses of Ty21a, yet this product is inexplicably not available in the United States. New genetically engineered live typhoid vaccines are actively being developed by mutation of aromatic biosynthesis pathway genes, the adenylate cyclase and cAMP regulatory genes, or other virulence genes or by combination of several genetic changes in the same candidate strain. These strains are being pursued not only for immunization against typhoid but also for development of live vectors into which extraneous genes can be cloned for oral delivery of protective antigens from unrelated species. In addition, Vi-protein conjugates are being made and evaluated as immunogens suitable for infants, especially in endemic regions where infantile typhoid is prevalent and remains a dangerous disease.

Typhoid is a reportable disease in the United States. Patients should be monitored for prolonged carriage and treated for it if necessary. Precautions in food handling by carriers and in disposal of their stools are obvious and important (see Chap. 98).

PROGNOSIS   Appropriate therapy of typhoid fever, especially if patients present for medical care in the early stage of disease, is highly successful. The mortality rate should be under 1 percent, and few complications should occur.

NONTYPHOIDAL SALMONELLOSIS

Infections caused by any *Salmonella* other than *S. typhi* are termed *nontyphoidal salmonellosis*. These infections can present as acute diarrhea, a septicemic syndrome, focal abscesses, meningitis, osteomyelitis, endocarditis, or mycotic aneurysm or can be asymptomatic.

EPIDEMIOLOGY   The species *S. cholerasuis* and *S. enteritidis* include a diverse group of organisms with both host-adapted and non-host-adapted serotypes. Two human-adapted serotypes, *S. paratyphi A* and *S. schottmuelleri* (more often called *S. paratyphi B*) mimic *S. typhi* and cause a milder form of typhoid fever. Of the more than 2200 known *S. enteritidis* serotypes, just 10 account for 75 percent of all human disease isolates in the United States, and 4 serotypes (*S. typhimurium, enteritidis, heidelberg,* and *newport*) cause about two-thirds of all disease. *S. typhimurium* has previously been the most frequent isolate, representing around 35 percent of all strains

reported to the CDC. In past surveillance studies, periodic increases in recovery of certain serotypes have represented either the introduction of a new transmission source or the occurrence of a large outbreak. For example, a fivefold increase in *S. enteritidis* isolates between 1976 and 1986 was due to ingestion of contaminated grade A eggs primarily in the northeastern United States. Infections from this source have continued to increase in North and South America, Europe, and probably Africa as well. By 1992, *S. enteritidis* overtook *S. typhimurium* as the most frequently isolated *Salmonella* in the United States and at least eight countries in Europe, suggesting a new global pandemic related primarily to infected poultry eggs.

Careful analysis of surveillance data in the United States has shown that not only is the number of nontyphoidal *Salmonella* isolates increasing, but the incidence appears to be increasing as well, from 8 per 100,000 of the general population in 1965 to 12 per 100,000 in 1975, peaking at around 18 per 100,000 in 1985, and dropping slightly to approximately 16 per 100,000 in 1991. While the incidence of disease in young children is five times higher than in older subjects, the rate is also somewhat higher in adults over 70 years. Between 1970 and 1986, the median age of infected individuals rose from 6 years to 20 years and has remained as high since then. The greatest increase has been in the 20- to 39-year-old population, suggesting that foods consumed by young adults are becoming important vehicles or that they are traveling more to endemic areas. For example, the emergence of serious systemic infections in southern California due to *S. dublin* carrying a large virulence plasmid has been associated with the ingestion of unpasteurized dairy products or nontraditional nutritional treatments using raw calf-liver extracts contaminated with this serotype. A reasonable estimate of the total incidence of symptomatic *Salmonella* infection in the United States is around 2 million cases per year. This degree of morbidity implies a significant economic impact in lost productivity and medical costs and, by extension, a serious and underestimated cause of mortality.

Because nontyphoidal *Salmonella* are so often non-host-adapted, many kinds of domestic animals can harbor the organism and serve as the source for human infection. From 50 to 75 percent of broiler and layer chicken flocks in Canada are infected with a large variety of *Salmonella* serotypes, many of which are virulent for humans. In one experimental setting, 10 percent of the intact eggs of a naturally infected layer flock were positive for a human virulent *S. enteritidis* phage type 4. Although the number of organisms per egg was less than 10 at laying, growth to large numbers quickly occurs if eggs are not kept at 4°C; after 2 days at room temperature, over 10^8 organisms per gram of yolk can be isolated. At this level of contamination, viable organisms will survive cooking by any method. The source of the *Salmonella* can be the surface of the shell if the egg rests for a short time on infected hen feces or even the dry bedding of an infected hen, since the bacteria can penetrate the intact egg through microscopic pores normally present in the shell. Because the epidemic is so profound and so unlike past problems of *Salmonella* associated with cracked eggs, and because it has involved free-range as well as commercial henhouse eggs, a transovarian route is more likely and presents a rather major problem for infection control. Conditions of raising, shipping, slaughtering, and marketing contribute to the spread of *Salmonella* in the food supply. Introduction of the organism into processed foods can result in widespread dissemination, and contamination of such common foods as eggs or milk leads to large-scale outbreaks, including nosocomial hospital epidemics. Dried or frozen foods preserve viable salmonellae. For these reasons, salmonellosis is more a disease of the industrialized world than of the developing world. Additional sources of human infection are animals sold as pets, including baby chicks or ducks and turtles, and medical products of animal origin, such as carmine dye (from insects), pancreatin, bile salts, or tissue extracts from thyroids, adrenals, stomaches, or rattlesnakes.

A potentially serious problem is the selection of antibiotic-resistant strains of salmonellae by unregulated drug use in animal husbandry.

There are a number of instances where transmission to humans has occurred. Persistent and severe salmonellosis also has been recognized as a problem among patients with AIDS (see Chap. 279).

PATHOGENESIS As with *S. typhi*, the events following ingestion of the organism are determined by environmental factors (dose), microbial factors (the ability to invade epithelial cells and multiply within mononuclear phagocytes and to resist intestinal peptide antibiotic defensins), and host resistance factors (gastric acid and the ability to rapidly mobilize phagocytic cells and to activate and expand clones of T cells involved in protection, such as V gamma 9–bearing gamma-delta T cells). As few as 10^3 virulent organisms may cause disease, especially in patients with achlorhydria or having recent antimicrobial therapy. Systemic invasion is more likely in patients with "reticuloendothelial blockade" due to hemolysis (malaria, bartonellosis, leptospirosis, sickle cell anemia) or intracellular infections (histoplasmosis). The incidence of documented bacteremia varies from 5 to 45 percent but is assumed to occur early in the course of many, and possibly all, *Salmonella* infections. Bacteremia is quickly cleared in patients infected with most *S. enteritidis* serotypes. Certain serotypes, such as *dublin*, *infantis*, *virchow*, *panama*, and *newport*, may be more invasive; this property is associated with an 80-kilobase virulence plasmid in *S. dublin*. *S. typhimurium* isolated from the bloodstream are significantly more likely (76 percent) to hybridize with a probe from the highly conserved EcoR1 fragment of the *S. dublin* plasmid than are fecal isolates (42 percent). *S. typhimurium* is the most frequent blood isolate, but the rate of isolation is no more than the average for all nontyphoidal *Salmonella*. Systemic and focal tissue infections are secondary to bacteremia. *S. cholerasuis* is a highly invasive serotype that usually causes a septicemia syndrome and is commonly isolated from blood but not from stool. Microbial factors, which determine the invasiveness of salmonellae, include motility and the presence of chromosomal and plasmid genes needed to invade and replicate within mononuclear phagocytes. Many of these genes are turned on by contact of the organism with host cells and are regulated by a two-component system, *PhoP/PhoQ*. Invasion is also associated with visible ruffling of the surface membrane and a major rearrangement of actin filaments, alpha-actinin, and tropomyosin to generate the force necessary for entry and appears to require host cell tyrosine kinase and phospholipase C activity, which results in a flux of inositol phosphate and release of intracellular calcium.

The pathogenesis of *Salmonella* enteritis is not clear. Virulent strains are invasive and able to induce inflammatory responses in the gut mucosa. Some strains produce a heat-labile enterotoxin which is structurally, functionally, and immunologically related to the cholera and *E. coli* LT toxins and/or heat-labile cytotoxins that act like Shiga toxins to inhibit intestinal protein synthesis.

CLINICAL MANIFESTATIONS **Gastroenteritis** The incubation period of *Salmonella* gastroenteritis is generally short, 24 to 48 h. Sporadic illness is likely to go undiagnosed because culture specimens are not taken. Large outbreaks, often considered as "food poisoning" and characterized by self-limited fever and diarrhea, are more likely to be investigated and diagnosed. Diarrhea may be associated with nausea, vomiting, and abdominal cramps and occasionally becomes bloody or even dysenteric when the colon becomes involved. Direct microscopic examination of stool shows many leukocytes, which are a clue to the invasive nature of the infection. The illness is generally mild and resolves without use of specific therapy, but it may cause severe dehydration or disseminate and lead to death in debilitated elderly patients or neonates. Blood cultures often become positive as the patient is improving. Treatment may be discontinued after identification of the organism unless there is an underlying immunosuppressive disease (e.g., sickle cell disease, AIDS, malignancy such as a lymphoma) or the patient is receiving glucocorticoid or immunosuppressive drug therapy. In these conditions, an appropriate antibiotic should be administered for 7 to 10 days. Carriage of salmonellae in the stool lasts several weeks after symptomatic disease but rarely exceeds 2 months.

Localization of systemic infections Bloodborne salmonellae can invade any tissue or organ. The most common isolates are *S. typhimurium*, *S. enteritidis*, *S. virchow*, and *S. cholerasuis*. Localized infections usually follow intestinal infection, although there may be no prior diarrhea. Endocarditis is rare, but when it occurs, there may be destructive cardiac lesions, including valve perforations or ring or septal abscesses. Therapy may require both appropriate antimicrobials and surgery (see Chap. 85).

Arterial infection generally occurs in preexisting arteriosclerotic infrarenal aortic aneurysms, especially in men older than 50. *S. cholerasius*, which accounts for about 20 percent of these infections, is isolated in fewer than 1 percent of patients with *Salmonella* diarrhea, thus reflecting its capacity to cause systemic invasive disease. *S. typhimurium* accounts for approximately 25 percent of isolates in arterial infections, consistent with its high prevalence in gastrointestinal salmonellosis. In addition to treatment with antimicrobials, eradication usually requires prompt excision and drainage with bypass through uninvolved tissue. The disease should be suspected when elderly men develop prolonged fever following gastroenteritis, accompanied by back, abdomen, or chest pain; when bacteremia is present or recurrent after therapy for the initial illness; or when bacteremia occurs in patients with vertebral osteomyelitis or in those with prosthetic valves.

Cholecystitis, other *hepatobiliary infection*, and *splenic abscess* are the most common intraabdominal localized infections due to *Salmonella*. In addition to *S. typhimurium* and *S. enteritidis*, *S. typhi* is an important cause.

Urinary tract infections due to *Salmonella* sometimes occur, especially in patients with urolithiasis, structural abnormalities, or immunosuppressive diseases or therapy, and can coexist with renal tuberculosis or *Schistosoma haematobium* infection.

Pneumonia or *empyema* caused by *Salmonella* is rare and usually seen in patients with preexisting abnormalities of the lungs or pleura or with conditions that predispose to infection, including malignancy, diabetes, glucocorticoid use, sickle cell disease, or alcohol abuse.

Meningitis caused by *Salmonella* is also rare and is most prevalent in infants and young children. Gram's stains of cerebrospinal fluid are usually positive. Mortality rates of 40 to 60 percent are reported in children and adults, respectively. In survivors, residua include seizures, hydrocephalus, subdural empyemas, and permanent disabilities such as retardation, paresis, athetosis, and visual disturbances.

Septic arthritis due to *Salmonella* is associated with positive joint fluid cultures and should not be confused with reactive arthritis (a culture-negative inflammatory joint disease occurring after invasive diarrheas, especially in HLA-B2– or -B7–positive patients). Underlying conditions that are often present include glucocorticoid or immunosuppressive drug therapy, sickle cell disease, prosthetic joints, or aseptic necrosis. Drainage may be needed in addition to appropriate antibiotics.

Salmonella osteomyelitis is predictably associated with sickle cell disease, sickle-C disease, and sickle thalassemia. It generally affects long bones and occurs primarily in young patients; blood cultures are often positive (the most common isolate is *S. typhimurium*).

Bacteremia Sepsis, with prolonged fever and positive blood cultures but generally without prior diarrhea, occurs most commonly with *S. cholerasuis* or *S. dublin* infection. While this presentation is "typhoidal," typical manifestations of typhoid (rose spots, relative bradycardia, leukopenia) are absent, and the illness is more acute in onset. *S. cholerasuis* or *S. dublin* sepsis is a severe disease, associated with high mortality.

Intermittent symptomatic *Salmonella* bacteremia is seen in patients with hepatosplenic or urinary schistosomiasis. Clinically severe *Salmonella* sepsis due to *S. typhimurium* also occurs in AIDS patients (see Chap. 279), is often recurrent, and may develop before the diagnosis of AIDS is made. The infection may be refractory to treatment or recurrent despite appropriate therapy. The incidence of salmonellosis in AIDS patients in the United States is now estimated to be between 46 and 384 per 100,000, which is 100- to 1000-fold greater than the incidence in the general population (0.3 per 100,000).

DIAGNOSIS　Specific diagnosis depends on the isolation of the organisms from stool, blood, or tissue fluids. All clinical laboratories should be able to make the initial isolation and identify common serotypes. Uncommon serotypes usually must be sent to reference laboratories for identification.

TREATMENT　Treatment for focal systemic infections requires selection of the most appropriate antibiotic and, at times, drainage or resection of infected tissue. Bactericidal antibiotics by the parenteral route are the usual choice and may include ampicillin in a dose of 6 to 12 g/d in adults or 100 mg/kg in young children in divided doses or appropriate doses of third-generation cephalosporins such as ceftriaxone. Chloramphenicol in a dose of 2 to 4 g/d in adults or 50 mg/kg in children in divided doses or a 4-fluoroquinolone such as ciprofloxacin or ofloxacin in patients older than 17 is also effective.

The proper treatment of *Salmonella* gastroenteritis is not clear; antibiotics do not shorten illness but do increase the duration of convalescent carriage. For this reason it is generally recommended that no treatment other than supportive care and fluid replacement be administered. Results suggest that 4-fluoroquinolones reduce the duration of illness and rapidly eradicate the organism from stool, although contradictory data have been published as well. Positive blood cultures in the setting of otherwise uncomplicated gastroenteritis do not require antibiotic therapy; treatment is usually reserved for patients with underlying immunosuppressive disease. In an infant under 3 months of age with diarrhea, the stool should be cultured, a workup to localize the septic process initiated, and presumptive treatment begun with a third-generation cephalosporin until culture results are available. Fever is often absent in very young infants and is not a reliable indicator of systemic infection. Asymptomatic patients with salmonellae other than *S. typhi* in the stool should *not* receive antimicrobial treatment, since active disease may be provoked and the carriage state prolonged.

PREVENTION AND CONTROL　It is probably not possible to eradicate nontyphoidal salmonellosis because the organisms are so widespread in nature. Reduction in the use in animal feed of antimicrobials employed for human infection and improved animal rearing and marketing practices would be useful. Vigilance in food preparation and in quality testing of the known and commonly contaminated foods should help as well. It is recommended that eggs not be eaten raw or partially cooked, especially in those at high risk, but even fully cooked eggs can harbor viable *Salmonella*. If universal body substance precautions are not routinely utilized, hospital staff caring for patients with salmonellosis should be placed on "enteric precautions," with gowning and gloving when handling stool and urine and careful handwashing after patient contact (see Chap. 98).

During outbreaks, food handlers may be responsible for transmission. Much effort is given to the identification by stool culture of asymptomatic food handlers who are carriers during food-borne outbreaks, and they are usually kept from work until they become culture-negative. However, it is more important that standards are maintained to ensure the environmental and personal hygiene of food handlers to prevent the problem in the first place, since carriage may be intermittent and is often not uniform within a single stool sample and foods contaminated with the organism require improper handling to permit the growth of a sufficient inoculum to cause disease. It may be truly justifiable to restrict carriers from the workplace only in the course of a hospital outbreak or when there are workers who refuse to improve their personal hygiene.

The development of effective vaccines may be difficult because of the great number of serotypes involved in infection. Some progress has been made with galactose epimerase and aroA vaccine mutants of *S. typhimurium* for use in animals, and these may ultimately be tested in humans. Of all the nontyphoidal salmonellae, it would be most useful to have vaccines for *S. cholerasuis*, *S. typhimurium*, and *S. enteritidis*. *S. dublin* and *S. virchow*, while quite virulent, are still uncommon causes of human disease.

REFERENCES

Aspergilla MO et al: Quinolone antibiotics in the treatment of *Salmonella* infections. Rev Infect Dis 12:873, 1990

Bhutta ZA: Multidrug-resistant typhoid in children: Presentation and clinical features. Rev Infect Dis 13:832, 1991

Cohen JI et al: Extra-intestinal manifestations of *Salmonella* infections. Medicine 66:349, 1987

Fang FC, Fierer J: Human infection with *Salmonella dublin*. Medicine 70:198, 1991

Finley BB, Falkow S: *Salmonella* as an intracellular parasite. Mol Microbiol 3:1833, 1989

Gotuzzo E et al: Association between the acquired immunodeficiency syndrome and infection with *Salmonella typhi* or *Salmonella paratyphi* in an endemic typhoid area. Arch Intern Med 151:381, 1991

Humphrey TJ et al: *Salmonella enteritidis* phage type 4 from the contents of intact eggs: A study involving naturally infected hens. Epidemiol Infect 103:415, 1989

Lasserre R et al: Three-day treatment of typhoid fever with two different doses of ceftriaxone, compared to 14-day therapy with chloramphenicol: A randomized trial. J Antimicrob Chemother 28:765, 1991

Levine WC et al: Epidemiology of nontyphoidal *Salmonella* bacteremia during the human immunodeficiency virus epidemic. J Infect Dis 164:81, 1991

Mock CN et al: Improvement in survival from typhoid ileal perforation: Results of 221 operative cases. Ann Surg 215:244, 1992

Naqvi SH et al: Therapy of multidrug resistant typhoid in 58 children. Scand J Invest Dis 24:175, 1992

Pavia AT et al: Epidemiologic evidence that prior antimicrobial exposure decreases resistance to infection by antimicrobial-sensitive *Salmonella*. J Infect Dis 161:255, 1990

Punjabi NH et al: Treatment of severe typhoid fever in children with high-dose dexamethasone. Pediatr Infect Dis J 7:598, 1988

Rodrigue DC et al: International increase in *Salmonella enteritidis*: A new pandemic? Epidemiol Infect 105:21, 1990

Rodriques-Noriega E et al: Quinolones in the treatment of *Salmonella* carriers. Rev Infect Dis 11(suppl 5):S1179, 1989

Ryan CA et al: *Salmonella typhi* infections in the United States, 1975–1984: Increasing role of foreign travel. Rev Infect Dis 11:1, 1989

St. Louis ME et al: The emergence of grade A eggs as a major source of *Salmonella enteritidis* infections: New implications for the control of salmonellosis. JAMA 259:2103, 1988

Woodruff BA et al: A new look at typhoid vaccination. Information for the practicing physician. JAMA 265:756, 1991

118　SHIGELLOSIS

GERALD T. KEUSCH

DEFINITION　*Shigellosis* is an acute infectious inflammatory colitis due to one of the members of the genus *Shigella*. Although the disease is often referred to as "bacillary dysentery," many patients have only mild watery diarrhea and never develop dysenteric symptoms. The less severe illness predominates in industrialized countries such as the United States, whereas more severe, often fatal dysentery occurs in patients in developing countries.

ETIOLOGY　*Shigella* are slender, gram-negative, nonmotile bacilli and are members of the family Enterobacteriaceae and tribe Escherichae. They are so closely related to *Escherichia coli* that the two genera cannot be distinguished by DNA hybridization methods. There are four *Shigella* species (*dysenteriae*, *flexneri*, *boydii*, and *sonnei*), defined on the basis of surface somatic O antigens and carbohydrate fermentation patterns. Most are lactose-negative (*S. sonnei* are late lactose fermenters) and produce acid but not gas from glucose, resulting in a typical acid butt and alkaline slant in triple sugar iron agar (TSI), without H_2S production, in contrast to *Salmonella*. The genus is characterized by its ability to invade intestinal epithelial cells and to produce highly potent protein toxins that irreversibly inhibit eukaryotic cell protein synthesis by a specific enzymatic action.

EPIDEMIOLOGY　It is estimated that at least 140 million cases and almost 600,000 deaths due to shigellosis occur annually in young children under the age of 5 years, primarily in developing countries. The organism is found everywhere in the world but is most common where poor environmental sanitation and crowding facilitate transmission from person to person. The reported incidence in the United States is around 15,000 cases each year. This is no doubt a gross underestimate, since organisms from most patients are neither cultured nor identified. In industrialized countries and developing countries alike, most patients are young children. In the United States from 1974 to 1980, 93,516 cases were identified by means of a nationwide passive surveillance system. While the overall isolation rate was 4.7 per 100,000 population per year, among children aged 1 to 4 the rate was 22.3 per 100,000 children per year. In the United States, the disease is most common in the urban poor, in infants in day-care centers, and in retarded children institutionalized for custodial care. One high-risk group has also been identified: male homosexuals, who transmit infection by anal-oral sexual practices.

Since the description of the genus, major global shifts in prevalence of the four species have been noted. Until World War I, S. dysenteriae type 1 was the predominant isolate, frequently occurring in devastating epidemics with high mortality until it was replaced by S. flexneri. Since World War II, however, S. flexneri has been steadily replaced by S. sonnei in the industrialized countries. The reasons for these shifts are not clear. S. boydii, the fourth species, has remained largely confined to the Indian subcontinent and is uncommon elsewhere.

The genus is highly host-adapted and is a natural pathogen of only humans and a few subhuman primates. Transmission is fecal-oral from person to person and is generally via direct contact, although contaminated food, water, flies, and fomites may serve as vectors. Direct contact is efficient, and only a few hundred organisms suffice to transmit disease so that even recreational water sports in contaminated pools or lakes are sufficient to transmit infection. Also for this reason, rapid spread can occur among confined populations kept in close contact, for example, in day-care centers, in institutions for the mentally retarded, on cruise ships, or among military personnel. Shigella is also one of several pathogens associated with gay bowel syndrome. These cases are almost always due to S. flexneri, and homosexual young men may be a major reservoir for these organisms in the United States (see Chap. 279).

Shigellosis is associated with a high secondary household transmission rate. As many as 40 percent of children and 20 percent of adult household contacts of a case (generally a preschool child) will develop Shigella infection, often symptomatic in children but asymptomatic in adults, who seem to have an acquired immunity. In contrast, epidemic disease affects all ages, with a clustering of severe and fatal cases in the very young and very old. Since 1969, epidemic S. dysenteriae type 1 has reappeared in Latin America, in the Indian subcontinent and elsewhere in Asia, and in central Africa and was accompanied by relatively high mortality rates until the cause was recognized and effective therapy initiated. Prolonged asymptomatic carriage is uncommon, and unless there is underlying malnutrition which is associated with prolonged fecal excretion, organisms are cleared in a few weeks.

PATHOGENESIS AND PATHOLOGY Shigella are orally ingested, and because they survive low pH better than other enteric pathogens (a genetically regulated property), they seem to have little difficulty in passing the gastric acid barrier. An essential step in pathogenesis is invasion of colonic epithelial cells and cell-to-cell spread of infection. Invasion and cell-to-cell spread involve the initial attachment of the organism to colonic cells, entry by an endocytic mechanism in which organisms are initially encased in and then escape from plasma membrane–enclosed vesicles, and a jet propulsion–like movement to the epithelial cell surface that is powered by bacteria-induced actin polymerization at the trailing end of the bacterium. This not only provides the organism with a means to evade host defenses but also allows effective local spread. Although invasion is initially innocuous, with subsequent intracellular multiplication, cell damage and death occur, resulting in characteristic mucosal ulcerations.

These processes are extremely complicated and require the functions of multiple genes and regulatory elements encoded on both chromosomal and plasmid DNA. Early studies on the genetics of Shigella virulence demonstrated that conjugal transfer of E. coli chromosomal DNA from the xyl-rha, his, or purE loci to virulent S. flexneri 2a recipients yielded hybrids able to invade but not survive within cells. The xyl-rha region is known to code for aerobactin and iron-regulated outer membrane proteins (OMPs), while the his region controls specific side chains of lipopolysaccharide, which respectively may help the organism compete for iron with the host and protect it from host defenses. However, transfer of these regions from S. flexneri to E. coli K12 does not confer virulence until other genes present on the large 120- to 140-MDa plasmids in all clinical Shigella isolates are transferred as well. These plasmids contain certain highly conserved regions common to all Shigella and invasive E. coli that encode a group of antigenic OMPs called invasion plasmid antigens (IPAs) and an operon called mxi, which controls insertion of the IPA proteins into the outer membrane of the organism. Mutation of some, but not all, IPAs inhibits invasiveness.

Invasion of epithelial cells by Shigella has been likened to the process of neutrophil phagocytosis. Internalization of Shigella by cells in culture or intestinal cells occurs within membrane-bounded vesicles associated with the polymerization of actin filaments. By use of transposon mutagenesis, a plasmid-encoded, acid pH–activated contact hemolysin has been found to mediate the rapid lysis of the phagocytic vacuole that allows the organisms to gain entry into the cytoplasm. While the basis for intracytoplasmic multiplication of Shigella is uncertain, another plasmid gene, icsA (for intraintercellular spread and formerly called virG), encodes a 120-kDa antigenic OMP that governs the ability of the organism to spread within the cytoplasm or to form plaques in HeLa cell monolayers indicative of cell-to-cell extension of infection. These intra- and intercellular migrations of Shigella occur along a network of actin stress fibers within the cells and are powered by actin polymerization induced by the organism after invasion and are blocked by the addition of cytochalasins.

Several plasmid and chromosomal genes regulate these virulence properties. A plasmid locus, virF, codes for a 30-kDa protein that activates the IPA genes and icsA. Another chromosomal locus, virR, is a temperature-dependent repressor of the plasmid invasion genes at 30°C but not at 37°C, while kcpA, originally defined as a locus essential for keratoconjunctivitis in guinea pigs, also controls the expression of icsA.

A second property of apparent importance in virulence, at least for S. dysenteriae type 1, is the ability to produce cytotoxic proteins. Shiga toxin, encoded by an iron-regulated chromosomal gene, stx, is composed of two distinct peptide subunits, each with highly conserved active regions. The first, located on the larger A subunit, is an N-glycosidase enzyme which hydrolyzes adenine from specific sites of ribosomal RNA of the mammalian 60-S ribosomal subunit, resulting in the irreversible inhibition of protein synthesis. The second common region is a binding site on the B subunit that recognizes glycolipids of target cell membranes that terminate in a galactose $\alpha 1 \rightarrow 4$-galactose disaccharide. The glycolipid Gb3, containing a gal-gal trisaccharide, is a specific receptor present on toxin-sensitive rabbit intestinal villus cells but not crypt cells, and toxin action is specific for the former.

In shigellosis, the epithelial surface of the human colon shows extensive ulcerations, with an exudate consisting of desquamated colonic cells, polymorphonuclear leukocytes, and erythrocytes; the ulcerations may resemble a pseudomembrane in severely affected areas. Marked mucus depletion and increased mitotic activity are seen in the crypt regions, presumably as a response to the loss of surface colonic cells. The lamina propria is edematous and hemorrhagic and infiltrated with neutrophils and plasma cells. There is also swelling of capillary and venular endothelial cells, with margination of neutrophils. The tropism of toxin for endothelial cells can explain this pathology, which may contribute to fluid losses and underlie the systemic complications of S. dysenteriae type 1 infection such as glomerular damage and microangiopathic hemolysis (hemolytic-uremic syndrome). At the ultrastructural level, bacteria can be seen within vesicles as well as free in the cytoplasm.

Epidemiologic evidence indicates that immunity develops and is serotype specific. The precise nature of this immunity, however, is not known. Common surface OMPs involved in invasion are known to elicit serum antibodies; however, these are cross-reactive among *Shigella* species and serotypes and do not seem to be protective. The serotype-specific determinants are likely to be somatic antigens, as serum antibody to O antigens predicts resistance to infection, and there is evidence of IgA-mediated mucosal anti-O antigen responses during convalescence from shigellosis. Cellular mechanisms also have been proposed that involve antibody-dependent cellular cytotoxicity responses by Fc receptor–positive lymphocytes and phagocytic cells.

CLINICAL MANIFESTATIONS The spectrum of clinical shigellosis was shown in a study in which human volunteers ingested 10,000 *S. flexneri* type 2a. While approximately one-quarter of the volunteers never became ill, over the first 24 to 48 h approximately 25 percent of volunteers developed a transient fever, another 25 percent had fever and a self-limited watery diarrhea, and the remaining 25 percent had fever and watery diarrhea that progressed to bloody diarrhea and dysentery. In young children, in particular, the temperature can rapidly rise to 40 to 41°C and sometimes result in generalized seizures. These rarely recur or result in serious sequelae. Dysentery is characterized by frequent (usually 10 to 30 times per day) small-volume stools consisting of blood, mucus, and pus, plus abdominal cramps and tenesmus, the painful straining with stooling that may lead to rectal prolapse, especially in young children. The likelihood of severe dysentery is greatest in *S. dysenteriae* type 1 and *S. flexneri* infection and least likely in *S. sonnei*. With mild disease, patients generally recover without specific therapy in a few days to a week. Severe shigellosis can progress to toxic dilatation and colonic perforation, which may be fatal.

Endoscopy shows the mucosa to be hemorrhagic with mucous discharge and focal ulcerations, sometimes with overlying exudate. The majority of the lesions are in the distal colon and progressively diminish in the more proximal segments of large bowel. Mild dehydration is common in patients with watery diarrhea; severe dehydration is very rare. With extensive colonic involvement, protein-losing enteropathy occurs and can have very important adverse nutritional consequences for the already poorly nourished child.

A variety of *extraintestinal complications* of shigellosis have been described. The majority of these occur in patients in developing countries and are related to both the prevalence of *S. dysenteriae* type 1 and *S. flexneri* infection as well as to the poor nutritional state of the patients. For example, bacteremia, thought to be relatively infrequent in the United States, occurs in up to 8 percent of patients hospitalized for shigellosis in Dacca, Bangladesh. The causative *Shigella* species is isolated in half the patients; other Enterobacteriaceae are found in the remainder. Bacteremia is associated with higher than usual mortality and is more common in infants under 1 year of age and in those with protein-energy malnutrition. Persistent and clinically severe *Shigella* bacteremia has been encountered in the United States in patients with AIDS (see Chap. 279).

Hemolytic-uremic syndrome (HUS) may occur with *S. dysenteriae* type 1 infection. In the United States, the more likely cause of HUS is a hemorrhagic colitis–causing strain of *E. coli* producing high levels of Shiga-family toxins, such as *E. coli* O157:H7. HUS usually develops toward the end of the first week of shigellosis, when the dysentery is already resolving. Oliguria and a marked drop in hematocrit (as much as a 10 percent decrease within 24 h) are the first signs and may progress to anuria and renal failure or severe anemia with congestive heart failure, respectively. With HUS, leukemoid reactions with leukocyte counts over 50,000 per microliter may occur; thrombocytopenia (30,000 to 100,000 platelets per microliter) is common. Profound hyponatremia and severe hypoglycemia may be present. Central nervous system abnormalities include encephalopathic symptoms, seizures, altered consciousness, and bizarre posturing.

Other less common extraintestinal manifestations include seizures in some patients and reactive arthritis in others, both usually due to

infection with *S. flexneri* strains. In patients expressing histocompatibility antigen HLA-B27, the full triad of Reiter's syndrome sometimes develops (see Chap. 289). Pneumonia, meningitis, vaginitis in prepubertal girls, keratoconjunctivitis, and "rose spot" rashes are rare events.

DIAGNOSIS AND LABORATORY FINDINGS Shigellosis is the principal bacterial cause of dysentery and should be considered in every patient presenting with bloody diarrhea. However, in the United States, because *S. sonnei* is the most common species, most patients will present with fever and a nonbloody watery diarrhea, indistinguishable from other bacterial or viral causes of mild to moderate diarrhea, while many patients with bloody diarrhea will have enterohemorrhagic *E. coli* as the cause. The specific diagnosis is made by culturing *Shigella* from the stool; however, polymerase chain reaction (PCR) diagnosis is possible. The yield of *Shigella* is increased by only culturing stool from patients with fecal leukocytes or bloody diarrhea. The organism is very labile and must be quickly transferred to plates or holding media (such as buffered glycerol saline) or it will not survive. Stool samples are preferable to swabs; when the latter are used, a rectal sample should be obtained. For culturing, more than one selective medium should be used, including MacConkey and one other, such as Hektoen enteric or xylose-lysine-deoxycholate.

Serology can be performed, since antibodies to somatic antigens develop early in the acute phase of disease; however, such tests are not generally available and are usually used only for epidemiologic studies.

The differential diagnosis includes other microbial causes of inflammatory colitis: enterohemorrhagic and enteroinvasive *E. coli*, *Campylobacter jejuni*, *Salmonella enteriditis* serotypes, *Yersinia enterocolitica*, *Clostridium difficile*, and the protozoan *Entamoeba histolytica*. Ulcerative colitis or Crohn's colitis are among the "noninfectious" causes (see Chap. 255). All except *E. histolytica* are associated with the presence of large numbers of fecal leukocytes. Amebiasis can be diagnosed by finding erythrophagocytic trophozoites in the stool (see Chap. 173).

Other laboratory studies are nonspecific and may disclose a moderate neutrophilic leukocytosis, anemia due to blood loss with hemorrhagic diarrhea, prerenal azotemia, or a hyperchloremic acidosis if watery diarrhea has been pronounced. Laboratory findings in shigellosis complicated by the HUS are discussed above.

TREATMENT The mild to moderate dehydration in shigellosis is readily corrected with oral rehydration solutions (see Chap. 120). The role of antibiotic therapy is variable and dependent on the organism and severity of disease. Since *S. sonnei* infection is usually self-limited, culture results generally do not become available until the patient is better and there is little clinical need for further therapy. The use of antibiotics in more severe cases with bloody diarrhea or dysentery will reduce the duration of illness and can shorten the duration of the carriage state. Resistance to sulfonamides, streptomycin, chloramphenicol, and tetracyclines is almost universal, and many *Shigella* are now also resistant to ampicillin and trimethoprim-sulfamethoxazole. Knowledge of the pattern of resistance in a given population, which can change with time, is useful. In the United States, multiresistant strains are most likely acquired during travel abroad, and either ampicillin, 50 to 100 mg/kg per day in children or 2 g/d in adults in divided doses, or trimethoprim-sulfamethoxazole, 8/40 mg/kg per day in children or 2 regular-strength tablets twice a day in adults, given for 5 days, is generally recommended. Amoxicillin should *not* be substituted for ampicillin because it is not effective treatment for shigellosis. In developing countries, where resistance to both these drugs is commonplace, the drug of choice for the treatment of multiresistant *S. dysenteriae* type 1 infections has been nalidixic acid, 55 mg/kg per day for 5 days; however, resistance is increasing in prevalence. The 4-fluoroquinolones (e.g., ciprofloxacin) are highly effective for all strains (see Chap. 100) but are currently too costly for the third world and in the United States are not yet approved for use in children under 17 because of the concern for cartilage toxicity. Alternative drugs shown to be effective include oral pivamdinocillin (but not yet available in the United States) and intravenous ceftriaxone, 50 mg/kg per day for 5 days. In small clinical trials, cephalexin has had no effect in limiting symptoms; single doses of ceftriaxone may be effective, but more information is needed. No antibiotic treatment is recommended for the convalescent carriage state, since this is usually limited to only several weeks' duration. Patients with AIDS may develop chronic carriage of shigella and be subject to relapsing infection with bacteremia (see Chap. 279). This cycle may be interrupted by prolonged (several weeks) treatment with a quinolone.

The role of antimotility agents such as atropine sulfate and diphenoxylate (Lomotil) and loperamide (Imodium) in the early phases of shigellosis remains unclear. They may reduce the diarrhea without provoking more severe disease through delayed excretion of organisms. There is no indication for their use in the dysenteric phase of disease, however, and they are not recommended.

Treatment of complications of shigellosis often differs in developed and developing countries. For example, antibiotic-unresponsive toxic megacolon, with or without perforation, is often managed by colectomy in the United States. Surgery is less often employed in developing countries because of lack of availability or difficulties in ileostomy management. Hemolytic-uremic syndrome often requires dialysis. In developing countries this may be less commonly needed because azotemia is slow to develop and the risk of significant hyperkalemia is often diminished because of the preexisting deficiency in total-body potassium with malnutrition and wasting of lean body mass. The management of hyponatremia, usually caused by inappropriate secretion of antidiuretic hormone (vasopressin), is governed by its severity and the symptomatic state of the patient as outlined in Chap. 45. Infusion of glucose can reverse clinical manifestations caused by hypoglycemia, and responses can be monitored by finger-stick blood glucose tests if no biochemistry laboratory is available. Optimal nutritional management is needed to correct the deficiencies due to underlying malnutrition and the superimposed catabolic stress and protein-losing enteropathy of shigellosis. This should begin during the acute illness and may require months of nutritional support afterwards (see Chap. 76).

PREVENTION Direct contact transmission of shigellosis can be prevented by appropriate environmental and personal hygiene. Hand washing with soap and water, decontamination of water supplies, use of sanitary latrines or toilets, and protection of food preparation and its storage can all reduce the primary and secondary transmission of *Shigella* infection. In the highly endemic developing countries, infants are protected during the period of exclusive breast feeding, and this should be encouraged. Any measures that also reduce the burden of malnutrition will have a favorable effect on the population as well. Hospitalized patients should be put on stool precautions to ensure safe disposal of infected excreta and linens, and hospital personnel must wash their hands and medical instruments such as stethoscopes after each contact with an infected patient. Cohorting of asymptomatic infected children, use of antibiotics to reduce infectiousness, and scrupulous attention to hygiene are usually successful in hospital outbreaks. Children in day-care must be kept at home while clinically ill and ideally should have a negative stool culture before returning to the group. Food handlers who develop shigellosis also should be required to be culture-negative before being allowed to return to work. Antibiotic treatment is not indicated for the asymptomatic carriage state. No effective vaccine is available.

REFERENCES

BASKIN DH et al: *Shigella* becteremia in patients with the acquired immune deficiency syndrome. Am J Gastroenterol 82:338, 1987

BENNISH ML: Potentially lethal complications of shigellosis. Rev Infect Dis 13(suppl):S319, 1991

—— et al: Hypoglycemia during diarrhea in childhood: Prevalence, pathophysiology, and outcome. N Engl J Med 322:1357, 1990

CLEMENTS JD et al: Breast feeding as a determinant of severity in shigellosis. Am J Epidemiol 123:710, 1986

COHEN D et al: Prospective study of the association between serum antibodies to lipopolysaccharide O antigen and the attack rate of shigellosis. J Clin Microbiol 29:386, 1991

GRIFFIN PM et al: Emergence of highly trimethoprim-sulfamethoxazole–resistant *Shigella* in a native American population: An epidemiologic study. Am J Epidemiol 129:1042, 1989

HALE TL: Genetic basis of virulence in *Shigella* species. Microbiol Rev 55:206, 1991

HALPERN Z et al: Shigellosis in adults: Epidemiologic, clinical, and laboratory features. Medicine 68:210, 1989

HOFFMAN RE, SHILLAM PJ: The use of hygiene, cohorting, and antimicrobial therapy to control an outbreak of shigellosis. Am J Dis Child 144:219, 1990

LEE LA et al: Hyperendemic shigellosis in the United States: A review of surveillance data for 1967–1988. J Infect Dis 164:894, 1991

LEVINE OS, LEVINE MM: Houseflies (*Musca domestica*) as mechanical vectors of shigellosis. Rev Infect Dis 13:688, 1991

SALAM MA, BENNISH ML: Antimicrobial therapy for shigellosis. Rev Infect Dis 13(suppl):S332, 1991

SANSONETTI PJ et al: *Pathogenesis of Shigellosis*. Berlin, Springer-Verlag, 1992

SORVILLO FJ et al: Shigellosis associated with recreational water contact in Los Angeles County. Am J Trop Med Hyg 38:613, 1988

TAUXE RV et al: Antimicrobial resistance of *Shigella* isolates in the USA: The importance of international travelers. J Infect Dis 162:1107, 1990

VARSANO I et al: Comparative efficacy of ceftriaxone and ampicillin for treatment of severe shigellosis in children. J Pediatr 118:627, 1991

ZVULUNOV A et al: The prognosis of convulsions during childhood shigellosis. Eur J Pediatr 149:293, 1990

119 CAMPYLOBACTER INFECTIONS

MARTIN J. BLASER

DEFINITION *Campylobacteriosis* refers to the group of pyogenic infections caused by bacteria of the genus *Campylobacter*. Although acute diarrheal illnesses are most common, these organisms may cause infections in virtually all parts of the body, especially in compromised hosts, and there may be late nonsuppurative sequelae. The designation *Campylobacter* comes from the Greek for "curved rod" and refers to the organism's vibrio-like morphology.

ETIOLOGY Campylobacters are motile, non-spore-forming, curved gram-negative rods. Originally known as *Vibrio fetus*, these bacilli were reclassified as a new genus in 1973 after it was recognized that they were quite dissimilar from other vibrios. Since then, more than 15 different *Campylobacter* species have been identified. However, not all these species are pathogens of humans. The human pathogens can be divided into two major groups: those that primarily cause diarrheal disease and those that cause extraintestinal infection. The principal diarrheal pathogen is *C. jejuni*, which accounts for 80 to 90 percent of all recognized illness due to campylobacters. Other organisms that cause diarrheal disease include *C. coli*, *C. upsaliensis*, *C. lari*, and *C. fetus*. The major species causing extraintestinal illnesses is *C. fetus;* however, any of the diarrheal agents may cause systemic or localized infection as well. Neither aerobes nor strict anaerobes, these microaerophilic organisms are adapted for survival in the gastrointestinal mucous layer. This chapter will focus on *C. jejuni* and *C. fetus* as the major pathogens and prototypes for their groups.

EPIDEMIOLOGY Campylobacters are found within the gastrointestinal tract of many animals used for food production (including poultry, cattle, sheep, and swine) and of household pets (including birds, dogs, and cats). However, these microorganisms usually do not cause illness in their animal hosts. In most cases, campylobacters are transmitted to humans in raw or undercooked food products or through direct contact with infected animals. In the United States and other developed countries, ingestion of contaminated poultry that has not been sufficiently cooked is the most common means of acquiring infection (50 to 70 percent of cases). Other modes of transmission include ingestion of raw (unpasteurized) milk or untreated water, contact with infected household pets, travel to developing countries (campylobacters being among the causes of traveler's diarrhea), and occasionally, contact with an index case who is incontinent of stool.

Campylobacter infections are not rare. Several studies indicate that in the United States diarrheal disease due to campylobacters is more common than that due to *Salmonella* and *Shigella* combined. Infections occur throughout the year, but their incidence peaks during summer and early autumn. Persons of all ages are affected; however, attack rates for *C. jejuni* are highest among young children and young adults, while those for *C. fetus* are highest at the extremes of ages. Systemic infections due to *C. fetus* (and other *Campylobacter* species) are most common in compromised hosts. Persons at increased risk include those with AIDS, hypogammaglobulinemia, neoplasia, liver disease, diabetes mellitus, and generalized atherosclerosis and pregnant women. However, apparently healthy, nonpregnant persons occasionally develop transient *Campylobacter* bacteremia.

In developing countries, *C. jejuni* infections are hyperendemic, with the highest rates in very young children (<2 years old). Infection rates fall with age, as does the illness-to-infection ratio; these observations suggest that frequent exposure to *C. jejuni* leads to the acquisition of immunity.

PATHOLOGY AND PATHOGENESIS   Many *C. jejuni* infections are subclinical, especially in partially immune hosts. Most illnesses occur within 2 to 4 days (range 1 to 7 days) of exposure to the organism in food or water. The sites of tissue injury include the jejunum, ileum, and colon. Biopsies show an acute nonspecific inflammatory reaction, with neutrophils, monocytes, and eosinophils in the lamina propria, as well as damage to the epithelium, including loss of mucus, glandular degeneration, and crypt abscesses. Biopsy findings may be consistent with Crohn's disease or ulcerative colitis, but these "idiopathic" chronic inflammatory diseases should not be diagnosed unless infectious colitis, *specifically including* that due to infection with *Campylobacter*, has been ruled out.

The high frequency of *C. jejuni* infections and their severity and recurrence among hypogammaglobulinemic patients suggest that antibodies are important in protective immunity. The pathogenesis of infection is uncertain. Motility and adherence of the strain to host tissues both appear to favor disease, but classic enterotoxins and cytotoxins (although described) do not appear to play a role in tissue injury or disease production. The documentation of a significant tissue response and occasionally of *C. jejuni* bacteremia suggests that tissue invasion may occur, but this point has not been resolved satisfactorily.

The pathogenesis of *C. fetus* infections is better defined. Virtually all clinical isolates of *C. fetus* possess a proteinaceous capsule-like structure (S-layer) that renders the organism resistant to complement-mediated killing and opsonization. As a result, *C. fetus* can be bacteremic beyond the intestinal tract and can seed systemic sites. The ability of the organism to switch S-layer proteins, a phenomenon that induces antigenic variability, may contribute to the chronicity and high rate of recurrence of these infections in compromised hosts.

CLINICAL MANIFESTATIONS OF C. JEJUNI AND C. FETUS INFECTIONS   The clinical features of infections due to all of the *Campylobacter* species causing enteric disease appear identical. There is often a prodrome with fever, headache, myalgia, and/or malaise 12 to 48 h before the onset of diarrheal symptoms. The most common symptoms of the intestinal phase are diarrhea, abdominal pain, and fever. The degree of diarrhea varies from several loose stools to grossly bloody stools; most patients presenting for medical attention have 10 or more bowel movements on the worst day of illness. Abdominal pain usually consists of cramping and may be the most prominent symptom. Pain usually is generalized but may become localized; *C. jejuni* infection may cause pseudoappendicitis. Fever may be the only initial manifestation of *C. jejuni* infection, a situation mimicking the early stages of typhoid fever. Febrile young children may develop convulsions. *Campylobacter* enteritis generally is self-limited; however, symptoms persist for longer than 1 week in 10 to 20 percent of patients seeking medical attention, and relapses occur in 5 to 10 percent of untreated patients.

C. fetus may cause a diarrheal illness similar to that due to *C.*

jejuni, especially in normal hosts, or may cause either intermittent diarrhea or nonspecific abdominal pain without localizing signs. Sequelae are uncommon, and outcome is benign. *C. fetus* also may cause a prolonged relapsing systemic illness (with fever, chills, and myalgias) that has no obvious primary source; this manifestation is especially common in compromised hosts. Secondary seeding of an organ (including meninges, brain, bone, urinary tract, and soft tissue) complicates the course, which may be fulminant. *C. fetus* infections have a tropism for vascular sites; endocarditis, mycotic aneurysm, and septic thrombophlebitis all may occur. Infection during pregnancy often leads to fetal death.

COMPLICATIONS   Bacteremia is uncommon, developing most often in immunocompromised hosts and at the extremes of age. Three patterns of extraintestinal infection have been noted: (1) Transient bacteremia in a normal host with enteritis. The course is benign, and no specific treatment is needed. (2) Sustained bacteremia or focal infection in a normal host. Bacteremia originates from enteritis, and patients respond well to antimicrobial therapy. (3) Sustained bacteremia or focal infection in a compromised host. Enteritis may not be present. Antimicrobial therapy, possibly prolonged, is necessary for suppression or cure of the infection.

Campylobacter infections in patients with AIDS or hypogammaglobulinemia may be severe, persistent, and extraintestinal; relapse after cessation of therapy is common. Hypogammaglobulinemic patients also may develop osteomyelitis and an erysipelas-like rash.

Local suppurative complications of infection include cholecystitis, pancreatitis, and cystitis, and distant complications include meningitis, endocarditis, arthritis, peritonitis, or septic abortion; all are rare. Hepatitis, interstitial nephritis, and the hemolytic-uremic syndrome occasionally complicate acute infection. Reactive arthritis and other rheumatologic complaints may develop several weeks after infection, especially in persons with the HLA-B27 phenotype. Guillain-Barré syndrome follows *Campylobacter* infection uncommonly (i.e., in 1 of every 1000 to 2000 cases). However, because of the high incidence of infection due to campylobacters, it is now estimated that *Campylobacter* infections may trigger 10 to 30 percent of all cases of Guillain-Barré syndrome.

LABORATORY FINDINGS   In patients with *Campylobacter* enteritis, peripheral leukocyte counts reflect the severity of the inflammatory process. However, stools contain leukocytes or erythrocytes in nearly all patients presenting for medical attention in the United States. Fecal smears should be stained with Gram's or Wright's stain and examined in all suspected cases. Diagnosis of *Campylobacter* enteritis is established by visualization of organisms with characteristic vibrioid morphology on direct microscopic examination of stools with Gram's staining (or the use of phase-contrast or dark-field microscopy to identify the characteristic "darting" motility) or by isolation of the organism from fecal culture. Confirmation of the diagnosis of *Campylobacter* infection is based on identification of an isolate from cultures of stool, blood, or another site. Since all *Campylobacter* species are fastidious, they will not be isolated unless selective media or other selective techniques are used. Not all media are equally useful for isolation of the broad array of campylobacters; therefore, failure to isolate campylobacters from stool does not entirely rule out their presence. The presence of the organism almost always implies infection; there is a brief period of postconvalescent fecal carriage and no commensalism. In contrast, *C. sputorum* and related organisms found in the oral cavity are commensals without known pathogenic significance.

DIFFERENTIAL DIAGNOSIS   The symptoms of *Campylobacter* enteritis are not unusual enough to distinguish this illness from that due to *Salmonella*, *Shigella*, or *Yersinia*, among other pathogens. The combination of fever and fecal leukocytes or erythrocytes is indicative of inflammatory diarrhea, and definitive diagnosis is based on culture. Similarly, extraintestinal *Campylobacter* illness is diagnosed by culture. Infection due to *Campylobacter* should be suspected in the setting of septic abortion and that due to *C. fetus* specifically in the setting of septic thrombophlebitis. It is important to reiterate that the presentation of *Campylobacter* enteritis may mimic that of ulcerative colitis or Crohn's disease, that *Campylobacter* enteritis is much more common than either of the latter (especially among young adults), and that biopsy may not distinguish among these entities. Thus a diagnosis of inflammatory bowel disease should not be made until *Campylobacter* infection has been ruled out, especially in persons with a history of foreign travel, significant animal contact, immunodeficiency, or practices incurring a high risk of transmission.

TREATMENT Fluid and electrolyte replacement is central to the treatment of diarrheal illnesses (see Chap. 87). Even among patients presenting for medical attention with *Campylobacter* enteritis, fewer than half will clearly benefit from specific antimicrobial therapy. Indications for such therapy include high fever, bloody diarrhea, severe diarrhea, persistence for more than 1 week, and worsening of symptoms. A 5- to 7-day course of erythromycin (250 mg PO four times daily, or 30 to 50 mg/kg per day in divided doses for children) is the regimen of choice. Although not studied in clinical trials, the in vitro susceptibility of *Campylobacter* species to macrolides, such as clarithromycin and azithromycin, suggest that they also would be useful therapeutic agents. An alternative regimen for adults is ciprofloxacin (500 mg PO twice daily) for 5 to 7 days. Other alternatives include tetracycline, norfloxacin, and furazolidone. Use of antimotility agents, which may prolong the duration of symptoms and have been associated with deaths, is not recommended.

For systemic infections, treatment with an aminoglycoside such as gentamicin, a third-generation cephalosporin such as cefotaxime, or chloramphenicol should be started empirically, but susceptibility testing should then be performed. Erythromycin and amoxicillin/clavulanate are alternative agents. For immunocompromised patients with systemic infections due to *C. fetus*, prolonged therapy is usually necessary.

PROGNOSIS Nearly all patients recover fully from *Campylobacter* enteritis, either spontaneously or after antimicrobial therapy. Volume depletion likely contributes to the few deaths that are reported. As stated above, occasional patients develop reactive arthritis or Guillain-Barré syndrome. Systemic infection with *C. fetus* is much more often fatal; this higher mortality reflects in part the population affected. Prognosis is dependent on the rapidity with which appropriate therapy is begun. Normal hosts usually survive *C. fetus* infections without sequelae.

REFERENCES

BLASER MJ et al: *Campylobacter* enteritis: Clinical and epidemiologic features. Ann Intern Med 91:179, 1979
—————— et al: *Campylobacter* enteritis in the United States: A multicenter study. Ann Intern Med 98:360, 1983
NACHAMKIN I et al (eds): *Campylobacter jejuni: Current Strategy and Future Trends.* Washington, American Society for Microbiology, 1992, pp 1–300
PERLMAN DM et al: Persistent *Campylobacter jejuni* infections in patients infected with the human immunodeficiency virus. Ann Intern Med 108:540, 1988

120 CHOLERA AND OTHER VIBRIOSES

GERALD T. KEUSCH / ROBERT L. DERESIEWICZ

Members of the genus *Vibrio* cause a number of important infectious syndromes. Classic among them is that caused by *V. cholerae* group O1, cholera, a devastating diarrheal disease responsible for seven world pandemics and much suffering over the past two centuries. Epidemic cholera remains a major public health concern and is dealt with at length in this chapter. Recently, other vibrioses have been described, including syndromes of diarrhea, soft-tissue infection, or primary sepsis caused by additional named species within the genus *Vibrio*. Those, too, are considered below.

All members of the genus are actively motile, facultatively anaerobic, curved gram-negative rods with one or more polar flagella. With the exception of *V. cholerae* and *V. mimicus,* all require salt for growth ("halophilic vibrios"). In nature they most commonly reside in tidal rivers and bays under conditions of moderate salinity. They proliferate in the summer months when water temperatures exceed about 20°C. As might be expected, the illnesses they cause also increase in frequency during the warm months. Some isolates of certain species within the genus share important determinants of virulence, in particular the ability to produce a potent protein enterotoxin (O1 and non-O1 *V. cholerae, V. mimicus,* and *V. fluvialis*).

CHOLERA

DEFINITION Cholera is an acute diarrheal disease that can, in a matter of hours, result in profound, rapidly progressive dehydration and death. Accordingly, cholera gravis (the severe form of cholera) is a much feared disease, particularly in its epidemic presentation. Fortunately, prompt, aggressive fluid repletion and supportive care can obviate the high mortality that it has historically wrought. The term *cholera* has occasionally been applied to any severely dehydrating secretory diarrheal illness whether due to *V. cholerae* or not and, indeed, whether infectious in etiology or not (including, for example, diarrhea due to endocrine syndromes such as vasoactive intestinal peptide–secreting tumors).

ETIOLOGY AND EPIDEMIOLOGY The species *V. cholerae* comprises a host of organisms classified on the basis of their somatic O antigen. Those which agglutinate in O group 1 antiserum cause the majority of cases of clinical cholera. Some 70 other members of the species are recognized and are collectively known as non-O1 *V. cholerae.* While some of the latter also can cause diarrhea, only rarely do they cause cholera gravis.

V. cholerae O1 exists in two biotypes, *classical* and *El Tor,* that are distinguished on the basis of a number of characteristics, including phage susceptibility and hemolysin production. Each biotype is further subdivided into two serotypes, termed *Inaba* and *Ogawa.* Serotyping is a useful tool in field epidemiologic studies.

Cholera is native to the Ganges delta in the Indian subcontinent. Since 1817, seven world pandemics have occurred. Before 1991, the last to reach the United States was in 1911, when the sixth pandemic made brief entry into New York and Massachusetts. In the past decade, sporadic endemic infection due to consumption of contaminated shellfish has been recognized along the Gulf Coasts of Louisiana and Texas. As well, small outbreaks associated with contaminated drinking water have been recognized aboard offshore oil rigs.

In January 1991, epidemic cholera struck in Latin America. Beginning in Peru, the disease was carried by fisherman to Ecuador and Colombia and then by travelers to virtually all of South and Central America, to Mexico, and to the United States. Nearly 400,000 cases were reported in the first year of the outbreak, greatly exceeding the number of cases reported to the World Health Organization (WHO) worldwide in any previous year of record keeping. The epidemic continues, although at a much lower incidence. While the overall mortality rate has been about 1 percent, it approached 20 to 30 percent in the communities first affected, where a lack of familiarity with the disease led initially to the employment of draconian and wholly ineffective therapeutic measures. Intensive education of health providers and of the community at large has enhanced awareness of the disease and its appropriate management and has greatly diminished mortality. Of note, the epidemic reached the United States via illegally transported boiled crab meat, affecting eight people at a family party in New Jersey. This underscores the need for vigilance among health professionals, even in locations remote from the epicenter of an outbreak.

As it did in Africa in the 1970s, the organism has proven capable of establishing itself in inland waters rather than in its classical niche of coastal salt waters and has already become endemic in many of the countries into which it was recently introduced.

In 1993, an outbreak of severe clinical cholera occurred in Bangladesh and in India, affecting all age groups. The organism turned out to be a non-O1 *V. cholerae* and was designated *O139 Bengal*. The initial characterization of O139 Bengal has demonstrated the same major virulence attributes as in O1 *V. cholera*, including the key virulence regulatory genes. The only apparent difference in epidemiologic behavior between O139 Bengal and O1 *V. cholerae* is that prior immunity to the latter seems not to be effective in protecting individuals against the former. Accordingly, the population at risk is behaving as a virgin population with respect to severe, lethal cholera, and the same devastating epidemiology and clinical outcome seen in prior global pandemics of O1 *V. cholerae*, including the epidemic in the Americas in 1991, is being repeated in Asia. The isolate is resistant to trimethoprim-sulfamethoxazole but, at least at the outset, is sensitive to tetracycline.

Ingestion of water soiled by infected human feces is the most common means of transmission, but consumption of contaminated food in the home, in restaurants, or from street vendors also can contribute to spread. There is no known animal reservoir. The infectious dose is relatively high but is markedly reduced in hypochlorhydric subjects, in those using antacids, and when gastric acidity is buffered by a meal. In endemic areas, cholera is predominantly a pediatric disease, but it affects adults and children equally when newly introduced into a population. In endemic areas the disease is more common in the summer and fall months. While not fully explained, this seasonality may be due to environmental conditions that affect the multiplication of vibrios or to seasonal alterations in human behavior that affect their contact with water. Asymptomatic infections are frequent and are more common with the El Tor than with the classical biotype. In endemic areas, children under 2 years of age are less likely to develop severe cholera than are older children, perhaps due to passive immunity acquired from breast milk. For unexplained reasons, susceptibility to cholera is significantly influenced by ABO blood group status; those with type O are at greatest risk, while those with group AB are at least risk.

PATHOGENESIS   Once ingested, the organism must safely traverse the acidic gastric environment. If successful, it next colonizes the upper small bowel. Attachment is mediated principally by the toxin coregulated pilus (TCP), so named because its synthesis is regulated in parallel with that of cholera toxin (CT). Several other properties of the organism enhance its ability to colonize, including its motility, chemotaxis, and hemagglutinin/protease production. The last, formerly termed *cholera lectin*, is closely related to the *Pseudomonas aeruginosa* elastase. It is both an agglutinin and a zinc-dependent protease and is able to cleave mucin and fibronectin, as well as the A subunit of cholera toxin. It also may serve to detach organisms so that they can attack distal intestinal sites or be excreted.

CT, TCP, and several other putative virulence factors, including an accessory colonization factor and various hemagglutinins, are coordinately regulated by the *tox*R gene product. ToxR protein is a "master switch" that modulates the expression of virulence genes in response to signals that it senses in the environment, the most important of which, at least in vitro, are changes in osmolarity, pH, and the presence of certain free amino acids. Coordinate regulation presumably enables the organism to tailor its repertoire of proteins to suit its needs as it passes from microenvironment to microenvironment. Regulation of the toxR type has become a paradigm for similar systems that have been discovered in a wide range of pathogenic bacteria.

Once established, the organism produces CT, a protein toxin that is the principal cause of the watery diarrhea characteristic of cholera. CT consists of a monomeric enzymatic moiety (the A subunit) and a pentameric binding moiety (the B subunit). The B pentamer binds to G_{M1} ganglioside, a glycolipid receptor on the surface of jejunal epithelial cells, and so delivers the A subunit to its cytosolic target. The activated A subunit (A_1) irreversibly transfers ADP-ribose from nicotinamide adenine dinucleotide (NAD) to its specific target protein, the GTP-binding regulatory component of adenylate cyclase in intestinal epithelial cells. When ADP-ribosylated, this so-called G protein up-regulates the cyclase catalytic subunit, which results in the intracellular accumulation of high levels of cyclic AMP (cAMP). cAMP, in turn, inhibits the absorptive sodium transport system in villus cells and activates the excretory chloride transport system in crypt cells, leading to the accumulation of sodium chloride in the intestinal lumen. Since water moves passively to maintain osmolality, isotonic fluid accumulates in the lumen. When the volume of that fluid exceeds the capacity of the rest of the gut to resorb it, watery diarhea results. Unless the wasted fluid and electrolytes are adequately replaced, shock (due to profound dehydration) and acidosis (due to loss of bicarbonate) follow.

The nature of the immune response to cholera is poorly understood. Protection seems to be mediated primarily by an antibacterial effect at the mucosal surface and secondarily by antitoxin antibodies of the secretory IgA class. Serum antibody, though a marker for prior exposure, is not protective.

CLINICAL MANIFESTATIONS   After a 24- to 48-h incubation period, cholera begins with the sudden onset of painless watery diarrhea that may quickly become voluminous and is often soon followed by vomiting. In severe cases, stool volume can exceed 250 mL/kg in the first 24 h. If fluids and electrolytes are not replaced, hypovolemic shock and death ensue. Fever is usually absent. Muscle cramps due to electrolyte disturbances are common. The stool has a characteristic appearance: a nonbilious, gray, slightly cloudy fluid with flecks of mucus, no blood, and a somewhat sweet, inoffensive odor. It has been referred to by the sobriquet "rice water" stool because of its resemblance to the water in which rice has been washed. Clinical symptoms parallel volume contraction: At losses of 3 to 5 percent of normal body weight, thirst occurs; at 5 to 8 percent, postural hypotension, weakness, tachycardia, and decreased skin turgor; above 10 percent, oliguria, weak to absent pulses, sunken eyes and (in infants) sunken fontanelles, wrinkled ("washerwoman") skin, somnolence, and coma. Complications derive exclusively from the effects of volume and electrolyte depletion and include, for example, renal failure due to acute tubular necrosis. Thus, if the patient is adequately treated with fluid and salt, complications are averted and the process self-limited, resolving in a few days.

Laboratory data usually reveal an elevated hematocrit in nonanemic patients (due to hemoconcentration); mild neutrophilic leukocytosis; elevations of BUN and creatinine consistent with prerenal azotemia; normal sodium, potassium, and chloride levels; a markedly reduced bicarbonate level (<15 mmol/L); and an elevated anion gap (due to coexistent increases in serum lactate, protein, and phosphate). Arterial pH is usually low (about 7.2).

DIAGNOSIS   The clinical suspicion of cholera can be confirmed by the identification of the organism in stool. In experienced hands, the organism can be detected directly by dark-field microscopy on a wet mount of fresh stool, and its serotype discerned by immobilization with Inaba- or Ogawa-specific antiserum. The best selective culture medium is thiosulfate–citrate–bile salts–sucrose (TCBS) agar, on which the organism grows as a flat yellow colony. If a delay in sample processing is expected, Carey-Blair transport medium and/or alkaline-peptone water-enrichment medium should be inoculated as well. In endemic areas there is little need for biochemical characterization, though it may be worthwhile in places where *V. cholerae* is an uncommon isolate. Standard microbiologic biochemical testing for Enterobacteriaceae will suffice for identification of *V. cholerae*. All vibrios are oxidase-positive. *V. cholerae* can be distinguished from the otherwise similar *V. mimicus* by its ability to ferment sucrose.

TREATMENT   Cholera is simple to treat, needing only the rapid and adequate replacement of fluids, electrolytes, and base. The mortality rate is usually less than 1 percent. It has been proven conclusively that fluid may be given orally, thereby taking advantage of the hexose-Na$^+$ cotransport mechanism to move Na$^+$ across the gut mucosa together with an actively transported molecule such as glucose. Since Na$^+$ losses in the stool are high, a fluid containing 90 mmol/L Na$^+$ has been recommended by the WHO (Table 120-1). That amount of Na$^+$ is higher than needed to treat diarrhea due to most other causes. The solution is safe, even in infants, if alternated with sodium-free fluid such as breast milk or water. For the sake of simplicity, WHO advises routine use of this single solution for diarrheal disease rather than attempting to select from multiple formulations according to etiology. In the future, cereal-based oral rehydration solutions may be more widely recommended. For severely dehydrated patients, the intravenous route of fluid replacement, if available, is preferable for initial management. Because profound acidosis (pH < 7.2) is common in that group, Ringer's lactate is the best choice among commercial products (Table 120-2). It requires the use of additional potassium supplements, preferably given by mouth. The total fluid deficit (usually estimated at 10 percent of body weight in severely dehydrated patients) can be replaced safely within the first 4 h of therapy, half within the first hour. Thereafter, oral therapy usually can be initiated, with the goal of maintaining fluid intake equal to output. However, patients with continued large-volume diarrhea may require prolonged intravenous treatment to keep up with gastrointestinal fluid losses. Severe hypokalemia can be present but will respond to potassium given either intravenously or orally. In the absence of adequate staff to monitor the patient's progress, the oral route of rehydration and potassium repletion is safer than the intravenous route and is physiologically regulated by thirst and urine output.

Though not necessary to achieve cure, the use of an antibiotic to which the organism is susceptible will diminish the duration and volume of fluid loss and will hasten clearance of the organism from the stool. Single-dose tetracycline (2 g) or doxycycline (300 mg) is effective in adults but is not recommended for children under 8 years of age because of possible deposition in bone and developing teeth. Trimethoprim-sulfamethoxazole (5 mg/kg of trimethoprim and 25 mg/kg of sulfamethoxazole given bid for 3 days) is a suitable alternative for young children. Other antibiotics, including ampicillin and the new 4-fluoroquinolones, are also active. Emerging drug resistance is a concern.

CONTROL In outbreaks, efforts should first be made to identify case contacts and to treat incubating carriers. Next, epidemiologic study should be undertaken to establish the modes of transmission in order to define the best strategy to interrupt them. Rehydration centers should be established and rehydration techniques taught, both of which are essential to reducing mortality.

PREVENTION Provision of safe water, facilities for sanitary disposal of feces, improved nutrition, and attention to food preparation and storage in the household could significantly reduce the incidence of cholera. Much effort has been devoted to the development of a cholera vaccine over the past two decades, focusing particularly on the use of live oral vaccine strains. Traditional killed cholera vaccine given intramuscularly provides little protection to nonimmune subjects

TABLE 120-2 Electrolyte composition of cholera stool and of intravenous rehydration solution

Substance	Concentration, mmol/L			
	Na$^+$	K$^+$	Cl$^-$	Base
Stool				
Adult	135	15	90	30
Child	100	25	90	30
Ringer's lactate	130	4*	109	28

* Potassium supplements, preferably administered by mouth, are required to replete the usual potassium losses from stool.

and predictably causes adverse effects, including pain at the injection site, malaise, and fever. A new approach, the oral administration of killed whole bacterial cells either with or without cholera toxin B subunit (BS-WC vaccine or WC vaccine), has shown promise. In trials in Bangladesh, both vaccines conferred about 50 percent protection compared with placebo over a 3-year evaluation period. Protective efficacy of BS-WC was superior to that of WC during the initial 8 months of follow-up (69 versus 41 percent) but equivalent or inferior thereafter. Immunity was relatively sustained in persons vaccinated above the age of 5 years but only poorly so in younger vaccinees. Several laboratories are now bringing the powerful techniques of molecular biology to bear on this problem and offer the hope that an inexpensive, easily administered, and broadly efficacious vaccine will one day be available. Although one case per week of travel-associated cholera is presently being reported in the United States, it is estimated that using the existing intramuscular vaccine and assuming 1 case per 500,000 trips, a routine vaccination program for travelers from North America to endemic areas would cost over $28 million for each case of cholera prevented and would produce over 100 vaccine-associated adverse events. Vaccine is therefore not recommended for Americans traveling in cholera-endemic areas unless mandated by the country to be visited. Travelers should observe careful hygiene and eating and drinking habits that reduce the likelihood of their encountering the organism.

OTHER *VIBRIO* SPECIES

In recent years, the taxonomic, epidemiologic, pathophysiologic, and clinical features of the non-O1 vibrios have been increasingly well understood. Ten human pathogens are currently recognized within the genus *Vibrio*. Included are species associated primarily with gastrointestinal illness (*V. parahaemolyticus*, non-O1 *V. cholerae*, *V. mimicus*, *V. fluvialis*, *V. hollisae,* and *V. furnissii*) and species associated primarily with soft tissue infections (*V. vulnificus, V. alginolyticus,* and *V. damsela*). As well, *V. vulnificus* has emerged as a cause of primary sepsis in certain compromised hosts. Vibrios are abundant in coastal waters the world over and tend to concentrate in the tissues of filter-feeding mollusks. Under optimal conditions some can double in as little as 9 minutes. Consequently, seawater and raw or undercooked shellfish are important sources of human infection (Table 120-3). Vibrios grow best at temperatures between about 28 and 44°C but not at all below 4°C or above 60°C. Most can be cultured on blood or MacConkey agar, each of which contains enough salt to support the growth of the halophilic organisms (≥0.5 percent). As with *V. cholerae*, TCBS is the best selective medium. The species can be differentiated in the laboratory by standard biochemical tests. The most important members of the group are *V. parahaemolyticus*, a major cause of gastroenteritis in the Far East, and *V. vulnificus,* a notable cause of sepsis in certain immunosuppressed patients in the United States. These and other select species are considered below in greater detail.

SPECIES ASSOCIATED PRIMARILY WITH GASTROINTESTINAL ILLNESS *V. parahaemolyticus* First implicated as a cause of enteritis by Japanese workers in 1953, *V. parahaemolyticus* is now

TABLE 120-1 Composition of World Health Organization oral rehydration solution (WHO ORS)*,†

	Concentration, mmol/L				
	Na$^+$	K$^+$	Cl$^-$	Citrate‡	Glucose
WHO ORS	90	20	80	10	111

* Contains NaCl 3.5 g, Na$_3$C$_6$H$_5$O$_7$·2H$_2$O 2.9 g, KCl 1.5 g, and glucose 20 g per package, to be added to 1 L of drinking water.

† If prepackaged ORS is unavailable, a simple homemade alternative can be prepared by combining 5 g NaCl (about 1 level teaspoon) and either 50 g precooked rice cereal or 40 g sucrose in 1 L of drinking water. In that case, potassium must be supplied separately (e.g., orange juice or coconut water).

‡ 10 mmol of citrate per liter, which supplies 30 mmol of HCO$_3$ per liter.

TABLE 120-3   Features of select noncholera vibrioses

Organism	Vehicle or activity	Host at risk	Syndrome
V. parahaemolyticus	Shellfish, seawater	Normal	Gastroenteritis
	Seawater	Normal	Wound infection
Non-O1 *V. cholerae*	Shellfish, travel	Normal	Gastroenteritis
	Seawater	Normal	Wound infection, otitis media
V. vulnificus	Shellfish	Immunosuppressed*	Sepsis, secondary cellulitis
	Seawater	Normal	Wound infection, cellulitis
V. alginolyticus	Seawater	Normal	Wound infection, cellulitis, otitis
	Seawater	Burn, other immunosuppressed	Sepsis

* Especially liver disease or hemochromatosis.

recognized as an important intestinal pathogen in many parts of the world. In one study from Japan, 24 percent of reported cases of food poisoning were attributed to it, presumably owing to the widespread consumption of raw seafood there. In the United States it has been responsible for several well-documented common-source outbreaks of diarrhea, typically linked to ingestion of undercooked or improperly handled seafood or to other foods that have been contaminated by seawater. Most reports have come from the Atlantic Coast, the Gulf of Mexico, or Hawaii. The organism is ubiquitous in marine environments and is able to grow in saline concentrations up to about 8 to 10 percent. The ability to cause hemolysis on Wagatsuma agar (the so-called Kanagawa phenomenon) is closely linked to enteropathogenicity. In one study, 96.5 percent of isolates from patients with diarrhea were hemolytic versus only about 1 percent of isolates from seawater. Hemolysis is attributed to a 42-kDa heat-stable protein, the exact pathophysiologic role of which is uncertain. The mechanism by which *V. parahaemolyticus* causes diarrhea is uncertain.

V. parahaemolyticus has been associated with two distinct gastrointestinal presentations. Most common is a syndrome of watery diarrhea, usually accompanied by abdominal cramps, nausea, and vomiting, and by fever and chills in about one-quarter of cases. The incubation period ranges from 4 h to 4 days, and the symptomatic period persists for a median duration of 3 days. The vast majority of North American cases have been of this type. A less common syndrome is one of dysentery described in India and Bangladesh and characterized by severe abdominal cramps, nausea, vomiting, and bloody or mucoid stools. Most cases of either type are self-limited and require neither antimicrobials nor hospitalization. The occasional severe case should be treated with fluid repletion and antibiotics, as described above for cholera. Mortality is very rare. There are no reliable differential diagnostic features. *V. parahaemolyticus* should be considered in all cases of diarrhea that can be epidemiologically linked to seafood consumption or to the sea.

In addition to gastrointestinal disease, *V. parahaemolyticus* is a rare cause of extraintestinal infections, including wound infections, otitis, and, very rarely, sepsis.

Non-O1 *V. cholerae* The non-O1 *V. cholerae* are a heterogeneous group of organisms that on routine testing are biochemically indistinguishable from *V. cholerae* O1 but that fail to agglutinate in O1 antiserum. They have been responsible for several well-described food-borne outbreaks of gastroenteritis, as well as sporadic cases of otitis media, wound infection, and bacteremia. About half the U.S. isolates are obtained from stool specimens. Like other vibrios, they are widely distributed in marine environments, but unlike most, they require only trace amounts of NaCl to survive (nonhalophilic). Recognized U.S. cases have invariably been associated either with the consumption of raw oysters or with recent travel, typically to Mexico. The clinical spectrum of diarrheal disease that they cause is broad and likely reflects the heterogeneous virulence attributes among members of the group. Occasional isolates make a protein enterotoxin very similar to cholera toxin. Others make cytotoxins, hemolysins, or invasins.

Gastroenteritis due to non-O1 *V. cholerae* typically has an incubation period of less than 2 days. Stools may be copious and watery and may leave the patient severely dehydrated, as with cholera, or they may be partly formed, of lesser volume, and bloody or mucoid. Abdominal cramps, nausea, vomiting, and fever are often present. In one series, 11 percent of patients were hospitalized; in another, 50 percent. The duration of illness ranges from about 2 to 7 days. As with cholera, patients with significant dehydration should be treated with oral or intravenous fluids. The role of antibiotics is uncertain.

Wound infections and otitis media each account for about 10 percent of non-O1 *V. cholerae* isolates. Bacteremias account for another 20 percent. Patients with extraintestinal infection often have a history of occupational or recreational exposure to seawater. Bacteremia is more likely in those with liver disease. Extraintestinal infections should be treated with antibiotics. There is a paucity of data by which to guide one's choice of a specific agent and schedule. Most strains are sensitive in vitro to tetracycline, chloramphenicol, and other agents.

SPECIES ASSOCIATED PRIMARILY WITH SOFT TISSUE INFECTIONS OR BACTEREMIA ***V. vulnificus*** Though it represents only a minority of the *Vibrio* species found in nature (4 percent of Atlantic coast isolates in one study), *V. vulnificus* is perhaps the most important cause of severe *Vibrio* infections in the United States (0.8 cases per 100,000 population in one study from Louisiana). Formerly grouped in the species *V. parahaemolyticus*, *V. vulnificus* was distinguished in the 1970s by its ability to ferment lactose and by recognition of the distinct clinical syndromes that it causes. Like most vibrios, it proliferates in the warm summer months. It requires saline for growth but prefers concentrations (range up to about 8 percent, optimal about 1 percent) lower than do *V. parahaemolyticus* and *V. alginolyticus*. Human infections typically occur in coastal states between the months of May and October, most often in men over age 40. It has been unequivocally linked to two distinct syndromes: primary sepsis, typically in patients with antecedent liver disease, and primary wound infections, usually in people without underlying disease. Some have suggested that it causes gastroenteritis, but the evidence for this is tenuous.

The organism is remarkably invasive in animal models. It is endowed with a number of virulence attributes, including an antiphagocytic capsule, serum resistance, a cytotoxin/hemolysin (it is Kanagawa-positive), collagenase, elastolytic protease, phospholipase, and siderophores. Its virulence, as measured by the 50 percent lethal dose (LD_{50}) in mice, is markedly enhanced under conditions of iron overload, a fact consonant with its propensity to infect patients with hemochromatosis.

Primary sepsis occurs most commonly in patients with cirrhosis or hemochromatosis but also has been observed in patients with hematopoietic disorders or chronic renal insufficiency, in those using immunosuppressive medications or alcohol, and rarely, in those without apparent underlying disease. Most have ingested raw oysters within 2 days of onset (median incubation period 16 h). The process begins precipitously with malaise, chills, fever (mean 39.8°C), and prostration. Hypotension develops in one-third of cases, often by the time of admission. Cutaneous manifestations, which develop in three-quarters of cases usually by 36 h after onset, typically are on the extremities, lower more often than upper. A common sequence is the evolution of erythematous patches followed by ecchymoses, vesicles, and bullae. (Indeed, the presence of sepsis and bullous skin lesions should suggest the diagnosis in the appropriate setting.) Necrosis and sloughing may occur. Laboratory study reveals leukopenia more often than leukocytosis, thrombocytopenia, and occasionally, elevated fibrin split products. The organism can be cultured from blood or cutaneous lesions. Mortality approaches 50 percent, usually due to uncontrolled sepsis. Accordingly, prompt treatment is critical and should include empirical antibiotics, aggressive debridement, and general supportive care. The organism is sensitive to a number of antimicrobials in vitro, including tetracycline, gentamicin, and third-generation cephalosporins. There are no compelling clinical data in humans to support the use of any particular one of these agents. Tetracycline is demonstrably superior in a murine model and is considered the drug of choice (0.5 to 1 g IV every 12 h), either alone or in combination with gentamicin. The duration of therapy is guided by the clinical response.

Wound infections occur in patients with or without underlying disease and invariably follow contact of seawater with either an existing or a fresh wound. The incubation period is brief (4 h to 4 days, mean 12 h). The disease begins with swelling, erythema, and often intense pain around the wound. A rapidly spreading cellulitis follows, with vesicular, bullous, or necrotic lesions developing in some. Metastatic events do not generally occur. Fever (median 38.9°C) and leukocytosis are present in most. The organism can be cultured from the skin lesions and occasionally from blood. Prompt antibiotic therapy and debridement are usually curative.

V. alginolyticus This species was first recognized as a human pathogen in 1973 and is now known to cause occasional wound, ear, and eye infections. It is the most salt-tolerant of the vibrios, able to grow in concentrations exceeding 10 percent. Most clinical isolates come from superinfected wounds presumably contaminated at the beach. Infection varies in severity but is generally not serious and responds well to antibiotics and drainage. A few reports describe otitis externa, otitis media, or conjunctivitis. Therapy with tetracycline is usually curative. The organism is a rare cause of bacteremia in immunocompromised hosts.

REFERENCES

BLAKE PA et al: Disease of humans (other than cholera) caused by vibrios. Annu Rev Microbiol 34:341, 1980

CARPENTER CCJ: The treatment of cholera: Clinical science at the bedside. J Infect Dis 166:2, 1992

CENTERS FOR DISEASE CONTROL: Update: Cholera—Western hemisphere, and recommendation for treatment of cholera. Morb Mort Week Rep 40:562, 1991

———: Cholera associated with international travel—1992. Morb Mort Week Rep 41:664, 1992

CLEMENS JD et al: ABO blood groups and cholera: New observations on specificity of risk and modification of vaccine efficacy. J Infect Dis 159:770, 1989

——— et al: Field trial of oral cholera vaccines in Bangladesh: Results from three-year follow-up. Lancet 335:270, 1990

GLASS RI et al: Epidemic cholera in the Americas. Science 256:1524, 1992

HIRSHHORN N, GREENOUGH WB: Progress in oral rehydration therapy. Sci Am 264:50, 1991

LEVINE MM, EDELMAN R: Future vaccines against enteric pathogens. Infect Dis Clin North Am 4:105, 1990

LOWRY PW et al: Cholera in Louisiana: Widening spectrum of seafood vehicles. Arch Intern Med 149:2079, 1989

MACPHERSON DW, TONKIN M: Cholera vaccination: A decision analysis. Can Med Assoc J 146:1947, 1992

MORRIS JG JR: Non-O1 V. cholerae: A look at the epidemiology of an occasional pathogen. Epidemiol Rev 12:179, 1990

MORRIS JG, BLACK RE: Cholera and other vibrioses in the United States. N Engl J Med 312:343, 1985

Prevention and treatment of cholera. Med Lett 33:107, 1991

SWERDLOW DL et al: Waterborne transmission of epidemic cholera in Trujillo, Peru: Lessons for a continent at risk. Lancet 340:28, 1992

TACKET CO et al: Cholera vaccines. Biotechnology 20:53, 1992

VANDEN BROUCKE JP et al: Who made John Snow a hero? Am J Epidemiol 133:967, 1991

121 BRUCELLOSIS

DONALD KAYE

DEFINITION Brucellosis is an infection caused by bacteria of the genus *Brucella*. Human infection results from occupational contact with an infected animal or from ingestion of infected milk, milk products, or tissues. The symptoms of brucellosis are often nonspecific and include fever, malaise, and weight loss, often without physical findings.

ETIOLOGY There are four species of *Brucella* that cause infection in humans. The most pathogenic is *B. melitensis*, followed by *B. suis*, *B. abortus*, and *B. canis*. While each of these tends to produce infection in a specific animal host (*B. melitensis* in sheep and goats, *B. suis* in swine, *B. abortus* in cattle, and *B. canis* in dogs), cross-species infection occurs (e.g., *B. abortus* in sheep) and other animals may become infected.

Brucella are small, nonmotile, nonencapsulated, gram-negative coccobacilli which do not form spores. *Brucella* grow best at 37°C under increased CO_2 tension and are separated from each other by biochemical and serologic techniques. Strains with decreased lipopolysaccharide in the outer membrane have reduced virulence.

EPIDEMIOLOGY Animals acquire brucellosis either sexually or by ingesting contaminated milk or other animal products. Humans develop disease following ingestion of contaminated animal food products, by contact of *Brucella* with abraded skin, through the conjunctivae, or by inhalation. Person-to-person transmission rarely, if ever, occurs.

While there are 500,000 new cases of brucellosis reported annually worldwide, it has become a rare disease in the United States, with fewer than 200 cases reported each year. However, it is estimated that only about 4 percent of cases are recognized and reported. *B. abortus* and *B. suis* cause most cases in the United States; *B. melitensis* and *B. canis* are rare. In the United States, brucellosis is mainly an occupational disease, with most cases occurring in working-age males who are abattoir workers, butchers, or farmers. Veterinarians may become infected by accidental inoculation of live attenuated *B. abortus* vaccine, which causes mild disease. In most instances of brucellosis acquired in the United States from ingestion of contaminated milk products, the foods came from other parts of the world (Mexico, Mediterranean countries, the Far East, and South America).

Worldwide, *B. melitensis* is the most frequent cause of brucellosis. There are tremendous differences in the yearly incidence of human brucellosis in different countries, mainly depending on the extent of animal brucellosis. The areas with the highest prevalence are the Mediterranean countries, Asia, and Central and South America.

PATHOGENESIS AND PATHOLOGY After invading the body, *Brucella* are phagocytized by polymorphonuclear leukocytes and macrophages. Some *Brucella* are killed, but others multiply within these cells and destroy them. *Brucella* are able to survive inside phagocytes by inhibiting degranulation of myeloperoxidase-containing granules and thus interfering with myeloperoxidase-dependent bactericidal mechanisms.

Organisms spread via lymphatics to regional lymph nodes and, if not contained, to the bloodstream. Bacteremia may result in foci in cells of the reticuloendothelial system in the liver, spleen, and bone marrow and in other organs such as the kidneys. *Brucella* inside phagocytic cells (as in the reticuloendothelial system and tissue macrophages) are protected against antibody and many antibiotics.

The reaction of tissues to *Brucella* is the formation of granulomas with epithelioid cells, giant cells, lymphocytes, and plasma cells. *B. abortus* usually causes mild disease with noncaseating granulomas in the liver and other reticuloendothelial organs. *B. suis* causes more severe disease with local suppurative complications and granulomas that may caseate. *B. melitensis* produces the most severe acute disease with symptoms that may be disabling. *B. canis* results in mild disease similar to that seen with *B. abortus*. Activated macrophages can kill *Brucella*, and this is the probable mechanism by which spontaneous cure and immunity occur. Granulomas in brucellosis eventually heal with fibrosis and often calcification.

Brucella localize to the placenta in pregnant ungulates due to the presence of erythritol, which enhances the growth of the bacteria. Abortion may ensue. However, erythritol is not found in significant concentrations in humans, and abortions do not occur any more frequently with this disease than with other bacteremias.

MANIFESTATIONS Brucellosis may be asymptomatic, with only serologic evidence of infection. Children are particularly prone to subclinical infection. The manifestations of symptomatic brucellosis may be divided into acute brucellosis, localized disease, and chronic brucellosis.

Acute brucellosis The incubation period of acute brucellosis usually varies between 7 and 21 days but may be months. The onset is often insidious, with a low-grade fever and no localizing complaints. Malaise, weakness, fatigue, headache, backache, myalgias, sweats, and chills are often prominent. Most patients are anorectic and lose weight. With *B. melitensis* infection, the onset may be acute with high fever.

Typically, there are a multitude of complaints but a paucity of physical findings. When physical findings occur, the major manifestations are splenomegaly (which occurs in 10 to 20 percent of patients), lymphadenopathy (15 percent of patients), and hepatomegaly (less than 10 percent).

Localized brucellosis Localized disease may occur at almost any anatomic location, but osteomyelitis, splenic abscess, genitourinary tract infection, pulmonary disease, and endocarditis are among the more common. Osteomyelitis usually occurs in the vertebrae, with the lumbosacral area the most frequent site. There is a disc space infection with involvement of both adjacent vertebrae. Bone scans are positive early, followed by roentgenographic evidence of osteoporosis, anterior vertebral plate erosion, and formation of "parrot-beaked" osteophytes. Arthritis, which is much less common than osteomyelitis, most often involves the knee. Splenic abscesses may occur and result in areas of calcification. Epididymoorchitis and less often clinically apparent prostatic or renal infection may be observed. Neurologic complications are uncommon and include meningoencephalitis, myelitis, radiculitis, and peripheral neuropathy. Pleural effusion and pneumonia are occasional manifestations.

Endocarditis is the most common cause of mortality among patients with brucellosis. It has been reported predominantly in males, most often involves the aortic valve, has an indolent onset, results in bulky and ulcerative vegetations, is accompanied by a high rate of congestive heart failure and arterial embolization, and has usually required both valve replacement and antibiotic therapy to achieve cure.

Chronic brucellosis Chronic brucellosis is defined as ill health for more than 1 year following onset of brucellosis. It has mixed manifestations and includes patients with relapsing illness, with or without localized infection, as well as those who have no objective signs of infection (e.g., no fever) and no evidence of active brucellosis (by serology or culture). While the former clearly have brucellosis, it is doubtful that the latter have active brucellosis. Their complaints, fatigue and weakness, are more likely functional.

An unusual complication that occurs in veterinarians removing placentas from infected animals consists of an erythematous macular, papular, or pustular rash on the hands and arms, which is presumed to be a hypersensitivity reaction to *Brucella* antigens.

DIAGNOSIS Brucellosis is a relatively rare disease, and there are many common illnesses that may mimic the most frequent presentation (i.e., fever without localizing symptoms or physical findings). Among them are infectious mononucleosis, toxoplasmosis, tuberculosis, hepatitis, systemic lupus erythematosus, typhoid fever, and many others. The clinical suspicion that the patient has brucellosis should be higher in farmers, abattoir workers, veterinarians, and others exposed to infected tissues or animal products. Most routine laboratory tests are not helpful. The white blood cell count is usually normal or low, and the erythrocyte sedimentation rate may be normal.

Cultures The definitive evidence of *Brucella* infection consists of isolating *Brucella* from the patient. However, culturing *Brucella* organisms may be dangerous to laboratory personnel. Therefore, specimens should be labeled as "suspected brucellosis" and should be processed only in laboratories that have biosafety level 3 facilities. Up to half the untreated patients studied early in the course of infection will have *Brucella* in the blood when a culture is grown in trypticase soy broth for 1 to 3 weeks in the presence of 5 to 10% CO_2. Optimally, Casteñeda's medium (a biphasic trypticase soy broth and agar medium) should be used and incubated for 4 weeks. Bone marrow cultures are often positive in acute brucellosis when blood cultures are not. They are also more likely to remain positive later in the course of the disease and in spite of administration of antimicrobial agents. As the illness progresses, bacteremia is less frequent, and organisms may then be isolated from infected lymph nodes or granulomas involving the spleen, liver, and bone. Altogether, only 15 to 20 percent of cases of brucellosis are confirmed by culture. In localized brucellosis, biopsy and isolation of *Brucella* may be necessary for diagnosis. In the majority of cases of brucellosis, the diagnosis is made serologically.

Serology The standard tube *Brucella* agglutination test (STA) has been used most in the diagnosis of brucellosis. It measures antibodies directed primarily at *Brucella* lipopolysaccharide antigens. A titer of $\geq$1:160 is considered positive and indicates past or present exposure to *Brucella* organisms or antigens that cross-react with *Brucella* species (*Brucella* skin tests, cholera vaccination, and infection with *Vibrio cholerae*, *Francisella tularensis*, or *Yersinia enterocolitica*). A fourfold or greater rise in titer of antibody in serum specimens drawn 1 to 4 weeks apart is indicative of recent exposure to *Brucella* or *Brucella*-like antigens. Paired specimens should be tested on the same day in the same laboratory. Most patients develop a rise in titer, as measured by the STA, within 1 to 2 weeks of illness, and by 3 weeks virtually all patients will show seroconversion. If there is strong clinical suspicion of brucellosis, dilutions as high as 1:1280 should be made, because false-negative tests due to blocking antibodies have been reported with blocking antibody titers as high as 1:640. True STA titers below 1:160 are strong evidence against active brucellosis.

The methods for serologic diagnosis of brucellosis use *B. abortus* antigens, because antibodies to *B. melitensis* and *B. suis* cross-react with *B. abortus*. However, antibodies to *B. canis* will not react with *B. abortus* antigen, and specialized serologic studies are necessary to detect these antibodies.

IgM antibody titers rise early in brucellosis (usually in the first week of infection), peak at about 3 months, and then fall gradually. However, high titers may persist for years. IgG antibodies appear 2 to 3 weeks after onset of illness, peak in about 8 weeks, and persist as long as the infection is active. With cure, IgG antibody titers decrease rapidly and usually disappear within 1 year. The persistence of IgG antibody indicates continuing active infection. With relapse, both IgM and IgG titers increase. Use of 2-mercaptoethanol (2-ME) in the STA destroys the agglutinating activity of IgM antibodies and allows measurement of only the IgG-agglutinating antibody. In contrast to elevated IgM antibodies, a single titer of $\geq$1:160 in the 2-ME STA is good evidence of either current or very recent infection.

The *Brucella* skin test is only a measure of past infection. Because it may cause a rise in antibody titers, confusing the interpretation of the STA, it should not be performed.

TREATMENT The combination of doxycycline 100 mg every 12 hours or tetracycline 30 mg/kg per day in four equally divided doses, orally, for 3 to 6 weeks plus streptomycin 15 mg/kg every 12 h intramuscularly for the first 2 weeks is considered the treatment of choice for brucellosis. The longer duration of a tetracycline is recommended for patients with localized brucellosis. Patients who relapse are usually cured with retreatment. Tetracyclines should not be used in pregnant women or children below the age of 8 because of the danger of staining developing teeth. Streptomycin may cause eighth-nerve toxicity, and the dose must be decreased in patients with renal insufficiency.

A variety of other regimens, including a tetracycline plus gentamicin or rifampin in lieu of streptomycin or trimethoprim-sulfamethoxazole alone, have been tried in an attempt to decrease relapses and toxicity, but none has been superior to the tetracycline-streptomycin combination. When a tetracycline plus streptomycin cannot be used, trimethoprim-sulfamethoxazole (480/2400 mg/d) for 4 weeks is a reasonable substitute, although relapses are common. Addition of rifampin (900 mg/d) to the basic tetracycline-streptomycin or trimethoprim-sulfamethoxazole regimen may improve results when response is poor or when meningitis or endocarditis is present. Despite in vitro activity against *Brucella*, ciprofloxacin has resulted in a high relapse rate and should not be used. Successful therapy of endocarditis has usually required valve replacement in addition to one of the above antimicrobial regimens. The role of the third-generation cephalosporins in brucellosis remains to be determined, despite their apparent in vitro activity against strains of *Brucella*.

Abscesses should be drained when indicated. Splenectomy has been performed in some patients with splenomegaly and multiple relapses and has apparently been successful in preventing further relapses. Headache, backache, and generalized aches and pains should be treated with analgesics.

PROGNOSIS Even before the advent of antimicrobial treatment, the mortality rate of brucellosis was less than 5 percent, and only 15 percent of patients had an illness exceeding 3 months in duration. With chemotherapy, the mortality rate is less than 2 percent, and long illnesses and complications are rare. When the morbidity exceeds 1 to 2 months, other causes, previously unsuspected underlying disease, or a complication of brucellosis should be considered.

PREVENTION The key to elimination of brucellosis in humans is the eradication of animal brucellosis. This can be accomplished by immunization of animals with a live attenuated *Brucella* vaccine, which produces immunity. No vaccine is available for human immunization in the United States. The risk of acquiring brucellosis can be decreased by use of pasteurized milk and pasteurized milk products, by guarding against exposure to tissue from infected animals, and by protecting potential portals of entry in high-risk individuals (veterinarians, meat inspectors, slaughterhouse workers) with protective bandages over cuts and the use of protective clothing, gloves, and goggles.

REFERENCES

CASTILLO JD et al: Comparative trial of doxycycline plus streptomycin versus doxycycline plus rifampin for the therapy of human brucellosis. Chemotherapy 35:146, 1989
CISNEROS JM et al: Multicenter prospective study of treatment of *Brucella melitensis* brucellosis with doxycycline for 6 weeks plus streptomycin for 2 weeks. Antimicrob Agents Chemother 34(5):881, 1990
GOTUZZO E et al: An evaluation of diagnostic methods for brucellosis—The value of bone marrow culture. J Infect Dis 153(1):122, 1986
JACOBS F et al: Brucella endocarditis: The role of combined medical and surgical treatment. Rev Infect Dis 12(5):740, 1990
LANG R et al: Failure of prolonged treatment with ciprofloxacin in acute infections due to *Brucella melitensis*. J Antimicrob Chemother 26:841, 1990
MIKOLICH, DJ, BOYCE, JM: Brucella species, in *Principles and Practice of Infectious Diseases*, 3d ed, GL Mandell et al (eds). New York, Churchill Livingstone, 1990
SHEHABI A et al: Diagnosis and treatment of 106 cases of human brucellosis. J Infect 20:5, 1990
SMITH LD, FICHT TA: Pathogenesis of brucella. Clin Rev Microbiol 17(3):209, 1990
STASZKIEWICZ J et al: Outbreak of *Brucella melitensis* among microbiology laboratory workers in a community hospital. J Clin Microbiol 29(2):287, 1991
YOUNG EJ: Serologic diagnosis of human brucellosis: Analysis of 214 cases by agglutination tests and review of the literature. Rev Infect Dis 13:359, 1991

122 TULAREMIA

DONALD KAYE

DEFINITION Tularemia (rabbit fever, deer fly fever) is an infection caused by *Francisella tularensis*. *F. tularensis* is found in many animals and is transmitted to human beings by direct contact or via an insect vector. The illness is characterized by an ulcerative lesion at the site of inoculation with regional lymphadenopathy, by pneumonia, or by fever without localizing findings.

ETIOLOGY *F. tularensis* is a small, nonmotile, pleomorphic, gram-negative, aerobic coccobacillus. It grows poorly in many media but will grow well in glucose-cysteine blood agar, thioglycolate broth, and other media supplemented with cysteine. *F. tularensis* is found only in the northern hemisphere. There are two types of *F. tularensis*. Type A is distributed solely in North America, is virulent for humans and rabbits, produces citrulline ureidase, and ferments glycerol. Type B is found in North America, Europe, and Asia, causes no or mild disease in humans and rabbits, does not produce citrulline ureidase, and does not ferment glycerol. *F. tularensis* cross-reacts serologically with *Brucella* species and *Yersinia pestis*.

EPIDEMIOLOGY *F. tularensis* has been found in many mammals, including rabbits, squirrels, muskrats, beavers, deer, cattle, and sheep; in birds; in amphibians; and in fish. Tularemia can result from skin contact with any of these species. Tularemia also has been caused by cat bite. Ticks and deer flies can transmit the bacterium. Ticks pass *F. tularensis* to their offspring via a transovarian route. The organism is found in tick feces but not in salivary glands. In the United States, the disease can be carried by *Dermacentor andersoni* (Rocky Mountain wood tick), *Dermacentor variabilis* (American dog tick), *Dermacentor occidentalis* (Pacific Coast dog tick), and *Amblyomma americanum* (Lone Star tick). *F. tularensis* also has been recovered from streams.

In the United States, most cases of tularemia result from skin contact with infected wild rabbits (especially cottontail rabbits) or tick feces. Infection occasionally results from ingestion or inhalation of infected material. Hunters and trappers are at greatest risk. Tularemia is most likely to occur in adult males, and person-to-person transmission rarely, if ever, occurs.

Tularemia has been reported from all parts of the United States, but mostly from Arkansas, Missouri, Texas, Oklahoma, and Tennessee. Fewer than 200 cases are reported annually in the United States. Arthropod-borne disease occurs mainly in the spring and summer, and rabbit-produced infection occurs mainly in the winter.

PATHOGENESIS AND PATHOLOGY In human infection, the most common portal of entry is through the skin or mucous membranes either directly through inapparent abrasions or via the bite of a tick or other arthropod. Inhalation or ingestion of *F. tularensis* also can result in infection. Fewer than 50 organisms will result in infection when injected into the skin or inhaled, whereas more than 10^8 are usually required to produce infection via the oral route.

Following inoculation into the skin, the bacteria multiply locally and after 2 to 5 days (occasionally 1 to 10 days) produce an erythematous, tender, or pruritic papule. The papule rapidly enlarges and forms an ulcer with a black base. The bacteria spread to regional lymph nodes, producing lymphadenopathy, and further spread with bacteremia may occur. With bacteremia, organisms are cleared from the blood by phagocytic cells of the reticuloendothelial system (mainly in the liver and spleen) and may survive intracellularly for long periods of time.

Affected organs (liver, spleen, lymph nodes) demonstrate areas of focal necrosis initially surrounded mainly by polymorphonuclear leukocytes. Subsequently, granulomas form with epithelioid cells and lymphocytes and sometimes multinucleated giant cells surrounding the areas of necrosis, which may resemble caseation necrosis.

Coalescence of granulomas can lead to formation of abscesses. Nodes may occasionally become fluctuant and even rupture. Healing occurs with fibrosis and calcification of the granulomas. While antibody to *F. tularensis* is formed, it probably plays a minor role in immunity and containment of infection. Cell-mediated immunity, which develops over a 2- to 4-week period, plays the major role. Macrophages, once activated, are capable of killing *F. tularensis*.

Contamination of the conjunctiva can result in infection of the eye with regional lymph node enlargement. Aerosolization and inhalation of *F. tularensis* can result in pneumonia. Pneumonia also can occur via the hematogenous route. There is an inflammatory reaction with foci of alveolar necrosis and initially polymorphonuclear leukocytic and later mononuclear cell infiltration with granuloma formation. Chest roentgenograms usually reveal bilateral patchy infiltrates rather than large areas of consolidation. Mediastinal or other regional lymphadenopathy may occur.

Pharyngitis with cervical lymphadenopathy or gastrointestinal tularemia with mesenteric lymphadenopathy may follow ingestion of large numbers of *F. tularensis*. Typhoidal tularemia, which is characterized by fever and no localizing signs, is uncommon; the portal of entry is unknown.

CLINICAL MANIFESTATIONS   Tularemia usually has an incubation period of 2 to 5 days, after which there is onset of one of a number of syndromes (listed below), all of which are usually associated with fever and chills and often with headache, myalgias, and malaise. Tender hepatosplenomegaly is common. About 20 percent of patients develop a generalized maculopapular rash which may occasionally become pustular, and some report erythema nodosum.

Ulceroglandular tularemia   Most patients with tularemia (75 to 85 percent) develop infection secondary to inoculation of the skin. In cases related to rabbits, the portal of entry is usually on the finger or hand. In tick-related cases, the site of inoculation is usually on the lower extremities, inguinal or axillary areas, scalp, abdomen, or chest.

At time of onset of illness the patient usually has an erythematous papule that may be tender or pruritic, or an ulcer is already present at the portal of entry of the organism. If there is a papule, it evolves over a period of several days to form a punched-out ulcer with sharply dermarcated edges and a yellow exudate. The ulcer gradually develops a black base. The patient has very tender, large regional lymphadenopathy (usually axillary or epitrochlear with tularemia from rabbits and inguinal or femoral lymphadenopathy with tick-borne disease). The nodes may become fluctuant and drain spontaneously. In 5 to 10 percent of patients, the skin lesion may be inapparent and the lymphadenopathy the only physical finding. This has been called "glandular tularemia."

Oculoglandular tularemia   In about 1 percent of patients, the conjunctiva serves as the portal of entry for the organism. Purulent conjunctivitis with regional lymphadenopathy (preauricular, submandibular, or cervical) is present. Corneal perforation may occur.

Oropharyngeal and gastrointestinal tularemia   Rarely, tularemia occurs after ingestion of *F. tularensis* (usually in undercooked meat), resulting in acute exudative or membranous pharyngitis associated with cervical lymphadenopathy or ulcerative intestinal lesions with associated mesenteric lymphadenopathy, diarrhea, abdominal pain, nausea, vomiting, and gastrointestinal bleeding.

Pulmonary tularemia   Tularemia pneumonia can present as an atypical pneumonia and must be considered in the differential diagnosis of atypical pneumonia. Involvement of the lung can result from inhalation of *F. tularensis* or as a part of the bacteremia caused by tularemia at another site. Inhalation pulmonary disease occurs most often in laboratory workers and is a serious infection with high mortality. Pulmonary involvement occurs in 10 to 15 percent of patients with ulceroglandular tularemia and in about half the patients with typhoidal tularemia. The patient has cough, which is usually nonproductive, and may have dyspnea or pleuritic chest pain. Most

often the physical examination is normal. Roentgenograms of the chest usually reveal bilateral patchy infiltrates which have been described as "ovoid densities." Lobar pneumonia may occur, and pleural effusion(s) with a polymorphonuclear leukocytic (rarely mononuclear) exudate may be present.

Typhoidal tularemia   In about 10 percent of cases of tularemia, fever develops without apparent skin lesion or lymphadenopathy. In the absence of a history of possible contact with a vector of the disease, diagnosis is extremely difficult.

Other manifestations   Meningitis, pericarditis, peritonitis, endocarditis, and osteomyelitis have been reported. The meningitis causes a lymphocytic response in the spinal fluid. Bacteremia may be associated with acute rhabdomyolysis.

DIAGNOSIS   Differential diagnosis   In patients with fever and large, tender lymphadenopathy, the possibility of tularemia should be strongly considered, and an attempt should be made to determine if there was an appropriate animal or arthropod vector contact. The suspicion of tularemia should be especially high in hunters, trappers, game wardens, veterinarians, and laboratory workers. However, in up to 40 percent of patients with tularemia, no history of epidemiologic contact with an animal or arthropod vector can be elicited.

Ulceroglandular tularemia is often so characteristic that it does not present a problem in differential diagnosis, but on occasion it must be differentiated from other diseases. The skin lesion may resemble those seen in sporotrichosis, skin infection with coagulase-positive staphylococci or group A streptococci, syphilis, anthrax, rat-bite fever (caused by *Spirillum minus*), rickettsial infections (such as scrub typhus), and *Mycobacterium marinum* infection. However, the regional lymphadenopathy in these diseases is usually not as impressive as in tularemia.

The lymphadenopathy of tularemia must be differentiated from that of plague (see Chap. 123), lymphogranuloma venereum (see Chap. 140), and cat-scratch disease (see Chap. 95). However, in these infections there is usually no local lesion resembling the ulcer of tularemia.

Typhoidal tularemia may resemble typhoid fever, other *Salmonella* bacteremias, rickettsial infections (such as Rocky Mountain spotted fever), brucellosis, infectious mononucleosis, toxoplasmosis, miliary tuberculosis, sarcoid, or hematologic malignancies. Tularemia pneumonia may resemble pneumonias caused by other bacteria as well as viral or *Mycoplasma* pneumonia.

Laboratory diagnosis   Blood cultures are usually negative, and the diagnosis is most frequently made serologically by agglutination methods. A significant rise in titer (i.e., fourfold or greater) in paired serum specimens over a 2- to 3-week period is diagnostic. Agglutinating antibody appears after 1 to 2 weeks of illness. Fifty percent of patients have antibody in the second week, and the rest develop antibody later in the course. Titers peak at 4 to 8 weeks and may remain elevated for years. A single agglutinating titer of $\geq$1:160 in a patient who has been ill for at least 2 weeks is highly suggestive of tularemia but may only indicate old infection. Antibodies to *F. tularensis* may cross-react with *Brucella*, but the titers to *Brucella* are usually much lower than the titers to *F. tularensis*. In the future, enzyme-linked immunosorbent assay (ELISA) tests may offer an advantage because they tend to turn positive earlier than agglutinating antibody tests.

F. tularensis is rarely observed on Gram stains of skin lesions, sputum, or aspirates of nodes. However, the organisms can often be demonstrated by staining with a modified Dieterle stain or by fluorescent antibody staining techniques. Cultures of these materials or blood may be positive if processed on appropriate media, but there is a major risk of infection in laboratory personnel. Cultivation of *F. tularensis* should only be attempted in laboratories with adequate isolation techniques and experienced personnel.

Isolation of *F. tularensis* can be achieved by inoculation intraperitoneally into guinea pigs, which will die within 10 days, and by direct plating onto glucose-cysteine blood agar. Agents such as cycloheximide, polymyxin B, and penicillin are frequently added to media to suppress other organisms in specimens that may overgrow *F. tularensis*.

A delayed-type skin test (similar to the tuberculin test) with *F. tularensis* antigen or killed whole bacilli turns positive during the first week of illness, prior to the appearance of agglutinating antibody, and persists for years. However, the skin test antigen is not available commercially and can boost titers of agglutinating antibodies.

The white blood cell count is usually normal, and the erythrocyte sedimentation rate may be normal as well. Pyuria is common.

TREATMENT   Streptomycin, in a dose of 7.5 to 10 mg/kg every 12 h intramuscularly, is considered the drug of choice. In severe infections, 15 mg/kg every 12 h may be used for the first 48 to 72 h. Therapy is continued for 7 to 10 days. Gentamicin, in a dose of 1.7 mg/kg, intramuscularly or intravenously, every 8 h, is also effective. Virtually all strains are susceptible to streptomycin and gentamicin. Temperature response occurs within 2 days, but skin lesions and lymph nodes may take 1 to 2 weeks to heal. When therapy is not initiated until several weeks of illness have elapsed, the temperature response may be delayed. Relapses are very uncommon with streptomycin therapy.

Tetracycline or chloramphenicol, 30 mg/kg per day in four divided doses for 14 days, also has been used to treat tularemia. While response to these agents is good, the relapse rate is unacceptably high, occurring in up to 20 percent of patients. The newer fluoroquinolones such as ciprofloxacin seem promising in preliminary reports.

If fluctuant nodes require aspiration or drainage, at least several days of antibiotic therapy should be given first to avoid exposure of medical personnel to aerosolization of infected material.

PREVENTION   Prevention of tularemia is based on avoidance of exposure and vaccination of high-risk populations. Avoidance of skinning wild mammals, especially rabbits, and wearing gloves while handling rabbit carcasses will decrease the risk of transmission. Use of insect repellents and prompt removal of ticks will help prevent transmission by ticks in tick-infested areas.

A multiple-puncture intradermal vaccine made from live attenuated *F. tularensis* and available from the Centers for Disease Control is effective in decreasing the frequency and severity of disease but will not totally prevent tularemia. Protection is long-lasting. Veterinarians, hunters, trappers, game wardens, and others who are likely to come in contact with infected wild mammals are candidates for immunization. Laboratory workers who handle specimens containing *F. tularensis* should be immunized. Prophylactic treatment with streptomycin will prevent development of clinical disease in patients who are incubating *F. tularensis*.

PROGNOSIS   If untreated, symptoms of tularemia usually last 1 to 4 weeks but may continue for months. The mortality of severe untreated infection (which includes all untreated tularemia pneumonia) can be as high as 30 percent. However, the overall mortality rate for untreated tularemia is less than 8 percent. Mortality is about 1 percent with appropriate therapy and is often associated with long delays in diagnosis and treatment. Following tularemia there is usually lifelong immunity.

REFERENCES

BOYCE JM: *Francisella tularensis* (Tularemia), in *Principles and Practice of Infectious Diseases*, 3d ed, GL Mandell et al (eds). New York, Churchill Livingstone, 1990

CRAVEN RB, BARNES AM: Plague and tularemia. Infect Dis Clin North Am 5(1):165, 1991

PENN RL, KINASEWITZ GT: Factors associated with a poor outcome in tularemia. Arch Intern Med 147:265, 1987

SYRJÄLÄ H et al: In vitro susceptibility of *Francisella tularensis* to fluoroquinolones and treatment of tularemia with norfloxacin and ciprofloxacin. Eur J Clin Microbiol Infect Dis 10:68, 1991

TAYLOR JP et al: Epidemiologic characteristics of human tularemia in the southwest-central states, 1981–1987. Am J Epidemiol 133(10):1032, 1991

TARNVIK A: Nature of protective immunity to *Francisella tularensis*. Rev Infect Dis 11(3):440, 1989

123   PLAGUE AND OTHER *YERSINIA* INFECTIONS

DARWIN L. PALMER

DEFINITION   Plague is an acute infectious illness of humans, rodents, and their ectoparasites which is caused by the gram-negative bacillus *Yersinia pestis*. The disease persists because of its firm entrenchment in both wild and domestic rodent-flea ecosystems throughout the world. In the United States, wild rodent contact leads to sporadic human disease; the historically explosive Asian and European urban epidemics resulted from transmission of disease by rats. Human plague follows bites by rodent fleas; after several days, painful febrile lymphadenitis (the bubo) occurs. If untreated, it results in death in more than 50 percent of cases with sepsis and multiorgan involvement. Primary plague pneumonia is transmitted between humans by cough-generated aerosols, has a fulminant course, and is almost universally fatal if untreated.

EPIDEMIOLOGY   Sylvatic plague involves more than 200 species of wild rodents and is found in the southwestern United States, Russia, India, Vietnam, and Africa. In the United States, field and burrowing rodents, especially ground squirrels, rock squirrels, wood rats, and prairie dogs, are potential carriers. Rodent disease is characterized by occurrence in the spring and summer, year-to-year variations in disease activity, chronicity in the populations involved, slow regional spread, and rare geographic regression. The epizootic disease results in cyclic rodent population die-offs, leaving both resistant survivors and infected fleas seeking another host. Disease also persists in natural foci because of latent infection during animal hibernation, by prolonged viability of *Y. pestis* in soil of rodent burrows, by survival of infected fleas (and possibly ticks), and by persistent infection in relatively resistant rodents. Rodent predators also may spread plague; felines, such as domestic cats, generally die when infected with *Y. pestis*, whereas canines (e.g., foxes, coyotes, dogs) and bears often recover and may serve as serologic sentinels of wild rodent disease. Human disease can be readily acquired from domestic pets when the pets become infected or catch and return plague-infected rodents or their fleas to rural homes. Hares and rabbits are occasional nonrodent sources of the disease in humans, especially during the winter hunting season.

Rodent fleas are critical to the natural plague cycle and are implicated in about 85 percent of human cases. After infection, fleas develop obstruction of the foregut, causing regurgitation of plague bacilli during the next blood meal. The rat flea, *Xenopsylla cheopis*, is an especially efficient plague vector both between rats and between rodents and humans. Transmission without fleas may occur by ingestion of infected carcasses by predators, possibly by contact with infected tissue through an open wound, or by inhalation of infected aerosols. Human body lice as well as ticks also are capable of interhuman or person-to-person transmission.

In the last four decades there has been a fluctuating incidence of sporadic human plague originating in the western United States, varying from 40 cases per year to none. An overall death rate of 16 percent is double that seen in large outbreaks and reflects delay in the diagnosis or incorrect therapy. Travel during the incubation period out of plague endemic areas and failure to elicit a history of animal exposure are common diagnostic problems. Sporadic human plague occurs most frequently in the spring and summer, especially in males, children, or youths under age 20, reflecting outdoor activities and risk of wild rodent contact. While urban rat-related human outbreaks are rare in the United States, they are still important sources of human disease in Asia and Africa. Spread from sylvatic rodents into urban rats was documented as recently as 1983 in Los Angeles. Primary plague pneumonia arises as a hematogenous disseminated pulmonary infection during bubonic/septicemic disease. It may thereafter result in person-to-person spread via infectious aerosols. In close quarters it is rapidly transmitted. A primary pneumonic plague outbreak in the United States last occurred in 1919, when 13 cases with 12 deaths (including two physicians and one nurse) developed before the disease was recognized and halted by case isolation. Cases of primary human pneumonic plague also have been acquired from domestic cats dying of plague pneumonia.

ETIOLOGY *Yersinia pestis* is a member of family Enterobacteriaceae. It is a pleomorphic, gram-negative, nonmotile, aerobic bacillus which grows optimally at 28°C. The organism is a facultative intracellular parasite, but it grows readily, although slowly, on routine media, and cultures should not be discarded before 72 h. Although weakly gram-negative, *Y. pestis* stains best with Giemsa's or Wayson's stains, with which it shows prominent bipolar "safety pin" microscopic morphology. Related virulence-associated plasmids are found in several *Yersinia* species which encode determinants for temperature requirements and calcium dependence. These plasmids appear to enable the organism to grow inside macrophages during the early incubation period. The same virulence plasmids encode for production of outer membrane proteins and V and W antigens which confer resistance to phagocytic intracellular killing. Other virulence factors include pesticin, fibrinolysin, coagulase, and lipopolysaccharide endotoxin. No separate serotypes are recognized, but biotypes *antigua*, *orientalis*, and *mediaevalis* have geographic distributions which presumably mark historic epidemic spread. The organism is relatively resistant to drying and may maintain its viability in cool, moist conditions, such as the soil of an animal burrow, for many months. Antibiotic resistance can be developed in the laboratory and has been noted in wild strains, but significant resistance to streptomycin and tetracycline has not been seen in clinical outbreaks.

PATHOGENESIS After *Y. pestis* is inoculated into the skin by a flea bite, bacteria migrate to local lymph nodes, where they are taken up but not killed by mononuclear cells. Intracellular multiplication results in development of capsular envelopes containing envelope antigen (fraction 1 protein); toxins are elaborated. An acute inflammatory response is provoked in the lymph node in the ensuing 2 to 6 days, resulting in the bubo. At this stage, the organisms are relatively resistant to phagocytosis by polymorphonuclear leukocytes because the bacteria are protected by increased elaboration of envelope antigen and the lack of specific opsonic antibody. Characteristically, hemorrhagic necrosis of lymph nodes with lysis of macrophages next occurs, from which large numbers of bacteria gain access to the bloodstream and other organs. Extensions along lymphatics involve superficial nodes at the site of inoculation, the spleen, and nodes in the abdomen, mediastinum, or perihilar areas. The lung is secondarily infected in 10 to 20 percent of patients, generally as a rapidly progressive, multilobar pneumonia, often with pleural exudate. The early acute inflammatory reaction is followed by lobar consolidation and hemorrhagic necrosis and, if death does not intervene, may progress to abscess formation. Fibrin thrombi may be extensive in the pulmonary vessels as well as in glomeruli and vessels of skin and other organs. Secondarily, the adult respiratory distress syndrome or a rise in pulmonary artery pressure may be seen. Pericarditis with a small amount of seropurulent exudate is frequent, and meningitis may occur late in partially or untreated bubonic plague. In 5 to 15 percent of patients, the skin, predominantly of the extremities, is involved with purpuric lesions due to thrombocytopenia and vasculitis. Late in the disease, buboes may become fluctuant and occasionally may become superinfected with other bacteria. Endotoxemia may result in both septic shock and disseminated intravascular coagulation.

MANIFESTATIONS Bubonic plague has an incubation period of 2 to 7 days from flea bite to onset of illness. Although many patients do not remember an insect contact, a small eschar may be found at the bite site. Patients present with a painful bubo and fever accompanied by headache, prostration, and abdominal distress. The bubo, a tender enlarged lymph node or nodes, ranges in size from 1 to 10 cm and is found in the groin in 70 percent of patients; alternatively, buboes may develop in axillary or cervical nodes or in several lymphatic chains simultaneously. Buboes are extremely tender and not fixed to skin or underlying structures, and overlying skin is often erythematous. Fever and rigors are prominent and occasionally precede appearance of a bubo by 1 to 3 days. Gastrointestinal symptoms are present in more than half the patients, with abdominal pain often extending from the groin bubo and accompanied by anorexia, nausea, vomiting, and diarrhea, which may be bloody. Cutaneous petechiae and hemorrhages occur in 5 to 50 percent of patients and may be extensive late in the disease. Disseminated intravascular coagulation occurs in subclinical form in as many as 86 percent of patients, 5 to 10 percent of whom have clinical manifestations, including gangrene of the skin, fingers, toes, and penis. If untreated, bubonic disease may proceed without other organ system involvement to generalized sepsis, prostration, hypotension, and death within the next 2 to 10 days. Some patients have very prominent early signs of sepsis with high-density bacteremia and no demonstrable bubo. This represents a form of bubonic plague in which lymphatic involvement is limited to deep structures or where the buboes are so small as to be overlooked in the presence of overwhelming signs of infection. Septicemic disease may progress rapidly with chills, fever, rapid pulse, severe headache, nausea, vomiting, delirium, and death within 48 h. The case fatality rate may exceed one-third. In such fulminant sepsis, bacteremia is so prominent that buffy coat blood smear may readily show *Y. pestis* on Gram stain.

Other than the lymphatics, the lung is the organ most commonly involved, with development of secondary pneumonia in 10 to 20 percent of all patients. Cough, fever, and tachypnea appear on days 2 to 3 of illness, accompanied by minimal pulmonary infiltrates. Later, or less commonly, from the start, symptoms worsen rapidly, with marked dyspnea, bloody sputum, and evidence of respiratory failure. There may be multilobar involvement, with variable degrees of consolidation, the sputum may teem with *Y. pestis* and is highly contagious when disseminated by cough-generated aerosols. Primary plague pneumonia is a fulminant illness; time from the initial contact to death ranges from 2 to 6 days. The adult respiratory distress syndrome (ARDS), characterized by noncardiac pulmonary edema, anoxia, and respiratory failure, also occurs as a manifestation of plague sepsis and may be indistinguishable from plague pneumonia except for absence of bacteria in respiratory secretions. Both *Y. pestis* pneumonia and the ARDS form of illness have a mortality in excess of 75 percent, despite appropriate antimicrobial and supportive therapy. Less commonly, marked perihilar adenopathy may present alone or accompany pneumonia.

Plague meningitis, as a late complication that occurs in 6 percent of untreated patients, is characterized by nuchal rigidity, headache, confusion, and coma and is often preceded or accompanied by bacteremia. Most meningitis cases have been described in patients treated with antibiotics that do not readily cross the blood-brain barrier, such as tetracycline and streptomycin. Other contributory factors seem to be late or inadequate therapy. Meningitis due to plague is indistinguishable from that caused by other bacteria.

Rarely, patients with plague have a very mild illness manifested chiefly by low-grade fever and adenopathy. In this group are patients with tonsillar plague, who have positive throat cultures, serologic conversion, and minimal illness. Other, less common late complications include persistent hectic fever despite appropriate therapy, fluctuance and spontaneous drainage from buboes, and pulmonary cavitation with abscess formation.

LABORATORY FINDINGS With the exception of definitive microbiologic studies, laboratory tests are of little diagnostic help. A polymorphonuclear leukocytosis of 15 to 20 cells $\times$ 10^9 per liter is common, and the white cells may show toxic changes. Rarely, a marked leukemoid reaction with more than 100×10^9 white cells per liter is seen. Modest elevations of serum aminotransferases are common, but otherwise, liver function studies are normal. Evidence of disseminated intravascular coagulation with low platelet counts, prolonged partial thromboplastin times, and positive fibrin degradation products in the serum is common. The electrocardiogram is usually normal but may show right axis deviation and peaked P waves indicative of acute cor pulmonale. The chest x-ray will show infiltrates, often with pleural effusion, in secondary or primary plague pneumonia or evidence of pulmonary edema in patients with ARDS. In meningitis, examination of cerebrospinal fluid demonstrates polymorphonuclear pleocytosis, low sugar, elevated protein, and gram-negative coccobacillary organisms, although culture may demonstrate *Y. pestis* more reliably.

Confirmation of the clinical suspicion of bubonic plague may be obtained by needle aspiration of a bubo with direct staining of the aspirated material. With either Wayson's or Giemsa's stain, the characteristic bipolar-staining, "safety pin" forms are seen. By fluorescent antibody staining, a presumptive diagnosis may be specifically confirmed in about 80 percent of cases. Cultures of aspirated material, as well as sputum, pleural fluid, and blood, will be positive in a high percentage of patients. Microscopic examination of buffy coat smear may show *Y. pestis* in septicemic cases. A serologic response with a fourfold or greater rise is detected in the second week of illness by complement fixation, hemagglutination, or indirect immunofluorescent antibody.

DIAGNOSIS Bubonic plague must be suspected in any febrile patient with painful adenopathy who has a history of wild animal exposure in a plague endemic area, but it may be confused with other illnesses. Presentation with fever and a painful groin bubo can mimic lymphogranuloma venereum or syphilis or, when more severe, an acute abdominal crisis such as incarcerated inguinal hernia, appendicitis, or a ruptured viscus. Abdominal pain and bloody diarrhea can be mistaken for shigellosis or other acute diarrheal processes. With an axillary or cervical bubo, acute streptococcal or staphylococcal lymphadenitis, tularemia, cat-scratch fever, lymphogranuloma venereum, or syphilis need to be considered. Bubonic/septicemic disease with an absent or small bubo suggests typhoid fever or bacteremia due to other causes. Primary or secondary pneumonic plague may mimic bacterial pneumonia from any cause.

When plague is suspected, diagnostic maneuvers must include aspiration of buboes with appropriate stains and cultures, as well as blood cultures and cultures from other sources. Cultures should not be discarded early because the organism grows slowly and may only appear in 48 to 72 h. A serologic rise by passive hemagglutination is evident by day 5 and peaks by day 14. Newer serologic methods such as enzyme-linked immunosorbent assay compare well in sensitivity with standard passive hemagglutination tests and are more rapid.

TREATMENT If plague is strongly suspected on clinical and/or epidemiologic grounds, therapy must be started immediately, prior to completion of diagnostic studies. Antibiotic and supportive treatment should reduce the 40 to 100 percent mortality of untreated bubonic or pneumonic plague to 5 to 10 percent. Effective antibiotics include streptomycin, tetracycline, and chloramphenicol. Streptomycin, the most effective therapy, should be given in a dosage of 7.5 to 15 mg/kg every 12 h intramuscularly for a total of 10 days. Streptomycin is in limited supply and is available only through state health departments. Tetracycline, for patients who cannot tolerate streptomycin, may be given orally or intravenously at 10 to 20 mg/kg every 6 h. Tetracycline may be started concurrently and streptomycin discontinued after 3 days without fever but should be continued for a total of 5 to 7 days after the fever has disappeared. In less severely ill patients, tetracycline alone at 5 to 10 mg/kg every 6 h may be given by mouth. Chloramphenicol in a dose of 12.5 to 25 mg/kg given intravenously every 6 h should be substituted for streptomycin or tetracycline in patients with meningitis (because of its better central nervous system penetration) or in hypotensive patients. In hypotensive patients, intravenous chloramphenicol or gentamicin are effective and rapidly distributed. Tetracycline or trimethoprim-sulfamethoxazole can be used for the prophylaxis of case contacts and should be given orally for 5 days. Local treatment of the bubo is not indicated unless fluctuance or spontaneous drainage occurs, when cultures should be obtained to detect staphylococci. Ventilatory support for patients with plague pneumonia or ARDS may be necessary and lifesaving.

PREVENTION AND CONTROL Individuals working in high-risk occupations in plague endemic areas or conducting laboratory work with *Y. pestis* should consider use of the formalin-killed whole-bacteria vaccine; however, the vaccine must be readministered every 6 months owing to rapidly waning immunity. Individuals briefly visiting a plague epidemic area should use insect repellant and garments to cover the arms and legs and may take tetracycline or trimethoprim-sulfamethoxazole prophylaxis. Following the presumptive diagnosis of pneumonic plague, patients should be placed in respiratory isolation; simple hand-washing precautions suffice for bubonic cases. Contacts of a patient with plague pneumonia should be given oral tetracycline prophylaxis, 250 mg four times daily by mouth, and should be advised to seek medical attention if respiratory symptoms or fever develop. Possibly due to such precautions, transmission of primary plague pneumonia has not occurred in the United States for many years.

The potential for spread of plague into urban rat populations from sylvatic rodent sources is an ever-present risk. Prevention depends on control of urban rat populations and their exclusion from dwellings, as well as surveillance of sylvatic rodents and of their local predators. Picnickers, hikers, and others traveling into plague endemic regions during the spring-summer seasons should be warned that plague is a potential danger. They should avoid touching carcasses or sick rodents and should restrain and treat pets with flea-repellent powders. No practical measures exist for eliminating plague from wild rodent sources. Reducing rodent harborage and use of insecticides around rural homes in endemic regions is important. Killing rodents around rural dwellings with rodenticides should be preceded by insect control to prevent displaced rodent fleas from seeking humans or domestic pets.

OTHER *YERSINIA* INFECTIONS (*Y. PSEUDOTUBERCULOSIS* AND *Y. ENTEROCOLITICA*)

ETIOLOGY *Y. enterocolitica* and *Y. pseudotuberculosis* are both non-lactose-fermenting, gram-negative, aerobic bacilli related to one another and to *Y. pestis* and are members of the Enterobacteriaceae. Other *Yersinia* species have been discovered but do not appear to be pathogenic for humans. Both organisms grow slowly on media used for the detection of other enteric bacteria, and their detection can be enhanced by cold enrichment incubation at 20 to 25°C. Strains can be distinguished from one another and from *Y. pestis* on the basis of serologic and biochemical reactions as well as by antibiotic sensitivities. As in *Y. pestis*, both organisms elaborate W and V virulence factors which confer dependency on calcium for growth at 37°C and enable the organisms to survive intracellularly. This requirement is transmitted by a 70-kilobase plasmid which is common to all invasive *Yersinia*. Invasive strains of *Y. enterocolitica* also carry a plasmid-mediated outer membrane protein which enhances both attachment and cell invasion. These strains evoke a keratoconjunctivitis of guinea pigs (Sereney test) and produce a suppurative infection of Peyer's patches and mesenteric lymph nodes. They invade further to cause systemic infection of lung, liver, and spleen, especially in the presence of excess iron, since they normally lack siderophores. Both organisms produce an endotoxin, and *Y. enterocolitica* elaborates a heat-stable enterotoxin which may be of significance in food-borne illness. A large number of serotypes of both organisms exist causing disease in many animal species, but most human infections are caused by a limited number of strains. Strain and disease differences exist between Europe and the United States; American strains appear more invasive but less likely to cause postinfectious sequelae.

MANIFESTATIONS Although recognized most commonly in northern Europe and North America, *Y. enterocolitica* causes enteric infection worldwide and accounts for approximately 1 to 3 percent of all cases of acute bacterial enteritis. The origin of the disease is often unclear, although the portal of entry is the oropharynx or gastrointestinal tract, and outbreaks traced to both food and water have been reported; person-to-person as well as animal-to-person transmission is common. Manifestations of the disease vary with age. In infants and young children, the predominant symptom is acute watery diarrhea lasting 3 to 14 days; 5 percent of children have blood in the stool. In older children and young adults, a syndrome of right lower quadrant pain accompanied by fever and moderate leukocytosis indistinguishable from acute appendicitis occurs. In adults, especially in women over age 40, erythema nodosum often follows enteritis by 1 to 2 weeks. Adults in Scandinavia may develop a monarticular arthritis of the knee, foot, or hand with or without preceding enteritis. Rarely, a severe, disabling suppurative arthritis is seen. Among patients with arthritis, 65 percent have histocompatibility group HLA-B27. A high prevalence of antibodies to *Y. enterocolitica* membrane antigens has been reported in individuals with Graves' disease. *Y. enterocolitica* also causes bacteremia, mostly in individuals with underlying illness such as diabetes mellitus, severe anemia, cirrhosis, or malignancy or in conditions of iron overload. Septicemic patients complain of headache, fever, and abdominal pain with or without diarrhea and frequently develop abscesses in multiple organs. Exudative pharyngitis with *Y. enterocolitica* was found in adult patients during the course of an outbreak of milk-borne yersiniosis.

Pseudotuberculosis is a rare illness acquired from humans or domestic and wild animals, presumably by fecal-oral contact. Most cases are sporadic and occur in the young, with males more commonly affected than females and with a peak in the winter months corresponding to the peak occurrence in animals. After ingestion, the organisms apparently penetrate the ileal mucosa, localize in the ileocecal lymph nodes, and produce an acute mesenteric adenitis which is generally accompanied by vomiting, abdominal pain, and diarrhea. Fever is usually high, and leukocytosis is common. At laparotomy, the appendix appears normal, but enlarged mesenteric lymph nodes and inflammation of the terminal ileum may be seen. Complications appear in adults less commonly than with *Y. enterocolitica* but include arthritis, erythema nodosum, and septicemia.

DIAGNOSIS   *Y. enterocolitica* is much more frequent as a human pathogen than *Y. pseudotuberculosis*. They cause similar signs and symptoms but may have different reservoirs; the first is characterized primarily by diarrhea and the second by mesenteric adenitis. Therefore, *Y. enterocolitica* causes disease similar to other bacterial diarrheas and must be distinguished from them by microbiologic means. Laboratory detection of the organism depends on special cultural techniques. The diagnosis is made best by isolation of the organism from stool in patients with enteritis or atypical cases of appendicitis, erythema nodosum, or reactive arthritis. Cultures of pharyngeal exudate, blood, peritoneal fluid, and other body fluids should be obtained where clinically indicated. Hemagglutination titers peak in 8 to 10 days and remain elevated for 18 months after infection. Cross-reactivity with some *Brucella*, *Salmonella*, and *Vibrio cholerae* antigens occurs. The diagnosis of *Y. pseudotuberculosis* is also made by culture of stool and mesenteric lymph nodes.

THERAPY AND PREVENTION   *Y. enterocolitica* organisms are susceptible in vitro to aminoglycosides, chloramphenicol, tetracycline, trimethoprim-sulfamethoxazole, and the third-generation cephalosporins but are generally resistant to the penicillins and first-generation cephalosporins. However, the value of antimicrobial therapy is unclear, because most cases of enteritis are self-limited. Patients with very severe illness or septicemia should be treated, because treatment may shorten both the duration of disease and the shedding of organisms. *Y. pseudotuberculosis* is usually sensitive to ampicillin, tetracycline, chloramphenicol, and cephalosporins. No controlled clinical trials demonstrate efficacy of treatment, although patients with septicemic disease should receive ampicillin or tetracycline because severe infection has a high mortality. Prevention depends on reducing contamination from animal reservoirs and hygienic measures such as careful food handling, availability of clean drinking water, and hand washing to prevent spread within families or other human contacts.

REFERENCES

Plague

CENTERS FOR DISEASE CONTROL: Human plague—United States, 1988. Morb Mort Week Rep 37:653, 1988

BECKER TB et al: Plague meningitis. A retrospective analysis of cases reported in the U.S., 1970–79. West J Med 147:554, 1987

BUTLER T: A clinical study of bubonic plague: Observations on the 1970 Vietnam epidemic with emphasis on coagulation studies, skin histology, and electrocardiograms. Am J Med 53:268, 1972

KAUFMAN AF et al: Public health implications of plague in domestic cats. Am J Vet Assoc 179:875, 1981

REED WP et al: Bubonic plague in the southwestern United States: A review of recent experience. Medicine 49:465, 1970

SIMPSON WJ et al: Recombinant capsular antigen (fraction 1) from *Yersinia pestis* induces a protective antibody response in *Balb/c* mice. Am J Trop Med Hyg b3:389, 1990

Other *Yersinia* infections

BUTLER T: *Yersinia* species (including plague), in *Principles and Practice of Infectious Diseases*, 3d ed, GL Mandell et al (eds). New York, Wiley, 1990, pp 1748–1756

MILLER VL, et al: Nucleotide sequence of the *Yersinia enterocolitica ail* gene and characterization of the Ail protein product. J Bacteriol 172:1062, 1990

COVER TL, ABER RC: *Yersinia enterocolitica*. N Engl J Med 321:16, 1989

TACKET CO et al: *Yersinia enterocolitica* pharyngitis. Ann Intern Med 99:40, 1983

TERTTI R et al: An outbreak of *Yersinia pseudotuberculosis* infection. J Infect Dis 149:245, 1984

124   BARTONELLOSIS AND BACILLARY ANGIOMATOSIS

LUCY STUART TOMPKINS

BARTONELLOSIS

DEFINITION   Bartonellosis consists of two clinical manifestations produced by infection with *Bartonella bacilliformis*, a member of the rickettsia group closely related to *Rochalimaea quintana* and *R. henselae*, the bacterial agent of bacillary angiomatosis. The disease occurs almost exclusively in the Andes Mountains of Peru, Ecuador, and Colombia. Initial infection in nonimmune persons produces Oroya fever, characterized by fever, profound anemia, and a high mortality rate; lesions called *verruga peruana* develop during the convalescent phase or during chronic infection. Daniel Carrion, a Peruvian medical student, inoculated himself with blood from a patient with verruga peruana and subsequently died from Oroya fever, thus proving that both diseases are caused by a single agent. As a result, bartonellosis is also known as *Carrion's disease*.

Carrion's disease is rarely seen outside South America because of the geographic localization of the arthropod vector. However, the disorder is similar in many ways to two disorders that do occur in the United States—cutaneous bacillary angiomatosis and the angiogenic response engendered by *Rochalimaea* species.

CLINICAL MANIFESTATIONS   Oroya fever occurs following the bite of the sandfly vector, *Phlebotomus*, an insect found in the river valleys of the Andes Mountains at altitudes from 600 to 2500 m. The disease has rarely been described in the United States. Onset of symptoms may be either insidious or abrupt after an incubation period of approximately 3 weeks. In the subacute presentation, low-grade fever, malaise, headache, and anorexia may be present. Sudden-onset disease characterized by high fever, chills, diaphoresis, headaches, and changes in mental status is followed by the sudden development of profound anemia due to a marked decrease in numbers of erythrocytes associated with macrocytic changes in poikilocytosis, Howell-Jolly bodies, nucleated erythrocytes, and immature myeloid cells. The leukocyte differential usually shifts to the left, although the total count may be normal. The erythrocyte count may fall to extremely low levels. Numerous microorganisms can be seen adhering to most erythrocytes in eosin/thiazine-stained peripheral blood smears.

During the acute phase, muscle and joint pain and headache may be severe; central nervous system changes also occur, including insomnia, delerium, and decreased level of consciousness. Thrombocytopenic purpura may develop. If the patient survives, a convalescent phase ensues characterized by the sudden disappearance of bacteria from blood smears, declining fever, and increase in erythrocyte count. While much of the mortality is due to profound anemia and toxicity, bacterial secondary infections, including salmonellosis and other enteric infections, malaria, and tuberculosis, often contribute substantially.

After convalescence from acute Oroya fever, verrugas may develop. The red or purple cutaneous lesions may be tiny and sessile or large, pedunculated, and nodular. They bear a marked resemblance to the lesions in bacillary angiomatosis. Both types of cutaneous lesion may resemble Kaposi's sarcoma.

PATHOLOGY During initial infection in the nonimmune host, *B. bacilliformis* cells adhere to erythrocytes and produce indentations in the cell membrane, with subsequent intracellular entry and persistent deformation of the cellular cytoskeleton. The parasitized erythrocytes are phagocytosed and destroyed. Although the life span of infected erythrocytes is markedly decreased, not all of this change can be attributed to the mechanical fragility induced by internalization, and decreased bone marrow erythropoiesis also contributes to the anemia. Bacteria can be cultured in vitro from the blood during acute infection. The hallmark of verruga peruana is the formation of new blood vessels (angiogenesis) at the sites of bacterial replication.

TREATMENT Oroya fever responds to a variety of antimicrobial agents, including chloramphenicol, tetracyclines, penicillin, and streptomycin. Chloramphenicol is most often used because of its efficacy against most *Salmonella* infections, which may occur intercurrently. Verruga peruana may respond similarly; failure of response or relapse is common.

BACILLARY ANGIOMATOSIS

DEFINITION Bacillary angiomatosis was initially described as an infectious complication of human immunodeficiency virus (HIV) diseases that causes cutaneous lesions resembling Kaposi's sarcoma. The infectious microorganism *Rochalimaea henselae* causes three clinical syndromes: chronic bacteremia, bacillary peliosis hepatis, and cutaneous or disseminated bacillary angiomatosis. Immunocompromised individuals, especially those with HIV infection or those with AIDS, are at particularly high risk of infection; rarely, patients are not obviously immunosuppressed. A recent study has shown that *Rochalimaea quintana*, the agent of trench fever, can also cause bacillary angiomatosis in HIV-positive patients. Several recently described studies have implicated *R. henselae* as a cause of typical cat scratch disease (CSD) in immunocompetent individuals.

CLINICAL MANIFESTATIONS The skin lesions of bacillary angiomatosis (also called *epithelioid angiomatosis*) are vascular nodules, papules, or tumors of variable size, ranging from tiny lesions resembling cherry angiomas or pyogenic granulomas to large, pedunculated, exophytic masses (Fig. 124-1). Characteristically, the lesions are red or purple, resembling Kaposi's sarcoma; they may be surrounded by an epithelial collarette, may be located anywhere on the skin, and also may involve mucous membranes. The overlying epidermis may be focally ulcerated, and underlying bone may be invaded and destroyed.

Dissemination of *R. henselae* infection occurs primarily in patients with cellular immune defects. The liver, spleen, bone marrow, and lymph nodes are primarily affected. In addition, HIV-infected patients may develop CNS abnormalities (including psychiatric disorders and brain lesions) responsive to antibiotic therapy. Skin lesions are usually not present in patients with disseminated infection. Involvement of

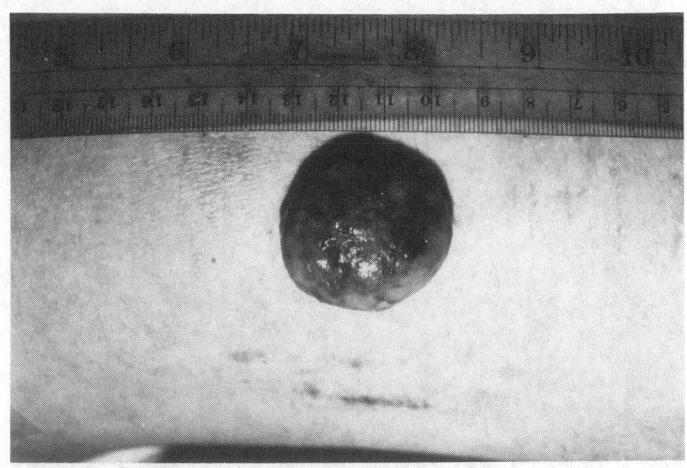

FIGURE 124-1 Characteristic skin lesion of bacillary angiomatosis in an HIV-positive young woman. This large, pedunculated tumor exhibits the typical angiomatous appearance. The patient was treated with oral erythromycin, with nearly complete resolution of the lesion; however, upon discontinuation of antibiotic therapy after a 4-week course, the lesion recurred.

the liver or spleen may produce bacillary peliosis hepatis. Clinical manifestations accompanying dissemination are often nonspecific and include persistent fever, abdominal pain, weight loss, and malaise. Patients with peliosis hepatis may have localized pain on palpation of the abdomen. Nodular lesions of variable size can be demonstrated by CT scan or MRI, with or without contrast agents.

Koehler and colleagues described three cases of bacillary angiomatosis caused by *R. quintana* in patients with HIV infection.

Infection also may present as prolonged fever and bacteremia in the absence of cutaneous lesions. Two patients reportedly developed chronic bacteremia following tick bites. Although symptoms generally abate after appropriate antibiotic therapy, relapse and recrudescence may occur. This clinical picture is quite similar to trench fever, a febrile illness initially described during World War I, which is caused by *R. quintana* transmitted by the human body louse.

Recent serologic studies demonstrated that most patients with typical CSD had antibodies which specifically reacted with *R. henselae*. Furthermore, *R. henselae* has been isolated from lymph nodes of patients with CSD. Therefore, the role of *Afipia felis*, the putative agent of CSD, is presently uncertain.

DIFFERENTIAL DIAGNOSIS The differential diagnosis of cutaneous lesions includes Kaposi's sarcoma, angiomas, and pyogenic granulomas. These can be distinguished by histopathologic examination of biopsied material. Cases of persistent fever following an insect bite must be differentiated from trench fever and other rickettsial infections by identification of bacteria from blood cultures and by negative results of appropriate serologic tests for rickettsial species.

MICROBIOLOGY The etiologic microorganisms can be demonstrated in tissue by Warthin-Starry silver stain and morphologically resemble *Apifia felis*, the agent of CSD. Clumps and clusters of small pleomorphic bacilli appear as purple deposits in tissue stained with hematoxylin and eosin. The nature of the bacilli was first recognized by Relman and colleagues, who used molecular techniques to analyze DNA extracted from tissue samples. The bacteria also have been isolated from blood and from other sites. Bacterial colonies develop after prolonged incubation; bacterial cells are gram-negative. Taxonomic studies have revealed that *R. henselae* is closely related to *R. quintana*, the agent of trench fever, and also to *B. bacilliformis*; it is less closely related to *A. felis* which was isolated from patients with CSD. Unlike other rickettsiae, *R. henselae* is not an obligate intracellular parasite and does not appear inside endothelial cells.

EPIDEMIOLOGY Most infections of bacillary angiomatosis occur in patients with HIV disease or other types of immunosuppression; thus an immune deficiency of T cells is implicated. Cutaneous

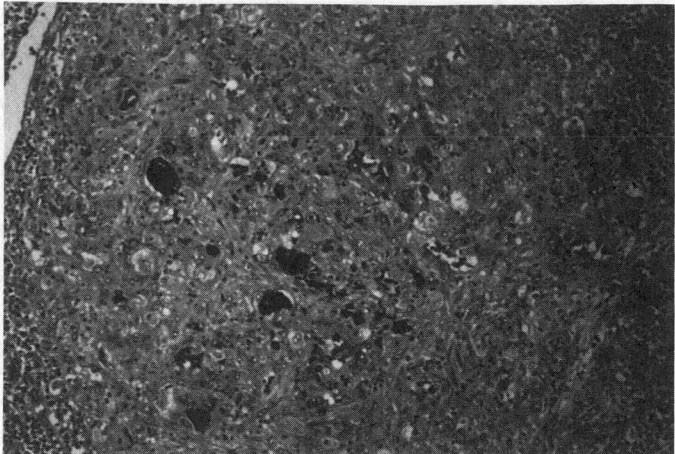

FIGURE 124-2 Histopathologic appearance of bacillary angiomatosis involving the skin. Characteristic features include nodules composed of epithelioid endothelial cells forming irregular, poorly formed vascular channels and large amounts of collagen. An neutrophilic inflammatory response is also present. Bacillary bacterial forms can be seen upon Warthin-Starry staining (hematoxylin and eosin; original magnification ×200).

infections occur primarily in urban areas of the United States in which HIV infection is most prevalent. However, tick-associated cases have been reported in Oklahoma. The prevalence of specific antibodies among healthy individuals is not established. Because of the tick-associated cases and the close taxonomic relationship of *R. henselae* to *R. quintana* and *Bartonella*, both of which are transmitted by insects, an insect vector has been postulated. Exposure to cats is a risk factor for bacillary angiomatosis and CSD.

PATHOGENESIS AND PATHOLOGY   Bacillary angiomatosis is characterized by a lobular proliferation of new blood vessels (angiogenesis) and a neutrophilic inflammatory response to myriad bacilli located within collagen-rich microscopic and macroscopic nodules (Fig. 124-2). The endothelial cells lining the vascular spaces have a typical epithelioid appearance, and the lesions may resemble Kaposi's sarcoma histopathologically, although the characteristic spindle cell of the latter disease is usually absent. Of note is the striking similarity between bacillary angiomatosis and verruga peruana. The bacterial and eucaryotic host factors that elicit the pathologic response are unknown. The pathologic response of immunocompetent patients with CSD consists of granulomas and microabscesses in lymph nodes draining the site of inoculation. Angiogenesis is not seen in CSD in otherwise healthy individuals.

TREATMENT   Cutaneous lesions have been treated with a wide variety of antimicrobial drugs, including macrolides and tetracyclines, and *R. henselae* is susceptible to most antibiotics in vitro. Erythromycin given orally over a 3-week course is usually efficacious; however, relapse may require prolonged therapy. Patients with peliosis hepatis should be treated with intravenous antibiotics, and those with disseminated disease or bacteremia should be treated with a prolonged course of oral antibiotics, such as macrolides, cephalosporins, or norfloxacin. Relapses may require prolonged treatment with antibiotics that reach an intracellular compartment, such as macrolides or floxacins. Cutaneous lesions may regress spontaneously, an event perhaps reflecting the status of the host's immunity.

REFERENCES

ARIAS-STELLA J et al: Histology, immunohistochemistry, and ultrastructure of the verruga in Carrion's disease. Am J Surg Pathol 10:595, 1986

BENSON LA et al: Entry of *Bartonella bacilliformis* into erythrocytes. Infect Immun 54:347, 1986

COCKERELL CJ, LEBOIT PE: Bacillary angiomatosis: A newly characterized, pseudoneoplastic, infectious, cutaneous vascular disorder. J Am Acad Dermatol 22:501, 1990

—— et al: Epithelioid angiomatosis: A distinct vascular disorder in patients with the acquired immunodeficiency syndrome of AIDS-related complex. Lancet 2:654, 1987

KEMPER CA et al: Visceral bacillary epithelioid angiomatosis: Possible manifestations of disseminated cat scratch disease in the immunocompromised host: A report of two cases. Am J Med 89:449, 1990

KOEHLER JE et al: Isolation of *Rochalimaea* species from cutaneous and osseous lesions of bacillary angiomatosis. New Engl J Med 327:1625, 1992

LEBOIT PE et al: Bacillary angiomatosis: The histopathology and differential diagnosis of pseudoneoplastic infection in patients with human immunodeficiency virus disease. Am J Surg Pathol 13:909, 1989

LUCEY D et al: Relapsing illness due to *Rochalimaea henselae* in immunocompetent hosts: Implication for therapy and new epidemiological associations. Clin Infect Dis 14:683, 1992

O'CONNOR SP et al: 16S rRNA sequences of *Bartonella bacilliformis* and cat scratch disease bacillus reveal phylogenetic relationships with the alpha-2 subgroup of the class *Proteobacteria*. J Clin Microbiol 29:2144, 1991

PERKOCHA LA et al: Clinical and pathological features of bacillary peliosis hepatis in association with human immunodeficiency virus infection. N Engl J Med 323:1581, 1990

REGNERY RL et al: Characterization of a novel *Rochalimaea* species, *R. henselae* sp. nov., isolated from blood of a febrile, human immunodeficiency virus-positive patient. J Clin Microbiol 30:265, 1992

—— et al: Serological response to "*Rochalimaea henselae*" antigen in suspected cat-scratch disease. Lancet 339:1443–45, 1992

RELMAN DA et al: The organism causing bacillary angiomatosis, peliosis hepatis, and fever and bacteremia in immunocompromised patients. N Engl J Med 324:1514, 1991

—— et al: The agent of bacillary angiomatosis: An approach to the identification of uncultured pathogens. N Engl J Med 323:1573, 1990

RICKETTS WE: Clinical manifestations of Carrion's disease. Arch Intern Med 84:751, 1949

SLATER LN et al: A newly recognized fastidious gram-negative pathogen as a cause of fever and bacteremia. N Engl J Med 323:1587, 1990

125   DONOVANOSIS (GRANULOMA INGUINALE)

KING K. HOLMES

DEFINITION   Donovanosis (granuloma inguinale) is a mildly contagious, chronic, indolent, progressive, autoinoculable, ulcerative disease involving the skin and lymphatics of the genital or perianal areas. The disease appears to be sexually transmitted and is associated with the presence in affected tissues of an intracellular microorganism, identified morphologically as the Donovan body.

ETIOLOGY   Donovanosis was described by McLeod in India in 1882, and in 1905 Donovan described the intracellular bodies which are thought to cause the disease. During the 1940s, encapsulated bacteria resembling Donovan bodies were recovered from pseudo-buboes of granuloma inguinale by inoculation of chick embryo yolk sacs or yolk-agar medium. These bacteria, which are known as *Calymmatobacterium granulomatis,* measure 1.5 by 0.7 μm. Such isolates are no longer available, *C. granulomatis* has not been cultivable in recent years, and the organism has not yet been characterized. Electron microscopic studies of Donovan bodies show their morphologic resemblance to gram-negative bacteria.

EPIDEMIOLOGY   Donovanosis is endemic in the tropics, particularly in Papua, New Guinea, southern India, and southern Africa. In the United States, the disease is rare. In reported cases, the sex ratio of males to females is nearly 10:1. The disease is uncommon in Caucasians. The frequency of donovanosis in sexual partners of chronically infected patients is highly variable, ranging from 1 to over 50 percent. Evidence for sexual transmission includes the age-specific incidence, which corresponds to that of other sexually transmitted diseases, the frequent concomitant presence of syphilis, the predilection for genital involvement in heterosexuals and for anorectal infection in homosexually active men, and the fact that outbreaks of clusters of cases of donovanosis have been traced to sexual exposure to a single-source contact. A significant association of HIV infection with donovanosis has been found among men in Durban, South Africa.

CLINICAL MANIFESTATIONS The incubation period ranges from 8 days to 12 weeks, but most lesions appear within 30 days after sexual exposure.

Donovanosis begins as a papule that ulcerates and develops into a painless elevated zone of clean, beefy-red, friable granulation tissue. The edges are irregular and spread by continuity or by autoinoculation of approximated skin surfaces. Secondary anaerobic infection may produce pain and a foul-smelling exudate. Less common complications of the disease include deep ulcerations, chronic cicatricial lesions, phimosis, lymphedema, and exuberant epithelial proliferation which grossly resembles carcinoma. In men, the lesions are usually located on the glans, prepuce, or shaft of the penis or the perianal area, while infection of the labia is most common in women. Lesions in women often arise at the fourchette and progress anteriorly in a V shape along the vulva. Extragenital lesions may occur, involving the face, neck, mouth, and other sites. The chronicity of the disease is of diagnostic importance, since several months often elapse before patients seek treatment. Extension to the inguinal region by autoinoculation, by continuity, or via the lymphatics results in a diffuse intradermal and subcutaneous swelling or suppuration known as a *pseudobubo* because involvement of the underlying lymph nodes is minimal. Locally destructive lesions and secondary infection may produce severe morbidity or death. Fatal disseminated disease, involving the bones, joints, or liver, has been reported. Disseminated infection apparently occurs more frequently during pregnancy. The relationship of donovanosis to subsequent carcinoma of the genitalia is uncertain.

DIAGNOSIS Early donovanosis may be mistaken for the primary chancre or condyloma latum of syphilis. Epithelial proliferation resembling carcinoma in the genital or perianal region in a young individual should always raise the suspicion of donovanosis if unnecessary destructive surgery is to be avoided. Chronic ulcerative or cicatricial changes may resemble lymphogranuloma venereum.

Amebiasis can produce penile lesions resembling donovanosis. In the United States, *Haemophilis ducreyi* frequently has been isolated from lesions resembling donovanosis, which have been termed *pseudo-granuloma inguinale–chancroid*. Histologic studies in donovanosis reveal marked acanthosis and pseudoepitheliomatous hyperplasia. The dermis contains an inflammatory infiltrate consisting mainly of plasma cells and histiocytes. Because Donovan bodies are seldom detectable in sections stained with hematoxylin and eosin, these changes may lead to an erroneous diagnosis of carcinoma and to unnecessary destructive surgery. Although silver impregnation techniques are useful for demonstration of Donovan bodies in sections, the diagnosis is best made by examination of impression smears prepared from specimens obtained by punch biopsy of granulation tissue from the periphery of a lesion; the deep portion of the specimen is removed, crushed between two slides which are air-dried and fixed in methanol, and stained with Wright-Giemsa stain. With this method, Donovan bodies appear as very rounded coccobacilli, 1 by 2 μm in size, which lie within cystic spaces in the cytoplasm of large mononuclear cells. The capsule stains as a dense acidophilic zone surrounding the bacterium, which resembles a closed safety pin because of bipolar condensation of chromatin. The pathognomonic mononuclear cell is 25 to 90 μm in diameter and has many cystic areas containing Donovan bodies. Donovan bodies also have been identified in histiocytes in cervical Papanicolaou smears.

Perianal donovanosis may resemble condylomata lata of secondary syphilis. Other venereal diseases, particularly syphilis, frequently coexist with donovanosis. Repeated negative dark-field examinations of lesions and negative serologic tests will exclude syphilis but should not be rigidly required while treatment is withheld from potentially noncompliant patients. In countries where donovanosis is endemic, the persistence of suspected condylomata lata after appropriate penicillin therapy for syphilis is highly suggestive of donovanosis.

TREATMENT The antimicrobials currently effective in the treatment of donovanosis in various parts of the world include trimethoprim-sulfamethoxazole, tetracycline, erythromycin, newer quinolones, gentamicin, and chloramphenicol or the related drug thiamphenicol (not available in the United States). Streptomycin, once commonly used for this condition, is not widely used today. Ampicillin is not recommended for donovanosis. Unfortunately, no comparative trials have been conducted with the currently used antimicrobials, and in vitro susceptibility testing is not possible. The minimum duration of treatment is not well established, and it is common protocol to continue therapy until lesions have completely healed over. Thus treatment for large lesions is generally more prolonged. Healing of small lesions is usually apparent within 3 weeks, as the lesions become pale and flatter and peripheral reepithelialization begins. Lack of objective clinical response within 7 days should lead to reassessment of the diagnosis and therapy. Donovan bodies disappear from lesions within a few days after onset of therapy. Typical dosages of the commonly used drugs include tetracycline or erythromycin, 500 mg four times daily, or trimethoprim-sulfamethoxazole (trimethoprim 160 mg, sulfamethoxazole 800 mg) twice daily.

REFERENCES

FREINKEL AL et al: A serologic test for granuloma inguinale. Genitourin Med 68:269, 1992

KRAUS SJ et al: Pseudogranuloma inguinale caused by *Haemophilus ducreyi*. Arch Dermatol 118:494, 1982

KUBERSKI T: Granuloma inguinale (donovanosis). Sex Transm Dis 7:29, 1980

O'FARRELL N: Clinico-epidemiological study of donovanosis in Durban, South Africa. Genitourin Med 69:108

———— et al: A rapid stain for the diagnosis of granuloma inguinale. Genitourin Med 66:200, 1990

———— et al: HIV-1 infection among heterosexual attendees of a sexually transmitted disease clinic in Durban. S Afr Med J 80:17, 1991

RICHENS J: The diagnosis and treatment of donovanosis (granuloma inguinale). Genitourin Med 67:441, 1991

ROSEN T et al: Granuloma inguinale. J Am Acad Dermatol 11:433, 1984

SCHNEIDER J et al: Extragenital donovanosis: Three cases from Western Australia. Genitourin Med 62:196, 1966

section 7 Miscellaneous bacterial infections

126 NOCARDIOSIS

GREGORY A. FILICE

DEFINITION *Nocardia* species are aerobic actinomycetes associated with several characteristic syndromes. Pneumonia and disseminated disease, both thought to follow inhalation of fragmented bacterial mycelia, are most common. Three syndromes follow transcutaneous inoculation: cellulitis, a lymphocutaneous syndrome, and mycetoma. Keratitis occurs after inoculation into the eye, usually after corneal trauma.

MICROBIOLOGY *Nocardia* species are common inhabitants of soil, where they contribute to decay of organic matter. Only three species are well-documented human pathogens, *N. asteroides*, *N. brasiliensis*, and *N. otitidiscaviarum* (formerly *N. caviae*). *N. farcinica* and *N. nova* are species of uncertain or controversial pathogenic status that have been isolated from humans. *N. transvalensis* has been reported in association with disseminated infection in three patients with host defense defects and has been isolated from a few cases of mycetoma.

EPIDEMIOLOGY Nocardiosis occurs throughout the world, and approximately 1000 cases of infection are diagnosed annually in the United States, 85 percent of them pulmonary and/or systemic. The disease is more common in adults and in males. Epidemics are rare, and person-to-person spread has not been established.

The risk for pulmonary or disseminated disease is increased in people with deficient cell-mediated immunity, especially deficiency associated with lymphoma or transplantation. Nocardiosis has been reported in people with AIDS, although nocardiosis is not as common as some other opportunistic infections in this group (see Chap. 279). Nocardiosis also has been associated with pulmonary alveolar proteinosis, tuberculosis, and chronic granulomatous disease.

Nocardia species are among several aerobic actinomycetes associated with mycetoma (see below). Cases of mycetoma occur mainly in tropical and subtropical regions, especially Mexico, Central and South America, Africa, and India. The most important risk factor for mycetoma is frequent contact with soil or vegetable matter.

PATHOLOGY The characteristic histologic feature of pulmonary or systemic *Nocardia* infection is an abscess infiltrated extensively with neutrophils. Granulation tissue usually surrounds the lesions, but extensive fibrosis or encapsulation is uncommon. Nocardial mycetoma is characterized by suppurative inflammation with sinus tract formation. Mycetoma lesions and their drainage contain granules composed of dense masses of bacterial filaments.

CLINICAL MANIFESTATIONS **Pulmonary disease** Nocardial infection typically presents as a subacute pneumonia with symptoms developing over a few days to several weeks. Nocardiosis may occur in a more acute form in immunosuppressed patients. Cough is prominent and is often productive of small amounts of thick, purulent nonmalodorous sputum. Fever, anorexia, weight loss, and malaise are common. Dyspnea, pleuritic pain, and hemoptysis occur in some patients. Tracheitis and bronchitis are rare. Remissions and exacerbations over periods of several weeks are frequent.

Roentgenographic patterns of pulmonary nocardiosis are variable. Infiltrates or nodules of varying size and density are typical, occurring in any lobe. Cavitation is common, and empyema is present in one-third of cases.

Pulmonary nocardiosis may spread directly from the lungs to involve adjacent tissue, causing pericarditis, mediastinitis, and superior vena caval obstruction. Spread through the chest wall is rare.

Nocardia species are sometimes isolated from respiratory secretions of patients without apparent nocardial disease. Most of these patients have underlying pulmonary disease with abnormal chest roentgenograms. A positive sputum culture in the presence of symptoms and signs of pulmonary infection must be considered indicative of nocardial pneumonia. In the absence of clear evidence of pneumonia, the presence of nocardiae on Gram stain and the ability to isolate nocardiae in multiple cultures are factors suggesting an increased likelihood of nocardial disease. A positive sputum culture in an immunosuppressed patient usually reflects disease, not colonization.

Extrapulmonary dissemination In one-half of cases of pulmonary nocardiosis, disease appears in disseminated form outside the lungs. One-fifth of patients present only with disease outside the lungs, which is assumed to have spread hematogenously from an inapparent or healed pulmonary focus. The most commonly infected sites outside the lungs are brain, skin and supporting structures, kidneys, bone, and muscle, but dissemination to nearly every organ has occurred. Peritonitis and endocarditis have been reported. The typical manifestation of extrapulmonary dissemination is a subacute or chronic abscess. A minority of abscesses outside the lungs or central nervous system (CNS) form fistulas and discharge small amounts of pus.

The CNS is the most common location for disseminated disease. Usually there are one or more supratentorial brain abscesses, often multiloculated. The symptoms and signs are somewhat more indolent than those of other cases of bacterial brain abscess. Brain abscesses sometimes burrow into the ventricles or out into the subarachnoid space and result in meningitis. Occasional patients present with meningitis, but many of these are found to have brain abscesses by careful clinical evaluation or by imaging studies. The organism is not easily recovered from cerebrospinal fluid (CSF) even in cases with meningitis.

Transcutaneous inoculation Infection following transcutaneous inoculation usually occurs in patients with intact immune systems and takes one of three forms: cellulitis, lymphocutaneous syndrome, or mycetoma. In the United States, cellulitis is most common, followed by the lymphocutaneous syndrome, and finally by mycetoma.

Cellulitis usually begins 1 to 3 weeks after a recognized breach of the skin. Often, there has been obvious contamination of the wound with soil. A subacute cellulitis with pain, swelling, erythema, and warmth develops over a period of days to weeks. The lesions are usually firm and nonfluctuant. The process may progress to involve underlying muscle, tendon, bones, and joints. Dissemination is rare. In colder climates, most cases are associated with *N. asteroides;* in warmer climates, *N. brasiliensis* is more common.

In the lymphocutaneous form, there is typically a pyodermatous lesion at the site of inoculation with central ulceration and purulent or honey-colored drainage. Subcutaneous nodules may appear along lymphatics that drain the primary lesion. The lymphangitic form closely resembles lymphocutaneous sporotrichosis (see Chap. 169). Most cases of the lymphocutaneous syndrome are associated with *N. brasiliensis*.

Mycetoma usually begins with a nodular swelling, sometimes with a history of local trauma. Lesions typically occur on the feet or the hands but may involve the posterior part of the neck, the upper back, the head, and other locations. The nodule eventually forms one or more fistulas. The fistulas tend to come and go, with new ones forming as old ones disappear. The discharge is serous or purulent and may be bloody; it often contains 0.1- to 2-mm white granules which consist of masses of mycelia. The lesions spread slowly along fascial planes to involve adjacent areas of skin, subcutaneous tissue, and bone. Over a period of months to years, there may be extensive deformation of the affected part. Pain is minimal in lesions involving soft tissues but may be severe if lesions affect bones or joints. Systemic symptoms of fever and malaise are absent or minimal. Infection rarely disseminates from a mycetoma, and lesions on the hands and feet usually cause only local disability. Lesions on the head, neck, and trunk can invade locally to involve deep organs and result in severe disability or death.

Keratitis *Nocardia* species, usually *N. asteroides,* are uncommon causes of subacute keratitis. The infection usually follows eye trauma. Nocardial infection of lacrimal glands has been reported. Disease involving deeper eye structures is usually a manifestation of disseminated disease.

DIAGNOSIS The first step is examination of sputum or pus for crooked, branching, beaded, gram-positive filaments 1 μm in width and up to 50 μm in length. Most nocardiae are acid-fast in direct smears if a weak acid is used for decolorization, as with the modified Kinyoun, Ziehl-Neelsen, or Fite-Faraco methods. Nocardiae often take up silver stains. Nocardiae grow relatively slowly; colonies may take up to 2 weeks to appear and may not develop their characteristic appearance for up to 4 weeks. Growth is so different from more common pathogens that the laboratory should always be alerted when *Nocardia* is suspected so that the likelihood of recovering it is maximized. In difficult cases, paraffin baiting can be employed, since nocardiae are among the few aerobic microorganisms that can use paraffin as a carbon source.

When smears are negative, it is often necessary to pursue the diagnosis by more invasive procedures. For pulmonary cases, bronchoscopy, needle aspiration, and open lung biopsy are all effective. Transtracheal aspiration should be avoided because it frequently leads to nocardial cellulitis in tissues around the puncture wound.

All patients with nocardial pneumonia should be evaluated for disseminated disease with a careful history and physical examination. Suggestive symptoms or signs should be pursued with further diagnostic tests. Computed tomography or magnetic resonance imaging of the head with and without contrast material should be done if there are signs or symptoms suggesting brain involvement.

Biphasic culture bottles (liquid medium over agar) incubated aerobically for up to 30 days often yield nocardiae, but routine blood cultures are usually negative. If clinically indicated, specimens of CSF or urine should be concentrated and then cultured. In mycetoma cases, an effort should be made to find granules in the discharge. Suspect particles should be washed in saline, examined microscopically, and cultured.

Several presumptive diagnostic tests have been studied, including tests for antibodies and nocardial metabolites in serum or CSF. None is ready for clinical use at this time.

THERAPY Sulfonamides are the drugs of choice. Sulfadiazine or sulfisoxazole, 6 to 8 g/d in four divided doses, is commonly administered, but doses from 4 to 12 g/d have been given. In difficult cases, sulfonamide blood levels should be measured and dosages adjusted to keep serum levels between 100 and 150 μg/mL. The combination of sulfamethoxazole and trimethoprim has been associated with similar success with a modestly increased risk of hematologic toxicity. Trimethoprim, 5 to 20 mg/kg, and sulfamethoxazole, 25 to 100 mg/kg, should be given each day in two divided doses. Nocardiosis has been rare among transplant recipients receiving sulfamethoxazole and trimethoprim for prophylaxis against other infectious diseases,

which has suggested that the combination may prevent nocardiosis as well.

Minocycline is the best-established alternative orally administered drug and should be given in doses of 100 to 200 mg twice a day. There is little clinical evidence that other tetracyclines are reliably effective. Amoxicillin and clavulanic acid have been effective in some cases and would be a reasonable choice in patients who cannot be treated with sulfonamides or minocycline. Other orally administered antimicrobials have been used, but there is less experience with them. Chloramphenicol (1 g four times a day), cycloserine (250 mg three times a day), and ampicillin (1 g four times a day) have appeared effective in some cases, often used together with sulfonamides. Ampicillin and erythromycin (500 to 750 mg four times a day) may be effective when used together, but erythromycin alone is not usually effective.

Amikacin is the best-established parental drug, given in doses of 5 to 7.5 mg/kg every 12 h. Serum levels should be monitored with prolonged therapy, in the face of diminished renal function, or in the elderly. Limited experience with newer β-lactam antibiotics, including cefotaxime, ceftizoxime, and imipenem, suggests that they may be helpful alone or in combination with other antimicrobials.

Antimicrobial susceptibility testing of *Nocardia* species has not been developed to the point where clinical relevance is ensured, and ordinarily, choices of antimicrobials should be based on published clinical experience. In cases in which the usual antimicrobials fail or cannot be used, susceptibility testing may be used to guide the choice of alternative agents. Sulfonamides, most aminoglycosides, minocycline, fusidic acid, and some newly developed β-lactam antibiotics appear active against most strains. Sulbactam and clavulanic acid inactivate nocardial β-lactamases, but the potential clinical effectiveness of combinations including β-lactamase inhibitors is unknown.

In many cases, two or more antimicrobials have been used to treat nocardiosis, often in combinations including a sulfonamide or minocycline. Whether therapy with two or more agents is better than therapy with a single agent is not known, and therapy with multiple drugs increases the risk of toxicity.

Brain abscesses should be treated surgically if the diagnosis is unclear, if an abscess is large and accessible, or if an abscess fails to respond to chemotherapy. Aspiration, excision, and drainage are all effective. Small abscesses and abscesses in inaccessible or critical locations should be treated medically. In cases managed medically, results should be monitored with repeated imaging.

Antimicrobial therapy usually suffices for treatment of nocardial mycetoma. In deep or extensive cases, drainage or excision of heavily involved tissue may facilitate healing, but structure and function should be preserved whenever possible.

Immunosuppressive therapy should be continued if necessary for treatment of an underlying disease or to prevent rejection of a transplanted organ. In other cases, it seems prudent to reduce or eliminate immunosuppressive therapy.

Nocardial infections tend to relapse, and long courses of antimicrobial therapy are necessary. Nocardiosis is particularly tenacious and likely to relapse in people with chronic granulomatous disease. For nonimmunosuppressed patients, treatment of pulmonary or systemic nocardiosis outside the CNS should be continued for 6 to 12 months. Ordinarily, treatment of CNS nocardiosis should be continued for 1 year. If all apparent disease has been excised, the duration of therapy may be reduced to 6 months. For immunosuppressed patients, treatment of pulmonary or systemic nocardiosis should be continued for 1 year. If nocardial disease is unusually extensive, or if the response to therapy is slow, these recommendations should be exceeded.

Patients with cellulitis or the lymphocutaneous syndrome should be treated for 2 months if infection is limited to soft tissues and for 4 months if bone is involved. Unusually extensive cases or cases in immunosuppressed people should be treated longer, depending on degrees of involvement and of immunosuppression. Therapy of mycetoma should be continued for 6 to 12 months after clinical cure. Keratitis should be treated with oral and topical sulfonamides until the infection appears cured and then with oral sulfonamides alone for an additional 2 to 4 months.

The mortality for pulmonary or disseminated nocardiosis outside the CNS should be less than 5 percent. CNS disease increases the risk of death. Patients should be followed carefully for at least 6 months after therapy has ended. Any child with nocardiosis and no known cause of immunosuppression should have tests performed to determine the adequacy of the child's phagocytic respiratory burst.

REFERENCES

BERKEY P, BODEY GP: Nocardial infection in patients with neoplastic disease. Rev Infect Dis 11:407, 1989

BROSS JE, GORDON G: Nocardial meningitis: Case reports and review. Rev Infect Dis 13:160, 1991

JAVALY K et al: Nocardiosis in patients with human immunodeficiency virus infection: Report of 2 cases and review of the literature. Medicine 71:128, 1992

KIM J et al: Nocardial infection as a complication of AIDS: Report of six cases and review. Rev Infect Dis 13:624, 1991

PALMER DL et al: Diagnostic and therapeutic considerations in Nocardia asteroides infection. Medicine 53:391, 1974

PETERSON EA et al: Minocycline treatment of pulmonary nocardiosis. JAMA 250:930, 1983

SATTERWHITE TK, WALLACE RJ JR: Primary cutaneous nocardiosis. JAMA 242:333, 1979

TIGHT RR, BARTLETT MS: Actinomycetoma in the United States. Rev Infect Dis 3:1139, 1981

WALLACE RJ et al: Antimicrobial susceptibility patterns of Nocardia asteroides. Antimicrob Agents Chemother 32:1776, 1988

127   ACTINOMYCOSIS

PHILLIP I. LERNER

Actinomycosis is caused by filamentous, gram-positive bacteria that are part of the normal oral flora. In this chronic, suppurative, fibrosing infection, external sinuses often discharge tiny colonies of organisms that are referred to as *sulfur granules* because of their resemblance to elemental pharmaceutical sulfur particles. After oral commensals have invaded the face, neck, lungs, and/or ileocecal region, infection spreads to contiguous structures, unrestricted by normal tissue plane barriers. The indolent course resembling that of fungal infection, tuberculosis, or malignancy can confound early diagnosis. In fact, the diagnosis can be stubbornly elusive, often being made only after months or even years. Between three and four times as many men as women develop actinomycosis. Prolonged antibiotic therapy coupled with removal of foreign bodies and drainage of suppurative sites is usually necessary for its eradication.

AGENTS OF ACTINOMYCOSIS   Classic actinomycosis is caused most often by *Actinomyces israelii* (78 percent) but also can be attributed to other anaerobic and microaerophilic oral commensals, including *A. naeslundii*, *A. viscosus*, *A. odontolyticus*, *A. meyeri*, and *Propionibacterium* (formerly *Arachnia*) *propionica*. In the microbiology laboratory, all species of *Actinomyces* (except *A. viscosus*) and *Propionibacterium propionica* require extended anaerobic or microaerophilic (6% to 10% CO_2) incubation. The best attainable culture sensitivity is only 50 percent for samples of frank pus or tissue free of contamination from mucosal surfaces. Thus laboratory personnel must be alerted when actinomycosis is suspected. Pathologists must be diligent in sectioning and examining resected tissues for diagnostic granules. In early or acute infections, organisms may appear as separate gram-positive, branching filaments rather than the characteristic colonies or granules typical of advanced lesions. Fluorescein isothiocyanate species-specific conjugate antisera can identify all major *Actinomyces* species, *P. propionica*, and even mixed species in granules.

Actinomycotic lesions characteristically include "associates"— other members of the endogenous oral or gastrointestinal flora that cannot be separated from the actinomycetes in culture. These organisms usually are not considered in the selection of antibiotic therapy. *Actinobacillus actinomycetemcomitans*, *Haemophilus* species, fusobacteria, streptococci, micrococci, staphylococci, *Eikenella corrodens*, and oral *Bacteroides* species can be found in cervicofacial and thoracic actinomycosis, while coliforms and intestinal anaerobes are the associated microbes in abdominal actinomycosis. Although there is probably an essential synergy between the actinomycetes and these associates, this relationship is not understood.

PATHOGENESIS AND PATHOLOGY   The species of *Actinomyces* and *Propionibacterium* that cause actinomycosis are endogenous oral saprophytes of low virulence that dwell in periodontal pockets, carious teeth, dental plaque, and tonsillar crypts; they also can be isolated from the lower gastrointestinal and female genital tracts. Thus the growth of actinomycetes in cultures from these sites is nondiagnostic. After trauma, surgery, or another infection that alters the host's mucosal barriers, these organisms advance to invade surrounding tissues. The process is usually chronic and fibrosing, and the frequent absence of clinical findings associated with bacterial infections (e.g., fever, leukocytosis, and anemia) raises suspicions of a fungal or mycobacterial infection or a malignancy. Lesions may be indurated masses or soft and loculated. Sinus tracts extending from these lesions to skin, mucous membranes, or internal organs permit further spread of the infection, particularly in the abdomen and pelvis. The actinomycetes are only rarely opportunists in immunocompromised states such as leukemia, solid tumor malignancies, renal failure, and AIDS.

Histologic examination generally reveals pus surrounded by acute or chronic fibrosing granulation tissue, although fibrosis may not be evident in pulmonary infections or any early process. In advanced lesions, classic yellow, brown, or dull white granules may form in pockets of suppuration or collect on gauze dressings over draining sinuses. These so-called sulfur granules occur only in vivo and are actually mineralized bacterial filaments encased in calcium phosphate as a result of alkaline phosphatase activity in inflamed host tissues. While other infectious agents, including fungi, *Nocardia*, *Streptomyces*, and *Staphylococcus*, can form similar aggregates, only the granules of actinomycosis feature surface "clubs" visible by light microscopy. Granules (diameter, 1 to 2 mm) from pus or surgical dressings can be stained and crushed between microscope slides. Upon staining with 1% methylene blue at low magnification, the distinctive cauliflower-like granules become visible; Gram staining at high magnification reveals the thin (diameter ≤ 1 μm), branching, gram-positive filaments of the organisms. These granules may be sparse; careful examination of multiple histologic sections of abscess wall, sinus tract, or tumor masses is often required for the diagnosis of actinomycosis.

CLINICAL SYNDROMES   Cervicofacial actinomycosis   Between 50 and 96 percent of cases of human actinomycosis affect the head and neck region. The clinician should suspect actinomycosis when a patient has acute, subacute, or chronic phlegmon of the skin or soft tissue or swelling of the head and neck, especially if a draining sinus develops. A dental portal is usually implicated; infection is often preceded by a tooth extraction, and evidence of poor dental hygiene, tooth decay or abscess, or periodontal disease is frequently found. Even a simple molar eruption or nonpenetrating jaw trauma can interrupt mucosal integrity enough to precipitate infection.

Clinically, there are two patterns of cervicofacial actinomycosis. In the more indolent form, a painless, fluctuant, bluish or purplish lesion enlarges slowly, often where the facial artery and vein cross the lower border of the mandible. In this slowly evolving form, patients eventually develop trismus and oral or cutaneous fistulas. The second form, which is more acute and painfully suppurative, can occur anywhere in the head and neck; it involves the submandibular area, the angle of the mandible, and the parotid region particularly often. Isolated infection, with or without fistulas, can appear in the scalp, orbit, lacrimal glands, middle ear, mastoid, paranasal sinuses, thyroid, or trachea, with no clue as to the original site of oral mucosal entry. Infection spreads without regard for fascial tissue planes or lymphatic channels. In this acute, rapidly progressive form, subcutaneous abscesses and trismus develop, and impressive edema of involved tissues is often documented. The incidence of spontaneous abscess rupture in acute cervicofacial disease has decreased in the antibiotic era. An acute abscess, inflammatory nodule, or infiltrating mass resembling a tumor may involve the pharyngeal and laryngeal structures. If the infection reaches the bone, periostitis is followed by lytic destruction with surrounding hyperdensity.

Thoracic and disseminated actinomycosis Actinomycosis can involve the lungs, pleura, and mediastinal structures. Infection at these sites follows aspiration, direct extension from the neck or esophagus, or retroperitoneal spread from the abdomen. Antecedent chronic lung disease predisposes to pulmonary actinomycosis. Diagnosis can be extremely difficult: symptoms such as fever or cough are often minimal or absent, and the common use of empirical antibiotic therapy may limit spread to the lungs, preventing the appearance of a classic granule-discharging sinus in the chest wall.

Pulmonary actinomycosis is usually a debilitating illness resembling tuberculosis or carcinoma. Chest radiography may show a fibrocavitary process with a loss of volume, an alveolar process, or a mass compressing or invading a bronchus. Actinomycosis and tuberculosis can coexist. Since *Actinomyces* species can proliferate in necrotic tumors, a positive sputum culture alone is not diagnostic.

Radiographic features suggestive of thoracic actinomycosis include (1) lung lesions eroding the chest wall, (2) periostitis or lysis of ribs, sternum, or shoulder girdle adjacent to a chronic lung process, (3) pulmonary infiltrate crossing an interlobar fissure, and (4) vertebral destruction with sparing of the disk space and erosion of both the body and the processes of the affected vertebra and adjacent ribs. Mediastinal infection can obstruct the superior vena cava or provoke a transesophageal or systemic-to-pulmonary venous fistula. Fewer than 2 percent of cases of actinomycosis include pleuropulmonary involvement, and massive empyema is rare.

Disseminated actinomycosis generally occurs in conjunction with thoracic disease and is quite unusual. Vasculitic lesions in the skin, subcutaneous tissue, or muscle can harbor both actinomycetes and associated microorganisms. Concomitant pulmonary disease may assume a miliary pattern. Rarely occurring primary actinomycosis of the extremity is preceded by trauma—e.g., a human bite or fist fight (punch actinomycosis)—in 60 percent of cases.

Abdominal and pelvic actinomycosis Most abdominal actinomycotic infections are preceded by surgery, e.g., laparotomy for acute appendicitis, perforated diverticulum or ulcer, cholecystitis, perforating trauma, or another abdominal catastrophe. Rarely, nonpenetrating trauma initiates the process. Infection usually begins in the gastrointestinal tract and spreads to the peritoneal cavity and abdominal wall or extends paracecally to the subphrenic space or pouch of Douglas. Sinus tracts are common; true bowel fistulas are not. The interval between inoculation and diagnosis can be months or even years. Actinomycotic lesions may be mistaken for Crohn's disease, malignancy, tuberculosis, amebiasis, or chronic appendicitis.

Gastric actinomycosis follows perforation of or surgery for gastric ulcer and can itself mimic peptic ulcer disease or carcinoma. Hepatic involvement, seen in 15 percent of cases, occurs via the portal vein, by direct extension from contiguous viscera, or (rarely) via the hepatic artery during disseminated infection; in turn, hepatic infection can extend to the abdominal wall or diaphragm, adjacent viscera, or retroperitoneum. Hepatic involvement may appear as single or multiple hepatic lesions or as a miliary process.

Pelvic actinomycosis may originate in an anal crypt and spread posterolaterally to the gluteal region or extend to the anorectal region from elsewhere in the pelvis, causing recurrent draining sinuses, anal fistulas, and rectal fissures. Endometrial infection is uncommon unless it is introduced directly during abortion, from an intrauterine device (IUD), or through infected pessaries or retained surgical sutures. IUD-associated actinomycosis ranges from vaginal discharge to pelvic inflammatory disease with tuboovarian abscess, ureteral obstruction, or a "frozen pelvis" mimicking malignancy. *Actinomyces*-like organisms seen in Papanicolaou smears from IUD users neither signal pathology nor mandate IUD removal. Five percent of healthy women without IUDs also harbor *Actinomyces*-like organisms in the genital tract.

Actinomycosis of the central nervous system The CNS is involved in 10 percent of all cases of actinomycosis. Infections spreading hematogenously from the mouth, lungs, abdomen, or pelvis numerically exceed those extending from a cervicofacial primary site. CNS disease usually presents as a single, multiloculated hemispheric abscess; multiple lesions occur in 15 percent of cases. A primary focus for CNS actinomycosis may not exist. Meningeal involvement may produce only chronic lymphocytic meningitis. Infection can reach the vertebral canal via the intervertebral foramina from a cervicofacial, thoracic, or abdominal focus and cause epidural abscess and cord compression.

THERAPY Actinomycosis should be suspected when a recurrent pattern of exacerbation and remission of infection develops during empirical antibiotic therapy. Since the 1960s, the treatment of choice has been a prolonged course of high-dose intravenous benzylpenicillin coupled with appropriate surgical drainage, bony curettage, foreign body removal, debridement, or radical sinus tract excision. Occasionally, a complete response of acute disease (particularly early cervicofacial infection) to therapy with intravenous penicillin alone eliminates the need for surgery or allows better definition of fascial planes and renders subsequent surgery less extensive. Penicillin G (10 to 20 million units per day for 2 to 6 weeks), followed by oral penicillin V (e.g., phenoxymethyl penicillin, 2 to 4 g/d, to the limits of the patient's tolerance for 3 to 6 additional months), is an accepted regimen for most deep-seated infections. The likelihood of relapse diminishes with at least 2 to 4 months of therapy in early or mild cases and with 6 to 12 months of antibiotic treatment in severe or chronic actinomycosis. Erythromycin and clindamycin also can be used. Tetracyclines are as effective as penicillin G for cervicofacial disease. Metronidazole, oral cephalosporins, oral antistaphylococcal penicillins, and quinolone antibiotics should not be used.

In vivo acquisition of resistance by *Actinomyces* species, particularly that to penicillin G, is not a problem. When the response to therapy is poor or a relapse occurs, an undrained abscess or resistant bacterial associate should be sought. In general, the susceptibility of associated organisms is not considered when antibiotics are prescribed, but some investigators prefer ampicillin or amoxicillin initially because associated bacteria are less susceptible to penicillin G. Metronidazole or clindamycin may be added to the regimen when *Bacteroides* species (e.g., *B. fragilis*, *B. thetaiotamicron*) are isolated.

REFERENCES

BERARDI RS: Abdominal actinomycosis. Surg Gynecol Obstet 149:257, 1979

BENNHOFF DF: Actinomycosis: Diagnostic and therapeutic considerations. Laryngoscope 94:1198, 1984

BURDEN P: Actinomycosis. J Infect 19:95, 1989

LERNER PI: The lumpy jaw: Cervicofacial actinomycosis. Infect Dis Clin North Am 2:203, 1988

PEABODY JW, SEABURY JH: Actinomycosis and nocardiosis. Am J Med 28:99, 1960

RICHTSMEIER WJ, JOHNS ME: Actinomycosis of the head and neck. CRC Crit Rev Clin Lab Sci 11:175, 1979

SCHAAL KP: The genera *Actinomyces, Arcanobacterium*, and *Rothia*, in *Prokaryotes 2*, A Balows et al (eds). New York, Springer-Verlag, 1992, chap 38

SMEGO RA JR: Actinomycosis of the central nervous system. Rev Infect Dis 9:855, 1987

128   INFECTIONS DUE TO MIXED ANAEROBIC ORGANISMS

DENNIS L. KASPER

DEFINITIONS   *Anaerobic* bacteria are organisms that require reduced oxygen tension for growth, failing to grow on the surface of solid media in 10% CO_2 in air. *Microaerophilic* bacteria can grow in 10% CO_2 in air or under anaerobic or aerobic conditions. *Facultative* bacteria can grow in the presence or absence of air. This chapter describes infections caused by nonsporulating anaerobic bacteria. In general, anaerobes associated with human infections are relatively aerotolerant. They can survive for as long as 72 h in the presence of oxygen, although generally they will not multiply in this environment. Many fewer pathogenic anaerobic bacteria, which are also part of the normal flora, die after brief contact with oxygen, even in low concentrations.

The nonsporulating anaerobic bacteria exist as normal flora on the mucosal surfaces of humans and animals. The major reservoirs of these bacteria are the mouth, gastrointestinal tract, skin, and the female genital tract. Of the oral flora, anaerobes are the predominant commensal organisms, ranging in concentrations from 10^9 per milliliter in saliva to 10^{12} in gingival scrapings. In the oral cavity the relative concentration of anaerobic to aerobic bacteria ranges from 1:1 on the surface of a tooth to 1000:1 in the gingival crevice. Anaerobic bacteria are not found in appreciable numbers in the normal intestine until the distal ileum. In the colon, the proportion of anaerobes increases significantly, as does the overall bacterial count. For example, in the colon there are 10^{11} to 10^{12} organisms per gram of stool, with a ratio of anaerobes to aerobes of approximately 1000:1. In the female genital tract there are approximately 10^9 organisms per milliliter of secretions, with a ratio of anaerobes to aerobes of approximately 10:1. Hundreds of species of anaerobic bacteria have been identified as part of the normal flora of humans. Identification of as many as 500 different anaerobic species in fecal specimens reflects the diversity of the anaerobic flora. Despite the complex array of bacteria which exist in the normal flora, relatively few species are isolated commonly from human infection.

Anaerobic infections occur when the harmonious relationship between the host and bacteria is disrupted. Any site in the body is susceptible to infection with these indigenous organisms when a mucosal barrier or the skin is compromised by surgery, trauma, tumor, or ischemia or necrosis, which reduces local tissue redox potentials. Because the sites that are colonized by anaerobic bacteria contain many species of bacteria, disruption of anatomic barriers allows penetration of many organisms, resulting in mixed infections involving multiple species of anaerobes combined with facultative or microaerophilic organisms. Such mixed infections are seen in the head and neck (chronic sinusitis, chronic otitis media, Ludwig's angina, and periodontal abscesses). Brain abscesses and subdural empyema are the most frequent anaerobic infections of the central nervous system. Anaerobes are responsible for pleuropulmonary diseases such as aspiration pneumonia, necrotizing pneumonia, lung abscesses, and empyema. Anaerobes play an important role in various intraabdominal infections such as peritonitis and intraabdominal and liver abscesses (see Chap. 86). They are isolated frequently in female genital tract infections such as salpingitis, pelvic peritonitis, tuboovarian abscess, vulvovaginal abscesses, septic abortions, and endometritis (see Chaps. 88 and 89). Anaerobic bacteria also are frequently found in infections of the skin, soft tissue, and bones and in bacteremia.

ETIOLOGY   The major anaerobic gram-positive cocci producing disease are *Peptostreptococcus* species. The major species involved in infections are *P. magnus*, *P. asaccharolyticus*, *P. anaerobius*, and *P. prevotii*. Clostridia are gram-positive rods which are isolated from

wounds, abscesses, abdominal infections, and bacteremias; they are discussed in Chap. 108. The principal anaerobic gram-negative bacilli are the *Bacteroides* "family," which includes the *Bacteroides fragilis* group, fusobacteria, *Prevotella*, and *Porphyromonas*. The *B. fragilis* group contains the anaerobic pathogens most frequently isolated from clinical infections. Members of this group are part of the normal bowel flora. The group comprises several distinct species, including *B. fragilis*, *B. thetaiotaomicron*, *B. distasonis*, *B. vulgatus*, *B. uniformis*, and *B. ovatus*. Of this group, *B. fragilis* is the most important clinical isolate. However, in the normal fecal flora, the frequency with which *B. fragilis* is isolated is low compared with other *Bacteroides* species. A second major group of phenotypically similar organisms is part of the indigenous oral flora. These are primarily pigment-producing bacteria which were previously classified under the species *B. melaninogenicus*, now known as *Prevatella melaninogenica*. The terminology of this group has changed so that several distinct species are recognized, including *Porphyromonas gingivalis*, *Porphyromonas asaccharolyticus*, and *P. melaninogenica*. In female genital tract infections, *Prevotella bivius* and *Prevotella disiens* are the most frequent isolates, although *B. fragilis* is not uncommon. Fusobacteria are also isolated from clinical infections, including necrotizing pneumonia and abscesses.

Infections due to anaerobic bacteria most frequently are mixed infections with more than one organism. They may be due to one or several anaerobic species or a combination of anaerobic organisms and aerobic bacteria acting synergistically.

APPROACH TO THE PATIENT WITH ANAEROBIC BACTERIAL INFECTIONS   There are several features to remember when approaching the patient with presumptive infection due to anaerobic bacteria. (1) Most of these organisms are harmless commensals, and very few cause disease. (2) In order for these organisms to cause infection, they must spread beyond the normal mucosal barriers. (3) Conditions favoring the propagation of these bacteria, particularly a lowered oxidation-reduction potential, are necessary. These include sites of trauma, tissue destruction, compromised vascular supply, or complication of preexisting infection that produces necrosis. (4) There is a complex array of infecting flora. For example, as many as 12 different types of organisms can be isolated from a suppurative site. (5) Anaerobic organisms tend to be found in abscess cavities or in necrotic tissue. The detection of an abscess in a patient which fails to yield organisms on routine culture is the clue that the abscess is likely to contain anaerobic bacteria. Often smears of this "sterile pus" are teeming with bacteria on Gram's stain. The malodorous nature of the pus should suggest anaerobic infections. Although some facultative organisms, such as *Staphylococcus aureus*, also are capable of causing abscesses, abscesses in organs or within deeper body tissues should call to mind anaerobic infection. (6) Treatment need not be directed at all the organisms in the infectious site. However, some species in particular require specific therapy. The best example of this principle is the need to treat the *B. fragilis* group. Many of these synergistic infections can be cured with antibiotics directed at some, but not all, of the organisms. Antibiotic therapy, combined with drainage, disrupts the interdependent relationship among the bacteria, and species which are resistant to the antibiotic do not survive without the coinfective organisms. (7) Manifestations of disseminated intravascular coagulation are unusual in patients with anaerobic infection.

EPIDEMIOLOGY   Difficulties in obtaining appropriate cultures, contamination of cultures by aerobic bacteria or normal flora, and the lack of readily available reliable culture techniques have made accurate incidence or prevalence data on anaerobic infections unavailable. However, these infections are encountered frequently in hospitals with active surgical, trauma, and obstetric and gynecologic services. In some centers, anaerobic bacteria, particularly *B. fragilis*, account for approximately 8 to 10 percent of positive blood cultures.

PATHOGENESIS   Anaerobic bacterial infections usually occur when an anatomic barrier becomes disrupted and the local flora enter a site which was previously sterile. The bacteria which are isolated from infected sites have survived changes in oxidation-reduction potential and exposure to host defenses. Because of the specific growth requirements of anaerobic organisms and their presence as commensals on mucosal surfaces, conditions must arise which allow these organisms to penetrate mucosal barriers and enter tissue with a lowered oxidation-reduction potential. Therefore, tissue ischemia, trauma, surgery, perforated viscus, shock, or aspiration provide environments conducive to the proliferation of anaerobes. Some highly fastidious anaerobes lack the enzyme superoxide dismutase (SOD) that in other organisms reduces toxic superoxide radicals, thereby lessening the potentially lethal effects of superoxide. In the case of a perforated viscus, hundreds of species of anaerobic bacteria are spilled into the peritoneal cavity, but many of these organisms are unable to survive because the highly vascularized tissue provides an adequate oxygen supply. The entry of oxygen into the environment results in selection of aerotolerant organisms.

The ability of an organism to adhere to host tissues is important to the establishment of infection. Some oral species adhere to crevicular epithelium in the oral cavity. *P. melaninogenica* actually attach to other microorganisms. *P. gingivalis* is a common isolate in periodontal disease. These organisms have been shown to have fimbriae which facilitate attachment. Some unencapsulated *Bacteroides* strains appear to be piliated, which may account for their ability to adhere.

The most extensively studied virulence factor of the nonsporulating anaerobes is the polysaccharide capsule of *B. fragilis*. These polysaccharides possess distinct biologic properties such as the ability to promote abscess formation in a rodent model of intraabdominal sepsis. Abscess induction is a T cell–dependent phenomenon requiring CD4+, CD8+ T cells. Immunization with the capsule confers protection against abscess induction following challenge with whole *B. fragilis* and is mediated by a non-major histocompatibility complex–restricted T cell circuit. Although some clinicians have viewed abscess formation as a protective host response to localize and contain infecting bacteria, abscess formation in patients with sepsis often results in severe and chronic illness that requires surgical drainage in combination with extensive antimicrobial therapy.

Anaerobic bacteria produce a number of exoenzymes which are capable of enhancing their virulence. These enzymes include a heparinase elaborated by *B. fragilis* which may contribute to intravascular clotting and lead to a requirement for increased doses of heparin in patients on heparin therapy. Collagenase, produced by *P. gingivalis*, may enhance tissue destruction. Both *B. fragilis* and *P. melaninogenica* possess lipopolysaccharides (endotoxins) which lack the biologic potency characteristic of endotoxins associated with aerobic gram-negative bacteria. The biologic inactivity of the endotoxin may account for the rarity of disseminated intravascular coagulation and purpura in *Bacteroides* bacteremia compared with facultative and aerobic gram-negative rod bacteremia.

CLINICAL MANIFESTATIONS   Anaerobic infections of the mouth, head, and neck (See Chap. 84)   Infections of the mouth can be divided into those infections which arise from the supragingival or subgingival dental plaque. Supragingival plaque formation begins with the adherence of gram-positive bacteria to the tooth surface. This form of plaque is influenced by salivary and dietary components, oral hygiene, and local host factors. Once established, the acquisition of pathogenic bacteria as well as an increase in the amount of plaque is responsible for the ultimate development of gingivitis. Early bacteriologic changes in the supragingival plaque initiate an inflammatory response in the gingiva, including edema, swelling, and increase in gingival fluid, and are responsible for the development of caries and endodontic (pulp) infections. Also, these changes contribute to the subsequent pathogenic alteration in the subgingival plaque which arises from poor or inadequate oral hygiene. Subgingival plaque is associated with periodontal disease and disseminated infection arising from the oral cavity. Bacteria that colonize the subgingival area are

primarily anaerobic. The black-pigmented gram-negative anaerobic bacilli, principally *P. gingivalis* and *P. melaninogenica*, are the most important. Infections in this area are frequently mixed and involve both anaerobic and aerobic bacteria. After establishment of local infection either in root canals or in the periodontal area, infection may extend into the mandible, causing osteomyelitis; to the maxillary sinuses; or to local tissues in the submandibular or submental spaces, depending on which teeth are involved. Periodontitis also may result in spreading infection that can involve adjacent bone or soft tissues.

GINGIVITIS   Gingivitis may become a necrotizing infection (trench mouth, Vincent's stomatitis). The onset of disease is usually sudden and is associated with tender bleeding gums, foul breath, and a bad taste. The gingival mucosa, especially the papillae between the teeth, become ulcerated and may be covered by a gray exudate which is removable with gentle pressure. These patients may become systemically ill, developing fever, cervical lymphadenopathy, and leukocytosis. Occasionally, ulcerative gingivitis can spread to the buccal mucosa, the teeth, and the mandible or maxilla, resulting in widespread destruction of bone and soft tissue. This infection is termed *acute necrotizing ulcerative mucositis* (cancrum oris, noma). It destroys tissue rapidly, causing the teeth to fall out and large areas of bone, even the whole mandible, to be sloughed. A strong putrid odor frequently is present, although the lesions are not painful. The gangrenous lesions eventually heal, leaving large disfiguring defects. This infection is seen most commonly following a debilitating illness or in severely malnourished children in underdeveloped areas. It has been known to complicate leukemia or to develop in individuals with a genetic deficiency of catalase.

ACUTE NECROTIZING INFECTIONS OF THE PHARYNX   These usually occur in association with ulcerative gingivitis. Symptoms include an extremely sore throat, foul breath, and a bad taste in the mouth, accompanied by a sensation of choking and fever. Examination of the pharynx demonstrates that the tonsillar pillars are swollen, red, and ulcerated and covered with a grayish membrane that peels easily. Lymphadenopathy and leukocytosis are common. The disease may last for only a few days or may persist for weeks if not treated. Lesions begin unilaterally but may spread to the other side of the pharynx or the larynx. Aspiration of the infected material by the patient can result in lung abscesses. Soft tissue infection of the oral-facial area may or may not be odontogenic in origin. *Ludwig's angina*, a periodontal infection usually arising from the third molar, may produce submandibular cellulitis that results in marked local swelling of tissues with pain, trismus, and superior and posterior displacement of the tongue. Submandibular swelling of the neck develops, which can impair swallowing and cause respiratory obstruction. In some cases tracheotomy may be life-saving.

FASCIAL INFECTIONS   These arise from the spread of organisms originating in the upper airways to potential spaces formed by the fascial planes of the head and neck. Perimandibular space infection most commonly involves the submandibular, peritonsillar, and parapharyngeal spaces. Peritonsillar abscesses occur in association with pharyngitis. Complicated dental infections spread to the submandibular and buccal spaces. Both portals of entry can result in parapharyngeal space infections. Although there are few well-documented reports on the microbiology of these syndromes, anaerobes from the oral flora have been implicated in many cases. *Staphylococcus aureus* and *Streptococcus pyogenes* infections may arise from boils or impetigo, whereas anaerobes are associated with space infections arising from diseases of the mucous membranes or dental manipulations or occurring spontaneously.

SINUSITIS AND OTITIS   The role of anaerobic bacteria in acute sinusitis may be underestimated because of improper collection of specimens. In chronic sinusitis, anaerobic bacteria were found in 52 percent of specimens collected during external frontoethmoidotomy or radical antrotomy. Anaerobic bacteria are much more easily implicated in chronic suppurative otitis media than in acute otitis media. Purulent exudate from chronically draining ears has been found to contain anaerobes, particularly *Bacteroides* species, in up to 50 percent of patients. In contrast to other infections of the head and neck, *B. fragilis* has been isolated from up to 28 percent of patients with chronic otitis media.

COMPLICATIONS OF ANAEROBIC HEAD AND NECK INFECTIONS Contiguous spread of these infections craniad may result in osteomyelitis of the skull or mandible or in intracranial infections such as brain abscesses and subdural empyema. Caudad spread can produce mediastinitis or pleuropulmonary infections. Hematogenous complications also may result from anaerobic infections of the head and neck. Bacteremia, which can occasionally be polymicrobial, can lead to endocarditis or other distant infections. When infections spread to produce suppurative thrombophlebitis of the internal jugular vein, a destructive syndrome with prolonged fever, bacteremia, septic emboli to both the lung and brain, and multiple metastatic foci of suppurative infection may develop. This syndrome has been reported with septicemia from species of *Fusobacterium* following exudative pharyngitis but is uncommon in this era of antimicrobial agents.

Central nervous system infections Brain abscesses are frequently associated with anaerobic bacteria (see Chap. 374). If optimal bacteriologic techniques are employed, as many as 85 percent of brain abscesses yield anaerobic bacteria. The anaerobic bacteria found most often in these infections are anaerobic gram-positive cocci, followed in frequency by fusobacteria and *Bacteroides* species. Frequently, facultative or microaerophilic streptococci and coliforms are involved in brain abscesses as mixed infections.

Pleuropulmonary infections Anaerobic pleuropulmonary infections result from the aspiration of oropharyngeal contents, which is often associated with an altered state of consciousness or absent gag reflex. There are four clinical syndromes associated with anaerobic pleuropulmonary infection produced by aspiration: simple aspiration pneumonia, necrotizing pneumonia, lung abscess, and empyema.

ASPIRATION PNEUMONITIS Aspiration pneumonitis must be distinguished from two other types of aspiration pneumonitis, neither of which is bacterial. One aspiration syndrome results from aspiration of solids, usually food. Obstruction of major airways with resulting atelectasis is typical. Moderate nonspecific inflammation occurs. Therapy consists of removal of the foreign body.

A second aspiration syndrome is more easily confused with bacterial aspiration. This is the so-called Mendelson's syndrome, resulting from regurgitation of stomach contents and aspiration of chemical material, usually gastric juices. Pulmonary inflammation including destruction of alveolar lining with transudation of fluid into the alveolar space occurs with remarkable rapidity. Typically this syndrome develops within hours, often following anesthesia when the gag reflex is depressed. The patient becomes tachypneic, hypoxic, and febrile. The leukocyte count may rise, and the chest x-ray may evolve suddenly from normal to a complete whiteout bilaterally within 8 to 24 h. Minimal sputum production occurs. The pulmonary signs and symptoms can resolve quickly with symptomatic therapy or result in respiratory failure with subsequent development of bacterial superinfection over a period of days. Antibiotic therapy is not indicated unless bacterial infection supervenes. The signs of bacterial infection include sputum, persistent fever, leukocytosis, and clinical evidence of sepsis.

In contrast to these syndromes, bacterial aspiration pneumonia develops more slowly. It is seen in patients who are hospitalized and have a depressed gag reflex, elderly patients, or those with transient impaired consciousness in the wake of seizures or alcoholic blackouts. Patients who enter the hospital with this syndrome typically have been ill for several days and generally complain of low-grade fever, malaise, and sputum production. Usually the history reveals a predisposition for aspiration, such as alcohol overdose or residence in a nursing home. Sputum characteristically is not malodorous unless the process has been present for at least a week. Mixed bacterial flora with many polymorphonuclear leukocytes are present on Gram's stain; reliable cultures can be obtained only by avoiding contamination with normal oral flora, i.e., by transtracheal aspiration. In general, this procedure is not indicated in the evaluation of these patients.

Chest x-rays show consolidation in dependent pulmonary segments. These are the basilar segments of the lower lobes if the patient aspirated while upright or sitting, or the posterior segment of the upper lobe, usually on the right side, or the superior segment of the lower lobe if aspiration has occurred in the supine position. Organisms isolated reflect the pharyngeal flora; *P. melaninogenica*, *Fusobacterium* species, and anaerobic cocci are the most frequent isolates. The patient who aspirates in a hospital setting also may have mixed infection involving enteric gram-negative rods.

NECROTIZING PNEUMONITIS This is a form of anaerobic pneumonitis characterized by numerous small abscesses which spread to involve several pulmonary segments. The process can be indolent or fulminating. This syndrome is less common than either aspiration pneumonia or lung abscess and includes features of both types of infection.

ANAEROBIC LUNG ABSCESSES These result from subacute anaerobic pulmonary infection. The clinical syndrome typically involves a history of constitutional symptoms including malaise, weight loss, fever, chills, and foul-smelling sputum which may occur over a period of weeks (see Chap. 220). Patients who develop lung abscesses characteristically have dental infection and periodontitis, but there are reports of lung abscesses in patients who are edentulous. Abscess cavities may be single or multiple and generally occur in dependent pulmonary segments. Anaerobic abscesses must be distinguished from tuberculosis, neoplasia, and other causes of lung abscess, despite the fact that the clinical syndrome is usually typical. Oral anaerobes predominate, although *B. fragilis* is isolated in up to 10 percent of cases. *S. aureus* may be found as well. For many years penicillin was considered the gold standard of therapy for lung abscesses. Recent clinical trials have shown that clindamycin therapy results in a better clinical outcome than penicillin, presumably because of the enhanced spectrum of activity of clindamycin against oral anaerobes. Thus a combination of penicillin and metronidazole or other antibiotic combinations that treat both oral anaerobes and aerobes are likely to be as effective as clindamycin. Bronchoscopy is indicated only to rule out the presence of airway obstruction but should be delayed until the antimicrobial has begun to affect the disease process so that it does not spread the infection. Bronchoscopy has no role in enhancing drainage. Surgery is almost never indicated because of the danger of spilling the abscess contents into the lungs.

Empyema Empyema is a manifestation of long-standing anaerobic pulmonary infection. The clinical presentation resembles other anaerobic pulmonary infections including the presence of foul-smelling sputum. Patients may complain of pleuritic chest pain and marked chest wall tenderness.

Empyema may be masked by overlying pneumonitis and should be considered especially in cases of persistent fever in a patient receiving antibiotic therapy. Diligent physical examination and the use of ultrasound to localize a loculated empyema are important diagnostic tools. The presence of a foul-smelling exudate obtained by thoracentesis is typical. Drainage is required. Defervescence, a return to a feeling of well-being, and resolution of the process may require several months.

Extension from a subdiaphragmatic infection also may result in an anaerobic empyema. Septic pulmonary emboli may originate from intraabdominal or female genital tract infections and can produce anaerobic pneumonia.

Intraabdominal infections (See Chap. 86)

Pelvic infections The vagina of a healthy woman is one of the major reservoirs of anaerobic and aerobic bacteria. In the normal flora of the female genital tract, anaerobes outnumber aerobes by a ratio of approximately 10:1 and include anaerobic gram-positive cocci and *Bacteroides* species. Anaerobes are isolated from the majority of patients with infections of the genital tract, when infection is not caused by a sexually transmitted pathogen. The major anaerobic pathogens are *B. fragilis*, *P. bivius*, *P. disiens*, *P. melaninogenica*, anaerobic cocci, and clostridial species. Anaerobes frequently are encountered in tuboovarian abscess, septic abortion, pelvic abscess, endometritis, and postoperative wound infection, particularly following hysterectomy. Although these infections are frequently mixed, involving both anaerobes and coliforms, pure anaerobic infections without coliform or other facultative bacterial species occur more often in pelvic infections than in intraabdominal infections and are characterized by drainage of foul-smelling pus or blood from the uterus, generalized uterine or local pelvic tenderness, and continued fever and chills. Suppurative thrombophlebitis of the pelvic veins may complicate the infections and lead to repeated episodes of septic pulmonary emboli. Anaerobic bacteria have been the presumed cause of bacterial vaginosis, but some observers believe it is the anaerobic gram-negative coccobacillus belonging to the genus *Mobiluncus*. This hypothesis is not universally accepted, and others believe that an imbalance in the normal microbial flora of the female genital tract is key.

Skin and soft tissue infections   Injury to skin, bone, or soft tissue by trauma, ischemia, or surgery creates a suitable environment for anaerobic infections. These infections are most frequently found when the site is prone to contamination with feces or upper airway secretions. Examples include wounds associated with intestinal surgery, decubitus ulcers, and human bites. Anaerobic bacteria can be isolated in cases of crepitant cellulitis, synergistic cellulitis, or gangrene and necrotizing fasciitis. These organisms have been isolated from cutaneous abscesses, rectal abscesses, and axillary sweat gland infections (hydradenitis suppurativa). Anaerobes frequently have been cultured from foot ulcers in diabetic patients.

These soft tissue or skin infections are usually polymicrobial. A mean of 4.8 bacterial species can be isolated with a roughly 3:2 ratio of anaerobes to aerobes. The most frequently isolated organisms include *Bacteroides* species, anaerobic streptococci, enterococci, clostridial species, and *Proteus* species. The presence of anaerobes in these types of infections is associated with a higher frequency of fever, foul-smelling lesions, or a visible foot ulcer.

Anaerobic bacterial *synergistic gangrene* (Meleney's) is exquisitely painful, red, and swollen, followed by induration. Erythema surrounds a central zone of necrosis. A granulating ulcer which may heal forms at the original center as necrosis and erythema extend outward. Symptoms are limited to pain. Fever is not typical. These infections usually involve a combination of anaerobic cocci and *S. aureus*. Treatment includes surgical removal of necrotic tissue and antimicrobial therapy.

NECROTIZING FASCIITIS   This is a rapidly spreading destructive disease of the fascia, usually attributed to group A streptococci, but it can be caused by anaerobic bacteria including *Peptostreptococcus* and *Bacteroides* species. Similarly, myonecrosis can be associated with mixed anaerobic infection. Fournier's gangrene is an anaerobic cellulitis involving the scrotum, perineum, and anterior abdominal wall in which mixed anaerobic organisms spread along deep external fascial planes and cause extensive loss of skin.

Bone and joint infections   Although *actinomycosis* (see Chap. 127) accounts on a worldwide basis for the majority of anaerobic infections in bone, other organisms, including anaerobic or microaerophilic cocci, *Bacteroides* species, *Fusobacterium*, and *Clostridium* species, can be found. These infections frequently arise adjacent to soft tissue infections. Hematogenous seeding of bone is uncommon. Oral *Bacteroides* are seen in infections involving the maxilla and mandible, whereas *Clostridium* species have been reported as anaerobic pathogens in cases of osteomyelitis of the long bones, following fracture or trauma. Fusobacteria have been isolated in pure culture from osteomyelitis adjacent to the perinasal sinuses. Anaerobic and microaerophilic cocci have been reported as significant pathogens in infections involving the skull or mastoid.

In cases of anaerobic septic arthritis, the most common isolates are *Fusobacterium* species. Most of these patients have uncontrolled peritonsillar infections progressing to septic cervical venous thrombophlebitis and resulting in hematogenous dissemination which shows a predilection for the joints. Following the introduction of antibiotics, the isolation of *Fusobacterium* species from joints has been less

common. Unlike anaerobic osteomyelitis, most cases of pyoarthritis caused by anaerobes are not polymicrobial and may be acquired hematogenously. Anaerobes are important pathogens in infections involving prosthetic joints; in these infections, the causative organisms are part of the normal skin flora, such as anaerobic gram-positive cocci and *P. acnes*.

In patients with osteomyelitis (see Chap. 92), the most reliable source of culture is a bone biopsy obtained free from normal uninfected skin and subcutaneous tissue. If mixed flora is isolated from a bone biopsy, all isolates should be treated. When an anaerobic isolate is recognized as a major or sole pathogen involving a joint, the duration of treatment should be similar to that for arthritis caused by aerobic bacteria. Therapy includes management of underlying disease states, appropriate antimicrobial therapy, temporary joint immobilization, percutaneous drainage of effusions, and usually removal of infected prostheses or internal fixation devices. Surgical drainage and debridement such as sequestrectomy are essential for removal of necrotic tissue that would sustain anaerobic infections.

Bacteremia   Transient bacteremia is a well-known event that occurs in healthy people when the anatomic mucosal barriers are injured (e.g., dental extractions or dental scaling). These bacteremic episodes, which are often due to anaerobes, have no pathologic consequences. However, anaerobic bacteria are found in blood cultures from clinically ill patients when proper culture techniques are used. *B. fragilis* is the single most frequent anaerobic isolate. In recent years, the isolation rate for anaerobic bacteria from blood cultures has been decreasing. Studies from the 1970s and early 1980s reported that 10 to 15 percent of positive blood cultures grew anaerobes. More recently, similar surveys have yielded lower rates. The cause of this change is not defined but may relate to antibiotic prophylaxis before intestinal surgery, earlier recognition of localized infections, and the empirical use of broad-spectrum antibiotics for presumed infection.

The portal of bloodstream entry can frequently be deduced along with the likely underlying problem that led to seeding of the bloodstream by identification of the organism and understanding its place of normal residence. For example, mixed anaerobic bacteremia including *B. fragilis* usually implies colonic pathology with mucosal disruption from neoplasia, diverticulitis, or some other inflammatory lesion. The initial manifestations are determined by the portal of entry and reflect the localized condition. When bloodstream invasion occurs, patients can become extremely ill with rigors and hectic fevers ranging up to 40.6°C (105°F). The clinical picture may be quite similar to that seen in sepsis with aerobic gram-negative bacilli. Although other complications of anaerobic bacteremia such as septic thrombophlebitis and septic shock have been reported, the incidence of these complications in association with anaerobic bacteremia is low. Anaerobic bacteremia is potentially fatal and requires rapid diagnosis and appropriate therapy. Mortality appears to increase with the age of the patient (reported over 66 percent in patients over 60 years of age), polymicrobial bloodstream isolates, and failure to surgically remove a focus of infection.

ENDOCARDITIS (See Chap. 85)   Endocarditis due to anaerobes is uncommon. However, anaerobic streptococci, which are often classified incorrectly, are responsible for this disease more frequently than is appreciated. Gram-negative anaerobes are unusual causes of endocarditis.

DIAGNOSIS   Because of the time and difficulty involved in the isolation of anaerobic bacteria, diagnosis of these infections must frequently be made on presumptive evidence. Certain clinical settings such as avascular, necrotic tissues with lowered oxidation-reduction potential favor the diagnosis of an anaerobic infection. When infections occur in proximity to mucosal surfaces normally harboring anaerobic flora, such as the gastrointestinal tract, female genital tract, or oropharynx, anaerobes should be considered as potential etiologic agents. A foul odor often is present, since anaerobes produce certain organic acids as they proliferate in necrotic tissue. Although the presence of these odors is nearly pathognomonic for anaerobic infection, the absence of odor does not exclude these organisms as potential etiologic agents. Because anaerobes often coexist with other bacteria to form a mixed or synergistic infection, Gram-stained exudate frequently reveals numerous pleomorphic cocci and bacilli suggestive of anaerobes. Sometimes these organisms will have morphologic characteristics associated with specific species.

The presence of gas in tissues is highly suggestive, but not diagnostic, of anaerobes. Culture reports from obviously infected sites which yield no growth or only streptococci or a single aerobic species such as *E. coli*, when a Gram's stain reveals mixed flora, imply that the anaerobic microorganisms failed to grow because of inadequate transport and/or culture techniques. Failure of a patient to respond to antibiotics that are not active against anaerobes, e.g., aminoglycosides and, in some circumstances, penicillin, cephalosporins, or tetracyclines, suggests the possibility of anaerobic infection.

There are three critical steps to diagnose anaerobic infection: (1) proper specimen collection, (2) rapid transportation of these specimens to the microbiology laboratory, preferably in anaerobic transport media, and (3) proper handling of these specimens by the laboratory. Collection of specimens must be performed by meticulously sampling infected sites and avoiding contamination with normal flora. When there is a likely contamination of a specimen with normal flora, the specimen is unacceptable for processing by the bacteriology laboratory. Examples of unacceptable specimens for anaerobic culture include (1) sputum collected by expectoration or nasal tracheal suction, (2) bronchoscopy specimens, (3) direct collections through the vaginal vault, (4) collections of urine by voided specimen, and (5) feces. Specimens which can be cultured for anaerobes include blood, pleural fluid, transtracheal aspirates, pus obtained by direct aspiration from an abscess cavity, fluid obtained by culdocentesis, suprapubic bladder aspirates, cerebrospinal fluid, and lung puncture specimens.

Because even brief exposure to oxygen may kill some anaerobic organisms and result in failure to isolate them in the laboratory, abscess cavities which are aspirated with a syringe should have the air expelled and the needle capped with a sterile rubber stopper. Proper precautions should be utilized when handling contaminated needles. Specimens can be injected into transport bottles containing a reduced medium or brought immediately in syringes to the laboratory for direct culture on anaerobic media. In general, swabs should not be used. If a swab must be used, it should be placed in a reduced semisolid carrying medium before transport to the laboratory. Delays in transportation may lead to failure to isolate anaerobes due to exposure to oxygen or overgrowth of facultative organisms, which may eliminate or obscure the anaerobes that are present. All clinical specimens from suspected anaerobic infections should be Gram-stained and examined for organisms with characteristic morphology. It is not unusual for organisms to be observed on Gram's stain but not isolated in culture. If purulent materials are found to be sterile or organisms are seen on Gram's stain but do not grow in the culture, suspicion should be raised that anaerobes are involved.

TREATMENT   Successful therapy of anaerobic infections involves a combination of appropriate antibiotics, surgical resection, and drainage. Perforations must be closed promptly, devitalized tissues removed, closed spaces drained, tissue compartments decompressed, and adequate blood supply established. Drainage of abscess cavities should be carried out as soon as fluctuation or localization occurs. While surgery was formerly required to establish drainage, with the advent of CT, MRI, and ultrasound, diagnostic radiologists now are able to perform percutaneous drainage of a number of abscess sites.

Patients with infections due to anaerobic bacteria require appropriate antibiotics. Antibiotic susceptibility testing of anaerobic bacteria has been difficult and controversial. The slow growth rate of many anaerobes, lack of standardized methodology, lack of clinically related standards for resistance, and generally good results with empirical therapy have resulted in susceptibility testing being recommended only for studying resistance patterns in regional centers or local hospitals, predicting efficacy of new antibiotics, and helping to manage selected patients. The selection of initial antibiotic therapy should be based on knowledge of the pathogens likely to be present in a specific clinical setting, in combination with the Gram-stain findings, which should suggest the likelihood of certain species of organisms. Because many anaerobic infections tend to be mixed with coliforms and other facultative organisms, it is advisable, in general, to use drugs active against both aerobic and anaerobic components. If anaerobes are suspected, the choice of empirical antibiotics can nearly always be made reliably, since patterns of antimicrobial susceptibility are usually predictable (see Chap. 100 and Table 128-1).

Organisms belonging to the *B. fragilis* group are resistant to penicillin. This clinically significant resistance mandates that anaerobic infections arising below the diaphragm be treated with specific therapy directed at *B. fragilis* (see Table 128-1). Recently, β-lactamase production has been reported in strains which are usually isolated from infections originating above the diaphragm. Forty to sixty percent of the clinical isolates classified at *Prevotella* and *Porphyromonas*, non–*B. fragilis* species of *Bacteroides*, and *Fusobacterium* species have been reported as producing β-lactamase. The clinical implications of this resistance has not been completely clarified, and most oral anaerobic infections and anaerobic pneumonia respond to penicillin therapy. However, clindamycin does appear to be superior to penicillin for the treatment of lung abscesses. Some infections due to oral organisms fail to respond to penicillin treatment, and in these cases the use of a drug which is effective against penicillin-resistant anaerobes is recommended (see Table 128-1). It is imperative that other appropriate antibiotics be used in conjunction with metronidazole in the treatment of mixed anaerobic and aerobic infections. Metronidazole is inactive against aerobic bacteria, *Actinomyces*, and *Propionibacterium*. The sensitivity of peptostreptococci to metronidazole is unpredictable. Therapy of intraabdominal sepsis (see Chap. 86) must include drugs active against the aerobic flora of the bowel. Combinations of antibiotics used in the treatment of mixed infections of oral origin must include antibiotics active against the aerobic flora of the mouth.

Infections arising from a colonic source are likely to contain *B. fragilis*. Many therapeutic failures have been noted in patients with documented *B. fragilis* infection who are treated with penicillin or first-generation cephalosporins. In intraabdominal sepsis, the use of antibiotics effective against anaerobes has clearly reduced the incidence of postoperative infection and serious infectious complications. The number of antimicrobial agents effective against *B. fragilis* has expanded, and there are currently several choices which are useful (see Table 128-1). In general, greater than 80 percent cure rates can be achieved in patients with *B. fragilis* infection when treated with appropriate antimicrobial therapy and drainage.

TABLE 128-1   Antimicrobial therapy for infections involving *Bacteroides fragilis* group, non–*B. fragilis Bacteroides*, and penicillin-resistant *Prevotella*, *Porphyromonas*, and *Fusobacterium* species, according to antimicrobial resistance

Group 1 (<1% resistance)	Group 2 (<15% resistance)	Group 3 (variable resistance)	Group 4 (resistant)
Metronidazole*	Clindamycin	Penicillin	Aminoglycosides
Ampicillin-sulbactam	Cefoxitin	Cephalosporins	Quinolones
or	High-dose	Tetracycline	Monobactams
Ticarcillin-clavulanic acid	antipseudomonal	Vancomycin	
	penicillins	Erythromycin	
Imipenem			
Chloramphenicol			

* Usually need to give in combination with aerobic bacterial coverage. For infections originating below the diaphragm, aerobic gram-negative coverage is essential. For infections from an oral source, aerobic gram-positive coverage is added. Metronidazole is also not active against *Actinomyces* or *Propionibacterium* and is unreliable against peptostreptococci.

Antibiotic recommendations for treatment of anaerobes is usually based on known resistance patterns in certain species and the likelihood of encountering a given species in the clinical setting at hand. Antibiotics active against the *B. fragilis* group, penicillin-resistant *Prevotella* and *Porphyromonas*, non–*B. fragilis* species of *Bacteroides*, and *Fusobacterium* species can be grouped into four categories based on their predicted activity against anaerobes (see Table 128-1).

Resistance of *B. fragilis* to metronidazole has been reported rarely. This well-tolerated drug achieves significant serum levels and also can be found in high levels within abscess cavities. It should be considered first-line therapy against *B. fragilis* infection. If a patient fails to respond to one of the group 1 or 2 drugs (Table 128-1), consideration should be given to alternative therapy and to determining the resistance patterns among *B. fragilis* group isolates. Although in vitro resistance to chloramphenicol has not been reported, this drug may not be as effective as other group 1 drugs. Among newer drugs, ampicillin-sulbactam, ticarcillin-clavulanic acid, and imipenem have been excellent in the treatment of *B. fragilis* infection. Penicillin remains the drug of choice for peptostreptococci.

Specific regimens must be tailored to the initial infecting site in clinical situations. In the treatment of intraabdominal sepsis, a group 1 drug must be included in the broad-spectrum coverage (see Chap. 86). If gram-positive bacteria are suspected, an appropriate penicillin should be added. Chloramphenicol can be used successfully in patients with anaerobic central nervous system infections at a dose of 30 to 60 mg/kg per day depending on the severity of illness. However, penicillin G and metronidazole also cross the blood-brain barrier and are bactericidal for many anaerobic organisms (see Chap. 374).

Nearly all the drugs mentioned have toxic side effects. These are described in detail in Chap. 100.

Anaerobic infections that have failed to respond to treatment or that relapse should be reassessed. Consideration should be given to additional surgical drainage or debridement. Superinfections with resistant gram-negative facultative or aerobic bacteria should be ruled out. Drug resistance also must be entertained; repeated cultures should yield the pathogenic organism.

Other supportive measures in the management of anaerobic infections include careful attention to fluid and electrolyte balance, since extensive local edema formation may lead to hypoalbuminemia; hemodynamic support for septic shock; immobilization of infected extremities; maintenance of adequate nutrition during chronic infections by parenteral hyperalimentation; relief of pain; and anticoagulation with heparin for thrombophlebitis. Hyperbaric oxygen therapy is advocated by some experts but is of no proven value.

REFERENCES

APPELBAUM PC et al: β-Lactamase production and susceptibilities to amoxicillin, amoxicillin-clavulanate, ticarcillin, ticarcillin-clavulanate, cefoxitin, imipenem, and metronidazole of 320 non–*Bacteroides fragilis Bacteroides* isolates and 129 fusobacteria from 28 U.S. Centers. Antimicrob Agents Chemother 34:1546, 1990

BARTLETT JG: Infections caused by anaerobic bacteria, in *Infectious Diseases*, SL Gorbach et al (eds). Philadelphia, Saunders, 1992

———, FINEGOLD SM: Anaerobic infections of the lung and pleural space. Am Rev Respir Dis 110:56, 1974

CRABB JH et al: T-cell regulation of *Bacteroides fragilis*–induced intraabdominal abscesses. Rev Infect Dis 12:S178, 1990

DORSHER CW et al: Anaerobic bacteremia: Decreasing rate over a 15-year period. Rev Infect Dis 13:633, 1991

FINEGOLD SM: Anaerobes: Problems and controversies in bacteriology, infections, and susceptibility testing. Rev Infect Dis 12:S223, 1990

———, GEORGE WL: *Anaerobic Infections in Humans*, San Diego, Academic, 1989

GIBBS RS: Microbiology of the female genital tract. Am J Obstet Gynecol 156:491, 1987

GORBACH SL: Anaerobic bacteria, in *Principles and Practices of Infectious Diseases*, 3d ed, GL Mandell et al (eds). New York, Wiley, 1990

HORN J et al: Role of anaerobic bacteria in permandibular space infections. Ann Otol Rhinol Laryngol Suppl 154:34, 1991

LEVIN S, GOODMAN LJ: Selected overview of nongynecologic surgical intraabdominal infections: Prophylaxis and therapy. Am J Med 79:146, 1985

MATHISEN GE et al: Brain abscess and cerebritis. Rev Infect Dis 6:5101, 1984

NAKATA MN, LEWIS RP: Anaerobic bacteria in bone and joint infections. Rev Infect Dis 6:5165, 1984

NEWMAN MG: Anaerobic oral and dental infections. Rev Infect Dis 6:5107, 1984

ONDERDONK AB et al: Animal model system for studying virulence of and host response to *Bacteroides fragilis*. Rev Infect Dis 12:S169, 1990

PANTOSTI A et al: Immunochemical characterization of two surface polysaccharides of *Bacteroides fragilis*. Infect Immun 59(5):1690, 1991

THORNSBERRY C: Antimicrobial susceptibility testing of anaerobic bacteria: Review and update on the role of the National Committee for Clinical Laboratory Standards. Rev Infect Dis 12:S218, 1990

TZIANABOS AO et al: Structural features of polysaccharides that induce intra-abdominal abscesses. Science 262:416, 1993

ZALEZNIK DF: Role of bacterial virulence factors in pathogenesis of anaerobic infections, in *Anaerobic Infections in Humans*, S. Finegold (ed). Orlando, Academic, 1989

———, KASPER DL: *Bacteroides* species, in *Principles and Practice of Infectious Diseases*, 3d ed, GL Mandell et al (eds). New York, Wiley, 1990

section 8 Mycobacterial diseases

129 ANTIMYCOBACTERIAL AGENTS

PAUL W. WRIGHT / RICHARD J. WALLACE

The physician is greatly challenged to provide optimal therapy for mycobacterial illnesses because of the advent of AIDS, the increase in both drug-susceptible and multidrug-resistant tuberculosis, and the plethora of new antibiotics with antimycobacterial potential. This chapter reviews the therapeutic agents used for treatment of tuberculosis, leprosy (Hansen's disease), and diseases caused by the pathogenic nontuberculous mycobacteria, including *M. avium-intracellulare* (MAI), *M. kansasii*, the rapidly growing mycobacteria, and *M. marinum*.

TUBERCULOSIS

Drugs used to treat tuberculosis have been classified into first-line and second-line agents. *First-line* antituberculous agents are the most effective and are considered essential for any short-course therapeutic regimen. The two drugs in this category are isoniazid and rifampin. First-line supplemental agents either can further shorten chemotherapy (e.g., pyrazinamide) or are considered highly effective, with infrequent toxicity (ethambutol and streptomycin). *Second-line* antituberculous drugs are clinically much less effective and have a much higher incidence of severe drug reactions. These drugs are used rarely in therapy and then only by individuals experienced in their use. They include *para*-aminosalicylic acid, ethionamide, cycloserine, kanamycin, amikacin, capreomycin, and thiacetazone.

FIRST-LINE ANTITUBERCULOUS DRUGS Isoniazid Perhaps the best antituberculous drug currently available, isoniazid should be included in all tuberculosis treatment regimens unless the organism is resistant. It is inexpensive, readily synthesized and available worldwide, very selective for mycobacteria, and well tolerated, with only 5 percent of patients exhibiting any adverse effects. In the United States it is usually given in combination form with rifampin.

MECHANISM OF ACTION Isoniazid is the hydrazide of isonicotinic acid, a small, water-soluble molecule that easily penetrates the cell. Its mechanism of action is inhibition of mycolic acid cell wall synthesis at unidentified sites. Isoniazid is bacteriostatic against resting bacilli and bactericidal against rapidly multiplying organisms, both extracellularly and intracellularly. Wild-type (untreated) strains of *M. tuberculosis* have minimal inhibitory concentrations (MICs) of <0.1 μg/mL, while *M. kansasii* usually has MICs in the range of 0.5 to 2.0 μg/mL. The MICs for other mycobacteria are much higher.

PHARMACOLOGY Both oral and intramuscular preparations are readily absorbed; a 300-mg oral dose produces peak serum levels that are usually within the 3 to 5 μg/mL range. Isoniazid diffuses well throughout the body and provides therapeutic concentrations in serum, cerebrospinal fluid (CSF), and infected tissue, including caseous granulomas. Isoniazid is metabolized in the liver via acetylation and hydrolysis, with the metabolites being excreted into the urine. The rate of acetylation is genetically controlled. The usual daily dosage for tuberculosis is 5 mg/kg for adults and 10 to 20 mg/kg for children, to a maximum daily dose of 300 mg for both groups. Even in moderate to severe renal failure, the adult dose rarely needs reduction below 200 mg/d.

ADVERSE EFFECTS (Table 129-1) The two most important adverse effects of isoniazid therapy are hepatotoxicity and peripheral neuropathy. Other adverse effects are either rare or less significant and include rash (2 percent), fever (1.2 percent), anemia, acne, arthritic symptoms, optic atrophy, seizures, and psychiatric symptoms. Isoniazid-associated hepatitis is idiosyncratic and increases in incidence with age. It occurs in 0.3 percent of those under 35 years of age, 1.2 percent of those under 49 years of age, and 2.3 percent of those over 50 years of age. An increased risk of isoniazid-related hepatitis is associated with daily alcohol consumption, concomitant rifampin administration, and slow acetylation of isoniazid (Table 129-2). Mortality from isoniazid-induced hepatitis has been reported to be 6 to 12 percent, but the real risk is certainly much lower, since this rate occurred in high-risk patients who continued taking the drug despite progressive symptoms of hepatitis and without monitoring of liver enzymes. Liver enzymes are routinely monitored in most current settings among all high-risk patients. No specific guidelines have been proposed, but a reasonable approach would be to determine serum AST or ALT at baseline, at 2 and 4 weeks, and monthly thereafter for up to 6 months. An ALT or AST level is mandatory, however, whenever a patient notices the onset of symptoms suggestive of isoniazid hepatitis (i.e., fever, anorexia, nausea, flulike syndrome, etc.), with immediate discontinuation of the drug until the relationship between the two is determined. Isoniazid also should be discontinued whenever an asymptomatic AST or ALT level exceeds 150 to 200 IU. When these guidelines are followed, death from isoniazid-associated hepatitis has occurred at a rate of only 14 per 100,000 treated patients. Twelve percent of patients taking isoniazid may experience transient elevations of AST. If the AST elevation persists, if AST is elevated more than three to five times normal, or if symptoms of hepatitis occur, drug withdrawal is required.

Peripheral neuritis associated with isoniazid occurs at a dose-dependent rate of 2 to 20 percent; this rate can be reduced to 0.2 percent with the prophylactic administration of 10 to 50 mg pyridoxine (vitamin B_6) daily.

RESISTANCE Isoniazid-resistant mutants of *M. tuberculosis* occur spontaneously at a rate of 1 in 10^5 to 10^6 organisms. The mechanism and molecular site of isoniazid resistance developed in the laboratory or in vivo are unknown. However, recent molecular genetic studies of some mycobacterial strains demonstrate an association of isoniazid resistance with reduced catalase and peroxidase activity. These studies demonstrated restored or increased bacterial sensitivities to isoniazid in an isoniazid-resistant strain of *M. smegmatis* and some strains of *Escherichia coli*, which were genetically engineered with a single *M. tuberculosis* gene encoding for both catalase and peroxidase. Conversely, they showed isoniazid resistance in two clinical isolates of *M. tuberculosis* from which this same gene was deleted. Primary drug resistance occurs in previously untreated patients at a rate of 7 percent in native U. S. populations but may approach 50 percent in immigrant populations from Southeast Asia. To prevent secondary drug resistance, isoniazid should be given in combination with one or more effective antituberculous drugs.

Rifampin Rifampin, a semisynthetic derivative of *Streptomyces mediterranei*, is the second most important antituberculous agent with efficacy against *M. tuberculosis* comparable with that of isoniazid. It is also active against a wide spectrum of other organisms, including some gram-positive and gram-negative bacteria, *Legionella* species, *M. kansasii*, *M. marinum*, and some strains of MAI.

PHARMACOLOGY Rifampin is a fat-soluble complex macrocyclic antibiotic that is absorbed readily either orally or intravenously. Serum levels of 10 to 20 μg/mL are achieved after a standard oral dose of 600 mg. Rifampin distributes well throughout most body tissues, including inflamed meninges. It turns body fluids (urine, saliva, sputum, tears) to a red-orange color, thereby providing a simple and inexpensive check on patient compliance. Rifampin is excreted primarily through the bile and enterohepatic circulation, while 30 to 40 percent is excreted via the kidneys. It is administered once daily, usually 600 mg for adults (10 mg/kg) and 10 to 20 mg/kg for children.

MECHANISM OF ACTION Rifampin has both intracellular and extracellular bactericidal activity. It blocks RNA synthesis by specifically binding and inhibiting DNA-dependent RNA polymerase. Susceptible strains of *M. tuberculosis* as well as *M. kansasii* and *M. marinum* are inhibited by 1 μg/mL or less.

ADVERSE EFFECTS (Table 129-1) Even though the drug is generally well tolerated, patients with chronic liver disease, especially alcoholism and old age, appear to be at higher risk for the most common adverse drug reaction, which is hepatotoxicity. Other adverse effects include a flulike syndrome (20 percent, primarily with intermittent therapy), nausea and vomiting (1.5 percent), rash (0.8 percent), hemolytic anemia (<1 percent), renal failure due to interstitial nephritis or acute tubular necrosis (<1 percent), and immunosuppression of questionable clinical importance. Rifampin induces hepatic microsomal enzyme production and thereby decreases the half-life of a number of drugs, including digoxin, warfarin, prednisone,

---

TABLE 129-1 Monitoring adverse effects of common antituberculosis drugs

Drug	Adverse effect	What to monitor/management
Isoniazid	Hepatitis	AST/limit alcohol consumption/ monitor for hepatitis symptoms
	Peripheral neuritis	Administer vitamin B_6
	Optic neuritis	Administer vitamin B_6
	Seizures	Administer vitamin B_6
Rifampin	Rash	Observation
	Liver dysfunction	AST/limit alcohol consumption/ monitor for hepatitis symptoms
	Flulike syndrome	Administer twice or more weekly
	Red-orange urine	Reassure patient
	Drug interaction	Consider monitoring drug levels, when possible, especially with contraceptives, anticoagulants, chloramphenicol, and digoxin.
Pyrazinamide	Hepatitis	AST/limit dosage to 15–30 mg/ kg per day
	Hyperuricemia	Monitor uric acid level only if symptomatic with gout or renal failure
Ethambutol	Optic neuritis	Use lower dose (15 g/kg per day) when possible; monitor visual acuity and color vision monthly; educate patient about this side effect.
Streptomycin	Ototoxicity	Limit dose and length of therapy as possible; BUN, serum creatinine, audiometry before and (as needed) during therapy; screen patients for tinnitus, nausea, and vertigo, and decreased hearing; Measure levels if possible.

propranolol, cyclosporine, methadone, oral contraceptives, and quinidine (Table 129-2).

RESISTANCE   Rifampin resistance occurs as a result of spontaneous mutations that presumably affect either cell wall transport (low-level resistance) or the RNA polymerase (high-level resistance). Recent studies with rifampin resistant *M. leprae* showed 8 of 9 strains to have a mutation involving a serine residue in the rpoB gene, which encodes the beta subunit of RNA polymerase.

FIRST-LINE SUPPLEMENTAL DRUGS   Pyrazinamide (PZA)   A derivative of nicotinic acid, pyrazinamide is an important bactericidal drug used in short-course chemotherapy of tuberculosis.

PHARMACOLOGY   Pyrazinamide is well absorbed after oral administration, with a plasma concentration of 45 μg/mL in 2 h and excellent distribution throughout the body. It is hydrolyzed in the liver into several metabolites, one of which, pyrazinoic acid, is considered the active form of the drug. Pyrazinoic acid is then hydroxylated to 5-hydroxypyrazinoic acid, which is subsequently excreted by renal glomerular filtration.

MECHANISM OF ACTION   Pyrazinamide is similar to isoniazid in its narrow spectrum of antibacterial activity against essentially only *M. tuberculosis*. The drug is considered primarily effective against slowly metabolizing organisms located within the acid environment of the phagocyte or caseous granuloma, since it is active only at a pH below 6.0. The mechanism of action is unknown.

ADVERSE EFFECTS (Table 129-1)   With the high dosages used in the past, hepatotoxicity was a major complication of pyrazinamide therapy. However, at the current recommended dosages of 15 to 30 mg/kg with a maximum of 2 g/d (may be given in one daily dose), the occurrence of hepatotoxicity is not increased over that observed with concomitant isoniazid and rifampin therapy. Hyperuricemia is a common adverse effect of pyrazinamide therapy that is probably reduced by concurrent rifampin therapy. Clinical gout is only rarely seen in patients receiving pyrazinamide; polyarthralgias are not uncommonly encountered but are not related to the hyperuricemia.

Ethambutol   A derivative of ethylenediamine, ethambutol is a water-soluble compound that is active only against mycobacteria. Susceptible species include *M. tuberculosis*, *M. marinum*, *M. kansasii*, and MAI. Among first-line drugs, it is the least potent against *M. tuberculosis*. It is used most often with rifampin in the treatment of tuberculosis in patients who are unable to tolerate isoniazid or who are suspected or known to be infected with isoniazid-resistant organisms.

MECHANISM OF ACTION   Ethambutol is bacteriostatic against rapidly growing mycobacteria. The mechanisms of action and resistance to ethambutol are unknown.

PHARMACOLOGY   After oral administration, 75 to 80 percent of the drug is absorbed from the gastrointestinal route and produces peak serum levels of 2 to 4 μg/mL 2 to 4 h after the usual 15 mg/kg dose. Distribution throughout the body is adequate except in the CSF, where it achieves only low levels. Almost all the drug is excreted by the kidneys within 24 h of ingestion, either unchanged or as metabolites. The usual adult dosage of ethambutol is 15 mg/kg (may be given in one daily dose) in initial treatment regimens and 25 mg/kg in retreatment regimens (usually 800 to 1600 mg daily) or for the initial 6 to 8 weeks on the four-drug regimen for suspected drug-resistant tuberculosis. These dosages must be lowered in patients with renal insufficiency (creatinine clearance of <25 mL/min) to prevent drug accumulation and toxicity.

ADVERSE EFFECTS (Table 129-1)   The drug is usually well tolerated, with optic neuritis (usually retrobulbar) being the most serious adverse effect. Axial or central neuritis, the only form of retrobulbar optic neuritis reported in patients taking daily doses of <30 mg/kg, involves the papillomacular bundle of fibers and results in reduced visual acuity, central scotoma, and loss of ability to see green. Symptoms of ocular toxicity typically occur several months after initiation of therapy, but rapid-onset optic neuritis has been reported. Optic neuritis is dependent on dose and duration of therapy and occurs in 5 percent of patients receiving 25 mg/kg but less than 1 percent of patients on a dose of 15 mg/kg. Patients should be tested monthly for visual acuity and red-green color discrimination. Optic neuritis with the associated visual loss is usually reversible, but recovery may take up to 6 months.

Other adverse effects with ethambutol are infrequent. Hyperuricemia occurs but is usually asymptomatic. The drug is not recommended for young children in whom visual complications would be difficult to monitor.

Streptomycin   Streptomycin is an aminoglycoside which was isolated from *Streptomyces griseus*. It is available for intramuscular administration only. In the United States it is the least used first-line supplemental drug for tuberculosis because of its toxicity, the difficulty in obtaining serum levels, and the inconvenience of intramuscular administration. In developing countries, however, it is frequently used because of its low cost. Streptomycin is active against untreated strains of *M. tuberculosis*, *M. kansasii*, and *M. marinum* and some strains of MAI at readily achievable serum levels.

PHARMACOLOGY   The drug achieves peak serum levels of 25 to 40 μg/mL after a 1.0-g dose. Streptomycin is bactericidal for rapidly dividing extracellular mycobacteria but is ineffective in the acid environment within the macrophage. It diffuses poorly into the meninges and achieves CSF levels in patients with meningitis that are only 20 percent of the serum drug level.

The usual adult dose is 0.5 to 1.0 g/d (10 to 15 mg/kg) or five times per week; the pediatric dose is 20 to 40 mg/kg per day, with a maximum of 1.0 g/d. Dosage must be lowered in most patients over 50 years of age and in any patient with renal impairment because streptomycin is almost exclusively eliminated by the kidneys.

MECHANISM OF ACTION   Streptomycin inhibits protein synthesis by disruption of ribosomal function.

ADVERSE EFFECTS (Table 129-1)   Adverse effects from streptomycin therapy occur in 10 to 20 percent of patients, with ototoxicity and renal toxicity being the most common and serious. Renal toxicity, usually manifested as nonoliguric renal failure, is less common with streptomycin than with other commonly used aminoglycosides such as gentamicin. Ototoxicity involves both hearing loss and vestibular dysfunction. The latter is more common and includes nausea, vertigo, and tinnitus. Patients receiving streptomycin must be monitored carefully for these adverse effects. Less serious effects include eosinophilia, rash, and drug fever.

TABLE 129-2   Major antituberculous drug interactions

Rifampin	Isoniazid	Pyrazinamide	Ethambutol	Streptomycin
Warfarin	Warfarin	Probenecid	Antacids	Methicillin
Glucocorticoids	Glucocorticoids			
Cyclosporine	Alcohol			
Digoxin	Antacids			
Quinidine	PAS			
Oral contraceptives	Oral contraceptives			
Oral hypoglycemic agents	Levodopa			
Ketoconazole	Ketoconazole			
Narcotics	Meperidine			
Halothane	Enflurane			
Barbiturates	Aspirin			
Diazepam	Benzodiazepines			
Beta blockers	Propranolol			
Analgesics				
Verapamil				
Clofibrate				
Progestins				
Disopyramide				
Mexiletine				
Theophylline				
Chloramphenicol				
Anticonvulsants				
Probenecid				
Dapsone				

RESISTANCE Streptomycin resistance in mycobacteria is believed to be similar in mechanism to resistance in other bacteria. It develops rapidly with one-drug therapy, and random mutational resistance occurs in 1 in 10^5 organisms. Low-level resistance can result from alterations in cellular transport, while high-level resistance is secondary to alteration in the ribosomal binding protein. Isolates of *M. tuberculosis* resistant to streptomycin are not cross-resistant to capreomycin or amikacin.

SECOND-LINE ANTITUBERCULOUS DRUGS Second-line antituberculous drugs are used either for drug-resistant tuberculosis or when first-line supplemental drugs are not available. The more important second-line drugs are discussed below.

***Para*-aminosalicylic acid (PAS)** PAS is rarely indicated because of its low antituberculous activity and its high gastrointestinal toxicity (consisting of nausea, vomiting, diarrhea) and occasional hepatitis. Adult dosage is 10 to 12 g/d in several doses and requires the patient to swallow 20 to 24 large and unpleasant-tasting tablets. PAS is well absorbed from oral administration and is distributed throughout the body, but it has low concentrations in the CSF. The drug has a short half-life of 1 h, and 80 percent is excreted in the urine.

Ethionamide Another derivative of isonicotinic acid (as are isoniazid and PZA), ethionamide exerts bactericidal activity against metabolizing *M. tuberculosis* and some nontuberculous mycobacteria. It is most useful in the therapy of multidrug-resistant tuberculosis. However, drug use is severely limited by its toxicity and frequent adverse effects that include intense gastrointestinal intolerance (anorexia, vomiting, and dysgeusia), serious neurologic reactions, reversible hepatitis (5 percent), hypersensitivity reactions, and hypothyroidism. It is well absorbed orally and widely distributed throughout the body, including the CSF. Ethionamide is excreted primarily through the kidneys, with 99 percent of the drug being excreted as a metabolite. Adult patients initially are given 250-mg tablets twice daily and then increased to 250 mg four times daily (15 mg/kg per day with 1 g/d maximum) as tolerated. Pyridoxine should be administered with ethionamide.

Cycloserine Cycloserine, D-4-amino-3-isoxazolidinone, is produced by *Streptomyces orchidaceus* and has activity against a broad spectrum of bacteria as well as *M. tuberculosis*. It has excellent oral absorption and is widely distributed throughout body fluids, including the CSF. Serious adverse effects limit the use of this drug and include psychosis even resulting in suicide, seizures, peripheral neuropathy, headaches, somnolence, and allergic reactions. Because excretion is primarily renal, dosage must be adjusted in patients with reduced renal function. The usual adult dose is 250 mg three times per day (15 to 20 mg/kg). Plasma concentrations should be maintained below 30 μg/mL to reduce toxicity. However, the assay for determination of plasma levels is not performed in most hospital laboratories. Pyridoxine should be administered with this drug. Cycloserine should not be given to patients with epilepsy, active alcohol abuse, severe renal insufficiency, or a history of depression or psychosis.

Capreomycin Capreomycin is a complex cyclic polypeptide antibiotic derived from *Streptomyces capreolus*. This drug is similar to streptomycin in dosing, mechanism of action, pharmacology, and toxicity. It is administered only by the intramuscular route in doses of 10 to 15 mg/kg per day or five times per week (maximum daily dose of 1 g), with peak blood levels of 20 to 40 μg/mL. Patients should be monitored closely for renal and eighth cranial nerve toxicity, which are of major concern with this drug. Dosage must be reduced in patients over 50 years of age and those with renal insufficiency. Cross-resistance with kanamycin and amikacin is common, but not with streptomycin. Capreomycin is the injectable drug of choice for tuberculosis in patients unable to tolerate streptomycin due to hypersensitivity or whose isolate is streptomycin-resistant.

Kanamycin and amikacin These are well-known aminoglycosides that are bactericidal to extracellular organisms. Kanamycin is rarely used because of greater toxicity. Amikacin is active against *M. tuberculosis* and several of the nontuberculous species, including the rapidly growing mycobacteria, *M. scrofulaceum*, MAI, and *M. leprae*.

The usual dosage is 10 mg/kg intramuscularly or intravenously three to five times a week, with a maximum daily dose of 0.5 g.

Thiacetazone This drug is not available in the United States but is widely used in combination with isoniazid to treat tuberculosis in the developing world because it is inexpensive and readily available. It is usually given in a dosage of 150 mg/d in combination with 300 mg isoniazid in a single tablet. Thiacetazone is structurally related to isoniazid but is bacteriostatic and more toxic.

Rifabutin This is a recently approved derivative of rifamycin that is related to rifampin. It is bactericidal against *M. tuberculosis*, MAI, and other nontuberculous mycobacteria. Rifabutin appears to have efficacy in treating both tuberculosis and nontuberculous mycobacterial infections. Usual adult dosage will probably be 300 to 600 mg/d. The drug produces much lower serum levels than rifampin but has a much longer half-life and is much more active against isolates of MAI. Isolates of *M. tuberculosis* resistant to rifampin are usually cross-resistant to rifabutin.

Quinolones Two newer fluorinated quinolones, ciprofloxacin and ofloxacin, show activity against many of the mycobacteria, especially *M. tuberculosis*, *M. marinum*, *M. kansasii*, and *M. fortuitum*. These two drugs are well absorbed orally, reach high serum levels, and distribute well to body tissues and fluid. Adverse effects, which are uncommon (0.5 to 3 percent), include gastrointestinal intolerance, skin rashes, or CNS problems such as headache, insomnia, and dizziness. The quinolones prevent DNA synthesis by inhibiting DNA gyrase. Resistance, from either a change in the permeability of the organism or a change in the DNA gyrase, develops rapidly with mycobacteria as with bacterial species.

LEPROSY (HANSEN'S DISEASE)

Therapy for leprosy remains difficult, especially in developing countries, because of the length of therapy required, the cost and availability of drugs, frequent adverse effects, acquired drug resistance, and the difficulty of susceptibility testing given the inability to grow the organism in vitro. While many drugs show activity against *M. leprae*, only dapsone, rifampin, and clofazimine are part of standard World Health Organization (WHO) therapy for paucibacillary and multibacillary leprosy.

DAPSONE (DDS) Dapsone (4,4'-diaminodiphenylsulfone), a sulfone, inhibits bacterial folic acid synthesis. It is considered the drug of first choice in most cases of Hansen's disease because of its availability, low cost, low toxicity, and the susceptibility of untreated strains of *M. lepra* to very low concentrations of the drug.

Pharmacology The drug is well absorbed orally and distributes well throughout the body. The usual adult daily dosage is 100 mg and 1.0 to 1.5 mg per kg for children. Peak plasma concentrations occur within 1 to 3 h, and the median half-life of elimination is 22 h. Dapsone is cleared by acetylation in the liver, with genetic variation similar to the acetylation of isoniazid. The drug is 70 percent bound to plasma protein. Usual daily doses produce serum concentrations of 10 to 15 μg/mL that far exceed the MIC for *M. leprae* of 0.01 to 0.001 μg/mL.

Adverse effects Hemolysis and methemoglobinemia are common untoward reactions to dapsone. Patients should be screened for glucose-6-phosphate dehydrogenase deficiency to prevent drug-induced hemolysis. However, most patients tolerate dapsone therapy well with adequate clinical and laboratory supervision. Other adverse effects include gastrointestinal intolerance, headache, pruritus, agranulocytosis, fever, and rash. In lepromatous leprosy, erythema nodosum leprosum (ENL) may occur and may be difficult to distinguish from allergic reactions to the drug (dapsone syndrome).

RIFAMPIN Rifampin, the second most useful drug in leprosy therapy, has the major limitation worldwide of cost. It is bactericidal against *M. leprae* and rapidly reduces the number of viable bacilli in patient tissue. It must be combined with other antileprosy drugs to prevent the development of resistance. For cost reasons the drug is given 600 mg once a month (supervised) outside the United States but is given daily in the United States.

CLOFAZIMINE A phenazine iminoquinone dye, clofazimine is weakly bactericidal against *M. leprae*. It is useful in treating dapsone-resistant leprosy and may lessen ENL. Clofazimine's mode of action is not well understood, but it may inhibit DNA binding. The drug is absorbed orally and distributed to the fatty tissues and the reticuloendothelial system. Its serum half-life is about 60 to 70 days, with only a small amount being excreted daily into the urine or bile. Bactericidal activity occurs very slowly and may be observed about 50 days after administration. Usual adult dosage is 50 to 100 mg/d, 100 mg three times a week, or 300 mg/d for treatment of ENL. Untoward effects include skin discoloration and, less commonly, gastrointestinal intolerance. Clofazimine also has in vitro activity against some of the nontuberculous mycobacterial species, including MAI, *M. kansasii*, *M. simiae*, and *M. abscessus*.

OTHER AGENTS A number of other drugs show significant activity against *M. leprae*, but clinical experience with these agents is lacking. Thalidomide may be useful in suppressing ENL but acts as a tranquilizer and is also extremely teratogenic; it is no longer available in the United States. Second-line drugs for the treatment of leprosy include ethionamide, prothionamide, and amithiozone (a thiosemicarbazone).

The newer macrolide antibiotics, particularly clarithromycin, and minocycline, a long-acting tetracycline, and a number of the fluoroquinolones have recently shown bactericidal activity against *M. leprae* in mice. Ofloxacin appears to be the most bactericidal agent among the newer quinolones. These new drugs show considerable promise for leprosy therapy because of their low toxicity and various modes of action that differ from the established drugs. Rifabutin has similar activity to rifampin, but its longer half-life may facilitate less frequent dosing.

NONTUBERCULOUS MYCOBACTERIA (NTM)

The nontuberculous mycobacteria are of low pathogenicity but cause pulmonary, skin, bone and joint, lymph node, and soft tissue infection and disseminated disease in immunocompromised hosts, including patients with AIDS. MAI and *M. kansasii* are the two most common causes of NTM pulmonary infection; up to 40 percent of AIDS patients develop disseminated disease with MAI.

MAI Therapy for MAI is controversial because of the lack of controlled clinical trials. First-line antituberculous drugs are much less active against MAI than against *M. tuberculosis*. Cycloserine and ethionamide show the best in vitro activity but are markedly limited by their toxicity. The American Thoracic Society recommends the following initial daily therapy for MAI lung disease (HIV-negative patients) for 18 to 24 months: isoniazid (300 mg), rifampin (600 mg), ethambutol (25 g/kg and 15 mg/kg from the third month on), with 0.5 to 1.0 g streptomycin. The streptomycin therapy should be 5 days per week for the first 6 to 12 weeks and then two to three times per week for a total of 3 to 6 months of therapy as tolerated. Because of the relatively poor in vivo and in vitro activity of isoniazid and its higher incidence of toxicity in the elderly population, replacement of isoniazid with one of the newer macrolides has been suggested by some experts but has not been studied by clinical trial. For disseminated disease in AIDS, commonly used drugs include one of the newer macrolides (clarithromycin or azithromycin) plus rifampin, ethambutol, and/or clofazimine. Alternative drugs include ciprofloxacin, amikacin, ethionamide, and cycloserine. Rifabutin at a dose of 300 mg/d was recently approved for prophylaxis of disseminated MAI in AIDS patients with CD4 counts of less than 100.

MYCOBACTERIUM KANSASII *M. kansasii* is usually sensitive to most antituberculous drugs, with the major exception of pyrazinamide. Current recommendations for therapy of pulmonary disease are 18 to 24 months of daily isoniazid (300 mg), rifampin (600 mg), and ethambutol (15 mg/kg).

RAPIDLY GROWING MYCOBACTERIA (RGM) *M. fortuitum*, *M. abscessus*, and *M. chelonae* account for more than 80 percent of clinical disease due to the RGM. They are resistant to antituberculous agents other than amikacin but are variably susceptible to several traditional antibiotics, including amikacin (80 to 100 percent), cefoxitin (80 percent of *M. abscessus* and *M. fortuitum*), doxycycline (50 percent of *M. fortuitum*), imipenem (100 percent of *M. fortuitum*, 70 percent of *M. chelonae* and *M. abscessus*), and the fluorinated quinolones (ciprofloxacin and ofloxacin, 100 percent of *M. fortuitum*), and sulfonamides (90 percent of *M. fortuitum*).

MYCOBACTERIUM MARINUM *M. marinum*, a photochromogen, is typically susceptible to minocycline, rifampin, ethambutol, clarithromycin, and trimethoprim/sulfamethoxazole.

CLARITHROMYCIN Clarithromycin, 6-O-methylerythromycin, is a new macrolide that is similar to erythromycin in mechanism of action. However, unlike erythromycin, it is well absorbed with or without meals and has little gastrointestinal intolerance at low doses. It distributes well into body tissues and fluids, but there are no data about its penetration into the CSF. The drug is metabolized in the liver, with approximately 30 percent excreted in the urine. Standard dosage for bacterial infections is 250 to 500 mg twice daily. Dosage should be reduced if the creatinine clearance is 30 mL/min or less. As with erythromycin, the drug binds with plasma proteins (65 to 70 percent) and can raise the levels of drugs such as theophylline and carbamazepine. Clarithromycin appears to be the best single drug for therapy of MAI infections, especially disseminated disease in AIDS patients. However, because the organism may acquire drug resistance, the drug should be combined with other amtimycobacterial agents such as ethambutol and rifampin. The drug is also highly active against *M. marinum*, *M. kansasii*, *M. chelonae*, and most isolates of *M. fortuitum*. Standard antimycobacterial drug doses have been 500 mg twice daily, with doses of 1000 mg twice daily generally being used in disseminated MAI disease in AIDS patients. The more common adverse effects seen with high doses include nausea, vomiting, a bitter taste, and occasionally abnormal liver function tests. The drug is teratogenic in laboratory animals and is rated category C for pregnancy. Azithromycin, another new macrolide, appears to have similar activity in vitro, but less is known about its clinical activity against mycobacteria.

REFERENCES

EDWARDS E, KIRKPATRICK CH: The immunology of mycobacterial disease. Am Rev Respir Dis 134:1062, 1986

HASTINGS RC et al: Leprosy. Clin Microbiol Rev 1:330, 1988

HEIFETS LB et al: Clarithromycin minimal inhibitory and bactericidal concentrations against *Mycobacterium avium*. Am Rev Respir Dis 145:856, 1992

JACOBS RF, ABERNATHY RS: Management of tuberculosis in pregnancy and the newborn. Clin Perinatol 15:305, 1988.

LEIBOLD JE: The ocular toxicity of ethambutol and its relation to dose. Ann NY Acad Sci 135:904, 1966

MACKAY AD, COLE RB: The problems of tuberculosis in the elderly. Q J Med 53:497, 1984

O'BRIEN RJ: Present chemotherapy of tuberculosis. Semin Respir Infect 4:216, 1989

REYNOLDS JEF (ed): *Martindale The Extra Pharmacopoeia*, 29th ed. London, The Pharmaceutical Press, 1989

SCHILD HS et al: Rapid reversible ocular toxicity from ethambutol therapy. Am J Med 90:404, 1991

STAKRE JR et al: Medical Progress: Resurgence of tuberculosis in children. J Pediatr 120:839, 1992

UNDERLIED CB: Antimycobacterial agents: in vitro susceptibility testing, spectrums of activity, mechanism of action and resistance, and assays for activity in biological fluid, in *Antibiotics in Laboratory Medicine*, 3d ed, V Lorian (ed). Baltimore, Williams & Wilkins, 1991, pp 134–197

WALLACE RJ JR et al: Diagnosis and treatment of disease caused by nontuberculous mycobacteria. Am Rev Respir Dis 142:940, 1990

WAYNE LG, SRAMEK HA: Agents of newly recognized or infrequently encountered mycobacterial diseases. Clin Microbiol Rev 5:1, 1992

WOLINSKY E: Nontuberculous mycobacteria and associated diseases. Am Rev Respir Dis 119:107, 1979

YODER LJ: Leprosy. Curr Opin Infect Dis 4:302, 1991

ZHANG Y et al: The catalase-peroxidase gene and isoniazid resistance of *Mycobacterium tuberculosis*. Nature 358:591, 1992

130   TUBERCULOSIS

THOMAS M. DANIEL

DEFINITION Tuberculosis is a chronic bacterial infection caused by *Mycobacterium tuberculosis* and characterized by the formation of granulomas in infected tissues and by cell-mediated hypersensitivity. The usual site of disease is the lungs, but other organs may be involved. In the absence of effective treatment for active disease, a chronic wasting course is usual, and death ultimately supervenes.

ETIOLOGY *Mycobacterium tuberculosis*, the tubercle bacillus, is one of more than 30 well-characterized and many unclassified members of the genus *Mycobacterium*. Along with the closely related *M. bovis*, it causes tuberculosis. *M. leprae* is the etiologic agent of leprosy (see Chap. 131). *M. avium* and a number of other mycobacterial species produce less common human diseases (see Chap. 132). Most mycobacteria are not pathogenic for humans, and many are readily isolated from environmental sources.

Mycobacteria are distinguished by their surface lipids, which render them acid-fast so that they cannot be decolorized with acid alcohol after staining. Because of this lipid, heat or detergents are usually necessary to accomplish primary staining.

Important to understanding the pathogenesis of tuberculosis is recognition that *M. tuberculosis* contains many immunoreactive substances. Surface lipids of mycobacteria and water-soluble components of cell wall peptidoglycan are important adjuvants that may exert their effects through their primary actions on host macrophages. Mycobacteria contain an array of protein and polysaccharide antigens, some probably species-specific but others clearly sharing epitopes broadly throughout the genus. Cell-mediated hypersensitivity is characteristic of tuberculosis and is an important determinant of the disease's pathogenesis.

EPIDEMIOLOGY Tuberculosis continues as an important cause of death. In 1991, a total of 26,283 cases of tuberculosis were reported in the United States, a case rate of 10.4 per 100,000 per year. The case rate had been falling at a rate of 5 to 6 percent per year, but since 1985 this trend has reversed, with the rate having increased by 15.8 percent in the ensuing 5 years. It is estimated that 10 million Americans have a positive tuberculin test but that fewer than 1 percent of American children are tuberculin reactors. Tuberculosis in North America tends to be a disease of the elderly, of the urban poor, of minority groups, and of patients with AIDS. At all ages, case rates among nonwhites tend to be twice those in whites. Hispanic, Haitian, and Southeast Asian immigrants may have case rates as high as those of the countries from which they come, and in these individuals the frequency of disease among younger persons reflects its occurrence in young individuals in those countries. The geographic distribution of tuberculosis in the United States reflects the distribution of the populations in which this disease is prevalent. New York, including New York City, has been particularly affected by the recent increase in tuberculosis in the United States, with a 30.4 percent increase from 1985 to 1990.

Because in the United States tuberculosis has become a disease of the elderly, it is frequently seen in nursing homes. Although transmission of infection can occur at any age, most disease in older persons represents a legacy of previous times. The elderly of today were children when transmission of tubercle bacilli occurred much more frequently. Of those who were infected, many developed disease in young adulthood. Some, especially males, did not and are only now developing reactivation disease in their late years. However, an increasing portion of elderly persons have never been infected and have acquired nosocomial new infections in nursing homes.

In much of the world, transmission of tuberculous infection is declining, but in many impoverished nations this is not true. In some countries, estimated new case rates are as high as 400 per 100,000 per year. As in North America and Europe, poverty and tuberculosis go hand in hand. In high-prevalence areas, tuberculosis is seen with equal prevalence in rural and urban settings and afflicts chiefly young adults. In countries where human immunodeficiency virus (HIV) infection is endemic, tuberculosis is commonly the single most important cause of morbidity and mortality in AIDS patients. A reasonable estimate of the magnitude of tuberculosis in the world is that one-third of the population of the world is infected with *M. tuberculosis*, that there are 30 million cases of active tuberculosis in the world, that 10 million new cases occur annually, and that 3 million people die of tuberculosis each year. Tuberculosis probably causes 6 percent of all deaths worldwide.

TRANSMISSION *M. tuberculosis* is transmitted from person to person via the respiratory route. Although other routes of transmission are possible and have been documented on occasion, none is of major importance. Tubercle bacilli in respiratory secretions form nuclei for liquid droplets expelled during coughing, sneezing, and vocalizing. Droplets evaporate within a short distance from the mouth, and thereafter desiccated bacilli remain airborne for long periods. Infection of a susceptible host occurs when a few of these bacilli are inhaled. The number of bacilli excreted by most infected persons is not large; typically, household contact of many months is required for transmission. However, patients with laryngeal tuberculosis, endobronchial disease, recent transbronchial spread of tuberculosis, and extensive cavitary pulmonary disease are often highly contagious. Infectiousness correlates with the number of organisms in the expectorated sputum, extent of pulmonary disease, and frequency of cough. Mycobacteria are susceptible to ultraviolet irradiation, and outdoor transmission of infection rarely occurs in daylight. Adequate ventilation is the most important measure to reduce the infectiousness of the environment. Fomites are not important in the transmission of tuberculosis. Most patients become noninfectious within 2 weeks after the institution of appropriate chemotherapy because of a decrease in the number of organisms excreted and a decrease in cough.

Transmission of infection with *M. bovis* has long been associated with the consumption of contaminated cow's milk. This organism is no longer a major cause of human disease in most of the world.

PATHOGENESIS The initial entry of tubercle bacilli into the lungs or another site in a previously uninfected individual elicits a nonspecific acute inflammatory response which is rarely noted and is usually accompanied by few or no symptoms. Bacilli are then ingested by macrophages and transported to the regional lymph nodes. If spread of the organism is not contained at the level of regional lymph nodes, then tubercle bacilli reach the bloodstream and widespread dissemination ensues. Most lesions of disseminated tuberculosis heal, as do most primary pulmonary lesions, although they remain potential foci of later reactivation. Dissemination may result in miliary or meningeal tuberculosis—illnesses with potential for major morbidity and mortality, especially in infants and young children.

During the 2 to 8 weeks after primary infection, while bacilli continue to multiply in their intracellular environment, cell-mediated hypersensitivity develops in the infected host. Immunologically competent lymphocytes enter areas of infection, where they elaborate chemotactic factors, interleukins, and lymphokines. In response, monocytes enter the area and undergo transformation into macrophages and subsequently into specialized histiocytic cells, which become organized into granulomas. Mycobacteria may persist within macrophages for many years despite increased lysozyme production within these cells, but their further multiplication and spread are usually confined. Healing then occurs, often with late calcification of the granulomas that sometimes leaves a residual lesion visible on chest radiograph. The combination of a calcified peripheral lung lesion and calcified hilar lymph node is known as a *Ghon complex*.

In the United States, 90 to 95 percent of immunocompetent individuals undergo complete healing of primary tuberculous lesions with no subsequent evidence of disease. In other populations, where infective inocula may be higher and where nutritional status and other host factors may be less propitious, failure of complete healing may occur in more than 5 to 10 percent of individuals. Famine and many intercurrent diseases adversely affect healing and threaten the stability of healed tuberculous lesions.

Tuberculosis—the clinical disease—develops in the minority who do not successfully contain their primary infections. In some individuals, tuberculosis develops within weeks after primary infection; in most, organisms lie dormant for many years before entering a phase of exponential multiplication leading to disease. Among many, age can be identified as a significant factor determining the course of tuberculosis. In infants, tuberculous infection frequently progresses rapidly to disease, and the risk of disseminated disease, including meningitis and miliary tuberculosis, is high. In children older than 1 or 2 years up to about the age of puberty, primary tuberculous lesions almost always heal; most of those destined to develop tuberculosis do so during adolescence or young adulthood. Individuals infected in adulthood are at greatest risk of developing tuberculosis within approximately 3 years following infection. Tuberculous disease is more common in young adult women, whereas it is more common in men later in life.

IMMUNOLOGY   Immunity   Humans display native immunity to tuberculosis, with substantial individual variation. Studies of twins have demonstrated that tuberculosis is more likely to occur in both members of monozygotic sibships than in dizygotic sibships or other family relationships. Attempts to link susceptibility to tuberculosis to HLA phenotype have produced conflicting data. Although susceptibility to tuberculosis has been associated with race, the evidence is largely anecdotal and is not convincing. As noted, age is an important determinant of native immunity to tuberculosis. Although specific data on nutrition and tuberculosis immunity are lacking, the association of tuberculosis with famine is clear.

Acquired immunity follows primary tuberculous infection. Disease due to exogenous reinfection is probably rare in North America and Europe; it may be more frequent in populations of high prevalence, where the risk of repeated exposure is great. It is useful to recall that *immunity*, in the classic sense of the word, refers to resistance to infection, whereas *hypersensitivity* describes a state of altered host reactivity. In this sense, immunity also may result from vaccination with bacillus Calmette-Guérin (BCG) or from infection with other species of mycobacteria.

In animal models, antigen-specific immunity is T lymphocyte–dependent and can be transferred adoptively with lymphocytes. It closely parallels cutaneous-type delayed hypersensitivity in its development.

Tuberculin hypersensitivity   Tuberculin hypersensitivity is antigen-specific in nature and follows primary infection. It is chiefly or perhaps entirely directed against protein antigens. It is mediated by T lymphocytes through secretion of lymphokines, which act on effector monocytes.

Mycobacterial antigens have been subjected to extensive immunochemical study. It is clear that there is no single dominant antigen and that infected and artificially sensitized hosts develop hypersensitivity to an array of mycobacterial proteins. Tuberculin purified protein derivative (PPD), the antigen preparation most frequently employed clinically and epidemiologically to demonstrate tuberculin hypersensitivity, is a crude mixture of largely denatured antigens and is a poor representative of native antigens. Nevertheless, its use has yielded much information.

Antigen recognition by the sensitized host follows processing by macrophages and depends on expression by the macrophage—at its surface—of antigen-specific epitopes in association with Ia antigen, a gene product of the major histocompatibility locus. This complex is recognized by specific T lymphocytes. Macrophage synthesis and secretion of interleukin 1 are also necessary for T lymphocyte response to the presented antigen. Following antigen presentation, T lymphocyte clonal expansion occurs. Specific subsets of T lymphocytes develop that have antigen-specific immunoregulatory functions and that modulate the immune response (see Chap. 277).

Immunoreactive lymphocytes secrete mediators, and in response macrophages become activated and serve as the principal effector cells of tuberculin hypersensitivity. Peripheral blood monocytes from tuberculous patients have been shown to have several features characteristic of activated macrophages, including increased hexose monophosphate shunt activity, augmented surface adhesiveness, expression of characteristic membrane structures, and increased bactericidal activity. Animal studies have demonstrated that these features are T lymphocyte–dependent. Activated monocytes/macrophages are important immunoregulatory cells possessing suppressor functions.

In tuberculosis, aberrations of this carefully modulated state of hypersensitivity occur with some frequency and are recognizable in 15 percent of acutely ill patients. This has given rise to the suggestion that tuberculosis may present with an immunologic spectrum similar to that seen in leprosy but more subtly expressed. At one pole are patients with chronic cavitary disease, relatively chronic courses, and florid expression of tuberculin hypersensitivity. At the other pole are the rarely seen patients with cutaneous anergy, a few of whom have absence of granuloma formation and all other manifestations of cellular hypersensitivity, pancytopenia, widely disseminated disease, and a progressive downhill course. Although the delayed tuberculin skin reaction is the best-known manifestation of tuberculin hypersensitivity (see below), granuloma formation is probably its central and most important expression because it is important in containing the spread of infection.

Production of antibodies to protein and polysaccharide antigens of mycobacteria is readily demonstrated in tuberculosis. There is no evidence that these antibodies play a role in immunity, hypersensitivity, or pathogenesis.

CLINICAL MANIFESTATIONS   Primary tuberculosis   Primary tuberculous infection is usually asymptomatic. A nonspecific pneumonitis typically occurs in the lower or midlung zones. Hilar lymph node enlargement is usual and in children is sometimes sufficient to produce bronchial obstruction. In low-prevalence areas, primary infection may not occur until adulthood. It may progress directly to clinical disease that has the pathologic features of reactivation disease. In these persons, presentation as subapical pneumonia is common.

Reactivation tuberculosis   Reactivation tuberculosis is a chronic wasting disease, and in pulmonary tuberculosis, constitutional manifestations are often more prominent than respiratory symptoms. Weight loss and low-grade fever are common. Many patients present with typical drenching night sweats over the upper half of the body several times a week.

Pulmonary tuberculosis   Reactivation-type pulmonary tuberculosis has a predilection for the apical posterior segments of the upper lobes and the superior segments of the lower lobes of the lungs. The extent of disease varies from minimal infiltrates that produce no clinical illness and that are barely discernible on chest radiographs to massive involvement with extensive cavitation and debilitating constitutional and respiratory symptoms. In the absence of effective therapy, pulmonary tuberculosis pursues a chronic and progressive course. There are often long periods of stability and relative well-being, but in most patients these give way to episodes of disease progression with increasing involvement of lung parenchyma.

The onset of pulmonary tuberculosis is usually insidious, and illness may not be noted by the patient for some time. However, it is incorrect to view this onset as one of slow progression. In fact, pulmonary tuberculosis usually reaches its full extent within a few weeks. About one-third of patients will live long lives with chronic illness interspersed with periods of relative well-being. The overall death rate of untreated pulmonary tuberculosis approaches 60 percent, and the median course to death is about $2\frac{1}{2}$ years.

As pulmonary lesions progress, central necrosis occurs with development of caseation, so named because of the cheesy nature of necrotic material that only partly liquefies. Satellite lesions develop concomitantly. They can usually be recognized on chest x-ray films and are often helpful in distinguishing tuberculosis from pulmonary neoplasms. Necrotic material may empty into bronchi, with resulting cavitation of the nodular disease. Other parts of the lung may be seeded transbronchially, with the development of exudative lesions. In some patients, tuberculous pneumonia develops in a lobar or segmental pulmonary distribution. Occasionally, transbronchial spread following rupture of a tuberculous peribronchial lymph node into a bronchus leads to tuberculous pneumonia in the absence of other obvious disease. With the progression of pulmonary tuberculosis, the normal pulmonary architecture is lost. Fibrosis, volume loss, and upward contraction are typical. However, recently diseased areas may heal with relatively little destruction when effective chemotherapy is administered.

Pulmonary cavities may persist even though effective chemotherapy has resulted in apparent cure. In the absence of therapy, persistence of cavities is to be expected. Cavities may be a source of major hemoptysis, especially in the presence of continued active disease. Persistent terminal pulmonary arteries within cavities may be a source of profound bleeding (Rasmussen's aneurysm). Another cause of bleeding is an aspergilloma in a chronic tuberculous cavity, and bleeding in this instance may occur without persisting tuberculous disease. Rupture of a tuberculous cavity into the pleural space may lead to tuberculous empyema and bronchopleural fistula.

Chronic cough is the principal respiratory symptom. Sputum is usually scant and nonpurulent. Hemoptysis is frequent and is usually limited to blood streaking of the sputum. Massive, life-threatening hemoptysis is rare.

Findings on physical examination of the lung in patients with pulmonary tuberculosis are typically few and generally can be appreciated only in the presence of extensive disease. Rales that are accentuated or heard only posttussively are characteristic of apical disease. With extensive cavitation, amphoric breath sounds may be present. Dullness to percussion may sometimes be recognized in Krönig's isthmus and at the clavicles, reflecting extensive apical disease.

Extrapulmonary tuberculosis PLEURISY WITH EFFUSION Pleurisy with effusion results when the pleural space is seeded with *M. tuberculosis*. Following a peripheral primary infection, the pleural space may be contaminated by organisms that are transported lymphogenously to the pleura and then across the surface of the lung to the hilum. Pleural effusion occurs, sometimes massively, usually with substantial pleuritic pain. The onset of symptoms is often abrupt. The effusion is most frequently, but not invariably, unilateral. Classically, tuberculous pleurisy with effusion occurs in younger individuals in the absence of pulmonary tuberculosis. However, in the United States this disease presents in many individuals past the age of 35, and simultaneous pulmonary tuberculosis is present in about one-third of patients. The effusion is exudative in nature, and a protein concentration greater than 3.0 g/dL is the most characteristic feature of the pleural fluid. Lymphocytes usually, but not invariably, predominate among the pleural fluid cells. Mesothelial cells are rare. Needle biopsy of the parietal pleura may reveal granulomas, confirming the diagnosis of tuberculous pleurisy. The tuberculin skin test is negative in one-third of patients, either because the disease presents early before tuberculin reactivity develops or because this form of tuberculosis is particularly prone to aberrations of immunoregulation. Untreated, tuberculous pleurisy usually remits, but active pulmonary tuberculosis develops within 5 years in two-thirds of cases. Response to chemotherapy is good. Complete removal of pleural fluid is not necessary. There is rarely a need for surgical decortication.

Bronchopleural fistula and tuberculous empyema are catastrophic complications of untreated tuberculosis resulting from rupture of a pulmonary lesion into the pleural space. The diagnosis is usually not difficult, and acid-fast bacilli are usually readily demonstrated in the pleural exudate. Treatment consists of adequate surgical drainage and chemotherapy.

TUBERCULOUS PERICARDITIS AND PERITONITIS The pericardium and peritoneum may be the sites of tuberculosis. Pericarditis sometimes occurs in association with pleurisy and may represent an extension of that process. More commonly, the pericardium is seeded by drainage from an infected lymph node. Exudative effusion occurs,

and patients present with fever and pericardial pain. A friction rub may be present. Cardiac tamponade occasionally occurs. Chronic constrictive pericarditis is a late sequel. The diagnosis of tuberculous pericarditis is often difficult and sometimes requires thoracotomy for pericardial biopsy.

Tuberculous peritonitis results from hematogenous seeding of the peritoneum or entry of bacilli from an abdominal lymphatic or genitourinary organ source. As with other serositis, an exudative effusion occurs. The onset is usually insidious, and the disease is often mistaken for hepatic cirrhosis in alcoholic patients. As with tuberculous pericarditis, the diagnosis is often difficult, and recovery of the organism from paracentesis fluid is possible only in a minority of cases. Surgical biopsy may be necessary for diagnosis.

LARYNGEAL AND ENDOBRONCHIAL TUBERCULOSIS Tuberculosis of the larynx is usually seen in association with far-advanced pulmonary disease. Occasionally it occurs with only minimal pulmonary involvement. It results from seeding of the mucosal surface during expectoration. The disease progresses from a superficial laryngitis to ulceration and granuloma formation. The epiglottis and hypopharynx are occasionally involved. Hoarseness is the principal symptom of tuberculous laryngitis. In a similar fashion, the bronchial mucosa may be seeded, with resultant tuberculous bronchitis. Indeed, localized bronchitis in segmental bronchi leading to diseased portions of lung is common. Cough and minor hemoptysis are the chief clinical manifestations. Patients with tuberculous laryngitis and extensive bronchitis are usually highly infectious. These forms of disease respond rapidly to chemotherapy and have a favorable prognosis with treatment.

TUBERCULOUS ADENITIS *Scrofula* is chronic tuberculous lymphadenitis of the cervical lymph nodes. Any of the cervical nodes may be involved, but the anterior triangle of the neck just below the mandible is the most frequent site of disease. Tuberculous nodes are usually rubbery and not tender. With progression, they become harder and matted. Chronic draining fistulas may develop, but these are rare, and the course of this form of tuberculosis is usually indolent. The diagnosis is commonly established by surgical biopsy. Lymph node biopsy specimens obtained for this purpose should always be submitted for culture as well as histologic examination, and chemotherapy should be instituted at or before the time of surgery to avoid postoperative fistulas in the surgical wound site. Lymph nodes other than those in the cervical regions are less commonly involved in tuberculosis and account for about 35 percent of tuberculous adenitis.

In children, *M. scrofulaceum* and *M. intracellulare* are frequently the cause of scrofula. The onset of this disease is usually before 5 years of age. As with tuberculosis, lymph nodes high in the neck are most frequently involved. A single enlarged node is commonly the presenting manifestation. Constitutional symptoms are absent, and the adenitis usually is not tender. Progression is common, with necrosis of the node and the development of fistulous sinus tracts. The organisms involved are usually not susceptible to drugs, and treatment, if necessary, is surgical excision. Spontaneous resolution is usual after puberty.

SKELETAL TUBERCULOSIS Bone and joint disease is a not-infrequent manifestation of tuberculosis. Pott's disease, tuberculosis of the spine, usually involves the midthoracic spine. Tubercle bacilli reach the spine hematogenously or through lymphatic channels from the pleural space to paravertebral lymph nodes. Anterior erosion of vertebral bodies leads to collapse. The result is a sharply angulated kyphosis without scoliosis (gibbus deformity). Paraplegia may result. If there is no neurologic compromise, Pott's disease can be treated with chemotherapy. If the spine is unstable, surgical stabilization may be necessary. In the face of new paraparesis, immediate orthopedic consultation should be obtained. Paravertebral "cold abcesses" are a frequent concomitant of tuberculous spondylitis. They usually do not need to be drained, if adequate chemotherapy is given, unless they are very large. They may extend along fascial planes and point in the inguinal region or in other remote sites.

Tuberculosis of joints most frequently affects large weight-bearing joints such as the hips and knees. It responds well to immobilization and chemotherapy. Tuberculous synovitis may occur alone or in association with tuberculous arthritis.

GENITOURINARY TUBERCULOSIS Genitourinary tuberculosis may involve any part of either the male or female genitourinary system. Renal tuberculosis usually presents initially as microscopic pyuria and hematuria with a sterile routine urine culture. The diagnosis may be established by finding tubercle bacilli on culture of the urine. As the disease progresses, cavitation of the renal parenchyma occurs. In the past, nephrectomy was often performed for renal tuberculosis. However, with adequate chemotherapy, surgical removal of a kidney is almost never necessary. The ureters and bladder may be infected by tubular spread of the organism, and ureteral stricture may result.

Tuberculous salpingitis often results in female sterility. Genital tuberculosis in the male most commonly involves the prostate, seminal vesicles, and epididymis. Prostatic and epididymal tuberculosis is characterized by nontender nodular induration detectable by physical examination. The presentation of genital tuberculosis in both males and females is insidious, with chronic or subacute symptoms. The diagnosis is usually made by culture of acid-fast bacilli.

MENINGEAL TUBERCULOSIS The leptomeninges are relatively frequently seeded by organisms that disseminate during primary infection. In young children, tuberculous meningitis may develop at this time. This chronic infection is manifested not only by meningeal signs but also frequently by cranial nerve signs, reflecting a tendency for basilar distribution of the infection. High protein content, low glucose, and lymphocytosis are characteristic of the cerebrospinal fluid. Prior to the advent of effective chemotherapy, this disease was almost always fatal. Chemotherapy with isoniazid, rifampin, and ethambutol is effective. Intrathecal drug administration is not necessary. Late reactivation of meningeal tuberculous foci may produce disease in adults who have no evidence of pulmonary tuberculosis. Tuberculomas of the meninges or brain may become evident in adult life many years after primary infection, and seizures are often their major clinical manifestation.

OCULAR TUBERCULOSIS Tuberculosis may involve almost any part of the eye. Chorioretinitis and uveitis are the most common manifestations. The diagnosis of tuberculosis of the eye is extremely difficult to establish, and most diagnoses are presumptive. The manifestations cannot be distinguished clinically from sarcoidosis or systemic mycoses, but phlyctenular keratitis strongly suggests tuberculosis. Phlyctenular lesions are thought to represent manifestations of tuberculin hypersensitivity rather than bacterial infection. Choroid tubercles are often present in patients with miliary tuberculosis, and their recognition may be helpful in the diagnosis of miliary tuberculosis. Ocular tuberculosis responds well to standard chemotherapy.

GASTROINTESTINAL TUBERCULOSIS The stomach is extremely resistant to tuberculous infection, and a large number of virulent tubercle bacilli can be swallowed without establishing an infection. Rarely, usually concomitantly with extensive cavitary pulmonary disease and severe debility, swallowed organisms reach the terminal ileum and cecum and tuberculous ileitis develops. Chronic diarrhea and fistula development are the principal manifestations, and the disease is difficult to distinguish from Crohn's disease. Tuberculosis of the liver can occur as an isolated event, but it is usually a manifestation of miliary tuberculosis.

ADRENAL TUBERCULOSIS Hematogenous seeding of the adrenal gland is probably fairly common, but disease due to this infection is rare and usually seen only in association with long-standing and extensive pulmonary tuberculosis. The cortex is most frequently involved, and adrenal insufficiency may result. In contrast, carcinomatous involvement of the adrenal cortex, even though very extensive, rarely produces clinical adrenal insufficiency.

CUTANEOUS TUBERCULOSIS Tuberculous infection of the skin is rare in the absence of long-standing, untreated disease elsewhere. Lupus vulgaris is a granulomatous disease of the skin, and it responds well to treatment. Diagnosis is made by skin biopsy. Tuberculin

hypersensitivity manifestations are common. Erythema nodosum may be present, although it much more commonly results from other granulomatous diseases, including sarcoidosis and systemic mycoses. Tuberculids are poorly understood papular lesions of tuberculin hypersensitivity.

MILIARY TUBERCULOSIS Miliary tuberculosis results from widespread hematogenous dissemination. It often presents as a perplexing fever, sometimes with a double quotidian curve, often accompanied by anemia and splenomegaly. Miliary tuberculosis is apt to be more fulminating in children than in adults.

Classically, miliary tuberculosis develops following hematogenous dissemination at the time of primary infection, and patients present with no antecedent history of tuberculosis. Lesions develop synchronously throughout the body. Patients become ill before radiographic changes, which take 4 to 6 weeks to become recognizable, appear. The typical radiologic findings are soft, uniformly distributed, fine nodules throughout both lung fields. They often can be recognized first on a lateral chest film or an underpenetrated posteroanterior radiograph. The diagnosis is difficult, and expectorated sputum rarely contains organisms. Transbronchial biopsy and liver biopsy are usually, but not invariably, positive. Bone marrow biopsy is positive in approximately two-thirds of patients.

When hematogenous dissemination occurs in a previously diseased individual, a much more fulminant course results. Prostration is common. Diffuse but ragged nodular infiltrates develop within a few weeks, and the sputum is often positive. The diagnosis is rarely difficult.

The subacute form and the rare chronic form of miliary tuberculosis often present major problems in diagnosis. These types of disease are usually attributed to repeated seeding of the bloodstream from a tuberculous focus. A very rare form of disseminated tuberculosis occurs with widespread dissemination of disease, a massive number of bacteria in tissues, complete absence of granuloma formation, and pancytopenia. It is termed *disseminated nonreactive tuberculosis* and has a poor prognosis, even with chemotherapy.

Tuberculin anergy is common in miliary tuberculosis, and a negative skin test should not be a deterrent to considering this diagnosis. Anergy may or may not extend to other delayed hypersensitivity antigens. In vitro cultured leukocyte studies also demonstrate hyporesponsiveness, and experimental data suggest that this anergy is mediated by monocytes with suppressor function. With treatment and stabilization of patients with miliary tuberculosis, tuberculin hypersensitivity is restored.

Without treatment, the prognosis for miliary tuberculosis is grave. This disease responds well to chemotherapy, however, and can be treated with the same drug regimens employed for other forms of tuberculosis.

SILICOTUBERCULOSIS Tuberculosis occurs with increased frequency in patients with silicosis and possibly in patients with some other pneumoconioses. The diagnosis is often difficult because of confounding radiographic changes due to the underlying pneumoconiosis. Even with therapy, the prognosis is less favorable than in other patients. Patients with silicotuberculosis should be treated for longer than customary periods. Patients with silicosis who are tuberculin-positive should be considered for isoniazid prophylaxis even when they do not meet other criteria for this form of therapy. Isoniazid prophylaxis may be less effective in persons with silicosis.

TUBERCULOSIS IN AIDS Tuberculosis is a major opportunistic infection of HIV-infected persons. For individuals infected first with *M. tuberculosis* and then with HIV, the risk of developing tuberculosis is 5 to 10 percent per year. When these infections are acquired in the reverse order, the association is even more dramatic: Tuberculosis develops in as many as half of HIV-infected persons following primary infection with *M. tuberculosis*, usually within a few months. In the United States, 3 to 4 percent of tuberculosis patients are HIV-seropositive. In a survey in New York City, 42 percent of hospitalized males with tuberculosis were HIV-seropositive; intravenous drug users made up the majority of these patients. In Africa, tuberculosis is the single most important infectious complication of AIDS, and in Kampala, Uganda, 66 percent of hospitalized tuberculosis patients are HIV-seropositive. In the Ivory Coast, death has been attributed to tuberculosis in 40 percent of autopsied patients with AIDS. The potential epidemiologic impact of the HIV pandemic on the incidence of tuberculosis in areas of high tuberculosis prevalence can scarcely be overstated. New case rates for tuberculosis may be as high as 2000 per 100,000 population by the end of the twentieth century in some parts of sub-Saharan Africa.

Lymphocytes and monocytes, the primary defense cells mustered against tuberculous infection, are destroyed by HIV. What is remarkable, however, is that the failure of antituberculous immunity is manifest early, before severe depletion of CD4 T lymphocytes. Tuberculin skin test reactivity may be lost by HIV-infected individuals who are still healthy and free of clinical AIDS, yet as many as two-thirds of HIV-infected patients with tuberculosis have positive tuberculin skin tests. Although tuberculosis may develop at any time during the course of HIV infection in persons also infected with *M. tuberculosis*, it commonly precedes the first other AIDS-defining opportunistic infection by 1 to 3 months. CD4 T lymphocyte counts in HIV-seropositive tuberculosis patients are typically in the range of 150 to 200 cells per cubic millimeter, with considerable individual variation.

Nearly half of AIDS patients with tuberculosis have extrapulmonary forms of the disease, with tuberculous lymphadenitis, usually in the anterior neck, predominating. Among AIDS patients with pulmonary tuberculosis, nearly half have atypical roentgenographic findings, with diffuse fine infiltrates, pneumonic infiltrates, hilar adenopathy and perihilar infiltrates, and pleural effusions frequently seen. Some AIDS patients with sputum-positive tuberculosis have normal chest radiographs. Mycobacterial infections other than tuberculosis are frequently seen in patients with AIDS. In the United States, approximately half of AIDS patients develop disseminated disease due to *M. avium*, usually late in the course of AIDS (see Chap. 279). *M. avium* disease is virtually unknown among AIDS patients in sub-Saharan Africa.

DIAGNOSIS Bacteriology The diagnosis of tuberculosis is established when tubercle bacilli are identified in the sputum, urine, body fluids, or tissues of the patient. For the majority of patients who have pulmonary tuberculosis, the diagnosis can be established most readily by sputum examination. The staining characteristics of *M. tuberculosis* allow its ready identification in clinical specimens, although it is usually present in small numbers so that prolonged study of stained slides is necessary. A slender (less than 0.5 μm diameter), sometimes curved, often polychromatically beaded rod, it frequently presents in clinical specimens as pairs or clumps of a few organisms lying side by side. When stained with fluorescent auramine-rhodamine, tubercle bacilli can be seen under usual high-dry (100×) magnification. A more definitive stain consists of carbolfuchsin; this stain requires meticulous scanning with oil-immersion (1000×) microscopy. Sputum culture adds to the diagnostic yield and also permits the specific identification of acid-fast bacilli and the determination of drug susceptibility. Primary isolation from clinical specimens usually requires 4 to 8 weeks on classical media. Radiometric techniques using highly selective media allow cultivation in 1 or 2 weeks, but confirmation of the identity of an isolated organism may require additional time. Mycobacteria are aerobes. Modern culture techniques are excellent, and there is no longer reason to inoculate guinea pigs for primary isolation. Niacin production characterizes *M. tuberculosis* and helps to distinguish it from other species. Nucleic acid hybridization probes have been developed for the rapid identification of mycobacteria in cultures.

If expectorated sputum is not readily available for examination, expectoration may be induced or samples obtained by nasotracheal aspiration. Early-morning gastric aspiration provides excellent material for culture and for smear examination. Although nonpathogenic mycobacteria are occasionally found in gastric aspirates, their number is so small as to preclude their appearance in smears of gastric

aspirates. Bronchoscopy has a high yield in the diagnosis of tuberculosis, but in the absence of other considerations, it should not be undertaken unless multiple attempts by simpler means have failed and the diagnosis remains obscure.

The diagnostic yield of sputum smear and culture is directly related to the extent of pulmonary disease. About one-third of patients in whom a positive sputum culture can be obtained will have acid-fast bacilli identified on an initial sputum smear. With repeated examinations on separate days, this figure rises to about two-thirds. There is rarely an indication for obtaining more than five sputum examinations. However, only about one-third of patients with minimal pulmonary tuberculosis will have a positive sputum smear, even after multiple examinations. If there is no lesion visible on the chest radiograph, then there is usually little reason to obtain sputum examinations for tubercle bacilli. Conversely, if a patient with extensive cavitary disease or an exudative pneumonic process has a negative sputum smear, diagnoses other than tuberculosis should be sought.

Newer methods of rapid diagnosis Serologic tests for the diagnosis of tuberculosis that are based on the recognition of serum IgG antibody to selected mycobacterial antigens and that use enzyme-linked immunosorbent (ELISA) techniques have been developed and appear to offer promise, with sensitivity similar to that of sputum microscopy. Serology may have its greatest application in children and in patients with extrapulmonary tuberculosis–i.e., in cases where sputum is not available. Gene amplification by the polymerase chain reaction (PCR) has been used with great sensitivity and specificity to identify mycobacterial DNA. If this technique can be applied successfully in routine clinical laboratories, it offers great promise for rapid diagnosis. In reference laboratories with sufficient instrumentation, high-performance chromatographic techniques are capable of rapidly identifying mycobacteria by their characteristic lipids.

Radiology The chest radiograph is an important tool for both diagnosis and evaluation of tuberculosis. Healed primary lesions may leave a small peripheral nodule that may calcify with the passing of years. The Ghon complex comprises a calcified peripheral nodule together with a calcified hilar lymph node. Similar lesions result from histoplasmosis and coccidioidomycosis, and it is not possible to distinguish radiologically between healed primary lesions of these diseases. Calcification of right paratracheal lymph nodes is seen more commonly in histoplasmosis.

Multinodular infiltration in the apical posterior segments of the upper lobes and superior segments of the lower lobes is the most typical lesion of pulmonary tuberculosis. Cavitation is frequently present and is usually accompanied by substantial amounts of infiltration in the same pulmonary segments. Laminagrams are often helpful in recognizing satellite nodular lesions, which are characteristic of tuberculosis and not usually seen in carcinoma. Lordotic views may be of help in evaluating disease obscured by the intersection of the third or fourth posterior rib, second anterior rib, and clavicle. They are of little use in evaluating disease located elsewhere. As tuberculosis becomes inactive or heals, fibrotic scarring becomes apparent on the chest radiograph. There is frequently volume loss in the involved upper lobes, and upward and medial retraction of hilar markings is common. Fibrotic lesions may develop calcifications. The activity of tuberculosis may be judged from serial films. It is never wise to judge tuberculosis to be inactive on the basis of a single chest radiograph.

Clinical pathology Other than bacteriologic examinations, clinical laboratory tests contribute relatively little to the diagnosis of tuberculosis. Peripheral blood monocytosis in the range of 8 to 12 percent is common. The erythrocyte sedimentation rate is usually elevated, and modest anemia may be present.

Tuberculin test The intracutaneous tuberculin skin test is a reliable means of recognizing prior mycobacterial infection. The preferred antigen is tuberculin purified protein derivative (PPD), and the intermediate-strength dose should be used. In North America this is 5 tuberculin units of material, which is standardized by bioassay (bioequivalent) against reference antigen designated PPD-S. In other parts of the world, PPD lot RT-23, prepared in Denmark and widely distributed by the World Health Organization, is available. A gravimetric unit has been assigned to this material, and 2 units of this PPD is equivalent to 5 units of PPD-S. Diluents for PPD should contain polysorbate 80, which decreases loss of potency due to adsorption onto glass and plastic surfaces. Multiple puncture devices offer much convenience but do so at the cost of decreased specificity. They can be recommended only as screening tests, and positive tests should be repeated using intracutaneous PPD.

The tuberculin test is usually applied on the forearm. Reactions should be read by measuring the transverse diameter of induration as detected by gentle palpation at 48 to 72 h. Patients with tuberculosis have normally distributed reaction sizes, with the mean and mode at 17 mm. Infected but healthy, nondiseased individuals have similarly distributed reactions. A reaction to PPD is presumptive evidence of current or prior mycobacterial infection.

Tuberculin hypersensitivity may result from contact with nonpathogenic environmental mycobacteria, and this nonspecific reactivity may confound the interpretation of tuberculin tests. Nonspecific tuberculin reactivity is rarely found in northern climates, and in such areas all reactivity to PPD can be considered to reflect infection with *M. tuberculosis*. In many warm and humid climatic zones, including all the coastal areas of the southeastern United States, nonspecific tuberculin reactivity is common. In such regions it is customary to consider reactions smaller than 10 mm as not significant and attribute them to cross reactivity with environmental mycobacterial antigens. However, considering smaller reactions as not significant always incurs the risk of missing some reactions which bespeak infection with *M. tuberculosis*. A reasonable and pragmatic approach to the interpretation of tuberculin skin test reactions is to consider any reaction positive in HIV-infected persons; any reaction of ≥5 mm positive in persons likely to be infected, especially household contacts of tuberculous patients; reactions of ≥10 mm positive in persons from population groups at elevated risk of tuberculosis; and reactions of ≥15 mm positive in persons from low-risk general populations, especially in geographic areas known to have a high prevalence of nonspecific tuberculin reactivity.

Repeated skin testing may boost reaction size, whether the primary reactivity was directed to *M. tuberculosis* or was nonspecific. Caution must be used in attributing a small increase in reactivity to new infection. It is well established, however, that repeated skin testing with PPD does not lead to positive reactions in uninfected persons. Positive reactions do not occur as a result of allergy to components of the diluent. Tuberculin reactivity wanes with advancing age, and the booster phenomenon may be useful in this situation. For example, if an older person fails to react to initial testing, repeat testing with intermediate-strength PPD may be done after 7 to 10 days. A reaction at this time should be accepted as significant.

PPD is also available in a second strength that contains 50 times the amount of PPD in intermediate-strength material. Except as a test for anergy, this product has little use. Because PPD at this strength so readily elicits nonspecific reactivity, a positive reaction to second-strength PPD is much more apt to give misinformation than to contribute to the correct diagnosis. A first-strength PPD is also available. It contains one-fifth the amount of PPD of intermediate PPD and is not useful clinically.

Anergy is the paradoxical absence of dermal tuberculin reactivity in infected persons. It occurs in association with a number of disease states and in immunosuppressed individuals. It also occurs in as many as 15 percent of tuberculous patients with newly active pulmonary disease. In these persons, tuberculin reactivity reappears with stabilization of the disease process. One-half of patients with miliary tuberculosis and one-third of patients with newly diagnosed tuberculous pleurisy have negative tuberculin tests. It has become common practice in many medical centers to use a battery of delayed hypersensitivity antigens as controls for tuberculin tests in demonstrating anergy. However, antigens standardized for this purpose are not available, and tuberculin anergy may be antigen-specific. False-negative tuberculin tests may result from technical errors, including subcutaneous injection, use of outdated PPD, and permitting PPD to remain in syringes before use. Such errors should not be mistaken for anergy.

TREATMENT The modern treatment of tuberculosis is based on the administration of effective drugs. In the presence of adequate chemotherapy, hospitalization, rest, and improved diet do not contribute to achieving cures. In order to prevent the emergence of drug-resistant mutants, which are present initially in very small numbers, at least two effective drugs are always required. Because of the long generation time of mycobacteria and their long periods of metabolic inactivity, prolonged courses of drug therapy are always necessary. Treatment regimens do not differ for pulmonary and extrapulmonary tuberculosis.

Table 130-1 presents dosage and toxicity information on drugs currently in use for the treatment of tuberculosis. Table 130-2 describes several effective treatment regimens. Daily therapy with regimens including isoniazid and rifampin for 9 to 12 months represents the most effective treatment available and is capable of achieving a favorable outcome in 99 percent of patients. Many experts add a third drug initially until the results of sensitivity tests become available; pyrazinamide is the optimal third drug, and ethambutol is also effective. In developing countries where drug costs are a limiting factor, the extremely low-cost combination of isoniazid and thioacetazone for 12 to 18 months provides a regimen that can achieve 80 to 90 percent cure rates.

An accepted hypothesis states that tubercle bacilli exist in tuberculous patients in three pools—a metabolically active extracellular pool and relatively metabolically inactive intracellular and necrotic caseum pools. Only rifampin is bactericidal for all these pools, and it may not be necessary to continue rifampin-containing regimens for as long as other regimens that rely on organisms entering the metabolically active pool to achieve sterilization. Isoniazid and streptomycin are both bactericidal against extracellular, metabolically active organisms. Against intracellular organisms, isoniazid and pyrazinamide are bactericidal and streptomycin is inactive. In clinical trials, pyrazinamide has been found to be particularly useful during the first 2 months of treatment. Ethambutol is only bacteriostatic.

TABLE 130-1 Drugs used in the treatment of tuberculosis

Drug	Usual daily adult dose	Major toxicity
Isoniazid	300 mg	Hepatitis, peripheral neuropathy, drug fever
Rifampin	600 mg	Hepatitis, influenza-like syndrome, thrombocytopenia (rare)
Streptomycin	0.75–1 g	Deafness, loss of vestibular function, loss of renal function
Pyrazinamide	1.5–2 g	Hepatitis, hyperuricemia
Ethambutol	15 mg/kg	Optic neuritis (extremely rare at this dose)
p-Aminosalicylic acid	12 g	Diarrhea, hepatitis, hypersensitivity reactions
Ethionamide	1 g	Hepatitis
Cycloserine	1 g	Depression, personality changes, psychosis, convulsions
Thioacetazone	150 mg	Exfoliative dermatitis, hepatitis
Kanamycin	1 g	Deafness, loss of renal function, loss of vestibular function (rare)
Capreomycin	1 g	Deafness, loss of vestibular function, loss of renal function
Viomycin	1 g	Deafness, loss of vestibular function, loss of renal function

TABLE 130-2　Effective drug regimens for the treatment of tuberculosis

Regimen (adult drug dose)	Comment
Isoniazid (300 mg) and rifampin (600 mg) daily for 9–12 months	An effective regimen for initial treatment of patients unless drug resistance is suspected.
Isoniazid (300 mg) and ethambutol (15 mg/kg) daily for 12–18 months	The least toxic effective regimen. Suitable for patients with minimal disease.
Isoniazid (300 mg) and thioacetazone (150 mg) daily for 12–18 months	The least expensive effective regimen. Streptomycin (0.75–1 g) may be added daily for the first 8 weeks to increase effectiveness, but this doubles both cost and toxicity.
Isoniazid (300 mg), rifampin (600 mg), pyrazinamide (2 g), with or without streptomycin (1 g) or ethambutol (15 mg/kg) daily for 2 months followed by one of the following:	Initial intensive phase for short-course regimens. Short-course regimens have only been demonstrated to be effective under conditions of close patient supervision.
a　Isoniazid (300 mg) and rifampin (600 g) daily for 4 months	
b　Isoniazid (300 mg), rifampin (600 mg), and streptomycin (1 g) twice weekly for 6 months	Suitable for fully supervised therapy.
c　Isoniazid (300 mg) and thioacetazone (150 mg) daily for 6 months	Inexpensive.
Isoniazid (300 mg) and rifampin (600 mg) daily for 1 month followed by isoniazid (900 mg) and rifampin (600 mg) twice weekly for 8 months	Effectiveness demonstrated in ambulatory treatment programs in Arkansas. Has not been compared with other regimens in clinical trials.

The major problem in tuberculosis treatment programs is patient default. It is unusual for a tuberculosis clinic to achieve a default rate of less than 15 percent, and default rates of 40 to 60 percent are common. Unfortunately, these rates tend to be highest in those parts of the world where high tuberculosis prevalence is coupled with limited resources. Default leads not only to treatment failure but also to the emergence and transmission of drug-resistant organisms. Since most patient defaults occur within the first 6 months of the treatment program, short-course therapy has been employed to mitigate the consequences of default. This strategy will be successful only if the resources conserved by shortening treatment are used to maintain patient compliance. Completely supervised regimens are often successful for noncompliant patients, but their widespread use is costly. Twice-weekly drug administration is effective and facilitates patient supervision.

Short-course treatment programs are best considered as consisting of two phases. An initial 2-month intensive phase of daily therapy should include isoniazid, rifampin, and pyrazinamide and also may include either streptomycin or ethambutol. A consolidation phase of daily therapy with isoniazid and one other drug should be continued for an additional 4 months, and preferably 6 months. In the United States, a regimen of isoniazid 300 mg and rifampin 600 mg daily for 1 month, followed by isoniazid 900 mg and rifampin 600 mg twice weekly for 8 months, has been highly effective. Patients with AIDS should be treated in the same manner as immunocompetent individuals with tuberculosis. Response to therapy is favorable in these patients, although they have more frequent drug reactions, particularly skin rashes. The optimal duration of therapy for these patients is not known, although it is probably wise to avoid short regimens. AIDS patients should be followed for relapse after therapy for the rest of their lives.

Relapses after successful therapy should be less than 1 percent. Since these few relapses usually present with symptoms and are almost never found by routine x-rays, patients may be discharged from follow-up at the completion of therapy. Relapses are more frequent after short-course therapy, usually occurring within the first year, and follow-up for such patients for 1 or 2 years is justified.

Symptomatic improvement occurs within the first 2 to 3 weeks in most patients. Clearing of infiltrates on the chest radiograph may not occur within the first month but usually is rapidly recognized between the second and fourth months. Most patients reach a point of radiologic stability between 3 and 6 months. Therapy usually should be continued for 6 months after this point of stability is reached, even if this means prolonging the planned period of treatment. Sputum conversion occurs in most patients within the first 2 months. The fact that an individual patient responds more slowly than the norm should not necessarily be a cause for concern, provided the patient is taking effective drugs.

Since there are alternative effective drug regimens, toxicity becomes a factor in choice of therapy. Major individual drug toxicities are listed in Table 130-1; the toxicity of greatest concern is hepatitis. Toxicity sufficient to require change in regimen occurs in 3 to 5 percent of patients taking isoniazid and rifampin and in about 1.5 percent of patients taking isoniazid and ethambutol. The toxicity of isoniazid and thioacetazone appears to vary with the racial characteristics of the patient population. It reaches about 30 percent in Oriental groups but is only 2 to 5 percent in other populations. It approaches 25 percent in HIV-infected persons. Routine monitoring of serum enzymes or other blood tests reflecting liver disease is of little use and is not recommended. Normal values do not predict absence of toxicity, and serum enzymes in patients taking isoniazid may rise transiently to three times normal values without the subsequent development of hepatitis. A well-educated patient and an alert treatment supervisor are the principal safeguards against drug hepatitis. If medication is discontinued during the prodromal phase or promptly with the onset of jaundice, drug hepatitis can be expected to resolve without untoward incident. Isoniazid toxicity is probably due to toxic metabolites of acetyl isoniazid. Induction of cytochrome P-450 enzymes by alcohol or long-acting barbiturates predisposes to isoniazid hepatitis. Isoniazid also causes a peripheral neuropathy that is preventable and reversible by the administration of pyridoxine. Patients with such predisposing factors as old age, diabetes, alcoholism, and malnutrition should be given pyridoxine concomitantly with isoniazid; the usual dose is 50 mg/d.

Isoniazid is safe in pregnant patients. Data are less complete for other drugs but suggest that both ethambutol and rifampin are acceptable. Rifampin should always be used if the tuberculosis is disseminated or very extensive. Streptomycin should not be used in pregnancy because of the risk of fetal ototoxicity. Tuberculosis often pursues an unfavorable course during and just after pregnancy, and treatment of a pregnant woman should never be deferred. It is reasonable, however, to postpone isoniazid prophylaxis until just after delivery.

Patients with chronic renal failure also present special treatment problems, and these patients have tuberculosis case rates approximately 10 times those of the general population. Isoniazid is acetylated to an inactive form by the liver and then excreted by the kidney. Acetyl isoniazid is the precursor of hydrazines, which are probably hepatotoxic. Both isoniazid and acetyl isoniazid are not bound by plasma proteins and are dialyzable. In patients with renal failure, isoniazid should be reduced to 5 mg/kg body weight (300 mg in adults) two or three times weekly. Patients on dialysis should receive the drug following each dialysis. Ethambutol behaves like isoniazid, except that it is excreted by the kidney as the active drug. As with isoniazid, the usual daily dose should be given at longer intervals, and administration should follow dialysis. Optic nerve toxicity of ethambutol appears to be related not to intermittent high drug levels but to sustained high drug levels. Patients with renal failure who are receiving ethambutol should have their color vision and visual acuity monitored regularly. Rifampin is protein-bound, nondialyzable, and excreted in the bile by the liver. No change in dose or interval is necessary in the presence of renal failure. Caution should be exercised in using rifampin in patients with hepatic failure.

Faced with relapse in a previously treated patient, a major concern should be the possibility of drug resistance, and resistance studies of the organism should be obtained in a competent reference laboratory. In one-third of patients who relapse after adequate regular drug therapy, the relapse is caused by drug-resistant organisms. If, however, the patient took the drug sporadically or the previous regimen was inadequate, then the likelihood of drug resistance is about two chances in three. Therapy for presumed drug-resistant tuberculosis should be instituted with two drugs that the patient has not taken previously, provided that one of these two new drugs is isoniazid or rifampin. Otherwise, four drugs should be used, including as many new drugs as possible. When resistance studies become available, the regimen should be modified appropriately. It is beneficial to continue isoniazid even when laboratory studies indicate drug resistance. In general, all retreatment regimens should be closely supervised and directed by physicians with special experience with this problem.

Primary drug resistance should be suspected in patients who appear to have contracted their infection from patients with known drug resistance or with known noncompliance and in patients who come from areas where drug resistance is common. In the United States, this group includes immigrants from Haiti, Southeast Asia, and many areas of Latin America. Multidrug-resistant strains of tuberculosis have been seen with increasing frequency in the United States, especially in New York City, where 20 to 25 percent of newly diagnosed patients with tuberculosis currently have organisms resistant to both isoniazid and rifampin. While laboratory resistance studies are pending, drug therapy should be dictated by the prior treatment of the suspected index case. In immigrant populations, most of the drug resistance of concern is to isoniazid. In this circumstance, therapy should be initiated with isoniazid, rifampin, pyrazinamide, and ethambutol. One or two of these drugs may be discontinued when resistance studies become available. Treatment of suspected multidrug-resistant tuberculosis is difficult and should only be made on consultation with local experts or public health authorities. Some experts recommend that a fluoroquinolone be added to initial regimens, with final decisions on therapy made when drug resistance studies are completed. Other possibilities for a fifth drug include streptomycin, cycloserine, or ethionamide.

PREVENTION Chemoprophylaxis In one of the largest controlled clinical trials ever conducted, 1 year of isoniazid has been shown to be effective in reducing the incidence of tuberculosis in tuberculin-positive individuals presumed to have been infected with *M. tuberculosis*. The benefit of isoniazid prophylaxis has been demonstrated so clearly that the question of its use now hinges primarily on the risk of drug toxicity, chiefly hepatitis.

In administering isoniazid prophylaxis, highest priority should be assigned to treating immunosuppressed and HIV-infected persons, household contacts of persons with active tuberculosis, and persons known to have become infected within the preceding year. The risks of developing tuberculosis in these three groups are, respectively, 5 to 10 percent per year, 0.5 percent per year, and 3 percent during the first year. Particular attention should be given to treating children in these categories. Prophylaxis of childhood household contacts with isoniazid should be started immediately. After 3 months of therapy, the child should be skin-tested with intermediate-strength PPD. If the skin test is negative at that time, isoniazid may be discontinued. If it is positive, 12 months of prophylaxis should be completed.

Younger individuals benefit most from isoniazid prophylaxis because the drug is most effective when the infection is recent and because older individuals often have already outlived a substantial part of their risk. The risk of hepatitis rises with age, reaching approximately 2 percent by the seventh decade. Cost-benefit analyses with large data bases have shown that there is a 1:1 ratio of cases of tuberculosis prevented and hepatitis caused at age 45 when individuals without added risks are considered. Based on this calculation, there is a general consensus that all persons younger than age 35 with a positive tuberculin reaction should receive isoniazid 300 mg/d for 1 year.

It is also possible to develop criteria for the prophylactic use of isoniazid in older persons with remote tuberculosis, either known historically or evident radiographically, who have never received adequate chemotherapy. The annual risk of tuberculosis in such persons is at least 0.5 percent. Isoniazid 300 mg/d should be given for 1 year to all persons in this category who have a life expectancy greater than 10 years. In compliant adults with fibrotic residuals of untreated tuberculosis visible on roentgenograms, 1 year of isoniazid prophylaxis reduced disease during the subsequent 5 years by 75 percent, and 6 months of isoniazid reduced disease by 65 percent. Others at high risk for the development of tuberculosis include tuberculin-positive individuals with AIDS or Hodgkin's disease (both of which alter T lymphocyte–mediated immunity), patients with silicosis (which affects macrophage function), and persons who are (1) receiving immunosuppressive agents or glucocorticoids chronically or (2) suffering from renal failure. As with therapy for active tuberculosis, monitoring serum enzymes is not useful in patients receiving isoniazid prophylaxis.

BCG vaccination Bacillus Calmette-Guérin (BCG) is an attenuated strain of *M. bovis* that has been given to more than 2 billion persons as a vaccine against tuberculosis. It is clearly safe, but its efficacy is in some dispute. In some controlled studies it offered little or no protection. However, even then, the disseminated forms of tuberculosis, which have such high mortalities among children, were virtually eliminated. While final judgment on the efficacy of BCG must be reserved, its continued use in high-prevalence areas appears justified.

BCG vaccination induces tuberculin hypersensitivity. However, the dermal reaction to PPD is usually not as large as that which follows natural infection, usually does not persist as long, and varies from strain to strain of vaccine. Individuals with large PPD reactions persisting for many years after vaccination should be viewed as infected and considered for isoniazid prophylaxis.

CONTROL PROGRAMS In most low-prevalence areas, such as North America, resources are relatively abundant and disease occurrence is mostly sporadic. Increasingly, tuberculosis is being seen in microepidemics, often centered in family groups or congregate housing facilities. Immigrant groups and residents and employees of nursing homes are at high risk. Homeless shelters and correctional institutions are frequent sites of transmission of infection. Central to any program is an efficient case-reporting and registry system. Contact investigation must be carried out effectively and is especially important when index cases occur in children. The major modality for decreasing the spread of infection is chemotherapy for all infectious patients. Chemoprophylaxis is necessary for contacts.

At the other end of the spectrum are high-prevalence areas with few or no resources for tuberculosis control. The single most effective measure in this setting is a network of ambulatory tuberculosis treatment centers that provide diagnosis by direct sputum smear and standardized drug therapy. Successful treatment must entail no cost to the patient. Tuberculosis diagnostic and treatment programs should be integrated into national health programs, under expert supervision. Treatment records should be maintained, but complex registries are of little value.

In high-prevalence areas, BCG vaccine should be offered to every individual under age 15 or 20 without prior tuberculin testing. Older individuals can be assumed to have been infected already. Before a mass BCG campaign is initiated, planning should begin for continuing vaccination of newborns or young schoolchildren. Community-wide isoniazid prophylaxis programs have not been successful.

REFERENCES

AMERICAN THORACIC SOCIETY: Treatment of tuberculosis and tuberculosis infection in adults and children. Am Rev Respir Dis 134:355, 1986

——: Mycobacterioses and the acquired immunodeficiency syndrome. Am Rev Respir Dis 136:492, 1987

——: Diagnostic standards and classification of tuberculosis. Am Rev Respir Dis 142:725, 1990

BRUDNEY K, DOBKIN J: Resurgent tuberculosis in New York City: Human immunodeficiency virus, homelessness, and the decline of tuberculosis control programs. Am Rev Respir Dis 144:745, 1991

COMSTOCK GW, EDWARDS PQ: The competing risks of tuberculosis and hepatitis for adult tuberculin reactors. Am Rev Respir Dis 111:573, 1975

———— et al: The tuberculin skin test. Am Rev Respir Dis 124:356, 1981

————: Epidemiology of tuberculosis. Am Rev Respir Dis 125(suppl):8, 1982

EDWARDS LB et al: An atlas of sensitivity to tuberculin, PPD-B, and histoplasmin in the United States. Am Rev Respir Dis 99(suppl):1, 1969

GLASSROTH J et al: Tuberculosis in the 1980s. N Engl J Med 302:1441, 1980

GROSSET J: Bacteriologic basis of short-course chemotherapy for tuberculosis. Clin Chest Med 1:231, 1980

GRZYBOWSKI S, ENARSON DA: The fate of cases of pulmonary tuberculosis under various treatment programmes. Bull Int Union Tuberc 53:70, 1978

MURRAY JF: The white plague: Down and out, or up and coming. Am Rev Respir Dis 140:1788, 1989

————: Cursed duet: HIV infection and tuberculosis. Respiration 57:210, 1990

SELWYN PA et al: A prospective study of the risk of tuberculosis among intravenous users with human immunodeficiency virus infection. N Engl J Med 320:545, 1989

SNIDER DE, JR: The tuberculin skin test. Am Rev Respir Dis 125(suppl):108, 1982

STEAD WW et al: Tuberculosis as an endemic and nosocomial infection among the elderly in nursing homes. N Engl J Med 312:1483, 1985

tenDAM HG et al: Present knowledge of immunization against tuberculosis. Bull WHO 54:255, 1976

131 LEPROSY (HANSEN'S DISEASE)

RICHARD A. MILLER

DEFINITION AND ETIOLOGY Leprosy (Hansen's disease) is a chronic granulomatous infection of humans which attacks superficial tissues, especially the skin and peripheral nerves. *Mycobacterium leprae* is the causal agent of leprosy. It is an acid-fast rod assigned to the family Mycobacteriaceae on the basis of morphologic, biochemical, antigenic, and genetic similarities to other mycobacteria. Although it has not been cultivated in artificial media or tissue culture, it can be propagated in armadillos and in the foot pads of mice. The bacillus multiplies exceedingly slowly, with an estimated optimal doubling time of 11 to 13 days during logarithmic growth in mouse foot pads. The mouse model has been used extensively for the study of antileprosy drugs, and the high bacterial yield from armadillos has been crucial for immunologic and genetic studies.

The cellular components of *M. leprae* which are responsible for its pathogenicity and ability to survive within the host are poorly understood. The best-characterized virulence factor is phenolic glycolipid I, a prominent surface lipid specific to *M. leprae*. Phenolic glycolipid I can bind to complement component C3, which in turn mediates phagocytosis of the bacterium by mononuclear phagocytes via CR1, CR3, and CR4 receptors on their cell surfaces. Once inside the phagocyte, phenolic glycolipid I helps to protect the bacterium from oxidative killing by chemically scavenging hydroxyl radicals and superoxide anions.

EPIDEMIOLOGY There are probably 10 to 20 million persons affected with leprosy in the world. The disease is more common in tropical countries, in many of which the prevalence rate is 1 to 2 percent of the population. A warm environment is not critical for transmission, and leprosy also occurs in certain regions with cooler climates, such as Korea and central Mexico. Distribution of infected individuals within countries is very nonhomogeneous, and districts in which 20 percent of the population is affected can be found. The distribution of cases across the spectrum of leprosy also varies between countries, with lepromatous disease predominating in some countries, such as Mexico, and tuberculoid disease in others, such as India. Ninety percent of the cases diagnosed in the United States in the past two decades have occurred in immigrants from leprosy-endemic countries. Indigenous transmission occurs primarily in Hawaii, the Pacific Island territories, and sporadically along the Gulf Coast. The incidence of leprosy in the United States has fallen from a peak of

360 cases in 1985, associated with the influx of immigrants from Southeast Asia, to 139 cases in 1991.

Leprosy can present at any age, although cases in infants less than 1 year of age are extremely rare. The age-specific incidence peaks during childhood in most developing countries; up to 20 percent of cases occur in children under 10. Since leprosy is most prevalent in poorer socioeconomic groups, this may simply reflect the age distribution of the high-risk population. The sex ratio of leprosy presenting during childhood is 1:1, but males predominate by a 2:1 ratio in adults.

It is humbling to realize how little is known concerning the modes of transmission and acquisition of leprosy, given that the communicable nature of the infection has been recognized for millennia and that the etiologic agent was identified over 100 years ago. Direct human-to-human transmission is believed responsible for most cases of leprosy, although a history of prior exposure can be elicited from fewer than half of all patients. Animal reservoirs exist among feral armadillos and possibly among nonhuman primates, but in only a few human cases has zoonotic transmission been implicated. Among close family contacts of untreated lepromatous patients, the risk of disease is increased approximately eightfold, and the attack rate can be as high as 10 percent. Development of clinical disease in contacts of tuberculoid patients is less common, although immunologic tests suggest that most of these contacts have been sensitized to *M. leprae*. The site of entry remains a matter of conjecture but is probably either the skin or the mucosa of the upper respiratory tract. The chief portal of exit is thought to be the nasal mucosa of untreated lepromatous patients.

The incubation period is frequently 3 to 5 years but has been reported to range from 6 months to several decades.

PATHOGENESIS The early events following the entry of *M. leprae* into the body have not been described in humans. The bacilli are surrounded by a dense, nearly inert lipid capsule, produce no exotoxins, and engender little inflammatory response. Immunologic and epidemiologic studies suggest that only a small fraction, possibly 10 to 20 percent, of those infected will develop signs of indeterminate leprosy and that only about 50 percent of those with indeterminate disease will progress to full-blown clinical leprosy.

The intensity of the specific cell-mediated immune response to *M. leprae* correlates with the clinical and histologic disease class. Individuals with polar tuberculoid disease have an intense cellular response to *M. leprae* and a low bacillary load, whereas patients with lepromatous leprosy have no detectable cellular immunity to the leprosy bacillus. There is evidence from family studies that specific HLA-associated genes may be linked to different classes of disease. HLA-DR2 is inherited preferentially by children with polar tuberculoid disease, whereas HLA-MT1 is associated with polar lepromatous disease. The effect of the HLA-associated genes is limited to influencing the type of leprosy; there is no association between HLA haplotypes and overall susceptibility to leprosy.

The defect in cell-mediated immunity in lepromatous patients is extremely specific. They do not suffer increased morbidity following infection by pathogens such as viruses, protozoa, or fungi for which cellular immunity is important, and they do not have an increased risk of neoplasia. Patients with lepromatous leprosy have been shown to have an increased number of circulating CD8+ ("suppressor") lymphocytes which can be specifically activated by *M. leprae* antigens, and the lymphocytes present in their cutaneous granulomas are almost exclusively CD8+. In contrast, CD4+4B4+ ("helper") cells predominate among the T cells in the cutaneous lesions of tuberculoid patients. In lepromatous leprosy, cells of the monocyte-macrophage family become engorged with *M. leprae* and are unable to kill or digest the organisms. However, when studied in vitro, monocytes from these patients respond normally to cytokines and display normal phagocytic and microbicidal activity. These results suggest that an underlying defect in regulation of T lymphocyte subpopulations is responsible for the immunologic tolerance characteristic of lepromatous leprosy.

Intense bacillemia is very common in lepromatous leprosy, and organisms can often be seen in stained smears of peripheral blood or buffy coats, but high fever and signs of systemic toxicity are absent. Even in the most advanced cases, destructive lesions are limited to the skin, peripheral nerves, anterior portions of the eyes, upper respiratory passages above the larynx, testes, and structures of the hands and feet. One feature common to these sites is that they are all usually several degrees cooler than 37°C. Two sites of preferential involvement are the ulnar nerves near the elbow and the peroneal nerves where they pass around the head of the fibula; above and below these areas, where these nerves take deeper courses, they are less severely involved. In patients with lepromatous leprosy, collections of bacilli are also found in the liver, spleen, and bone marrow, but no visceral organ system dysfunction has been associated with the presence of these bacilli.

CLINICAL AND HISTOPATHOLOGIC MANIFESTATIONS The variable immune response to infection with *M. leprae* results in a wide spectrum of histologic and clinical manifestations. There is a strong concordance between the clinical findings and the dermal histopathology, and they will be discussed together.

Early or indeterminate leprosy The first signs of leprosy are usually cutaneous. The lesions of indeterminate leprosy are very subtle and are most commonly diagnosed in examination of contacts of known leprosy patients. One or more hypopigmented or hyperpigmented macules or plaques may be seen. Often an anesthetic or paresthetic patch is the first symptom noted by the patient, but on careful examination, skin involvement can be found. Sensation is often preserved in these early lesions, particularly those on the face. The lesions may clear spontaneously in a year or two, but specific treatment is recommended.

Tuberculoid leprosy The initial lesion of tuberculoid leprosy, one of the "poles" of the clinical and immunologic spectrum, is often a hypopigmented macule which is sharply demarcated and hypesthetic. Later the lesions enlarge by peripheral spread, and the margins become elevated and circinate or gyrate (Fig. 131-1). The central area in turn becomes atrophic and depressed. Fully developed lesions are densely anesthetic and have lost the normal skin organs (sweat glands and hair follicles). The lesions are single or few in

FIGURE 131-1 Tuberculoid leprosy. Large, solitary lesion with a raised, indurated border. The central clear area of the lesion is hypesthetic with thinning of the dermis and loss of dermal structures such as sweat glands and hair follicles.

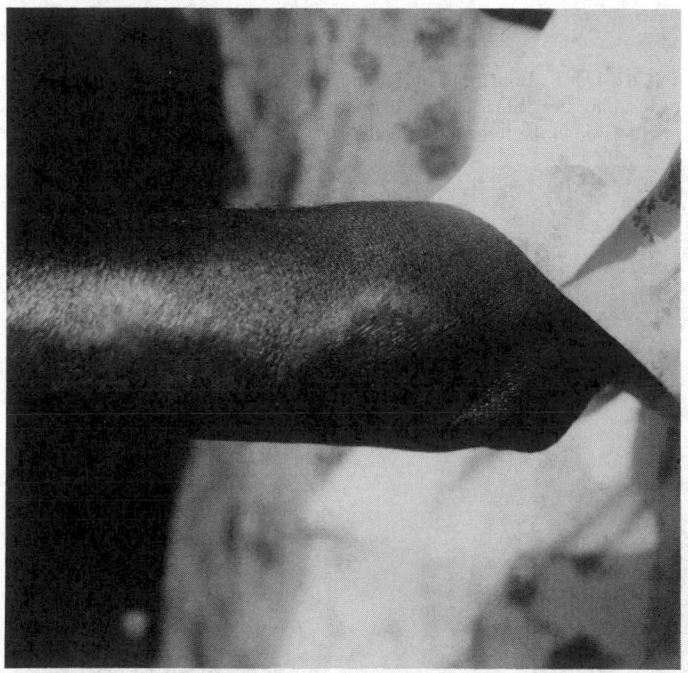

number. Nerve involvement occurs early, and the superficial nerves leading from the lesions may be enlarged. The larger peripheral nerves (especially the ulnar, peroneal, and greater auricular nerves) may be palpably and visibly enlarged, particularly those closest to the skin lesion. There may be severe neuritic pain. Neural involvement leads to muscle atrophy, especially of the small muscles of the hand. Contractures of the hand and foot are frequent. Trauma, especially from burns and splinters and from excessive pressure, leads to secondary infection of the hands and to plantar ulcers. Later, resorption and loss of phalanges may supervene. When the facial nerves are involved, there may be lagophthalmos, exposure keratitis, and corneal ulceration leading to blindness.

The histologic picture consists of noncaseating granulomas comprising lymphocytes, epithelioid cells, and perhaps giant cells; bacilli are frequently absent or difficult to demonstrate.

Lepromatous leprosy Lepromatous leprosy is the other polar form. The cutaneous involvement is extensive and roughly bilaterally symmetric across the midline of the host. Individual skin lesions are highly variable and can include macules, nodules, plaques, or papules. The borders of the lesions are ill defined, and the centers of raised lesions are indurated and convex (rather than concave, as in tuberculoid disease). There is diffuse infiltration of the dermis between discrete lesions, and apparently normal skin will usually contain bacilli demonstrable by staining. The sites of predilection are the face (cheeks, nose, brows), ears, wrists, elbows, buttocks, and knees. At times, involvement with infiltration and little or no nodulation may progress so subtly that the disease goes unnoticed. Loss of the lateral portions of the eyebrows is common. Much later the skin of the face and forehead becomes thickened and corrugated (leonine facies), and the earlobes become pendulous.

Nasal "stuffiness," epistaxis, and obstructed breathing are common early symptoms. Complete nasal obstruction, laryngitis, and hoarseness also occur. Septal perforation and nasal collapse lead to saddlenose. Invasion of the anterior portion of the eye can result in keratitis and iridocyclitis. Painless inguinal and axillary lymphadenopathy occurs. In adult males infiltration and scarring of the testes lead to sterility. Gynecomastia is common.

Involvement of the major nerve trunks is less prominent in the lepromatous form, but diffuse hypesthesia involving the peripheral portions of the extremities is common in advanced disease. Pathologically, the peripheral nerves are heavily infected but often better preserved than in the tuberculoid form.

Histologically, there is a diffuse granulomatous reaction with macrophages, large foam (Virchow or lepra) cells, and many intracellular bacilli, frequently in spheroidal masses (globi). Epithelioid cells and giant cells are not found.

Borderline leprosy The borderline portion of the spectrum lies between the tuberculoid and lepromatous poles and is usually subdivided into borderline tuberculoid, borderline (or dimorphous), and borderline lepromatous classes. Classification within the borderline region of the spectrum is less precise than at the poles. Lesions tend to increase in number and heterogeneity but decrease in individual size as the lepromatous pole is approached. The skin lesions of borderline tuberculoid leprosy generally resemble those of tuberculoid disease but are greater in number and have less well defined borders. Involvement of multiple peripheral nerve trunks is more common than in polar tuberculoid disease.

Increasing variability in the appearance of the skin lesions is characteristic of borderline leprosy. Papules and plaques may coexist with macular lesions. Anesthesia is less prominent than in tuberculoid disease. The earlobes may be slightly thickened, but the eyebrows and nasal regions are spared. Skin lesions become even more numerous in borderline lepromatous disease, but the distribution lacks the bilateral symmetry typical of polar lepromatous disease (Fig. 131-2).

The histopathology of the granulomas in borderline leprosy changes from an epithelioid cell predominance in borderline tuberculoid disease to a macrophage predominance as the lepromatous pole is approached. The presence and number of lymphocytes are variable

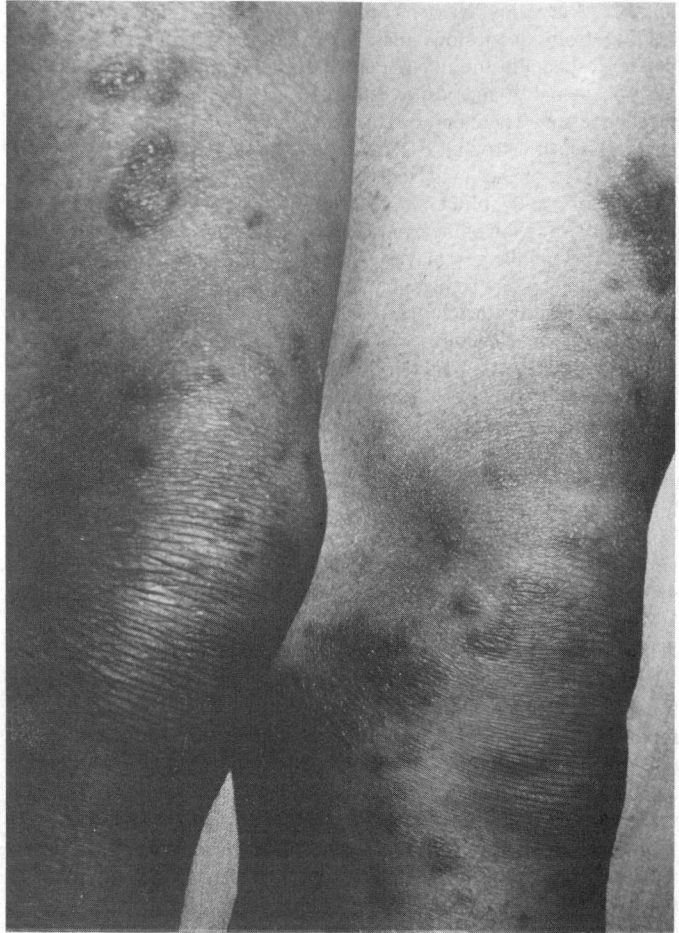

FIGURE 131-2 Borderline lepromatous leprosy. Multiple macules, papules, and nodules with an asymmetric distribution. Individual lesions are small but may become confluent.

and correlate poorly with the disease class. Bacilli are present in large numbers in the skin granulomas of borderline and borderline lepromatous patients. For this reason, these groups, together with polar lepromatous leprosy, are referred to as *multibacillary leprosy*. Borderline tuberculoid, polar tuberculoid, and indeterminate classes are grouped together as *paucibacillary leprosy*.

The borderline disease states are unstable and may shift toward the lepromatous form in the untreated patient or toward the tuberculoid pole during treatment. Change of either polar type to the other is exceedingly rare.

In all forms of leprosy, peripheral nerve involvement is a constant feature. In any histologic section, involvement of nerves will tend to be more severe than involvement of other tissues. Much of the neural destruction appears to result from the granulomatous reaction of the host rather than from an innate neurotoxic property of the bacillus. Though uncommon, neural involvement can occur in the absence of cutaneous lesions (pure neural leprosy).

REACTIONAL STATES The general course of leprosy is indolent, but it may be interrupted by two types of reaction. Both forms of reactions can occur in untreated patients but more often emerge as complications of chemotherapy.

Erythema nodosum leprosum Erythema nodosum leprosum (ENL), or type 2 lepra reaction, occurs in lepromatous and borderline lepromatous patients, most frequently in the latter half of the initial year of treatment. Tender, inflamed subcutaneous nodules develop, usually in crops. Each nodule lasts a week or two, but new crops may appear. ENL may last only a week or two, or it may persist for long periods. Fever, lymphadenopathy, and arthralgias can accompany severe ENL. Histologically, ENL is characterized by polymorphonu-

clear infiltration and deposits of IgG and complement, resembling an Arthus reaction.

Reversal reaction Reversal reaction, or type 1 lepra reaction, can complicate all three borderline categories. Existing skin lesions develop erythema and swelling, and new lesions may appear. An early influx of lymphocytes into existing lesions is followed by edema and a shift toward tuberculoid histology. Cellular immunity increases. Reversal reactions can be differentiated from disease progression or relapse by mouse inoculations to test bacillary viability and by histologic studies. Downgrading reactions, which clinically mimic reversal reactions, are most common in untreated patients and in women during the third trimester of pregnancy. Skin biopsies reveal a shift toward lepromatous histology and reflect a decrease in cellular immunity.

COMPLICATIONS Leprosy is probably the most frequent cause of crippling of the hand in the world (Fig. 131-3). Trauma and secondary chronic infections can lead to loss of digits or distal extremities. Blindness is also common.

The *Lucio phenomenon*, characterized by arteritis, is limited to patients with diffuse, infiltrative, nonnodular lepromatous disease. Severe cases clinically resemble other forms of necrotizing vasculitis and are associated with a high mortality rate.

Secondary amyloidosis is a complication of severe lepromatous disease, especially in chronic ENL.

Leprosy and human immunodeficiency virus (HIV) infection Surprisingly, given the experience with other mycobacterial diseases and the intricate immune response to *M. leprae*, concurrent infection with HIV appears to have little effect on the clinical manifestations or natural history of leprosy. Anecdotal reports suggest that the relapse rate after completion of therapy for paucibacillary disease may be slightly increased in HIV-infected patients, and HIV-positive patients with early or subclinical leprosy may be more likely to develop overt disease. Concurrent leprosy also may accelerate the course of HIV disease.

DIAGNOSIS The demonstration of acid-fast bacilli in skin smears made by the scraped-incision method is strong evidence for leprosy, but in tuberculoid disease bacilli may not be demonstrable. Wherever possible, a skin biopsy specimen from the affected area should be sent to a pathologist knowledgeable in leprosy. The histologic involvement of peripheral nerves is pathognomonic, even in the absence of bacilli. Work is underway on the development of tests using genetic probes for the rapid identification and speciation of mycobacteria in clinical specimens.

FIGURE 131-3 Borderline tuberculoid leprosy. Bilateral claw hand deformities resulting from ulnar and median nerve damage. Note the severe loss of muscle tissue in the forearms secondary to neuropathic and disuse atrophy.

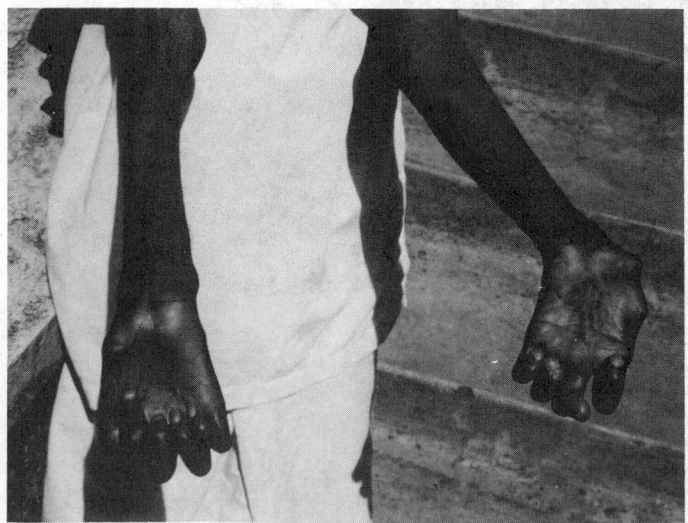

Hematologic and blood chemistry tests are of little help in establishing the diagnosis. Lepromatous patients frequently have mild anemia, an elevated erythrocyte sedimentation rate, and hyperglobulinemia. Between 10 and 20 percent of lepromatous patients have low-titer false-positive serologic tests for syphilis or autoantibodies directed against nuclear or cellular antigens.

Lepromin is a suspension of killed *M. leprae* prepared from heavily infected human or armadillo tissue. Intradermal injection elicits, somewhat variably, a tuberculin-like reaction at 48 h (Fernandez's reaction) and, more consistently, a papular reaction at 3 to 4 weeks (Mitsuda's reaction). The Mitsuda reaction is usually positive in tuberculoid patients and is always negative in lepromatous patients. However, because it is also positive in nearly all normal adults, even those residing in areas free of endemic leprosy, it has no diagnostic value. Lepromin is not commercially available.

A specific serodiagnostic test for leprosy has been developed. Based on the detection of antibody to phenolic glycolipid I, this assay has a sensitivity of over 95 percent in polar lepromatous disease and about 30 percent in tuberculoid disease. The level of antibody appears to correlate with the bacillary load, which explains the high false-negative rate in polar tuberculoid disease. Despite this limitation, the near 100 percent specificity of this assay makes it potentially useful for confirming the diagnosis of leprosy and as an epidemiologic tool for studying disease incubation and transmission.

The differential diagnosis includes lupus erythematosus, lupus vulgaris, sarcoidosis, yaws, dermal leishmaniasis, and a host of banal skin diseases. The skin lesions of leprosy, especially of turberculoid disease, are characterized by hypesthesia, and peripheral nerve involvement can always be demonstrated. Peripheral neuropathy from other causes and syringomyelia may be confused with leprosy, although skin involvement is not a feature of other diseases causing peripheral neuropathy. The combination of a chronic skin disease and peripheral nerve involvement should always lead to the consideration of leprosy.

TREATMENT The management of leprosy involves a broad, multidisciplinary approach, including consultative services such as orthopedic surgery, ophthalmology, and physical therapy in addition to antimicrobial chemotherapy.

Specific chemotherapy *Dapsone* (4,4′-diaminodiphenylsulfone, DDS, diphenylsulfone), a folate antagonist, is the mainstay of therapy. The daily dosage is 50 to 100 mg in adults. Dapsone is very inexpensive, safe in pregnancy, and has a long serum half-life of about 24 h, allowing once daily administration. Major side effects, which are relatively uncommon, include hemolysis, agranulocytosis, hepatitis, and potentially fatal exfoliative dermatitis. In lepromatous disease, enough bacilli are killed during the first 10 to 12 weeks of dapsone monotherapy to render mouse foot pad inoculations negative. However, in this form of the disease nonviable bacilli disappear slowly and may be found in the tissues for 5 to 10 years. Moreover, a few viable bacilli (persisters) may survive in the tissues for many years and cause a relapse if treatment is discontinued.

Years of dapsone monotherapy led to the emergence of dapsone-resistant strains of *M. leprae*. Secondary resistance occurs in 2 to 30 percent of lepromatous patients receiving dapsone monotherapy. It presents as a clinical and bacteriologic relapse after several years of apparently successful, regular therapy. Primary dapsone resistance in previously untreated patients has complicated empiric therapy in many parts of the world but remains uncommon (less than 3 percent) in the United States. To counteract this problem, the World Health Organization, in 1982, recommended the use of multiple-drug therapy for all leprosy patients.

Rifampin is the most rapidly mycobactericidal drug known for *M. leprae*. The viability of skin bacilli falls to undetectable levels within 5 days following a single 1500-mg dose of oral rifampin. The usual dosage is 600 mg/d. The high cost of rifampin has limited its use in the developing world and has led to regimens in which it is given at a dosage of 600 or 900 mg once per month. Many leprologists prefer to treat with daily or twice-weekly rifampin if cost is not a

crucial issue. Rare cases of rifampin-resistant *M. leprae* have been reported. Rifampin has not been approved for the intermittent treatment of leprosy by the Food and Drug Administration.

Clofazimine is a compound derived from a phenazine dye. It is highly lipophilic and accumulates in the skin, the gastrointestinal tract, and macrophages and monocytes. It is usually given in a dosage of 50 to 200 mg/d and has an apparent half-life of over 70 days. Major toxicity is restricted to the skin and the intestinal tract. The reddish skin pigmentation, often accompanied by ichthyosis, is unacceptable to many light-skinned patients and can lead to poor compliance. The intestinal toxicity is also dose-related and is reflected in diarrhea and cramping abdominal pain. Clofazimine is not safe for use during pregnancy.

There are several older agents with limited activity against *M. leprae* which have been used in certain clinical situations, including ethionamide, prothionamide, thiambutosine, and amithiozone. All these drugs have significant toxicities, and none has been approved for this purpose by the Food and Drug Administration. An extremely important and exciting development in the last few years has been the identification of several new antimicrobials with impressive activity against *M. leprae*. The most promising agents are minocycline, ofloxacin, and clarithromycin. Fusidic acid, ampicillin/clavulanic acid, and brodimoprim also have shown activity against *M. leprae* in vitro or in mice. Clinical trials of many of these new drugs are now underway, but all should be considered investigational, and none has been approved for the treatment of leprosy by the Food and Drug Administration.

Therapy for multibacillary disease should consist of three drugs, usually dapsone, rifampin, and clofazimine. If the organism is known to be dapsone-sensitive, the combination of dapsone and rifampin may be adequate for borderline and borderline lepromatous cases, but the likelihood of secondary dapsone resistance makes the addition of a third drug advisable in lepromatous disease. Objective measures of response to therapy, including skin scrapings and biopsies, should be monitored and therapy continued at least until morphologically intact bacilli are consistently absent and the inflammatory cell infiltrate has resolved. The optimal duration of therapy is unknown, but a minimum of 2 years is recommended. Indefinite therapy may be required in some cases of lepromatous disease.

Therapeutic regimens containing two drugs, usually dapsone and rifampin, are adequate for paucibacillary leprosy. The World Health Organization recommends a 6-month course and reports an annual failure rate after completion of only 0.1 percent. Standard practice in the United States is to treat with dapsone and rifampin for the first 6 to 12 months (depending on the clinical response), followed by dapsone alone to complete a total of 24 months of therapy.

Evidence of clinical improvement should be visible by the second or third month of treatment. The clinical response to therapy may be confused by intercurrent reactional states, but the disease stops progressing and the skin lesions gradually improve. Recovery from neurologic impairment is limited.

Treatment of reactional states Mild ENL is managed with antipyretics and analgesics. Severe cases can be rapidly controlled with high dosages of prednisone (60 to 120 mg/d). Antimicrobial therapy should be continued, since glucocorticoid therapy promotes the viability of *M. leprae* in mice not given antileprosy drugs. Rifampin enhances the metabolism of glucocorticoids by the liver, necessitating administration of larger doses to achieve a given therapeutic effect. Thalidomide is the most effective drug for ENL. The usual initial dosage is 200 mg twice a day, which can be gradually tapered to a maintenance dosage of 50 to 100 mg/d for patients with chronic ENL. Thalidomide is absolutely contraindicated in women of childbearing age because of its teratogenicity but has proved relatively free of major side effects in other leprosy patients. This drug has not been approved by the Food and Drug Administration but is available through the Hansen's Disease Center, Carville, Louisiana, as an investigational agent. Clofazimine has anti-inflammatory properties as well as antimycobacterial activity and can be valuable in the treatment of chronic ENL, but it requires at least 3 to 4 weeks to reach effective levels, making it of little use in acute attacks. Other anti-inflammatory agents, including chloroquine, cyclosporine, and cytotoxic drugs, have been used in difficult cases; in general, these unusual situations should be managed in consultation with a leprosy specialist.

Reversal reactions are often acute and can lead to rapid and irreversible neurologic damage. Glucocorticoids are indicated for severe reversal reactions. Clofazimine is of some use in chronic situations, but it is generally necessary to continue glucocorticoids as well. Reversal reactions do not respond to thalidomide.

Other measures Many of the deformities and disabilities of leprosy are preventable. Plantar ulcers, which are very common, may be prevented by rigid-soled footwear or walking plaster casts, and contractures of the hand may be prevented by physical therapy and application of casts. Reconstructive surgery is sometimes helpful. Nerve and tendon transplants and release of contractures can give patients more functional ability. Vocational retraining is often necessary for those with permanent disability. Plastic repair of facial deformities assists acceptance of patients in society. The psychological trauma which resulted from prolonged segregation is now minimized by home therapy in virtually all cases.

CONTROL Case finding and chemotherapy form the present basis of control. Infectiousness can be quickly suppressed with chemotherapy, making early detection of cases important. In endemic countries, this means establishing local clinics or traveling teams. Family and other close contacts need to be examined regularly for leprosy. A benefit of the short (6- to 24-month) multidrug treatment regimens is that patients can be certified disease-free much sooner than was possible with dapsone monotherapy. This permits leprosy case workers to devote proportionately more effort to contact screening and case detection. In the United States, patients are eligible for treatment by the Public Health Service, and special clinics are located in several major cities. Risk of transmission is very low, even in untreated patients, and no unusual infection control precautions are required when patients are hospitalized. Chemoprophylaxis with lowered doses of dapsone may be effective, but contact screening by yearly physical examinations is preferred to empiric therapy in most situations. Vaccine trials with bacillus Calmette-Guérin in endemic areas have yielded conflicting results with, at most, modest efficacy. At least four new experimental vaccines are currently in field trials in India and South America.

REFERENCES

BLAKE LA et al: Environmental nonhuman sources of leprosy. Rev Infect Dis 9:562, 1987

BLOOM BR, GODAL T: Selective primary health care: Strategies for the control of disease in the developing world. V. Leprosy. Rev Infect Dis 5:765, 1983

BULLOCK WE: *Mycobacterium leprae* (leprosy), in *Principles and Practice of Infectious Diseases*, 3d ed, GL Mandell et al (eds). New York, Wiley, 1990, pp 1906–1914

EDITORIAL: Serological tests for leprosy. Lancet 1:533, 1986

GOODLESS DR et al: Reactional states in Hansen's disease: Practical aspects of emergency management. South Med J 84:237, 1991

HASTINGS RC (ed): *Leprosy*. New York, Churchill Livingstone, 1985

JACOBSON R: The face of leprosy in the United States today. Arch Dermatol 126:1627, 1990

MASTRO TD et al: Leprosy in the United States, 1971–1988. Am J Public Health 82:1127, 1992

MILLER RA: Leprosy and AIDS. Int J Lepr Other Mycobact Dis 59:639, 1991

SCHLESINGER LS et al: Phenolic glycolipid-1 of *Mycobacterium leprae* binds complement component C3 in serum and mediates phagocytosis by human monocytes. J Exp Med 174:1031, 1991

SHIELDS ED et al: Genetic epidemiology of the susceptibility to leprosy. J Clin Invest 79:1139, 1987

132　MYCOBACTERIUM AVIUM COMPLEX AND OTHER NONTUBERCULOUS MYCOBACTERIAL INFECTIONS

FERRIC C. FANG / STANLEY D. FREEDMAN

Mycobacteria other than the tubercle bacillus have been known to be agents of human disease since the 1950s. A classification of these organisms based on colonial morphology and growth characteristics was provided by Runyon. He classified mycobacteria as photochromogens (pigment production induced by light), scotochromogens (constitutive pigment production), nonchromogens (absent pigment production), or rapid growers. These bacteria are widely distributed in nature as saprophytes, primarily in soil and water. Animals can be infected and may serve as reservoirs for infection of humans. Person-to-person transmission occurs rarely, if at all. Skin tests with tuberculins from the various species have demonstrated the extent of infection in the United States and other countries, as well as notable geographic variability among species. These bacteria have been referred to as *atypical mycobacteria* or *anonymous mycobacteria*, reflecting the emphasis of earlier microbiologists on *Mycobacterium tuberculosis*. Currently preferred designations are *nontuberculous mycobacteria* (NTM), *mycobacteria other than tuberculosis* (MOTT), and *environmental mycobacteria*. The frequency with which they are found in the environment requires that repeated isolation from a diseased site or isolation from blood or bone marrow be achieved before nontuberculous mycobacteria can be definitively identified as the cause of disease. In some cases, pathologic evidence of a granulomatous inflammatory process also may be required before a disease process can be attributed unequivocally to a nontuberculous mycobacterium. With recent improvements in laboratory techniques, such as radiometric culture systems and nucleic acid probes, species designations are becoming increasingly familiar (Table 132-1). Although of lesser virulence than the tubercle bacillus, these organisms may be important pathogens in compromised individuals, particularly those with impaired cellular immunity or underlying lung disease. The recognition of serious disseminated nontuberculous mycobacterial infections in patients with AIDS has given new significance to the nontuberculous mycobacteria. Although infections with *M. asiaticum*, *M. flavescens*, *M. fortuitum*/*M. chelonae*, *M. gordonae*, *M. haemophilum*, *M. kansasii*, *M. malmoense*, *M. marinum*, *M. scrofulaceum*, *M. simiae*, *M. smegmatis*, *M. szulgai*, *M. ulcerans*, and *M. xenopi* have

TABLE 132-1　Human mycobacterial pathogens other than *M. tuberculosis* and *M. leprae*

Mycobacterium	Pigmentation*	Usual site of disease	Environmental source
M. avium complex	N	Disseminated, lungs, lymph nodes	Water, soil, ? Animals
M. fortuitum/ *M. chelonae*	N	Skin, lungs	Water, soil
M. haemophilum	N	Skin	Unknown
M. kansasii	P	Lungs	? Water, ? animals
M. marinum	P	Skin	Water, fish
M. scrofulaceum	S	Lymph nodes	Water, soil
M. szulgai	S†	Lungs	? Fish
M. ulcerans	N	Skin	Tropical grasses
M. xenopi	S	Lungs	Water, animals
M. asiaticum	P	Lungs	? Animals
M. malmoense	N	Lungs	Unknown
M. shimoidei	N	Lungs	Unknown
M. simiae	P (weak)	Lungs	Water, ? animals

* P = photochromogen, N = nonchromogen, S = scotochromogen
† Scotochromogen at 37°C, photochromogen at 25°C

been reported in association with AIDS, more than 95 percent of nontuberculous mycobacterial infections in AIDS are caused by *M. avium* complex (MAC).

MYCOBACTERIUM AVIUM COMPLEX   Although a variety of technical methods can distinguish *M. avium* from *M. intracellulare*, species distinction by routine culture methods is difficult, and they are often considered as a complex (MAC); alternatively, this group of organisms may be referred to collectively as *Mycobacterium avium-intracellulare* (MAI). Commercially available specific nucleic acid probes now permit rapid and convenient differentiation of *M. avium* and *M. intracellulare*. These ubiquitous organisms are particularly prevalent in the southeastern United States and, overall, are the most commonly isolated mycobacteria. They can be isolated from soil, water (including tap water), house dust, food, and animals. MAC organisms are classified as nonchromogens, but some strains are lightly pigmented.

The lungs are the most important site of localized infection due to MAC. Aerosols are thought to be an important mode of acquisition of respiratory disease. Colonization and inapparent infection are common. When the lungs are involved, the clinical picture frequently resembles pulmonary tuberculosis. Alternatively, patients may present with lower zone nodular subpleural shadowing, bronchiectasis, or solitary nodules. Underlying pulmonary disease, collagen-vascular disease, a possible genetic predilection, and advanced age are risk factors. When a MAC organism is isolated from a patient with pulmonary disease, it is important to be certain of the pathogenic role of the organism in the disease process, because chemotherapy is often associated with morbidity.

Skin involvement and musculoskeletal infections including vertebral osteomyelitis that resembles Pott's disease have been described. MAC is the major mycobacterial cause of cervical lymphadenitis in American children and is especially common between 1 and 5 years of age. Genitourinary disease, meningitis, gastrointestinal ulcers, panniculitis, pericarditis, and otomastoiditis also have been reported. Disseminated MAC infection can occur in children and adults, mostly in association with severe underlying diseases.

MAC in AIDS   There is a striking association between disseminated *Mycobacterium avium* complex infection and AIDS (see Chap. 279). MAC infection is diagnosed in 10 to 30 percent of AIDS patients antemortem and in 50 percent at autopsy. MAC infection occurs fairly uniformly among different AIDS risk groups; the most important risk factor appears to be a CD4 count less than 100 cells per microliter of blood. Massive involvement of the gastrointestinal tract has suggested the possibility of an oral route of infection from contaminated water, and experimental evidence supporting this hypothesis has been obtained in the beige mouse model. Nevertheless, the relationship between colonization and the development of disseminated infection remains uncertain at present, and respiratory colonization appears to precede disseminated illness in some cases. The organism burden is extremely high, with up to 10^6 bacteria per milliliter of blood and 10^{10} bacteria per gram of tissue. The cellular inflammatory response, granulomatous or otherwise, is minimal. It has been speculated that the fibrillar peptidoglycolipid sheath of MAC organisms both protects the microbe from host defenses and prevents activation of inflammatory mediators by shielding toxic sulfatides and cord factor in the organism's cell wall.

Fever, weight loss, and cytopenias are common. Involvement of the small intestine may produce watery diarrhea and malabsorption. The histopathology resembles that of Whipple's disease; acid-fast stains reveal that the macrophages filling the intestinal lamina propria are packed with mycobacteria. In other organs these macrophages may resemble lepra cells. Colonic involvement may produce severe abdominal pain. Hepatic infiltration is frequent and may result in marked elevation of the serum alkaline phosphatase. The findings of hepatosplenomegaly, thickening of the small bowel wall, and bulky lymphadenopathy on abdominal CT scan suggest MAC infection. Although endobronchial lesions with airway narrowing may occur and bacteria are frequently present in the respiratory secretions

of infected patients, pulmonary parenchymal disease is curiously uncommon.

The diagnosis of disseminated MAC infection is made by isolation of organisms from blood, bone marrow, or liver tissue. Radiometric blood culture systems can quickly confirm the diagnosis in the vast majority of patients with disseminated disease, and nucleic acid probes can facilitate rapid speciation. MAC organisms may be recovered from the blood in as few as 5 to 14 days. The compound NAP (p-nitro-α-acetylamino-β-hydroxypropiophenone) selectively inhibits species of the *M. tuberculosis* complex in culture, and its inclusion in radiometric cultures may aid in presumptive identification. Bone marrow biopsy, liver biopsy, or intestinal biopsy also may provide a diagnosis of disseminated MAC infection. Culture of MAC organisms from these tissues by routine methods usually takes 4 weeks. The presence of heavy acid-fast bacilli on touch preparations of tissue or stool smear is highly suggestive. It has been reported that buffy coat acid-fast smears are positive in approximately one-third of patients. MAC organisms also have been found in the lymph nodes, eye, thyroid, esophagus, mediastinum, pericardium, pancreas, adrenal, kidney, muscle, brain, joint, bone, and skin of infected patients. The usual survival is only 4 to 10 months once the diagnosis of disseminated MAC infection has been made in a patient with AIDS, but therapy reduces morbidity in some patients and may extend survival.

Both microbial and host factors appear to be critical to the development of disseminated MAC infection in AIDS. *M. avium* is isolated from 97 percent of AIDS patients with MAC infection, whereas *M. intracellulare* accounts for 40 percent of MAC infections in patients without AIDS. Furthermore, strains of *M. avium* from patients with AIDS are more likely to be from serovars 1, 4, and 8; produce pigment; contain plasmids; and have a particular RFLP (restriction fragment length polymorphism) pattern. MAC organisms have been demonstrated to inhibit phagosome-lysosome fusion and superoxide production by macrophages. Although no difference has been found in the ability of normal or AIDS-infected macrophages to phagocytose and kill MAC organisms, the characteristic pathologic finding of macrophages stuffed with acid-fast bacilli is consistent with the idea that impaired T cell function results in an inability of host macrophages to control MAC replication. MAC growth is suppressed in macrophages cocultivated with sensitized T cells or natural killer cells. Recent studies have indicated that MAC growth in macrophages also may be modulated by cytokines and serum factors that are deficient in some patients with AIDS.

Treatment of MAC infections   Treatment of these infections is difficult and often unsatisfactory. The organisms are usually resistant to most conventional antimycobacterial agents. Multiple-drug therapy sometimes appears to be of benefit, possibly reflecting synergy between agents which are not individually very active. The value of in vitro susceptibility studies is controversial. Nonetheless, it seems prudent to select an antimicrobial regimen that includes drugs to which an isolate is susceptible. For pulmonary disease thought to warrant treatment, the American Thoracic Society has recommended isoniazid, rifampin, ethambutol, and the initial use of streptomycin. These recommendations were made on the basis of limited clinical studies but may require modification as experience with newer antimycobacterial agents accumulates. Surgical excision is the treatment of choice for lymphadenitis and is a reasonable alternative for a few other localized infections.

Because it has been difficult to demonstrate clinical benefit of antimicrobial therapy in many AIDS patients with disseminated MAC infection, treatment usually has been reserved for highly symptomatic patients. Agents which may be useful in this setting include ethambutol, rifampin, rifabutin (ansamycin), ciprofloxacin, clofazimine, streptomycin, amikacin, clarithromycin, azithromycin, and sparfloxacin. Ethionamide and cycloserine also have activity against some MAC isolates but are often poorly tolerated. The new macrolides clarithromycin and azithromycin appear to be particularly useful against MAC organisms and have shown encouraging results in early clinical trials. Among the attractive features of these agents is their ability to be concentrated within phagocytic cells. When used as monotherapy, the new macrolides give rise to resistance fairly rapidly. This is not surprising in view of the organism load in infected patients and underscores the importance of using multiple agents in the treatment of mycobacterial infections. The new fluoroquinolone sparfloxacin is also active against MAC in vitro, but clinical studies are pending. Clarithromycin, sparfloxacin, and, to a lesser extent, azithromycin slow intracellular MAC replication in macrophages in vitro; the addition of ethambutol or rifampin provides synergy. Other investigational agents such as rifapentine, WIN57273, thiacetazone, and liposomal amikacin are undergoing evaluation.

Therapy of symptomatic patients with disseminated MAC infection may improve the quality of their lives. Until studies define the optimal regimen, initial therapy with one of the newer macrolides plus two other agents, e.g., ethambutol and rifampin, should be considered. Rifabutin (ansamycin) is active against the majority of *M. avium* isolates and is being evaluated as a prophylactic agent in AIDS patients with less than 200 CD4 cells per microliter. Early results from these studies are promising. Use of combination therapy for prophylaxis is also under investigation.

Other MAC organisms *M. avium* ssp. *paratuberculosis* is the etiologic agent of Johne's disease in ruminants. It is dependent on mycobactin, an iron-chelating factor, for in vitro growth. A mycobactin-dependent mycobacterium resembling *M. avium* ssp. *paratuberculosis* has been isolated from the terminal ileum of a small number of patients with Crohn's disease, but the significance of this finding remains highly controversial.

MYCOBACTERIUM FORTUITUM/CHELONAE AND OTHER RAPID GROWERS The distinguishing feature of these acid-fast bacteria is their rapid growth. Initial growth may take as long as 1 to 5 weeks, but subsequent subcultures generally grow within 1 to 3 days. Their distinction from more slowly growing mycobacteria has been supported by rRNA sequence analysis. These gram-positive, nonpigmented organisms are readily cultured on most media and may be confused with diphtheroids. Unlike other mycobacteria, they may not stain with auramine-rhodamine used in fluorescence microscopy. Although geographically widespread, these organisms are isolated most frequently in the southern United States from Georgia to Texas.

M. fortuitum and *M. chelonae* account for more than 95 percent of the reported infections due to rapid growers. Rare infections have been reported with other rapid-growing mycobacteria such as *M. smegmatis*, *M. thermoresistibile*, *M. flavescens*, and *M. neoaurum*. *M. smegmatis* can be part of the normal urogenital flora and is sometimes responsible for misleading positive acid-fast smears of urine. *M. fortuitum* is frequently associated with posttraumatic and postoperative skin and soft tissue infection. Most pulmonary infections and disseminated disease have been attributed to *M. chelonae*. Three biovars of *M. fortuitum* and three subspecies of *M. chelonae* have been described, but subspeciation is not necessary for clinical purposes. Since they are widespread in nature and in hospital environments and are highly resistant to antibiotics, antiseptics, and disinfectants, rapid growers are important nosocomial pathogens. Contamination of equipment, solutions, or water in the hospital setting also may lead to "pseudoepidemics."

Most skin infections are associated with interruption of the integument and injury or alteration of the soft tissues. Surgery, accidental trauma, or injections are important risk factors. Cutaneous infection may result in pyogenic abscesses, chronic ulcers, or sporotrichoid lesions. Although a chronic granulomatous reaction with caseation may occur, the typical pathologic process is suppurative with formation of microabscesses, and diphtheroid-like organisms may be seen on Gram's stain. In contrast to patients with lung infection caused by other nontuberculous mycobacteria, most patients with *M. chelonae* or *M. fortuitum* pulmonary infections have no underlying lung disease. The majority of these patients are women over 50 years of age. Cavitation is less frequent than in other mycobacterial lung infections. Other reported clinical manifestations include bone and joint infection, otitis media, intravascular or peritoneal catheter infection, shunt infection, lymphadenitis, ocular infection, intraoral or facial infection, pericarditis, mediastinitis, hepatitis, gastrointestinal infection, prostatitis, meningitis, and endocarditis involving porcine, prosthetic, or natural valves. Hematogenous dissemination is uncommon and affects primarily those with impaired host defenses. Infections have followed cardiothoracic surgery, augmentation mammaplasty, arthroplasty, ocular surgery, and dialysis.

Adequate debridement and drainage with removal of foreign bodies are indicated whenever possible. Many of these organisms are highly resistant to antimicrobial agents, but antimicrobial susceptibility testing is indicated because it may be a more reliable determinant of appropriate chemotherapy than it is in infections with other nontuberculous mycobacteria. *M. chelonae* tends to be more drug-resistant than *M. fortuitum* but is generally sensitive to cefoxitin and amikacin. Other drugs sometimes useful in the treatment of infections caused by rapidly growing mycobacteria include erythromycin, doxycycline, minocycline, ciprofloxacin, ofloxacin, ethionamide, tobramycin, imipenem, sulfonamides, and rifabutin. Relapses are not unusual, and prolonged therapy (12 to 16 weeks) is often recommended. Clarithromycin and other new macrolides are active in vitro, and preliminary anecdotal clinical reports are encouraging.

MYCOBACTERIUM HAEMOPHILUM This organism is a very fastidious, slow-growing, nonpigmented mycobacterium which requires hemin (factor X) or ferric ammonium citrate for in vitro growth. Optimal growth occurs at 30°C in 10% CO_2. *M. haemophilum* has been associated principally with chronic nodular skin lesions of the extremities, most often in immunocompromised patients (AIDS, lymphoma, transplant patients). The skin lesions may ulcerate. Arthritis, tenosynovitis, osteomyelitis, and occasionally lymphadenitis also have been reported. Some isolates have been susceptible to rifampin, rifabutin, PAS (*para*-amino salicylate), ciprofloxacin, cycloserine, kanamycin, minocycline, doxycycline, and trimethoprim-sulfamethoxazole. Surgical debridement has been helpful in some instances.

MYCOBACTERIUM KANSASII *M. kansasii* is nearly always photochromogenic, grows optimally at 37°C, and characteristically appears long and thick with prominent transverse banding on acid-fast smear. Infections are most common in the central United States, Japan, England, and Wales; most patients in the United States have originated in Louisiana, Texas, California, Illinois, or Florida. The reasons for these geographic variations are unknown but likely relate to subtle ecologic preferences of these organisms. *M. kansasii* has been isolated from tap and natural water sources, as well as from cattle and swine. Person-to-person spread is not recognized. The incidence of infection is highest in white adult males.

Pulmonary disease is the most frequent manifestation of infection with this organism, and the clinical picture closely resembles pulmonary tuberculosis, although signs and symptoms are milder. Pneumoconiosis and chronic obstructive pulmonary disease (COPD) are important predisposing conditions. Thin-walled cavities with minimal inflammatory reaction are typical roentgenographic findings. Pleural effusions are uncommon. Abnormalities usually progress slowly in the absence of therapy. As with other nontuberculous mycobacteria, isolation of *M. kansasii* does not necessarily indicate the presence of disease; 25 to 50 percent of positive sputum cultures are thought to represent colonization.

Skin and soft tissue involvement may mimic *M. marinum* infections. Tenosynovitis, osteomyelitis, lymphadenitis, pericarditis, and genitourinary tract infections have been reported. Disseminated disease is now recognized as an important manifestation of *M. kansasii* infections. Hematogenous spread is associated with hairy cell leukemia, malignancies, AIDS, and bone marrow and renal transplantation. Fever and signs and symptoms of multiple organ system involvement occur. Pancytopenia has been reported in disseminated infection.

Localized disease due to *M. kansasii* responds well to treatment. Rifampin appears to be the most effective drug and should be used in all initial regimens. Ethambutol and isoniazid are usually the other drugs administered. Typical strains demonstrate low-level resistance to isoniazid and streptomycin, but approximately 95 percent of patients respond to a 15- to 18-month course of isoniazid, rifampin, and ethambutol. The addition of ethambutol is important because the acquisition of rifampin resistance greatly complicates management. Other potentially active agents include sulfonamides, ciprofloxacin, ofloxacin, ethionamide, cycloserine, erythromycin, rifabutin, amikacin, and minocycline. Surgery is occasionally useful but seldom required.

MYCOBACTERIUM MARINUM This organism, previously known as *M. balnei*, is a photochromogen which inhabits fresh and salt water, grows best at 30°C, and causes disease in fish. Human infections are usually associated with some aquatic activity, such as working with fish tanks or swimming. *M. marinum* is relatively common along the Gulf Coast of the United States. The organism enters abraded skin and may form a nodule, which can spread along lymphatics in a pattern suggesting sporotrichosis, cause verrucous lesions, or, less commonly, ulcerate. The pathology consists of a granulomatous lesion which lacks caseation—the so-called swimming pool or fishtank granuloma. On acid-fast smear, *M. marinum* are relatively long organisms with frequent cross-barring, but primary smears reveal organisms in only a minority of patients. Infection is frequently associated with a positive tuberculin test reflecting shared antigens with *M. tuberculosis*. Because the differential diagnosis includes sporotrichosis as well as other mycobacterial infections, appropriate cultures at an incubation temperature of 28 to 32°C are critical. As with other mycobacteria associated with cutaneous disease (e.g., *M. haemophilum*, *M. ulcerans*), the inability of *M. marinum* to grow at 37°C explains its limitation to superficial tissues. Infections of tendon sheaths, bone, and synovium have been described in association with penetrating injuries. An unusual case involving the eye and a possible case of visceral involvement have been reported. Cutaneous ulcerations similar to those caused by *M. ulcerans*, as well as disseminated skin lesions, have been reported in immunocompromised patients. Minor lesions may resolve spontaneously. The organism is often sensitive in vitro to rifampin and ethambutol, and these drugs have been curative.

Tetracyclines, especially minocycline, and trimethoprim-sulfamethoxazole also have been used with favorable results. Prior steroid injections into infected sites are associated with an unfavorable prognosis. Surgical debridement is sometimes required.

MYCOBACTERIUM SCROFULACEUM This bacillus, which forms yellow-orange pigment even in the dark (scotochromogenic), is a cause of lymphadenitis in children. Environmental isolation has been reported from soil, water, raw milk, and oysters. *M. scrofulaceum* appears to be decreasing in incidence in the United States. Submandibular nodes are typically involved, in contrast to *M. tuberculosis*, which more frequently involves tonsillar, anterior cervical, or supraclavicular nodes, and associated systemic symptoms are rare. Definitive diagnosis requires culture, and definitive therapy requires total excision of the node and sinus tract, if present. There are a few reports of pulmonary disease, osseous and soft tissue infections, conjunctivitis, meningitis, and hepatitis. Dissemination usually is associated with serious underlying conditions. Surgery remains the mainstay of therapy. *M. scrofulaceum* is typically resistant to many drugs in vitro, and multiple-drug regimens have been used. Some isolates are sensitive to isoniazid, rifampin, streptomycin, cycloserine, sulfonamides, erythromycin, ethambutol, or ethionamide.

MYCOBACTERIUM SZULGAI At 37°C this organism is scotochromogenic and can be confused with more common tap water contaminants; at 25°C it is photochromogenic. It has been isolated from snails and tropical fish. *M. szulgai* is more than 99 percent homologous to *M. malmoense* at the RNA sequence level. *M. szulgai* was initially recognized as an uncommon pulmonary pathogen producing disease similar to *M. tuberculosis*. Bursitis, lymphadenitis, tenosynovitis, skin lesions, osteomyelitis, and disseminated disease also have been reported. Most isolates are sensitive to rifampin and

ethionamide. Isoniazid, ethambutol, streptomycin, erythromycin, tetracycline, trimethoprim-sulfamethoxazole, cefoxitin, and amikacin also may be active. As with other mycobacterial infections, combination therapy is advisable. Surgery may be required for definitive management.

MYCOBACTERIUM ULCERANS *M. ulcerans* is the etiologic agent of the Buruli or Bairnsdale ulcer. It is a nonchromogen which grows only at 30 to 33°C. Colonies may require 6 to 12 weeks to appear; isolation may be enhanced by inoculation of mouse footpads. A disease of the tropics, it is concentrated in Australia and Africa; foci in Malaysia, Papua (New Guinea), Guyana, and Mexico also have been recognized. The organism may be cultured from grass and is believed to be introduced into the skin via grass cuts. The first sign of infection with *M. ulcerans* is a small painless nodule developing into an extensive granulomatous ulceration, usually affecting the extensor surfaces of the extremities. Characteristically, the ulcer is deep with a necrotic base and undermined edges. Satellite lesions may develop. Tissue destruction may be mediated by a soluble bacterial toxin that appears to mute the host response. Patients do not exhibit constitutional symptoms. Wide surgical excision with skin grafting is curative; there are no clear data regarding chemotherapy. Dapsone and streptomycin with or without ethambutol may be used as adjunctive therapy. Isoniazid, trimethoprim-sulfamethoxazole, rifampin, oxytetracycline, minocycline, and clofazimine also may be active, but treatment failures have been reported despite in vitro drug susceptibility.

MYCOBACTERIUM XENOPI *M. xenopi* is a slow-growing scotochromogen. Although the mycobacterium was first isolated from a toad, birds may be an important reservoir in nature. Geographic foci with increased rates of isolation have been described in Ontario, southeast England, and Scandinavia. Although *M. xenopi* may grow in hot or cold water, it grows optimally at 42°C, and some strains will grow only at 42 to 45°C. Clusters of cases have occurred in association with contaminated hot water generators. *M. xenopi* infrequently causes tuberculosis-like pulmonary disease in humans, usually in association with underlying diseases. Cavitary disease is particularly common. Extrapulmonary disease is rare, but prosthetic joint, sinus tract, epididymis, osseous, and lymph node isolates have been described. Reports of disseminated disease are becoming more common, notably in patients with AIDS. Unlike a number of nontuberculous mycobacteria, it is sensitive to most of the antituberculous drugs in vitro, but some pulmonary infections have not responded well to antimicrobial therapy. Active agents include isoniazid, rifampin, ethambutol, streptomycin, ethionamide, cycloserine, and ciprofloxacin; some isolates are susceptible to vancomycin, cefuroxime, and erythromycin.

OTHER MYCOBACTERIA *M. asiaticum* is a photochromogen first isolated from monkeys. It is an uncommon cause of lung disease which resembles pulmonary tuberculosis but occurs predominantly in individuals with preexisting lung disease. The first reports of human disease due to *M. asiaticum* originated in Australia, and the organism is rarely isolated in the United States. Agents used in treatment have included isoniazid, rifampin, ethambutol, pyrazinamide, capreomycin, PAS, and streptomycin. Some isolates have been reported to be susceptible in vitro to cycloserine, kanamycin, and ciprofloxacin, although *M. asiaticum* appears to be somewhat less sensitive to fluoroquinolones than other nontuberculous mycobacteria.

M. malmoense is nonpigmented, microaerophilic, and slow growing. It grows poorly on conventional mycobacterial media; isolation can be facilitated by adjusting the pH to 6 to 6.5 and substituting 0.4% sodium pyruvate for glycerol. The organism can be confused microbiologically with nonpathogenic *M. terrae* or *M. gastri* species. Although a rare isolate in the United States, *M. malmoense* has been reported as a cause of chronic pulmonary disease in Scandinavia, Switzerland, Germany, Belgium, and the United Kingdom. Cases of lymphadenitis and dissemination in patients with AIDS or leukemia also have been described. Some isolates are susceptible to ethambutol, ethionamide, kanamycin, cycloserine, and erythromycin, but in vitro

in 1978, when infectious syphilis was most prevalent in homosexual and bisexual men. The dramatic increase in primary and secondary syphilis in women from 1986 to 1990 has resulted in a proportional increase in the number of infants born with congenital syphilis, to 2899 infants in 1990. It is important to note, however, that the case definition for congenital syphilis was broadened in 1989 and now includes all live or stillborn infants delivered to women with untreated or inadequately treated syphilis at delivery.

Approximately one of two individuals named as sexual contacts of persons with infectious syphilis becomes infected. Many sexual contacts will have already developed manifestations of syphilis when they are first seen, and about 30 percent of apparently uninfected contacts who are examined within 30 days of exposure will actually be in the incubation stage and will themselves develop infectious syphilis if not treated. Because of this, the identification and "epidemiologic" treatment of all recently exposed sexual contacts has become an important aspect of syphilis control. For every sex partner notified of exposure to syphilis during 1991, the CDC estimates that approximately 0.2 developed new previously untreated syphilis and received treatment and that 0.5 were exposed but seronegative and received prophylactic treatment. Also important is the identification of infected persons by serologic testing of pregnant women, hospital admissions, military inductees, and persons undergoing examination in physicians' offices. More controversial are laws and regulations requiring routine premarital serologic testing for syphilis, where the yield is undoubtedly lower, though national data are not available.

NATURAL COURSE AND PATHOGENESIS OF UNTREATED SYPHILIS *T. pallidum* rapidly penetrates intact mucous membranes or abraded skin and within a few hours enters the lymphatics and blood to produce systemic infection and metastatic foci long before the appearance of a primary lesion. Blood from a patient with incubating or early syphilis is infectious. The generation time of *T. pallidum* during early active disease in vivo is estimated to be 30 to 33 h, and the incubation period of syphilis is inversely proportional to the number of organisms inoculated. The concentration of treponemes generally reaches at least 10^7 per gram of tissue before the appearance of a clinical lesion. In experimental infection in rabbits or humans, very low numbers of treponemes can initiate infection which leads to a discernible lesion only after several weeks, although histopathologic changes are evident earlier; intradermal injection of 10^6 organisms usually produces a lesion within 72 h. The number of organisms required for production of symptomatic infection in humans was determined by intradermal injection of three graded doses of *T. pallidum* simultaneously at separate inoculation sites into each of eight volunteers; based on these results, the 50 percent infectious dose (ID_{50}) was calculated to be 57 organisms. The median incubation period in humans of about 21 days suggests an average inoculum of 500 to 1000 infectious organisms for naturally acquired disease. Experimental inoculations of humans and rabbits show that the period from inoculation until the primary lesion is discernible rarely exceeds 6 weeks. Subcurative therapy during the incubation period may delay the onset of the primary lesion, but it is not certain that this treatment reduces the probability of ultimate development of symptomatic disease.

The primary lesion appears at the site of inoculation, usually persists for 2 to 6 weeks, and then heals spontaneously. Histopathology of primary lesions shows perivascular infiltration, chiefly by lymphocytes (including CD8+ and CD4+ cells), plasma cells, and histiocytes, with capillary endothelial proliferation and subsequent obliteration of small blood vessels. At this time *T. pallidum* is demonstrable in the chancre in spaces between epithelial cells as well as within invaginations or phagosomes of epithelial cells, fibroblasts, plasma cells, and the endothelial cells of small capillaries, within lymphatic channels, and in the regional lymph nodes. Phagocytosis of organisms by macrophages ultimately causes their destruction, resulting in spontaneous resolution of the chancre.

The generalized parenchymal, constitutional, and mucocutaneous manifestations of secondary syphilis usually appear about 6 to 8 weeks after healing of the chancre, although 15 percent of patients with secondary syphilis have persisting or healing chancres. In other patients, secondary lesions may appear several months after the chancre has healed, and some patients may enter the latent stage without ever developing secondary lesions. Secondary maculopapular skin lesions show histopathologic features of hyperkeratosis of the epidermis, capillary proliferation with endothelial swelling in the superficial corium, and dermal papillae with transmigration of polymorphonuclear leukocytes and, in the deeper corium, perivascular infiltration by monocytes, plasma cells, and lymphocytes. Treponemes are found in many tissues, including the aqueous humor of the eye and the cerebrospinal fluid. Invasion of the central nervous system by *T. pallidum* occurs during the first weeks or months of infection, and cerebrospinal fluid abnormalities are detected in as many as 40 percent of patients during the secondary stage. Clinical hepatitis and immune complex–induced membranous glomerulonephritis are relatively rare but recognized manifestations of secondary syphilis; abnormal liver function tests may be demonstrated in up to a quarter of patients with early syphilis. Generalized lymphadenopathy is present in 85 percent of patients with secondary syphilis and is characterized by marked follicular hyperplasia, with histiocytic infiltration and lymphocyte depletion of the paracortical areas, where treponemes are present in greatest numbers. The reason for the paradoxical appearance of secondary manifestations in the face of high antibody titers (including immobilizing antibody) to *T. pallidum* is unknown. The secondary lesions subside within 2 to 6 weeks, and the patient enters the latent stage, which is detectable only by serologic testing. In the preantibiotic era, up to 25 percent of untreated patients experienced one or more subsequent generalized or localized mucocutaneous relapses at some time during the first 2 to 4 years after infection. Since 50 percent of such infectious relapses occur during the first year, identification and examination of sexual contacts are most important for patients with syphilis of less than 1 year's duration. Recurrent generalized rash is now rare.

In the preantibiotic era, about one-third of patients with untreated latent syphilis developed clinically apparent tertiary disease; today specific treatment and coincidental therapy of early and latent syphilis have greatly reduced the apparent incidence of tertiary disease. In the past, the most common type of tertiary disease was the gumma, a usually benign granulomatous lesion. Today, gummas are very uncommon. The tertiary lesions are caused by obliterative small-vessel endarteritis, which usually involves the vasa vasorum of the ascending aorta and, less often, the central nervous system. Asymptomatic CNS involvement is demonstrable in up to 25 percent of patients with late latent syphilis. Factors which determine development and progression of tertiary disease are unknown.

The course of untreated syphilis has been studied retrospectively in a group of nearly 2000 patients with primary or secondary syphilis diagnosed clinically, before the dark-field and Wassermann tests came into use (the Oslo Study, 1891–1951); prospectively in 431 black men with seropositive latent syphilis of 3 or more years' duration (the Tuskegee Study, 1932–1972); and retrospectively in a review of 198 autopsies of patients with untreated syphilis (the Rosahn Study, 1917–1942).

In the Oslo Study, 24 percent of the patients developed relapsing secondary lesions within 4 years, and 28 percent eventually developed one or more manifestations of late syphilis. Cardiovascular syphilis, including aortitis, was detected in 10 percent, with no cases occurring in those infected before age 15; symptomatic neurosyphilis occurred in 7 percent, and 16 percent developed benign tertiary syphilis (gumma of the skin, mucous membranes, and skeleton). Syphilis was the primary cause of death in 15 percent of males and 8 percent of females. Cardiovascular syphilis was found in 35 percent of men and 22 percent of women who eventually came to autopsy. In general, serious late complications were nearly twice as common in men as in women.

The Tuskegee Study showed that the death rate of untreated black men with syphilis, 25 to 50 years of age, was 17 percent greater than in uninfected subjects and that 30 percent of all deaths were attributable to cardiovascular or CNS syphilis. The ethical issues raised by this study, begun in the preantibiotic era but continuing into the early 1970s, had a major influence on development of current guidelines for human medical experimentation. By far the most important factor in increased mortality was cardiovascular syphilis. Anatomic evidence of aortitis was found in 40 to 60 percent of autopsied subjects with syphilis (versus 15 percent of controls), while CNS syphilis was found in only 4 percent. Hypertension also was increased in the infected subjects. These studies each show that about one-third of patients with untreated syphilis develop clinical or pathologic evidence of tertiary syphilis, about one-fourth die as a direct result of tertiary syphilis, and additional excess mortality not directly attributable to tertiary syphilis is also seen.

MANIFESTATIONS Primary syphilis The typical primary chancre usually begins as a single painless papule which rapidly becomes eroded and usually, but not always, is indurated, with a characteristic cartilaginous consistency on palpation of the edge and base of the ulcer (Fig. 133-3). Histologic examination of the ulcer shows lymphocytic and histiocytic infiltrates with obliterative endarteritis and periarteritis of small vessels. *T. pallidum* is seen by electron microscopy to lie in interstitial perivascular spaces and within invaginations or phagosomes of macrophages, neutrophils, endothelial cells, and plasma cells.

The chancre is usually located on the penis in heterosexual men, whereas in homosexual men it is often found in the anal canal or rectum, within the mouth, or on the external genitalia. In women, common primary sites are the cervix and labia. Consequently, primary syphilis may go unrecognized in women and homosexual men.

Atypical primary lesions are common. The clinical appearance depends on the number of treponemes inoculated and on the immunologic status of the patient. A large inoculum produces a dark-field–positive ulcerative lesion in nonimmune volunteers but may produce a small dark-field–negative papule, an asymptomatic but seropositive latent infection, or no response at all in individuals with a history of syphilis. A small inoculum usually produces only a papular lesion, even in nonimmune humans. Therefore, syphilis should be considered even in the evaluation of trivial or atypical, dark-field–negative genital lesions. The most common genital lesions which must be differentiated from primary syphilis include traumatic superinfected lesions, genital herpes simplex virus infection (see Chap. 143), and chancroid (see Chap. 112). *Primary genital herpes* may produce inguinal adenopathy, but the nodes are tender and associated with multiple painful vesicles, which later ulcerate and which are often accompanied by systemic symptoms including fever; *recurrent genital herpes* typically begins with a cluster of painful vesicles, usually without associated adenopa-thy. *Chancroid* produces painful, superficial exudative, nonindurated, more often multiple ulcers; adenopathy is either unilateral or bilateral, is tender, and may suppurate.

Regional lymphadenopathy usually accompanies the primary syphilitic lesion, appearing within 1 week of the onset of the lesion. The nodes are firm, nonsuppurative, and painless. Inguinal lymphadenopathy is bilateral and may occur with anal as well as with external genital chancres, since lymphatic drainage of the anus involves inguinal nodes. Rectal chancres result in perirectal lymphadenopathy, while chancres of the cervix and vagina result in iliac or perirectal adenopathy. The chancre generally heals within 4 to 6 weeks (range 2 to 12 weeks), but the lymphadenopathy may persist for months.

Secondary syphilis The manifestations of the secondary stage are protean but usually include localized or diffuse symmetric mucocutaneous lesions and generalized nontender lymphadenopathy. The healing primary chancre is still present in 15 percent of cases. The skin rash consists of macular, papular, papulosquamous, and occasionally pustular syphilides, often with one or more forms present simultaneously. The eruption may be very subtle, and approximately 25 percent of patients with a discernible rash of secondary syphilis may be unaware that they have dermatologic manifestations. Initial lesions are bilaterally symmetric, pale red or pink, nonpruritic, discrete, round macules, 5 to 10 mm in diameter, distributed on the trunk and proximal extremities (Fig. 133-4). After several days or weeks, red papular lesions 3 to 10 mm in diameter also appear. These may progress to necrotic lesions (resembling pustules) in association with increasing endarteritis and perivascular mononuclear infiltration. These lesions are distributed widely, frequently involve the palms and soles (Fig. 133-5), and may occur on the face and scalp. Tiny papular *follicular syphilides* involving hair follicles may result in patchy alopecia (alopecia areata) and loss of scalp hair, eyebrows, or beard in up to 5 percent of patients. Nonpatchy hair loss also occurs

FIGURE 133-4 Maculopapular rash of secondary syphilis. (*Reprinted, with permission, from Sexually Transmitted Diseases, Prof. Dr. E. Stolz, Rotterdam, ©Boehringer Ingelheim International, 1977.*)

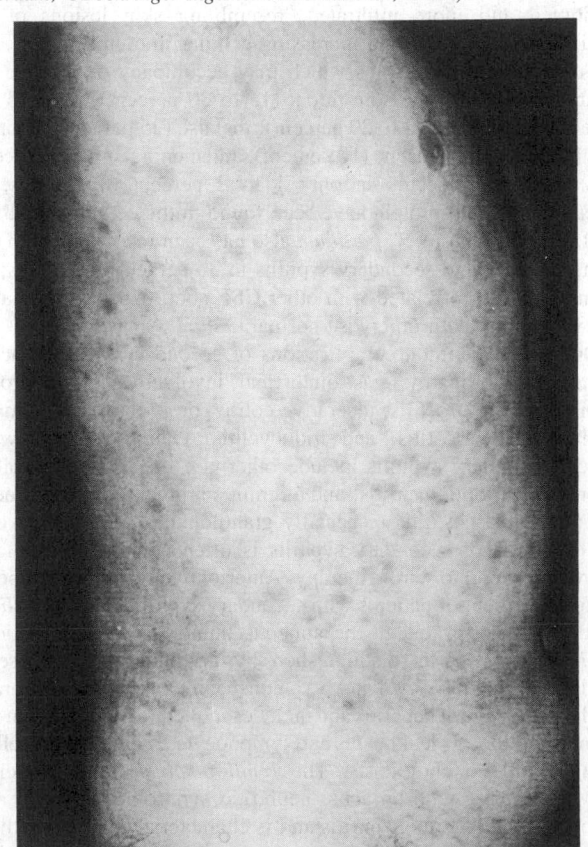

FIGURE 133-3 Primary chancre on the penis. (*Reprinted, with permission, from Sexually Transmitted Diseases, Prof. Dr. E. Stolz, Rotterdam, ©Boehringer Ingelheim International, 1977.*)

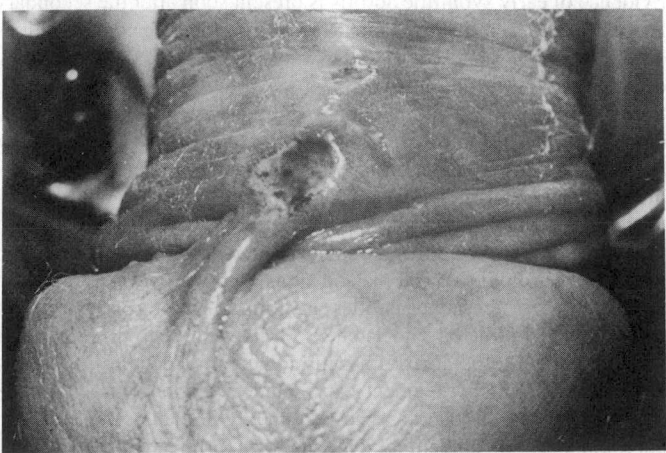

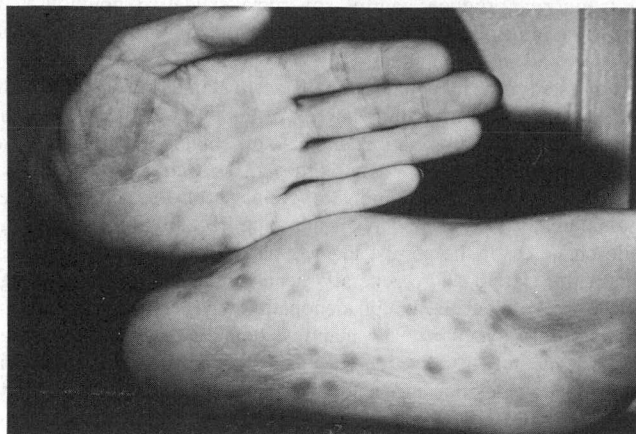

FIGURE 133-5   Secondary rash on palms and soles. (*From Ronald Roddy; reprinted, with permission, from Gynecology and Obstetrics, JW Sciarra (ed), New York, Harper & Row, 1985.*)

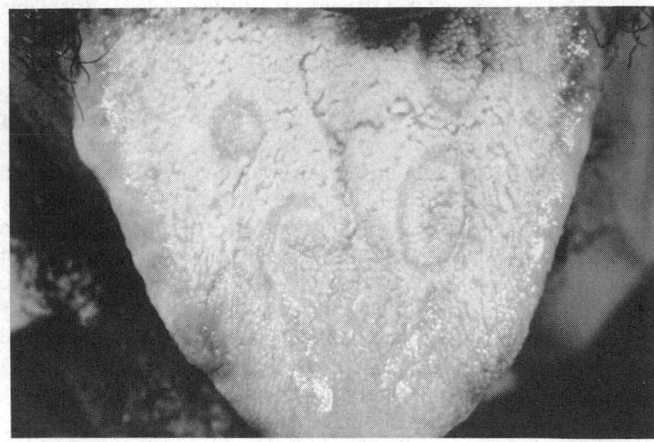

FIGURE 133-6   Mucous patches on the tongue. (*From Ronald Roddy; reprinted, with permission, from Sexually Transmitted Diseases, 2d ed, KK Holmes et al (eds), New York, McGraw-Hill, 1990.*)

in secondary syphilis. Progressive endarteritis obliterans and ischemia result in superficial scaling of papules (*papulosquamous syphilides*) and eventually may lead to central necrosis (*pustular syphilides*). In warm, moist, intertriginous areas, including the perianal area, vulva, scrotum, inner thighs, axillae, and the skin under pendulous breasts, papules enlarge and become eroded to produce broad, moist, pink or gray-white, highly infectious lesions called *condylomata lata*, which are seen in 10 percent of patients with secondary syphilis. Superficial mucosal erosions, called *mucous patches*, occur in 10 to 15 percent of patients and may involve lips, oral mucosa, tongue (Fig. 133-6), palate, pharynx, vulva and vagina, glans penis, or inner prepuce. The typical mucous patch is a silver-gray erosion surrounded by a red periphery and is usually painless.

During relapses of secondary syphilis, condylomata lata are particularly common, and skin lesions tend to be asymmetrically distributed and more infiltrated, resembling skin lesions of late syphilis, perhaps reflecting increasing cellular immunity.

Constitutional symptoms which may accompany or precede secondary syphilis include sore throat (15 to 30 percent), fever (5 to 8 percent), weight loss (2 to 20 percent), malaise (25 percent), anorexia (2 to 10 percent), headache (10 percent), and meningismus (5 percent). *Acute meningitis* occurs in only 1 to 2 percent of patients, but increased cells and protein have been found in the cerebrospinal fluid in 30 percent or more. *T. pallidum* also has been recovered from CSF during primary and secondary syphilis in 30 percent of patients; this finding is often correlated with other CSF abnormalities but may be seen in patients with otherwise normal CSF.

Other less common complications of secondary syphilis include hepatitis, nephropathy, gastrointestinal involvement (hypertrophic gastritis, patchy proctitis, ulcerative colitis, or a rectosigmoid mass), arthritis and periostitis, and iridocyclitis. Ocular findings which suggest secondary syphilis include otherwise unexplained pupillary abnormalities, optic neuritis, and a retinitis pigmentosa syndrome, as well as the classic iritis (especially granulomatous iritis) or uveitis. The diagnosis of secondary syphilis is often considered only after failure to respond to steroid therapy. Anterior uveitis has been reported in 5 to 10 percent of patients with secondary syphilis, and *T. pallidum* has been demonstrated in the aqueous humor from these patients. *Syphilitic hepatitis* is distinguished by an unusually high serum alkaline phosphatase level and by a nonspecific histologic appearance which is unlike viral hepatitis and includes moderate inflammation with polymorphonuclear leukocytes and lymphocytes, some hepatocellular damage, and no cholestasis. The *renal involvement* is associated with proteinuria, with an acute nephrotic syndrome, or rarely with hemorrhagic glomerulonephritis and is characterized by subepithelial electron-dense deposits and glomerular immune complexes—findings

suggesting that this complication is a form of immune-complex glomerulonephritis.

Latent syphilis   A diagnosis of latent syphilis is established by the finding of a positive specific treponemal antibody test for syphilis together with a normal CSF examination and the absence of clinical manifestations of syphilis on physical examination and chest films. The diagnosis is often suspected on the basis of a history of primary or secondary lesions, history of exposure to syphilis, or delivery of an infant with congenital syphilis. A previous negative serologic test and a history of lesions or exposure may help establish the duration of latent infection. *Early latent* syphilis encompasses the first year after infection, while *late latent* syphilis beginning 1 year after infection in the untreated patient is associated with relative immunity to infectious relapse and with increasing resistance to reinfection. *T. pallidum* may still intermittently seed the bloodstream during this stage; pregnant women with latent syphilis may infect the fetus in utero; and transfusion syphilis has been transmitted from patients with latent syphilis of many years' duration. It was thought that untreated late latent syphilis had three possible outcomes: (1) it could persist throughout the life of the infected individual, (2) it could end in development of late syphilis, or (3) it could end with spontaneous cure of infection, with reversion of serologic tests to negative. It is now apparent, however, that the more sensitive treponemal antibody tests rarely, if ever, become negative. About 70 percent of untreated patients with latent syphilis never develop clinically evident late syphilis, but the occurrence of spontaneous cure is in doubt.

Late syphilis   The onset of slowly progressive inflammatory disease leading to the tertiary stage begins early during the pathogenesis of syphilis, although it may not be clinically apparent for years. Evidence of early syphilitic aortitis is present soon after the secondary lesions subside, and it is patients who develop CSF abnormalities during the early stages of syphilis who appear to be at highest risk of late neurologic complications.

ASYMPTOMATIC NEUROSYPHILIS   Central nervous system syphilis represents a continuum of early invasion, usually within the first weeks or months of infection, and asymptomatic involvement, which may or may not result in neurologic manifestations. Traditionally, the diagnosis of asymptomatic neurosyphilis has been made in patients who no longer have manifestations of primary or secondary syphilis, who lack neurologic symptoms and signs, and who have certain CSF abnormalities. Such abnormalities are found in up to one-quarter of patients with untreated late latent syphilis, and it is these patients who are known to be at risk for neurologic complications. However, evidence of CNS involvement can include isolation of *T. pallidum* from CSF even in the absence of other CSF abnormalities, and approximately 40 percent of patients with primary and secondary syphilis have had *T. pallidum* isolated from the CSF, abnormalities of the CSF consistent with asymptomatic neurosyphilis, or both. Although the therapeutic implications of these findings in early syphilis are uncertain, it seems appropriate to conclude that patients with early syphilis who have such findings do indeed have asymptomatic neurosyphilis. In patients with untreated asymptomatic neurosyphilis, the overall cumulative probability of progression to clinical neurosyphilis is about 20 percent in the first 10 years but increases with passing time and is highest in those who show the greatest degree of pleocytosis or protein elevation. Patients with untreated latent syphilis and normal CSF probably have no future risk of subsequently developing neurosyphilis.

SYMPTOMATIC NEUROSYPHILIS   Although mixed features are common, the major clinical categories of symptomatic neurosyphilis include meningeal, meningovascular, and parenchymatous syphilis. The last category includes general paresis and tabes dorsalis. The interval from infection to onset of symptoms is a few months to 20 years for meningeal syphilis (usually in the first year) and for meningovascular syphilis (average 7 years), 20 years for general paresis, and 25 to 30 years for tabes dorsalis. However, many patients with symptomatic neurosyphilis, particularly in the antibiotic era, do not present a classic picture but have mixed and subtle or incomplete syndromes. *Meningeal syphilis* may involve either the brain or spinal cord, and patients may present with headache, nausea, vomiting, neck stiffness, cranial nerve palsies, seizures, and changes in mental status. *Meningovascular syphilis* is associated with diffuse inflammation of the pia and arachnoid, together with evidence of focal or widespread arterial involvement of small, medium, or large vessels. The most common presentation is a stroke syndrome in a relatively young adult involving the middle cerebral artery; however, unlike the usual thrombotic or embolic stroke syndrome of sudden onset, meningovascular syphilis often presents after a subacute encephalitic prodrome with headaches, vertigo, insomnia, and psychological abnormalities followed by a gradually progressive vascular syndrome. The manifestations of *general paresis* reflect widespread parenchymal damage and include abnormalities corresponding to the mnemonic *paresis* [*p*ersonality, *a*ffect, *r*eflexes (hyperactive), *e*ye (e.g., Argyll Robertson pupils), *s*ensorium (illusions, delusions, hallucinations), *i*ntellect (decreased recent memory, orientation, calculations, judgment, insight), and *s*peech]. *Tabes dorsalis* presents symptoms and signs of demyelination of the posterior columns, dorsal roots, and dorsal root ganglia. Symptoms include ataxic wide-based gait and footslap, paresthesias, bladder disturbances, impotence, areflexia, and loss of position, deep pain, and temperature sensation. Trophic joint degeneration (Charcot's joints) and perforating ulceration of the feet can result from loss of pain sensation. The Argyll Robertson pupil, seen in both tabes dorsalis and paresis, is a small, irregular pupil which reacts to accommodation but not to light. *Optic atrophy* also occurs frequently in association with tabes.

CARDIOVASCULAR SYPHILIS   Cardiovascular manifestations are limited to the large vessels in which the blood supply is provided by vasa vasorum. Endarteritis obliterans of the vasa vasorum produces medial necrosis with destruction of elastic tissue, particularly in the ascending and transverse segments of the aortic arch, resulting in uncomplicated aortitis, aortic regurgitation, saccular aneurysm, or coronary ostial stenosis. The onset of symptoms occurs from 10 to 40 years after infection. Cardiovascular complications are more common and occur at an earlier age in men than in women and may be more common in blacks than in whites. In the preantibiotic era, the incidence of symptomatic cardiovascular complications in late untreated syphilis was approximately 10 percent, with aortic regurgitation being two to four times as common as aneurysm. However, syphilitic aortitis was demonstrated at autopsy in about one-half of black men with untreated syphilis.

Asymptomatic syphilitic aortitis may be suspected if linear calcification of the ascending aorta is demonstrated on chest x-ray films, since arteriosclerotic disease seldom produces this sign. Aortic dilatation and a tambour quality of the sound of aortic closure are unreliable signs of aortitis. Syphilitic aneurysms are usually saccular, occasionally fusiform, and do not lead to dissection. Approximately 1 in 10 aortic aneurysms of syphilitic origin may involve the abdominal aorta, but these aneurysms tend to occur above the renal arteries, whereas arteriosclerotic abdominal aneurysms usually are found below the renal arteries. With increasing age, the nervous system is also affected in up to 40 percent of patients with cardiovascular syphilis.

LATE LESIONS OF THE EYES   Iritis associated with pain, photophobia, and dimness of vision or chorioretinitis occurs not only during secondary syphilis but also as a relatively common manifestation of late syphilis. Adhesions of the iris to the anterior lens may produce a fixed pupil, not to be confused with Argyll Robertson pupil.

LATE BENIGN SYPHILIS (GUMMA)   Gummas may be multiple or diffuse but are usually solitary lesions which range from microscopic size to several centimeters in diameter and histologically consist of granulomatous inflammation with central necrosis surrounded by mononuclear, epithelioid, and fibroblastic cells, occasional giant cells, and perivasculitis. Although *T. pallidum* is rarely demonstrated microscopically, it has reportedly been recovered from the lesions. The most commonly involved sites are the skin and skeletal systems, mouth and upper respiratory tract, larynx, liver, and stomach, although any organ may be involved. Gummas of skin produce painless nodular, papulosquamous, or ulcerative lesions, which are indurated and form characteristic circles or arcs, with peripheral hyperpigmentation. The lesions are usually indolent and may heal spontaneously with scarring, but they also may be explosive in onset and are often destructive. These lesions may resemble many other chronic granulomatous conditions, including tuberculosis and sarcoidosis, leprosy, and deep fungal infections. Skeletal gummas involve long bones of the legs with greatest frequency, although any bone may be affected. Trauma may predispose to involvement of a specific site. Presenting symptoms usually include focal pain and tenderness. When sufficiently advanced to produce radiographic abnormalities, the findings may include periostitis or destructive or sclerosing osteitis. Gummas of the upper respiratory tract can lead to perforation of the nasal septum or palate. Gummatous hepatitis may produce epigastric pain and tenderness and low-grade fever and may be associated with splenomegaly and anemia.

The histopathology and extensive tissue necrosis associated with gummas suggest that delayed hypersensitivity to *T. pallidum* produces these lesions. Certain individuals appear to develop an exaggerated delayed-hypersensitivity response to *T. pallidum*, presumably mediated by sensitized T lymphocytes and macrophages. Since the histologic changes may be suggestive but are nonspecific, the diagnosis of late benign syphilis is confirmed by serologic testing and by therapeutic trial. Treatment with penicillin results in rapid healing of active gummatous lesions.

Congenital syphilis   Transmission of *T. pallidum* from a syphilitic woman to her fetus across the placenta may occur at any stage of pregnancy, but the lesions of congenital syphilis develop generally after the fourth month of gestation, when immunologic competence begins to develop. This timing suggests that the pathogenesis of congenital syphilis may depend on the immune response of the host rather than on a direct toxic effect of *T. pallidum*. The risk of infection of the fetus during untreated early maternal syphilis is estimated to be 75 to 95 percent, decreasing to about 35 percent for maternal syphilis of longer than 2 years' duration, with the risk of fetal infection apparently continuing throughout late latent maternal syphilis. Adequate treatment of the mother before the sixteenth week of pregnancy should prevent fetal damage. Untreated maternal infection may result in up to 40 percent fetal loss (stillbirth is more common than abortion, because of the late onset of fetal pathology), prematurity, neonatal death, or nonfatal congenital syphilis. Of mothers with untreated syphilis of less than 2 years' duration, 21 percent aborted or had a stillbirth, 13 percent had infants who died within 2 months, 43 percent had infants with syphilis alive at 2 months, and 23 percent had nonsyphilitic infants. Only fulminant cases of congenital syphilis are clinically apparent in live infants at birth, and these babies have a very poor prognosis. The most common clinical problem is the healthy-appearing baby born to a mother who has a positive serologic test. Routine serologic testing in early pregnancy is considered cost-effective in virtually all populations, even in areas of low prenatal prevalence of syphilis. In noncompliant individuals, rapid plasma reagin (RPR) screening should be performed when pregnancy is detected to ensure prompt treatment. Where the prevalence of syphilis is high, and in high-risk patients, syphilis serology should be repeated in the third trimester and at delivery.

The manifestations of congenital syphilis can be divided into (1) early manifestations, which appear within the first 2 years of life, often between 2 and 10 weeks of age, are infectious, and resemble severe secondary syphilis in the adult; (2) late manifestations, which appear after 2 years and are noninfectious; and (3) the residual stigmata of congenital syphilis. During 1990, 87 percent of reported cases of congenital syphilis were diagnosed during the first year of life.

The earliest sign of congenital syphilis is usually rhinitis ("snuffles"), soon followed by other mucocutaneous lesions. These may include bullae (syphilitic pemphigus), vesicles, superficial desquamation, petechiae, and later, papulosquamous lesions, mucous patches, and condylomata lata. The most common early manifestations are osteochondritis and osteitis, particularly involving the metaphyses of long bones, progressing in severity during the first 6 months of life and then spontaneously subsiding; and periostitis, which continues to progress after the first 6 months. Hepatosplenomegaly, lymphadenopathy, anemia, jaundice, thrombocytopenia, and leukocytosis are common. The anemia is usually hypoproliferative but may be hemolytic (paroxysmal cold hemoglobinuria due to Donath-Landsteiner antibody, an IgG antibody that binds to the P antigen of red cells at low temperatures). The nephrotic syndrome in early congenital syphilis, as in adult secondary syphilis, represents an immune-complex–induced glomerulonephritis. A compilation of clinical presentations of congenital syphilis in nine studies involving a total of 212 infants included abnormal bone x-rays (61 percent), hepatomegaly (51 percent), splenomegaly (49 percent), petechiae (41 percent), other skin rash (35 percent), anemia (34 percent), lymphadenopathy (32 percent), jaundice (30 percent), pseudoparalysis (28 percent), and snuffles (23 percent).

Neonatal congenital syphilis must be differentiated from other generalized congenital infections, including rubella, cytomegalovirus or herpes simplex virus infection, and toxoplasmosis, as well as from erythroblastosis fetalis. Neonatal death is usually due to pulmonary hemorrhage, secondary bacterial infection, or severe hepatitis. Pathologic findings include interstitial and perivascular inflammation, followed by variable fibroblastic proliferation, involving skin, bones, liver, kidneys, pancreas, spleen, lungs, and intestines, and by extramedullary hematopoiesis.

Late congenital syphilis is defined as congenital syphilis which remains untreated after 2 years of age. In perhaps 60 percent of cases, the infection remains subclinical, while the clinical spectrum in the remainder differs in certain respects from that of acquired late syphilis in the adult. For example, cardiovascular syphilis rarely develops in late congenital syphilis, whereas interstitial keratitis is much more common and occurs between ages 5 and 25. The onset is acute, with photophobia, pain, and circumcorneal injection, followed by superficial and deep vascularization of the cornea, which progresses despite antibiotic therapy and eventually becomes bilateral. The symptoms and signs may be suppressed with glucocorticoid therapy. Although treponemes have occasionally been demonstrated in aqueous humor in interstitial keratitis, the pathogenesis is obscure and is ascribed to "hypersensitivity." Other manifestations associated with interstitial keratitis are eighth-nerve deafness and recurrent arthropathy. Bilateral knee effusions are known as *Clutton's joints*. Examination of CSF discloses asymptomatic neurosyphilis in about one-third of untreated patients without other late clinical manifestations, and clinical neurosyphilis occurs in a quarter of untreated individuals with

congenital syphilis over 6 years of age. The clinical manifestations of congenital neurosyphilis correspond to those seen in adult neurosyphilis. Gummatous periostitis occurs between ages 5 and 20 and, as in nonvenereal endemic childhood syphilis, tends to cause destructive lesions of the palate and nasal septum.

Characteristic stigmata include *Hutchinson's teeth*, the centrally notched, widely spaced, peg-shaped upper central incisors and "mulberry" molars, sixth-year molars which have multiple, poorly developed cusps, numbering more than the usual four. The abnormal facies of congenital syphilis, which includes frontal bossing, saddlenose, and poorly developed maxillae, also may be seen in congenital ectodermal dysplasia. Saber shins, or anterior tibial bowing, are rare but were probably more common in the past when syphilitic periostitis of the anterior tibia was accompanied by vitamin D deficiency. *Rhagades* are linear scars at the angles of the mouth and nose caused by secondary bacterial infection of the early facial eruption. Other stigmata include unexplained nerve deafness, old chorioretinitis, optic atrophy, and corneal opacities due to past interstitial keratitis.

LABORATORY EXAMINATIONS Dark-field examination technique Dark-field examination is essential in evaluating cutaneous lesions, such as the chancre of primary syphilis or condylomata lata of secondary syphilis. Although it is often difficult to demonstrate *T. pallidum* in dry maculopapular lesions in secondary syphilis by dark-field examination, the organism may be demonstrated by saline aspiration of lymph nodes during this stage. The surface of the suspected ulcerated lesion should be cleaned with saline and gauze and then gently abraded further with dry gauze without production of bleeding. The lesion is then squeezed to express a serous transudate, and a drop of the transudate is picked up on the surface of a glass slide. A drop of saline (without bacteriostatic additives) may be mixed with the transudate if necessary, and this preparation is then covered with a coverslip and examined immediately for *T. pallidum* with a dark-field or phase-contrast microscope by an experienced individual. The identification of a single characteristic motile organism by a trained observer is sufficient for diagnosis. Examination of oral lesions by this method is not recommended, and it is also difficult to differentiate *T. pallidum* from other spirochetes that may be present in anal ulcers. A single negative examination does not exclude syphilis, since at least 10^4 treponemes per microliter of transudate must be present to be seen, and prior use of topical antiseptic or cleansing by the patient may obfuscate the results. Cleansing or use of topical medication should therefore be avoided, and ideally, the dark-field examination should be repeated on three successive days before being considered negative.

Direct immunofluorescence Most syphilis is diagnosed in private physicians' offices where dark-field microscopy is not available; alternative methods for the identification of *T. pallidum* in exudate are needed. The direct fluorescent antibody *T. pallidum* (DFA-TP) test, available at central laboratories, uses fluorescein-conjugated polyclonal antitreponemal antibody for detection of *T. pallidum* in fixed smears prepared from suspect lesions. Because of cross-reactive antibodies which also will stain commensal nonpathogenic spirochetes, the antiserum is extensively absorbed with cultured treponemes in an effort to produce a specific reagent.

A refinement of this technique using a monoclonal antibody which is specific only for the pathogenic treponemes has been developed but is not yet commercially available. It has been shown in clinical trials to be as sensitive and specific as dark-field microscopy for examination of suspicious lesions. A new monoclonal antibody–based ELISA test, which detects *T. pallidum* in swab specimens from primary and secondary lesions, is currently being evaluated.

Demonstration of *T. pallidum* in tissue It is often necessary to demonstrate *T. pallidum* in tissue when clinical or histopathologic features suggest the diagnosis of syphilis. Although the organism can be found in tissue by appropriate silver stains, these results should be interpreted with caution, because artifacts resembling *T. pallidum* are often seen. Treponemes can be demonstrated more reliably in tissue by immunofluorescence or immunohistochemistry using specific monoclonal or polyclonal antibodies to *T. pallidum*.

Serologic tests for syphilis The profusion of serologic tests for syphilis causes much unnecessary confusion. Syphilitic infection produces two types of antibodies, the nonspecific *reaginic* antibody and specific antitreponemal antibody, which are measured by the nontreponemal and treponemal tests, respectively (Table 133-1). The treponemal tests, as well as the nontreponemal tests, are reactive in persons with any treponemal infection, including yaws, pinta, and endemic syphilis.

The nontreponemal antibodies produced in syphilis contain both IgG and IgM immunoglobulins directed against a lipoidal antigen that results from the interaction of *T. pallidum* with host tissues and possibly against a lipoidal antigen of *T. pallidum* itself. The term *reagin* is unfortunate, since the unrelated IgE antibody involved in certain allergic phenomena is also known as reagin. The most widely used nontreponemal or reagin antibody tests for syphilis are the RPR test, which can be automated (ART), and the Venereal Disease Research Laboratory (VDRL) slide test. Other, less frequently used nontreponemal tests include the unheated serum reagin (USR) and the reagin screen test (RST). In these tests, antibody is detected by the microscopic (VDRL, USR) or macroscopic (RPR, RST) flocculation of the antigen suspension (see Table 133-1).

The RPR is often more expensive than the VDRL test but is easier to perform and uses unheated serum; it is the test of choice for rapid serologic diagnosis in a clinic or office setting. The VDRL reagents are less expensive but must be prepared fresh daily. Although the development of the simpler macroscopic tests has resulted in the replacement of the VDRL by the RPR test for examination of serum in many laboratories, the VDRL test remains the standard for use with CSF.

RPR and VDRL tests are equally sensitive and may be used for initial screening or for quantitation of serum reagin antibody titer. The reagin titer reflects the activity of the disease. A fourfold or greater rise in titer may be seen during the evolution of primary syphilis; VDRL titers usually reach 1:32 or higher in secondary syphilis; a persistent fall in titer following treatment of early syphilis provides essential evidence of an adequate response to therapy. VDRL titers do not correspond directly to RPR titers, and sequential quantitative testing (as for response to therapy) must employ a single test.

There are two standard treponemal tests: the fluorescent treponemal antibody–absorption (FTA-ABS) test and the microhemagglutination assay for antibodies to *T. pallidum* (MHA-TP). Another hemagglutination test, the TPHA, is widely used in Europe but is not available in the United States.

For the FTA-ABS test, the patient's serum is first diluted with a substance containing nonpathogenic treponemal antigens (sorbent) to bind group-specific antibodies which may be produced against saprophytic oral and genital treponemes. The patient's absorbed serum is then placed on a slide which contains fixed *T. pallidum*. If specific antibody to *T. pallidum* is present in the patient's serum, it is bound to the dried treponemes and is then detected by the addition of fluorescein-labeled antihuman gamma globulin and subsequent examination of the slide by fluorescence microscopy. The *T. pallidum*

hemagglutination tests (MHA-TP and TPHA) also use a sorbent-like diluent for binding treponemal group antibodies. *T. pallidum*–specific antibody is detected by agglutination of *T. pallidum*–coated sheep or turkey erythrocytes. These hemagglutination tests are more commonly used than the FTA-ABS test. The *T. pallidum* immobilization (TPI) test, in which immobilization of live *T. pallidum* is produced by immune serum plus complement, is the most specific treponemal test but is more laborious and, in the United States, is available only in research laboratories. Both the hemagglutination and FTA-ABS tests are very specific and, when used for confirmation of positive reaginic antibody tests, have a very high positive predictive value for the diagnosis of syphilis. However, even these tests give false-positive rates as high as 1 to 2 percent when used for screening normal populations.

The relative sensitivities of the VDRL, FTA-ABS, and MHA-TP tests in the various stages of syphilis are shown in Table 133-2. The nontreponemal tests are nonreactive in nearly one-third of patients with primary or late syphilis. In early primary syphilis, the detection of antibody can be maximized either by performing an FTA-ABS test or simply by repeating a VDRL test after 1 to 2 weeks if the initial VDRL was negative. However, obtaining a reagin antibody test alone is not sufficient in evaluating late symptomatic syphilis; the more sensitive FTA-ABS test should be obtained routinely in suspected late syphilis. The hemagglutination tests are even less sensitive than the reagin tests in primary syphilis but are as sensitive as the FTA-ABS test in other stages. All treponemal and nontreponemal tests are reactive during secondary syphilis, and a nonreactive result virtually excludes syphilis in a patient with otherwise compatible mucocutaneous lesions. (Less than 1 percent of patients with secondary syphilis have a nonreactive or weakly reactive VDRL test with undiluted serum which becomes positive in higher dilutions—the *prozone* phenomenon.) While the nontreponemal tests will become negative or decline in titer following therapy for early syphilis, the treponemal tests will often remain reactive after therapy and are not helpful in determining the infection status in persons with past syphilis.

The presence of specific IgM antibody has been proposed as a marker for active syphilis, with the claim that IgM disappears following adequate therapy. The rate at which IgM declines after therapy is quite variable from patient to patient, and the use of this criterion for cure is not universally accepted. A new 19S IgM FTA-ABS test for syphilis has been approved for use by the Centers for Disease Control and is recommended for evaluation of infants with suspected congenital syphilis.

False-positive serologic tests for syphilis Because the antigen used in the nontreponemal tests is found in other tissues, the tests may be reactive in persons without treponemal infection, although rarely in titers exceeding 1:8. In a population which has been selected for screening because of clinical suspicion, history of exposure, or increased risk for sexually transmitted infections, <2 percent of reactive tests are falsely positive. False-positive reagin tests are classified as acute if they become negative within 6 months and may occur during a variety of acute infections, such as viral diseases, *Mycoplasma* pneumonia, and malaria, and following certain immuni-

---

TABLE 133-1 Common serologic tests for syphilis

Nontreponemal (reagin) tests
  Microscopic flocculation: Venereal Disease Research Laboratory (VDRL)
  Macroscopic flocculation: rapid plasma reagin (RPR)

Treponemal tests
  Immunofluorescence: fluorescent treponemal antibody-absorption (FTA-ABS)
  Hemagglutination: *T. pallidum* hemagglutination assay (MHA-TP, TPHA)

TABLE 133-2 Reactivity of serodiagnostic tests in untreated syphilis

Test	Stage of disease, % positive*			
	Primary	Secondary	Latent	Tertiary
VDRL	59–87	100	73–91	37–94
FTA-ABS	86–100	99–100	96–99	96–100
MHA-TP	64–87	96–100	96–100	94–100

* Percentage figures provided should not be interpreted as absolute values because there are small numbers in certain categories and test results vary from study to study.
SOURCE: Modified (with permission) from H Jaffe, D Musher, Management of the reactive syphilis serology, in *Sexually Transmitted Diseases*, KK Holmes et al (eds), 2d ed. New York, McGraw-Hill, 1990, p 935.

zations. Chronic reactions, which persist 6 months or longer, occur in intravenous drug addiction, in autoimmune diseases, and with aging. False-positive reagin tests occur in 25 percent of narcotic addicts and in 10 to 20 percent of patients with active systemic lupus erythematosus. The autoimmune nature of the false-positive reagin test is suggested by the occurrence of systemic lupus erythematosus or other connective tissue diseases in 15 to 45 percent of chronic false-positive reactors. Other antibodies which have been found with great frequency in sera from chronic false-positive reactors include antinuclear, antithyroid, and antimitochondrial antibodies as well as rheumatoid factor and cryoglobulins. The Donath-Landsteiner antibody responsible for paroxysmal cold hemoglobinuria is an autoimmune hemolysin which appears in syphilis. The prevalence of false-positive reagin tests increases with advancing age, and 10 percent of people over 70 years of age have false-positive reactions. Other diseases associated with hyperglobulinemia, such as leprosy, also may produce chronic false-positive reactions.

In the patient with a false-positive reagin test, syphilis is excluded by obtaining a nonreactive treponemal test. A typical *reactive* FTA-ABS test occurs infrequently in conditions other than syphilis. Although false-positive FTA-ABS tests have been reported in 15 percent of patients with active systemic lupus erythematosus, the fluorescent staining is often weak or has an atypical "beaded" appearance which is recognized by the technician. For practical purposes, most clinicians need to be familiar with the three uses of serologic tests for syphilis: (1) for testing large numbers of sera for screening or diagnostic purposes (e.g., RPR or VDRL), (2) for quantitative measurement of reaginic antibody titer in order to assess the clinical activity of syphilis or to follow the reagin titer in response to therapy (e.g., VDRL or RPR), and (3) for confirmation of the diagnosis of syphilis in a patient with a positive reagin antibody test or with a suspected clinical diagnosis of syphilis (e.g., FTA-ABS or MHA-TP).

Evaluation for asymptomatic neurosyphilis Asymptomatic involvement of the central nervous system is detected by examination of cerebrospinal fluid. CSF abnormalities are very infrequent in the primary stage, but pleocytosis or elevated protein can be demonstrated in CSF from up to 40 percent of patients with secondary or latent syphilis. *T. pallidum* has been recovered by rabbit inoculation from up to 40 percent of those with primary and secondary syphilis but rarely from those with latent syphilis. The demonstration of *T. pallidum* in CSF is often associated with other CSF abnormalities; however, organisms can be recovered from patients without pleocytosis or elevated protein. In the prepenicillin era, the risk of developing clinical neurosyphilis was roughly proportional to the intensity of CSF changes in early syphilis. CSF examination is essential in any seropositive patient with neurologic signs and symptoms and is recommended in all patients with untreated syphilis of unknown duration or of greater than 1 year's duration. The possibility that asymptomatic neurosyphilis is present in some patients with secondary and early latent disease is not addressed by these recommendations. Because standard penicillin G benzathine (benzathine benzylpenicillin) therapy for early syphilis fails to result in treponemicidal levels in the CSF, some experts advise lumbar puncture in secondary and early latent syphilis, with follow-up examinations for patients with abnormalities.

CSF is examined for pleocytosis, increased protein concentration, and VDRL reactivity. The CSF VDRL test is very specific if the fluid is not contaminated with blood. The CSF VDRL test is relatively insensitive, however, and may be nonreactive even in progressive symptomatic neurosyphilis. Highest sensitivities are seen in meningovascular syphilis and paresis; lower sensitivities are seen in asymptomatic neurosyphilis and tabes dorsalis. The unabsorbed FTA test on CSF is reactive far more often than the CSF VDRL test in all stages of syphilis, but FTA reactivity may reflect passive transfer of serum antibody into the CSF. Most specialists do not recommend performing an FTA test on CSF. Similarly, the finding of a reactive CSF FTA-ABS test without other CSF abnormalities in a patient with nonspecific neurologic findings does not prove a diagnosis of neurosyphilis. Even in the absence of confirmatory CSF examination, a therapeutic trial of penicillin in doses adequate for neurosyphilis is warranted in any patient with a positive serum treponemal antibody test who also has neurologic findings consistent with neurosyphilis.

Attempts to identify a more sensitive and specific marker for neurosyphilis have included CSF oligoclonal banding and measurement of intrathecal production of antitreponemal IgM and IgG. CSF from 80 percent of patients with multiple sclerosis and approximately 40 percent of patients with other inflammatory CNS diseases (including neurosyphilis, bacterial meningitis, viral encephalitis, subacute sclerosing panencephalitis) has discrete oligoclonal immunoglobulin bands in the gamma globulin region following agarose gel electrophoresis. These antibodies are thought to be intrathecally produced and have specificity for the etiologic agent (e.g., *T. pallidum* in syphilis and measles virus in subacute sclerosing panencephalitis); however, an oligoclonal banding pattern per se is not specific for neurosyphilis in a seropositive patient.

Evaluation for syphilis in patients concurrently infected with human immunodeficiency virus (HIV) Because persons at highest risk for acquiring syphilis (inner-city populations and homosexually active men) are also at high risk for acquisition of HIV, these infections are frequently found in the same patient. There is evidence that syphilis and other genital ulcer diseases may be important risk factors for acquisition and transmission of HIV infection. Several studies propose that the manifestations of syphilis may be altered in patients with concurrent HIV infection, and multiple cases of neurologic relapse following standard therapy have been reported in HIV-infected patients. *T. pallidum* has been isolated from the CSF of patients following therapy for early syphilis with penicillin G benzathine. One case of VDRL and FTA-ABS seronegative secondary syphilis has been reported in a patient with AIDS; this patient finally seroconverted prior to therapy after weeks of secondary manifestations. In contrast, HIV-infected patients with unusually high VDRL or RPR titers also have been described. It should be emphasized that the nature and extent of the interaction between HIV infection and syphilis have not been well defined. The frequency of unusual clinical and laboratory manifestations of syphilis in patients coinfected with HIV is unknown, and such changes may be dependent on the stage of HIV infection and degree of immunosuppression. There is no clear evidence that the sensitivity of serologic tests for syphilis or the serologic response to therapy is different in the vast majority of HIV-infected patients, and interpretation of serologic results in these patients should be the same as for HIV-uninfected individuals.

The evaluation of all syphilis patients should include serologic testing for HIV, with the patient's consent. Conversely, persons with newly diagnosed HIV infection should be tested for syphilis. Examination of CSF for evidence of neurosyphilis is recommended by some authorities for all coinfected patients, regardless of the clinical stage of syphilis. If CSF abnormalities are found, or if CSF examination is not performed, therapy adequate for neurosyphilis should be administered regardless of the apparent stage of infection. Serologic testing following treatment is important for all patients with syphilis and particularly for those also infected with HIV.

TREATMENT OF ACQUIRED SYPHILIS Penicillin G is the drug of choice for all stages of syphilis. *T. pallidum* is killed by very low concentrations of penicillin G, although a long period of exposure to penicillin is required for treatment because of the unusually slow rate of multiplication of the organism. The efficacy of penicillin for syphilis remains undiminished after nearly 50 years of use. Other antibiotics which are effective in syphilis include the tetracyclines, erythromycin, and the cephalosporins. Aminoglycosides and spectinomycin inhibit *T. pallidum* only in very large doses, and the sulfonamides and the quinolones are inactive. The optimal dose and duration of therapy have not been established definitively for any antimicrobial for any stage of syphilis.

It is necessary to achieve serum levels of penicillin G of 0.03 µg/mL or more for at least 7 days to cure early syphilis. Recurrence rates for a given regimen increase as infection progresses from incubating syphilis to seronegative primary to seropositive primary to secondary to late syphilis. Therefore, it is probable, but unproved, that a longer duration of therapy is required to effect cure as the infection progresses. For these reasons, some authorities use more prolonged penicillin therapy than that recommended by the U.S. Public Health Service when treating secondary, latent, or late syphilis.

The treatment regimens recommended for syphilis are summarized in Table 133-3 and are described below.

Early syphilis Preventive (abortive, "epidemiologic") treatment is recommended for seronegative individuals without signs of syphilis who have been exposed to infectious syphilis within the previous 3 months. Before treatment is given, every effort should be made to establish a diagnosis by examination and serologic testing. *The regimens recommended for preventive treatment are the same as those recommended for early syphilis.*

For patients who have no known exposure to syphilis but who are undergoing treatment for other sexually transmitted diseases, most currently recommended STD regimens involving β-lactam or tetracycline antibiotics are probably also effective for very early incubating syphilis. It is likely that the regimen currently recommended for treating gonorrhea [ceftriaxone 250 mg intramuscularly followed by doxycycline or tetracycline orally for 1 week (see Chap. 110)] is effective against incubating syphilis.

Penicillin G benzathine is the most widely used form of treatment for early syphilis, including primary, secondary, and early latent syphilis, although it is more painful on injection than penicillin G procaine. A single dose of 2.4 million units cures over 95 percent of cases of primary syphilis. Because efficacy for secondary syphilis may be slightly lower, some physicians administer a second dose of 2.4 million units 1 week after the initial dose for secondary syphilis. There are reports of treatment failure following penicillin G benzathine in patients coinfected with HIV and early syphilis. Therapeutic recommendations should be guided by knowledge of CSF abnormalities in such patients. CSF examination in HIV-seropositive individuals with syphilis of any stage is recommended. Patients without HIV infection also may benefit from CSF examination. Some experts recommend treatment with regimens effective against neurosyphilis for all HIV-seropositive individuals with syphilis of any stage.

Late latent and late syphilis Lumbar puncture should be performed in the evaluation of latent syphilis of more than 1 year's duration, in suspected neurosyphilis, and also in late complications other than symptomatic neurosyphilis, since asymptomatic neurosyphilis may coexist with other late complications. In older asymptomatic individuals, the yield of lumbar puncture is relatively low. CSF examination is most clearly indicated in the following situations: neurologic signs or symptoms, treatment failure, serum reagin titer ≥ 1:32; HIV antibody positivity, other evidence of active syphilis (e.g., aortitis, gumma, visual or hearing changes), or nonpenicillin therapy planned. Recommended treatment for late latent syphilis with normal CSF, for cardiovascular syphilis, and for late benign syphilis (gumma) is penicillin G benzathine, 2.4 million units intramuscularly once a week for 3 successive weeks (7.2 million units total). If CSF abnormalities are found, the patient should be treated for neurosyphilis.

No studies of penicillin G benzathine for cardiovascular syphilis have been reported, and the efficacy of penicillin therapy in any form for cardiovascular syphilis has not been proved. The response of cardiovascular syphilis to penicillin is seldom dramatic because aortic aneurysm and aortic regurgitation cannot be reversed by antibiotic treatment, although further progression of these lesions may be arrested. In contrast, the response of benign tertiary syphilis and of meningovascular syphilis to penicillin G is usually impressive. The response of parenchymal neurosyphilis has been variable. In a cooperative study of the treatment of 1086 general paretics with penicillin, the frequency of clinical improvement or termination of progression ranged from 38 percent of those with severe involvement to 81 percent of those with mild involvement. Tabes dorsalis or optic atrophy responds less often. In general, treatment of inactive neurosyphilis in which neurologic damage has already occurred may not produce any clinical change, and retreatment of such cases is not warranted. However, persistence of CSF pleocytosis or recurrence of pleocytosis following initial response to treatment indicates continuing active infection, which should respond to additional treatment. The 1989 Centers for Disease Control treatment guidelines for neurosyphilis are presented in Table 133-3. Because penicillin G benzathine given in doses of up to 7.2 million units to adults or 50,000 units per kilogram to infants does not produce detectable concentrations of penicillin G in CSF, this form of penicillin is unreliable for the treatment of neurosyphilis in the adult or infant, and asymptomatic neurosyphilis has been found to relapse in up to one-quarter of patients treated with 2.4 million units of penicillin G benzathine. Therefore, use of penicillin G benzathine alone for treatment of neurosyphilis is not recommended. On the other hand, administration of intravenous penicillin G in doses of 12 million units or more per day for 10 days or longer ensures treponemicidal concentrations of penicillin G in CSF and occasionally cures patients who failed to respond to other therapy. There are no data to support the use of antibiotics other than penicillin G for the treatment of

---

TABLE 133-3   Recommendations for therapy of syphilis*

Stage of syphilis	Patients without penicillin allergy	Patients with confirmed penicillin allergy
Primary, secondary, or early latent	Benzathine penicillin G, 2.4 million units single dose IM (1.2 million units in each buttock)	Tetracycline hydrochloride, 500 mg PO 4 times daily; or doxycycline, 100 mg PO twice daily, for two weeks

Late latent (or latent of uncertain duration), cardiovascular, or benign tertiary	Lumbar puncture
	  CSF normal: Benzathine penicillin G, 2.4 million units IM weekly for 3 weeks
	  CSF abnormal: Treat as neurosyphilis
		Lumbar puncture
		  CSF normal: Tetracycline hydrochloride, 500 mg PO 4 times daily; or doxycycline, 100 mg PO twice daily, for 4 weeks
		  CSF abnormal: Treat as neurosyphilis

Neurosyphilis[†] (asymptomatic or symptomatic)	Aqueous penicillin G, 12–24 million units per day IV for 10–14 days *Or* Aqueous procaine penicillin G, 2.4 million units IM daily, plus oral probenecid, 500 mg 4 times each day, both for 10–14 days	Confirm penicillin allergy by skin-testing; if confirmed, desensitize and treat with penicillin
Syphilis in pregnancy	According to stage	Confirm penicillin allergy by skin-testing; if confirmed, desensitize and treat with penicillin

* See text for discussion of syphilis therapy in HIV-infected individuals.
† Some authorities recommend following these regimens with three doses of 2.4 million units of benzathine penicillin G, given IM one week apart. Benzathine penicillin G alone has given inferior results for treatment of neurosyphilis. Drugs other than penicillin are not recommended. Many patients who give a history of penicillin allergy prove negative when skin-tested for immediate hypersensitivity to penicillin and could be given aqueous crystalline penicillin G for CNS syphilis under close supervision in the hospital.
SOURCE: These recommendations are modified from Centers for Disease Control, 1989.

neurosyphilis; however, some of the third-generation cephalosporins may deserve further evaluation. In patients with penicillin allergy documented by skin testing, desensitization may be the best course (see Chap. 85).

Management of syphilis in pregnancy Every pregnant woman should undergo a nontreponemal test at her first prenatal visit, and women who are at high risk for acquiring STDs should have a repeat test in the third trimester and at delivery. In the pregnant patient with presumed syphilis (evidenced by a reactive serology, with or without clinical manifestations) and with no history of treatment for syphilis, expeditious evaluation and initiation of treatment are essential. Therapy should be administered according to stage of the disease, as for nonpregnant patients. Patients should be warned of the risk of a Jarisch-Herxheimer reaction, which may be associated with mild premature contractions but rarely results in premature delivery.

Penicillin is the only recommended therapy for syphilis in pregnancy. If the patient has well-documented penicillin allergy, and this is confirmed by demonstration of an immediate wheal-and-flare response to skin testing with penicilloyl polylysine or penicillin G minor determinant mixture, desensitization and penicillin treatment should be carried out in a hospital using the 1989 STD guidelines issued by the Centers for Disease Control. After treatment, a quantitative reagin test should be repeated monthly throughout pregnancy, and if a fourfold rise in titer occurs, treatment should be repeated. Treated women who do not show a fourfold decrease in titer in a 3-month period also should be retreated.

Evaluation and management of congenital syphilis Newborn infants of mothers with reactive VDRL or FTA-ABS tests may themselves have reactive tests, whether or not they have become infected, because of transplacental transfer of maternal IgG antibody. Rising or persistent titers indicate infection, and the infant should be treated. If the seropositive mother received inadequate penicillin treatment or treatment other than penicillin, if her treatment status is unknown, or if the infant may be difficult to follow, the infant should be treated at birth. It is unwise to require proof of diagnosis before treatment in such cases. The CSF should be examined as a baseline before treatment of such infants. Penicillin is the only recommended drug for syphilis in infants. The calculation of penicillin dosage for treatment of late congenital syphilis is the same as that used in the infant, until dosage based on weight reaches that used for adult neurosyphilis. Specific recommendations for treatment of infants can be found in the 1989 Centers for Disease Control treatment guidelines. Neonatal IgM antibody can be detected in cord or neonatal sera in the 19S IgM FTA-ABS test, in which IgM is enriched by column chromatography (to remove IgG) and detected by fluorescein-labeled antihuman IgM. This test avoids the specificity and sensitivity problems associated with earlier versions of the IgM FTA-ABS test. Alternatively, monthly quantitative reagin tests may be performed on asymptomatic infants born to women who were treated adequately with penicillin during pregnancy.

Jarisch-Herxheimer reaction A dramatic, though usually mild, reaction consisting of fever (average temperature elevation 1.5°C), chills, myalgias, headache, tachycardia, increased respiratory rate, increased circulating neutrophil count (average total white blood cell count 12,500 per microliter), and vasodilatation with mild hypotension may occur following initiation of treatment for syphilis. This reaction occurs in approximately 50 percent of patients with primary syphilis, 90 percent with secondary syphilis, and 25 percent with early latent syphilis. The onset occurs within 2 h of treatment, the peak temperature occurs at about 7 h, and defervescence takes place within 12 to 24 h. The reaction is more delayed in neurosyphilis, with peak fever occurring after 12 to 14 h. In patients with secondary syphilis, an increase in erythema and edema of the mucocutaneous lesions occurs; occasionally, subclinical or early mucocutaneous lesions may first become apparent during the reaction. The pathogenesis of this reaction is undefined. Patients should be warned to expect such symptoms, which can be managed by bed rest and aspirin. Adjunctive steroid

therapy has not been shown to prevent the Jarisch-Herxheimer reaction in syphilis and is not recommended.

Follow-up evaluation of responses to therapy for all stages of syphilis The response of early syphilis to treatment should be determined by following the quantitative VDRL or RPR titer 1, 3, 6, and 12 months after treatment. More frequent serologic examination (1, 2, 3, 6, 9, and 12 months) is recommended for patients concurrently infected with HIV. Because the FTA-ABS and hemagglutination tests remain positive in most patients treated for seropositive early syphilis, these tests are not useful in following the response to therapy. After successful treatment of seropositive first-episode primary or secondary syphilis, the VDRL titer progressively declines, becoming negative by 12 months in 40 to 75 percent of seropositive primary cases and 20 to 40 percent of secondary cases. Two years after treatment for first-episode primary syphilis, ≥60 percent of patients have a negative VDRL, although 25 to 58 percent of patients with secondary disease and a higher proportion of those treated for early latent syphilis maintain low reagin titers. Patients with a history of syphilis have less rapid declines in titer and are less likely to become VDRL- or RPR-negative. If the VDRL becomes negative or reaches a fixed low titer within 1 or 2 years, performing a lumbar puncture is unnecessary at that time, since the CSF examination is almost invariably normal and there is little risk of subsequent neurosyphilis. However, if a VDRL titer of 1:8 or more fails to fall at least fourfold within 12 months, if the VDRL titer rises fourfold, or if clinical symptoms persist or recur, retreatment is indicated. Every effort should be made to differentiate treatment failure from reinfection, and the CSF should be examined. Patients with suspected treatment failure, especially those with abnormal CSF, should be treated as described for neurosyphilis. If the patient remains seropositive but asymptomatic after such retreatment, no further therapy is necessary. Patients treated for late latent syphilis frequently have a low-titered VDRL test prior to therapy and may not demonstrate a fourfold drop following therapy with penicillin; about half of these patients remain seropositive in low titer for years following therapy. Retreatment is not warranted unless the titer rises or signs and symptoms of syphilis recur.

The activity of neurosyphilis correlates best with the degree of CSF pleocytosis. Changes in the CSF cell count and, to a lesser extent, in CSF protein concentration provide the most sensitive index of response to treatment. CSF examination should be performed every 3 to 6 months for 3 years after treatment of asymptomatic or symptomatic neurosyphilis. An elevated CSF cell count falls to 10 or fewer per microliter within 3 to 12 months in 95 percent of adequately treated cases and becomes normal in all cases within 2 to 4 years. Elevated levels of CSF protein fall more slowly, and the CSF reagin titer declines slowly over a period of several years.

Persistence of treponemal forms The persistence of *T. pallidum* in the aqueous humor, CSF, lymph nodes, brain, inflamed temporal arteries, and other tissues following "adequate" penicillin treatment of latent or late syphilis has been suggested by dark-field microscopy, immunofluorescent antibody and silver staining techniques, and rabbit inoculation. Because the data on persisting treponemes are scanty, no modification of the treatment recommendations for latent or late syphilis seems warranted. Adherence to recommendations regarding CSF examination prior to selection of therapy should minimize the possibility of *T. pallidum* persistence.

IMMUNITY AND PREVENTION OF SYPHILIS About 50 percent of the named contacts of patients with primary and secondary syphilis become infected, but the actual risk of infection from a single exposure is probably much lower. The rate of development of acquired resistance to *T. pallidum* following natural or experimental infection is quantitatively related to the amount of the antigenic stimulus, which depends on both the size of the infecting inoculum and the duration of infection prior to treatment. The role of serum antibody in conferring immunity to syphilis remains controversial. Reagin (VDRL) antibody is not protective. Passively administered antibody from rabbits recovering from experimental syphilis prevents or delays appearance of clinical manifestations of syphilis; it does not prevent infection. Cellular immunity is considered to be of major importance in the healing of early lesions and control of syphilis infection. The cellular infiltration of early lesions is predominantly composed of T lymphocytes and macrophages, and specifically sensitized T lymphocytes develop early in the course of infection in humans and experimentally infected rabbits. Clearance of organisms from early lesions is mediated by macrophages. Specific antibody enhances phagocytosis and is required for macrophage-mediated killing of *T. pallidum*.

Inability to cultivate pathogenic treponemes in vitro has hindered analysis, purification, and concentration of treponemal antigens. Attempts to induce immunity to syphilis by vaccination have shown limited promise, although several specific antigens have been identified and characterized. The outer membrane of *T. pallidum* contains few integral membrane proteins, and no surface-exposed antigens have been definitively identified. Many of the major antigens are lipoproteins, which are probably associated via their lipid tail with the inner membrane, projecting into the periplasmic space. Repeated injection of rabbits with gamma-irradiated motile strains has conferred immunity to a rechallenge. Until a practical and effective vaccine is developed, the prevention of syphilis will depend on use of condoms and antiseptic prophylactic agents and the detection and treatment of infectious cases.

REFERENCES

BAKER-ZANDER et al: Macrophage-mediated killing of opsonized *T. pallidum*. J Infect Dis 165:69, 1992

BERRY CD et al: Neurologic relapse after benzathine penicillin therapy for secondary syphilis in a patient with HIV infection. N Engl J Med 316:1587, 1987

CENTERS FOR DISEASE CONTROL: Guidelines for the prevention and control of congenital syphilis. Morb Mort Week Rep (Suppl) 37(S-1):1, 1988

————: Recommendations for diagnosing and treating syphilis in HIV-infected individuals. Morb Mort Week Rep 37:600, 1988

————: Regional and temporal trends in the surveillance of syphilis, United States 1986–1990. Morb Mort Week Rep 40 (SS-3):29, 1991

————: 1989 Sexually transmitted diseases treatment guidelines. Morb Mort Week Rep 38(Suppl 8):1, 1989

CHAPEL T: The signs and symptoms of secondary syphilis. Sex Trans Dis 7:161, 1980

GREENE BM et al: Failure of penicillin G benzathine in the treatment of neurosyphilis. Arch Intern Med 140:1117, 1980

HOOK EW III et al: Detection of *Treponema pallidum* in lesion exudate with a pathogen-specific monoclonal antibody. J Clin Microbiol 22:241, 1985

HOTSON JR: Modern neurosyphilis: A partially treated chronic meningitis. West J Med 135:191, 1981

KATZ DA et al: Neurosyphilis in acquired immunodeficiency syndrome. Arch Neurol 46:895, 1989

LUGER A et al: Diagnosis of neurosyphilis by examination of the cerebrospinal fluid. Br J Vener Dis 57:232, 1981

LUKEHART SA et al: Invasion of the central nervous system by *Treponema pallidum*: Implications for diagnosis and treatment. Ann Intern Med 109:855, 1988

McLEISH WM et al: The ocular manifestations of syphilis in the human immunodeficiency virus type I–infected host. Ophthalmology 97:196, 1990

MOHR JA et al: Neurosyphilis and penicillin in cerebrospinal fluid. JAMA 236:2208, 1976

MULLER F, MOSKOPHIDIS M: Estimation of the local production of antibodies to *Treponema pallidum* in the central nervous system of patients with neurosyphilis. Br J Vener Dis 59:80, 1983

MUSHER DM et al: Effect of human immunodeficiency virus infection on the course of syphilis and on the response to treatment. Ann Intern Med 113:872, 1990

RADOLF JD et al: Outer membrane ultrastructure explains the limited antigenicity of virulent *Treponema pallidum*. Proc Natl Acad Sci 86:2051, 1989

RIVIERE GR et al: Identification of spirochetes related to *Treponema pallidum* in necrotizing ulcerative gingivitis and chronic periodontitis. N Engl J Med 325:539, 1991

ROMANOWSKI B et al: Serologic response to treatment of infectious syphilis. Ann Intern Med 114:1005, 1991

SIMON RP: Neurosyphilis. Arch Neurol 42:606, 1985

WENDEL GD et al: Penicillin allergy and desensitization in serious infections during pregnancy. N Engl J Med 312:1229, 1985

134   ENDEMIC TREPONEMATOSES

PETER L. PERINE

GENERAL CONSIDERATIONS   Nonvenereal treponematoses occur in remote, impoverished areas of the world. Yaws, pinta, and endemic syphilis are distinguished from venereal syphilis solely by clinical and epidemiologic features. Yaws, pinta, and endemic syphilis are caused by treponemes which have no demonstrated significant morphologic or genetic differences from *T. pallidum*. The etiologic agents of endemic syphilis and yaws are generally held to be identical with *T. pallidum* and have been designated as *T. pallidum* ssp. *endemicum* and ssp. *pertenue*, respectively. Pinta is caused by *T. carateum* and involves the skin alone; yaws affects skin and bones; and endemic syphilis involves the skin, bone, and mucous membranes. Each disease tends to progress by stages, but these are neither as distinct nor as predictable as in syphilis. Congenital infections and cardiovascular and central nervous system involvement occur rarely, if ever, in the nonvenereal treponematoses but are common in syphilis. It is unclear whether the clinical and epidemiologic differences among yaws, pinta, endemic syphilis, and venereal syphilis are solely determined by environmental and host factors or are attributable to undefined biologic differences among the causal treponemes. The relationship of the treponematoses is summarized in Table 134-1.

EPIDEMIOLOGY   Treponemal antibodies are demonstrable in some proportion of nonhuman primates in regions of Africa where human yaws and endemic syphilis are common, and pathogenic treponemes have been found in skin lesions and lymph nodes of seropositive animals. These treponemes have produced yawslike lesions in susceptible monkeys and hamsters. There is no epidemiologic evidence to indicate that these treponemes play a significant role in the epidemiology of yaws in humans.

Yaws and endemic syphilis are diseases of young children. Yaws occurs throughout the world between the Tropics of Cancer and Capricorn in humid, warm environments. Transmission of yaws among children is favored by scanty clothing, poor hygiene, and frequent skin trauma. Spread occurs by direct contact with infected lesions and perhaps by passive transfer of treponemes by insects. Endemic syphilis occurs in arid subtropical or temperate climates in Africa, the eastern Mediterranean, the Arabian peninsula, and central Asia. It is not observed in the Western Hemisphere. Skin-to-skin transmission is less important than in yaws; instead, infection of mucous membranes results from direct mouth-to-mouth contact or from contaminated fomites, such as shared drinking or eating utensils. Venereal syphilis can spread by nonvenereal contact among children and cause household outbreaks in modern cities when crowding and poverty favor transmission of *T. pallidum*.

Although cutaneous pigmentary changes resembling late stages of pinta occur in yaws or endemic syphilis, pinta is a separate, more benign disease which occurs only in the Western Hemisphere. The onset is typically later than in yaws or endemic syphilis, usually when the person is between 10 and 20 years of age. Pinta is not very contagious, and its mode of transmission is not well defined.

The WHO/UNICEF-assisted mass campaign for eradication of endemic nonvenereal treponematosis from 1948 to 1969 was an unusually successful public health campaign. Over 160 million people were examined in 46 countries, and approximately 50 million cases, contacts, and latent infections were treated. The impact of this program was remarkable. The prevalence of active yaws lesions was reduced from over 20 percent to less than 1 percent in many rural areas. In Bosnia, formerly part of Yugoslavia, endemic syphilis was eradicated—the only example of eradication of an endemic treponematosis.

Relaxation of active surveillance activities after the mass campaigns has led to a resurgence of yaws, particularly in Africa. Yaws has not

TABLE 134-1   Etiology, epidemiology, and clinical manifestations of the treponematoses

	Venereal syphilis	Endemic syphilis	Yaws	Pinta
Organism	*T. pallidum* ssp. *pallidum*	*T. pallidum* ssp. *endemicum*	*T. pallidum* ssp. *pertenue*	*T. carateum*
Transmission	Sexual, transplacental*	Household contacts: mouth-to-mouth or via drinking, eating utensils	Skin-to-skin ? Insect vector	Skin-to-skin ? Insect vector
Usual age	Adult	Early childhood	Early childhood	Adolescent
Primary lesion	Cutaneous ulcer (chancre)	Rarely seen	Framboise (raspberry), or "mother yaw"	Nonulcerating papule with satellites
Secondary lesion	Mucocutaneous; occasional periostitis	Florid mucocutaneous lesions (mucous patch, split papule, condyloma latum); osteoperiostitis	Cutaneous papulosquamous lesions; osteoperiostitis	Pintides
Tertiary	Gumma, cardiovascular, and CNS lues	Destructive cutaneous osteoarticular gummas	Destructive cutaneous osteoarticular gummas	Dyschromic, achromic macules

* Since the nonvenereal treponematoses are usually acquired in childhood and treponemal bacteremia ceases with time, only in adult-onset venereal syphilis is there any likelihood of a mother giving birth to an infected child.

been eradicated in any large area. A large reservoir of yaws persists in West Africa which includes the Ivory Coast, Ghana, Togo, Benin, and the pygmies of Zaire and the Central African Republic. Yaws is also prevalent in Indonesia; Papua, New Guinea; and the Solomon Islands of the western Pacific. The Sahelian African nations of Mali, Niger, Burkina Faso, and Senegal have prevalence rates in some areas of 10 to 15 percent for endemic syphilis. These rates exceed those reported before the mass treatment campaigns. Seroactivity and late manifestations of endemic syphilis continue to occur among nomads in Saudi Arabia. The resurgence of yaws and endemic syphilis led to a new yaws campaign in Ghana in 1980, and other national campaigns are planned to control resurgent yaws and endemic syphilis in Africa.

Antitreponemal and reaginic seroreactivity has been detected in a small percentage of children without clinical disease born after the mass campaigns in some areas (e.g., Nigeria, New Guinea, and Bosnia). This may represent attenuated or asymptomatic infection or may simply reflect the decreased predictive value of serologic tests (probability that disease is present if the test is positive) when the prevalence of disease is sharply reduced.

In the Americas, foci of yaws persist in Haiti; Dominica, St. Lucia, and St. Vincent; Peru, Colombia, and Ecuador; a few areas of Brazil; and Guyana and Surinam. Pinta is confined to Central America and northern South America, where it appears to have regressed to remote Indian villages. Its prevalence today is probably less than 1 percent of that found 20 years ago.

BIOLOGIC RELATIONSHIPS   Specific humoral antibodies to *T. pallidum* are produced in individuals with yaws, pinta, or endemic syphilis, but the time of appearance of antibodies after onset of infections is variable. The fluorescent treponemal antibody absorption (FTA-ABS) test, the *T. pallidum* hemagglutination test (TPHA), and the *T. pallidum* immobilization (TPI) test cannot differentiate among the treponematoses.

In addition to the clinical and epidemiologic differences among the treponematoses in humans, the range of susceptible animal hosts and some manifestations of experimental infection are also different. In particular, *T. carateum* has produced an infection in chimpanzees which resembles pinta, but attempts to infect other experimental animals have been unsuccessful. Individuals who have had yaws or pinta are considered relatively immune to syphilis, and persons with active pinta or syphilis cannot be superinfected with *T. pallidum* ssp. *pertenue* by experimental inoculation.

CLINICAL MANIFESTATIONS   Yaws   Also known as *pian*, *framboesia*, or *bubas*, yaws is a chronic infectious disease of childhood caused by *T. pallidum* ssp. *pertenue*. The disease is characterized by an initial skin lesion(s) followed by relapsing, nondestructive,

secondary lesions of skin and bone. In the late stages, destructive lesions of skin, bone, and joints occur.

The incubation period following experimental inoculation of susceptible human beings is 3 to 4 weeks. Disruption of the skin by insect bites, abrasions, or injuries promotes acquisition of natural infection from infected contacts, most likely by fingers contaminated directly or indirectly with material from early yaws lesions. The initial early lesion is a single papule which is usually located on a leg. The lesion enlarges and becomes papillomatous (Fig. 134-1). This lesion also is known as a *framboesioma* (raspberry), or "mother yaw." It becomes superficially eroded and covered by a thin yellow crust of serous exudate containing *T. pallidum* ssp. *pertenue*. Erythema and induration do not occur. The lesion is mildly pruritic, and regional lymphadenopathy occurs. The initial lesion usually heals in 6 months. As a result of treponemal bacteremia and autoinoculation, a generalized secondary eruption of similar lesions appears either before or after the initial lesion has healed and is most extensive on the exposed surfaces of the body. These early cutaneous lesions of yaws have a variety of forms, including desquamative macular and papular as well as papillomatous types. Painful papillomata on the soles of the feet result in a crablike gait referred to as "crab yaws." Early lesions are infectious and heal slowly; they may result in scarring, hyperpigmentation, or depigmentation, resembling the pigmentary changes seen in pinta. Histologic findings are mononuclear cell infiltration, acanthosis, hyperkeratosis, and the presence of many treponemes.

Other manifestations of early yaws include lymphadenopathy and nocturnal bone pain and polydactylitis due to periostitis. Fever and other constitutional symptoms are rare, however, unless lesions become secondarily infected. Infectious cutaneous relapses are characteristic during the first 5 years after infection. Late yaws lesions occur in about 10 percent of cases, starting 5 years or more after infection, and differ histologically from early lesions in showing endarteritis. Late lesions include gummas of the skin and long bones, particularly of the legs, hyperkeratoses of the soles and palms, osteitis, periostitis, juxtaarticular fibromatous nodes, and hydrarthrosis.

Late lesions of yaws are characteristically extensive and usually destructive. Destruction of the nose, maxilla, palate, and pharynx, termed *gangosa*, or *rhinopharyngitis mutilans*, occurs in late yaws, as well as in leprosy and leishmaniasis. Hypertrophic paranasal maxillary osteitis produces distinctive facies known as *goundou*.

The clinical features of yaws have become less reliable for diagnosis as the prevalence of yaws has decreased, necessitating the use of easily performed serologic tests, such as the rapid plasma reagin (RPR) card test. *T. pallidum* ssp. *pertenue* can be demonstrated by dark-field examination in early cutaneous lesions but should not be confused with other spirochetes found in tropical ulcers. The serum

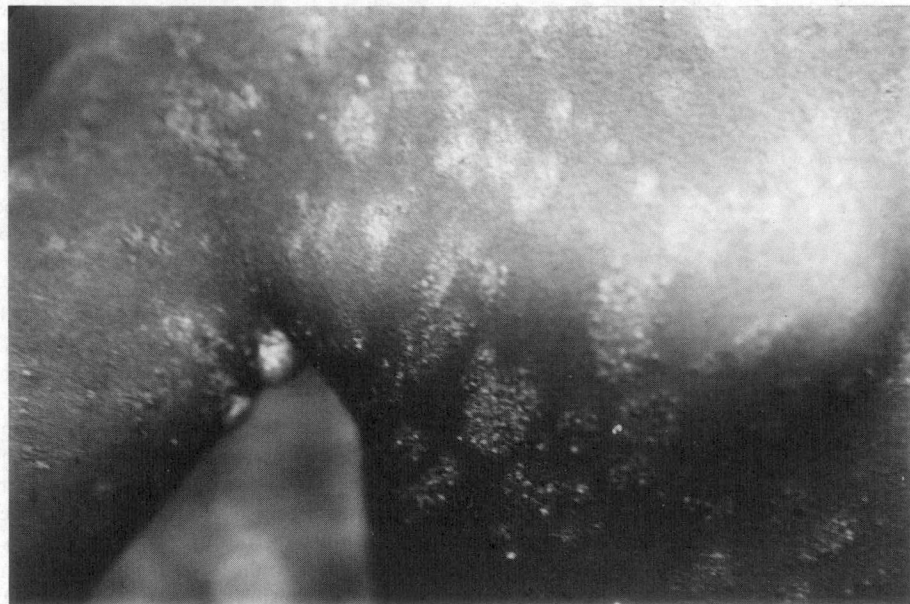

FIGURE 134-1 Young man with squamous micropapules of early yaws with papillomas in the left axilla and scapular area.

reagin antibody tests become positive after 1 month, and the FTA-ABS test is also positive.

Endemic syphilis Synonyms for endemic syphilis are Bejel, Siti, Dichuchwa, Njovera, and Skerljevo. It is a chronic nonvenereal treponemal infection of childhood characterized by early mucous membrane or mucocutaneous lesions, a latent period of indeterminate duration, and late complications including gummas of bone and skin. The causative organism, *T. pallidum* ssp. *endemicum*, is indistinguishable from *T. pallidum* ssp. *pallidum*. Endemic syphilis differs from congenital syphilis in that dental changes, interstitial keratitis, and neurosyphilis rarely, if ever, occur. Cardiovascular complications are considered rare in both endemic and congenital syphilis.

Primary cutaneous lesions are infrequent and, when present, are extragenital. The earliest manifestation of endemic syphilis is usually an intraoral mucous patch or mucocutaneous lesion resembling the split papules or condylomata of secondary syphilis. Periostitis is common. Regional lymphadenopathy occurs, but generalized lymphadenopathy is unusual. Treponemes are abundant in the moist early lesions and in aspirates from regional lymph nodes. After a variable latent period, late lesions may develop and are the most frequent clinical manifestations. These resemble the lesions of late benign syphilis and include osseous or cutaneous gummas. Destructive gummas, osteitis, and gangosa are more common than in late yaws. Gummas occur on the nipples of mothers who have themselves previously had endemic syphilis and who breastfeed infants with oral lesions. Both early and late forms of endemic syphilis thus may coexist in the same family. The tertiary lesions of endemic syphilis sometimes may be a consequence of repeated exposure of a previously sensitized host to reinfection.

Pinta Also known as *mal del pinto*, *carate*, *azul*, or *purupuru*, pinta is an infectious disease of the skin caused by *T. carateum*. This disease has three cutaneous stages characterized by marked changes in the skin color, does not involve osseous tissue or viscera, and causes no disability other than that associated with cosmetic disfigurement.

The initial lesion is a small papule which appears 7 to 30 days after exposure and is located most often on the extremities, face, neck, or buttocks. It increases in size slowly by peripheral extension and by coalescing with smaller satellite papules. Regional lymphadenopathy occurs. A secondary eruption not associated with generalized lymphadenopathy appears 1 month to 1 year after the appearance of the initial lesion. The secondary lesions are termed *pintides*, may be numerous, and evolve into a psoriatic or circinate configuration.

Pintides are initially red but become deeply pigmented, reaching a slate-blue color after a period of time which is related to exposure to sun. Pigmentation occurs most rapidly on the exposed parts of the body. These pigmented lesions are known as dyschromic macules and contain treponemes which are located principally in the epidermis in older lesions. Histologically, there is deposition of pigment in the dermis with decreased melanin pigment in the basal cell layer. Within 3 months to a year, most of the pintides show varying degrees of depigmentation, becoming brown and finally white and giving the skin a mottled appearance. The porcelain-white achromic lesions represent the "late" stage of the disease in which the epidermis is atrophic, and melanocytes and melanin are absent. *T. carateum* can be demonstrated in transudates from initial, early secondary, or dyschromic lesions. Reaginic and antitreponemal antibody tests are positive but may take four times longer to become positive in pinta than in venereal syphilis.

TREATMENT Treatment is similar for all the endemic treponematoses. Intramuscular injection of 2.4 million units of benzathine penicillin G in adults and half this dose in children results in rapid resolution of lesions and prevents recurrence. Procaine penicillin G in oil and 2% aluminum monostearate (PAM) has been used extensively. In persons who are allergic to penicillin, tetracycline hydrochloride in a dose similar to that used for infectious syphilis (see Chap. 133) is effective. In areas where less than 5 percent of the population has active disease, cases are managed on an individual basis, and all contacts of infected persons are treated with antibiotics.

PREVENTION Although the nonvenereal treponematoses are less amenable to eradication than smallpox, the resurgence of yaws has led some authorities to suggest that the application of *selective epidemiologic control* as used in smallpox eradication be applied to yaws control. This strategy would emphasize ongoing active surveillance, investigation of outbreaks, and treatment of active cases and their contacts rather than mass treatment. There is concern that the epidemiology and course of yaws and endemic syphilis will be adversely affected by the HIV pandemic in Africa and Asia. Cutaneous lesions may be prolonged, be more easily secondarily infected, and serve as a portal for nonvenereal transmission of HIV.

REFERENCES

BURKE JP et al (eds): International symposium on yaws and other endemic treponematoses. Rev Infect Dis 7:S217, 1985
ENGELKENS HJH et al: Endemic treponematosis. Int J Dermatol 30:77, 1991

GUTHE T: Clinical, serological and epidemiological features of framboesia tropica (yaws) and its control in rural communities. Acta Dermatol Venereol 49:343, 1969

NOORDHOEK GT, VAN EMBDEN JDA: Yaws, an endemic treponematosis reconsidered in the HIV era. Eur J Clin Microbiol Infect Dis 10:4, 1991

MEHEUS A, ANTAL GM: Endemic treponematoses: Not yet eradicated. World Health Stat Q 45:228, 1992

PERINE PL et al: Handbook of Endemic Treponematoses. Geneva, WHO, 1984

Treponematoses Research: Report of a WHO Scientific Group, WHO Technical Report Series 674, 1982

135 LEPTOSPIROSIS

JAY P. SANFORD

DEFINITION *Leptospirosis* is a term applied to disease caused by all leptospiras regardless of specific serotype. Correlation of clinical syndromes with infection by differing serotypes leads to the conclusion that a single serotype of *Leptospira* may be responsible for a variety of clinical features; conversely, a single syndrome, e.g., aseptic meningitis, may be caused by multiple serotypes. Hence there is a preference for the general term *leptospirosis* rather than the synonyms such as *Weil's disease* and *canicola fever*.

ETIOLOGY The genus *Leptospira* contains only one species, *L. interrogans*, which may be subdivided into two complexes, interrogans and biflexa. The interrogans complex includes the pathogenic strains, while the biflexa complex includes saprophytic strains. Within each complex the organisms show antigenic variations that are stable and allow them to be classed as serotypes (serovars). Serotypes with common antigens are arranged in serogroups (varieties). Despite contrary common usage, an example of the correct designation of *Leptospira* is as follows: Pomona serogroup of *L. interrogans* or *L. interrogans* var. pomona, not *L. pomona*. The interrogans complex now contains about 240 serotypes arranged in 23 serogroups (the number in parentheses refers to number of serotypes within the serogroup): Icterohemorrhagiae (18), Hebdomadis (30), Autumnalis (17), Canicola (12), Australis (12), Tarassovi (17), Pyrogenes (12), Bataviae (10), Javanica (8), Pomona (8), Ballum (3), Cynopteri (3), Celledoni (3), Grippotyphosa (5), Panama (2), Shermani (1), Ranarum (2), and Bufonis (1). At least 27 serotypes of *Leptospira* occur naturally in the United States.

EPIDEMIOLOGY Leptospirosis is thought to be the most widespread zoonosis in the world. Cases are regularly reported from all continents except Antarctica and are especially prevalent in the tropics. Although leptospirosis is not a common disease, it has been reported from all regions of the United States, including arid areas such as Arizona. Between 1987 and 1992, 43 to 93 cases were reported annually. Infection in humans is an incidental occurrence and is not essential to the maintenance of leptospirosis. The disease occurs in a wide range of domestic and wild animal hosts, including poikilothermic vertebrates. In many species, such as opossums, skunks, raccoons, and foxes, infectivity ratios in the range of 10 to 50 percent are not unusual. Interspecies spread of specific serotypes of leptospiras between animal hosts is frequent; e.g., Pomona, a serotype principally associated with livestock, has been demonstrated in dogs. Infection in animals may vary from inapparent illness to severe, fatal disease. Even asymptomatic animals may carry high numbers ($>10^{10}$ organisms per gram) in their kidneys. The carrier state, in which the host may shed leptospiras in its urine for months to years, may develop in many animals. Immunization of dogs may not prevent the carrier, or shedder, state.

Survival of pathogenic leptospiras in nature is governed by such factors as pH of the urine of the host, pH of soil or water into which they are shed, and ambient temperature. Leptospiras in most "urine spots" in soil retain infectivity for 6 to 48 h. Acid urine permits only limited survival; however, if the urine is neutral or alkaline and is shed into a similar moist environment which has low salinity, is not badly polluted with microorganisms or detergents, and has a temperature above 22°C, leptospiras may survive for several weeks. Human infections can occur either by direct contact with urine or tissue of an infected animal or indirectly through contaminated water, soil, or vegetation. The usual portals of entry in humans are abraded skin, particularly about the feet, and exposed conjunctival, nasal, and oral mucous membranes. Swallowing contaminated water during immersion has been associated with high attack rates. The previously held concept that organisms could penetrate intact skin has been questioned. While leptospiras have been isolated from ticks, these arthropods appear to be unimportant in transmission.

With the ubiquitous infection of animals, leptospirosis in human beings can occur in all age groups, at all seasons, and in both sexes. However, it is primarily a disease of teenage children and young adults (about one-half of patients are between the ages of 10 and 39), occurs predominantly in males (80 percent), and develops most frequently in hot weather (in the United States one-half of infections occur from July to October). The wide spectrum of animal hosts results in both urban and rural human disease. Leptospirosis has been considered an occupational disease; however, improved methods of rat control and better standards of hygiene have reduced the incidence among occupational groups such as coal miners and people who work in sewers. The epidemiologic pattern has changed; in the United States, the United Kingdom, Europe, and Israel, water-associated and cattle-associated leptospirosis is most common. Fewer than 20 percent of patients have had direct contact with animals; they are mostly farmers, trappers, or abattoir workers. In the majority of patients, exposure is incidental; two-thirds of cases occur in children, students, or housewives. Swimming or partial immersion in contaminated water, e.g., riding motorcycles through contaminated pools of water, has been implicated in one-fifth of patients and has accounted for most of the recognized common-source outbreaks. In Hawaii, one-fourth of cases have been associated with aquaculture industries; in the United Kingdom, fish; while in Italy, farm workers are at increased risk; leptospirosis remains common in the rice-growing areas of the Po River Valley (a serologic survey of railway workers in the area showed an antibody prevalence of 10 percent).

PATHOLOGY In patients who have died with hepatorenal involvement (Weil's syndrome), the significant gross changes include hemorrhages and bile staining of tissues. The hemorrhages, which vary from petechial to ecchymotic, are widespread and are most prominent in skeletal muscle, kidneys, adrenals, liver, stomach, spleen, and lungs.

In skeletal muscle, focal, necrotic, and necrobiotic changes typical of leptospirosis occur. Biopsies early in the illness demonstrate swelling and vacuolation. Leptospiral antigen has been demonstrated in these lesions by the fluorescent antibody technique. Healing ensues by the formation of new myofibrils with minimal fibrosis. The renal lesions in the acute phase involve predominantly the tubules and vary from simple dilatation of distal convoluted tubules to degeneration, necrosis, and basement membrane rupture. Interstitial edema and cellular infiltrates consisting of lymphocytes, neutrophilic leukocytes, histiocytes, and plasma cells are uniformly present. Glomerular lesions either are absent or consist of mesangial hyperplasia and focal foot process fusion, which are interpreted as representing nonspecific changes associated with acute inflammation and protein filtration. Microscopic alterations in the liver are not diagnostic and correlate poorly with the degree of functional impairment. The changes include cloudy swelling of parenchymal cells, disruption of liver cords, enlargement of Kupffer cells, and bile stasis in biliary canaliculi. The changes in the brain and meninges are also minimal and are not diagnostic. Microscopic evidence of myocarditis has been recorded. Pulmonary findings consist of a patchy, localized hemorrhagic pneumonitis. Special staining techniques utilizing silver impregnation methods have demonstrated organisms in the lumina of renal tubules but rarely in other organs.

PATHOGENESIS Leptospirosis is one of the recognized human spirochetal diseases; other diseases in this group include syphilis, pinta, yaws, bejel, relapsing fever (due to *Borrelia* species), Lyme disease, and rat-bite fever (due to *Spirillum minus*). Despite differences in epidemiology, there are many similarities among these entities. Spirochetemia develops soon after the entry of leptospiras through the skin or mucous membranes, with wide dessemination throughout tissue and body fluid. Coincident with an immune response (both humoral and cellular), spirochetemia either terminates or is greatly reduced; however, organisms may persist in immunologically isolated areas. With leptospirosis, persistence in the kidney and shedding of leptospiras in urine are integral to epidemiology. Later manifestations, e.g., aseptic meningitis and iridocyclitis, are thought to be immunopathologically mediated. Such occurrences are features in each of the spirochetal diseases.

The cell wall of *L. interrogans* contains lipopolysaccharide (endotoxin). With initiation of antimicrobial therapy in leptospirosis, a Jarisch-Herxheimer–like reaction (J-HR) similar to that seen with other spirochetal diseases may occur. It had been postulated that the J-HR was due to release of endotoxin; however, in the clinically most predictable and severe J-HR (that associated with louse-borne relapsing fever), limulus amebocyte lysate (LAL) assays for endotoxin were negative, and it was concluded that endotoxin, if present, had leaked into the circulation from intestinal gram-negative organisms.

Watt and associates studied 24 patients with proven leptospirosis who were treated with penicillin. While none had J-HR, 78 percent had endotoxemia, as measured by LAL assays. Patients with positive LAL specimens had significantly higher leukocyte counts and levels of serum creatinine and bilirubin than did patients with negative LAL assays. The authors postulated delayed hepatic clearance of endotoxin due to hepatic dysfunction. Recently, in patients with proven *Borrelia recurrentis* infection who experienced J-HR with penicillin treatment, the peak of the J-HR was strongly associated with high plasma levels of tumor necrosis factor (TNF). Peaks of interleukin 6 and interleukin 8 occurred just after that of TNF. Extrapolation of these data to leptospirosis suggests that cytokine release through rapid phagocytosis of *L. interrogans* in response to antibody or therapy may mediate many of the symptoms, especially in the secondary phase.

CLINICAL MANIFESTATIONS General features The incubation period following immersion or accidental laboratory exposure has shown extremes of 2 to 26 days, the usual range being 7 to 13 days and the average 10 days.

Leptospirosis is a typically biphasic illness. *During the leptospiremic, or first, phase*, leptospiras are present in the blood and cerebrospinal fluid (CSF). The onset is typically abrupt, and initial symptoms include headache, which is usually frontal, is less often retroorbital, but occasionally may be bitemporal or occipital. Severe muscle aching occurs in most patients, the muscles of the thighs and lumbar areas being most prominently involved, and often is accompanied by severe pain on palpation. Patients often complain of leg pain with walking. The myalgia may be accompanied by extreme cutaneous hyperesthesia (causalgia). Chills followed by a rapidly rising temperature are prominent. Following the abrupt onset, the leptospiremic phase typically lasts 4 to 9 days. Features during this interval include recurrent chills, high spiking temperatures [usually 38.9°C (102°F) or greater], headache, and continued severe myalgia. Involvement of one organ system may predominate, often leading to initial misdiagnosis. Such symptom complexes most commonly include hepatitis, nephritis, atypical pneumonia, influenza, or "viral" gastroenteritis. Anorexia, nausea, and vomiting are encountered in one-half or more of patients. Occasional patients have diarrhea. Pulmonary manifestations, usually either cough or chest pain, have varied in frequency of occurrence from less than 25 percent to 86 percent. Hemoptysis occurs uncommonly in the United States and Europe but is a common feature in Korea and China, being noted in 40 percent of patients. Examination during this phase reveals an acutely ill, febrile patient, with a relative bradycardia and normal blood pressure. Disturbances in sensorium may be encountered in up

to 25 percent of all patients and in one-half of patients with icteric disease. Transient cerebral ischemic attacks in children associated with leptospiral arteritis have been reported from China.

The most characteristic physical sign is conjunctival suffusion, which usually first appears on the third or fourth day. It may be lacking in some patients but more often is overlooked. It may be associated with photophobia, but serous or purulent secretion is unusual. Less common findings may include pharyngeal injection, cutaneous hemorrhages, and skin rashes that, even when they occur, are not prominent. The rashes may be macular, maculopapular, or urticarial and usually occur on the trunk. Uncommon findings are splenomegaly, hepatomegaly, lymphadenopathy, or jaundice. The first phase terminates after 4 to 9 days, usually with defervescence and improvement in symptoms. This coincides with the disappearance of leptospiras from the blood and CSF.

The second phase has been characterized as the "immune" phase and correlates with the appearance of circulating IgM antibodies; the concentration of C3 in serum remains normal. The clinical manifestations of this phase show greater variability than those during the first phase. After a relatively asymptomatic period of 1 to 3 days, the fever and earlier symptoms recur, and meningismus may develop. The fever rarely exceeds 38.9°C (102°F) and is usually of 1 to 3 days' duration. It is not uncommon for fever to be absent or quite transient. Even when symptoms or signs of meningeal irritation are absent, routine examination of CSF after the seventh day has revealed pleocytosis in 50 to 90 percent of patients. Less common features include iridocyclitis, optic neuritis, and other nervous system manifestations, including encephalitis, myelitis, and peripheral neuropathy. Leptospirosis during pregnancy may be associated with an increased risk of fetal loss.

Specific features WEIL'S SYNDROME *Weil's syndrome*, which may be due to serotypes other than Icterohemorrhagiae, is defined as severe leptospirosis with jaundice, usually accompanied by azotemia, hemorrhages, anemia, disturbances in consciousness, and continued fever. It occurs in 1 to 6 percent of patients with leptospirosis, although the figure may have been as high as 62 percent in a recent series from Portugal. There is uncertainty as to the pathogenesis of the syndrome, i.e., whether it represents direct toxic damage due to leptospiras or is the consequence of immune response to leptospiral antigens. The consensus favors toxic damage.

The onset and first stage are identical with the less severe forms of leptospirosis. The distinctive features of Weil's syndrome appear from the third to the sixth days but do not reach their peak until well into the second stage. As in milder forms of leptospirosis, there is a tendency for defervescence about the seventh day; however, with recurrence, fever is marked and may persist for several weeks. Either renal or hepatic manifestations may predominate. Hepatic disturbances include tenderness in the right upper quadrant and hepatic enlargement, both of which are common when jaundice is present. Serum aspartate aminotransferase (AST) values are rarely increased more than fivefold regardless of the degree of hyperbilirubinemia (in which conjugated bilirubin predominates). The predominant mechanism appears to be an intracellular block to bilirubin excretion.

Renal manifestations of Weil's syndrome consist primarily of proteinuria, pyuria, hematuria, and azotemia. Dysuria is rare. Serious renal damage usually occurs in the form of acute tubular necrosis associated with oliguria. The peak elevation of blood urea nitrogen usually is seen on the fifth to seventh day. Hemorrhagic manifestations are most prevalent in this group of patients and include epistaxis, hemoptysis, gastrointestinal bleeding, hemorrhage into the adrenal glands, hemorrhagic pneumonitis, and subarachnoid hemorrhage. These have been explained on the basis of diffuse vasculitis with capillary injury. In addition, in some patients hypoprothrombinemia, thrombocytopenia, and thrombotic thrombocytopenic purpura have been observed.

HEMORRHAGIC FEVER WITH RENAL SYNDROME Studies on the epidemiology of Hantavirus (Chap. 159) have shown that for the initial 24 to 72 h there is significant overlap in the clinical features of leptospirosis, hemorrhagic fever with renal syndrome (HFRS), and scrub typhus (H.W. Lee, personal communication). In Korea, where all three diseases are prevalent, 21 percent of the blood samples submitted for Hantavirus serology had antibody to *Leptospira* antigens and 6 percent to *Rickettsia tsutsugamushi*. Conversely, among 261 patients in Singapore clinically suspected of having leptospirosis, 3 percent had serologic evidence of Hantavirus infection. Hantavirus disease, which varies from mild (nephropathica epidemica) to severe (Balkan nephropathy), is common in Europe and Scandinavia. Because of the similarity in epidemiology and clinical presentation and the potential for dual infections, it has been recommended that blood be submitted for Hantavirus serology in all cases of suspected leptospirosis. Clinically, the term *lepthangamushi syndrome* has been used to describe this overlap syndrome.

ATYPICAL PNEUMONIA SYNDROME Pulmonary symptoms and signs are common in patients with leptospirosis; even the adult respiratory distress syndrome (ARDS) has been reported. While this association is not fully appreciated in the United States, leptospirosis is recognized in other parts of the world as an important differential diagnostic consideration in the patient with fever, chills, headache, severe myalgia, and bilateral bronchopneumonia, with or without an associated "active" urine sediment. In Italy, respiratory or influenza-like symptoms were the only clinical signs of illness in 21 percent of more than 300 patients with confirmed leptospirosis. In a group of 37 Korean patients with pulmonary radiographic findings, 21 had small nodular densities, 10 had a diffuse ground glass pattern, and 6 had large confluent areas of consolidation. Abnormalities were bilateral and nonlobar in all. In surviving patients, resolution occurred within 15 days. Given appropriate epidemiologic circumstances, leptospirosis should be added to the differential diagnosis of "atypical" pneumonia.

ASEPTIC MENINGOENCEPHALITIS A leptospiral etiology has been incriminated in 5 to 13 percent of sporadic cases of aseptic meningitis. Pleocytosis is not present before the immune phase but then develops rapidly. There are usually tens to hundreds of leukocytes, occasionally 1000, per microliter, among which neutrophils or mononuclear cells may predominate. CSF glucose concentration is almost always normal, but occasional instances of lowered glucose levels have been recorded. CSF protein may exceed 1 g/L (100 mg/dL) early in the course. Xanthochromic CSF has been observed in the presence of jaundice. Neurologic manifestations may include encephalitis and, in rare cases, hemiparesis. Each of the serotypes of *Leptospira* that is pathogenic for humans is probably capable of causing aseptic meningitis. The most prevalent serotypes have been Canicola, Icterohemorrhagiae, and Pomona.

MYOCARDITIS Cardiac arrhythmias, including paroxysmal atrial fibrillation, atrial flutter, ventricular tachycardia, and premature ventricular contractions, have been described but are usually of little clinical significance. However, on rare occasions pericarditis and definite cardiac dilatation with acute left ventricular failure have been observed. Associated manifestations have included jaundice (occurring in 95 percent of cases described in a recent report), pulmonary infiltrates, arthritis, and skin rashes. The serotypes thus far incriminated have included Icterohemorrhagiae, Autumnalis, Pomona, and Grippotyphosa.

CHILDREN Several clinical features that are not seen or are very rare in adults occur in children: hypertension, acalculous cholecystitis (five of nine children in one series), pancreatitis, abdominal causalgia, and peripheral desquamation of a rash that may be associated with gangrene and cardiopulmonary arrest. The features of desquamation, myocardial involvement, and hydrops of the gallbladder suggest Kawasaki syndrome [mucocutaneous lymph node syndrome (see Chap. 58)].

LABORATORY FEATURES Leukocyte counts vary from leuko-penic levels to mild elevations in the anicteric patients. In patients with jaundice, leukocytosis—with as many as 70,000 cells per microliter—may be present. However, regardless of the total leukocyte count, neutrophilia (greater than 70 percent neutrophils) is very frequently encountered during the first stage.

Hemolytic substances have been demonstrated in cultures of pathogenic leptospiras. In contrast to many hemolysins of bacterial origin which are not hemolytic in vivo, the leptospiral hemolysins appear to be active in vivo. In patients with jaundice, anemia may be severe and is most characteristically due to intravascular hemolysis. Other mechanisms of anemia include azotemia and blood loss secondary to hemorrhage. Anemia due to leptospirosis is unusual in anicteric patients.

Thrombocytopenia sufficient to be associated with bleeding (less than 30,000 platelets per microliter) may be encountered. Additional hematologic abnormalities include elevation of the erythrocyte sedimentation rate in over one-half of patients (usually less than 50 mm/h).

Urinalysis during the leptospiremic phase reveals mild proteinuria, casts, and an increase in cellular elements. In anicteric infections, these abnormalities rapidly disappear after the first week. Proteinuria and abnormalities in the urine sediment usually are not associated with elevations in blood urea nitrogen. Since the anicteric form of the disease often has gone undiagnosed, estimates of the frequency of azotemia and jaundice are probably high. Azotemia has been reported in approximately one-fourth of patients. In three-fourths of these patients, the blood urea nitrogen level is less than 36 mmol/L (100 mg/dL). Azotemia is usually associated with jaundice. The serum bilirubin levels may reach 1110 µmol/L (65 mg/dL); however, in two-thirds of patients the levels are less than 340 µmol/L (20 mg/dL). During the first phase, one-half of patients have increased serum creatine phosphokinase (CK) levels, with mean values of five times normal. Such increases are not seen in viral hepatitis, and a slight increase in transaminase with a definite increase in CK suggests leptospirosis rather than viral hepatitis.

DIAGNOSIS Diagnosis is based on culture of the organism or serologic proof of its existence. The most common initial diagnostic impressions in patients with leptospirosis are meningitis, hepatitis, nephritis, fever of undetermined origin (FUO), influenza, Kawasaki syndrome, toxic shock syndrome, and Legionnaires' disease. Leptospiras may be isolated quite readily during the first phase from blood and CSF or during the second phase from the urine. Leptospiras may be excreted in the urine for up to 11 months after the onset of illness and may persist despite antimicrobial therapy. Whole blood should be inoculated immediately into tubes containing semisolid medium, such as Fletcher's or EMJH medium. If culture medium is not available, leptospiras reportedly will remain viable up to 11 days in blood to which anticoagulants, preferably sodium oxalate, have been added. Animal inoculation (preferably either suckling hamsters or guinea pigs) may be used and is of particular value if specimens are contaminated. Direct examination of blood or urine by dark-field methods has been employed; *however, this method so frequently results in failure or misdiagnosis that it should not be employed.* Serologic methods are applicable during the second phase; antibodies appear from the sixth to the twelfth days of illness. Two serologic methods are commonly used: a macroscopic or slide agglutination test, which is easy to perform but lacks specificity and sensitivity and hence is suitable for screening only, and the microscopic agglutination test, which is more complicated but also more specific. An IgM-specific dot-ELISA has been effective in diagnosing leptospirosis in an endemic area. Serologic criteria for diagnosis include a fourfold or greater rise in titer during the course of illness. Cross-agglutination reactions between various serotypes commonly occur so that the infection serotype often cannot be determined with certainty without isolation of leptospiras.

PROGNOSIS The prognosis is dependent on both the virulence of the organism and the general condition of the patient. The mortality rate in reported cases in the United States has varied annually between 2.5 and 16.4 percent, averaging 7.1 percent. Age is the most significant host factor related to increased mortality. In a representative series, the mortality rate rose from 10 percent in men less than 50 years of age to 56 percent in those over 51 years of age. The virulence of the infecting leptospiras correlates best with the development of jaundice. In anicteric patients, death is extremely rare, but with the development of jaundice, the mortality rate in various series has ranged from 15 to 48 percent. Death is usually secondary to hemorrhage (especially gastrointestinal) or to renal failure. The long-term prognosis following the acute renal lesion of leptospirosis is good. Glomerular filtration rates have returned to normal, usually within 2 months; however, a few patients show residual tubular dysfunction such as a defect in concentrating capacity.

TREATMENT A variety of antimicrobial drugs, including penicillin, streptomycin, the tetracycline congeners, chloramphenicol, erythromycin, and ciprofloxacin, have been effective in vitro and in experimental leptospiral infections. Data concerning the efficacy of antibiotics in human beings have been conflicting. Within 4 to 6 h after initiation of penicillin G therapy, a Jarisch-Herxheimer type of reaction, which suggests antileptospiral activity, may occur. A controlled trial of intravenous penicillin (1.5 million units every 6 h for 7 days) clearly demonstrated shortening of duration of fever and creatinine elevation, shortening of hospitalization, and prevention of leptospiruria, even when treatment was started after the fifth day of illness. In contrast, a randomized trial of high-dose penicillin was not beneficial in jaundiced patients. Doxycycline (100 mg orally taken twice daily for 7 days), when started within 4 days of onset of symptoms, significantly shortened the duration of fever and most other symptoms and decreased the frequency of leptospiruria in patients with mild illness. Doxycycline (200 mg orally taken once per week) is also highly effective in preventing disease in an area of high prevalence. Azotemia and jaundice require meticulous attention to fluid and electrolyte therapy. Since the renal damage is reversible, patients with azotemia should be considered for peritoneal hemodialysis. Exchange transfusion may be beneficial in the management of patients with extreme hyperbilirubinemia.

REFERENCES

CICERONI L et al: Recent trends in human leptospirosis in Italy. Eur J Epidemiol 4:49, 1988
CORWIN A et al: Waterborne outbreak of leptospirosis among United States military personnel in Okinawa, Japan. Int J Epidemiol 19:743, 1990
EDWARDS CN et al:Leptospirosis in Barbados: A clinical study. West Indian Med J 39:27, 1990
FEIGIN RD, ANDERSON DC: Human leptospirosis. CRC Crit Rev Clin Lab Sci 5:413, 1975
GILKS CF et al: Failure of penicillin prophylaxis in laboratory acquired leptospirosis. Postgrad Med J 64:236, 1988
GRIFFIN GE: New insights into the pathophysiology of the Jarisch-Herxheimer reaction. J Antimicrob Chemother 29:613, 1992
HINDRICHSEN S et al: Hantavirus infection in Brazilian patients from Recife with suspected leptospirosis. Lancet 341:50, 1993
IM JG et al: Leptospirosis of the lung: Radiographic findings in 58 patients. AJR 152:955, 1989
JACKSON LA et al: Outbreak of leptospirosis associated with swimming. Pediatric Infect Dis J 12:48, 1993
JOHNSON WD JR et al: Serum creatine phosphokinase in leptospirosis. JAMA 233:981, 1975
KUDESRI G et al: Dual infection with Leptospira and Hantavirus. Lancet 1:1397, 1988
LECOUR H et al: Human leptospirosis—A review of 50 cases. Infection 17:8, 1989
MCCLAIN JB et al: Doxycycline therapy for leptospirosis. Ann Intern Med 100:696, 1984
PARK SK et al: Leptospirosis in Chonbuk Province of Korea in 1987: A study of 97 patients. Am J Trop Med Hyg 41:345, 1989
SCHMID GP: Epidemiology and clinical similarities of human spirochetal disease. Rev Infect Dis 11(suppl 6):S1460, 1989
TAKAFUJI ET et al: An efficacy trial of doxycycline chemoprophylaxis against leptospirosis. N Engl J Med 310:497, 1984
TURNER JS, WILLCOX PA: Respiratory failure in leptospirosis. Q J Med 72:841, 1989
WATT G: Leptospirosis. Curr Opin Infect Dis 5:659, 1992
—— et al: Placebo-controlled trial of intravenous penicillin for severe and late leptospirosis. Lancet 1:433, 1988
—— et al: Rapid diagnosis of leptospirosis: Prospective comparison of dot-ELISA and genus specific microscopic agglutination test at different stages of illness. J Infect Dis 157:840, 1988
—— et al: Central nervous system leptospirosis in the Philippines. Southeast Asian J Trop Med Public Health 20:265, 1989
—— et al: Limulus lysate positivity and Herxheimer-like reactions in leptospirosis: A placebo-controlled study. J Infect Dis 162:564, 1990
WINEARLS CG et al: Acute renal failure due to leptospirosis: Clinical features and outcome in six cases. Q J Med 53:487, 1984
WONG ML et al: Leptospirosis: A childhood disease. J Pediatr 90:532, 1977

136 RELAPSING FEVER

BAYU TEKLU / PETER L. PERINE

DEFINITION Relapsing fever is an acute spirochetal infection characterized by recurrent episodes of fever alternating with apyrexial intervals. The disease is caused by spirochetes of the genus *Borrelia* and has two epidemiologic varieties—louse-borne and tick-borne.

ETIOLOGY Borreliae are motile, spiral-shaped organisms 8 to 20 μm long and 0.2 to 0.45 μm thick. Their length may vary, but their thickness remains constant. They have an inner and an outer cell membrane with an interposed flagellum, which makes them unique morphologically. They are microaerophilic and grow and multiply easily in their vertebrate and invertebrate hosts. Several species can be cultured in embryonated eggs or Kelly's medium. After several passages in the laboratory, cultured strains may lose their infectivity. While *B. recurrentis* is the sole cause of louse-borne relapsing fever, there are over a dozen species of borreliae causing tick-borne relapsing fever.

EPIDEMIOLOGY The body louse is the only vector of louse-borne relapsing fever, and humans are the only known host, although other primates may be experimentally infected. The louse ingests blood from an infected person, and the spirochetes multiply in its tissues. Body lice travel from one person to another in conditions of crowding and poor hygiene and cause intense itching. Infection takes place when the louse is crushed intentionally or accidentally and its body fluids enter the bloodstream through the bite site, skin abrasions caused by scratching, or occasionally through mucous membranes. Accidental touching of the conjunctivae with contaminated fingernails is also known to produce infection.

Louse-borne relapsing fever is endemic in Central and East Africa and is thought to exist in Peru and China. In this century, epidemics destroyed large populations in Africa, Asia, and Europe during both world wars. Louse-borne relapsing fever is endemic in the highlands of Ethiopia and neighboring Sudan, where there is a steep increase in the incidence during the rainy season when the poor and louse-ridden huddle together in crowded shelters; an estimated 10,000 cases of louse-borne relapsing fever occur annually. Imported cases of louse-borne relapsing fever are seen occasionally in Europe and North America.

Tick-borne relapsing fever has a worldwide distribution, occurring in all the continents except Australasia. Soft-shelled argasid ticks belonging to the genus *Ornithodoros* are the vectors of the spirochetes, and small rodents act as their natural host. These ticks are nocturnal feeders and become infected by taking a blood meal from an infected rodent or human. The spirochetes multiply in the midgut and then enter the salivary glands and reproductive organs, where they remain alive and infective for years. Ticks of both sexes transmit the spirochetes, and female ticks infect their progeny transovarially. Humans become infected by a tick bite when the salivary and coxal secretions containing spirochetes are injected into the bloodstream. Urine and milk of infected rodents also contain live spirochetes, and contact of their infected urine with the mucous membranes of the mouth, nose, or conjunctivae also can cause infection.

B. duttoni is the most common species of borreliae causing tick-borne disease in Africa. In North America, the main species responsible are *B. hermsii*, *B. parkeri*, and *B. turicatae*, each species being named for the species of tick that transmits the spirochete. In North America, relapsing fever is prevalent in spring and summer in the western states, when people are out of doors and ticks and rodents are active. Most infections are acquired by staying overnight in log cabins infested with *Borrelia*-infected ticks. In Africa and Asia, borreliae are transmitted by domestic ticks living in the cracks of walls and mud floors. Once established, a reservoir of *Borrelia*-infected ticks can last for decades unless eradicated by insecticides.

PATHOGENESIS AND PATHOLOGY   The spirochetes live and multiply with ease in the arthropods, which are devoid of an immune system. Spirochetes have survived throughout the years in their rodent reservoirs through *serologic mutation*. In this phenomenon, spirochetes constantly change their surface antigens to avoid destruction by the immune system. By the time spirochetemia peaks, antibodies have developed to clear the blood of opsonized parasites by phagocytosis. However, a few organisms with spontaneously derived mutant surface antigens escape phagocytosis, rapidly multiply, and produce another relapse in 5 to 10 days.

A large number of different *Borrelia* serotypes emerge spontaneously by multiphasic antigenitic variation during the course of untreated relapsing fever. Serotype specificity is determined by variable antigens in the outer membrane of *Borrelia* called *Vmp lipoproteins*. A variant spirochete carrying a new Vmp appears spontaneously at a frequency of 10^{-4} to 10^{-3} per cell generation and will flourish until the host responds with serotype-specific antibodies. There are at least 25 different serotypes of HSI strain of *B. hermsi* prevalent in the western United States.

Once spirochetes enter the bloodstream, they rapidly multiply and reach 10^5 to 10^8 per cubic milliliter of blood. Fever is the first clinical manifestation and begins 3 to 12 days after infection. The severity of illness and injury is proportional to the number of spirochetes in the blood. Most injury occurs intravascularly with extensive endothelial damage, extravasation of blood into the mucous membranes and skin, and disseminated intravascular coagulation. Spirochetes also invade the brain and kidneys and may appear in the cerebrospinal fluid and urine.

At autopsy, splenic microabscesses, serosal petechiae, intracranial hemorrhages, diffuse histiocytic myocarditis, and hepatitis with focal necrosis are common. Spirochetes cross the placenta and may cause abortion or relapsing fever in the neonate.

CLINICAL MANIFESTATIONS   Louse-borne relapsing fever runs a more severe clinical course than tick-borne fever. After an incubation period of 3 to 18 days, those with louse-borne relapsing fever experience an abrupt onset of rigors with fever, usually remittent, headaches, arthralgia, and myalgias. Abdominal pain, nausea, vomiting, and mental confusion are common. Dry cough and signs of heart failure may develop. Epistaxis occurs in 10 to 40 percent of cases, jaundice in 15 to 45 percent, and skin petechiae or ecchymoses in up to 60 percent. Subconjunctival and retinal hemorrhages occur rarely, and hemoptysis and hematuria are infrequent. Meningismus is seen in 40 percent of cases.

The first attack lasts 3 to 6 days and ends by crisis characterized by rigors, with abruptly rising body temperature, blood pressure, pulse, and respiratory rate lasting 10 to 20 minutes. Peak core body temperature rapidly increases and may reach 44°C. This is followed by profuse sweating, falling temperature, and hypotension which may last several hours. The patient either recovers or dies during crisis from a combination of hyperpyrexia, severe hypotension, and intractable heart failure due to myocarditis. If recovery occurs, the patient may feel reasonably well for 5 to 10 days until less severe relapse occurs; additional relapses are rare. The decreased number of spirochetes during relapses is attributed to the increasingly effective host immune response. Although fewer in number, the spirochetes producing relapses are as virulent as those producing first attacks in a susceptible host.

In tick-borne relapsing fever, neurologic sequelae occur more frequently. Deafness and unilateral blindness secondary to panophthal-mitis or iridocyclitis and other neurologic deficits are seen in subsequent relapses. Splenomegaly occurs in 41 percent, hepatomegaly in 18 percent. Jaundice or neurologic features are seen in 8 percent. Skin rash is seen in 28 percent and epistaxis in only 2 percent. Convulsions occur frequently in children. Up to 10 relapses have been documented; each tends to be less severe and symptomatic. In pregnant women, relapsing fever can cause abortion and stillbirth.

LABORATORY FINDINGS   A mild anemia and thrombocytopenia are frequent findings. The white cell count is usually normal. Transient elevations of blood urea and creatinine are seen. Elevations in alanine aminotransferase, serum bilirubin, prothrombin time, and activated partial thromboplastin time are common. The majority of patients develop agglutinins to *Proteus* OXK and OX19. Proteinuria and microscopic hematuria may occur. A chest x-ray may show cardiomegaly and pulmonary edema. The ECG shows a prolongation of QTc interval and premature ventricular contractions.

Definitive diagnosis is made by demonstrating borreliae in peripheral blood films, thin or thick, stained with Wright's, Giemsa, or Leishman's stain. Motile borreliae also may be demonstrated in wet preparations with dark-field or phase-contrast microscopy. If spirochetemia is light, a peripheral blood smear may be negative, and repeated examinations are usually necessary, especially of samples collected during spikes of fever. If the smear is negative and there is a strong suspicion of the tick-borne disease, blood may be injected into mice and their blood examined subsequently for spirochetes. In patients with meningeal signs, the cerebrospinal fluid may show increased protein and mononuclear pleocytosis; in rare cases borreliae are seen by dark-field or phase-contrast microscopy.

DIFFERENTIAL DIAGNOSIS   In both varieties of relapsing fever, the differential diagnosis includes malaria, typhoid fever, typhus, Lyme disease, rat-bite fever, leptospirosis, meningococcal disease, and hepatitis. In tick-borne relapsing fever, brucellosis, tularemia, juvenile rheumatoid arthritis, dengue fever, and Rocky Mountain spotted fever also should be considered.

TREATMENT   Borreliae are highly susceptible to a variety of antimicrobials, including penicillins, tetracycline, chloramphenicol, and erythromycin, but are resistant to rifampicin and sulfonamides. Before administration of intravenous antibiotic, a good peripheral or preferably a central venous line should be secured. In louse-borne relapsing fever, the drug of choice is tetracycline, 500 mg, intravenously or orally, as a single dose, which clears the blood of spirochetes within a few hours. The same dose may be used for chloramphenicol or erythromycin with similar results. All antibiotics precipitate the Jarisch-Herxheimer reaction (J-HR). If intravenous tetracycline is used, patients with louse-borne relapsing fever invariably develop a severe J-HR within 1 h of drug administration. The initial "chill" phase, in which the patient abruptly becomes agitated with severe rigors, lasts about 1 h. During this phase, blood pressure, pulse, and respiratory rate rise sharply and the patient develops hyperpyrexia, usually over 40°C and lasting up to 1 h. Severe abdominal pain, vomiting, and diarrhea with urinary incontinence also may occur. Serial blood films show that spirochetes rapidly decrease in number, accompanied by leukopenia and thrombocytopenia. Hyperpyrexia should be treated promptly with tepid sponging or acetaminophen. A "flush" phase follows that is characterized by profound vasodilation, drenching sweats, and falling vital signs. Systolic blood pressure may reach 70 mmHg or less, and congestive heart failure or pulmonary edema may ensue. Failure can be managed by judicious use of saline infusions and digoxin, 0.5 mg intravenously. Hypotension and listlessness may last several hours and, rarely, contribute to multiple organ failure and death.

The crisis and Jarisch-Herxheimer reaction in louse-borne relapsing fever have recently been shown to be temporally associated with high circulating levels of the monokines tumor necrosis factor α, interleukin 6 (IL-6), and IL-8. It may be possible to block the reaction by pretreatment with human anti-TNF antibody.

Aspirin, acetaminophen, high-dose oral or intravenous corticosteroids, or intravenous naloxone administered during the reaction or before antibiotic administration do not prevent or ameliorate the J-HR. Meptazinol, an opioid antagonist with some agonist properties, in a dose of 300 to 500 mg intravenously, reduces the severity of the J-HR. Since relapses have occasionally been noted after ampicillin or penicillin treatment, this treatment should be followed by a single 500-mg oral dose of tetracycline, chloramphenicol, or erythromycin after the crisis has ended. If the peripheral smear is negative for *Borrelia* and there is a strong clinical suspicion of louse-borne relapsing fever, 500 mg tetracycline either intravenously or orally can be given as a therapeutic trial. Occurrence of the crisis confirms the diagnosis, while its absence virtually excludes the disease. Typhoid fever, typhus, malaria, Kala-azar, rickettsiosis, and tuberculosis may occur concomitantly.

The treatment of choice for tick-borne relapsing fever is tetracycline, 500 mg, orally every 6 h for 10 days, or in those not tolerating tetracycline, erythromycin in the same dose may be substituted. Doxycycline, 100 mg, twice daily for 10 days, is equally effective. J-HR occurs in one-third of cases of tick-borne relapsing fever following administration of antibiotics.

Improved personal hygiene and living conditions should eradicate louse-borne relapsing fever. Because patients with the disease are usually infected with lice, they should be bathed, their scalp hair shaved, and 1% lindane or lysol solution or DDT powder applied. Cohabitants should be deloused in a similar manner. If buildings and cracks in walls are sprayed with 2% benzene hydrochloride, and if campers avoid tick-infested areas, the incidence of tick-borne relapsing fever can be reduced. Camping in tents is safer than sleeping in rodent-infested log cabins. A novel means of eradicating ticks in rodent burrows is to scatter pyrethrin-impregnated cotton balls on the ground around dwellings known to harbor *Borrelia*-infected ticks; rodents collect these cotton balls and carry them back to their burrows as nesting material. The insecticide-impregnated cotton kills ticks living in the borrow.

PROGNOSIS The mortality from louse-borne relapsing fever in the preantibiotic era was 30 to 70 percent, but with antibiotic therapy, mortality in hospitals and at refugee camps ranges from 0 to 5 percent. Poor prognostic signs include coma, deep jaundice, hemorrhage, and evidence of myocarditis.

In tick-borne relapsing fever, mortality varies from 0 to 8 percent. Fatalities usually occur in young children and congenitally infected neonates.

REFERENCES

BARBOUR AG: Antigenic variation of a relapsing fever borrelia species. Annu Rev Microbiol 44:155, 1990

HORTON JM, BLASER MJ: The spectrum of relapsing fever in Rocky Mountains. Arch Intern Med 145:871, 1985

JUDGE DM et al: Louse-borne relapsing fever in man. Arch Pathol 97:136, 1974

NEGUSSIE Y et al: Detection of plasma tumor necrosis factor, interleukins 6 and 8 during the Jarisch-Herxheimer reaction of relapsing fever. J Exp Med 175:1207, 1992

TEKLU B et al: Meptazinol diminishes the Jarisch-Herxheimer reaction of relapsing fever. Lancet 1:835, 1983

137 LYME BORRELIOSIS

ALLEN C. STEERE

DEFINITION Lyme borreliosis, a tick-transmitted spirochetal illness, usually begins with a characteristic expanding skin lesion, erythema migrans (EM) (stage 1, localized infection). After several days to weeks, the spirochete may spread hematogenously to many different sites (stage 2, disseminated infection). Possible manifestations of disseminated infection include secondary annular skin lesions,

meningitis, cranial or peripheral neuritis, carditis, or migratory musculoskeletal pain. Months to years later, usually following periods of latent infection, intermittent or chronic arthritis or chronic neurologic or skin abnormalities may develop (stage 3, persistent infection). Although there are regional variations, the basic stages of the illness are similar worldwide.

ETIOLOGY *Borrelia burgdorferi*, the causative agent of the disease, is a fastidious, microaerophilic bacterium that grows best at 33°C in a complex liquid medium called Barbour, Stoenner, Kelly (BSK) medium. Except in the case of erythema migrans skin lesions, culture of the spirochete from clinical specimens has been difficult. Three genomic subgroups of *B. burgdorferi* have recently been defined. To date, American isolates have been genomic subgroup 1, whereas European isolates have included all 3 subgroups. These differences probably account for the clinical variations in the disease in different geographic regions.

EPIDEMIOLOGY The distribution of Lyme disease correlates primarily with the geographic ranges of certain ixodid ticks—*Ixodes dammini*, *I. pacificus*, *I. ricinus*, and *I. persulcatus*. *I. dammini* is the principal vector in the northeastern United States (from Massachusetts to Maryland) and in the Midwest (Wisconsin and Minnesota). In surveys of *I. dammini* in these states, 20 percent or more of the ticks have been infected with *B. burgdorferi*, and most cases of Lyme disease in the United States have occurred in these areas. *I. pacificus* is the vector in the western United States. The disease may be acquired throughout Europe—from Great Britain to Scandinavia to Russia—where *I. ricinus* is the vector; in Asia, where *I. persulcatus* is the vector; and in Australia. The ticks have different animal hosts; for *I. dammini*, the white-footed mouse is the preferred host of the immature tick and the white-tailed deer of the mature tick.

Most new cases have onsets during the summer months. Cases have occurred in association with hiking, camping, and hunting trips or among people living in wooded or rural areas. Patients of any age and both sexes are affected. Cases have been reported in 47 states, and more than 1000 people now acquire the infection in the United States each summer.

PATHOGENESIS After injection into the skin, *B. burgdorferi* may migrate outward, producing EM, and may spread hematogenously to other organs. The spirochete has been cultured from blood, skin (EM), cerebrospinal fluid, and joint fluid and has been seen in most affected tissues. These findings and the response of all stages of the disease to antibiotic therapy suggest that the organism invades and persists in affected tissues throughout the illness.

Initially, the immune response seems to be suppressed. The mononuclear cells of patients respond minimally to *B. burgdorferi* antigens and less than normally to mitogens. After the first several weeks of infection, mononuclear cells generally have heightened responsiveness to *B. burgdorferi* antigens and to mitogens, and evidence of B cell hyperactivity—elevated total serum IgM levels, cryoprecipitates, and circulating immune complexes. The specific antibody response to the spirochete develops gradually over months to years and is directed at an increasing array of spirochetal polypeptides. Specific IgM antibody titers to *B. burgdorferi* peak between the third and sixth week after disease onset; specific IgG antibody titers rise slowly and are generally highest months or years later, when arthritis is present. By that time, antigen-reactive mononuclear cells and immune complexes are found in the joint fluid. Patients with chronic arthritis have an increased frequency of the class II major histocompatibility complex alleles HLA-DR4 and, secondarily, HLA-DR2. These alleles may determine a host immune response to *B. burgdorferi* that has autoreactive features.

CLINICAL MANIFESTATIONS Early infection: Stage 1 (localized infection) After an incubation period of 3 to 32 days, EM, which occurs at the site of the tick bite, usually begins as a red macule or papule that expands to form a large annular lesion, most often with a bright-red outer border and partial central clearing. Because of the small size of ixodid ticks, most patients do not remember the preceding tick bite. The center of the lesion sometimes becomes intensely erythematous and indurated, vesicular, or necrotic. In other instances, the expanding lesion remains an even, intense red; several red rings are found within the outside one; or the central area turns blue before it clears. Although the lesion can be located anywhere, the thigh, groin, and axilla are particularly common sites. The lesion is warm but not often painful. Skin biopsies show perivascular infiltrates or lymphocytes and histiocytes. Perhaps as many as 25 percent of patients lack this characteristic skin manifestation of the disorder.

Early infection: Stage 2 (disseminated infection) Within days after the onset of EM, the organism often spreads hematogenously to many different sites. Such patients frequently develop secondary annular skin lesions which are similar in appearance to the initial lesion. Skin involvement is often accompanied by severe headache, mild neck stiffness, fever, chills, migratory musculoskeletal pain, arthralgias, and profound malaise and fatigue. Less common manifestations include generalized lymphadenopathy or splenomegaly, hepatitis, sore throat, nonproductive cough, conjunctivitis, iritis, or testicular swelling. Except for fatigue and lethargy, which are often constant, the early signs and symptoms of Lyme disease are typically intermittent and changing. Even in untreated patients, the early symptoms usually improve or disappear within several weeks.

Symptoms suggestive of meningeal irritation may occur early in Lyme disease, when EM is present, but are usually not associated with a spinal fluid pleocytosis or objective neurologic deficit. After several weeks to months, about 15 percent of patients develop frank neurologic abnormalities, including meningitis, subtle encephalitic signs, cranial neuritis (including bilateral facial palsy), motor or sensory radiculoneuropathy, mononeuritis multiplex, chorea, or myelitis, alone or in various combinations. The usual pattern consists of fluctuating symptoms of meningitis accompanied by facial palsy and peripheral radiculoneuropathy. Cerebrospinal fluid shows a lymphocytic pleocytosis (about 100 cells per microliter), often with elevated protein, and normal or slightly low glucose. In Europe, the first-neurologic sign is characteristically radicular pain, which is followed by the development of a cerebrospinal fluid pleocytosis (called Bannwarth's syndrome), but meningeal or encephalitic signs are frequently absent. These early neurologic abnormalities usually resolve completely within months, but chronic neurologic disease may occur later.

Within several weeks after the onset of illness, about 8 percent of patients develop cardiac involvement. The most common abnormality is fluctuating degrees of atrioventricular block (first-degree, Wenckebach, or complete heart block). Some patients have more diffuse cardiac involvement, including electrocardiographic changes of acute myopericarditis, left ventricular dysfunction on radionuclide scans, or, rarely, cardiomegaly or pancarditis. Cardiac involvement usually lasts only a few weeks but may recur. One case of chronic cardiomyopathy caused by *B. burgdorferi* has been reported.

During this stage, musculoskeletal pain is common. The typical pattern is migratory pain in joints, tendons, bursae, muscle, or bone, usually without joint swelling, lasting hours or days in one or two locations at a time.

Late infection: Stage 3 (persistent infection) Months after the onset of infection, about 60 percent of patients in the United States who have received no antibiotic treatment develop frank arthritis. The typical pattern is intermittent attacks of oligoarticular arthritis in large joints, especially knees, lasting weeks to months in a given joint. Small joints and periarticular sites also may be affected, primarily during early attacks. The number of patients who continue to have recurrent attacks decreases each year. However, in a small percentage of patients, involvement in large joints, usually one or both knees, becomes chronic and may lead to erosion of cartilage and bone. The involvement of joints seems to be a more frequent manifestation of the illness in the United States than in Europe.

Joint fluid white cell counts range from 500 to 110,000 cells per microliter (average, 25,000 cells per microliter), mostly polymorpho-nuclear leukocytes. Tests for rheumatoid factor or antinuclear antibodies are usually negative. Synovial biopsies show fibrin deposits, villous hypertrophy, vascular proliferation, microangiopathic lesions, and a heavy infiltration of lymphocytes and plasma cells.

Although less common, chronic neurologic or skin involvement (acrodermatitis chronica atrophicans) also may occur months to years after the onset of infection, sometimes following long periods of latent infection. This late skin manifestation of the disorder has been observed primarily in Europe. The most common form of chronic central nervous system involvement is a subtle encephalopathy affecting memory, mood, or sleep. These patients often have evidence of memory impairment on neuropsychological tests and abnormal CSF analyses. The encephalopathy is frequently accompanied by an axonal polyneuropathy manifested as either distal paresthesias or spinal or radicular pain. Electromyography generally shows extensive abnormalities of proximal and distal nerve segments. Leukoencephalitis, a rare manifestation of Lyme borreliosis, is a severe neurologic disorder that may include spastic parapareses, upper motor neuron bladder dysfunction, and lesions in the periventricular white matter. Acrodermatitis begins with red-violaceous lesions that become sclerotic or atrophic over a period of years. This chronic skin disorder has been observed primarily in elderly women.

DIAGNOSIS Lyme disease is diagnosed by recognition of a characteristic clinical picture with serologic confirmation. Although serologic testing may be negative during the first several weeks of infection, most patients have a positive antibody response to *B. burgdorferi*, determined by ELISA, after that time. Western blotting is often helpful in sorting out false-positive results in patients who have indeterminate responses by ELISA. However, patients with previous Lyme disease often remain seropositive, and a small percentage of patients have asymptomatic infection. If these patients develop another illness, the positive serologic test for Lyme disease may cause diagnostic confusion. In about 5 percent of patients who receive antibiotic therapy during the first several weeks of infection, the spirochete may still survive in protected niches and cause subtle joint or neurologic symptoms. In these patients, the humoral immune response may be aborted, but a cellular immune response to the spirochete can usually be demonstrated by proliferative assay.

TREATMENT The various manifestations of Lyme disease can usually be treated successfully with oral antibiotic therapy, except for objective neurologic abnormalities, which seem to require intravenous therapy. For early Lyme disease, doxycycline, 100 mg twice a day, or amoxicillin, 500 mg four times a day, is effective therapy, but doxycycline should not be given to children or pregnant women. Cefuroxime, 500 mg twice a day, seems to be an equally effective alternative in patients with penicillin allergy. Erythromycin, 250 mg four times a day, is less effective clinically but is another alternative in patients with allergies to the other medications. In children, amoxicillin is effective (50 mg/kg per day); in cases of penicillin allergy, erythromycin (30 mg/kg per day) can be given. For patients with infection localized to the skin, 10 days of therapy is generally sufficient. For patients with disseminated infection, a course of 20 to 30 days may be needed. Approximately 15 percent of patients experience a Jarisch-Herxheimer–like reaction during the first 24 h of therapy.

These oral antibiotic regimens, when given for 30 days, also may be effective for the treatment of Lyme arthritis. However, the response to therapy may be slow. A small percentage of patients with arthritis, particularly those with the HLA-DR4 allele and an immune response to the OspA or OspB proteins of the spirochete, do not respond to antimicrobial therapy. Synovectomy may be successful in these patients.

For objective neurologic abnormalities, with the possible exception of facial palsy alone, parenteral antibiotic therapy seems to be necessary. Intravenous ceftriaxone, 2 g/d for 2 to 4 weeks, is most commonly used for this purpose, but intravenous penicillin G, 20 million units/d in divided doses, also may be effective. In patients with high-degree atrioventricular block or a PR interval of greater than 0.3 s, intravenous ceftriaxone, 2 g/d, or intravenous penicillin, 10 to 20 million units/d for at least 10 days, and cardiac monitoring are recommended. In patients with complete heart block or congestive heart failure, glucocorticoids may be of benefit if the patient does not improve on antimicrobial therapy alone within 24 h.

In a small percentage of patients, infection with *B. burgdorferi* may trigger fibromyalgia, which is thought to be a variant of the chronic fatigue syndrome. It is important to distinguish this diffuse pain syndrome from active Lyme disease, since the pain syndrome does not respond to antibiotic therapy. The risk of infection with *B. burgdorferi* after a recognized tick bite is so low that prophylactic antimicrobial treatment is not routinely indicated. If the patient is quite anxious or if the tick is engorged, 10 days of amoxicillin or doxycycline therapy is likely to prevent the occurrence of Lyme disease.

PROGNOSIS The response to treatment is best early in the illness. Treatment of Lyme borreliosis later in the course of illness often results in months of convalescence. Eventually, complete recovery ensues in the majority of patients.

REFERENCES

BARANTON G et al: Delineation of *Borrelia burgdorferi* sensu stricto, *Borrellia garinii* sp. nov., and group VS461 associated with Lyme borreliosis. Int J Sys Bact 42:378, 1992

BARBOUR AG, HAYES SF: Biology of *Borrelia* species. Microbiol Rev 50:381, 1986

LOGIGIAN EL et al: Chronic neurologic manifestations of Lyme disease. N Engl J Med 323:1438, 1990

MASSAROTTI EM et al: The treatment of early Lyme disease. Am J Med 92:396, 1992

PACHNER AR, STEERE AC: The triad of neurologic manifestations of Lyme disease: Meningitis, cranial neuritis, and radiculoneuritis. Neurology 35:47, 1985

———: Lyme disease. N Engl J Med 321:586, 1989

——— et al: Lyme carditis: Cardiac abnormalities of Lyme disease. Ann Intern Med 93:8, 1980

——— et al: The early clinical manifestations of Lyme disease. Ann Intern Med 99:76, 1983

——— et al: The clinical evolution of Lyme arthritis. Ann Intern Med 107:725, 1987

section 10 *Rickettsia, Mycoplasma, and Chlamydia*

138 RICKETTSIAL DISEASES

THEODORE E. WOODWARD

The rickettsial diseases of humans consist of a variety of clinical entities caused by microorganisms of the family Rickettsiaceae. The rickettsias are obligate intracellular parasites about the size of bacteria and are usually seen microscopically as pleomorphic coccobacilli. Each of the rickettsias pathogenic for humans is capable of multiplying in one or more species of arthropod as well as in animals and humans. Indeed, the majority of the rickettsias are maintained in nature by a cycle which involves an insect vector and an animal reservoir, and infection of humans is unimportant in the cycle. Epidemic typhus presents a number of points of dissimilarity to most of the other rickettsioses. Until recently, the natural cycle of infection was thought to involve only humans and lice. The finding of a sylvatic reservoir in flying squirrels associated with a human illness which resembles classic typhus emphasizes that there are other mechanisms.

A compendium of information on the rickettsial diseases is given in Table 138-1.

Of all the afflictions of the human race, the rickettsial diseases, particularly epidemic typhus, rank among the foremost as a cause of suffering and death. The record of deaths from epidemic typhus in this century in the Balkan countries and in Poland and Russia reached astounding figures. Typhus ravaged Russia and eastern Poland from 1915 to 1922, infecting 30 million inhabitants and causing an estimated 3 million deaths. It is currently quite prevalent in Ethiopia.

The past two decades have seen the development of excellent methods for the prevention and treatment of rickettsioses. In fact, these measures have been so successful that the rickettsioses have become of minor importance in the United States and in many other countries. Although conquered, these infections have not been eliminated, and they could again become rampant if the will to control them, the present high standards of sanitation, and the necessary industrial capacities for production of effective insecticides and therapeutic agents should be compromised.

PATHOGENESIS Rickettsial diseases develop after infection through the skin or the respiratory tract. Agents of the typhus and spotted fever groups are introduced through the bite of the infected arthropod vector. Ticks and mites, which transmit the agents of spotted fever and scrub typhus, inoculate the rickettsias directly into the dermis during feeding. The louse and flea, which transmit epidemic and murine typhus, respectively, deposit infected feces on the skin; infection occurs when organisms are rubbed into the puncture wound made by the arthropod. The rickettsias of Q fever gain entry through the respiratory tract when infected dust is inhaled; the respiratory route is also occasionally implicated in epidemic typhus when infection results from inhalation of dried infected louse feces.

Although organisms probably multiply at the original site of entry in all instances, local lesions appear with regularity only in certain diseases, namely, the initial cutaneous lesions of scrub typhus, rickettsialpox, and boutonneuse fever and the pneumonitis which develops in about half the persons with Q fever.

Volunteers infected with either scrub typhus or Q fever develop rickettsemia late in the incubation period, often some hours before the onset of fever. Similar events probably occur in all the rickettsial diseases; circulating rickettsias can be detected during the early febrile period in practically all patients. Little is known about the pathogenesis of infection during the midportion of the incubation period. However, it is reasonable to assume that during this time, in patients with typhus or spotted fever, a transient low-grade rickettsemia results from release of organisms multiplying at the initial site of infection and that this seeds infection in the endothelial cells of the vascular tree. Vascular lesions developing at such sites account for the pathologic changes, including the rash.

Rickettsias apparently invade and proliferate in the endothelial cells of small blood vessels. Raoult separated endothelial cells from the blood of patients with Mediterranean spotted fever. By means of antiendothelial antibody, endothelial cells were bound to magnetized beads; the rickettsias were identified by the immunofluorescence technique. Endothelial cell destruction results from the proliferation of organisms and eventual disruption. Rickettsias may exert a cytotoxic effect on endothelial cells; in mice the rickettsial toxin causes a remarkable increase in capillary permeability, independent of

TABLE 138-1 Rickettsial diseases

Disease Type	Agent	Geographic distribution	Natural cycle Arthropod	Natural cycle Mammal	Principal means of transmission to humans	Serologic diagnosis Weil-Felix reaction	Serologic diagnosis CF, MA, and IFA reactions*
SPOTTED FEVER GROUP							
Rocky Mountain spotted fever	R. rickettsii	Western hemisphere	Ticks	Wild rodents, dogs	Tick bite	Positive OX-19 OX-2	Positive Group- and type-specific
Boutonneuse fever	R. conorii	Africa, Europe, Middle East, India	Ticks	Rodents, dogs	Tick bite	Positive OX-19 OX-2	Positive Group- and type-specific
Queensland tick typhus	R. australis	Australia	Ticks	Marsupials, wild rodents	Tick bite	Positive OX-19 OX-2	Positive Group- and type-specific
North Asian tick-borne rickettsiosis	R. sibirica	Siberia, Mongolia	Ticks	Wild rodents	Tick bite	Positive OX-19 OX-2	Positive Group- and type-specific
Rickettsialpox	R. akari	United States, Russia, Africa	Blood-sucking mites	House mice, other rodents	Mite bite	Negative	Positive Group- and type-specific
TYPHUS GROUP							
Endemic (murine)	R. typhi	Worldwide	Fleas	Small rodents	Infected flea feces into broken skin	Positive OX-19	Positive Group- and type-specific
Epidemic	R. prowazekii	Worldwide	Body lice	Humans, flying squirrels	Infected louse feces into broken skin	Positive OX-19	
	R. canada	North America	Ticks			Positive OX-19	
Brill-Zinsser disease	R. prowazekii	Worldwide	Recurrence years after original attack of epidemic typhus			Usually negative	Positive
Scrub	R. tsutsugamushi	Asia, Australia, Pacific islands	Trombiculid mites	Wild rodents	Mite bite	Positive OX-K	Positive in about 50% of patients
OTHER RICKETTSIAL DISEASES							
Q fever	R. burnetii	Worldwide	Ticks	Small mammals, cattle, sheep, goats	Inhalation of dried infected material	Negative	Positive
Trench fever	R. quintana†	Europe, Africa, North America	Body lice	Humans	Infected louse feces into broken skin	Negative	None available

* CF = complement fixation; MA = microscopic agglutination; IFA = immunofluorescent antibody.
† Some authorities no longer place the agent in the genus *Rickettsia* because it can be cultured on artificial media.

proliferation. The anatomic location of multiple microscopic lesions and the numerous foci of rickettsial vascular changes with rickettsias present coincide well with the organs examined microscopically such as the kidney, lung, heart, and liver. These findings confirm Wolbach's original conclusion that "the lesions of the blood vessel are due to the presence of the parasite." Absence of inflammatory cell reactions in fulminant Rocky Mountain spotted fever tends to exclude several host-mediated immunopathogenetic mechanisms. The underlying cause of the toxic-febrile state which characterizes the rickettsial diseases remains unknown. Several rickettsial species contain type-specific toxins which are lethal for mice, and these may play a role in humans. Careful studies of *Rickettsia*-infected cells and macrophages maintained in tissue culture may help explain the mechanisms of the increased permeability which typifies Rocky Mountain spotted fever and severe typhus fever. Increased release of prostaglandins (PG_1 and PG_2) and leukotrienes (LTB_4) by damaged endothelial cells and macrophages has suggested a possible mechanism to explain capillary leakage. If confirmed, corrective strategies might be developed to diminish production of arachidonate metabolites.

PATHOLOGIC PHYSIOLOGY Peripheral vascular collapse results in death in fulminating cases during the first week, with capillary dilatation and pooling of blood without increased capillary permeability or loss of fluid into extravascular spaces. Proliferative and thrombotic lesions develop in small vessels, resulting in necrosis and increased capillary permeability, with loss of water, electrolytes, proteins, and erythrocytes. These events in turn result in a decrease in blood volume, together with an increase in the extravascular space and clinical edema, particularly during the later stages of illness (stage III). Edema, anoxia of the myocardium, and histologic evidence of myocarditis are disclosed by electrocardiographic abnormalities, including serious arrhythmias. Liver function is impaired. The azotemia which develops in seriously ill patients late in illness appears to be prerenal. Clinical manifestations resulting from the peripheral vascular collapse are oliguria and anuria, azotemia, anemia, hypoproteinemia, hyponatremia, edema, and coma. In spotted fever and typhus patients with hemorrhagic skin lesions, consumptive coagulopathy is present. All these alterations are absent or minimal in patients with mild cases or in those who are given specific treatment early.

PATHOLOGY The basic changes in the spotted and typhus fever groups are vascular, with resultant widespread lesions in adjacent parenchymatous organs. They are most common in the skin, muscles, heart, lung, and brain. The most conspicuous and diverse are found in Rocky Mountain spotted fever, where swelling, proliferation, and degeneration of the endothelial cells occur, frequently with thrombus formation which partially or completely occludes the lumen. The muscle cells of the arterioles undergo swelling and fibrinoid changes. The adventitial tissues are infiltrated with mononuclear leukocytes, lymphocytes, and plasma cells. The vascular damage is scattered along arteries, veins, and capillaries, with normal architecture prevailing throughout most of the vascular bed. The changes in murine, epidemic, and scrub typhus fevers resemble those in Rocky Mountain spotted fever, but thrombosis is uncommon and involvement of the musculature is rare.

Interstitial myocarditis occurs in each of these diseases but is usually most extensive in Rocky Mountain spotted fever and scrub typhus. In the brain, glial nodules are found in all members of the group, but microinfarcts in the brain tissue or in the myocardium are most often observed in spotted fever. By immunofluorescence techniques, rickettsias can be identified in brain, lung, myocardium, and other tissues.

Rickettsial pneumonitis occurs, at least to some extent, in many patients with spotted or typhus fever and is characteristic in patients with Q fever. The process is patchy and consists microscopically of areas of congestion and edema. Within the consolidated areas the alveoli are filled with compact fibrinocellular exudate containing lymphocytes, plasma cells, large mononuclear cells, and erythrocytes but few, if any, polymorphonuclear leukocytes.

Rickettsias can occasionally be observed microscopically in sections of tissue such as brain, myocardium, and lung. Failure to demonstrate them is of no diagnostic significance. They are readily identifiable by the immunofluorescence technique, even after 50 years of fixation.

LABORATORY DIAGNOSIS Diagnostic procedures which depend on isolation of the etiologic agent from blood or other clinical material are expensive, time-consuming, and hazardous to laboratory personnel. Primary isolation of rickettsias by chick embryo inoculation or tissue culture usually fails because of the small number of organisms in the patient's blood. Rickettsias have been identified in stained cultured monocytes of infected monkeys and by direct or indirect immunofluorescence of infected animal tissues. Except in unusual circumstances, however, currently available serologic tests are adequate for laboratory confirmation of the clinical diagnosis in each of the rickettsial diseases. The demonstration of a rise in titer of specific antibody during convalescence is of prime importance in establishing laboratory confirmation. Table 138-2 summarizes the serologic results usually encountered in persons who have rickettsial diseases in the United States. The Weil-Felix test employing Proteus strains OX-19 and OX-2 gives positive results in patients with spotted fever and murine typhus and negative results in those with rickettsialpox and Q fever. It is useful as a screening procedure but cannot be relied on to differentiate spotted fever from murine typhus. In patients with Brill-Zinsser disease, the Proteus OX-19 reaction is usually negative or low in titer.

Serologic tests employing group-specific rickettsial antigens provide data which clearly differentiate the most common infections, i.e., epidemic typhus, murine typhus, Rocky Mountain spotted fever, and Q fever. Type-specific rickettsial antigens generally make it possible to distinguish rickettsialpox from spotted fever and Brill-Zinsser disease from murine typhus.

The type of immunoglobulin in acute (IgM) and late or recurrent (IgG) illness is helpful in identifying recrudescent typhus (Brill-Zinsser disease). In general, the Weil-Felix and complement fixation tests are useful for routine diagnosis; microscopic agglutination, immunofluorescent antibody, and hemagglutination reactions are valuable for specific identification.

Specific antibiotic therapy has little effect on the time of appearance of antibodies or on their ultimate titer, provided treatment is instituted some days after onset of the illness. However, if the illness is cut short by early and vigorous treatment, antibody production may be delayed for a week or so, and the maximum titers attained may be below those illustrated in Table 138-2. Under these circumstances, a sample of blood taken 4 to 6 weeks after onset of illness also should be tested.

The immunofluorescent antibody test is very useful for detecting Rickettsia in the tissues of patients with the typhus group of rickettsioses, the spotted fevers, and Q fever. Identifiable rickettsias have been visualized in skin lesions of patients with Rocky Mountain spotted fever as early as the fourth day of illness and as late as the tenth day. Rickettsias may be visualized in human tissues several days after administration of chloramphenicol or tetracycline. The technique also visualizes rickettsias in ticks and in animal tissues, including those fixed with paraffin.

Normochromic anemia occurs in patients severely ill with rickettsial diseases. The white blood cell count in Rocky Mountain spotted fever, rickettsialpox, murine and epidemic typhus, Brill-Zinsser disease, Q fever, and other rickettsial diseases is usually within the normal range: 6000 to 10,000 cells per microliter. Leukopenia is occasionally observed, and in the presence of complications, such as

TABLE 138-2 Serologic diagnosis of rickettsial diseases in the United States

Group	Disease	Proteus	Weil-Felix reaction 10th day	20th day	Cases with diagnostic titer	Rickettsial antigen	CF 10th day	20th day	30th day	Cases with diagnostic titer
Spotted fever	Rocky Mountain spotted fever	OX-19 / OX-2	40 / 20	320 / 160	Most	R. rickettsii	20	160	80	Most
	Rickettsialpox	OX-19 / OX-2	0 / 0	0 / 0	None	R. akari	0	64	128	Most
Typhus	Murine typhus	OX-19 / OX-2	160 / 10	640 / 40	Most	R. typhi	0	160	160	Most
	Epidemic typhus, squirrel related	OX-19 / OX-2	160 / 10	640 / 40	Most	R. prowazekii	0	160	160	Most
	Brill-Zinsser disease	OX-19 / OX-2	160 / 0	20 / 0	Few	R. prowazekii	1280	640	320	Most
	Q fever	OX-19 / OX-2	0 / 0	0 / 0	None	R. burnetii	10	80	160	Most

superimposed infections and extensive vascular lesions, moderate leukocytosis occurs. The differential blood cell count is usually normal. Thrombocytopenia occurs in severely ill patients with spotted and scrub typhus fever and extensive vascular lesions; hypofibrinogenemia, prolonged prothrombin and partial thromboplastin times, and other clotting abnormalities occur.

TREATMENT Patients seriously ill with one of the diseases of the typhus–spotted fever group may show circulatory collapse, coma, oliguria and anuria, azotemia, anemia, hypoproteinemia, hypochloremia and hyponatremia, and edema. These alterations are often absent in the mildly ill, and in them management is much less complicated. The therapeutic principles necessary for treatment of all rickettsioses are (1) specific chemotherapy and (2) supportive care. Attention to both is mandatory for the seriously ill patient first recognized late in the disease. During the first week in the moderately ill patient, supportive therapy may need to be less energetic, because specific chemotherapy usually suffices. The early mild case may be successfully treated at home; more severely ill patients should receive hospital care because manifestations can progress rapidly in fulminant cases.

Specific therapy Specific therapy is most effective when initiated during the early stages of disease coincident with the appearance of the rash. When therapy is delayed until the rash has become hemorrhagic and widespread, the response is less dramatic. The antibiotics of choice are chloramphenicol and the tetracyclines, which are effective because of their rickettsiostatic properties. They are not rickettsiocidal. Ciprofloxacin therapy is effective in patients with Western Mediterranean spotted fever. Its value for other rickettsial diseases is unknown.

The following antibiotic regimen is considered optimal: for chloramphenicol, an initial dose of 50 mg/kg of body weight, and for tetracycline, 25 mg/kg. Subsequent daily doses are the same as the initial loading dose, with the requirement divided equally and given at 6- to 8-h intervals. Antibiotic treatment is continued until the patient has improved and has been afebrile approximately 24 h. The decision to stop specific therapy is based on careful assessment of the patient's status coupled with good clinical judgment. In patients too ill to take oral medication, an intravenous preparation of one of the antimicrobials should be employed.

Adrenal cortical hormones may be needed for their antitoxemic effects in patients first observed late in the course of severe illness. Large doses for brief periods of about 3 days, in combination with specific antibiotics, are recommended in critically ill patients.

In uncomplicated cases of spotted fever, there is symptomatic improvement within 24 h, and the temperature becomes normal in 60 to 72 h.

Supportive care Frequent turning of the patient relieves pressure from prominent bony parts and also militates against the development of aspiration pneumonia. Proper mouth care, with frequent swabbing of the oral cavity, may avert the development of parotitis and gingivitis. Sucking of the juice of a lemon or the oral use of glycerin or mineral oil is helpful. Usually food is well tolerated by patients with rickettsial disease, and the daily diet should provide 1 to 2 g protein per kilogram of normal body weight; the diet may need to be supplemented with oral or parenteral hyperalimentation (see Chap. 76).

When indicated, red cell transfusions given slowly are helpful. The support of the hypotensive patient with rickettsial disease is similar to that of other patients with shock (see Chap. 83). Dialysis is indicated when there is clear-cut evidence of acute renal failure.

ROCKY MOUNTAIN SPOTTED FEVER Definition Rocky Mountain spotted fever is an acute febrile illness caused by *Rickettsia rickettsii*. It is transmitted to humans by ticks. The disease is characterized by sudden onset with headache and chills and by fever which persists for 2 to 3 weeks. A characteristic exanthem appears on the extremities and trunk about the fourth day of illness. Delirium, shock, and renal failure occur in severely ill patients.

Etiology and epidemiology The causative microbe, *R. rickettsii*, is the prototype for the rickettsial group of agents. The minute organisms are purple when stained by Giemsa's method or red by Macchiavello's technique; most of them are gram-negative. These organisms often occur in pairs and possess a cell wall similar in structure and chemical composition to that of gram-negative bacteria; there are a cell membrane, cytoplasmic granules corresponding to ribosomes, and prokaryotic organization of nuclear material. The cell membrane is selectively permeable; the cell wall is the focus of important antigens and an endotoxin-like substance.

The rickettsias grow in the nucleus and the cytoplasm of infected cells of ticks, mammals, and embryonated eggs; the intranuclear situation of the organisms is shared by the other members of the spotted fever group but not by rickettsias of the typhus group. *Rickettsia rickettsii* is readily distinguishable from the agents of the typhus fevers by cross-immunity tests in guinea pigs and by complement fixation tests employing antigens prepared from infected yolk sac tissues. The differentiation of *R. rickettsii* from closely related members of the spotted fever group frequently requires elaborate procedures. Strains of the agent of Rocky Mountain spotted fever vary considerably in their virulence for humans and animals.

The first reports of spotted fever in Idaho and Montana during the final decade of the last century led to the name *Rocky Mountain spotted fever*. However, the disease has been reported from all states (except Maine, Alaska, and Hawaii), as well as from Canada, Mexico, Colombia, and Brazil. Although related diseases are found on other continents, this particular infection is limited to the Western Hemisphere. From 1981 to 1986, an average of 933 cases per year were reported in the United States, while more recently (1987–1990), the yearly average has decreased to 621 cases. Why this decrease has occurred is not known. The mortality rate was about 20 percent in the days before specific therapy but has decreased to about 7 percent. More than half the cases occur in the South Atlantic and South Central states, with the greatest number in North Carolina, Virginia, Georgia, Maryland, Tennessee, and Oklahoma.

An unusual outbreak of "urban" spotted fever occurred in New York City's Bronx borough during the summer of 1987. Eight percent of dog ticks were positive for *R. rickettsii*.

A number of species of ticks are found infected with *R. rickettsii* in nature, but only two are important in transmitting spotted fever to humans. These are *Dermacentor andersoni*, the wood tick, which is the principal vector in the West, and *D. variabilis*, the dog tick, which assumes this role in the East. *Amblyomma americanum*, the lone star tick, and *D. variabilis* are the common vectors in the west South Central states. Infected female ticks transmit the agent transovarially to at least some of their offspring. Ticks which become infected, either through the egg or at one of the stages during their development cycle by feeding on an infected mammal, harbor the rickettsias throughout their lifetime, which may be several years; thus the tick is a reservoir as well as a vector. Small wild mammals are suspected of playing an important role in spreading the rickettsias in nature by infecting ticks which feed on them during rickettsemia.

Disease in humans is generally acquired from the bite of an infected tick. Transmission is unlikely unless the tick remains attached for a number of hours. Infection also may be acquired through abrasions in the skin which become contaminated with infected tick feces or tissue juices, hence the hazard associated with crushing ticks between the fingers when removing them from persons or animals. The agent of Rocky Mountain spotted fever has been transmitted accidentally to humans by transfusion of blood taken from a donor just before onset of illness.

There are seasonal variations in the incidence of cases of spotted fever, as well as differences in age and sex distribution of cases. In each instance these differences are related to exposure to ticks. Most cases are seen during the period of maximal tick activity, i.e., April to September, and 60 percent of cases occur in individuals under 20 years of age. This age distribution is undoubtedly influenced by propinquity to the wood and dog ticks. The mortality rate increases with the age of the patient.

Rocky Mountain spotted fever has been acquired by laboratory workers via aerosol transmission, and special precautions are necessary when the agent is handled in the laboratory.

Clinical manifestations INCUBATION PERIOD AND PRODROMATA A history of tick bite is elicited in approximately 80 percent of patients. The incubation period varies between 3 and 12 days, with a mean of 7 days. A short incubation period usually indicates a more serious infection.

ONSET In nonvaccinated persons, the onset is usually abrupt, with severe headache, a sudden shaking rigor, prostration, generalized myalgia (especially in the back and leg muscles), nausea with occasional vomiting, and fever which reaches 39.4 to 40°C (103 to 104°F) within the first 2 days. Pain in the abdominal muscles may be severe, and arthralgia is not uncommon. Deep muscle palpation often elicits tenderness. Occasionally, the debut of illness in children and adults is mild, accompanied by lethargy, anorexia, headache, and low-grade fever. These symptoms are similar to those of many acute infectious diseases, and specific diagnosis is therefore difficult during the first few days. The course of illness is occasionally rapid, with death 6 or 7 days after onset.

PYREXIA Fever continues for approximately 15 to 20 days in untreated cases. The febrile course in children may be shorter. Hyperthermia of 40.5°C (105°F) or greater is of unfavorable prognostic significance, although fatalities may occur when the patient is hypothermic, with concurrent vasomotor collapse. Fever generally terminates by lysis over a period of several days but rarely does so by crisis. Recurrent fever is uncommon except in the presence of secondary pyrogenic complications.

The *headache* is generalized and excruciating and frequently most intense over the frontal area. It persists throughout the first and second weeks of illness in untreated cases. Occasionally, headache is mild. Malaise continues for the first week; irritability is notable, and the patient shuns distractions such as questioning and examination.

CUTANEOUS MANIFESTATIONS The rash which is present in practically all cases is the most characteristic and helpful diagnostic sign. It usually appears on the fourth febrile day; the range is 2 to 6 days. Faint-pink macules which fade on pressure have been noted on the first febrile day. The initial lesions are on the wrists, ankles, palms, soles, and forearms. The first lesions are macular, nonfixed, pink, irregularly defined, and measure 2 to 6 mm. A warm compress applied to the extremity accentuates the rash in the early stages. The exanthem is most prominent when the temperature is elevated. After 6 to 12 h, the rash extends centripetally to the axilla, buttocks, trunk, neck, and face. (This is in contrast to the eruption of typhus fever, which begins on the trunk and spreads centrifugally, rarely involving the face, palms, or soles.) The rash becomes maculopapular after 2 to 3 days (it may be felt by light palpation) and assumes a deeper red hue. By about the fourth day it is petechial and fails to fade on pressure. Not uncommonly, the hemorrhagic lesions coalesce to form large ecchymotic blemishes; these lesions tend to form over bony prominences and may ultimately slough to form indolent, slow-healing ulcers. Patients who have had the typical rash show brownish discolorations at the site for several weeks during convalescence. In milder cases, the rash does not become purpuric and may disappear within a few days. Antibiotic therapy may abort the early exanthem; the later fixed lesion fades less rapidly with specific therapy. Occasionally, a rash does not occur or is unnoticed, particularly in dark-skinned patients.

The application of tourniquets for several minutes or the occasional taking of the blood pressure may provoke additional petechiae (Rumpel-Leede phenomenon), further evidence of capillary abnormalities.

CARDIOVASCULAR AND RESPIRATORY FEATURES During the early stages, the pulse is full and regular and is accelerated in proportion to the height of the temperature, and the blood pressure is well sustained. During the peak of illness in seriously ill patients, the pulse is rapid and feeble, and hypotension of 90 mmHg or less is common. If circulatory failure is sustained, the resultant hypoxia and shock lead to agitation and delirium and contribute to the formation of ecchymoses and gangrene of fingers, toes, genitalia, buttocks, earlobes, and nose. Cyanosis of the peripheral parts of the body is common. A reduction of the total blood volume is found occasionally, late in the course of illness. The ECG shows low voltage, minor ST-segment deflections, and, occasionally, delay in atrioventricular conduction. These changes are transient and nonspecific. Severely ill patients have a puffy appearance of the face, hands, ankles, feet, and lower parts of the sacrum. Occasionally, a severe arrhythmia associated with myocarditis results in sudden death.

Respirations are either normal or slightly accelerated. Cough may be harassing and nonproductive, and localized pneumonitis may occur, but pulmonary consolidation is extremely rare. Pulmonary edema may develop after injudicious use of intravenous fluids.

HEPATIC AND RENAL MANIFESTATIONS In the majority of patients there is little alteration in renal or hepatic function. The liver may be enlarged, but jaundice is unusual. Oliguria and anuria commonly occur in seriously ill patients. Azotemia is common; when marked, it is a very unfavorable sign. Abnormalities in liver function include hypoproteinemia, with reduction in the albumin fraction.

NEUROLOGIC MANIFESTATIONS The principal neurologic manifestations are headache, restlessness, and varying degrees of insomnia. Stiffness of the back is common. The cerebrospinal fluid (CSF) is clear, with normal dynamics and normal chemical constituents. Occasionally, the CSF pressure is elevated; there may be a slight increase in mononuclear cells. Coma and muscular rigidity may occur. Athetoid movements, convulsive seizures, and hemiplegia are grave manifestations. Deafness during the active stages of the disease is not uncommon. As a rule, all neurologic signs abate without residua. Findings based on follow-up examinations and electroencephalograms may be interpreted as indicative of minor residual brain damage for a year or more following recovery of some patients from Rocky Mountain spotted fever.

OTHER PHYSICAL MANIFESTATIONS Patients become dehydrated, with extreme dryness of the lips, gums, tongue, and pharynx. The skin is hot and dry; the conjunctivae are frequently injected and the eyes suffused. Photophobia is common in the early stages of illness. Petechial hemorrhages may be noted in the conjunctivae or in the retina. The spleen is enlarged in approximately one-half the cases and is firm and nontender. Usually there is abdominal distention and some degree of intestinal ileus. Occasionally, the severity of abdominal discomfort associated with muscle spasm may suggest the diagnosis of acute appendicitis, cholecystitis, and localized peritonitis. An elevated leukocyte count suggests an inflammatory reaction. Vasculitis involving small vessels is probably responsible for the conflicting symptoms.

Course In patients with mild and moderately severe cases who are given no specific antibiotic therapy, the disease abates within 2 weeks, and convalescence is rapid. In fatal cases, death usually occurs during the latter part of the second week as a result of toxemia, vasomotor collapse and shock, or renal failure. In a few patients, the course is fulminant, with death occurring as early as the sixth day of illness.

In vaccinated individuals who contract the disease, the illness is mild, with a short febrile course and an atypical rash.

Prognosis If the serious manifestations of spotted fever are regarded as intrinsic parts of the disease, then complications are uncommon and consist mainly of secondary bacterial infections such as bronchopneumonia, otitis media, and parotitis. Thrombosis of major blood vessels may result in gangrene of a portion of an extremity. Hemiplegia and peripheral neuritis are rare sequelae.

The overall mortality rate for spotted fever was formerly about 20 percent. Death occurred in more than half of persons over 40 years of age, but the mortality rate was much lower in children and young adults. Since the introduction of the broad-spectrum antibiotics and the development of more precise knowledge regarding correction of the physiologic abnormalities which develop during the disease, fewer deaths occur. Some of the fatalities can be attributed to failure to consider spotted fever in the differential diagnosis and resultant delay in instituting appropriate treatment.

Differential diagnosis During the early stages of infection, before the rash has appeared, differentiation from other acute infections is difficult. A history of tick bite while living or traveling in wooded or bushy sites known to be in a highly endemic area is helpful. The rash of meningococcemia (see Chap. 109) resembles Rocky Mountain spotted fever in certain aspects, because it is macular, maculopapular, or petechial in the chronic form and petechial, confluent, or ecchymotic in the fulminant type. The meningococcal skin lesion is tender and develops with extreme rapidity in the fulminant form, whereas the rickettsial rash occurs on about the fourth day of disease and gradually becomes petechial. *Spotted fever is often confused with measles.* The exanthem of rubeola rapidly becomes confluent, while that of rubella *usually remains discrete.* In boutonneuse fever, Mediterranean spotted fever, and related diseases, there is often an eschar along with enlarged glands at the site of the tick attachment; the rash is typically red, is distinctly maculopapular, and may become hemorrhagic.

Murine typhus is a milder disease than Rocky Mountain spotted fever; the rash is less extensive, nonpurpuric, and nonconfluent, and renal and vascular complications are uncommon. Not infrequently, differentiation of these two rickettsial infections must await the results of specific serologic tests. Epidemic typhus fever is capable of causing all the pronounced clinical, physiologic, and anatomic alterations seen in patients with Rocky Mountain spotted fever, i.e., hypotension, peripheral vascular collapse, cyanosis, skin necrosis and gangrene of digits, renal failure and azotemia, and neurologic manifestations. However, the rash of classic typhus is noted initially in the axillary folds of the trunk and later extends peripherally, rarely involving the palms, soles, or face. The serologic patterns in these two diseases are distinctive when specific rickettsial antigens are employed. Moreover, louse-borne typhus is now recognized in the United States as a flying squirrel–related illness which occurs sporadically and as Brill-Zinsser disease (recrudescent typhus fever). Rickettsialpox, although caused by a member of the spotted fever group, is usually readily differentiated from Rocky Mountain spotted fever by the initial lesion, the relative mildness of the illness, and the early vesiculation of the maculopapular rash. The Weil-Felix reaction is positive in Rocky Mountain spotted fever and in murine and epidemic typhus but is negative in rickettsialpox. Agglutinins against *Proteus* OX-19 and OX-2 appear in the sera of patients with spotted fever, but only those against OX-19 are generally found in murine and epidemic typhus. In Lyme disease, the typical skin lesion, erythema chronicum migrans, consists of concentric annular rings with clear centers.

Complications *Pyogenic complications,* including otitis media and parotitis, are encountered in patients severely ill with Rocky Mountain spotted fever and other rickettsioses. These localized infections respond to therapy with appropriate antibiotics combined with surgical measures.

Pneumonitis may develop as a result of specific rickettsial action or as a bacterial superinfection. The sputum is scanty and should be examined to determine whether superimposed bacterial infection is present. Specific therapy is guided by the results of these laboratory studies. The pneumonitis generally responds to the antibiotic therapy the patient is receiving, but if staphylococcal pneumonia is suspected, a penicillinase-resistant penicillin or a cephalosporin should be added to the tetracycline or chloramphenicol.

Circulatory failure of peripheral or central origin is treated with careful administration of plasma expanders and fluids (see Chaps. 34 and 83). When the clinical signs reveal unmistakable evidence of cardiac failure, digitalis, diuretics, and other cardiac drugs should be employed as indicated (see Chap. 195).

Prevention Prevention is attained primarily by avoidance of tick-infested areas. When this is impractical, prophylactic measures include (1) spraying the ground with dieldrin or chlordane for area control of ticks (although there are environmental objections to the use of residual insecticides in area control of ticks, under special conditions such procedures may be warranted), (2) application of repellents such as diethyltoluamide or dimethylphthalate to clothing and exposed parts of the body or in very heavily infested areas the wearing of clothing which interferes with the attachment of ticks, i.e., boots and a one-piece outer garment, preferably impregnated with repellent, and (3) daily inspection of the entire body, including the hairy parts, to detect and remove attached ticks. In removing attached ticks, great care should be taken to avoid crushing the arthropod with resultant contamination of the bite wound. Gentle traction with tweezers applied close to the mouthparts may be necessary; the skin area should be disinfected with soap and water or other antiseptics. Similarly, precautions should be employed in removing engorged ticks from dogs and other animals, because infection through minor abrasions on the hands is possible. Improved vaccines containing inactivated *R. rickettsii* are under development and when available commercially should be used for those at great risk, namely, persons frequenting highly endemic areas and laboratory workers exposed to the agent. Because the broad-spectrum antibiotics are such excellent therapeutic agents in spotted fever, there has been less impetus for vaccination of persons who run only a minor risk of infection.

After a tick bite in a known endemic area, an exposed person should be observed for signs of fever, headache, prostration, and rash; therapy is very effective early in the infection.

MURINE (ENDEMIC) TYPHUS FEVER Definition Murine typhus fever is an acute febrile disease caused by *Rickettsia typhi (mooseri)* and transmitted to humans by fleas. The clinical illness is characterized by fever of 9 to 14 days, headache, a maculopapular rash appearing on the third to fifth day, and myalgia.

Etiology and epidemiology *R. typhi* resembles other rickettsias in morphologic properties, staining characteristics, and intracellular parasitism. Under the electron microscope, *R. typhi* is seen to contain dense masses of nuclear material in a less dense homogeneous protoplasmic substance, the whole of which is surrounded by a limiting membrane. It differs from *R. rickettsii* in that it always multiplies within the cytoplasm of cells, in contrast to the intranuclear and cytoplasmic positions of spotted fever rickettsias.

Invasion of the body by *R. typhi* provokes specific and nonspecific immunologic responses. With highly purified antigens, specific antibodies may be demonstrated readily by complement fixation, microscopic agglutination, and immunofluorescent antibody reactions. The positive Weil-Felix reaction that occurs in this disease is nonspecific because it is attributable to the presence of common carbohydrate antigens.

The common vector of *R. typhi* for rats and humans is the rat flea (*Xenopsylla cheopis*). In nature, the rat louse (*Polypax spinulosis*) may transmit the agent among rodents. Customarily, rat fleas become infected on ingestion of blood from diseased rats; the rickettsias multiply within the intestinal cells of the arthropod and are excreted in the feces. Infection in humans occurs after the flea bite and contamination of the broken skin by *Rickettsia*-laden feces. Dried flea feces also may infect via the conjunctivae or the upper part of the respiratory tract.

Rats and mice are naturally infected with murine typhus, and although the rodent disease is nonfatal, viable rickettsias persist in the brain for variable periods.

Murine typhus is one of the most benign and widespread of the rickettsioses in the United States. Prevalent in the southeastern and Gulf Coast states, it has been identified in most of the other states and in harbor centers throughout the world wherever rats and fleas abound. In the early 1940s, 2000 to 5000 cases of murine typhus were reported annually. This contrasts with between 50 and 69 cases reported in the United States yearly between 1986 and 1990. This sharp reduction was achieved by control of rats and their fleas in known areas of high prevalence. In urban areas the disease is more prevalent during the summer and fall and occurs predominantly among persons working in proximity to granaries or food depots. There has been an extension to certain rural areas when changing agricultural practices have provided rats with ready access to adequate food supplies. Endemic typhus has been reported in laboratory workers. This emphasizes the importance of taking special precautions when working with rickettsial organisms in the laboratory.

Clinical manifestations INCUBATION PERIOD AND PRODROMATA The incubation period ranges from 8 to 16 days, with a mean of 10 days. Common prodromata are headache, backache, arthralgia, and chilly sensations. Nausea, malaise, and transient temperature rises may precede the true onset of disease.

ONSET AND GENERAL SYMPTOMS A frank shaking chill and repeated rigors are present at the onset, associated with a severe frontal headache and fever. This triad of headache, chill, and pyrexia is usually followed within a few hours by nausea and vomiting. Prostration, malaise, and weakness are sufficient to enforce cessation of activity in adults, in contrast to children, whose illness is less severe. Occasionally, mild symptoms make it difficult to define the actual onset.

PYREXIA The usual febrile course in murine typhus lasts for about 12 days in adults; the temperature ranges from 38.8 to 40°C (102 to 104°F) but may reach 40.5 to 41.1°C (105 to 106°F) in children. The temperature may reach high levels abruptly after onset or ascend in a stepwise manner during the first few days. With the appearance of the rash, fever is usually sustained, with partial daily remissions which occasionally reach normal levels in the morning. Defervescence is generally by lysis over several days but sometimes occurs by crisis. Transient mild fever of 37.7°C (100°F) is not uncommon during early convalescence. A few patients experience only low-grade fever throughout, but this does not necessarily connote a mild illness.

CUTANEOUS MANIFESTATIONS The early lesions, which are sparse and discrete, are hidden in the axillae and inner surface of the arm. Most patients then develop with surprising suddenness a generalized, dull-red macular rash of the upper part of the abdomen, shoulders, chest, arms, and thighs. The individual lesions are discrete and pea-sized, with an ill-defined border, and fade on pressure during the first 24 h. They later become maculopapular, in contrast to the exanthem of epidemic typhus, which is persistently macular. The distribution over the trunk with sparse involvement of the extremities, palms, soles, and face differs from the peripheral distribution and facial involvement of Rocky Mountain spotted fever. The murine rash generally appears initially on the fifth febrile day, but rarely it is seen concurrently with the onset of fever or develops as late as the seventh day.

Eighty percent of patients develop a rash which persists for 4 to 8 days and fades before defervescence. The cutaneous manifestations vary greatly in intensity and duration and may be fleeting. They are readily overlooked in dark-skinned patients, in whom they should be sought by light palpation and indirect lighting.

CARDIOVASCULAR AND RESPIRATORY FEATURES An irritating, nonproductive cough is frequent and is occasionally associated with moderate hemoptysis. Early in the second week, rales may be detected in the basilar lung areas. These changes are generally a result of the primary rickettsial infection rather than bacterial superinfection. Pulmonary congestion occurs in extremely ill and elderly patients.

Accelerated pulse and hypotension occur, although less frequently than in patients with epidemic typhus or Rocky Mountain spotted fever. Rickettsial endocarditis is thought, by some, to be a rare complication of murine typhus.

NEUROLOGIC MANIFESTATIONS Headache is the most common neurologic manifestation of murine typhus and may dominate the clinical picture. It is frontal and continues into the second week of illness. Stupor and prostration may occur in the second week, and in severe cases there may be delirium, extreme agitation, or coma.

Coma in elderly patients after 2 weeks of illness presages death. Nuchal rigidity and general spasticity often suggest meningitis, although the CSF is normal except for slight increases in pressure and the presence of lymphocytes (5 to 30 per microliter). Transient partial deafness occurs occasionally, but rarely is there localized neuritis or hemiplegia. Neurologic sequelae are unusual. Children experience minimal neurologic changes.

OTHER PHYSICAL MANIFESTATIONS During the first 2 days of illness the patient may be nauseated and vomit, but vomiting later in the illness should arouse suspicion of a complication. Abdominal pain is bothersome; when associated with diarrhea or ileus, it responds to intravenous alimentation. Hepatomegaly and jaundice are unusual. There is splenomegaly in approximately 25 percent of patients.

Photophobia, retroocular pain, and suffusion of the conjunctivae are common but are less severe than in the other typhus and spotted fevers.

Renal function is usually unaltered except in elderly patients with prolonged hypotension. Under these circumstances, azotemia may develop to the degree observed in epidemic typhus. In severe murine typhus, as in the epidemic typhus, hyponatremia and hypoalbuminemia are encountered.

Course After defervescence, murine typhus patients recover rapidly. Fatalities occur between the ninth and twelfth days in elderly or debilitated patients, usually as a result of circulatory and renal failure or intercurrent bacterial infection.

Prognosis The mortality rate in murine typhus was low even before the introduction of specific therapy (<1 percent).

Differential diagnosis Because murine typhus and Rocky Mountain spotted fever occur in many of the same states, the problem of differential diagnosis often arises. Flea-borne murine typhus, which is predominantly an urban disease, is more likely to occur in late summer and autumn. In contrast, spotted fever is a rural and suburban disease in which exposure to ticks is important. Most cases occur in the spring and summer.

Treatment and prevention Both chloramphenicol and the tetracycline antibiotics have controlled the disease (see above). Prevention of murine typhus in humans is attained by reducing the natural reservoir and vector by applying measures for eliminating rodents and employing appropriate insecticides in rat-infested areas to control fleas. Spraying of rat burrows with DDT effectively reduces the population of the vector.

EPIDEMIC (LOUSE-BORNE) TYPHUS FEVER Definition Classic epidemic typhus is a severe, febrile disease caused by R. prowazekii and transmitted to humans by the body louse. Intense headache, continuous pyrexia of about 2 weeks, a macular skin eruption appearing on about the fifth febrile day, malaise, and vascular and neurologic disturbances represent the principal clinical features. Confirmation of the diagnosis is made by demonstration of Proteus OX-19 agglutinins and of specific complement-fixing antibodies in convalescence. The broad-spectrum antibiotics are specific therapeutic agents.

Etiology and epidemiology The causative microbe, R. prowazekii, is closely related to R. typhi, which causes murine typhus; indeed, the two have a number of common antigens.

Human beings generally are infected when Rickettsia-laden louse feces are rubbed into the broken skin; scratching the louse bite facilitates this process. Pediculus humanus corporis, which is peculiarly adapted to humans, is the only important vector of epidemic typhus. It dies of its infection and fails to transmit rickettsias to its offspring. R. prowazekii has been isolated from flying squirrels, and the organism probably infests their ectoparasites. Generally, however, the organism is maintained by a cycle involving human-louse-human. New epidemics apparently originate from patients with Brill-Zinsser disease (recurrent epidemic typhus). Flying squirrels can serve as a potential host to initiate an outbreak of epidemic typhus, provided an avid human vector, such as the body louse, is prevalent. Pathogenic rickettsias reside for long periods in patients with epidemic typhus as well as Rocky Mountain spotted fever and scrub typhus. Lice readily become infected when they feed on patients with recurrent typhus. Inhalation of dust containing dried louse feces may cause infection. An established nonhuman reservoir such as flying squirrels poses a serious threat.

If uncontrolled, epidemic typhus behaves as a cyclic disease in a susceptible population, extending over a 3-year period. During the first year there is a gradual seeding of cases throughout the group, during the second there is epidemic spread, and during the third the epidemic tapers off, because the majority of persons have become immune. Outbreaks of epidemic typhus last occurred in the United States in the nineteenth century, and its presence is now recognized in the form of Brill-Zinsser disease and flying squirrel–related typhus. Cases of epidemic typhus now occur in significant numbers in Ethiopia and probably in highland areas of other impoverished countries.

Clinical manifestations Epidemic typhus resembles murine typhus but is more severe. After an incubation period of about 7 days, an abrupt onset of headache, chill, and rapidly mounting fever ushers in the illness. Headache, malaise, and prostration continue unabated until the rash appears on the fifth febrile day. It is initially macular in the axillary folds but ultimately invades the trunk and extremities as a pink, irregular macular lesion which becomes fixed, petechial, and confluent in the later stages.

Neurologic features range from headache and general spasticity to extreme agitation, stupor, and coma. Circulatory disturbances consisting of tachycardia, hypotension, and cyanosis are more profound than those observed in murine typhus and are almost as severe as in Rocky Mountain spotted fever. Ultimately, in untreated cases, azotemia often reaches high levels as a result of vascular and renal failure, and death occurs late in the second week of illness. Thrombosis of major blood vessels and cutaneous gangrene develop in a manner similar to that seen in the virulent form of Rocky Mountain spotted fever.

The complications and sequelae of epidemic typhus are more severe than those in murine typhus but not as severe as those in Rocky Mountain spotted fever. However, during certain outbreaks, epidemic typhus was fatal in 60 percent of those infected, and convalescence in survivors was prolonged. The use of chloramphenicol or tetracycline has almost eradicated mortality in this dread disease, provided therapy is instituted before irreversible organ system changes occur.

Differential diagnosis Differentiation of epidemic typhus from the various rickettsioses and other diseases with which it may be confused was described earlier. The disease is not known to occur in epidemic form in the absence of louse infestation in the general population. Under the conditions in which typhus epidemics are likely to occur, other diseases which may cause confusion include malaria, relapsing fever, pneumonia, and tuberculosis. Classic typhus contracted by a previously vaccinated person is usually mild and may be clinically indistinguishable from murine typhus except by serologic methods.

Treatment and prevention Both chloramphenicol and the tetracycline antibiotics have been found to be highly efficient therapeutic agents in epidemic typhus. Usually the patient becomes afebrile after 2 days of treatment. Under field conditions, 100 mg doxycycline in a single oral dose resulted in abatement of clinical manifestations and defervescence in epidemic typhus.

The most effective measures for controlling epidemic typhus are those which eliminate lice. DDT or lindane powder when dusted into clothing is suitable for this purpose. If resistant lice are found, malathion or carbaryl may prove effective.

A commercially available vaccine prepared from formalin-treated suspensions of infected yolk sac tissue is an effective immunizing agent.

BRILL-ZINSSER DISEASE (RECRUDESCENT TYPHUS) Brill-Zinsser disease is a recrudescent episode of epidemic typhus fever that occurs years after the initial attack. *R. prowazekii* has been isolated from lice feeding on patients during the active stages of illness.

The clinical entity, not always mild, resembles epidemic typhus in the character of the rash, circulatory disturbances, and hepatic, renal, and nervous system changes. Recovery is the rule. The Weil-Felix reaction with the various *Proteus* antigens is usually negative or positive in very low titer. The specific complement fixation, microscopic agglutination, and immunofluorescent antibody reactions are valuable in establishing the diagnosis. In Brill-Zinsser disease the specific complement-fixing antibodies appear as early as the fourth day after the onset of illness; antibodies are IgG, and the peak response is attained by the eighth to tenth days. Specific antibody titers in the primary attack of epidemic typhus begin later, about the eighth to twelfth day, with maximum titers on about the sixteenth day after onset. Treatment is the same as for other rickettsial infections.

SCRUB TYPHUS **Definition** Scrub typhus is limited to eastern and southeastern Asia, India, northern Australia, and the adjacent islands. It is common in northern Thailand. It is caused by *R. tsutsugamushi* and is characterized by a primary lesion at the site of the bite of an infected mite, a fever of about 2 weeks' duration, a cutaneous rash which develops about the fifth day, and the appearance late in the second week of agglutinins against the OX-K strain of *Proteus* bacillus. Antibiotics similar to those used for other rickettsial infections are specific therapeutic agents.

Etiology The agent of scrub typhus resembles other rickettsias in its physical properties but differs from them in antigenic structure, vector, and reservoir. The disease is transmitted by larvae of several species of mites, especially *Leptotrombidium* (*Trombicula*) *akamushi* and *L. deliense*. These tiny chiggers attach themselves to the skin and during the process of obtaining a meal of tissue juice may acquire infection from the host or transmit rickettsias to the vertebrate. The infection is maintained in nature by a cycle involving mites and small rodents and by transovarial transmission in mites; human infection represents an accident attributable to propinquity.

Clinical manifestations About 10 to 12 days after infection, illness begins abruptly with chilliness, severe headache, fever, conjunctival injection, and moderate generalized lymphadenopathy, which is most prominent in the nodes draining the area of the primary lesion. The initial lesion at the beginning of fever is evidenced by an erythematous indurated area 1 cm in diameter, surmounted by a multiloculated vesicle; within a few days the vesicle ulcerates and becomes covered with a black crust.

Fever increases progressively during the first week, generally reaching 40 to 40.5°C (104 to 105°F), but the pulse remains relatively slow, 70 to 100 beats per minute. The red macular rash, which begins on the trunk about the fifth day and spreads to the extremities, sometimes becomes maculopapular but usually fades in a few days. The course of the disease and the complications resemble those of endemic and epidemic typhus; however, interstitial myocarditis is more prominent than in the other typhus fevers.

Prognosis Before the introduction of chloramphenicol and tetracycline, the mortality rate varied from 1 to 60 percent, depending on the geographic area and the virulence of the local strains of *R. tsutsugamushi*, and convalescence was prolonged. With modern therapeutic methods, deaths are rare and convalescence is short.

Differential diagnosis Scrub typhus must be differentiated from the other members of the typhus and spotted fever group of diseases as well as from measles, typhoid fever, and the meningococcal infections. The geographic localization of scrub typhus, the primary lesion, and the occurrence of OX-K agglutinins are especially useful in establishing the diagnosis.

Treatment and prevention Chloramphenicol and the tetracycline antibiotics are extremely effective in scrub typhus. Scrub typhus is more amenable to drugs than are the other rickettsial infections, and patients with this disease regularly become afebrile and are decidedly improved within 24 to 36 h after beginning treatment, irrespective of the stage of disease. Antibiotic treatment may be discontinued after several afebrile days.

Relapse of clinical illness is unusual unless specific treatment is initiated early, such as before the fifth febrile day. Under these circumstances, recrudescence is prevented by giving the antibiotic for several days and resuming treatment about 5 days after cessation of the initial course of therapy.

Prevention of disease in the individual is accomplished by the application of miticidal chemicals (dibutyl phthalate, benzyl benzoate, diethyltoluamide, and others) to clothing and the skin. There is no satisfactory vaccine. Chemoprophylactic studies conducted in highly endemic infested areas of scrub typhus showed that single oral doses of chloramphenicol or tetracycline given every 5 days for a total of 35 days (seven doses with 5-day nontreatment intervals) prevent scrub typhus and result in active immunity. This procedure is recommended under special circumstances. A long-acting tetracycline (doxycycline) serves the same purpose.

TRENCH FEVER Trench fever is a rare febrile disease transmitted between humans by the body louse, *Pediculus humanus corporis*. It is characterized by a sudden onset with headache and severe pain in the muscles, bones, and joints. In most cases the fever and other symptoms assume a relapsing character. Fatalities are rare. The disease is also known as shin bone fever, Volhynia fever, His-Werner disease, and quintan fever. Because of its rarity in the United States, textbooks of rickettsiology should be consulted for a detailed description.

RICKETTSIALPOX Definition Rickettsialpox is a mild, nonfatal, self-limited, febrile illness caused by *R. akari*, which is transmitted from mice to humans by mites. It is characterized by an initial skin lesion at the mite bite, a week's febrile course, and a papulovesicular rash.

Etiology and epidemiology Rickettsialpox was first recognized in New York City in 1946, and about 180 cases were reported annually for several years thereafter. It has been diagnosed in several other areas of the United States, and outbreaks have been reported in European Russia. A possible new focus has been identified in Baltimore, Md. The vector is a small, colorless mite, *Allodermanyssus sanguineus* (Hirst), which infests small mice and rodents. House mice serve as the reservoir of infection.

R. akari is morphologically and biologically similar to other rickettsias and is antigenically related to, but distinct from, *R. rickettsii*, the cause of Rocky Mountain spotted fever.

Clinical manifestations The initial skin lesion appears about 7 to 10 days after the mite bite as a firm red papule 1 to 1.5 cm in diameter. In a few days, the center vesiculates, and the papule is surrounded by an area of erythema. The regional lymph glands are moderately enlarged. The primary lesion, which is not painful, becomes covered with a black scab; it heals slowly, and a small scar is visible on separation of the crust.

The febrile phase begins 3 to 7 days after the initial lesion, and an exanthem may accompany the fever or begin several days later. The onset of fever is sudden, with chilly sensations or frank chills, headache, sweats, myalgia, anorexia, and photophobia. The pyrexia ranges from 39.4 to 40°C (103 to 104°F) and continues for about a week, occasionally with morning remissions.

The exanthem is maculopapular-vesicular, is generalized in distribution, and may be abundant or scant. The lesions may involve the oral cavity but not the palms or soles. In a week, the vesicles dry and form scabs which eventually scale but leave no scar.

The constitutional symptoms are generally mild, and the course of illness is uncomplicated. No fatal cases have been reported.

The disease may be confused with chickenpox, which is different because it occurs usually in childhood and has no initial lesion and the papular cutaneous lesion is entirely transformed into a vesicle. Variola (smallpox) is accompanied by a more severe constitutional reaction, and the vesicles become pustules. The skin lesions of the other rickettsioses differ in their lack of vesiculation. The Weil-Felix reaction is usually negative in this rickettsial disease, but specific complement fixation, microscopic agglutination, and immunofluorescence antibody reactions are useful diagnostic aids even though there is considerable antigenic crossing with Rocky Mountain spotted fever.

Treatment and prevention Chloramphenicol and the tetracycline antibiotics are all effective for treating patients with rickettsialpox. The temperature reaches normal levels in about 2 days, and recovery is rapid.

Control measures should be directed toward elimination of house mice and the vector mites responsible for transmitting the disease.

OTHER TICK-BORNE RICKETTSIAL DISEASES Definition Boutonneuse fever, North Asian tick-borne rickettsiosis, and Queensland tick typhus, three diseases occurring in the Eastern Hemisphere, are caused by rickettsias closely related to one another and to the agent of Rocky Mountain spotted fever. Each is transmitted by the bite of an ixodid tick. These mild to moderately severe illnesses are characterized by an initial lesion (called *tache noire* in boutonneuse fever), a fever of several days to 2 weeks, and a generalized maculopapular erythematous rash which appears on about the fifth day and usually involves the palms and soles. Specific complement-fixing antibodies appear in the patients' sera during convalescence, but agglutinins to *Proteus* OX-19 (Weil-Felix reaction) are frequently found only in low titer.

Etiology and epidemiology The etiologic agents of these three diseases are all members of the spotted fever group of rickettsias. Together with *R. rickettsii* and *R. akari* they possess common group antigens which are readily demonstrated by agglutination, complement fixation, microscopic agglutination, and immunofluorescent antibody reactions.

Boutonneuse fever (Mediterranean spotted fever), which may be regarded as the prototype of the three, is caused by *R. conorii*. Modern serologic methods employing specific rickettsial antigens have shown this *Rickettsia* to be the causative agent for a single widely disseminated disease known by various local names. Information on the distribution and etiology of the various tick-borne rickettsial diseases is contained in Table 138-1.

In general, the epidemiology of these tick-borne rickettsioses resembles that of spotted fever in the Western Hemisphere. Ixodid ticks and small wild animals maintain the rickettsias in nature; if humans intrude accidentally into the cycle, they become a dead end in the transmission chain. In certain areas, the cycle of boutonneuse fever involves domiciliary environments, with the brown dog tick, *Rhipicephalus sanguineus*, as the dominant vector.

Clinical manifestations These three tick-borne rickettsioses resemble one another closely. The clinical course is usually milder than that of spotted fever, with a shorter febrile period and fewer severe complications; fatalities are rare and generally limited to the aged and debilitated. Boutonneuse fever is not always mild; fulminant cases with death are reported. The initial lesion, which is present in most cases at the onset of fever, heals slowly; the regional lymph nodes are enlarged. The rash usually remains papular and only in severe cases becomes hemorrhagic.

The clinical picture (including the primary lesion), the geographic location, and epidemiologic considerations are helpful in establishing the diagnosis. The typhus fevers, meningococcal infections, leptospirosis, and measles must be considered in the differential diagnosis; the Weil-Felix and complement fixation tests are of value here.

Treatment and prevention Chloramphenicol and the tetracyclines are effective therapeutic agents, patients generally become afebrile after 2 to 3 days of treatment, and recovery is rapid. Ciprofloxacin is effective but is not regarded as the first choice.

The major effective methods of control are concerned with avoidance of tick bites; these include application of repellents and prompt removal of attached ticks. Effective vaccines are not available commercially.

Q FEVER Definition Q fever is an acute infectious disease caused by *Coxiella burnetii* and characterized by a sudden onset of fever, malaise, headache, weakness, anorexia, and interstitial pneumonitis. Rickettsemia occurs during the febrile period, and specific complement-fixing antibodies are present during convalescence. In contrast to the other rickettsioses, the disease is not associated with a cutaneous exanthem or agglutinins for the *Proteus* bacteria (Weil-Felix reaction).

Etiology and epidemiology   *C. burnetii* possesses the general properties of other rickettsias but is somewhat more resistant to inactivation in unfavorable environments and more pleomorphic than the others. Its infectivity after drying under natural conditions is of importance in the spread of infection to humans. *C. burnetii* has a wide host range in nature, but guinea pigs and embryonated eggs are the common laboratory hosts employed for its propagation.

C. burnetii undergoes antigenic phase variation similar to the rough-smooth dissociation of bacteria. Phase I organisms are found in nature; they possess a cell wall–associated surface antigen that is probably related to virulence and is antiphagocytic. The phase II variant is a laboratory artifact that follows adaptation of phase I in chick embryos. Complement-fixing antibodies to phase I antigen reflect a recent acute infection; they appear in 7 to 10 days, peak at about 20 days, and slowly decline.

Human Q fever is contracted by inhalation of infected dusts, by handling infected materials, possibly by drinking milk contaminated with *C. burnetii*, and, in one instance, by blood transfusion. The disease in Australia is enzootic in animals, especially bandicoots, and is transmitted in nature by ticks. *Rickettsia*-laden tick feces may contaminate cattle hides, and inhalation of this material has caused infection in humans. In the United States, a number of species of ticks are naturally infected, among them *Dermacentor andersoni* and *Amblyomma americanum*, and in North Africa, transovarial transmission of the agent in indigenous ticks has been demonstrated. Sheep, goats, and cows have been found to be naturally infected in North America and in Europe, and *C. burnetii* has been recovered from the milk of such animals. Both milk and infected excretions from livestock probably account for certain outbreaks of human disease following inhalation by cows of infected dust from barns and pens. The airborne route of dried contaminated material is the most likely method of spread. A number of epidemics have occurred among laboratory workers engaged in studies on *C. burnetii*. The disease is not transmitted between humans.

Slaughterhouse workers are often exposed to infected aerosols; in 1985, five cases of hepatitis occurred at a meat packing plant that processed sheep in California. A serologic survey of approximately 100 employees, conducted to identify the extent of the outbreak, revealed a total of 31 persons with evidence of infection. The primary reservoirs of *C. burnetii* are cattle, sheep, goats, and ticks. Many wild and domestic animals are susceptible to infection. In Uruguay, there were 14 outbreaks of Q fever between 1975 and 1985, comprising 1358 clinically suspected cases, all of which occurred in workers at meat processing plants; 814 were serologically confirmed.

An "urban" outbreak of Q fever occurred in 12 poker players in Halifax, Nova Scotia. Presumably the disease was transmitted by a parturient cat.

Clinical manifestations   After incubation for approximately 19 days (range 14 to 26 days), the disease begins with headache, chilly sensations, fever, malaise, myalgia, and anorexia. For several days, the temperature ranges from 38.3 to 40°C (101 to 104°F); the entire course rarely exceeds 2 weeks and usually ranges from 3 to 6 days. There may be wide fluctuations in the fever. Respiratory and gastrointestinal symptoms are not conspicuous in the early stages. Headache and fever predominate. A dry cough and chest pain occur after about 5 days, when rales are usually audible. Roentgenographic findings indistinguishable from those of primary atypical pneumonia are present usually by the third to fourth day of disease, first as patchy areas of consolidation involving a portion of one lobe, giving a homogeneous ground-glass appearance. Occasionally, a homogeneous localized infiltration may resemble a tumor mass. These manifestations

persist beyond the febrile period and may appear in patients who are unaware of pulmonary involvement. Complications are rare, and coincident with defervescence the appetite begins to return. Convalescence progresses slowly for several weeks, during which time the principal disability is weakness. It is not uncommon for patients to lose 7 to 9 kg during the active stages of disease. The disease may be protracted in approximately 20 percent of cases, with fever persisting for longer than 4 weeks, particularly in elderly patients. Occasionally, relapse occurs, especially in patients treated with antibiotics during the first several days of disease.

Hepatitis, with the development of clinically detectable icterus, occurs in approximately one-third of patients with the protracted form. This form of Q fever is characterized by fever, malaise, absence of headache or respiratory signs, and hepatomegaly with right upper quadrant pain. Liver biopsy specimens show diffuse granulomatous changes with multinucleated giant cells and scattered infiltrations of polymorphonuclear leukocytes, lymphocytes, and macrophages. *C. burnetii* may be demonstrated in such specimens with the fluorescent antibody technique. Q fever must be included in the differential diagnosis of patients with hepatitis and those with hepatic granulomas such as tuberculosis, sarcoidosis, histoplasmosis, brucellosis, tularemia, syphilis, and others.

Endocarditis with *C. burnetii* has been identified by smear and isolation of the *Rickettsia* in vegetations on the heart valves obtained at operation or autopsy. The aortic valve is most commonly involved, often with large vegetations. It is important to suspect Q fever in cases of apparent subacute bacterial endocarditis with persistently negative blood cultures. Operative intervention with replacement of damaged valves is usually necessary for recovery because the available antibiotics are not rickettsicidal. In some instances, long-term antibiotic therapy has been successful.

A high complement-fixing antibody titer to phase I antigen is present in patients with endocarditis and granulomatous hepatitis.

Prognosis   Few fatalities have been recorded, and except for the patient with protracted illness and hepatic involvement or endocarditis, the course of disease is generally uncomplicated and benign.

Treatment and control   The tetracycline antibiotics and chloramphenicol are effective in the treatment of patients with Q fever. Most patients, when treated early in the course of disease, respond promptly and recover without relapses. The therapeutic procedures are comparable with those used in spotted fever.

Control of Q fever depends primarily on immunization of susceptible persons with specific vaccines. Vaccines made from phase I rickettsias are potent and afford considerable protection to slaughterhouse and dairy workers, herders, rendering-plant workers, wool sorters, tanners, laboratory workers, and others at risk. To avoid side reactions, it is important that the vaccine be given only to persons who are skin test negative. Measures should be taken to avoid exposure to infected aerosols; milk from infected domestic livestock must be pasteurized or boiled.

EHRLICHIOSIS   Clinical manifestations range from the asymptomatic to an abrupt onset illness with fever, chills, headache, and malaise present in most cases. Some patients exhibit a maculopapular or petechial rash involving the trunk and extremities. Abdominal pain, vomiting, and diarrhea may occur. Important hematologic and hepatic abnormalities include leukopenia, thrombocytopenia, and elevated levels of transaminase and alkaline phosphatase. In severe cases, disseminated intravascular coagulation, renal and bone marrow failure, hepatitis and disorientation can develop.

The causative agents, *Ehrlichia*, are *Rickettsia*-like bacteria transmitted to humans by ticks. Often specific confirmation is made only by serologic procedures using the indirect fluorescent antibody test (IFA) to detect IgG antibodies against *Ehrlichia*. Patients with ehrlichiosis respond well to the tetracycline antibiotics and chloramphenicol, similar to the response in Rocky Mountain spotted fever. Hence the physician who cannot distinguish clearly between the two diseases should initiate treatment in order to ensure against late sequelae.

REFERENCES

BOZEMAN FM et al: Serologic evidence of *Rickettsia canada* infection in man. J Infect Dis 121:367, 1970

———— et al: Epidemic typhus rickettsiae isolated from flying squirrels. Nature 255:545, 1975

CENTERS FOR DISEASE CONTROL: Summary of notifiable diseases, United States, 1987. Morb Mort Week Rep 36:54, 1987

DERRICK EH: The epidemiology of Q fever: A review. Med J Aust 1:245, 1953

DUMLER JS et al: Rapid immunoperoxidase demonstration of *Rickettsia rickettsii* in fixed cutaneous specimens from patients with Rocky Mountain spotted fever. Am J Clin Pathol 93:410, 1990

FERGUSON IC et al: Clinical, virological and pathological findings in a fatal case of Q fever endocarditis. Br J Clin Pathol 15:235, 1962

GAMBRILL MR, WISSEMAN CL JR: Mechanisms of immunity in typhus infections. Infect Immun 8:519, 1973

HARRELL GT: Rickettsial involvement of the nervous system. Med Clin North Am 37:395, 1953

HATTWICK MAW et al: Rocky Mountain spotted fever: Epidemiology of an increasing problem. Ann Intern Med 84:732, 1976

KOSTER FT et al: Cellular immunity in Q fever: Specific lymphocyte unresponsiveness in Q fever endocarditis. J Infect Dis 152:1283, 1985

LANGLEY J et al: Poker player's pneumonia: An urban outbreak of Q fever following exposure to a parturient cat. N Engl J Med 319:354, 1988

MURRAY ES et al: Brill's disease: I. Clinical and laboratory diagnosis. JAMA 142:1059, 1950

————, Snyder JC: Brill's disease: II. Etiology. Am J Hyg 53:22, 1951

ORMSBEE RA et al: The influence of phase on the protective potency of Q fever vaccine. J Immunol 92:404, 1964

———— et al: Serologic diagnosis of epidemic typhus fever. Am J Epidemiol 105:261, 1977

PEDERSEN CE et al: Demonstration of *Rickettsia rickettsii* in Rhesus monkeys by immune fluorescence microscopy. J Clin Microbiol 2:121, 1975

PERINE PL et al: A clinico-epidemiological study of epidemic typhus in Africa. Clin Infect Dis 14:1149, 1992

PHILIP RN et al: A comparison of serologic methods for diagnosis of Rocky Mountain spotted fever. Am J Epidemiol 105:56, 1977

RAOULT D et al: Ciprofloxacin therapy for Mediterranean spotted fever. Antimicrob Agents Chemother 30:606, 1986

ROSE HM: The clinical manifestations and laboratory diagnosis of rickettsialpox. Ann Intern Med 31:871, 1949

SALGO MP et al: A focus of Rocky Mountain Spotted Fever within New York City. N Engl J Med 318:345, 1988

SMADEL JE: Influence of antibiotics on immunologic responses in scrub typhus. Am J Med 17:246, 1954

———— (ED): *Symposium on Q Fever*, Medical Science Publication 6. Washington, DC, Walter Reed Army Institute of Research, 1959

SOMENSHINE DE et al: Epizootiology of epidemic typhus (*Rickettsia prowazekii*) in flying squirrels. Am J Trop Med Hyg 27:339, 1978

SOMMA-MOREIRA RE et al: Analysis of Q fever in Uruguay. Rev Infect Dis 9:386, 1987

VINSON JW: Etiology of trench fever in Mexico, in *Industry and Tropical Health*, vol V. Boston, Harvard School of Public Health, 1964, p 109

WALKER DH, CAIN BG: A method for specific diagnosis of Rocky Mountain spotted fever on fixed, paraffin-embedded tissue by immunofluorescence. J Infect Dis 137:206, 1978

————, BRADFORD WD: Rocky Mountain spotted fever in childhood, in *Perspectives in Pediatric Pathology*, vol 6, HS Rosenberg, J Bernstein (eds). New York, Masson Publishing, 1981, pp 35–61

———— et al: Histopathology and immunohistologic demonstration of the distribution of *Rickettsia typhi* in fatal murine typhus. Am J Clin Pathol 91:720, 1989

WOODWARD TE: A historical account of the rickettsial diseases with a discussion of unsolved problems. J Infect Dis 127:583, 1973

————: Identification of *Rickettsia* in skin tissues. J Infect Dis 134:297, 1976

———— et al: The remarkable contributions of S. Burt Wolbach on rickettsial vasculitis updated. Trans Am Clin Climatol Assoc vol CIII, pp 78–94 1992

139 MYCOPLASMA INFECTIONS

WALLACE A. CLYDE, JR.

The mycoplasmas are a heterogeneous group of unusual bacteria belonging to microbial class Mollicutes ("soft skin"). They differ from classical bacteria by lacking rigid cell wall structures, being contained instead by trilaminar unit membranes. This property confers on mycoplasmas an inability to react with organic dyes, such as those in the Gram stain, and an absolute insensitivity to the penicillins, since there are no cell wall receptor sites for these antibiotics.

The mycoplasma genome is roughly one-sixth the size of that in *Escherichia coli*, making the mycoplasmas fastidious species requiring many precursor substances for growth in artificial media. With maximum dimensions of 0.15 to 0.5 μm, less than some of the larger viruses, mycoplasmas are the smallest organisms known that are capable of extracellular existence.

Mycoplasmas are ubiquitous in nature and cause a wide variety of diseases among animals, birds, plants, and insects. In humans the most important pathogen is *Mycoplasma pneumoniae*, a common cause of respiratory tract infections. *M. hominis* and *Ureaplasma urealyticum* also are implicated in disease involving mainly the genitourinary system. A newly described species having many pathogenic properties, *M. genitalium*, is of uncertain significance. In addition to these organisms, there are eight other distinct species that are components of the normal microflora on the oropharyngeal and genital mucosal surfaces.

MYCOPLASMA PNEUMONIAE

DEFINITION *M. pneumoniae* produces an influenza-like respiratory illness of gradual onset with headache, malaise, fever, and cough. When pneumonia is present, physical findings may be minimal despite extensive changes seen in chest x-rays. Synonyms include Eaton agent pneumonia, cold hemagglutinin–positive pneumonia, atypical or primary atypical pneumonia, and "walking" pneumonia. Asymptomatic infections also occur, especially in young children and partially immune adults.

ETIOLOGY *M. pneumoniae* was discovered by Eaton in 1941 and related to the syndrome of atypical pneumonia. It is a minute, motile filament, measuring approximately 0.1 by 2 μm, that has one differentiated pole where a specialized adhesin (P1) mediates attachment to respiratory epithelial cells. Production of peroxide and an inhibitor of host cell catalase are thought to be major mediators of parasitized cell injury. The organism may be isolated from respiratory secretions using complex artificial media, requiring usually 1 to 3 weeks or more for growth and identification procedures. New rapid diagnostic techniques, based on antigen detection or nucleic acid probes used directly on specimens, appear promising.

Invasive disease caused by *M. pneumoniae* has been reported—albeit only rarely—in severe or complicated cases. The usual clinical manifestations thus are mediated by surface parasitism of respiratory epithelial cells. Peribronchial accumulations of lymphoid and plasma cells develop, and intraluminal recruitment of macrophages and polymorphonuclear leukocytes takes place. In addition to sIgA, IgA, IgM, and IgG antibodies, a variety of autoantibodies develop in many patients. These include antibodies reactive with brain, heart, and muscle; erythrocyte I antigen; intermediate filaments; and mitotic spindles of dividing cells. Polyclonal B cell activation and suppression of delayed hypersensitivity also have been described. It is not clear that any of the various nonrespiratory complications of *M. pneumoniae* disease are due to these immunologic aberrations.

EPIDEMIOLOGY Communicability of *M. pneumoniae* infections is thought to be via large droplets of respiratory secretions; close indoor contact such as in household, institutional, or dormitory settings facilitates spread. The incubation period has been estimated at 2 to 3 weeks. Disease occurs most commonly in elementary school children, adolescents, and young adults. Infections can be found during any season of the year, although epidemic disease tends to occur during the fall and early winter months in temperate countries. Many studies have shown a periodicity of 3 to 5 years in the occurrence of major outbreaks. In Seattle, Washington, it was found that the average incidence of disease across all years and age groups was 2 per 1000 population per year. This occurrence doubled during epidemic years and was higher in the age groups between 5 and 40 years. In adolescent patients, 15 to 20 percent of all pneumonias could be attributed to *M. pneumoniae*. The organism has been implicated in up to 50 percent of pneumonia episodes in college students and in 20 to 30 percent of cases occurring in military recruits.

CLINICAL MANIFESTATIONS The most common clinical syndrome associated with *M. pneumoniae* infection is that of an acute or subacute tracheobronchitis. Symptoms appearing over several days' time include headache, malaise, feverishness, scratchy sore throat, and dry cough. The cough may be paroxysmal, often disturbing sleep, and gradually becomes productive of mucoid or mucopurulent sputum. Physical findings may be minimal, other than temperature elevation rarely exceeding 38.9°C (102°F). If pneumonia is present, isolated crackles or areas of wheezing may be heard, usually over one of the lower lobes. Areas of subsegmental atelectasis and small pleural effusions that may be seen on chest x-rays rarely are detectable by physical examination.

Most *M. pneumoniae* disease is mild and self-limited, running its course in 2 to 4 weeks without treatment. Appropriate antibiotics in controlled clinical trials have been shown to shorten significantly the duration of fever, hospitalization, and x-ray manifestations. Rarely, severe, life-threatening, or fatal episodes can occur.

A wide variety of respiratory and nonrespiratory tract complications may be encountered. Otitis media may be seen in children, while sinusitis is commonly present in adults. Occasional patients develop the syndrome of bullous myringitis. Nondescript maculopapular skin rashes are frequent in children, and *M. pneumoniae* infections have been associated with erythema multiforme and the Stevens-Johnson syndrome. Central nervous system complications of meningoencephalitis, cerebellar ataxia, and various radiculopathies have been described. Other rare complications include monarticular arthritis, myocarditis, pericarditis, coagulopathies, hemolytic anemia, and noncardiogenic pulmonary edema.

ROENTGENOGRAPHIC FINDINGS X-ray manifestations of *M. pneumoniae* pneumonia are protean and nonspecific. The most frequent pattern is one of bronchial thickening with areas of interstitial infiltration and subsegmental atelectasis involving one of the lower lobes. Another common finding is the occurrence of "platelike" atelectasis, often seen to best advantage on lateral views. Other changes include areas of small nodular densities, which can be confused with tuberculosis, and hilar adenopathy suggesting a variety of other entities. Lobular or lobar consolidation and massive pleural effusions are uncommon.

LABORATORY FINDINGS Total blood leukocyte and differential cell counts are usually normal, but the erythrocyte sedimentation rate is often elevated and C-reactive proteins may be demonstrated. There are no characteristic findings in urinalysis, liver or renal function tests, serum electrolytes, or electrocardiograms, although abnormalities may be seen with some of the disease complications. Specific diagnostic tests include recovery of *M. pneumoniae* from respiratory secretions or demonstration of fourfold titer changes between paired sera using a variety of methods, of which the complement fixation technique is the most widely available. However, these test results are not available promptly enough to assist therapeutic decision making. New rapid diagnostic tests of four types have been marketed. One depends on detection of *M. pneumoniae* rRNA by a nucleic acid hybridization technique. A second detects a major protein present in the organisms. The polymerase chain reaction has been applied—with promising results—to the diagnosis of *M. pneumoniae* infection and may prove useful clinically if costs and difficulties caused by in-laboratory contamination can be controlled. The fourth test detects *M. pneumoniae*-specific IgM antibody by agglutination. False-positive results may be obtained if antibody from a prior infection is detected; false-negative results may be obtained if the test is done too early in the course of infection or in an adult in whom prior infection has elicited a predominantly IgG response. The usefulness of these rapid tests will be determined as greater clinical experience with them accrues.

Another helpful test is cold hemagglutination serology, because of its rapidity and simplicity. These IgM class antibodies directed toward the I antigen of erythrocyte membranes develop during the first or second week of illness in up to 80 percent of patients with pneumonia (95 percent of those below age 20) and may be present in high or rising titers when patients first present. Single titers of ≥64 or fourfold or greater titer changes in sera collected ≥5 days apart are considered significant. False-positive cold hemagglutinin reactions may be seen in rubeola, infectious mononucleosis, adenovirus pneumonias, and several tropical diseases, and, more rarely, in collagen vascular disease. As in some of these entities, polyclonal B lymphocyte activation and T cell suppression occurring during *M. pneumoniae* infections may explain the appearance of various host tissue autoantibodies and of transient anergy in some patients.

DIFFERENTIAL DIAGNOSIS Because of its common occurrence, *M. pneumoniae* should be considered in all cases of pneumonia. Generally, patients with mycoplasma pneumonia have milder illnesses than are caused by classical bacteria, less dense pulmonary infiltrations on x-rays, and normal blood leukocyte values. Epidemiologic data are especially useful: age (5 to 40 years), season (fall months predominantly), year (3- to 5-year epidemic cycles), and contact history with other cases. Other infections requiring special consideration are influenza virus pneumonia or its secondary bacterial complications (during epidemic periods) (see Chap. 152), adenovirus pneumonias (see Chap. 150) (particularly in military recruits), and mild forms of community-acquired *Legionella pneumophila* (see Chap. 113) pneumonia. The agent *Chlamydia pneumoniae* (TWAR) may produce disease clinically indistinguishable from that due to *M. pneumoniae*. TWAR infection is estimated to occur half as frequently as mycoplasma pneumonia.

TREATMENT Erythromycin and tetracycline derivatives are effective in reducing the morbidity of *M. pneumoniae* disease. For adults, erythromycin (0.5 g every 6 h orally), tetracycline (250 mg every 6 h orally), or doxycycline (100 mg once daily orally) in 10- to 14-day courses is usually prescribed. In severely ill patients, intravenous erythromycin may be selected, but tetracycline is not recommended by this route. For children less than 8 to 10 years old, erythromycin (30 to 50 mg/kg per day orally for 14 days) is the primary choice; tetracycline and doxycycline are alternatives for older patients. Relapses occasionally occur upon cessation of therapy but respond to retreatment. In cases where *Legionella* infection cannot be excluded, erythromycin should be chosen for therapy. If *Chlamydia pneumoniae* pneumonia is a consideration, the use of tetracycline or doxycycline is recommended.

OTHER MYCOPLASMAL INFECTIONS

A growing body of literature documents evidence of other human mycoplasma infections, including a variety of genitourinary syndromes in both sexes and perinatal diseases. Mycoplasma infection should be considered in suppurative processes where classical bacterial cultures are negative; examples include urethritis, salpingitis, amnionitis, pyelonephritis, postpartum sepsis, and neonatal pneumonia or meningitis. Mycoplasmal abcesses or arthritis may occur in immunocompromised patients. Recent interest has focused on isolation of fastidious strains of *M. fermentans* from some patients with AIDS; the significance of this association is presently unknown. Sexually transmitted diseases associated with mycoplasmas are considered in Chaps. 88 and 89.

In these infections, the species most commonly encountered are *M. hominis* and *U. urealyticum*. Standard bacteriologic media may support growth of *M. hominis* as minute colonies, especially media for anaerobic bacteria that are incubated for several days. Selective media for *Ureaplasma* species are available that may permit their identification in 24 to 48 h. Cultural facilities for *Mycoplasma* species are available in some diagnostic microbiology laboratories, whereas serodiagnosis of infections other than those due to *M. pneumoniae* is not routine. Specimens may be transported on wet ice (within 24 h) or dry ice (greater than 24 h) to reference laboratories for assistance. For *M. hominis* infections, tetracycline and clindamycin are effective antibiotics; this species is insensitive to erythromycin. Erythromycin or tetracycline may be used for *Ureaplasma* infections. Resistance of both species to the recommended antibiotics occurs and is a problem requiring special laboratory guidance. It has been shown in vitro that *M. hominis* is sensitive to ciprofloxacin, but ureaplasmas have limited susceptibility to quinolones currently on the market. Since mycoplasmas do not synthesize folic acid, they are insensitive to trimethoprim-sulfamethoxazole.

REFERENCES

BROUGHTON RA: Infections due to *Mycoplasma pneumoniae* in childhood. Pediatr Infect Dis J 5:71, 1986

CASSELL GH (ed): Ureaplasmas of humans: With emphasis upon maternal and neonatal infections. Pediatr Infect Dis J 5:S221, 1986

CLYDE WA JR: Mycoplasmal infections, in *Diagnostic Procedures for Bacterial Infections*, 7th ed, BB Wentworth (ed). Washington, DC, American Public Health Association, 1987, pp 391–405

GRAYSTON JT et al: A new respiratory pathogen: *Chlamydia pneumoniae* strain TWAR. J Infect Dis 161:618, 1990

MÅRDH P-A et al (eds): International symposium on *Mycoplasma hominis*—a human pathogen. Sex Transm Dis 10(Suppl):225, 1983

McCRACKEN GH JR: Current status of antibiotic treatment for *Mycoplasma pneumoniae* disease. Pediatr Infect Dis J 5:167, 1986

NAGAYAMA Y et al: Isolation of *Mycoplasma pneumoniae* from children with lower-respiratory-tract infections. J Infect Dis 157:911, 1988

140 CHLAMYDIAL INFECTIONS

WALTER E. STAMM / KING K. HOLMES

The genus *Chlamydia* contains three species: *C. psittaci, C. trachomatis,* and *C. pneumoniae* (formerly the TWAR agent). *C. psittaci* is widely distributed in nature, producing genital, conjunctival, intestinal, or respiratory infections in many mammalian and avian species. Genital infections with *C. psittaci* have been well characterized in several species and cause complications such as abortion and infertility. Although mammalian strains of *C. psittaci* are not known to infect humans, avian strains occasionally infect humans, causing pneumonia and the systemic illness known as psittacosis.

C. pneumoniae is a fastidious chlamydial species that appears to be a frequent cause of upper respiratory tract infection and pneumonia, primarily in children and young adults. No animal reservoir has been identified for *C. pneumoniae,* and it appears to be a human pathogen spread by close personal contact.

C. trachomatis is exclusively a human pathogen and was recognized as the cause of trachoma in the 1940s. Since then, *C. trachomatis* has been recognized as a major cause of sexually transmitted and perinatal infection.

Chlamydiae are obligate, intracellular parasites. They possess both DNA and RNA, have a cell wall and ribosomes similar to those of gram-negative bacteria, and are inhibited by antibiotics such as tetracycline. Chlamydiae are classified as bacteria belonging to their own order (Chlamydiales).

A unique feature of all chlamydiae is their complex reproductive cycle. Two forms of the microorganism—the extracellular elementary body and the intracellular reticulate body—participate in this cycle. The elementary body is adapted for extracellular survival and is the infective form transmitted from one person to another. Elementary bodies attach to susceptible target cells (usually columnar or transitional epithelial cells) and enter the cells within a phagosome. Within 8 h, the elementary bodies reorganize into reticulate bodies. These forms are adapted to intracellular survival and multiplication. They undergo binary fission, eventually producing numerous replicates contained within the membrane-bound ''inclusion body,'' which occupies much of the infected host cell. Chlamydial inclusions resist lysosomal fusion until late in the developmental cycle. After 24 h, the reticulate bodies condense and form elementary bodies still contained within the inclusion. The inclusion then ruptures, releasing elementary bodies from the cell to initiate infection of adjacent cells.

C. psittaci, C. pneumoniae, and *C. trachomatis* share a genus-specific or group lipopolysaccharide antigen. Antibody to this antigen is measured in the complement fixation (CF) serologic test available in most state health departments. With a microimmunofluorescence test, *C. trachomatis* strains can be further characterized serologically on the basis of antibody to their major outer-membrane protein (MOMP). Recent studies using monoclonal antibodies to MOMP and nucleotide sequencing of MOMP have delineated at least 20 serotypes of *C. trachomatis.* According to the serovar classification system of Wang and Grayston, strains associated with trachoma have generally been those of the A, B, Ba, and C serovars, while serovars D through K have been largely associated with sexually transmitted and perinatally acquired infections. Serovars L_1, L_2, and L_3 produce lymphogranuloma venereum (LGV) and hemorrhagic proctocolitis. The LGV strains demonstrate unique biologic behavior in that they are more invasive than the other serovars, produce disease in lymphatic tissue, grow readily in cell culture systems and macrophages, and are fatal when inoculated intracerebrally into mice and monkeys. Non-LGV strains of *C. trachomatis* characteristically produce superficial infections involving the columnar epithelium of the eye, genitalia, and respiratory tract.

C. trachomatis has been reported as an infrequent cause of subacute endocarditis, peritonitis, pleuritis, and possibly periappendicitis and may occasionally cause respiratory infections in older children and adults. Immunosuppressed patients with pneumonia have had, in some cases, either serologic or cultural evidence of *C. trachomatis* infection, but more data are necessary to define the role of *Chlamydia* in these patients.

SEXUALLY TRANSMITTED AND PERINATAL INFECTIONS DUE TO *C. TRACHOMATIS*

SPECTRUM OF *C. TRACHOMATIS* GENITAL INFECTIONS Genital infections caused by *C. trachomatis* represent the most common bacterial sexually transmitted disease (STD) in the United States. An estimated 3 to 4 million cases occur each year. In adults the clinical spectrum of sexually transmitted *C. trachomatis* infections parallels the spectrum of gonococcal infections (Table 140-1). Chlamydial and gonococcal infections have been associated with urethritis, proctitis, and conjunctivitis in both sexes; with epididymitis in men; and with mucopurulent cervicitis, acute salpingitis, bartholinitis, and the Fitz-Hugh–Curtis syndrome (perihepatitis) in women. Moreover, both types of infection can be associated with systemic complications, particularly arthritis. In general, however, chlamydial infections produce fewer symptoms and signs than corresponding gonococcal infections at the same site; in fact, the former are often totally asymptomatic. Increasing evidence suggests that many chlamydial infections of the genital tract, especially in women, persist for months without producing symptoms. Simultaneous infection with *C. trachomatis* occurs in up to 30 to 50 percent of women with cervical gonococcal infection and in up to 25 percent of heterosexual men with gonococcal urethritis.

EPIDEMIOLOGY Infections due to *C. trachomatis* have been made reportable in many states, and national incidence data show steadily rising numbers of reported infections, probably reflecting both increased testing and reporting. The annual occurrence of nongonococcal urethritis (NGU) has been measured by surveys of diagnoses made by physicians in private practice and has been used as a surrogate measure of trends in chlamydial infection. The incidence of NGU increased dramatically during the 1960s and 1970s, a period when chlamydiae caused 30 to 50 percent of such cases. Even as the incidence of gonococcal urethritis fell during the 1980s, the incidence of NGU stabilized in the United States, probably reflecting the relative

TABLE 140-1   Clinical parallels between sexually transmitted infections due to *Neisseria gonorrhoeae* and *Chlamydia trachomatis*

Site of infection	Resulting clinical syndrome	
	N. gonorrhoeae	*C. trachomatis*
MEN		
Urethra	Urethritis	Nongonococcal or post-gonococcal urethritis
Epididymis	Epididymitis	Epididymitis
Rectum	Proctitis	Proctitis
Conjunctiva	Conjunctivitis	Conjunctivitis
Systemic	Disseminated gonococcal infection	Reiter's syndrome
WOMEN		
Urethra	Acute urethral syndrome	Acute urethral syndrome
Bartholin's gland	Bartholinitis	Bartholinitis
Cervix	Cervicitis	Cervicitis
Endometrium	Endometritis	Endometritis
Fallopian tube	Salpingitis	Salpingitis
Conjunctiva	Conjunctivitis	Conjunctivitis
Liver capsule	Perihepatitis	Perihepatitis
Systemic	Disseminated gonococcal infection	Reiter's syndrome

lack of implementation of programs to control chlamydial infections. More recently, implementation of chlamydial control programs in some regions has been associated with a decline in the proportion of NGU cases caused by chlamydiae; thus trends in NGU may be less reliable as a surrogate for trends in the incidence of chlamydial infection.

The age of peak incidence of genital *C. trachomatis* infections is the late teens and early twenties, as in other sexually transmitted infections. The prevalence of chlamydial urethral infection in young men ranges from 3 to 5 percent of men seen in general medical settings, to over 10 percent of asymptomatic soldiers undergoing routine physical examination, to 15 to 20 percent of heterosexual men seen in STD clinics. Urethral chlamydial infection is less common among homosexual than among heterosexual men, but rectal infections occur in homosexual men who practice receptive anorectal intercourse without condoms. The ratio of chlamydial to gonococcal urethritis is highest for heterosexual men and for those with high socioeconomic status and is lowest for homosexual men and indigent populations.

The incidence of cervical infection in women has ranged from approximately 5 percent among asymptomatic college students or prenatal patients in the United States, to over 10 percent of women seen in family planning clinics, to over 20 percent of women seen in STD clinics. In the United States, the prevalence of *C. trachomatis* in the cervix of pregnant women is 5 to 10 times higher than that of *Neisseria gonorrhoeae*. The prevalence of genital infection with either agent is highest in individuals who are single, nonwhite (primarily black or hispanic), and between ages 18 and 24. Oral contraceptive use also confers an increased risk of chlamydial infection. The proportion of infections that are asymptomatic appears to be higher for *C. trachomatis* than for *N. gonorrhoeae,* and symptomatic *C. trachomatis* infections are clinically less severe. It is suspected that mild or asymptomatic chlamydial infections of the fallopian tubes may nonetheless cause ongoing tubal damage and infertility. Furthermore, because the total number of *C. trachomatis* infections exceeds that of *N. gonorrhoeae* infections in industrialized countries, the total morbidity caused by *C. trachomatis* genital infections in these countries equals or exceeds that caused by *N. gonorrhoeae*. The prevalence of *C. trachomatis* is higher than that of *N. gonorrhoeae* in industrialized countries, in part because measures such as treatment

of sex partners and routine cultures for case detection in asymptomatic individuals have been applied much more effectively to the control of gonorrhea than to that of *C. trachomatis* infection.

CLINICAL MANIFESTATIONS   Nongonococcal and postgonococcal urethritis   Nongonococcal urethritis is a diagnosis of exclusion that is applied to men with symptoms and/or signs of urethritis who do not have gonorrhea. Postgonococcal urethritis (PGU) refers to nongonococcal urethritis developing 2 to 3 weeks after treatment of gonococcal urethritis in men with single-dose regimens such as amoxicillin or cephalosporins that lack sufficient activity against chlamydia. Since treatment for gonorrhea now also includes 7 days of tetracycline or doxycycline for concomitant chlamydial infection, both the incidence of PGU and the causative role of chlamydiae in this syndrome have declined. *C. trachomatis* causes 20 to 50 percent of the cases of NGU and PGU in heterosexual men but is less commonly isolated from homosexual men with these syndromes. The cause of most of the remaining cases is uncertain, although considerable evidence suggests that *Ureaplasma urealyticum* causes many of these infections, while *Trichomonas vaginalis* and herpes simplex virus cause some cases of NGU.

Nongonococcal urethritis is diagnosed by documentation of a leukocytic urethral exudate and by exclusion of gonorrhea by Gram's stain or culture. *C. trachomatis* urethritis is generally less severe than gonococcal urethritis, although in an individual patient these two forms of urethritis cannot be reliably differentiated solely on clinical grounds. Symptoms include urethral discharge, dysuria (often whitish and mucoid rather than frankly purulent), and urethral itching. The examination may show meatal erythema and tenderness and a urethral exudate that is often demonstrable only by stripping of the urethra. At least one-third of males with *C. trachomatis* urethral infection have no demonstrable signs or symptoms of urethritis. Asymptomatic chlamydial urethritis has been demonstrated in 5 to 10 percent of sexually active adolescent males screened in teen clinics. Such patients frequently have first-glass pyuria (≥ 15 leukocytes per $400\times$ microscopic field in the sediment of first-voided urine), a positive leukocyte esterase test, or an increased number of leukocytes on Gram-stained smear prepared from a urogenital swab inserted 1 to 2 cm into the anterior urethra. For the enumeration of leukocytes, the smear is first scanned at low power to identify areas of the slide containing the highest concentration of leukocytes. These areas are then examined under oil-immersion ($1000\times$). An average of four or more leukocytes in at least three of five $1000\times$ (oil-immersion) fields is indicative of urethritis and correlates with recovery of *C. trachomatis*. To differentiate between true urethritis and functional symptoms among symptomatic patients or to make a presumptive diagnosis of *C. trachomatis* infection in asymptomatic men (e.g., male patients in STD clinics, sex partners of women with nongonococcal salpingitis or mucopurulent cervicitis, fathers of children with inclusion conjunctivitis), the examination of an endourethral specimen for increased leukocytes is useful if specific diagnostic tests for chlamydiae are not available. Alternatively, noninvasive screening for urethritis can be accomplished by testing a first-void urine sample for pyuria either by microscopy or by the leukocyte esterase test.

Epididymitis   *C. trachomatis* is the major cause of epididymitis in sexually active heterosexual men under 35 years of age, accounting for about 70 percent of cases. *N. gonorrhoeae* causes most of the remaining cases, and some men have simultaneous infections with both pathogens. Asymptomatic urethritis as defined above is usually present in these patients. In homosexual men, sexually transmitted coliform infection acquired via rectal intercourse may cause epididymitis. Coliform bacteria and *Pseudomonas aeruginosa* are the most common causes of epididymitis in men over 35, usually in association with preceding urologic instrumentation or surgery. These men typically present with unilateral scrotal pain, fever, and epididymal tenderness or swelling on examination. The illness may be mild enough to treat in the outpatient setting or severe enough to require hospitalization. Testicular torsion should be promptly excluded by radionuclide scan, Doppler flow study, or surgical exploration in a teenager or young adult who presents with acute unilateral testicular pain without urethritis. Testicular tumor or chronic infection (e.g., tuberculosis) should be excluded in the patient with unilateral intrascrotal pain and swelling who does not respond to appropriate antimicrobial therapy.

Reiter's syndrome Reiter's syndrome consists of conjunctivitis, urethritis (or cervicitis in females), arthritis, and characteristic mucocutaneous lesions (see Chap. 289). *C. trachomatis* has been recovered from the urethra of up to 70 percent of men with untreated nondiarrheal Reiter's syndrome and associated urethritis. In the absence of overt urethritis, it is important to exclude subclinical urethritis in the men in whom this diagnosis is suspected.

The pathogenesis of Reiter's syndrome remains obscure. However, since more than 80 percent of affected patients have HLA-B27 and since other mucosal infections (*Salmonella*, *Shigella*, or *Campylobacter*, for example) produce an identical syndrome, chlamydial infection is thought to initiate an aberrant and hyperactive immune response that produces inflammation at the involved target organs in these genetically predisposed individuals. Evidence of exaggerated cell-mediated and humoral immune responses to chlamydial antigens in Reiter's syndrome supports this hypothesis. The presumptive demonstration of chlamydial elementary bodies and chlamydial DNA in the joint fluid and synovial tissue of patients with Reiter's syndrome suggests that chlamydiae may actually spread from genital to joint tissues in these patients.

Proctitis *C. trachomatis* of either the genital immunotypes D through K or the LGV immunotype L₂ causes proctitis in homosexual men who practice receptive anorectal intercourse. The vast majority of cases are due to immunotypes D through K and present either as asymptomatic infection or as mild proctitis not unlike gonococcal proctitis. These infections may be seen in heterosexual women as well. Clinically, these patients present with mild rectal pain, mucous discharge, tenesmus, and occasionally bleeding. Nearly all have neutrophils in their rectal Gram's stain. Anoscopy in these non-LGV cases of chlamydial proctitis reveals mild, patchy mucosal friability and mucopurulent discharge, and the disease process is limited to the distal rectum. LGV strains produce a more severe ulcerative proctitis or proctocolitis that can be confused clinically with herpes simplex virus proctitis (severe rectal pain, bleeding, discharge, and tenesmus) and that histologically resembles Crohn's disease in that giant-cell formation and granulomas can be seen (see Chap. 255). In the United States, these cases occur almost exclusively in homosexual men.

Mucopurulent cervicitis *C. trachomatis* has been isolated from the cervix of 20 percent or more of women with gonorrhea or a history of contact with men who have gonorrhea or NGU and from the cervix of 10 to 20 percent of women attending STD clinics who do not have a history of contact with a partner with urethritis. Women who have cervical ectopy or who use oral contraceptives appear to have an increased prevalence of cervical infection with *C. trachomatis*.

Although many women with *C. trachomatis* infection of the cervix have no symptoms or signs, a careful speculum examination will demonstrate evidence of mucopurulent cervicitis in 30 to 50 percent. As discussed more fully in Chap. 89, mucopurulent cervicitis is associated with yellow mucopurulent discharge from the endocervical columnar epithelium and with ≥20 neutrophils per 1000× microscopic field within strands of cervical mucus on a thinly smeared, Gram-stained preparation of endocervical exudate. Other characteristic findings include edema of the zone of cervical ectopy and a propensity of the mucosa to bleed on minor trauma, e.g., when specimens are collected with a swab. Pap smear shows increased numbers of neutrophils as well as a characteristic pattern of mononuclear inflammatory cells, including plasma cells, transformed lymphocytes, and histiocytes. Cervical biopsy shows predominantly a mononuclear infiltrate of the subepithelial stroma, often with a follicular cervicitis.

Pelvic inflammatory disease (PID) *C. trachomatis* plays an important causative role in salpingitis. *C. trachomatis* infection has been demonstrated in laparoscopically verified salpingitis, the organism has been recovered from the fallopian tubes in the absence of other pathogens, and serologic evidence of recent *C. trachomatis* infection has been found in women with PID. In the United States *C. trachomatis* has been identified in the fallopian tubes or endometrium in up to 50 percent of women with PID, and its role as an important etiologic agent in this syndrome is well accepted.

Pelvic inflammatory disease occurs via ascending intraluminal spread of *C. trachomatis* from the lower genital tract. Mucopurulent cervicitis is thus followed by endometritis, endosalpingitis, and finally pelvic peritonitis. Evidence of mucopurulent cervicitis is usually present in women with laparoscopically verified salpingitis. Similarly, endometritis, demonstrated by endometrial biopsy showing plasma cell infiltration of the endometrial epithelium, is present in most women with laparoscopically verified chlamydial (or gonococcal) salpingitis. Chlamydial endometritis also can occur in the absence of clinical evidence of salpingitis: approximately 40 to 50 percent of women with mucopurulent cervicitis have plasma cell endometritis. Histologic evidence of endometritis has been correlated with an "endometritis syndrome," consisting of vaginal bleeding, lower abdominal pain, and uterine tenderness in the absence of adnexal tenderness, and with peripheral blood leukocytosis. It is not known what proportion of those with chlamydial endometritis without adnexal tenderness had salpingitis. However, chlamydial salpingitis may produce milder symptoms than does gonococcal salpingitis and may be associated with less marked adnexal tenderness. The presence of mild adnexal or uterine tenderness in sexually active women with cervicitis suggests PID.

Infertility associated with fallopian tube scarring has been strongly linked to antecedent *C. trachomatis* infection in serologic studies. Since many infertile women with tubal scarring and antichlamydial antibody have no history of PID, is appears that subclinical tubal infection ("silent salpingitis") may produce scarring. Ectopic pregnancy, which occurs in over 70,000 women in the United States annually, is also thought to be related to *Chlamydia*-induced tubal scarring in many cases.

Perihepatitis, or the Fitz-Hugh–Curtis syndrome, was originally described as a complication of gonococcal PID. However, cultural and/or serologic evidence of *C. trachomatis* infection is found in three-quarters of women with this syndrome. *C. trachomatis* has also been cultured from exudate on the hepatic capsule in laparoscopically verified cases. This syndrome should be suspected whenever a young, sexually active woman presents with an illness resembling cholecystitis (fever and right upper quadrant pain of subacute or acute onset). Symptoms and signs of salpingitis may be minimal. High titers of antichlamydial antibodies are generally present.

Urethral syndrome in women In the absence of infection with uropathogens such as coliforms or *Staphylococcus saprophyticus*, *C. trachomatis* is the pathogen most commonly isolated from college women with dysuria, frequency, and pyuria (see Chap. 90). *Chlamydia* also can be isolated from the urethra of women without symptoms of urethritis, and up to 25 percent of female STD clinic patients with chlamydial urogenital infection have had positive *C. trachomatis* cultures from the urethra only.

C. trachomatis infection in pregnancy *C. trachomatis* in pregnancy has been associated in some studies (but not in others) with premature delivery and with postpartum endometritis. Whether these complications are in part attributable to *C. trachomatis* is not clear.

PERINATAL INFECTIONS: INCLUSION CONJUNCTIVITIS AND PNEUMONIA Epidemiology Studies in the United States have demonstrated that 5 to 25 percent of pregnant women have *C. trachomatis* infections of the cervix. In these studies, approximately one-half to two-thirds of the children who were exposed during birth acquired *C. trachomatis* infection. Roughly half of the infected infants (or 25 percent of the group exposed) developed clinical evidence of inclusion conjunctivitis. In addition to being found in eye infection, *C. trachomatis* has been isolated frequently and persistently from the nasopharynx, the rectum, and the vagina, occasionally for periods exceeding 1 year in the absence of treatment. Pneumonia occurs in about 10 percent of children infected perinatally, and otitis media may in some cases result from perinatally acquired chlamydial infection.

Inclusion conjunctivitis of the newborn (neonatal chlamydial conjunctivitis)   Neonatal chlamydial conjunctivitis has an acute onset and often produces a profuse mucopurulent discharge. In the newborn, chlamydial conjunctivitis generally has a longer incubation period than gonococcal conjunctivitis (usually 5 to 14 days vs. 1 to 3 days); however, this guideline is not reliable for the diagnosis of individual cases, and in any event it is impossible to differentiate chlamydial conjunctivitis from other forms of neonatal bacterial conjunctivitis clinically. Instead, laboratory diagnosis is required. Besides *C. trachomatis* and *N. gonorrhoeae*, the other important infectious causes of conjunctivitis in newborns include *Haemophilus influenzae*, *Streptococcus pneumoniae*, and herpes simplex virus. Inclusions within epithelial cells often can be demonstrated in Giemsa-stained conjunctival smears, but these smears are less sensitive than cultures or antigen detection tests. Gram-stained smears may show gonococci or occasional small gram-negative coccobacilli in *Haemophilus* conjunctivitis, but smears should be accompanied by cultures for these agents. Very rarely a trachoma-like eye disease occurs in children who have chlamydial infection and live in areas that do not have endemic trachoma. If neonatal chlamydial conjunctivitis is not treated appropriately with oral antimicrobials, it may be followed by chlamydial pneumonia.

Infant pneumonia   *C. trachomatis* causes a distinctive pneumonia syndrome in infants. Recent epidemiologic studies have linked chlamydial pulmonary infection in infants with increased occurrence of subacute lung disease (bronchitis, asthma, wheezing) in later childhood. For details, consult standard textbooks of pediatrics.

LYMPHOGRANULOMAVENEREUM   Definition   Lymphogranuloma venereum is a sexually transmitted infection caused by *C. trachomatis* strains of the L_1, L_2, and L_3 serovars. Most cases are caused by L_2 organisms. Acute LGV in heterosexual men is characterized by a transient primary genital lesion followed by multilocular suppurative regional lymphadenopathy. Women, homosexual men, and—in occasional instances—heterosexual men may develop hemorrhagic proctitis with regional lymphadenitis. Acute LGV is almost always associated with systemic symptoms such as fever and leukocytosis and is rarely associated with systemic complications such as meningoencephalitis. After a latent period of years, late complications include genital elephantiasis due to lymphatic involvement, strictures, and fistulas of the penis, urethra, and rectum.

EPIDEMIOLOGY   LGV is usually sexually transmitted, but occasional transmission by nonsexual personal contact, fomites, or laboratory accidents has been documented. Laboratory work involving creation of aerosols of the causative organisms (e.g., sonication, homogenization) must be conducted with appropriate biologic containment.

The peak incidence of LGV corresponds to the age of greatest sexual activity, the second and third decades of life. The worldwide incidence of LGV is falling, but the disease is still endemic and a major cause of morbidity in Asia, Africa, South America, and parts of the Caribbean. In the Bahamas, an apparent outbreak of LGV has been described in association with a concurrent increase in heterosexual human immunodeficiency virus (HIV) infection. However, only 277 cases were reported in the United States in 1990.

The frequency of infection following exposure is believed to be much lower than that associated with gonorrhea and syphilis. Early manifestations are recognized far more often in men than in women, who usually present with late complications. In the United States, where the reported sex ratio is 3.4 males to 1 female, most cases have involved homosexually active men and travelers, seamen, and military personnel returning from abroad. The main reservoir of infection is presumed to be asymptomatically infected individuals, although such a reservoir has not been directly demonstrated.

Clinical manifestations   In heterosexuals, a *primary genital lesion* develops from 3 days to 3 weeks after exposure. It is a small, painless vesicle or nonindurated ulcer or papule located on the penis

in men and on the labia, posterior vagina, or fourchette in women. The primary lesion is noticed by less than one-third of men with LGV and only rarely by women. It heals in a few days without scarring and, even when noticed, is usually not recognized as LGV except in retrospect. LGV strains of *C. trachomatis* have occasionally been recovered from genital ulcers, and also from the urethra of men and the endocervix of women who present with inguinal adenopathy; these areas may be the primary site of infection in some cases.

In women and homosexual men, *primary anal or rectal infection* develops following receptive anorectal intercourse. In women, rectal infection with LGV (or non-LGV) strains of *C. trachomatis* presumably can also arise either via contiguous spread of infected secretions along the perineum (as with rectal gonococcal infection in women) or perhaps by spread to the rectum via the pelvic lymphatics.

From the site of the primary urethral, genital, anal, or rectal infection, the organism spreads via the regional lymphatics. Penile, vulvar, and anal infection can lead to inguinal and femoral lymphadenitis. Rectal infection produces hypogastric and deep iliac lymphadenitis. Upper vaginal or cervical infection results in enlargement of the obturator and iliac nodes.

The most common presenting picture in heterosexual men is the *inguinal syndrome*, which is characterized by painful inguinal lymphadenopathy beginning 2 to 6 weeks after presumed exposure; rarely the onset occurs after a few months. The inguinal adenopathy is unilateral in two-thirds of cases, and palpable enlargement of the iliac and femoral nodes is often evident on the same side as the enlarged inguinal nodes. The nodes are initially discrete, but progressive periadenitis results in a matted mass of nodes that becomes fluctuant and suppurative. The overlying skin becomes fixed, inflamed, and thinned and finally develops multiple draining fistulas. Extensive enlargement of chains of inguinal nodes above and below the inguinal ligament ("the sign of the groove") is common but not specific and is documented in only a minority of cases. Histologically, infected nodes initially show characteristic small stellate abscesses surrounded by histiocytes. These abscesses coalesce to form large, necrotic, suppurative foci. Spontaneous healing usually occurs after several months; inguinal scars or granulomatous masses of varying size persist for life. Massive pelvic lymphadenopathy in women or homosexual men may lead to exploratory laparotomy.

As cultures and serologic tests for *C. trachomatis* are being used more often, increasing numbers of cases of LGV proctitis are being recognized in homosexual men. Such patients present with anorectal pain and mucopurulent, bloody rectal discharge. Although patients may complain of diarrhea, the condition usually represents frequent, painful, unsuccessful attempts at defecation (tenesmus). Sigmoidoscopy reveals ulcerative proctitis or proctocolitis, with purulent exudate and mucosal bleeding. The histopathologic findings in the rectal mucosa include granulomas with giant cells, along with crypt abscesses and extensive inflammation. These clinical, sigmoidoscopic, and histopathologic findings may closely resemble Crohn's disease of the rectum.

Constitutional symptoms are common during the stage of regional lymphadenopathy and, in the presence of proctitis, may include fever, chills, headache, meningismus, anorexia, myalgias, and arthralgias. These findings in the presence of lymphadenopathy are sometimes mistaken for malignant lymphoma. Other systemic complications are infrequent but include arthritis with sterile effusion, aseptic meningitis, meningoencephalitis, conjunctivitis, hepatitis, and erythema nodosum. Chlamydiae have been recovered from the cerebrospinal fluid and in one case were isolated from the blood of a patient with severe constitutional symptoms, indicating the occurrence of disseminated infection. Laboratory-acquired infections suspected of being due to inhalation of aerosols have been associated with mediastinal lymphadenitis, pneumonitis, and pleural effusion.

Complications of untreated anorectal infection include perirectal abscess, fistula in ano, and rectovaginal, rectovesical, and ischiorectal fistulas. Secondary bacterial infection probably contributes to these complications. Rectal stricture is a late complication of anorectal infection and usually occurs 2 to 6 cm from the anal orifice, within reach on digital rectal examination. Proximal extension of the stricture for several centimeters may lead to a mistaken clinical and radiographic diagnosis of carcinoma.

A small percentage of cases of LGV in men present as chronic progressive infiltrative, ulcerative, or fistular lesions of the penis, urethra, or scrotum. Associated lymphatic obstruction may produce elephantiasis. When urethral stricture occurs it usually involves the posterior urethra and causes incontinence or difficulty with urination.

APPROACH TO THE DIAGNOSIS AND TREATMENT OF *C. TRACHOMATIS* GENITAL INFECTIONS

Four types of laboratory procedures are available to confirm *C. trachomatis* infection. These are direct microscopic examination of tissue scrapings for typical intracytoplasmic inclusions; isolation of the organism in cell cultures; detection of chlamydial antigens or nucleic acid by immunologic or hybridization methods; and detection of antibody in the serum or in local secretions.

Except in conjunctivitis, direct microscopic examination of Giemsa-stained cell scrapings for typical inclusions has an unacceptably low sensitivity, and false-positive interpretations by inexperienced observers are common. But even for conjunctivitis this approach has been replaced by direct fluorescent antibody staining of conjunctival smears to identify chlamydial elementary bodies (see below).

Cell culture techniques are available in most large medical centers for isolation of *C. trachomatis*. While LGV strains grow well in many cell lines, the other *C. trachomatis* strains are much more difficult to culture. Although culture remains the gold standard for diagnosis of chlamydial infection, it is expensive, technically demanding, and not available to most clinicians. Therefore, nonculture methods utilizing antigen detection or nucleic acid hybridization have been developed that can be used instead of cultures. In the immunofluorescent slide test, potentially infected genital or ocular secretions are smeared on a slide, fixed, and stained with fluorescein-conjugated monoclonal antibody specific for chlamydial antigens. The observation of fluorescing elementary bodies confirms the diagnosis. Compared with culture, this test is 80 to 90 percent sensitive, and it is quite specific when used for confirmation of urethral, cervical, or ocular infection in high-risk patients with suspected *C. trachomatis* infection. The apparently lower sensitivity of the test in low-risk populations, along with its relatively labor-intensive nature, limits its value as a screening tool.

Enzyme-linked immunosorbent assay (ELISA) techniques for chlamydial antigen detection provide another alternative to culture. The reported sensitivity and specificity of these tests for genital infections have been 70 to 95 percent and 94 to 99 percent, respectively, in high-risk populations. Sensitivities have generally been higher in cervical infection (80 to 90 percent) and lower in urethritis among males (70 to 85 percent). Like the direct fluorescence antibody slide test, ELISA is less accurate in low-prevalence populations. ELISAs are better suited than culture to screening because large numbers of specimens can be easily processed. Newer diagnostic tests in which the polymerase chain reaction (PCR) is used to amplify small amounts of chlamydial DNA in samples are now being investigated and may offer greater sensitivity than current nonculture diagnostic methods for some purposes (e.g., for diagnosis of asymptomatic urethral infection in men). However, as such tests become commercially available, they are expected to be expensive, and their role remains to be defined.

Serologic tests have limited usefulness in the diagnosis of chlamydial oculogenital infections. The CF test with the heat-stable genus-specific antigen has been used to diagnose LGV with some success, but it is insensitive in non-LGV *C. trachomatis* infections. The microimmunofluorescence (micro-IF) test with *C. trachomatis* antigens is more sensitive but is generally available only in research laboratories. The test measures antibodies by serovar specificity and by immunoglobulin class (IgM, IgG, IgA, secretory IgA) in both serum and local secretions. Serologic diagnosis using the micro-IF test may be useful in infant pneumonia (in which high-titer IgM antibody and/or fourfold titer rises can often be demonstrated), in chlamydial salpingitis (especially Fitz-Hugh–Curtis syndrome), and in LGV.

Table 140-2 summarizes the diagnostic tests of choice for patients with suspected chlamydial infection. With few exceptions, the most suitable method for diagnosis is demonstration of the agent in cell culture or by antigen detection methods. Selection of the most appropriate of these tests depends upon local availability and expertise. In patients in whom medico-legal considerations may apply (victims of sexual or child abuse), cultures should always be used. Since *C. trachomatis* is an intracellular pathogen, adequate specimens for chlamydial culture must include epithelial cells. Cultures of pus result in fewer isolations of the organism. In urethritis, a thin-shafted urogenital swab should be inserted at least 2 cm into the urethra to obtain an appropriate specimen. Although cultures of urine for chlamydiae are less sensitive than urethral cultures, recent studies suggest that an ELISA for chlamydial antigen or a PCR test on a first-void urine specimen from men may be a reasonably sensitive diagnostic alternative to the more invasive urethral swab-based tests. When a cervical sample is taken for culture, the external os should first be cleaned of debris and purulent material; a plastic-shafted swab should then be inserted into the cervix, rotated slowly several times, and withdrawn. When conjunctival specimens are sought, the epithelium should be swabbed to remove cells rather than simply purulent material. All specimens for chlamydial culture should be placed immediately into transport medium and then either refrigerated (if they will reach the laboratory within 12 to 18 h) or frozen at $-70°C$ (if longer storage is anticipated). A major advantage of antigen detection techniques is their less rigid transport requirements.

From a public health viewpoint, the most effective use of chlamydial diagnostic testing has not been established and will vary depending upon clincial population, local resources, and laboratory expertise. The Centers for Disease Control and Prevention have recommended empiric treatment (without diagnostic testing if resources are not available for testing) of selected high-risk groups. These include men with NGU or sexually transmitted epididymitis; women with mucopurulent cervicitis (MPC) or PID; asymptomatic sex partners of patients with these syndromes; women and heterosexual men with gonorrhea (because of the high proportion of these patients who also have *C. trachomatis* infection); and sexual contacts of men or women with gonorrhea. Diagnostic testing has several potential benefits in these patients, including confirmation of infection and support of the clinical diagnosis (especially in women with MPC and PID), enhancement of sex partner referral and compliance with drug therapy, determination of prognosis, and education of physicians regarding the correlation of signs and symptoms with culture results. As chlamydial diagnostic testing becomes more widely available, its use for specific diagnosis in such patients should be promoted. Where diagnostic testing must be rationed because of limited resources, the highest priority should be given to the screening of asymptomatic high-risk women who would not otherwise receive treatment for presumptive chlamydial infection, especially those seen in high-risk settings (i.e., STD clinics, abortion clinics) and those with a high-risk profile (e.g., sexually active and ≤21 years of age, new sex partner within past 2 months, or more than one current sex partner).

ANTIMICROBIAL SUSCEPTIBILITY In laboratory tests that evaluate the growth of chlamydiae in cell cultures, the tetracyclines, erythromycin, rifampin, certain fluoroquinolones (especially ofloxacin), and the new macrolide azithromycin are all highly active against these organisms. Sulfonamides and clindamycin are also active against *C. trachomatis*, but to a lesser degree. Penicillin and ampicillin suppress chlamydial multiplication but do not eradicate the organism in vitro. The cephalosporins also appear relatively ineffective against *C. trachomatis*. Streptomycin, gentamicin, neomycin, kanamycin, vancomycin, ristocetin, spectinomycin, and nystatin are not effective

TABLE 140-2   Diagnostic tests in *C. trachomatis* infection

Infection	Suggestive signs/symptoms	Presumptive diagnosis*	Confirmatory test of choice
MEN			
Nongonococcal urethritis, postgonococcal urethritis	Discharge, dysuria	Gram's stain with more than four neutrophils per oil-immersion field, no gonococci	Urethral culture or antigen detection test for *C. trachomatis*
Epididymitis	Unilateral intrascrotal swelling, pain, tenderness; fever; nongonococcal urethritis	Gram stain with more than four neutrophils per oil immersion field, no gonococci	Urethral culture or antigen detection test for *C. trachomatis*
WOMEN			
Cervicitis	Mucopurulent cervical discharge, bleeding and edema of the zone of cervical ectopy	Cervical Gram's stain with ≥20 neutrophils per oil-immersion field in cervical mucus	Cervical culture or antigen detection test for *C. trachomatis*
Salpingitis	Lower abdominal pain, cervical motion tenderness, adnexal tenderness or masses	*C. trachomatis* always potentially present in salpingitis	Cervical culture or antigen detection test for *C. trachomatis*
Urethritis	Dysuria and frequency without urgency or hematuria	Mucopurulent cervicitis, sterile pyuria, negative routine urine culture	Urethral and cervical cultures or antigen detection test for *C. trachomatis*
ADULTS OF EITHER SEX			
Proctitis	Rectal pain, discharge, tenesmus, bleeding; history of receptive anorectal intercourse	Negative gonococcal culture and Gram's stain; at least one neutrophil in rectal Gram's stain	Rectal culture or direct immunofluorescence test for *C. trachomatis*
Reiter's syndrome	Nongonococcal urethritis, arthritis, conjunctivitis, typical skin lesions	Gram's stain with more than four neutrophils per oil-immersion field, no gonococci indicates nongonococcal urethritis	Urethral culture or antigen detection test for *C. trachomatis*
LGV	Regional adenopathy, primary lesion, proctitis, systemic symptoms	None	Isolation of LGV strain from node or rectum, occasionally from urethra or cervix; LGV CF titer, ≥1:64; micro-IF titer, ≥1:512
NEONATES			
Conjunctivitis	Purulent conjunctival discharge 6 to 18 days postdelivery	Negative cultures and Gram stains for gonococci, *Haemophilus* sp., pneumococci, staphylococci	Conjunctival culture or antigen detection test for *C. trachomatis*; Giemsa-stained scraping of conjunctival material can provide more rapid diagnosis but is less sensitive
Infant pneumonia	Afebrile, staccato cough, diffuse rales, bilateral hyperinflation, interstitial infiltrates	None	Chlamydial culture of sputum, pharynx, eye, rectum; micro-IF antibody to *C. trachomatis*—fourfold change in IgG or IgM antibody

* A presumptive diagnosis of chlamydial infection is often made in the syndromes listed when gonococci are not found. A positive test for *Neisseria gonorrhoeae* does not exclude *C. trachomatis*, which often is also present in patients with gonorrhea.

at concentrations inhibitory for most bacteria and fungi. There does not appear to be much strain-to-strain variation in susceptibility to antibiotics, and clinically significant antimicrobial resistance in chlamydiae has not been described. Thus antimicrobial susceptibility testing is not needed in the routine management of patients with chlamydial infection.

TREATMENT   Until the introduction of azithromycin, chlamydial infections could not be eradicated by single-dose or short-term antimicrobial regimens. In most situations in adults, 7 days of treatment with doxycycline or tetracycline should be given for uncomplicated genital infections, but 2 weeks of therapy is recommended for complicated chlamydial infections (e.g., PID, epididymitis) and for LGV. Failure after treatment of genital infections with a tetracycline usually indicates poor compliance or reinfection.

Therapy for *C. trachomatis* urethritis is more effective than therapy for other forms of NGU. *C. trachomatis* is eradicated from the urethra by treatment with tetracycline hydrochloride, 500 mg qid for 7 days, or doxycycline, 100 mg by mouth bid for 7 days. An effective alternative regimen is erythromycin, 500 mg qid for 7 days.

Eradiction of *C. trachomatis* from the cervix has been demonstrated with similar doses and durations of tetracycline, doxycycline, and

erythromycin. Erythromycin base, 500 mg qid for 10 to 14 days, is the regimen of choice for pregnant women with *C. trachomatis* infection. Amoxicillin, 500 mg tid for 10 days, has also been used successfully in one study of pregnant women. Tetracycline hydrochloride, 500 mg qid, or doxycycline, 100 mg bid, for 14 days, produces clinical and microbiologic cure of epididymitis and PID associated with *C. trachomatis* infection, but in this situation tetracycline should always be used together with a drug that is highly effective against gonorrhea.

Two relatively new antimicrobial agents have recently been approved for treatment of uncomplicated chlamydial genital infections in men and women. Ofloxacin, 300 mg orally twice daily for 7 days, is as effective as doxycycline for treatment of chlamydial infection and appears to be safe and well tolerated. It cannot be used in pregnancy. Azithromycin, a macrolide, has been effective in uncomplicated chlamydial infection as a 1-g single dose. It causes fewer adverse gastrointestinal reactions than do older macrolides like erythromycin. Both ofloxacin and azithromycin offer alternatives for treatment that may be of value in selected patients allergic to or intolerant of tetracyclines and erythromycin, but they are considerably more expensive than these standard regimens. The single-dose regimen of azithromycin has great appeal for the treatment of patients with a history of poor compliance, particularly those seen in urgent-care settings (e.g., emergency rooms), where follow-up is not assured.

Treatment of sex partners The continued high prevalence of chlamydial infections in most parts of the United States is due primarily to the failure to diagnose—and therefore treat—patients with symptomatic or asymptomatic infection and their sex partners. Cases of NGU, epididymitis, Reiter's syndrome, and mucopurulent endocervicitis are sometimes not treated with antimicrobials, and sex partners are treated even less often. *C. trachomatis* urethral or cervical infection has been well documented in a high proportion of the sex partners of patients with NGU, epididymitis, Reiter's syndrome, salpingitis, or endocervicitis. If possible, confirmatory laboratory tests for *Chlamydia* should be undertaken in such patients, but even those without evidence of clinical disease who have recently been exposed to proven or possible chlamydial infection (for example, NGU) should be offered therapy.

In neonates with conjunctivitis or infants with pneumonia, erythromycin ethylsuccinate or estolate can be given orally in a dose of 50 mg/kg per day, preferably as 122.5 mg/kg qid, for 2 weeks. Careful attention must be given to compliance with therapy—a frequent problem. Relapses of eye infection are common following treatment with topical erythromycin or tetracycline opthalmic ointment and may also occur after oral erythromycin therapy. Thus follow-up cultures should be obtained after treatment. Both parents should be examined for *C. trachomatis* infection and, if diagnostic tests are not readily available, should be treated with a tetracycline.

PREVENTION Early diagnosis and treatment shorten the duration of infectiousness of the carrier and therefore constitute primary prevention of chlamydial infection. By the early 1990s, one of the 10 regions of the United States (region X, the Pacific Northwest) had formally undertaken a chlamydial control program utilizing widespread testing. Approximately 500,000 tests per year were undertaken in 150 family planning clinics throughout the region in women meeting criteria for high risk. Within 5 years, the prevalence of chlamydial infection had fallen from 10 percent to 5 percent. It is appalling that, as of 1992, no other U.S. region had attempted a similar control effort. Moreover, throughout the nation, many public STD clinics still were not offering chlamydial testing, which has been performed for as little as $5 per test in region X.

TRACHOMA AND ADULT INCLUSION CONJUNCTIVITIS

DEFINITION Trachoma is a chronic conjunctivitis associated with infection by *C. trachomatis* serovars A, B, Ba, and C. It has produced an estimated 20 million cases of blindness throughout the world and remains an important preventable cause of blindness. Inclusion conjunctivitis is an acute ocular infection caused by sexually transmitted *C. trachomatis* strains (usually serovars D through K) in adults exposed to infected genital secretions and in their newborn offspring.

EPIDEMIOLOGY Epidemiologically, two types of eye disease are caused by *C. trachomatis*. In trachoma-endemic areas where the classic eye disease is seen, transmission is from eye to eye via hands, flies, towels, and other fomites and usually involves serovar A, B, Ba, or C. In nonendemic areas, organisms of serovars D through K can be transmitted from the genital tract to the eye, usually causing only the inclusion conjunctivitis syndrome, occasionally with keratitis. Rarely the eye disease acquired in this way progresses with the development of pannus and scars similar to those seen in endemic trachoma. These cases may be referred to as paratrachoma to differentiate them epidemiologically from eye-to-eye-transmitted endemic trachoma.

The worldwide incidence and severity of trachoma have decreased dramatically during the past 35 years in areas with improving hygienic and economic conditions. Endemic trachoma is still the major cause of preventable blindness in north Africa, sub-Saharan Africa, the Middle East, and parts of Asia. Transmission of the endemic disease occurs primarily through close personal contact, particularly among young children in rural communities with limited water supplies. In endemic areas, trachoma is associated with repeated exposure and reinfection, but the infection can also be latent. In the United States a mild form of endemic trachoma still occurs in Mexican Americans as well as in immigrants from areas where trachoma is endemic. Acute relapse of old trachoma occasionally follows treatment with cortisone eye ointment or develops in very old persons who were exposed in their youth.

CLINICAL MANIFESTATIONS Both endemic trachoma and adult inclusion conjunctivitis present initially as a conjunctivitis characterized by small lymphoid follicles in the conjunctiva. In regions with hyperendemic classic blinding trachoma, the disease usually starts insidiously before the age of 2 years. Reinfection is common and probably contributes to the pathogenesis of trachoma. Studies using PCR techniques indicate that chlamydial DNA is often present in the ocular secretions of patients with trachoma, even in the absence of positive cultures. Thus persistent infection may be more common than was previously thought.

The cornea becomes involved with inflammatory leukocytic infiltrations and superficial vascularization (pannus formation). As the inflammation continues, conjunctival scarring eventually distorts the eyelids, causing them to turn inward so that the inturned lashes constantly abrade the eyeball (trichiasis and entropion); eventually the corneal epithelium is abraded and may ulcerate, with subsequent corneal scarring and blindness. Destruction of the conjunctival goblet cells, lacrimal ducts, and lacrimal gland may produce a "dry-eye" syndrome, with resultant corneal opacity due to drying (xerosis) or secondary bacterial corneal ulcers.

Communities with blinding trachoma often experience seasonal epidemics of conjunctivitis due to *Haemophilus influenzae* that contribute to the intensity of the inflammatory process. In such areas the active infectious process usually resolves spontaneously in affected persons between 10 and 15 years of age, but the conjunctival scars continue to shrink, producing trichiasis and entropion and subsequent corneal scarring in adults. In areas with milder and less prevalent disease, the process may be much slower, with active disease continuing into adulthood; blindness is rare in these cases.

Eye infection with genital *C. trachomatis* strains in sexually active young adults presents as the acute onset of unilateral follicular conjunctivitis and preauricular lymphadenopathy similar to that seen in acute adenovirus or herpesvirus conjunctivitis. If untreated, the disease may persist for 6 weeks to 2 years. It is frequently associated with corneal inflammation in the form of discrete opacities ("infiltrates"), punctate epithelial erosions, and minor degrees of superficial corneal vascularization. Very rarely conjunctival scarring and eyelid distortion occur, particularly in patients treated for many months with topical glucocorticoids. Recurrent eye infections develop most often in patients whose sexual consorts are not treated with antimicrobials.

DIAGNOSIS The clinical diagnosis of classic trachoma can be made if two of the following signs are present:

1 Lymphoid follicles on the upper tarsal conjunctiva
2 Typical conjunctival scarring
3 Vascular pannus
4 Limbal follicles or their sequelae, Herbert's pits

The clinical diagnosis of endemic trachoma should be confirmed by laboratory tests in children with more marked degrees of inflammation. Intracytoplasmic chlamydial inclusions are found in 10 to 60 percent of Giemsa-stained conjunctival smears in such populations, but isolation in cell cultures, newer antigen detection tests, or chlamydial PCR is more sensitive. Follicular conjunctivitis in adult Europeans or Americans living in trachomatous regions is rarely due to trachoma.

Sporadic cases of adult inclusion conjunctivitis must be differentiated from adenovirus and herpes simplex virus keratoconjunctivitis during the first 15 days after onset and from other forms of chronic follicular conjunctivitis later. Demonstration of chlamydial infection by Giemsa- or immunofluorescent-stained smears or by isolation in cell cultures constitutes definitive evidence of infection. Genital examination and tests for genital chlamydial infection are indicated. Serum antibody does not constitute evidence of chlamydial eye infection since many sexually active adults have acquired serum antibody from genital infection. A practical diagnostic procedure in cases with chronic follicular conjunctivitis is treatment for 6 days with an oral tetracycline or erythromycin; a marked response of symptoms within 3 to 4 days is highly suggestive of inclusion conjunctivitis, and treatment should be continued for at least 3 weeks.

DIFFERENTIAL DIAGNOSIS OF CONJUNCTIVITIS AND KERATOCONJUNCTIVITIS   The eye and its adnexa may be infected during the course of many cutaneous and systemic viral diseases. Sometimes these ocular infections produce minor manifestations, such as the transient loss of accommodation in dengue and the milder forms of conjunctivitis in systemic adenovirus infections. Other virus infections, however, such as herpes simplex (see Chap. 143), herpes zoster (see Chap. 144), measles (see Chap. 155), and vaccinia (see Chap. 147), occasionally produce serious and permanent visual loss. In addition, congenital infections are an important cause of blindness, particularly rubella, which leads to cataracts and microphthalmus; cytomegalic inclusion disease with retinal involvement; and syphilis with interstitial keratitis or optic neuritis. Among the viral infections limited to the outer eye and manifested as a follicular conjunctivitis are epidemic keratoconjunctivitis, herpes simplex keratoconjunctivitis, Newcastle disease virus conjunctivitis, and acute hemorrhagic conjunctivitis.

TREATMENT   Public health control programs for endemic trachoma have consisted of the mass application of tetracycline or erythromycin ointment to the eyes of all children in affected communities for 21 to 60 days or on an intermittent schedule. These programs also include surgical correction of inturned eyelids by a mobile surgical team that visits each locality. Oral erythromycin, but none of the oral tetracyclines, offers an alternative method of mass antibiotic treatment for trachoma of young children and pregnant women.

Adult inclusion conjunctivitis responds well to treatment with full doses of systemic tetracycline or erythromycin for 3 weeks. Treating all sexual consorts of the patient simultaneously is also necessary to prevent ocular reinfection and to avoid the genital diseases due to chlamydial infection. Topical antibiotic treatment is not required for patients treated with systemic antibiotics.

PREVENTION   Efforts to develop a trachoma vaccine have not yet been successful. General hygienic measures associated with improved living standards are effective in the elimination of endemic trachoma. Adequate water supply for personal cleanliness may be a key factor. In some areas the reduction of flies in the household is important.

PSITTACOSIS

DEFINITION   Psittacosis is primarily an infectious disease of birds that is caused by *Chlamydia psittaci*. Transmission of infection from birds to humans results in a febrile illness characterized by pneumonitis and systemic manifestations. Inapparent infections or mild influenza-like illnesses may also occur. The term *ornithosis* is sometimes applied to infections contracted from birds other than parrots or parakeets, but *psittacosis* is the preferred generic term for all forms of the disease.

EPIDEMIOLOGY   Almost any avian species can harbor *C. psittaci*. Psittacine birds (parrots, parakeets, budgerigars) are most commonly infected, but human cases have been traced to contact with pigeons, ducks, turkeys, chickens, and many other birds. Psittacosis may be considered an occupational disease of pet-shop owners, poultry workers, pigeon fanciers, taxidermists, veterinarians, and zoo attendants. During the past 20 years, there has been an increase in incidence, with cases and outbreaks occurring primarily among employees of poultry processing plants. It is suspected that many cases are undiagnosed and not reported. The disease appears to be more common in England, where budgerigars are popular household pets and where restrictions on the importation of these birds have been eased.

The agent is present in nasal secretions, excreta, tissues, and feathers of infected birds. Although the disease can be fatal, infected birds frequently show only minor evidence of illness, such as ruffled feathers, lethargy, and anorexia. Asymptomatic avian carriers are common, and complete recovery may be followed by continued shedding of the organism for many months.

Psittacosis is almost always transmitted to humans by the respiratory route. On rare occasions the disease may be acquired from the bite of a pet bird. Prolonged contact is not essential for transmission of the disease; a few minutes spent in an environment previously occupied by an infected bird has resulted in human infection. The severity of the disease in humans bears no apparent relationship to closeness or duration of contact, although sick birds are more likely to transmit infection than healthy ones. A psittacosis-like agent has been transmitted among hospital personnel, with severe and sometimes fatal infections. There is evidence that these "human" strains are more virulent than avian organisms. There is no record of infection acquired by eating poultry products.

PATHOGENESIS   The psittacosis agent gains entrance to the body through the upper part of the respiratory tract, spreads via the bloodstream, and eventually localizes in the pulmonary alveoli and in the reticuloendothelial cells of the spleen and liver. Invasion of the lung probably takes place by way of the bloodstream rather than by direct extension from the upper air passages. A lymphocytic inflammatory response occurs on both the interstitial and the respiratory surfaces of the alveoli as well as in the perivascular spaces. The alveolar walls and interstitial tissues of the lung are thickened, edematous, necrotic, and occasionally hemorrhagic. Histologically, the affected areas show alveolar spaces filled with fluid, erythrocytes, and lymphocytes. The picture is not pathognomonic of psittacosis unless macrophages containing characteristic cytoplasmic inclusion bodies (LCL bodies) can be identified. The respiratory epithelium of the bronchi and bronchioles usually remains intact.

CLINICAL MANIFESTATIONS   The clinical manifestations and course of psittacosis are extremely variable. After an incubation period of 7 to 14 days or longer, the disease may start abruptly with shaking chills and fever ranging as high as 40.5°C (105°F), but the onset is often gradual with fever increasing over a 3- to 4-day period. Headache is almost always a prominent symptom; it is usually diffuse and excruciating and is often the patient's chief complaint.

Many patients present with a dry hacking cough that is usually nonproductive, but small amounts of mucoid or bloody sputum may be raised as the disease progresses. Cough may begin early in the course of the disease or as late as 5 days after the onset of fever. Chest pain, pleurisy with effusion, or a friction rub may all occur but are rare. Pericarditis and myocarditis have been reported. Most patients have a normal or slightly increased respiratory rate; marked dyspnea with cyanosis occurs only in severe psittacosis with extensive pulmonary involvement. In psittacosis, as in most nonbacterial pneumonias, the physical signs of pneumonitis tend to be less prominent than symptoms and x-ray findings would suggest. The initial examination may reveal fine sibilant rales, or clinical evidence of pneumonia may be completely lacking. Rales usually become audible and more numerous as the illness progresses. Signs of frank pulmonary consolidation are usually absent. Symptoms of upper respiratory tract infection are not prominent, although mild sore throat, pharyngitis, and cervical adenopathy are often present; on occasion the last may be the only manifestations of illness. Epistaxis is encountered early in the course of nearly one-fourth of cases. Photophobia is also a common complaint.

Patients often report generalized myalgia, and spasm and stiffness of the muscles of the back and neck may lead to an erroneous diagnosis of meningitis. Lethargy, mental depression, agitation, insomnia, and disorientation have been prominent features of the illness in some epidemics but not in others; delirium and stupor develop near the end of the first week in severe cases. Occasional patients are comatose when first seen, and the diagnosis of psittacosis may be elusive in these cases. Gastrointestinal problems such as abdominal pain, nausea, vomiting, or diarrhea are noted in some cases; constipation and abdominal distention sometimes occur as late complications. Icterus, the result of severe hepatic involvement, is a rare and ominous finding. A faint macular rash (Horder's spots) simulating the rose spots of typhoid fever has been described.

Patients without cough or other clinical evidence of respiratory involvement present with fever of unknown origin (see Chap. 16). The pulse rate is slow in relation to the fever. When splenomegaly is present in a patient with acute pneumonitis, psittacosis should be considered; the reported incidence of splenomegaly in this disease ranges from 10 to 70 percent. Nontender hepatic enlargement also occurs, but jaundice is rare. Thrombophlebitis is not unusual during convalescence; indeed, pulmonary infarction is sometimes a late complication and may be fatal.

In untreated cases of psittacosis, sustained or mildly remittent fever persists for 10 days to 3 weeks or occasionally for as long as 3 months. Over this period, the respiratory manifestations gradually abate. Psittacosis contracted from parrots or parakeets is more likely to be a severe, prolonged illness than infection acquired from pigeons or barnyard fowl. Relapses occur but are rare. Occasional patients develop endocarditis, and C. psittaci infection should be considered in cases of culture-negative endocarditis. Secondary bacterial infections are uncommon. Immunity to reinfection is probably permanent.

LABORATORY FINDINGS The chest x-ray in psittacosis mimics that in a great variety of pulmonary diseases. The pneumonic lesions are usually patchy in appearance but can be hazy, diffuse, homogeneous, lobar, atelectatic, wedge-shaped, nodular, or miliary. The white blood cell count is normal or moderately decreased in the acute phase of the disease but may rise in convalescence. The erythrocyte sedimentation rate is frequently not elevated. Transient proteinuria is common. The cerebrospinal fluid sometimes contains a few mononuclear cells but is otherwise normal. Despite hepatomegaly, the results of liver function tests are generally normal.

The diagnosis can be confirmed only by isolation of the causative microorganism or by serologic studies. The agent is present in the blood during the acute phase of the disease and in the bronchial secretions for weeks or sometimes years after infection, but it is difficult to isolate. Further, the organism is hazardous to work with in the laboratory, and most clinical laboratories do not offer culture for C. psittaci. Thus psittacosis is most readily diagnosed by the demonstration of a rising titer of CF antibody in the serum of a patient with a compatible clinical syndrome. Both an acute-phase and a convalescent-phase specimen should always be tested. C. trachomatis, C. psittaci, and C. pneumoniae all share a genus-specific "group" antigen, which is the basis of the CF test. Thus acute infections with C. trachomatis or C. pneumoniae can also produce titer rises in the CF test. However, these three species have different MOMPs that are the principal antigens in the micro-IF test. If there is doubt as to the interpretation of the CF test, the micro-IF test can therefore be used to differentiate among them. The prompt initiation of treatment with tetracycline has been shown to delay an antibody rise in convalescence for several weeks or months.

DIFFERENTIAL DIAGNOSIS A history of exposure to birds may be the only clinical basis for differentiating psittacosis from a variety of infectious and noninfectious febrile disorders. A partial list of pulmonary diseases that may be confused with psittacosis includes Mycoplasma pneumonia, C. pneumoniae pneumonia, legionellosis, viral pneumonia, Q fever, coccidioidomycosis, tuberculosis, enteroviral infection, carcinoma of the lung with bronchial obstruction, and common bacterial pneumonias. In the early stages, before pneumonitis

appears, psittacosis may be mistaken for influenza, typhoid fever, miliary tuberculosis, and infectious mononucleosis.

TREATMENT The tetracyclines are consistently effective in the treatment of psittacosis. Defervescence and alleviation of symptoms usually take place within 24 to 48 h after the institution of therapy with 2 g daily in four divided doses. To avoid relapse, treatment should probably be continued for at least 7 to 14 days after defervescence. In severe cases, hospitalization and pulmonary intensive care may be indicated. Sulfonamides are not active against C. psittaci. Erythromycin can be used in patients allergic to or intolerant of tetracyclines.

C. PNEUMONIAE INFECTIONS

A third chlamydial species, C. pneumoniae, has been described. C. pneumoniae can be distinguished from the other two species on the basis of DNA hybridization and restriction endonuclease analyses. Although C. pneumoniae can be grown in a variety of cell cultures, it is considerably more difficult to culture than other chlamydiae, especially from clinical specimens. Fewer than 50 isolates have been obtained from patients worldwide. HL cells appear to be the most effective cell line for isolation of C. pneumoniae.

Knowledge of the epidemiology of C. pneumoniae infections has been derived primarily from serologic studies. Infections begin to occur in late childhood and adolescence and continue throughout adult life. Seroprevalence in the many adult populations that have been tested throughout the world exceeds 40 percent—a figure suggesting that C. pneumoniae infections are ubiquitous. Secondary episodes (reinfections) appear to occur in older adults throughout life. In Scandinavia, C. pneumoniae produces epidemics of pneumonia and respiratory illness followed by periods of infrequent infection. The incidence of infections outside of epidemics remains poorly defined. Transmission appears to be from person to person, probably primarily in schools and family units.

The clinical spectrum of C. pneumoniae infection includes acute pharyngitis, sinusitis, bronchitis, and pneumonitis, primarily in young adults. The clinical manifestations seen in primary infection appear to be more severe and prolonged than those seen in reinfection. The pneumonitis resembles Mycoplasma pneumoniae pneumonia in that leukocytosis is frequently absent and patients often have prominent antecedent upper respiratory tract symptoms, fever, nonproductive cough, mild to moderate degree of illness, minimal findings on chest auscultation, and small segmental infiltrates on chest x-ray. In elderly patients, pneumonia due to C. pneumoniae can be especially severe and may necessitate hospitalization and respiratory support.

Epidemiologic studies have demonstrated an association between serologic evidence of C. pneumoniae infection and coronary atherosclerotic disease. In addition, C. pneumoniae has been identified in atherosclerotic plaques by electron microscopy, DNA hybridization, and immunostaining. The clinical significance of these findings is not yet clear.

Diagnosis of C. pneumoniae infection is currently difficult because cell culture techniques are not available for routine clinical use and noncultural tests using antigen detection methods or DNA probes have not been developed. Acute- and convalescent-phase sera can be tested for chlamydial CF antibody to make a retrospective diagnosis. However, this test does not distinguish C. pneumoniae infection from infection due to C. trachomatis or C. psittaci. Although controlled treatment trials have not been conducted, C. pneumoniae is inhibited in vitro by erythromycin and tetracycline. Recommended therapy is 2 g/d of either agent for 10 to 14 days.

REFERENCES

CATES W JR, WASSERHEIT JN: Genital chlamydial infections: Epidemiology and reproductive sequelae. Am J Obstet Gynecol 164:1771, 1991

CENTERS FOR DISEASE CONTROL: Chlamydia trachomatis infections: Policy guidelines for prevention and control. MMWR 34:535, 1985

CHERNESKY M et al: Detection of *Chlamydia trachomatis* antigens in urine as an alternative to swabs and cultures. J Infect Dis 161:124, 1989

COULTS II et al: Clinical and radiographic features of psittacosis infection. Thorax 40:530, 1985

GRAYSTON JT: Infections caused by *Chlamydia pneumoniae*, strain TWAR. Clin Infect Dis 15:757, 1992

—— et al: A new *Chlamydia psittaci* strain, TWAR, isolated in acute respiratory tract infections. N Engl J Med 315:161, 1986

HANDSFIELD HH et al: Criteria for selective screening for *Chlamydia trachomatis* infection in women attending family planning clinics. JAMA 255:1730, 1986

HOLMES KK: Lower genital tract infections in women: Cystitis, urethritis, vulvovaginitis, and cervicitis, in *Sexually Transmitted Diseases*, 2d ed, KK Holmes et al (eds). New York, McGraw-Hill, 1990

JONES RB: Treatment of *Chlamydia trachomatis* infections of the urogenital tract, in *Chlamydial Infections*, WE Bowie et al (eds). London, Cambridge University Press, 1990, pp 509–519

MARTIN DH et al: A controlled trial of a single dose of azithromycin for the treatment of chlamydial urethritis and cervicitis. N Engl J Med 327: 921, 1992

RETTIG PJ: Perinatal infections with *Chlamydia trachomatis*. Clin Perinatol 15:321, 1988

SCHACHTER J et al: Experience with the routine use of erythromycin for chlamydial infections in pregnancy. N Engl J Med 314:276, 1986

SHAFER MA et al: Urinary leukocyte esterase test for asymptomatic chlamydia and gonococcal infections in males. JAMA 262:2562, 1989

STAMM WE: Diagnosis of *Chlamydia trachomatis* genitourinary infections. Ann Intern Med 108:710, 1988

——, HOLMES KK: *Chlamydia trachomatis* infections in adults, in *Sexually Transmitted Diseases*, 2d, ed KK Holmes et al (eds). New York, McGraw-Hill, 1990

—— et al: *Chlamydia trachomatis* urethral infections in men. Prevalence, risk factors, and clinical manifestations. Ann Intern Med 100:47, 1984

TOOMEY KE, BARNES RC: Treatment of *Chlamydia trachomatis* genital infections. Rev Infect Dis 12 (suppl 6):S645, 1990

section 11　Viral diseases

141　THE BIOLOGY OF VIRUSES

KENNETH L. TYLER / BERNARD N. FIELDS

STRUCTURE AND CLASSIFICATION OF VIRUSES　A typical virus particle (*virion*) contains a core of nucleic acid of either DNA or RNA. There is considerable variability in the structure and size of animal viruses and their associated nucleic acids (Table 141-1 and Fig. 141-1). The genomes of smallest molecular weight, such as those of the Parvoviridae, encode three or four proteins, whereas the larger genomes, such as those of the Poxviridae, encode more than 100 structural proteins and enzymes. The number of proteins encoded by a viral genome may be greater than predicted from the genome's molecular weight because of the presence of multiple open reading frames and/or overlapping regions of nucleic acid that can be transcribed into several distinct messenger RNAs. Extensive nucleotide sequence data are available for part or all of the genomes of many viruses.

The viral nucleic acid is surrounded by either a single or double protein shell (*capsid*). The viral nucleic acid plus the capsid are referred to as the *nucleocapsid*. The viral capsids are composed of smaller repetitive subunits (*capsomers*) arranged in symmetric constructions. The repeating subunits facilitate assembly of viral proteins into mature virions and reduce the amount of genomic information required to encode structural proteins. Capsids are formed by self-assembly of their structural subunits.

The two fundamental patterns of capsid structural symmetry are icosahedral and helical. Some of the largest viruses, such as the poxviruses, have more complex structural patterns. The retroviruses appear to have icosahedral capsid symmetry and helical core symmetry. Viruses with icosahedral capsid symmetry generally follow principles of physical organization that specify the total allowable number of structural subunits. The nucleic acid in icosahedral viruses is usually in a condensed form and is geometrically independent of the surrounding capsid structure.

Animal viruses with helical symmetry have RNA genomes. A general feature of animal viruses is the binding of protein subunits of the capsid in a regular, periodic fashion along the viral RNA. This close interaction between the capsid proteins and nucleic acid is in sharp contrast to the loose interactions in viruses with icosahedral symmetry and imposes different constraints for viral assembly.

Many viruses have an envelope surrounding the nucleocapsid. The viral envelope is composed of virus-specific proteins and of lipids and carbohydrates derived from host cell membranes. The host cell components are added as the virus buds through the host cell nuclear membrane, endoplasmic reticulum, Golgi apparatus, or cytoplasmic membrane. Different viruses utilize distinctive types of host cell membranes for budding. The factors that determine this specificity are incompletely understood. In some cases, virus-specific envelope proteins may include a matrix protein (*M protein*), which lines the inner side of the envelope and is in contact with the nucleocapsid. Virus-specific glycoproteins protrude from the outer surface of the envelope (e.g., as ''spikes'') and may in some cases contain hydrophobic domains, which span the lipid bilayer of the envelope, as well as internal domains, which may contact the M proteins.

Viral proteins, referred to as *structural* or *virion proteins*, can form the viral capsid, can be a major component of viral envelopes, or can be associated with the viral nucleic acid (*core proteins*). A number of viruses contain surface glycoproteins that agglutinate red blood cells (*hemagglutinins*) by binding to receptors on the red cell surface. Many viruses contain proteins with enzymatic activity. In many cases these enzymes are required for the synthesis of messenger RNA (mRNA) of the appropriate (+) polarity for translation into protein or for replication of the viral genome.

The earliest classifications of viruses were based solely on their ability to pass through filters with small pore sizes. Subsequent classifications stressed pathogenic properties, specific organ tropisms (e.g., enteroviruses), or epidemiologic characteristics (e.g., arboviruses). Current classifications of viruses are based on a combination of genetic, physicochemical, and biologic factors. These include the type and structure of the viral nucleic acid; the nature of virion ultrastructure, including size, type of capsid symmetry, capsid composition; and the presence or absence of an envelope; as well as the strategy used by the virus for genome replication. The reliance on morphologic criteria often means that electron-micrographic studies provide sufficient information to identify both the family and the genus to which a virus belongs. Subdivisions within major viral taxonomic groups may be based on immunologic, cytopathologic, pathogenetic, or epidemiologic features. The application of recombinant DNA techniques will require revision of these classifications based on degrees of genetic relatedness.

REPLICATION　*Replication* refers to the process by which viruses infect susceptible cells, reproduce their genomic material and proteins, and assemble and release infectious progeny. The diversity among viruses in terms of structure and type of genomic material is reflected by the large number of replicative strategies.

The first stage of viral infection of target cells begins with adsorption of the virus particles and ends when the infectious progeny

TABLE 141-1   Structure of viral nucleic acid

Family	Example	Type of nucleic acid	Genome size, kilobases or kilobase pairs	Envelope	Capsid symmetry
Picornaviridae	Poliovirus	ss(+)RNA	7.2–8.4	No	I
Caliciviridae	Norwalk virus	ss(+)RNA	8	No	I
Togaviridae	Rubella virus	ss(+)RNA	12	Yes	I
Flaviviridae	Yellow fever virus	ss(+)RNA	10	Yes	UNK
Coronaviridae	Coronaviruses	ss(+)RNA	16–21	Yes	H
Rhabdoviridae	Rabies virus	ss(−)RNA	13–16	Yes	H
Filoviridae	Marburg virus	ss(−)RNA	13	Yes	H
Paramyxoviridae	Measles virus	ss(−)RNA	16–20	Yes	H
Orthomyxoviridae	Influenza viruses	8 ss(−)RNA segments*	14	Yes	H
Bunyaviridae	California encephalitis virus	3 circular ss(−)RNA segments	13–21	Yes	H
Arenaviridae	Lymphocytic choriomeningitis virus	2 circular ss(−)RNA segments	10–14	Yes	H
Reoviridae	Rotaviruses	10–12 dsRNA† segments	16–27	No	I
Retroviridae	HIV-1	2 identical ss(+)RNA segments	3–9	Yes	I-capsid H-nucleocapsid (probable)
Hepadnaviridae	Hepatitis B virus	dsDNA with ss portions	3	Yes	UNK
Parvoviridae	Human parvovirus B-19	ss(+) or (−) DNA	5	No	I
Papovaviridae	JC virus	Circular dsDNA	5–8	No	I
Adenoviridae	Human adenoviruses	dsDNA	36–38	No	I
Herpesviridae	Herpes simplex virus	dsDNA	120–200	Yes	I
Poxviridae	Vaccinia virus	dsDNA with covalently closed ends	130–280	Yes	Complex

* Influenza C = 7 segments.
† Reovirus, orbivirus = 10 segments; rotavirus = 11 segments; Colorado tick fever virus = 12 segments.
NOTE: ds = double-stranded; ss = single-stranded; (+) = message sense; (−) = anti-message sense; I = icosahedral; H = helical; UNK = unknown.
SOURCE: FA Murphy, DW Kingsbury, in *Fields' Virology*, BN Fields, DM Knipe (eds), New York, Raven Press, 1990.

virus begins to form. This stage is often referred to as the *eclipse period* and may last from a few hours (picornaviruses) to more than 72 h (some herpesviruses). From the beginning of this period (adsorption) to the end (formation of infectious progeny virus), there is a dramatic drop in the amount of infectious virus that can be recovered from disrupted cells.

Adsorption appears to be a process that is initially reversible, resulting from random collisions between viruses and target cells. It has been estimated that only 1 in 10^3 to 10^4 such collisions leads to tighter binding (*attachment*). Attachment is facilitated by the appropriate ionic and pH conditions but is largely temperature-independent and does not require energy. Adsorption of virus to a target cell may involve specific binding of viral proteins to receptors on the cell surface. The virion structure mediating cell attachment has been identified for a number of viruses. For enveloped viruses, the viral attachment protein is typically one of the "spikes" inserted on the outer surface of the viral envelope such as the hemagglutinin (HA) of influenza viruses or the gp120 protein of human immunodeficiency virus (HIV). For some enveloped viruses, such as the herpesviruses and vaccinia virus, attachment may be mediated by several proteins acting together. In nonenveloped viruses, surface polypeptides, such as the fiber protein of adenovirus and the hemagglutinin (σ1) protein of reovirus, often function as attachment proteins.

The exact nature of the cellular receptors for animal viruses is known in only a few specific cases. Among the putative cell surface receptors for viruses are sialic acid residues (influenza virus), epidermal growth factor receptor (vaccinia virus), lymphocyte antigen CD4 (HIV), complement receptor CR2 (Epstein-Barr virus), intercellular adhesion molecule ICAM-1 (human rhinovirus 14), heparan sulfate (herpes simplex virus), and an immunoglobulin superfamily protein (poliovirus) (Table 141-2). Even when the specific receptor

is still unknown, it has been possible to identify "families" or classes of viral receptors using competition binding studies. Viruses of the same species but different serotypes may compete for the same receptor class (e.g., poliovirus serotypes 1, 2, 3) or for different receptor classes (e.g., human rhinovirus 2 and 14). Viruses from

TABLE 141-2   Putative viral receptors

Virus	Receptor
Cytomegalovirus	Beta-2-microglobulin/MHC
Echovirus 1	Integrin VLA-2
Ecotropic murine leukemia virus	y+, membrane amino acid transporter
Encephalomyocarditis virus	Glycophorin A (RBCs)
Epstein-Barr virus	C3d receptor (CR2) (CD21)
Herpes simplex virus	Heparan sulfate proteoglycans
Human coronavirus 229E	Human aminopeptidase N
Human immunodeficiency virus	CD4 (T4 antigen)
Human rhinovirus 14	ICAM-1 (CD54)
Influenza virus	Glycophorin A (RBCs) Sialic acid
Lactate dehydrogenase elevating virus	Ia
Mouse hepatitis virus	CEA family glycoprotein
Poliovirus	Immunoglobulin superfamily protein
Rabies virus	Acetylcholine receptor
Reovirus type 3 (Dearing)	Glycophorin A (RBCs), sialic acid residues
Semliki Forest virus	HLA, H-2 antigens
Sendai virus	Sialic acid
Sindbis virus	Laminin receptor
SV40	Class I MHC
Vaccinia virus	Epidermal growth factor receptor
Vesicular stomatitis virus	Phospho- or glycolipids

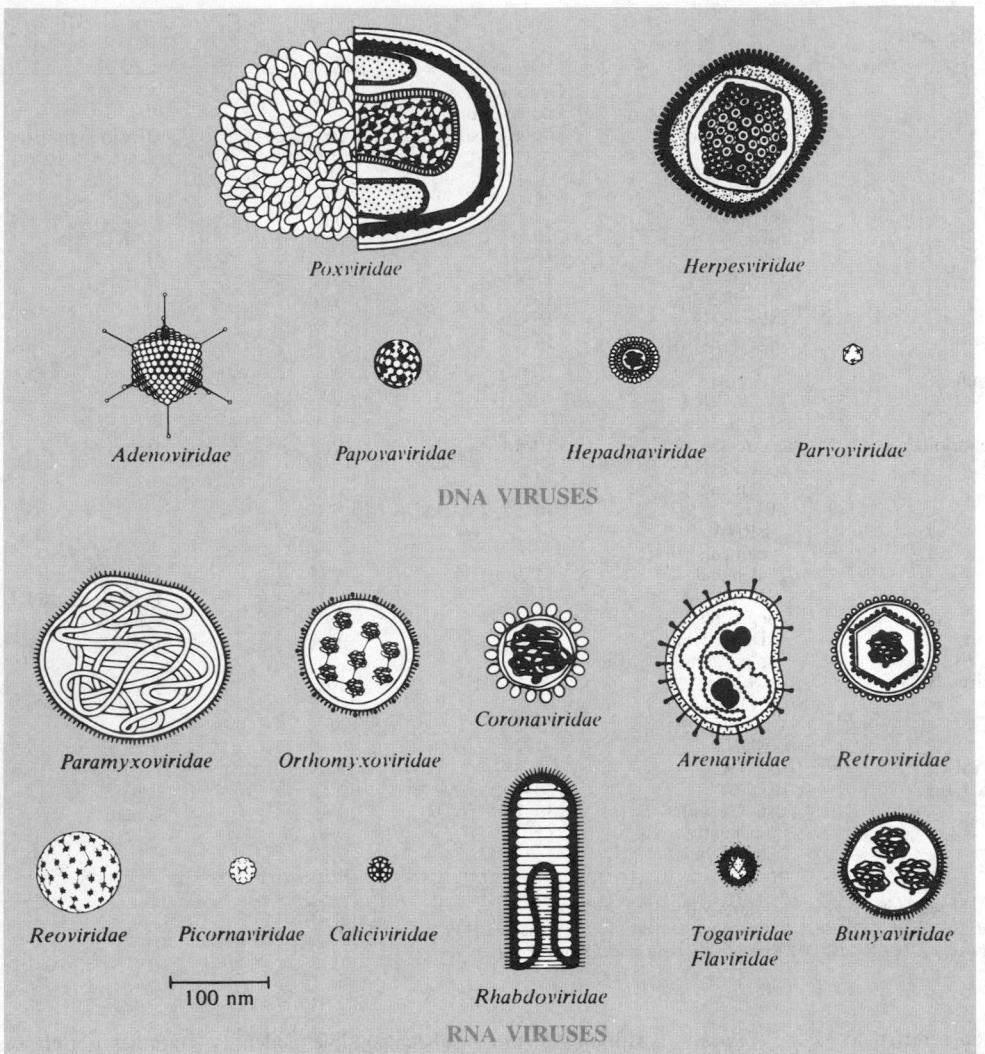

Poxviridae   *Herpesviridae*

Adenoviridae   *Papovaviridae*   *Hepadnaviridae*   *Parvoviridae*

DNA VIRUSES

Paramyxoviridae   *Orthomyxoviridae*   *Coronaviridae*   *Arenaviridae*   *Retroviridae*

Reoviridae   *Picornaviridae*   *Caliciviridae*   *Togaviridae*   *Bunyaviridae*
Flaviridae

100 nm

Rhabdoviridae

RNA VIRUSES

FIGURE 141-1 Structure of DNA and RNA viruses. (*From White DO, Fenner FJ: Medical Virology, 3d ed. Orlando, Academic Press, 1986. Reprinted by permission.*)

different families (e.g., coxsackievirus B3 and adenovirus 2) also may compete for the same class of receptor. These types of binding studies suggest that there are generally 10^4 to 10^6 viral binding sites (receptors) per cell.

Once attachment has occurred, the entire virion or a substructure containing the viral genome and any virion polymerases required for its initial transcription must be translocated across the plasma membrane of the cell. The rate of penetration varies depending on the nature of the virus, the type of cells being infected, and environmental factors such as temperature. Some nonenveloped viruses such as poliovirus and reovirus undergo a process of receptor-mediated endocytosis (*viropexis*) and appear in the cytoplasm inside endocytic vesicles. Other nonenveloped viruses may be able to cross the plasma membrane directly and appear free in the cytoplasm without entering endocytic vesicles.

Enveloped viruses also utilize at least two strategies for penetration. The first is exemplified by Semliki Forest virus (SFV). SFV, a togavirus, binds to specific cell surface receptors, which then aggregate at distinct sites on the plasma membrane (*coated pits*) and are internalized by receptor-mediated endocytosis. They subsequently appear inside clathrin-coated vesicles within the cell cytoplasm. Fusion between the viral envelope and the endosomal membrane causes release of the viral nucleocapsid into the cytoplasm. A second mechanism for penetration of enveloped viruses occurs with paramyxoviruses (e.g., Sendai). The viral envelope fuses directly with the cell plasma membrane, and the viral nucleocapsid is discharged free into the cytoplasm.

Uncoating is the process of removing or disaggregating part or all of the viral protein capsid in preparation for transcription and translation of the viral genome. In many cases penetration and uncoating are part of a single process. Some picornaviruses, for example, seem to undergo an alteration in capsid structure and integrity and loss of an internal protein as they are translocated across the plasma membrane. The structural alterations associated with loss of the protein may facilitate entry of the viral RNA into the cytoplasm.

Nonenveloped viruses which enter endosomes, such as adenovirus, may induce fusion of lysosomes with the endosome and have their capsid removed by lysosomal enzymes. In the case of reoviruses, intraendosomal proteases sequentially remove the three outer capsid proteins to produce an "infectious subviral particle." Further proteolytic processing to a "core particle" leads to activation of the viral transcriptase. Uncoating of poxviruses, such as vaccinia virus, may require virus-induced uncoating proteins with trypsin-like activity.

A number of strategies have evolved for *transcription* of viral genomes into mRNA and *translation* of mRNA into protein. One approach is for viruses to contain mRNA that is translated into a large precursor polyprotein, which is then cleaved to produce the various virion proteins (e.g., in picornaviruses). In the case of both the picornaviruses and the togaviruses, a virally encoded RNA polymerase synthesizes a complementary RNA using the genomic RNA as template. In turn, the newly synthesized RNA serves as template for the synthesis of more genomic RNA.

Viruses which contain linear or segmented RNA produce unique mRNAs for each viral protein rather than a single large mRNA molecule. A transcriptase enzyme contained in the virion (the virion polymerase) is required to produce mRNAs from the genomic RNA. The presence of multiple mRNAs allows regulation of the amount of each protein synthesized. A single region of genomic RNA may have multiple reading frames, each of which is transcribed into unique mRNAs, which are in turn translated into distinct proteins. Genomic (−) single-stranded (ss)RNA is replicated via a (+)ssRNA intermediate, which then serves as a template to synthesize more (−)ss genomic RNA.

Reoviruses contain an RNA-dependent RNA polymerase that transcribes (+)ssRNAs from the (−) strand of each double-stranded (ds) RNA segment. These (+)ssRNAs are extruded from the viral core through channels in the core spike and serve as mRNAs for translation into viral proteins. The viral RNA polymerase also synthesizes (+)ssRNAs, which in turn serve as templates for the complementary (−) strand during replication of the viral genome.

The retroviruses utilize a unique replicative strategy. Viral (+)ssRNA serves as a template for the virion RNA-dependent DNA polymerase (reverse transcriptase) and primer transfer RNAs (tRNAs). An ssDNA copy is produced which is initially hydrogen bonded to its complementary (+)ssRNA. A virally encoded ribonuclease digests the ssRNA, and a complementary DNA strand is synthesized. Then dsDNA is integrated into chromosomal DNA in the host cell nucleus. Transcription of this integrated viral DNA is under the control of the host cell transcriptases.

DNA viruses such as papovaviruses, adenoviruses, and herpesviruses use replicative strategies in which transcription of viral DNA into mRNA occurs in the nucleus of the host cell and depends on host cell enzymes. The viral mRNA encodes a DNA polymerase that replicates the viral DNA. Protein synthesis occurs in a series of sequential stages in which the first (early) proteins synthesized include regulatory proteins and proteins involved in DNA replication. Viral structural proteins are synthesized subsequently.

Poxviruses are the most complicated of the known animal viruses, and their replicative cycle is correspondingly complex. All the initial steps of transcription and translation appear to occur in the host cell cytoplasm; thus the virus must contain its own DNA-dependent RNA polymerase to initiate transcription. Replication, transcription, and later viral assembly all occur in virus-initiated "factories" within the host cell cytoplasm. Sequential groups of virus-specified proteins can be detected in infected cells. Early proteins include a number of enzymes (e.g., a DNA polymerase and a thymidine kinase), as well as some structural proteins. As infection proceeds, DNA replication begins, the synthesis of the early nonstructural proteins ceases, and the synthesis of late proteins begins. Many of the late proteins are structural proteins; other late proteins include enzymes and proteins that may play a role in viral assembly.

Once replication of the viral genome and synthesis of the viral proteins have been completed, intact virions must then be assembled and released from the host cells. Assembly of the nonenveloped viruses and the nucleocapsid of enveloped viruses often appears to proceed in a crystallization-like fashion which depends on the self-assembly of viral capsomers.

In most cases, nonenveloped virions accumulate within the infected cell and are released together when the cell lyses. The events leading to cell disruption include inhibition of the synthesis of host cell protein, lipid, and nucleic acids; disorganization of the host cell cytoskeleton; and alteration of host cell membrane structure. Membrane disruption may result in increased cell permeability and the release of proteolytic enzymes from lysosomes. The failure to replenish energy-rich substrate molecules inhibits the function of ion transport pumps and disturbs transport of essential nutrients and cellular waste products.

Enveloped viruses are typically released from infected cells by budding. This process may be lethal to the cell. In all cases, virus-specified proteins are inserted into host cell membranes in a fashion that restructures the membrane by displacing some of its normal protein components. Viral capsids may then bind to virus-specified matrix proteins which line the cytoplasmic side of these altered patches of membrane. In the case of the smallest enveloped viruses, the togaviruses, the capsids bind to the intracytoplasmic domains of viral proteins inserted in the host cell membrane rather than to matrix proteins.

Release of certain enveloped and nonenveloped viruses occurs preferentially from particular surfaces of certain types of polarized cells, such as epithelial cells. In the case of enveloped viruses, selective insertion of envelope glycoproteins into either the apical or the basolateral cell membrane precedes polarized release. Recent studies suggest that specific amino acid sequences within the viral envelope proteins may determine their insertion at a particular cell surface. The mechanisms responsible for polarized release of nonenveloped viruses remain to be determined. Polarized release may have important implications for pathogenesis. Release of virus at apical surfaces may facilitate local spread of infection, whereas release at the basolateral surface may facilitate systemic invasion.

PATHOGENESIS The signs and symptoms of disease are the result of the culmination of a series of interactions between the virus and the host. A virus must first be able to enter the host, then undergo a period of primary replication, followed by spread to its final target tissue. Once a virus reaches its target organs, it must then infect and successfully replicate in a susceptible population of host cells. The outcome of this last step may be a productive infection with or without cell injury, latent infection, or persistent infection. To transmit infectious virus to the next host, the virus must successfully avoid or overcome the host immune response and a wide variety of other host defense mechanisms. A great deal of viral replication can occur before any signs or symptoms of clinical illness are detectable. This "incubation period" can vary from a few days (e.g., influenza) to weeks (e.g., measles, varicella) to months (e.g., rabies, hepatitis) to years (e.g., slow viruses).

Most viral diseases result from exposure to exogenous virus. However, in some cases disease results from the reactivation of endogenous virus that has been latent within specific host cells. Examples of infections caused by reactivated endogenous viruses include shingles (herpes zoster), progressive multifocal leukoencephalopathy (JC or BK papovaviruses), recurrent labial and genital herpes (herpes simplex), and some types of cytomegalovirus (CMV) infections.

In the majority of cases, transmission of viral illnesses occurs between members of a susceptible host population (*horizontal spread*). *Vertical spread* of infection occurs when the fetus becomes infected in utero through virus carried in the germ cell line, virus infecting the placenta, or virus in the maternal birth canal. HIV, rubella virus, CMV, herpes simplex virus, varicella-zoster virus, and hepatitis B virus can all produce vertically transmitted congenital infections.

The age and genetic background of the host can have important implications for the outcome of viral infections. Newborns, for example, are particularly susceptible to severe, disseminated herpes simplex virus infections. In contrast, many of the exanthematous illnesses, poliovirus infection, and EBV infection are typically more severe in older individuals than in children. In mice, specific genes help determine susceptibility to certain viral infections. These genes may act through effects on the immune system, interferon production, or viral receptors. Inadequate host nutritional status may increase susceptibility to infections such as measles, perhaps by depressing cell-mediated immunity. The host also can influence viral infections in ways that are still poorly understood. Stress may trigger recurrent herpes labialis. Strenuous exercise may have an adverse effect on the course of polio.

Viral infection begins with *entry* into the host, which may occur via a number of routes. The stratum corneum of the skin provides both a physical and a biologic barrier against the entry of viruses. Some viruses overcome the skin barrier by being directly inoculated via insect or animal bites or mechanical devices such as needles. The arthropod-borne viruses are directly inoculated into the bloodstream when an infected tick or mosquito takes a blood meal. Rabies virus and herpesvirus simiae (monkey B virus) enter tissues after an animal bite. Iatrogenic inoculation allows entry of a large number of viruses. Hepatitis B virus, CMV, and HIV-1 may all be present in contaminated blood products used for transfusion. Parenteral vaccination using live attenuated virus represents another category of iatrogenic inoculation.

A large number of viruses enter the host by crossing mucosal barriers in the respiratory and gastrointestinal tracts. Respiratory infection can be transmitted by means of aerosol droplets, nasal secretions, or saliva. Entry via either the respiratory or the enteric route requires that the virus overcome a formidable series of host defenses. In the lung, immunologic defenses include secretory IgA, natural killer (NK) cells, and macrophages. Nonspecific glycoprotein viral inhibitors are present in tracheobronchial mucus. Ciliated respiratory epithelial cells continually move mucus away from the lower respiratory tract. The harsh acidic environment of the stomach inactivates acid-labile viruses such as rhinoviruses. Bile salts, present in the lumen of the small intestine, can destroy the lipid envelope of many viruses and may account for the fact that entry via the gastrointestinal route is limited largely to nonenveloped viruses. Proteolytic enzymes and secretory IgA contribute to host antiviral defenses in the gastrointestinal tract. Specific viral capsid proteins may allow some viruses to withstand proteolytic digestion in the gut.

For some enteric viruses, passage across the mucosal barrier of the gut is mediated by a specific population of cells overlying Peyer's patches known as *microfold (M) cells*. These cells, and perhaps their analogues in bronchial lymphoid tissue, facilitate transport of some viruses, including reoviruses and polioviruses, to the abluminal surface of the small intestine.

Venereal transmission with entry across the genitourinary or rectal mucosa appears to be important for herpes simplex virus type 2, CMV, hepatitis B virus, and HIV-1.

For some viruses, the processes of entry, primary replication, and tissue tropism all occur at the same anatomic site. Examples of this type of viral illness include the upper and lower respiratory infections caused by the rhinoviruses, orthomyxoviruses, and paramyxoviruses; the enteritis caused by rotaviruses; and the dermatologic lesions induced by human papillomavirus (warts) and paravaccinia virus (milker's nodules). In other cases, a virus enters at one site and must subsequently spread to a distant area, such as the central nervous system, to produce disease. Enteroviruses enter via the gastrointestinal tract but must spread to the CNS to produce meningitis, encephalitis, and poliomyelitis. Measles virus and varicella virus enter the body through the respiratory tract but then spread to produce skin disease (exanthem) and often generalized organ involvement.

Neural, hematogenous, and lymphatic pathways are all utilized by viruses to spread to target tissues. Rabies virus, herpes simplex virus, herpesvirus simiae (monkey B), varicella-zoster virus, reovirus type 3, and certain coronaviruses spread via nerves. Herpes simplex virus appears to enter nerves via receptors located primarily near synaptic endings rather than on the nerve cell body. Rabies virus accumulates at the motor end plate of the neuromuscular junction (NMJ), as do La Crosse bunyavirus and the togavirus Sindbis. Rabies virus can infect muscle and then spread via motor and sensory nerves to the spinal cord. The kinetics of neural spread for rabies virus, herpes simplex virus, reovirus, and poliovirus strongly suggest that these agents utilize intraneuronal mechanisms involved with fast axonal transport. Infection of Schwann cells may provide another "neural" pathway to the CNS. Axonal transport also provides a pathway for spread of viruses within the CNS and from it to the periphery.

The olfactory pathway represents a special category of neural spread. The rod processes of olfactory receptor cells lie exposed in the olfactory mucosa. These cells synapse directly with the mitral cells in the olfactory bulb within the CNS. Under experimental conditions, intranasal or aerosol inoculations of rabies virus, herpes simplex virus, poliovirus, and some togaviruses can lead to CNS infection via the olfactory route. This route may provide a pathway to the CNS in humans for rabies and possibly other viruses in circumstances where high-titer aerosols are present, such as in caves

occupied by large numbers of rabid bats or in accidental laboratory-acquired infections. An olfactory route of spread might be one explanation for the localization of herpes simplex virus to the orbitofrontal and medial temporal cortex in cases of herpes simplex encephalitis.

Hematogenous spread is important for many viruses. A period of primary replication usually precedes the initial viremia and can be asymptomatic or result in prodromal symptoms. For enteric viruses, primary replication occurs in Peyer's patches and peritonsillar lymphatic tissue. Primary replication of respiratory viruses occurs in epithelial or alveolar cells and for many enteroviruses and togaviruses in skeletal muscle. In some cases virus travels from the site of initial multiplication via lymphatics to regional lymph nodes before entering the bloodstream. The initial (*primary*) viremia often disseminates virus to tissues such as the spleen and liver, where continued multiplication in parenchymal cells leads to an amplified secondary viremia. Growth in endothelial cells may help sustain the viremic phase in some togavirus infections. Sustained secondary amplification of the viremia is required if a virus is to overcome clearance by reticuloendothelial cells.

Blood-borne virus can travel free or in association with cellular elements. Hepatitis B virus, picornaviruses, and togaviruses all travel free within plasma; Colorado tick fever virus and Rift Valley fever virus are associated with red blood cells; EBV, CMV, rubella virus, and HIV are lymphocyte- or monocyte-associated.

In some cases, viruses use different pathways of spread at different stages in the infectious cycle. Varicella-zoster virus disseminates to the skin by the hematogenous route to produce chickenpox. The virus then spreads centripetally along nerves from the skin to the dorsal root ganglion, where it remains latent. Reactivation results in centrifugal spread of virus down sensory nerves to their skin dermatome and the production of shingles (zoster).

Once a virus has spread from its site of primary replication to a target organ, it must infect a population of susceptible cells. This requires the interaction between specific viral structures (*viral attachment proteins*) and viral receptors on cells. Virus-encoded tissue-specific enhancers may in part mediate viral injury to specific cell populations. Lytic infection also requires that all the subsequent steps in the viral replicative cycle be successfully completed.

HOST FACTORS   The antibody response   Most viruses make good antigens for stimulating the immune response because they contain a large number of foreign proteins, each of which may contain multiple antigenic sites. In addition, although the amount of viral antigenic material may initially be quite small, there is amplification in its quantity due to viral replication. Few of the antibodies play a significant role in protecting the host against infection, and in some cases they may themselves be implicated in disease pathogenesis.

The immunogenicity of viruses depends on the nature of the virus itself and on a variety of host factors. The route of viral infection also may play a role in immunity. In experimental influenza infections, intravenous inoculation is more immunogenic than intraperitoneal inoculation, which in turn exceeds the subcutaneous route.

Antibodies which destroy the infectivity of virus are referred to as *neutralizing antibodies (Nab)*. The binding of Nab to virus is generally a reversible reaction. Viral infectivity may be reduced because Nab inhibits attachment, penetration, or uncoating of virus; produces aggregation of virions; accelerates viral degradation in vesicles; or enhances viral opsonization and subsequent phagocytosis. In the case of poliovirus, Nab binding appears to induce a conformational rearrangement of the viral outer capsid which blocks viral uncoating but not attachment. It is important to recognize that some antibodies which fail to neutralize viral infectivity in vitro may still protect against viral infection in vivo and that, conversely, not all Nab is protective in vivo.

Complement   Viruses can trigger activation of both the alternate and classical pathways of complement in the absence of an antibody response. Activated complement components (e.g., C3b) may act as opsonins that enhance phagocytosis of viruses. Activation of the alternate complement pathway, in combination with antibody, may produce lysis of enveloped viruses or virus-infected cells. Although the complement system plays a role in the protection against viral infection in animals, human complement-deficiency states are not typically associated with an increase in the frequency or severity of viral illnesses.

Cell-mediated immunity Virus-infected cells can be lysed by lymphocytes and other cells through both antibody-dependent and antibody-independent pathways. NK cells are large granular lymphocytes that bind to infected target cells and then secrete cytotoxic molecules contained in azurophilic granular vesicles. NK activity is increased by interferons and possibly by some viral glycoproteins and does not require antibody. NK cytotoxicity provides one of the earliest host defenses against viral infection (peak activity at 2 to 3 days) and precedes the appearance of antibody (7 days), cytotoxic T lymphocytes (CTLs), and delayed-type hypersensitivity (DTH). Activated NK cells have been identified in human viral infections caused by CMV, EBV, measles virus, and mumps virus.

Antibody-dependent lysis of infected cells can occur via antibody-dependent cell-mediated cytotoxicity (ADCC). In ADCC reactions, virus-specific antibody bound to antigens on an infected cell interacts with Fc receptors for IgG on the surface of leukocytes, and this interaction results in the activation of these leukocytes and their subsequent killing of the target cell.

Lysis of infected cells mediated by CTLs is typically class I histocompatibility antigen–restricted, although examples of class II–restricted CTLs have been described. CTLs must be activated by antigen presented by macrophages or other antigen-presenting cells (APCs). The nature of the specific epitopes expressed on the surface of infected cells that CTLs recognize has been defined for some viruses, such as influenza. In contrast to the specificity of neutralizing antibodies, which typically recognize epitopes on intact viral surface proteins, CTLs recognize antigens presented as short peptides derived from both viral surface and internal proteins. The pathways by which these peptides are processed, appear on the surface of infected cells, and interact with major histocompatibility complex (MHC) antigens are subjects of active investigation.

Interferons Leukocytes produce more than a dozen alpha (''leukocyte'') interferons that share about 77 percent amino acid sequence homology. Beta (''fibroblast'') interferon is produced by fibroblasts and epithelial cells and has 30 percent homology to α-interferons. Both α- and β-interferons are acid-stable (pH = 2) and relatively heat resistant. ''Immune'' (γ-) interferon is produced by both sensitized and unsensitized lymphocytes, has different physicochemical properties and different inducers, and uses a different cellular receptor from α- and β-interferons. Genes encoding interferons are located on human chromosomes 9(α and β) and 12(γ).

Interferons can be induced by both active and inactivated viruses, by dsRNA, and by a number of other compounds. The amount of interferon produced may vary with different viruses. All the interferons have extremely high specific activity and are generally most active in cells of the species in which they are induced (''species-specific''), presumably because of variation in the nature of the interferon receptor. Interferon production appears to involve a derepression of cellular genes induced by the presence of viral nucleic acid in the host cell cytoplasm. This results in the rapid production of mRNAs for interferon and subsequent interferon synthesis.

Newly produced interferon is released into extracellular fluid and then binds to a specific receptor on adjacent cells. The gene encoding the glycoprotein receptor for α- and β-interferon is on human chromosome 21, and that for γ-interferon is on chromosome 6. Binding of interferon to its receptor results in a complex variety of subsequent events. A protein kinase is synthesized and phosphorylates a protein synthesis initiation factor (eIF_2), resulting in inhibition of initiation complex formation and hence of viral protein synthesis. An induced 2,5-oligoisoadenylate synthetase produces 2,5-oligoadenylates, which in turn activate a cellular ribonuclease (RNase L) that cleaves viral mRNAs. Inhibition of methyltransferase reactions decreases methylation of mRNAs and thereby interferes with viral protein synthesis. In addition to these actions, changes in target cell surface antigens result in enhanced expression of both class I and class II histocompatibility antigens. Interferons also increase the activity of NK cells, CTLs, and cells involved in ADCC reactions. The relative importance of each of these activities in creating the interferon-induced antiviral state is not established.

Virus-induced immunopathology Viruses can combine with virus-specific antibodies to produce circulating immune complexes which may be involved in immunopathogenesis. Virus stimulation of B lymphocytes may result in the production of polyclonal antibodies to antigens unrelated to the inciting virus. Viruses also can induce cross-reacting antibodies to normal host structures which contain antigenic regions similar to those of the virus (*molecular mimicry*). These types of autoantibodies also may lead to immune-complex formation. Immune complexes can become trapped in basement membranes at a variety of sites, including the skin, the kidney, the choroid plexus, and the walls of blood vessels. These immune complexes result in tissue injury by attracting and activating a variety of inflammatory mediators.

Autoantibodies produced by virus infection also may result in direct tissue injury. Autoantibodies to lymphocytes, platelets, smooth muscle, intermediate filaments, immunoglobulins, and myelin basic protein are usually transient and of low titer. These autoantibodies could result from a variety of mechanisms, including (1) incorporation of host antigens into viral structures or virus-induced alteration of host antigens, (2) virus-induced alterations in immunoregulatory systems, (3) cross reactivity between virus antigens and normal host cell structures (molecular mimicry), and (4) elicitation of anti-idiotypic antibodies which stimulate host cell receptors.

EPIDEMIOLOGY Viral epidemiology includes the study of the causes, distribution, frequency, modes of transmission, and spread of viral diseases. Accurate enumeration of the incidence and prevalence of viral diseases is an important aspect of epidemiology. *Incidence* can be defined as the number of *new* cases of a particular disease that appear during a defined period of time, and *prevalence* as the *total* number of cases. It is often useful to refer to incidence and prevalence *rates*, which are obtained by dividing incidence or prevalence numbers by the size of the total population at risk. Terms such as *epidemic* and *outbreak* are arbitrary and simply indicate that a greater than expected number of cases of a particular disease has occurred in a specific population, geographic location, or time period.

The appearance of an acute viral disease indicates that an infected host has come into contact with a susceptible individual under conditions that permit the transmission of a particular viral agent. The time interval between exposure to a virus and the development of signs and symptoms of disease is referred to as the *incubation period* and can vary from a few days (e.g., influenza) to years (slow virus diseases). Viral infection does not always lead to overt clinical disease. The percentage of those infected who develop overt disease ranges from 100 percent (e.g., rabies, measles) to 0 percent (BK, JC papovaviruses). In most cases, symptomatic disease is less common in children than in adults (e.g., EBV mononucleosis, paralytic poliomyelitis, hepatitis A virus).

Transmission of a virus from an infected host to a susceptible individual can take a variety of forms. Human-to-human transmission can occur from an acutely ill individual, from a chronic carrier, or from mother to fetus. The method of spread can involve respiratory aerosols, fecal-oral contamination, sexual contact, or direct inoculation via infected needles or blood products.

Respiratory aerosolization usually occurs via coughing or sneezing. A sneeze may generate up to 2 million aerosol particles and a cough up to 90,000. The fate of these particles depends on both ambient environmental conditions (e.g., humidity, wind currents) and particle size. Small particles remain airborne longer and can escape the filtering action of the nose, which traps particles larger than 6 μm in diameter. The number of viral particles aerosolized may vary for different strains of the same virus.

For most viruses it is unclear how many viral particles are required to initiate a respiratory infection. For influenza A virus, adenovirus, or coxsackievirus A21, as few as 10 particles may be sufficient. Aerosolization is not the only possible route of respiratory transmission. EBV is typically spread by saliva during kissing. A critical pathway of spread for rhinoviruses, which cause the common cold, is from hands to eyes, nose, or mouth—a cycle which can be interrupted by hand washing.

Gastrointestinal transmission occurs when virus shed in feces contaminates food or water and is then ingested by a susceptible individual (fecal-oral spread). Stool-tainted hands, resulting from poor personal hygiene, provide another vehicle of spread for enteric viruses. The high incidence of enteric virus infections in infant day-care centers and institutions for the mentally retarded reflects the difficulty of maintaining hygiene in these settings.

In many types of viral disease the vector is an insect or infected animal. In dengue fever there is a continuing cycle between humans and infected mosquitoes. Dengue virus multiplies in the gut of the *Aedes aegypti* mosquito, spreads to its salivary glands, and is injected into a human during the mosquito's blood meal. The infected person develops a high-titer viremia which is sufficient to transmit virus to an uninfected mosquito during biting. In other arbovirus infections the human being is a "dead-end host" because the degree of viremia in infected individuals is insufficient to transmit infection to a new group of insect vectors. Examples of this type of cycle are provided by togaviruses, such as eastern, western, and St. Louis encephalitis viruses. The normal animal reservoirs for arboviruses include small birds and mammals. The horse, like humans, is usually a dead-end host, although in Venezuelan equine encephalitis, horses may be a reservoir of virus.

Some arthropod-borne infections do not require a viremic vertebrate intermediate host. Virus can be passed in transovarian fashion to the progeny of an infected tick or mosquito or by venereal transmission between male and female mosquitoes. Transovarian transmission may allow survival of arthropod viruses through the winter months.

Zoonotic infections illustrate another mechanism of disease transmission. In the case of rabies, transmission results from the bite of an infected animal. Many human infections occur when humans are exposed to the excreta (feces, urine, saliva) of infected rodents. Examples include arenavirus infections and the hemorrhagic fevers with renal disease caused by the bunyaviruses.

DIAGNOSIS OF VIRAL DISEASES   A reasonably accurate diagnosis of some viral illnesses, such as measles, can be made on clinical grounds alone. In other cases the best that can be done clinically is to identify a group of viruses that are likely pathogens for specific categories of illness. More definitive diagnosis is often necessary because of availability of antiviral agents with activity limited only to certain types of viruses. Definitive diagnosis requires isolation of the virus in animals or in tissue culture, identification of the virus or detection of virus-specified antigens or viral nucleic acids in tissues or body fluids, or documentation of specific serologic responses. The physician must ensure that the appropriate specimens are obtained for diagnostic studies during a suitable phase of the illness, that they are rapidly transported, and that adequate clinical information is provided to the diagnostic laboratories.

In the case of diarrheal or gastrointestinal illness where a viral etiology is suspected, a fresh *stool sample* is the specimen of choice for virus isolation. In diseases of the respiratory system, including pharyngitis, croup, bronchiolitis, and pneumonia, nasopharyngeal or tracheal *aspirates* provide the best specimens. Nasopharyngeal and throat *swabs* are less satisfactory. When a vesicular rash is present, a needle aspirate of vesicular fluid provides the optimal specimen. When the rash is petechial or maculopapular, both nasopharyngeal aspirates and a stool sample should be obtained. In patients with CNS diseases of suspected viral etiology, including meningitis, encephalitis, myelitis, and Guillain-Barré syndrome, a nasopharyngeal aspirate and stool and cerebrospinal fluid specimens should be

obtained. A urine sample may be helpful when infection due to CMV, measles virus, mumps virus, or papovaviruses is suspected. Blood specimens may be useful for the detection of some arboviruses, herpesviruses, and lymphocytic choriomeningitis (LCM) virus. Saliva has been used for the detection of rabies and mumps viruses. A brain biopsy specimen is often required for the definitive diagnosis of herpes simplex encephalitis, progressive multifocal leukoencephalopathy, subacute sclerosing panencephalitis (SSPE), and progressive rubella panencephalitis.

Nasopharyngeal or rectal swab specimens should be placed in an appropriate transport medium. In general, this consists of a few milliliters of a neutral isotonic salt solution to which a small amount of protein or animal serum has been added. Antibiotics should be added to inhibit bacterial contaminants. Specimens can be placed in a thermos flask filled with crushed ice if any delay in transport is anticipated. Ideally, specimens should be inoculated into the appropriate culture systems on arrival in the virology laboratory. Storage up to 48 h can often be done safely at refrigerator temperature (4°C), and longer storage should be at −70°C. Many viruses quickly lose infectivity if repeatedly frozen and thawed.

Isolation of virus from clinical specimens is done in cell cultures, embryonated eggs, and animals such as suckling mice. Cell culture techniques involve the use of primary cultures of cells prepared from organs of freshly killed animals (e.g., monkey kidney cells), human diploid cell lines such as WI-38 embryo fibroblasts, and continuous (heterodiploid) cell lines such as HeLa, HEp-2, BHK-21, and Vero. Some viruses grow better on certain cell lines than others. Inoculation into the amniotic cavity or the allantoic cavity of embryonated chicken eggs is useful in the isolation of influenza virus. Intraperitoneal and intracerebral inoculation into neonatal mice may be necessary for isolation of coxsackievirus A and may help in the isolation of many arboviruses, rabies virus, arenaviruses, and orbiviruses. Adult mice or guinea pigs can be used to isolate LCM virus. Special isolation techniques using brain tissue explants are required to identify measles virus in cases of SSPE or rubella virus in cases of progressive rubella panencephalitis.

Once cell culture inoculation has been performed, the specimens are examined for distinctive patterns of cytopathic effect (CPE). Viruses such as HSV and many enteroviruses produce early CPE, whereas cultures may need to be followed for weeks and even subcultured to detect CPE due to CMV, rubella virus, and some adenoviruses. Cultured cells are examined for cell lysis and vacuolization. The presence of syncytia suggests HSV, respiratory syncytial virus (RSV), measles virus, or mumps virus. Cytomegaly is seen with HSV, varicella-zoster virus (VZV), and CMV. Detection of inclusion bodies is aided by the use of Giemsa or other stains. Immunocytochemical staining of cell cultures to detect viral antigens using fluorescein or enzyme-conjugated specific antiviral antibodies can aid in the detection and identification of many viruses. Some viruses produce minimal or no detectable CPE. Orthoviruses and paramyxoviruses (influenza, parainfluenza, measles, mumps) can be detected by the ability of infected cultures to adsorb certain red blood cells (*hemadsorption*). Infection with rubella virus can be detected by the ability of infected cultures to block the CPE produced by infection with a second challenge virus (*interference*).

Identification of virus particles or antigens in tissue specimens provides another important method of viral diagnosis. Skin scrapings from the base of vesicles can be stained with Wright or Giemsa stain according to the Tzanck method to help identify HSV or VZV. Similar techniques may help identify CMV-infected cells in urine sediment or measles virus–infected cells in scrapings from Koplik spots. In some cases, examination of appropriately prepared specimens by electron microscopy (EM) is of diagnostic value; high concentrations of virus must be present. A special technique which concentrates virus in specimens by adsorbing excess fluid and salts on an agarose surface may enable detection of as few as 10^4 particles per milliliter (pseudoreplica technique). EM easily distinguishes between vaccinia virus and VZV in vesicular fluid negatively stained with phosphotungstic acid and may be extremely useful in identifying skin viruses such as human papilloma virus, orf virus, and molluscum contagiosum virus. The use of specific antisera to aggregate virus in prepared stool specimens facilitates EM detection of rotaviruses, hepatitis A virus, and the Norwalk agent. EM examination of brain biopsy specimens may allow identification of herpes simplex encephalitis, progressive multifocal leukoencephalopathy (PML), and SSPE.

Detection of virus-specific antigens is facilitated by immunofluorescence and immunocytochemical techniques. These procedures are particularly valuable in diagnosing rabies, herpes infection, PML, and SSPE from brain biopsy specimens; herpes keratitis from corneal scrapings; HSV, VZV, and vaccinia virus infections from vesicle scrapings; parainfluenza virus, influenza virus, and RSV infections from nasopharyngeal aspirates; hepatitis B virus infections from liver biopsy specimens; and Colorado tick fever virus infection from blood clots. Radioimmunoassays and immunoassays in which viral antibody coupled to a solid support (ELISA) is used to detect viral antigens have proved useful in the diagnosis of hepatitis A and B virus, rotavirus, and adenovirus infections.

The detection of a fourfold or greater increase in antibody titer to a specific viral agent in a patient's acute and convalescent (3 to 4 weeks later) sera can usually be considered diagnostic of acute infection. A single serum specimen is only occasionally useful in viral diagnosis. A high antibody titer against a rare agent in a typical clinical setting or a distinct pattern of antibody titers to viral antigens of specific types may provide presumptive evidence of acute infection. Blood for serology should be collected in anticoagulant- and preservative-free glass tubes and allowed to clot. Serum should be separated out and stored frozen. A number of different types of antibodies, including neutralizing (N), complement-fixing (CF), and hemagglutination-inhibiting (HI) antibodies, are routinely assayed. The time course of these antibody responses and their sensitivity and specificity differ greatly.

Restriction enzyme analysis of the genomes of DNA viruses (e.g., HSV, VZV, CMV) and oligonucleotide fingerprinting of ribonuclease T_1 cleaved genomes of RNA viruses (e.g., influenza virus, dengue enterovirus) are valuable in epidemiologic studies and in establishing the origin of certain types of viral isolates. In situ hybridization and the polymerase chain reaction technique may enable the detection of even single copies of virus genomes in tissue samples or cells from body fluids.

VACCINES FOR THE PREVENTION OF VIRAL ILLNESS Currently available vaccines utilize inactivated virus, attenuated virus, or virus subunits to induce active immunization. Formalin-inactivated vaccines are available for rabies virus, influenza virus, and poliovirus. A highly purified subunit vaccine preparation containing the surface antigen of hepatitis B virus is also available. Strains used in the inactivated influenza whole-virus vaccine are specified yearly by the FDA. The vaccine is composed of formalin-inactivated natural isolates of influenza virus and laboratory-designed reassortant strains containing the hemagglutinin and neuraminidase genes of the influenza viruses that are currently circulating. As many as 60 to 80 percent of those immunized show a reduction in the frequency or severity of influenzal illness. Guillain-Barré syndrome occurred in 1 in 100,000 individuals vaccinated with the swine influenza vaccine in 1976 to 1977 but has not been associated with subsequent influenza vaccine preparations. Killed polio vaccine is widely used in Sweden, Finland, and the Netherlands; is used in combination with live vaccine in Denmark; but in the United States is reserved for immunization of immunodeficient individuals and their household contacts, immunization of pregnant women, and adult primary immunization in certain other instances.

Inactivated virus vaccines have advantages and disadvantages compared with live vaccines. The absence of live virus results in immunization without active infection. Since there is no live virus present, reversion to virulence does not occur, although improperly prepared vaccines can contain virulent virus or adventitious viral contaminants (e.g., SV40, avian leukosis virus). Effective local immunity does not develop, so vaccinated individuals may still transmit virus to the community. In rare cases (measles virus, RSV), inactivated vaccines have resulted in atypical immunologic responses which potentiated rather than prevented subsequent natural infections.

The attenuated live virus vaccines in current use have been developed either from naturally occurring attenuated viruses (e.g., poliovirus type 2 strain 712) or from viruses after serial passage in tissue culture cells or embryonated eggs. These passage-selected viruses have mutations when compared with their wild-type parents. For example, the vaccine strain of poliovirus type 1 differs in 21 amino acids from the original parent virus. On some vaccine viruses, the largest number of mutations are located in genes coding for viral surface proteins such as VP1 (polio) or V3 (yellow fever). However, in the case of the type 1 polio vaccine strain, mutations responsible for attenuation appear to be distributed throughout the viral genome, including the 5'noncoding region. In other cases (e.g., mumps virus) a clear marker for the vaccine virus strain has not been identified.

Following immunization with the oral Sabin polio vaccine, the vaccinated person excretes virus which can infect other individuals in the community. In rare cases, the excreted virus appears to be more virulent than the vaccine strain and may account for some of the rare cases of paralytic polio in close contacts of vaccinees. Reversion to virulence by the vaccine strain of virus also may cause paralytic polio in vaccinees. Approximately 1 in 10 million vaccinated individuals develops paralytic polio, and there are 3 cases of paralytic polio per 10 million household and community contacts of recent vaccinees. These risks are small and are probably overestimates which include coincidental as well as causal associations. In rare settings, where exposure to polio occurs at a very young age, a combined program using both inactivated (killed) and attenuated vaccines may be of benefit (see also Chap. 154).

Live attenuated measles, mumps, and rubella vaccines can be administered together (MMR) without any loss in immunizing capacity (>90 percent). Of individuals who receive the measles vaccine alone (Schwarz strain), 10 to 30 percent have mild clinical reactions, and there are rare cases of encephalitis (<1 in 1 million). Widespread use of measles vaccine has been associated with a dramatic reduction in the incidence of SSPE. Children and nonimmune adults (except for pregnant women and immunocompromised individuals) should be vaccinated. The attenuated Jeryl Lynn B strain is used in the live mumps virus vaccine, which should be given to all children except those with immunodeficiency or a history of anaphylactic reactions to eggs. Adverse effects are rare and include allergic reactions as well as CNS complications. The most commonly used rubella vaccine strain (RA 27/3) was attenuated by multiple passages through the WI-38 line of cultured human diploid fibroblasts. The most notable complications are transient arthralgia and rare cases of arthritis. The vaccine is extremely effective, and all immunocompetent children should be immunized. It is essential to ensure that women of childbearing age are immune; nonpregnant women should be revaccinated if there is any ambiguity concerning their immune status.

A live attenuated vaccine for yellow fever has been prepared using virus derived from passage through chicken embryos. Of those vaccinated intradermally, 95 percent develop an immune response. Serious adverse reactions occur in fewer than 1 in 1 million cases. The vaccine is currently indicated only for travelers going to yellow fever-endemic areas.

A novel approach to vaccination is illustrated by the adenovirus vaccine. In this case, the live vaccine virus strains (4, 7) are not attenuated, but the route of administration (via oral ingestion of an enteric coated tablet) results in an asymptomatic infection with subsequent immunity. Ingested virus does not reach the respiratory tract but produces an intestinal infection that stimulates an immune response against subsequent adenovirus-induced respiratory infections. This vaccine is extremely effective, and side effects are very rare. It is used primarily in military recruits to prevent outbreaks of acute respiratory disease.

Two vaccines utilize virus subunits rather than whole virus to induce immunity. The influenza subunit vaccine is composed of purified envelope glycoproteins. It appears to be less toxic than live whole virus vaccine but also less antigenic. The hepatitis B vaccine uses HBsAg protein derived from cloned viral DNA expressed in yeast. The vaccine appears to be extremely effective, with few associated adverse effects. It should be given to people at high risk of exposure to hepatitis B, including health care workers, hemodialysis patients, certain institutionalized individuals, intimate contacts of hepatitis B chronic carriers, and intravenous drug users.

With the eradication of smallpox, routine vaccination with live attenuated vaccinia virus is no longer necessary. Its use should be limited to researchers working with vaccinia or related viruses.

ANTIVIRAL THERAPY   Immune globulins   The role in antiviral therapy of immunoglobulins extracted from pooled lots of adult plasma is limited. Antibody titers to specific viruses in different pooled lots of gamma globulin vary over a tenfold range. Intramuscular administration of immune globulin at the time of exposure to hepatitis A virus can prevent infection or decrease the severity of subsequent illness. A similar beneficial effect has been reported for measles virus infection and possibly for hepatitis B virus infection.

Specific immune globulins are made from plasma with high antibody titer against specific viruses. When given within 72 h of exposure to VZV, varicella-zoster immune globulin can prevent or modify subsequent infection. Such therapy is of value in exposed immunocompromised individuals, pregnant women, and newborn infants of mothers who develop chickenpox or of nonimmune mothers exposed to chickenpox. Hepatitis B immune globulin is useful in preventing infection of individuals exposed to HBsAg-positive material (e.g., a needle stick) or of infants born to hepatitis B–infected mothers. Rabies immune globulin is an integral part of postexposure prophylaxis of rabies. Other immune globulins are available but are not widely used.

Antiviral chemotherapy   See Chap. 142.

REFERENCES

Evans AS (ed): *Viral Infections of Humans: Epidemiology and Control*, 3d ed. New York, Plenum Press, 1989

Fields BN et al (eds): *Virology*, 2d ed. New York, Raven Press, 1990

Galasso GJ et al (eds): *Antiviral Agents and Viral Diseases of Man*, 3d ed. New York, Raven Press, 1990

Lennette EH et al (eds): *Laboratory Diagnosis of Infectious Diseases, Principles and Practice*, vol 2, *Viral, Rickettsial and Chlamydial Diseases*. New York, Springer-Verlag, 1988

Mandell GL et al (eds): *Principles and Practice of Infectious Diseases*, 3d ed. New York, Churchill Livingstone, 1990

Mims CA, White DO: *Viral Pathogenesis and Immunology*. Oxford, Blackwell, 1984

Notkins AL, Oldstone MBA (eds): *Concepts in Viral Pathogenesis*. New York, Springer-Verlag, 1984

———: *Concepts in Viral Pathogenesis II*. New York, Springer-Verlag, 1986

———: *Concepts in Viral Pathogenesis III*. New York, Springer-Verlag, 1989

142   ANTIVIRAL CHEMOTHERAPY

RAPHAEL DOLIN

The use of antiviral compounds for chemotherapy and chemoprophylaxis of viral diseases is a relatively new development in the field of infectious diseases, particularly when compared with the more than 45 years of experience with antibacterial antibiotics. The principles which underlie the use of antiviral compounds have been modeled after those successfully employed in the treatment of bacterial

infections, as outlined in Chap. 100. However, application of these principles to antiviral chemotherapy and chemoprophylaxis presents a number of unique problems.

First, antiviral compounds must possess a high degree of selectivity because of the biologic properties of viruses. Bacteria can replicate extracellularly and have evolved metabolic and structural features which differ considerably from those of mammalian cells. However, viruses must replicate intracellularly and often employ host cell enzymes, macromolecules, and organelles for the synthesis of virus particles. Therefore, safe and effective antiviral compounds must be able to discriminate with a high degree of efficiency between cellular and virus-specific functions. Inhibitors of virus replication which lack this selectivity are likely to be too toxic for clinical use.

Second, because of the nature of virus replication, evaluation of the in vitro sensitivity of virus isolates to antiviral compounds must be carried out in a complex culture system consisting of living cells (e.g., tissue culture). The results from such assay systems vary widely according to the type of tissue culture cells which are employed and the conditions of assay. Furthermore, the precise relationship between the in vitro sensitivity of an isolate and the outcome of antiviral therapy is not well worked out for many viral infections.

Third, information regarding the pharmacokinetics of antiviral compounds, particularly in diverse clinical settings, is limited, particularly when compared with that available for antibacterial antibiotics. For compounds such as acyclovir, considerable detailed pharmacokinetic data are available, while for others such as amantadine, relatively little information exists. Assays to determine concentrations of antivirals, particularly of active moieties within cells, are not widely available. There are few guidelines with which to adjust dosage levels to maximize antiviral activity and to minimize toxicity. Therefore, clinical use of antiviral compounds must be accompanied by particular vigilance for unanticipated side effects or toxicities.

Fourth, it is clear that highly complex host defense systems play critical roles in the course of viral infections. The presence or absence of preexisting immunity and the ability to mount humoral and/or cell-mediated immune responses are especially important determinants in the outcome of viral infections. For example, profound "immunosuppression" may result in infections in which prolonged viral replication is present, and inhibition of such replication by antiviral compounds may be particularly useful. On the other hand, if host defenses are severely depressed, as in bone marrow transplants, antiviral therapy may be relatively ineffective. The state of host defenses and their interactions with antiviral compounds need to be considered when antivirals are utilized or evaluated.

Finally, as with antibacterial antibiotics, the optimal use of antiviral compounds requires that a specific and timely diagnosis be made. For some viral infections, such as herpes zoster, the clinical manifestations are so characteristic that a diagnosis can be made on clinical grounds alone. For other viral infections, such as influenza A, epidemiologic information (i.e., community-wide outbreaks) can be utilized to make a presumptive diagnosis with a high degree of accuracy. However, for most other viral infections, including herpes simplex encephalitis, cytomegalovirus infections, and acute viral gastroenteritis, diagnosis on clinical grounds alone cannot be accomplished with certainty. For such infections, rapid, noninvasive viral diagnostic techniques are sorely needed, and considerable effort is being expended to develop such tests.

Despite the preceding complexities, the efficacy of several antiviral compounds has been clearly established in rigorously conducted and controlled studies. The compounds which are currently licensed or likely to be licensed in the immediate future for clinical use are discussed below and summarized in Table 142-1.

AMANTADINE AND RIMANTADINE   Amantadine (1-adamantanamine hydrochloride) and the closely related compound rimantadine (α-methyl-1-adamantanemethylamine hydrochloride) are primary symmetric amines with antiviral activity limited to influenza A viruses. They inhibit influenza A virus replication by interfering with uncoating of virus after infection of the cell has occurred through interaction with the influenza A M2 matrix protein. A substitution of a single amino acid in the M2 protein can result in a virus which is resistant to amantadine and rimantadine.

Amantadine and rimantadine have been demonstrated to be effective in the prophylaxis of influenza A in large-scale studies in young adults and in less extensive studies in children and elderly subjects. In such studies, efficacy rates of 55 to 80 percent in prevention of influenza-like illness were noted, and even higher rates were reported when virus-specific attack rates were calculated. Amantadine and rimantadine also have been demonstrated to be effective in the treatment of influenza A infection in studies carried out predominantly in young adults and, to a lesser extent, in children. Administration of these compounds within 24 to 72 h after the onset of illness has resulted in a reduction of duration of signs and symptoms by approximately 50 percent when compared with a placebo-treated group. The effect on signs and symptoms of illness has been demonstrated to be superior to that of commonly used antipyretic-analgesics. Only anecdotal reports are available concerning the efficacy of amantadine or rimantadine in the prevention or treatment of complications of influenza (e.g., pneumonia).

Amantadine and rimantadine are available only in oral formulations and are ordinarily administered in a dose of 200 mg/d for adults, given once or twice daily. Despite their structural similarities, the pharmacokinetics of the two compounds are different. Amantadine is not metabolized and is excreted almost entirely by the kidney, with a half-life of 12 to 17 h and peak plasma concentrations of 0.4 µg/mL. Rimantadine is extensively metabolized to hydroxylated derivatives and has a half-life of 30 h. Only 30 percent of an orally administered dose is recovered in the urine. The peak plasma levels of rimantadine are approximately one-half those of amantadine, but rimantadine is concentrated in respiratory secretions to a greater extent than amantadine. For prophylaxis, the compounds must be administered daily for the period at risk (i.e., the peak duration of the outbreak). For therapy, amantadine or rimantadine is generally administered for 5 to 7 days.

Although these compounds are generally well tolerated, 5 to 10 percent of amantadine recipients experience mild central nervous system side effects, consisting primarily of dizziness, anxiety, insomnia, and difficulty in concentrating. These side effects are rapidly reversible upon cessation of the drug. In a dose of 200 mg/d, rimantadine is better tolerated than amantadine, and in a large-scale study in young adults, side effects were no more frequent in rimantadine recipients than in placebo recipients. Seizures and worsening of congestive heart failure also have been reported in patients treated with amantadine, although a causal relationship has not been established. Because amantadine is excreted primarily by the kidney, dosage should be reduced in patients with renal failure and in the elderly, for whom a dose of 100 mg/d is recommended.

Resistance to amantadine and rimantadine can be induced readily in vitro. The emergence and probable transmission of virus resistance to these drugs also have been noted in vivo after treatment of children or adults with rimantadine or amantadine. Amantadine is licensed for the prophylaxis and therapy of influenza A in the United States, while rimantadine remains experimental.

RIBAVIRIN Ribavirin is a synthetic nucleoside analogue that inhibits a wide range of RNA and DNA viruses. The mechanism of action of ribavirin is not completely defined and may be different for different groups of viruses. Ribavirin-5'-monophosphate blocks the conversion of inosine-5'-monophosphate to xanthosine-5'-monophosphate and interferes with the synthesis of guanine nucleotides and both RNA and DNA synthesis. Ribavirin-5'-monophosphate also inhibits capping of virus-specific messenger RNA in certain viral systems. In studies demonstrating the effectiveness of ribavirin, the compound has been administered as a small-particle aerosol. It has been utilized to treat respiratory syncytial virus (RSV) infection in infants and, to a lesser extent, parainfluenza infections in children and influenza A and B infection in young adults. In RSV infection in infants, ribavirin administered by continuous aerosol for 3 to 6 days resulted in more rapid resolution of illness, lower respiratory tract signs, and less arterial oxygen desaturation when compared with placebo-treated groups. It also has had beneficial clinical effect in infants with RSV who required mechanical ventilation. Aerosolized ribavirin has been administered to adults with severe RSV infections, but the benefit, if any, is unclear. Orally administered ribavirin has not been effective in the treatment of influenza A infections. Intravenous or oral ribavirin has reduced mortality in patients with Lassa fever, particularly when given within the first 6 days of illness.

Large doses of ribavirin administered orally (800 to 1000 mg/d) have been associated with reversible hematopoietic toxicity, but this has not been observed with aerosolized ribavirin, apparently because little drug is absorbed systemically. Aerosolized administration of ribavirin is generally well tolerated but can be associated with occasional bronchospasm, rash, or conjunctival irritation. Aerosolized ribavirin has been licensed for treatment of RSV infection in infants. Because of the need for aerosolized administration, the drug can only be given for this indication under close supervision. Health care workers exposed to the drug have experienced minor toxicity, including eye and respiratory tract irritation.

ACYCLOVIR Acyclovir, 9-[(2-hydroxyethoxy)methyl]guanine, is a highly potent and selective inhibitor of replication of certain herpesviruses, including herpes simplex 1 (HSV-1), herpes simplex 2 (HSV-2), varicella-zoster virus (VZV), and Epstein-Barr virus (EBV). It is relatively ineffective in human cytomegalovirus (CMV) infections.

The high degree of selectivity of acyclovir is related to its mechanism of action, which requires that the compound first be phosphorylated to acyclovir monophosphate. This phosphorylation occurs efficiently in herpesvirus-infected cells by means of a virus-coded thymidine kinase. In uninfected mammalian cells, little phosphorylation of acyclovir occurs, and therefore, the drug is concentrated in herpesvirus-infected cells. Acyclovir monophosphate is subsequently converted by host cell kinases to a triphosphate which is a potent inhibitor of virus-induced DNA polymerase but has relatively little effect on host cell DNA polymerase. Acyclovir triphosphate also can be incorporated into viral DNA, with early chain termination.

Acyclovir is available in intravenous, oral, and topically administered forms. Intravenous acyclovir has been demonstrated to be markedly effective in the therapy of mucocutaneous HSV infections in immunocompromised hosts, reducing time to healing, duration of pain, and virus shedding. When administered prophylactically during periods of intense immunosuppression such as chemotherapy for leukemia or transplantation, but before lesions are present, intravenous acyclovir also has reduced the frequency of HSV-associated disease. After prophylaxis was discontinued, recurrent HSV lesions developed. Intravenous acyclovir also has been demonstrated to be effective in the treatment of HSV encephalitis, and two comparative trials have indicated that acyclovir is more effective than vidarabine for treatment of the latter infection (see below). Varicella-zoster virus (VZV) is generally less sensitive to acyclovir than is HSV, so higher doses of acyclovir must be used to treat VZV infections. In immunocompromised patients with herpes zoster, intravenous acyclovir reduced the frequency of cutaneous dissemination and visceral complications and was more effective than vidarabine in one comparative trial. Acyclovir administered orally at doses of 800 mg five times a day had a modest beneficial effect on localized herpes zoster lesions in both immunocompromised and immunocompetent patients and is being further evaluated in large-scale collaborative trials. Orally administered acyclovir (600 mg five times a day) reduced complications of herpes zoster ophthalmicus in a placebo-controlled trial.

In normal children with chickenpox, acyclovir administered at 20 mg/kg four times a day up to a maximum of 800 mg four times a day within 24 h of the onset of rash resulted in a modest overall clinical benefit. Intravenous acyclovir also has been reported to be effective in the therapy of immunocompromised children with chickenpox.

The most widespread use of acyclovir is in the therapy of

TABLE 142-1   Antiviral chemotherapy and chemoprophylaxis

Infection	Antiviral drug	Administration	Dosage	Comment
Influenza A (prophylaxis)	Amantadine	Oral	Adults: 200 mg/d for period at risk Children ≤9 yrs: 4.4–8.8 mg/kg per day not to exceed 150 mg/d	Needs to be administered for the duration of the outbreak. Dosage should be reduced in renal failure and in the elderly. Can be administered along with vaccine.
Influenza A (therapy)	Amantadine	Oral	As above for 5–7 days	Both amantadine and rimantadine are effective in uncomplicated influenza. Neither drug has been demonstrated to be effective in complicated influenza (e.g., pneumonia).
Respiratory syncytial virus	Ribavirin	Aerosol	Administered continuously by small-particle aerosol from a reservoir containing 20 mg/mL for 3–6 days	Utilized for treatment of infants and young children hospitalized with RSV pneumonia and bronchiolitis.
Herpes simplex encephalitis	Acyclovir or vidarabine	IV IV	10 mg/kg q 8 h for 10 days 15 mg/kg per day as a continous infusion for 12 h for 10 days	Acyclovir is the drug of choice for this infection on the basis of comparative trials vs. vidarabine. Optimal results are obtained when therapy is initiated early in illness.
Neonatal herpes simplex	Vidarabine or acyclovir	IV IV	30 mg/kg per day given as a continuous infusion over 12 h per day for 14–21 days 10 mg/kg q 8 h for 14–21 days	Vidarabine and acyclovir are equivalent in clinical efficacy. Serious morbidity is frequent despite therapy.
Genital herpes simplex: primary infection	Acyclovir	IV Oral Topical	5 mg/kg q 8 h for 5–10 days 200 mg 5 times per day for 10 days 5% ointment; 4–6 applications per day for 7–10 days	IV route is preferred if infection is of sufficient severity to warrant hospitalization, or if neurologic complications are present. Preferred route of administration for patients who do not warrant hospitalization. Adequate hydration should be maintained. Largely supplanted by oral therapy. May be of use in pregnant women in order to avoid systemic therapy. Systemic symptoms and untreated areas are not affected.
Genital herpes simplex: recurrent infections (therapy)	Acyclovir	Oral	200 mg 5 times per day for 5 days	Clinical effect is modest and is enhanced if therapy is initiated early. No effect on subsequent recurrence rates.
Genital herpes simplex: recurrent infections (suppression)	Acyclovir	Oral	400 mg 2 times per day for 12 months or longer	Suppressive therapy is recommended only for patients with frequent recurrences, at least 6 to 10 per year. Occasional "breakthrough" may occur, and asymptomatic shedding of virus occurs. Need for suppressive therapy should be reevaluated after 1 year.
Mucocutaneous herpes simplex in immunocompromised patients (treatment)	Acyclovir or vidarabine	IV Oral Topical IV	250 mg/m² q 8 h for 7 days 400 mg PO 5 times per day for 10 days 5% ointment; 4–6 applications per day for 7 days or until healed 10 mg/kg per day for 7 days given as a 12-h infusion	Choice of intravenous or oral route will depend on severity of infection and whether patient can take oral medication. Oral or IV administration has supplanted topical therapy except for small, easily accessible lesions. Efficacy has been demonstrated in HSV-1 infections and in patients who were older than 40. Appears to be less useful than acyclovir in this setting.
Herpes zoster ophthalmicus	Acyclovir	Oral	600 mg PO 5 times a day for 10 days	Reduces ocular complications including ocular keratitis and uveitis.
Cytomegalovirus retinitis in immunosuppressed patients	Ganciclovir or foscarnet	IV IV	5 mg/kg twice a day for 14–21 days, then 5 mg/kg per day as maintenance 60 mg/kg q 8 h for 14–21 days, then 90–120 mg/kg per day as maintenance	Both ganciclovir and foscarnet are licensed for treatment of CMV retinitis in immunosuppressed patients, including those with AIDS. Effectiveness in colitis, pneumonia, or "wasting" syndromes associated with CMV is uncertain. Foscarnet is not myelosuppressive and is active against acyclovir- and ganciclovir-resistant strains of herpesviruses.
HIV infection	Zidovudine or didanosine or	Oral Oral	200 mg PO q 8 h 125–200 mg (tablets) PO twice per day.	Licensed for treatment of patients with HIV infection and CD4 counts less than 500 per microliter. Lower doses (500–600 mg/d) are equally effective and less toxic than higher doses. ddI is licensed for patients with HIV infection who are intolerant of or failing on ZDV. Studies comparing ddI and ZDV are underway.

TABLE 142-1 Antiviral chemotherapy and chemoprophylaxis (*continued*)

Infection	Antiviral drug	Administration	Dosage	Comment
	zalcitabine	Oral	0.75 mg PO q 8 h	Licensed for use in combination with ZDV in patients with advanced infection who are failing on ZDV alone.
Mucocutaneous herpes simplex in immunocompromised patients (prevention of recurrences during periods of intense immunosuppression)	Acyclovir	Oral	200 mg 4 times per day	Acyclovir is administered during periods when intense immunosuppression is expected, e.g., antitumor chemotherapy, after transplantation. After therapy is discontinued, lesions recur.
		IV	5 mg/kg q 12 h	
Herpes simplex keratitis	Trifluorothymidine or	Topical	One drop of 0.1% ophthalmic solution every 2 h while awake (maximum 9 drops per day)	Therapy should be undertaken in consultation with an ophthalmologist.
	vidarabine	Topical	0.5-in ribbon of 3% ophthalmic ointment 5 times per day	As above
Varicella in normal hosts	Acyclovir	Oral	20 mg/kg (up to a maximum of 800 mg), 4 times per day for 5 days.	Modest clinical benefit when administered within 24 h of onset of rash.
Varicella in immunocompromised patients	Acyclovir or	IV	500 mg/m² every 8 h for 7 days	Studies comparing IV acyclovir with vidarabine in the treatment of varicella have not been performed. Limited placebo-controlled studies suggest the effects of both drugs on varicella are similar.
	vidarabine	IV	10 mg/kg per day in a 12-h infusion for 5 days	
Herpes zoster in immunocompromised patients	Acyclovir or	IV	500 mg/m² q 8 h for 7 days	Efficacy of acyclovir and vidarabine are established for localized zoster, particularly when treated early, and acyclovir appears to be more effective. Studies of the effectiveness of the two drugs in treatment of disseminated zoster are underway. Oral acyclovir (4 g/d) is under study in herpes zoster in immunosuppressed patients.
	vidarabine	IV	10 mg/kg per day in a 12-h infusion for 5 days.	
Herpes zoster in immunocompetent hosts	Acyclovir	Oral	800 mg 5 times per day for 7–10 days	Acyclovir accelerated resolution of skin lesions and provided some acute symptomatic relief.
Condyloma acuminatum	Interferon α2b or	Intralesional	1 million units per wart (maximum of 5) 3 times per week for 3 weeks	Intralesional treatment results in frequent clearance of warts, but lesions often recur. Parenteral administration may be useful if lesions are numerous.
	interferon αn3	Intralesional	250,000 units per wart (maximum of 10) 2 times per week for up to 8 weeks.	
Chronic hepatitis, non-A, non-B/C	Interferon α2b	SC or IM	3 million units 3 times/week for 24 weeks	Normalization of serum ALT values occur in 40 percent, but half will relapse when treatment is stopped. Optimal duration and regimens of treatment are under study.
Chronic hepatitis B	Interferon α2b	SC or IM	5 million units per day for 16 weeks	Loss of HBeAg and HBV DNA occurs in 40 to 50 percent of patients. Histopathologic improvement is also seen.

genital HSV infections. Both intravenous and oral formulations have shortened the duration of symptoms, reduced virus shedding, and accelerated healing when employed for the treatment of primary genital HSV infections. Oral acyclovir also had a modest effect in the therapy of recurrent genital HSV infections. However, treatment of either primary or recurrent disease did not reduce the frequency of subsequent recurrences, indicating that acyclovir was ineffective in elimination of latent infection. Chronically administered oral acyclovir for periods ranging from 1 to 6 years has been shown to reduce the frequency of recurrences markedly while on therapy, although once the drug was discontinued, lesions recurred. In AIDS patients, chronic or intermittent administration of acyclovir has been associated with the development of HSV and VZV strains resistant to the action of the drug and with clinical failures. The most common mechanism of resistance is a deficiency of the virus-induced thymidine kinase. Patients with HSV or VZV infections resistant to acyclovir have frequently responded to foscarnet.

With the availability of the oral and intravenous forms, there are few indications for topical acyclovir, although treatment with this formulation has shown modest beneficial effects in the therapy of primary genital HSV infections and of mucocutaneous HSV infections in immunocompromised hosts.

Overall, acyclovir is remarkably well tolerated and generally free of toxicity. The most frequently encountered toxicity has been occasional renal dysfunction, particularly after rapid intravenous administration or when patients have been inadequately hydrated. Central nervous system changes, including lethargy and tremors, occasionally have been reported, primarily in immunosuppressed patients. However, whether these changes are related to acyclovir, to concurrent administration of other therapy, or to underlying infection remains unclear. Acyclovir is excreted primarily unmetabolized by the kidney, by both glomerular filtration and tubular secretion. Approximately 15 percent of a dose of acyclovir is metabolized to 9-[(carboxymethoxy)methyl]guanine or other minor metabolites. Reduction in dosage is indicated in patients with creatinine clearance less than 50 mL/min per 1.73 m². The half-life of acyclovir is approximately 3 h in normal adults, and the peak plasma concentration after a 1-h infusion employing a 5 mg/kg dose is 9.8 μg/mL. Approximately 22 percent of acyclovir administered orally is absorbed, and peak plasma concentrations of 0.3 to 0.9 μg/mL are attained after administration of a 200-mg dose. Acyclovir penetrates relatively well into the cerebrospinal fluid, with CSF concentrations approaching one-half of those found in plasma.

GANCICLOVIR   An analogue of acyclovir, ganciclovir, 9-[(1,3-dihydroxy-2-propoxy)methyl]guanine, has activity against all herpesviruses but markedly increased activity against CMV. Ganciclovir triphosphate inhibits CMV DNA polymerases and can be incorporated into CMV DNA with eventual termination of elongation of viral DNA. CMV, unlike HSV, does not code for its own thymidine kinase, but ganciclovir is phosphorylated by a virus-coded protein kinase and/or cellular kinases. Ganciclovir triphosphate is present in tenfold greater concentrations in CMV-infected cells than in uninfected cells. Ganciclovir has been utilized extensively in the treatment of CMV infection in AIDS and otherwise immunosuppressed patients and has been licensed for the treatment of CMV retinitis in immunocompromised patients. It also has been used to treat other CMV-associated syndromes, such as CMV colitis, ''wasting'' syndrome, and pneumonitis, but its efficacy for these infections remains to be established.

Ganciclovir is available only for intravenous administration. It has a plasma half-life of 2.9 ± 1.3 h and is excreted primarily by the kidney, unmetabolized. The most commonly employed dosage for initial therapy is 5 mg/kg twice a day for 14 to 21 days, followed by a maintenance dose of 5 mg/kg per day or 5 times per week, possibly for as long as the immunosuppression persists. Administration of ganciclovir has been associated with profound bone marrow suppression, particularly neutropenia, which represents a major limitation of its use in many patients. Bone marrow toxicity is potentiated when other bone marrow suppressants such as zidovudine are used concomitantly. CMV isolates resistant to ganciclovir have been reported in AIDS patients receiving the drug.

FOSCARNET   Foscarnet (phosphonoformic acid) is a pyrophosphate-containing compound which is a potent inhibitor of herpesviruses, including CMV. It inhibits viral DNA polymerases at the pyrophosphate binding site at concentrations which have relatively little effect on cellular polymerases. Because foscarnet does not require phosphorylation to exert its antiviral activity, it is active against herpesviruses that are resistant to acyclovir because of deficiencies in thymidine kinase and against ganciclovir-resistant strains of CMV. Foscarnet also inhibits the reverse transcriptase of HIV and is active against HIV in vivo.

Foscarnet is poorly soluble and must be administered intravenously in a dilute solution infused over 1 to 2 h. The plasma half-life of foscarnet is 3 to 5 h and increases with decreasing renal function, since the drug is primarily eliminated by the kidneys. It has been estimated that 10 to 28 percent of a dose may be deposited in bone, where it can persist for months. The most common initial dosage of foscarnet is 60 mg/kg every 8 h for 14 to 21 days, followed by a maintenance dose of 90 to 120 mg/kg given once a day.

Foscarnet is licensed for the treatment of CMV retinitis in patients with AIDS. In a comparative clinical trial, it appeared to have efficacy similar to that of ganciclovir against CMV retinitis but was associated with a longer survival, which is as yet unexplained. It also has been used to treat acyclovir-resistant HSV and VZV infections and ganciclovir-resistant CMV infections.

The major toxicity of foscarnet is renal impairment, and renal function should be monitored closely, particularly during the initial phase of therapy. Since foscarnet binds divalent metal ions, hypocalcemia, hypomagnesemia, hypokalemia, and hypo- or hyperphosphatemia can occur. Although hematologic abnormalities also have been observed, foscarnet is not generally myelosuppressive and may be administered concomitantly with myelosuppressive medications such as zidovudine.

ZIDOVUDINE   Zidovudine (ZDV), also known as azidothymidine (AZT), inhibits the replication of HIV through a competitive inhibition of HIV reverse transcriptase by AZT triphosphate, and through chain termination of viral DNA synthesis as well. ZDV is administered orally and has a plasma half-life of approximately 1 h. Ninety percent of a dose is recovered as ZDV or its metabolite in urine. A large-scale placebo-controlled trial carried out in 1987 in patients with AIDS or with advanced AIDS-related complex (ARC) demonstrated that administration of ZDV was associated with prolonged survival and with a decreased frequency and severity of opportunistic infections. Subsequently, placebo-controlled trials in patients with less advanced HIV disease, including patients with early symptomatic disease (CD4 counts of 200 to 800 per microliter and oral thrush, hairy leukoplakia, or intermittent diarrhea) and asymptomatic patients with CD4 counts of less than or equal to 500 per microliter demonstrated lower rates of progression of HIV disease in ZDV recipients. Studies in asymptomatic patients with CD4 counts greater than 500 per microliter are currently underway.

ZDV is currently licensed for treatment of patients with HIV infection who have 500 or fewer CD4 lymphocytes per microliter in peripheral blood. In patients with advanced disease, the beneficial clinical effects of ZDV appear, for unclear reasons, to wane after 12 to 18 months of therapy. HIV isolates obtained from patients with advanced disease who have received ZDV for more than 6 months show high rates of resistance to ZDV in vitro, which may play a role in clinical failures of ZDV. The development of resistance appears to be less frequent in asymptomatic patients or in patients with less advanced disease. ZDV resistance is associated with specific amino acid substitutions in the HIV reverse transcriptase.

The most frequently employed dosage of ZDV is 200 mg by mouth every 8 h, and comparative dosage studies indicate that total daily doses of 500 to 600 mg are as effective and less toxic than higher doses which had been previously recommended. The major toxicities of ZDV are hematopoietic, particularly anemia and granulocytopenia, which occur more frequently in patients with more advanced HIV disease. Nausea, headache, and malaise are also encountered frequently, and a ZDV-related myopathy also can occur.

DIDANOSINE   Didanosine (or ddI) is a nucleoside analogue with antiviral activity against HIV-1 and HIV-2. It is an inhibitor of the HIV reverse transcriptase and also can act as a chain terminator for viral DNA elongation. ddI is phosphorylated and converted to ddATP, which is the active antiviral moiety. ddI is active in vitro against most HIV isolates which are resistant to ZDV.

ddI is given orally and is highly acid labile, so it must be administered with buffers against stomach acidity. These buffers are incorporated into the powder or tablet preparations. ddI in tablets is 20 to 25 percent more bioavailable than in powder. The plasma half-life of ddI is 1.5 h, and approximately 50 percent of a dose is cleared by renal mechanisms. The intracellular half-life of ddATP is considerably longer (8 to 24 h) and provides the rationale for the recommended dosing schedule of every 12 h.

ddI has been carefully studied in phase I trials and has received extensive use in a large-scale ''expanded access'' program under which more than 22,000 patients with HIV infection have received the drug. On the basis of a favorable effect on circulating CD4 counts and serum p24 concentrations in the phase I studies and of an interim analysis of an ongoing phase II study, ddI has been licensed for patients who are intolerant of ZDV therapy or who are failing clinically or immunologically on ZDV treatment. Controlled studies comparing ddI and ZDV are nearing completion and should provide important information regarding the clinical efficacy and appropriate use of this drug.

The major toxicities encountered in the use of ddI have been pancreatitis and peripheral neuropathy. Overall rates of pancreatitis in recipients of ddI have been estimated to be 5 to 9 percent, and cases occur more frequently in patients with advanced HIV disease.

Most cases are mild to moderate in severity, but fatal cases have occurred, though rarely. Painful peripheral neuropathy, primarily involving the lower extremities, also may develop and is generally reversible if recognized early and if drug administration is stopped. Medications or other factors which can cause pancreatitis or peripheral neuropathy should be avoided in patients who are taking ddI. ddI has not been associated with consistent hematopoietic toxicity, and in fact, hemoglobin, white blood cell, and platelet counts frequently improve on ddI therapy. Thus ddI may be particularly useful in the setting where hematopoietic suppression is present or anticipated, either from drugs or from underlying diseases.

ZALCITABINE AND OTHER ANTIRETROVIRAL DRUGS Zalcitabine (or ddC) is a nucleoside analogue which is a potent inhibitor of HIV. The triphosphate of ddC (ddCTP) inhibits HIV reverse transcriptase activity and also acts as a chain terminator. ddC is administered orally, has a plasma half-life of 1.2 h, and is excreted primarily by the kidney. A recently concluded study comparing ddC with ZDV in patients who had received less than 3 months of ZDV showed that ddC was less effective than ZDV in prevention of opportunistic infections and neoplasms. The major toxicities of ddC are a dose-related peripheral neuropathy and aphthous stomatitis. Hematologic toxicities, as manifested by anemia and neutropenia, were not major problems. Recently, phase I studies of combinations of ZDV and ddC have demonstrated a favorable effect on CD4 counts and p24 concentrations, and large-scale clinical trials of this combination are underway. ddC has recently been licensed for use in combination with ZDV to treat patients with advanced HIV infection who are failing clinically or immunologically on ZDV alone.

A variety of other antiretroviral drugs are at various stages of preclinical and early (phase I) clinical development. These include reverse transcriptase inhibitors of the nucleoside analogue class such as d4T and nonnucleoside inhibitors such as TIBO or BI-RG-587. Compounds that interfere with HIV binding or with replication at other sites such as inhibitors of viral protease, inhibitors of protein glycosylation (N-butyl-deoxynojirimycin), and inhibitors of HIV tat protein are also under development.

VIDARABINE Vidarabine (9-β-D-arabinofuranosyladenine) is a purine nucleoside analogue with activity against HSV-1, HSV-2, VZV, and EBV. Vidarabine inhibits viral DNA synthesis through its 5′-triphosphorylated metabolite, although the precise molecular mechanisms of action are not completely understood. In the therapy of herpes zoster in immunosuppressed patients, vidarabine, administered in a dose of 10 mg/kg per day for 5 days, resulted in reduction of rates of cutaneous and visceral dissemination and of postherpetic neuralgia but was less effective overall than acyclovir in a comparative trial. Beneficial effects also have been observed in the treatment of varicella in immunosuppressed patients. Vidarabine administered in a higher dose (15 mg/kg per day for 10 days) was demonstrated to be effective in the therapy of herpes simplex encephalitis in a placebo-controlled study, but comparative studies indicate that acyclovir (30 mg/kg per day) is the drug of choice for this infection. Vidarabine appears to be equal in efficacy to acyclovir in the treatment of neonatal herpes simplex infection. The ophthalmic ointment of vidarabine (3%) is effective in the treatment of HSV keratitis.

For systemic administration, vidarabine is available only as an intravenous preparation with poor solubility and is administered as a constant 12-h infusion, so a substantial fluid load can result which may be a significant problem in central nervous system infections. Vidarabine at doses of 10 to 15 mg/kg per day is generally well tolerated, but at somewhat higher doses (20 mg/kg per day) the drug has been associated with hematopoietic side effects, including anemia, leukopenia, and thrombocytopenia. Neurotoxicity also has been reported, particularly with high dosages and in patients with hepatic or renal insufficiency.

TOPICAL ANTIVIRALS IUdR (5′-iodo-2′-deoxyuridine) is an inhibitor of DNA virus replication, including herpesviruses and poxviruses. It was formerly used systemically to treat herpesvirus infections, including HSV encephalitis, but because of associated toxicity and lack of demonstrated efficacy, its systemic use has largely been abandoned. Topical IUdR has been effective in the treatment of HSV keratitis, particularly in superficial epithelial infections, but has been largely supplanted by topically applied trifluorothymidine or vidarabine.

Trifluorothymidine (TFT) is an analogue of deoxythymidine, which is also effective against herpesvirus infections. Because of bone marrow suppression, its use is restricted to topical application in the eye, where it appears to be somewhat more effective and better tolerated than IUdR and at least as effective as vidarabine. TFT also has been effective in some patients who had not responded clinically to topical IUdR or vidarabine.

INTERFERONS From its earliest descriptions, considerable interest has existed in the application of interferon to the prophylaxis and/ or therapy of viral infections. Interferons are cytokines with broad antiviral activities, as well as immunomodulating and antiproliferative properties. Early studies with human leukocyte interferon demonstrated an effect in the prophylaxis of experimentally induced rhinovirus infections in humans and in the treatment of varicella-zoster infections in immunosuppressed patients. DNA recombinant technology has made available highly purified α-, β-, and γ-interferons, which have been evaluated in a variety of viral infections. Results of such trials have confirmed the effectiveness of intranasally administered interferon in the prophylaxis of rhinovirus infections, although its use has been associated with nasal mucosal irritation. Recent studies also have demonstrated a beneficial effect of parenterally administered interferons on genital warts, primarily in reduction of size of lesions, and this mode of therapy may be useful in individuals who have numerous warts which cannot easily be treated by individual intralesional injection. However, lesions frequently recur after intralesional or parenteral interferon therapy is discontinued.

Interferons also have received extensive study in the therapy of chronic hepatitis B infection. Interferon α2b administered to patients with stable chronic hepatitis B infection resulted in loss of markers of HBV replication, such as HBeAg and HBV DNA, in 40 to 50 percent of patients who received daily doses of 5 million units for 16 weeks; 10 to 20 percent of patients also became HBsAg negative. More than 80 percent of patients who lose HBeAg and HBV DNA markers will have return of serum aminotransferases to normal levels, and both short- and long-term improvement in liver histopathology has been described. Predictors of a favorable response to therapy include low pretherapy HBV DNA levels, high pretherapy serum ALT levels, short duration of chronic hepatitis B infection, and active liver histopathology. Adverse effects of the preceding dose of interferon are common and include fever, chills, myalgia, and fatigue. Approximately 25 percent of patients receiving a daily dose of 5 million units will require dose reduction, but fewer than 5 percent will require discontinuation of therapy.

Several interferon preparations, including α2a, α2b, and αL (lymphoblastoid) have been studied as therapy for chronic non-A, non-B/C infections. A variety of dose regimens have been employed, of which the most common is 1 or 3 million units three times per week for 6 months. A complete response, defined as a return to normal serum ALT values at the end of treatment, has been observed in approximately 40 percent of patients. Liver biopsies also showed decrease of lobular and periportal inflammation. However, relapse occurred in half or more of the patients when therapy was discontinued. Relapses have generally responded quickly to retreatment. Additional clinical studies to develop more effective regimens of therapy and to define prognostic variables in this patient population are currently underway.

Interferon is licensed in the United States for the treatment of chronic hepatitis B (α2b), chronic hepatitis non-A, non-B/C infection (α2b), condyloma acuminatum (α2b, αn3), hairy-cell leukemia (α2a, α2b) and Kaposi's sarcoma (α2a, α2b). Interferon-γ (γ1b) is licensed for the treatment of patients with chronic granulomatous disease.

REFERENCES

DAVIS GL et al: Treatment of chronic hepatitis with recombinant interferon alfa: A multicenter randomized, controlled trial. N Engl J Med 32:1501, 1989

DOLIN R et al: A controlled trial of amantadine and rimantadine in the prophylaxis of influenza A infection. N Engl J Med 307:580, 1982

FAULDS D, HEEL RC: Ganciclovir: A review of its antiviral activity, pharmacokinetic properties, and therapeutic efficacy in cytomegalovirus infections. Drugs 39:597, 1990

FISCHL M et al: The efficacy of azidothymidine (AZT) in the treatment of patients with AIDS and AIDS-related complex; a double blind placebo-controlled trial. N Engl J Med 317:185, 1987

HALL CB et al: Aerosolized ribavirin treatment of infants with respiratory syncytial viral infection: A randomized double blind study. N Engl J Med 308:1443, 1983

MERTZ GJ et al: Double blind placebo-controlled trial of oral acyclovir in first episode genital herpes simplex infection. JAMA 252:147, 1984

PALESTINE AG et al: A randomized, controlled trial in the treatment of cytomegalovirus retinitis in patients with AIDS. Ann Intern Med 115:669, 1991

PERILLO RP et al: A randomized, controlled trial of interferon alfa-2b alone and after prednisone withdrawal, in the treatment of chronic hepatitis B infection. N Engl J Med 323:295, 1990

REICHMAN RL et al: Treatment of condyloma acuminatum with three different interferons administered intralesionally: A double-blind, placebo-controlled trial. Ann Intern Med 108:675, 1988

VOLBERDING P et al: Zidovudine in asymptomatic human immunodeficiency virus infection: A controlled trial in persons with fewer than 500 CD4-positive cells per cubic millimeter. N Engl J Med 322:941, 1990

WHITLEY RJ et al and the NIAID Collaborative Antiviral Study Group: Herpes simplex encephalitis: Adenine arabinoside versus acyclovir therapies. N Engl J Med 314:144, 1986

YARCHOAN R et al: Long term toxicity/activity profile of 2'3'-dideoxyinosine in AIDS and AIDS related complex. Lancet 336:526, 1990

section 12   DNA viruses

143   HERPES SIMPLEX VIRUSES

LAWRENCE COREY

DEFINITION Herpes simplex viruses (HSV-1, HSV-2; *Herpesvirus hominis*) produce a variety of infections involving mucocutaneous surfaces, the central nervous system, and occasionally visceral organs. The advent of effective antiviral chemotherapy for HSV infections has made prompt recognition of these syndromes of clinical importance.

ETIOLOGY The genome of herpes simplex virus is a linear, double-stranded DNA molecule (about 100×10^6 in molecular weight) that encodes for more than 60 gene products. The genomic structures of the two HSV subtypes are similar, and the overall sequence homology between HSV-1 and HSV-2 is about 50 percent. The homologous sequences are distributed over the entire genome map, and most of the polypeptides specified by one viral type are antigenically related to polypeptides of the other viral type. Many type-specific regions unique to HSV-1 and HSV-2 proteins do exist, however, and many of these regions appear to be important in host immunity. Restriction endonuclease analysis of viral DNA can be utilized to distinguish between the two subtypes and among strains of the two subtypes. The variability of nucleotide sequences from clinical strains of HSV-1 and HSV-2 is such that HSV isolates obtained from two individuals can be differentiated by restriction enzyme patterns unless the isolates are from epidemiologically related sources, such as sexual partners, mother-infant pairs, or common-source outbreaks.

The viral genome is packaged within a regular icosahedral protein shell (capsid) composed of 162 capsomers. The outer covering of the virus is a lipid-containing membrane (envelope) derived from modified cell membrane and acquired as the DNA-containing capsid buds through the inner nuclear membrane of the host cell. Between the capsid and lipid bilayer of the envelope is the tegument, composed of a number of viral proteins whose properties and functions are largely unknown. Viral replication has both nuclear and cytoplasmic phases. The initial steps of replication include attachment, fusion between the viral envelope and a cell membrane to liberate the nucleocapsid into the cytoplasm of the cell, and disassembly of the nucleocapsid to release the viral DNA. Replication of HSV is highly regulated. Following fusion of the virion envelope with the host cell membrane, two proteins are released from the HSV virion. HSV shuts off host protein synthesis, and α TIF, a γ gene product, "turns on" transcription of the α genes (immediate early). The presence of the α-gene products is required for synthesis of the subsequent polypeptide group, the β polypeptides, many of which are regulatory proteins and enzymes required for DNA replication. Most current antiviral drugs interrupt β proteins such as the viral DNA polymerase enzyme. The third (γ) class of HSV genes requires viral DNA replication for expression and constitutes most of the structural proteins specified by the virus.

Following replication of the viral genome and synthesis of structural proteins, nucleocapsids are assembled in the nucleus of the cell. Envelopment occurs as the nucleocapsids bud through the inner nuclear membrane into the perinuclear space. In some cells, viral replication within the nucleus forms two types of inclusion bodies: type A basophilic Feulgen-positive bodies that contain viral DNA and an eosinophilic inclusion body that is devoid of viral nucleic acid or protein and represents a "scar" of viral infection. Virions are then transported via the endoplasmic reticulum and the Golgi apparatus to the cell surface.

HSV infection of some neuronal cells does not result in cell death. Instead, viral genomes are maintained by the cell in a repressed state compatible with survival and normal activities of the cell, a process called *latency*. Subsequently, activation of the viral genome may occur, resulting in viral replication and, in some cases, the redevelopment of herpetic lesions, a process termed *reactivation*. Whereas infectious virus rarely can be recovered from sensory or autonomic nervous system ganglia dissected from cadavers, maintenance and growth of the neural cells in tissue culture result in production of infectious virions, a process called *explantation*, and subsequent permissive infection of susceptible cells, a process called *cocultivation*. Virus replication was first detected in neurons during reactivation in vitro, suggesting that the neuron harbors the latent virus in vivo. Subsequently, viral DNA has been found in neural tissue at times when infectious virus cannot be isolated. HSV DNA extracted from latently infected neural tissue differs from HSV DNA in cells with actively replicating virus. In latently infected cells, only partial transcription of viral proteins occurs. Two RNA transcripts which overlap the immediate early (α) gene product, called ICP-o, are found in abundance in the nuclei of latently infected neurons. The coding of these RNA transcripts in an "antisense" direction suggests that they may be a factor in inhibiting the subsequent transcription of β and γ proteins. Deletion mutants of this region have been made. While these viruses can become latent, the efficiency of their subsequent reactivation is reduced; thus the "antisense" transcripts may play a role in maintaining rather than in establishing latency. Understanding molecular mechanisms of latency may lead to new therapies to prevent reactivation of HSV.

PATHOGENESIS Exposure to virus at mucosal surfaces or abraded skin permits entry of virus and initiation of replication in cells of the epidermis and dermis. Whether or not clinically apparent lesions develop, sufficient viral replication to permit infection of either sensory or autonomic nerve endings may occur. Whether latency always results from peripheral mucosal infection is unclear. Virus—or, more likely, nucleocapsid—is then thought to be transported intraaxonally to the nerve cell bodies in ganglia. In humans, the time from inoculation of virus in peripheral tissue to spread to the ganglia is unknown. During the initial phase of infection, viral replication occurs in ganglia and contiguous neural tissue. Virus then spreads to other mucosal skin surfaces through centrifugal migration of infectious virions via peripheral sensory nerves. This spread of virus to the skin from peripheral sensory nerves helps explain the large surface area, the high frequency of new lesions distant from the initial crop of vesicles which are characteristic in patients with primary genital or oral-labial HSV infection, and the recovery of virus from neural tissue distant from neurons innervating the inoculation site. Contiguous spread of locally inoculated virus also may occur and allow further mucosal extension of disease.

Following resolution of primary disease, infectious virus can no longer be recovered in the ganglia. The mechanisms by which various stimuli cause reactivation of HSV infection are unknown. Ultraviolet light, immunosuppression, and trauma to the skin or ganglia are associated with reactivation.

Analysis of the HSV DNA from sequentially isolated strains of HSV or from multiple infected ganglia in any one individual has revealed identical restriction endonuclease patterns in most persons. Occasionally, and more frequently in immunocompromised persons, multiple strains of the same viral subtype can be detected in the same person. This finding suggests that exogenous infection with different strains of the same subtype is possible.

IMMUNITY Host responses to infection influence the acquisition of disease, severity of infection, resistance to development of latency, maintenance of latency, and frequency of HSV recurrences. Both antibody-mediated and cell-mediated reactions are clinically important. Immunocompromised patients with defects in cell-mediated immunity experience more severe and extensive HSV infections than those with deficits in humoral immunity such as agammaglobulinemia. Experimental ablation of lymphocytes indicates that T cells play a major role in preventing lethal disseminated disease, although antibodies help reduce virus titers in neural tissue. Some aspects of the pathogenesis of disease also may be related to the host immune response, e.g., stromal opacities associated with recurrent herpetic keratitis. The surface viral glycoproteins have been shown to be antigens recognized by antibodies mediating neutralization and immune-mediated cytolysis (antibody-dependent cell-mediated cytotoxicity, ADCC). Monoclonal antibodies specific for each of the known viral glycoproteins have, in experimental infections, conferred protection against subsequent neurologic disease or ganglionic latency. Multiple cell populations, including natural killer (NK) cells, macrophages, a variety of T lymphocyte populations, and lymphokines generated by these cells, play a role in host defenses to HSV infections. In animals, passive transfer of primed lymphocytes confers protection from subsequent challenge. Maximum protection usually requires the activation of multiple T cell subpopulations, including cytotoxic T cells and T cells responsible for delayed hypersensitivity. The latter cells may confer protection by the antigen-stimulated release of lymphokines (e.g., interferons), which may have a direct antiviral effect or activate other nonspecific effector cells.

EPIDEMIOLOGY Seroepidemiologic studies have shown that HSV infections are found worldwide. Because much of the humoral immune response to HSV is to type-common antigenic determinants, it is difficult to detect HSV-2 antibodies in persons with prior HSV-1 infection and HSV-1 antibodies in those with prior HSV-2 infections. Serologic assays which utilize whole-virus antigen preparations, such as complement fixation, neutralization, indirect immunofluorescence assay (IFA), passive hemagglutination (PHA), radioimmunoassay

(RIA), and enzyme-linked immunosorbent assay (ELISA), do not reliably distinguish between the two viral subtypes. Recently, serologic assays which identify antibodies to type-specific surface proteins of the two viruses have been developed. These assays can reliably distinguish the human antibody response between HSV-1 and HSV-2. These assays are based on demonstrating antibodies to type-specific epitopes of the virus; the most commonly utilized are those which measure antibodies to glycoprotein G of HSV-1 (gGl) and HSV-2 (gG2). At present, these assays are available only in a limited number of laboratories.

Infection with HSV-1 is acquired more frequently and earlier than infection with HSV-2. Over 90 percent of adults have antibodies to HSV-1 by the fifth decade. In lower socioeconomic populations, most persons will acquire HSV-1 infection before the third decade.

Antibodies to HSV-2 are not routinely detected until puberty. Antibody prevalence rates correlate with past sexual activity and vary greatly among different population groups. In most routine obstetrical and family planning clinics, 20 to 30 percent of women possess HSV-2 antibodies, although only 10 percent report a history of genital lesions. As many as 50 percent of heterosexual adults attending STD clinics possess HSV-2 antibodies. In university clinics, HSV antibody prevalence may be as low as 3 to 8 percent. Antibody prevalence rates average about 5 percent higher in women than in men. The large reservoir of unidentified carriers of HSV-2 and the frequent asymptomatic reactivation of virus from the genital tract have fostered the continued spread of genital herpes throughout the world. HSV-2 infection has been shown to be a risk factor for the acquisition and transmission of infection with human immunodeficiency virus type 1 (HIV-1).

HSV infections occur throughout the year. The incubation period ranges from 1 to 26 days (median 6 to 8 days). Contact with active ulcerative lesions or asymptomatically excreting patients can result in transmission. Asymptomatic salivary excretion of HSV-1 has been reported in 2 to 9 percent of adults and 5 to 8 percent of children. HSV-2 has been isolated from the genital tract of 0.3 to 6 percent of males and 1.5 to 13 percent of females attending STD clinics. The titer of HSV in cultures from lesions is 100 to 1000 times higher than from salivary or genital tract secretions in asymptomatically excreting persons. The efficiency of transmission is greater during symptomatic than asymptomatic periods of viral excretion.

CLINICAL SPECTRUM HSV has been isolated from nearly all visceral or mucocutaneous sites. The clinical manifestations and course of HSV depend on the anatomic site of the infection, the age and immune status of the host, and the antigenic type of the virus. First episodes of HSV disease, especially primary infections (i.e., first infections with either HSV-1 or HSV-2 in which the host lacks HSV antibodies in acute-phase sera), are frequently accompanied by systemic signs and symptoms, involve both mucosal and extramucosal sites, and have a longer duration of symptoms, a longer time during which virus is isolated from lesions, and a higher rate of complications than recurrent episodes of disease. Both viral subtypes can cause genital and oral-facial infections, and these infections are clinically indistinguishable. However, the frequency of future reactivations of infection is influenced by the anatomic site and virus type. Genital HSV-2 infection is twice as likely to reactivate and will recur 8 to 10 times more frequently than genital HSV-1 infection. Conversely, oral-labial HSV-1 infections will recur more frequently than oral-labial HSV-2 infections.

Oral-facial HSV infections Gingivostomatitis and pharyngitis are the most frequent clinical manifestations of first-episode HSV-1 infection, while recurrent herpes labialis is the most frequent clinical manifestation of reactivation HSV infection. HSV pharyngitis and gingivostomatitis usually result from primary infection and are most commonly seen in children and young adults. Clinical symptoms and signs include fever, malaise, myalgias, inability to eat, irritability, and cervical adenopathy, which may last from 3 to 14 days. Lesions may involve the hard and soft palate, gingiva, tongue, lip, and facial area. HSV-1 or HSV-2 infection of the pharynx usually results in exudative or ulcerative lesions of the posterior pharynx and/or tonsillar pillars. Concomitant lesions of the tongue, buccal mucosa, or gingiva may occur later in the course in one-third of cases. Fever lasting from 2 to 7 days and cervical adenopathy are common. The clinical differentiation of HSV pharyngitis from bacterial pharyngitis, *Mycoplasma pneumoniae* infections, and noninfectious causes of pharyngeal ulcerations such as Stevens-Johnson syndrome may be difficult. No substantial evidence suggests that reactivation oral-labial HSV infection is associated with symptomatic recurrent pharyngitis.

Reactivation of HSV from the trigeminal ganglia may be associated with asymptomatic excretion in the saliva, development of intraoral mucosal ulcerations, or herpetic ulcerations on the vermilion border of the lip or external facial skin. About 50 to 70 percent of seropositive patients undergoing trigeminal nerve root decompression and 10 to 15 percent of those undergoing dental extraction will develop oral-labial HSV infection a median of 3 days after these procedures.

In immunosuppressed patients infection may extend into mucosal and deep cutaneous layers. Friability, necrosis, bleeding, severe pain, and inability to eat or drink may result. HSV mucositis is clinically similar to mucosal lesions due to cytotoxic drug therapy, trauma, or fungal or bacterial infections. Persistent ulcerative HSV infections are among the most common infections in patients with AIDS. Concomitant HSV and *Candida* infections also occur commonly. Systemic acyclovir therapy speeds the rate of healing and relieves the pain of mucosal HSV infections in immunosuppressed patients. Patients with atopic eczema also may develop severe oral-facial HSV infections (eczema herpeticum) which may rapidly involve extensive areas of skin and occasionally disseminate to visceral organs. Prompt resolution of extensive eczema herpeticum has been achieved with the administration of intravenous acyclovir. Erythema multiforme (EM) also may be associated with HSV infections, and some evidence suggests that HSV infection is the precipitating event in about 75 percent of cases of cutaneous EM. HSV antigen has been demonstrated both in circulatory immune complexes and in skin lesion biopsy of these patients. Patients with severe HSV-associated EM are candidates for chronic suppressive oral acyclovir therapy.

Genital HSV infections First-episode primary genital herpes is characterized by fever, headache, malaise, and myalgias. Pain, itching, dysuria, vaginal and urethral discharge, and tender inguinal lymphadenopathy are the predominant local symptoms. Characteristically, widely spaced bilateral lesions of the external genitalia are seen. Lesions may be present in varying stages, including vesicles, pustules, or painful erythematous ulcers. Involvement of the cervix and urethra is seen in over 80 percent of women with first-episode infections. First episodes of genital herpes in patients who have had prior HSV-1 infection are associated with less frequent systemic symptoms and faster healing than primary genital herpes. The clinical courses of acute first-episode genital herpes among patients with HSV-1 and HSV-2 infections are similar. However, the recurrence rates of genital disease differ. About 90 percent of patients with first-episode HSV-2 infection will have a recurrence within 12 months (median number of recurrences, four) compared with 55 percent of those with primary HSV-1 infections (median number of recurrences, less than one). Recurrence rates of genital HSV-2 infections vary greatly between individuals and over time within the same individual. HSV has been isolated from the urethra and urine of men and women without concomitant external genital lesions. A clear mucoid discharge and dysuria are characteristics of symptomatic HSV urethritis. HSV has been isolated from the urethra of 5 percent of women with the dysuria-frequency syndrome. Occasionally, genital tract disease manifested by HSV endometritis and salpingitis in women and HSV prostatitis in men may occur.

Both HSV-1 and HSV-2 can cause symptomatic or asymptomatic rectal and perianal infections. Symptoms of HSV proctitis include anorectal pain, anorectal discharge, tenesmus, and constipation. Sigmoidoscopy reveals ulcerative lesions of the distal 10 cm of the rectal mucosa. Rectal biopsies show mucosal ulceration, necrosis, polymorphonuclear and lymphocytic infiltration of the lamina propria,

and occasionally multinucleated intranuclear inclusion–bearing cells. Perianal herpetic lesions are also seen in immunosuppressed patients receiving cytotoxic therapy. Either HSV-1 or HSV-2 can cause perianal herpes. The HSV-1 strains isolated from perianal lesions are often identical to those found in the oropharynx. This finding suggests that the mode of spread is autoinoculation of the perianal area from HSV-infected saliva and/or finger lesions. Replication of HSV-2 from sacral nerve root ganglia may lead to extensive perianal herpetic lesions and/or HSV proctitis among patients with HIV infection or those undergoing transplantation. Chronic acyclovir therapy is often used to suppress such recurrences.

Herpetic whitlow Herpetic whitlow, HSV infection of the finger, may occur as a complication of primary oral or genital herpes by inoculation of virus via a break in the epidermal surface or by direct introduction of virus into the hand through occupational or other exposure. Clinical signs and symptoms include the abrupt onset of edema, erythema, and localized tenderness of the infected finger. Vesicular or pustular lesions of the fingertip indistinguishable from pyogenic bacterial infection are seen. Fever, lymphadenitis, and epitrochlear and axillary lymphadenopathy are common. The infection may recur. Prompt diagnosis to avoid unnecessary and potentially exacerbating surgical therapy and/or transmission is essential.

Herpes gladiatorum HSV may infect almost any area of skin. Mucocutaneous HSV infections of the thorax, ears, face, and hands have been described among wrestlers. Transmission of these infections is facilitated by trauma to the skin sustained during wrestling. Prompt diagnosis and therapy are required to contain spread of this infection.

Herpetic eye infections HSV infection of the eye is the most frequent cause of corneal blindness in the United States. HSV keratitis presents with acute onset of pain, blurring of vision, chemosis, conjunctivitis, and characteristic dendritic lesions of the cornea. Use of topical corticosteroids may exacerbate symptoms and lead to involvement of deep structures of the eye. Debridement, topical antiviral treatment, and/or interferon therapy hastens healing. However, recurrences are common, and immunopathologic injury of the deeper structures of the eye may occur. Chorioretinitis, usually as a manifestation of disseminated HSV infection, may occur in neonates or in patients with HIV infection. Acute necrotizing retinitis due to HSV is an uncommon but severe manifestation of HSV infection.

Central and peripheral nervous system infections with HSV-1 and HSV-2 HSV encephalitis is the most common identified cause of acute, sporadic viral encephalitis in the United States, comprising 10 to 20 percent of all cases. The estimated incidence is about 2.3 cases per million persons per year. Cases are distributed throughout the year, and the age distribution appears biphasic, with peaks at 5 to 30 and >50 years of age. HSV-1 accounts for more than 95 percent of cases. The pathogenesis of HSV encephalitis varies. In children and young adults, primary HSV infection may result in encephalitis; presumably, exogenously acquired virus enters the CNS by neurotropic spread from the periphery via the olfactory bulb. However, most adults with HSV encephalitis have clinical or serologic evidence of mucocutaneous HSV-1 infection prior to the onset of the CNS symptoms. In about 25 percent of the cases examined, the HSV-1 strains from the oropharynx and brain tissue of the same patient differ; thus some cases may result from reinfection with another strain of HSV-1 that reaches the CNS. Two theories have been proposed to explain the development of actively replicating HSV in localized areas of the CNS in persons from whom the ganglionic and CNS isolates are similar. Reactivation of latent trigeminal or autonomic nerve root HSV-1 infection may be associated with extension of virus into the CNS via nerves innervating the middle cranial fossa. HSV DNA has been demonstrated by DNA hybridization in human autopsy brain tissue. Reactivation of long-standing latent CNS infection may be another potential mechanism for the development of HSV encephalitis.

The clinical hallmark of HSV encephalitis has been the acute onset of fever and focal neurologic, especially temporal lobe, symptoms. Differentiation of HSV encephalitis from other viral encephalitides, as well as from other focal infections and noninfectious processes, is difficult. An increase in CSF and serum antibodies to HSV does occur with most cases of HSV encephalitis. However, these increased antibody titers rarely are present prior to 10 days into the illness and, while useful retrospectively, are usually not helpful in establishing the clinical diagnosis early in the course of disease. Demonstration of HSV antigen or DNA in brain biopsy has a high sensitivity and a low complication rate and also provides the best opportunity to diagnose and establish alternative, potentially treatable causes of encephalitis. The most sensitive early noninvasive method for diagnosing HSV encephalitis is the demonstration of HSV DNA in CSF by polymerase chain reaction (PCR). Antiviral chemotherapy reduces the mortality of HSV encephalitis, and intravenous acyclovir is more effective than vidarabine. Even with therapy, however, neurologic sequelae are frequent, especially in those over 35 years of age. Most authorities recommend initiating intravenous acyclovir treatment in patients with presumed HSV encephalitis until the diagnosis is confirmed or an alternative diagnosis is made.

HSV has been isolated from the cerebrospinal fluid (CSF) of 0.5 to 3 percent of patients presenting to the hospital with aseptic meningitis. HSV meningitis is usually seen in association with primary genital HSV infection. HSV meningitis is an acute, self-limited disease manifested by headache, fever, and mild photophobia and lasting from 2 to 7 days. A lymphocytic pleocytosis in the CSF is characteristic. Neurologic sequelae are rare. Recurrent bouts of aseptic meningitis related to reactivation of HSV have been reported.

Autonomic nervous system dysfunction, especially of the sacral region, has been reported in association with both HSV and varicella-zoster infections. Numbness, tingling of the buttock or perineal areas, urinary retention, constipation, CSF pleocytosis, and impotence in males may occur. Symptoms appear to resolve slowly over a period of days to weeks. Occasionally, hypesthesia and/or weakness of the lower extremities may persist for many months. Rarely, transverse myelitis manifested by a rapidly progressive symmetric paralysis of the lower extremities or a Guillain-Barré syndrome may occur after HSV infection. Similarly, peripheral nervous system involvement [idiopathic facial paralysis (Bell's palsy)] or cranial polyneuritis also may be related to reactivation of HSV-1 infection. Transitory hypesthesia of the area of skin innervated by the trigeminal nerve and vestibular system dysfunction as measured by electronystagmography are the predominant signs of disease. Studies to determine if antiviral chemotherapy may abort or alleviate the frequency and severity of these signs are unavailable.

Visceral infections HSV infection of visceral organs usually results from viremia, and multiple organ involvement is common. Occasionally, however, the clinical manifestations of HSV infection may involve only the esophagus, lung, or liver. HSV esophagitis may result from direct extension of oral-pharyngeal HSV infection into the esophagus or may occur de novo by reactivation of HSV and spread of virus to the esophageal mucosa via the vagus nerve. The predominant symptoms of HSV esophagitis are odynophagia, dysphagia, substernal pain, and weight loss. There are multiple oval ulcerations on an erythematous base with or without a patchy white pseudomembrane. The distal esophagus is most commonly involved. With extensive disease, diffuse friability may spread to the entire esophagus. Neither endoscopic nor barium examination can differentiate HSV esophagitis from *Candida* esophagitis or from esophageal ulcerations due to thermal injury, radiation, and corrosives. Endoscopically obtained secretions for cytologic examination and culture provide the most useful material for diagnosis. Systemic antiviral chemotherapy usually reduces symptoms and heals esophageal ulcerations.

HSV pneumonitis is uncommon except in severely immunosuppressed patients and may result from extension of herpetic tracheobronchitis into lung parenchyma. Focal necrotizing pneumonitis usually results. Hematogenous dissemination of virus from oral or genital mucocutaneous disease also may occur and produce a bilateral interstitial pneumonitis. Concomitant bacterial, fungal, and parasitic pathogens are common in HSV pneumonitis. Since the mortality of HSV pneumonia in immunosuppressed patients is high (>80 percent), these patients should be candidates for antiviral chemotherapy. HSV also has been isolated from the lower respiratory tract of persons with acute respiratory distress syndrome (ARDS). However, the relationship between isolation of HSV and the pathogenesis of the respiratory distress syndrome is unclear.

HSV is an uncommon cause of hepatitis in immunocompetent patients. HSV infection of the liver is associated with fever, abrupt elevations of bilirubin and the serum transaminases, and leukopenia (white blood cells <4000 per microliter). Disseminated intravascular coagulation also may be present.

Other isolated but reported complications of HSV include monarticular arthritis, adrenal necrosis, idiopathic thrombocytopenia, and glomerulonephritis. Disseminated HSV infection in the immunocompetent patient is rare. In immunocompromised, burn, or malnourished patients, dissemination of HSV to other visceral organs such as adrenal glands, pancreas, small and large intestine, and bone marrow may occur occasionally. Rarely, primary HSV infection in pregnancy may disseminate and may be associated with mortality in both mother and fetus. This uncommon event is usually associated with acquisition of primary infection in the third trimester.

Neonatal HSV infection Neonates (<6 weeks of age) have the highest frequency of visceral and/or CNS infection of any HSV-infected patient population. Untreated, over 70 percent of neonatal herpes cases will disseminate or develop into CNS infection. Without therapy, the overall mortality of neonatal herpes is 65 percent, and less than 10 percent of neonates with CNS infection experience normal development. While skin lesions are the most commonly recognized features of disease, many infants do not develop lesions until well into the course of disease. Seventy percent of neonatal HSV cases are caused by HSV-2 infection, almost all of which result from contact via infected genital secretions at the time of delivery. However, congenitally infected infants have been reported, usually from mothers who acquired primary HSV infection during pregnancy. Neonatal HSV-1 infections may be acquired from genital HSV-1 infection in the mother, through postnatal contact with immediate family members with symptomatic or asymptomatic oral-labial HSV-1 infection, or from nosocomial transmission within the hospital. Antiviral chemotherapy has reduced the mortality of neonatal herpes to 25 percent. However, the morbidity, especially in infants with HSV-2 CNS involvement, is still very high.

DIAGNOSIS Both clinical and laboratory criteria are useful for establishing the diagnosis of HSV infections. Clinical diagnosis can be made accurately where characteristic multiple vesicular lesions on an erythematous base are present. Scrapings of the base of the lesions and subsequent staining with Wright, Giemsa (Tzanck preparation), or Papanicolaou's stain will demonstrate characteristic giant cells or intranuclear inclusions of a herpesvirus infection. These cytologic techniques are often useful as a quick office procedure to confirm the diagnosis. Limitations of this method are that it does not differentiate between HSV and varicella-zoster infections and is only about 60 percent as sensitive as viral isolation. The laboratory confirmation of HSV infection is best performed by isolation of virus in tissue culture or demonstration of HSV antigens in scrapings from lesions. HSV causes a discernible cytopathic effect in a variety of cell culture systems, and most specimens can be identified within 48 to 96 h after inoculation. Spin-amplified culture with subsequent staining for HSV antigen has shortened the time needed to identify HSV to less than 24 h. The sensitivity of viral isolation varies with the stage of lesions (higher in vesicular than in ulcerative lesions), whether the patient has a first or recurrent episode of the disease (higher in first episodes), and whether the sample is from an immunosuppressed or immunocompetent patient (more antigen in immunosuppressed). IFA, ELISA, and some DNA hybridization procedures have approached the sensitivity of viral isolation for detecting HSV from genital or oral-labial lesions but appear only about 50 percent as sensitive as viral isolation for the detection of asymptomatic HSV in cervical or salivary secretions. HSV PCR techniques may be more sensitive than viral isolation. Laboratory confirmation allows for subtyping the virus, which may be useful epidemiologically as well as in helping to predict the frequency of reactivation after first-episode oral-labial or genital HSV infection. Restriction endonuclease analysis of viral DNA can be used to differentiate between HSV-1 and HSV-2 as well as to differentiate between strains within the same subtypes; the latter information may be very useful in identifying common-source outbreaks of HSV.

Acute and convalescent serum can be useful in documenting seroconversion during primary HSV-1 or HSV-2 infection. However, only 5 percent of patients with recurrent mucocutaneous HSV infections show a fourfold or greater rise in anti-HSV antibodies between acute and convalescent sera. Serologic assays, especially type-specific assays, should be utilized to identify asymptomatic carriers of HSV-1 or HSV-2 infection, and such carriers should be counseled about the risk of transmission.

THERAPY Many aspects of mucocutaneous and visceral HSV infections are amenable to antiviral chemotherapy. For mucocutaneous infections, acyclovir has been the mainstay of therapy. Several antivirals are available for topical use in HSV eye infections: idoxuridine, trifluorothymidine, and topical vidarabine. For HSV encephalitis, intravenous acyclovir is the treatment of choice. For neonatal HSV infections, high-dose intravenous vidarabine and acyclovir are effective.

Acyclovir has been shown to be effective in shortening the duration of symptoms and lesions of mucocutaneous HSV infections in immunocompromised patients and first-episode genital herpes in immunocompetent patients (Table 143-1). Intravenous and oral acyclovir also will prevent reactivation of HSV in seropositive immunocompromised patients during induction chemotherapy for acute leukemia or in the period immediately following bone marrow transplantation.

Oral acyclovir also has been shown to speed the healing and resolution of symptoms in first and recurrent episodes of genital HSV-1 and HSV-2 infections. The benefit of treating acute episodes of recurrent genital disease with oral acyclovir is modest, and thus routine use for recurrent episodes of disease, especially for mild episodes, is not recommended. Chronic daily suppressive therapy reduces the frequency of reactivation disease among patients with frequent genital herpes. Chronic suppressive oral acyclovir does not eliminate sacral ganglionic latency, and reactivation of genital herpes occurs after discontinuation of therapy. Oral acyclovir is of benefit in primary gingivostomatitis but has limited benefit in the treatment of recurrent oral-labial lesions; lesions are not aborted and total healing time is not reduced. If started early, the duration of the ulcerative stage of the lip lesion may be reduced.

Both intravenous vidarabine 15 mg/kg per day over 12 h and intravenous acyclovir 30 mg/kg per day given as 10 mg/kg infusion over 1 h at 8-hourly intervals have been shown to be effective in reducing the mortality of HSV encephalitis. Primary determinants of outcome include young age and early therapy. Comparative trials of the two drugs for the treatment of HSV encephalitis have indicated a lower mortality rate and fewer neurologic sequelae with intravenous acyclovir. The major side effect associated with intravenous acyclovir is transient renal insufficiency, usually due to crystallization of the compound in the renal parenchyma. This can be avoided if the medication is given slowly over 1 h and the patient is well-hydrated. Because CSF levels of acyclovir average only 30 to 50 percent of plasma levels, the dosage of acyclovir used for treatment of CNS infection (30 mg/kg per day) is double that used for treatment of mucocutaneous or visceral disease (15 mg/kg per day). Vidarabine at doses of 15 mg/kg per day tends to produce more hematopoietic and hepatic toxicity than acyclovir, but this is usually not a limiting problem in treating severe neonatal or CNS infections.

Acyclovir-resistant strains are being identified with increasing frequency, especially in HIV-infected persons. Almost all clinically significant acyclovir resistance has been seen in immunocompromised

TABLE 143-1 Antiviral chemotherapy of HSV infection

Mucocutaneous HSV infections
A Immunosuppressed patients
  1 Acute symptomatic first or recurrent episodes: IV acyclovir (5 mg/kg every 8 h) or oral acyclovir (400 mg PO 4 times per day for 7 to 10 days) relieves pain and speeds healing. With localized external lesions 5% topical acyclovir ointment applied 4 to 6 times daily may be beneficial.
  2 Suppression of reactivation disease: IV (5 mg/kg every 8 h) or oral acyclovir (400 mg PO 3 to 5 times per day) will prevent recurrences during high-risk periods, e.g., the immediate posttransplantation period.
B 1 Genital herpes
    a First episodes: Oral acyclovir (200 mg PO 5 times per day for 10 to 14 days) is the treatment of choice. IV acyclovir (5 mg/kg every 8 h for 5 days) is given for severe disease or neurologic complications such as aseptic meningitis. Topical 5% ointment or cream applied 4 to 6 times daily for 7 to 10 days may be beneficial in patients without cervical, urethral, or pharyngeal involvement.
    b Symptomatic recurrent genital herpes: Oral acyclovir (200 mg PO 5 times per day for 5 days) has modest benefit in shortening lesion duration and viral excretion time. Routine use for all episodes is not recommended.
    c Suppression of recurrent genital herpes: Daily oral acyclovir (200-mg capsules 2 or 3 times daily, 400 mg PO 2 times daily, or 800 mg PO once daily) will prevent reactivation of symptomatic recurrences.
    d Suppression of reactivation of oral-labial HSV: Oral acyclovir (400 mg PO 2 times per day), if started before exposure and continued for the duration of exposure (usually 5 to 10 days), will prevent reactivation of recurrent oral-labial HSV associated with severe sun exposure.
  2 Oral-labial HSV infections
    a First episode: Oral acyclovir 200 mg is given 4 or 5 times per day.
       Recurrent episodes: Topical acyclovir ointment is of no clinical benefit. Oral acyclovir has minimal benefit.
  3 Herpetic whitlow: Oral acyclovir 200 mg is given 5 times daily for 7 to 10 days.
  4 HSV proctitis: Oral acyclovir (400 mg PO 5 times per day) is useful in shortening course of infection. In immunosuppressed patients or in patients with severe infection, IV acyclovir 5 mg/kg every 8 h may be useful.
C Herpetic eye infections: In acute keratitis, topical trifluorothymidine, vidarabine, idoxuridine, acyclovir, and interferon are all beneficial. Debridement may be required; topical steroids may worsen disease.
CNS HSV infections
A HSV encephalitis: Intravenous acyclovir 10 mg/kg every 8 h (30 mg/kg per day) for 10 days or vidarabine (15 mg/kg per day) decreases mortality; acyclovir is the preferred agent.
B HSV aseptic meningitis: No studies of systemic antiviral chemotherapy exist. If therapy is to be given IV, acyclovir at 15 to 30 mg/kg per day should be utilized.
C Autonomic radiculopathy: No studies are available.
Neonatal HSV infections: Intravenous vidarabine (30 mg/kg per day) or acyclovir (30 mg/kg per day) is given. Neonates appear to tolerate this high dose of vidarabine.
Visceral HSV infections
A HSV esophagitis: Systemic acyclovir (15 mg/kg per day) should be considered. In some patients with milder forms of immunosuppression, 800 mg 3 times daily will relieve symptoms.
B HSV pneumonitis: No controlled studies exist. Systemic acyclovir (15 mg/kg per day) should be considered.
Disseminated HSV infections: No controlled studies exist. Intravenous acyclovir or vidarabine should be attempted. Because of reduced side effects, acyclovir is preferred. No definite evidence indicates that therapy will decrease mortality.
Erythema multiforme associated with HSV: Anecdotal observations suggest that oral acyclovir capsules 2 to 3 times daily will suppress EM.
Infections due to acyclovir-resistant viruses: Foscarnet 40 mg/kg IV every 8 h should be given until lesions heal. The optimal duration of therapy and the usefulness of its continuation to suppress lesions are unclear. Some patients may benefit from cutaneous application of trifluorothymidine.

patients who have received multiple intermittent courses of therapy. The frequent reactivation of virus and high virus titers in the lesions of immunocompromised patients in combination with the use of the medication selects out these resistant variants. Most acyclovir-resistant strains of HSV have an altered substrate specificity for phosphorylating acyclovir. Thus intracellular levels of acyclovir triphosphate are low. In some patients, higher doses of acyclovir will be associated with clearing of lesions. In others, clinical disease will progress despite high-dose therapy. Isolation of HSV from persisting lesions despite adequate dosages and blood levels of acyclovir should raise the suspicion of acyclovir resistance. Therapy with the antiviral drug foscarnet is useful (see Chap. 142). Because of its toxicity and cost, this drug is usually reserved for patients with extensive mucocutaneous infections.

PREVENTION   The large reservoir of persons with asymptomatic HSV-1 and HSV-2 infections indicates that control of HSV disease through suppressive antiviral chemotherapy and/or educational programs will be limited. Control of HSV infection will require prevention of infection, a goal most likely achievable by vaccination. Effective HSV vaccines are not currently available. Heterologous vaccines such as smallpox, bacillus Calmette-Guérin, and influenza, which have been used as therapies for genital HSV infection, have been ineffective.

Barrier forms of contraception, especially condoms, decrease transmission of disease, especially during periods of asymptomatic viral excretion. When lesions are present, the disease may be transmitted despite the use of a condom, and patients should be instructed to avoid sexual activity during these intervals.

REFERENCES

ASHLEY R et al: Inability of enzyme immunoassays to accurately discriminate between infections with herpes simplex virus types 1 and 2. Ann Intern Med 115:520, 1991
BROWN ZA et al: Neonatal herpes simplex virus infection in relation to asymptomatic maternal infection at the time of labor. N Engl J Med 324:1247, 1991
COREY L, SPEAR P: Infections with herpes simplex viruses. N Engl J Med 314:686, 1986
ERLICH KS et al: Acyclovir-resistant herpes simplex virus infections in patients with the acquired immunodeficiency syndrome. N Engl J Med 320:293, 1989
HOOK EW et al: Herpes simplex virus infection as a risk factor for human immunodeficiency virus infection in heterosexuals. J Infect Dis 165:251, 1992
MERTZ GJ et al: Risk factors for the sexual transmission of genital herpes. Ann Intern Med 116:197, 1992
SAFRIN S et al: A controlled trial comparing foscarnet with vidarabine for acyclovir-resistant mucocutaneous herpes simplex in the acquired immunodeficiency syndrome. N Engl J Med 325:551, 1991
STONE KM, WHITTINGTON WL: Treatment of genital herpes. Rev Infect Dis 12:S610, 1990
WHITLEY R, GNANN JW: Acyclovir: A decade of experience. N Engl J Med (in press)

144   VARICELLA-ZOSTER VIRUS INFECTIONS

RICHARD J. WHITLEY

DEFINITION   Varicella-zoster virus (VZV) causes two distinct clinical entities: varicella, or chickenpox, and herpes zoster, or shingles. Chickenpox, a ubiquitous and extremely contagious infection, is usually a benign illness of childhood characterized by an exanthematous, vesicular rash. With reactivation of latent VZV, more common after the sixth decade of life, the disease presents as a dermatomal, vesicular rash which is usually associated with severe pain.

ETIOLOGY   A clinical association between varicella and herpes zoster has been recognized for nearly 100 years. Early in the twentieth century, similarities in the histopathologic findings of skin lesions resulting from varicella and herpes zoster were demonstrated. Viral isolates from patients with chickenpox and herpes zoster produced similar alterations in tissue culture, specifically the appearance of eosinophilic intranuclear inclusions and multinucleated giant cells, suggesting that the viruses were biologically similar. Restriction endonuclease analyses of viral DNA from a patient with chickenpox who subsequently developed herpes zoster verified the molecular identity of the two viruses responsible for these differing clinical

presentations. Varicella-zoster virus is a member of the herpesvirus family, sharing such similar structural characteristics as a lipid envelope surrounding a nucleocapsid with icosahedral symmetry, a total size of approximately 150 to 200 nm, and centrally located double-stranded DNA with a molecular weight of approximately 80 million. Only enveloped virions are infectious.

PATHOGENESIS AND PATHOLOGY   Primary infection   Transmission is most likely by the respiratory route, followed by localized replication at an undefined site, presumably the nasopharynx, and leading to seeding of the reticuloendothelial system with, ultimately, viremia. The occurrence of viremia in patients with chickenpox is supported by the diffuse and scattered nature of the skin lesions and can be verified in selected cases by the recovery of virus from the blood. Vesicles involve the corium and dermis, with degenerative changes characterized by ballooning, multinucleated giant cells, and eosinophilic intranuclear inclusions. Infection may involve localized blood vessels of the skin, resulting in necrosis and epidermal hemorrhage. With disease evolution, vesicular fluid becomes cloudy with the recruitment of polymorphonuclear leukocytes, degenerated cells, and fibrin. Ultimately, the vesicles rupture and release their fluid contents, which include infectious virus, or are gradually reabsorbed.

Recurrent infection   The mechanism of reactivation of VZV that results in herpes zoster is unknown. It is presumed that virus infects the dorsal root ganglia during chickenpox, where it remains latent until reactivated. Histopathologic examination of the representative dorsal root ganglia during active herpes zoster demonstrates hemorrhage, edema, and lymphocytic infiltration.

Active VZV replication can occur in other organs, such as the lung or brain, during either chickenpox or herpes zoster but is uncommon in the immune-competent host. Lung involvement is characterized by interstitial pneumonitis, multinucleated giant cell formation, intranuclear inclusions, and pulmonary hemorrhage. Central nervous system (CNS) infection leads to histopathologic evidence of perivascular cuffing similar to that encountered with measles and other viral encephalitides. Focal hemorrhagic necrosis of the brain, characteristic of herpes simplex virus encephalitis, is uncommon with VZV infection.

EPIDEMIOLOGY AND CLINICAL PRESENTATION   Chickenpox   Humans are the only known reservoir for VZV. Chickenpox is highly contagious, with an attack rate of at least 90 percent among susceptible or seronegative individuals. Both sexes and individuals of all races are infected equally. The virus is endemic in the population at large; however, it becomes epidemic among susceptible individuals during seasonal periods, namely, late winter and early spring in the temperate zone. Children between the ages of 5 and 9 are most commonly affected and account for 50 percent of all cases. Most other cases occur between the ages of 1 to 4 and 10 to 14. Over the age of 15, approximately 10 percent of the population of the United States is susceptible to infection.

The incubation period of chickenpox ranges between 10 and 21 days but is usually between 14 and 17 days. Secondary attack rates in susceptible siblings within a household are between 70 and 90 percent. Patients are infectious approximately 48 h prior to the onset of the vesicular rash, during the period of vesicle formation (generally 4 to 5 days), and until all vesicles are crusted.

Clinically, chickenpox presents as a rash, low-grade fever, and malaise, although a few patients will develop a prodrome 1 to 2 days prior to the onset of the exanthem. In the immune-competent, this is usually a benign illness that is associated with lassitude and fever from 37.8 to 39.4°C (100 to 103°F) of 3 to 5 days' duration. The skin lesions, the hallmark of the infection, consist of maculopapules, vesicles, and scabs in varying stages of evolution. The evolution of lesions from maculopapules to vesicles occurs over a matter of hours to days. The lesions appear on the trunk and face and rapidly involve other areas of the body. Most are small and have an erythematous base with a diameter of 5 to 10 mm. Successive crops appear over a 2- to 4-day period. Lesions also can be found on the mucosa of the pharynx or the vagina. Their severity varies from individual to individual. Some individuals have very few lesions, while others can have as many as 2000. Younger children tend to have fewer vesicles than older individuals. Immunocompromised individuals, both children and adults, particularly those with leukemia, have more numerous lesions, often with a hemorrhagic base, and the lesions take longer to heal. These individuals also are at greater risk for visceral complications, which occur in 30 to 50 percent of cases and which are fatal in 15 percent.

The most common infectious complication of varicella is secondary bacterial superinfection of the skin, which is usually caused by *Streptococcus pyogenes* or *Staphylococcus aureus*. This may result from excoriation of skin lesions following scratching. Gram stain of skin lesions should help clarify the etiology of unusually erythematous and pustulated lesions.

The most common extracutaneous site of involvement in children is the central nervous system. The syndrome consists of acute cerebellar ataxia and meningeal irritation which generally appears approximately 21 days after the onset of the rash and rarely occurs in the preeruptive phase. The cerebrospinal fluid contains lymphocytes and elevated levels of protein. This is a benign complication of VZV infection in children and does not generally require hospitalization. Aseptic meningitis, encephalitis, transverse myelitis, Guillain-Barré syndrome, and Reye's syndrome also can occur. Encephalitis is reported in 0.1 to 0.2 percent of children with chickenpox. No specific therapy, other than supportive care, is available for patients with CNS involvement caused by VZV.

Varicella pneumonia is the most serious complication following chickenpox, occurring more commonly in adults (up to 20 percent) than in children. It usually appears 3 to 5 days into the course of illness and is associated with tachypnea, cough, dyspnea, and fever. Cyanosis, pleuritic chest pain, and hemoptysis are frequent. Roentgenographic evidence of disease consists of nodular infiltrates and an interstitial pneumonitis. Resolution of pneumonitis parallels improvement of skin rash; however, patients may have persistent fever and compromised pulmonary function for weeks.

Other complications of chickenpox include myocarditis, corneal lesions, nephritis, arthritis, bleeding diatheses, acute glomerulonephritis, and hepatitis. Hepatic involvement, distinct from Reye's syndrome, is common in chickenpox and is usually characterized by an elevation of liver enzymes, particularly aspartate aminotransferase (AST) and alanine aminotransferase (ALT). Hepatic involvement is usually asymptomatic.

Perinatal varicella is associated with a high mortality rate when maternal disease develops within 5 days before delivery and 48 h post partum. Because the newborn does not receive protective transplacental antibodies and has an immature immune system, illness may be exaggerated. The mortality rate has been reported as high as 30 percent in this group. Congenital varicella with clinical manifestations at birth is extremely uncommon.

Herpes zoster Herpes zoster, a sporadic disease, is the consequence of reactivation of latent virus from the dorsal root ganglia. It occurs at all ages but mainly among the elderly. Most patients have no history of exposure to other individuals with VZV infection. The highest incidence is between 5 and 10 cases per 1000 persons for individuals in the sixth through the eighth decades of life. It has been suggested that approximately 2 percent of herpes zoster patients will develop a second episode of infection.

Herpes zoster, or "shingles," is characterized by a unilateral vesicular eruption within a dermatome, often associated with severe pain. The dermatomes from T3 to L3 are most frequently involved. If the ophthalmic branch of the trigeminal nerve is involved, zoster ophthalmicus results. The factors responsible for reactivation of virus are not known. In children, reactivation is usually benign, whereas in adults, acute neuritis and postherpetic neuralgia can be particularly debilitating. The onset of disease is heralded by pain within the dermatome that may precede lesions by 48 to 72 h, followed by an erythematous maculopapular rash which evolves rapidly to vesicular

lesions. In the normal host, these lesions may remain few in number and continue to form only for a period of 3 to 5 days. The total duration of disease is generally between 7 and 10 days; however, it may take as long as 2 to 4 weeks before the skin returns to normal. In a few patients, characteristic localization of pain to a dermatome with serologic evidence of herpes zoster has been reported in the absence of skin lesions. When branches of the trigeminal nerve are involved, lesions may appear on the face, in the mouth, in the eye, or on the tongue. Lesions appear on the ear canal and tongue when the sensory branch of the facial nerve is involved (Ramsay Hunt syndrome).

The most debilitating complication of herpes zoster, in both the normal and the immunocompromised host, is pain associated with acute neuritis and postherpetic neuralgia. Postherpetic neuralgia is uncommon in young individuals; however, at least 50 percent of patients over age 50 with zoster will report pain in the involved dermatome months after resolution of cutaneous disease. Changes in sensation within the dermatome, resulting in either hypo- or hyperesthesia, are common.

Central nervous system involvement following localized herpes zoster may occur. Many patients without signs of meningeal irritation will have cerebrospinal fluid pleocytosis and moderately elevated levels of CSF protein. Symptomatic meningoencephalitis is characterized by headache, fever, photophobia, meningitis, and vomiting. A rare manifestation of CNS involvement is granulomatous angiitis with contralateral hemiplegia, which can be diagnosed by cerebral arteriography. Other neurologic manifestations include transverse myelitis with or without motor paralysis.

As with chickenpox, herpes zoster in the immunocompromised host is more severe than in the normal individual. Lesion formation continues for over a week, and total scabbing does not develop in the majority of patients until 3 weeks into the course of illness. Patients with Hodgkin's disease and non-Hodgkin's lymphoma are at greatest risk for progressive herpes zoster because cutaneous dissemination develops in about 40 percent of these patients. Among patients with cutaneous dissemination, there is a 5 to 10 percent increased risk of pneumonitis, meningoencephalitis, hepatitis, and other serious complications. However, even in immunocompromised patients, disseminated zoster is rarely fatal.

Patients who have had a bone marrow transplant are at particular risk of VZV infection. Thirty percent of cases of posttransplant VZV infections occur within 1 year (50 percent of these within 9 months), and 45 percent of such patients have cutaneous or visceral dissemination. The mortality rate is 10 percent, and postherpetic neuralgia, scarring, and bacterial superinfection are more frequent in VZV infections occurring within 9 months of a transplant. Among infected patients, concomitant graft-versus-host disease increases the chance for dissemination and/or a fatal outcome.

TABLE 144-1 Recommendations for VZIG utilization

Exposure
  A Both exposure to person with chickenpox or zoster as:
      1 Continuous household contact
      2 Playmate for >1 h indoors
      3 Hospital contact (same room or prolonged face-to-face)
      4 Newborn exposure whereby mother had onset of chickenpox <5 days before delivery to 48 h post partum
  B And time elapsed ≤96 h (preferably sooner)
Candidates (provided significant exposure) include
  A Immunocompromised susceptible children
  B Normal susceptible adolescents (>15 years) and adults, especially pregnant women
  C Newborn infants of mothers with onset of chickenpox 5 days before or 2 days after delivery
  D Hospitalized premature infants
      1 ≥28 weeks' gestation when mother has no history of chickenpox
      2 <28 weeks' gestation and/or birth weight of ≤1000 g regardless of maternal history

SOURCE: Adapted from *1991 Redbook*, American Academy of Pediatrics.

DIFFERENTIAL DIAGNOSIS The diagnosis of chickenpox is not difficult. The characteristic rash of chickenpox and the epidemiologic history of recent exposure should lead to prompt diagnosis. Other viral infections which can mimic chickenpox include disseminated herpes simplex virus infection in patients with atopic dermatitis and the disseminated vesiculopapular lesions sometimes associated with coxsackievirus, echovirus, or atypical measles infections. These rashes are more commonly morbilliform with a hemorrhagic component rather than vesicular or vesiculopustular. Rickettsialpox can be confused with chickenpox; however, it can be easily distinguished by finding the "herald spot" at the site of the mite bite and a more pronounced headache. Serologic testing is useful in differentiating rickettsialpox from varicella.

Unilateral vesicular lesions in a dermatomal pattern should lead rapidly to the diagnosis of herpes zoster. Both herpes simplex virus and coxsackievirus infections can be a cause of dermatomal vesicular lesions. In such situations, a Tzanck smear with supportive diagnostic virology will be helpful in ensuring the proper diagnosis. In the prodromal stage of herpes zoster, the diagnosis can be exceedingly difficult and may only be achieved once lesions have appeared or by retrospective serologic assessment.

LABORATORY FINDINGS Unequivocal confirmation of the diagnosis is possible only through the isolation of virus in susceptible tissue culture cell lines or by the demonstration of seroconversion or a fourfold or greater antibody rise in convalescent versus acute specimens. A rapid impression can be obtained by a Tzanck smear, performed by scraping the base of the lesions in an attempt to demonstrate multinucleated giant cells. Direct immunofluorescent staining of cells from the skin base or detection of viral antigens by other assays (immunoperoxidase) also can be utilized, although such tests are not commercially available. The most frequently employed serologic tools for assessing host response are immunofluorescent detection of antibodies to VZV membrane antigens, the fluorescent antibody to membrane antigen (FAMA) test, immune adherence hemagglutination, and enzyme-linked immunosorbent assay (ELISA). The FAMA and ELISA tests appear to be the most sensitive.

PROPHYLAXIS In the normal host, prophylaxis and treatment of chickenpox are of relatively little value because the disease is usually benign. However, the immunocompromised individual is at significant risk for developing progressive varicella; modalities of prevention include passive immunization or experimental administration of a live attenuated vaccine. Immune prophylaxis can be accomplished by the administration of specific zoster immune globulin (ZIG) derived from patients with herpes zoster, varicella-zoster immune globulin (VZIG), or the intravenous formulation of zoster immune plasma (ZIP). Both ZIG and VZIG should be given within 96 h, but preferably within 72 h, of exposure in order to be effective. It is likely that ZIP can be given somewhat later. Indications for the administration of ZIG or VZIG are summarized in Table 144-1. VZIG should be administered to immunodeficient patients under age 15 who have a negative or unknown history of chickenpox, who have not been vaccinated against VZV, and who have had a contact in a household, with a playmate for more than 1 h indoors, or in a shared hospital room. It also should be administered to the newborn whose mother had an onset of chickenpox within less than 5 days before delivery and 48 h post partum. VZIG should be administered to normal susceptible adolescents (≥15 years of age) and adults, especially pregnant women; however, serologic evaluation of immune status is advised. Finally, AZIG is recommended for hospitalized premature infants of ≥28 weeks' gestation whose mother has no history of chickenpox and those of <28 weeks' gestation regardless of maternal history when exposure is significant.

Clinical trials in Japan and the United States have demonstrated the efficacy of live attenuated vaccine (OKA) both in normal individuals and in immunocompromised hosts. This live attenuated VZV vaccine may be licensed in the United States in the near future.

TREATMENT Medical management of chickenpox in the normal host is directed toward preventing avoidable complications. Obvi-ously, good hygiene should include daily bathing and soaks. Secondary bacterial infection of the skin can be avoided by meticulous skin care, particularly with close cropping of fingernails. Pruritus can be decreased with topical dressings or the administration of antipruritic drugs. Tepid water baths and wet compresses are better than drying lotions for the relief of itching. Domeboro soaks for the management of herpes zoster can be both soothing and cleansing. Administration of aspirin should be avoided in children with chickenpox because of the recent association between aspirin derivatives and the development of Reye's syndrome. In addition, acyclovir therapy (800 mg PO five times daily for 5 to 7 days) is recommended for adolescents and adults with chickenpox of ≤24 h duration. Acyclovir therapy for children <12 years of age may be of benefit if initiated early in the disease (<24 h) at a dose of 20 mg/kg every 6 h.

Patients with varicella pneumonia may require removal of bronchial secretions and ventilatory support. Zoster ophthalmicus should be referred promptly and immediately to an ophthalmologist. Therapy consists of administration of analgesics for severe pain and the use of atropine. The administration of acyclovir in the management of zoster ophthalmicus will accelerate healing. Patients with herpes zoster may benefit from acyclovir therapy, as evidenced by accelerated cutaneous healing and decreased postherpetic neuralgia. The dose is 800 mg PO five times daily for 7 to 10 days.

Both chickenpox and herpes zoster in the immunocompromised host should be treated with intravenous vidarabine or, preferably, acyclovir. Acyclovir is used preferentially over vidarabine because of decreased toxicity, especially in immunocompromised patients. Intravenous acyclovir leads to the decreased occurrence of visceral complications but has no effect on healing of skin lesions or pain. The dose is 500 mg/m^2 every 8 h for 7 days. These treatment recommendations apply to immunocompromised patients with disseminated herpes zoster as well. Oral acyclovir therapy is not recommended for treatment of VZV infections in immune-compromised patients. Concomitant with the administration of intravenous acyclovir to the immunosuppressed host, it is desirable to attempt to wean patients from immunosuppressive treatment.

Management of acute neuritis and/or postherpetic neuralgia can be particularly difficult. In addition to the judicious use of analgesics, ranging from nonnarcotic to narcotic derivatives, drugs such as amitriptyline hydrochloride and fluphenazine hydrochloride have been reported to be beneficial for pain relief. Glucocorticoids have been reported in some studies to be useful when administered early in the course for prevention of postherpetic neuralgia. This approach remains controversial.

REFERENCES

BRUNELL PA et al: Prevention of varicella by zoster immune globulin. N Engl J Med 280:1191, 1969

BALFOUR HH JR et al: Acyclovir treatment of varicella in otherwise healthy adolescents. J Pediatr 120:627–633, 1992

DUNKLE LM et al: A controlled trial of acyclovir for chickenpox in normal children. N Engl J Med 325:1539, 1991

ESSMAN V et al: Prednisone does not prevent postherpetic neuralgia. Lancet 2:126, 1987

GERSHON AA et al: Live attenuated varicella vaccine. JAMA 252:355, 1984

HOPE-SIMPSON RE: The nature of herpes zoster: A long-term study and a new hypothesis. Proc R Soc Med 58:9, 1965

LOCKSLEY RM et al: Infection with varicella-zoster virus after marrow transplantation. J Infect Dis 152:1172, 1985

PROBER CG et al: Acyclovir therapy of chickenpox in immunosuppressed children—a collaborative study. J Pediatr 101:622, 1982

SHEPP D et al: Treatment of varicella-zoster virus in severely immunocompromised patients: A randomized comparison of acyclovir and vidarabine. N Engl J Med 314:208, 1987

WEIBEL RE et al: Live attenuated varicella versus vaccine: Efficacy trail in healthy children. N Engl J Med 310:1409, 1984

WELLER TH: Varicella and herpes zoster: Changing concepts of the natural history, control, and importance of a not-so-benign virus. N Engl J Med 309:1362, 1983

WHITLEY RJ et al: Early vidarabine therapy to control the complications of herpes zoster in immunosuppressed patients. N Engl J Med 307:971, 1982

——— et al: Vidarabine therapy of varicella in immunosuppressed patients. J Pediatr 1:125, 1982

——— et al: Varicella-zoster virus infections, in *Antiviral Agents and Viral Diseases of Man*, vol 2, GJ Galasso et al (eds). New York, Raven, 1984, pp 517–542

——— et al: Disseminated herpes zoster in the immunocompromised host: A comparative trial of acyclovir and vidarabine. J Infect Dis 165:450, 1992

ZAIA JA et al: Evaluation of varicella-zoster immune globulin: Protection of immunosuppressed children after household exposure to varicella. J Infect Dis 147:737, 1983

145   EPSTEIN-BARR VIRUS INFECTIONS, INCLUDING INFECTIOUS MONONUCLEOSIS

ROBERT T. SCHOOLEY

DEFINITION   Epstein-Barr virus (EBV) is a B lymphotropic human herpesvirus which is worldwide in distribution. Primary infection with EBV during childhood is usually subclinical. Between 25 and 70 percent of adolescents and adults who undergo a primary EBV infection develop the clinical syndrome of infectious mononucleosis. Infectious mononucleosis is defined by the clinical triad of fever, lymphadenopathy, and pharyngitis combined with the transient appearance of heterophil antibodies and an atypical lymphocytosis. EBV is also associated with nasopharyngeal carcinoma and certain B cell lymphomas.

EPIDEMIOLOGY OF EBV INFECTIONS   EBV is a ubiquitous agent that has been found in all population groups surveyed to date. The virus was initially described by Epstein, Achong, and Barr, who noted, by electron microscopy, the presence of particles similar in morphology to herpes simplex virus in continuous cell lines which had arisen from tumor tissue obtained from patients with Burkitt's lymphoma. Following an observation by the Henles of antibodies to EBV in a patient with infectious mononucleosis, large-scale serologic surveys confirmed EBV as the etiologic agent for infectious mononucleosis.

EBV is transmitted primarily in saliva or, less commonly, by blood transfusion. Primary infection tends to occur at an earlier age among lower socioeconomic groups and in developing countries. In industrialized countries, approximately 50 percent of individuals have experienced a primary EBV infection by adolescence. These early infections are usually mild and nonspecific or clinically inapparent. A second wave of seroconversions to EBV occurs with the onset of the social activity associated with adolescence and young adulthood. Primary EBV infection among this age group accounts for most cases of infectious mononucleosis. The peak incidence of infectious mononucleosis occurs between 14 and 16 years of age for girls and between 16 and 18 years of age for boys. By adulthood, most individuals are EBV-seropositive.

EBV is shed from the oropharynx for up to 18 months following primary infection; thereafter it is shed intermittently by all EBV-seropositive individuals in the absence of a clinical illness. EBV can be isolated from the oropharyngeal washings of 15 to 25 percent of healthy EBV-seropositive individuals. Immunosuppressed individuals shed the virus more frequently. EBV can be isolated from 25 to 50 percent of the oropharyngeal washings obtained from renal allograft recipients and from virtually all patients with AIDS. Asymptomatic shedding of EBV by healthy individuals accounts for most of the spread to uninfected members of the population despite the fact that it is not highly contagious. Transmission is largely dependent on salivary contact (e.g., kissing). It is not likely to be transmitted by aerosol or fomites. Thus isolation restrictions on patients with mononucleosis or individuals likely to be shedding EBV are not appropriate.

ETIOLOGY AND PATHOGENESIS OF INFECTIOUS MONONUCLEOSIS   By electron microscopy, EBV appears as an icosahedral nucleocapsid surrounded by a complex envelope and is indistinguishable from other members of the human herpesvirus group. The double-stranded EBV DNA has a molecular weight of approximately 101×10^6 and encodes for at least 30 polypeptides. Two types of EBV (types A and B) have been recognized on the basis of divergence of several of the Epstein-Barr nuclear antigens (see below). Type B virus is less efficient at transforming B lymphocytes and was initially thought to be prevalent primarily in central Africa and New Guinea. Type A virus is found in a greater number of individuals worldwide and is the type most frequently isolated from throat washings obtained from healthy members of the western community. Recent work suggests that type B virus is found more widely geographically than was previously appreciated and is found more frequently in immunocompromised individuals, especially those with HIV-1 infection. In such individuals, dual infection with both types of EBV has been demonstrated. There is currently no evidence that type differences account for the wide range of clinical conditions associated with EBV infection.

When EBV is transmitted by saliva, the initial site of replication is the oropharynx. EBV grows productively in B lymphocytes and oropharyngeal epithelial cells of patients with infectious mononucleosis; both cell types have specific surface receptors for EBV. During the acute phase of the illness, EBV antigens can be demonstrated within the nuclei of up to 20 percent of circulating B lymphocytes. After the infection subsides, the virus can be isolated from a small number of B lymphocytes of EBV-seropositive individuals and also resides within nasopharyngeal epithelial cells.

Virus-host interactions   EBV infection has both direct and indirect effects on the cellular and humoral immune responses. Within 18 to 24 h after entry of EBV into B lymphocytes by means of the C3d receptor (also known as CD21), Epstein-Barr nuclear antigens (EBNA) are detectable within the nucleus of the infected cell. The six antigens which comprise EBNA (EBNA 1, 2, 3a, 3b, 3c, and leader protein) are responsible for conferring the transformed phenotype on EBV-infected B lymphocytes. Immortalized B lymphocytes can be propagated continuously in vitro and are polyclonally stimulated by EBV to produce immunoglobulin. Antibodies reactive with sheep red blood cells (heterophil) and antibodies with several other specificities are manifestations of polyclonal immunoglobulin production and may mediate several of the complications of infectious mononucleosis. A minority of EBV-infected B lymphocytes enter the lytic cycle (production of mature progeny virus and death of the host cell) and produce EBV antigens that are detected during virus replication. These are divided into the early antigen (EA) complex and viral capsid antigens (VCA). The EA complex consists of two groups of antigens: (1) diffuse (EA-D), which are detectable in both the cytoplasm and the nucleus of cells in the lytic cycle, and (2) restricted (EA-R), which are demonstrable only in the cytoplasm. These antigens serve as markers of infection at the cellular level; the pattern of the antibody response to these antigens is useful diagnostically in the identification of EBV-associated disease states (Table 145-1). After the appearance of VCA, the host cell dies and virions are released, which can infect and transform additional B lymphocytes.

An effective immune response to EBV involves humoral and cellular components. Neutralizing antibodies which inactivate cell-free virus and antibodies to VCA and EBNA appear during primary infection in all patients; antibodies to EA-D appear in most patients. The cellular immune response is largely responsible for controlling B cell proliferation and polyclonal immunoglobulin production triggered by EBV and is composed primarily of T lymphocytes having functional and surface phenotypic characteristics of activated, suppressor-cytotoxic T lymphocytes (CD8+, Ia+). These EBV-specific cytotoxic T lymphocytes appear to be directed primarily at several epitopes within the EBNA complex. As the illness progresses, memory T lymphocytes capable of limiting proliferation of autologous EBV-infected B lymphocytes are demonstrable. These memory T lymphocytes persist for life. However, latent EBV remains in a small

TABLE 145-1 EBV-specific antibodies

Antibody specificity	Time of appearance in IM	Persistence	Percent of IM patients with antibody	Comments
VCA:				
IgM	At clinical presentation	1–2 months	100	Best indicator of primary infection; not present with reactivation
IgG	At clinical presentation	Lifelong	100	Standard "EBV titer" reported by most commercial and state labs; major utility is as a marker for prior or current infection in epidemiologic studies
EA:				
EA-D	Peaks 3–4 weeks after onset	3–6 months	70	Presence correlates with more severe disease in patients with IM; present in nasopharyngeal carcinoma; IgA anti-EA-D antibodies useful for prediction of NPC in high-risk populations
EA-R	Several weeks after onset	Months to years		Present in high titer in African Burkitt's lymphoma; may be useful as an indicator of reactivation of EBV in immunosuppressed patients
EBNA	3–6 weeks after onset	Lifelong	100	Late appearance of anti-EBNA antibodies in IM makes seroconversion a useful marker for primary infection if IgM anti-VCA antibody studies are not available

NOTE: IM = infectious mononucleosis; VCA = viral capsid antigen; EA = early antigens; EA-D = diffuse early antigens; EA-R = restricted early antigens; EBNA = Epstein-Barr nuclear antigens; NPC = nasopharyngeal carcinoma.

proportion of B lymphocytes and also in epithelial cells in the oropharynx.

During the primary immune response to EBV, global cellular immune hyporesponsiveness is readily demonstrable. This resolves after resolution of the illness, but reactivation of EBV is facilitated by conditions which interfere with the cellular immune response (immunosuppressive drugs, especially cyclosporin A, and disorders associated with cellular immunodeficiency, such as HIV-1 infection). EBV and cytomegalovirus (CMV) reactivation in immunosuppressed patients is frequently associated with a return of the immunoregulatory abnormalities characteristic of the primary immune response to these viruses. In the case of CMV particularly, this hyporesponsiveness may contribute to many of the superinfections which frequently accompany CMV infections in immunocompromised hosts. The cellular hyporesponsiveness associated with EBV reactivation is generally less intense and less prolonged than that associated with CMV but also may contribute to morbidity in immunocompromised individuals.

CLINICAL MANIFESTATIONS   Symptoms and signs   After an incubation period of 4 to 8 weeks, prodromal symptoms of malaise, anorexia, and chills frequently precede the onset of pharyngitis, fever, and lymphadenopathy by several days. Severe pharyngitis is the symptom which most frequently prompts patients to seek medical attention. Occasionally, patients will note only fever or lymphadenopathy or will present with one of the complications of infectious mononucleosis. Most patients also complain of headache and malaise. Abdominal pain is infrequent in the absence of splenic rupture.

Physical examination   Fever is present in 90 percent of patients and may reach 39 to 40°C. Periorbital edema may be seen. The pharyngitis is usually diffuse; an exudate is observed in one-third of patients. Palatal petechiae also may be observed. Posterior and/or anterior cervical adenopathy is noted in 90 percent of patients with infectious mononucleosis. Individual nodes are rarely painful but may be moderately tender to palpation. Hepatomegaly is infrequent, although mild hepatic tenderness is present in up to half the patients. Approximately half of all patients have splenomegaly, which is usually maximal in the second or third week of illness. In 5 percent of patients, a macular, petechial, scarlatiniform, urticarial, or erythema multiforme–like rash may appear. Administration of ampicillin results in a pruritic, maculopapular eruption in 90 to 100 percent of patients.

Clinical course   Infectious mononucleosis is a self-limited illness in the vast majority of cases. The pharyngitis is maximal for 5 to 7 days and then resolves over the subsequent 7 to 10 days. Fever usually persists for 7 to 14 days but occasionally may continue somewhat longer. The course of the lymphadenopathy is variable but rarely exceeds 3 weeks. The most persistent symptom is malaise. Most patients are well enough to return to work or school within 3 to 4 weeks, but occasional patients remain exhausted, have difficulty concentrating, and are unable to return to full activities for months. This subgroup is often found among those who present with a less acute onset without severe pharyngitis and high fever.

Occasional patients have been reported in whom recurrent pharyngitis and fever are accompanied by persistent or resurgent heterophil antibodies. A group of patients has been described with nonspecific symptoms which may include malaise, fatigue, pharyngitis, fever, lymphadenopathy, and difficulty with higher cognitive function. These patients are usually heterophil-negative. The demonstration that some of these patients have anti-VCA and anti-EA-R titers which are higher and anti-EBNA titers which are lower than median titers for the general population has led to the speculation that this symptom complex may be a manifestation of ongoing replication of EBV. However, since healthy members of the general population may have antibodies to EA-R antigens, there is no reason to apply the diagnosis of chronic active EBV infection to patients with these nonspecific symptoms simply on the basis of the presence of anti-EA-R antibodies. Several studies have demonstrated the lack of utility of EBV-specific antibodies in the evaluation of patients with chronic fatigue and malaise. A blinded, placebo-controlled crossover study demonstrated no benefit from acyclovir therapy in this patient population. The group of patients formerly given the diagnosis of chronic active EBV infection has been included in a larger diagnostic category termed the *chronic fatigue syndrome* (see Chap. 388) to reflect the uncertain pathogenesis of this illness. Occasional patients have been reported in whom mortality or severe morbidity (pneumonitis, fever, pancytopenia) is associated with evidence of ongoing EBV replication. Such patients are extremely rare, and specific antiviral therapy may be useful in their management.

Complications   Complications of infectious mononucleosis occur infrequently but may be so dramatic as to be the predominant manifestation of the illness (Table 145-2). Hematologic complications

TABLE 145-2   Complications of infectious mononucleosis

Hematologic complications:
   Autoimmune hemolytic anemia
   Thrombocytopenia
   Granulocytopenia
Splenic rupture
Neurologic complications:
   Encephalitis
   Cranial nerve palsies, especially Bell's palsy
   Meningoencephalitis
   Guillain-Barré syndrome
   Seizures
   Mononeuritis multiplex
   Transverse myelitis
   Psychosis
Hepatic complications:
   Hepatitis
Cardiac complications:
   Pericarditis
   Myocarditis
Pulmonary complications:
   Airway obstruction
   Interstitial pneumonitis

include autoimmune hemolytic anemia, which may be mediated by IgM antibodies with anti-i specificity. Hemolytic anemia usually subsides over a 1- to 2-month period. Mild thrombocytopenia occurs in up to 50 percent of cases; profound thrombocytopenia is a rare but well-recognized complication and is frequently antibody-mediated. Mild granulocytopenia is frequently observed in uncomplicated infectious mononucleosis, and severe granulocytopenia associated with infection or death has been reported. Antibodies which react with granulocytes have been detected in up to 80 percent of patients and may contribute to the profound granulocytopenia which is occasionally observed. Both the thrombocytopenia and the granulocytopenia are usually self-limited and resolve over 3 to 6 weeks. Glucocorticoids have been advocated for treatment of both hemolytic anemia and thrombocytopenia associated with infectious mononucleosis, but efficacy has not been proved in controlled studies. Splenic rupture is an infrequent complication of infectious mononucleosis, often accompanied by the insidious or abrupt onset of abdominal pain, and is usually observed during the second or third week of illness. Surgery, usually splenectomy or splenorrhaphy, is the only effective management.

Neurologic complications of infectious mononucleosis may be the presenting or sole manifestation of the illness. Heterophil antibodies may be absent, and atypical lymphocytes may not be present at the onset of the neurologic event. The most frequent neurologic complications are cranial nerve palsies and encephalitis which may present initially with cerebellar findings. The onset of the encephalitis is usually abrupt. Cerebrospinal fluid findings are not diagnostic, and localization by noninvasive neurodiagnostic studies may suggest herpes simplex encephalitis. Eighty-five percent of patients with EBV-associated neurologic findings recover spontaneously.

Hepatitis is a common component of infectious mononucleosis. Almost 90 percent of patients have mild elevation of hepatic transaminases. Although more serious hepatic sequelae have been reported, severe or permanent hepatic dysfunction is exceedingly rare.

Cardiac abnormalities are uncommon but may include pericarditis, myocarditis, coronary artery spasm, and electrocardiographic abnormalities.

Airway obstruction from pharyngeal or paratracheal adenopathy can occur. This may require surgical intervention but is usually quite sensitive to glucocorticoid therapy. Pulmonary parenchymal abnormalities such as interstitial infiltrates are noted infrequently in adults but appear to be more common among children.

Infectious mononucleosis is rarely fatal. Neurologic complications, airway obstruction, and splenic rupture are the most frequent causes of death in previously healthy individuals with primary EBV infection. Sporadic or X-linked cases of overwhelming EBV infection accom-

panied by lymphoproliferation and hepatic dysfunction have been reported.

The X-linked condition known as *X-linked lymphoproliferative (XLP)* or *Duncan's syndrome* (see Chap. 278) results in the death of 40 percent of affected males during primary EBV infection. In addition to overwhelming lymphoproliferation, XLP patients may manifest severe immunologic or hematologic sequelae such as agammaglobulinemia, aplastic anemia, or lymphocytic lymphoma. The pathophysiology of the XLP syndrome has not yet been completely elucidated, but an X-linked defect in the immune response to EBV may result in failure to control EBV replication or in disordered immunoregulation which leads to the other immunologic sequelae observed in this syndrome.

LABORATORY MANIFESTATIONS Heterophil antibodies Antibodies to sheep erythrocytes which can be removed by prior absorption with beef red blood cells, but not with guinea pig kidney, are termed *heterophil antibodies*. Heterophil antibodies are demonstrated in 50 percent of children and 90 to 95 percent of adolescents and adults with mononucleosis. Although the classic tube heterophil titer is still performed in many laboratories, the "monospot" test using a commerical kit is sensitive, specific, easily performed, and more routinely employed. The frequency of heterophil positivity associated with infectious mononucleosis depends on the test used, the age of the patient population, and the time during the illness at which the test is performed. Monospot tests may be slightly more sensitive than heterophil titers. Ten to fifteen percent of patients with mononucleosis may be heterophil-negative if tested only during the first week of the illness. If the clinical suspicion of mononucleosis is high enough, retesting for heterophil antibodies during the second or third week of illness is warranted. Heterophil antibodies decline in titer after the acute illness has resolved but may be detectable for up to 9 months after the onset of the illness.

Atypical lymphocytosis A relative and absolute lymphocytosis is present in about 75 percent of cases of infectious mononucleosis. The lymphocytosis usually peaks in the second or third week of illness and is characterized by cells with atypical morphology. These atypical lymphocytes, which are primarily activated T lymphocytes, are larger than mature lymphocytes and often contain eccentrically placed lobulated nuclei with nucleoli and vacuolated cytoplasm with rolled up edges. Mild neutropenia and thrombocytopenia are frequent. Other laboratory abnormalities include a mild polyclonal increase in immunoglobulins of the IgM, IgG, and IgA classes and mild elevations of hepatocellular enzymes.

EBV-specific antibody response Antibodies to several EBV-specific antigens arise during primary EBV infection (see Table 145-1). Proper utilization of EBV-specific antibody studies may facilitate the diagnosis of primary EBV infection in clinically atypical or heterophil-negative cases. IgM antibodies to the VCA are diagnostic of a primary EBV infection. IgG anti-VCA antibodies are present at clinical presentation in almost all patients and remain detectable for life. IgG anti-VCA antibodies are useful mainly as a test for susceptibility to EBV and are not useful for the diagnosis of primary infection. Approximately 70 percent of patients with infectious mononucleosis make antibodies to EA-D. Anti-EA-D antibodies usually peak 3 to 4 weeks after the onset of illness and usually disappear after recovery. Antibodies to EBNA appear 6 to 8 weeks into the illness and persist for life. The presence of IgM anti-VCA antibodies and seroconversion to EBNA are diagnostic of a primary EBV infection. Patients with defects in cellular immunity may fail to make antibodies to EBNA.

DIAGNOSIS The diagnosis of infectious mononucleosis is not difficult in the vast majority of cases. The constellation of fever, pharyngitis, and lymphadenopathy coupled with an atypical lymphocytosis and heterophil antibodies is virtually always due to primary EBV infection and requires no further laboratory studies. Certain patients with EBV-induced mononucleosis, particularly preadolescents or those with neurologic complications, may be heterophil-negative or may lack an atypical lymphocytosis. Primary EBV infection can be diagnosed with certainty in these patients with the proper use of EBV-specific serologic studies (see above). Culturing EBV from oropharyngeal washings or peripheral blood mononuclear cells is laborious, and because of the ubiquity of the virus among EBV-seropositive individuals, it is not diagnostic of primary EBV infection.

Primary CMV infection is the illness most frequently confused with EBV-induced infectious mononucleosis. About two-thirds of adults with heterophil-negative mononucleosis have CMV-induced mononucleosis. Patients with CMV mononucleosis are, on average, slightly older than those with EBV-induced infectious mononucleosis and usually have an illness characterized predominantly by fever and malaise. Pharyngitis and lymphadenopathy are less common than with infectious mononucleosis. CMV-induced mononucleosis is usually more insidious in onset and slower to resolve than EBV-induced mononucleosis. The diagnosis can be made by the isolation of CMV from the peripheral blood and the demonstration of seroconversion or a fourfold or greater rise in antibody titer to CMV. Although CMV is also shed in saliva and urine by patients with CMV mononucleosis, demonstration of the agent in the blood is a more specific, but less sensitive, indicator of CMV-induced morbidity.

Severe pharyngitis also may be caused by another virus (e.g., herpes simplex) or by group A beta-hemolytic streptococci. Since group A beta-hemolytic streptococci can be isolated from the throat of up to 30 percent of patients with infectious mononucleosis, isolation of this organism does not rule out the diagnosis of infectious mononucleosis. Atypical lymphocytes also may be observed in a number of other conditions, including rubella, hepatitis, toxoplasmosis, mumps, and drug reactions. These conditions rarely pose major differential diagnostic problems when careful attention is paid to the other clinical and laboratory features of these illnesses.

TREATMENT Infectious mononucleosis usually requires only supportive management. Patients should be advised to obtain adequate rest; there is no evidence that forced bed rest hastens recovery. Fever and pharyngitis are usually ameliorated by acetaminophen. Because of the infrequent complication of splenic rupture, patients should be advised to avoid contact sports for 6 to 8 weeks after the onset of illness. The timing of return to school or work is determined solely by symptoms. Patients with mild illness may not require any major changes in routine. Occasional patients with protracted illness may not return to a full school or work schedule for several months. Recovery from mononucleosis is often gradual, and the malaise may wax and wane for some time.

Although glucocorticoids may hasten defervescence and the resolution of pharyngitis, they are indicated only for certain specific complications of mononucleosis; airway obstruction usually responds dramatically to parenteral glucocorticoids. Glucocorticoids also may hasten the recovery of patients with severe hemolytic anemia or thrombocytopenia. There is no evidence that glucocorticoids are beneficial for the neurologic complications of the illness. Occasional selected patients with protracted illness may benefit from a short course of prednisone, but glucocorticoids should be avoided in the majority of patients with infectious mononucleosis.

Acyclovir, α-interferon, and 9-[2-hydroxy-1-(hydroxymethyl)ethoxy]methyl guanine (ganciclovir) are active inhibitors of EBV replication in vitro. α-Interferon has antiviral activity and can decrease shedding of EBV by renal allograft recipients treated with antithymocyte globulin. Administration of intravenous or high-dose oral acyclovir halts oropharyngeal shedding of EBV in patients with acute infectious mononucleosis; however, clinical benefits are minimal or inapparent.

EBV-ASSOCIATED MALIGNANCY Since the initial description of EBV in patients with African Burkitt's lymphoma, the virus has been detected in association with several other malignancies. EBV DNA sequences have been detected in tumor tissue from more than 90 percent of patients with African Burkitt's lymphomas. American Burkitt's lymphoma, which often affects older children and more often presents as an intraabdominal tumor, is EBV-associated in only 15 percent of cases. Anaplastic nasopharyngeal carcinoma, a common neoplasm in southeast China, is highly associated with EBV; virtually all adequately studied patients with this malignancy have evidence of EBV in tumor tissue.

There is increasing evidence that implicates EBV in the pathogenesis of certain cases of lymphocytic lymphoma in the immunoincompetent host (see Chap. 311). B cell lymphoma is greatly overrepresented among malignancies developing in immunosuppressed individuals such as organ allograft recipients, patients with ataxia telangiectasia, and patients with AIDS. Immunologically privileged areas such as the central nervous system also appear to be particularly susceptible to EBV-associated B cell lymphomas. Cardiac allograft recipients treated with cyclosporin A appear to be particularly susceptible to B cell lymphoma. EBV sequences are detectable in up to half the B cell malignancies encountered in immunosuppressed individuals. The pathogenesis of B cell lymphoma is complex. In some cases, EBV-driven B cell transformation may be an early event; in others, transformation may be driven primarily by cytokines such as interleukin 6. The process, which may be polyclonal initially, becomes oligoclonal or monoclonal with a second-step chromosomal translocation made more likely by the increased number of proliferating B lymphocytes. The biologic behavior of these tumors does not always correlate with clonality as defined by conventional techniques. Patients have been described who have succumbed to lymphoproliferative processes which appear to be polyclonal by surface immunoglobulin studies. More sensitive techniques of defining clonality, such as that utilizing immunoglobulin gene rearrangement, may reveal that a larger proportion of the polyclonal lymphomas are in fact oligo- or monoclonal. The response of these B cell lymphomas to conventional chemotherapy is often disappointing. On occasion, these lymphoproliferative syndromes are reversible if the immunosuppression is decreased. There are case reports of apparent responses to acyclovir therapy; in most cases, however, such tumors do not respond to acyclovir, and conventional combination chemotherapy is required. Studies of larger numbers of these patients for the presence of EBV sequences and for the progression from a polyclonal to an oligoclonal or monoclonal disorder will shed more light on the role of EBV in oncogenesis in both immunoincompetent and immunologically normal hosts.

REFERENCES

GROSE C et al: Primary Epstein-Barr virus infections in acute neurologic diseases. N Engl J Med 292:392, 1975

HENLE W et al: Epstein-Barr virus specific diagnostic tests in infectious mononucleosis. Hum Pathol 5:551, 1974

HOLMES GP et al: Chronic fatigue syndrome: A working case definition. Ann Intern Med 108:387, 1989

MEEKER TC et al: Evidence for molecular subtypes of HIV-associated lymphoma: Division into peripheral monoclonal, polyclonal, and central nervous system lymphoma. AIDS 5:669, 1991

MILLER G et al: Selective lack of antibody to a component of EB nuclear antigen in patients with chronic active Epstein-Barr virus infection. J Infect Dis 156:26, 1987

MURRAY RJ et al: Human cytotoxic T-cell responses against Epstein-Barr virus nuclear antigens demonstrated by using recombinant vaccinia vectors. Proc Natl Acad Sci USA 87:2906, 1990

SCHOOLEY RT et al: Chronic Epstein-Barr virus infection associated with fever and interstitial pneumonitis. Ann Intern Med 104:636, 1986

SCULLEY TB et al: Coinfection with A-type and B-type Epstein-Barr virus in human immunodeficiency virus–positive subjects. J Infect Dis 162:643, 1990

SIXBY JW et al: Epstein-Barr virus replication in oropharyngeal epithelial cells. N Engl J Med 310:1225, 1984

STRAUS SE et al: Treatment of the chronic fatigue syndrome with acyclovir: Lack of efficacy in a placebo-controlled trial. N Engl J Med 319:1692–1698, 1988

146 CYTOMEGALOVIRUS INFECTION

MARTIN S. HIRSCH

DEFINITION Cytomegalovirus (CMV), which was initially isolated from patients with congenital cytomegalic inclusion disease, is now recognized as an important pathogen in all age groups. In addition to inducing severe birth defects, CMV causes a wide spectrum of disorders in older children and adults, ranging from an asymptomatic, subclinical infection to a mononucleosis syndrome in healthy individuals to disseminated disease in the immunocompromised. Human CMV is one of several related species-specific viruses that cause similar diseases in various animals. All are associated with the production of characteristic enlarged cells, hence the name *cytomegalovirus.*

ETIOLOGY CMV is a member of the beta herpesvirus group and contains double-stranded DNA, a protein capsid, and a lipoprotein envelope. Like other members of the herpesvirus group, CMV demonstrates icosahedral symmetry, replicates in the cell nucleus, and can cause either a lytic and productive or a latent infection. CMV can be distinguished from other herpesviruses by certain biologic properties such as host range and the type of cytopathology induced. Virus replication is associated with the production of large intranuclear inclusions and smaller cytoplasmic inclusions. The virus appears to replicate in a variety of cell types in vivo; in tissue culture it grows preferentially in fibroblasts. It is unclear whether CMV is oncogenic in vivo. However, the virus can rarely transform fibroblasts, and genomic transforming fragments have been identified.

EPIDEMIOLOGY CMV has a worldwide distribution. Approximately 1 percent of newborns in the United States are infected with CMV, and the percentage is higher in many less-developed countries. Communal living and poor personal hygiene facilitate early spread. Perinatal and early childhood infections are common. Virus may be present in milk, saliva, feces, and urine. Transmission of CMV has been identified among young children in day-care centers and has been traced from infected toddler to pregnant mother to developing fetus. When an infected child introduces CMV into a household, 50 percent of susceptible family members seroconvert within 6 months.

The virus is not readily spread by casual contact but requires repeated or prolonged intimate exposure for transmission. In late adolescence and young adulthood, CMV is often transmitted sexually, and asymptomatic viral carriage in semen or cervical secretions is common. The rate of detectable CMV antibody titers approaches 100 percent in female prostitutes and in sexually active homosexual men. Sexually active adults may harbor several strains of CMV simultaneously. Transfusion of whole blood or certain blood products containing viable leukocytes also may transmit CMV with a frequency of 0.14 to 10 percent per unit transfused.

Once infected, an individual probably carries the virus for life. Most commonly these infections remain latent. However, with compromise of T lymphocyte–mediated immunity, as occurs following organ transplantation or in association with lymphoid neoplasms and certain acquired immunodeficiencies (in particular, that caused by infection with the human immunodeficiency virus, or HIV; see Chap. 279), CMV reactivation syndromes develop frequently. Most primary CMV infections in organ transplant recipients result from transmission of the virus in the graft itself. In CMV-seropositive transplant recipients, infection results from reactivation of latent virus or, less commonly, from reinfection by a new strain of CMV.

PATHOGENESIS Congenital CMV infection can follow either primary or reactivation infection of the mother. However, clinical disease in the fetus or newborn is almost exclusively related to primary maternal infections (Table 146-1). Factors determining the severity of congenital infection are unknown; a deficient capacity to produce precipitating antibodies and to mount T cell responses to CMV is associated with more severe disease.

Primary infection in late childhood or adulthood is often associated with a vigorous T lymphocyte response that may contribute to the development of a mononucleosis syndrome similar to that observed following Epstein-Barr virus infection (see Chap. 145). The hallmarks of such infections are the appearance of atypical lymphocytes in the peripheral blood; these cells are predominantly activated T lymphocytes of cytotoxic-suppressor phenotype. Polyclonal activation of B cells by the virus contributes to the development of rheumatoid factors and other autoantibodies during CMV mononucleosis.

Once acquired during symptomatic or asymptomatic primary infection, CMV persists indefinitely in tissues of the host. The sites of persistent or latent infection are unclear but probably include multiple cell types and various organs. Transmission following blood transfusion or organ transplantation is due to silent infections in these tissues. Autopsy studies suggest that salivary glands and bowel also may be areas of latent infection.

If T cell responses of the host become compromised by disease or by iatrogenic immunosuppression, latent virus can be reactivated to cause a variety of syndromes. Chronic antigenic stimulation (as occurs following tissue transplantation) in the presence of immunosuppression appears to be an ideal setting for CMV activation and CMV-induced disease. Certain particularly potent suppressants of T cell immunity, such as antithymocyte globulin, are associated with a high rate of clinical CMV syndromes, which may follow either primary or reactivation infection. CMV may itself contribute to further T lymphocyte hyporesponsiveness, which often precedes superinfection with other opportunistic pathogens, such as *Pneumocystis carinii.* CMV and pneumocystis are frequently found together in immunosuppressed patients with severe interstitial pneumonia. CMV may function as a cofactor to activate latent HIV infection.

PATHOLOGY Cytomegalic cells in vivo are presumed to be infected epithelial cells. They are two to four times larger than

---

TABLE 146-1   CMV in the immunocompromised host

Population	Risk factors	Principal syndromes	Treatment	Prevention
Fetus	Primary maternal infection/ early pregnancy	Cytomegalic inclusion disease	None	Avoidance of exposure
Organ transplant recipient	Seropositive donor, seronegative recipient; intensive immunosuppression, particularly with antilymphocyte globulins, cyclosporine	Febrile leukopenia; pneumonia; gastrointestinal disease	Ganciclovir	Donor-matching; CMV immunoglobulin; ganciclovir or high-dose acyclovir
Bone marrow transplant recipient	Graft-vs-host disease; older age; seropositive recipient; viremia	Pneumonia; gastrointestinal disease	Ganciclovir plus CMV immunoglobulin	Ganciclovir or high-dose acyclovir
Person with AIDS	<100 CD4 cells/mm^3; CMV seropositivity	Retinitis; gastrointestinal disease	Foscarnet or ganciclovir	Trials under way

surrounding cells and often contain an 8- to 10-μm intranuclear inclusion that is eccentrically placed and surrounded by a clear halo resulting in an "owl's eye" appearance. Smaller granular cytoplasmic inclusions also may be demonstrated occasionally. Cytomegalic cells are found in a wide variety of organs, including salivary glands, lung, liver, kidney, intestines, pancreas, adrenal glands, and the central nervous system.

The cellular inflammatory response to infection consists of plasma cells, lymphocytes, and monocyte-macrophages. Granulomatous reactions are occasionally observed, particularly in the liver. Immunopathologic reactions may contribute to CMV disease. Immune complexes have been described in infected infants, sometimes associated with CMV-related glomerulopathies. Immune-complex glomerulopathy has been observed in some CMV-infected patients following renal transplantation.

CLINICAL MANIFESTATIONS **Congenital CMV infection** Fetal infections range from inapparent to severe and disseminated. Cytomegalic inclusion disease develops in approximately 5 percent of infected fetuses and is seen almost exclusively in infants born to mothers who develop primary infections during pregnancy. Petechiae, hepatosplenomegaly, and jaundice are the most common presenting features (60 to 80 percent). Microcephaly with or without cerebral calcifications, intrauterine growth retardation, and prematurity are noted in 30 to 50 percent of patients. Inguinal hernias and chorioretinitis occur less commonly. Laboratory abnormalities, in decreasing order of frequency, include an increase in serum IgM to >0.20 g/L (>20 mg/dL), atypical lymphocytosis, elevated liver transaminases, thrombocytopenia, hyperbilirubinemia, and an increase in cerebrospinal fluid protein to >0.20 g/L (>20 mg/dL). Prognosis among severely infected infants is poor, with mortality rates of 20 to 30 percent; few patients escape intellectual or hearing difficulties in later years. Differential diagnoses of cytomegalic inclusion disease in infants include syphilis, rubella, toxoplasmosis, herpes simplex or enterovirus infection, and bacterial sepsis.

Most congenital CMV infections are clinically inapparent at birth. Between 5 and 25 percent of asymptomatically infected infants develop significant psychomotor, hearing, ocular, or dental abnormalities over the next several years.

Perinatal CMV infection The newborn may acquire CMV at the time of delivery by passage through an infected birth canal or by postnatal contact with maternal milk or other secretions. Approximately 40 to 60 percent of infants who are breast-fed for over 1 month by seropositive mothers will become infected. Iatrogenic transmission also can result from neonatal blood transfusion. Screening of blood products prior to transfusion into low-birth-weight seronegative infants or seronegative pregnant women will decrease the risk of infection. The great majority of infants infected at or after delivery will remain asymptomatic. However, protracted interstitial pneumonitis has been associated with perinatally acquired CMV infection, particularly in premature infants, occasionally associated with *Chlamydia trachomatis, P. carinii,* or *Ureaplasma urealyticum* infections. Poor weight gain, adenopathy, rash, hepatitis, anemia, and atypical lymphocytosis also may be present, and CMV excretion often persists for months to years.

CMV mononucleosis The most common clinical manifestation of CMV infection in normal hosts beyond the neonatal period is a heterophil-antibody-negative mononucleosis syndrome. This may occur spontaneously or following the transfusion of leukocyte-containing blood products. Although the syndrome occurs at all ages, sexually active young adults are most often involved. Incubation periods range from 20 to 60 days, and the illness generally lasts 2 to 6 weeks. Prolonged high fevers, sometimes accompanied by chills, profound fatigue, and malaise, characterize this disorder. Myalgias, headache, and splenomegaly are frequent, but in CMV mononucleosis (as opposed to infectious mononucleosis caused by Epstein-Barr virus), exudative pharyngitis and cervical lymphadenopathy are rare. Occasional patients will develop rubelliform rashes, often after exposure to ampicillin. Less commonly observed are interstitial or segmental pneumonia, myocarditis, pleuritis, arthritis, or encephalitis. Rarely, Guillain-Barré syndrome may complicate CMV mononucleosis. The characteristic laboratory abnormality is a peripheral blood relative lymphocytosis with greater than 10 percent atypical lymphocytes. Total leukocyte counts may be low, normal, or markedly elevated. Although significant jaundice is uncommon, moderately elevated serum transaminase and alkaline phosphatase levels are often present. Heterophil antibodies are absent; however, transient immunologic abnormalities are common. These may include the presence of cryoglobulins, rheumatoid factors, cold agglutinins, and antinuclear antibodies. Rarely, hemolytic anemia, thrombocytopenia, and granulocytopenia complicate recovery.

Most patients recover without sequelae, although postviral asthenia may persist for months. CMV excretion in urine, genital secretions, or saliva often continues for months to years. Rare patients have recurrent episodes of fever and malaise, sometimes associated with autonomic nervous system dysfunction, e.g., attacks of sweating or flushing.

CMV infection in the immunocompromised host (See also Table 146-1) CMV appears to be the most frequent and important viral pathogen complicating organ transplantation. In renal, cardiac, lung, and liver transplant recipients, CMV induces a variety of syndromes, including fever and leukopenia, hepatitis, pneumonitis, esophagitis, gastritis, colitis, and retinitis. The maximal period of risk is between 1 and 4 months after transplantation, although retinitis may be a later complication. The risk of disease appears greater following primary infection. In addition, molecular studies indicate that seropositive transplant recipients are susceptible to reinfection with donor-derived, genotypically variant CMV, which often results in disease. Reactivation infection, although frequent, is less likely to be important clinically. Clinical disease is related to various factors (see Table 146-1), such as the degree of immunosuppression; patients receiving certain immunosuppressive agents, such as antithymocyte globulin, appear more likely to have severe infections than those receiving other agents, such as cyclosporin A. The transplanted organ is particularly vulnerable as a target for CMV infection; i.e., CMV hepatitis follows liver transplantation, and CMV pneumonitis more commonly follows lung transplantation.

CMV pneumonia occurs in nearly 15 to 20 percent of bone marrow transplant recipients, with a case-fatality rate of 84 to 88 percent. The risk is greatest between 5 and 13 weeks after transplantation, and several risk factors have been identified. These include type of immunosuppression, acute graft-versus-host disease, older age, viremia, and seropositivity before transplantation.

CMV has become recognized as an important pathogen in patients with AIDS (see Chap. 279). CMV infection is nearly ubiquitous in patients with AIDS and often causes retinitis or disseminated disease, contributing to death. CMV-induced immunosuppression probably also contributes to the T lymphocyte deficiency initiated by the etiologic retrovirus.

CMV syndromes in the immunocompromised host often begin with prolonged fever, malaise, anorexia, fatigue, night sweats, and arthralgias or myalgias. Liver function abnormalities, leukopenia, thrombocytopenia, and atypical lymphocytosis may be observed during these episodes. The development of tachypnea, hypoxia, and unproductive cough signals respiratory involvement. Radiologic examination of the lung often demonstrates bilateral interstitial or reticulonodular infiltrates, beginning in the periphery of the lower lobes and spreading centrally and superiorly; localized segmental, nodular, or alveolar patterns are less commonly observed. Diagnosis requires lung biopsy or bronchoalveolar lavage, since neither peripheral virus excretion nor high antibody titers provide sufficient information to prove etiology. The differential diagnoses include *P. carinii*; other viral, bacterial, or fungal pathogens; pulmonary hemorrhage; and injury secondary to radiation or cytotoxic drugs.

Gastrointestinal CMV involvement may be localized or extensive and occurs almost exclusively in compromised hosts. Ulcers of the esophagus, stomach, small intestine, or colon may result in bleeding or perforation. CMV infection may lead to exacerbations of underlying ulcerative colitis. Hepatitis occurs frequently, particularly following liver transplantation, and CMV-associated acalculous cholecystitis has been described.

CMV rarely causes meningoencephalitis in otherwise healthy individuals. Although CMV antigens and inclusions are observed occasionally in brains of patients dying from AIDS encephalopathy, the relative roles and interactions of CMV and HIV in this disorder are unclear. In immunocompromised patients, CMV can cause a subacute progressive polyradiculopathy, which is often reversible if recognized and treated promptly.

CMV retinitis is an important cause of blindness in immunocompromised patients, particularly patients with AIDS. Early lesions consist of small, opaque, white areas of granular retinal necrosis that spread in a centrifugal manner and are later accompanied by hemorrhages, vessel sheathing, and retinal edema (see Fig. A8-14). CMV must be distinguished from other causes of retinopathy, including toxoplasmosis, candidiasis, and herpes simplex virus infection.

Fatal CMV infections are often associated with persistent viremia and multiple organ system involvement. Progressive pulmonary infiltrates, pancytopenia, hyperamylasemia, and hypotension are characteristic, often with a terminal bacterial, fungal, or protozoan superinfection. Extensive adrenal necrosis with CMV inclusions is often present at autopsy, as is CMV involvement of many other organs.

DIAGNOSIS The diagnosis of CMV infection usually cannot be made reliably on clinical grounds alone. Virus isolation from appropriate clinical specimens, together with demonstration of a fourfold or greater antibody rise or persistently elevated antibody titers, is the preferred diagnostic approach. Virus excretion or viremia is readily detected by culture of appropriate specimens on human fibroblast monolayers. If virus titers are high, as is frequently the case in congenital disseminated infection or in patients with AIDS, characteristic cytopathic effects may be detected within a few days. However, in some situations, e.g., CMV mononucleosis, virus titers are low, and cytopathic effects may take several weeks to appear. Many laboratories expedite diagnosis by using an overnight tissue culture method (shell vial assay) involving centrifugation and an immunocytochemical detection technique employing monoclonal antibodies to an immediate early CMV antigen. Virus isolation from urine or saliva by itself does not prove acute infection, since excretion from these sites may continue for months to years following illness. Detection of CMV viremia is a better predictor of acute infection. Detection of CMV immediate-early antigens or DNA in peripheral blood leukocytes may hasten the diagnosis of CMV disease in certain populations, e.g., organ transplant recipients. Positivity in such assays may antedate culture positivity by several days.

A variety of serologic assays (complement fixation, immunofluorescence, indirect hemagglutination, ELISA) are available to detect antibody rises to CMV antigens. Antibody rises may not be detectable for up to 4 weeks after primary infection, and titers often remain high for years after infection. For this reason, single-sample antibody determinations are of no value in assessing the acuteness of infection. Detection of CMV-specific IgM is sometimes useful in the diagnosis of recent or active infection; circulating rheumatoid factors may result in occasional false-positive IgM tests.

PREVENTION AND TREATMENT Several prophylactic measures are useful to prevent CMV infection in patients at high risk. The use of blood from seronegative donors or blood that was frozen, thawed, and deglycerolized greatly decreases transfusion-associated transmission of CMV. Similarly, matching of organ or bone marrow transplants by CMV serology, using only organs from seronegative donors for seronegative recipients, reduces primary infections following transplantation.

CMV immune globulin has been reported to reduce CMV-associated syndromes and fungal or parasitic superinfections in seronegative renal transplant recipients. Similar studies in bone marrow transplant recipients have produced conflicting results. Pro-

phylactic acyclovir has been demonstrated to reduce CMV infection and disease in seronegative renal transplant recipients; acyclovir is not effective in treatment of active CMV disease, however.

Ganciclovir (dihydroxypropoxymethyl guanine, DHPG) is a guanosine derivative with considerably more activity against CMV than its congener, acyclovir. After intracellular conversion, ganciclovir triphosphate is a selective inhibitor of CMV DNA polymerase. Several clinical studies have indicated response rates of 70 to 90 percent among patients with AIDS given ganciclovir for the treatment of CMV retinitis or colitis. In bone marrow transplant recipients with CMV pneumonia, ganciclovir is less effective when given alone, but a favorable clinical response occurs 50 to 70 percent of the time when it is combined with CMV immune globulin. Prophylactic or suppressive ganciclovir may be useful in high-risk bone marrow or organ transplant recipients e.g., those who are CMV-seropositive pretransplant or who are CMV culture-positive posttransplant. In many patients with AIDS and CMV disease, clinical and virologic relapses occur if treatment with ganciclovir is discontinued. Therefore, prolonged maintenance regimens are recommended. Resistance to ganciclovir is common in patients treated for more than 3 months. Usual induction courses for CMV retinitis are 5 mg/kg IV twice daily for 14 to 21 days followed by 5 mg/kg daily for 5 to 7 days per week. Peripheral blood neutropenia, the major toxic effect of ganciclovir, often can be ameliorated by the concomitant use of granulocyte colony-stimulating factor or granulocyte-macrophage colony-stimulating factor.

Foscarnet (sodium phosphonoformate) also acts against CMV infection by inhibiting the viral DNA polymerase. Because this agent does not require phosphorylation to be active, it is also effective against ganciclovir-resistant CMV isolates. A comparative trial of foscarnet and ganciclovir in 234 patients with AIDS and CMV retinitis demonstrated equivalent activity against retinitis but longer survival (12.6 versus 8.5 months) in the foscarnet group. Although the reasons for the survival differences are unclear, the antiretroviral activity of foscarnet and the greater use of zidovudine in foscarnet recipients are strong possibilities. Foscarnet exhibits considerable toxicity, including renal dysfunction, hypomagnesemia, hypokalemia, hypocalcemia, seizures, fever, and rash, each occurring in more than 5 percent of recipients. Moreover, foscarnet administration requires the use of an infusion pump and close clinical monitoring. The recommended regimen of foscarnet for CMV retinitis is induction with 60 mg/kg IV every 8 h for 14 to 21 days, followed by daily maintenance infusions of 90 to 120 mg/kg.

REFERENCES

BALFOUR HH et al: A randomized, placebo-controlled trial of oral acyclovir for the prevention of cytomegalovirus disease in recipients of renal allografts. N Engl J Med 320:1381, 1989

BOWDEN RA et al: Cytomegalovirus (CMV)-specific intravenous immunoglobulin for the prevention of primary CMV infection and disease after marrow transplant. J Infect Dis 164:483, 1991

BUHLES WC et al: Ganciclovir treatment of life- or sight-threatening cytomegalovirus infection: Experience in 314 immunocompromised patients. Rev Infect Dis 10:S495, 1988

CHOU S: Newer methods for diagnosis of cytomegalovirus infection. Rev Infect Dis 12:5727, 1990

DREW WL: Cytomegalovirus infection in patients with AIDS. J Infect Dis 158:449, 1988
——— et al: Prevalence of resistance in patients receiving ganciclovir for serious cytomegalovirus infection. J Infect Dis 163:716, 1991

EMMANUEL D et al: Cytomegalovirus pneumonia after bone marrow transplantation successfully treated with the combination of ganciclovir and high-dose intravenous immunoglobulin. Ann Intern Med 109:777, 1988

GERNA G et al: Monitoring of human cytomegalovirus infections and ganciclovir treatment in heart transplant recipients by determination of viremia, antigens and DNA emia. J Infect Dis 164:488, 1991

GRUNDY JE et al: Symptomatic cytomegalovirus infection in seropositive kidney recipients: Reinfection with donor virus rather than reactivation of recipient virus. Lancet 2:132, 1988

HIRSCH MS: Cytomegalovirus and its role in the pathogenesis of acquired immunodeficiency syndrome. Transplant Proc 23:S118, 1991
———: The treatment of cytomegalovirus in AIDS: More than meets the eye. N Engl J Med 326:264, 1992

Ho M: *Cytomegalovirus: Biology and Infection*. New York, Plenum Press, 1982

HORWITZ CA et al: Clinical and laboratory evaluation of cytomegalovirus-induced mononucleeosis in previously healthy patients. Medicine 65:124, 1986.

JACOBSON MA, MILLS J: Serious cytomegalovirus disease in the acquired immunodeficiency syndrome (AIDS). Ann Intern Med 108:585, 1988

MERIGAN TC et al: A controlled trial of ganciclovir to prevent cytomegalovirus disease after heart transplantation. N Engl J Med 326:1182, 1992

MEYERS JD et al: Cytomegalovirus excretion as a predictor of cytomegalovirus disease after marrow transplantation: Importance of cytomegalovirus viremia. J Infect Dis 162:373, 1990

MILLER, RG et al: Ganciclovir in the treatment of progressive AIDS-related polyradiculopathy. Neurology 40:569, 1990

ONORATO IM et al: Epidemiology of cytomegaloviral infections: Recommendations for prevention and control. Rev Infect Dis 7:479, 1985

PASS RF et al: Young children as a probable source of maternal and congenital cytomegalovirus infection. N Engl J Med 316:1366, 1987

PREIKSAITIS JK et al: The risk of cytomegalovirus infection in seronegative transfusion recipients not receiving exogenous immunosuppression. J Infect Dis 157:523, 1988

REED EC et al: Treatment of cytomegalovirus pneumonia with ganciclovir and intravenous cytomegalovirus immunoglobulin in patients with bone marrow transplants. Ann Intern Med 109:783, 1988

SCHMIDT GM et al: A randomized controlled trail of prophylactic ganciclovir for cytomegalovirus pulmonary infection in recipients of allogeneic bone marrow transplants. N Engl J Med 324:1005, 1991

SCHOOLEY RE: Cytomegalovirus in the setting of the infection with human immunodeficiency virus. Rev Infect Dis 12:5811, 1990

SMYTH RL et al: Cytomegalovirus infection in heart-lung transplant recipients: Risk factors, clinical associations, and response to treatment. J Infect Dis 164:1045, 1991

SNYDMAN DR et al: Use of cytomegalovirus immune globulin to prevent cytomegalovirus disease in renal transplant recipients. N Engl J Med 317:1049, 1987

STUDIES OF OCULAR COMPLICATION OF AIDS RESEARCH GROUP, AIDS CLINICAL TRIALS GROUP: Mortality in patients with the acquired immunodeficiency syndrome treated with either foscarnet or ganciclovir for cytomegalovirus retinitis. N Engl J Med 326:213, 1992

VAN DEN BERG AP et al: Antigenemia in the diagnosis and monitoring of active cytomegalovirus infection after liver transplantation. J Infect Dis 164:265, 1991

147 SMALLPOX, VACCINIA, AND OTHER POXVIRUSES

HARVEY M. FRIEDMAN

Poxviruses that infect humans share the common feature of producing cutaneous vesicular eruptions. They are brick-shaped, double-stranded DNA viruses and are the largest of the animal viruses. Human pathogens include variola, vaccinia, monkeypox, cowpox, milker's node virus, and molluscum contagiosum. These viruses can be distinguished from one another by antigenic differences, clinical manifestations of infection, and pox morphology when inoculated onto chick embryo chorioallantoic membranes. Global eradication of smallpox and the concomitant reduction in smallpox vaccination programs have changed the epidemiology of variola and vaccinia and have modified their importance in modern medicine.

SMALLPOX

DEFINITION Smallpox (variola major) is a highly contagious disease characterized by fever, a vesicular and pustular eruption, and a high mortality rate. A milder form (variola minor) may be caused by the same virus.

The global eradication of smallpox was officially announced in 1979, marking one of the greatest achievements of modern medicine. Smallpox has not reappeared for over a decade. If this pattern persists, a disease that once accounted for 10 percent of all deaths will become an illness mainly of historical interest.

ETIOLOGY Variola virus, the causative agent of smallpox, is an orthopoxvirus within the Poxviridae family. Variola is a large (200 to 400 nm) DNA virus differing from other DNA viruses in that it lacks icosahedral symmetry. When viewed by electron microscopy, it has a complex structure and appears brick-shaped. It has an outer membrane, two lateral bodies, and a dumbbell-shaped core that contains a single molecule of double-stranded DNA.

PATHOGENESIS AND PATHOLOGY The oropharynx of infected patients serves as the main source for virus spread. Contacts become infected by inhaling virus which enters the respiratory tract and multiplies locally, probably within macrophages. Virus is carried within macrophages into the circulation and to regional lymph nodes. Multiplication occurs within lymphoid organs, and a secondary viremia develops. Virus localizes within small dermal blood vessels, leading to endothelial swelling and infection of epidermal cells. Intraepidermal vesicles form in skin and mucous membranes. When stained with hematoxylin and eosin, the cytoplasm of infected cells contains faintly basophilic or acidophilic inclusions (Guarnieri bodies). Extension of infection into the corium and sebaceous glands produces pockmarks, or scars, which, upon healing, are characteristic of smallpox infection.

Virus infection stimulates cytotoxic T cell responses, neutralizing antibodies, and the production of interferons. These responses restrict viral replication and induce prolonged immunity if the patient recovers. The infection is likely to be most severe in impaired hosts, particularly those with T cell deficits. Milder forms of the infection have been observed in immunized patients, although it remains unclear why variola minor may be produced by the same virus in the unimmunized.

EPIDEMIOLOGY Smallpox was described in Asia during the first century A.D., in Europe and Africa around 700 A.D., and in Central, South, and North America during the sixteenth and seventeenth centuries. Endemic variola major was eradicated from the United States in 1926, and variola minor during the 1940s. Eradication was slower in Asia, Africa, and parts of the Americas. The last naturally occurring smallpox infection occurred in Somalia, Africa, in October 1977. The last known case developed 1 year later in Birmingham, England, in September 1978, and was the result of a laboratory accident. The ability to eradicate this disease by an effective worldwide vaccination program appears to be centrally related to the facts that human beings were the only known reservoir for the variola virus; that no asymptomatic carrier state existed, facilitating surveillance; and that early diagnosis and prevention of disease or modification of the course by rapid vaccination of contacts were possible.

In temperate climates, endemic smallpox occurred in winter and spring. It was mainly a disease of children and young adults. Spread in unvaccinated family contacts was approximately 58 percent, compared with 4 percent in vaccinees. Patients were usually severely ill and confined to bed, which restricted transmission to immediate family contacts. Index cases rarely infected more than five patients, most commonly those sharing living quarters. Transmission intervals were 2 to 3 weeks apart, and new cases would appear in a community or region over many months.

CLINICAL FEATURES Smallpox was endemic in every country of the world and existed as two forms, variola major, which was a serious illness with a mortality rate of >20 percent in the unvaccinated, and variola minor, which was a milder infection with a mortality of <1 percent. Both were caused by the same virus. On an individual case basis, it may be difficult to distinguish variola minor from a mild case of variola major. The severity of an entire outbreak is generally required to differentiate the two. The evolution of rash in variola minor is more rapid, similar to accelerated smallpox.

Variola major has been classified into five clinical categories:

1 *Ordinary type:* This comprised >70 percent of cases. It is characterized by raised pustular skin lesions which can be divided into three categories: (a) *confluent* rash present on face and forearms, (b) *semiconfluent* rash present on face with discrete rash elsewhere, and (c) *discrete* rash on all involved areas with normal skin between pustules. In unvaccinated patients, mortality was 62 percent for confluent infection, 37 percent for semiconfluent, and 9 percent for discrete infection.

2 *Modified type:* This form of smallpox is similar to ordinary disease, except that the course is accelerated and pustular lesions are

smaller. Modified smallpox was common in vaccinated patients who developed lesions, in health care workers exposed by accidental inoculation, and in those intentionally infected by variolation, a procedure once widely used as a method of vaccination.

3 *Variola sine eruptione:* Patients have fever but no rash. This was seen in vaccinated patients or those previously infected. Laboratory testing is required for confirmation of the diagnosis.

4 *Flat type:* Pustules remain flat and are usually confluent or semiconfluent in distribution. This form of infection occurred mainly in children and was often fatal.

5 *Hemorrhagic type:* Skin lesions and mucous membranes become hemorrhagic. Pregnant women were predisposed to this form of smallpox, which was rare but severe. Profound prostration, heart failure, diffuse bleeding, and bone marrow suppression resulted, and most infections were fatal within 3 to 4 days, earning the name "sledgehammer smallpox."

In a typical case of ordinary type smallpox, the incubation period is 7 to 19 days, with a mean of 12. A preeruptive phase lasting 2 to 4 days is characterized by sudden onset of fever, severe headache, backache, and malaise. Vomiting occurs in 50 percent and diarrhea in 10 percent of patients. The rash first appears as minute red spots on the tongue and palate and as small macules (herald spots) on the face. Spread is centrifugal, involving the face, proximal extremities, trunk, and then distal extremities. Intraoral rash evolves from papules to vesicles, which break down and release large amounts of virus. The enanthem is an important source of virus spread. On the skin, macules evolve to papules by day 2, vesicles by days 4 to 5, and pustules by day 7 of rash. Fever may recur during the pustular phase. Lesions, which range from few to thousands, have a shotty, hard feel to them. Crusts develop by day 14 and heal leaving depigmented areas.

LABORATORY FINDINGS Virus isolation Virus can be isolated from skin lesions (until scabs form), oropharynx, conjunctiva, and urine. Viremia precedes the rash and clears in most patients when the rash appears. Virus particles can be seen by negative-staining electron microscopy performed on fluid obtained from skin lesions. This form of diagnosis was used to identify cases during the intensified eradication programs carried out in the 1960s and 1970s.

Serology Antibodies appear by days 6 to 8 of infection. Antibody titer rises can be detected by testing paired serum samples drawn 2 to 3 weeks apart. Methods used to measure antibodies include hemagglutination inhibition, complement fixation, neutralization, and gel precipitation.

Hematology Granulocytopenia, thrombocytopenia, and lymphocytosis are common during the prodromal and early rash phase. Leukocytosis occurs with pustulation of the vesicles. A profile consistent with disseminated intravascular coagulation is seen in patients with hemorrhagic smallpox.

DIFFERENTIAL DIAGNOSIS Distinguishing varicella from smallpox was particularly difficult during epidemics of variola minor or when mild smallpox infection developed in vaccinated patients. Dense rash on the trunk and appearance of lesions in crops are features of varicella not seen in smallpox. Human monkeypox, seen in western and central Africa, is difficult to distinguish from smallpox. Monkeypox is associated with more lymphadenopathy than smallpox. In the past, virus isolation was required to differentiate the two. On occasion, virus isolation also was required to distinguish disseminated vaccinia infection from smallpox.

COMPLICATIONS AND SEQUELAE Complications include secondary bacterial infections of the skin, keratitis and corneal ulcerations, viral arthritis and osteomyelitis, bacterial pneumonia, orchitis, and encephalitis. Sequelae include blindness from corneal scarring, limb deformities, and pockmarks, which appear hypopigmented in dark-skinned individuals and hyperpigmented in light-skinned patients.

TREATMENT AND OUTCOME In the past, mortality was highest in infants and the elderly. Infection in pregnant women led to abortion rates of >60 percent. Vaccination during the first week of incubation modified the course of disease by protecting many and reducing the severity of infection in others. This constituted an important method for control of smallpox. Immunotherapy with vaccinia immune globulin given during the incubation period of infection modified disease; however, supplies were too limited for this form of therapy to be widely applicable. Several different thiosemicarbazones, a class of antiviral compounds, were tried for treatment, but no benefit was detected in controlled human trials. One thiosemicarbazone, metisazone, was found to be useful as preventive therapy following exposure. Vaccinia immune globulin also was effective in postexposure prophylaxis without the side effects of metisazone. The mainstay of treatment was good nursing care, which was often provided by family members at home or in hospitals.

CONTROL Attempts at control of smallpox began once it was noted that accidental exposure to smallpox by scratch on the skin resulted in less severe infection. This led to the practice of variolation, which began in China and India in the tenth century. Variolation involved intentional administration of pustular fluids or scabs to uninfected persons. In 1796, Edward Jenner showed that inoculation with cowpox virus protected against smallpox and carried less risk of illness than variolation. Subsequently, vaccination was modified to use of vaccinia virus for smallpox control. The origins of vaccinia virus are uncertain, but many strains existed which were apparently derived from either variola or cowpox virus. Successful vaccination provided high levels of protection for 5 years and some protection for 20 years. Periodic revaccination was necessary for optimal protection. Postexposure vaccination lowered the incidence and reduced the severity of infection when administered within 1 week after exposure.

In 1959, the World Health Assembly adopted a program aimed at global eradication of smallpox. The development of stable freeze-dried vaccine meant that vaccination programs could reach less developed tropical countries. Efforts were intensified by 1967 and were built on the principles of surveillance and containment involving case detection, quarantine of infected patients, and vaccination of contacts and others living in the immediate area. Surveillance and contact vaccination were extremely important for the eventual success of the program. This approach was successful because smallpox has a long incubation period that allows vaccination to modify the course of the illness. The lack of a reservoir for variola, other than humans, the ease of clinical diagnosis; and the fact that variola does not establish latent or persistent infection were important contributors to the success of the eradication program.

VACCINIA

DEFINITION AND ETIOLOGY Vaccinia is a localized skin infection caused by inoculation of vaccinia virus. In immunosuppressed patients it may occasionally disseminate and produce severe disease. Vaccinia virus is thought to be derived from either variola, cowpox, or perhaps a hybrid of the two. "Vaccination" with vaccinia induces immunity to variola and was the method used to control or prevent smallpox. Endemic smallpox was eradicated from the United States in 1949, which led to the eventual discontinuation of routine childhood immunization by 1972. Evidence of immunization against smallpox is no longer required for international travel.

COMPLICATIONS OF VACCINATION Vaccine is applied to the skin, which is punctured several times by a sterile needle to penetrate the epidermis. Primary vaccination results in formation of a papule in 4 to 5 days that becomes a vesicle 2 to 3 days later. Mild fever and localized lymphadenopathy are often present at this stage. Within 2 weeks, a scab forms that leaves a scar when healing is complete. The response during revaccination is accelerated and generally is not associated with fever or lymphadenopathy.

Vaccinia virus never underwent controlled trials to establish safety and efficacy before licensing. Nevertheless, the vaccine was highly effective, despite considerable adverse effects. *Complications* included: (1) *Progressive vaccinia* (vaccinia gangrenosum) developed in patients who were agammaglobulinemic, T cell deficient, or receiving immunosuppressive therapy. Destruction of local areas of skin, subcutaneous tissue, and other underlying structures occurred, with metastatic lesions appearing at other cutaneous sites and in viscera and bone. This complication developed in approximately 1 patient per million during primary or revaccination and was usually fatal over a period of several months. (2) *Eczema vaccinatum* involved wide cutaneous spread of vaccinia virus in vaccinees and their contacts who had eczema or other chronic skin diseases. It developed in 1 per 100,000 primary vaccinations or 1 per million revaccinations and was sometimes fatal; bacterial superinfection often complicated eczema vaccinatum. (3) *Generalized vaccinia*, characterized by satellite lesions around the inoculation site or more widely disseminated pox, occasionally occurred in immunocompetent individuals and developed in 3 per 100,000 primary vaccinations or 1 per million revaccinations. This complication had a good prognosis. (4) *Accidental inoculation*, especially of eyelids, perineum, and vulva, occurred in 3 per 100,000 to 1 million vaccinees. The consequences were generally not serious. (5) *Postvaccinial encephalitis* was a serious complication which occurred in 3 per million patients after primary vaccination. It usually developed 6 to 15 days after vaccination and had a violent onset. Features included convulsions, hemiplegia, and aphasia. Spinal fluid analysis was normal except for increased pressure. Recovery was often incomplete, and neurologic sequelae ensued.

Contraindications to vaccination include B or T cell immune disorders, neoplasms of the reticuloendothelial system, concomitant use of immunosuppressive drugs, eczema, pregnancy, and disorders of the central nervous system. When complications developed due to uncontrolled or progressive vaccinia infection, some were treated effectively with vaccinia immune globulin. This treatment is not effective for postvaccinial encephalitis. A role for antivirals, such as thiosemicarbazones, has not been definitely established.

Interest has reemerged in vaccinia as a vehicle for vaccination. Genes from herpes simplex virus, hepatitis B virus, human immunodeficiency virus, and malaria have been introduced into the vaccinia genome. Proteins encoded by these genes are expressed during vaccinia infection, which indicates that this virus potentially could serve as a vector for multiple vaccines. Should this approach prove successful, then the same precautions should be followed as in vaccination to prevent smallpox.

OTHER POXVIRUSES

HUMAN MONKEYPOX The monkeypox virus is a member of the *Orthopoxvirus* genus. Human monkeypox is a rare zoonosis that occurs in tropical rain forests of west and central Africa. This disease was first recognized in the 1960s during smallpox eradication efforts. Identification resulted from attempts to confirm suspected cases of smallpox by laboratory methods. Infection does not spread from person to person, which accounts for the low number of cases, less than 100, identified so far. The clinical features of infection are similar to smallpox, except that cervical and inguinal lymphadenopathy are more prominent in human monkeypox. The diagnosis can be established by the characteristic pox morphology when virus is inoculated onto chorioallantoic membrane cultures.

COWPOX Cowpox virus is another member of the genus *Orthopoxvirus*. Infection develops by hand contact with infected ulcers on the teats of cows. The virus is also found in wild rodents, which may serve as a reservoir for some human infections. After exposure, one or more skin lesions develop, most often on the hands. The evolution of a lesion is similar to that seen during primary smallpox vaccination: a vesicle progresses to a pustule that later scabs. The rash does not become generalized. It is often associated with lymphangitis and localized lymphadenopathy. The disease may be confused with milker's nodule (see below). Laboratory confirmation can be estab-

lished by the characteristic pox that develop when virus is isolated on chorioallantoic membranes.

MILKER'S NODE VIRUS This infection is caused by a parapoxvirus and is sometimes referred to as pseudocowpox or paravaccinia. It is acquired by contact with infected cows. Lesions appear as red nodules that progress to firm purple papules. The lack of vesicles or pustules distinguishes it from cowpox. Lesions are relatively painless and generally resolve in 4 to 6 weeks.

ORF This is a disease of sheep that is sometimes referred to as contagious pustular dermatitis. It is caused by a parapoxvirus. Human infection is acquired by contact with sheep infected around the mouth, nose, or eyes. Human infection usually occurs at abrasion sites on the hands. Single or multiple painful large vesicles develop and are often associated with lymphadenopathy. Resolution occurs within several weeks.

MOLLUSCUM CONTAGIOSUM This infection occurs only in humans and is caused by an unclassified poxvirus that cannot be cultured in vitro. Lesions occur anywhere on the body, except on the palms and soles, and appear as pearly, flesh-colored, raised, umbilicated nodules 2 to 5 mm in diameter. Lesions develop in crops, are painless, and resolve over a period of weeks to several years. Spread is probably by direct contact, which accounts for the commonly observed genital distribution of lesions in sexually active adults. An increased incidence of molluscum contagiosum is seen in patients infected with the human immunodeficiency virus. No specific therapy is available, although lesions can be removed by curettage.

REFERENCES

BAXBY D: The origins of vaccinia virus. J Infect Dis 136:453, 1977

BREMAN JG, ARITA I: The confirmation and maintenance of smallpox eradication. N Engl J Med 303:1263, 1980

FENNER F: Poxviruses, in *Virology*, 2d ed, BN Fields et al (eds). New York, Raven, 1990, pp 2113–2133

——— et al: *Smallpox and Its Eradication*. Geneva, World Health Organization, 1988

Moss B: Poxviridae and their replication, in *Virology*, 2d ed, BN Fields et al (eds). New York, Raven, 1990, pp 2079–2111

———: Vaccinia virus: A tool for research and vaccine development. Science 252:1662, 1991

148 PARVOVIRUS

NEIL R. BLACKLOW

DEFINITION The parvovirus group includes several species-specific viruses of animals. One parvovirus, designated B19, is known to be a human pathogen. B19 is a small (diameter 20 to 25 nm), icosahedral, nonenveloped, single-stranded DNA virus with an outer capsid formed by two structural proteins. Individual virus particles contain DNA strands of positive or negative polarity. The virus is stable and retains infectivity after incubation at 60°C for 16 h. It has failed to grow in conventional cell culture lines and animal model systems but does replicate in vitro in erythroid progenitor cells derived from human bone marrow, umbilical cord, peripheral blood, or fetal liver sources.

During the 1980s, it was discovered that B19 causes a variety of disorders ranging from erythema infectiosum and acute arthropathy in otherwise healthy hosts to transient aplastic crisis and chronic anemia in compromised patients to fetal infection manifested by death or hydrops fetalis. Many of the severe manifestations of B19 viremia relate to the propensity of the virus to infect and lyse erythroid precursor cells in the bone marrow. The name B19 is derived from the code number of the human serum in which the virus was discovered.

PATHOGENESIS   Two studies of adult volunteers have provided a basis for understanding the pathogenesis of B19 infection, which has two phases. The first phase is characterized by viremia that develops approximately 6 days after intranasal inoculation of B19 into susceptible individuals who lack serum antibodies to the virus. The viremia lasts about 1 week; its clearance is correlated with the development of IgM antibodies to B19 that remain detectable for up to a few months. IgG antibodies develop several days later and persist indefinitely. Nonspecific systemic symptoms lasting 2 or 3 days occur early during the viremic phase; these symptoms include headache, malaise, myalgia, fever, chills, and pruritus and are accompanied by reticulocytopenia and excretion of the virus from the respiratory tract. Several days after the onset of symptoms, a clinically insignificant decline in hemoglobin concentration is noted; the decreased level is maintained for 7 to 10 days, during which time examination of bone marrow samples reveals a marked depletion of erythroid precursor cells. Transient mild lymphopenia, neutropenia, and a drop in platelet count also may be documented. A second phase of illness begins around 17 or 18 days after virus inoculation (after the clearance of viremia, the cessation of viral shedding in throat secretions, and the resolution of reticulocytopenia). This illness mimics erythema infectiosum in adults, with 2 to 3 days of fine maculopapular rash accompanied by arthralgias and arthritis that last another 1 or 2 days. This phase occurs in the presence of rising serum titers of antibody to B19.

The studies just described indicate that B19 disease in the otherwise *healthy host*, manifested by self-limited erythema infectiosum and/or arthropathy, is almost certainly an immune-complex disorder. This concept is supported by the induction of erythema infectiosum through the infusion of immunoglobulins into chronically viremic patients. In contrast, B19 disease in the *compromised host* (chronic hemolytic disease or immunodeficiency syndromes) is often serious, resulting from the destruction by B19 of erythroid precursor cells. Normal hosts can tolerate 7 to 10 days of shutoff of erythropoiesis; however, patients with hemolytic disease who require increased production of erythrocytes do not tolerate erythroid cell destruction and thus usually develop severe transient aplastic crisis. Patients who are immunodeficient may fail to clear B19 viremia, the results being persistent infection of red blood cells and chronic severe anemia. The fetus requires increased production of red blood cells and possesses an immature immune system; both these factors could explain B19-induced hydrops fetalis.

EPIDEMIOLOGY   Although B19 infections occur year round, they appear most commonly as outbreaks of erythema infectiosum in schools during winter and spring months. Between 20 and 60 percent of children in outbreaks are symptomatic, and 10 percent have asymptomatic infection. Seroepidemiologic studies indicate that approximately half of adults possess serum antibodies to B19, with antibody prevalence (reflecting prior exposure and probable immunity to the virus) rising rapidly between the ages of 5 and 18. B19 can be detected in throat swabbings, respiratory tract secretions, and serum, and its detection at these sites probably correlates with infectiousness. Thus patients with transient aplastic crisis are highly infectious. Their infectivity has been well documented as the source of one well-defined nosocomial outbreak of erythema infectiosum among nurses. In contrast, individuals with erythema infectiosum are much less infectious. The usual route of viral transmission under natural conditions is unknown but may be respiratory or through direct contact. B19 can be transmitted during therapy with clotting factor concentrate, even after exposure to steam or dry heat.

CLINICAL MANIFESTATIONS   Erythema infectiosum   Erythema infectiosum is the most common manifestation of B19 infection and occurs predominantly in children. This entity is also called *fifth disease* because it was classified in the late nineteenth century as the fifth in a series of six exanthems of childhood. Normally a mild illness, erythema infectiosum typically presents as a facial rash with a "slapped-cheek" appearance that is sometimes preceded by low-grade fever. The rash may develop quickly on the arms and legs and usually has a lacy, reticular, erythematous appearance. The trunk, palms, and soles are less commonly involved. Occasionally, the rash appears with maculopapular, morbilliform, vesicular, purpuric, or pruritic characteristics. The typical rash resolves in about a week but can recur intermittently for several weeks, particularly after stress, exercise, exposure to sunlight, bathing, or change in environmental temperature. Arthralgia and arthritis are uncommon among children but are frequent among adults, in whom the rash is often absent or nonspecific, with a lack of the characteristic facial erythema.

Arthropathy   B19 infection in adults most commonly presents as acute arthralgias and arthritis, sometimes accompanied by rash. The arthritis is characteristically symmetric and peripheral, involving the wrists, hands, and knees most frequently. It normally resolves in about 3 weeks and is nondestructive. However, a small percentage of patients have arthritis persisting for months or even (in rare cases) for years. It is not known whether these individuals have persistent infection or an abnormal immune response to the virus. Several case reports have suggested a link—as yet unproven—between B19 and vascular purpura and vasculitis, idiopathic thrombocytopenic purpura, virus-associated hemophagocytic syndrome with pancytopenia, Lyme-like arthritis, recurrent paresthesias, rheumatoid arthritis, fibromyalgia, periarteritis nodosa, and systemic lupus erythematosus.

Transient aplastic crisis   B19 infection is the cause in most instances of transient aplastic crisis developing suddenly in patients with chronic hemolytic disease. Nearly all hemolytic conditions can be affected by B19 infection, including sickle cell disease, erythrocyte enzyme deficiencies, hereditary spherocytosis, thalassemias, paroxysmal nocturnal hemoglobinuria, and autoimmune hemolysis. B19-induced aplastic crisis also can occur in the setting of acute blood loss. Patients present with weakness, lethargy, pallor, and severe anemia, a syndrome often preceded by a few days of nonspecific symptoms. These patients have intense reticulocytopenia lasting 7 to 10 days, and their bone marrow contains no erythroid precursor cells despite a normal myeloid series. Transient aplastic crisis can produce life-threatening anemia and may require urgent transfusion therapy. Unlike patients with erythema infectiosum or arthropathy, those with transient aplastic crisis are viremic and can readily transmit B19 virus infection to other people.

Chronic anemia in immunodeficient patients   Immunodeficient patients may be unable to eliminate B19 infection, probably because they cannot produce adequate levels of virus-specific IgG antibodies. The result is persistent infection with destruction of erythroid precursor cells in the bone marrow and chronic transfusion-dependent anemia. This condition has been described in patients with immunodeficiency related to infection with human immunodeficiency virus, congenital immunodeficiencies, and acute lymphocytic leukemia during maintenance chemotherapy, as well as in recipients of bone marrow transplants. B19-induced chronic anemia also may be the presenting finding of an otherwise unrecognized immunodeficiency. Chronic anemia may fluctuate in intensity over time and may be cured or controlled by immunoglobulin therapy. Both the spectrum of immunodeficiencies associated with B19-induced chronic anemia and the frequency of the association remain to be determined.

Fetal infection   Maternal B19 infections usually do not adversely affect the fetus; more often than not, in fact, the fetus remains uninfected. It is estimated that fewer than 10 percent of maternal B19 infections lead to fetal death; when fetal death does occur, it is usually attributable to the development of nonimmune hydrops fetalis, wherein the fetus succumbs to severe anemia and congestive heart failure. B19 virus can be detected in fetal tissues, with predominant infection of erythroblasts. Some hydropic fetuses survive B19 infection and appear normal at delivery. There is no evidence that B19 infection produces congenital abnormalities. A pregnant woman is not likely to become infected with B19 after exposure to a child with erythema infectiosum because the infectious stage of this disease is probably over by the time the classic rash develops.

DIAGNOSIS   Diagnosis most commonly relies on measurements of B19 virus–specific IgM and IgG antibodies. The virus, its DNA, or its antigens are also detected in the serum or infected tissues of some patients. Acute infection can be proven by B19-compatible symptoms and the presence of IgM antibodies or virus itself, whereas past infection is documented by IgG antibodies. Individuals with erythema infectiosum and acute arthropathy usually have IgM antibodies without detectable virus in serum. Those with transient aplastic crisis may have IgM antibodies but typically possess high titers of virus and its DNA in serum. Immunodeficient patients with anemia often lack readily detectable antibodies but have viral particles and DNA in serum. Fetal infection may be recognized by hydrops fetalis and the presence of B19 DNA in amniotic fluid or fetal blood. Until recently, serologic tests required the use of B19 virus itself (collected from the blood of infected patients); this requirement restricted the use of these assays to a few laboratories, such as those at the Centers for Disease Control and Prevention. The expression of genetically engineered B19 capsids in infected cell cultures should lead to an ample supply of reagents and the ready availability of immunoassay kits for IgM antibodies.

TREATMENT AND PREVENTION Erythema infectiosum usually requires no treatment; the same is true for many cases of arthropathy. More severe cases of arthritis, particularly those involving chronic symptoms, can be treated with nonsteroidal anti-inflammatory agents. Transient aplastic crisis is usually treated with erythrocyte transfusions. In immunodeficient anemic patients, B19 infection should be treated with commercial intravenous immunoglobulin, which is known to contain IgG antibodies to B19. This therapy controls and may cure B19 infection. Prophylaxis of B19 infection should be considered for patients with chronic hemolysis or immunodeficiency and for pregnant women. The risk of infection for these persons may be reduced by hand washing before eating or after contact with respiratory or other secretions when B19 is known to be present in a community. Patients with transient aplastic crisis or chronic B19 infection (but not those with erythema infectiosum or arthropathy) pose a serious risk for nosocomial transmission of infection. They should be hospitalized in a private room with contact and respiratory isolation precautions. It is not known whether pre- or postexposure administration of immunoglobulin prevents infection. No vaccine for B19 is available; however, a baculovirus-infected insect cell line that expresses noninfectious B19 capsid proteins could serve as a prototype vaccine candidate.

REFERENCES

ANAND A et al: Human parvovirus infection in pregnancy and hydrops fetalis. N Engl J Med 316:183, 1987

ANDERSON LJ: Human parvoviruses. J Infect Dis 161:603, 1990

ANDERSON MJ et al: Experimental parvoviral infection in humans. J Infect Dis 152:257, 1985

BELL LM et al: Human parvovirus B19 infection among hospital staff members after contact with infected patients. N Engl J Med 321:485, 1989

BLACKLOW NR: Adeno-associated viruses of man, in *Parvoviruses and Human Disease*, JR Pattison (ed). Boca Raton, CRC Press, 1988, pp 165–174

CENTERS FOR DISEASE CONTROL: Risks associated with human parvovirus B19 infection. Morb Mort Week Rep 38:81, 1989

FRICKHOFEN N et al: Persistent B19 parvovirus infection in patients infected with human immunodeficiency virus type 1 (HIV-1): A treatable cause of anemia in AIDS. Ann Intern Med 113:926, 1990

HARRIS JW: Parvovirus B19 for the hematologist. Am J Hematol 39:119, 1992

KAJIGAYA S et al: Self-assembled B19 parvovirus capsids, produced in a baculovirus system, are antigenically and immunologically similar to native virions. Proc Natl Acad Sci USA 88:4646, 1991

KURTZMAN G et al: Pure red-cell aplasia of 10 years' duration due to persistent parvovirus B19 infection and its cure with immunoglobulin therapy. N Engl J Med 321:519, 1989

NAIDES SJ et al: Rheumatologic manifestations of human parvovirus B19 infection in adults: Initial two-year clinical experience. Arthritis Rheum 33:1297, 1990

PLUMMER FA et al: An erythema infectiosum-like illness caused by human parvovirus infection. N Engl J Med 313:74, 1985

POTTER CG et al: Variation of erythroid and myeloid precursors in the marrow and peripheral blood of volunteer subjects infected with human parvovirus (B19). J Clin Invest 79:1486, 1987

TOROK TJ et al: Prenatal diagnosis of intrauterine infection with parvovirus B19 by the polymerase chain reaction technique. Clin Infect Dis 14:149, 1992

149 HUMAN PAPILLOMAVIRUS INFECTIONS

RICHARD C. REICHMAN

DEFINITION Human papillomaviruses (HPV) selectively infect the epithelium of skin or mucous membranes. These infections may be asymptomatic, produce warts, or be associated with a variety of both benign and malignant neoplasias.

ETIOLOGY HPV, members of the A genus of the family Papovaviridae, are nonenveloped viruses, 50 to 55 nm in diameter, with icosahedral capsids composed of 72 capsomers. They contain a double-stranded, circular DNA genome of about 7900 base pairs. Papillomaviruses (PV) are species-specific, and HPV have not been propagated in tissue culture or in standard experimental animals. Although virus particles of HPV types 1 and 11 can be produced in human tissues implanted beneath the renal capsule of athymic mice, significant quantities of other HPV types are difficult to obtain. At least partly because of these problems, HPV have been only incompletely characterized. Structural viral proteins make up 88 percent of the mass of PV virions. A major capsid protein with a molecular weight of 56,000 and a minor capsid protein which migrates at 76,000 have been identified by sodium dodecyl sulfate–polyacrylamide gel electrophoresis. Viral DNA is complexed with cellular histones. Type-specific antigenic determinants appear to be located on the virion surface. Antisera produced by immunization of experimental animals with disrupted PV virions are broadly cross-reactive.

The genomic organization of all PV is similar. Types and subtypes are defined by degree of DNA hybridization under stringent conditions. DNA of a distinct PV type cross-hybridizes less than 50 percent with DNAs of other classified viruses. More than 60 types of HPV are recognized. Individual types are associated with specific clinical manifestations (Table 149-1).

EPIDEMIOLOGY There are few good studies of the incidence or prevalence of human warts in well-defined populations. Common warts are found in as many as 25 percent of some groups and are most prevalent among young children. Plantar warts are also widely prevalent and occur most commonly among adolescents and young adults. The incidence of venereal warts (condylomata acuminata) has risen dramatically in the last 15 to 20 years, and condyloma acuminatum is one of the most common sexually transmitted diseases

TABLE 149-1 Correlation of human papillomavirus (HPV) type with disease

Disease	Associated HPV type(s)*
Deep plantar warts	1, 2, 4
Common warts	1, 2, 4, 26, 27, 29, 41, 57
Common warts of meat handlers	7
Flat warts	3, 10, 27, 28, 41, 49
Intermediate warts	10, 26, 28
Epidermodysplasia verruciformis	5, 8, 9, 12, 14, 15, 17, 19–25, 36, 46, 47, 50
Condylomata acuminata	6, 11, 30, 42–45, 51, 54
Intraepithelial neoplasias, unspecified	30, 33–35, 39, 40, 42–45, 51–53, 56–59, 66
Bowen's disease	16, 31, 34
Bowenoid papulosis	16, 34, 39, 42, 55
High-grade dysplasias	16, 18
Low-grade dysplasias	6, 11, 31, 42, 45, 51
Cervical carcinoma	16, 18, 31, 33, 35, 39, 45, 51, 52, 56, 58
Laryngeal papillomas	6, 11, 30
Focal epithelial hyperplasia of Heck	13, 32
Conjunctival papillomas	6, 11
Others	36–38, 41, 46, 48, 60

*Types 61 to 65 have been identified but have not yet been described in the literature.

in the United States. HPV infection of the uterine cervix produces the most commonly detected squamous cell abnormalities on Papanicolaou smears.

DNA hybridization analyses of specimens from patients have provided important insights into the epidemiology and clinical spectrum of genital tract HPV infection. DNA of HPV can be detected in a significant proportion of cytologically normal cervical specimens obtained from sexually active women. This finding suggests that many HPV infections are latent. Seroepidemiologic studies of HPV infections have been hampered severely by lack of appropriate antigens. However, recent studies using intact HPV type 11 particles in an ELISA have demonstrated specific antibodies in sera of patients with condyloma acuminatum or recurrent respiratory papillomatosis.

CLINICAL MANIFESTATIONS   Until the mid-1970s, it was generally believed that there was only one type of HPV and that clinical and pathologic differences among warts were a function of the nature of the squamous epithelium at the site of infection. With the discovery of multiple HPV types, it has become clear that the specific HPV is an important determinant of the nature of the lesion. Thus clinical manifestations of HPV infection depend on location of lesions and virus type. Common warts (verrucae vulgaris) usually occur on the hands and are flesh-colored to brown, exophytic, hyperkeratotic papules. Plantar warts (verrucae plantaris) may be quite painful and can be differentiated from callus by paring the surface to reveal thrombosed capillaries. Flat warts (verrucae plana) are most common among children and occur on the face, neck, chest, and flexor surfaces of forearms and legs.

Anogenital warts (condylomata acuminata, or venereal warts) occur on skin and mucosal surfaces of external genitalia and perianal areas. The differential diagnosis of anogenital warts includes condylomata lata of secondary syphilis, molluscum contagiosum, pearly penile papules, fibroepitheliomas, and a variety of benign and malignant mucocutaneous neoplasms. Anogenital warts are sexually transmitted and have an incubation period of 1 to 6 months. In men, condylomata are found most frequently at the frenum or coronal sulcus, but they may affect any part of the penis. They occur commonly at the urethral meatus and may extend proximally. Perianal warts are common among homosexual men but appear in heterosexual men as well. In women, warts appear first at the posterior introitus and adjacent labia. They then spread to other parts of the vulva and commonly involve the perineum and anus. Condylomata frequently involve the vagina and cervix. These lesions may be present in the absence of external warts. Respiratory papillomatosis is uncommon, occurs predominantly in preschool children, and may result from acquisition of virus at the time of delivery through an infected birth canal. These lesions are typically multiple and may produce life-threatening airway obstruction. Disease in adults may be acquired by orogenital sexual contact.

Immunosuppressed patients, particularly those undergoing organ transplantation, often develop pityriasis versicolor–like lesions from which DNA of several HPV types has been extracted. Occasionally, such lesions appear to undergo malignant transformation. Patients infected with human immunodeficiency virus (HIV) have more severe clinical manifestations of HPV infection and appear to be at higher risk of developing cervical and anal malignancies.

Epidermodysplasia verruciformis is a rare, autosomal recessive disease characterized by the inability to control HPV infection. The patients involved often are infected with unusual HPV types and frequently develop cutaneous squamous cell malignancies, particularly in sun-exposed areas. Lesions resemble flat warts or macules similar to those of pityriasis versicolor.

Complications of warts include itching and occasionally bleeding. Rarely, warts may become secondarily infected with bacteria or fungi. Large masses of warts may produce mechanical problems such as obstruction of the birth canal.

Epidemiologic, cytopathologic, virologic, and histologic data have established a strong association of HPV infection with dysplasia and carcinoma of the uterine cervix. HPV nucleic acids have been detected in cervical scrapings and biopsy specimens from patients with these diseases. In addition, squamous carcinomas and dysplasias of the penis, anus, vagina, and vulva have been associated with HPV infection. HPV types 16 and 18 are the most frequently detected types in dysplasias and carcinomas of the genital tract, whereas HPV types 6 and 11 are most commonly associated with condyloma acuminatum.

PATHOGENESIS   HPV infection is transmitted by close personal contact and is facilitated by minor trauma at the site of inoculation. It may result from direct contact with another individual or, less commonly, from autoinoculation or contact with fomites. All types of squamous epithelium may be infected by HPV, and gross and histologic appearances of individual lesions vary with site of infection and virus type. Exophytic warts are characterized by papillomatosis, hyperkeratosis, and parakeratosis. Acanthosis, an increase in cellularity, occurs in the prickle cell layer in association with viral DNA synthesis. Late gene expression, manifested by the appearance of structural proteins and assembled virions, is evident within nuclei of cells in the granular layer, where koilocytosis develops. Koilocytes are large round cells with pyknotic nuclei and large areas of perinuclear vacuolization surrounded by a ring of dense amphophilic cytoplasm. Histologically normal epithelium may contain HPV DNA. The presence of residual DNA after treatment may produce recurrent disease.

Host defense responses to HPV infection are poorly understood. Most immunologic studies are difficult to interpret because of a lack of standardized antigen preparations and assay techniques. The relative importance of type-specific and genus-specific responses in resolution of and protection from disease has not been adequately evaluated. Virus-specific IgM and IgG antibodies have been demonstrated in patients with and without clinical evidence of active infection. Cell-mediated immune responses to HPV antigens also have been measured, and patients with defects in cell-mediated immunity appear to be more susceptible than normal individuals to HPV infections. Such patients occasionally develop extensive HPV disease.

DIAGNOSIS   Most warts that are visible to the naked eye can be diagnosed correctly by history and physical examination alone. Colposcopy is invaluable in assessing vaginal and cervical lesions and is helpful in the diagnosis of oral and cutaneous HPV disease as well. Papanicolaou smears prepared from cervical scrapings often show cytologic evidence of HPV infection. Persistent or atypical lesions should be biopsied and examined by routine histologic methods. In addition, genus-specific capsid antigens can be identified in tissue sections by immunohistochemical techniques, and virus type can be determined by nucleic acid hybridization.

TREATMENT   Therapy should be initiated with the knowledge that no treatment of proven safety and efficacy is currently available and that many HPV lesions resolve spontaneously. Frequently used therapies include cryosurgery, application of caustic agents, electrodesiccation, surgical excision, and ablation with laser. Topical antimetabolites such as 5-fluorouracil also have been used. Failure as well as recurrence have been well-documented following all these methods of treatment. The high frequency of recurrence may be explained by the presence of HPV DNA in normal-appearing tissue adjacent to lesions and in previously involved areas during periods of remission. Cryosurgery is the initial treatment of choice for condyloma acuminatum. Topically applied podophyllum preparations also have been used, and recently, a well-characterized preparation of the active ingredient, podophyllotoxin, has become available in the United States. Different interferon preparations have been employed with modest success in the treatment of respiratory papillomatosis and condyloma acuminatum. Two α-interferon preparations are currently licensed in the United States for intralesional therapy of anogenital warts.

At the present time, no effective methods of prevention are available for HPV infections other than avoiding contact with infectious lesions. Barrier methods of contraception may be helpful in preventing transmission of condyloma acuminatum and other HPV-associated diseases of the genital tract.

REFERENCES

Bonnez W et al: Antibody response to human papillomavirus (HPV) type 11 in children with juvenile-onset recurrent respiratory papillomatosis (RRP). Virology 188:384, 1992

de Villiers E-M: Heterogeneity of the human papillomavirus group. J Virol 63:4898, 1989

────── et al: Human papillomavirus infections in women with and without abnormal cervical cytology. Lancet 2:703, 1987

Koutsky LA, Wolner-Hanssen P: Genital human papillomavirus infections: Current knowledge and future prospects. Obstet Gynecol Clin North Am 16:541, 1989

Reichman RC et al: Treatment of condyloma acuminatum with three different alpha interferon preparations administered parenterally: A double-blind, placebo-controlled trial. J Infect Dis 162:1270, 1990

────── , Bonnez W: Papillomaviruses, in *Principles and Practice of Infectious Diseases*, GL Mandell et al (eds). New York, Wiley, 1990

Rose RC et al: Expression of the full-length products of the HPV-6b and HPV-11 L2 open reading frames by recombinant baculovirus, and antigenic comparisons with HPV-11 whole virus particles. J Gen Virol 71:2725, 1990

Shah KV, Howley PM: Papillomaviruses, in *Virology*, BN Fields (ed). New York, Raven Press, 1990

Stoler MH et al: Infectious cycle of human papillomavirus type 11 in human foreskin xenografts in *nude* mice. J Virol 64:3310, 1990

section 13 DNA and RNA respiratory viruses

150 COMMON VIRAL RESPIRATORY INFECTIONS

RAPHAEL DOLIN

GENERAL CONSIDERATIONS Acute viral respiratory illnesses are among the most common of human diseases, accounting for one-half or more of all acute illnesses. The incidence of acute respiratory disease in the United States is from 3 to 5.6 cases per person per year. The highest rates occur in children under 1 (6.1 to 8.3 cases per year), and the rates remain high until age 6, when a progressive decrease is noted. Adults have 3 to 4 cases per person per year. Morbidity from acute respiratory illnesses accounts for 30 to 50 percent of time lost from work by adults and from 60 to 80 percent of time lost from school by children.

It has been estimated that two-thirds to three-fourths of cases of acute respiratory illnesses are caused by viruses. More than 200 antigenically distinct viruses from 8 different genera have been reported to cause acute respiratory illness, and it is likely that additional agents will be described in the future. The vast majority of these viral infections involve the upper respiratory tract, but lower respiratory tract disease also can occur, particularly in younger age groups and in certain epidemiologic settings.

The illnesses caused by respiratory viruses traditionally have been divided into multiple distinct syndromes, such as the "common cold," pharyngitis, croup (laryngotracheobronchitis), tracheitis, bronchiolitis, bronchitis, and pneumonia. These general categories of illnesses have a certain epidemiologic and clinical utility; e.g., croup occurs exclusively in very young children and has a characteristic clinical course. Some types of respiratory illnesses are more likely to be associated with certain viruses, e.g., the "common cold" with rhinoviruses, while others occupy characteristic epidemiologic niches, such as adenoviruses in military recruits. The syndromes most commonly associated with infection with the major respiratory virus groups are summarized in Table 150-1. Despite these associations, it is clear that most respiratory viruses have the potential to cause more than one type of respiratory illness, and frequently features of several types of illness may be present in the same patient. Moreover, the clinical illnesses induced by these viruses are rarely sufficiently distinctive to enable an etiologic diagnosis to be made on clinical grounds alone, although the epidemiologic setting increases the likelihood that one group of viruses rather than another may be involved. In general, laboratory methods must be relied on to establish a specific viral diagnosis.

This chapter will review viral infections caused by five of the major groups of respiratory viruses: rhinoviruses, coronaviruses, respiratory syncytial viruses, parainfluenza viruses, and adenoviruses. Influenza viruses, which are a major cause of mortality as well as morbidity, are reviewed in Chap. 152. Herpesviruses, which occasionally cause pharyngitis and which also cause lower respiratory

TABLE 150-1 Illnesses associated with respiratory viruses

Frequency of respiratory syndromes associated with virus groups

Virus	Most frequent	Occasional	Infrequent
Rhinoviruses	Common cold	Exacerbation of chronic bronchitis and asthma	Pneumonia (children)
Coronaviruses	Common cold	Exacerbation of chronic bronchitis and asthma	Pneumonia and bronchiolitis
Respiratory syncytial virus	Pneumonia and bronchiolitis in young children	Common cold in adults	Pneumonia in elderly
Parainfluenza viruses	Croup and lower respiratory tract disease in young children	Pharyngitis and common cold	Tracheobronchitis in adults
Adenoviruses	Common cold and pharyngitis in children	Outbreaks of ARD in military recruits*	Pneumonia in children and immunosuppress patients
Influenza A viruses	"Influenza-like illness"†	Pneumonia and excess mortality in "high-risk" patients	Pneumonia in healthy individuals
Influenza B viruses	"Influenza-like illness"†	Rhinitis and pharyngitis alone	Pneumonia
Enteroviruses	Acute undifferentiated febrile illnesses‡	Rhinitis and pharyngitis	Pneumonia
Herpes simplex viruses	Gingivostomatitis (children) Pharyngotonsillitis (adults)	Tracheitis and pneumonia in immuno-compromised patients	Disseminated infection in immuno-compromised patients

* Serotypes 4 and 7.
† Fever, cough, myalgia, malaise.
‡ May or may not have a respiratory component.

tract disease in immunosuppressed patients, are reviewed in Chap. 143. Enteroviruses, which account for occasional respiratory illnesses during the summer months, are reviewed in Chap. 154.

RHINOVIRUS INFECTIONS

ETIOLOGY Rhinoviruses are members of the Picornaviridae family, which are small (15 to 30 nm), nonenveloped viruses which contain a single-stranded RNA genome. In contrast to other members of the picornavirus family, such as enteroviruses, rhinoviruses are acid-labile and are almost completely inactivated at pH 3 or lower. Rhinoviruses grow preferentially at 33 to 34°C, which is the temperature of nasal passages in humans, rather than the higher temperature (37°C) of the lower respiratory tract. One hundred distinct serotypes and one subtype of rhinoviruses are recognized.

EPIDEMIOLOGY Rhinoviruses are a major cause of the common cold and have been isolated from 15 to 40 percent of adults with common cold–like illnesses. Overall infection rates with rhinoviruses are higher among infants and young children and decrease with increasing age. Rhinovirus infections occur throughout the year, but seasonal peaks occur in early fall and spring in temperate climates. Rhinovirus infections are most often introduced into families by preschool or grade school children below 6 years of age. Between 25 and 70 percent of initial illnesses in family settings are followed by secondary cases, with the highest attack rates occurring in the youngest siblings at home. Attack rates also increase with increasing size of families.

The spread of rhinoviruses appears to be by direct contact with infected secretions, usually respiratory droplets. In some volunteer studies, transmission was most efficient by hand-to-hand contact, with subsequent self-inoculation of the conjunctival or nasal mucosa. In other studies, aerosol transmission appeared to be more important. Virus also can be recovered from plastic surfaces inoculated 1 to 3 h previously, suggesting that environmental surfaces also may contribute to transmission. In studies conducted in married couples in which serum antibody was not present in either partner, transmission was associated with prolonged contact (122 h or more) during a 7-day period. Transmission was infrequent unless virus was recoverable from the donor's hands and nasal mucosa, at least 1000 TCID$_{50}$ of virus was present in nasal washes of the donor, and the donor was at least moderately symptomatic with the "cold." Despite anecdotal observations, exposure to cold temperatures, fatigue, or sleep deprivation has not been associated with increased rates of rhinovirus-induced illness in volunteers.

Infection with rhinoviruses is worldwide in distribution, and by the time they reach adulthood, nearly all individuals have neutralizing antibodies to multiple serotypes, although the prevalence of antibody to any one serotype varies widely. Multiple serotypes circulate simultaneously, and generally no single serotype or group of serotypes has emerged as being more prevalent than others.

PATHOGENESIS Rhinoviruses infect cells via attachment to specific cellular receptors; the major group of such receptors has been recently recognized to be intercellular adhesion molecule 1(ICAM-1). Relatively limited information is available on the histopathology and pathogenesis of acute rhinovirus infections in humans. Biopsies performed in experimentally induced and in naturally occurring illness indicate that the nasal mucosa is edematous, often hyperemic, and, during acute illness, is covered by a mucoid discharge. There is a mild infiltrate with inflammatory cells, including neutrophils, lymphocytes, plasma cells, and eosinophils. Mucus-secreting glands in the submucosa appear hyperactive; the nasal turbinates are engorged, which may lead to obstruction of nearby openings of sinus cavities.

The incubation period for rhinovirus illness is short, generally ranging from 1 to 2 days. Virus shedding coincides with the onset of illness or may begin shortly before symptoms develop. The mechanisms of immunity to rhinovirus are not well worked out. In some studies, the presence of homotypic antibody significantly reduced the rates of subsequent infection and illness, but conflicting data exist as to the relative importance of serum and local antibody in protection from rhinovirus infection.

CLINICAL MANIFESTATIONS The most common clinical manifestations of rhinovirus infections are those of the common cold. Initially, illness begins with rhinorrhea and sneezing, accompanied by nasal congestion. Sore throat is frequently present and in some cases may be the initial complaint. Systemic signs and symptoms, such as malaise and headache, are mild or absent, and fever is unusual. Illness generally lasts for 4 to 9 days and resolves spontaneously without sequelae. In children, bronchitis, bronchiolitis, and bronchopneumonia have been reported, although it appears that rhinoviruses are not major causes of lower respiratory tract disease in children. Rhinoviruses also may cause exacerbations of asthma and chronic pulmonary disease in adults. The vast majority of rhinovirus infections resolve without sequelae, but complications related to obstruction of the eustachian tubes or sinus ostia, including otitis media or acute sinusitis, can occur.

DIAGNOSIS Although rhinoviruses are the most frequently recognized cause of the common cold, similar illnesses may be caused by a variety of other viruses, and the etiologic diagnosis cannot be made on clinical grounds alone. The diagnosis of rhinovirus infection is made by isolation of virus from nasal washes or nasal secretions in tissue culture. In practice, this procedure is rarely carried out because of the benign, self-limited nature of the illness. Because of the large number of serotypes of rhinovirus, diagnosis of rhinovirus infections by serum antibody tests is currently not practical. Common laboratory tests such as white cell count and sedimentation rate are not helpful in the diagnosis of rhinovirus infection.

TREATMENT AND PREVENTION Rhinovirus infections are generally mild and self-limited, so treatment is not necessary. Some patients may benefit from the use of analgesics and nasal decongestants, and reduction of activity is prudent if significant discomfort or fatigability is present. Antibacterial antibiotics should only be used if bacterial complications such as otitis media or sinusitis develop. Specific antiviral therapy is not available. Application of interferon sprays intranasally has been effective in the prophylaxis of rhinovirus infections but is also associated with local irritation of nasal mucosa. Prevention of rhinovirus infection by antibodies directed against rhinovirus receptors or by the use of the soluble purified receptors themselves is under study. Experimental vaccines to certain rhinovirus serotypes have been prepared, but their utility is questionable because of the existence of the large number of serotypes and the uncertainty regarding the mechanisms of immunity. Thorough hand washing or barrier protection against autoinoculation may help to reduce transmission of infection.

CORONAVIRUS INFECTIONS

ETIOLOGY Coronaviruses are pleomorphic, single-stranded RNA viruses, 80 to 160 nm in diameter, with clublike projections emanating from the virus envelope, resulting in an appearance which resembles that of the solar "corona," from which their name is derived. Three distinct coronavirus serotypes, designated B814, 229E, and OC43, have been isolated from humans. Coronaviruses are fastidious and are difficult to culture in vitro. Some strains will grow only in human tracheal organ cultures rather than in tissue culture.

EPIDEMIOLOGY Only limited seroepidemiologic studies have been carried out in coronavirus infections. Seroprevalence studies of two of the serotypes, 229E and OC43, have yielded variable rates of serum antibodies, ranging from 12 to more than 80 percent in various populations. Overall, coronaviruses account for 10 to 20 percent of common colds. Coronavirus infections appear to be particularly prevalent in late fall, winter, and early spring, at a time when rhinovirus infections are less common. Depending on the serotype, a cyclical pattern for outbreaks of coronavirus infection has been suggested, which ranges from every 2 years for OC43 to every 2 to 4 years with 229E.

CLINICAL FEATURES The clinical features of illness caused by coronaviruses are similar to those caused by rhinoviruses. In volunteer studies, the mean incubation period of illness induced by coronaviruses (3 days) is somewhat longer than that caused by rhinoviruses, and the duration of illness is somewhat shorter, with a mean of 6 to 7 days. In some studies, the amount of nasal discharge was somewhat greater in colds induced by coronaviruses than in those induced by rhinoviruses. Coronaviruses also have been recovered from infants with pneumonia and from military recruits with lower respiratory tract disease and also have been associated with worsening of chronic bronchitis. However, the overall significance of coronaviruses in lower respiratory tract disease in humans is unclear.

TREATMENT AND PREVENTION The approach to the treatment of common colds caused by coronaviruses is similar to that discussed above for rhinovirus-induced illnesses. Because of the uncertainty regarding the number and relative importance of coronavirus serotypes and the mechanisms of immunity, vaccines against coronaviruses have not been developed.

RESPIRATORY SYNCYTIAL VIRUS INFECTIONS

ETIOLOGY Respiratory syncytial virus (RSV) is a member of the Paramyxoviridae family and comprises the genus *Pneumovirus*. RSV is an enveloped virus, approximately 150 to 300 nm in size, so named because virus replication leads to fusion of neighboring cells into large multinucleated syncytia. The single-stranded RNA genome codes for 10 virus-specific proteins. Viral RNA is contained in a helical nucleocapsid surrounded by a lipid envelope bearing two glycoproteins, one of which is the G protein by which the virus attaches to cells, and the other is the F, or fusion, protein which facilitates entry of virus into the cell by fusing host and viral membranes. Respiratory syncytial viruses have been considered to be of a single antigenic type, but it has been found that two distinct subtypes (A and B) exist. The epidemiologic and clinical significance of subtype differences are being investigated.

EPIDEMIOLOGY RSV is the major respiratory pathogen of young children and is the major cause of lower respiratory disease in infants. Infection with RSV is seen throughout the world in annual epidemics which occur in either late fall, winter, or spring and can last up to 5 months. The virus is rarely encountered during the summer. The highest rates of illness occur in infants between 1 and 6 months of age, with peak rates occurring between 2 and 3 months of age. The attack rates among susceptibles are extraordinarily high, approaching 100 percent in settings such as day-care centers where large numbers of susceptible infants are present. RSV accounts for 20 to 25 percent of hospital admissions for pneumonia of young infants and children and up to 75 percent of cases of bronchiolitis in this age group. It has been estimated that more than half of infants who are at risk will become infected during an RSV epidemic.

In older children and adults, reinfection with RSV is frequent, but disease is milder than in infancy. A "common cold–like syndrome" is the illness most commonly associated with RSV infection in adults. Severe lower respiratory tract disease with pneumonitis can occur in elderly, often institutionalized, adults or those with immunocompromising disorders or treatment. RSV infection is more severe and prolonged in immunocompromised children. RSV is also an important nosocomial pathogen and can infect pediatric patients and up to 25 to 50 percent of the staff on pediatric wards during an RSV outbreak. The spread of virus among families is also efficient, and up to 40 percent of siblings may become infected when RSV is introduced into the family setting.

RSV is transmitted primarily by close contact with contaminated fingers or fomites and by self-inoculation of the conjunctiva or anterior nares. Virus also may be spread by coarse aerosols produced by coughing or sneezing but is inefficiently spread by fine-particle aerosols. The incubation period of illness is approximately 4 to 6 days, and virus shedding may last for 2 weeks or longer in children and for shorter periods of time in adults.

PATHOGENESIS Little is known about the histopathology of minor RSV infection. In severe bronchiolitis or pneumonia, there is necrosis of the bronchiolar epithelium and a peribronchiolar infiltrate of lymphocytes and mononuclear cells. Interalveolar thickening and filling of alveolar spaces with fluid also can occur. The characteristics of the immune response to RSV are not well elucidated. Because reinfection occurs frequently and is often associated with illness, the immunity that develops after single episodes of infection is not complete or long-lasting. However, the cumulative effect of multiple reinfections ameliorates subsequent disease and provides some temporary measure of protection against infection. Studies of experimentally induced disease in normal volunteers indicate that the presence of nasal IgA neutralizing antibody correlates more closely with protection than does the presence of serum antibody. Studies in infants, however, suggest that maternally acquired antibody provides some protection from lower respiratory tract disease, although severe illness also may occur in infants who have moderate levels of maternally derived serum antibody.

CLINICAL MANIFESTATIONS RSV infection leads to a wide spectrum of respiratory illnesses. In infants, 25 to 40 percent of infections result in lower respiratory tract involvement, including pneumonia, bronchiolitis, and tracheobronchitis. In infants, illness begins most frequently with rhinorrhea, low-grade fever, and mild systemic symptoms, often accompanied by cough and wheezing. Most patients gradually recover in 1 to 2 weeks. In more severe illness, tachypnea and dyspnea develop, and eventually frank hypoxia, cyanosis, and apnea can ensue. Physical examination may reveal diffuse wheezing, rhonchi, and rales. Chest x-ray shows hyperexpansion, peribronchial thickening, and variable infiltrates ranging from diffuse interstitial infiltrates to segmental or lobar consolidation. Illness may be particularly severe in children with congenital cardiac disease, bronchopulmonary dysplasia, or immunosuppression. One study documented a 37 percent mortality rate for infants with RSV pneumonia and congenital cardiac disease.

In adults, the most common symptoms of RSV infection are those of the common cold, with rhinorrhea, sore throat, and cough. Illness may occasionally be associated with moderate systemic symptoms such as malaise, headache, and fever. RSV also has been reported to cause febrile lower respiratory tract disease in adults, including severe pneumonia in the elderly.

LABORATORY FINDINGS AND DIAGNOSIS The diagnosis of RSV infection can be suspected on the basis of the epidemiologic setting, i.e., severe illness in infants during an outbreak of RSV in the community. Infections in older children and adults cannot be differentiated with certainty from those caused by other respiratory viruses. The specific diagnosis is established by isolation of RSV from respiratory secretions, including sputum, throat swabs, or nasopharyngeal washes. Virus is detected in tissue culture and identified specifically by immunologic reactions employing immunofluorescence, enzyme-linked immunosorbent assay (ELISA), or other techniques. Immunofluorescence microscopy of nasal scrapings or washings provides a rapid diagnostic method that is in use in many diagnostic virology laboratories. Serologic tests which depend on fourfold or greater rises in complement fixing or neutralizing antibody titers are useful for diagnosis in older children and adults but are less sensitive in children under 4 months of age. Compared with complement fixation or neutralization tests, ELISA detects serum antibody with more sensitivity. As with other serologic tests, diagnosis requires comparison of acute and convalescent serum specimens and is therefore not useful during the acute illness.

TREATMENT AND PREVENTION Treatment of upper respiratory tract RSV infection consists primarily of symptomatic therapy similar to that for other upper respiratory tract viral infections. For lower respiratory tract infections, treatment consists of respiratory therapy, including hydration, suctioning of secretions, and administration of humidified oxygen and antibronchospastic agents as needed. If severe hypoxia is present, intubation and ventilatory assistance may be required. Studies of infants with RSV infection who were given aerosolized ribavirin, a nucleoside analogue which is active in vitro against RSV, have demonstrated a beneficial effect on the resolution of lower respiratory tract illness, including improvement of blood gases. Similar studies have not been performed in adults with RSV pneumonitis, and the benefit of ribavirin in these patients is unknown.

Considerable interest exists in the development of an effective vaccine against RSV. Inactivated whole-virus vaccines have either been ineffective or, in one study, potentiated the disease in infants. Other approaches to vaccine development include immunization with purified F and G surface glycoproteins of RSV or generation of stable, live attenuated virus vaccines. In the settings where high rates of transmission occur, such as pediatric wards, barrier methods of protection of hands and conjunctivae may be useful in reducing the spread of virus.

PARAINFLUENZA VIRUS INFECTIONS

ETIOLOGY   Parainfluenza viruses are members of the Paramyxoviridae family and comprise the genus *Paramyxovirus*. Parainfluenza viruses are 150 to 250 nm in diameter, enveloped, and contain a single-stranded RNA genome. The envelope is studded with two glycoproteins, one of which possesses both hemagglutinin and neuraminidase activity, while the other glycoprotein contains the fusion activity. The viral RNA genome is enclosed in a helical nucleocapsid and codes for eight or nine virus-specific proteins. There are four distinct serotypes of parainfluenza viruses, all of which share certain common antigens with other members of the Paramyxoviridae family, including mumps and Newcastle disease virus.

EPIDEMIOLOGY   Parainfluenza viruses are distributed throughout the world, although type 4 has been reported less widely, probably because it is more difficult to grow in tissue culture. Infection occurs in early childhood so that by 8 years of age most children show antibodies to serotypes 1, 2, and 3. Parainfluenza types 1 and 2 cause epidemics during the fall, primarily in odd-numbered years. Type 3 infection has been detected during all seasons of the year, but epidemics of type 3 virus have occurred annually in the spring.

The contribution of parainfluenza infections to respiratory disease is variable according to both the location and year. In studies carried out in the United States, parainfluenza virus infections accounted for 4.3 to 22 percent of respiratory illnesses in children. In adults, parainfluenza infections are generally mild and account for less than 5 percent of respiratory illnesses. The major importance of parainfluenza viruses is as a cause of respiratory illness in young children, where they are second only to RSV as causes of lower respiratory tract illness. Parainfluenza type 1 is the most frequent cause of croup (laryngotracheobronchitis) in children, while serotype 2 causes similar, although generally less severe, disease. Parainfluenza type 3 is an important cause of bronchiolitis and pneumonia in infants, while illnesses associated with parainfluenza type 4 have been generally mild. Parainfluenza type 3, but not types 1 and 2, frequently causes illness during the first month of life, while passively acquired maternal antibody is still present. Parainfluenza viruses are spread through infected respiratory secretions, primarily by person-to-person contact and/or by large droplets. In experimental studies, the incubation period has varied from 3 to 6 days but may be somewhat shorter in naturally occurring disease in children.

PATHOGENESIS   Immunity to parainfluenza viruses is incompletely understood, but there is suggestive evidence that immunity to infections with serotypes 1 and 2 is mediated by local IgA antibodies in the respiratory tract. Passively acquired serum-neutralizing antibodies also confer some protection against infection with parainfluenza types 1, 2, and, to a lesser degree, 3.

CLINICAL MANIFESTATIONS   Parainfluenza virus infections occur most frequently in children, in whom initial infection with serotypes 1, 2, or 3 is associated with an acute febrile illness in 50 to 80 percent of cases. Children may present with coryza, sore throat, hoarseness, and cough, which may or may not be croupy. In severe croup, fever persists, with worsening coryza and sore throat. A brassy or barking cough may be noted and may progress to frank stridor. In most children, recovery will occur over the next 1 to 2 days, although progressive airway obstruction and hypoxia may ensue occasionally. If bronchiolitis or pneumonia develops, progressive cough accompanied by wheezing, tachypnea, and intercostal retractions may be present. In this setting, a moderate increase in sputum production can be seen. Physical examination shows nasopharyngeal discharge and oropharyngeal injection, along with rhonchi, wheezes, or coarse breath sounds. Chest x-rays can show air trapping and, occasionally, interstitial infiltrates.

In older children and adults, parainfluenza infections tend to be milder, presenting most frequently as the common cold or hoarseness, with or without cough. Lower respiratory tract involvement in older children and adults is uncommon, but tracheobronchitis in adults has been reported. More severe and prolonged parainfluenza infection has been reported in children with severe immunosuppression.

LABORATORY FINDINGS AND DIAGNOSIS   As with other respiratory viral diseases, the clinical syndromes caused by parainfluenza viruses are not sufficiently distinctive to permit a diagnosis to be made on clinical grounds alone, with the possible exception of croup in young children. A specific diagnosis is established by detection of virus in respiratory tract secretions, throat swabs, or nasopharyngeal washings. Virus is detected by growth in tissue culture, either by hemagglutination or by cytopathic effect, or by immunofluorescence of viral antigens in exfoliated cells from the respiratory tract. Serologic diagnosis can be made by fourfold or greater rises in acute and convalescent serum specimens as detected by hemagglutination inhibition or complement fixation or neutralization tests. However, frequent heterotypic responses occur among the parainfluenza serotypes, so identification of the serotype which causes the illness often cannot be made by serologic techniques alone.

Acute epiglottitis caused by *Haemophilus influenzae* type B (bacterial croup) must be differentiated from viral croup. Influenza A virus also is a common cause of croup during epidemic periods.

TREATMENT AND PREVENTION   For upper respiratory tract illness, symptomatic therapy can be employed as discussed for other viral respiratory tract illnesses. If complications such as sinusitis, otitis, or superimposed bacterial bronchitis develop, appropriate antibiotics should be administered. Mild cases of croup should be treated with bed rest and moist air as generated by vaporizers. More severe cases require hospitalization and close observation for the development of respiratory distress. If acute respiratory distress develops, humidified oxygen and intermittent racemic epinephrine are usually administered. High-dose systemic glucocorticoids also may be of benefit. There is no specific antiviral therapy available, although ribavirin has activity against parainfluenza viruses in vitro and is being evaluated clinically. Effective vaccines against parainfluenza viruses have not been developed.

ADENOVIRUS INFECTIONS

ETIOLOGY   Adenoviruses are complex DNA viruses which are 70 to 80 nm in diameter. Human adenoviruses belong to the genus *Mastadenovirus*, of which 47 serotypes are recognized. Adenoviruses have a characteristic morphology consisting of an icosahedral shell composed of 20 equilateral triangular faces and 12 vertices. The protein coat (''capsid'') consists of hexon subunits with group-specific and type-specific antigenic determinants and penton subunits at each vertex primarily containing group-specific antigens. From each penton, a fiber with a knob at the end projects, which contains type-specific and some group-specific antigens. Adenoviruses have been divided into six or seven subgroups based on the homology of DNA genomes. The adenovirus genome is a linear double-stranded DNA which codes for structural and nonstructural polypeptides. The replicative cycle of adenovirus may result either in lytic infection of cells or in the establishment of a latent infection (primarily involving lymphoid cells). Some adenovirus types can induce oncogenic transformation, and tumor formation has been observed in rodents, but despite intensive investigation, adenoviruses have not been associated with tumors in humans.

EPIDEMIOLOGY Adenovirus infections occur most frequently in infants and children. Infections occur throughout the year but are most commonly noted from fall to spring. Large-scale surveys have shown that adenoviruses account for 3 to 5 percent of acute respiratory infections in children. Infections are less frequent in adults and account for less than 2 percent of respiratory illness in civilians. Nearly 100 percent of adults have serum antibody against multiple serotypes, indicating that infection is common in childhood. Types 1, 2, 3, and 5 are the most frequent isolates obtained from children. Certain adenovirus serotypes, particularly 4 and 7, but also 3, 14, and 21, are associated with outbreaks of acute respiratory disease (ARD) in military recruits which occur in winter and spring. Transmission of adenovirus infection can occur by inhalation of aerosolized virus, by inoculation of virus in conjunctival sacs, and probably by the fecal-oral route as well. Type-specific antibody generally develops after infection and is associated with protection against infection with the same serotype.

CLINICAL MANIFESTATIONS In children, adenoviruses cause a variety of clinical syndromes. The most common is an acute upper respiratory tract infection, with prominent rhinitis. On occasion, lower respiratory tract disease, including bronchiolitis and pneumonia, also can be seen. Adenoviruses, particularly types 3 and 7, cause pharyngoconjunctival fever, a characteristic acute febrile illness of children which occurs in outbreaks, most often in summer camps. The syndrome is marked by bilateral conjunctivitis in which the bulbar and palpebral conjunctiva have a granular appearance. Low-grade fever is frequently present, along with rhinitis, sore throat, and cervical adenopathy. The illness generally lasts for 1 to 2 weeks and resolves spontaneously. Febrile pharyngitis without conjunctivitis also has been associated with adenovirus infection. Adenoviruses also have been isolated from cases of whooping cough with or without *Bordetella pertussis;* the significance of adenovirus in that disease is unknown.

In adults, the most frequently reported illness has been ARD in military recruits caused by adenovirus types 4 and 7. This illness is marked by a prominent sore throat and the gradual onset of fever, often reaching 39°C on the second or third day of illness. Cough is almost always present, and coryza and regional lymphadenopathy are also frequently seen. Physical examination may show pharyngeal edema, injection, and tonsillar enlargement with little or no exudate. If pneumonia is present, auscultation of the chest and x-ray may indicate areas of patchy infiltration.

Adenoviruses also have been associated with a number of non-respiratory tract diseases, including acute diarrheal illness in young children caused by adenovirus types 40 and 41 and hemorrhagic cystitis caused by adenoviruses 11 and 21. Epidemic keratoconjunctivitis, caused most frequently by adenovirus types 8, 19, and 37, has been associated with contaminated common sources such as ophthalmic solutions and roller towels. Adenoviruses also have been associated with disseminated disease and pneumonia in immunosuppressed patients, including patients with acquired immunodeficiency syndrome (AIDS).

LABORATORY FINDINGS AND DIAGNOSIS Adenovirus infection should be suspected in the epidemiologic setting of ARD and in certain of the clinical syndromes such as pharyngoconjunctival fever or epidemic keratoconjunctivitis in which outbreaks of characteristic illnesses occur. In the majority of cases, however, illnesses caused by adenovirus infection cannot be differentiated from those caused by a number of other viral respiratory agents and *Mycoplasma pneumoniae.* A definitive diagnosis of adenovirus infection is established by culture or detection of virus from sites such as the conjunctiva and oropharynx or from sputum, urine, or stool. Virus may be detected in tissue culture by cytopathic changes and specifically identified by immunofluorescence or other immunologic techniques. Adenovirus types 40 and 41, which have been associated with diarrheal disease in children, require special tissue culture cells for isolation, and these serotypes are most commonly detected by direct ELISA of stool. Serum antibody rises can be demonstrated by complement fixation or neutralization, ELISA, or radioimmunoassays. Hemagglutination inhibition tests also may be done for those adenoviruses which hemagglutinate red cells.

TREATMENT AND PREVENTION Only symptomatic and supportive therapy is available for adenovirus infections, and no clinically useful antiviral compounds have emerged. Live vaccines have been developed against adenovirus types 4 and 7 and are widely utilized to control this illness in military recruits. These vaccines consist of live, unattenuated virus which is administered in enteric coated capsules. Infection of the gastrointestinal tract with types 4 and 7 does not cause disease but stimulates local and systemic antibodies which protect against subsequent ARD with those serotypes. Vaccines prepared from purified subunits of adenovirus are currently under investigation.

REFERENCES

Rhinoviruses

GREVE JM et al: The major human rhinovirus receptor is ICAM-1. Cell 56:809, 1989

GWALTNEY JM: Rhinoviruses, in *Principles and Practice of Infectious Diseases*, 3d ed, GF Mandell et al (eds). New York, Churchill Livingstone, 1990, pp 1399–1404

ROSSMAN MG et al: Structure of a human common cold virus and functional relationships to other picornaviruses. Nature 317:145, 1985

TYRRELL DAJ: Common colds. Intervirology 25:177, 1986

Coronaviruses

BRADBURNE AF et al: Effects of a "new" human respiratory virus in volunteers. Br Med J 3:767, 1967

LARSON HE et al: Isolation of rhinoviruses and coronaviruses from 38 colds in adults. J Med Virol 5:221, 1980

MCINTOSH K: Coronaviruses, in *Virology*, 2d ed, BN Fields (ed). New York, Raven, 1989, pp 857–864

Respiratory syncytial virus

ENGLUND JA et al: Respiratory syncytial virus infection in immunocompromised adults. Ann Intern Med 109:203, 1988

GLEZEN WP et al: Risk of primary infection and reinfection with respiratory syncytial virus. Am J Dis Child 140:543, 1986

HALL CB et al: Aerosolized ribavirin treatment of infants with respiratory syncytial viral infection. A randomized double blind study. N Engl J Med 308:1443, 1983

HENDERSON FW et al: Respiratory syncytial virus infections, reinfections and immunity. N Engl J Med 300:530, 1979

MUFSON MA et al: Respiratory syncytial virus epidemics: Variable dominance of subgroups A and B strains among children, 1981–1986. J Infect Dis 1:143, 1988

SMITH DW et al: A controlled trial of aerosolized ribavarin in infants receiving mechanical ventilation for severe respiratory syncytial virus infection. N Engl J Med 325:24, 1991

Parainfluenza viruses

DENNY FW et al: Croup: An 11 year study in a pediatric practice. Pediatrics 71:871, 1983

HEILMAN CA: Respiratory syncytial and parainfluenza viruses. J Infect Dis 161:402, 1990

WRIGHT PF: Parainfluenzaviruses, in *Textbook of Human Virology*, 2d ed, RB Belshe (ed). St. Louis, Mosby, 1991, pp 342–350

Adenoviruses

BAUM SG: Adenoviruses, in *Principles and Practice of Infectious Diseases*, 3d ed, G Mandell et al (eds). New York, Churchill Livingstone, 1990, pp 1185–1190

FOX JP et al: The Seattle virus watch. VII. Observations of adenovirus infections. Am J Epidemiol 105:362, 1977

WIGAND R et al: Adenoviridae: Second report. Intervirology 18:169, 1982

ZAHRADNIK JM et al: Adenovirus infection in the immunosuppressed patient. Am J Med 68:725, 1980

section 14   RNA viruses

151   THE HUMAN RETROVIRUSES

ROBERT C. GALLO / ANTHONY S. FAUCI

Retroviruses were first described at the beginning of the century as filterable agents that caused transmissible tumors in chickens; the first recognized mammalian retroviruses were isolated from mice with leukemia in the 1950s. However, despite extensive investigation, the first human retrovirus, HTLV-I, was not isolated until 1978. Isolation became possible only after the discovery of RNA-to-DNA transcription by viruses and through the use of reverse transcriptase (RT) as a sensitive "footprint" for these viruses. In addition, the obligate requirement of a T cell growth factor, interleukin 2 (IL-2) (see Chap. 277), for growth of T cells in culture helped make isolation possible. There are now four well-characterized pathogenic human retroviruses belonging to two distinct groups: the human T cell leukemia retroviruses, HTLV-I and HTLV-II, and the human immunodeficiency viruses, HIV-1 and HIV-2.

Although retroviruses are sometimes categorized as oncogenic viruses, lentiviruses, and spumaviruses, they also may be grouped by the disease they cause, their electron-microscopic appearance, and their biologic effects. In contrast to the infectious retroviruses, some, called *endogenous retroviruses,* are transmitted in the germ line. Although there is limited homology of the genomes of animal retroviruses to some sequences in the human genome, there are no known human endogenous viruses. The spumaviruses are known for their ability to produce a characteristic foamy cytopathic effect in tissue culture, but their existence and biologic role in human beings are still debatable. The lentiviruses, first recognized in ungulates, until recently were associated only with nonmalignant disease, particularly neurologic disorders (visna virus), immune-complex disease (equine infectious anemia virus), encephalitis and arthritis (caprine arthritis encephalitis virus), and immunodeficiencies (feline immunodeficiency virus, simian immunodeficiency virus, HIV). These viruses are "slow-acting" only by comparison with viruses that cause acute infections, such as influenza virus, but not by comparison with other retroviruses. Retroviruses associated with malignant disease include HTLV-I and HTLV-II, some of the closely related simian viruses (STLV-I), feline leukemia virus (FeLV), bovine leukemia virus (BLV), gibbon ape leukemia virus (GaLV), and many avian and murine viruses. These viruses also may induce nonmalignant disease. For example, FeLV, which can cause T cell leukemia, more frequently causes immunodeficiency in cats, mimicking human AIDS. It appears that a change in the envelope of the virus is correlated with a change in the kind of disease induced by the virus.

When retroviruses cause malignant disease, they do so by one of several molecular mechanisms; in each case, however, the mechanism is direct in that the DNA proviral sequences are integrated in clonal fashion in each cell of the tumor. Recent evidence indicates that retroviruses sometimes greatly facilitate the development of certain neoplasms by indirect mechanisms wherein the virus-infected cell is not transformed but influences tumor development in some uninfected cell. HIV-1–associated B cell lymphomas and Kaposi's sarcoma are examples.

GENERAL BIOLOGY OF RETROVIRUSES   Retroviruses are enveloped viruses, usually about 100 nm in diameter, that form by budding from cell membranes (Fig. 151-1). An electron-dense central core surrounds two identical copies of the single-stranded viral RNA genome; thus retroviruses are diploid—a structure unusual among viruses (see Chap. 141). However, it is the DNA polymerase, known as *reverse transcriptase,* that is the distinguishing feature of a retrovirus. Complexed to an RNA in the viral core, this enzyme catalyzes the transcription of the RNA genome into a double-stranded DNA form that migrates from the cytoplasm to the nucleus and integrates into the host cell DNA. In this form, known as the *provirus,* the viral genes remain integrated for the lifetime of the cell. They are duplicated with the cell DNA during the S phase of the cell cycle. Therefore, once established, infection of an organism is generally lifelong. When the provirus is expressed, viral RNA and proteins are

FIGURE 151-1   Electron micrographs of the characterized human retroviruses. The viruses are shown as they replicate by budding from a cell membrane *(upper panels)* and as mature infectious extracellular virions *(lower panels).*

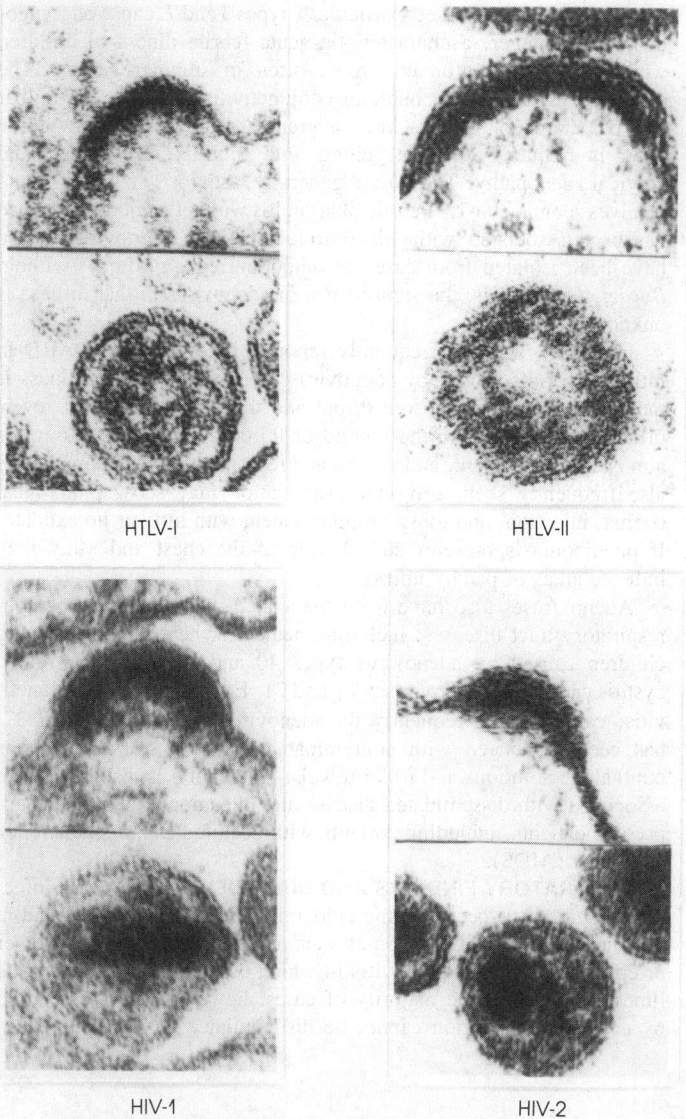

HTLV-I   HTLV-II

HIV-1   HIV-2

found in the cell cytoplasm and assembled at the cell membrane, where budding and release of infectious virions complete the replication cycle (Fig. 151-2).

The molecular mechanisms by which retroviruses alter the life cycle of infected cells are strikingly diverse and often depend on the organization of the viral genome. All retroviruses contain three essential genes for virus replication: *gag, pol,* and *env* (Fig. 151-3). *Gag* codes for a polyprotein precursor that is cleaved by a viral protease into three or four structural proteins; *pol* codes for RT and the viral protease and integrase; *env* codes for the transmembrane and outer glycoprotein of the virus. The properties of the envelope have a major influence on the kind of cell the virus can infect (though they are not the sole determinant of infectivity), and production of antibodies to the envelope is one of the essential features sought in a vaccine. At either end of the provirus, the long terminal repeats (LTRs) are covalently joined to the cellular DNA; they contain regulatory elements that influence the expression of the viral genes and sometimes nearby cellular genes. The LTRs share features in common with movable genetic elements such as retrotransposons.

Examples of retroviruses that contain only these three genes are FeLV, murine leukemia virus (MuLV), GaLV, and avian leukosis virus (ALV). These are the chronic leukemia viruses. They are all replication competent, take a long time to cause disease, and are relatively common in nature. There is some evidence that they cause leukemia by integration into a specific region of a chromosome so that the associated LTRs act to promote continual expression of a nearby cellular gene involved in growth (a proto-oncogene) (see Chap. 63). The best-studied examples of this *cis* mechanism is in chickens, where the LTRs of avian leukosis virus promote expression of the cellular proto-oncogene *myc,* believed to be the first step in the induction of B cell leukemia by this virus. Since integration by retroviruses is random, a high rate of replication increases the chance of integration into regions sufficiently near the cellular oncogene to effect its expression. There are no known human viruses of this type.

When a retrovirus acquires a host cell gene that rapidly transforms cells and induces acute malignancies, the virus is often called an *acute leukemia* or *sarcoma virus,* and the acquired gene (i.e., host proto-oncogene) is called a *viral onc gene.* This type of change almost always leads to an incomplete viral genome that forms defective viral particles. The virus then needs the addition of a helper virus and in vitro manipulation by the virologist for its propagation. Viruses with *onc* genes are thought to be rare in nature and are of interest in animals chiefly as tools for investigating mechanisms of neoplastic transformation rather than as causes of naturally occurring cancer. An example relates to FeLV. In addition to the mechanism of specific integration near a proto-oncogene and subsequent activation of this gene, the relatively frequent acquisition of cell-derived oncogenes may enable FeLV to cause malignancies. Every cell infected by these viruses can be transformed (giving rise to polyclonal tumors) because the product of the viral *onc* gene directly transforms the cells. Therefore, a common site of integration or a second genetic event to trigger transformation is not needed. The development of the malignancy is usually rapid and sometimes occurs within months of infection. Human viruses of this type have not been found.

FEATURES OF HUMAN RETROVIRUSES   The known human and some related animal retroviruses can be regarded as unique categories of retroviruses. Human T lymphotropic (or leukemia) viruses (HTLV-I and HTLV-II) transform cells in culture, while human immunodeficiency viruses (HIV-1 and -2) are cytopathic in culture. While the two groups have little sequence homology and major differences, they also have some striking similarities.

Shown in Fig. 151-4 is the structure of an HIV-1 virion, or virus particle, with the location of the virion proteins as indicated. The envelope proteins can be seen as a rod and sphere protruding from the viral lipid bilayer. Just inside the lipid shell is the matrix protein. The major capsid protein, p24, makes up the outer surface of the core, which contains the viral genome and the proteins necessary for replication and integration of the viral genome, such as RT.

In addition to the usual viral structural genes, all the human retroviruses contain extra genes that provide regulatory signals essential to the replication and biologic activities of the virus. Such genes were found first in HTLV-I and HTLV-II and more recently in HIV-2 and HIV-1, the well-known causes of AIDS.

One of these genes, called *tax*-1 in HTLV-I and *tat*-1 in HIV-1, codes for proteins that activate the expression of viral and some cellular genes. Another gene, *rex* in HTLV-I and *rev* in HIV-1, codes

FIGURE 151-2 Life cycle of a retrovirus (as represented by HIV-1). Intact virions are endocytosed via a specific cellular receptor. The uncoated viral single-stranded RNA is then transcribed into double-stranded DNA, enters the cell nucleus, and integrates into the host genome. The DNA provirus in some conditions is unexpressed. In other cases it is transcribed, giving rise to viral RNA encoding viral proteins and genome-length viral RNA molecules, which then reassemble with viral proteins to make complete virions. These progeny are released by budding from the cell membrane. All known infectious retroviruses follow these steps. The specific molecules described pertain only to HIV-1 (the CD4 receptor with Vif, Tat, and Rev viral proteins).

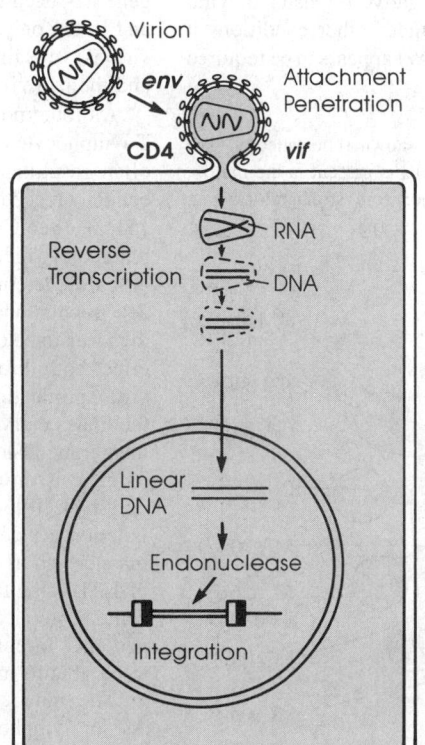
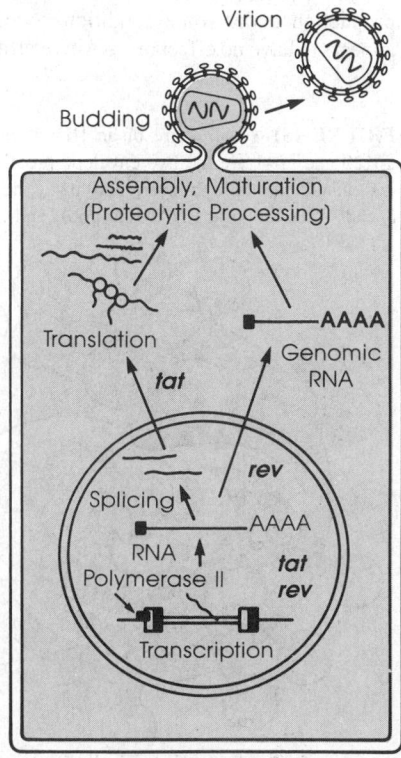

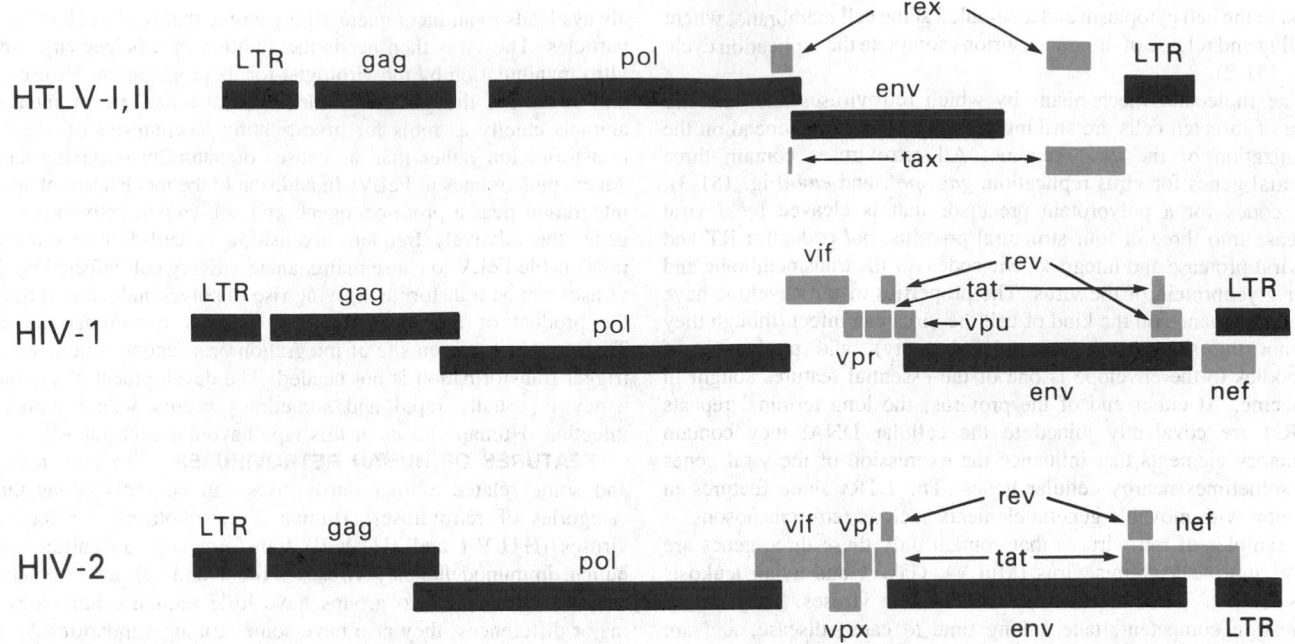

FIGURE 151-3 Genomic structure of human retroviruses. Viral proteins may be translated in each of three reading frames. RNA is transcribed from viral DNA and processed by viral and cellular enzymes, giving rise to both genomic viral RNA and mRNA. Arrows indicate double-spliced mRNA. LTR, long terminal repeat; *gag,* core proteins; *pol,* polymerase (RT); *env,* envelope. Viral genes shown in color code for regulatory proteins.

for proteins that favor the expression of unspliced or single-spliced viral mRNA; in their absence only small, double-spliced or multiply spliced mRNAs are made. The *rev/rex* proteins are localized in the nucleus and appear to increase transport of the larger mRNAs, which encode structural proteins, to the cytoplasm. Conversely, they diminish the availability of the mRNA for *rev* or *rex* and for the other regulatory proteins. For each virus these proteins are structurally distinct but have similar functions.

HIV-1 follows many of the same regulatory strategies as HTLV-I, but its genome is even more complex. By deletion analysis the function of several other genes has been evaluated.

The *nef* gene product appears to be a negative regulator of viral production under some conditions, while under other conditions it appears to have no effect or a positive effect. *Nef* appears to be required

FIGURE 151-4 Structure of an HIV-1 virion, shown schematically. The gp120 and gp41 are the two envelope proteins; p17 is present in the matrix, just inside the lipid bilayer; and p24, the major core structural protein, encapsulates the viral RNA, RT (p66), and integrase (p32).

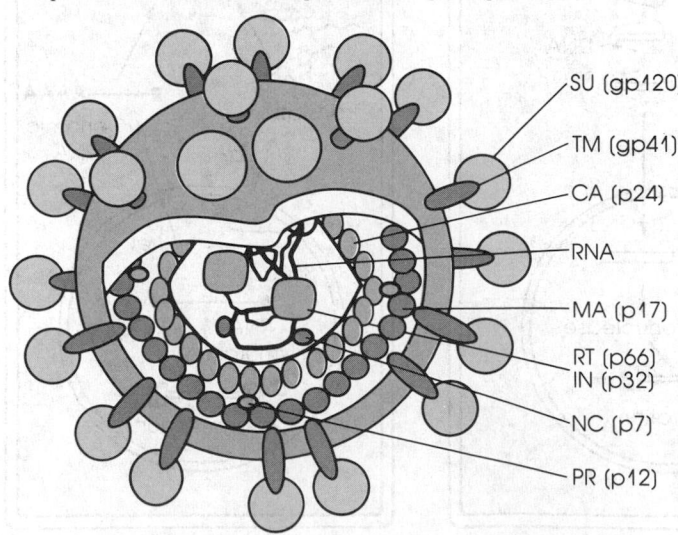

for the maintenance of a high load of simian immunodeficiency virus (SIV), an HIV-related virus of monkeys, in vivo and for the production of disease by this virus. The *vif* gene affects the ability of virus particles to infect target cells but does not affect viral expression or transmission by cell-to-cell contact. The *vpu* gene has been reported to modestly enhance the exit of virus from the cell in vitro and to destabilize the complex formed in the endoplasmic reticulum between newly synthesized envelope-protein precursor and intracellular CD4, the cell surface receptor for incoming virus (see below). This destabilization appears to facilitate envelope precursor processing, which may be how *vpu* enhances transmission by virions. The *vpr* gene has been reported to stimulate the promoter region of the virus and is the only one of these extra gene products to be contained in virions. In reality, the functions of these genes are poorly understood and their in vivo relevance is unclear.

All four known human retroviruses preferentially infect the CD4 + T lymphocyte (T4 cell), and the diseases they cause involve this cell, often resulting in profound biologic consequences. Ironically, the cellular receptor for HIV is the CD4 molecule itself (see Fig. 151-2). (See Chap. 277 for discussion of the function of CD4.) The remarkably high affinity of gp120 envelope protein for this molecule probably determines the host range of the virus, the nature of target cell populations, the mode of virus transmission, and the ability of the virus to be efficiently transmitted and contributes to the cytopathic effect both through the formation of syncytia and through effects on virus production. A region of the transmembrane protein gp41 facilitates entry of the virus into the cell by fusing with the target cell membrane. The cellular receptor(s) for the HTLVs is not known, but its gene is on chromosome 17. HTLV-I usually can be transmitted only by cell-to-cell contact, probably because its envelope does not function efficiently, while the HIVs can be transmitted both in this manner and as extracellular virus. The limited mode of transmission of HTLV-I suffices because the virus is able to immortalize its host cell, the replication of which is sufficient to propagate the HTLV-I genome. In contrast, HIV-1 sometimes kills its host cell and needs to be able to infect new cells efficiently.

The monocyte-macrophage is also a major target for HIV-1. As for lymphocytes, entry requires attachment to CD4 molecules expressed on the cell surface and may be enhanced by Fc receptor–

mediated endocytosis, although this point has been disputed. Infected monocytes are believed to play a major role in the disease by acting as reservoirs for the virus, as vehicles for its spread, and as inappropriate producers of growth factors and other cytokines. Related cells are infected in the brain, lymph node, skin, lung, and gastrointestinal tract. HIV infection induces certain cytokines. Cytokine production by infected monocytes and T cells may play a direct role in the induction of malignancy, neurologic disease, and perhaps other clinical manifestations such as enteritis, arthritis, and lymphoid interstitial pneumonitis. Moreover, many cytokines are able to induce virus production from latently infected cells (see Chap. 279).

DISEASES ASSOCIATED WITH HTLV-I INFECTION HTLV-I rapidly induces transformation of human T cells in vitro; it has neither an *onc* gene nor a single integration site, yet it results in monoclonal malignancies. The majority of HTLV-I-induced leukemias or lymphomas involve the CD4 + cell. Infection of CD4 + cells by HTLV-I or HTLV-II leads to the transformation of some of the infected cells, and the properties of such transformed cells are similar. The infected cells often exhibit extensive "cerebriform" lobulation of the nuclei and form giant multinucleated cells in culture. They constitutively express increased numbers of receptors for IL-2 (IL-2R), which can be found on circulating CD4 + cells. Increased receptor expression may be due to the *tax* gene product, which can up-regulate the receptor, transform T cells when transfected, and induce tumors in transgenic animals. The maintenance of malignancy is not believed to require additional viral gene products since the HTLV-I genes are not highly expressed in the leukemic cells in vivo by the time the leukemia is clinically evident. The reason that only some individuals develop malignancy is not known. Since cells other than T4 lymphocytes can be infected, the reason for the frequency of transformation of the CD4 + cell is unclear. The relatively high incidence of adult T cell leukemia/lymphoma (ATLL) (lifetime risk of 1 to 3 percent) independent of geographic location suggests that a specific environmental cofactor is not necessary to produce disease. In contrast, lymphoma associated with Epstein-Barr virus (EBV) develops at a much lower rate and only in certain areas such as the "Burkitt lymphoma belt" in Africa, where specific environmental cofactors are present.

Leukemias/lymphomas caused by HTLV-I are characterized by an aggressive course, frequent hypercalcemia (associated with tumor necrosis factor β and parathyroid hormone induction by the Tax protein), opportunistic infection, and in over one-half of cases, leukemic skin infiltrates. HTLV-I also may be involved in T4 cell leukemias/lymphomas that exhibit a more chronic course (15 to 20 percent of cases) involving progression from polyclonal T cell proliferation to an expansion of a particular clone to frank clinical malignancy. The latter malignancies, in contrast to adult T cell leukemia (ATL), may be indistinguishable pathologically or clinically from chronic T cell lymphocytic leukemia (CLL), diffuse histiocytic lymphoma, large and mixed cell lymphomas, and mycosis fungoides or Sézary leukemias (see Chaps. 310 and 311). Typical ATL cases recognized worldwide are almost always HTLV-I–positive. In the United States, only a small percentage of T cell malignancies are HTLV-I–positive. In contrast, in endemic areas, almost all T4 cell malignancies are virus-positive.

In areas of the world where HTLV-I is endemic, some B cell lymphoid malignancies and certain other cancers are associated with HTLV-I infection more frequently than would be expected from the prevalence of the virus in the general population. In contrast to virus-positive T cell leukemias, where the viral genes are integrated into the DNA of the leukemic cell, these B cell tumors have no HTLV-I in their DNA. Instead, the virus is present in the normal T cells of these patients, and the role of the virus must be indirect, as in HIV-1 and B cell lymphomas and Kaposi's sarcoma. Several of these B cell neoplasms have been shown to make specific antibody to HTLV-I; thus years of stimulation of some B cell populations by HTLV-I proteins may be involved in their malignant transformation.

The etiologic association of HTLV-I with ATL was firmly established by the epidemiology and serology in endemic areas and by the presence of proviral DNA integrated in the host chromosomes in a monoclonal manner in the tumor. The integration of proviral DNA indicated that the first transformed cell contained the provirus rather than the tumor being infected later in an opportunistic manner. The ability of HTLV-I to immortalize target T cells in vitro is also consistent with its role in vivo as a transforming virus. Considerable data in animals show that exogenous type C retroviruses are usually leukemogenic. This finding predicted that HTLVs also would be leukemogenic in human beings.

An interesting aspect of HTLV-I is the association of this virus with a demyelinating disorder, tropical spastic paraparesis (TSP) (see Chap. 375). This syndrome also has been referred to as *HTLV-I–associated myelopathy* (HAM). It is a chronic progressive encephalomyelopathy with symmetric upper motor neuron disease, prominent lower extremity weakness, and hyperreflexia, with sphincter and sensory abnormalities that may resemble a spinal cord variant of multiple sclerosis. Central nervous system lesions are seen on magnetic resonance imaging (MRI) scans. The pathogenesis is not certain, but the high antibody responses to HTLV-I, the presence of spontaneously proliferating ("activated") CD8 + cytotoxic T lymphocytes directed against HTLV-I Env, Tax, and Rex proteins in peripheral blood, and the improvement with glucocorticoids suggest an autoimmune disease mechanism. A few individuals have both ATL and neurologic disease. While the lifetime risk of developing ATL appears to be between 1 and 3 percent in HTLV-I–infected individuals, the attack rate of TSP in some areas such as Colombia may be higher. Several other diseases may be associated with HTLV-I infection in endemic areas, including infectious dermatitis, polymyositis, Bell's palsy, Guillain-Barré syndrome, and rheumatoid arthritis.

HTLV-II, which is 55 percent identical to HTLV-I at the nucleotide sequence level, was first isolated from a cell line derived from a patient with hairy cell leukemia. In contrast to HTLV-I, HTLV-II has been associated only with several cases of T cell variants of hairy cell leukemia and an increase in bacterial infections. The difference from HTLV-I is surprising, since HTLV-II appears to have the same biologic properties in vitro as HTLV-I. This difference suggests that host factors are more successful in preventing pathogenesis by HTLV-II than by HTLV-I.

There are two major considerations in the treatment of HTLV-I infection. First, the time from infection to disease may be 20 years or more. Second, when ATL develops, the virus is often transcriptionally silent in the peripheral blood leukemic cells. Treatment for asymptomatic seropositive individuals at present is limited to periodic evaluation for neurologic and hematologic disease, screening of family members at risk, and avoidance of infection transmitted by breast feeding, sexual activity, and transfusion. Thus far, no regimen of chemotherapy has been demonstrated to increase survival in ATL, though there are case reports of remission obtained with zidovudine (AZT) combined with interferon-α. Several experimental approaches are currently being evaluated in clinical trials, including targeting of the IL-2 receptor on leukemic cells with toxin-coupled antibody. Since virus is generally not replicating, antiviral chemotherapy seems unlikely to be effective. Thus the success in a few cases of ATL with AZT and interferon-α is puzzling. Several reports have indicated that high-dose glucocorticoids benefit TSP patients, but well-controlled trials have not been done.

ORIGIN AND EPIDEMIOLOGY OF HTLV-I AND HTLV-II Originally discovered in two black patients with T cell malignancies in the United States, HTLV-I was, within a year, associated with clusters of a newly described T cell malignancy (ATL) in some southwestern islands of Japan and in Caribbean-born blacks. It may have been brought to both areas from Africa centuries ago by merchants and slave traders. HTLV-I occurs worldwide but tends to be highly restricted or clustered geographically. Recent studies show evidence of ancient infections of some South Pacific tribal bush populations, but the HTLV-I of these regions appears to be of a unique subtype that differs significantly from cosmopolitan HTLV-I found in cities all over the world, which is highly conserved (Fig. 151-5). In endemic areas the fraction of infected individuals ranges from 5 to 25 percent. Transmission is by sexual contact, by blood or blood products, and by breast feeding (and perhaps by infection of the developing fetus in utero). Because of increased travel, changes in sexual habits, intravenous drug abuse (blood-contaminated needles), and wide use of blood and blood products, the prevalence of HTLV in nonendemic areas may be increasing.

Until recently, it has been difficult to distinguish HTLV-II from HTLV-I in seropositive individuals. With the advent of polymerase chain reaction (PCR) amplification technology, it has become relatively simple to amplify the viral DNA sequences in peripheral blood and to distinguish whether the amplified DNA is derived from HTLV-I or HTLV-II. Data obtained with this technique have shown that much of the HTLV-I seropositivity in drug addict populations is due to HTLV-II. HTLV-II seems to be the major infecting type among seropositive new world indians, including those from Alaska, New Mexico, and Central America and nonacculturated tribes from South America. HTLV-II thus appears to be primarily a new world virus and, in light of its wide prevalence, has likely been so for a long time. It is apparently far less pathogenic than HTLV-I, a characteristic suggesting that it is well adapted to its hosts.

It was through analyses of PCR-amplified DNA from HTLV-I–infected people that variants of HTLV-I that were much more divergent than previously reported strains were discovered in parts of the South Pacific, such as Papua New Guinea. The discovery of these viruses raises the possibility that in some areas viruses equally related to HTLV-I and HTLV-II may exist—or even that a continuous genetic spectrum of these viruses exists.

DISEASES ASSOCIATED WITH HIV INFECTION (See also Chap. 279) Just as the discovery of the tuberculosis bacillus or the spirochete of syphilis unified diverse disease manifestations, the

FIGURE 151-5 Phylogenetic tree of HTLV-I and HTLV-II. This dendrogram was constructed on the basis of the DNA sequence of the HTLV-I and HTLV-II envelope encompassing the carboxy terminus of gp46 and almost all of gp21. The cosmopolitan HTLV-I group includes most of the HTLV-I strains from the Americas, West Africa, Europe, and Japan, with an average nucleotide divergence among themselves of approximately 2 percent. HTLV-I from the equatorial region of Zaire constitutes a quasi-species, since a discrete divergence is found among the genotypes present in the same host. The members of this group of viruses diverge from the cosmopolitan HTLV-I by 3 percent. HTLV-I variants from Melanesia and Australia are another quasi-species whose members differ among themselves by approximately 4 percent and diverge from the two other HTLV-I groups by 8 percent. HTLV-II strains can be divided genetically in two subgroups and diverge from all HTLV-I strains by approximately 30 percent.

spectrum of disease associated with AIDS has been interpreted in the context of the biology and epidemiology of HIV-1 infection. HIV-2, the most recently described human retrovirus, has about 40 percent genetic identity with HIV-1. It is even more closely related to some members of a group of viruses causing immune deficiency in simians (SIV). HIV-2 has been isolated from patients with immunodeficiency and has been detected serologically in western Africa in populations (different from those with HIV-1 infection) in whom AIDS is not endemic. It appears to be a relatively uncommon and inefficient cause of AIDS and is not spreading with the rapidity of HIV-1.

HIV-1–infected patients have an increased incidence of certain B cell lymphomas, Hodgkin's disease, certain carcinomas, and Kaposi's sarcoma (KS) (see Chap. 279). The reason for the increase in these malignancies is not completely understood, but it is not necessarily associated with the degree of immune impairment, especially in the case of KS. HIV-1 is not the direct cause of any of these tumors because viral sequences are not found in the DNA from the majority of tumor cells. For the B cell lymphomas, the mechanism may be similar to the indirect role described above for HTLV-I.

Infection with HIV-1 induces a variety of cytokines, and various protein factors have been shown to augment the growth of cells in cultures of tissue from KS lesions. HIV-1 also may play a more direct role. Viral Tat protein has been shown to be secreted by HIV-1–infected cells and taken up in an active form by other cells. Tat appears to act as a growth promoter for KS-derived cells and could play a similar role in vivo. Additional support for this concept is the appearance of KS-like lesions in transgenic male mice expressing the Tat protein. Thus the role of HIV-1 in KS may be dual: it may augment the production of a number of cytokine growth factors [e.g., tumor necrosis factor (TNF), IL-1, IL-6, oncostatin, platelet-derived growth factor (PDGF), and basic fibroblast growth factor (bFGF)] that facilitate growth of KS spindle cells and angiogenesis, and it may exert effects similar to those of the HIV-1 protein Tat.

MOLECULAR HETEROGENEITY OF HIV Analysis at the molecular level of various HIV isolates reveals variation of nucleotide sequences of certain parts of the genome, especially in the envelope gene. In different isolates the amino acid sequence of the envelope proteins ranges from very closely related (1 to 2 percent variation) to variation by 25 to 30 percent. These changes tend to cluster in hypervariable regions. One such region, called *V3*, is a target for neutralizing antibodies and contains recognition sites for T cell responses. Variability in this region is almost certainly due to selective pressure from the host immune system.

A single individual (and perhaps intimate contacts) is usually infected with a "swarm" of closely related viruses that may constitute a single "strain." Shown in Fig. 151-6 is a dendrogram, or genetic tree, graphically representing the relative genetic differences among strains of HIV-1. The group encompassing the LW strains and the HXB2, HXB3, BH8, and BH10 strains include virus isolates from a single individual. The BAL-1, JRFL, SC, MN, NY5CG, and RF strains, which are isolates from different individuals in the United States, are more distant on the tree. The African isolates are yet more distant, reflecting increased variability. SIV$_{cpz}$, and HIV-1–related virus from a chimpanzee, is least related to the other HIV-1 strains. Even a very small difference, called *microheterogeneity,* may exert a profound influence on the biology of the virus. Variation within an individual appears to increase with time, perhaps as a result of selective pressure exerted by the host immune response. Transmission from one individual to another also appears to select subpopulations from the virus swarm in the transmitter. Both prolonged duration of infection and multiple rounds of person-to-person transmission contribute to the diversity seen in HIV-1. The greater interstrain variability in Africa than in Europe or the United States suggests an earlier origin from a limited focus of infection in Africa. Variation does not occur to any great extent during prolonged tissue culture of a single molecularly cloned virus; thus these changes may occur during transcription of the viral RNA genome to the DNA form and/or during the recombinational process when the DNA provirus

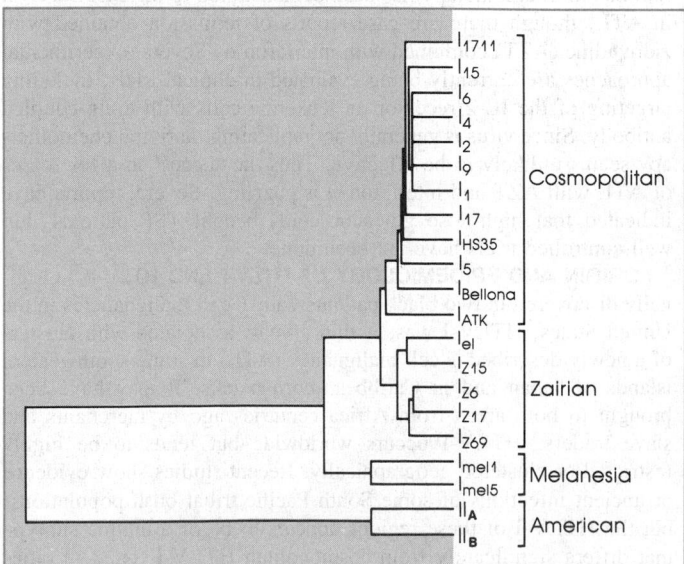

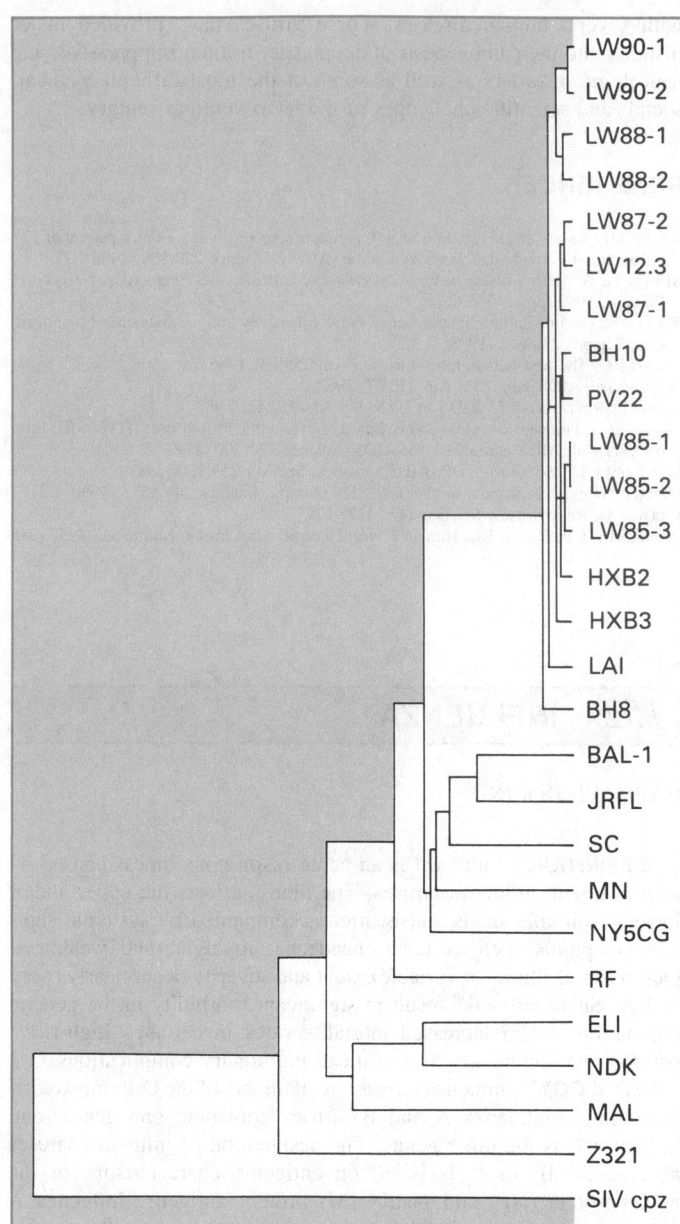

FIGURE 151-6 Dendrogram showing the relative genetic distances of HIV-1 isolates. The LW isolates and BH8, BH10, HXB2, HXB3, PV22, and LAI are variants within the same strain. BAL-1, JRFL, SC, MN, NY5CG, and RF are U.S. strains, and ELI, NDK, MAL, and Z321 are African strains. SIV$_{cpz}$ is an HIV-1–related isolate from a chimpanzee and is the most distant from the HIV-1 isolates.

integrates into the host cell DNA. RT tends to be error-prone because, unlike cellular DNA polymerases, it lacks a proofreading mechanism. The RT of HIV may be particularly error-prone. Variation of other genes is generally far less frequent than that of the envelope. It is possible that strain variation may account for a difference in the clinical course of an HIV-infected person; experimental studies have revealed significant biologic variations among strains, including target cell tropism and response to neutralizing antibody. A variant that can avoid elimination by antibodies or cytotoxic CD8+ T cells could lead more easily to progressive disease. For example, selection pressure on cultured viruses in the presence of human neutralizing antisera has resulted in viruses with one amino acid change that is no longer neutralized by the selecting sera.

PREVENTION AND TREATMENT OF RETROVIRUS INFECTION

There are three major approaches to the control of human retroviral disease: vaccination, antiviral therapy, and education and public health measures (see Chap. 279). Vaccines have proved to be the least costly and most effective way of preventing infectious disease, especially those caused by viruses, but there are special problems with HIV: (1) Because of the integration of viral genes, a limited number of viral particles may be sufficient to establish infection, and therefore, the demands on a vaccine may be very stringent. (2) CD4+ T cells are the principal cells that induce protection against a virus, and these are the cells destroyed by the virus. (3) Envelope heterogeneity, as mentioned above, allows the escape from neutralizing antibodies; several conserved areas of the envelope gene are being studied as subunit vaccines. (4) The nature of a protective immune response is not yet clear. Most infected individuals develop progressive disease despite the presence of neutralizing antibodies and cytotoxic T cells. The expectation is that immunization prior to infection may prevent disease. Some encouragement comes from the finding that for most infections of a single individual only one strain of the virus has been found. This fact suggests that an individual is infected only once despite repeated exposure. (5) Animal models for vaccine development against HIV are limited, but the development of animal systems with SIV, which can produce AIDS in macaques, is likely to be very helpful. Protection against infection by low doses of the strain of killed virus used for vaccination has been achieved with SIV in monkeys. Chimpanzees similarly have been protected from HIV-1 by a regimen of inoculations with native viral envelope proteins and peptides representing the V3 loop. The protection of chimps by passive immunization with neutralizing antibodies suggests that such antibodies are effective if they are already present at the time of infection. Indeed, in most of the successful animal vaccine studies to date, the protected animal was challenged only at the time of the peak immune response following vaccination and only with a single virus strain. The difficulty of maintaining a high-level immune response and the variability of the virus remain major obstacles.

Another issue that needs to be taken into account in vaccine design is the extent to which mucosal transmission takes place, particularly during sexual activity. One piece of evidence that this issue may prove important is the high rate of heterosexual transmission in Africa and Thailand. Heterosexual contact is less likely to produce trauma leading to exposure of the blood than is homosexual contact; heterosexual transmission is thus more likely to be purely mucosal. The argument that heterosexual contact may be less risky is weakened by the higher rate of venereal diseases associated with genital lesions in these areas than in the United States and Europe. Transmission of SIV by swabbing of virus onto the vaginal mucosa of monkeys also has been demonstrated. This transmission, however, required a high dose of virus. The preceding information suggests that mucosal transmission may occur but that it is inefficient. If this should be a common route, vaccines will have to be designed so that they elicit mucosal immunity.

Antiviral therapy is based on a detailed understanding of the viral replication cycle, and almost every definable step offers the possibility of interfering with replication of virus (see Chap. 279). Approaches are available, beginning with HIV binding to the cell. Recombinant CD4 is being tested that acts as a "molecular decoy" for the virus by competing with cellular receptors for binding viral gp120 envelope proteins. This approach has been effective in vitro but has not been of any clinical benefit. Two likely reasons are the very short half-life of recombinant CD4 in the circulation and the greater resistance of field strains of HIV-1 than of laboratory strains to inhibition by CD4. The most successful agents to date affect the next stage, formation of the DNA provirus, by inhibiting RT. These agents include zidovudine and other nucleoside analogues such as dideoxyinosine (ddI) and dideoxycytidine (ddC). The next targets are the synthesis, maturation, and transport from nucleus to cytoplasm of viral RNA from proviral DNA, for which inhibitors of *tat* and *rev* function are being studied. Viral mRNA must be translated, and on an experimental basis this step can be inhibited specifically with antisense DNA. Lastly, viral proteins must assemble to form new virus, and this step depends on a specific viral protease. This protein has been crystallized, and inhibitors have been shown to be effective in vitro.

Because infection with HIV probably always means integration of the viral genes into the DNA of the infected cells, it is likely that lifelong treatment will be required. To minimize toxicity and reduce the chance for viral resistance, it may be necessary to use a combination of compounds with different mechanisms of action. Another approach would be to kill infected cells; success would depend on elimination of all infected cells. However, this may not be possible with human retroviruses because most infected cells do not express viral proteins and are therefore not distinguishable from uninfected cells. Moreover, infected macrophages appear to act as reservoirs for the virus and may release additional virions from intracellular vacuolar membranes when killed.

A different approach to treating people who are already infected involves the genetic alteration of uninfected target cells so that they are no longer susceptible to infection or of infected cells so that they are incapable of producing virus. For example, CD4 + peripheral blood cells altered ex vivo could be placed back into the patient, comprising an HIV-1–resistant population whose presence might slow the decline in the immune system. A more attractive possibility would be to do the same thing with pluripotent hematopoietic stem cells in the bone marrow so that the immune system might be able to reconstitute itself. To date, however, only stem cells from mice have been sufficiently well studied to permit their unambiguous isolation from mouse marrow.

There are a number of genes whose products have been shown to interfere with the production of HIV-1 in vitro and could thereby protect target cells. One such gene produces an RNA transcript containing multiple tandem copies of a region on viral RNA, called the *tat activation region* (TAR), that must bind with the HIV-1 Tat protein for efficient RNA expression. In vitro, the multiple TAR outcompetes viral RNA for Tat and strongly inhibits virus production. Another gene makes a defective copy of one of the viral structural core proteins. Even a few copies of this protein inserted into an otherwise-normal virus core prevent the formation of infectious virus. There are also mutants of *rev* and *tat* that not only are nonfunctional but actually interfere with normal *rev* and *tat* function and inhibit virus expression. These are called *trans*-dominant negative mutants. All these genes have been shown to be effective in vitro.

OTHER DISEASES ASSOCIATED WITH HUMAN RETROVIRAL INFECTION   The possibility that several well-described human diseases are associated with retroviral infection should be considered carefully. While the potential of many candidate viruses to cause disease has not been realized, the number of retroviruses with diverse mechanisms of disease found in other species suggests a wide range of possibilities. A report of RT activity in non-A, non-B hepatitis has not been substantiated, and a new flavivirus has been discovered as the probable cause. T activity has been detected in patients with Kawasaki disease, but neither a virus nor viral sequences have been found, and there has been no confirmation of the original reports. Mammary tumors in mice have been transmitted via breast milk infected with mammary tumor virus. Despite sporadic reports of electron-micrographic evidence of virus in human tumors, no human equivalent has been isolated and characterized. Retroviruses are known to produce neurologic disease in some species (e.g., visna in sheep and murine leukemia in some mice); HIV-1 infects the central nervous system; and HTLV-I is associated with a demyelinating disease. A retroviral etiology of multiple sclerosis has been considered. Sequences related to HTLV-I have been reported in the peripheral blood of patients with multiple sclerosis by in situ hybridization or polymerase chain reaction. Differentiation of these sequences from those endogenous to cells and recovery of intact virus are needed to confirm the significance of these associations. An HTLV-II–related retrovirus has been reported to be linked to the chronic fatigue syndrome by nucleic acid and serologic studies. This link has not been confirmed, and no virus has been isolated.

The discovery of the HTLV-I occurred at a time when many thought that there would be no human retroviruses. In the ensuing decade, four human retroviruses have been discovered and associated with several human diseases. These viruses have provided major insights into the pathogenesis of neoplastic, immunosuppressive, and neurologic disorders as well as some of the most difficult medical, social, and scientific challenges of the late twentieth century.

REFERENCES

Baare-Sinoussi F et al: Isolation of a T lymphotropic retrovirus from a patient at risk for acquired immune deficiency syndrome (AIDS). Science 220:868, 1983

Blattner W: Retroviruses, in *Viral Infections of Humans*, AS Evans (ed). New York, Plenum, 1989, pp. 545–592

Fauci AS: The human immunodeficiency virus: Infectivity and mechanisms of pathogenesis. Science 239:617, 1988

Gallo RC: The first human retrovirus. Sci Am 255:88, 1986

———: The AIDS virus. Sci Am 256:47, 1987

———, Montagnier L: AIDS in 1988. Sci Am 259:41, 1988

——— et al: Frequent detection and isolation of cytopathic retroviruses (HTLV-III) from patients with AIDS and at risk for AIDS. Science 224:500, 1984

Matthews TJ, Bolognesi DP: AIDS vaccines. Sci Am 259:120, 1988

Mitsuya H et al: Molecular targets for AIDS therapy. Science 249:1533, 1990

Varmus H: Retroviruses. Science 240:1427, 1988

Wong-Staal F, Gallo RC: Human T-lymphotropic retroviruses. Nature 317:395, 1985

152   INFLUENZA

RAPHAEL DOLIN

DEFINITION   Influenza is an acute respiratory illness caused by infection with influenza viruses. The illness affects the upper and/or lower respiratory tracts and is often accompanied by systemic signs and symptoms such as fever, headache, myalgia, and weakness. Outbreaks of illness of variable extent and severity occur nearly every winter. Such outbreaks result in significant morbidity in the general population and in increased mortality rates in certain "high-risk" patients, predominantly as a result of pulmonary complications.

ETIOLOGY   Influenza viruses are members of the Orthomyxoviridae family. Influenza A and B viruses constitute one genus, and influenza C is the other genus. The designation of influenza viruses as type A, B, or C is based on antigenic characteristics of the nucleoprotein (NP) and matrix (M) protein antigens. Influenza A viruses are further subdivided (subtyped) on the basis of the surface hemagglutinin (H) and neuraminidase (N) antigens (see below). Individual strains are also designated according to the site of origin, isolate number, year of isolation, and subtype (e.g., influenza A/Victoria/3/79 H3N2). Influenza B and C viruses are similarly designated, but H and N antigens from these viruses do not receive subtype designations, since intratypic variations in H and N antigens of influenza B and C viruses are less extensive.

Most of the information regarding the molecular biology of influenza viruses has been generated from studies of influenza A viruses, and less is known about the replicative cycle of influenza B and C viruses. Morphologically, influenza viruses A, B, and C are similar. The virions are irregularly shaped spherical particles, 80 to 120 nm in diameter, that contain a lipid envelope from whose surface the hemagglutinin and neuraminidase glycoproteins project. The hemagglutinin serves as the site by which virus binds to cell receptors, while the neuraminidase degrades the receptor and probably plays a role in release of virus from infected cells after replication has taken place. Antibodies directed against the H antigen are the major determinants of immunity against influenza virus, while antineuraminidase antibodies limit viral spread and contribute to reduction of the infection. The inner surface of the lipid envelope contains the matrix proteins (M1 and M2), whose functions are incompletely understood but which may be involved in virus assembly and stabilization of the lipid envelope. The virion also contains the nucleoprotein (NP) with which the genome of the virus is associated, as well as three polymerase (P) proteins which are essential for transcription and synthesis of viral RNA. Two nonstructural (NS) proteins of unknown function are also present in infected cells.

The genome of influenza A virus consists of eight single-stranded segments of viral RNA, which code for the structural and nonstructural proteins. Because the genome is segmented, the opportunity for reassortment of genes during infection is high, and reassortment has been noted to occur frequently during infection of cells with more than one influenza A virus.

EPIDEMIOLOGY   Influenza outbreaks occur virtually every year, although the extent and severity of such outbreaks vary widely. Localized outbreaks occur at variable intervals, usually every 1 to 3 years. Global epidemics or pandemics have occurred approximately every 10 to 15 years since the 1918–1919 pandemic (Table 152-1).

The most extensive and severe outbreaks are caused by influenza A viruses. In part, this is a result of the remarkable propensity of the hemagglutinin and neuraminidase antigens of influenza A virus to undergo periodic antigenic variation. Major antigenic variations are referred to as *antigenic shifts*, which most likely occur from reassortment of genome segments between viral strains. Antigenic shifts may be associated with pandemics and are restricted to influenza A viruses. Minor variations are called *antigenic drifts* and likely arise from point mutations. These antigenic changes may involve the hemagglutinin alone or both the hemagglutinin and the neuraminidase. In human infections, three major antigenic subtypes of hemagglutinins (H1, H2, and H3) and two neuraminidases (N1, N2) have been recognized. The hemagglutinins formerly designated as H0 and Hsw1 are now classified as variants of H1. An example of an antigenic shift which involved both the hemagglutinin and neuraminidase occurred in 1957, when the predominant influenza A virus subtype shifted from H1N1 to H2N2, and resulted in a severe pandemic, with an estimated 70,000 *excess deaths*, i.e., deaths in excess of the number expected without an influenza epidemic, in the United States alone. In 1968, an antigenic shift occurred which involved only the hemagglutinin (H2N2 to H3N2), and the subsequent pandemic was less severe than that seen in 1957. In 1977, an A/H1N1 virus emerged which caused a pandemic that primarily affected younger individuals, i.e., those born after 1957. As can be seen in Table 152-1, H1N1 viruses circulated from 1918 to 1956, so individuals born prior to 1957 would be expected to possess some degree of immunity to H1N1 viruses. During most outbreaks of influenza A, a single subtype has circulated at a time. However, since 1977, both A/H1N1 and A/H3N2 viruses have circulated simultaneously, resulting in outbreaks of varying severity. In some outbreaks influenza B viruses also circulated simultaneously with influenza A viruses.

The origin of pandemic strains is unknown. Because of the marked differences between the primary structures of the hemagglutinins of different subtypes of influenza A viruses (H1, H2, or H3), it is believed unlikely that antigenic shifts result from spontaneous mutations in the hemagglutinin gene. Because the segmented genome of influenza viruses may result in high rates of reassortment, it has been suggested that pandemic strains may emerge by reassortment of genes between human and animal influenza viruses. Influenza B viruses do not have an animal reservoir and do not undergo antigenic shifts, although antigenic drifting occurs.

Although pandemics provide the most dramatic evidence of the impact of influenza, illnesses that occur between pandemics account for an even greater total in mortality and morbidity, albeit over a longer period of time. Since 1957, interpandemic illness has been associated with 10,000 or more excess deaths on 20 occasions in the United States, resulting in an accumulated mortality of more than 500,000 over that period of time. Influenza A viruses that circulate between pandemics demonstrate antigenic drifts in the hemagglutinin antigen. These antigenic drifts apparently result from point mutations which involve the RNA segment that codes for the hemagglutinin. Amino acid analysis of "drifted" hemagglutinins indicates that changes in a single amino acid have little effect on the antigenic properties of the hemagglutinin. Epidemiologically significant strains, i.e., those which have potential for causing widespread outbreaks, have changes in amino acids in at least two of the four major antigenic sites in the HA molecule. Since two-point mutations are unlikely to occur simultaneously, it is believed that antigenic drifts result from point mutations which occur sequentially during the spread of virus from person to person. Antigenic drifts have occurred nearly annually since 1977 for A/H1N1 viruses and since 1968 for A/H3N2 viruses.

Influenza A epidemics begin abruptly, reach a peak over a 2- to 3-week period, generally last for 2 to 3 months, and often subside almost as rapidly as they began. The first indication of influenza activity in a community is an increase in the number of children with febrile respiratory illnesses who present for medical attention. This is followed by increases in influenza-like illnesses among adults and eventually by an increase in hospital admissions for patients with pneumonia, worsening of congestive heart failure, and exacerbations of chronic pulmonary disease. Rises in industrial and school absenteeism also occur at this time. An increase in the number of deaths caused by pneumonia and influenza is generally a late observation in an outbreak. Attack rates have been highly variable from outbreak to outbreak but most commonly are in the range of 10 to 20 percent of the general population. During the pandemic of 1957, it was estimated that the attack rate of clinical influenza exceeded 50 percent in urban populations and that an additional 25 percent or more may have been subclinically infected with influenza A virus. Among institutionalized populations and in semiclosed settings where a large number of susceptible individuals are present, even higher attack rates have been reported.

Epidemics of influenza occur almost exclusively during the winter months in the Northern and Southern Hemispheres. It is highly unusual to detect influenza A virus at times other than those in which an outbreak occurs, although rarely serologic rises have been noted at other times of the year. Where or how influenza A virus persists between outbreaks is unknown. A possible explanation is that influenza A viruses are maintained in the human population on a worldwide basis by person-to-person transmission and that large population clusters might be able to support a low level of interepidemic transmission. Alternatively, human strains may persist in animal reservoirs, but convincing evidence to support either explanation is not available. In the modern era, rapid modes of transportation may contribute to the transmission of viruses from widespread geographic locales.

The factors which result in the inception and termination of outbreaks of influenza are also incompletely understood. A major determinant of the extent and severity of an outbreak is the level of immunity present in the population at risk. When an antigenically novel influenza virus emerges to which little or no antibody is present in a community, extensive outbreaks may occur. When the absence of antibody is worldwide, epidemic disease may spread around the globe, resulting in a pandemic. Such pandemic waves can occur for

TABLE 152-1   Emergence of antigenic subtypes of influenza A associated with pandemic or epidemic disease

Year	Subtype of influenza A	Extent of outbreak
1889–90	H2N8*	Severe pandemic
1900–03	H3N8*	?Moderate epidemic
1918–19	H1N1† (formerly HswN1)	Severe pandemic
1933–35	H1N1† (formerly H0N1)	Mild epidemic
1946–47	H1N1	Mild epidemic
1957–58	H2N2	Severe pandemic
1968–69	H3N2	Moderate pandemic
1977–78‡	H1N1	Mild pandemic

* As determined by retrospective serologic survey of individuals alive during those years ("seroarcheology").

† Hemagglutinins formerly designated as Hsw and H0 are now classified as variants of H1.

‡ From this time until the present (1991–92), new antigenic subtypes of influenza A have not emerged. Rather, viruses of H1N1 or H3N2 subtypes have circulated either in alternating years or concurrently.

several years, until immunity in the population reaches a high level. In the years following pandemic influenza, antigenic drifts among influenza viruses result in outbreaks of variable severity in populations that have high levels of immunity to the pandemic strain which circulated earlier. This situation persists until another antigenically novel pandemic strain emerges. On the other hand, outbreaks also may terminate despite the persistence of a large pool of susceptible individuals in the population. Occasionally, the emergence of a significantly different antigenic variant will result only in a localized outbreak. The "swine influenza outbreak" of 1976 in the United States, caused by an A/H1N1 virus antigenically similar to the virus which circulated in 1918–1919 (see Table 152-1), may be an example of this, although this outbreak may simply represent the introduction of a swine influenza virus into a crowded human population without spread beyond that setting. It also has been suggested that certain viruses, such as recently circulating A/H1N1 strains, may be intrinsically less virulent and cause less severe disease, even in immunologically virgin subjects, suggesting that other undefined factors besides the level of preexisting immunity play a role in the epidemiology of influenza.

Influenza B causes outbreaks which are generally less extensive and are associated with less severe disease than those caused by influenza A virus. The hemagglutinin and neuraminidase of influenza B virus undergo less frequent and less extensive variation than is seen in influenza A viruses, which may account, in part, for the observation of less extensive disease. Influenza B outbreaks are seen most frequently in schools and military camps, although occasional outbreaks in institutions in which elderly individuals reside also have been noted. The most serious complication of influenza B virus infection is Reye's syndrome (see below). Influenza C has been infrequently associated with human disease, although the prevalence of serum antibody to influenza C virus is widespread, which indicates that asymptomatic infection may be common.

The morbidity and mortality of influenza outbreaks continue to be substantial. Mortality occurs primarily in individuals with underlying diseases who have been characterized as being at "high risk" for complications of influenza. Excess hospitalizations for adults with "high risk" medical conditions have reached rates of 800 per 100,000 during recent outbreaks of influenza. These high-risk conditions are primarily chronic cardiac and pulmonary diseases, as well as increased age. Increased mortality rates also have been observed among individuals with chronic metabolic, renal, and certain immunosuppressive diseases, although to a lesser extent than among those with chronic cardiopulmonary diseases. In addition to the excess mortality, the morbidity of influenza in the general population is also extensive. For each of three outbreaks in the United States that were studied during the 1960s, it has been estimated that direct and indirect economic costs ranged from 1.5 to 3.5 billion dollars and that today such costs would be much greater.

PATHOGENESIS   The initial event in influenza is infection of the respiratory epithelium with influenza virus, which is acquired from respiratory secretions of acutely infected individuals. In all likelihood, this occurs via aerosols generated by coughs and sneezes, although hand-to-hand, other personal contact, and even fomite transmission may occur. Experimental evidence suggests that infection by small-particle aerosol (less than 10 μm in diameter) is more efficient than that produced by larger droplets. Initially, viral infection involves the ciliated columnar epithelial cells, but it also may involve other respiratory tract cells, including alveolar cells, mucous gland cells, and macrophages. In infected cells, virus replication takes place within 4 to 6 h, after which infectious virus is released to infect adjacent or nearby cells. This results in spread of infection from a few foci to a large number of respiratory cells over several hours. In experimentally induced infection, the incubation period of illness has ranged from 18 to 72 h, depending on the size of the virus inoculum. Histopathologically, degenerative changes can be seen in infected ciliated cells, including granulation, vacuolization, swelling, and pyknotic nuclei. The cells eventually become necrotic and desquamate, and in some areas, previously columnar epithelium is replaced by flattened and metaplastic epithelial cells. The severity of illness is correlated with the quantity of virus shed in secretions, suggesting that the degree of viral replication itself may be an important mechanism in the pathogenesis of illness. Despite the frequent presence of systemic signs and symptoms such as fever, headache, and myalgias, influenza virus has only rarely been detected in extrapulmonary sites, including the bloodstream, and the pathogenesis of systemic symptoms in influenza remains unknown.

The host response to influenza infections involves a complex interplay of humoral antibody, local antibody, cell-mediated immune responses, interferon, and other host defenses. Serum antibody responses may be measured by a variety of techniques and can be detected by the second week after primary infection with influenza virus. Such antibodies may be measured by hemagglutination inhibition (HAI), complement fixation (CF), neutralization, enzyme-linked immunosorbent assays (ELISA), and antineuraminidase antibody assays. Antibodies directed against the hemagglutinin appear to be the most important mediators of immunity, and in several studies, HAI titers of 40 or greater have been associated with protection from infection. Secretory antibodies produced in the respiratory tract are predominantly of the IgA class and also play a major role in protection against infection. Secretory antibody neutralization titers of 4 or higher also have been associated with protection. A variety of cell-mediated immune responses, both antigen-specific and non-antigen-specific, can be detected early after infection, depending on prior immunity of the host. These responses include T cell proliferative, T cell cytotoxic, and natural killer cell activity. Interferons have been detected in respiratory secretions shortly after shedding of virus has begun, and rises in interferon titers coincide with decreases in virus shedding.

The host defense factors responsible for cessation of virus shedding and resolution of illness have not been defined specifically. Virus shedding generally stops within 2 to 5 days after symptoms first appear, at a time when serum and local antibody responses are often not detectable by conventional techniques, although antibody rises may be detected earlier by use of highly sensitive techniques, particularly in individuals with previous immunity to the virus. It has been suggested that interferon, cell-mediated immune responses, or nonspecific inflammatory responses may be important in the resolution of illness.

MANIFESTATIONS   Influenza has been most frequently described as an illness characterized by the abrupt onset of systemic symptoms such as headache, feverishness, chilliness, myalgia, or malaise, accompanied by respiratory tract signs, particularly cough and sore throat. In many cases, the onset is so abrupt that patients can recall the precise time of the onset of illness. A typical case of naturally occurring influenza is depicted in Fig. 152-1. However, a wide spectrum of clinical presentations may occur. These can range from mild, afebrile respiratory illnesses similar to the common cold, with either gradual or abrupt onset, to illnesses in which severe prostration with relatively few respiratory signs and symptoms may be present. In the majority of cases which come to a physician's attention, fever is present, and temperatures can range from 38°C to as high as 41°C. The temperature rises rapidly within the first 24 h of illness and is generally followed by a gradual defervescence over a 2- to 3-day period, although, on occasion, fever may last for as long as a week. Patients complain of a feverish feeling and chilliness, but true rigors are rare. Headache, either generalized or frontal, is often a particularly troublesome complaint. Myalgias may involve any part of the body but are most common in the legs and lumbosacral area. Arthralgias also may be present.

Respiratory complaints often become more prominent as systemic symptoms subside. Many patients complain of a sore throat or persistent cough, which may last for a week or more and which is often accompanied by substernal discomfort. Ocular signs and

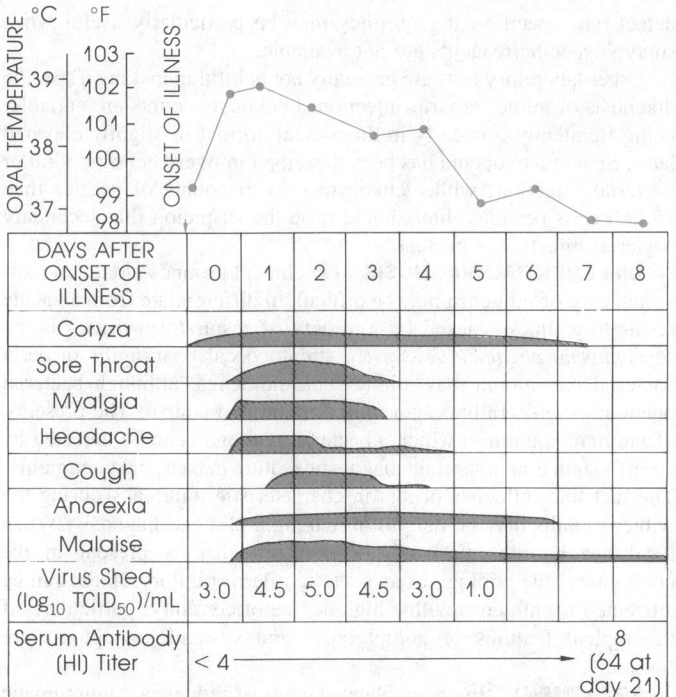

FIGURE 152-1 Clinical characteristics of a naturally occurring case of influenza A in an otherwise healthy 28-year-old male. (*From R Dolin, Am Fam Phys 14:74, 1976.*)

symptoms include pain on motion of the eyes, photophobia, and burning of the eyes.

Physical findings are usually minimal in cases of uncomplicated influenza. Early in the illness, the patient appears flushed, and the skin is hot and dry, although diaphoresis and mottled extremities, particularly in older patients, may occur. Examination of the pharynx may be surprisingly unremarkable despite a severe sore throat, but injection of the mucous membranes and postnasal discharge can be present. Mild cervical lymphadenopathy may be noted, particularly in younger individuals. Chest examination is largely negative in uncomplicated influenza, although rhonchi, wheezes, and scattered rales have been reported with variable frequency in different outbreaks. Frank dyspnea, hyperpnea, cyanosis, diffuse rales, and signs of consolidation are evidence of pulmonary complications. Patients with apparently uncomplicated influenza have been reported to have a variety of mild ventilatory defects and increased alveolar-capillary diffusion gradients, indicating that subclinical pulmonary involvement may be more frequent than is appreciated.

In uncomplicated influenza, the acute illness generally resolves over a 2- to 5-day period, and most patients have largely recovered in 1 week. In a significant minority, however, symptoms of weakness or lassitude ("postinfluenzal asthenia") may persist for several weeks, particularly in the elderly, and may prove troublesome for those who wish to return to full activity promptly. The pathogenetic basis for this "asthenia" is unknown, although pulmonary function abnormalities may persist for several weeks after uncomplicated influenza.

COMPLICATIONS OF INFLUENZA The most common complication of influenza is pneumonia, which may occur either as "primary" influenza viral pneumonia, secondary bacterial pneumonia, or mixed viral and bacterial pneumonia. Primary influenza viral pneumonia is the least common but most severe of the pneumonic complications. It presents as acute influenza which does not resolve but instead relentlessly progresses with persistent fever, dyspnea, and eventual cyanosis. Sputum production is generally scanty but can contain blood, and few physical signs may be present early in the illness. In more advanced cases, diffuse rales may be noted, and chest x-ray

findings consistent with diffuse interstitial infiltrates and/or acute respiratory distress syndrome may be present. In such cases, arterial blood gases show marked hypoxia. Viral cultures, particularly if taken early in illness, show high titers of virus in respiratory secretions and in the lung parenchyma. Histopathology of fatal cases of primary viral pneumonia shows a marked inflammatory reaction in the alveolar septa, with edema and infiltration with lymphocytes, macrophages, occasional plasma cells, and variable numbers of neutrophils. Fibrin thrombi in alveolar capillaries, along with necrosis and hemorrhage, also have been noted. Eosinophilic hyaline membranes also can be found lining alveoli and alveolar ducts.

Primary influenza viral pneumonia has a predilection for individuals with cardiac disease, particularly those with mitral stenosis, but also has been reported in otherwise healthy young adults, as well as in older individuals with chronic pulmonary disorders. In some epidemics of influenza (notably 1918 and 1957), pregnancy increased the risk of the development of primary influenza pneumonia.

Secondary bacterial pneumonia is a complication in which bacterial infection develops following a case of acute influenza. With this illness, patients experience a period of improvement for 2 to 3 days after acute influenza, followed by a reappearance of fever, along with clinical signs and symptoms of bacterial pneumonia. These include cough, production of purulent sputum, and physical and x-ray signs of consolidation. The most common bacterial pathogens in this setting are *Streptococcus pneumoniae*, *Staphylococcus aureus*, and *Haemophilus influenzae*, organisms that can colonize the nasopharynx and that cause infection in the wake of changes in bronchopulmonary defenses. The etiology can often be determined by Gram's stain and culture of an appropriately obtained sputum specimen. Secondary bacterial pneumonia occurs most frequently in high-risk individuals with chronic pulmonary and cardiac disease and in elderly individuals. Patients with secondary bacterial pneumonias will often respond to antibiotic therapy when it is instituted promptly.

Perhaps the most common of the pneumonic complications that occur during outbreaks of influenza are mixed viral and bacterial pneumonias. The clinical course of this complication contains features of both primary and secondary pneumonias. Patients may have a gradual progression of their acute illness or may show a transient improvement followed by a clinical worsening, with eventual manifestion of the clinical features of a bacterial pneumonia. Sputum cultures may contain both influenza A virus and one of the bacterial pathogens described above. Patchy infiltrates or areas of consolidation may be noted by physical examination and chest x-ray. Patients with mixed viral and bacterial pneumonias generally have less widespread involvement of the lung than those with primary viral pneumonia, and their bacterial infections may respond to appropriate antibiotics. Mixed viral and bacterial pneumonias occur primarily in patients with chronic cardiovascular and pulmonary diseases.

In addition to the pulmonary complications of influenza, a number of extrapulmonary complications may occur. *Reye's syndrome* is a serious complication of influenza B and to a lesser extent of influenza A virus infection, as well as of varicella-zoster virus infection. It occurs in children most commonly between the ages of 2 and 16 and follows several days after a generally unremarkable viral illness. Reye's syndrome is marked by the onset of nausea and vomiting for 1 to 2 days, after which central nervous system symptoms appear. These are most frequently changes in mental status, ranging from lethargy to coma, and can include delirium and seizures. Hepatomegaly is noted, along with a marked elevation of AST, ALT, and LDH levels. Bilirubin values are only moderately elevated, so the children are not jaundiced, but blood ammonia levels are elevated in virtually all patients. Hypoglycemia can occur, especially after varicella-zoster virus infection or after viral gastrointestinal illnesses. Children are usually afebrile, and while lumbar puncture generally shows an elevated pressure, the cerebrospinal fluid is quite unremarkable, indicating that an encephalopathy rather than a meningoencephalitis is present. The mortality of the syndrome is related to the state of consciousness on admission and has decreased from more than 40 percent, when the syndrome was originally described, to approximately 10 percent, reflecting earlier recognition and improved management of cerebral edema and hypoglycemia. Histopathology demonstrates little in the way of inflammatory changes in either the liver or the central nervous system. Liver biopsy shows diffuse fatty infiltration of hepatocytes and swelling and pleomorphism in mitochondria. Cerebral edema and anoxic changes in neurons are the only pathologic changes detected in the central nervous system. The pathogenesis of Reye's syndrome is unknown, but the virus is almost never found in the affected liver and brain. An epidemiologic association with aspirin therapy for the antecedent viral infection has been noted, and the incidence of Reye's syndrome has decreased markedly with widespread warnings regarding the use of aspirin in children with acute viral respiratory infections.

Myositis, rhabdomyolysis, and myoglobinuria also have been reported as occasional complications of influenza infection. Although myalgias are exceedingly common in influenza, true myositis is rare. Patients with acute myositis have exquisite tenderness of the affected muscles, most commonly in the legs, and may not be able to tolerate even the slightest pressure, such as the touch of bed sheets. In the most severe cases, there is frank swelling and bogginess of muscles. Markedly elevated serum creatine phosphokinase and aldolase levels are present, and an occasional patient has developed renal failure from myoglobinuria. The pathogenesis of influenza-associated myositis is also unclear, although the presence of influenza virus in affected muscles has been reported.

Myocarditis and pericarditis in association with influenza virus infection was reported during the 1918–1919 pandemic, based largely on histopathologic findings, and has been documented infrequently since that time. Electrocardiographic changes during acute influenza are commonly noted in patients who have cardiac disease, but these have been most often ascribed to exacerbations of the underlying cardiac disease rather than to direct involvement of the myocardium with influenza virus.

Central nervous system disease also has been reported during influenza, including encephalitis, transverse myelitis, and Guillain-Barré syndrome. The etiologic relationship of influenza virus to such CNS illnesses remains unestablished. "Toxic shock" syndrome caused by *S. aureus* infection following acute influenza infection has been reported recently (see Chap. 102).

In addition to complications involving the specific organ systems described above, every influenza outbreak includes a number of elderly and other high-risk individuals who develop influenza and who subsequently experience a gradual deterioration of underlying cardiovascular, pulmonary, or renal function, occasionally leading to irreversible changes and death. These fatalities contribute to the overall toll of excess mortality associated with influenza A outbreaks.

LABORATORY FINDINGS   Laboratory diagnosis is accomplished during the acute illness by isolation of virus from throat swabs, nasopharyngeal washes, or sputum. Virus is usually detected in tissue culture or less commonly in the amniotic cavity of chick embryos within 48 to 72 h after inoculation. Viral antigens may be detected somewhat earlier by use of immunodiagnostic techniques in tissue culture or directly in exfoliated nasopharyngeal cells obtained by washings, although this technique is less sensitive than isolation of virus in tissue culture. The type of influenza virus (A or B) may be identified by either immunofluorescence or hemagglutination inhibition techniques, and the hemagglutinin subtype of influenza A virus (H1, H2, or H3) may be identified by hemagglutination inhibition using subtype-specific antisera. Serologic methods for diagnosis require comparison of antibody titers in sera obtained during the acute illness with those obtained 10 to 14 days after the onset of illness and are useful primarily in retrospect. Fourfold or greater titer rises as detected by hemagglutination inhibition or complement fixation or significant rises in antibody levels as measured by ELISA techniques are diagnostic of acute infection. Complement fixation tests are generally less sensitive than other serologic techniques, but since they

detect type-specific antigens, they may be particularly useful when subtype-specific reagents are not available.

Other laboratory tests are generally not helpful in making a specific diagnosis of influenza virus infection. Leukocyte counts are variable, being frequently low early in illness and normal or slightly elevated later. Severe leukopenia has been described in overwhelming viral or bacterial infection, while leukocytosis with counts of greater than 15,000 cells per microliter should raise the suspicion that secondary bacterial infection is present.

DIFFERENTIAL DIAGNOSIS   On clinical grounds alone, an individual case of influenza may be difficult to differentiate from an acute respiratory illness caused by a variety of respiratory viruses or by *Mycoplasma pneumoniae*. Severe streptococcal pharyngitis or early bacterial pneumonia may mimic acute influenza, although bacterial pneumonias generally do not run a self-limited course. The presence of purulent sputum in which a bacterial pathogen can be detected by Gram's stain is an important diagnostic feature in bacterial pneumonia. The fact that influenza occurs in characteristic outbreaks during the winter months may be helpful in making a clinical diagnosis. When local health authorities indicate that influenza is present in the community, the etiology of an acute febrile respiratory illness can be attributed to influenza with a high degree of certainty, particularly if the typical features of abrupt onset and systemic symptoms are present.

TREATMENT   In uncomplicated cases of influenza, symptomatic therapy for headache, myalgia, and fever may be considered, employing either acetaminophen or salicylates, but salicylates should be avoided in children below 18 years of age because of the possible association of salicylates with Reye's syndrome. Since cough is ordinarily self-limited, treatment with cough suppressants generally is not indicated, although codeine-containing compounds may be employed if the cough is particularly troublesome. Patients should be advised to rest and maintain hydration during acute illness and should return to full activity only gradually after the illness has resolved, particularly if illness has been severe.

The only specific antiviral therapy available for influenza is amantadine. Amantadine is active only against influenza A viruses and has been licensed for the prophylaxis and therapy of influenza A virus infections in the United States. If begun within 48 h of the onset of illness, amantadine reduces the duration of systemic and respiratory symptoms of influenza by approximately 50 percent, and in one study, it was superior to aspirin. From 5 to 10 percent of individuals who receive amantadine will experience mild central nervous system side effects, primarily jitteriness, anxiety, insomnia, or difficulty in concentrating. These side effects disappear promptly upon cessation of the drug. The dose of amantadine for adults is 200 mg/d for 3 to 5 days or up to 48 h after illness has resolved. Because amantadine is excreted almost entirely by the kidneys, the dose should be reduced in individuals with renal insufficiency. Rimantadine, an experimental drug which is a closely related analogue of amantadine, appears to be equally efficacious and is associated with less frequent central nervous system side effects than is amantadine. Ribavirin, a nucleoside analogue with activity against a variety of viral agents, has been reported to be effective against both influenza A and B virus infections when administered as an aerosol, although it is relatively ineffective when administered orally.

Studies demonstrating the therapeutic efficacy of antiviral compounds in influenza have been carried out almost exclusively in uncomplicated disease in young adults, and it is not known whether such compounds are effective in the treatment of complications such as influenza pneumonia. Therapy for primary influenza pneumonia is directed at maintaining oxygenation and is most appropriately managed in an intensive care unit, with aggressive respiratory and hemodynamic support as needed. Bypass membrane oxygenators have been employed in this setting with variable results. When an acute respiratory distress syndrome develops, fluids must be administered cautiously, with close monitoring of blood gases and hemodynamic function.

Antibacterial drugs should be reserved for the therapy of bacterial complications of acute influenza such as secondary bacterial pneumonia. The choice of antibiotics should be guided by Gram's stain and culture of appropriate specimens of respiratory secretions, such as sputum or transtracheal aspirates. If the etiology of a bacterial pneumonia is unclear from examination of respiratory secretions, empiric antibiotics should be selected which are effective against the most common bacterial pathogens in this setting, namely, *S. pneumoniae*, *S. aureus*, and *H. influenzae* (see Chaps. 101, 102, and 119).

PROPHYLAXIS The major public health measure for prevention of influenza has been the use of inactivated influenza vaccines. These vaccines are derived from influenza A and B viruses which circulated during the previous influenza season. If the vaccine and currently circulating viruses are closely related, such vaccines would be expected to provide 50 to 80 percent protection against influenza. Currently available vaccines have been highly purified and are associated with few reactions. Up to 5 percent of individuals will experience low-grade fever and mild systemic symptoms 8 to 24 h after vaccination, and up to one-third may have mild redness or tenderness at the vaccination site. Since the vaccine is produced in eggs, individuals with true hypersensitivity to egg products either should be desensitized or should not receive vaccine. Although the 1976 swine influenza vaccine appears to have been associated with an increased frequency of Guillain-Barré syndrome, influenza vaccines administered since 1976 have not been associated with Guillain-Barré syndrome. Live attenuated ("cold-adapted") influenza A vaccines also have been developed and appear to be promising in ongoing studies in adults and children. Such vaccines are administered intranasally and stimulate local antibody production more efficiently than conventional inactivated vaccines.

The U.S. Public Health Service recommends influenza vaccination for any individual older than 6 months of age who is at an increased risk for complications of influenza. These include individuals with chronic cardiovascular or pulmonary disorders (including asthma) and residents of nursing homes and other chronic care facilities. Other populations for whom the vaccine is recommended include otherwise healthy individuals over 65 years of age and individuals who have required regular medical attention for diabetes mellitus, renal disease, hemoglobinopathies, or immunosuppression. Individuals who provide care for high-risk patients or who come into frequent contact with such patients, including household members, also should receive vaccine to reduce the likelihood of transmission of infection. Since commercially available vaccines are inactivated ("killed"), they may be administered safely to immunocompromised patients. Influenza vaccination is not associated with exacerbations of chronic nervous system diseases such as multiple sclerosis. Vaccination should be administered early in the autumn before influenza outbreaks occur and should be administered on an annual basis to maintain immunity against the most current influenza virus strains.

Amantadine and rimantadine also have been demonstrated to be effective in the prophylaxis of influenza A. Studies have demonstrated 70 to 100 percent effectiveness of these drugs in preventing illness associated with influenza A virus infection. The major use for prophylaxis with amantadine or rimantadine is likely to be for high-risk individuals who have not received influenza vaccine or when the vaccines previously administered are relatively ineffective because of antigenic changes in the circulating virus. If vaccination is performed during an outbreak, amantadine can be administered simultaneously with inactivated vaccine, since it will not interfere with an immune response to the vaccine. There is also evidence that the protective effects of amantadine and vaccine may be additive. Amantadine also has been employed to control nosocomial outbreaks of influenza A. For prophylaxis, amantadine or rimantadine should be instituted promptly when influenza A activity is detected and must be administered daily for the duration of the outbreak. The dosage most frequently employed has been 200 mg/d for adults, but the dose of amantadine should be reduced in patients with renal insufficiency and in the elderly. Viruses resistant to both amantadine and rimantadine can emerge quickly after therapy with these drugs.

REFERENCES

CENTERS FOR DISEASE CONTROL: Prevention and control of influenza. Morb Mort Week Rep 40:1, 1991

DOLIN R et al: A controlled trial of amantadine and rimantadine in the prophylaxis of influenza A infection. N Engl J Med 307:580, 1982

DOUGLAS RG JR (ed): Prevention, management, and control of influenza: A mandate for the 1980s. Am J Med 82 (suppl 6A), 1987

GLEZEN WP: Serious morbidity and mortality associated with influenza epidemics. Epidemiol Rev 4:25, 1982

MURPHY BR, WEBSTER RG: Orthomyxoviruses, in *Virology*, 2d ed, BN Fields (ed). New York, Raven Press, 1990, pp 1091-1152

YINNON AM, DOLIN R: Using antivirals to fight influenza in 1991–1992. J Respir Dis 12:1146, 1991

153 VIRAL GASTROENTERITIS

HARRY B. GREENBERG

In less developed countries, acute infectious diarrheal disease is a leading cause of morbidity in all age groups and of mortality in infants and young children. In developed countries, acute diarrheal illness remains an important cause of morbidity among both children and adults. Two distinct groups of viruses—the rotaviruses and the enteric caliciviruses such as Norwalk virus—as well as a variety of bacterial pathogens (see Chap. 87) have emerged as important etiologic agents of gastroenteritis. The rotaviruses are primarily pathogens of young children. The Norwalk and related enteric caliciviruses affect predominantly older children and adults.

ROTAVIRUS   Classification and characterization   Rotaviruses are members of the Reoviridae family. The rotavirus virion consists of a 70-nm double-shelled icosahedral capsid which surrounds a genome composed of 11 segments of double-stranded RNA. The virus has two surface proteins which are both involved with viral neutralization. Because rotaviruses have a segmented genome, they are capable of undergoing gene reassortment at very high frequency. The role of gene reassortment in generating rotavirus antigenic diversity is not known. In humans, rotavirus infection is characterized by replication that is localized almost exclusively in the small intestinal epithelial cells.

Epidemiology   Rotavirus infection occurs worldwide. By the age of 3, virtually every individual has been infected by rotaviruses at least once. In areas with a temperate climate, rotavirus infection is seasonal, occurring in the cooler winter months. In the United States, the annual seasonal rotavirus epidemic tends to spread from West to East, starting in California and ending in New England. In tropical areas, rotavirus infection tends to occur throughout the year, with some increase in incidence during the cooler rainy season. Rotaviruses are the single most important cause of severe dehydrating diarrhea in infants and young children under age 3 in both developed and less developed countries and account for between 30 and 50 percent of all cases of diarrhea requiring hospitalization or intensive rehydration therapy. Although rotavirus infections are primarily confined to infants and small children, they are frequently associated with diarrhea in adults, particularly family members of affected infants, geriatric patients, and immunocompromised hosts. They account for up to 10 percent of traveler's diarrhea (see Chap. 87). Rotaviruses also may be responsible for some cases of acute and chronic diarrhea in patients with AIDS. Subclinical infections or mild gastrointestinal illnesses which do not require hospitalization account for the majority of rotavirus infections. Subclinical infections also have been documented in neonates; these infections were shown to protect against severe rotavirus gastroenteritis for up to 3 years. At least eight distinct serotypes of human rotavirus have been described, but only four types are commonly encountered. The relationship of the frequency of infection with these serotypes to host immune status is unclear. A large variety of other mammals and avian species can be infected by rotavirus, but it does not appear that these animal rotavirus strains cause disease in humans under most conditions. Rotaviruses are shed in very large numbers (up to 10^{10} particles per gram of feces) in the stool; it is presumed that transmission occurs via fecal-oral spread.

Pathophysiology   Rotavirus infects and kills the mature villous tip cells of the small intestine. The mature epithelial cells are replaced by immature absorptive cells that cannot absorb carbohydrates or other nutrients efficiently. Rotavirus infection leads to an osmotic diarrhea due to nutrient malabsorption. Changes in intracellular cyclic adenosine monophosphate or guanosine monophosphate are not involved in the etiology of rotavirus diarrhea.

Manifestations   These range from subclinical infections to mild diarrhea to severe, occasionally fatal illness. Most information concerning the signs and symptoms of rotavirus infection has been derived from studies of hospitalized young children. The onset of illness is usually abrupt. Vomiting, followed by diarrhea, occurs in over 80 percent of affected children. About one-third of hospitalized children will have a temperature greater than 39°C (102.2°F). Gastrointestinal symptoms usually last between 2 and 6 days. Mucus is commonly found in the stool, but white and red blood cells are present in less than 15 percent of cases. Rotavirus infection frequently occurs in conjunction with respiratory tract symptoms, but there is little evidence to indicate that rotavirus replicates in the respiratory tract. Rotavirus infection has been observed in association with a wide variety of other clinical syndromes, including sudden infant death syndrome, Reye's syndrome, encephalitis, aseptic meningitis, pneumonia, exanthem subitum, Kawasaki's syndrome, necrotizing enterocolitis, intussusception, Schönlein-Henoch purpura, hemolytic uremic syndrome, disseminated intravascular coagulation, and Crohn's disease. The etiologic relationship between these clinical syndromes and rotavirus infection is probably coincidental rather than causal. Rotavirus infection may be especially severe, and even fatal, in immunocompromised children.

Clinical immunity   Relative immunity to rotavirus illness is acquired following infection early in childhood. Immunity is not complete, and adults with low levels of antibody can be symptomatically infected. Local immunity appears to be a critical determinant in protection, and cellular immune mechanisms appear to be involved as well.

Diagnosis   Because rotavirus is shed in large amounts in the stool, detection is relatively easy. A variety of specific commercial immunoassays are available to detect rotavirus antigen in fecal specimens. DNA probe diagnosis also appears to be sensitive and specific. There are no pathognomonic signs or symptoms of rotavirus infection, but rotavirus infection is more frequently associated with severe dehydration than are infections caused by other enteric bacterial or viral pathogens.

Treatment and prevention   Despite the fact that rotavirus diarrhea is caused by intestinal epithelial cell lysis and death, it can be adequately treated by standard oral rehydration therapy. Only rarely is intravenous rehydration required. Since rotavirus infections have persisted in developed countries with advanced sanitation facilities and widely available clean water, it is unlikely that the viral infection will be preventable by hygienic measures alone. Progress with a number of candidate live attenuated vaccines suggests that prevention through vaccination may be feasible in the future.

NORWALK AND RELATED ENTERIC CALICIVIRUSES   Classification and characterization   A variety of round 27- to 32-nm particles, some with clearly defined ultrastructure, have been identified in the stools of individuals with acute nonbacterial gastroenteritis. These agents have not been definitely classified because they are shed in the stool in small amounts for only a few days, and they have not been adapted to cell culture or to animal models. The Norwalk virus represents the most extensively studied and best characterized member of this group of agents, which also includes such serologically distinct viruses as the Hawaii agent, the Snow Mountain agent, the W-Ditchling agent, and a number of agents described as calicivirus-like.

The Norwalk virus and the Snow Mountain virus appear to have a protein structure similar to that of typical caliciviruses. Recently, the genome of Norwalk virus has been cloned and partially sequenced. It is a plus-stranded RNA molecule of approximately 7.5 kilobases.

Epidemiology   Norwalk infection occurs year round and is common. From 58 to 70 percent of adults in both developed and less developed countries have antibodies to this virus. Antibody acquisition occurs at a considerably younger age in children in less developed countries than in those in developed areas, consistent with the presumption that Norwalk virus is spread by the fecal-oral route. In developed countries, the virus is responsible for approximately one-third of all epidemics of nonbacterial gastroenteritis. Norwalk virus has been incriminated in a variety of food-borne epidemics, and transmission vehicles have included oysters, green salad, and chocolate icing. The virus is a common cause of waterborne epidemics of gastroenteritis and has been shown to be the etiologic agent in nursing home, cruise ship, and institutional (summer camps and schools) outbreaks. Norwalk virus is also responsible for a small proportion of cases of traveler's diarrhea.

In less developed countries, the role of Norwalk virus infection in the etiology of diarrhea has not been thoroughly investigated. Preliminary studies indicate that Norwalk virus can cause mild diarrhea in young children, but it does not appear to cause severe illness in infants in either developed or less developed countries. The other serologically distinct calicivirus-like gastroenteritis agents must be studied in more detail before their epidemiology can be distinguished from that of Norwalk virus. It appears, however, that some human caliciviruses, especially those with well-defined ultrastructure, are primarily pathogens of young children rather than adults.

Pathophysiology   Following infection with Norwalk or Hawaii virus, the proximal small intestinal architecture is altered, with villus shortening, crypt hyperplasia, and lamina propria infiltration by polymorphonuclear and mononuclear cells. Changes are not observed in the stomach or colon. The cells in which viral replication occurs have not been identified. The histologic alterations are accompanied by mild steatorrhea, carbohydrate malabsorption, and decreased levels of some brush border enzymes. Changes in adenylate cyclase activity have not been observed.

Manifestations   Norwalk illness has an incubation period of between 18 and 72 h. Disease is characterized by the abrupt onset of nausea and abdominal cramps followed by vomiting and/or diarrhea. Vomiting occurs more frequently in children than adults. Low-grade fever [above 37.5°C (99.5°F)] is seen in about half of affected individuals. Headache, myalgias, and abdominal pain are common. The white blood cell count is normal; rarely, there is leukocytosis with a relative lymphopenia. Red and white cells are not found in the stool. The illness is usually mild and self-limited, lasting 24 to 48 h.

Clinical immunity   For most people, long-term (2 years or greater) resistance to Norwalk reinfection does not occur. In volunteers challenged with Norwalk agent, there is a paradoxical relationship between the level of antibody to Norwalk virus and susceptibility to illness. Low levels of Norwalk antibody in the serum and intestine are associated with clinical resistance to illness. It appears, therefore, that immune mechanisms are not the primary determinants of protection from Norwalk virus.

Diagnosis, treatment, and prevention   Radioimmunoassays and an enzyme-linked immunosorbent assay (ELISA) have been developed for Norwalk virus and several other 27- to 30-nm gastroenteritis agents. These tests are not yet available commercially. Recently, detection assays based on nucleic acid probing and the polymerase chain reaction also have been developed. Norwalk illness is acute and self-limited; treatment is not usually required. In the rare case of severe vomiting or diarrhea, oral or intravenous rehydration is indicated. Because long-term immunity to Norwalk illness does not usually follow natural infection, it seems unlikely that a vaccine will be developed.

MISCELLANEOUS ENTERIC VIRAL PATHOGENS   Enteric adenoviruses are a minor (10 percent) cause of diarrheal illness in infants and children. These viruses differ from other adenovirus strains in a variety of ways, including neutralization serotype, restriction endonuclease digestion pattern, and ability to grow in tissue culture. The role of enteric adenovirus illness in adults or in persons in less developed countries is not known.

Several strains of antigenically distinct rotaviruses, presently called "atypical rotaviruses" or group B and C rotaviruses, have been identified as the cause of occasional episodes of diarrhea in humans and animals.

Preliminary epidemiologic studies have indicated that astroviruses are a relatively frequent cause of mild to moderate diarrhea in young children in developed and less developed countries, accounting for about half as much illness as group A rotaviruses. Astroviruses are 27 to 32 nm in diameter, have a characteristic icosahedral ultrastructure, and contain a plus-stranded RNA genome with a size of approximately 7.8 kilobases. The recent availability of sensitive and specific diagnostic assays should facilitate more complete assessment of the importance of these agents.

Coronaviruses are frequent causes of diarrheal disease in a variety of animals. Several investigators, using electron microscopy, have identified putative coronavirus-like particles in the stools of patients with diarrhea. In most cases, however, these particles do not have the typical morphologic features of coronaviruses and may represent bacterial breakdown products or cellular fragments.

REFERENCES

BLACK RE et al: A two-year study of bacterial, viral and parasitic agents associated with diarrhea in rural Bangladesh. J Infect Dis 142:660, 1980

BLACKLOW NR, GREENBERG HB: Viral gastroenteritis. N Engl J Med 325:252, 1991

HO M et al: Rotavirus as a cause of diarrheal morbidity and mortality in the United States. J Infect Dis 158:1112, 1988

JIANG X et al: Norwalk virus genome cloning and characterization. Science 250:1580, 1990

KAPIKIAN AZ, CHANOCK RM: Rotaviruses, in Virology, vol 2, 2d ed, BN Fields, DM Knipe, RM Chanock, MS Hirsch, JL Melnick, TP Monath (eds). New York, Raven, 1990, p 1353

LeBARON CW et al: Annual rotavirus epidemic patterns in North America. JAMA 264:983, 1990

MATSUI SM et al: The isolation and characterization of a Norwalk virus-specific cDNA. J Clin Invest 87:1456, 1991

154 ENTEROVIRUSES AND REOVIRUSES

C. GEORGE RAY

GENERAL CONSIDERATIONS

Enteroviruses consist of a major subgroup of picornaviruses that include the polioviruses, coxsackieviruses, echoviruses, and more recently discovered agents that are simply designated enteroviruses. The number of serotypes that infect humans is nearly 70, and more are likely to be found in the future. Their name is derived from their ability to infect intestinal tract epithelial and lymphoid tissues and to be shed into the feces.

Enteroviruses can cause paralytic disease, encephalitis and acute aseptic meningitis syndromes, pleurodynia, exanthems, pericarditis, myocarditis, nonspecific febrile illness, and occasional fulminant disease in the newborn. The spectrum of disease may be even broader. Some infections can lead to permanent damage, and others may trigger chronic, active disease processes.

Since these viruses have many features in common, they will first be considered as a group. Some of the special features of important serotypes will be discussed in detail later in this chapter.

CHARACTERISTICS OF ENTEROVIRUSES As a group, the picornaviruses are extremely small (22 to 30 nm in diameter), single-stranded RNA viruses with icosahedral symmetry. In contrast to the rhinoviruses, the enterovirus subgroup is resistant to ether, acid pH (3.0), and bile. Another feature is cationic stability; in the presence of magnesium chloride, the viruses become more resistant to thermal inactivation. They can survive for prolonged periods in sewage and even in chlorinated water if sufficient organic debris is present. Although some of the enterovirus serotypes share antigens, there are no significant serologic relationships between the major classes listed in Table 154-1; however, a single, highly conserved epitope may be shared by virtually all serotypes. Genetic variation within specific strains occurs, and mutants which exhibit antigenic drift and altered tropism for specific cell types have been recognized. Definitive identification of isolates usually requires neutralization tests.

Most of these agents can be isolated in primate (human or simian) cell cultures; however, some strains, such as several coxsackievirus group A serotypes, are grown with difficulty in vitro, and inoculation of newborn mice may be necessary for detection. This latter procedure was one basis for the original classification of group A and B coxsackieviruses. After the mice have been inoculated, at 24 h of age or less, and observed for 2 to 12 days, group A viruses primarily have a widespread, inflammatory, necrotic effect on skeletal muscle, leading to flaccid paralysis and usually death; similar inoculation of group B viruses causes encephalitis, resulting in spasticity and occasionally convulsions. Other organs are variably affected, and histopathologic examination is sometimes helpful in distinguishing the two. Echoviruses and polioviruses rarely have an adverse effect on mice, unless special adaptation procedures are employed. The higher-numbered enteroviruses (types 68 to 71), which have overlapping growth and host characteristics, have been classified separately.

Humans are the major natural host for the polioviruses, coxsackieviruses, and echoviruses. There are enteroviruses of other animals with limited host ranges that do not appear to extend to humans. Conversely, viruses thought to be identical or related to human enteroviruses have been isolated from dogs and cats. Whether these agents cause disease in the animals is debatable, and there is no evidence of spread from animals to humans.

EPIDEMIOLOGY The enteroviruses have a worldwide distribution, and asymptomatic infection is common. The proportion of infected individuals who will develop illness varies from 2 to 100 percent depending on the serotype or strain involved, prior immune status, and age of the patient. Secondary infections in households are common and range as high as 40 to 70 percent depending on factors such as family size, crowding, and sanitary conditions.

There is a seasonal predilection; epidemics are usually observed during the summer and fall. In subtropical and tropical climates, the duration of greatest transmission sometimes extends into the winter. Certain serotypes emerge as dominant strains during some years; they then may wane, only to reappear in epidemics years later.

Direct or indirect fecal-oral transmission is considered the most common mode of spread. After infection, the virus persists in the oropharynx for 1 to 4 weeks, and it can be shed in the feces for 1 to 18 weeks. Sewage-contaminated water, contaminated foods, or insect

TABLE 154-1 Enteroviruses that infect humans

Class	Number of serotypes
Poliovirus	3
Coxsackievirus	
Group A	23*
Group B	6
Echovirus	31
Enterovirus	Types 68–71†

* Includes several subtypes; coxsackievirus A23 is the same as echovirus 9.
† The classification of the more recently described enteroviruses is based on overlapping biologic characteristics. These are identified numerically.

vectors (flies, cockroaches) may occasionally be the source of infection. More commonly, however, spread is directly from person to person. Approximately two-thirds of all isolates are from children 9 years of age or younger.

Incubation periods vary, but relatively short intervals (2 to 10 days) are the rule. Illness is often seen concurrently in more than one family member, and the clinical features may vary within the household.

PATHOGENESIS AND PATHOLOGY After primary replication in the epithelial cells and lymphoid tissues in the upper respiratory and gastrointestinal tracts, viremic spread to other sites can occur. Potential target organs vary according to the virus strain and its tropism but may include the central nervous system, heart, vascular endothelium, liver, pancreas, gonads, lungs, skeletal muscles, synovial tissues, skin, and mucous membranes. Histopathologic findings include cell necrosis and mononuclear cell inflammatory infiltrates; in the central nervous system, the inflammatory cells are localized most prominently in perivascular sites. The initial tissue damage is thought to result from the lytic cycle of virus replication. Viremia is usually undetectable when symptoms appear, and termination of virus replication commences with the appearance of circulating interferon, neutralizing antibody, and mononuclear cell infiltrations of infected tissue. The early antibody response is mainly immunoglobulin M–specific and usually wanes 6 to 12 weeks after onset to be replaced by IgG-specific antibodies.

Although initial acute tissue damage may be caused by the lytic effects of the virus on the cell, many of the secondary sequelae appear to be immunologically mediated. Enterovirus-caused poliomyelitis, disseminated disease of the newborn, aseptic meningitis, encephalitis, exanthems, and acute respiratory illnesses, thought to represent primary lytic infections, can usually be identified through routine methods of virus isolation and determination of specific antibody titer changes. On the other hand, syndromes such as myopericarditis, nephritis, and myositis have been associated with enteroviruses primarily by serologic evidence and the use of cDNA probes to detect viral RNA in tissues. Viral isolation is the exception. The pathogenesis of these illnesses involves cell-mediated immunologic responses to tissue injury by the virus or to viral or virus-induced antigens that persist in the affected tissues.

Infection by a specific serotype in an immunologically normal host is followed by a humoral antibody response, which can often be detected by neutralization methods for many years thereafter. There is relative immunity to reinfection by the same serotype; however, reinfection has been reported, usually resulting in subclinical infection or mild illness. Although there is some antigenic sharing between serotypes in some of the enterovirus classes (e.g., group B coxsackieviruses), there is no evidence of significant heterotypic immunity to infection by different serotypes.

LABORATORY DIAGNOSIS In acute enteroviral infections, the diagnosis is most readily established by virus isolation from throat swabs, stool or rectal swabs, body fluids, and occasionally tissues. Except in young infants, viremia is usually not detected. When there is central nervous system involvement, cerebrospinal fluid (CSF) cultures taken during the acute phase of the disease may be positive in 10 to 85 percent of cases (except in poliovirus infections, in which virus recovery from this site is rare) depending on the stage of illness and the serotype involved. Direct isolation of virus from affected tissues or body fluids in enclosed spaces (e.g., pleural, pericardial, or CSF) usually confirms the diagnosis. Isolation of an enterovirus from the throat is suggestive of an etiologic association because the virus is usually detectable at this site for only 2 days to 2 weeks after infection; isolation of virus from fecal specimens only must be interpreted more cautiously because asymptomatic shedding from the bowel may persist for as long as 4 months.

The diagnosis may be further supported by a fourfold or greater neutralizing antibody titer increase in paired acute and convalescent serum samples. This method is expensive and cumbersome, requiring careful selection of serotypes for use as antigens. Serodiagnosis is generally reserved for critical situations in which the etiology is questionable, such as isolation of a virus only from a peripheral source such as the feces or, in illnesses such as myopericarditis, in which the yield on routine culture is low and the number of serotypes that might be expected to be involved is limited. Quantitative interpretations of antibody titers on single serum samples are rarely helpful because of the high prevalence and wide range of titers to different serotypes that can be found in healthy individuals. In acute poliovirus infections, complement-fixing antibody titer determinations on acute and convalescent sera can aid in diagnosis.

Recently, it has been shown that common enteroviral RNA sequences can be revealed by the polymerase chain reaction, enhancing and often speeding detection in tissue and CSF. However, routine diagnostic testing for enterovirus infections by this method is not currently available.

White blood cell counts and the erythrocyte sedimentation rates are usually only mildly elevated. If there is necrosis (e.g., liver, lung), a neutrophilic reaction may be noted. Hyperbilirubinemia and elevated transaminase and alkaline phosphatase levels may be seen in patients with hepatitis. Albuminuria often occurs transiently, but hematuria is rare.

PROPHYLAXIS AND TREATMENT Vaccines, which are available only for the prevention of poliovirus infections, will be discussed in detail below. Although proper disposal of feces and careful personal hygiene are recommended, the usual quarantine or isolation measures are relatively ineffective in controlling the spread of enteroviruses in the family or community.

None of the currently available antiviral agents or immune serum globulins has been effective in treatment or prophylaxis of enterovirus infections. The only exception may be the intravenous or intraventricular use of high-titered immunoglobulin in the treatment of chronic enteroviral encephalitis in antibody-deficient patients. Otherwise, treatment is entirely symptomatic and supportive. Glucocorticoids are contraindicated.

POLIOVIRUS INFECTIONS

The most important enteroviruses are the three poliovirus serotypes (types 1, 2, and 3). They first emerged as important causes of disease in developed temperate-zone countries during the latter part of the nineteenth century and continue to be a serious public health problem in some developing countries. In 1988, the World Health Organization committed itself to the global elimination of poliomyelitis by the year 2000. Thus far, eradication efforts have been particularly successful in the Western Hemisphere, where reported cases of wild-type poliovirus infections dropped to a low of 9 in 1991 and none during the first 9 months of 1992; most recently, these have all been localized in areas of Colombia and Peru.

The particular tropism of polioviruses for the central nervous system, which they usually reach by passage across the blood-CNS barrier, is perhaps favored by reflex dilatation of capillaries supplying the affected motor centers of the anterior horn of the brainstem or spinal cord. An alternate pathway may be via entry into motor neurons at peripheral neuromuscular junctions. Motor neurons are particularly vulnerable to infection and variable degrees of destruction. The histopathologic findings in the brainstem and spinal cord include necrosis of neuronal cells and perivascular "cuffing" by infiltration with mononuclear cells, primarily lymphocytes.

CLINICAL MANIFESTATIONS Most infections (perhaps 90 percent) are either subclinical or extremely mild. When disease does result, the incubation period can be from 4 to 35 days but is usually between 7 and 14 days. The disease falls into three classes: The first, *abortive poliomyelitis*, is a nonspecific febrile illness of 2- to 3-day duration with no signs of CNS localization. A second group of patients will additionally develop *aseptic meningitis*. Recovery is rapid and complete, usually within a few days. The third class, *paralytic poliomyelitis*, is the major possible outcome of infection and is often preceded by a period of fever and "minor illness." Classically, after several days, symptoms disappear. In 5 to 10 days fever recurs, and signs of meningeal irritation and asymmetric flaccid paralysis ensue. Cramping muscle pain and spasm as well as coarse twitching in affected parts follows. The maximum extent of involvement is apparent within a few days after first paralysis. In children under 5 years, paralysis of one leg is most common. In patients 5 to 15 years of age, weakness of one arm or paraplegia is frequent, while in adults, quadriplegia is more likely to occur. Urinary bladder and respiratory muscle dysfunction are also frequent in adults. Encephalitis is rare.

Tendon reflexes are diminished or absent. Sensation is intact, in contrast to the usually symmetric paralysis and mild sensory disturbance of the Guillain-Barré syndrome. Paralysis due to heavy metal poisoning also may be difficult to distinguish clinically from poliomyelitis.

Among paralytic cases, 6 to 25 percent may be bulbar. Myocarditis, hypertension, pulmonary edema, shock, nosocomial gram-negative or staphylococcal pneumonias, urinary tract infections, and emotional problems are among the complications of severe paralytic disease. Treatment is supportive. About 2 to 5 percent of children and 15 to 30 percent of adults with paralyzing infection die. As temporarily damaged neurons regain their function, recovery begins and may continue for as long as 6 months. Paralysis persisting beyond that time is permanent and may be associated with complaints of severe pain in the affected areas that sometimes recurs years after the illness.

Some patients develop progressive muscle weakness, usually beginning 20 to 30 years later. This is called *postpoliomyelitis neuromuscular atrophy*, or the *postpolio syndrome*. Symptoms vary from mild to moderate deterioration of function, with fatigue, muscle pain, fasciculations, and weakness that may stabilize or progress to muscle atrophy. The limbs are often affected; in addition, clinical or subclinical involvement of the bulbar and respiratory musculature can sometimes lead to severe dysphagia, choking episodes, aspiration, or sleep apnea. The pathogenesis is usually considered to involve a dysfunction of surviving motor neurons with slow disintegration of axon terminals, leading to late denervation of muscle. There is also evidence suggesting that reactivation of latent or persistent poliovirus in the central nervous system may occur in some patients.

PREVENTION Two types of poliovirus vaccines are currently licensed in the United States: inactivated polio vaccine and live, oral, attenuated virus vaccine. Each contains the three serotypes of poliomyelitis virus.

Inactivated polio vaccine (IPV) has been used extensively in some countries, notably Sweden, Finland, and the Netherlands, and its efficacy has been excellent. The current product is considered safe, with no significant deleterious side effects. In 1988, a more potent IPV, which is produced in human diploid cells, was licensed. This enhanced-potency IPV has been shown to produce 99 to 100 percent seropositivity for all three poliovirus types after two doses in infants. Primary vaccination with three subcutaneous doses (two doses 4 to 8 weeks apart and the third 6 to 12 months later) is recommended for unimmunized children and adults. A booster dose at the time of school entry is recommended for children. The duration of protection is at least 5 years and may be considerably longer.

Oral polio vaccine (OPV) is composed of live, attenuated viruses. The vaccine is given as a primary series of three doses (the first two doses usually 6 to 8 weeks apart and the third 8 to 12 months later) and produces antibodies to all three serotypes in more than 95 percent of recipients. As with IPV, recall boosters are recommended to maintain adequate antibody levels. Like wild poliovirus, OPV viruses infect and replicate in the oropharynx and intestinal tract and may be shed into the feces for 6 weeks or longer.

One disadvantage of OPV is the remote risk of vaccine-associated paralytic disease in some recipients, such as immunocompromised persons; susceptible adults are at a higher risk than children. The incidence of vaccine-associated paralytic poliomyelitis is estimated to be approximately 1 per 2.6 million doses distributed and 1 per 520,000 after the first dose. Of the 138 cases of paralytic poliomyelitis

reported in the United States from 1973 through 1984, 105 were vaccine-associated (35 in healthy recipients, 50 in close contacts, 14 with immune-deficiency conditions, and 6 with no history of vaccination or contact).

The major advantages of OPV include ease of administration and secondary immunization of nonimmune contacts through shedding of vaccine virus into the intestinal tract, resulting in more widespread immunity in the population. It is also theorized that during outbreaks, transient vaccine virus colonization results in the induction of mucosal immunity (primarily through secretory IgA), which may interfere with subsequent acquisition and spread of wild poliovirus.

The choice between IPV and OPV for routine primary immunization is widely debated; however, it is clear that both are highly effective vaccines and that immunization with one or the other is important in the prevention of disease. Ideally, immunization should commence in infancy. A susceptible adult at risk of exposure to infection because of occupation or travel to an endemic area should receive complete immunization, preferably with IPV. Persons with immunodeficiency or altered immune status should not be exposed to OPV, either directly or by household contact, because of the increased risk of vaccine-associated paralysis. Other situations where IPV immunization is specifically indicated include persons with compromised immunity who are unimmunized or partially immunized, human immunodeficiency virus–infected patients, whether or not symptomatic, household contacts of either of the above groups, and partially immunized or unimmunized adults (or other close contacts) in households of children to be given OPV, but only if timely immunization of the child can be ensured.

Although there are no currently recognized areas of wild poliovirus prevalence in the United States, importation of these strains can occur from endemic areas in developing nations. Once introduced into a community, the virus can spread rapidly among susceptible individuals. For this reason, continuing immunization programs are of utmost importance in preventing spread of this disease.

COXSACKIEVIRUSES AND ECHOVIRUSES

The coxsackieviruses and echoviruses are widespread throughout the world. The basic features of their epidemiology and pathogenesis are the same as those of the polioviruses. Unlike polioviruses, they have a tendency to affect the meninges and occasionally the cerebrum, and only rarely do they affect anterior horn cells.

The consequences of infection with these agents are highly variable and related only in part to virus subgroup and serotype. Up to 60 percent of infections are subclinical. The main interest in these agents stems from their ability to cause more serious illness, which becomes most evident during epidemics.

Inapparent infection is common, but it varies with the infecting strain and the host involved. The manifestations of illness range from mild to lethal and from acute to chronic. Table 154-2 lists the major syndromes and serotypes commonly associated with each. Considerable overlap occurs, however, and it is not surprising to find different enteroviral serotypes associated with any specific syndrome. The group B coxsackieviruses generally have the greatest latitude with regard to tissue tropism.

ASEPTIC MENINGITIS (See Chap. 375) In terms of relative frequency, aseptic meningitis is the most important illness associated with enterovirus infections. This syndrome can be mild and self-limiting; however, it is occasionally accompanied by encephalitis, which can lead to permanent sequelae, particularly in infants. Overall, enteroviruses cause the majority of all nonbacterial CNS infections now observed in the United States.

There may be a mild prodromal malaise, but major illness usually begins with fever, headache, and stiff neck. Kernig's and Brudzinski's signs may be present. Localizing sensory or motor deficits are unusual. Confusion and delirium are common. These acute findings may persist for 4 to 7 days. Cerebrospinal pleocytosis is usually less than 500

TABLE 154-2 Clinical syndromes reported to be commonly associated with enterovirus serotypes

Syndrome	Coxsackievirus Group A	Coxsackievirus Group B	Echovirus and enterovirus (E)
Aseptic meningitis, encephalitis	2,4,7,9,10	1,2,3,4,5	4,6,9,11,16,30; E70,E71
Muscle weakness and paralysis (poliomyelitis-like disease)	7,9	2,3,4,5	2,4,6,9,11,30;E71
Cerebellar ataxia	2,4,9	3,4	4,6,9
Generalized disease (infants)	——	1,2,3,4,5	3,6,9,11,14,17,19
Exanthems and enanthems	4,5,6,9,10,16	2,3,4,5	2,4,5,6,9,11,16,18, 25;E71
Pericarditis, myocarditis	4,16	2,3,4,5	1,6,8,9,19
Epidemic myalgia (pleurodynia), orchitis	9	1,2,3,4,5	1,6,9
Respiratory symptoms	9,16,21,24	1,3,4,5	4,9,11,20,25
Conjunctivitis	24	1,5	7;E70

cells per microliter. Early, there may be as many as 90 percent polymorphonuclear leukocytes, but within 48 h the cellular response usually becomes predominantly or totally mononuclear. Persistence of polymorphonuclear leukocytes in the CSF suggests pyogenic meningitis or intracerebral, subdural, or epidural abscess. Gram's stain and appropriate CSF cultures must be done to exclude bacterial meningitis, tuberculosis, or mycotic meningitis. Protein concentration in the CSF is moderately elevated, but glucose is usually normal. Early in the illness enteroviruses may be isolated from CSF, even in the absence of significant pleocytosis. It usually takes several weeks before the CSF reverts to normal. An occasional patient may develop a transient syndrome of inappropriate secretion of antidiuretic hormone. In hypo- or agammaglobulinemic syndromes echoviruses have persisted in CSF for months to years, producing a progressive encephalitis or polymyositis.

For attempts at virus isolation, throat, stool, and CSF specimens should be collected as early in the course as possible. Acute and convalescent sera also can be studied for rises in type-specific neutralizing antibodies in patients in whom viral isolation results are negative or equivocal.

It is often not possible to distinguish clinically between aseptic meningitis due to various enteroviruses, arboviruses, Epstein-Barr virus, human immunodeficiency virus type 1, or mumps. Localizing findings, hemiplegia, oculogyric crises, coma, and bloody CSF favor the diagnosis of type 1 herpes simplex virus encephalitis (see Chap. 143). Although enterovirus aseptic meningitis most often is self-limited and recovery in persons afflicted after the first year of life is usually complete within 1 to 2 weeks, about 10 percent of patients have more serious involvement of the central nervous system. Minor muscle weakness with reflex changes may persist for weeks to months, but over 90 percent of patients recover completely within a year. Occasionally, choreiform movements, ataxia, nystagmus, transverse myelitis, Guillain-Barré syndrome, poliomyelitis-like symptoms, coma, bulbar involvement, and death occur.

OTHER ENTEROVIRAL ILLNESSES *Generalized disease of the newborn* is a highly lethal expression of enteroviral infection in which the infant may be overwhelmed by simultaneous virus infection of the heart, liver, adrenals, brain, and other organs.

Acute myocarditis and/or pericarditis can be caused by a variety of viral agents; however, it is estimated that as many as 50 percent of cases are associated with infection by coxsackievirus B. Such infections are usually self-limited, but they can lead to a fatal outcome (arrhythmia or heart failure) or cause chronic heart disease (see Chaps. 205 and 206).

The exanthems may or may not be associated with CNS inflammation. The rashes can resemble rubella, roseola infantum, or adenovirus exanthems. They are usually macular or maculopapular, with sparing of the palmar and plantar surfaces. This latter feature contrasts with the frequently prominent distal extremity involvement seen with otherwise similar-appearing eruptions caused by some drugs, Kawasaki disease, syphilis, rickettsial infections, staphylococcal and streptococcal toxins, and rat-bite fevers. Vesicular or hemangioma-like lesions also have been associated with enterovirus infections. Hand-foot-and-mouth disease usually affects children and is characterized by a vesicular eruption over the extremities and the anterior oral cavity. Coxsackievirus A16 is the specific agent most frequently implicated, but others, such as enterovirus 71, can cause a similar illness.

Herpangina is an enanthematous (mucous membrane) disease characterized by the acute onset of fever and sore throat. Characteristic small vesicles or white papules (lymphonodules) surrounded by a red halo are seen over the posterior half of the palate, pharynx, and tonsillar areas. This mild, self-limiting (1 to 2 weeks) illness usually has been associated with infection by several different group A coxsackievirus serotypes.

Epidemic myalgia (pleurodynia, or Bornholm disease) is characterized by fever and sudden onset of intense upper abdominal or lower thoracic pain, often accompanied by a frontal headache. The pain may be aggravated by movement, such as breathing or coughing, and usually persists for 3 to 14 days. Group B coxsackieviruses are most frequently implicated.

A variety of other illnesses also may result from infections by this subgroup. Epidemic acute hemorrhagic keratoconjunctivitis associated with enterovirus 70 has been reported in Asia and the United States, and outbreaks of disease resembling paralytic poliomyelitis caused by enterovirus 71 infection have occurred in Bulgaria, Australia, and the United States. Sporadic cases of poliomyelitis-like disease also have been reported with other enterovirus infections, notably coxsackievirus A7 and several echovirus serotypes. There is some evidence that certain enteroviruses may participate in the pathogenesis of at least some cases of insulin-dependent diabetes mellitus, acute arthritis, polymyositis, hemolytic-uremic syndrome, and idiopathic acute nephritis.

REOVIRUS INFECTIONS

The reoviruses (respiratory enteric orphans) are naked virions that contain double-stranded RNA. They have been found in humans, simians, cattle, rodents, and a variety of other hosts. Three serotypes are known to infect humans; however, their role and relative importance in causing disease remain uncertain. Sporadic cases of febrile upper respiratory infections, exanthems, pneumonia, hepatitis, encephalitis, and gastroenteritis have all been reported to be associated with these viruses. Reovirus type 3 has been implicated as a possible cause of biliary atresia and neonatal hepatitis, but this relationship remains uncertain. Asymptomatic shedding of reoviruses often makes it difficult to prove association with disease. Reoviruses can be isolated in cell cultures, particularly primary monkey kidney or human kidney monolayers.

REFERENCES

BARAK Y, SCHWARTZ JF: Acute transverse myelitis associated with echo type 5 infection. Am J Dis Child 142:128, 1988

BOWLES NE et al: Detection of coxsackie-B-virus-specific RNA sequences in myocardial biopsy samples from patients with myocarditis and dilated cardiomyopathy. Lancet 1:1120, 1986

—— et al: Dermatomyositis, polymyositis, and coxsackie-B-virus infection. Lancet 1:1004, 1987

BROWN WR et al: Lack of correlation between infection with reovirus 3 and extrahepatic biliary atresia or neonatal hepatitis. J Pediatr 113:670, 1988

HAYWARD JC et al: Outbreak of poliomyelitis-like paralysis associated with enterovirus 71. Pediatr Infect Dis J 8:611, 1989

JOSSELSON J et al: Acute rhabdomyolysis associated with an echovirus infection. Arch Intern Med 140:1671, 1980

KAPLAN MH et al: Group B coxsackievirus infections in infants younger than three months of age: A serious childhood illness. Rev Infect Dis 5:1019, 1983

MCKINNEY RE JR et al: Chronic enteroviral meningoencephalitis in agammaglobulinemia patients. Rev Infect Dis 9:334, 1987

ONORATO IM et al: Mucosal immunity induced by enhanced-potency inactivated and oral polio vaccines. J Infect Dis 163:1, 1991

QUERFURTH H, SWANSON PD: Vaccine-associated paralytic poliomyelitis: Regional case series and review. Arch Neurol 47:541, 1990

REN R, RACANIELLO VR: Poliovirus spreads from muscle to the central nervous system by neural pathways. J Infect Dis 166:747, 1992

ROTBART HA: Diagnosis of enteroviral meningitis with the polymerase chain reaction. J Pediatr 117:85, 1990

SHARIEF MK et al: Intrathecal immune response in patients with the post-polio syndrome. N Engl J Med 325:749, 1991

SHARPE AH, FIELDS BN: Pathogenesis of viral infections: Basic concepts derived from the reovirus model. N Engl J Med 312:486, 1985

SONIES BC, DALAKOS MD: Dysphagia in patients with the post-polio syndrome. N Engl J Med 324:1162, 1991

WRIGHT PF et al: Strategies for the global eradication of poliomyelitis by the year 2000. N Engl J Med 325:1774, 1991

155 MEASLES (RUBEOLA)

C. GEORGE RAY

DEFINITION Measles, or rubeola, is an acute febrile eruption which has been one of the most common diseases of civilization. Despite the development of an effective vaccine, it remains a worldwide health problem.

ETIOLOGY The measles virion is composed of a central core of ribonucleic acid with a helically arranged protein coat surrounded by a lipoprotein envelope with small, spikelike structures. The virion is 120 to 200 nm in diameter and is classified as a morbillivirus in the paramyxovirus family. There are at least six virion structural proteins, three of which are in the envelope. These latter include the matrix (M) protein that is important in virus assembly and two glycoprotein projections (peplomers); the hemagglutinin (H) mediates attachment to host cells, and the other (F) mediates cell fusion and viral entry into cells.

EPIDEMIOLOGY Measles occurs naturally only in human beings, although infection with the virus can be demonstrated in laboratory colonies of monkeys exposed to infected individuals. Before active immunization was available, epidemics of measles occurred in 2- to 3-year cycles, usually during the spring months, and about 95 percent of urban dwellers developed the disease before the age of 15. The virus is transmitted by transfer of nasopharyngeal secretions, either directly or in airborne droplets, to the respiratory mucous membranes or conjunctivae of susceptible individuals. Persons infected with the virus may transmit the disease during a period which extends from 5 days after exposure until 5 days after skin lesions have appeared. The virus is highly contagious, with secondary attack rates among susceptible household contacts usually exceeding 90 percent; asymptomatic primary infections are rare. In the United States, the number of reported measles cases reached an all-time low of 1492 in 1983. However, this has since increased substantially, particularly in 1990, when nearly 28,000 cases occurred. This rise has been associated with outbreaks among unvaccinated infants and preschool children; other outbreaks have involved groups of high school and college students, where the immunization rates were often 95 percent or greater. Recent data also indicate shifts in age-specific attack rates away from the previous high frequency among children in the 5- to 14-year age group. In 1990, 22 percent of cases occurred in adults 20 years of age or older, and nearly half were in unvaccinated preschool children, mostly minorities.

PATHOGENESIS AND PATHOLOGY Once access has been gained to the respiratory tract epithelium, virus replication com-

mences. This process damages or destroys susceptible cells and promotes cell fusion with formation of syncytia, disruption of the cellular cytoskeleton, chromosomal disorganization, and appearance of nuclear and cytoplasmic inclusion bodies. Initial replication is followed by viremic (and probably lymphatic) dissemination to other sites, including lymphoid tissues, bone marrow, liver and other viscera, eyes, and skin. Viremia is detectable during the prodromal phase, and viruria persists for as long as 4 days after onset of the rash. Virus replication in thymic Hassall's corpuscles, capillary endothelium, and hepatic endothelium also occurs. During viremia, measles can infect T and B lymphocytes, macrophages, and polymorphonuclear leukocytes. These latter events do not cause significant cytolysis but can impair critical general defense functions such as immunoglobulin synthesis and generation of oxygen radicals by polymorphonuclear leukocytes and macrophages. In the early stages of infection, natural killer cells and cytotoxic T cells play a role in limiting virus replication. These, and cytokines produced as a result of immune activation, also play a role in mediating the inflammatory responses observed in the early acute phase. At rash onset, specific antibody becomes detectable, and effector lymphocytes are found in areas of viral replication in the skin and mucosal lesions. This event usually heralds the onset of viral clearance and clinical recovery, as well as the development of anergy; there is depressed hypersensitivity to skin test antigens such as tuberculin and reduced in vitro lymphoproliferation and cytokine production in response to mitogenic stimuli. Anergy can persist for several weeks and is also seen in recipients of live, attenuated measles virus vaccine.

The mucous membrane lesions (Koplik's spots) consist of vesicle formation and epithelial necrosis. Histology of the Koplik's spots reveals cytoplasmic and intranuclear inclusions, giant cells, and intercellular edema. Large multinucleated epithelial giant cells that show inclusion bodies within the nucleus and cytoplasm can be found during the prodrome and acute stages of illness in the buccal mucosa, pharynx, tracheobronchial mucosa, and occasionally the urine. In addition, reticuloendothelial giant cells (Warthin-Finkeldey cells) are found in hyperplastic lymphoid tissues, including lymph nodes, tonsils, spleen, and thymus. The epithelium of the respiratory passages can become necrotic and slough off, leading to secondary bacterial infection; interstitial pneumonia with giant cell infiltration may be observed. Changes in the brain of patients with encephalomyelitis resemble those seen in other postviral encephalitides and consist of focal hemorrhage, congestion, and perivenous demyelination. Levels of soluble CD8 are elevated in the cerebrospinal fluid during the acute phase of postmeasles encephalomyelitis, but virus cannot be detected. The pathogenesis is probably related to infiltration of CD8 + cytotoxic T cells in the brain, which react with target cells—either myelin-forming cells or virus-infected cells.

MANIFESTATIONS The time from exposure to the development of the first symptoms of measles infection is usually 8 to 12 days and from exposure to the appearance of rash about 2 weeks. The initial manifestations of the disease are malaise, irritability, temperature as high as 40.6°C (105°F), conjunctivitis with excessive lacrimation, edema of the eyelids and photophobia, moderately severe hacking cough, and nasal discharge. The prodromal period usually lasts 3 to 4 days, with a range of 1 to 8 days before the onset of a rash. Koplik's spots—small, red, irregular lesions with blue-white centers—appear 1 or 2 days before the onset of the rash on the mucous membranes of the mouth and occasionally on the conjunctivae or intestinal mucosa. The findings of the prodromal illness subside or disappear within 1 or 2 days after the appearance of skin lesions, although the cough may persist throughout the course of the disease.

The red maculopapular rash of measles breaks out first on the forehead, spreads downward over the face, neck, and trunk, and appears on the feet on the third day. The density of lesions is greatest on the forehead, face, and shoulders, where coalescence of individual spots usually occurs. The lesions in each area persist for about 3 days and disappear in the same order in which they appeared, resulting in total duration of rash of about 6 days. As the maculopapules fade, a brown discoloration of the skin may be noticed, and finely granular desquamation may occur. In adults the duration of fever may be longer, the rash more prominent, and the incidence of complications higher.

The course of measles can be altered by the administration of gamma globulin soon after exposure. The incubation period may be prolonged for as long as 20 days. The prodromal period of the modified disease may be shorter; the fever, respiratory symptoms, and conjunctivitis milder; the rash less marked; and Koplik's spots may not be present.

COMPLICATIONS Measles, usually a benign self-limited disease, may be complicated by a number of illnesses. Viral involvement of the respiratory tract may lead to croup, bronchitis, bronchiolitis, or rarely to *interstitial giant cell pneumonia*. The last is seen most often in children suffering from severe systemic disease such as leukemia, congenital or acquired immunodeficiency, or severe malnutrition and is characterized by severe respiratory symptoms, pulmonary infiltration, and multinucleated giant cells in the pulmonary parenchyma. Pneumonitis may occur in the absence of the typical measles exanthem. *Conjunctivitis*, which is seen regularly in the course of uncomplicated measles, may occasionally progress to corneal ulceration, keratitis, and blindness. *Myocarditis*, characterized by transient changes in the electrocardiogram, occurs in about 20 percent of patients with measles, but clinical evidence of cardiac dysfunction is rare. Viral involvement of the mesenteric lymph nodes and appendix may result in abdominal pain and signs of peritoneal inflammation so severe that surgical exploration is considered. The situation is especially confusing if evidence of appendiceal involvement becomes manifest during the preeruptive phase of the disease. *Hepatitis*, usually without clinical signs, also frequently occurs. It is usually detected by the presence of a transient elevation of AST or ALT values during the acute phase of illness. Transient *acute glomerulonephritis* also has been observed during the acute phase of illness. In adults, mild to moderate hypocalcemia and musculoskeletal symptoms with elevated CPK levels have each been reported to occur in one-third or more of cases. Measles infection of pregnant women can be particularly severe and also results in death of the fetus in about 20 percent of the cases; however, a teratogenic effect such as that observed in rubella has not been demonstrated.

Superimposed bacterial pneumonia caused by streptococci, pneumococci, staphylococci, or *Haemophilus influenzae* is considerably more common than giant cell pneumonia and occasionally may progress to empyema or lung abscess. Bacterial otitis media is a frequent sequel of measles infection in children. In tropical areas, stomatitis, probably of bacterial origin, progressing to cancrum oris may be encountered during the course of the disease.

Clinically apparent *encephalomyelitis* occurs in 1 of 1000 patients with measles. It usually begins 4 to 7 days after the appearance of the eruption but may precede the rash by 10 days or follow it by 24 days. It is characterized by high fever, headache, drowsiness, and coma and in some patients by focal brain or spinal cord involvement. Death occurs in about 10 percent of affected individuals, and persistent signs of central nervous system damage, including mental changes, epilepsy, and paralysis, are encountered. Electroencephalographic abnormalities without other signs of CNS dysfunction have been detected in 50 percent of patients with otherwise uncomplicated measles. A progressive, fatal encephalitis has been described in children with lymphatic malignancies treated with immunosuppressive drugs, with onset 1 to 6 months after an episode of measles. Other, more unusual neurologic complications include transverse myelitis and ascending myelitis. An extremely rare condition, *subacute sclerosing panencephalitis* (see Chap. 375), is probably a late complication of measles. *Thrombocytopenia* may occur 3 to 15 days after the onset of symptoms and results in purpura as well as bleeding from mouth, intestine, and genitourinary tract. Measles is also associated with exacerbation of existing tuberculosis and an increased incidence of new tuberculous infections.

LABORATORY FINDINGS Leukopenia is frequent in the prodromal phase of measles, and the appearance of leukocytosis suggests bacterial superinfection or another complication. Extreme lymphopenia (fewer than 2000 lymphocytes per microliter) is considered to be a poor prognostic sign. During the prodrome and in the early eruptive phase, multinucleated giant cells can be identified in stained preparations of sputum, nasal secretions, or urine, and the measles virus can be isolated by inoculation of the same materials onto appropriate cell cultures. Measles antigen can often be detected quickly by fluorescent antibody staining of infected respiratory or urinary epithelial cells. Complement fixation, enzyme immunoassay, immunofluorescent, and hemagglutination inhibition tests are available for serologic confirmation of measles. Spinal fluid protein of patients with encephalomyelitis ranges from 48 to 240 mg/dL, and lymphocyte counts are usually in a range of 5 to 99 cells per microliter, although counts as high as 1000 cells per microliter have been reported. Bacterial infection can be identified by appropriate cultures.

DIFFERENTIAL DIAGNOSIS With its prodrome, Koplik's spots, and characteristic rash, measles is infrequently confused with other diseases. Rubella is a milder disease of shorter duration with mild or no respiratory complaints. Infectious mononucleosis and toxoplasmosis can be identified by the presence of atypical lymphocytes and by serologic tests. Secondary syphilis may show skin lesions similar to the measles rash. Other infections which can sometimes mimic measles include those caused by adenoviruses, enteroviruses, *Mycoplasma pneumoniae*, *Staphylococcus aureus* (toxic shock syndrome), and *Streptococcus pyogenes* (scarlet fever). Drug reactions, particularly those associated with ampicillin and phenytoin, and Kawasaki syndrome also can produce a morbilliform rash.

ATYPICAL MEASLES During the period 1963–1967, a formalin-inactivated ("killed") measles vaccine was given to an estimated 600,000 to 900,000 recipients in the United States. Distribution of this vaccine was discontinued after 1967, but use continued in Canada through 1970. Between 1965 and 1968, there were multiple reports of a severe, atypical illness in children exposed to wild virus who had received killed measles vaccine 2 to 4 years earlier. Subsequently, a similar, although somewhat more variable, syndrome has been described among young adults who were immunized with killed measles vaccine 20 or more years previously. There are also reports of atypical measles among a few individuals who had received live measles vaccine.

The pathogenesis of atypical measles is thought to be related to formalin inactivation of F glycoprotein with preservation of H antigenicity. The resultant lack of antibodies to F may allow cell-to-cell spread of virus by fusion, and the antigens produced could generate immune complexes, cytotoxic cell-mediated responses, or both.

In atypical measles, the incubation period is similar to that of typical measles, but the prodromal period often develops abruptly. High fever, headaches, myalgias, abdominal pain, and a nonproductive cough usually last for 1 to 3 days, followed by an eruption which can be urticarial, maculopapular, hemorrhagic, and/or vesicular. In contrast to natural measles, the rash begins on the hands and feet and progresses toward the head. It is especially prominent on the legs and in the body creases. Koplik's spots are rarely seen. Pneumonia, often associated with extremity edema, frequently occurs. The pneumonia is lobar or segmental; hilar lymphadenopathy and pleural effusion are common. Ill-defined nodular shadows may persist at the periphery of the lung for as long as 2 years. Symptoms often last for 2 weeks or longer. The severity of illness, abruptness of onset, and unique clinical findings that are variably observed have sometimes suggested diagnoses such as Rocky Mountain spotted fever, varicella pneumonia, scarlet fever, or meningococcemia; in the prodromal phase, acute appendicitis and bacterial pneumonia have been considered.

The diagnosis of atypical measles is based on clinical, epidemiologic, and serologic grounds. Unlike typical measles, virus-isolation attempts are generally unsuccessful. Antibodies rapidly increase from undetectable or low levels to very high titers that usually exceed those observed in convalescence from typical measles.

PROPHYLAXIS Active immunity can be induced by the use of live, attenuated measles virus, which does not spread to contacts of vaccinated individuals. The vaccine of choice, even in adults, is measles-mumps-rubella (MMR). Vaccination induces immunity in more than 95 percent of individuals inoculated at 15 months of age or older; this immunity extends for more than 20 years and is probably lifelong. The vaccine also usually provides protection if given within 3 days after exposure. Routine immunization in infancy is begun at 15 months of age; a second dose is recommended at ages 11 to 12 years. Most persons born before 1957 can be considered immune and usually do not need to be vaccinated; however, a small portion of such persons are in fact susceptible and should be considered for immunization unless there is documented proof of immunity, particularly if they are involved in a high-risk outbreak setting. Entrants into colleges and universities and health care workers who do not have clear proof of immunity (physician-diagnosed measles or laboratory evidence of immunity) should be required to provide documentation of two doses of measles vaccine commencing on or after their first birthday; if there has been no previous measles immunization, then the second dose should follow the first by no less than 1 month.

Persons who received killed measles vaccine in the past should be considered unprotected and, in fact, at high risk of severe atypical measles if exposed to wild virus. At least one dose of live vaccine should be given to them as well as to anyone who received vaccine of unknown type in 1963–1967. Measles reimmunization is also recommended for persons who received killed vaccine followed in 3 months by live vaccine, were immunized before their first birthday, or received further attenuated (Schwartz or Moraten strains) or unknown vaccine with immunoglobulin. Asymptomatic (and probably also symptomatic) HIV-infected persons also should be immunized if they are susceptible.

Live measles vaccine should not be given to pregnant women, to patients with untreated tuberculosis, to patients with leukemia or lymphoma, or to those whose immune responsiveness is depressed. However, persons with leukemia who are in remission and have not received chemotherapy for at least 3 months and HIV-infected persons can be vaccinated. All children infected with HIV should be immunized on schedule; the degree of protection is uncertain. Hypersensitivity reactions to the vaccine even among egg-sensitive individuals have been rare; however, extreme caution should be observed in persons with a history of anaphylactic reactions following egg ingestion or receipt of neomycin. Except in unusual circumstances, vaccination should not be given in the first 13 months of life. If epidemiologic circumstances suggest a risk to infants less than 15 months of age, monovalent vaccine or MMR may be given as early as 6 months of age, followed by a dose of MMR vaccine at 15 months of age.

Approximately 5 to 15 percent of nonimmune vaccinees will develop temperatures of 103°F (39.4°C) or higher, usually beginning 5 to 12 days after vaccination and lasting 1 to 2 days; rarely, fever can continue for up to 5 days. The prevalence of vaccine-induced rash is approximately 5 percent. Encephalitis after measles vaccination is extremely rare; it has not been possible to discern its risk from the background prevalence of encephalitis of unknown cause. Prior recipients of killed measles vaccine have a risk of up to 50 percent for reactions to live vaccine. Most such reactions are mild, consisting of local swelling, erythema, and low-grade fever for 1 to 2 days. Rarely, more severe reactions such as lymphadenopathy, prolonged fever, and extensive local Arthus-like reactions are seen. However, recipients of killed measles vaccine are likely to have significantly more serious illness when exposed to natural measles than that which may occur with live vaccine. There is no evidence suggesting an increased risk of adverse effects from measles or MMR vaccines among persons who are already immune.

Measles can be modified or prevented by the intramuscular administration of gamma globulin, 0.25 mL/kg (not to exceed 15 mL), within 6 days of exposure. This approach is not recommended for outbreak control but is useful in situations where measles vaccine is contraindicated (e.g., susceptible pregnant women, persons receiving cancer chemotherapy) or where vaccine-induced immunity cannot be ensured (e.g., HIV-infected patients). If measles immunoglobulins are administered, in either gamma globulin or other blood products, vaccination should be deferred for at least 3 months.

TREATMENT No therapy is indicated for uncomplicated measles. Gamma globulin, although effective in prophylaxis, is of no value once symptoms are evident. In areas where nutritional deficiencies and severe measles are common, vitamin A supplementation (400,000 IU orally) on two successive days as soon as measles is diagnosed may reduce the risk of delayed mortality and blindness. Patients should be monitored for the development of bacterial superinfections, which require appropriate antibiotics on the basis of clinical and bacteriologic findings. Aerosolized ribavirin also has been used for treatment of severe measles pneumonia; however, reports of efficacy have thus far been anecdotal.

REFERENCES

ATMAR RL et al: Complications of measles during pregnancy. Clin Infect Dis 14:217, 1992

BLOCH AB et al: Measles outbreak in a pediatric practice: Airborne transmission in an office setting. Pediatrics 75:676, 1985

CENTERS FOR DISEASE CONTROL: Update on adult immunization: Recommendations of the Immunization Practices Advisory Committee (ACIP). Morb Mort Week Rep 40(no. RR-12):19, 1991

CHERRY JD et al: Atypical measles in children previously immunized with attenuated measles virus vaccines. Pediatrics 50:712, 1972

DERMSTADT GL, HALSEY NA: Measles in mother-infant pairs. Pediatr Infect Dis J 11:492, 1992

FULGINITI VA, HELFER RE: Atypical measles in adolescent siblings 16 years after killed measles virus vaccine. JAMA 244:804, 1980

GAVISH D et al: Hepatitis and jaundice associated with measles in young adults. Arch Intern Med 143, 1983

GILADI M et al: Measles in adults: A prospective study of 291 consecutive cases. Br Med J 295:1314, 1987

GRIFFIN DE et al: Immune activation in measles. N Engl J Med 320:1667, 1989

GUSTAFSON TL et al: Measles outbreak in a fully immunized secondary-school population. N Engl J Med 317:771, 1987

HUSSEY GD, KLEIN M: A randomized, controlled trial of vitamin A in children with severe measles. N Engl J Med 323:160, 1990

LAVI S et al: Administration of measles, mumps, and rubella virus vaccine (live) to egg-allergic children. JAMA 263:269, 1990

MARKOWITZ LE et al: Persistence of measles antibody after revaccination. J Infect Dis 166:205, 1992

MINNICH LL et al: Use of immunofluorescence to identify measles virus infections. J Clin Microbiol 29:1148, 1991

MOUALLEM M et al: Measles epidemic in young adults. Arch Intern Med 147:1111, 1987

NATIONAL VACCINE ADVISORY COMMITTEE: The measles epidemic: The problems, barriers, and recommendations. JAMA 266:1547, 1991

RIVERA ME et al: Nosocomial measles infection in a pediatric hospital during a community-wide epidemic. J Pediatr 119:183, 1991

156 RUBELLA ("GERMAN MEASLES") AND OTHER VIRAL EXANTHEMS

C. GEORGE RAY

RUBELLA

DEFINITION Rubella ("German measles," "3-day measles") is usually a benign febrile exanthem, but when it occurs in pregnant women, it may lead to serious chronic fetal infection and malformations.

ETIOLOGY   In the late 1930s and 1940s rubella was transmitted experimentally to humans and monkeys, and in 1962 a viral agent was recovered in cell cultures inoculated with nasopharyngeal secretions of infected persons. The rubella virion, 60 to 70 nm in diameter, is a somewhat spheroidal RNA virus which has been classified in the togavirus family.

PATHOGENESIS AND PATHOLOGY   Rubella can be induced in susceptible persons by the instillation of virus into the nasopharynx, and natural infection is probably induced in the same way. Initial replication of the virus in the respiratory tract is followed by spread via the bloodstream. Viremia has been detected for as long as 8 days before and up to 2 days after appearance of the rash, and shedding of virus from the oropharynx persists for up to 8 days after the onset of symptoms.

Congenital rubella results from transplacental transmission of virus to the fetus from an infected mother and may be associated with growth retardation, infiltration of liver and spleen by hematopoietic tissue, interstitial pneumonia, a decreased number of megakaryocytes in the bone marrow, and various structural malformations of the cardiovascular and central nervous systems. The virus can persist in the fetus during intrauterine life and may be excreted for 6 to 31 months after birth.

EPIDEMIOLOGY   Rubella is not as contagious as measles, and immunity to the disease is not so widespread. Estimates of susceptibility to rubella among young adults now range from 6 to 11 percent. The number of reported rubella cases in the United States steadily declined from more than 56,000 in 1969, when routine vaccination began, to a low of 225 in 1988. Of the more than 900 cases reported in 1990, approximately 57 percent occurred in persons $\geq$15 years of age. In addition, at least 20 cases of congenital rubella syndrome were diagnosed among infants born in 1990. Limited outbreaks continue to occur in colleges and work environments (e.g., hospitals), further reflecting an epidemiologic shift away from young children.

MANIFESTATIONS   The time from exposure to the appearance of the rash of rubella is 14 to 21 days, usually about 18 days. In adults there may be a prodromal illness preceding the exanthem by 1 to 7 days. The prodrome consists of malaise, headache, fever, mild conjunctivitis, and lymphadenopathy. In children the rash may be the first manifestation of disease. It is apparent from serologic studies that 25 to 50 percent of infections are subclinical or result in only lymph node enlargement without skin lesions; however, rash without lymphadenopathy is uncommon. Respiratory symptoms are mild or absent. Small, red lesions (Forschheimer spots) occasionally appear on the soft palate but are not pathognomonic of the disease.

The rash begins on the forehead and face and spreads downward to the trunk and extremities. The small maculopapular lesions, of lighter hue than those of measles, are usually discrete but can coalesce to form a diffuse erythema suggestive of scarlet fever. The rash may last from 1 to 5 days but is most commonly present for 3 days. Enlarged, tender lymph nodes appear before the rash, are most impressive during the early eruptive phase, and often persist several days after the rash has disappeared. Splenomegaly or generalized lymphadenopathy may occur, but the postauricular and suboccipital nodes are most strikingly involved. Arthralgias and slight joint swellings sometimes accompany rubella, especially in young women. The pain and swelling, involving wrists, fingers, and knees, are most marked during the period of rash and may persist for 1 to 14 days after other manifestations of rubella have disappeared. Recurring joint symptoms for a year or more also have been reported. Purpura with or without thrombocytopenia may occur and can be associated with hemorrhage. Encephalomyelitis following rubella resembles other postinfectious encephalitides but is much less common than encephalitis following measles. Testicular pain is also occasionally reported in young adults.

Congenital rubella   The syndrome of congenital rubella has conventionally been thought to consist of heart malformations—patent ductus arteriosus, interventricular septal defect, or pulmonic stenosis; eye lesions—corneal clouding, cataracts, chorioretinitis, and micro-

phthalmia; microcephaly; mental retardation; and deafness. In the American epidemic of 1964, thrombocytopenic purpura, hepatosplenomegaly, intrauterine growth retardation, interstitial pneumonia, myocarditis or myocardial necrosis, and metaphyseal bone lesions were encountered frequently in association with the previously recognized manifestations, leading to the term *expanded rubella syndrome.* Some infants also have been found to have significant humoral and/or cellular immunodeficiency, which generally resolves as chronic viral excretion diminishes and eventually ceases. Any combination of lesions may be seen in an individual infant, and the severity is highly variable.

Later complications include an apparent higher risk of development of diabetes mellitus. There are reports of patients with congenital rubella who develop a progressive, subacute panencephalitis, with onset in the second decade of life. It is characterized by intellectual deterioration, ataxia, seizures, and spasticity. T cell abnormalities, including slightly decreased T4/T8 ratios and other minor subset defects, sometimes persist into adulthood.

Congenital rubella is usually the result of maternal infection during the first trimester of pregnancy, although well-documented cases have resulted from infection several days before conception; deafness may occur as a result of infection in the fourth month. The greatest risk to the fetus is when maternal infection develops 3 to 6 weeks after conception. Asymptomatic maternal rubella can result in severe fetal disease. It is therefore desirable to ascertain the immune status of every woman either before conception or as early in the pregnancy as possible by history of previous immunization or by serologic testing. If rubella antibodies are present before or within 10 days after exposure, the patient is considered immune, and the risk of fetal damage is virtually nil. If antibodies are not detectable and exposure has occurred, acute and convalescent antibody titers should be determined simultaneously on sera obtained 2 to 4 weeks apart, with the exact interval depending on the time after exposure when the acute sample was drawn.

DIAGNOSIS   Rubella is frequently confused with other diseases associated with maculopapular exanthems, with infectious mononucleosis (see Chap. 145), as well as with drug eruptions and scarlet fever. *A certain diagnosis of rubella can be made only by virus isolation and identification or by changes in antibody titers.* Rubella antibodies may be detectable by the second day of rash and increase in titer over the next 10 to 21 days. A variety of serologic tests are available for diagnosis or determination of immune status. The presence of IgM-specific antibodies suggests recent rubella infection (within 2 months); however, they have been known to persist as long as 1 year in some cases. There are no other laboratory findings helpful in the diagnosis of rubella, although lymphocytosis with atypical lymphocytes often occurs.

Patients with the congenital rubella syndrome may lose antibodies at age 3 or 4 years. Therefore, a negative serologic test in a child over 3 years of age does not exclude the possibility of congenital rubella. Congenital rubella should be differentiated from congenital syphilis by appropriate serologic tests (see Chap. 133), toxoplasmosis (see Chap. 177), and cytomegalic inclusion virus disease (see Chap. 146). IgM-specific antibodies are often found early in the first year of life in infants with congenital rubella, but virus isolation is the most reliable way to confirm the diagnosis.

PREVENTION   In adults and children, rubella is usually a mild disease with infrequent complications. However, the severity of congenital infection has prompted efforts to prevent the disease. Administration of gamma globulin to exposed persons can abort the clinical disease, but seroconversion and transmission of the disease from mother to fetus may occur despite the administration of large amounts of gamma globulin soon after exposure.

Active immunization with live, attenuated rubella vaccines has been practiced in this country since 1969, especially among young children. The aim has been to decrease the frequency of the infection in the population and to decrease the chance that susceptible pregnant women will be exposed. Vaccination is strongly recommended for adolescents and adults, particularly females, unless there is proof of immunity (i.e., positive results in serologic tests or documentation of rubella vaccination on or after the first birthday). The only exceptions are persons in whom vaccination is specifically contraindicated, as noted below. Persons working in hospitals or clinics who might contract rubella from infected patients or who, if infected, might transmit the infection to pregnant patients should be required to have proof of immunity.

The attenuated virus can be detected in the respiratory secretions of vaccinees for as long as 4 weeks after immunization, but transmission to other susceptible individuals has never been documented during more than 20 years of experience. The vaccine induces detectable antibodies that persist at least 16 years and probably for a lifetime in about 95 percent of recipients. After heavy exposure in closed populations, vaccinated individuals sometimes develop subclinical infections (diagnosed by antibody rises and virus isolation). However, the failure to demonstrate viremia in immunized persons suggests that previously vaccinated pregnant women will not infect their fetuses even if they acquire subclinical rubella.

Side effects of fever, rash, lymphadenopathy, polyneuropathy, or arthralgias occur very seldom in vaccinated children; joint pain and swelling or paresthesias are seen in less than 2 percent of women with vaccines prepared in human embryonic fibroblast cell cultures (RA 27/3 vaccine). The joint symptoms usually begin 1 to 3 weeks after vaccination and may be confused with other forms of arthritis. *Rubella vaccine must never be given to pregnant women or to those who may become pregnant within 3 months of immunization.* Although no infant with the congenital rubella syndrome has been reported to have been born to a woman inadvertently vaccinated during pregnancy, the theoretical risk of vaccine virus–induced fetal damage remains. Vaccine is contraindicated in patients who have immune-deficiency diseases or who are taking immunosuppressive drugs. One exception is HIV infection. Rubella vaccination should be provided to asymptomatic HIV-infected children and adults. Furthermore, the presence of HIV-related symptoms is not a contraindication with regard to rubella vaccination (or, more commonly, mumps-measles-rubella vaccination) of children, and vaccination also should be considered for symptomatic adults. If immunoglobulin (Ig) is being used, the vaccine should be given at least 14 days before Ig administration or deferred until a minimum of 6 weeks (preferably 3 months) afterward. Postpartum rubella immunization is not contraindicated when whole-blood or human anti-Rho(D)Ig has recently been used, but follow-up testing 6 to 8 weeks later is advised to ensure that seroconversion has occurred.

OTHER VIRAL EXANTHEMS

In addition to the diseases such as measles, rubella, and chickenpox that historically have been associated with prominent skin lesions, there are other virus infections in which skin manifestations may occur. Table 156-1 lists the most commonly recognized causes of maculopapular eruptions. Some of them, particularly the enteroviruses, also can occasionally cause papulovesicular or petechial rashes; others are capable of provoking erythema multiforme–like eruptions. One helpful aspect of the physical examination is the observation that virus-caused maculopapular (not vesicular) exanthems usually *relatively* spare the palms and soles. This is in contrast to eruptions associated with drug reactions, bacteria, *Mycoplasma*, and *Rickettsia*, in which a prominent palmar or plantar eruption is often noted.

EXANTHEM SUBITUM (ROSEOLA INFANTUM) Exanthem subitum is a benign disease of infants 6 months to 4 years of age that is characterized by a high fever and rash. Several different agents, such as enteroviruses and adenoviruses, may produce a similar illness; however, human herpesvirus type 6 (HHV-6) has been implicated as the major cause. The first manifestations of disease, after an estimated incubation period of 5 to 15 days, are the abrupt onset of irritability and fever, which last for 3 to 5 days; the temperature can be as high

TABLE 156-1   Causes of maculopapular eruptions

Viral	Other
Measles	*Mycoplasma pneumoniae*
Rubella	Syphilis
Exanthem subitum: human herpes-virus type 6	Typhoid fever
Erythema infectiosum: human parvovirus B19	Bacterial toxins: streptococci and staphylococci
Enteroviruses	Rat-bite fever
Epstein-Barr virus	*Rickettsia*
Adenoviruses	Live-virus vaccines
Reoviruses	Drug eruptions
Arboviruses	Mucocutaneous lymph node syndrome

as 40.6°C (105°F). There may be mild pharyngitis and slight lymph node enlargement; convulsions sometimes occur during the height of the fever. On the fourth to fifth day of illness, there is a sudden drop in temperature to normal or below normal; several hours before or after defervescence, the rash suddenly appears. It is characterized by faint 2- to 3-mm macules or maculopapules over the neck and trunk and may extend to the thighs and buttocks; it lasts for a few hours to 1 to 2 days. Leukopenia is frequently noted later in the febrile period. The disease is benign and very rarely associated with complications. In the early, preeruptive phase, the disease may be difficult to differentiate from an acute bacteremia, particularly one associated with *Streptococcus pneumoniae*. Although a leukocytosis with an increase in band forms is often seen in bacteremias presenting in this fashion, blood cultures are necessary to make the diagnosis.

Recent laboratory and clinical studies indicate that HHV-6 infection is widespread; by 3 to 5 years of age, up to 95 percent of children have serologic evidence of infection. Seroprevalence rates decline to ≤55 percent after the fourth decade of life. The virus has been found in saliva from more than 90 percent of healthy adults studied; this reservoir is very likely a major source of transmission. In immunocompetent older children and adults, HHV-6 infection has been associated with mononucleosis-like symptoms, afebrile lymphadenopathy, and acute hepatitis. The virus also has been implicated in interstitial pneumonitis in bone marrow transplant recipients. Further investigations are necessary to clearly define the pathogenesis of HHV-6–related illnesses. At present, the infection is most commonly diagnosed by serologic testing; molecular and immunologic probe methods are also being employed increasingly.

ENTEROVIRAL EXANTHEMS Many individual enteroviruses have been associated with rash. Most commonly implicated have been echovirus serotypes 1–7, 9, 11, 12, 14, 16, 18–20, 25, and 30 and coxsackievirus serotypes A4–A6, A9, A10, A16, B2, B3, and B5. Except in hand-foot-and-mouth disease, usually associated with coxsackievirus A16 or enterovirus 71 infection (see Chap. 154), there is no set of clinical or epidemiologic features that aids in differentiating the specific enteroviral agent involved in a specific case. All are capable of producing maculopapular rashes which vary in intensity and duration and also can occasionally produce petechial or papulovesicular exanthems and enanthems. In community and household outbreaks, younger children and infants are usually more likely to have exanthems, while other features of enteroviral infection, such as fever, myalgia, and aseptic meningitis, are more prominent among older children and young adults. Two enterovirus serotypes that have been particularly associated with outbreaks of febrile exanthems are echoviruses 9 and 16.

ERYTHEMA INFECTIOSUM (FIFTH DISEASE)   See Chap. 148.

REFERENCES

ASANO Y et al: Viremia and neutralizing antibody response in infants with exanthem subitum. J Pediatr 114:535, 1989

CARRIGAN DR et al: Interstitial pneumonitis associated with human herpesvirus-6 infection after marrow transplantation. Lancet 338:147, 1991

CENTERS FOR DISEASE CONTROL: Update on adult immunization: Recommendations of the Immunization Practices Advisory Committee (ACIP). Morb Mort Week Rep 40:1, 1991

ENDERS G et al: Outcome of confirmed periconceptional rubella. Lancet 1:1445, 1988

HERRMANN KL: Available rubella serologic tests. Rev Infect Dis 7:S108, 1985

LEE SH et al: Resurgence of congenital rubella syndrome in the 1990s. JAMA 267:2616, 1992

LEVY JA et al: Frequent isolation of HHV-6 from saliva and high seroprevalence of the virus in the population. Lancet 335:1047, 1990

MCINTOSH EDG, MENSER MA: A fifty-year follow-up of congenital rubella. Lancet 340:414, 1992

NAIDES SJ et al: Human parvovirus B19-induced vesiculopustular skin eruption. Am J Med 84:968, 1988

STEEPER TA et al: The spectrum of clinical and laboratory findings resulting from human herpesvirus-6 (HHV-6) in patients with mononucleosis-like illnesses not resulting from Epstein-Barr virus or cytomegalovirus. Am J Clin Pathol 93:776, 1990

TOWNSEND JJ et al: Progressive rubella panencephalitis: Late onset after congenital rubella. N Engl J Med 292:990, 1975

157   MUMPS

C. GEORGE RAY

DEFINITION   Mumps is an acute communicable disease of viral origin characterized by painful enlargement of the salivary glands and sometimes by involvement of the gonads, meninges, pancreas, and other organs.

ETIOLOGY   The causative agent of mumps is a paramyxovirus of intermediate size (120 to 200 nm in diameter). It has a tight helical inner core (single-stranded RNA) enclosed in an outer envelope of lipid and glycoproteins. Only one antigenic type is known.

EPIDEMIOLOGY   Human beings are the only natural host for mumps. The disease is worldwide in distribution and is endemic in urban communities. Epidemics are relatively infrequent and are usually confined to closely associated groups who live in orphanages, army camps, or schools. The disease is most frequent in the spring, particularly during April and May. Although mumps is generally considered less "contagious" than measles and chickenpox, this difference may be more apparent than real because many mumps infections (at least 25 percent) tend to be inapparent clinically. In some surveys, 80 to 90 percent of an adult population had serologic evidence of previous mumps. Approximately 5000 mumps cases were reported annually in the United States in 1988, 1989, and 1990. There has been an apparent upward shift in the age groups affected. In 1989, 38 percent of patients were ≥15 years of age; in 1977, the figure was only 12 percent.

Infections are rare before the age of 2 years. The virus is transmitted in infected salivary secretions, although its isolation from urine suggests that it also may spread via this route. The saliva is infectious for approximately 6 days prior to the onset of parotitis, and virus has been recovered from this site for as long as 2 weeks after onset of parotid swelling. Viruria also persists for 2 to 3 weeks in some patients. Despite this prolonged secretion of virus, the period of greatest infectivity is from a day or two before onset of parotitis to 5 days after the appearance of glandular enlargement. Patients are usually no longer contagious 9 days after onset of parotid swelling.

One attack of clinical or subclinical mumps confers lasting immunity, and second attacks are most unusual. Unilateral parotitis affords protection just as effectively as does bilateral disease.

PATHOGENESIS   The virus enters via the respiratory route; during the incubation period of 12 to 25 days, it presumably replicates in the upper respiratory tract and cervical lymph nodes, from which it is disseminated via the bloodstream to target tissues such as the parotid glands and meninges. After initial replication in these sites, a secondary viremia may occur, resulting in variable involvement of organs such as the gonads, pancreas, thyroid, breasts, liver, heart, and kidneys. The salivary adenitis is thought by many to be secondary to initial viremia, but direct spread from the respiratory tract has not been ruled out as an alternative mechanism. Viruria is common; nearly all infections are associated with discernible impairment of renal function.

Immunity is correlated with the presence of neutralizing antibody. Cellular immune mechanisms are thought to contribute both to the pathogenesis of the acute disease and to recovery. Like other systemic viral infections, mumps can cause a transient suppression of delayed-type hypersensitivity to previously recognized antigens, such as tuberculin protein.

MANIFESTATIONS   Salivary adenitis   The onset of parotitis is usually sudden, although it may be preceded by a prodromal period of malaise, anorexia, chilly sensations, feverishness, sore throat, and tenderness at the angle of the jaw. In many cases, however, parotid swelling is the first indication of illness. The glands enlarge progressively over a period of 1 to 3 days, and the swelling resolves within a week after maximal enlargement. The swollen gland extends from the ear to the lower portion of the mandibular ramus and to the inferior portion of the zygomatic arch, often displacing the ear upward and outward. The skin over the gland is usually not warm or erythematous, in contrast to the findings in bacterial parotitis. There may be reddening and pouting of the orifice of Stensen's duct. Usually, pain and tenderness are marked, although at times they are absent. The edema of mumps has been described as "gelatinous," and when the involved gland is tweaked, it rolls like jelly. Swelling may involve only the submaxillary and sublingual glands and may extend over the anterior part of the chest, producing *presternal edema*. Involvement of submaxillary glands alone can cause difficulty in distinguishing mumps from acute cervical adenitis. Swelling of the glottis occurs rarely but may require tracheostomy. Parotitis is bilateral in two-thirds of cases and remains confined to one side in the remainder. The second gland tends to swell as the first is subsiding, usually 4 to 5 days after onset. In general, parotitis is accompanied by a temperature of 37.8 to 39.4°C (100 to 103°F), malaise, headache, and anorexia, but systemic symptoms may be virtually absent, particularly in children. In most patients, the chief complaints are difficulty in eating, swallowing, and talking.

Epididymoorchitis   Mumps is complicated by orchitis in 20 to 30 percent of postpubertal males. Testicular involvement usually appears 7 to 10 days after onset of parotitis, although it may precede it or appear simultaneously. Occasionally, orchitis occurs in the absence of parotitis. Gonadal involvement is bilateral in 3 to 17 percent of patients with epididymoorchitis. Orchitis is heralded by recrudescence of malaise and appearance of chilly sensations, headache, nausea, and vomiting. Shaking chills and high fevers, with temperatures between 39.4 and 41.1°C (103 and 106°F), are frequent. The testicle becomes greatly swollen and acutely painful. The epididymis is often palpable as a swollen tender cord. Occasionally there may be epididymitis without orchitis. Swelling, pain, and tenderness persist for 3 to 7 days and gradually subside; lysis of fever usually parallels abatement of swelling. The temperature occasionally falls by crisis. Mumps orchitis is followed by progressive atrophy of the testicle in one-half of cases. Even after bilateral orchitis, sterility is unusual, provided no significant atrophy has taken place. However, if bilateral testicular atrophy occurs after mumps, sterility or subnormal sperm counts are quite common. Plasma testosterone levels are depressed during acute orchitis but return to normal with recovery. *Pulmonary infarction* has been noted to follow mumps orchitis. This may be the result of thrombosis of the veins in the prostatic and pelvic plexuses in association with the testicular inflammation. Priapism is a rare but painful complication of mumps orchitis.

Pancreatitis   Pancreatic involvement is a potentially serious manifestation of mumps, which may rarely be complicated by shock or pseudocyst formation. It should be suspected in patients with abdominal pain and tenderness together with clinical or epidemiologic evidence of mumps. It is difficult to document, since hyperamylasemia, the hallmark of pancreatitis, is also often present in parotitis.

Many times the symptoms resemble those of gastroenteritis. Although diabetes or pancreatic insufficiency rarely follows mumps pancreatitis, several children have developed "brittle" diabetes a few weeks after mumps.

Central nervous system involvement Approximately 60 percent of patients with clinical mumps have an increased number of cells, usually lymphocytes, in the cerebrospinal fluid (CSF), while 10 percent have symptoms of meningitis: stiff neck, headache, and drowsiness. In typical cases, the onset of overt central nervous system signs and symptoms occurs 3 to 10 days after the onset of parotitis; however, CNS mumps may develop prior to the parotitis or 2 to 3 weeks later. In approximately 30 to 40 percent of laboratory-proven cases, there is *no* associated salivary gland involvement at any time in the course of illness. The CSF protein is moderately elevated, and CSF glucose tends to be normal, although in as many as 10 percent of patients low CSF glucose concentrations, in the range of 1.1 to 2.8 mmol/L (20 to 50 mg/dL), may be seen. True encephalitis is unusual, although it is responsible for most of the CNS sequelae, including behavioral disturbances, headaches, seizures, deafness (usually unilateral), and visual disturbances. Mumps also should be recognized as capable of presenting a picture of mild paralytic poliomyelitis; definition of the cause depends on isolation of virus or serologic confirmation of mumps in the absence of changing antibody titers to poliomyelitis viruses. Rarely, mumps may produce a transverse myelitis, cerebellar ataxia, or the Guillain-Barré syndrome. Mumps meningitis, without clinical encephalitis, is generally benign.

Other manifestations Mumps virus tends to involve glandular tissues; inflammation of the lacrimal glands, thymus, thyroid, breasts, and ovaries occurs occasionally. *Oophoritis* may be recognized by persistence of pain in the lower part of the abdomen and fever. It does not result in sterility. Mumps virus has been implicated in the causation of subacute thyroiditis; occasionally the virus can be isolated from the thyroid gland. Myxedema following mumps thyroiditis has been reported. Ocular manifestations of mumps include dacryoadenitis, optic neuritis, keratitis, iritis, conjunctivitis, and episcleritis. Although these conditions may transiently interfere with vision, complete resolution is the rule. Mumps *myocarditis* is evidenced primarily by transient abnormalities in the electrocardiogram. It does not usually produce symptomatic disease or impair cardiac function, but rare deaths have been reported. Similarly, *hepatic* involvement may be manifested by mild abnormalities in liver function, but icterus and other clinical signs of hepatic damage are extremely rare. *Thrombocytopenic purpura* as a complication of mumps has been described, and an occasional patient has a leukemoid reaction involving predominantly lymphocytes. Tracheobronchitis and interstitial pneumonia also have been associated with mumps infection, particularly among young children.

Other rare but interesting manifestations of mumps include *polyarthritis* which is often migratory. Monarticular arthritis is most common in males between the ages of 20 and 30. Joint symptoms begin 1 to 2 weeks after subsidence of parotitis; usually the large joints are involved, especially the hip or knee. The illness lasts 1 to 12 weeks, and complete recovery is the rule. The pathogenesis of mumps-associated arthritis is unclear. The usual delayed onset after parotitis and the failure to isolate the virus from synovial fluid suggest an immunologically mediated mechanism.

Acute hemorrhagic glomerulonephritis in the absence of streptococcosis has been reported after mumps. The relationship of these two diseases is not clear.

Late complications With the exception of the rare CNS complications and occasional sterility following bilateral testicular involvement, mumps leaves no sequelae. However, persistent mumps infection may be a cause of inclusion-body myositis, a chronic inflammatory myopathy that occurs primarily in the sixth decade. There is no firm evidence that offspring with congenital defects are more common among mothers who have mumps during pregnancy. Mumps illness during the first trimester of pregnancy has been associated with an increased risk of spontaneous abortion, however.

LABORATORY FINDINGS In uncomplicated parotitis, the blood leukocyte count is normal, although there may be mild leukopenia with relative lymphocytosis. Patients with mumps orchitis, however, may have a marked leukocytosis with a shift to the left. In meningoencephalitis, the white blood cell count is usually within normal limits. The erythrocyte sedimentation rate is usually normal but may rise with testicular or pancreatic involvement. The serum amylase level is elevated both in pancreatitis and in salivary adenitis. It also may be elevated in some patients in whom the sole evidence of mumps is meningoencephalitis, and such elevation probably reflects subclinical involvement of the salivary glands. In contrast to the amylase level, the serum lipase level is elevated only in pancreatitis, in which hyperglycemia and glucosuria also may occur. The CSF contains up to 2000 cells per microliter, almost all mononuclear, although occasionally polymorphonuclear cells will predominate in the early stages. The pleocytosis in mumps meningitis tends to be greater than in aseptic meningitides caused by the enteroviruses. There is no relationship between the cell count and the severity of CNS involvement. Transient hematuria and mild reversible abnormalities in renal function, including inability to concentrate the urine maximally and to clear creatinine, occur in association with the viruria of mumps.

DIAGNOSIS The definitive diagnosis of mumps depends on isolation of the virus from blood, throat swabs, secretions from Stensen's duct, CSF, or urine. In addition, immunofluorescence can be utilized for rapid detection of the viral antigen directly in oropharyngeal cells. Serologic determination of acute infection or susceptibility can be done by a variety of methods. The best test is the enzyme-linked immunosorbent assay (ELISA). Immunofluorescent assays also can be used for identification of IgM- and IgG-specific antibody responses. The complement fixation test can be employed to quantitate antibody responses to the S and V antigenic components for the diagnosis of acute or recent mumps infection. Antibodies to the S antigen develop rather rapidly, often reaching a peak within 1 week after the onset of symptoms, and usually disappear in 6 to 12 months. Complement-fixing antibodies to the V antigen reach a peak titer within 2 to 3 weeks after onset, remain elevated for at least 6 weeks, and then persist at lower levels for years afterward. Paired sera obtained 2 to 3 weeks apart are recommended. A fourfold increase in titer by any standard assay confirms recent infection. When an acute serum is not obtained until later in the course of illness, either an elevation of antibodies to the S antigen to a titer that exceeds the V antibody titer or the presence of IgM-specific antibody suggests recent infection. The *skin test* consists of intradermal injection of killed mumps virus; previous exposure will result in a delayed reaction of the tuberculin type and an anamnestic antibody titer rise to mumps. The skin test is unreliable for determining the mumps immune status of an individual; if this information is needed, ELISA or neutralization assays should be used.

The diagnosis of mumps during an epidemic is usually obvious. Sporadic cases, however, must be distinguished from other causes of parotid enlargement. Parotitis may be caused by other viruses, notably parainfluenza, influenza, and coxsackieviruses. *Bacterial parotitis* usually occurs in debilitated patients with severe underlying diseases. The parotid glands are swollen, warm, and tender, and pus can be expressed from the orifices of Stensen's ducts. Marked polymorphonuclear leukocytosis is present. *Staphylococcus aureus* is the usual causative organism. Dehydration followed by inspissation of secretions in the salivary ducts is an important predisposing factor. *Calculus* in a salivary duct is usually detectable by palpation or by injection of radiopaque media into Stensen's duct. *Drug reactions* may produce tender swelling of the parotid and other salivary glands. "Iodine mumps" is the most common type; it may follow such procedures as intravenous urography. The antihypertensive agent guanethidine also may cause parotid enlargement and tenderness. A careful history usually serves to clarify the cause of these reactions. *Cervical adenitis* caused by streptococci, "bullneck" diphtheria, infectious mononucleosis, cat-scratch disease, sublingual cellulitis (Ludwig's angina), or cellulitis of the external auditory canal is usually easy to distinguish from mumps by careful examination. Parotid tumors and chronic infections such as actinomycosis tend to follow a more indolent course, with slowly progressive swelling. The common "mixed tumor" of the parotid is well-circumscribed, nontender, and very firm (almost cartilaginous) on palpation. Parotid swelling and fever, often accompanied by lacrimal adenitis and uveitis (Mikulicz's syndrome), may occur in tuberculosis, leukemia, Hodgkin's disease, and lupus erythematosus. The onset may be sudden, but the process is usually painless and of long duration. Uveoparotid fever of similar type may be the first manifestation of sarcoidosis; in this disease, parotid swelling is frequently accompanied by single or multiple palsies of cranial nerves, particularly the facial nerve, and is referred to as *Heerfordt's syndrome*. Presternal edema also may be a manifestation of malignant lymphoma involving retrosternal lymph nodes. Bilateral painless parotid swelling unassociated with fever is found in patients with Laennec's cirrhosis, chronic alcoholism, malnutrition, diabetes mellitus, pregnancy and lactation, and hypertriglyceridemia.

Sjögren's syndrome (see Chap. 288) is a chronic inflammation of the parotid and other salivary glands which is often associated with atrophy of the lacrimal glands and occurs most commonly in women past the menopause. With cessation of lacrimal and salivary function, there may be striking dryness of the conjunctiva and the cornea (keratoconjunctivitis sicca) and of the mouth (xerostomia). These patients also may have a variety of systemic manifestations, including rheumatoid arthritis, splenomegaly, leukopenia, and hemolytic anemia. The chronicity of the process and its occurrence in elderly women make confusion with mumps unlikely. Finally, benign hypertrophy of both masseter muscles, presumably due to habitual clenching and grinding of teeth, may be confused with painless parotid swelling.

The causes of aseptic meningitis are discussed in Chap. 375.

Orchitis occurring in the absence of parotitis is likely to remain undiagnosed. Serologic testing may later confirm the diagnosis of mumps. Orchitis may occur in association with acute bacterial prostatitis and seminal vesiculitis. It is a rare complication of gonorrhea. Occasionally, testicular inflammation accompanies pleurodynia, leptospirosis, melioidosis, tuberculosis, relapsing fever, chickenpox, brucellosis, and lymphocytic choriomeningitis. *Chlamydia trachomatis* also should be considered in the differential diagnosis of epididymitis, particularly among young adults.

TREATMENT There is no specific treatment for infections with the mumps virus. Patients with parotitis should receive mouth care, analgesics, and a bland diet. Bed rest is advisable only as long as the patient is febrile; contrary to popular belief, physical activity has no influence on the development of orchitis or other complications. Patients with epididymoorchitis may be acutely ill and in great pain. Many forms of treatment, including surgical decompression of the testicle, infiltration of the spermatic cord with local anesthetics, and administration of estrogens, convalescent serum, and broad-spectrum antibiotics, have not been regularly effective. Despite failure to document their effectiveness in controlled studies, glucocorticoids have been of apparent benefit in diminishing fever and testicular pain and swelling. A large daily dose corresponding to 60 mg of prednisone is given initially; then the dose is tapered over 7 to 10 days. Glucocorticoids have not exerted an adverse effect on concomitant pancreatitis or meningitis, although they have not benefited patients with meningeal involvement, and their withdrawal usually has been accompanied by a recrudescence of symptoms. They have not prevented the appearance of parotid involvement on the contralateral side. Mumps arthritis is usually responsive to ibuprofen but not to salicylates. Mumps thyroiditis may subside spontaneously, but excellent relief has been obtained with glucocorticoids.

PREVENTION A live, attenuated mumps virus vaccine (Jeryl Lynn strain) has been highly effective in producing significant rises in mumps antibody in individuals who are seronegative prior to vaccination and has afforded 75 to 95 percent protection to individuals subsequently exposed to mumps. The vaccine also has boosted antibody levels in vaccinated individuals who are seropositive. The vaccine produces an inapparent, noncommunicable infection. Parotitis

or fever after vaccination has been reported only rarely, and CNS dysfunction has not been proved to be a complication in the United States. The vaccine has conferred excellent protection for at least 17 years and has not interfered with vaccines against measles, rubella, and poliomyelitis or with smallpox vaccine given simultaneously.

Live mumps vaccine can be administered at any time after 1 year of age, and vaccination should be considered particularly for children approaching puberty, adolescents, and adults born after 1956 who have not had clinical mumps or live mumps vaccine in the past. Individuals living in groups or in institutions should be vaccinated, particularly because it has been shown that physical isolation of mumps patients does not effectively prevent transmission of the infection. Vaccination is also recommended for asymptomatic HIV-infected persons and may be considered for those who are symptomatic. Killed mumps vaccine was available from 1950 until 1978; persons who received this vaccine might benefit from revaccination with a live-virus product. There is no evidence for an increased risk of adverse reactions to live mumps vaccine among persons who are already immune to mumps.

Vaccination is contraindicated in babies under the age of 1 year because of the interfering effect of maternal antibody; in individuals with a history of hypersensitivity to vaccine components; in patients with febrile illnesses, leukemia, lymphoma, or generalized malignancies; in those receiving glucocorticoids, alkylating drugs, antimetabolites, or irradiation; and in pregnant women.

It is not known whether the vaccine will prevent infection when administered after exposure, but no contraindication to its use in this situation exists. Neither mumps immune globulin nor ordinary gamma globulin has been shown to be effective in postexposure prophylaxis, and neither is recommended.

REFERENCES

BEARD CM et al: The incidence and outcome of mumps orchitis in Rochester, Minnesota, 1935 to 1974. Mayo Clin Proc 52:3, 1977

CENTERS FOR DISEASE CONTROL: Update on adult immunization: Recommendations of the Immunization Practices Advisory Committee (ACIP). Morb Mort Week Rep 40:22, 1991

CHAUDARY S, JASKI BE: Fulminant mumps myocarditis. Ann Intern Med 110:569, 1989

CHOU SM: Inclusion body myositis: A chronic persistent mumps myositis? Hum Pathol 17:765, 1986

COHEN AA et al: Mumps-associated acute cerebellar ataxia. Am J Dis Child 146:930, 1992

GORDON SC, LAUTER CB: Mumps arthritis: Unusual presentation as adult Still's disease. Ann Intern Med 97:45, 1982

HAREL L et al: Mumps arthritis in children. Pediatr Infect Dis J 9:928, 1990

HERSH BS et al: Mumps outbreak in a highly vaccinated population. J Pediatr 119:187, 1991

LEVITT LP et al: Central nervous system mumps: A review of 64 cases. Neurology 20:829, 1970

McDONALD JC et al: Clinical and epidemiologic features of mumps meningoencephalitis and possible vaccine-related disease. Pediatr Infect Dis J 8:751, 1989

158   RABIES, RHABDOVIRUSES, AND MARBURG-LIKE AGENTS

LAWRENCE COREY

RABIES

DEFINITION Rabies is an acute viral disease of the central nervous system that affects all mammals and that is transmitted by infected secretions, usually saliva. Most exposures to rabies are through the bite of an infected animal, but on occasion a virus aerosol or the ingestion or transplantation of infected tissues may initiate the disease process.

ETIOLOGY The rabies virus is a bullet-shaped, enveloped, single-stranded ribonucleic acid virus of 75- to 80-nm diameter belonging to the rhabdovirus group. The envelope glycoproteins are arranged in knoblike structures which cover the surface of the virion. The viral glycoproteins bind to acetylcholine receptors, contribute to the neurovirulence of rabies virus, elicit neutralizing and hemagglutination-inhibiting antibodies, and stimulate T cell immunity. The nucleocapsid antigen induces a complement-fixing antibody. Neutralizing antibodies to the surface glycoproteins appear to be protective. Antirabies antibodies used in diagnostic immunofluorescence assays are generally directed against the nucleocapsid antigens. Isolates of rabies virus from different animal species and locales differ in their antigenic and biologic properties. These variations may account for differences in virulence between isolates. Interferon is induced by rabies virus, particularly in those tissues with high virus concentrations, and may play some role in retarding progressive infection.

EPIDEMIOLOGY Rabies exists in two epidemiologic forms: *urban*, propagated chiefly by unimmunized domestic dogs and/or cats, and *sylvatic*, propagated by skunks, foxes, raccoons, mongooses, wolves, and bats. Infection in domestic animals usually represents a "spillover" from sylvatic reservoirs of infection, and human beings can be infected by either. Hence human infection tends to occur in locales where rabies is enzootic or epizootic, where there is a large population of unimmunized domestic animals, and where human contact with the outdoors is common. While only about 1000 rabies deaths are reported to the World Health Organization (WHO) each year, the worldwide incidence of rabies is approximated at over 30,000 cases per year. Southeast Asia, the Philippines, Africa, the Indian subcontinent, and tropical South America are areas where the disease is especially common. In some endemic areas 1 to 2 percent of autopsied patients show evidence of rabies. Increased spread of terrestrial rabies and increased travel to countries where urban rabies is present have made recognition of clinical rabies and its prevention of increasing importance. In the United States, human rabies is exceedingly rare, and most cases now originate from animal bite exposures in countries where canine rabies is endemic.

In most areas of the world, the dog is the important vector of rabies virus for humans. However, the wolf (eastern Europe, arctic regions), the mongoose (South Africa, the Caribbean), the fox (western Europe), and the vampire bat (Latin America) also may be prominent vectors of the disease. In the United States, cat rabies is now reported more frequently than dog rabies; thus the vaccination of domestic cats is extremely important. Rodents and lagomorphs are rarely infected with rabies. In the United States, rabies in wildlife accounts for about 85 percent of the reported animal rabies, with dogs and cats comprising only about 2 and 3 percent, respectively. However, most cases of postexposure prophylaxis are associated with dog or cat bites.

Several cases of human-to-human transmission of rabies through corneal transplantation also have been documented.

PATHOGENESIS The first event is the introduction of live virus through the epidermis or onto a mucous membrane. Initial viral replication appears to occur within striated muscle cells at the site of inoculation. The peripheral nervous system is exposed at the neuromuscular and/or neurotendinal spindles. The virus then spreads centripetally up the nerve to the central nervous system, probably via peripheral nerve axoplasm. Experimentally, viremia has been shown to occur but is not thought to play a role in naturally acquired disease. Once the virus reaches the central nervous system, it replicates almost exclusively within the gray matter and then passes centrifugally along autonomic nerves to reach other tissue—the salivary glands, adrenal medulla, kidney, lung, liver, skeletal muscle, skin, and heart. Passage into the salivary glands facilitates further transmission of the disease via infected saliva. The incubation period of rabies is exceedingly variable, ranging from 10 days to over 1 year (mean 1 to 2 months). The time period appears to depend on the amount of virus introduced, the amount of tissue involved, host defense mechanisms, and the actual distance that the virus has to travel from the site of inoculation to the central nervous system. Cases of human rabies with an extended incubation period (2 to 7 years) have been reported, but they are rare. Host immune responses and viral strains also may influence disease expression. Cell-mediated immune responses were noted in patients with rabies encephalitis but were absent in patients with paralytic rabies.

The neuropathology of rabies resembles other viral diseases of the central nervous system: hyperemia, varying degrees of chromatolysis, nuclear pyknosis, and neuronophagia of the nerve cells; infiltration by lymphocytes and plasma cells of the Virchow-Robin space; microglial infiltration; and parenchymal areas of nerve cell destruction. In experimental animal models, adenohypophyseal infection with rabies virus, with reduction in growth hormone and vasopressin release, is common. The pathognomonic lesion of rabies is the Negri body. This eosinophilic mass, approximately 10 nm in size, is made up of a finely fibrillar matrix and rabies virus particles. Negri bodies are distributed throughout the brain, particularly in Ammon's horn, the cerebral cortex, the brainstem, the hypothalamus, the Purkinje cells of the cerebellum, and the dorsal spinal ganglia. Negri bodies are not demonstrated in at least 20 percent of cases of rabies, and their absence from brain material does not rule out the diagnosis.

MANIFESTATIONS The clinical manifestations of rabies can be divided into four stages: (1) a nonspecific prodrome, (2) an acute encephalitis similar to other viral encephalitides, (3) a profound dysfunction of brainstem centers that produces the classic features of rabies encephalitis, and (4) rarely, recovery.

The prodromal period usually persists for 1 to 4 days and is marked by fever, headache, malaise, myalgias, increased fatigability, anorexia, nausea and vomiting, sore throat, and a nonproductive cough. The prodromal symptom suggestive of rabies is the complaint of paresthesias and/or fasciculations at or about the site of inoculation of virus and may be related to the multiplication of virus in the dorsal root ganglion of the sensory nerve supplying the area of the bite. This symptom is present in 50 to 80 percent of patients.

The encephalitic phase is usually ushered in by periods of excessive motor activity, excitation, and agitation. Quickly, confusion, hallucinations, combativeness, bizarre aberrations of thought, muscle spasms, meningismus, opisthotonic posturing, seizures, and focal paralysis appear. Characteristically, the periods of mental aberration are interspersed with completely lucid periods, but as the disease progresses, the lucid periods get shorter until the patient lapses into coma. Hyperesthesia, with excessive sensitivity to bright light, loud noise, touch, and even gentle breezes, is very common. On physical examination, the temperature may be found to be as high as 40.6°C (105°F). Abnormalities of the autonomic nervous system include dilated irregular pupils, increased lacrimation, salivation, perspiration, and postural hypotension. Evidence of upper motor neuron paralysis with weakness, increased deep tendon reflexes, and extensor plantar responses is the rule. Paralysis of the vocal cords is common.

The manifestations of brainstem dysfunction begin shortly after the onset of the encephalitic phase. Cranial nerve involvement causes diplopia, facial palsies, optic neuritis, and the characteristic difficulty with deglutition. The combination of excessive salivation and difficulty in swallowing produces the traditional picture of "foaming at the mouth." Hydrophobia, the painful, violent, involuntary contraction of the diaphragm, accessory respiratory, pharyngeal, and laryngeal muscles initiated by swallowing liquids, is seen in about 50 percent of cases. Involvement of the amygdaloid nucleus may result in priapism and spontaneous ejaculation. The patient lapses into coma, and involvement of the respiratory center produces an apneic death. The prominence of early brainstem dysfunction distinguishes rabies from other viral encephalitides and accounts for the rapid downhill course. The median survival after the onset of symptoms is 4 days, with a maximum of 20, unless artificial supporting measures are instituted.

If intensive respiratory support is used, a number of late complications may appear and include inappropriate secretion of antidiuretic hormone, diabetes insipidus, cardiac arrythmias, vascular instability, adult respiratory distress syndrome, gastrointestinal bleeding, thrombocytopenia, and paralytic ileus. Recovery is very rare and, when it occurs, gradual.

Occasionally, rabies may present as an ascending paralysis resembling the Landry-Guillain-Barré syndrome (dumb rabies, *rage tranquille*). This clinical pattern occurs most frequently in those who are bitten by vampire bats or who have received postexposure rabies prophylaxis.

The difficulty of suspecting rabies when it is associated with ascending paralysis is illustrated by the documentation of person-to-person transmission of the virus by tissue transplantation. Corneal transplants from two donors who died of presumed Landry-Guillain-Barré syndrome produced clinical rabies and death in the recipients. Retrospective pathologic examinations of the brains of both recipients demonstrated Negri bodies, and rabies virus was subsequently isolated from each donor's frozen eye.

LABORATORY FINDINGS Early in the disease the hemoglobin and routine blood chemistries are normal, but abnormalities occur as hypothalamic dysfunction, gastrointestinal bleeding, and other complications ensue. The peripheral white blood cell count is usually slightly elevated (12,000 to 17,000 cells per microliter) but may be normal or as high as 30,000 cells per microliter.

As in any viral infection, the specific diagnosis of rabies depends on (1) the isolation of virus from infected secretions [saliva, rarely cerebrospinal fluid (CSF), or tissue (brain)], (2) the serologic demonstration of acute infection, or (3) the demonstration of viral antigen in infected tissue, e.g., corneal impression smears, skin biopsies, or brain. Samples of brain obtained either on postmortem examination or at brain biopsy should be subjected to (1) mouse inoculation studies for virus isolation, (2) fluorescent antibody (FA) staining for viral antigen, and (3) histologic and/or electron-microscopic examination for Negri bodies. While the mouse inoculation studies for virus isolation and direct FA staining for viral antigen are quite reliable and sensitive, "autosterilization" may occur and these tests may be negative if the patient's life has been prolonged and high levels of neutralizing antibody are present in serum and CSF. The use of FA staining of skin biopsies, corneal impression smears, and saliva for evidence of rabies antigen has been helpful in diagnosing rabies during life. Confirmation of these findings either serologically or by demonstration of virus in brain should be sought.

If the patient has not received antirabies immunization, a fourfold rise in neutralizing antibody to rabies virus in serial serum samples is diagnostic. If the patient has received rabies vaccination, a clue to the diagnosis may be obtained from the absolute titers of serum-neutralizing antibody and the presence of neutralizing antibody to rabies in CSF. Postexposure rabies prophylaxis rarely produces CSF-neutralizing antibody to rabies. If present, it is usually in low titer, e.g., less than 1:64, whereas CSF titers in human rabies may vary from 1:200 to 1:160,000.

DIFFERENTIAL DIAGNOSIS There is little to distinguish rabies from other viral encephalitides, and the most helpful point in diagnosis is the history of exposure. Other problems to be considered include hysterical reactions to animal bites (pseudohydrophobia), Landry-Guillain-Barré syndrome, poliomyelitis, and allergic encephalomyelitis to rabies vaccine. The latter occurs most commonly after use of nerve tissue–derived vaccine and usually begins 1 to 4 weeks after vaccination.

PREVENTION AND TREATMENT Each year more than 1 million Americans are bitten by animals. In each instance, a decision must be made whether to initiate postexposure rabies prophylaxis. When deciding whether to institute rabies prophylaxis, the following considerations apply: (1) whether the individual came into physical contact with saliva or another substance likely to contain rabies virus, (2) whether rabies is known or suspected in the species and area associated with the exposure (e.g., all persons within the continental United States bitten by a bat that then escapes should receive postexposure prophylaxis), (3) the circumstances surrounding the exposure, and (4)

the treatment alternative and complications. A guide for postexposure rabies prophylaxis is illustrated in Fig. 158-1.

If rabies is known to be present or suspected to be present in the animal species involved in a human exposure, the animal should be captured, if possible. Wild animals or any ill, unvaccinated, or stray domestic animal involved in a rabies exposure, particularly any animal involved in an unprovoked bite, exhibiting abnormal behavior, or suspected of being rabid, should be humanely killed, and the head should be sent immediately to an appropriate laboratory for rabies FA examination. If examination of the brain by the FA technique is negative for rabies, it can be assumed that the saliva contains no virus, and the exposed person need not be treated. Persons exposed to escaped wild animals capable of carrying rabies (bats, skunks, coyotes, foxes, raccoons, etc.) in an area where rabies is known or suspected to be present should receive both passive and active immunization against rabies.

If a healthy dog or cat bites a person, the animal should be captured, confined, and observed for 10 days. If any illness or abnormal behavior develops in the animal during the observation period, it should be killed for FA examination. Experimental and epidemiologic evidence suggests that animals that remain healthy for 10 days after a bite will not have transmitted rabies virus at the time of the bite.

Postexposure prophylaxis Once a decision regarding the necessity to initiate postexposure rabies prophylaxis has been made, the general principle of postexposure therapy is to minimize the amount of virus at the site of inoculation with local treatment of the wound and to establish an early and long-lasting neutralizing antibody titer to rabies virus. In most instances, postexposure therapy includes administration of globulin and vaccines. The following is a therapeutic regimen:

1 *Local wound therapy*. This is an important part of rabies prevention. The wound should be scrubbed with soap and then flushed with water. Both mechanical and chemical cleansing are important. Quaternary ammonium compounds such as 1 to 4% benzalkonium chloride or 1% cetrimonium bromide are useful because they inactivate the rabies virus. However, 0.1% benzalkonium solutions

FIGURE 158-1 Postexposure rabies prophylaxis algorithm.

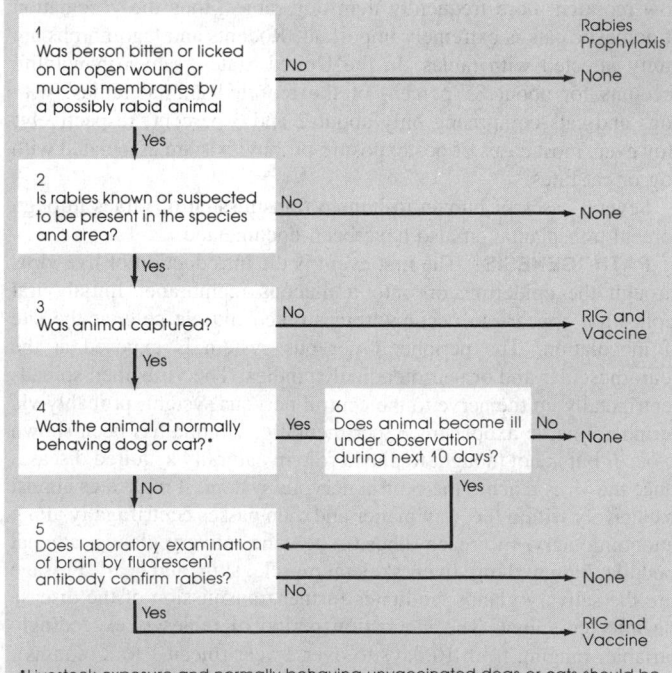

*Livestock exposure and normally behaving unvaccinated dogs or cats should be considered individually and local and state public health officials should be consulted.

are less effective than 20% soap solutions. Usually tetanus toxoid and antibiotics should be administered.

2 *Passive immunization with antirabies antiserum* of either equine or human origin. Human rabies immune globulin (HRIG) is preferred because equine antiserum may cause serum sickness. Fifty percent of the total dose of 20 units per kilogram for HRIG and 40 units per kilogram for the equine antiserum is given by local infiltration of the wound, and the rest is administered intramuscularly into the gluteal region.

3 *Active immunization with antirabies vaccine.* Human diploid cell vaccine (HDCV) is the recommended rabies vaccine. In the United States, two products are licensed. One vaccine contains the Pitman-Moure strain of virus (Pasteur-Meriux; Imovax) that is grown on human diploid cell cultures and inactivated with β-propiolactone. The other vaccine, rabies vaccine absorbed (RVA), is distributed by the Biologics Products Program, Michigan Department of Public Health, and is prepared from the Kissling strain of virus adapted to fetal rhesus lung diploid cells. Both vaccines are considered equally efficacious and safe. Severe reactions to HDCV are uncommon. Immediate hypersensitivity responses such as urticaria have been reported in approximately 1 in 650 recipients. Systemic reactions such as fever, headache, and nausea are generally mild and are reported in 1 to 4 percent of recipients. Local reactions such as swelling, erythema, and induration at the injection site occur in 15 to 20 percent of vaccinees.

Five 1-mL doses of HDCV are given intramuscularly, preferably in the deltoid or anterolateral thigh area, as soon as possible after exposure. The first dose (day 0) also should be accompanied by antirabies serum (HRIG) in the gluteal area. Five doses should be administered within 28 days on the following schedule: days 0, 3, 7, 14, and 28. The WHO also recommends a 21- and 90-day course.

The combination of HRIG and HDCV produces high titers of neutralizing antibodies in almost all recipients. Only rarely has this regimen proved unsuccessful in preventing the subsequent development of rabies. The administration of vaccine alone appears to be associated with a higher failure rate than HRIG and HDCV, especially in severe bite exposures. The combination of HRIG plus 0.1-mL intradermal doses at eight sites on day 0, four sites on day 7, and one site on days 28 and 91 produces good antibody responses, although the clinical experience with this regimen is less than with intramuscular administration.

Preexposure prophylaxis Individuals with a high risk of contact with rabies virus—veterinarians, cave explorers, laboratory workers, and animal handlers—should have preexposure prophylaxis with rabies vaccine. HDCV is the preferred vaccine for preexposure prophylaxis; three IM or three 0.1-mL intradermal injections on days 0, 7, and 28 should be administered. RVA should not be used intradermally. A neutralizing antibody titer should be checked after vaccination. Concomitant chloroquine administration interferes with the antibody response to vaccine. Depending on risk, serologic testing should be done at 2- to 6-year intervals. When neutralizing titers fall below 1:5, booster doses should be given. Booster doses may be administered either as a single 1-mL intramuscular or 0.1-mL intradermal injection. Postexposure prophylaxis in individuals previously given preexposure therapy consists of HDCV alone (two IM doses of HDCV on days 0 and 3 are usually adequate).

Booster doses of HDCV are associated with fever, headache, muscle aches, and joint pains in about 20 percent of recipients. Up to 6 percent of persons receiving IM booster doses of HDCV have developed an immune-complex–like reaction characterized by urticaria, arthritis, nausea, vomiting, and, occasionally, angioedema. These reactions have been self-limited and appear to be associated with the presence of β-propriolactone-altered human serum albumin in the vaccine and the development of IgE antibodies to this antigen. Persons who work in high-risk areas should undergo periodic measurement of antibodies, and booster doses are recommended for

those with low antibody titers. Those at very low risk may elect not to receive routine booster doses but only to receive active immunization with any substantive exposure.

MOKOLA VIRUS

Mokola virus was first isolated from wild shrews captured in Nigeria and subsequently was shown to be related morphologically and serologically to rabies virus. However, neither of the two reported cases of human disease (both in children) demonstrated classic clinical features of rabies. One patient had a nonfatal illness characterized by fever, pharyngitis, and convulsions. Mokola virus was recovered from her cerebrospinal fluid (CSF). The second patient initially had fever, cough, and vomiting, followed in several days by drowsiness, confusion, and generalized flaccid weakness. Her CSF was normal. She progressed to deep coma and died within 10 days of onset. Mokola virus was isolated from her brain, and histopathologic sections revealed finely granular cytoplasmic inclusions that were distinguishable from Negri bodies in many neurons.

VESICULAR STOMATITIS VIRUS

Vesicular stomatitis is a viral illness of animals that occasionally affects humans. It presents as an acute, self-limited, influenza-like disease. The disease in animals is found in the United States and South America and affects chiefly domestic cattle, horses, swine, wild deer, raccoons, skunks, and bobcats.

In animals, vesicular stomatitis is characterized by the development of vesicles on the oral mucosa, particularly the tongue, udders, and heels. The mode of spread is probably by direct contact; however, epidemics tend to occur in warm weather, and isolation of the virus from *Phlebotomus* sandflies in Panama and *Aedes* species in New Mexico suggests these as possible vectors. Two distinct serotypes, New Jersey and Indiana, have been recognized, and most of the outbreaks in North America have been attributed to the New Jersey strain. The disease is most common in laboratory workers, and in one report, three-fourths of laboratory personnel handling experimentally infected animals or manipulating the virus developed neutralizing antibodies. The disease is transmissible, however, under natural conditions among workers having direct contact with infected animals, especially cattle. The incubation period ranges from 1 to 6 days. This is followed by the sudden onset of fever up to 40°C (104°F), chills, profuse sweating, myalgias, malaise, headache, and pain on ocular movement. One-third to one-half of patients have sore throat and cervical and/or submandibular adenopathy. Small raised vesicular lesions may appear on the buccal mucosa. Conjunctivitis and coryza are present in about 20 percent of cases. Occasionally, small subcorneal, intraepithelial vesicles may appear on the fingers, usually associated with direct inoculation of the virus. Symptoms generally last 3 to 4 days, but occasionally a diphasic course may occur. Inapparent infection is common, and among laboratory workers with serologic evidence of infection, only about one-half reported clinical symptoms. In some areas of Panama, 17 to 35 percent of the population have neutralizing antibodies against vesicular stomatitis virus.

The differential diagnosis includes hand-foot-and-mouth disease, herpangina, primary herpetic pharyngitis and other mucocutaneous syndromes, and influenza. Viral isolation from patients is not common; however, a rise in complement fixation and/or neutralizing antibodies to vesicular stomatitis virus between acute and convalescent sera will help to confirm the diagnosis. Treatment is nonspecific.

MARBURG VIRUS DISEASE

DEFINITION Marburg virus causes an acute systemic febrile illness characterized by the abrupt onset of headache, myalgias, pharyngitis, rash, and hemorrhagic manifestations. It was recognized first in 1967 when it caused simultaneous outbreaks in the Federal Republic of Germany and Yugoslavia among laboratory workers exposed to imported African green monkeys (*Cercopithecus aethiops*). Outbreaks have been reported from Kenya. The clinical manifestations are similar to those of other hemorrhagic fevers of the arenavirus class or flavivirus group (Argentinian and Bolivian hemorrhagic fever; Chap. 160). The high case-fatality rate and demonstrated ability for nosocomial spread have made recognition of this rare agent an important worldwide public health concern.

ETIOLOGY   The Marburg virus has been isolated in guinea pig and various cell culture systems such as vervet monkey kidney. The virus particle contains lipid and RNA, and under the electron microscope the virus appears as an 80- to 100-nm elongated filamentous particle with occasional "blister-like excrescences." Marburg and Ebola viruses have been included in a new family of viruses called Filoviridae. These viruses are biosafety level 4 pathogens, and maximum biologic containment facilities are recommended.

EPIDEMIOLOGY   The initial outbreak affected 31 patients in Marburg and Frankfurt, Germany, and Belgrade, Yugoslavia, and was epidemiologically linked to monkeys imported from the same source in Uganda. Virus was isolated from the blood and tissue of these monkeys. Of the 25 primary infections, there were seven deaths and six secondary cases, most of which appeared related to accidental needle sticks or abrasions. The wife of one patient developed Marburg virus disease. Marburg virus was demonstrated in semen of the original patient, despite the presence of circulating antibody, and this secondary case is believed to have been acquired through sexual intercourse. Recently, Marburg and Ebola viruses have been isolated from cynomolgus monkeys imported into the United States; these isolates are morphologically similar but genetically distinct from the viruses isolated in Europe in 1967. Human disease has not yet been associated with these latter strains.

PATHOLOGY   Marburg virus appears "pantropic" and produces lesions in almost all organs, including lymphoid tissue, liver, spleen, pancreas, adrenals, thyroid, kidney, testes, skin, and brain. In lymphoid tissue, focal necrosis with degeneration is apparent. In the liver, eosinophilic cytoplasmic bodies resembling the Councilman bodies of yellow fever have been noted. The lungs may show interstitial pneumonitis, as well as vascular lesions in small arterioles, indicative of endarteritis. Neuropathologic changes consist of multiple small hemorrhagic infarcts with glial proliferation.

CLINICAL MANIFESTATIONS   After an incubation period of 3 to 9 days, patients develop frontal and temporal headache, malaise, myalgias (especially in the lumbar area), nausea, and vomiting. Fever of 39.4 to 40°C (103 to 104°F) is characteristic, and about half the patients have conjunctivitis. Between 1 and 3 days after onset, watery diarrhea (often severe), lethargy, and a change in mentation are noted. An enanthem of the palate and tonsils and cervical lymphadenopathy also may be noted during the first week of illness. The most reliable clinical feature is the appearance of nonpruritic maculopapular rash, which begins on the fifth to seventh day on the face and neck and spreads centrifugally to involve the extremities. A fine desquamation of the affected skin, especially the palms and soles, appears 4 to 5 days later. Hemorrhagic manifestations, including gastrointestinal, renal, vaginal, and/or conjunctival hemorrhages, generally develop between days 5 and 7 of disease.

During the first week, the temperature continues in the vicinity of 40°C (104°F), falling by lysis during the second week, to increase again between the twelfth and fourteenth days. Other clinical signs apparent in the second week of disease include splenomegaly, hepatomegaly, facial edema, and scrotal or labial reddening. Complications include orchitis, which may lead to testicular atrophy; myocarditis with irregular pulse and electrocardiographic abnormalities; and pancreatitis. The overall case-fatality rate has been about 25 percent, with death usually occurring during the eighth to sixteenth days of illness. Recovery is often protracted over a 3- to 4-week period, and during this period, loss of hair, intermittent abdominal

pain, poor appetite, and prolonged psychotic disturbances have been noted. Late sequelae, including transverse myelitis and uveitis, have been reported. Marburg virus has been isolated from the anterior eye chamber and semen nearly 3 months after onset of disease.

LABORATORY FINDINGS   Abnormalities in granulocyte function are found, and leukopenia is detected as early as the first day, with leukocyte counts as low as 1000 cells per microliter and a neutrophilia by the fourth day. Subsequently, atypical lymphocytes, as well as neutrophils exhibiting the characteristic of the Pelger-Huët anomaly, may appear. Thrombocytopenia appears early and is most marked, often less than 10,000 cells per microliter, between the sixth and twelfth days. In fatal cases, evidence of disseminated intravascular coagulation can be demonstrated. Hypoproteinemia, proteinuria, and azotemia may occur. Elevations in aspartate aminotransferase (SGOT) and alanine aminotransferase (SGPT) are usual. Lumbar puncture may be normal or reveal a minimal pleocytosis. The erythrocyte sedimentation rate is usually low.

DIAGNOSIS   The characteristic clinical course and epidemiologic features are the basis of the diagnosis. Specific diagnosis requires isolation of the virus or serologic evidence of infection in paired serum samples. Viremia coincides with the febrile state of disease, and virus has been isolated from tissue as well as urine, semen, and throat and rectal swabs. Attempts to isolate virus must be carried out only in *specialized high-security laboratories*. All patients should be kept in strict isolation, and all specimens should be handled and shipped according to World Health Organization guidelines.

TREATMENT   Patients have received a multiplicity of drugs without apparent influence on the course of the illness. Convalescent serum was administered to four patients, whose subsequent disease followed a mild course. However, similarly benign outcomes were observed in patients who did not receive serum.

EBOLA VIRUS

Between July and November 1976, simultaneous outbreaks of an acute febrile hemorrhagic disease occurred in southern Sudan and northern Zaire. "Secondary and tertiary" spread of infection, particularly among hospital staff, was noted. In the Sudan over 300 cases with 151 deaths and in Zaire 237 cases with 211 fatalities were reported. The virus isolated from these patients was morphologically similar to but antigenically distinct from the Marburg agent. The name *Ebola virus*, after the river in Zaire located near the epidemic, has been proposed. Biologic and antigenic differences between strains of Ebola viruses isolated in Zaire and the Sudan may account for the differences in mortality between the two outbreaks. Sporadic cases of disease also appear to occur, and a serosurvey revealed a prevalence rate of 7 percent for antibodies to Ebola virus in endemic areas. As with other hemorrhagic fevers, neutrophil leukocytosis, hypofibrinogenemia, thrombocytopenia, and microangiopathic hemolytic anemia are features of the illness.

Ebola virus has been propagated in tissue culture (Vero cells) and in suckling mice and guinea pigs. The source of the outbreak in both the Sudan and Zaire is unknown; however, as with other viral hemorrhagic fevers, peridomestic rodents are suspected as being a reservoir of the infection, and serologic evidence of Ebola virus infection was detected in a domestic guinea pig trapped in Zaire. More recently, the isolation of Ebola virus from Asian macaques has suggested that these animals are the natural reservoir of infection. Once established, nosocomial as well as community-acquired cases occur, especially among persons who have close and prolonged contact with infected individuals. Parenteral exposure to the virus through disinfected rather than sterilized needles may have played a role in transmission. Barrier nursing and strict isolation precautions with use of protective clothing appeared to decrease the number of nosocomial cases.

CLINICAL MANIFESTATIONS   Clinically, the disease is similar to Marburg virus disease. The incubation period ranges from 4 to 6 days. Patients usually present on the fifth day of illness with a history of abrupt onset of headache, malaise, myalgias, high fever, diarrhea, abdominal pain, dehydration, and lethargy. Pleuritic chest pain, a dry hacking cough, and a pronounced pharyngitis also have been noted. A maculopapular eruption develops between days 5 and 7 of illness. On black skins the rash is often faint and not recognized until desquamation occurs. Hematemesis, melena, and bleeding from the nose, gums, and vagina are common. Abortion and massive metrorrhagia are frequent complications among pregnant women. Death usually occurs in the second week of illness and is preceded by severe blood loss and shock.

TREATMENT Patients should be isolated until virologic studies indicate they are free of virus, usually 21 days from onset of illness. The frequent detection of malaria parasites in blood films of patients with Ebola virus infection in the Sudan indicated that parasitemia does not rule out concomitant viral illness. Treatment with plasma containing Ebola virus–specific antibodies has resulted in diminished levels of viremia; however, further tests are required to establish the effectiveness of this form of therapy. Requests for viral isolation as well as convalescent plasma should be addressed to WHO Regional Centers in Atlanta or Geneva.

REFERENCES

Rabies

BAER GM: Research towards rabies prevention: Overview. Rev Infect Dis 10(suppl 4):S576, 1988

———, FISHBEIN DB: Rabies post exposure prophylaxis. N Engl J Med 316:1270, 1987

BERNARD KW et al: Preexposure immunization with intradermal human diploid cell rabies vaccine. JAMA 257:1059, 1987

HOUFF SA et al: Human-to-human transmission of rabies virus by a corneal transplant. N Engl J Med 300:603, 1979

NICHOLSON KG: Rabies. Lancet 335:1201, 1990

PAPPAIVANOU M et al: Antibody response to preexposure diploid-cell rabies vaccine given concurrently with chloroquine. N Engl J Med 314:280, 1986

Recommendations of the Public Health Service, Immunization Practices Advisory Committee (ACIP): Rabies prevention. United States, 1991. Morb Mort Week Rep 40(RR-3):1, 1991

SMITH JS et al: Unexplained rabies in three immigrants to the United States. N Engl J Med 324:205, 1991

WARRELL DA, WARRELL MJ: Human rabies and its prevention: An overview. Rev Infect Dis 10 (Suppl 4):S726, 1988

Mokola virus

FAMILUSI JB: Fatal human infection with Mokola virus. Am J Trop Med Hyg 21:959, 1972

Marburg virus

Filovirus infections among persons with occupational exposure to nonhuman primates. Morb Mort Week Rep 39:266, 1990

SIMPSON DH: Marburg and Ebola virus infections: A guide for their diagnosis, management and control. Geneva, WHO Offset Publication 36, 1977

SMITH DH et al: Marburg-virus disease in Kenya. Lancet 1:816, 1982

Ebola virus

JAHRLING PB: Preliminary report: Isolation of Ebola virus from monkeys imported to USA. Lancet 335:502, 1990

McCORMICK JB et al: Biologic differences between strains of Ebola virus from Zaire and Sudan. J Infect Dis 147:264, 1983

STANSFIELD SK: Antibody to Ebola virus in guinea pigs: Tandala, Zaire. J Infect Dis 146:483, 1982

159 ARBOVIRUS INFECTIONS

JAY P. SANFORD

DEFINITION AND CLASSIFICATION The definition of an arthropod-borne virus (arbovirus) was published in 1967 by the World Health Organization:

Arboviruses are viruses which are maintained in nature principally, or to an important extent, through biological transmission between susceptible vertebrate hosts by hematophagous arthropods; they multiply and produce viremia in the vertebrates, multiply in the tissues of arthropods, and are passed on to new vertebrates by the bites of arthropods after a period of extrinsic incubation.

From this definition it can be appreciated that the term *arbovirus* is used in the ecologic sense. Transmission by vectors is not correlated with virus architecture. Current approaches to taxonomy are based on viral morphology, structure, and function. As a result, for taxonomic purposes, the term *arbovirus* has been eliminated. The purpose of this chapter is to define viral illness transmitted to humans by biting insects. Because the number of agents is large, mention will be made of those which have been best documented, have demonstrated unusual features, or seem to be of greatest potential public health importance.

The more than 530 antigenically distinct "arboviruses" are now grouped into six families (Table 159-1). The majority of agents contain single-stranded RNA, although some, such as the Reoviridae, contain double-stranded RNA. Sixty arboviruses have been isolated in the United States and Canada, of which 16 are associated with human disease.

"Arboviruses" are of importance in both temperate and tropical zones. Representative viruses have been isolated in almost every geographic area outside the polar regions.

"Arbovirus" infection of vertebrates is usually asymptomatic. The viremia stimulates an immune response which sharply limits the duration of the viremia. In "arbovirus" infections other than urban yellow fever, phlebotomus fever, chikungunya, o'nyong-nyong, mayaro, oropouche, and dengue, infection of humans represents an incidental occurrence which is tangential to the basic maintenance cycle of the virus. Hence the isolation of virus from arthropod vectors or the detection of infection in the natural vertebrate host may provide a means for early detection and enable control of epizootic infection before significant spread to humans occurs.

Most human "arbovirus" infections are asymptomatic. When disease is produced, the spectrum of clinical illness is varied both in predominant features and in severity. Most commonly, disease is self-limited with symptoms of fever, headache, malaise, and myalgia. Associated rash and lymphadenopathy may be features. "Arboviruses" which may cause three major clinical syndromes—arthralgia-arthritis, encephalitis–aseptic meningitis, or hemorrhagic disease—are tabulated in Table 159-2.

INFECTIONS PRESENTING CHIEFLY WITH FEVER, MALAISE, HEADACHE, AND MYALGIA

VENEZUELAN EQUINE ENCEPHALITIS Venezuelan equine encephalitis (VEE) was first noted in equines in Colombia in 1935.

Etiology Like other alphaviruses, the causative agent of VEE is a 40- to 45-nm, single-stranded RNA virus. Based on serologic tests and oligonucleotide fingerprints, a complex of Venezuelan encephalitis viruses has been established: VE subtypes IA to IE, II (Everglades), III (Mucambo), and IV (Pixuna). IA was the original epidemic strain which occurred in Venezuela, and IB, which was recognized in Ecuador in 1963, spread through Central America into Mexico and was responsible for the epidemic in Mexico in 1971 which spread into southern Texas, with the occurrence of at least 76 laboratory-

TABLE 159-1 Virus taxonomy and arboviruses-arenaviruses*

Family	Genus	Virus "English vernacular name"†	Family	Genus	Virus "English vernacular name"†
Reoviridae	Orbivirus	Colorado tick fever‡ Orungo Kemerovo Lipovnik Tribec	Rhabdoviridae	Vesiculovirus	Vesicular stomatitis Indiana‡ Vesicular stomatitis New Jersey‡ Chandipura Piry Isfahan

Togaviridae	Alphavirus (group A)	*Associated with encephalitis*
		Eastern equine encephalitis‡
		Venezuelan encephalitis‡
		Western equine encephalitis‡
		Associated with acute arthropathy
		Sindbis
		  Okelbo (Pogosta and Karelian
		  fevers)
		  Babanki
		Semliki Forest complex
		  Chikungunya‡
		  O'nyong-nyong
		  Igbo Ora
		  Ross River‡
		  Barmah Forest
		  Mayaro
				Lyssavirus	Rabies‡
					Mokola
					Duvenhage

			Filoviridae		Marburg‡ Ebola‡ Reston strain

			Bunyaviridae	Bunyavirus (16 serogroups)	Twenty-four agents may cause fever, fever-rash. None cause death. None in United States.
					California serogroup
					  LaCrosse‡
					  Snowshoe hare
					  Jamestown Canyon
					  California encephalitis
					  Tahyna

Flavivirdae	Flavivirus (group B)	*Associated with encephalitis*
		St. Louis encephalitis‡
		Japanese encephalitis‡
		Murray Valley encephalitis‡
		Tick-borne encephalitis complex‡
		  Russian spring-summer encepha-
		  litis
		  Central European encephalitis
		Negishi
		Powassan‡
		Louping-ill
		Rocio
		Associated with fever-arthralgia-rash
		Dengue fever‡
		West Nile fever‡
		Ten other agents—of less public
		  health importance
		Associated with hemorrhagic fever
		Yellow fever‡
		Dengue fever‡
		  Omsk hemorrhagic fever
		Kyasanur Forest disease
				Phlebovirus	Thirty-seven phleboviruses iso-lated from human beings; none cause death except Rift Valley fe-ver virus.
					Sandfly fever–Naples‡
					Sandfly fever–Sicilian‡
					Toscana
					Rift Valley fever‡

				Nairovirus	Crimean-Congo hemorrhagic fever‡
				Hantavirus	Hantaan‡ Puumala‡ Seoul‡ Porogia‡
			Arenaviridae	Arenavirus	Lymphocytic choriomeningitis‡ Lassa‡ Machupo‡ Junin‡ Guanarito‡

* Only agents which have been shown to naturally infect humans are tabulated.
† Virus species have not yet been designated formally. The International Committee on Taxonomy of Viruses lists species under the term "English vernacular name."
‡ Viruses found in the United States and/or of major public health importance.

confirmed human cases. In early 1973, almost 4000 cases occurred in Peru.

Epidemiology VEE has been primarily a disease of equines and other mammals, although occasionally the agent has infected humans. Evidence of human infection (virus isolation or specific neutralizing antibodies) has been found in Colombia, Ecuador, Panama, Surinam, Guyana, French Guiana, Mexico, Brazil, Curaçao, Trinidad, Argentina, Peru, Florida, and Texas. Each subtype of VE virus is unique to its enzootic vector and does not replicate well in other vectors. Most common is an enzootic cycle between *Culex* mosquitoes and forest rodents. Enzootic VEE infects people who enter the rain forest or swamps, rubber tappers, forestry workers, and military personnel on jungle maneuvers. During an epizootic, many species of mosquitoes can transmit virus, especially *Aedes*, *Mansonia*, and *Psorophora*. The virus has a wide host range in wild mammals, with at least 20 genera, including capuchin monkeys, rats, mice, opossum, jackrabbit, fox, and bats, being naturally infected. Domestic animals other than equines which have been shown to be infected include cattle and pigs in Mexico and goats and sheep in Venezuela. VEE appears to multiply well in mammals with high titers of virus in the blood; e.g., infected horses may have titers of up to $10^{7.5}$ mouse intraperitoneal lethal doses per milliliter of blood. Although 29 species of wild birds have been shown to be naturally infected with VEE (20 percent of which

are colonial nestling herons and related species), whether the VEE-viremia levels in birds are high enough to infect vector mosquitoes is not known. During the initial 3 days of illness, viremia has been detected in approximately two-thirds of patients. The levels of viremia are sufficiently high that humans could serve as a reservoir. VEE virus also has been isolated by pharyngeal swab in a few patients, suggesting the potential for person-to-person transmission. The available observations make it reasonable to consider that the natural vector is a mosquito, with the primary reservoir being either wild or domestic terrestrial mammals. However, natural infection can probably take place without an arthropod vector. Laboratory infections have occurred and are probably due to inhalation of aerosols.

Clinical manifestations In humans, infection with VEE virus usually results in a mild acute febrile illness without neurologic complications. No age is spared, and there is no sex preponderance. The incubation period is 2 to 5 days, followed by the abrupt onset of headache, fever often associated with rigors, malaise, and myalgia. Other common symptoms may include nausea, vomiting, diarrhea, and sore throat. Uncommon features include photophobia, seizures, mental confusion, coma, tremors, and diplopia. Lymphadenopathy occurs in one-third of patients. On laboratory examination initial leukocyte counts are normal with 80 percent neutrophils. By the third day leukopenia occurs in two-thirds of patients. The cerebrospinal

TABLE 159-2 Major clinical syndromes,* associated arboviruses-arenaviruses, and major geographic distribution

Virus	Geographic distribution	Virus	Geographic distribution
FEVER, MALAISE, MYALGIA		**ENCEPHALITIS/ASEPTIC MENINGITIS** (*continued*)	
Phlebotomus (Sandfly) fever	Mediterranean, Middle East, northwest India, Central and South America, East Africa, southern China	Japanese encephalitis	Japan, Korea, China, India, Philippines, Southeast Asia, Thailand, Former Soviet Union
		Murray Valley encephalitis	Australia, New Guinea
Colorado tick fever	Rocky Mountain region of United States and Canada	Rocio	Brazil
		Omsk hemorrhagic fever	Former Soviet Union
Venezuelan equine encephalitis	South and Central America, Florida and Texas	Kyasanur Forest disease complex	India
		Negishi	Japan
Rift Valley fever	Eastern and South Africa, Egypt	Powassan	New York, eastern Canada
		Louping ill	United Kingdom, Ireland
FEVER, MALAISE, LYMPHADENOPATHY, AND RASH		Russian spring-summer encephalitis	Western Siberia
		Central European encephalitis	Eastern Europe, Scandinavia, France, Switzerland
Dengue	Tropical Asia, Oceania, Africa, Australia, Americas	California group (except Tahyna)	North America
West Nile fever	Africa, Middle East, former Soviet Union, France, India, Indonesia	Tahyna	Europe
		Rift Valley fever	Eastern and South Africa, Senegal, Mauritania
FEVER, ACUTE ARTHOPATHY		Lymphocytic choriomeningitis	United States, Germany, Hungary, Argentina
Chikungunya	Africa, Southeast Asia		
O'nyong-nyong	Eastern Africa (? central Africa)	**HEMORRHAGIC FEVER**	
Ross River	Australia, Papua, New Guinea, Fiji, Somoa, Cook Islands	Yellow fever	South America, Africa
Barmah Forest	Eastern Australia	Dengue	Caribbean, Southeast Asia, China
Mayaro	South and Central America	Chikungunya	Southeast Asia
Sindbis	Africa, former Soviet Union, Finland, Sweden, South and Central America	Kyasanur Forest disease	India
		Omsk hemorrhagic fever	Former Soviet Union
Igbo Ora	Central Africa, Nigeria, Ivory Coast	Crimean-Congo hemorrhagic fever	Africa, eastern Europe, Middle East, Asia
ENCEPHALITIS/ASEPTIC MENINGITIS		Hantaan	Korea, Japan, eastern China, Manchuria, former Soviet Union, central Europe
Kemerovo	Central Europe, former Soviet Union	Seoul	Korea, Japan
Eastern equine encephalitis	Atlantic, Gulf coasts, United States, upper New York, Caribbean, western Michigan	Puumala	Scandinavia, central Europe
		Porogia	Balkan area of Europe
		Marburg	Uganda, Kenya, Zimbabwe (consider sub-Saharan Africa)
Venezuelan equine encephalitis	Northern South America, Central America, Mexico, Florida	Ebola	Zaire, Sudan (under sub-Saharan Africa)
Western equine encephalitis	United States, Canada, Central and South America	Lassa fever	West Africa
		Machupo	Bolivia
St. Louis encephalitis	United States, Caribbean	Junin	Argentina
		Guanarito	Venezuela

* Most agents are more often associated with undifferentiated febrile illness than with the specific syndromes. See text for exceptions.

fluid (CSF) may reveal pleocytosis with modest increases in protein and normal glucose concentration. Virus may be isolated both from blood and from CSF. The symptoms usually last 3 to 5 days in mild cases and up to 8 days in more severe cases. A biphasic course of illness may be encountered, with recrudescence of symptoms on the sixth to the ninth day. In an epidemic in Venezuela in 1962, almost 16,000 cases of acute disease were evaluated; 38 percent were classified as encephalitis, but only 3 to 4 percent had severe neurologic abnormalities: convulsions, nystagmus, drowsiness, delirium, or meningitis. The mortality rate was estimated to be less than 0.5 percent, and nearly all deaths occurred in young children.

PHLEBOTOMUS FEVER Phlebotomus (sandfly, pappataci, or 3-day) fever is an acute, relatively mild, self-limited infection caused by at least seven immunologically distinct phleboviruses (Naples, Sicilian, Punta Toro, Alenquer, Toscana, Chagres, and Candiru). Humans, the only known host, probably serve as a dead-end host. The virus is likely maintained by transovarial transmission in sandflies, with vertebrate hosts having little role in the transmission cycle.

Prevalence The disease occurs throughout the Mediterranean basin, the Balkans, the Near and Middle East, the eastern part of Africa, the former Soviet republics of central Asia, Pakistan, parts of India, Panama, Brazil, and possibly certain parts of southern China. In the Middle East and central Asia, native populations acquire the disease at an early age and develop and maintain high levels of immunity. Cases in Panama and Brazil are sporadic, occurring mainly in persons entering the forest. The apparent absence of phlebotomus

fever in indigenous adult populations residing in areas where sandflies are abundant may present a deceptive picture of the actual risk to susceptible persons.

Epidemiology In the Middle East and central Asia, the disease occurs during the hot, dry season (summer or autumn months) and is transmitted to human beings by the bite of infected sandflies (*Phlebotomus* spp.), which are small (2- to 3-mm) urban flies, highly anthropophilic, that can penetrate ordinary house screens. Only the female bites and usually does so during the night. In persons who are not sensitive, there is neither pain nor local irritation after the bite; hence only about 1 percent of patients will remember having been bitten. In contrast, most of the human-biting sandflies (*Lutzomyia* spp.) of tropical America are sylvan in their habits, infrequently entering houses to bite people. In humans, the incubation period averages 3 to 5 days. Viremia is present for at least 24 h before the onset of fever but is not detectable for more than 2 days after the onset of illness. Following recovery, the patient has lifelong immunity to the infecting virus but not to heterologous serotypes. Hence an individual can have illnesses several times.

Clinical manifestations The onset of symptoms is abrupt in over 90 percent of patients, with the temperature rapidly rising to its highest point, which may vary from 37.8 to 40.1°C (100 to 105°F). Headache is nearly always present and often is accompanied by pain on moving the eyes and retroorbital pain. Myalgia is common and may be localized to the chest, resembling pleurodynia, or to the abdomen. Other symptoms may include vomiting, photophobia, giddiness, neck stiffness, alteration or loss of taste, and arthralgia. Conjunctival injection is present in approximately one-third of patients. Small vesicles may be seen on the palate, and macular or urticarial rashes occur. The spleen is rarely palpable, and lymphadenopathy is absent. The pulse rate may be elevated in proportion to the temperature on the first day; thereafter, bradycardia is often present. The fever persists 3 days in most patients, with gradual defervescence. Giddiness, weakness, and feelings of depression are frequently encountered during convalescence. Second attacks 2 to 12 weeks after the first occur in 15 percent of cases.

In common with other "arbovirus" infections, phlebotomus fever may be associated with *aseptic meningitis*. In one series, 12 percent of patients had symptoms and signs sufficient to warrant a lumbar puncture. Findings in these patients included pleocytosis, with an average cell count of 90 per microliter and a predominance of either polymorphonuclear or mononuclear leukocytes. CSF protein concentration ranged from 0.2 to 1.3 g/L (20 to 130 mg/dL). In another series, mild papilledema was observed in a few patients with severe illness.

Laboratory findings   The changes in leukocyte count constitute the only positive laboratory findings. Total leukocyte counts of less than 5000 cells per microliter are observed in 90 percent of patients if daily counts are done during the febrile period and convalescence. The leukopenia may not appear until the last day of fever or even after defervescence. The differential leukocyte count will reveal an absolute decrease in lymphocytes on the first day, accompanied by an increase in nonsegmented neutrophils. During the second or third day, the number of lymphocytes begins to return to normal and may constitute 40 to 65 percent of the total count. Concurrently, there is a reversal in proportion of segmented and band neutrophils. The differential count usually returns to normal within 5 to 8 days after defervescence. Erythrocyte values and urinalyses are usually normal.

Diagnosis   In the absence of a readily available serologic test, the diagnosis must be made on clinical and epidemiologic grounds.

Treatment   The disease is self-limited, and no specific therapy is available. Symptomatic care, including bed rest, adequate fluid intake, and analgesia with aspirin, is recommended. Convalescence may require a week or longer.

Prognosis   No fatalities have been recorded among tens of thousands of cases.

COLORADO TICK FEVER   Colorado tick fever is one of the two tick-transmitted viral diseases of humans recognized in the United States and Canada, Powassan virus being the other. Though "mountain fever" had been described ever since the advent of immigrants to the Rocky Mountain region, it must be differentiated from mild Rocky Mountain spotted fever. Once the clinical picture of disease had been established, it was renamed Colorado tick fever. A second serotype of the Colorado tick fever serogroup (Eyach virus) was isolated from *Ixodes ricinus* ticks near the village of Eyach in Germany and in France. This agent has not been clearly associated with human disease.

Etiology   Colorado tick fever virus is grouped as an "arbovirus" because it replicates in ticks. It is a double-stranded RNA virus belonging to the orbivirus genus of the Reoviridae family (see Table 159-1).

Prevalence   The disease has been contracted in mountain forest areas at 4000 to 10,000 ft in the Rocky Mountain region of the United States and Canada. The possibility exists that Colorado tick fever may occur over a wider geographic area. Mild and clinically inapparent forms of the disease occur. Up to 15 percent of perennial campers have neutralizing antibodies. The number of cases of Colorado tick fever reported in Colorado is 20 times greater than that of Rocky Mountain spotted fever. In fact, almost one-half of the patients diagnosed as having Rocky Mountain spotted fever in Utah were subsequently shown to have Colorado tick fever.

Epidemiology   Colorado tick fever is transmitted to humans by the adult hard-shelled wood tick, *Dermacentor andersoni*. The virus has been found in 10 to 25 percent of this species of ticks collected in endemic areas. Transovarial transmission of the virus in the tick has been established. Illness occurs from late March through

September, mostly in May and June. Virus can be recovered from blood for 2 weeks in most patients, for at least 1 month in nearly one-half, and from CSF during the acute illness. The virus persists within erythrocytes of convalescent patients for as long as 120 days and can be readily isolated from washed erythrocytes 100 days following infection. Transfusion-associated Colorado tick fever has been reported.

Clinical manifestations   The incubation period is usually 3 to 6 days, and in 90 percent a history of tick contact within 10 days of onset of illness can be obtained. Failure to obtain such a history militates against the diagnosis. Persons affected usually are those whose occupational or recreational activities bring them in contact with ticks. The disease may occur at any age, although 40 percent in one series were 20 to 29 years of age. The clinical picture is characterized by the sudden onset of severe aching of the muscles of the back and legs, chilliness without true rigors, a rapid increase in temperature, which usually reaches 38.9 to 40°C (102 to 104°F), headache with pain on ocular movement, retroorbital pain, and photophobia. Abdominal pain and vomiting occur in one-fourth of patients; diarrhea is rare. The physical findings are not specific. Tachycardia in proportion to the temperature, flushed facies, and variable conjunctival injection may be present. Occasionally, the spleen is palpable. Rash occurs in 5 to 12 percent of patients, but on occasion, a petechial rash involving primarily the arms and legs or a maculopapular rash over the entire body may occur. Rarely, punched-out ulcers may form at the site of tick bite. The fever with the associated symptoms lasts about 2 days and then abruptly lyses to normal or subnormal, leaving the patient very weak. After an afebrile period of about 2 days, the fever recurs, may be higher than in the first phase, and may last as long as 3 days. One-half of patients show this saddleback pattern of temperature. Rarely there may be three febrile phases. Convalescence of more than 3 weeks is reported in 70 percent of patients over age 30, while symptoms last less than 1 week in 60 percent of patients under 20. Prolonged convalescence has no relationship to persistent viremia.

Evidence of central nervous system involvement has been recorded in a few patients (3 to 7 percent). The findings are those of either an aseptic meningitis with stiffness of the neck or encephalitis with clouding of the sensorium, delirium, and coma. Hemorrhagic fever with epistaxis, gastrointestinal bleeding, and purpura have been observed in children. Rarer complications include epididymoorchitis and patchy pneumonitis.

Laboratory findings   The most important laboratory feature is moderate to marked leukopenia, although in one-third of confirmed cases leukocyte counts remain about 4500 cells per microliter. On the first day of illness, the total leukocyte count may be at normal levels, but usually by the fifth or sixth day there has been a decrease to 2000 to 3000 cells per microliter. Characteristically, there is a proportionate decrease in lymphocytes and granulocytes. Toxic changes in neutrophils are often conspicuous, and "virocyte" types of lymphocytes are frequently observed. Bone marrow examination reveals "maturation arrest" in the granulocytic series. Erythrocyte values remain normal. The blood picture returns to normal within a week after the fever subsides. Mild elevations in serum aspartate aminotransferase and creatine phosphokinase are reported.

Diagnosis   The diagnosis of Colorado tick fever is suspected on the basis of the epidemiologic history and clinical findings. Because of the infrequency of rash, patients who develop fever and rash after tick bites should be suspected of having Rocky Mountain spotted fever. The usual methods for confirming Colorado tick fever are mouse inoculation and fluorescent antibody (FA) staining of patients' erythrocytes; a combination of the two is best. Special handling of blood is not necessary for the FA test, which remains positive for several weeks after clinical illness.

Prognosis   Three deaths have been reported, all with hemorrhagic signs.

RIFT VALLEY FEVER   Rift Valley fever is an acute disease principally of livestock, sheep, goats, cattle, and camels which is widespread throughout eastern and South Africa. It was first described in humans during an extensive epizootic of hepatitis in sheep in the Rift Valley in Kenya. During an epizootic in South Africa in 1950–1951, an estimated 20,000 humans became infected. Fatal human disease, four cases of hemorrhagic illness and hepatitis, was first reported during an epizootic in South Africa in 1975. In 1977 Rift Valley fever jumped the Sahara to Egypt with a major outbreak. Cases occurred in subsequent years until 1980; an estimated 200,000 cases with 598 reported deaths occurred in 1977.

Virus has been found in several species of mosquitoes: *Culex pipiens*, *Eretmapodites chrysogaster*, *Aedes caballus*, *Aedes circumluteolus*, and *Culex theileri*. *Culex pipiens* has been suggested as the vector in Egypt. While antibodies to Rift Valley fever have been found in wild field rats in Uganda, the reservoir is unknown. It has been suggested that the virus may be maintained by transovarial transmission in floodwater *Aedes*. Although humans presumably can be infected by arthropods, many infections occur as a result of handling infected animal tissues. In addition, laboratory-acquired infections have been common, suggesting a respiratory route of transmission.

The incubation period is usually 3 to 6 days. The onset is abrupt, with malaise, chilly sensation or rigors, headache, retroorbital pain, and generalized aching and backache. The temperature rises rapidly to 38.3 to 40°C (101 to 104°F). Later complaints include anorexia, loss of taste, epigastric pain, and photophobia. Findings on examination are usually unremarkable except for flushing of the face and conjunctival injection. The temperature curve is often saddleback in type, with an initial elevation lasting 2 to 3 days, followed by a remission and second febrile period. Convalescence is typically rapid. Prior to the outbreak in Egypt, Rift Valley fever was a benign illness with almost no fatalities. In Egypt, approximately 1 percent of patients developed severe complications, such as encephalitis, retinopathy, or hemorrhagic manifestations. Encephalitis appeared as the acute infection waned and was severe with serious residua in some survivors. Generalized hemorrhages and icterus appeared as the disease evolved. Deaths from massive hepatic necrosis occurred 7 to 10 days after onset of illness. The fatality rate in severely ill patients may exceed 50 percent. Visual loss, including light perception, occurred 2 to 7 days after the onset of fever. Macular edema, hemorrhage, vasculitis, retinitis, and vascular occlusion were noted. One-half of patients had some permanent loss of visual acuity. A characteristic finding is an initial normal total leukocyte count followed by leukopenia with a decrease in neutrophils associated with an increase in band forms. The diagnosis is made by isolating the virus from the blood by inoculation of mice. Three-fourths of patients are viremic (up to 10^8 mouse intraperitoneal lethal doses per milliliter blood) when first seen. Neutralizing antibodies have been demonstrated as early as 4 days after onset. There is no specific treatment. A killed vaccine which had been stockpiled in the United States is being utilized.

HANTAVIRUS DISEASE—UNITED STATES Acute hantavirus infection was recognized in at least 30 people in 1993 in the New Mexico-Arizona-Colorado region. Patients presented with fever, myalgia, headache, and cough followed by rapid development of respiratory failure and noncardiogenic pulmonary edema. Approximately two-thirds of the cases were fatal. Examination of trapped rodents indicated that *Peromyscus maniculatis* (deer mouse) was the most likely vector through exposure to its excreta. Diagnosis can be confirmed by serologic (IgM) response, polymerase chain reaction, or immunohistochemical stains of infected tissues.

INFECTIONS PRESENTING CHIEFLY WITH FEVER, MALAISE, LYMPHADENOPATHY, AND RASH

DENGUE FEVER Dengue is endemic over large areas of the tropics and subtropics, Asia, Oceania, Africa, Australia, and the Americas. Outbreaks of dengue have occurred in the Caribbean, including Puerto Rico and the U.S. Virgin Islands, since 1969. Indigenous infection occurred in the United States for the first time in 35 years in 1980. Eleven cases have been recognized in residents of the Rio Grande Valley of Texas. In the summer of 1981, almost 350,000 cases of dengue with 158 deaths occurred in Cuba. *Aedes aegypti*, the vector, has reappeared along the U.S. Gulf Coast; hence the threat of dengue along the Gulf Coast is real. Dengue is emerging as an important disease of travelers, with 102 cases reported in U.S. residents in 1990.

Etiology There are four serotypes of dengue viruses, all of which are flaviviruses. In the Caribbean, type 1 was associated with the 1977–1978 outbreak, type 2 in 1968–1969, type 3 in 1963–1964, and type 4 was documented in the Western Hemisphere for the first time in 1981.

Epidemiology Dengue infections in nature involve primarily humans and *Aedes* mosquitoes. Dengue transmission involving monkeys and forest *Aedes* spp. has been documented in Malaysia and West Africa. *Aedes aegypti* is the most important worldwide vector species. This species, as well as the less common vector species, is peridomestic, biting humans readily or even preferentially and breeding in small collections of water such as cisterns and backyard litter. Surveys in Texas have revealed containers with water in which *A. aegypti* were breeding in up to 25 percent of premises. They fly during the day. Humans appear to be uniformly susceptible, and susceptibility is not influenced by age, sex, or race. During outbreaks, attack rates may be very high; in Puerto Rico and the U.S. Virgin Islands, the overall rate of clinical illness was 20 percent, with infection rates as determined by serologic survey as high as 79 per 100.

Clinical manifestations Dengue viruses frequently produce inapparent infections in humans. When symptoms develop, three broad clinical patterns may be encountered: classic dengue, hemorrhagic fever (see below), and a mild atypical form. Classic dengue (breakbone fever) occurs primarily in nonimmune individuals, specifically nonindigenous adults and children. The usual incubation period is 5 to 8 days. Prodromal symptoms such as mild conjunctivitis or coryza may occur, followed in hours by the abrupt onset of a severe splitting headache, retroorbital pain, backache, especially in the lumbar area, and leg and joint pains. The headache is aggravated by movement. At least three-fourths of patients have ocular soreness, with pain on moving the eyes. A few have mild photophobia. Though true rigors are common during the course, they are usually not present at the onset. Additional symptoms include insomnia, anorexia with loss of taste or bitter taste, and weakness. Mild transient rhinopharyngitis occurs in as many as one-quarter of the individuals. Cough is almost never seen. Some patients present with epistaxis, gingival bleeding, hematuria, or melena. In a study of 26 patients with upper gastrointestinal bleeding, 13 percent had gastric or duodenal ulcers and hemorrhagic gastritis on endoscopy. Examination reveals scleral injection (90 percent), tenderness upon pressure on the ocular globe, and nontender posterior cervical, epitrochlear, and inguinal lymphadenopathy. Over one-half of patients have an enanthem characterized initially by pinpoint-sized vesicles over the posterior half of the soft palate. The tongue is often coated. Skin rashes, varying from diffuse flushing to scarlatiniform and morbilliform, are frequently present over the thorax and inner aspects of the arms. These are transient and fade, only to be followed by a more definite maculopapular rash which appears on the trunk on the third to the fifth day and spreads peripherally. The rash may be pruritic and generally terminates with desquamation. Extreme bradycardia is not observed. Within 2 to 3 days after the onset, the temperature may decrease to nearly normal and other symptoms disappear. The remission typically lasts 2 days and is followed by return of fever and the other symptoms, although they are generally less severe than during the initial phase. This saddleback diphasic febrile course is considered characteristic but often is not encountered. The febrile illness usually lasts 5 to 6 days and terminates abruptly. Complaints of fatigue for several weeks after infection are common.

In addition to this "classic" syndrome, an atypically mild illness may occur. Symptoms include fever, anorexia, headache, and myalgia. On examination, evanescent rashes may be seen, but lymphadenopathy is usually absent. The course is usually less than 72 h in duration.

At the onset both in classic and in mild dengue, the leukocyte counts may be low or normal; however, by the third to the fifth day, leukopenia, usually with counts of less than 5000 leukocytes per microliter, and neutropenia are the rule. Occasionally albuminuria of moderate degree occurs.

Diagnosis Inoculation of blood obtained within the first 3 to 5 days onto mosquito tissue cell cultures or inoculation into mosquitoes is used for primary viral isolation. Diagnosis can be made by serologic tests employing paired serums for hemagglutination inhibition tests and complement fixation tests. IgM antibodies are produced in primary dengue infections. Specific serologic diagnosis is complicated by cross-reactions with other flavivirus antibodies such as those following immunization with yellow fever vaccine.

Treatment Treatment is entirely symptomatic.

Prognosis In the absence of the dengue hemorrhagic fever or dengue shock syndrome, mortality is nil.

Prevention An attenuated vaccine for dengue type 2 is undergoing experimental evaluation. Control depends on mosquito abatement.

WEST NILE FEVER West Nile virus is distributed throughout Africa, the Middle East, parts of Europe (Camargue, France), the former Soviet Union, India, and Indonesia. It produces a clinical picture closely resembling dengue. Outbreaks of disease involving several hundred patients occurred in Israel in 1950 to 1952. In one outbreak, over 60 percent of the population developed overt disease.

Epidemiology The disease is highly endemic in Egypt but goes largely unrecognized. Presumably most of the adult population is immune, and the infection in childhood is an undifferentiated mild febrile illness, whereas in Israel it mainly affects adults. The infection occurs in the summer both in Israel and in Egypt. The transmission cycle in the Middle East is bird-mosquito-bird, with *Culex univittatus* and *Culex pipiens molestus* being the principal vectors. *Culex tritaeniorhynchus* is an important vector in Asia. Although humans and a variety of other vertebrates are infected by the virus, their involvement is tangential.

Clinical manifestations The incubation period is 1 to 6 days. Most of the patients in Israel have been young adults, with neither sex predominating. The onset is usually abrupt and without prodromal symptoms. The temperature quickly rises to 38.3 to 40°C (101 to 104°F), with chills occurring in one-third of patients. Symptoms include drowsiness, severe frontal headache, ocular pain, and pain in the abdomen and back. A small number of patients have anorexia, nausea, and dryness of the throat. Cough is uncommon. There are flushing of the face, conjunctival injection, and coating of the tongue. The prominent finding is general enlargement of lymph nodes, which are of moderate size but are not hard and are only slightly tender. Occipital, axillary, and inguinal nodes are usually involved. The spleen and liver are slightly enlarged in a small proportion of patients. In one-half of patients a rash may appear from the second to the fifth day of illness and may persist for several hours or until defervescence. The rash occurs predominantly over the trunk and consists of pale roseolar maculopapular lesions. The illness is self-limited and lasts 3 to 5 days in 80 percent of patients.

In a few patients, transitory meningeal involvement may be encountered. CSF examinations may reveal a pleocytosis and some increase in protein concentration.

Leukopenia occurs in the majority of patients, and total leukocyte counts are lower than 4000 cells per microliter in one-third. Differential counts vary from a moderate shift to the left to a slight lymphocytosis.

Convalescence is often prolonged, lasting 1 to 2 weeks, with prominent symptoms of fatigue. Enlargement of lymph nodes subsides over several months. Only rarely have complications, sequelae, or fatalities been seen in natural infections, although in one outbreak in a group of elderly patients a high proportion of patients developed meningoencephalitis, and four fatalities ensued.

Accurate diagnosis rests on virus isolation, which can be accomplished because viremia persists for as long as 6 days, or the demonstration of a rising specific antibody titer.

The treatment is symptomatic.

INFECTIONS PRESENTING CHIEFLY WITH FEVER, ACUTE ARTHROPATHY, AND RASH

CHIKUNGUNYA This term is a local tribal word meaning "that which bends up" which was used to describe an epidemic of acute arthropathy in Tanzania in 1952–1953 shown to be caused by a togovirus of the alphavirus genus (Table 159-1). It is likely that chikungunya (CHIK) virus caused epidemics in Southeast Asia, India, Africa, and possibly the southern United States in the 1800s and early 1900s. Today, CHIK is responsible for extensive *A. aegyti*–transmitted disease in cities in Africa and Asia. With the increase in *A. aegypti* and introduction of *A. albopictus* in the United States, the possibility of CHIK exists today.

Clinical manifestations The incubation period is usually 2 to 3 days (range 1 to 12 days) followed by the abrupt onset of fever (often to 40°C), rigors, and acute joint pain. The arthalgias are polyarticular and predominantly affect the smaller joints of the hands, wrists, ankles, and feet. Swelling (periarticular) is common, but joint effusions are not. Generalized myalgia is frequent. The acute phase typically lasts 2 to 3 days, with the fever remitting. A maculopapular rash involving the trunk and limbs is typical, usually appearing with defervescence. The rash lasts 1 to 5 days. Constitutional symptoms and signs are common but do not dominate the clinical picture. Conjunctival suffusion is common. Two-thirds of patients will have joint symptoms for several weeks. About 5 percent, usually older patients, have persistent joint pain for 3 to 5 years. In Asia, the clinical syndrome differs, being seen predominantly in children who present with fever, headache, pharyngitis, vomiting, abdominal pain, constipation, or diarrhea, and cough. A maculopapular rash and conjunctival injection are common, but arthritis and arthralgia are not seen. In Bangkok, about 10 percent of patients with the dengue–hemorrhagic fever syndrome have CHIK infection.

O'NYONG-NYONG FEVER O'nyong-nyong fever was first noted as an epidemic illness characterized by joint pains, rash, and lymphadenopathy in the northern province of Uganda in 1959. The agent is an alphavirus which shows close antigenic relationships with chikungunya viruses. The original outbreak was associated with an explosive epidemic which spread to Tanzania and other areas in east Africa. By 1961, 2 million cases were recorded. In some areas, 78 percent of the population had either clinical disease or inapparent infection. Local outbreaks extended over the entire year. All age groups were affected. The most likely vectors are *Anopheles funestus* and *Anopheles gambiae*. The clinical features are similar to those of chikungunya virus infection. The disease disappeared in 1962. While the virus was isolated from *A. funestus* in Kenya in 1978, no further outbreaks have been recongized.

SINDBIS VIRUS Sindbis virus, once thought rarely to present as clinical disease, has been recognized in Africa (Uganda, Zimbabwe, central Africa, and South Africa), Australia, Malaysia, and Europe (former Soviet Union, Finland, and Sweden). In the former Soviet Union it is known as Karelian fever, in Sweden as Okelbo disease, and in Finland as Pogosta disease. Clinically, fever is low-grade and accompanied by malaise, myalgia, and arthralgia involving joints and tendons. The most striking feature is a maculopapular rash appearing on the trunk and extremities but usually sparing the face. Unlike the rash of chikungunya or o'nyong-nyong, the rash often becomes vesicular, especially on the feet and hands. Joint disease is usually multiple—ankles, knees, and wrists. Periarticular involvement is common. Persistent or recurrent joint pains lasted for 2 years in one-third of patients in a Swedish series. Permanent joint deformity is not described.

ROSS RIVER VIRUS   Epidemics of polyarthritis associated with rashes have been observed in Australia since 1928. Outbreaks occur almost entirely in the period December to June. Ross River virus infection was limited to Australia, New Guinea, and the Solomon Islands until 1979, when a major outbreak occurred in Fiji which spread to the Samoan, Cook, and some Melanesian Islands. In the Fiji outbreak in 1979, infection rates were equal at all ages and in both sexes, but clinical attack rates were 4 percent in patients under 20 years and 42 percent in adults, and the clinical attack rate of males to females was 1:1.7. The onset is usually sudden and the initial symptom usually joint pain. Initially, fever may be absent or minimal [highest 38°C (100.4°F)]. In about one-half of patients, arthritis, involving mainly the small joints, wrists, and ankles and sometimes associated with swelling, and paresthesias precede a rash by 1 to 15 days. In the other half, the rash precedes the arthralgia. The rash, which lasts 2 to 10 days, is usually maculopapular, appears on the cheeks and forehead, occasionally spreads to the trunk, or may be restricted to the limbs. The rash may be pruritic. Vesicles occur rarely. Tender lymphadenopathy occurs in one-fifth of the patients. Joint symptoms persist for 3 weeks to 3 months. The virus has been isolated from *Culex annulirostris* and *Aedes vigilax*. Animals may serve as reservoir hosts in Australia. In the Pacific, person-mosquito-person transmission seems likely.

BARMAH FOREST VIRUS   Barmah Forest virus is an alphavirus in Australia (Queensland, New South Wales, Victoria) which recently has been recognized as a cause of fever (two-thirds of patients), chills (one-third), arthritis/arthralgia (three-quarters), rash (one-half, occasionally vesicular), myalgia (two-thirds), and respiratory symptoms (one-fifth). Desquamation has been noted as the rash resolves. The virus has been isolated from the same vector mosquitoes as Ross River virus. There is serologic evidence of extensive infection in Queensland (0.23 percent of the population per year). It is likely that Barmah Forest virus has been misdiagnosed as Ross River virus as one of the causes of epidemic polyarthritis.

MAYARO VIRUS   Three epidemics have been described, two in Brazil in the Amazon region and one in Bolivia. In the outbreak in Belterra, Brazil, the attack rate was high (20 percent), with a high proportion of individuals having symptomatic disease. The symptoms and signs were similar in occurrence and frequency to those noted with other alphavirus infections.

INFECTIONS WITH CNS INVOLVEMENT

Four "arboviruses" are presently recognized as numerically important causes of central nervous system disease in the United States: St. Louis encephalitis virus (SLE), eastern equine encephalitis virus (EEE), western equine encephalitis virus (WEE), and the California serogroup (CE) viruses. The spectrum of infection caused by these agents includes inapparent infection, fever with headache, aseptic meningitis, and encephalitis. Some 1500 to 2000 cases of encephalitis are reported in the United States each year. In the absence of epidemics, 5 to 10 percent of these (75 to 200 cases) are confirmed as "arboviral" in cause. In nonepidemic years, California serogroup viruses (predominantly LaCrosse virus) represent two-thirds to three-fourths of the cases.

Etiology   Despite the diversity of specific viral causes (see Table 159-2), in individual patients the clinical manifestations of aseptic meningitis and encephalitis are very similar and preclude an etiologic diagnosis without ancillary information regarding epidemiologic and serologic features (Table 159-3). The clinical features of aseptic meningitis due to "arboviruses" are indistinguishable from those due to the more prevalent enteroviruses. Since transmission to humans in the United States and Canada involves arthropods, specifically mosquitoes, except for Powassan and Colorado tick fever, indigenously acquired disease occurs at times when mosquitoes are prevalent, such as late spring through early fall.

Clinical manifestations   The clinical features of "arbovirus" encephalitis differ among age groups. In infants under 1 year of age, the only consistently noted symptoms are sudden onset of fever, which is often accompanied by convulsions. Convulsions may be generalized or focal. Typically, fever ranges between 38.9 and 40°C (102 and 104°F). Other physical findings may include bulging of the fontanelle, rigidity of the extremities, and abnormal reflexes.

In children between 5 and 14 years of age, subjective symptoms are more easily elicited. Headache, fever, and drowsiness of 2 to 3 days' duration before medical attention is sought are common. The symptoms may then subside or become more intense and may be associated with nausea, vomiting, muscular pain, photophobia, and, less frequently, convulsions (less than 10 percent except in California encephalitis). The child is found to be acutely ill, febrile, and lethargic. Nuchal rigidity and intention tremors are often present, and on occasion muscular weakness can be demonstrated.

In adults, the initial symptoms commonly include the fairly abrupt onset of fever, nausea with vomiting, and severe headache. The headache is most often frontal but may be occipital or diffuse. Mental aberrations, represented by confusion and disorientation, usually appear within the subsequent 24 h. Other symptoms may include diffuse myalgia and photophobia. The abnormalities found on physical examination predominantly relate to the neurologic examination, although conjunctival suffusion is frequently seen and skin rashes may occur. Disturbances in mentation are among the most outstanding clinical features. These range from coma through severe disorientation to subtle abnormalities detected only by cerebral function tests such as the subtraction of serial 7s. A small proportion of patients show only lethargy, lying quietly, apparently asleep unless stimulated.

TABLE 159-3   Features of arboviral encephalitides common in the United States

	Geographic predominance in the United States	Urban/ rural	Age, years	Sex	Unique clinical features	Mortality, %	Residua
California encephalitis	Midwest	Rural	5–10	M	Seizures	2	Seizures (one-fourth who had them in acute phase), behavioral problems (15%)
Eastern equine encephalitis	Eastern seaboard	Both	<5 >55	=	CSF may have >1000 WBC/μL	50	Children <10 years have emotional lability, retardation, convulsions
St. Louis encephalitis	Eastern and midwest	Both	>35	=	Dysuria	2–12	Ataxia, speech difficulties (5%)
Western equine encephalitis	Entire	Both	<1 >55	=	None	3	Children <3 months have behavioral problems, convulsions

Tremor is common and is observed more frequently in individuals over 40 years of age. The tremors vary in location and may be continuous or intention in type. Cranial nerve abnormalities resulting in oculomotor muscle paresis and nystagmus, facial weakness, and difficulty in deglutition may occur and are usually present within the initial several days. Objective sensory changes are unusual. Hemiparesis or monoparesis may occur. Reflex abnormalities are also common; these include exaggerated palmomental reflexes and suck and snout reflexes. Superficial abdominal and cremasteric reflexes are usually absent. Changes in the tendon reflexes are variable and inconstant. The plantar response may be extensor and fluctuates almost hourly. Dysdiadochokinesia often exists.

The duration of the fever and neurologic symptoms and signs varies from several days to a month but usually ranges from 4 to 14 days. Clinical improvement generally follows the subsidence of the fever within several days unless irreversible anatomic changes have occurred.

Laboratory findings Erythrocytes are usually normal. Total leukocyte counts often reveal both a slight to moderate leukocytosis (occasionally greater than 20,000 leukocytes per microliter) and neutrophilia. Examination of the CSF usually reveals several hundred cells per microliter, but on occasion cloudy CSF with cells in excess of 1000 per microliter may be seen. Within the first several days of illness, polymorphonuclear neutrophils may predominate. The initial CSF protein is usually only slightly elevated but on occasion may exceed 1.0 g/L (100 mg/dL). The level of CSF sugar is normal; a significant decrease should raise serious consideration of an alternative diagnosis. As the illness progresses, mononuclear cells in the CSF tend to increase so that they predominate and the protein concentration may increase. Other laboratory studies have been reported only sporadically, but abnormalities may include hyponatremia, often due to the inappropriate secretion of antidiuretic hormone, and elevations in serum creatine phosphokinase.

Diagnosis Specific diagnosis requires the isolation of the virus or detection of antibodies with a rising titer between the acute phase of disease and convalescence. Antibodies can be detected by hemagglutination inhibition, complement fixation, or virus neutralization techniques.

Treatment Treatment is entirely supportive and requires meticulous attention in the comatose patient.

LACROSSE ENCEPHALITIS A previously undescribed virus was isolated in 1943 from mosquitoes in Kern County, California. Since 1963, a large number of agents now designated as the California group of viruses have been isolated (see Table 159-1). LaCrosse, Snowshoe hare, Jamestown Canyon, California encephalitis, and Trivittatus viruses cause human encephalitis in North America. Tahyna and Inkoo viruses are associated with febrile and, rarely, encephalitic disease in Europe. Since 1966 in midwestern United States, LaCrosse virus (California) encephalitis has been incriminated in 5 to 6 percent of cases of acute central nervous system disease, ranking above all agents except the enteroviruses.

Epidemiology LaCrosse virus infection occurs in the North Central states, in New York, in wooded areas of eastern Texas and Louisiana, and along the Eastern Seaboard. The virus is maintained by transovarial transmission in woodland mosquitoes, *Aedes triseratus*, which breed in tree holes in hardwood forests and have adapted to discarded tires. The virus is present in seminal fluid of male mosquitoes and is transmitted to the female. The virus overwinters in eggs of *A. triseratus*. Chipmunks and gray squirrels serve as amplifier hosts. LaCrosse virus (California) encephalitis occurs during the summer months (June to October), most often involving boys (60 percent) 5 to 10 years of age (60 percent) who live in rural areas.

Clinical manifestations Two clinical patterns of LaCrosse virus disease have been defined. One is a mild form with a 2- to 3-day prodrome of fever, headache, malaise, and gastrointestinal symptoms. About the third day the temperature increases to 40°C (104°F), and the patient becomes lethargic and develops meningeal signs. These findings abate gradually over a 7- to 8-day period without overt

sequelae. The second pattern, a severe form which occurs in at least one-half of patients, begins abruptly with fever, headache, and vomiting, followed shortly by lethargy and disorientation. During the first 2 to 4 days, the course is rapidly progressive, with the occurrence of seizures (50 to 60 percent), focal neurologic signs (20 percent), pathologic reflexes (10 percent), and coma (10 percent). Focal neurologic signs may include asymmetric flaccid paralysis. Uncommon findings have included arthralgia and rash. Clinical laboratory features include peripheral leukocyte counts ranging from 7000 to 30,000 cells per microliter (median 16,000 cells per microliter) with neutrophilia. CSF examination reveals 10 to 500 cells per microliter, usually with a predominance of mononuclear cells, protein concentrations of less than 1.0 g/L (100 mg/dL), and normal sugar concentrations. Electroencephalograms (EEGs) are abnormal in at least 80 percent of patients, revealing slow delta-wave activity. In one-half of patients the abnormality is asymmetric, suggesting focal destructive lesions. Brain scans using ^{99m}Tc-pertechnetate and computed tomography (CT) also may be abnormal, and temporal lobe localization has been observed. Beginning about the fourth day and proceeding over the next 3 to 7 days, there is progressive improvement, with almost all patients becoming afebrile, seizure-free, and ready for discharge from the hospital within 2 weeks after onset.

Diagnosis Serum and CSF should be tested for LaCrosse virus IgM antibodies. Serum capture IgM enzyme-linked immunosorbent assay (ELISA) tests detected 83 percent of cases on admission in LaCrosse encephalitis. Early specific diagnosis eliminates the need for brain biopsy to exclude herpes encephalitis, which is suggested by the temporal lobe localization.

Treatment Initial seizure activity is frequently prolonged and difficult to control. The most effective anticonvulsant medication has been parenteral diazepam. Patients with the severe form of disease should be discharged on anticonvulsants such as phenobarbital for 6 to 12 months.

Prognosis The case-fatality ratio is low (2 percent or less); however, one-third of patients may have abnormal neurologic findings at the time of discharge. During the early convalescent period, emotional lability and irritability are common. In one series, recurrent seizures occurred in one-quarter of the patients who had seizures during the acute phase. In this same series, EEGs were abnormal in one-third of patients evaluated 1 to 8 years after their acute illness. In another series, 15 percent had sequelae, predominantly personality or behavioral problems.

OTHER CALIFORNIA GROUP ENCEPHALITIDES Jamestown Canyon encephalitis is uncommon but, in contrast to LaCrosse encephalitis, usually occurs in adults. Snowshoe hare virus has been isolated from mosquitoes throughout Canada and from Alaska. Encephalitis has been reported from the eastern provinces. In the Midwest, antibodies to Trivittatus virus are common, but only one case of human illness has been reported. Clinical features of Tahyna virus disease, which has been seen in children in Europe, include fever, pharyngitis, pneumonitis, gastrointestinal symptoms, and aseptic meningitis. Neither mortality nor sequelae are reported.

EASTERN EQUINE ENCEPHALITIS Eastern equine encephalitis (EEE), an alphavirus, was first isolated in 1933 from the brain tissue of horses during an outbreak of equine illness in New Jersey. The first recognized human outbreak occurred in Massachusetts in 1938.

Epidemiology The virus is distributed along the East Coast of the Americas from northeastern United States to Argentina. Foci have been found in the Syracuse region of New York, Ontario, Canada, western Michigan, and South Dakota. Viral isolations also have been reported in the Philippines, Thailand, Czechoslovakia, Poland, and the former Soviet Union, but the question of type specificity has not been resolved. In the northeastern United States, epidemics occur in the late summer and early fall. Epizootics in horses precede the occurrence of human cases by 1 to 2 weeks. The disease affects mainly infants, children, and adults over 55 years of age. There is no sex preponderance. Inapparent infection occurs in all age groups, suggesting that the decreased likelihood of developing overt infection in the 15- to

54-year age group is not the result of decreased exposure. The ratio of inapparent infection to overt encephalitis approximates 25:1.

The transmission of EEE involves *Culiseta melanura* mosquitoes and swamp-dwelling birds, e.g., red-winged blackbirds, sparrows, pheasants. Transmission by pecking has been shown in domestic pheasant flocks. *C. melanura* rarely feed on horses or humans, and other mosquitoes, especially *Aedes sollicitans*, a salt-marsh mosquito which is an avid human feeder, have been postulated as the epidemic vector. In June 1991, EEE virus was isolated from *A. albopictus* in Florida. *A. albopictus* has the potential for becoming an important epidemic vector. The epidemiology of overwintering and maintenance between outbreaks remains unknown. Equine animals and human beings are "dead ends" in the transmission cycle, and infection in them is accidental.

Clinical manifestations Though human infections have been thought usually to result in serious, if not fatal, central nervous system involvement, the detection of inapparent infection as well as relatively mild disease establishes the occurrence of milder forms. In many patients, the CSF is cloudy and contains in excess of 1000 cells per microliter.

Diagnosis ELISA tests for the detection of specific IgM antibodies in CSF or serum permit early diagnosis, although absence of IgM does not exclude infection. Confirmation can be obtained by a fourfold or more rise or fall in complement fixation (CF), hemagglutination inhibition, or virus neutralization tests.

Prognosis The mortality rate in clinical infection exceeds 50 percent. In the most severe cases, death occurs between the third and fifth days. Children under 10 years of age have a greater likelihood of surviving the acute illness, but they also have a greater likelihood of developing severe disabling residuals: mental retardation, convulsions, emotional lability, blindness, deafness, speech disorders, and hemiplegia.

ST. LOUIS ENCEPHALITIS St. Louis encephalitis (SLE) was first recognized as an entity during a major outbreak in St. Louis, Missouri, in 1933. Subsequently, sporadic, unpredictable outbreaks have occurred in the Ohio-Mississippi Valley, eastern Texas, Florida, Kansas, Colorado, and California. The attack rate in Greenville, Mississippi, in 1975 was the highest which has been encountered, 10 per 10,000 population.

Epidemiology In the United States, epidemics of SLE fall into two epidemiologic patterns. One pattern is found in the West, where mixed outbreaks of western equine encephalitis and SLE have occurred primarily in irrigated rural areas. The vector has been *Culex tarsalis*. The second pattern occurred in the original St. Louis outbreak and the numerous subsequent epidemics in the Midwest, Texas, New Jersey, and Florida. These outbreaks have been more urban in location and are characterized by occurrence of encephalitis in older persons. In such urban-suburban epidemics, the epidemic vectors have been mosquitoes of the *Culex pipiens-quinquefasciatus* complex with the exception of the Florida epidemic, in which *Culex nigripalpus* was incriminated. The presence of SLE virus outside the United States has been proved by isolations in Trinidad, Panama, Jamaica, Brazil, and Argentina. However, except for Jamaica, SLE has not been reported outside the United States. The basic transmission cycle is that of wild bird–mosquito–wild bird. The virus survives the winter in female mosquitoes which ingest a blood meal from a viremic bird before overwintering. The disease in humans usually appears in midsummer to early fall. In urban epidemics, there is no sex predominance, while among sporadic cases in the West, men predominate 2:1 due to greater occupational exposure. The human represents an accidental host and plays no role in the basic transmission cycle. Serologic studies following most urban epidemics indicate that infection rates are similar in all age groups and that the increasing age-specific attack rate for clinical encephalitis which is typical of urban St. Louis encephalitis is probably due to age differences in host susceptibility to overt disease rather than to a higher rate of infection.

Clinical manifestations Infection with SLE virus most commonly results in an inapparent infection. Of the patients with confirmed disease, approximately three-fourths have clinical encephalitis; the remainder present with aseptic meningitis, febrile headaches, or nonspecific illness. Virtually all patients over 40 years have encephalitic manifestations. Urinary frequency and dysuria have been symptoms in approximately 20 percent of patients despite sterile routine aerobic urine cultures. SLE virus antigen has been demonstrated in urine; viruria may account for the occurrence of urinary tract symptoms.

Diagnosis The occurrence of either encephalitis or aseptic meningitis as manifested by febrile illness with CSF pleocytosis in the months of June through September in an adult, especially over 35 years of age, should raise the suspicion of St. Louis encephalitis. Because approximately 40 percent of patients with SLE have antibodies detectable by hemagglutination inhibition at the onset of illness, acute serum for serologic studies should be submitted promptly to a competent laboratory. ELISA tests for the detection of specific IgM antibodies in CSF or serum provide a means of early specific diagnosis.

Prognosis The case-fatality ratio in the original St. Louis epidemic was 20 percent. In most subsequent outbreaks the mortality rate has varied from 2 to 12 percent. Subjective complaints, including nervousness, headaches, and easy fatigability and excitability, appear to be the most common residuals. Late organic defects such as speech defects, difficulty in walking, and disturbances in vision were demonstrated in approximately 5 percent of patients 3 years following infection.

WESTERN EQUINE ENCEPHALITIS Western equine encephalitis (WEE) virus is an alphavirus that was isolated in 1930 in California from horses with encephalitis. In 1938 it was recovered from a fatal human infection.

Epidemiology WEE virus has been isolated in the United States, Canada, Brazil, Guyana, and Argentina. Human disease has been diagnosed in the United States, Canada, and Brazil. In the United States, the virus is found in virtually all geographic areas. The central valley of California represents an important endemic area. The disease occurs mainly in early and midsummer. Wild birds, which develop viremia of sufficiently high titer to be able to infect mosquitoes that feed on them, are the basic reservoir. *Culex tarsalis* is the principal vector in the western United States. In areas east of the Appalachian Mountains, the virus has been repeatedly isolated from *Culiseta melanura;* however, the importance of this species has been questioned, since it is not primarily a human-biting mosquito. The overwintering mechanism is not known. The ratio of inapparent infection to disease, as evidenced by serologic survey studies, varies from 1:1 in infants to 58:1 in children to 1150:1 in adults. Approximately one-fourth of patients are less than 1 year of age. The highest attack rates occur in persons 55 years or older.

Prognosis The case-fatality rate approximates 3 percent in laboratory-confirmed cases. The incidence and severity of sequelae are related to age. Sequelae among very young infants are frequent (appearing in 61 percent of a group of patients less than 3 months old) and severe; they consist of upper motor neuron impairment, involving the pyramidal tracts, extrapyramidal structures, and cerebellum, and result in behavioral problems and convulsions. Both the incidence and severity of sequelae diminish rapidly after 1 year of age. Adults may complain of nervousness, irritability, easy fatigability, and tremulousness for 6 months or longer after the acute illness. Probably not more than 5 percent of adults have sequelae which are sufficiently severe to be of practical significance. Postencephalitic seizures are rare.

JAPANESE ENCEPHALITIS The name *Japanese B encephalitis* was employed during an epidemic which occurred in 1924 to distinguish it from von Economo's disease, which was designated as type A encephalitis. The designation as Japanese B no longer seems useful, and the term *Japanese encephalitis* (JE) is used.

Epidemiology JE virus infection is known to occur in eastern Siberia, China, Korea, Japan, all of Southeast Asia, Guam, Nepal, and India. Since the late 1960s, JE has virtually disappeared in Japan

(<20 cases annually) and is declining in China (still >10,000 cases annually). JE remains a major problem in northern Thailand (attack rates of 10 to 20 per 100,000 annually). In temperate climates, the disease shows a late-summer–early-fall seasonal incidence. In tropical climates, epidemics occur mainly in the summer monsoon months. The mosquito *Culex tritaeniorhynchus* is the major vector species. It is a rural mosquito which breeds in rice fields and preferentially bites large domestic animals, such as pigs, but also feeds on birds and humans. The human is an accidental host in the transmission cycle. In endemic areas, children ages 3 to 15 are primarily affected. Epidemics in nonendemic areas have affected all age groups, but young children and older adults predominate. The ratio of inapparent infection, as evidenced by a serologic survey study of Australian troops in Vietnam, was 210:1.

Clinical manifestations The incubation period is 5 to 15 days. As with SLE, illness may present as encephalitis, aseptic meningitis, or febrile headache. The occurrence of severe rigors at the onset has been noted in almost 90 percent of patients. On admission, most patients are alert, but deterioration of mental status occurs in about three-fourths of patients within 3 to 4 days. Localized paresis is found more often than with other "arboviral" encephalitides, e.g., in 31 percent of cases, with predominantly upper extremity involvement; however, it resolves rapidly with defervescence. Convulsions are frequent in children but occur in less than 10 percent of adults. Severe hyperthermia may occur and require treatment. A peripheral leukocytosis with 50 to 90 percent neutrophils is common. Weight loss has been very striking. The failure of the temperature to lyse, appearance of diaphoresis, tachypnea, and the accumulation of bronchial secretions are grave prognostic signs.

Prognosis The immediate mortality rate has varied from 7 to 50 percent and is highest in young children and persons over 65. The occurrence of sequelae varies inversely with the case-fatality rate; in those series with high case-fatality rates (33 percent), sequelae occurred in 3 to 14 percent. In another series with a case-fatality rate of 7.4 percent, the rate of adverse sequelae was 32 percent. Individuals who had neurologic abnormalities during the acute phase but survived have no more than an 80 percent chance for complete recovery. Sequelae consist of seizures, persistent paralysis, ataxia, mental retardation, and behavioral disorders.

Prevention Cases have been reported among U.S. citizens traveling to endemic areas (Southeast Asia, China). In 1983, the Centers for Disease Control obtained an investigational new drug exemption from the Food and Drug Administration to evaluate the BIKEN JE vaccine. The vaccine is inactivated and prepared in mouse brain. Protective efficacy has been 80 percent or more, with adverse effects occurring in fewer than 1 percent of vaccinees. Millions of doses have been administered. In non-Asian adults, a three-dose immunization schedule probably affords the best protection. JE vaccine is still not licensed and available in the United States, but it is available in Canada and many European countries. Vaccine should be considered for travelers during summer monsoon months whose activities will include travel into rural farming areas or sleeping in unscreened quarters.

OTHER "ARBOVIRUSES" WITH CENTRAL NERVOUS SYSTEM INVOLVEMENT A large number of additional "arboviruses" have been associated with encephalitis or aseptic meningitis. Some of these agents are listed in Table 159-2. Though the epidemiologic picture of each of these agents is unique, the general features are sufficiently similar to require laboratory support for their differentiation.

DISEASES PRESENTING CHIEFLY WITH HEMORRHAGIC MANIFESTATIONS

For 300 years, yellow fever was the only epidemic viral disease known to be accompanied by grave hemorrhagic manifestations. Since the 1930s, diverse viral etiologies of the hemorrhagic fever syndrome have been recognized (see Table 159-2). Additional agents include members of several families and genera: flavivirus, Filoviri-

dae, phlebovirus, Nairovirus, Hantavirus, and arenavirus (see Chap. 160). Despite diverse causes, there are many similar clinical manifestations. The onset is usually sudden, with headache, backache, generalized myalgia, conjunctivitis, and prostration. From approximately the third day, the initial stage is followed by hypotension, and hemorrhagic manifestations may occur; these are characterized by bleeding gums, epistaxis, hemoptysis, hematemesis, melena, petechiae, ecchymoses, and hemorrhages into most visceral organs. Mild leukopenia develops early, but with the appearance of hemorrhagic manifestations, leukocytosis may occur. The pathophysiology of the cardinal signs is attributable to hematopoietic and capillary damage, with variable localization of lesions. On the basis of limited confirmatory observations, variable degrees of disseminated intravascular coagulation may be in part responsible for the pathophysiology of the hemorrhagic fever syndromes. Death usually occurs in the second week of disease, at which time a high titer of antibody has developed and the patient may have become afebrile. Death is usually associated with coma, which is due not to encephalitis but to an encephalopathy. The pathologic changes may be similar despite diverse viral causes, with midzonal hepatic necrosis and acidophilic cytoplasmic inclusions similar to the Councilman bodies of yellow fever.

YELLOW FEVER Yellow fever is an acute infectious disease of short duration and extremely variable severity; it is caused by a flavivirus and is followed by lifelong immunity. The classic triad of symptoms—jaundice, hemorrhages, and intense albuminuria—is present only in severe infections, which make up only a small proportion of the total.

Prevalence For more than 200 years, after the first identifiable outbreak occurred in Yucatan in 1648, yellow fever was one of the great plagues of the world. As late as 1905, New Orleans and other southern United States ports experienced at least 5000 cases and 1000 deaths. Because of the existence of the sylvatic form of the disease, protective measures must be maintained against human disease. During the past 20 years, outbreaks and extensive epidemics have occurred in South America (Bolivia, Brazil, Colombia, Ecuador, Peru, Venezuela) and Africa (Burkino Faso, Gambia, Ghana, Nigeria, Senegal). In southern Ethiopia from 1962 to 1964 there were over 100,000 cases with some 30,000 deaths. In Gambia the attack rate was 2.6 to 4.4 percent, with a case-fatality rate of 19 percent. Yellow fever has never occurred in Asia.

Epidemiology Human infection results from two different cycles of virus transmission, urban and sylvatic. The urban cycle is human-mosquito-human, i.e., *Aedes aegypti*–transmitted yellow fever. After a 2-week extrinsic incubation period, mosquitoes can transmit infection. Sylvan yellow fever differs under various ecologic circumstances. In the rain forests of South and Central America, species of treetop *Haemagogus* or *Sabethes* mosquitoes maintain transmission in wild primates. Once infected, the mosquito vector remains infectious for life; hence it may serve as a reservoir as well as a vector. When humans come into proximity with the forest-canopy mosquitoes, sporadic cases or focal outbreaks may occur. With sylvan yellow fever, males predominate. Focal outbreaks may be quite extensive; in Brazil in 1973 at least 21,000 persons out of 1.5 million (1.4 percent) were infected. In east Africa, the mosquito-primate cycle is maintained by the forest-canopy mosquito *A. africanus*, which seldom feeds on humans. The peridomestic mosquito *A. simpsoni* feeds on primates entering the village gardens and can then in turn transmit the virus to humans. Once yellow fever is reintroduced into urban areas, the *A. aegypti*–borne urban cycle can be reinitiated, with the potential for epidemic disease. In the Americas, *A. aegypti* outbreaks have not occurred for 30 years, while in Africa, both sylvan and urban epidemics have occurred.

Clinical manifestations The incubation period is usually 3 to 6 days. In accidental laboratory- or hospital-acquired infections, longer incubation periods (10 to 13 days) have been reported. In mild yellow fever the only symptoms may be the abrupt onset of fever and headache. Additional symptoms may include nausea, epistaxis, relative bradycardia known as *Faget's sign* [e.g., with a temperature of 38.9°C (102°F) the pulse may be only 48 to 52 beats per minute], and slight albuminuria. The mild illness lasts only 1 to 3 days and resembles influenza except that coryzal symptoms are lacking.

Moderately severe and malignant attacks of yellow fever are characterized by three distinct clinical periods: the period of infection, the period of remission, and the period of intoxication. Prodromal symptoms are usually absent. The onset is characteristically sudden, with headache, dizziness, and temperature elevations to 40°C (104°F) without a relative bradycardia. Young children may have febrile convulsions. The headache is followed quickly by pains in the neck, back, and legs. Often there is nausea with vomiting and retching. Examination reveals a flushed face and injection of the conjunctivae. The congestion of the eyes persists until the third day. The tongue characteristically shows bright-red margins and tip and a white furred center. Faget's sign appears by the second day. Epistaxis and gingival bleeding are common. On the third day of illness the fever may fall by crisis and the patient enters remission, or in the malignant form, copious hemorrhages, anuria, or delirium may occur. The stage of remission lasts from several hours to several days. In the third stage, the "classic" symptoms develop; the fever returns, but the pulse remains slow. Jaundice becomes detectable about the third day; however, jaundice often is not prominent even in fatal illnesses. Increased epistaxis, melena, and uterine hemorrhages are common, but gross hematuria is rare. Of the classic signs, "black vomit" is more characteristic than is jaundice. Hematemesis usually does not occur before the fourth day and is often associated with a fatal outcome. Albuminuria, which rarely develops before the third day, occurs in 90 percent of patients and may be quite marked (3 to 20 g albumin per liter). Despite this massive albuminuria, edema or ascites has not been reported. In malignant infections, coma frequently occurs 2 to 3 days before death. Shortly before death, which usually occurs between the fourth and the sixth days, the patient becomes delirious and wildly agitated. Though the duration of fever in the third stage is usually 5 to 7 days, the period of intoxication is the most variable of the stages and may last up to 2 weeks. Yellow fever is relatively free from complications, suppurative parotitis being the most striking of those which do occur. Clinical relapses are not characteristic of yellow fever.

Laboratory findings Early in the disease, progressive leukopenia may occur. By the fifth day, total leukocyte counts of 1500 to 2500 cells per microliter often are found, the decrease being due mostly to a decrease in neutrophils. Total leukocyte counts return to normal by the tenth day, and in fatal cases there may be a marked terminal leukocytosis. Hemoglobin values remain normal except terminally, when hemoconcentration or bleeding may occur. Platelet counts are normal or decreased. Prolongation of clotting, prothrombin, and partial thromboplastin times is marked in patients with jaundice. Increases in total and conjugated bilirubin occur. In icteric patients, marked elevations of serum glutamic oxaloacetic transaminase occur. Hypoglycemia has been seen in patients with severe hepatic damage. Electrocardiograms may show T-wave changes. The CSF is normal.

Diagnosis Inoculation onto mosquito cell cultures and intrathoracically into mosquitoes are methods of choice for virus isolation from blood. Isolation is most likely from specimens obtained during the first 3 days of illness. Serologic methods include plaque reduction neutralization tests on paired sera and detection of yellow fever IgM antibodies and antigen usually by ELISA methods. The ELISA method enables confirmation in the field within 3 h.

Treatment The management has been symptomatic and supportive and should be based on assessment and correction of the circulatory abnormalities. Close attention to fluids and electrolytes is essential. As with all the hemorrhagic fevers, aspirin is contraindicated. Ribavirin has in vitro antiviral activity against yellow fever virus, but trials in experimentally infected monkeys showed no therapeutic effect.

Prognosis The overall fatality rate in yellow fever is between 5 and 10 percent of clinical cases; it may be even less, since many infections are mild or inapparent.

Prevention Effective control measures are available. Immunization with the 17 Da vaccine has been effective in the prevention of outbreaks. With the occurrence of sylvatic outbreaks, work in the area of epizootic activity should be discontinued, and intensive mosquito abatement measures should be instituted. These measures may provide the time necessary for a mass immunization program.

DENGUE HEMORRHAGIC FEVER All four dengue virus serotypes can cause dengue hemorrhagic fever (DHF) and dengue shock syndrome (DSS). Infection with dengue 1, 3, or 4 followed within a few years by dengue 2 may be especially important in the pathogenesis. There is consensus that DHF is an immunologically mediated disease. Enhanced growth of dengue 2 virus occurs in peripheral blood mononuclear phagocytes obtained from dengue immune donors or in cells from normal donors in the presence of subneutralizing concentrations of dengue or cross-reacting heterotypic flavivirus antibodies. Infectious virus-antibody complexes attach and enter mononuclear phagocytes by way of Fc receptors. Increased replication of virus in macrophages may result in clinical "sepsis" due to excessive production of tumor necrosis factor, interleukins, and platelet-activiting factor.

Prevalence The reasons for the apparent sudden "appearance" of the syndrome in the past 40 years are completely obscure. However, during the 1922 epidemic of dengue fever in Louisiana, hemorrhagic manifestations, including epistaxis, bleeding gums, melena, menorrhagia, and even "black vomit," were observed. DHF is now a leading cause of morbidity and mortality in tropical Asia. Over 500,000 cases of DHF have been officially reported, with major epidemics in the People's Republic of China, Vietnam, Indonesia, Thailand, and Cuba. In the Cuban outbreak in 1981, almost 350,000 persons developed dengue, approximately 10,000 had hemorrhagic manifestations, and 158 died (1.6 percent mortality). DHF in Asia is a disease of childhood, with one peak observed in children under 1 year and a second in children ages 3 to 5. The disease in infants is associated with primary infection in the presence of maternal antibody. Studies in Thailand have estimated the frequency of DSS as 11 cases per 1000 secondary dengue infections. DSS occurs more frequently in girls than in boys. Dengue hemorrhagic fever occurs almost exclusively in indigenous populations; it has been observed only rarely in whites of European descent, despite the frequent occurrence of classic dengue in this group.

Clinical manifestations Illness begins abruptly, with a minor stage characterized by fever, cough, pharyngitis, headache, anorexia, nausea, vomiting, and abdominal pain which is often severe. This continues for 2 to 4 days. In contrast to classic dengue, myalgia, arthralgia, and bone pain are unusual. Physical signs include fever varying from 38.3 to 40.6°C (101 to 105°F), injection of the tonsils and pharynx, and palpable lymph nodes and liver. The initial state is followed by abrupt deterioration, with the rapid onset of lassitude and weakness (Table 159-4). On examination, the child is found to be restless and to have cold clammy extremities with a warm trunk and a pallid face with circumoral cyanosis. Petechiae, most frequently

TABLE 159-4 World Health Organization's clinical classification of dengue hemorrhagic fever

	Grade	Clinical features	Laboratory findings
DHF* {	I	Fever, constitutional symptoms, positive tourniquet test	Hemoconcentration Thrombocytopenia
	II	Grade I plus spontaneous bleeding (e.g., skin, gums, gastrointestinal tract)	Hemoconcentration Thrombocytopenia
DSS* {	III	Grade II plus circulatory failure, agitation	Hemoconcentration Thrombocytopenia
	IV	Grade II plus profound shock (blood pressure = 0)	Hemoconcentration Thrombocytopenia

* DHF, dengue hemorrhagic fever; DSS, dengue shock syndrome.

located on the forehead and distal extremities, are seen in half the cases. Occasionally there may be a macular or maculopapular rash. The extremities are frequently cyanotic. Hypotension, with narrowing of the pulse pressure, and tachycardia occur. Pathologic reflexes may be present. Most fatalities occur in the fourth or fifth day of illness; melena, hematemesis, coma, or unresponsive shock are poor prognostic signs. Cyanosis, dyspnea, and convulsions are terminal manifestations. Following this critical period, survivors show steady and rapid improvement.

Laboratory findings In one study, hemoconcentration was found in one-fifth of the children. The majority had leukocyte counts between 5000 and 10,000 cells per microliter, with one-third showing a leukocytosis. Only 10 percent of children had a true leukopenia. The most characteristic findings were thrombocytopenia, rarely with blood platelets under 75,000 cells per microliter, positive tourniquet test, and prolonged bleeding time. Prothrombin time and partial thromboplastin times were usually near normal values. Depression of clotting factors V, VII, IX, and X may be present. Bone marrow examination may reveal maturation arrest of megakaryocytes. In Manila or Bangkok, hematuria has been infrequent even with other serious bleeding manifestations; however, in Tahiti, gross hematuria was common. CSF examinations are usually normal. Other abnormal laboratory findings may include hyponatremia, acidosis, elevated blood urea nitrogen levels, elevation in serum glutamic oxalacetic transaminase levels, mild hyperbilirubinemia, and hypoproteinemia. Electrocardiograms may reveal diffuse myocardial abnormalities. Two-thirds of patients have radiologic evidence of bronchopneumonia, with many showing pleural effusions. Ultrasonography is useful in detecting pleural effusions, ascites, and thickening of the gallbladder wall.

Diagnosis The World Health Organization (WHO) has established criteria for the diagnosis of DHF: fever—acute onset, high, continuous, and lasting for 2 to 7 days; hemorrhagic manifestations, including at least a positive tourniquet test and any of the following: petechiae, purpura, ecchymoses, epistaxis, bleeding gums, hematemesis, or melena; enlargement of the liver; thrombocytopenia, ≤100,000 cells per microliter; hemoconcentration, hematocrit increased by ≥20 percent. Criteria for DSS are a rapid, weak pulse with narrowing of the pulse pressure (≤20 mmHg) or hypotension with cold, clammy skin and restlessness. The WHO classification includes a grading of severity (see Table 159-4). Minor hemorrhagic manifestations may be seen during the course of classic dengue fever without meeting WHO criteria for DHF. These cases should be termed *dengue fever with hemorrhage*, not DHF.

Treatment The mainstay is correction of circulatory collapse while avoiding fluid overload. Administration of 5% glucose in 0.5 *N* saline at a rate of 40 mL/kg restored blood pressure within 1 to 2 h in one-half of patients. When stable, the rate of administration of intravenous fluids was slowed to 10 mL/kg per hour. If improvement did not occur, plasma or a plasma expander (20 mL/kg) was administered. Transfusion of whole blood is not recommended. Oxygen should be administered. Glucocorticoids have been used, but doses of 25 mg/kg have not resulted in significant improvement. Since the evidence for severe disseminated intravascular coagulation is questionable, use of heparin is not clear-cut, although in a group of Filipino children with type 3 dengue virus, administration of heparin (1 mg sodium heparin per kilogram) was associated with a dramatic rise in number of platelets and level of plasma fibrinogen. Antibiotics are not indicated; sympathomimetic amines and salicylates are contraindicated. Recovery from vascular collapse usually occurs within 24 to 48 h, at which time diuretics and digitalis may be necessary. An uncontrolled trial of interferon was conducted during the 1981 epidemic in Cuba with some indication of efficacy.

Prognosis Mortality has varied from 1 to 23 percent. Deaths have been most common in infants under 1 year of age.

Prevention At present, vector control is the only method available to prevent hemorrhagic fever.

TICK-BORNE HEMORRHAGIC FEVERS   Crimean-Congo hemorrhagic fever

At the close of World War II, a new disease entity was recognized in the Crimea region of the former Soviet Union. Retrospective studies demonstrated that an almost identical syndrome had been recognized in the south central Asian republics of the former Soviet Union for many years. Soviet workers repeatedly isolated virus strains during 1967 to 1969.

The virus of Crimean hemorrhagic fever (CHF) is antigenically identical with Congo virus, which was isolated from patients, cattle, and ticks in Kenya, Uganda, Zaire, and Nigeria. Crimean-Congo hemorrhagic fever (CCHF) virus is now known in South Africa, throughout most of subsaharan Africa, eastern Europe, the Middle East, and Asia as far as the Xinjiang Province of China. CCHF occurs where *Hyalomma* ticks are found.

The cases occur between April and September. The sex distribution of CCHF is equal, and 80 percent of the cases occur in the 20- to 60-year age group, with the majority occurring in dairy and agricultural workers. The major arthropod vectors for transmission to humans are ticks which belong to the genus *Hyalomma*. Cattle and wild hares appear to be important reservoirs, and rooks and other birds have been implicated. Once a case of human CCHF occurs, person-to-person transmission is possible. Nosocomial outbreaks have occurred in the former Soviet Union, Pakistan, India, and Iraq. Transmission is presumed to occur through direct contact with infected blood. There are no data to suggest airborne transmission.

After an incubation period of 3 to 6 days, the onset is abrupt, with temperatures to 40°C (104°F), dizziness, headache, and diffuse myalgia. The course of fever is occasionally biphasic, with an average duration of 8 days. Findings include flushing of the face, conjunctival injection, vomiting, and, on occasion, epigastric pain. Hepatomegaly occurs in half the patients. Splenomegaly has been reported in 2 to 25 percent of patients. Respiratory symptoms or signs are unusual. Hemorrhagic manifestations generally begin on the fourth day, with petechiae on the oral mucosa and skin, epistaxis, gingival bleeding, hematemesis, and melena. Neurologic abnormalities, seen in 10 to 25 percent of patients, include nuchal rigidity, excitation, and coma. Laboratory findings show leukopenia, with the number of white blood cells falling as low as 1000 cells per microliter, and thrombocytopenia, which is often severe. Proteinuria and microscopic hematuria are common, but azotemia and oliguria are not. Convalescence may be prolonged. Death is usually attributed to shock or intercurrent infection. Sequelae include transient alopecia and mono- or polyneuritis.

The major approach to therapy has been supportive. Convalescent immune serum has shown promise if administered during the first 3 days of illness. Patients should be isolated, with contact restricted to hospital staff and immediate family. Masks and gowns should be worn, and blood and body fluids should be handled as infectious. The reported mortality rate has varied between 9 and 50 percent.

Omsk hemorrhagic fever Omsk hemorrhagic fever (OHF) is an acute febrile disease which occurs in the Omsk and Novosibirsk oblasts in the former Soviet Union and is caused by a flavivirus. OHF is transmitted to humans either by the bite of infected ticks, *Ixodes apronophorus*, or by the handling of infected muskrats. Epidemics occurred from 1945 to 1948, but recently the disease has been less prevalent.

Following an incubation interval of 3 to 8 days, illness begins abruptly with fever, headache, and hemorrhagic manifestations, which include epistaxis and gastrointestinal and uterine bleeding. OHF has a low case-fatality rate (0.5 to 3.0 percent).

Kyasanur Forest disease Kyasanur Forest disease was shown to be due to a flavivirus. Kyasanur Forest disease occurs following occupational exposure to *Haemaphysalis spinigera* ticks in the tropical forests of western Mysore in southern India. Laboratory-associated infections have been common.

The major symptoms include abrupt onset of fever, headache, fatigue, myalgia (especially of the lumbar area and calf muscles), and retroorbital pain. Cough and abdominal pain occur in half the patients. On examination, findings include relative bradycardia, conjunctival injection, and generalized lymphadenopathy. Fine and coarse rales are frequently heard. The fever usually lasts from 6 to 11 days. After an afebrile period of 9 to 21 days, approximately half the patients may develop a second phase, which lasts from 2 to 12 days. This is manifested by recurrence of fever, severe headache, neck stiffness, mental disturbance, coarse tremors, giddiness, and abnormalities in reflexes, as well as by recurrence of many of the initial symptoms. No sequelae have been observed, but convalescence is often prolonged.

Only limited laboratory studies have been reported. During the initial phase, leukopenia is a constant feature. During the second phase, there is a mild leukocytosis. Lumbar puncture during the second phase has shown a pattern of aseptic meningitis. Diagnosis is based upon virus isolation from blood. Serologic tests of paired sera also can be performed. The management is supportive. The mortality rate is approximately 5 percent.

HEMORRHAGIC FEVER WITH RENAL SYNDROME

Synonyms for this disease (HFRS) include *Korean hemorrhagic fever*, *Far Eastern hemorrhagic fever*, *endemic* or *epidemic nephroso-nephritis*, *Manchurian epidemic hemorrhagic fever*, *Songo fever*, and *Churilov's disease*. A similar but milder disease in Scandinavia has been called *nephropathia epidemica* or *epidemic nephritis* (EN).

ETIOLOGY In 1976, the antigen of HFRS was demonstrated in the lungs of the rodent *Apodemus agrarius coreae*. Diagnostic increases in immunofluorescent antibodies were demonstrated in 113 of 116 cases of severe HFRS. The agent designated *Hantaan virus* is a single-stranded RNA virus belonging to the family Bunyaviridae, genus Hantavirus (see Table 159-1). The genus consists of at least five species: Hantaan virus (Korean hemorrhagic fever), Seoul virus, Puumala virus (nephropathia epidemica), Porogia virus (Balkan HFRS), and Prospect Hill virus (isolated from meadow voles in Maryland and associated with human infection, not disease).

PREVALENCE In Korea between April 1951 and January 1953, 2070 cases of epidemic hemorrhagic fever were reported among United Nations personnel. In a recent analysis of sera collected in 1951–1954 from 245 clinically diagnosed patients, 94 percent had specific IgM antibody against Hantaan virus. The disease usually occurs as an isolated event; hence overall attack rates have relatively less meaning. With this reservation, attack rates in two United States Army divisions stationed in Korea varied between 1.9 and 2.9 cases per 1000 persons per epidemic season. Approximately 800 cases per year have continued to occur; however, most cases are now seen in Korean civilians and military, with less than 10 cases per year in U.S. military personnel. During the past 15 years, the disease has increased in prevalence in Korea, urban Japan, and China. In the People's Republic of China, over 100,000 cases of HFRS are reported annually; the incidence is increasing. Hundreds of cases of EN have occurred annually in Finland and other Scandinavian countries since the 1930s. In 1953 a severe form of HFRS was recognized in the Balkan countries, and in 1982, in Greece and France. Antibody studies indicate worldwide distribution. Antibodies in human sera have been found in Argentina, Brazil, Colombia, Europe, Canada, the United States (including Hawaii and Alaska), Southeast Asia, Egypt, and central Africa.

EPIDEMIOLOGY In Korea, the majority of cases occur in May to June and in October to November. These peaks coincide with rodent population density. Hantaan virus is present in rodent urine, feces, and saliva in high titer. Transmission from rodent to rodent is primarily respiratory, with transmission to people through inhalation of virus-containing dried excreta. There is no evidence for person-to-person transmission. The urban reservoir appears to be the house rat. Laboratory-acquired cases have occurred in the former Soviet Union,

Korea, Japan, and Europe, with rats implicated in Korea, Japan, and the United Kingdom.

CLINICAL MANIFESTATIONS There are two forms of disease, a mild illness characteristically diagnosed in Scandinavia as epidemic nephritis (EN) and the more severe HFRS seen especially in the Far East and central Europe.

EN is characterized by sudden onset of high fever, backache, headache, and abdominal pain. On the third or fourth day, hemorrhagic manifestations may occur, and conjunctival hemorrhages, palatine petechiae, and a petechial rash appear on the trunk. About one patient in five is "toxic" and mentally obtunded. Oliguria and azotemia develop. Urinalysis reveals proteinuria, hematuria, and leukocyturia. After about 3 days the rash subsides, the patient develops polyuria, and recovers in several weeks.

Hemorrhagic fever with renal syndrome (HFRS) The incubation period in HFRS is usually 10 to 25 days, with possible extremes of 7 and 36 days. Visitors who contract the disease in an endemic area may not develop illness until after their return home.

The clinical course of HFRS may be divided into phases on the basis of the underlying physiologic aberrations: febrile, hypotensive, oliguric, diuretic, and convalescent. There is considerable variation among patients in the severity of the illness. In one study, two-thirds of the 264 cases studied were classified as mild, while 14 percent were termed severe.

FEBRILE (INVASIVE) PHASE From 10 to 20 percent of patients describe vague prodromal symptoms resembling mild upper respiratory infections. The onset is then usually abrupt, often initiated by a chill and accompanied by fever, headache, backache, abdominal pain, and generalized myalgia. Anorexia and thirst are almost universal, while nausea and vomiting are common, although not constant, symptoms. The headache is most commonly frontal or retroorbital. Eye symptoms, especially mild photophobia and pain on movement of the eyes, are characteristic. Diarrhea is not a feature. Fever is present in almost all patients; the temperature ranges from 37.8 to 41.1°C (100 to 106°F), reaches a peak on the third or fourth day after onset, and falls by lysis on the fourth to seventh day. There is a relative bradycardia. Initially the blood pressure is normal. One of the most typical early findings is a diffuse reddening of the skin, most marked over the face and V area of the neck, that may resemble a severe sunburn. The erythema blanches on pressure. Dermographism can be demonstrated in over 90 percent of patients at the same time as the flush. Slight edema of the upper eyelids causes a bleary-eyed appearance. Bulbar and palpebral conjunctivae show injection. Conjunctival petechiae may develop by the third or fifth day of illness. Subconjunctival hemorrhages may be striking. Intense pharyngeal reddening without significant sore throat is typical. The first location for petechiae is usually the palate, where they occur in half the patients. Within 12 to 24 h, petechiae appear at pressure areas such as the axillary folds, lateral chest wall, belt line, hips, and thighs. Retinal hemorrhages occur rarely. Cervical, axillary, and inguinal nodes are moderately enlarged but nontender. Abdominal and costovertebral tenderness is almost a constant finding. Splenomegaly is unusual. The degree of flush, fever, and conjunctival injection and the number of petechiae correlate quite well with the overall severity of illness.

Laboratory studies during this phase are often not striking. Initial hemoglobin and hematocrit values are usually normal. Prior to the fourth day, leukocyte counts range from 3600 to 6000 cells per microliter but are associated with neutrophilia. Early in the course urine specific gravity may be high. Albuminuria, which is an almost universal finding, appears, often abruptly, between the second and fifth days of illness. The urinary sediment reveals microscopic hematuria and hyaline, granular, red blood cell casts, and/or white blood cell casts. Erythrocyte sedimentation rates are normal during the first week. Capillary fragility tests are usually positive at the time of admission and become most abnormal by the ninth day. Electrocardiographic abnormalities may be seen in 15 to 30 percent of patients; these include sinus bradycardia and low or inverted T waves. Lumbar punctures may reveal gross blood in the spinal fluid.

HYPOTENSIVE PHASE   On about the fifth day of illness, during the last 24 to 48 h of the febrile phase, hypotension or shock may occur. In mild cases, only a transient fall in blood pressure occurs; among moderately and severely ill patients, shock may persist for 1 to 3 days. In 828 patients, 16.5 percent had clinical shock, and another 14 percent had hypotension without shock. Headache often diminishes, but thirst persists. In the beginning of the hypotensive phase, most patients have warm, dry skin and extremities. As the systolic blood pressure decreases and pulse pressure narrows, the skin becomes cool and moist. Tachycardia replaces the relative bradycardia.

At this stage an increase in hematocrit with no change in total serum protein level is found. This is thought to reflect a loss of plasma through damaged capillaries. On about the fifth day, all patients develop marked proteinuria. The previously normal urine specific gravity begins to fall and in 2 to 3 days is usually around 1.010. Blood urea nitrogen concentrations begin to increase. Other laboratory findings include leukocytosis with white blood cell counts of 10,000 to 56,000 per microliter with neutrophilia and toxic granulation. The number of platelets often decreases to less than 70,000 per microliter.

OLIGURIC PHASE (HEMORRHAGIC OR TOXIC PHASE)   About the eighth day of illness, blood pressure returns to the normal range and in some instances increases to hypertensive levels. While oliguria may have appeared during the shock phase, it now becomes a prominent feature. Oliguria develops even though hypotension was not recognized. Symptomatically, patients continue to feel weak and thirsty and have more severe backache. Protracted vomiting and hiccups may ensue.

Blood urea nitrogen levels increase rapidly and are associated with hyperkalemia, hyperphosphatemia, and hypocalcemia. Metabolic acidosis is rarely severe. Although platelets begin to return to normal, hemorrhagic manifestations become more prominent and include petechiae, hematemesis (analogous to "black vomit" in yellow fever), melena, hemoptysis, gross hematuria, and hemorrhages into the central nervous system. The enlarged lymph nodes may now become tender.

With the onset of diuresis on about the seventh to the eleventh day, symptoms of fluid and electrolyte abnormalities and central nervous system or pulmonary complications may appear. Central nervous system symptoms include disorientation, extreme restlessness, lethargy, paranoid delusions, and hallucinations. Grand mal seizures, pulmonary edema, and pulmonary infection occur in some patients.

DIURETIC PHASE   With the onset of diuresis, progressive improvement is the rule. Most patients begin to eat and regain their strength. In fatal cases, the diuretic phase is associated with a daily urine output of less than 4 L and often less than 2 L, in contrast to larger volumes in surviving patients.

CONVALESCENT PHASE   The convalescent phase lasts 3 to 6 weeks. Weight is regained slowly. Complaints include muscular weakness, intention tremor, and lack of stamina. Hyposthenuria and polyuria are present; however, within 2 months most patients are able to concentrate their urine to a specific gravity of 1.023 or greater after a 12-h period of water deprivation.

DIAGNOSIS   Diagnosis is based on demonstration of specific IgM antibodies by ELISA or a fourfold change in immune adherence hemagglutination titers in paired sera. Studies on the epidemiology of Hantavirus have shown that during the initial 24 to 72 h (febrile phase) there is significant overlap in the clinical features of leptospirosis, HFRS, and scrub typhus. In Korea, where all three diseases are prevalent, of blood samples submitted for Hantavirus serology, 21 percent had antibody to leptospira antigens and 6 percent to *Rickettsia tsutsugamushi*. Because of the similarity in epidemiology and clinical presentation and the potential for dual infections, it has been recommended that blood be submitted for Hantavirus serology in all cases of suspected leptospirosis (see Chap. 135).

TREATMENT   Clinical management primarily revolves around meticulous supportive care. Trials with a variety of agents, including antibiotics, glucocorticoids, antihistamines, convalescent serum, and interferon-α, were without significant beneficial effect during the Korean epidemics. In a controlled U.S./Chinese clinical trial in the People's Republic of China, ribavirin was shown to have efficacy.

PROGNOSIS   The experience in the former Soviet Union indicates a mortality rate of 3 to 32 percent; in China, the case-fatality ratio was 7 to 15 percent. Between April 1951 and December 1976, the overall case-fatality ratio in Korea was 6.6 percent.

Residua are uncommon. Of 783 surviving patients cared for at the Hemorrhagic Fever Center in Korea between April and December 1952, only 16 were unable to return to duty within a period of 4 months. Fifteen of these individuals still had hyposthenuria. Follow-up studies on patients 3 to 5 years later showed that they had many more subsequent hospital admissions for urologic problems than did a control group and that the relative frequency correlated with the severity of the acute episode of HFRS.

REFERENCES

"Arboviruses": Definition, classification, and general review

FIELDS BN et al (eds): *Virology*, 2d ed. New York, Raven, 1990

HALSTEAD SB: Dengue fever, viral hemorrhagic fever, and rabies. Curr Opin Infect Dis. 5:332, 1992

MONATH TP (ed): *The Arboviruses: Epidemiology and Ecology*, vols 2 to 4. Boca Raton, CRC Press, 1988, 1989

TSAI TF: Arboviral infections in the United States. Infect Dis Clin North Am 5:73, 1991

Infections characterized by fever, malaise, headaches, and myalgia

BOWEN GS et al: Clinical aspects of human Venezuelan equine encephalitis in Texas, 1971. Bull Pan Am Health Org 10:46, 1976

BRICENO ROSSIE AL: Rural epidemic encephalitis in Venezuela caused by a group A arbovirus (VEE). Prog Med Virol 9:176, 1967

DIETZ WH JR et al: Ten clinical cases of human infection with Venezuelan equine encephalomyelitis virus, subtype I–D. Am J Trop Med Hyg 28:329, 1979

FLEMING J et al: Sandfly fever. Review of 664 cases. Lancet 1:443, 1947

GOODPASTURE HC et al: Colorado tick fever: Clinical, epidemiologic and laboratory aspects of 228 cases in Colorado in 1973–1974. Ann Intern Med 88:303, 1978

HUGHES LE et al: Persistence of Colorado tick fever virus in red blood cells. Am J Trop Med Hyg 23:530, 1974

LAUGHLIN LW et al: Epidemic Rift Valley fever in Egypt: Observations of the spectrum of human illness. Trans R Soc Trop Med Hyg 73:630, 1979

LENNETTE EH, KOPROWSKI H: Human infection with Venezuelan equine encephalomyelitis virus. JAMA 123:1088, 1943

SCHERER WF et al: Ecologic studies of Venezuelan encephalitis virus in Southeastern Mexico: VII. Infection of man. Am J Trop Med 21:79, 1972

SIAM AL et al: Rift Valley fever ocular manifestations: Observations during 1977 epidemic in Egypt. Br J Ophthalmol 64:366, 1980

Infections presenting chiefly with fever, malaise, lymphadenopathy, and rash

ALVAREZ MD, RAMÍREZ-RONDA CH: Dengue and hepatic failure. Am J Med 79:670, 1985

CENTERS FOR DISEASE CONTROL: Dengue epidemic, Peru 1990. Morb Mort Week Rep 40:145, 1991

MICKS DW, MOON WB: *Aedes aegypti* in a Texas coastal county as an index of dengue fever receptivity and control. Am J Trop Med Hyg 29:1382, 1980

TSAI CJ et al: Upper gastrointestinal bleeding in Dengue fever. Am J Gastroenterol 86:33, 1991

Infections presenting chiefly with fever, acute arthropathy, and rash

AASKOV JG et al: An epidemic of Ross River virus infection in Fiji, 1979. Am J Trop Med Hyg 30:1053, 1981

CLARK JA et al: Annually recurrent epidemic polyarthritis and Ross River virus activity in a coastal area of New South Wales. I. Occurrence of the disease. Am J Trop Med Hyg 22:543, 1973

DELLER JJ JR, RUSSELL PK: Chikungunya disease. Am J Trop Med 17:107, 1968

PHILLIPS DA et al: Clinical and subclinical Barmah Forest virus infection in Queensland. Med J Aust 152:463, 1990

PINHEIRO FP et al: An outbreak of Mayaro virus disease in Belterra, Brazil: I. Clinical and virological findings. Am J Trop Med Hyg 30:674, 1981

ROBINSON MC: An epidemic of virus disease in Southern Province, Tanganyika territory in 1952–53: I. Clinical features. Trans R Soc Trop Med Hyg 49:28, 1955

SHORE H: O'nyong-nyong fever: An epidemic virus disease in East Africa: III. Some clinical and epidemiological observations in the Northern Province of Uganda. Trans R Soc Trop Med Hyg 55:361, 1961

Infections presenting chiefly with central nervous system involvement

BALFOUR HH JR et al: California arbovirus (LaCrosse) infections. Pediatrics 52:680, 1973

BURKE DS, LEAKE CJ: Japanese encephalitis, in *Arboviruses: Epidemiology and Ecology*, vol 3, TP Monath (ed). Boca Raton, CRC Press, 1998, p 63

CENTERS FOR DISEASE CONTROL: Eastern equine encephalitis virus associated with *Aedes albopictus*, Florida, 1991. Morb Mort Week Rep 41:115, 1992

DICKERSON RB et al: Diagnosis and immediate prognosis of Japanese B encephalitis. Observations based on more than 200 patients with detailed analysis of 65 serologically confirmed cases. Am J Med 12:277, 1952

FINLEY KH et al: Western equine and St. Louis encephalitis. Preliminary report of a clinical follow-up study in California. Neurology 5:223, 1955

GRABOW JD et al: The electroencephalogram and clinical sequelae of California arbovirus encephalitis. Neurology 19:394, 1969

HILTY MD et al: California encephalitis in children. Am J Dis Child 124:530, 1972

KETEL WB, OGNIBENE AJ: Japanese B encephalitis in Vietnam. Am J Med Sci 261:271, 1971

LUBY JP et al: The epidemiology of St. Louis encephalitis (SLE): A review. Ann Rev Med 20:329, 1969

————: Antigenemia in St. Louis encephalitis. Am J Trop Med Hyg 29:265, 1980

POLAND JD et al: Evaluation of potency and safety of inactivated Japanese encephalitis vaccine in U.S. inhabitants. J Infect Dis 161:878, 1990

SCHNEIDER RJ et al: Clinical sequelae after Japanese encephalitis: One year follow-up study in Thailand. Southeast Asian J Trop Med Public Health 5:560, 1974

Diseases presenting primarily with hemorrhagic manifestations

BRUNO P et al: Hemorrhagic fever with renal syndrome imported to Hawaii from West Germany. Am J Med 89:232, 1990

BURNEY MI et al: Nosocomial outbreak of viral hemorrhagic fever caused by Crimean hemorrhagic fever—Congo virus in Pakistan, January 1976. Am J Trop Med Hyg 29:941, 1980

CENTERS FOR DISEASE CONTROL: Viral hemorrhagic fever. Initial management of suspected and confirmed cases. Ann Intern Med 101:73, 1984

————: Korean hemorrhagic fever. JAMA 259:1622, 1988

DENNIS LH et al: The original hemorrhagic fever: Yellow fever. Blood 30:858, 1967

GARTNER L: Hantaan virus infection (Korean hemorrhagic fever) as a cause of acute renal failure. Dtsch Med Wochenschr 113:937, 1988

HALSTEAD SB, O'ROURKE EF: Dengue viruses and mononuclear phagocytes: I. Infection enhancement by non-neutralizing antibody. J Exp Med 146:201, 1977

————: The pathogenesis of dengue: Molecular epidemiology in infectious disease. Am J Epidemiol 114:632, 1981

KLIKS SC et al: Antibody-dependant enhancement of dengue virus growth in human monocytes as a risk factor for dengue hemorrhagic fever. Am J Trop Med Hyg 40:444, 1989

KUDESIA G et al: Dual infection with leptospira and Hantavirus. Lancet 1:1397, 1988

LEDUC JW et al: A retrospective analysis of sera collected by the Hemorrhagic Fever Commission during the Korean Conflict. J Infect Dis 162:182, 1990

LEE HW et al: Isolation of the etiologic agent of Korean hemorrhagic fever. J Infect Dis 137:298, 1978

MONATH TP et al: Yellow fever in the Gambia, 1978–1979: Epidemiologic aspects with observations on the occurrence of Orongo virus infections. Am J Trop Med Hyg 29:912, 1980

NELSON ER: Hemorrhagic fever in children in Thailand: Report of 69 cases. J Pediatr 56:101, 1960

PILASKI J et al: Haemorrhagic fever with renal syndrome in Germany. Lancet 337:111, 1991

PINHEIRO FP et al: An epidemic of yellow fever in Central Brazil 1972–1973: I. Epidemiological studies. Am J Trop Med Hyg 27:125, 1978

WORLD HEALTH ORGANIZATION: *Dengue hemorrhagic fever: Diagnosis, treatment and control*. Geneva, 1986

————: Hemorrhagic fever with renal syndrome: Memorandum from a WHO meeting. Bull WHO 61:269, 1983

---

160   ARENAVIRUS INFECTIONS

JAY P. SANFORD

DEFINITION AND CLASSIFICATION   The term *arenavirus* is the designation for a group of RNA viruses which have unique morphology. The virions are pleomorphic, with diameters between 50 and 300 nm, and contain an electron-dense membrane with projections and 2 to 10 inclusion-like dense particles (resembling ribosomes) that give the virion an appearance of having been sprinkled with sand (Latin *arenaceus*, "sandy"). Fifteen distinct arenaviruses have been described (Table 160-1). All except Tacaribe are parasites of rodents, and most are unique to tropical America. A special property of arenaviruses that cause disease in humans is the capacity of congenitally or newborn acquired infections to persist in their reservoir hosts with no ill effects and in the absence of an immune response.

LYMPHOCYTIC CHORIOMENINGITIS   The first-recognized arenavirus was lymphocytic choriomeningitis (LCM) virus. It was recognized early that LCM was carried by apparently healthy laboratory mice. Clinically, LCM has been considered primarily in the context of aseptic meningitis; however, it is associated with at least two clinical syndromes in humans: central nervous system (CNS) and influenza-like illness which may be associated with rash, arthritis, or orchitis. LCM virus has provided a valuable model for the study of chronic, persistent, and generally symptomless viral infections in laboratory animals.

Prevalence   In the United States, human infection with LCM virus is rare; however, seroepidemiologic studies on specimens obtained in 1935 to 1940 from persons with no history of CNS disease

TABLE 160-1   Classification of arenaviruses

Virus	Clinical disease	Reservoir	Known geographic range
OLD WORLD SPECIES			
Lymphocytic choriomeningitis	Aseptic meningitis, meningoencephalitis, influenzal syndrome, orchitis, arthritis	Mice, hamsters	Worldwide except Australia
Lassa	Lassa fever	*Mastomys natalensis*	Nigeria, Liberia, Sierra Leone, Republic of Guinea, Central African Republic
Ippy		*Arvicanthis* spp.	Central African Republic
Mobala		*Praomys jacksoni*	Central African Republic
Mopeia		*Mastomys natalensis*	Mozambique
NEW WORLD SPECIES: TACARIBE COMPLEX			
Tacaribe		Bats	Trinidad
Junin	Argentinian hemorrhagic fever	*Calomys musculinus*	Argentina
Machupo	Bolivian hemorrhagic fever	*Calomys callosus*	Northeast Bolivia
Guanarito	Venezuelan hemorrhagic fever	*Sigmodon hispidus* (cotton rat) *Oryzomys* spp. (rice rat)	Northwest Venezuela
Amapari			Brazil
Latino			Bolivia
Parana			Paraguay
Pichinde			Colombia
Tamiami			Florida
Flexal		*Orzomys* spp.	Brazil

from all parts of the United States revealed neutralizing antibodies in 10 to 28 percent. In recent years, the prevalence of infection seems to have decreased markedly.

Epidemiology The virus of LCM is worldwide in distribution. Foci of LCM virus have been defined in Germany, Hungary, and elsewhere in Europe. Scandinavia appears to be LCM virus–free, as are most of the Americas except Argentina. Although infection can be induced in a variety of animals, mice are the major natural reservoir as well as the primary host in which latent, asymptomatic infection occurs. The latency of infection in the mouse depends on immunologic tolerance. Animals infected in utero or shortly after birth excrete LCM virus for life without overt disease. Human infections are secondary to contact with an infected rodent. The mode of transmission is thought to be via airborne spread or contact with excrement from infected animals. In the past, most cases have arisen in persons living in rodent-infested houses, but lately outbreaks of LCM virus disease in humans have been reported from Germany and the United States in which the source of infection was traced to laboratory animals and household pets, specifically hamsters, which, like mice, can shed LCM virus in urine and stool. LCM occurs throughout the year but has been more frequent in the colder months. Person-to-person transmission has not been demonstrated.

Pathogenesis In natural infection, the portal of entry of the LCM virus is probably the respiratory tract. Virus multiplication occurs initially in the respiratory epithelium, and an influenza-like illness develops. Dissemination of virus to extrapulmonary sites, presumably to reticuloendothelial cells with multiplication, and viremia occur. LCM virus crosses the blood-brain barrier. In mice, the resulting meningitis is attributed to a cell-mediated immune reaction. Support for this hypothesis derives from observations that disease but not infection can be prevented in experimental animals by neonatal thymectomy, irradiation, or immunodepressant drugs such as cyclophosphamide. Similar pathogenetic mechanisms may operate in humans, although isolation of LCM virus from the cerebrospinal fluid (CSF) of patients with aseptic meningitis is quite common.

Clinical manifestations The exact incubation period is not known. Following experimental inoculation of LCM virus into volunteers, fever occurred in $1\frac{1}{2}$ to 3 days, while an influenza-like constellation of symptoms developed 5 to 10 days after exposure. An influenza-like illness is the most common clinical pattern. In some patients the illness may be biphasic, with subsequent aseptic meningitis or encephalomyelitis. Fever, usually from 38.3 to 40°C (101 to 104°F), associated with rigors, is uniformly noted. Other symptoms which are encountered in over one-half of patients include malaise, weakness, myalgia (especially lumbar aching), retroorbital headache, photophobia, anorexia, nausea, and light-headedness. Symptoms which occur in one-fourth to one-half of patients include sore throat, vomiting, and dysesthesias. Later, arthralgias, especially in the hands, occur. Less common complaints (up to one-quarter of patients) include aching pain in the chest, associated with pneumonitis; increased hair loss progressing to generalized alopecia, 2 or 3 weeks after the onset of illness; testicular pain or frank orchitis, usually unilateral, 1 to 3 weeks after onset; and parotid pain, which may lead to a misdiagnosis of mumps. Physical findings in the first week of illness are few. Patients often have a relative bradycardia. Pharyngeal injection without exudate is common (60 percent). Mild nontender cervical or axillary lymphadenopathy may occur. The initial phase lasts from 5 days to 3 weeks, followed by improvement. After a remission of 1 to 2 days, many patients relapse with recurrent fever and more prominent headache. Physical signs may include skin rashes, swelling of metacarpophalangeal and proximal interphalangeal joints, meningeal signs, orchitis, parotitis, and alopecia. Convalescence generally is of 1 to 4 weeks' duration, characterized by easy fatigability, an excessive need for sleep, dysesthesias, and occasional dizziness. Patients with aseptic meningitis almost always recover without sequelae. With encephalitis, 25 to 30 percent of patients have neurologic residua.

Laboratory findings Leukopenia and thrombocytopenia are almost uniform during the first week of illness. Although leukocyte counts usually vary between 2000 and 3000 cells per microliter, counts as low as 600 cells per microliter have been recorded. Differential counts generally show slight relative lymphocytosis. Platelet counts are usually between 50,000 and 100,000 per microliter. Anemia is not encountered. The erythrocyte sedimentation rate often is normal. Mild elevations of serum aspartate aminotransferase and lactic dehydrogenase (LDH) may occur. Chest radiographs may suggest basilar pneumonias. In patients with meningeal signs, examination of the CSF usually reveals several hundred cells per microliter, although cell counts in excess of 1000 per microliter are reported in half the patients in some series. Lymphocytes predominate (greater than 80 percent) even early. The initial CSF protein is usually slightly elevated, but on occasion levels may exceed 1.5 g/L (150 mg/dL). Although a normal CSF glucose level is considered the hallmark of viral meningitides, low CSF glucose has been observed in up to 27 percent of patients with LCM.

Diagnosis The diagnosis of LCM can be established with certainty by recovery of the virus from blood or spinal fluid; however, this procedure requires a biosafety level 3 facility. The simplest method is a direct immunofluorescent assay (IFA) of infected cells fixed on a microscopic slide. ELISA or radioimmunoassay also may be used. IgG antibodies appear by 7 to 10 days. Neutralizing antibodies appear after 6 to 8 weeks, increase in titer slowly, and remain high for years. The clinical manifestations of LCM cannot be differentiated from those produced by numerous other viruses.

Treatment There is no specific treatment.

ARGENTINIAN AND BOLIVIAN HEMORRHAGIC FEVERS The first cases of a new American hemorrhagic disease were seen near the Argentinian town of Junin near Buenos Aires in 1953. A virus was isolated from patients' blood and from local rodents and their mites. In 1959, cases of a disease thought to resemble severe epidemic typhus were noted among rural workers in northeastern Bolivia. The similarity between these syndromes was recognized. In 1963, the causal virus was isolated from patients and rodents and named the *Machupo virus*. Machupo virus is serologically related to but distinct from Junin virus.

Prevalence Junin virus infections, Argentinian hemorrhagic fever (AHF), have occurred in epidemic form since 1958, with between 100 and 3500 cases reported annually. Since initial recognition, AHF has spread more widely. In contrast, Bolivian hemorrhagic fever (BHF) has not spread to other geographic areas, and virtually no cases have been reported in the past 10 years.

Epidemiology AHF occurs in sharply endemic seasonal form (February to August), mostly among male rural workers, especially those exposed to fields at the time of the maize harvest. Virus is transmitted in the urine of rodents with chronic infection and viruria. Humans acquire the virus through contact with items or foodstuffs which have been contaminated with infected rodent urine. The main reservoir is two species of rodents, *Calomys laucha* and *C. musculinus*.

BHF is similarly transmitted by the urine of *C. callosus* (a mouselike rodent) chronically infected with Machupo virus. Direct person-to-person transmission is possible and may have occurred in the outbreak in Cochabamba. Disease has not occurred in medical personnel attending infected patients.

Clinical features AHF presents manifestations of renal, cardiovascular, and hematologic involvement. Inapparent infections are rare. The incubation period is estimated to be 7 to 16 days, followed by a gradual onset of chills, fever, headache, malaise, myalgia, anorexia, nausea, and vomiting. The temperature reaches 38.9 to 40°C (102 to 104°F), facial flushing may be prominent, and there is a painless enanthem of the pharynx. Lymphadenopathy and splenomegaly are not present. From 3 to 5 days after the onset, the signs and symptoms worsen, with the appearance of dehydration, relative bradycardia, hypotension to 50 to 100 mmHg, and oliguria. In the more severe cases, hemorrhagic manifestations, including bleeding from the gums, hematemesis, hematuria, and melena, occur. At this phase, one-half of patients will have neurologic symptoms: cranial nerve weakness, oculogyric crises, and tremor of the tongue and extremities. Some patients develop psychic manifestations, with agitation, delirium, or stupor. Progressive shock, hypothermia, gallop rhythm, or gastrointestinal bleeding may occur from the seventh to tenth days. In fatal cases, pulmonary edema usually is the cause of death. During convalescence, temporary alopecia has been noted. Erythrocyte counts are normal or elevated. The total leukocyte counts drop to less than 1000 cells per microliter, and platelet counts of less than 100,000 per microliter are invariable. Disseminated intravascular coagulation does not seem to be the mechanism responsible for the hemorrhagic manifestations. Intense proteinuria is common, and microscopic hematuria also occurs. Blood urea nitrogen levels rise rapidly.

The clinical picture of BHF is similar to that of AHF, although epistaxis and hematemesis at the onset are more common in BHF.

Diagnosis IgG antibodies, which appear within 7 to 10 days, are detected by IFA.

Treatment Treatment consists of supportive measures, including peritoneal dialysis or hemodialysis-filtration to correct both the azotemia and the pulmonary edema. In AHF, a double-blind trial with immune plasma reduced mortality from 16 to 1 percent. However, 10 percent of treated patients developed neurologic symptoms 4 to 6 weeks after treatment. The neurologic syndrome included fever, headache, ataxia, and intention tremors but lasted less than 1 week. Preliminary studies suggest that ribavirin may be effective in both experimental BHF and AHF. Treatment protects against the acute hemorrhagic phase but does not prevent the late neurologic disease. Since Junin virus is seldom isolated from the CNS in fatal human AHF, evaluation of ribavirin in humans with AHF seems justified.

Prognosis The mortality rate among patients with AHF is usually 3 to 15 percent, while that in BHF is 5 to 30 percent.

Prevention In Bolivia, rodent control measures directed primarily against *C. callosus* populations in the houses has resulted in a prompt and dramatic cessation of human cases. In Argentina, the wide dispersal of infected hosts renders rodent control measures futile.

VENEZUELAN HEMORRHAGIC FEVER An outbreak of severe hemorrhagic illness occurred in Guanarito, Venezuela, in September 1989.

Epidemiology Although preliminary transmission through contact with infected rodents or their excretions is likely, a newly identified agent, Guanarito virus, a new member of the Tacaribe complex of Arenaviridae, was isolated from the cotton rat, and antibodies were identified in the rice rat. Infection rate was low in family contacts (10 percent had antibodies), and illness was not recognized in hospital personnel who cared for over 100 patients with the disease. Transmission seems to occur in and around houses, as with BHF and Lassa fever.

Clinical features Patients range in age from 6 to 54 years, with sexes equally affected. Duration of illness at the time of admission to hospital was 3 to 12 days. The most common presenting symptoms included fever (93 percent), headache (60 percent), diarrhea (46 percent), cough (40 percent), and hemorrhagic manifestations (86 percent): epistaxis, bleeding gums, menorrhagia, and melena. Clinical signs included pharyngitis (some with tonsillar exudate), marked conjunctival injection, facial edema, cervical lymphadenopathy, scattered pulmonary rales, and petechiae. Among 104 presumed cases there were 26 deaths, while 9 (60 percent) of 15 patients with confirmed cases died. Among the 6 survivors, one had temporary alopecia and one a mild hearing loss. Convalescence was lengthy, lasting several months.

Laboratory features Hemoglobin and hematocrit values were normal. Leukopenia (1100 to 3900 cells per microliter) was noted in two-thirds of patients. Platelet counts were less than 100,000 per microliter in one-half; serum creatinine levels were elevated in one-third.

Diagnosis The virus was isolated from serum and spleen by tissue culture on vero cells. In surviving patients, antibodies were measured by IFA tests.

Treatment While treatment is still undefined, an approach similar to that for AHF seems appropriate.

LASSA FEVER A virus disease which is both highly contagious and virulent occurred in a missionary nurse in Lassa, a town in northeast Nigeria, in 1969.

Epidemiology Since the initial outbreak at Lassa in 1969, during which one of the patients was transferred to New York City, there have been other outbreaks near Jos in northern Nigeria in 1970 (32 suspected cases with 10 deaths), in Zorzor, Liberia, in 1972 (11 cases with 4 deaths), and in the eastern province of Sierra Leone with 63 suspected cases admitted to two hospitals between 1970 and 1972. Lassa fever occurs as an endemic disease in eastern Sierra Leone. Population surveys showed more than one-half of older adults had antibodies. Other countries in west Africa having clinical or serologic evidence of Lassa fever include Senegal, Gambia, Guinea, Ghana, Burkina Faso (formerly Upper Volta), Mali, and Ivory Coast. Lassa-related viruses (Mopeia, Mobala) have been isolated from rodents in Mozambique, Zimbabwe, and the Central African Republic; however, they have not been associated with human illness. In Jos and Zorzor, outbreaks apparently resulted from person-to-person nosocomial spread from the index case to hospital workers or other patients. In Sierra Leone, the great majority of cases were acquired outside the hospital, although hospital workers were at risk. *Mastomys natalensis*, a multimammate rat widespread in Africa, is the animal reservoir, and primary human cases result from contamination of foodstuffs with rodent urine. Human-to-human transmission may occur through contact with urine, feces, vomitus, or saliva through droplets, and particularly through wounds contaminated with blood. Intrafamilial outbreaks have occurred around several cases. There are a number of cases which have been acquired through accidental autoinoculation with needles while starting intravenous fluids. At least one laboratory-acquired infection has occurred. In Sierra Leone 6 percent of the population surveyed had complement fixing antibody against Lassa virus, while only 0.2 percent had recognized disease, suggesting mild disease or inapparent infection. In Liberia 10 percent of hospital personnel had antibodies. In west Africa the incidence is estimated to be greater than 250,000 cases per year.

Clinical features The incubation period is usually 7 to 18 days. Patients have ranged from 5 months to 46 years of age; approximately two-thirds are women. Three of eight women in one series were 22 to 28 weeks pregnant during their illness. The apparent predilection for women may relate to exposure to contaminated food or work in hospitals rather than to differences in susceptibility. The onset of illness was described by most patients as insidious. The most frequent initial symptoms were fever (100 percent), chilliness and true rigors, headache (50 percent), malaise (100 percent), and myalgia (50 percent). Most patients did not seek medical attention for 4 to 9 days after onset. Symptoms of a systemic viral illness then developed with anorexia, nausea, vomiting, myalgia, and pain in the chest, epigastrium, and lumbar area. Headache was usually present. Two-thirds of patients developed a dry nonproductive cough. Early examination revealed fever and flushing of the face and V area of the neck. Pharyngitis developed in 70 percent and became progressively more severe during the first week; patients expectorated saliva because swallowing was so painful. Examination often revealed raised patches of whitish exudate occurring on the palatine arches, which occasionally coalesced into a pseudomembrane. Oral ulcerations have been noted in up to one-half of cases. Generalized nontender lymphadenopathy occurred in one-half of patients. During the second week, severe lower abdominal pain and intractable vomiting were common, and facial and neck swelling with conjunctival edema and infection frequently developed. Occasionally patients had tinnitus, epistaxis, bleeding from the gums and venipuncture sites, maculopapular rashes, and dizziness. During the acute stage, systolic blood pressures of less than 90 mmHg, with pulse pressures less than 20 mmHg, occurred in 60 to 80 percent of patients. Initially, relative bradycardia was common. During the second week, the patients who recovered defervesced, while the patients who died often developed signs of shock, clouding of the sensorium, rales, signs of pleural effusion, agitation, and, on occasion, grand mal seizures. The duration of illness in surviving patients ranged from 7 to 31 days (average 15 days), while that in fatal cases was 7 to 26 days (average 12 days). The mortality rates in Jos and Zorzor were 52 and 36 percent, respectively, while in Sierra Leone the rate was 8 percent. During convalescence, occasional flurries of rapid involuntary eye movement (oculogyric crises) occurred. Late sequelae included deafness (29 percent) and alopecia.

Laboratory features   The hematologic findings include relatively normal hematocrit values and early leukopenia (less than 4000 cells per microliter in 36 percent) with a relative neutrophilia and immature forms of leukocytes. In two cases in which it was recorded, the erythrocyte sedimentation rate was normal. Urinalyses revealed proteinuria, which was often massive. Chest radiographs may suggest basilar pneumonitis and pleural effusions. Electrocardiographic abnormalities compatible with diffuse myocardial disease have been encountered. Levels of serum enzymes, SGOT, creatinine phosphokinase (CPK), and LDH have been elevated. An SGOT of > 150 IU/L is associated with a case-fatality rate of 50 percent. A viremia of $> 1 \times 10^{3.0}$ TCID$_{50}$ per milliliter is associated with increased mortality. Both factors together carry a risk of death of 80 percent. Lassa virus may be recovered from CSF.

Diagnosis   Diagnosis can be made by demonstrating a fourfold rise in antibody titer to Lassa virus between acute-phase and convalescent-phase serum specimens with the IFA technique or with Lassa IgM antibodies. The diagnosis is unlikely if IgM antibodies are absent by the fourteenth day of illness.

Treatment   The management has been supportive. Infusion of immune plasma from convalescent patients resulted in a dramatic effect in three of four patients. Because of the self-limited nature of the disease, these results cannot be assessed easily. In a study of the

antiviral agent ribavirin, 19 of 20 patients treated intravenously within 6 days of onset with a 2.0-g loading dose, followed by 1.0 g every 6 h for 4 days, then 0.5 g every 8 h for another 6 days, survived, whereas 11 of 18 who received no therapy and 10 of 16 who received convalescent plasma died. In view of the hospital association and the presence of virus in pharyngeal secretions and urine, respiratory and enteric isolation and blood precautions are required. With reasonable isolation practices, nosocomial spread need not be as feared as previously.

OTHER HEMORRHAGIC FEVERS   Ebola hemorrhagic fever and Marburg virus disease are caused by members of the family Filoviridae and are discussed in Chap. 158 and summarized in Table 159-1.

REFERENCES

BAUM SG et al: Epidemic non-meningitic lymphocytic-choriomeningitis virus infection. N Engl J Med 274:934, 1966

CASALS J: Arenaviruses. Yale J Biol Med 48:115, 1975

CENTERS FOR DISEASE CONTROL: Viral hemorrhagic fever. Initial management of suspected and confirmed cases. Ann Intern Med 101:73, 1984

CUMMINS D et al: Acute sensorineural deafness in Lassa fever. JAMA 264:2093, 1990

FIELDS BN et al (eds): Virology, 2d ed. New York, Raven, 1990

FRAME JD et al: Lassa fever, a new virus disease of man from West Africa: I. Clinical description and pathological findings. Am J Trop Med Hyg 19:670, 1970

JOHNSON KM et al: Hemorrhagic fever of Southeast Asia and South America. A comparative approach. Prog Med Virol 9:105, 1967

McCORMICK JB et al: Lassa fever: Effective therapy with ribavirin. N Engl J Med 314:20, 1986

McKEE KT JR et al: Ribavirin prophylaxis and therapy for experimental Argentine hemorrhagic fever. Antimicrob Agents Chemother 32:1304, 1988

MacKENZIE RB et al: Epidemic hemorrhagic fever in Bolivia: 1. A preliminary report of the epidemiologic and clinical findings in a new epidemic area in South America. Am J Trop Med Hyg 13:620, 1964

MERTENS PE et al: Clinical presentation of Lassa fever cases during the hospital epidemic at Zorzor, Liberia, March–April 1972. Am J Trop Med Hyg 22:780, 1973

MONATH TP et al: Lassa fever in the Eastern Province of Sierra Leone, 1970–1972: II. Clinical observations and virological studies on selected hospital cases. Am J Trop Med Hyg 23:1140, 1974

SALAS R et al: Venezuelan hemorrhagic fever. Lancet 338:1033, 1991

VANZEE BE et al: Lymphocytic choriomeningitis in University hospital personnel. Clinical features. Am J Med 58:803, 1975

---

section 15 Fungal infections

161 DIAGNOSIS AND THERAPY OF FUNGAL INFECTIONS

JOHN E. BENNETT

DIAGNOSIS

Many fungi can be identified as to genus or even species by microscopic examination of smears or biopsies. Calcofluor white stain with fluorescent microscopy is a sensitive technique for smear of sputum, bronchoalveolar lavage, or pus. India ink smear remains the choice for detecting cryptococci in cerebrospinal fluid (CSF). Smears of vaginal or oral lesions for *Candida* pseudohyphae can be done by wet mount or Gram's stain. For histopathology slides, Gomori methenamine silver and a neutral counterstain are preferred.

Methodology has a marked effect on rapidity and sensitivity of blood cultures for fungi, except that *Candida* species are relatively easy to grow. For most other fungi, concentrating blood by lysis centrifugation and culturing on solid medium constitute the optimal

technique. Commercially available nucleic acid hybridization techniques can speed the identification of slow-growing molds, such as *Histoplasma capsulatum*. Serology has limited value, but testing serum or CSF for cryptococcal antigen or antibody to *Coccidioides immitis* can be diagnostic. Skin testing with fungal antigens is not useful in detecting active infection.

ANTIFUNGAL THERAPY

TOPICAL AGENTS   Imidazoles and triazoles   These synthetic compounds act by inhibiting ergosterol synthesis in the fungal cell wall and when given topically may cause direct damage to the cytoplasmic membrane. Drug resistance rarely arises in the previously sensitive strains. Imidazoles available for cutaneous application include clotrimazole, econazole, ketoconazole, sulconazole, oxiconazole, and miconazole. Vaginal formulations include four imidazoles—miconazole, clotrimazole, tioconazole, and butoconazole—and one triazole—terconazole. Miconazole lotion and vaginal preparations of both miconazole and clotrimazole are available without prescription. As yet, no substantial difference in efficacy or local intolerance among the topical azoles has appeared. All are effective in treatment of cutaneous candidiasis, tinea versicolor, and mild to moderately severe ringworm of the glabrous skin. Vaginal formulations are effective in vulvovaginal candidiasis. Clotrimazole is poorly absorbed from the gastrointestinal tract, but the oral troche is useful as a topical treatment for oral and esophageal candidiasis.

Polyene macrolide antibiotics These broad-spectrum antifungal agents combine with sterol in the fungal cytoplasmic membrane, increasing membrane permeability. Topically, they are not active against ringworm but are effective against candidiasis of the skin and mucous membranes. Nystatin suspension is effective in oral thrush, and vaginal troches are effective in vulvovaginal candidiasis. Both nystatin and amphotericin B are available in topical preparations for cutaneous candidiasis. Natamycin ophthalmic suspension is marketed in some countries (but not in the United States) for mycotic keratitis and conjunctivitis.

Other topical antifungals Ciclopirox olamine, haloprogin, and naftifine have the same clinical spectrum among the cutaneous mycoses as the imidazoles. Tolnaftate and undecylenic acid are effective against ringworm but not candidiasis. Keratolytic agents, such as salicylic acid, are helpful as accessory drugs for some hyperkeratotic skin lesions.

SYSTEMIC ANTIFUNGALS Griseofulvin Griseofulvin is a useful drug in treating certain kinds of ringworm; however, it is ineffective in treating candidiasis. The microcrystalline and ultramicrocrystalline preparations differ in dose but not in efficacy. Absorption of both is enhanced when ingested with fat-containing foods. Griseofulvin interacts with phenobarbital and coumarin-type anticoagulants.

Imidazoles and triazoles KETOCONAZOLE Absorption of ketoconazole is variable among individuals, is not affected by food, and is poor in patients with AIDS and those taking cimetidine or other H-2 blocking agents. Simultaneous administration of antacids also can impair absorption. Metabolism is chiefly hepatic, but substantial liver disease has minimal effect on plasma ketoconazole concentrations. Ketoconazole plasma levels are decreased in patients taking rifampin and also in some taking isoniazid. Ketoconazole administration can elevate cyclosporine blood levels, can increase the likelihood of terfenadine or astemizole cardiotoxicity, and, occasionally, can enhance the anticoagulant effect of warfarin. The drug is contraindicated during pregnancy and, because it appears in breast milk, during breast-feeding. Neither renal disease nor hemodialysis affects the metabolism of ketoconazole. The most common toxicities of ketoconazole are dose-related nausea, anorexia, and occasionally, vomiting. Hepatotoxicity is idiosyncratic and usually mild but rarely can be serious and fatal. Several dose-related, temporary endocrine effects have been observed: decreased adrenal cortical reserve; gynecomastia; decreased serum testosterone, libido, and potency in males; and menstrual irregularity in females. Pruritus or rash also may occur. Ketoconazole is effective in blastomycosis, histoplasmosis, paracoccidioidomycosis, chronic mucocutaneous candidiasis, esophageal candidiasis, and some forms of disseminated coccidioidomycosis and pseudallescheriasis. The usual adult dose is 400 mg, taken once daily. Partial improvement may be seen in cutaneous sporotrichosis and chromoblastomycosis. Although vulvovaginal candidiasis, ringworm, and tinea versicolor are responsive to the drug, the toxicity of oral ketoconazole makes topical imidazoles or other drugs preferable for these indications.

ITRACONAZOLE This triazole analogue of ketoconazole is superior to the parent compound in safety and efficacy. Hormonal suppression and hepatotoxicity are less with itraconazole than with ketoconazole. Clinical indications for itraconazole include all those for ketoconazole but also selected patients with sporotrichosis, cryptococcosis, and aspergillosis. The drug is marketed as 100-mg capsules. No parenteral formulation is available. The usual dose is 200 mg, once or twice a day by mouth. Itraconazole is metabolized in the liver, with the hydroxy metabolite retaining antifungal activity. Concurrent therapy with rifampin, carbamazepine, and H-2 receptor antagonists or phenytoin decreases itraconazole blood levels. Cardiotoxicity due to terfenadine or astemizole and cyclosporine nephrotoxicity may occur during concomitant itraconazole therapy.

FLUCONAZOLE This triazole can be administered as oral tablets or intravenous infusion. With a half-life of about 31 h, fluconazole can be given once a day. Bioavailability by the oral route is excellent and unimpaired by lack of gastric acid or presence of food. Fluconazole therapy can elevate blood levels of phenytoin, cyclosporine, warfarin, and sulfonylureas. Approximately 80 percent of the drug is excreted unchanged in the urine. Patients with creatinine clearance of 21 to 50 and 11 to 20 mL/min should have their fluconazole dose reduced by 50 and 75 percent, respectively. Penetration of drug into the CSF and other body fluids is very good. Aside from nausea and allergic reactions, toxicity has been unusual. Fluconazole is useful in certain forms of candidiasis, cryptococcosis, and coccidioidomycosis.

Amphotericin B A colloidal preparation of this drug is available for intravenous or intrathecal administration. The drug cannot be given intramuscularly and is not absorbed orally. Sodium or potassium salts must not be added to the infusion solutions because the colloidal drug will precipitate out of solution. In-line filters with 0.22-μm pore diameter may trap some of the colloid. Catabolism is extremely slow and is not influenced by renal failure, hepatic failure, or hemodialysis. Penetration into CSF and vitreous humor is poor; however, concentrations in pleural, peritoneal, and articular exudates are adequate for many mycoses. Histoplasmosis, blastomycosis, paracoccidioidomycosis, candidiasis, and cryptococcosis are the most responsive mycoses. Coccidioidomycosis, extraarticular sporotrichosis, aspergillosis, and mucormycosis are less responsive; chromoblastomycosis, mycetoma, and pseudallescheriasis show little, if any, response. The usual course is 8 to 10 weeks of 0.4 to 0.6 mg/kg daily. Infusions are generally given in 5% dextrose over 2 to 4 h. Severe febrile reactions to initial doses generally prompt use of an initial test dose with 1 mg, followed by escalating doses based on the gravity of the patient's infection and tolerance of the drug. Virtually all patients show toxic reactions that are related to the dose and duration of therapy. These side effects include azotemia, anemia, hypokalemia, nausea, anorexia, weight loss, phlebitis, and occasionally, hypomagnesemia. Intrathecal amphotericin B is indicated in coccidioidal meningitis and refractory cryptococcal meningitis, although this therapy is associated with considerable toxicity. Doses of 0.1 to 0.5 mg are given three times per week initially, then with decreasing frequency. Several new intravenous formulations of amphotericin B with reduced nephrotoxicity are in clinical trial, but their efficacy is as yet unknown.

Flucytosine Flucytosine (5-fluorocytosine) is a synthetic oral drug useful in cryptococcosis, candidiasis, and chromoblastomycosis. Within the fungal cell, flucytosine is converted to the antimetabolite 5-fluorouracil. Drug resistance appears rather rapidly when flucytosine is used alone. For this reason, the drug is generally used in combination with amphotericin B, permitting a lower dose of the latter. The usual regimen is amphotericin B 0.3 mg/kg daily and flucytosine 37.5 mg/kg every 6 h. Flucytosine is well absorbed from the gastrointestinal tract, even in the presence of food. The drug penetrates well into the CSF and is excreted unchanged in the urine. Hemodialysis results in significant drug removal. Even modest reductions in renal function may elevate flucytosine blood levels into the toxic range, $\geq$100 to 125 μg/mL. Elevated levels are associated with a significant incidence of neutropenia and thrombocytopenia. Elevated flucytosine blood levels also seem to predispose to colitis, the other major toxicity of this drug. Hepatotoxicity is idiosyncratic and uncommon. An allergic rash also may occur.

REFERENCES

General

KWON-CHUNG KJ, BENNETT JE: *Medical Mycology.* Philadelphia, Lea & Febiger, 1992

Therapy

Bennett JE: Antifungal agents, in *Goodman and Gilman's The Pharmacological Basis of Therapeutics*, AG Gilman et al (eds). New York, Pergamon, 1990, pp 1165–1181

Goodman JL et al: A controlled trial of fluconazole to prevent fungal infections in patients undergoing bone marrow transplantation. N Engl J Med 326:845, 1992

Lazar JD, Hilligoss DM: The clinical pharmacology of fluconazole. Semin Oncol 17:14, 1990

Tucker RM et al: Adverse events associated with itraconazole in 189 patients on chronic therapy. J Antimicrob Chemother 26:561, 1991

Wingard JR et al: Increase in *Candida krusei* infection among patients with bone marrow transplantation and neutropenia treated prophylactically with fluconazole. N Engl J Med 325:1274, 1991

162   HISTOPLASMOSIS

JOHN E. BENNETT

ETIOLOGY *Histoplasma capsulatum* is a dimorphic fungus that grows as a mold in nature or on Sabouraud's agar at room temperature. Hyphae bear both large and small spores, which are used for identification. *H. capsulatum* grows as a small budding yeast in host tissue and on enriched agar, such as blood cysteine glucose, at 37°C. Despite the name, the fungus is unencapsulated. Coculture of isolates with the opposite mating type can produce the perfect state called *Ajellomyces capsulatus*.

PATHOGENESIS AND PATHOLOGY Infection with *H. capsulatum* has been encountered in many areas of the world but is much more frequent in certain areas. Within the United States, infection is most common in the southeastern, midatlantic, and central states. Endemic areas are probably determined by the availability of proper conditions in nature for growth of the fungus. *H. capsulatum* prefers moist surface soil, particularly when it is enriched by droppings of certain birds and bats. The fungus has not only been isolated repeatedly from such sites, but many case clusters have occurred 5 to 18 days after groups were exposed to such dust, e.g., by raking, cleaning dirt-floored chicken coops, bulldozing, or cave exploring. Judging by skin test reactivity in many endemic areas, 80 percent or more of residents over age 16 have been exposed.

Microconidia, or small spores, of *H. capsulatum* are small enough to reach the alveoli on inhalation and are transformed to budding forms. With time, an intense granulomatous reaction occurs. Caseation necrosis or calcification may mimic tuberculosis. The primary infection in children usually heals completely but may leave spotty calcification in the hilar nodes or lung. Transient dissemination may leave calcified granulomas in the spleen. In adults, a rounded mass of scar tissue, with or without central calcification, may remain in the lung. This has been called a *histoplasmoma*. Previous exposure is thought to confer some protection against reinfection, but infection in persons with prior positive skin tests clearly has occurred.

In a small proportion of patients, histoplasmosis becomes a progressive, potentially fatal infection. The disease occurs either as chronic fibrocavitary pneumonia or, less commonly, as disseminated infection. Patients with either form lack a history of acute primary pulmonary histoplasmosis. Chronic pulmonary infection favors otherwise healthy males over the age of 40. A history of cigarette use can be elicited from nearly all patients with chronic progressive pulmonary histoplasmosis. An acute, rapidly fatal course is most likely to be encountered in young children and immunosuppressed patients, including those with AIDS. A more chronic but equally lethal disseminated infection is more common in previously healthy adults.

CLINICAL MANIFESTATIONS The vast majority of infections are either asymptomatic or mild, and the diagnosis is elusive. Cough, fever, malaise, and chest x-ray findings of hilar adenopathy with or without one or more areas of pneumonitis occur. Erythema nodosum and erythema multiforme have been reported in a few outbreaks.

Hilar adenopathy may cause temporary compression of the right middle lobe bronchus in children and young adults. Subacute pericarditis may occur, probably by extension from contiguous lymph nodes. Rarely, hilar nodes undergo a caseous, granulomatous reaction with perinodal fibrosis. Mediastinal structures become encased by progressive fibrosis, and over many years, compression of the pulmonary veins, superior vena cava, pulmonary arteries, and esophagus may occur. Late in mediastinal disease only rare nonviable histoplasma can be found in caseous residua of lymph nodes.

Patients with *chronic pulmonary histoplasmosis* have a gradual onset over weeks or months of increasing productive cough, weight loss, and sometimes night sweats. Chest x-ray reveals uni- or bilateral fibronodular apical infiltrates. Approximately one-third of cases will stabilize or improve spontaneously early in the course. The remainder show insidious progression. Retraction and cavitation of the upper lobes occur with spread to the apex of the lower lobes and other areas of the lung. Emphysema and bullae formation further compromise pulmonary function. Death from cor pulmonale, bacterial pneumonia, or histoplasmosis occurs after months or years.

Acute disseminated histoplasmosis may be mistaken for miliary tuberculosis (see Chap. 130). Common findings include fever, emaciation, hepatosplenomegaly, lymphadenopathy, jaundice, anemia, leukopenia, and thrombocytopenia. All these features may occur in chronic dissemination as well, but the disease tends to be more localized. Indurated ulcers of the mouth, tongue, nose, or larynx occur in about a fourth of patients. Other focal findings include granulomatous hepatitis, Addison's disease, gastrointestinal ulceration, endocarditis, and chronic meningitis. Chest x-ray abnormalities occur in half the cases and show discrete nodules or a miliary pattern.

The presumed *ocular histoplasmosis* syndrome is a distinct clinical form of uveitis. Although a positive histoplasmin skin test is a requisite for diagnosis, none of these patients has had active histoplasmosis.

Infection with *H. capsulatum var. duboisii* is rare outside of Africa. The yeast form is larger in tissue than *H. capsulatum*. Clinical manifestations resemble blastomycosis more than histoplasmosis because skin and bone lesions are very common.

DIAGNOSIS Histoplasmosis may be suspected by serologic tests and clinical manifestations, but definitive diagnosis requires demonstration of the organism by culture or histology. Serologic tests are performed on serum or cerebrospinal fluid (CSF) using either a culture filtrate called *histoplasmin* or whole yeast form cells. The results are interchangeable. Complement fixation is quantifiable and is the best test. An agar gel diffusion test with histoplasmin is useful but not quantifiable. An H band on agar gel testing is more diagnostic of active histoplasmosis than an M band. Frequent false-negative and false-positive results limit all current serologic tests. Serologic conversion is helpful but occurs rarely except in acute pulmonary histoplasmosis. High complement fixation titers, such as 1:32 or greater, are suggestive of the diagnosis, but no titer is diagnostic. Cross-reactions with serologic tests for blastomycosis are common. A 5-mm or more diameter area of induration 24 to 48 h after skin testing with histoplasmin has been very helpful in identifying prior exposure to *Histoplasma*, but false-negative and false-positive results are so frequent that skin testing has little value in the study of ill patients. Further, a positive skin test can cause seroconversion.

Culture of *H. capsulatum* from sputum is difficult but is the procedure of choice in chronic pulmonary histoplasmosis. Digestion by proteolytic enzymes and centrifugation of sputum are helpful.

In patients with chronic pulmonary histoplasmosis, organisms may be infrequent in lung biopsies and lead to a mistaken diagnosis of lymphomatoid granulomatosis or Wegener's granulomatosis. Examination of several sections stained with methenamine silver may be necessary.

Acute disseminated histoplasmosis is difficult to diagnose in AIDS patients because fever, weight loss, leukopenia, and thrombocytopenia may occur with either infection. These patients also may have a diffuse pulmonary infiltrate resembling *Pneumocystis carinii* pneumonia. Patients may no longer be living in the endemic area, so the diagnosis may not be considered. Culture of blood by the lysis centrifugation technique, culture of bone marrow aspirate or bronchoalveolar lavage fluid, and Giemsa-stained smears of these specimens are important in detecting histoplasmosis. Radioimmunoassay for *Histoplasma* antigen in urine and serum has been helpful in diagnosis and in following results of therapy, but the test is not commercially available. Histologic examination of mucosal, skin, liver, or lymph node biopsy specimens can expedite diagnosis.

TREATMENT Acute pulmonary histoplasmosis requires no therapy. Patients with mediastinal fibrosis may benefit by surgery, but the ultimate prognosis is poor. All patients with disseminated or chronic fibronodular pulmonary histoplasmosis should receive chemotherapy. The indications for using ketoconazole or itraconazole, as well as the treatment regimen, are the same as those given in Chap. 164 for blastomycosis. Amphotericin B is given as 0.4 to 0.5 mg/kg per day or double that on alternate days and is continued for at least 10 weeks. AIDS patients with disseminated histoplasmosis respond poorly to ketoconazole and should be treated with amphotericin B. After an initial intensive course, these patients are given amphotericin B, 1 mg/kg once a week, or itraconazole, 200 mg once daily, to prevent relapse. In chronic pulmonary histoplasmosis, chest x-ray abnormalities improve somewhat, but pulmonary function improves very little. Successful therapy prevents progression. Addisonian crisis is a preventable cause of death in disseminated histoplasmosis.

REFERENCES

McKinsey DS et al: Long-term amphotericin B therapy for disseminated histoplasmosis in patients with the acquired immunodeficiency syndrome (AIDS). Ann Intern Med 111:655, 1989

Wheat JL et al: Disseminated histoplasmosis in the acquired immune deficiency syndrome: Clinical findings, diagnosis and treatment, and review of the literature. Medicine 69:361, 1990

163 COCCIDIOIDOMYCOSIS AND PARACOCCIDIOIDOMYCOSIS

JOHN E. BENNETT

COCCIDIOIDOMYCOSIS

ETIOLOGY *Coccidioides immitis* has two forms, growing as a white fluffy mold on most culture media but as a nonbudding spherical form, a spherule, in host tissue or under specialized conditions. Reproduction in the host tissue is by formation of small endospores within mature spherules. After rupture of the spherule, the released endospores enlarge, become spherules, and repeat the cycle. The fungus is identified by its appearance and by formation of thick-walled, barrel-shaped spores, called *arthrospores*, in the hyphae of the mold form.

PATHOGENESIS AND PATHOLOGY *C. immitis* is a soil saprophyte in certain arid regions of the United States, Mexico, Central America, and South America. Within the United States, most cases are acquired in California, Arizona, western Texas, and New Mexico. A few cases are acquired in bordering areas and by exposure to fomites from endemic areas, such as in cotton bales.

Infection in humans and animals results from inhalation of wind-borne arthrospores arising from soil sites. This primary pulmonary infection is symptomatic in only 40 percent of individuals, with symptoms ranging from a mild, influenza-like illness to severe pneumonia. Mild, self-limited infections may come to medical attention because of case clusters or hypersensitivity reactions:

erythema nodosum, erythema multiforme, toxic erythema, arthralgia, arthritis, conjunctivitis, or episcleritis. Case clusters occur 10 to 14 days after a group of susceptible individuals is exposed to dust in an endemic area through such activities as unearthing Indian relics, rock hunting, military maneuvers, or construction. Wind storms can carry spores to adjacent nonendemic areas and cause case clusters. The usual course of primary pulmonary infection is complete healing, although an area of pneumonitis on x-ray may heal by forming a coinlike lesion, or *coccidioidoma*. Less commonly, a single thin-walled cavity remains as a chronic sequela in the area of consolidation. The consolidation may persist as a chronic pneumonia or progress to fibronodular, cavitary disease.

Pleural effusion may be the only manifestation of primary infection. Self-healing of this form is common.

An uncommon but dreaded complication of coccidioidomycosis is dissemination beyond the lung and hilar lymph nodes. Dissemination is more frequent in blacks, Filipinos, Native Americans, Mexican-Americans, and pregnant or immunosuppressed patients, including those with AIDS.

C. immitis incites a chronic granulomatous reaction in host tissue, often with caseation necrosis. Lung and hilar node lesions may show calcification. Both IgM and IgG antibodies against *C. immitis* are induced by infection, but neither appears protective. The amount of specific IgG antibody is a rough measure of the antigenic mass, i.e., of the amount of infection, and a high titer is a poor prognostic sign. Appearance of delayed hypersensitivity to antigens of *C. immitis* is most common in those clinical forms of disease with a good prognosis, such as self-limited primary pulmonary disease. Negative skin tests to *Coccidioides* antigens occur in roughly half the patients with disseminated disease and portend a poor prognosis.

CLINICAL MANIFESTATIONS Symptomatic primary pulmonary infection is manifested by fever, cough, chest pain, malaise, and sometimes hypersensitivity reactions. Chest x-ray may show an infiltrate, hilar adenopathy, or pleural effusion. Peripheral blood may show a mild eosinophilia. Spontaneous improvement begins after several days to 2 weeks of illness and usually culminates in complete recovery.

The symptoms of a chronic thin-walled cavity include cough or hemoptysis in half the cases; the other patients are asymptomatic. Chronic progressive pulmonary coccidioidomycosis produces cough, sputum, variable degrees of fever, and weight loss. The first indications of dissemination usually appear during the primary infection. Reactivation with dissemination in later years occurs occasionally, especially if Hodgkin's disease, non-Hodgkin's lymphoma, renal transplantation, AIDS, or other immunosuppression has supervened. Dissemination should be suspected when fever, malaise, hilar or paratracheal lymphadenopathy, elevated sedimentation rate, and high complement fixation titers show abnormal persistence in patients with primary pulmonary coccidioidomycosis. With time, lesions appear in the bone, skin, subcutaneous tissue, meninges, joints, and other sites. Without therapy, dissemination may progress rapidly to death or wax and wane for years.

DIAGNOSIS When coccidioidomycosis is suspected, sputum, urine, and pus should be examined for *C. immitis* by wet smear and culture. *The laboratory request should indicate clearly that coccidioidomycosis is suspected because the mold form must be handled with extreme care to prevent infection of laboratory personnel.* On biopsy, smaller spherules must be distinguished from nonbudding forms of *Blastomyces* and *Cryptococcus*, but appearance of the mature spherule is diagnostic.

Serologic tests are very helpful in coccidioidomycosis. Latex agglutination and agar gel diffusion tests are useful in screening sera for antibody to *Coccidioides*. The complement fixation test is used on cerebrospinal fluid (CSF) and to confirm and quantitate serum antibody detected by screening tests. The number of cases with a positive complement fixation test will depend on the severity of disease and on the laboratory performing the test. Positive tests are least common in patients with solitary pulmonary cavities or primary pulmonary infection, while sera from patients with multiorgan disseminated disease are nearly all positive. Seroconversion is helpful in primary pulmonary coccidioidomycosis but may not occur for up to 8 weeks after onset. A positive complement fixation test in unconcentrated CSF is diagnostic of meningitis. Rarely, a parameningeal focus will cause a positive CSF serology.

Conversion of the skin test from negative to positive ($\geq$5 mm induration at 24 or 48 h) with either coccidioidin or spherulin, the two commercially available antigens, may occur between the third and twenty-first days of symptoms in primary pulmonary coccidioidomycosis. Skin testing also can be helpful in epidemiologic studies, such as investigation of case clusters or definition of endemic areas. The utility of skin testing as a diagnostic tool is limited by the presence of persistent positive tests resulting from remote exposures to *Coccidioides* and by the frequency of negative skin tests in many patients with either thin-walled cavities or disseminated coccidioidomycosis.

TREATMENT Primary pulmonary coccidioidomycosis usually resolves spontaneously. Some physicians give a few weeks of intravenous amphotericin B when patients show an unusually severe or protracted primary infection, hoping to abort disseminated or chronic pulmonary disease. There is no solid evidence to support this practice, but the stronger the suspicion of dissemination becomes in any given patient, the more logical this approach appears. Once evidence for dissemination becomes incontrovertible, amphotericin B may be palliative rather than curative.

Patients with severe or rapidly progressing disseminated coccidioidomycosis are begun on intravenous amphotericin B, 0.5 to 0.7 mg/kg daily. Patients who have improved after amphotericin B or who have more indolent disseminated infection are given ketoconazole, 400 to 800 mg/d, or itraconazole, 200 to 400 mg/d. These oral agents are useful for long-term suppression of infection and should be continued for years. Patients with coccidioidal meningitis are usually begun on fluconazole 400 mg daily but may require intrathecal amphotericin B. Hydrocephalus is a frequent complication of uncontrolled meningitis. Surgical debridement of bone lesions or drainage of abscesses can be helpful. Prognosis for ultimate cure of disseminated coccidioidomycosis is guarded.

Resection of chronic progressive pulmonary lesions is a helpful adjunct to chemotherapy when infection is confined to the lung and to one lobe. A single thin-walled cavity tends to close spontaneously and ordinarily is not resected. Such a cavity responds poorly to chemotherapy.

PARACOCCIDIOIDOMYCOSIS

ETIOLOGY Formerly called *South American blastomycosis*, this is the mycosis caused by *Paracoccidioides brasiliensis*. A dimorphic fungus, *P. brasiliensis* grows as a budding yeast in tissue but may be grown as either yeast or mold on a culture medium. Identification is by gross and microscopic appearance. A superficial resemblance to *Blastomyces dermatitidis* may cause misdiagnosis.

PATHOGENESIS AND PATHOLOGY Infection is thought to be acquired by inhalation of spores from environmental sources, but the reservoir in nature remains obscure. Pulmonary infection produces few symptoms initially. Hematogenous spread to the mucous membranes of the mouth and nose, the lymph nodes, and other sites brings the patient to medical attention. Fatal cases show spread to the adrenal, the gastrointestinal tract, and many other viscera.

CLINICAL MANIFESTATIONS Common symptoms include indurated ulcers of the mouth, oropharynx, larynx, and nose; enlarged and draining lymph nodes; lesions of the skin and genitalia; and productive cough, weight loss, dyspnea, and sometimes fever. Acquisition of infection is restricted to South America, Central America, and Mexico, but the extreme indolence of this infection may lead to recognition many years after the patient has left the endemic area. Chest x-ray most often shows a bilateral patchy pneumonia.

DIAGNOSIS Cultures of sputum, pus, and mucosal lesions are often diagnostic. The diagnosis can be made by smear or histologic section, though confirmation by culture is preferable. Serologic tests are useful in suggesting the diagnosis and monitoring therapy.

TREATMENT Milder cases may be cured by one year's treatment with oral ketoconazole, 200 to 400 mg daily. Itraconazole appears to give comparable results. More advanced cases are given intravenous amphotericin B, followed by ketoconazole.

REFERENCES

AMPEL NM et al: Coccidioidomycosis: Clinical update. Rev Infect Dis 11:897, 1989

BAKOS I et al: Disseminated paracoccidioidomycosis with skin lesions in a patient with acquired immunodeficiency syndrome. Am Acad Dermatol 20:854, 1989

GALGIANI JN et al: Ketoconazole therapy of progressive coccidioidomycosis. Comparison of 400 and 800 mg doses and observations at higher doses. Am J Med 84:603, 1988

GRAYBILL JR et al: Itraconazole treatment of coccidioidomycosis. Am J Med 89:282, 1990

RESTREPO A et al: Itraconazole in the treatment of paracoccidioidomycosis: A primary report. Rev Infect Dis 9(suppl 1):51, 1987

SUGAR AM et al: Paracoccidioidomycosis in the immunosuppressed host: Report of a case and review of the literature. Am Rev Respir Dis 129:340, 1984

TUCKER RM et al: Treatment of coccidioidal meningitis with fluconazole. Rev Infect Dis 12:S380, 1990

164   BLASTOMYCOSIS

JOHN E. BENNETT

ETIOLOGY *Blastomyces dermatitidis* is a dimorphic fungus that grows at room temperature as a white or tan mold but grows within the host or at 37°C as budding, round yeastlike cells. The fungus is identified by its appearance, its dimorphism, and the appearance of small spores borne on hyphae of the mold form. When isolates of the two opposite mating types are grown closely together on specialized culture media, sporulating structures appear which characterize the perfect form, *Ajellomyces dermatitidis*.

PATHOGENESIS AND PATHOLOGY The infection is restricted by geography and age. Blastomycosis is uncommon in any locality, but the majority of cases occur in the southeast, central, and midatlantic areas of the United States, with occasional cases in other localities in the United States and Canada. Cases also have been encountered in Africa, Mexico, Central America, and, rarely, South America. Most patients are between 20 and 69 years old. The male/female ratio is about 10:1. There is no occupational predisposition.

Infection appears to be acquired by inhalation of the fungus from soil, decomposed vegetation, or rotting wood. Several case clusters have occurred during recreational activities in wooded areas along waterways. Infection is not transmissible from person to person. The initial pulmonary infection may heal spontaneously or become chronic. Spread to other portions of the lung, cavitation, or endobronchial lesions may appear in chronic cases. Whether or not the lung lesion resolves spontaneously, infection commonly spreads hematogenously to skin, subcutaneous tissue, bone, prostate, epididymis, or mucosa of the nose, mouth, or larynx. Less commonly, infection spreads to the brain, meninges, liver, lymph nodes, or spleen. Dissemination may not be evident for weeks or years after the appearance of the lung lesion. Progressive infection is only rarely attributable to an underlying disease or immunosuppressive treatment. The inflammatory response includes lymphocytes, giant cells, and neutrophils. Pseudoepitheliomatous hyperplasia may be striking and lead to a mistaken diagnosis of squamous cell carcinoma.

CLINICAL MANIFESTATIONS A small number of patients have an acute, self-limited pneumonia. Fever, productive cough, myalgia, and malaise usually have resolved within a month. Pulmonary infiltrates have cleared slowly as *B. dermatitidis* disappeared from the sputum.

The vast majority of patients with blastomycosis have an indolent onset and a chronically progressive course. Fever, cough, weight loss, lassitude, skin lesions, and chest ache are common symptoms. Skin lesions favor exposed areas and enlarge over many weeks from a pimple to a well-circumscribed, verrucous, crusted, or ulcerated lesion. Pain and regional lymphadenopathy are minimal. Large chronic lesions may show central healing with scarring and contracture. Mucous membrane lesions resemble squamous cell carcinoma. Chest x-ray is abnormal in two-thirds of cases, with one or more pneumonic or nodular infiltrates. Calcification, hilar adenopathy, and large pleural effusions are rare. Osteolytic lesions may occur in nearly any bone and present as cold abscess or a draining sinus. Extension to a contiguous joint may cause indolent swelling, pain, and restricted motion. Prostatic and epididymal lesions resemble tuberculosis clinically.

DIAGNOSIS The diagnosis is made by demonstrating the fungus in culture of sputum, pus, or urine. In experienced hands, diagnosis by appearance of the organism in wet smear or histopathologic section is adequate. The fungus may be visible in a sputum cytology smear but is easily overlooked.

TREATMENT A few patients have been observed with transitory lung lesions, but no guidelines are known to distinguish these patients from those whose disease will progress locally or disseminate. Therefore, every patient should receive treatment. Intravenous amphotericin B is the drug of choice for patients with rapidly progressive infections, severe illness, or meningitis. Skin and noncavitary lung lesions should be treated for about 8 to 10 weeks. The recommended total dose for an adult is about 2.0 g. Cavitary lung disease or infection beyond the lung and skin should be treated for about 10 to 12 weeks with 2.5 g or more. Ketoconazole is an effective drug in patients with indolent nonmeningeal blastomycosis of mild to moderate severity and who take the drug reliably. The initial adult dose is 400 mg once daily, raised after a month to 600 or 800 mg daily if improvement is suboptimal. Itraconazole, 200 mg PO once or twice daily, is an effective alternative agent. Therapy is continued for 6 to 12 months. The mortality rate in appropriately treated cases is 15 percent or less.

REFERENCES

Bradsher RW: Blastomycosis: Fungal infections of the lung. Update 1989. Semin Respir Infect 5:105, 1990

Klein BS et al: Serological tests for blastomycosis: Assessments during a large point-source outbreak in Wisconsin. J Infect Dis 155:262, 1989

165 CRYPTOCOCCOSIS

JOHN E. BENNETT

ETIOLOGY Cryptococcosis is an infection caused by the yeastlike fungus *Cryptococcus neoformans*. *C. neoformans* reproduces by budding and forms round, yeastlike cells 4 to 6 μm in diameter. Within the host and on certain culture media, a large polysaccharide capsule surrounds each yeast cell. The fungus grows well as smooth, creamy white colonies on Sabouraud's or other simple media at 20 to 37°C. Certain culture media for ringworm contain cycloheximide, which inhibits *C. neoformans*. Identification is based on gross and microscopic appearance, biochemical tests, and growth at 37°C. The fungus has four capsular serotypes, designated A, B, C, and D. There

are also two mating types. Coculture of opposite mating types creates a transient diploid state called *Filobasidiella neoformans* for serotypes A or D and *Filobasidiella bacillispora* for serotypes B or C.

Weathered pigeon droppings commonly contain serotype A or D *Cryptococcus neoformans*. Serotypes B or C have been rarely found in nature, with the exception of flowering *Eucalyptus camaldulensis* trees in Australia. Transmission of infection to man from a specific natural site or from another patient has never been clearly documented, except for transplantation of an infected kidney, cornea, or other organ. Currently, more than half the cases in the United States are in AIDS patients. Cryptococcosis is a grave complication of late HIV infection at a time when the CD4 count is below 200 per cubic microliter. Among the cryptococcosis patients who are not infected with HIV, more than half are immunosuppressed. Corticosteroid therapy, but not neutropenia or immunoglobulin deficiency, predisposes to cryptococcosis. The male-to-female ratio in the non-AIDS patients is 2:1. Infection before puberty is uncommon.

PATHOGENESIS AND PATHOLOGY Infection is thought to be acquired by inhalation of fungus into the lungs. Pulmonary infection has a tendency toward spontaneous resolution and is frequently asymptomatic. Silent hematogenous spread to the brain leads to clusters of cryptococci in the perivascular areas of cortical gray matter, basal ganglia, and, to a lesser extent, other areas of the central nervous system. Inflammatory response around these foci is usually scant. In the more chronic cases, a dense basilar arachnoiditis occurs. Lung lesions show an intense granulomatous inflammation. Cryptococci are best seen in tissue by staining with methenamine silver or periodic acid Schiff. A strongly positive mucicarmine stain of the organism in tissue is diagnostic, but staining varies from intense to absent.

CLINICAL MANIFESTATIONS The majority of patients have *meningoencephalitis* at the time of diagnosis. This form of the infection is invariably fatal without appropriate therapy, and death occurs anywhere from 2 weeks to several years from onset of symptoms. Early manifestations include headache, nausea, staggering gait, dementia, irritability, confusion, and blurred vision. Both fever and nuchal rigidity are often mild or absent. Papilledema is present in one-third of patients at the time of diagnosis. Cranial nerve palsies, typically asymmetric, occur in about one-fourth of the patients. Other lateralizing signs are rare. With progression of the infection, deepening coma and signs of brainstem compression appear. Autopsy often reveals cerebral edema in the more acute cases or hydrocephalus in more chronic cases.

Pulmonary cryptococcosis causes chest pain in about 40 percent of patients and cough in 20 percent. Chest x-ray shows one or more dense infiltrates, which are often well circumscribed. Cavitation, pleural effusions, and hilar adenopathy are infrequent. Calcification is not present, and fibrotic stranding is rarely noticeable.

Skin lesions are present in 10 percent of patients with cryptococcosis, and the vast majority of patients with skin lesions have disseminated infection. One or a few asymptomatic tiny papular lesions appear, slowly enlarge, and tend to show central softening leading to ulceration. Osteolytic bone lesions occur in 4 percent of patients and usually present as a cold abscess. Rare manifestations of cryptococcosis include prostatitis, endophthalmitis, hepatitis, pericarditis, endocarditis, and renal abscess.

DIAGNOSIS Fever and headache in a patient with AIDS or with risk factors for HIV infection should suggest the possibility of cryptococcosis, toxoplasmosis, or central nervous system lymphoma. Presence of a focal lesion on magnetic resonance imaging (MRI) is unusual in cryptococcosis. In patients without AIDS, meningitis due to *C. neoformans* resembles that due to *M. tuberculosis*, *Histoplasma capsulatum*, *Coccidioides immitis*, or metastatic cancer. Lumbar puncture is the single most useful test. An india ink smear of centrifuged spinal fluid sediment reveals encapsulated yeast in more than half the cases, although artifacts can cause confusion. In patients without AIDS, cerebrospinal fluid glucose is reduced in half the cases, protein is usually increased, and a lymphocytic pleocytosis is usually present. CSF abnormalities are less pronounced in patients with AIDS, though india ink smear is more often positive.

Approximately 90 percent of patients with cryptococcal meningoencephalitis, including all those with a positive CSF smear, will have capsular antigen detectable in CSF or serum by latex agglutination. False-positive tests occur occasionally, making culture the definitive diagnostic test. *C. neoformans* is often present in urine from patients with meningoencephalitis. Fungemia occurs in 10 to 30 percent of patients and is particularly common in AIDS patients.

Pulmonary cryptococcosis mimics malignancy by x-ray and symptoms. Sputum culture is positive in only 10 percent, and serum antigen tests are positive in only a third. Occasionally, *C. neoformans* appears in one or multiple sputum specimens as an endobronchial saprophyte. Biopsy is usually required for diagnosis of pulmonary cryptococcosis. Cutaneous cryptococcosis may be mistaken for a comedo, basal cell carcinoma, or sarcoidosis. In AIDS patients, skin lesions may be numerous and mistaken for molluscum contagiosum. Biopsy reveals a myriad of cryptococci. Osseous cryptococcosis resembles tuberculosis.

TREATMENT   Patients with AIDS and cryptococcosis are treated initially with intravenous amphotericin B with or without flucytosine and then changed to fluconazole. During active infection, fluconazole, 400 mg, is given once daily. After infection is controlled, fluconazole, 200 mg daily, is continued indefinitely. Itraconazole is being evaluated for maintenance therapy as an alternative to fluconazole.

In patients without AIDS cryptococcosis may be treated with amphotericin B alone or in combination with flucytosine. Amphotericin B is given as 0.5 to 0.6 mg/kg per day when used alone or as 0.3 mg/kg per day in combination therapy. With either regimen, double-dose therapy on alternate days may be employed. Flucytosine is given initially as 37.5 mg/kg every 6 h to patients with normal renal function. Although nomograms are available for adjusting flucytosine dosage in the presence of reduced renal function, frequent measurement of serum levels and maintenance between 50 and 100 μg/mL offer the best chance of preventing toxicity.

Duration of therapy is based on the results of lumbar punctures. These are best done weekly until culture conversion is clearly documented. Six weeks of therapy may be adequate for patients with at least four weekly cultures of 2 to 4 mL CSF, whose india ink smear has become negative, and whose CSF glucose is normal. Approximately 50 to 70 percent of non-AIDS patients are cured.

Hydrocephalus may be an early or late complication of cryptococcosis. Blindness, dementia, and personality change are other sequelae.

Patients with extraneural cryptococcosis most often require intravenous amphotericin B, with or without flucytosine. Observation or excision of lesions may suffice for some patients who are previously normal, who have a single focus in lung, skin, or bone, and who have no cryptococci in the cerebrospinal fluid, urine, or blood.

REFERENCES

CHUCK SL, SANDE MA: Infections with *Cryptococcus neoformans* in the acquired immunodeficiency syndrome. N Engl J Med 321:794, 1989

POWDERLY WG et al: A controlled trial of fluconazole or amphotericin B to prevent relapse of cryptococcal meningitis in patients with the acquired immunodeficiency syndrome. N Engl J Med 326:793, 1992

SAAG MS et al: Comparison of amphotericin B with fluconazole in the treatment of acute AIDS-associated cryptococcal meningitis. N Engl J Med 326:83, 1992

SUGAR AM et al: Overview: Treatment of cryptococcal meningitis. Rev Infect Dis 12:S338, 1990

166   CANDIDIASIS

JOHN E. BENNETT

ETIOLOGY   *Candida albicans* is the most common cause of candidiasis, but *C. tropicalis, C. parapsilosis, C. guilliermondii, C. glabrata, C. krusei,* and a few other species can cause deep candidiasis and may even be fatal. *C. parapsilosis* is particularly notable for its ability to cause endocarditis. *C. tropicalis* accounts for about one-third of the cases of deep candidiasis in neutropenic patients. All *Candida* species pathogenic for humans are also encountered as commensals of humans, particularly in the mouth, stool, and vagina. These species grow rapidly at 25 to 37°C on simple media as oval, budding cells. In specialized culture media, hyphae or elongated branching structures called *pseudohyphae* are formed. *C. glabrata,* formerly called *Torulopsis glabrata,* differs from other members of the genus in that no true hyphae or pseudohyphae are formed in vitro or in infected tissue. *C. albicans* can be identified presumptively by its ability to form germ tubes in serum or by the formation of thick-walled large spores, called *chlamydospores.* Final identification of all species requires biochemical tests.

PATHOGENESIS AND PATHOLOGY   Either local or systemic factors may lead to tissue invasion by *Candida.* Chronic maceration predisposes to cutaneous candidiasis, as in diaper rash, intertrigo in obese patients, or paronychia in bartenders or cannery workers. Age is important because neonatal colonization often leads to oral candidiasis (thrush). Women in the third trimester of pregnancy are prone to vulvovaginal thrush. Patients with diabetes mellitus or hematologic malignancy or those receiving broad-spectrum antibiotics or high doses of adrenal corticosteroids are especially susceptible to candidiasis. Oral thrush is common any time in the course of HIV infection. As the number of CD4 cells declines, *Candida* esophagitis is also common. Breaks in the integrity of the skin or mucous membranes may provide access to deeper tissues. Examples include perforation of the gastrointestinal tract by trauma, surgery, and peptic ulceration; indwelling catheters for intravenous alimentation, peritoneal dialysis, and urinary tract drainage; severe burns; and intravenous drug abuse. In many hospitals, candidemia is the sixth most common cause of sepsis due to intravenous catheters.

Candida species, except *C. glabrata,* appear in tissue as both yeast and pseudohyphae. In any single lesion, only one form may be present. With *C. glabrata,* only yeast cells are present. Visceral lesions are characterized by necrosis and a neutrophilic inflammatory response. Neutrophils kill *Candida* yeast cells and damage segments of pseudohyphae in vitro, and visceral candidiasis complicates neutropenia, suggesting a major role for the neutrophil in host defense against this fungus. Visceral lesions show a preference for kidney, brain, spleen, heart, eye, and liver.

CLINICAL MANIFESTATIONS   *Oral thrush* presents as discrete and confluent adherent white plaques on the oral and pharyngeal mucosa, particularly in the mouth and tongue. These lesions are usually painless, but fissuring at the corners of the mouth can be painful. *Cutaneous candidiasis* presents as red, macerated intertriginous areas, paronychia, balanitis, or pruritus ani. Candidiasis of the perineal and scrotal skin may be accompanied by discrete pustular lesions on the inner aspects of the thighs. *Chronic mucocutaneous candidiasis* or *Candida granuloma* typically presents as circumscribed hyperkeratotic skin lesions, crumbling dystrophic nails, partial alopecia in areas of scalp lesions, and both oral and vaginal thrush. Systemic infection is very rare, but disfigurement of the face and hands can be severe. Other findings may include chronic epidermophytosis, dental dysplasia, and hypofunction of the parathyroid, adrenal, or thyroid glands. A variety of defects in T cell function have been described in these patients. Vulvovaginal thrush causes pruritus, discharge, and sometimes pain on intercourse or urination. Speculum examination reveals an inflamed mucosa and a thin exudate, often with white curds.

From one to multiple small shallow ulcerations due to *Candida* may appear in the esophagus or gastrointestinal tract. Esophageal lesions favor the distal third and may cause dysphagia or substernal pain. Other such lesions tend to be asymptomatic but assume importance in the leukemic patient as a portal for disseminated candidiasis. Within the urinary tract, the most common lesions are either hematogenous renal abscesses, which can cause azotemia, or bladder thrush. Bladder invasion usually follows catheterization or instrumentation of a patient with diabetes mellitus or who is receiving broad-spectrum antibiotics. This lesion generally is asymptomatic and benign. Rarely, retrograde invasion of the renal pelvis leads to renal papillary necrosis.

Hematogenous dissemination of Candida presents with fever and toxicity but with few localizing findings. One or more retinal abscesses may appear and extend slowly into the vitreous humor. The patient may note orbital pain, blurred vision, scotoma, or opacities floating across the visual field. Pulmonary candidiasis is almost always hematogenous and is visible on chest x-ray only when the abscesses are numerous enough to cause a diffuse, vaguely nodular infiltrate. Candidiasis of the endocardium or around intracardiac prostheses resembles bacterial infection of these sites. Chronic *Candida* meningitis or arthritis may occur, from either disseminated disease or insertion of a prosthesis in the case of arthritis or ventriculoperitoneal shunt infection. Rare focal manifestations of disseminated disease include osteomyelitis, pustular skin lesions, myositis, and brain abscess.

DIAGNOSIS Demonstration of pseudohyphae on wet smear with confirmation by culture is the procedure of choice for diagnosing superficial candidiasis. Scrapings for the smear may be obtained from skin, nails, and oral and vaginal mucosa. Culture alone is not diagnostic; however, recovery of *Candida* species from multiple superficial sites in immunosuppressed patients may portend visceral invasion.

Deeper lesions of *Candida* may be diagnosed by histologic section of biopsy specimens or by culture of cerebrospinal fluid, blood, joint fluid, or surgical specimens. Blood cultures are very useful in *Candida* endocarditis and intravenous catheter–induced sepsis but are positive less often in other forms of disseminated disease. Serologic tests for antibody or antigen are not useful.

TREATMENT Cutaneous candidiasis of macerated areas responds to measures which reduce moisture and chafing plus a topically applied antifungal agent in a nonocclusive base. Nystatin powder or a cream with ciclopirox or an azole is useful. Clotrimazole, miconazole, econazole, ketoconazole, sulconazole, and oxiconazole are available as creams or lotions. *Candida* vulvovaginitis responds better to an azole than to nystatin suppositories. There is little difference in efficacy among miconazole, clotrimazole, tioconazole, butoconazole, and terconazole vaginal formulations. Systemic treatment of *Candida* vulvovaginitis with ketoconazole or fluconazole is more convenient that topical treatment, but the potential for adverse effects is higher. Clotrimazole troches, used five times a day, are more effective in oral and esophageal candidiasis than nystatin suspension. Ketoconazole, 200 to 400 mg daily, is also useful in *Candida* esophagitis, but many of the patients absorb the drug poorly because they are receiving H-2 receptor antagonists or have AIDS. In AIDS patients, fluconazole, 100 to 200 mg daily, is the most effective azole for oral and esophageal candidiasis.

When esophageal symptoms are pronounced, a 5- to 10-day course of intravenous amphotericin B, 0.3 mg/kg per day, may be beneficial. Bladder thrush responds to bladder irrigations with amphotericin B, 50 μg/mL for 5 days. If no bladder catheter is present, oral fluconazole can be used to control candiduria. In all forms of superficial candidiasis, relapse after successful treatment is common unless the underlying factor can be eliminated.

Intravenous amphotericin B is the drug of choice in disseminated candidiasis. The drug is usually given as 0.4 to 0.5 mg/kg every day or as a double dose on alternate days for several weeks. In patients with no contraindication to the use of flucytosine, administration of that drug in dosage of 100 to 150 mg/kg per day plus amphotericin B, 0.3 mg/kg per day, is an effective alternative. Ketoconazole in an adult dose of 200 mg daily is probably the drug of choice for chronic mucocutaneous candidiasis.

Candida isolated from a properly obtained blood culture should be considered significant; true false-positives are rare. All patients with *Candida* cultured from peripheral blood should receive intravenous amphotericin B to treat acute infection and prevent late sequelae. In patients without neutropenia, endocarditis, or other deep focus, treatment for 2 weeks is often adequate. Funduscopic examination through a dilated pupil is invaluable in detecting endophthalmitis before permanent loss of vision has occurred. Removal of an infected intravenous catheter is usually required to effect cure. If a catheter has caused suppurative phlebitis of a peripheral vein, excision of the infected portion of the vein is usually required.

In one study of bone marrow transplant recipients, daily prophylaxis with fluconazole, 400 mg, appeared to decrease the number of cases of deep candidiasis. Fluconazole also can be used to complete treatment of chronic disseminated ("hepatosplenic") candidiasis if amphotericin B is given until the patient is no longer neutropenic. A comparison of fluconazole with intravenous amphotericin B in the nonneutropenic patient with catheter-acquired candidemia is currently underway. *C. krusei* appears to be resistant to fluconazole.

REFERENCES

AHONEN P et al: Clinical variation of autoimmune polyendocrinopathy-candidiasis-ectodermal dystrophy in a series of 68 patients. N Engl J Med 322:1829, 1991

ANAISSIE E et al: Fluconazole therapy for chronic disseminated candidiasis in patients with leukemia and prior amphotericin B therapy. Am J Med 91:142, 1991

DUPONT B, DROUHET E: Fluconazole in the management of oropharyngeal candidosis in a predominantly HIV antibody-positive group of patients. J Med Vet Mycol 26:67, 1988

MEUNIER F: Candidiasis. Eur J Clin Microbiol Infect Dis 8:438, 1989

ODD FC: *Candida and Candidosis*. Philadelphia, Saunders, 1988

THALER M et al: Hepatic candidiasis in cancer patients: The evolving picture of the syndrome. Ann Intern Med 198:88, 1988

167   ASPERGILLOSIS

JOHN E. BENNETT

ETIOLOGY *Aspergillus fumigatus* is the most common pathogen, but *A. flavus, A. niger*, and several other species can cause disease. *Aspergillus* is a mold with septate hyphae about 2 to 4 μm in diameter. The fungus is identified by its gross and microscopic appearance in culture.

PATHOGENESIS AND PATHOLOGY All the common species of *Aspergillus* which cause disease in humans are ubiquitous in the environment, growing on dead leaves, stored grain, compost piles, hay, and other decaying vegetation. Inhalation of *Aspergillus* spores must be extremely common, but disease is rare. Invasion of lung tissue is almost entirely confined to immunosuppressed patients. Roughly 90 percent will have two of these three conditions: fewer than 500 granulocytes per microliter of peripheral blood, supraphysiologic doses of adrenal corticosteroids, and a history of cytotoxic drugs such as azathioprine. Invasive aspergillosis is an occasional complication of HIV infection, usually concurrent with neutropenia and CD4 cell depletion. Infection is characterized by hyphal invasion of blood vessels, thrombosis, necrosis, and hemorrhagic infarction. Chronic granulomatous disease of childhood also predisposes to invasive pulmonary aspergillosis, but here the inflammatory response is granulomatous and blood vessel invasion is rare.

Massive inhalation of *Aspergillus* spores by normal persons can lead to an acute, diffuse, self-limited pneumonitis. Epithelioid granulomas with giant cells and central pyogenic areas containing hyphae are seen. Spontaneous recovery taking several weeks is the usual course.

Aspergillus can colonize the damaged bronchial tree, pulmonary cysts, or cavities of patients with underlying lung disease. Balls of hyphae within cysts or cavities may reach several centimeters in diameter and be visible on chest x-ray. Tissue invasion does not occur. The term *allergic bronchial aspergillosis* denotes the condition of patients with preexisting asthma who have eosinophilia, IgE antibody to *Aspergillus*, and fleeting pulmonary infiltrates from bronchial plugging (see Chap. 218).

CLINICAL MANIFESTATIONS *Endobronchial pulmonary aspergillosis* presents as chronic productive cough and often hemoptysis in a patient with prior chronic lung disease, such as tuberculosis, sarcoidosis, bronchiectasis, or histoplasmosis. *Aspergilloma* refers to a ball of hyphae within a lung cyst or cavity, usually in the upper lobe. *Aspergillus* may be spread from its endocavitary or endobronchial site to the pleura during the course of bacterial lung abscess or surgery.

Invasive aspergillosis in the immunosuppressed host presents as an acute pneumonia and has a tendency to cavitation. Infection progresses by hematogenous spread as well as extension to surrounding lung and other contiguous structures. Occasionally, the portal of infection in the immunosuppressed host is the paranasal sinus, gastrointestinal tract, skin, or palate.

Aspergillus sinusitis in nonimmunosuppressed patients may take two forms. A ball of hyphae may form in a chronically obstructed paranasal sinus, without tissue invasion. Much less commonly, a chronic, fibrosing granulomatous inflammation with *Aspergillus* hyphae within tissue may begin in the sinus and spread slowly to the orbit and brain.

Growth of *Aspergillus* on cerumen and detritus within the external auditory canal is termed *otomycosis*. Trauma to the cornea may cause *Aspergillus* keratitis. Endophthalmitis follows introduction of *Aspergillus* into the globe by trauma or surgery. *Aspergillus* may infect intracardiac or intravascular prostheses.

DIAGNOSIS Repeated isolation of *Aspergillus* from sputum or demonstration of hyphae in sputum or bronchial brushing specimens suggests endobronchial colonization or infection. Even a single isolation of *Aspergillus* from the sputum of a neutropenic patient with pneumonia, particularly a child or nonsmoker, suggests the diagnosis of invasive aspergillosis. Fungus ball of the lung is usually detectable by chest x-ray. Antibody of the IgG class to *Aspergillus* antigens is demonstrable in the serum of many colonized patients and of virtually all patients with fungus ball.

Biopsy is usually required to diagnose invasive aspergillosis of the lung, paranasal sinus, or sites of dissemination. Blood cultures are rarely positive, even in patients with infected cardiac prosthetic valves. *Aspergillus* hyphae can be identified presumptively by histology, but culture is required for confirmation and determination of species.

TREATMENT Patients with severe hemoptysis due to fungus ball of the lung may benefit by lobectomy. Poor pulmonary function in residual lung and dense pleural adhesions around the lesion can complicate the resection. Systemic chemotherapy is of no value in endobronchial or endocavitary aspergillosis.

Intravenous amphotericin B has resulted in arrest or cure of invasive aspergillosis when immunosuppression is not severe. Combined flucytosine–amphotericin B may be useful in nonneutropenic patients with invasive aspergillosis. Itraconazole, 200 mg bid, is useful in some of the less immunosuppressed patients with indolent or slowly progressive invasive aspergillosis.

REFERENCES

DENNING DW, STEVENS DA: Antifungal and surgical treatment of invasive aspergillosis: Review of 2121 published cases. Rev Infect Dis 12:1147, 1990

——— et al: Treatment of invasive aspergillosis with itraconazole. Am J Med 86:791, 1989

SHIRAKUSA T et al: Surgical treatment of pulmonary aspergilloma and *Aspergillus* empyema. Ann Thorac Surg 48:779, 1989

TALBOT GH et al: Invasive *Aspergillus* rhinosinusitis in patients with acute leukemia. Rev Infect Dis 13:219, 1991

168　MUCORMYCOSIS

JOHN E. BENNETT

ETIOLOGY Species of *Rhizopus, Rhizomucor,* and *Cunninghamella* are most common, but species of *Apophysomyces, Saksenaea, Mucor,* and *Absidia* occasionally cause mucormycosis. These molds have broad, rarely septate hyphae of uneven diameter, ranging from 6 to 50 μm. The fungus is inexplicably difficult to grow from infected tissue. When it occurs, growth is rapid and profuse on most media at room temperature. Identification is based on gross and microscopic appearance of the mold.

Zygomycosis is a term that includes mucormycosis and entomophthoramycosis. The latter is a tropical infection of the subcutaneous tissue or paranasal sinuses caused by species of *Basidiobolus* or *Conidiobolus.*

PATHOGENESIS AND PATHOLOGY *Rhizopus* and *Rhizomucor* species are ubiquitous, appearing on decaying vegetation, dung, and foods of high sugar content. Infection is uncommon and is largely confined to patients with serious preexisting diseases. Mucormycosis originating in the paranasal sinuses and nose occurs predominantly in patients with poorly controlled diabetes mellitus. Patients with organ transplantation, hematologic malignancy, or who are receiving long-term deferoxamine therapy are predisposed to mucormycosis of either sinus or lung. Gastrointestinal mucormycosis occurs in a variety of conditions, including uremia, severe malnutrition, and diarrheal diseases. Infection is acquired from nature, with no person-to-person spread. In all forms of mucormycosis, vascular invasion by hyphae is prominent. Ischemic or hemorrhagic necrosis is the predominant histologic finding.

CLINICAL MANIFESTATIONS Mucormycosis originating in the nose and paranasal sinuses produces a characteristic clinical picture. Low-grade fever, dull sinus pain, and sometimes nasal congestion or a thin, bloody nasal discharge are followed in a few days by double vision, increasing fever, and obtundation. Examination reveals a unilateral generalized reduction of ocular motion, chemosis, and proptosis. The nasal turbinates on the involved side may be dusky red or necrotic. A sharply delineated area of necrosis, strictly respecting the midline, may appear in the hard palate. The skin of the cheek may become inflamed. Fungal invasion of the globe or ophthalmic artery leads to blindness. Opacification of one or more sinuses is found on CT scan or by magnetic resonance imaging. Carotid arteriogram may show invasion or obstruction of the carotid siphon. Coma is due to direct invasion of the frontal lobe. Early symptoms mimic bacterial sinusitis. Clouding of the sensorium may be attributed to diabetic acidosis. Cavernous sinus thrombosis may be considered when orbital invasion occurs. Without treatment, death may occur in a few days to a few weeks.

Pulmonary mucormycosis is a progressive severe pneumonia, accompanied by high fever and toxicity. The necrotic center of large infiltrates may cavitate. Hematogenous spread to other areas of the lung, as well as to brain and other organs, is common. Survival beyond 2 weeks is unusual. Gastrointestinal invasion presents as one or more ulcers which tend to perforate. Hematogenous dissemination can originate from the gastrointestinal tract, lung, or paranasal sinuses. Sometimes no portal of entry can be found.

DIAGNOSIS Lesions of the lung and craniofacial structures are best diagnosed by biopsy and histologic section. Cultural confirmation should be attempted. Wet smear of crushed tissue can provide rapid diagnosis. Cultures of blood and cerebrospinal fluid are negative. Smear and culture of sputum may be positive during cavitation of a lung lesion.

TREATMENT Regulation of diabetes mellitus and decreasing the dose of immunosuppressive drugs aid in the treatment. Extensive debridement of craniofacial lesions appears to be very important. Orbital exenteration may be required. Intravenous amphotericin B is clearly of value in craniofacial mucormycosis and should be employed in the other forms of mucormycosis as well. Maximum tolerated doses are given until progression is halted. The drug is continued for a total of 10 to 12 weeks. Appropriate management results in cure of about half the craniofacial infections. Survival of patients with pulmonary, gastrointestinal, or disseminated mucormycosis is rare.

REFERENCES

GALETTA SL et al: Rhinocerebral mucormycosis: management and survival after carotid occlusion. Ann Neurol 28:103, 1990

INGRAM CW et al: Disseminated zygomycosis: Report of four cases and review. Rev Infect Dis 11:741, 1989

VLASVELD TL, VAN ASBECK BS: Treatment with deferoxamine: A real risk factor for mucormycosis? Nephron 571:487, 1991

169 MISCELLANEOUS MYCOSES

JOHN E. BENNETT

CHROMOBLASTOMYCOSIS This chronic subcutaneous mycosis is rarely seen in the United States but presents as a verrucoid, ulcerated, or crusted skin lesion. Disease originates when thorns or bits of vegetation introduce the fungus into the subcutaneous tissue. Infection spreads over ensuing months and years to contiguous tissue, causing very few symptoms. Appearance of the thick-walled dark-colored rounded forms (''copper pennies'') in tissue is diagnostic. No satisfactory treatment is available.

DERMATOPHYTOSIS **Definition** Dermatophytosis, also known as ringworm or tinea, is a chronic fungal infection of the skin, hair, or nails.

Etiology Species of *Trichophyton*, *Microsporum*, and *Epidermophyton* are called *dermatophytes*. They grow in and remain confined to the keratinous structures of the body. Other mycoses can show fungal invasion of keratinous structures, such as candidiasis, pityriasis versicolor, and tinea nigra, but are traditionally not termed *dermatophytoses*.

Pathology and pathogenesis Dermatophyte species are called *anthropophilic*, *zoophilic*, or *geophilic* depending on whether their usual reservoir within nature appears to be humans, animals, or soil. Infectivity of all these sources is low, and group outbreaks are largely confined to an occasional case clustering of scalp infections in children. Acquisition of a dermatophytosis appears to be favored by minor trauma, maceration, and poor hygiene of the skin. Infection does not seem to confer solid immunity. Repeated infection with the same species is common, particularly with anthropophilic species. Infrequency of scalp infection in adults has been attributed to local factors rather than immunity.

Invasion of the stratum corneum by dermatophytes may cause little inflammation or, particularly with zoophilic fungi, inflammation

can be intense. Shedding of the stratum corneum is increased by inflammation. To the extent that fungal growth cannot keep up with shedding, inflammation may help terminate infection. Conversely, infection is probably favored when shedding is reduced by glucocorticoids and cytotoxic drugs. Antifungal drugs interfere with the ability of fungal growth to keep up with shedding.

Clinical manifestations The disease varies with the site of infection and fungal species. Foot infection (athlete's foot, tinea pedis) may present as fissuring of the toe webs, scaling of the plantar surfaces, or vesicles around the toe webs and soles. Interdigital lesions may be pruritic or, when bacterial superinfection occurs, may be painful. Hand infection is less common but resembles foot infection. Scalp dermatophytosis (tinea capitis) is characterized by areas of alopecia and scaling. In so-called endothrix infection, the hair shaft breaks off at the skin surface, leaving the hairs visible as black dots in the scalp. With some forms of scalp infection, an intense boggy suppuration occurs, called a *kerion*. Dermatophytosis of the glabrous skin (tinea corporis) presents as circumscribed lesions with a wide variety of appearances. Scales, vesicles, or pustules may appear. Inflammation may be minimal or intense. Central healing of less inflamed lesions may be seen. The serpiginous border of inflammation is the source of the name *ringworm*. Dermatophytosis of the bearded area (tinea barbae) appears as a pustular folliculitis. Onychomycosis (tinea unguium) presents as white discolored nails or thickened, chalky, crumbling nails. Peeling and fissuring of the paronychia or keratotic debris under the nail edge also may be seen.

Diagnosis Discolored hairs, scales, and keratotic debris under infected nails should be collected for KOH smear and culture. In the scraping of skin lesions, a drop of water on the skin site may keep the removed scales from flying off and aid in their collection. Culture is important in distinguishing dermatophytes from *Candida* and fungal saprophytes growing in keratinaceous debris.

Treatment Noninflammatory lesions of the trunk, groin, hands, and feet usually respond to twice-daily applications of clotrimazole, miconazole, ketoconazole, econazole, or ciclopirox olamine cream. Hyperkeratotic lesions of the palms and soles respond slowly to these agents and may benefit from Whitfield's ointment initially to thin the keratin. Ointment should not be used between the toes or in the groin or gluteal crease because maceration permits bacterial infection.

Ringworm that is moderately severe, that is unresponsive to topical therapy, or that involves the scalp, nails, or bearded area should be treated systemically. The drug of choice is griseofulvin. Either 500 mg of the microcrystalline form or 375 mg of the ultramicrocrystalline form is given once daily or divided into two doses, given with meals. Double this amount has been recommended for refractory infections. Treatment must be continued until all infected keratin is gone. Cutting of infected hair, epilating nails, and cleansing interdigital webs can expedite cure. Secondary bacterial infection of the foot may require soaks or antibacterial agents. Relapse of dermatophyte foot infections may be decreased by measures to keep the feet clean and dry. Griseofulvin-resistant cases may respond to oral ketoconazole, 200 to 400 mg daily.

FUSARIOSIS Fusarium species can cause localized or hematogenously disseminated infection. Almost all patients with the latter have had hematopoietic malignancy and neutropenia. Abrupt onset of fever, sometimes with myalgia, is followed by distinctive skin lesions in two-thirds of cases. The lesions resemble ecthyma gangrenosum, tend to be multiple, progressively expand in size, and favor the extremities. A portal of infection is not usually apparent. Blood cultures have been positive in 59 percent of cases. Amphotericin B is probably the drug of choice, but recovery depends on diminution of neutropenia.

MALASSEZIA INFECTION (PITYRIASIS) *Malassezia furfur* is part of the normal human skin flora but can cause tinea (pityriasis) versicolor or catheter-acquired sepsis. Tinea versicolor appears as asymptomatic well-delineated hyperpigmented or hypopigmented macules, centered on the upper trunk and upper arms. Confluence of lesions may cover large areas, making the border difficult to find. A fine branny scale or folliculitis is sometimes visible. Skin scrapings examined microscopically by KOH mount show characteristic round and elongated cells. On inspection with Wood's light, lesions either do not fluoresce or appear yellow-green. Erythrasma resembles tinea versicolor but has gram-positive bacilli on smear and fluoresces coral red. Azole creams are effective treatment for small areas of tinea versicolor, but application of selenium sulfide shampoo (Selsun) for 10 min daily, followed by showering to remove the shampoo, is more practical for large areas. Oral ketoconazole is also effective. Catheter-acquired sepsis occurs in patients receiving intravenous lipid, particularly neonates, requires special culture conditions for growth, and is cured by catheter removal.

MYCETOMA Etiology *Actinomycetoma* refers to infection by actinomycetes of the genera *Nocardia, Nocardiopsis, Streptomyces,* and *Actinomadura. Eumycetoma* is caused by true fungi of many different genera. The most common agent varies with the locality.

Pathogenesis and pathology The pathogens live in the soil and enter the skin through minor trauma. The most common site of infection is the foot. Infection runs a relentless course over many years, with destruction of contiguous bone and fascia. Grains are found in purulent foci, surrounded by fibrosis and a mononuclear cell inflammatory response.

Clinical manifestations *Mycetoma* is a chronic suppurative infection originating in subcutaneous tissue and characterized by the presence of grains, which are tightly clumped colonies of the causative agent. The infected site shows painless swelling, woody induration, and sinus tracts which discharge pus intermittently. Systemic symptoms and spread to distant sites in the body are not seen.

Diagnosis The clinical picture is characteristic, but confusion with chronic osteomyelitis or botryomycosis may occur. The diagnosis requires demonstration of grains in pus from the draining sinus or in biopsy sections. Many histologic sections may need to be examined to locate a grain.

Treatment Actinomycetoma may respond to prolonged combination chemotherapy, such as streptomycin and either dapsone or trimethoprim-sulfamethoxazole. Eumycetoma rarely has responded to chemotherapy. As a possible exception, some cases infected with *Madurella mycetomatis* have appeared to respond to ketoconazole.

PHAEOHYPHOMYCOSIS This is the name given to infections caused by fungi with dark-walled hyphae, excluding those infections which can be given conventional names such as chromoblastomycosis. Although an extraordinary variety of fungi and clinical syndromes are encompassed by this definition, the majority of patients have brain abscess, subcutaneous abscess, or allergic fungal sinusitis. Most of the brain abscesses are due to *Cladosporium trichoides* and occur in previously normal persons. Subcutaneous abscesses are usually single, arise at the site of minor trauma, and occur in both immunosuppressed and previously normal persons.

Allergic fungal sinusitis occurs in patients with allergic rhinitis and presents as an expanding mucoid mass in one or more paranasal sinuses. The tenacious mucus contains eosinophils, Charcot-Leyden crystals, and occasional hyphae. Surgical excision of phaeohyphomycotic lesions is important; response to antifungal therapy is often unsatisfactory.

PSEUDALLESCHERIASIS Etiology Also called *Petriellidium boydii, Pseudallescheria boydii* is a mold frequently found in soil. When the fungus is isolated in the imperfect state, it is called *Scedosporium apiospermum.*

Pathogenesis and pathology Wind-borne spores of *P. boydii,* arising in soil, are the presumed source of infection. The fungus grows as a mold within tissue, causing necrosis and abscess formation.

Clinical manifestations *P. boydii* resembles *Aspergillus* in its ability to colonize the endobronchial tree, to form fungus balls in the lung or paranasal sinuses, and to invade the cornea or globe following trauma or surgery and by its propensity to invade the immunosuppressed host. Hyphae of *P. boydii* in tissue may be difficult to distinguish from *Aspergillus.* Infection with *P. boydii* is much less common than with *Aspergillus. P. boydii* is the single most common

cause in the United States of mycetoma. Intravascular hyphae, a hallmark of invasive aspergillosis, also can be found in pseudallescheriasis. Occasional normal patients have developed necrotizing pneumonia or abscesses in brain or other organs due to *P. boydii.*

Diagnosis Demonstration of hyphae in tissue and culture confirmation are required for diagnosis.

Treatment Intravenous miconazole, itraconazole, or ketoconazole is recommended, but therapeutic response to all drugs has been poor.

SPOROTRICHOSIS Etiology *Sporothrix schenckii* lives as a saprophyte on plants in many areas of the world. In nature and on culture at room temperature the fungus grows as a mold, but within host tissue or at 37°C on enriched media it grows as a budding yeast. Identification is by appearance of the fungus in mold and yeast forms.

Pathogenesis and pathology Infection results when minor trauma inoculates the fungus into subcutaneous tissue. Nursery workers, florists, and gardeners acquire the illness from roses, sphagnum moss, and other plants. Infection may be limited to the site of inoculation (plaque sporotrichosis) or extend along proximal lymphatic channels (lymphangitic sporotrichosis). Spread beyond an extremity, the usual site of infection, is rare, and hematogenous dissemination from the skin remains unproven. The portal for osteoarticular, pulmonary, and other extracutaneous forms of sporotrichosis is unknown but is likely the lung.

Untreated sporotrichosis shows little evidence of self-healing and is capable of extreme chronicity. The inflammatory response contains both clusters of neutrophils and a marked granulomatous response with epithelioid cells and giant cells.

Clinical manifestations Lymphangitic sporotrichosis, by far the most common manifestation, forms a nearly painless red papule at the site of inoculation. Over the next several weeks, similar nodules form along proximal lymphatic channels. Nodules intermittently discharge small amounts of pus. Ulceration may occur. The proximal extension of these lesions, often with skip areas, is quite distinctive but may be mimicked by lesions of *Nocardia brasiliensis, Mycobacterium marinum,* or, on rare occasions, by *Leishmania brasiliensis* or *M. kansasii.*

Plaque sporotrichosis is a nontender red maculopapular granuloma confined to the site of inoculation. Osteoarticular sporotrichosis presents as mono- or polyarticular arthritis of indolent onset and progression over months or years involving the elbows, knees, wrists, ankles, and, rarely, smaller joints of the extremities. Periarticular bone develops areas of demineralization on x-ray, and draining sinuses may appear over joints and bursae. Hematogenous spread to the skin may be observed during polyarticular disease, but none of the skin lesions shows lymphangitic spread. Immunosuppression, including advanced HIV infection, predisposes to hematogenous spread. Pulmonary sporotrichosis usually presents as a single chronic cavitary upper-lobe lung lesion.

Diagnosis Culture of pus, joint fluid, sputum, or skin biopsy specimen is the preferred method of diagnosis. Appearance of *S. schenckii* in tissue is quite variable. In skin lesions, the organisms are hard to find.

Treatment Cutaneous sporotrichosis can be cured with oral administration of a saturated solution of potassium iodide given in increasing divided daily doses up to 4.5 to 9 mL/d for adults, as tolerated. Gastrointestinal disturbance or acneiform rash over the cape area and face is common, but therapy should be continued for 1 month after resolution of all lesions. Patients with serious allergic reactions to iodides may respond to local heat, particularly when plaque sporotrichosis is the only form of disease. Itraconazole, an experimental drug, may be of value. Extracutaneous sporotrichosis rarely responds to iodides, but cures have been obtained in over half such patients with prolonged courses of intravenous amphotericin B. Itraconazole is effective in lymphocutaneous sporotrichosis and in some cases of extracutaneous sporotrichosis.

TRICHOSPORONOSIS *Trichosporon beigelii* causes asymptomatic small white concretions on hair shafts, a condition called *white* *piedra*, but can cause hematogenously disseminated infection in neutropenic patients, mostly leukemics. Multiple erythematous or purpuric papules accompany the fungemia. The lesions can evolve into large, tense hemorrhagic bullae. Blood cultures are usually positive. Prosthetic valve endocarditis due to *T. beigelii* is also well described. Intravenous amphotericin B is the drug of choice.

REFERENCES

Chromoblastomycosis

TUFFANELLI L, MILBURN PB: Treatment of chromoblastomycosis. J Am Acad Dermatol 23:728, 1990

Dermatophytosis

WRIGHT DC et al: Generalized chronic dermatophytosis in patients with human immunodeficiency virus type I infection and CD4 depletion. Arch Dermatol 127:265, 1991

Fusariosis

ANAISSIE E et al: New spectrum of fungal infections in patients with cancer. Rev Infect Dis 11:369, 1989
GAMIS AS et al: Disseminated infection with *Fusarium* in recipients of bone marrow transplants. Rev Infect Dis 13:1077, 1991

Malassezia infection (pityriasis)

DANKER WM et al: *Malassezia* fungemia in neonates and adults: Complication of hyperalimentation. Rev Infect Dis 9:743, 1987

Mycetoma

GUMAA SA et al: Mycetoma of the head and neck. Am J Trop Med Hyg 35:594, 1986
TIGHT RR, BARTLETT MS: Actinomycetoma in the United States. Rev Infect Dis 3:1139, 1981

Phaeohyphomycosis

WASHBURN RG et al: Chronic fungal sinusitis in apparently normal hosts. Medicine 67:231, 1988

Pseudallescheriasis

BERENGUER J et al: Central nervous system infection caused by *Pseudallescheria boydii*: Case report and review. Rev Infect Dis 11:890, 1989
GALGIANI JN et al: *Pseudallescheria boydii* infections treated with ketoconazole. Chest 86:219, 1984
TRAVIS LB et al: Clinical significance of *Pseudallescheria boydii*: A review of 10 years' experience. Mayo Clin Proc 60:531, 1985

Sporotrichosis

BULLPITT P, WEEDON D: Sporotrichosis: A review of 39 cases. Pathology 10:249, 1978
ENGLAND DM, HOCHHOLZER L: Primary pulmonary sporotrichosis. Am J Surg Pathol 9:193, 1985
FRIEDMAN SJ, DOYLE JA: Extracutaneous sporotrichosis. Int J Dermatol 22:171, 1983
PLUSS JL, OPAL SM: Pulmonary sporotrichosis: Review of treatment and outcome. Medicine 65:143, 1986
SHAW JC et al: Sporotrichosis in the acquired immunodeficiency syndrome. J Am Acad Dermatol 21:1145, 1989

Trichosporonosis

WALSH TJ et al: Trichosporonosis in patients with neoplastic disease. Medicine 65:268, 1986

(Pityrosporum)

JACINTO-JAMORA S et al: *Pityrosporum* folliculitis in the Philippines: Diagnosis, prevalence and management. J Am Acad Dermatol 24:693, 1991

section 16   Protozoal and helminthic infections: General considerations

170   MOLECULAR BIOLOGY AND IMMUNOLOGY OF PARASITIC INFECTIONS

JOHN R. DAVID / LEO X. LIU

Protozoan and helminthic parasites have caused incalculable human suffering and death through the ages, and their global impact on human health remains enormous today. Every year several hundred million people contract malaria, the most serious human protozoal disease, and close to a million children die of falciparum malaria in Africa alone. Another protozoan, *Trypanosoma cruzi*, is a major cause of heart disease in South America. Protozoal parasites such as *Toxoplasma* and *Cryptosporidium* have emerged as important opportunistic pathogens in patients with AIDS and other immunocompromised conditions. Schistosomiasis, a helminthic fluke disease transmitted via snails, affects 200 to 300 million persons worldwide. Filarial nematode parasites infect a similar number of people, and one of these, *Onchocerca volvulus,* is the second most common infectious cause of blindness in the world. Over one *billion* people harbor intestinal nematode parasites, including *Ascaris*, hookworm, and *Trichuris*.

Many traditional control measures have failed to curb the magnitude of parasitic infections. Nowhere is this more evident and serious than in the case of malaria. In the middle of this century there was widespread optimism that malaria could be eradicated by spraying homes with DDT against mosquitoes and by treating infected people with chloroquine. However, the development of widespread insecticide resistance in mosquitoes and chloroquine resistance in *Plasmodium falciparum* has contributed to an alarming resurgence of malaria in the last two decades. For example, in Sri Lanka, the annual number of reported malaria cases in the 1960s rose from 18 to over half a million! Furthermore, modernization efforts in many developing countries have paradoxically increased the spread of certain parasitic infections. Dams constructed in Egypt and Ghana to provide industrial energy have vastly expanded the amount of lake coastline available for the transmission of schistosomiasis to local residents by infected snails. Irrigation schemes in Asia for rice cultivation have multiplied the number of breeding sites for mosquitoes that carry malaria. Clearing of the Amazon rainforest has greatly increased human contact with indigenous sandflies that transmit leishmaniasis.

PARASITE BIOLOGY   The term *parasite* derives from the Greek παρασιτοσ, meaning literally "one who eats at the table of another." In a broad sense, all infectious microorganisms can be considered parasites, since they depend on the host organism for essential nutrients and impart some degree of harm. Nevertheless, by convention, *parasitic infections* refer to those caused by protozoa and helminths. What distinguish these eukaryotic parasites are complex life cycles and long-lived chronic infections of the human host. A typical parasite life cycle comprises sequential developmental stages which can include parasitic life-styles in more than one host and in some instances a period of free-living existence. Nonhuman hosts involved in the rather bewildering variety of parasite life cycles include insects, mollusks, and mammals. Transmission by these biologic vectors or infected intermediate hosts is a crucial feature of

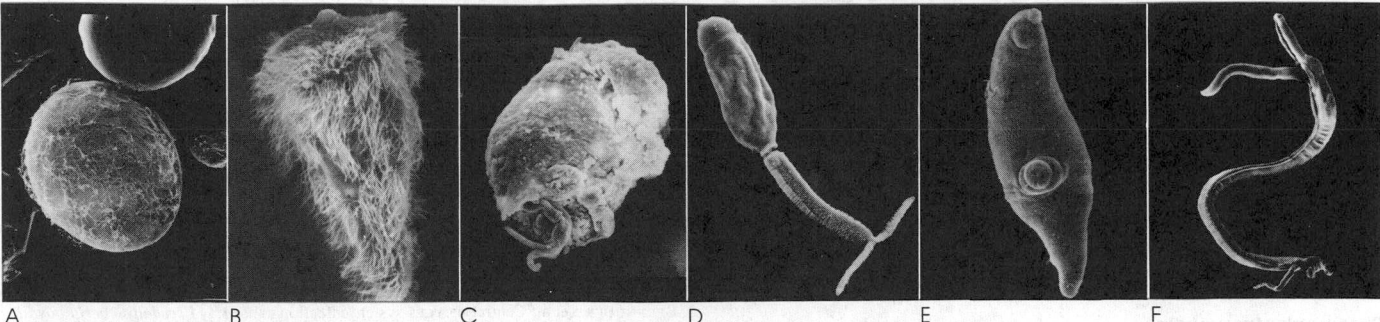

A   Egg in human tissues and stool   D   Cercaria in water and human skin

B   Miracidium in water   E   Schistosomulum in human tissues and blood

C   Sporocyst in snail   F   Adult worms in mesenteric veins

FIGURE 170-1 Morphologic transformations of schistosome parasites in the course of their life cycle. (*Scanning electron micrographs of Schistosome* *japonicum and S. mekongi courtesy of Prasert Sobhon, Ph.D., Mahidol University, Thailand.*)

many parasitic infections. The functional adaptations required of a parasite to negotiate completely different environments results in parasite stages which are morphologically and biochemically distinct from one another. Each transition from one parasite stage to another should be envisioned as an all-encompassing transformation no less radical than the metamorphosis of a caterpillar to a butterfly (Fig. 170-1). Compared with viruses and bacteria, parasites are antigenically complex. Each developmental stage is antigenically different, which has direct implications for the nature of immune responses in parasitic infections.

GENERAL FEATURES OF PARASITIC INFECTIONS There are important differences between protozoal and helminthic parasites. Protozoal parasites are unicellular and replicate directly within the human host by asexual division. Helminthic parasites, on the other hand, are relatively large, multicellular worms which (with rare exceptions) cannot directly multiply in humans. Protozoans, being of small size, can be intracellular or extracellular parasites, whereas helminths are almost exclusively extracellular parasites of tissue, blood, or the gastrointestinal tract. Like viruses and bacteria, protozoal parasites replicate directly within the host, without having to pass through the outside environment or through intermediate hosts. In malaria, for example, infective sporozoites multiply as merozoites in the liver, and merozoites subsequently infect host erythrocytes with repeating amplification cycles of parasite replication and reinvasion. Thus even a single infectious mosquito bite can ultimately result in severe morbidity or death from malaria. In contrast, helminth parasites typically reproduce sexually in the host to generate eggs or larvae which must be passed out (via the feces, urine, or a biting insect vector) in order to continue development. Further parasite development in the environment or an intermediate host is then required to reach a stage infective for humans. Thus many helminthic infections, unlike malaria, require repeated exposures to infectious larvae or eggs in order for a heavy burden of parasites to develop. This usually entails prolonged residence in an area of ongoing transmission. Even in an endemic area, most individuals are only lightly infected and often asymptomatic, whereas helminthic *disease* develops mainly in those individuals who bear heavy worm burdens.

Chronicity is a predominant characteristic of infections with protozoa and helminths and is related to the remarkable ability of parasites to counteract or evade host immune responses. Immediate mortality is unusual in parasitic infections except for severe malaria, visceral leishmaniasis and trypanosomiasis. Some parasites (such as *Toxoplasma* and *Trichinella*) become latent after the initial phase of invasion. Pathologic changes and clinical disease take years to develop in many parasitic infections, such as Chagas' disease and most helminthic infections.

Whereas in many instances, immunity to viruses and bacteria can be complete and lifelong after only a single exposure to the pathogen, such sterilizing immunity is rare among protozoa and nonexistent for helminth parasites. For many protozoal and helminthic infections, protection from serious infection is rarely, if ever, complete, becomes maximal only after repeated infection, and declines in the absence of further exposure. For certain parasites such as the intestinal nematodes, naturally acquired immunity does not appear to develop at all. Finally, detrimental host immune responses can lead to immunopathologic tissue damage that typifies some parasitic diseases such as schistosomiasis and lymphatic filariasis.

The scientific understanding of parasitic protozoa and helminths has lagged behind that of viruses and bacteria in part because their complex structures and life cycles make parasites more difficult to study in the laboratory. Furthermore, most serious parasitic infections are largely confined to the developing countries of Africa, Asia, and South America. The last two decades, however, have witnessed a resurgence of scientific interest in medically important parasites, leading to impressive progress in understanding their biology. The development of DNA cloning techniques and monoclonal antibodies, as well as in vitro culture methods for certain protozoa such as malaria, has made it possible to study parasites at a molecular level. The enormous public health impact of parasitic infections and the failure of classic control programs have stimulated a search for better ways to treat and control these diseases using modern immunologic and molecular biology methods.

MOLECULAR MECHANISMS OF PARASITE INVASION

Parasites can enter the human body by only a few infective routes, including oral ingestion, skin penetration, and bites of insect vectors. Virtually any host organ or tissue can become parasitized, however, and most parasites are highly specific in the selection of host sites in which they become established. Parasitic protozoa and helminths have evolved a variety of exquisite adaptations to recognize, invade, and survive in specific host cells and tissues (Table 170-1). For intracellular protozoa such as *Plasmodium* and *Leishmania* spp., attachment to a specific host cell is followed by membrane invagination or endocytosis that allows the parasite to enter that cell. Attachment to host cell membranes is also vital to extracellular protozoal parasites such as *Entamoeba histolytica,* which uses an adherence protein (a galactose-inhibitable lectin) that binds to colonic mucins. Other extracellular parasites have developed specialized structures, such as the adhesive ventral disk of *Giardia* trophozoites, to affix themselves to host tissues.

TABLE 170-1 Some molecular mechanisms of parasite invasion and establishment

Parasite	Cell or tissue target	Proposed mediators Host cell organelle or molecule	Parasite-derived factors
INTRACELLULAR PARASITES			
Leishmania promastigote	Macrophage	Complement receptors CR1 and CR3	LPG (lipophosphoglycan, gp63)
		Mannose-fucose receptor advance glycosylation end-product receptor	
Plasmodium sporozoite	Liver hepatocyte	Basolateral membrane	CSP (circumsporozoite protein)
P. vivax merozoite	Reticulocytes only		PvRBP 1 and 2 (reticulocyte-binding proteins)
	Duffy (+) erythrocytes only	Duffy group antigen	PvDAP-1 (Duffy adhesion protein)
P. falciparum merozoite	All erythrocytes	Glycophorins	SABP (sialic acid–binding protein)
			MSP-I (merozoite surface protein-I)
P. falciparum–infected RBCs	Endothelium	ICAM-1, CD36, thrombospondin	PfEMP-1, PfHRP-2
Trypanosoma cruzi	Macrophage	Vacuolar membrane	TC-TOX, a C9-like pore-forming protein
	Fibroblast	Surface adhesion	Penetrin, a heparin-binding protein
	Many cell types	Membrane surface glycoproteins	*trans*-Sialidase
	Many cell types	Fibronectin	GP85, a fibronectin receptor
Trichinella spiralis	Skeletal muscle	Induction of muscle cell dedifferentiation	Unknown
EXTRACELLULAR PARASITES			
Entamoeba histolytica	Colonic mucosa	Surface mucinous glycoproteins	Galactose-inhibitable lectin
Giardia lamblia	Gut epithelium	Surface glycans	Trypsin-activated lectin
Schistosoma cercariae	Skin		Elastase
Hookworms	Skin penetration, anticoagulant		Metalloproteinase

MOLECULAR PARASITE-HOST INTERACTIONS IN MALARIA

Malarial parasites furnish elegant examples of host cell recognition, attachment, and invasion by successive parasite stages. Malaria is transmitted by the bite of an infected anopheline mosquito. Malarial sporozoites injected into the bloodstream from the mosquito salivary gland soon invade the liver, where each parasite divides asexually to produce many merozoites. These burst out of the hepatocytes into the bloodstream and invade erythrocytes. The parasite further divides within the erythrocyte to generate more merozoites, which eventually rupture the cell and invade other erythrocytes in repeating cycles that are responsible for much of the clinical disease. Some merozoites develop into gametocytes that are taken up by another mosquito when it bites an infected person, leading to the development of sporozoites which are infective for humans.

The surface membrane of the malarial sporozoite is covered by a stage-specific protein called the *circumsporozoite protein* (CSP), which has been intensively investigated in the quest for a malaria vaccine (see below). In addition to an immunogenic central domain, CSP also contains a carboxyl-terminal region (termed *region II*) whose amino acid sequence is similar to a known cell adhesion domain of the bridging protein thrombospondin. Recent studies have shown that CSP binds exclusively to hepatocytes and not to other cells or organs and in particular attaches to the basolateral segment of the hepatocyte membrane which is exposed to the bloodstream. Synthetic region II peptides can block not only the binding of recombinant CSP to hepatocytes but also the penetration of live sporozoites into liver cells, indicating that this adhesive motif of the parasite molecule is critical for recognition and invasion of the target host cell.

Bloodstream infection begins when *Plasmodium* merozoites invade red blood cells. In addition to adhering to the erythrocyte surface, the merozoite must orient itself so that its apical end (containing key organelles for invasion) faces the host cell membrane. After the parasite and erythrocyte membranes form a tight junction, the erythrocyte membrane invaginates to form a parasitophorous vacuole that engulfs the merozoite. Different malarial species prefer different types of erythrocytes; for example, *P. vivax* primarily invades the reticulocyte (immature) subpopulation, whereas *P. falciparum* invades all types of red blood cells. How do these species recognize different types of erythrocytes? In the case of *P. falciparum*, the merozoites

appear to exploit sialic acid residues of glycophorins (which are integral membrane proteins of *all* erythrocytes) as cell-surface receptors. Two *P. falciparum* proteins have been discovered to date that bind erythrocyte sialic acid. *P. vivax* merozoites, on the other hand, require Duffy blood group glycoproteins for erythrocyte attachment and entry. Indeed, the resistance of most black Africans to *P. vivax* malaria can be explained by the absence of Duffy group antigens on their erythrocytes. Research into this phenomenon has uncovered merozoite apical complex proteins which mediate specific binding to Duffy glycoproteins, as well as others which bind only to reticulocytes.

Malaria has exerted a more profound influence on human genetics than any other infectious disease, as is evident from the variety of genetic polymorphisms (such as the thalassemias and hemoglobin S) that confer protection against fatal falciparum malaria in heterozygous individuals. Recently, specific HLA haplotypes also have been shown to confer protection against severe falciparum malaria; these are the first known examples of immune-response genes that protect against a fatal infectious agent. One reason *P. falciparum* is so dangerous is that parasitized erythrocytes are sequestered in deep vascular beds of the brain, giving rise to cerebral malaria. This sequestration is caused by the adherence of parasite-derived proteins on the surface of infected erythrocytes to endothelial cells. Intercellular adhesion molecule-1 (ICAM-1, which also binds leukocytes and human rhinoviruses) has been identified as an endothelial cytoadhesion receptor for *P. falciparum*–infected erythrocytes. Other endothelial molecules which bind parasitized red blood cells include CD36, an integral membrane glycoprotein, and thrombospondin, a protein thought to bridge cells together by linking membrane-associated proteins.

INVASION STRATEGIES OF OTHER INTRACELLULAR PARASITES

Many other remarkable tactics are used by parasites to invade host cells. *Leishmania* parasites occupy what is seemingly the most inhospitable site for any infectious organism, namely, the phagolysosome of macrophages. To reach this unusual niche, infective *Leishmania* promastigotes actually activate serum complement and become opsonized with C3b, which promotes their uptake into macrophages. How do these parasites manage to avoid being killed by the activated complement pathway? *Leishmania* promastigotes are covered by a complex polysaccharide called *lipophosphoglycan* (LPG), which is the major C3 acceptor on the parasite surface. In virulent promastigotes, an elongated form of LPG (created by the addition of repeated oligosaccharide subunits) prevents the insertion of the terminal C5–C9 membrane attack complex into the parasite membrane. Both LPG and a surface protease called *gp63* mediate the in vitro uptake of promastigotes via complement receptors on the macrophage surface. Once inside the phagolysosome, the parasite appears to survive by inactivating lysosomal enzymes and toxic oxidative metabolites. Here again, LPG plays an important role by inhibiting the macrophage oxidative burst and by scavenging oxygen radicals.

T. cruzi, the cause of Chagas' disease, can invade many different types of host cells. The invasive trypomastigote stage possesses a surface enzyme, required for host cell entry, which has the unique ability to transfer sialic acid residues from host glycoproteins to the parasite's own surface. Shortly after entering the host cell inside a parasitophorous vacuole, the parasite disrupts the vacuolar membrane to reach the cytoplasm, where it multiplies. This escape may be effected by another *T. cruzi* protein that forms a pore in the vacuolar membrane and is structurally similar to C9, the terminal pore-forming complement component.

The ancient disease known as *trichinosis* is caused by *Trichinella spiralis* larvae ingested by humans when they eat infected meat. These multicellular worms have the extraordinary ability to invade a skeletal muscle cell and completely transform the host cell morphology and gene expression, with an increase in cell size and nuclei numbers coupled with the loss of contractile proteins. *Trichinella* appears to have evolved mechanisms to take over the transcriptional machinery of myocytes, causing the muscle cell to redifferentiate into a nurse cell which sustains the larva.

INVASION OF HOST TISSUES BY HELMINTH PARASITES Helminth parasites elaborate a complex variety of enzymes and other substances which allow them to penetrate host tissues. Invasive larvae of nematodes and trematodes, such as hookworm larvae or schistosome cercariae, secrete proteolytic enzymes which help to penetrate the skin. Once inside the host, helminth parasites use a variety of mechanisms to remain fixed in their preferred anatomic locale. *Trichuris* whipworms, for example, thread themselves into the superficial colonic epithelium, whereas *Ancylostoma* hookworms use buccal teeth to fasten onto small bowel mucosa. Worms which live in a vascular or gut lumen presumably "swim" by active motility to resist being swept downstream. These include adult filariae in the lymphatic channels and *Ascaris* roundworms in the gut. Still other parasites, such as *Trichinella* larvae and *Onchocerca* adult worms, envelop themselves with a specialized structure which protects them from immune attack. The molecular basis of locating an appropriate host, tissue tropism, and tissue invasion by helminth parasites remains largely unexplored, however. In vitro culture systems like those taken for granted in the study of viruses and bacteria have not yet been realized for parasitic helminths, which can be experimentally propagated only through host animals and invertebrate vectors. Once parasitic helminths do invade the host, they unveil a sophisticated array of mechanisms to evade host immune responses, and some of these have been elucidated as described below.

PARASITE BIOCHEMISTRY

DRUG RESISTANCE The development of drug resistance in parasites, as for pathogenic viruses and bacteria, has become a serious issue. The situation is most grave for the treatment and prophylaxis of malaria. Chloroquine resistance in *P. falciparum,* the most malignant form of human malaria, is so widespread that it is no longer the exception but the rule. Resistance to chloroquine appears to be due to enhanced efflux of the drug out of the malarial cell. *Leishmania* spp. can become resistant to antimetabolite drugs by a process of gene amplification, in which they overproduce the target parasite enzymes to overcome inhibition by the drugs. Other known mechanisms by which parasites become resistant include reduced drug

uptake, increased drug inactivation, and alteration and loss of receptor sites and target molecules for a drug. Drug resistance has already developed to relatively new antiparasitic agents such as mefloquine for malaria, praziquantel for schistosomiasis, and ivermectin for nematode infections. Unfortunately, the actual site and mechanism of action of these and many other useful drugs are still unknown, which hinders the understanding of drug resistance and attempts to overcome it by chemical modifications to the parent compound.

DRUG DESIGN A better understanding of parasite biochemistry also may suggest new targets for antiparasite chemotherapy. Because many parasites by their nature depend on host metabolism, some of their own biochemical pathways have degenerated. For example, parasitic protozoa and helminths are unable to synthesize their own purines and must depend on intricate purine salvage pathways. In other cases, parasites may have evolved unique enzymes which are employed exclusively in essential parasitic behaviors. It may be possible to rationally exploit such differences between parasite and host biochemistry and metabolism to develop new drugs which act selectively against a parasite without incurring host toxicity. Unfortunately, there are limited commercial incentives to develop drugs that are most needed in poor tropical countries. For example, only a few new drugs are undergoing clinical testing for malaria (a disease that causes 1 to 3 million deaths yearly), and none of these is being developed by U.S. pharmaceutical companies. In contrast, almost 100 drugs are currently in testing for AIDS, a disease of rich countries as well as poor.

DIAGNOSTIC TESTS Contemporary molecular and immunologic techniques provide a new generation of sensitive tools suitable for clinical diagnosis and epidemiologic studies. Immunodiagnostic assays can be designed to detect either parasite antigens or host antiparasite antibodies. The enzyme-linked immunosorbent assay (ELISA), for example, is useful for detecting tissue parasites, such as *Toxoplasma* and cysticerci, that cannot be isolated readily from body fluids of patients. Serologic cross-reactions are common in parasitic infections, a fact which limits the usefulness of immunoassays in endemic areas where people are commonly exposed to many kinds of parasites. This problem can be overcome by the use of monoclonal antibodies to parasite antigens which are species-specific. Extremely sensitive detection of parasite DNA is possible with DNA hybridization techniques and the polymerase chain reaction. For example, using specific DNA probes, it is possible not only to detect *Leishmania* in skin biopsies but also to determine the particular species involved. Other clinical applications of parasite DNA detection include the diagnosis of low-grade malaria or screening of donor blood in areas where *T. cruzi* is endemic. Such methods are also useful in epidemiologic field surveys of infected humans or vectors as part of mass control programs.

IMMUNE EVASION BY PARASITES

Parasites have evolved a variety of ingenious ways to evade immune responses of the host. Some of these are listed in Table 170-2. For intracellular pathogens such as those discussed above, invasion and immune evasion are often two sides of the same coin, for seclusion within a host cell can provide a privileged site inaccessible to immunologic surveillance. Other protozoa besides *Leishmania* manage to avoid lysis by complement. The virulent trypomastigotes of *T. cruzi,* for example, release an inhibitor of C3 convertase activity, thereby limiting complement activation on the parasite surface. *Toxoplasma* parasites, after being engulfed by a macrophage, block fusion of the phagosome with lysosomes and prevent the acidification of the phagosome. A number of parasites induce suppressor mechanisms which dampen or eliminate an effective host immune response. Other parasites can destroy mediators of inflammation involved in an effective immune response. For example, *Taenia* cestodes destroy complement components, and amebae produce factors that neutralize macrophage chemotaxis. Nematodes possess metabolically active

TABLE 170-2 Some mechanisms of parasite immune evasion

Parasite	Mechanism
Trypanosoma brucei, Giardia, Plasmodium merozoites	Antigenic variation
Plasmodium, Leishmania, T. cruzi	Escape into host cells
Toxoplasma gondii	Prevention of lysosome-phagosome fusion
Leishmania, Toxoplasma, T. brucei, T. cruzi	Inhibition of complement
Leishmania amastigotes	Prevention of lysosomal toxic action
Schistosomes	Acquisition of host molecules
Schistosomes	Antigenic mimicry
Schistosomes, *Trichinella*	Shedding of surface antigens
Schistosomes, filariae	Immune suppression
Schistosomes, *Fasciola, T. cruzi*	Cleavage of bound immunoglobulins
Schistosomes, parasitic nematodes	Surface and secreted antioxidant enzymes
Many tissue nematodes	Shedding of mucinous surface coat
Taenia, amebae	Inactivation of inflammatory mediators

cuticles which can absorb extrinsic molecules and secrete abundant quantities of parasite enzymes which may be important in evading innate and antibody-mediated host defenses. Many nematode parasites are also covered by an outermost surface glycocalyx which is rapidly turned over and can be sloughed off in the event of antibody-mediated leukocyte attachment.

ANTIGENIC VARIATION IN AFRICAN TRYPANOSOMES The protozoa that cause African sleeping sickness display a particularly fascinating and formidable mechanism of immune evasion. *T. brucei* possesses a thick surface coat made up of $>10^7$ molecules of a single antigenic glycoprotein. When laboratory animals are experimentally injected with cloned trypanosomes, all bearing the same surface antigen, successive waves of parasites appear in the blood similar to those seen when a human is bitten by an infected tsetse fly. Each wave consists mainly of organisms expressing a single variant surface glycoprotein (VSG) antigen that is different from VSGs expressed in previous peaks in the same infection. Each peak of parasitemia induces soluble antibody directed at the major VSG. However, the parasites escape immune destruction by periodically switching from one surface VSG to another VSG. A single trypanosome clone can sequentially produce hundreds of different VSGs! VSGs are linked to the parasite membrane by a glycosylphosphotidyl inositol (GPI) anchor, which allows rapid turnover of the exposed protein by the cleavage action of a specific phospholipase. Indeed, GPI anchoring of membrane surface proteins was first discovered in these parasite antigens. Molecular studies have shown that each VSG is encoded by a distinct gene and that only one VSG gene is usually expressed at a time from the hundreds available in the trypanosome genome. A VSG gene can be expressed following several different types of novel gene rearrangements. For example, a particular VSG gene to be expressed can be copied and transposed to a telomeric site on another chromosome which is used for expression. Only the duplicate gene, referred to as an *expression-linked copy,* is then expressed. If each VSG gene is visualized as a tape cassette in a library, then a selected VSG gene cassette is duplicated, and the duplicate cassette is removed from the library and inserted into a genetic tape deck to be played. Basic research on trypanosomes has led to the discovery of other unique molecular mechanisms that have expanded existing concepts of eukaryotic gene expression, including *trans* splicing and RNA editing. In the phenomenon of *trans* splicing, mRNAs from two noncontiguous segments of nuclear DNA, an invariant miniature exon and the protein-coding exon, are spliced together to produce a chimeric mRNA. RNA editing, which occurs in mitochondrial (kinetoplast) transcripts, entails the addition or deletion of uridine bases to mRNA, which results in the modification of noncoding primary transcripts (specified in the DNA) to mature mRNA molecules which do code

for proteins. Whether these novel molecular processes contribute to parasitism or could provide specific targets for antiparasite drug development is as yet unknown.

IMMUNE EVASION BY SCHISTOSOMES In schistosomiasis, the adult worms can live for decades in the human vasculature despite direct exposure to effector elements of the immune system, such as B and T lymphocytes and myelocytes. Schistosomes provide the most intensively studied examples of immune evasion among helminth parasites. Their battery of evasion strategies includes molecular mimicry, antigenic disguise, suppression of immune responses, and blocking antibodies. Following invasion, schistosomes can disguise themselves by acquiring host antigens that are incorporated into the outer lipid bilayer of the parasite tegument. These include blood group antigens, MHC glycoproteins, fibronectin, immunoglobulins, a C1q receptor, antiproteases, and a molecule resembling human decay accelerating factor. Schistosomes also produce a surface protein that mimics host alpha$_2$-macroglobulin. Their tegumental membrane is periodically turned over, and areas containing bound immunoglobulin can be shed. Schistosomes also produce immunomodulatory molecules such as β-endorphin as well as proteases that cleave immunoglobulins and interfere with complement action. Finally, ongoing antigenic stimulation by schistosome molecules can result in the preferential generation of IgM and irrelevant IgG antibodies (blocking antibodies) that may down-regulate effective humoral or cytotoxic cellular responses against the parasite.

IMMUNOLOGIC RESPONSES TO PARASITIC INFECTIONS

A variety of humoral and cell-mediated immune mechanisms have been found to be effective against parasites in vitro. However, the nature of protective immunity in vivo against most parasites is highly elusive. Protozoal and helminthic parasites present a complex panoply of antigens to the host. Different stages of the same parasite usually occupy different sites in the body, and each stage displays a distinct repertoire of antigens so that the parasite in effect presents a moving target to the host immune system. Furthermore, as discussed above, parasites have evolved numerous ways of escaping host defenses. In a typical chronic parasitic infection, the host mounts a series of immunologic responses which are unable to eliminate the parasite and in some cases lead to immunopathologic damage to host tissues. Few if any of these diverse host immune responses may prevent reinfection or limit the expression of clinical disease. For many parasitic infections, the evidence for acquired immunity rests on empirical epidemiologic observations. For example, population studies suggest that age-related resistance develops in schistosomiasis because adults have less intense infections and are less likely to become reinfected than children following curative chemotherapy. The dissection of protective immune responses, i.e., those which parasites *cannot* evade, is the central challenge of parasite immunology.

IMMUNE EFFECTOR MECHANISMS AGAINST PARASITES These include antibodies, antibody-dependent cell-mediated cytotoxicity, activated macrophages, CD8+ cytotoxic T cells, and possibly natural killer cells. Antibodies can be effective against intracellular protozoa by blocking receptors involved in host cell entry. For example, antibodies against some of the malarial merozoite proteins mentioned above can block erythrocyte invasion, and antibodies against gp63 can prevent *Leishmania* from infecting macrophages in vitro. Antibodies are also an integral component of the classical complement pathway, in which lytic killing of target cells follows opsonization by antibody. African trypanosomes can be lysed in vitro by serum complement in the presence of antibodies against VSG, but complement-mediated killing is probably not significant in actual human infection with trypanosomes and most other parasites.

In the laboratory, purified eosinophils will kill schistosomules of *S. mansoni* if the schistosomules have been coated previously with specific antiparasite IgG antibodies, a phenomenon known as *antibody-dependent cell-mediated cytotoxicity* (ADCC). This mechanism entails the attachment of eosinophils to the Fc portion of the IgG via an Fc receptor, followed by the release of toxic eosinophil granule proteins which kill the schistosome larvae. If antibodies contact the parasite surface, macrophages and even platelets can be shown in vitro to attach to these antibodies through their Fc receptors and kill parasites. Interferon-γ (IFN-γ) and other cytokines such as migration inhibitory factor (MIF) and tumor necrosis factor α (TNFα) can activate effector cells to enhance antibody-dependent parasite killing.

IMMUNOREGULATION BY T CELLS AND CYTOKINES Some of the most exciting new developments in immunology research concern T lymphocytes and their secreted cytokines, which have been shown to strongly influence both protective immunity and immunopathology in parasitic infections. CD4+ helper T cells can be classified into two major subsets, T_{H1} and T_{H2}, based on differential profiles of cytokine secretion, according to evidence derived from murine models and recently extended to cultured human T cells. T_{H1} cells produce IFN-γ and interleukin 2 (IL-2) and are responsible for cell-mediated immune reactions such as delayed-type hypersensitivity. IFN-γ provides a key signal that activates macrophages to kill intracellular organisms by reactive oxygen intermediates and nitric oxide. Animals injected with antibodies to IFN-γ or transgenic mice with disrupted genes for IFN-γ or the IFN-γ receptor are highly susceptible to *Leishmania*, mycobacteria, and other intracellular pathogens. T_{H2} cells, on the other hand, release IL-4, IL-5, and other cytokines which result in eosinophilia, elevated serum IgE, and mastocytosis, which are seen in both allergic reactions and helminthic infections.

Experimental infections with *L. major*, a cause of cutaneous leishmaniasis, have provided the strongest evidence of genetically controlled T cell–mediated resistance to a parasitic infection. Cutaneous infection of most inbred mouse strains with *L. major* provides a T_{H1} response with abundant local generation of IFN-γ, which in turn results in a limited skin lesion that heals spontaneously and confers resistance to reinfection. Certain other inbred mouse strains instead mount a T_{H2}-type response upon infection, with very little production of IFN-γ, and here the infection progresses to a disseminated and ultimately fatal form of leishmaniasis. CD8+ T cells, which produce high levels of IFN-γ and can kill infected host cells, also appear to play an important role in protecting against certain intracellular protozoa. In experimental models CD8+ T cells have recently been shown to confer resistance against *T. cruzi, T. gondii,* and the preerythryocytic liver stages of malaria. Whereas T_{H1} cells play a protective role against *Leishmania* and shistosomes, T_{H2} cells protect against certain nematodes.

EOSINOPHILS, IgE, AND IMMUNITY IN HELMINTHIC INFECTIONS The immunologic hallmarks of chronic infection with parasitic helminths include eosinophilia, elevated IgE levels, and in certain cases mastocytosis. These responses appear to be induced mainly by T_{H2} cytokines: IL-5 stimulates eosinophilopoiesis, IL-4 induces immunoglobulin isotype switching to IgE, and IL-4 and other cytokines stimulate mastocytosis. Eosinophils have been thought to play a protective function in helminthic infections because of their potency in killing schistosomes and other helminths via ADCC. Helminthic parasites also can be killed in vitro by IgE-mediated activation of macrophages and other cytotoxic cells. It is unclear, however, whether eosinophils and IgE protect against helminthic infections in vivo. Field studies of schistosomiasis in Africa showed that adults, who had high levels of antiparasite IgE, were far less likely to become reinfected following chemotherapy than children, who had low levels of antischistosome IgE, despite comparable exposure to infection through cercariae-infested waters. Rats made specifically IgE-deficient by repeated injections of antiepsilon chain antibodies show a markedly impaired resistance to *Trichinella* infection. However, the depletion in rodents of IgE by injection of monoclonal antibodies to IL-4 does not influence resistance to *S. mansoni* and other helminthic infections. Similarly, administration of

monoclonal antibodies to IL-5 drastically reduces blood and tissue eosinophils in rodents but does not alter their worm burden or resistance to reinfection with schistosomes or *Trichinella*.

In animals that have established chronic infections with adult schistosome worms, new invading cercariae are destroyed while the adult worms remain unaffected—an unusual form of immunity called *concomitant immunity*. Of note, T_{H1}-type responses, characterized by high IFN-γ and IL-2 levels, predominate early in schistosome infection and are also associated with protective immunity induced by vaccination with irradiated cercariae. On the other hand, a T_{H2} pattern of response (with high levels of IL-4 but low levels of IFN-γ) characterizes the granulomatous reaction to schistosome eggs in the liver and may thus contribute to the immunopathology of hepatosplenic schistosomiasis. These disparate immunologic features of the same disease may be somewhat reconciled by considering that different parasite stages, localized to different organs, may stimulate different T cell–mediated immune responses that can result in organ-specific sequelae ranging from true protection to tolerance to immunopathology.

IMMUNOPATHOLOGY Schistosomiasis can be considered an immunologic disease, i.e., host immune responses to the parasite are largely responsible for disease manifestations. Cercarial dermatitis is believed to be due to a hypersensitivity reaction to cercarial proteins. Acute schistosomiasis or Katayama fever is a serum sickness–like syndrome characterized by fever, hepatosplenomegaly, and urticaria. The intense eosinophilia, complement activation, and immune-complex formation in this syndrome are due to immediate hypersensitivity reactions to egg antigens once adult worms begin to lay eggs. Local and systemic allergic reactions are encountered in the course of many other tissue helminthic infections, including hydatid cyst rupture, tropical pulmonary eosinophilia (occult filariasis), pulmonary ascariasis, acute trichinosis, and the larva migrans syndromes. Compelling evidence indicates that the lesions of chronic hepatosplenic schistosomiasis are due to T cell–mediated granulomatous reactions to schistosomal egg antigens. Indeed, tumor necrosis factor alpha (TNFα), a T cell–derived cytokine, has recently been found to trigger the granulomatous response to schistosome eggs in severe combined immunodeficiency mice (which lack functional B and T cells). Interestingly, egg output by adult female worms increases dramatically both in vitro and vivo upon administration of TNFα, suggesting that schistosomes exploit the cytokine network for their own reproduction. Chronic delayed-type hypersensitivity responses are also the basis of lymphatic destruction leading to elephantiasis in filarial infection. Host responses may be further modified by anti-idiotypic antibodies or anti-idiotypic T cells, which arise when the antigen binding site (idiotype) of the original antiparasite antibody induces antibodies or T cells whose antigen combining site recognizes the idiotype.

VACCINES AGAINST PARASITIC DISEASES?

The reawakening of scientific interest in parasite biology has stimulated immunologic approaches to the control of parasitic infections. The preceding discussion makes it clear that the development of antiparasite vaccines will not be an easy task, and in fact, no vaccine against any human parasitic disease has yet been successfully produced. Because the nature of protective immunity in parasitic infections is poorly understood, approaches to vaccine development have been essentially empirical. Such approaches must consider the entire repertoire of stage-specific parasite antigens and host immune responses to those antigens. Development of a vaccine against filariasis, for example, must take into account the fact that the disease largely results from deleterious host immune responses rather than toxic effects of the parasite itself. The use of killed or attenuated organisms, as for many viral and bacterial vaccines, is not practicable for human parasites because they cannot be produced in the industrial quantities necessary for mass immunization. Subunit vaccines based on parasite protein or carbohydrate antigens are therefore desirable and could be produced with use of recombinant DNA or peptide synthesis technologies. Some of these scientific issues are illustrated in the ongoing saga of vaccine development for malaria.

MALARIA VACCINE Intensive work is under way on vaccines for *P. falciparum,* the most malignant malaria parasite. Following initial infection, humoral immune responses are minimal until the merozoite stage. These asexual blood stages are antigenically diverse and can undergo antigenic variation with each successive erythrocytic cycle. It is unclear whether any of the antibodies generated to merozoite antigens are protective or correlate with less severe disease. The best evidence for the existence of immunity in humans is in areas that are highly endemic for malaria. Here, repeatedly infected individuals develop a more chronic, benign infection with low parasitemia and often no symptoms, in contrast to severe parasitemia and attendant complications that occur in young children or immigrants and travelers to the area.

Sporozoite vaccine The cardinal impetus for the development of a sporozoite vaccine was the demonstration that humans and experimental animals can be protected against sporozoite infection by prior vaccination with irradiated sporozoites. This "vaccination" was accomplished by allowing irradiated infected mosquitoes (containing irradiated sporozoites incapable of dividing) to bite volunteers. Laboratory studies showed that antibodies from protected individuals neutralized sporozoites by binding specifically to the CSP. Furthermore, monoclonal antibodies to CSP could passively transfer protection against malaria in naive mice and monkeys. Molecular cloning of the CSP gene revealed the target epitopes of protective antibodies to be a central domain consisting of 23 repeats of the amino acid sequence NANP or NVDP. However, trials of recombinant or synthetic sporozoite vaccines in humans have been disappointing because the vaccines elicited poor antibody responses, and parasitemia was prevented in only a few individuals who had high titers of antibody. Efforts are underway to enhance immunogenicity by using new adjuvants and by combining the CSP repeat sequence with potent T cell epitopes found elsewhere in the molecule.

Accumulating experimental evidence indicates that cell-mediated immune responses are important in protection against malaria. For example, IFN-γ and CD8+ cytotoxic T cells inhibit the early liver stages of malarial parasites. Furthermore, an oral vaccine consisting of an attenuated strain of *Salmonella typhimurium* transfected with the CSP gene induced cellular and not humoral responses in mice and yet protected them from challenge with live sporozoites. Incorporating T cell immunogens into a genetically engineered peptide vaccine also would allow natural boosting of immunity in endemic areas by infective mosquito bites. However, individual T cell epitopes may be limited by the MHC-restricted responsiveness to peptide epitopes in human populations. Finally, an antisporozoite vaccine would have to be virtually 100 percent effective to prevent disease, since a person can still develop malaria even if only a few sporozoites manage to escape immune destruction.

Blood-stage vaccine Other potential targets for a malaria vaccine are the asexual blood stages that are responsible for the clinical symptoms and pathology. Unlike a sporozoite vaccine, a vaccine directed against blood stages would still be beneficial if parasitemia were only partially reduced. A large number of merozoite and infected erythrocyte antigens have been identified and cloned. Monoclonal antibodies to some of these blood-stage antigens confer passive protection in rodent malaria, and antigens purified with use of these antibodies can induce protective immunity. Some success has been achieved in protecting primates with blood-stage vaccines by the use of recombinant or synthesized antigens combined with complete Freund's adjuvant.

In an unconventional approach pioneered in Colombia, a blood-stage vaccine was chemically synthesized by polymerization of three different merozoite antigens together with the NANP repeat peptide of CSP. This polymeric vaccine, known as SPf66, substantially reduced the risk of falciparum malaria in immunized volunteers in a recent large Colombian field trial and will undergo further trials in Africa and Southeast Asia. Of note, there was no correlation between antibody levels and protection, and continual natural boosting by mosquito bites in the malarious region was necessary to establish strong immunity, thus strongly suggesting a key role for cell-mediated immune mechanisms. This exciting new development represents one of the most encouraging results to date of prototype malaria vaccines.

Gametocyte vaccine Gametocytes, the sexual stages of malaria, do not cause clinical symptoms but are responsible for malaria transmission via mosquitoes in the population at large. Antibodies to gametocytes would be taken up in the mosquito blood meal and block further sexual development within the mosquito. Several monoclonal antibodies to isolated gametocyte antigens do prevent the fertilization of gametocytes in the mosquito. Transmission-blocking vaccines will not protect the individual but could substantially reduce the incidence and prevalence of malaria in certain endemic areas.

Antidisease vaccine Host cytokines that are generated in response to specific malarial antigens can contribute to the clinical manifestations of malaria. In particular, TNFα, produced by activated macrophages, has been found to potentiate many of the complications of malaria such as anemia and cytoadherence. Thus an "antidisease" vaccine directed against TNF-inducing antigens, as opposed to an "antiparasite" vaccine, might be effective in preventing such pathologic consequences. Indeed, animals immunized with a *P. falciparum* antigen responsible for TNF production survive high levels of parasitemia that kill unvaccinated animals. Alternatively, a vaccine that could block the cytoadherence of *P. falciparum*–infected erythrocytes to endothelium might prevent cerebral malaria, which is often lethal.

Conclusion An effective malaria vaccine will probably have to comprise a cocktail of antigens from several stages of the parasite life cycle, together with epitopes that stimulate T cells and possibly immunomodulators that stimulate protective cytokines. A highly successful recombinant vaccine has recently been developed against a veterinary parasite, the cestode *Taenia ovis* in sheep. In this case, a fusion protein consisting of a recombinant defined cestode antigen linked to a schistosome glutathione-*S*-transferase proved to be highly protective against challenge infection. This achievement demonstrates the feasibility of employing modern immunologic and molecular approaches in the development of antiparasite vaccines. Such vaccines could prove a highly cost-effective means of protecting the great masses of humanity who are exposed to serious parasitic infections.

REFERENCES

Ash C, Gallagher RB (eds): *Immunoparasitology Today.* Cambridge, Elsevier Trends Journals, 1991

David JR: Host-parasite interface: immune invasion, in *Tropical and Geographic Medicine,* 2d ed, KS Warren, AAF Mahmoud (eds). New York, McGraw-Hill, 1990, p 117

Englund PT, Sher A (eds): *The Biology of Parasitism.* New York, Liss, 1988

Mahmoud AAF: Parasitic protozoa and helminths: Biological and immunological challenges. Science 246:1015, 1989

Maizels RM et al: Immunological modulation and evasion by helminth parasites in human populations. Nature 365:797, 1993

Mendis KN: Malaria vaccine research: a game of chess, in *Malaria: Waiting for the Vaccine,* GAT Targett (ed). New York, Wiley, 1992, p 183

Sher A, Coffman RL: Regulation of immunity to parasites by T cells and T cell-derived cytokines. Annu Rev Immunol 10:385, 1992

Wang CC (ed): *Molecular and Immunological Aspects of Parasitism.* Washington, American Association for the Advancement of Science, 1991

Warren KS (ed): *Immunology and Molecular Biology of Parasitic Infections,* 3d ed. Oxford, Blackwell, 1993

Wyler DJ (ed): *Modern Parasite Biology: Cellular, Immunological, and Molecular Aspects.* New York, Freeman, 1990

171   LABORATORY DIAGNOSIS OF PARASITIC INFECTIONS

CHARLES E. DAVIS

The cornerstone for the diagnosis of parasitic infections is a careful history of the patient's illness. Epidemiologic aspects of the illness are especially important because the risks of acquiring many parasites are closely related to occupation, recreation, or travel to areas of high endemicity. Without a basic knowledge of the epidemiology and life cycles of the major parasites, it is difficult to approach the diagnosis of parasitic infections systematically. Accordingly, the medical classification of important human parasites in this chapter emphasizes their geographic distribution, their transmission, and the anatomic location and stages of the life cycle that occur in people. The text and tables are intended to serve as a guide to the correct diagnostic procedures for the major parasitic infections and to direct the reader to subsequent chapters which contain more comprehensive information about each infection. Tables 171-1 to 171-3 summarize the geographic distributions, anatomic locations, and the laboratory methods employed for the diagnosis of parasitic infections.

In addition to selecting the correct diagnostic procedures, physicians also must counsel their patients to ensure that specimens are collected properly and arrive at the laboratory promptly. For example, the diagnosis of Bancroftian filariasis is unlikely to be confirmed by laboratory personnel unless blood is drawn near midnight when the nocturnal microfilariae are active. The motile, erythrophagocytic trophozoites of *Entamoeba histolytica* are fragile and will not be detected in fecal specimens that arrive at the laboratory several hours after collection. Laboratory personnel and surgical pathologists should be notified in advance when a parasitic infection is suspected. Continuing interaction with the laboratory staff and the surgical pathologists helps to ensure that parasites in body fluids or biopsy specimens are examined carefully by the most capable individuals.

INTESTINAL PARASITES   Most helminths and protozoa exit the body in the fecal stream. The patient or attendant should be instructed

TABLE 171-1   Flatworm infections

Parasite	Geographic distribution	Life-cycle hosts Intermediate (transmission)	Definitive	Parasite stage	Diagnosis Body fluid or tissue	Serologic test	Other
TAPEWORMS (CESTODES)							
Intestinal tapeworms							
Taenia saginata (beef tapeworm)	Worldwide	Beef	Humans	Ova, segments	Feces	—	Motile segments
Hymenolepis nana (dwarf tapeworm)	Worldwide	Grain beetle	Humans, mouse*	Ova	Feces	—	—
Diphyllobothrium latum (fish tapeworm)	Worldwide	Copepods–fish‡	Humans, other mammals	Ova, segments	Feces	—	Megaloblastic anemia in 1%
Taenia solium† (pork tapeworm)	Worldwide	Swine	Humans	Ova, segments	Feces	WB	Esp. Mexico, C. and S. America, Africa
Somatic tapeworms							
Echinococcus granulosus (hydatid disease)	Sheep raising and hunting areas	Sheep, camels, humans, others	Dogs	Hydatid	Lung, liver	WB	Chest x-ray, CT, MRI
Echinococcus multilocularis (hydatid disease)	Subarctic	Rodents, humans	Fox, dog, cat	Hydatid	Liver	—	May resemble cholangiocellular Ca
Taenia solium† (pork tapeworm)	Worldwide	Swine, humans	Humans	Cysticercus	Muscles, CNS	WB	CT, MRI, x-ray
FLUKES (TREMATODES)							
Intestinal flukes							
Fasciolopsis buski	China, India	Snail–water chestnut	Humans	Ova	Feces	—	—
Heterophyes heterophyes	Far East, India	Snail–fish	Humans	Ova	Feces	—	—
Metagonimus yokogawai	Focal in Europe and N. Africa	Snail–fish	Humans	Ova	Feces	—	—
Liver flukes							
Clonorchis sinensis	China, S.E. Asia	Snail–fish	Humans	Ova	Feces, bile	—	Recurrent bacterial cholangitis
Fasciola hepatica	Sheep raising areas	Snail–watercress	Humans, sheep	Ova	Feces, bile	—	Cirrhosis, portal hypertension
Lung flukes							
Paragonimus spp.	Orient, Africa, S. America	Snail–crabs/crayfish	Humans, other mammals	Adults, ova	Lung, sputum, CNS	WB	Chest x-ray, CT, MRI
Blood flukes							
Schistosoma mansoni	Africa, C. and S. America, W. Indies	Snail	Humans	Ova, adults	Feces	EIA	Rectal snips, liver biopsy
Schistosoma haematobium	Africa	Snail	Humans	Ova, adults	Urine	EIA	Liver, urine, or bladder biopsy
Schistosoma japonicum	Far East	Snail	Humans	Ova, adults	Feces	EIA	Liver biopsy

NOTE: WB = Western blot; CF = complement fixation; EIA = enzyme immunoassay; serologic tests listed in Tables 171-1, 171-2, and 171-3 are available from the Centers for Disease Control and Prevention (CDC), Atlanta, Ga.
* Larvae also can mature in intestinal villi of humans and mice.
† *Taenia solium* can cause either intestinal infections or cysticercosis. Ova are identical to *T. saginata;* scolices and segments differ.
‡ When there are two intermediate hosts, the first is separated from the second by a hyphen. Definitive hosts are infected by the second intermediate host.

TABLE 171-2 Roundworm infections

| Parasite | Geographic distribution | Life-cycle hosts | | Diagnosis | | | |
		Intermediate (transmission)	Definitive	Parasite stage	Body fluid or tissue	Serologic tests	Other
INTESTINAL ROUNDWORMS							
Enterobius vermicularis (pinworm)	Temperate and tropical zones	Fecal-oral	Humans	Ova	Perianal skin	—	"Scotch tape" test
Trichuris trichiura (whipworm)	Temperate and tropical zones	Soil, fecal-oral	Humans	Ova	Feces	—	Rectal prolapse
Ascaris lumbricoides (roundworm of man)	Temperate and tropical zones	Soil, fecal-oral	Humans	Ova	Feces		Sx of pulmonary migration
Ancylostoma duodenale (old world hookworm)	EuroAsia, Africa, Pacific	Soil→skin	Humans	Ova/larvae	Feces	—	Sx of pulmonary migration, anemia
Necator americanus (new world hookworm)	U.S., Africa, worldwide	Soil→skin	Humans	Ova/larvae	Feces	—	Sx of pulmonary migration, anemia
Strongyloides stercoralis (strongylodiasis)	Moist tropics and subtropics	Soil→skin	Humans	Larvae	Feces, sputum, duodenal fluid	EIA	Dissemination in immunodeficiency
TISSUE ROUNDWORMS							
Trichinella spiralis (trichinosis)	Worldwide	Swine/humans	Swine/humans	Larvae	Muscle	BF	Muscle biopsy
Wuchereria bancrofti (filariasis)	Coastal in tropics and subtropics	Mosquito	Humans	Microfilariae	Blood, lymph nodes	—	Nocturnal periodicity*
Brugia malayi (filariasis)	Asia, Indian subcontinent	Mosquito	Humans	Microfilariae	Blood	—	Nocturnal
Loa loa (African eye worm)	West and Central Africa	Mango fly (chrysops)	Humans	Microfilariae	Blood	—	May be visible in eye, diurnal
Onchocerca volvulus (river blindness)	Africa, Mexico, C. and S. America	Black flies	Humans	Adults/larvae	Skin/eye	—	Examine nodules or skin snips
Dracunculus medinensis (guinea worm)	Orient, Africa, W. Indies, Brazil	Cyclops	Humans	Adults/larvae	Skin	—	May be visible in lesion
LARVA MIGRANS SYNDROMES							
Ancylostoma braziliensis (creeping eruption)	Tropical and temperate zones	Soil→skin	Dog/cat, humans	Larvae	Skin	—	Dog and cat hookworm
Toxocara canis and *cati* (visceral larva migrans)	Tropical and temperate zones	Soil, fecal-oral	Dog/cat, humans	Larvae	Viscera, CNS, eye	EIA	Also caused by roundworms of other spp.

NOTE: BF = bentonite flocculation
* Blood should be drawn at midnight, except for infection acquired in the South Pacific.

to collect feces in a clean cardboard container and to record the time of collection on the container. Contamination with water, which could contain free-living protozoa, or urine should be avoided. Fecal samples should be collected before ingestion of barium or other contrast agents for radiologic procedures and before treatment with antidiarrheal agents and antacids because these substances change the consistency of the feces and interfere with microscopic detection of parasites. Cyclic shedding of most parasites in the feces requires examination of a minimum of three samples collected on alternate days. When delays in transport to the laboratory are unavoidable or specimens must be shipped by mail, fecal samples should be kept in polyvinyl alcohol to preserve protozoal trophozoites. Refrigeration also will preserve trophozoites for a few hours and protozoal cysts and helminth ova for several days.

Analysis of fecal samples consists of both a macroscopic and a microscopic examination. Watery or loose stools are more likely to contain protozoal trophozoites, but protozoal cysts and all stages of helminths may be found in formed feces. If adult worms or tapeworm segments are observed in the physician's office or on the wards, they should be transported promptly to the laboratory or washed and preserved in fixative for later examination. The only tapeworm with

motile segments is *Taenia saginata*, the beef tapeworm, which patients will sometimes bring to the physician. Motility is an important distinction, because the ova of *T. saginata* and *T. solium*, the cause of cysticercosis, are indistinguishable.

Microscopic examination of the feces (See also Table 171-4) Microscopic examination of feces is not complete until direct wet mounts, concentration techniques, and permanent stains have been examined. The physician should insist that the laboratory conduct each of these procedures before accepting the final report as negative for ova and parasites. Some intestinal parasites are more readily detected in anatomic locations other than feces. For example, the string test or its commercial substitutes to sample duodenal contents is sometimes necessary to detect *Giardia lamblia* and *Cryptosporidium*. The "Scotch tape" technique to detect pinworm ova on the perianal skin will sometimes reveal ova of *T. saginata* deposited perianally when the motile segments disintegrate (see Table 171-4).

Two routine solutions are used to make wet mounts for the identification of the various life stages of helminths and protozoa: physiologic saline for trophozoites, cysts, ova, and larvae and dilute iodine solution for staining protozoal cysts and ova. Iodine solution

TABLE 171-3   Protozoal infections

Parasite	Geographic distribution	Life-cycle hosts Intermediate (transmission)	Definitive	Diagnosis Parasite stage	Body fluid or tissue	Serologic tests	Other
INTESTINAL PROTOZOANS							
Entamoeba histolytica (amebiasis)	Worldwide, esp. tropics	Fecal-oral	Humans	Troph, cyst	Feces, liver	ID,* IHA	Ultrasound, CT liver
Giardia lamblia (giardiasis)	Worldwide	Fecal-oral	Humans	Troph, cyst	Feces	AG detection	String test
Isospora belli	Worldwide	Fecal-oral	Humans	Oocysts	Feces	—	Acid-fast
Cryptosporidium	Worldwide	Fecal-oral	Humans and animals	Oocysts	Feces	AG detection	Acid-fast, biopsy
Enterocytozoon bieneusi (microsporidiosis)	Worldwide?	?	Animals, humans	Spores	Feces	—	Modified trichrome, biopsy
FREE-LIVING AMEBAS							
Naegleria	Worldwide	Warm water	Humans	Troph, cyst	CNS, nares	—	Biopsy, nasal swab
Acanthamoeba	Worldwide	Soil, water	Humans	Troph, cyst	CNS, skin, cornea	—	Biopsy, scrapings
BLOOD AND TISSUE PROTOZOANS							
Plasmodium spp. (malaria)	Subtropics and tropics	Mosquito	Humans	Asexual	Blood	Little use	—
Babesia microti (babesiosis)	U.S., esp. New England	Tick	Rodents, humans	Asexual	Blood	IIF	Animal spp. in asplenia
Trypanosoma rhodesiense (Afr. sleeping sickness)	Subsaharan E. Africa	Tsetse fly	Humans, herbivores	Tryp	Blood, CSF	Card agglut., IIF†	Also chancre, lymph nodes
Trypanosoma gambiense (Afr. sleeping sickness)	Subsaharan W. Africa	Tsetse fly	Humans, swine	Tryp	Blood, CSF	Card agglut., IIF†	Also chancre, lymph nodes
Trypanosoma cruzi (Chagas' disease)	Mexico→S. America	Reduviid bugs (triatomes)	Humans, dogs and wild animals	Amastigotes, Tryp	Multiple organs/ blood	CF, IIF	Reactivation in immunosuppressed
Leishmanis tropica, etc.	Widespread in tropics and subtropics	Sand flies (phlebotomus)	Humans, dogs, rodents	Amastigotes	Skin	EIA‡	Biopsy, scraping, culture
Leishmania braziliensis (mucocutaneous)	Mexico→S. America	Sand flies (lutzomyia)	Humans, dogs, rodents	Amastigotes	Skin mucous membranes	EIA‡	Biopsy, scraping, culture
Leishmania donovani (kala-azar)	Widespread in tropics and subtropics	Sand flies (phlebotomus)	Humans, dogs, wild animals	Amastigotes	RE system	EIA‡	Biopsy, culture
Toxoplasma gondii (toxoplasmosis)	Worldwide	Humans, other mammals	Cats	Cyst, troph	CNS, eye, muscles, other	EIA, IIF	Reactivation in immunosuppressed
Pneumocystis carinii	Worldwide	?	Humans	Cyst, troph	Lung, Other	—	Induced sputum, biopsy

* ID = immunodiffusion by commerical kit (not available at the CDC); IHA = indirect hemagglutination; AG = antigen; CF = complement fixation; Troph = trophozoite; Tryp = trypomastigote form; IIF = indirect immunofluorescence
† Card agglutination provided to endemic countries by the World Health Organization; IIF available intermittently—contact the WHO or CDC.
‡ Limited specificity.

must never be used to examine specimens for trophozoites because it kills the parasites and destroys their characteristic motility.

The two most common concentration procedures for detecting small numbers of cysts and ova are formalin-ether sedimentation and zinc sulfate flotation. The formalin-ether technique is preferable because all parasites sediment, but not all float. Permanently stained slides for trophozoites should be prepared before concentration. Additional stained slides for cysts and ova may be made from the concentrate.

In many instances, especially in differentiation of *E. histolytica* from other amebae, identification from wet mounts or concentrates must be considered tentative. Permanently stained smears allow study of the cellular detail necessary for definitive identification. The iron-hematoxylin stain is excellent for critical work, but the trichrome stain, which can be completed in 1 h, is a satisfactory alternative that also stains parasites in specimens preserved in PVA fixative.

BLOOD AND TISSUE PARASITES   Protozoa and helminths invading the tissues present a more difficult problem in the choice of

diagnostic techniques. For example, physicians must understand that aspiration of an amebic liver abscess rarely reveals *E. histolytica* because the trophozoites are located primarily in the abscess wall. They must remember to order an examination of the sputum for ova of *Paragonimus westermani* in the Southeast Asian immigrant with a cystic lung lesion (Table 171-5) and know that the urine sediment offers the best opportunity to detect *Schistosoma haematobium* in the Ethiopian youngster or American traveler who returns from Africa with hematuria (Table 171-6). Tables 171-1, 171-2, and 171-3, which offer a quick guide to the geographic distribution and anatomic locations of the major tissue parasites, should help the physician to select the appropriate body fluid or biopsy site for microscopic examination. Tables 171-5 through 171-8 provide additional information about identification of parasites in samples from specific anatomic locations. The laboratory procedures for detection of parasites from other body fluids are similar to those used in the examination of feces. The physician should insist on wet mounts, concentration techniques, and permanent stains of all body fluids. The trichrome or iron-

TABLE 171-4 Laboratory diagnosis of parasites found in feces*

Parasites and fecal stages	Alternative diagnostic procedures
TAPEWORMS (CESTODES)	
Taenia saginata ova and segments	Perianal "Scotch tape" test for ova
Hymenolepis nana ova	None
Diphyllobothrium ova and segments	None
Taenia solium ova and segments	Brain bx for neurocysticercosis; serology
FLUKES (TREMATODES)	
Fasciolopsis buski ova	None
Heterophyes heterophyes ova	None
Metagonimus yokogawai ova	None
Clonorchis sinensis ova	Examine bile for ova and adults in cholangitis
Fasciola hepatica ova	Examine bile for ova and adults in cholangitis
Paragonimus spp. ova	Sputum, lung bx, or brain bx for ova; serology
Schistosoma ova	Rectal snips (esp. *S. mansoni*), urine (*S. haematobium*), liver bx, and serology for all
ROUNDWORMS	
Enterobius vermicularis ova and adults	Perianal "Scotch tape" test for ova and adults
Trichuris trichiura ova	None
Ascaris lumbricoides ova and adults	Examine sputum for larvae in lung disease
Hookworm ova and occasional larvae	Examine sputum for larvae in lung disease
Strongyloides larvae	Duodenal asp. or jejunal bx‡; sputum or lung bx for filariform larvae in disseminated disease; serology
Capillaria phillipinensis ova†	None
PROTOZOANS	
Entamoeba histolytica trophs and cysts	Liver bx for trophs; serology
Giardia lamblia trophs and cysts	Duodenal aspirate or jejunal bx‡
Isospora belli oocysts	Duodenal aspirate or jejunal bx‡
Cryptosporidium oocysts	Duodenal aspirate or jejunal bx‡
Enterocytozoon bieneusi spores	Duodenal aspirate or jejunal bx‡

* Stains and concentration techniques are discussed in the text.
† Can be confused with *Trichuris trichiura*.
‡ Commercial string test or Crosby capsule are satisfactory: *Isospora* and *Cryptosporidium* are acid-fast.

TABLE 171-5 Laboratory diagnosis of parasitic infections of the lungs

	Parasite stage(s)	Stains
SPUTUM*/BRONCHOALVEOLAR LAVAGE		
Pneumocystis carinii	Trophs and cysts	Methenamine silver, toluidine blue, indirect immunofluorescence test
Ascaris lumbricoides	Third-stage larvae	Wet mount, trichrome, iron-hematoxylin, Giemsa
Hookworms	Filariform larvae	Same as *Ascaris*
Strongyloides	Filariform larvae	Same as *Ascaris*
Paragonimus spp.	Ova	Same as *Ascaris*
Entamoeba histolytica	Trophozoites	Same as *Ascaris*
Echinococcus	Scolices	Wet mount, acid-fast
Toxocara species	Larvae	Same as *Ascaris*
LUNG BIOPSY (OPEN OR TRANSBRONCHIAL)		
Pneumocystis carinii	Trophs and cysts	H&E‡ and as above
Paragonimus spp.	Adults and ova	H&E, iron-hematoxylin
Entamoeba histolytica	Trophozoites	Same as *Paragonimus*
Echinococcus	Hydatid, scolices	H&E‡, iron-hematoxylin, acid-fast
Schistosoma spp.	Ova	H&E, iron-hematoxylin
Brugia and *Wuchereria*†	Microfilariae	H&E, Giemsa
Toxocara spp.	Larvae	Same as *Paragonimus*

* Induced sputum for *Pneumocystis*. There are no data for the efficacy of induced sputum or BAL in the diagnosis of the other parasites. Transbronchial brush may be included in BAL.
† In lymphatic filariasis and tropical pulmonary eosinophilia.
‡ Hematoxylin and eosin for typical histopathology and for detection of all parasites except *Pneumocystis*.

TABLE 171-6 Identification of parasites in blood and other body fluids

	Enrichment/stain	Culture technique
BLOOD		
Plasmodium spp.	Thick and thin smears/ Giemsa or Wright's	Not useful for diagnosis
Leishmania spp.	Buffy coat/Giemsa	Media available from CDC
African trypanosomes*	Buffy coat, anion column/wet mount, and Giemsa	Mouse or rat inoculation*
Trypanosoma cruzi†	As for African species	As above and xenodiagnosis
Toxoplasma gondii	Buffy coat/Giemsa	Fibroblast cell lines
Microfilariae‡	Nuclepore filtration/ wet mount, and Giemsa	None
URINE§		
Schistosoma haematobium	Centrifugation/wet mount	None
Microfilariae (in chyluria)	As for blood	None
SPINAL FLUID		
African trypanosomes	Centrifugation, anion column/wet mount, and Giemsa	As for blood
Naegleria fowleri	Centrifugation/wet mount, and Giemsa or trichrome	Nonnutrient agar overlaid with *E. coli*

* *T. rhodesiense* and *T. gambiense*. Inject mice intraperitoneally with 0.2 mL whole heparinized blood (0.5 mL for rats). After 5 days, tail blood should be checked daily for trypanosomes as described above.
† Detectable in blood by conventional techniques only during acute disease. Xenodiagnosis is successful in about 50 percent of patients with chronic Chagas' disease.
‡ Day (1000–1400) and night (2200–0200) blood should be drawn to maximize the chance of detecting *Wuchereria* (nocturnal except for Pacific strains), *Brugia* (nocturnal), and *Loa Loa* (diurnal).
§ *Trichomonas vaginalis* is often detectable in urine, but examination of vaginal secretions is probably the preferable technique.

hematoxylin stains are satisfactory for all tissue helminths in body fluids other than blood, but microfilarial worms and the blood protozoa are more easily visualized when stained with Giemsa or Wright's stain.

The most common parasites detected in Giemsa-stained blood smears are the plasmodia, microfilariae, and African trypanosomes (see Table 171-6). Most patients with Chagas' disease present in the chronic phase when *T. cruzi* is no longer microscopically detectable in blood smears. Wet mounts are sometimes more sensitive than stained smears for the detection of microfilariae and the African trypanosomes because these active parasites cause noticeable movement of the erythrocytes in the microscopic field. Nuclepore filtration of blood facilitates detection of microfilariae. The intracellular amastigote forms of *Leishmania* spp. and *T. cruzi* can sometimes be visualized in stained smears of peripheral blood, but aspirates of the bone marrow, liver, and spleen are the best sources for microscopic detection and culture of *Leishmania* in kala-azar and *T. cruzi* in chronic Chagas' disease.

The diagnosis of malaria and the critical differentiation among the *Plasmodium* spp. is made by microscopic examination of stained thick and thin blood films (see Table 171-7). Most malariologists

TABLE 171-7   Differential diagnosis of *Plasmodium* species in blood smears

	Falciparum	*Vivax*	*Malariae*	*Ovale*
FEATURE OF RBC				
Size	All sizes	Large (young)	Small (old)	Large (young)
Shape	Round; may be crenated	Round or oval	Round	Round or pear-shaped, fimbriated
Stippling	Maurer's clefts: large, red (up to 20)	Schuffner's dots: numerous, small red dots	None	Schuffner's dots
FEATURE OF PARASITE				
Ring trophozoite	Thread-like, multiple infections, double chromatin dots, accole forms*	Thicker	Compact	Compact
Mature trophozoites	Absent	Ameboid, may fill cell	More regular, smaller, band forms†	Less ameboid and smaller than vivax
Schizonts	Absent	12 to 24 merozoites	8 to 12 merozoites often rosetted around pigment	8 to 12 merozoites
Gametocytes	Banana-shaped, central chromatin (female) or diffuse (male)	Round, fills cell, pigment often central	Round, large, coarse pigment	Smaller and oval, but similar to vivax
DIAGNOSTIC KEYS				
	Gametocyte, multiple rings, double chromatin dots, accole forms, heavy infections	Schizont, large RBCs, ameboid forms	Schizont, small RBCs, band forms	Schizont and large RBCs, pear-shaped, fimbriated RBCs

* At periphery of RBC; may be flattened into rod shape.
† Stretch across RBC, but not banana-shaped.

prefer Giemsa stain because of its overall high quality, suitability for staining both thick and thin smears, and stability in tropical climates. Wright's stain can produce high-quality thin smears and is widely used in the Americas, but it deteriorates rapidly in the tropics because its methanol base is highly hygroscopic. Specimens of capillary or venous blood should be obtained every 4 to 12 h until a diagnosis is established. The thin smear is made on clean slides exactly like a blood film for a white blood cell differential. The thick film is made by placing one drop of blood on the slide and stirring it in a circular motion to a diameter of about 2 cm. The erythrocytes in the thick film are lysed with water, but the thin film is fixed in methanol to preserve erythrocyte morphology.

Although most tissue parasites stain with the traditional hematoxylin and eosin stain, surgical biopsy specimens also should be stained with appropriate special stains. The surgical pathologist who is accustomed to staining induced sputum and transbronchial biopsies with silver stains for *Pneumocystis carinii* may have to be reminded to examine wet mounts and iron-hematoxylin stains of pulmonary specimens for helminth ova and *E. histolytica* (see Table 171-5). The clinician also should be able to advise the surgeon and pathologist about optimal techniques for identification of parasites from specimens obtained by certain specialized minor procedures (see Table 171-8). For example, the excision of skin snips for the diagnosis of onchocerciasis, rectal snips for the diagnosis of schistosomiasis, and punch biopsies of skin lesions for the identification and culture of cutaneous and mucocutaneous species of *Leishmania* are simple procedures, but the diagnosis can be missed if the specimens are improperly obtained or processed.

NONSPECIFIC TESTS   Eosinophilia is a common accompaniment of infections with most of the tissue helminths and may reach high absolute numbers in trichinosis and the migratory phases of filariasis (Table 171-9). Intestinal helminths provoke eosinophilia only during pulmonary migration of the larval stages. Eosinophilia is not a manifestation of protozoal infections, with the possible exceptions of *Isospora* and *Dientamoeba fragilis*.

Like the hypochromic, microcytic anemia of heavy hookworm

TABLE 171-8   Minor procedures for diagnosis of parasitic infections

Procedure	Parasite(s) and stage
Skin snips: Lift skin with a needle and excise about 1 mg to a depth of 0.5 mm from several sites. Weigh each, place in 0.5 mL saline for 4 h, and examine wet mounts and Giemsa stains of the saline either directly or after filtration. Count microfilariae.*	*Onchocerca volvulus* and *Mansonella streptocerca* microfilariae
Biopsies of subcutaneous nodules: Giemsa stains of routine histopathologic sections and impression smears.	*Loa loa* adults and *Onchocerca volvulus* adults and microfilariae
Muscle biopsies: Excise about 1.0 g of deltoid or gastrocnemius m. and squash between two glass slides for direct microscopic examination.	*Trichinella spiralis* larvae (*Taenia solium* cysticerci may be detected)
Rectal snips: From four areas of mucosa take 2-mg snips, tease onto a glass slide, and flatten with a second slide before direct exam at 10X. May be fixed in alcohol or stained.	*Schistosoma* ova of all species, but esp. *S. mansoni*
Aspirate of chancre or lymph node†: Aspirate center with 18-gauge needle, place a drop on a slide, and examine for motile forms. Insufficient material may be Giemsa stained.	*Trypanosoma gambiense* and *Trypanosoma rhodesiense* trypomastigotes
Corneal scrapings: Obtain sample from opthalmologist for immediate Giemsa stain and culture on nutrient agar overlaid with *E. coli*.	*Acanthamoeba* species trophozoites or cysts
Swabs, aspirates, or punch biopsies of skin lesions: Obtain specimen from margin of lesion for Giemsa stain of impression smears and section and culture on special media from CDC.	Cutaneous and mucocutaneous species of *Leishmania*

* Counts of >100 per milligram are associated with significant risk of complications.
† Lymph node aspiration is contraindicated in some infections and should be used judiciously.

TABLE 171-9 Parasites frequently associated with eosinophilia*

Parasite	Comment
TAPEWORMS (CESTODES)	
Echinococcus granulosus	When hydatid cyst leaks
Taenia solium	During muscle encystation and in CSF with neurocysticercosis
FLUKES (TREMATODES)	
Paragonimus spp.	Uniformly high in acute stage
Fasciola hepatica	May be high in acute stage
Clonorchis sinensis	Variable
Schistosoma mansoni	50% of infected travelers
Schistosoma haematobium	25% of infected travelers
Schistosoma japonicum	Up to 6000 per microliter in acute infection
ROUNDWORMS	
Ascaris lumbricoides	During larval migration
Hookworm species	During larval migration
Strongyloides stercoralis	Profound during migration and early years of infection
Trichinella spiralis	Up to 7000 per microliter
Wuchereria bancrofti	From normal to 2500 per cubic microliter[†]
Brugia spp.	Similar to *Wuchereria*[†]
Loa loa	Varies but can reach 5000 to 8000 per microliter
Onchocerca volvulus	May exceed 5000 per microliter
Toxocara spp.	>3000 per microliter
Ancylostoma braziliensis	With extensive cutaneous eruption
Gnathostoma spinigerum	In VLM and eosinophilic meningitis
Angiostrongylus cantonensis	In eosinophilic meningitis
Angiostrongylus costaricensis	During larval migration in mesenteric vessels
POSSIBLE PROTOZOAL CAUSES	
Isospora belli	A few reports of profound eosinophilia
Dientamoeba fragilis	Possible pathogenicity and eosinophilia

* Virtually every helminth has been associated with eosinophilia. This table includes both common and uncommon parasites that frequently elicit eosinophilia during infection.
† Also in tropical pulmonary eosinophilia, where eosinophilia, fleeting infiltrates, and asthma may be the only manifestations of filariasis.

TABLE 171-10 Serologic tests for parasitic infections

Infections with	Antibody tests	Antigen tests
TAPEWORMS		
Echinococcosis	WB, IHA	
Cysticercosis	WB	
FLUKES		
Paragonimiasis	WB	
Schistosomiasis	EIA, WB	
ROUNDWORMS		
Strongyloidiasis	EIA	
Trichinellosis	BF	
Toxocariasis	EIA	
PROTOZOANS		
Amebiasis	IHA	
Giardiasis		EIA, IIF
Cryptosporidiosis		IIF
Malaria (all species)*	IIF	
Babesiosis (*B. microti*)	IIF	
Chagas' disease	IIF, CF	
Leishmaniasis	IIF, CF	
Toxoplasmosis	IIF, EIA-IgM	
Pneumocystosis		IIF

NOTE: BF = bentonite flocculation; CF = complement fixation; EIA = enzyme immunoassay; WB = western blot; IHA = indirect hemagglutination; IIF = indirect immunofluorescence. All antibody tests listed are available from the CDC. Antigen and parasite detection kits are available commercially.
* Of use primarily for screening blood donors.

infections, other nonspecific laboratory abnormalities may suggest parasitic infection in patients with appropriate geographic and/or environmental exposures. Biochemical evidence of cirrhosis or an abnormal urine sediment in an African immigrant certainly raises the possibility of schistosomiasis. Megaloblastic anemia can be the presenting manifestation of the fish tapeworm (*Diphyllobothrium latum*), and anemia and thrombocytopenia in a febrile traveler or immigrant are among the hallmarks of malaria. Computed tomography and magnetic resonance imaging also contribute to the diagnosis of infections with many tissue parasites and have become invaluable adjuncts to the diagnosis of neurocysticercosis and cerebral toxoplasmosis.

ANTIBODY AND ANTIGEN DETECTION As shown in Table 171-10, there are useful antibody assays for many of the important tissue parasites. The filarial worms are a notable exception. Although filariae provoke a strong immune response and many antibody assays have been used, none has proved sensitive and specific enough for universal adoption. The detection of antibody to plasmodia is primarily an epidemiologic tool of limited use for the diagnosis of malaria in individual patients. The limited geographic distribution of many of the tropical parasites increases the usefulness of antibody detection as a means of establishing diagnoses in travelers from industrialized countries. On the other hand, a large proportion of the world has been exposed to *T. gondii*, and the presence of IgG antibody does not establish the presence of active disease. One or more of the antibody assays listed in the tables are available at the Centers for Disease Control and Prevention (CDC) in Atlanta, Georgia. The results of most serologic tests not listed in the tables nor offered by the CDC should be interpreted with caution.

Many fewer antibody assays are available for the diagnosis of intestinal parasites. Although most stimulate coproantibodies and humoral antibodies, problems of cross-reactivity between parasites, lack of efficient cultivation techniques, and the ability to establish diagnoses without invasive procedures have discouraged intensive investigation. *E. histolytica* is the major exception. The availability of sensitive specific serologic tests is an invaluable aid in the diagnosis of amebiasis. Commercial kits for the detection of antigen by ELISA and whole organisms by fluorescent antibody are now available for the diagnosis of giardiasis and cryptosporidiosis.

MOLECULAR TECHNIQUES DNA hybridization with probes that are repeated many times in the genome of a specific parasite and amplification of a specific DNA fragment by the polymerase chain reaction (PCR) are promising techniques for the diagnosis of infections with parasites and other infectious agents. DNA probes for hybridization to *P. falciparum*, *T. cruzi*, the African trypanosomes, and lymphatic filariae are already being used for detection of these agents in infected insect vectors and are being applied investigationally in animal models and human trials. Although none is available for routine use in patients at this time, DNA probes and PCR should become important additions to our future diagnostic armamentarium.

REFERENCES

DESPOMMIER DD, KARAPELEU JW: *Parasite Life Cycles.* New York, Springer-Verlag, 1987

FLECK SL, MOODY AH: *Diagnostic Techniques in Medical Parasitology.* London, Wright, 1988

GUTIERREZ V, LITTLE MD (eds): *Clinics in Laboratory Medicine: Diagnosis of Important Parasitic Diseases,* vol 11. Philadelphia, Saunders, 1991

TOMECKI KJ (ed): *Dermatologic Clinics: Systemic Mycoses and Parasitic Diseases,* vol 7. Philadelphia, Saunders, 1989

WEBER R et al: Improved light-microscopical detection of microsporidia spores in stool and duodenal aspirates. N Engl J Med 326:161, 1992

WELLER PF: Eosinophilia in travelers, in *The Medical Clinics of North America: Travel Medicine,* vol 76, MS Wolfe (guest ed). Philadelphia, Saunders, 1992

WILSON M, SCHANTZ P: Nonmorphologic diagnosis of parasitic infections, in *Manual of Clinical Microbiology,* 5th ed, A Balows (ed). Washington, American Society of Microbiology, 1991

172   THERAPY FOR PARASITIC INFECTIONS

LEO X. LIU / PETER F. WELLER

Chemotherapy for parasitic diseases is beset with potential problems. Knowledge of the fundamental biology and metabolism of eukaryotic parasites is still rudimentary. Many essential antiparasitic drugs, such as chloroquine or diethylcarbamazine, have been used for decades without our having a full understanding of their mechanisms of action. For a disease such as falciparum malaria, which causes tremendous suffering and death worldwide, the emergence of drug resistance poses an urgent problem. Because most parasitic infections primarily affect populations in poor developing countries, commercial incentives to develop and market antiparasitic drugs are limited. Nevertheless, the introduction in recent years of several new agents such as mefloquine, praziquantel, and ivermectin has improved the therapy for several parasitic infections. Table 172-1 summarizes drug therapy for the more common parasitic diseases. Information regarding indications, adverse effects, and contraindications of selected drugs follows below. Drugs considered investigational by the Food and Drug Administration (FDA) for a given parasitic indication are marked with an asterisk (*). Other drugs, marked with a dagger (†), may not be generally available in the United States but may be obtained through the Centers for Disease Control and Prevention Drug Service, Atlanta, GA 30333 (telephone 404-639-3670). Antiparasitic drug treatment for children and pregnant women or in certain unusual circumstances is detailed in the references.

Albendazole* This new benzimidazole derivative is active against a variety of helminthic parasites but is currently available only from the manufacturer (Smith-Kline Beecham). Albendazole is the drug of choice for the medical treatment of hydatid cysts and is also useful as an adjunct to surgical therapy. It is effective for cysticercosis, is also promising for many intestinal and tissue nematode infections, and is less toxic than the older benzimidazoles. Adverse reactions to albendazole include occasional diarrhea and abdominal pain, and its use during pregnancy is contraindicated.

Benznidazole* This nitroimidazole derivative, not presently available in the United States, can ameliorate the course of acute

TABLE 172-1   Treatment of parasitic infections

Infection	Treatment of choice	Alternative regimen
Amebiasis *(Entamoeba histolytica)*		
Asymptomatic	Diloxanide furoate 500 mg tid for 10 days	Iodoquinolol 650 mg tid for 20 days; **or** paromomycin 25–30 mg/kg/d in 3 doses for 7 days
Mild to moderate disease	Metronidazole 750 mg tid for 10 days followed by iodoquinolol 650 mg tid for 20 days	Paromomycin as above **or** tinidazole 2 g/d; either followed by iodoquinolol as above
Severe intestinal disease	Metronidazole as above **or** tinidazole 600 mg bid for 5 days followed by iodoquinolol as above	Dehydroemetine 1–1.5 mg/kg/d (max 90 mg/d) IM up to 5 days; **or** paromomycin as above; either followed by iodoquinolol as above
Hepatic abscess	Metronidazole as above **or** tinidazole 800 mg tid for 5 days followed by iodoquinolol as above	Dehydroemetine as above, followed by chloroquine phosphate 600 mg base (1 g)/d for 2 days, then 300 mg base (500 mg)/d for 2–3 weeks plus iodoquinolol as above
Amebic meningoencephalitis *(Naegleria)*	Amphotericin B 1 mg/kg/d IV for uncertain duration	
Angiostrongyliasis *(Angiostrongylus cantonensis)*	Supportive therapy and glucocorticoids as needed	
(Angiostrongylus costaricensis)	Thiabendazole 75 mg/kg/d in 3 doses for 3 days (max 3 g/d)	
Anisakiasis *(Anisakis)*	Surgical or endoscopic removal	
Ascariasis *(Ascaris lumbricoides)*	Mebendazole 100 mg bid for 3 days; **or** piperazine 75 mg/kg (max 3.5 g) for 2 days	Pyrantel pamoate 11 mg/kg (max 1 g); **or** albendazole 400 mg once
Babesiosis *(Babesia)*	Clindamycin 1.2 g bid IV; **or** 600 mg tid PO for 7 days, plus quinine 650 mg tid PO for 7 days	
Balantidiasis *(Balantidium coli)*	Tetracycline 500 mg qid for 10 days	Metronidazole 750 mg tid for 5 days
Capillariasis *(Capillaria philippinensis)*	Mebendazole 200 mg bid for 20 days	Albendazole 200 mg bid for 10 days; **or** thiabendazole 25 mg/kg/d in 2 doses for 30 days
Cryptosporidiosis *(Cryptosporidium)*	No effective specific therapy; self-limited in normal hosts	
Cutaneous larva migrans (creeping eruption)	Thiabendazole 10% suspension topically qid; **or** 25 mg/kg for 2–5 days	Cryotherapy
Cysticercosis *(Cysticercus cellulosae)*	Praziquantel 50 mg/kg/d in 3 doses for 15 days; **or** albendazole 15 mg/kg/d in 3 doses for 8 days, repeated as necessary, with concurrent glucocorticoids for CNS disease	Surgery
Dracunculiasis *(Dracunculus medinensis)*	Metronidazole 250 mg tid for 10 days plus worm removal	Thiabendazole 50–75 mg/kg/d in 2 doses for 3 days plus worm removal

TABLE 172-1 Treatment of parasitic infections (*continued*)

Infection	Treatment of choice	Alternative regimen
Echinococcosis		
Echinococcus granulosus (hydatid cyst)	Surgical excision plus preoperative albendazole	Albendazole 400 mg bid for 28 days, repeated as necessary
Echinococcus multilocularis	Surgical excision	
Enterobiasis		
(*Enterobius vermicularis*, pinworm)	Pyrantel pamoate 11 mg/kg once (max 1 g) **or** mebendazole 100 mg once **or** albendazole 400 mg once; each repeated after 2 weeks	
Filariasis		
Lymphatic filariasis (*Wuchereria bancrofti, Brugia malayi*)	Diethylcarbamazine Day 1: 50 mg PO Day 2: 50 mg tid Day 3: 100 mg tid Days 4–21: 6 mg/kg/d in 3 doses	
Loaisis (*Loa loa*)	Diethylcarbamazine Day 1: 50 mg PO Day 2: 50 mg tid Day 3: 100 mg tid Days 4–21:9 mg/kg/d in 3 doses	
Mansonella ozzardi	Ivermectin 25–200 μg/kg single dose	
Mansonella perstans	Mebendazole 100 mg bid for 30 days	Ivermectin 25–200 μg/kg single dose
Mansonella streptocerca	Diethylcarbamazine as for lymphatic filariasis	
Tropical pulmonary eosinophilia	Diethylcarbamazine 6 mg/kg/d in 3 doses for 21 days	
Onchocerciasis *Onchocerca volvulus*	Ivermectin 150 μg/kg once, repeated every 6–12 months	
Fluke infections		
Liver flukes (*Clonorchis sinensis; Opisthorchis viverrini*)	Praziquantel 75 mg/kg/d in 3 doses for 1 day	
Sheep liver fluke (*Fasciola hepatica*)	Bithionol 30–50 mg/kg on alternate days for 10–15 doses	
Intestinal flukes (*Fasciolopsis buski, Heterophyes heterophyes, Metagonimus yokogawai*)	Praziquantel 75 mg/kg/d in 3 doses for 1 day	
Lung fluke (*Paragonimus westermani*)	Praziquantel 75 mg/kg/d in 3 doses for 2 days	Bithionol 30–50 mg/kg on alternate days for 10–15 doses
Giardiasis		
(*Giardia lamblia*)	Metronidazole 250 mg tid for 5 days; **or** quinacrine HCl 100 mg tid for 5 days	Tinidazole 2 g once; **or** paromomycin 25–30 mg/kg/d in 3 doses for 7 days; **or** furazolidone 100 mg qid for 7–10 days
Gnathostomiasis		
(*Gnathostoma spinigerum*)	Surgical removal; **or** mebendazole 200 mg q3h for 6 days	
Hookworm		
(*Ancylostoma duodenale, Necator americanus*)	Mebendazole 100 mg bid for 3 days; **or** pyrantel pamoate 11 mg/kg (max 1 g) for 3 days	Albendazole 400 mg once
Isosporiasis		
(*Isospora belli*)	Trimethoprim-sulfamethoxazole (160/800 mg) qid for 10 days, then bid for 3 weeks	Pyrimethamine 5075 mg once daily for 3 weeks
Leishmaniasis		
—cutaneous, mucocutaneous, or visceral (*L. braziliensis, L. mexicana, L. tropica, L. major, L. donovani*)	Stibogluconate sodium 20 mg/kg/d (max 800 mg/d) IV or IM for 28 days; **or** meglumine antimoniate 20 mg/kg/d for 20–28 days; may be repeated or continued until response	Amphotericin B 0.25—1 mg/kg slow infusion daily or every 2 days for up to 8 weeks; **or** pentamidine isethionate 2–4 mg/kg/d IM up to 15 doses
Malaria treatment (*Plasmodium falciparum, P. ovale, P. vivax, P. malariae*)		
All except chloroquine-resistant *P. falciparum*		
Oral	Chloroquine phosphate 600 mg base (1 g) then 300 mg base (500 mg) at 6, 24, and 48 h	
Parenteral	Quinidine gluconate 10 mg/kg loading dose (max 600 mg) over 1 h followed by continuous infusion of 0.02 mg/kg/min for 3 d maximum	Chloroquine HCl 200 mg base (250 mg) IM q6h if oral therapy cannot be started
Followed by (for *P. vivax & P. ovale* only)	Primaquine phosphate 15 mg base (26.3 mg)/d for 14 days or 45 mg base (79 mg)/wk for 8 weeks	
Chloroquine-resistant *P. falciparum*		
Oral	Quinine sulfate 650 mg tid for 3 days plus pyrimethamine-sulfadoxine 3 tablets at once on last day of quinine; **or** plus tetracycline 250 mg qid for 7 days; **or** plus clindamycin 900 mg tid for 3 days	Mefloquine 1250 mg once; **or** halofantrine 500 mg q6h for 3 doses
Parenteral	Quinidine gluconate as above	
Malaria prophylaxis		
Chloroquine-sensitive areas	Chloroquine phosphate 300 mg base (500 mg salt) orally, once/wk beginning 1 wk before and continuing for 4 weeks after last exposure	

(*continued*)

TABLE 172-1 Treatment of parasitic infections (*continued*)

Infection	Treatment of choice	Alternative regimen
Chloroquine-resistant areas	Mefloquine 250 mg oral once/week continuing for 4 weeks after last exposure; **or** doxycycline 100 mg daily during exposure and for 4 weeks afterwards; **or** chloroquine phosphate as above plus pyrimethamine-sulfadoxine for presumptive treatment **or** plus proguanil 200 mg daily for sub-Saharan Africa during exposure and for 4 weeks afterward	
***Pneumocystis* pneumonia** (*Pneumocystis carinii*)	Trimethoprim-sulfamethoxazole (20/100 mg/kg/d) oral or IV in 4 doses for 14–21 days; **or** pentamidine isethionate 4 mg/kg/d IV for 14–21 days plus prednisone for severe pneumonia	Trimethoprim 5 mg/kg PO q6h for 21 days plus dapsone 100 mg PO once daily for 21 days; **or** primaquine 15 mg base PO once daily for 21 days plus clindamycin 300–450 mg PO q6h for 21 days; **or** trimetrexate 45 mg/m^2 IV once daily for 21 days plus folinic acid 20 mg/m^2 PO or IV q6h for 21 days
Schistosomiasis		
S. mansoni	Praziquantel 40 mg/kg/d in 2 doses for 1 day	Oxamniquine 15 mg/kg once; 30 mg/kg once for East Africa; 30 mg/kg once daily for 2 days for Egypt and South Africa
S. haematobium	Praziquantel 40 mg/kg/d in 2 doses for 1 day	
S. japonicum, S. mekongi	Praziquantel 60 mg/kg/d in 3 doses for 1 day	
Strongyloidiasis (*Strongyloides stercoralis*)	Thiabendazole 50 mg/kg/d in 2 doses (max 3 g/d) for 2 days; for disseminated disease continue for 7d, or longer if immunocompromised	Ivermectin 200 μg/kg/d for 1–2 days; **or** Albendazole 400 mg once daily for 3 days
Tapeworm intestinal infections *Diphyllobothrium latum*—fish; *Taenia saginata*—beef; *T. solium*—pork; *Dipylidium caninum*—dog	Praziquantel 10–20 mg/kg once; **or** niclosamide single dose of 4 tablets (2 g), chewed thoroughly	
Hymenolepis nana (dwarf tapeworm)	Praziquantel 25 mg/kg once; **or** niclosamide, single dose of 4 tablets (2 g) chewed thoroughly then 2 tablets daily for 6 days	
Toxoplasmosis (*Toxoplasma gondii*)	Pyrimethamine 75 mg/d plus sulfadiazine 2–4 g/d	Clindamycin 450 g/d tid plus pyrimethamine 75 mg/d
Trichinosis (*Trichinella spiralis*)	Glucocorticoids for severe symptoms plus mebendazole 200–400 mg tid for 3 days, then 400–500 mg tid for 10 days	
Trichomoniasis (*Trichomonas vaginalis*)	Metronidazole 2 g once or 250 mg tid PO for 7 days; **or** tinidazole 2 g once	
Trichostrongyliasis (*Trichostrongylus*)	Pyrantel pamoate 11 mg/kg once (max 1 g)	Mebendazole 100 mg bid for four days; **or** albendazole 400 mg once
Trichuriasis (whipworm) (*Trichuris trichiura*)	Mebendazole 100 mg bid for 3 days; **or** albendazole 400 mg once	
Trypanosomiasis		
T. cruzi (Chagas' disease)	Nifurtimox 8–10 mg/kg/d PO in 4 doses for 120 days	Benznidazole 5–7 mg/kg/d for 30–120 days
T. brucei gambiense, T.b. rhodesiense (sleeping sickness)		
Hemolymphatic stage	Suramin 100–200 mg test dose IV, then 1 g IV on days 1, 3, 7, 14, 21; **or** eflornithine 100 mg/kg qid for 14 days, then 300 mg/kg/d PO for 3–4 weeks	Pentamidine isethionate 4 mg/kg/d for 10 days
Late stage with CNS involvement	Melarsoprol 2–3.6 mg/kg/d IV for 3 doses; after 1 week 3.6 mg/kg/d IV for 3 doses; repeat after 10–21 days; **or** eflornithine 100 mg/kg qid for 14 days, then 300 mg/kg/d PO for 3–4 weeks	Tryparsamide 30 mg/kg (max 2 g) IV q5d to total of 12 injections; may repeat after 1 month, plus suramin 10 mg/kg IV q5d to total of 12 injections; may be repeated after 1 month
Visceral larva migrans (toxocariasis)	Supportive therapy and glucocorticoids	Diethylcarbamazine 2 mg/kg tid for 7–10 days; **or** mebendazole 100–200 mg bid for 5 doses; **or** thiabendazole 50 mg/kg/d in 2 doses for 5 days (max 3 g/d)

Chagas' disease. Frequent side effects include rashes, nausea, and peripheral neuritis.

Bithionol† This drug is used for the treatment of fascioliasis and paragonimiasis. Adverse cutaneous and gastrointestinal effects are common.

Chloroquine This mainstay oral antimalarial drug is a 4-amino-

quinolone that rapidly kills schizonts and gametocytes of *Plasmodium vivax, P. ovale, P. malariae,* and susceptible strains of *P. falciparum.* Unfortunately, in many areas *P. falciparum* is resistant to chloroquine, and in Oceania resistance has emerged in *P. vivax.* Chloroquine is still effective in the treatment and prophylaxis of malaria in areas where resistance is not yet established. Chloroquine phosphate is available as generic and commercial tablets in the United States; chloroquine sulfate is also available outside the United States. Hydroxychloroquine sulfate, more familiarly used as an antiarthritic agent, also has been used effectively. Chloroquine is safe in children and pregnant women. Side effects may include abdominal discomfort, headache, and dizziness.

Dehydroemetine† This is an ipecac alkaloid used as an alternative treatment for invasive amebiasis. Dehydroemetine is highly irritating and should only be administered by intramuscular injection. Pain, cellulitis, or abscess formation at the injection site is frequent. Cardiac arrhythmias, chest pain, and hypotension are common and limit the use of this drug to a monitored setting. Dehydroemetine is contraindicated in pregnancy.

Diethylcarbamazine† This piperazine derivative remains the drug of choice for lymphatic filariasis despite adverse reactions and a cumbersome dosage schedule. The mechanism of action of diethylcarbamazine is unclear, but it is microfilaricidal in vivo. Side effects are generally proportional to the microfilarial burden and include fever, headache, dizziness, and transient exacerbation of lymphangitis. In onchocerciasis, the drug elicits prominent pruritus and ocular and constitutional symptoms (Mazzotti reaction) and has been supplanted by ivermectin. Diethylcarbamazine is effective for treatment and prophylaxis of *Loa loa* infection and has been used for visceral larva migrans. The drug is not commercially available in the United States; limited amounts may be obtained from the manufacturer (Lederle).

Diloxanide furoate† This amebicidal agent is poorly absorbed and is active only against luminal amebas. Its mode of action is unknown. Mild side effects include flatulence and gastrointestinal discomfort.

Eflornithine Commonly known as difluoromethylornithine or DFMO, this drug is effective in both hemolymphatic and central nervous system stages of *Trypanosoma brucei gambiense* infections (African trypanosomiasis). Eflornithine is available in the United States only from the manufacturer (Merrell Dow). It acts by irreversible inhibition of the trypanosomal ornithine decarboxylase, although *Trypanosoma brucei rhodesiense* is relatively insensitive. Side effects of diarrhea, anemia, and leukopenia are frequent but reversible.

Furazolidone This nitrofuran derivative is used as an alternative drug for giardiasis. Unlike other drugs for giardiasis, it is not bitter and is available in a liquid form useful for young children. Nausea, vomiting, and allergic reactions occur. The drug is a monoamine oxidase (MAO) inhibitor and also produces a disulfiram-like reaction when taken with alcohol.

Halofantrine This new oral antimalarial drug, recently available in the United States, has been used to treat malaria due to chloroquine-resistant *P. falciparum.* Adverse effects include abdominal pain, diarrhea, and pruritus. It should not be used in pregnancy.

Iodoquinol This halogenated oxyquinolone is used for noninvasive amebiasis and *Dientamoeba fragilis* infection and as an alternative for *Balantidium coli* infection. Adverse effects are uncommon, but optic neuritis has been observed with prolonged use of excessively high doses.

Ivermectin† This semisynthetic derivative of avermectin is now the drug of choice for *Onchocerca volvulus* infections. A single oral dose of ivermectin is active against microfilariae but has no effect on the adult worms. Its mechanism of action has not been conclusively identified. Ivermectin also is active against a range of intestinal nematodes and is under investigation for the treatment of lymphatic filariasis. The drug is safe and well-tolerated in children and adults, but its safety in pregnancy has not been specifically addressed.

Mebendazole This benzimidazole derivative is effective against a spectrum of intestinal and tissue nematodes, including *Ascaris,* hookworm, *Enterobius,* and *Trichuris,* and is an investigational drug for *Capillaria.* Benzimidazoles may act by binding β-tubulin to disrupt microtubule formation and glucose uptake. Side effects include mild abdominal pain and diarrhea. Benzimidazoles can be teratogenic in experimental animals and so are avoided during pregnancy.

Mefloquine This new antimalarial agent is active against the blood stages of all malarial species and the schizonts of *P. falciparum.* A 4-aminoquinolone derivative, mefloquine is the currently preferred agent for the prophylaxis and oral treatment of chloroquine-resistant malaria. Adverse effects are generally dose-related and include nausea and dizziness and, more rarely, vomiting, diarrhea, psychosis, and seizures. Because it has been associated with sinus bradycardia, mefloquine is contraindicated in persons taking beta-adrenoreceptor and calcium-channel blocking agents and should not be given concurrently with quinine or quinidine. Mefloquine resistance of *P. falciparum* occurs in parts of Southeast Asia and Africa and will present a growing problem. Since its safety in pregnancy has not been established, mefloquine should be avoided during pregnancy.

Melarsoprol† This organic arsenical compound is used only to treat late-stage African trypanosomiasis involving the central nervous system. Only after intravenous administration does enough drug enter the cerebrospinal fluid to kill the trypanosomes. Severe adverse effects are common, including myocarditis, encephalopathy, and Herxheimer reactions.

Metrifonate This organophosphate compound is active against *Schistosoma haematobium.* Adverse effects include abdominal pain, nausea, vomiting, diarrhea, headache, and vertigo. It should not be used during pregnancy.

Metronidazole This 5-nitroimidazole has potent activity against anaerobic bacteria and several protozoa, including *Entamoeba histolytica, Giardia lamblia, Trichomonas vaginalis,* and *Balantidium coli.* Metronidazole is the drug of choice for giardiasis (although not FDA approved for this indication) and the initial treatment of invasive amebiasis. It is generally well tolerated, but mild abdominal pain, headache, nausea, and a persistent metallic taste are common. The drug is teratogenic in animals and should be avoided in early pregnancy. Because it produces a disulfiram-like reaction, abstinence from alcohol is advisable.

Niclosamide Niclosamide is safe and highly effective against intestinal tapeworms when given as a single oral dose and chewed thoroughly before it is washed down with water. Intestinal reactions are minimal, and there are no contraindications to its use. Since it is not absorbed from the gastrointestinal tract, niclosamide is not active against larval cestodes.

Nifurtimox† This is a synthetic nitrofuran compound active in acute *Trypanosoma cruzi* infection. Response rates are variable, and the drug has little effect in chronic Chagas' disease. Adverse reactions, including nausea, vomiting, insomnia, headache, vertigo, tremor, paresthesias, and convulsions, are common and dose-dependent.

Oxamniquine This tetrahydroquinolone derivative is used as an alternative agent for *Schistosoma mansoni* infection. Higher doses are needed in Egypt and South Africa, and resistant strains also have been encountered. Oxamniquine is well tolerated, with occasional side effects of headache, dizziness, drowsiness, and gastrointestinal disturbances. It should not be used in pregnancy.

Paromomycin This oral, poorly absorbed aminoglycoside is used as an alternative treatment for noninvasive amebiasis. Though not approved for the purpose, paromomycin also has been used in lieu of metronidazole to treat amebiasis and giardiasis in pregnant women.

Pentamidine isethionate This is a stable aromatic diamine compound active against *Pneumocystis carinii* and several protozoal pathogens, including *Leishmania* spp. and *T. brucei gambiense.* Its mechanism of action remains uncertain. Adverse reactions to parenteral pentamidine are common, including reversible nephrotoxicity, acute hypotension, pancreatitis, hypoglycemia, cardiac arrhythmias, blood dyscrasias, and sterile abscesses at the injection site. Aerosolized pentamidine used for the prophylaxis of *Pneumocystis* pneumonia in susceptible patients is associated with local adverse effects, including sore throat, oral paresthesias, metallic taste, cough, and bronchospasm.

Piperazine This inexpensive drug, widely used in developing countries for the treatment of ascariasis and enterobiasis, is an anticholinergic agent that acts by paralyzing the worms, allowing them to be flushed out by peristalsis. Intestinal disturbances, hypersensitivity reactions, and dizziness are occasional adverse reactions. Piperazine and pyrantel pamoate have antagonistic modes of action and should not be administered together.

Praziquantel   This novel agent is the drug of choice for most trematode (fluke) and many cestode infections. Its mechanism of action is unknown, but in schistosomes it causes paralysis and tegumental disruption, which may then permit a synergistic host immune response. Praziquantel is highly active against all human schistosome parasites, intestinal tapeworms, cysticercosis, and other flukes exclusive of *Fasciola hepatica*. Side effects include headache, dizziness, drowsiness, and abdominal discomfort. Higher doses and adjunctive anti-inflammatory corticosteroids are recommended for neurocysticercosis.

Primaquine   This 8-aminoquinolone derivative is the only standard drug active against the intrahepatic hypnozoite forms of malarial species and is used for the radical cure of *P. vivax* and *P. ovale* malaria following schizonticidal therapy. It is also an effective gametocidal agent. A potent oxidant, primaquine causes acute hemolysis in the presence of glucose-6-phosphate dehydrogenase deficiency, and at-risk patients should be screened before such therapy is instituted. Primaquine is contraindicated during pregnancy.

Proguanil*   This pyrimidine derivative is active against the preerythrocytic intrahepatic forms of *P. falciparum* and possibly *P. vivax*. Its use is largely limited to malaria prophylaxis, in combination with chloroquine, in parts of Africa where chloroquine-resistant *P. falciparum* is not yet widely prevalent. However, foci of proguanil resistance also exist in many regions, and clinical failures with proguanil are common. Proguanil is not licensed in the United States but is sold in Europe and Africa.

Pyrantel   This well-tolerated pyrimidine derivative acts against intestinal nematodes by inducing neuromuscular paralysis in the worms, allowing them to be expelled. A single dose is usually curative for ascariasis, enterobiasis, and trichostrongyliasis, but several doses are recommended for hookworm infection. It is safe for use in pregnancy.

Pyrimethamine-sulfonamides   Pyrimethamine combined with sulfadiazine is used in the treatment of toxoplasmosis. The high doses required for the latter often result in significant folate deficiency, necessitating folinic acid replacement. Abdominal symptoms and rashes are also common. Pyrimethamine combined with sulfadoxine is active against most strains of *P. falciparum*, although drug resistance is becoming more widespread. Pyrimethamine-sulfadoxine, as an adjunct to quinine, is still useful in the oral treatment of chloroquine-resistant *P. falciparum* malaria, but it is no longer recommended for malarial prophylaxis because of occasional severe and fatal skin hypersensitivity reactions and hepatitis.

Quinacrine   This acridine dye used to treat giardiasis is well absorbed and may impart a yellow color to the urine and, rarely, to the skin or sclerae. Adverse effects include headache, dizziness, vomiting, diarrhea, and, less commonly, psychotic episodes. Distribution of this drug has ceased within the United States.

Quinine and quinidine   These cinchona alkaloids have reemerged as first-line drugs for treatment of falciparum malaria because of widespread chloroquine resistance. Quinine plus a second orally active drug (to reduce the likelihood of recurrence) is recommended

for oral therapy for *P. falciparum* malaria. For severe infections requiring intravenous therapy, only quinidine gluconate (which is at least as effective as parenteral quinine) is available in the United States. Cardiac monitoring during quinidine infusion is mandatory, and oral quinine should be substituted as soon as the patient is able to take it. Both quinine and quinidine can cause hypoglycemia. Symptoms of cinchonism, including tinnitus, headache, visual disturbances, nausea, and abdominal pain, often develop with treatment but are rarely grounds for discontinuing the drug. Oral quinine also is used with clindamycin to treat babesiosis.

Spiramycin   This is an alternative to antifolates in the treatment of toxoplasmosis, particularly for pregnant women, in whom it is safe. This agent is available from the FDA.

Stibogluconate sodium† (sodium antimony gluconate)   This pentavalent antimonial parenteral solution is the drug of choice for all forms of leishmaniasis. Its mechanism of action is unknown. Adverse effects include muscle pain, joint stiffness, nausea, vomiting, and, less commonly, rash and cardiac or hepatic toxicity. Meglumine antimoniate, another pentavalent antimonial drug, is used in many French- and Spanish-speaking countries.

Suramin†   This complex derivative of urea is the drug of choice for treating early African trypanosomiasis and is the only available drug active against adult *Onchocerca volvulus* worms. It must be given intravenously and is excreted very slowly. Adverse effects are common and can be severe, including vomiting, pruritus, urticaria, paresthesias, photophobia, peripheral neuropathy, anaphylaxis, and renal damage.

Tetracycline, doxycycline   Tetracycline is effective against *Balantidium coli* and *Dientamoeba fragilis* and also is used as an adjunct to quinine in treating chloroquine-resistant falciparum malaria. Doxycycline, a once-daily form, may be used for chemoprophylaxis of chloroquine-resistant falciparum malaria. Tooth staining in children and photosensitivity are potential hazards.

Thiabendazole   This older benzimidazole derivative is active against a variety of nematode parasites, but frequent and severe side effects limit its primary systemic use to treatment of strongyloidiasis. These adverse reactions include dizziness, nausea, vomiting, drowsiness, pruritus, headache, neuropsychiatric disturbances, hepatitis, and hypersensitivity reactions, including Stevens-Johnson syndrome. A topical suspension of thiabendazole is used for cutaneous larva migrans.

Tinidazole*   This nitroimidazole is available only outside the United States for the treatment of amebiasis, giardiasis, and vaginal trichomoniasis. Tinidazole appears to be more effective and better tolerated than metronidazole.

Trimethoprim-sulfamethoxazole   This antifolate combination is active in *P. carinii* pneumonia and *Isospora belli* infection in immunocompromised patients. Adverse effects are predominantly due to the sulfamethoxazole and include skin, liver, and bone marrow toxicity.

REFERENCES

Drugs for parasitic infections. Med Lett Drugs Ther 34:17, 1992
ROSENBLATT JE: Antiparasitic agents. Mayo Clin Proc 67:276, 1992
WORLD HEALTH ORGANIZATION: *Model Prescribing Information: Drugs Used in Parasitic Diseases*. Geneva: WHO, 1990

section 17   Protozoal infections

173   AMEBIASIS AND INFECTION WITH FREE-LIVING AMEBAS

SHARON L. REED

AMEBIASIS

DEFINITION   Amebiasis is an infection with the intestinal protozoan *Entamoeba histolytica*. About 90 percent of infections are asymptomatic, and the remaining 10 percent display a spectrum of clinical syndromes ranging from dysentery to abscesses of the liver or other organs.

LIFE CYCLE AND TRANSMISSION   *E. histolytica* is acquired by ingestion of viable cysts from fecally contaminated water, food, or hands. Food-borne exposure is most prevalent, particularly when handlers are shedding cysts or food is grown in fecally contaminated soil, fertilizer, or water. Less common sources include waterborne transmission, oral and anal sexual practices, and, rarely, direct rectal inoculation through colonic irrigation devices. Motile trophozoites are released from cysts in the small intestine, where they remain as harmless commensals in the bowel of most patients. After encystation, infectious cysts are shed in the stool and can survive for several weeks in a moist environment. In some patients, the trophozoites invade either the bowel mucosa, causing symptomatic colitis, or the bloodstream, causing distant abscesses of the liver, lungs, or brain. The trophozoites may not encyst in patients with active dysentery, and motile, hematophagous trophozoites are frequently present in fresh stools. Trophozoites are rapidly killed by exposure to air or stomach acid, however, and therefore cannot cause infection.

EPIDEMIOLOGY   About 10 percent of the world's population is infected with *E. histolytica*; amebiasis is the third cause of death from parasitic disease after schistosomiasis and malaria. Areas of highest incidence include most developing countries in the tropics due to inadequate sanitation and crowding, particularly in Mexico, Central and South America, India, tropical Asia, and Africa. The main groups at risk in developed countries are travelers, recent immigrants, homosexual men, and inmates of institutions.

All *E. histolytica* trophozoites and cysts are morphologically identical, but the wide spectrum of clinical disease is determined by the virulence of the infecting strain. Isolates of *E. histolytica* from patients with invasive amebiasis have unique isoenzymes, surface antigens, DNA markers, and virulence properties (including the production of extracellular proteinases and resistance to complement-mediated lysis).

Most asymptomatic carriers, including homosexual men and AIDS patients, harbor nonpathogenic strains and have self-limited infections. These findings suggest that nonpathogenic strains of *E. histolytica* are incapable of causing invasive disease, since *Cryptosporidium* and *Isospora belli*, which also cause only self-limited illnesses in immunocompetent people, cause devastating diarrhea in AIDS patients. Some asymptomatic individuals are infected with strains that are pathogenic, as shown by isoenzyme patterns. In one study, 10 percent of asymptomatic patients who were colonized with pathogenic strains went on to develop amebic colitis, while the rest remained asymptomatic and cleared the infection within 1 year. Host factors play a role as well, since some patients infected with pathogenic strains do not develop invasive amebiasis.

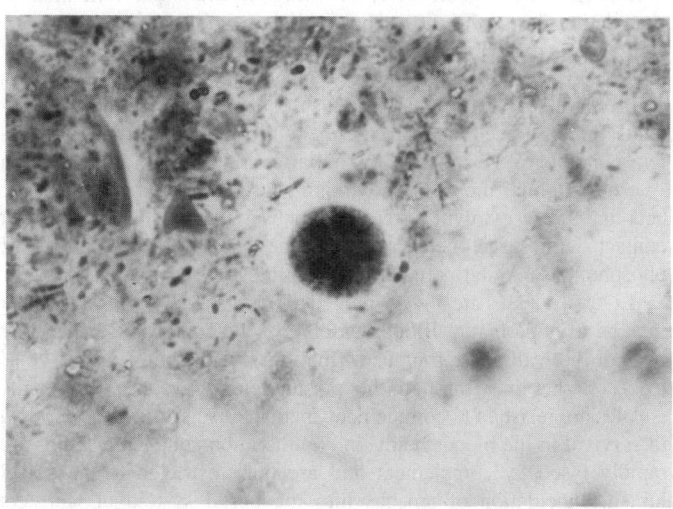

FIGURE 173-1   Cyst of *E. histolytica* showing three of the four nuclei (trichrome stain).

PATHOGENESIS AND PATHOLOGY   Both cysts (Fig. 173-1) and trophozoites (Fig. 173-2) are found in the intestinal lumen, but only trophozoites invade tissue. The trophozoite is 20 to 60 μm in diameter and contains vacuoles and a nucleus with a characteristic central karyosome. In animals, depletion of intestinal mucus, diffuse inflammation, and disruption of the epithelial barrier occur before trophozoites actually come into contact with the colonic mucosa. Trophozoites attach to the interglandular epithelium by surface lectins. The earliest intestinal lesions are microulcerations of the mucosa of the cecum, sigmoid colon, or rectum that release erythrocytes, inflammatory cells, and epithelial cells. Proctoscopy reveals small ulcers with heaped up margins and normal intervening mucosa. Submucosal extension of ulcerations under viable-appearing surface mucosa causes the classic "flask-shaped" ulcer containing trophozoites at the margins of dead and viable tissues. Although neutrophilic

FIGURE 173-2   Trophozoite of *E. histolytica* demonstrating a single nucleus with a central, dotlike karyosome (trichrome stain).

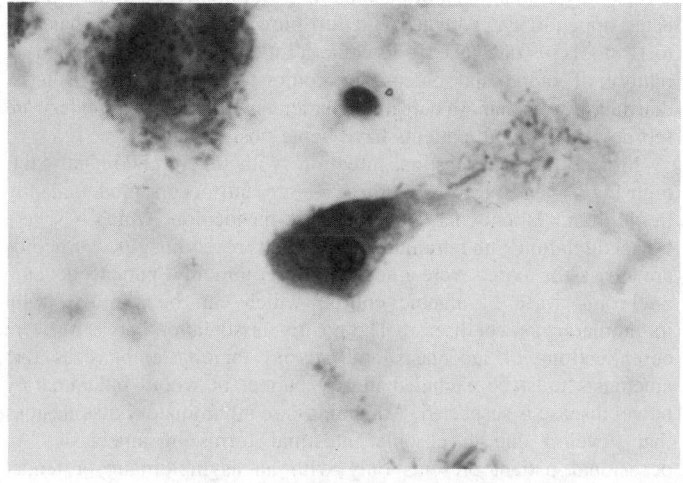

infiltrates may accompany the early lesions in animals, human intestinal infection is marked by a paucity of inflammatory cells, probably in part because of the killing of neutrophils by trophozoites. Treated ulcers characteristically heal with little or no scarring. Occasionally, however, full-thickness necrosis and perforation occur.

Rarely, intestinal infection results in the formation of a mass lesion or ameboma in the bowel lumen. The overlying mucosa is usually thin and ulcerated, while other layers of the wall are thickened, edematous, and hemorrhagic, resulting in exuberant formation of granulation tissue with little fibrous tissue response.

A number of virulence factors have been linked to the ability of amebas to invade through the interglandular epithelium. One is an extracellular proteinase that degrades collagen, elastin, and components of the extracellular matrix. Other enzymes may disrupt glycoprotein bonds between mucosal epithelial cells in the gut. Amebas can lyse neutrophils, monocytes, lymphocytes, and colonic and hepatic cell lines. The cytolytic effect of amebas appears to require direct contact with target cells and may be linked to the release of phospholipase A and pore-forming peptides.

Liver abscesses are always preceded by intestinal colonization that may be asymptomatic. Blood vessels may be compromised early by lysis of the wall and thrombus formation. Trophozoites invade veins to reach the liver through the portal venous system. Pathogenic isolates are resistant to complement-mediated lysis, a property critical to survival in the bloodstream. In contrast, nonpathogenic strains are rapidly lysed by complement and are thus restricted to the bowel lumen. Inoculation of amebas into the portal system of hamsters results in an acute cellular infiltrate consisting predominantly of neutrophils. Later, the neutrophils are lysed by contact with amebas, and the release of neutrophil toxins may contribute to necrosis of hepatocytes. The liver parenchyma is replaced by necrotic material that is surrounded by a thin rim of congested liver tissue. The necrotic contents of a liver abscess are classically described as "anchovy paste," although the fluid is variable in color and is composed of bacteriologically sterile granular debris with few or no cells. Amebas, if seen, tend to be found only near the capsule of the abscess.

Clinical infection does not induce immunity to recurrent colonization with E. histolytica, but repeated episodes of colitis or liver abscess are unusual. Antibody is not protective; titers correlate with the length of illness rather than with the severity of disease. Studies of animals suggest that cell-mediated immunity may be important for protection, although patients with AIDS do not appear to be predisposed to more severe disease.

CLINICAL SYNDROMES **Intestinal amebiasis** The most common type of amebic infection is that of asymptomatic cyst passage. Even in highly endemic areas, most patients harbor nonpathogenic strains.

Symptomatic amebic colitis develops 2 to 6 weeks after the ingestion of infectious cysts. Lower abdominal pain and mild diarrhea develop gradually and are followed by malaise, weight loss, and diffuse lower abdominal or back pain. Cecal involvement may mimic acute appendicitis. Patients with full-blown dysentery may have 10 to 12 stools per day. The stools contain little fecal material and consist mainly of blood and mucus. In contrast to those with bacterial diarrhea, fewer than 40 percent of patients with amebic dysentery are febrile. Virtually all patients have heme-positive stools.

More fulminant intestinal infection, with severe abdominal pain, high fevers, and profuse diarrhea, is rare and occurs predominantly in children. Patients may develop toxic megacolon, which is severe bowel dilatation with intramural air. Patients receiving glucocorticoids are at risk for more severe amebiasis. Uncommonly, patients develop a chronic form of amebic colitis, which can be confused with inflammatory bowel disease. The positive association between severe complications of amebiasis and steroid therapy emphasizes that amebiasis must be excluded in any patient in whom inflammatory bowel disease is suspected. Amebomas are inflammatory mass lesions that develop due to chronic intestinal forms of amebiasis. An occasional patient presents only with an asymptomatic or tender abdominal mass caused by an ameboma, which is easily confused with cancer on barium studies. A positive serologic test or biopsy can prevent unnecessary surgery in this setting. The syndrome of postamebic colitis, persistent diarrhea following documented cure of amebic colitis, is controversial; no evidence of recurrent amebic infection can be found, and retreatment usually has no effect.

Amebic liver abscess Extraintestinal infection by E. histolytica most often involves the liver. Of travelers who develop an amebic liver abscess after leaving an endemic area, 95 percent do so within 5 months. Young patients with an amebic liver abscess are more likely to present acutely with prominent symptoms of less than 10 days' duration. The majority of patients are febrile and have right upper quadrant pain, which may be dull or pleuritic in nature and radiate to the shoulder. Point tenderness over the liver and right pleural effusion are common. Jaundice is rare. Although the initial site of infection is the colon, fewer than one-third of patients with an amebic abscess have active diarrhea. Older patients from endemic areas are more likely to have a subacute course lasting 6 months, with weight loss and hepatomegaly. About one-third of patients with chronic presentations are febrile. Thus the clinical diagnosis of an amebic liver abscess may be difficult to establish because the symptoms and signs are often nonspecific. Since 10 to 15 percent of patients present only with fever, amebic liver abscess must be considered in the differential diagnosis of fever of unknown origin.

Complications of amebic liver abscess Pleuropulmonary involvement, which occurs in 20 to 30 percent of patients, is the most frequent complication of amebic liver abscess. Manifestations include sterile effusions, contiguous spread from the liver, and rupture into the pleural space. Sterile effusions and contiguous spread usually resolve with medical therapy, but frank rupture into the pleural space requires drainage. An hepatobronchial fistula may cause cough productive of large amounts of necrotic material that may contain amebas. This dramatic complication carries a good prognosis. Abscesses that rupture into the peritoneum may present as an indolent leak or an acute abdomen and require both percutaneous catheter drainage and medical therapy. Rupture into the pericardium, usually from abscesses of the left lobe of the liver, carries the gravest prognosis, can occur during medical therapy, and requires surgical drainage.

Other extraintestinal sites Involvement of the genitourinary tract may occur by direct extension from the colon or hematogenous spread. Painful genital ulcers, characterized by a punched-out appearance and profuse discharge, may develop secondary to extension from either the intestine or the liver. Both these conditions respond well to medical therapy. Cerebral involvement occurs in fewer than 0.1 percent of patients in large clinical series. Symptoms and prognosis depend on the size and location of the lesion.

DIAGNOSTIC TESTS **Laboratory diagnosis** Stool examinations, serology, and noninvasive imaging of the liver are the most important tests to establish the diagnosis. Fecal findings suggestive of amebic colitis include a positive test for heme, a paucity of neutrophils, and the presence of Charcot-Leyden crystal protein (double pyramid-shaped crystals normally found in the cytoplasm of eosinophils). The cornerstone of the diagnosis of amebic colitis, however, is the demonstration of the hematophagous trophozoites or the cysts of E. histolytica (Figs. 173-1 and 173-2). Because trophozoites are rapidly killed by water, drying, or barium, it is important to examine at least three fresh stool specimens. Examination of a combination of wet mounts, iodine-stained concentrates, and trichrome stains of fresh stool and concentrates confirms the diagnosis in 75 to 95 percent of cases. Cultures of amebas are more sensitive but are not routinely available. If stool examinations are negative, sigmoidoscopy with biopsy of the edge of ulcers may increase the yield but is risky during fulminant colitis because of the risk of perforation. Trophozoites in the biopsy of a colonic mass confirm the diagnosis of ameboma, but trophozoites are rare in liver aspirates. Accurate diagnosis requires experience, since trophozoites may be confused with neutrophils and the cysts must be differentiated

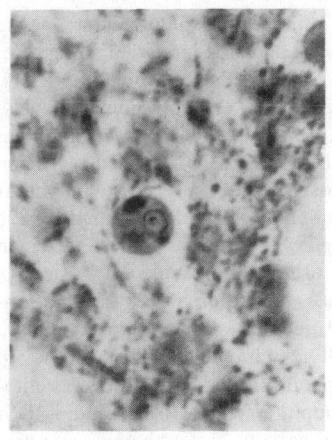
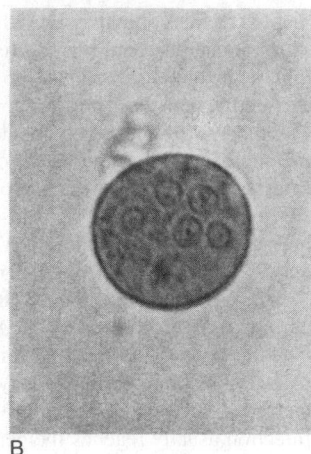

A   B

FIGURE 173-3 *A.* Cyst of *E. hartmanni* showing the smaller size with a single nucleus and eccentric karyosome. *B.* Cyst of *E. coli* showing five of the seven nuclei. *(A and B from FM Spencer, LS Monroe, Color Atlas of Intestinal Parasites, Springfield, Ill, Charles C Thomas, 1982.)*

morphologically from *E. hartmanni* and *E. coli* (Fig. 173-3 *A* and *B*) and from *Endolimax nana*, which do not cause clinical disease and do not warrant therapy. Unfortunately, the cysts of pathogenic and nonpathogenic *E. histolytica* cannot be distinguished microscopically.

Serology is helpful in the diagnosis of invasive amebiasis. Kits for the performance of counterimmunodiffusion, agar gel diffusion, and ELISA assays are commercially available, and the results of these tests are positive in more than 90 percent of patients with colitis, amebomas, or liver abscess. Positive results suggest active disease because serologies usually revert to negative within 6 to 12 months. Even in highly endemic areas such as South Africa, fewer than 10 percent of asymptomatic people have a positive amebic serology. The interpretation of the indirect hemagglutination (IHA) test is more difficult because titers may remain positive for as long as 10 years. Up to 10 percent of patients with acute amebic liver abscess may have a negative serology; in suspected cases, testing should be repeated in a week. In contrast to carriers of nonpathogenic strains, most asymptomatic carriers of pathogenic strains develop antibodies. Thus serologic tests are helpful in assessing the risk of invasive amebiasis in an asymptomatic patient. Serologies also should be assessed in patients with ulcerative colitis before the institution of steroid therapy to prevent the development of severe colitis or toxic megacolon during unsuspected amebiasis.

Routine hematology and chemistry tests are usually not very helpful in the diagnosis of invasive amebiasis. About three-fourths of patients with an amebic liver abscess have leukocytosis (>10,000 cells per cubic millimeter); this condition is particularly likely if symptoms are acute or complications have developed. Invasive amebiasis does not elicit eosinophilia. Anemia, if present, is usually multifactorial. Even with large liver abscesses, liver enzymes are normal or minimally elevated. The alkaline phosphatase level is most often elevated and may remain so for months. Transaminase elevations suggest acute disease or a complication.

Radiographic studies Radiographic barium studies are potentially dangerous in acute amebic colitis. Amebomas are usually identified first by a barium enema, but biopsy is necessary for differentiation from carcinoma.

Newer radiographic techniques have improved the detection of amebic liver abscesses. Liver scans, ultrasonography, computed tomography, and magnetic resonance imaging are all useful for detection of the round or oval hypoechoic cyst. More than 80 percent of patients who have had symptoms for more than 10 days have a single abscess of the right lobe of the liver. Approximately 50 percent of patients who have had symptoms for less than 10 days have multiple abscesses. Findings associated with complications include large abscesses (>10 cm) in the superior part of the right lobe, which

may rupture into the pleural space; multiple lesions, which must be differentiated from pyogenic abscesses; and lesions of the left lobe, which may rupture into the pericardium. Because abscesses resolve slowly and may increase in size in patients who are responding clinically to therapy, frequent follow-up ultrasonography may prove confusing. Complete resolution of a liver abscess within 6 months can be anticipated in two-thirds of patients, but 10 percent may have persistent abnormalities for a year.

DIFFERENTIAL DIAGNOSIS The differential diagnosis of intestinal amebiasis includes bacterial diarrheas caused by *Campylobacter*, enteroinvasive *Escherichia coli*, and *Shigella*, *Salmonella*, and *Vibrio* species. Although the typical patient with amebic colitis has less prominent fever and heme-positive stools with few neutrophils, bacterial cultures, microscopic examination of stools, and amebic serology are essential for correct diagnosis. Amebiasis must be ruled out in any patient thought to have inflammatory bowel disease.

Because of the variety of presenting signs and symptoms, amebic liver abscess can easily be confused with pulmonary or gallbladder disease or with any febrile illness with few localizing signs, e.g., malaria or typhoid fever. The diagnosis should be considered in high-risk groups with a history of recent travel outside the United States and in inmates of institutions. Once radiographic studies have identified an abscess in the liver, the most important differential is between amebic and pyogenic abscess. The patient with pyogenic abscess typically is older and has a history of underlying bowel disease or recent surgery. Amebic serology is helpful, but aspiration of the abscess, with Gram stains and cultures of the material, may be required to differentiate the two diseases.

TREATMENT **Intestinal disease** Drugs to treat amebiasis can be classified according to their primary site of action. Luminal amebicides are poorly absorbed and reach high concentrations within the bowel, but their activity is limited to cysts and trophozoites close to the mucosa. Three luminal drugs are available in the United States: iodoquinol, paromomycin, and diloxanide furoate (Table 173-1). Indications for the use of luminal agents include eradication of cysts in patients with colitis or a liver abscess and treatment of asymptomatic carriers. Until probes are available for differentiating nonpathogenic from pathogenic cysts, it is prudent to treat asymptomatic individuals who pass cysts.

Tissue amebicides reach high concentrations in the blood and tissue after oral or parenteral administration. The development of nitroimidazole compounds, especially metronidazole, was a major advance in the treatment of invasive amebiasis. Patients with amebic colitis should be treated with metronidazole, 750 mg, three times daily, IV or orally, for 10 days. Side effects include nausea, vomiting,

TABLE 173-1   Drug therapy for amebiasis

	Dosage
ASYMPTOMATIC CARRIER (LUMINAL AGENTS)	
Iodoquinol (650-mg tablets)	650 mg tid for 20 days
Diloxanide furoate* (500-mg tablets)	500 mg tid for 10 days
Paromomycin (250-mg tablets)	500 mg tid for 10 days
ACUTE COLITIS	
Metronidazole (250- or 500-mg tablets)	750 mg PO or IV tid for 5–10 days
plus	
Luminal agent as above	
AMEBIC LIVER ABSCESS	
Metronidazole	750 mg PO or IV tid for 5–10 days
Tinidazole†	2 g PO
Ornidazole†	2 g PO
plus	
Luminal agent as above	

* Available only through the CDC at telephone number (404) 639-3356.
† Not available in the United States.

abdominal discomfort, and a disulfiram-like effect. Other imidazole compounds such as tinidazole and ornidazole are as effective but are not available in the United States. All patients should receive a full course of therapy with a luminal agent, since metronidazole does not eradicate cysts. Resistance to metronidazole has not been identified. Relapses probably represent reinfection or failure to eradicate amebas from the bowel because of inadequate dosage or duration of therapy.

Amebic liver abscess   Metronidazole is the drug of choice for amebic liver abscess. The usefulness of nitroimidazoles in single-dose or abbreviated regimens is important in endemic areas with limited access to hospitalization. With early diagnosis and therapy, mortality from uncomplicated amebic liver abscess is less than 1 percent. Second-line therapeutic agents such as emetine and chloroquine should be avoided if possible because of the potential cardiovascular and gastrointestinal side effects of the former and the higher relapse rates with the latter. There is no evidence that combined therapy with two drugs is more effective than the single-drug regimen. Studies of South Africans with liver abscesses demonstrated that 72 percent of patients without intestinal symptoms were colonized asymptomatically with pathogenic strains; thus all treatment regimens should include a luminal agent to eradicate cysts and prevent further transmission. Amebic liver abscess recurs rarely.

Aspiration of liver abscesses   More than 90 percent of patients respond dramatically to metronidazole therapy with decreases in both pain and fever within 72 h. Indications for aspiration of liver abscesses are (1) the need to rule out a pyogenic abscess, particularly in patients with multiple lesions, (2) the failure to respond clinically in 3 to 5 days, (3) the threat of imminent rupture, and (4) the prevention of rupture of left lobe abscesses into the pericardium. There is no evidence that aspiration, even of large abscesses (up to 10 cm), leads to more rapid healing. Percutaneous drainage may be successful even if the liver abscess has already ruptured. Surgery should be reserved for instances of bowel perforation and rupture into the pericardium.

PREVENTION   Amebic infection is spread by ingestion of food or water contaminated with cysts. Since an asymptomatic carrier may excrete up to 15 million cysts a day, prevention of infection requires adequate sanitation and eradication of cyst carriage. In high-risk areas, infection can be minimized by avoiding unpeeled fruits and vegetables and using bottled water. Because cysts are resistant to readily attainable levels of chlorine, disinfection by iodination (tetraglycine hydroperiodide) is recommended. There is no effective prophylaxis.

INFECTION WITH FREE-LIVING AMEBAS

EPIDEMIOLOGY   Free-living amebas of the genera *Acanthamoeba* and *Naegleria* are distributed throughout the world and have been isolated from a wide variety of fresh and brackish water, including that from lakes, taps, hot springs, swimming pools, and heating and air-conditioning units, and even from the nasal passages of healthy children. Encystation may protect the protozoa from desiccation and food deprivation. The persistence of *Legionella pneumophila* in water supplies may be attributable in part to chronic infection of free-living amebas, particularly *Naegleria*.

NAEGLERIA INFECTIONS   More than 100 cases of primary amebic meningoencephalitis from *Naegleria fowleri* have been reported. Infection follows the aspiration of water contaminated with trophozoites or cysts or the inhalation of dust leading to invasion of the olfactory neuroepithelium. After an incubation period of 2 to 15 days, severe headache, high fever, nausea, vomiting, and meningismus occur. Photophobia and palsies of the third, fourth, and sixth cranial nerves are common. Rapid progression to seizures and coma may follow, and most patients die within a week. Infection is most common in otherwise healthy children or young adults, who often report recent swimming in lakes or heated swimming pools, particularly in July and August.

Diagnosis depends on the detection of motile trophozoites in wet mounts of fresh spinal fluid. Other laboratory findings resemble those of fulminant bacterial meningitis, with elevated intracranial pressure, high white blood cell counts (up to 20,000 cells per cubic millimeter), elevated spinal fluid protein concentration, and low glucose levels. The diagnosis should be considered in any patient who has purulent meningitis without evidence of bacteria by Gram stain, antigen detection, and culture. The prognosis is uniformly poor. Only four survivors, treated with high-dose amphotericin B and rifampin, have been reported. Antibodies to *Naegleria* spp. have been detected in normal adults, and serology is not useful in the acute diagnosis.

ACANTHAMOEBA INFECTIONS   Granulomatous amebic encephalitis   Infection with *Acanthamoeba* species follows a more indolent course and occurs typically in chronically ill or debilitated patients. Risk factors include lymphoproliferative disorders, chemotherapy, glucocorticoid therapy, lupus erythematosus, and AIDS. Infection usually reaches the central nervous system hematogenously from a primary focus in the skin or lungs. The onset is insidious and often mimics a space-occupying lesion. Altered mental status, headache, and stiff neck may be accompanied by focal findings such as cranial nerve palsies, ataxia, and hemiparesis. Cutaneous ulcers or hard nodules containing amebas were detected in 9 of the 30 patients reported in the United States.

Examination of the cerebrospinal fluid for trophozoites may be helpful, but lumbar puncture may be contraindicated because of increased intracerebral pressure. Computed tomography frequently reveals cortical and subcortical lesions of decreased density consistent with embolic infarcts. Demonstration of the trophozoites and cysts of *Acanthamoeba* in biopsies establishes the diagnosis. Fluorescein-labeled antiserum is available from the Centers for Disease Control to be used in detecting protozoa in biopsy specimens. At least nine cases of granulomatous amebic encephalitis have been reported in patients with AIDS, who may have an accelerated course because of their difficulty in forming granulomas. Although studies in animals suggest that rifampin may be useful, the infection is almost uniformly fatal. A similar syndrome may be caused by a leptomyxid ameba.

Keratitis   The incidence of keratitis caused by *Acanthamoeba* has increased in the past 15 years; more than 250 infections have been reported to the Centers for Disease Control. The first recognized infections were associated with trauma to the eye and exposure to contaminated water. At present, most infections are linked to extended-wear contact lenses. Risk factors include the use of homemade saline, wearing lenses while swimming, and inadequate disinfection. Since contact lenses presumably cause microscopic trauma, the early corneal findings may be nonspecific. The first symptoms usually include tearing and the painful sensation of a foreign body. Once infection is established, progression is rapid, and the characteristic clinical sign is an annular, paracentral corneal ring representing a corneal abscess. Deeper corneal invasion and loss of vision may follow.

The differential diagnosis includes bacterial, mycobacterial, and herpetic infection. The irregular, polygonal cysts of *Acanthamoeba* may be identified in corneal scrapings or biopsy material, and trophozoites can be grown on special media. Cysts are resistant to available drugs, and the results of medical therapy are disappointing. Some reports have suggested partial responses to the combination of propamidine isethionate eyedrops and topical steroids. Severe infections usually require keratoplasty.

REFERENCES

Amebiasis

ALLASON-JONES E et al: *Entamoeba histolytica* as a commensal intestinal parasite in homosexual men. N Engl J Med 315:353, 1986

IRUSEN EM et al: Asymptomatic intestinal colonization by pathogenic *Entamoeba histolytica* in amebic liver abscess: Prevalence, response to therapy, and pathogenic potential. Clin Infect Dis 14:889, 1992

KATZENSTEIN D et al: New concepts of amebic liver abscess derived from hepatic imaging, serodiagnosis, and hepatic enzymes in 67 consecutive cases in San Diego. Medicine 61:237, 1982

RAVDIN JL (ed): *Amebiasis: Human Infection by Entamoeba histolytica*. New York, Wiley, 1988

REED SL: Amebiasis: an update. Clin Infect Dis 14:385, 1992

———— et al: *Entamoeba histolytica* infection and AIDS. Am J Med 90:269, 1991

SARGEAUNT PG: The reliability of *Entamoeba histolytica* zymodemes in clinical diagnosis. Parasitol Today 3:40, 1987

THOMPSON JE et al: Amebic liver abscess: A therapeutic approach. Rev Infect Dis 7:171, 1985

Acanthamoeba and Naegleria

MA P et al: *Naegleria* and *Acanthamoeba* infections: Review. Rev Infect Dis 12:490, 1990

STEHR-GREEN JK et al: *Acanthamoeba* keratitis in soft contact lens wearers: A case-control study. JAMA 258:57, 1987

VISVESVARA GS, STEHR-GREEN JK: Epidemiology of free-living ameba infections. J Protozool 37:25S, 1990

WILEY CA et al: Acanthamoeba meningoencephalitis in a patient with AIDS. J Infect Dis 155:130, 1987

174 MALARIA AND BABESIOSIS

NICHOLAS J. WHITE / JOEL G. BREMAN

MALARIA

Malaria is a protozoan disease transmitted by the bite of *Anopheles* mosquitoes. It is the most important of the parasitic diseases of humans, affecting 103 endemic countries with a population of over 2.5 billion people and causing between 1 and 3 million deaths each year. Malaria has now been eradicated from North America, Europe, and Russia; however, despite enormous control efforts, there has been a resurgence of the disease in many parts of the tropics. In addition, drug resistance poses increasing problems in most malarious areas. Malaria remains today, as it has for centuries, a major burden on tropical communities and a danger to travelers.

ETIOLOGY   Four species of the genus *Plasmodium* infect humans. These are *P. vivax, P. ovale, P. malariae,* and *P. falciparum* (Table 174-1). Almost all deaths from malaria are caused by *P. falciparum.* Human infection begins when a female anopheline mosquito inoculates sporozoites from its salivary glands during a blood meal (Fig. 174-1). These small motile forms are carried rapidly via the bloodstream to the liver, where they target hepatic parenchymal cells, invade, and begin a period of asexual reproduction. By this amplification process (known as *intrahepatic* or *pre-erythrocytic merogony*), a single sporozoite eventually produces several thousand daughter merozoites. The swollen liver cell eventually bursts, discharging merozoites into the bloodstream—an event that initiates the symptomatic stage of the infection. In *P. vivax* and *P. ovale* infections, a proportion of the intrahepatic forms do not divide immediately but remain dormant for months before reproduction begins. These

"sleeping" forms, or hypnozoites, are the cause of the relapses that characterize infection with these two species.

After entering the bloodstream, merozoites rapidly invade erythrocytes. Attachment is mediated by a specific erythrocyte surface receptor. In *P. vivax* this receptor is related to the Duffy blood group antigen Fy^a or Fy^b. Most West Africans (or people with origins in that region) carry the Duffy-negative Fy phenotype and are therefore resistant to *P. vivax* malaria. The glycophorins, a family of membrane sialoglycoproteins, are the red cell attachment sites for the merozoites of *P. falciparum.* During the early stage of development, the small "ring forms" of the four parasite species appear similar under light microscopy. As the trophozoites enlarge, species-specific characteristics become evident, pigment becomes visible, and the parasite assumes an irregular or ameboid shape. By the end of the 48-h cycle (72 h for *P. malariae*), the parasite has grown to occupy most of the red cell. Multiple nuclear fission (merogony) then takes place, and the red cell ruptures to release 6 to 32 daughter merozoites, each of which is capable of invading a new red cell and repeating the cycle. After a period of asexual reproduction, a proportion of the parasites develop into morphologically distinct sexual forms (gametocytes) that are long-lived and are not associated with illness.

After ingestion of a blood meal by a biting female anopheline mosquito, male and female gametocytes fuse in the insect's midgut to form a zygote. This stage matures to form an ookinete, which penetrates and encysts in the mosquito's gut wall. The resulting oocyst expands by asexual division until it bursts to liberate myriad motile sporozoites, which migrate to the mosquito's salivary gland to await inoculation into humans at the next feeding.

The disease in humans is attributable to the direct effects of red cell invasion and destruction and the host's reaction to this process.

EPIDEMIOLOGY   Malaria occurs throughout most of the tropical regions of the world. *P. falciparum* predominates in sub-Saharan Africa, New Guinea, and Haiti. While *P. vivax* is more common in Central America and the Indian subcontinent, an increase in *P. falciparum* infections has occurred in India over the past decade. The prevalence of these two species is approximately equal in South America, eastern Asia, and Oceania. *P. malariae* is found in most areas (particularly in West and Central Africa) but is less common. *P. ovale* infection is relatively unusual outside Africa.

The epidemiology of malaria may vary even within small geographic areas. Major epidemiologic determinants are the immunologic and genetic makeup of the population, the species of parasite and mosquito in the community at risk, the level of rainfall, the temperature, the distribution of mosquito breeding sites, the use of antimalarial drugs, and the application of other control measures that could decrease transmission.

Endemicity has been defined in terms of prevalence of parasitemia and a palpable spleen in children less than 9 years of age, although these figures can vary with the season and with the presence of other endemic diseases causing splenomegaly. An area is considered to be hypoendemic if fewer than 10 percent of children have parasitemia

TABLE 174-1   **Characteristics of *Plasmodium* species infecting humans**

Characteristic	*P. falciparum*	*P. vivax*	*P. ovale*	*P. malariae*
Duration of intrahepatic phase (days)	5–7	7–8	9	14–16
Duration of erythrocytic cycle (hours)	48	48	50	72
Red cell preference	Younger cells, but can invade cells of all ages	Reticulocytes	Reticulocytes	Older cells
Morphology	Usually only ring forms; parasitemia level may exceed 2 percent, with multiple infections of a single erythrocyte; banana-shaped gametocytes	Irregularly shaped, large rings and trophozoites; enlarged erythrocytes; Schüffner's dots	Infected erythrocytes enlarged and oval; Schüffner's dots	Band or rectangular forms of trophozoites common
Pigment color	Black	Yellow-brown	Dark brown	Brown-black
Relapses	No	Yes	Yes	No

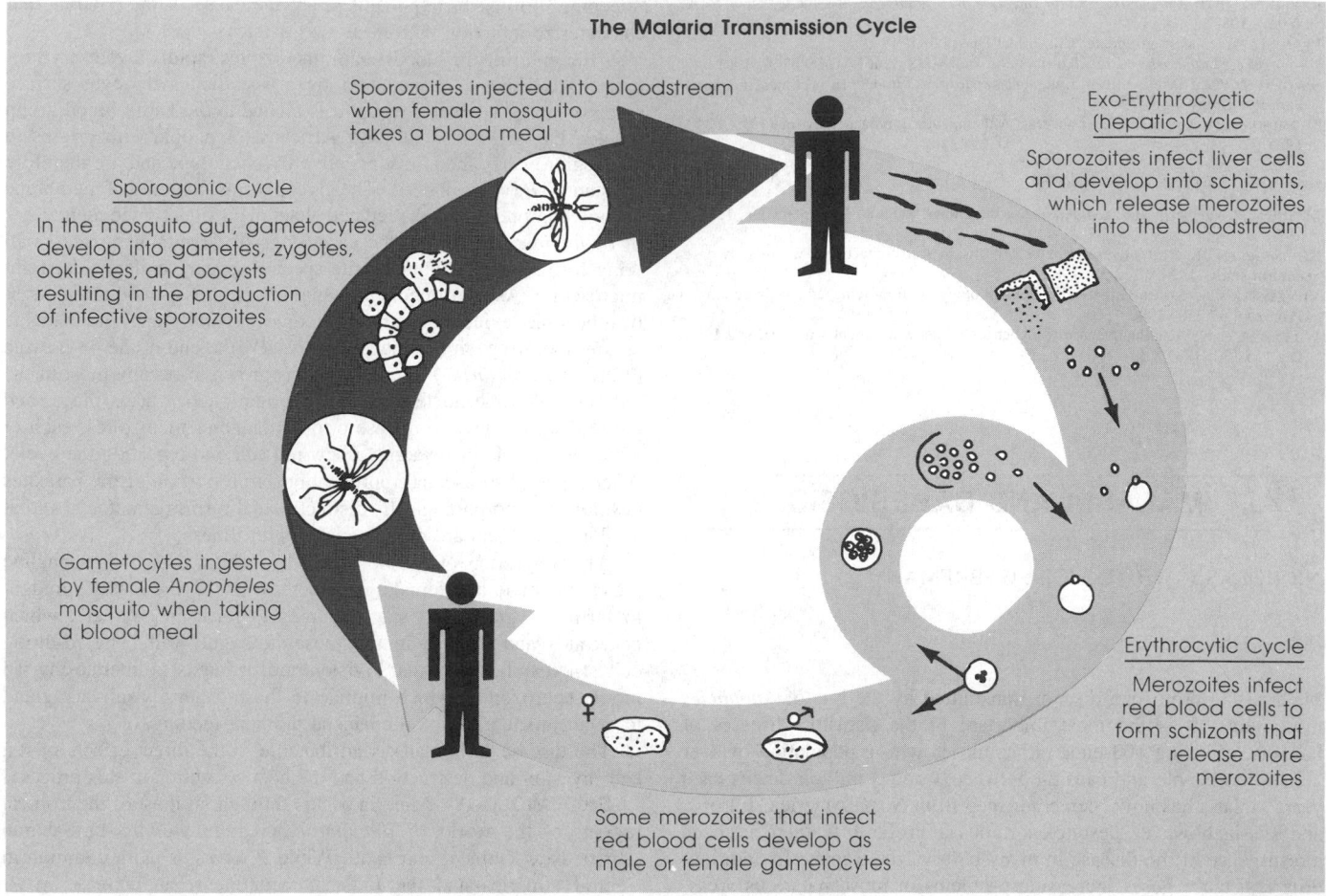

FIGURE 174-1 The malaria transmission cycle. (From Breman and Steketee.)

and a palpable spleen, mesoendemic if the figures are 11 to 50 percent, hyperendemic if they are 51 to 75 percent, and holoendemic if they are greater than 75 percent. In holo- and hyperendemic areas (e.g., much of tropical Africa and coastal New Guinea), where *P. falciparum* transmission is intense, persons are infected repeatedly throughout their lives. Malaria causes illness and death during childhood. The development of immunity is perilous, but by adulthood malaria infections are largely asymptomatic. This situation is termed *stable malaria*. In areas in which transmission is low, erratic, or focal, the chance that one infected person will transmit malaria to another is relatively small, full immunity is not acquired, and symptomatic disease may occur at any age. This situation is termed *unstable malaria*. Even in areas with stable malaria, seasonal variations in disease coincide with increased breeding of mosquitoes during the rainy season. Malaria can behave like an epidemic disease in some areas (such as northern India, Sri Lanka, Madagascar, and northwestern Brazil) when refugees or workers migrate from a nonmalarious region to areas of high transmission or when malaria control measures (mainly household spraying with insecticides) are stopped abruptly. Epidemics of falciparum malaria can produce considerable mortality at all ages.

The principal determinants of malaria transmission are the sporozoite rates, (proportion of potential vectors with sporozoites in the salivary glands), biting habits, longevity, and density of the mosquito vectors. In general, the rate of malaria transmission is directly proportional to (1) the density of the vector, (2) the square of the number of human bites per day per mosquito, and (3) the tenth power of the probability of a mosquito surviving for 1 day. Because the extrinsic cycle from gametocyte ingestion to subsequent sporozoite inoculation takes a minimum of 7 days (with the exact interval depending on ambient temperature), mosquito longevity is particularly important.

Therefore, the most effective mosquito vectors are long-lived, occur in high densities, and bite humans frequently (e.g., *Anopheles gambiae* in West Africa). The entomologic inoculation rate, which is used as a measure of the intensity of malaria transmission, is the number of sporozoite-positive mosquito bites per person per unit time.

ERYTHROCYTE CHANGES   After invasion, the growing parasite progressively consumes and degrades intracellular proteins, principally hemoglobin, and alters the red cell membrane by changing its transport properties, exposing cryptic surface antigens, and inserting new parasite-derived proteins. The red cell becomes more spherical and less deformable. In *P. falciparum* infections, membrane protuberances appear on the erythrocyte surface in the second 24 h of the asexual cycle. These "knobs" overlie accretions of electron-dense, histidine-rich parasite proteins. They extrude a strain-specific, adhesive-variant protein of high molecular weight that mediates red cell attachment to receptors on venular and capillary endothelium, causing a phenomenon called *cytoadherence*. *P. falciparum*–infected red cells also adhere to uninfected red cells to form rosettes. This event occurs at the same stage of parasite development as cytoadherence and has been linked to cerebral malaria. Cytoadherence and rosetting are central to the pathogenesis of falciparum malaria. These processes result in the formation of red cell aggregates and the intravascular sequestration of red cells that contain mature forms of the parasite in vital organs (particularly the brain and heart). Aggregated and sequestered red cells interfere with microcirculatory flow and metabolism and allow parasite development away from the principal host defense, splenic processing and filtration. As a consequence, only the younger ring forms of the asexual parasites are seen in the peripheral blood in falciparum malaria, and the peripheral parasitemia (which can reach high levels) is an underestimate of the true number of parasites within the body. With *P. vivax, P. malariae,* and *P. ovale,* sequestration does not take place, all stages of parasite development may be seen on peripheral blood smears, and levels of parasitemia seldom exceed 1 to 2 percent. These species show a marked predilection for either old red cells *(P. malariae)* or reticulocytes *(P. vivax)* (see Table 174-1).

HOST RESPONSE The initial response to infection in a nonimmune person is the activation of nonspecific host defense mechanisms. Immunologic and filtrative functions of the spleen are augmented, with accelerated removal of both parasitized and uninfected erythrocytes. The parasitized cells that escape splenic removal are destroyed when the schizont (meront) ruptures. The material released induces the activation of macrophages and the release of mononuclear cell–derived cytokines (including tumor necrosis factor) and, in succession, interleukins 1, 6, and 8, which cause fever and other pathologic effects. High serum concentrations of tumor necrosis factor are associated with a poor prognosis in severe malaria, although whether or not tumor necrosis factor is directly lethal in malaria remains to be determined. Temperatures of 40°C or higher are schizontocidal, leading to the synchronization of the parasite cycle and to production of the regular fever spikes and rigors that were once used to characterize the different malarias (quotidian, daily fever spike; tertian, every 2 days; quartan, every 3 days). These regular fever patterns are seldom seen in patients who receive prompt, effective antimalarial treatment.

The distribution of sickle cell disease, thalassemia, and glucose-6-phosphate dehydrogenase (G6PD) deficiency in the world closely resembles that of malaria before the introduction of control measures. This correlation implies that these genetic disorders may confer protection against death from malaria. This has been confirmed in the case of sickle cell trait, but the mechanism of protection has not been elucidated, except in Melanesian ovalocytosis, in which the rigid erythrocytes resist merozoite invasion and the intraerythrocytic electrolyte milieu is hostile to the parasite.

The specific immune response to malaria limits the level of parasitemia and, with repeated exposure to a sufficient number of strains, eventually confers protection from disease but not from infection. This state of premunition is specific for both the species and the strain of the infecting malaria parasite. Both humoral and cellular immune systems participate, but the mechanisms are incompletely understood. Immune individuals have a polyclonal increase in serum IgM, IgG, and IgA, although much of this antibody is unrelated to protection. Antibodies and cellular immune responses to parasite antigens expressed both on the merozoite surface (leading to agglutination) and on the erythrocyte surface (leading to parasite killing and erythrophagocytosis) presumably act in concert to limit in vivo parasite replication. Passive transfer IgG from immune mothers reduces the level of parasitemia in children. Passive transfer of maternal antibody also contributes to the relative protection of the infant from severe malaria during the first months of life.

Factors that retard the development of cellular immunity include the absence of major histocompatibility antigens on the surface of infected red cells, which precludes direct α and β T cell recognition; malaria antigen–specific immune unresponsiveness coupled with nonspecific parasite-induced mitogenic activity that produces an "immunologic smokescreen"; and the diversity of malarial strains and their ability to express antigens on the erythrocyte surface that change during the course of infection. Hence no individual is ever immune to all strains. Parasites may persist in the blood for months—or, in the case of *P. malariae,* for years—if untreated. Because of the complex immune response in malaria, the diversity of the parasites' evasive mechanisms, and the lack of a good means of in vitro assessment of clinical immunity, no effective vaccine is available yet.

GENERAL CLINICAL FEATURES The first symptoms are nonspecific and similar to those of a minor viral illness, with malaise, headache, fatigue, abdominal discomfort, and muscle aches, followed by fever and chills. In some cases, a prominence of headache, chest pain, nausea, vomiting, abdominal pain, arthralgia, myalgia, or diarrhea may suggest other illnesses. The classic malarial paroxysms in which fever spikes, chills, and rigors (tremors induced by chills) occur at regular intervals are rare. True rigors are more common with *P. vivax* and *P. ovale* than with *P. falciparum.* More often, the fever is irregular at first; in nonimmune adults or children, nausea, vomiting, and orthostatic hypotension are common. Most patients with uncomplicated acute infections have few abnormal physical findings other than mild anemia and in some cases a palpable spleen.

SEVERE FALCIPARUM MALARIA (See Table 174-2) **Cerebral malaria** Coma is a characteristic and ominous feature of severe falciparum malaria and, despite treatment, is associated with a mortality of approximately 20 percent in adults and 15 percent in children. Lesser degrees of obtundation, delirium, or abnormal behavior also should be addressed with urgency because deterioration can be rapid. The onset of coma may be gradual or sudden following a convulsion. Cerebral malaria is a diffuse symmetric encephalopathy; focal neurologic signs are unusual. Although there may be passive resistance to head flexion, signs of meningeal irritation are absent. The eyes may be divergent, and a pout reflex is common, but other primitive reflexes are usually absent. The corneal reflexes are preserved except in deep coma. Muscle tone may be increased or decreased. The tendon reflexes are variable, and the plantar reflexes may be flexor or extensor; abdominal and cremasteric reflexes are absent. Flexor or extensor posturing may occur. Approximately 15 percent of patients have retinal hemorrhages. Anemia and jaundice are common. Convulsions, which are usually generalized, are common in children with cerebral malaria and in about half of adults. Seizures are associated with high temperatures (≥40°C). Approximately 10 percent of children who survive cerebral malaria, particularly those

---

TABLE 174-2 Manifestations of severe malaria

MAJOR SIGNS

Unarousable coma/ cerebral malaria	Failure to localize or respond appropriately to noxious stimuli; coma should persist for >30 min after generalized convulsion
Severe normochromic, normocytic anemia	Hematocrit <15 percent or hemoglobin <5 g/dL with parasitemia level >10,000 per microliter
Renal failure	Urine output <400 mL/24 h in adults or 12 mL/kg per 24 h in children; no improvement with rehydration; serum creatinine >265 μmol/L (>3.0 mg/dL)
Pulmonary edema/ adult respiratory distress syndrome	
Hypoglycemia	Glucose <2.2 mmol/L (<40 mg/dL)
Hypotension/shock	Systolic blood pressure <50 mmHg in children 1–5 years or <80 mmHg in adults; core skin temperature difference >10°C.
Bleeding/disseminated intravascular coagulation	Significant bleeding and hemorrhage from the gums, nose, gastrointestinal tract, and/or evidence of disseminated intravascular coagulation.
Convulsions	More than two generalized seizures in 24 h
Acidemia/acidosis	Arterial pH <7.25 or plasma bicarbonate <15 mmol/L, venous lactate >6 mmol/L
Hemoglobinuria	Macroscopic black, brown, or red urine; not associated with effects of oxidant drugs and red blood cell enzyme defects (such as G6PD deficiency)

OTHER SIGNS

Impaired consciousness/ arousable	
Extreme weakness	
Hyperparasitemia	Parasitemia >5 percent in nonimmune patients
Jaundice	Serum bilirubin level >50 mmol/L (>3.0 mg/dL)
Hyperpyrexia	Rectal temperature >40°C.

with hypoglycemia, severe anemia, repeated seizures, and deep coma, have persistent neurologic deficits. Residual deficits are unusual in adults (< 3 percent).

Hypoglycemia Hypoglycemia is associated with a poor prognosis. Children and pregnant women are at special risk. Hypoglycemia results from failure of hepatic gluconeogenesis and increased consumption of glucose by the host and the parasites. Plasma concentrations of the principal gluconeogenic substrates, lactate and alanine, are increased. To compound the situation, quinine and quinidine, the drugs of choice for the treatment of severe chloroquine-resistant malaria, are powerful stimulants to pancreatic insulin secretion; pregnant women who receive quinine are especially prone to hypoglycemia. Clinical diagnosis of severe hypoglycemia is difficult because the adrenergic signs (sweating, gooseflesh, tachycardia) may be absent and neurologic impairment attributable to hypoglycemia cannot be distinguished from that of malaria itself.

Lactic acidosis Anaerobic glycolysis occurs in tissues where sequestered parasitized erythrocytes interfere with microcirculatory flow. This phenomenon, together with hypotension and a failure of hepatic lactate clearance, causes lactic acidosis. Hyperventilation is usually followed by circulatory failure refractory to volume expansion and to inotropic drugs. The prognosis of lactic acidosis is poor.

Noncardiogenic pulmonary edema Adult respiratory distress syndrome (ARDS) may develop in adults with severe falciparum malaria, even after several days of antimalarial therapy and clearance of parasites. The pathogenesis is unclear, but the mortality rate of established ARDS is over 80 percent.

Renal impairment Renal impairment is common among adults with severe falciparum malaria but rare among children. Renal failure is associated with high mortality. The pathogenesis is unclear but may be related to sequestration of parasitized erythrocytes and reduction of renal microcirculatory flow. Clinically and pathologically, malaria-induced renal failure resembles acute tubular necrosis; if the anuric patient survives the acute phase and effective dialysis is undertaken, the flow of urine usually recommences in about 4 days, and the serum creatinine level returns to normal in 2 to 3 weeks (see Chap. 236).

Hematologic abnormalities Anemia is caused by accelerated destruction and removal of red cells by the spleen and by suppression of the bone marrow with ineffective erythropoiesis. Anemia can develop rapidly, and transfusion is often required. Anemia is a particular problem in children. In some patients with *P. falciparum*, massive hemolysis causes hemoglobinemia, black urine, and renal failure (blackwater fever). Coagulation defects occur in falciparum malaria. Bleeding is significant in fewer than 5 percent of patients with cerebral malaria and is usually associated with disseminated intravascular coagulation. Hematemesis, presumably from stress ulceration or acute gastric erosions, also may occur.

Other complications People with malaria are predisposed to bacterial superinfection. Aspiration pneumonia following convulsions is an important cause of death in cerebral malaria. Pneumonia and catheter-induced urinary tract infections are common in unconscious patients. In Africa, falciparum malaria has been associated with *Salmonella* septicemia.

MALARIA IN PREGNANCY *P. falciparum* infection of the placenta of pregnant women is associated with low birth weight, particularly in the primigravida. In areas with stable and intense transmission, pregnant women generally remain asymptomatic despite sequestration of parasitized erythrocytes in the placental microcirculation. In areas that have unstable transmission (hypo- or mesoendemic), pregnant women are prone to severe infections and are particularly vulnerable to the development of high levels of parasitemia, anemia, hypoglycemia, and acute pulmonary edema. Fetal distress, premature labor, spontaneous abortion, and stillbirth are common. Congenital malaria occurs in fewer than 5 percent of newborns whose mothers are infected and is related directly to the parasite density in the placenta.

MALARIA IN CHILDREN Most of the 1 to 3 million who die each year from falciparum malaria are children, mainly in Africa. Convulsions, coma, hypoglycemia, metabolic acidosis, and severe anemia are relatively common among children with severe malaria, whereas severe jaundice, acute renal failure, and acute pulmonary edema are unusual. In general, children tolerate antimalarial drugs well and respond rapidly to treatment.

TRANSFUSION MALARIA Malaria can be transmitted by blood transfusion or by needle sharing between infected intravenous drug users. *P. malariae* and *P. falciparum* are the most common etiologic agents in such cases. The incubation period is often short because there is no pre-erythrocytic development. Clinical features and management are similar to those of naturally acquired infections, although falciparum malaria tends to be especially severe in drug addicts. Radical chemotherapy with primaquine in infections due to *P. vivax* or *P. ovale* is unnecessary because intrahepatic merogony does not take place in transfusion-induced malaria.

TROPICAL SPLENOMEGALY (HYPERREACTIVE MALARIOUS SPLENOMEGALY) Some residents of endemic areas exhibit an abnormal immunolological response to repeated malarial infections that results in massive splenomegaly, hepatomegaly, marked elevations in serum levels of IgM and malaria antibody, hepatic sinusoidal lymphocytosis, and—in Africa—10 percent develop peripheral (B cell) lymphocytosis. This immune response is associated with the production of cytotoxic IgM antisuppressor lymphocyte (CD8+) antibodies, which leads to uninhibited B cell production of IgM and the formation of cryoglobulins (IgM aggregates and immune complexes). This process then stimulates reticuloendothelial hyperplasia and clearance activity and eventually produces splenomegaly. Patients with hyperactive malarial splenomegaly have an abdominal mass or experience a dragging sensation in the abdomen with occasional sharp abdominal pains that suggests perisplenitis. Patients are usually anemic and exhibit some degree of pancytopenia. In most cases, malaria parasites cannot be found in peripheral blood smears. Patients with hyperreactive malarious splenomegaly are particularly vulnerable to infections, and have an increased mortality. Hyperreactive malarious splenomegaly usually responds to antimalarial prophylaxis. In patients who are refractory to therapy, clonal lymphoproliferation may occur, resulting in a malignant lymphoproliferative disorder.

QUARTAN MALARIAL NEPHROPATHY Chronic or repeated infections with *P. malariae* may cause soluble immune-complex injury to the renal glomeruli, resulting in the nephrotic syndrome. Other factors contribute because only a small proportion of infected persons develops renal disease. The histologic appearance of the glomeruli is of focal or segmental glomerulonephritis with splitting of the capillary basement membrane. Dense subendothelial deposits are seen on electron microscopy, and immunofluorescence reveals deposits of complement and immunoglobulins; in children, *P. malariae* antigens are often seen. Patients who have a coarse granular pattern of basement-membrane immunofluorescent deposits (predominantly IgG3) and selective proteinuria have a better prognosis than those with a fine, granular, predominantly IgG2 pattern and nonselective proteinuria. Quartan nephropathy usually does not respond to treatment with either antimalarial agents or glucocorticoids and cytotoxic drugs.

DIAGNOSIS The diagnosis of malaria rests on the demonstration of asexual form of the parasite in peripheral blood smears stained preferably with Giemsa (see Chap. 171). Other Romanowsky stains (Wright's, Field's or Leishman's) are less reliable. Both thin and thick blood smears should be made with great care on clean slides. The thin smear should be air dried rapidly, fixed in anhydrous methanol, and stained. The red cells in the tail of the film should be examined under oil immersion microscopy. The level of parasitemia is expressed as the number of parasitized erythrocytes per 1000 red blood cells, and this figure is then converted to the number per microliter of blood.

The thick smear should be dried thoroughly and stained (also with Giemsa) without alcohol fixation. Since many layers of erythrocytes overlie one another and are lysed during the staining procedure, the thick film concentrates the parasites up to 40 times that of the thin smear, thereby increasing the sensitivity of diagnosis. Both parasites and white blood cells are counted, and the number of parasites per unit volume is calculated from the total leukocyte count. A minimum of 200 white cells should be counted. Interpretation of thick films requires experience because artifacts are common. Phagocytosed malaria pigment may be visible inside peripheral blood monocytes or polymorphonuclear leukocytes and may provide a clue to recent infection if malaria parasites are not seen. Occasionally, parasites and pigment are evident in bone marrow aspirates or smears obtained from fluid expressed after intradermal puncture, but not on peripheral blood smears. Staining of the parasites with the fluorescent dye acridine orange allows a more rapid diagnosis when levels of parasitemia are low. Compared with microscopy, this technique is less accurate for species identification and for quantitation of parasitemia. The relation between the level of parasitemia and the prognosis is complex; in general, patients with parasitemia levels in excess of 10^5 per microliter (~2 percent) are more likely to die. However, nonimmune patients may die with relatively low parasite densities, and partially immune persons may tolerate relatively high levels with minor symptoms. At any level of parasitemia, a predominance of more mature parasites (i.e., >20 percent of parasites with visible pigment) or circulating *P. falciparum* schizonts (meronts) carries a poor prognosis.

LABORATORY FINDINGS Normochromic, normocytic anemia is the rule. The leukocyte count is low to normal, although it may be elevated in severe infections. The erythrocyte sedimentation rate, plasma viscosity, and C-reactive protein level are high. The platelet count is usually moderately reduced (to about 100,000 per microliter). In severe infections, the prothrombin and partial thromboplastin times may be prolonged, and thrombocytopenia may be severe. Levels of antithrombin III are reduced even in mild infection. In uncomplicated malaria, plasma concentrations of electrolytes, blood urea nitrogen, and creatinine are usually normal. In severe falciparum malaria, metabolic acidosis may be present with low plasma concentrations of glucose, sodium, bicarbonate, calcium, phosphate, and albumin and elevated plasma levels of lactate, blood urea nitrogen, creatinine, urate, muscle and liver enzymes, and conjugated and unconjugated bilirubin. Hypergammaglobulinemia is usual in immune and semi-immune patients. In adults with cerebral malaria, the mean opening pressure at lumbar puncture is normal or mildly elevated. Approximately 20 percent of adult patients have elevated CSF pressure (>200 mm of CSF); in contrast, approximately 80 percent of children have raised CSF pressure (>100 mm H_2O; the normal range is lower than in adults). The CSF protein level is usually normal or slightly elevated (<100 mg/dL). In cerebral malaria, the white blood cell count often varies between 9000 and 11,000 per microliter but can be higher than 20,000 per microliter; the differential count is usually normal. The CSF glucose level in cerebral malaria is about two-thirds of the blood glucose level, which, in about 10 percent of patients, is low. Low glucose [<2.2 mmol/L(40mg/dL] and high lactate [>6mmol/ L(54 mg/dL)] concentrations in blood or CSF indicate a poor prognosis.

PREVENTION In most of the rural tropics, eradication of malaria is not feasible because of the paucity of resources and the incomplete understanding of the biologic and epidemiologic features of the infection and the disease. Over the past decade, there has been an increased focus on the reduction of malaria mortality by effective management of patients rather than by prevention, particularly in tropical Africa, where most malaria cases occur. Where practical, the disease is contained by judicious use of insecticides to kill the mosquito vector and of chemoprophylaxis in high-risk groups (e.g., pregnant women, nonimmune travelers, military personnel, and workers on priority economic projects). Treating bed nets with permethrin, a residual synthetic pyrethroid, reduces the incidence of malaria and reduces overall mortality in West Africa. Despite massive investment aimed at the development of a malaria vaccine, and despite major advances in understanding the biology and immunology of malaria, a safe, effective, and long-lasting vaccine is unlikely to be available in the near future.

PERSONAL PROTECTION AGAINST MALARIA Measures to reduce the frequency of mosquito bites can be effective. These include avoiding exposure at peak mosquito feeding times (usually from dusk to dawn), wearing clothing that covers the skin, and using insect repellents. Sleeping in areas that are distant from breeding sites and in rooms that are air-conditioned and screened against mosquitoes is also advised. Use of bed nets, especially those impregnated with insecticide, is advised for persons in endemic areas, as is the use of insecticide spray for flying insects in sleeping quarters.

CHEMOPROPHYLAXIS (See also Table 174-3) Recommendations for prophylaxis rely on knowledge of the drug sensitivity of local parasites and the likelihood of acquiring infection. Chemoprophylaxis is never entirely effective, and malaria should always be considered in the differential diagnosis of fever in patients who have traveled to endemic areas, even if they have taken prophylactic antimalarial drugs.

With chloroquine-resistant *P. falciparum* present throughout most of the malarious world (Fig. 174-2), mefloquine (250 mg weekly for adults) is the drug of choice for prophylaxis for nonimmune individuals traveling to such areas. Mefloquine is effective and well tolerated, although nausea, dizziness, and abdominal pain may occur. Rarely (1:10,000), prophylaxis with mefloquine is associated with an acute reversible neuropsychiatric reaction manifested by confusion, psychosis, convulsions, or encephalopathy. Large-scale assessments of the side effects experienced by Swiss travelers who took mefloquine indicated that these effects are similar to those of chloroquine. The safety of mefloquine prophylaxis in pregnancy has not been established. Daily administration of doxycycline (100 mg maximum) is an effective alternative. Doxycycline is generally well tolerated but may cause *Candida* infections, diarrhea, and photosensitivity. Doxycycline cannot be used during pregnancy or given to children less than 8 years of age. Women who are pregnant or intending to become so should avoid travel to areas with chloroquine-resistant *P. falciparum* because there is no completely safe and effective antimalarial prophylaxis in pregnancy.

Because of the increasing spread and intensity of chloroquine resistance in Africa and other areas of the world, the Centers for Disease Control and Prevention (CDC, which recommend weekly mefloquine for all travelers to such areas except for pregnant women) maintain an updated 24-h malaria information audiotape that can be accessed by touch-tone telephone (404-332-4555) and an interactive international travel information service that responds by fax (404-332-4565).

Chloroquine (5 mg of base per kilogram per week, 300 mg maximum) is the drug of choice for the prevention of infection with drug-sensitive *P. falciparum* (in the few areas where such sensitivity still exists; see Fig. 174-2) and with other species. Chloroquine is generally well tolerated, although some patients cannot take the drug because of dysphoria, headache, or (in black patients) pruritus. Chloroquine is considered relatively safe in pregnancy. In adults, cumulative prophylactic doses of more than 100 g are associated with retinopathy; this complication is rare and occurs more often with treatment for rheumatoid arthritis than with prophylaxis of malaria. Skeletal and cardiac myopathy may occur but are also more likely with the high doses of 4-aminoquinoline drugs (e.g., hydroxychloroquine) used in the treatment of rheumatoid arthritis. Neuropsychiatric reactions and skin rashes are unusual. Another 4-aminoquinoline drug, amodiaquine, can cause agranulocytosis and is not recommended. The recent reports of chloroquine-resistant strains of *P. vivax* from Papua New Guinea and Indonesia indicate that no drug is 100 percent effective against malaria.

TABLE 174-3 Recommended regimens for malaria prophylaxis

Drugs	Adult dosage	Pediatric dosage
AREAS WITH CHLOROQUINE-RESISTANT *P. falciparum*		
Mefloquine*	250 mg (250 mg base, 1 tablet), once weekly for 1 week before exposure, during exposure, and for 4 weeks after exposure	15–19 kg: ¼ tab per week 20–30 kg: ½ tab per week 31–45 kg: ¾ tab per week >45 kg: 1 tab per week
Alternatives (1) Doxycycline† *or* (2) Chloroquine	100 mg daily for 1–2 days before exposure, during exposure, and for 4 weeks after exposure 300 mg of base once weekly for 1 week before exposure, during exposure, and for 4 weeks after exposure	>7 years: 2 mg/kg daily up to adult dose 5 mg of base per kilogram once weekly up to 300 mg of base
plus (a) Proguanil‡	200 mg daily for 1–2 days before exposure, during exposure, and for 4 weeks after exposure	<2 years: 50 mg/d 2–6 years: 100 mg/d 7–9 years: 150 mg/d >9 years: 200 mg/d
Carry (b) Pyrimethamine-sulfadoxine	Carry single dose of 3 tablets (25 mg pyrimethamine and 500 mg sulfadoxine per tab) for self-treatment of febrile illness when medical treatment is not immediately available	<1 year: ¼ tab 1–3 years: ½ tab 4–8 years: 1 tab 9–14 years 2 tabs >14 years: 3 tabs
AREAS WITH CHLOROQUINE-SENSITIVE *P. falciparum*		
Chloroquine	300 mg of base once weekly for 1 week before exposure, during exposure and for 4 weeks after exposure	5 mg of base per kilogram once weekly up to 300 mg of base

* Mefloquine should not be used by children who weigh <15 kg, by pregnant women, or by patients with a history of psychiatric or seizure disorders (see Table 174-4). Caution should be used in administering mefloquine to persons with underlying cardiac conduction abnormalities who are taking beta blockers, or to persons requiring critical motor skills, such as pilots.
† Doxycycline should not be given to pregnant women or children <8 years of age.
‡ Proguanil is not available in the United States but may be obtained in the United Kingdom and some disease-endemic countries.

FIGURE 174-2 Distribution of malaria and chloroquine-resistant *Plasmodium falciparum*, 1993.

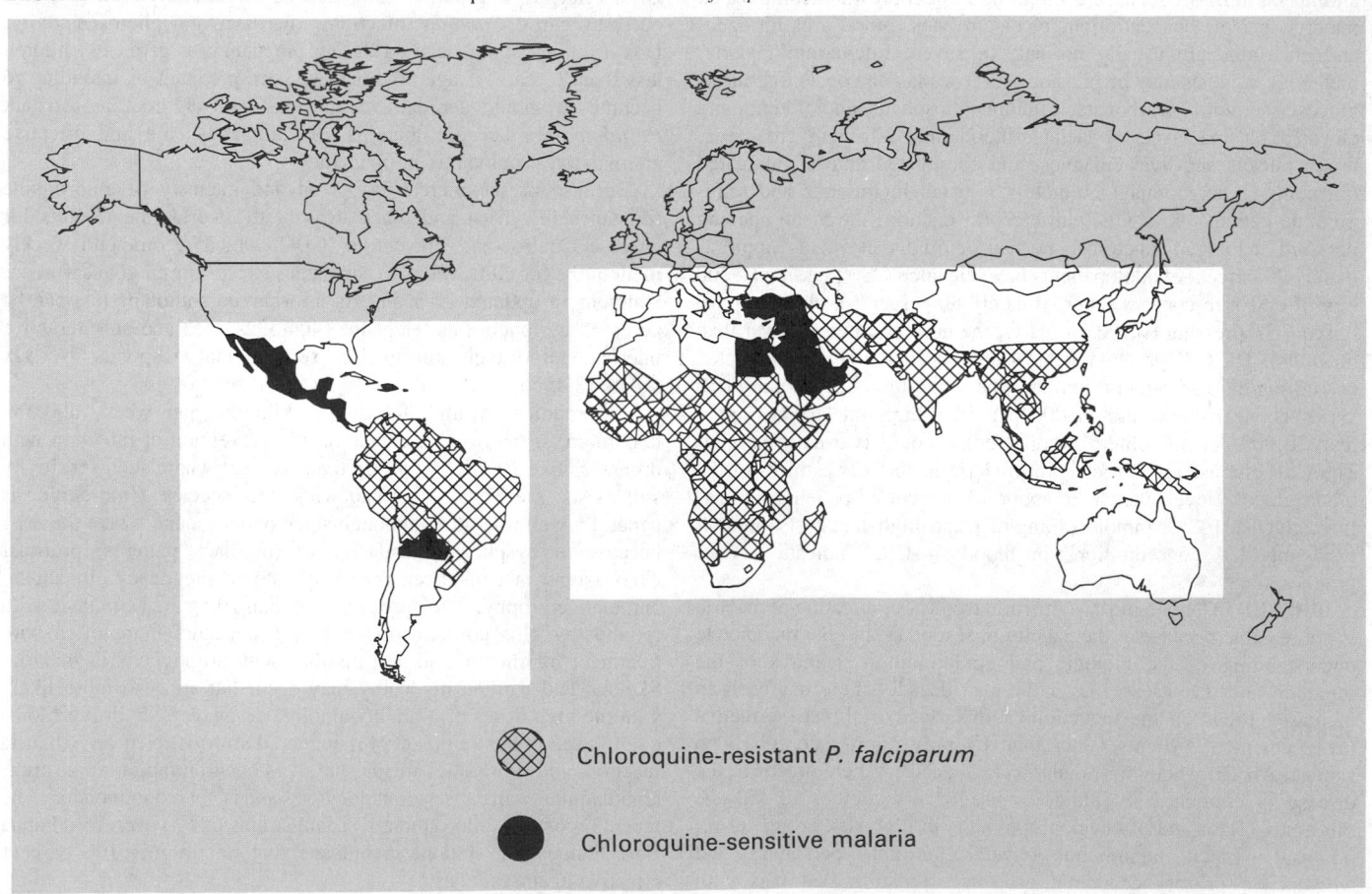

⊞ Chloroquine-resistant *P. falciparum*

● Chloroquine-sensitive malaria

In the past, the dihydrofolate reductase inhibitors pyrimethamine and proguanil (chloroguanide) were used for malaria prophylaxis, but resistant strains of both *P. falciparum* and *P. vivax* limit their efficacy. Whereas the quinoline antimalarials, such as chloroquine, act only on the erythrocyte stage of parasite development, the dihydrofolate reductase inhibitors also inhibit pre-erythrocytic growth in the liver (causal prophylaxis) and development in the mosquito (sporontocidal activity). The prophylactic use of the combination of pyrimethamine and sulfadoxine is not recommended because of severe toxicity, including exfoliative dermatitis and other skin rashes, agranulocytosis, hepatitis, and pulmonary eosinophilia. An alternative for persons who cannot take mefloquine or doxycycline is chloroquine weekly and proguanil (3 mg/kg daily, 200 mg maximum), but this regimen appears to be failing increasingly, particularly in East Africa. The combination of pyrimethamine with dapsone (0.2/1.5 mg/kg weekly, 25/200 mg maximum) is also used in areas with chloroquine-resistant *P. falciparum*. The combination is generally well tolerated, although resistance is increasing and dapsone may cause methemoglobinemia, allergic reactions, and (with higher doses) agranulocytosis.

Travelers should start taking antimalarial drugs at least 1 week (1 to 2 days for doxycycline) before arrival in an endemic area to allow time for the detection of untoward reactions and for the attainment of therapeutic blood levels; prophylaxis should continue for 4 weeks after departure from this area. Individuals who were born in malarious countries but live away from these areas for many years lose their immunity. These persons, particularly children, are at risk when they return to their homeland; thus they should receive chemoprophylaxis and take other preventive measures against malaria.

TREATMENT Patients in or from malarious areas who develop fever should have thick and thin blood smears made promptly to confirm the diagnosis and identify the species of infecting parasite. In endemic areas, uncomplicated infections may be treated on an outpatient basis. Patients with severe malaria or those unable to take oral drugs should receive parenteral antimalarial treatment. If there is any doubt about drug resistance, then quinine or quinidine should be given. Several drugs are available for oral treatment, and the choice of drug depends on the likely sensitivity of the infecting parasites. Despite recent reports of chloroquine-resistant *P. vivax* from Oceania and Indonesia, chloroquine is still the treatment of choice for *P. vivax, P. malariae,* and *P. ovale.* Recommended regimens are detailed in Table 174-4, and the characteristics of various agents are given in Table 174-5.

Uncomplicated malaria Infections due to *P. vivax, P. malariae, P. ovale,* or known sensitive strains of *P. falciparum* (Table 174-4) should be treated with oral chloroquine (25 mg of base per kilogram) given over 48 h. Where there is resistance to chloroquine, either quinine plus tetracycline or quinine plus pyrimethamine-sulfadoxine should be used; tetracycline should not be given to pregnant women or children less than 8 years of age. Oral quinine is extremely bitter and regularly produces the symptom complex of cinchonism which comprises tinnitus, high-tone deafness, nausea, vomiting, and dysphoria. Therefore, a 7-day course of quinine given with a 7-day course of tetracycline or a single dose of pyrimethamine-sulfadoxine. Chloroquine-resistant strains are sensitive to a single dose of pyrimethamine-sulfadoxine in some areas (e.g., Africa). All the quinoline antimalarials (chloroquine, mefloquine, and quinine) may exacerbate the orthostatic hypotension of malaria, and all are tolerated better by children than by adults. Symptomatic treatment with tepid sponging and acetaminophen lowers fever and reduces the propensity to vomit the oral antimalarial drugs. While mefloquine is effective against multidrug-resistant strains of *P. falciparum,* therapeutic doses (25 mg/kg) cause neuropsychiatric reactions in about 0.01–0.1 percent of patients. In addition, significant resistance of *P. falciparum* to mefloquine has been reported in Thailand, Burma, and Cambodia. Halofantrine, which is also effective against multidrug-resistant strains of *P. falciparum,* is used in some parts of Europe, Africa, and Asia but is not available in the United States. Although the drug is generally

well tolerated, it has variable bioavailability, and the optimal regimen remains to be determined. The principal adverse effects of halofantrine are diarrhea and a quinidine-like effect on the myocardium (prolonged electrocardiographic QT_c interval).

The Chinese compound artemisinin (quinghaosu) and its derivatives artemether and artesunate are being used increasingly in Asia. These drugs are effective against multidrug-resistant infections with *P. falciparum* and are rapid acting and appear to be safe. They are not available in the United States.

Pregnant women, young children, patients unable to tolerate oral therapy, and nonimmune persons (e.g., travelers) with malaria should be hospitalized. If the identity of the malaria species is doubtful, treatment should be given for chloroquine-resistant falciparum malaria. Since one negative smear does not rule out malaria, repeat thick blood films should be taken at least every 6 to 12 h at least 2 days to exclude the diagnosis. Following treatment, nonimmune persons with malaria should have daily parasite counts until thick films are negative. If the level of parasitemia does not fall below 25 percent of the admission value in 48 h, or if parasitemia has not cleared by 7 days, drug resistance is likely, and treatment should be changed.

Primaquine (0.3 mg of base per kilogram, 15 mg maximum) should be given daily for 14 days in *P. vivax* or *P. ovale* infection after G6PD deficiency is excluded. If the patient has a mild variant of G6PD deficiency, then primaquine can be given in a dose of 0.6 mg of base per kilogram (45 mg maximum) once weekly for 6 weeks.

Severe malaria Severe falciparum malaria (see Table 174-4) is a medical emergency that requires intensive nursing care and careful management. Patients should be weighed; if comatose, their blood glucose should be checked, and they should be positioned on their side and given a single intramuscular dose of phenobarbital (5 to 7 mg/kg) to prevent convulsions. Frequent evaluation is essential. Ancillary drugs such as high-dose glucocorticoids, mannitol, urea, heparin, and dextran are of no value.

The choice of drug dosage and route of administration depend on the prevailing sensitivity of *P. falciparum* to antimalarial drugs, the condition of the patient, and the place where treatment is given. The cinchona alkaloids (quinidine or quinine) are the mainstays of treatment because of their activity against chloroquine-resistant strains of *P. falciparum.* Quinidine gluconate is as effective as quinine and is more readily available outside tropical areas. In the United States, quinidine has replaced quinine for the parenteral treatment of severe malaria. Because quinidine is more cardiotoxic than quinine, its administration must be closely monitored if dysrhythmia or hypotension is to be avoided. A blood level in excess of 22 μmol/L (7 mg/L), an electrocardiographic QT interval of >0.55 s, or a QRS prolongation of >50 percent or QT_c >25 percent of baseline is an indication for slowing infusion rates. If arrhythmia or saline-unresponsive hypotension develops, quinidine should be discontinued. The dosage for quinidine is provided in Table 174-4.

Cardiovascular monitoring is not required routinely during quinine treatment. An initial loading dose (Table 174-4) should be given so that therapeutic concentrations are reached as soon as possible, but such a dose is not necessary if adequate treatment is started before admission to the hospital. The clearance and volume of distribution of these alkaloids are reduced in severe malaria, but plasma protein binding is increased and blood concentrations after a given dose are raised in proportion to disease severity. If the patient remains seriously ill or in acute renal failure for 3 days, the maintenance doses should be reduced by one-third to one-half to prevent accumulation of the drugs to toxic levels. (The initial doses should not be reduced.) If chloroquine is given, dose reduction is unnecessary even in renal failure.

In unconscious patients, the blood glucose value should be measured every 4 to 6 h; if the blood glucose value falls below 2.2 mmol/L (40 mg/dL), the patient should receive intravenous dextrose (0.3 g/kg). All patients given intravenous quinine or quinidine should receive a continuous infusion of 5% to 10% dextrose. The parasite

TABLE 174-4 Recommended regimens for the treatment of uncomplicated and severe malaria

Chloroquine-resistant *P. falciparum*	Chloroquine-sensitive *P. falciparum*, *P. vivax*, *P. malariae*, and *P. ovale*
UNCOMPLICATED, CAN BE TREATED ANYWHERE	
Quinine sulfate, 650 mg (salt) tid orally for 7 days; pediatric dosage, 10 mg (salt)/kg tid for 7 days *plus either* Tetracycline, 250 mg qid orally for 7 days; pediatric dosage, 5 mg/kg qid for 7 days[a] *or* Pyrimethamine/sulfadoxine, 3 tablets (25 mg pyrimethamine and 500 mg sulfadoxine per tab) in single dose; pediatric dose 6–11 months, ¼ tab; 1–3 years, ½ tab; 4–8 years, 1 tab; 9–14 years, 2 tabs; >14 years, 3 tabs *Alternative treatments:* Mefloquine, 15–25 mg of base per kilogram, single dose (maximum 1500 mg)[c] Halofantrine, 8 mg of base per kilogram every h for 3 doses (maximum 500 mg per dose); dosage repeated after 7 days for nonimmune persons[d]	Chloroquine, 10 mg of base per kilogram (maximum 600 mg), followed by 5 mg of base per kilogram (maximum 300 mg) at 6, 24, and 48 h (or 10 mg of base per kilogram daily for 3 days) *plus* Primaquine phosphate, 0.3 mg of base per kilogram (maximum 15 mg) daily for 14 days for *P. vivax* or *P. ovale* infections[b]
SEVERE, AT HOSPITALS (WITH NURSING FACILITIES)	
Quinidine gluconate, 10 mg of base per kilogram infused IV as loading dose over 1–2 h, followed by 0.02 mg/kg per min, keeping quinidine blood levels at 3–7 mg/L until parasitemia is <1 percent and patient can take drugs orally[e]; complete with quinine sulfate tablets for 3–7 days and tetracycline or pyrimethamine-sulfadoxine as indicated above *or* Quinine, 7 mg of salt per kilogram infused IV at a constant rate over 30 min as a loading dose, followed immediately by 10 mg of salt per kilogram over 4 h; after a 4-h interval, infusions of 10 mg of salt per kilogram over 8 h or until patient can complete 3–7 days of treatment orally with quinine sulfate tablets; tetracycline or pyrimethamine-sulfadoxine also should be given as indicated above *Alternative treatment* Artemether and related compounds, 3.2 mg/kg IM, followed by 1.6 mg/kg IM every 12–24 h until patient awakes[f,g] *plus* Exchange transfusion for very high parasitemia (>10 percent) and altered mental status	Chloroquine, 10 mg of base per kilogram (maximum 600 mg) infused IV at a constant rate over 8 h, followed by 15 mg of base per kilogram (maximum 900 mg) infused over 24 h[e] *plus* Exchange transfusion as for chloroquine-resistant malaria
SEVERE, AT RURAL CLINICS (NO NURSING FACILITIES)[h]	
Quinine, 20 mg of salt per kilogram IM, followed by 10 mg of salt per kilogram every 8 h given by deep IM injection Quinine concentration should be 60–100 mg of salt per milliliter, and first dose should be split, with one-half the dose given deep IM in each thigh. Evacuate patient as soon as possible (when stable). When patient can take drugs orally, complete 3–7 days with quinine sulfate and tetracycline or pyrimethamine-sulfadoxine as indicated above	Chloroquine, 3.5 mg of base per kilogram (maximum 200 mg) every 6 h or 2.5 mg of base per kilogram every 4 h (maximum 150 mg) by either SC or IM injection; when patient can take medicines orally, complete treatment with chloroquine as above; total doses, 25 mg/kg of base (maximum 1500 mg)

[a]Tetracycline should not be given to pregnant women or to children <8 years of age.
[b]Patients who require primaquine should be screened for G6PD deficiency before treatment; patients with mild variants of G6PD deficiency can receive primaquine phosphate 0.75 mg of base per kilogram (maximum 45 mg) once weekly for 6 weeks. Primaquine should not be given during pregnancy.
[c]Treatment with mefloquine is associated with very infrequent neuropsychiatric side effects; this drug should not be used by children who weigh <15 kg, by pregnant women, by persons with underlying cardiac conduction abnormalities who are taking beta blockers, or by patients with a history of psychiatric or seizure disorders. Caution should be used in administering mefloquine to persons requiring critical motor skills, such as pilots.
[d]Halofantrine should not be given to persons with underlying cardiac conduction abnormalities or a long ECG QT interval.
[e]Infusion should be stopped temporarily if the electrocardiograph QRS interval is prolonged by >50 percent of the baseline or the QT_c instead is prolonged by >25 percent of the baseline; oral treatment should be substituted for parenteral treatment when the patient can swallow satisfactorily.
[f]This drug has not been approved by the Food and Drug Administration at the time of this publication.
[g]Artemether is only available in some countries in Asia, Africa, and South America.
[h]Nasogastric administration of oral antimalarials should be attempted if parenteral treatment is not possible, pending transfer to a hospital.

count and hematocrit should be measured every 12 h. If the hematocrit falls below 15 to 20 percent, then whole blood (preferably fresh) or packed cells should be transfused slowly, with careful attention to circulatory status; judicious use of diuretics may be required to prevent fluid overload. Renal function should be assessed daily. Management of fluid balance is difficult in severe malaria because there is a thin dividing line between overhydration, which can lead to pulmonary edema, and underhydration, which can contribute to renal impairment. If necessary, pulmonary arterial wedge pressure should be measured and maintained in the low to normal range. As soon as the patient can take fluids, oral antimalarials should be substituted.

COMPLICATIONS Acute renal failure If blood urea nitrogen or creatinine levels rise despite adequate rehydration, fluid administration should be restricted to prevent volume overload. The indications for dialysis are the same as those in other forms of hypercatabolic acute renal failure (see Chap. 236). Although peritoneal dialysis is adequate, hemodialysis is preferable when available and where secondary bacterial infections are common. Some patients pass small volumes of urine sufficient to allow control of fluid balance and may be managed conservatively if other indications for dialysis do not arise. Renal function usually improves within days but may not recover fully for weeks.

Acute pulmonary edema Patients should be positioned in bed at a 45° angle and given oxygen and intravenous diuretics. Their pulmonary arterial wedge pressure may be normal, indicating increased pulmonary capillary permeability. Positive-pressure ventilation should be started if these immediate measures fail (see Chap. 231).

TABLE 174-5 Characteristics of antimalarial drugs

Drug	Pharmacokinetic properties	Antimalarial activity	Minor toxicity	Major toxicity
Quinidine and quinine	Absorption: *Oral*: good. *Intramuscular*: good. Cl* and V_d† decreased, but plasma protein binding increased (90%) in malaria. $t_{1/2}$: 16 h in malaria, 11 h in healthy persons.	Acts mainly on mature trophozoite blood stage. Gametocytocidal against *P. vivax, P. ovale,* and *P. malariae*; no action on liver stages.	Bitter tasting. *Common:* "Cinchonism," tinnitus, high-tone hearing loss, nausea, vomiting, dysphoria, postural hypotension. prolonged electrocardiographic QT_c interval. *Rare:* Diarrhea, visual disturbance, rashes.	*Common:* Hypoglycemia. *Rare:* Hypotension, blindness, deafness, cardiac arrhythmias, thrombocytopenia, hemolysis, cholestatic hepatitis, neuromuscular paralysis. Quinidine more cardiotoxic.
Chloroquine	Absorption: *Oral*: good. *Intramuscular* and *subcutaneous*: very rapid. Complex pharmacokinetics. Enormous Cl and V_d (unaffected by malaria). Distribution processes determine blood concentration profile in malaria. $t_{1/2}$: 1–2 months.	Acts on ring-stage parasites. As for quinine	Bitter tasting. Well-tolerated. *Common:* Nausea, dysphoria, pruritus in dark-skinned patients, postural hypotension. *Rare:* Accommodation difficulties, rash.	*Acute:* Hypotensive shock (parenteral), cardiac arrhythmias, neuropsychiatric reactions. *Chronic:* Rare retinopathy (cumulative dose >100 g), skeletal and cardiac myopathy.
Mefloquine	Absorption: *Oral*: good. No parenteral preparation. $t_{1/2}$: 20 days.	As for quinine.	*Common:* Nausea, giddiness, dysphoria, postural hypotension.	Neuropsychiatric reactions infrequent; convulsions, encephalopathy.
Halofantrine‡	Absorption: variable, increased by fats. $t_{1/2}$: 1–3 days. Active desbutyl metabolite. $t_{1/2}$ 3–7 days.	As for quinine but more rapid.	Diarrhea, prolonged electrocardiographic QT_c interval.	Cardiac arrhythmias
Artemisinin and derivatives (artemether, artesunate)‡	Absorption: good. Rapid biotransformation to active metabolite dihydroartemisinin, which is eliminated rapidly.	Broader stage specificity and more rapid than other drugs; no action on liver stages.	Drug-induced pyrexia.	Neurotoxicity documented in animals.
Pyrimethamine	Absorption: *Oral*: good. *Intramuscular*: variable. $t_{1/2}$: 4 days.	For blood stages acts mainly on mature forms.	Well-tolerated.	Megaloblastic anemia, pancytopenia, pulmonary infiltration.
Proguanil (chloroguanide)	Absorption: *Oral*: good. biotransformed to active metabolite, cycloguanil. $t_{1/2}$: 16 h.	Causal prophylactic; not used for treatment.	Well-tolerated. *Rare:* Mouth ulcers, hair loss.	Megaloblastic anemia in renal failure.
Primaquine	Absorption: *Oral*: complete. Active compound not known. $t_{1/2}$:7 h.	Radical cure eradicates exoerythrocytic forms of *P. vivax* and *P. ovale.* Gametocytocidal against *P. falciparum.*	Nausea, vomiting, diarrhea, abdominal pain, hemolysis, methemoglobinemia.	Massive hemolysis in subjects with severe G6PD deficiency.

*Cl = systemic clearance.
†V_d = total apparent volume of distribution.
‡Not been approved by the U.S. Food and Drug Administration at the time of this publication.

Hypoglycemia An initial slow injection of 50% dextrose (0.5 g/kg) should be followed by an infusion of 10% dextrose (0.10 g/kg per hour). The blood glucose value should be monitored regularly thereafter, since recurrent hypoglycemia is common, particularly in patients who are receiving quinine or quinidine. In severely ill patients, hypoglycemia commonly occurs with lactic acidosis and may prove fatal.

Other complications Patients who develop spontaneous bleeding should be given fresh blood and intravenous vitamin K. Convulsions should be treated with intravenous (or rectal) diazepam. Aspiration pneumonia should be suspected in any unconscious patient with convulsions, particularly if he or she has persistent hyperventilation (see Chap. 100). Hypoglycemia or gram-negative septicemia should be suspected in any patient whose condition deteriorates for no obvious reason during antimalarial treatment. Exchange transfusion should be considered for patients with a parasitemia level of greater than 10 percent and deteriorating neurologic status.

Physicians who have questions about the management of patients with malaria can call the Malaria Branch, CDC, 404-488-4046 (nights and weekends, 404-639-2888).

BABESIOSIS

Babesiosis is a protozoan disease of animals that is transmitted by ticks; humans are infected incidentally and develop initially a nonspecific febrile illness. *Babesia* organisms enter red blood cells and resemble malaria parasites morphologically, thus posing a diagnostic problem.

ETIOLOGY AND NATURAL CYCLE Of the more than 70 species of *Babesia, B. microti* and *B. divergens* cause most human infections. Ixodid (or hard-bodied) ticks, in particular *Ixodes dammini* and *I. ricinus,* are vectors. Ticks ingest *Babesia* while feeding, and the parasites multiply within the gut wall of the vector. The organisms then spread to the salivary glands; their inoculation into a vertebrate host by a tick larva, nymph, or adult completes the transmission cycle. Asexual reproduction of *Babesia* within red blood cells produces two to four parasites. Transovarial transmission occurs in *I. ricinus* infected with *B. bovis,* a parasite of cattle that is slightly larger than *B. divergens* and is usually located on the margin of the red blood cell.

EPIDEMIOLOGY While *Babesia* infections in wild and domestic animals are distributed globally, almost all *B. microti* infections in the United States occur along the northeastern coast, including Nantucket Island and Martha's Vineyard in Massachusetts, Long Island and Shelter Island in New York, and the nearby mainland, including Connecticut. Cases also have been reported from California and Wisconsin. The deer tick, *I. dammini,* is the vector associated with *B. microti.*

Transfusions also have been the source of babesiosis. In several such cases, parasites were not detected in the donors, but serologic testing of the donor's blood for *Babesia* gave a positive result.

B. divergens infections have occurred sporadically in previously splenectomized patients in several countries of Europe. *I. ricinus* is probably the vector in these cases, as it is for transmission of this organism among cattle. The infected persons had been splenectomized and thus were predisposed to illness.

I. dammini feeds on rodents during its larval and nymphal stages and on deer as an adult; nymphs are abundant during the spring and summer and feed on humans readily. In some endemic areas, the seroprevalence in the human population may be greater than 2 percent, which indicates that asymptomatic infection is more frequent than is generally thought.

CLINICAL PRESENTATION   The incubation period for *B. microti* is about 1 to 4 weeks. Splenectomized individuals and the elderly have the most severe illness. The clinical presentation varies widely; symptoms and signs include gradual onset of irregular fever, chills, sweating, muscle pain, and fatigue. Mild hepatosplenomegaly and mild hemolytic anemia may occur. The level of parasitemia may exceed 10 percent. The illness may continue for weeks or months.

Patients infected with *B. divergens* have a more severe illness, with rapid onset of chills, fever, nausea, vomiting, and hemolytic anemia progressing to jaundice, hemoglobinemia, and renal failure. *B. divergens* infections are often fatal.

DIAGNOSIS   Whether or not they have a history of exposure to ticks or tick bites, febrile persons living in endemic areas should have Giemsa-stained thick and thin blood films made and examined for small intraerythrocytic parasites. *B. microti* appears as a small ring form similar to *P. falciparum.* Unlike infection with *Plasmodium,* that with *Babesia* does not cause the production of pigment in red blood cells, nor are schizonts or gametocytes formed. *B. microti,* dividing within red blood cells, can form four daughter parasites attached by strands of cytoplasm; these "tetrad" forms are seen infrequently in human blood films but are a distinguishing feature. An immunofluorescence antibody test is useful for the diagnosis of infection with *B. microti* but does not replace the blood smear. The serum antibody titer rises 2 to 4 weeks after the onset of illness and then wanes over 6 to 12 months; cross-reactions can occur with other species of *Babesia* and with *Plasmodium.* About half of patients infected with *B. microti* have antibody to *Borrelia burgdorferi,* the agent of Lyme disease (Chap. 137). Mixed infections occur, since both organisms are transmitted by *I. dammini.* Intraperitoneal inoculation of blood from patients with babesiosis into hamsters or gerbils has resulted in detectable parasitemia within 2 to 4 weeks.

TREATMENT   *B. microti* infections in patients with intact spleens are generally self-limiting without treatment. The combination of quinine sulfate (650 mg of salt PO tid) and clindamycin (600 mg PO tid or 1.2 g parenterally bid) for 7 to 10 days is effective in some cases but may not eliminate parasites. Symptoms may persist for months with or without treatment, although there are no permanent sequelae. More severe infections with high levels of *B. microti* parasitemia in asplenic patients have been successfully treated with exchange transfusions in addition to quinine and clindamycin.

Massive exchange transfusion, intravenous clindamycin, and oral chloroquine have been used successfully for the treatment of infection caused by *B. divergens,* a species that has been most refractory to therapy. Pentamidine (not approved by the Food and Drug Administration for this use) may be an alternative agent, since it is effective against several species of *Babesia* in animals.

REFERENCES

BREMAN JG, STEKETEE RW: Malaria, in *Maxcy-Rosenau-Last Public Health and Preventive Medicine,* 13th ed, JM Last, RB Wallace (eds). Norwalk, Conn, Appleton and Lange, 1992, pp 240–253

BRUCE CHWATT LJ: *Essential Malariology,* 2d ed. New York, Wiley, 1985

CENTERS FOR DISEASE CONTROL: Information for International Travelers. Washington, Public Health Service, U.S. Department of Health and Human Services, Publication No. 93-8280, 1993

GARNHAM PCC: Malaria parasites of man: Life cycles and morphology (excluding ultrastructure) in malaria, in *Principles and Practice of Malariology,* WH Wernsdorfer, I McGregor (eds). Edinburgh, Churchill Livingstone, 1988, pp. 61–96

HEALY G, RISTIC M: Human babesiosis, in *Babesiosis of Domestic Animals and Man,* M Ristic (ed). Boca Raton, Fla, CRC Press, 1988, pp 209–225

HOWARD RJ, GILLADOGGA AD: Molecular studies related to the pathogenesis of cerebral malaria. Blood 74:2603, 1989

KITCHEN SF: Symptomatology: General considerations and falciparum malaria, in *Malariology,* Vol 2. MF Boyd (ed). Philadelphia, Saunders, 1949, pp 966–1016

MILLER KD et al: Treatment of severe malaria in the United States with a continuous infusion of quinidine gluconate and exchange transfusion. N Engl J Med 321:65, 1989

MOLINEAUX L, GRAMICCIA G: *The Garki Project: Research on the Epidemiology and Control of Malaria in the Sudan Savannah of West Africa.* Geneva, World Health Organization, 1980

OAKS SC JR et al (eds): *Malaria: Obstacles and Opportunities,* CS Carpenter, CS Oaks (eds). Washington, National Academy Press, 1991

ROSNER F et al: Babesiosis in splenectomized adults: Review of 22 reported cases. Am J Trop Med Hyg 76:696, 1984

SPITZ S: Pathology of acute falciparum malaria. Military Med 99:555, 1946

STEFFEN R et al: Mefloquine compared with other malaria chemoprophylactic regimens in tourists visiting East Africa. Lancet 341:1299, 1993

WARRELL DA et al: Dexamethasone proves deleterious in cerebral malaria: A double-blind trial in 100 comatose patients. N Engl J Med 306:313, 1982

WHITE NJ: Drug treatment and prevention of malaria. Eur J Clin Pharmacol 34:1, 1988

———, Ho M: The pathophysiology of malaria. Adv Parasitol 31:84, 1992

WORLD HEALTH ORGANIZATION, DIVISION OF CONTROL OF TROPICAL DISEASES: Severe and complicated malaria. Trans R Soc Trop Med Hyg 84(suppl 2): 1, 1990

175   LEISHMANIASIS

RICHARD M. LOCKSLEY

DEFINITION   *Leishmaniasis* denotes disease caused by any of a number of species of protozoa in the genus *Leishmania.* There are four major clinical syndromes—visceral leishmaniasis (kala azar), cutaneous leishmaniasis of the old and new worlds, mucocutaneous leishmaniasis (espundia), and diffuse cutaneous leishmaniasis. Most commonly, these parasites are transmitted from animal reservoirs to human hosts by the bite of phlebotomine sandflies.

ETIOLOGY   Different *Leishmania* species appear identical and are generally distinguished by clinical and geographic characteristics. Modern speciation by isoenzyme patterns, monoclonal antibodies, DNA hybridization, DNA restriction endonuclease fragment analysis, and chromosomal karyotyping is continuing to delineate new species, particularly in the new world, and to demonstrate the capacity of different species to cause similar clinical syndromes.

In the sandfly and in culture media, *Leishmania* exist as motile, spindle-shaped promastigotes (1.5 to 4 μm by 14 to 20 μm) with a single anterior flagellum. On inoculation into a mammalian host, the organisms enter mononuclear phagocytes, lose their flagella, and multiply as small (2 by 5 μm), oval, obligate intracellular amastigotes (Leishman-Donovan bodies).

EPIDEMIOLOGY   Leishmaniasis is a zoonotic infection which involves the rodents, canines, and various forest mammals of every inhabited continent except Australia. The disease is spread when female sandflies of the genus *Phlebotomus* (old world) or *Lutzomyia* (new world) ingest amastigotes while taking a blood meal from an infected mammal. These transform into promastigotes within the insect's gut, migrate to the salivary glands, and are deposited on the skin of the new host when the insect next engorges. Phlebotomines breed in warm, humid microclimates and are typically found in rodent burrows, termite hills, and rotting vegetation. Humans may acquire the disease when they encroach on this sylvatic cycle. Establishment of infection in the domestic dog provides an important urban reservoir of leishmaniasis. Animal reservoirs have not been identified in the central East African and Indian forms of kala azar. It is estimated that worldwide over 12 million people are infected.

PATHOGENESIS Promastigotes are deposited on the skin into a small pool of blood drawn by the probing sandfly. Products from the fly salivary gland promote vasodilation and infectivity, in part via peptides that deactivate host macrophages. Complement is activated by the classical and/or alternative pathways, depending on the species, and is deposited onto the major outer membrane molecules of the promastigote—a 63-kDa molecular weight glycoprotein protease (gp63) and lipophosphoglycan (LPG). LPG and gp63 either directly or through bound C3b or C3bi target the organisms to macrophages via the complement receptors CR3 and CR1. The promastigotes transform into amastigotes within phagolysosomes and replicate by binary fission. They eventually rupture the cell and invade adjacent macrophages.

The course of the subsequent disease is determined by the host's cellular immunity as well as the species of the parasite. In cutaneous leishmaniasis, there is a marked lymphocytic infiltration associated with a reduction in the number of parasites, the development of a delayed skin test (leishmanin or Montenegro) reaction, and frequently, spontaneous cure. In mucocutaneous disease, the complete or partial resolution of the primary lesion may be followed by metastatic mucocutaneous lesions at a later date. In diffuse cutaneous leishmaniasis there is no infiltration by lymphocytes or reduction in the number of parasites, the leishmanin reaction remains negative, and the skin lesions become chronic, progressive, and disseminated. The patients have a selective anergy to *Leishmania* antigens. In visceral leishmaniasis, the parasites spread to macrophages throughout the body, perhaps due to the greater resistance of *L. donovani* to the spontaneous cidal activity present in normal serum.

Cure of visceral leishmaniasis has been correlated with the capacity of sensitized T lymphocytes from the patient to release macrophage-activating cytokines, particularly interferon-γ (IFN-γ). Macrophage activation results in induction of nitric oxide synthase and the production of nitric oxide, which is toxic for the intracellular amastigotes. Cure is thought to confer immunity to the infecting strain. Failure to cure has been related not only to the absence of production of IFN-γ but also to the release of macrophage-deactivating cytokines, such as interleukins 4 and 10 and transforming growth factor beta, in response to *Leishmania* antigens. Antibodies reach high levels in disseminated disease but are not protective against the intracellular organisms. In mucosal leishmaniasis, IFN-γ is produced, but concurrent production of deactivating cytokines leads to the inability to completely clear the parasite and to continuous inflammation, thus contributing to severe tissue destruction.

DIAGNOSIS Diagnosis of leishmaniasis requires demonstrating the organism by smear or culture of aspirates or tissue. Although Novy-MacNeal-Nicolle (NNN) medium traditionally has been used to culture *Leishmania*, several commercially available liquid media offer improved storage capability and enhanced recovery of organisms. Cultures are maintained at 22 to 28°C for 21 days and examined microscopically for the presence of the motile promastigotes. Inoculation of hamsters with infected clinical material results in infections after a period of weeks.

Species-specific diagnosis of human cutaneous new world isolates has been achieved by use of monoclonal antibodies or by hybridization of tissue touch blots with radiolabeled kinetoplast DNA probes.

Antibodies are detectable in all forms of leishmaniasis but are most useful in visceral leishmaniasis where cutaneous lesions are not present. The direct agglutination test detects IgM antibody and is a sensitive indicator of acute disease. The test is group-specific, but the titer is generally greatest to the homologous strain. A positive test

(> 1:32) varies from 97 percent in visceral leishmaniasis to 81 percent in new world cutaneous leishmaniasis. Direct agglutination antibodies decline and may disappear with cure. ELISAs also have been developed that are highly sensitive and specific in visceral leishmaniasis.

The Montenegro skin test using promastigote antigens is negative in visceral leishmaniasis. It is generally nonstandardized and is used only for epidemiologic purposes.

VISCERAL LEISHMANIASIS (KALA AZAR) *Leishmania donovani* causes kala azar, a disease that may be endemic, epidemic, or sporadic. *African kala azar* is found in the eastern half of Africa from the Sahara in the north to the equator in the south. Sporadic cases have been reported from West Africa. It is a disease of older children and young adults (10 to 25 years); males are involved more commonly than females. It is endemic in dogs and several wild carnivores in many areas and is more resistant to therapy with antimony compounds than the forms of kala azar found in the rest of the world.

Mediterranean, or infantile, kala azar is seen primarily in the Mediterranean area, China, and Latin America. It is a disease of children under the age of 4, but adults, particularly travelers to endemic areas, are not spared. Dogs, jackals, and foxes serve as reservoirs. Rats have been identified as a potential reservoir in Italy. The strains responsible for the Mediterranean and American disease are sometimes referred to as *L. infantum* and *L. chagasi*, respectively.

Indian kala azar has an age and sex distribution similar to African kala azar. Humans are the only known reservoir, and transmission is carried out by anthropophilic sandflies.

Manifestations The incubation period is generally about 3 months (3 weeks to 18 months). A primary cutaneous lesion (leishmanioma) is not uncommon in Africa. The onset of disease may be insidious or abrupt; the latter occurs more frequently in individuals from nonendemic areas. Failure to thrive is common among infected infants and children. Fever, typically nocturnal and occasionally double-quotidian, is almost universal and is accompanied by tachycardia without signs of toxemia. Diarrhea and cough are frequent. Nontender splenomegaly becomes dramatic by the third month. The liver enlarges less conspicuously. Cirrhosis and portal hypertension occur in about 10 percent of patients. Lymphadenopathy accompanies some cases of African kala azar. Asymptomatic and prolonged, subclinical forms of infection are common in endemic areas; malnutrition is a risk factor for the progression to full-blown disease. Fulminant kala azar has been described in patients with AIDS.

Pancytopenia is characteristic. Anemia is multifactorial: autoimmune hemolysis, splenomegaly, and gastrointestinal blood loss all contribute. The latter is exacerbated by thrombocytopenia. Agranulocytosis, cancrum oris, and superinfections complicate untreated cases. Extensive leishmanial infiltration of the gastrointestinal tract may lead to malabsorption. Hypoalbuminemia and polyclonal hypergammaglobulinemia (IgG and IgM) are constant features. Circulating immune complexes are frequently present. Immune-complex glomerulonephritis and interstitial nephritis have been described. Edema, cachexia, and hyperpigmentation (*kala azar* means "black fever") are late manifestations. Without treatment, death occurs within 3 to 20 months in 90 to 95 percent of adults and 75 to 85 percent of children, usually from superinfections or gastrointestinal hemorrhage.

After successful treatment, 3 to 10 percent of cases develop post–kala azar dermal leishmaniasis (PKDL), characterized by a spectrum of lesions ranging from depigmented macules to wartlike nodules over the face and extensor surfaces of the limbs. PKDL appears shortly after symptoms subside in African cases and typically disappears after several weeks. In the Indian disease, PKDL appears after a latent period of 1 to 2 years and may last for years, creating a persistent human reservoir. A clinical variant of *L. chagasi* causing papular cutaneous lesions without visceral involvement occurs in Honduras.

Diagnosis Bone marrow aspirate and biopsy are positive in over 85 percent of cases. In Brazil and Africa, splenic aspiration (95 percent) has proved quite safe and has been used serially to assess the response to therapy. In general, however, aspiration of the spleen or liver (75 percent) is not recommended because of the risk of hemorrhage. Aspirates or biopsy of enlarged lymph nodes will show parasites in 60 percent of cases. Suspicious skin lesions should be biopsied as well. The direct agglutination test is positive early in the disease. The leishmanin skin test becomes positive 6 to 8 weeks after recovery. Other causes of fever in the tropics, including malaria, brucellosis, tuberculosis, typhoid, and hepatic abscess, can be distinguished by appropriate testing. PKDL must be differentiated from leprosy, syphilis, and yaws.

Treatment   Transfusions and treatment of complicating superinfections must supplement specific therapy. Pentavalent antimonials are highly effective against *Leishmania* and are relatively nontoxic. Sodium antimony gluconate (Pentostam; 100 mg Sb^{5+} per milliliter) is given intravenously or intramuscularly in a single daily dose of 20 mg/kg for 28 days. Meglumine antimoniate (Glucantime; 85 mg Sb^{5+} per milliliter) also can be used. Therapy should be repeated using 20 mg/kg for 40 to 60 days in patients with relapses or incomplete responses. Periodic electrocardiographic monitoring is recommended during prolonged therapy. The addition of oral allopurinol (20 to 30 mg/kg per day in three divided doses) has been effective. Incomplete therapy of the initial illness remains the major risk factor for relapse with drug-resistant organisms. Such cases must be treated with intravenous amphotericin B (0.5 to 1 mg/kg on alternate days) or pentamidine (3 to 4 mg/kg three times per week for 5 to 25 weeks, depending on the response). Adjunctive splenectomy has been successful in some cases of drug-resistant kala azar. Mortality remains 15 to 25 percent in advanced cases, although the cure rate is over 90 percent when therapy is given early. Follow-up at 3 and 12 months is recommended to detect relapses. PKDL should be treated in the same fashion as the initial illness. Recombinant human interferon-γ has shown promise as adjunctive therapy with pentavalent antimony in previous treatment failures or in seriously ill patients with kala azar.

Prevention   Preventive measures include early treatment of human cases, elimination of diseased dogs, and the use of DDT against sandflies. Application of insect repellents and the use of permethrin-coated fine netting are important for travelers. There are no useful prophylactic agents.

CUTANEOUS AND MUCOCUTANEOUS LEISHMANIASIS   This form of leishmaniasis is caused by a number of species in both the old world and the new world. Disease is characterized by the development of single or multiple localized lesions on exposed areas of skin that typically ulcerate. Although spontaneous healing is the rule for old world cutaneous leishmaniasis, this is less common in new world disease.

Old world cutaneous leishmaniasis   *L. tropica* causes anthroponotic (urban, chronic, dry) cutaneous leishmaniasis, an endemic disease of children and young adults in areas bordering the Mediterranean, the Middle East, The Republic of Georgia, and India. The principal reservoirs are humans, although domestic dogs are synanthropic hosts. The incubation period ranges from 2 to 24 months. Usually the lesion begins as a single, red pruritic papule on the face (oriental sore). The central area ulcerates and slowly enlarges centrifugally, reaching a size of approximately 2 cm. Lymphadenopathy is unusual. Healing occurs over 1 to 2 years and leaves a small depigmented scar. The disease can be complicated by the development of leishmaniasis recidiva, a condition marked by persistent facial lesions containing a scant number of parasites and by an exaggerated delayed hypersensitivity response to parasite antigens. Rarely, the organism may spread to the viscera and present as fever of unknown origin (viscerotropic leishmaniasis) or as typical kala azar.

L. major causes zoonotic (rural, acute, moist) cutaneous leishmaniasis, which is endemic across the desert areas of the Middle East to Afghanistan and in Africa. The reservoir is maintained in burrowing rodents. The incubation period ranges from 2 to 6 weeks. The initial lesions are often multiple and located on the lower extremities. Regional lymphadenopathy and satellite lesions are common. Healing

with scarring occurs within 3 to 6 months. *L. major* has been implicated in cases of mucocutaneous leishmaniasis in Saudi Arabia.

L. aethiopica, maintained in rock hyraxes of the Ethiopian and Kenyan highlands, causes cutaneous leishmaniasis which may pursue a relatively prolonged course and can be complicated by the development of diffuse cutaneous leishmaniasis (see below).

DIAGNOSIS   Lesions should first be cleansed with alcohol to reduce bacterial contamination, which hinders recovery of the organisms. Aspirates should be obtained from the outer edge of the ulcer. If the aspirated smears are negative, full-thickness skin biopsies from the ulcer margin should be taken for touch smears, histology, and culture. The direct agglutination test and the leishmanin skin test become positive within 4 to 6 weeks.

TREATMENT   Specific therapy should be withheld in endemic areas until ulceration takes place, thereby conferring immunity. Exceptions include disfiguring or disabling lesions and lesions persisting for longer than 6 months. Imidazoles have some efficacy, and ketoconazole (600 mg/d orally for 4 weeks) has been recommended prior to use of antimonials when possible. Treatment with antimonials is as described for kala azar, although shorter courses (20 days) are effective. Higher doses of antimony may be required for *L. aethiopica* infections (20 mg/kg twice a day for 30 days). Ulcers should be covered to prevent infection of vectors and other canine and human hosts.

New world cutaneous and mucocutaneous leishmaniasis   Leishmanias causing new world cutaneous disease are divided into numerous subspecies within the *L. mexicana* and *L. braziliensis* groups (Table 175-1). Spontaneous healing occurs more commonly in disease due to *L. mexicana*. The natural reservoirs for these organisms include a wide variety of mammals inhabiting the forests of South and Central America. Disease is most prevalent in the Amazon basin but occurs throughout the Americas as far north as south-central Texas.

L. mexicana causes chiclero's ulcer, or bay sore. Chicle gatherers who work in forests during the rainy season when sandflies are abundant develop isolated cutaneous lesions on the hand or head. These show little tendency to ulcerate and generally heal spontaneously within 6 months. Ear lesions, however, may persist and cause extensive destruction of the pinna.

L. venezuelensis causes indolent nodular lesions. *L. amazonensis* causes persistent lesions that may be multiple and seldom heal spontaneously. *L. amazonensis* also may cause diffuse cutaneous leishmaniasis (see below), visceral leishmaniasis, and mucocutaneous leishmaniasis.

L. peruviana causes uta, a disease consisting of single or multiple ulcers typically on the face. Spontaneous healing within 3 months to a year is the rule. The reservoir is the domestic dog. The disease occurs on the western slopes of the Peruvian Andes at altitudes above 600 m (2000 ft). Species of *L. mexicana* and new world *L. major*–like organisms also have been implicated in uta.

Mucocutaneous leishmaniasis, or espundia, is caused primarily by *L. braziliensis*, which typically produces one or several lesions on the lower extremities that undergo extensive ulceration; complete healing may or may not occur spontaneously. After months to years, metastatic lesions appear in the nasopharynx in 2 to 5 percent of patients. Less frequently, lesions occur in the perineum. Multiple, large antecedent skin lesions and insufficient antimony therapy for the primary infection are risk factors. Nasal obstruction and epistaxis are frequent presenting symptoms. Extensive destruction of soft tissue structures ensues, with painful mutilating erosions (espundia). Fever, anemia, and weight loss are common. Death is caused by bacterial infection, inanition, aspiration, and respiratory obstruction.

L. panamensis causes nonhealing ulcerative lesions, and *L. guyanensis* causes nodular lesions that persist and metastasize along lymphatics (pian bois). These strains can cause mucocutaneous leishmaniasis.

DIAGNOSIS   Speciation of the infecting organism should be attempted for prognostic and epidemiologic purposes. Regional interna-

TABLE 175-1 New world *Leishmania* Species

Species	Geographic distribution	Reservoir	Clinical syndrome*
L. chagasi	Mexico, Honduras, Guatemala, Surinam, El Salvador, Colombia, Venezuela, Ecuador, Brazil, Bolivia, Paraguay, Argentina, Martinique, Guadeloupe	Canines	VL, CL, PKDL
L. mexicana complex			
L. mexicana	Mexico, Guatemala, Belize, Costa Rica, Panama, Colombia, Ecuador, Texas (U.S.A.)	Forest rodents	CL, DCL
L. amazonensis	Brazil, Costa Rica, Panama, Colombia, French Guyana, Ecuador, Peru, Bolivia, Venezuela	Rodents, marsupials	CL, VL, PKDL, MCL, DCL
L. venezuelensis	Venezuela	?	CL
L. braziliensis complex			
L. braziliensis	Brazil, Guatemala, Honduras, Belize, Colombia, Venezuela, Peru, Bolivia, Paraguay, Ecuador	Forest rodents	CL, MCL
L. guyanensis	Colombia, Brazil, Surinam, French Guyana, Guyana, Ecuador	Sloths, anteaters	CL, MCL
L. panamensis	Panama, Honduras, Colombia, Ecuador	Sloths	CL, MCL
L. peruviana	Peru	Canines	CL
L. lainsoni	Brazil	?	CL
L. naiffi	Brazil	?	CL
L. colombiensis	Colombia, Panama, Venezuela	Sloths	CL
L. major–like isolates	Venezuela, Ecuador	?Canines	CL, DCL

* VL = visceral leishmaniasis; CL = cutaneous leishmaniasis; PKDL = post–kala azar dermal leishmaniasis; MCL = mucocutaneous leishmaniasis; DCL = diffuse cutaneous leishmaniasis.

tional reference laboratories for speciation have been identified by the World Health Organization (Geneva). Skin biopsies are the preferred means of obtaining tissue for stains and culture. Parasites may be scant, particularly in mucocutaneous lesions. The direct agglutination test and the leishmanin skin test become positive within 4 to 6 weeks. Syphilis, yaws, blastomycosis, paracoccidioidomycosis, sporotrichosis, leprosy, and carcinoma must be considered in the differential diagnosis.

TREATMENT In general, cutaneous lesions should be treated with systemic antimonials for 20 days in order to decrease the subsequent risk of mucocutaneous disease. Local heat (40 to 41°C) may accelerate healing. Oral ketoconazole (600 mg/d for 28 days) has been efficacious in cutaneous lesions caused by *L. mexicana.*

Espundia should be treated with antimonials (20 mg/kg per day) for 28 days, although long-term cure may be difficult, particularly among patients with severe disease. Failures should be treated with amphotericin. Reconstructive facial prostheses should not be used until the disease has been in remission for at least 1 year without therapy. A rising antibody titer may predict relapse and indicate that further therapy is required.

Diffuse cutaneous leishmaniasis Diffuse cutaneous leishmaniasis is found in Venezuela, Peru, Brazil, Mexico, and the Dominican Republic in the new world and in Ethiopia in the old world. Patients display a specific deficiency of cell-mediated immunity to leishmanial antigens. Organisms from the *L. mexicana* complex have been implicated in the Americas, and *L. aethiopica* in Africa. Disease is characterized by massive dissemination of skin lesions without visceral involvement. The clinical picture often bears a striking resemblance to lepromatous leprosy. The diagnosis is not difficult, because the lesions contain large numbers of organisms. In contrast to all other types of cutaneous leishmaniasis, the leishmanin skin test remains negative. The disease is progressive and very refractory to treatment. High doses of antimony (20 mg/kg twice a day for 30 days) and multiple courses of amphotericin or pentamidine are often required to produce remission, but cures are rare. Immunotherapy with a combination of BCG and *Leishmania* antigens and administration of recombinant IFN-γ have been promising.

REFERENCES

BADARO R et al: Treatment of visceral leishmaniasis with pentavalent antimony and interferon-gamma. N Engl J Med 322:16, 1990

BARRAL A et al: Leishmaniasis in Bahia, Brazil: Evidence that *Leishmania amazonensis* produces a wide spectrum of clinical disease. Am J Trop Med Hyg 44:536, 1991

CARVALHO EM et al: Immunologic markers of clinical evolution in children recently infected with *Leishmania donovani chagasi.* J Infect Dis 165:535, 1992

FRANKE ED et al: Efficacy and toxicity of sodium stibogluconate for mucosal leishmaniasis. Ann Intern Med 113:934, 1990

GRIMALDI G JR et al: A review of the geographic distribution and epidemiology of leishmaniasis in the new world. Am J Trop Med Hyg 41:687, 1989

HERWALDT BL et al: The natural history of cutaneous leishmaniasis in Guatemala. J Infect Dis 165:518, 1992

HERWALDT BL, BERMAN JD: Recommendations for treating leishmaniasis with sodium stibogluconate (Pentostam) and review of pertinent clinic studies. Am J Trop Med Hyg 46:296, 1992

MELBY PC et al: Cutaneous leishmaniasis: Review of 59 cases seen at the National Institutes of Health. Clin Infect Dis 15:924, 1992

NAVIN TR et al: Placebo-controlled clinical trial of sodium stibogluconate (Pentostam) versus ketoconazole for treating cutaneous leishmaniasis in Guatemala. J Infect Dis 165:528, 1992

176 TRYPANOSOMIASIS

LOUIS V. KIRCHHOFF

CHAGAS' DISEASE

DEFINITION Chagas' disease, or American trypanosomiasis, is a zoonosis caused by the protozoan parasite *Trypanosoma cruzi.* Acute Chagas' disease is generally a mild, febrile illness that results from initial infection with the organism. Following spontaneous resolution of the acute illness, most infected individuals remain for life in the indeterminate phase of chronic Chagas' disease, which is characterized by subpatent parasitemia, high levels of anti-*T. cruzi* antibodies, and an absence of symptoms. In a minority of chronically infected individuals, cardiac and gastrointestinal lesions develop that can result in serious morbidity and even death.

LIFE CYCLE AND TRANSMISSION *T. cruzi* is transmitted among its mammalian hosts by hematophagous triatomine insects, or reduviid bugs. The insects become infected by sucking blood from animals or humans who have circulating parasites. Ingested organisms multiply in the gut of the reduviids, and infective forms are discharged with the feces at the time of subsequent blood meals. Transmission to a second vertebrate host occurs when breaks in the skin, mucous membranes, or conjunctivae are contaminated with bug feces that contain infective parasites. *T. cruzi* also can be transmitted by transfusion of blood donated by infected persons, and congenital infections occur as well.

PATHOLOGY   An indurated inflammatory lesion called a *chagoma* often appears at the site of the parasite's entry. Local histologic changes include intracellular parasites in leukocytes and cells of subcutaneous tissues, interstitial edema, lymphocytic infiltration, and reactive hyperplasia of adjacent lymph nodes. After dissemination through the lymphatics and the bloodstream, muscles, including the myocardium, may be heavily parasitized. The characteristic pseudocysts seen in sections of infected tissues are intracellular aggregates of multiplying parasites.

The pathogenesis of chronic Chagas' disease is poorly understood. The heart is the organ most commonly affected, and changes include biventricular enlargement, thinning of the ventricular walls, apical aneurysms, and mural thrombi. Widespread lymphocytic infiltration, diffuse interstitial fibrosis, and atrophy of myocardial cells are often present, but parasites are rarely demonstrated in myocardial tissue. Conduction system involvement most frequently affects the right branch and the left anterior branch of the bundle of His. In chronic Chagas' disease of the gastrointestinal tract (megadisease), the esophagus and colon may be enormously dilated and hypertrophied. On microscopic examination, focal inflammatory lesions with lymphocytic infiltration are seen, and the number of neurons in the myenteric plexus is reduced.

EPIDEMIOLOGY   *T. cruzi* is found only in the Americas. Wild and domestic mammals harboring *T. cruzi* and infected reduviids are found in spotty distributions from the southern United States to southern Argentina. Humans become involved in the cycle of transmission when infected vectors take up residence in the primitive wood, adobe, and stone houses common in much of Latin America. Thus human *T. cruzi* infection is primarily a health problem among the poor in rural areas of Central and South America. Most new *T. cruzi* infections in rural settings occur in children, but the incidence is unknown because most go undiagnosed. Thousands of individuals also become infected every year through blood transfusions in urban areas. Currently, it is estimated that 16 million people, more than a third of whom live in Brazil, are chronically infected with *T. cruzi*. Chronic Chagas' disease is a major cause of morbidity and mortality in many Latin American countries, including Mexico, since many chronically infected individuals eventually develop symptomatic cardiac lesions or gastrointestinal disease.

Acute Chagas' disease is rare in the United States. Four cases of autochthonous transmission have been described, and recently, three instances of transmission by blood transfusion have occurred. In addition, between 1971 and 1992, seven laboratory-acquired infections and nine imported cases of acute Chagas' disease have been reported to the Centers for Disease Control and Prevention. In contrast, the prevalence of chronic *T. cruzi* infections in the United States has increased considerably in recent years. Since the mid-1970s enormous numbers of Central Americans have emigrated to the United States, and in one study done in Washington, D.C., 5 percent of Salvadoran and Nicaraguan immigrants were found to have chronic *T. cruzi* infections. Conservative estimates place the total number of infected immigrants now living here at more than 50,000. The presence of these carriers of *T. cruzi* poses a significant risk of transmission by blood transfusion, as evidenced by the occurrence of the three transfusion-associated cases.

CLINICAL COURSE   The first signs of acute Chagas' disease occur at least 1 week after invasion by the parasites. When the organisms have entered through a break in the skin, an indurated area of erythema and swelling, the *chagoma*, may appear, accompanied by local lymphadenopathy. Romaña's sign, the classic finding in acute Chagas' disease, consists of unilateral painless edema of the palpebrae and periocular tissues that can result when the conjunctiva

is the portal of entry. These initial local signs are followed by malaise, fever, anorexia, and edema of the face and lower extremities. Generalized lymphadenopathy and mild hepatosplenomegaly may appear. Severe myocarditis develops rarely, and most deaths in acute Chagas' disease are due to heart failure. Neurologic signs are not common, but meningoencephalitis has been reported. The acute symptoms resolve spontaneously in virtually all patients, who then enter the asymptomatic or indeterminate phase of chronic *T. cruzi* infection.

Symptomatic chronic Chagas' disease becomes apparent years or even decades after the initial infection. The heart is commonly involved, and symptoms are caused by rhythm disturbances, cardiomyopathy, and thromboembolism. Right bundle branch block is the most common electrocardiographic abnormality, but other types of atrioventricular block, premature ventricular contractions, and tachy- and bradyarrhythmias are seen frequently. Cardiomyopathy often results in right-sided or biventricular heart failure. Embolization of mural thrombi to the brain or other areas may occur. Patients with megaesophagus suffer from dysphagia, odynophagia, chest pain, and regurgitation. Aspiration can occur, especially during sleep, and repeated episodes of aspiration pneumonitis are common. Weight loss, cachexia, and pulmonary infection can result in death. Patients with megacolon are plagued by abdominal pain and chronic constipation, and advanced megacolon can cause obstruction, perforation, septicemia, and death.

DIAGNOSIS   The diagnosis of Chagas' disease requires the detection of parasites. Microscopic examination of fresh anticoagulated blood or of the buffy coat is the simplest way to see the motile organisms. Parasites also can be seen in Giemsa-stained thin and thick blood smears. When repeated attempts to visualize the organisms are unsuccessful, mouse inoculation and culture of blood in specialized media should be performed. As a last resort, xenodiagnosis should be attempted. In this technique, uninfected reduviid bugs are allowed to feed on the patient's blood. Approximately 30 days after the blood meal, the intestinal contents of the bugs are examined for parasites. When done properly, this method is positive in virtually all patients with acute Chagas' disease and in approximately half of those with chronic infections. Since early treatment of acute Chagas' disease is extremely important, however, the decision to initiate anti-*T. cruzi* therapy in a patient with negative wet preparations and smears must be made on clinical and epidemiologic grounds before the results of these indirect methods become available. Serologic testing is of limited usefulness in diagnosing acute Chagas' disease.

The diagnosis of chronic Chagas' disease is made by detecting antibodies that bind to *T. cruzi* antigens. Demonstration of the parasite is not of primary importance. Several highly sensitive serologic tests for the detection of anti-*T. cruzi* antibodies are used widely in Latin America, including complement fixation and immunofluorescence assays and enzyme-linked immunosorbent assay (ELISA). However, a persistent problem with these conventional assays is the occurrence of false-positive reactions, typically with sera from patients with diseases such as leishmaniasis. For this reason, it is generally recommended that positivity in one assay be confirmed in two other tests and that well-characterized positive and negative comparison sera be included in each run. A highly sensitive and specific method for detecting anti-*T. cruzi* antibodies that employs immunoprecipitation of radiolabeled *T. cruzi* antigens has been described. This assay effectively deals with the problem of false-positive reactions and is available in the author's laboratory, but it has not been adapted for mass screening. Serodiagnostic assays that employ recombinant *T. cruzi* proteins as target antigens are being developed, as are tests based on polymerase chain reaction amplification of *T. cruzi* DNA sequences, but they are not yet available for general use.

TREATMENT   Therapy for Chagas' disease is unsatisfactory. Nifurtimox is the only drug active against *T. cruzi* that is available in the United States. In acute Chagas' disease, nifurtimox markedly reduces the duration of symptoms and parasitemia and decreases mortality. Nevertheless, its ability to eradicate parasites is limited, since patients treated with nifurtimox during the acute phase may have positive xenodiagnoses after full courses of the drug. Nifurtimox treatment should be initiated as early as possible in acute Chagas' disease. Moreover, when laboratory accidents occur in which it appears likely that *T. cruzi* infection could become established, nifurtimox therapy should be initiated without waiting for clinical or parasitologic indications of infection.

The usefulness of nifurtimox in individuals with indeterminate phase or symptomatic chronic Chagas' disease has not been established. There is no evidence that patients in the indeterminate phase are less likely to develop symptomatic disease after treatment with nifurtimox, and likewise, it has not been shown to have any effect on symptomatic chronic disease. Moreover, posttreatment xenodiagnoses are also positive in a large proportion of chronically infected patients given this drug. Hence there is no indication for treating individuals with chronic *T. cruzi* infections with nifurtimox.

Common adverse effects of nifurtimox include abdominal pain, anorexia, nausea, vomiting, and weight loss. Neurologic symptoms may include restlessness, disorientation, insomnia, twitching, paresthesia, polyneuritis, and seizures. These symptoms usually disappear when the dosage is reduced or treatment is discontinued. The recommended dosage for adults is 8 to 10 mg/kg body weight per day. The dosage for adolescents is 12.5 to 15 mg/kg per day, and for children 1 to 10 years of age, 15 to 20 mg/kg per day. The drug should be given orally in four divided doses each day, and therapy should be continued for 90 to 120 days. Nifurtimox is available from the Drug Service of the CDC, Atlanta, Georgia (telephone no. 404-639-3670).

Benznidazole is a second agent used to treat Chagas' disease. Its efficacy is similar to that of nifurtimox, and adverse effects include peripheral neuropathy, rash, and granulocytopenia. The recommended oral dosage is 5 mg/kg per day for 60 days. Benznidazole is used widely in Latin America, but it is not available in the United States.

Limited studies in experimental systems and in humans have suggested that allopurinol may be useful for treating chronic Chagas' disease. Currently, its efficacy is being evaluated in trials in humans. In addition, studies in mice have shown that recombinant interferon-γ decreases the duration and severity of acute *T. cruzi* infection, but its usefulness in persons with acute Chagas' disease has not been evaluated systematically.

PREVENTION Since drug therapy is unsatisfactory and vaccines are not available, the control of *T. cruzi* transmission in endemic countries must depend on reduction of domiciliary vector populations by spraying of insecticides and improvement in housing. Also, in endemic areas, expansion and improvement of programs for screening donated blood for the presence of *T. cruzi* are necessary to reduce transmission by transfusion. Tourists traveling in endemic areas should avoid sleeping in dilapidated houses outside urban areas. Mosquito nets and insect repellent will provide additional protection.

In the United States, blood donations should not be accepted from immigrants from regions in which Chagas' disease is endemic, unless serologic assays indicate that the donor is not infected with *T. cruzi*. Moreover, all immigrants from endemic regions should be screened for serologic evidence of infection with the parasite. Identification of infected individuals in this group is important not only to prevent transmission by blood transfusion but also to enable physicians who care for these patients to undertake appropriate diagnostic monitoring and supportive therapy when indicated. Laboratory personnel should wear gloves and eye protection when working with *T. cruzi* and infected vectors. Patients with end-stage chagasic cardiopathies should not undergo cardiac transplantation because the immunosuppression required after surgery often leads to reactivation of *T. cruzi* infection with serious consequences and even death.

SLEEPING SICKNESS

DEFINITION Sleeping sickness, or African trypanosomiasis, is caused by flagellated protozoan parasites belonging to the *Trypano-soma brucei* complex that are transmitted to humans by tsetse flies. In untreated patients, the trypanosomes first cause a febrile illness that is followed months or years later by progressive neurologic impairment and death.

THE PARASITES AND THEIR TRANSMISSION The East African (*rhodesiense*) and the West African (*gambiense*) forms of sleeping sickness are caused, respectively, by two trypanosome subspecies, *T. brucei rhodesiense* and *T. brucei gambiense*. These subspecies are indistinguishable morphologically but cause illnesses that are epidemiologically and clinically distinct. The parasites are transmitted by blood-sucking tsetse flies of the genus *Glossina*. The insects acquire the infection when they ingest blood from infected mammalian hosts. After many cycles of multiplication in the midgut of the vector, the parasites migrate to the salivary glands, and transmission takes place when they are inoculated during a subsequent blood meal. The injected trypanosomes multiply in the blood and other extracellular spaces and evade immune destruction in mammalian hosts for long periods by undergoing antigenic variation, a process by which the antigenic structure of their surface coat of glycoproteins changes periodically.

PATHOGENESIS AND PATHOLOGY A self-limited inflammatory lesion (trypanosomal chancre) may appear a week or so after the bite of an infected tsetse fly. A systemic febrile illness then evolves as the parasites are disseminated through the lymphatics and bloodstream. Systemic African trypanosomiasis without central nervous system (CNS) involvement is generally referred to as *stage I disease*. In this stage, there is widespread lymphadenopathy and splenomegaly, reflecting marked lymphocytic and histocytic proliferation and invasion of morular cells, which are plasmacytes that may be involved in the production of IgM. An endarteritis with perivascular infiltration of both parasites and lymphocytes may develop in lymph nodes and spleen. Myocarditis develops frequently in patients with stage I disease, especially with *T. b. rhodesiense* infections.

Hematologic manifestations that accompany stage I trypanosomiasis include a moderate leukocytosis, thrombocytopenia, and anemia. High levels of immunoglobulins, consisting primarily of polyclonal IgM, are a constant feature, and heterophile antibodies, anti-DNA antibodies, and rheumatoid factor are often detected. High levels of antigen-antibody complexes may play a role in the tissue damage and increased vascular permeability that facilitate dissemination of the parasites.

Stage II trypanosomiasis involves invasion of the CNS. The presence of trypanosomes in perivascular areas is accompanied by intense infiltration of mononuclear cells. Cerebrospinal fluid (CSF) abnormalities include increased pressure, elevated total protein concentration, and pleocytosis. Trypanosomes also are frequently present in the CSF.

EPIDEMIOLOGY The trypanosomes that cause sleeping sickness are found only in Africa. Approximately 20,000 new cases are reported each year, but this number is surely an underestimate. Humans are the only reservoir of *T. b. gambiense*, and infections occur in widely distributed foci in tropical rain forests of Central and West Africa. Gambiense trypanosomiasis is primarily a problem in rural populations, and tourists rarely become infected. Trypanotolerant antelope species in savanna and woodland areas of Central and East Africa are the principal reservoir of *T. b. rhodesiense*. Cattle also can become infected but generally succumb to the parasite. Humans acquire *T. b. rhodesiense* infection only incidentally, since for the most part risk results from contact with tsetse flies that feed on wild animals. Thus the disease is an occupational hazard for persons who work in areas where infected game and vectors are present. In addition, occasional cases of *T. b. rhodesiense* infection occur among visitors to game parks in East Africa. During the past two decades, 16 cases of imported African trypanosomiasis have been reported to the CDC, most of which were caused by *T. b. rhodesiense*.

CLINICAL COURSE A painful trypanosomal chancre appears in some patients at the site where parasites were inoculated. Hematogenous and lymphatic dissemination (stage I disease) is marked by the onset of fever, and typically, bouts of high temperatures lasting several days are separated by afebrile periods. Lymphadenopathy is prominent in *T. b. gambiense* trypanosomiasis. The nodes are discrete, movable, rubbery, and nontender. Cervical nodes are often visible, and enlargement of the nodes of the posterior cervical triangle, or Winterbottom's sign, is a classic finding in individuals infected with *T. b. gambiense*. Pruritus is frequent, and a circinate rash is often present. Inconstant findings include malaise, headache, arthralgias, weight loss, edema, hepatosplenomegaly, and tachycardia.

CNS invasion (stage II disease) is characterized by the insidious development of protean neurologic manifestations, accompanied by progressive abnormalities in the CSF. A picture of progressive indifference and daytime somnolence (sleeping sickness) develops, sometimes alternating with restlessness and insomnia at night. A listless gaze accompanies a loss of spontaneity, and speech may become halting and indistinct. Extrapyramidal signs may include choreiform movements, tremors, and fasciculations. Ataxia is frequent, and the patient may appear to have Parkinson's disease with a shuffling gait, hypertonia, and tremors. In the final phase, progressive neurologic impairment ends in coma and death.

The most striking difference between the West African and East African trypanosomiases is that the latter illness tends to follow a more acute course. Typically, in tourists, systemic signs of infection such as fever, malaise, and headache may appear before the end of the trip or shortly after their return home. Persistent tachycardia unrelated to fever is common early in the course of *T. b. rhodesiense* trypanosomiasis, and death may result from arrhythmias and congestive heart failure before CNS disease develops. In general, untreated East African trypanosomiasis leads to death in a matter of weeks to months, often without a clear distinction between the hemolymphatic and CNS stages.

DIAGNOSIS A definitive diagnosis of African trypanosomiasis requires detection of the parasite. If a chancre is present, fluid should be expressed and examined directly by light microscopy for the highly motile trypanosomes. The fluid also should be fixed and stained with Giemsa. Material obtained by needle aspiration of lymph nodes early in the course of the illness should be examined similarly. Examination of wet preparations and Giemsa-stained thin and thick films of serial blood samples is also useful. If parasites are not found by these methods, the buffy coat from 10 to 15 mL anticoagulated blood or the pellet obtained by centrifugation of the eluate from 25 to 50 mL blood passed through a DEAE-cellulose column should be examined. Trypanosomes also may be seen in material aspirated from the bone marrow, and the aspirate can be inoculated into liquid culture medium, as can blood, buffy coat, lymph node aspirates, and CSF. Finally, *T. b. rhodesiense* infection can be detected by inoculation of these specimens into mice or rats, resulting in patent parasitemias in a week or two. This is a highly sensitive method for the detection of *T. b. rhodesiense*, but unfortunately, due to host specificity, *T. b. gambiense* cannot be detected by this technique.

Examination of the CSF is mandatory in all patients suspected of having African trypanosomiasis. An increase in the CSF cell count is the first abnormality to be detected, and increased opening pressure, as well as total protein and IgM levels, develops later. Trypanosomes may be seen in the sediment of centrifuged CSF. Any CSF abnormality in a patient in whom trypanosomes have been found in specimens from other sites must be viewed as pathognomonic for CNS involvement, and thus specific treatment for CNS disease must be given.

A number of serologic assays are available to aid in the diagnosis of African trypanosomiasis, but their variable sensitivity and specificity mandate that treatment decisions be based on demonstration of the parasite. These tests are of value for epidemiologic surveys.

TREATMENT The drugs traditionally used for treatment of African trypanosomiasis are suramin, pentamidine, and organic arsenicals. A recent addition to this list is eflornithine (difluoromethylornithine), which was approved by the U.S. Food and Drug Administration (FDA) in November 1990 for treatment of West African trypanosomiasis. In the United States these drugs can be obtained from the CDC. Therapy for African trypanosomiasis must be individualized on the basis of the infecting organism (*T. b. gambiense* or *T. b. rhodesiense*), the presence or absence of CNS disease, adverse reactions, and occasionally, drug resistance. The choices of drugs for treatment of African trypanosomiasis are summarized as follows.

Stage I (normal CSF) West African trypanosomiasis (*T. b. gambiense*) should be treated with either suramin or eflornithine. Pentamidine can be used as an alternative drug. Stage II West African trypanosomiasis (abnormal CSF) should be treated with eflornithine.

Stage I East African trypanosomiasis (*T. b. rhodesiense*) should be treated with suramin, and pentamidine can be used as an alternative drug. Since suramin and pentamidine do not penetrate the CNS well and eflornithine has variable efficacy against *T. b. rhodesiense*, stage II East African trypanosomiasis should be treated with melarsoprol, and patients who cannot tolerate the latter drug should be treated with tryparsamide plus suramin.

Suramin is highly effective against stage I disease, but it can cause serious adverse effects and must be administered under the close supervision of a physician. A 100- to 200-mg intravenous test dose should be administered to detect hypersensitivity. The dosage for adults is 1 g intravenously on days 1, 3, 7, 14, and 21. The regimen for children is 20 mg/kg body weight (maximum dose is 1 g) intravenously on days 1, 3, 7, 14, and 21. The drug is given by slow intravenous infusion of a freshly prepared 10% aqueous solution. Approximately 1 patient in 20,000 has an immediate, severe, and potentially fatal reaction to the drug consisting of nausea, vomiting, shock, and seizures. Less severe reactions include fever, photophobia, pruritus, arthralgias, and skin eruptions. Renal damage is the most common important adverse effect of suramin. Transient proteinuria often appears during treatment. Urinalysis should be done before each dose, and the drug should be discontinued if proteinuria increases or casts and red cells appear in the sediment. Suramin should not be used in patients with renal insufficiency.

Eflornithine is highly effective for treatment of both stages of West African trypanosomiasis. In the trials on which the FDA based its approval, it cured more than 90 percent of 600 stage II patients. The recommended treatment schedule is 400 mg/kg per day intravenously in four divided doses for 2 weeks. This should be followed by oral treatment with 300 mg/kg per day for 3 to 4 weeks. Adverse effects include diarrhea, anemia, thrombocytopenia, seizures, and hearing loss. The efficacy of eflornithine in *T. b. rhodesiense* infection has not been determined. The high dosage and long duration of therapy are disadvantages that may make widespread use of eflornithine difficult.

Pentamidine isoethionate is the alternative drug for patients with stage I African trypanosomiasis, but it should be kept in mind that some *T. b. rhodesiense* infections are unresponsive to this drug. The dose for both adults and children is 4 mg/kg per day intramuscularly or intravenously for 10 days. Frequent, immediate adverse reactions include nausea, vomiting, tachycardia, and hypotension. These reactions are usually transient and do not warrant cessation of therapy. Other adverse reactions include nephrotoxicity, abnormal liver function tests, neutropenia, rashes, hypoglycemia, and sterile abscesses.

The arsenical melarsoprol is the drug of choice for therapy of East African trypanosomiasis with CNS involvement. Melarsoprol will cure both stages of the disease, and thus it is also indicated for treatment of stage I patients in whom suramin and/or pentamidine have failed or are not tolerated. However, melarsoprol should never be the first choice for therapy of stage I disease because of its relatively high toxicity. In adults the drug should be given in three courses of 3 days each. The dosage is 2 to 3.6 mg/kg per day intravenously in three divided doses for 3 days, followed 1 week later by 3.6 mg/kg per day, also in three divided doses and for 3 days. The latter course is then repeated 10 to 21 days later. In debilitated patients, 2 to 4 days of suramin treatment are administered before starting melarsoprol, and an 18-mg initial dose of the latter drug, followed by progressive increases to the standard dose, has been recommended. For children, a total of 18 to 25 mg/kg should be given over 1 month. A starting dose of 0.36 mg/kg intravenously should be increased gradually to a maximum of 3.6 mg/kg at 1- to 5-day intervals for a total of 9 to 10 doses.

Melarsoprol is highly toxic and should be administered with great care. The incidence of reactive encephalopathy has been reported to be as high as 18 percent in some series. Clinical manifestations of reactive encephalopathy include high fever, headache, tremor, impaired speech, seizures, and even coma and death. Melarsoprol should be discontinued at the first sign of encephalopathy but may be restarted cautiously with small doses a few days after the signs have resolved. Extravasation of the drug results in intense local reactions, and vomiting, abdominal pain, nephrotoxicity, and myocardial damage can occur.

The treatment for patients with stage II East African disease who cannot tolerate melarsoprol is problematic. The combination of the arsenical tryparsamide and suramin is one possible approach, but its efficacy is limited because suramin does not penetrate the CNS and tryparsamide is much less effective against *T. b. rhodesiense* than it is against *T. b. gambiense*. The dose of tryparsamide is 30 mg/kg body weight (maximum 2 g) in a single intravenous dose every 5 days for a total of 12 doses, and that for suramin is 10 mg/kg every 5 days, also for a total of 12 injections. Tryparsamide can cause encephalopathy, fever, vomiting, abdominal pain, rash, tinnitus, and a variety of ocular symptoms. Alternatively, eflornithine can be administered as outlined above to patients who cannot tolerate melarsoprol, but as noted, its effectiveness against *T. b. rhodesiense* is variable.

PREVENTION The trypanosomiases constitute complex public health and epizootic problems in Africa. Considerable progress has been made in some areas through control programs that focus on eradication of vectors and drug treatment of infected humans, but there is no consensus on the best approach to solving the overall problem. Individuals can reduce the risk of acquiring trypanosomiasis by avoiding areas known to harbor infected insects, by wearing protective clothing, and by using insect repellent. Chemoprophylaxis is not recommended, and no vaccine is available to prevent transmission of the parasites.

REFERENCES

Chagas' disease

BRENER Z: Biology of *Trypanosoma cruzi*. Annu Rev Microbiol 27:347, 1973

HAGAR JM, RAHIMTOOLA SH: Chagas' heart disease in the United States. N Engl J Med 325:763, 1991

KIRCHHOFF LV: Is *Trypanosoma cruzi* a new threat to our blood supply? Ann Intern Med 111:773, 1989

———: American trypanosomiasis (Chagas disease): A persistent problem in Latin America now affects the United States. N Engl J Med (in press)

——— et al: American trypanosomiasis (Chagas' disease) in Central American immigrants. Am J Med 82:915, 1987

——— et al: Increased specificity of serodiagnosis of Chagas' disease by detection of antibody to the 72- and 90-kilodalton glycoproteins of *Trypanosoma cruzi*. J Infect Dis 155:561, 1987

MARR JJ et al: Chemotherapy for Chagas' disease: A perspective on current therapy and considerations for future research. Rev Infect Dis 8:884, 1986

SALAZAR SCHETTINO PM et al: Chagas disease in Mexico. Parasitol Today 4:348, 1988

SCHIFFLER RJ et al: Indigenous Chagas' disease (American trypanosomiasis) in California. JAMA 251:2983, 1984

SCHMUNIS GA: *Trypanosoma cruzi*, the etiologic agent of Chagas' disease: Status in the blood supply in endemic and nonendemic countries. Transfusion 31:547, 1991

Sleeping sickness

BRYAN RT et al: African trypanosomiasis in American travelers: A 20 year review, in *International Travel Medicine*, R Steffen (ed). Berlin, Springer-Verlag, 1990

DONELSON JE et al: Molecular biology of trypanosome antigenic variation. Microbiol Rev 49:107, 1985

DOUA F et al: Treatment of human late-stage gambiense trypanosomiasis with alpha-difluoromethylornithine (eflornithine): Efficacy and tolerance in 14 cases in Cote D'Ivoire. Am J Trop Med Hyg 37:525, 1987

JORDAN AM: *Trypanosomiasis Control and African Rural Development*. London, Longmans, 1986

POLTERA AA: Pathology of human African trypanosomiasis with reference to experimental African trypanosomiasis and infections of the central nervous system. Br Med Bull 41:169, 1985

VICKERMAN K: Developmental cycles and biology of pathogenic trypanosomes. Br Med Bull 41:105, 1985

177 TOXOPLASMA INFECTION AND TOXOPLASMOSIS

LLOYD H. KASPER

DEFINITION Toxoplasmosis is the disease caused by infection with the obligate intracellular parasite *Toxoplasma gondii*. *Toxoplasma* infection refers to the presence of the parasite in the infected person. Acute *Toxoplasma* infection acquired after birth is usually asymptomatic. This condition should be distinguished from chronic *Toxoplasma* infection, which describes the persistence of tissue cysts containing parasites in clinically asymptomatic individuals. Both acute and chronic toxoplasmosis are conditions in which the parasite is responsible for the development of clinical signs and symptoms (i.e., encephalitis, myocarditis, pneumonitis). Acute toxoplasmosis in the immunocompetent host usually is self-limited, is of short duration, and results in chronic toxoplasmosis. This condition is generally asymptomatic but can result in the recrudescence of clinical signs and symptoms if the immune response is compromised. Congenital toxoplasmosis is an infection of newborns resulting from the transplacental passage of parasites from an infected mother to the fetus. These infants usually are asymptomatic at birth but later manifest a wide range of signs and symptoms, including chorioretinitis, strabismus, epilepsy, and psychomotor retardation.

ETIOLOGY *T. gondii*, is an intracellular coccidian that infects both birds and mammals. There are two distinct aspects of the life cycle of *T. gondii*: a nonfeline and a feline cycle. The nonfeline, asexual tachyzoite form of this parasite occurs within intermediate hosts such as humans, mice, sheep, and swine. *T. gondii* are able to grow in all mammalian cells except red blood cells, which they enter but do not divide in. During acute infection, parasites can be found in many organs of the body. Once the parasite attaches to and actively penetrates the host cell, it forms a parasitophorous vacuole and begins to divide by endodyogeny, a process akin to binary fission. Division time is usually 6 to 8 h for the more virulent strains. When the number of parasites within the infected cell approaches the critical mass (usually 64 to 128 in culture), the cell ruptures, releasing tachyzoites that infect adjoining cells. In this manner, an infected organ soon shows evidence of a cytopathic process. Most of the tachyzoites are eliminated by means of humoral and cell-mediated immune responses of the host. Tissue cysts containing many bradyzoites develop 7 to 10 days after the systemic tachyzoite infection. These tissue cysts occur in a variety of host organs but principally within the central nervous system (CNS) and muscle, where they may exist for the lifetime of the host. When cysts are ingested (e.g., humans eat undercooked meat products), the cyst membrane undergoes rapid digestion in the presence of acidic pH gastric secretions. In nonfeline hosts, the ingested bradyzoites enter the small intestinal epithelium and transform into rapidly dividing tachyzoites. This acute, systemic tachyzoite infection is followed by the formation of tissue cysts that contain slowly replicating bradyzoites. The development of this chronic stage completes the nonfeline cycle. Active infection in the immunocompromised host is most likely due to the spontaneous release of encysted parasites that undergo rapid transformation into tachyzoites within the CNS.

The principal life cycle of the parasite is in the cat (the definitive host) and its prey. The sexual life cycle of the parasite is defined by the formation of oocysts within the feline host. This enteroepithelial cycle begins with the ingestion of the bradyzoite tissue cysts and culminates after several intermediate stages in the production of micro- and macrogametes. The microgamete is flagellated, which allows the parasite to seek a macrogamete. Gamete fusion produces a zygote, which envelopes itself in a rigid wall and is secreted in the feces as an unsporulated oocyst. After 2 to 3 days of exposure to air at ambient temperature, the noninfectious oocyst sporulates to produce eight sporozoite progeny. The sporulated oocyst can be ingested by an intermediate host such as a pregnant woman emptying a cat's litter box, a pig rummaging in the barnyard, or perhaps a mouse. Once freed from the oocysts by digestion, the released sporozoites infect the intestinal epithelium of the nonfeline host, producing rapidly growing asexual tachyzoites and ultimately bradyzoites.

EPIDEMIOLOGY   Because of its ability to infect virtually any nucleated host cell, *T. gondii* is able to infect a wide range of mammals and birds. The seroprevalence is dependent on locale and age of the population. Generally, hot, arid climatic conditions are associated with a low prevalence of infection. In the United States and most European countries, the prevalence of seroconversion increases with age and exposure. For example, in the United States, 5 to 30 percent of individuals 10 to 19 years old and 10 to 67 percent of those over the age of 50 years show serologic evidence of prior exposure. The increase in seroprevalence is approximately 1 percent per year. In Central America, France, Turkey, and Brazil, the seroprevalence is much higher, approaching 90 percent by the time adults reach age 40.

ORAL TRANSMISSION   The principal source of transmission in human *Toxoplasma* infection remains uncertain. Transmission in acquired infection is primarily oral and can occur by ingestion of either sporulated oocysts from contaminated soil or bradyzoites from undercooked meat. During acute feline infection, a cat may excrete as many as 100 million parasites per day. About 1 percent of the cat population sheds oocysts in their feces. These very stable sporozoite-containing oocysts are highly infectious and may remain viable for many years in the soil. Humans infected during a well-documented outbreak of oocyst-transmitted infection develop stage-specific antibodies to the oocyst/sporozoite.

Children and adults also can acquire infection from tissue cysts containing bradyzoites. The ingestion of a single cyst is all that is required for human infection. Underprepared meat or insufficient freezing is an important source of infection in the developed world. In the United States, 10 to 20 percent of lamb and 25 to 35 percent of pork meat products show evidence of cysts that contain bradyzoites. The incidence in beef is much lower and may be as low as 1 percent. Direct ingestion of bradyzoite cysts in these various meat products will lead to acute infection. The recent identification of stage-specific bradyzoite antigens may allow for better determination of the source for oral transmission.

In addition to oral transmission, there is a low incidence of direct transmission of the parasite by blood or organ products during transplantation. Viable parasites can be cultured from refrigerated, anticoagulated blood and may be a source of infection in individuals receiving blood transfusions. *T. gondii* infection also has been reported to occur in kidney and heart transplant recipients who were uninfected before transplantation.

TRANSPLACENTAL TRANSMISSION   *T. gondii* can be transmitted to the fetus if the mother acquires primary infection during pregnancy. About one-third of all women infected during pregnancy will transmit the parasite to the fetus. Of the various factors that may determine fetal outcome, gestational age at the time of infection is most critical. There are few data to support a role for recrudescent maternal infection as the source of congenital disease. Thus women who are seropositive before pregnancy usually are protected against acute infection and do not give birth to congenitally infected neonates.

The following general guidelines can be used to evaluate congenital infection. There is essentially no risk if the mother is infected 6 months or more before conception. If infection occurs less than 6 months before conception, the likelihood of transplacental infection increases as the interval between infection and conception decreases. Most women infected during pregnancy give birth to normal, uninfected babies. About one-third of women infected during pregnancy will transmit the infection to their offspring. If infection occurs during the first trimester, the incidence of transplacental infection is lowest (about 15 percent), but the disease in the neonate is the most severe. If infection occurs during the third trimester, the incidence of transplacental infection is greatest (65 percent), but the infant is usually asymptomatic at birth. Recent evidence, however, suggests that those infants which are infected and normal at birth may have a higher incidence of learning disabilities and chronic neurologic sequelae than uninfected children. Only a small number of women (20 percent) infected with *T. gondii* show clinical signs of infection. Often the diagnosis is first appreciated when routine postconception serologic tests show evidence of specific antibody.

PATHOGENESIS   Upon the ingestion by the host of either tissue cysts containing bradyzoites or oocysts containing sporozoites, the parasites are released from the cyst by a digestive process. Bradyzoites are resistant to the effect of pepsin and quickly invade and multiply within the gastrointestinal tract of the host. Within the enterocytes, the parasites undergo morphologic transformation, giving rise to invasive tachyzoites. In mice, these tachyzoites are able to induce host secretory immunity, as evidenced by increased levels of parasite-specific IgA. These asexual parasites soon rupture the invaded host cell and then are disseminated to a variety of organs, particularly lymphatic tissue, skeletal muscle, myocardium, retina, placenta, and most frequently, the CNS. In these organs, the parasite infects host cells, replicates by endodyogeny, ruptures the cells, and goes on to invade the adjoining cells. In this fashion, cell death and focal necrosis surrounded by an acute inflammatory response become the hallmarks of infection. In the normal immune host, both the humoral and cellular immune responses are important in controlling infection. Tachyzoites are sequestered by a variety of immune mechanisms, including induction of parasiticidal antibody, activation of macrophages, production of interferon-γ (IFN-γ), and stimulation of cytotoxic T cells (CTLs) of the CD8+ phenotype. These antigen-specific CTLs are capable of killing both extracellular parasites and target cells infected with parasites. Once the tachyzoites are cleared from the acutely infected host, tissue cysts containing bradyzoites begin to appear, usually within the CNS and retina. A number of immune factors, including altered antibody levels within the CNS, IFN-γ, and CD4+ and CD8+ T cells, have been implicated in modulating the persistence of infection within the normal host. In the immunocompromised or fetal host, the immune factors necessary to control the spread of tachyzoite infection are lacking. This altered immune state gives rise to a progression of focal destruction that results in organ failure (i.e., necrotizing encephalitis, pneumonia, and myocarditis).

Persistence of infection in the normal host by cysts containing bradyzoites is common. This lifelong infection usually remains subclinical. Although bradyzoites are in a slow metabolic phase, degeneration and rupture of cysts do occur within the CNS. This degenerative process, with the development of new bradyzoite-containing cysts, is the most likely source of persistent antibody titers in the normal host. Degeneration of these cysts is the most probable source of recrudescent infection in immunocompromised individuals.

PATHOLOGY   Cell death and focal necrosis by replicating tachyzoites induce an intense mononuclear inflammatory response in any tissue or cell type infected. Tachyzoites rarely can be visualized by routine histopathologic staining of these inflammatory lesions. However, immunofluorescence staining with parasite antigen–specific antibodies can be positive for the organism or reveal evidence of antigenemia. In contrast to this inflammatory process caused by tachyzoites, the bradyzoite-containing cysts exhibit evidence of inflammation only at the early stages of development, perhaps in response to the presence of tachyzoite antigens. Once the cyst reaches maturity, the inflammatory process can no longer be detected, and the cysts remain immunologically quiescent within the brain matrix until they rupture.

Lymph nodes During acute infection, lymph node biopsy will demonstrate characteristic findings, including follicular hyperplasia and irregular clusters of tissue macrophages with eosinophilic cytoplasm. Granulomas rarely are seen in these specimens. Although tachyzoites are not usually observed, their presence can be assessed either by subinoculation of infected tissue into mice, with resultant disease, or by the polymerase chain reaction (PCR). PCR amplification of DNA fragments representing either the p30 (SAG-1) or p22 (SAG-2) antigens has been shown to be an effective and sensitive assay for establishing infection of lymph node tissue by tachyzoites.

Ocular In the eye, infiltrates of monocytes, lymphocytes, and plasma cells may produce uni- or multifocal lesions. Granulomatous lesions and retinochoroiditis can be observed in the posterior chamber following acute necrotizing retinitis. Other ocular complications of infection include iridocyclitis, cataracts, and glaucoma.

Central nervous system During CNS involvement, both focal and diffuse meningoencephalitis can be observed, with evidence of necrosis and microglial nodules. Necrotizing encephalitis in the patient without AIDS is characterized by small, diffuse lesions with perivascular cuffing in contiguous areas. In the AIDS population, polymorphonuclear leukocytes may be present in addition to monocytes, lymphocytes, and plasma cells. Cysts containing bradyzoites frequently are found contiguous with the necrotic tissue border. In the mouse model, parasite DNA has been detected by PCR amplification in association with reactivation of CNS toxoplasmosis.

Pulmonary Among patients with AIDS who die of toxoplasmosis, 40 to 70 percent have involvement of the heart and lung. Interstitial pneumonitis can occur in the neonate and the immunocompromised patient. Thickened and edematous alveolar septa infiltrated with mononuclear and plasma cells are observed. This inflammation may extend to the endothelial walls. Tachyzoites and bradyzoite-containing cysts have been observed within the alveolar membrane. A superimposed bronchopneumonia can be caused by other microbial agents.

Heart Cysts and aggregates of parasites in cardiac muscle tissue can be seen in patients with AIDS who die of toxoplasmosis. Focal necrosis surrounded by inflammatory cells is associated with hyaline necrosis and disrupted myocardial cells. Pericarditis is an infrequent but reported condition associated with toxoplasmosis in some patients.

Pathologic changes during disseminated infection are similar to those described for the lymph nodes, eye, and CNS. In patients with AIDS, involvement of the skeletal muscle, pancreas, stomach, and kidneys consists of necrosis, invasion by inflammatory cells, and the rare observation of tachyzoites by routine staining. Large necrotic lesions may cause direct tissue destruction. In addition, secondary effects from acute infection of these various organs, including pancreatitis, myositis, and glomerulonephritis, have been reported.

HOST IMMUNE RESPONSE Acute *Toxoplasma* infection evokes a cascade of protective immune responses in the normal host. *Toxoplasma* enter the host at the gut mucosal level and evoke the production of IgA antibody. This isotype, which constitutes more than 80 percent of all antibody in the mucosa, has now been shown to be a potentially important modulator of protection and indicator of infection. Titers of serum IgA antibody directed at p30 (SAG-1) have been shown to be useful human serum markers of congenital and acute toxoplasmosis. Milk whey IgA from acutely infected mothers shows a high titer of antibody to *T. gondii* and is able to block infection of enterocyte cells in vitro. The predominant parasite antigen recognized by the whey IgA is p30. In mice, IgA intestinal secretions directed at the parasite are abundant and associated with the induction of mucosal T cells.

If the parasite is able to evade the host mucosal response, both humoral and cellular immunity is evoked. *T. gondii* rapidly induces detectable levels of both IgM and IgG antibodies in serum. Monoclonal gammopathy of the IgG class can occur in congenital infected infants. IgM levels may be increased in the newborn with congenital infection. The polyclonal IgG antibodies evoked by infection are parasiticidal in vitro in the presence of serum complement and are the basis for the Sabin-Feldman dye test. However, cell-mediated immunity is the

major protective response evoked by the parasite during host infection. Macrophages are activated following phagocytosis of antibody-opsonized parasites. This activation can lead to death of the parasite by either an oxygen-dependent or an oxygen-independent process. In addition, T cells are activated by a variety of parasite antigens. These antigens can be either membrane-associated or cytoplasmic. The CD4+ and CD8+ T cell responses are antigen-specific and further stimulate the production of a variety of important lymphokines that expand the T cell and natural killer cell repertoire. Studies in mice indicate that INF-γ is an important factor in eliciting host immune protection against *Toxoplasma* infection. Antibody to this molecule converts an avirulent infection into a lethal one. T cells exhibiting both T_{H1} (IFN-γ) and T_{H2} (interleukin 4) have been identified during murine infection. The role of CD8+ cells appears critical to host immunity in experimental toxoplasmosis. In humans, prolonged alteration in T cell subpopulations is associated with *T. gondii* infection. Both asymptomatic patients and those with active infection may show a depression in the ratio of helper to suppressor lymphocytes. This shift may be correlated with disease syndrome but is not necessarily correlated with disease outcome. Several human T cell clones of both CD4+ and CD8+ phenotype have recently been isolated and characterized. Some of the human CD8+ T cell clones have been shown to be cytolytic against parasite-infected target cells. These T cell clones produce a wide range of cytokines, including INF-γ, interleukin 2 (IL-2), and tumor necrosis factor (TNF). In mice IL-12, a modulator of NK cells, appears to be important during acute infection by upregulating the production of IFN-γ.

In patients with AIDS, both the humoral and cellular responses to *T. gondii* are altered. Although infection in the patient with AIDS is believed to be recrudescent, determination of antibody titers is not helpful in establishing reactivation. Because of the severe depletion in CD4+ T cells, quite frequently there is no observed increase in antibody titer during exacerbation of infection. In regard to cytokines, T cells from AIDS patients with reactivation of toxoplasmosis fail to secrete both INF-γ and IL-2. This alteration in the production of these critical immune cytokines contributes to the persistence of infection. *Toxoplasma* infection frequently occurs late in the course of AIDS, when the loss of T cell–dependent protective mechanisms, particularly CD8+ T cells, becomes most pronounced.

CLINICAL MANIFESTATIONS In the person whose immune system is intact, acute toxoplasmosis is usually asymptomatic and self-limited. This condition can go unrecognized in 80 to 90 percent of adults and children with acquired infection. The asymptomatic nature of this infection makes diagnosis difficult in mothers infected during pregnancy. The wide range of clinical manifestations observed in congenitally infected children includes severe neurologic complications such as hydrocephalus, microcephaly, mental retardation, and retinochoroiditis. If prenatal infection is severe, multiorgan failure and subsequent intrauterine fetal death can occur. In children and adults, chronic infection can persist throughout life, with little consequence to the immunocompetent host.

Toxoplasmosis in the immunocompetent person The most common manifestation of acute toxoplasmosis is cervical lymphadenopathy. The nodes may be single or multiple, are usually nontender, are discrete, and vary in firmness. Lymphadenopathy also may be found in suboccipital, supraclavicular, inguinal, and mediastinal areas. Generalized lymphadenopathy occurs in 20 to 30 percent of symptomatic patients. Between 20 and 40 percent of patients with lymphadenopathy have headache, malaise, fatigue, and fever (usually <40°C). A smaller number of symptomatic individuals have myalgia, sore throat, abdominal pain, maculopapular rash, meningoencephalitis, and confusion. Rare complications associated with infection in the normal immune host include pneumonia, myocarditis, encephalopathy, pericarditis, and polymyositis. Symptoms associated with acute infection usually resolve within several weeks, although the lymphadenopathy may persist for some months. In a recent epidemic, toxoplasmosis was diagnosed correctly in only 3 of the 25 patients who consulted physicians. If toxoplasmosis is considered in the differential diagnosis, routine laboratory and serologic screening should be performed before node biopsy.

Routine laboratory studies are usually unremarkable, except for minimal lymphocytosis, elevated sedimentation rate, and nominal increase in liver transaminases. Evaluation of cerebrospinal fluid (CSF) in the patient with evidence of encephalopathy or meningoencephalitis shows an elevation of intracranial pressure, mononuclear pleocytosis (10 to 50 cells per milliliter), a slight increase in protein concentration, and occasionally an increase in the gamma globulin level. PCR amplification of the *Toxoplasma* DNA target sequence in the CSF may be beneficial. The CSF in chronically infected individuals is normal.

Ocular infection   Infection with *T. gondii* is estimated to cause 35 percent of all cases of chorioretinitis in the United States and Europe. Although most ocular involvement is believed to be due to congenital infection, there is a very low incidence following acquired infection. Individuals with AIDS also can develop debilitating chorioretinitis. A variety of ocular manifestations can be observed, including blurred vision, scotoma, photophobia, and eye pain. Macular involvement occurs with loss of central vision, and nystagmus is secondary to poor fixation. Involvement of the extraocular muscles may lead to disorders of convergence and to strabismus. Ophthalmologic examination should be undertaken in newborns with suspected congenital infection. As the inflammation resolves, vision improves, but episodic flare-ups of chorioretinitis, which progressively destroy retinal tissue and lead to glaucoma, are common.

The ophthalmologic examination will reveal lesions of yellow-white, cotton-like patches with indistinct margins of hyperemia. As the lesions age, white plaques with distinct borders and black spots within the retinal pigment become more apparent. Lesions usually are located near the posterior pole of the retina; they may be single but are more commonly multiple. Congenital lesions may be unilateral or bilateral and will show evidence of massive chorioretinal degeneration with extensive fibrosis. Surrounding these areas of involvement will be normal retina and vasculature. In patients with AIDS, retinal lesions are often large with diffuse necrosis of the retina and reveal both free tachyzoites and cysts containing bradyzoites.

Infection of the immunocompromised person   Patients with AIDS and those receiving immunosuppressive therapy for lymphoproliferative disorders are the most at risk for developing acute toxoplasmosis. This predilection may be due either to reactivation of latent infection or to acquisition of parasites from exogenous sources such as blood or transplanted organs. In individuals with AIDS, more than 95 percent of cases of *Toxoplasma* encephalitis are believed to be due to recrudescent infection. In most of these cases, encephalitis develops when the CD4+ cell count falls below 100 cells per cubic millimeter. In the immunocompromised individual, the disease may be rapidly fatal if untreated. Thus accurate diagnosis and initiation of appropriate therapy are necessary to prevent fulminant infection.

Toxoplasmosis is the major opportunistic infection of the CNS in persons with AIDS. Between 20,000 and 40,000 patients with AIDS will have developed *Toxoplasma* encephalitis by 1993. Although geographic origin may be related to frequency of infection, it has no correlation with the severity of disease in the immunocompromised host. Individuals with AIDS who are seropositive for *T. gondii* are at a very high risk for developing encephalitis. In the United States, about one-third of the 15 to 40 percent of adult patients with AIDS who are latently infected with the parasite will develop *Toxoplasma* encephalitis.

The signs and symptoms of acute toxoplasmosis in the immunocompromised patient are principally within the CNS. Over 50 percent of patients with clinical manifestations have intracerebral involvement. Clinical findings at the time of presentation can range from nonfocal to focal dysfunction. These findings include encephalopathy, meningoencephalitis, and mass lesions. Patients may present with altered mental status (75 percent), fever (10 to 72 percent), seizures (33 percent), headaches (56 percent), and focal neurologic findings (60 percent), including motor deficits, cranial nerve palsies, movement

disorders, dysmetria, visual-field loss, and aphasia. Patients who present with evidence of diffuse cortical dysfunction develop evidence of focal neurologic disease as the infection progresses. This altered condition is due not only to the necrotizing encephalitis caused by direct invasion of the parasite but also to secondary effects, including vasculitis, edema, and hemorrhage. Onset of infection can range from an insidious onset over several weeks to an acute confusional state with fulminant focal deficits, including hemiparesis, hemiplegia, visual-field defects, localized headache, and focal seizures.

Although lesions within the CNS can occur anywhere, the areas most involved appear to be the brainstem, basal ganglia, pituitary gland, and corticomedullary junction. Brainstem involvement will give rise to a variety of neurologic dysfunctions, including cranial nerve palsy, dysmetria, and ataxia. With basal ganglia infection, patients may develop hydrocephalus, choreiform movements, and choreoathetosis. Because *Toxoplasma* usually causes encephalitis, meningeal involvement is unusual, and thus CSF findings may be unremarkable or perhaps show a modest increase in cell count and protein—but not in glucose—concentration.

Cerebral toxoplasmosis needs to be differentiated from other opportunistic infections or tumors within the CNS of those afflicted with AIDS. This would include herpes simplex encephalitis, cryptococcal meningitis, progressive multifocal leukoencephalopathy, and primary CNS lymphoma. Involvement of the pituitary gland can give rise to panhypopituitarism and hyponatremia from inappropriate secretion of vasopressin (antidiuretic hormone). AIDS-dementia complex may present as cognitive impairment, attention loss, and altered memory. Brain biopsy in those patients who have been treated for *Toxoplasma* encephalitis but who continue to exhibit neurologic dysfunction often fails to identify organisms.

Autopsies of patients infected with *Toxoplasma* have demonstrated multiple organ involvement with or without CNS disease. The organs infected include the lungs, gastrointestinal tract, pancreas, skin, eyes, heart, and liver. *Toxoplasma* pneumonia can occur and can be confused with *Pneumocystis carinii* infection. Respiratory involvement usually will present as dyspnea, fever, and a nonproductive cough, which may rapidly progress to acute respiratory failure with hemoptysis, metabolic acidosis, hypotension, and occasionally disseminated intravascular coagulation. Histopathologic studies will demonstrate necrosis and a mixed cellular infiltrate. The presence of organisms is a helpful diagnostic indicator, but organisms can also be found in healthy tissue. Most commonly, myocardial infection is asymptomatic. However, infection of the heart can be associated with cardiac tamponade or biventricular failure. As discussed previously, ocular involvement can occur without concomitant encephalitis. This infection should be distinguished from chorioretinitis caused by cytomegalovirus, which is usually more hemorrhagic in character. Toxoplasmic retinochoroiditis may be a prodrome to the development of encephalitis.

A presumptive clinical diagnosis of toxoplasmic encephalitis in patients with AIDS is based on clinical presentation, history of exposure as evidenced by positive serology, and radiologic evaluation. When these criteria are used, the predictive value is as high as 80 percent. More than 97 percent of patients with AIDS and toxoplasmosis have IgG antibody to the parasite in their sera. IgM serum antibody is usually not demonstrable. Intrathecal antibody to *T. gondii* may be present. Neuroradiologic evaluation should include a double-dose contrast computed tomographic (CT) scan of the head. By this test, single and frequently multiple contrast-enhancing lesions (<2 cm) may be identified. Magnetic resonance imaging (MRI) usually will demonstrate multiple lesions and will provide a more sensitive evaluation of efficacy of therapy. Patients with primary CNS lymphoma are four times more likely than patients with *Toxoplasma* encephalitis to have solitary lesions on an MRI scan. A therapeutic trial of anti-*Toxoplasma* medications frequently is used to assess the diagnosis. Recent studies have shown that treatment of presumptive *Toxoplasma* encephalitis with pyrimethamine-clindamycin results in a quantifiable clinical improvement in more than 50 percent of patients by day 3. By day 7, over 90 percent of patients successfully treated show evidence of improvement. In contrast, if patients fail to respond or have lymphoma, clinical signs and symptoms worsen by day 7. Thus patients in this category require brain biopsy with or without a change in therapy. This procedure can now be performed by a stereotactic CT-guided method that can reduce potential complications. Brain biopsy for the presence of *T. gondii* identifies organisms in 50 to 75 percent of cases. More recent studies indicate that PCR amplification of target genes significantly increases the sensitivity for detection of parasites.

DIAGNOSIS Tissue and body fluid The diagnosis of acute toxoplasmosis can be made by isolation of the parasite from either blood or other body fluids after subinoculation of the body fluid into the peritoneal cavity of mice. Mice should be tested for organisms in the peritoneal fluid 6 to 10 days postinfection. If no parasites are found in the mouse's peritoneal fluid, its anti-*Toxoplasma* serum titer can be evaluated 4 to 6 weeks following inoculation. Isolation of *T. gondii* from the patient's body fluids reflects acute infection, whereas isolation from biopsy tissue is an indication only of the presence of tissue cysts and should not be misinterpreted as acute toxoplasmosis. Persistent parasitemia in patients with latent, asymptomatic infection is rare. Histologic examination of lymph nodes may suggest the characteristic changes described above. Demonstration of tachyzoites in lymph nodes will establish the diagnosis of acute toxoplasmosis. As with subinoculation into mice, demonstration of cysts containing bradyzoites in histologic specimens confirms only prior infection with *T. gondii* but is nondiagnostic for acute infection.

Serology The preceding procedures have great diagnostic value but are limited because of the difficulty either in growing parasites in vivo or in identifying tachyzoites by histochemical methods. Serologic diagnosis has become the routine method. A wide range of serologic tests that can be used to measure antibody to *T. gondii* are available commercially. The reader is referred to the excellent review by Remington and McLeod discussing the various serologic tests currently available.

Diagnosis of acute infection with *T. gondii* can be established by determining the simultaneous presence of IgG and IgM antibody to *Toxoplasma* in the patient. The presence of circulating IgA favors the diagnosis of an acute infection. The Sabin-Feldman dye test, indirect fluorescent antibody test (IFA), and enzyme linked immunoassay (ELISA) all satisfactorily measure the presence of circulating IgG antibody to *Toxoplasma*. Positive IgG titers (>1:10) can be detected as early as 2 to 3 weeks after infection. These titers usually peak at 6 to 8 weeks and slowly decline to a new baseline, which remains elevated for life. It is necessary to obtain a serum IgM titer in concert with the IgG titer to better establish the time of infection. The methods currently available for this determination are the double-sandwich ELISA-IgM and the IgM-immunosorbent assay (IgM-ISAGA). Both these assays are specific, sensitive, and avoid false-positive results associated with rheumatoid factor and antinuclear antibody. The double-sandwich IgA-ELISA is more sensitive than the IgM-ELISA for detecting congenital infection in the fetus and newborn.

The immunocompetent adult or child For the patient who presents with lymphadenopathy only, a positive IgM titer is an indication of acute infection and for therapy if that is clinically warranted (see "Treatment," below). The serum titer should be determined again in 3 weeks. An elevation in the IgG titer without an increase in the IgM titer suggests that infection is present, but that it is not acute. If there is a borderline increase in either IgG or IgM, the titers should be assessed again in 3 to 4 weeks.

Ocular toxoplasmosis Because of the congenital nature of this infection, the serum titer may not correlate with presence of active lesions in the fundus. In general, if there is a positive IgG titer (on undiluted serum if necessary) and typical lesions, the diagnosis is established. If lesions are atypical and the titer is in the low-positive range, the diagnosis is presumptive.

Immunocompromised host As discussed above, in patients with AIDS, the presence of IgG and radiologic findings consistent with toxoplasmosis determine a presumptive diagnosis. Evaluation of rising IgG titers or attempts at identifying whether IgM is present are unreliable. Serologic evidence of infection is present in virtually all patients before they develop *Toxoplasma* encephalitis. It is therefore important to determine antibody status in all HIV-infected patients. Antibody titers may range from negative to 1:1024 in patients with AIDS and *Toxoplasma* encephalitis. Fewer than 3 percent of patients have no demonstrable antibody to *Toxoplasma* at the time of diagnosis. Determination of intrathecal antibody titer may be useful in identifying prior infection. PCR amplification of genetic material of the parasite found within the CSF may prove beneficial in the future.

Patients with toxoplasmic encephalitis will have focal or multifocal abnormalities demonstrable on CT or MRI scan. These findings are not pathognomonic of *Toxoplasma* infection since 40 percent of CNS lymphomas are multifocal and 50 percent are ring-enhancing. Lesions on CT scan are multiple and located in both hemispheres, with the basal ganglia and corticomedullary junction most commonly involved. A CT scan may underestimate the degree of inflammation during early disease. Double-dose contrast enhancement may increase the sensitivity of diagnosis. For both MRI and CT scans, the rate of false-negative results is approximately 10 percent. The finding of a single lesion on an MRI scan increases the suspicion of primary lymphoma and strengthens the argument for performing a brain biopsy. An MRI should be performed if the CT scan shows only a single lesion. CT and MRI scans are important for the assessment of response to therapy. As with other conditions, the radiologic response may lag behind the clinical response. Resolution of lesions may take from 3 weeks to 6 months. Some patients may show clinical improvement in the presence of worsening radiographic findings.

A presumptive diagnosis of *Toxoplasma* encephalitis should initiate prompt therapy. Patients should be monitored for neurologic deterioration during the first 7 days. After this time, successful therapy should result in stabilization or improvement in clinical status. After 3 weeks, repeat radiologic studies should identify improvement. If glucocorticoids have been administered, radiologic studies should be repeated at the time of discontinuation to determine if exacerbation of disease has occurred. If the patient's clinical conditions becomes worse, performance of a biopsy must be a strong consideration.

Congenital infection Serologic diagnosis of acute toxoplasmosis in the neonate is based either on persistence of IgG antibody or on a positive IgM titer (after the first week to exclude the possibility of placental leak). The determination of IgG titer should be repeated every 6 to 12 weeks to establish the pattern of response. An increase in IgM titer that extends beyond the first week is indicative of acute infection (the half-life of maternal IgM is 3 to 5 days).

TREATMENT Immunologically competent adults and older children who have only lymphadenopathy do not require specific therapy unless they have persistent and severe symptoms. Because of the high virulence of *Toxoplasma* strains used in the laboratory, it is advisable to treat patients with laboratory acquired infections. Patients with ocular toxoplasmosis should be treated for 1 month with sulfadiazine and pyramethamine. A large percentage of patients with chorioretinitis have shown clinical improvement. The alternative therapeutic agents for patients with ocular involvement include a combination of clindamycin and pyrimethamine.

Patients with AIDS should be treated for acute toxoplasmosis. Current therapeutic protocols are directed at folate metabolism, protein synthesis, or nucleic acid synthesis of the parasite. Pyrimethamine and trimethoprim are directed at the enzyme dihydrofolate reductase. The gene encoding this molecule has been cloned recently and expressed in vitro, making rational development of other folate inhibitors feasible. Inhibitors of protein synthesis, including clindamycin, chlortetracycline, and azithromycin, have been shown to affect growth of the parasite. Inhibitors of purine synthesis, such as arprinocid, may prove to be important. The antimicrobial agent hydroxynaphthoquinone (BW566C80), which blocks pyrimidine salvage, has demonstrated potent toxoplasmacidal activity against both the tachyzoite and cyst.

In the immunocompromised patient, toxoplasmosis is rapidly fatal if untreated. The mainstay of treatment for *Toxoplasma* encephalitis is combination therapy. Pyrimethamine and sulfadiazine administered together block folic acid metabolism and successfully reduce the parasite burden. Folinic acid (leucovorin) is given as an adjunct to prevent the bone marrow toxicity associated with pyrimethamine. Both pyrimethamine and sulfadiazine cross the blood-brain barrier. A major consequence of dual therapy is the high incidence of associated toxicity (40 percent). Rash may occur during the first 3 weeks in up to 20 percent of patients but does not preclude the use of this combination. Other complications include hematologic effects, crystalluria, hematuria, radiolucent renal stones, and nephrotoxicity. During therapy, serum levels of these drugs may be erratic, but such fluctuations have not been correlated with these potential complications. The current medication regimen includes pyrimethamine, a 200-mg loading dose followed by 50 to 75 mg/d, plus sulfadiazine, 4 to 6 g/d in four divided doses. In addition, the administration of calcium folinate, 10 to 15 mg/d for 6 weeks, is required. These agents are active only against the tachyzoite stage of the parasite. Thus, after these patients complete the initial course (4 to 6 weeks or until the radiologic improvement), they must receive lifelong suppressive therapy with pyramethamine (25 to 50 mg) and sulfadiazine (2 to 4 g). If sulfadiazine cannot be tolerated, a combination of pyrimethamine (75 mg/d) plus clindamycin (450 mg tid) can be used. It is possible that pyrimethamine (50 to 75 mg/d) is sufficient for chronic suppressive therapy. Congenitally infected neonates are treated with oral pyrimethamine (0.5 to 1 mg/kg) and sulfadiazine (100 mg/kg). In addition, therapy with spiramycin (100 mg/kg) plus prednisone (1 mg/kg) has been shown to be efficacious for congenital infection.

Alternative therapies have been established because of the toxicity associated with the long-term antimicrobial therapy necessary for many individuals infected with *T. gondii*. Although effective in animal models, trimethoprim-sulfamethoxazole has not yet been fully established as beneficial for humans. Dapsone (diamino-diphenyl sulfone) is a potent sulfone effective against murine toxoplasmosis. As with pyrimethamine, dapsone has no effect on the tissue cyst. Dapsone, because of its longer serum half-life and decreased toxicity, may be an effective alternative to sulfadiazine. Spiramycin has been used in Europe to treat pregnant women. Presumably, this medication is able to reduce transplacental transmission, although supporting evidence is not yet conclusive. Spiramycin has been ineffective as primary prophylaxis in patients with AIDS. Clindamycin is effective in treating murine toxoplasmosis. It is well absorbed from the gastrointestinal tract, and peak serum levels occur 1 to 2 h after administration. Recent data suggest that the combination of oral pyrimethamine (25 to 75 mg/d) plus intravenous clindamycin (1200 to 4800 mg/d) is effective in treating patients with AIDS who have *Toxoplasma* encephalitis. It is not clear if this treatment regimen is superior to that of pyrimethamine and sulfadiazine. Toxic effects from clindamycin include nausea, vomiting, neutropenia, rash, and pseudomembranous colitis. Macrolides in addition to spiramycin that have been evaluated in the murine system include roxithromycin, clarithromycin, and azithromycin. A combination of pyrimethamine and clarithromycin appears to be effective in a small number of patients evaluated to date. There is no evidence suggesting that the macrolides are beneficial by themselves. The agent hydroxynaphthoquinone (BW566C80) may be effective against the cysts containing bradyzoites and has sustained prolonged remission of the disease in an experimental model. Glucocorticoids can be used to treat intracerebral edema, but their benefit is not yet established. It is difficult to assess the benefit of glucocorticoids when they are administered in conjunction with anti-*Toxoplasma* medication. Anticonvulsants are sometimes necessary for treatment of seizures, but attention should be given to the potential interaction between sulfadiazine and phenytoin. There is currently no indication for primary prophylactic treatment in those who are seropositive for *T. gondii* and are at risk of developing *Toxoplasma* encephalitis.

PREVENTION Primary infection with *Toxoplasma* can be reduced by not eating undercooked meat and by avoiding oocyst-contaminated material (i.e., the cat's litter box). Meat should be heated to 60°C or frozen to kill cysts. Hands should be washed thoroughly after work in the garden, and all fruits and vegetables should be washed. Blood intended for transfusion into seronegative immunocompromised individuals should be screened for antibody to *T. gondii*. Although such serologic screening is not routinely performed, seronegative women should be screened for evidence of infection several times during pregnancy if they are exposed to environmental conditions that put them at risk for infection with *T. gondii*.

REFERENCES

BROOKS RG et al: Role of serology in the diagnosis of toxoplasmic lymphadenopathy. Rev Infect Dis 9:1055, 1987

BURG JL et al: Direct and sensitive detection of a pathogenic protozoan, *Toxoplasma gondii*, by polymerase chain reaction. J Clin Microbiol 27:1787, 1989

DAFFOS F et al: Prenatal management of 746 pregnancies at risk for congenital toxoplasmosis. N Engl J Med 318:271, 1988

DECOSTER A et al: IgA antibodies against P30 as markers of congenital and acute toxoplasmosis. Lancet 2:1104, 1988

GROVER CM et al: Rapid prenatal diagnosis of congenital *Toxoplasma* infection by using polymerase chain reaction and amniotic fluid. J Clin Microbiol 10:2297, 1990

KASPER LH et al: Antigen-specific (p30) mouse CD8+ T cells are cytotoxic against *Toxoplasma gondii*–infected peritoneal macrophages. J Immunol 148:1493, 1992

KHAN IA et al: Induction of antigen-specific human cytotoxic T cells by *Toxoplasma gondii*. J Clin Invest 85:1879, 1990

LUFT BJ, REMINGTON JS: Toxoplasmic encephalitis in AIDS. Clin Infect Dis 15:211, 1992

MCCABE RE, REMINGTON JS: Toxoplasmosis: The time has come. N Engl J Med 318:313, 1988

MACK DG, MCLEOD R: Human *Toxoplasma gondii*–specific secretory immunoglobulin A reduces *T. gondii* infection of enterocytes in vitro. J Clin Invest 90:2585, 1992

Prophylaxis for toxoplasma encephalitis. Infect Dis Alert 11:164, 1992

REMINGTON JS, MCLEOD R: Toxoplasmosis, in *Infectious Diseases in Medicine and Surgery*, J Bartlett, S Gorbach, N Blacklow (eds). Philadelphia, Saunders, 1992

178   PNEUMOCYSTIS CARINII PNEUMONIA

PETER D. WALZER

DEFINITION *Pneumocystis carinii* is an opportunistic pathogen whose natural habitat is the lung. The organism is an important cause of pneumonia in the compromised host.

The taxonomy of *P. carinii* has long been controversial; however, recent studies favor placement in the fungal kingdom. Analysis of gene sequences of ribosomal RNA, mitochondrial proteins, and major enzymes (thymidylate synthase, dihydrofolate reductase) has demonstrated that *P. carinii* is more closely related to fungi than to protozoa. Biochemical studies have suggested that the cell wall of *P. carinii* contains glucans; drugs which inhibit 1,3-β-glucan synthesis in fungi are highly active against *P. carinii* in animal models.

ETIOLOGY Knowledge of the basic biology of *P. carinii* has been severely hampered by the lack of a reliable in vitro cultivation system. Major developmental stages of the organism include the small (1- to 4-μm) pleomorphic trophozoite or trophic form; the 5- to 8-μm cyst, which has a thick cell wall and contains up to eight intracystic bodies; and the precyst, an intermediate stage. The life cycle of *P. carinii* probably involves asexual replication by the trophic form and sexual reproduction by the cyst which ends in release of the intracystic bodies; an intracellular stage has not been identified. Ultrastructurally, *P. carinii* has a primitive organelle system, but little is known about its metabolism.

P. carinii has two major groups of antigens: a 110- to 120-kDa surface glycoprotein (gp120), which appears to mediate adherence to host cells, and a moiety of 35 to 45 kDa in human-derived and of 45 to 55 kDa in rat-derived organisms, respectively, which is the antigen most commonly recognized by the host.

EPIDEMIOLOGY *P. carinii* has a worldwide distribution among humans and has been found in a variety of animals. Organisms for these hosts are morphologically identical, but species or strain differences exist. Data about the fungal nature of *P. carinii* raise intriguing questions about new developmental stages and environmental sources of the organism. Serologic surveys indicate that most normal children have been exposed to the organism by 3 to 4 years of age. Animal model experiments have demonstrated that *P. carinii* is transmitted by the airborne route. Human-to-human transmission has been suggested by the occurrence of outbreaks of pneumocystosis among institutionalized debilitated infants and in hospitals caring for immunosuppressed patients. On the basis of animal studies, the incubation period is thought to be 4 to 8 weeks.

PATHOGENESIS AND PATHOLOGY *P. carinii* pneumonia occurs in the following hosts: premature, malnourished infants; children with primary immunodeficiency diseases; patients receiving immunosuppressive therapy (particularly corticosteroids) for cancer, organ transplantation, and other disorders; and people with AIDS. Pneumocystosis is a leading opportunistic infection and cause of death in AIDS patients in the United States and other industrialized countries, but it is less common in AIDS patients in tropical and developing countries. The reasons for this difference are unclear but may relate to the occurrence of more virulent infections (e.g., tuberculosis) in populations from the developing world.

The major host factor which predisposes to *P. carinii* pneumonia is impaired cellular immunity. The incidence of pneumocystosis among HIV patients can be correlated with the number of circulating CD4 cells. However, there is increasing evidence that antibodies also play a role in host defenses against this organism. It is generally thought that *P. carinii* pneumonia develops by reactivation of latent infection with immunosuppressive drugs or progressive breakdown of the immune system in AIDS. An alternative view is that the host is periodically exposed to new sources of *P. carinii*. Resolution of this argument awaits the development of better markers of the organism.

Within the lung, *P. carinii* attaches firmly to the alveolar type I pneumocyte. In vitro studies suggest several possible mechanisms of adherence to host cells, including the binding of gp120 to fibronectin or to mannose receptors. Animal models have shown that *P. carinii* organisms propagate slowly, gradually filling the alveoli; this phenomenon is accompanied by a series of complex changes in the microenvironment, such as increased alveolar-capillary permeability and alterations in surfactant constituents, which culminate in damage to the type I cell.

On hematoxylin and eosin–stained lung sections, the alveoli are filled with the typical foamy, vacuolated exudate. With severe disease there may be interstitial edema, fibrosis, and hyaline membrane formation. The host inflammatory changes usually consist of hypertrophy of alveolar type II cells, a typical reparative response, and a mild mononuclear cell interstitial infiltrate. Malnourished infants display an intense plasma cell infiltrate which gave the disease its early name of "interstitial plasma cell pneumonia."

CLINICAL FEATURES Patients with *P. carinii* pneumonia complain of dyspnea, fever, and nonproductive cough. Symptoms in non-AIDS patients often begin after the glucocorticoid dose has been tapered and typically last 1 to 2 weeks. AIDS patients are usually ill for several weeks or longer and have more subtle manifestations. However, the clinical picture in individual patients is quite variable, and thus a high index of suspicion and careful history are key features to early detection.

Physical findings include tachypnea, tachycardia, and cyanosis, but lung auscultation reveals few abnormalities. The white blood count is variable and usually governed by the patient's underlying disease. Arterial blood gases demonstrate hypoxia, increased alveolar-arterial oxygen gradient ($PA_{O_2} - Pa_{O_2}$), and respiratory alkalosis.

There also may be changes in pulmonary function tests (diffusing capacity) and increased uptake with nuclear imaging techniques (gallium scan). Elevated serum lactate dehydrogenase (LDH) has been reported, probably reflecting lung parenchymal damage, but is not specific for *P. carinii*. In general, the laboratory abnormalities are less severe in AIDS patients.

The classic findings on chest radiograph consist of bilateral diffuse infiltrates beginning in the perihilar regions, but a variety of atypical manifestations (nodular densities, cavitary lesions) also have been reported. Patients who receive aerosol pentamidine have an increased frequency of upper lobe infiltrates and pneumothorax. Early in the course of pneumocystosis, the chest radiograph may be normal.

DIAGNOSIS Since the clinical picture of *P. carinii* can be produced by many different infectious and noninfectious agents, diagnosis must be made by specific identification of the organism. Definitive diagnosis is made by histopathologic staining. Traditional stains have included reagents (methenamine silver, toluidine blue, cresyl echt violet) which selectively stain the wall of *P. carinii* cysts and reagents (Wright-Giemsa) which stain the nuclei of all developmental stages. Immunofluorescence and immunoperoxidase staining, which are somewhat more sensitive, have gained in popularity as monoclonal antibodies to *P. carinii* became commercially available. Other reagents include nonspecific fluorochrome stains (calofluor white) and the Papanicolaou stain. Selection of these staining techniques is largely a matter of personal preference; frequently, more than one reagent is used to make the diagnosis. Molecular probes and the polymerase chain reaction offer promise in *P. carinii* diagnosis, but little progress has been made with culture or antigen and antibody detection techniques.

Successful diagnosis of pneumocystosis requires an aggressive approach to obtain proper specimens. In general, the yield from different diagnostic procedures is higher in AIDS patients than in non-AIDS patients; this probably reflects the higher organism burden in people with AIDS. In recent years, induced sputum has gained popularity as a simple, noninvasive technique; this procedure requires trained and dedicated personnel, and success in using it has varied at different institutions. Fiberoptic bronchoscopy with bronchoalveolar lavage (BAL), which is more sensitive and invasive than induced sputum, is the mainstay of *P. carinii* diagnosis. This procedure provides information about the organism burden, host inflammatory response, and the presence of other opportunistic infections. Transbronchial biopsy and open lung biopsy, which are the most invasive procedures, are reserved for situations when a diagnosis cannot be made by lavage.

COURSE AND PROGNOSIS Although *P. carinii* usually remains confined to the lungs, cases of disseminated infection have occurred in AIDS and non-AIDS patients. Estimates of the frequency of extrapulmonary pneumocystosis have ranged from <1 to 3 percent in different series. One risk factor in HIV patients appears to be the administration of aerosol pentamidine. The most common sites of involvement have been lymph nodes, liver, spleen, and bone marrow. Disseminated *P. carinii* infection can occur without clinical evidence of pneumonia.

In the typical case of untreated *P. carinii* pneumonia, there is progressive respiratory embarrassment leading to death. Therapy is most effective when instituted early in the course of the disease, before there is extensive alveolar damage. The most widely used prognostic indicators have been the arterial oxygen pressure and alveolar-arterial oxygen gradient. Other factors which may influence survival include the organism burden, percentage of neutrophils in BAL fluid, chest radiograph abnormalities, serum LDH and albumin levels, and the expertise of the hospital in caring for AIDS patients. Concurrent pulmonary infections also complicate management, but the presence of cytomegalovirus does not affect the outcome of pneumocystosis.

TREATMENT The two major drugs used in the treatment of *P. carinii* pneumonia have been trimethoprim-sulfamethoxazole (TMP-SMX) and pentamidine isethionate. These agents are equally effective, with an overall success rate of 70 to 80 percent. TMP-SMX acts by inhibiting folic acid synthesis, but the mode of action of pentamidine against *P. carinii* is unclear. TMP-SMX is administered orally or intravenously in a dose of 15 to 20 mg/kg per day TMP and 75 to 100 mg/kg per day SMX in three or four divided doses. Pentamidine is given as a single dose of 4 mg/kg per day by slow intravenous infusion; a lower (3 mg/kg per day) dose has been used to treat milder forms of pneumocystosis in limited studies and causes fewer adverse effects. Aerosol pentamidine is not as effective as the parenteral drug and cannot be recommended for therapy. The duration of treatment is 14 days in non-AIDS patients and 21 days for persons with AIDS. Since AIDS patients usually respond more slowly to therapy than non-AIDS patients, it is prudent to wait at least 7 days before switching these individuals to another drug. The combination of TMP-SMX and pentamidine is no more effective than either agent used alone.

TMP-SMX is well tolerated by non-AIDS patients, but over half of the AIDS patients experience serious adverse reactions, including fever, rash, neutropenia, thrombocytopenia, and hepatitis. Pentamidine is a toxic drug for all recipients; major side effects include cardiovascular abnormalities, dysglycemias, azotemia, neutropenia, and sterile abscesses if intramuscular injection is used.

There are several promising alternative regimens. The combination of TMP and dapsone appears to be as effective as TMP-SMX in milder forms of pneumocystosis and causes fewer adverse effects. Clindamycin and primaquine have been helpful in patients who cannot tolerate sulfonamides. Other agents undergoing clinical evaluation include trimetrexate, an inhibitor of *P. carinii* dihydrofolate reductase; 566C80, a hydroxynaphthoquinone; and eflornithine, a polyamine inhibitor.

There is increasing evidence that the host's inflammatory or immune response contributes to the lung damage in *P. carinii* pneumonia, but the mechanisms involved are poorly understood. Several studies have shown that the administration of corticosteroids to AIDS patients with moderate to severe pneumocystosis (i.e., $P_{O_2} \leq 70$ mmHg or $P_{A_{O_2}} - P_{a_{O_2}} \geq 35$ mmHg) can prevent the early deterioration in respiratory function which frequently occurs after antimicrobial therapy and improve survival. The steroids should be started early in the course of the illness (usually when antimicrobial drugs are begun) to achieve the maximum benefit; the recommended dose is prednisone 40 mg orally twice daily, tapering to a dose of 20 mg/d over a 3-week period. This regimen has generally proven to be safe, but there is concern about its effects on other opportunistic infections and Kaposi's sarcoma. The use of steroids as adjunctive therapy in non-AIDS patients remains to be evaluated.

Other important supportive measures include maintaining adequate oxygenation, nutrition, and fluid and electrolyte balance. The use of mechanical ventilation and intensive care in *P. carinii* patients with respiratory failure was once considered controversial; however, the improved survival in recent years with these measures has encouraged their use.

PREVENTION   People with AIDS who recover from pneumocystosis commonly experience recurrent episodes of the disease. Recurrences are less frequent among non-AIDS patients but can occur as long as the underlying immunosuppressive conditions persist. Some of these recurrences are probably due to relapse of *P. carinii* pneumonia, and patients with large numbers of organisms in BAL fluid following therapy appear to be at increased risk. Other recurrent episodes may represent new *P. carinii* infection. TMP-SMX and aerosol pentamidine have been the most widely used drugs to prevent these recurrences (i.e., secondary prophylaxis); recent data have demonstrated the superiority of TMP-SMX in terms of effectiveness and cost. The recommended dose of TMP-SMX is one double-strength tablet (160 mg TMP, 800 mg SMX) per day, although other dose regimens also may be effective. The major limitation of TMP-SMX is the high frequency of adverse effects in AIDS patients. The dose schedules of aerosol pentamidine vary among manufacturers; the most common regimen is a monthly dose of 300 mg administered

in a Respirgard II nebulizer. Problems associated with aerosol pentamidine include bronchospasm and increased risk of spreading pulmonary tuberculosis.

Primary prophylaxis of *P. carinii* pneumonia is indicated for HIV patients at high risk of developing the disease: persons with CD4 counts less than 200 cells per cubic millimeter or the presence of constitutional symptoms such as thrush or prolonged fever of unknown cause. Drug recommendations are the same as for secondary prophylaxis, and all agents should be continued for life. Since *P. carinii* is communicable, it is prudent to separate patients with pneumocystosis from direct contact with other susceptible hosts.

REFERENCES

COLANGELO G et al: Follow-up bronchoalveolar lavage in AIDS patients with *Pneumocystis carinii* pneumonia. Am Rev Respir Dis 143:1067, 1991

CUSHION MT et al: Cellular and molecular biology of *Pneumocystis carinii* pneumonia. Int Rev Cytol 131:59, 1991

DAVEY RT JR, MASUR H: Recent advances in the diagnosis, treatment, and prevention of *Pneumocystis carinii* pneumonia. Antimicrob Agents Chemother 34:499, 1990

LEVINE SJ et al: Effect of aerosolized pentamidine prophylaxis on the diagnosis of *Pneumocystis carinii* pneumonia by induced sputum examination in patients infected with the human immunodeficiency virus. Am Rev Respir Dis 144:760, 1991

LUNDGREN B et al: Antibody responses to a major *Pneumocystis carinii* antigen in HIV infected patients with and without *P. carinii* pneumonia. J Infect Dis 165:1151, 1992

MEDINA I et al: Oral therapy for *Pneumocystis carinii* in the acquired immunodeficiency syndrome. N Engl J Med 323:776, 1990

NATIONAL INSTITUTES OF HEALTH–UNIVERSITY OF CALIFORNIA EXPERT PANEL FOR CORTICOSTEROIDS AS ADJUNCTIVE THERAPY FOR PNEUMOCYSTIS PNEUMONIA: Consensus statement on the use of corticosteroids as adjunctive therapy for *Pneumocystis* pneumonia in the acquired immunodeficiency syndrome. N Engl J Med 323:1500, 1990

PEGLOW SL et al: Serologic responses to *Pneumocystis carinii* antigens in health and disease. J Infect Dis 161:296, 1990

PHAIR J et al: The risk of *Pneumocystis carinii* pneumonia among men infected with human immunodeficiency virus type 1. N Engl J Med 322:161, 1990

POTTRATZ ST et al: *Pneumocystis carinii* attachment to cultured lung cells by pneumocystis gp120, a fibronectin binding protein. J Clin Invest 88:403, 1991

ROTHS JB, SIDMAN CL: Immunity and hyperresponsiveness to *Pneumocystis carinii* resulting from CD4+ but not CD8+ cells. J Clin Invest 90:673, 1992

SMULIAN AG et al: Isolation and characterization of a recombinant antigen of *Pneumocystis carinii*. Infect Immun 60:907, 1992

TELZAK EE et al: Extrapulmonary *Pneumocystis carinii* infections. Rev Infect Dis 12:380, 1990

U.S. PUBLIC HEALTH SERVICE TASK FORCE ON ANTIPNEUMOCYSTIS PROPHYLAXIS IN PATIENTS WITH HUMAN IMMUNODEFICIENCY VIRUS INFECTION: Guidelines for prophylaxis against *Pneumocystis carinii* for persons infected with human immunodeficiency virus. Morb Mort Week Rep 41(no. RR-4):1, 1992

WACHTER RM et al: *Pneumocystis carinii* pneumonia and respiratory failure in AIDS. Am Rev Respir Dis 143:251, 1991

WAKEFIELD AE et al: Detection of *Pneumocystis carinii* with DNA amplification. Lancet 336:451, 1990

WALZER PD: Immunopathogenesis of *Pneumocystis carinii* infection. J Lab Clin Med 118:206, 1991

179   PROTOZOAL INTESTINAL INFECTIONS: GIARDIASIS, CRYPTOSPORIDIOSIS, TRICHOMONIASIS, AND OTHERS

THEODORE E. NASH / PETER F. WELLER

GIARDIASIS   *Giardia lamblia* is a cosmopolitan protozoal parasite that inhabits the small intestines of humans and other mammals. Giardiasis is one of the most common parasitic diseases worldwide and causes both endemic and epidemic intestinal disease and diarrhea.

Life cycle and epidemiology   Infection occurs following ingestion of environmentally hardy cysts that excyst in the small intestine, releasing trophozoites which multiply by binary fission, occasionally to enormous numbers. *Giardia* remains a proximal small bowel pathogen and does not disseminate hematogenously. Trophozoites are present within the lumen or are attached to the mucosal epithelium by means of a ventral sucking disk and only rarely have been detected below the intestinal mucosa. As a trophozoite encounters unfavorable or altered conditions, such as changes in pH, osmolality, and bile salt concentration, it forms a morphologically distinct cyst, which is the stage of the parasite usually found in the feces. In loose or watery stools, trophozoites may be present and even predominate, but it is the resistant cyst that survives outside the body and is responsible for transmission. Cysts do not tolerate heating, desiccation, or continued exposure to feces but do remain viable for months in cold fresh water. The number of cysts excreted varies widely but can approach 10^7 cysts per gram of stool.

Giardia infections are common in both developed and developing countries because enormous numbers of cysts are excreted, which contaminates both the environment and close personal contacts. Transmission is facilitated because ingestion of a small number of cysts, even as few as 10, is sufficient to cause infection in humans. Because cysts are infectious when excreted or shortly thereafter, person-to-person transmission occurs in settings with poor fecal hygiene. Giardiasis, as a symptomatic or asymptomatic infection, is especially prevalent in day-care centers; person-to-person spread also occurs in other institutional settings with poor fecal hygiene and between homosexuals. If food is contaminated with *Giardia* cysts after cooking or preparation, food-borne transmission can occur, although it has been documented infrequently. Waterborne transmission accounts for episodic infections, as occur in backpackers and travelers, and massive epidemics in metropolitan settings. Surface water, ranging from mountain streams to large municipal reservoirs, is at risk of contamination with fecally derived *Giardia* cysts; such contamination also can occur in older or outmoded water systems due to cross-contamination from leaking sewer lines. The efficacy of water as a means of transmission is enhanced by *Giardia*'s low infectious inoculum, the prolonged survival of cysts in cold water, and the resistance of cysts to killing by routine chlorination methods adequate for controlling bacteria. Viable cysts can be eradicated from water by either boiling or filtration. In the United States, *Giardia* is the most common agent identified in waterborne epidemics of gastroenteritis. Although prevalences in unselected populations throughout the United States are not available, cross-sectional studies in selected populations show prevalences from a few tenths of a percent to 50 percent or higher. In developing countries, infections can be extremely common, with cumulative rates of infection close to 100 percent by 2 years of age and prevalences of 20 to 30 percent or higher in adults.

The importance of animal reservoirs as sources of infection for humans is unclear. *Giardia* parasites morphologically similar to those in humans are found in a large number of mammals, including beavers from reservoirs implicated in epidemics, dogs, cats, and ruminants. Although the high degree of isolate heterogeneity noted in humans is consistent with infections originating from different animal sources, animals have not been directly established as sources of human infection.

Giardiasis creates a significant economic burden because water purification systems that employ filtration are required to prevent waterborne epidemics. There are also the costs of epidemics which involve large communities and costs associated with evaluation and treatment of endemic infections. In the United States, giardiasis results in about the same number of hospitalizations as shigellosis.

Pathophysiology The reasons why some, but not all, infected patients develop clinical manifestations and the mechanisms by which this parasite causes alterations in small bowel function are largely unknown. While trophozoites adhere to the epithelium, they do not cause invasive or locally destructive alterations. The development of lactose intolerance and the significant malabsorption that develops in a minority of infected adults or children are clinical signs of the loss of brush border enzyme activities. In most infections, the morphology of the bowel is unaltered, but in a few, usually chronically infected symptomatic patients, the histopathologic findings and clinical mani-

festations resemble those of tropical sprue and gluten-sensitive enteropathy. The villi are flattened, and varying inflammation is found in the lamina propria. The pathogenesis of diarrhea in giardiasis is not known.

The natural history of *Giardia* infection is not well defined and varies markedly. Infections may be aborted, transient, recurrent, or chronic. Both parasite and host factors may be important in determining the course of infection and disease. Protective immunity has not been demonstrated conclusively in humans, although it occurs in experimental infections. Both cellular and humoral responses develop in human infections, but their precise roles in the control of infection and/or disease are unknown. Because patients with hypogammaglobulinemia commonly suffer from prolonged, severe infections poorly responsive to chemotherapeutic regimens, humoral responses appear to be important in the development of immunity. The greater susceptibility of the young than the old and of newly exposed persons than chronically exposed populations also suggests that immunity develops. Although strains of the parasite that are clearly nonpathogenic have not yet been identified, *Giardia* isolates vary biochemically and biologically. The marked biochemical differences between some isolates may help account for the different courses of infection noted in experimentally infected humans and animals. The surface of trophozoites is covered by a family of related cysteine-rich proteins which undergo surface antigenic variation and may contribute to prolonged and/or repeated infections.

Clinical manifestations Disease manifestations of giardiasis vary and range from asymptomatic carriage to fulminant diarrhea and malabsorption. Most infected persons identified in cross-sectional studies are asymptomatic, but in epidemics the proportion of symptomatic cases may be higher. Symptoms may develop acutely or gradually. In those with acute giardiasis, symptoms develop after an incubation period that is minimally 5 to 6 days but usually is 1 to 3 weeks. Prominent early symptoms include diarrhea, abdominal pain, bloating, belching, flatus, nausea, and vomiting. Although diarrhea is common, upper intestinal manifestations such as nausea, vomiting, bloating, and abdominal pain may predominate. The duration of acute giardiasis is usually in excess of 1 week, although diarrhea will often subside. Those with chronic giardiasis may present with or without having experienced an antecedent acute episode of symptomatic giardiasis. Diarrhea is not necessarily prominent, but increased flatus, loose stools, sulfurous burping, and in some weight loss occur. Symptoms may be continual or episodic and can persist for years. Some who experience relatively mild symptoms for long periods of time only recognize the extent of their discomfort retrospectively. The presence of fever or blood and/or mucus in the stools, as well as other signs and symptoms of colitis, is uncommon and should suggest another or concomitant illness. Most commonly, symptoms tend to be intermittent, recurrent, annoying, chronic, and gradually debilitating compared with the acute systemic disabling symptoms associated with many enteric bacterial infections. Because of the less severe illness and the propensity for chronic infections, patients may seek medical advice late in the course of the illness; however, disease can be severe, consisting of malabsorption, weight loss, growth retardation, dehydration, and rarely even death. A number of extraintestinal manifestations have been described such as urticaria, anterior uveitis, and arthritis, but whether these are caused by giardiasis or concomitant processes is unclear.

Patients with hypogammaglobulinemia are frequently infected, and their infections are more refractory to treatment. Giardiasis in this population can be life-threatening and is typically difficult to treat and eradicate. Although *Giardia* is one of the pathogens that can cause enteric illness in those with AIDS, neither the course of infection nor the response to treatment differs for patients with and without AIDS. *Giardia* infections, which are common, can complicate other preexisting intestinal diseases such as cystic fibrosis.

Diagnosis The diagnosis is established by identifying cysts in the feces or trophozoites in the feces or small intestines. Cysts are oval, measure 8 to 12 μm × 7 to 10 μm, and characteristically contain four nuclei. Trophozoites are readily recognized as pear-shaped, dorsally convex, flattened parasites with two nuclei and four pairs of flagella. The diagnosis is sometimes difficult to establish. Direct examination of fresh or properly preserved stools as well as concentration methods should be used. Because cyst excretion is variable and may be undetectable at times, repeated stool examinations, sampling of duodenal fluid, and small intestinal biopsy may be required to detect the parasite. Tests to detect parasite antigen in stool, now commercially available, are as sensitive and specific as good microscopic examinations and easier to perform but are relatively expensive. All of these methods may uncommonly yield false-negative results.

Treatment   Metronidazole (250 mg tid for 5 days) and quinacrine (100 mg bid for 5 days) treatments are equally effective, but furazolidone (100 mg qid for 7 to 10 days) is somewhat less effective. Cure rates are usually greater than 80 percent. Those who fail initial treatment can be retreated with another drug or a longer course of the same drug. Almost all patients respond to therapy and are cured, although some with chronic giardiasis experience delayed resolution of symptoms even after eradication of *Giardia*. Those who remain infected after repeated treatments should be evaluated for the possibility of reinfection from family members, close personal contacts, and environmental sources, as well as for the presence of hypogammaglobulinemia. In cases refractory to multiple treatment courses, combined therapy with metronidazole (750 mg tid for 21 days) and quinacrine (100 mg bid for 21 days) has been successful. Tinidazole, not available in the United States, is considered more effective than metronidazole or quinacrine. Frequently, children attending day care centers infect the entire family, and in this situation, treatment of all infected family members, including asymptomatic carriers, may be required to prevent reinfection. Paromomycin, an oral aminoglycoside that is not well absorbed, can be used in symptomatic pregnant women, although sufficient experience is not available to judge how frequently this agent either eradicates infection or ameliorates symptoms.

Prevention   Although *Giardia* is extremely infectious, disease can be prevented by eating and drinking noncontaminated food and water. Cooking food adequately or boiling or filtering potentially contaminated water prevents infection. Transmission between heterosexual adults is not common when hygienic practices are employed.

CRYPTOSPORIDIOSIS   The coccidian parasite *Cryptosporidium* has become recognized in the last decade to cause human diarrheal disease in normal hosts and especially those with AIDS or other forms of immunodeficiency.

Life cycle and epidemiology   Infections are acquired by consumption of oocysts, which excyst to liberate sporozoites, which in turn enter and infect intestinal epithelial cells. Further development occurs by both asexual and sexual cycles, which produce forms capable of infecting other epithelial cells and of generating oocysts that are passed in the feces. *Cryptosporidium* spp. infect a number of animals and can spread from infected animals to humans. Oocysts are infectious when passed in feces, so person-to-person transmission occurs within day-care centers and among household contacts and medical providers. As with giardiasis, waterborne transmission accounts for infections in travelers and for common-source epidemics. Oocysts are quite hardy and resist killing by routine chlorination.

Pathophysiology   Although intestinal epithelial cells harbor the parasite in an intracellular vacuole, the means by which secretory diarrhea is elicited remain uncertain. No characteristic pathologic changes are found on biopsies. The distribution of infection can be spotty within the principal site of infection, the small bowel. In some patients, cryptosporidia are found in the pharynx, stomach, and large bowel and have been recovered from the respiratory tract, although the pathogenicity of the infection for human respiratory epithelium has not been determined. Involvement of the biliary tract can cause papillary stenosis, sclerosing cholangitis, or cholecystitis.

Clinical manifestations   Asymptomatic infections can occur in both normal and immunocompromised hosts. In normal hosts, symp-toms develop after an incubation period of about a week and consist principally of watery, nonbloody diarrhea at times with abdominal pain, nausea, anorexia, fever, or weight loss. In these hosts, the illness usually subsides after 1 to 2 weeks, whereas in immunocompromised hosts, especially those with AIDS, diarrhea can be chronic, persistent, and remarkably profuse, leading to clinically significant fluid and electrolyte depletion. Stool volumes may range from 1 to 25 L/d. Weight loss, wasting, and abdominal pain may be severe. Biliary tract involvement can manifest as midepigastric or right upper quadrant pain.

Diagnosis   Evaluation usually starts with fecal examination for the small oocysts 4 to 5 μm in diameter. While these are smaller than the fecal stages of most other parasites, experienced microscopists can recognize them. Detection is enhanced by evaluation of stools obtained on multiple days and by several staining techniques, including modified acid-fast stains. If low numbers of oocysts are being excreted, Sheather's cover-slip flotation method concentrates oocysts for examination. Cryptosporidia also can be identified by light and electron microscopy at the apical surfaces of intestinal epithelium from biopsies of small bowel and less frequently large bowel. Serologic tests are available but have as yet undefined value in diagnosing either acute infections or infections in immunocompromised patients.

Treatment and prevention   To date, no effective chemotherapeutic agents have been identified. Treatment therefore consists of supportive care with fluid and electrolyte replacement and antidiarrheal agents. Biliary tract obstruction may require papillotomy or T-tube placement. Prevention requires minimizing exposure to infectious oocysts in human or animal feces.

TRICHOMONIASIS

Although different species of trichomonads can be found in the mouth in association with periodontitis and occasionally in the gastrointestinal tract, *Trichomonas vaginalis,* one of the most prevalent protozoal parasites in the United States, is a pathogen of the genitourinary tract and a major cause of symptomatic vaginitis.

Life cycle and epidemiology   *T. vaginalis* is a pear-shaped, actively motile organism, about 10 by 7 μm in size, that replicates by binary fission and inhabits the lower genital tract in females and the urethra and prostate in males. In the United States, it accounts for about 3 million infections per year in women. While the organism can survive for a few hours in moist environments and could be acquired by direct contact, person-to-person venereal transmission accounts for virtually all cases of trichomoniasis. Its prevalence is greatest among those with multiple sexual partners and those with other sexually transmitted diseases.

Clinical manifestations   Most men are asymptomatic, although a few will experience urethritis and rarely epididymitis or prostatitis. In contrast, following an incubation period of 5 to 28 days, infection develops in women that is usually symptomatic and manifest by an often yellow-colored malodorous vaginal discharge, vulvular erythema and itching, dysuria or urinary frequency (in 30 to 50 percent), and dyspareunia. These manifestations, however, do not clearly distinguish trichomoniasis from other causes of infectious vaginitis.

Diagnosis   Detection of motile trichomonads by microscopy of wet mounts of vaginal or prostatic secretions has been the conventional means of diagnosis, and although such microscopy has the advantage of providing an immediate diagnosis, the sensitivity of detecting *T. vaginalis* is only about 50 to 60 percent in routine evaluations of vaginal secretions. Culture of the parasite is the most sensitive means of detection but is not readily available and takes 3 to 7 days. Direct immunofluorescence antibody staining is more sensitive (70 to 90 percent) than wet mount examinations. *T. vaginalis* can be recovered from the urethra of both males and females and is detectable in males following prostatic massage.

Treatment and prevention   Metronidazole is the mainstay of treatment and may be given as either a single 2-g dose or 250 mg tid for 7 days. It is important that all sexual partners be treated concurrently to prevent reinfection, especially from asymptomatic males. Metronidazole should be avoided in the first trimester of pregnancy and if possible later in pregnancy. Alternative therapies during pregnancy are not readily available, although use of 100-mg clotrimazole vaginal suppositories nightly for 2 weeks may cure some infections during pregnancy. Although reinfection often accounts for apparent treatment failures, strains of *T. vaginalis* exhibiting high-level resistance to metronidazole have been encountered. Successful treatment of these resistant infections has been achieved with metronidazole given in higher oral doses, in parenteral doses, or in concurrent oral and vaginal doses.

OTHER INTESTINAL PROTOZOA Balantidiasis *Balantidium coli* is a large ciliated protozoal parasite which can produce a spectrum of large intestinal disease analogous to amebiasis. The parasite is widely distributed in the world. Since the parasite infects pigs, human cases are more common where pigs are raised; in Muslim countries, rodents may be important carriers. Transmission of infective cysts can occur by person-to-person contact and by waterborne transmission, but many cases are recognized as being due to ingestion of cysts derived from porcine feces, as may occur in association with slaughtering, with use of pig feces for fertilizer, or when pig feces contaminate water supplies.

Ingested cysts liberate trophozoites which reside and replicate in the large bowel. Many patients remain asymptomatic, but some will have persisting intermittent diarrhea and a few may develop more fulminant dysentery. In those with symptoms, the pathology in the bowel both grossly and microscopically is similar to that with amebiasis, with varying degrees of mucosal invasion, focal necrosis, and ulceration. Balantidiasis, unlike amebiasis, does not spread hematogenously to other organs. The diagnosis is made by detecting usually the trophozoite stage in stool or sampled colonic tissue. Tetracycline (500 mg qid for 10 days) is effective therapy.

Blastocystis hominis infection *Blastocystis hominis,* long considered a nonpathogenic yeast, is believed by some to be a protozoan capable of causing intestinal disease, although its taxonomy and inherent pathogenicity remain areas of uncertainty. Some patients found to be passing *B. hominis* in their stools will be asymptomatic, whereas others will have diarrhea and associated intestinal symptoms. Among those with symptoms, diligent evaluation can detect other potential bacterial, viral, or protozoan causes of diarrhea in some but not all patients. Because of the uncertainty of whether *B. hominis* is pathogenic, and because therapy of *Blastocystis* is neither specific nor uniformly effective, patients with prominent intestinal symptoms should be fully evaluated for other infectious etiologies for diarrhea. If diarrheal symptoms associated with *Blastocystis* are prominent, either metronidazole (750 mg tid for 10 days) or iodoquinol (650 mg tid for 20 days) can be used.

Dientamoeba fragilis infection *Dientamoeba fragilis* is unique among intestinal protozoa in that it has a trophozoite, but not a cyst, stage. The means by which trophozoites survive to transmit infection are not known, but heightened prevalence of *D. fragilis* in those with pinworm infection raises the possibility that eggs or larvae of *Enterobius* may facilitate transmission of *D. fragilis*. When symptoms are present with *D. fragilis,* they are generally mild and include intermittent diarrhea, abdominal pain, and anorexia. Diagnosis is made by finding trophozoites in stool, but the lability of these forms accounts for the greater yield found when fecal samples are preserved immediately after collection. Fecal excretion rates vary so that examination of several samples obtained on alternate days increases detection. Treatment can be with iodoquinol (650 mg tid for 20 days), paromomycin (25 to 30 mg/kg per day in three doses for 7 days), or tetracycline (500 mg qid for 10 days).

Isosporiasis The coccidian parasite *Isospora belli* causes human intestinal disease. Infections are acquired by consumption of oocysts, after which the parasite invades intestinal epithelium cells and undergoes both sexual and asexual cycles of development. Oocysts excreted in stool are not immediately infectious but must undergo further maturation. Although *I. belli* infects many animals, little is yet known about the epidemiology or prevalence of this parasite in humans. It appears to be more common in tropical and subtropical countries. Acute infections can begin abruptly with fever, abdominal pain, and watery nonbloody diarrhea and may last for weeks or months. In patients with AIDS or other immunocompromise, infections are often not self-limited but rather may resemble cryptosporidiosis with chronic, profuse watery diarrhea. Eosinophilia, not found with other enteric protozoan infections, may be present. The diagnosis is usually made by detecting in stool the large (~25 μm diameter) oocysts, which stain with modified acid-fast stains. Oocyst excretion may be low and intermittent, and if repeated stool examinations are unrevealing, sampling of duodenal contents by aspiration or a string test (Enterotest) or a small bowel biopsy often with electron microscopic examination may be necessary.

In contrast to cryptosporidiosis, isosporiasis responds to chemotherapy. Trimethoprim-sulfamethoxazole (160/800 mg qid for 10 days and then bid for 3 weeks) has been effective; for those intolerant of sulfonamides, pyrimethamine (50 to 75 mg/d) can be used. Relapses occur in those with AIDS and necessitate maintenance therapy with trimethoprim-sulfamethoxazole (160/800 mg 3 times a week) or combined sulfadoxine (500 mg) and pyrimethamine (25 mg) once weekly.

Microsporidiosis Microsporidia are obligate intracellular spore-forming protozoa known to infect many animals. Only recently have four genera of microsporidia, *Encephalitozoon, Pleistophora, Nosema,* and *Enterocytozoon,* been recognized as causes of human disease, especially in those immunocompromised with AIDS. The different microsporidia are distinguished on the basis of size, nuclear morphology, mode of division, and whether intracellular proliferating forms are sequestered within membrane-bound vacuoles or are in direct contact with the cytoplasm. Little is known about how humans become infected and whether microsporidia cause self-limited disease in normal hosts. In patients with AIDS, intestinal infections with *Enterocytozoon bieneusi* are increasingly recognized in association with chronic diarrhea. Patients with AIDS also have developed keratoconjunctivitis with a coarse punctate epithelial keratopathy due to *Encephalitozoon* spp., whereas stromal keratitis due to *Nosema* spp. has been identified in a few HIV-seronegative patients. Peritonitis and hepatitis due to *Encephalitozoon* microsporidia have occurred in patients with AIDS, and an HIV-seronegative immunocompromised patient developed myositis with a *Pleistophora* species.

Microsporidia are small gram-positive organisms with mature spores measuring 0.5 to 2 μm by 1 to 4 μm. Diagnosis of microsporidial infections within tissue often has required electron microscopy, although on light microscopy intracellular spores can be visualized with hematoxylin-eosin, Giemsa, or tissue Gram's stains. For diagnosing intestinal microsporidiosis, recently developed chromotrope-based staining enables spores to be detected in smears of feces or duodenal aspirates. Specific therapy for microsporidial infections has not been established.

Sarcosporidiosis Various *Sarcocystis* spp. of coccidian parasites are widely distributed causative agents of infections in numerous animals. These parasites have an obligatory cycle of development involving two hosts. Sexual reproduction occurs in the intestine and leads to passage of sporocysts in feces. Asexual multiplication leads to development of muscle cysts. Humans, apparently infrequently, can develop intestinal infections by ingesting muscle-stage cysts present in undercooked pork or beef. While the full spectrum of the intestinal disease is not defined, a diarrheal illness can ensue, and sporocysts are found in the stool. Alternatively, ingestion of fecally derived sporocysts can lead to development of muscle cysts found in human striated or cardiac muscle. Some patients have experienced muscle pain and swelling, but the frequency and nature of symptoms elicited by muscle involvement are not clear, and these cysts, measuring 100 to 325 μm in size, also have been found incidentally in muscle specimens. Muscle-stage infections do not lead to further spread within the infected human. Specific therapy for either intestinal or muscle-stage *Sarcocystis* infections in humans is not available.

REFERENCES

Giardiasis

ADAM RD: The biology of *Giardia* spp. Microbiol Rev 55:706, 1991
ERLANDSEN SL, MEYER EA (eds): *Giardia* and Giardiasis: Biology, Pathogenesis, and Epidemology, New York, Plenum, 1984

Cryptosporidiosis

WOLFSON JS et al: Cryptosporidiosis in immunocompetent patients. N Engl J Med 312:1278, 1985

FAYER R, UNGAR BLP: *Cryptosporidium* spp. and cryptosporidiosis. Microbiol Rev 50:458, 1986

Trichomoniasis

LOSSICK JG, KENT HL: Trichomoniasis: Trends in diagnosis and management. Am J Obstet Gynecol 165:1217, 1991
WØLNER-HANSSEN P et al: Clinical manifestations of vaginal trichomoniasis. JAMA 261:571, 1989

Other intestinal protozoa

WEBER R et al: Improved light-microscopical detection of microsporidia spores in stool and duodenal aspirates. N Engl J Med 326:161, 1992

section 18 Helminthic infections

180 TRICHINOSIS AND TISSUE NEMATODES

LEO X. LIU / PETER F. WELLER

Nematodes are elongated symmetric roundworms that constitute one of the largest phyla in the animal kingdom. Most nematode species are free-living, but some have evolved into parasites of plants and animals, including humans. Parasitic nematodes of medical significance may be broadly classified into intestinal and tissue nematodes, but such a classification system is imperfect. This chapter covers trichinosis, visceral and ocular larva migrans, cutaneous larva migrans, cerebral angiostrongyliasis, and gnathostomiasis. All are zoonotic infections caused by incidental exposures to infectious parasites; clinical symptoms are largely due to invasive larval stages that (with the exception of *Trichinella*) do not reach maturity in humans.

TRICHINOSIS   Trichinosis develops after the ingestion of infected pork or other meat of carnivores containing cysts of *Trichinella spiralis*. While most infections are mild and asymptomatic, heavy infections can cause severe enteritis, periorbital edema, myositis, and (in rare cases) death.

Life cycle and epidemiology   *T. spiralis* is found worldwide in a great variety of carnivorous and omnivorous animals. After the consumption of trichinous meat, encysted larvae are liberated by digestive acid and pepsin. The larvae invade the small bowel mucosa and mature rapidly into adult worms. After about 1 week, female worms release newborn larvae that migrate via the circulation to striated muscle cells. The larvae then encyst by inducing a radical transformation of the muscle cell architecture. Although host immune responses may help to expel the adult worms, they have little effect on the encysted larvae.

Most human trichinosis is caused by the ingestion of infected pork products and thus can occur in almost any location where domestic or wild swine meat is eaten. Human trichinosis also may be acquired from the meat of other animals, including dog meat in parts of Asia and Africa, horse meat in Italy and France, and bear and walrus meat in northern regions. Although cattle (being herbivores) are not natural hosts of *Trichinella*, beef has been implicated in outbreaks when contaminated or adulterated with trichinous pork. Laws that prohibit the feeding of uncooked garbage to pigs have greatly reduced the transmission of the disease in the United States. About 50 to 100 cases of trichinosis are reported annually in the United States, but most mild cases probably remain undiagnosed. Recent American outbreaks have been attributable to undercooked ethnic pork dishes, homemade and commercial sausage, wild boar meat, and walrus meat.

Pathogenesis and clinical features   Clinical symptoms of trichinosis arise from the successive phases of parasite enteric invasion, larval migration, and muscle encystment. Most light infections (<10 larvae per gram of muscle) are asymptomatic, whereas heavy infections (which can involve >50 larvae per gram of muscle) can be life-threatening. Parasites invading the gut in the first week after infection occasionally provoke diarrhea in heavy infections. Abdominal pain, constipation, nausea, or vomiting also may be prominent. Prolonged and fulminant diarrhea has been noted with arctic trichinosis, probably reflecting a response to repeated infection.

Symptoms due to larval migration and muscle invasion begin to appear in the second week after infection. The migrating *Trichinella* larvae provoke a marked local and systemic hypersensitivity reaction with fever and hypereosinophilia. Periorbital and facial edema is common, as are hemorrhages in the subconjunctivae, retina, and nail beds ("splinter" hemorrhages). A maculopapular rash, headache, cough, dyspnea, or dysphagia is sometimes present. Myocarditis with tachyarrhythmias or heart failure—and, less commonly, encephalitis or pneumonitis—may develop and account for most fatalities in trichinosis.

Upon onset of larval encystment in muscle about 2 to 3 weeks after infection, symptoms of myositis with myalgias, muscle edema, and weakness develop, usually overlapping with the inflammatory reactions to migrating larvae. The most commonly involved muscle groups include the extraocular muscles, jaw, neck, biceps, lower back, and diaphragm. Peaking about 3 weeks after infection, symptoms subside only gradually during a prolonged convalescence.

Laboratory findings and diagnosis   Blood eosinophila develops in more than 90 percent of patients with symptomatic trichinosis and may peak at a level of greater than 50 percent between 2 and 4 weeks after infection. Serum levels of IgE and muscle enzymes, including creatine phosphokinase, lactate dehydrogenase, and aspartate amino-transferase, are elevated in most symptomatic patients. Patients should be thoroughly questioned regarding their consumption of pork and wild animal meat and whether other individuals became ill after eating a common meat. A presumptive clinical diagnosis can be based on fevers, eosinophilia, periorbital edema, and myalgias after a suspect meal. A rise in titers of parasite-specific antibody (assayed in the bentonite flocculation test), which is usually delayed until after the third week of infection, confirms the diagnosis. Alternatively, a definitive diagnosis requires surgical biopsy of at least 1 g of involved muscle, with the highest yields near tendinous insertions. The fresh muscle tissue should be compressed between glass slides and examined microscopically because routine histopathologic sectioning alone may miss larvae.

Treatment Current anthelmintic drugs are ineffective against *Trichinella* larvae in muscle. Fortunately, most lightly infected patients recover uneventfully with bed rest, antipyretics, and analgesics. Glucocorticoids like prednisone (1 mg/kg daily for 5 days) are beneficial for severe myositis and myocarditis. Mebendazole, like thiabendazole, appears to be active against enteric stages of the parasite, but its efficacy against encysted larvae has not been conclusively demonstrated.

Prevention Larvae may be killed by cooking pork until it is no longer pink or by freezing at −15°C for 3 weeks. However, arctic strains (*T. spiralis* var. *nativa*) in walrus or bear meat are more resistant and may remain viable despite freezing.

VISCERAL AND OCULAR LARVA MIGRANS Visceral larva migrans is a syndrome caused by nematodes that are normally parasitic for other host species. In humans, the nematode larvae do not typically develop into adult worms but instead migrate through host tissues and elicit eosinophilic inflammation. The most common form of visceral larva migrans is toxocariasis due to larvae of the canine ascarid *Toxocara canis* and less commonly the feline ascarid *T. cati*. Rare cases with eosinophilic meningoencephalitis have been caused by the raccoon ascarid *Baylisascaris procyonis*.

Life cycle and epidemiology The canine roundworm *T. canis* is distributed among dogs worldwide. Ingestion of infective eggs by dogs is followed by liberation of *Toxocara* larvae. Some larvae pass through tissues and return to the intestinal tract to develop into adult worms, which produce eggs released in the feces. The progress of other larvae is arrested. These organisms become dormant in canine tissues; they resume migration in pregnant bitches and infect puppies prenatally (via transplacental transmission) and after birth (via suckling). As a result, most puppies and lactating bitches shed *T. canis* eggs in their stools. Humans acquire toxocariasis mainly by eating soil contaminated by puppy feces containing infective eggs. Visceral larva migrans is most common among children with the habit of eating dirt, but most toxocaral infections are subclinical. Reported rates of *Toxocara* seropositivity range from 2 percent in an unselected American population to greater than 20 percent among kindergarten children in the United States and England.

Pathogenesis and clinical features Clinical disease most commonly afflicts preschool children. After humans ingest *Toxocara* eggs, the larvae hatch and penetrate the intestinal mucosa to be carried by the circulation to a wide variety of organs and tissues. The larvae invade the liver, lungs, central nervous system, and other sites, releasing toxic products and provoking intense local eosinophilic granulomatous responses. The degree of clinical illness depends on larval number and tissue distribution, reinfection, and host immune responses. Most light infections are asymptomatic and may be manifest only by blood eosinophilia. Characteristic symptoms of visceral larva migrans include fever, malaise, anorexia and weight loss, cough, wheezing, and rashes. Hepatosplenomegaly is common. These features are often accompanied by extraordinary peripheral eosinophilia that may approach 90 percent. Uncommonly, seizures or behavioral disorders may occur. The rare deaths in this disease are due to severe neurologic, pneumonic, or myocardial involvement.

Diagnosis and treatment In addition to prominent eosinophilia, leukocytosis and hypergammaglobulinemia are usually evident. Transient pulmonary infiltrates on chest x-ray are found in about half of patients with symptoms of pneumonitis. The clinical diagnosis can be confirmed by ELISA for toxocaral antibodies. Stool examination, while important in the evaluation of unexplained eosinophilia, is worthless for toxocariasis, since the larvae do not develop into egg-producing adults in humans. The vast majority of infections are self-limited and resolve without specific therapy. In patients with severe myocardial, central nervous system, or pulmonary involvement, glucocorticoids may be employed to reduce inflammatory complications. Available anthelmintic drugs, including diethylcarbamazine and thiabendazole, have not been conclusively shown to alter the course of larva migrans. Control measures include prohibiting dog excreta in public parks and playgrounds, deworming dogs, and preventing pica in children.

The ocular form of the larva migrans syndrome occurs when *Toxocara* larvae invade the eye. An eosinophilic granulomatous mass, most commonly in the posterior pole of the retina, develops around the entrapped larva. The retinal lesion can mimic retinoblastoma in appearance, and mistaken diagnosis of the latter condition can lead to unnecessary enucleation. The spectrum of eye involvement also includes endophthalmitis, uveitis, and chorioretinitis. Unilateral visual disturbances, strabismus, and eye pain are the most common presenting symptoms. In contrast to visceral larva migrans, ocular toxocariasis usually develops in older children or young adults with no history of pica; these patients seldom have eosinophilia or visceral manifestations. Treatment is unsatisfactory, and the role of glucocorticoids or anthelmintic drugs in management is controversial.

CUTANEOUS LARVA MIGRANS Cutaneous larva migrans ("creeping eruption") is a serpiginous skin eruption caused by burrowing larvae of animal hookworms, usually the dog and cat hookworm *Ancylostoma braziliense*. The larvae hatch from eggs passed in dog and cat feces and mature in the soil. Humans become infected after skin contact with soil in areas frequented by dogs and cats, such as underneath house porches or scrub vegetation. Cutaneous larva migrans is more prevalent among children and in warm, humid climates, including the southeastern United States.

After larvae penetrate the skin, erythematous lesions form along the tortuous tracts of larvae migrating through the dermal-epidermal junction, advancing several centimeters in a day. These intensely pruritic lesions may occur anywhere on the body and can be numerous if the patient has lain on the ground. Vesicles and bullae may form later. The animal hookworm larvae do not mature in humans and left untreated will die out after several weeks, with resolution of skin lesions. The diagnosis is made readily on clinical grounds, and a skin biopsy only rarely yields diagnostic parasite material. Symptoms can be alleviated by thiabendazole administered orally (25 mg/kg bid) or topically (10% aqueous or petroleum jelly suspension) for 2 to 5 days.

***ANGIOSTRONGYLUS CANTONENSIS* INFECTION** *Angiostrongylus cantonensis*, the rat lungworm, is the most common cause of human eosinophilic meningitis.

Life cycle and epidemiology This infection occurs principally in Southeast Asia and the Pacific Basin. *A. cantonensis* larvae produced by adult worms in the rat lung migrate to the gastrointestinal tract and are expelled with the feces. They develop into infective larvae within land snails and slugs. Humans acquire the infection by ingesting raw infected mollusks, vegetables contaminated by mollusk slime, or crabs, freshwater shrimp, and certain marine fish that have themselves eaten infected mollusks. The larvae then migrate to the brain.

Pathogenesis and clinical features The parasites eventually die in the central nervous system, but not before initiating pathologic consequences which in heavy infections can result in permanent neurologic sequelae or death. Migrating larvae cause proteolytic damage and marked local eosinophilic inflammation and hemorrhage, with subsequent necrosis and granuloma formation around dying worms. Clinical symptoms develop between 2 and 35 days after ingestion of larvae. Patients usually present with an insidious or abrupt excruciating frontal, occipital, or bitemporal headache. Neck stiffness, nausea and vomiting, and paresthesias are also common. Fever is usually absent. Cranial and extraocular nerve palsies, seizures, paralysis, and lethargy are uncommon.

Laboratory findings and treatment Examination of the cerebrospinal fluid is mandatory in suspected cases and usually reveals an elevated opening pressure, a white blood cell count of 150 to 2000 cells per microliter, and an eosinophilic pleocytosis of >20 percent. The protein concentration is usually elevated and the glucose level normal. The motile larvae of *A. cantonensis* are only rarely seen in the cerebrospinal fluid. Peripheral blood eosinophilia may be mild.

The diagnosis is generally based on the clinical presentation of eosinophilic meningitis together with a compatible epidemiologic history. Specific chemotherapy has not been shown to be of benefit in angiostrongyliasis, in part because larvicidal agents may exacerbate inflammatory brain lesions. Management consists of supportive measures, including the administration of analgesics, sedatives, and—in severe cases—glucocorticoids. In most patients, in fact, cerebral angiostrongyliasis has a self-limited course, and recovery is complete. The infection may be prevented by adequately cooking snails, crabs, and prawns and inspecting vegetables for mollusk infestation. Other parasitic causes of eosinophilic meningitis in endemic areas may include gnathostomiasis, paragonimiasis, schistosomiasis, and neurocysticercosis.

GNATHOSTOMIASIS Infections of human tissues with larvae of *Gnathostoma spinigerum* can cause eosinophilic meningoencephalitis, migratory cutaneous swellings, or invasive masses of the eye and visceral organs.

Life cycle and epidemiology Human gnathostomiasis is endemic in Southeast Asia and parts of China and Japan. In nature, the mature adult worms parasitize the gastrointestinal tract of dogs and cats. First-stage larvae hatch from eggs passed into water and are ingested by *Cyclops* species (water fleas). Infective third-stage larvae develop in the flesh of many animal species (including fish, frogs, eels, snakes, chickens, and ducks) that have eaten either infected *Cyclops* or another infected second intermediate host. Humans typically acquire the infection by eating raw or undercooked fish or poultry. The raw fish dishes of *somfak* in Thailand and *sashimi* in Japan account for most cases of human gnathostomiasis. Some cases in Thailand result from the local practice of applying frog or snake flesh as a poultice.

Pathogenesis and clinical features Clinical symptoms are due to the aberrant migration of a single larva in cutaneous, visceral, neural, or ocular tissues. After invasion, larval migration may cause local inflammation, with pain, cough, or hematuria accompanied by fever and eosinophilia. Painful, itchy, migratory swellings may develop in the skin, particularly in the distal extremities or periorbital area. Cutaneous swellings usually last about a week but often recur intermittently over many years. Larval invasion of the eye can provoke a sight-threatening inflammatory response. Finally, invasion of the central nervous system results in eosinophilic meningitis with myeloencephalitis, a serious complication due to ascending larval migration along a large nerve track. Patients characteristically present with agonizing radicular pain and paresthesias in the trunk or a limb, which are followed shortly by paraplegia. Cerebral involvement, with focal hemorrhages and tissue destruction, is often fatal.

Diagnosis and treatment Cutaneous migratory swellings with marked peripheral eosinophilia, supported by an appropriate geographic and dietary history, generally constitute an adequate basis for a clinical diagnosis of gnathostomiasis. However, patients may present with ocular or cerebrospinal involvement without antecedent cutaneous swellings. In the latter case, eosinophilic pleocytosis will be documented (usually along with hemorrhagic or xanthochromic cerebrospinal fluid), but worms will almost never be recovered from the cerebrospinal fluid. Surgical removal of the parasite from subcutaneous or ocular tissue, though rarely feasible, is both diagnostic and therapeutic. A prolonged course of mebendazole may alleviate cutaneous swellings but is not curative. At present, cerebrospinal involvement is managed with supportive measures and generally a course of glucocorticoids. Gnathostomiasis can be prevented by adequate cooking of fish and poultry in endemic areas.

REFERENCES

Jaroonvesama N: Differential diagnosis of eosinophilic meningitis. Parasitol Today 4:262, 1988

Koo J et al: *Angiostrongylus (Parastrongylus)* eosinophilic meningitis. Rev Infect Dis 10:1155, 1988

Landry SM et al: Trichinosis: Common source outbreak related to commercial pork. South Med J 85:428, 1992

Lewis JM, Maizels RM (eds): *Toxocara and Toxocariasis: Clinical, Epidemiological, and Molecular Perspectives*. London, Institute of Biology, 1993

MacLean JD et al: Epidemiologic and serologic definition of primary and secondary trichinosis in the Arctic. J Infect Dis 165:908, 1992

McAuley JB et al: Trichinosis surveillance, United States, 1987–1990. Morb Mort Week Rep CDC Surveill Summ 40:35, 1992

Shields JA: Ocular toxocariasis: A review. Surv Ophthalmol 28:361, 1984

Taylor MRH et al: The expanded spectrum of toxocaral disease. Lancet 1:692, 1988

181   INTESTINAL NEMATODES

LEO X. LIU / PETER F. WELLER

Over 1 billion people worldwide are infected with one or more species of intestinal nematodes. Table 181-1 summarizes biological and clinical features of the major intestinal parasitic nematodes. These parasites are most common in regions with poor fecal sanitation, particularly in developing countries in the tropics and subtropics but also in the United States. Although nematode parasites do not usually cause fatal infections, they contribute to malnutrition and diminished work capacity. Humans may on occasion be infected with nematode parasites that ordinarily infect animals; these zoonotic infections include trichostrongyliasis, anisakiasis, capillariasis, and abdominal angiostrongyliasis.

Intestinal nematodes are roundworms ranging in length from 1 mm to many centimeters when mature (see Table 181-1). Their life cycles are complex and highly varied; some species, including *Strongyloides* and pinworm, can be transmitted directly from person to person, while others, such as *Ascaris* and hookworm, require a soil phase for development. Because most helminthic parasites do not self-replicate, a large burden of adult worms requires repeated exposure to the parasite in its infectious stage, whether larvae or eggs. Hence clinical disease, as opposed to asymptomatic infection, generally requires prolonged residence in an endemic area. Eosinophilia and elevated serum IgE levels are features of many helminthic infections and, when unexplained, should always prompt a search for an occult helminthiasis. Significant protective immunity to intestinal nematodes does not appear to develop, although mechanisms of parasite immune evasion and host immune responses to these infections have not been elucidated in detail.

ASCARIASIS *Ascaris lumbricoides* is the largest intestinal nematode parasite of humans, reaching up to 40 cm in length. An estimated 1 billion people are infected. Most infected individuals have low worm burdens and are asymptomatic. Clinical disease arises from pulmonary hypersensitivity and intestinal complications.

Life cycle Adult worms live in the lumen of the small intestine. Mature female *Ascaris* worms are extraordinarily fecund, each producing up to 200,000 eggs a day, which pass with the feces. Ascarid eggs, which are remarkably resistant to environmental stresses, become infective after several weeks of maturation in the soil and can remain infective for years. After infective eggs are swallowed by fecal-oral passage, larvae hatched in the intestine invade the mucosa, migrate via the circulation to the lungs, break into the alveoli, ascend the bronchial tree, and return via swallowing to the small intestine, where they develop into adult worms. Between 2 and 3 months elapse between initial infection and egg production. The adult worms live for approximately 1 to 2 years.

Epidemiology *Ascaris* is widely distributed in tropical and subtropical climates, including the rural southeastern United States. Transmission typically occurs via fecally contaminated soil due either to the lack of sanitary facilities or to use of human manure ("night soil") as fertilizer. With their propensity for hand-to-mouth fecal carriage, younger children in impoverished rural areas are most affected. Infection outside endemic areas, though uncommon, can occur via eggs borne on transported vegetables.

TABLE 181-1 Major human intestinal nematode parasites

	Ascaris lumbricoides (roundworm)	Necator americanus Ancylostoma duodenale (hookworm)	Strongyloides stercoralis	Trichuris trichiura (pinworm)	Enterobius vermicularis (whipworm)
Global prevalence (millions)	1000	900	50	500	300
Endemic areas	Worldwide	Tropics and subtropics	Tropics and subtropics	Worldwide	Worldwide
Infective stage	Egg	Filariform larvae	Filariform larvae	Egg	Egg
Route of infection	Oral	Percutaneous	Percutaneous or autoinfection	Oral	Oral
GI location of worms	Jejunum lumen	Jejunum mucosa	Small bowel mucosa	Cecum, colon mucosa	Cecum, appendix
Adult worm size	15–40 cm	7–12 mm	2 mm	30–50 mm	8–13 mm (female)
Pulmonary passage of larvae	Yes	Yes	Yes	No	No
Incubation* (days)	60–75	40–100	17–28	70–90	35–45
Longevity	1 y	N. americanus 2–5 y A. duodenale 6–8 y	Unknown	5 y	2 months
Fecundity (eggs/day/ worm)	240,000	N. americanus 4000–10,000 A. duodenale 10,000–25,000	5000–10,000	3000–7000	2000
Principal symptoms	Rarely GI or biliary obstruction	Iron deficiency anemia in heavy infection	GI symptoms; malabsorption or sepsis in hyperinfection	GI symptoms, anemia	Perianal pruritus
Diagnostic stage	Eggs in stool	Eggs in fresh stool larvae in old stool	Larvae in stool or duodenal aspirate; sputum in hyperinfection	Eggs in stool	Eggs from perianal skin on cellulose acetate tape
Treatment	Mebendazole Albendazole† Pyrantel pamoate Piperazine citrate	Mebendazole, Pyrantel pamoate Albendazole†	Thiabendazole Albendazole†	Mebendazole Albendazole†	Mebendazole Pyrantel pamoate Piperazine citrate

* Time from infection to egg production by mature female worm.
† Not approved by the Food and Drug Administration.

Clinical features During the lung phase of larval migration, about 9 to 12 days after egg ingestion, patients may develop an irritating, nonproductive cough and burning substernal discomfort, aggravated by coughing or deep inspiration. Dyspnea and blood-tinged sputum are less common. Fever is usually present and may exceed 38.5°C. Eosinophilia occurs during this symptomatic phase and subsides slowly over weeks. Chest x-rays may reveal evidence of eosinophilic pneumonitis (Loeffler's syndrome), with round or oval infiltrates a few millimeters to several centimeters in size. These infiltrates may be transient and intermittent, clearing after several weeks. Where there is seasonal transmission of the parasite, *Ascaris* may cause seasonal pneumonitis with eosinophilia in previously infected and sensitized hosts.

In mature infections, adult worms within the small intestine are usually asymptomatic. In heavy infections, particularly in children, a large bolus of entangled worms can cause pain and small bowel obstruction, which may be complicated by perforation, intussusception, or volvulus. Single worms may cause disease when they migrate into aberrant sites. A large worm can enter and occlude the biliary tree, causing biliary colic, cholecystitis, cholangitis, pancreatitis, and rarely intrahepatic abscesses. Migration of an adult worm up the esophagus can provoke coughing and oral expulsion of the worm. In highly endemic areas, intestinal and biliary ascariasis can rival acute appendicitis and gallstones as causes of surgical acute abdomen.

Laboratory findings Most cases of ascariasis are diagnosable by stool examination, upon microscopic detection of characteristic mammillated *Ascaris* eggs (65 by 45 μm) in fecal samples. Occasionally, patients present after passing an adult worm, identifiable by its large size and smooth cream-colored surface, in the stool or rarely through the mouth or nose. During the early transpulmonary migratory phase when eosinophilic pneumonitis occurs, larvae can be found in sputum or gastric aspirates before diagnostic eggs appear in the stool. The prominent eosinophilia during this early stage usually decreases to minimal levels in established infection. The large adult worms may be visualized, occasionally serendipitously, on contrast studies of the gastrointestinal tract. A plain abdominal film may reveal masses of worms in gas-filled loops of bowel in patients with intestinal obstruction. Pancreaticobiliary worms can be detected by ultrasound and endoscopic retrograde cholangiopancreatography; the latter method also has been used to extract biliary *Ascaris* worms.

Treatment *Ascaris* should always be treated to prevent potentially serious complications. Mebendazole or albendazole (which is not yet approved by the Food and Drug Administration) are effective. These benzimidazoles are contraindicated in pregnancy and in heavy infections, where they may provoke ectopic migration. Pyrantel pamoate and piperazine citrate are safe in pregnancy. Mild diarrhea and abdominal pain are uncommon side effects of these agents. Partial intestinal obstruction should be managed with nasogastric suction, intravenous fluids, and piperazine instillation through the nasogastric tube, but complete obstruction and its severe complications require immediate surgical intervention.

HOOKWORM One-fourth of the world's population is infected with one of the two hookworm species *Ancylostoma duodenale* or *Necator americanus*. Most infected individuals are asymptomatic. Hookworm disease develops from a combination of heavy worm burden, prolonged duration of infection, and inadequate iron intake and results in iron deficiency anemia and, on occasion, hypoproteinemia.

Life cycle Adult hookworms, which are about 1 cm long, use buccal teeth (*Ancylostoma*) or cutting plates (*Necator*) to attach to the small bowel mucosa and suck blood (0.2 mL/d per adult *Ancylostoma*) and interstitial fluid. The adult hookworms produce thousands of eggs daily. The eggs are deposited with feces in soil, where rhabditiform larvae hatch and develop over a 1-week period into infectious filariform larvae. Infective larvae penetrate the skin and reach the lungs by way of the bloodstream. There they invade alveoli and ascend the airways before being swallowed to reach the small intestine. The prepatent period from skin invasion to appearance of eggs in the feces is about 6 to 8 weeks but may be longer with *A. duodenale*. Larvae of *A. duodenale*, if swallowed, can survive and develop directly in the intestinal mucosa. Adult hookworms may survive over a decade but usually live about 6 to 8 years for *A. duodenale* and 2 to 5 years for *N. americanus*.

Epidemiology *A. duodenale* is prevalent in southern Europe, North Africa, and northern Asia, and *N. americanus* is the predominant species in the Western Hemisphere and equatorial Africa. The two species overlap in many tropical regions, particularly Southeast Asia. In most areas, older children have the greatest incidence and intensity of hookworm infection. In rural areas where fields are fertilized with "night soil," older working adults also may be heavily affected.

Clinical features Most hookworm infections are asymptomatic. Infective larvae may provoke a pruritic maculopapular dermatitis ("ground itch") at the site of skin penetration, as well as serpiginous tracts of subcutaneous migration (similar to cutaneous larva migrans) in previously sensitized hosts. Larvae migrating through the lungs occasionally can cause a mild transient pneumonitis, but this is less frequent than with *Ascaris*. In the early intestinal phase, infected persons may develop epigastric pain (often with postprandial accentuation), inflammatory diarrhea, or other abdominal symptoms accompanied by eosinophilia. The major consequence of chronic hookworm infection is iron deficiency. Symptoms are minimal if iron intake is adequate, but marginally nourished individuals develop symptoms of progressive iron-deficiency anemia and hypoproteinemia, including weakness, shortness of breath, and skin depigmentation. Intercurrent infections may precipitate frank cardiac failure. Changes in the intestinal mucosa are minimal, and malabsorption is uncommon.

Laboratory findings The diagnosis is established by finding the characteristic 40 by 60 µm oval hookworm eggs in the feces. Stool concentration procedures may be required to detect light infections. Eggs of the two species are indistinguishable. If a stool sample is not freshly examined, the eggs may hatch to release rhabditiform larvae, which should be differentiated from those of *Strongyloides stercoralis*. A hypochromic, microcytic anemia, occasionally with eosinophilia or hypoalbuminemia, is characteristic of hookworm disease.

Treatment Eradication of the parasite can be achieved with several safe and highly effective antihelminthic drugs, including mebendazole and pyrantel pamoate (see Chap. 172). Mild iron-deficiency anemia often can be treated with oral iron alone. Severe hookworm disease with protein loss and malabsorption necessitates nutritional support and oral iron replacement along with deworming.

STRONGYLOIDIASIS *Strongyloides stercoralis* is distinguished by a capacity, unusual among helminths to replicate within the human host, thereby permitting ongoing cycles of autoinfection due to internal production of infective larvae. Strongyloidiasis can thus persist for decades without further exposure to exogenous infective larvae. In immunocompromised hosts, large numbers of invasive *Strongyloides* larvae can disseminate widely and be fatal.

Life cycle In addition to a parasitic cycle of development, *Strongyloides* also can undergo a free-living cycle of development in the soil, which facilitates parasite survival in the absence of mammalian hosts. Rhabditiform larvae passed in feces can transform into infectious filariform larvae either directly or after a free-living phase of development. Humans acquire strongyloidiasis following contact with fecally contaminated soil, when filariform larvae penetrate the skin or mucous membranes. The larvae then travel through the bloodstream to the lungs, where they break into the alveolar spaces, ascend the bronchial tree, and are swallowed to reach the small intestine. There larvae mature into adult worms that penetrate the mucosa of the proximal small bowel. The minute (2 mm long) parasitic adult female worms reproduce by parthenogenesis; parasitic adult males do not exist. Eggs hatch locally within the intestinal mucosa, releasing rhabditiform larvae that migrate to the lumen and pass with the feces into soil. Alternatively, rhabditiform larvae within the bowel can develop directly into filariform larvae that penetrate the colonic wall or perianal skin and enter the circulation to repeat the migration that establishes ongoing internal reinfection. This autoinfection cycle allows strongyloidiasis to persist for decades after the host has left an endemic area.

Epidemiology *S. stercoralis* is spottily distributed in tropical, humid regions, particularly in Southeast Asia, sub-Saharan Africa, and Brazil. In the United States, it is endemic in parts of the south and is found in residents of mental institutions who have poor hygiene and in immigrants and military veterans who have lived in endemic areas abroad.

Clinical features In uncomplicated strongyloidiasis, many patients are asymptomatic or have mild cutaneous abdominal symptoms. Recurrent urticaria, often involving the buttocks and wrists, is the most common cutaneous manifestation. Migrating larvae can elicit a pathognomonic serpiginous eruption, *larva currens* ("running larva"), a pruritic, raised, erythematous lesion that advances as rapidly as 10 cm/h along the course of larval migration. Adult parasites burrow into the duodenojejunal mucosa and can cause abdominal, usually midepigastric, pain that resembles peptic ulcer pain except that it is aggravated by food ingestion. Nausea, diarrhea, gastrointestinal bleeding, mild chronic colitis, and weight loss can occur. Pulmonary symptoms are rare in uncomplicated strongyloidiasis. Eosinophilia is common, with levels fluctuating over time.

The ongoing autoinfection cycle of strongyloidiasis is normally contained by unknown factors of the host immune system. Abrogation of host immunity, following immunosuppressive therapy or concomitant malignancy or malnutrition, leads to hyperinfection strongyloidiasis with the generation of large numbers of filariform larvae. Colitis, enteritis, or malabsorption may develop. In disseminated strongyloidiasis, larvae may invade not only gastrointestinal tissues and the lungs but also the central nervous system, peritoneum, liver, and kidney. Moreover, bacteremia may develop due to enteric flora entering through disrupted mucosal barriers. Gram-negative sepsis, pneumonia, or meningitis may complicate or dominate the clinical course. Eosinophilia is often absent in severely infected patients. Disseminated strongyloidiasis, particularly in patients with unsuspected strongyloidiasis given immunosuppressive drugs, can be fatal. Although strongyloidiasis has been associated with both HIV and HTLV-1 infection, disseminated strongyloidiasis is uncommon in these conditions.

Diagnosis In uncomplicated strongyloidiasis, the finding of rhabditiform larvae in feces is diagnostic. The eggs are almost never detectable because they hatch in the intestine. Rhabditiform larvae are 200 to 250 µm long, with a short buccal cavity that distinguishes them from hookworm rhabditiform larvae. Single stool examinations will detect only about one-third of uncomplicated infections, in which few larvae are passed. Serial examinations or the Baermann concentration method improves the sensitivity of stool diagnosis. If stool examination is negative, *Strongyloides* can be detected by sampling the duodenojejunal contents by aspiration, biopsy, or the Enterotest string method. An ELISA test for antibodies to excretory-secretory antigens of *Strongyloides* is also a sensitive method of diagnosing uncomplicated infections. In disseminated strongyloidiasis, filariform larvae (550 µm long) should be sought on stool examinations as well as in samples obtained from other sites of potential larval migrations, including sputum, bronchoalveolar lavage fluid, or surgical drainage fluid.

Treatment Even in the asymptomatic state, strongyloidiasis must be treated because of the potential for fatal hyperinfection. Thiabendazole (25 mg/kg bid) is generally administered for 2 days, but in disseminated strongyloidiasis, treatment should be extended for at least 5 to 7 days or until the parasites are eradicated. Common adverse effects of thiabendazole include nausea, vomiting, diarrhea, dizziness, and neuropsychiatric disturbances. Because thiabendazole is not uniformly effective, stool examinations and eosinophil counts as well as clinical symptoms should be monitored following treatment. Albendazole and ivermectin are promising agents for intestinal disease, but to date only thiabendazole has demonstrated efficacy in disseminated strongyloidiasis.

Strongyloides fülleborni This unusual species, which has been encountered in Africa and Papua, New Guinea, is thought to be transmitted person-to-person and via maternal milk. *S. fülleborni* releases membranous sacs filled with eggs into the stool. Most commonly affected are infants and young children, who present with abdominal distention, respiratory distress, vomiting, or diarrhea.

TRICHURIASIS Most infections with the whipworm *Trichuris trichiura* are asymptomatic, but heavy infections may cause gastrointestinal symptoms. Like the other soil-transmitted helminths, whipworm is distributed globally in the tropics and subtropics and is most common in poor children.

Life cycle   A broad posterior section and a thin anterior portion give *Trichuris* its characteristic whiplike shape. The adult worms reside in the colon and cecum, the anterior portions threaded into the superficial mucosa. Thousands of eggs laid daily by adult female worms pass via the feces and mature in the soil. After ingestion, infective eggs hatch in the duodenum, releasing larvae that mature before migrating to the large bowel. The entire cycle takes about 3 months, and adult worms may live for several years.

Clinical features   Tissue reactions to whipworms are mild. Most infected individuals have no symptoms or eosinophilia. Heavy infections may result in abdominal pain, anorexia, and bloody or mucoid diarrhea resembling inflammatory bowel disease. Rectal prolapse can occur from massive infections in children, who often suffer from malnourishment and other diarrheal illnesses. Moderately heavy whipworm burdens also contribute to growth retardation.

Diagnosis and treatment   The characteristic 50 by 20 μm lemon-shaped whipworm eggs are readily detected on stool examination. Adult worms, which measure 3 to 5 cm long, occasionally can be seen on proctoscopy. Mebendazole is safe and effective for treatment (see Chap. 172).

ENTEROBIASIS (PINWORM)   *Enterobius vermicularis* is more common in temperate countries than in the tropics. Over 40 million Americans, particularly school children, are estimated to be infected with pinworms.

Life cycle and epidemiology   *Enterobius* adult worms measure about 1 cm long and dwell in the bowel lumen. The gravid female worm migrates nocturnally out into the perianal region and releases up to 10,000 immature eggs. The eggs become infective within hours and are transmitted via hand-to-mouth passage. The larvae hatch and mature entirely within the intestine. This life cycle takes about 1 month, and adult worms survive for about 2 months. Self-infection occurs by perianal scratching and transport of infective eggs on the hands or under the nails to the mouth. Given the ease of person-to-person spread, pinworm infections are common among family members and institutionalized populations.

Clinical features   Most pinworm infections are asymptomatic. Perianal pruritus is the cardinal symptom. The itching is often worse at night due to the nocturnal migration of the female worms and may lead to excoriation and bacterial superinfection. Heavy infections have been claimed to cause abdominal pain and weight loss. Pinworms may rarely invade the female genital tract, causing vulvovaginitis and pelvic or peritoneal granulomas. Eosinophilia or elevated serum IgE levels are rare.

Diagnosis and treatment   Since pinworm eggs are not usually released in the bowel, the diagnosis cannot be made by looking for eggs in the feces. Instead, eggs deposited in the perianal region are detected by applying clear cellulose acetate tape in the morning to the perianal region. After transferring the tape to a microscope slide, low power examination will reveal the characteristic oval (55 by 25 μm) pinworm eggs. All affected individuals should be treated with a dose of mebendazole or pyrantel pamoate, repeated after 10 to 14 days (see Chap. 172). Treating household members is also advocated to eliminate asymptomatic reservoirs for reinfection.

TRICHOSTRONGYLIASIS   *Trichostrongylus* spp. that are normally parasites of herbivorous animals may occasionally infect humans, particularly in Asia and Africa. This parasite has been termed *pseudohookworm* because of similarities in life cycle and egg morphology. Humans acquire the infection by accidentally ingesting *Trichostrongylus* larvae on contaminated leafy vegetables. The larvae do not migrate in humans but mature directly in the small bowel into adult worms. These worms ingest far less blood than hookworms; most infected people are asymptomatic, but heavy infections may give rise to mild anemia and eosinophilia. *Trichostrongylus* eggs encountered on stool examination resemble those of hookworm but are larger (85 by 115 μm). Treatment is with mebendazole (see Chap. 172).

ANISAKIASIS   Anisakiasis is a gastrointestinal infection caused by the accidental ingestion in uncooked saltwater fish of nematode larvae belonging to the family of Anisakidae. The incidence of anisakiasis in the United States has increased as a result of the growing popularity of raw fish dishes. Most cases occur in Japan, the Netherlands, and Chile, where the raw fish in the form of sushi, pickled green herring, and ceviche, respectively, are national culinary staples. Anisakid nematodes parasitize large sea mammals such as whales, dolphins, and seals. As part of a complex parasite life cycle involving marine food chains, infectious larvae migrate to the musculature of a variety of fish. Both *Anisakis simplex* and *Pseudoterranova decipiens* have been implicated in human anisakiasis, but an identical gastric syndrome may be caused by the red larvae of eustrongylides parasites of fish-eating birds. When humans consume infected raw fish, live larvae may be coughed up within 48 h. Alternatively, larvae may immediately penetrate the mucosa of the stomach. Within hours violent upper abdominal pain ensues, accompanied by nausea and occasionally vomiting, mimicking an acute abdomen. The diagnosis can be established by direct visualization on upper endoscopy, outlining of the worm by contrast radiographic studies, or histopathology of extracted tissue. In experienced hands, the first technique is preferable because extraction of the burrowing larva by endoscopic technique is curative. Larvae also may pass instead to the small bowel, where they penetrate the mucosa and provoke a vigorous eosinophilic granulomatous response. Symptoms may appear 1 or 2 weeks after the infective meal, with intermittent abdominal pain, diarrhea, nausea, and fever resembling Crohn's disease. The diagnosis may be suggested by barium studies and confirmed by curative surgical resection of a granuloma in which the worm is embedded. Anisakid eggs will not be found in the stool, since the larvae do not mature in humans. Anisakid larvae in saltwater fish are killed by cooking to 60°C, freezing at −20°C for 3 days, or commercial blast freezing but not usually by salting, marinating, or cold smoking the fish.

CAPILLARIASIS   Intestinal capillariasis is caused by ingestion of raw fish infected with *Capillaria philippinensis*. Subsequent autoinfection can lead to a severe wasting syndrome. The disease occurs in the Philippines and Thailand and on occasion elsewhere in Asia. The natural cycle of *C. philippinensis* involves fish from fresh and brackish water. When humans eat infected raw fish, the larvae mature in the intestine to adult worms, which directly produce invasive larvae that cause intestinal inflammation and villus loss. Capillariasis has an insidious onset with nonspecific abdominal pain and watery diarrhea. If untreated, progressive autoinfection can lead to a protein-losing enteropathy and severe malabsorption, leading to death from cachexia, cardiac failure, or superinfection. The diagnosis is established by identifying the characteristic peanut-shaped (20 × 40 μm) eggs on stool examination. Severely ill patients require hospitalization and supportive therapy in addition to prolonged antihelminthic treatment with mebendazole or albendazole (see Chap. 172).

ABDOMINAL ANGIOSTRONGYLIASIS   Abdominal angiostrongyliasis is found in Latin America and Africa. The zoonotic parasite *Angiostrongylus costaricensis* causes eosinophilic ileocolitis following the ingestion of contaminated vegetation. *A. costaricensis* normally parasitizes the cotton rat and other rodents, with slugs and snails serving as intermediate hosts. Humans become infected by accidentally ingesting infective larvae in mollusk slime deposited on fruits and vegetables; children are at highest risk. The larvae penetrate the gut wall and migrate to the mesenteric artery, where they develop into adult worms. Eggs deposited in the gut wall provoke an intense eosinophilic granulomatous reaction, and adult worms may cause mesenteric arteritis, thrombosis, or frank bowel infarction. Symptoms may mimic appendicitis, including abdominal pain and tenderness, fever, vomiting, and a palpable mass in the right iliac fossa. Leukocytosis and eosinophilia are prominent. A barium enema may reveal ileocecal filling defects, but definitive diagnosis is usually made surgically with partial bowel resection. Pathology reveals thickened bowel wall with eosinophilic granulomas surrounding the

Angiostrongylus eggs. In nonsurgical cases, the diagnosis rests solely on clinical grounds because larvae and eggs cannot be detected in the stool. Medical therapy for abdominal angiostrongyliasis is unsatisfactory. Careful observation and surgical resection for severe symptoms are the mainstays of treatment.

REFERENCES

ASH LR, ORIHEL TC: *Atlas of Human Parasitology,* 3d ed. Chicago, ASCP Press, 1990

COOPER ES, BUNDY DAP: Trichuris is not trivial. Parasitol Today 4:301, 1988

CROSS JH: Intestinal capillariasis. Clin Microbiol Rev 5:120, 1992

GENTA RM et al: Strongyloidiasis in US veterans of the Vietnam and other wars. JAMA 258:49, 1987

KHUROO MS et al: Hepatobiliary and pancreatic ascariasis in India. Lancet 335:1503, 1990

LEIGHTON PM, MACSWEEN HM: *Strongyloides stercoralis:* The cause of an urticarial-like eruption of 65 years' duration. Arch Intern Med 150:1747, 1990

LONGWORTH DL, WELLER PF: Hyperinfection syndrome with strongyloidiasis, in *Current Clinical Topics in Infectious Diseases,* vol 7, JS Remington, MN Swartz (eds). New York, McGraw-Hill, 1986, p 1

OCHOA B: Surgical complications of ascariasis. World J Surg 15:222, 1991

SCHAD GA, WARREN KS (eds): *Hookworm Disease: Current Status and New Directions.* London, Taylor and Francis, 1990

SCHANTZ PM: The dangers of eating raw fish (editorial). N Engl J Med 320:1143, 1989

182 FILARIASIS AND RELATED INFECTIONS (LOIASIS, ONCHOCERCIASIS, AND DRACUNCULIASIS)

THOMAS B. NUTMAN / PETER F. WELLER

Filarial worms are nematodes that dwell in the subcutaneous tissues and the lymphatics. Eight filarial species infect humans (Table 182-1); of these, four—*Wuchereria bancrofti, Brugia malayi, Onchocerca volvulus,* and *Loa loa*—are responsible for most serious filarial infections. Filarial parasites, which infect an estimated 140 million persons worldwide, are transmitted by specific species of mosquitoes or other arthropods and have a complex life cycle that includes infective larval stages that are carried by insects and adult worms that reside in either lymphatic or subcutaneous tissues of humans. The offspring of adults are microfilariae, which, depending on their species, are 200 to 250 μm long and 5 to 7 μm wide, may or may not be enveloped in a loose sheath, and either circulate in the blood or migrate through the skin (see Table 182-1). To complete the life cycle, microfilariae are ingested by the arthropod vector and develop over 1 to 2 weeks into new infective larvae. Adult worms live many years, whereas microfilariae survive from 3 to 36 months.

Usually, infection is only established with repeated and prolonged exposures to infective larvae. Since the clinical manifestations of filarial diseases develop relatively slowly, these infections should be considered chronic diseases with possible long-term debilitating effects. In terms of the nature, severity, and timing of clinical manifestations, patients with filariasis who are native to endemic areas and have lifelong exposures may differ significantly from those who are travelers or who have recently moved to these same areas. Characteristically, the disease is more acute and intense in newly exposed individuals than in natives of endemic areas.

LYMPHATIC FILARIASIS

Lymphatic filariasis is caused by *W. bancrofti, B. malayi,* or *B. timori.* The threadlike adult parasites reside in either lymphatic channels or lymph nodes, where they may remain viable for more than two decades.

EPIDEMIOLOGY *W. bancrofti,* the most widely distributed human filarial parasite, affects an estimated 80 million people and is found throughout the tropics and subtropics, including Asia and the Pacific Islands, Africa, areas of South America, and the Caribbean basin. Humans are the only definitive host for the parasite. Nocturnally periodic forms of microfilariae are scarce in peripheral blood by day and increase at night, whereas with subperiodic forms microfilariae are present in peripheral blood at all times and reach maximal levels in the afternoon. Generally, the subperiodic form is found only in the Pacific Islands; elsewhere, *W. bancrofti* is nocturnally periodic. Natural vectors are *Culex fatigans* mosquitoes in urban settings and anopheline or aedean mosquitoes in rural areas.

Brugian filariasis due to *B. malayi* occurs primarily in China, India, Indonesia, Korea, Japan, Malaysia, and the Philippines. *B. malayi* also has two forms distinguished by the periodicity of microfilaremia. The more common nocturnal form is transmitted in areas of coastal rice fields, while the subperiodic form is found in forests. *B. malayi* naturally infects cats as well as human hosts. *B. timori* exists only on two islands in Indonesia.

TABLE 182-1 Characteristics of the filariae

Organism	Periodicity	Distribution	Vector	Location of adult	Microfilarial location	Sheath
Wuchereria bancrofti	Nocturnal	Cosmopolitan Mainly India China, Indonesia	*Culex* (mosquitoes) *Anopheles* (mosquitoes) *Aedes* (mosquitoes)	Lymphatic	Blood	+
	Subperiodic	Eastern Pacific	*Aedes* (mosquitoes)	Lymphatic	Blood	+
Brugia malayi	Nocturnal	Southeast Asia, Indonesia, India	*Mansonia, Anopheles* (mosquitoes)	Lymphatic	Blood	+
	Subperiodic	Indonesia, Southeast Asia	*Coquilletidia* (mosquitoes) *Mansonia* (mosquitoes)	Lymphatic	Blood	+
Brugia timori	Nocturnal	Indonesia	*Anopheles* (mosquitoes)	Lymphatic	Blood	+
Loa loa	Diurnal	West and Central Africa	*Chrysops* (deerflies)	Subcutaneous	Blood	+
Mansonella ozzardi	None	South and Central America Carribean	*Culicoides* (midges) *Simulium* (blackflies)	Undetermined	Blood	−
Mansonella perstans	None	South and Central America, Africa	*Culicoides* (midges)	Body cavities, mesentery, perirenal	Blood	−
Mansonella streptocerca	None	West and Central Africa	*Culicoides* (midges)	Subcutaneous	Skin	−
Onchocerca volvulus	None	South and Central America, Africa	*Simulium* (blackflies)	Subcutaneous	Skin, eye	−

PATHOLOGY The principal pathologic changes result from inflammatory damage to the lymphatics caused by adult worm and not by microfilariae. Adult worms live in afferent lymphatics or sinuses of lymph nodes and cause lymphatic dilatation and thickening of the vessel walls. Plasma cells, eosinophils, and macrophages infiltrate in and around the infected vessels and, with endothelial and connective tissue proliferation, lead to tortuosity of the lymphatics and damaged or incompetent lymph valves. Lymphedema and chronic stasis changes with hard or brawny edema develop in the overlying skin. These consequences of filariasis are not due to simple lymphatic obstruction by resident adult worms but rather to the immune response of the host to the parasite. These immune responses are believed to cause the granulomatous and proliferative processes that precede lymphatic obstruction. It is thought that as long as the worm remains viable, the vessel remains patent and that death of the worm leads to an enhanced granulomatous reaction and fibrosis. Lymphatic obstruction results, and despite collateralization of the lymphatics, lymphatic function is compromised.

CLINICAL FEATURES The common manifestations of lymphatic filariasis are asymptomatic microfilaremia, filarial fevers, and lymphatic obstruction. Asymptomatic microfilaremia is found in the majority of infected individuals who are clinically well. Filarial fevers are acute episodes in which high fever is often accompanied by shaking chills, lymphatic inflammation (lymphangitis and lymphadenitis), and transient local edema. Episodes can recur as frequently as 10 times per year and usually abate spontaneously after 7 to 10 days. The lymphangitis characteristically develops in a retrograde or descending fashion, extending peripherally from the draining node where the parasite presumably resides. Regional lymph nodes are often enlarged, and the entire lymphatic channel can become indurated and inflamed. Concomitant local thrombophlebitis can develop. In brugian filariasis, a local abscess may form over a lymphatic tract and rupture. Lymphadenitis and lymphangitis occur in both upper and lower extremities with bancroftian and brugian filariasis, but genital lymphatic involvement develops almost exclusively with *W. bancrofti* infection. Genital involvement can be manifested by funiculitis, epididymitis, and scrotal pain and tenderness.

If lymphatic damage progresses into lymphatic obstruction, the permanent changes associated with elephantiasis may follow. Brawny edema follows early pitting edema. With thickening of subcutaneous tissues, hyperkeratosis, fissuring of the skin, and hyperplastic changes develop. Bacterial superinfection of the poorly vascularized tissues is common. In bancroftian filariasis, scrotal lymphedema or hydrocele formation can occur. If the retroperitoneal lymphatics become obstructed, increased pressure leads to the rupture of renal lymphatics and the development of chyluria, which is usually intermittent and most prominent in the morning.

The clinical manifestations of filarial infections in travelers or transmigrants who have recently entered an endemic region are distinctive. Given a sufficient number of bites by infected vectors, usually over a 3- to 6-month period, recently exposed patients can develop acute lymphatic or scrotal inflammation with or without urticaria and localized angioedema. Lymphadenitis of epitrochlear, axillary, femoral, or inguinal lymph nodes is often followed by retrogradely evolving lymphangitis. Acute attacks are short-lived and, in contrast to filarial fevers in patients native to endemic areas, are usually not accompanied by fever. With prolonged exposures to infected mosquitoes, these attacks, if untreated, become more severe and lead to permanent lymphatic inflammation and obstruction.

DIAGNOSIS The definitive diagnosis can be made only by detection of the parasites and hence can be problematic. Adult worms localized in lymphatic vessels or nodes are largely inaccessible, and biopsies usually are not revealing and therefore are not indicated. Microfilariae can be found in blood, in hydrocele fluid, or (occasionally) in other body fluids. Such fluids can be examined microscopically—either directly or with greater sensitivity after concentration of the parasites by filtration of fluids through a polycarbonate cylindrical pore filter (pore size 3 μm) or by centrifugation of fluid fixed in 2% formalin (Knott's concentration technique). Many infected individuals do not have microfilaremia, and definitive diagnosis in such patients can be difficult; in some instances, the diagnosis must be made on clinical grounds. In acute episodes, lymphatic filariasis must be distinguished from thrombophlebitis, infection, and trauma. Retrogradely evolving lymphangitis is a characteristic feature that helps distinguish filarial lymphangitis from typically ascending bacterial lymphangitis. Chronic filarial lymphedema must be distinguished from the lymphedema of malignancy, postoperative scarring, trauma, chronic edematous states, and congenital lymphatic-system abnormalities. Eosinophilia and elevations of serum IgE and antifilarial antibody concentrations support the diagnosis of lymphatic filariasis. There is, however, extensive cross-reactivity between filarial antigens and antigens of other helminths, including the common intestinal roundworms; thus interpretations of serologic findings can be difficult. In addition, residents of endemic areas can become sensitized to filarial antigens through exposure to infected mosquitoes without having patent filarial infections. Thus most serologic and skin tests are of less diagnostic value in individuals native to endemic areas than in travelers or short-term visitors.

TREATMENT Treatment for lymphatic filariasis is currently limited to diethylcarbamazine (DEC) given at 6 mg/kg per day in either single or divided doses for 2 to 3 weeks. This regimen clears microfilariae from the blood and has a limited but definite effect on adult parasites. If at least some adult parasites survive, as is often the case, microfilaremia along with clinical symptoms can recur within months after therapy. There is some evidence that several courses of DEC or chronic administration of low-dose DEC may effect a cure. Ivermectin, a drug active in onchocerciasis, has been used in trials of therapy for lymphatic filariasis; in a single dose (not approved by the FDA), it appears to be as effective as DEC at clearing microfilariae. Side effects of DEC (or ivermectin) treatment include fever, chills, arthralgia, headaches, nausea, and vomiting. Both the development and the severity of these reactions, which may reflect an acute reaction to antigens released by dying parasites, are related directly to the number of microfilariae circulating in the blood. To avoid these side effects, one can either initiate treatment with a small dose of DEC and increase to a full dose over a few days or premedicate the patient with glucocorticoids.

Treatment of chronic lymphatic obstruction is difficult but may be helpful. Elevation of the infected limb, use of elastic stockings, and local foot care eliminate some of the associated symptoms. Surgical decompression with a nodovenous shunt may provide relief for severely affected limbs. Hydroceles can be drained or managed surgically. The management of filarial chyluria is unsatisfactory; neither surgical intervention nor sclerosis of infected lymphatics is effective.

PREVENTION Avoidance of mosquito bites usually is not feasible for residents of endemic areas, but visitors should use insect repellent and mosquito nets. DEC can kill developing filarial larvae and is useful as a prophylactic agent, although the optimal regimen for prophylaxis has not been ascertained. Mass treatment with DEC may reduce community levels of microfilariae so as to interrupt vector-borne transmission among humans.

TROPICAL PULMONARY EOSINOPHILIA

Tropical pulmonary eosinophilia (TPE) is a distinct syndrome that develops in some individuals infected with lymphatic filarial species. This syndrome affects males and females at a ratio of 4:1, often during the third decade of life. The majority of cases have been reported from India, Pakistan, Sri Lanka, Brazil, and Southeast Asia.

CLINICAL FEATURES The main features include a history of residence in filarial endemic regions, paroxysmal cough and wheezing that are usually nocturnal (and probably related to the nocturnal periodicity of microfilariae), weight loss, low-grade fever, adenopathy, and pronounced blood eosinophilia (>3000 per microliter). Chest x-rays may be normal but generally show increased bronchovascular markings; diffuse miliary lesions or mottled opacities may be present in the middle and lower lung fields. Tests of pulmonary function show restrictive abnormalities in half and obstructive defects in most. Total serum IgE levels (10,000 to 100,000 ng/mL) and antifilarial antibody titers are characteristically elevated.

PATHOLOGY In TPE there is rapid immune-mediated clearance of microfilariae from the bloodstream into the lungs, and the clinical symptoms result from allergic and inflammatory reactions elicited by the cleared parasites. In some subjects, microfilarial trapping in other reticuloendothelial organs can cause hepatomegaly, splenomegaly, or lymphadenopathy. A prominent, eosinophil-enriched, intraalveolar infiltrate is often present. In the absence of successful treatment, interstitial fibrosis can lead to progressive pulmonary damage.

DIFFERENTIAL DIAGNOSIS TPE must be distinguished from asthma, Löffler's syndrome, allergic bronchopulmonary aspergillosis, allergic granulomatosis with angiitis (Churg-Strauss syndrome), the systemic vasculitides (most notably periarteritis nodosa and Wegener's granulomatosis), chronic eosinophilic pneumonia, and the idiopathic hypereosinophilic syndrome. In addition to a geographic history of filarial exposure, useful features for distinguishing TPE include wheezing that is solely nocturnal, very high levels of antifilarial antibodies, and a rapid initial response to treatment with DEC.

TREATMENT DEC is used at a dosage of 4 to 6 mg/kg of body weight per day for 14 days. Symptoms usually resolve within 3 to 7 days after initiating therapy. Relapse, which occurs in approximately 12 to 25 percent of individuals (sometimes after an interval of years), requires retreatment.

ONCHOCERCIASIS

Onchocerciasis ("river blindness") is caused by the filarial nematode *Onchocerca volvulus*, which infects an estimated 13 million individuals, primarily in equatorial Africa and Latin America. Onchocerciasis is the second leading cause of infectious blindness worldwide.

ETIOLOGY AND EPIDEMIOLOGY Infection in humans begins with the deposition of infective larvae onto the skin by the bite of an infected blackfly. Infected larvae develop into adults that are typically found in subcutaneous nodules. About 7 months to 3 years after infection, the gravid female releases microfilariae that migrate out of the nodule and throughout the tissues, concentrating in the dermis. Infection is transmitted to other persons when a female fly ingests microfilariae from the host's skin and these microfilariae then develop into infective larvae. Adult *O. volvulus* females and males are about 40 to 60 cm and 3 to 6 cm in length, respectively. The life span of adults can be up to 18 years, with an average of approximately 9 years. Because the blackfly vector breeds along free-flowing rivers and streams (particularly in rapids) and generally restricts its flight to within several kilometers from these breeding sites, both biting and disease transmission are most intense at these locations. The majority of individuals infected with *O. volvulus* are in the equatorial region of Africa extending from the Atlantic coast to the Red Sea. About 70,000 persons are infected in Guatemala and Mexico, with smaller foci in Venezuela, Colombia, Brazil, Ecuador, Yemen, and Saudi Arabia.

PATHOLOGY Onchocerciasis affects primarily the skin, eyes, and lymph nodes. In contrast to lymphatic filariasis, the damage in onchocerciasis is elicited by microfilariae and not by adults. In the skin, there are mild but chronic inflammatory changes that can eventuate in loss of elastic fibers, atrophy, and fibrosis. The subcutaneous nodules, or onchocercomata, consist primarily of fibrous tissues surrounding the adult worm, often with a peripheral ring of inflammatory cells. In the eye, neovascularization and corneal scarring lead to corneal opacities and blindness. Inflammation in the anterior and posterior chambers frequently can result in anterior uveitis, chorioretinitis, and optic atrophy. Although punctate opacities are due to an inflammatory reaction surrounding dead or dying microfilariae, the pathogenesis of most manifestations of onchocerciasis is still unclear.

CLINICAL FEATURES Skin Pruritus, the most frequent manifestation of onchocercal dermatitis, can be incapacitating even when skin microfilariae are rare. Long-term infection results in exaggerated and premature wrinkling of the skin, loss of elastic fibers, and epidermal atrophy that can lead to loose, redundant skin and hypo- or hyperpigmentation. A localized eczematoid dermatitis can cause hyperkeratosis, scaling, and pigmentary changes. Such lesions are often seen in the lower extremities but can be distributed more extensively.

Onchocercomata These subcutaneous nodules, which can be palpable or visible, contain the adult worm. In Africa they are common over the coccyx and sacrum, the trochanter of the femur, the lateral anterior crest, and other bony prominences. In Latin America, the subcutaneous nodules tend to be found preferentially in the upper part of the body, particularly the head, neck, and shoulders. Nodules vary in size and characteristically are firm and not tender. It has been estimated that for every palpable nodule there are four deeper, nonpalpable ones.

Ocular tissue Visual impairment is the most serious complication of onchocerciasis and usually affects only those persons with moderate or heavy infections. Lesions may be present in all parts of the eye. The most common early finding is conjunctivitis with photophobia. In the cornea, punctate keratitis—acute inflammatory reactions surrounding dying microfilariae manifested as "snowflake" opacities—is frequent in younger age groups and resolves without apparent complications. Sclerosing keratitis occurs in approximately 5 percent of persons infected with savannah strains and 1 percent of those infected with forest strains and is the leading cause of onchocercal blindness in Africa. Anterior uveitis and iridocyclitis develop in about 5 percent of infected persons in Africa. In Latin America, complications of the anterior uveal tract (pupillary deformity) may cause secondary glaucoma. Characteristic chorioretinal lesions develop as a result of atrophy and hyperpigmentation of the retinal pigment epithelium and the choriopapillaris. Constriction of the visual field and frank optic atrophy may occur.

Lymph nodes Mild to moderate lymphadenopathy is frequent, particularly in the inguinal and femoral areas, where enlargement of nodes may be gravitationally dependent ("hanging groin") and may predispose to inguinal and femoral hernias.

Systemic manifestations Some heavily infected individuals develop cachexia with loss of adipose tissue and muscle mass. In adults who become blind, there is a three- to fourfold increase in the mortality rate.

DIAGNOSIS Definitive diagnosis depends on the detection of an adult worm in an excised nodule or, more commonly, microfilariae in a skin snip. Skin snips are most readily obtained with a corneal-scleral punch, which collects a blood-free skin biopsy sample extending just below the epidermis. The biopsy tissue is incubated in tissue culture medium or in saline on a glass slide or flat-bottomed microtiter plate. After incubation for 2 to 4 h (or occasionally overnight in light infections), microfilariae emergent from the skin can be seen under a microscope.

TREATMENT The major goals of therapy are to prevent irreversible lesions and alleviate symptoms. Surgical excision is recommended when nodules are located on the head because of the proximity of microfilaria-producing adult worms to the eye, but chemotherapy is the mainstay of management. Ivermectin, a semisynthetic macrocyclic lactone active against microfilariae, is the first-line agent for the treatment of onchocerciasis. It is given orally in a single dose of 150 µg/kg, either yearly or semiannually. After treatment, most individuals have few or no reactions. Pruritus, cutaneous edema, and/or maculopapular rash occurs in approximately 1 to 10 percent of treated individuals. Contraindications to treatment include pregnancy, breast feeding, central nervous system disorders that may increase the penetration of ivermectin into the CNS (e.g., meningitis), and an age of less than 5 years. Although ivermectin treatment results in a marked drop in microfilarial density, its effect may last only 6 months. Suramin, a potent but potentially toxic macrofilaricidal agent, is recommended only if total cure is necessary. First, ivermectin is given to reduce the microfilarial load; then suramin is administered intravenously after a test dose. Weekly doses are started at 200 mg and increased by 200-mg increments until a total dose of 60 to 70 mg/kg is reached. Because of the drug's nephrotoxicity, renal function must be monitored closely. After suramin therapy, an additional course of ivermectin is customarily given to eliminate any remaining microfilariae.

PREVENTION Vector control has been beneficial in highly endemic areas with breeding sites that are vulnerable to insecticide spraying, but most endemic areas for onchocerciasis are not suited for this type of control. While persons working in fly-infested areas can minimize the number of bites they sustain by wearing protective garments, this approach is not feasible for the large majority of individuals in endemic foci. No drug has been shown to prevent infection with *O. volvulus*.

LOIASIS

ETIOLOGY AND EPIDEMIOLOGY Loiasis (the African eye worm) is caused by *Loa loa*, which is present in the rain forests of West and Central Africa. Adult parasites (females, 50 to 70 mm long and 0.5 mm wide; males, 25 to 35 mm long and 0.25 mm wide) live in subcutaneous tissues; microfilariae circulate in the blood with a diurnal periodicity that peaks between 12:00 noon and 2:00 P.M.

CLINICAL FEATURES Manifestations in natives of endemic areas may differ from those in temporary residents or visitors. Among the indigenous population, loiasis is often an asymptomatic infection with microfilaremia. Infection may be recognized only after subconjunctival migration of an adult worm (the so-called eye worm) or manifested as episodic Calabar swellings, evanescent localized areas of angioedema and erythema on the extremities and less frequently elsewhere. Nephropathy, encephalopathy, and cardiomyopathy are rare. In nonresidents, allergic symptoms predominate. The episodes of Calabar swelling tend to be more frequent and debilitating; microfilaremia is rare, and eosinophilia and increased levels of antifilarial antibodies are characteristic.

PATHOLOGY The pathogenesis of the manifestations is poorly understood. Calabar swellings are thought to result from a hypersensitivity reaction to the adult worm.

DIAGNOSIS Definitive diagnosis requires detection of microfilariae in the peripheral blood or isolation of the adult worm from the eye or from a subcutaneous biopsy at a site of swelling developing after treatment. In practice, the diagnosis must often be based on a characteristic history and clinical presentation, blood eosinophilia, and elevated levels of antifilarial antibodies, particularly in travelers to the endemic region, who are usually a microfilaremic. Other clinical findings in the latter individuals include hypergammaglobulinemia, elevated levels of serum IgE, and elevated leukocyte and eosinophil counts.

TREATMENT AND PREVENTION DEC (8 to 10 mg/kg per day for 21 days) is effective against both the adult and the microfilarial forms of *L. loa*, but multiple courses are frequently necessary before disease resolves completely. In cases of heavy microfilaremia, allergic or other inflammatory reactions can occur during treatment, including CNS involvement with coma and encephalitis. Heavy infections are treated initially with low doses of DEC (0.5 mg/kg per day) and glucocorticoids (40 to 60 mg prednisone per day). If there are no adverse effects from the antifilarial treatment, prednisone can be rapidly tapered and the dose of DEC gradually increased to 4 to 8 mg/kg per day.

STREPTOCERCIASIS

Mansonella streptocerca, found mainly in the tropical forest belt of Africa from Ghana to Zaire, is transmitted by biting midges. The

major clinical manifestations involve the skin and include pruritus, papular rashes, and pigmentation changes. Many infected individuals have inguinal adenopathy, although the majority are asymptomatic. The diagnosis is made by detection of the characteristic microfilariae in skin snips. DEC (6 mg/kg per day in divided doses for 14 to 21 days) is effective in killing both microfilariae and adults. As in onchocerciasis, urticaria, arthralgias, myalgias, headaches, and abdominal discomfort may accompany treatment.

MANSONELLA PERSTANS INFECTION

Mansonella perstans, distributed across the center of Africa and in northeastern South America, is transmitted by midges. Adult worms reside in serous cavities—pericardial, pleural, and peritoneal—as well as in the mesentery and the perirenal and retroperitoneal tissues. Microfilariae circulate in the blood without periodicity. The clinical and pathologic features are poorly defined. Most patients appear to be asymptomatic, but manifestations may include transient angioedema and pruritus of the arms, face, or other parts of the body (analogous to Calabar swellings of loiasis), fever, headache, arthralgias, and right upper quadrant pain. Occasionally, pericarditis and hepatitis occur. The diagnosis is based on the demonstration of microfilariae in blood or serosal effusions. Perstans filariasis is often associated with peripheral blood eosinophilia and antifilarial antibody elevations. Although DEC (8 to 10 mg/kg per day for 21 days) is the standard therapy, there is little evidence that it is efficacious. If cure is obtained, symptoms and eosinophilia disappear; multiple courses of therapy are usually required. Mebendazole (100 mg twice daily for 30 days) also has been reported to be effective.

MANSONELLA OZZARDI INFECTION

The distribution of *Mansonella ozzardi* is restricted to Central and South America and certain Caribbean islands. Adult worms are rarely recovered from humans. Microfilariae circulate in the blood without periodicity. Although many consider this organism to be nonpathogenic, headache, articular pain, fever, pulmonary symptoms, adenopathy, hepatomegaly, pruritus, and eosinophilia have been ascribed to *M. ozzardi* infection. Diagnosis is made by the detection of microfilariae in peripheral blood. No drug is proven to be effective; ivermectin was effective in a single case report.

DRACUNCULIASIS (GUINEA WORM INFECTION)

ETIOLOGY AND EPIDEMIOLOGY Dracunculiasis, caused by *Dracunculus medinensis*, affects approximately 5 million people in the Middle East, Africa, India, and Pakistan. Humans acquire this infection when they ingest water containing infective larvae derived from the *Cyclops*, a crustacean that is the intermediate host. Larvae penetrate the stomach or intestinal wall, mate, and mature. The adult male probably dies; the female *Dracunculus* develops over a year and migrates to subcutaneous tissues, usually in the lower extremity. As the thin female *Dracunculus*, ranging in length from 300 cm to 1 m, approaches the skin, a blister forms that, over days, breaks down and forms an ulcer. When the blister opens, large numbers of motile, rhabditiform larvae can be released into stagnant water; ingestion by the *Cyclops* completes the life cycle.

CLINICAL FEATURES Few or no clinical manifestations are evident until just before the blister forms, when there is the onset of fever and generalized allergic symptoms, including periorbital edema, wheezing, and urticaria. The emergence of the worm is associated with local pain and swelling. When the blister ruptures (usually as a result of immersion in water), the adult releases larva-rich fluid, and this release is associated with a relief of symptoms. The shallow ulcer surrounding the emerging adult worm heals over weeks to months.

Such ulcers, however, can become secondarily infected, the result being cellulitis, local inflammation, abscess formation, or (uncommonly) tetanus. Occasionally, the adult worm does not emerge but becomes encapsulated and calcified.

DIAGNOSIS The diagnosis is based on the findings developing with the emergence of the adult worm.

TREATMENT AND PREVENTION Gradual extraction of the worm by winding of a few centimeters on a stick each day remains the common and effective practice. Worms may be excised surgically. Thiabendazole (25 mg/kg twice daily for 3 days) or metronidazole (250 mg three times daily for 10 days) may relieve symptoms but have no proven activity against the worm. Prevention, which remains the only real control measure, depends on the provision of safe drinking water.

ZOONOTIC FILARIAL INFECTIONS

Dirofilariae that affect primarily dogs, cats, and raccoons and *Brugia* parasites that affect small mammals occasionally infect humans incidentally. Because humans are an abnormal host, the parasites never fully develop. Pulmonary dirofilarial infection caused by the canine heartworm *Dirofilaria immitis* generally presents in humans as a solitary pulmonary nodule. Chest pain, hemoptysis, or cough is uncommon. Infections with *D. repens* (from dogs) or *D. tenuis* (from raccoons) can cause local subcutaneous nodules in humans. Zoonotic *Brugia* infection can produce isolated lymph node enlargement. Eosinophilia and antifilarial antibodies are not commonly elevated. Excisional biopsy is both diagnostic and curative; these infections usually do not respond to chemotherapy.

REFERENCES

Eberhard ML, Lammie PJ: Laboratory diagnosis of filariasis. Clin Lab Med 11:977, 1991

Lymphatic filariasis

Filariasis. Ciba Found Symp 127:1, 1985
WHO Expert Committee on Lymphatic Filariasis: Fifth report. Technical Report Series No. 821, Geneva, WHO 1993

Tropical pulmonary eosinophilia

Ottesen EA, Nutman TB: Tropical pulmonary eosinophilia. Annu Rev Med 43:417, 1992

Onchocerciasis

WHO Expert Committee on Onchocerciasis: Third report. Technical Report Series No. 752, Geneva, WHO, 1987

Loiasis

Klion AD et al: Loiasis in endemic and non-endemic populations: Immunologically mediated differences in clinical presentation. J Infect Dis 163:1318, 1991

Other filarial infections

Adolph PE et al: Diagnosis and treatment of *Acanthocheilonema perstans* filariasis. Am J Trop Med Hyg 11:76, 1962
Marinkelle CJ, German E: Mansonelliasis in the Comisaria del Vaupes of Colombia. Trop Georgr Med 22:101, 1970
Meyers WM et al: Human streptocerciasis: A clinicopathologic study of 40 Africans (Zairians) including identification of the adult filaria. Am J Trop Med Hyg 21:528, 1972

Dracunculiasis

Ranque P, Hopkins D: Current status of the global campaign to eradicate dracunculiasis (guinea worm disease) Ann Parasitol Hum Comp 66(suppl 1):37, 1991

Zoonotic filarial infections

Ro JY et al: Pulmonary dirofilariasis: The great imitator of primary or metastatic lung tumor. A clinicopathologic analysis of seven cases and a review of the literature. Hum Pathol 20:69, 1989

183 SCHISTOSOMIASIS AND OTHER TREMATODE INFECTIONS

THEODORE E. NASH

The trematodes (flukes) that commonly infect humans live in the intestines, biliary tract, lungs, and venules of intestines or genitourinary tract. With the exception of the intestinal schistosomes, which cause a unique type of liver fibrosis, disease is limited primarily to the organs where the parasites reside. The pathophysiology of disease differs among the trematodes. Schistosomiasis is the best understood, and some of the factors important in disease development in this infection appear to apply to infections caused by many of the other trematodes. In endemic areas, large proportions of the population are infected but asymptomatic; the disease is mostly limited to heavily infected persons. Distinct acute and chronic syndromes are recognizable, as are predictable pathologic changes over time. Eosinophilia and fever are common findings in acute disease. Because many of these parasites follow complicated migration routes and/or are poorly adapted to suvival in a human host, infections in ectopic locations are an important cause of morbidity.

Infections in humans are limited to digenetic trematodes, i.e., those which undergo sexual reproduction and produce eggs in mammalian definitive hosts and asexual reproduction in snails. After eggs reach water, they either hatch immediately or undergo maturation before releasing a free-swimming *miracidium* which seeks out the appropriate intermediate snail host or is ingested by the snail. After a number of cycles of multiplication in the snail, free-swimming *cercariae* are released and, depending on the species, can (1) infect the definitive host, (2) seek out a second intermediate host such as fish or crustacea, or (3) encyst on vegetation. The encysted cercaria, or *metacercaria*, is a dormant, relatively resistant form which infects the host following ingestion. With the exception of schistosomes, most trematodes are flat, leaf-shaped parasites that vary in length from 1 mm to 7 cm. They possess two grasping organs called *suckers* and lack a body cavity. The gut usually lacks an anus, and digested food is regurgitated through the oral opening. The surfaces of trematodes are covered by a syncytium of cells or tegument through which nutrients are absorbed. Schistosomes differ from the other trematodes infecting humans in a number of important ways. Most trematodes are hermaphroditic, but the sexes are separate in the schistosomes, and completion of the sexual cycle requires the presence of male and female worms. The adult schistosomes reside in the bloodstream, whereas the other trematodes dwell in the liver, lung, or intestines. In schistosomiasis, humans become infected by freeswimming cercariae that invade the skin; in contrast, in the other trematode infections, humans become infected after ingestion. The eggs of hermaphroditic trematodes possess a characteristic operculum, or caplike structure. The morphology of schistosome ova differs from that of other trematode ova, as described below.

A large number of trematodes can infect humans. With the exception of some species of schistosomes, most trematodes have domestic or wild animals as definitive hosts, and humans are accidentally infected. In highly endemic situations or under particularly advantageous circumstances, humans are able to maintain the life cycle in the absence of the usual definitive host. Some infections are rare or occur in populations in limited geographic areas, while others affect large numbers of persons over extensive areas or produce recognizable syndromes.

A pertinent history is important to determine the diagnosis. Persons from endemic areas; travelers who are exposed to fresh water or ingest undercooked fish, crustacea, or potentially contaminated vegetation; or others who ingest locally obtained but potentially contaminated vegetation such as watercress or undercooked, pickled, or smoked fish can be infected. Eosinophilia is common in acute invasive trematode infections. The definitive diagnosis is established by demonstrating eggs in stool or sputum or by biopsy of the affected tissue. Serologic tests are available for schistosomiasis, fascioliasis, and paragonimiasis; a positive test is indicative of infection. Serologic tests for other trematode infections may be available in endemic areas or research laboratories.

SCHISTOSOMIASIS

Three major schistosome species, *Schistosoma mansoni, Schistosoma haematobium*, and *Schistosoma japonicum*, and a number of less prevalent species of the genus *Schistosoma* infect humans. Both *S. mansoni* and *S. japonicum* adults reside in the venules of the intestine, and the major disease manifestations of these parasites are hepatic. *S. mansoni* is found in parts of South America (Brazil, Venezuela, and Surinam), some Caribbean islands, Africa, and the Middle East, while infections with *S. japonicum* occur in the Far East, mostly in China and the Philippines. *S. haematobium* adults are found mostly in the venules of the urinary tract and cause lesions primarily of the ureters and bladder. Infections with this species occur in Africa and the Middle East. Of lesser importance are *S. mekongi*, a parasite related to *S. japonicum* which is found along the Mekong River in Indochina, and *S. intercalatum*, found in certain areas of central West Africa. Worldwide, as many as 200 million persons may be infected, and infection of entire communities is common. However, most infected persons experience few, if any, signs and symptoms, and only a small minority develop significant disease.

LIFE CYCLE   The schistosome species infecting humans all share the same basic life cycle but are unique in ways which account for some of the different clinical and pathologic findings. Important differences include the length of time before egg laying begins (prepatent period), location of the adult worms, number of eggs produced by each pair of worms, response by the host to the ova, and eventual fate of retained eggs. The morphology of the parasites and the types of intermediate host snail are also distinct. Humans become infected after contact with water containing the infective stage of the parasite, called a *cercaria*, which is a microscopic form of the schistosome possessing a forked tail used for swimming and a head which is the anlage of the worm. Cercariae penetrate the unbroken skin, with the help of secreted enzymes, and in the skin transform into *schistosomules*, or developing schistosomes. After 2 to 3 days, the schistosomules migrate to the lungs and then to the portal vein, probably by an intravascular route. In the portal vein the maturing male and female schistosomes pair and migrate to the venules of the mesentery, bladder, or ureters, depending on the species of schistosome, and begin to deposit eggs. The time spent in migration and maturation differs. *S. mansoni* and *S. japonicum* begin depositing eggs around 4 to 5 weeks after infection, while egg deposition begins after 2 to 3 months for *S. haematobium*. Adult worms are about 1 to 2 cm in length and migrate in the blood vessels without eliciting a local inflammatory reaction. Adult worms do not multiply in humans, and immunosuppressive therapy does not result in increased numbers of worms. Once released, eggs are either retained in the tissues at the site of deposition or swept back, mostly to the liver, by way of the venous portal system in the case of the intestinal schistosomes. Eggs are deposited mainly in the bladder and ureters by *S. haematobium*. A portion of the mature schistosome ova are extruded into the lumen of the intestines, bladder, or ureters and, after contact with water, hatch, releasing a miracidium. This free-swimming ciliated stage seeks out the proper intermediate snail vector and burrows into the soft tissues of the snail. After 1 to 2 months, depending on the species, the miracidium develops into a primary and then secondary sporocyst which, after further development, begins releasing cercariae into the surrounding water. Thousands of cercariae can be released daily from each infected snail. Therefore, one miracidium produces many cercariae, and this amplifies the number of infective parasites and the risk of infection. Cercariae are most infectious immediately after shedding and are not viable 48 h

after release, so storing water for 48 h before contact prevents exposure and infection. Unlike most other trematodes, the sexes are separate in schistosomes, but this is only evident in the adult stage. Ova are laid only when males and females infect the same individual.

PATHOPHYSIOLOGY   A number of factors govern the disease manifestations. These include the duration and intensity of infection, location of egg deposition, host genetics, concurrent infections, and other still undefined factors.

In individuals from endemic areas, initial infection goes unnoticed. There are a number of possible reasons for this, including age at initial exposure, manner of exposure, and transfer of antigens, antibodies, and anti-idiotypes from the mother. In visitors to endemic areas, initial infection with schistosomes commonly results in an acute febrile illness (Katayama fever or acute schistosomiasis) which is most likely a manifestation of the immune response to the developing schistosomes and eggs. There is a vigorous hypersensitivity response which becomes modulated. These individuals have elevated levels of eosinophils and immune complexes and react markedly to schistosome antigens, as measured by lymphocyte blastogenesis. Despite ongoing infection, symptoms subside, as do blastogenic responses to schistosome antigens but not to unrelated antigens such as purified protein derivative of tuberculin (PPD). The exudative acute granulomatous response to schistosome eggs is also modulated.

A major factor in determining the development of disease in humans is the worm burden of the host, which determines the number of eggs produced. The inflammatory and fibrotic response to these eggs is responsible for most of the morbidity and mortality associated with schistosomiasis. Factors which limit parasite survival will limit the development of disease. Immunity exists in experimental animals, but in human schistosome infections it has not been clearly established that protective immunity develops; however, immunity is thought to develop because reinfection rates in previously treated humans are reduced in older populations despite similar amounts of water contact. In the first few days after infection, the schistosomule is relatively susceptible to immune attack. A number of systems employing antibody and/or eosinophils, neutrophils, macrophages, and complement have been used to kill schistosomules in vitro. However, as the schistosomules mature, they become refractory to these immune responses. In addition, schistosomes coat their tegument with host proteins and evade recognition by the host. A number of antibodies which block effective killing also may result in enhanced parasite survival. Schistosomule and adult antigens have been defined with the hope of developing vaccines; the administration of murine monoclonal antibodies to some of these antigens has reduced worm burdens in challenge infections by about 50 percent, and immunization of rodents with a number of defined antigens produced similar levels of protection. Successful vaccination with anti-idiotypes also has been reported.

All schistosome eggs elicit a granulomatous response which is best understood in *S. mansoni* infections. The host becomes sensitized to the egg proteins by a T cell–mediated mechanism which induces a larger granuloma. However, with continued infection the granuloma decreases in size due to the recruitment of suppressor T cells, while antibody has no effect on granuloma size. The regulation of granulomas due to *S. japonicum* eggs differs from that of granulomas from *S. mansoni* eggs. Immune modulation is mediated by serum factors, including anti-idiotype networks, at least in the chronic stage of infection. Both eggs and granulomas release factors which induce fibroblast proliferation in vitro. The early cellular response induced by granulomas is followed by fibrosis in vivo; however, liver fibrosis in humans probably involves more than simple fusion of fibrotic granulomas. After years of continued infection, some heavily infected individuals develop end-stage fibrotic lesions, mainly portal fibrosis (Symmers' fibrosis), sometimes resulting in esophageal varices and splenomegaly in *S. mansoni, S. japonicum*, and *S. mekongi* infections and fibrosis of the ureters and bladder in *S. haematobium* infections. After the development of portal fibrosis, eggs are shunted to the lungs via portal-systemic collateral veins, resulting in cor pulmonale in

TABLE 183-1　Clinical manifestations of schistosomiasis from various *Schistosoma* species*

Manifestation	*S. mansoni*	*S. japonicum*	*S. haematobium*
Acute toxemic schistosomiasis	+	+	+
Chronic asymptomatic schistosomiasis	+	+	+
Hepatosplenic schistosomiasis	+	+	0
Cor pulmonale	+	+	±
Glomerulonephritis (clinically significant)	+	+	0[†]
Colonic polyposis	+	+	±
Ectopic lesions			
Brain	±	+	±
Spinal cord	+	±	+
Skin	+	+	+
Chronic cystitis and ureteritis	0	0	+
Mass lesions, bladder and ureters	0	0	+
Bladder cancer	0	0	+
Association with *Salmonella*	+	+	+
Prolonged fever	+	+	+
Urinary carrier stage	?	?	+
Swimmer's itch[‡]	+	+	+

* + = recognized complications of infections by this species; ± = findings much less prominent in individuals infected by this species; 0 = complications not present in infections by this species.
† Except with associated *Salmonella* infections.
‡ Usually from schistosomes that do not infect humans.

about 15 percent of patients with Symmers' fibrosis. Immune complexes shunted to the systemic circulation cause glomerulonephritis.

Host genetic factors have been found to influence the development of Symmers' fibrosis, although there is no general agreement as to which are important. Schistosomes even of the same species are also genetically diverse, as shown by endonuclease restriction analysis, but the effect of this on disease in humans is unknown.

CLINICAL SYNDROMES (See Table 183-1)　**Acute schistosomiasis**　Acute schistosomiasis, or Katayama fever, occurs following initial exposure and infection with *S. mansoni* and *S. japonicum*. It rarely follows infection with *S. haematobium*. Acute schistosomiasis is seldom recognized in endemic populations and therefore is noted primarily in visitors to endemic areas. Immediately following exposure, patients frequently complain of intense transient itching. From 2 to 6 weeks or longer after exposure the patient may complain of a variety of symptoms, including fever, chills, headache, hives or angioedema, weakness, weight loss, nonproductive cough, abdominal pain, and diarrhea. Sometimes symptoms abate but return with increased intensity about the time egg laying commences. These symptoms gradually diminish but may last as long as 2 to 3 months. Other newly infected individuals may be asymptomatic or have only minimal symptoms. In these individuals, the diagnosis is established only after further evaluation prompted by suggestive laboratory test results or exposure history. More severe symptoms occur with heavier infections, but light infections may cause severe illness. Central nervous system lesions may occur during acute schistosome infection. The diagnosis of acute schistosomiasis is suggested by the clinical findings and the presence of eosinophilia, which is sometimes greater than 50 percent. Leukocytosis, increased immune complexes, and elevated IgM, IgG, and IgE immunoglobulins are found commonly. Although immune complexes have been suggested to play a role in the pathophysiology of acute schistosomiasis, glomerulonephritis and vasculitis are not present. The specific diagnosis can be established, even before the shedding of ova, by the detection of antibodies to adult schistosome gut antigens or, after egg excretion (5 to 6 weeks following exposure), by appropriate serologic testing and the finding

of eggs in the stool or rectal biopsy. Clinically, acute schistosomiasis is frequently misdiagnosed as typhoid fever, but it can be confused with any prolonged febrile illness. Although these patients seem to tolerate chemotherapy well, whether therapy shortens the course of disease or decreases symptoms is unclear. Glucocorticoids may be useful, but this has not been demonstrated in controlled studies.

Liver fibrosis　The most important complication of intestinal schistosome infection is the development of periportal or Symmers' fibrosis and portal hypertension (hepatosplenic schistosomiasis). This pathognomonic finding occurs in *S. mansoni*, *S. japonicum*, and *S. mekongi* infections but has been best studied in *S. mansoni* infections, where it normally develops after 10 to 15 years of prolonged exposure and infection. The liver may be enlarged but in many cases is small, firm, and nodular, and the left lobe is characteristically prominent. Macroscopically, finger-sized bands of fibrosis (''pipe-stem'' fibrosis) encompass the large portal tracts. The portal venous tracts are replaced with fibrous tissue, sometimes leading to presinusoidal blockage, portal hypertension, splenomegaly, and esophageal and gastric varices. The intrahepatic pressure is normal. Hepatic function is generally well preserved, and patients commonly present with hematemesis and/or signs and symptoms of splenomegaly. Ascites, hepatic coma, edema, spider angiomas, gynecomastia, and other signs of liver failure occur less frequently than in alcoholic and postnecrotic cirrhosis. Despite repeated episodes of hematemesis, patients may do reasonably well.

In the past, the diagnosis of periportal fibrosis required a wedge biopsy of the liver; needle biopsy specimens are frequently inadequate. Ultrasonograms of the liver show characteristic findings. The fibrotic bands appear as dense echogenic areas surrounding the portal vein and its tributaries. Studies comparing wedge biopsies of the liver with ultrasonographic examination showed that the latter technique had a specificity and sensitivity of 100 percent. Ultrasonography should replace invasive biopsies as the method of choice to diagnose hepatic schistosomiasis.

Ultrasonographic evaluation of *S. mansoni*–infected populations in the Sudan revealed a much higher prevalence of periportal fibrosis than could be determined by physical examination. As many as half the patients studied lacked palpable splenomegaly, and a majority did not give a history of hematemesis. Treatment resulted in regression of periportal fibrosis in some patients.

Patients with periportal fibrosis may not have schistosome eggs in the feces because of previous treatment and/or attrition of adult worms without subsequent reinfection. Since schistosome infections are practically universal in many populations, the mere presence of schistosome eggs in the feces does not establish the diagnosis of schistosomal periportal fibrosis; other liver diseases may be present. It is not clear whether there is any benefit from shunting procedures or splenectomy, although these procedures are used commonly. The mortality of patients with portal fibrosis has not been well studied, but in one group it was 8.2 percent after 3.6 years.

Glomerulonephritis and pulmonary hypertension　These two complications occur almost exclusively in patients with periportal fibrosis and portal hypertension. Pulmonary hypertension appears to be due to obliteration of pulmonary arterioles by granulomatous inflammation induced by shunted and embolized schistosome eggs. This is most frequently recognized with *S. mansoni* and *S. japonicum* infections but also occurs with *S. haematobium*. The association of glomerulonephritis and schistosomiasis has been noted in humans and in experimentally infected animals. This complication is manifested clinically as proteinuria and/or renal failure. Schistosome-specific antibodies and antigens have been detected in the glomeruli of infected patients.

Other complications　Focal dense deposits of eggs of *S. mansoni* in the large intestine (and less commonly of *S. haematobium* and probably of *S. japonicum*) incite an exudative granulomatous response resulting in the formation of inflammatory polyps. Histologically, these consist of masses of eggs, inflammatory cells, and fibrosis. The major clinical presentation is bloody diarrhea, sometimes associated with protein-losing enteropathy and anemia. This type of involvement of the bowel is recognized primarily in Egypt and the Sudan. Gastrointestinal symptoms are not greater in most chronically infected patients than in control populations, although blood in the stool is found more frequently in some studies. Granulomatous masses involving the bowel wall may mimic carcinoma of the bowel. Central nervous system involvement with S. mansoni and S. haematobium has a predilection for the spinal cord, while the brain is involved more commonly in S. japonicum infections.

Patients infected with the three major species of schistosomes and subsequently infected with Salmonella may develop a prolonged intermittent febrile illness. In S. haematobium infections, prolonged excretion of Salmonella in the urine is common. Many times treatment of the Salmonella infection alone is not effective, and specific antischistosomal chemotherapy is also required. Salmonella may be protected from host immune responses by residing in schistosome gut or by adhering to the surface of the schistosome.

SCHISTOSOMA MANSONI **Epidemiology and manifestations** S. mansoni is found in South America and certain islands of the Caribbean, Africa, and the Middle East. The prepatent period is about 4 to 5 weeks. The intermediate hosts are various species in the genus Biomphalaria.

Although infection is frequent and sometimes universal in endemic areas, the development of disease is relatively uncommon and depends on a number of factors which include the duration and intensity of infection. In endemic populations chronic infections are usual, many times lasting decades, and disease manifestations develop in a predictable manner. For the most part, the initial infection of persons living in endemic areas goes unnoticed. In endemic populations, throughout the first decade of life the intensity of infection, as measured by the number of eggs excreted in the feces, increases, and prevalence rates often approach 100 percent in highly endemic communities. Few, if any, symptoms are attributable to schistosomiasis during this time. The liver, particularly the left lobe, gradually enlarges and becomes firm. Between 10 and 15 years of age, some heavily infected persons develop splenomegaly, which partly reflects the presence of portal fibrosis and portal hypertension. About the same time, the number of eggs in the feces decreases, and there is evidence to suggest that immune factors as well as decreased water contact are responsible for this. During the next three decades, persons with portal fibrosis and hypertension may experience repeated bouts of hematemesis secondary to esophageal varices or symptoms secondary to a massively enlarged spleen. Not infrequently, because of prior chemotherapy, decreased exposure, or increased host immunity, patients with end-stage portal fibrosis no longer excrete eggs. Adult schistosomes can survive 20 years or more in the human host but usually live 5 to 8 years. The prognosis and the potential for reversing complications of infection after appropriate chemotherapy depend on the stage of disease. Some regression of periportal fibrosis occurs after chemotherapy, as judged by ultrasound examination, but in most individuals with periportal fibrosis and clinical manifestations, regression does not occur. Glomerulonephritis and cor pulmonale secondary to schistosomiasis occur exclusively in patients with portal fibrosis. Central nervous system involvement can occur at any stage of the infection and is not related to the intensity of infection.

Diagnosis The diagnosis of S. mansoni is established by identification of ova in the feces or tissues. The ova are 114 to 175 μm in length and 45 to 68 μm in width and have a prominent lateral spine. In light infections with fewer than 50 eggs per gram of feces, ova may not be detected in the stool without the use of techniques which sample large quantities of stool. Even in light infections, ova can usually be detected in rectal biopsies and are best identified by squashing a small amount of tissue between two glass slides and searching for ova microscopically.

Many serologic tests have been employed in the diagnosis of schistosomiasis. These tests are not standardized and differ in sensitivity and specificity. Most current tests have greater than 90 percent sensitivity, and a positive serology is indicative of a present or past infection. An immunofluorescent antibody test employing sections of adult schistosomes to determine the presence of antibodies to schistosome gut antigens has been extremely useful in identifying recently infected persons or those with acute schistosomiasis. Recently, antigen detection assays have been developed that appear to be useful in diagnosing infections and determining treatment response.

Treatment In the past, chemotherapy was offered only to more heavily infected individuals who were more likely to develop disease. Although the risks of continued infection have not been clearly defined, with the availability of easily administered and safe drugs, most infected persons are likely to benefit from treatment. Patients with active infections have live eggs, which can be identified microscopically by experienced parasitologists or by the presence of flame cells or their ability to hatch after contact with water. Although a number of drugs are available for the treatment of S. mansoni infection, praziquantel and oxamniquine are the drugs of choice (Table 183-2). Both drugs are equally safe and effective in S. mansoni infections found in the Caribbean and South America. Because some strains of S. mansoni in Africa are relatively resistant to oxamniquine, praziquantel is the better drug. Both drugs can be used in patients with portal fibrosis. The side effects of praziquantel and oxamniquine are frequent but transient and mild. For praziquantel, they include abdominal pain, lethargy, diarrhea, and fever, and for oxamniquine, dizziness, tiredness, nausea and vomiting, neuropsychiatric manifestations, and rarely convulsions.

SCHISTOSOMA JAPONICUM **Epidemiology and clinical manifestations** S. japonicum is found in Southeast Asia and is an important health concern in areas of China and the Philippines. The intermediate hosts are amphibious snails of the genus Oncomelania. Besides humans, numerous mammals such as cattle and water buffalo are naturally infected and serve as reservoirs of infection. The prepatent period is about 4 weeks.

The course of infection and clinical manifestations of S. japonicum are similar to those of S. mansoni, but the epidemiology and disease manifestations are less well studied. Experimental infections are more virulent, probably because each worm pair produces 10 times as many eggs as S. mansoni. The granulomas contain clusters of eggs and are larger and frequently show central necrosis. As in S. mansoni

TABLE 183-2 **Treatment of schistosomiasis**

Species	Drug	Total dose* (mg/kg body weight)	Regimen
S. haematobium	Praziquantel	40	Single dose or two 20 mg/kg doses
	Metrifonate[†]	22.5–30	Single dose of 7.5 to 10 mg/kg body weight given every other week $\times$ 3
S. mansoni			
Americas and Caribbean	Oxamniquine	15	Single oral dose with food
	Praziquantel	40	Single or two 20 mg/kg doses 4 h apart with food
Africa and Middle East	Oxamniquine	60	15 mg/kg body weight twice a day for 2 days with food
	Praziquantel	40	Single dose or two 20 mg/kg doses 4 h apart with food
S. japonicum or S. mekongi	Praziquantel	60	20 mg/kg body weight every 4 h with food

* All recommended drugs are given orally.
[†] Available from the Parasitic Diseases Division, Centers for Infectious Diseases, Centers for Disease Control, Atlanta, GA 30333.

infections, periportal fibrosis is the major clinical manifestation. The other clinical syndromes described in *S. mansoni* also occur as complications of this infection. However, there are some notable differences in disease manifestations, particularly central nervous system (CNS) involvement. In acute schistosomiasis associated with *S. japonicum* infections, about 2 to 3 percent of patients experience CNS symptoms and signs that mimic acute encephalitis or a focal neurologic process. Computed tomography shows multiple enhancing lesions. In chronic infections, patients may present with focal lesions of the brain which mimic brain tumors. These lesions contain masses of eggs and granulomas. Uncontrolled studies suggest that treatment with antischistosomal drugs and glucocorticoids is effective.

Diagnosis　The principles of diagnosis are similar to those of *S. mansoni* and require the demonstration of the typical ova in the tissues or feces of infected individuals. The eggs are oval in shape, 70 to 100 μm by 50 to 65 μm, and have a vestigial spine. Old, calcified, dead eggs are commonly retained in the tissues for long periods of time and do not indicate active infection.

Treatment　Most infected persons should be treated. The only safe and effective therapy for *S. japonicum* infections is praziquantel (see Table 183-2).

SCHISTOSOMA MEKONGI　*S. mekongi* occurs in the Mekong River in Indochina (Laos, Cambodia, and Thailand). The intermediate host is an aquatic snail, *T. aperta*. The eggs are similar to *S. japonicum*'s but are slightly smaller and round, about 56 by 64 μm. Dogs and human beings are frequently naturally infected. The prepatent period is about 5 weeks. The disease manifestations appear to be similar to those of *S. japonicum* but are not fully documented. Praziquantel is effective therapy for this infection (see Table 183-2).

SCHISTOSOMA HAEMATOBIUM　**Epidemiology and clinical manifestations**　*S. haematobium* infections occur in extensive areas of Africa and in the Middle East. The intermediate hosts are of the genus *Bulinus*. The prepatent period is 2 to 3 months. Natural infection is primarily limited to human beings.

As in *S. mansoni* infections, the prevalence and intensity of infection in endemic areas increases until 10 to 15 years of age. Thereafter, the intensity decreases markedly while the prevalence rate falls moderately. The signs and symptoms due to *S. haematobium*, owing to its predilection for the veins of the urinary tract, result from involvement of the ureters and bladder. In contrast to the asymptomatic period following initial infection with the intestinal schistosomes, dysuria and hematuria are frequently noted 2 to 3 months after infection. These findings may continue throughout the course of active infection. Initially, the eggs evoke an intense inflammatory and granulomatous response which may cause anatomic and/or functional obstruction, hydroureter and hydronephrosis, and masses in the bladder or ureters. Cystoscopic examination may reveal friable masses extending into the bladder, ulceration, petechiae, and granulomas. These early lesions are reversible after antischistosomal chemotherapy. Eggs shed into the urine are usually easily demonstrable. As the infection progresses, the inflammatory component lessens, possibly due to a modulating effect of the host's immune response, and fibrosis increases, most likely due to the accumulation of many old and some new lesions. Later, most lesions consist of masses of dead and calcified eggs in fibrous tissue. When the concentration of calcified eggs in the tissues is large enough, radiographic opacification of the affected areas of the urinary tract becomes evident. Fibrotic lesions which cause hydroureter and hydronephrosis are not reversible by antischistosomal chemotherapy. Renal failure occurs in a surprisingly small proportion of infected individuals.

Portal fibrosis and clinically significant glomerulonephritis are not complications of this infection, but passage of eggs into the lungs may result in pulmonary hypertension. Prolonged excretion of *Salmonella* in the urine and intermittent bacteremias are well documented. Urinary tract infections with other bacteria do not appear to be increased in frequency unless there is instrumentation of the urinary tract; however, they may be difficult to eradicate once established. CNS infection most commonly involves the spinal cord, as in *S.*

mansoni infections. Although eggs of *S. haematobium* are frequently detected in the feces in low numbers and are often found in rectal biopsies, intestinal polyposis is uncommon. In certain geographic areas squamous cell cancer of the bladder is felt to be associated with *S. haematobium* infection and is a significant cause of morbidity and mortality.

Diagnosis　The diagnosis of *S. haematobium* infection is established by demonstrating the characteristic eggs in the tissues or urine. These are 112 to 170 μm by 40 to 70 μm, have a prominent terminal spine, and are easily seen in the urine. An increased number of eggs is excreted around midday, and microscopic examination of a centrifuged urine specimen collected at this time usually reveals ova. In light infections, examination of increased quantities of urine is sometimes required. Gross or microscopic hematuria is common in endemic populations, and its presence should always suggest the diagnosis in exposed individuals. Antibodies to *S. haematobium* can be detected using *S. mansoni* antigen preparations. Ultrasonographic examinations reveal anatomic alteration of the genitourinary tract.

Treatment　Infected persons should be treated. Dead and calcified eggs are common in tissue, are often seen in urine specimens, and should be differentiated from viable eggs. Although a number of drugs have been used to treat *S. haematobium*, praziquantel is the treatment of choice (see Table 183-2). Metrifonate, a safe, orally administered agent, is also effective. Its major advantage is low cost, and the major disadvantage is that in order to cure infection it needs to be given in three doses 2 weeks apart.

SCHISTOSOMA INTERCALATUM　*S. intercalatum* infection is limited to areas of West Africa. Eggs, 140 to 240 μm by 50 to 85 μm, are found in the stool and have a terminal spine. Few symptoms are attributable to this infection, and no cases of portal fibrosis have been reported. Praziquantel is effective treatment (see Table 183-2).

SCHISTOSOME DERMATITIS (SWIMMER'S ITCH)　When cercariae penetrate the skin, they may provoke a reaction known as *schistosome dermatitis*. Symptoms occur most commonly after penetration of nonhuman schistosomes of birds and mammals. In previously unexposed persons, the initial invasion causes transient itching and uncommonly urticaria followed by the development of macules within 24 h and papules after 24 h. Following repeated exposures, the signs and symptoms increase dramatically and occur earlier. Large pruritic, erythematous papules and, uncommonly, vesicles develop within 24 h. The lesions are most intense 2 to 3 days following exposure and subside after a few days. These lesions represent a delayed hypersensitivity reaction to the invading schistosome. Nonhuman schistosomes do not fully develop in humans, and the signs and symptoms are limited to the skin. A similar dermatitis also occurs after infection with human schistosomes.

Schistosome dermatitis occurs after exposure to fresh water in many areas of the world but is particularly common in the north central and western United States. A dermatitis following seawater exposure (clam digger's itch) also has been described.

Treatment is symptomatic. Since cercariae need some time to invade the skin (15 min or less), rapid removal of cercariae-containing droplets after water contact will decrease exposure. Limiting the numbers of the intermediate host snail in frequented areas can effectively control exposure.

CONTROL OF SCHISTOSOMIASIS　Theoretically, schistosome infections can be controlled by a variety of methods, but their application has generally been only partially successful. Simple and effective health education measures such as the elimination of indiscriminate urination and defecation are difficult to implement in endemic areas. Elimination of the intermediate molluscan host can be accomplished with the use of molluscicides or by destroying the habitat of the snail. Both methods require dedication of resources and personnel often not readily available. Mass chemotherapy of populations has been tried, and repeated treatments will be needed depending on the degree of reinfection. Some advocate the treatment of those likely to develop serious disease (e.g., those heavily infected).

The methods employed will depend on the nature of the endemic area and the resources available.

OTHER TREMATODES

BILIARY DUCT–DWELLING TREMATODES, *CLONORCHIS SINENSIS*, *OPISTHORCHIS VIVERRINI*, AND *OPISTHORCHIS FELINEUS* These closely related trematodes commonly infect the biliary system of humans, have similar life cycles and routes of infection, appear to have similar pathophysiology and disease manifestations, and produce eggs which closely resemble one another. They are responsible for symptoms and signs related to obstruction of the biliary tract or pancreatic duct and the increased risk of developing cholangiocarcinoma. *C. sinensis* is endemic in China, Taiwan, Korea, Japan, and Vietnam; *O. viverrini* is found in Laos and Thailand; and *O. felineus* is found in parts of eastern Europe and the former U.S.S.R.

Life cycle Humans become infected after ingesting metacercariae in poorly cooked, pickled, or smoked fish. The metacercariae excyst in the small intestine and migrate through the ampulla of Vater into the biliary ducts, where they mature in 3 to 4 weeks. Worms are 7 to 20 mm by 1.5 to 3 mm (depending on the species) and may live for 20 to 25 years (*C. sinensis*).

Pathophysiology Disease manifestations (mostly described for *O. viverrini* and *C. sinensis*) depend on the duration of infection, worm burden, and location of the parasites. Flukes reside in the biliary system mostly in the small to medium-sized ducts but at times also can be found in the larger biliary ducts as well as the gallbladder. They do not invade the parenchyma of the liver, and most of the disease manifestations are direct or indirect effects of the adult trematodes on the biliary ducts. Their presence leads to adenomatous hyperplasia and varying amounts of periductal inflammation followed by periductal fibrosis. Diffuse and localized dilation of ducts is frequently found due to obstruction by worms, stones, or strictures. Remnants of parasites have been found in biliary stones. The number of persons with disease in a given population increases with the worm burden (thousands of flukes in heavy infections), and manifestations include the findings noted above as well as enlarged gallbladder, cholelithiasis, cholecystitis, and chlolangiocarcinoma. The last is found in much greater frequency in *O. viverini* and *C. sinensis* endemic areas and is an important cause of mortality. In heavy infections, flukes are also found in the pancreatic duct and may be associated with pancreatitis.

Clinical manifestations Acute infections are infrequently recognized and are characterized by fever, eosinophilia, and hepatomegaly. In endemic areas, almost the entire population may be infected; however, most are lightly infected and asymptomatic. More heavily infected persons suffer vague constitutional complaints and symptoms associated with cholelithiasis and pancreatitis. An enlarged and tender liver may be present. Ascending cholangitis is a serious complication. Cholangiocarcinomas usually are associated with proximal obstruction and subsequent massive dilation of the biliary ducts. Ultrasonography reveals varying degrees of peripheral dilation of the biliary ducts without proximal obstruction. Biliary stones and flukes also may be noted ultrasonographically. Endoscopic cholangiopancreatography reveals ductal dilation, proliferation, irregularities, and blunting of the terminal branches in a majority of cases. Adult worms are visualized as multiple filling defects.

Diagnosis and treatment Diagnosis is made by the clinical presentation and the detection of the characteristic ova in the feces or bile. Worms can be visualized by a number of techniques and are frequently noted at surgery. Eggs are about 30 by 12 μm and are ovoid in shape. At the smaller end, an operculum, a sort of cap, appears to rest on a rim which protrudes slightly away from the eggs. The other end is broader and has a median knob. The eggs of *C. sinensis* and *O. viverrini* are difficult to distinguish, but those of *O. felineus* are somewhat longer and thinner. The treatment of choice is praziquantel, 25 mg/kg tid for 1 day.

LUNG-DWELLING TREMATODES, *PARAGONIMUS WESTERMANI* AND OTHER RELATED SPECIES Over 30 species of *Paragonimus* have been described, and a number of these infect humans. Adult flukes reside mainly in the lungs, but ectopic localization is relatively common. *P. westermani*, found in the Far East, is the most common infection in humans. Others include *P. skrjabini (szechuanensis)* (China), *P. heterotrema* (Southeast Asia), *P. philipinensis* (Philippines), *P. mexicanus* (Central America and parts of South America), *P. africanus* (Nigeria and Cameroon), and *P. uterobilateralis* (Nigeria and other areas of West Africa). *P. kellicotti* is indigenous to the United States but has rarely been documented in humans.

Life cycle Humans become infected primarily by ingesting poorly cooked or pickled crabs or crayfish. Metacercariae excyst in the duodenum and within 1 h pass through the intestinal wall into the peritoneal cavity. After 3 to 6 h they migrate into the abdominal wall and then through the diaphragm and into the pleura and lung tissue, where they become encapsulated, usually in pairs or triplets. It takes 65 to 90 days for the flukes to fully develop, although symptoms may begin earlier. Eggs are shed around the worm and, with rupture of the contents of the encapsulated cyst into the bronchioles, are excreted in the sputum or swallowed and found in the feces. Adults are 7.5 to 12 mm by 4 to 6 mm by 3.5 to 5 mm and may live for 20 years.

Pathophysiology Disease is caused by the inflammation and fibrosis elicited by the worms in the lungs or in ectopic locations. Manifestations depend on the duration of infection and probably the intensity of infection, although the latter fact is not well documented. Flukes and eggs initially elicit an acute inflammatory response mostly consisting of eosinophils followed by the formation of a fibrous capsule. In the lung parenchyma, the cysts rupture into the bronchioles, extruding blood, eggs, and inflammatory exudate. Pleural-based lesions cause eosinophilic empyemas which are clinically confused with tuberculosis. Lesions in long-standing infections show increased fibrosis and decreased inflammatory responses, and some eventually calcify. Flukes are found not uncommonly in abnormal locations, including the pleura, abdominal wall, viscera, and brain, where they elicit inflammation and fibrosis. Brain involvement is a particularly serious complication. Although frequent and severe bacterial infections may be associated with paragonimiasis, this relationship has not been substantiated. Ectopic lesions of the abdominal wall and liver are a hallmark of *P. skrjabini* infections.

Clinical manifestations Both acute and chronic manifestations occur. Acute disease is infrequently noted but may include fever, hepatosplenomegaly, cough, eosinophilia, pleural effusions, pulmonary abnormalities, pneumothorax, and signs and symptoms referable to ectopic locations. The findings in chronic infections frequently include cough, expectoration of rusty or pigmented sputum, and hemoptysis. Dyspnea, chest pain, fever, and constitutional complaints occur less frequently. Chest x-ray findings are varied, nondiagnostic, and often confused with those of tuberculosis. Localized or multisegmental infiltrates, usually poorly defined, are most common, but nodular, cystic, cavitary, ring shadow patterns are also found. Other findings include pleural effusions, empyemas, pleural thickening, and calcification of lesions. In contrast to tuberculosis, apical lesions do not predominate, cavities are smooth and regular, and infiltrates less well defined. Although lung involvement alone appears to cause little mortality, significant morbidity and mortality occur with ectopic lesions. In one series, 30.7 and 8.4 percent of hospitalized patients had ectopic lesions and brain involvement, respectively. Both acute and chronic forms of brain involvement are recognized, the former associated with the sudden onset of neurologic symptoms, usually in the presence of pulmonary disease, and the latter usually associated with seizures and long-term deficits. "Soap bubble" calcifications are a characteristic x-ray pattern in chronic neuroparagonimiasis.

Diagnosis and treatment The diagnosis is established by detecting the characteristic ova in stool or sputum. The golden-brown eggs are unembryonated and measure 80 to 118 μm by 48 to 60 μm. Concentration techniques may be needed to detect eggs in lightly infected patients. Serologic tests are available and may be particularly useful in lightly infected individuals or those with suspected ectopic lesions. In acute disease, the presence of eggs may not be detected until 2 to 3 months after exposure. Praziquantel is the treatment of choice at 25 mg/kg tid, for 2 days. Bithionol is also effective but more toxic.

LIVER-DWELLING TREMATODES, *FASCIOLA HEPATICA* Humans are accidently infected with this parasite of sheep, cattle, and other ruminants. Acute manifestations are a combination of systemic symptoms and signs and manifestations directly referable to invasion of the liver. Chronic disease has many features indistinguishable from that caused by the other liver flukes.

Life cycle Ruminants become infected after ingestion of metacercariae encysted on aquatic vegetation. Watercress is commonly implicated in human infections. Metacercariae excyst in the duodenum, pass through the intestine into the peritoneum, invade the liver through Glisson's capsule, and eventually reside in the biliary ducts. In humans, the flukes require at least 3 to 4 months to mature, but eggs may not be detected in stool. Adults are relatively large, measuring 30 by 13 mm. Infections occur worldwide in areas where sheep and cattle are raised, including Europe, Australia, and other developed countries. Endogenously acquired infections are rare in the continental United States but occur in Puerto Rico.

Pathophysiology The severity of infection depends on the intensity and duration of infection and responses of the host. Early manifestations are due to migration of the flukes through the tissues. Punctuate hemorrhages, tracts, and nodules are seen on the surface of the liver and are points of entry, migration routes, and areas of encapsulated eosinophilic abscesses, respectively. Granulomatous reactions also occur around eggs themselves. In chronic infections, worms reside in the biliary system, and the anatomic changes caused by the worms generally resemble those of the other liver flukes. However, intermittent obstruction of the biliary passages by worms appears more common in fascioliasis and leads to periods of jaundice.

Clinical findings Fever, hepatomegaly and/or abdominal pain, and eosinophilia are the hallmark of acute fascioliasis, which usually begins within 2 to 3 months following ingestion. Nausea, diarrhea, cough, and urticaria are also frequent. Elevation of liver function tests is inconstant, anemia is usually present, and the erythrocyte sedimentation rate is commonly elevated. Untreated, the disease lasts from months to years, but the manifestations change and with time more closely resemble those of other liver flukes, including intermittent obstruction, gallbladder and biliary duct thickening, cholecystitis, lithiasis, and the development of strictures. Ectopic localizations of flukes is also relatively common and leads to findings related to the invaded tissue. In contrast to the other liver flukes, there is no apparent association with cholangiocarcinoma. Because exposure is sometimes long-standing, acute and chronic manifestations may occur at the same time. Computed tomographic scans show multiple, hypodense, irregular lesions in the liver; ultrasonography fails to detect these lesions but is helpful in detecting resulting biliary duct pathology.

Diagnosis and treatment The presence of fever, eosinophilia, and hepatomegaly or liver pain in the proper clinical setting should suggest the diagnosis. Definitive diagnosis is established by detecting ova in the feces and/or by serologic tests. Ova may not be detected in the feces because disease manifestation occurs before patency, because of the inability of ova to pass into the biliary system, or because of ectopic location or low level of ova excretion. Therefore, stool concentration methods should be employed. The ova are immature in the feces, measure 130 to 150 μm by 90 μm, and are indistinguishable from those of *Fasciolopsis buski*. Although effective in other trematode infections, praziquantel does not appear to be very effective in *F. hepatica* infection, and bithionol at 30 to 50 mg/kg on alternate days for 10 to 15 doses is the treatment of choice. Infections also have been treated successfully with the experimental drugs triclabendazole and albendazole.

INTESTINE-DWELLING TREMATODES *Fasciolopsis buski* One of the largest parasites that infect humans, *F. buski* measures 20 to 70 mm by 8 to 20 mm by 0.5 to 3 mm and resides in the small intestine and occasionally in the colon or pylorus. It is confined to the Far East. The adults attach to the intestinal epithelium, causing ulcerations and localized inflammation. Light infections are generally asymptomatic, but persons heavily infected complain of diarrhea, fever, and abdominal pain and may develop ascites, anasarca, and intestinal obstruction. The pathophysiology has not been well studied. The diagnosis is established by detecting ova (indistinguishable from those of *F. hepatica*) in the feces. The treatment of choice is praziquantel, 25 mg/kg tid for 1 day.

Heterophyes heterophyes and Metagonimus yokogawai Both are tiny (about 1 mm) intestine-dwelling parasites whose major clinical manifestation is diarrhea. Humans acquire infection after the ingestion of undercooked freshwater fish. *H. heterophyes* and *M. yokogawai* are found in the Far East, but the former is also common in the Nile Delta and present in other areas of the Middle East. The worms attach to and at times burrow into the intestinal mucosa, eliciting inflammatory responses. Ova of *H. heterophyes* have been found in the heart and other organs and have reportedly caused clinically significant myocarditis. The diagnosis is established by detecting ova in the feces; the ova of both species are identical and resemble those of *C. sinensis* and related parasites. Praziquantel is the drug of choice, at 25 mg/kg tid for 1 day.

Nanophyetus salmincola This tiny small-intestine–dwelling trematode has recently infected humans in the Pacific Northwest. It was previously known to infect humans in eastern Siberia. Infections occur after ingestion of undercooked, smoked, or raw fish, usually salmon or trout. Symptoms vary from asymptomatic carriage to watery diarrhea, abdominal pain, bloating, and other gastrointestinal complaints. Eosinophilia is found in a majority but is not universal. Unembryonated ova (64 to 97 μm by 34 to 55 μm) appear in the feces after 1 week but are excreted in low numbers so that concentration techniques are needed. The treatment of choice is praziquantel, 20 mg/kg tid for 1 day.

REFERENCES

Schistosomes

CHEEVER AW, ANDRADE ZA: Pathological lesions associated with *Schistosoma mansoni* infection in man. Trans R Soc Trop Med Hyg 61:626, 1968

FORSYTH DM: A longitudinal study of endemic urinary schistosomiasis in a small East African community. Bull WHO 40:771, 1969

HAGAN P: Reinfection, exposure and immunity in human schistosomiasis. Parasitol Today 8:12, 1992

HIAT RA et al: Factors in the pathogenesis of acute schistosomiasis mansoni. J Infect Dis 139:659, 1979

HOMEIDA M et al: Morbidity associated with *Schistosoma mansoni* infection as determined by ultrasound: A study in Gezira, Sudan. Am J Trop Med Hyg 39:196, 1988

———: Diagnosis of pathologically confirmed Symmers' periportal fibrosis by ultrasonography: A prospective blinded study. Am J Trop Med Hyg 39:86, 1988

HOMEIDA MA et al: Association of the therapeutic activity of praziquantel with the reversal of Symmers' fibrosis induced by *Schistosoma mansoni*. Am J Trop Med Hyg 45:360, 1991

JORDAN P, WEBBE G (eds): *Schistosomiasis, Epidemiology, Treatment and Control*. London, Heinemann Medical, 1982

LEHMAN JS et al: Urinary schistosomiasis in Egypt: Clinical, radiological, bacteriological, and parasitological correlations. Trans R Soc Trop Med Hyg 67:384, 1973

NASH TE et al: Schistosome infections in humans: Perspective and recent findings. Ann Intern Med 97:740, 1982

ROLLINSON O, SIMPSON AJG (eds): *The Biology of Schistosomes. From Genes to Latrines*. New York, Academic, 1987

SAAD AMA et al: Oesophageal varices in region of the Sudan endemic for *Schistosoma mansoni*. Br J Surg 78:1252, 1991

Other trematodes

BEAVER PC et al: *Clinical Parasitology*, 9th ed. Philadelphia, Lea & Febiger, 1984

ELKINS DB et al: A high frequency of hepatobiliary disease and suspected cholangiocarcinoma associated with heavy *Opisthorchis viverrini* infection in a small community in northeast Thailand. Trains R Soc Trop Med Hyg 84:715, 1990

FACEY MB et al: Fascioliasis in man: An outbreak in Hampshire. Br Med J ii:619, 1960

FRITSCHE TR et al: Praziquantel for treatment of human *Nanophyetus salmincola* (*Troglotrema salmincola*) infection. J Infect Dis 160:896, 1989

GUTIERREZ Y: *Diagnostic Pathology of Parasitic Infections with Clinical Correlations*. Philadelphia, Lea & Febiger, 1990

Hou P-C: The pathology of *Clonorchis sinensis* infestation of the liver. J Pathol Bacteriol 70:53, 1955

Koenigstein RP: Observations on the epidemiology of infections with *Clonorchis sinensis*. Trans R Soc Trop Med Hyg 42:503, 1949

Sadun EH, Buck AA: Paragonimiasis in South Korea—Immunodiagnostic, epidemiologic, clinical, roentgenologic and therapeutic studies. Am J Trop Med Hyg 9:562, 1960

———, Maiphoom C: Studies in the epidemiology of the human intestinal fluke, *Fasciolopsis buski* (Lankester) in Central Thailand. Am J Trop Med Hyg 2:1084, 1953

Singh TS et al: Pulmonary paragonimiasis: Clinical features, diagnosis and treatment of 39 cases in Manipur. Trans R Soc Trop Med Hyg 80:967, 1986

Sithithaworn P et al: Quantitative post-mortem study of *Opisthorchis viverrini* in man in northeast Thailand. Trans R Soc Trop Med Hyg 85:765, 1991

Takeyama N et al: Computed tomography findings of hepatic lesions in human fascioliasis: Report of two cases. Am J Gastroenterol 81:1078, 1986

Yokogawa M: Epidemiology and control of paragonimiasis, in *Parasitic Diseases*, EM Sasa (ed). Tokyo, International Medical Foundation of Japan, 1974, pp 137–149

184 CESTODES

THOMAS B. NUTMAN / PETER F. WELLER

Cestodes, or tapeworms, are segmented worms. The adults reside in the gastrointestinal tract, but the larvae can be found in almost any organ. Human tapeworm infections can be divided into two major clinical groups. In one group, humans are the definitive hosts, and the adult tapeworms live in the gastrointestinal tract (*Taenia saginata, Diphyllobothrium, Hymenolepis,* and *Dipylidium caninum*). In the other, humans are intermediate hosts, and larval-stage parasites are present in the tissues. Diseases in this category include echinococcosis, sparganosis, and coenurosis. For *Taenia solium,* the human may be either the definitive or the intermediate host.

The ribbon-shaped tapeworm attaches to the intestinal mucosa by means of sucking cups or grooves located on the head (scolex). Behind the scolex is a short, narrow neck from which proglottids (or segments) form. As each proglottid matures, it is displaced further back from the neck by new, less mature segments. The progressively elongated chain of attached proglottids, called the *strobila,* constitutes the bulk of the tapeworm and may contain over 1000 proglottids and be several meters in length. As each proglottid becomes gravid, eggs are released. Since eggs of different *Taenia* spp. are morphologically identical, differences in the morphology of the scolex or proglottids provide the only basis for diagnostic identification of the tapeworm species. Most human tapeworms require at least one intermediate host for complete larval development. After ingestion by an intermediate host, an egg develops into a larval oncosphere capable of penetrating the intestinal mucosa. The oncosphere migrates to tissues and develops into an encysted form known as a *cysticercus* (single scolex), a *coenerus* (multiple scolices), or a *hydatid* (cyst with daughter cysts each containing several scolices). Ingestion by the definitive host of tissues containing a cyst enables a scolex to develop into a tapeworm.

TAENIASIS SAGINATA The beef tapeworm, *Taenia saginata,* occurs in all countries where raw or undercooked beef is eaten and is more prevalent in sub-Saharan African and Middle Eastern countries.

Etiology and pathogenesis Humans are the only definitive host for the adult stage of *T. saginata.* This 3- to 10-meter-long tapeworm inhabits the upper jejunum and has a scolex with four prominent suckers and 1000 to 2000 proglottids. Each gravid segment has 15 to 30 uterine branches (in contrast to 8 to 12 with *T. solium*). The eggs are indistinguishable from those of *T. solium,* each measuring 30 to 40 μm, with a thick, brown striated shell containing a fully developed embryo. Eggs deposited on vegetation can live for months to years until they are ingested by cattle or other herbivores. The embryo released after ingestion invades the intestinal wall and is carried to striated muscle predominantly in the hindlimbs, diaphragm,

and tongue, where it transforms into a cysticercus. When ingested in raw or undercooked beef, this form can infect humans. After the cysticercus is ingested, it takes about 2 months for an adult worm to develop.

Clinical manifestations Patients become aware of the infection most commonly by noting passage of proglottids in their feces, and they may experience a discomforting perianal sensation when proglottids are discharged. Although usually minimal or mild, abdominal pain or discomfort, nausea, change in appetite, weakness, and weight loss can occur with *T. saginata* infection.

Diagnosis The diagnosis is made by detecting eggs or proglottids in the stool as soon as about 3 months after infection. Eggs also may be present on the perianal area, so if proglottids or eggs are not found in the stool, the perianal region should be examined with use of a cellophane-tape swab, as is done for pinworm infection. Separation of this infection from *T. solium* requires examination of mature proglottids or the scolex. Serologic tests are not helpful diagnostically. Eosinophilia and elevations of serum IgE may be present.

Treatment and prevention Either niclosamide (a single dose of four 0.5-g tablets chewed thoroughly) or a single dose of praziquantel (10 to 20 mg/kg) is highly effective therapy. The major means of preventing beef tapeworm infection involves the adequate cooking of beef; temperatures as low as 56°C for 5 min will destroy cysticerci. Refrigeration or salting for long periods or freezing at −10°C for 9 days also kills cysticerci in beef. General preventive measures include beef inspection and proper disposal of human feces.

TAENIASIS SOLIUM AND CYSTICERCOSIS The pork tapeworm, *Taenia solium,* can cause two distinct forms of infection, depending on whether humans are infected with adult tapeworms in the intestine or with larval forms in the tissues (cysticercosis). Humans are the only definitive hosts for *T. solium,* and pigs are the usual intermediate hosts, although dogs, cats, and sheep may harbor the larval forms. *T. solium* exists worldwide but is most prevalent in Mexico, Africa, Southeast Asia, eastern Europe, and South America. Cysticercosis occurs in industrialized nations largely as a result of the immigration of infected persons from endemic areas.

Etiology and pathogenesis The adult tapeworm generally resides in the upper jejunum, and its globular scolex attaches by both sucking disks and two rows of hooklets. Often only one adult worm is present but may live for up to 25 years. The tapeworm, usually about 3 m in length, may have as many as 1000 proglottids, each of which produces up to 50,000 eggs. Groups of 3 to 5 proglottids generally are released and excreted into the feces, and the eggs in these proglottids are infective for both humans and animals. The eggs survive in the environment for several months. After ingestion by the intermediate host, eggs embryonate, penetrate the intestinal wall, and are carried to many tissues, with a predilection for striated muscle of the neck, tongue, and trunk. Within 60 to 90 days, the encysted larval stage develops. These cysticerci can survive for long periods. Infections of humans that lead to intestinal tapeworms occur by ingestion of undercooked pork containing cysticerci. Infections that cause human cysticercosis occur after the ingestion of *T. solium* eggs, usually from fecally contaminated food. Autoinfection may occur if an individual with an egg-producing tapeworm unhygienically ingests eggs derived from his or her own feces or potentially if eggs reflux from the intestine into the stomach.

Clinical manifestations Intestinal infections with *T. solium* may be asymptomatic. Complaints of epigastric discomfort, nausea, sensation of hunger, weight loss, and diarrhea are infrequent. Fecal passage of proglottids may be noted by patients.

In cysticercosis, the clinical manifestations are entirely different. Since cysticerci can be found anywhere in the body (most commonly in the brain and the skeletal muscle), the location and size of cysticerci determine the clinical presentation. The manifestations of cysticercosis reflect two distinct processes, the local inflammatory response induced by the parasite and the local effect of the space-occupying lesions. Neurologic manifestations are the most common presentation. When inflammation surrounds lesions, seizures and focal neurologic deficits are frequent, and communicating and noncommunicating hydrocephalus and meningitis also can be seen. Generalized, focal, or Jacksonian seizures occur in most. Signs of increased intracranial pressure, including headache, nausea, vomiting, changes in vision, dizziness, ataxia, and confusion, often are present. In patients with hydrocephalus, papilledema and alteration in mental status may occur. An unusual form of cyticercosis is the racemose form, which consists of grapelike clusters of proliferating larval membranes. Characteristically, this form occurs at the base of the brain or in the subarachnoid space and causes chronic meningitis and arachnoiditis. Communicating or noncommunicating hydrocephalus frequently develops. The clinical presentation of neurocysticercosis, therefore, depends on the number, form, and location of cysticerci, the extent of cyst-associated inflammatory responses, and the duration of disease.

Diagnosis   The diagnosis of intestinal *T. solium* infection is made by finding eggs or proglottids, as described for *T. saginata*. For cysticercosis, definitive diagnosis requires examination of the cysticercus within an involved tissue, but a diagnosis often can be based on the clinical presentation and results of compatible radiographic, especially computed tomographic (CT) and magnetic resonance imaging (MRI), studies and serologic tests.

For soft-tissue involvement, plain films may reveal multiple calcified "puffed-rice" lesions. For cerebral cysticercosis, CT studies demonstrate parenchymal lesions of varying number and size that are either cystic or solid and may exhibit contrast enhancement. On CT studies, some or many of the lesions may be calcified, so multiple punctate calcifications are common findings in neurocysticercosis. Ventricular dilatation may be demonstrable, but the CT finding of multiple calcified or noncalcified cystic lesions is strongly suggestive of cerebral cysticercosis. MRI detects cystic structures on T_1- and T_2-weighted images and high-intensity rims around cysts, particularly on T_2-weighted images. Because CT is more sensitive in identifying calcified lesions and MRI is better at identifying small cystic lesions, both techniques are useful in evaluating neurocysticercosis.

Most patients with cerebral cysticercosis show a cerebrospinal fluid (CSF) pleocytosis with a mononuclear cell predominance. In CSF, glucose is often decreased, and protein is elevated. Serologic tests of CSF and sera are helpful in establishing the diagnosis. A variety of serologic assays have been used, but many were complicated by cross-reactivity with other tapeworm, filarial and echinococcal infections. However, an immunoblotting technique has improved specificity to 98 percent, with sensitivities reaching 91 percent. Even with this technique, however, patients with single intracranial neurocysticercotic lesions may be seronegative.

Treatment and prevention   Intestinal *T. solium* infection is treated with niclosamide or praziquantel, as specified for *T. saginata* infection. With the latter drug, however, there is the possible risk of evoking an inflammatory response in the central nervous system if concomitant cryptic cysticercosis is present. Preventive measures regarding pork are similar to those for beef and *T. saginata* above.

The therapy for cysticercosis can involve chemotherapy, surgery, and supportive medical treatment. Asymptomatic patients with calcified soft tissue or neural lesions generally require no treatment. For symptomatic patients with neurocysticercosis, both praziquantel (50 mg/kg per day in three doses for 15 days) and albendazole (15 mg/kg per day in three doses for 8 days) are effective. Because both agents provoke inflammatory responses around dying cysticerci, patients receiving either drug should be hospitalized and given high doses of glucocorticoids during treatment. Efficacy of therapy can be monitored by radiographic imaging, with a decrease in the size of active lesions expected within 3 to 6 months. For ocular and spinal lesions, drug-induced inflammation may cause irreversible damage; thus these lesions, as well as those within the ventricles, are best managed by surgical resection. Ventricular obstruction may require a ventriculostomy or ventriculoperitoneal shunting. Not all neurologic deficits resolve after therapy, and some patients may require continued anticonvulsive therapy. Prevention of cysticercosis involves minimizing the opportunities for ingestion of fecally derived eggs by

means of good personal hygiene, improvements in fecal disposal, and treatment and prevention of human intestinal infections.

ECHINOCOCCOSIS   Echinococcosis is an infection of humans caused by the larval stage of *Echinococcus granulosus, E. multilocularis,* or *E. vogeli. E. granulosus,* which produces unilocular cystic lesions, is prevalent in areas where livestock is raised in association with dogs. It is found in Australia, Argentina, Chile, Africa, eastern Europe, the Middle East, New Zealand, and the Mediterranean, particularly Lebanon and Greece. *E. multilocularis,* which causes multilocular, alveolar lesions which are locally invasive, is found in subarctic or arctic regions, including Canada, the United States, and northern Europe and Asia. *E. vogeli* causes polycystic hydatid disease and is found only in Central and South America. As with other cestode infections, echinococcal species have both intermediate and definitive hosts. The definitive hosts are dogs that pass eggs in their feces. When the intermediate hosts—sheep, cattle, humans, goats, camels, and horses for *E. granulosus* and mice or other rodents for *E. multilocularis*—ingest the eggs, cysts develop within these hosts. When a dog ingests beef or lamb containing cysts, the life cycle is completed.

Etiology   The small, 5-mm-long adult *E. granulosus* worm, which is resident with a 5- to 20-month lifespan in the jejunum of dogs, has only three proglottids—one immature, one mature, and one gravid. The gravid segment splits to release eggs morphologically indistinguishable from *Taenia* eggs and extremely hardy. After humans ingest the eggs, embryos escape from the eggs, penetrate the intestinal mucosa, enter the portal circulation, and are carried to various organs, most commonly the liver and lungs. Larvae develop into fluid-filled unilocular hydatid cysts which consist of an external membrane and an inner germinal layer. Daughter cysts develop from the inner aspect of the germinal layer, as do germinating cystic structures called *brood capsules*. New larvae, called *scolices*, develop in large numbers within the brood capsule. The cysts expand slowly over a period of years. The life cycle of *E. multilocularis* is similar except that small rodents serve as intermediate hosts. The cyst, however, is quite different, in that the larval form remains in the proliferative phase, the hydatid cyst is always multilocular, and vesicles progressively invade the host tissue by peripheral extension of processes from the germinal layer.

Clinical manifestations   Slowly enlarging echinococcal cysts generally remain asymptomatic until their expanding size or their space-occupying effect in an involved organ elicits symptoms. Liver and lung are the most common sites. Since 5 to 20 years often elapses before cysts enlarge sufficiently to cause symptoms, the cysts may be discovered as an incidental finding on a routine x-ray or ultrasound study. Patients with hepatic echinococcosis who are symptomatic most often present with abdominal pain or a palpable mass in the right upper quadrant. Compression of a bile duct or leakage of cyst fluid into the biliary tree may mimic recurrent cholelithiasis, and biliary obstruction can result in jaundice. Rupture or episodic leakage from an hydatid cyst may produce fever, pruritus, urticaria, eosinophilia, or fatal anaphylaxis. Pulmonary hydatid cysts may rupture into the bronchial tree or peritoneal cavity and produce cough, chest pain, or hemoptysis. Rupture of hydatid cysts, by spreading the multitude of infectious scolices, leads to multifocal dissemination of new cyst-forming elements and can occur spontaneously or at surgery, especially when a cyst is not recognized to be of echinococcal etiology. Cysts may involve any organ, and other presentations are due to those in bone (invasion of the medullary cavity with slow bone erosion producing pathologic fractures), the central nervous system (space-occupying lesions), and the heart (conduction defects, pericarditis).

The cysts of *E. multilocularis* characteristically present as a slowly growing hepatic tumor with progressive destruction of the liver and extension into vital structures. Patients commonly complain of upper quadrant and epigastric pain, and obstructive jaundice may be present. A minority of patients will have metastatic lesions to the lung and brain.

Diagnosis Radiographic and related imaging studies are important in detecting and evaluating echinococcal cysts. Plain films will define pulmonary cysts, usually as rounded, irregular masses of uniform density, but may miss other cysts in other organs unless there is cyst wall calcification, as occurs in the liver. CT scans and ultrasound reveal well-defined cysts with thick or thin walls. If older cysts contain a layer of hydatid sand that is rich in accumulated scolices, these imaging methods may detect this fluid layer of different density, but the most pathognomonic finding, if demonstrable, is the visualization of daughter cysts within the larger cyst. This finding, as well as eggshell, or mural, calcification, indicates *E. granulosus* infection and helps to distinguish the cyst from carcinomas, bacterial or amebic liver abscesses, or hemangiomas. With alveolar hydatid cysts, CT reveals indistinct solid masses with central necrosis and plaquelike calcifications.

Specific diagnosis could be made by examination of aspirated fluids for the presence of scoliceal hooklets, but diagnostic aspiration is not conventionally recommended because of the risks from fluid leakage either by disseminating infection or provoking anaphylactic reactions. However, CT-guided aspiration of hydatid cysts for diagnosis has been utilized successfully in some centers in conjunction with installation of ethanol after aspiration. Pretreatment with albendazole (1-month course) is believed to minimize possible biopsy complications. Serodiagnostic assays can be useful, although a negative test does not exclude the diagnosis of echinococcosis. While cysts in the liver are more likely to elicit positive antibody responses than those in the lungs, up to 50 percent of infected individuals may have negative serology. Detection of antibody to a specific echinococcal antigen (antigen 5 or arc 5) has the highest degree of specificity, although false-positive findings may be present in cysticercosis.

Treatment Therapy for echinococcosis is based on considerations of the size, location, and manifestations of cysts and the overall health of the patient. Surgery, when feasible, is the principal definitive method of treatment by excising *E. granulosus* cysts or resecting tissue containing *E. multilocularis* cysts. Risks at surgery from leakage of fluid include anaphylaxis and dissemination of infectious scolices. The latter has been minimized by instilling scolicidal solutions such as hypertonic saline or ethanol. These may cause hypernatremia, ethanol intoxication, or possibly sclerosing cholangitis. Albendazole, which has antiechinococcal activity, can be administered adjunctively in the perioperative period and may be useful for medical treatment of echinococcosis. While albendazole has shown efficacy, the exact role of chemotherapy, potentially combined with percutaneous drainage, remains to be defined. As medical therapy, albendazole, given at 400 mg twice a day for 28 days and repeated from 1 to 8 times, separated by drug-free intervals of 2 to 3 weeks, is most efficacious for those with hepatic and/or pulmonary cysts.

Prevention In endemic areas, echinococcosis can be prevented by praziquantel treatment of infected dogs and by denying dogs access to butchering sites or offal of infected animals. Limitation of the number of stray dogs is helpful in reducing the prevalence of human infection.

HYMENOLEPIASIS NANA *Hymenolepis nana*, the dwarf tapeworm, is the most common of all the cestode infections. *H. nana* is endemic in both temperate and tropical regions of the world. Infection is spread by fecal/oral contamination and is common in institutionalized children.

Etiology and pathogenesis *H. nana* is the only cestode of humans that does not require an intermediate host. Both the larval and adult phases occur in the human. The adult, the smallest tapeworm parasitizing humans, is about 2 cm long and dwells in the proximal ileum. Proglottids, which are quite small and rarely seen in the stool, release spherical eggs 30 to 44 μm in diameter that each contain an oncosphere with six hooklets. The eggs are immediately infective and are unable to survive in the external environment for more than 10 days. *H. nana* also can be acquired by the ingestion of insects (especially larval meal worms and larval fleas) infected with the

parasite. When the egg is ingested by a new host, the oncosphere is freed and penetrates the intestinal villi, becoming a cysticercoid larva. Larvae migrate back into the intestinal lumen, attach to the mucosa, and mature over 10 to 12 days into adult worms. Eggs also may hatch before passing into the stool, causing internal autoinfection with increasing numbers of intestinal worms. Although the lifespan of adult *H. nana* is only about 4 to 10 weeks, the autoinfection cycle perpetuates the infection.

Clinical manifestations *H. nana* infection, even with many intestinal worms, is usually asymptomatic. When infection is intense, anorexia, abdominal pain, and diarrhea occur.

Diagnosis, treatment, and prevention Infection is diagnosed by finding eggs in the stool. Praziquantel (25 mg/kg once) is the treatment of choice, since it acts against both the adult worms and the cysticercoids in the intestinal villi. The alternative, niclosamide (2 g on day 1 and 1 g/d for 6 more days), must be given over a week, since it is ineffective against the cysticercoid stage. The dosage for children must be adjusted for body weight. Good personal hygiene and improved sanitation can eradicate the disease. Epidemics have been controlled by the use of mass chemotherapy coupled with improved hygiene.

HYMENOLEPIASIS DIMINUTA *Hymenolepis diminuta*, a cestode of rodents, occasionally infects small children, who become infected with the adult worm after ingesting uncooked cereal foods contaminated by fleas and other insects in which larval development occurs. Infection is usually asymptomatic and is diagnosed by finding the eggs in the stool. Niclosamide or praziquantel results in cure in most individuals.

DIPHYLLOBOTHRIASIS *Diphyllobothrium latum* and other *Diphyllobothrium* spp. can be found in the lakes, rivers, and deltas of the Northern Hemisphere, Central Africa, and Chile.

Etiology and pathogenesis The adult worm, the longest tapeworm, reaches lengths up to 25 m. It attaches to the ileal and occasionally to the jejunal mucosa by its suckers, which are located on its elongated scolex. The adult worm has 3000 to 4000 proglottids, which release approximately 1 million eggs daily into the feces. If an egg reaches water, it hatches and releases a free-swimming embryo that can be eaten by small freshwater crustaceans (*Cyclops* or *Diaptomus* spp.). After this infected crustacean containing a developed procercoid is swallowed by a fish, the larva migrate into the fish's flesh and grows into a plerocercoid, or sparganum larva. Humans acquire the infection by ingesting infected raw fish. Within 3 to 5 weeks, the tapeworm matures in the human intestine into an adult.

Clinical manifestations The majority of *D. latum* infections are asymptomatic, although manifestations may include transient abdominal discomfort, diarrhea, vomiting, weakness, and weight loss. Occasionally, infection can cause acute abdominal pain and intestinal obstruction; in rare cases cholangitis or cholecystitis may be caused by migrating proglottids. Because the tapeworm absorbs large quantities of vitamin B_{12} and interferes with ileal B_{12} absorption, vitamin B_{12} deficiency can develop. Up to 2 percent of infected patients, especially the elderly, have a megaloblastic anemia resembling pernicious anemia and may exhibit neurologic sequelae of B_{12} deficiency.

Diagnosis The diagnosis is made readily by detecting in the stool the characteristic eggs, which possess a single shell with an operculum at one end and a knob on the other. Mild to moderate eosinophilia may be present.

Treatment and prevention Praziquantel (10 to 20 mg/kg once) and niclosamide (a single 2-g dose) are highly effective. Parenteral vitamin B_{12} should be given if B_{12} deficiency is manifest. Infection can be prevented by heating fish to 54°C for 5 min or by freezing it at −18°C for 24 h. Placing fish in brine with a high salt concentration for long periods kills the eggs.

DIPYLIDIASIS *Dipylidium caninum*, a common tapeworm of dogs and cats, may accidentally infect humans. Dogs, cats, and occasionally humans become infected by ingesting fleas harboring cysticercoids. Children are more likely to become infected than adults.

Most infections are asymptomatic, but abdominal pain, diarrhea, anal pruritus, urticaria, and eosinophilia can occur. Diagnosis is made by detecting proglottids in the stool. Therapy is with praziquantel or niclosamide as for *D. latum* infection. Prevention requires antihelminthic treatment and flea control for pet dogs or cats.

SPARGANOSIS   Humans can be infected by sparganum, or plerocercoid larva, of another diphyllobothrid tapeworm of the genus *Spirometra*. Infection can be acquired by drinking water containing infected *Cyclops*, by ingesting infected snakes, birds, or other mammals, or by the application of infected flesh as poultices. The worm will migrate slowly in tissues, and infection commonly presents as a subcutaneous swelling. Periorbital tissues can be involved, and ocular sparganosis may destroy the eye. Surgical excision is used to treat localized sparganosis.

COENUROSIS   This rare infection of humans by the larval (or coenurus) stage of the dog tapeworm *Taenia multiceps* results in a space-occupying cystic lesion. As in cysticercosis, involvement of the central nervous system and subcutaneous tissue is most common. Both definitive diagnosis and treatment require surgical excision of the lesion. Chemotherapeutic agents are not effective.

REFERENCES

HORTON RJ: Chemotherapy of *Echinococcus* infection in man with albendazole. Aust NZ J Surg 59:665, 1989

RICHARDS F JR, SCHANTZ PM: Laboratory diagnosis of cysticercosis. Clin Lab Med 11:1011, 1991

SCHAEFER JW, KHAN MY: Echinococcosis (hydatid disease): Lessons from experience with 59 patients. Rev Infect Dis 13:243, 1991

SCHANTZ PM, OKELO GBA: Echinococcosis (hydatidosis), in *Tropical and Geographical Medicine*, 2d ed, KS Warren, AAF Mahmoud (eds). New York, McGraw-Hill, 1990, p 505

SCHARF D: Neurocysticercosis: Two hundred thirty eight cases from a California hospital. Arch Neurol 46:77, 1989

TEITELBAUM GP et al: MR imaging of neurocysticercosis. AJR 153:857, 1989

section 19   Ectoparasites

<table>
<tr><td>

185   ECTOPARASITE INFESTATIONS

</td></tr>
</table>

JAMES H. MAGUIRE / ANDREW SPIELMAN

Ectoparasites are arthropods or helminths that *infest* the skin of other animals from which they derive sustenance. They may penetrate beneath the surface of the host or attach superficially by their mouthparts. These organisms damage their hosts by direct injury, by eliciting a hypersensitivity reaction, or by inoculating toxins or pathogens. The main medically important ectoparasites are arachnids (including mites and ticks), insects (including lice, fleas, and flies), pentastomes (tongue worms), and leeches.

SCABIES

The human itch mite, *Sarcoptes scabiei*, which infests some 300 million persons each year, is one of the most common causes of itching dermatoses throughout the world. Gravid female mites measuring 0.3 to 0.4 mm in length burrow for a month superficially beneath the stratum corneum, where they deposit two to three eggs a day. Larvae that hatch from these eggs mature in a series of molts in about 2 weeks and then emerge to the surface of the skin, where they mate and subsequently reinvade the skin of the same or another host. Transfer of newly fertilized female mites from person to person occurs by intimate personal contact and is facilitated by crowding, uncleanliness, and sexual promiscuity. Medical practitioners are at particular risk of infestation. Transmission via sharing of contaminated bedding or clothing occurs only infrequently because these mites cannot survive much more than a day without host contact. In the United States, scabies may account for 2 to 5 percent of visits to dermatologists, particularly involving children, immigrants from developing countries, and close household contacts. Outbreaks occur in nursing homes, mental institutions, and hospitals.

The itching and rash associated with scabies derive from a sensitization reaction directed against the excreta that the mite deposits in its burrow. For this reason, an initial infestation remains asymptomatic for 4 to 6 weeks, and a reinfestation produces a hypersensitivity reaction without delay. Scratching generally destroys the burrowing mite, but symptoms remain even in its absence. Burrows become surrounded by infiltrates of eosinophils, lymphocytes, and histiocytes, and a generalized hypersensitivity rash later develops in remote sites. By destroying these pathogens, immunity and associated scratching limit most infestations to less than 15 mites per person. Hyperinfestation with thousands or millions or mites, a condition known as *crusted* (or *Norwegian*) *scabies*, may result from glucocorticoid use, immunodeficiency disease including AIDS, and neurologic and psychiatric illnesses that interfere with itching and scratching.

Patients with scabies complain of intense itching that worsens at night and after a hot shower. Typical burrows may be difficult to find because they are few in number and may be obscured by excoriations. Burrows appear as dark wavy lines in the epidermis measuring 3 to 15 mm and ending in a small pearly bleb which contains the female mite. In the majority of patients they occur on the volar wrists, between the fingers, on the elbows, and on the penis. Small papules and vesicles, often accompanied by eczematous plaques, pustules, or nodules, are symmetrically distributed in these sites and in skin folds under the breasts and around the navel, axillae, belt line, buttocks, upper thighs, and scrotum. Except in infants, the face, scalp, neck, palms, and soles are spared. Burrows and other typical lesions may be sparse in persons who wash frequently, and topical corticosteroids and bacterial superinfection may alter the appearance of the rash. Superinfection with nephritogenic strains of streptococci has led to acute glomerulonephritis. Crusted scabies resembles psoriasis because of the widespread erythema, thick keratotic crusts, scaling, and dystrophic nails. Characteristic burrows are not seen, and patients usually do not itch, although they are highly contagious and have been responsible for outbreaks of classic scabies in hospitals.

Diagnosis of scabies should be considered in patients with pruritus and symmetric polymorphic skin lesions in characteristic locations, particularly if there is a history of household contact. Burrows should be sought and unroofed with a sterile needle or scalpel blade, and the scrapings should be examined microscopically for the mite, its eggs, or its fecal pellets. A drop of mineral oil facilitates removal of the sample. Biopsies or scrapings of papulovesicular lesions also may be diagnostic. In the absence of identifiable mites or mite products, the diagnosis is based on the clinical presentation and history. Other sexually transmitted diseases should be excluded in adults with scabies.

The 5% permethrin cream that is the treatment of choice for

scabies is less toxic than the commonly used 1% lindane preparations and is effective against lindane-tolerant infestations. Both scabicides are applied from the neck down after bathing and are removed 8 h later by means of soap and water. Lindane is absorbed through the skin, and its overuse has led to seizures and aplastic anemia. It should not be applied to pregnant women or infants. Alternatives include topical crotamiton cream, benzyl benzoate, and sulfur ointments.

Although effectively treated scabies infestations become noninfectious within a day, itching and rash due to hypersensitivity frequently persist for weeks or months. Unnecessary retreatment of such patients may provoke a contact dermatitis. Antihistamines, salicylates, and calamine lotion relieve itching during treatment, and topical glucocorticoids are useful for the pruritus that lingers after effective treatment. An oral antibiotic may be necessary for bacterial superinfections that fail to resolve with antiscabietic therapy. To prevent reinfestations, bedding and clothing should be washed in hot water, and close contacts, even if asymptomatic, should be treated simultaneously.

SARCOPTIC MANGE (ANIMAL SCABIES)

Persons who have close contact with dogs and to a lesser extent cats and horses may become transiently infested by zoonotic scabies. Such mites are unable to propagate on the human host or to produce their elongate burrows, and the characteristic pruritic papulovesicular rash is self-limited.

CHIGGERS AND OTHER MITE INFESTATIONS

Chiggers are the larvae of trombiculid (harvest) mites that normally feed on mice in grassy or brush-covered sites in the tropics and subtropics. They quest for hosts on low vegetation and attach themselves to passing animals or to people. The larva then pierces the skin of its host and deposits a tubelike structure in the dermis through which it imbibes lymph and tissue juices. This highly antigenic "stylosotome" serves as the focus of an exceptionally pruritic papule that may be 2 cm in diameter and that develops within hours of attachment in persons previously sensitized to mite antigen. Scratching invariably destroys the body of a mite attached to a person. These lesions generally vesiculate and develop a hemorrhagic base. Itching and burning last for weeks. The rash is most common on the ankles or near tight-fitting clothes that obstruct the mites' movements.

Certain mesostigmatid mites that infest the nests of mice or birds feed on human beings when their normal hosts have been displaced. Intense episodes of itching dermatitis, for example, may follow removal of trash from a human residence or departure of pigeons that have been nesting on a window air-conditioner. Other mites that infest grain, straw, cheese, or other animal products occasionally produce similar episodes. Diagnosis of mite-induced dermatitides (including chiggers) leans heavily on a history of exposure to the source of the mite, since the tiny mite may escape notice or may already have fallen off or been scratched off the lesions. Antihistamines or topical steroids effectively reduce mite-induced pruritus.

Chiggers are the agents of scrub typhus in tropical and subtropical parts of Asia, and mouse mites are the agents of rickettsialpox in the cities of the northeastern United States. Repellants are useful for preventing chigger bite and sanitary measures for rickettsialpox.

TICK INFESTATIONS AND TICK PARALYSIS

Hard ticks (Ixodidae), including dog ticks and deer ticks, have become increasingly abundant since the mid-1900s, and their bites have come to be associated with diverse debilitating diseases. Because soft ticks (Argasidae) rarely attack human hosts in the United States, the following discussion deals with hard ticks. Ticks attach and feed painlessly; blood is their only food. Their secretions, however,

produce local reactions, a febrile illness, or paralysis. Local reactions to tick bites vary from small pruritic papules to chronic nodules, or "tick granulomas," reaching several centimeters in diameter. Tick-induced fever, associated with headache, nausea, and malaise, usually resolves within 24 to 36 h after the tick is removed. Tick paralysis is an ascending flaccid paralysis believed to be caused by a toxin in tick saliva that causes neuromuscular block and decreased nerve conduction. This rare complication has occurred following bites of the dog and wood ticks (*Dermacentor variabilis* and *D. andersoni*) in the United States and various other kinds of ticks elsewhere in North America and the world. Weakness begins in the lower extremities 5 to 6 days after the tick has been attached and ascends symmetrically over several days to result in complete paralysis of the extremities and cranial nerves. Deep tendon reflexes are diminished or absent, but sensory examination and findings on lumbar puncture are typically normal. Removal of the tick results in improvement within an hour and usually complete recovery after several days. Failure to remove the tick may lead to death from aspiration or respiratory paralysis. Diagnosis depends on finding the tick, which often is hidden beneath hair. Ticks should be removed by firm traction with a forceps placed near their point of attachment. Rupture of their bodies may permit the escape of fluids containing pathogenic viruses, rickettsiae, borelliae, or the agent of tularemia. An antiserum to saliva of *Ixodes holocyclus*, the usual cause of tick paralysis in Australia, effectively reverses paralysis caused by these ticks.

PEDICULOSIS (LICE INFESTATIONS)

All three species of human lice feed at least once a day on human blood. *Pediculus humanus* var. *capitis* infests the head, *P. humanus* var. *corporis* the clothing, and *Pthirus pubis* mainly the hair of the pubis. Females firmly cement their eggs to hair or clothing. The saliva of lice produces an intensely irritating maculopapular or urticarial rash in sensitized persons.

Head lice are transmitted directly from person to person and occasionally by shared headgear and grooming implements. Prevalence is greatest in school-aged girls who wear long hair; black children are less frequently infested than other children. Excoriations of pruritic lesions on the scalp, neck, and shoulders lead to oozing, crusting, matting of hair, bacterial infections, and regional lymphadenopathy.

Body lice remain in clothing except when feeding and are unable to survive more than a few hours away from the human host. It follows, therefore, that *P. humanus* var. *corporis* mainly infests disaster victims or indigent persons who do not change their clothes. Transmission by direct contact or sharing of clothing and beds is enhanced under crowded conditions. Body lice leave febrile persons or corpses as they become cold, thus facilitating transmission of typhus, louse-borne relapsing fever, and trench fever (see Chap. 138). Pruritic lesions are particularly common around the neckline. Chronic infestations result in postinflammatory hyperpigmentation and thickening of skin known as *vagabond disease*.

The cosmopolitan crab or pubic louse is transmitted mainly by sexual contact but can infest eyelashes, axillary hair, and hair in other sites as well as pubic hair. Intensely pruritic lesions and 2- to 3-mm blue macules (maculae ceruleae) develop at the site of bites. Blepharitis commonly accompanies infestations of the eyelashes.

A suspected diagnosis of pediculosis is confirmed by the finding of nits or adult lice on hairs or in clothing. The preferred treatment is topical permethrin (1%) or 0.5% malathion, which kills both eggs and lice. Alternative agents such as the more toxic 1% lindane and pyrethrins with piperonyl butoxide are not ovicidal and require a second application 1 week later to kill hatching nymphs. Lindane-resistant head lice have been reported. After louse infestations have been treated with insecticide, the hair should be combed with a fine-toothed nit comb to remove nits. Combs and brushes should be disinfected in hot water at 65°C for 5 min or soaked in insecticide for 1 h. Body lice can be eliminated by bathing and topical pediculicides applied from head to foot. Clothes and bedding are deloused by heat sterilization in a dryer at 65°C for 30 min or by fumigation. Pubic lice are treated with topical pediculicides except on the eyelashes, where a coating of petrolatum should be applied for 3 to 4 days.

FLEA INFESTATIONS AND TUNGIASIS

Fleas are wingless insects 2 to 4 mm long that feed on the blood of human beings and other warm-bodied animals. Common human-biting fleas include the dog and cat fleas (*Ctenocephalides* spp.) and the rat flea (*Xenopsylla cheopis*), which inhabit the nests and resting sites of their hosts. Larval fleas feed on pellets of dried host blood that the adult fleas eject from their rectums while feeding. The high-jumping adults attack human beings or other available warm-bodied animals when the usual host abandons or is driven from its nest. The human flea (*Pulex irritans*) infests human bedding and furniture but mainly in relatively humid buildings that lack central heating. Sensitized persons develop erythematous, pruritic papules, urticaria, and occasionally vesicles and bacterial superinfection at the site of the bite. Treatment consists of antihistamines and antipruritics.

Fleas transmit plague, murine typhus, and rat and dog tapeworms. Infestations by fleas are eliminated by frequent cleaning of the nesting sites and bedding of the host or judicious dusting or spraying of insecticides such as pyrethrin, DDT, or malathion.

Human infestations with *Tunga penetrans*, the chigoe flea, sand flea, or jigger, occur in tropical regions of Africa and the Americas. Adults live in sandy soil and burrow under the skin between toes, under nails, or on the soles of bare feet. The fleas engorge on blood and grow from pinpoint to pea size over a 2-week period. The lesions resemble a white pustule with a central black depression and may be pruritic or painful. Occasional complications include tetanus, bacterial infections, and autoamputation of toes. Tungiasis is treated by removal of the intact flea with a sterile needle or scalpel.

MYIASIS

Myiasis refers to infestations by maggots, mainly due to the larvae of metallic-colored screw-worm flies or botflies. Maggots invade living or necrotic tissue or body cavities and produce different clinical syndromes depending on the species of fly.

FURUNCULAR MYIASIS In forested parts of Central and South America, larvae of *Dermatobia hominis*, the human botfly, produce boil-like subcutaneous nodules 2 to 3 cm in diameter. The adult female captures a mosquito or other bloodsucking insect and deposits her eggs beneath its abdomen. When the carrier insect attacks a human or bovine host several days later, the warmth and moisture of the host's surface stimulate the larvae to hatch and penetrate the skin. After 6 to 12 weeks, the larvae mature and drop to the ground, where they pupate. The African tumbu fly, *Cordylobia anthropophaga*, produces similar lesions. Dozens of eggs are deposited on sand or drying laundry that is contaminated with urine or sweat. Larvae hatch on contact with the body, penetrate the skin, and produce boils from which they emerge 8 or 9 days later. Diagnosis of furuncular myiasis is suggested by discomforting lesions with a central breathing pore that emits bubbles when submerged in water. Tumbu fly larvae can be removed by manual expression after the air pore is coated with petrolatum to suffocate the larvae and induce them to emerge. *Dermatobium* larvae often require surgical excision.

CREEPING DERMAL MYIASIS Maggots of the horse botfly, *Gasterophilus intestinalis*, do not mature after penetrating human skin but migrate for weeks in the epidermis. The resulting pruritic and serpiginous eruption resembles cutaneous larva migrans caused by *Ancylostoma braziliense*. Horseback riders become infested when eggs deposited on the flank of the horse hatch against their bare legs. The black spines of the larvae can be identified after mineral oil is smeared over the lesion. Larva are removed with a needle. The larvae of the cattle botfly (*Hypoderma* spp.) invade more deeply and produce boil-like swellings.

WOUND AND BODY CAVITY MYIASIS Certain flies are attracted to blood and pus, and their newly hatched larvae enter wounds or diseased skin. Some larvae remain superficial and confined to necrotic tissue and were used in the past to debride purulent wounds. Other species, including the screw-worms, *Chrysomyia bezziana* in Asia and Africa and *Cochliomyia hominivorax*, and the flesh fly, *Wohlfahrtia vigil*, in the Americas, invade more deeply into viable tissue and produce large, suppurating lesions. Larvae that infest wounds also may infest body cavities such as the mouth, nose, ears, sinuses, anus, vagina, and lower urinary tract, particularly in unconscious or otherwise debilitated patients. The consequences range from harmless colonization to destruction of the nose, meningitis, and deafness. Treatment involves removal of maggots and debridement of tissue.

OTHER FORMS OF MYIASIS The maggots responsible for furuncular and wound myiasis also may cause ophthalmomyiasis. Sequelae include nodules in the eyelid, retinal detachment, and destruction of the globe. In addition, the adult sheep botfly, *Oestrus ovis*, may oviposit larvae into the eyes of persons tending sheep and goats and produce a conjunctival infestation and acute conjunctivitis. True intestinal myiasis occurs when fly eggs or larvae of the drone fly, *Eristalis tenax*, are ingested with contaminated food and mature in the gut and cause an enteritis. Most instances in which maggots are found in human feces are the result of larviposition by flesh flies on recently passed stools.

PENTASTOMIASIS

Pentastomids, or tongue worms, are parasites with characteristics of both helminths and arthropods and are classified in a separate phylum. The wormlike adults inhabit the respiratory passages of reptiles and carnivorous mammals. Human infestation with *Linguatula serrata* is common in the Middle East and occurs in the Sudan following ingestion of encysted larval stages in raw liver or lymph nodes of sheep and goats, the intermediate hosts. The larvae migrate to the nasopharynx and produce an acute self-limiting syndrome known as halzoun (Marrara in the Sudan), which is characterized by pain and itching of the throat and ears, coughing, hoarseness, dysphagia, and dyspnea. Severe edema may cause obstruction and necessitate tracheostomy, and ocular invasion has been described. Diagnostic larvae measuring 5 to 10 mm in length are found in the copious nasal discharge or vomitus. Human beings become infected with *Armillifer armillatus* by ingestion of eggs in contaminated food or drink or after handling the definitive host, the African python. Larvae encyst in various organs and rarely cause symptoms unless they compress vital structures or perforate an organ during migration. Cysts occasionally require surgical removal as they enlarge while molting, but they are usually encountered as an incidental finding at autopsy. There are reports of the cutaneous larva migrans syndrome due to other pentastomes (*Reighardia* and *Sebekia* spp.) in Southeast Asia and Central America.

LEECH INFESTATIONS

Medically important leeches are annelid worms that attach to their hosts with chitinous cutting jaws and draw blood with muscular suckers. The medicinal leech, *Hirudo medicinalis*, is still occasionally used to reduce venous congestion in surgical flaps or replanted body parts. This practice has been complicated by wound infections, myonecrosis, and sepsis due to *Aeromonas hydrophila*, which colonizes the gullets of commercially available leeches.

Ubiquitous aquatic leeches that parasitize fish, frogs, and turtles readily attach to the skin of human beings and avidly suck blood. More notorious are the land leeches (*Haemadipsa*) that live in moist vegetation of tropical rain forests. Attachment is usually painless. Hidrudinin, a powerful anticoagulant secreted by the leech, causes continued bleeding after the leech has fallen off. Healing of the wound is slow, and bacterial infections are not uncommon. Several species of aquatic leeches in Africa, Asia, and southern Europe can enter through the mouth, nose, and genitourinary tract and attach to mucosal surfaces as deep as in the esophagus and trachea. Bleeding may be intense. Externally attached leeches are removed by steady gentle traction. Removal is hastened by application of alcohol, salt, vinegar, or a flame to the leech. Internal attachments may be relieved by saline gargles or removal by forceps.

REFERENCES

CHODOSH J, CLARRIDGE J: Ophthalmomyiasis: A review with special reference to *Cochliomyia hominivorax*. Clin Infect Dis 14:444, 1992

DONABEDIAN H, KHAZAN U: Norwegian scabies in a patient with AIDS. Clin Infect Dis 14:162, 1992

DRABICK JJ: Pentastomiasis. Rev Infect Dis 9:1087, 1987

HARWOOD RF, JAMES MT: *Entomology in Human and Animal Health*. New York, Macmillan, 1979.

LINEAWEAVER WC: *Aeromonas hydrophila* infections following clinical use of medicinal leeches: A review of published cases. Blood Coag Fibrinol 2:201, 1991

MEINKING TL, TAPLIN D: Advances in pediculosis, scabies, and other mite infestations. Adv Dermatol 5:131, 1990

SANUSI ID et al: Tungiasis: Report of one case and review of the 14 reported cases in the United States. J Am Acad Dermatol 20:941, 1989

SCHULTZ MW et al: Comparative study of 5% permethrin cream and 1% lindane lotion for the treatment of scabies. Arch Dermatol 126:167, 1990

STRICKLAND GT (ed): *Hunter's Tropical Medicine*, 7th ed. Philadelphia, Saunders, 1991

section 1 Disorders of the heart

186 APPROACH TO THE PATIENT WITH HEART DISEASE

EUGENE BRAUNWALD

The symptoms caused by heart disease result most commonly from myocardial ischemia, from disturbance of the contraction and/or relaxation of the myocardium, from obstruction to blood flow, or from an abnormal cardiac rhythm or rate. Ischemia is manifest most frequently as chest discomfort, while reduction of the pumping ability of the heart commonly leads to weakness and fatigability or, when severe, produces cyanosis, hypotension, syncope, and elevated intravascular pressure behind a failing ventricle; the latter results in abnormal fluid accumulation, which in turn leads to dyspnea, orthopnea, and systemic or pulmonary edema. Obstruction to blood flow, as in valvular stenosis, can cause symptoms resembling those resulting from congestive heart failure, despite normal or near-normal myocardial function. Cardiac arrhythmias often develop suddenly, and the resulting signs and symptoms—palpitation, dyspnea, angina, hypotension, and syncope—generally occur abruptly and may disappear as rapidly as they develop.

A cardinal principle useful in the evaluation of the patient with suspected heart disease is that myocardial or coronary function which may be adequate at rest may be inadequate during exertion. Thus a history of chest discomfort and/or dyspnea which appears only during activity is characteristic of heart disease, while the opposite pattern, i.e., the appearance of these symptoms at rest and their remission during exertion, is rarely observed in patients with organic heart disease.

Patients with cardiocirculatory disease also may be asymptomatic, both at rest and during exertion, but may present an abnormal physical finding, such as a heart murmur, elevated systemic arterial pressure, or an abnormality of the electrocardiogram or of the cardiac silhouette on the chest roentgenogram. Patients may exhibit asymptomatic ischemia on an exercise stress test or an ambulatory electrocardiogram.

Diseases of the heart and circulation are so common and the laity is so well acquainted with the major symptoms resulting from these disorders that patients, and occasionally physicians, erroneously attribute many noncardiac complaints to organic cardiovascular disease. The combination of the widespread fear of heart disease with the deep-seated emotional connotations concerning this organ's function results in the frequent development of symptoms which mimic those of organic disease in persons with normal cardiovascular systems. Sometimes it is difficult to interpret correctly the symptoms of patients with recognized organic cardiovascular disturbances. Such patients, in addition to having symptoms resulting from their disease, also may develop functional complaints referable to the cardiovascular system. The unraveling of symptoms and signs due to organic heart disease from those which are not directly related is an important and challenging task in these patients.

Dyspnea, one of the cardinal manifestations of diminished cardiac reserve, is not limited to disease of the heart but is also characteristic of conditions as diverse as pulmonary disease, marked obesity, and anxiety (Chap. 31). Similarly, chest discomfort may result from a variety of causes other than myocardial ischemia (Chap. 12). Whether heart disease is responsible for these symptoms can frequently be determined by carrying out a careful clinical examination. Noninvasive testing using electrocardiography at rest and during exercise (Chap. 189), echocardiography, roentgenography, and myocardial imaging (Chap. 190) usually provides important additional information to permit the correct interpretation of symptoms; more specialized invasive examinations (catheterization and angiography) are occasionally necessary.

DIAGNOSIS   In every branch of medicine the development of a rational plan of management and the assessment of prognosis are based on a correct diagnostic appraisal. In patients with disorders of the cardiocirculatory system, particular care must be taken to establish not only a correct but also a *complete* diagnosis. As outlined by the New York Heart Association, the elements of a complete cardiac diagnosis include consideration of

1 *The underlying etiology.* Is the disease congenital, infectious, hypertensive, or ischemic in origin?
2 *The anatomic abnormalities.* Which chambers are involved? Which valves are affected? Is there pericardial involvement? Has there been a myocardial infarction?
3 *The physiologic disturbances.* Is an arrhythmia present? Is there evidence of congestive heart failure or of myocardial ischemia?
4 *The extent of functional disability.* How strenuous is the physical activity required to elicit symptoms? The latter should be evaluated in the light of the intensity of therapy.

Two simple examples may serve to illustrate the importance of establishing a complete diagnosis: (1) The identification of myocardial ischemia as the cause of exertional chest discomfort is of great clinical importance. However, the recognition of ischemia is insufficient to develop either a therapeutic strategy or prognosis until the underlying disease process responsible for the myocardial ischemia, e.g., coronary atherosclerosis or aortic stenosis, is identified and a judgment made as to whether other factors which cause an imbalance between myocardial oxygen supply and demand, such as severe anemia, thyrotoxicosis, or supraventricular tachycardia play a contributory role. (2) Determining that heart disease is congenital provides an important starting point, but the decision about whether surgical treatment is advisable depends on the specific anatomic defect present and often on the nature of the physiologic disturbance and the functional impairment as well.

The establishment of a correct and complete cardiac diagnosis often requires the use of six different methods of examination: (1)

history, (2) physical examination (Chap. 188), (3) electrocardiogram (Chap. 189), (4) chest roentgenogram (Chap. 190), (5) noninvasive graphic examinations (echocardiogram, radionuclide and other noninvasive imaging techniques) (Chaps. 190 and 191), and occasionally (6) specialized invasive examinations, i.e., cardiac catheterization, angiocardiography, and coronary arteriography (Chap. 192). In order to be most effective, the results obtained from each of these six modalities should be analyzed independently of one another as well as with the information derived from the other methods clearly in mind. Only in this way can one avoid overlooking a subtle, though important, finding. For example, an electrocardiogram should be obtained in every patient suspected of having heart disease. It may provide the critical clue in establishing the correct diagnosis, e.g., the finding of a moderate atrioventricular conduction disturbance in a patient with unexplained syncope, even when all other methods of examination reveal no abnormal findings. On the other hand, when combined intelligently with the results of other methods of examination, the electrocardiogram may provide essential confirmatory data. Thus the knowledge that a patient has an apical diastolic rumbling murmur may direct particular attention to the P waves, and the recognition of left atrial enlargement electrocardiographically supports the suggestion that the murmur is caused by mitral stenosis. Under these circumstances, the additional finding on the electrocardiogram of right ventricular hypertrophy suggests that pulmonary hypertension is present and that the mitral stenosis is severe.

Family history　In obtaining the history of a patient with known or suspected cardiovascular disease, particular attention should be directed to the family history. Familial clustering is common in many forms of heart disease. Genetic transmission may occur, as in hypertrophic cardiomyopathy (Chap. 205), the Marfan syndrome (Chap. 351), and sudden death associated with a prolonged QT syndrome (Chap. 198). In patients with essential hypertension or coronary atherosclerosis, the genetic component may be less obvious but is also of considerable importance. Familial clustering of cardiovascular diseases may occur not only on a genetic basis but also may be related to familial dietary or behavior patterns, such as excessive ingestion of salt or calories or cigarette smoking.

Assessment of functional impairment　When an attempt is made to ascertain the severity of functional impairment in a patient with heart disease, it is helpful to ascertain the level of activity and the rate at which it is performed before symptoms develop. Thus breathlessness which occurs after running up two long flights of stairs denotes far less functional impairment than similar symptoms occurring after taking a few steps on the level. Also, the degree of customary physical activity at work and during recreation should be considered. The development of two-flight dyspnea in a marathon runner may be far more significant than the development of one-flight dyspnea in a previously sedentary person. Similarly, the history must include a detailed consideration of the patient's therapeutic regimen. For example, the persistence or development of edema, breathlessness, and other manifestations of heart failure in a patient whose diet is rigidly restricted in sodium content and who is receiving optimal doses of diuretics must be interpreted quite differently from the development of similar manifestations of heart failure in the absence of these measures. In an effort to ascertain the rate of progression of symptoms, and thereby of the severity of the underlying illness, it may be useful to ascertain what, if any, specific tasks the patient could carry out 1 year earlier which he or she cannot carry out now.

Electrocardiogram　Although the electrocardiogram is an invaluable aspect of every cardiovascular examination, with the exception of the identification of arrhythmias and of many instances of acute myocardial infarction, it rarely permits establishment of a specific diagnosis. In the absence of other abnormal findings, electrocardiographic changes must not be overinterpreted. The range of normal electrocardiographic findings is wide, and the tracing can be affected significantly by many noncardiac factors, such as age, body habitus, and serum electrolyte concentrations.

Natural history　The natural history of cardiovascular disease must be appreciated. Cardiovascular disorders often present acutely, as in a previously asymptomatic patient with extensive coronary atherosclerosis who develops an acute myocardial infarction or the previously asymptomatic patient with hypertrophic cardiomyopathy whose first clinical manifestation is syncope or even sudden death. However, in both instances, the alert physician may recognize the patient at risk of these complications long before they occur and can often take measures to prevent their occurrence. For example, the patient with acute myocardial infarction may well have had risk factors for atherosclerosis for many years. Had these been recognized, their elimination or reduction might have delayed or even prevented the infarction. Similarly, the patient with hypertrophic cardiomyopathy may have had the familial form of this disorder, and a careful family history might have led to an echocardiographic examination and the recognition of the condition long before the acute manifestations.

PITFALLS IN CARDIOVASCULAR MEDICINE　Increasing subspecialization in internal medicine and the perfection of advanced diagnostic techniques in cardiology can lead to several undesirable consequences, which can be summarized as follows:

1 Failure by the *noncardiologist* to recognize cardiac manifestations of systemic illnesses. Examples of the latter are (*a*) the Down syndrome (associated with endocardial cushion defect); (*b*) gonadal dysgenesis, i.e., the Turner syndrome (associated with a variety of congenital cardiovascular defects, particularly coarctation of the aorta); (*c*) bony abnormalities of the upper extremities (associated with atrial septal defect in the Holt-Oram syndrome); (*d*) muscular dystrophies (associated with cardiomyopathy); (*e*) hemochromatosis and glycogen storage disease (associated with myocardial infiltration and restrictive cardiomyopathy); (*f*) congenital deafness (associated with prolonged QT interval and serious cardiac arrhythmias); (*g*) Raynaud's disease (associated with primary pulmonary hypertension and coronary vasospasm); (*h*) connective tissue disorders, i.e., the Marfan syndrome, Ehlers-Danlos and Hurler syndromes, and related disorders of mucopolysaccharide metabolism (aortic dilatation, prolapsed mitral valve, a variety of arterial abnormalities); (*i*) chronic hemolytic anemia (cardiac dilatation); (*j*) Refsum's disease (myocardial failure and conduction defects); (*k*) acromegaly (hypertension, accelerated coronary atherosclerosis, conduction defects, cardiomyopathy); (*l*) hyperthyroidism (heart failure, atrial fibrillation); (*m*) hypothyroidism (pericardial effusion, coronary artery disease); (*n*) rheumatoid arthritis (pericarditis, aortic valve disease); (*o*) Whipple's disease (pericarditis and endocarditis); (*p*) scleroderma (cor pulmonale, myocardial fibrosis, pericarditis); (*q*) systemic lupus erythematosus (valvulitis, myocarditis, pericarditis); (*r*) polymyositis (pericarditis, myocarditis); (*s*) sarcoidosis (arrhythmias, cardiomyopathy); (*t*) Fabry's disease (myocardial ischemia, heart failure); and (*u*) exfoliative dermatitis (high-output heart failure). In patients with these and other systemic disorders a detailed clinical and noninvasive examination of the cardiovascular system should be carried out to identify cardiovascular involvement.

2 Failure by the cardiologist to recognize an underlying systemic illness, such as those listed above, among patients with a cardiac disorder. Patients known or suspected of having heart disease require a detailed general assessment and a search for the frequent *noncardiac* manifestations of systemic disorders with cardiovascular manifestations. For example, infective endocarditis should be considered in patients with known congenital or valvular heart disease with fever, anemia, or albuminuria. A cardiovascular abnormality may provide the clue critical to the recognition of some systemic disorders. For instance, in an elderly person, unexplained atrial fibrillation may provide the first clue to the diagnosis of thyrotoxicosis.

3 Overreliance on and overutilization of laboratory tests, particularly invasive techniques for the examination of the cardiovascular system. Catheterization of the right and left sides of the heart,

selective angiography, and coronary arteriography (Chap. 192) provide precise diagnostic information under many circumstances. For example, they aid in establishing a specific anatomic diagnosis and in determining the physiologic consequences of the abnormalities in patients with chest pain of uncertain cause in whom ischemic heart disease is suspected, and in determining the functional significance of valvular abnormalities in patients with rheumatic heart disease being considered for surgical treatment. Although a great deal of attention has been lavished on these specialized examinations, it should be recognized that they serve to *supplement*, not *supplant*, a careful examination carried out by clinical and noninvasive examination. There is an unfortunate tendency to carry out procedures such as coronary arteriography in patients with chest pain suspected of having ischemic heart disease instead of taking a detailed and thoughtful history; although coronary arteriography may establish whether the coronary arteries are obstructed, the results often do not provide a definite answer to the question of whether a patient's complaint of chest pain is clearly attributable to coronary arteriosclerosis. Coronary arteriography is also often carried out unnecessarily in patients with symptoms and signs of mild myocardial ischemia and normal left ventricular function who are not likely to be candidates for coronary bypass surgery. Similarly, catheterization of the left side of the heart is all too frequently employed to determine whether operative treatment of valvular disease is indicated, even before the patient has had a trial of medical therapy.

Despite the enormous value of these invasive tests it must not be overlooked that they entail some small risk to the patient, involve discomfort and substantial cost, and place a strain on existing medical facilities. Therefore, *they should be carried out not as part of a "fishing expedition" or as evidence to the patient and the family that "everything is being done," but only if, after detailed clinical examination and assessment by noninvasive tests, the results of the invasive examination can be expected to modify or aid in the patient's management.*

MANAGEMENT After a complete diagnosis has been established, a number of therapeutic options are usually available. Several examples may be used to demonstrate some of the principles of modern cardiovascular therapeutics:

1 In the absence of evidence for the existence of heart disease, a clear, definitive statement to that effect should be made and the patient should *not* be asked to return at intervals for repeated examinations. If there is no evidence for disease, such attention may lead to the patient developing inappropriate anxiety and fixation on the heart.

2 If there is no evidence of cardiovascular disease but the patient has one or more risk factors for the development of ischemic heart disease (Chap. 208), a plan for their reduction should be developed and the patient should be retested at intervals to assess that he or she is complying and that these risk factors are in fact being reduced.

3 Asymptomatic or mildly symptomatic patients with established valvular heart disease should be evaluated periodically, every 6 to 12 months, by clinical and noninvasive examinations (Chap. 190). Early signs of deterioration of ventricular function can be detected in this manner and in appropriate patients may signify the need for cardiac catheterization and surgical treatment before the development of disabling symptoms, irreversible myocardial damage, and an excessive risk of surgical treatment (Chap. 201).

4 It is critical to establish clear criteria for deciding on the form of treatment (medical, angioplasty, or surgical revascularization) in patients with ischemic heart disease (Chap. 203). Surgical treatment represents a major therapeutic advance in the treatment of this most common form of heart disease, but operation has probably been employed too widely in the United States; the mere presence of angina pectoris and/or the demonstration of critical coronary arterial narrowing at angiography should not reflexly evoke a decision to treat the patient surgically. Instead, this form of treatment should be limited to those patients with ischemic heart disease in whom it has been demonstrated that surgical treatment is superior to medical treatment.

REFERENCES

BRAUNWALD E (ED): *Heart Disease*, 4th ed. Philadelphia, Saunders, 1992

CHRISTIE LG, CONTI CR: Systematic approach to the evaluation of angina-like chest pain. Am Heart J 102:897, 1981

GOLDMAN L et al: Pitfalls in the serial assessment of cardiac functional status. How a reduction in "ordinary" activity may reduce the apparent degree of cardiac compromise and give a misleading impression of improvement. J Chronic Dis. 35:763, 1982

NEW YORK HEART ASSOCIATION, CRITERIA COMMITTEE: *Nomenclature and Criteria for Diagnosis of Diseases of the Heart and Great Vessels*, 8th ed. Boston, Little, Brown, 1981

PERLOFF K (ED): *Physical Examination of the Heart and Circulation*, 2d ed. Philadelphia, Saunders, 1990.

SAPIRA JD: The history, in *The Art and Science of Bedside Diagnosis*. Baltimore, Urban Schwartzenberg, 1990, pp 9–45

SCHMITT BP et al: The diagnostic usefulness of the history of the patient with dyspnea. J Gen Intern Med 1:386, 1986

SUTTON GC: Symptoms of heart disease, in *Diseases of the Heart*, DG Julian (ed). London, Balliere Tindall, 1989, pp 89–99

187 CELLULAR AND MOLECULAR BIOLOGY OF CARDIOVASCULAR DISEASE

EUGENE BRAUNWALD

Because the principal function of the heart is to serve as a pump, clinical cardiology, since the era of William Harvey, has been deeply rooted in physiology and hemodynamics. The development of electrocardiography at the beginning of this century and the recognition of clinical disturbances of cardiac rhythm led to increasing interest in electrophysiology. Since both the mechanical and the electrical properties of the heart can be altered profoundly by drugs, pharmacology also has provided strong scientific underpinnings to clinical cardiology.

A fuller understanding of cardiac function and dysfunction will ultimately require studies at the cellular, molecular, and genetic levels. However, such investigations have been retarded by the absence of any cell line of adult, fully differentiated myocytes that can be readily grown in vitro, manipulated, and studied. Perhaps for this reason, cellular biology and molecular genetics have been slower to have an impact on cardiovascular disease than on some other branches of medicine, such as hematology, oncology, endocrinology, and infectious diseases. However, application of these techniques to cardiovascular science has now gained momentum, and these efforts are beginning to influence the care of patients with cardiovascular disease. Several examples of this influence are considered in this chapter and include advances in understanding the process of myocardial hypertrophy, the constituents of the bloodstream such as apolipoproteins, and noncardiac cells, including vascular smooth-muscle cells, endothelial cells, and platelets. Discussed elsewhere (Chap. 316) are advances in thrombolytic therapy which also have resulted from studies at the cellular and molecular levels.

HYPERTROPHY

MYOCARDIAL HYPERTROPHY One of the most remarkable and important capacities of the heart is to adapt both acutely and chronically to changes in hemodynamic load. *Acute* adaptations are mediated by the two mechanisms discussed in Chap. 194: (1) an alteration in the number of cross-bridges that cycle between the actin and myosin myofilaments, which in turn is dependent on the length of the myocardial sarcomeres (this adaptation expresses, at the molecular level, Starling's law of the heart), and (2) changes in contractility mediated by the adrenergic neurotransmitter norepinephrine via adrenergic receptors. The degree of activation of these receptors ultimately regulates the concentration of calcium ions near the contractile proteins and, thereby, myocardial contractility. In contrast, with *chronic* hemodynamic overload, as in hypertension, valvular heart disease, and many forms of congenital heart disease, *myocardial hypertrophy* is the major adaptive response. As the ventricle hypertrophies, new sarcomeres are added to each myocyte, protein synthesis is augmented, and sometimes protein degradation declines. The fraction of total cardiac protein composed of myofibrillar proteins increases in hypertrophy and subsequently declines as heart failure supervenes. Exactly how mechanical load is converted into growth, a process that might be termed *mechanogrowth coupling*, is not fully understood. When myocytes are stretched in vitro, an increase in mRNA and protein synthesis takes place. Thus myocytes appear to be able to *sense* external load and to undergo hypertrophy, perhaps involving a release of growth factors.

The imposition of a pressure load on the ventricle is accompanied by an increase in the expression of messenger RNA (mRNA) that codes for various contractile proteins, and these increased levels of mRNA are responsible for the increase in myocardial protein synthesis. Proteins often occur in families of closely related isoforms, the expression of which is regulated in a tissue-specific and developmentally specific manner. In experimental animals, the hypertrophic response to pressure overload involves the reappearance in the adult heart of contractile protein isoforms characteristic of the fetus such as the V_3 form of beta-myosin heavy chain ("slow myosin"), which has a low ATPase activity and promotes a slower, more sustained contraction requiring less energy than the V_1 form ("fast myosin"). The fetal isoforms of alpha actin and tropomyosin and the mRNA of atrial natriuretic peptide (ANP) are also reexpressed when left ventricular hypertrophy is induced. This reexpression of fetal protein genes appears to represent a general adaptive response to hemodynamic overload in experimental animals.

The mechanisms of hypertrophy depend on the inciting stimulus. In contrast to the cardiac hypertrophy resulting from hemodynamic overload, the hypertrophy of hyperthyroidism is *not* accompanied by the induction of fetal forms of contractile protein genes or of the ANP gene. Thyroid hormone acts directly via nuclear receptors to regulate myosin heavy chain gene expression at the transcriptional level, causing an accumulation of alpha-myosin heavy chain mRNA, and inhibits the expression of beta-myosin heavy chain mRNA, thereby increasing the level of myosin isoenzyme V_1 and bringing about a more rapid contraction. Hypothyroid hearts have higher levels of beta-myosin heavy chain mRNA and the V_3 myosin isoform and lower levels of the mRNA encoding Ca^{2+} ATPase and Ca^{2+} release channels of sarcoplasmic reticulum.

Some of the changes in gene expression in ventricular hypertrophy may involve proto-oncogenes, which are normal cellular homologues of transforming genes carried by oncogenic retroviruses (Chap. 63). Three major classes of proto-oncogenes are induced rapidly by pressure overload: (1) proto-oncogenes such as c-*cis* that encode peptide growth factors, such as the beta chain of platelet-derived growth factor (PDGF), (2) proto-oncogenes such as c-*myc* and c-*fos*, which code for nuclear proteins that regulate transcription of a variety of genes which influence cell growth, and (3) proto-oncogenes such as c-*ras*, which code for cytoplasmic proteins that bind to guanine nucleotides and regulate other intracellular signaling systems. The reinduction of genes normally expressed in fetal life, such as the fetal isoforms of myosin and ANP (in the ventricle), is a later event.

Stimuli that increase intracellular cyclic AMP (cAMP) and intracellular Ca^{2+} (such as beta-adrenergic agonists) or those which enhance the turnover of inositol phospholipids (such as angiotensin II and alpha-adrenergic agonists) have direct trophic effect on cardiac myocytes when studied in vitro. Norepinephrine and angiotensin II augment expression of proto-oncogenes, stimulate protein synthesis, and induce the synthesis of fetal isoforms of actin and myosin. This action of the alpha-adrenergic agonists and angiotensin II occurs though G protein–coupled receptors and the subsequent activation of phospholipases and the protein kinase cascade (see below).

In addition to the growth of myocytes, the interstitium also participates in pressure-overload hypertrophy, which is associated with hyperplasia of fibroblasts and the deposition of excess and altered types of extracellular collagen. The relief of hemodynamic overload, either surgically or pharmacologically, usually results in partial regression of myocyte hypertrophy but not necessarily in regression of interstitial proliferation.

There are many potential applications to cardiology of the growing understanding of the mechanisms involved in myocyte hypertrophy. For example, overexpression of the c-*myc* proto-oncogene in the heart of transgenic mice results in cardiac enlargement due to myocyte hyperplasia. Treatment of animals with angiotensin-converting enzyme (ACE) inhibitors has been shown to cause regression of cardiac hypertrophy and interstitial fibrosis induced by hemodynamic overload. Investigation of these phenomena also might reveal the mechanism by which compensatory hypertrophy sometimes leads to myocardial failure and could suggest measures to prevent this complication. Ultimately, this knowledge also could lead to the development of a method for stimulating myocardial hypertrophy or even myocyte hyperplasia after cell death has occurred consequent to myocardial infarction or viral myocarditis.

VASCULAR WALL   The renin-angiotensin system in the vascular wall may be involved in the development of hypertrophy of vascular smooth muscle. Angiotensinogen mRNA in blood vessel walls may be elevated in chronic hypertension. The addition of angiotensin II to cultures of vascular smooth-muscle cells causes the rapid activation of the c-*fos* proto-oncogene, which may mediate angiotensin II–induced hypertrophy in smooth-muscle cells in vivo. Indeed, angiotensin II induces hypertrophy of arterial smooth-muscle cells in vitro, in association with rapid induction in c-*fos*, c-*myc*, and c-*jun* mRNA levels followed by marked increases in the expression of the α chain of PDGF. This hypertrophy of vascular smooth muscle can be blocked by ACE inhibitors. The gene for the PDGF receptor has been cloned; the PDGF receptor mediates the mitogenic effects of this substance on vascular smooth-muscle (and other) cells. The PDGF receptor has a structure similar to a family of growth factor receptors that have tyrosine kinase activity. The PDGF receptor interacts with the c-*ras* proto-oncogene product and activates phospholipase C.

Many growth factors for vascular smooth muscle, such as angiotensin II, vasopressin, PDGF, and epidermal growth factor, are also vasoconstrictors. These considerations may be of significance in selecting or designing antihypertensive drugs. Indeed, ACE inhibitors are more potent in causing regression of left ventricular hypertrophy than are direct-acting vasodilators such as hydralazine.

INHERITED DISORDERS OF THE CARDIOVASCULAR SYSTEM

A number of disorders of the cardiovascular system are inherited as single-gene disorders, but many more are multigene disorders. Efforts are underway to identify the genes responsible for hypertrophy using the technique of genetic linkage (or cosegregation) analysis (see Chap. 61). This technique is used to map the loci of genes that are tightly linked to a specific phenotype by making use of restriction fragment length polymorphisms (RFLPs) which are due to DNA sequence differences between individuals.

HYPERTROPHIC CARDIOMYOPATHY   (See Chap. 205) This condition is familial in slightly more than half of all patients; it is transmitted as an autosomal dominant trait with almost complete

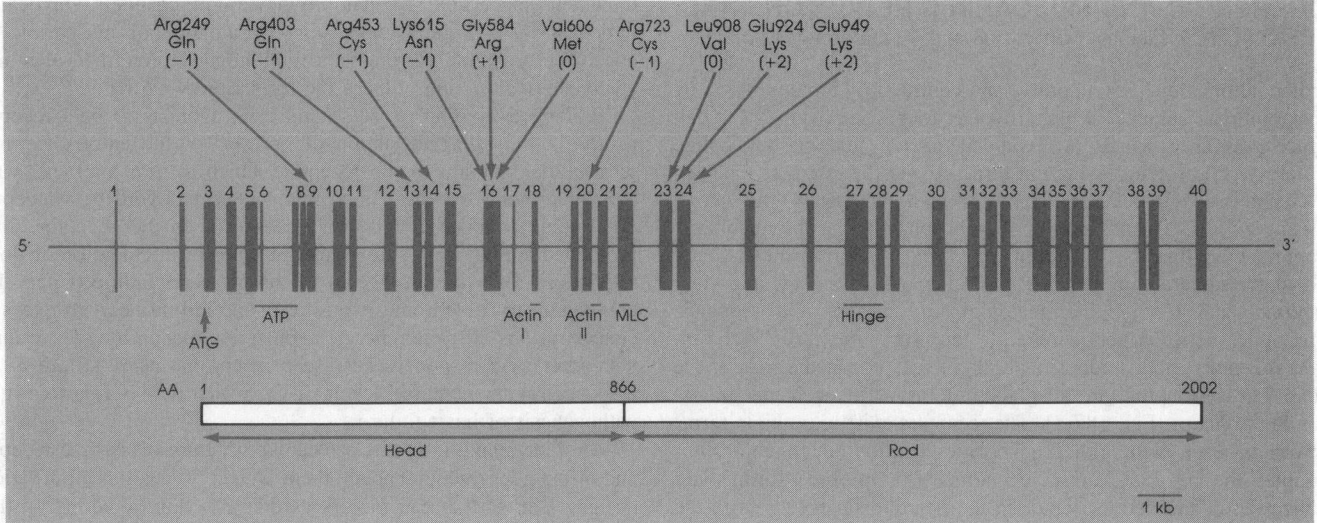

FIGURE 187-1 A diagram of the beta cardiac (myosin heavy chain) gene and the location of ten different missense mutations that cause (familial hypertrophic cardiomyopathy). The gene is divided into 40 exons (*small boxes*), and the locations of the exons that encode the head and rod regions of the myosin heavy chain polypeptide are indicated. Sequences that encode the initiation of gene transcription (ATG), ATPase activity (ATP), actin binding (actin I and actin II), myosin light chain binding (MLC), and hinge function (Hinge) are indicated. Mutations result in amino acid substitutions (designated by triple-letter code) and usually result in a change in charge (indicated). The ban above exon 40 represents a deletion. (*Modified from CE Seidman et al, in E Braunwald (ed), Heart Disease: Clinical Update 4, 4th ed, Philadelphia, Saunders, 1992; modified from H Watkins et al, N Engl J Med 326:1108, 1992.*)

penetrance. Linkage analysis for markers of variations in DNA sequence in affected family members has identified mutations in band 1 of chromosome 14 in about half of all patients with familial hypertrophic cardiomyopathy (FHC). One of the principal genes that encodes adult ventricular myosin heavy chain (MHC), the cardiac MHC gene, is also located in band 1 of chromosome 14, and it appears that mutations in this gene are associated with those cases of FHC linked to this chromosome (Fig. 187-1). Eight missense mutations involving a change of a single nucleotide base pair that alters an amino acid in the beta cardiac MHC have been described. When found in one family member, the same mutation occurs in all affected family members, and identical mutations have been observed in different family members. FHC is genetically heterogeneous; approximately one-half of the cases of FHC are *not* linked to mutations of the beta cardiac MHC gene on chromosome 14, and the absence of a mutation in this gene does not exclude the diagnosis of FHC. There is a wide range of phenotypic expressions of FHC, and genetic typing using circulating lymphocytes has identified mutations of the beta cardiac MHC gene associated with more serious clinical outcomes, including early death.

FHC with clinical features indistinguishable from those with mutations in the beta cardiac MHC gene also has been mapped to chromosome 1. Three genes encoding contractile proteins on the short arm of chromosome 1 (isoforms of actin, tropomyosin, and troponin) are possible genes for this FHC locus.

Genetic typing of FHC should make possible prenatal diagnosis, the identification of asymptomatic persons with FHC, prognostic stratification, genetic counseling, and ultimately, the early initiation of treatment.

DUCHENNE'S MUSCULAR DYSTROPHY (See also Chap. 385) This X-linked recessive skeletal muscle disorder is sometimes associated with cardiomyopathy and heart failure, as well as with atrioventricular and interventricular conduction disorders and a variety of arrhythmias and sudden death. The gene responsible for this disorder has been mapped to the X chromosome; it is large, spans more than 2.5×10^6 base pairs, and encodes a large (427 kDa) protein termed *dystrophin*. Mutations of this gene may cause dystrophin to be absent from the transverse tubules of skeletal and cardiac muscle of patients with Duchenne's muscular dystrophy. Its absence in the myocardium is directly or indirectly responsible for the cardiomyopathy that frequently occurs in this condition.

MYOTONIC MUSCULAR DYSTROPHY (See also Chap. 385) This autosomal dominant defect is frequently associated with replacement of the cardiac conduction system with fatty and fibrous tissue resulting in cardiac conduction disturbances and sudden death and occasionally in a cardiomyopathy. The responsible gene has been mapped to chromosome 19. The abnormal protein responsible for myotonic dystrophy has not yet been isolated, but its identification should provide new insights into the mechanism of conduction disturbances in the Purkinje tissue.

LONG QT SYNDROME (See also Chap. 198) This autosomal dominant disorder predisposes to ventricular tachycardia and fibrillation, episodes of syncope, and sudden death. In one large family the syndrome has been linked to the Harvey *ras*-1 gene located on chromosome 11. This gene is involved in the regulation of cardiac potassium channels and may thereby be responsible for delayed repolarization, the hallmark of this syndrome.

MARFAN SYNDROME (See also Chap. 351) This condition exhibits simple Mendelian autosomal dominant inheritance with variable expression; approximately 15 percent of patients represent de novo mutations. This disorder of connective tissue is associated with numerous life-threatening cardiovascular manifestations, including aortic dissection, aortic aneurysm, myxomatous degeneration, and regurgitation of the aortic and mitral valves.

The connective tissue of patients with the Marfan syndrome has reduced content of microfibrils, of which a large (350 kDa) connective tissue glycoprotein *fibrillin* is an important constituent. The gene for fibrillin has been mapped to chromosome 15 and is tightly linked to the Marfan syndrome. There appears to be genetic heterogeneity of fibrillins, which may be responsible for the phenotypic variations in the Marfan syndrome. Mutation of a second gene for fibrillin, on chromosome 5, is responsible for a condition resembling the Marfan syndrome.

The identification of the genetic defects in the Marfan syndrome should allow genetic diagnosis and the commencement of therapy prior to the development of clinical manifestations.

ADRENERGIC AND MUSCARINIC RECEPTORS AND G PROTEINS (See also Chaps. 68 and 69 and Fig. 187-2)

Cardiac automaticity, excitability, and contractility are controlled by transmembrane signals, which involve four components: (1) cell surface receptors which are coupled to (2) guanine nucleotide regulatory (G) proteins, which in turn activate (3) effectors, such as ion channels or intracellular enzymes, which generate (4) the second messengers cAMP and inositol trisphosphate. Plasma membrane receptors bind ligands, including drugs and neurotransmitters, and mediate their interaction with cells (see Chap. 69). There are important functional and topographic analogies and amino acid sequence homologues between beta-adrenergic receptors, muscarinic (cholinergic) receptors, and rhodopsin, the light receptor in the rods of the retina. These receptors are all glycoproteins with seven membrane-spanning domains (Fig. 187-3). The receptors exist in multiple forms (isoforms), each with either a specific location or function. For example, the beta-adrenergic receptor exists in three forms with localization of the beta$_1$ receptor in the heart, beta$_2$ receptors in the airways, and beta$_3$ receptors in adipocytes. The genes coding for all three isoforms of beta-adrenergic receptors and the five muscarinic receptors have been cloned.

Beta-adrenergic and alpha$_1$-adrenergic receptors are coupled to different classes of G proteins. The binding of agonists such as norepinephrine released by adrenergic neurons or of infused dobutamine to the beta-adrenergic receptor--G protein complex results in a conformational change of the G stimulatory protein (G$_s$). This change in turn activates effectors such as adenylate cyclase that increase cAMP, a stimulant of myocardial contractility. G proteins couple alpha$_1$-adrenergic receptors to the activation of phospholipase C, which in turn breaks down a cell membrane phospholipid (PIP$_2$) into inositol trisphosphate (IP$_3$) and diacylglycerol. IP$_3$ in turn liberates calcium ions from intracellular stores and thereby stimulates cardiac contractility. Diacylglycerol activates a Ca^{2+}-sensitive protein kinase

C which appears to regulate myocyte ion channels, myocardial hypertrophy, and gene expression. Stimulation of muscarinic and adenosine receptors [through the inhibitory G protein (G$_i$)] inhibits adenylate cyclase and reduces the formation of cAMP.

Prolonged binding of beta-adrenergic agonists to beta receptors results in the phosphorylation of portions of the carboxy-terminal intracellular domain of the receptor, which in turn interacts with a cellular protein, *arrestin;* this protein interferes with beta receptor–G protein association and hence desensitizes the receptor. More prolonged agonist exposure results in receptor degradation or down-regulation. This process occurs in chronic heart failure (Chap. 194) consequent to the chronic exposure of the failing heart to excessive concentrations of the adrenergic agonist norepinephrine. The reduced beta-adrenergic responsiveness seen in chronic heart failure is also associated with increased levels of G$_i$, which may play a role in the pathogenesis of heart failure.

An understanding of the molecular structure of cardiac receptors and of the genes which encode them is likely to lead to more rational design of drugs that can modify cardiac function by acting on these receptors.

CALCIUM CHANNELS Calcium ions play a unique role in a variety of cellular functions, in particular contraction of cardiac and vascular smooth muscle (Chap. 194). Calcium enters cardiac cells through voltage-sensitive calcium channels (see Fig. 187-2) that are controlled by transmembrane electrical potentials and open during depolarization of the sarcolemma. Interaction of the Ca^{2+} channel with the catalytic subunit of cAMP-dependent protein kinase results in activation of the calcium channels, increasing the probability of their opening and thereby increasing influx of calcium into myocytes and enhancing the force of cardiac contraction. This explains, in part, the positive inotropic actions of the beta-adrenergic agonists and of the phosphodiesterase inhibitors, both of which enhance levels of cAMP.

The (L-type) cardiac calcium channels appear to be large aqueous

---

FIGURE 187-2 Ion transport through the sarcolemma of a myocyte. The Na$^+$ channel of the heart muscle cell opens briefly at the start of an action potential, permitting an influx of Na$^+$. The Na$^+$ channel can be blocked by tetrodotoxin (TTX) or by type I antiarrhythmic agents (see Chap. 198). Depolarization of the sarcolemma leads to Ca^{2+} influx through the Ca^{2+} channel, which is sensitive to the change in potential. The Ca^{2+} channel can be blocked by the calcium entry blockers. D, diltiazem; V, verapamil; DHP, dihydropyridines. Repolarization of the membrane results principally from the opening of K$^+$ channels and the efflux of K$^+$. Ca^{2+} is removed from the cell by the Na$^+$/Ca^{2+} exchanger and by a Ca^{2+}-ATPase (an energy-requiring process). The Na$^+$ pump (Na$^+$,K$^+$-ATPase) removes Na$^+$ which has flowed into the cell and returns K$^+$ to the cell by an energy-requiring process; it may be blocked by digitalis (DIG).

Two types of receptors modulate ionic pathways. Beta-adrenergic receptors (which are one kind of type 2 receptor) stimulate the production of the second messenger cyclic AMP which by causing phosphorylation (P) allows the Ca^{2+} channel to open. Muscarinic cholinergic receptors (one kind of type 1 receptor) inhibit cyclic AMP production and also activate phospholipase C, the enzyme producing the second messenger inositol trisphosphate (IP$_3$), which in smooth-muscle cells mobilizes intracellular calcium.

Abbreviations: DIG, digitalis glycoside (Na$^+$,K$^+$-ATPase inhibitor); R$_1$ and R$_2$, binding proteins for the respective receptor types; AC, adenylate cyclase; Ni (AC-inhibiting) and Ns (AC-stimulating) nucleotide binding G proteins (G$_i$ and G$_s$, respectively); PhC, phospholipase C; PIP$_2$, phosphotidyli-nositol diphosphate, a membrane phospholipid. *(Reproduced with permission from U Ruegg, Sandorama 2:5, 1987.)*

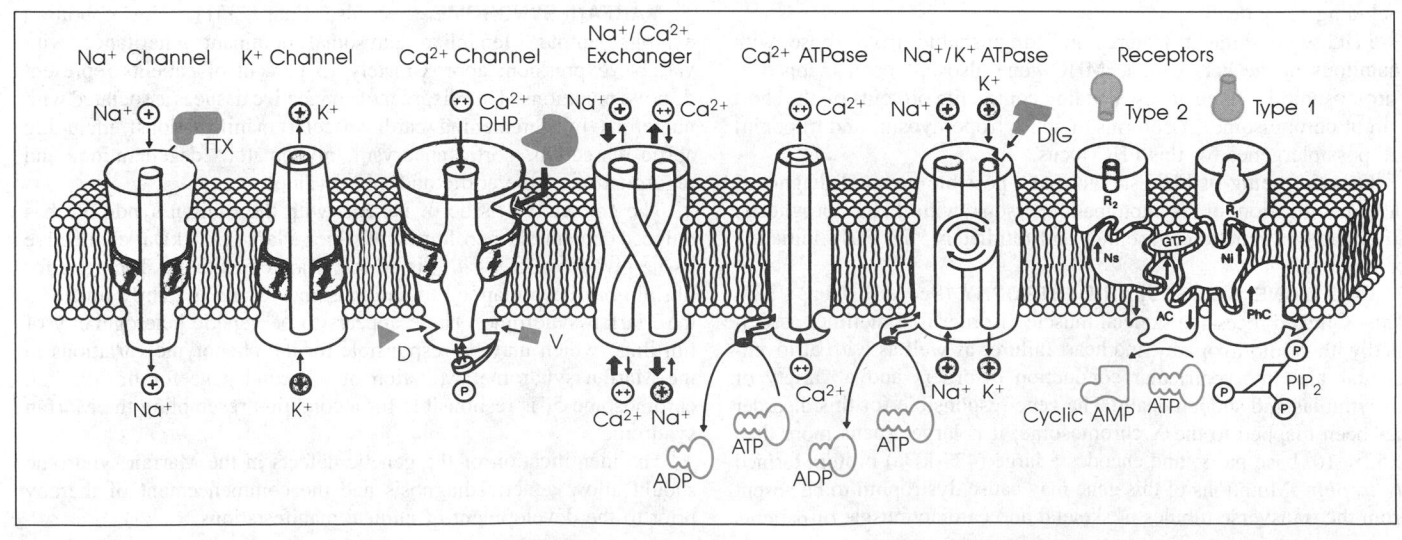

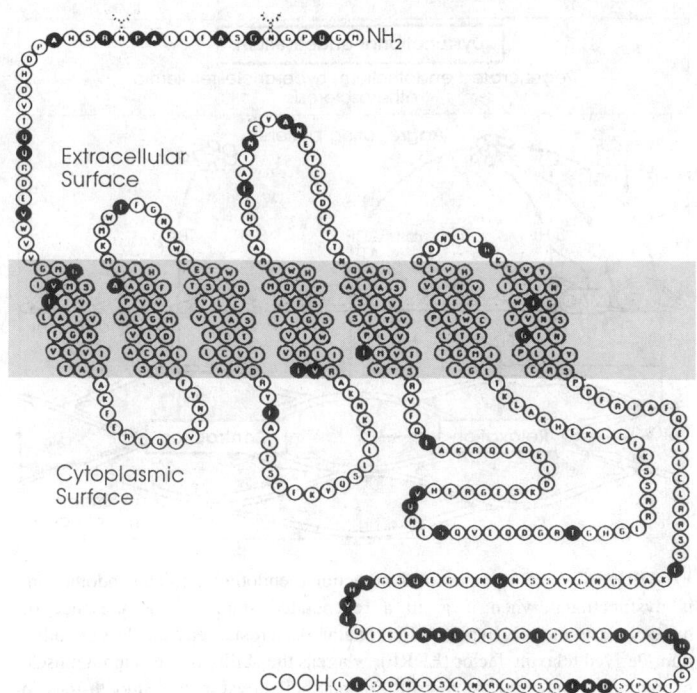

FIGURE 187-3 Structure of the human beta₂-adrenergic receptor as it may be organized within the membrane. Open circles represent amino acids that are identical to those of hamster beta₂-adrenergic receptor. *(Reproduced with permission from Dohlman et al, Biochemistry 26:2664, 1987.)*

pores through which the calcium ions move, probably in single file. Their primary structure has been elucidated by cDNA cloning. These channels are quite selective for calcium ions under physiologic conditions and are composed of several subunits, the largest of which has a molecular weight of 243 kDa and binds calcium channel antagonists. Prolongation of the action potential occurs often in hypertrophied myocytes and may be responsible for arrhythmias in patients with heart failure. This prolongation may be due to delays in the inactivation of the L-type calcium channels. Three physically associated but distinct sites in the channels bind the three classes of calcium antagonists—nifedipine, verapamil, and diltiazem (Chap. 203). The cDNAs (DNAs complementary to their mRNA) encoding the calcium channels have been cloned, and their predicted sequences have been determined. This new understanding of the structure and function of calcium channels should make possible the design of drugs to influence the function of these channels with greater specificity, thereby increasing the ability to control function of the myocardium and of vascular smooth muscle.

SARCOLEMMAL ATPase One of the most important membrane proteins is the Na⁺,K⁺-ATPase (see Fig. 187-2) which plays a critical role in establishing sodium and potassium gradients across cell membranes. This enzyme catalyzes the reaction that extrudes sodium and transports potassium into the cell against concentration gradients. This process requires the hydrolysis of ATP and is critical to the function of cardiac (and other excitable) tissue by controlling membrane potentials. Phosphorylation and ATP binding sites are on the cytoplasmic component of the enzyme, and the cardiac glycoside binding site is located on the extracellular component. Knowledge of the primary structure of the enzyme may allow the design of inhibitors perhaps more potent and/or more selective than the cardiac glycosides.

APOLIPOPROTEINS AND ATHEROGENESIS

Abnormalities in the number or function of the low-density lipoprotein (LDL) receptors are responsible for some forms of atherosclerosis (Chaps. 208 and 344). Abnormalities of the *apolipoproteins*, many

of which are genetic, may play more frequent roles in atherogenesis. At least 10 apolipoproteins are embedded in the surface of the spherical lipoprotein particles that carry the lipids in the bloodstream and are encoded by genes localized to chromosomes 1, 2, 6, 11, and 19 (the LDL receptor gene is also on chromosome 19). Amino acid sequences suggest that several of these apolipoproteins are derived from a common ancestral gene. The major functions of apolipoproteins are to serve as (1) ligands that interact with cellular receptors for the lipoprotein particles, (2) cofactors of enzymes involved in lipid metabolism, and (3) structural components of the lipoproteins.

High-density lipoproteins (HDL) take up excess cholesterol from cells, and the risk of the development of ischemic heart disease is related inversely to the concentration of circulating HDL (Chaps. 208 and 344). Apolipoproteins (apo) AI, CIII, and AIV are three HDL apolipoproteins encoded by genes clustered on chromosome 11. Several disorders are associated with mutations of these apolipoproteins, leading to a defect in the synthesis or function of HDL and the development of premature atherosclerosis. For example, apo AI serves as a cofactor for the enzyme lecithin cholesterol acyl transferase (LCAT) which catalyzes the reaction that converts cholesterol taken up by the HDL particle into the form in which it is transported, i.e., cholesteryl ester. Some variants of apo AI are defective for this cofactor activity, thereby preventing the normal function of HDL and causing premature atherosclerosis.

Apo E is one of the principal constituents of very low density lipoproteins (VLDL) and of chylomicron remnants, the latter particles having potential atherogenic activity. Three alleles of the apo E gene, located on chromosome 19, have been described. Subjects who are homozygous for the E^2 allele, which encodes apo E^2, have decreased clearance of VLDL and chylomicron remnants from the circulation, presumably because apo E^2 fails to bind normally to lipoprotein receptors. In addition, persons with an E^2 allele have reduced lipolytic conversion of VLDL to LDL with lower plasma concentrations of the latter. Since apo E^3 and apo E^4 normally activate lipoprotein lipase, normolipidemic persons with the apo E phenotype E^2/E^2 or E^2/E^3 have higher VLDL and lower LDL levels than persons with E^3/E^3 phenotype. The E^4 allele enhances conversion of VLDL to LDL, leading to decreased VLDL and increased LDL levels in phenotypes E^3/E^4 and E^4/E^4. Epidemiologic studies have found that apo E^4 rather than apo E^2 is associated with coronary heart disease. The E^2 allele plays a permissive role in the development of type 3 hyperlipoproteinemia, a condition associated with the development of xanthomas and premature atherosclerosis (Chap. 208).

Elevation of the plasma concentration of Lp(a) (referred to as "lipoprotein little a") appears to be another risk factor for the development of premature atherosclerosis. Its protein components consist of apo B100 linked to apo(a). It shares similarities with LDL as a B100 cholesterol-rich lipoprotein. Six inherited apo(a) isoproteins and a series of alleles at a single gene locus control the apo(a) phenotypes and appear to determine the Lp(a) concentration. An interesting clue to the mechanism by which Lp(a) accelerates atherosclerosis has emerged. Through cDNA cloning and the deduced protein structure, it has been shown that apo(a) is a deformed relative of plasminogen, the precursor of the proteolytic enzyme plasmin, which dissolves fibrin clots (Chap. 316). Apo(a) contains multiple copies of kringle 4 (a portion of the plasminogen molecule in the shape of the Danish pastry known as *kringle*) followed by kringle 5 and the protease domain. This strong resemblance between a lipoprotein and plasminogen may provide a link between lipids, the clotting system, and atherogenesis. Microthrombi containing fibrin on the vessel wall become incorporated into atherosclerotic plaques. Kringle 4 of plasminogen normally binds to fibrin during fibrinolysis. Apo(a), with many copies of this kringle, also could bind to fibrin in microthrombi in the vessel wall. Following endothelial damage, Lp(a) may insinuate itself into the arterial wall, inhibiting the cleavage of fibrin in microthrombi by competing with plasminogen for access to fibrin.

Discussed above are just three of many possible examples showing how the genes encoding apolipoproteins can play a critical role in determining the risk for the development of atherosclerosis. Eventually, it may prove to be cost-effective to attempt to identify genetic defects of apolipoproteins (as well as of the LDL receptor) in childhood and to use a preventive approach on these subjects.

ENDOTHELIUM

For many years the endothelium, the monolayer of cells in direct contact with blood, was considered to be a relatively inert, smooth boundary between the blood and the vascular wall (Fig. 187-4). In fact, endothelial cells are quite active metabolically and normally produce a number of substances that affect the vascular lumen as well as platelets.

The first and best known of the endothelial vasodilators is prostacyclin (PGI_2) (see Chap. 70), which also inhibits the aggregation of platelets. The action of PGI_2 involves the activation of adenylyl cyclase and formation of cAMP. When stimulated by a large number of substances, including ATP and ADP, acetylcholine, thrombin, neurotransmitters, and serotonin, the normal endothelium also releases a labile, highly diffusible vasodilator termed *endothelium-derived relaxing factor* (EDRF), which appears to be nitric oxide (NO) or a relatively more stable adduct thereof. Normal endothelium also releases EDRF when stimulated by the shear stress of flowing blood, thereby controlling the lumen of arteries and arterioles in relation to the blood flow through the vessel. EDRF stimulates soluble guanylyl cyclase, which catalyzes the formation of cyclic GMP (cGMP) and, in turn, relaxes vascular smooth muscle. EDRF also inhibits adhesion

FIGURE 187-4 Current concepts of endothelium-derived factors and their modulation of vascular smooth-muscle contraction: Endothelium-derived relaxing factor (EDRF), a potent vasodilator of the underlying smooth muscle, increases cyclic GMP (cGMP) levels through activation of soluble guanylate cyclase. Prostacyclin (PGI_2) is another vasodilator released from the endothelium but whose effects depend on elevation of cyclic AMP (cAMP) through activation of adenylate cyclase. EDRF and PGI_2 may act synergistically in relaxing vascular smooth muscle and inhibiting platelet aggregation. The endothelial cells also secrete a hyperpolarizing factor (EDHF), the exact nature of which is unknown and which also has a vasodilator action. There are at least two endothelium-derived contracting factors; one is indomethacin-insensitive ($EDCF_1$) and may be endothelin, while the other is indomethacin-sensitive ($EDCF_2$) and may be superoxide anion. ACh, acetylcholine; 5-HT, 5-hydroxytryptamine (serotonin); ADP, adenosine diphosphate; AA, arachidonic acid; +, synergism or facilitation; −, inhibition; ?, exact nature unknown; M, muscarinic receptor; S, serotoninergic receptor; P, purinergic receptor; T, thrombin receptor; V, vasopressinergic receptor. *(Reproduced with permission from P Vanhoutte and Shimokawa, Circulation 80:1, 1989.)*

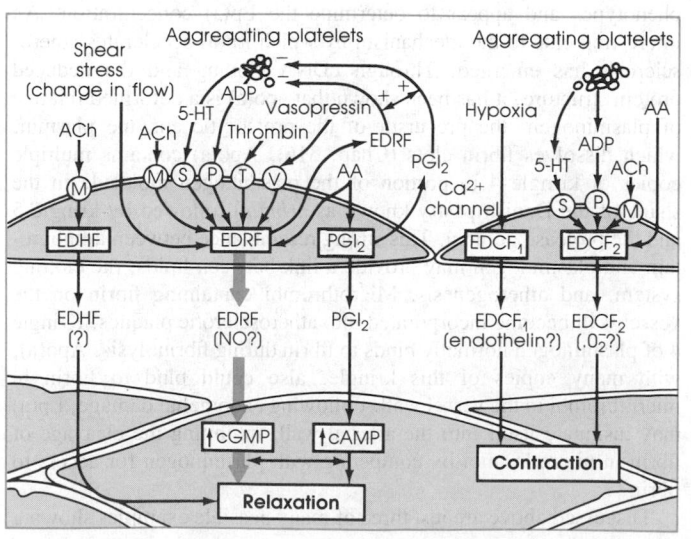

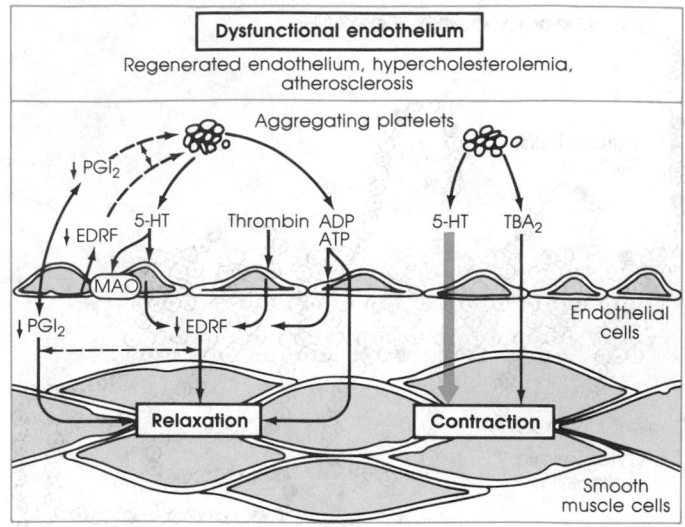

FIGURE 187-5 Responses of dysfunctional endothelium. The endothelium is dysfunctional when it is in a regenerated state, in the presence of hypercholesterolemia, hypertension, or atherosclerosis, releasing less endothelium-derived relaxing factor (EDRF), whereas the ability of the smooth muscle to contract is unaltered. As a result, in endothelial dysfunction smooth-muscle contraction predominates. In atherosclerosis, the production of both EDRF and prostacyclin (PGI_2) are reduced, and their synergistic actions against aggregating platelets may not occur, enhancing platelet aggregation. This may lead to thrombus formation, enhanced vascular contraction, and atherogenesis. 5-HT, 5-hydroxytryptamine (serotonin); ADP, adenosine diphosphate; ATP, adenosine triphosphate; TBA2, thromboxane A_2; MAO, monomine oxidase; ms, inhibition; +, synergism. *(Reproduced with permission from Vanhoutte and Shimokawa, Circulation 80:1, 1989.)*

and aggregation of platelets, an action apparently also mediated by cGMP. EDRF and prostacyclin interact synergistically to dilate blood vessels and inhibit platelet aggregation.

When the endothelium is destroyed or damaged (Fig. 187-5), as in atherosclerotic plaques, EDRF production may be impaired, thereby permitting coronary vasoconstriction in the vicinity of such plaques. Moreover, subtle damage to the endothelium, as in hypertension, some forms of hyperlipidemia, reperfusion after ischemia, and regenerating endothelium after mechanical trauma, leads to defective release of EDRF. On the other hand, the eicosapentaenoic and docosahexaenoic acids in fish oils stimulate the production of EDRF, perhaps explaining the putative antiatherogenic properties of these substances. A third endothelial product with antiplatelet properties is the ectoADPase located on the luminal surface. This enzyme degrades ADP, thereby limiting its access to and activation of platelets.

Endothelium also synthesizes *thrombomodulin*, a glycoprotein with a molecular weight of 105 kDa which is localized to the luminal side of the vascular endothelium and which serves as an endothelial receptor for thrombin. When bound to thrombomodulin, thrombin loses its hemostatic activity (conversion of fibrinogen to fibrin, stimulation of platelets), the rate at which it is inactivated by antithrombin is accelerated, and its activation of protein C, a naturally occurring anticoagulant and profibrinolytic substance, is enhanced.

Endothelium releases at least two vasoconstrictors. One is a product of cyclooxygenase activity that appears to be responsible for hypoxia-induced vascular contraction, while the other is an extremely potent 21-amino-acid peptide called *endothelin*. The expression of the gene for endothelin appears to be inhibited by the shear stress of flowing blood, a mechanism that acts in concert with the release of EDRF by the same stimulus to enhance vessel diameter as flow increases. In hypertension, EDRF release is impaired, whereas the release of endothelin may be augmented, presumably aggravating this condition. Like PDGF, endothelin is both a vasoconstrictor and a smooth-muscle mitogen.

In early atherosclerosis, endothelial injury or dysfunction leads to attenuated vasodilator responses and to enhanced platelet deposition on the arterial wall. If unopposed by EDRF and prostacyclin, serotonin and thromboxane A_2 released from the deposited platelets cause arterial constriction and spasm in the coronary arterial system. The adhesion and aggregation of platelets and the enhancement of the atherosclerotic process are also promoted by the release of these platelet products.

ANGIOGENESIS

Endothelial cells also secrete a group of growth factors that are mitogenic for endothelium and can induce formation of new blood vessels (angiogenesis). Angiogenic stimuli cause the elongation and proliferation of endothelial cells and the generation of new vessels. A group of angiogenic mitogens, which are heparin-binding peptides related to endothelial cell growth factors, has been identified. The amino acid sequences of several of these growth factors have been deduced by cloning and analysis of their genes.

Angiogenesis is of considerable pathogenic significance. Folkman has postulated that the growth of tumors depends on an adequate blood supply, which in turn is dependent on the growth of new vessels into the tumors; the latter is stimulated by angiogenesis factor(s) secreted by the tumor. Inhibition of angiogenesis can cause tumor regression in animal models. Abnormal angiogenesis may be involved in diverse disease states, including diabetic retinopathy, neovascular glaucoma, rheumatoid arthritis, and psoriasis.

The development of new vessels in the heart, i.e., of the coronary collateral circulation, is of critical importance in protecting the myocardium from the consequences of coronary obstruction. The extent of the collateral circulation varies enormously among patients with similar degrees of coronary arterial narrowing, and this difference may be related in part to differences in the production of angiogenic factors. It has been speculated that the introduction of purified angiogenic factors directly into ischemic myocardium might enhance the development of collaterals, accelerate the healing of the necrotic tissue, and prevent infarct expansion and cardiac dilatation. Angiogenesis also may be deleterious. Coronary atheroma are highly vascularized by a fragile capillary network, and rupture of these newly formed capillaries when they are exposed to high intravascular pressures may lead to hemorrhage into atherosclerotic plaques and coronary occlusion.

CONCLUSIONS

The applications of cellular and molecular biology to studies of the myocardium, vascular wall, platelets, and lipoproteins have already increased greatly our understanding of the fundamental abnormalities in cardiovascular disease. In the future these approaches are likely to improve the diagnosis of patients with genetic disorders causing cardiac disease, help to identify individuals at risk of developing these disorders, thereby leading to the institution of preventive measures, and provide new agents for the treatment and prevention of cardiovascular diseases.

REFERENCES

BOHELER KR, SCHWARTZ K: Gene expression in cardiac hypertrophy. Trends Cardiovasc Med 2:176, 1992

BRAUNWALD E: On future directions for cardiology: The Paul Dudley White lecture. Circulation 77:13, 1988

CHIEN KR: Molecular advances in cardiovascular biology. Science 260:916, 1993

COHEN SA, BARCHI RL: Cardiac sodium channel structure and function. Trends Cardiovasc Med 2:133, 1992

DIETZ HC et al: Marfan syndrome caused by a recurrent de novo missense mutation in the fibrillin gene. Nature 352:337, 1991

FOLKMAN J, WEISZ PB: Control of angiogenesis, in Biocatalysis and Biometrics, JD Burrington, DS Clark (eds). Washington, American Chemical Society, ACS Symposium Series 392, 1989, pp 19–32

GENEST J JR: Genetic lipid disorders in cardiovascular disease. Trends Cardiovasc Med 2:140, 1992

KEATING M et al: Linkage of a cardiac arrhythmia, the long QT syndrome, and the Harvey ras-1 gene. Science 252:704, 1991

KLUG D et al: Role of mechanical and hormonal factors in cardiac remodeling and the biologic limits of myocardial adaptation. Am J Cardiol 71:46A, 1993

NADAL-GINARD B, MAHDAVI V: General principles of cardiovascular cellular and molecular biology, in Heart Disease, 4th ed, E Braunwald (ed). Philadelphia, Saunders, 1992

NEER EJ, CLAPHAM DE: Signal transduction through G proteins in the cardiac myocyte. Trends Cardiovasc Med 2:6, 1992

PETTERSSON K et al: Endothelial integrity and injury in atherogenesis. Transplant Proc 25:2054, 1993

ROBERTS R (ed): Molecular Basis of Cardiology. Boston, Blackwell Scientific, 1992

SOLOMON SD et al: Left ventricular hypertrophy and morphology in familial hypertrophic cardiomyopathy associated with mutations of the β-myosin heavy chain gene. J Am Coll Cardiol (in press)

THOMPSON WG: Apoproteins, lipoprotein subfractions, and the risk of coronary artery disease. South Med J 86:194, 1993

188 PHYSICAL EXAMINATION OF THE CARDIOVASCULAR SYSTEM

ROBERT A. O'ROURKE / EUGENE BRAUNWALD

A careful physical examination is a relatively low cost method for an accurate assessment of the cardiovascular system and often provides important information for the appropriate selection of additional tests. First, the general physical appearance should be evaluated. The patient may appear tired because of a chronic low cardiac output; the respiratory rate may be rapid, indicating pulmonary venous congestion. Central cyanosis, often associated with clubbing of the fingers and toes, indicates right-to-left cardiac or extracardiac shunting or inadequate oxygenation of blood by the lungs. Cyanosis in the distal extremities, cool skin, and increased sweating result from vasoconstriction in patients with severe heart failure (Chap. 32). Noncardiovascular details can be equally important. For example, the diagnosis of infective endocarditis is highly likely in patients with petechiae, Osler's nodes, and Janeway lesions (Chap. 85).

The blood pressure should be taken in both arms and with the patient supine and upright; the heart rate should be timed for 1 min. Orthostatic hypotension and tachycardia may indicate a reduced blood volume, while resting tachycardia may be a clue to the presence of severe heart failure.

Careful examination of the optic fundi is essential (Chap. 209), and the retinal vessels may show evidence of systemic hypertension, arteriosclerosis, or embolism. The latter may result from atherosclerosis in larger arteries (e.g., carotid) or may represent a complication of valvular heart disease (e.g., endocarditis).

Palpation of the peripheral arterial pulses in the upper and lower extremities is necessary to define the adequacy of systemic blood flow and to detect the presence of occlusive arterial lesions. It is also important to examine both legs for evidence of edema, varicose veins, or thrombophlebitis (Chap. 211). The cardiovascular examination includes careful evaluation of both the carotid arterial and the jugular venous pulses, as well as deliberate precordial palpation and attentive cardiac auscultation. An understanding of the events of the cardiac cycle is vital to performing an accurate cardiovascular examination.

ARTERIAL PRESSURE PULSE The normal central aortic pulse wave is characterized by a fairly rapid rise to a somewhat rounded peak (Fig. 188-1). The anacrotic shoulder, present on the ascending limb, occurs at the time of peak rate of aortic flow just before maximum pressure is reached. The less steep descending limb is interrupted by a sharp downward deflection, synchronous with aortic valve closure, called the incisura. As the pulse wave is transmitted peripherally, the initial upstroke becomes steeper, the anacrotic shoulder becomes less apparent, and the incisura is replaced by the smoother dicrotic notch. Accordingly, palpation of a peripheral

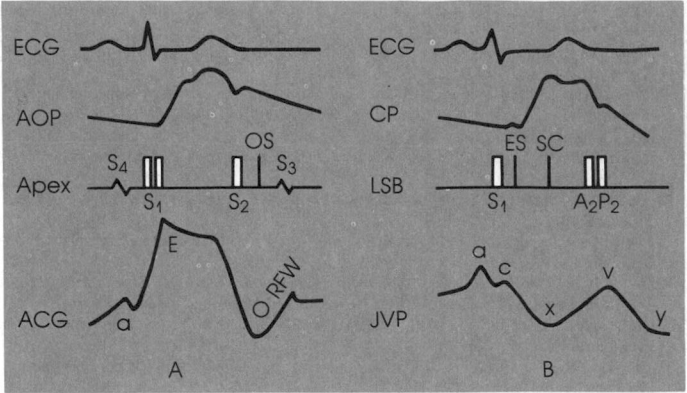

FIGURE 188-1 *A.* Schematic representation of electrocardiogram, aortic pressure pulse (AOP), phonocardiogram recorded at the apex, and apexcardiogram (ACG). On the phonocardiogram, S_1, S_2, S_3, and S_4 represent the first through fourth heart sounds; OS represents the opening snap of the mitral valve, which occurs coincident with the O point of the apexcardiogram. S_3 occurs coincident with the termination of the rapid-filling wave (RFW) of the ACG, while S_4 occurs coincident with the a wave of the ACG. *B.* Simultaneous recording of electrocardiogram, indirect carotid pulse (CP), phonocardiogram along the left sternal border (LSB), and indirect jugular venous pulse (JVP). ES, ejection sound; SC, systolic click.

arterial pulse (e.g., radial) frequently gives less information than examination of a more central pulse (e.g., carotid) regarding alterations in left ventricular ejection or aortic valve function. However, certain findings such as the hyperkinetic pulse of aortic regurgitation or pulsus alternans are more readily evident in peripheral than in central arteries (Fig. 188-2). The carotid pulse usually is best examined with the sternocleidomastoid muscle relaxed and with the head rotated slightly toward the examiner. In palpating the brachial arterial pulse, the examiner can support the subject's relaxed elbow with the right arm while compressing the brachial pulse with the thumb. The usual technique for palpating the pulse is to compress the artery with the thumb or forefinger until the maximum pulse is sensed. Varying degrees of pressure should then be applied while concentrating on the separate phases of the pulse wave. This method, known as *trisection*, is useful for assessing the sharpness of the upstroke, systolic peak, and diastolic slope of the arterial pulse. In most normal persons a dicrotic wave is not palpable.

A small weak pulse, *pulsus parvus*, is frequently present in conditions with a diminished left ventricular stroke volume, a narrow pulse pressure, and increased peripheral vascular resistance (Fig. 188-2). A *hypokinetic* pulse may be due to hypovolemia, to left ventricular failure secondary to myocardial disease or myocardial infarction, to restrictive pericardial disease, or to mitral valve stenosis. In aortic valve stenosis the delayed systolic peak, *pulsus tardus*, is the result of mechanical obstruction to left ventricular ejection and is often accompanied by the transmission of a coarse systolic thrill. In contrast, a large bounding, or *hyperkinetic*, pulse is usually associated with an increased left ventricular stroke volume, a wide pulse pressure, and a decrease in peripheral vascular resistance. This occurs characteristically in patients with abnormally elevated stroke volumes, as in complete heart block, hyperkinetic circulation due to anxiety, anemia, exercise, or fever, or in patients with an abnormally rapid runoff of blood from the arterial system (patent ductus arteriosus, peripheral arteriovenous fistula). Patients with mitral regurgitation or a ventricular septal defect also may have a bounding pulse, since vigorous left ventricular ejection produces a rapid upstroke in the arterial pulse even though the duration of systole and the forward stroke volume may be diminished. In aortic regurgitation, the rapidly rising, bounding arterial pulse results from increased left ventricular stroke volume and the associated increased rate of ventricular ejection.

The *bisferiens pulse*, which consists of two systolic peaks, is characteristic of aortic regurgitation (with or without accompanying stenosis) and of hypertrophic cardiomyopathy (Chap. 205). In the latter the pulse wave upstroke rises rapidly and forcefully, producing the first systolic peak ("percussion wave"). A brief decline in pressure follows because of the sudden decrease in the rate of left ventricular ejection during midsystole, when severe obstruction often develops. This pressure trough is followed by a smaller and more slowly rising positive pulse wave ("tidal wave") produced by continued ventricular ejection and by reflected waves from the periphery. The *dicrotic pulse* has two palpable waves, one in systole and one in diastole. It occurs most frequently in patients with a very low stroke volume, particularly in those with dilated (congestive) cardiomyopathy.

Pulsus alternans refers to a pattern in which there is regular alteration of the pressure pulse amplitude, despite a regular rhythm (Fig. 188-2). It is due to alternating left ventricular contractile force, usually denotes severe impairment of left ventricular function, and commonly occurs in patients who also have a loud third heart sound. Pulsus alternans also may occur during or following paroxysmal tachycardia or for several beats following a premature beat in patients without heart disease. In *pulsus bigeminus* there is also regular alteration of pressure pulse amplitude, but it is caused by a premature ventricular contraction that follows each regular beat. *Pulsus paradoxus* is an accentuation of the decrease in systolic arterial pressure accompanying the reduced amplitude of the arterial pulse which normally occurs during inspiration. In patients with pericardial tamponade (Chap. 206), airway obstruction, or superior vena cava obstruction, the decrease in systolic arterial pressure frequently exceeds the normal of 10 mmHg (1.33 kPa) and the peripheral pulse may disappear completely during inspiration.

Simultaneous palpation of the radial and femoral arterial pulses, which normally are virtually coincident, is important to rule out aortic coarctation, in which the latter is weaker and delayed (Chap. 199).

JUGULAR VENOUS PULSE (JVP)   The two main objectives of the bedside examination of the neck veins are inspection of their waveform and estimation of the central venous pressure (CVP). In

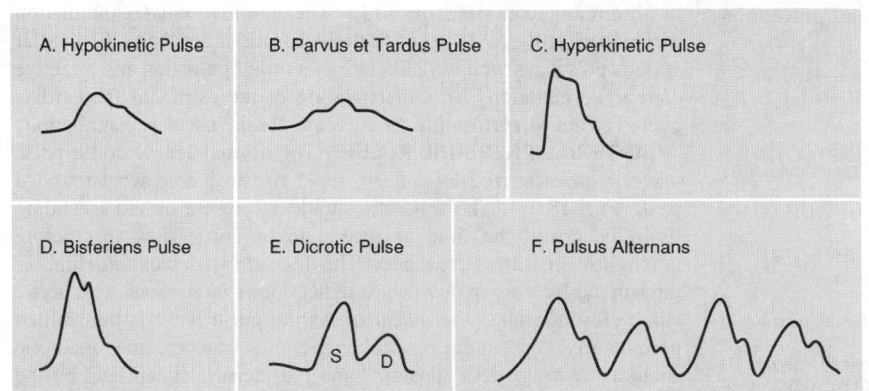

FIGURE 188-2 Schematic representation of arterial pulse waveforms that occur with alterations in cardiac hemodynamics which may result from normal physiologic responses or may be due to cardiac disease. S, systole; D, diastole. (*Modified from RA O'Rourke, in JW Hurst et al, eds. The Heart, 7th ed, New York, McGraw-Hill, 1990, with permission.*)

most patients, the right internal jugular vein is superior for both purposes. Usually, the maximum pulsation of the internal jugular vein is observed when the trunk is inclined by less than 30°. In patients with elevated venous pressure it may be necessary to elevate the trunk further, sometimes to as much as 90°. When the neck muscles are relaxed, shining a beam of light tangentially across the skin overlying the vein exposes the pulsations of the internal jugular vein. Simultaneous palpation of the left carotid artery aids the examiner in deciding which pulsations are venous and in relating the venous pulsations to their timing in the cardiac cycle.

The normal JVP reflects phasic pressure changes in the right atrium and consists of two or sometimes three positive waves and two negative troughs (Fig. 188-1). The positive presystolic *a* wave is produced by venous distention due to right atrial contraction and is the dominant wave in the JVP, particularly during inspiration. Large *a* waves indicate that the right atrium is contracting against an increased resistance (Fig. 188-3), such as occurs with tricuspid stenosis or more commonly with increased resistance to right ventricular filling (pulmonary hypertension or pulmonic stenosis). Large *a* waves also occur during arrhythmias whenever the right atrium contracts while the tricuspid valve is closed by right ventricular systole. Such "cannon" *a* waves may occur regularly (as during junctional rhythm) or irregularly (as in atrioventricular dissociation with ventricular tachycardia or complete heart block). The *a* wave is absent in patients with atrial fibrillation, and there is an increased temporal delay between the *a* wave and the carotid arterial pulse in patients with first-degree atrioventricular block.

The *c* wave, often but not invariably observed in the JVP, is a positive wave produced by the bulging of the tricuspid valve into the right atrium during right ventricular isovolumetric systole and by the impact of the carotid artery adjacent to the jugular vein. The *x* descent is due to a combination of atrial relaxation and the downward displacement of the tricuspid valve during ventricular systole. In patients with constrictive pericarditis (Fig. 188-3), there is often increased prominence of the *x* descent wave during systole, but this wave is reduced with right ventricular dilatation and often is reversed in tricuspid regurgitation. The positive, late systolic *v* wave results from the increasing volume of blood in the venae cavae and right atrium during ventricular systole when the tricuspid valve is closed. With tricuspid regurgitation the *v* wave is more prominent, and when tricuspid regurgitation becomes severe, the combination of a prominent *v* wave and obliteration of the *x* descent results in a single large positive systolic wave. After the peak of the *v* wave is reached, the right atrial pressure falls because of the decreased bulging of the tricuspid valve into the right atrium as right ventricular pressure declines and the tricuspid valve opens (Fig. 188-3).

This negative descending limb, referred to as the *y* descent of the JVP, is produced mainly by the tricuspid valve opening and the

subsequent rapid inflow of blood into the right ventricle. A rapid, deep *y* descent in early diastole occurs with severe tricuspid regurgitation. A venous pulse characterized by a sharp *y* descent, a deep *y* trough, and a rapid ascent to the baseline is seen in patients with constrictive pericarditis or with severe failure of the right side of the heart and a high venous pressure. A slow *y* descent in the JVP suggests an obstruction to right ventricular filling, as occurs with tricuspid stenosis or right atrial myxoma.

For accurate estimation of the central venous pressure, the right internal jugular vein is best utilized, with the sternal angle as the reference point, since in the average patient the center of the right atrium lies approximately 5 cm below the sternal angle, regardless of body position. The patient is examined at the optimal degree of trunk elevation for visualization of venous pulsations. The vertical distance between the top of the oscillating venous column and the level of the sternal angle is determined and generally found to be less than 3 cm (3 cm + 5 cm = 8 cm blood). The most common cause of an elevated venous pressure is an elevated right ventricular diastolic pressure. In patients suspected of having right ventricular failure who have a normal CVP at rest, the abdominojugular reflux test may be helpful. The palm of the hand is placed over the abdomen, and firm pressure is applied for 10 s or more. Normally, the jugular venous pressure is not significantly altered, but with impaired function of the right side of the heart the upper level of venous pulsation usually increases. A positive abdominojugular test is best defined as an increase in JVP during 10 s of firm midabdominal compression followed by a rapid drop in pressure of 4 cm blood on release of the compression. The most common cause of a positive test is right-sided heart failure secondary to elevated left heart filling pressures. Also, abdominal compression may elicit the typical JVP of tricuspid regurgitation when the resting pulse wave is normal. Kussmaul's sign, an increase rather than the normal decrease in the CVP during inspiration, is most commonly caused by severe right-sided heart failure; it is a frequent finding in patients with constrictive pericarditis or right ventricular infarction.

PRECORDIAL PALPATION The location, amplitude, duration, and direction of the cardiac impulse usually can be best appreciated with the fingertips. The normal left ventricular apex impulse is located at or medial to the left midclavicular line in the fourth or fifth intercostal space and is a tapping, early systolic outward thrust localized to a point not more than 3 cm in diameter. It is due primarily to recoil of the heart as blood is ejected and should be evaluated with the patient supine and in the left lateral decubitus position. Left ventricular hypertrophy results in an exaggerated amplitude, duration, and often size of the normal left ventricular thrust. The impulse may be displaced laterally and downward into the sixth or seventh interspace, particularly in patients with a left ventricular volume load such as occurs in aortic regurgitation and in those with a dilated cardiomyopathy.

Additional abnormal features of the left ventricular apex include marked presystolic distention of the left ventricle, often accompanying a fourth heart sound in patients with an excessive left ventricular pressure load or myocardial ischemia/infarction, and a prominent early diastolic rapid-filling wave, often accompanying a third heart sound in patients with left ventricular failure or mitral valve regurgitation (Fig. 188-1). A double systolic apical impulse is frequently palpable in patients with hypertrophic cardiomyopathy.

Right ventricular hypertrophy results in a sustained systolic lift at the lower left parasternal area which starts in early systole and is synchronous with the left ventricular apical impulse. In patients with chronic obstructive pulmonary disease, a right ventricular impulse often may be detected by sliding the fingers up under the rib cage just beneath the sternum. The enlarged right ventricle strikes the ends of the fingertips as an inferiorly directed movement.

Abnormal precordial pulsations occur during systole in patients with left ventricular dyssynergy due to ischemic heart disease or to diffuse myocardial disease from some other cause. These pulsations often occur in patients with a recent transmural myocardial infarction

FIGURE 188-3 Abnormal jugular venous pulse waveforms commonly present in patients with cardiac disease and/or arrhythmias. See text. (*Modified from RA O'Rourke, in JW Hurst et al, eds. The Heart, 7th ed, New York, McGraw-Hill, 1990, with permission.*)

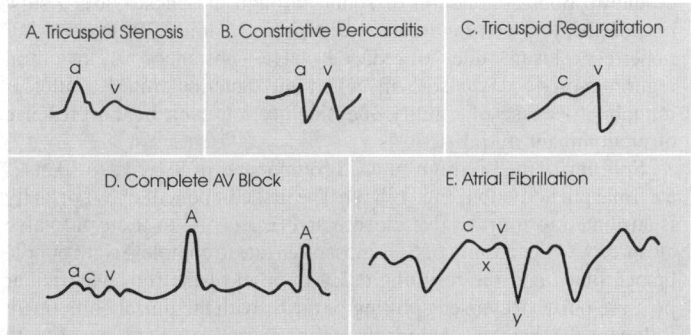

and may be present in some patients only during episodes of anginal pain. They are most commonly felt in the left midprecordium one or two interspaces above and/or 1 to 2 cm medial to the left ventricular apex. When a systolic bulge occurs in the region of the apex, it is difficult to distinguish from the impulse of left ventricular hypertrophy.

A left parasternal lift is present frequently in patients with severe mitral regurgitation. This pulsation occurs distinctly later than the left ventricular apical impulse, is synchronous with the *v* wave in the left atrial pressure curve, and is due to anterior displacement of the right ventricle by an enlarged, expanding left atrium. A similar impulse occurs to the right of the sternum in some patients with severe tricuspid regurgitation and a giant right atrium. Pulsation of the right sternoclavicular joint may indicate a right-sided aortic arch or aneurysmal dilatation of the ascending aorta. Pulmonary artery pulsation is often visible and palpable in the second left intercostal space and may be normal in children or thin young adults. However, this pulsation usually denotes pulmonary hypertension, increased pulmonary blood flow, or poststenotic pulmonary artery dilatation. Abnormally forceful valve closure can be palpated as a tap, and it occurs most commonly in the second left intercostal space in patients with pulmonary hypertension, in the second right intercostal space in patients with systemic hypertension, and at the cardiac apex in patients with mitral stenosis.

Thrills are palpable, low-frequency vibrations associated with heart murmurs. The systolic murmur of mitral regurgitation may be palpated at the cardiac apex. When the palm of the hand is placed over the precordium, the thrill of aortic stenosis crosses the palm of the hand toward the right side of the neck, while the thrill of pulmonic stenosis radiates more often to the left side of the neck. The thrill due to a ventricular septal defect is usually located in the third and fourth intercostal spaces near the left sternal border.

Percussion should be performed in each patient to identify normal or abnormal position of the heart, stomach, and liver. However, in patients with a normal cardiac situs, percussion adds little to careful inspection and palpation in the recognition of cardiac enlargement.

CARDIAC AUSCULTATION

To obtain maximal information from cardiac auscultation, the observer should keep in mind several principles: (1) It should be carried out in a quiet room to avoid the distractions caused by the noises of normal activity. (2) In order to hear a faint heart sound or murmur, attention must be focused on that phase of the cardiac cycle during which the auscultatory event may be expected to occur. (3) The accurate timing of a heart sound or murmur necessarily involves determining its relation to other observable events in the cardiac cycle—the carotid arterial pulse, the apical impulse, or the JVP. (4) To define the significance of a cardiac sound or murmur, it is often necessary to observe alterations in its timing or intensity during various physiologic and/or pharmacologic interventions (Table 188-1).

HEART SOUNDS   The major components of heart sounds are vibrations associated with the abrupt acceleration or deceleration of blood within the cardiovascular system, but there is continuing controversy regarding the relative significance of the vibrations of valves, muscles, vessels, and supporting structures in the production of the heart sounds. Studies using simultaneous echocardiographic-phonocardiographic recordings indicate that the first and second heart sounds are produced primarily by the closure of the AV and semilunar valves and the events that accompany these closures. The intensity of the *first heart sound* (S_1) is influenced by (1) the position of the mitral leaflets at the onset of ventricular systole, (2) the rate of rise of the left ventricular pressure pulse, (3) the presence or absence of structural disease of the mitral valve, and (4) the amount of tissue, air, or fluid between the heart and the stethoscope. S_1 is louder if diastole is shortened because of tachycardia, if atrioventricular flow is increased because of high cardiac output or prolonged because of

---

TABLE 188-1   Effects of physiologic and pharmacologic interventions on the intensity of heart murmurs and sounds*

RESPIRATION

Systolic murmurs due to TR or pulmonic blood flow through a normal or stenotic valve and diastolic murmurs of TS or PR generally increase with inspiration as do right-sided S_3 and S_4. Left-sided murmurs and sounds usually are louder during expiration.

VALSALVA MANEUVER

Most murmurs decrease in length and intensity. Two exceptions are the systolic murmur of HCM, which usually becomes much louder, and that of MVP, which becomes longer and often louder. Following release of the Valsalva, right-sided murmurs tend to return to control intensity earlier than left-sided murmurs.

POST VPB OR AF

Murmurs originating at normal or stenotic semilunar valves increase in the cardiac cycle following a VPB or in the cycle after a long cycle length in AF. By contrast, systolic murmurs due to AV valve regurgitation do not change, diminish (papillary muscle dysfunction), or become shorter (MVP).

POSITIONAL CHANGES

With *standing* most murmurs diminish, two exceptions being the murmur of HCM, which becomes louder, and that of MVP, which lengthens and often is intensified. With *squatting* most murmurs become louder but those of HCM and MVP usually soften and may disappear.

EXERCISE

Murmurs due to blood flow across normal or obstructed valves (e.g., PS, MS) become louder with both isotonic and submaximal isometric (handgrip) exercise. Murmurs of MR, VSD, and AR also increase with handgrip exercise. However, the murmur of HCM often decreases with near maximum handgrip exercise. Left-sided S_4 and S_3 are often accentuated by exercise, particularly when due to ischemic heart disease.

PHARMACOLOGIC INTERVENTIONS

During the initial relative hypotension following amyl nitrite inhalation, murmurs of MR, VSD, and AR decrease while murmurs of aortic stenosis or sclerosis increase. During the later tachycardia phase, murmurs of MS and right-sided lesions also increase. The response in MVP often is biphasic (softer then louder than control). The arterial constrictor phenylephrine tends to produce the opposite effects.

TRANSIENT ARTERIAL OCCLUSION

Transient external compression of both arms by bilateral cuff inflation to 20 mmHg > peak systolic pressure augments the murmurs of MR, VSD, and AR but not murmurs due to other causes.

* TR, tricuspid regurgitation; TS, tricuspid stenosis; PR, pulmonic regurgitation; HCM, hypertrophic cardiomyopathy; MVP, mitral valve prolapse; PS, pulmonic stenosis; MS, mitral stenosis; MR, mitral regurgitation; VSD, ventricular septal defect; AR, aortic regurgitation; VPB, ventricular premature beat; and AF, atrial fibrillation.

---

mitral stenosis, or if atrial precedes ventricular contraction by an unusually short interval, reflected in a short PR interval. The loud S_1 in mitral stenosis usually signifies that the valve is pliable and that it remains open at the onset of isovolumetric contraction because of the elevated left atrial pressure. A reduction in the intensity of S_1 may be due to poor conduction of sound through the chest wall, a slow rise of the left ventricular pressure pulse, a long PR interval, or imperfect closure due to reduced valve substance, as in mitral regurgitation. S_1 is also soft when the anterior mitral leaflet is immobile because of rigidity and calcification even in the presence of predominant mitral stenosis.

Splitting of the two high-pitched components of S_1 by 10 to 30 ms is a normal phenomenon (Fig. 188-1). The first component of S_1 normally is attributed to mitral valve closure and the second to tricuspid valve closure. A widened split of S_1 is most often due to complete right bundle branch block and the resulting delay in onset of the right ventricular pressure pulse. Reversed splitting of the S_1 with the mitral component following the tricuspid component may be present in patients with severe mitral stenosis, left atrial myxoma, and complete left bundle branch block.

Splitting of S_2 into audibly distinct aortic (A_2) and pulmonic (P_2) components occurs normally during inspiration when augmented inflow into the right ventricle increases its stroke volume and ejection period and delays closure of the pulmonic valve. P_2 is coincident with the incisura of the pulmonary artery pressure curve, which is separated from the right ventricular pressure tracing by an interval termed the "hangout time." The absolute value of this interval reflects the resistance to pulmonary blood flow and the impedance characteristics of the pulmonary vascular bed. This interval is prolonged and physiologic splitting of S_2 is accentuated in conditions associated with right ventricular volume overload and a distensible pulmonary vascular bed. However, in patients with an increase in pulmonary vascular resistance, the hangout time is markedly reduced and narrow splitting of S_2 is present. Splitting that persists with expiration, heard best at the pulmonic area or left sternal border, is usually abnormal when the patient is in the upright position. Such splitting may be due to a number of causes: delayed activation of the right ventricle (right bundle branch block); left ventricular ectopic beats; a left ventricular pacemaker; prolongation of right ventricular contraction with an increased right ventricular pressure load (pulmonary embolism or pulmonic stenosis); or delayed pulmonic valve closure because of right ventricular volume overload associated with right ventricular failure or diminished impedance of the pulmonary vascular bed and a prolonged hangout time (atrial septal defect).

In pulmonary hypertension, P_2 is increased in intensity, and splitting of the second heart sound may be diminished, normal, or accentuated depending on the cause of the pulmonary hypertension, the pulmonary vascular resistance, and the presence or absence of right ventricular decompensation. Early aortic valve closure, occurring with mitral regurgitation or a ventricular septal defect, also may produce splitting that persists during expiration. It also may occur with constrictive pericarditis. In patients with atrial septal defect the proportion of right atrial filling contributed by the left atrium and the venae cavae varies reciprocally during the respiratory cycle so that right atrial inflow remains relatively constant. Therefore, the volume and duration of right ventricular ejection are not significantly increased by inspiration, and there is little inspiratory exaggeration of the splitting of S_2. This phenomenon, termed *fixed splitting* of the second heart sound, is of considerable diagnostic value.

A delay in aortic valve closure causing P_2 to precede A_2 results in so-called reversed (paradoxic) splitting of S_2. Splitting is then maximal in expiration and decreases during inspiration with the normal delay of pulmonic valve closure. The most common causes of reversed splitting of S_2 are left bundle branch block and delayed excitation of the left ventricle from a right ventricular ectopic beat. Mechanical prolongation of left ventricular systole, resulting in reversed splitting of S_2, also may be caused by severe aortic outflow obstruction, a large aorta-to-pulmonary artery shunt, systolic hypertension, and ischemic heart disease or cardiomyopathy with left ventricular failure. P_2 is normally softer than A_2 in the second left intercostal space; when P_2 is greater than A_2 in this area, it suggests pulmonary hypertension, except in patients with atrial septal defect.

The *third heart sound* (S_3) is a low-pitched sound produced in the ventricle 0.14 to 0.16 s after A_2, at the termination of rapid filling. This sound is frequent in normal children and in patients with high cardiac output. However, in patients over 40 years of age, an S_3 usually indicates impairment of ventricular function, AV valve regurgitation, or other conditions which increase the rate or volume of ventricular filling. The left-sided S_3 is best heard with the bell piece of the stethoscope at the left ventricular apex during expiration and with the patient in the left lateral position. The right-sided S_3 is best heard at the left sternal border or just beneath the xiphoid and is increased with inspiration. Often it is accompanied by the systolic murmur of functional tricuspid regurgitation. Third heart sounds often disappear with treatment of heart failure.

An earlier (0.10 to 0.12 s after A_2), higher-pitched third heart sound (pericardial knock) often occurs in patients with constrictive pericarditis; its presence is dependent on the restrictive effect of the adherent pericardium, which halts diastolic filling abruptly.

The *opening snap* (OS) is a brief, high-pitched, early diastolic sound which is usually due to stenosis of an AV valve, more commonly the mitral valve. It is usually heard best at the lower left sternal border and radiates well to the base of the heart. The A_2-OS interval is inversely related to the height of the mean left atrial pressure and ranges from 0.04 to 0.12 s. In the second intercostal space an OS is often confused with P_2. However, careful auscultation at the upper left sternal border will reveal both components of S_2, followed by the OS. The OS of tricuspid stenosis occurs later in diastole than the mitral OS. Since most patients with tricuspid stenosis also have severe mitral valve disease, the tricuspid OS is often overshadowed by the diastolic rumble and OS originating in the stenotic mitral valve. An OS also may occur when there is increased flow across an AV valve, such as exists with left-to-right intracardiac shunts and mitral or tricuspid regurgitation.

The *fourth heart sound* (S_4) is a low-pitched, presystolic sound produced in the ventricle during ventricular filling; it is associated with an effective atrial contraction and is heard best with the bell piece of the stethoscope. The sound is absent in patients with atrial fibrillation. The S_4 occurs when diminished ventricular compliance increases the resistance to ventricular filling, and it is present frequently in patients with systemic hypertension, aortic stenosis, hypertrophic cardiomyopathy, ischemic heart disease, and acute mitral regurgitation. Most patients with an acute myocardial infarction and sinus rhythm have an audible S_4. The fourth heart sound is frequently accompanied by visible and palpable presystolic distention of the left ventricle. It is maximal in intensity at the left ventricular apex with the patient in the left lateral position and is accentuated by mild isotonic or isometric exercise in the supine position. The right-sided S_4 is present in patients with right ventricular hypertrophy secondary to either pulmonic stenosis or pulmonary hypertension and frequently accompanies a prominent presystolic *a* wave in the JVP.

An S_4 frequently accompanies delayed AV conduction even in the absence of clinically detectable heart disease. The incidence of an audible S_4 increases with increasing age. Whether an audible S_4 in adults without other evidence of cardiac disease is abnormal remains controversial.

The *ejection sound* is a sharp, high-pitched event occurring in early systole closely following the first heart sound. Ejection sounds occur in the presence of semilunar valve stenosis, when there are opening snaps of the aortic or pulmonic valves, and in conditions associated with dilation of the aorta or pulmonary artery. The aortic ejection sound is usually heard best at the left ventricular apex and the second right interspace; the pulmonary ejection sound is of maximal intensity at the upper left sternal border. The latter, unlike most other right-sided acoustical events, is heard better during expiration.

Nonejection or midsystolic clicks, occurring with or without a late systolic murmur, often denote prolapse of one or both leaflets of the mitral valve. They also may be caused by tricuspid valve prolapse. They probably result from functionally unequal length of the chordae tendineae of either or both AV valves and are heard best along the lower left sternal border and at the left ventricular apex. Systolic clicks may be single or multiple, and they may occur at any time in systole but usually later than the systolic ejection sound. Frequently the midsystolic click is misinterpreted as S_2, and the actual second heart sound is called an OS or S_3.

HEART MURMURS Cardiac murmurs result from vibrations set up in the bloodstream and the surrounding heart and great vessels as a result of turbulent blood flow, the formation of eddies, and cavitation (bubble formation as a result of sudden decrease in pressure).

The intensity (loudness) of murmurs may be graded from I to VI. A grade I murmur is so faint that it can be heard only with special effort, a grade IV murmur is commonly accompanied by a thrill, and a grade VI murmur is audible with the stethoscope removed from

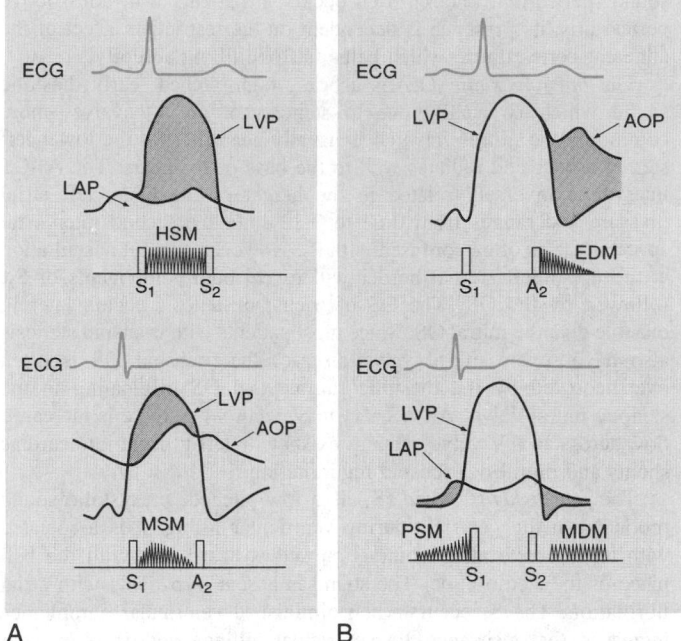

A   **B**

FIGURE 188-4 *A*. Schematic representation of ECG, aortic pressure (AOP), left ventricular pressure (LVP), and left atrial pressure (LAP). The striped areas indicated a transvalvular pressure difference during systole. HSM, holosystolic murmur; MSM, midsystolic murmur. *B*. Graphic representation of ECG, aortic pressure (AOP), left ventricular pressure (LVP) and left atrial pressure (LAP) with striped areas indicating transvalvular diastolic pressure difference. EDM, early diastolic murmur; PSM, presystolic murmur; MDM, middiastolic murmur.

contact with the chest. The configuration of a murmur may be crescendo, decrescendo, crescendo-decrescendo (diamond-shaped), or plateau. The precise time of onset and time of cessation of a murmur depend on the instant in the cardiac cycle at which an adequate pressure difference between two chambers appears and disappears (Fig. 188-4).

The location on the chest wall where the murmur is best heard and the areas to which it radiates can be helpful in identifying the cardiac structure from which the murmur originates. For example, the murmur of aortic valve stenosis usually is loudest in the second right intercostal space and radiates to the carotid arteries. By contrast, the murmur of mitral regurgitation most often is loudest at the cardiac apex. It may radiate to the left sternal border and base of the heart when the posterior mitral leaflet is predominantly involved or to the axilla and back when the anterior leaflet is more severely affected. In the former case, the regurgitant blood is directed toward the posterior left atrial wall.

Often it is difficult to classify with certainty a cardiac murmur based on its timing, configuration, location, radiation, pitch, or intensity. However, by noting changes in the characteristics of the murmur during maneuvers that alter cardiac hemodynamics, the auscultator often can identify its correct origin and significance (Table 188-1).

Accentuation of a murmur during inspiration, a maneuver which augments systemic venous return, implies that it originates on the right side of the circulation; expiratory exaggeration has less significance. Prolonged expiratory pressure against a closed glottis, i.e., the Valsalva maneuver, reduces the intensity of most murmurs by diminishing both right and left ventricular filling (i.e., ventricular preload). The systolic murmur associated with *hypertrophic cardiomyopathy* and the late systolic murmur due to *mitral valve prolapse* are exceptions and may be paradoxically accentuated during the Valsalva maneuver. Murmurs due to flow across a normal or obstructed semilunar valve increase in intensity in the cycle following a premature ventricular beat or a long RR interval in atrial fibrillation. In contrast,

murmurs due to AV valve regurgitation or a ventricular septal defect do not change appreciably during the beat following a prolonged diastole. Standing, which decreases left ventricular volume, accentuates the murmur of hypertrophic cardiomyopathy and occasionally the murmur due to mitral valve prolapse. Squatting, which increases both venous return and systemic arterial resistance and thus ventricular afterload, increases most murmurs, except those due to hypertrophic cardiomyopathy and mitral regurgitation due to a prolapsed mitral valve, which often decrease. Sustained handgrip exercise, which increases systemic arterial pressure and heart rate, often accentuates the murmurs of mitral regurgitation, aortic regurgitation, and mitral stenosis but usually diminishes those due to aortic stenosis or hypertrophic cardiomyopathy. Pharmacologic interventions include inhalation of amyl nitrite, which reduces systemic arterial pressure and increases blood flow, thereby increasing the intensity of murmurs due to valvular stenosis while diminishing those due to aortic or mitral regurgitation (Table 188-1). Transient external arterial occlusion by the inflation of bilateral arm cuffs to 20 mmHg (2.66 kPa) above systolic blood pressure for 5 s has been shown to intensify murmurs due to left-sided regurgitant lesions; this method is applicable to almost all patients and does not require administration of any drug.

Systolic murmurs *Holosystolic (pansystolic) murmurs* are generated when there is a flow between two chambers which have widely different pressures throughout systole, such as the left ventricle and either the left atrium or the right ventricle (Fig. 188-4). The pressure gradient is established early in contraction and lasts until relaxation is almost complete. Therefore, holosystolic murmurs begin before aortic ejection, and at the area of maximal intensity they begin with S_1 and end after S_2. Holosystolic murmurs accompany mitral or tricuspid regurgitation, ventricular septal defect, and under certain circumstances aortopulmonary shunts. Although the typical high-pitched murmur of mitral regurgitation usually continues throughout systole, the shape of the murmur may vary considerably. The holosystolic murmurs of mitral regurgitation and ventricular septal defect are augmented by transient exercise and are diminished by lowering the left ventricular systolic pressure by inhalation of amyl nitrite. The murmur of tricuspid regurgitation associated with pulmonary hypertension is holosystolic and frequently increases during inspiration. Not all patients with mitral or tricuspid regurgitation or ventricular septal defect have holosystolic murmurs (Chap. 201).

Midsystolic murmurs, also called *systolic ejection murmurs*, often crescendo-decrescendo in shape, occur when blood is ejected across the aortic or pulmonic outflow tracts (Fig. 188-4). The murmur starts shortly after S_1 when the ventricular pressure rises sufficiently to open the semilunar valve. Ejection then begins and with it the onset of the murmur; as ejection increases, the murmur is augmented, and as ejection declines, it diminishes. The murmur ends before the ventricular pressure falls enough to permit closure of the aortic or pulmonic leaflets. In the presence of normal semilunar valves, an increased flow rate, as occurs in states of elevated cardiac output, ejection into a dilated vessel beyond the valve, or increased transmission of sound through a thin chest wall, may be responsible for the production of this murmur. Most benign, functional murmurs are midsystolic and originate from the pulmonary outflow tract. Valvular or subvalvular obstruction to either ventricle also may cause such a midsystolic murmur, the intensity being related to the flow.

The murmur of aortic stenosis is the prototype of the left-sided midsystolic murmur. The location and radiation of this murmur are influenced by the direction of the high-velocity jet within the aortic root. In *valvular aortic stenosis* the murmur is usually maximal in the second right intercostal space, with radiation into the neck. In *supravalvular aortic stenosis* the murmur is occasionally loudest even higher, with disproportionate radiation into the right carotid artery. In hypertrophic cardiomyopathy, the midsystolic murmur originates within the left ventricular cavity and is usually maximal at the lower left sternal edge and apex, with relatively little radiation to the carotids. When the aortic valve is immobile (calcified), the aortic closure sound (A_2) may be soft and inaudible so that the length and configuration of the murmur are difficult to determine. Midsystolic murmurs also occur in patients with mitral regurgitation or, less frequently, tricuspid regurgitation resulting from papillary muscle dysfunction. Such murmurs due to mitral regurgitation are often confused with those originating in the aorta, particularly in elderly patients.

The patient's age and the area of maximal intensity aid in determining the significance of midsystolic murmurs. Thus, in a young adult with a thin chest and high velocity of blood flow, a faint or moderate midsystolic murmur heard only in the pulmonic area is usually without clinical significance, while a somewhat louder murmur in the aortic area may indicate congenital aortic stenosis. In elderly patients, pulmonic flow murmurs are rare, while aortic systolic murmurs are frequent and may be due to aortic dilatation, to a significant degree of valvular aortic stenosis, or to nonstenotic deformity of the aortic valve. Midsystolic aortic and pulmonic murmurs are intensified by amyl nitrite inhalation and during the cardiac cycle following a premature ventricular beat, while those due to mitral regurgitation are unchanged or softer. Aortic systolic murmurs are diminished by interventions which increase aortic impedence, such as intravenous phenylephrine. Echocardiography or cardiac catheterization may be necessary to separate a prominent and exaggerated functional murmur from one due to congenital semilunar valve stenosis.

Early systolic murmurs begin with the first heart sound and end in midsystole. They may be due to a very small *ventricular septal defect, a large defect with pulmonary hypertension*, or *severe acute mitral* or *tricuspid regurgitation*. In large ventricular septal defects with pulmonary hypertension, the shunting at the end of systole may be small or absent, resulting in an early systolic murmur. A similar murmur may occur with very small muscular ventricular septal defects, the shunt being interrupted in late systole. An early systolic murmur is a feature of tricuspid regurgitation occurring in the absence of pulmonary hypertension. This lesion is common in drug addicts with infective endocarditis, in whom a tall regurgitant right atrial *v* wave reaches the level of the normal right ventricular pressure in late systole, confining the murmur to early systole. In patients with acute mitral regurgitation and a large *v* wave in a noncompliant left atrium, a loud early systolic murmur is frequently heard which diminishes as the pressure gradient between left ventricle and left atrium decreases in late systole (Chap. 201).

Late systolic murmurs are faint or moderately loud, high-pitched apical murmurs which start well after ejection and do not mask either heart sound. They are probably related to papillary muscle dysfunction caused by infarction or ischemia of these muscles or to their distortion by left ventricular dilatation. They may appear only during angina but are common in patients with myocardial infarction or diffuse myocardial disease. Late systolic murmurs following midsystolic clicks are associated with late systolic mitral regurgitation caused by prolapse of the mitral valve into the left atrium (Chap. 201).

Diastolic murmurs *Early diastolic murmurs* (Fig. 188-4) begin with or shortly after S_2 as soon as the corresponding ventricular pressure falls sufficiently below that in the aorta or pulmonary artery. The high-pitched murmurs of aortic regurgitation or pulmonic regurgitation due to pulmonary hypertension are generally decrescendo, since there is a progressive decline in the volume or rate of regurgitation during diastole. Faint, high-pitched murmurs of aortic regurgitation are difficult to hear unless they are specifically sought by applying firm pressure with the diaphragm over the left midsternal border while the patient sits, leans forward, and holds a breath in full expiration. The diastolic murmur of aortic regurgitation is enhanced by an acute elevation of the arterial pressure such as occurs with handgrip exercise; it diminishes with a decrease in arterial pressure, as with amyl nitrite inhalation. The diastolic murmur of congenital pulmonic regurgitation without pulmonary hypertension is low- to medium-pitched. The onset of this murmur is delayed because at the onset of pulmonic valve closure the regurgitant flow is minimal, since the reverse pressure gradient responsible for the regurgitation is negligible at this time.

Middiastolic murmurs usually arise from the AV valves (Fig. 188-4), occur during early ventricular filling, and are due to disproportion between valve orifice size and flow rate. Such murmurs may be quite loud (grade III) despite only slight AV valve stenosis when there is normal or increased blood flow. Conversely, the murmur may be soft or even absent despite severe obstruction if the cardiac output is markedly reduced. When stenosis is marked, the diastolic murmur is prolonged and the duration of the murmur is more reliable than its intensity as an index of the severity of valve obstruction.

The low-pitched, middiastolic murmur of mitral stenosis characteristically follows the OS. It should be specifically sought by placing the bell of the stethoscope at the site of the left ventricular impulse, which is best localized with the patient on the left side. Frequently the murmur of mitral stenosis is present only at the left ventricular apex, and it may be increased in intensity by mild supine exercise or by inhalation of amyl nitrite. In tricuspid stenosis the middiastolic murmur is localized to a relatively limited area along the left sternal edge and may increase in intensity during inspiration.

Middiastolic murmurs may be generated across the mitral valve in ventricular septal defect, patent ductus arteriosus, or mitral regurgitation and across the tricuspid valve in atrial septal defect or tricuspid regurgitation. These murmurs are related to the torrential flow across an AV valve, usually follow an S_3, and tend to occur with large left-to-right shunts or severe AV valve regurgitation. A soft middiastolic murmur may sometimes be heard in patients with acute rheumatic fever (Carey-Coombs murmur). It has been attributed to inflammation of the mitral valve cusps or excessive left atrial blood flow as a consequence of mitral regurgitation.

In acute, severe regurgitation, the left ventricular diastolic pressure may exceed the left atrial pressure, resulting in a middiastolic murmur due to "diastolic mitral regurgitation." In severe, chronic aortic regurgitation, a murmur is frequently present which may be either middiastolic or presystolic (Austin Flint murmur). This murmur appears to originate at the anterior mitral valve leaflet when blood simultaneously enters the left ventricle from both the aortic root and the left atrium.

Presystolic murmurs begin during the period of ventricular filling that follows atrial contraction and therefore occur in sinus rhythm. They are usually due to AV valve stenosis and have the same quality as the middiastolic filling rumble but are usually crescendo, reaching peak intensity at the time of a loud S_1. The presystolic murmur corresponds to the AV valve gradient, which may be minimal until the moment of right or left atrial contraction. It is the presystolic rather than the middiastolic murmur which is most characteristic of tricuspid stenosis and sinus rhythm. A right or left *atrial myxoma* may occasionally cause either middiastolic or presystolic murmurs that resemble the murmurs of mitral or tricuspid stenosis.

Continuous murmurs begin in systole, peak near S_2, and continue into all or part of diastole. These murmurs result from continuous flow due to a communication between high- and low-pressure areas which persists through the end of systole and the beginning of diastole. A *patent ductus arteriosus* causes a continuous murmur as long as the pressure in the pulmonary artery is much below that in the aorta. The murmur is intensified by elevation of the systemic arterial pressure and is reduced by amyl nitrite inhalation. When pulmonary hypertension is present, the diastolic portion may disappear, leaving the murmur confined to systole. A continuous murmur is uncommon in aortopulmonary septal defects, since this malformation is generally associated with severe pulmonary hypertension. Surgically produced connections and the subclavian–pulmonary artery anastomosis result in murmurs similar to that of a patent ductus.

Continuous murmurs may result from congenital or acquired *systemic arteriovenous fistula, coronary arteriovenous fistula*, anomalous origin of the left coronary artery from the pulmonary artery, and communications between the *sinus of Valsalva and the right side of the heart*. Continuous murmurs also may occur in patients with a small atrial septal defect with a high left atrial pressure. Murmurs associated with *pulmonary arteriovenous fistulas* may be continuous but are usually only systolic. Continuous murmurs may also be due to disturbances of flow pattern in constricted systemic (e.g., renal) or pulmonary arteries when marked pressure differences between the two sides of the narrow segment persist; a continuous murmur in the back may be present in *coarctation of the aorta; pulmonary embolism* may cause continuous murmurs in partially occluded vessels.

In nonconstricted arteries, continuous murmurs may be due to rapid flow through a tortuous bed. Such murmurs typically occur within the bronchial arterial collateral circulation in cyanotic patients with severe pulmonary outflow obstruction. The "mammary souffle," an innocent murmur heard over the breasts during late pregnancy and early postpartum, may be systolic or continuous. The innocent cervical venous hum is a continuous murmur usually audible over the medial aspect of the right supraclavicular fossa with the patient upright. The hum is usually louder during diastole and can be instantaneously abolished by digital compression of the ipsilateral internal jugular vein. Transmission of a loud venous hum to the area below the clavicles may result in a mistaken diagnosis of patent ductus arteriosus.

The *pericardial friction rub*, which may have presystolic, systolic, and early diastolic scratchy components, may be confused with a murmur or extracardiac sound when heard only in systole. It is best appreciated with the patient upright and leaning forward and may be accentuated during inspiration.

REFERENCES

ABRAMS J: *Essentials of Cardiac Physical Diagnosis*. Philadelphia, Lea & Febiger, 1987

BRAUNWALD E: Physical examination, in *Heart Disease*, 4th ed, E Braunwald (ed). Philadelphia, Saunders, 1992, p. 13

CRAWFORD MH: *Examination of the Heart*, part 2: *Inspection and Palpation of Venous and Arterial Pulses*. Chicago, American Heart Association, 1990

EILEN SD, CRAWFORD MH, O'ROURKE RA: Accuracy of precordial palpation for detecting increased left ventricular volume. Ann Intern Med 99:628, 1983

EWY GA: The abdominojugular test: Technique and hemodynamic correlates. Ann Intern Med 109:456, 1988

GREWE K et al: Differentiation of cardiac murmurs by auscultation. Curr Probl Cardiol 13(10):699, 1988

LEMBO NJ ET AL: Bedside diagnosis of systolic murmurs. N Engl J Med 318:1572, 1988

PERLOFF JK (ED): *Physical Examination of the Heart and Circulation*, 2d ed. Philadelphia, Saunders, 1990

———: Heart sounds and murmurs: Physiological mechanisms, in *Heart Disease*, 4th ed, E Braunwald (ed). Philadelphia, Saunders, 1992, p 43

SHAVER JA et al: Normal and abnormal heart sounds in cardiac diagnosis, Part I: Systolic sounds. Curr Probl Cardiol 10(3):1, 1985

189 ELECTROCARDIOGRAPHY

ARY L. GOLDBERGER

The electrocardiogram (ECG or EKG) is a graphic recording of electric potentials generated by the heart. The signals are detected by means of metal electrodes attached to the extremities and chest wall and are then amplified by a sensitive voltmeter such as the electrocardiograph. ECG *leads* actually record the instantaneous *differences* in potential between these electrodes.

The clinical utility of the ECG derives from its immediate availability as a noninvasive, inexpensive, and highly versatile test. In addition to the detection of arrhythmias, conduction disturbances, and myocardial ischemia, electrocardiography may reveal other findings related to life-threatening metabolic disturbances (e.g., hyperkalemia) or increased susceptibility to sudden cardiac death (e.g., QT prolongation syndromes). The advent of coronary thrombolysis in the early therapy of acute myocardial infarction (Chap. 189) has refocused particular attention on the sensitivity and specificity of ECG signs of myocardial ischemia.

ELECTROPHYSIOLOGY (See also Chaps. 197 and 198) Depolarization of the heart is the initiating event for cardiac contraction. The electric currents which spread through the heart are produced by three components: cardiac pacemaker cells, specialized conduction tissue, and the heart muscle itself. The ECG, however, records only the depolarization (stimulation) and repolarization (recovery) potentials generated by the atrial and ventricular myocardium. Under resting conditions, myocardial cells are *polarized*; i.e., they carry an electric charge on their surface due to transmembrane ion concentration differences. The charge measured across atrial and ventricular cell membranes is about 90 mV, with the inside negative relative to the outside. When these cells are stimulated above a critical threshold potential, they rapidly depolarize and transiently reverse their membrane polarity. This depolarization process spreads in a wavelike manner through the atria and ventricles. The return of myocardial fibers to their original resting state occurs during repolarization.

The depolarization stimulus for the normal heartbeat originates in the *sinoatrial* (SA) or *sinus node*, a collection of *pacemaker* cells which fire spontaneously; i.e., they exhibit *automaticity* (Fig. 189-1). The first phase of cardiac electrical activation is spread of the depolarization wave through the right and left atria, followed by atrial contraction. Next, the impulse stimulates pacemaker and specialized conduction tissues in the atrioventricular (AV) nodal and His-bundle areas; together, these two regions constitute the AV junction. The bundle of His bifurcates into two main branches, the right and the left bundles, that rapidly transmit depolarization wavefronts to the right and left ventricular myocardium by way of Purkinje fibers. The main left bundle bifurcates into two primary subdivisions, a left anterior fascicle and a left posterior fascicle. The depolarization wavefronts then spread through the ventricular wall, from endocardium to epicardium, triggering ventricular contraction.

Since the cardiac depolarization and repolarization waves have direction and magnitude, they can be represented by vectors. *Vectorcardiograms* that measure and display these instantaneous potentials are no longer used much in clinical practice. However, the general principles of vector analysis remain fundamental to understanding the genesis of normal and pathologic ECG waveforms. Vector analysis illustrates a central concept of electrocardiography—namely, that the ECG records the complex spatial and temporal summation of electrical potentials from multiple myocardial fibers conducted to the surface of the body. This principle accounts for inherent limitations in both ECG *sensitivity* (activity from certain cardiac regions may be canceled out or not of sufficient magnitude to be recorded) and *specificity* (the

FIGURE 189-1 Schematic of the cardiac conduction system.

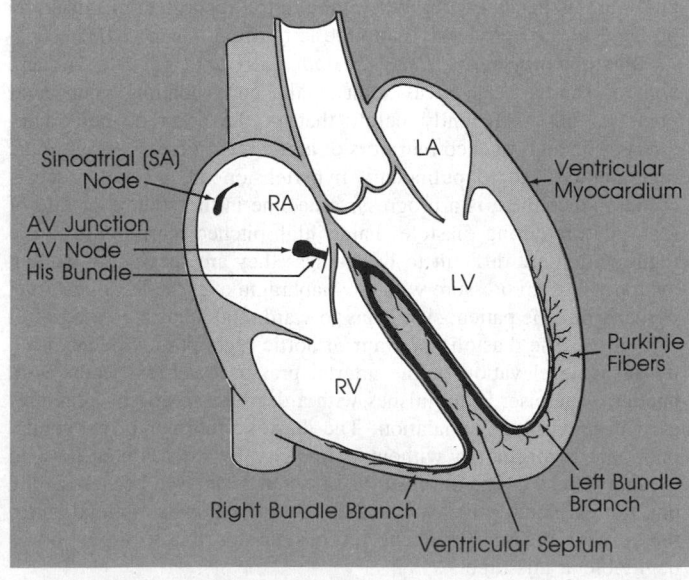

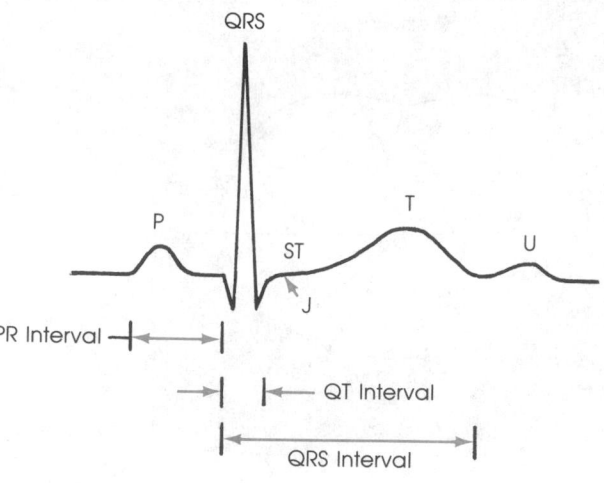

FIGURE 189-2 Basic ECG waveforms and intervals. Not shown is the R-R interval, the time between consecutive QRS complexes.

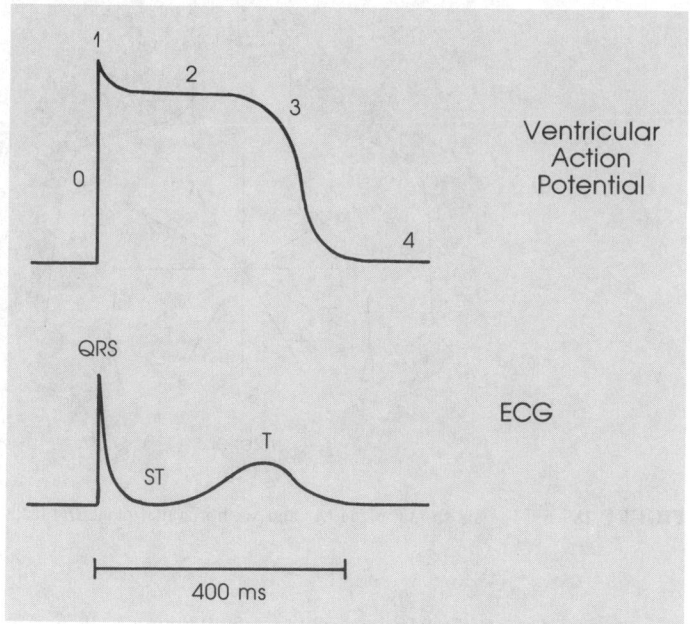

FIGURE 189-3 The QRS-T cycle corresponds to different phases of the ventricular action potential.

same vectorial sum can result from either a selective gain or loss of forces in opposite directions).

ECG WAVEFORMS AND INTERVALS The ECG waveforms are labeled alphabetically beginning with the P wave, which represents atrial depolarization (Fig. 189-2). The QRS complex represents ventricular depolarization, and the ST-T-U complex (ST segment, T wave, and U wave) represents ventricular repolarization. The J point is the junction between the end of the QRS complex and the beginning of the ST segment. Atrial repolarization is usually of too low an amplitude to be detected, but it may become apparent in such conditions as acute pericarditis or atrial infarction.

The QRS-T waveforms of the surface (extracellular) ECG correspond in a general way with the different phases of simultaneously obtained ventricular *action potentials*, the intracellular recordings from single myocardial fibers (Fig. 189-3) (see also Chap. 197). The rapid upstroke (phase 0) of the action potential corresponds to the onset of QRS. The plateau (phase 2) corresponds to the isoelectric ST segment and active repolarization (phase 3) to the inscription of the T wave. Factors that decrease the slope of phase 0 by impairing the influx of Na^+ (e.g., drugs such as quinidine or procainamide, or hyperkalemia) tend to increase QRS duration. Conditions that prolong

phase 2 (amiodarone, hypocalcemia) increase the QT interval. In contrast, shortening of ventricular repolarization (phase 2), by digitalis or hypercalcemia, abbreviates the ST segment.

The electrocardiogram is ordinarily recorded on special graph paper which is divided into 1-mm² gridlike boxes (Fig. 189-4). Since the ECG paper speed is generally 25 mm/s, the smallest (1 mm) horizontal divisions correspond to 0.04 s (40 ms), with heavier lines at intervals of 0.20 s (200 ms). Vertically, the ECG graph measures the amplitude of a given wave or deflection (1 mV = 10 mm with standard calibration; the voltage criteria for hypertrophy mentioned below are given in millimeters). There are four major ECG intervals: R-R, PR, QRS, and QT (Fig. 189-2). The heart rate (beats per minute) can be readily computed from the interbeat (R-R) interval by dividing the number of large (0.20 s) time units between consecutive R waves into 300 or the number of small (0.04 s) units into 1500. The PR interval (normally 120 to 200 ms) measures the time (normally 120 to 200 ms) between atrial and ventricular depolarization, which

FIGURE 189-4 The ECG graph paper records the time (interval) between cardiac electrical events along the horizontal axis and their amplitude (voltage) along the vertical axis.

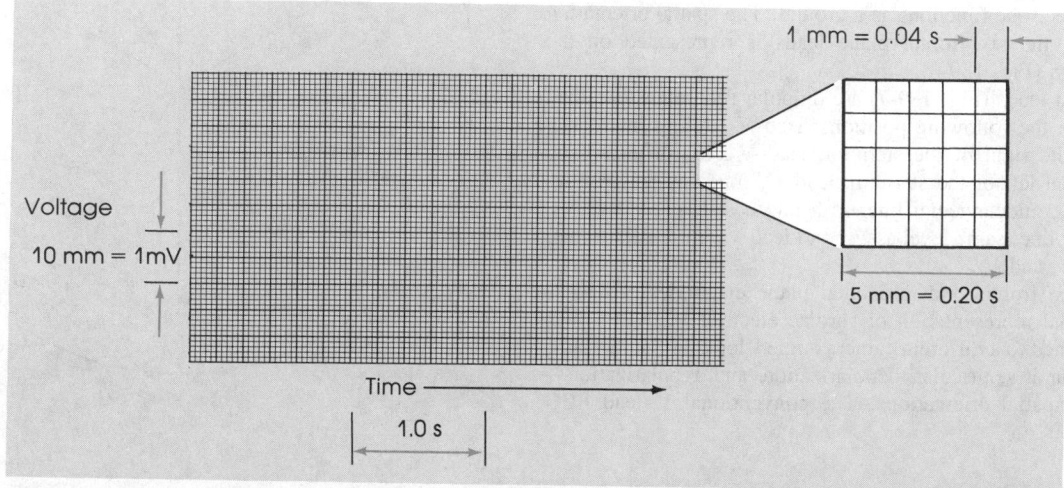

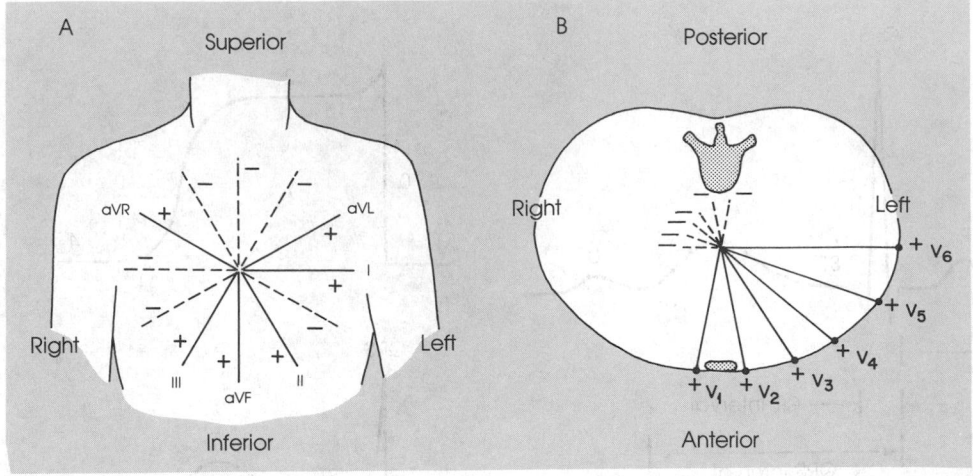

FIGURE 189-5   The six frontal plane (*A*) and six horizontal plane (*B*) leads provide a three-dimensional representation of cardiac electrical activity.

includes the physiologic delay imposed by stimulation of cells in the AV junction area. The QRS interval (normally 100 ms or less) reflects the duration of ventricular depolarization. The QT interval includes both ventricular depolarization and repolarization times and varies inversely with the heart rate. A rate-related ("corrected") QT interval, or QT_c, can be calculated as $QT/\sqrt{R\text{-}R}$ and normally is ≤ 0.44 s.

The QRS complex is subdivided into specific deflections or waves. If the initial QRS deflection in a given lead is negative, it is termed a *Q wave*; the first positive deflection is termed an *R wave*. A negative deflection after an R wave is an *S wave*. Subsequent positive or negative waves are labeled R' and S', respectively. Lowercase letters (qrs) are used for relatively small amplitude waves. An entirely negative QRS complex is termed a *QS wave*.

ECG LEADS   The 12 conventional ECG leads record the difference in potential between electrodes placed on the surface of the body. These leads are divided into two groups; six extremity (limb) leads and six chest (precordial) leads. The extremity leads record potentials transmitted onto the *frontal plane* (Fig. 189-5*A*), and the chest leads record potentials transmitted onto the *horizontal plane* (Fig. 189-5*B*). The six extremity leads are further subdivided into three *bipolar* leads (I, II, and III) and three *unipolar* leads (aVR, aVL, and aVF). Each bipolar lead measures the difference in potential between electrodes at two extremities: lead I = left arm − right arm voltages, lead II = left leg − right arm, and lead III = left leg − left arm. The unipolar leads measure the voltage (V) at one locus relative to an electrode (called the *central terminal* or *indifferent electrode*) that has approximately zero potential. Thus aVR = right arm, aVL = left arm, and aVF = left leg (foot). The lower case *a* indicates that these unipolar potentials are electrically augmented by 50 percent. The right leg electrode functions as a ground. The spatial orientation and polarity of the six frontal plane leads is represented on the hexaxial diagram (Fig. 189-6).

The six chest leads (Fig. 189-7) are unipolar recordings obtained by electrodes in the following positions: lead V_1, fourth intercostal space, just to the right of the sternum; lead V_2, fourth intercostal space, just to the left of the sternum; lead V_3, midway between V_2 and V_4; lead V_4, midclavicular line, fifth intercostal space; lead V_5, anterior axillary line, same level as V_4; and lead V_6, midaxillary line, same level as V_4 and V_5.

Together, the frontal and horizontal plane electrodes provide a three-dimensional representation of cardiac electrical activity. Each lead can be likened to a different camera angle "looking" at the same events—atrial and ventricular depolarization and repolarization—from different spatial orientations. The conventional 12-lead ECG

can be supplemented with additional leads under special circumstances. For example, right precordial leads V_3R, V_4R, etc. are useful in detecting evidence of acute right ventricular ischemia. Esophageal leads may reveal atrial activity not detectable on the surface ECG. Bedside telemetry units and ambulatory ECG (Holter) recordings usually employ only one or two modified leads, respectively. Intracardiac electrocardiography and electrophysiologic testing are discussed in Chaps. 197 and 198.

The ECG leads are configured so that a positive (upright) deflection will be recorded in a lead if a wave of depolarization spreads toward the positive pole of that lead and a negative deflection if the wave spreads toward the negative pole. If the mean orientation of the

FIGURE 189-6   The frontal plane (extremity or limb) leads are represented on a hexaxial diagram. Each ECG lead has a specific spatial orientation and polarity. The positive pole of each lead axis (*solid line*) and negative pole (*hatched line*) are designated by their angular position relative to the positive pole of lead I (0^0). The mean electrical axis of the QRS complex is measured with respect to this display.

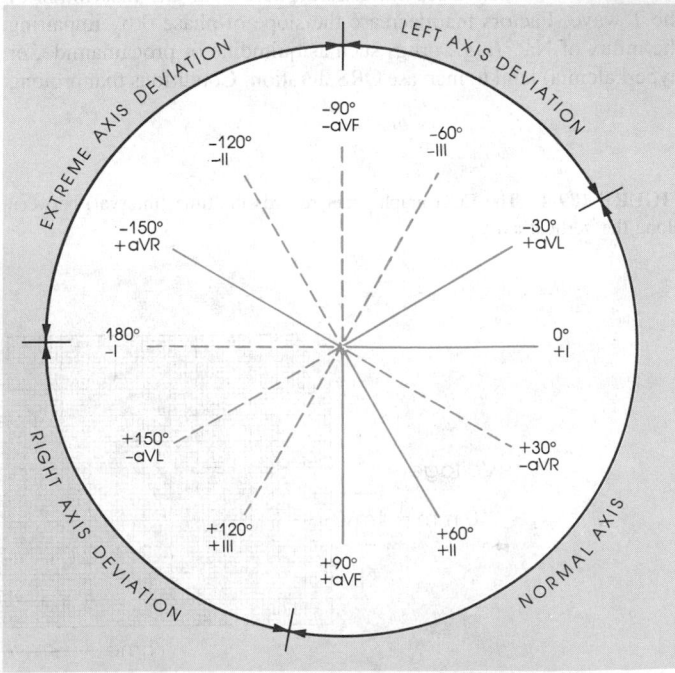

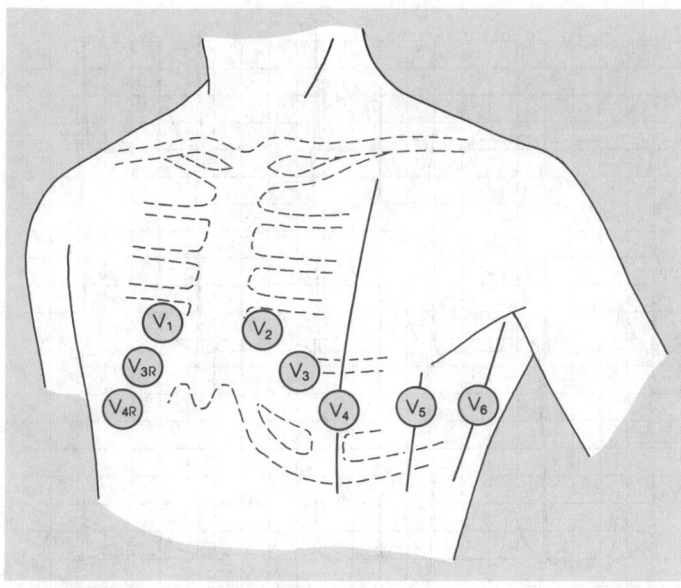

FIGURE 189-7 The horizontal plane (chest or precordial) leads are obtained with electrodes in the designated locations.

depolarization vector is at right angles to a given lead axis, a small biphasic (equally positive and negative) deflection will be recorded.

GENESIS OF THE NORMAL ECG

P WAVE The normal atrial depolarization vector is oriented downward and toward the subject's left, reflecting the spread of depolarization from the sinus node to the right and then the left atrial myocardium. Since this vector points toward the positive pole of lead II and toward the negative pole of lead aVR, the normal P wave will be positive in lead II and negative in lead aVR. By contrast, activation of the atria from an ectopic pacemaker in the lower part of either atrium or in the AV junction region may produce retrograde P waves (negative in lead II, positive in lead aVR).

QRS COMPLEX Normal ventricular depolarization proceeds as a rapid, continuous spread of activation wavefronts. This complex process can be divided into two major, sequential phases, and each phase can be represented by a mean vector (Fig. 189-8). The first phase is depolarization of the interventricular septum from the left to the right (vector 1). The second results from the simultaneous depolarization of the main mass of the right and left ventricles and is normally dominated by the more massive left ventricle so that vector 2 points leftward and posteriorly. Therefore, a right precordial lead (V_1) will record this biphasic depolarization process with a small positive deflection (septal r wave) followed by a larger negative deflection (S wave). A left precordial lead, e.g., V_6, will record the

FIGURE 189-8 Ventricular depolarization can be divided into two major phases, each represented by a vector. *A.* The first phase (*arrow 1*) denotes depolarization of the ventricular septum, beginning on the left side and spreading to the right. This process is represented by a small "septal" r wave in lead V_1 and a small septal q wave in lead V_6. *B.* Simultaneous depolarization of the left and right ventricles (LV and RV) constitutes the second phase. Vector 2 is oriented to the left and posteriorly, reflecting the electrical predominance of the LV. *C.* Vectors (*arrows*) representing these two phases are shown in reference to the horizontal plane leads. *(After Goldberger and Goldberger.)*

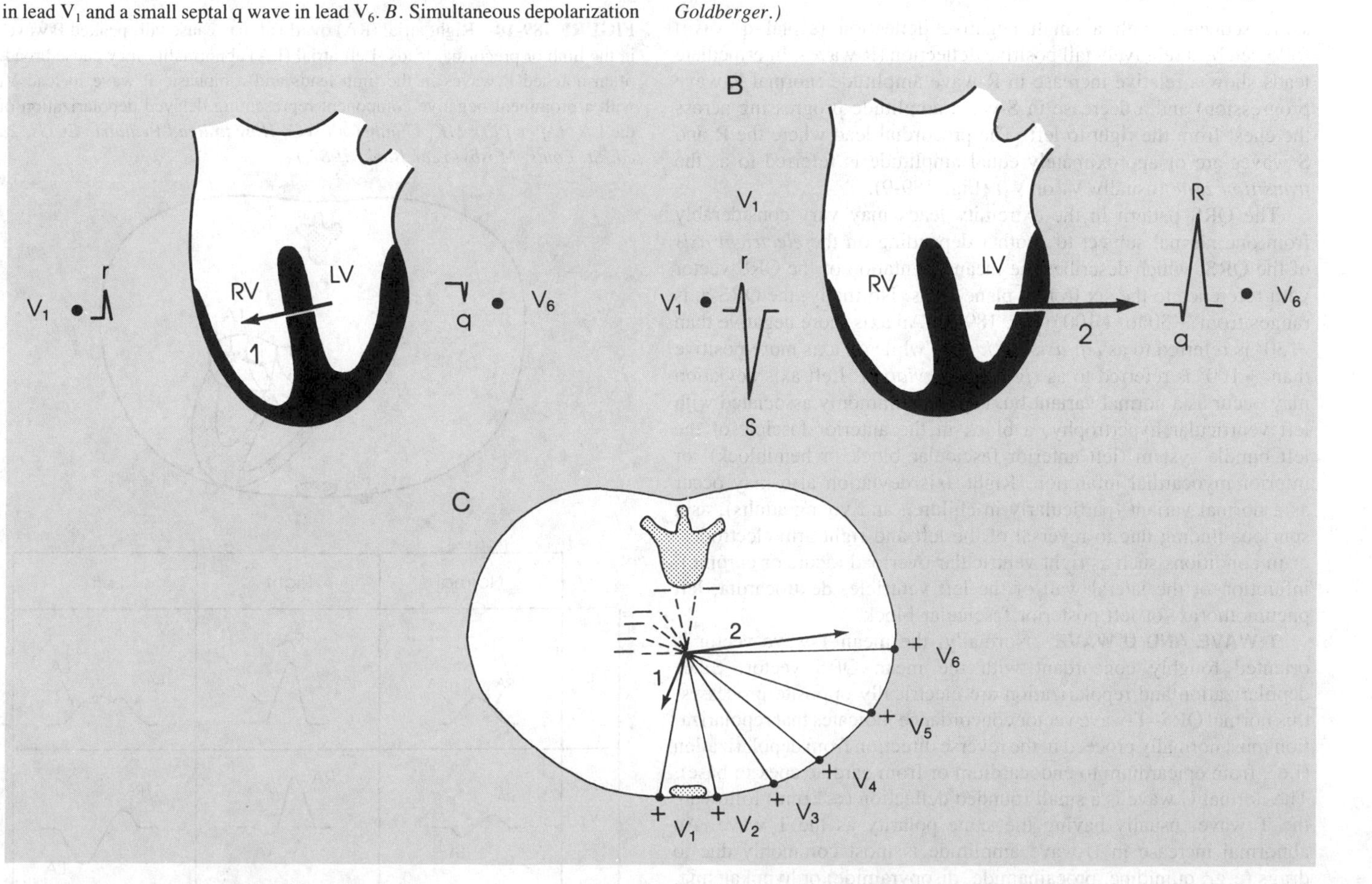

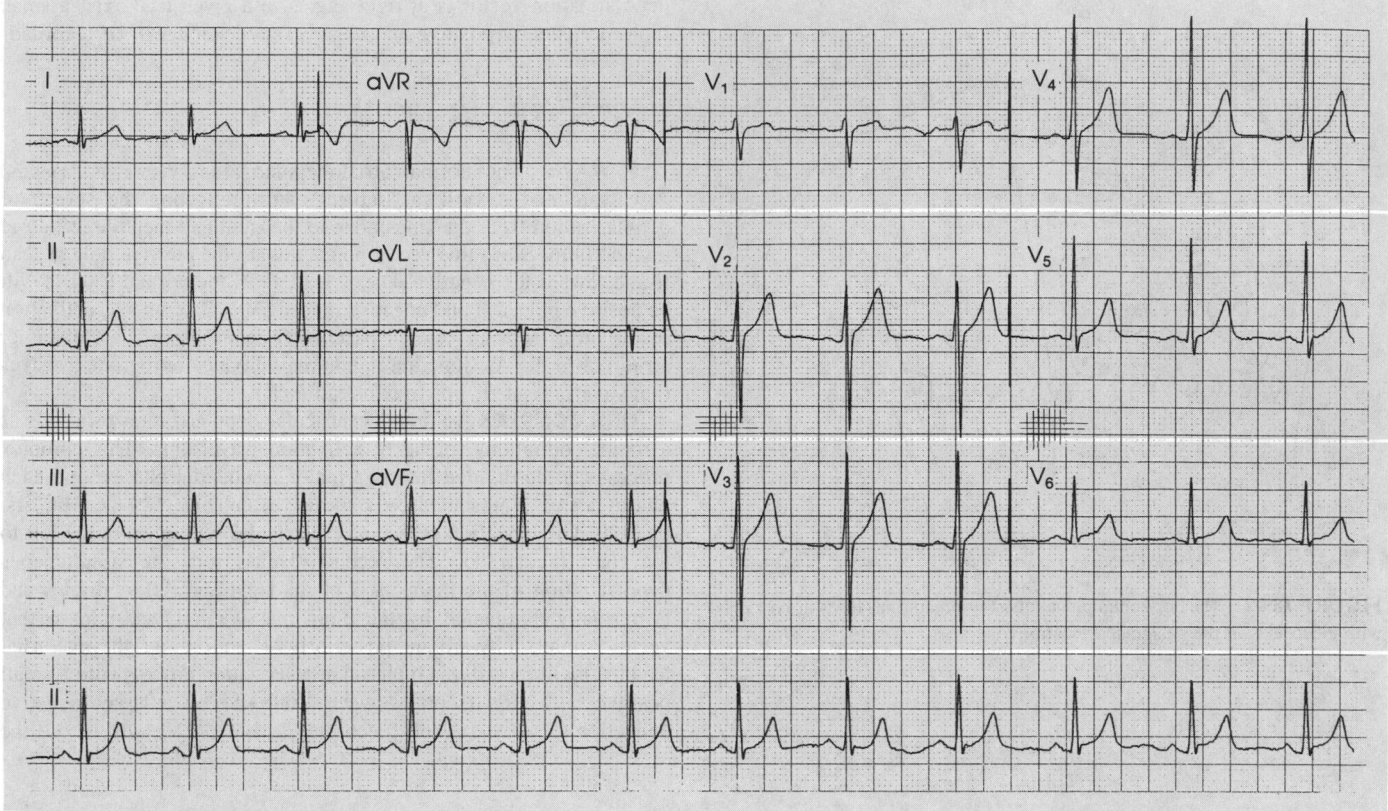

FIGURE 189-9 Normal electrocardiogram from a healthy subject. Sinus rhythm is present with a heart rate of 75 beats per minute. PR interval is 0.16 s; QRS interval (duration) is 0.08 s; QT interval is 0.36 s; the mean QRS axis is about +70°. The precordial leads show normal R-wave progression with the transition zone (R wave = S wave) in lead V_3.

same sequence with a small negative deflection (septal q wave) followed by a relatively tall positive deflection (R wave). Intermediate leads show a relative increase in R-wave amplitude (normal R-wave progression) and a decrease in S-wave amplitude progressing across the chest from the right to left. The precordial lead where the R and S waves are of approximately equal amplitude is referred to as the *transition zone* (usually V_3 or V_4) (Fig. 189-9).

The QRS pattern in the extremity leads may vary considerably from one normal subject to another depending on the *electrical axis* of the QRS, which describes the mean orientation of the QRS vector with reference to the six frontal plane leads. Normally, the QRS axis ranges from −30 to +100° (Fig. 189-7). An axis more negative than −30° is referred to as *left axis deviation*, while an axis more positive than +100° is referred to as *right axis deviation*. Left axis deviation may occur as a normal variant but is more commonly associated with left ventricular hypertrophy, a block in the anterior fascicle of the left bundle system (left anterior fascicular block or hemiblock), or inferior myocardial infarction. Right axis deviation also may occur as a normal variant (particularly in children and young adults), as a spurious finding due to reversal of the left and right arm electrodes, or in conditions such as right ventricular overload (acute or chronic), infarction of the lateral wall of the left ventricle, dextrocardia, left pneumothorax, or left posterior fascicular block.

T WAVE AND U WAVE Normally, the mean T-wave vector is oriented roughly concordant with the mean QRS vector. Since depolarization and repolarization are electrically opposite processes, this normal QRS–T-wave vector concordance indicates that repolarization must normally proceed in the reverse direction from depolarization (i.e., from epicardium to endocardium or from cardiac apex to base). The normal U wave is a small rounded deflection (≤1 mm) following the T wave, usually having the same polarity as the T wave. An abnormal increase in U-wave amplitude is most commonly due to drugs (e.g., quinidine, procainamide, disopyramide) or hypokalemia. Very prominent U waves are a marker of increased susceptibility to

FIGURE 189-10 Right atrial (RA) overload may cause tall, peaked P waves in the limb or precordial leads. Left atrial (LA) abnormality may cause broad, often notched P waves in the limb leads and a biphasic P wave in lead V_1 with a prominent negative component representing delayed depolarization of the LA. *(After Park MK, Guntheroth WG, How to Read Pediatric ECGs, 2d ed, St. Louis, Mosby–Year Book, 1987.)*

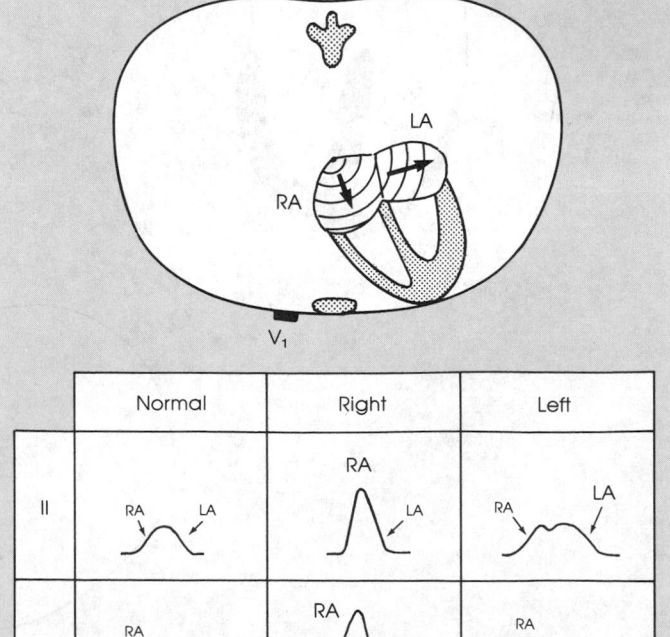

the *torsades de pointes* type of ventricular tachycardia (Chap. 198). Inversion of the U wave in the precordial leads is abnormal and may be a subtle sign of ischemia.

MAJOR ECG ABNORMALITIES

CARDIAC ENLARGEMENT AND HYPERTROPHY Right atrial overload (acute or chronic) may lead to an increase in P-wave amplitude (≥ 2.5 mm) (Fig. 189-10). Left atrial overload typically produces a biphasic P wave in V_1 with a broad negative component or a broad (≥ 120 ms), often notched P wave in one or more limb leads (Fig, 189-10). This pattern also may occur with left atrial conduction delays in the absence of actual atrial enlargement, leading to the more general designation of *left atrial abnormality*.

Right ventricular hypertrophy due to a pressure load (e.g., pulmonic valve stenosis or pulmonary artery hypertension) is characterized by a relatively tall R wave in lead V_1 (R $\geq$ S wave) usually with right axis deviation (Fig. 189-11); alternatively, there may be a qR pattern in V_1 or V_3R. ST depression and T-wave inversion in the right to midprecordial leads are also often present. This so-called ventricular strain pattern is attributed to repolarization abnormalities in hypertrophied muscle. Right ventricular hypertrophy due to ostium secundum type atrial septal defects, with the accompanying right ventricular volume overload, is commonly associated with an incomplete or complete right bundle branch block pattern with a rightward QRS axis.

Acute cor pulmonale due to pulmonary embolism, for example, may be associated with a normal ECG or a variety of abnormalities.

Sinus tachycardia is the most common arrhythmia, although other tachyarrhythmias such as atrial fibrillation or flutter may occur. The QRS axis may shift to the right, sometimes in concert with the so-called $S_1Q_3T_3$ pattern (prominence of the S wave in lead I, Q wave in lead III, with T-wave inversions in lead III). Acute right ventricular dilatation also may be associated with poor R-wave progression and T-wave inversions in V_1 to V_4 (right ventricular strain) simulating acute anterior infarction. A right ventricular conduction disturbance may appear.

Chronic cor pulmonale due to obstructive lung disease usually does not produce the classic ECG patterns of right ventricular hypertrophy noted above. Instead of tall right precordial R waves, chronic lung disease more typically is associated with small R waves in right to midprecordial leads (poor R-wave progression) due in part to downward displacement of the diaphragm and the heart. Low-voltage complexes are commonly present due to hyperaeration of the lungs.

A number of different voltage criteria for *left ventricular hypertrophy* (Fig. 189-11) have been proposed based on the presence of tall left precordial R waves and deep right precordial S waves (e.g., SV_1 + RV_5 or $RV_6 \geq 35$ mm; or RV_5 or $V_6 \geq 25$ mm). Repolarization abnormalities (ST depression with T-wave inversions) also may appear (left ventricular strain pattern) in leads with prominent R waves. However, prominent precordial voltages may occur as a normal variant, especially in athletic or thin-chested individuals. Left ventricular hypertrophy may increase limb lead voltage (e.g., RaVL ≥ 11 to 13 mm, RaVF ≥ 20 mm; R_1 + $S_{III} \geq 25$ mm) with or without increased precordial voltage. The presence of left atrial abnormality increases the likelihood of underlying left ventricular hypertrophy in

FIGURE 189-11 Left ventricular hypertrophy (LVH) increases the amplitude of electrical forces directed to the left and posteriorly. In addition, repolarization abnormalities may cause ST-segment depression and T-wave inversion in leads with a prominent R wave strain pattern. Right ventricular hypertrophy (RVH) may shift the QRS vector to the right, usually associated with an R, RS, or qR complex in lead V_1. T-wave inversions may be present in right precordial leads (''strain'' pattern).

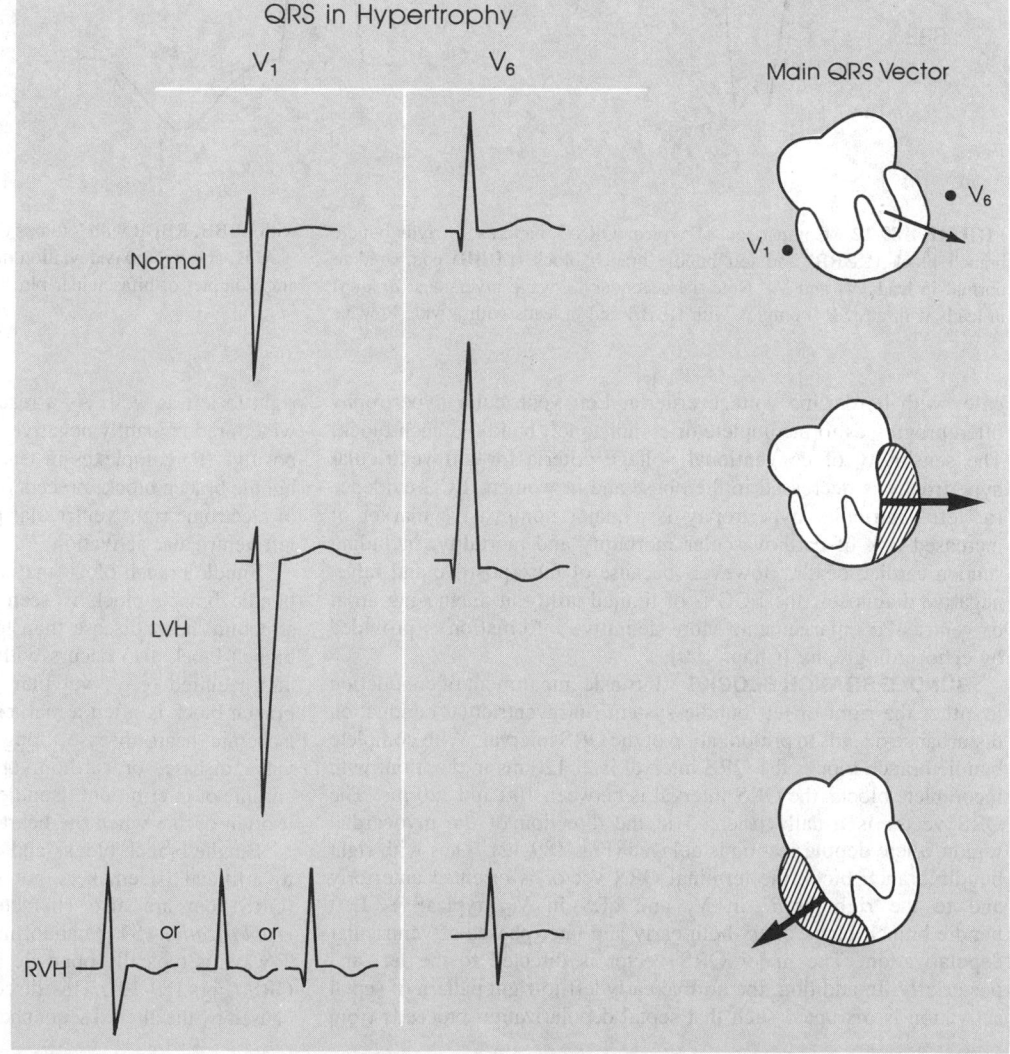

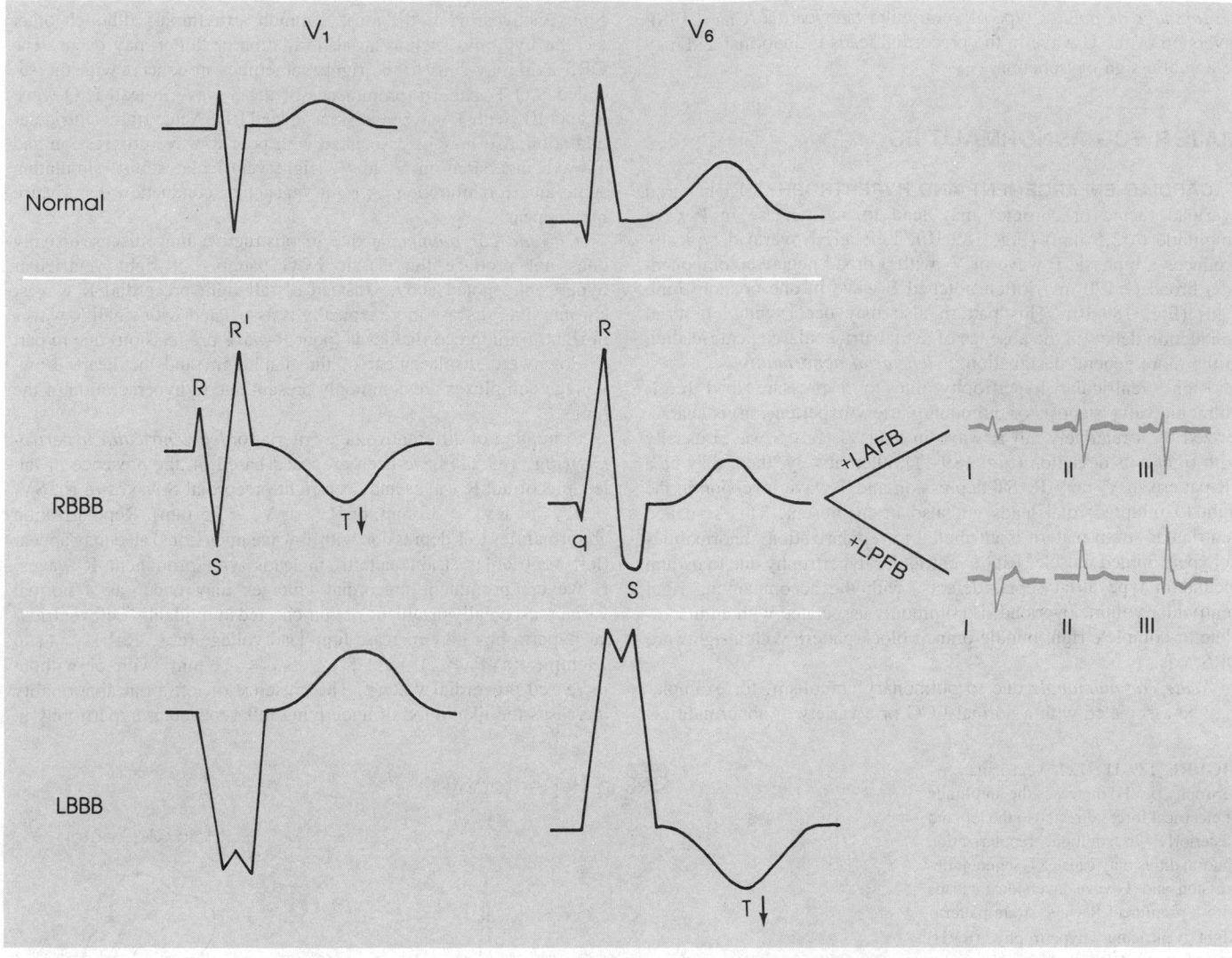

FIGURE 189-12 Comparison of typical QRS-T patterns in right bundle branch block (RBBB) and left bundle branch block (LBBB) compared to normal in leads V_1 and V_6. Note the secondary T-wave inversions (*arrows*) in leads with an rSR′ complex with RBBB and in leads with a wide R wave with LBBB. RBBB with left axis deviation due to left anterior fascicular block (LAFB) and right axis deviation due to left posterior fascicular block (LPFB) are examples of bifascicular block.

cases with borderline voltage criteria. Left ventricular hypertrophy often progresses to incomplete or complete left bundle branch block. The sensitivity of conventional voltage criteria for left ventricular hypertrophy is decreased in the obese and in women. ECG evidence for left ventricular hypertrophy is a major noninvasive marker of increased risk of cardiovascular morbidity and mortality, including sudden cardiac death. However, because of false-positive and false-negative diagnoses, the ECG is of limited utility in diagnosing atrial or ventricular enlargement. More definitive information is provided by echocardiography (Chap. 190).

BUNDLE BRANCH BLOCKS Intrinsic impairment of conduction in either the right or left bundle system (intraventricular conduction disturbances) leads to prolongation of the QRS interval. With complete bundle branch blocks the QRS interval is ≥ 120 ms in duration; with incomplete blocks the QRS interval is between 100 and 120 ms. The QRS vector is usually oriented in the direction of the myocardial region where depolarization is delayed (Fig. 189-12). Thus with right bundle branch block the terminal QRS vector is oriented anteriorly and to the right (r*SR*′ in V_1 and q*RS* in V_6, typically). Left bundle branch block alters both early and later phases of ventricular depolarization. The major QRS vector is directed to the left and posteriorly. In addition, the normal early left-to-right pattern of septal activation is disrupted such that septal depolarization proceeds from

right to left as well. As a result, left bundle branch block generates wide, predominantly negative (QS) complexes in lead V_1 and entirely positive (R) complexes in lead V_6. A pattern identical to that of left bundle branch block, preceded by a sharp spike, is seen in most cases of electronic right ventricular pacing because of the relative delay in left ventricular activation.

Bundle branch block may occur in a variety of conditions. Right bundle branch block is seen more commonly in subjects without structural heart disease than left bundle branch block. Right bundle branch block also occurs with congenital (e.g., atrial septal defect) and acquired (e.g., valvular, ischemic) heart disease. Left bundle branch block is often a marker of one of four underlying conditions: ischemic heart disease, long-standing hypertension, severe aortic valve disease, or cardiomyopathy. Bundle branch blocks may be chronic or intermittent. Bundle branch block may be rate-related; e.g. it often occurs when the heart rate exceeds some critical value.

Bundle branch blocks and depolarization abnormalities secondary to artificial pacemakers not only affect ventricular depolarization (QRS) but are also characteristically associated with *secondary repolarization* (ST-T) abnormalities. With bundle branch blocks, the T wave is typically opposite in polarity to the last deflection of the QRS (Fig. 189-12). This discordance of the QRS–T-wave vectors is caused by the altered sequence of repolarization that occurs secondary

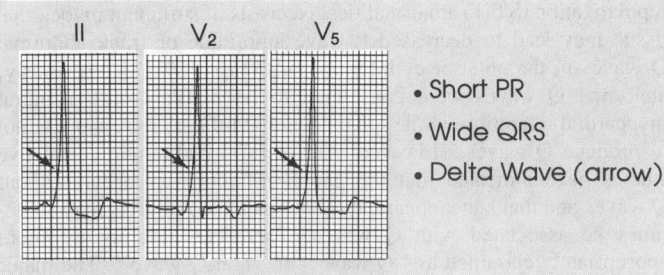

- Short PR
- Wide QRS
- Delta Wave (arrow)

FIGURE 189-13 Wolff-Parkinson-White pattern, due to ventricular preexcitation, causes a characteristic ECG triad.

TABLE 189-1 Differential diagnosis of a wide QRS complex

Intrinsic intraventricular delay (IVCD)*
  A Left bundle branch block and variants
  B Right bundle branch block and variants
  C Other nonspecific IVCD patterns
Extrinsic IVCD
  A Hyperkalemia
  B Drug-induced: type I antiarrhythmias and related agents (tricyclics, phenothiazines)
Ventricular beat (premature, escape, paced)
Ventricular preexcitation Wolff-Parkinson-White (WPW) pattern and variants

---

* Bundle branch block patterns may occur transiently. Note also that a spuriously wide QRS will occur if the ECG is unintentionally recorded at fast paper speeds (50 or 100 mm/s).

to altered depolarization. In contrast, *primary repolarization* abnormalities are independent of QRS changes and are related instead to actual alterations in the electrical properties of the myocardial fibers themselves (e.g., resting membrane potential or action potential duration), not just to changes in the sequence of repolarization. Ischemia, electrolyte imbalance, and drugs such as digitalis all cause such primary ST–T-wave changes. Primary and secondary T-wave changes may coexist. For example, T-wave inversions in the right precordial leads with left bundle branch block or in the left precordial leads with right bundle branch block may be important markers of underlying ischemia or other abnormalities.

Partial blocks ("hemiblocks") in the left bundle system (left anterior or posterior fascicular blocks) generally do not prolong QRS duration substantially but instead are associated with shifts in the frontal plane QRS axis (leftward or rightward, respectively). More complex combinations of fascicular and bundle branch blocks may occur involving the left and right bundle system. Examples of *bifascicular block* include right bundle branch block and left posterior fascicular block, right bundle branch block with left anterior fascicular block, and complete left bundle branch block. Chronic bifascicular block in an asymptomatic individual is associated with a relatively low risk of progression to high-degree AV heart block. In contrast, new bifascicular block with acute anterior myocardial infarction carries a much greater risk of complete heart block. Alternation of right and left bundle branch block is a sign of *trifascicular disease*. However, the presence of a prolonged PR interval and bifascicular block does not necessarily indicate trifascicular involvement, since this combination may arise with AV node disease and bifascicular block. Intraventricular conduction delays also can be caused by extrinsic (toxic) factors that slow ventricular conduction, particularly hyperkalemia or drugs (type 1 antiarrhythmic agents, tricyclic antidepressants, phenothiazines).

Prolongation of QRS duration does not necessarily indicate a conduction delay but may be due to *preexcitation* of the ventricles via a bypass tract, as in the Wolff-Parkinson-White (WPW) syndrome (Fig. 189-13) and related variants. The diagnostic triad of WPW consists of a wide QRS complex associated with a relatively short PR interval and slurring of the initial part of the QRS (delta wave), the latter due to aberrant activation of ventricular myocardium. The presence of a bypass tract predisposes to reentrant supraventricular tachyarrhythmias (Chap. 198). The differential diagnosis of a wide QRS complex is summarized in Table 189-1.

MYOCARDIAL ISCHEMIA AND INFARCTION The ECG is a cornerstone in the diagnosis of acute and chronic ischemic heart disease. The findings depend on several key factors: the nature of the process [reversible (i.e., ischemia) versus irreversible (i.e., infarction)], the duration (acute versus chronic), extent (transmural versus subendocardial), and localization (anterior versus inferoposterior), as well as the presence of other underlying abnormalities (ventricular hypertrophy, conduction defects).

Ischemia exerts complex time-dependent effects on the electrical properties of myocardial cells. Severe, acute ischemia lowers the resting membrane potential and shortens the duration of the action potential. Such changes cause a voltage gradient between normal and ischemic zones. As a consequence, current flows between these regions. These so-called currents of injury are represented on the surface ECG by deviation of the ST segment (Fig. 189-14). When the acute ischemia is *transmural*, the ST vector is usually shifted in the direction of the outer (epicardial) layers, producing ST elevations and sometimes, in the earliest stages of ischemia, tall, positive so-called hyperacute T waves over the ischemic zone. With ischemia confined primarily to the *subendocardium*, the ST vector typically shifts toward the subendocardium and ventricular cavity so that overlying (e.g., anterior precordial) leads show ST-segment depression (with ST elevation in lead aVR). Multiple factors affect the amplitude of acute ischemic ST deviations. Profound ST elevation or depression in multiple leads usually indicates very severe ischemia. Complete resolution of ST elevation promptly following thrombolytic therapy is a relatively specific, though not sensitive, marker of successful reperfusion.

The ECG leads are more helpful in localizing regions of Q wave than non-Q wave ischemia. For example, acute anterior wall ischemia leading to Q wave infarction is reflected by ST elevations or increased T-wave positivity (Fig. 189-15) in one or more of the precordial leads (V_1 to V_6) and leads I and aVL. Anteroseptal ischemia produces these changes in leads V_1 to V_3, apical or lateral ischemia in leads V_4 to V_6. Inferior wall ischemia produces changes in leads II, III, and aVF. Posterior wall ischemia may be indirectly recognized by *reciprocal* ST depressions in leads V_1 to V_3. Prominent reciprocal ST depressions in these leads also occur with certain inferior wall infarcts, particularly those with posterior or lateral wall extension. Right ventricular ischemia usually produces ST elevations in right-sided chest leads

FIGURE 189-14 Acute ischemia causes a current of injury. With predominant subendocardial ischemia, the resultant ST vector will be directed toward the inner layer of the affected ventricle and the ventricular cavity. Overlying leads therefore will record ST depression. With ischemia involving the outer ventricular layer (transmural or epicardial injury), the ST vector will be directed outward. Overlying leads will record ST elevation.

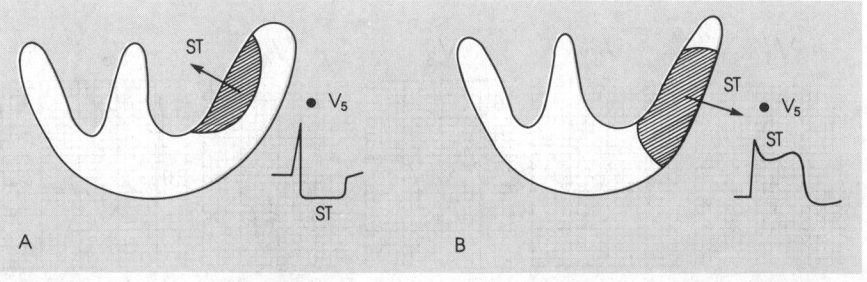

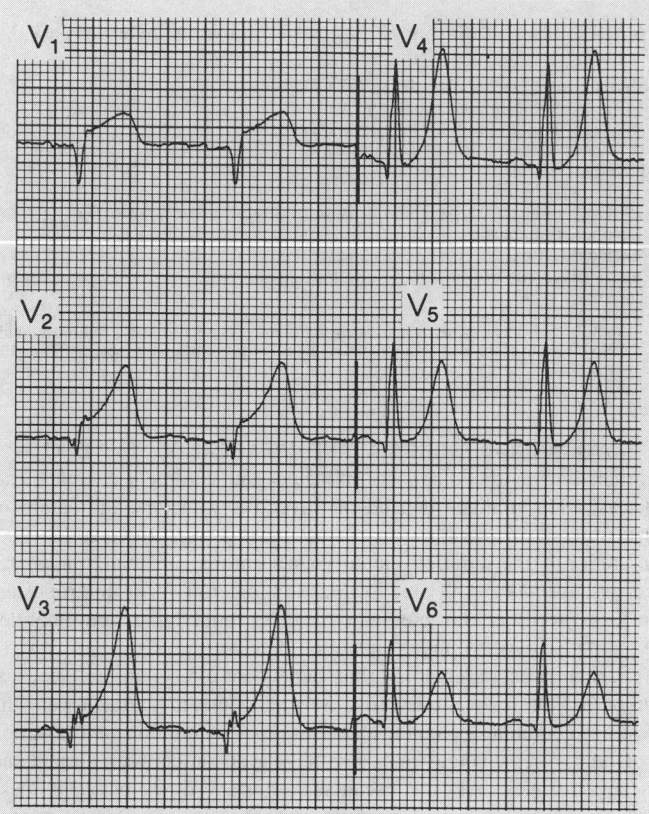

FIGURE 189-15 Hyperacute phase of anteroseptal myocardial infarction (MI). Note the tall positive T waves (V_2 to V_3) along with ST-segment elevations and Q waves (V_1 to V_3).

repolarization (ST-T) abnormalities. Necrosis of sufficient myocardial tissue may lead to decreased R-wave amplitude or frank abnormal Q waves in the anterior or inferior leads (Fig. 189-17). Previously, abnormal Q waves were considered to be markers of transmural myocardial infarction, while subendocardial infarcts were thought not to produce Q waves. However, careful ECG-pathologic correlative studies have indicated that transmural infarcts may occur without Q waves and that subendocardial (nontransmural) infarcts may sometimes be associated with Q waves. Therefore, infarcts are more appropriately classified as "Q-wave" or "non-Q-wave". The major acute ECG changes in syndromes of ischemic heart disease are schematically summarized in Fig. 189-18. Loss of depolarization forces due to posterior or lateral infarction may cause reciprocal increases in R-wave amplitude in leads V_1 and V_2 without diagnostic Q waves in any of the conventional leads. Atrial infarction may be associated with PR-segment deviations due to an atrial current of injury, changes in P-wave morphology, or atrial arrhythmias. In the weeks and months following infarction, these ECG changes may persist or begin to resolve. Complete normalization of the ECG following Q-wave infarction is uncommon but may occur, particularly with smaller infarcts. In contrast, persistent ST-segment elevations several weeks or more after a Q-wave infarct usually correlate with a severe underlying wall motion disorder (akinetic or dyskinetic zone), although not necessarily a frank ventricular aneurysm.

ECG changes due to ischemia may occur spontaneously or may be provoked by various exercise protocols (stress electrocardiography) (Chap. 203). In patients with severe ischemic heart disease, exercise testing is most likely to elicit signs of subendocardial ischemia (horizontal or downsloping ST depression in multiple leads). ST-segment elevation during exercise is most often observed after a Q-wave infarct. This repolarization change does not necessarily indicate active ischemia but correlates strongly with the presence of an underlying ventricular wall motion abnormality. However, in patients *without* prior infarction, transient ST-segment elevation with exercise is a reliable sign of transmural ischemia.

The ECG has important limitations in both sensitivity and specificity in the diagnosis of ischemic heart disease. Although a single normal ECG does not exclude ischemia or even acute infarction, a normal ECG *throughout* the course of an acute infarct is distinctly uncommon. Prolonged chest pain without diagnostic ECG changes, therefore, should always prompt a careful search for other noncoronary causes of chest pain (see Chap. 12). Furthermore, the diagnostic changes of acute or evolving ischemia are often masked by the presence of left bundle branch block, electronic ventricular pacemaker patterns, and WPW preexcitation. On the other hand, clinicians may overdiagnose ischemia or infarction based on the presence of ST-segment elevations or depressions, T-wave inversions, tall positive T waves, or Q waves *not* related to ischemic heart disease (pseudoinfarct patterns). For example, ST-segment elevations simulating ischemia may occur with acute pericarditis (Fig. 189-19) or myocarditis or as a normal variant ("early repolarization" pattern). Similarly, tall positive T waves do not invariably represent hyperacute ischemic changes but also may be due to normal variants, hyperkalemia, cerebrovascular injury, and left ventricular volume overload due to mitral or aortic regurgitation, among other causes. ST-segment elevations and tall, positive T waves are common findings in leads

(Fig. 189-7). When ischemic ST elevations occur as the earliest sign of acute infarction, they are typically followed within a period ranging from hours to days by evolving T-wave inversions and often by Q waves occurring in the same lead distribution. (T-wave inversions due to evolving or chronic ischemia correlate with prolongation of repolarization and are often associated with QT lengthening.) Reversible transmural ischemia, e.g., due to coronary vasospasm (Prinzmetal's variant angina), may cause transient ST-segment elevations without development of Q waves. Depending on the severity and duration of such ischemia, the ST elevations may either resolve completely within minutes or be followed by T-wave inversions that persist for hours or even days. Patients with ischemic chest pain who present with deep T-wave inversions in multiple precordial leads (e.g., V_1 to V_4) with or without cardiac enzyme elevations typically have severe obstruction in the left anterior descending coronary artery system (Fig. 189-16). In contrast, patients whose baseline ECG already shows abnormal T-wave inversions may develop T-wave normalization (pseudonormalization) during episodes of acute transmural ischemia.

With infarction, depolarization (QRS) changes often accompany

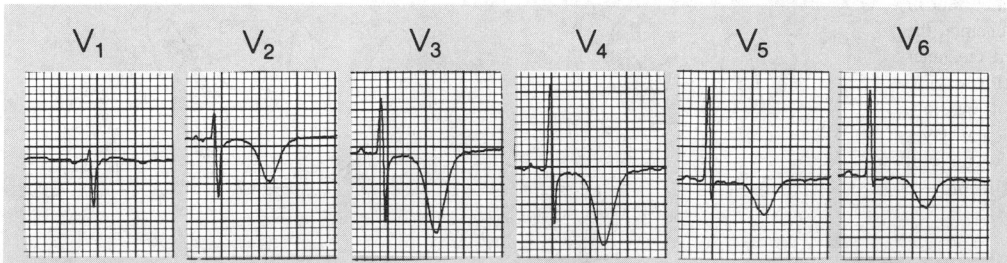

FIGURE 189-16 Severe anterior wall ischemia (with or without infarction) may cause prominent T-wave inversions in the precordial leads. This pattern is usually associated with a high-grade stenosis of the left anterior descending coronary artery.

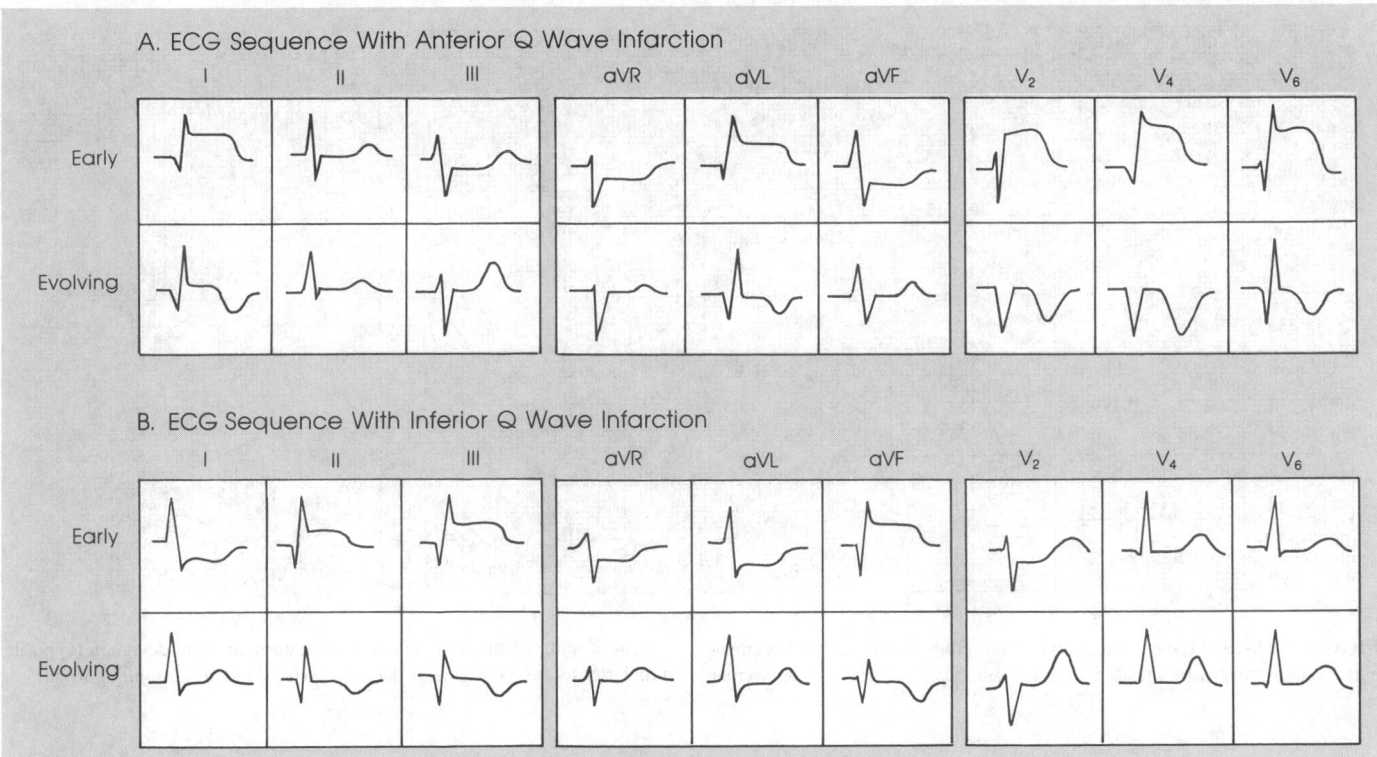

A. ECG Sequence With Anterior Q Wave Infarction

I II III aVR aVL aVF V₂ V₄ V₆

Early

Evolving

B. ECG Sequence With Inferior Q Wave Infarction

I II III aVR aVL aVF V₂ V₄ V₆

Early

Evolving

FIGURE 189-17 Sequence of depolarization and repolarization changes with (*A*) acute anterior and (*B*) acute inferior wall Q-wave infarctions. With anterior infarcts, ST elevation in leads I, aVL, and the precordial leads may be accompanied by reciprocal ST depressions in leads II, III, and aVF. Conversely, acute inferior (or posterior) infarcts may be associated with reciprocal ST depressions in leads V₁ to V₃. (*After Goldberger and Goldberger.*)

V₁ and V₂ in left bundle branch or left ventricular hypertrophy in the absence of ischemia. The differential diagnosis of Q waves (Table 189-2) includes physiologic or positional variants, ventricular hypertrophy, acute or chronic noncoronary myocardial injury, hypertrophic cardiomyopathy, and ventricular conduction disorders. Digitalis, ventricular hypertrophy, hypokalemia, and a variety of other factors may cause ST-segment depression mimicking subendocardial ischemia. Prominent T-wave inversion may occur with ventricular hypertrophy, cardiomyopathy, myocarditis, and cerebrovascular injury (particularly intracranial bleeds; Fig. 189-20), among many other conditions.

METABOLIC FACTORS AND DRUG EFFECTS A variety of metabolic and pharmacologic agents alter the ECG and in particular cause changes in repolarization (ST-T-U) and sometimes QRS prolongation (Table 189-1). Certain life-threatening electrolyte disturbances may be diagnosed initially and monitored from the ECG. *Hyperkalemia* produces a sequence of changes usually beginning with narrowing and peaking (tenting) of the T waves. Further elevation of extracellular K⁺ leads to AV conduction disturbances, diminution in P-wave amplitude, and widening of the QRS interval. Severe hyperkalemia eventually causes cardiac arrest with a slow sinusoidal type of mechanism ("sinewave" pattern) followed by asystole. *Hypokalemia* (Fig. 189-20) prolongs ventricular repolarization, often with prominent U waves. Prolongation of the QT interval (Fig. 189-20) is also seen with drugs that increase the duration of the ventricular action potential: type 1A antiarrhythmic agents and related drugs (e.g., quinidine, disopyramide, procainamide, tricyclic antidepressants, phenothiazines) and type III agents (amiodarone, sotalol). Marked QT prolongation, sometimes with deep, wide T-wave inversions, may occur with intracranial bleeds, particularly subarachnoid hemorrhage ("CVA T-wave" pattern) (Fig. 189-20). Systemic *hypothermia* (Fig. 189-20) also prolongs repolarization, usually with a distinctive convex elevation of the J point (Osborn wave). *Hypocalcemia* typically prolongs the QT interval (ST portion),

FIGURE 189-18 Variability of ECG patterns with myocardial ischemia. The ECG also may be normal or nonspecifically abnormal. Furthermore, these categorizations are not mutually exclusive. For example, a non-Q-wave infarct may evolve into a Q-wave infarct, ST elevations may be followed by a non-Q-wave infarct, or ST depressions and T-wave inversions may be followed by a Q wave infarct. (*After Goldberger.*)

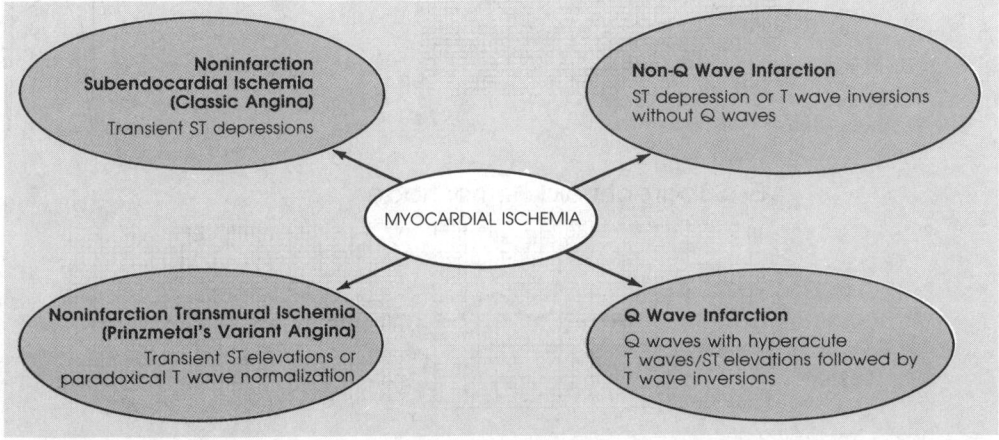

Noninfarction
Subendocardial Ischemia
(Classic Angina)
Transient ST depressions

Non-Q Wave Infarction
ST depression or T wave inversions
without Q waves

MYOCARDIAL ISCHEMIA

Noninfarction Transmural Ischemia
(Prinzmetal's Variant Angina)
Transient ST elevations or
paradoxical T wave normalization

Q Wave Infarction
Q waves with hyperacute
T waves/ST elevations followed by
T wave inversions

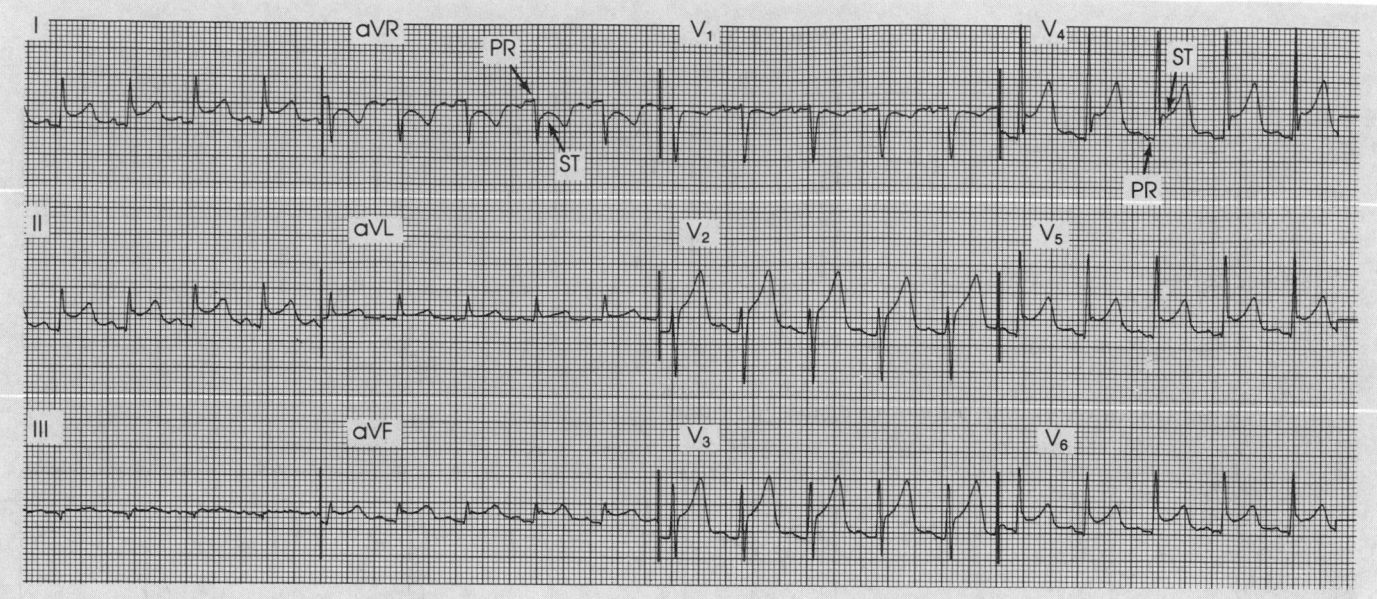

FIGURE 189-19 Acute pericarditis often produces diffuse ST-segment elevations (in this case in leads I, II, aVF, and V_2 to V_6) due to a ventricular current of injury. Note also the characteristic PR-segment deviation (opposite in polarity to the ST segment) due to a concomitant atrial injury current.

FIGURE 189-20 A variety of metabolic derangements, drug effects, and other factors may prolong ventricular repolarization with QT prolongation or prominent U waves. Repolarization prolongation, particularly due to hypokalemia or pharmacologic agents, indicates increased susceptibility to torsades de pointes type ventricular tachycardia. Hypothermia is associated with a distinctive convex "hump" at the J point (Osborn wave, *arrow*). Note QRS and QT prolongation along with sinus tachycardia in tricyclic antidepressant overdose.

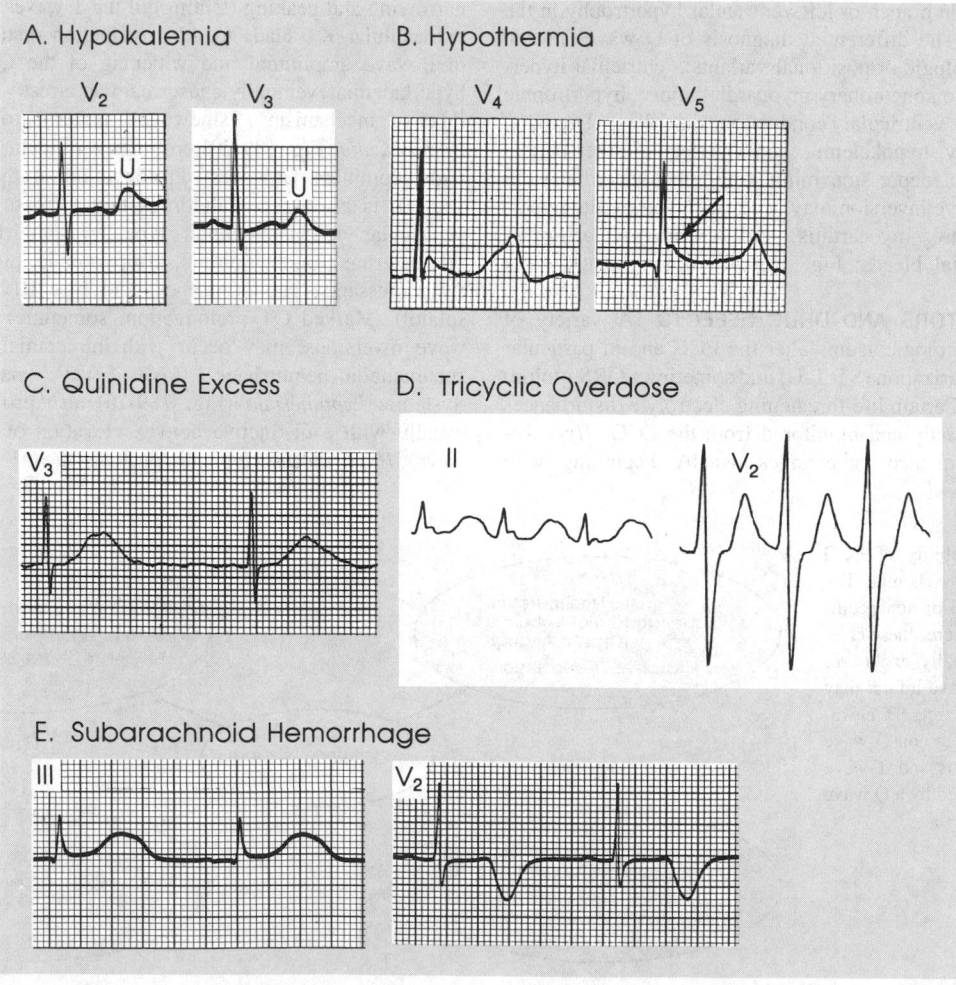

A. Hypokalemia

B. Hypothermia

C. Quinidine Excess

D. Tricyclic Overdose

E. Subarachnoid Hemorrhage

TABLE 189-2   Differential diagnosis of Q waves (with selected examples)

Physiologic or positional factors
 A Normal variant "septal" q waves
 B Normal variant Q waves in V_1 to V_2, aVL, III, and aVF
 C Left pneumothorax or dextrocardia: loss of lateral R-wave progression
Myocardial injury or infiltration
 A Acute processes: myocardial ischemia or infarction, myocarditis, hyperkalemia
 B Chronic processes: myocardial infarction, idiopathic cardiomyopathy, myocarditis, amyloid, tumor, sarcoid, scleroderma, Chagas' disease, echinococcus cyst
Ventricular hypertrophy/enlargement
 A Left ventricular (poor R-wave progression*)
 B Right ventricular (reversed R-wave progression[†] or poor R-wave progression, particularly with chronic obstructive lung disease)
 C Hypertrophic cardiomyopathy (may simulate anterior, inferior, posterior or lateral infarcts)
Conduction abnormalities
 A Left bundle branch block (poor R-wave progression*)
 B Wolff-Parkinson-White patterns

* Small or absent R waves in the right to midprecordial leads.
[†] Progressive decrease in R-wave amplitude from V_1 to the mid- or lateral precordial leads.
SOURCE: *After Goldberger.*

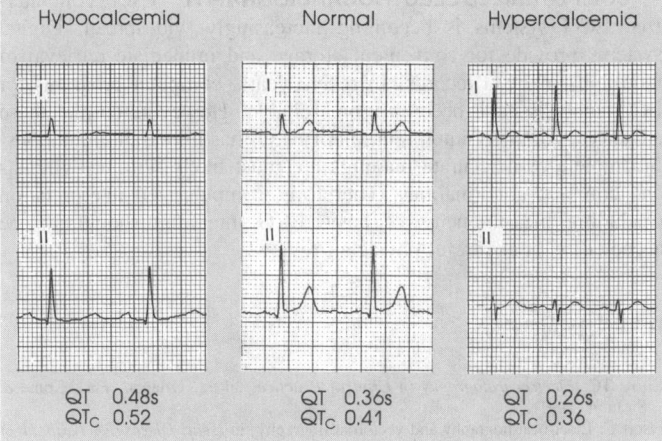

FIGURE 189-21 Prolongation of the Q-T interval (ST-segment portion) typical of hypocalcemia. Hypercalcemia may cause abbreviation of the ST segment and shortening of the QT interval.

while *hypercalcemia* shortens it (Fig. 189-21). Digitalis glycosides also shorten the QT interval, often with a characteristic "scooping" of the ST–T-wave complex (*digitalis effect*).

ELECTRICAL ALTERNANS   Electrical alternans, i.e., a beat-to-beat alternation in one or more components of the ECG signal, is a common type of nonlinear cardiovascular response to a variety of perturbations. For example, total electrical alternans (P-QRS-T) with sinus tachycardia is a relatively specific sign of pericardial effusion, often with cardiac tamponade (Fig. 189-22). The mechanism relates to a periodic swinging motion of the heart in the effusion at a frequency exactly one-half the heart rate. Alternation of the QRS complex (and sometimes R-R intervals) has been reported with rapid paroxysmal supraventricular tachycardias, usually involving a concealed bypass tract (Chap. 198). ST-segment alternans is a specific sign of severe transmural myocardial ischemia and may precede ventricular fibrillation. U-wave alternans may occur with idiopathic or acquired QT prolongation syndromes prior to the onset of *torsades de pointes* tachycardia (Chap. 198).

Many other factors are associated with ECG changes, particularly alterations in ventricular repolarization. T-wave flattening, minimal T-wave inversions or slight ST-segment depression ("nonspecific ST–T-wave changes") may occur with a variety of electrolyte and acid-base disturbances, a variety of infectious processes, central nervous system disorders, endocrine abnormalities, many drugs, ischemia, hypoxia, and virtually any type of cardiopulmonary abnormality. While subtle ST–T-wave changes may be markers of ischemia, transient nonspecific repolarization changes also may occur following a meal or with postural (orthostatic) change, hyperventilation, or exercise in healthy individuals.

CLINICAL INTERPRETATION OF THE ECG   Accurate analysis of ECGs require thoroughness and care. Interpretation should always be done in the context of the patient's age, gender, and clinical status. For example, T-wave inversions in leads V_1 to V_3, are more likely to represent a normal variant in a healthy, young adult woman ("persistent juvenile T-wave pattern") than similar findings in an elderly male with chest discomfort. Similarly, the likelihood that ST-segment depression during exercise testing represents ischemia must be considered in light of the prior probability of coronary artery disease (Chap. 10).

Many mistakes in ECG interpretation are errors of omission. Therefore, a systematic approach is desirable. The following 14 points should be analyzed carefully in every ECG: (1) standardization (calibration) and technical features (including lead placement and artifact), (2) heart rate, (3) rhythm, (4) PR interval, (5) QRS interval, (6) QT interval, (7) P waves, (8) QRS voltages, (9) mean QRS electrical axis, (10) precordial R-wave progression, (11) abnormal Q waves, (12) ST segments, (13) T waves, and (14) U waves.

Only after analyzing all these points should the interpretation be formulated. Where appropriate, important clinical correlates or inferences should be mentioned. For example, prolonged ventricular repolarization with prominent U waves should suggest hypokalemia or drug toxicity (e.g., due to quinidine or procainamide) (see Fig. 189-20). The combination of left atrial abnormality (enlargement) and signs of right ventricular hypertrophy suggests mitral stenosis. Low voltage with sinus tachycardia raises consideration of pericardial tamponade or chronic obstructive lung disease. Sinus tachycardia with QRS and QT (U) prolongation suggests tricyclic antidepressant overdose (Fig. 189-20). Comparison with previous ECGs is essential. The diagnosis and management of specific cardiac arrhythmias and conduction disturbances are discussed in Chaps. 197 and 198.

FIGURE 189-22 Beat-to-beat alternation in QRS axis/amplitude with sinus tachycardia is a highly specific, though not particularly sensitive, sign of pericardial effusion with cardiac tamponade.

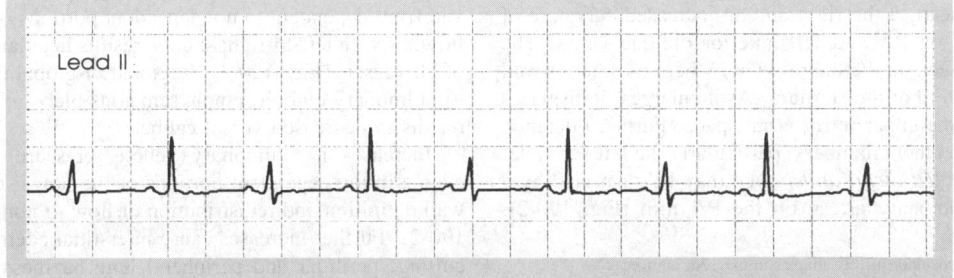

COMPUTERIZED ELECTROCARDIOGRAPHY   Use of computerized ECG systems is becoming increasingly widespread. Digital systems provide for convenient storage and immediate retrieval of thousands of ECG records. In recent years, computer programs for ECG analysis have become more reliable. However, despite these advances, computer interpretation of ECGs has important limitations. Incomplete or inaccurate readings are most likely with arrhythmias and complex abnormalities. Therefore, computerized interpretation (including measurements of basic ECG intervals) should not be accepted without careful physician review.

REFERENCES

Chou TC: *Electrocardiography in Clinical Practice*, 3d ed. Orlando, Fla., Grune & Stratton, 1991

Fisch C: Electrocardiography and vectorcardiography, in *Heart Disease: A Textbook of Cardiovascular Medicine*, 4th ed, E Braunwald (ed). Philadelphia, Saunders, 1992, pp 116–160

Goldberger AL: *Myocardial Infarction: Electrocardiographic Differential Diagnosis*, 4th ed. St. Louis, Mosby–Year Book, 1991

———, Goldberger E: *Clinical Electrocardiography: A Simplified Approach*, 4th ed. St. Louis, Mosby–Year Book, 1990

Hecht HS et al: Digital supine bicycle stress echocardiography: A new technique for evaluating coronary artery disease. J Am Coll Cardiol 21:950, 1993

Levy D et al: Determinants of sensitivity and specificity of electrocardiographic criteria for left ventricular hypertrophy. Circulation 81:815, 1990

MacFarland PW, Lawrie TDV: *Comprehensive Electrocardiography: Theory and Practice in Health and Disease*. New York, Pergamon Press, 1989

Marriott HJC: *Practical Electrocardiography*, 8th ed. Baltimore, Williams & Wilkins, 1988

190 NONINVASIVE METHODS OF CARDIAC EXAMINATION
Roentgenography, echocardiography, and radionuclide techniques

PATRICIA C. COME / RICHARD T. LEE / EUGENE BRAUNWALD*

ROENTGENOGRAPHY

The chest roentgenogram provides information about the size and configuration of the heart and great vessels and about pulmonary arterial and venous pressures and flow. Chamber dilatation usually produces changes in cardiac size and contour. Myocardial hypertrophy, in contrast, often results in wall thickening at the expense of cavity size, producing only a slight alteration of the cardiac silhouette. Posteroanterior (PA) and lateral chest roentgenograms are obtained routinely (Fig. 190-1). A full cardiac series, also including right and left anterior oblique views, and image-intensification fluoroscopy may be used to better assess chamber sizes, shapes, and movement; detect calcification; recognize pericardial effusion or thickening if epicardial fat can be identified; and assess movement of radiopaque valvular prostheses.

CARDIAC SILHOUETTE   Enlargement of the right atrium may cause bulging of the heart to the right and an increased curvature of the right heart border on PA and left anterior oblique views. The *right ventricle* is best seen on the lateral view, where its anterior wall lies behind the lower third of the sternum. As it enlarges, it displaces lung tissue, filling in the upper retrosternal space. Further dilatation may passively displace other chambers, particularly the left ventricle.

Enlargement of the *left atrial appendage* may be suspected by a bulge beneath the pulmonary artery on the PA film (Fig. 190-2).

* Dr. Joshua Wynne was a coauthor of this chapter in the 12th edition.

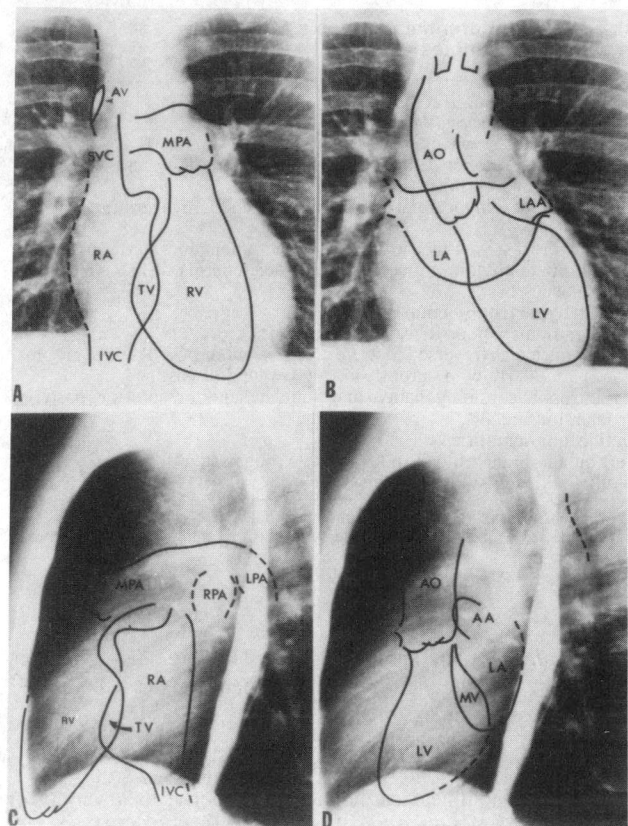

FIGURE 190-1   Posteroanterior (A,B) and lateral (C,D) views of the heart, demonstrating the positions of the cardiac chambers, valves, and interatrial and interventricular septa. Since these views were part of a larger cardiac series, the patient had swallowed barium (note the position of the barium-filled esophagus on the lateral view). AV = azygos vein; SVC = superior vena cava; RA = right atrium; IVC = inferior vena cava; TV = tricuspid valve; RV = right ventricle; MPA = main pulmonary artery; RPA = right pulmonary artery; LPA = left pulmonary artery; AO = aorta; LA = left atrium; LAA = left atrial appendage; LV = left ventricle; MV = mitral valve. [*From PC Come (ed), Diagnostic Cardiology. Reprinted with permission of Robert E. Dinsmore, M.D., and J.B. Lippincott Company, 1985*]

Dilatation of the body of the *left atrium* is best demonstrated by posterior displacement of the barium-filled esophagus in the lateral or right anterior oblique view. As the left atrium dilates further, its right border contacts right lung posteriorly, forming a second border or "double density" adjacent to the right atrial wall. The left bronchus may be displaced posteriorly and superiorly. The *left ventricle* enlarges inferiorly, posteriorly, and to the left, often increasing the cardiothoracic ratio (maximal cardiac diameter divided by maximal internal thoracic diameter, normally less than 0.50). The chest roentgenogram is a useful screening or initial test, but other imaging techniques, such as echocardiography, provide more definitive assessment of individual cardiac chambers.

PULMONARY VASCULATURE   Since pulmonary vessel size is proportional to flow, vessels normally taper from central to peripheral and from dependent to nondependent portions of the lungs. Increased flow, as with left-to-right shunts, results in enlargement and tortuosity of all vessels (Fig. 190-3). Regional or global reduction of flow, due to pulmonary emboli, emphysematous blebs, or a right-to-left shunt, results in decreased vessel caliber.

Increases in pulmonary venous pressure produce perivascular edema in the dependent portions of the lungs, causing loss of vessel wall definition and redistribution of flow to nondependent areas (Fig. 190-2). Further increases cause interstitial edema, with peribronchial cuffing, perihilar and peripheral lung haziness, and linear densities

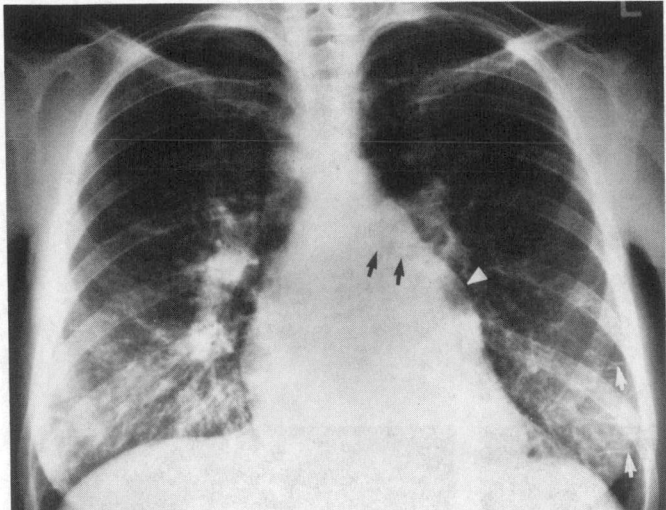

FIGURE 190-2 Posteroanterior chest roentgenogram from a patient with mitral stenosis and a mean pulmonary capillary wedge pressure of 38 mmHg. There is enlargement of the left atrial appendage (white arrowhead), uplifting of the left bronchus (black arrows) by an enlarged left atrium, multiple Kerley B lines (two of which are indicated by the white arrows in the left lower lung field), and redistribution of blood flow from the lung bases to the apices. The borders of the lower zone vessels have been obscured by the presence of interstitial pulmonary edema.

(Kerley B lines) perpendicular to the pleura. They represent fluid collection in the dependent interlobular septa. Alveolar pulmonary edema, with air bronchograms, may ultimately develop. There may be considerable temporal delay between hemodynamic changes and roentgenographic findings.

Pulmonary artery hypertension produces dilatation of the main pulmonary artery and its central branches. When associated with conditions increasing pulmonary arteriolar resistance, such as primary pulmonary hypertension, the distal pulmonary arteries often appear small (''pruned'').

Computed tomography, *magnetic resonance imaging*, and *positron emission tomography* are other noninvasive techniques used to provide information about the heart and vessels (see Chap. 191).

ECHOCARDIOGRAPHY

Echocardiography uses ultrasound to image the heart and great vessels. A transducer containing a piezoelectric crystal, which interconverts electrical and mechanical (i.e., sound) energy, functions both as the transmitter of sound and as the receiver of reflected waves. Three types of studies are performed: M-mode, two-dimensional, and Doppler. In *M-mode echocardiography*, a single transducer, emitting 1000 to 2000 pulses per second along a single line, provides an ''ice-pick'' view of the heart, with excellent *temporal* resolution. When beam direction is changed, the heart can be scanned from the ventricles to the aorta and left atrium. *Two-dimensional echocardiography* (Figs. 190-4, 190-5, and 190-6) produces an image in two dimensions by steering the sound beam through an arc of up to 90° some 30 times per second. It provides excellent *spatial* resolution, permitting analysis of structural movement in real time from multiple transducer positions on the chest and upper abdomen. Commonly assessed views are the parasternal long and short axis, apical four- and two-chamber, and subcostal views. It is also possible to obtain imaging and Doppler echocardiographic studies via the esophagus using a probe mounted at the tip of a flexible gastroscope. Because of the proximity of the esophagus to the heart (especially the left atrium) and to the descending aorta, and also because of the lack of interposed lung or bone between the esophagus and these structures, excellent images can be obtained

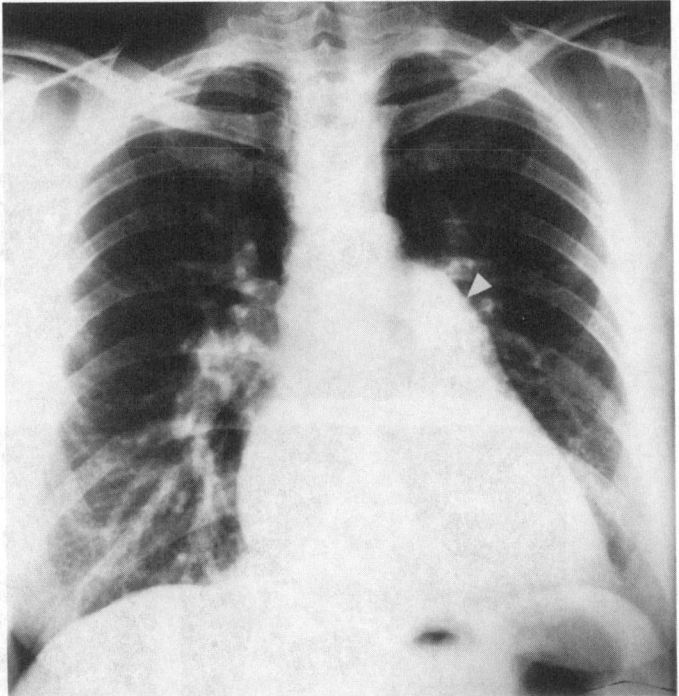

FIGURE 190-3 Posteroanterior chest roentgenogram from a patient with an atrial septal defect resulting in a large left-to-right shunt (pulmonic to systemic flow ratio by radionuclide ventriculogram of 3:1). The main pulmonary artery is enlarged (white arrowhead), as are all peripheral pulmonary vessels, reflecting the increase in pulmonary blood flow. The lateral borders of the lower zone vessels remain distinct, because there is no interstitial pulmonary edema. (*Courtesy of Sven Paulin, M.D.*)

FIGURE 190-4 Two-dimensional long- and short-axis views in diastole from patients with marked reduction of effective mitral valve orifice area (MVO) due to mitral stenosis (MS) and left atrial (LA) myxoma (MYX). In the MS patient, the valve leaflets are thickened, particularly at their tips, and there is markedly reduced diastolic separation of the anterior and posterior leaflets. The LA is enlarged. The LA MYX is seen to prolapse into the MVO during diastole, causing obstruction. RV = right ventricle; LV = left ventricle; AoV = aortic valve.

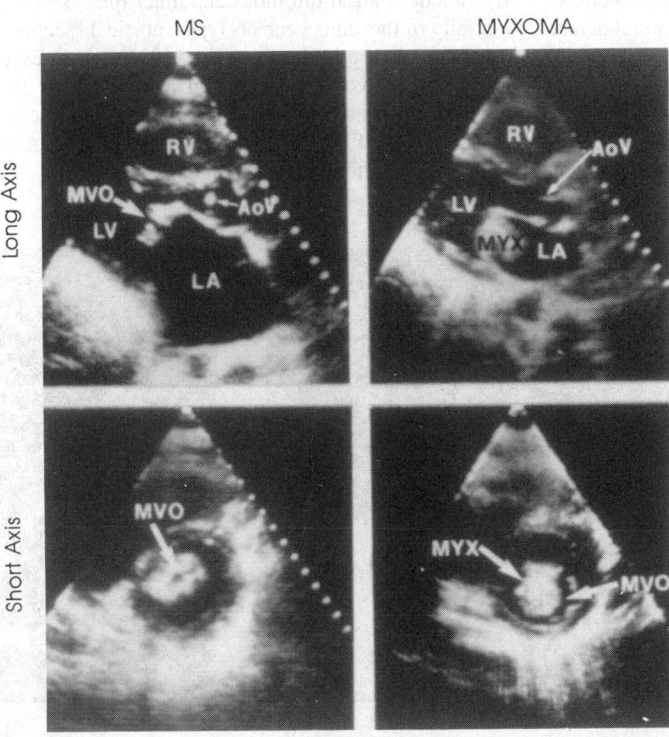

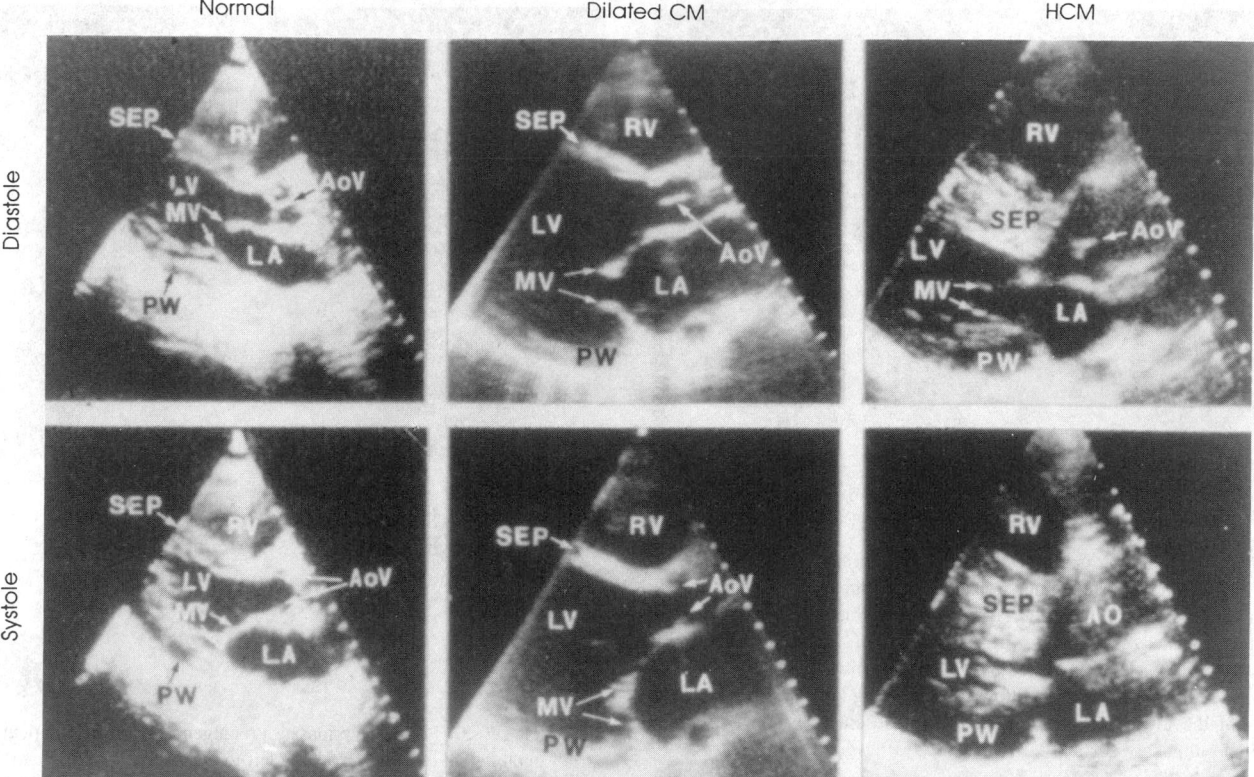

FIGURE 190-5 Long-axis parasternal views of the left ventricle in diastole and systole in a normal individual and in patients with dilated cardiomyopathy (CM) and hypertrophic cardiomyopathy (HCM). Normal diastolic wall thicknesses and normal systolic wall thickening and excursion are illustrated in the left panels. In the patient with dilated CM, left ventricular (LV) and left atrial (LA) diameters are increased, and there is markedly reduced systolic thickening and excursion of the septum (SEP) and posterior wall (PW). In the patient with HCM, the SEP is abnormally thick and highly echogenic. The LV cavity is small in diastole and almost disappears during systolic contraction. RV = right ventricle; MV = mitral valve; AoV = aortic valve.

with high-frequency transducers. Transesophageal echocardiography, therefore, may facilitate cardiac evaluation of patients with suboptimal transthoracic scans, such as ventilated patients or those with obesity or emphysema. Compared with transthoracic echocardiography, transesophageal echocardiography is more sensitive for detection of prosthetic valve dysfunction, atrial thrombus and other masses, atrial septal defects (especially of the sinus venosus type), aortic dissection, and complications of infective endocarditis (Fig. 190-6). It is used intraoperatively to monitor myocardial function and to assess the results of valvular repair and correction of congenital heart defects.

Doppler echocardiography (Fig. 190-7) detects blood flow velocity and turbulence. When sound encounters moving red blood cells, the frequency of its reflected signal is altered. The magnitude of the change *(Doppler shift)* indicates the velocity V of blood flow with respect to the sound beam:

$$V = \frac{C \times (\text{Doppler shift})}{(2 \times \text{emitted frequency}) \cos \theta}$$

where C is the speed of sound in tissue, and θ is the angle between the Doppler beam and the mean axis of blood flow. An upward shift (increased frequency of the reflected sound) indicates blood motion toward the transducer and a downward shift, motion away.

There are several types of Doppler studies, all of which can be performed using a single probe. Pulsed Doppler echocardiography,

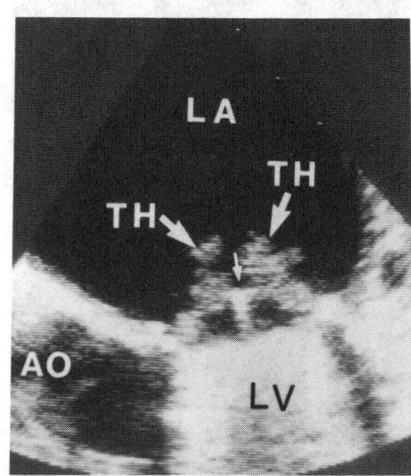

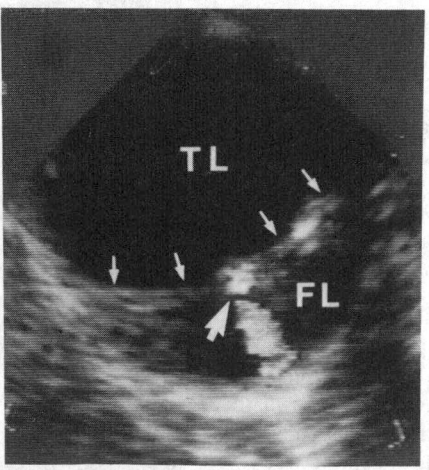

FIGURE 190-6 Transesophageal echocardiograms. *A.* An image in systole from a patient with a Medtronic Hall mitral valve prosthesis who presented with a cerebral embolus. Thrombi (TH) are seen to arise from the annular insertion points of the prosthesis. The small white arrow indicates part of the prosthesis. LA = left atrium; LV = left ventricle; AO = aortic root.

B. Transverse view of the descending thoracic aorta in a patient presenting with aortic dissection. Color flow imaging (white) demonstrates flow from the true lumen (TL) into the false lumen (FL). The site of an initimal tear is indicated by the larger white arrow. The small white arrows indicate the intimal flap.

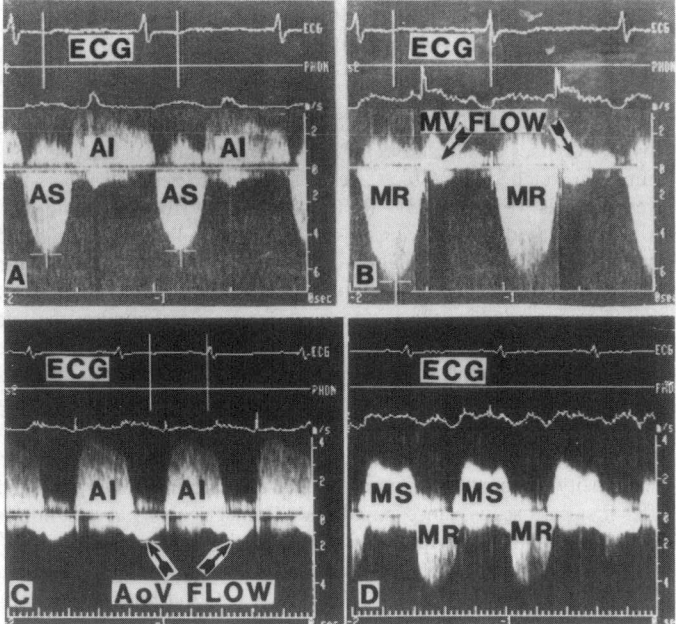

FIGURE 190-7 Continuous-wave Doppler studies, performed with the probe positioned at the apex, from one patient (*A, B*) with aortic stenosis (AS), aortic insufficiency (AI), and mitral regurgitation (MR) and from another patient (*C, D*) with mital stenosis (MS), severe MR, and AI. Flow away from the transducer, in the AS and MR jets, is depicted below the center (zero flow) line, while flow toward the transducer, in the AI and MS jets, is depicted above the center line. Flow velocity (*V*) in meters per second is given on the right side of each panel. As expected from knowledge of points of crossover between aortic, left ventricular, and left atrial pressures, the AS signal is shorter in duration than the MR signal and has a lower velocity. The AI signal is of longer duration than the MS signal. Instantaneous pressure gradients (*P*) across the valves can be calculated using the equation, $P = 4V^2$. Peak *V* of 5.1 m/s in the AS jet indicates a peak left ventricular to aortic *P* of 104 mmHg, while the peak *V* of 6.8 m/s in the MR jet indicates a left ventricular to left atrial systolic *P* of 185 mmHg. Peak aortic to left ventricular diastolic *P* in the AI jet is 81 mmHg, and peak left atrial to left ventricular *P* in the MS jet is 40 mmHg. Mean gradient, calculated using an off-line computer system, in the MS jet was markedly elevated at 26 mmHg.

which uses a single crystal to assess flow velocity and turbulence within operator-selected areas of interest in the heart and great vessels, permits excellent spatial localization of flow disturbances resulting from valvular stenosis and regurgitation and from shunts. Quantitation of high-flow velocity requires a continuous-wave transducer with two separate, adjacent crystals, one that continuously transmits sound and one that continuously receives reflected sound. Since continuous-wave transducers cannot spatially localize flow disturbances, optimal assessment of flow within the heart and vessels generally requires both pulsed- and continuous-wave technology. Combined two-dimensional echocardiography and pulsed Doppler techniques permit calculation of flow volumes across cardiac valves and, therefore, of cardiac output, pulmonic-to-systemic flow ratios, and regurgitant fractions. Pressure gradients (*P*) across restrictive orifices such as cardiac valves can be calculated using the modified Bernoulli equation, $P = 4V^2$, where *P* is the pressure gradient in mmHg and *V* the velocity in m/s.

Doppler color flow imaging is a complicated, combined imaging and Doppler technique in which blood flow direction, relative velocity, and turbulence are depicted by various colors superimposed on a two-dimensional image of the heart. It should be recognized, however, that color Doppler is extremely sensitive for regurgitation. Small signs of mitral, tricuspid, and pulmonic insufficiency are imaged in the majority of even normal individuals.

VALVULAR HEART DISEASE Imaging echocardiography can detect abnormalities of valve thickness and movement responsible for stenosis and regurgitation. In addition, the heart's response to pressure

or volume overload can be assessed in terms of chamber dilatation, hypertrophy, and wall movement. Doppler techniques permit evaluation of regurgitation and stenosis (see also Chap. 201.)

Mitral stenosis The echocardiographic appearance of a restricted valve opening, due to leaflet thickening and commissural fusion, and of shortened, thickened chordae is virtually diagnostic of rheumatic deformity (Fig. 190-4, *left*). Planimetry of the mitral area in the diastolic short-axis view and evaluation of the rate of falloff of the estimated transmitral diastolic pressure gradient by Doppler permit quite reliable estimation of valve area. Using the Doppler technique, mitral valve area (MVA) in square centimeters can be estimated with the equation MVA = 220 divided by duration of time (in milliseconds) necessary for the peak diastolic pressure gradient to decrease by 50 percent. Other causes of inflow obstruction, such as atrial myxoma (Fig. 190-4, *right*) or thrombus, massive annular calcification, supravalvular ring, cor triatriatum, and parachute mitral valve also may be detected.

Mitral regurgitation Systolic mitral competence depends on normal function of the mitral leaflets and their supporting structures, including the annulus, chordae tendineae, papillary muscles, and surrounding myocardium. Two-dimensional transthoracic or transesophageal techniques are useful for recognizing the etiology of mitral regurgitation, which includes rheumatic disease, prolapse, flail leaflets resulting from chordal or papillary muscle rupture, annular calcification, atrioventricular canal defects, myxomas, endocarditis, hypertrophic cardiomyopathy, and ventricular dysfunction. Doppler mapping provides a gross estimate of the severity of regurgitation.

Aortic stenosis Subvalvular, valvular, and supravalvular obstruction can generally be detected by two-dimensional echocardiography. Systolic leaflet doming and an unusual number or size of cusps (two in a bicuspid valve) suggest congenital valve disease. Acquired fibrosis and calcification cause valve thickening. Doppler detection of high-flow velocity across the valve, corresponding to a high transvalvular gradient, indicates the presence of stenosis. Lesser flow velocities do not, however, exclude stenosis because both reduced stroke volume and inability to position the Doppler beam parallel to flow may appreciably decrease measured velocities. If velocity can be reliably measured, aortic valve area (AVA) can be quantitated.

Aortic regurgitation Dilatation of the aortic root and aortic dissection can be distinguished from valve leaflet abnormalities causing regurgitation, including congenital disease, sclerosis, endocarditis, prolapse, and flail cusps. The presence and spatial extent of regurgitation is evaluated by Doppler study.

Tricuspid and pulmonary valve disease Two-dimensional echocardiography allows visualization of right-sided valves and can detect changes in structure and movement due to rheumatic deformity, Ebstein's malformation, prolapse, flail cusps, endocarditis, congenital dysplasia, and thickening due to carcinoid, amyloid, Loeffler's endocarditis, or endocardial fibrosis. Systolic doming of the pulmonic valve is characteristic of pulmonic stenosis. Stenosis and regurgitation are assessed by Doppler techniques. The flow velocity in a tricuspid regurgitant jet can be used to estimate right ventricular and pulmonary arterial systolic pressures.

Prosthetic valves (Fig. 190-6) Mechanical prostheses are difficult to evaluate, because their intrinsically high echogenicity often interferes with recognition of valve motion, vegetations, thrombi, and regurgitation. Abnormalities of bioprostheses, including fibrosis, calcification, vegetations, tears, and regurgitation, are more easily recognized. Transesophageal echocardiography should be considered strongly in patients with suspected prosthetic mitral valve dysfunction when transthoracic evaluation is nonrevealing. Angiography and hemodynamic study may be necessary for full evaluation.

Endocarditis Valvular vegetations, characterized by masses of shaggy-appearing echoes, are evident in most patients with native valve endocarditis (Chap. 85). They are less commonly identified in prosthetic valve endocarditis. Transesophageal techniques are more sensitive and, additionally, can readily detect perivalvular abscesses.

Left ventricle A combination of M-mode and two-dimensional echocardiography is widely used to measure left ventricular size, wall thickness, and function. The rate of wall thinning in diastole may permit assessment of diastolic function, and the percentage of shortening of the minor axis, normally greater than 28 percent, and the mean velocity of circumferential fiber shortening are useful measurements of systolic performance. These indexes of systolic performance are influenced, however, by preload and afterload as well as by myocardial contractility. Analyses of end-systolic pressure-dimension relations, which are independent of preload and incorporate afterload, provide better information regarding contractile function. Estimates of global ventricular performance, based on icepick M-mode views, are useful, however, only when ventricular shape is normal and systolic movement relatively symmetric in extent and timing. Two-dimensional echocardiography, which images the ventricle in a number of different planes, improves assessment of volumes and function, particularly in patients with asymmetric contraction resulting from ischemic heart disease, in whom localized regional wall motion can be present. The left ventricular apex can be visualized only by two-dimensional techniques. Complications of infarction, including wall movement abnormalities, true and false aneurysms, myocardial rupture (septal, papillary muscle, or free wall), thrombi, and mitral regurgitation, may be detected. In patients being evaluated for ischemic heart disease, two-dimensional images can be recorded during exercise or pacing stress or during pharmacologic challenge with vasodilators (adenosine or dipyridamole) or with the beta agonist dobutamine. The development of one or more wall movement abnormalities, not present at rest, provides a highly sensitive and specific means of recognizing ischemia.

Echocardiography permits recognition of *cardiomyopathy* (Chap. 205), and classification into dilated, hypertrophic, and restrictive-obliterative types (Fig. 190-5). In dilated cardiomyopathy, both ventricles are generally enlarged and poorly contracting, and wall thicknesses are normal or only slightly increased. In contrast, appreciable ventricular hypertrophy (usually involving the septum asymmetrically), small ventricular size, enhanced systolic performance, and impaired diastolic relaxation characterize hypertrophic cardiomyopathy. Systolic anterior movement of the mitral valve to abut the septum, partial midsystolic aortic valve closure, and increased left ventricular outflow tract velocity correlate with dynamic obstruction. Increased wall thickness, biatrial enlargement, mitral and tricuspid regurgitation, and slowed diastolic filling characterize infiltrative disorders. In patients presenting with heart failure, echocardiographic recognition of whether ventricular dysfunction is predominantly systolic or diastolic has important prognostic and therapeutic implications.

Pericardial effusion Echocardiography can detect effusions as small as 15 mL. Diastolic compression of heart chambers, usually the right atrium and ventricle, and exaggerated respiratory variation in transvalvular flow velocities may suggest tamponade.

Cardiac masses Most masses involving the heart and pericardium are easily recognized. They include myxomas (Fig. 190-4), other primary and secondary tumors, and thrombi. The left atrium and its appendage are best studied by transesophageal echocardiography.

Congenital heart disease Since valvular abnormalities and relationships of atria, valves, ventricles, and great vessels can easily be recognized by two-dimensional echocardiography, this technique has revolutionized the diagnosis of congenital heart disease. Contrast and Doppler echocardiography, especially color flow mapping, facilitate detection of shunts and of valvular stenosis and regurgitation.

RADIONUCLIDE IMAGING OF THE HEART

There are five major clinical indications for radionuclide study of the heart: (1) assessment of systolic and diastolic ventricular function using radionuclide ventriculography, (2) identification and quantification of intracardiac shunts using radioangiocardiography, (3) assessment of myocardial perfusion using ionic tracers, principally thallium 201, (4) detection of acute myocardial necrosis with infarct-avid radionuclides, and (5) assessment of myocardial metabolism by means of positron emission tomography (see Chap. 191).

VENTRICULAR PERFORMANCE Radionuclide ventriculography (RVG) uses a radioactive intravascular indicator, usually technetium 99m attached to red blood cells, to delineate heart chambers and great vessels (Fig. 190-8). RVGs may be performed using two different methods. In the *first-pass* technique, radiotracer is injected intravenously, and a scintillation camera tracks its transit through the right heart, lungs, and left heart. In the *equilibrium*, or *gated*, method, counts are recorded in at least two views from several hundred cardiac cycles following uniform distribution of radiotracer throughout the blood pool. The scintigraphic information in each cycle is divided into multiple frames (often 30 or more), using the ECG as a timing reference. Counts from corresponding frames of each cycle are then summed by computer to provide images of the spatial distribution and density of counts over time. Gated scans are frequently obtained after first-pass scans, since no additional injection of radionuclide is required. Because detected counts, after background subtraction, are proportional to blood volume, these studies permit accurate estimation of chamber volumes, rates of ventricular ejection and filling, left-to-right ventricular stroke volume ratios, and ventricular ejection fractions. Using a time-activity curve generated from a region of interest over the left ventricle, left ventricular ejection fraction (LVEF), a widely used index of left ventricular function (Chap. 194), can be calculated as $LVEF = EDC - ESC/EDC$, where EDC is end-diastolic counts and ESC is end-systolic counts. Repeated scans can be obtained up to 20 h after injection, permitting assessment of the effects of interventions, such as exercise and drugs, on ventricular performance.

RVG may be used to detect patients with chronic ischemic heart disease. Since resting function may be normal, exercise is often used to provoke ischemia. Scans are obtained at rest and at peak exercise.

FIGURE 190-8 End-diastolic and end-systolic gated blood pool images from a normal individual (with estimated left and right ventricular ejection fractions of 69 and 45 percent, respectively) and from a patient with idiopathic dilated cardiomyopathy and marked, global reduction of left ventricular systolic function (left ventricular ejection fraction of 23 percent). In the patient with cardiomyopathy, there is very little change in left ventricular cavity size or count density from diastole to systole. The right ventricle, however, shows normal function, with an ejection fraction of 57 percent. RV = right ventricle; LV = left ventricle.

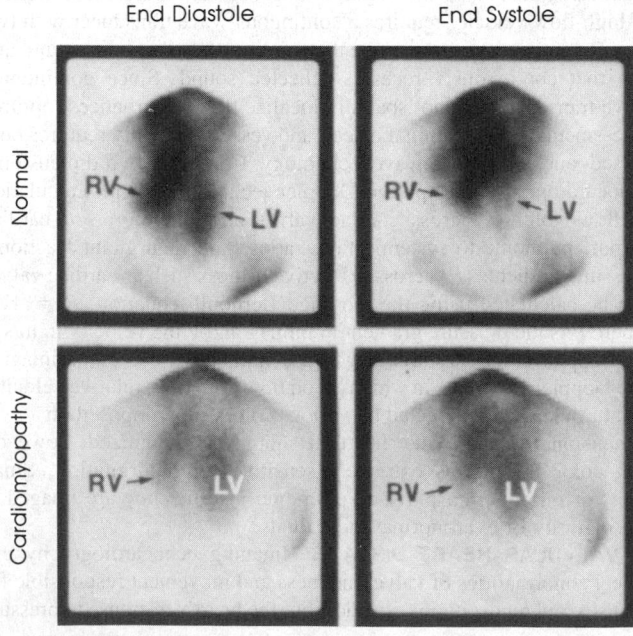

End Diastole   End Systole

Failure to increase left ventricular ejection fraction by at least 5 units (e.g., from 40 to 45 percent) and development of one or more regional wall movement abnormalities have a sensitivity and specificity of approximately 90 and 60 percent, respectively, for detection of significant ischemic heart disease. The test is most helpful in patients with an intermediate pretest probability of disease. Low resting ejection fractions after acute infarction have been correlated with increased short- and long-term morbidity and mortality. Mitral regurgitation, septal rupture, and aneurysms resulting from infarction also may be detected. RVG can assess systolic and diastolic function in patients with cardiomyopathy (Fig. 190-8) or volume overload. A reduced resting ejection fraction correlates with a poor prognosis in patients with mitral or aortic regurgitation, even after valve replacement. The added value of exercise RVG in detecting reduced myocardial reserve due to volume overload remains controversial. Thrombi and other tumors may be recognized, but RVG is less sensitive than echocardiography.

SHUNT SCINTIGRAPHY Assessment of left-to-right shunts utilizes a modification of the first-pass RVG in which the "region of interest" is focused over an area of lung. Following rapid injection of radiotracer into a large vein, usually the external jugular, the pulmonary time-activity curve is recorded by a gamma camera–computer system. Normally, counts increase sharply as the bolus reaches the lung underlying the detector. Following peak activity, there is a smooth descent and a later, smaller increase in counts representing normal recirculation of the radiotracer following systemic circulation. Left-to-right shunts cause premature interruption of the descent due to early reappearance of radioactivity within the lung. Computer analysis of the areas under the curve permits reliable determination of the ratio of pulmonic-to-systemic blood flow. Right-to-left shunts also may be recognized and quantified.

MYOCARDIAL PERFUSION IMAGING The potassium analogue thallium 201, cyclotron-produced with a half-life of 72 h, is the most commonly used agent to assess myocardial perfusion. Its active uptake by normal myocardial cells is proportional to regional blood flow. Areas of myocardial necrosis, fibrosis, and ischemia show reduced thallium accumulation ("cold spots") on images obtained soon after injection. Following its initial accumulation within cells, however, thallium 201 continues to exchange with the systemic pool. After several hours, equilibration occurs; viable myocardial cells having intact membrane function contain nearly equal concentrations.

Thallium 201 scintigraphy is used most commonly to detect exercise-induced ischemia (Fig. 190-9). Thallium is injected intravenously at peak exercise, and images are obtained 5 to 10 minutes later in several projections using either planar imaging or single photon emission computed tomography (SPECT). The images may be analyzed qualitatively or quantitatively using computer algorithms. Normal scans show relatively homogeneous distribution of activity, while those of patients with infarction or ischemia typically demonstrate one or more "cold spots." Because of continued exchange of thallium between viable cells and the systemic pool, however, most initial defects due to ischemia "fill in" on repeat imaging several hours later. Some, however, require up to 24 h for redistribution or are best identified following reinjection of thallium 4 h after exercise, but areas of infarction demonstrate persistent reduction of uptake.

Compared with routine exercise electrocardiography, exercise thallium scintigraphy increases the sensitivity for detection of coronary disease from approximately 60 to 80 percent and increases specificity slightly from about 80 to 90 percent. It is most useful in patients with atypical chest pain in whom the exercise ECG is nondiagnostic or uninterpretable due to baseline ST abnormalities, left bundle branch block, ventricular hypertrophy, or drug and electrolyte effects; in patients who fail to achieve 85 percent of predicted maximal heart rate; and in patients with a high likelihood of a false-positive exercise ECG study. Thallium scanning improves localization of ischemia and provides prognostic information, since the presence and number of redistributing defects correlate with the incidence of future cardiac events. Thallium scintigraphy also has been used to detect ischemia

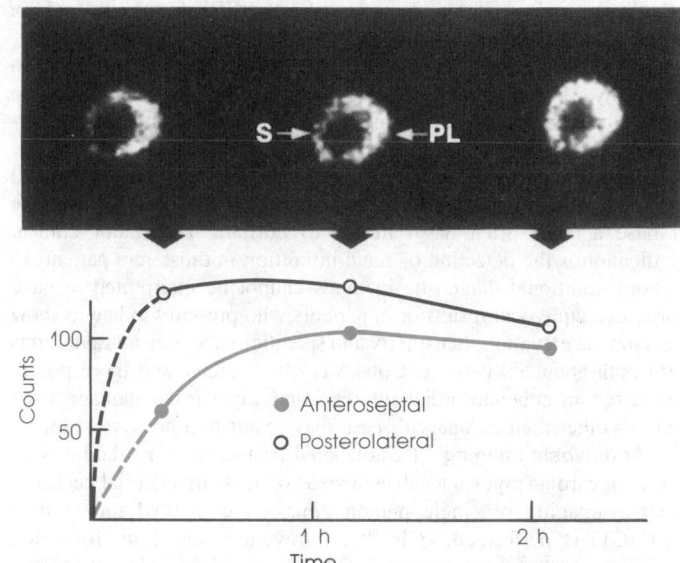

FIGURE 190-9 Serial thallium 201 scintigrams obtained in the 45° LAO projection in a patient undergoing exercise testing for evaluation of chest pain. The immediate postexercise image (*left*) demonstrates decreased perfusion of the septum. The 1- and 2-h delayed images (*middle and right*) demonstrate "filling in" of the defect, reflecting redistribution. The computer-derived time-activity curves (*bottom*) confirm the significant reduction in initial counts in the septum, relative to the posterolateral wall, and demonstrate near equalization of activity by 2 h. S = septum; PL = posterolateral wall. [*From PC Come (ed), Diagnostic Cardiology. Reprinted with permission of George A. Beller, M.D., and J.B. Lippincott Company,* 1985]

during spontaneous pain, pacing, and adenosine- and dipyridamole-induced coronary vasodilation. Dipyridamole thallium imaging appears to be as sensitive and specific as exercise thallium scintigraphy for detection of ischemic heart disease. It should be considered for patients unable to exercise, including those with peripheral vascular disease who have an increased risk of cardiac morbidity and mortality with vascular surgery.

Thallium scanning does not distinguish new from old infarcts and is less accurate than serum enzyme analysis in detecting acute necrosis. It does, however, offer prognostic information. Patients with smaller defects have better survival rates. On submaximal exercise thallium tests following infarction, the presence of multiple fixed or redistributing defects and/or increased lung uptake of thallium (probably representing transudation into the lung during periods of high pulmonary capillary pressure) identifies patients at higher risk for postinfarction morbidity and mortality.

The new perfusion imaging agents technetium 99m Sesta-MIBI and technetium 99m teboroxime offer some advantages over thallium 201. They are generator-produced, permitting continuous on-site availability. Image resolution is enhanced by both the ideal energy of technetium 99m for standard gamma camera imaging and its shorter half-life, which permits use of higher doses of radioactivity. Given the high count rates achieved, first-pass imaging for assessment of ejection fraction can be performed in addition to perfusion imaging. Redistribution of Sesta-MIBI is minimal, allowing scanning to be performed for up to 6 h after injection. Patients suspected of having acute infarction can therefore be injected at the bedside and stabilized or even treated with a thrombolytic agent prior to imaging. The image, of course, reflects the distribution of coronary blood flow at the time of injection, not at the time of imaging. However, separate injections are required to differentiate perfusion abnormalities due to ischemia from those due to infarction. Teboroxime has rapid washout from the myocardium, permitting dual-injection rest and exercise studies to be completed within 1 h. Alternatively, taking advantage of the different energy spectra of thallium 201 and technetium 99m, thallium can be injected at rest and Sesta-MIBI during exercise for dual postexercise imaging.

IMAGING OF NECROTIC MYOCARDIUM   Pyrophosphate scintigraphy   Pyrophosphate labeled with technetium 99m binds to calcium and organic macromolecules in irreversibly damaged myocardial cells, producing an image with increased uptake ("hot spot"). Scans are most likely to be positive when injections are performed 48 to 72 h after suspected infarction, when the elevated creatine kinase activity often has returned to normal. The major clinical indication is the detection of acute infarction in those rare patients in whom traditional diagnostic methods cannot be interpreted or have provided equivocal results or in patients who present too late to show an enzyme elevation. Sensitivity and specificity for transmural infarcts are both about 90 percent. Uptake is often fainter and more poorly localized in subendocardial infarcts, and myocardial damage from causes other than coronary disease may result in a positive scan.

Antimyosin imaging   Radiolabeled fragments of antibodies specific for cardiac myosin localize in areas of acute myocardial necrosis. Planar imaging or single photon emission computed tomography (SPECT) is performed 48 h after intravenous injection, following disappearance of the radionuclide from the blood pool. This technique can detect, localize, and quantitate acute myocardial infarction and also appears promising for detection of acute myocarditis and for prediction of cardiac transplant rejection.

POSITRON EMISSION TOMOGRAPHY   See Chap. 191.

REFERENCES

BANSAL RC et al: Biplane transesophageal echocardiography: Technique, image orientation, and preliminary experience in 131 patients. J Am Soc Echocardiogr 3:348, 1990

FREEMAN MR et al: Role of resting thallium 201 perfusion in predicting coronary anatomy, left ventricular wall motion, and hospital outcome in unstable angina pectoris. Am Heart J 117:306, 1989

MARCUS ML et al (eds): *Cardiac Imaging: A Companion to Braunwald's Heart Disease.* Philadelphia, Saunders, 1991

PACE L et al: Evaluation of myocardial perfusion and function by technetium-99m methoxy isobutyl isonitrile before and after percutaneous transluminal coronary angioplasty. Preliminary results. Clin Nucl Med 18:286, 1993

ROSE EL et al: Prognostic value of noninvasive cardiac tests in the assessment of patients with peripheral vascular disease. Am J Cardiol 71:40, 1993

SCHECHTER D et al: Left ventricular thrombus identification. A scintigraphic and echocardiographic correlation. Clin Nucl Med 18:353, 1993

SEWARD JB et al: Biplanar transesophageal echocardiography: Anatomic correlations, image orientation, and clinical applications. Mayo Clin Proc 65:1193, 1990

191   NEW CARDIAC IMAGING TECHNIQUES

CHARLES B. HIGGINS

The strategy for applying cardiac imaging techniques to the diagnosis of cardiovascular disease is currently in transition. Echocardiography and cardiac scintigraphy (Chap. 190) have been used with increasing frequency during the past decade. Initially, these techniques were used for preliminary diagnosis, but definitive therapy was generally based upon cardiac catheterization and angiography. Echocardiographic findings now have been accepted as sufficiently reliable and definitive for preoperative evaluation of most cardiac lesions. The emergence of the new noninvasive tomographic techniques, which include cine computed tomography (cine-CT), magnetic resonance imaging (MRI), and positron emission tomography (PET), should further encourage the trend away from catheterization as a requisite for definitive therapy. The strength of cine-CT and MRI lies in their being comprehensive cardiac imaging techniques for evaluation of both cardiac anatomy and function. Because of the good contrast and spatial resolution and the capacity to image the entire heart in a tomographic fashion, quantitation of dimensions and function is achieved by cine-CT and MRI to a degree even exceeding that possible with cardiac angiography. Each technique can be applied in a manner that produces a three-dimensional data set from which precise and reproducible volumetric and functional measurements can be done. Myocardial metabolism can now be assessed with PET and magnetic resonance spectroscopy (MRS). Because these new techniques are still in the stage of development and evaluation, they are not available at many hospitals at the current time. The most readily available of the new techniques is MRI, but many of these instruments are still not fully adapted for cardiac diagnosis.

ULTRAFAST COMPUTED TOMOGRAPHY (CINE-CT)

The unique design of the cine-CT scanner accomplishes the x-ray exposure for a complete tomogram in 50 ms. This short exposure time offsets the degrading effects of cardiac motion. Moreover, tomograms at the same level can be obtained sequentially after a delay of only 8 ms and initiated by, as well as related precisely to, the time in the cardiac cycle. The multiple sequential images can all be obtained within a single cardiac cycle and thus provide a true real-time image; these images are laced together in a closed-loop cinematic format, termed a *cine-CT display.*

The tomograms are approximately 10 mm in thickness, so that 12 to 14 adjacent tomograms are required to encompass the average adult heart. Eight tomographic levels can be acquired during a single imaging sequence. The maximum number of images is 80 per sequence. When tomographic images encompassing the entire heart are required, cine-CT becomes a three-dimensional imaging technique. Consequently, highly accurate and reproducible measurements of ventricular volume are possible. Such precision is possible because chamber volumes can be measured directly by planimetry of the blood pool on each tomogram encompassing the various cardiac chambers, rather than estimating volumes through assumed geometric models derived from measurements in one or two planes. Cine-CT and MRI are the only techniques that can quantify right ventricular as well as left ventricular mass.

Several other types of fast CT scanners have been introduced in the past few years. These scanners are called *spiral* CT scanners; this name derives from the continuous clockwise rotation of the scanner gantry. Standard scanners rotate in one direction during the transmission and detection of x-rays and then rotate back to the initial position before another scan is acquired. The standard scanner acquires a tomogram at a single anatomic level in 2 to 4 s and the time between scans is 2.5 s, whereas the spiral (helical) CT scanner obtains a tomogram in 1 s with virtually no interscan delay. Although the spiral CT scanner lacks the temporal resolution for the evaluation of cardiac function, the images of the heart and great vessels are adequate for the assessment of cardiovascular morphology. The spiral CT scanners are more readily available than the cine-CT scanners, and in a few years will be present in most large hospitals.

The blood pool is distinguished from the myocardium after the intravenous injection of iodinated contrast medium. Because the latter and ionizing radiation are used, cine-CT is not a true noninvasive cardiac imaging technique, like echocardiography and MRI. Cine-CT is effective for the diagnosis of many congenital and acquired cardiac abnormalities, but its role is limited because of the high diagnostic yield achieved by other totally noninvasive techniques.

INDICATIONS   The principal indications for the use of cine-CT in the diagnosis of heart disease are given in Table 191-1. In ischemic heart disease, cine-CT demonstrates regional wall thinning and absence of systolic wall thickening at the site of prior myocardial infarction. It is most effective for demonstrating complications of infarction such as mural thrombi and true and false aneurysms of the left ventricle. A mural thrombus produces a filling defect projecting into the left ventricular blood pool; it is usually attached to the wall thinned by prior infarction. An aneurysm produces a regional evagination of the left ventricular wall in diastole and paradoxical motion during systole.

TABLE 191-1 Principal indications for the new imaging modalities for cardiovascular diagnosis

FAST COMPUTED TOMOGRAPHY

Thoracic aortic diseases
  Dissection
  Aneurysm
Pulmonary arterial disease
  Pulmonary embolism
  Pulmonary arterial aneurysm
  Intrinsic and extrinsic tumors
Pericardial disease
  Constrictive diseases
  Pericardial cysts, tumors
Paracardiac and intracardiac masses
  Primary tumors
  Secondary tumors
  Intracardiac thrombus
Coronary artery bypass graft patency
Complications of myocardial infarctions
  Left ventricular aneurysms
  Left ventricular thrombus
Identification of coronary arterial calcification as an indicator of
  atherosclerotic disease
Analysis of ventricular function
  Global and regional left ventricular function (volume and wall thickness)
  Global right ventricular function (volume and wall thickness)
  Distribution of ventricular hypertrophy (assessment of hypertrophic
   cardiomyopathy)
  Ventricular function during interventions (exercise, drug interventions)
  Regional myocardial perfusion (under evaluation)

MAGNETIC RESONANCE IMAGING

Thoracic aortic diseases
  Dissection
  Aneurysm
  Thrombus
  Aortitis
  Aortic hemorrhage
Pericardial diseases
  Constrictive disease
  Effusion, hemorrhagic vs. nonhemorrhagic
  Pericardial cyst, tumor
Paracardiac and intracardiac masses
  Primary tumors (myxoma, etc.)
  Secondary tumors (lung, mediastinal, metastatic)
  Intracardiac thrombus
Hypertrophic cardiomyopathy
  Variant forms (distribution of hypertrophy)
Complications of myocardial infarction
  Left ventricular aneurysm and pseudoaneurysm
  Left ventricular thrombus
Regional myocardial perfusion using fast cine-MRI and MR constant media
  (under evaluation)
Congenital heart disease
  Thoracic aortic anomalies
   Arch anomalies
   Coarctation
  Pulmonary arterial anomalies
   Pulmonary atresia (presence and size of central pulmonary arteries)
   Unilateral absence (atresia)
   Peripheral pulmonary stenoses
  Complex lesions
   Univentricular atrioventricular connections
   Volume of ventricles
   Presence and size of ventricular septum
   Status of extracardiac operative procedures: Fontan, Rastelli, Jatene,
    etc.
Analysis of ventricular function
  Ventricular volumes and mass
  Regional left ventricular function
  Detection and quantities of valvular regurgitation
Obstructive arterial disease
  Intracranial and extracranial carotid arteries
  Renal arterial stenosis (under evaluation)
  Aortoiliac and lower limb arteries
  Coronary arteries (under evaluation)

POSITRON EMISSION TOMOGRAPHY

Ischemic heart disease
  Recognition of viable myocardium
  Regional myocardial perfusion

Cine-CT has a diagnostic accuracy of greater than 90 percent in the determination of patency of coronary arterial bypass grafts (Fig. 191-1). After intravenous injection of contrast medium, scans are exposed sequentially; the bypass grafts are opacified simultaneously with the ascending aorta. The technique is not usually capable of identifying stenosis of the graft or adequacy of blood flow through the graft, but there is hope that flow abnormalities might be detectable by analysis of contrast-dilution curves or contrast transit times in the grafts.

Computed tomography is considerably more sensitive and specific than x-ray fluoroscopy in both the identification and precise localization of vascular calcification. Consequently, cine-CT has been used to detect coronary arterial calcification (Fig. 191-2) as a screening test to identify patients at increased risk for obstructive coronary arterial disease (CAD). Cine-CT can quantify the density and the extent of coronary calcification. A three-dimensional map of the extent of coronary arterial calcification can be produced. Studies using fluoroscopy and cine-CT have shown that coronary arterial calcification increases with age. However, a recent report has indicated that the total calcium score, a product of density and volume of calcium, on cine-CT is substantially higher in patients with significant CAD when compared with those without CAD at each decade of age extending from 30 to 70 years. At each decade of age nearly all patients with significant CAD, demonstrated by angiography, had calcification detected by cine-CT. Calcification, though to a lesser extent, was also detected in patients without hemodynamically significant CAD. The absence of coronary arterial calcification indicates that the risk of significant CAD is very low. These early results have now led to the proposal that cine-CT might be used as a screening test to identify patients at increased risk for the presence of significant CAD and future coronary events.

Cine-CT can be used in the evaluation of hypertrophic and congestive cardiomyopathies by quantitating ventricular volumes and myocardial mass. Because of the wide field of view and three-

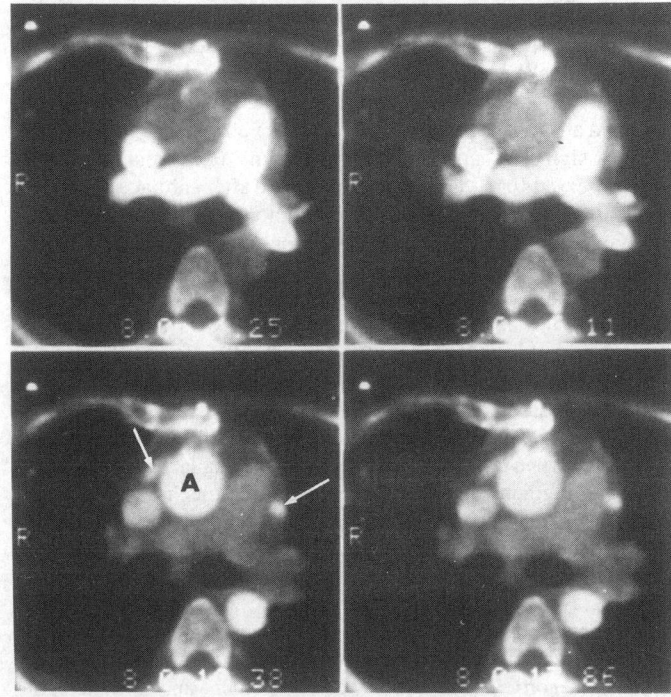

FIGURE 191-1 Cine-CT images at the level of the proximal ascending aorta acquired on sequential heart beats during passage of contrast medium throughout the central cardiovascular structures. The bypass grafts to the right (arrow) and left anterior descending (arrow) coronary arteries opacify simultaneously with the ascending aorta (A). Images from upper left to lower right display sequential opacification from pulmonary artery to the aorta.

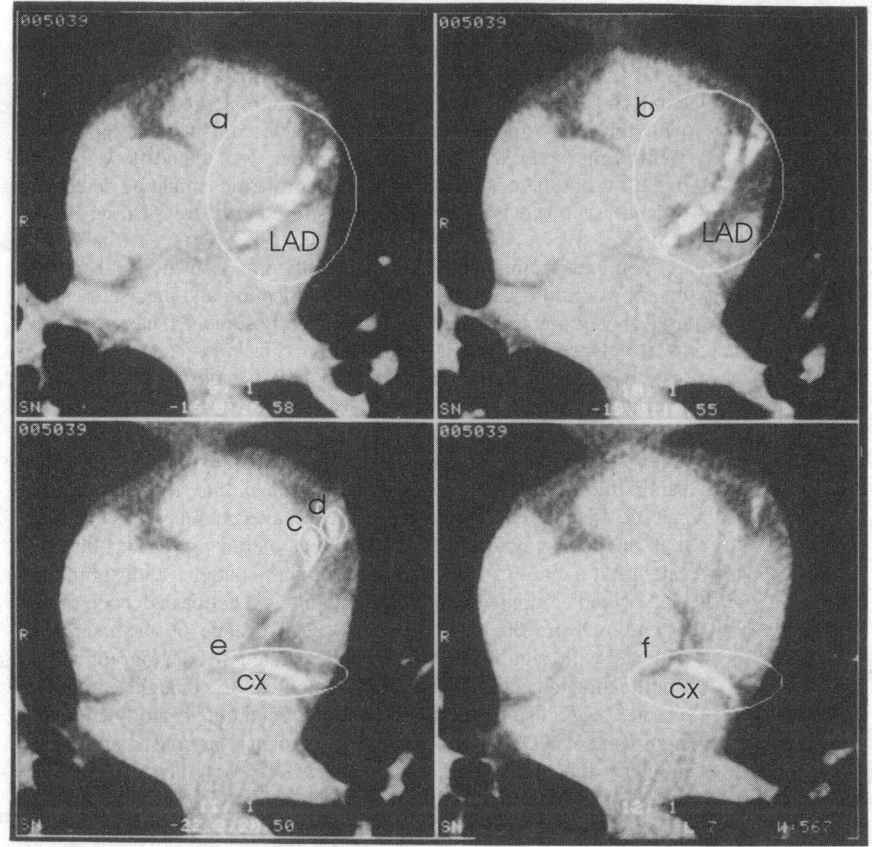

FIGURE 191-2   Cine-CT scans at four adjacent levels at the base of the heart. No contrast medium was used, and tomograms are 3 mm in thickness. Heavy calcification (circled) is identified at multiple sites in the left anterior descending (a,b,c,d) and circumflex coronary arteries (e,f).

dimensional scope of this technique, it can depict the distribution of ventricular hypertrophy. This is particularly useful for depiction of the various forms of hypertrophic cardiomyopathy and for quantifying the increase in myocardial mass.

The role of cine-CT in valvular heart disease is limited when compared to echo Doppler and color flow mapping and cine-MRI. Although both cine-MRI and echo Doppler can demonstrate the regurgitant flow, estimate its volume, and estimate the gradient across valvular stenoses, cine-CT can evaluate only indirectly the severity of regurgitation (see below).

For the evaluation of pericardial disease, standard CT or cine-CT can be used to visualize and measure the thickness of the pericardium. The diagnosis of constrictive pericarditis is supported by demonstrating pericardial thickness exceeding 4 mm and, sometimes, calcification (Fig. 191-3). Other indirect signs of this disease shown by CT are: (1) dilated atria and inferior vena cava; (2) small ventricular chambers; and (3) a sigmoid-shaped ventricular septum. Pericardial thickening is also observed for a variable period of time after cardiac surgery and in patients experiencing the postpericardiotomy syndrome (Dressler's syndrome). CT can also be used to demonstrate pericardial effusions and pericardial masses. Standard CT has been used to evaluate intracardiac and paracardiac masses and to define possible cardiac involvement by mediastinal and lung tumors. The capability is considerably enhanced by cine-CT, although MRI seems to be superior to both standard and cine-CT for the evaluation of intra- and paracardiac masses.

The role of CT for the evaluation of congenital heart disease is very limited when considered in relation to the availability and success of echocardiography and MRI. Encouraging results have been shown for cine-CT, but the results add little to echocardiography in the display of intracardiac anatomy and seem to be inferior to MRI for defining congenital abnormalities of the thoracic aorta and pulmonary artery.

Standard CT as well as cine-CT are effective for the diagnosis of diseases of the aorta (Chap. 210). The accuracy of CT for the diagnosis of aortic dissection exceeds 90 percent and in some series is nearly 100 percent. The definitive diagnosis of aortic dissection is based upon the demonstration of displacement of the inner portion of the aortic wall into the lumen (intimal flap) and/or differential enhancement of the true and false aortic channels.

FIGURE 191-3   CT image shows calcification (arrow) and thickening of the pericardium in a patient with constrictive pericarditis.

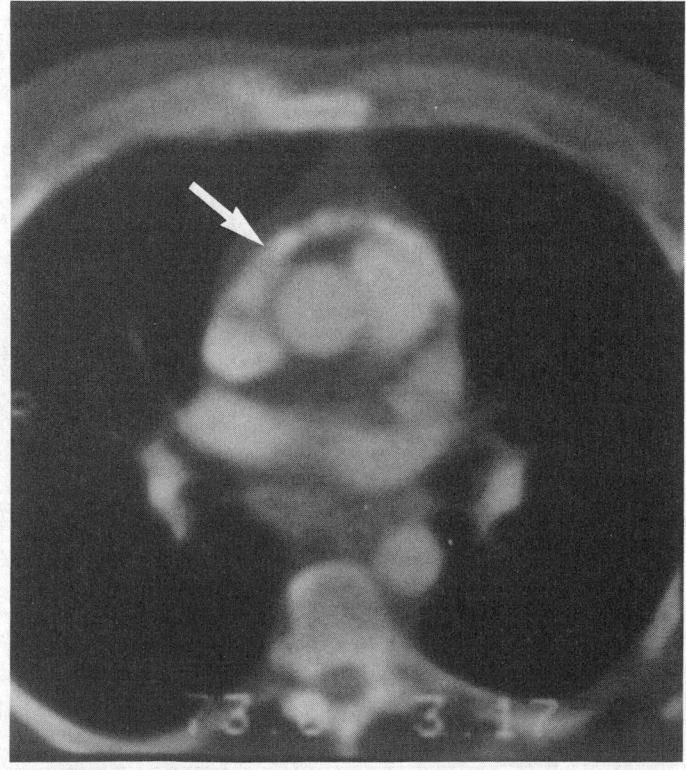

EVALUATION OF CARDIAC FUNCTION WITH CINE-CT The exposure time of 50 ms attained by cine-CT is adequate for quantitating many aspects of cardiac function. The three-dimensional nature of the technique permits precise measurement of chamber volume. Right and left ventricular volumes can be assessed with equal accuracy. A disparity in the stroke volumes of the two ventricles is caused by shunts and valvular regurgitation, which can be measured by cine-CT. Cine-CT can also be used for monitoring the effect of interventions on the right and left ventricles. Cine-CT performed at peak effort during supine bicycle exercise has been used to identify the *abnormal* response in patients with suspected coronary arterial stenoses. Most patients with severe lung disease and pulmonary arterial hypertension also display an abnormal response to exercise. Cine-CT has also been proposed as a method for measuring regional myocardial perfusion at rest and following interventions that increase myocardial blood flow, such as exercise and vasodilators. Perfusion is estimated by monitoring density values of the myocardium over time on CT scans exposed sequentially during peak opacification and wash-out of contrast medium from the myocardium.

MAGNETIC RESONANCE IMAGING

This noninvasive technique uses no ionizing radiation or contrast medium for cardiovascular imaging. MR images are based upon the radiofrequency (RF) signal emitted by hydrogen nuclei of tissues after they have been perturbed by RF pulses in the presence of a strong magnetic field. The RF signal emitted has certain characteristics called *relaxation times*, consisting of T1 relaxation time (longitudinal magnetization) and T2 relaxation time (transverse magnetization). These properties are variable among tissues and are the predominant factors responsible for contrast among tissues. The signal intensity of one tissue compared to another (contrast) can be manipulated by varying the elapsed time between application of RF pulses (repetition time) and the time between an RF pulse and sampling the emitted signal (echo delay time).

The techniques used in MR imaging of the heart depend upon the primary goal of the procedure. When the evaluation of anatomic abnormalities is paramount, the use of ECG-gated spin echo technique provides static images with high signal-to-noise ratio. When the primary goal is to assess cardiac contractile function, cine gradient echo imaging (cine-GRE) is used. The cardiac cycle can be divided into more than 60 time frames with this latter technique, although the framing rate used is usually no greater than 30. By lacing these together in a cinematic format, tomograms of the beating heart (cine-MRI) are obtained.

The blood pool has a unique signal on both spin echo and gradient echo images. The blood pool on the ECG-gated spin echo images is generally a signal void, which provides high contrast between blood and the myocardial wall (Fig. 191-4). On the other hand, the blood pool produces a very bright signal when the gradient echo technique is used (Fig. 191-5). This also causes high contrast between the blood pool and the myocardial wall.

Blood flow velocity can be measured using a technique called flow velocity mapping because of the existence of a linear relationship between the motion of protons in blood and the magnitude of the shift in phase of the signal of moving protons relative to stationary ones. When this sequence is applied as part of the cine-GRE technique, a series of images is acquired at evenly spaced intervals (usually 15 to 20 time segments) throughout the cardiac cycle. This sequence, called *velocity-encoded cine-MRI*, can be used to produce velocity vs. time curves and volume flow vs. time curves as the product of velocity and cross-sectional areas of the flow region. Integration of the flow values measured on cross-sectional images of the proximal aorta and pulmonary artery provides a direct measurement of stroke volume of the right and left ventricles and the disparity between the two stroke volumes in left-to-right shunts. Because the technique distinguishes between antegrade and retrograde flow, it can be used

to quantify pathologic flow, such as valvular regurgitation. The technique has many practical similarities to Doppler echocardiography and, like Doppler, can be applied for estimating the gradient across valvular stenoses using the modified Bernoulli equation. The peak velocity (V) beyond the valvular stenosis is measured from the flow channel distal to the valve and used in the formula: peak gradient $= 4V^2$.

EVALUATION OF PATHOANATOMY MRI has been shown to be effective and useful in the diagnosis of a wide variety of cardiovascular abnormalities (Table 191-1). Patients with congenital heart disease are evaluated initially with the use of two-dimensional echocardiography, and in many congenital lesions MR is a secondary diagnostic technique in which the anatomy is displayed with the precision of angiography. In anomalies of the aortic arch and

FIGURE 191-4 *A*. ECG gated spin echo MRI in the cardiac short axis plane. Arrows = papillary muscles; L = left ventricle; RO = right ventricular outflow tract. *(From Higgins CB et al with permission) B*. Transaxial spin echo MR image demonstrates a mass in the left atrium (arrow). The wide area of attachment of the mass to the left atrial wall suggests a sarcoma rather than a benign myxoma. A = aorta; LA = left atrium; RA = right atrium; RV = right ventricle.

A

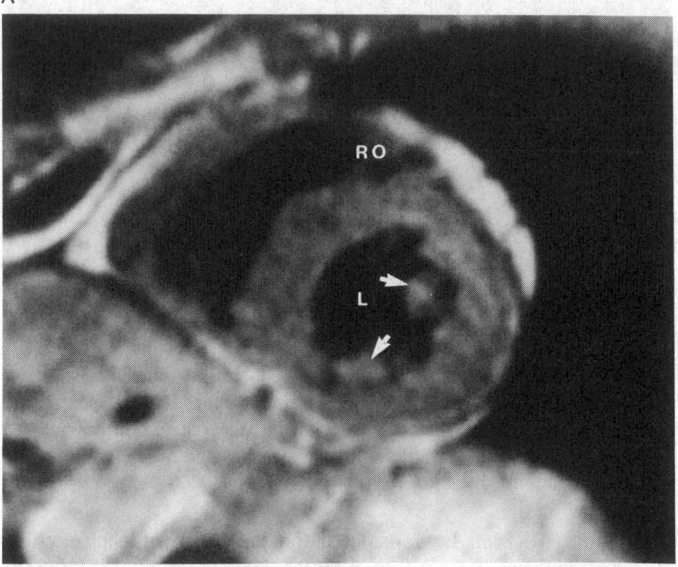

B

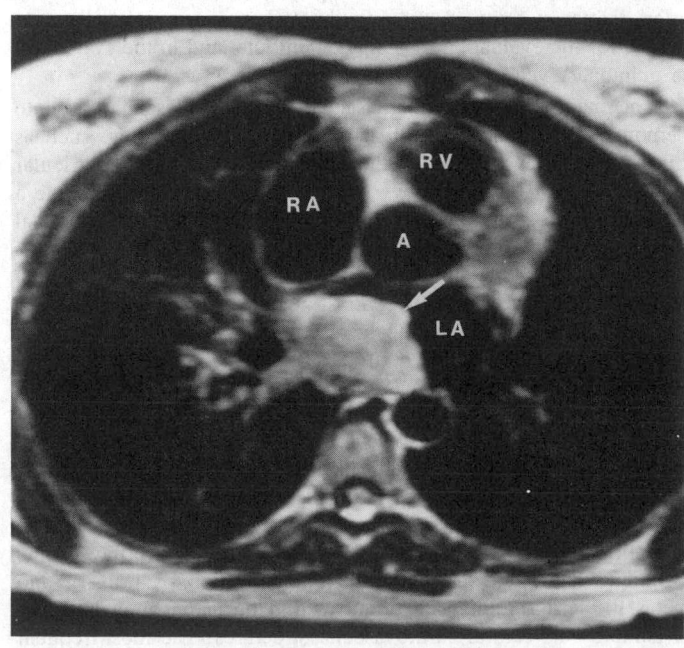

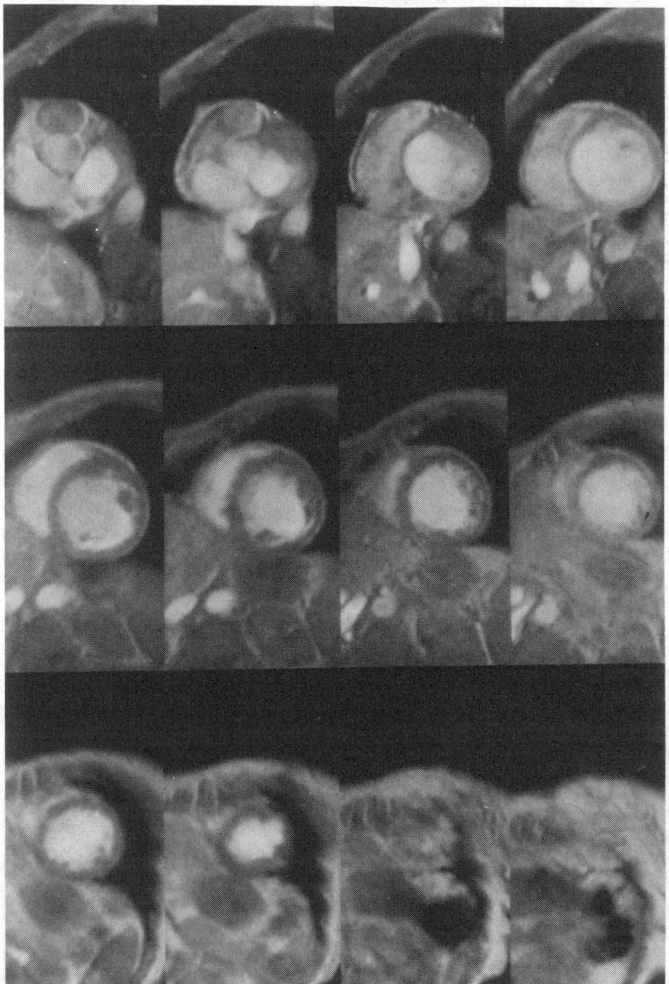

FIGURE 191-5 Series of cine gradient echo images at end-diastole for sequential anatomic levels extending from base (upper left) to apex (lower right) of the left ventricle. These tomograms provide a three-dimensional data set for measuring right and left ventricular volumes and masses.

coarctation, MR can be considered the procedure of choice. Also MRI is often the most useful study for the demonstration of pulmonary arterial abnormalities; for evaluating the status of the pulmonary arteries after systemic-pulmonary shunts have been surgically produced; for the evaluation of a single ventricle; and in the evaluation of pulmonary venous abnormalities.

The major use of MRI in ischemic heart disease has been to demonstrate complications of acute myocardial infarction, such as true and false aneurysms of the left ventricle and intraventricular thrombi (Fig. 191-6). However, in the future, MRI may assume a broader role in ischemic heart disease by demonstrating: (1) residual viable myocardium in a region involved by a previous infarct; (2) patency (or lack thereof) of coronary artery bypass grafts; and (3) regional perfusion using MR contrast media.

MRI has been used to define the extent and distribution of abnormal muscle in patients with hypertrophic cardiomyopathy. It provides accurate and reproducible measurement of myocardial mass, which can be used in monitoring response to therapy. It provides direct imaging of the pericardium, so that a diagnosis of abnormal pericardial thickness can be made. MRI is the procedure of choice for establishing the diagnosis of constrictive pericarditis.

MRI has been found to be effective for demonstrating intracardiac thrombi and tumors (Figs. 191-4B and 191-6). The utility of the technique has been shown in the demonstration of primary and metastatic cardiac tumors and tumors within the mediastinum invading or compressing central cardiovascular structures. The most frequent

indication for the use of MRI in evaluating an intracardiac mass is when echocardiography raises a question regarding abnormal echogenicity within the cardiac chambers.

Thoracic aortic diseases are evaluated best with MR. In patients with aortic dissection, MRI displays the intimal flap and the extent of the dissection within the aorta (Fig. 191-7). It can also identify a thrombus in the false channel and involvement of the arch and visceral arterial branches. In the search for the source of arterial embolism, MRI can be applied to identify a thrombus in the left atrium, left ventricle, or aorta.

EVALUATION OF CARDIAC FUNCTION   Functional evaluation of the cardiovascular system is now practical using cine-MRI. By achieving a temporal resolution of 30 images per cardiac cycle, cine-MRI successfully captures end diastole and end systole, such that end-diastolic and end-systolic volumes, stroke volume, and ejection

FIGURE 191-6 ECG-gated spin echo MR images acquired in transverse plane demonstrate complications of myocardial infarctions. True aneurysm and mural thrombus (T) *(top).* False aneurysm (A) *(bottom).* The ostium is nearly as wide as the fundus of the true aneurysm, while the ostium is smaller than the fundus for the false aneurysm.

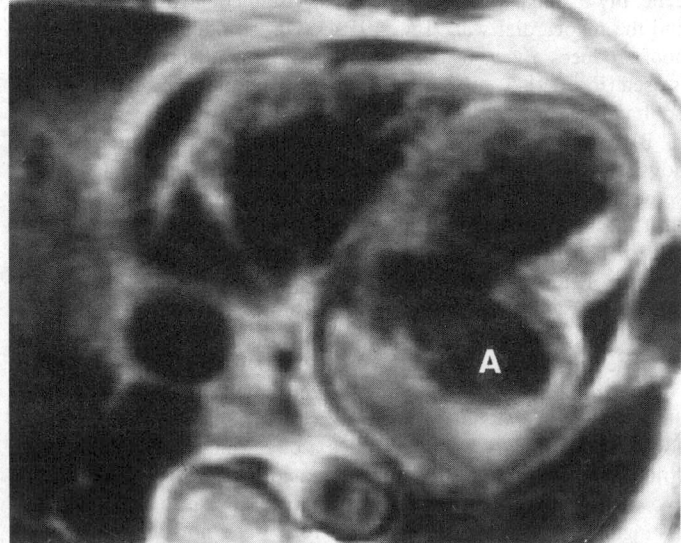

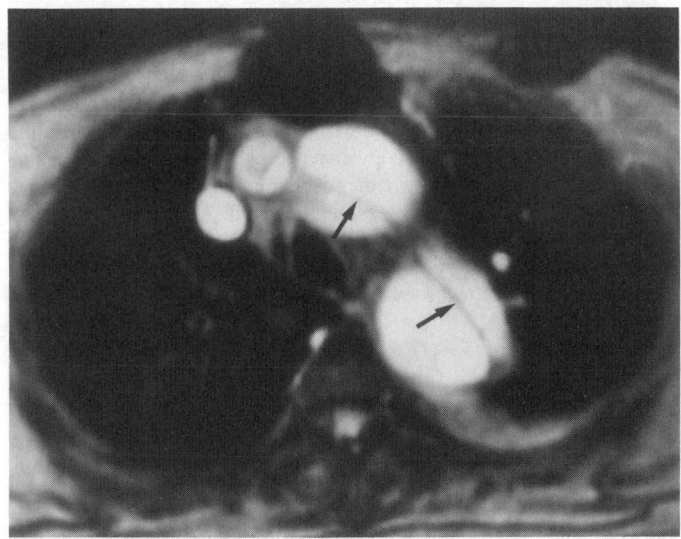

FIGURE 191-7 ECG-referenced gradient echo image in transaxial plane at the level of the aortic arch demonstrates an intimal flap (arrows) in the ascending and descending aorta. *(From Higgins CB et al, with permission)*

fraction can be calculated accurately. The temporal resolution of cine-MRI does not capture a single cardiac cycle, but rather separates an "average" cycle, acquired over 256 cardiac cycles, into many component images. A good correlation has been found between left ventricular volumes calculated from cine-MRI and those measured by angiography. Measurement of left ventricular mass using MRI has shown a close correlation with postmortem measurements in animals and estimates from angiography in human beings. Accurate measurement of left ventricular mass is important, as changes in mass may be the most effective way to monitor the response to therapy in diseases causing left ventricular hypertrophy. MRI has also been shown to provide measurement of right ventricular mass. Functional evaluation in ischemic heart disease by MRI is achieved by monitoring wall thickening during the cardiac cycle. The site of previous myocardial infarction can be recognized by the absence or diminution of wall thickening during systole.

Faster gradient echo techniques have been developed in recent years so that it is now possible to obtain 15 or more images evenly spaced throughout a cardiac cycle during a single breath-hold period. Another new technique called *echoplanar imaging* acquires an image in 30 to 50 ms, so that images at multiple phases of the cardiac cycle can be obtained during a single heart beat, which constitutes real-time imaging of the heart. These innovations should extend the capability of MRI for the evaluation of cardiac function.

QUANTITATION OF VALVULAR LESIONS The blood pool usually has a homogeneous high signal intensity throughout most of the cardiac cycle on cine-MR. Stenosis of or regurgitation through either the atrioventricular or semilunar valves is associated with a high-velocity jet that causes a signal void within the otherwise high-signal-intensity chamber (Fig. 191-8). This void can be used to identify the presence of valvular regurgitation. In aortic regurgitation, the signal void is in continuity with the closed aortic valve, whereas in mitral regurgitation it is in continuity with the closed mitral valve. Quantitation of the severity of valvular regurgitation can be accomplished by measuring the right and left ventricular stroke volumes and using these measurements to calculate regurgitant fraction or regurgitant volume. The volume of the signal void caused by regurgitation can also be measured on the images and used to estimate the severity of regurgitation. The velocity-encoded cine-MRI technique can be used to measure the volume of valvular regurgitation and to estimate the peak gradient across valvular stenosis (see below).

Velocity-encoded cine-MRI has been applied for the quantification of blood flow in the heart and great vessels in a variety of diseases. It has been used to measure the retrograde flow in the ascending aorta in diastole in order to directly quantify the regurgitant volume in aortic regurgitation. It has also been shown to provide an accurate measurement of the stoke volume of the right and left ventricles by quantifying systolic flow in the main pulmonary artery and aorta, respectively. The volume of regurgitant lesions is calculated as the difference in stroke volume of the two ventricles. Valvular and arterial stenoses can be estimated from the modified Bernoulli equation by measuring the peak flow velocity across the stenosis. This technique can be used to measure flow separately in the right and left pulmonary arteries; such measurements may be useful in the assessment of pulmonary blood flow in treated and untreated patients with congenital heart disease.

FIGURE 191-8 Coronal cine-MR images in a patient with aortic regurgitation (*A*) and another with aortic stenosis (*B*). Regurgitation causes a signal void in the left ventricle during diastole. Aortic stenosis causes a signal void (arrow) starting at the valve level (arrow) and extending into the ascending aorta in systole. A = aorta; LV = left ventricle; P = pulmonary artery; RA = right atrium.

A

B

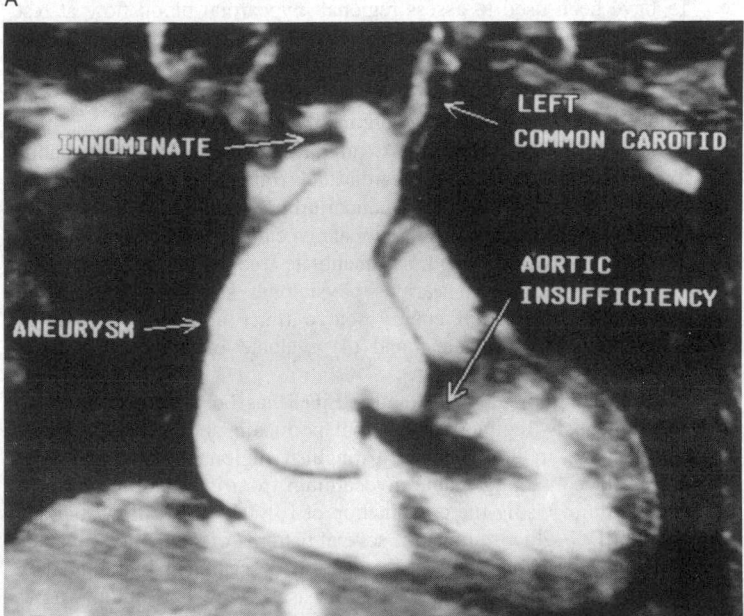

MR SPECTROSCOPY

MR spectroscopy is used for the evaluation of myocardial metabolism. It may eventually be used to assess the early response of the myocardium to various therapeutic and pharmacologic interventions, establish myocardial viability, assess beneficial or detrimental effects of reperfusion on the ischemically injured myocardium, and investigate the link between myocardial function and metabolism.

MR spectroscopy operates upon the same principle as MRI in that the nuclei of some atoms (those with an odd number of nuclear particles) resonate when radiofrequency energy is applied at a frequency specific for a particular atom. After this energy is applied, the nuclei resonate at a characteristic frequency so that the presence of a particular atom within a chemical compound or tissue can be identified by MR. In distinction to imaging, which is usually only sensitive to the presence of a certain atom within a compound, MR spectroscopy can provide a map of the various sites where an atom exists within a compound. MR spectroscopy depicts the very slight difference in resonant frequencies of the same nuclei when they exist in different compounds. This slight variation in resonant frequencies is called *chemical shift*, and the graphic display of the various frequencies is the MR spectrum of the nuclei. An example of this is the MR spectrum of phosphorus 31 (^{31}P), where the multiple spectral peak represent ^{31}P in the compounds inorganic phosphate, creatine phosphate, adenosine triphosphate, etc. (Fig. 191-9). The MR spectra are displayed in a convention whereby the position of the peak in the spectrum (horizontal axis) indicates the specific compounds, e.g., creatine phosphate, and the height of the peak (vertical axis) indicates the relative concentration of the compound.

The nuclei for which MR spectroscopy seems to be the most useful for diagnostic purposes are hydrogen 1, carbon 13, and phosphorus 31. Hydrogen 1 (proton) spectroscopy has been used to detect lactate in ischemic tissue and lipid accumulation in ischemically injured tissue. Metabolism of energy substrates in the myocardium has been approached using carbon 13; the technique has the potential for monitoring the utilization of fat and glucose by the myocardium and the manner in which ischemia influences their utilization. At this time most attention has been devoted to phosphorus 31 MR spectroscopy as a method for studying high-energy phosphate stores in various myocardial disease states and alterations of high-energy phosphate stores in response to therapeutic interventions.

FIGURE 191-9 Phosphorus 31 magnetic resonance spectrum from a normal subject. The important spectral peaks are inorganic phosphate, not seen; creatine phosphate (PCr); and the three for ATP, labeled α, β, and γ. The 2,3-diphosphoglycerate (DPG) peak indicates that the signal is partially derived from intracavitary blood as well as from myocardium. PD = phosphodiester.

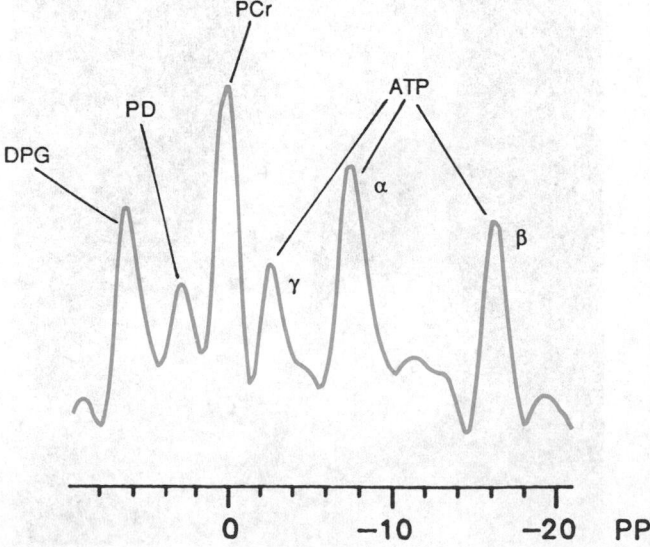

In experimental preparations, phosphorus 31 spectroscopy has been used to evaluate the influence of potentially toxic agents, such as adriamycin and ethanol, on the myocardium. Calcium channel antagonists have been found to enchance recovery of both function and high-energy phosphate stores of the ischemically injured myocardium. Phosphorus 31 MR spectroscopy may be used also in experimental preparations to determine whether ischemic myocardium which is reperfused is reversibly or irreversibly damaged. Abnormal ^{31}P spectra have been observed in patients with myocardial disease. However, the sensitivity, specificity, and, indeed, the clinical utility of ^{31}P MR spectroscopy has yet to be established.

POSITRON EMISSION TOMOGRAPHY

PET is a technique in which tomographic images are produced in relation to the concentration and position of positron emitters within the heart or any other organ. The positron is a positively charged electron produced during positron decay of a nucleus. After the positron interacts with a neighboring electron, a pair of photons are emitted in opposite directions. Because the photons simultaneously travel at equal speeds along paths at 180° to one another, photon detectors arrayed in a circle around the body can compute the precise site of origin of the pair. A substantial number of positron emitters are available for evaluating blood flow and various aspects of metabolic activity of the myocardium. Blood flow can be measured with ammonia labeled with nitrogen 13 (^{13}N), rubidium 82 (^{82}Rb), or oxygen 15 (^{15}O). Glucose utilization, fat utilization and metabolism, and myocardial oxygen consumption can be assessed by fluorine 18 (^{18}F)-labeled deoxyglucose (DG), carbon 11 (^{11}C)-labeled palmitate, and ^{11}C-labeled acetate, respectively.

PET can evaluate regional myocardial blood flow and metabolism. The transverse tomograms provide distinct spatial separation between various regions of the left ventricle, so that the uptake of metabolic markers can be assigned to the various myocardial regions. This technique may provide the capability of distinguishing between reversibly and irreversibly injured ischemic myocardium and predicting its response to reperfusion. By monitoring changes in metabolic patterns or substrate uptake, it may also prove capable of monitoring early response to therapy.

ASSESSMENT OF REGIONAL MYOCARDIAL BLOOD FLOW Because the various regions of the left ventricle are separated from one another on the transverse tomographic images, PET scans using perfusion markers can be used to detect and localize coronary artery disease. Nitrogen 13 ammonia ([^{13}N]H$_3$), rubidium 82, and oxygen 15 have been used to assess regional myocardial blood flow at rest and in a hyperemic state induced by strong vasodilators such as dipyridamole and adenosine. This technique has shown regional reduction of the positron emitter in the presence of stenoses that reduce luminal diameter by more than 40 to 50 percent.

Myocardial metabolism An unique feature of PET is the capability to measure regional myocardial substrate uptake and metabolic kinetics in a noninvasive and nonperturbing fashion. Specifically, it has been used to (1) measure regional myocardial uptake of exogenous glucose and free fatty acid; (2) quantitate free fatty acid metabolism in the myocardium in various physiologic states; (3) define the preferential myocardial energy source (fatty acid vs. glucose) in various physiologic states; and (4) evaluate myocardial chemical receptor sites.

PET employing [^{13}N]H$_3$ and [^{18}F]DG has been used to evaluate simultaneously regional myocardial perfusion and glucose uptake, respectively, in an effort to distinguish regions with a perfusion defect but containing viable myocardium from irreversibly infarcted myocardium. Using the combination of [^{13}N]H$_3$ (blood flow marker) and [^{18}F]DG (glucose uptake), several patterns of segmental myocardial metabolic abnormalities have been described in patients with various forms of ischemic heart disease. One is a "blood flow-metabolism match," in which a defect in the regional myocardial

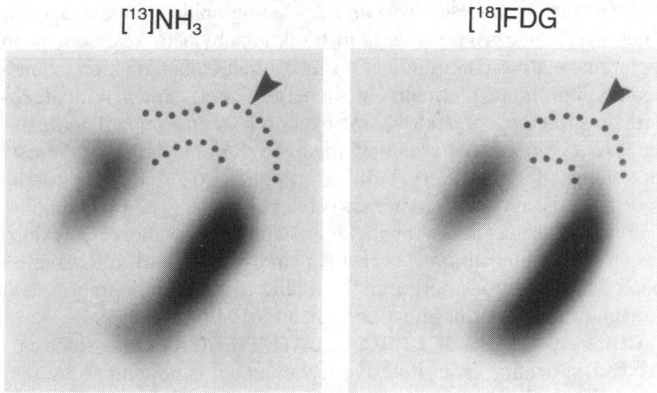

$[^{13}N]NH_3$ $[^{18}F]DG$ $[^{13}N]NH_3$ $[^{18}F]DG$

FIGURE 191-10 Positron emission tomograms in two subjects: matched defects (*left*) and mismatched defects (*right*). Images show distribution for [^{13}N]ammonium and [^{18}F]deoxyglucose. The matched defects (arrowheads) in the anterior regions indicate a scar from a transmural infarct. The mismatched

defects show reduced perfusion (arrow) but persistent glucose uptake (arrow) consistent with viable (salvageable) myocardium. (*Images provided courtesy of Heinrich Schelbert, MD.*)

distribution of both isotopes is present. This pattern is usually caused by myocardial scar or nonviable myocardium (Fig. 191-10*A*). A second pattern is a "blood flow–metabolism mismatch," in which there is a segmental defect in [^{13}N]H without a deficit in [^{18}F]DG (Fig. 191-10*B*). This indicates reduced perfusion to a myocardial region but continued uptake of glucose. Both patterns have been observed in patients with wall motion abnormalities in the left ventricular region displaying the perfusion defects. This mismatch pattern is considered to be associated with ischemic but viable myocardium as surgical revascularization of patients with this pattern causes improved wall motion in a majority of such segments. Moreover, a substantial percentage of patients showing the mismatch pattern after acute myocardial infarction have demonstrated some recovery of regional function. On the other hand, the match pattern has been associated with no recovery of function after revascularization of akinetic segments.

PET using the positron emitter [^{11}C]palmitic acid has identified the consequences of myocardial ischemia and infarction on myocardial free fatty acid metabolism. These studies revealed that exogenous ^{11}C-labeled palmitic acid can enter two metabolic pools within the myocardium: a rapidly metabolized pool in which the fatty acid is immediately oxidized to CO_2 or a storage pool of triglycerides. During myocardial ischemia, myocardial uptake of [^{11}C]palmitic acid and its distribution into the two pools are altered. The free fatty acid pathway most vulnerable to ischemia is β oxidation, and consequently the amount of [^{11}C]palmitic acid entering this pathway is decreased initially.

Prediction of successful salvage of myocardium after thrombolysis has been achieved by PET imaging of [^{11}C]palmitic acid uptake in the jeopardized myocardium. Successful thrombolysis is associated with resumption of uptake of [^{11}C]palmitic acid in the jeopardized region. The principal indications for PET at the current time are to detect ischemic myocardium and to demonstrate potentially salvageable (viable) myocardium in the presence of acute or chronic myocardial ischemia.

REFERENCES

Cine-CT

AGATSON AS et al: Quantification of coronary arterial calcium using ultrafast computed tomography. J Am Coll Cardiol 1:827, 1990

MARCUS ML, WEISS RM: Evaluation of cardiac structure and function with ultrafast computed tomography, in *Cardiac Imaging*, ML Marcus et al (eds). Philadelphia, Saunders, 1991, p 669

STANFORD W et al: Sensitivity and specificity of assessing coronary bypass graft patency with ultrafast computed tomography. Results of a multicenter study. J Am Coll Cardiol 12:1, 1988

MR imaging

BARAKOS JA et al: Magnetic resonance imaging of cardiac and paracardiac masses. Pictorial essay. Am J Roentgenol 153:47, 1989

HIGGINS CB: MR of the heart: Anatomy, physiology and metabolism. Am J Roentgenol 151:239, 1988

———: Evaluation of valvular heart disease using cine GRE magnetic resonance imaging. Circulation (suppl) 84(3):I-194, 1991

——— et al: Magnetic resonance imaging in hypertrophic cardiomyopathy. Am J Cardiol 55:1121, 1985

——— et al: *Congenital Heart Disease. Echocardiography and Magnetic Resonance Imaging*. New York, Raven Press, 1990

——— et al (eds): *Magnetic Resonance Imaging of the Body*, 2d ed. New York, Raven Press, 1991

MACMILLAN RM: Cardiac magnetic resonance imaging. Cardiovasc Clin 23:125, 1993

SOMMERHOFF BA et al: Aortic dissection: Sensitivity and specificity of MR imaging. Radiology 3:651, 1988

UNDERWOOD R, FIRMIN D: *Magnetic Resonance of the Cardiovascular System*. Oxford, Blackwell Scientific, 1991

MR spectroscopy

MEYERHOFF DJ et al: Magnetic resonance spectroscopy, in *Magnetic Resonance Imaging of the Body*, 2d ed, CB Higgins et al (eds). New York, Raven Press, 1991

WEISS RG et al: Regional myocardial metabolism of high energy phosphates during isometric exercise in patients with coronary artery disease. N Engl J Med 323:1593, 1990

Positron Emission Tomography

ISADA L et al: Physiologic evaluation of coronary flow: The role of positron emission tomography. Cleve Clin J Med 60:19, 1993

SCHELBERT HR, BUXTON D: Insights into coronary artery disease gained from metabolic imaging. Circulation 78:496, 1988

SCHELBERT HR et al: Principles of positron emission tomography, in *Cardiac Imaging*, ML Marcus et al (eds). Philadelphia, Saunders, 1991, p 1140

192 DIAGNOSTIC CARDIAC CATHETERIZATION AND ANGIOGRAPHY

WILLIAM GROSSMAN / DONALD S. BAIM

Cardiac catheterization and angiography remain the gold standard for the assessment of both anatomy and physiology of the heart and vasculature. Initially developed in the animal laboratory, cardiac catheterization was first applied to humans in 1929 by Werner Forssmann, who at age 25 performed a right heart catheterization on himself. Forssmann's primary goal was to develop a therapeutic technique for the direct delivery of drugs into the heart. The potential

---

TABLE 192-1   Relative contraindications to cardiac catheterization and angiography

1 Uncontrolled ventricular irritability: increased risk of ventricular tachycardia and fibrillation during catheterization if ventricular irritability is uncontrolled
2 Uncorrected hypokalemia or digitalis toxicity
3 Uncorrected hypertension: predisposes to myocardial ischemia and/or heart failure during angiography
4 Intercurrent febrile illness
5 Decompensated heart failure: especially acute pulmonary edema, unless catheterization can be done with patient sitting up
6 Anticoagulated state: prothrombin time >18 s
7 Severe allergy to radiographic contrast agent
8 Severe renal insufficiency and/or anuria: unless dialysis is planned to remove fluid and radiographic contrast load

---

of Forssmann's technique as a diagnostic tool was appreciated by others, especially André Cournand and Dickinson Richards in New York, who shared the Nobel Prize with Forssmann in 1956 for the development of cardiac catheterization. Today, cardiac catheterization and angiography are performed as a combined procedure for diagnostic purposes, therapeutic intervention, or both. This chapter deals with cardiac catheterization as a diagnostic tool.

INDICATIONS AND CONTRAINDICATIONS   Cardiac catheterization is recommended when there is a need to confirm the presence of a clinically suspected condition, define its anatomic and physiologic severity, and determine whether important associated conditions are present. This need most commonly arises when a patient is experiencing significant or increasing symptoms of cardiac dysfunction or when objective measures suggest that rapid deterioration, myocardial infarction, or other adverse events are imminent.

While there is debate as to whether cardiac catheterization is necessary in all patients being considered for cardiac surgery, cardiac catheterization and coronary arteriography remain the only techniques currently capable of defining coronary anatomy with sufficient precision to provide the data for decisions regarding coronary surgery or balloon angioplasty. In patients with other forms of heart disease (e.g., dilated cardiomyopathy, valvular heart disease), cardiac catheterization can provide hemodynamic characterization essential to the design of an appropriate medical regimen as well as assessment of prognosis. In some instances, however, decisions regarding cardiac surgery can be made without cardiac catheterization and angiography. Examples of such instances include children with simple congenital heart disease (e.g., patent ductus arteriosus, atrial septal defect), for whom a definitive diagnosis can be established by clinical examination and noninvasive studies.

Relative contraindications to cardiac catheterization are listed in Table 192-1.

TABLE 192-2   Patient characteristics associated with increased mortality from cardiac catheterization

1 *Age:* Infants (<1 month old) and the elderly (>80 years old) are at increased risk of death during cardiac catheterization. Elderly women appear to be at higher risk than elderly men.
2 *Functional class:* Mortality in class IV patients is more than 10 times greater than in class I–II patients.
3 *Severity of coronary obstruction:* Mortality for patients with left main disease is more than 10 times greater than in patients with one- or two-vessel disease.
4 *Valvular heart disease:* Especially when severe and combined with coronary disease is associated with a higher risk of death at cardiac catheterization than coronary artery disease alone.
5 *Left ventricular dysfunction:* Mortality in patients with left ventricular ejection < 30 percent is more than 10 times greater than in patients with ejection fraction ≥ 50 percent.
6 *Severe noncardiac disease:* Patients with renal insufficiency, insulin-requiring diabetes, advanced cerebrovascular and/or peripheral vascular disease, and severe pulmonary insufficiency have an increased incidence of death and other major complications from cardiac catheterization.

A history of *allergic reaction* to radiographic contrast agents, which may range from urticaria to frank anaphylactic reaction, is an important relative contraindication to cardiac catheterization, which requires appropriate pretreatment. Generally, pretreatment with glucocorticoids (prednisone 20 to 40 mg every 6 h), conventional antihistamines (e.g., diphenhydramine 25 mg every 6 h), and H-2 antagonists (cimetidine 300 mg every 6 h), starting 18 to 24 h prior to the procedure, is adequate. Alternatively, one of the newer nonionic contrast agents may be used with less risk of a severe allergic reaction. Despite these precautions, occasional individuals will still develop anaphylactic reactions during radiographic contrast angiography, and intravenous epinephrine must be at hand in such instances.

COMPLICATIONS OF CARDIAC CATHETERIZATION   Since cardiac catheterization is an invasive technique, it is not surprising that potential complications include death, myocardial infarction, stroke, perforation of the heart or great vessels, and local vascular problems. Table 192-2 lists those characteristics associated with increased risk of death from cardiac catheterization.

TECHNIQUES

Cardiac catheterization is performed with the patient in the fasting state and awake, although sedated. Typical sedatives include diazepam (Valium 5 to 10 mg orally) and diphenhydramine (Benadryl 25 to 50 mg orally). Prophylactic antibiotics are not necessary. If patients have been anticoagulated chronically with warfarin, this agent must be discontinued for at least 48 h prior to the procedure, and the prothrombin time must be less than 18 s if the study is to be done safely. The technique of cardiac catheterization involves either direct exposure of artery and vein (usually the brachial artery and vein in the antecubital fossa) or catheterization by percutaneous approach (usually via the femoral artery and vein). Either technique can be used for right and/or left heart catheterization with coronary arteriography, but many procedures (e.g., intraaortic balloon pumping, mitral valve valvuloplasty, coronary atherectomy) require the femoral approach. For a procedure where either approach would be possible, the brachial approach has advantages in the patient with perpipheral vascular disease involving the abdominal aorta and iliac or femoral arteries and suspected thrombosis of the femoral or iliac vein or inferior vena cava. Advantages of the percutaneous femoral approach are that arteriotomy and arterial repair are not required; the procedure can be performed repeatedly in the same patient at intervals; infection and thrombophlebitis at the catheterization site are quite rare, and no scar is left.

RIGHT HEART CATHETERIZATION   This is most commonly performed under fluoroscopic guidance utilizing a balloon flotation catheter which is advanced from a suitable vein (femoral, brachial, subclavian, or internal jugular) into the superior vena cava, where blood is sampled for oximetry. The catheter is then positioned in the right atrium, where pressure is measured. The balloon is inflated with air or carbon dioxide and advanced into the right ventricle, pulmonary artery, and pulmonary artery wedge positions. Pressures are recorded in each position, and the balloon is then deflated so that pulmonary artery pressure is monitored and blood sampled from the catheter tip. With a thermistor-tipped balloon catheter, cardiac output can be measured utilizing cold saline injection and a small computer (thermodilution technique). Comparison of oxygen saturations in the venae cavae, chambers of the right heart, and pulmonary artery blood permits assessment of the presence of a left-to-right shunt at the atrial, ventricular, or pulmonary artery level which will be manifested as an increase ("step-up") in oxygen saturation of blood as it traverses these vessels and chambers. As discussed below, measurements of the pulmonary artery and aortic oxygen content and oxygen consumption allow calculation of the cardiac output by the Fick principle as an alternative to use of thermodilution.

The experienced operator will be alert to abnormalities in the course of the catheter during its passage through the right heart chambers, potentially providing information concerning the presence of congenital heart disease. For example, the catheter may pass directly from the right to the left atrium through an atrial septal defect, may enter an anomalous pulmonary vein draining into the right atrium, or may pass from the pulmonary artery directly into the aorta through a patent ductus arteriosus.

LEFT HEART CATHETERIZATION When left heart catheterization is done from the *brachial approach*, surgical cut-down is performed in the right (or left) antecubital fossa, with exposure of the brachial artery. An arteriotomy is made, and an appropriate catheter (e.g., Sones catheter) is advanced under fluoroscopic guidance to the central aorta, where pressure is measured and recorded. Next, the catheter is advanced in retrograde fashion across the aortic valve into the left ventricle, where pressure is measured. If a right heart catheter is in place, this is an appropriate time for simultaneous measurement and recording of left heart, right heart, and peripheral arterial pressures together with determination of cardiac output by either thermodilution or Fick principle. These measures allow assessment of possible pressure gradients across the mitral and aortic valves, and catheter pullback on the right side permits assessment of possible gradients across pulmonic and tricuspid valves. Simultaneous measurement of pressures and cardiac output provides the data for calculation of systemic and pulmonary vascular resistances.

The *percutaneous femoral approach* to left heart catheterization involves puncture of the right (or left) femoral artery with a Seldinger needle, passage of a J-tipped guidewire retrograde to the abdominal aorta under fluoroscopic guidance, and placement of an intraarterial sheath with a side arm port for flushing. An appropriate catheter (e.g., pigtail catheter) is then advanced over a guidewire to the descending aorta, at which time the guidewire is removed and the catheter aspirated and flushed vigorously. Under pressure monitoring and fluoroscopic guidance, the catheter is advanced to the ascending aorta, where pressure is recorded simultaneously with peripheral arterial pressure. Subsequent steps in the procedure are identical to those listed for the brachial approach.

An additional method of left heart catheterization is the *transseptal approach*. This approach, which is not commonly employed today except for special diagnostic problems or for purposes of therapeutic intervention (especially mitral valvuloplasty), involves a controlled puncture of the interatrial septum with a long stainless steel needle and advancement of a Teflon catheter or sheath over the needle into the left atrium. Rarely, direct catheterization of the left heart through the chest wall is necessary, by *left ventricular puncture* using a needle inserted into the cardiac apex.

CARDIAC ANGIOGRAPHY

Cardiac angiography involves injection of radiopaque contrast agent into a specific cardiac chamber or vessel using either hand injection or power injection through an automated syringe. Contrast agents utilized today are either nonionic or ionic; the nonionic contrast agents (and the ionic dimer ioxaglate) have less myocardial depressant effect but are substantially more expensive than traditional high-osmolar ionic agents. During injection, these low-osmolar contrast agents usually produce less vasodilatation and less sensation of marked warmth throughout the distribution of the injection than earlier high-osmolar agents.

CORONARY ANGIOGRAPHY This common procedure involves selective injection of radiographic contrast agent into the coronary arteries. Placement of the catheter tips into the right and left coronary arteries is carried out under fluoroscopic guidance, and contrast agent is injected by hand during recording of the radiographic image. Each coronary artery is usually viewed in several projections to permit assessment of severity of stenosis and to minimize overlap of adjacent vessels. In addition to the detection of coronary artery stenoses, coronary angiography is useful for the detection of congenital abnormalities of the coronary circulation, coronary arteriovenous fistulas, and patency of coronary artery bypass grafts. Examples of normal and abnormal coronary anatomy are seen in Figs. 192-1 to 192-3.

FIGURE 192-1 Representation of coronary anatomy relative to the interventricular and atrioventricular valve planes. Coronary branches are indicated as L Main (left main), LAD (left anterior descending), D (diagonal), S (septal), CX (circumflex), OM (obtuse marginal), RCA (right coronary artery), CB (conus branch), SN (sinus node), AcM (acute marginal), PD (posterior descending, PL (posterolateral left ventricular). RAO, right anterior oblique, LAO, left anterior oblique. *(From DS Baim, W Grossman, in W Grossman, DS Baim (eds), 1991, with permission.)*

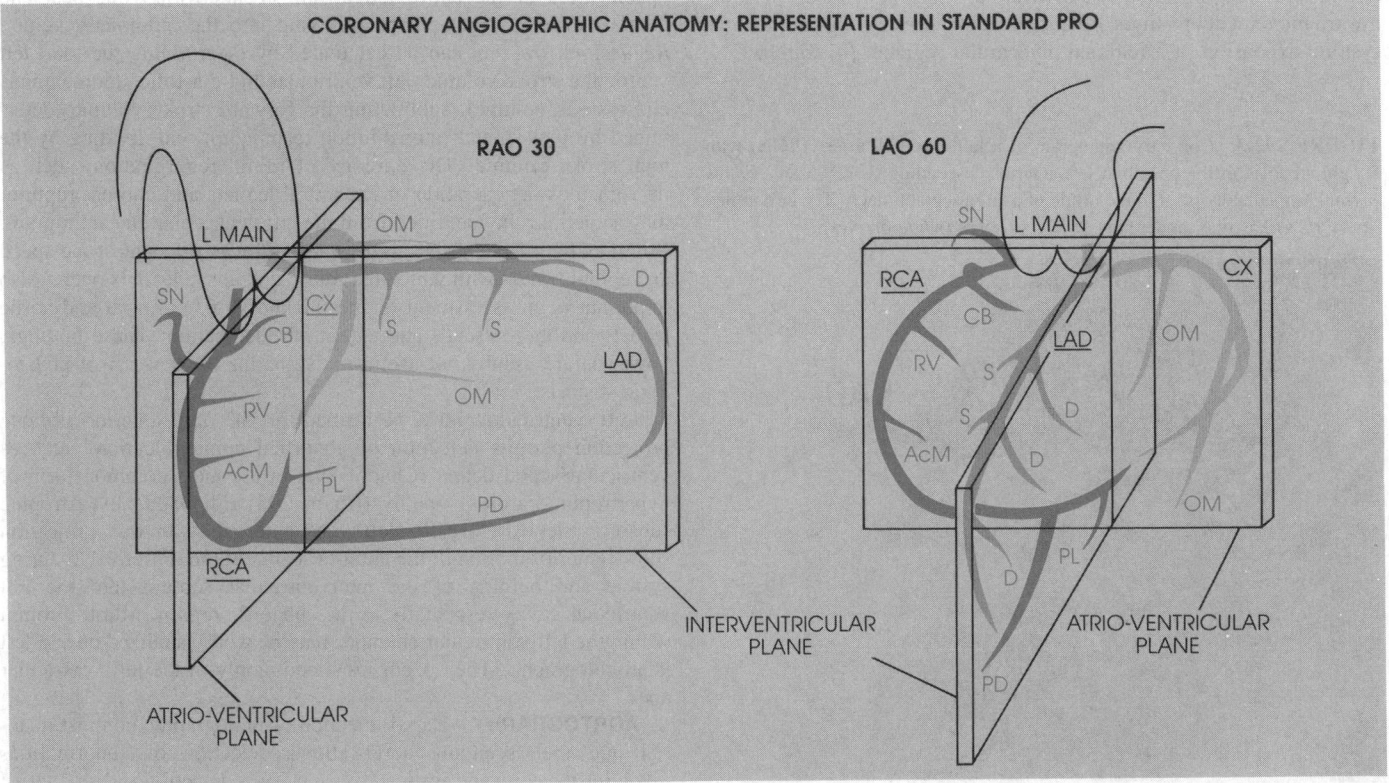

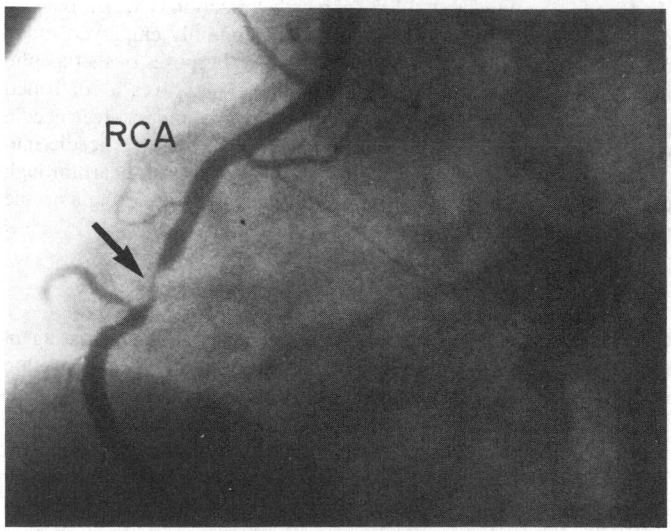

FIGURE 192-2   Coronary angiogram showing a right coronary artery (RCA) with a severe (95 percent) stenosis at its midpoint (*arrow*).

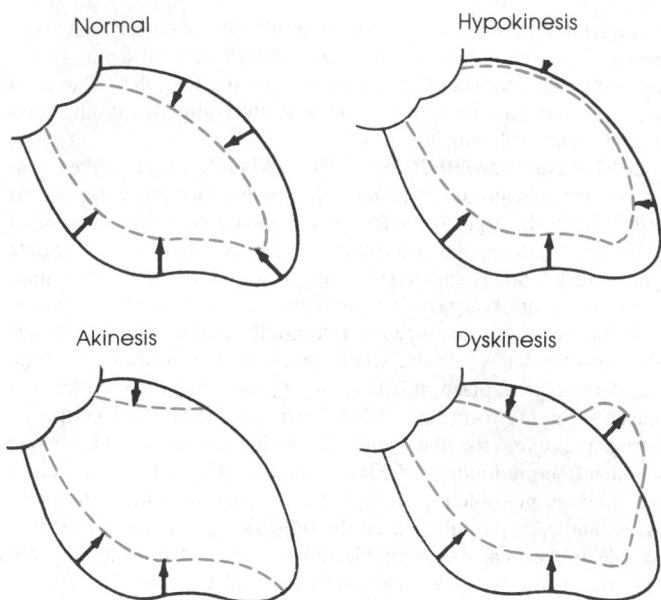

FIGURE 192-4   Diagrammatic representation of end-diastolic (*solid line*) and end-systolic (*dashed line*) silhouettes of left ventricular cineangiograms in various forms of localized wall motion disorder in patients with coronary heart disease. Normal wall motion is symmetric; a patient with *hypokinesis* exhibits reduced contraction, seen here over the anterior and apical surfaces; a patient with *akinesis* exhibits absent wall motion, seen here over the anteroapical surface; the patient with *dyskinesis* exhibits paradoxic bulging of a small portion of the anterior wall with systole.

LEFT VENTRICULOGRAPHY   Injection of radiographic contrast material directly into the left ventricular cavity is an important part of routine left heart catheterization and yields important diagnostic information. Usually, a power injector is utilized to inject 30 to 45 mL of radiographic contrast material into the left ventricular chamber at an injection rate appropriate for the particular catheter being used. Angiographic assessment of the left ventricular silhouette at end-diastole and end-systole permits calculation of left ventricular chamber volumes and ejection fraction, as well as assessment of regional wall motion abnormalities. The normal left ventricle ejects 50 to 80 percent of its end-diastolic volume with each beat; i.e., its *ejection fraction* is 0.50 to 0.80. In adults, normal values for left ventricular volumes are end-diastolic volume, 72 ± 15 mL/m^2 (mean $\pm$ standard deviation), and end-systolic volume, 20 ± 8 mL/m^2. Regional abnormalities of wall motion are illustrated in Fig. 192-4 and include diminished inward motion of a myocardial segment (*hypokinesis*), no inward movement of a myocardial segment (*akinesis*), and paradoxical systolic expansion of a regional myocardial segment (*dyskinesis*).

FIGURE 192-3   Coronary angiogram of a left coronary artery (LCA) with a tight stenosis in the proximal left anterior descending (LAD) artery (*black arrow*) immediately prior to the origin of a large septal branch. The circumflex artery (CX) has two moderately severe stenoses (*white arrows*).

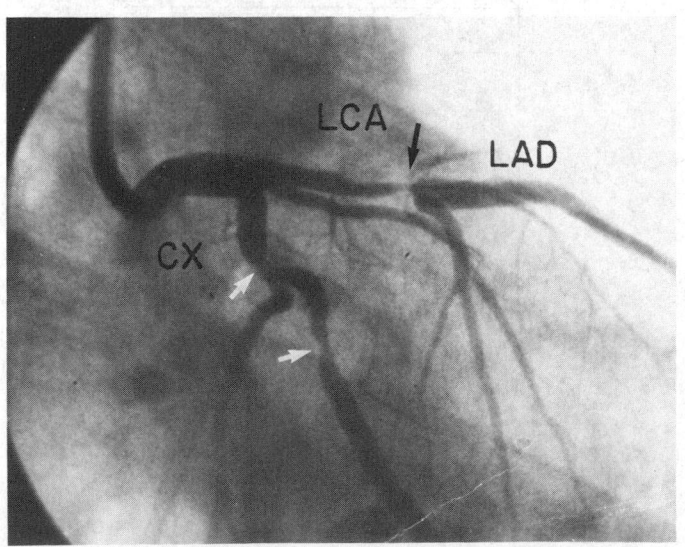

Left ventriculography is usually performed in the right anterior oblique projection, which allows assessment of the mitral and aortic valves. Mitral regurgitation is easily visualized as the appearance of radiographic contrast material in the left atrium during left ventricular systole. Its severity can be estimated qualitatively using a grading system of 1+ (mild, radiographic contrast material clears with each beat and never opacifies the entire left atrium) to 4+ (severe, opacification of the entire left atrium occurs within one beat and contrast material can be seen refluxing into the pulmonary veins). *Regurgitant fraction* can be calculated by determining the total left ventricular stroke volume (left ventricular end-diastolic volume minus end-systolic volume), subtracting the forward stroke volume (determined by Fick or indicator-dilution technique), and dividing by the total stroke volume. The etiology of mitral regurgitation, such as myxomatous degeneration of the mitral leaflets and chordal rupture, may sometimes be identified from the left ventricular cineangiogram. Mitral and aortic stenosis can be *detected* by assessment of the speed and completeness with which the mitral and aortic leaflets open. Also important is an assessment of the thickness of the mitral and aortic leaflets and the presence and extent of calcification. These findings, however, are usually not useful in estimating the *severity* of physiologic stenosis.

Left ventriculography performed in the left anterior oblique projection permits detection of abnormal communications such as ventricular septal defect (Chap. 199). In the most common form of hypertrophic cardiomyopathy (Chap. 205) (idiopathic hypertrophic subaortic stenosis, IHSS), left ventriculography in this projection shows anterior motion of the anterior leaflet of the mitral valve during systole and bulging of the interventricular septum into the left ventricular cavity, especially in the subaortic region. Mural thrombi within the left ventricular chamber may be well visualized during left ventriculography. They occur most commonly in the left ventricular apex.

AORTOGRAPHY   Rapid injection of radiographic contrast material into the ascending aorta allows detection of abnormalities involving the aorta and aortic valve. It permits detection and qualitative

TABLE 192-3   Normal values for hemodynamic parameters

1	Pressures (mmHg)	
	A Systemic arterial	
	(*1*) Peak systolic/end-diastolic	100–140/60–90
	(*2*) Mean	70–105
	B Left ventricle	
	(*1*) Peak systolic/end-diastolic	100–140/3–12
	C Left atrium (or pulmonary capillary wedge)	
	(*1*) Mean	2–10
	(*2*) *a* wave	3–15
	(*3*) *v* wave	3–15
	D Pulmonary artery	
	(*1*) Peak systolic/end-diastolic	15–30/4–12
	(*2*) Mean	9–18
	E Right ventricle	
	(*1*) Peak systolic/end-diastolic	15–30/2–8
	F Right atrium	
	(*1*) Mean	2–8
	(*2*) *a* wave	2–10
	(*3*) *v* wave	2–10
2	Resistances [(dyn•s)/cm^5]	
	(*1*) Systemic vascular resistance	700–1600
	(*2*) Pulmonary vascular resistance	20–130
3	Cardiac index [(L/min)/m^2]	2.6–4.2
4	Oxygen consumption index [(L/min)/m^2]	110–150
5	Arteriovenous oxygen difference (mL/L)	30–50

assessment of the severity of aortic regurgitation utilizing a 1+ to 4+ scale, as for mitral regurgitation. Abnormal communications between the aorta and right side of the heart, such as patent ductus arteriosus or ruptured aneurysm of a sinus of Valsalva, may be visualized. Aortography can permit identification of aortic aneurysm

and of aortic dissection (Chap. 210) and may visualize an intimal flap within the aortic lumen.

PRESSURE MEASUREMENTS

Pressures within the cardiac chambers and great vessels are recorded routinely during cardiac catheterization and provide important information concerning function of ventricular myocardium and cardiac valves. Normal values for pressures measured during cardiac catheterization are summarized in Table 192-3.

Simultaneous measurement of pressures in the left ventricle, aorta, and left atrium (or pulmonary capillary wedge position) permits assessment of mitral and aortic valve function. As seen in Fig. 192-5, left ventricular and aortic pressures are essentially equal during systole, while left atrial (pulmonary capillary wedge) and left ventricular pressures are equal during diastole in the normal heart. A pressure gradient between the left ventricle and aorta during systole may be due to obstruction at the level of the aortic valve (e.g., *calcific aortic stenosis*) or at the subaortic level (e.g., *hypertrophic obstructive cardiomyopathy*). A gradient between the left atrium (pulmonary capillary wedge) and left ventricle in diastole generally indicates *mitral stenosis*, although it also may be seen in rare conditions such as cor triatriatum and left atrial myxoma. An example of a large diastolic pressure gradient in a patient with mitral stenosis is seen in Fig. 192-6. As seen in Fig. 192-7, a prominent *v* wave in the pulmonary capillary wedge pressure will often increase substantially during modest exercise in a patient with significant mitral regurgitation. Severe *aortic regurgitation* produces a widening of the aortic pulse pressure, with equilibration of aortic and left ventricular pressures in diastole (Fig. 192-8). Right-sided pressures exhibit

FIGURE 192-5 Left ventricular (LV), radial artery, and pulmonary capillary wedge (PCW) pressures in a patient with normal cardiovascular function. Note the absence of a pressure gradient between the LV and radial artery in systole and between the LV and PCW in diastole.

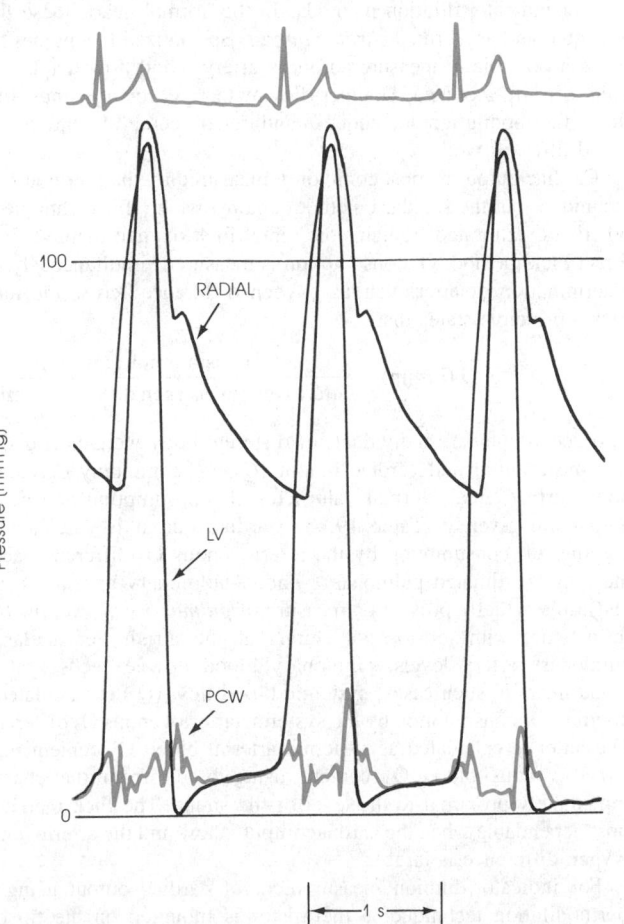

FIGURE 192-6 Pulmonary capillary wedge (PCW) and left ventricular (LV) pressure tracings in a 40-year-old woman with mitral stenosis. This patient also had systemic hypertension and significant elevation of her LV diastolic pressure. *(From BA Carabello, W Grossman, in W Grossman, DS Baim (eds), 1991, with permission.)*

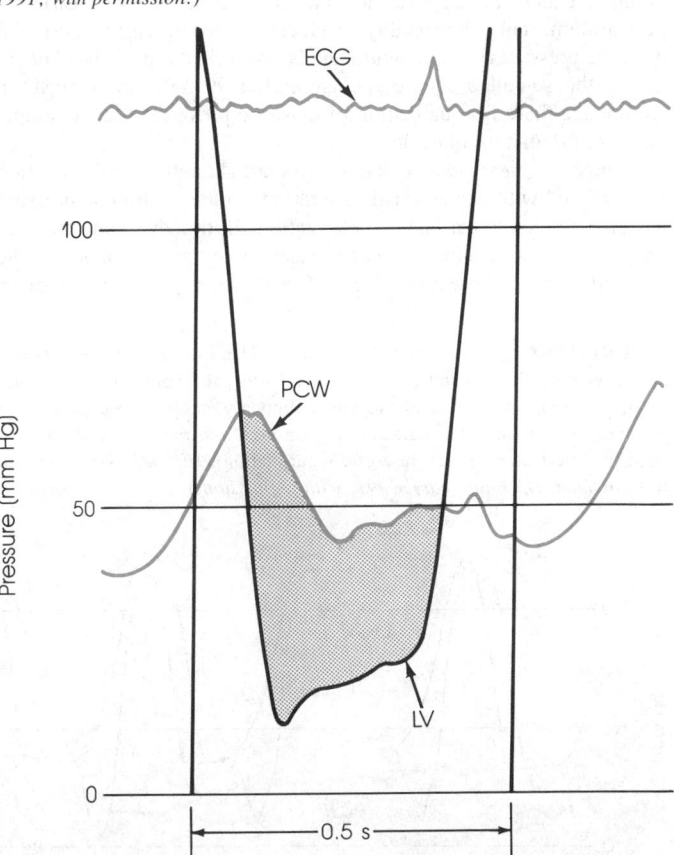

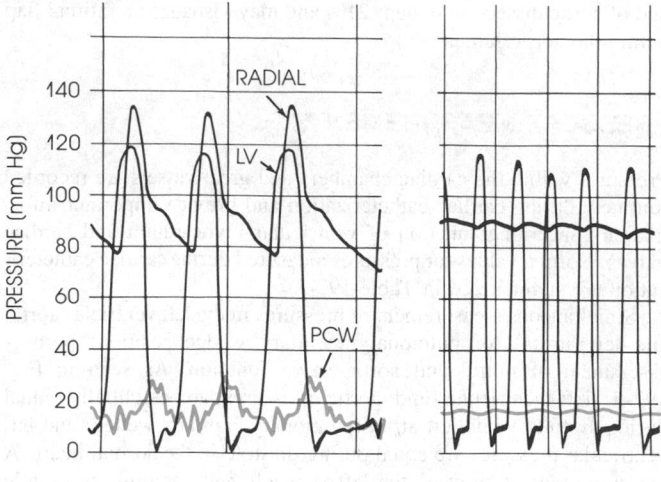

FIGURE 192-7 Hemodynamic findings at rest and during exercise in a patient with mitral regurgitation. Left ventricular (LV), pulmonary capillary wedge (PCW), and radial artery pressure tracings are shown before (*left*) and during (*right*) the sixth minute of supine bicycle exercise. PCW mean pressure and *v* wave increase substantially with exercise. *(From BH Lorell, W Grossman, in W Grossman, DS Baim (eds), 1991, with permission.)*

characteristic deformity in the presence of valvular heart disease affecting the tricuspid or pulmonic valves. In patients with severe *tricuspid regurgitation*, right atrial pressure resembles closely in appearance the right ventricular pressure. Mean right atrial pressure and right ventricular end-diastolic pressure are both elevated in tricuspid regurgitation. In *tricuspid stenosis* there is a pressure gradient between right atrium and ventricle during diastole.

Characteristic deformities of right and left ventricular diastolic pressures occur in patients with *cardiac tamponade* or *pericardial constriction*. In both conditions there is equalization of left and right ventricular diastolic pressures. However, in constrictive pericarditis, nearly all ventricular filling occurs shortly after mitral and tricuspid valve opening; following this period of rapid filling, ventricular volumes cannot increase further due to the limit of the constricting pericardium. This abnormality produces an abrupt early ventricular diastolic pressure rise with a mid and late ventricular pressure plateau, giving the so-called square root sign (Fig. 192-9). In contrast, in tamponade there is equalization of diastolic pressures with a gradual increase throughout diastole.

Congestive heart failure due to myocardial contractile dysfunction is associated with characteristic alterations in the ventricular pressure waveforms seen at cardiac catheterization. Both isovolumic pressure rise and pressure decline are not as steep as in the normal heart. The reduced slopes of pressure rise and decline are associated with an

FIGURE 192-8 Severe aortic regurgitation. There is equilibration between the left ventricular (LV) and aortic or femoral artery (FA) pressures in diastole. Also, LV diastolic pressure exceeds pulmonary capillary wedge (PCW) pressure early in diastole, indicating premature closure of the mitral valve (a characteristic feature of severe aortic regurgitation). *(From W Grossman, in W Grossman, DS Baim (eds), 1991, with permission.)*

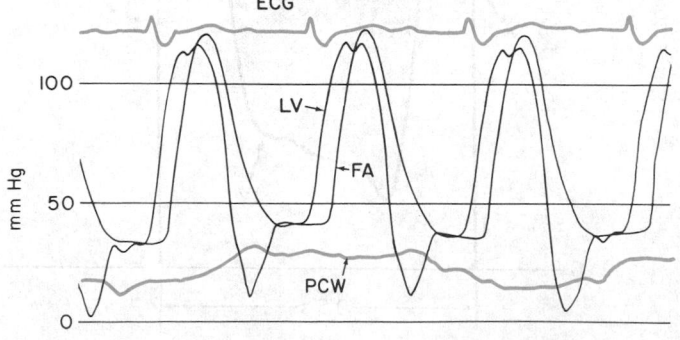

abbreviated ejection period, giving the left ventricular pressure tracing a triangular appearance (Fig. 192-10). Also, the pressure decline does not continue to zero, so the minimal left ventricular diastolic pressure may be elevated. This hemodynamic finding correlates with an increased ventricular end-systolic volume, which is a sign of depressed contractile function of the left ventricular myocardium.

MEASUREMENT OF FLOW

Systemic and pulmonary blood flows may be measured by either the Fick or indicator-dilution methods. In the normal heart, these flows are equal and are termed *cardiac output*. Specialized techniques have made it possible to measure coronary artery blood flow (catheter- or guidewire-tip-mounted Doppler flowmeter), coronary sinus blood flow (thermodilution technique), and renal, cerebral, and femoral blood flows as well.

Cardiac output is most commonly measured by the thermodilution technique, but the standard method, against which this technique and others are calibrated, remains the direct Fick oxygen method. In the direct Fick method, O_2 consumption is measured simultaneously with determination of arteriovenous oxygen difference across the lungs. Fick's principle states that

$$Q \text{ (L/min)} = \frac{O_2 \text{ consumption (mL/min)}}{\text{arteriovenous oxygen difference (mL/L)}}$$

In order to compare individuals of different body weights and sizes, O_2 consumption and cardiac output (Q) are commonly divided by body surface area. Normal values for O_2 consumption and cardiac output are given in Table 192-3. Cardiac output is calculated by dividing O_2 consumption by the arteriovenous O_2 difference across the lungs (estimated pulmonary venous–pulmonary arterial O_2 content); this actually provides a measure of *pulmonary blood flow* (Q_p). In patients with left-to-right shunts at the atrial, ventricular, or pulmonary artery levels, pulmonary blood flow exceeds systemic blood flow. In such cases, systemic blood flow (Q_s) is calculated by dividing O_2 consumption by the systemic arteriovenous O_2 difference. The latter is calculated as systemic arterial blood O_2 content minus mixed venous blood O_2 content using blood from the chamber immediately proximal to the level of the shunt. The Fick method is most dependable when the cardiac output is low and the arteriovenous oxygen difference is large.

For indicator-dilution measurement of cardiac output using the thermodilution technique, a thermistor is mounted on the tip of a

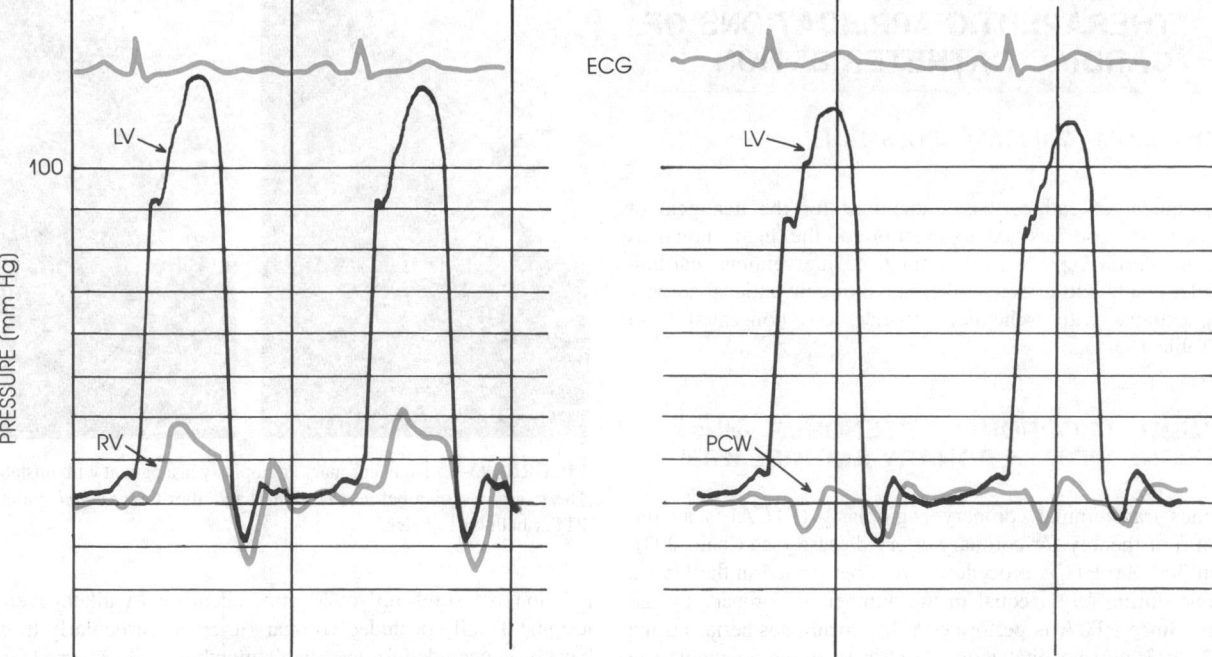

FIGURE 192-9 Left ventricular (LV), right ventricular (RV), and pulmonary capillary wedge (PCW) pressure tracings in a patient with severe constrictive pericarditis. Note the diastolic dip and plateau ("square root sign") pattern for left and right ventricular diastolic pressures (*left*). The wedge pressure (*right*) shows early systolic and early diastolic dips.

balloon-flotation catheter, and the catheter is advanced so that the balloon tip and thermistor are located in the pulmonary artery. Cold dextrose solution or saline is injected via a proximal port on the catheter into the vena cava or right atrium, and the change in temperature monitored at the thermistor is integrated mathematically. This integral is inversely proportional to the volume flow rate past the thermistor, and if the temperatures of the injectate and pulmonary artery blood are measured, cardiac output (actually pulmonary blood flow) can be calculated. In contrast to the Fick method, the indicator-dilution method is least reliable when the cardiac output is low.

FIGURE 192-10 Left ventricular (LV) and aortic (Ao) pressures in a patient with advanced dilated cardiomyopathy. Marked slowing of the rates of left ventricular pressure rise and fall (impairment of contractility and relaxation) give the LV pressure pulse a triangular appearance. Also, the minimal value for left ventricular diastolic pressure is markedly elevated, suggesting an increased end-systolic volume and a reduced LV ejection fraction. *(From W Grossman, in W Grossman, DS Baim (eds), 1991, with permission.)*

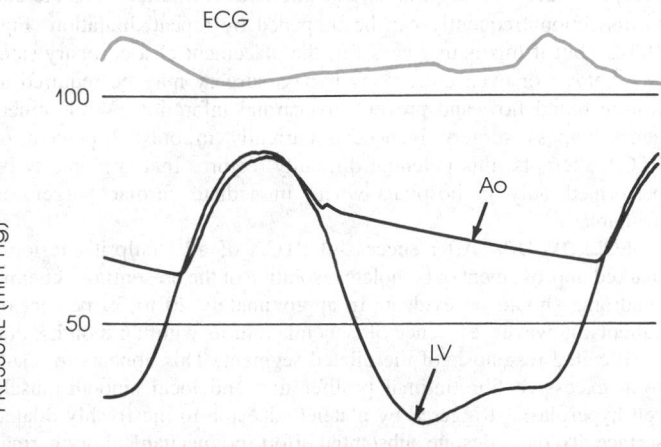

Valve areas and resistances Using simultaneous measures of pressure and flow, the resistance to blood flow across cardiac valves as well as the pulmonary and systemic arteriolar beds may be estimated. Valve areas are calculated using the Gorlin formula:

$$A = \frac{\text{flow}}{K\sqrt{\Delta P}}$$

where A = valve orifice area (cm²), *flow* is the blood flow (mL/s) across the stenotic valve, ΔP is the mean pressure gradient (mmHg) during the period of blood flow, and K is a constant (44.3 for the aortic valve and 37.7 for the mitral valve).

The resistance to blood flow through the systemic vascular bed is

$$SVR = 80(MAP - RA)/SBF$$

where SVR is systemic vascular resistance [(dyn·s)/cm⁵], MAP and RA are mean aortic and right atrial pressures (mmHg), 80 is a constant for converting to metric units, and SBF is systemic blood flow (L/min).

Resistance to blood flow through the pulmonary vascular bed is

$$PVR = 80(PA - PCW \text{ or } LA)/PBF$$

where PVR is pulmonary vascular resistance [(dyn·s)/cm⁵]; PA, PCW, and LA are pulmonary artery, pulmonary capillary wedge, and left atrial mean pressures (mmHg); and PBF is pulmonary blood flow (L/min). Normal values for pulmonary and systemic vascular resistances are given in Table 192-3.

REFERENCES

GODLEWSKI KJ et al: Interpretation of cardiac pathophysiology from pressure waveform analysis: Acute aortic insufficiency. Cathet Cardiovasc Diagn 28:244, 1993

GROSSMAN W: Cardiac catheterization, in *Heart Disease*, 4th ed, E Braunwald (ed). Philadelphia, Saunders, 1992, p 180

———, BAIM DS (eds): *Cardiac Catheterization, Angiography, and Intervention*, 4th ed. Philadelphia, Lea & Febiger, 1991

JOHNSON LW, KRONE R: Cardiac catheterization 1991: A report of the Registry of the Society for Cardiac Angiography and Interventions (SCA&I). Cathet Cardiovasc Diagn 28:219, 1993

KERN MJ et al: Interpretation of cardiac pathophysiology from pressure waveform analysis: Simultaneous left and right ventricular pressure measurements. Cathet Cardiovasc Diagn 28:51, 1993

193 THERAPEUTIC APPLICATIONS OF CARDIAC CATHETERIZATION

DONALD S. BAIM / WILLIAM GROSSMAN

The development of catheter-based therapies for the treatment of cardiovascular disease has led to creation of the field known as *interventional cardiology*. In current practice, interventional cardiology provides a safe and effective alternative to conventional surgery for many patients with ischemic, valvular, and congenital heart disease (Table 193-1).

TREATMENT OF CORONARY STENOSES AND OCCLUSIONS WITH CORONARY ANGIOPLASTY

Percutaneous transluminal coronary angioplasty (PTCA) is an important form of therapy for coronary artery disease (see Chap. 203). More than 300,000 PTCA procedures were performed in the United States alone during 1991, equal to the number of coronary bypass operations. Since PTCA is performed using local anesthesia, during a short (2- to 3-day) hospitalization, its use in suitable patients can greatly decrease expense and recovery time compared to coronary bypass surgery, although it carries a 0.4 to 1.0 percent procedure-related mortality, similar to that of elective coronary bypass surgery.

INDICATIONS The main indication for PTCA is the presence of one or more coronary stenoses that are approachable by balloon catheters and that are felt to be responsible for a clinical syndrome warranting revascularization (Fig. 193-1). Moreover, the risks and benefits for revascularization by PTCA should compare favorably with those of conventional surgery. Significant left main stenosis and multivessel disease in which vessels supplying significant areas of viable myocardium are not approachable by PTCA (due to chronic total occlusion or other unfavorable anatomic features) constitute relative contraindications to PTCA if surgery is technically possible.

For most patients, the clinical syndrome being treated is moderately severe, chronic, stable angina that persists despite medical antianginal therapy. Approximately 15 percent of current PTCA patients, however, have only mild anginal symptoms despite suitable coronary anatomy and objective evidence of ischemia (i.e., an abnormal exercise test). At the other extreme, many patients have more pressing indications for PTCA, including unstable angina or even acute myocardial infarction (with or without prior thrombolytic therapy).

As the clinical indications for PTCA have broadened, so have its anatomic capabilities. Thus PTCA is no longer restricted to proximal, discrete, subtotal, concentric, noncalcified lesions, as was the case initially. Angioplasty catheters with smaller deflated profiles, controlled by highly steerable guidewires, are now available and can be advanced successfully across severe stenoses located virtually anywhere in the coronary tree. These balloon catheters tolerate

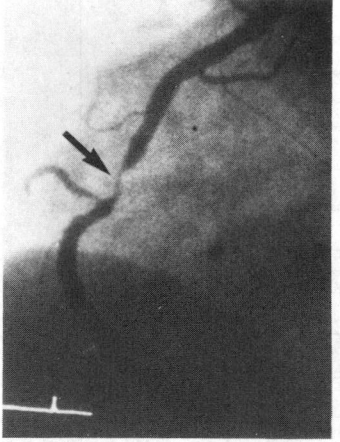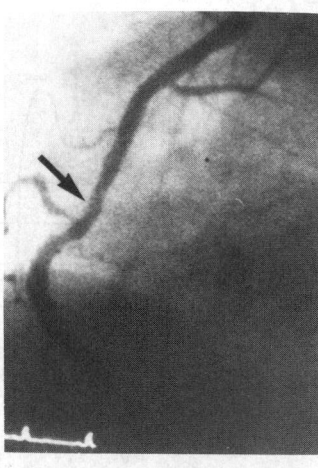

FIGURE 193-1   Right coronary angioplasty in a patient with unstable angina. The lesion is shown before (*left panel*) and after (*right panel*) inflation of the PTCA balloon catheter.

inflation pressures up to 20 atm, adequate to dilate even calcific lesions. Totally occluded coronary arteries (particularly those which have been occluded for less than 6 months) can be crossed and dilated effectively, although the success rate remains somewhat lower than for subtotal lesions (i.e., 60 percent versus 90 percent for subtotal stenotic lesions). In addition to lesions in the native coronary tree, obstructions in saphenous vein or internal mammary artery bypass grafts also can be dilated successfully to treat postbypass angina. If multiple lesions are responsible for the clinical syndrome, most or all such lesions can generally be dilated during a single procedure.

RESULTS The current PTCA success rate (for reducing a target stenosis to <50 percent of its original diameter without producing an associated complication) exceeds 90 percent. About half the failures result from inability to cross the target lesion with the guidewire or balloon catheter, particularly when that target lesion is a chronic total occlusion. The remaining failures are due to excessive local dissection (separation of coronary artery intima from media) resulting from attempted dilatation. While some local dissection is present in virtually all successful PTCA procedures, more extensive dissection (particularly in association with local thrombus formation or vasospasm) can lead to abrupt closure of the dilated segment soon after withdrawal of the balloon catheter. Routine use of vasodilators (nitrates and calcium channel antagonists), anticoagulation (heparin 10,000 to 15,000 units during the procedure), and antiplatelet therapy (acetylsalicylic acid, 325 mg/d starting at least 24 h prior to PTCA and continued for 3 to 6 months after the procedure) helps to prevent abrupt closure due to spasm and/or thrombus formation. Closure due to dissection frequently can be reopened by repeat dilatation (Fig. 193-2), but if this is unsuccessful, the placement of a coronary stent (see below) or even emergency bypass surgery may be required to restore blood flow and prevent myocardial infarction. While emergency bypass surgery is needed currently in only 2 percent of PTCA attempts, this potential difficulty requires that angioplasty be performed only in hospitals where immediate cardiac surgery is available.

FOLLOW-UP After successful PTCA of all "culprit" lesions, marked improvement or complete resolution of the presenting ischemic syndrome should be evident. In approximately 20 to 30 percent of patients, however, evidence of ischemia returns within 6 months, due to so-called restenosis of the dilated segment. This appears to result from excessive fibrointimal proliferation and local smooth-muscle cell hyperplasia, triggered by platelet adhesion to the freshly dilated surface. To date, despite substantial effort, no mechanical or pharmacologic strategy has substantially reduced this restenosis rate. When recurrent ischemia develops more than 6 months after PTCA, it usually reflects progression of disease at another site, rather than restenosis. With use of repeat PTCA to treat either restenosis or

---

TABLE 193-1   Therapeutic applications of cardiac catheterization

Treatment of coronary stenoses and occlusions
  Percutaneous transluminal coronary angioplasty (PTCA)
  Laser techniques
  Intravascular stents
  Atherectomy
Treatment of valvular stenoses
  Balloon valvuloplasty (aortic, mitral, pulmonic)
Treatment of congenital defects
  Atrial septostomy
  Umbrella closure of patent ductus arteriosus and defects in atrial or ventricular septum
  Coil closure of undesired collateral vessels

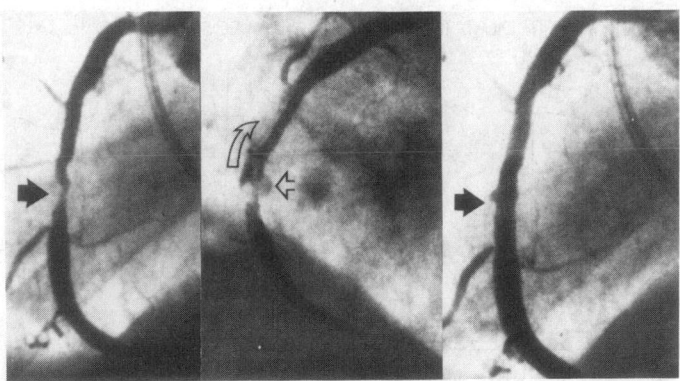

FIGURE 193-2 Abrupt closure of a mid-right coronary artery lesion after attempted dilatation in a patient with recurrent ischemia following rt-PA therapy for inferior wall infarction. The involved lesion is shown before dilatation (*left panel*), during abrupt closure immediately after initial dilatation (*center panel*, arrows indicate local dissection), and following stabilization by redilatation (*right panel*).

disease progression, only about 10 percent of patients require bypass surgery during the 5 years following a successful PTCA procedure.

NEWER NONBALLOON TECHNIQUES In an attempt to circumvent the existing limitations of balloon angioplasty, intensive evaluation of a variety of nonballoon techniques is currently under way. One or more of these newer techniques may aid in crossing total occlusions, dilating rigid or elastic lesions, stabilizing dissections, or reducing the incidence of restenosis.

Laser Laser energy (at wavelengths from the ultraviolet to the infrared) can be delivered to coronary lesions through 50-μm optical fibers bundled into wire-guided catheters from 1.2 to 2.5 mm in diameter. Depending on the specific delivery parameters, this energy, associated with various degrees of acoustic (blast) or local thermal injury, can produce direct ablation of atherosclerotic plaques. Laser ablation can provide partial lumen enlargement of even diffuse or calcified lesions. However, given the small diameter of the current catheters (and hence the resulting lumen), postlaser balloon dilatation is almost always required. Since no ablative laser technologies distinguish plaque from normal vessel wall, careful case selection (avoiding curves and bifurcations) is required to minimize the risk of laser-induced vessel perforation of the coronary artery. Lasers also have been used to deliver controlled thermal energy to atherosclerotic plaque. Laser heating of a metal cap (the thermal probe) was used successfully to cross occlusions in the peripheral circulation but has proven impractical in the coronary arteries due to excessive vasospasm and thrombosis.

Intravascular stents Permanent metallic endoprostheses (stents) of several designs can be delivered into the peripheral and coronary arteries (Fig. 193-3). Since a successfully deployed stent scaffolds the vessel lumen, it provides excellent acute luminal patency. Over a period of 8 weeks stents become covered by endothelial cells and incorporated into the vessel wall. Until that time, however, intense anticoagulation, generally with warfarin and acetylsalicylic acid, is needed to minimize the risk of developing an occlusive thrombus within the stent. Because of this risk, stenting is used in only the small percentage (5 to 10 percent) of angioplasties where it is beneficial in improving suboptimal luminal appearance, managing elastic lesions or stenoses in vein grafts, and reversing abrupt closure. Since stenting does not reduce the amount of local intimal hyperplasia, any reduction in restenosis is therefore based on the larger lumen provided by stenting in comparison with conventional balloon angioplasty.

Mechanical atherectomy Unlike balloon angioplasty—which merely *redistributes* plaque to improve luminal caliber—atherectomy seeks to *remove* plaque material. Several catheter designs have been developed, including side-cutting (directional) atherectomy (Fig. 193-4), end-cutting (extraction) atherectomy, and abrasive (rotational) atherectomy. Each has been employed in both the peripheral and coronary circulations, demonstrating that safe enlargement of lumen is possible without vessel perforation. Directional atherectomy is currently used in 10 percent of angioplasty procedures, where it provides a more predictable result than conventional balloon angioplasty in treating ostial, eccentric, and bifurcation lesions. In addition, directional atherectomy is unique in its ability to recover plaque samples for histologic and biochemical evaluation, improving the understanding of plaque formation and restenosis.

TREATMENT OF VALVULAR STENOSIS: BALLOON VALVULOPLASTY

Following successful balloon dilatation of vascular stenoses, both pediatric and adult cardiologists applied balloon dilatation to the treatment of stenotic cardiac valves. While the initial use was in patients with congenital pulmonic and aortic stenosis, this technique has now been extended to patients with acquired rheumatic and calcific stenoses of the mitral and aortic valves.

PULMONIC VALVULOPLASTY Although congenital pulmonic stenosis is predominantly a pediatric disease, it is sometimes encountered in adults (see Chap. 199). Transvalvular pressure gradients >50 mmHg may produce exertional symptoms or lead to progressive right ventricular hypertrophy or failure. Using a guidewire placed into the pulmonary artery from the femoral vein, one or more valvuloplasty balloons with a combined cross-sectional area as much as 20 percent larger than the pulmonic valve annulus are positioned within the stenotic valve and inflated with liquid contrast medium at pressures of 3 to 5 atm. This typically reduces the transvalvular gradient from

FIGURE 193-3 Severe eccentric stenosis of the right coronary artery (*left*) with partial response to conventional angioplasty (*left center*) but larger lumen after placement of a stent (*right center*) and preservation of patency at 6-month restudy (*right*). The collapsed and expanded Palmar Schatz stents are shown in the bottom panel. (*From MJ Levine et al, J Am Coll Cardiol 16:332, 1990.*)

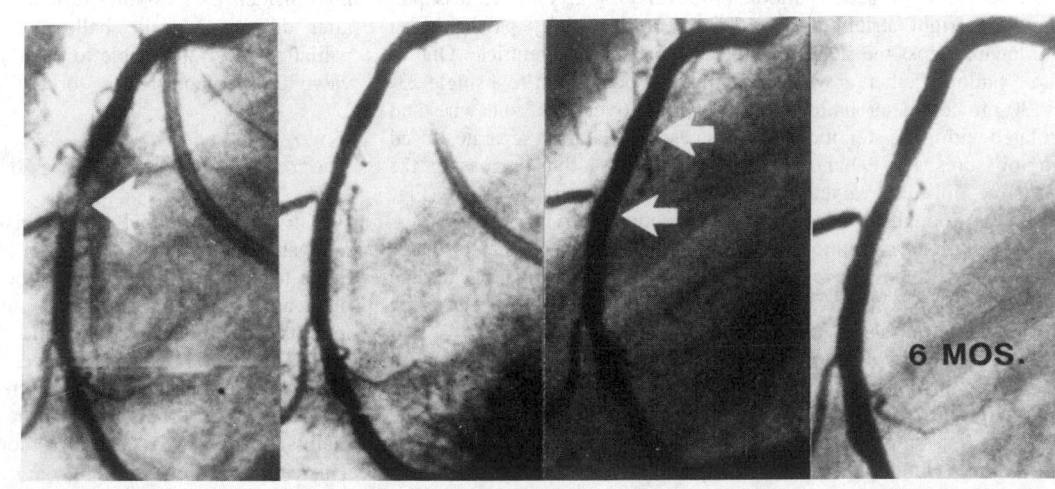

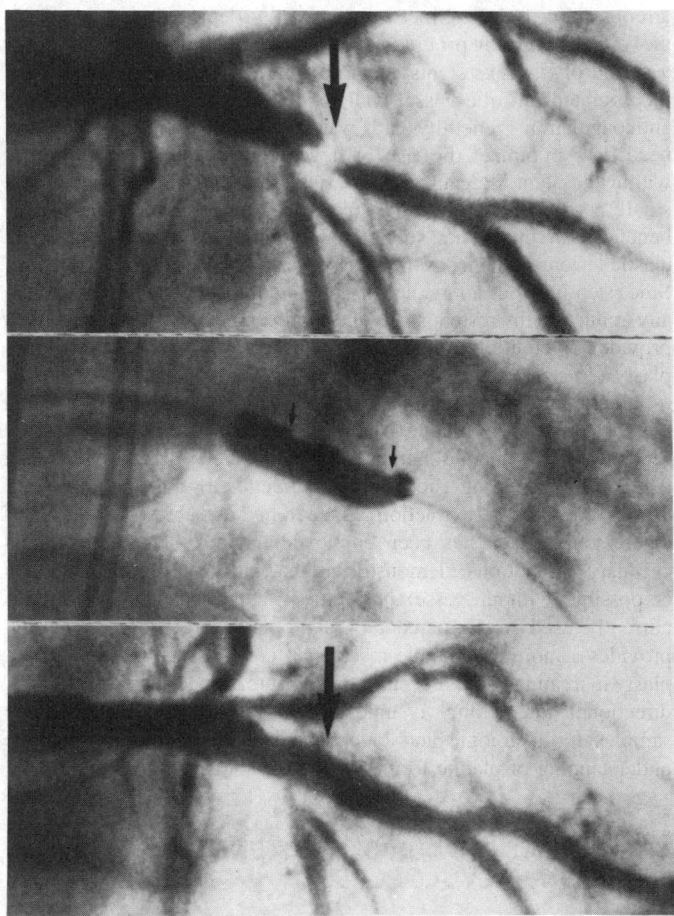

FIGURE 193-4 Eccentric, ulcerated lesion in the mid-left anterior descending coronary artery (*top*), being treated by directional atherectomy (*middle*), with a large and smooth luminal result (*bottom*).

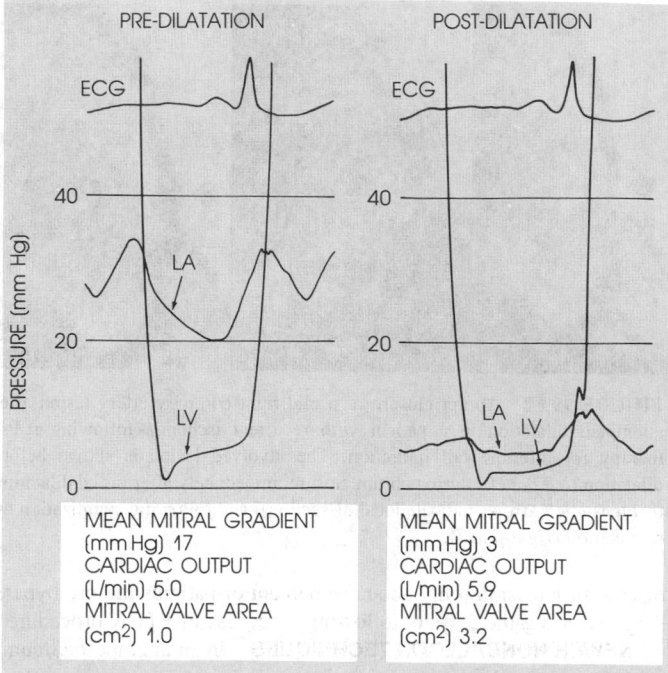

FIGURE 193-5 Hemodynamic results of mitral valvuloplasty in a 38-year-old woman with mitral stenosis. The transmitral [left atrium (LA)–to–left ventricle (LV)] gradient, cardiac output, and calculated mitral valve area are shown before (*left panel*) and after (*right panel*) balloon dilatation.

75 to 15 mmHg. Balloon pulmonary valvuloplasty now stands as the preferred therapy for this lesion.

MITRAL VALVULOPLASTY   The predominant application of balloon mitral valvuloplasty is in patients with rheumatic mitral stenosis, in whom stenosis results primarily from commissural fusion with associated leaflet thickening. Such patients previously would have undergone open or closed surgical commissurotomy but are now treated almost exclusively by balloon valvuloplasty. Other patients (with left atrial thrombus, mitral regurgitation, subvalvular disease, or leaflet thickening or rigidity) have less satisfactory results with either surgical commissurotomy or balloon valvuloplasty and are better treated by surgical valve replacement.

The usual approach to balloon mitral valvuloplasty is via transseptal puncture (right atrium to left atrium), followed by passage of a guidewire across the stenotic valve and into the left ventricle. One or more balloon catheters with a dilating area equivalent to a single 23- to 30-mm diameter balloon are advanced over this guidewire and inflated within the stenotic valve. Successful dilatation separates fused commissures and enhances leaflet compliance, thus increasing the effective diastolic valve area from 0.9 to 2.0 cm^2 or more (Fig. 193-5). Although this is still restricted compared with the 3.5- to 5-cm^2 area of a normal mitral valve, this increase in valve area provides excellent symptomatic relief and is equivalent to or approaches the increase in orifice size resulting from surgical mitral commissurotomy or prosthetic mitral valve replacement.

The main complications of balloon mitral valvuloplasty relate to the potential for cardiac perforation during transseptal puncture (approximately 2 percent of patients) and the chance of systemic embolization (approximately 1 percent of patients) despite preprocedure echocardiographic exclusion of patients with left atrial thrombus.

AORTIC VALVULOPLASTY   Balloon aortic valvuloplasty may be performed in children with congenital aortic stenosis and in adults with rheumatic or acquired calcific aortic stenosis. Some patients with rheumatic aortic stenosis have leaflet fusion, but the problem in acquired calcific aortic stenosis is due more to rigidity of the valve leaflets themselves. In this latter group of patients, balloon valvuloplasty fractures leaflet calcium (providing new hinge points along which the valve leaflets can open) and temporarily expands the aortic annulus.

The most prevalent approach to balloon aortic valvuloplasty consists of femoral arterial puncture with retrograde passage of a guidewire and balloon (inflated diameter 18 to 23 mm) across the valve. Overdilatation of the valve annulus may cause leaflet avulsion and is generally avoided. Balloon aortic valvuloplasty typically increases the effective systolic valve area from 0.6 to 1.0 cm^2. The resultant valve area is still small compared with the area of a normal aortic valve (3 to 4 cm^2) or with the effective area of an inflated 20-mm balloon (3.1 cm^2), but it does relieve symptoms at rest or during mild to moderate exertion in most patients with critical aortic stenosis. Unfortunately, the relatively small effective orifice achieved and the high incidence of valvular restenosis (up to 50 percent within 1 year after dilatation) make balloon aortic valvuloplasty a temporary palliation most applicable to elderly patients who are poor risks for valve replacement or as a ''bridge'' to valve replacement.

TREATMENT OF CONGENITAL MALFORMATIONS

Pediatric interventional cardiologists have developed a number of innovative techniques to correct or palliate congenital cardiac lesions. Some techniques are those described above—i.e., balloon dilatation of stenotic pulmonary arteries, surgical shunts, or balloon valvuloplasty—but others are unique to the pediatric population.

ATRIAL SEPTOSTOMY   In certain patients with cyanotic congenital heart disease, such as some with transposition of the great vessels, it is desirable to produce or enlarge an atrial septal defect in order to facilitate passage of oxygenated blood into the right side of the heart. This can be achieved by passage of a balloon catheter from right to left atrium across a patent foramen ovale, followed by forceful withdrawal of the inflated balloon. Alternatively, a catheter with a concealed blade can be passed across the septum. The blade can then be deployed in the left atrium to incise the septum as the catheter is withdrawn. The resulting septal incision can be widened by conventional balloon septostomy.

CLOSURE OF UNDESIRED SHUNTS OR COLLATERAL VESSELS A variety of appliances have been developed to close undesired intracardiac shunts, including defects in the atrial or ventricular septum and patent ductus arteriosus. These devices resemble a double (back-to-back) umbrella, which can be folded into a cylinder for containment in a catheter. Under fluoroscopic guidance, the delivery catheter can be positioned across the target defect so that the umbrella can be deployed to block undesired flow.

Smaller vascular shunts can be closed using special coils. These coils can be placed within a catheter and delivered to the undesired vessel. Once in place, the coil interferes with blood flow and promotes local thrombotic occlusion of the target vessel.

REFERENCES

BAIM DS: Interventional catheterization techniques: Percutaneous transluminal angioplasty, valvuloplasty and related procedures, in *Heart Disease*, 4th ed, E Braunwald (ed). Philadelphia, Saunders, 1992, p 1365

CARROZZA JP et al: Angiographic and clinical outcome of intracoronary stenting: Immediate and long-term results from a large single-center experience. J Am Coll Cardiol 20:328, 1992

DE FEYTER PJ et al: Balloon angioplasty for the treatment of lesions in saphenous vein bypass grafts. J Am Coll Cardiol 21:1539, 1993

FISHMAN R et al: Long-term results of coronary atherectomy—predictors of restenosis. J Am Coll Cardiol 20:1101, 1992

HANDENSCHILD CC: Pathobiology of restenosis after angioplasty. Am J Med 94:40S, 1993

JOHNSON MC et al: Repair of coarctation of the aorta in infancy. Comparison of surgical and balloon angioplasty. Am Heart J 125:464, 1993

KUNTZ RE et al: Predictors of event-free survival after balloon aortic valvuloplasty. N Engl J Med 325:17, 1991

LOCK JE et al: Transcatheter umbrella closure of congenital heart defects. Circulation 75:593, 1987

O'LAUGHLIN MP et al: Transcatheter closure of residual atrial septal defect following cardiac transplantation. Cathet Cardiovasc Diagn 28:162, 1993

194 NORMAL AND ABNORMAL MYOCARDIAL FUNCTION

EUGENE BRAUNWALD

CELLULAR BASIS OF CARDIAC CONTRACTION

The *myocardium* is composed of individual striated muscle cells (fibers), normally 10 to 15 μm in diameter and 30 to 60 μm in length (Fig. 194-1*A*). Each fiber contains multiple cross-banded strands (myofibrils) that run the length of the fiber and are, in turn, composed of serially repeating structures, the sarcomeres. The cytoplasm between the myofibrils contains other cell constituents, such as the single centrally located nucleus, numerous mitochondria, and intracellular membrane system, the sarcoplasmic reticulum.

The *sarcomere,* the structural and functional unit of contraction, is delimited by two adjacent dark lines, the Z lines (Fig. 194-1). The distance between Z lines varies with the degree of contraction or stretch of the muscle and ranges between 1.6 and 2.2 μm. Within the confines of the sarcomere are alternating light and dark bands, giving the myocardial fibers their striated appearance under the light microscope. At the center of the sarcomere is a dark band of constant width (1.5 μm), the A band, which is flanked by two lighter bands,

the I bands, which are of variable width. The sarcomere of heart muscle, like that of skeletal muscle, is made up of two sets of interdigitating myofilaments. Thicker filaments, composed principally of the protein myosin, traverse and are limited to the A band. They are about 10 nm (100 Å) in diameter, with tapered ends, and measure 1.5 to 1.6 μm in length. Thinner filaments, composed primarily of actin, course from the Z line through the I band into the A band. They are approximately 5 nm (50 Å) in diameter and 1.0 μm in length. Thus there is overlapping of thick and thin filaments only within the A band, while the I band contains only thin filaments (Fig. 194-1). On electron-microscopic examination, bridges may be seen to extend between the thick and thin filaments within the A band.

THE CONTRACTILE PROCESS The "sliding" model for muscle rests on the fundamental observation that the thick and thin filaments are constant in overall length during both contraction and relaxation. With activation, repeated interactions take place at the bridges between the actin and myosin filaments, and the actin filaments are propelled further into the A band. In the process, the A band remains constant in width, whereas the I band becomes more narrow and the Z lines move toward one another.

The myosin molecule is a complex, asymmetric fibrous protein with a molecular weight of about 500,000; it has a rod-like portion that is about 150 nm (1500 Å) in length with a globular portion at its end. This globular portion of the myosin is the site of adenosine triphosphatase (ATPase) activity and also forms the bridges between the myosin and actin. In forming the thick myofilament, which is composed of 300 longitudinally stacked myosin molecules, the rod-like segments of the myosin molecules are laid down in an orderly, polarized manner, leaving the globular portions projecting outward so that they can interact with actin to generate force and shortening (Fig. 194-2*A*). Actin has a molecular weight of 47,000. The thin filament is composed of a double helix of two chains of actin molecules wound about each other, intimately associated with two regulatory proteins, tropomyosin and troponin (Fig. 194-2*B*); the latter can be separated into three components, troponins C, I, and T (Fig. 194-2*C*). In contrast to myosin, actin has no intrinsic enzymatic activity, but it has the ability to combine reversibly with myosin in the presence of ATP and Mg^{2+}, which activates the myosin ATPase. In relaxed muscle this interaction is inhibited by tropomyosin.

During activation Ca^{2+} becomes attached to troponin C, which results in a conformational change in the regulatory protein tropomyosin, which in turn exposes the actin cross-bridge interaction sites. This results in sliding of the actin along the myosin filaments, ultimately causing muscle shortening and/or the development of tension. The splitting of ATP then dissociates the myosin cross-bridge from the actin. In the presence of ATP linkages between actin and myosin filaments are made and broken cyclically as long as sufficient Ca^{2+} is present; these linkages are broken when Ca^{2+} concentration falls below a critical level, and the troponin-tropomyosin complex once more prevents interactions between the myosin cross-bridges and the actin filaments. Ionic calcium is a principal mediator of the inotropic state of the heart; most positive inotropic drugs, including the digitalis glycosides and catecholamines, act by increasing the concentrations of Ca^{2+} in the vicinity of the myofilaments.

The *sarcoplasmic reticulum* (Fig. 194-1*B*) is a complex network of anastomosing intracellular channels that invests the myofibrils. It is less profuse in cardiac than in skeletal muscle. Its longitudinally disposed membrane-lined tubules are closely applied to the surfaces of individual sarcomeres but have no direct continuity with the outside of the cell. However, closely related to the sarcoplasmic reticulum, both structurally and functionally, are the transverse tubules or T system, formed by tubelike invaginations of the sarcolemma that extend into the myocardial fiber along the Z lines, i.e., the ends of the sarcomeres.

CARDIAC ACTIVATION At rest, the cardiac cell is polarized; i.e., the interior has a negative charge relative to the outside of the cell, with a transmembrane potential of -80 to -100 mV (Chap. 197). The sarcolemma, which in the resting state is largely imperme-

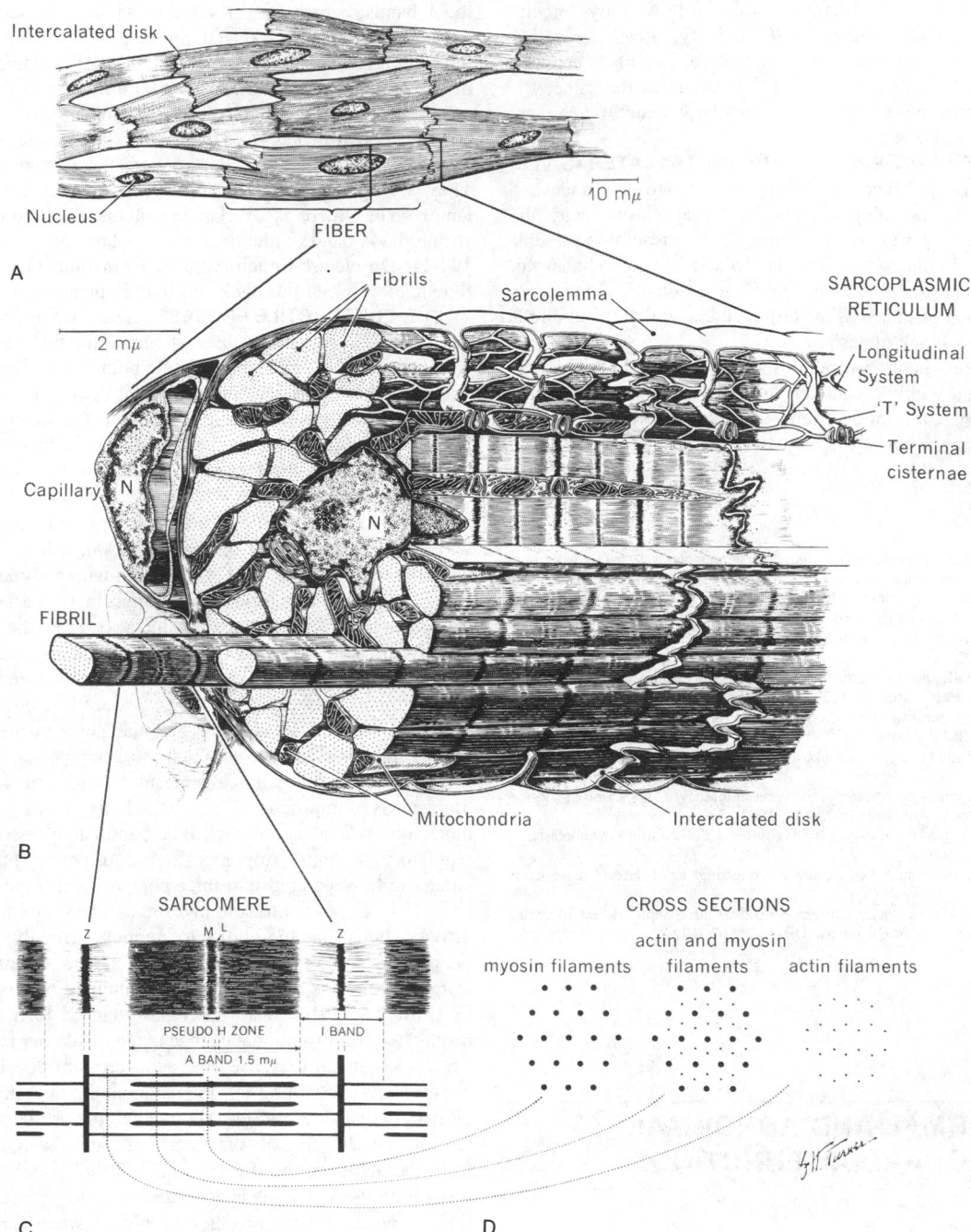

FIGURE 194-1 Microscopic structure of heart muscle. *A.* Myocardium as seen under the light microscope. Branching of fibers is evident. Each fiber, or cell, contains a centrally located nucleus. *B.* Myocardial cell, reconstructed from electron micrographs. Each cell is composed of multiple parallel fibrils. Each fibril is composed of serially connected sarcomeres (N, nucleus). *C.* Sarcomere from a myofibril, with diagrammatic representation of myofilaments. Thick filaments (1.5 μm long, composed of myosin) form the A band, and thin filaments (1 μm long, composed primarily of actin) extend from the Z line through the I band into the A band. The overlapping of thick and thin filaments is seen only in the A band. *D.* Cross sections of the sarcomere indicate the specific lattice arrangements of the myofilaments. In the center of the sarcomere only the thick, or myosin, filaments arranged in a hexagonal array are seen. In the distal portions of the A band, both thick and thin, or actin, filaments are found, with each thick filament surrounded by six thin filaments. In the I band only thin filaments are present. *(From Braunwald E, ed, Heart Disease, 4th ed, 1992, p 353.)*

able to Na⁺, has a Na⁺- and K⁺-stimulating pump requiring ATP that extrudes Na⁺ from the cell; the pump plays a critical role in establishing this resting potential. Thus on the inside of the cell $[K^+]$ is relatively high and $[Na^+]$ is far lower, while in the extracellular milieu $[Na^+]$ is high and $[K^+]$ is low. At the same time, in the resting state, the extracellular $[Ca^{2+}]$ greatly exceeds the free intracellular $[Ca^{2+}]$.

During the plateau of the action potential (phase 2) there is a slow inward current which reflects primarily a movement of Ca^{2+} into the cell (Fig. 194-3), although the absolute quantity of Ca^{2+} that crosses the surface membrane is relatively small and itself appears to be incapable of bringing about full activation of the contractile apparatus. The depolarizing current not only extends across the surface of the cell but penetrates deeply into the cell by way of the ramifying T system; this current triggers the release of much larger quantities of Ca^{2+} from the sarcoplasmic reticulum, a process termed "regenerative release" of Ca^{2+}. This rise in intracellular Ca^{2+} is the key step in initiating contraction.

The Ca^{2+} released from the sarcoplasmic reticulum then diffuses toward the sarcomere, and as already described, combines with

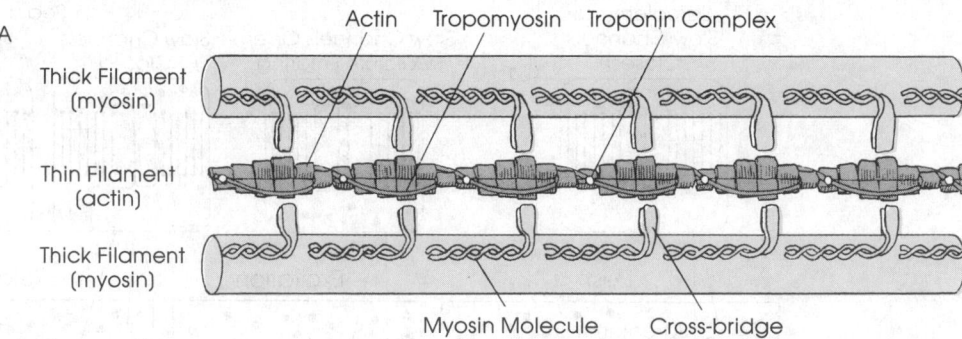

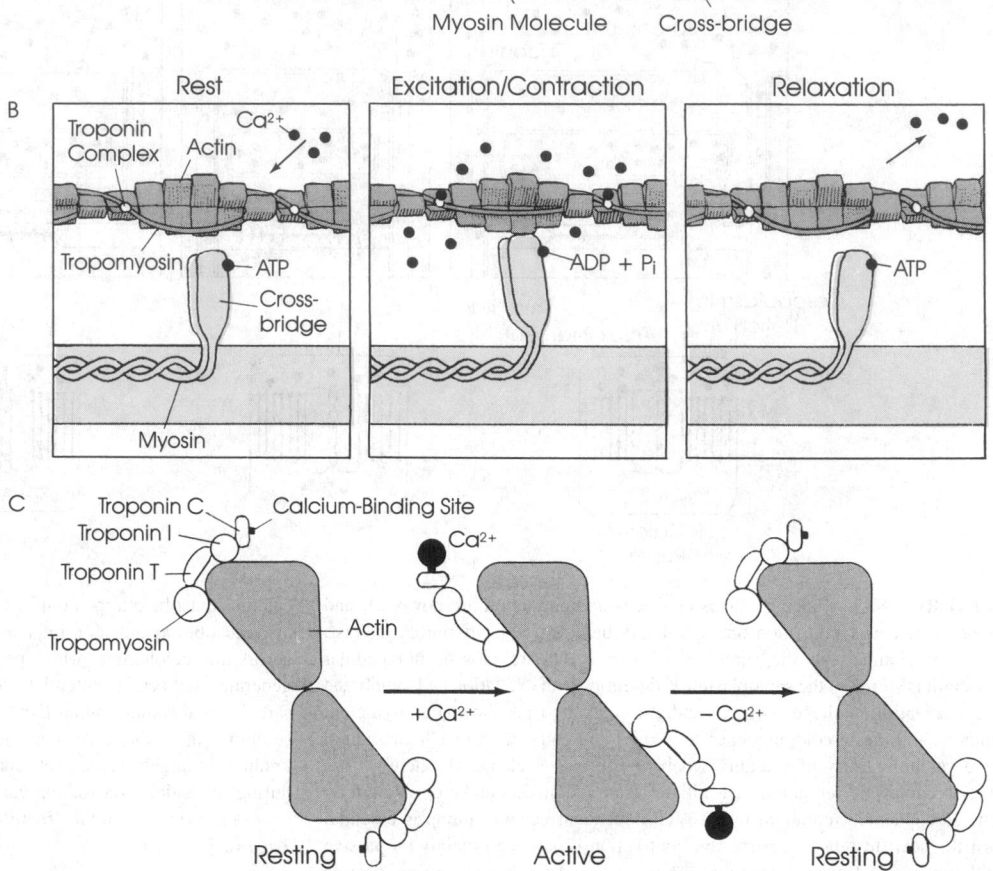

FIGURE 194-2 Contractile protein inter-actions and the role of calcium as activator messenger are shown schematically: *A.* Contractile proteins (myosin and actin) and regulatory proteins (troponin complex and tropomyosin) are shown in relative positions on myofilaments. *B.* Contraction takes place when the heads of myosin molecules, which form cross-bridges of thick filament, bind to actin, followed by shift in orientation of cross-bridge that pulls thin filament toward center of sarcomere. Activation requires calcium binding to troponin complex, reversing inhibition of interaction between myosin and actin. In the cycle of chemical reactions underlying contraction, hydrolysis of ATP produces the cross-bridge motion. Relaxation occurs when calcium becomes dissociated from troponin. *C.* Molecular rearrangements at the level of the thin filament involve regulatory proteins (tropomyosin and troponins C, I, T) in an allosteric effect. Calcium binding to troponin C loosens bond linking troponin I to actin; resulting dissociation of troponin T from actin backbone of thin filament displaces tropomyosin, exposing active sites for interaction with myosin. [*Reproduced by permission, from AM Katz, VE Smith, Hosp Prac, 19(1):69, 1984. Illustration by Bunji Tagawa.*]

troponin C. By repressing this inhibitor of contraction Ca^{2+} activates the myofilaments to produce contraction. During repolarization the sarcoplasmic reticulum reaccumulates Ca^{2+} against a concentration gradient. This is an energy-requiring process which lowers the concentration of Ca^{2+} in the vicinity of the myofibrils to a level that inhibits the actin-myosin interaction responsible for contraction and in this manner leads to relaxation. Thus, the cell membrane, transverse tubules, and sarcoplasmic reticulum, with their ability to transmit an action potential, to release and then reaccumulate Ca^{2+}, appear to play a fundamental role in the rhythmic contraction and relaxation of heart muscle.

The ATP formed from substrate oxidation is the principal source of energy for almost all of the mechanical work of contraction performed by the myocardial cell. The high-energy phosphate stores in ATP are in equilibrium with those in the form of creatine phosphate. The activity of myosin ATPase determines the rate of forming and breaking of the actin-myosin cross-bridges and ultimately the velocity of muscle contraction.

THE ROLE OF MUSCLE LENGTH In all striated muscle, including cardiac muscle, the force of contraction depends on initial muscle length. The sarcomere length associated with the most forceful contraction is approximately 2.2 μm. At this length the two sets of myofilaments of the sarcomere are situated to provide the greatest area for their interaction. In support of the sliding-filament hypothesis,

force development diminishes in direct proportion to the decrease in the overlap between thick and thin filaments and the resultant reduction in the number of reactive sites. The length of the sarcomere also appears to regulate the extent of activation of the contractile system, i.e., its sensitivity to Ca^{2+}, which is also greatest at approximately 2.2 μm. When sarcomere length is increased to 3.65 μm, the thin filaments are entirely withdrawn from the A band, and no tension can be developed. Similarly, when the sarcomeres are shorter than 2.0 μm, the thin filaments bypass one another, doubly overlapping each other and so reducing both the sensitivity of the contractile sites to Ca^{2+} and the capacity for force development.

The relation between the initial length of the muscle fibers and the developed force is of prime importance for the function of heart muscle. This forms the basis of the Frank-Starling relation (Starling's law of the heart), which states that, within limits, the force of ventricular contraction is a function of the end-diastolic length of the cardiac muscle, which in turn is closely related to the ventricular end-diastolic volume. In heart muscle, operating along the ascending limb of the length-active tension curve sarcomere length is directly proportional to muscle length. As muscle length decreases to the point at which sarcomere length approaches 1.5 μm and at which developed tension approaches zero, the I bands at first narrow, then disappear while the A band remains constant in length. At this latter point, the Z lines abut the edges of the A bands. Thus the sarcomere

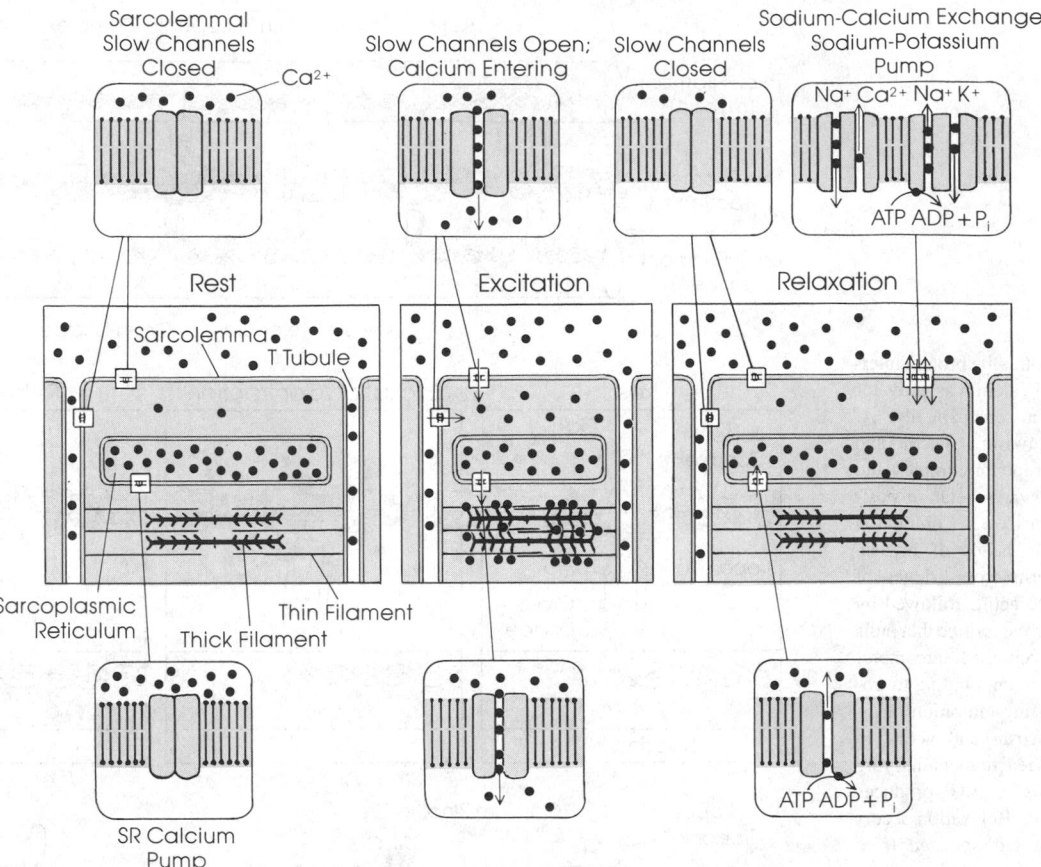

FIGURE 194-3 Calcium fluxes that activate contraction are downhill, and those that cause relaxation are uphill. As depicted in heart muscle at rest, calcium channels in the sarcolemmal membrane are closed; intracellular calcium is stored in the sarcoplasmic reticulum. With excitation and membrane depolarization, voltage-sensitive sodium channels (not shown) and calcium channels in the sarcolemma open to allow rapid entry of extracellular sodium and calcium. Entry of calcium is believed to cause release of calcium from the sarcoplasmic reticulum that initiates contraction. Reuptake of calcium by the sarcoplasmic reticulum by an ATP-dependent calcium pump is essential for the heart to relax. Importantly, contraction is activated mainly by passive calcium fluxes from the sarcoplasmic reticulum. By contrast, during diastole calcium must be pumped out of the cytosol to accomplish relaxation. Energy also must be expended during diastole to restore sodium and calcium gradients across the sarcolemma, which provide for the depolarizing ionic currents that generate the action potential. Sodium transport is accomplished by the sarcolemmal sodium pump (Na^+, K^+-ATPase), which utilizes ATP to pump sodium out of the cell in exchange for potassium. The resultant sodium gradient is largely responsible for active transport of calcium out of the cell during relaxation, via sodium-calcium exchange. [*Reproduced by permission from AM Katz, VE Smith, Hosp Prac, 19(1):69, 1984. Illustration by Bunji Tagawa.*]

length–active tension curve forms the ultrastructural basis of Starling's law of the heart.

MYOCARDIAL MECHANICS

THE FORCE-VELOCITY CURVE The mechanical activity of all muscle may be expressed externally in two ways: shortening and the development of tension. Hill showed in skeletal muscle that the velocity of shortening is inversely related to the magnitude of tension development, an expression of the so-called force-velocity relation, now recognized to be a fundamental property of muscle. Expressed simply, the greater the load the muscle is called upon to lift, the lower the velocity of shortening and vice versa. The force-velocity relation also applies to cardiac muscle. However, in this respect there is a basic difference between skeletal and cardiac muscle. Skeletal muscle fibers have a single, essentially fixed, force-velocity curve; i.e., at any given muscle length, force and velocity are always related to each other in the same manner. The contractile activity of skeletal muscle is increased by the recruitment of additional muscle fibers, i.e., motor units, and by increasing the frequency of nerve impulses, while the contractile properties of each individual fiber, expressed in the force-velocity curve, remain constant. Although resting length also influences the characteristics of contraction, this variable remains essentially fixed in vivo because of the skeletal muscles' skeletal attachments. In contrast, the number of cardiac cells and within them the myofibrils and sarcomeres which become activated during each contraction is constant. However, the contractile activity of the myocardium may be readily altered under physiologic conditions by changes in resting fiber length and by changes in the inotropic state, i.e., the contractility, both of which shift the myocardial force-velocity curve.

Cardiac muscle exhibits an inverse relation between the force against which it contracts, i.e., the afterload, and the extent and velocity of shortening. The myocardial force-velocity curve obtained in isolated heart muscle represents this inverse relation and can be used to describe myocardial performance. A change in the initial length of heart muscle shifts the force-velocity curve primarily by altering the total force which can be developed by the muscle without a change in the maximum velocity of contraction of unloaded muscle, i.e., V_{max}. This type of shift in the force-velocity curve may be contrasted with that obtained when a positive inotropic agent, such as Ca^{2+}, digitalis, or norepinephrine (which act ultimately by increasing the concentration of Ca^{2+} in the vicinity of the myofilaments) is added to the muscle while the initial length is held constant. These agents increase not only the force which the muscle is capable of developing but also V_{max}.

VENTRICULAR EJECTION AND FILLING

Analysis of the heart as a pump has classically centered on the relation between the end-diastolic volume of the ventricle (which is related to the length of the muscle fibers) and its stroke volume (the Frank-Starling relation). The end-diastolic or "filling" pressure of the ventricle is sometimes used as a surrogate for the end-diastolic volume. In the heart-lung preparation the stroke volume is a function of diastolic fiber length at any given level of arterial resistance (afterload), and the failing heart delivers a smaller-than-normal stroke volume from a normal or elevated end-diastolic volume. The relation between the mean atrial or the ventricular end-diastolic pressure and the stroke work of the corresponding ventricle (the ventricular function curve) provides a useful definition of the level of the contractile, or inotropic, state of the ventricle. An increase in ventricular contractility is accompanied by a shift of the ventricular function curve upward and to the left, depression of contractility by a shift downward and to the right.

It has been observed that during the adrenergic stimulation of the myocardium accompanying a stress such as exercise, relatively little change in ventricular end-diastolic volume occurs, while cardiac output, aortic flow velocity, stroke work, and the rate of ventricular pressure development are all augmented, sometimes greatly. Thus, neural and humorally mediated changes in myocardial contractility, heart rate, venous return, and peripheral vascular resistance may be of greater importance in circulatory adaptation than changes in ventricular end-diastolic volume and may mask the operation of the Frank-Starling mechanism.

The important influence of the adrenergic neurotransmitter, norepinephrine (Chap. 68), on the mechanical properties of the myocardium has long been recognized. Direct stimulation of the cardiac adrenergic nerves augments ventricular function as a consequence of the release of norepinephrine from adrenergic nerve endings in the heart. These adrenergic effects are evidenced by tachycardia, a reduction in cardiac dimensions, increased velocity of ejection, and an enhanced rate of tension development.

ASSESSMENT OF CARDIAC PERFORMANCE Several techniques are available for defining impaired cardiac performance in intact humans. With the patient at rest, the cardiac output and stroke volume may be depressed, but not uncommonly these variables are within normal limits. A more sensitive index is the ejection fraction, i.e., the ratio of stroke volume to end-diastolic volume, which may be estimated by standard radiocontrast or radionuclide angiography (Chaps. 190 and 192), and which is frequently depressed in heart failure even when the stroke volume itself is normal. A limitation of the ejection fraction (and of cardiac output) in the assessment of cardiac function is that these variables are influenced strongly by ventricular loading conditions. Thus, a depressed ejection fraction and lowered cardiac output may be observed in patients with normal ventricular function but reduced preload, as occurs in hypovolemia, or with acutely elevated arterial pressure. A useful technique for evaluating ventricular performance involves the measurement of the circulatory changes occurring during stresses such as exercise or increased afterload. Thus, left ventricular performance may be estimated accurately by measuring the left ventricular end-diastolic pressure, cardiac output, and total body O_2 consumption at rest and during exercise. In normal persons, the cardiac output rises by more than 500 mL/min for each 100-mL increase in minute O_2 consumption. The left ventricular end-diastolic pressure at rest is less than 12 mmHg and rises slightly, remains unchanged, or decreases slightly during exercise, while stroke volume usually rises, especially when exercise is carried out in the upright position. The failing left ventricle, on the other hand, is characterized by an elevation of end-diastolic pressure during exercise, which reaches a value exceeding 12 mmHg, accompanied by either no change or a fall in stroke volume and a subnormal increase in cardiac output related to the increase in minute O_2 consumption. Various degrees of impairment intermediate between the normal response and that of the failing left ventricle during the stress of exercise may occur.

The potential value of stressing the left ventricle in assessing its performance is emphasized by the fact that the normal range of left ventricular end-diastolic pressure, cardiac index, and ventricular stroke work in the resting state is wide, with values that frequently overlap those seen in patients with ventricular dysfunction. The response to stress may prove useful not only in the detection of the impairment of myocardial function but also in expressing the severity of this impairment quantitatively.

The end-systolic left ventricular pressure-volume relationship is a particularly useful index of ventricular performance since it is independent of both preload and afterload. At any level of myocardial contractility left ventricular end-systolic volume varies inversely with end-systolic pressure; as contractility declines, end-systolic volume (at any level of end-systolic pressure) rises. Noninvasive techniques, particularly echocardiography and radionuclide angiography (Chap. 190), are of great value in the clinical assessment of myocardial function.

CONTROL OF CARDIAC PERFORMANCE AND OUTPUT

The extent of shortening of mammalian heart muscle and, therefore, the stroke volume of the intact ventricle are, in the final analysis, determined by three influences: (1) the length of the muscle at the onset of contraction, i.e., the preload; (2) the inotropic state of the muscle, i.e., the position of its force-velocity-length relation; and (3) the tension which the muscle is called upon to develop during contraction, i.e., the afterload. Heart rate determines the cardiac output at any stroke volume as long as the other three influences are maintained. Ventricular filling is influenced by the extent and speed of myocardial relaxation, which in turn is determined by the rate of uptake of Ca^{2+} by the sarcoplasmic reticulum; the latter may be augmented by positive inotropic stimuli and reduced by ischemia. Filling may be impeded by the stiffness of the ventricular wall, which may be increased by ventricular hypertrophy and conditions that infiltrate the myocardium, or by an extrinsic constraint (e.g., pericardial compression).

VENTRICULAR END-DIASTOLIC VOLUME (PRELOAD) At any level of its inotropic state, the performance of the myocardium is influenced profoundly by ventricular end-diastolic fiber length and therefore by diastolic ventricular volume, i.e., by operation of the Frank-Starling mechanism discussed above. The following are the major determinants of ventricular preload in the intact organism:

Total blood volume When this is depleted, as in hemorrhage, dehydration, or prolonged vomiting, venous return to the heart declines (Chap. 34) and ventricular end-diastolic volume (preload) falls, as does ventricular performance, as reflected in ventricular work.

Distribution of blood volume At any given total blood volume, the ventricular end-diastolic volume is influenced by the distribution of blood between the intra- and extrathoracic compartments. This distribution in turn is influenced by the following:

1 *Body position.* Gravitational forces tend to pool blood in dependent portions. The upright posture augments extrathoracic at the expense of intrathoracic blood volume, and reduces ventricular work.

2 *Intrathoracic pressure.* Normally, mean intrathoracic pressure during the respiratory cycle is negative, a factor that acts to increase thoracic blood volume and ventricular end-diastolic volume and to enhance the return of blood to the heart, particularly during inspiration, when this pressure becomes more negative. Elevation of intrathoracic pressure, as occurs in a tension pneumothorax, during the Valsalva maneuver, in prolonged bouts of coughing, or with positive-pressure ventilation, tends to impede venous return to the heart and diminish intrathoracic blood volume and ultimately reduces stroke volume and ventricular work.

3 *Intrapericardial pressure.* When this pressure is elevated, as in pericardial tamponade (Chap. 206), there is interference with

cardiac filling, and the resultant reduction in ventricular diastolic volume lowers stroke volume and ventricular work.

4 *Venous tone.* The venous system is not a simple system of passive conduits between the systemic capillary bed and the right atrium. Instead, the smooth muscle in the walls of the venules and veins responds to a variety of neural and humoral stimuli. Venoconstriction occurs during muscular exercise, deep respiration, fright, or marked hypotension, tending to diminish extrathoracic and to augment intrathoracic and intraventricular blood volumes and ventricular performance.

5 *The pumping action of skeletal muscle.* During muscular exercise the contracting skeletal muscles squeeze blood out of the venous bed and, with the aid of the venous valves, displace it centrally, thereby increasing intrathoracic blood volume, ventricular end-diastolic volume, and ventricular work.

Atrial contraction   Vigorous, appropriately timed atrial contraction augments ventricular filling and end-diastolic volume. The atrial contribution to ventricular filling is of particular importance in patients with concentric ventricular hypertrophy, in whom the loss of atrial systole (as in atrial fibrillation) tends to reduce ventricular end-diastolic pressure and volume, ultimately lowering myocardial performance. The atrial contribution to ventricular filling may be reduced by atrioventricular dissociation, prolongation or abbreviation of the P-R interval, and depression of the inotropic state of the atrium.

INOTROPIC STATE (MYOCARDIAL CONTRACTILITY)   A number of factors determine the level of ventricular performance at any given ventricular end-diastolic volume, i.e., the position of the ventricular function curve. These influences may be considered to operate by modifying myocardial force-velocity-length relations. In the final analysis, most of these influences act by altering the concentration of Ca^{2+} in the vicinity of the myofilaments.

Adrenergic nerve activity (See also Chap. 68)   The quantity of norepinephrine released by adrenergic nerve endings in the heart is, under ordinary circumstances, dependent on the adrenergic nerve impulse traffic, and alterations in the frequency of nerve impulses modify the quantity of norepinephrine released and acting on the beta-adrenergic receptors in the myocardium. This mechanism is the most important one which acutely modifies the position of the force-velocity and ventricular function curves under physiologic conditions.

Circulating catecholamines (See also Chap. 68)   The adrenal medulla and other sympathetic ganglia outside the heart, when stimulated by adrenergic nerve impulses, release catecholamines, which, when they reach the heart, augment the inotropic state and the frequency of contraction.

The force-frequency relation   The position of the myocardial force-velocity curve also is influenced by the rate and rhythm of cardiac contraction; e.g., ventricular extrasystoles result in post-extrasystolic potentiation, presumably by increasing the Ca^{2+} which enters the cardiac cell.

Exogenously administered inotropic agents   The cardiac glycosides, isoproterenol, dopamine, dobutamine, and other sympathomimetic agents, calcium, caffeine, theophylline, and their derivatives, all improve the myocardial force-velocity relation and therefore may be used therapeutically to augment ventricular performance at any given ventricular end-diastolic volume.

Physiologic depressants   Included among these are severe myocardial hypoxia, hypercapnia, ischemia, and acidosis. Acting either singly or in combination, these influences exert a depressant effect on the myocardial force-velocity curve and depress left ventricular work at any given ventricular end-diastolic volume.

Pharmacologic depressants   These include quinidine, procainamide, disopyramide, high doses of certain calcium antagonists, barbiturates, alcohol, and other local and general anesthetics, as well as many other drugs.

Loss of ventricular substance   When a sufficiently large portion of ventricular myocardium becomes nonfunctional or necrotic, as occurs transiently during ischemia (Chap. 203) and permanently in

myocardial infarction (Chap. 202), total ventricular performance at any given level of end-diastolic volume may become depressed.

Intrinsic myocardial depression   Although the fundamental mechanisms responsible for depression of myocardial contractility in most cases of chronic congestive heart failure remain to be elucidated, it is now apparent that in this condition the inotropic state of each unit of myocardium is depressed and that the level of ventricular performance at any ventricular end-diastolic volume is thereby lowered.

VENTRICULAR AFTERLOAD   The stroke volume is ultimately a function of the extent of ventricular fiber shortening. In the intact heart, as in isolated cardiac muscle, the velocity and extent of shortening of ventricular muscle fibers at any given level of diastolic fiber length and myocardial inotropic state are inversely related to the load which opposes shortening, i.e., the afterload. The afterload on the intact heart may be defined as the tension or stress developed in the wall of the ventricle during ejection. Therefore, the afterload on the ventricular muscle fibers also is dependent on the level of aortic pressure as well as on the volume and thickness of the ventricular cavity, since Laplace's law indicates that the tension of the myocardial fiber is a function of the product of the intracavitary ventricular pressure and ventricular radius divided by the wall thickness. Thus, at the same level of aortic pressure, the afterload faced by a dilated left ventricle is higher than that encountered by a ventricle of normal size. Conversely, at the same aortic pressure and ventricular diastolic volume the afterload of a thick-walled ventricle is lower than of a thin-walled chamber. The aortic pressure, in turn, is influenced largely by the peripheral vascular resistance, the physical characteristics of the arterial tree, and the volume of blood it contains at the onset of ejection. At any given ventricular end-diastolic volume and level of the inotropic state, the left ventricular stroke volume is related inversely to the afterload.

The critical role played by the ventricular afterload in cardiovascular regulation is shown in Fig. 194-4. As already noted, increases in both preload and contractility increase myocardial fiber shortening, while increases in afterload reduce it. The extent of myocardial fiber shortening and left ventricular size are the determinants of stroke volume. Arterial pressure, in turn, is related to the product of cardiac output and systemic vascular resistance, while afterload is a function of left ventricular volume, wall thickness, and arterial pressure. An increase in arterial pressure induced by vasoconstriction, for example, augments afterload, which opposes myocardial fiber shortening, reducing stroke volume, and cardiac output; this in turn tends to restore arterial pressure to its previous level.

When left ventricular function becomes impaired and the chamber dilates, i.e., when there is little or no preload reserve, left ventricular afterload becomes increasingly important in determining cardiac performance. Increases in afterload may result from the influence on the arterial bed of neural, humoral, or structural changes which can occur in response to a fall in cardiac output. This increased afterload may reduce cardiac output further while myocardial oxygen requirements are increased. Treatment with vasodilators (Chap. 195) has the opposite effect. In this way, alterations in the peripheral vascular bed probably play an important role in the hemodynamic and metabolic events which usually are attributed to progressive impairment of the myocardium.

All of the influences acting on cardiac performance enumerated above interact in a complex fashion to maintain cardiac output at a level appropriate to the requirements of the metabolizing tissues, and in a normal person interference with one of these mechanisms may not influence the cardiac output. For example, a moderate reduction of blood volume *or* the loss of the atrial contribution to ventricular contraction can ordinarily be sustained without a reduction in the resting cardiac output. Other factors, such as an increase in the frequency of adrenergic nerve impulses to the heart and an increase in heart rate, will, in a normal individual, augment contractility and sustain cardiac output. Mechanisms are also available that prevent elevation of the cardiac output when there is no physiologic demand

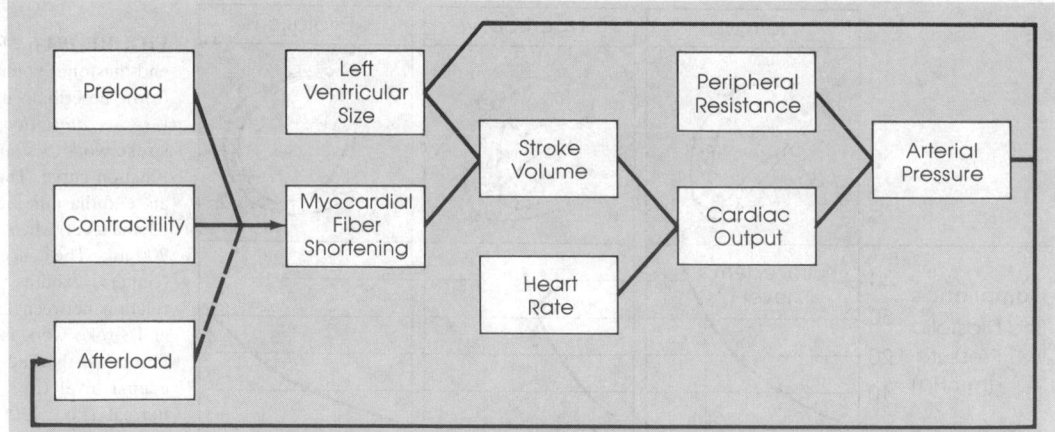

FIGURE 194-4 Scheme of interactions among various components that regulate cardiac activity. Solid lines indicate an augmenting effect; broken line represents an inhibiting effect. *(From Braunwald E: Regulation of the Circulation. N Engl J Med 290:1124–1129, 1420–1425, 1974.)*

for augmented flow. For example, augmentation of myocardial contractility by means of cardiac glycosides does not increase the cardiac output in normal humans. Thus, in analyzing the effect of an intervention on cardiac output, it is important to recognize that it is the preload, which in turn is related to the volume of blood available for filling the heart, rather than the inotropic state of the myocardium or the afterload which limits cardiac output in the normal individual. An improvement of myocardial contractility by a drug such as digitalis or the reduction of afterload with nitroprusside would not be expected to elevate the output in a normal subject. On the other hand, in the presence of congestive heart failure, the cardiac output usually is limited by the depressed contractile state of the myocardium, and a

FIGURE 194-5 Diagram showing the interrelations among influences on ventricular end-diastolic volume (EDV) through stretching of the myocardium and the contractile state of the myocardium. Levels of ventricular EDV associated with filling pressures that result in dyspnea and pulmonary edema are shown on the abscissa. Levels of ventricular performance required when the subject is at rest, while walking, and during maximal activity are designated on the ordinate. The broken lines are the descending limbs of the ventricular-performance curves, which are rarely seen during life but which show the level of ventricular performance if end-diastolic volume could be elevated to very high levels. For further explanation see text. *(From Braunwald E, ed, Heart Disease, 4th ed, 1992, p 413).*

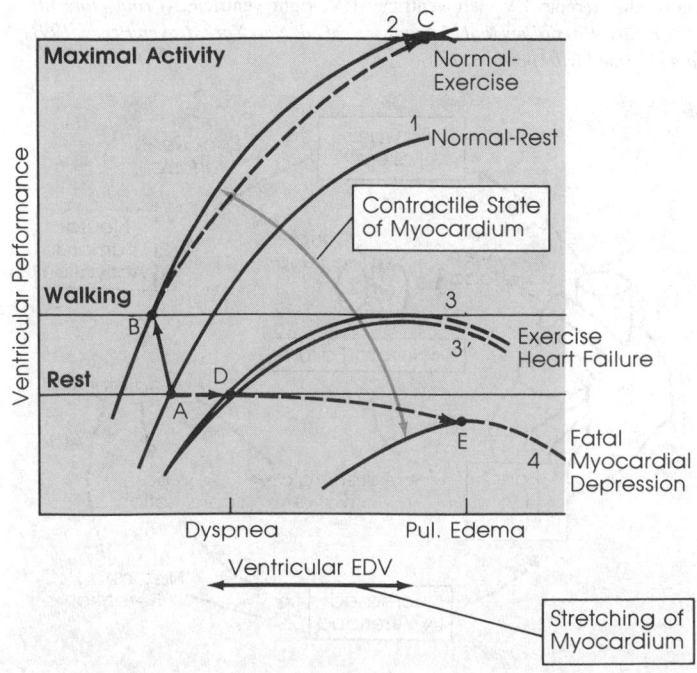

positive inotropic drug and/or reduction of afterload raises cardiac output (Chap. 195).

EXERCISE The hemodynamic changes which normally occur during exercise in the upright position are complex (Fig. 194-5). The hyperventilation, the pumping action of the exercising muscles, and the venoconstriction which occur all tend to augment venous return and hence ventricular filling and preload. Simultaneously, the increase in the adrenergic nerve impulses to the myocardium, the increased concentration of circulating catecholamines, and the tachycardia which occur during exercise all combine to augment the contractile state of the myocardium (Fig. 194-5, curves 1 and 2) and lead to an elevation of stroke work and stroke volume, with no change or even a decrease of end-diastolic pressure and volume (Fig. 194-5, points A and B). Vasodilation occurs in the exercising muscles, thus tending to counteract the marked increase in arterial pressure which would otherwise occur as cardiac output rises. This ultimately allows the achievement of a greatly elevated cardiac output during exercise, at an arterial pressure only moderately higher than in the resting state.

THE FAILING HEART

Though heart failure may be readily described as a clinical syndrome, characterized by well-known symptoms and physical signs, a precise physiologic or biochemical definition is far more difficult. However, from the clinical point of view, heart failure may be considered to be the condition in which *an abnormality of cardiac function is responsible for the inability of the heart to pump blood at a rate commensurate with the requirements of the metabolizing tissues and/or can do so only from an abnormally elevated ventricular diastolic volume.* Abnormalities during systole and/or diastole may be present in heart failure (Fig. 194-6). In so-called *systolic heart failure*, i.e., classic heart failure, an impaired inotropic state causes weakened systolic contraction, which leads, ultimately, to a reduction in stroke volume, inadequate ventricular emptying, cardiac dilatation, and often elevation of ventricular diastolic pressure. Idiopathic dilated cardiomyopathy (Chap. 205) is the prototype of systolic heart failure.

In *diastolic heart failure* (p. 1000) the principal abnormality involves impaired relaxation of the ventricle and leads to an elevation of ventricular diastolic pressure at any given diastolic volume. Failure of relaxation can be functional, i.e., as during transient ischemia, or it can be caused by a stiffened, thickened ventricle. Typical conditions in which diastolic failure occurs are restrictive cardiomyopathy secondary to infiltrative conditions, such as amyloidosis or hemochromatosis, as well as hypertrophic cardiomyopathy (Chap. 205). In many patients with cardiac hypertrophy and dilatation, systolic and diastolic failure coexist; the ventricle both empties and fills abnormally. There may be cardiac dilatation, but the ventricle's pressure-volume relation is shifted, raising the ventricular diastolic pressure at any given volume.

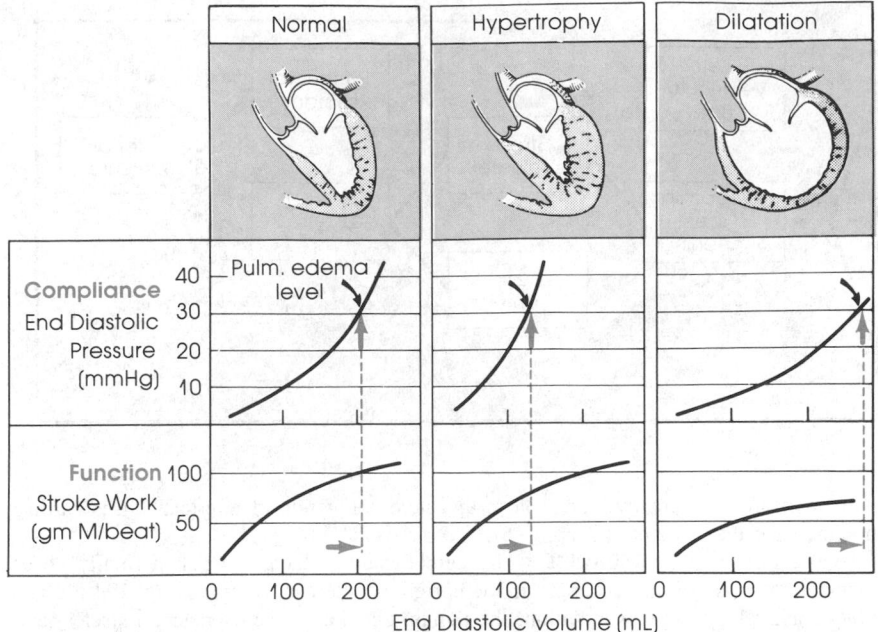

FIGURE 194-6 Relationship between left ventricular end-diastolic volume and (1) end-diastolic pressure (top), describing the *compliance* of the left ventricle, i.e., its *diastolic* properties; and (2) left ventricular stroke work (bottom), describing the ventricle's *systolic* function curve. The normal left ventricle (left) reaches an end-diastolic pressure of 30 mmHg (pulmonary edema level) when its end-diastolic volume is elevated to 200 mL. The concentrically hypertrophied left ventricle (center), exhibits normal systolic function since the relation between left ventricular end-diastolic volume and stroke work is unchanged, but there is "diastolic failure" in that end-diastolic pressure reaches pulmonary edema level (i.e., 30 mmHg) at a lower level than normal (i.e., 130 mL). The dilated ventricle (right) exhibits "systolic failure" in that the maximal stroke work and the stroke volume at any level of end-diastolic volume are depressed. The left ventricle displays increased diastolic compliance, i.e., distensibility, with a higher than normal end-diastolic volume (280 mL) required to reach the pulmonary edema level. *(Reprinted with permission from Gorlin R, Prim Cardiol 6:84, 1980.)*

Though a defect in myocardial contraction is characteristic of systolic heart failure, this defect may result from a primary abnormality in the heart muscle, as in cardiomyopathy, or it may be secondary to a chronic excessive work load as in hypertension and valvular heart disease. In ischemic heart disease systolic heart failure results from a loss in the quantity of normally contracting cells.

It is important to distinguish heart failure from (1) states of circulatory insufficiency in which myocardial function is not primarily impaired, such as cardiac tamponade or hemorrhagic shock; (2) conditions in which there is circulatory congestion because of abnormal salt and water retention but in which there is no serious disturbance of the heart's function, and (3) conditions in which a normal myocardium is suddenly presented with a load which exceeds its capacity, e.g., accelerated hypertension or rupture of a valve cusp secondary to infective endocarditis.

Adaptive mechanisms A series of mechanisms aid the heart faced with an increased hemodynamic burden, such as pressure or volume overload, or which has lost myocardial substance. These adaptive mechanisms include: (1) the Frank-Starling mechanism operating through an increase in preload (p. 991); (2) the development of myocardial hypertrophy, which restores elevated ventricular wall stress to normal; (3) redistribution of a subnormal cardiac output away from the skin, skeletal muscle, and kidneys with maintenance of blood flow to vital organs such as the brain and the heart itself; and (4) neurohumoral adjustments, which tend to maintain arterial pressure and are discussed on p. 997 and in Chap. 68.

The intrinsic contractile state of myocardium removed from failing animal hearts has been shown to be depressed soon after the imposition of a pressure overload. The laying down of more myofibrils often restores contractility to normal, but when the overload is maintained for prolonged periods, intrinsic myocardial contractility again declines. This state is often characterized by a relative reduction in the ratio of mitochondria to myofibrils.

In papillary muscles removed from the left ventricles of patients with heart failure the maximum degree of active tension which they can develop is reduced. Electron-microscopic analysis of failing cat papillary muscles fixed at the apexes of the length–active tension curves revealed sarcomere lengths averaging 2.2 μm. Thus, the abnormalities of contractility do *not* appear to be produced by an alteration in the overlap of filaments within the sarcomere.

The failing ventricle may still eject a normal or nearly normal stroke volume despite considerable depression of function, when its end-diastolic volume increases, i.e., through the operation of the

Frank-Starling mechanism. As outlined above, an increase in the initial volume of the ventricle is associated with stretching of the sarcomere, a process that augments the number of sites at which the actin and myosin filaments can interact and/or which increases their sensitivity to Ca^{2+}. Furthermore, the development of ventricular hypertrophy may be considered to provide additional contractile units and thereby constitutes an important compensatory mechanism when the myocardium's intrinsic inotropic state is depressed.

CARDIAC METABOLISM IN HEART FAILURE There is no unifying theory providing a biochemical basis for heart failure. The common forms of low-output heart failure, secondary to coronary atherosclerosis, hypertension, cardiomyopathy, and certain valvular

FIGURE 194-7 Features of forward and backward failure. Note association of forward failure with hypotension and neurohumoral activation with consequent afterload increase. Note also the association of backward failure with pulmonary congestion. Backward failure is associated with abnormalities of left atrial emptying or LV relaxation. α, alpha adrenergic; β, beta adrenergic; aldo, aldosterone; LV, left ventricle; RV, right ventricle. *(From Opie LH: The Heart: Physiology and Metabolism, 2d ed, New York, Raven Press, 1991, p 411. Used with permission.)*

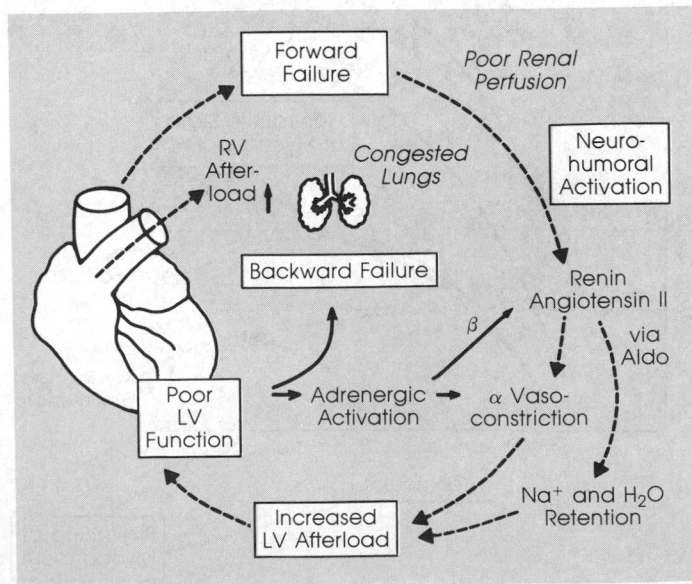

and congenital lesions, are characterized by an absolute or a relative reduction in the external work delivered by the heart, although myocardial oxygen consumption remains normal. Therefore, the external efficiency, i.e., the ratio of external work performed to energy consumed, is often depressed. When heart failure occurs in the absence of myocardial ischemia, there appears to be no abnormality of ATP generation or ATP use. When heart failure occurs in the presence of acute or chronic ischemia it can be attributed to reduced myocardial energy supplies.

Although some controversy concerning myocardial metabolism in heart failure persists, it now appears that severe impairment of myocardial performance may occur *without* disturbances of mitochondrial function or reduction of high-energy phosphate stores, although abnormalities in these processes have been shown to occur in some forms of experimental (and perhaps of clinical) heart failure.

Substantial evidence supports the view that in many forms of heart failure there is an *abnormality of excitation-contraction coupling*, which reduces the delivery of Ca^{2+} to the contractile sites, thereby impairing cardiac performance. However, the molecular basis of this abnormality, indeed the subcellular structures involved, i.e., the sarcolemma, T tubules, and/or sarcoplasmic reticulum, have yet to be defined. One attractive hypothesis involves reduced uptake of Ca^{2+} by the sarcoplasmic reticulum. This can impair myocardial relaxation and contribute to the development of diastolic heart failure. In addition, a reduction of Ca^{2+} in the sarcoplasmic reticulum can also lower Ca^{2+} released to the myofilaments during activation, thereby causing systolic heart failure.

NEUROHUMORAL ADJUSTMENTS A reduction in cardiac performance evokes a series of neurohumoral adjustments which may be considered to be "two-edged swords" (Fig. 194-7). Although they are useful because they maintain arterial perfusion pressure in the face of a reduction of cardiac output, they increase the hemodynamic burden and oxygen requirements of the failing ventricle.

The renin-angiotensin-aldosterone system When cardiac output declines, the renin-angiotensin-aldosterone system (Chap. 335) is activated. Concentrations of circulating angiotensin II and aldosterone are both increased, the former contributing to excess vasoconstriction and the latter to the retention of salt and water. Patients with chronic heart failure are usually improved by blocking this system with angiotensin-converting enzyme inhibitors and by aldosterone antagonists (Chap. 195).

The adrenergic nervous system In patients with heart failure the levels of circulating norepinephrine may be markedly elevated, indicating that the activity of adrenergic neurons is augmented; the prognosis varies inversely with the concentration. This increased activity of the adrenergic neurons supports ventricular contractility in congestive heart failure. Heart failure is intensified when large doses of beta-adrenergic blocking agents are administered to such patients.

The density of adrenergic receptors and concentration of cardiac norepinephrine (NE) are both reduced in chronic, severe heart failure.

FIGURE 194-8 Schematic representation of influences on intramyocardial Ca^{2+} concentration and excitation-contraction coupling. The action potential is associated with intracellular entry of Na^+ and the extrusion of K^+ (not shown) and the entry of Ca^{2+} (shown). The Na^+-Ca^{2+} exchanger depends on concentration gradients and does not require ATP. Not shown is the energy-dependent sarcolemmal Ca^{2+} pump which extrudes Ca^{2+} from the cell. Isoproterenol and norepinephrine, the latter shown intraneuronally, stimulate the beta-adrenergic receptor in the outer sarcolemma. The beta receptor is coupled to G (guanine nucleotide–binding regulatory) proteins (GR), which in turn activate the catalytic adenylate cyclase (AC). The latter catalyzes the production of cyclic AMP from ATP. AC can be stimulated directly by the administration of forskolin, which bypasses both the beta receptor and the G proteins. Cyclic AMP activates protein kinase, which in turn enhances the phosphorylation of the Ca^{2+} channel, increasing transarcolemmal Ca^{2+} influx. Activated protein kinase also phosphorylates phospholamban, which in its phosphorylated form enhances the uptake of Ca^{2+} by the sarcoplasmic tubular network. Phosphodiesterase catalyzes the breakdown of cyclic AMP to AMP while milrinone, caffeine, and isobutylmethylxanthine inhibit phosphodiesterase, thereby augmenting cyclic AMP concentration. Digoxin inhibits the Na^+, K^+-ATPase in the sarcolemma, inhibiting Na^+ efflux from and K^+ influx into the cell. As a consequence the intracellular Na^+ concentration falls and Na^+-Ca^{2+} exchange is reduced, thereby raising intracellular Ca^{2+}. P represents phosphorylation. *(From Feldman AMD et al, by permission of the American Heart Association, Inc.)*

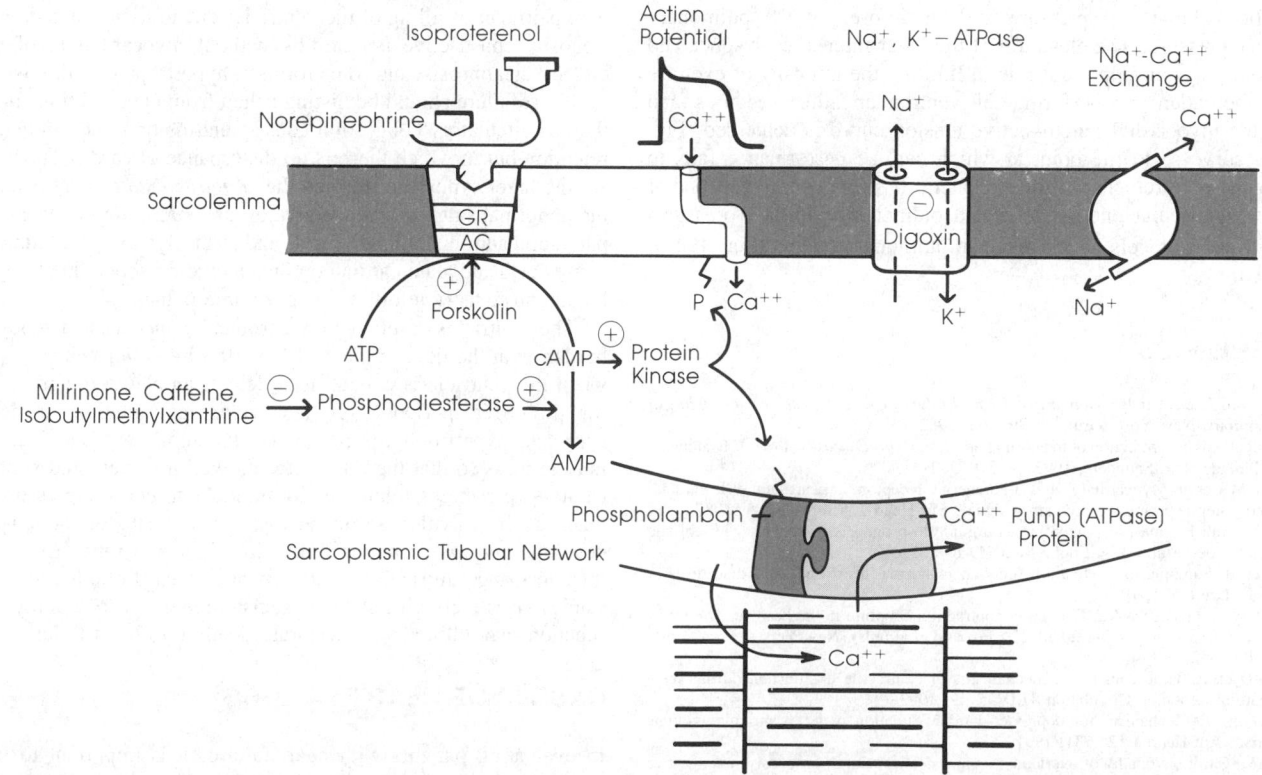

These changes are accompanied by a reduction in the activity of adenylate cyclase, which may lower the intracellular concentration of cyclic AMP. The latter in turn reduces the activation of protein kinase, the phosphorylation of Ca^{2+} channels, transarcolemmal Ca^{2+} entry, as well as the phosphorylation of phospholamban, a protein in the sarcoplasmic reticulum, thereby depressing the reuptake of Ca^{2+} by the latter (Fig. 194-8). Changes in the G (guanine regulatory) proteins, which couple the beta receptor to the catalytic adenylate cyclase (which is responsible for the production of cyclic AMP), may also occur in heart failure, with increased activity of the inhibitory subunit and/or reduced activity of the stimulatory subunit of the G proteins. The reduction of cardiac NE stores and the down-regulation of myocardial beta receptors in heart failure may be responsible for loss of the much-needed adrenergic support in the failing heart. On the other hand, the increased adrenergic stimulation and rise in circulating catecholamines may exert undesirable side effects by elevating vascular resistance and thereby presenting the heart with an afterload which is higher than optimal. It may also enhance the likelihood of ventricular arrhythmias. The survival of patients with congestive heart failure varies inversely with the concentration of circulating NE.

In the final analysis, in heart failure, the fundamental abnormality resides in depressions of the myocardial force-velocity relationship and of the length–active tension curve, reflecting reductions in the contractile state of the myocardium (Fig. 194-5, curves 1 to 3). In many instances, cardiac output and external ventricular performance at rest are within normal limits but are maintained at these levels only by an increased end-diastolic fiber length and an elevated ventricular end-diastolic volume, i.e., through the operation of the Frank-Starling mechanism (Fig. 194-5, points A to D). The elevation of left ventricular preload is associated with similar changes in the pulmonary capillary pressure, contributing to the dyspnea experienced by patients with heart failure. The normal improvement of contractility due to augmented adrenergic activity during exercise is attenuated or even prevented by NE depletion which occurs in severe heart failure (Fig. 194-5, curves 3 and 3'). The factors which tend to augment ventricular filling during exercise in the normal subject push the failing myocardium along its flattened length–active tension curve, and although the left ventricle may perform somewhat better, this occurs only as a consequence of an inordinate elevation of ventricular end-diastolic volume and pressure and, therefore, of the pulmonary capillary pressure. The elevation of the latter intensifies dyspnea and therefore plays an important role in limiting the intensity of exercise which the patient can perform. Left ventricular failure becomes fatal when the myocardial length–active tension curve is depressed (Fig. 194-5, curve 4) to the point at which cardiac performance fails to satisfy the requirements of the peripheral tissues even at rest, and/or the left ventricular end-diastolic and pulmonary capillary pressures are elevated to levels which result in pulmonary edema (Fig. 194-5, point E).

REFERENCES

BRAUNWALD E et al (eds): *Congestive Heart Failure: Current Research and Clinical Applications.* New York, Grune & Stratton, 1982
——— et al (eds): Contraction of the normal heart, in *Heart Disease,* 4th ed, E Braunwald (ed). Philadelphia, Saunders, 1992, pp 370–382
BRISTOW MR et al: Myocardial α and β-adrenergic receptors in heart failure: Is cardiac-derived norepinephrine the regulatory signal? Eur Heart J 9(Suppl H):35, 1988
COHN JN et al: Plasma norepinephrine as a guide to prognosis in patients with chronic congestive heart failure. N Engl J Med 311:819, 1984
EDES I et al: Sarcoplasmic reticulum function in normal heart and in cardiac disease. Heart Failure 6:221, 1991
GIBBONS WR, ZYGMUNT AC: Excitation-contraction coupling in the heart, in *The Heart and Cardiovascular System,* 2d ed, HA Fozzard et al (eds). New York, Raven, 1991, pp 1249–1352
GUTH BD et al: Time course and mechanisms of contractile dysfunction during acute myocardial ischemia. Circulation 87:IV35–42, 1993
HOLT W et al: Mechanism for depressed cardiac function in left ventricular volume overload. Am Heart J 121:531, 1991
KATZ AM: Cardiomyopathy of overload: A major determinant of prognosis in congestive heart failure. N Engl J Med 322:100, 1990
———: Heart failure, in *Physiology of the Heart,* 2d ed. New York, Raven, 1992, pp 638–668
OM A, HESS ML: Inotropic therapy of the failing myocardium. Clin Cardiol 16:5, 1993
SMITH V-E, ZILE MR: Relaxation and diastolic properties of the heart, in *The Heart and Cardiovascular System,* 2d ed, HA Fozzard et al (eds). New York, Raven, 1991, pp 1353–1368

195   HEART FAILURE

EUGENE BRAUNWALD

While a number of definitions of heart failure are commonly employed, here we consider heart failure to be the pathophysiologic state in which an abnormality of *cardiac* function is responsible for the failure of the heart to pump blood at a rate commensurate with the requirements of the metabolizing tissues *and/or* its ability to do so requires an abnormally elevated filling pressure. Heart failure is frequently, but not always, caused by a defect in myocardial contraction, and then the term *myocardial failure* is appropriate. The latter may result from a primary abnormality in heart muscle, as occurs in the cardiomyopathies (Chap. 205). Myocardial failure also may result from extramyocardial abnormalities, such as coronary atherosclerosis which leads to myocardial ischemia and infarction, as well as from abnormalities of the heart valves in which the heart muscle is damaged by the long-standing excessive hemodynamic burden imposed by the valvular abnormality, and/or by the rheumatic process (Chap. 200). In patients with chronic constrictive pericarditis, myocardial damage resulting from infiltration of the heart muscle by pericardial inflammation and calcification is common (Chap. 206).

In other patients with heart failure, however, a similar clinical syndrome is present, but without any detectable abnormality of *myocardial* function. In some of these patients the normal heart is suddenly presented with a load that exceeds its capacity, such as an acute hypertensive crisis, rupture of an aortic valve cusp, or massive pulmonary embolism. Heart failure, in the presence of normal myocardial function, also occurs in chronic conditions in which there is impairment of filling of the ventricles due to tricuspid and/or mitral stenosis, constrictive pericarditis without myocardial involvement, endocardial fibrosis, and some forms of hypertrophic cardiomyopathy.

Heart failure should be distinguished from (1) conditions in which there is circulatory congestion consequent to abnormal salt and water retention but in which there is no disturbance of cardiac function per se (the latter syndrome, termed the *congested state,* may result from the abnormal salt and water retention of renal failure or from excess parenteral administration of fluids and electrolytes) and (2) noncardiac causes of inadequate cardiac output, including shock due to hypovolemia and redistribution of blood volume (Chap. 34).

The ventricles respond to a chronically increased hemodynamic burden with the development of hypertrophy. With volume overload when the ventricle is called on to deliver an elevated cardiac output for prolonged periods, as in valvular regurgitation, it develops *eccentric* hypertrophy, i.e., cavity dilatation, with an increase in muscle mass so that the ratio between wall thickness and ventricular cavity size remains relatively constant. With chronic pressure overload, as in valvular aortic stenosis or untreated hypertension, it develops *concentric* hypertrophy, in which the ratio between wall thickness and ventricular cavity size increases. In both conditions, a stable hyperfunctioning state may exist for many years, but myocardial function may ultimately deteriorate, leading to heart failure.

CAUSES OF HEART FAILURE

In evaluating patients with heart failure, it is important to identify not only the *underlying cause* of the heart disease but also the *precipitating cause* of heart failure. The cardiac abnormality produced by a congenital or acquired lesion such as valvular aortic stenosis may exist for many years and produce no clinical disability. Frequently, however, clinical manifestations of heart failure appear for the first time in the course of some acute disturbance which places an additional load on a myocardium that chronically is excessively burdened. The heart may be compensated but have no additional reserve, and a precipitating cause results in further deterioration of cardiac function. Identification of such precipitating causes is of critical importance because their prompt alleviation may be lifesaving. However, in the absence of underlying heart disease, these acute disturbances do not usually, by themselves, lead to heart failure.

PRECIPITATING CAUSES

1 *Pulmonary embolism.* Physically inactive patients with low cardiac output are at increased risk of developing thrombi in the veins of the lower extremities or the pelvis. Pulmonary emboli may result in further elevation of pulmonary arterial pressure, which in turn may produce or intensify ventricular failure. In the presence of pulmonary vascular congestion, such emboli also may cause pulmonary infarction (Chap. 226).

2 *Infection.* Patients with pulmonary vascular congestion are also more susceptible to pulmonary infections; any infection may precipitate heart failure. The resulting fever, tachycardia, and hypoxemia and the increased metabolic demands may place a further burden on the overloaded, but compensated myocardium of a patient with chronic heart disease.

3 *Anemia.* The oxygen needs of the metabolizing tissues can be met only by an increase in the cardiac output in the presence of anemia (Chap. 56); though such an increase in cardiac output can be sustained by a normal heart, a diseased, overloaded, but otherwise compensated heart may be unable to augment sufficiently the volume of blood which it delivers to the periphery. In this manner, the combination of anemia and previously compensated heart disease can lead to inadequate oxygen delivery to the periphery and precipitate heart failure.

4 *Thyrotoxicosis and pregnancy.* As in anemia and fever, in thyrotoxicosis and pregnancy, adequate tissue perfusion requires an increased cardiac output. The development or intensification of heart failure may actually be one of the first clinical manifestations of hyperthyroidism in a patient with underlying heart disease which was previously compensated (Chap. 334). Similarly, heart failure not infrequently occurs for the first time during pregnancy in women with rheumatic valvular disease, in whom cardiac compensation may return following delivery.

5 *Arrhythmias.* In patients with compensated heart disease, arrhythmias are among the most frequent precipitating causes of heart failure. They exert a deleterious effect for a variety of reasons: (*a*) Tachyarrhythmias reduce the time period available for ventricular filling. In patients with ischemic heart disease, tachyarrhythmias also may cause ischemic myocardial dysfunction. (*b*) The dissociation between atrial and ventricular contractions characteristic of many arrhythmias results in the loss of the atrial booster pump mechanism, thereby raising atrial pressures. (*c*) In any arrhythmia associated with abnormal intraventricular conduction, myocardial performance may become further impaired because of the loss of normal synchronicity of ventricular contraction. (*d*) Marked bradycardia associated with complete atrioventricular block or other severe bradyarrhythmias will reduce cardiac output unless stroke volume rises reciprocally; this compensatory response cannot occur with serious myocardial dysfunction even in the absence of heart failure.

6 *Rheumatic and other forms of myocarditis.* Acute rheumatic fever and a variety of other inflammatory or infectious processes affecting the myocardium may impair myocardial function in patients with or without preexisting heart disease (Chaps. 200 and 205).

7 *Infective endocarditis.* The additional valvular damage, anemia, fever, and myocarditis which often occur as a consequence of infective endocarditis may, singly or in concert, precipitate heart failure (Chap. 85).

8 *Physical, dietary, fluid, environmental, and emotional excesses.* The augmentation of sodium intake, the inappropriate discontinuation of medications to treat heart failure, blood transfusions, physical overexertion, excessive environmental heat or humidity, and emotional crises all may precipitate heart failure in patients with heart disease who were previously compensated.

9 *Systemic hypertension.* Rapid elevation of arterial pressure, as may occur in some instances of hypertension of renal origin or upon discontinuation of antihypertensive medication, may result in cardiac decompensation (Chap. 209).

10 *Myocardial infarction.* In patients with chronic but compensated ischemic heart disease, a fresh infarct, sometimes otherwise silent clinically, may further impair ventricular function and precipitate heart failure (Chap. 202).

A systematic search for these precipitating causes should be made in every patient with the new development or recent intensification of heart failure, particularly if it is refractory to the usual methods of therapy. If properly recognized, the precipitating cause of heart failure usually can be treated more effectively than the underlying cause. Therefore, the prognosis in patients with heart failure in whom a precipitating cause can be identified, treated, and eliminated is more favorable than in patients in whom the underlying disease process has advanced to the point of producing heart failure.

FORMS OF HEART FAILURE

Heart failure may be described as *high-output* or *low-output*, *acute* or *chronic*, *right-sided* or *left-sided*, *forward* or *backward*, and *systolic* or *diastolic*. These descriptors are often useful in a clinical setting, particularly early in the patient's course, but late in the course of chronic heart failure the differences between them often become blurred.

HIGH-OUTPUT VERSUS LOW-OUTPUT HEART FAILURE It is useful to classify patients with heart failure into those with a low cardiac output, i.e., *low-output heart failure*, and those with an elevated cardiac output, i.e., *high-output heart failure*. The former occurs secondary to ischemic heart disease, hypertension, dilated cardiomyopathy, valvular and pericardial disease, but the latter is seen in patients with heart failure and hyperthyroidism, anemia, pregnancy, arteriovenous fistulas, beriberi, and Paget's disease. In clinical practice, however, low-output and high-output heart failure cannot always be readily distinguished. The normal range of cardiac output is wide [2.5 to 3.8 $(L/min)/m^2$], and in many patients with so-called low-output heart failure the cardiac output may actually be just within the normal range at rest (although it is lower than it had been previously), but it fails to rise normally during exertion. On the other hand, in patients with so-called high-output heart failure the output may not exceed the upper limits of normal (although it would have been elevated had it been measured before heart failure supervened), but rather it may be close to the upper limit of normal. Regardless of the *absolute* level of the cardiac output, however, cardiac failure may be said to be present when the characteristic clinical manifestations described below are accompanied by a depression of the curve relating ventricular end-diastolic volume to cardiac performance (see Fig. 194-5, p. 995).

An integral physiologic component of *systolic* heart failure (p. 995) is the finding that the heart does not deliver the quantity of oxygen required by the metabolizing tissues. In the absence of peripheral shunting of blood, such inadequate delivery of oxygen to the metabolizing tissues is reflected in an abnormal widening of the normal arterial–mixed venous oxygen difference (35 to 50 mL/L in the basal state). In mild cases, such an abnormality may not be present at rest but becomes evident only during exertion or other hypermetabolic states. In patients with high cardiac output states, such as those associated with arteriovenous fistula, beriberi, thyrotoxicosis,

Paget's disease, etc., the arterial–mixed venous oxygen difference is normal or low. The mixed venous oxygen saturation is raised by the admixture of blood which has been diverted from the metabolizing tissues, and it may be presumed that even in these patients the delivery of oxygen to the latter is reduced despite the normal or even elevated mixed venous oxygen saturation. When heart failure occurs in such patients, the arterial–mixed venous oxygen difference, regardless of the absolute value, still exceeds the level which existed prior to the development of heart failure, and therefore, the cardiac output, though normal or elevated, is lower than before heart failure supervened.

The mechanisms responsible for the development of heart failure in patients whose cardiac outputs are initially high are complex and depend on the underlying disease process. In most of these conditions the heart is called on to pump abnormally large quantities of blood in order to deliver the normal quota of oxygen to the metabolizing tissues. The burden placed on the myocardium by the increased flow load resembles that produced by chronic regurgitant valvular lesions. In addition, thyrotoxicosis and beriberi also may impair myocardial metabolism directly, while severe anemia may interfere with myocardial function by producing myocardial anoxia, especially in the presence of underlying obstructive artery disease.

ACUTE VERSUS CHRONIC HEART FAILURE The prototype of acute heart failure is the patient who was entirely well previously but who suddenly develops a large myocardial infarction or rupture of a cardiac valve. Chronic heart failure is typically observed in patients with dilated cardiomyopathy or multivalvular heart disease which develops or progresses slowly. Acute heart failure is usually largely systolic, and the sudden reduction in cardiac output often results in systemic hypotension without peripheral edema. In chronic heart failure, arterial pressure tends to be well maintained, but there is often accumulation of edema. Despite these obvious differences in clinical presentation, there is no fundamental distinction between acute and chronic heart failure. For example, intensive efforts to prevent expansion of blood volume by means of dietary sodium restriction and the administration of diuretics will frequently delay the development of exertional dyspnea and edema in patients with chronic valvular heart disease (i.e., it will mask the clinical manifestations of chronic heart failure) until an acute episode, such as an arrhythmia or infection, precipitates acute heart failure. Without intensive efforts to restrict blood volume, the same patients would have been considered to have been suffering from chronic heart failure, even though their underlying myocardial disease was no further advanced.

RIGHT-SIDED VERSUS LEFT-SIDED HEART FAILURE Many of the clinical manifestations of heart failure result from the accumulation of excess fluid behind either one or both ventricles (Chaps. 31 and 33). This fluid usually localizes upstream to (behind) the specific cardiac chamber which is initially affected. For example, patients in whom the left ventricle is mechanically overloaded (e.g., aortic stenosis) or weakened (e.g., postmyocardial infarction) develop dyspnea and orthopnea as a result of pulmonary congestion, a condition referred to as *left-sided heart failure*. In contrast, when the underlying abnormality affects the right ventricle primarily (e.g., valvular pulmonic stenosis or pulmonary hypertension secondary to pulmonary thromboembolism), symptoms resulting from pulmonary congestion such as orthopnea or paroxysmal nocturnal dyspnea are less common, and edema, congestive hepatomegaly, and systemic venous distention, i.e., clinical manifestations of *right-sided heart failure*, are more prominent. However, when heart failure has existed for months or years, such localization of excess fluid behind the failing ventricle may no longer exist. For example, patients with long-standing aortic valve disease or systemic hypertension may have ankle edema, congestive hepatomegaly, and systemic venous distention late in the course of their disease, even though the abnormal hemodynamic burden initially was placed on the left ventricle. This occurs in part because of the secondary pulmonary hypertension and resultant right-sided heart failure but also because of the persistent retention of salt and water. It is also useful to recall that the muscle

bundles composing both ventricles are continuous and both ventricles share a common wall, the interventricular septum. Also, biochemical changes which occur in heart failure and which may be involved in the impairment of myocardial function, such as norepinephrine depletion and alterations in the activity of myosin ATPase, occur in the myocardium of *both* ventricles, regardless of the specific chamber on which the abnormal hemodynamic burden is placed initially.

BACKWARD VERSUS FORWARD HEART FAILURE For many years a controversy has revolved around the question of the mechanism of the clinical manifestations resulting from heart failure. The concept of *backward heart failure* contends that in heart failure, one or the other ventricle fails to discharge its contents or fails to fill normally. As a consequence, the pressures in the atrium and venous system behind the failing ventricle rise, and retention of sodium and water occurs as a consequence of the elevation of systemic venous and capillary pressures and the resultant transudation of fluid into the interstitial space (Chap. 33). In contrast, the proponents of the *forward heart failure* hypothesis maintain that the clinical manifestations of heart failure result directly from an inadequate discharge of blood into the arterial system. According to this concept, salt and water retention is a consequence of diminished renal perfusion and excessive proximal tubular sodium reabsorption and of excessive distal tubular reabsorption through activation of the renin-angiotensin-aldosterone system.

A rigid distinction between *backward* and *forward heart failure* (like a rigid distinction between right and left heart failure) is artificial, since both mechanisms appear to operate to varying extents in most patients with heart failure. However, the rate of onset of heart failure often influences the clinical manifestations. For example, when a large portion of the left ventricle is suddenly destroyed, as in myocardial infarction, although stroke volume and blood pressure are suddenly reduced (both manifestations of forward failure), the patient may die of acute pulmonary edema, a manifestation of backward failure. If the patient survives the acute insult, clinical manifestations resulting from a chronically depressed cardiac output, including the abnormal retention of fluid within the systemic vascular bed, may develop. Similarly, in the case of massive pulmonary embolism, the right ventricle may dilate and the systemic venous pressure may rise to high levels (backward failure), or the patient may develop shock secondary to low cardiac output (forward failure), but this low-output state may have to be maintained for some days before sodium and water retention sufficient to produce peripheral edema occurs.

SYSTOLIC VERSUS DIASTOLIC FAILURE The distinction between these two forms of heart failure, described on p. 991 and in Fig. 194-6, relates to whether the principal abnormality is the inability to contract normally and expel sufficient blood (systolic failure) or to relax and fill normally (diastolic failure). The major clinical manifestations of systolic failure relate to an inadequate cardiac output with weakness, fatigue, reduced exercise tolerance, and other symptoms of hypoperfusion, while in diastolic failure they relate principally to an elevation of filling pressures. In many patients, particularly those who have both ventricular hypertrophy *and* dilatation, abnormalities both of contraction and relaxation coexist.

Diastolic heart failure may be caused by increased resistance to ventricular inflow and reduced ventricular diastolic capacity (constrictive pericarditis and restrictive, hypertensive, and hypertrophic cardiomyopathy), impaired ventricular relaxation (acute myocardial ischemia, hypertrophic cardiomyopathy), and myocardial fibrosis and infiltration (dilated, chronic ischemic, and restrictive cardiomyopathy).

REDISTRIBUTION OF CARDIAC OUTPUT The redistribution of cardiac output serves as an important compensatory mechanism. This redistribution is most marked when a patient with heart failure exercises, but as heart failure advances, redistribution occurs even in the basal state. Blood flow is redistributed so that the delivery of oxygen to vital organs, such as the brain and myocardium, is maintained at normal or near-normal levels, while flow to less critical areas, such as the cutaneous and muscular beds and viscera, is reduced. Vasoconstriction mediated by the adrenergic nervous system is largely responsible for this redistribution, which in turn may be responsible for many of the clinical manifestations of heart failure, such as fluid accumulation (reduction of renal flow), low-grade fever (reduction of cutaneous flow), and fatigue (reduction of muscle flow).

SALT AND WATER RETENTION (See also Chap. 33)

When the volume of blood pumped by the left ventricle into the systemic vascular bed is reduced, and/or when one or both ventricles fail to expel the normal fraction of their end-diastolic volumes, a complex sequence of adjustments occurs which ultimately results in the abnormal accumulation of fluid. On the one hand, many of the troubling clinical manifestations of heart failure are secondary to this excessive retention of fluid; on the other, this abnormal fluid accumulation and the expansion of blood volume which accompanies it also constitute an important compensatory mechanism which tends to maintain cardiac output and therefore perfusion of the vital organs. Except in the terminal stages of heart failure, the ventricle operates on an ascending, albeit depressed and flattened, function curve (Fig. 194-5), and the augmented ventricular end-diastolic volume and pressure characteristic of heart failure must be regarded as helping to maintain the reduced cardiac output, despite causing pulmonary and/or systemic venous congestion.

Congestive heart failure is also characterized by a complex series of neurohumoral adjustments. The activation of the adrenergic nervous system is discussed on p. 414; there is also activation of the renin-angiotensin-aldosterone system and release of antidiuretic hormone. These influences increase systemic vascular resistance and enhance sodium and water retention and potassium excretion. These actions are, to a minor extent, opposed by the release of atrial natriuretic peptide, which also occurs in congestive heart failure. Patients with severe heart failure may exhibit a reduced capacity to excrete a water load, which may result in dilutional hyponatremia. In the presence of heart failure, effective filling of the systemic arterial bed is reduced, a condition which initiates the renal and hormonal changes mentioned above.

The elevation of systemic venous pressure and the alterations of renal and adrenal function characteristic of heart failure vary in their relative importance in the production of edema in different patients with heart failure. The renin-angiotensin-aldosterone axis is activated most intensely by acute heart failure, and its activity tends to decline as heart failure becomes chronic. In patients with tricuspid valve disease or constrictive pericarditis, the elevated venous pressure and the transudation of fluid from systemic capillaries appear to play the dominant role in edema formation. On the other hand, severe edema may be present in patients with ischemic or hypertensive heart disease, in whom systemic venous pressure is within normal limits or is only minimally elevated. In such patients, the retention of salt and water is probably due primarily to a redistribution of cardiac output and a concomitant reduction in renal perfusion, as well as activation of the renin-angiotensin-aldosterone axis. Regardless of the mechanisms involved in fluid retention, untreated patients with chronic congestive heart failure have elevations of total blood volume, interstitial fluid volume, and body sodium. These abnormalities diminish after clinical compensation has been achieved by treatment.

CLINICAL MANIFESTATIONS OF HEART FAILURE

Dyspnea   Respiratory distress which occurs as the result of increased effort in breathing is the most common symptom of heart failure (Chap. 31). In early heart failure, dyspnea is observed only during activity, when it may simply represent an aggravation of the breathlessness which occurs normally under these circumstances. As heart failure advances, however, dyspnea appears with progressively less strenuous activity. Ultimately, breathlessness is present even when the patient is at rest. The principal difference between exertional dyspnea in normal persons and in cardiac patients is the degree of activity necessary to induce the symptom. Cardiac dyspnea is observed most frequently in patients with elevations of pulmonary venous and capillary pressures. Such patients usually have engorged pulmonary vessels and interstitial pulmonary edema, which may be evident on radiologic examination and which reduces the compliance of the lungs and thereby increases the work of the respiratory muscles required to inflate the lungs. The activation of receptors in the lungs results in the rapid, shallow breathing characteristic of cardiac dyspnea. The oxygen cost of breathing is increased by the excessive work of the respiratory muscles. This is coupled with the diminished delivery of oxygen to these muscles, which occurs as a consequence of the reduced cardiac output and which may contribute to fatigue of the respiratory muscles and the sensation of shortness of breath.

Orthopnea   Dyspnea in the recumbent position is usually a later manifestation of heart failure than exertional dyspnea. Orthopnea occurs because of the redistribution of fluid from the abdomen and lower extremities into the chest causing an increase in the pulmonary capillary hydrostatic pressure, as well as elevation of the diaphragm. Patients with orthopnea must elevate their heads on several pillows at night and frequently awaken short of breath or coughing (the so-called nocturnal cough) if their heads slip off the pillows. The sensation of breathlessness usually is relieved by sitting upright, since this position reduces venous return and pulmonary capillary pressure, and many patients report that they find relief from sitting in front of an open window. As heart failure advances, orthopnea may become so severe that patients cannot lie down at all and must spend the entire night in a sitting position. On the other hand, in other patients with long-standing, severe left ventricular failure, symptoms of pulmonary congestion may actually diminish with time as the function of the right ventricle becomes impaired.

Paroxysmal (nocturnal) dyspnea   This term refers to attacks of severe shortness of breath and coughing which generally occur at night, usually awaken the patient from sleep, and may be quite frightening. Though simple orthopnea may be relieved by sitting upright at the side of the bed with legs dependent, in the patient with paroxysmal nocturnal dyspnea, coughing and wheezing often persist even in this position. The depression of the respiratory center during sleep may reduce ventilation sufficiently to lower arterial oxygen tension, particularly in patients with interstitial lung edema and reduced pulmonary compliance. Also, ventricular function may be further impaired at night because of reduced adrenergic stimulation of myocardial function. *Cardiac asthma* is closely related to paroxysmal nocturnal dyspnea and nocturnal cough and is characterized by wheezing secondary to bronchospasm—most prominent at night. *Acute pulmonary edema* (Chap. 31) is a severe form of cardiac asthma due to marked elevation of pulmonary capillary pressure leading to alveolar edema, associated with extreme shortness of breath, rales over the lung fields, and the transudation and expectoration of blood-tinged fluid. If not treated promptly acute pulmonary edema may be fatal.

Cheyne-Stokes respiration   Also known as *periodic* or *cyclic respiration*, Cheyne-Stokes respiration is characterized by diminished sensitivity of the respiratory center to arterial P_{CO_2}. There is an apneic phase, during which the arterial P_{O_2} falls and the arterial P_{CO_2} rises. These changes in the arterial blood stimulate the depressed respiratory center, resulting in hyperventilation and hypocapnia, followed in turn by apnea. Cheyne-Stokes respiration occurs most often in patients with cerebral atherosclerosis and other cerebral lesions, but the prolongation of the circulation time from the lung to the brain which occurs in heart failure, particularly in patients with hypertension and coronary artery disease and associated cerebral vascular disease, also appears to precipitate this form of breathing.

Fatigue, weakness, and reduced exercise capacity   These non-specific but common symptoms of heart failure are related to the reduction of perfusion of skeletal muscle. Exercise capacity is reduced by the limited ability of the failing heart to increase its output and deliver oxygen to the exercising muscle. Anorexia and nausea associated with abdominal pain and fullness are frequent complaints which may be related to the congested liver and portal venous system.

Cerebral symptoms   In severe heart failure, particularly in elderly patients with accompanying cerebral arteriosclerosis, reduced cerebral perfusion, and arterial hypoxemia, there may be alterations in the mental state characterized by confusion, difficulty in concentration, impairment of memory, headache, insomnia, and anxiety. *Nocturia* is common in heart failure and may contribute to insomnia.

PHYSICAL FINDINGS (See Chap. 188)   In moderate heart failure, the patient appears to be in no distress at rest except that he or she may be uncomfortable when lying flat for more than a few minutes. In more severe heart failure, the pulse pressure may be diminished, reflecting a reduction in stroke volume, and occasionally, the diastolic arterial pressure is elevated as a consequence of generalized vasoconstriction. In acute heart failure, hypotension may be prominent. There may be cyanosis of the lips and nail beds and sinus tachycardia, and the patient may insist on sitting upright. *Systemic venous pressure* is often abnormally elevated in heart failure and may be recognized by observing the extent of distention of the jugular veins. In the early stages of heart failure, the venous pressure may be normal at rest but may become abnormally elevated during and immediately after exertion as well as with sustained pressure on the abdomen (positive abdominojugular reflux).

Third and fourth heart sounds are often audible but are not specific for heart failure, and *pulsus alternans*, i.e., a regular rhythm in which there is alternation of strong and weak cardiac contractions and therefore alternation in the strength of the peripheral pulses, may be present. Pulsus alternans may be detected by sphygmomanometry and in more severe instances by palpation; it frequently follows an extrasystole and is observed most commonly in patients with cardiomyopathy or hypertensive or ischemic heart disease. It is a sign of severe heart failure and is caused by a reduction in the number of contractile units during weak contractions and/or by alternation in the ventricular end-diastolic volume.

Pulmonary rales   Moist, inspiratory, crepitant rales and dullness to percussion over the lung bases are common in patients with heart failure and elevated pulmonary venous and capillary pressures. In patients with pulmonary edema, rales may be heard widely over both lung fields; they are frequently coarse and sibilant and may be accompanied by expiratory wheezing. Rales may, however, be caused by many conditions other than left ventricular failure. Some patients with long-standing heart failure have no rales because of increased lymphatic drainage of alveolar fluid.

Cardiac edema   Cardiac edema is usually dependent, occurring in the legs symmetrically, particularly in the pretibial region and ankles in ambulatory patients, in whom it is most prominent in the evening, and in the sacral region of individuals at bed rest. Pitting edema of the arms and face occurs rarely and then only late in the course of heart failure.

Hydrothorax and ascites   Pleural effusion in congestive heart failure results from the elevation of pleural capillary pressure and transudation of fluid into the pleural cavities. Since the pleural veins drain into *both* the systemic and pulmonary veins, hydrothorax occurs most commonly with marked elevation of pressure in both venous systems but also may be seen with marked elevation of pressure in either venous bed. It is more frequent in the right pleural cavity than in the left. *Ascites* also occurs as a consequence of transudation and results from increased pressure in the hepatic veins and the veins draining the peritoneum (Chap. 43). Marked ascites occurs most frequently in patients with tricuspid valve disease and constrictive pericarditis.

Congestive hepatomegaly   An enlarged, tender, pulsating liver also accompanies systemic venous hypertension and is observed not only in the same conditions in which ascites occurs but also in milder forms of heart failure from any cause. With prolonged, severe hepatomegaly, as in patients with tricuspid valve disease or chronic constrictive pericarditis, enlargement of the spleen, i.e., congestive splenomegaly, also may occur.

Jaundice   This is a late finding in congestive heart failure and is associated with elevations of both the direct- and indirect-reacting bilirubin; it results from impairment of hepatic function secondary to hepatic congestion and the hepatocellular hypoxia associated with central lobular atrophy. Serum transaminase concentrations are frequently elevated. If hepatic congestion occurs acutely, the jaundice may be severe and the enzymes strikingly elevated.

Cardiac cachexia   With severe chronic heart failure there may be serious weight loss and cachexia because of (1) elevation of circulating concentrations of tumor necrosis factor, (2) elevation of the metabolic rate, which results in part from the extra work performed by the respiratory muscles, the increased oxygen needs of the hypertrophied heart, and/or the discomfort associated with severe heart failure, (3) anorexia, nausea, and vomiting due to central causes, to digitalis intoxication, or to congestive hepatomegaly and abdominal fullness, (4) impairment of intestinal absorption due to congestion of the intestinal veins, and (5) rarely, in patients with particularly severe failure of the right side of the heart, a protein-losing enteropathy.

Other manifestations   With reduction of blood flow, the extremities may be cold, pale, and diaphoretic. Urine flow is depressed, and the urine contains albumin and has a high specific gravity and a low concentration of sodium. In addition, prerenal azotemia may be present. In patients with long-standing severe heart failure, impotence and depression are common.

ROENTGENOGRAPHIC FINDINGS   In addition to the enlargement of the particular chambers characteristic of the lesion responsible for heart failure, distention of pulmonary veins and redistribution to the apices is common in patients with heart failure and elevated pulmonary vascular pressures (Chap. 190). Also, pleural effusions may be evident and associated with interlobar effusions.

DIFFERENTIAL DIAGNOSIS   The diagnosis of congestive heart failure may be established by observing some combination of the clinical manifestations of heart failure described above, together with the findings characteristic of one of the etiologic forms of heart disease. Since chronic heart failure is often associated with cardiac enlargement, the diagnosis should be questioned, but is by no means excluded, when all chambers are normal in size. Two-dimensional echocardiography is particularly useful in assessing the dimensions of each cardiac chamber. Heart failure may be difficult to distinguish from pulmonary disease, and the differential diagnosis is discussed in Chap. 31. Pulmonary embolism also presents many of the manifestations of heart failure, but hemoptysis, pleuritic chest pain, a right ventricular lift, and the characteristic mismatch between ventilation and perfusion on lung scan should point to this diagnosis (see Chap. 226).

Ankle edema may be due to varicose veins, cyclic edema, or gravitational effects (Chap. 33), but in these patients there is no jugular venous hypertension at rest or with pressure over the abdomen. Edema secondary to renal disease can usually be recognized by appropriate renal function tests and urinalysis and is rarely associated with elevation of venous pressure. Enlargement of the liver and ascites occur in patients with hepatic cirrhosis and also may be distinguished from heart failure by normal jugular venous pressure and absence of a positive abdominojugular reflux.

TREATMENT OF HEART FAILURE

The treatment of heart failure may be divided logically into three components: (1) removal of the precipitating cause, (2) correction of the underlying cause, and (3) control of the congestive heart failure state. The first two are discussed in other chapters together with each specific disease entity or complication. An example is the treatment of pneumococcal pneumonia and acute heart failure (removal of the precipitating cause) followed by mitral valvotomy (correction of the underlying cause) in a patient with mitral stenosis. In many instances, surgical treatment will correct or at least alleviate the underlying cause. The third component of the treatment of heart failure, i.e., control of the congestive heart failure state, may, in turn, be divided into three categories: (1) reduction of cardiac work load, including both the preload and the afterload, (2) control of excessive retention of salt and water, and (3) enhancement of myocardial contractility. The vigor with which each of these measures is pursued in any individual patient should depend on the severity of heart failure. Following effective treatment, recurrence of the clinical manifestations of heart failure can often be prevented by continuing those measures which were originally effective.

While a simple rule for the treatment of all patients with heart failure cannot be formulated because of the varied etiologies, hemodynamic features, clinical manifestations, and severity of heart failure, insofar as the treatment of chronic congestive failure is concerned, simple measures such as moderate restriction of activity and sodium intake should be tried first. If these are insufficient, therapy with a combination of a diuretic; a vasodilator, preferably an angiotensin-converting enzyme inhibitor; and usually a digitalis glycoside is then begun. The next step is more rigorous restriction of salt intake and higher doses of loop diuretics, sometimes accompanied by other diuretics. If heart failure persists, hospitalization with rigid salt restriction, bed rest, intravenous vasodilators, and positive inotropic agents comes next. In some patients, the order in which these measures are applied may be altered.

REDUCTION OF CARDIAC WORK LOAD This consists of reducing physical activity, instituting emotional rest, and reducing afterload. Modest restriction of physical activity in mild cases and rest in bed or in a chair in severe failure remain cornerstones in the treatment of heart failure. Meals should be small in quantity but perhaps more frequent, and every effort should be made to diminish the patient's anxiety; sometimes drugs such as diazepam (2–5 mg tid) for several days are useful. Physical and emotional rest tends to lower arterial pressure and reduce the load on the myocardium by diminishing the requirements for cardiac output. These influences act in concert to diminish the need for redistribution of the cardiac output, and in many patients, particularly those with mild heart failure, simple bed rest and mild sedation often result in an effective diuresis.

Rest at home or in the hospital should be maintained for 1 to 2 weeks in patients with overt congestive failure and should be continued for several days after the patient's condition has stabilized. The hazards of phlebothrombosis and pulmonary embolism which occur with bed rest may be reduced with anticoagulants, leg exercises, and elastic stockings. *Absolute* bed rest rarely is required or advisable and the patient should be encouraged to sit in a chair and be given toilet privileges unless heart failure is extreme. Heavy sedation should be avoided, but small doses of tranquilizers may be helpful in calming the emotionally disturbed patient during the first few days of therapy and in permitting much-needed sleep. In patients with chronic, moderately severe heart failure, additional periods of bed rest on weekends will frequently allow continuation of gainful employment. Following recovery from heart failure, the patient's activities must be carefully assessed, and often, professional, community, and/or family responsibilities must be curtailed. Intermittent rest during the day (e.g., a scheduled 1-h nap or rest following lunch) and the avoidance of strenuous exertion are often helpful once compensation has been restored. Weight reduction by restriction of caloric intake in obese patients with heart failure also diminishes cardiac work load and is an essential component of the therapeutic program. Vasodilator therapy (p. 1004) may be considered a form of reduction of the cardiac work load. This form of therapy has been shown not only to ameliorate heart failure but also to retard its development in patients with left ventricular dysfunction.

CONTROL OF EXCESSIVE FLUID Many of the clinical manifestations of heart failure result from hypervolemia and expansion of the interstitial fluid volume. By the time fluid retention due to heart failure becomes clinically evident, most commonly as edema, considerable expansion of the extracellular space has already occurred, and heart failure usually is already advanced. Exertional dyspnea and orthopnea may be caused by displacement of fluid from the systemic to the pulmonary vascular bed. Treatment aimed at reducing extracellular fluid volume is dependent primarily on lowering total-body sodium stores, while fluid restriction is of less importance. A negative sodium balance can be achieved by reducing the dietary intake and increasing the urinary excretion of this ion with the aid of diuretics. In severe heart failure, mechanical removal of extracellular fluid by means of thoracentesis, paracentesis, and rarely hemodialysis or peritoneal dialysis also may be employed.

Diet In patients with mild heart failure, considerable improvement in symptoms may result simply from reducing the sodium intake, particularly if accompanied by periods of physical rest. In patients with more severe heart failure, the sodium intake must be controlled more rigidly, and other measures, such as diuretics, vasodilators, and glycosides, are used. Even following recovery from a bout of heart failure, if the underlying cause has not been corrected, at least moderate sodium restriction should be maintained. The normal diet contains approximately 6 to 10 g sodium chloride; this intake can be reduced by half simply by excluding salt-rich foods and salt which is added at the table. Reduction of the ordinary dietary intake to approximately one-fourth of normal may be achieved if, in addition, all salt is omitted from cooking. In patients with severe heart failure, in whom the daily sodium chloride intake should be reduced to between 500 and 1000 mg, milk, cheese, bread, cereals, canned vegetables and soups, some salted cuts of meat, and some fresh vegetables, including spinach, celery, and beets, must be eliminated. A variety of fresh fruit, green vegetables, specially processed breads and milk, and salt substitutes are permissible, but it is difficult to keep such diets palatable over the long term. Water intake may be ad libitum in all but the most severe forms of congestive heart failure. Late in the course of heart failure, dilutional hyponatremia may develop in patients who are unable to excrete a water load, sometimes because of excessive secretion of antidiuretic hormone. In such cases, water intake as well as sodium intake must be restricted.

Attention also must be directed to the caloric content of the diet. Calories should be restricted in obese patients with heart failure. On the other hand, in patients with severe heart failure and cardiac cachexia, an attempt must be made to maintain nutritional intake and to avoid caloric and vitamin deficiencies; nutritional supplements may be in order.

Diuretics A variety of diuretic agents is available, and in patients with mild heart failure, almost all are effective. However, in the more severe forms of heart failure, the selection of diuretics is more difficult, and any existing abnormalities in serum electrolytes must be taken into account. Overtreatment must be avoided, since the resultant hypovolemia may reduce cardiac output, interfere with renal function, and produce profound weakness and lethargy.

THIAZIDE DIURETICS These agents are used widely in clinical practice because of their effectiveness when administered orally. In patients with chronic heart failure of mild or moderate severity, the continued administration of a thiazide diuretic abolishes or diminishes the need for rigid dietary sodium restriction, although salty foods and table salt still should be avoided. Thiazides are well absorbed following oral administration; chlorothiazide and hydrochlorothiazide reach their peak action in 4 h, and diuresis persists for approximately 12 h. Thiazide diuretics reduce the reabsorption of sodium and chloride in the first half of the distal convoluted tubule and a portion of the cortical ascending limb of the loop of Henle, and water follows the unreabsorbed salt. Thiazides fail to increase free water clearance, and in some instances reduce it, supporting the hypothesis that these drugs inhibit selective reabsorption of sodium chloride in the distal cortical diluting segment, at a site where the urine is normally diluted (Chap. 235). This may result in the excretion of a hypertonic urine and may contribute to dilutional hyponatremia. As a consequence of increased delivery of sodium to the distal nephron, sodium-potassium ion exchange is enhanced, and kaliuresis results. In contrast to the loop diuretics which enhance calcium excretion, the thiazides have the opposite effect. These drugs are effective and useful in the treatment of heart failure as long as the glomerular filtration rate exceeds approximately 50 percent of normal.

Chlorothiazide is administered in doses of up to 500 mg every 6 h. Many derivatives of this compound are available but differ principally in dosage and duration of action and therefore offer few, if any, significant advantages over the parent compound, except for chlorthalidone, which may be administered once daily. Potassium depletion and metabolic alkalosis (the latter due to increased H^+ secretion as a substitute for the depleted intracellular stores of potassium and increased proximal tubular reabsorption of filtered HCO_3^- when there is relative depletion of the extracellular fluid volume) are the chief adverse metabolic effects following prolonged administration of the thiazides, of metolazone, and of the loop diuretics. Hypokalemia may enhance seriously the dangers of digitalis intoxication, induce fatigue and lethargy, and may be prevented by the oral supplementation of potassium chloride. However, the solution is not palatable and may be hazardous in patients with renal failure. Therefore, to prevent potassium depletion in patients receiving thiazide diuretics, intermittent dosage schedules, e.g., omitting the diuretic every third day, and the addition of a potassium-retaining diuretic, such as a spironolactone or triamterene, may be preferable. Other side effects of thiazides include reduction of the excretion of uric acid, which may lead to hyperuricemia, and a hyperglycemic effect, which rarely may precipitate hyperosmolar coma in the poorly regulated diabetic. Skin rashes, thrombocytopenia, and granulocytopenia also have been reported.

METOLAZONE   This quinethazone derivative has a site of action and potency similar to those of the thiazides but has been reported to be effective in the presence of moderate renal failure. The usual dose is 5 to 10 mg/d.

FUROSEMIDE, BUMETANIDE, AND ETHACRYNIC ACID   These "loop" diuretics are similar physiologically but differ chemically. These extremely powerful diuretics reversibly inhibit the reabsorption of sodium, potassium, and chloride in the thick ascending limb of Henle's loop, apparently by blocking a cotransport system in the luminal membrane. They may induce renal cortical vasodilatation and can produce rates of urine formation which may be as high as one-fourth of the glomerular filtration rate. While other diuretics lose their effectiveness as blood volume is restored to normal levels, the loop diuretics remain effective despite the elimination of excessive extracellular fluid volume. The major side effects of these agents are due to this marked diuretic potency, which on rare occasions may result in contraction of the plasma volume, circulatory collapse, reductions in the renal blood flow and glomerular filtration rate, and the development of prerenal azotemia. Metabolic alkalosis is produced by a large increase in the urinary excretion of chloride, hydrogen, and potassium ions. Hypokalemia (see discussion of thiazides, above) and hyponatremia may occur, and hyperuricemia and hyperglycemia are observed occasionally, as with thiazide diuretics. The reabsorption of free water is decreased.

All three drugs are readily absorbed orally and are excreted in the bile and urine. They are usually effective by mouth and intravenously. Weakness, nausea, and dizziness may complicate the administration of all loop diuretics; ethacrynic acid has been associated with transient or even permanent deafness as well as with skin rash and granulocytopenia.

These extremely effective diuretics are useful in all forms of heart failure, particularly in otherwise refractory heart failure and pulmonary edema. They have been shown to be effective in patients with hypoalbuminemia, hyponatremia, hypochloremia, hypokalemia, and reductions in the glomerular filtration rate and to produce a diuresis in patients in whom thiazide diuretics and aldosterone antagonists, alone and in combination, are ineffective.

In patients with refractory heart failure, the action of furosemide, bumetanide, and ethacrynic acid may be potentiated by intravenous administration and the addition of all other diuretics, i.e., thiazides, carbonic anhydrase inhibitors, osmotic diuretics, and the potassium-sparing diuretics—spironolactone, triamterene, and amiloride. These latter agents act on the cortical collecting ducts, are relatively weak, and therefore are rarely indicated as sole agents. However, their potassium-sparing properties make them particularly useful in conjunction with the more potent kaliuretic agents, the loop diuretics and thiazides. The potassium-sparing agents fall into two classes, as noted below.

ALDOSTERONE ANTAGONISTS   The 17-spironolactones resemble aldosterone structurally and act on the distal half of the convoluted tubule and the cortical portion of the collecting duct by competitive inhibition of aldosterone, thereby blocking the exchange between sodium and both potassium and hydrogen in the distal tubules and collecting ducts. These agents produce a sodium diuresis, and in contrast to the thiazides, ethacrynic acid, and furosemide, they result in potassium retention. Although secondary hyperaldosteronism exists in some patients with congestive heart failure, the spironolactones are effective even in patients in whom the serum aldosterone concentration is within normal limits. Aldactone A may be administered in doses of 25 to 100 mg three to four times daily by mouth. The maximal effect of this regimen is not observed for approximately 4 days. Spironolactones are most effective when administered in combination with thiazide and/or loop diuretics. The opposing action of these drugs on urine and serum potassium makes possible a sodium diuresis without either hyper- or hypokalemia when spironolactone and one of these other agents are administered in combination. Also, since spironolactone, triamterene, and amiloride act on the distal tubule, they are particularly effective when used in combination with one of these other diuretics which acts more proximally.

Spironolactone, triamterene, and amiloride should not be administered alone to patients with hyperkalemia, renal failure, or hyponatremia. Reported complications include nausea, epigastric distress, mental confusion, drowsiness, gynecomastia, and erythematous eruptions.

TRIAMTERENE AND AMILORIDE   These two drugs exert renal effects similar to those of the spironolactones; i.e., they block sodium reabsorption and secondarily inhibit potassium secretion in the distal tubules. However, their fundamental mechanism of action differs from that of the spironolactones, since they are active in adrenalectomized animals and their action does not depend on the presence of aldosterone. The effective dose of triamterene is 100 mg once or twice daily, and that of amiloride is 5 mg daily. Side effects include nausea, vomiting, diarrhea, headache, granulocytopenia, eosinophilia, and skin rash. Both triamterene and the chemically unrelated diuretic amiloride resemble Aldactone A in that their diuretic potency is not great, but they are effective in preventing the hypokalemia characteristic of the administration of thiazides, furosemide, and ethacrynic acid. A number of diuretic preparations contain a combination of a thiazide and either triamterene or amiloride in a single capsule. They may be useful in patients who develop hypokalemia with a thiazide but should not be used in patients with impaired renal function and/or hyperkalemia.

CHOICE OF DIURETICS   Orally administered thiazides and metolazone are the agents of choice in the treatment of chronic cardiac edema of mild to moderate degree in patients without hyperglycemia, hyperuricemia, or hypokalemia. Spironolactones, triamterene, and amiloride are not potent diuretics when used alone, but they potentiate other diuretics, particularly the thiazide and loop diuretics. However, in patients with heart failure and severe secondary hyperaldosteronism, spironolactone may be quite effective. Ethacrynic acid, bumetanide, and furosemide, given alone or with spironolactone or triamterene, are the agents of choice in patients with severe heart failure refractory to other diuretics. In very severe heart failure, the combination of a thiazide, a loop diuretic, and a potassium-sparing diuretic is required.

VASODILATOR THERAPY   In many patients with heart failure, left ventricular afterload is increased as a consequence of the several neural and humoral influences which act to constrict the peripheral vascular bed. These include the previously mentioned increased activity of the adrenergic nervous system, elevation of circulating catecholamines, and activation of the renin-angiotensin system, and perhaps increased circulating antidiuretic hormone. In addition to the vasoconstriction, the ventricular end-diastolic volume rises in heart failure. As a consequence of the operation of Laplace's law, which relates myocardial wall tension to the product of intraventricular pressure and radius (both of which may become elevated in heart failure), the aortic impedance, i.e., the force which opposes left ventricular ejection, or the ventricular afterload, rises. Vasoconstriction is generally considered to be a useful compensatory mechanism that allows blood flow to vital organs to persist in the presence of hypovolemia and many forms of shock associated with reduction of the total cardiac output (Chap. 34). However, in the presence of severely impaired cardiac function, the increase in afterload may reduce cardiac output further.

As shown in Fig. 194-4, afterload is a major determinant of cardiac function. When cardiac function is normal, a moderate elevation in afterload does not reduce stroke volume significantly, because the resultant increase in left ventricular end-diastolic volume, i.e., preload, can be tolerated easily. However, when myocardial function is impaired, such an increase in preload evoked by an elevation of afterload may raise ventricular end-diastolic and pulmonary capillary pressures to levels that may produce severe pulmonary congestion or even pulmonary edema. In many patients with heart failure, the ventricle is already operating at the peak, flat portion of its Frank-Starling curve (Fig. 194-5), and any additional increase in aortic impedance (afterload) will reduce stroke volume (p. 994). Conversely, a modest reduction of afterload will not have a significant effect on stroke volume in normal subjects, but in patients with heart failure it will tend to restore hemodynamics to normal by elevating the stroke volume of the failing ventricle and may reduce the elevated ventricular filling pressure.

The pharmacologic reduction of impedance to left ventricular ejection with vasodilator drugs represents an important adjunct in the management of heart failure. This approach may be particularly helpful but is by no means limited to patients with acute heart failure due to myocardial infarction (Chap. 202), valvular regurgitation (Chap. 201), elevated systemic vascular resistance and/or arterial pressure, and marked cardiac dilatation. The reduction of afterload by means of a variety of vasodilators reduces left ventricular end-diastolic pressure, volume, and oxygen consumption while raising stroke volume and cardiac output and causing only modest reduction in aortic pressure. Vasodilators should, of course, not be used in patients with hypotension.

In patients with both acute and chronic heart failure secondary to ischemic heart disease, cardiomyopathy, or valvular regurgitation who are treated with vasodilators, cardiac output increases, the pulmonary wedge pressure falls, the signs and symptoms of heart failure are relieved, and a new steady state is achieved in which cardiac output is higher and afterload lower with no or only mild reduction of arterial pressure (Fig. 195-1). Furthermore, the reduction of an elevated left end-diastolic pressure may improve subendocardial perfusion.

Vasodilator therapy is useful in the treatment of all forms of heart failure, ranging from the mild-chronic to the severe-acute forms.

The several available vasodilators vary in their hemodynamic effects, locus and duration of action, and mode of administration. Some vasodilators, such as hydralazine, minoxidil, and the alpha-adrenergic blocking agents, such as prazosin, act predominantly on the arterial bed and primarily increase stroke volume; others, such as nitroglycerin and isosorbide dinitrate, act almost entirely on the venous side of the circulation. The latter agents cause pooling of blood in the venous bed and act primarily to reduce ventricular filling pressures. Angiotensin-converting enzyme inhibitors, prazosin, and sodium nitroprusside are "balanced vasodilators" i.e., they act on both the arterial and venous beds. Some agents, such as sodium nitroprusside, must be administered by continuous intravenous infusion; nitroglycerin requires administration in ointment patch or intravenous forms when a prolonged effect is desired; and isosorbide

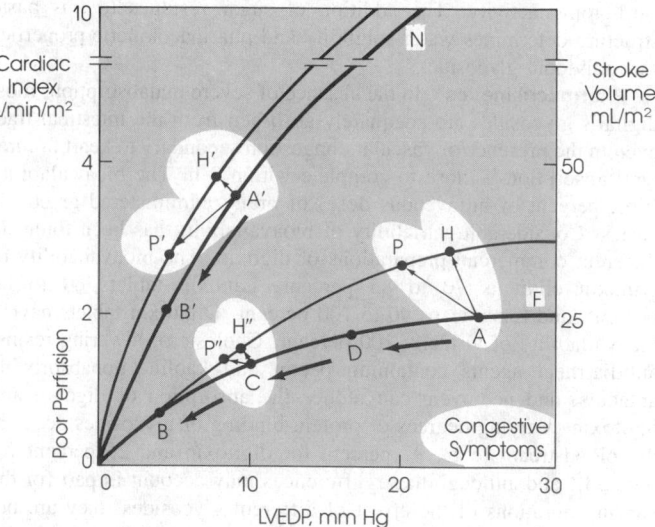

FIGURE 195-1 Effects of various vasodilators on the relationship between left ventricular end-diastolic pressure (LVEDP) and cardiac index or stroke volume in normal (N) and failing (F) hearts. H represents hydralazine or any other pure arterial dilator. It produces only a minimal increase in cardiac index in the normal subject (A' → H') or in the patient with heart failure with normal LVEDP (C → H''). In contrast, it elevates output in the patient with heart failure and elevated LVEDP (A → H). P represents a balanced vasodilator, such as sodium nitroprusside or an ACE inhibitor. It reduces filling pressure in all patients, elevates cardiac output in patients with heart failure and elevated LVEDP (A → P), lowers cardiac output in normal subjects (A' → P'), and has little effect on cardiac output in heart failure patients with normal filling pressures (C → P''). *(Reprinted with permission from TW Smith et al.)*

dinitrate is most effective when it is administered by the sublingual route.

The ideal vasodilator for the treatment of *acute* heart failure should have a rapid onset and brief duration of action when administered by intravenous infusion; sodium nitroprusside qualifies as such a drug, but its use requires careful monitoring of the arterial pressure and electrocardiogram and, if possible, of the pulmonary artery wedge pressure in an intensive care unit. For the treatment of chronic congestive heart failure, the agent should be effective on oral administration, and its action should persist for at least 6 h. Angiotensin-converting enzyme (ACE) inhibitors satisfy these requirements and have, quite properly, become the most useful and widely used vasodilators. It is advisable to commence therapy with very low doses, particularly in patients receiving diuretics, in order to avoid hypotension and gradually increase the dose.

Vasodilators are potent and effective in acutely improving the deranged hemodynamics of heart failure, and there is evidence in favor of a beneficial chronic effect as well. Studies with ACE inhibitors have demonstrated a favorable long-term reduction of symptoms and enhancement of exercise tolerance. Importantly, these drugs and, to a lesser extent, the combination of hydralazine and isosorbide dinitrate prolong survival of patients with heart failure. The administration of ACE inhibitors has been shown to prevent or retard the development of heart failure in patients with left ventricular dysfunction but without heart failure and to reduce long-term mortality when it is begun in such patients shortly after acute myocardial infarction.

ENHANCEMENT OF MYOCARDIAL CONTRACTILITY—DIGITALIS The improvement of myocardial contractility by means of cardiac glycosides is an important component in the control of heart failure. The basic molecular structure of digitalis glycosides is a steroid nucleus to which an unsaturated lactone ring is attached at C-17. These two elements together are called *aglycone* or *genin*, and it is this portion of the molecule which is responsible for the cardiotonic activity. The addition of sugar residues to this basic structure determines water solubility and pharmacokinetic properties for individual glycosides.

Pharmacokinetics In the absence of severe malabsorption, most digitalis glycosides are adequately absorbed from the intestinal tract even in the presence of vascular congestion secondary to heart failure. Oral absorption is close to complete within 2 h. The bioavailability (i.e., percent of intravenous dose) of orally administered glycoside varies. Considerable variability of bioavailability has been found in different commercial preparations of digoxin. The bioavailability of Lanoxin elixir is 70 to 85 percent, Lanoxin tablets 60 to 80 percent, and Lanoxicaps 90 to 100 percent. Digitoxin tablets have a bioavailability of virtually 100 percent. Cholesterol-lowering resins, antidiarrheal agents containing pectin and kaolin, nonabsorbable antacids, and neomycin can reduce the absorption of digoxin and digitoxin. Varying degrees of protein-binding of glycosides occur in the bloodstream (e.g., 97 percent for digitoxin and 25 percent for digoxin), and although these differences may account in part for the varying durations of the effect of different glycosides, they are not related to the speed of action of these drugs. The plasma contains only approximately 1 percent of the body stores of digoxin; therefore, digoxin is not effectively removed from the body by dialysis, exchange transfusions, or during cardiopulmonary bypass, presumably because of tissue binding. The major fraction of the glycosides is directly bound by various tissues, including the heart, in which the concentration is approximately 30 times that in the plasma for digoxin and 7 times for digitoxin; the latter is less polar and more lipid-soluble than digoxin.

Digoxin, which has a half-life of 1.6 days, is filtered in the glomeruli and secreted by the renal tubules; 85 percent is excreted in the urine, most in unchanged form; only 10 to 15 percent of digoxin is eliminated in the stool through biliary excretion in the presence of normal renal function. The ratio of digoxin clearance to endogenous creatinine clearance is 0.8, and the percentage of the body's total stores of digoxin lost per day can be calculated as $(14 \pm 0.2) \times$ creatinine clearance in milliliters per minute. In patients with normal renal function, a plateau concentration in the blood and tissue is reached after 5 days of daily maintenance treatment without a loading dose (see Fig. 66-2). Therefore, significant reductions of the glomerular filtration rate reduce the elimination of digoxin (but not of digitoxin) and, therefore, may prolong digoxin's effect, allowing it to accumulate to toxic levels if it is administered in patients with impaired renal function. The administration of most diuretics does not alter the excretion of digoxin significantly, but spironolactone can inhibit tubular secretion of digoxin, resulting in significant accumulation of the drug. *Digitoxin*, with a half-life of approximately 5 days, is metabolized chiefly in the liver; only 15 percent is excreted in the urine unchanged and an equal fraction in the stool. Drugs such as phenobarbital and phenylbutazone that increase the activity of hepatic microsomal enzymes accelerate the metabolism of digitoxin. To reach a steady state, digitoxin requires maintenance doses for 3 to 4 weeks. *Ouabain* is very rapidly acting, exhibiting an onset of action in 5 to 10 min and a peak effect within 60 min following intravenous injection. It is poorly and irregularly absorbed from the gastrointestinal tract, is excreted by the kidneys, has a half-life of 21 h, and is useful in emergencies.

Mechanism of action The cardiac actions of all digitalis glycosides are alike. The clinical effects result from augmenting myocardial contractility and from prolonging the refractory period of the atrioventricular node.

The most important effect of digitalis on cardiac muscle is to shift its force-velocity relation upward (Chap. 194). This positive inotropic effect is exhibited in normal, nonfailing hypertrophied, and failing hearts. In the absence of heart failure, however, when cardiac output is not limited by cardiac contractility, the drug does not elevate the output.

Excitation-contraction coupling is the membrane and intracellular process most likely involved in producing the positive inotropic effect

of digitalis glycosides. These drugs inhibit transmembrane sodium and potassium movement by inhibition of the monovalent cation transport enzyme–coupled Na^+,K^+-ATPase. The latter, localized to the sarcolemma, appears to be the receptor for cardioactive glycosides, whose action results in an increase in intracellular sodium content; this, in turn, increases intracellular calcium concentration through a Na^+-Ca^{2+} exchange carrier mechanism. The increased myocardial uptake of calcium augments calcium released to the myofilaments during excitation (p. 989) and, therefore, invokes a positive inotropic response. There is a correlation between the degree of Na^+,K^+-ATPase inhibition and the inotropic potency of the glycoside.

Cardiac glycosides also produce alterations in the electrical properties of both the contractile cells and the specialized automatic cells. While low concentrations of glycosides produce little effect on the action potential, high concentrations result in a reduction in the resting potential (phase 4, see Fig. 197-2) and an augmented rate of diastolic depolarization. The reduction in the resting potential brings the cell closer to the threshold for depolarization. These two effects lead to increased automaticity and ectopic impulse activity. With the lowering of the resting potential, the rate of rise of the action potential is reduced, resulting in a slowing of conduction velocity, which is conducive to the development of reentry. Thus the known electrophysiologic effects of digitalis glycosides are capable of explaining the development of both reentry and ectopic foci and the resultant arrhythmias associated with digitalis intoxication.

The glycosides also prolong the effective *refractory period* of the atrioventricular node, largely as a result of an enhanced vagal effect. Digitalis also shortens the refractory period of the atrial and ventricular muscle. Small action potentials are propagated in a decremental fashion in the atrioventricular junction. Most do not reach the ventricles but leave some of the atrioventricular junctional cells in a refractory state. This helps to explain the slowing of ventricular rate produced by digitalis in supraventricular tachycardias. In atrial fibrillation, the slowing of ventricular rate is explained by prolongation of the effective refractory period of the atrioventricular node and increased concealed conduction. These actions reduce the frequency at which impulses penetrate the atrioventricular junction owing to both vagal and possibly direct effects of glycosides on junctional tissue.

Digitalis exerts a clinically significant negative chronotropic action, usually only in the setting of ventricular failure. In heart failure, slowing of the sinus rate following the administration of digitalis results also from withdrawal of sympathetic activity secondary to general improvement in circulatory status due to the positive inotropic effect of the glycoside. In the nonfailing heart, the slowing effect is negligible, and digitalis should not be used for the treatment of sinus tachycardia unless heart failure is present. The apparent suppression of pacemaker activity which may take place following large doses of digitalis is probably due not to arrest of the pacemaker but rather to a sinoatrial block related to a depression of conduction of impulses out of the sinus node.

In addition, the digitalis glycosides also exert an action on the peripheral vasculature, causing venous and arterial constriction in normal individuals and reflex dilatation resulting from withdrawal of sympathetic constrictor activity in patients with congestive heart failure.

Use in heart failure By stimulating myocardial contractility moderately, digitalis improves ventricular emptying; i.e., it increases cardiac output, augments the ejection fraction, promotes diuresis, and reduces the elevated diastolic pressure and volume and end-systolic volume of the failing ventricle with consequent reduction of symptoms resulting from pulmonary vascular congestion and elevated systemic venous pressure. It is most beneficial in patients in whom ventricular contractility is impaired secondary to chronic ischemic heart disease or when hypertensive, valvular, or congenital heart disease imposes an excessive volume or pressure load. It is particularly helpful in the treatment of heart failure accompanied by atrial flutter and fibrillation and a rapid ventricular rate. It is of relatively little value in most forms of cardiomyopathy, myocarditis, beriberi with heart failure, mitral stenosis, thyrotoxicosis (all with sinus rhythm), cor pulmonale when the lung disease is not being treated concurrently (Chap. 204), and chronic constrictive pericarditis (Chap. 206). Nonetheless, when used in proper doses, it is not contraindicated in these disorders and is frequently used because it may exert a beneficial effect, albeit not a striking one.

Digitalis intoxication Although digitalis is one of the cornerstones of the treatment for heart failure, it is a two-edged sword, because intoxication due to digitalis excess is a serious and potentially fatal complication. The therapeutic-to-toxic ratios are similar for all cardiac glycosides. In most patients with heart failure, the lethal dose of most glycosides is probably 5 to 10 times the minimal effective dose and only about twice the dose which leads to minor toxic manifestations. In addition, advanced age, acute myocardial infarction or ischemia, hypoxemia, magnesium depletion, renal insufficiency, hypercalcemia, electrical cardioversion, and hypothyroidism all may reduce the tolerance of the patient to the digitalis glycosides or provoke latent digitalis intoxication. The most common precipitating cause of digitalis intoxication, however, is depletion of potassium stores, which often occurs as a result of diuretic therapy and secondary hyperaldosteronism. Since it is not necessary for a patient to receive a maximally tolerated dose of digitalis to derive a beneficial effect, even small doses provide some therapeutic action; this point should be considered if these drugs are to be used in patients prone to toxicity, particularly the elderly.

Anorexia, nausea, and vomiting, which are among the earliest signs of digitalis intoxication, are caused by direct stimulation of centers in the medulla and are not of gastrointestinal origin. The most frequent disturbance of cardiac rhythm caused by digitalis is premature ventricular beats, which may take the form of bigeminy because of increased myocardial irritability or facilitation of reentry. Atrioventricular block of varying degrees of severity may occur. Nonparoxysmal atrial tachycardia with variable atrioventricular block is quite characteristic of digitalis intoxication. Sinus arrhythmia, sinoatrial block, sinus arrest, and atrioventricular junctional and multifocal ventricular tachycardia also may occur. These arrhythmias are due to action of the glycoside both on cardiac tissues and on the central nervous system. Chronic digitalis intoxication may be insidious in onset and characterized by exacerbations of heart failure, weight loss, cachexia, neuralgias, gynecomastia, yellow vision, and delirium. Digitalis-toxic cardiac arrhythmias precede extracardiac (gastrointestinal or central nervous system) toxicity in about one-half of cases.

The administration of quinidine to patients receiving digoxin raises the serum concentration of the latter by reducing both the renal and nonrenal elimination of digoxin and by reducing its volume of distribution and thereby increasing the propensity to digitalis intoxication. The calcium channel antagonist verapamil and the antiarrhythmic agent amiodarone also appear to raise serum digoxin levels. Therefore, serum digoxin concentrations and electrocardiograms should be followed carefully when these drugs are administered to digitalized patients. The radioimmunoassays for digoxin and digitoxin make possible the correlation of serum glycoside levels with the presence of toxicity. In patients receiving standard maintenance doses of digoxin and digitoxin and in whom no sign of intoxication is present, serum concentrations approximate 1 to 1.5 and 20 to 25 ng/mL, respectively. When signs of intoxication are present, serum levels of more than 2 and 30 ng/mL, respectively, of these glycosides are often found. Since many factors other than the serum concentration determine digitalis intoxication, and since there is considerable overlap in serum glycoside concentrations in patients with and without toxicity, these levels cannot be used as a sole guide to digitalis dosage. However, when taken together with findings on the clinical examination and electrocardiogram, they add useful information to the clinical evaluations of digitalis intoxication. In addition, they will indicate whether a patient for whom the history of digitalis intake is in doubt has, in fact, been receiving the drug.

Treatment of digitalis intoxication When tachyarrhythmias result from digitalis intoxication, withdrawal of the drug and treatment

with potassium, phenytoin, a beta-adrenoceptor blocker, or lidocaine are indicated. Potassium should be administered cautiously and by the oral route whenever possible if hypokalemia is present, but *small* doses also may be helpful when serum potassium levels are normal; *potassium must not be employed in the presence of atrioventricular block or hyperkalemia.* A beta-adrenoceptor should not be used to treat digitalis toxicity in the presence of severe heart failure or atrioventricular block but may be useful otherwise; lidocaine is effective in the treatment of digitalis-induced ventricular tachyarrhythmias in the absence of preceding atrioventricular block. A cardiac pacemaker may be required in digitalis-induced atrioventricular block. Electrical conversion may not only be ineffective in treating digitalis-caused tachyarrhythmias but also may induce more serious arrhythmias. However, it may be lifesaving in digitalis-induced ventricular fibrillation. Quinidine and procainamide are of limited value in the treatment of digitalis intoxication. Fab fragments of purified, intact digitalis antibodies are a potentially lifesaving approach to the treatment of severe intoxication.

SYMPATHOMIMETIC AMINES (See also Chap. 68) Five sympathomimetic amines which act largely on beta-adrenergic receptors—norepinephrine, epinephrine, isoproterenol (isoprenaline), dopamine, and dobutamine—improve myocardial contractility in various forms of heart failure. The latter two agents appear to be most effective in the management of heart failure; they must be administered by constant intravenous infusion and are useful in patients with intractable heart failure, particularly those with a reversible component, such as exists in patients who have undergone cardiac surgery, and in some instances of myocardial infarction and shock or pulmonary edema. While they improve the hemodynamics in these conditions, it is not clear that they improve survival. Their administration should be accompanied by careful and continuous monitoring of the electrocardiogram, arterial pressure, and, if possible, pulmonary artery wedge pressure.

Dopamine (p. 420), the naturally occurring immediate precursor of norepinephrine, has a combination of actions which makes it particularly useful in the treatment of a variety of hypotensive states and congestive heart failure. At very low doses, i.e., 1 to 2 (μg/kg)/min, it dilates renal and mesenteric blood vessels through stimulation of specific dopaminergic receptors, thereby augmenting renal and mesenteric blood flow and sodium excretion. In the range of 2 to 10 (μg/kg)/min, dopamine stimulates myocardial beta receptors but induces relatively little tachycardia, while at higher doses it also stimulates alpha-adrenergic receptors and elevates arterial pressure.

Dobutamine is a synthetic catecholamine which acts on $beta_1$, $beta_2$, and alpha receptors. It exerts a potent inotropic action, has only a modest cardioaccelerating effect, and lowers peripheral vascular resistance, but since it simultaneously raises cardiac output, it has little effect on systemic arterial pressure. Dobutamine, given in continuous infusions of 2.5 to 10 (μg/kg)/min, is useful in the treatment of acute heart failure without hypotension. Like the other sympathomimetic amines, it may be particularly valuable in the management of patients requiring relatively short-term inotropic support—up to 1 week—in conditions which are reversible, such as the cardiac depression which sometimes follows open-heart surgery, or in patients with acute heart failure who are being prepared for operation. Adverse effects include sinus tachycardia, tachyarrhythmias, and hypertension.

A major problem with all sympathomimetics is the loss of responsiveness, apparently due to "downregulation" of adrenergic receptors, which becomes evident within 8 h of continuous administration. This problem may be managed by intermittent therapy.

Amrinone This bipyridine, a noncatecholamine, nonglycoside exerts both positive inotropic and vasodilator actions by inhibiting a specific phosphodiesterase. It is suitable for intravenous use only, and by simultaneously stimulating cardiac contractility and dilating the systemic vascular bed it reverses the major hemodynamic abnormalities associated with heart failure.

REFRACTORY HEART FAILURE   When the response to ordinary treatment is inadequate, heart failure is considered to be refractory. Before assuming that this condition simply reflects advanced, perhaps preterminal, myocardial depression, careful consideration must be given to several possibilities: (1) an underlying and overlooked cause of the heart disease that may be amenable to specific surgical or medical therapy, such as silent aortic or mitral stenosis, constrictive pericarditis, infective endocarditis, hypertension, or thyrotoxicosis, (2) one or a combination of the precipitating causes of heart failure, such as pulmonary or urinary tract infection, recurrent pulmonary emboli, arterial hypoxemia, anemia, or arrhythmia, and (3) complications of overly vigorous therapy, such as digitalis intoxication, hypovolemia, or electrolyte imbalance.

Recognition and proper treatment of the aforementioned complications are likely to make the patient responsive to therapy again. Perhaps the most common complication results from overzealous treatment with diuretics. When administered too rapidly, these drugs can produce sudden hypovolemia before edema fluid can be mobilized to replace the loss of blood volume, the result being a shocklike state with evidence of systemic hypoperfusion in the presence of edema. The chronically excessively diuresed patient may have exchanged the hazards of pulmonary edema and the inconvenience of systemic edema for a persistently depressed cardiac output with its associated weakness, lethargy, prerenal azotemia, and sometimes cardiac cachexia. Temporarily easing up on salt restriction and diuretic administration may overcome this difficulty, but as heart failure worsens, this course of action may lead to increased pulmonary congestion, which is equally unacceptable.

Hyponatremia is a late manifestation of refractory heart failure. It, too, may be a complication of overaggressive diuresis leading to reduced glomerular filtration rate and decreased delivery of NaCl to the diluting sites in the distal tubule. Hyponatremia also may result from nonosmotic stimuli for the continued secretion of antidiuretic hormone. Therapy involves improvement of the cardiovascular status, if possible (sometimes requiring the administration of a sympathomimetic amine such as dopamine or dobutamine), as well as temporary cessation of diuretic therapy and restriction of oral water intake. Hypertonic saline is very rarely indicated because total-body sodium is usually elevated, not depressed, in heart failure.

The combination of an intravenously administered vasodilator, such as sodium nitroprusside, along with a potent sympathomimetic amine, such as dopamine or dobutamine, often results in an additive effect, raising cardiac output and lowering filling pressure. Intravenous amrinone, sometimes accompanied by the administration of a converting enzyme inhibitor, also may be useful in patients with refractory heart failure.

Cardiac transplantation   When patients with heart failure become unresponsive to a combination of all the aforementioned therapeutic measures, are in New York Heart Association class IV, and are deemed unlikely to survive 1 year, they should be considered for cardiac transplantation (see Chap. 196).

TREATMENT OF ACUTE PULMONARY EDEMA   Pulmonary edema secondary to left ventricular failure or mitral stenosis is described in Chap. 31. It is life-threatening and must be considered a medical emergency. As is the case for the more chronic forms of heart failure, in the treatment of pulmonary edema, attention must be directed to identifying and removing any precipitating causes of decompensation, such as an arrhythmia or infection. However, because of the acute nature of the problem, a number of additional nonspecific measures are necessary. If it does not delay treatment unduly, recording pulmonary vascular pressures through a Swan-Ganz catheter and intraarterial pressure directly is advisable. The first six measures listed below are ordinarily applied simultaneously or nearly so.

1 Morphine is administered intravenously repetitively, as needed, in doses from 2 to 5 mg. This drug reduces anxiety, reduces adrenergic vasoconstrictor stimuli to the arteriolar and venous beds, and thereby helps to break a vicious cycle. Naloxone should be available in case respiratory depression occurs.

2 Because the alveolar fluid interferes with oxygen diffusion, resulting in arterial hypoxemia, 100% oxygen should be administered, preferably under positive pressure. The latter increases intraalveolar pressure and therefore reduces transudation of fluid from the alveolar capillaries and impedes venous return to the thorax, reducing pulmonary capillary pressure.

3 The patient should be maintained in the sitting position, with the legs dangling along the side of the bed, if possible, which also tends to reduce venous return.

4 Intravenous loop diuretics, such as furosemide or ethacrynic acid (40 to 100 mg), or bumetanide (1 mg) will, by rapidly establishing a diuresis, reduce circulating blood volume and thereby hasten the relief of pulmonary edema. In addition, when given intravenously, furosemide also exerts a venodilator action, reduces venous return, and reduces pulmonary edema even before the diuresis commences.

5 Afterload reduction is achieved with intravenous sodium nitroprusside at 20 to 30 μg/min in patients whose systolic arterial pressures exceed 100 mmHg.

6 If digitalis has not been administered previously, three-fourths of a full dose of a rapidly acting glycoside, such as ouabain, digoxin, or lanatoside C, should be administered intravenously.

7 Sometimes, aminophylline (theophylline ethylenediamine), 240 to 480 mg intravenously, is effective in diminishing bronchoconstriction, increasing renal blood flow and sodium excretion, and augmenting myocardial contractility.

8 If the above-mentioned measures are not sufficient, rotating tourniquets should be applied to the extremities.

After these emergency therapeutic measures have been instituted and the precipitating factors treated, the diagnosis of the underlying cardiac disorder responsible for the pulmonary edema must be established if it is not already known. After stabilization of the patient's condition, a long-range strategy for prevention of future episodes of pulmonary edema must be established, and this may require surgical treatment.

PROGNOSIS

The prognosis in heart failure depends primarily on the nature of the underlying heart disease and on the presence or absence of a precipitating factor which can be treated. When one of the latter can be identified and removed, the outlook for immediate survival is far better than if heart failure occurs without any obvious precipitating cause. In the latter situation, survival usually ranges between 6 months and 4 years depending on the severity of the heart failure. Also, the long-term prognosis for heart failure is most favorable when the underlying forms of heart disease can be treated. The prognosis also can be estimated by observing the response to treatment. When clinical improvement occurs with only modest dietary sodium restriction and small doses of diuretics or digitalis, then the outlook is far better than if, in addition to these measures, intensive diuretic therapy and vasodilators are necessary. Other factors which have been shown to be associated with a poor prognosis in heart failure include short (<3 min) exercise time, reduced (<133 meq/L) serum sodium concentration, reduced (<3 meq/L) serum potassium concentration, elevated circulating atrial natriuretic peptide and norepinephrine concentrations, as well as frequent ventricular extrasystoles on Holter monitoring. A large fraction of patients with congestive heart failure die suddenly, presumably of ventricular fibrillation. Unfortunately, there is no evidence that this complication can be prevented by the administration of antiarrhythmic agents.

REFERENCES

BONOW RO, UDELSON JE: Left ventricular diastolic dysfunction as a cause of congestive heart failure: mechanisms and management. Ann Intern Med 117: 502, 1992

BRAUNWALD E: ACE inhibitors: A cornerstone of the treatment of heart failure. N Engl J Med 325:351, 1991

———, GROSSMAN W: Clinical aspects of heart failure, in *Heart Disease*, 4th ed, E Braunwald (ed). Philadelphia, Saunders, 1992, pp 444–463

CODY RJ: Optimising ACE inhibitor therapy of congestive heart failure. Clin Pharmacokinet 24:59, 1993

COHN JN et al: A comparison of enalapril with hydralazine-isosorbide dinitrate in the treatment of chronic congestive heart failure. N Engl J Med 325:303, 1991

FRANCIS GS et al: Comparison of neuroendocrine activation in patients with left ventricular dysfunction with and without congestive heart failure: A substudy of the Studies of Left Ventricular Dysfunction (SOLVD). Circulation 82:1724, 1990

——— et al: Neurohumoral activation in preclinical heart failure. Remodeling and the potential for intervention. Circulation 87 (suppl 5):IV90, 1993

GILMAN A (ed): Cardiovascular drugs, in *Goodman and Gilman's The Pharmacological Basis of Therapeutics*, 8th ed. New York, Macmillan, 1990, pp 749–896

GRODEN DL: Vasodilator therapy for congestive heart failure. Lessons from mortality trials. Arch Intern Med 153:445, 1993

ISKANDRIAN AS et al: Predicting left ventricular function: Bedside examination. Prim Cardiol (Suppl) 10:3A, 1984

KANNEL WB: Epidemiologic aspects of heart failure, in *Heart Failure: Current Concepts and Management*, Cardiology Clinics Series 7/1, Weber KT (ed). Philadelphia, Saunders, 1989

PACKER P: The neurohormonal hypothesis: A theory to explain the mechanism of disease progression in heart failure. J Am Coll Cardiol 20:248, 1992

SMITH TW et al: Management of heart failure, in *Heart Disease*, 4th ed, E Braunwald (ed). Philadelphia, Saunders, 1992, p. 464

SOLVD INVESTIGATORS: Effect of enalapril on survival in patients with reduced left ventricular ejection fractions and congestive heart failure. N Engl J Med 325:293, 1991

SWEDBERG K: Reduction in mortality by pharmacological therapy in congestive ehart failure. Circulation 87 (suppl 5):IV126, 1993

WILCOX CS: Diuretics, in *The Kidney*, 4th ed., BM Brenner, FC Rector Jr (eds). Philadelphia, Saunders, 1991, pp 2123–2148

196 CARDIAC TRANSPLANTATION

JOHN S. SCHROEDER

Orthotopic allograft cadaver cardiac transplantation as a treatment for end-stage cardiac disease achieved its twenty-fifth anniversary on December 7, 1992. On that day in 1967 Dr. Christiaan Barnard accomplished the first successful cardiac transplant in man, quickly followed by Drs. Norman Shumway and Richard Lower at Stanford University. After an initial early wave of enthusiasm, the problems of immunosuppression slowed application of the procedure until the introduction of cyclosporine in 1980. A subsequent worldwide expansion of cardiac transplantation has resulted in approximately 2500 cardiac transplants per year, with further increases limited only by the donor supply. Current 1- and 5-year survival rates of 95 and 70 percent indicate that cardiac transplantation is the therapy of choice in patients with end-stage heart disease who are unlikely to survive the next 6 to 12 months. This chapter reviews the procedure, indications, short- and long-term immunosuppressive therapy, and complications.

Since the introduction of cyclosporine in 1980 and the development of "low-dose" triple immunosuppressive regimens using azathioprine and prednisone, 1-year survival is reported at 80 to 90 percent and 5-year survival at 60 to 70 percent. The longest survivor has now lived 22 years after transplantation. Therefore, these survival statistics must be compared with those for other medical or surgical therapies in considering alternative therapies for end-stage heart disease.

INDICATIONS AND SELECTION OF CANDIDATES The limited donor supply and relatively high cost of cardiac transplantation have restricted it to patients most likely to survive and resume a functional life after transplantation. It is estimated that only 2000 potential donors in the United States, for a pool of at least 20,000 candidates

based on current guidelines, become available yearly. Attempts to increase donor awareness in both physicians and the public are being made. Optimal candidates for this procedure are those who would be expected to return to a functional life if their hearts were replaced. This requires a mentally vigorous, medically compliant person who has not suffered extensive other end-stage organ damage from cardiac failure or does not have other systemic disease such as severe diabetes mellitus, collagen vascular disease, or HIV positivity. Long-standing pulmonary hypertension or recurrent pulmonary emboli and infarction may result in irreversible pulmonary hypertension leading to intraoperative death. Several heart transplant centers have initiated cardiac transplantation for newborns with left ventricular hypoplasia, but long-term survival experience is still very limited.

Timing of the recommendation to undergo cardiac transplantation can be difficult and requires assessment of the patient's current disability, stability of course, and likelihood of surviving the next 6 to 12 months. Generally, left ventricular ejection fractions under 15 to 20 percent and presence of serious ventricular arrhythmias indicate a 1-year survival rate of 50 percent or less. The increasing acceptance of cardiac transplantation as a treatment modality for heart failure without a corresponding increase in donor availability has led to prolonged waiting times of as much as 2 years or more. This longer waiting time has led to more rigorous medical care of the patient awaiting transplant with meticulous monitoring of electrolytes, fluid status, and overall well-being. Recurrent hospitalizations may be required. Patients may become dopamine/dobutamine-dependent to maintain adequate cardiac output. This dependency moves the patient to the highest ("status I") priority for a donor heart.

In addition to these pharmacologic bridges to transplantation, mechanical bridges are occasionally used where pharmacologic therapy is no longer effective. Three approaches are currently used. The first is intraaortic balloon pumping, which can increase cardiac output by 15 to 20 percent. The second is a left ventricular assist device (LVAD), which empties blood via a tube placed in the apex of the left ventricle and pumps it with an electrically driven "bellows-type" mechanism into the abdominal aorta. This approach is highly effective and has been used for up to 60 days with successful subsequent transplantation. Limitations include right ventricular failure and/or high pulmonary vascular resistance, since the LVAD does not "unload" the right ventricle. Blood clotting in the device remains a problem, in addition to the obvious problems of infection. Finally, total mechanical heart replacement is also applied in some transplant centers. This complete replacement circumvents the problem of right ventricular failure but is limited by the greater complexity of the device, which can lead to clotting and systemic emboli. Patients who underwent mechanical assistance *and* received a donor heart have 1-year survival statistics similar to those who went directly to transplantation. Tissue cross-matching between donor and recipient has generally not been done because of difficulty in obtaining good matches and lack of correlation between match and outcome. Size, ABO matching, negative lymphocyte cross-match, and avoidance of a transplantation from a cytomegalovirus (CMV)–positive donor to a CMV-negative recipient are more important.

OPERATIVE PROCEDURE The operative technique for orthotopic transplantation developed in animals in the early 1960s by Shumway and Lower remains little changed. In this technique, the surgeon removes the diseased heart but leaves the posterior wall of the right atrium in place and the superior and inferior venae cavae intact. The posterior wall of the left atrium is also left in situ with pulmonary veins intact. The donor heart is then removed in toto with the posterior wall of the right and left atria incised, which allows suturing of left atrial donor rim to recipient rim and right atrial donor rim to recipient rim, with anastomosis of the aorta and pulmonary artery.

IMMUNOSUPPRESSION AND REJECTION Controlling rejection while avoiding the adverse side effects of immunosuppressive agents is pivotal to successful transplantation. Rejection is characterized by perivascular infiltration of killer T lymphocytes, which migrate into the myocardium and cause cellular necrosis if not checked. Since early rejection can be silent, it is important to detect it before necrosis occurs. Immunologic monitoring of activated T lymphocytes in peripheral blood offers clues to the timing of a rejection process but has not been sufficiently reliable to dictate antirejection therapy. Therefore, repeated percutaneous transvenous right ventricular endo-myocardial biopsies via the right internal jugular vein are required for histologic determination of the state of immunosuppression and rejection.

Billingham and associates have graded the stages of rejection as cannot rule out rejection, mild early rejection, moderate rejection, and severe rejection. Serial biopsies are taken every 1 to 2 weeks early after transplantation, with gradually widening intervals depending on the patient's course and rejection history. Prolongation of isovolumic relaxation time measured by echocardiography also may provide early clues to rejection.

Immunosuppressive therapy regimens vary but usually include triple therapy with cyclosporine, azathioprine, and prednisone. Pro-phylactic courses of monoclonal antibody OKT3 or antithymocyte globulin also may be given early after transplantation. Careful monitoring of the adverse side effects of these agents is extremely important because they include nephrotoxicity, bone marrow suppres-sion, and opportunistic infections.

EARLY COURSE AND COMPLICATIONS   It is rare for a cardiac transplant patient to have a completely uncomplicated postoperative course. In the immediate postoperative period, right-sided heart failure due to pulmonary vascular disease is most life-threatening. During the 2 to 3 weeks after transplantation, the patient is hospitalized with meticulous monitoring for evidence of rejection and infections, repeated percutaneous transvenous endomyocardial biopsies, and adjustment of immunosuppressive drugs. During the ensuing 4 to 6 weeks, infectious complications, including bacterial, viral, and protozoan infections, are common. A successful transplant program requires a highly aggressive and sophisticated approach to diagnosis and therapy of infections in the immunocompromised host. Depending on the degree of cardiac cachexia preoperatively, the patient is usually functional at 1 week and discharged from the hospital at 2 to 3 weeks if no major complication occurs.

The average first-year cost ranges from $100,000 to $150,000, depending on the need for repeated hospitalization and cardiac biopsies, and is occasionally much higher. Yearly costs for immuno-suppressive agents range from $5000 to $10,000, in addition to the expense of medical surveillance for rejection or complications.

PHYSIOLOGY AND FUNCTION   Since the allografted heart re-mains denervated, cardiac function differs from that of the innervated heart during both rest and exercise. The electrocardiogram in Fig. 196-1 shows two P waves. The P wave of the recipient's heart reflects the residual sinus node and posterior walls of the remaining native atria but is dissociated from the QRS, since the depolarization impulse does not cross the suture line. Although it does not control donor heart rate, the recipient's sinus node remains innervated and under the influence of the autonomic nervous system. The donor sinus node controls the rate of the transplanted heart. The donor heart's P wave has a regular PR interval, reflecting conduction to the ventricles. Since the controlling sinus node is denervated, it maintains a heart rate of 100 to 110 beats per minute, and rate increase depends on alterations in chronotropic agents perfusing the sinus node. Partial reinnervation may occur in some patients late after transplantation. This is manifested primarily by the occurrence of angina-like symp-toms in patients who have developed accelerated graft atherosclerosis (see below).

Ventricular function in response to isometric and isotonic exercise has been studied extensively. The early response to exercise is more dependent on the Frank-Starling mechanism and change in ventricular volume and filling pressure. As exercise proceeds and catecholamines are released with their positive inotropic effects, cardiac output begins to rise. The cardiac transplant recipient can achieve approximately

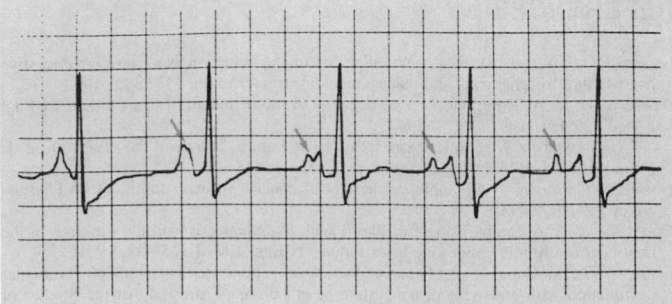

FIGURE 196-1   Electrocardiogram in a patient with a transplanted heart. The arrows denote the P wave generated by the recipient's atrium. The P wave just preceding the QRS complex is generated by the donor heart.

70 percent of the maximal cardiac output expected for his or her age, easily sufficient for the stresses of everyday life.

LATE COURSE AND COMPLICATIONS   Although the rejection process partially subsides, lifelong administration of immunosup-pressive drugs, albeit at lower doses, is still required and remains a hazard. Infectious complications and unsuspected rejection continue to occur, requiring ongoing surveillance and monitoring. Cardiac biopsies are performed at 3-month intervals to assess the response to rejection treatment. Figure 196-2 shows the causes of death by time posttransplantation from the Registry of the International Society for Heart and Lung Transplantation: Eighth Official Report, 1991. Acute rejection or infection predominates in the first year after transplantation. Subsequently, chronic rejection (i.e., accelerated coronary vascular disease) becomes the most important cause of death. In addition to the well-known hazards of long-term glucocorti-coid usage, the immunosuppressed patient is at increased risk for neoplasia. Angina is rare, and patients may present with sudden death or silent myocardial infarction. This diffuse accelerated vascular process affects both distal and proximal coronary vessels so that standard approaches, such as angioplasty or coronary artery bypass grafting, are not generally useful.

Accelerated coronary vascular disease appears to be one of the major factors limiting longer-term survival. The process is a fibrointimal hyperplasia which can go undetected by coronary arteriography at first and then cause diffuse atherosclerotic changes. Risk factors for its development may include number of rejection episodes and elevated lipids. An unusual form of lymphoma can occur frequently in extranodal locations, which is linked to prior Epstein-Barr viral infection. This lymphoma may be polyclonal or monoclonal, is associated with excessive immunosuppression, and

FIGURE 196-2   Relationship between cause of death and survival interval in heart recipients. (*From Kreitt and Kaye.*)

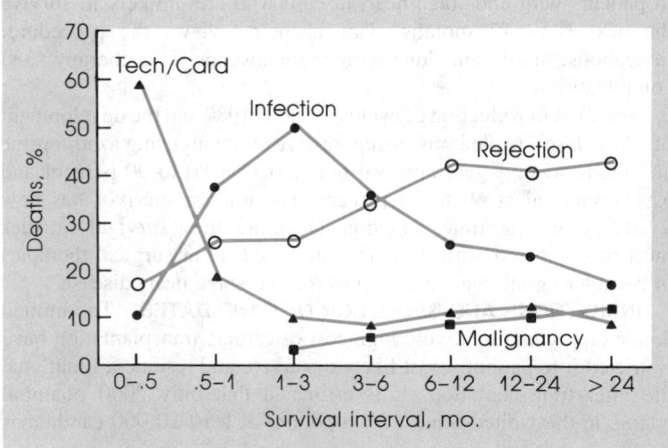

may respond to simply lowering doses of cyclosporine and administration of acyclovir rather than requiring more aggressive chemo- or radiotherapy. Many cases regress fully and do not recur. Retransplantation has been employed for some patients with severe graft atherosclerosis but it is limited by the scarcity of donors and poorer survival expectations after the second transplant. Dilitazem has been reported to reduce the severity and occurrence of this accelerated vascular process when started at the time of transplantation. CMV infections also have been associated with higher frequency of this disease. Uncontrolled trials with anticoagulation, aspirin, and improved immunosuppression with cyclosporine have done little to lower this frequency; 40 to 50 percent of patients show arteriographic evidence of coronary vascular disease 5 years after transplantation.

HEART-LUNG TRANSPLANTATION

Patients with congenital heart disease with Eisenmenger's complex (Chap. 199) or primary pulmonary hypertension (Chap. 225) are now considered for heart-lung transplantation. The surgical technique is similar to that for heart transplantation, except that the pulmonary venous attachments to the left atrium are left intact, and a tracheal anastomosis is required. The postoperative period is more complex, since the lungs may be rejected separately from the heart, requiring repeated endobronchoscopic biopsies when rejection is suspected. The immunosuppressive regimen is similar to that for heart transplants. Long-term survival has in the past been limited by obliterative bronchiolitis due to chronic unrecognized rejection; survival rates have been approximately 60 percent at 1 year and 50 percent at 2 years but appear to be improving. Heart-lung transplants also have been applied to primary pulmonary hypertension, but more recent experience with single-lung transplants for these patients has been satisfactory, thus utilizing scarce donors more effectively. Single-lung transplants are also being applied increasingly for patients with advanced emphysema. Double-lung transplants for patients with cystic fibrosis also have become the operation of choice for this group (see also Chap. 232).

REFERENCES

CAREY NR: Diagnostic criteria of chronic rejection in transplanted hearts. Transplant Proc 25:2026, 1993

COPELAND JG et al: Orthotopic total artificial heart bridge to transplantation: Preliminary results. J Heart Transplant 8:124, 1989

GAO S-Z et al: Progressive coronary luminal narrowing after cardiac transplantation. Circulation 82(suppl IV):IV-269, 1990

GRATTAN MT et al: Cytomegalovirus infection is associated with cardiac allograft rejection and atherosclerosis. JAMA 261:3561, 1989

KRIETT JM, KAYE MP: The Registry of the International Society for Heart and Lung Transplantation: Eighth Official Report, 1991. J Heart Lung Transplant 10:491, 1991

LEVENSON JL, OLSBRISCH ME: Psychiatric aspects of heart transplantation. Psychosomatics 34:114, 1993

REEDY JE et al: Bridge to heart transplantation: Importance of patient selection. J Heart Transplant 9:475, 1990

SCHROEDER JS, HUNT SA: Cardiac transplantation: Update 1987. JAMA 258:3142, 1987
—— et al: A preliminary study of diltiazem in the prevention of coronary artery disease in heart-transplant recipients. N Engl J Med 328:30, 1993

STEVENSON LW et al: Poor survival of patients with idiopathic cardiomyopathy considered too well for transplantation. Am J Med 83:871, 1987

TANIO JW, EISEN HJ: Medical aspects of cardiac transplantation. Hosp Pract 28:61, 1993

197   THE BRADYARRHYTHMIAS: DISORDERS OF SINUS NODE FUNCTION AND AV CONDUCTION DISTURBANCES

MARK E. JOSEPHSON / FRANCIS E. MARCHLINSKI / ALFRED E. BUXTON

ANATOMY OF THE CONDUCTING SYSTEM   Under normal conditions, the pacemaker function of the heart resides in the sinoatrial (SA) node, which lies at the junction of the right atrium and superior vena cava. The SA node is approximately $1\frac{1}{2}$ cm long and 2 to 3 mm wide and is supplied by the sinus node artery, which arises from either the right coronary artery (60 percent of cases) or the left circumflex coronary artery (40 percent). Once the impulse exits the sinus node and perinodal tissue, it traverses the atrium until it reaches the atrioventricular (AV) node. The blood supply of the AV node is derived from the posterior descending coronary artery (90 percent of cases), which lies at the base of the interatrial septum just above the tricuspid annulus and anterior to the coronary sinus. The electrophysiologic properties of the AV node result in slow conduction, which is responsible for the normal delay in AV conduction, i.e., the PR interval.

The bundle of His emerges from the AV node, enters the fibrous skeleton of the heart, and courses anteriorly across the membranous interventricular septum. It has a dual blood supply from the AV nodal artery and a branch of the anterior descending coronary artery. The branching (distal) portion of the bundle of His gives rise to a broad sheet of fibers that course over the left side of the interventricular septum to form the left bundle branch and a narrow cable-like structure on the right side that forms the right bundle branch. The arborization of both the right and left bundle branches gives rise to the distal His-Purkinje system, which ultimately extends throughout the endocardium of the right and left ventricles.

The sinus node, atrium, and AV node are significantly influenced by autonomic tone. Vagal influences depress automaticity of the sinus node, depress conduction, and prolong refractoriness in the tissue surrounding the sinus node; inhomogeneously decrease atrial refractoriness and slow atrial conduction; and prolong AV nodal conduction and refractoriness. Sympathetic influences exert the opposite effect.

ELECTROPHYSIOLOGIC PRINCIPLES

In the resting state, the interior of most cardiac cells, with the exception of the sinus and AV nodes, is approximately -80 to -90 mV, negative with respect to a reference extracellular electrode. The resting membrane potential is determined primarily by the concentration gradient of potassium across the cell membrane. Activation of cardiac cells results from movement of ions across the cell membrane, causing a transient depolarization known as the *action potential*. The ionic species responsible for the action potential varies among the cardiac tissues, and the configuration of the action potential is therefore unique to each tissue (Fig. 197-1).

The action potential of the His-Purkinje system and ventricular myocardium has five phases (Fig. 197-2). The rapid depolarizing current (phase 0) is mainly determined by an influx of sodium into myocardial cells followed by a secondary (slower) influx of calcium which produces a slow inward current. The repolarization phases of the action potential (phases 1 to 3) are primarily related to outward flux of potassium. The resting membrane potential is phase 4.

The bradyarrhythmias result from abnormalities either of impulse formation, i.e., automaticity, or of conduction. *Automaticity*, which is normally observed in the sinus node, the specialized fibers of the His-Purkinje system, and some specialized atrial fibers, is the property

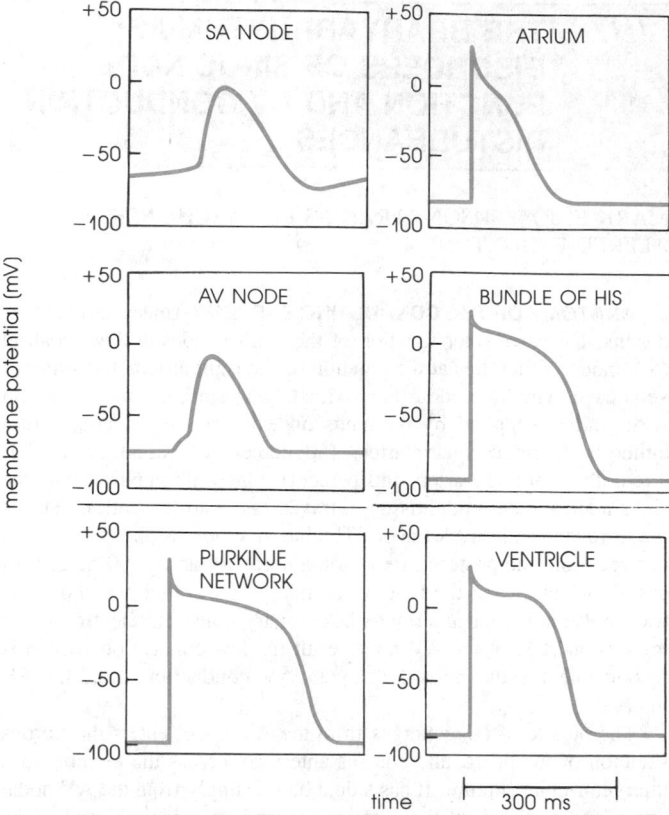

FIGURE 197-1   Action potential configurations in different regions of the mammalian heart. (*From AM Katz, Physiology of the Heart, New York, Raven, 1977.*)

of a cardiac cell which causes it to depolarize spontaneously during phase 4 of the action potential, leading to the generation of an impulse. To exhibit automaticity, the resting membrane potential must decrease spontaneously until threshold potential is reached and an all-or-none regenerative response occurs. The ionic components producing spontaneous diastolic depolarization appear to involve the inward current of either sodium or calcium. The velocity of *conduction*, i.e., impulse propagation through cardiac tissues, depends on

FIGURE 197-2   Schematic representation of the action potential in normal ventricle depicting the direction, strength, and period of flow of the ionic currents underlying the action potential. The arrow's direction and size indicate whether current is inward- or outward-directed and the approximate current strength of the ion identified at the arrow's base. The horizontal position of the arrow corresponds to the same moment in the time course of action potential (see text). The five phases of the action potential are indicated by the numerals placed along the waveform. (*From Ten Eick et al, Progress in Cardiovascular Diseases 24(2):157, 1981; used with permission.*)

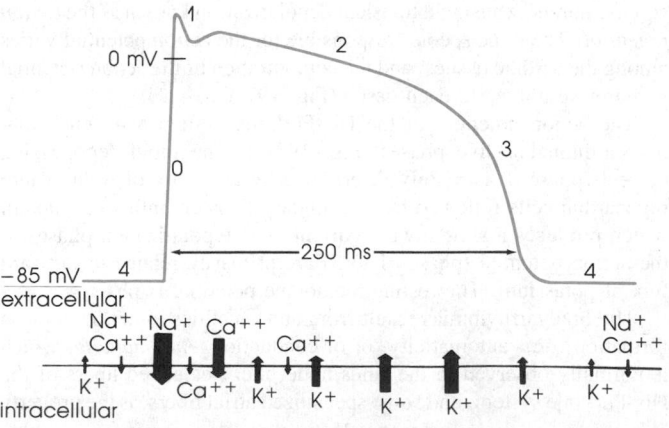

the magnitude of inward current, which is directly related to the rate of rise and amplitude of phase 0 of the action potential. The more positive the threshold potential and the slower the rate of depolarization toward threshold, the slower is the rate of rise of phase 0 of the action potential and the slower is the conduction velocity. Disease states or drugs may result in lower rates of rise of phase 0 at any given membrane potential. Passive membrane properties (e.g., intracellular resistance and intercellular coupling) also can affect impulse propagation. Propagation is more rapid parallel to fiber orientation than transverse to it, a property termed *anisotropic conduction*.

Refractoriness is a property of cardiac cells which defines the period of recovery that cells require after being discharged before they can be reexcited by a stimulus. The *absolute refractory period* is defined by that portion of the action potential during which no stimulus, regardless of its strength, can evoke another response. The *effective refractory period* is that part of the action potential during which a stimulus can evoke only a local, nonpropagated response. The *relative refractory period* extends from the end of the effective refractory period to the time that the tissue is fully recovered. During this time, a stimulus of greater than threshold strength is required to evoke a response which is propagated more slowly than normal. In the normal His-Purkinje system or ventricular myocytes, excitability is recovered following completion of the action potential, and evoked responses have characteristics similar to the spontaneous normal response. In the AV node, recovery of excitability occurs well after completion of the action potential.

INTRACARDIAC RECORDINGS OF THE SPECIALIZED CONDUCTING SYSTEM   Electrode catheters allow the recording of activation of portions of the specialized conducting system, including the bundle of His. To obtain a recording from the bundle of His, the electrode catheter is positioned across the tricuspid valve (Fig. 197-3). The interval from local atrial depolarization in the His bundle recording to the onset of depolarization of the His bundle deflection is called the *AH interval* (normal = 60 to 125 ms) and represents an indirect method of assessing AV nodal conduction time. The interval from the beginning of the His bundle deflection to the earliest onset of ventricular activation, as measured from any of multiple-surface electrocardiogram (ECG) leads or the intracardiac ventricular electrogram, is called the *HV interval* (normal = 35 to 55 ms) and represents conduction time through the His-Purkinje system. Electrode catheters can be positioned in the area of the sinus node to record high right atrial activity. Left atrial activity may be recorded directly via a catheter placed across a patent foramen ovale or indirectly using a catheter inserted into the coronary sinus. The atrial activation sequence may be "mapped", and sites of intra- and interatrial conduction abnormalities may be ascertained.

SINUS NODE DYSFUNCTION

The sinus node is normally the dominant cardiac pacemaker because its intrinsic discharge rate is the highest of all potential cardiac pacemakers. Its responsiveness to alterations in autonomic nervous system tone is responsible for the normal acceleration of heart rate during exercise and the slowing that occurs during rest and sleep. Increases in sinus rate normally result from an increase in sympathetic tone acting via beta-adrenergic receptors and/or a decrease in parasympathetic tone acting via muscarinic receptors. Slowing of the heart rate is normally due to opposite alterations. In adults, the normal sinus rate under basal conditions is 60 to 100 beats per minute. Sinus bradycardia is said to exist when the sinus rate is less than 60 beats per minute, and sinus tachycardia when it exceeds 100 beats per minute. However, there is wide variation among individuals, and rates less than 60 beats per minute do not necessarily indicate pathologic states. For example, trained athletes often exhibit resting rates under 50 beats per minute due to increases in vagal tone. Normal elderly individuals also may show marked sinus bradycardia at rest.

ETIOLOGY   Sinus node dysfunction most often is found in the elderly as an isolated phenomenon. Although interruption of the blood

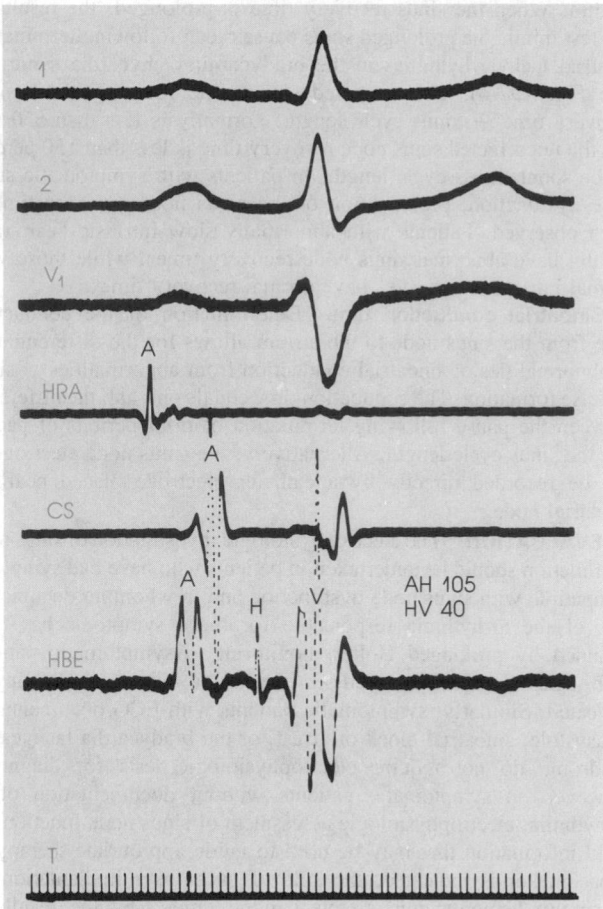

FIGURE 197-3 Normal intracardiac recording. Surface ECG leads I, II, and V₁ are displayed with intracardiac ECGs from the high right atrium (HRA), left atrium from the coronary sinus (CS), and AV junction to obtain a His bundle electrogram (HBE). T = time lines. A = atrial activation; H = His bundle activation; V = ventricular activation. Atrial activation begins in the high right atrium and spreads inferiorly to the low atrial septum, as recorded in the HBE, and the left atrium, as recorded in the CS. The AH and HV intervals represent AV nodal and His-Purkinje conduction times, respectively. Vertical lines = 0.10 s. (*From ME Josephson, SF Seides, Clinical Cardiac Electrophysiology: Techniques and Interpretations. Philadelphia, Lea & Febiger, 1979.*)

supply to the sinus node may produce dysfunction, the correlation between obstruction of the sinus node artery and clinical evidence of sinus node dysfunction is poor. Specific disease states associated with sinus node dysfunction include senile amyloidosis and other conditions associated with infiltration of the atrial myocardium. Sinus bradycardia is associated with hypothyroidism, advanced liver disease, hypothermia, typhoid fever, and brucellosis; it occurs during episodes of hypervagotonia (vasovagal syncope), severe hypoxia, hypercapnia, acidemia, and acute hypertension. However, in most cases of sinus node dysfunction a specific cause cannot be identified.

MANIFESTATIONS Although marked (≤50 beats per minute) sinus bradycardia may cause fatigue and other symptoms due to

inadequate cardiac output, more commonly sinus node dysfunction is manifest as paroxysmal dizziness, presyncope, or syncope. These symptoms usually result from abrupt, prolonged sinus pauses caused by failure of sinus impulse formation (sinus arrest) or block of conduction of sinus impulses to the surrounding atrial tissue (sinus exit block). In either case, the ECG manifestation is a prolonged period (>3 s) of atrial asystole. In some patients, sinus node dysfunction is accompanied by abnormalities in AV conduction. In addition to the absence of atrial activity, lower pacemakers fail to emerge during the sinus pauses, resulting in periods of ventricular asystole and syncope. Occasionally, sinus node dysfunction is manifested initially by the failure of the sinus rate to accelerate in response to conditions such as exercise or fever that normally cause increases in the sinus rate. In some patients, sinus node dysfunction may become manifest only in the presence of certain cardioactive drugs: cardiac glycosides, beta-adrenergic blocking drugs, verapamil, quinidine, and other antiarrhythmic agents. These agents, which do not cause sinus node dysfunction in normal people, may unmask evidence of sinus node dysfunction in susceptible individuals.

The *sick sinus syndrome* refers to a combination of symptoms (dizziness, confusion, fatigue, syncope, and congestive heart failure) caused by sinus node dysfunction and manifested by marked sinus bradycardia, sinoatrial block, or sinus arrest. Because these symptoms are nonspecific, and because ECG manifestations of sinus node dysfunction are not infrequently intermittent, it may be difficult to prove that such symptoms are actually caused by sinus node dysfunction.

Atrial tachyarrhythmias such as atrial fibrillation, atrial flutter, or atrial tachycardia may be accompanied by sinus node dyfunction. The *bradycardia-tachycardia syndrome* refers to paroxysmal atrial arrhythmia which upon termination is followed by prolonged sinus pauses (Fig. 197-4) or in which there are alternating periods of tachyarrhythmia and bradyarrhythmia. Syncope or presyncope may result from failure of the sinus node to recover function following suppression of automaticity by atrial tachyarrhythmia.

DIAGNOSIS *First-degree sinoatrial exit block* denotes a prolonged conduction time from the sinus node to the surrounding atrial tissue. It cannot be recognized on a standard (surface) ECG but requires invasive intracardiac recordings (see below). *Second-degree sinoatrial exit block* denotes the intermittent failure of conduction of sinus impulses to the surrounding atrial tissue; it is manifested as the intermittent absence of P waves (Fig. 197-5). *Third-degree*, or *complete, sinoatrial block* is characterized by a lack of atrial activity or by the presence of an ectopic subsidiary atrial pacemaker. On the standard ECG it cannot be distinguished from sinus arrest, but direct intracardiac recordings of sinus node activity permit this distinction. The *bradycardia-tachycardia syndrome* is manifested on the standard ECG as tachyarrhythmias (see Fig. 197-4). Most often these are atrial flutter or fibrillation, although any tachycardia with retrograde conduction to the atria may cause overdrive suppression of the sinus node resulting in clinical appearance of this syndrome.

The most important step in the diagnosis is to correlate symptoms with ECG evidence of sinus node dysfunction. While ambulatory ECG (Holter) monitoring remains a mainstay in evaluating sinus node function, most episodes of syncope are paroxysmal and unpredictable. Single and even multiple 24-h Holter monitor recordings may fail to include a symptomatic episode. Therefore, noting the response to carotid sinus pressure and pharmacologic autonomic "denervation"

FIGURE 197-4 Tachycardia-bradycardia syndrome. Rhythm strip of ECG lead II showing spontaneous cessation of supraventricular tachycardia followed by a 5.6-s pause prior to resumption of sinus activity. The patient was

asymptomatic during supraventricular tachycardia, but the sinus pause caused severe light-headedness.

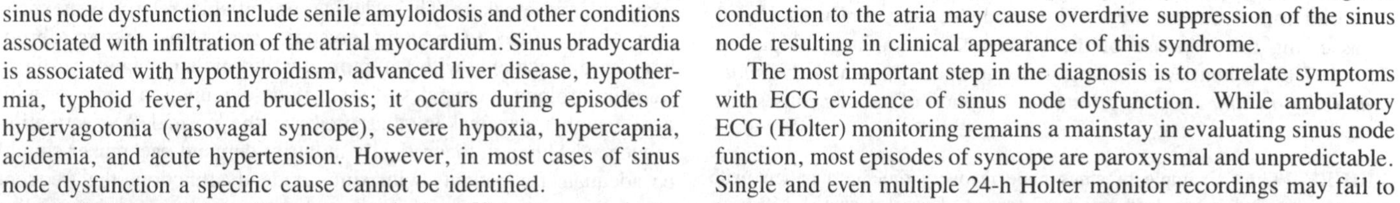

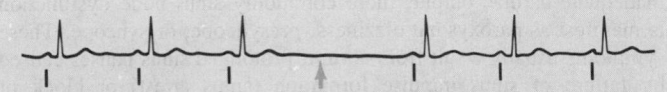

FIGURE 197-5 Second-degree sinoatrial exit block. Surface ECG denoting abrupt absence of P wave during sinus rhythm. Prior to the pause, the sinus rate is regular. The interval of the pause is exactly twice the basal sinus cycle length. The arrow marks the appropriate location for the absent P wave.

of the heart is frequently helpful. Carotid sinus pressure is particularly useful in patients in whom paroxysmal dizziness or syncope is compatible with the hypersensitive carotid sinus syndrome (see Chap. 17). In such patients, the response can be dramatic, and sinus pauses in excess of 5 s may occur. Normally, a sinus pause of ≤3 s results from 5 s of unilateral carotid sinus massage. However, in elderly patients, pauses >3 s are common and do not necessarily signify a diagnostic response. In all individuals it is important to correlate symptoms with such ECG phenomena. If atropine can prevent the effects of carotid sinus pressure, autonomic dysfunction, not primary (intrinsic) sinus node dysfunction, is responsible. The other noninvasive test of sinus node function involves the use of pharmacologic agents to manipulate the autonomic nervous system and assess the balance of parasympathetic and sympathetic activity on the sinus node. Physiologic or pharmacologic maneuvers which are vagomimetic (Valsalva maneuver or phenylephrine-induced hypertension), vagolytic (atropine), sympathomimetic (isoproterenol or hypotension by nitroprusside), or sympatholytic (beta-adrenergic blocking agents) can be utilized, singly and in combination. These studies are designed to test the response of the sinus node to autonomic stimulation and inhibition and thereby characterize the status of autonomic regulation of the sinus node. Abnormalities of the autonomic control of sinus function are particularly common in patients in whom the only presenting arrhythmia is sinus bradycardia.

Intrinsic heart rate   This is a manifestation of the primary activity of the sinus node, and its determination requires chemical autonomic blockade of the heart. Complete autonomic blockade is achieved with 0.2 mg/kg propranolol intravenously, followed after 10 min by 0.04 mg/kg atropine sulfate intravenously. Normal values of intrinsic heart rate (in beats per minute) are calculated by the formula $118.1 - (0.57 \times age)$. The use of autonomic blockade can separate patients with asymptomatic sinus bradycardia into a group with primary sinus node dysfunction (slow intrinsic heart rate) and a group with autonomic imbalance (normal intrinsic heart rate). Autonomic blockade is particularly useful when combined with invasive assessment of sinus node function (see below). Autonomic blockade may depress conduction in patients with intrinsic disease of the conduction system and should be carried out only in a setting where arrhythmias can be monitored and rapidly treated.

Sinus node recovery time   Sinus node recovery time is evaluated by assessing the response of the sinus node to rapid atrial pacing (Fig. 197-6). When atrial pacing is discontinued, a pause, the *sinus node recovery time*, occurs prior to resumption of spontaneous sinus

FIGURE 197-6 Example of sinus node recovery time in a patient with symptomatic sinus node dysfunction. Cessation of atrial pacing at 150 beats per minute (cycle length 400 ms) results in a prolonged sinus pause (2.8 s). Surface ECG leads V_1 and V_6 are shown in addition to intracardiac recordings at the high right atrium (A), which demonstrates atrial pacing rate.

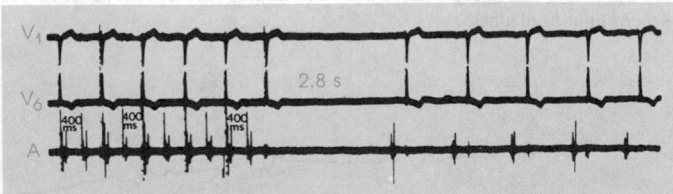

rhythm. When the sinus recovery time is prolonged, the results of this test mimic the prolonged sinus pauses seen following termination of atrial tachyarrhythmias in the bradycardia-tachycardia syndrome (see Fig. 197-4). The corrected sinus node recovery time (sinus recovery time − sinus cycle length) normally is less than 550 ms, and the uncorrected sinus node recovery time is less than 150 percent of the spontaneous cycle length. In patients with symptomatic sinus node dysfunction, prolongation of the sinus node recovery time is often observed. Patients with abnormally slow intrinsic heart rates usually have abnormal sinus node recovery times, while those with normal intrinsic heart rates have normal recovery times.

Sinoatrial conduction time   Determination of the conduction time from the sinus node to the atrium allows for the differentiation of abnormalities of sinoatrial conduction from abnormalities of sinus impulse formation. The conduction time equals one-half the difference between the pause following termination of brief periods of pacing and the sinus cycle length. Alternatively, the sinus node electrogram can be recorded directly by a catheter electrode placed near the sinoatrial node.

EVALUATION   The electrophysiologic investigation of sinus node dysfunction should be undertaken in patients who have had symptoms compatible with sinus node dysfunction and in whom no documentation of the arrhythmia responsible for these symptoms has been obtained by prolonged Holter monitoring. Asymptomatic patients with sinus bradycardia need *not* be tested, since no therapy is indicated. Similarly, symptomatic patients with ECG documentation of asystole, sinoatrial block or arrest, or the bradycardia-tachycardia syndrome do not require electrophysiologic tests for diagnosis. However, in symptomatic patients without documentation of an arrhythmia, electrophysiologic assessment of sinus node function can yield information that may be used to guide appropriate therapy. If a pacemaker is indicated, the side of pacemaker implantation for maximum hemodynamic effects can be guided by the results of electrophysiologic investigation. However, the results of tests of sinus node function must be interpreted with caution. Sinus node dysfunction coexists frequently with other disorders such as AV conduction disturbances which may cause symptoms such as syncope. Electrophysiologic evaluation of patients with symptoms such as undiagnosed syncope must not stop with the demonstration of abnormalities of sinus node dysfunction or carotid sinus hypersensitivity. Instead, complete evaluation, including His bundle recordings and programmed atrial and ventricular stimulation (see Chap. 198), is necessary to search for additional electrophysiologic abnormalities which could be responsible for symptoms.

TREATMENT   Permanent pacemakers (see p. 1017) are the mainstay of therapy for patients with symptomatic sinus node dysfunction. Patients with intermittent paroxysms of bradycardia or sinus arrest and with the cardioinhibitory form of the hypersensitive carotid sinus syndrome are usually adequately treated by demand ventricular pacemakers. These devices are reliable, relatively inexpensive, and suffice to prevent episodic symptoms due to abrupt bradycardia. Patients with symptomatic chronic sinus bradycardia or frequent prolonged episodes of sinus node dysfunction do better with dual-chamber pacemakers that preserve the normal AV activation sequence. Although theoretically an atrial demand pacemaker should be adequate for patients with sinus node dysfunction, the frequent accompaniment of dysfunction in other portions of the cardiac conduction system usually mandates placement of a pacemaker capable of ventricular pacing. Recent studies suggest that AV sequential pacing also may be useful in preventing atrial fibrillation, an important component of the bradycardia-tachycardia syndrome.

AV CONDUCTION DISTURBANCES

The specialized cardiac conducting system normally ensures synchronous conduction of each sinus impulse from the atria to the ventricles. Abnormalities of conduction of the sinus impulse to the ventricles may portend the development of heart block, which can ultimately lead to syncope or cardiac arrest. In order to evaluate the clinical significance of conduction abnormalities, the physician must assess (1) the site of conduction disturbance, (2) the risk of progression to complete block, and (3) the probability that a subsidiary escape rhythm arising distal to the site of block will be electrophysiologically and hemodynamically stable. This latter point is perhaps the most important, since the rate and stability of the escape pacemaker determine what symptoms result from heart block. The escape pacemaker following AV nodal block is usually in the His bundle, which generally has a stable rate of 40 to 60 beats per minute and is associated with a QRS complex of normal duration (in the absence of a preexisting intraventricular conduction defect). This contrasts with escape rhythms arising in the distal His-Purkinje system, which have lower intrinsic rates (25 to 45 beats per minute), manifest wide QRS complexes with prolonged duration, and are unstable. Although prolonged QRS complexes are invariable when the distal His-Purkinje pacemakers form the escape mechanism, wide QRS complexes also can coexist with AV nodal block and a His bundle rhythm. Therefore, QRS morphology alone may not be adequate to identify the site of block.

ETIOLOGY The AV node is supplied by the parasympathetic and sympathetic nervous systems and is sensitive to variations in autonomic tone. Chronic slowing of AV nodal conduction may be seen in highly trained athletes who have hypervagotonia at rest. A variety of diseases also can influence AV nodal conduction. These include acute processes such as myocardial infarction (particularly inferior), coronary spasm (usually of the right coronary artery), digitalis intoxication, excesses of beta and/or calcium blockers, acute infections such as viral myocarditis, acute rheumatic fever, infectious mononucleosis, and miscellaneous disorders such as Lyme disease, sarcoidosis, amyloidosis, and neoplasms, particularly cardiac mesotheliomas. AV nodal block also may be congenital.

Two degenerative diseases are commonly responsible for damage to the specialized conducting system and produce AV block usually associated with bundle branch block (see Chap. 189). In *Lev's disease*, there is calcification and sclerosis of the fibrous cardiac skeleton, which frequently involves the aortic and mitral valves, the central fibrous body, and the summit of the ventricular septum. *Lenegre's disease* appears to be a primary sclerodegenerative disease within the conducting system itself with no involvement of the myocardium or the fibrous skeleton of the heart. These two diseases are probably the most common causes of isolated chronic heart block in adults. Hypertension and aortic and/or mitral stenosis are specific disorders that either accelerate the degeneration of the conducting system or have a direct effect by calcification and fibrosis involving the conducting system.

First-degree AV block, more properly termed *prolonged AV conduction*, is characterized by a PR interval >0.20 s. Since the PR interval is determined by atrial, AV nodal, and His-Purkinje activation, delay in any one or more of these structures can contribute to a prolonged PR interval. In the presence of a QRS complex of normal duration, a PR interval >0.24 s almost invariably is due to a delay within the AV node. If the QRS is prolonged, delays may be present at any of the levels mentioned above. Delay within the His-Purkinje system is always accompanied by a prolonged QRS duration in addition to a prolonged PR interval. However, as indicated below, it is only with intracardiac recordings that the exact site of delay can be determined.

Second-degree heart block (intermittent AV block) is present when some atrial impulses fail to conduct to the ventricles. Mobitz type I second-degree AV block (AV Wenckebach block) is characterized by progressive PR interval prolongation prior to block of an atrial impulse (Fig. 197-7A). The pause that follows is less than fully compensatory (i.e., is less than two normal sinus intervals), and the PR interval of the first conducted impulse is shorter than the last conducted atrial impulse prior to the blocked P wave. This type of block is almost always localized to the AV node and associated with a normal QRS

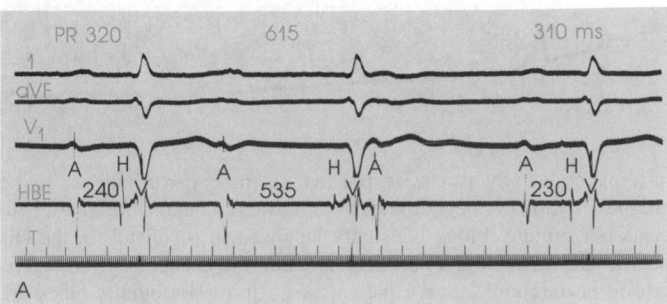

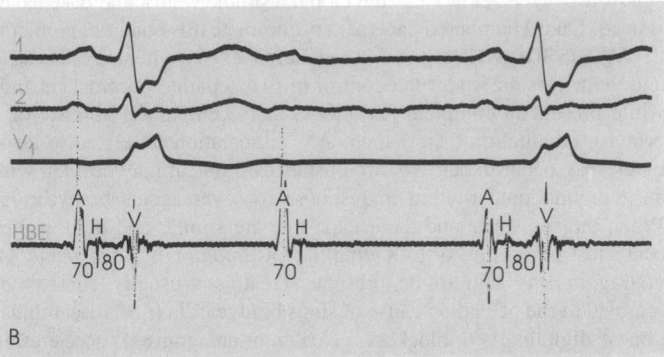

FIGURE 197-7 *A.* Mobitz type I second-degree AV block. Intracardiac recordings demonstrate that the PR prolongation (320, 615 ms) is localized to the AV node (AH 240, 535 ms, respectively). HBE = His bundle electrogram; A = atrium; H = His; V = ventricle. Time lines (T) = 100 ms (*From ME Josephson, SF Seides, Clinical Cardiac Electrophysiology: Techniques and Interpretations. Philadelphia, Lea & Febiger, 1979.*) *B.* Mobitz type II second-degree AV block. Intracardiac recordings document block below the His bundle.

duration. It is seen most often as a transient abnormality with inferior wall infarction or with drug intoxication, particularly digitalis, beta blockers, and occasionally calcium channel antagonists. This type of block also can be observed in normal individuals with heightened vagal tone. Although Mobitz type I block can progress to complete heart block, this is uncommon. Even when it does, however, the heart block is usually well tolerated because the escape pacemaker usually arises in the proximal His bundle and provides a stable rhythm. As a result, the presence of Mobitz type I second-degree AV block usually does not mandate aggressive therapy. Therapeutic decisions depend on the ventricular response and the symptoms of the patient. If the ventricular rate is adequate and the patient is asymptomatic, observation is sufficient.

In Mobitz type II second-degree AV block, conduction fails suddenly and unexpectedly without a preceding change in PR intervals (Fig. 197-7B). It is usually due to disease of the His-Purkinje system and is most often associated with a prolonged QRS duration. It is important to recognize this type of block because it has a high incidence of progression to complete heart block with an unstable, slow, lower escape pacemaker. Therefore, pacemaker implantation is necessary in this condition. Mobitz type II block may occur in the setting of anteroseptal infarction or in the primary or secondary sclerodegenerative or calcific disorders of the fibrous skeleton of the heart. In so-called high-degree AV block there are periods of two or more consecutively blocked P waves. Regardless of the site of origin of the escape rhythm, if it is slow and the patient is symptomatic, a cardiac pacemaker is mandatory.

Third-degree AV block is present when no atrial impulse propagates to the ventricles. If the QRS complex of the escape rhythm is of normal duration, occurs at a rate of 40 to 55 beats per minute, and increases with atropine or exercise, AV nodal block is probable. Congenital complete AV block is usually localized to the AV node (Fig. 197-8). If the block is within the His bundle, the escape

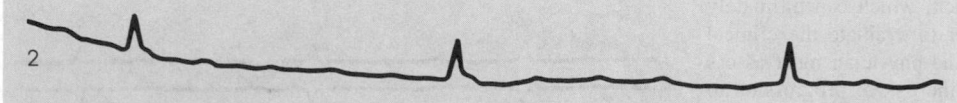

FIGURE 197-8 Third-degree AV block. Complete heart block with a slow, wide complex escape rhythm is present. Block in this instance is usually intra-His.

pacemaker usually is less responsive to these perturbations. If the escape rhythm of the QRS is wide and associated with rates ≤40 beats per minute, block is usually localized in, or distal to, the His bundle and mandates a pacemaker, since the escape rhythm in this setting is unreliable. Some patients with infra-His bundle block are capable of retrograde conduction. In such patients, a ''pacemaker syndrome'' (see below) may develop if a simple ventricular pacemaker is used. Dual-chambered pacemakers eliminate this potential problem.

AV DISSOCIATION AV dissociation exists whenever the atria and ventricles are under the control of two separate pacemakers and, while present in complete AV block, can occur in the absence of a primary conduction disturbance. AV dissociation unrelated to heart block may occur under two circumstances: First, it may develop with an AV junctional rhythm in response to severe sinus bradycardia. When the sinus rate and the escape rate are similar and the P waves occur just before, in, or following the QRS complex, *isorhythmic AV dissociation* is said to be present. Treatment usually consists of removal of the offending cause of sinus bradycardia (i.e., discontinuation of digitalis, beta blockers, or calcium antagonists), accelerating the sinus node by vagolytic agents, or insertion of a pacemaker if the escape rhythm is slow and results in symptoms. Second, AV dissociation can be caused by an enhanced lower (junctional or ventricular) pacemaker which competes with normal sinus rhythm and frequently exceeds it. This has been called *interference AV dissociation* because the rapid lower pacemaker results in bombardment of the AV node in a retrograde fashion, rendering it refractory to the normal sinus impulses. Thus failure of antegrade conduction is a physiologic response in this circumstance. Interference dissociation commonly occurs during ventricular tachycardia, accelerated junctional or ventricular rhythms seen with digitalis intoxication, myocardial ischemia and/or infarction, or local irritation following cardiac surgery. The accelerated rhythm should be treated with either antiarrhythmic drugs (see Chap. 198), removal of an offending drug, or correction of the metabolic abnormality or ischemia.

INTRACARDIAC ELECTROCARDIOGRAPHIC RECORDINGS IN DIAGNOSIS AND MANAGEMENT The main therapeutic decision in patients with AV conduction disturbance is whether or not a permanent pacemaker is required, and a number of circumstances exist in which His bundle electrocardiography can be a useful diagnostic tool upon which to base this decision. It is unquestionable that patients with *symptomatic* second- or third-degree AV block should be paced, and therefore, these patients do not require electrophysiologic study. However, intracardiac ECG recordings can be useful in at least the following three groups of patients:

1 Patients with syncope and bundle branch or bifascicular block without documentation of AV block. In such patients, the demonstration of marked infra-His bundle conduction disturbances, i.e., a prolonged HV interval (>100 ms), may usually be taken as an indication of the need for the insertion of the permanent pacemaker. With intervals ranging from 60 to 100 ms, the indications for pacing are equivocal. Block below the His bundle developing during atrial pacing at rates of less than 150 beats per minute and the development of an infra-His bundle block or HV prolongation >100 ms following 1 g procainamide intravenously also signify that the patient is at high risk for the development of subsequent AV block and that a pacemaker is indicated. Complete electrophysiologic evaluation, including atrial and ventricular programmed stimulation, is indicated to help identify other possible cardiac etiologies for the syncope. Since the incidence of significant advanced AV block is low in *asymptomatic* patients who have bifascicular block, electrophysiologic evaluation or permanent

pacemakers are not cost-effective. In this group, observation appears most reasonable.

2 Patients with 2:1 atrioventricular conduction. Intracardiac recordings are necessary to ascertain the site of the conduction disturbance because the typical ECG features of Mobitz type I or Mobitz type II block cannot be discerned during a 2:1 pattern of AV conduction on the surface ECG. Intracardiac recordings may demonstrate that AV nodal block, intra-His bundle block, infra-His bundle block, or combinations of block may be responsible. A surface electrocardiogram finding that suggests an infra-His bundle lesion is the presence of alternating bundle branch block associated with changing PR intervals. Intracardiac recordings in such patients confirm that the block is almost always in the His-Purkinje system. The finding of infra-His bundle block in patients with asymptomatic second-degree AV block mandates pacemaker therapy because of the high likelihood of their developing symptomatic high-grade AV block and syncope.

3 Asymptomatic patients with third-degree AV block. In such patients, electrophysiologic studies may be useful in assessing the stability of the junctional pacemaker. Pacing is indicated when the His bundle escape pacemaker is shown to be unstable by an inadequate response to exercise, atropine, or isoproterenol or by a prolonged junctional recovery time following ventricular pacing.

MANAGEMENT OF BRADYARRHYTHMIAS

PHARMACOLOGIC THERAPY Pharmacologic therapy is usually reserved for acute situations. Atropine (0.05 to 2.0 mg intravenously) and isoproterenol (1 to 4 μg/min intravenously) are useful in increasing heart rate and decreasing symptoms in patients with sinus bradycardia or AV block localized to the AV node. They have an insignificant effect on lower pacemakers. In patients with neurovascular syncope, beta blockers and disopyramide have been suggested as methods to depress left ventricular function and decrease mechanoreceptor-related reflexes. Mineralocorticords, ephedrine, and theophylline also have been reported to be of benefit to occasional patients. Unfortunately, no controlled study has shown that any of these pharmacologic modalities works in a predictable fashion in all patients. Further work on delineating different mechanisms in different patient groups may allow us to apply pharmacologic agents more appropriately. Recently, theophylline has been suggested in patients with vasovagal syncope. Long-term therapy of bradyarrhythmias is best accomplished by pacemakers.

PACEMAKERS External energy sources can be used to stimulate the heart when disorders in impulse formation and/or transmission lead to symptomatic bradyarrhythmias. Pacer stimuli can be applied to the atria and/or ventricles. Indications for pacemaker insertion are listed in Table 197-1.

Temporary pacing This is usually instituted to provide immediate stabilization prior to permanent pacemaker placement or to provide pacemaker support when a bradycardia is precipitated by what is presumed to be a transient event such as ischemia or drug toxicity. Temporary pacing is usually achieved by the transvenous insertion of an electrode catheter with the catheter positioned in the right ventricular apex and attached to an external generator. This procedure is associated with a small risk of cardiac perforation, infection at the insertion site, and thromboembolism; the risk of the latter two complications increases markedly if the pacing wire is left in place for more than 48 h. The development of an entirely external transthoracic cardiac pacing system may preclude the need for transvenous pacing in selected patients. However, occasional failure

TABLE 197-1   Indications for permanent pacing*

ACQUIRED AV BLOCK IN ADULTS

Class I

A Complete heart block, permanent or intermittent, at any anatomic level, associated with any anatomic level, associated with any one of the following complications:

 1 Symptomatic bradycardia. In the presence of complete heart block, symptoms must be presumed to be due to the heart block unless proved to be otherwise.

 2 Congestive heart failure.

 3 Ectopic rhythms and other medical conditions that require drugs that suppress the automaticity of escape pacemakers and result in symptomatic bradycardia.

 4 Documented periods of asystole ≥ 3.0 s or any escape rate < 40 beats per minute in symptom-free patients.

 5 Confusional states that clear with temporary pacing.

 6 Post-AV junction ablation, myotonic dystrophy.

B Second-degree AV block, permanent or intermittent, regardless of the type or the site of block, with symptomatic bradycardia.

C Atrial fibrillation, atrial flutter, or rare cases of supraventricular tachycardia with complete heart block or advanced AV block, bradycardia, and any of the conditions described under *IA*. The bradycardia must be related to digitalis or drugs known to impair AV conduction.

Class II

A Asymptomatic complete heart block, permanent or intermittent, at any anatomic site, with ventricular rates of 40 beats per minute or faster.

B Asymptomatic type II second-degree AV block, permanent or intermittent.

C Asymptomatic type I second-degree AV block at intra-His or intra-His levels.

Class III

A First-degree AV block.

B Asymptomatic type I second-degree AV block at the supra-His (AV node) level.

AFTER MYOCARDIAL INFARCTION

Class I

A Persistent advanced second-degree AV block or complete heart block after acute myocardial infarction with block in the His-Purkinje system (bilateral bundle branch block).

B Patients with transient advanced AV block and associated bundle branch block.

Class II

A Patients with persistent advanced block at the AV node.

Class III

A Transient AV conduction disturbances in the absence of intraventricular conduction defects.

B Transient AV block in the presence of isolated left anterior hemiblock.

C Acquired left anterior hemiblock in the absence of AV block.

D Patients with persistent first degree AV block in the presence of bundle branch block not demonstrated previously.

BIFASCICULAR AND TRIFASCICULAR BLOCK

Class I

A Bifascicular block with intermittent complete heart block associated with symptomatic bradycardia.

B Bifascicular or trifascicular block with intermittent type II second-degree AV block without symptoms attributable to the heart block.

Class II

A Bifascicular or trifascicular block with syncope that is not proved to be due to complete heart block, but other possible causes for syncope are not identifiable.

B Markedly prolonged HV (>100 ms).

C Pacing-induced infra-His block.

Class III

A Fascicular block without AV block or symptoms.

B Fascicular block with first-degree AV block without symptoms.

SINUS NODE DYSFUNCTION

Class I

A Sinus node dysfunction with documented symptomatic bradycardia. In some patients this will occur as a consequence of long-term (essential) drug therapy of a type and dose for which there are no acceptable alternatives.

Class II

A Sinus node dysfunction, occurring spontaneously or as a result of necessary drug therapy, with heart rates < 40 beats per minute when a clear association between significant symptoms consistent with bradycardia and the actual presence of bradycardia has not been documented.

SINUS NODE DYSFUNCTION (*continued*)

Class III

A Sinus node dysfunction in asymptomatic patients, including those in whom substantial sinus bradycardia (heart rate < 40 beats per minute) is a consequence of long-term drug treatment.

B Sinus node dysfunction in patients in whom symptoms suggestive of bradycardia are clearly documented not to be associated with a slow heart rate.

HYPERSENSITIVE CAROTID SINUS AND NEUROVASCULAR SYNDROMES

Class I

A Recurrent syncope associated with clear, spontaneous events provoked by carotid sinus stimulation; minimal carotid sinus pressure induces asystole of >3 s duration in the absence of any medication that depresses the sinus node or AV conduction.

Class II

A Recurrent syncope without clear, provocative events and with a hypersensitive cardioinhibitory response.

B Syncope with associated bradycardia reproduced by a head-up tilt with or without isoproterenol or other forms of provocative maneuvers and in which a temporary pacemaker and a second provocative test can establish the likely benefits of a permanent pacemaker.

Class III

A A hyperactive cardioinhibitory response to carotid sinus stimulation in the absence of symptoms.

B Vague symptoms, such as dizziness, light-headedness, or both, with a hyperactive cardioinhibitory response to carotid sinus stimulation.

C Recurrent syncope, light-headedness, or dizziness in the absence of a cardioinhibitory response.

SOURCE: Dreifus LS et al.

* Class I: agreement that permanent pacemaker should be implanted. Class II: divergence of opinion regarding need for implantation. Class III: agreement that pacemaker is unnecessary.

of ventricular capture and significant discomfort related to the large current required for effective transthoracic ventricular stimulation preclude the uniform use of this approach.

Permanent pacing   This mode of pacing is instituted for persistent or intermittent symptomatic bradycardia not related to a self-limiting precipitating factor or for documented infranodal second- or third-degree AV block. Permanent pacing leads are usually inserted transvenously through the subclavian or cephalic vein with the leads positioned in the right atrial appendage for atrial pacing and the right ventricular apex for ventricular pacing. The leads are then attached to the pulse generator, which is inserted into a subcutaneous pocket below the clavicle. Epicardial lead placement is used when (1) transvenous access cannot be obtained, (2) the chest is already open, i.e., in the course of a cardiac operation, and (3) adequate endocardial lead placement cannot be achieved. Most pacemaker generators are powered by lithium batteries. The life expectancy of the generator is related to (1) current output required for capture, (2) requirement for incessant or intermittent pacing, and (3) number of cardiac chambers paced. Life expectancy of the simple ventricular demand pacemaker can exceed 10 years.

Pacing code   A code consisting of three to five letters has been developed for describing pacemaker type and function (Table 197-2). The first letter indicates the chamber(s) paced and is designated *V* for ventricular pacing, *A* for atrial pacing, or *D* for dual-chamber (both atrial and ventricular) pacing. The second letter indicates the chamber in which electrical activity is sensed and is also indicated by *A, V,* or *D*. An additional designation, *O*, has been used when pacemaker discharge is not dependent on a sensed electrical activity. The third letter refers to the response to a sensed electric signal. The letter *O* represents no response to an underlying electric signal, usually related to the absence of associated sensing function; *I* represents inhibition of pacing function; *T* represents triggering of pacing function; and *D* indicates a dual response, i.e., spontaneous atrial and ventricular activity inhibiting atrial and ventricular pacing and

TABLE 197-2   The NASPE/BPEG generic pacemaker code

Position category	I Chamber(s) paced	II Chamber(s) sensed	III Response to sensing	IV Programmability, rate modulation	V Antitachyarrhythmia function(s)

	O = None
	A = Atrium
		O = None
		A = Atrium
			O = None
			T = Triggered
				O = None
				P = Simple
				  programmable
					O = None
					P = pacing
					  (antitachyarrhythmia)

	V = Ventricle D = Dual (A + V)	V = Ventricle D = Dual (A + V)	I = Inhibited D = Dual (T + I)	M = Multiprogrammable C = Communicating R = Rate modulation	S = Shock D = Dual (P + S)
Manufacturer's designation	S = single (A or V)	S = (A or V)			

SOURCE: Zipes DP

atrial activity triggering a ventricular response. Additional fourth and fifth letters of the pacing code have been recommended to indicate whether the pacemaker is programmable and has rate modulation (fourth) and whether special antitachycardia functions are available (i.e., antitachycardia pacing, *T*, and delivery of high- or low-energy shocks). In the fourth category, *M* represents multiprogrammability and *R* represents rate response ("physiologic") pacing. It follows from the described code that the standard VVIR (ventricular demand pacemaker) paces the ventricle, senses the ventricle, is inhibited by sensed spontaneous ventricular activity, and has rate modulation, while the DDDR pulse generator is capable of sensing and pacing both the atria and ventricles and has a dual response to the sensed atrial and ventricular activity as described above (Fig. 197-9). Both pacemakers have rate modulation (*R*). "Physiologic" pacemakers use sensors (e.g., muscular activity, respiratory rate, temperature, O_2 saturation, QT interval, etc.) as methods to allow the pacemaker to increase the heart rate in response to physiologic demands, i.e., exercise. These pacemakers are essential when chronotropic incompetence is present and an increase in heart rate is required to enhance physiologic performance. Studies have shown that such "physiologic" pacemakers improve exercise tolerance and relieve symptoms to a greater degree than fixed-rate pacemakers.

FIGURE 197-9   Normally functioning DDD pacemaker. All three panels show a lead II rhythm strip at 50 mm/s. The programmed lower rate is approximately 55 beats per minute. (*Top*) AV sequential pacing with a paced AV interval of 160 ms is shown for the first two complexes. A VPC occurs and is sensed, resetting the cycle. (*Middle*) The first beat is AV paced, but spontaneous sinus P waves and APC trigger a ventricular paced complex with a sensed P to QRS of 120 ms. (*Bottom*) After the first AV paced complex, a paced atrial complex conducts to the ventricle with a PR of 120 ms, inhibiting the ventricular pacemaker.

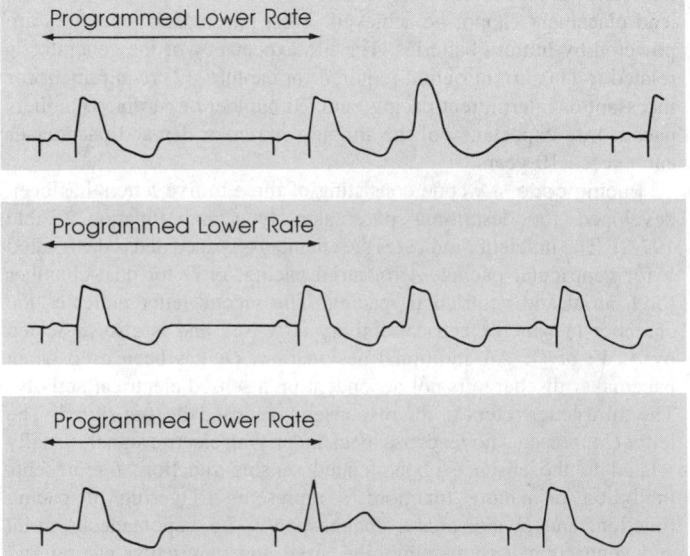

Selection of the appropriate pacemaker and pacing mode depends on the clinical condition and the type of bradyarrhythmia being treated. The two most common pacing mode selections are DDD and VVI. DDD provides AV sequential pacing, which is ideally suited for the relatively young and active patient who has intact sinus node function or intermittent dysfunction and high-grade persistent or intermittent AV block. The DDD mode will allow for physiologic atrial sensed and ventricular paced rates and improve exercise tolerance. AV synchrony and dual-chamber pacing also may be desirable in patients with borderline hemodynamic reserve who are dependent on atrial contribution to cardiac output and in those patients who develop the pacemaker syndrome (see below) in response to ventricular demand pacing. Rate-responsive DDD (i.e., DDDR) pacing is indicated when chronotropic incompetence is present in a patient who requires AV synchrony. The DDD pacing mode is contraindicated in chronic atrial fibrillation or flutter, because rapid and irregular ventricular pacing will occur to the upper rate limit. In some cases this will produce a more rapid ventricular rate than the patient's own rate in the absence of a pacemaker. DDD pacemakers must either automatically switch or be reprogrammed to the VVI mode. Almost all such pacemakers are now combined with some form of rate responsiveness so that when the device functions in the VVI mode, it also will respond to physiologic demands (VVIR). Chronotropic insufficiency is a contraindication, since a DDD pacemaker will act as a "fixed-rate" pacemaker at the upper rate cutoff. In these situations, a rate-adaptive or "physiologic" pacemaker is indicated (VVIR or DDDR). In patients with impaired sinus node function or chronic atrial fibrillation, a sensor-driven, rate-adaptive pacemaker must be implanted. As mentioned earlier, these pacemakers automatically adjust ventricular pacing rates to a sensed indicator of exertion. The DDD pacing mode also may be contraindicated in patients with intermittent or persistent ventriculoatrial (VA) conduction, who may develop pacemaker-mediated tachycardia (see below).

Programmability of pacemakers   This allows for modification of pacing function after implantation and for adaptation to changes in clinical needs. Pacemaker programming is accomplished by activation of the programming head positioned over the implanted pulse generator after making the desired changes in programmable parameters (see Table 197-2). A radio frequency system is routinely used to communicate the program to the pacemaker. A high degree of sophistication is required to recognize the presence and causes of pacemaker malfunction and their treatment.

Complications   Adverse effects of permanent pacing are usually associated with failure or malfunction of the pacing system. These problems are usually secondary to over- or undersensing, output failure, and/or lead fracture or displacement. Two other problems may occur. The *pacemaker syndrome* consists of fatigue, dizziness, syncope, and distressing pulsations in the neck and chest and can be associated with adverse hemodynamic effects. The pathophysiologic contributors to the pacemaker syndrome include (1) loss of atrial contribution to ventricular systole, (2) vasodepressor reflex initiated by cannon *a* waves which are caused by atrial contractions against a closed tricuspid valve and observed in the jugular venous pulse (Chap.

188), and (3) systemic and pulmonary venous regurgitation due to atrial contraction against a closed AV valve. The symptoms associated with the pacemaker syndrome can be prevented by maintaining AV synchrony by dual-chamber pacing or, in the case of a ventricular demand pacemaker, by programming a hysteresis escape rate 15 to 20 beats per minute below that of the paced rate. As a result of this programming, sinus activity and thus atrial contraction will be less likely to occur at the same time as ventricular pacing and ventricular contraction. The second major problem peculiar to dual-chamber pacemakers is the development of *pacemaker-mediated tachycardia.* In this instance, retrograde depolarization of the atria, resulting from a premature ventricular depolarization or a paced ventricular complex, is sensed and leads to subsequent triggering of ventricular pacing. This, in turn, can result in repetition of the phenomenon of ventriculoatrial conduction with the development of an endless-loop, pacemaker-mediated tachycardia. It may be corrected by reprogramming the atrial refractory period.

REFERENCES

BAROLD SS et al: Electrocardiography of contemporary DDD pacemakers. Basic concepts: Upper rate response, retrograde ventriculoatrial conduction and differential diagnosis of pacemaker tachycardias, in *Electrical Therapy for Cardiac Arrhythmias: Pacing, Antitachycardia Devices, Catheter Ablation*, S Saksena, N Goldschlager (eds). Philadelphia, Saunders, 1990, p 225

BERNSTEIN AD et al: The NASPE/BPEG generic pacemaker code for antibradyarrhythmias and adaptive-rate pacing and antitachyarrhythmia devices. PACE 10:794, 1987

DREIFUS LS et al: Guidelines for implantation of cardiac pacemakers and antiarrhythmic devices: A report of the American College of Cardiology/American Heart Association Task Force on Assessment of Diagnostic and Therapeutic Cardiovascular Procedures (Committee on Pacemaker Implantation). J Am Coll Cardiol 18:1, 1991

ELLENBOGEN KA et al: New insights into pacemaker syndrome gained from hemodynamic, humoral and vascular responses during ventriculo-atrial pacing. Am J Cardiol 65(1):53, 1990

HUANG SK et al: Carotid sinus hypersensitivity in patients with unexplained syncope: Clinical, electrophysiologic and long-term follow-up observations. Am Heart J 116:989, 1988

JOSEPHSON ME: *Clinical Electrophysiology*, 2d ed. Philadelphia, Lea and Febiger, 1992, chaps 4, 5, 6, 13

MENDES LA, DAVIDOFF R: Cardiogenic seizure with bradyarrhythmia: Documentation of the mechanism during asystole. Am Heart J 125:1786, 1993

SRA JS et al: Comparison of cardiac pacing with drug therapy in the treatment of neurocardiogenic (vasovagal) syncope with bradycardia or asytole,. N Engl J Med 328:1085, 1993

WALLER BF et al: Anatomy, histology and pathology of the cardiac conduction system: Part II. Clin Cardiol 16:347, 1993

ZIPES DP: Cardiac pacemakers and antiarrhythmia devices, in *Heart Disease: A Textbook of Cardiovascular Medicine*, 4th ed, E Braunwald (ed). Philadelphia, Saunders, 1992, p 726

198 THE TACHYARRHYTHMIAS

MARK E. JOSEPHSON / ALFRED E. BUXTON / FRANCIS E. MARCHLINSKI

MECHANISMS OF TACHYARRHYTHMIAS

Tachyarrhythmias may be divided into disorders of impulse propagation and disorders of impulse formation. Disorders of impulse propagation (reentry) are generally considered to be the most common mechanism of sustained paroxysmal tachyarrhythmia. The requirements for initiating reentry include (1) electrophysiologic inhomogeneity (i.e., differences in conduction and/or refractoriness) in two or more regions of the heart connected with each other to form a potentially closed loop, (2) unidirectional block in one pathway, (3) slow conduction over an alternative pathway, allowing time for the initially blocked pathway to recover excitability, and (4) reexcitation of the initially blocked pathway to complete a loop of activation (Fig. 198-1). Repetitive circulation of the impulse over this loop can

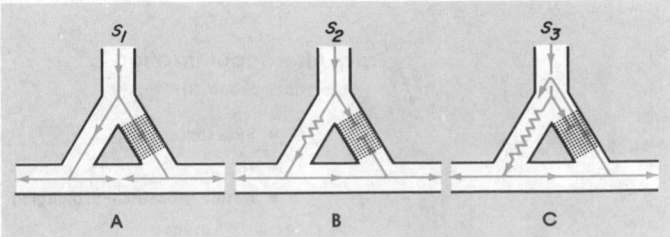

FIGURE 198-1   Schema of reentry. Y branching of the Purkinje system to ventricular muscle is shown in panels *A* through *C*. The right limb (*hatched area*) of the Purkinje system has a longer refractory period than the left. *A.* During a slow stimulated rate (S_1), conduction proceeds normally over both Purkinje fibers, resulting in collision in the ventricular muscle. *B.* An early premature stimulus (S_2) results in block in the Purkinje fiber on the right and slow conduction down the left. The impulse conducts through the ventricle and attempts to reenter the initial site of block but fails because this site has not fully recovered excitability. *C.* An earlier stimulus (S_3) again results in block on the left. The resulting slower propagation down the left fiber provides enough time for the initial site of block to recur and allows the impulse to conduct through it to produce a reentrant circuit.

produce a sustained tachyarrhythmia. While anatomic obstacles may underlie reentry and provide an inexcitable center around which the impulse can circulate, they are not essential. Reentrant arrhythmias can be reproducibly initiated and terminated by premature complexes and rapid stimulation. The response of these arrhythmias to stimulation can help distinguish them from arrhythmias caused by triggered activity.

Disorders of impulse formation can be subdivided into tachyarrhythmias caused by enhanced automaticity and those caused by triggered activity. In addition to the sinus node, automatic pacemaker activity can be observed in specialized atrial fibers, fibers of the atrioventricular (AV) junction, and Purkinje fibers (see Chap. 197). Myocardial cells do not normally possess pacemaker activity. Enhancement of normal automaticity in latent pacemaker fibers or the development of abnormal automaticity due to partial depolarization of the resting membrane occurs as a consequence of a variety of pathophysiologic states, which include (1) increased endogenous or exogenous catecholamines, (2) electrolyte disturbances (e.g., hyperkalemia), (3) hypoxia or ischemia, (4) mechanical effects (e.g., stretch), and (5) drugs (e.g., digitalis). Tachycardia caused by automaticity cannot be started or stopped by pacing.

Triggered activities are events that do not occur spontaneously but require a change in cardiac frequency as a trigger. Triggered activity may be caused by early afterdepolarizations, which occur during phases 2 and 3 of the action potential, or delayed afterdepolarizations, which occur following completion of phase 3 of the action potential (Fig. 198-2). Triggered activity has been observed in atrial, ventricular, and His-Purkinje tissue under conditions such as increased local catecholamine concentration, hyperkalemia, hypercalcemia, and digitalis intoxication (delayed afterdepolarizations) or during bradycardia, hypokalemia, or other situations prolonging action potential duration (early afterdepolarizations). All these conditions produce an accumulation of intracellular calcium, which causes depolarizations during phase 2 or 3 of the action potential or following the action potential, termed *afterdepolarizations* (see Fig. 198-2). With increasing amplitude of the afterdepolarizations, threshold can be reached and repetitive activity produced. The exact role of triggered activity in spontaneous clinical arrhythmias is unknown, but tachyarrhythmias associated with digitalis intoxication, accelerated idioventricular rhythm in acute infarction, and exercise-induced ventricular tachycardia (VT) may be caused by triggered activity due to delayed afterdepolarizations. Torsades de pointes (polymorphic VT associated with long QT intervals) may be caused by triggered activity due to early afterdepolarizations.

The use of electrophysiologic studies, i.e., intracardiac recordings and programmed stimulation, has greatly expanded the understanding

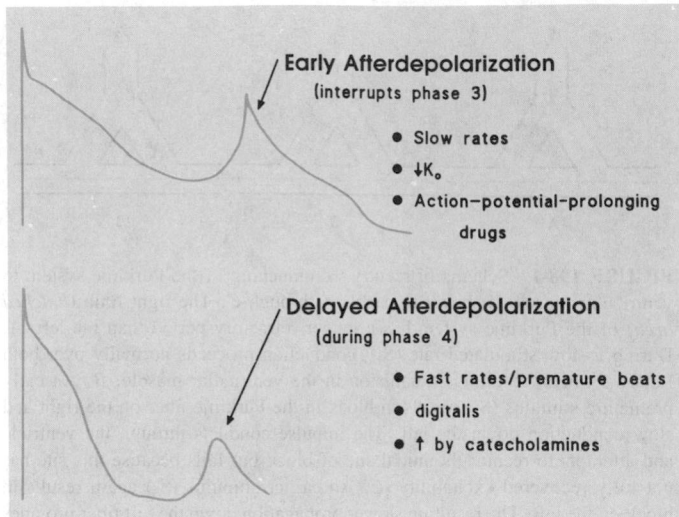

FIGURE 198-2 Early and late afterdepolarizations.

of the mechanisms of tachyarrhythmias. In addition to helping diagnose arrhythmias, these techniques may be of value in determining the most appropriate types of therapy because they allow the physician to observe the hemodynamic and symptomatic consequences of the arrhythmia in the presence or absence of therapy. EP studies of tachycardias require the positioning of multiple electrode catheters at critical areas within the heart. These electrodes must be capable of both stimulating and recording from multiple sites in the atria and/or ventricles.

PREMATURE COMPLEXES

ATRIAL PREMATURE COMPLEXES (APCs) APCs can be found on 24-h Holter monitoring in over 60 percent of normal adults. APCs are usually asymptomatic and benign, although at times they may be associated with palpitations. In susceptible patients, they can initiate paroxysmal supraventricular tachycardias. APCs may originate from

any location in either atrium, and they are recognized on the ECG as early P waves with a morphology which differs from the sinus P wave (Fig. 198-3A). While APCs usually conduct to the ventricles when they occur late in the cardiac cycle, early APCs may reach the AV conduction system while it is still in its relative refractory period, resulting in a conduction delay manifested by prolonged PR interval following the premature P wave (Fig. 198-3A). Very early APCs may even block in the AV node if this structure is encountered during its effective refractory period. APCs, whether conducted or not, are usually followed by a pause before a return to sinus activity. Most commonly, an APC enters and resets the sinus node, so the sum of the pre- and postextrasystolic PP intervals is less than the sum of two sinus PP intervals (Fig. 198-3A). In this case, the pause is said to be less than fully compensatory. The QRS complex following most APCs is normal, although early APCs may be followed by aberrantly conducted QRS complexes due to the premature complex falling within the relative refractory period of the His-Purkinje system.

Since most APCs are asymptomatic, treatment is not required. When they cause palpitations or trigger paroxysmal supraventricular tachycardias (see below), treatment may be useful. Factors that precipitate APCs, such as alcohol, tobacco, or adrenergic stimulants, should be identified and eliminated, and in their absence, mild sedation or the use of a beta blocker may be tried. If this fails, quinidine or other type I agents may be used.

AV JUNCTIONAL COMPLEXES The site of origin of these complexes is thought to be in the bundle of His, since the normal AV node in vivo possesses no automaticity (p. 1012). AV junctional complexes are less common than either atrial or ventricular premature complexes and are more often associated with cardiac disease or digitalis intoxication. Junctional premature impulses can conduct both antegradely to the ventricles and retrogradely to the atrium and, on rare occasions, may fail to conduct in either direction. Premature AV junctional complexes can be recognized by normal-appearing QRS complexes that are not preceded by a P wave. Retrograde P waves (inverted in leads II, III, and aVF) may be observed after the QRS complex.

While often asymptomatic, junctional premature complexes may be associated with palpitations and cause cannon *a* waves which may result in distressing pulsations in the neck. When symptomatic, they should be treated like APCs.

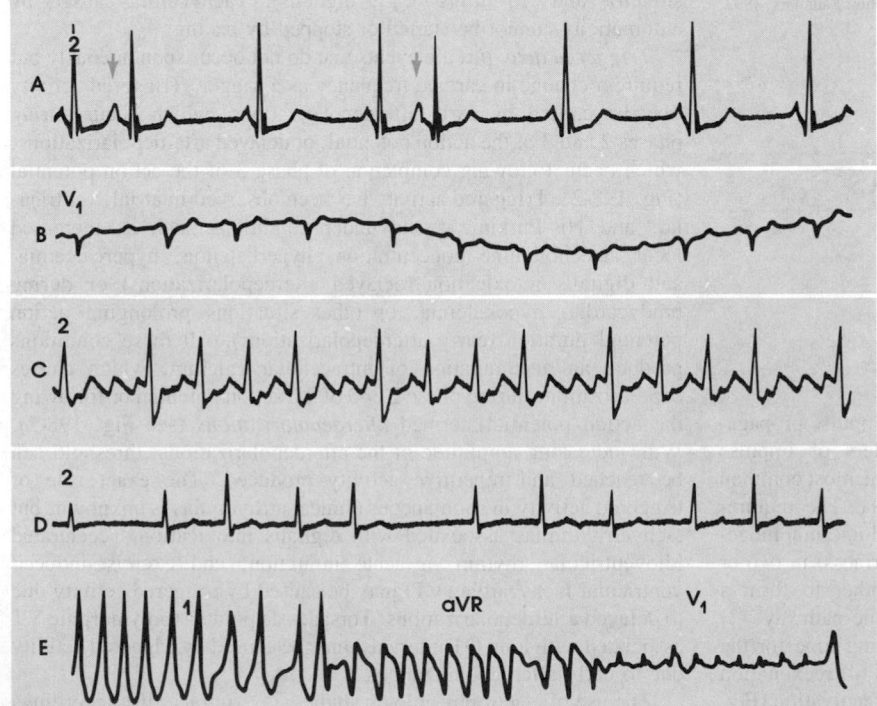

FIGURE 198-3 *A*. ECG lead II. Sinus rhythm with two atrial premature complexes (*arrows*). Note the difference in P-wave configuration between sinus and the premature atrial complexes. In addition, note that the PR interval of the premature complexes is prolonged, due to slowed conduction of the premature impulse through the AV conduction system. *B*. ECG lead V_1. Atrial tachycardia with varying degrees of AV block, typical of digitalis toxicity. *C*. ECG lead II. Atrial flutter. Note the characteristic sawtooth baseline seen in the inferior ECG leads during atrial flutter. Variable degrees of AV conduction block are present. *D*. ECG lead II. Atrial fibrillation. Note the irregular wavy baseline without discrete atrial activity. The ventricular response is irregularly irregular. *E*. ECG leads I, aVR, and V_1. Atrial fibrillation in a patient with Wolff-Parkinson-White syndrome. Note the extremely rapid, grossly irregular ventricular rate with wide, bizarre QRS complexes.

VENTRICULAR PREMATURE COMPLEXES (VPCs) These are among the most common arrhythmias and occur in patients with and without heart disease. Of adult males ≥60 percent will exhibit VPCs during a 24-h Holter monitoring. In patients without heart disease, VPCs have not been shown to be associated with any increased incidence in mortality or morbidity. VPCs may occur in up to 80 percent of patients with previous myocardial infarction, and in this setting, if frequent (>10 per hour) and/or complex (occurring in couplets), they have been associated with increased mortality. However, cardiac mortality in such patients usually occurs in association with significantly impaired ventricular function. While frequent and complex ventricular ectopy is an independent risk factor, it is not as strong a risk factor as is impaired ventricular function. Moreover, even though ventricular tachycardia and/or fibrillation may be the basis for the sudden death in these patients, this does not a priori establish a cause-and-effect relation between spontaneous ectopy and life-threatening ventricular tachycardia or fibrillation. Very early cycle (R or T) VPCs have been stated by some to increase the risk of sudden death. Although this has been observed during acute ischemia and in the setting of QT prolongation, frequently, ventricular tachycardia or fibrillation is precipitated by VPCs which occur after the T wave of the prior beat.

VPCs are recognized by wide (usually >0.14 s), bizarre QRS complexes that are not preceded by P waves (Fig. 198-4A). Often they bear a relatively fixed relationship to the preceding sinus complex and are thus considered fixed coupled VPCs. When fixed coupling is not present and the interval between VPCs has a common denominator, *ventricular parasystole* is said to be present (Fig. 198-5). Under these circumstances, the VPCs are a manifestation of abnormal automaticity of a protected ventricular focus; because it is not penetrated by sinus impulses, it is not reset by them, and the interectopic intervals remain relatively fixed (≤120 ms variation of mean RR cycle length).

VPCs may occur singly; in patterns of bigeminy, in which every sinus beat is followed by a VPC; in trigeminy, in which two sinus beats are followed by a VPC; in quadrigeminy, etc. Two successive VPCs are termed *pairs* or *couplets*, while three or more consecutive VPCs are termed *ventricular tachycardia* when the rate exceeds 100 beats per minute. VPCs may have similar morphologies (monomorphic, or uniform) or different morphologies (polymorphic, or multiformed) (Fig. 198-4C).

Most commonly, VPCs are not conducted retrogradely to the atrium to reset the sinoatrial node. Thus they produce a fully compensatory pause; i.e., the interval between conducted sinus beats which bracket the VPC equals two basic RR intervals. Ventricular impulses also may manifest retrograde conduction to the atrium and cause inverted P waves in leads II, III, and aVF. The pause that results may therefore be less than compensatory. In many instances, the QRS complex will not be associated with retrograde ventriculoatrial (VA) conduction but may block in the AV node. This renders the AV node refractory to the subsequent sinus beat and causes slowed conduction (i.e., prolonged PR interval) or block of the next sinus P wave. This prolonged PR interval is said to be a manifestation of concealed retrograde conduction of the ventricular impulse into the AV node. A VPC that does not produce any manifestation of retrograde concealed conduction and fails to influence the oncoming sinus impulse is termed an *interpolated VPC*.

VPCs can cause palpitations or neck pulsations secondary to either the occurrence of cannon *a* waves or the increased force of contraction due to postextrasystolic potentiation of ventricular contractility. Patients with frequent VPCs or bigeminy may rarely develop syncope because the VPCs do not result in an adequate stroke volume and the cardiac output is reduced by the "halving" of the heart rate.

Management In the absence of cardiac disease, isolated asymptomatic VPCs, regardless of configuration and frequency, need no treatment. When arrhythmias are symptomatic, the symptoms should first be addressed by either allaying the patient's anxiety or, if this is not successful, reducing the frequency of the VPCs with antiarrhythmic agents. Beta-adrenergic blockers may be successful in managing

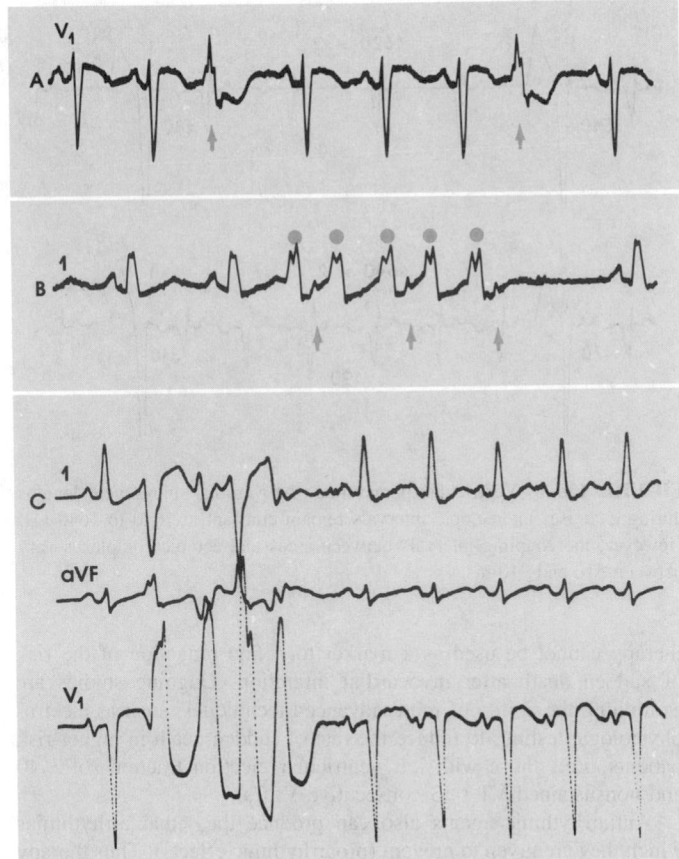

FIGURE 198-4 *A.* Single ventricular ectopy. During sinus rhythm, two premature ventricular complexes (*arrows*) occur. Note that the QRS configuration is bizarre, different from that during sinus rhythm. The premature ventricular complexes are not preceded by P waves. The QRS width of the premature complexes is approximately 160 ms. The pause surrounding the premature complexes is fully compensatory, the sinus beat after the premature complex occurring on time. *B.* A 5-beat run of nonsustained ventricular tachycardia having a uniform morphology (*dots*). Although intraventricular conduction during sinus rhythm is slightly prolonged, during the run of ventricular tachycardia the QRS duration is further prolonged. Note that 2:1 VA conduction is present during ventricular tachycardia. Retrograde P waves are denoted by the arrows. *C.* Simultaneous recordings of ECG leads I, aVF, and V₁. A 4-beat run of polymorphic nonsustained ventricular tachycardia is demonstrated. No two consecutive QRS complexes are the same. Polymorphic VT is not associated with a prolonged QT interval in this case.

VPCs that occur primarily in the daytime or under stressful situations and in specific settings such as mitral valve prolapse and thyrotoxicosis. Quinidine or quinidine-like agents may be tried should this be unsuccessful. In patients with cardiac disease, frequent VPCs are often associated with an increased risk of sudden and nonsudden cardiac death, and many physicians have attempted to eliminate or reduce the frequency of these VPCs in an attempt to reduce this risk. However, the cause-and-effect relationship of the VPCs to fatal events has never been established. The ability of pharmacologic antiarrhythmic therapy guided by continuous ECG monitoring to reduce the risk of sudden death in patients with frequent (≥6 per minute) VPCs was tested by the Cardiac Arrhythmia Suppression Trial (CAST). This study compared mortality in patients whose ectopy was suppressed by one of three agents (encainide, flecainide, or moricizine) and then randomized to treat with either the "effective" drug or placebo. After a mean follow-up of 2 years, the study was discontinued because both the sudden death and overall mortality rate was significantly increased in patients receiving antiarrhythmic agents. This study has shown that in patients having the characteristics of the study population, abolition of ventricular ectopy by pharmacologic

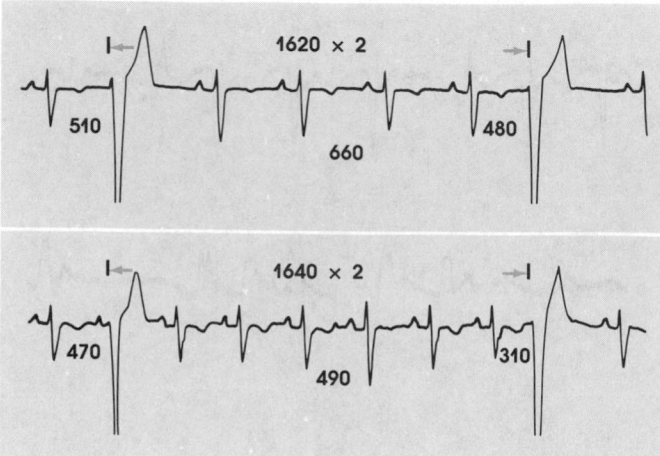

FIGURE 198-5 Ventricular parasystole. At varying sinus cycle lengths during exercise, interectopic intervals remain constant at 1620 to 1640 ms. However, the coupling intervals between sinus and ectopic complexes vary between 510 and 310 ms.

therapy cannot be used as a marker to define reduction of the risk of sudden death after myocardial infarction. Ongoing studies are examining the ability of more advanced techniques, such as electrophysiologic testing, to reduce the rate of sudden death in higher-risk patients, i.e., those with left ventricular ejection fractions of ≤40 and nonsustained VT (≥3 consecutive VPCs).

Antiarrhythmic agents also can produce the lethal arrhythmias which they are given to prevent (proarrhythmic effects). Thus therapy directed toward VPCs in the setting of chronic cardiac disease may result in an inappropriate and costly use of agents without proven efficacy and with potential side effects in many patients. The high incidence of side effects and the frequent exacerbation of arrhythmias caused by all antiarrhythmic drugs make it mandatory to monitor patients being treated with such agents.

In acute myocardial infarction, the greatest incidence of primary ventricular fibrillation occurs within the first 24 h (Chap. 202). Temporary prophylactic antiarrhythmic therapy with lidocaine has therefore been recommended for all patients with acute infarction, regardless of the presence or degree of spontaneous ectopy. However, recently, recognition of the toxicity of lidocaine has led to a reevaluation of this practice. Most physicians now recommend prophylactic lidocaine administration only to young patients with complicated infarctions, where a favorable risk-benefit ratio may be obtained. Other studies have shown that intravenous beta blockers also may reduce the incidence of primary ventricular fibrillation.

TACHYCARDIAS

Tachycardias refer to arrhythmias with three or more complexes at rates exceeding 100 beats per minute; they occur more often in structurally diseased than in normal hearts. Those paroxysmal tachycardias that are initiated by APCs or VPCs are considered to be due to reentry, except some of the digitalis-induced tachyarrhythmias, which are probably due to triggered activity (see below).

If the patient is hemodynamically stable, an attempt should be made to determine the mechanism and origin of the tachycardia, since this will usually lead to an appropriate therapeutic decision. Information to be obtained from the ECG includes (1) the presence, frequency, morphology, and regularity of P waves and QRS complexes, (2) the relationship between atrial and ventricular activity, (3) a comparison of the QRS morphology during sinus rhythm and during the tachycardia, and (4) the response to carotid sinus massage or other vagal maneuvers. It is useful first to compare the ECG during the tachycardia with one recorded during sinus rhythm, and it is often

desirable to record long rhythm strips using surface leads with the largest P waves, usually leads II or V_1. One also can utilize the electrodes situated at the end of a flexible pacing catheter inserted into the esophagus behind the left atrium to record atrial activity.

Carotid sinus pressure should only be applied while the patient is electrocardiographically monitored with resuscitative equipment available to manage the rare episode of asystole and/or ventricular fibrillation associated with this procedure. Carotid sinus massage should not be performed in patients with carotid arterial bruits. The patient should be positioned flat with the neck extended. Massage of one carotid bulb at a time should be performed by applying firm pressure just underneath the angle of the jaw for up to 5 s. Alternative vagomimetic maneuvers include the Valsalva maneuver, immersion of the face in cold water, and administration of 5 to 10 mg edrophonium.

Observation of the jugular venous pulse can provide clues to the presence of atrial activity and its relationship to ventricular ectopy. Intermittent cannon *a* waves suggest AV dissociation, while persistent cannon *a* waves suggest 1:1 VA conduction. Flutter waves may be seen or no atrial activity may be apparent, as in the presence of atrial flutter and fibrillation, respectively. The arterial pulse also may manifest AV dissociation or atrial fibrillation by demonstrating variations in amplitude. A first heart sound of variable intensity during a regular rhythm also suggests AV dissociation or atrial fibrillation.

SINUS TACHYCARDIA In the adult, sinus tachycardia is said to be present when the heart rate exceeds 100 beats per minute; sinus tachycardia rarely exceeds 200 beats per minute and is not a primary arrhythmia; instead, it represents a physiologic response to a variety of stresses, such as fever, volume depletion, anxiety, exercise, thyrotoxicosis, hypoxemia, hypotension, or congestive heart failure. Sinus tachycardia has a gradual onset and offset. The ECG demonstrates P waves with sinus contour preceding each QRS complex. Carotid sinus pressure usually produces modest slowing with a gradual return to the previous rate upon cessation. This contrasts with the response of paroxysmal supraventricular tachycardias, which may slow slightly and terminate abruptly.

Sinus tachycardia should not be treated as a primary arrhythmia, since it is almost always a physiologic response to a demand placed on the heart. As such, the therapy should be directed to the primary disorder. This may involve institution of digitalis and/or diuretics for heart failure and oxygen for hypoxemia, treatment of thyrotoxicosis, volume repletion, aspirin for fever, or tranquilizers for emotional upset.

ATRIAL FIBRILLATION (AF) This common arrhythmia may occur in paroxysmal and persistent forms. It may be seen in normal subjects, particularly during emotional stress or following surgery, exercise, or acute alcoholic intoxication. It also may occur in patients with heart or lung disease who develop acute hypoxia, hypercapnia, or metabolic or hemodynamic derangements. Persistent AF usually occurs in patients with cardiovascular disease, most commonly rheumatic heart disease, nonrheumatic mitral valve disease, hypertensive cardiovascular disease, chronic lung disease, atrial septal defect, and a variety of miscellaneous cardiac abnormalities. AF may be the presenting finding in thyrotoxicosis. So-called lone AF, which occurs in patients without underlying heart disease, is considered to represent the tachycardia phase of the tachycardia-bradycardia syndrome (p. 1013).

The morbidity associated with AF is related to (1) excessive ventricular rate, which in turn may lead to hypotension, pulmonary congestion, or angina pectoris in susceptible individuals, (2) the pause following cessation of AF, which can cause syncope, (3) systemic embolization, which occurs most commonly in patients with rheumatic heart disease, (4) loss of the contribution of atrial contraction to cardiac output, which may cause fatigue, and (5) anxiety secondary to palpitations. In patients with severe cardiac dysfunction, particularly those with hypertrophied, noncompliant ventricles, the combination of the loss of the atrial contribution to ventricular filling and the abbreviated filling period due to the rapid ventricular rate in AF can produce marked hemodynamic embarrassment, resulting in hypotension, syncope, or heart failure. In patients with mitral stenosis, in whom ventricular filling time is critical, development of AF with a rapid ventricular rate may precipitate pulmonary edema (see Chap. 201).

AF is characterized by disorganized atrial activity without discrete P waves on the surface ECG (Fig. 198-3*D*). Atrial activation is manifested by an undulating baseline or by more sharply inscribed atrial deflections of varying amplitude and frequency ranging from 350 to 600 beats per minute. The ventricular response is irregularly irregular. This results from the large number of atrial impulses which penetrate the AV node, making it partially refractory to subsequent impulses. This effect of nonconducted atrial impulses to influence the response to subsequent atrial impulses is termed *concealed conduction*. As a result, the ventricular response is relatively slow, considering the actual atrial rate. AF may convert to atrial flutter, especially in response to antiarrhythmic drugs like quinidine or flecainide. If AF converts to atrial flutter, which has a slower atrial rate, the effect of concealed conduction may be diminished, and a paradoxic increase in the ventricular response may occur. The main factor determining the rate of the ventricular response is the functional refractory period of the AV node or the most rapid paced rate at which 1:1 conduction through the AV node can be observed.

If, in the presence of AF, the ventricular rhythm becomes regular and slow (e.g., 30 to 60 beats per minute), complete heart block is suggested, and if the ventricular rhythm is regular and rapid (e.g., ≥100 beats per minute), a tachycardia arising in the AV junction or ventricle should be suspected. Digitalis intoxication is a common cause of both phenomena.

Patients with AF exhibit a loss of *a* waves in the jugular venous pulse and variable pulse pressures in the carotid arterial pulse. The first heart sound usually varies in intensity. On echocardiography, the left atrium is frequently enlarged, and in patients in whom the left atrial diameter exceeds 4.5 cm, it may not be possible to convert AF to sinus rhythm or to maintain the latter despite therapy.

Management In acute AF, a precipitating factor such as fever, pneumonia, alcoholic intoxication, thyrotoxicosis, pulmonary emboli, congestive heart failure, or pericarditis should be sought. When such a factor is present, therapy should be directed toward the primary abnormality. If the patient's clinical status is severely compromised, electrical cardioversion is the treatment of choice. In the absence of severe cardiovascular compromise, slowing of ventricular rate becomes the initial therapeutic goal. This may be accomplished with digitalis, calcium channel antagonists, or beta-adrenergic blockers, all of which prolong the refractory period of the AV node and slow conduction within it. Intravenous verapamil usually gives the most rapid response. However, in cases where catecholamine levels or sympathetic nervous system tone is likely to be elevated, beta blockers may be favored. Conversion to sinus rhythm may then be attempted, using quinidine-like (type IA) drugs or flecainide or other type IC drugs (Table 198-1). It is important to increase AV node refractoriness prior to administering such drugs because their vagolytic effect and their ability to convert AF to atrial flutter may reduce the concealed conduction and lead to an excessively rapid ventricular response. Beta-adrenergic blockers are especially useful in this regard. If medical therapy fails to convert AF, electrical cardioversion is useful; it generally requires 100 to 200 W·s of energy. Anticoagulation should be started at least 2 weeks prior to and continued for 2 weeks following any attempt at cardioversion, either pharmacologic or electrical, in patients with long-standing AF. Anticoagulation appears to decrease the incidence of systemic embolization associated with cardioversion. It is less likely for chronic AF to convert to or remain in sinus rhythm in the presence of long-standing rheumatic heart disease and/or when the atria are markedly enlarged. It is also unlikely for patients with lone AF to be converted to and maintained in sinus rhythm.

The goal of therapy in patients in whom AF cannot be converted to sinus rhythm is control of the ventricular response. This can usually

TABLE 198-1 Classification of antiarrhythmic drugs

Type I   Drugs that reduce maximal velocity of phase of depolarization (V_{max}) due to block of inward Na^+ current in tissue with fast response action potentials

    A $\downarrow V_{max}$ at all heart rates and $\uparrow$ action potential duration, e.g., quinidine, procainamide, disopyramide

    B Little effect at slow rates on V_{max} in normal tissue; $\downarrow V_{max}$ in partially depolarized cells with fast response action potentials
       Effects increased at faster rates
       No change or $\downarrow$ in action potential duration, e.g., lidocaine, phenytoin, tocainide, mexiletine

    C $\downarrow V_{max}$ at normal rates in normal tissue
       Minimal effect on action potential duration, e.g., flecainide, propafenone, moricizine

Type II Antisympathetic agents, e.g., propranolol and other beta-adrenergic blockers: $\downarrow$ SA nodal automaticity, $\uparrow$ AV nodal refractoriness, and $\downarrow$ AV nodal conduction velocity

Type III Agents that prolong action potential duration in tissue with fast-response action potentials, e.g., bretylium, amiodarone, sotalol

Type IV Calcium (slow) channel blocking agents: $\downarrow$ conduction velocity and $\uparrow$ refractoriness in tissue with slow-response action potentials, e.g., verapamil, diltiazem

Drugs that cannot be classified by this schema:
  Digitalis
  Adenosine

---

be accomplished by digitalis, beta blockers, or calcium channel blockers singly or in combination. In occasional patients, the ventricular response cannot be controlled by pharmacologic therapy alone. In such patients, the creation of complete heart block by radiofrequency catheter ablation of the AV junction followed by permanent pacemaker implantation is appropriate. Surgical or direct-current catheter ablation of the AV junction is rarely required to achieve AV block.

If sinus rhythm is restored electrically or pharmacologically, quinidine or related agents as well as the type IC agents (e.g., flecainide) or amiodarone may be used to prevent recurrence. In patients in whom cardioversion is unsuccessful or in whom AF is likely to recur, it is probably wisest to allow the patient to remain in AF and to control the ventricular response with calcium antagonists, beta-adrenergic blockers, or digitalis glycosides. Since such patients are always at risk of systemic embolization, chronic anticoagulation must be considered. Several studies have now demonstrated conclusively that the incidence of embolization in patients with AF not associated with valvular heart disease is reduced by chronic anticoagulation with warfarin-like agents. Aspirin also may be effective for this purpose, but the data supporting its use are less extensive.

ATRIAL FLUTTER This arrhythmia occurs most often in patients with organic heart disease. Flutter may be paroxysmal, in which case there is usually a precipitating factor, such as pericarditis or acute respiratory failure, or it may be persistent. Atrial flutter (as well as AF) is very common during the first week following open heart surgery. Atrial flutter is usually less long-lived than is AF, although on occasion it may persist for months to years. Most commonly, if it lasts for more than a week, atrial flutter will convert to AF. Systemic embolization is less common in atrial flutter than in AF.

Atrial flutter is characterized by an atrial rate between 250 and 350 beats per minute. Typically, the ventricular rate is half the atrial rate, i.e., approximately 150 beats per minute. If the atrial rate is slowed to <220 beats per minute by antiarrhythmic agents such as quinidine, which also possess vagolytic properties, the ventricular rate may rise suddenly because of the development of 1:1 AV conduction. Classically, flutter waves are seen as regular sawtooth-like atrial activity, most prominent in the inferior leads (Fig. 198-3*C*). When the ventricular response is regular and not a simple fraction of the atrial rate, complete AV block is present, which may be a manifestation of digitalis toxicity. Activation mapping suggests that atrial flutter is a form of atrial reentry localized to the low right atrium.

Management The most effective treatment of atrial flutter is direct-current cardioversion, which can be accomplished at low energy

(10 to 50 W·s) under mild sedation. In patients who develop atrial flutter following open-heart surgery or recurrent flutter in the setting of acute myocardial infarction, particularly when they are being treated with digitalis, atrial pacing (using temporary pacing wires implanted at the time of operation or a pacing lead inserted into the atrium pervenously) at rates of 115 to 130 percent of the atrial flutter rate can usually convert the atrial flutter to sinus rhythm. Atrial pacing also may result in the conversion of atrial flutter to AF, which allows for easier control of the ventricular response. If immediate conversion of atrial flutter is not mandated by the patient's clinical status, the ventricular response should first be slowed by blocking the AV node with a beta blocker, calcium antagonist, or digitalis; the last drug occasionally converts atrial flutter into AF. Once AV nodal conduction is slowed with any of these drugs, an attempt to convert flutter to sinus rhythm using quinidine or quinidine-like agents should be made. Increasing doses of the drug selected are administered until the rhythm converts or side effects occur.

Quinidine, quinidine-like drugs, flecainide, propafenone, and amiodarone (Table 198-2) may be useful in preventing recurrences of both atrial flutter and atrial fibrillation.

PAROXYSMAL SUPRAVENTRICULAR TACHYCARDIAS (PSVT)

In most cases, functional differences in conduction and refractoriness in the AV node or the presence of an AV bypass tract provide the substrate for the development of PSVT (previously termed *paroxysmal atrial tachycardia*). Electrophysiologic studies have demonstrated that reentry is the mechanism responsible for the vast majority of cases of PSVT (Fig. 198-6). Reentry has been localized to the sinus node, atrium, AV node, or a macroreentrant circuit involving conduction in the antegrade direction through the AV node and retrograde through an AV bypass tract. Such a bypass tract also may conduct antegradely, in which case the Wolff-Parkinson-White (WPW) syndrome is said to be present. More frequently, however, the bypass tract manifests only retrograde conduction, and therefore it is termed a *concealed bypass tract* (Fig. 198-6*B*). In these cases, the QRS complex during sinus rhythm is normal. In the absence of the WPW syndrome, reentry through the AV node or through a concealed bypass tract makes up more than 90 percent of all PSVTs.

AV NODAL REENTRANT TACHYCARDIA

There is no age or disease predisposition for the development of AV nodal reentrant tachycardia, the most common cause of supraventricular tachycardia. It is, however, more commonly observed in women. It usually presents as a narrow QRS complex with regular rates ranging from 120 to 250 beats per minute. APCs that initiate the arrhythmia are almost always associated with a prolonged PR interval. Retrograde P waves may be absent, buried in the QRS complex, or appear as distortions at the terminal parts of the QRS complex (Fig. 198-6*A*).

AV nodal reentrant PSVT (Fig. 198-7) can be reproducibly initiated and terminated by appropriately timed atrial premature extrastimuli. The onset of the tachycardia is almost always associated with prolongation of the PR interval due to marked AV nodal conduction delay (prolonged AH interval) following the APC that is critical for the genesis of the arrhythmia. The sudden prolongation of the AH interval is consistent with the concept of dual AV nodal pathways: (1) a beta (fast) pathway, which exhibits rapid conduction and a long refractory period, and (2) an alpha (slow) pathway, which has a short refractory period but conducts slowly. During sinus rhythm, only conduction over the fast pathway is manifest, resulting in a normal PR interval. The normal sinus impulse, which simultaneously conducts down the slow pathway, reaches the His bundle after it has been depolarized and is therefore refractory. Atrial extrastimuli at a

critical coupling interval are blocked in the beta pathway because of its longer refractory period and are conducted slowly through the alpha pathway. If conduction down the alpha pathway is slow enough to allow the previously refractory beta pathway time to recover excitability, a single atrial echo or sustained tachycardia ensues. A critical balance between conduction velocity and refractoriness within the node is required to sustain AV nodal reentry. Retrograde atrial and antegrade ventricular activation occur simultaneously, explaining why P waves may not be apparent on the surface ECG.

Clinical features   AV nodal reentry may produce palpitations, syncope, and heart failure depending on the rate and duration of the arrhythmia and the presence and severity of any underlying heart disease. Hypotension and syncope may occur because of the sudden loss of the atrial contribution to ventricular filling; this also can lead to a marked increase in atrial pressure, acute pulmonary edema, and a reduction in ventricular filling. Simultaneous atrial and ventricular contraction produces cannon *a* waves with each heartbeat.

Treatment   In patients without hypotension, vagal maneuvers, particularly carotid sinus massage, can terminate the arrhythmia in 80 percent of cases. If hypotension is present, raising the blood pressure by the cautious use of intravenous phenylephrine in 0.1-mg increments may terminate the arrhythmia alone or in combination with carotid sinus pressure. If these maneuvers are unsuccessful, verapamil (2.5 to 10 mg intravenously) or adenosine (6 to 12 mg intravenously) is the agent of choice. We prefer to use adenosine because of its extremely short half-life, lessening the consequences of any side effects. Propranolol (0.05 to 0.2 mg/kg intravenously) or other beta blockers also may be used to slow or terminate the tachycardia but are agents of second choice. Digitalis glycosides have a slower onset of action and should not be used for acute therapy. When these drugs fail to terminate the tachycardia, or when the tachycardia is recurrent, atrial or ventricular pacing via a temporary pacemaker inserted pervenously may be used to terminate the arrhythmia. However, if severe ischemia and/or hypotension is caused by the tachycardia, dc cardioversion should be considered.

AV nodal reentry can usually be prevented by the use of drugs that act primarily on the antegrade slow pathway (such as digitalis, beta blockers, or calcium channel antagonists) or on the fast pathway (such as quinidine-like agents and newer drugs such as flecainide, propafenone, and amiodarone). We favor as initial therapy digitalis, beta blockers, or calcium channel antagonists because the risk-benefit ratio associated with treatment with these agents is more favorable than that of IA or IC agents. Drugs most likely to avert recurrences prevent induction of the arrhythmias by programmed stimulation. This technique utilizes temporary pacemaker catheters connected to a physiologic stimulator capable of variable rate pacing and stimulation with one or more precisely timed premature impulses. In symptomatic patients who require chronic therapy, radiofrequency catheter modification of AV nodal function has recently acquired first-line treatment status. This technique can cure AV nodal reeentry in >90 percent of cases and has been proven to be safe, although a 1 to 5 percent risk of AV block requiring a permanent pacemaker exists.

AV REENTRANT TACHYCARDIA

PSVT due to AV reentry incorporates a concealed AV bypass tract (i.e., one that conducts only retrogradely) as part of the tachycardia circuit. Thus the impulse passes antegradely from the atria through the AV node and His-Purkinje system to the ventricles and then retrogradely through the (concealed) bypass tract back to the atrium. Patients with this disorder manifest the same type of PSVT as do patients with the WPW syndrome (see below), but the bypass tract cannot conduct in an

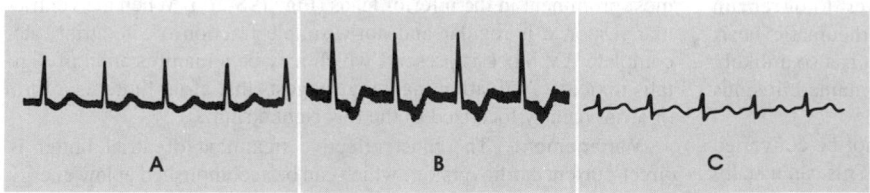

FIGURE 198-6 Examples of reentrant PSVT. *A*. AV nodal reentry. No P waves are visible. *B*. AV reentry using a concealed bypass tract. Inverted retrograde P waves are superimposed on the T wave. *C*. Intraatrial reentry. P waves precede the QRS complex.

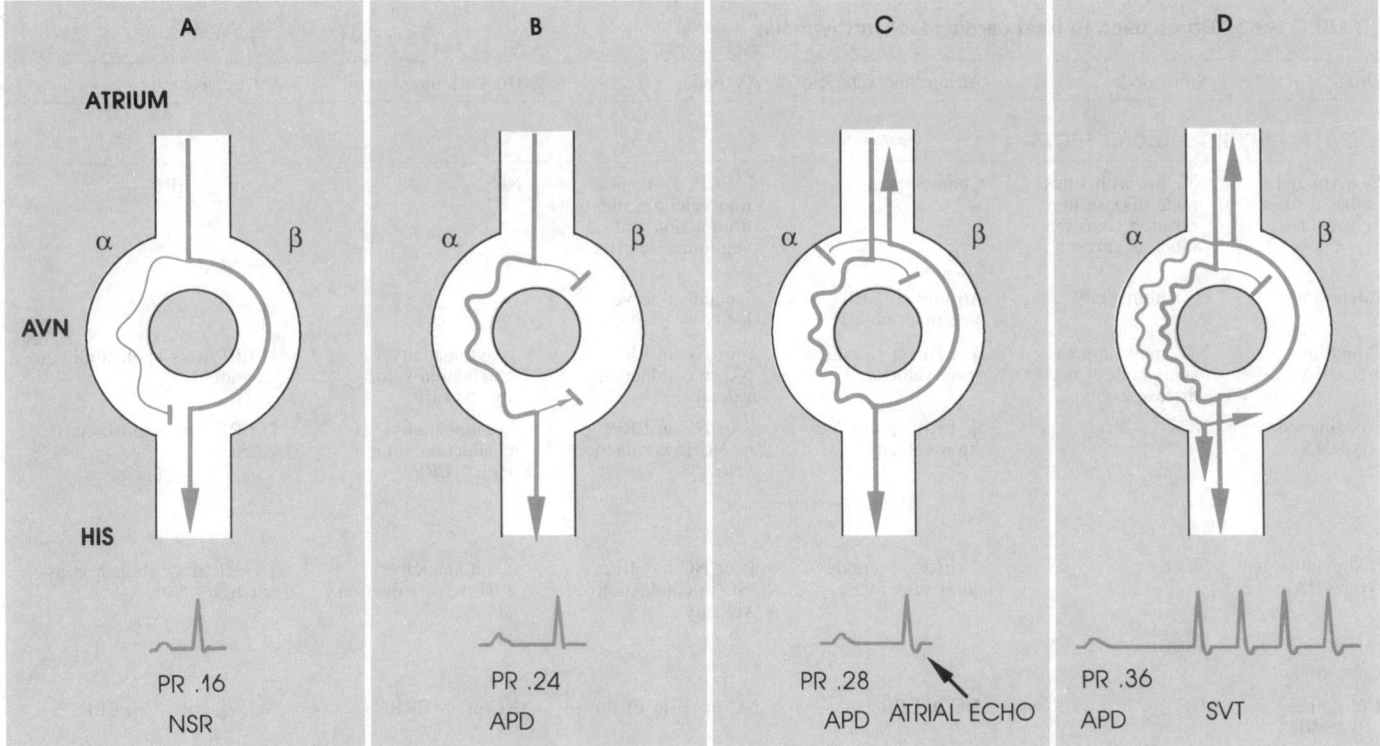

FIGURE 198-7 Mechanism of AV nodal reentry: The atrium, AV node (AVN), and His bundle are shown schematically. The AV node is longitudinally dissociated into two pathways, with different functional properties. The alpha pathway conducts relatively slowly while the beta pathway conducts rapidly (see text). In each panel of this diagram, heavy lines denote excitation in the AV node which is manifest on the surface electrocardiogram, while light lines denote conduction which is concealed and not apparent on the surface electrocardiogram. *A.* During sinus rhythm (NSR) the impulse from the atrium conducts down both pathways. However, only conduction over the fast (beta) pathway is manifest on the surface ECG, producing a normal PR interval of 0.16 s. *B.* An atrial premature depolarization (APD) blocks in the beta pathway. The impulse conducts over the alpha pathway to the His bundle and

ventricles, producing a PR interval of 0.24 s. Because the impulse is premature, conduction over the alpha pathway occurs more slowly than it would during sinus rhythm. *C.* A more premature atrial impulse blocks in the beta pathway, conducting with increased delay in the alpha pathway, producing a PR interval of 0.28 s. The impulse conducts retrogradely up the beta pathway producing a single atrial echo. Sustained reentry is prevented by subsequent block in the alpha pathway. *D.* A still more premature atrial impulse blocks initially in the beta pathway, conducting over the alpha pathway with increasing delay producing a PR interval of 0.36 s. Retrograde conduction occurs over the beta pathway and reentry occurs, producing a sustained tachycardia (SVT). (*After Josephson.*)

antegrade direction during sinus rhythm or other atrial tachyarrhythmias.

AV reentrant tachycardia can be initiated and terminated by either APCs or VPCs. Alternation of the QRS complexes and/or T wave occurs in approximately one-third of such tachycardias. Since atrial activation must follow ventricular activation during AV reentry, the P wave usually occurs after the QRS complex (see Fig. 198-6*B*).

Atrial activation mapping is of major value in evaluating the origin of these tachycardias. Most concealed bypass tracts are left-sided. Thus, during supraventricular tachycardia or during ventricular pacing, the earliest activation sequence is recorded in the left atrium, usually via a catheter in the coronary sinus (Fig. 198-8). This eccentric atrial activation is quite distinct from the normal retrograde activation sequence in which the earliest activation of the atria is in the area of the AV junction. The ability of a ventricular stimulus to conduct to the atrium at a time when the bundle of His is refractory and the termination of the tachycardia by a ventricular stimulus that does not reach the atrium are diagnostic of retrograde conduction over a concealed bypass tract.

Treatment is similar to that for AV nodal reentry tachycardia. Although pharmacologic agents may be used, at this time, patients who require chronic therapy should be considered candidates for radiofrequency catheter ablation of the bypass tract. This requires detailed electrophysiologic study to exclude other arrhythmias which may be responsible for patients' symptoms and to determine the location of the bypass tract(s). The efficacy of this procedure exceeds 90 percent, with minimal risks. In the remaining small number

of patients failing catheter ablation, surgical ablation should be considered.

SINUS NODE REENTRY AND OTHER ATRIAL TACHYCARDIAS
Reentry in the region of the sinus node or within the atria is invariably initiated by APCs. These arrhythmias are less common than AV nodal or AV reentry and are more often associated with underlying cardiac disease. During sinus node reentry, the P-wave morphology is identical to that occurring in sinus rhythm, but the PR interval is prolonged. This is in contrast to sinus tachycardia, in which the PR interval tends to shorten. With intraatrial reentry, the P-wave configuration differs from that during sinus rhythm, and the PR interval is prolonged (see Fig. 198-6*C*).

Treatment Sinus node and atrial reentrant arrhythmias are managed like other reentrant PSVTs except that catheter ablation is less successful because multiple foci may be present.

NONREENTRANT ATRIAL TACHYCARDIAS These may be a manifestation of digitalis intoxication or may be associated with severe pulmonary or cardiac disease, with hypokalemia, or with the administration of theophylline or adrenergic drugs. The last frequently present as multifocal atrial tachycardias (MAT) (Fig. 198-9). By definition, MAT requires three or more consecutive P waves of different morphologies at rates greater than 100 beats per minute. MAT usually has an irregular ventricular rate because of varying AV conduction. There is a high incidence of atrial fibrillation (50 to 70 percent) in patients with MAT. Treatment should be directed at the underlying disorder. The digitalis-induced arrhythmias may be caused by triggered activity and/or enhanced automaticity. In such atrial

TABLE 198-2   Drugs used to treat cardiac tachyarrhythmias

Drug	Sinus node	Atrium and ventricle	AV node	His-Purkinje system	AV bypass tracts
ELECTROPHYSIOLOGIC EFFECTS					
Digoxin and other cardiac glycosides	NC; pts with sinus node disease may develop sinus exit block or arrest	Controversial	↑ ERP, ↓ conduction velocity, due to drug action and vagomimetic effects	NC	NC or ↓ ERP
Adenosine	↓ automaticity	Atrium: ↓ ERP Ventricle: no effect	↓ conduction velocity		
Quinidine (type IA)	NC; may suppress sinus node if node disease exists	↑ ERP; ↓ conduction velocity	↓ or NC in ERP; NC in conduction velocity	↓ automaticity; ↓ conduction velocity; ↑ ERP	↑ ERP may abolish all conduction
Procainamide (type IA)	NC	↑ ERP; ↓ conduction velocity	↓ or NC in ERP; ↓ or NC in conduction velocity	↓ automaticity; ↓ conduction velocity; ↑ ERP	↑ ERP may abolish conduction
Disopyramide (type IIA)	NC	↑ ERP; ↓ conduction velocity	↓ or NC in ERP; NC in conduction velocity	↓ automaticity; ↑ ERP; ↓ conduction velocity	↑ ERP may abolish conduction
Lidocaine (type IB)	NC	NC in ERP	NC or ↓ in ERP	NC or ↓ ERP	NC, ↓, or ↑ in ERP
Phenytoin (type IB)	NC	NC in ERP	NC or ↓ in ERP; NC or ↑ in conduction velocity	↓ in ERP; ↓ automaticity	
Tocainide (type IB)	NC	NC	NC	NC; ↓ automaticity	↑ ERP
Mexiletine (type IB)	NC; pts with sinus node disease may develop sinus arrest	NC	Variable and inconsistent effects on conduction and refractoriness	↑ ERP; NC or ↓ conduction velocity	
Flecainide (type IC)	NC; pts with sinus node disease may develop exit block or arrest	↓ conduction velocity; ↑ ERP	↓ conduction velocity; ↑ ERP	↓ conduction velocity	↓ conduction velocity; ↑ ERP; may abolish all conduction
Propafenone (type IC) (also beta blocker)	No significant effect	↓ conduction velocity; ↑ ERP	↓ in conduction velocity; ↑ ERP	↓ conduction velocity; ↑ ERP	↑ ERP
Moricizine (type 1C)	No significant effect	Atrium: NC in ERP; ↓ conduction velocity Ventricle: slight increase in ERP; ↓ conduction velocity	↓ conduction velocity	↓ conduction velocity	
Propranolol (type II)	↓ sinus rate; ↑ sinus node recovery time	NC	↑ ERP; ↓ conduction velocity	NC	NC
Bretylium (type III)	Initial increase in sinus rate, followed by decrease	↑ ERP	NC	NC	
Amiodarone (type III)	↓ sinus rate	↑ ERP	↑ ERP; ↓ conduction velocity	↑ ERP; ↓ conduction velocity	↑ ERP
Sotalol (type III) (also beta blocker)	↓ sinus rate	↑ ERP	↑ ERP; ↓ conduction velocity	↑ ERP	↑ ERP

ABBREVIATIONS: NC = no change; ↑ = increase; ↓ = decrease.

TABLE 198-2   Drugs used to treat cardiac tachyarrhythmias *(continued)*

Indications	Side effects and toxicity

CLINICAL EFFECTS

Slowing of ventricular rate during AF, flutter, and other atrial tachycardias in the absence of preexcitation; slowing, termination and/or prevention of SVT due to AV nodal reentry and AV reentry utilizing bypass tracts; may terminate or prevent intraatrial reentrant tachycardias; ineffective in prevention of automatic atrial tachycardias	Atrial tachycardia, VT, AV nodal block, accelerated junctional rhythms, atrial and ventricular premature depolarizations, VT, VF, anorexia, nausea, vomiting, acceleration of ventricular rate during AF/flutter in the presence of preexcitation causing VF
Acute termination of regular reentrant SVT involving the AV node	Transient atrial standstill following termination of SVT; transient hypotension
Atrial and ventricular extrasystoles; atrial and ventricular tachyarrhythmias; all types of SVT; control of ventricular rate in pts with preexcitation and AF and flutter	
Same as quinidine	Anorexia, nausea, vomiting, diarrhea, cinchonism, tinnitus, confusion, hearing and visual changes; thrombocytopenia, hemolytic anemia, rash, drug interactions, elevation of digoxin levels; phenytoin and phenobarbital will decrease quinidine levels; QT prolongation associated with polymorphic VT (torsades de pointes); conversion of nonsustained to sustained acceleration of ventricular response to atrial flutter and fibrillation
Same as quinidine	Anorexia, nausea, confusion, hallucinations, agranulocytosis, and lupus erythematosus–like syndrome; QT prolongation associated with polymorphic VT (torsades de pointes); marked elevations in the primary metabolic rate (NAPA); may be more likely to cause polymorphic VT; conversion of nonsustained to sustained VT; acceleration of ventricular response to atrial flutter and fibrillation
Same as quinidine	Anticholinergic actions, including dry mouth, blurred vision, urinary retention, hesitancy, constipation, narrow-angle glaucoma, congestive heart failure, especially in patient with abnormal ventricular function and QT prolongation associated with polymorphic VT (torsades de pointes)
VT and VF, especially during acute ischemia and myocardial infarction	Dizziness, parasthesias, confusion, delirium, seizures, coma; may depress sinus node in pts with underlying sinus node disease; may suppress escape foci in pts with complete heart block; congestive heart failure or liver disease increases risk of side effects
Tachyarrhythmias induced by digitalis; occasionally effective for ventricular tachyarrhythmias not induced by digitalis, alone or in combination with other antiarrhythmic agents; polymorphic VT associated with increased QT	Gingival hypertrophy, rash, blood dyscrasias, nystagmus, ataxia, stupor, coma, lupus erythematosus syndrome, lymph node hyperplasia, peripheral neuropathy, hypocalcemia, hyperglycemia, phlebitis, and hypotension during IV administration
VT, VF, frequent VPCs	Ataxia, tremor, paresthesias, light-headedness, nausea, rash, lupus erythematosus syndrome, pulmonary fibrosis, bone marrow suppression; may exacerbate heart failure in pts with ventricular dysfunction
Refractory atrial and ventricular tachyarrhythmias; SVT due to AV node reentry and AV bypass tracts	Nausea, vomiting, ataxia, tremor, gait disturbances, rash
Refractory atrial and ventricular tachyarrhythmias; SVT due to AV node reentry and AV bypass tracts	Refractory polymorphic VT without increased QT if dose is increased too rapidly or in pts with abnormal conduction system; sinus arrest in pts with normal sinus node function; nausea, dizziness, blurred vision; may precipitate heart failure in pts with ventricular dysfunction
Atrial tachyarrhythmias including AF, SVT (not approved by the FDA for therapy of these arrhythmias), ventricular tachycardias	May exacerbate arrhythmias (increase frequency, convert nonsustained to sustained tachycardias); negative inotropic actions may worsen CHF; beta-blocking activity may worsen asthma, AV block, visual blurring, dizziness, paresthesias, taste disturbances
Slowing of ventricular rate during AF, atrial flutter, and other atrial tachycardias in the absence of preexcitation; SVT due to AV nodal reentry, reentry utilizing bypass tracts; arrhythmias induced by exercise; arrhythmias occurring in the presence of hyperthyroidism; polymorphic VT associated with congenital long QT syndrome.	Sinus bradycardia, AV node block, congestive heart failure, bronchospasm, masking symptoms of hypoglycemia
Atrial and ventricular tachyarrhythmias (not FDA approved for atrial arrhythmias)	May exacerbate ventricular tachycardia; dizziness, nausea
Refractory VT and VF, especially due to acute ischemia	Initially, transient hypertension; subsequent hypotension increased in upright position; the hypotensive effect can be prevented by tricyclic drugs; nausea, vomiting
Refractory atrial and ventricular tachyarrhythmias; refractory SVT due to AV nodal reentry and AV reentry utilizing bypass tracts; not approved by FDA for atrial arrhythmias; atrial and ventricular extrasystoles and tachyarrhythmias (not yet approved by the FDA)	Marked sinus bradycardia, complete heart block; IV administration may cause hypotension; increased QT associated with polymorphic VT; increased T_4, hypo- and hyperthyroidism; peripheral neuropathy; proximal myopathy, pulmonary fibrosis; increased liver enzymes; hepatitis; blue-gray skin discoloration; corneal microdeposits; elevation of digoxin levels; potential of oral coagulants; exacerbation of CHF, polymorphic VT associated with QT prolongation

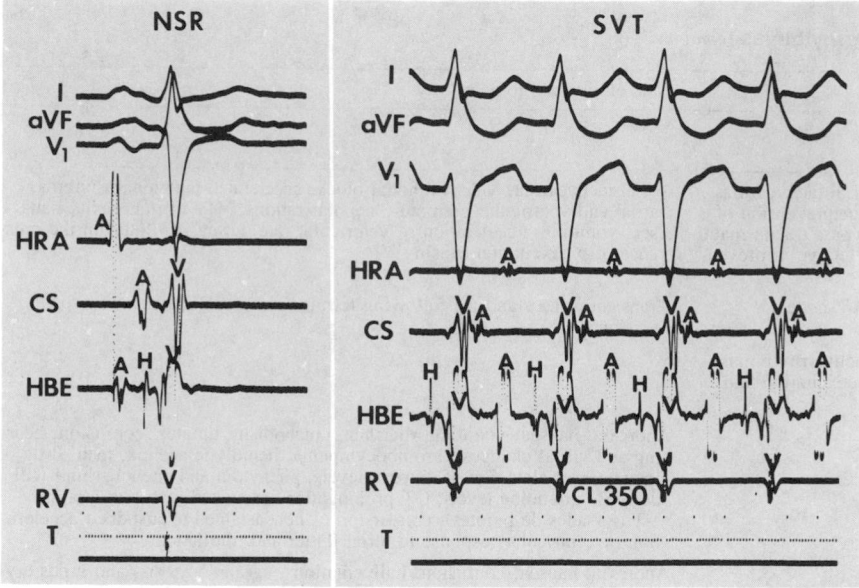

FIGURE 198-8 Intracardiac recordings during supraventricular tachycardia using a left-sided AV bypass tract. Intracardiac recordings during sinus rhythm (NSR) and in supraventricular tachycardia (SVT) are shown. ECG leads I, aVF, and V₁ are displayed with electrograms from the high right atrium (HRA), coronary sinus (CS), His bundle (HBE), and right ventricle (RV). During NSR, the QRS complex and the AH and HV intervals are normal. During SVT the retrograde atrial activation sequence is abnormal. The earliest site of atrial activation is in the CS, which is followed by activation in the HBE and HRA. This activation sequence is diagnostic of a left-sided AV bypass tract conduction retrogradely from ventricle to atrium *[From ME Josephson, in Update IV, Harrison's Principles of Internal Medicine, KJ Isselbacher et al (eds), New York, McGraw-Hill, 1983; used with permission.]*

tachycardias with AV block secondary to digitalis intoxication (see Fig. 198-3*B*), the atrial rate rarely exceeds 180 beats per minute, and typically 2:1 block is present. Atrial arrhythmias precipitated by digitalis usually can be treated by withdrawal of the drug.

Automatic atrial tachycardias not caused by digitalis are difficult to terminate, and in such cases the main goal of therapy should be to control the ventricular response, either by drugs which affect the AV node, such as digitalis, beta blockers, or calcium channel antagonists, or by ablation techniques. Catheter ablation and surgery have been employed to eradicate the arrhythmia's focus or create heart block for rate control.

PREEXCITATION (WPW) SYNDROME The most frequently encountered type of ventricular preexcitation is that associated with AV bypass tracts. These connections are composed of strands of atrial-like muscle which may occur almost anywhere around the AV rings. The term *Wolff-Parkinson-White (WPW) syndrome* is applied to patients with both preexcitation on the ECG and paroxysmal tachycardias. AV bypass tracts can be associated with certain congenital abnormalities, the most important of which is Ebstein's anomaly.

AV bypass tracts that conduct in an antegrade direction produce a typical ECG pattern of a short PR interval (<0.12 s), a slurred upstroke of the QRS complex (delta wave), and a wide QRS complex. This pattern results from a fusion of activation of the ventricles over both the bypass tract and the AV nodal His-Purkinje system (Fig. 198-10). The relative contribution of activation over each system determines the amount of preexcitation.

During PSVT in WPW, the impulse is usually conducted antegradely over the normal AV system and retrogradely through the bypass tract. The characteristics are identical to those described on p. 1024. Rarely (approximately 5 percent), tachycardias occurring in patients with WPW will exhibit a reverse pattern with antegrade conduction through the bypass tract and retrograde conduction through the normal AV system. This produces a tachycardia with a wide QRS complex in which the ventricles are totally activated by the bypass

tract. Atrial flutter and AF also occur commonly in patients with WPW syndrome. Since the bypass tract does not have the same decremental conducting properties as the AV node, the ventricular responses during atrial flutter or fibrillation may be unusually rapid (see Fig. 198-3*E*) and may cause ventricular fibrillation.

The goals of electrophysiologic evaluation in patients suspected of having the WPW syndrome are (1) to confirm the diagnosis, (2) to localize the bypass tract and determine how many bypass tracts are present, (3) to demonstrate the role of the bypass tract in the genesis of the arrhythmias, (4) to determine the potential for the development of possibly life-threatening rates during atrial flutter or fibrillation, and (5) to evaluate therapeutic options.

Management Pharmacologic therapy is aimed at altering the electrophysiologic properties (i.e., refractoriness or conduction velocity) of one or more components of the reentrant circuit. This is most often accomplished by agents such as beta blockers or calcium channel blockers that slow conduction and increase refractoriness of the AV node or by agents such as quinidine or flecainide that slow conduction and increase refractoriness primarily in the bypass tract. Some drugs may affect multiple sites (Fig. 198-11).

Acute management of episodes of PSVT in patients with WPW syndrome is similar to that of PSVT in patients with concealed bypass tracts.

In patients with the WPW syndrome and AF, dc cardioversion should be carried out if there is a life-threatening, rapid ventricular response. Alternatively, lidocaine (3 to 5 mg/kg) or procainamide (15 mg/kg) administered intravenously over 15 to 20 min will usually slow the ventricular response. Caution should be employed when using digitalis or intravenous verapamil in patients with the WPW syndrome and AF, since these drugs can shorten the refractory period of the accessory pathway and can increase the ventricular rate, thereby placing the patient at increased risk for ventricular fibrillation. Chronic oral therapy with verapamil is not associated with this risk. In addition to these drugs, beta-blocking agents are of no utility in controlling

FIGURE 198-9 Multifocal atrial tachycardia. A lead I rhythm strip demonstrates a multifocal atrial tachycardia defined by ≥3 consecutive P waves of variable morphology and rate >100 beats per minute (*arrows*).

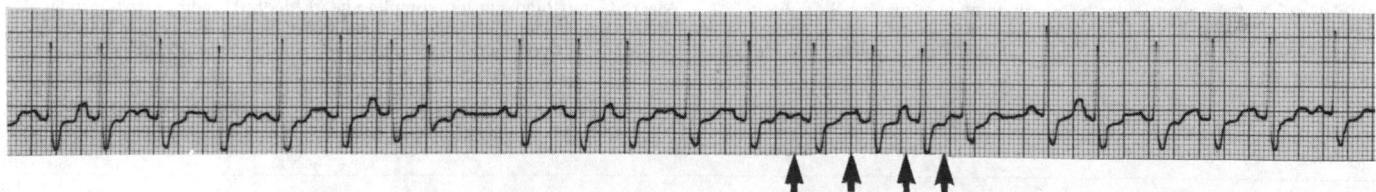

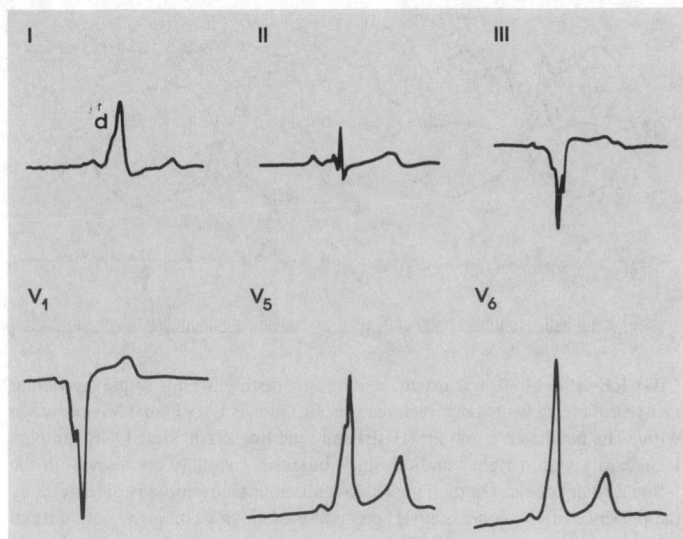

FIGURE 198-10 ECG in WPW syndrome. There is a short PR interval (0.11 s), a wide QRS complex (0.12 s), and slurring on the upstroke of the QRS produced by early ventricular activation over the bypass tract (delta wave, d in lead I). The negative delta waves in V$_1$ are diagnostic of a right-sided bypass tract. Note the Q wave (negative delta wave) in lead III, mimicking myocardial infarction.

the ventricular response during AF when conduction proceeds over the bypass tract. Although atrial or ventricular pacing can almost always terminate PSVT in patients with the WPW syndrome, they can induce AF. As such, chronic pacemaker therapy is to be discouraged.

Successful surgical ablation of bypass tracts is possible in more than 90 percent of cases and offers a permanent cure of SVT and most AFs associated with SVT. However, with the advent of radiofrequency catheter ablation, the need for surgery has been virtually eliminated. Catheter ablation of bypass tracts is possible in more than 90 percent of patients and is the treatment of choice in patients with symptomatic arrhythmias. It is safer, more cost-effective, and just as successful as surgery. Nevertheless, surgical ablation may be required in the occasional patient in whom catheter ablation fails.

NONPAROXYSMAL JUNCTIONAL TACHYCARDIA This rhythm usually results from conditions that produce enhanced automaticity or triggered activity in the AV junction and is most commonly due to digitalis intoxication, inferior wall myocardial infarction,

FIGURE 198-11 Site of action of antiarrhythmic agents in the WPW syndrome. The atrium, ventricle, antegrade conduction through the AV node (↓), retrograde conduction through the AV node (↑), and the bypass tract are shown. Drugs on the left affect antegrade AV nodal conduction. Type IA drugs on the upper right affect retrograde conduction over the node and antegrade conduction over the bypass tract. Drugs on the lower right affect conduction in both directions in the AV node and the bypass tract.

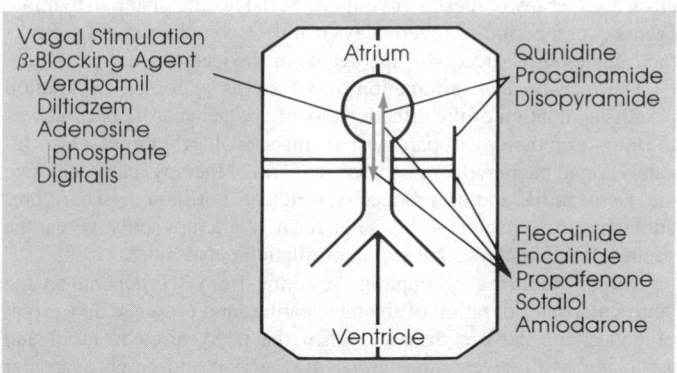

myocarditis, endogenous or exogenous catecholamine excess, acute rheumatic fever, or aftereffects of valve surgery.

The onset of nonparoxysmal junctional tachycardia is usually gradual, with a "warm-up" period prior to stabilization of the rate, which can range from 70 to 150 beats per minute, faster rates usually being associated with digitalis intoxication. Nonparoxysmal junctional tachycardia is recognized by a QRS complex identical to that of sinus rhythm. The rate can be influenced by autonomic tone and can be increased by catecholamines, vagolytic agents, or exercise and slowed somewhat by carotid sinus pressure. When this rhythm is due to digitalis intoxication, it usually is associated with AV block and/or dissociation. Soon after cardiac surgery, retrograde conduction is more likely to be present because of the heightened sympathetic state.

Management This is directed toward elimination of the underlying etiologic factors. Since digitalis is the most common cause of this rhythm, discontinuation of this drug is indicated. If the rhythm is associated with other serious manifestations of digitalis intoxication, such as ventricular or atrial irritability, active intervention with lidocaine or a beta blocker may be useful, and in some instances, use of digitalis antibodies (Fab fragments) should be considered. Cardioversion of this rhythm should not be attempted, particularly in the setting of digitalis intoxication. When AV conduction is intact, atrial pacing can capture and override the junctional focus and provide the AV synchrony necessary to maximize cardiac output. Nonparoxysmal junctional tachycardia usually is not a chronic, recurrent problem, and attention to the acute precipitating events can often resolve the tachycardia.

VENTRICULAR TACHYCARDIA (VT) *Sustained VT* is defined as *ventricular tachycardia* that persists for more than 30 s or requires termination because of hemodynamic collapse. VT generally accompanies some form of structural heart disease, most commonly chronic ischemic heart disease associated with a prior myocardial infarction. Sustained VT also may be associated with nonischemic cardiomyopathies, metabolic disorders, drug toxicity, or prolonged QT syndrome, and it occurs occasionally in the absence of heart disease or other predisposing factors. Nonsustained VT (three beats per 30 s) is also associated with cardiac disease but occurs in its absence more often than the sustained arrhythmia. While nonsustained VT usually does not produce symptoms, sustained VT is almost always symptomatic and is often associated with marked hemodynamic embarrassment and/or the development of myocardial ischemia. A fixed anatomic substrate, not acute ischemia, is responsible for most recurrent episodes of sustained uniform VT. Acute ischemia appears to have little role in the genesis of sustained uniform VT associated with chronic infarction but may play a role in the degeneration of stable VT into ventricular fibrillation (VF) or initiation of polymorphic VT. Most episodes of VF begin with VT.

The ECG diagnosis of VT is suggested by a wide-complex QRS tachycardia at a rate exceeding 100 beats per minute. The QRS configuration during any episode of VT may be uniform (monomorphic) (Figs. 198-4*B* and 198-12), or it may vary from beat to beat (polymorphic) (Fig. 198-4*C*). *Bidirectional tachycardia* refers to VT that shows an alternation in QRS amplitude and axis. Typically this appears as a QRS with a right bundle branch block pattern with alternating superior and inferior axes. While the rhythm is usually quite regular, slight irregularity may exist. Atrial activity may be dissociated from ventricular activity (Fig. 198-13), or the atria may be depolarized retrogradely. The onset of the tachycardia is generally abrupt, but in nonparoxysmal tachycardias it can be gradual. Paroxysmal VT is usually initiated by a VPC.

It is important to distinguish supraventricular tachycardia with aberration of intraventricular conduction from VT because the clinical implications and management of these two arrhythmias are totally different (Fig. 198-14). The most important clinical predictor of VT is the presence of structural heart disease. In a majority of cases, the diagnosis can and should be made by close examination of the 12-lead ECG. Pharmacologic maneuvers, such as administration of intravenous verapamil or adenosine, can be hazardous and should be

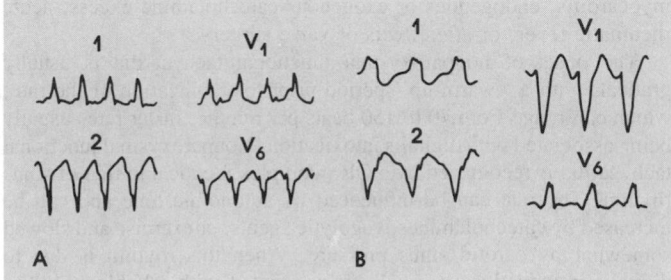

FIGURE 198-12 *A.* Sustained ventricular tachycardia having a uniform morphology. The QRS configuration in V_1 is a right bundle branch block type of configuration. Marked leftward frontal plane axis is present, denoted by the QS complex in lead II. The R/S ratio in lead V_6 is less than 1. The QRS width is greater than 140 ms. Note that 2:1 VA conduction is present with retrograde P waves present after every other QRS complex (best seen in leads I and V_1). *B.* Sustained ventricular tachycardia with a uniform, left bundle branch block type morphology (lead V_1). The QRS width is greater than 160 ms, and there are a Q wave in lead V_6 and a broad initial R wave in V_1, all favoring ventricular tachycardia rather than supraventricular tachycardia with aberrant conduction.

avoided. It is always useful to have a 12-lead ECG recorded during sinus rhythm for comparison with that during tachycardia. When the tracing obtained during sinus rhythm demonstrates a bundle branch block pattern with the same morphologic features as those during the tachycardia, the diagnosis of supraventricular tachycardia is favored. An infarction pattern on the sinus rhythm tracing suggests the potential presence of the anatomic substrate necessary for VT. Characteristics of the 12-lead ECG during the tachycardia that suggest a ventricular origin for the arrhythmia are (1) a QRS complex >0.14 s in the absence of antiarrhythmic therapy, (2) AV dissociation (with or without fusion or captured beats) or variable retrograde conduction, (3) a superior QRS axis in the presence of a right bundle branch block pattern, (4) concordance of the QRS pattern in all precordial leads (i.e., all positive or all negative deflections), and (5) other QRS patterns with prolonged duration that are inconsistent with typical right or left bundle branch block patterns. A wide, complex, bizarre tachycardia that is very irregular suggests AF with conduction over an AV bypass tract (see Fig. 198-3*E*). Similarly, a QRS complex in excess of 0.20 s is uncommon during VT in the absence of drug therapy and is more common with preexcitation. Intravenous verapamil will stop most recalcitrant supraventricular tachycardias involving the AV junction, but it is rarely effective for ventricular tachycardia. Because of this property, verapamil has been utilized to attempt to differentiate supraventricular tachycardia with aberrant conduction from ventricular tachycardia. However, this is extremely hazardous, since intravenous verapamil frequently precipitates cardiac arrest in patients with ventricular tachycardias.

FIGURE 198-13 Ventricular tachycardia with AV dissociation. P waves which are totally dissociated from the underlying ventricular rhythm are noted in lead III by arrows. AV dissociation is highly suggestive of ventricular tachycardia. In V_1 fusion complexes are present and denoted by arrows, confirming AV dissociation.

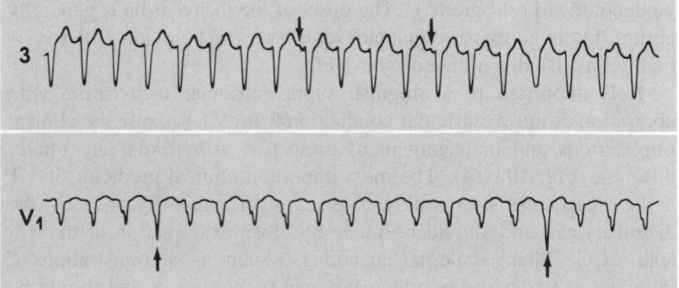

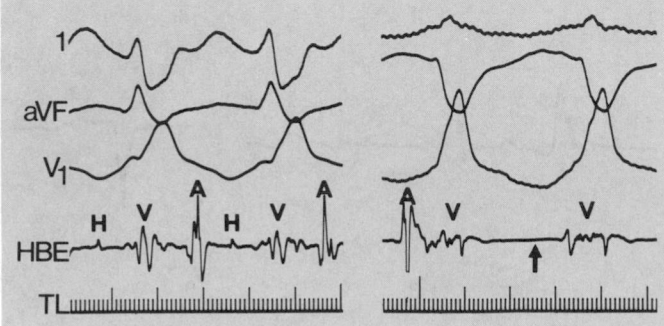

FIGURE 198-14 Intracardiac recordings distinguishing supraventricular tachycardia from ventricular tachycardia. ECG leads I, aVF, and V_1 are shown with a His bundle electrogram (HBE) and time line (TL). Wide QRS complex tachycardia with a right bundle branch block morphology are shown on the left and right panels. On the left, supraventricular tachycardia is diagnosed by the presence of His deflection (H) preceding each QRS complex, with normal HV interval. On the right, during ventricular tachycardia no His bundle deflections can be seen (*arrow*) and AV dissociation is observed (note single atrial deflection, A). *(From JA Kastor et al, N Engl J Med 304:1004, 1981; reprinted by permission.)*

The diagnosis of VT can be confirmed by analyzing the relationship between the electrogram recording from the His bundle and ventricular activity. In most cases of VT, the His deflection is not easily seen, but when visible, the interval from the His deflection to the onset of ventricular activation (HV interval) is less than that recorded during sinus rhythm, or negative due to retrograde activation over the His-Purkinje system, or is dissociated from ventricular activation (see Fig. 198-14). During SVT with aberrant conduction, the HV interval is greater than or equal to that recorded during sinus rhythm. In patients with a wide QRS complex tachycardia, the diagnosis of VT is confirmed when atrial pacing at rates equal to or greater than that of the tachycardia produces normalization of the QRS complex with a normal HV interval. Regardless of QRS morphology [left or right bundle branch block patterns (see Fig. 198-12)], VT due to ischemic heart disease arises from the *left* ventricle, in most instances near the subendocardium.

It has been possible to replicate sustained uniform VT in more than 95 percent of patients with this arrhythmia using programmed stimulation. In most patients the tachycardia is initiated with ventricular premature stimuli. A sustained monomorphic VT with a morphology identical to that of the spontaneous arrhythmia is the rule. The clinical significance of polymorphic VT initiated by programmed stimulation is not clear. It has been shown that when more aggressive stimulation is performed (i.e., the use of three or four extrastimuli), polymorphic VT and even VF can be induced in some normal subjects and in patients who have never had a clinical arrhythmia.

Sustained uniform VT can be terminated by programmed stimulation or rapid pacing in at least 75 percent of patients; the remainder require cardioversion. The ability to initiate and terminate a sustained, uniform VT reproducibly permits assessment of pharmacologic and electrical therapy of these arrhythmias. Serial testing of antiarrhythmic agents over a period of several days can be accomplished and predicts the likelihood of success of the agents or devices tested.

The reproducible termination of VT by programmed stimulation permits evaluation of the effectiveness of antitachycardia pacemakers for long-term therapy of paroxysmal episodes of arrhythmia. Unfortunately, rapid pacing, the most effective form of therapy, can accelerate the tachycardia and/or produce ventricular fibrillation. Therefore, antitachycardia pacing is a viable form of therapy only when the pacing device includes backup defibrillation capabilities.

Clinical features Symptoms resulting from VT depend on the ventricular rate, duration of the tachycardia, and presence and extent of underlying cardiac disease. When the tachycardia is rapid and associated with severe myocardial dysfunction and cerebrovascular disease, hypotension and syncope are common. However, the presence of hemodynamic stability does not preclude a diagnosis of VT. The loss of the atrial contribution to ventricular filling and an abnormal sequence of ventricular activation are important factors producing a decreased cardiac output during VT.

The *prognosis* of VT depends on the underlying disease state. If sustained VT develops within the first 6 weeks following acute myocardial infarction, the prognosis is poor, with a 75 percent mortality rate at 1 year. Patients with nonsustained VT following myocardial infarction have a threefold greater risk of death than a comparable group of patients without this arrhythmia. However, a cause-and-effect relationship between the nonsustained tachycardia and subsequent sudden death has not been established. Patients without heart disease who have uniform VT have a good prognosis and have an extremely low risk of sudden death.

Management The risk-benefit ratio of treating each specific type of VT should be considered before beginning therapy. This is important because antiarrhythmic agents can produce or exacerbate the very arrhythmias which they are given to prevent. In general, patients with VT but without organic heart disease have a benign course; such patients with asymptomatic, nonsustained VT need not be treated because their prognosis will not be affected. An exception is the patient with congenital long QT syndrome. Such patients have recurrent polymorphic VT and a high mortality from sudden death if untreated. Patients with sustained VT in the absence of heart disease usually require therapy because the arrhythmia causes symptoms. These tachycardias may respond to beta blockers, verapamil, or quinidine-like agents. In patients with VT and organic heart disease, if marked hemodynamic embarrassment is present or if there is evidence of ischemia, congestive heart failure, or central nervous system hypoperfusion, the rhythm should be promptly terminated by dc cardioversion (see below). If the patient with organic heart disease tolerates the VT well, pharmacologic therapy may be tried. Procainamide is probably the most effective agent for acute therapy. It may or may not terminate the tachycardia but almost always slows the rate. In stable patients in whom these drugs do not terminate the arrhythmia, a pacing catheter can be inserted pervenously into the right ventricular apex, and the tachycardia can be terminated by overdrive pacing.

Programmed stimulation is probably the most efficacious way to select the appropriate antiarrhythmic agent to prevent recurrent, sustained VT. After demonstrating that the tachycardia can be initiated reproducibly in the absence of antiarrhythmic agents, drugs can be studied serially, and the drug that prevents initiation of the tachycardia can be selected; long-term successful prevention of the arrhythmia can than be expected in 90 percent of patients. Drug levels demonstrated to be successful in the laboratory need to be maintained chronically. Unfortunately, prevention of inducible VT is expected in only 50 percent of cases.

Antitachycardia pacing has been used as a means to terminate drug-resistant tachycardia. This usually requires that the tachycardia be stable and slow and that the patient be aware of it. Automatic antitachycardia pacing devices are not used alone because pacing during VT may accelerate tachycardia, converting a stable arrhythmia into an unstable one and resulting in severe hemodynamic compromise. However, devices combining antitachycardia pacing with an implantable cardioverter defibrillator (ICD) (see below) afford a "backup" means of terminating unstable arrhythmias. Radiofrequency pacemakers, which are best activated by a physician, have been used in occasional patients.

The advent of endocardial catheter and intraoperative mapping led to the development of surgical techniques for the management of VT. Activation mapping permits localization of the site of origin of the arrhythmia. In centers in which expertise in mapping is available, operation has been successfully employed to cure tachycardias in the majority of patients in whom it has been undertaken. Even though most patients with VT and ischemic heart disease have markedly impaired left ventricular function and multivessel coronary artery disease, the operative mortality rate has ranged between 8 and 15 percent. Following operation, more than 90 percent of survivors are controlled either off (two-thirds of patients) or on (one-third) antiarrhythmic agents that were previously ineffective in controlling these rhythms.

Specific types of VT TORSADES DE POINTES *Torsades de pointes* ("twisting of the points") (Fig. 198-15) refers to VT characterized by polymorphic QRS complexes that change in amplitude and cycle length, giving the appearance of oscillations around the baseline. This rhythm is, by definition, associated with QT prolongation. The latter may result from electrolyte disturbances (particularly hypokalemia and hypomagnesemia), use of a variety of antiarrhythmic drugs (especially quinidine), phenothiazines and tricyclic antidepressants, liquid protein diets, intracranial events, and bradyarrhythmias, particularly third-degree AV block. It also may occur as an isolated idiopathic congenital or acquired anomaly.

The electrocardiographic hallmark is polymorphic VT preceded by marked QT prolongation, often in excess of 0.60 s. These patients often have multiple episodes of nonsustained polymorphic VT associated with recurrent syncope, but they also may develop VF and sudden cardiac death.

Therapy should be directed at removing the precipitating factors, i.e., correcting metabolic abnormalities and removing drugs which have induced the prolonged QT interval. In the setting of drug-induced torsades de pointes, atrial or ventricular overdrive pacing and the administration of magnesium also have been useful in terminating and preventing the arrhythmia. For patients with the congenital prolonged QT interval syndrome, beta-adrenergic blocking agents have been the mainstay of therapy; agents which shorten the QT interval also may be useful (e.g., phenytoin). Cervicothoracic sympathectomy has been proposed as a form of therapy for congenital prolonged QT syndrome, but it is not often effective as the sole therapy.

Polymorphic tachycardias associated with normal QT intervals in patients with ischemic heart disease that are initiated by "R-on-T" VPCs are probably caused by reentry, and their treatment is totally different. This is not true torsades de pointes. In such cases, quinidine-like agents may be the most effective form of therapy and should be administered in full antiarrhythmic doses. However, these arrhythmias also may result from acute, severe ischemia and will only respond to abolition of the ischemia, usually by revascularization.

ACCELERATED IDIOVENTRICULAR RHYTHM This arrhythmia, also termed slow VT, with a rate which ranges from 60 to 120 beats per minute, usually occurs in acute myocardial infarction, often during reperfusion. It also may be seen following cardiac operations, in patients with cardiomyopathy, rheumatic fever, or digitalis intoxication, as well as in patients with no evidence of heart disease. The rhythm is usually transient and rarely causes significant hemodynamic compromise or symptoms.

Treatment is rarely necessary and should usually be considered only if symptoms arise due to impaired hemodynamics, most commonly due to AV dissociation. In most cases, atropine can accelerate the sinus rate to overdrive the ventricular rhythm.

FIGURE 198-15 Torsades de pointes. During sinus rhythm (lead II) a markedly prolonged QT interval was present. Lead V_1 shows polymorphic VT.

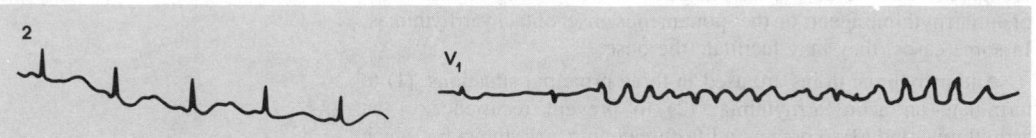

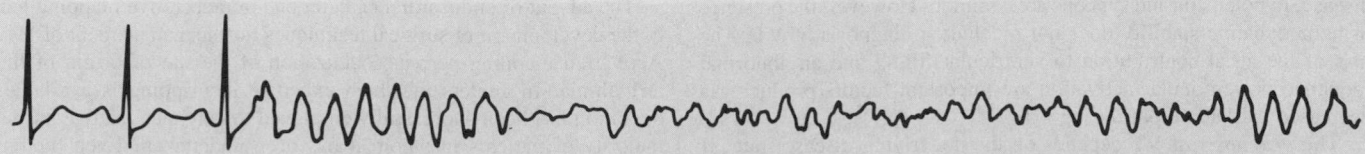

FIGURE 198-16   Ventricular fibrillation. In a patient with coronary disease ventricular fibrillation is initiated by a VPC that produces a rapid polymorphic ventricular tachycardia which rapidly degenerates to ventricular fibrillation (note the undulating baseline with indistinguishable systole and diastole).

VENTRICULAR FLUTTER AND VENTRICULAR FIBRILLATION

(VF) (See Fig. 198-16; see also Chap. 35)   These arrhythmias occur most often in patients with ischemic heart disease. They also occur following administration of antiarrhythmic drugs, particularly those which induce prolonged QT intervals and torsades de pointes (see above), in patients with severe hypoxia or ischemia, and in those with WPW who develop AF with an extremely rapid ventricular response (see p. 1028). Electrical accidents frequently cause cardiac arrest due to the development of VF. The onset of these arrhythmias is rapidly followed by loss of consciousness and, if untreated, death. Episodes of cardiac arrest recorded during Holter monitoring reveal that approximately three-fourths of the sudden deaths are due to VT or VF.

In patients with VF, the onset almost always begins with a short run of rapid VT, which is initiated by a relatively late coupled VPC. In patients with acute myocardial infarction or ischemia, however, VF is usually precipitated by a single early ventricular complex beat falling on the T wave (the vulnerable period), which produces a rapid VT which degenerates into VF (see Fig. 198-16).

The clinical setting in which VF occurs is important. Most patients who have primary VF within the first 48 h of the onset of acute infarction have a good long-term prognosis, with a very low rate of recurrence or sudden cardiac death. Their short-term mortality may, however, be slightly increased. In contrast, patients who experience VF unassociated with the development of acute myocardial infarction have a recurrence rate of 20 to 30 percent in the year following the event (see Chap. 35).

Ventricular flutter usually appears as a sine wave with a rate between 150 and 300 beats per minute. These oscillations make it impossible to assign a specific morphology to the arrhythmia and in some cases to distinguish it from rapid VT. VF is recognized by grossly irregular undulations of varying amplitudes, contours, and rates (see Fig. 198-16). Electrophysiologic studies have demonstrated that regardless of the apparent gross irregularity on the surface ECG, VF usually starts out with a rapid repetitive sequence of VT which ultimately breaks down into multiple wavelets of reentry.

Electrophysiologic studies have been useful in patients who have been resuscitated from cardiac arrest. Programmed stimulation has demonstrated that in approximately 70 percent of such patients one can reproducibly initiate a sustained VT. Treatment is discussed in Chap. 35.

PHARMACOLOGIC ANTIARRHYTHMIC THERAPY

Prior to initiation of pharmacologic antiarrhythmic therapy, potential aggravating factors such as transient metabolic abnormalities, congestive heart failure, or acute ischemia must be corrected; in some cases this may suffice to control arrhythmias. In addition, the potential role of drugs as a cause or exacerbating factor in the development of the arrhythmia must be considered. Despite their name, it must be recognized that we do not have a good understanding of the effects of antiarrhythmic agents on the spontaneous onset of tachyarrhythmias. In some cases, they may facilitate the onset.

Antiarrhythmic drugs are used in three principal situations: (1) to terminate an acute arrhythmia, (2) to prevent recurrence of an arrhythmia, and (3) to prevent a life-threatening arrhythmia for which the patient is perceived to be at risk but which has never occurred. (The acute pharmacologic therapy of tachyarrhythmias is summarized in Table 198-3.)

Most currently available antiarrhythmic agents have a relatively low toxic/therapeutic ratio; all can exert proarrhythmic effects, and

TABLE 198-3   Acute pharmacologic therapy of tachyarrhythmias

Arrhythmia	Drug	Dose
Atrial tachyarrhythmias (including AF and atrial flutter) in patients without pre-excitation	Initially verapamil or beta-blocking agent to control ventricular response, then procainamide or quinidine	Verapamil: IV, 2.5–10 mg bolus (may precede by IV calcium gluconate or chloride to prevent hypotension) Propranolol: IV, 1-mg increments until desired effect achieved or side effects Metoprolol: IV, 5–10 mg Esmolol: IV, loading dose of 500 µg/kg/min for 1 min, followed by maintenance infusion of 50 µg/kg/min for 4 min; if effect is inadequate, repeat load followed by maintenance of 100 µg/kg/min, up to maximum maintenance of 200 µg/kg/min Procainamide: IV, up to 15 mg/kg at 25–50 mg/min until arrhythmia terminates; monitor BP q 5 min Quinidine sulfate: PO, 200–400 mg
Atrial tachyarrhythmias (including AF and atrial flutter) in patients with preexcitation	Procainamide	IV up to 15 mg/kg at 25–50 mg/min; monitor BP q 5 min
SVT with regular rate and narrow QRS complex	Adenosine	IV, 6-mg bolus initially; if no effect within 60 s, give 12 mg; onset of action immediate
	Verapamil	IV, 5–10 mg over 2–3 min; onset of action within 12 min; peak effect in 10–15 min
Sustained monomorphic VT	Procainamide	IV, infusion at 25–50 mg/min up to 15 mg/kg; monitor BP q 5 min
	Lidocaine	IV, bolus of 1 mg/kg followed by a second bolus of 0.5 mg/kg 5 min later; at time of initial bolus, begin maintenance infusion of 1–4 mg/min

therefore they may exacerbate underlying arrhythmias. Serum levels can be determined for most currently available antiarrhythmic agents. Standards for therapeutic and toxic levels can serve only as a rough guide for selecting the appropriate dose in any individual patient. In the final analysis, the therapeutic level in a given patient is that concentration which achieves the desired antiarrhythmic effect, and the toxic level for each patient is that concentration at which undesirable side effects occur. Since many adverse effects are directly related to drug concentrations, the lowest serum level which achieves an effective antiarrhythmic response should be chosen.

In order to determine the therapeutic level for a patient, one must have a standard to judge drug efficacy. For a patient with an incessant arrhythmia, antiarrhythmic drugs may be administered empirically until the arrhythmia is suppressed. If a reproducible precipitating factor such as exercise can be identified, serial drug testing during such a provocative maneuver may be performed. Unfortunately, most arrhythmias are sporadic and occur unpredictably without identifiable precipitating factors. In these cases, if one waits to observe spontaneous recurrences on each antiarrhythmic drug, assessment of drug efficacy may require months. This type of assessment of efficacy may be adequate for arrhythmias which are not life-threatening. However, this mode of assessment is inadequate for arrhythmias that compromise hemodynamic stability, result in syncope, or cause cardiac arrest. In such cases, two methods for determination of arrhythmic drug efficacy have been utilized. The first, which consists of continuous ECG monitoring in the control state and then in the presence of antiarrhythmic drugs, has been used in order to determine the effect that each drug has on spontaneous atrial or ventricular ectopy. This method presupposes that the mechanism responsible for sustained arrhythmias is the same as that causing isolated premature depolarizations (which may or may not be true) and that therefore eradication of isolated ectopy will correlate with prevention of sustained arrhythmias. This method has a number of limitations. First, patients frequently show marked degrees of spontaneous variation in frequency of ectopy, which may mimic antiarrhythmic drug effects. Second, 25 to 30 percent of patients with sustained ventricular arrhythmias such as VT or VF demonstrate only rare spontaneous ectopy. Finally, many patients demonstrate a dissociation between the effects of antiarrhythmic agents on spontaneous ectopy and the effects of the same agent on sustained arrhythmias.

An alternative method to assess drug efficacy is programmed stimulation. Numerous studies have demonstrated that most clinically occurring supraventricular and ventricular tachyarrhythmias may be reproducibly initiated and terminated safely using this technique. Studies are performed initially in a baseline state in the absence of antiarrhythmic drugs (Fig. 198-17). If the patient's clinical arrhythmia can be reproducibly initiated, then the ability of individual antiarrhythmic drugs to prevent reinduction of the arrhythmia can be assessed either after the drug is administered intravenously or after several days of oral loading in order to achieve a steady state serum concentration. Use of this method assumes that (1) the induced and spontaneous arrhythmias are identical and (2) prevention of induction of arrhythmias will correlate with prevention of recurrent spontaneous tachycardias on the same drug regimen. This technique has been validated in patients with a variety of reentrant PSVTs, VT, and VF. The technique is safe when carefully performed, the potential complications being those of any intravascular catheterization. Appropriate interpretation of the results of programmed stimulation is critically dependent on correlating the patient's spontaneous arrhythmias with those induced in the laboratory, with regard to rate and morphology, in order to be certain that the arrhythmia induced in the laboratory represents the same arrhythmia that occurred spontaneously and caused symptoms.

Classification of antiarrhythmic drugs A number of classifications of antiarrhythmic drugs have been proposed, the most frequently used of which is a modification of one proposed by Vaughan-Williams (see Table 198-1). This classification is based in part on the ability of antiarrhythmic drugs to modify the cardiac cellular (1) excitatory

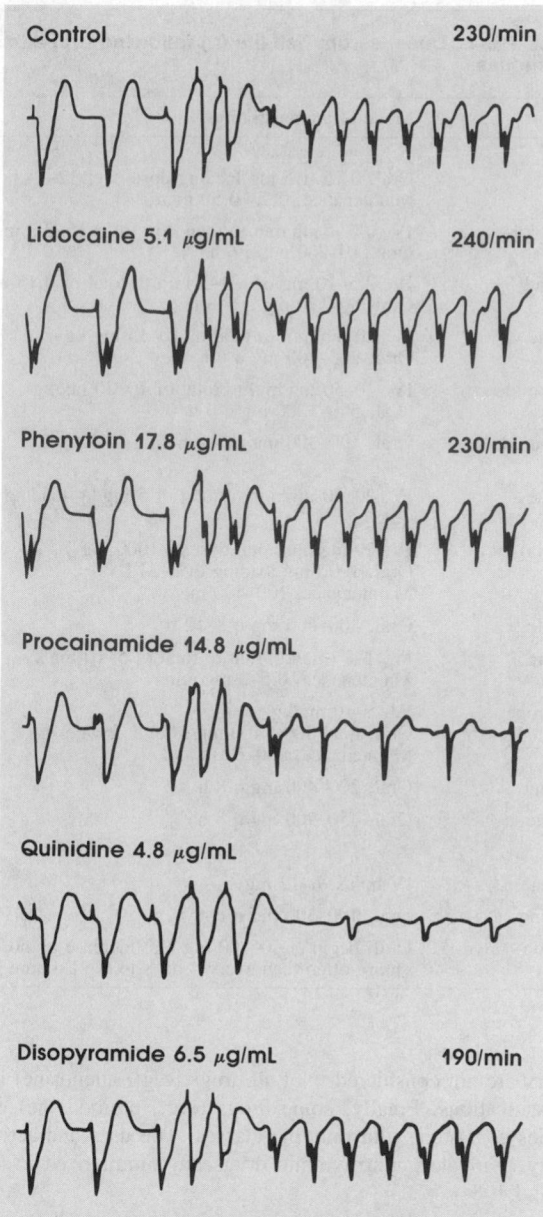

FIGURE 198-17 Selections of an effective antiarrhythmic drug for ventricular tachycardia by programmed stimulation. From top to bottom, the effects of programmed stimulation during the control state and following administration of several antiarrhythmic agents. During the control state two ventricular extrastimuli initiate the ventricular tachycardia at a rate of 230 per minute. Lidocaine, phenytoin, and disopyramide at the plasma levels shown failed to prevent induction of the tachycardia. Both procainamide and quinidine at the plasma levels shown prevented initiation of sustained tachycardia. Chronic oral quinidine therapy effectively prevented recurrences of the arrhythmia. *(From JA Kastor et al, N Engl J Med 304:1004, 1981; reprinted by permission.)*

currents (Na^+ or Ca^{2+}), (2) action potential duration, and (3) automaticity (phase 4 depolarization). These effects of the drugs on isolated cardiac cells are thought to account for some of the antiarrhythmic properties of the drugs. Thus depression of excitatory currents by type I and type IV antiarrhythmics results in slowing of conduction velocity and may interrupt arrhythmias by blocking conduction in areas of marginal excitability, where conduction velocity is already slow. Type III antiarrhythmics allegedly exert their action by increasing refractoriness through prolongation of the action potential duration. However, this classification has a number of limitations. The electrophysiologic effects of these drugs in vivo may differ from their effects on isolated cells. Also, the effects of heart rate and fiber

TABLE 198-4   Dose, serum half-life ($t_{\frac{1}{2}}$) following oral administration, and route of metabolism of drugs used in treatment of arrhythmias

Drug	Mode of administration	$t_{\frac{1}{2}}$ (oral), h	Route of metabolism
Digoxin	IV, 0.25–1.5 mg Oral, 0.75–1.5 mg loading dose over 12–24 h Maintenance, 0.23–0.50 mg/d	36	Renal
Propranolol	IV, 0.5–1 mg/min to total dose of 0.15–0.2 mg/kg Oral, 10–200 mg q 6 h	3–6	Hepatic
Verapamil	IV, 2.5–10 mg over 1–2 min to total of 0.15 mg/kg Oral, 80–120 mg q 6–8 h	3–8	Hepatic
Quinidine	IV, 20 mg/min to total of 10–15 mg/kg Oral, 200–400 mg q 6 h	5–9	Hepatic: 80% Renal: 20%
Procainamide	IV, 40–50 mg/min to total of 10–20 mg/kg Oral, 500–1000 mg q 4 h	3–5	Hepatic: 50% Renal: 50%
Disopyramide	Oral, 100–300 mg q 6–8 h	8–9	Renal: 50% Hepatic: 50%
Lidocaine	IV, 20–50 mg/min to total of 5-mg/kg loading dose followed by 1–4 mg/kg	1–2	Hepatic: 100%
Phenytoin	IV, 20 mg/min total dose to 1000 mg Oral, 1000-mg loading over 24 h Maintenance, 100–400 mg/d	18–36	Hepatic
Tocainide	Oral, 400–600 mg q 8–12 h	10–17	Hepatic-renal
Bretylium	IV, 1–2 (mg/kg)/min to total of 5–10 mg/kg Maintenance, 0.5–2 mg/min	8–14	Renal
Amiodarone	IV, 5–10 mg/kg Oral, load 800–1400 mg/d for 1–2 weeks Maintenance, 100–600 mg/d	Unknown	Unknown
Moricizine	Oral, 200–400 mg q 8 h	2–6	Hepatic
Propafenone	Oral, 450–900 mg q 8 h	5–8	Hepatic
Sotalol			
Adenosine	IV bolus, 6–12 mg	< 10 s	
Mexiletine	Oral, 100–300 mg q 6–8 h	9–12	Hepatic: 100%
Flecainide	Oral, begin at 50–100 mg bid; increase by no more than 50 mg not more often than every 4 days to a maximum of 400 mg daily	7–23	Hepatic: 75% Renal: 25%

geometry are not considered. Not all drugs (e.g., adenosine) fit into the classifications. Finally, some drugs (e.g., amiodarone) exhibit properties consistent with multiple classes. The uses and actions of currently available antiarrhythmic drugs are summarized in Tables 198-2 and 198-4.

ELECTRICAL THERAPY OF TACHYARRHYTHMIAS

PACEMAKERS Cardiac pacing can be used to terminate and in selected cases prevent recurrent supraventricular and ventricular arrhythmias. Because many tachyarrhythmias appear to be due to a reentrant mechanism with the impulse traveling in a circuit, a properly timed paced impulse can penetrate and prematurely depolarize part of the circuit, rendering it refractory to the next circulating wavefront and thereby interrupting the circus movement. Pacing therapy for arrhythmias is generally reserved for patients whose arrhythmias are refractory to drug therapy and who remain hemodynamically stable during the tachycardia. All forms of pacing therapy require repeated demonstration of their effectiveness and reliability in terminating the arrhythmias during electrophysiologic testing prior to implantation of the pacing device.

The type of pacing device and modality selected for arrhythmia termination depends on (1) the rate of the tachycardia (rates >160 beats per minute are rarely terminated by a single premature stimulus), (2) the type of the arrhythmia (atrial flutter and VT are rarely terminated by single extrastimuli), and (3) concomitant drug therapy. Underdrive pacing, i.e., pacing at a rate slower than the tachycardia, can be used when a single premature stimulus has been demonstrated to reproducibly terminate a tachycardia. It is rarely used today because

pacemakers are available which can deliver timed stimuli or an increasing number of stimuli.

Because many tachycardias cannot be terminated by single premature stimuli, pacemakers have been developed which allow for multiple extrastimuli (burst pacing) to be introduced. In reentrant tachycardias involving an accessory AV connection, sequential, near-simultaneous activation of the heart from both the atria and the ventricle using a dual-chamber pacemaker will increase the likelihood of bidirectional block and termination of the tachycardia. However, the use of antitachycardia pacing for supraventricular arrhythmias has been rendered almost obsolete by the advent of radiofrequency catheter ablation.

Cardiac pacing also has been used to prevent ventricular tachyarrhythmias. Polymorphic VT associated with a long QT interval and bradycardia (torsades de pointes, p. 1021) is most likely to respond. Pacing the atrium and/or ventricle at rates between 90 and 120 beats per minute appears to increase the homogeneity of electrical recovery and markedly reduces the propensity for a recurrence of arrhythmias.

Pacemakers may be self-contained or energized by an external radiofrequency source. The self-contained pacemaker may function automatically [i.e., it incorporates an arrhythmia recognition program (circuit)], or it may be activated by an external magnet. The major advantage of a fully automatic system is that there is no need for the patient to recognize the arrhythmia in order for termination to occur. The advantages of the externally activated system include (1) the decreased risk of unnecessary treatment because of faulty sensing and (2) the opportunity to initiate monitoring at the time of attempted termination of arrhythmia. This type of monitoring is frequently helpful if pacing techniques are employed to terminate VT, given the risk of acceleration of the arrhythmia by pacing.

The limitations of pacing therapy are primarily related to (1) the changes in the characteristics of the arrhythmia over time such that programmed pacing parameters no longer terminate the tachycardia, (2) the risk of acceleration of the tachycardia with the development of AF when stimulating the atrium and the development of rapid VT and VF when stimulating the ventricles, and (3) inappropriate recognition of supraventricular tachyarrhythmias as ventricular tachycardias, leading to delivery of therapy unnecessarily, which can initiate VT or VF. Future pacing generators which also can deliver a larger amount of energy and perform cardioversion and defibrillation of accelerated arrhythmias have been approved by the U.S. Food and Drug Administration and will increase the applicability of pacing therapy for the treatment of arrhythmias (see below).

CARDIOVERSION AND DEFIBRILLATION Electrical cardioversion and defibrillation remain the most reliable methods for terminating arrhythmias. By depolarizing all or at least a large portion of excitable myocardium in a near homogeneous fashion, the electrical shock can interrupt reentrant arrhythmias. External cardioversion is routinely performed by placing two paddles 12 cm in diameter in firm contact with the chest wall, with one paddle usually located to the right of the sternum at the level of the second rib and the other in the left midclavicular line in the fifth intercostal space. If the patient is conscious, a short-acting barbiturate to act as an anesthetic or an amnesic drug such as diazepam should be administered to prevent patient discomfort. A person skilled in maintaining an airway should be present.

Energy is delivered synchronously with the QRS complex for all arrhythmias except ventricular flutter and VF, since asynchronous shocks can produce VF. The amount of energy used will vary with the type of tachycardia being treated. With the exception of AF, supraventricular tachycardias can frequently be terminated with energy levels in the range of 25 to 50 W·s, while AF usually requires ≥100 W·s for termination. For terminating VT, energy levels ≥100 W·s should probably be employed. While energies as low as 25 W·s may be used successfully, they also have a higher incidence of producing VF. At least 200 W·s of energy should be used for initial attempts at terminating VF. If the initial shock fails, all repeated attempts at defibrillation should be with the maximum energy that the defibrillator is capable of delivering (320 to 400 W·s).

Indications for cardioversion depend on the clinical setting and the patient's general condition. Any tachycardia (except sinus tachycardia) that produces hypotension, myocardial ischemia, or heart failure warrants consideration of prompt termination using external cardioversion. Arrhythmias that fail to terminate with pharmacologic therapy also may be terminated by electrical cardioversion. Transient bradycardias and supraventricular and ventricular irritability following cardioversion are common and usually do not warrant antiarrhythmic intervention.

IMPLANTED CARDIOVERSION/DEFIBRILLATION Implantable cardioverter/defibrillator devices have been developed that will promptly recognize and terminate life-threatening ventricular arrhythmias. These devices can deliver <1 to 40 W·s, the amount of which can be programmed. Newer devices have antitachycardia pacing capabilities such that VT can be sensed and terminated without resorting to a painful shock. In such devices, high-energy shocks are reserved for hypotensive VT, acceleration of VT, or failure to terminate VT after a programmed duration (see Fig. 198-18). Clinical trials testing the function of these devices in patients with drug-refractory ventricular arrhythmias have demonstrated survival from sudden death at 1 year ranging between 92 and 100 percent. At the time of writing, use of the FDA-approved devices should be reserved for patients with VT which is not hemodynamically tolerated or for patients with VF whose arrhythmias are refractory to drug therapy. The most frequent problem with the device has been its inappropriate discharge in the absence of sustained ventricular arrhythmias. Additional potential problems include an increase in defibrillation threshold and decrease in tachycardia rates below the rate cut-off of the device in response to many antiarrhythmic drugs. Permanently implanted

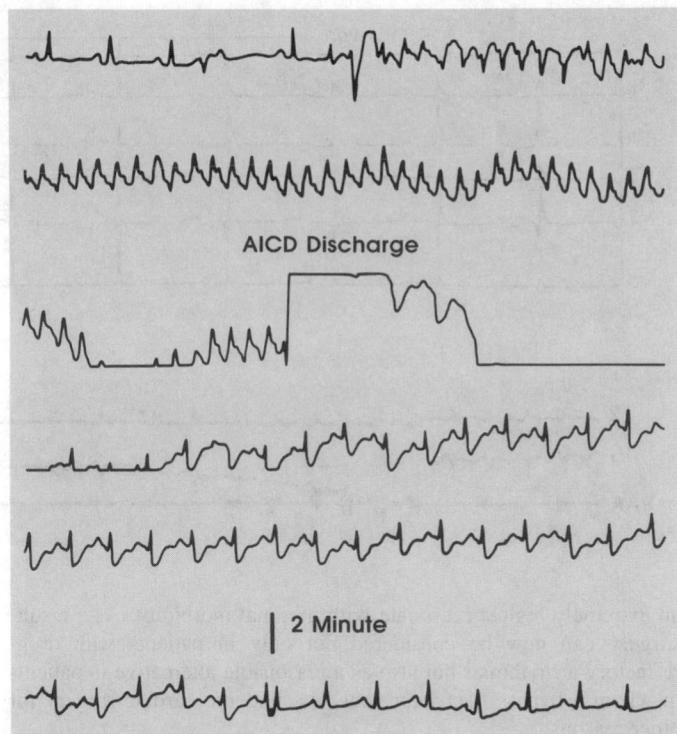

FIGURE 198-18 Normally functioning implantable defibrillators. A continuous Holter monitoring tracing is shown. On the top strip, a rapid polymorphic tachycardia is initiated which beats more uniformly. The automatic implantable cardioverter-defibrillator (AICD) senses the rhythm and delivers a shock which restores sinus rhythm.

ventricular pacemakers may interfere with the device's ability to sense VF. Many of these problems will be circumvented by advanced devices which are currently under investigation. These newer devices have the capability to take a "second look" prior to shock delivery and thus may abort delivery for self-terminating arrhythmias. In addition, the range of candidates suitable for implantation will be expanded because the newer devices have the capability of shock therapy for patients whose arrhythmias do not cause loss of consciousness. More advanced systems are being developed which can be implanted transvenously, thus avoiding the need to perform thoracotomy.

CATHETER ABLATION FOR ARRHYTHMIAS Catheter ablation techniques are now the procedures of choice for symptomatic patients with (1) concealed or manifest (WPW) bypass tracts, (2) AV nodal reentrant SVT, and (3) poorly controlled ventricular responses to atrial tachyarrhythmias, most commonly atrial fibrillation. Successful ablation of bypass tracts and modifications of the AV node by radiofrequency energy are extremely successful and cost-effective and are the procedure of choice for patients with recurrent episodes (see Figs. 198-19 and 198-20). The creation of AV block with implantation of a pacemaker is the method of choice in managing patients with atrial fibrillation and poorly controlled ventricular response.

SURGICAL TREATMENT OF ARRHYTHMIAS

Programmed stimulation and endocardial activation mapping have provided a better understanding of the mechanisms and sites of origin of many supraventricular and ventricular tachyarrhythmias so that in selected patients surgical treatment may be considered.

WOLFF-PARKINSON-WHITE SYNDROME Until the development of catheter ablation, surgery was the preferred form of therapy in patients with recurrent arrhythmias. However, advances made in the localization and surgical ablation of bypass tracts now allow for

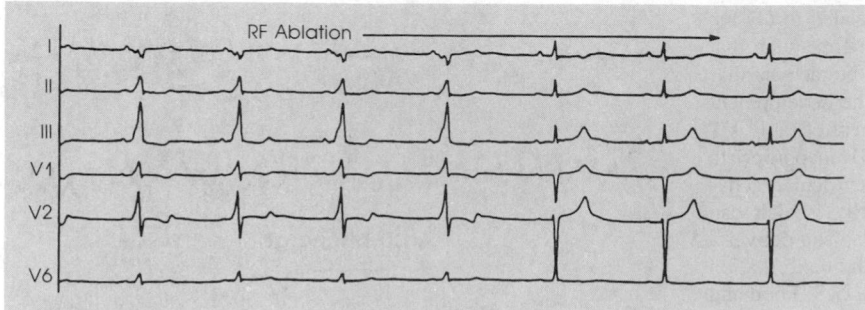

FIGURE 198-19 Radiofrequency ablation in Wolff-Parkinson-White syndrome. Leads I, II, III, V$_1$, V$_2$, and V$_6$ are shown. Preexcitation using a left lateral bypass tract is present in the final four complexes. Following the third complex, radiofrequency energy is applied. By the second beat, preexcitation is lost as the bypass tract is destroyed.

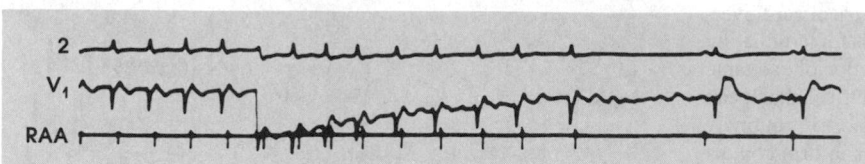

FIGURE 198-20 Ablation of AV nodal reentrant tachycardia. Leads II and V$_1$, along with a right append-age electrode (RAA), are shown. AV nodal reentry is present at the time radiofrequency energy is delivered between the coronary sinus and tricuspid valve. The tachycardia slows and is terminated by block in the slow pathway. *(After Calkins et al.)*

an extremely high success rate with minimal morbidity. As a result, surgery can now be considered not only in patients with drug-refractory arrhythmias but also as a reasonable alternative in patients in whom a bypass tract is present who undergo cardiac surgery for other reasons.

SUPRAVENTRICULAR TACHYCARDIA AND OTHER ATRIAL ARRHYTHMIAS   Although atrial flutter, AF, and PSVT are usually not life-threatening, they may be refractory to pharmacologic or pacing interventions. In such cases, surgery may be considered as a method of removing the abnormal focus, interrupting the reentry circuits, and curing the tachycardia or controlling the ventricular response by creating AV block. However, radiofrequency catheter ablation is now the therapy of choice for these arrhythmias. In atrial flutter and AF, the pathophysiologic substrate cannot be identified; thus the only option is to destroy the AV node–His bundle region by cryosurgery or transvenous catheter electroablation. Surgery, cryoablation, or electrode catheter ablation requires concomitant implantation of a permanent pacemaker. Focal atrial tachycardias have been treated surgically by discrete resection or ablation by cryothermal injury. Mapping the tachycardia is mandatory if a primary direct approach on the arrhythmia is to be performed. Surgery is for patients with arrhythmias refractory to other treatments and only when the tachycardia has been localized.

VENTRICULAR TACHYCARDIA   The demonstration that VT due to ischemic heart disease can often be reliably induced by programmed stimulation and that the arrhythmia is localized to a small region of endocardium in the area of prior infarction has permitted the development of specific surgical techniques for the cure of the arrhythmia.

Preoperatively, all morphologically distinct tachycardias that occur spontaneously are induced by programmed stimulation, and their respective sites of origin are determined by catheter activation mapping. Catheter mapping may be supplemented by intraoperative mapping, involving similar techniques. These studies have shown that tachycardias arise in the scar tissue near the endocardium.

Subendocardial resection and endocardial encircling ventriculotomy or cryoablation, the surgical techniques that have been applied to the management of ventricular tachycardia, are aimed at removing or isolating the pathophysiologic substrate of the arrhythmia, as identified by mapping. The major criterion for surgical success is the ability to localize the site from which the arrhythmias arise.

BRUGADA J et al: The complexity of mechanisms in ventricular tachycardia. PACE Pacing Clin Electrophysiol 16:680, 1993

CALKINS H et al: Diagnosis and cure of the Wolff-Parkinson-White syndrome or paroxsymal supraventricular tachycardias during a single electrophysiologic test. N Engl J Med 324:1612, 1991

COX JL: Surgical management of cardiac arrhythmias, in *Cardiac Pacing and Electrophysiology*. N El-Sherif, P Samet (eds). Philadelphia, Saunders, 1991, p 436

DREIFUS LS: Guidelines for implantation of cardiac pacemakers and antiarrhythmic devices: A report of the American College of Cardiology/American Heart Association Task Force on Assessment of Diagnostic and Therapeutic Cardiovascular Procedures (Committee on Pacemaker Implantation). J Am Coll Cardiol 18:1, 1991

ECHT DS et al: Mortality and morbidity in patients receiving encainide, flecainide, or placebo: The Cardiac Arrhythmia Suppression Trial (CAST). N Engl J Med 324:781, 1991

GUARDIAN MULTICENTER INVESTIGATORS GROUP: Long term multicenter experience with a second-generation implantable pacemaker-defibrillator in patients with malignant ventricular tachyarrhythmias. J Am Coll Cardiol 19:490, 1992

GUIRAUDON GM et al: Surgery for atrial flutter, atrial fibrillation, and atrial tachycardia, in *Cardiac Electrophysiology: From Cell to Bedside*, DP Zipes, J Jalife (eds). Philadelphia, Saunders, 1990, p 915

JACKMAN WM et al: Catheter ablation of accessory atrioventricular pathways (Wolff-Parkinson-White syndrome) by radiofrequency current. N Engl J Med 324: 1605, 1991

JOSEPHSON ME: *Clinical Cardiac Electrophysiology*, 2d ed. Philadelphia, Lea & Febiger, 1993

KIM YH et al: Nonpharmacologic therapies in patients with ventricular tachyarrhythmias. Catheter ablation and ventricular tachycardia surgery. Cardiol Clin 11:85, 1993

KUTALEK SP, DREIFUS LS: Implantable cardioverter-defibrillators. Adv Intern Med 38:421, 1993

PRITCHETT ELC: Management of atrial fibrillation. N Engl J Med 326:1264, 1991

RODEN DM: Treatment of cardiovascular diseases: Arrhythmias, in *Clinical Pharmacology: Basic Principles in Therapeutics*, KL Melmon et al (eds). New York, McGraw-Hill, 1992, pp 151–185

SCHEINMAN MM et al: Current role of catheter ablation procedures in patients with cardiac arrhythmias: A report for health professionals from the Subcommittee on Electrocardiography and Electrophysiology, American Heart Association. Circulation 83:2146, 1991

WYSE DG: Pharmacologic therapy in patients with ventricular tachyarrhythmias. Cardiol Clin 11:65, 1993

ZIPES DP: Specific arrhythmias: Diagnosis and treatment, in *Heart Disease: A Textbook of Cardiovascular Medicine*, 4th ed, E Braunwald (ed). Philadelphia, Saunders, 1992, pp 667–725

———: Genesis of cardiac arrhythmias: Electrophysiological considerations, in *Heart Disease: A Textbook of Cardiovascular Medicine*, 4th ed, E Braunwald (ed). Philadelphia, Saunders, 1992, pp 588–627

———: Management of cardiac arrhythmias: Pharmacological, electrical, and surgical techniques, in *Heart Disease: A Textbook of Cardiovascular Medicine*, 4th ed, E Braunwald (ed). Philadelphia, Saunders, 1992, pp 628–667

———: Cardiac pacemakers and antiarrhythmic devices, in *Heart Disease: A Textbook of Cardiovascular Medicine*, 4th ed, E Braunwald (ed). Philadelphia, Saunders, 1992, pp 726–755

REFERENCES

ALMENDRAL J et al: The importance of antitachycardia pacing for patients presenting with ventricular tachycardia. PACE Pacing Clin Electrophysiol 16:535, 1993

199 CONGENITAL HEART DISEASE IN THE ADULT

WILLIAM F. FRIEDMAN / JOHN S. CHILD

Congenital heart disease complicates approximately 1 percent of all live births. Substantial numbers of affected infants reach adulthood because of successful medical and/or surgical management, or because the alteration caused in cardiovascular physiology is well tolerated.

GENERAL CONSIDERATIONS

ETIOLOGY AND PREVENTION Congenital cardiovascular malformations are generally the result of aberrant embryonic development of a normal structure, or failure of such a structure to progress beyond an early stage of embryonic or fetal development. Malformations are due to complex multifactorial genetic and environmental causes. Recognized chromosomal aberrations and mutations of single genes account for less than 10 percent of all cardiac malformations (Table 199-1).

The presence of a cardiac malformation as one component of the multiple system involvement in Down's, Turner's, and the trisomy 13-15(D_1) and 17-18 (E) syndromes may be anticipated in occasional pregnancies by detection of abnormal chromosomes in fetal cells obtained from amniotic fluid or chorionic villus biopsy. Identification in such cells of the enzyme disorders characteristic of Hurler's syndrome, homocystinuria, or type II glycogen storage disease may also allow one to predict cardiac disease.

The feasibility of preventive programs will depend upon what is learned in the future about the cause of the majority of cardiovascular anomalies for which no cause is known. An effective rubella vaccine is available, and immunization of children with this vaccine may lessen maternal rubella and its cardiac consequences. Strict testing in animals of new drugs that can be teratogenic when taken early in pregnancy may reduce the chances of another thalidomide tragedy. In this regard, no medications should be taken during pregnancy without prior consultation with a physician. Physicians should be aware of known teratogens, as well as of drugs for which inadequate information exists as to teratogenic potential. Appropriate use of radiologic equipment and techniques for reducing gonadal and fetal radiation exposure should always be employed to reduce the hazards of birth defects.

PATHOPHYSIOLOGY The anatomic and physiologic changes in the heart and circulation due to any specific congenital cardiocirculatory lesion are not static, but rather progress from prenatal life to adulthood. Thus, malformations which are benign, or escape detection in childhood, may become clinically significant in the adult. For example, the functionally normal, congenitally bicuspid aortic valve may thicken and calcify with time, resulting in significant aortic stenosis; or the well-tolerated left-to-right shunt of an atrial septal defect may not result in cardiac decompensation, with or without pulmonary hypertension, until the fourth or fifth decade.

There are issues of particular concern to the *adult* with congenital heart disease that we will discuss separately in this chapter, including pulmonary hypertension and Eisenmenger syndrome of pulmonary vascular obstruction, the hematologic consequences of cyanotic heart disease, the special considerations of pregnancy in the woman with congenital heart disease, and problems involving employability and insurability.

Pulmonary hypertension This is a common accompaniment of many congenital cardiac lesions, and the status of the pulmonary vascular bed is often the principal determinant of the clinical manifestations, the course, and the feasibility of surgical repair. Increases in pulmonary arterial pressure result from elevation of pulmonary blood flow and/or resistance, the latter due sometimes to an increase in vascular tone but usually the result of obstructive, obliterative structural changes within the pulmonary vascular bed. Because pulmonary vascular obstructive disease can be the determining factor in assessing the advisability of operation, it is important to quantify and compare pulmonary to systemic flows and resistances in patients with severe pulmonary hypertension. The causes of pulmonary vascular obstructive disease are unknown, although increased pulmonary blood flow, increased pulmonary arterial blood pressure, elevated pulmonary venous pressure, polycythemia, systemic hypoxemia, acidosis, and the bronchial circulation have been implicated. The designation *Eisenmenger syndrome* is applied to patients with a large communication between the two circulations at the aortopulmonary, ventricular, or atrial levels and bidirectional or predominantly right-to-left shunts because of high-resistance and obstructive pulmonary hypertension. No specific treatment has proved beneficial for obstructive pulmonary vascular disease, although single lung transplantation and intracardiac defect repair, or total heart-lung transplantation show promise (see Chaps. 196 and 232).

Erythrocytosis The chronic hypoxemia in cyanotic congenital heart disease results in *erythrocytosis* due to increased erythropoietin production (see Chap. 32). The commonly used term *polycythemia* is a misnomer because white cell counts are normal and platelet counts are normal to decreased. Cyanotic patients with erythrocytosis may have compensated or decompensated hematocrits. Compensated erythrocytosis with iron-replete equilibrium hematocrits rarely results in symptoms of hyperviscosity at hematocrits less than 65 percent and occasionally with hematocrits of 70 percent or more. Therapeutic phlebotomy is rarely required in compensated erythrocytosis. In contrast, patients with decompensated erythrocytosis fail to establish equilibrium with unstable, rising hematocrits and recurrent hyperviscosity symptoms. Therapeutic phlebotomy, a two-edged sword, allows temporary relief of symptoms but begets instability of the hematocrit and compounds the problem by iron depletion. Iron-deficiency symptoms are usually indistinguishable from those of hyperviscosity; progressive symptoms after recurrent phlebotomy are usually due to iron depletion with hypochromic microcytosis. Iron depletion results in a larger number of smaller (microcytic) hypochromic red cells that are less capable of carrying oxygen and less deformable in the microcirculation. Because these microcytes are less deformable in the microcirculation and there are more of them relative to the plasma volume, the viscosity is greater than for an equivalent hematocrit with fewer, larger, iron-replete, deformable cells. As such, iron-depleted erythrocytosis results in increasing symptoms due to decreased oxygen delivery to the tissues.

Hemostasis is abnormal in cyanotic congenital heart disease, due in part to the increased blood volume and engorged capillaries, abnormalities in platelet function and sensitivity to aspirin or nonsteroidal anti-inflammatory agents, and abnormalities of the extrinsic and intrinsic coagulation system. Oral contraceptives are contraindicated for cyanotic women because of the enhanced risk of vascular thrombosis.

The risk of stroke is greatest in children less than 4 years old with cyanotic heart disease and iron deficiency, often with dehydration as an aggravating cause. In contrast, adults with cyanotic congenital heart disease do not appear to be at increased risk for stroke, unless there are excessive, injudicious phlebotomies or inappropriate use of aspirin or anticoagulants.

Symptoms of hyperviscosity can be produced in any cyanotic patient with erythrocytosis if dehydration causes a reduction of plasma volume. Phlebotomy, when required for symptoms of hyperviscosity not due to dehydration or iron deficiency, is a simple outpatient removal of 500 mL of blood over 45 min with isovolumetric replacement with isotonic saline (5% dextrose if congestive heart failure exists). Acute phlebotomy without volume replacement is contraindicated. Iron repletion in decompensated iron-depleted erythrocytosis ameliorates iron-deficiency symptoms but must be done gradually to avoid a sudden excessive rise in hematocrit and resultant hyperviscosity.

TABLE 199-1   Syndromes with associated cardiovascular involvement

Syndrome	Major cardiovascular manifestations	Major noncardiac abnormalities
HERITABLE AND POSSIBLY HERITABLE		
Ellis–van Creveld	Single atrium or atrial septal defect	Chondrodystrophic dwarfism, nail dysplasia, polydactyly
TAR (thrombocytopenia-absent radius)	Atrial septal defect, tetralogy of Fallot	Radial aplasia or hypoplasia, thrombocytopenia
Holt-Oram	Atrial septal defect (other defects common)	Skeletal upper limb defect, hypoplasia of clavicles
Kartagener	Dextrocardia	Situs inversus, sinusitis, bronchiectasis
Laurence-Moon-Biedl	Variable defects	Retinal pigmentation, obesity, polydactyly
Noonan	Pulmonary valve dysplasia, cardiomyopathy (usually hypertrophic)	Webbed neck, pectus excavatum, cryptorchidism
Tuberous sclerosis	Rhabdomyoma, cardiomyopathy	Phakomatosis, bone lesions, hamartomatous skin lesions
Multiple lentigines (leopard) syndrome	Pulmonic stenosis	Basal cell nevi, broad facies, rib anomalies
Rubenstein-Taybi	Patent ductus arteriosus (others)	Broad thumbs and toes, hypoplastic maxilla, slanted palpebral fissures
Familial deafness	Arrhythmias, sudden death	Sensorineural deafness
Osler-Rendu-Weber	Arteriovenous fistulas (lung, liver, mucous membranes)	Multiple telangiectasia
Apert	Ventricular septal defect	Craniosynostosis, midfacial hypoplasia, syndactyly
Incontinentia pigmenti	Patent ductus arteriosus	Irregular pigmented skin lesions, patchy alopecia, hypodontia
Alagille (arteriohepatic dysplasia)	Peripheral pulmonic stenosis, pulmonic stenosis	Biliary hypoplasia, vertebral anomalies, prominent forehead, deep-set eyes
DiGeorge	Interrupted aortic arch, tetralogy of Fallot, truncus arteriosus	Thymic hypoplasia or aplasia, parathyroid aplasia or hypoplasia, ear anomalies
Friedreich's ataxia	Cardiomyopathy and conduction defects	Ataxia, speech defect, degeneration of spinal cord dorsal columns
Muscular dystrophy	Cardiomyopathy	Pseudohypertrophy of calf muscles, weakness of trunk and proximal limb muscles
Cystic fibrosis	Cor pulmonale	Pancreatic insufficiency, malabsorption, chronic lung disease
Sickle cell anemia	Cardiomyopathy, mitral regurgitation	Hemoglobin SS
Conradi-Hünermann	Ventricular septal defect, patent ductus arteriosus	Asymmetric limb shortness, early punctate mineralization, large skin pores
Cockayne	Accelerated atherosclerosis	Cachectic dwarfism, retinal pigment abnormalities, photosensitivity dermatitis
Progeria	Accelerated atherosclerosis	Premature aging, alopecia, atrophy of subcutaneous fat, skeletal hypoplasia
CONNECTIVE TISSUE DISORDERS		
Cutis laxa	Peripheral pulmonic stenosis	Generalized disruption of elastic fibers, diminished skin resilience, hernias
Ehlers-Danlos	Arterial dilatation and rupture, mitral regurgitation	Hyperextensible joints, hyperelastic and friable skin
Marfan	Aortic dilatation, aortic and mitral incompetence	Gracile habitus, arachnodactyly with hyperextensibility, lens subluxation
Osteogenesis imperfecta	Aortic incompetence	Fragile bones, blue sclera
Pseudoxanthoma elasticum	Peripheral and coronary arterial disease	Degeneration of elastic fibers in skin, retinal angioid streaks
INBORN ERRORS OF METABOLISM		
Pompe's disease	Glycogen storage disease of heart	Acid maltase deficiency, muscular weakness
Homocystinuria	Aortic and pulmonary arterial dilatation, intravascular thrombosis	Cystathionine synthetase deficiency, lens subluxation, osteoporosis
Mucopolysaccharidosis: Hurler, Hunter	Multivalvular and coronary and great artery disease, cardiomyopathy	Hurler: Deficiency of α-l-iduronidase, corneal clouding, coarse features, growth and mental retardation Hunter: Deficiency of l-iduranosulfate sulfatase, coarse facies, clear cornea, growth and mental retardation
Morquio, Scheie, Maroteaux-Lamy	Aortic incompetence	Morquio: Deficiency of N-acetylhexosamine sulfate sulfatase, cloudy cornea, normal intelligence, severe bony changes involving vertebrae and epiphyses Scheie: Deficiency of α-l-iduronidase, cloudy cornea, normal intelligence, peculiar facies Maroteaux-Lamy: Deficiency of arylsulfatase B, cloudy cornea, osseous changes, normal intelligence
CHROMOSOMAL ABNORMALITIES		
Trisomy 21 (Down's syndrome)	Endocardial cushion defect, atrial or ventricular septal defect, tetralogy of Fallot	Hypotonia, hyperextensible joints, mongoloid facies, mental retardation
Trisomy 13 (D)	Ventricular septal defect, patent ductus arteriosus, double-outlet right ventricle	Single midline intracerebral ventricle with midfacial defects, polydactyly, nail changes, mental retardation

TABLE 199-1	Syndromes with associated cardiovascular involvement *(continued)*	
Syndrome	Major cardiovascular manifestations	Major noncardiac abnormalities
CHROMOSOMAL ABNORMALITIES *(continued)*		
Trisomy 18 (E)	Congenital polyvalvular dysplasia, ventricular septal defect, patent ductus arteriosus	Clenched hand, short sternum, low-arch dermal-ridge pattern on fingertips, mental retardation
Cri-du-chat (short-arm deletion-5)	Ventricular septal defect	Cat cry, microcephaly, antimongoloid slant of palpebral fissures, mental retardation
XO (Turner)	Coarctation of aorta, bicuspid aortic valve	Short female, broad chest, lymphedema, webbed neck
XXXY and XXXXX	Patent ductus arteriosus	XXXY: hypogenitalism, mental retardation, radial-ulnar synostosis XXXXX: small hands, incurving of fifth fingers, mental retardation
SPORADIC DISORDERS		
VATER association	Ventricular septal defect	Vertebral anomalies, anal atresia, tracheo-esophageal fistula, radial and renal anomalies
CHARGE association	Tetralogy of Fallot (other defects common)	Colobomas, choanal atresia, mental and growth deficiency, genital and ear anomalies
Williams	Supravalvular aortic stenosis, peripheral pulmonic stenosis	Mental deficiency, ''elfin'' facies, loquacious personality, hoarse voice
Cornelia de Lange	Ventricular septal defect	Micromelia, synophrys, mental and growth deficiency
Shprintzen (velocardiofacial)	Ventricular septal defect, tetralogy of Fallot, right aortic arch	Cleft palate, prominent nose, slender hands, learning disability
TERATOGENIC DISORDERS		
Rubella	Patent ductus arteriosus, pulmonic valvular and/or arterial stenosis, atrial septal defect	Cataracts, deafness, microcephaly
Alcohol-induced	Ventricular septal defect (other defects)	Microcephaly, growth and mental deficiency, short palpebral fissures, smooth philtrum, thin upper lip
Phenytoin-induced	Pulmonic stenosis, aortic stenosis, coarctation, patent ductus arteriosus	Hypertelorism, growth and mental deficiency, short phalanges, bowed upper lip
Thalidomide-induced	Variable	Phocomelia
Lithium-induced	Ebstein's anomaly, tricuspid atresia	None

PREGNANCY The presence of congenital heart disease or its consequences may pose special problems for the pregnant woman. Thus, pregnant women with pulmonary vascular obstruction, whether pre- or postoperative, are at risk of dying during delivery or in the immediate postpartum period. The cause of the increased mortality rate is poorly understood. A particularly high mortality rate has been reported for those undergoing a cesarean section, although such surgery should cause less cardiovascular stress than that of labor and vaginal delivery. Irrespective of approach to delivery, some simple guidelines include both continuous administration of oxygen and avoidance of inhalant anesthetic agents. Arterial blood gases and, if possible, pulmonary arterial and systemic blood pressure should be monitored serially throughout delivery and the early postpartum period. Some physicians advise early abortion in women with marked pulmonary vascular obstruction because of the risks of pregnancy, and all such women should receive counseling on birth control. Intrauterine devices should be avoided because of the risks of bleeding and infection; oral contraceptive agents are contraindicated because they are associated with a tendency to develop pulmonary vascular or cerebrovascular thrombosis. Use of a barrier method of birth control is preferable. Prevention of pregnancy is safer than any form of management during pregnancy, labor, delivery, and the postpartum period.

In women with regurgitant or obstructive left-side valvular lesions, the increased volume and/or pressure load on the left atrium or left ventricle imposed by the augmentation in blood volume during pregnancy may result in pulmonary edema, requiring vigorous cardiac decongestive measures (Chap. 31). With medical control of the pulmonary edema, a normal vaginal delivery with careful local and epidural anesthesia is preferable to nonvaginal delivery.

A unique problem exists in women whose congenital heart disease has been corrected with the use of a prosthetic cardiac valve and/or conduit. Such women are at risk for thromboembolism and/or obstruction of their conduits or valves, and are thus, usually, on anticoagulants. Early in pregnancy, coumarin derivatives cause an increase in abortion and stillbirth and in craniofacial, neurologic, and other birth defects. Moreover, the transplacental passage of oral anticoagulants places the fetus at risk of intracranial hemorrhage during delivery. Accordingly, coumarin derivatives should be avoided early (before 10 weeks) and late (after 32 weeks) in pregnancy, and subcutaneous or intravenous heparin should be substituted, although heparin, to a lesser degree, also has been associated with adverse fetal outcome.

INFECTIVE ENDOCARDITIS (See also Chap. 85) Routine antimicrobial prophylaxis is recommended for all patients with congenital heart disease and for the majority of patients after operative repair of the lesion, but it should be recognized that antibiotic prophylaxis is not uniformly effective. Nonetheless, it is recommended for all dental procedures, gastrointestinal and genitourinary surgery, and diagnostic procedures such as proctosigmoidoscopy and cystoscopy. The clinical and bacteriologic profile of infective endocarditis in patients with congenital heart disease has changed with the advent of intracardiac surgery and of prosthetic devices. Two major predisposing causes of infective endocarditis are a susceptible cardiovascular substrate and a source of bacteremia. Prophylaxis includes both chemotherapeutic (antimicrobial) and nonchemotherapeutic (hygienic) measures. Meticulous dental and skin care is required.

EXERCISE Advice on athletics and exercise is governed by the nature of the exercise and by the type and severity of the congenital cardiovascular lesion. Patients with lesions characterized by left ventricular outflow tract obstruction, if more than mild to moderate, or pulmonary vascular disease risk syncope or even sudden death. In Fallot's tetralogy, isotonic exercise–induced decrease in systemic vascular resistance relative to the right ventricular outflow obstruction augments the right-to-left shunt, increases hypoxemia, and causes an increase in subjective breathlessness due to the response of the respiratory center to the changes in blood gases and pH.

INSURABILITY AND EMPLOYABILITY Most patients with congenital heart disease must pay significantly more than standard life insurance rates, assuming their anomaly places them in a category that companies have determined is eligible for insurance. There is a paucity of actuarial survival data beyond adolescence for most cardiac lesions that have undergone operative repair. Accordingly, it is often difficult to convince insurance companies to offer insurance at reasonable cost to individual patients whose long-term prognosis is quite good.

Employment is affected by the patient's physical capacity relative to the type of job sought. Job discrimination exists, often because the employer is reluctant to accept health insurance responsibilities. Further, eligibility for some occupations is governed by public safety regulations, e.g., airline pilots, bus drivers.

SPECIFIC CARDIAC DEFECTS

Various classifications of congenital cardiovascular lesions have been proposed, depending on hemodynamic, anatomic, and radiographic factors. Table 199-2 provides a classification of cardiac anomalies that recognizes the general categories of clinical presentation, functional consequences, and site of origin of congenital defects. The text of this section focuses selectively on the more common or important congenital cardiac malformations in adults, whereas Table 199-2 presents a comprehensive list of lesions. Cardiac lesions are organized into those that do or do not result in cyanosis. The acyanotic group is subdivided into malformations with and without a left-to-right shunt. The shunt lesions are segregated by the principal site of communication between the systemic and pulmonary circulations. The acyanotic lesions without a shunt are distinguished by the location of the lesion in the left or right heart and by inflow versus outflow regions on either side of the circulation. Cyanotic lesions are classified with respect to pulmonary blood flow because the radiographic determination of its magnitude provides an insight into whether the cyanosis is the result of an obligatory admixture of systemic and pulmonary venous return (increased pulmonary blood flow), or of reduced pulmonary blood flow (pulmonary stenosis), or of pulmonary hypertension due to pulmonary vascular obstruction.

Categorizing the defect(s) in an individual patient requires an answer to a number of basic questions. Is the patient acyanotic or cyanotic? Is pulmonary arterial blood flow increased or not? Does the malformation originate in the left or right side of the heart? Which is the dominant ventricle? Is pulmonary hypertension present or not? With the above information as a foundation, using more refined diagnostic techniques such as transthoracic (precordial) and transesophageal echocardiography and Doppler imaging, magnetic resonance imaging, and/or hemodynamic study and angiocardiography leads to a precise anatomic and functional assessment.

ACYANOTIC CONGENITAL HEART DISEASE WITH A LEFT-TO-RIGHT SHUNT

ATRIAL SEPTAL DEFECT This is a commonly recognized cardiac anomaly in adults and occurs more frequently in females than in males. Defects of the *sinus venosus* type occur high in the atrial septum near the entry of the superior vena cava and are associated frequently with anomalous connection of pulmonary veins from the right lung to the junction of the superior vena cava and right atrium. Sinus venosus defects may also occur low in the atrial septum near the inferior vena cava orifice, associated with anomalous connection of the right inferior pulmonary vein to the right atrium. *Ostium primum* anomalies are a form of atrioventricular septal defect that lie immediately adjacent to the atrioventricular valves, either of which

---

TABLE 199-2 Classification of congenital heart disease

ACYANOTIC WITH LEFT-TO-RIGHT SHUNT

Atrial level shunt:
1 Atrial septal defect
  a Ostium primum
  b Ostium secundum
  c Sinus venosus
2 Atrial septal defect with mitral stenosis (Lutembacher's syndrome)
3 Partial anomalous pulmonary venous connection
Ventricular level shunt:
1 Ventricular septal defect
  a Inlet septum
  b Muscular septum
  c Perimembranous septum
  d Infundibular septum
2 Ventricular septal defect with aortic regurgitation
3 Ventricular septal defect with left ventricular to right atrial shunt
Aortic root to right heart shunt:
1 Ruptured sinus of Valsalva aneurysm
2 Coronary arteriovenous fistula
3 Anomalous origin of the left coronary artery from the pulmonary trunk
Aortopulmonary level shunt:
1 Aortopulmonary window
2 Patent ductus arteriosus
Multiple level shunts:
1 Complete common atrioventricular canal
2 Ventricular septal defect with atrial septal defect
3 Ventricular septal defect with patent ductus arteriosus

ACYANOTIC WITHOUT A SHUNT

Left heart malformations:
1 Congenital obstruction to left atrial inflow
  a Pulmonary vein stenosis
  b Mitral stenosis
  c Cor triatriatum
2 Mitral regurgitation
  a Atrioventricular septal (endocardial cushion)
  b Congenitally corrected transposition of the great arteries
  c Anomalous origin of the left coronary artery from the pulmonary trunk
  d Miscellaneous (double-orifice mitral valve, congenital perforations, accessory commissures with anomalous chordal insertion, congenitally short or absent chordae, cleft posterior leaflet, parachute mitral valve, etc.)
3 Primary dilated endocardial fibroelastosis
4 Aortic stenosis
  a Discrete subvalvular
  b Valvular
  c Supravalvular
5 Aortic valve regurgitation
6 Coarctation of the aorta
Right heart malformations:
1 Acyanotic Ebstein's anomaly of the tricuspid valve
2 Pulmonic stenosis
  a Subinfundibular
  b Infundibular
  c Valvular
  d Supravalvular (stenosis of pulmonary artery and its branches)
3 Congenital pulmonary valve regurgitation
4 Idiopathic dilatation of the pulmonary trunk

CYANOTIC

Increased pulmonary blood flow:
1 Complete transposition of the great arteries
2 Double-outlet right ventricle of the Taussig-Bing type
3 Truncus arteriosus
4 Total anomalous pulmonary venous connection
5 Single ventricle without pulmonic stenosis
6 Common atrium
7 Tetralogy of Fallot with pulmonary atresia and increased collateral arterial flow
8 Tricuspid atresia with large ventricular septal defect and no pulmonic stenosis
9 Hypoplastic left heart (aortic atresia, mitral atresia)
Normal or decreased pulmonary blood flow:
1 Tricuspid atresia
2 Ebstein's anomaly with right-to-left atrial shunt
3 Pulmonary atresia with intact ventricular septum
4 Pulmonic stenosis or atresia with ventricular septal defect (tetralogy of Fallot)

TABLE 199-2 Classification of congenital heart disease (*continued*)

CYANOTIC (*continued*)

5 Pulmonic stenosis with right-to-left atrial shunt
6 Complete transposition of the great arteries with pulmonic stenosis
7 Double-outlet right ventricle with pulmonic stenosis
8 Single ventricle with pulmonic stenosis
9 Pulmonary arteriovenous fistula
10 Vena caval to left atrial communication

OTHER

Congenitally corrected transposition of the great arteries
The cardiac malpositions
Congenital complete heart block

SOURCE: Modified from JK Perloff, 1987.

may be deformed and incompetent. Ostium primum defects occur commonly in patients with Down's syndrome, although the more complex atrioventricular septal defects with a common atrioventricular valve and a posterior defect of the basal portion of the interventricular septum are more characteristic of this chromosomal defect. Most often an atrial defect involves the fossa ovalis, is midseptal in location, and is of the *ostium secundum* type. This type of defect should not be confused with a *patent foramen ovale*. Anatomic obliteration of the foramen ovale ordinarily follows its functional closure soon after birth, but residual "probe patency" is a normal variant; atrial septal defect denotes a true deficiency of the atrial septum and implies functional and anatomic patency. *Lutembacher's syndrome* is the term applied to the rare combination of atrial septal defect and mitral stenosis, usually due to acquired rheumatic valvulitis.

The magnitude of the left-to-right shunt through an atrial septal defect depends on the defect size, the diastolic properties of both ventricles, and the relative impedance in the pulmonary and systemic circulations. The left-to-right shunt causes diastolic overloading of the right ventricle and increased pulmonary blood flow.

Patients with atrial septal defect are usually asymptomatic in early life, although there may be some physical underdevelopment and an increased tendency for respiratory infections; cardiorespiratory symptoms occur in many older patients. Beyond the fourth decade, a significant number of patients develop atrial arrhythmias, pulmonary arterial hypertension, bidirectional and then right-to-left shunting of blood, and cardiac failure. Patients exposed to the chronic environmental hypoxia of high altitude tend to develop pulmonary hypertension at younger ages. In some older patients, left-to-right shunting across the defect increases as progressive systemic hypertension and/or coronary artery disease result in reduced compliance of the left ventricle.

Physical examination Examination usually reveals a prominent right ventricular cardiac impulse and palpable pulmonary artery pulsation. The first heart sound is normal or split, with accentuation of the tricuspid valve closure sound. Increased flow across the pulmonic valve is responsible for a midsystolic pulmonary ejection murmur. The second heart sound is widely split and is relatively fixed in relation to respiration. A middiastolic rumbling murmur, loudest at the fourth intercostal space and along the left sternal border, reflects increased flow across the tricuspid valve. In patients with ostium primum defects, an apical thrill and holosystolic murmur indicate associated mitral or tricuspid incompetence or a ventricular septal defect.

The physical findings are altered when an increase in the pulmonary vascular resistance results in diminution of the left-to-right shunt. Both the pulmonary and tricuspid murmurs decrease in intensity, the pulmonic component of the second heart sound and a systolic ejection sound are accentuated, the two components of the second heart sound may fuse, and a diastolic murmur of pulmonic incompetence appears. Cyanosis and clubbing accompany the development of a right-to-left shunt.

In adults with atrial fibrillation and an atrial septal defect, the physical findings may be confused with the findings of mitral stenosis with pulmonary hypertension because the tricuspid flow murmur and widely split second heart sound may be mistakenly thought to represent the diastolic murmur of mitral stenosis and the mitral "opening snap," respectively.

Electrocardiogram In patients with an ostium secundum defect the ECG usually shows right axis deviation and an rSr' pattern in the right precordial leads representing delayed posterobasal activation of the ventricular septum and enlargement of the right ventricular outflow tract. An ectopic atrial pacemaker or first-degree heart block occurs occasionally in patients with defects of the sinus venosus type. In patients with an ostium primum defect, the right ventricular conduction defect is characteristically accompanied by left axis deviation and by superior orientation and counterclockwise rotation of the QRS loop in the frontal plane. Varying degrees of right ventricular and right atrial hypertrophy may occur with each type of defect, depending on the height of the pulmonary artery pressure; prolongation of the PR interval is most common with ostium primum defects. *Chest roentgenograms* reveal enlargement of the right atrium and ventricle, dilatation of the pulmonary artery and its branches, and increased pulmonary vascular marking. Left atrial enlargement is uncommon in the absence of atrial fibrillation.

Echocardiogram This shows pulmonary arterial and right ventricular dilatation, and anterior systolic (paradoxical) or flat interventricular septal motion if a significant right ventricular volume overload is present. The defect may be visualized directly from subcostal, right parasternal, or apical echocardiographic windows. In most institutions, two-dimensional echocardiography, supplemented by conventional or color Doppler flow examination, has supplanted cardiac catheterization as the confirmatory test for atrial septal defect. Transesophageal echocardiography is indicated if the transthoracic echocardiogram is ambiguous, which is often the case with sinus venosus defects. Cardiac catheterization is then employed if inconsistencies exist in the clinical data, if significant pulmonary hypertension or associated malformations are suspected, or if coronary artery disease is a possibility.

Management Operative repair, ideally in children between 3 and 6 years of age, should be advised for all patients with uncomplicated atrial septal defects in whom there is significant left-to-right shunting, i.e., with pulmonary-to-systemic flow ratios exceeding approximately 2.0:1.0. Excellent results may be anticipated, at low risk, even in patients beyond 40 years of age in the absence of pulmonary hypertension. The defect is closed, usually with a patch of pericardium or of prosthetic material with the patient on cardiopulmonary bypass. In patients with ostium primum defects cleft, deformed, and incompetent valves often require repair. Intraoperative transesophageal echocardiography is used to monitor the surgical results of mitral valve repair. Operation should not be carried out in patients with small defects and trivial left-to-right shunts, or in those with severe pulmonary vascular disease without a significant left-to-right shunt.

Atrioventricular septal defects more complex than the ostium primum defect are associated with failure to thrive, heart failure, and pulmonary hypertension early in life and require operative correction in infancy. Patients with atrial septal defect of the sinus venosus or ostium secundum types rarely die before the fifth decade. During the fifth and sixth decades the incidence of progressive symptoms, often leading to severe disability, increases substantially. Medical management should include prompt treatment of respiratory tract infections, antiarrhythmic medications for atrial fibrillation or supraventricular tachycardia, and the usual measures for hypertension, coronary disease, or heart failure (see Chap. 195), if these complications occur. The risk of infective endocarditis is quite low unless the defect is complicated by valvular regurgitation or has recently been repaired with a patch (see Chap. 85).

VENTRICULAR SEPTAL DEFECT Defects of the ventricular septum are common as isolated defects and as one component of a combination of anomalies. The opening is usually single and situated in the membranous portion of the septum. The functional disturbance is dependent primarily on its size and on the status of the pulmonary vascular bed, rather than on the location of the defect. Only small or moderate-size defects are usually seen initially in adulthood as the vast majority of patients with isolated large defects come to medical and, often, surgical attention very early in life.

A wide spectrum exists in the natural history of ventricular septal defect, ranging from spontaneous closure to congestive cardiac failure and death in early infancy. Within this spectrum is the possible development of pulmonary vascular obstruction, right ventricular outflow tract obstruction, aortic regurgitation, and infective endocarditis. Spontaneous closure is more common in patients born with a small ventricular septal defect and occurs in early childhood in most patients.

Patients with large ventricular septal defects and pulmonary hypertension are those at greatest risk for developing pulmonary vascular obstruction. Thus, large defects should be corrected surgically early in life when pulmonary vascular disease is still reversible or not yet developed. In patients with severe pulmonary vascular obstruction (Eisenmenger syndrome), symptoms in adult life consist of exertional dyspnea, chest pain, syncope, and hemoptysis. The right-to-left shunt leads to cyanosis, clubbing, and erythrocytosis. In all patients, the degree to which pulmonary vascular resistance is elevated before operation is a critical factor determining prognosis. If the pulmonary vascular resistance is one-third or less of the systemic value, progression of pulmonary vascular disease after operation is unusual. However, if a moderate to severe increase in pulmonary vascular resistance exists preoperatively, either no change or a progression of pulmonary vascular disease is common post-operatively.

Right ventricular outflow tract obstruction develops in approximately 5 to 10 percent of patients who present in infancy with a moderate to large left-to-right shunt. With time, as subvalvular right ventricular outflow tract obstruction progresses, the findings in these patients begin to resemble more closely those of the cyanotic tetralogy of Fallot.

In approximately 5 percent of patients, incompetence of the aortic valve results from insufficient cusp tissue or prolapse of the cusp through the interventricular defect; the aortic regurgitation then complicates and usually dominates the clinical course.

Two-dimensional *echocardiography* with conventional or color Doppler examination can usually define the number and location of defects in the ventricular septum and detect associated anomalies. Hemodynamic and angiographic study may be employed to assess the status of the pulmonary vascular bed and clarify details of the altered anatomy.

Management Surgery is not recommended for patients with normal pulmonary arterial pressures with small shunts (pulmonary-to-systemic flow ratios of less than 1.5 to 2.0:1.0). Operative correction is indicated when there is a moderate to large left-to-right shunt with a pulmonary-to-systemic flow ratio that exceeds 1.5:1.0 or 2.0:1.0, in the absence of prohibitively high levels of pulmonary vascular resistance.

PATENT DUCTUS ARTERIOSUS The ductus arteriosus is a vessel leading from the bifurcation of the pulmonary artery to the aorta just distal to the left subclavian artery. The vascular channel is open normally in the fetus but closes immediately after birth. The flow across the ductus is determined by the pressure and resistance relationships between the systemic and pulmonary circulations and by the cross-sectional area and length of the ductus. In most adults with this anomaly, pulmonary pressures are normal and a gradient and shunt from aorta to pulmonary artery persist throughout the cardiac cycle, resulting in a characteristic thrill and a continuous "machinery" murmur with a late systolic accentuation at the upper left sternal edge. In adults who were born with a large left-to-right shunt through the ductus arteriosus, pulmonary vascular obstruction (Eisenmenger syndrome) with pulmonary hypertension, right-to-left shunting, and cyanosis have usually developed. Severe pulmonary

vascular disease results in reversal of flow through the ductus, unoxygenated blood is shunted to the descending aorta, and the toes, but not the fingers, become cyanotic and clubbed, a finding termed *differential cyanosis*. The leading causes of death in adults with patent ductus are cardiac failure and infective endocarditis; occasionally severe pulmonary vascular obstruction may cause aneurysmal dilatation, calcification, and rupture of the ductus. In the absence of severe pulmonary vascular disease and predominant left-to-right shunting of blood, the patent ductus should be surgically ligated or divided. Operation should be deferred for several months in patients treated successfully for infective endocarditis, because the ductus may remain somewhat edematous and friable.

AORTIC ROOT TO RIGHT HEART SHUNTS The three most common causes of aortic root to right heart shunts are congenital aneurysm of an aortic sinus of Valsalva with fistula, coronary arteriovenous fistula, and anomalous origin of the left coronary artery from the pulmonary trunk. *Aneurysm of an aortic sinus of Valsalva* consists of a separation or lack of fusion between the media of the aorta and the annulus fibrosis of the aortic valve. Rupture usually occurs in the third or fourth decade of life; most often the aorticocardiac fistula is between the right coronary cusp and the right ventricle, but occasionally, when the noncoronary cusp is involved, the fistula drains into the right atrium. Abrupt rupture causes chest pain, bounding pulses, a continuous murmur accentuated in diastole, and volume overload of the heart. Diagnosis is confirmed by two-dimensional and Doppler echocardiographic studies; cardiac catheterization quantifies the left-to-right shunt, and thoracic aortography visualizes the fistula. Medical management is directed at cardiac failure, arrhythmias, or endocarditis. At operation, the aneurysm is closed and amputated, and the aortic wall is reunited with the heart, either by direct suture or with a prosthesis.

Coronary arteriovenous fistula, an unusual anomaly, consists of a communication between a coronary artery and another cardiac chamber, usually the coronary sinus or right atrium or ventricle. The shunt is usually of small magnitude, and myocardial blood flow is not usually compromised. Potential complications include infective endocarditis, thrombus formation with occlusion or distal embolization, rupture of an aneurysmal fistula, and rarely, pulmonary hypertension and congestive failure. A loud, superficial, continuous murmur at the lower or midsternal border usually prompts a further evaluation of asymptomatic patients. Doppler echocardiography demonstrates the site of drainage; if the site of origin is proximal, it may be detectable by two-dimensional echocardiography. Retrograde thoracic aortography or coronary arteriography permits identification of the size and anatomic features of the fistulous tract, which may be closed by suture obliteration.

The third anomaly causing a shunt from the aortic root to the right heart is *anomalous origin of the left coronary artery from the pulmonary artery*. As the elevated pulmonary vascular resistance declines immediately after birth, perfusion of the left coronary artery from the pulmonary artery ceases, and the direction of flow in the anomalous vessel reverses. Total myocardial perfusion must pass through the right coronary artery and may be sufficient if adequate collateral channels develop between the two coronary circulations. Myocardial infarction and fibrosis commonly lead to death within the first year, though up to 20 percent of patients survive to adolescence and beyond without surgical correction. In older children or adults, mitral regurgitation may result from dysfunction of ischemic or infarcted papillary muscles. The diagnosis of anomalous origin of the coronary artery is supported by the electrocardiographic findings of an anterolateral myocardial infarction. Aortic root or coronary angiography demonstrates the retrograde drainage of the coronary vessel into the pulmonary artery and the presence of a single right coronary artery arising from the aorta. Operative management of adults consists of coronary artery bypass with an internal mammary artery graft or saphenous vein–coronary artery graft. The outcome and prognosis are determined largely by the degree of preoperative myocardial damage.

ACYANOTIC CONGENITAL HEART DISEASE WITHOUT A SHUNT

CONGENITAL AORTIC STENOSIS Malformations that cause obstruction to left ventricular outflow include congenital valvular aortic stenosis, discrete subaortic stenosis, supervalvular aortic stenosis, and hypertrophic obstructive cardiomyopathy (Chap. 205).

Valvular aortic stenosis Valvular aortic stenosis occurs three to four times more often in males than in females. The congenital bicuspid aortic valve, which is not necessarily stenotic, is one of the most common congenital malformations of the heart, although it may go undetected in early life. Because bicuspid valves may become stenotic with time or be the site of infective endocarditis, the lesion may be difficult to distinguish in adults from acquired rheumatic or degenerative calcific aortic stenosis.

The dynamics of blood flow associated with a congenitally deformed, rigid aortic valve commonly lead to thickening of the cusps and, in later life, to calcification. Hemodynamically significant obstruction causes concentric hypertrophy of the left ventricular wall and dilatation of the ascending aorta.

The hemodynamic abnormalities are discussed in Chap. 201. A peak systolic pressure gradient exceeding 70 mmHg, in association with abnormal cardiac output, or an effective aortic orifice less than 0.6 cm^2 per square meter of body surface, is considered to represent critical obstruction to left ventricular outflow. In adults, the resting cardiac output is generally normal but often fails to rise normally during muscular exercise.

Many patients with congenital aortic stenosis are asymptomatic. Usually, a murmur is detected on a routine examination. Moderately severe obstruction should be suspected if there is a history of fatigability and exertional dyspnea. With severe obstruction, the inability of the left ventricle to increase its output and maintain cerebral flow during exercise may result in exertional syncope, and the disparity between the oxygen supply and myocardial oxygen requirements may cause angina. The symptomatic patient with valvular aortic stenosis generally has critical stenosis, although a lack of symptoms does not preclude the presence of moderately severe obstruction. Sudden death occurs in patients with critical stenosis, and ventricular arrhythmias, perhaps initiated by acute myocardial ischemia, may be responsible.

Hemodynamically significant obstruction is associated with a sustained left ventricular apical impulse and a precordial systolic thrill over the base of the heart with transmission to the jugular notch and along the carotid arteries. Presystolic apical expansion is often palpable. A systolic aortic ejection sound, signifying opening of the aortic valve, is typically heard best at the cardiac apex when the valve is mobile, particularly with mild to moderate stenosis. A fourth heart sound is generally associated with severe obstruction. The systolic murmur starts after the completion of left ventricular isometric contraction, is crescendo-decrescendo or diamond-shaped, loud, harsh, and best heard at the base of the heart. The murmur, like the thrill, radiates to the jugular notch and carotid vessels and to the apex. An early diastolic blowing murmur of aortic regurgitation may be present, but unless the valve has been eroded by infective endocarditis the regurgitation is usually not hemodynamically significant; rarely, in patients with a congenital bicuspid valve, severe aortic regurgitation may be the dominant hemodynamic lesion.

Electrocardiographic evidence of left ventricular hypertrophy tends to reflect the severity of obstruction, although a normal or near-normal electrocardiogram does not exclude severe aortic stenosis. The left ventricular "strain pattern" generally indicates that severe aortic stenosis is present. Two-dimensional echocardiography demonstrates the aortic valve morphology; Doppler echocardiography is the most accurate means of noninvasively estimating the magnitude of obstruction and valvular regurgitation if present. Cardiac catheterization and coronary angiography are indicated particularly if coronary artery disease is suspected.

TREATMENT The medical management of congenital valvular aortic stenosis includes prophylaxis against infective endocarditis and, in patients with diminished cardiac reserve, the administration of digitalis and diuretics and sodium restriction while awaiting operation. If severe aortic stenosis is present, strenuous physical activity should be avoided even when the patient is asymptomatic, and participation in competitive sports should probably be restricted in patients with milder degrees of obstruction. Aortic valve replacement is indicated in asymptomatic adults with severe obstruction or in patients who are symptomatic with an aortic valve area less than 1.0 cm^2. If surgery is contraindicated because of a complicating medical problem such as malignancy or renal or hepatic failure, balloon valvuloplasty may provide short-term improvement.

Subaortic stenosis The most common form of subaortic stenosis is the *idiopathic hypertrophic* variety, also termed *hypertrophic cardiomyopathy*, which is present at birth in about one-third of the patients and is discussed in Chap. 205. Both clinically and physiologically, the *discrete* form of subaortic stenosis resembles valvular aortic stenosis. The lesion usually consists of a membranous diaphragm or fibrous ring encircling the left ventricular outflow tract just beneath the base of the aortic valve. Echocardiography demonstrates the subaortic obstruction; Doppler studies show turbulence proximal to the aortic valve and also detect and quantify the pressure gradient and severity of aortic regurgitation. Treatment consists of excision of the membrane or fibrous ridge.

Supravalvular aortic stenosis This anomaly consists of a localized or diffuse narrowing of the ascending aorta originating just above the level of the coronary arteries at the superior margin of the sinuses of Valsalva. In contrast to other forms of aortic stenosis, the coronary arteries are subjected to the elevated pressures that exist within the left ventricle and are often dilated and tortuous.

COARCTATION OF THE AORTA Narrowing or constriction of the lumen of the aorta may occur anywhere along its length but is most common distal to the origin of the left subclavian artery near the insertion of the ligamentum arteriosum. Coarctation occurs in about 7 percent of patients with congenital heart disease and is twice as common in males as in females, although the lesion occurs frequently in patients with gonadal dysgenesis. Clinical manifestations depend on the site and extent of obstruction and the presence of associated cardiac anomalies, most commonly a bicuspid aortic valve. Aneurysmal arterial dilatation of the circle of Willis produces a high risk of sudden rupture and death.

Most children and young adults with isolated, discrete coarctation are asymptomatic. Headache, epistaxis, cold extremities, and claudication with exercise may occur, and attention is usually directed to the cardiovascular system when a heart murmur or hypertension in the upper extremities and absence, marked diminution, or delayed pulsations in the femoral arteries are detected on physical examination. Enlarged and pulsatile collateral vessels may be palpated in the intercostal spaces anteriorly, in the axillae, or posteriorly in the interscapular area. The upper extremities and thorax may be more developed than the lower extremities. A midsystolic murmur over the anterior part of the chest, back, and spinous processes may become continuous if the lumen is narrowed sufficiently to result in a high-velocity jet across the lesion throughout the cardiac cycle. Additional systolic and continuous murmurs over the lateral thoracic wall may reflect increased flow through dilated and tortuous collateral vessels. The electrocardiogram reveals left ventricular hypertrophy of varying degree. Roentgenograms may show a dilated left subclavian artery high on the left mediastinal border and a dilated ascending aorta. Indentation of the aorta at the site of coarctation and pre- and poststenotic dilatation (the "3" sign) along the left paramediastinal shadow are almost pathognomonic. Notching of the ribs, an important radiographic sign, is due to erosion by dilated collateral vessels. Two-dimensional echocardiography from para- or suprasternal windows identifies the site and length of coarctation, while Doppler studies record and quantify the pressure gradient. Transesophageal echocardiography and magnetic resonance imaging or digital angiography allow visualization of the length and severity of the obstruction and the associated collateral arteries. In adults, cardiac catheterization is indicated primarily to evaluate the coronary arteries.

The chief hazards result from severe hypertension and include the development of cerebral aneurysms and hemorrhage, rupture of the aorta, left ventricular failure, and infective endocarditis.

Management   This is usually surgical; resection and end-to-end anastomosis or subclavian flap angioplasty are employed commonly, although it may be necessary to use a tubular graft, patch, or bypass conduit if the narrowed segment is long. Systemic hypertension postoperatively, in the absence of residual coarctation, appears to be related to the duration of preoperative hypertension. Postsurgical recoarctation may be successfully treated with percutaneous balloon dilatation.

PULMONARY STENOSIS WITH INTACT VENTRICULAR SEPTUM
Obstruction to right ventricular outflow may be localized to the supravalvular, valvular, or subvalvular levels or occur at a combination of these sites. Multiple sites of narrowing of the peripheral pulmonary arteries are a feature of *rubella embryopathy* and may occur with both the familial and sporadic forms of supravalvular aortic stenosis. Valvular pulmonic stenosis is the most common form of isolated right ventricular obstruction.

The severity of the obstructing lesion, rather than the site of narrowing, is the most important determinant of the clinical course. In the presence of a normal cardiac output, a peak systolic transvalvular pressure gradient between 50 and 80 mmHg is considered to be moderate stenosis; levels below and above that range are classified as mild and severe, respectively. Patients with mild pulmonic stenosis are generally asymptomatic and demonstrate little or no progression in the severity of obstruction with age. In patients with more significant stenosis, the severity may increase with time. Symptoms vary with the degree of obstruction. Fatigue, dyspnea, right ventricular failure, and syncope may limit the activity of older patients, in whom moderate or severe obstruction may prevent an augmentation of cardiac output with exercise. In patients with severe obstruction, the systolic pressure in the right ventricle may exceed that in the left ventricle, since the ventricular septum is intact. Right ventricular ejection is prolonged with moderate or severe stenosis, and the sound of pulmonary valve closure is delayed and soft. Right ventricular hypertrophy reduces the compliance of that chamber, and a forceful right atrial contraction is necessary to augment right ventricular filling. A fourth heart sound, prominent *a* waves in the jugular venous pulse, and, occasionally, presystolic pulsations of the liver reflect vigorous atrial contraction. The clinical diagnosis is supported by a right parasternal lift and harsh systolic ejection murmur and thrill at the upper left sternal border, typically preceded by a systolic ejection sound, if the obstruction is valvular. The holosystolic decrescendo murmur of tricuspid regurgitation may accompany severe pulmonic stenosis, especially in the presence of congestive heart failure. Cyanosis usually reflects venoarterial shunting through a patent foramen ovale or atrial septal defect. In patients with supravalvular or peripheral pulmonary arterial stenosis, the murmur is systolic or continuous and is best heard over the area of narrowing, with radiation to the peripheral lung fields.

The *electrocardiogram* may be helpful in assessing the degree of right ventricular obstruction. In mild cases, the electrocardiogram is often normal, whereas moderate and severe stenoses are associated with right axis deviation and right ventricular hypertrophy. A ventricular strain pattern, as well as high-amplitude P waves in leads II and V_1, indicating right atrial enlargement, is associated with severe stenosis. The chest roentgenogram with mild or moderate pulmonic stenosis often shows a heart of normal size and normal vascularity of the lungs. In the presence of valvular stenosis, poststenotic dilatation of the main and left pulmonary arteries may be evident. With severe obstruction and resultant right ventricular failure, right atrial and ventricular enlargement are generally evident. The pulmonary vascularity may be reduced with severe stenosis, right ventricular failure, and/or a venoarterial shunt at the atrial level. Two-dimensional *echocardiography* visualizes pulmonary valve morphology; the out-

flow tract pressure gradient can be estimated by Doppler ultrasonography.

Management   The cardiac catheter technique of balloon valvuloplasty (Chap. 192) is usually effective. Direct surgical relief of moderate and severe obstruction may be accomplished at a low risk. Multiple stenoses of the peripheral pulmonary arteries are usually inoperable, but narrowing of a single branch or at the bifurcation of the main pulmonary trunk may be corrected.

CYANOTIC CONGENITAL HEART DISEASE WITH INCREASED PULMONARY BLOOD FLOW

COMPLETE TRANSPOSITION OF THE GREAT ARTERIES   In this condition the aorta arises from the right ventricle to the right of and anterior to the pulmonary artery, which emerges from the left ventricle. This results in two separate and parallel circulations, and some communication between the two circulations must exist after birth to sustain life. Most patients have an interatrial communication, two-thirds have a patent ductus arteriosus, and about one-third have an associated ventricular septal defect. Transposition is more common in males and accounts for approximately 10 percent of cyanotic heart disease.

The course is determined by the degree of tissue hypoxia, the ability of each ventricle to sustain an increased work load in the presence of reduced coronary arterial oxygenation, the nature of the associated cardiovascular anomalies, and the status of the pulmonary vascular bed. Severe morphologic alterations develop in the pulmonary vascular bed by 1 to 2 years of age in most patients who also have an associated large ventricular septal defect or large patent ductus arteriosus in the absence of obstruction to left ventricular outflow.

Surgical treatment   The creation or enlargement of an interatrial communication is the simplest procedure for providing increased intracardiac mixing of systemic and pulmonary venous blood; it may be achieved surgically or, preferably, by rupturing the valve of the foramen ovale with a balloon catheter during cardiac catheterization (Rashkind procedure). Systemic–pulmonary artery anastomosis may be indicated in the patient with severe obstruction to left ventricular outflow and diminished pulmonary blood flow. Intracardiac repair may be accomplished by rearranging the venous returns so that the systemic venous blood is directed to the mitral valve and thence to the left ventricle and pulmonary artery, while the pulmonary venous blood is diverted through the tricuspid valve and right ventricle to the aorta (Mustard or Senning operation). Many surgeons now prefer to correct this malformation in infancy by transposing both coronary arteries to the posterior artery and transecting, contraposing, and anastomosing the aorta and pulmonary arteries (Jatene or arterial switch operation). For those patients with a ventricular septal defect in whom it is necessary to bypass a severely obstructed left ventricular outflow tract, corrective operation employs an intracardiac ventricular baffle and extracardiac prosthetic conduit to replace the pulmonary artery (Rastelli procedure). Patients with a large ventricular septal defect require closure of the ventricular septal defect and the atrial switch operation early in infancy. There are now many adults who underwent venous switch repair early in life who are experiencing the long-term complications of that operation, including arrhythmias, baffle leaks, or obstruction and reduced performance of the systemic right ventricle.

TOTAL ANOMALOUS PULMONARY VENOUS CONNECTION   In this malformation all the pulmonary veins connect either to the right atrium directly or to the systemic veins or their tributaries. Because all venous blood returns to the right atrium, an interatrial communication is an integral part of this malformation. Most unoperated patients surviving to adult life have pulmonary vascular obstructive disease, a reduction in pulmonary blood flow, and cyanosis.

SINGLE VENTRICLE   This designation applies to a family of complex lesions with both atrioventricular valves or a common atrioventricular valve opening to a single ventricular chamber. In most patients, the single ventricle morphologically resembles a left ventricular chamber that is separated from an infundibular outlet chamber by a bulboventricular septum; in these cases the anomaly is often referred to as double-inlet left ventricle. Associated anomalies are common and include abnormal great artery positional relationships, pulmonic valvular or subvalvular stenosis, and subaortic stenosis.

Depending upon the associated anomalies, the clinical presentation of single ventricle mimics other conditions in which cyanosis and decreased (or increased) pulmonary blood flow coexist, e.g., tetralogy of Fallot in the former instance and complete transposition of the great arteries in the latter. Survival to adulthood depends upon a relatively normal pulmonary blood flow and good ventricular function. Correction of the defect usually consists of creation of a right atrial–pulmonary conduit (the Fontan procedure); some patients are candidates for a septation operation in which the single ventricle is partitioned with a prosthetic patch.

CYANOTIC CONGENITAL HEART DISEASE WITH DECREASED PULMONARY BLOOD FLOW

TRICUSPID ATRESIA Atresia of the tricuspid valve, an interatrial communication, and, frequently, hypoplasia of the right ventricle and pulmonary artery exist in this malformation. Because of the small or nearly absent right ventricle, this anomaly is basically a "univentricular" heart with a single inlet (mitral) to the left ventricle. The clinical picture is usually dominated by severe cyanosis due to obligatory admixture of systemic and pulmonary venous blood in the left ventricle. The electrocardiogram characteristically shows right atrial enlargement, left axis deviation, and left ventricular hypertrophy.

Atrial septostomy and palliative operations to increase pulmonary blood flow, often by anastomosis of a systemic artery or vein to a pulmonary artery, may allow survival to the second or third decade. A Fontan atriopulmonary connection may then allow functional correction in those patients with normal or low pulmonary arterial resistance pressure and good left ventricular function.

EBSTEIN'S ANOMALY This malformation is characterized by a downward displacement of the tricuspid valve into the right ventricle, due to anomalous attachment of the tricuspid leaflets. Tricuspid valve tissue is dysplastic; a variable portion of the septal and inferior cusps adhere to the right ventricular wall some distance away from the atrioventricular junction. The abnormally situated tricuspid orifice produces a portion of the right ventricle lying between the atrioventricular ring and the origin of the valve, which is continuous with the right atrial chamber. This proximal segment is "atrialized," and the distal ventricular chamber is small. The degree of impairment of right ventricular function depends primarily on the extent to which the right ventricular inflow portion is atrialized and on the magnitude of tricuspid valve regurgitation. Most patients survive at least to the third decade. Although the clinical manifestations are variable, some patients come to initial attention because of progressive cyanosis from right-to-left atrial shunting, or symptoms due to tricuspid regurgitation and right ventricular dysfunction, or paroxysmal atrial tachyarrhythmias with or without bypass tracts (type B Wolff-Parkinson-White syndrome is common). Diagnostic findings by two-dimensional echocardiography include the abnormal positional relation between the tricuspid and mitral valves with apical displacement of the septal tricuspid leaflet. Tricuspid regurgitation is detected and quantified by Doppler examination. Surgical approaches have included prosthetic replacement of the tricuspid valve when the leaflets are tethered, or, in patients with an elongated mobile anterior leaflet, creation of a competent, unicuspid valve by insertion of the elongated anterior leaflet into the original tricuspid annulus and plication of the atrialized right ventricle. Transection of bypass tracts may be necessary to abolish atrial tachyarrhythmias.

TETRALOGY OF FALLOT This malformation accounts for about 10 percent of all forms of congenital heart disease and is the most common cause of cyanotic forms. The four components of the tetralogy of Fallot are ventricular septal defect, obstruction to right ventricular outflow, aortic override (straddle) of the ventricular septal defect, and right ventricular hypertrophy. The basic anomaly results from an anterior and superior deviation of the infundibular ventricular septum away from its usual location in the heart between the limbs of the trabecular septum. This displacement causes subpulmonary obstruction, aortic "override," and a large, nonrestrictive, malalignment-type ventricular septal defect.

The severity of right ventricular outflow obstruction determines the clinical presentation. The severity of hypoplasia of the right ventricular outflow tract varies from mild to complete (pulmonary atresia). Pulmonary valve stenosis and supravalvular and peripheral pulmonary arterial obstruction may coexist; rarely there is unilateral absence of a pulmonary artery (usually the left). A right-sided aortic arch and descending aorta occur in about 25 percent of patients with tetralogy. The coronary arteries may have variations that are surgically important. The anterior descending artery sometimes originates from the right coronary artery, which may also give rise to a left branch coursing anterior to the infundibulum; a single left coronary artery may give rise to a branch that crosses the outflow tract of the right ventricle.

The relationship between the resistance to blood flow from the ventricles into the aorta and into the pulmonary vessels plays a major role in determining the hemodynamic and clinical picture. Thus, the severity of obstruction to right ventricular outflow is of fundamental significance. In many infants and children the obstruction is mild but progressive. When the obstruction is severe, the pulmonary blood flow is reduced markedly, and a large volume of desaturated systemic venous blood is shunted from right to left across the ventricular septal defect. Severe cyanosis and erythrocytosis occur, and symptoms and sequelae of systemic hypoxemia are prominent.

The *electrocardiogram* ordinarily shows right ventricular and, less often, right atrial hypertrophy. Radiologic examination characteristically reveals a normal-sized, boot-shaped heart (*coeur en sabot*) with prominence of the right ventricle and a concavity in the region of the pulmonary conus. The pulmonary vascular markings are typically diminished, and the aortic arch and knob may be on the right side. Two-dimensional echocardiography from the parasternal or subcostal windows demonstrates the malalignment of the ventricular septal defect and the subpulmonary stenosis. The presence or absence of stenoses at the origins of the main branch pulmonary arteries can also be assessed. Selective angiocardiography with right ventricular injection provides architectural details of the right ventricular outflow tract, pulmonary valve and annulus, and caliber of the main branches of the pulmonary artery; coronary arteriography identifies the anatomy and course of the coronary arteries.

Management Factors that may complicate the treatment of patients with tetralogy of Fallot include infective endocarditis, paradoxic embolism, excessive erythrocytosis, coagulation defects, and cerebral infarction or abscess. Corrective operation is advisable at some point for almost all patients with this anomaly. Successful correction avoids progressive infundibular obstruction, delayed growth, and complications due to hypoxemia and excessive erythrocytosis. The size of the pulmonary arteries rather than the age or size of the infant or child is the most important determinant in establishing candidacy for primary repair. Pronounced hypoplasia of the pulmonary arteries is a relative contraindication for an early corrective surgical procedure. When this problem is present, a palliative operation, such as creation of a systemic arterial–pulmonary arterial shunt, is carried out and is usually followed by complete correction, which can be carried out at a lower risk later in childhood.

OTHER FORMS OF CONGENITAL HEART DISEASES

CONGENITALLY CORRECTED TRANSPOSITION The two fundamental anatomic abnormalities in this malformation are transposition of the ascending aorta and pulmonary trunk and inversion of the ventricles. This arrangement results in desaturated systemic venous blood passing from the right atrium through the mitral valve to the left ventricle and into the pulmonary trunk, whereas arterialized pulmonary venous blood flows from the left atrium through the tricuspid valve to the right ventricle and into the aorta. Thus, the circulation is corrected functionally. The clinical presentation, course, and prognosis of patients with congenitally corrected transposition vary depending on the nature and severity of any complicating intracardiac anomalies. Ebstein-type anomalies of the left-side tricuspid atrioventricular valve, ventricular septal defect, obstruction to outflow from the venous ventricle, and congenital heart block are often associated with corrected transposition. The diagnosis of the malformation and associated lesions can often be established by two-dimensional echocardiography and Doppler examination.

MALPOSITIONS OF THE HEART Positional anomalies refer to conditions in which the cardiac apex is in the right side of the chest (dextrocardia), or at the midline (mesocardia), or in which there is a normal location of the heart in the left side of the chest but abnormal position of the viscera (isolated levocardia). Knowledge of the position of the abdominal organs and of the branching pattern of the main stem bronchi is important in categorizing these malpositions. When dextrocardia occurs *without* situs inversus, when the *visceral situs is indeterminate,* or if *isolated levocardia* is present, associated, often complex, multiple cardiac anomalies are usually present. In contrast, mirror-image dextrocardia is usually observed with complete situs inversus, which occurs most frequently in individuals whose hearts are otherwise normal.

SURGICALLY MODIFIED CONGENITAL HEART DISEASE

Because of the enormous strides in cardiovascular surgical techniques that have occurred in the past 15 years, a large number of long-term survivors of corrective operations in infancy and childhood have reached adulthood. These patients are often challenging because of the diversity of anatomic, hemodynamic, and electrophysiologic residua and sequelae of cardiac operations.

The proper care of the survivor of operation for congenital heart disease requires that the clinician understand the details of the malformation prior to operation, pay meticulous attention to the details of the operative procedure, and recognize the postoperative residua (conditions left totally or partially uncorrected), sequelae (conditions caused by surgery), and the complications that may have resulted from the operation. With the exception of ligation and division of an uncomplicated patent ductus arteriosus, almost every other surgical repair of an anomaly leaves behind or causes some abnormality of the heart and circulation that may range from trivial to serious. Intraoperative transesophageal echocardiography assists in detecting unsuspected lesions, in monitoring the repair, and in verifying a satisfactory result or directing further repair. Thus, even with results that are considered clinically to be good to excellent, continued long-term postoperative follow-up is advisable.

Table 199-3 lists the categories of common late postoperative problems. Several of these residua, sequelae, and complications deserve special mention. Thus, cardiac operations importantly involving the atria, such as closure of atrial septal defect, repair of total or partial anomalous pulmonary venous return, or venous switch corrections of complete transposition of the great arteries (the Mustard or Senning operations), may be followed years later by sinus node or atrioventricular node dysfunction or by atrial arrhythmias. Intraventricular surgery may also result in electrophysiologic consequences, including complete heart block necessitating pacemaker insertion to avoid sudden death. In addition, valvular problems may arise late after initial cardiac operation. An example is the progressive stenosis of an initially nonobstructive bicuspid aortic valve in the patient who underwent aortic coarctation repair. Such aortic valves may also be

TABLE 199-3 **Potential late postoperative problems**
Residual shunts
Residual ventricular outflow obstruction
Residual valvular anomalies
Systemic arterial hypertension
Pulmonary vascular obstruction
Arrhythmias and conduction defects
Myocardial dysfunction
Prosthetic valve malfunction
Prosthetic conduit obstruction
Infective endocarditis

the site of infective endocarditis. After repair of the ostium primum atrial septal defect, the cleft mitral valve may become progressively incompetent. Low-pressure pulmonary regurgitation is common and well tolerated in most patients with repaired tetralogy of Fallot. However, in such patients with significant residual peripheral pulmonary arterial stenoses, severe pulmonary valvular regurgitation may result in right ventricular failure and tricuspid regurgitation. Tricuspid regurgitation may also be progressive in the postoperative patient with tetralogy of Fallot if right ventricular outflow tract obstruction was not relieved adequately at initial surgery. In many patients, inadequate relief of an obstructive lesion, or a residual regurgitant lesion, or a residual shunt will cause or hasten the onset of clinical signs and symptoms of myocardial dysfunction. In many patients, particularly those who were cyanotic for many years before operation, a preexisting compromise in ventricular performance is due to the original underlying malformation. A final category of postoperative problems involves the use of prosthetic valves, patches, or conduits in the operative repair. The special risks in such patients include infective endocarditis, thrombus formation, and premature degeneration and calcification of the prosthetic materials. There are many patients in whom extracardiac conduits are required to correct the circulation functionally and often to carry blood to the lungs from the right atrium or right ventricle. These conduits may develop intraluminal obstruction and, if they include a prosthetic valve, it may show progressive calcification and thickening.

REFERENCES

CHILD JS: Echo-Doppler and color-flow imaging in congenital heart disease. Cardiol Clin 8:289, 1990

CROWLEY JJ et al: Telltale signs of congential heart disease. Radiol Clin North Am 31:573, 1993

FRIEDMAN WF: Congenital heart disease in infancy and childhood, in *Heart Disease,* 4th ed, E Braunwald (ed). Philadelphia, Saunders, 1992, p 887

NORA JJ: Causes of congenital heart diseases: Old and new modes, mechanisms and models. Am Heart J 125:1409, 1993

PERLOFF JK: *The Clinical Recognition of Congenital Heart Disease,* 3d ed. Philadelphia, Saunders, 1987

——, CHILD JS: *Congenital Heart Disease in Adults.* Philadelphia, Saunders, 1991

—— et al: 22nd Bethesda Conference: Congenital heart disease after childhood; an expanding patient population. J Am Coll Cardiol 18:311, 1991

WEIDMAN WH: Second natural history study of congenital heart defects. Circulation 87:II, 1993

WEINTRAUB R et al: Transesophageal echocardiography in infants and children with congenital heart disease. Circulation 86:711, 1992

200 RHEUMATIC FEVER

GENE H. STOLLERMAN

DEFINITION Rheumatic fever is an inflammatory disease which occurs as a delayed sequel to pharyngeal infection with group A streptococci. It involves principally the heart, joints, central nervous system, skin, and subcutaneous tissues. The usual manifestations in the acute form are migratory polyarthritis, fever, and carditis.

Sydenham's chorea, subcutaneous nodules, and erythema marginatum may occur as other typical manifestations. No single symptom, sign, or laboratory test is pathognomonic of rheumatic fever, although several combinations of them are diagnostic. Although the name *acute rheumatic fever* emphasizes involvement of the joints, rheumatic fever owes its importance to the involvement of the heart, which can be fatal during the acute stage or lead to rheumatic heart disease, a chronic condition due to scarring and deformity of the heart valves.

ETIOLOGY AND PATHOGENESIS The etiologic relationship of group A streptococci to rheumatic fever can be summarized briefly as follows: (1) Numerous clinical and epidemiologic studies have shown a close association of group A streptococcal infections and rheumatic fever. (2) Antecedent streptococcal infection can almost always be demonstrated immunologically in the acute stage of rheumatic fever by increased titers of antibodies to streptococcal antigens. Moreover, in long-term prospective follow-up studies, rheumatic fever recurs only as a result of intercurrent streptococcal infections. (3) Both primary and secondary attacks of the disease can be prevented by prompt treatment or prevention of streptococcal infections with antimicrobial therapy. (4) The site of infection is critical. The pharyngeal route of infection is necessary to initiate the rheumatic process. Streptococcal skin or soft tissue infections do not do so. (5) Not all strains of group A streptococci cause the disease. The so-called skin strains that cause streptococcal pyoderma do not cause rheumatic fever, even when infecting the throat. The strains that have been clearly associated with rheumatic fever outbreaks have distinct virulence properties when freshly isolated from the pharynx. They are very rich in the extractable serotypic surface M protein and contain large hyaluronic acid capsules that are responsible for the formation of mucoid colonies on blood agar plates. Such strains usually belong to certain serotypes, notably M types 3, 5, 18, 19, 24, and others. All strains within these serotypes, however, are not always in this phase of virulence and are not always rheumatogenic. The M protein of rheumatogenic strains forms an unusually large, extended molecule consisting of repeating peptide subunits not found in other strains of group A streptococci so far studied.

The mechanism by which the group A streptococcus initiates the disease process remains unknown. A relatively small percentage of persons who suffer from streptococcal sore throats subsequently develop rheumatic fever. The organism is not demonstrable in the lesions when rheumatic fever appears after a characteristic latent period of 1 to 5 weeks after the acute pharyngeal streptococcal infection. No one product of the streptococcus has been incriminated as a cause of the lesions, either as a direct tissue toxin or as an antigen inducing hypersensitivity. Several streptococcal antigens have demonstrated cross-reactivity with cardiac and other tissues. Notably, epitopes within the non-type-specific peptides of the M protein of rheumatogenic strains cross-react immunologically with myosin, keratin, and other coiled proteins found in cardiac tissues. Although the hyaluronic acid of group A streptococcal capsules and that of human host tissues are chemically identical, autoantibodies to this substance are demonstrable. Such findings suggest that a "molecular mimicry" type of autoimmunity may relate to the pathogenesis of rheumatic fever, perhaps induced by the strong immunologic adjuvant properties of some parts of the M protein molecule that have superantigen-like activity, i.e., the capability of activating lymphocyte receptors directly. Such properties may invoke autoimmune responses in susceptible hosts and also may explain the finding that all streptococcal antibodies so far studied tend to be higher in patients with acute rheumatic fever than in those who do not develop the disease following a bout of streptococcal pharyngitis.

INCIDENCE AND EPIDEMIOLOGY Although rheumatic fever may occur at any age, it is extremely rare in infancy; it appears most commonly between the ages of 5 and 15 years, when streptococcal infection is most frequent and intense. Similarly, the geographic distribution, incidence, and severity of rheumatic fever are, in general, a reflection of the frequency and severity of streptococcal pharyngitis. The attack rate of rheumatic fever following exudative streptococcal pharyngitis in epidemics averages approximately 3 percent. When streptococcal pharyngitis is sporadic and mild or due to strains of lesser or no rheumatic potential, the attack rate of rheumatic fever may be very much lower. Strains of group A streptococci that cause epidemics of streptococcal pharyngitis are most likely to be rheumatogenic. Following such infections, the attack rate of rheumatic fever is directly correlated with the magnitude of the streptococcal immune response. Analysis of reported epidemics of acute rheumatic fever caused by a variety of serotypes shows some, such as type 5, to be overrepresented and others to be conspicuously absent. In some populations, such as in Trinidad, strains responsible for rheumatic fever and acute glomerulonephritis are serotypically distinct.

Environmental, bacterial, and host factors which appear to play a role in the development of rheumatic fever are important primarily because they are related to the incidence and severity of preceding streptococcal infection. Such factors as latitude, altitude, dampness, economic factors, and age all affect the incidence of rheumatic fever because they are related to the incidence of streptococcal infection in general. Crowding is, however, the major environmental factor relating to the occurrence of this disease because, regardless of other variables, it promotes interpersonal spread of the most virulent group A streptococcal strains. Such crowding as occurs in military barracks, closed institutions, large families in small quarters, and those massed in the densely populated core of major urban centers is most likely to be associated with an increase in incidence of rheumatic fever.

The attack rate of rheumatic fever following streptococcal infections by rheumatogenic strains in patients who have had previous attacks of rheumatic fever is increased to as high as 5 to 50 percent and is also related to the virulence of the reactivating infection. Furthermore, the frequency of rheumatic recurrences following streptococcal infection is consistently greater in those with rheumatic heart disease than in those who escaped cardiac injury during prior attacks. The tendency to suffer recurrences of rheumatic fever following streptococcal infections declines with the passage of years since the preceding attack. It appears, therefore, that certain host variables, as well as qualitative and quantitative differences in the nature of the antecedent streptococcal infection, also influence the development of rheumatic fever. To what extent such variables are genetic or acquired has not been settled. It is common to obtain a family history of rheumatic fever as well as to encounter multiple cases among siblings of a single family. However, the concordance of rheumatic fever in identical twins is approximately 20 percent, suggesting only a limited penetrance of genetic predisposition to rheumatic fever. Although investigations of the distribution of haplotypes in rheumatic hosts have been limited in scope and number, there have been so far no class I and somewhat limited class II HLA-DR associations occurring along racial lines, particularly in those who have developed rheumatic carditis. Recently, B lymphocyte allotypic antigens have been found to be strikingly overrepresented in patients with rheumatic heart disease. Their nature and relation to pathogenesis, however, are not yet known.

The mortality of acute rheumatic fever has been declining steadily for the past 30 years. It is still, however, a major cause of death and disability in children and adolescents in socioeconomically depressed areas of the world. The incidence of rheumatic fever has been decreasing dramatically in countries where housing and economic conditions have been improving steadily. The rate of decrease in rheumatic fever may have been accelerated by the wide use of antimicrobial therapy. The decrease also may be due to a change in the prevalence of rheumatogenic streptococcal strains, which seemed to have disappeared in affluent societies, whereas the prevalence of streptococcal pharyngitis in school children remains the same. In recent years, however, local outbreaks of rheumatic fever have occurred in the United States in two military populations, one at the San Diego Naval Base, California, and the other at Fort Leonard Wood, Missouri. Outbreaks also have occurred among school children in Utah, Ohio, and Pennsylvania. Middle-class communities with relatively high standards of living and medical care have been affected.

Further investigations of the streptococcal strains causing pharyngitis in these communities have resulted in the recovery of "mucoid" strains of group A streptococci belonging to serotype M types 3 and 18. These strains were once prevalent in well-studied epidemics of rheumatic fever in the 1940s and 1950s, particularly in military populations. They have rarely been seen since then. The explanation for the reappearance of these strains in middle-class communities and in widely separated military bases is unclear and has caused a resurgence of interest in proper diagnosis and treatment of streptococcal sore throat. Rheumatic fever remains, however, a worldwide disease having its greatest incidence wherever poor economic conditions, overcrowding, and substandard housing are most common and where such conditions promote the transmission of rheumatogenic streptococci.

PATHOLOGY The lesions of rheumatic fever are disseminated widely throughout the body, with special predilection for connective tissues. Focal inflammatory lesions occur particularly around small blood vessels.

Cardiovascular lesions The heart is the site of the most characteristic and consequential involvement, and all its layers—endocardium, myocardium, and pericardium—may be involved. This generalized involvement gives rise to the term *rheumatic pancarditis*. The most characteristic and specific pattern of rheumatic inflammation is found in the *myocardial Aschoff body*, a submiliary granuloma. This lesion, when present in its classic form, is generally considered to be pathognomonic of rheumatic fever. In many areas the inflammatory lesion is accompanied by swelling and fragmentation of the collagen fibers and alteration in the staining properties of the ground substances of the connective tissues. This change is described as *fibrinoid degeneration of collagen*, but its chemical basis has not been established. Aschoff bodies with less exudative and more productive changes may persist for many years as the lingering traces of chronic rheumatic inflammation in patients with rheumatic heart disease, long after rheumatic fever has become clinically quiescent. The persistence of such lesions is most common in patients who develop severe mitral stenosis. Eventually, the Aschoff body is converted into a spindle-shaped or triangular scar lying between the muscle bundles and surrounding blood vessels.

Rheumatic endocarditis produces the verrucous valvulitis of acute rheumatic fever which leads to the most serious permanent cardiac damage. It may heal with fibrous thickening and adhesion of the valve commissures and chordae tendineae, leading to variable degrees of valvular regurgitation and stenosis. Deformity resulting in functional impairment of the heart occurs most commonly in the mitral and aortic valves, less frequently in the tricuspid valve, and almost never in the pulmonic valves. *Rheumatic pericarditis* (see Chap. 206) produces a serofibrinous effusion, with the deposit of shaggy elements of fibrin on the surface of the heart. The pericardium may become calcified, but pericardial constriction does not occur.

Extracardiac lesions Involvement of the *joints* is characterized by exudative rather than proliferative changes, and healing of these structures occurs without significant scarring or deformity. *Subcutaneous nodules*, seen during the acute phase of the disease, are composed of granulomas with localized areas of "fibrinoid" swelling of subcutaneous collagen bundles and perivascular collections of large cells with pale nuclei and prominent nucleoli. Synovitis is usually mild and nonspecific. *Pulmonary* and *pleural* lesions are less definite and less characteristic. Fibrinous pleurisy and rheumatic pneumonitis may occur with exudative and proliferative lesions but without definite Aschoff bodies. Patients with active *chorea* rarely die. The pathologic findings which have been reported in the central nervous system are not consistent, and no characteristic lesion has been reported to explain this clinical manifestation. During active chorea, the spinal fluid remains normal, being free of cells, with no increase in total protein and no change in the relative concentration of various proteins.

CLINICAL FEATURES The major clinical manifestations by which rheumatic fever can be recognized are polyarthritis, carditis, chorea, erythema marginatum, and subcutaneous nodules.

TABLE 200-1 Jones criteria, 1992 update

Major manifestations	Minor manifestations	Supporting evidence of antecedent group A streptococcal infection
Carditis	Clinical findings	Positive throat culture
Polyarthritis	Arthralgia	or rapid streptococcal
Chorea	Fever	antigen test
Erythema marginatum	Laboratory findings	Elevated or rising strep-
Subcutaneous nodules	Elevated acute phase reactants	tococcal antibody titer
	Erythrocyte sedimentation rate	
	C-reactive protein	
	Prolonged PR interval	

If supported by evidence of preceding group A streptococcal infection, the presence of two major manifestations or of one major and two minor manifestations indicates a high probability of acute rheumatic fever.

SOURCE: American Heart Association, 1992.

Arthritis The classic attack of rheumatic fever appears as an acute migratory polyarthritis accompanied by signs and symptoms of an acute febrile illness. The large joints of the extremities are most frequently affected, but no joint is impervious to the inflammatory process; one may find arthritis of the hands and feet but only rarely of the spine or of the sternoclavicular or temporomandibular joints. Joint effusions occur but are not persistent. As pain and swelling subside in one joint, others tend to become involved. Although such "migratory" involvement is characteristic, it is not invariable, and several large joints may be inflamed at one time. To be acceptable as a criterion for the diagnosis of rheumatic fever, the polyarthritis should involve two or more joints, should be associated with at least two minor manifestations such as fever and elevation of sedimentation rate, and should be associated with high titer of antistreptolysin O or some other streptococcal antibody (Table 200-1). There is nothing distinctive about the arthritis of rheumatic fever, and other causes of migratory polyarthritis that may be associated only coincidentally with high streptococcal antibody levels must, of course, be excluded.

Acute rheumatic carditis Acute rheumatic carditis first becomes manifest by the appearance of the heart murmurs of either mitral or aortic regurgitation, the former most frequently. Signs and symptoms of pericarditis and of congestive heart failure may supervene in more severe cases. Death may result from heart failure during the acute stage of the disease, or permanent valvular damage may be sustained which results ultimately in serious disability. Carditis may vary from a fulminating, fatal course to a low-grade, inapparent inflammation. *It is well to bear in mind that the vast majority of patients with carditis do not have symptoms referable to the heart.* The latter occur only in more severe cases when heart failure or pericardial effusions produce characteristic symptoms. For this reason, unless extracardiac manifestations, such as polyarthritis and chorea, are present, patients whose rheumatic fever is manifested only by carditis are frequently not diagnosed and in later life may be discovered to have rheumatic heart disease without a definite history of rheumatic fever.

When carditis is manifest, there is usually tachycardia disproportionate to the degree of fever, gallop rhythms are often heard, and the heart sounds may become fetal in character due to the loss of the muscular quality of the first heart sound. Occasionally, arrhythmias and/or a pericardial friction rub may be present. Prolongation of the conduction time may lead to dropped beats with varying degrees of heart block. Prolongation of the PR interval and other changes in the electrocardiogram are very common, but these findings, in the absence of clinical manifestations of carditis, have a benign prognosis. Therefore, changes in the electrocardiogram alone, unassociated with significant murmurs or cardiac enlargement, do not by themselves constitute an acceptable criterion for the diagnosis of rheumatic carditis. Pericarditis may cause precordial pain, and a friction rub may be audible.

A definite clinical diagnosis of carditis can be made if one or more of the following can be demonstrated: (1) the appearance of, or change in the character of, organic heart murmurs, (2) definite increase in heart size demonstrated by radiogram or fluoroscopy, (3) pericardial friction rub or effusion best demonstrated by echocardiography, or (4) signs of congestive heart failure. Rheumatic carditis is almost always associated with a significant murmur. The most common murmurs of acute rheumatic carditis are those due to mitral and aortic regurgitation caused by valvular inflammation. The former is usually a high-pitched holosystolic blowing murmur which must be carefully distinguished from the functional low-pitched, musical, apical flow murmur commonly heard with increased cardiac output in children and other thin-chested individuals. When more severe, mitral inflammation and left ventricular dilatation may produce, in addition to a blowing systolic murmur, a very low pitched, vibratory middiastolic murmur which often follows an accentuated third heart sound—the so-called Carey Coombs murmur. Aortic regurgitation murmurs are often associated with those of mitral origin, and in acute rheumatic fever, occasionally cooing or screeching (''seagull'') murmurs are heard that reflect the turbulence formed around swollen and distorted valves during the acute inflammatory phase of carditis.

Subcutaneous nodules These are usually small, pea-sized, painless swellings over bony prominences and therefore frequently go unnoticed by the patient. The skin moves freely over them. Characteristic locations are the extensor tendons of the hands and feet, the elbows, margins of the patellae, the scalp, over the scapulae, and over the spinous processes of the vertebrae.

Chorea (Sydenham's chorea, chorea minor, Saint Vitus' dance) This is a disorder of the central nervous system characterized by sudden, aimless, irregular movements, often accompanied by muscle weakness and emotional instability. Chorea is a delayed manifestation of rheumatic fever, and other manifestations may or may not still be present at the time it appears. Polyarthritis, when part of the same attack, almost always subsides before chorea appears. Carditis is often discovered for the first time when the presenting feature of rheumatic fever is chorea. Chorea usually appears after a long latent period (up to several months) from the antecedent streptococcal infection and at a time when all other manifestations of rheumatic fever have abated. When no previous rheumatic manifestations are noted, such cases are called *pure chorea*.

The clinical onset of chorea is often gradual. Patients may be unusually nervous and fidgety and may have difficulty in writing, drawing, and handiwork. They may stumble or fall, drop things, and grimace. As symptoms become more severe, spasmodic movements extend to all parts of the body, and muscular weakness may become so marked that patients cannot walk, talk, or sit up. Often the weakness is severe enough to simulate paralysis. The irregular, jerky, spasmodic movements may become so violent that cribs and beds must be padded to prevent injury. Symptoms are exaggerated by excitement, effort, or fatigue but subside during sleep. Emotional instability is almost invariable in patients with chorea. All degrees of speech disturbance are seen. Central nervous system stimulants exacerbate and sedatives suppress choreiform activity.

Erythema marginatum This evanescent pink rash is characteristic of rheumatic fever. The erythematous areas often have clear centers and round or serpiginous margins. They vary greatly in size and occur mainly on the trunk and proximal part of the extremities, never on the face. The erythema is transient, migratory, and may be brought out by the application of heat; it is nonpruritic, not indurated, and blanches on pressure.

Minor clinical criteria These include fever, arthralgia, abdominal pain, tachycardia, and epistaxis, clinical features which occur frequently in rheumatic fever but are also common to many other diseases and are therefore of minor diagnostic value.

LABORATORY FINDINGS There is no specific laboratory test to indicate the presence of rheumatic fever. The appraisal of rheumatic activity by laboratory findings is, however, of value, since various tests may indicate *continued* rheumatic inflammation when clinical features are not apparent.

Streptococcal antibody tests to disclose preceding streptococcal infection Streptococcal antibody titers differentiate preceding streptococcal from other acute respiratory infections and are increased following asymptomatic as well as symptomatic streptococcal infections. These antibody levels are increased in the early stages of acute rheumatic fever. They may be declining or low if the interval between the acute streptococcal infection and the detection of rheumatic fever has been longer than 2 months, a situation which occurs most often in patients whose presenting rheumatic manifestation is chorea. However, patients whose only major manifestation is rheumatic carditis also may have low antibody titers when first seen. Their rheumatic attack may have been in progress several months before becoming symptomatic and recognized. Except in these two instances, *one should be reluctant to make the diagnosis of acute rheumatic fever in the absence of serologic evidence of a recent streptococcal infection.* The antistreptolysin O (ASO) test is the most widely used and best-standardized streptococcal antibody test. In general, single titers of at least 250 Todd units in adults and at least 333 units in children over 5 years of age are considered to be increased. Depending on the general prevalence of streptococcal infections, a varying percentage of the normal population may show titers of this magnitude.

About 20 percent of patients in the early stages of acute rheumatic fever, and most patients who present with chorea, have a low or borderline ASO titer. In these instances, it is advisable to obtain a different streptococcal antibody test such as anti-DNase B or antihyaluronidase (AH). The antistreptozyme (ASTZ) test is a hemagglutination reaction to a concentrate of extracellular streptococcal antigens absorbed to red blood cells. It is a very sensitive indicator of recent streptococcal infection; virtually all patients with acute rheumatic fever have titers greater than 200 units per milliliter. A rise in titer of two dilution tubes or more can be demonstrated for at least one of the specific streptococcal antibodies in almost all recurrent as well as primary attacks of rheumatic fever. Increased streptococcal antibodies, however, do not reflect rheumatic activity per se, and their rate of decline is independent of the course of the rheumatic attack. Because it almost always occurs within the first 4 to 5 weeks of the antecedent streptococcal pharyngitis, polyarthritis is the clinical manifestation most promptly recognized and therefore most reliably associated with rising streptococcal antibody titers. The absence of increased or increasing streptococcal antibody titers in patients with acute polyarthritis therefore makes rheumatic fever a very unlikely cause.

Isolation of group A streptococci Some patients continue to harbor group A streptococci at the onset of acute rheumatic fever, but these organisms are usually present in small numbers and may be difficult to isolate by a single throat culture. The administration of penicillin or other antibiotics also may result in failure to isolate the infecting organism. In addition, a significant number of *normal* individuals, particularly children, may harbor group A streptococci in the upper respiratory tract. For these reasons, throat cultures are less satisfactory than antibody tests as supporting evidence of recent streptococcal infection.

Acute phase reactants These tests offer objective but nonspecific confirmation of the presence of an inflammatory process. The *erythrocyte sedimentation rate* (ESR) and the test for *C-reactive protein* (CRP) in serum are used most commonly. Unless the patient has received glucocorticoids or salicylates, these reactions are almost always abnormal in patients presenting with polyarthritis or acute carditis, whereas they are often normal in patients with ''pure'' chorea. Other laboratory findings which reflect inflammation include reactions such as leukocytosis and increases in serum complement, mucoproteins, and alpha$_2$ and gamma globulins. Prolongation of the PR interval of the electrocardiogram, although neither specific for rheumatic fever nor diagnostic of serious cardiac involvement, is frequent in acute rheumatic fever (about 25 percent of all cases), and other nonspecific electrocardiographic changes are also common. Anemia, due to the suppression of erythropoiesis characteristic of chronic inflammatory diseases, is another feature of rheumatic activity.

COURSE AND PROGNOSIS   The course of rheumatic fever varies greatly and is impossible to predict at the onset of the disease. In general, however, approximately 75 percent of acute rheumatic attacks subside within 6 weeks, 90 percent within 12 weeks, and less than 5 percent persist more than 6 months. These last usually consist of severe, intractable forms of rheumatic carditis or stubborn, prolonged attacks of Sydenham's chorea, both of which may persist for as long as several years. Once acute rheumatic fever has subsided and more than 2 months has elapsed after withdrawal of treatment with salicylates or glucocorticoids, rheumatic fever does not recur in the absence of new streptococcal infections. Recurrences are most common within the first 5 years of the initial attack and tend to decline with increasing duration of freedom from rheumatic activity. The frequency of recurrences is dependent on the frequency and severity of streptococcal infection with strains of rheumatogenic potential, the presence or absence of rheumatic heart disease following an attack, and the duration of the interval since the last attack.

Approximately 70 percent of patients who develop carditis do so within the first week of the disease, 85 percent within the first 12 weeks of the disease, and almost all within 6 months from the onset of the acute attack. Thereafter, if significant murmurs have not appeared, the prognosis for a patient in whom recurrences are prevented is excellent.

Chronic rheumatic carditis and the course of rheumatic heart disease   The remarkable variability in the course of rheumatic carditis and rheumatic valvular disease stems from several factors: (1) the variability in the duration and severity of the rheumatic inflammation, (2) the amount of scarring of the valves and myocardium following the abatement of the acute inflammation, (3) the location and severity of the hemodynamic lesion due to valvular insufficiency or stenosis, (4) the frequency of recurrent bouts of carditis, and (5) the progression of valvular calcification and sclerosis, which occurs as a secondary phenomenon in a deformed or injured valve without recurrent or persistent rheumatic inflammation (as seen in congenital valvular disease or following healed acute bacterial endocarditis). These factors, and possibly others not yet appreciated, produce striking variations in the clinical syndromes of rheumatic heart disease.

Chronic rheumatic myocarditis   In this syndrome, the presenting picture is one of chronic heart failure in a patient with a markedly dilated heart and with physical, roentgenographic, and electrocardiographic findings of mitral and/or aortic and sometimes tricuspid regurgitation. The differentiation of this syndrome from other forms of chronic myocarditis may be very difficult, if not impossible, when the associated extracardiac features of rheumatic fever (chorea, polyarthritis, and so forth) are not present (Chap. 205). Although rheumatic fever does not produce *isolated* myocarditis and is almost invariably a pancarditis, the pericardial inflammation may not be clearly evident, and the mitral valvulitis may not be distinguishable from mitral regurgitation due to dilation of the mitral ring. In such cases, one must search diligently for an evanescent friction rub, evidence of pericardial effusion, appearance of a soft aortic regurgitation murmur, and extracardiac clues such as fever responding promptly to salicylates, arthralgias, transient subcutaneous nodules, evanescent erythema marginatum, and subtle signs of chorea.

The course of chronic rheumatic carditis may be intractable and end fatally after months or even several years. Often, however, the patient improves rather suddenly and even recovers cardiac reserve dramatically in association with the disappearance of systemic manifestations of the inflammatory process. The heart may remain large, may decrease somewhat in size, or in occasional instances may return to normal size with varying degrees of residual valvular deformity. Such a course signals the termination of the "toxic" phase of the rheumatic process, and thereafter the course of rheumatic heart disease depends on the variables in healing cited above.

DIFFERENTIAL DIAGNOSIS   Early cases of rheumatic fever may be confused with other diseases which begin with acute polyarthritis. It is wise to exclude *bacteremia* by blood cultures, particularly because such infections may be masked by penicillin given for

presumed acute rheumatic fever. Polyarthritis due to *infective endocarditis* in a patient with preexisting rheumatic heart disease may be mistaken for a recurrence of acute rheumatic fever. If streptococcal antibodies are not increased, polyarthritis should be attributed to some cause other than rheumatic fever. Gonococcal polyarthritis may be distinguished from rheumatic fever by the dramatic response of the former to a therapeutic trial of penicillin. In rheumatoid arthritis, joint involvement will persist and characteristic joint deformities may appear. The latter are not seen in rheumatic fever. The rheumatoid factor so characteristic of rheumatoid arthritis is not present in rheumatic fever. Antibodies against nuclear components and against IgG are absent in rheumatic fever. Rheumatic pericarditis and myocarditis, associated with cardiac enlargement and heart failure, are both almost invariably associated with valvular lesions which produce significant murmurs.

Overdiagnosis of rheumatic fever is a danger. Unless ill-defined febrile syndromes are clearly associated with a major manifestation of rheumatic fever, the diagnosis of rheumatic fever should not be made. A common error is the premature, vigorous administration of glucocorticoids or salicylates before the signs and symptoms of rheumatic fever are unmistakable. In the absence of a curative agent, one should not suppress the signs and symptoms of rheumatic fever until they are clearly expressed.

Particularly confusing in the differential diagnosis of rheumatic fever is the drug sensitivity with fever and polyarthritis which may occur after administration of penicillin for a previous pharyngitis. Urticaria or angioedema, if present, helps identify penicillin sensitivity in such cases. The abdominal pain of rheumatic fever may be mistaken for appendicitis, and the crisis of sickle cell anemia also may be associated with joint pain, enlargement of the heart, and cardiac murmurs. The rapidity with which the arthritis symptoms of rheumatic fever are controlled with salicylates is characteristic of this disease. Dramatic response to salicylates does not in itself, however, establish a diagnosis of rheumatic fever.

In order to help clarify the diagnosis of acute rheumatic fever, the American Heart Association has accepted and modified criteria usually referred to as the *Jones criteria* (see Table 200-1). They are not to be used as a substitute for good medical judgment but are recommended as a guide for careful study of questionable cases. The finding of two major criteria or of one major and two minor criteria indicates a high probability of the presence of rheumatic fever if supported by evidence of a preceding streptococcal infection. The absence of the latter should always make the diagnosis questionable, except in the situation in which rheumatic fever is first discovered after a long latent period from the antecedent infection (Sydenham's chorea or low-grade carditis). Because the prognosis may differ according to the major manifestations, for recording purposes the diagnosis of rheumatic fever should be followed by a list of the major manifestations present, e.g., rheumatic fever manifested by polyarthritis and carditis (Table 200-2). An indication of the severity of carditis in terms of presence or absence of congestive heart failure and cardiomegaly is also advisable.

TABLE 200-2   Ninety-nine cases of acute rheumatic fever indicated by three major manifestations of Jones Criteria

Major manifestations*	Percent
Carditis	14
Polyarthritis	14
Chorea	4
Carditis and polyarthritis	44
Carditis and chorea	14
Carditis, chorea, and polyarthritis	6
Polyarthritis and chorea	4
Total	**100**

* Categories are mutually exclusive.
SOURCE: Acute rheumatic fever—Utah. Morb Mort Week Rep 36:109, 1988

TREATMENT   There is no specific cure for rheumatic fever, and no known measures change the course of the attack. Good supportive therapy, however, can reduce the mortality and morbidity of the disease.

Antibiotic therapy   After rheumatic fever is first diagnosed, a course of penicillin should be given to eliminate group A streptococci. This course is advisable even if bacteriologic examination yields throat cultures negative for streptococci, since the organisms may be present in areas inaccessible to swabs. It is preferable to administer penicillin parenterally. An effective course is a single injection of 1.2 million units of benzathine penicillin intramuscularly or 600,000 units of procaine penicillin intramuscularly daily for 10 days. Attempts to reduce ultimate heart damage by administering larger doses of penicillin early in the acute rheumatic attack have not been successful. After completion of the therapeutic course of penicillin, continuous protection from reinfection with streptococci should be provided by instituting one of the prophylactic regimens described below.

Suppressive therapy   For patients without carditis, treatment with glucocorticoids is unnecessary. Acute arthritis can be relieved with codeine or salicylate, the latter being preferable to reduce fever and joint inflammation. When salicylate is used in the therapy of rheumatic fever, the dosage should be increased until the drug produces either a clinical effect or systemic toxicity characterized by tinnitus, headache, or hyperpnea. A starting dose of 100 to 125 mg/ kg per day in children and 6 to 8 g in adults given in four or five divided doses is recommended. Of the various salicylate preparations, ordinary aspirin is cheapest and most effective.

Many physicians prefer glucocorticoids to salicylates for the treatment of carditis, despite the lack of a demonstrated advantage of these adrenal hormones in controlled clinical trials. Glucocorticoids are more potent anti-inflammatory agents but are more likely to be followed by posttherapeutic "rebounds," and they have the additional disadvantage of more frequent side effects, particularly acne, hirsutism, and cushingoid changes in facies and habitus. For this reason it is preferable to begin treatment of patients who have carditis with salicylates; if these drugs fail to reduce fever and to ameliorate heart failure, therapy with glucocorticoids may be initiated promptly. Prednisone is administered in doses of 60 to 120 mg or higher when necessary in four divided doses daily. After the inflammation has been brought under control by either salicylates or glucocorticoids, treatment should be continued until the sedimentation rate approaches near-normal values and should be maintained for several weeks thereafter. To prevent poststeroid rebounds, an "overlap" course of salicylate therapy may be added when steroids are tapered off over a 2-week period. A useful method for tapering steroids is outlined in Chap. 335. Salicylates may then be continued for an additional 2 to 3 weeks. Rebounds of rheumatic activity are usually of short duration and, when mild, are best managed without resuming anti-inflammatory treatment because a second or even a third rebound may occur when suppressive therapy is discontinued. About 5 percent of rheumatic attacks persist for 6 months or longer, either in the form of spontaneous acute recrudescences or as posttherapeutic rebounds. These "chronic" attacks are most likely to occur in patients with cardiac damage and with previous rheumatic episodes. Weekly tests for C-reactive protein in blood and for erythrocyte sedimentation rate are useful in following the healing process, particularly while treatment with glucocorticoids or salicylates is gradually withdrawn.

Treatment of chorea   The signs and symptoms of chorea usually do not respond well to treatment with antirheumatic agents. Because the patient with chorea is frequently emotionally unstable, and because the manifestations of chorea may be exaggerated by emotional trauma, complete mental and physical rest is essential. Patients with chorea should be kept in a quiet room and cared for by sympathetic attendants. Glucocorticoids or salicylates have little or no effect on chorea. Sedatives and tranquilizers, particularly diazepam and chlorpromazine, are useful. Chorea, no matter how severe, disappears during sleep, which should therefore be ensured by adequate sedation. Padded sideboards for the bed may be necessary to avoid injury to the patient. In the absence of other evidence of acute rheumatic disease, it is advisable to allow gradual resumption of physical activity when improvement is apparent rather than waiting for all choreiform movements to disappear, which may require many months.

Because of the great variability in the course of chorea, evaluating the effectiveness of various therapeutic measures is difficult. It is well to remember that chorea is a self-limited disease which is usually not followed by significant neurologic sequelae and that good results are almost invariably obtained by patient, attentive nursing care and conservative medical management.

PREVENTION OF RECURRENCE   The resurgence of localized outbreaks of rheumatic fever in the United States in recent years has been blamed, in part, on less than faithful adherence to conventional recommendations for rigorous penicillin regimens known to be highly effective in the prevention of both primary and secondary rheumatic attacks. It is recommended, therefore, that these regimens continue to be employed. The most efficient regimen for continuous prophylaxis against group A streptococci is a monthly intramuscular injection of 1.2 million units of benzathine penicillin G. The disadvantages and discomfort of this regimen have to be weighed against the individual patient's susceptibility to recurrences. Those with rheumatic heart disease, recent rheumatic fever, and exposure to an environment in which the incidence of streptococcal infection is frequent deserve the most effective protection. As a second choice, prophylaxis may be administered orally with either 1 g sulfadiazine daily in a single dose or 200,000 units of penicillin given twice daily on an empty stomach. The duration of continuous prophylaxis cannot be fixed arbitrarily. Certainly, those under the age of 18 years should receive a continuous prophylactic regimen. A minimum period of 5 years is recommended for patients who develop rheumatic fever without carditis over the age of 18 years. The decision to continue prophylaxis beyond this period should take into account a number of variables. Patients with rheumatic heart disease are more susceptible to reactivation of rheumatic fever if they contract a streptococcal infection. Moreover, patients who have had carditis in a previous attack are much more likely to suffer carditis again in a subsequent attack. Climate, age, occupation, household situation, cardiac status, and length of time since the previous attack are all significant variables which influence the risk of recurrence. The decline in recurrence rates with increasing age is due to (1) decreased rate of rheumatogenic streptococcal infection and (2) decrease in the rate of rheumatic reactivation following streptococcal infection in older rheumatic subjects. Despite this decreased rate, however, the risk of rheumatic recurrence in adults remains relatively high when the streptococcal disease encountered is severe or epidemic and particularly when rheumatic fever, and thus rheumatogenic streptococci, are known to be extant in the population to which a rheumatic subject is exposed.

PREVENTION OF INITIAL RHEUMATIC ATTACKS   Early and adequate treatment of pharyngeal infection due to group A streptococci will prevent initial attacks of rheumatic fever. If clinical streptococcal disease were properly detected by throat cultures and adequately treated, the spread of infection in a given population would be prevented, the epidemiology of streptococcal disease would be modified markedly, and the incidence of rheumatic fever in the community would be diminished. In communities where group A streptococcal disease has been diagnosed early and treated well and where socioeconomic standards are high, the group A organisms cultured frequently from school children's throats may be of relatively low virulence and may either not cause rheumatic fever at all or do so less frequently than more virulent strains prevalent in many epidemics. The appearance of rheumatic fever in a community, however, signals the presence of rheumatogenic streptococci whose spread must be interrupted by use of effective penicillin regimens. In a closed population, such as a military base or an institution, an outbreak of rheumatic fever is best treated by mass penicillin prophylaxis, i.e., treatment of all exposed individuals, whether or not symptomatic.

Streptococcal pharyngitis is adequately treated by a single intramuscular injection of 600,000 units of benzathine penicillin in children less than 10 years of age or 1.2 million units in older children and adults. Any alternative plan of parenteral therapy or combined parenteral and oral therapy should provide for treatment over a period of 10 days. If oral penicillin is employed, at least 800,000 units per day in four divided doses must be given for no less than 10 days to achieve results comparable with a single injection of benzathine penicillin. Erythromycin in daily doses of 1 g for 10 days may be substituted in penicillin-sensitive individuals. Tetracycline is not recommended because some strains of group A streptococci have acquired resistance to it. All group A streptococci have so far remained extremely sensitive to penicillin. When erythromycin has been used extensively in place of penicillin as the drug of choice to treat pharyngitis, erythromycin-resistant group A streptococci have emerged with high frequency. Penicillin therefore remains the treatment of choice for streptococcal sore throat.

REFERENCES

AMERICAN HEART ASSOCIATION COMMITTEE ON RHEUMATIC FEVER, ENDOCARDITIS AND KAWASAKI DISEASE OF THE COUNCIL ON CARDIOVASCULAR DISEASE: Prevention of rheumatic fever. Circulation 78:1082, 1988

BISNO AL: Group A streptococcal infections and acute rheumatic fever. N Engl J Med 35(11):783, 1991

BURGE DJ, DeHORATIUS RJ: Acute rheumatic fever. Cardiovasc Clin 23:3, 1993

FELDMAN T: Rheumatic mitral stenosis. On the rise again. Postgrad Med 93:93, 99, 1993

Guidelines for the diagnosis of rheumatic fever—Jones criteria, 1992 update. JAMA 268(15):2069, 1992

KAPLAN EL et al: Group A streptococcal serotypes isolated from patients and sibling contacts during the resurgence of rheumatic fever in the United States in the mid-1980s. J Infect Dis 159:101, 1989

STOLLERMAN GH: Rheumatogenic group A streptococci and the return of rheumatic fever. Adv Intern Med 35:1, 1990.

201   VALVULAR HEART DISEASE

EUGENE BRAUNWALD

The role of physical examination in the evaluation of patients with valvular disease is also considered in Chap. 188; of electrocardiography in Chap. 189; of roentgenography, echocardiography, and other noninvasive techniques in Chap. 190; of cardiac catheterization and angiography in Chap. 192; and of balloon valvuloplasty in Chap. 193.

MITRAL STENOSIS

ETIOLOGY AND PATHOLOGY   Two-thirds of all patients with mitral stenosis (MS) are females. MS is generally rheumatic in origin; rarely, it is congenital. Pure or predominant MS occurs in approximately 40 percent of all patients with rheumatic heart disease. The valve leaflets are diffusely thickened by fibrous tissue and/or calcific deposits. The mitral commissures fuse, the chordae tendineae fuse and shorten, the valvular cusps become rigid, and these changes, in turn, lead to narrowing at the apex of the funnel-shaped valve. While the initial insult to the mitral valve is rheumatic, the later changes may be a nonspecific process resulting from trauma to the valve caused by altered flow patterns due to the initial deformity. Calcification of the stenotic mitral valve immobilizes the leaflets and narrows the orifice further. Thrombus formation and arterial embolization may arise from the calcific valve itself.

PATHOPHYSIOLOGY   In normal adults the mitral valve orifice is 4 to 6 cm^2. In the presence of significant obstruction, i.e., when the orifice is less than approximately 2 cm^2, blood can flow from the left atrium to the left ventricle only if propelled by an abnormally elevated left atrioventricular pressure gradient (Fig. 192-6), the hemodynamic hallmark of MS. When the mitral valve opening is reduced to 1 cm^2, a left atrial pressure of approximately 25 mmHg is required to maintain a normal cardiac output. The elevated left atrial pressure, in turn, raises pulmonary venous and capillary pressures, reducing pulmonary compliance and causing exertional dyspnea. The first bouts of dyspnea are usually precipitated by clinical events which increase the rate of blood flow across the mitral orifice, which results in further elevation of the left atrial pressure (see below). In order to assess the severity of obstruction, it is essential to measure both the transvalvular pressure gradient and the flow rate (Chap. 192). The latter is dependent not only on the cardiac output but on the heart rate as well. An increase in heart rate shortens diastole proportionately more than systole and diminishes the time available for flow across the mitral valve. Therefore, at any given level of cardiac output, tachycardia augments the transvalvular gradient and elevates further the left atrial pressure.

The left ventricular diastolic pressure is normal in isolated MS; coexisting aortic valve disease, systemic hypertension, mitral regurgitation, ischemic heart disease and perhaps the residua of damage produced by rheumatic myocarditis are sometimes responsible for elevations which reflect impaired left ventricular function and/or reduced left ventricular compliance. Left ventricular dysfunction, as reflected in reduced ejection fraction and circumferential fiber shortening rate, occurs in about one-fourth of patients with severe MS. This may be a consequence of chronic reduction of preload and extension of the scarring from the valve into the adjacent myocardium. In pure MS and sinus rhythm, the mean left atrial and pulmonary artery wedge pressures are usually elevated, and the pressure pulse shows a prominent atrial contraction (*a* wave) and a gradual pressure decline after mitral valve opening (*y* descent). In patients with mild to moderate MS without elevation of the pulmonary vascular resistance, the pulmonary arterial pressure may be near the upper limits of normal at rest and may rise with exercise. In severe MS and whenever the pulmonary vascular resistance is significantly increased, the pulmonary arterial pressure is elevated even when the patient is at rest, and in extreme cases it may exceed the systemic arterial pressure. Further elevations of left atrial, pulmonary capillary, and pulmonary arterial pressures occur during exercise. When the pulmonary arterial systolic pressure exceeds approximately 50 mmHg in patients with MS, or for that matter with any lesion affecting the left side of the heart, the increased right ventricular afterload impedes the emptying of this chamber, and right ventricular end-diastolic pressure and volume usually rise as a compensatory mechanism.

Cardiac output   This varies considerably; the hemodynamic response to a given degree of mitral obstruction may range from a normal cardiac output at rest and a high left atrioventricular pressure gradient to a reduced cardiac output and low transvalvular pressure gradient at the opposite end of the hemodynamic spectrum. In a minority of patients with moderately severe MS, the cardiac output is normal at rest and rises normally during exertion; under these circumstances, the high atrioventricular pressure gradient elevates the left atrial and pulmonary capillary pressures markedly, and this elevation is responsible for symptoms of severe pulmonary congestion. In the majority of patients with moderate MS, however, the cardiac output is normal or almost so at rest but rises subnormally during exertion. In patients with severe MS, particularly those in whom the pulmonary vascular resistance is strikingly elevated, the cardiac output is subnormal at rest and may fail to rise or may even decline during activity. The depressed cardiac output in patients with MS is related primarily to the obstruction of the mitral orifice but also may be due to the impairment of the function of either ventricle.

Pulmonary hypertension   The clinical and hemodynamic features of MS are influenced importantly by the level of the pulmonary artery pressure. Pulmonary hypertension results from (1) the passive backward transmission of the elevated left atrial pressure, (2) pulmonary arteriolar constriction, which presumably is triggered by left atrial and pulmonary venous hypertension (reactive pulmonary hypertension), and (3) organic obliterative changes in the pulmonary vascular bed. The elevation of pulmonary vascular resistance may be considered to be a complication of long-standing and severe MS; in time, the resultant severe pulmonary hypertension results in tricuspid and pulmonary incompetence as well as right-sided heart failure. However, the changes in the pulmonary vascular bed also may be considered to exert a protective effect; the elevated precapillary resistance reduces the likelihood of symptoms of pulmonary congestion by reducing the surge of blood into the pulmonary capillary bed during activity which then dams up behind the stenotic mitral valve. However, this protection occurs at the expense of a decreased cardiac output.

SYMPTOMS AND COMPLICATIONS In temperate climates the latent period between the initial attack of rheumatic carditis (in the increasingly rare circumstances in which a history of one can be elicited) and the development of symptoms due to MS is generally on the order of two decades; most patients begin to experience disability in the fourth decade. Studies carried out prior to the development of mitral valvuloplasty revealed that once a patient with MS becomes seriously symptomatic, continuous progression of the disease to death usually occurs in 2 to 5 years. In economically deprived areas, particularly on the Indian subcontinent, in Central America, and the Middle East, MS tends to progress more rapidly and frequently causes serious symptoms before the age of 20 years. On the other hand, slowly progressive MS in the elderly is being recognized with increasing frequency in the United States and western Europe.

When valvular obstruction is mild, many of the physical signs of MS may be present in the absence of any symptoms. However, even in those patients whose mitral orifices are large enough to accommodate a normal blood flow with only mild elevations of left atrial pressure, extreme exertion, excitement, fever, severe anemia, paroxysmal tachycardia, sexual intercourse, pregnancy, and thyrotoxicosis all may precipitate elevations of pulmonary capillary pressure and lead to dyspnea and cough. As stenosis progresses, lesser stresses precipitate dyspnea, and the patient becomes limited in his or her daily activities. Redistribution of blood from the dependent portions of the body to the lungs, which occurs when the recumbent position is assumed, leads to orthopnea and paroxysmal nocturnal dyspnea. *Pulmonary edema* develops when there is a sudden surge in flow across a markedly narrowed mitral orifice (Chap. 31). When moderately severe MS has existed for several years, *atrial arrhythmias*—premature contractions, paroxysmal tachycardia, flutter, and fibrillation—occur with increasing frequency. The rapid ventricular rate associated with untreated or inadequately treated atrial fibrillation is frequently responsible for acute exacerbations of dyspnea. The development of permanent atrial fibrillation often marks a turning point in the patient's course and is generally associated with acceleration of the rate at which symptoms progress.

Hemoptysis (Chap. 30) results from rupture of pulmonary-bronchial venous connections secondary to pulmonary venous hypertension. It occurs most frequently in patients who have elevated left atrial pressures *without* markedly elevated pulmonary vascular resistances and is almost never fatal. True hemoptysis must be distinguished from the bloody sputum that occurs with pulmonary edema, pulmonary infarction, and bronchitis, three conditions that occur with increased frequency in the presence of MS.

As the condition progresses and the pulmonary vascular resistance rises or when tricuspid stenosis or regurgitation develops, symptoms secondary to pulmonary congestion sometimes diminish, and the episodes of acute pulmonary edema and hemoptysis become reduced in frequency and severity. Elevation of pulmonary vascular resistance further increases right ventricular systolic pressure, leading to right ventricular failure, fatigue, abdominal discomfort due to hepatic congestion, and edema.

Recurrent pulmonary emboli, sometimes with infarction (Chap. 226), are an important cause of morbidity and mortality late in the course of MS, occurring most frequently in patients with right ventricular failure. *Pulmonary infections*, i.e., bronchitis, bronchopneumonia, and lobar pneumonia, commonly complicate untreated MS. *Infective endocarditis* (Chap. 85) is rare in *pure* MS but is not uncommon in patients with combined stenosis and regurgitation. *Chest pain* occurs in about 10 percent of patients with severe MS; it may be due to pulmonary hypertension or myocardial ischemia secondary to coronary atherosclerosis; often the cause cannot be discovered.

Pulmonary and pulmonary vascular changes In addition to the aforementioned changes in the pulmonary vascular bed, fibrous thickening of the walls of the alveoli and pulmonary capillaries occurs commonly in MS. The vital capacity, total lung capacity, maximal breathing capacity, and oxygen uptake per unit of ventilation are reduced (Chap. 214), and in patients with severe MS, the latter fails to rise normally during exertion. The reduction of pulmonary compliance that occurs generally correlates directly with the severity of the dyspnea and with the heightened pulmonary capillary pressure, and these changes are intensified during exercise. In some patients, airway resistance is abnormally increased. These alterations in pulmonary mechanics contribute to an increase in the work of breathing and play an important role in the genesis of dyspnea. The changes in the lungs are due, in part, to increased transudation of fluid from the pulmonary capillaries into the interstitial and alveolar spaces as a consequence of the elevated pulmonary capillary pressure. The distribution of blood flow and ventilation may be uneven; as in other conditions in which left atrial pressure is elevated, pulmonary blood flow in the erect position is displaced from the basal to the apical segments of the lung (Chap. 214). The diffusing capacity may be reduced, particularly during exertion, as a result of structural changes in the diffusing surface and reduction of the pulmonary capillary blood volume. The thickening of the alveolar and capillary walls impedes the transudation of fluid into the alveoli and the development of pulmonary edema at times when the pulmonary capillary pressure exceeds the plasma oncotic pressure. The increased capacity of the pulmonary lymphatic system to drain excess fluid also retards the development of pulmonary edema.

Thrombi and emboli *Thrombi* may form in the left atria, particularly in the enlarged atrial appendages of patients with MS. If they *embolize*, they do so most commonly to the brain, kidneys, spleen, and extremities. Embolization occurs much more frequently in patients with atrial fibrillation or unstable rhythms, in older patients, and in those with a reduced cardiac output, and it is seen in patients with relatively mild, as well as in those with severe, obstruction. Thus systemic embolization may be the presenting complaint in otherwise asymptomatic patients with mild MS. At operation, thrombi are *not* found more frequently in the left atria of patients with a past history of embolization than in those without this complication, indicating that it is usually the freshly formed clots that dislodge. Patients who have had one or more systemic emboli have an increased predilection for further embolic episodes compared with patients with stenosis of comparable severity without previous embolization. Rarely, a large pedunculated thrombus or a free-floating clot may suddenly obstruct the stenotic mitral orifice. Such "ball valve" thrombi produce syncope, angina, and changing auscultatory signs with alterations in position, findings that resemble those produced by a left atrial myxoma (Chap. 207).

PHYSICAL FINDINGS (See also Chap. 188) **Inspection** Peripheral and facial *cyanosis* may occur in patients with extremely severe MS. In advanced cases there is a malar flush and the facies appear pinched and blue. The jugular venous pulse reveals prominent *a* waves due to vigorous right atrial systole in patients with sinus rhythm who have severe pulmonary hypertension or associated tricuspid stenosis. When atrial fibrillation is present, the jugular pulse reveals only a single expansion during systole (*c-v* wave). The systemic arterial pressure is usually normal or slightly low.

Palpation   A right ventricular tap along the left sternal border signifies an enlarged right ventricle. The first heart sound may be palpable in patients with pliable valve leaflets. In patients with pulmonary hypertension, the impact of pulmonary valve closure can usually be felt in the second and third left intercostal spaces just left of the sternum; the left ventricle is not palpable in severe, pure MS. A diastolic thrill is frequently present at the cardiac apex, particularly if the patient is turned into the left lateral recumbent position.

Auscultation   The first heart sound (S_1) is generally accentuated and snapping, and since the mitral valve does not close until the left ventricular pressure reaches the level of the elevated left atrial pressure, this sound is often slightly delayed on phonocardiography, causing a prolonged Q-S_1 interval, particularly in patients with severe stenosis. In patients with pulmonary hypertension, the pulmonary component of the second heart sound (P_2) is often accentuated, and the two components of the second heart sound are closely split. A pulmonary systolic ejection click may be heard in patients with severe pulmonary hypertension and marked dilatation of the pulmonary artery. The opening snap (OS) of the mitral valve is most readily audible in expiration at, or just medial to, the cardiac apex but also may be easily heard along the left sternal edge or at the base of the heart. This sound generally follows the sound of aortic valve closure (A_2) by 0.05 to 0.12 s; that is, it follows P_2. Since the OS occurs when the left ventricular pressure falls below the left atrial pressure, the time interval between A_2 closure and OS varies inversely with the severity of the MS. It tends to be short (0.05 to 0.07 s) in patients with severe obstruction, and long (0.10 to 0.12 s) in patients with mild MS. The intensities of the OS and S_1 correlate with the mobility of the anterior mitral leaflet.

The OS usually ushers in a low-pitched, rumbling, diastolic murmur, heard best at the apex with the patient in the left lateral recumbent position. It is accentuated by exercise carried out just before auscultation and reduced during the strain of a Valsalva maneuver. In general, the duration of this murmur correlates with the severity of the stenosis. In patients with sinus rhythm, the murmur often reappears or becomes reaccentuated during atrial systole, as atrial contraction reelevates the rate of blood flow across the narrowed orifice. Soft (grade I or II/VI) systolic murmurs are commonly heard at the apex or along the left sternal border in patients with pure MS and do not necessarily signify the presence of mitral regurgitation. Hepatomegaly, ankle edema, ascites, and pleural effusion, particularly in the right pleural cavity, may occur in patients with MS and right ventricular failure.

Associated lesions   With severe pulmonary hypertension, a pansystolic murmur produced by functional tricuspid regurgitation may be audible along the left sternal border. Characteristically, this murmur is accentuated by inspiration, diminishes during forced expiration or during performance of the Valsalva maneuver, diminishes or disappears as pulmonary artery pressure declines, and should not be confused with the apical pansystolic murmur of mitral regurgitation, since management of the two valvular lesions is quite different.

The recognition of associated mitral regurgitation is of considerable clinical importance in patients with MS. A presystolic murmur and an accentuated first heart sound speak against the presence of serious associated mitral regurgitation, but when the first heart sound and/or the opening snap are soft or absent in a patient with mitral valve disease who also has an apical systolic murmur, it is likely that significant mitral regurgitation and/or serious calcification of the deformed mitral valve leaflets are present. A third heart sound at the apex often signifies that the mitral regurgitation is serious; this sound is generally duller, lower pitched, and follows the opening snap. Occasionally, in patients with pure MS, physical signs may falsely suggest mitral regurgitation. Thus, in the presence of severe pulmonary hypertension and right ventricular failure, a third heart sound may originate from the right ventricle. The enlarged right ventricle may rotate the heart in a clockwise direction and form the cardiac apex, giving the examiner the erroneous impression of left ventricular enlargement. Under these circumstances, the rumbling diastolic murmur and the other auscultatory features of MS become less prominent or may even disappear and be replaced by the systolic murmur of functional tricuspid regurgitation which is mistaken for mitral regurgitation. When cardiac output is markedly reduced in a patient with MS, the typical auscultatory findings, including the diastolic rumbling murmur, may not be detectable (silent MS), but they may reappear as compensation is restored. Associated tricuspid stenosis also tends to obscure many of the physical signs of MS.

The Graham Steell murmur of pulmonary regurgitation, a high-pitched, diastolic, decrescendo blowing murmur along the left sternal border, results from dilatation of the pulmonary valve ring and occurs in patients with mitral valve disease and severe pulmonary hypertension. This murmur may be indistinguishable from the more common murmur produced by aortic regurgitation except that it is rarely audible at the second right intercostal space and may disappear following successful surgical treatment of the MS.

Electrocardiogram   In MS and sinus rhythm, the P wave usually suggests left atrial enlargement (Chap. 189). It may become tall and peaked in lead II and upright in lead V_1 when severe pulmonary hypertension or tricuspid stenosis complicates MS and right atrial enlargement occurs. The QRS complex may be normal, even in patients with critical MS. However, with severe pulmonary hypertension, right axis deviation and right ventricular hypertrophy are usually found. When left ventricular hypertrophy is present in patients with MS, it generally indicates that an additional lesion which places a significant burden on the left ventricle, such as mitral regurgitation, aortic valve disease, or hypertension, is present.

Echocardiogram   (See also Chap. 190)   The echocardiogram is the most sensitive and specific noninvasive method for diagnosing MS. Two-dimensional color Doppler flow echocardiographic imaging and Doppler echocardiography (see Figs. 190-4 and 190-7) provide critical information, including an estimate of the transvalvular gradient and of mitral orifice size, the presence and severity of accompanying mitral regurgitation, the extent of restriction of valve leaflets, their thickness, and the degree of distortion of the subvalvular apparatus. In addition, echocardiography provides an assessment of the size of the cardiac chambers, an estimation of the pulmonary artery pressure, and an indication of the presence and severity of associated tricuspid and pulmonic regurgitation.

Roentgenogram   (Chap. 190)   The earliest changes are straightening of the left border of the cardiac silhouette, prominence of the main pulmonary arteries, dilatation of the upper lobe pulmonary veins, and backward displacement of the esophagus by an enlarged left atrium. In patients with mild or moderate MS, the heart is not grossly enlarged. In severe MS, however, all chambers and vessels upstream to the narrowed valve are prominent, including the two atria, the pulmonary arteries and veins, right ventricle, and superior vena cava. Kerley B lines are fine, dense, opaque, horizontal lines which are most prominent in the lower and midlung fields and which result from distention of interlobular septa and lymphatics with edema when the resting mean left atrial pressure exceeds approximately 20 mmHg. As the pulmonary arterial pressure rises, the smaller pulmonary arteries become attenuated, at first in the lower, then in the middle, and finally in the upper lung fields. In patients who have had multiple hemoptyses, hemosiderin-containing macrophages fill the air spaces, and if they become confluent, they result in a fine, diffuse nodulation most prominent in the lower lung fields.

DIFFERENTIAL DIAGNOSIS   Significant mitral regurgitation may be associated with a prominent diastolic murmur at the apex, but this murmur commences slightly later than in patients with MS, and there is often clear-cut evidence of left ventricular enlargement on physical examination, roentgenography, and electrocardiography. In addition, an apical pansystolic murmur of at least grade III/VI intensity as well as a third heart sound should arouse the suspicion of significant associated regurgitation. Similarly, the apical middiastolic murmur associated with aortic regurgitation (Austin Flint murmur) may be mistaken for MS. However, in a patient with aortic regurgitation, the absence of an opening snap or of presystolic accentuation if sinus rhythm is present points to the *absence* of MS. Tricuspid stenosis, a valvular lesion that occurs very rarely in the absence of MS, may mask many of the clinical features of MS. Echocardiography is particularly useful in detecting MS in patients who have or are suspected of having other valve lesions and in defining the severity of the various lesions.

Exertional dyspnea and recurrent pulmonary infections may be falsely ascribed to pulmonary emphysema in patients with both *chronic lung disease* and MS. Careful auscultation, however, will generally reveal the characteristic opening snap and rumbling diastolic murmur. Similarly, the hemoptysis that occurs in many otherwise asymptomatic patients with MS may be improperly attributed to bronchiectasis or tuberculosis; the latter condition is uncommon in patients with significant mitral obstruction.

Primary pulmonary hypertension (Chap. 225) results in a number of the clinical and laboratory features observed in MS. It occurs most frequently in young women; however, the OS and diastolic rumbling murmur are absent, there is no left atrial enlargement, and the pulmonary artery wedge and left atrial pressures are normal, as is the size of the left atrium on echocardiography. *Atrial septal defect* (Chap. 199) also may be mistaken for MS; in both conditions there is often clinical, electrocardiographic, and roentgenographic evidence of right ventricular enlargement and accentuation of the pulmonary vascularity. The widely split S_2 of atrial septal defect may be confused with the mitral OS, and the diastolic flow murmur across the tricuspid valve may be mistaken for the mitral diastolic murmur. However, the absence of left atrial enlargement and of Kerley B lines and the demonstration of fixed splitting of S_2 favor atrial septal defect over MS. *Cor triatriatum* is an unusual congenital malformation that consists of a fibrous ring within the left atrium. It results in elevation of the pulmonary venous, capillary, and arterial pressures. This lesion can be recognized most readily by means of left atrial angiography.

Left atrial myxoma (Chap. 207) may obstruct left atrial emptying, causing dyspnea, a diastolic murmur, and hemodynamic changes resembling those of MS. However, patients with left atrial myxoma often demonstrate findings suggestive of a systemic disease, with weight loss, fever, anemia, systemic emboli, and elevated erythrocyte sedimentation rate and serum IgG concentration. Usually an OS is not audible, there is no clinical evidence of associated aortic valve disease, and the auscultatory findings frequently change with body position. The diagnosis can be established by demonstrating a characteristic echo-producing mass in the left atrium by two-dimensional echocardiography.

CARDIAC CATHETERIZATION AND ANGIOCARDIOGRAPHY Catheterization of the left side of the heart (Chap. 192) is extremely helpful in deciding whether valvulotomy is necessary in patients in whom it is difficult to estimate the severity of obstruction by clinical means and noninvasive tests. When combined with aortography and left ventricular angiocardiography, this procedure serves as the ultimate method for detecting and estimating associated mitral regurgitation and coexisting lesions such as aortic stenosis and regurgitation as well as left ventricular dysfunction. These "invasive" methods are also helpful in the detection of accompanying conditions, such as coronary artery disease, that impair left ventricular function and would thereby contraindicate or reduce the effectiveness of mitral valvulotomy. Catheterization is not usually necessary to aid in the decision regarding surgery in relatively young (<45 years for males, <50 for females) patients with typical findings of severe obstruction on clinical examination and echocardiography. In older patients, coronary angiography is usually advisable preoperatively, in order to detect patients with critical coronary obstructions which should be bypassed at the time of operation. Catheterization and left ventricular angiography are also indicated in most patients who have undergone previous mitral valve operations and who have redeveloped serious symptoms; in such patients, clinical assessment may be particularly difficult, and the hemodynamic studies allow determination of the severity of the lesion, intelligent planning of the operative procedure when it is indicated, and a more accurate estimate of the risk.

MANAGEMENT In the asymptomatic adolescent with mitral valve disease, penicillin prophylaxis of beta-hemolytic streptococcal infections (Chap. 200) and prophylaxis for infective endocarditis (Chap. 85) are important. In symptomatic patients, some improvement usually occurs with restriction of sodium intake and maintenance doses of oral diuretics. Digitalis glycosides do not alter the hemodynamics and usually do not benefit patients with pure stenosis and sinus rhythm, but they are necessary for slowing the ventricular rate of patients with atrial fibrillation and for reducing the manifestations of right-sided heart failure in the advanced stages of the disease. Small doses of beta blockers (e.g., atenolol 25 to 50 mg/d) may be added when cardiac glycosides fail to control ventricular rate in patients with atrial fibrillation or flutter. Particular attention should be directed toward detecting and treating any accompanying anemia and infections. Hemoptysis is treated by measures designed to diminish pulmonary venous pressure, including bed rest, the sitting position, salt restriction, and diuresis. Anticoagulants should be administered for at least 1 year in patients with MS who have suffered systemic and/or pulmonary embolization and continuously in those with atrial fibrillation.

If atrial fibrillation is of relatively recent origin in a patient whose MS is not severe enough to warrant surgical treatment, reversion to sinus rhythm pharmacologically or by means of electrical countershock is indicated. Usually this should be undertaken following 3 weeks of anticoagulant treatment. Conversion to sinus rhythm is rarely helpful in patients with severe MS, particularly those in whom the left atrium is especially enlarged or in whom atrial fibrillation has been present for more than 1 year, since reversion to atrial fibrillation is common.

Mitral valvulotomy Unless there is a specific contraindication, mitral valvulotomy is indicated in the symptomatic patient with pure MS whose effective orifice is less than approximately 1.3 cm^2 (or 0.8 cm^2/m^2 of body surface area). Operation usually not only results in striking symptomatic and hemodynamic improvement but also prolongs survival. In uncomplicated cases, the surgical mortality rate should be 0 to 3 percent. However, there is no evidence that surgical treatment improves the prognosis of patients with slight or no functional impairment. Therefore, unless recurrent systemic embolization has occurred, valvulotomy is *not* recommended for patients who are entirely asymptomatic, regardless of hemodynamic findings. When there is little symptomatic improvement following valvulotomy, it is likely that the procedure was ineffective, that it induced mitral regurgitation, or that associated valvular or myocardial disease was present. The recurrence of symptoms several years after what appeared to be a satisfactory initial result is usually due to an inadequate valvulotomy, but progression of other valvular lesions, restenosis of the mitral valve, or some combination of these conditions also may be responsible. More than half of all patients undergoing mitral valvulotomy require reoperation by 10 years. In the *pregnant patient* with MS, operative treatment should be carried out if pulmonary congestion occurs despite intensive medical treatment.

An "open" operation using cardiopulmonary bypass is usually preferable to closed commissurotomy for patients with pure MS who have not been operated on previously. In addition to opening the valve commissures, it is important to loosen any subvalvular fusion of papillary muscles and chordae tendineae and to remove large deposits of calcium, thereby improving valvular function, and to remove atrial thrombi. In patients with significant associated mitral regurgitation, those in whom the valve has been severely distorted by previous operative manipulation, or those in whom the surgeon does not find it possible to improve valve function significantly, the valve may have to be replaced with a prosthesis. Since the operative mortality of replacement of the mitral valve is still approximately 5 percent, and since there are long-term complications of valve replacement, patients in whom preoperative evaluation suggests the possibility that replacement may be required should be operated on only if they have *critical* mitral stenosis, i.e., an orifice <1.0 cm^2, and are in the New York Heart Association class III, i.e., symptomatic with ordinary activity, despite optimal medical therapy.

Percutaneous balloon valvuloplasty, described on p. 987, is an alternative to surgical mitral valvuloplasty in patients with pure or predominant rheumatic mitral stenosis. Young patients without extensive valvular calcification or thickening or subvalvular deformity are the best candidates for this procedure; in them the results approach those of closed surgical commissurotomy with similar low mortality. It is particularly useful in pregnant women but also may be used in older patients with severe valvular deformity with serious extracardiac disease who are poor operative candidates.

VALVE REPLACEMENT The results of replacement of any valve are dependent primarily on (1) the patient's myocardial function at the time of operation, (2) the technical abilities of the operative team and the quality of the postoperative care, and (3) the durability, hemodynamic characteristics, and thrombogenicity of the prosthesis. Increased operative mortality is associated with the degree of preoperative functional disability and pulmonary hypertension. Late complications of replacement of any valve, which fortunately are declining in incidence, include paravalvular leakage, thromboemboli, bleeding due to anticoagulants, mechanical dysfunction of the prosthesis, and infective endocarditis.

The considerations regarding the choice between a bioprosthetic (tissue) and artificial mechanical valve are similar in the mitral and aortic positions and in the treatment of stenotic, regurgitant, or mixed lesions. All patients who have undergone replacement of any valve with a mechanical prosthesis must be maintained permanently on anticoagulants. The primary advantage of bioprostheses over mechanical prostheses is the reduction of thromboembolic complications, and except for patients with chronic atrial fibrillation, few such instances have been associated with their use. The major disadvantage of bioprosthetic valves is their mechanical deterioration. This results in the need to replace the prosthesis in 30 percent of patients by 10 years and 50 percent by 15 years. Bioprostheses are ordinarily not used in younger patients (<35 years) because of accelerated deterioration but are particularly useful in the elderly (>70 years), in whom there is more concern about chronic anticoagulation than about long-term (>15 years) valve durability. These valves are also indicated in women who expect to become pregnant, as well as others in whom anticoagulation may be contraindicated. In patients without such contraindications, particularly those under 65 years, a mechanical prosthesis may be preferable. Many surgeons now select the St. Jude prosthesis, a double-disk tilting prosthesis, for replacement of both aortic and mitral valves because of somewhat more favorable hemodynamic characteristics and a suggestion of lower thrombogenicity.

The overall 10-year survival of operative survivors following mitral valve replacement is approximately 60 percent. Long-term prognosis is worse in older patients and those with marked disability and striking depression of the cardiac index preoperatively.

MITRAL REGURGITATION

ETIOLOGY Chronic rheumatic heart disease is the cause of severe mitral regurgitation (MR) in about one-third of cases. In contrast to MS, rheumatic MR occurs more frequently in males. The rheumatic process produces rigidity, deformity, and retraction of the valve cusps and commissural fusion, as well as shortening, contraction, and fusion of the chordae tendineae. MR also may occur as a congenital anomaly (Chap. 199), most commonly as (1) a defect of the endocardial cushions or in association with (2) corrected transposition, (3) endocardial fibroelastosis, and (4) the "parachute" mitral valve deformity. MR may occur with fibrosis of a papillary muscle in patients with healed myocardial infarction as well as in patients with infarction involving the base of a papillary muscle. Transient regurgitation also may occur during periods of ischemia involving a papillary muscle or the adjacent myocardium and may accompany bouts of angina pectoris. MR may occur with marked left ventricular enlargement of any cause in which dilatation of the mitral annulus and lateral displacement of the papillary muscles interfere with coaptation of the valve leaflets. In hypertrophic cardiomyopathy, the anterior leaflet of the mitral valve is displaced anteriorly during systole, leading to regurgitation (Chap. 205). Massive calcification of the mitral annulus of unknown cause, presumably degenerative, which occurs most commonly in elderly women, also can be responsible for significant MR. Systemic lupus erythematosus, rheumatoid arthritis, and ankylosing spondylitis are less common causes. *Acute* MR may occur secondary to infective endocarditis involving the valve or chordae tendineae, in acute myocardial infarction with rupture of a papillary muscle or one of its heads, as a consequence of trauma, or following apparently spontaneous chordal rupture.

Abnormal elongation of chordae tendineae and/or redundant posterior cusps of the mitral valve with prolapse of the cusps into the left atrium, the so-called floppy valve, leading to the syndrome of midsystolic click and midsystolic murmur, also referred to as the *prolapsing mitral valve leaflet syndrome* (see below), is another important cause of MR.

Regardless of cause, severe MR is often progressive, since enlargement of the left atrium places tension on the posterior mitral leaflet, pulling it away from the mitral orifice and thereby aggravating the valvular dysfunction. Similarly, the dilatation of the left ventricle increases the regurgitation, which in turn enlarges further the left atrium and ventricle, causing chordal rupture and resulting in a vicious cycle; hence the aphorism, "mitral regurgitation begets mitral regurgitation."

PATHOPHYSIOLOGY Since the regurgitant mitral orifice is in parallel with the aortic orifice, the resistance to left ventricular emptying is reduced in patients with MR. As a consequence, the left ventricle is decompressed into the left atrium during ejection, and with the reduction in left ventricular size there is a rapid decline in left ventricular tension, i.e., a progressive reduction in left ventricular afterload, allowing a greater proportion of the contractile activity of the left ventricle to be expended in shortening. The initial compensation to MR consists of more complete systolic emptying of the left ventricle. However, left ventricular volume increases progressively as the severity of the regurgitation increases and the function of the left ventricle deteriorates. This is often accompanied by a depressed forward cardiac output. The regurgitant volume varies directly with the left ventricular systolic pressure and the size of the regurgitant orifice; the latter, in turn, is influenced profoundly by the degree of left ventricular dilatation.

The atrial contraction wave in the left atrial pressure pulse (*a* wave) is not as prominent as it is in MS, but the *v* wave is usually taller, since it is inscribed during ventricular systole, when the left atrium fills from the pulmonary veins as well as from the left ventricle. During early diastole, as the distended left atrium suddenly empties, there is a particularly rapid *y* descent as long as there is no associated MS (Fig. 192-7, p. 984). Left ventricular end-diastolic pressure may be slightly elevated. However, in chronic MR, there is often an increase in left ventricular compliance, so ventricular volume may be increased with little elevation in end-diastolic pressure. The effective (forward) cardiac output usually declines in seriously symptomatic patients. Although a left atrioventricular pressure gradient persisting throughout diastole signifies the presence of significant associated MS, a brief, early diastolic gradient may occur in patients with pure regurgitation as a result of the torrential flow of blood across a normal-sized mitral orifice.

The prompt appearance of contrast material in the left atrium following its injection into the left ventricle signifies the presence of MR. The regurgitant volume can be measured by determining the difference between the total left ventricular stroke volume estimated angiocardiographically and the effective forward stroke volume determined by the Fick method (Chap. 192). The results of such studies suggest that in patients with severe regurgitation the regurgitant volume may be of the same magnitude as the effective forward stroke volume or may even exceed it. Qualitative, but clinically useful, estimates of the severity of regurgitation may be made by Doppler echocardiography, color Doppler flow echocardiographic imaging, and observation on cineangiograms of the degree of left atrial opacification following the injection of contrast material into the left ventricle.

The compliance, i.e., the pressure-volume relationship, of the left atrium and pulmonary venous bed affects the clinical picture. Patients with *normal or reduced compliance* usually have *acute* MR, little enlargement of the left atrium, but marked elevation of the left atrial pressure, particularly of the *v* wave. Pulmonary edema is common. After several months, the pulmonary vascular resistance may become markedly elevated, presumably as a consequence of the left atrial hypertension, and right-sided heart failure also may occur; sinus rhythm is usually present.

Patients with a *marked increase in left atrial compliance* are the opposite end of the spectrum, having severe long-standing severe MR, marked enlargement of the left atrium, and normal or only slightly elevated left atrial pressure, pulmonary artery pressure, and pulmonary vascular resistance. These patients usually complain of severe fatigue and exhaustion secondary to a low cardiac output, while symptoms resulting from pulmonary congestion are less prominent; atrial fibrillation is almost invariably present.

By far the most common group are patients whose clinical and hemodynamic features are between those in the other two groups with variable degrees of enlargement of the left atrium and with significant elevation of the left atrial pressure. Symptoms are secondary to both reduced cardiac output and pulmonary congestion.

SYMPTOMS Fatigue, exertional dyspnea, and orthopnea are the most prominent complaints in patients with chronic, severe MR. Since fluctuations of the mean pulmonary capillary pressure are less marked, symptoms resulting from pulmonary congestion tend to be less episodic in nature than in patients with chronic severe MR. Hemoptysis and systemic embolism also occur less frequently in MR than in MS. Right-sided heart failure, with painful hepatic congestion, ankle edema, distended neck veins, ascites, and tricuspid regurgitation, may be observed in patients with MR who have associated pulmonary vascular disease and marked pulmonary hypertension. In patients with *acute*, severe MR, left ventricular failure with acute pulmonary edema and/or cardiovascular collapse is common.

PHYSICAL FINDINGS The arterial pressure is usually normal, and in severe MR the arterial pulse is often characterized by a sharp upstroke. The jugular venous pulse shows abnormally prominent *a* waves in patients with sinus rhythm and marked pulmonary hypertension and prominent *v* waves in those with accompanying severe tricuspid regurgitation.

Palpation A systolic thrill is often palpable at the cardiac apex, the left ventricle is hyperdynamic with a brisk systolic impulse and a palpable rapid-filling wave, and the apex beat is often displaced laterally. When the left atrium is markedly enlarged, it may extend anteriorly, and its expansion may be palpable along the sternal border late during ventricular systole, resembling a right ventricular lift. The combination of retraction of the left ventricle and expansion of the left atrium during systole may produce a characteristic rocking motion of the chest with each cardiac cycle. A right ventricular tap and the shock of pulmonary valve closure may be palpable in patients with marked pulmonary hypertension.

Auscultation The first heart sound is generally absent, soft, or buried in the systolic murmur; an accentuated mitral closure sound is useful in excluding severe regurgitation. A pulmonary ejection sound is often audible in patients with associated pulmonary hypertension. In patients with severe MR, the aortic valve may close prematurely, resulting in wide splitting of the second heart sound. An OS indicates associated MS but does not exclude predominant regurgitation. A low-pitched third heart sound (S_3) occurring 0.12 to 0.17 s after the aortic valve closure sound, i.e. at the completion of the rapid-filling phase of the left ventricle, is believed to be caused by the sudden tensing of the papillary muscles, chordae tendineae, and valve leaflets and is an important auscultatory feature of severe MR. The absence

of an S_3 indicates that if MR exists, it may not be severe. The S_3 may be followed, often after a brief interval, by a short, rumbling, diastolic murmur, even in the absence of MS. A fourth heart sound is often audible in patients with acute, severe MR of recent onset who are in sinus rhythm. A presystolic murmur is not ordinarily heard in patients with pure MR and sinus rhythm but is present when there is significant associated MS.

A systolic murmur of at least grade III/VI intensity, is the most characteristic auscultatory finding in severe MR. It is usually holosystolic (Chap. 188), but it may be decrescendo in patients with acute, severe MR when the tall *v* wave in the left atrial pressure pulse reduces the late systolic left ventricular–atrial pressure gradient. In MR due to papillary muscle dysfunction or mitral valve prolapse, the systolic murmur commences in midsystole (see below). Although the systolic murmur is usually most prominent at the apex and radiates into the axilla, in a minority of patients, particularly those with ruptured chordae tendineae or primary involvement of the posterior mitral leaflet, the regurgitant jet strikes the left atrial wall adjacent to the aortic root, and the systolic murmur is transmitted to the base of the heart and therefore may be confused with the murmur of aortic stenosis. In patients with ruptured chordae tendineae the systolic murmur may have a cooing or "sea gull" quality; in patients with a flail leaflet the murmur may have a musical quality. The systolic murmur of MR is intensified by isometric strain but is reduced by the strain of the Valsalva maneuver.

Electrocardiogram In patients with sinus rhythm there is evidence of left atrial enlargement, but right atrial enlargement also may be present when pulmonary hypertension is severe. Chronic, severe MR with left atrial enlargement is generally associated with atrial fibrillation. In many patients there is no clear-cut electrocardiographic evidence of enlargement of either ventricle. In others the signs of left ventricular hypertrophy are often present, although in patients with pulmonary hypertension, combined ventricular hypertrophy may be noted.

Echocardiogram Doppler echocardiography and color Doppler flow echocardiography imaging are the most accurate noninvasive techniques for the detection and estimation of MR (see Fig. 190-7). The left atrium is usually enlarged and/or exhibits increased pulsations; the left ventricle may be hyperdynamic. With ruptured chordae tendineae or a flail leaflet coarse, erratic motion of the involved leaflets may be noted. Findings which help to determine the etiology of MR can often be identified. These include vegetations associated with infective endocarditis, incomplete coaptation of the anterior and posterior mitral leaflets, and annular calcification, as well as left ventricular dilatation, aneurysm, or dyskinesis. The echocardiogram in patients with mitral valve prolapse is described below.

Roentgenogram The left atrium and left ventricle are the dominant chambers; in chronic cases, the former may be massively enlarged and forms the right border of the cardiac silhouette. Pulmonary venous congestion, interstitial edema, and Kerley B lines are sometimes noted. Marked calcification of the mitral leaflets occurs commonly in patients with long-standing combined MR and MS. Calcification of the mitral annulus may be visualized. Contrast left ventriculography is useful in the quantification of MR.

TREATMENT Medical The nonsurgical management of MR is directed toward restricting those physical activities that regularly produce dyspnea and excessive fatigue, reducing sodium intake, and enhancing sodium excretion with the appropriate use of diuretics (Chap. 195). Vasodilators and digitalis glycosides increase the forward output of the failing left ventricle. Intravenous nitroprusside (Chap. 195) or nitroglycerin to reduce afterload and thereby the volume of regurgitant flow are useful in stabilizing patients with acute and/or severe MR. Angiotensin-converting enzyme inhibitors are given in chronic MR. The same considerations as in patients with MS apply to the reversion of atrial fibrillation to sinus rhythm. In the late stages of heart failure anticoagulants and leg binders are used to diminish the likelihood of venous thrombi and pulmonary emboli.

Surgical In the selection of patients for surgical treatment, the chronic, often slowly progressive nature of the disease must be balanced against the immediate risks and long-term uncertainties attendant on valve reconstruction or replacement. Patients with MR who are asymptomatic or who are limited only during strenuous exertion are not considered to be candidates for surgical treatment, since their condition may remain stable for many years. On the other hand, unless there are contraindications, surgical treatment should be offered to patients with severe MR whose limitations do not allow them to work full time or to perform normal household activities despite optimal medical management. Even in patients with mild symptoms, surgical treatment is indicated when left ventricular dysfunction is progressive. In patients with chronic heart failure, the risks of surgery rise sharply, the recovery of impaired left ventricular function is incomplete, and the long-term survival is reduced. However, conservative management has little to offer these patients, so operative treatment may be indicated even at an advanced stage of the disease, and occasionally, the clinical and hemodynamic improvement following surgical treatment in patients with advanced disease is dramatic. Though most patients who survive operation appear to be greatly improved, some degree of myocardial dysfunction may persist.

When surgical treatment is contemplated, right- and left-sided heart catheterization and left ventricular angiocardiography are generally indicated. These studies are helpful in confirming the presence of severe regurgitation and aid in the identification of patients with primary myocardial disease and relatively mild, functional MR, who usually do not benefit from operation. Hemodynamic studies are also helpful in detecting and assessing the severity of any associated valve lesions, which may have to be dealt with at the time of operation or which may limit the patient's ultimate improvement if they are left untreated. Coronary angiography identifies patients who require concomitant coronary revascularization.

Surgical treatment of MR, especially that caused by valves that are markedly deformed, with shrunken, calcified leaflets secondary to rheumatic fever, requires replacement of the valve with a prosthesis, although in an increasing fraction of patients, particularly those with severe annular dilatation, flail leaflets, mitral valve prolapse, ruptured chordae, or infective endocarditis, reconstruction of the mitral valve apparatus (mitral valvuloplasty) and/or mitral annuloplasty may be successful. Valve reconstruction should be carried out whenever feasible since the operative risk is about half (2 to 4 percent) of that associated with valve replacement. Also, reconstruction spares the patient the long-term adverse consequences of valve replacement (i.e., thromboembolic and hemorrhagic complications in the case of mechanical prostheses and late valve failure necessitating repeat valve replacement in the case of bioprostheses). In addition, by preserving the integrity of the papillary muscles and subvalvular apparatus, mitral valvuloplasty maintains left ventricular function.

MITRAL VALVE PROLAPSE

Mitral valve prolapse (MVP), also variously termed the *systolic click-murmur syndrome, Barlow's syndrome, floppy-valve syndrome*, and *billowing mitral leaflet syndrome*, is a common, but highly variable, clinical syndrome resulting from diverse pathogenic mechanisms of the mitral valve apparatus. Among these are excessive or redundant mitral leaflet tissue, which is commonly involved with myxomatous degeneration and greatly increased concentration of acid mucopolysaccharide. It is a frequent finding in patients who have the typical features of the Marfan syndrome or cystic medial necrosis (Chap. 210), although in most patients with MVP myxomatous degeneration is confined to the mitral valve leaflets without other clinical or pathologic manifestations of disease; the posterior leaflet is usually more affected than the anterior, and the mitral valve annulus is often greatly dilated. In many patients, elongated redundant chordae tendineae cause or contribute to the regurgitation.

In the majority of patients with MVP, the cause is unknown, but in some it appears to be a genetically determined collagen tissue

disorder. A reduction in the production of type III collagen has been incriminated and electron microscopy has revealed fragmentation of collagen fibrils. MVP may be associated with thoracic skeletal deformities similar to but not as severe as those in the Marfan syndrome, including a high arched palate and alterations of the chest and thoracic spine. MVP also may occur as a sequel of acute rheumatic fever, in chronic rheumatic heart disease and following mitral valvulotomy, in ischemic heart disease, and in cardiomyopathies, as well as in 20 percent of patients with ostium secundum atrial septal defect.

MVP may lead to excessive stress on the papillary muscles, which in turn leads to dysfunction and ischemia of the papillary muscles and subjacent ventricular myocardium; rupture of chordae tendineae and progressive annular dilatation and calcification also contribute to valvular regurgitation, which then places more stress on the diseased mitral valve apparatus, thereby creating a vicious cycle. The electro-cardiographic changes (see below) and ventricular arrhythmias appear to result from regional ventricular dysfunction related to increased stress placed on the papillary muscles.

MVP is more common in females and has been noted in a wide age range but most commonly between the ages of 14 and 30 years. There is an increased familial incidence in some patients suggesting an autosomal dominant form of inheritance. In many patients the echocardiographic abnormality is not accompanied by any other clinical manifestation of cardiac disease, and the significance of this finding is uncertain.

MVP encompasses a broad spectrum of severities, ranging from patients with only a systolic click and murmur and mild prolapse of the posterior leaflet of the mitral valve to those with severe MR due to chordal rupture and massive prolapse of both leaflets. In many patients, this condition progresses over years or decades.

Most patients are asymptomatic and remain so for their entire lives. Although severe MR is a relatively uncommon complication of MVP, the latter has become the most common cause of isolated *severe* MR. Arrythmias, most commonly ventricular premature contractions and paroxysmal supraventricular and ventricular tachycardia, have been reported and may cause palpitations, light-headedness, and syncope. Sudden death is a very rare complication. Many patients have chest pain which is difficult to evaluate. It is often substernal, prolonged, poorly related to exertion, and rarely resembles typical angina pectoris. Transient cerebral ischemic attacks secondary to emboli from the mitral valve with endothelial disruption have been reported. Infective endocarditis may occur in patients with MR associated with MVP.

PHYSICAL EXAMINATION   Auscultation   The most important finding is the mid- or late (nonejection) systolic click, which occurs 0.14 s or more after the first heart sound and is thought to be generated by the sudden tensing of slack, elongated chordae tendineae or by the prolapsing mitral leaflet when it reaches its maximum excursion. Systolic clicks may be multiple and may be followed by a high-pitched late systolic crescendo-decrescendo murmur, occasionally "whooping" or "honking," which is heard best at the apex. The click and murmur occur earlier with standing, the Valsalva maneuver, or inhalation of amyl nitrate, interventions which decrease left ventricular volume, exaggerating the propensity of mitral leaflet prolapse. Conversely, squatting and isometric exercise, which increase left ventricular end-diastolic volume, diminish the propensity for the mitral valve leaflets to prolapse, and the click-murmur complex is delayed and may even disappear. Some patients have a midsystolic click without the murmur; others have the murmur without a click.

LABORATORY EXAMINATION   The *electrocardiogram* most commonly is normal but may show biphasic or inverted T waves in leads II, III, and aVF and occasionally supraventricular or ventricular premature contractions. Two-dimensional echocardiography is particularly useful in identifying the abnormal position and prolapse of the mitral valve leaflets; a useful echocardiographic definition of MVP is systolic displacement (in the parasternal view) of the mitral valve leaflets into the left atrium with coaptation superior to the plane of the mitral annulus. Thickening of the mitral valve leaflets identifies a subgroup of patients at higher risk of infective endocarditis and the development of severe MR. Doppler studies are helpful in revealing and evaluating accompanying MR. *Angiocardiography* generally shows prolapse of the posterior and sometimes of both mitral valve leaflets and, rarely, severe MR. Some patients have bulging of the posteroinferior wall of the left ventricle into the left ventricular cavity during systole and/or hypokinesis of the anterolateral left ventricular wall. Others display prolapse of other valves, particularly the tricuspid, in addition to the mitral.

TREATMENT   The management of patients with MVP consists of reassurance of the asymptomatic patient without severe MR or arrhythmias, the prevention of infective endocarditis with antibiotic prophylaxis in patients with a systolic murmur and/or the typical echocardiographic features, and the relief of the atypical chest pain; beta blockers have been found to be helpful in this regard, although their use is empirical. Antiarrhythmic agents may be administered if frequent ventricular premature contractions or tachyarrhythmias have caused symptoms. If the patient is symptomatic from severe MR, mitral valve repair (or rarely, replacement) is indicated. Antiplatelet aggregation agents such as aspirin should be given to patients with transient ischemic attacks, and if these are not effective, anticoagulants should be employed.

AORTIC STENOSIS

Aortic stenosis (AS) occurs in about one-fourth of all patients with chronic valvular heart disease; approximately 80 percent of adult patients with symptomatic valvular AS are male.

ETIOLOGY   AS may be congenital in origin, it may be secondary to rheumatic inflammation of the aortic valve, or it may be due to degenerative calcification of the aortic cusps of unknown cause. The *congenitally affected valve* may already be stenotic at birth (see Chap. 199) and may become progressively more fibrotic, calcified, and stenotic. In others the valve may be congenitally deformed, usually bicuspid, without serious narrowing of the aortic orifice during childhood; its abnormal architecture makes its leaflets susceptible to otherwise ordinary hemodynamic stresses, which ultimately lead to valvular thickening, calcification, increased rigidity, and narrowing of the aortic orifice.

Rheumatic endocarditis of the aortic leaflets produces commissural fusion, resulting sometimes in a bicuspid valve. This, in turn, makes the leaflets more susceptible to trauma and ultimately leads to calcification and further narrowing. By the time the obstruction to left ventricular outflow causes serious clinical disability, the valve is usually a rigid calcified mass, and careful examination may make it difficult or even impossible to determine whether the underlying process was rheumatic or congenital. Rheumatic AS is almost always associated with rheumatic involvement of the mitral valve. A rheumatic etiology is favored by a history of active rheumatic fever and by associated severe aortic regurgitation.

Idiopathic calcific AS occurs most often in the elderly and may be associated with fibrosis and fusion of the valve cusps; the pathologic process is considered to be a degenerative one—a "wear-and-tear" phenomenon. It may produce many of the characteristic systolic murmurs of AS. However, the valvular obstruction is usually relatively mild and of little, if any, hemodynamic significance; it may, on occasion, produce critical obstruction.

OTHER FORMS OF OBSTRUCTION TO LEFT VENTRICULAR OUTFLOW   Besides valvular AS, three other lesions may be responsible for obstruction to left ventricular outflow.

1 Hypertrophic cardiomyopathy. This condition is characterized by marked hypertrophy of the left ventricle, involving in particular the interventricular septum of the left ventricular outflow tract, and may cause subaortic obstruction, as described in Chap. 205.

2 Discrete congenital subvalvular AS. This congenital anomaly is produced by either a membranous diaphragm or a fibrous ridge just below the aortic valve (Chap. 199).

3 Supravalvular AS. This uncommon congenital anomaly is produced by narrowing of the ascending aorta or by a fibrous diaphragm with a small opening just above the aortic valve (Chap. 199).

PATHOPHYSIOLOGY   The primary hemodynamic abnormality is obstruction to left ventricular outflow which causes a systolic pressure gradient between the left ventricle and aorta. When severe obstruction is suddenly produced experimentally, the left ventricle responds by dilatation and reduction of stroke volume. However, in patients the obstruction may be present at birth and/or increases gradually over the course of many years, and left ventricular output is maintained by the presence of left ventricular hypertrophy. This serves as a useful compensatory mechanism because it reduces toward normal the systolic stress developed by each segment of myocardium. A large transaortic valvular pressure gradient may exist for many years without a reduction of cardiac output, left ventricular dilatation, or the development of symptoms.

A peak systolic pressure gradient exceeding 50 mmHg in the face of a normal cardiac output or an effective aortic orifice less than approximately 0.5 cm²/m² of body surface area, i.e., less than approximately one-third of the normal orifice, is generally considered to represent critical obstruction to left ventricular outflow. The left ventricular pressure pulse exhibits a rounded summit as the contraction of this chamber becomes progressively more isometric. The elevated left ventricular end-diastolic pressure observed in many patients with severe AS does not necessarily signify the presence of left ventricular dilatation or failure but may reflect diminished compliance of the hypertrophied left ventricular wall.

A large *a* wave in the left atrial pressure pulse is usually present in severe AS. Loss of an appropriately timed, vigorous atrial contraction, as occurs in atrial fibrillation or atrioventricular dissociation, may result in a rapid aggravation of symptoms.

Although the cardiac output at rest is within normal limits in the majority of patients with severe AS, it may fail to rise normally during exercise. Late in the course the cardiac output and left ventricular–aortic pressure gradient decline, and the mean left atrial, pulmonary artery wedge, pulmonary arterial, and right ventricular pressures rise.

The hypertrophied left ventricular muscle mass elevates myocardial oxygen requirements. In addition, even in the absence of obstructive coronary artery disease, there may be interference with coronary blood flow, because the pressure compressing the coronary arteries exceeds the coronary perfusion pressure. Metabolic evidence of myocardial ischemia can be demonstrated in patients with AS both in the presence and in the absence of coronary arterial narrowing.

A significant fraction of patients with rheumatic AS has associated mitral valve disease. AS intensifies the severity of mitral regurgitation by increasing the pressure driving blood from the left ventricle to the left atrium.

SYMPTOMS   AS is rarely of hemodynamic or clinical importance until the valve orifice has narrowed to approximately one-third of normal, i.e., to 1 cm² in adults. Even critical AS may exist for many years without producing any symptoms because of the ability of the hypertrophied left ventricle to generate the elevated intraventricular pressures.

Most patients with pure or predominant AS have gradually increasing obstruction for years but do not become symptomatic until the fifth to seventh decades. Exertional dyspnea, angina pectoris, and syncope are the three cardinal symptoms. Often there is a history of insidious progression of fatigue and dyspnea associated with gradual curtailment of activities. *Dyspnea* results primarily from elevation of the pulmonary capillary pressure; the latter is caused by elevations of left atrial and left ventricular end-diastolic pressures secondary to reduced compliance and/or left ventricular dilatation. *Angina pectoris* usually develops somewhat later and reflects an imbalance between the augmented myocardial oxygen requirements and reduced oxygen availability; the former results from the increased myocardial mass and intraventricular pressure, while the latter may result from accompanying coronary artery disease, which is not uncommon in patients with AS, as well as from compression of the coronary vessels by the hypertrophied myocardium. Therefore, angina may occur in severe AS even without obstructive epicardial coronary artery disease. *Exertional syncope* may result from a decline in arterial pressure caused by vasodilatation in the exercising muscles and inadequate vasoconstriction in nonexercising muscles in the face of a fixed cardiac output or from a sudden fall in cardiac output produced by an arrhythmia.

Since the cardiac output at rest is usually well maintained until late in the course, marked fatigability, weakness, peripheral cyanosis, and other clinical manifestations of a low cardiac output are usually not prominent until this stage is reached. Orthopnea, paroxysmal nocturnal dyspnea, and pulmonary edema, i.e., symptoms of left ventricular failure, also occur only in the advanced stages of the disease. Severe pulmonary hypertension leading to right ventricular failure and systemic venous hypertension, hepatomegaly, atrial fibrillation, and tricuspid regurgitation are usually preterminal findings.

When AS and MS coexist, the latter lesion masks many of the clinical findings of the former. The reduction of cardiac output induced by MS lowers the pressure gradient across the aortic valve, diminishes the frequency of anginal episodes, and retards the development of severe left ventricular hypertrophy. On the other hand, symptoms considered more characteristic of MS, such as pulmonary congestion and hemoptysis, may be present. Physical, electrocardiographic, radiologic, and echocardiographic examinations in patients with combined AS and MS generally reveal more evidence of left ventricular enlargement than in patients with pure MS, and left heart catheterization is helpful in defining the relative importance of each valvular abnormality.

PHYSICAL FINDINGS   The systemic arterial pressure is usually within normal limits. In the late stages, however, when stroke volume declines, the systolic pressure may fall and the pulse pressure narrow. Systemic hypertension is unusual in patients with marked AS, and a basal systolic arterial pressure exceeding 200 mmHg practically excludes severe narrowing of this valve. The peripheral arterial pulse, as palpated in the carotid or brachial arteries, rises slowly to a delayed sustained peak. Indirect recordings of the carotid pulse exhibit a gradually ascending limb, often with a prominent anacrotic notch or shoulder on the upstroke, as well as a delayed peak, with coarse systolic vibrations. The left ventricular ejection period is prolonged, the preejection period is abbreviated, and the ratio of these two, i.e., the preejection period/systolic ejection period, is characteristically reduced. Late in the course of the disease, in the presence of heart failure, the ratio may return to normal. A palpable double systolic arterial pulse, the so-called bisferiens pulse, excludes pure or predominant AS and signifies dominant or pure aortic regurgitation or obstructive hypertrophic cardiomyopathy (Chap. 205). In the late stages of valvular AS, when the pulse pressure is reduced, the pulse amplitude may be so small that the anacrotic nature of the pulse and the delay in its upstroke may become difficult to appreciate. In many patients the *a* wave in the jugular venous pulse is accentuated. This results from the diminished distensibility of the right ventricular cavity caused by the bulging, hypertrophied interventricular septum and/or the presence of pulmonary hypertension.

Palpation   The apex beat is usually active and displaced laterally, reflecting the presence of left ventricular hypertrophy. A double apical impulse may be appreciated, particularly with the patient in the left lateral recumbent position; the first outward expansion occurs during atrial systole and reflects the important contribution made by atrial contraction to ventricular filling, while the second occurs during ventricular systole and usually is forceful and sustained during ejection. The right ventricle is palpable only when pulmonary hypertension develops in the late stages. A systolic thrill is generally present at the base of the heart, in the jugular notch, and along the carotid arteries, but occasionally it is palpable only during expiration and with the patient leaning forward. In patients who do not have marked pulmonary emphysema, a thick chest wall, thoracic deformity, or heart failure, the absence of a systolic thrill suggests that the aortic stenosis is relatively mild.

Auscultation   The rhythm is generally regular until very late in the course; at other times, atrial fibrillation should suggest the possibility of associated mitral valve disease. An early systolic ejection sound, actually the OS of the aortic valve, is frequently audible in children and adolescents with congenital *noncalcific* valvular AS. This sound usually disappears when the valve becomes calcified and rigid. The sound of aortic valve closure can also be identified most frequently in patients with AS who have pliable valves, and calcification diminishes the intensity of this sound as well. As AS increases in severity, left ventricular systole may become prolonged so that the aortic valve closure sound no longer precedes the pulmonic valve closure sound, and the two components may become synchronous, or aortic valve closure may even follow pulmonic valve closure, causing paradoxic splitting of the second heart sound (Chap. 188). The latter finding usually signifies severe obstruction to left ventricular outflow. Frequently, a fourth heart sound is audible at the apex in many patients with severe AS and reflects the presence of left ventricular hypertrophy and an elevated left ventricular end-diastolic pressure; a third heart sound generally occurs when the left ventricle dilates and fails.

The murmur of AS is characteristically an ejection systolic murmur which commences shortly after the first heart sound, increases in intensity to reach a peak toward the middle of ejection, and ends just before aortic valve closure (Chap. 188). It is usually low-pitched, rough, and rasping in character, loudest at the base of the heart, most commonly in the second right intercostal space. It is transmitted to the jugular notch and upward along the carotid arteries. Occasionally, it is transmitted downward and to the apex and may be confused with the systolic murmur of MR; however, the latter is usually holosystolic. In almost all patients with severe obstruction, the murmur is at least grade III/VI. In patients with mild degrees of obstruction or in those with severe stenosis with heart failure in whom the stroke volume and therefore the transvalvular flow rate are reduced, the murmur may be relatively soft and brief.

Electrocardiogram   This reveals left ventricular hypertrophy in the majority of patients with severe AS (Chap. 189). In advanced cases, ST-segment depression and T-wave inversion (left ventricular "strain") in standard leads I and aVL and in the left precordial leads are evident. However, there is no close correlation between the electrocardiogram and the hemodynamic severity of obstruction, and the absence of electrocardiographic signs of left ventricular hypertrophy does not exclude severe obstruction. The presence of left atrial enlargement should suggest the possibility of associated mitral valve disease.

Echocardiogram   The key findings are left ventricular hypertrophy and in patients with valvular calcification, multiple, bright, thick, echoes from within the aortic root. Eccentricity of the aortic valve cusps is characteristic of congenitally bicuspid valves. Left ventricular dilatation and reduced systolic shortening reflect impairment of left ventricular function. The transaortic valvular gradient can be estimated by Doppler echocardiography. Echocardiography is particularly useful for identifying valvular abnormalities such as MS and aortic regurgitation which sometimes accompany AS (Fig. 190–7), and for differentiating valvular from obstructive hypertrophic cardiomyopathy.

Roentgenogram   The chest roentgenogram may show no or little overall cardiac enlargement for many years, since the development of concentric left ventricular hypertrophy is the initial response to obstruction to left ventricular outflow. Hypertrophy without dilatation may produce some rounding of the cardiac apex in the frontal projection and slight backward displacement in the lateral view; critical AS is often associated with poststenotic dilatation of the ascending aorta. Aortic calcification is usually readily apparent on fluoroscopic examination with an image intensifier or by echocardiography; *the absence of valvular calcification in an adult suggests that severe valvular AS is not present.* In later stages of the disease as the left ventricle dilates, there is increasing evidence of left ventricular enlargement, roentgenographic signs of pulmonary congestion, as well as enlargement of the left atrium, pulmonary artery, and right side of the heart.

Catheterization and angiocardiography Catheterization of the left side of the heart and coronary arteriography should generally be carried out in patients suspected of having severe AS, particularly before a final decision concerning operative treatment is made. The goals are to (1) determine the severity of the aortic obstruction, often previously estimated by Doppler echocardiography, (2) assess the status of left ventricular function, and (3) determine the location of the left ventricular outflow obstruction. These investigations are especially indicated in the following:

1 Young, asymptomatic patients with noncalcific congenital AS (Chap. 199), in order to define the severity of obstruction to left ventricular outflow, since operation or balloon valvuloplasty may be indicated in them if severe AS is present, even in the absence of symptoms.
2 Patients in whom it is suspected that the obstruction to left ventricular outflow may not be at the aortic valve but rather in the sub- or supravalvular regions.
3 Patients with clinical signs of AS and symptoms of myocardial ischemia, in whom associated coronary artery disease is suspected. An effort should be made to determine whether aortic stenosis or coronary atherosclerosis is primarily responsible for the symptoms, and coronary arteriography should be carried out in addition to catheterization of the left side of the heart.
4 Patients with multivalvular disease, in whom the role played by each valvular deformity should be defined before operative treatment is planned.

Angiographic studies, while not mandatory, are helpful in defining the size of the left ventricular cavity, the thickness of the left ventricle, the site of obstruction, the degree of deformity and mobility of the aortic valve cusps, the diameter of the ascending aorta, and the presence and degree of accompanying mitral and aortic regurgitation and of obstructive coronary disease.

NATURAL HISTORY Death in patients with severe AS occurs most commonly in the seventh and eighth decades. Based on data obtained at postmortem examination in patients *not treated surgically*, the average time to death after the onset of various symptoms was as follows: angina pectoris, 3 years; syncope, 3 years; dyspnea, 2 years; and congestive heart failure, 1.5 to 2 years. Moreover, in more than 80 percent of patients who died with AS, symptoms had existed for less than 4 years. Congestive heart failure was considered to be the cause of death in one-half to two-thirds of patients. Among adults dying with valvular AS, sudden death, which presumably results from an arrhythmia, occurred in 10 to 20 percent and at an average age of 60 years.

TREATMENT All patients with moderate or severe AS require careful periodic follow-up. In patients with *severe* AS, strenuous physical activity should be avoided even in the asymptomatic stage. Digitalis glycosides, sodium restriction, and the cautious administration of diuretics are indicated in the treatment of congestive heart failure, but care must be taken to avoid volume depletion. While nitroglycerin is helpful in relieving angina pectoris, vasodilator therapy for heart failure is usually of little value. The most critical decision in the management of AS concerns the advisability of surgical treatment. The indications and results of operation, as well as the techniques, differ considerably, depending on the patient's age and the nature of the valvular deformity.

In children and adolescents with noncalcific congenital AS, considerable hemodynamic improvement can be anticipated from simple commissural incision under direct vision. This operation is recommended not only for symptomatic patients but also for asymptomatic children and adolescents with hemodynamic evidence of critical obstruction to left ventricular outflow, with a peak systolic pressure gradient exceeding 50 mmHg when the cardiac output is normal, or a calculated effective orifice less than 0.5 cm²/m² of body surface area.

In the majority of adults with calcific AS and critical obstruction, replacement of the valve is necessary. In most instances, it is prudent to postpone operation in patients with severe calcific AS who are asymptomatic, since their future course is difficult to predict and they may continue to do well for many years. However, they should be followed carefully by clinical examination for the development of symptoms and by serial echocardiograms (Chap. 190) for evidence of deteriorating left ventricular function; operation is generally indicated in patients with severe AS and left ventricular dysfunction, even if they are asymptomatic. In patients without heart failure, the operative risk is approximately 5 percent. It is likely that as the results of surgical replacement of the aortic valve continue to improve, many asymptomatic patients with severe AS will become candidates for operation before their left ventricular function deteriorates. At present, replacement of the aortic valve should be undertaken in patients with hemodynamic evidence of severe obstruction and symptoms, even when these are relatively mild, or in those with progressive left ventricular dysfunction regardless of the presence or absence of symptoms. In such patients, the operative risk is relatively low (<5 percent) in experienced centers.

When angina pectoris, syncope, or left ventricular decompensation develops in adults with severe valvular AS, the outlook, despite medical treatment, is very poor and can be improved significantly by replacement of the aortic valve with an artificial valve. The operative risk in this group of patients, although relatively high (approximately 10 percent), is still considerably lower than the risk involved by nonoperative treatment; moreover, the symptomatic improvement in some survivors of operation has been remarkable.

Operation should, if possible, be carried out before frank left ventricular failure develops; at this late stage, the operative risk is high (15 to 20 percent), and evidence of myocardial disease may persist even when the operation is technically successful. Furthermore, long-term postoperative survival also correlates inversely with preoperative left ventricular dysfunction. Nonetheless, in view of the very poor prognosis of such patients when they are treated medically, there is usually little choice but to advise immediate surgical treatment. In patients in whom severe AS and coronary artery disease coexist, relief of the AS and revascularization of the myocardium by means of aortocoronary bypass grafting may result in striking clinical and hemodynamic improvement. Since many patients with calcific AS are elderly, particular attention must be directed to the adequacy of hepatic, renal, and pulmonary function before valve replacement is recommended. The mortality rate depends to a substantial extent on the patient's preoperative clinical and hemodynamic state. The 10-year survival rate of patients with aortic valve replacement is approximately 67 percent. Approximately 15 percent of bioprosthetic valves evidence primary valve failure in 10 years, requiring re-replacement, and an approximately equal percentage of patients with mechanical prostheses develop significant hemorrhagic complications as a consequence of treatment with anticoagulants. Fortunately, there is evidence that regression of left ventricular hypertrophy may occur following relief of obstruction.

Percutaneous balloon aortic valvuloplasty, described in Chap. 193, is an alternative to surgery in children and young adults with congenital aortic stenosis. It is not commonly employed in elderly patients with severe calcific aortic stenosis because of a high restenosis rate. Nonetheless, this procedure may be useful in patients who are too ill or frail to undergo surgery, in patients with life-threatening aortic stenosis and advanced extracardiac disease, and as a "bridge to surgery" in patients with severe left ventricular dysfunction.

AORTIC REGURGITATION

ETIOLOGY Approximately three-fourths of patients with pure or predominant aortic regurgitation (AR) are males; females predominate among patients with AR who have associated mitral valve disease. In approximately two-thirds of patients with AR the disease is rheumatic in origin, resulting in thickening, deformation, and shortening of the individual aortic valve cusps, changes which prevent their proper opening during systole and closure during diastole. A rheumatic origin is less common in patients with isolated AR. Acute AR also may result from infective endocarditis, which may attack a valve previously affected by rheumatic disease, a congenitally deformed valve, or rarely a normal aortic valve, and perforate or erode one or more of the leaflets. Patients with discrete membranous subaortic stenosis often develop thickening of the aortic valve leaflets, which in turn leads to mild or moderate degrees of AR and makes these valves particularly susceptible to endocarditis. AR also may occur in patients with congenital bicuspid aortic valves. Prolapse of an aortic cusp, resulting in progressive chronic AR, occurs in approximately 15 percent of patients with ventricular septal defect (Chap. 199). Congenital fenestrations of the aortic valve occasionally produce mild AR. Although traumatic rupture of the aortic valve is an uncommon cause of acute AR, it does represent the most frequent serious lesion observed in patients surviving nonpenetrating cardiac injuries. In patients with AR due to primary valvular disease, dilatation of the aortic annulus may occur secondarily and intensify the regurgitation.

AR, both acute and chronic, also may be due entirely to marked aortic dilatation, i.e., aortic root disease, without primary involvement of the valve leaflets; widening of the aortic annulus and separation of the aortic leaflets are responsible for the AR. Syphilis and ankylosing rheumatoid spondylitis may be associated with cellular infiltration and scarring of the media of the thoracic aorta, leading to aortic dilatation, aneurysm formation, and severe regurgitation. In syphilis of the aorta (Chap. 210), the involvement of the intima may narrow the coronary ostia, which in turn may be responsible for myocardial ischemia. Cystic medial necrosis of the ascending aorta, which may or may not be associated with other manifestations of the Marfan syndrome, idiopathic dilatation of the aorta, osteogenesis imperfecta, and severe hypertension all may widen the aortic annulus and lead to progressive AR. Occasionally, AR is caused by retrograde dissection of the aorta involving the aortic annulus.

The coexistence of hemodynamically significant AS with AR usually excludes all the rarer forms of AR because it occurs almost exclusively in patients whose AR is on a rheumatic or congenital basis.

PATHOPHYSIOLOGY The total stroke volume expelled by the left ventricle (i.e., the sum of the effective forward stroke volume and the volume of blood which regurgitates back into the left ventricle) is increased in AR. In patients with wide-open (*free*) AR, the volume of regurgitant flow may equal the effective forward stroke volume. In contrast to MR, in which a fraction of the left ventricular stroke volume is delivered into the low-pressure left atrium, in AR the entire left ventricular stroke volume must be ejected into a high-pressure zone, the aorta. However, the low aortic diastolic pressure (low afterload) facilitates early ventricular emptying. An increase in the left ventricular end-diastolic volume (increased preload) constitutes the major hemodynamic compensation for AR. The dilatation of the left ventricle allows this chamber to expel a larger stroke volume without requiring any increase in the relative shortening of each myofibril. Therefore, severe AR may occur with a normal effective forward stroke volume and a normal ejection fraction [total (forward plus regurgitant) stroke volume/end-diastolic volume], together with an elevated left ventricular end-diastolic pressure and volume. However, through the operation of Laplace's law (which indicates that myocardial wall tension is the product of intracavitary pressure and left ventricular radius), left ventricular dilatation increases the left ventricular systolic tension required to develop any given level of systolic pressure. As left ventricular function deteriorates, the end-

diastolic volume and the ejection fraction and forward stroke volume decline. Deterioration of left ventricular function often precedes the development of symptoms. Considerable thickening of the left ventricular wall also occurs with chronic AR, and at autopsy the hearts of these patients may be among the largest encountered, sometimes exceeding 1000 g in weight.

The reverse pressure gradient from aorta to left ventricle, which is responsible for the aortic regurgitant flow, falls progressively during diastole, accounting for the decrescendo nature of the diastolic murmur. Equilibration between aortic and left ventricular pressures may occur toward the end of diastole in patients with severe AR, particularly when the heart rate is slow, and the left ventricular end-diastolic pressure may be elevated, occasionally to extremely high levels (>40 mmHg). Rarely, the left ventricular pressure exceeds the left atrial pressure toward the end of diastole, and this reversed pressure gradient closes the mitral valve prematurely or causes diastolic mitral regurgitation.

In patients with free AR, the effective forward cardiac output usually is normal or only slightly reduced at rest, but often it fails to rise normally during exertion. Early signs of left ventricular dysfunction include reductions in the fraction of systolic shortening and in the ejection fraction, determined by echocardiography or radionuclide or contrast angiography. In advanced stages there may be considerable elevation of the left atrial, pulmonary artery wedge, pulmonary arterial, and right ventricular pressures and lowering of the forward cardiac output at rest.

Myocardial ischemia may occur in patients with AR because myocardial oxygen requirements are elevated by both left ventricular dilatation and elevated left ventricular systolic tension. However, the major portion of coronary blood flow occurs during diastole, when arterial pressure is subnormal, thereby reducing coronary perfusion pressure. The combination of increased oxygen demand and reduced supply may cause myocardial ischemia.

HISTORY A family history may frequently be elicited from patients with AR associated with the Marfan syndrome. Patients with AR of obscure cause should be questioned about a positive serologic test for syphilis and about prior chest trauma; a history compatible with infective endocarditis may sometimes be elicited from patients with rheumatic or congenital involvement of the aortic valve, and the infection often precipitates or seriously aggravates preexisting symptoms. Ankylosing spondylitis is usually self-evident.

Patients with severe AR may remain asymptomatic for as long as 10 to 15 years.

In chronic, severe AR, uncomfortable awareness of the heartbeat, especially on lying down, may be an early complaint. Sinus tachycardia during exertion or with emotion or premature ventricular contractions may produce particularly uncomfortable palpitations, as well as head pounding. These complaints may persist for many years before the development of exertional dyspnea, usually the first symptom of diminished cardiac reserve. This is followed by orthopnea, paroxysmal nocturnal dyspnea, and excessive diaphoresis. Chest pain occurs frequently, even in younger patients, and it is not necessary to invoke the presence of coronary artery disease to explain this symptom in patients with AR. It may be due to myocardial ischemia, or it may originate from excessive cardiac pounding on the chest wall. Anginal pain may develop at rest as well as during exertion. Nocturnal angina may be a particularly troublesome symptom, and it may be accompanied by marked diaphoresis. The anginal episodes can be prolonged and often do not respond satisfactorily to sublingual nitroglycerin. Late in the course of the disease, evidence of systemic fluid accumulation, including congestive hepatomegaly, ankle edema, and ascites, may develop. Patients with severe AR tolerate high fevers, infections, or cardiac arrhythmias poorly and may die in pulmonary edema as a result of one of these complications.

In patients with acute, severe AR, as may occur in trauma or infective endocarditis, the left ventricle rapidly exhausts its ability to dilate, and left ventricular diastolic pressure rises rapidly with associated elevations of left atrial and pulmonary capillary pressures.

PHYSICAL FINDINGS Even prior to the examination of the heart of the patient with free AR, the jarring of the entire body and the bobbing motion of the head with each systole can be appreciated, and the abrupt distention and collapse of the larger arteries are easily visible. The examination should be directed toward the detection of conditions predisposing to AR, such as the Marfan syndrome, rheumatoid spondylitis, syphilis, essential hypertension, and ventricular septal defect.

Arterial pulse A rapidly rising "water-hammer" pulse, which collapses suddenly as arterial pressure falls rapidly during late systole and diastole (Corrigan's pulse), and capillary pulsations, an alternate flushing and paling of the skin at the root of the nail while pressure is applied to the tip of the nail (Quincke's pulse), are characteristic of free AR. A booming, "pistol-shot" sound can be heard over the femoral arteries (Traube's sign), and a to-and-fro murmur (Duroziez's sign) is audible if the femoral artery is lightly compressed with a stethoscope.

The arterial pulse pressure is widened, with an elevation of the systolic pressure, sometimes to as high as 300 mmHg, and a depression of the diastolic pressure. The measurement of arterial diastolic pressure with a sphygmomanometer may be complicated by the fact that systolic sounds are frequently heard with the cuff completely deflated. However, the level of cuff pressure at the time of muffling of the Korotkoff sounds generally corresponds fairly closely to the true intraarterial diastolic pressure. The severity of AR does not always correlate directly with the arterial pulse pressure, and severe regurgitation may exist in patients with arterial pressures in the range of 140/60. As the disease progresses and the left ventricular end-diastolic pressure rises markedly, the arterial diastolic pressure may actually rise also, since the aortic diastolic pressure cannot fall below the left ventricular end-diastolic pressure.

Palpation The apex beat is heaving and displaced laterally and inferiorly. The systolic expansion and diastolic retraction of the apex are prominent and contrast sharply with the sustained systolic thrust characteristic of severe AS. A diastolic thrill is often palpable along the left sternal border, and a prominent systolic thrill may be palpable in the jugular notch and transmitted upward along the carotid arteries. This thrill and the accompanying systolic murmur are due to the markedly increased blood flow across the aortic orifice and do not necessarily signify the coexistence of AS. In many patients with pure AR or with combined AS and AR, palpation or recording of the carotid arterial pulse reveals it to be bisferiens, i.e., with two systolic waves separated by a trough.

Auscultation In patients with severe AR, the aortic valve closure sound is usually diminished or absent. A third heart sound is common, and occasionally, a fourth heart sound also may be heard. A loud systolic ejection sound is frequently audible; presumably it results from the sudden dilatation of the aorta by a greatly increased stroke volume. The murmur of AR is typically a high-pitched, blowing, decrescendo diastolic murmur which is usually heard best in the third left intercostal space. In patients with mild regurgitation, this murmur is brief, but as the severity increases, the murmur generally becomes louder and longer, and in patients with free AR it is usually holodiastolic. When the murmur is soft, it can be heard best with the diaphragm of the stethoscope and with the patient sitting up, leaning forward, and with the breath held in forced expiration. As it increases in intensity, it tends to radiate widely, particularly along the lower sternal edge. In patients in whom the AR is caused by primary valvular disease, the diastolic murmur is usually louder along the left than the right sternal border. However, when the decrescendo diastolic murmur is heard best along the right sternal border, it suggests that the AR is caused by aneurysmal dilatation of the aortic root. "Cooing" or musical diastolic murmurs suggest eversion of an aortic cusp vibrating in the regurgitant stream. Unless it is trivial in magnitude, the AR is usually accompanied by peripheral signs such as a widened pulse pressure or a collapsing pulse. On the other hand, with the Graham Steell murmur of pulmonary regurgitation, there usually is clinical evidence of severe pulmonary hypertension, in-

cluding a loud and palpable pulmonary component of the second heart sound.

A midsystolic ejection murmur is frequently audible in AR. It is generally heard best at the base of the heart and is transmitted to the jugular notch and along the carotid vessels. This murmur may be quite loud without signifying organic obstruction; it is often higher pitched, shorter, and less rasping in quality than the ejection systolic murmur heard in patients with predominant AS. A third murmur which is frequently heard in patients with AR is the Austin Flint murmur, a soft, low-pitched, rumbling middiastolic or presystolic bruit. It is probably produced by the displacement of the anterior leaflet of the mitral valve by the aortic regurgitant stream but does not appear to be associated with hemodynamically significant mitral obstruction. Both the Austin Flint murmur and the rumbling diastolic murmur of MS are loudest at the apex, but the murmur of MS is usually accompanied by a loud first heart sound and immediately follows the opening snap of the mitral valve, while the Austin Flint murmur is often shorter in duration than the murmur of MS, and in patients with sinus rhythm the latter exhibits presystolic accentuation. The auscultatory features of AR are intensified by isometric exercise such as strenuous handgrip, which augments systemic resistance, and reduced by inhalation of amyl nitrite. A blowing holosystolic murmur at the apex, which is transmitted to the axilla, also may be heard in patients with AR who have marked left ventricular dilatation and functional mitral regurgitation.

In *acute*, severe AR, the elevation of left ventricular end-diastolic pressure may lead to early closure of the mitral valve, an associated middiastolic sound, a soft or absent S_1, a pulse pressure that is not particularly wide, and a soft, short diastolic murmur.

Electrocardiogram In patients with mild AR, there may be no electrocardiographic abnormalities, but with severe, chronic AR, the electrocardiographic signs of left ventricular hypertrophy become manifest (Chap. 189). In addition, these patients frequently exhibit ST-segment depressions and T-wave inversions in leads I, aVL, V_5, and V_6 ("left ventricular strain"). Left axis deviation and/or QRS prolongation denote diffuse myocardial disease, generally associated with patchy fibrosis, and usually signify a poor prognosis.

Echocardiogram This reveals increased systolic excursion of the posterior left ventricular wall; the extent and velocity of wall motion are normal or even supernormal, until myocardial contractility declines. A rapid, high-frequency fluttering of the anterior mitral leaflet produced by the impact of the aortic regurgitant jet is a characteristic finding. The echocardiogram is also useful in determining the cause of AR, by detecting dilatation of the aortic annulus. Thickening of the aortic valve and failure of coaptation of the leaflets also may be noted. Color Doppler flow echocardiographic imaging is very sensitive in the detection of AR, and Doppler echocardiography is helpful in assessing its severity (Fig. 190-7). Serial two-dimensional echocardiography is valuable in evaluating left ventricular performance and in detecting progressive myocardial dysfunction.

Roentgenogram In severe chronic AR the apex is displaced downward and to the left in the frontal projection, and frequently the cardiac shadow extends below the left diaphragm. Left ventricular enlargement also may be apparent in the left anterior oblique and lateral projections, in which the left ventricle is displaced posteriorly and encroaches on the spine. In patients in whom primary valvular disease is responsible for the AR, the ascending aorta and aortic knob may be moderately dilated. When AR is caused by primary disease of the aortic wall, aneurysmal dilatation of the aorta may be noted, and the aorta may fill the retrosternal space in the lateral view.

Cardiac catheterization and angiography These tests should be carried out to aid in the decision regarding surgical treatment. In addition to providing an accurate measurement of the magnitude of regurgitation and the status of left ventricular function, the condition of the coronary arterial bed may be evaluated.

TREATMENT Although operation constitutes the principal treatment of aortic regurgitation, and should be carried out before the development of heart failure, the latter usually does respond initially to treatment with digitalis glycosides, salt restriction, diuretics, and vasodilators, especially angiotensin-converting enzyme inhibitors. Digitalis also may be indicated in patients with severe regurgitation and dilated left ventricles without symptoms of frank left ventricular failure. Cardiac arrhythmias and infections are poorly tolerated in patients with free AR and must be treated promptly and vigorously. Although nitroglycerin and long-acting nitrates are not as helpful in relieving anginal pain as in patients with ischemic heart disease, they are worth a trial. Patients with syphilitic aortitis should receive a full course of penicillin therapy (Chap. 133).

In deciding on the advisability and proper timing of surgical treatment, two points should be kept in mind: (1) patients with chronic AR usually do not become symptomatic until *after* the development of myocardial dysfunction, and (2) surgical treatment often does not restore normal left ventricular function. Therefore, in patients with severe AR, careful clinical follow-up and noninvasive testing with echocardiography at approximately 6-month intervals are necessary if operation is to be undertaken at the optimal time, i.e., after the onset of left ventricular dysfunction but prior to the development of severe symptoms. Operation can be deferred as long as the patient remains asymptomatic *and* retains normal left ventricular function.

Replacement of the aortic valve with a suitable mechanical or tissue prosthesis is generally necessary in patients with rheumatic AR and in many patients with other forms of regurgitation. Rarely, when a leaflet has been perforated during an episode of infective endocarditis or torn from its attachments to the aortic annulus, surgical repair may be possible. When AR is due to aneurysmal dilatation of the annulus and ascending aorta rather than to primary valvular involvement, it may be possible to reduce the regurgitation by narrowing the annulus or by excising a portion of the aortic root without replacing the valve. More frequently, however, regurgitation can be eliminated only by replacing the aortic valve, excising the aneurysm responsible for the regurgitation, and replacing the latter with a graft. This formidable procedure entails a higher risk than aortic valve replacement alone.

As in patients with other valvular abnormalities, both the operative risk of aortic valve replacement and late mortality are largely dependent on the stage of the disease and on myocardial function at the time of operation; patients with marked cardiac enlargement and prolonged left ventricular dysfunction experience an operative mortality of approximately 10 percent and a late mortality of approximately 5 percent per year despite a technically satisfactory operation. Nonetheless, because of the poor prognosis with medical management, even patients with left ventricular failure should be considered for operation.

ACUTE AORTIC REGURGITATION Infective endocarditis, aortic dissection, and trauma are the most common causes of severe, acute AR. Since the left ventricle has not had time to dilate, stroke volume declines and ventricular diastolic pressure rises markedly; the arterial pulse pressure is often not markedly widened, and the physical signs characteristic of severe chronic AR may be absent. Premature closure of the mitral valve is common and can be recognized by echocardiography. The first heart sound is soft or absent; the aortic diastolic murmur is characteristically brief. Patients present with pulmonary congestion and edema, as well as hypotension secondary to a low cardiac output. Acute, severe regurgitation requires prompt surgical treatment, which may be lifesaving.

TRICUSPID STENOSIS

Tricuspid stenosis (TS), a relatively uncommon valvular lesion in North America and western Europe, is more common on the Indian subcontinent. It is generally rheumatic in origin and is more common in women than in men. It does not usually occur as an isolated lesion or in patients with pure MR but is usually observed in association with MS. Hemodynamically significant TS occurs in 5 to 10 percent of patients with severe MS; rheumatic TS is commonly associated with some degree of regurgitation.

PATHOPHYSIOLOGY A diastolic pressure gradient between the right atrium and ventricle can be recorded with a double-lumen cardiac catheter. It is augmented when the transvalvular blood flow increases during inspiration and is reduced during expiration. A *mean* diastolic pressure gradient exceeding 4 mmHg is usually sufficient to elevate the mean right atrial pressure to levels which result in systemic venous congestion and, unless sodium intake has been restricted and diuretics administered, it is associated with ascites and edema. In patients with sinus rhythm, the right atrial *a* wave may be extremely tall and may even approach the level of the right ventricular systolic pressure. The resting cardiac output is usually quite low and fails to rise during exercise. The low cardiac output is responsible for the normal or only slightly elevated left atrial, pulmonary arterial, and right ventricular systolic pressures despite the presence of MS.

SYMPTOMS Since the development of MS generally precedes that of TS, many patients initially have symptoms of pulmonary congestion. Amelioration of the latter should raise the possibility that TS may be developing. Characteristically, patients complain of relatively little dyspnea for the degree of hepatomegaly, ascites, and edema which they present. Fatigue secondary to a low cardiac output and discomfort due to refractory edema, ascites, and marked hepatomegaly are common in patients with TS and/or regurgitation. In some patients, TS may be suspected for the first time when symptoms of right ventricular failure persist after an adequate mitral valvulotomy.

PHYSICAL FINDINGS Since TS usually occurs in the presence of other obvious valvular disease, the diagnosis may be missed unless it is specifically considered and searched for. Severe TS is associated with marked hepatic congestion, often resulting in cirrhosis, jaundice, serious malnutrition, anasarca, and ascites. Congestive hepatomegaly and, in cases of severe tricuspid valve disease, splenomegaly are present. The jugular veins are distended, and in patients with sinus rhythm there may be giant *a* waves. The *v* waves are less conspicuous, and since tricuspid obstruction impedes right atrial emptying during diastole, there is a slow *y* descent. In patients with sinus rhythm there may be prominent presystolic pulsations of the enlarged liver as well.

The right ventricle and the shock of pulmonic valve closure are usually not palpable. Indeed, a giant *a* wave in the jugular venous pulse without palpatory evidence of pulmonary hypertension or right ventricular enlargement should suggest the possibility of TS. On auscultation, the pulmonic closure sound is not accentuated, and occasionally, an OS of the tricuspid valve may be heard approximately 0.06 s after pulmonic valve closure. The diastolic murmur of TS has many of the qualities of the diastolic murmur of MS, and since TS almost always occurs in the presence of MS, the less common valvular lesion may be missed. However, the tricuspid murmur is generally heard best along the left lower sternal margin and over the xiphoid process and is most prominent during presystole in patients with sinus rhythm. The diastolic murmur is reduced in amplitude as the stethoscope is inched laterally, only to intensify or reappear as the mitral murmur at the apex. The murmur is augmented during inspiration, and it is reduced during expiration and particularly during the Valsalva maneuver, when tricuspid blood flow is reduced. This finding (Carvallo's sign) is often most easily elicited when the patient is in the erect position.

Noninvasive examinations The features of right atrial enlargement (Chap. 189) include tall, peaked P waves in lead II, as well as prominent, upright P waves in lead V_1. The *absence* of electrocardiographic evidence of right ventricular hypertrophy in a patient with right-sided heart failure who is believed to have MS should suggest associated tricuspid valve disease. The chest roentgenograms in patients with combined TS and MS show particular prominence of the right atrium and superior vena cava without much enlargement of the pulmonary artery and with less evidence of pulmonary vascular congestion than occurs in patients with isolated MS. On echocardiographic examination, the tricuspid valve is usually thickened; the transvalvular gradient can be estimated by Doppler echocardiography.

TREATMENT Patients with TS generally exhibit marked systemic venous congestion; intensive salt restriction and diuretic therapy are required during the preoperative period. Such a preparatory period may diminish hepatic congestion and thereby improve hepatic function sufficiently so that the risks of operation are diminished. Surgical treatment of the tricuspid valve is not ordinarily indicated at the time of mitral valve surgery in patients with *mild* TS. On the other hand, definitive surgical relief of the TS should be carried out, preferably at the time of mitral valvulotomy, in patients with moderate or severe TS who have mean diastolic pressure gradients exceeding 4 to 5 mmHg and tricuspid orifices less than 1.5 to 2.0 cm². TS is almost always accompanied by significant tricuspid regurgitation. Open-heart operations utilizing cardiopulmonary bypass may permit substantial improvement of tricuspid valve function. If this cannot be accomplished, the tricuspid valve may have to be replaced with a prosthesis, preferably a tissue valve.

TRICUSPID REGURGITATION

Most commonly, tricuspid regurgitation (TR) is functional and secondary to marked dilatation of the right ventricle and the tricuspid annulus. Functional TR may complicate right ventricular enlargement of any cause, including inferior wall infarcts that involve the right ventricle, and it is commonly seen in the late stages of heart failure due to rheumatic or congenital heart disease with severe pulmonary hypertension, as well as in ischemic heart disease, cardiomyopathy, and cor pulmonale. It is in part reversible if pulmonary hypertension is relieved. Rheumatic fever may produce organic TR, often associated with TS. Less commonly, regurgitation results from congenitally deformed tricuspid valves, and it occurs with defects of the atrioventricular canal, as well as with Ebstein's malformation of the tricuspid valve (Chap. 199). Infarction of right ventricular papillary muscles, tricuspid valve prolapse, carcinoid heart disease, endomyocardial fibrosis, infective endocarditis, and trauma all may produce TR.

As is the case for TS, the clinical features of TR result primarily from systemic venous congestion and reduction of cardiac output. With the onset of TR in patients with pulmonary hypertension, symptoms of pulmonary congestion diminish, but the clinical manifestations of right-sided heart failure become intensified. The neck veins are distended with prominent *v* waves, and marked· hepatomegaly, ascites, pleural effusions, edema, systolic pulsations of the liver, and positive hepatojugular reflux are common. A prominent right ventricular pulsation along the left parasternal region and a blowing holosystolic murmur along the lower left sternal margin which may be intensified during inspiration and reduced during expiration or the Valsalva maneuver are characteristic findings; atrial fibrillation is usually present.

The electrocardiogram usually shows changes characteristic of the lesion responsible for the enlargement of the right ventricle which leads to TR and therefore is helpful in elucidating its cause. In the rare instances of isolated TR, the electrocardiogram often shows incomplete right bundle branch block. Roentgenographic examination usually reveals enlargement of both the right atrium and ventricle. Echocardiography may be helpful by demonstrating right ventricular dilatation and prolapsing or flail tricuspid leaflets; the diagnosis of tricuspid regurgitation can be made by color flow echocardiography and the severity estimated by Doppler examination. The latter is also useful in estimating pulmonary artery pressure.

In patients with severe TR, the cardiac output is usually markedly reduced, and the right atrial pressure pulse may exhibit no *x* descent during early systole but a prominent *c-v* wave with a rapid *y* descent. The mean right atrial and the right ventricular end-diastolic pressures are often elevated.

Isolated TR, without pulmonary hypertension, such as that occurring as a consequence of infective endocarditis or trauma, is usually well tolerated and does not require operation. Indeed, even total excision of an infected tricuspid valve is often well tolerated if the pulmonary artery pressure is normal. Treatment of the underlying cause of heart failure usually reduces the severity of functional TR. In patients with mitral valve disease and TR due to pulmonary hypertension and massive right ventricular enlargement, effective surgical correction of the mitral valvular abnormality results in lowering of the pulmonary vascular pressures and gradual reduction or disappearance of the TR without direct treatment of the tricuspid valve. However, recovery may be much more rapid in patients with severe secondary TR if, at the time of mitral valve replacement, tricuspid annuloplasty (often with the insertion of a plastic ring) or, in the rare instance of severe organic tricuspid valve disease, tricuspid valve replacement is performed. Surgical treatment of the TR also should be carried out in patients with severe regurgitation secondary to deformity of the tricuspid valve due to rheumatic fever, particularly those *without* severe pulmonary hypertension.

PULMONIC VALVE DISEASE

The pulmonic valve is affected by rheumatic fever far less frequently than are the other valves, and it is uncommonly the seat of infective endocarditis. The most common acquired abnormality affecting the pulmonic valve is regurgitation secondary to dilatation of the pulmonic valve ring as a consequence of severe pulmonary hypertension. This produces the Graham Steell murmur, a high-pitched, decrescendo, diastolic blowing murmur along the left sternal border, which is difficult to differentiate from the far more common murmur produced by aortic regurgitation. It is usually of little hemodynamic significance; indeed, surgical removal or destruction of the pulmonic valve by infective endocarditis does not produce heart failure unless serious pulmonary hypertension is also present. The *carcinoid syndrome* may cause pulmonic stenosis and/or regurgitation.

Congenital pulmonic stenosis is discussed in Chap. 199.

REFERENCES

BLOOMFIELD P et al: Twelve year comparison of a Bjork-Shiley mechanical heart valve with porcine bioprostheses. N Engl J Med 324:573, 1991

BOUDOULAS H, WOOLEY CF (eds): *The Mitral Valve Prolapse Syndrome*. Futura, Mount Kisco, NY 1988

BRAUNWALD E: Valvular heart disease, in *Heart Disease*, 4th ed, E Braunwald (ed). Philadelphia, Saunders, 1992, p 1007

FELDMAN T: Rheumatic mitral stenosis. On the rise again. Postgrad Med 93:93, 99, 1993

GRAY RJ, HELFANT RH: Timing of surgery for valvular heart disease. Casrdiovasc Clin 23:209, 1993

GRUNKEMEIER GL et al: Prosthetic heart valve performance: Long-term follow-up. Curr Probl Cardiol 17:331, 1992

HESS OM et al: Diastolic dysfunciotn in aortic stenosis. Circualtion 87(Suppl 5):IV73, 1993

JAMIESON WR: Modern cardiac valve devices—bioprostheses and mechanical prostheses: State of the art. J Card Surg 8:89, 1993

KIRKLIN JW, BARRATT-BOYES BG: Part III. Acquired valvular heart disease, in *Cardiac Surgery*, 2d ed, JW Kirklin, BG Barratt-Boyes (eds). New York, Wiley, 1993, p 425

KLUES HG, HANRATH P: Echocardiography in valvular heart disease. Curr Opin Cardiol 7:209, 1992

NAIR CK et al: Ten-year results with the St. Jude Medical Prosthesis. Am J Cardiol 65(3):217, 1990

PAN M et al: Factors determining late success after mitral balloon valvulotomy. Am J Cardiol 71:1181, 1993

RAVKILDE JL, HANSEN PS: Late results following closed mitral valvotomy in isolated mitral valve stenosis: Analysis of 35 years of follow-up in 240 patients using Cox regression. Thorac Cardiovasc Surg 39:133, 1991

REED D et al: Prediction of outcome after mitral valve replacement in patients with symptomatic chronic mitral regurgitation. Circ 84:23, 1991

RODRIGUEZ A et al: Factors influencing the outcome of balloon aortic valvuloplasty in the elderly. Am Heart J 120:373, 1990

SLATER J et al: Comparison of cardiac catheterization and Doppler echocardiography in the decision to operate in aortic and mitral valve disease. J Am Coll Cardiol 17:1026, 1991

STRONG MD 3d, BROCKMAN SK: Mitral valve reconstruction. Cardiovasc Clin 23:255, 1993

202 ACUTE MYOCARDIAL INFARCTION

RICHARD C. PASTERNAK / EUGENE BRAUNWALD

Myocardial infarction is one of the most common diagnoses occurring in hospitalized patients in western countries. In the United States, approximately 1.5 million myocardial infarctions occur each year. Mortality with acute infarction is approximately 30 percent, with more than half of the deaths occurring before the stricken individual reaches the hospital. Although survival following hospitalization has improved over the last two decades, an additional 5 to 10 percent of survivors die in the first year following myocardial infarction and the number of myocardial infarctions each year in the United States has remained largely unchanged since the early 1970s. Risk of excess mortality and recurrent nonfatal myocardial infarction persists in patients who recover.

Myocardial infarction generally occurs with the abrupt decrease in coronary blood flow that follows a thrombotic occlusion of a coronary artery previously narrowed by atherosclerosis. Progression of the atherosclerotic lesion to the point where thrombus formation occurs is a complex process related to vascular injury. This injury is produced or facilitated by factors such as cigarette smoking, hypertension, and lipid accumulation. In the majority of cases, infarction occurs when an atherosclerotic plaque fissures, ruptures, or ulcerates, and, with conditions favoring thrombogenesis (factors which may be local or systemic), a mural thrombus forms leading to coronary artery occlusion. In rare cases, infarction may be due to coronary artery occlusion secondary to coronary emboli, congenital abnormalities, coronary spasm, and a wide variety of systemic—particularly inflammatory—diseases. Ultimately, the amount of myocardial damage caused by coronary occlusion depends upon the territory supplied by the affected vessel, whether or not the vessel becomes totally occluded, native factors which can produce early spontaneous lysis of the occlusive thrombus, the quantity of blood supplied by collateral vessels to the affected tissue, and the demand for oxygen of the myocardium whose blood supply has been suddenly limited.

Patients at increased risk of developing acute myocardial infarction include those with unstable angina, multiple coronary risk factors (Chap. 208) and Prinzmetal's variant angina (Chap. 203). Less common etiologic factors include hypercoagulability, coronary emboli, collagen vascular disease, and cocaine abuse.

CLINICAL PRESENTATION

Although in roughly one-half of cases no precipitating factor appears to be present prior to myocardial infarction, triggers such as physical exercise, emotional stress, and medical or surgical illnesses can often be identified. The onset of myocardial infarction may be at any time of the day or night, but a higher frequency of onset occurs in the morning within a few hours of awakening. *Pain* is the most common presenting complaint in patients with myocardial infarction. In some instances, the discomfort may be severe enough to be described as the worst pain the patient has ever experienced (Chap. 12). The pain of myocardial infarction is deep and visceral; adjectives commonly used to describe it are *heavy, squeezing,* and *crushing.* It is similar in character to the discomfort of angina pectoris but is usually more severe and lasts longer. Typically the pain involves the central portion of the chest and/or epigastrium, and in about 30 percent of cases it radiates to the arms. Less common sites of radiation include the abdomen, back, lower jaw, and neck. The location of the pain beneath the xiphoid and patients' denial that they may be suffering a heart attack are chiefly responsible for the mistaken diagnosis of indigestion. The pain of myocardial infarction may radiate as high as the occipital area but not below the umbilicus. The pain is often accompanied by weakness, sweating, nausea, vomiting, giddiness, and anxiety. The discomfort usually commences with the patient at rest. When the pain begins during a period of exertion, in contrast to angina pectoris, it does not usually subside with cessation of activity. Approximately one-half of patients with myocardial infarction exhibit the prodrome of unstable angina (Chap. 203).

Although pain is the most common presenting complaint, it is by no means always present; a minimum of 15 to 20 percent of myocardial infarcts are *painless.* The incidence of painless infarcts is greater in women and patients with diabetes mellitus, and it increases with age. In the elderly, myocardial infarction may present as sudden-onset breathlessness, which may progress to pulmonary edema. Other less common presentations, with or without pain, include sudden loss of consciousness, a confusional state, a sensation of profound weakness, the appearance of an arrhythmia, evidence of peripheral embolism, or merely an unexplained drop in arterial pressure. The pain of myocardial infarction can be similar to pain from acute pericarditis (Chap. 206), pulmonary embolism (Chap. 226), acute aortic dissection (Chap. 210), or costochondritis. These conditions should be considered in the differential diagnosis.

PHYSICAL FINDINGS Most patients are anxious and restless, attempting to relieve the pain by moving about in bed, squirming, and stretching. Pallor is common and is often associated with perspiration and coolness of the extremities. The combination of substernal chest pain persistent for more than 30 min and diaphoresis strongly suggests acute myocardial infarction. Although many patients have a normal pulse rate and blood pressure, within the first hour of infarction about one-fourth of patients with anterior infarction have manifestations of sympathetic nervous system hyperactivity (tachycardia and/or hypertension), and up to one-half with inferior infarction show evidence of parasympathetic hyperactivity (bradycardia and/or hypotension).

The precordium is usually quiet, and the apical impulse may be difficult to palpate. In about one-fourth of patients with anterior wall infarction, an abnormal systolic pulsation caused by dyskinetic bulging of infarcted myocardium develops in the periapical area within the first days of the illness and then may resolve. Other physical signs of ventricular dysfunction that may be present include, in decreasing incidence, fourth (S_4) and third (S_3) heart sounds, decreased intensity of heart sounds, and, rarely, paradoxical splitting of the second heart sound (Chap. 188). A transient apical systolic murmur, presumably due to mitral regurgitation secondary to papillary muscle dysfunction during acute infarction, may be midsystolic or late systolic in timing. A pericardial friction rub is heard in many patients with transmural myocardial infarction at some time in their course if they are examined frequently. Jugular venous distention occurs commonly in patients with right ventricular infarction. The carotid pulse is often decreased in volume, reflecting reduced stroke volume. Temperature elevations up to 38°C may be observed during the first week following acute myocardial infarction; however, a temperature exceeding 38°C should prompt a search for other causes. The arterial pressure is variable; in most patients with transmural infarction systolic pressure declines approximately 10 to 15 mmHg from the preinfarction state.

LABORATORY FINDINGS

The laboratory tests of value in confirming the diagnosis of myocardial infarction may be divided into four groups: (1) nonspecific indexes of tissue necrosis and inflammation, (2) the electrocardiogram, (3) serum enzyme changes, and (4) cardiac imaging.

The *nonspecific reaction* to myocardial injury is associated with polymorphonuclear leukocytosis, which appears within a few hours after the onset of pain, persists for 3 to 7 days, and often reaches levels of 12,000 to 15,000 leukocytes per microliter. The erythrocyte sedimentation rate rises more slowly than the white blood cell count, peaking during the first week, and sometimes remaining elevated for 1 or 2 weeks.

The *electrocardiographic manifestations* of acute myocardial infarction are described in Chap. 189. Although electrocardiographic-pathologic correlations are not excellent, transmural infarction is often present if the electrocardiogram demonstrates Q waves or loss of R waves; nontransmural infarction may be present if the electrocardiogram shows only transient ST-segment and sustained T-wave changes. However, the latter changes are variable and nonspecific and should not form the sole basis for the diagnosis of infarction. Therefore, a more rational nomenclature for designating electrocardiographic infarction is now commonly in use, with the terms *Q-wave* or *non-Q-wave infarction* in place of the terms *transmural* or *nontransmural infarction*, respectively. In the past, the Q-wave/non-Q-wave dichotomy was held to be particularly useful for prognostic and management reasons; however, today this is widely recognized as an oversimplified distinction, useful primarily for descriptive purposes.

SERUM ENZYMES Enzymes are released in large quantities into the blood from necrotic heart muscle following myocardial infarction. The rate of liberation of specific enzymes differs following infarction, and the temporal pattern of enzyme release is of diagnostic importance. Creatine phosphokinase (CK) rises within 8 to 24 h and generally returns to normal by 48 to 72 h, except in the case of large infarctions, when CK clearance is delayed. Lactic dehydrogenase (LDH) rises later (24 to 48 h) and remains elevated for as long as 7 to 14 days. The serum aminotransferase enzymes AST and ALT (previously designated SGOT and SGPT) were utilized in the diagnosis of myocardial infarction for many years but have fallen out of favor because it has been recognized that their time course of elevation is intermediate between CK and LDH, thus offering little advantage, and because of lack of tissue specificity. The MB isoenzyme of CK has the advantage over CK and LDH in that it is not present in significant concentrations in extracardiac tissue and therefore is more specific. CK-MB isoenzymes are particularly useful when skeletal muscle and/or brain damage are suspected since both of these tissues contain large quantities of the CK enzyme but none of the MB isoenzyme. The myocardial specificity of the MB isoenzyme determination depends on the technique used for measurement. Radioimmunoassay techniques are most specific, but the more commonly employed gel electrophoresis technique is significantly less specific and therefore prone to more frequent false positives. Tissues differ with respect to the five specific LDH isoenzyme patterns. The isoenzyme which predominates in the heart is referred to as LDH_1, which rises before total LDH in patients with myocardial infarction and may rise when there is no change in total LDH. Therefore, increased LDH_1 is a more sensitive indicator of myocardial infarction than total LDH; sensitivity exceeds 95 percent. However, LDH isoenzymes need to be measured only when the initial CK or CK-MB elevation might have been missed (after 48 h), for they are not more sensitive than CK-MB and therefore only increase cost without increasing diagnostic accuracy.

A two- to threefold elevation of total CK (not CK-MB) may follow an intramuscular injection. This may lead to the erroneous diagnosis of myocardial infarction in a patient who has been given an intramuscular injection of a narcotic for chest pain of noncardiac origin. Other potential sources of total CK elevation worthy of note are (1) muscular diseases including muscular dystrophy, myopathies, and polymyositis, (2) electrical cardioversion, (3) cardiac catheterization, (4) hypothyroidism, (5) stroke, (6) surgery, and (7) skeletal muscle damage secondary to trauma, convulsions, and prolonged immobilization. Cardiac surgery, myocarditis, and electrical cardioversion often result in elevation of serum levels of MB isoenzyme.

While it has long been recognized that the *total* quantity of enzyme released correlates with the size of the infarct, the *peak* enzyme concentration is only weakly correlated with infarct size. Thus while the *area* under the CK-MB time curve is related to infarct size, the *absolute* value of the peak CK-MB and its time to peak are related to the kinetics of CK-MB washout from myocardium. The opening of a coronary artery occlusion (either spontaneously, or by mechanical or pharmacologic means) in the early hours of myocardial infarction will cause early and higher peaking (at about 8 to 12 h following

reperfusion) of both the CK and CK-MB time curves. Without reperfusion, the CK peak occurs at about 24 h.

Characteristic rises occur in serum enzyme concentration in more than 95 percent of patients with clinically proven myocardial infarction. CK and LDH levels generally do not rise in unstable angina. Many patients with suspected infarction have baseline enzyme levels that are normal and increase threefold in a pattern consistent with infarction, although the absolute level of enzyme in the blood never exceeds the upper limits of normal. These have been termed "microinfarctions," and such patients have a prognosis intermediate between that of unstable angina and that of proven myocardial infarction. Isoenzyme studies are particularly helpful in this situation.

CARDIAC IMAGING Several radionuclide imaging techniques are of value in the diagnosis or assessment of the patient with acute myocardial infarction (Chap. 190). Acute infarct scintigraphy ("hot-spot" imaging) is carried out with an infarct-avid imaging agent such as [^{99m}Tc]stannous pyrophosphate. Scans are usually positive 2 to 5 days after infarction, particularly in patients with transmural infarcts; although they aid in *localizing* infarcts and provide a measure of infarct size (Chap. 190), these scans are less sensitive than CK determination for making the *diagnosis* of myocardial infarction. Myocardial perfusion imaging with thallium 201 or technetium 99m Sesta-Mibi, which are distributed in proportion to myocardial blood flow and concentrated by viable myocardium, reveals a defect ("cold spot") in most patients during the first few hours after development of a transmural infarct (p. 971). However, since it is not possible to distinguish acute infarcts from chronic scars, perfusion scanning, although extremely *sensitive*, is not *specific* for the diagnosis of *acute* myocardial infarction. Through sequential [^{99m}Tc]Sesta-Mibi imaging (e.g., before and after thrombolysis) the area of myocardium at risk may be estimated; likewise, sequential scanning may permit assessment of the area of successful reperfusion and comparison of infarct size (late) with the area at risk (early). Radionuclide ventriculography, carried out with ^{99m}Tc-labeled red blood cells (p. 970), frequently demonstrates wall motion disorders and reduction in ventricular ejection fraction in patients with acute myocardial infarction. While of value in assessing the hemodynamic consequences of infarction, and in aiding in the diagnosis of right ventricular infarction when the right ventricular ejection fraction is depressed, this technique is also quite nonspecific, since many cardiac abnormalities other than myocardial infarction alter the radionuclide ventriculogram.

Two-dimensional echocardiography (Chap. 190) can also be of value in patients with acute myocardial infarction. Abnormalities of wall motion are almost universally present. Even with nontransmural myocardial infarction nearly two-thirds of patients have echocardiographically detectable wall motion abnormalities. Although acute infarction cannot be distinguished from old myocardial scar or from acute severe ischemia by an echocardiogram, the ease and safety of the procedure make its use appealing as a screening tool. In the emergency room setting, the early use of echocardiography can aid in management decisions such as whether or not thrombolytic agents should be administered (see later). Echocardiographic estimation of left ventricular function is relatively accurate and can be useful prognostically. Echocardiography may be particularly useful in the diagnosis of right ventricular infarction, ventricular aneurysm, pericardial effusion, and left ventricular thrombus. Additionally, Doppler echocardiography is useful in the detection of a ventricular septal defect and mitral regurgitation, complications of acute myocardial infarction.

Cardiac imaging employing newer technologies such as ultrafast computed tomography and magnetic resonance imaging (Chap. 191) is likely to be useful for many of the above-noted purposes in the future.

MANAGEMENT

The prognosis in acute myocardial infarction is largely related to the occurrence of two general classes of complications: (1) electrical (arrhythmias) and (2) mechanical ("pump failure"). Ventricular fibrillation is the most common form of arrhythmic death in acute myocardial infarction. The vast majority of deaths due to ventricular fibrillation occur within the first 24 h of the onset of symptoms, and of these deaths, over half occur in the first hour. Most out-of-hospital deaths from myocardial infarction are due to ventricular fibrillation. It may occur without warning symptoms or arrhythmias. Over the last 30 years, with careful monitoring and prompt attention to arrhythmias, the in-hospital mortality for acute myocardial infarction has been reduced from about 30 to between 10 and 15 percent, and death from in-hospital ventricular arrhythmia is now unusual.

Pump failure is now the primary cause of in-hospital death from acute myocardial infarction. The extent of ischemic necrosis correlates well with the degree of pump failure and with mortality, both early, i.e., within 10 days of infarction, and later as well. A classification dependent on the status of cardiac pump function, estimated clinically, originally proposed by Killip divides patients into four groups as follows: class I, no signs of pulmonary or venous congestion; class II, moderate heart failure as evidence by rales at the lung bases, S_3 gallop, tachypnea, or signs of failure of the right side of the heart including venous and hepatic congestion; class III, severe heart failure, pulmonary edema; and class IV, shock with systolic pressure less than 90 mmHg and evidence of peripheral vasoconstriction, peripheral cyanosis, mental confusion, and oliguria. The expected hospital mortality rate of patients in these clinical classes when this classification was established was as follows: class I, 0 to 5 percent; class II, 10 to 20 percent; class III, 35 to 45 percent; and class IV, 85 to 95 percent. With recent advances in management, mortality has fallen, perhaps by as much as one-third to one-half, in each class.

Given the information summarized above, the principal objectives of management of the patient with myocardial infarction are to prevent death from arrhythmia and to minimize the mass of infarcted tissue.

Arrhythmias can usually be managed successfully if trained personnel and appropriate equipment are available when this complication develops. Since mortality from arrhythmia is greatest during the first few hours after infarction, it is obvious that the effectiveness of treatment relates directly to the speed with which patients come under medical observation. The biggest delay usually is not in transportation to the hospital but rather between the onset of pain and the patient's decision to call for help. This delay can best be reduced by education of the public concerning the significance of chest pain and the importance of seeking early medical attention. Increasingly, monitoring and treatment are carried out by trained personnel in the ambulance, shortening even further the time between the onset of the infarction and appropriate care.

CORONARY CARE UNITS These have resulted in improved care of patients with myocardial infarction, reduction in mortality rates, and major increases in knowledge about myocardial infarction. These units are routinely equipped with a system which permits continuous monitoring of the cardiac rhythm of *each* patient and hemodynamic monitoring in *selected* patients. Defibrillators, respirators, noninvasive transthoracic pacemakers, and facilities for introducing pacing catheters and flow-directed balloon-tipped catheters should be available. Equally important is the organization of a highly trained team of nurses who can recognize arrhythmias, adjust the dosage of antiarrhythmic, vasoactive, and anticoagulant drugs, and perform cardiac resuscitation, including electroshock, when necessary.

Patients should be admitted to these units early in their illness when they may expect to derive maximum benefit from the care provided. In the past, all patients with suspected myocardial infarction were admitted to the coronary care unit. Currently, however, several factors have led to a change in this rule. The availability of electrocardiographic monitoring and trained personnel in "intermediate care units" has allowed admission of lower-risk patients (e.g., those not hemodynamically compromised or without active arrhythmias) to such units. For economic reasons, and to utilize limited facilities optimally, many institutions have developed guidelines to aid in triaging patients with suspected myocardial infarction. While most such patients in the United States are admitted to the hospital, in other countries, such as the United Kingdom, the patients at lowest risk may be cared for at home. Once admitted to the hospital the fraction of patients actually admitted to the coronary care unit may depend on a balance between the clinical status of the patient and bed availability. In some units beds are utilized primarily for patients with a complicated course, particularly those who require hemodynamic monitoring.

REPERFUSION Thrombolysis One of the most important developments in the care of patients with acute myocardial infarction derives from the recognition that early reperfusion of ischemic myocardium can potentially salvage tissue before it becomes irreversibly injured. Since most infarctions are caused by a relatively sudden thrombotic occlusion overlying an atherosclerotic plaque in a major epicardial coronary vessel, recent attention has been appropriately directed at techniques to pharmacologically or mechanically recanalize the "culprit" vessel. The thrombolytic agents streptokinase, anisoylated plasminogen streptokinase activator complex (APSAC), and tissue plasminogen activator (tPA) have been approved by the Federal Drug Administration for intravenous use in the setting of acute myocardial infarction. These agents, as well as other investigational ones, have been extensively studied in many clinical trials from which emerge important conclusions about the management of patients with acute myocardial infarction. Thrombolytic therapy can reduce in-hospital mortality for myocardial infarction by up to 50 percent when administered within the first hour of the onset of symptoms, with much of this benefit maintained for one or more years. Appropriately employed thrombolytic therapy appears to reduce infarct size and limit left ventricular dysfunction as well. Since salvage of myocardium can only occur before the myocardium is irreversibly injured, timing of thrombolytic therapy is of extreme importance in achieving maximum benefit. While an upper time limit depends on specific factors in individual patients, it is clear that "every minute counts" and that patients treated within 1 to 3 h of the onset of symptoms stand to benefit most. Although the reduction of mortality is more modest, institution of therapy remains of benefit in many patients seen 3 to 6 h after the onset of infarction, and some benefit appears possible up to 12 h, especially if chest discomfort is ongoing and ST segments remain elevated in electrocardiographic leads that do not yet demonstrate new Q waves. In addition to the possibility of early treatment, clinical factors that favor proceeding with thrombolytic therapy include: anterior wall injury, hemodynamically complicated infarction, and widespread ECG evidence of myocardial jeopardy.

tPA is more effective than streptokinase or APSAC at restoring coronary artery flow, and has a small edge in improving survival as well. The current recommended total dose of tPA is 100 mg, beginning with a 5 to 10 mg bolus followed by 60 mg intravenously over the first hour, followed by 20 mg each in the second and third hours. "Front-loaded" regimens utilizing a larger initial bolus, and weight-adjusted doses to minimize complications in smaller individuals, are being tested but thus far a consensus about an alternative to the FDA approved dose of tPA has not been reached. Streptokinase is administered as 1.5 million units intravenously over 1 h. APSAC has the benefit of being administered as a single dose of 30 mg over 2 to 5 min, making it an ideal agent when given out of the hospital. Anticoagulant and platelet regimens appear to aid in establishing and maintaining vessel patency, and aspirin has been shown to lower mortality when given with thrombolytic therapy. Recent studies suggest that 160 to 325 mg of aspirin and 5000 units of I.V. heparin should be given with the institution of thrombolytic therapy. This should be followed by 325 mg of aspirin daily and a continuous infusion of heparin for 2 to 5 days.

Clear contraindications to the use of thrombolytic agents include a history of cerebrovascular accident, a recent (within 2 weeks) invasive or surgical procedure (or prolonged cardiopulmonary resuscitation), marked hypertension (systolic arterial pressure greater than 180 mmHg and/or diastolic pressure greater than 100 mmHg) at any time during the acute presentation, and active peptic ulcer disease.

Other clinical reasons for an increased risk of bleeding should be sought and the potential benefit of such therapy weighed against expected risk before the decision to administer a thrombolytic agent is made. While advanced age is associated with an increase in hemorrhagic complications, the benefit of thrombolytic therapy in the elderly appears to merit its use in most cases, particularly if no other contraindications are present and the amount of myocardium in jeopardy appears to be substantial. Following thrombolytic therapy cardiac catheterization and coronary angiography should be carried out if there is evidence of coronary artery reocclusion (reelevation of ST segments and/or recurrent chest pain) or if recurrent ischemia develops (such as recurrent angina in the early hospital course or a positive exercise stress test prior to discharge). Under these circumstances, and if the coronary anatomy is suitable, coronary angioplasty should be performed. Coronary artery bypass surgery should be reserved for a small minority of patients whose coronary anatomy is unsuitable for angioplasty but in whom revascularization appears to be advisable because of extensive jeopardized myocardium or recurrent ischemia.

Repeat administration of a thrombolytic agent is an alternative to early mechanical revascularization. Although there is little to suggest how this might be best undertaken, one reasonable strategy is to give a half dose of tPA (50 mg over 4 h) if reocclusion occurs 12 to 24 h after the agent is initially given and a repeat full dose (100 mg over 3 h) if such an event occurs more than 24 h later. Both APSAC and streptokinase are antigenic; once one has been used, repeat administration with either agent should be avoided.

Allergic reactions to streptokinase or APSAC occur in approximately 2 percent of cases. While a minor degree of hypotension occurs in 4 to 10 percent of patients given these agents, marked hypotension occurs, though rarely, in association with severe allergic reactions. In such cases, in addition to specific treatment of the allergic response and stopping the infusion of the thrombolytic agent initially used, consideration should be given to the rapid additional use of tPA. Hemorrhage is the most frequent and potentially the most serious complication. Since bleeding episodes which require transfusion are more common when patients require invasive procedures, unnecessary venous or arterial intervention should be avoided in patients receiving thrombolytic agents. Hemorrhagic stroke is the most serious complication and occurs in approximately 0.4 percent of cases. This rate increases with advancing age, with patients greater than 70 years of age experiencing roughly twice the rate of intracranial hemorrhage as those less than 65 years of age. Large-scale intervention trials have suggested that the rate of intracranial hemorrhage with APSAC or tPA is slightly higher than that seen with streptokinase.

Primary percutaneous transluminal coronary angioplasty Primary PTCA without preceding thrombolysis is also effective in restoring perfusion in acute myocardial infarction. It has the advantages of being applicable to patients with contraindications to thrombolytic therapy; it appears to be more effective than thrombolysis in opening occluded coronary arteries and may be associated with a somewhat better clinical outcome. Subgroups of patients in which direct PTCA may provide a special benefit over thrombolytic therapy include patients with cardiogenic shock and others at high risk because of advanced age (>70 years) or hemodynamic compromise (systolic arterial pressure <100 mmHg). However, this technique is expensive in terms of personnel and facilities, and its applicability is seriously limited by logistic considerations.

The quantity of myocardium that becomes necrotic secondary to a coronary artery occlusion is determined by factors other than just the site of occlusion. One such important factor is the status of collateral blood supply to ischemic tissue. Myocardium well supplied by collaterals clearly has the capacity to survive hours longer than poorly collateralized areas following coronary occlusion. Infarct size is affected by a number of therapeutic agents currently in use. The balance between myocardial oxygen supply and demand in areas rendered ischemic determines the ultimate fate of these areas of jeopardized myocardium. While no routine therapeutic approach to reduce infarct size in all patients is currently recommended, the realization that infarct size may be increased by interventions which adversely alter the supply-demand balance has prompted the reevaluation of previously accepted therapeutic maneuvers in the management of patients with acute infarction. Cardioactive sympathomimetic amines must be used sparingly and only for clear-cut indications. The early administration of nitrates and beta blockers, with or without thrombolytic therapy, appears to be of benefit.

ROUTINE TREATMENT OF THE PATIENT WITH MYOCARDIAL INFARCTION

ANALGESIA Since myocardial infarction usually presents with severe pain, one of the important initial therapeutic objectives is the relief of pain. Morphine is an extremely effective analgesic for the pain associated with myocardial infarction. However, it may reduce sympathetically mediated arteriolar and venous constriction. The resultant venous pooling may produce a reduction in cardiac output and arterial pressure. This must be recognized but does not necessarily contraindicate its use. Hypotension associated with venous pooling usually responds promptly to elevation of the legs, but in some patients volume expansion with intravenous saline is required. The patient may experience diaphoresis and nausea, but these events usually pass and are replaced by a feeling of well-being associated with the relief of pain. Morphine also has a vagotonic effect and may cause bradycardia or advanced degrees of heart block, particularly in patients with posteroinferior infarction. These side effects of morphine usually respond to atropine (0.5 mg intravenously). Morphine is routinely administered by repetitive (every 5 min) intravenous injection of small doses of drug (2 to 4 mg) rather than by administration of a larger quantity by the subcutaneous route, by which absorption may be unpredictable. Meperidine hydrochloride or hydromorphone hydrochloride may be effectively employed in place of morphine.

Prior to administering morphine, sublingual nitroglycerin can be given safely to most patients with myocardial infarction. As long as hypotension does not occur, up to three 0.4-mg doses should be administered at about 5-min intervals. In addition to diminishing or abolishing chest discomfort, this form of therapy, once considered contraindicated in the setting of acute myocardial infarction, may be capable of both decreasing myocardial oxygen demand (by lowering preload) and increasing myocardial oxygen supply (by dilating infarct-related coronary vessels or collateral vessels). However, therapy with nitrates should be avoided in patients who present with a low systolic arterial pressure (<100 mmHg). The potential for an idiosyncratic reaction to nitrates, consisting of sudden marked hypotension and bradycardia, should be recognized. This problem, occurring more frequently in patients with inferior wall infarction, can usually be promptly reversed by the rapid administration of intravenous atropine. In patients whose initially favorable response to sublingual nitroglycerin is followed by the return of chest pain, particularly if accompanied by other evidence of ongoing ischemia such as further ST-segment or T-wave shifts, the use of intravenous nitroglycerin should be considered.

Intravenous beta blockers are also useful in the control of the pain of acute myocardial infarction. These drugs have been shown to control pain effectively in some patients, presumably by diminishing ischemia consequent to lowering myocardial oxygen demand. More importantly, there is some evidence that intravenous beta blockers reduce in-hospital mortality, particularly in high-risk patients. Dosing similar to that used to treat the hyperdynamic state may be utilized.

Glucocorticoids and nonsteroidal anti-inflammatory agents, with the exception of aspirin, should be avoided in the setting of acute myocardial infarction. They can impair infarct healing and increase the risk of myocardial rupture, and may produce a larger infarct scar. Additionally, they can increase coronary vascular resistance, thereby potentially reducing flow to ischemic myocardium.

OXYGEN The routine use of oxygen is supported by the observation that the arterial P_{O_2} is reduced in many patients with myocardial infarction and that oxygen inhalation reduces the area of ischemic injury in experimental animals. Oxygen should be administered by face mask or nasal prongs for the first day or two after infarction.

ACTIVITY Factors which increase the work of the heart during the initial hours of infarction may increase the size of the infarct. Circumstances in which heart size, cardiac output, or myocardial contractility are increased should be avoided. It has been demonstrated that 6 to 8 weeks are required for complete healing, i.e., replacement of the infarcted myocardium by scar tissue. The purpose of a graded increase in physical activity is to provide the most favorable possible circumstances for this healing.

Most patients with myocardial infarction should be admitted to a coronary care unit or suitable monitoring facility and remain there, under constant observation by trained personnel utilizing continuous electrocardiographic monitoring, until clinical stability has been demonstrated (usually 1 to 3 days). A catheter should be introduced into a peripheral vein, firmly fixed so that it is not easily dislodged, and be kept open either by the slow infusion of isotonic glucose solution or by a closed heparin lock. In the absence of heart failure or other complications during the first 1 to 3 days, the patient should be in bed most of the day, with one or two periods of 15 to 30 min in a bedside chair. The patient should be bathed but may eat unassisted. Bedside commode privileges are given to all hemodynamically stable patients with a stable rhythm from the first day. The bed should be equipped with a footboard, against which the patient should push both feet regularly to prevent venous stasis and thromboembolism and to maintain muscle tone in the legs.

By the third or fourth day the patient with an uncomplicated course should be spending at least 30 to 60 min in a chair twice a day. At this time the patient's blood pressure should be measured when standing in order to be aware of postural hypotension, which may be a problem when ambulation is begun. Standing and gradual ambulation are usually begun between the second and fourth days post infarction in patients with uncomplicated myocardial infarction. Ambulation is progressively increased, eventually including walks about the hospital floor. In many hospitals a cardiac rehabilitation program with progressive exercise is initiated in the hospital and continued after discharge. Ideally, such programs should include an educational component which provides patients with information about their disease and its risk factors. The total duration of hospitalization in uncomplicated cases (Killip class I, see p. 1068) is usually 6 to 11 days. Patients in Killip class II or higher may require 2 or more weeks of hospitalization depending upon the rapidity with which heart failure resolves and the home situation to which the patient is returning. Many physicians perform heart rate–limited exercise tolerance tests just prior to discharge in the majority of patients with myocardial infarction. In some centers, symptom-limited (maximal) exercise tests are performed, as preliminary evidence suggests that this approach poses no increase in risk and it may be more sensitive for the detection of ischemia. Testing identifies high-risk patients as those who develop angina, S-T segment change, hypotension, or serious ventricular ectopic activity during or immediately following exercise. Such patients require special attention including measures such as beta-adrenoceptor blocking agents, long-acting nitrates, and/or calcium antagonists for evidence of ischemia. Selected patients may require further evaluation for possible antiarrhythmic therapy (p. 1072).

If ischemia occurs at rest, or if ischemia and/or hypotension occur during limited exercise, coronary arteriography should be carried out, except in the very elderly or in those for whom contraindications to invasive procedures exist. If a large quantity of viable myocardium, perfused by critically narrowed vessel(s), is found at angiography, then revascularization (either by angioplasty or by operation) may be required. Exercise tests also aid in formulating an individualized exercise prescription, which can be much more vigorous in patients who tolerate exercise without any of the above-mentioned adverse signs. Additionally, predischarge stress testing may provide an important psychological benefit related to building the patient's confidence through the demonstration of reasonable exercise tolerance.

Furthermore, particularly when no arrhythmias or signs of ischemia are identified, the patient benefits by the physician's reassurance that objective evidence suggests no immediate jeopardy.

The remainder of the convalescent phase of myocardial infarction may be accomplished at home. From 2 to 6 weeks, the patient should be encouraged to increase activity by walking about the house and outdoors in good weather. Patients should still spend 8 to 10 h in bed each night. Additional rest periods in the morning and afternoon may be advisable for selected patients. Normal sexual activity may be resumed during this period.

From 6 to 8 weeks onward, the physician must regulate the patient's activity on the basis of his or her exercise tolerance. It is during this period of increasing activity that the patient may become aware of profound fatigue. Postural hypotension may still be a problem. Most patients will be able to return to work after 12 weeks, and many patients much earlier. If not performed earlier, a maximal exercise test is frequently performed after 6 to 8 weeks or prior to returning to work. A trend toward earlier ambulation, hospital discharge, and resumption of full activity for patients recuperating from acute myocardial infarction has developed in recent years.

DIET During the first 4 or 5 days, a low-calorie diet divided into multiple small feedings is preferred. Cardiac output increases following ingestion of food, and therefore the quantity of individual feedings should be kept low. If heart failure is present, sodium intake should be restricted. Since constipation is common, it is reasonable to give average or even increased amounts of bulk in the diet. In addition, the ingestion of potassium-rich foods should be encouraged in patients receiving diuretics. During the second week, increasing amounts of food may be introduced into the diet. At this time, the importance of restriction of calories, cholesterol, and saturated fat may be explained to the patient, and he or she can be started on an appropriate diet. Willingness to accept dietary restriction and to discontinue cigarette smoking is usually never greater than it is during this early period of convalescence.

BOWELS Bed rest of 3 to 5 days and the effect of the narcotics utilized for the relief of pain often lead to constipation. A bedside commode, rather than a bed pan, a diet rich in bulk, and the routine use of a stool softener such as dioctyl sodium sulfosuccinate, 200 mg daily, are recommended. If the patient remains constipated despite these measures, a laxative can be safely used. It is safe to perform a gentle rectal examination on patients with acute myocardial infarction.

SEDATION Most patients require sedation during hospitalization in order to withstand the period of enforced inactivity with tranquility. Diazepam, 5 mg, oxazepam, 15 to 30 mg, or lorazepam, 0.5 to 2 mg, given three or four times daily, is usually effective. An additional dose of any of the above medications may be given at night to ensure adequate sleep. Attention to this problem is especially important during the first few days in the coronary care unit, where the atmosphere of 24-h vigilance may interfere with the patient's sleep. However, sedation is no substitute for reassuring, quiet surroundings.

ANTICOAGULANTS AND ANTIPLATELET AGENTS The use of anticoagulant therapy to retard the process of coronary occlusion during the initial phases of the illness is of accepted importance as a result of the recognition that thrombosis plays an important role in the pathogenesis of acute myocardial infarction. Data from trials employing aspirin and/or thrombolytic agents have led to increased consensus about the appropriate treatment regimens. At the time of thrombolytic therapy, unless contraindications exist, most patients with possible or probable myocardial infarction should be started on aspirin, 160 or 325 mg daily. This should be started immediately, e.g., by chewing an aspirin in the Emergency Room as thrombolytic therapy is begun. In the patient who is to receive a thrombolytic agent, conventional therapy in the United States includes a 5000-unit bolus of intravenous heparin, followed by a constant intravenous infusion beginning at 1000 units per hour adjusted to keep the partial thromboplastin time (PTT) at 1.5 to 2 times normal. Patients with acute myocardial infarction not undergoing thrombolytic therapy should also generally receive aspirin. This strategy has been shown to prevent some patients who present with unstable angina from progressing to myocardial infarction, and data suggest that in-hospital mortality is lowered even among patients who do develop myocardial infarction if they are given aspirin early in their course. Additionally, in order to prevent venous thrombosis in patients *not* treated with thrombolytic therapy, either intravenous heparin or small subcutaneous doses of heparin (5000 units every 8 to 12 h) should be employed as well.

Controversy persists about the use of oral anticoagulants once the patient is out of the intensive care area. Warfarin should be used for patients with congestive heart failure which persists for more than 3 to 4 days or for those with large anterior infarctions in whom the risk of developing a left ventricular thrombus is greater. The incidence of arterial embolism from a clot originating in the ventricle at the site of an infarction is small but definite. Two-dimensional echocardiography allows for the early detection of left ventricular thrombi in about one-third of patients with anterior wall infarction but rarely in patients with inferior or posterior infarction. Arterial embolism often presents as a major complication, such as hemiparesis when the cerebral circulation is involved, or hypertension if the renal circulation is compromised. The low incidence of these complications, contrasted with their severity, renders it impractical to establish firm guidelines for the use of anticoagulant drugs as prophylaxis against arterial embolism in acute myocardial infarction. The likelihood of arterial embolism appears to increase with the extent of infarction and the resultant inflammation and endocardial stasis due to akinesis. Therefore the indication for anticoagulation as prophylaxis against arterial embolism increases with the extent of infarction. When a thrombus has been clearly demonstrated by echocardiographic or other techniques, systemic anticoagulation should be undertaken (in the absence of contraindications), for the incidence of embolic complications appears to be markedly lowered by such therapy. The appropriate duration of therapy is unknown, but probably should be carried out for 3 to 6 months.

Evidence suggests that warfarin lowers late mortality and the incidence of reinfarction after an acute myocardial infarction. Since studies comparing aspirin and warfarin therapy separately or in combination have not yet been completed, the final choice of agents must be based on physician preferences, experience, and patient characteristics.

BETA-ADRENOCEPTOR BLOCKERS The chronic routine use of oral beta-adrenoceptor blockers for at least 2 years following acute myocardial infarction is supported by well-conducted placebo-controlled trials which have convincingly demonstrated reductions in total mortality, sudden death, and in some instances, reinfarction rate. While beta blockers are of benefit, even when started as late as 28 days following the acute event, additional benefit probably accrues to those patients who are started earlier, including patients receiving thrombolytic therapy. For patients presenting with the clear picture of a hyperdynamic state, in the absence of contraindications such as congestive heart failure, hypotension, bradycardia, atrioventricular block, or a history of asthma, an intravenous dose of a beta blocker such as metoprolol may be given (5 mg every 5 to 10 min for a total dose of 15 mg, stopping between doses if any complications arise). This is usually followed by an oral dose regimen of metoprolol (50 to 100 mg bid). Later in the hospital course, a long-acting beta blocker, such as atenolol (50 to 100 mg qd) can be prescribed. Beta blocker therapy is probably indicated for most patients after myocardial infarction, except those for whom its use is specifically contraindicated (patients with heart failure, heart block, orthostatic hypotension, or severely compromised left ventricular function, but without symptoms of heart failure or a history of asthma) and perhaps those whose excellent long-term prognosis (defined as mortality less than 1 percent per year) markedly diminishes any potential benefit (patients with normal ventricular function, no complex ventricular ectopy, no angina, and a negative maximal exercise stress test).

OTHER AGENTS On the basis of the recently completed SAVE trial, the administration of *angiotensin-converting enzyme (ACE)*

inhibitors can now be recommended for improvement in mortality as well as for prevention of heart failure and recurrent myocardial infarction in patients with ejection fractions of 40 percent or less. In such cases, captopril (target dose 50 mg tid) should be started once hemodynamic stability has been demonstrated. In pharmacologically equivalent doses, other ACE inhibitors are likely to be of benefit as well, but these agents have not yet been tested. However, the early (within 24 h) use of intravenous enalaprilat has been shown to be of no benefit, and should be avoided as excessive hypotension may be produced.

Magnesium appears to have favorable effects on cardiac arrhythmias, coronary blood flow, platelet aggregation, as well as myocardial metabolism. One relatively large trial and meta-analyses of many smaller trials strongly suggest that the early use of intravenous magnesium (8 mmol $MgSO_4$ over 15 min, followed by 65 mmol over the next 24 h) significantly reduces serious arrhythmias and total mortality after myocardial infarction. Such therapy is inexpensive, causes few side effects, and is easy to administer.

As noted earlier, *nitrates* (intravenous or oral) may be useful in the relief of pain associated with acute myocardial infarction. Favorable effects on the ischemic process and ventricular remodeling (see below) has led many physicians to routinely use intravenous nitroglycerin (5 to 10 µg/min initial dose and up to 200 µg/min as long as hemodynamic stability is maintained) for the first 24 to 48 h after the onset of infarction.

Results of multiple trials of different *calcium antagonists* have failed to convincingly establish a role for these agents in the treatment of most patients with myocardial infarction. Unlike the more consistent data which exists for other drugs (e.g., beta blockers, aspirin, thrombolytic therapy, and magnesium) the routine use of calcium antagonists cannot be recommended. They should be reserved for patients who develop recurrent myocardial ischemia.

COMPLICATIONS OF MYOCARDIAL INFARCTION AND THEIR TREATMENT

ARRHYTHMIAS (See also Chaps. 197 and 198) The prompt management of arrhythmias constitutes a most significant advance in the treatment of myocardial infarction.

Ventricular premature systoles Infrequent, sporadic ventricular premature depolarizations occur in almost all patients with infarction and do not require therapy. Whereas in the past, frequent, multifocal, or early diastolic ventricular extrasystoles (so-called warning arrhythmias) were routinely treated, pharmacologic therapy is now reserved for patients with sustained or symptomatic ventricular arrhythmias. Prophylactic antiarrhythmic therapy (either intravenous lidocaine early or oral agents later), in the absence of clinically important ventricular tachyarrhythmias, is contraindicated as such therapy may actually increase late mortality. Beta-adrenoceptor blocking agents are effective in abolishing ventricular ectopic activity in infarction patients and in the prevention of ventricular fibrillation. They should be used routinely in patients without contraindications. In addition, hypokalemia is a risk factor for ventricular fibrillation in patients with acute myocardial infarction, and the serum potassium concentration should be adjusted to approximately 4.5 mmol/L.

Ventricular tachycardia and ventricular fibrillation Within the first 24 h of myocardial infarction ventricular tachycardia and fibrillation can occur without prior warning arrhythmias. The occurrence of such primary arrhythmias can be reduced by prophylactic administration of intravenous lidocaine. However, use in this manner has never been shown to reduce overall mortality with acute myocardial infarction. In fact, in addition to noncardiac complications that may occur with lidocaine use, lidocaine may predispose to bradycardia and asystole. This may explain the trend toward increased mortality with lidocaine in meta-analyses of its prophylactic use. Furthermore, over the past 20 years the incidence of primary ventricular fibrillation appears to have fallen dramatically, perhaps by as much as a factor of 10. For these reasons, and with earlier treatment of active ischemia, more frequent use of beta-blocking agents, and the nearly universal success of electrical cardioversion or defibrillation, routine *prophylactic* antiarrhythmic drug therapy is no longer recommended. It should be reserved for patients who cannot reach a hospital or those treated in hospitals that lack the constant presence in the coronary care unit of a physician or nurse trained in the recognition and treatment of ventricular fibrillation. Sustained ventricular tachycardia is treated first with lidocaine, and if it cannot be terminated by one or two 50- to 100-mg doses, electroconversion should be employed (Chap. 198). Electroshock is used immediately in patients with ventricular fibrillation, or when ventricular tachycardia causes hemodynamic deterioration. If fibrillation has persisted for more than a few seconds, the first shock may be unsuccessful, and in this situation it is advisable to administer closed-chest massage and mouth-to-mouth respiration before attempting electroconversion again. Improvement of oxygenation and perfusion increase the likelihood of successful defibrillation. Bretylium is useful in the treatment of both refractory ventricular fibrillation and ventricular tachycardia. For ventricular fibrillation, bretylium is given as a 5-mg/kg bolus and defibrillation is again attempted. If the latter fails, a second bolus of 10 mg/kg is given to facilitate electroconversion of ventricular fibrillation. Ventricular tachycardia can be treated with bretylium 5 to 10 mg/kg injected slowly over 10 min. In either situation, the initial dose of bretylium may be followed by a continuous infusion of 2 mg/min if the arrhythmia is recurrent. Severe postural hypotension occurs after intravenous bretylium administration; therefore, patients should always be supine when and immediately after the drug is given, and intravenous fluids should be available for rapid administration if needed. Ventricular arrhythmias, including the unusual form of ventricular tachycardia known as *torsades de pointes* (Chap. 198) may occur in infarct patients as a consequence of other concurrent problems (such as hypoxia, hypokalemia, or other electrolyte disturbances) or due to the toxic effects of agents already being administered to the patient (such as digoxin or quinidine). A search for such secondary causes should always be undertaken.

Long-term survival is good (generally better than 90 percent at 1 year) in patients with *primary* ventricular fibrillation, i.e., ventricular fibrillation resulting as a primary response to acute ischemia and not associated with predisposing factors such as congestive heart failure, shock, bundle branch block, or ventricular aneurysm. This prognosis is in sharp contrast to that for patients who develop ventricular fibrillation *secondary* to severe pump failure. In patients who develop ventricular tachycardia or ventricular fibrillation late in their hospital course, the mortality in 1 year may be as high as 85 percent. Such patients may warrant electrophysiologic study (Chap. 198).

Accelerated idioventricular rhythm   Accelerated idioventricular rhythm (AIVR, "slow ventricular tachycardia"), a ventricular rhythm with a rate of 60 to 100 beats per minute, occurs in 25 percent of patients with myocardial infarction. It is especially frequent in inferoposterior infarction, where it is usually associated with sinus bradycardia. It often occurs transiently during thrombolytic therapy at the time of reperfusion. The rate of AIVR is usually similar to that of the sinus rhythm which precedes and follows it, and this similarity of rate and the relatively minor hemodynamic effects make this rhythm difficult to detect other than by electrocardiographic monitoring. For the most part, this rhythm is benign and does not presage the development of classic ventricular tachycardia. Most AIVR does not require treatment if the patient is monitored carefully since degeneration into a more serious arrhythmia is rare, and if it occurs, the AIVR can generally be readily treated with a drug which decreases the ventricular escape rate, such as mexiletine, and/or one that increases the sinus rate (atropine).

Supraventricular arrhythmias   Sinus tachycardia is the most common arrhythmia of this type. If it occurs secondary to other causes (such as anemia, fever, heart failure, or a metabolic derangement), the primary problem should be treated first. However, if sinus tachycardia appears to be due to sympathetic overstimulation, such

as is seen as part of a hyperdynamic state, then treatment with a relatively short acting beta blocker such as propranolol should be considered. Other common arrhythmias in this group are junctional rhythm and tachycardia, atrial tachycardia, atrial flutter, and atrial fibrillation. These rhythm disturbances are often secondary to left ventricular failure. The administration of digoxin is usually the treatment of choice for supraventricular arrhythmias if heart failure is present. If heart failure is absent, verapamil is an ideal alternative, as this agent may also help control ischemia. If the abnormal rhythm persists for more than 2 h with a ventricular rate in excess of 120 beats per minute, or at any time when tachycardia induces heart failure, shock, or ischemia (as manifested by recurrent pain or ECG changes), electroshock should be utilized.

Junctional arrhythmias are of diverse etiology, are not indicative of any specific abnormality, and from a therapeutic viewpoint must be considered on an individual basis. Digitalis excess must be ruled out as a cause of junctional tachycardia. In some patients with severely compromised left ventricular function, the loss of appropriately timed atrial systole results in a marked decrease in cardiac output. Right atrial or coronary sinus pacing is indicated in such instances.

Sinus bradycardia   Treatment of sinus bradycardia is indicated if hemodynamic compromise results from the slow heart rate. Elevation of the legs and/or the foot of the bed is frequently helpful in the treatment of sinus bradycardia. Atropine is the most useful drug for increasing heart rate and should be given intravenously in doses of 0.5 mg initially. If the rate remains below 60 beats per minute, additional doses of 0.2 mg, up to a total of 2.0 mg, may be given in divided doses. Persistent bradycardia (<40 beats per minute) despite atropine may be treated with electrical pacing. Isoproterenol should be avoided.

Atrioventricular and intraventricular conduction disturbances (See also Chap. 197)   The in-hospital mortality rate of patients with complete AV block in association with anterior infarction is markedly higher (60 to 75 percent) than that of patients who develop AV block with inferior infarction (25 to 40 percent), and the risk of subsequent death in those who survive to leave the hospital is also increased in the former group. This difference is related to the fact that heart block in inferior infarction is usually caused by AV nodal ischemia. The AV node is a small discrete structure, and thus a small amount of ischemia or necrosis can result in AV nodal dysfunction. In anterior wall infarction, heart block is usually related to ischemic malfunction of all three fascicles of the conduction system and thus commonly results only from extensive myocardial necrosis.

Electrical pacing provides an effective means of increasing the heart rate of patients with bradycardia due to AV block, but it is not possible to be sure that such acceleration is always beneficial. For example, in patients with anterior wall infarction and complete heart block, the large size of the infarct is the major factor determining the outcome, and correction of the conduction deficit may not improve the poor prognosis in this group. It should, however, be carried out if it improves hemodynamics. But pacing does appear to be beneficial in patients with inferoposterior infarction who have complete heart block associated with heart failure, hypotension, marked bradycardia, or significant ventricular ectopic activity. A subgroup of these patients, those with right ventricular infarction, often respond poorly to ventricular pacing because of the loss of the atrial "kick." In such patients, dual chamber, atrioventricular sequential pacing may be required.

In the past, prophylactic placement of a pacing catheter has been advocated for patients with conduction disturbances known to be precursors of complete heart block. However, the availability of reliable noninvasive (external) temporary pacing devices makes it possible to pace conscious patients without insertion of a transvenous pacemaker lead. Therefore, routine, prophylactic insertion of a pacing catheter is no longer necessary in most situations. Permanent pacing has been advocated for patients who develop combined persistent bifascicular and transient third-degree heart block during the acute phase of myocardial infarction. Retrospective studies in such patients suggest that the incidence of sudden death is decreased in those in whom permanent pacing was instituted.

HEART FAILURE Some degree of transient impairment of left ventricular function occurs in over half of patients with myocardial infarction. The most common clinical signs are pulmonary rales and S_3 and S_4 gallop rhythms. Pulmonary congestion is also frequently seen on the chest roentgenogram. Elevation of left ventricular filling pressure and pulmonary artery pressure are the characteristic hemodynamic findings, but it should be appreciated that these findings may result from a reduction of diastolic ventricular compliance (diastolic failure) and/or a reduction of stroke volume with secondary cardiac dilatation (systolic failure) (Chap. 194). The management of heart failure in association with myocardial infarction is similar to that of acute heart failure secondary to other forms of heart disease, with a few exceptions (Chap. 195). The major difference concerns the use of cardiac glycosides. The benefit following the administration of digitalis in acute myocardial infarction is unimpressive. This is not surprising since the function of the noninfarcted tissue may be normal and digitalis would not be expected to improve the systolic or diastolic dysfunction of infarcted or ischemic tissue. On the other hand, diuretic agents are extremely effective since they diminish pulmonary congestion in the presence of systolic and/or diastolic heart failure. A fall in left ventricular filling pressure and an improvement in orthopnea and dyspnea follow the intravenous administration of furosemide. This drug should be used with caution, however, as it can result in a massive diuresis with associated decrease in plasma volume, cardiac output, systemic blood pressure, and hence coronary perfusion. Nitrates in various forms may be used to decrease preload and congestive symptoms. Oral isosorbide dinitrate, topical nitroglycerin ointment, or intravenous nitroglycerin, all have the advantage over a diuretic of lowering preload through venodilatation without decreasing the total plasma volume. Additionally, nitrates may improve ventricular compliance if concurrent ischemia is present, since ischemia causes an elevation of left ventricular filling pressure. The patient with pulmonary edema is treated in the manner described in Chap. 195, but vasodilators must be used with caution to prevent serious hypotension.

Ventricular remodeling Soon after myocardial infarction, the left ventricle begins to dilate. Acutely, this occurs as the result of expansion of the infarct. Later, lengthening of the noninfarcted segments occurs as well. Overall chamber enlargement is related to the size of the infarction, with greater degrees of dilatation causing more marked hemodynamic impairment, more frequent heart failure, and a poorer prognosis as well. Progressive dilatation and its clinical consequences may be attenuated by afterload-reducing therapy such as vasodilatation induced by an ACE inhibitor. Thus, in patients with a depressed ejection fraction (less than 40 percent), regardless of whether or not heart failure is present, consideration should be given to captopril therapy (beginning with 6.25 mg tid and advancing to 25 to 50 mg tid as tolerated). Equivalent doses of other ACE inhibitors are probably of benefit as well.

Hemodynamic monitoring Hemodynamic evidence of abnormal left ventricular function becomes apparent when contraction is seriously impaired in 20 to 25 percent of the left ventricle. Infarction of 40 percent or more of the left ventricle usually results in the syndrome of cardiogenic shock (see below). Positioning of a balloon flotation catheter in the pulmonary artery permits monitoring of left ventricular filling pressure, a technique which is useful in patients who exhibit clinical evidence of hemodynamic abnormalities or instability. However, in view of the complications that can occur, insertion of a pulmonary artery catheter should be limited to those patients with hemodynamic instability. Cardiac output can also be determined with a pulmonary artery catheter. With the addition of intraarterial pressure monitoring, systemic vascular resistance can be calculated as a guide to adjusting vasopressor and vasodilator therapy. Some patients with acute myocardial infarction have markedly elevated left ventricular filling pressures (>22 mmHg) and normal cardiac indexes [>2.6 and <3.6 (L/min)/m²], while others have relatively low filling pressures

(<15 mmHg) and reduced cardiac indexes. The former usually benefit from diuresis, while the latter respond to volume expansion by means of intravenous administration of colloid-containing solutions.

Cardiogenic shock—power failure In recent years efforts to reduce infarct size and prompt treatment of ongoing ischemia and other complications of myocardial infarction appear to have reduced the incidence of cardiogenic shock.

It is useful to consider cardiogenic shock as a form of severe left ventricular failure. This syndrome is characterized by marked hypotension with systolic arterial pressure <80 mmHg and a marked reduction of cardiac index [<1.8 (L/min)m²] in the face of elevated left ventricular filling (pulmonary capillary wedge) pressure >18 mmHg. Hypotension alone is not a basis for the diagnosis of cardiogenic shock, because many patients who make an uneventful recovery will have serious hypotension (systolic pressure <80 mmHg) for several hours. Such patients often have low left ventricular filling pressures, and their hypotension usually resolves with the administration of intravenous fluids. In contrast to hypovolemic hypotension (see below) cardiogenic shock is generally associated with a mortality rate of >70 percent; however, recent efforts to restore coronary blood flow early in the course of infarction (with coronary angioplasty or surgical revascularization), suggests that this high mortality rate can be lowered by as much as one-half.

Cardiogenic shock may develop during the first hours of the infarct and be present at the time of initial hospitalization. Alternatively, it may appear after hospitalization—most commonly during the first day but sometimes as late as the sixth day. Risk factors for the in-hospital development of shock include advanced age, depressed left ventricular ejection fraction on admission, large infarct, history of diabetes mellitus, and previous myocardial infarction. Patients with several of these risk factors may be considered for cardiac catheterization and mechanical reperfusion (angioplasty or surgery) *before* the development of shock.

Pathophysiology of pump failure Marked reduction in the quantity of contracting myocardium is the cause of cardiogenic shock in myocardial infarction. The initial insult results in a decrease in arterial pressure and hence in coronary blood flow because of its dependence on aortic perfusion pressure (Fig. 202-1). The reduction in coronary perfusion pressure and myocardial blood flow further impairs myocardial function and may increase the size of the myocardial infarction. Arrhythmias and metabolic acidosis also contribute to this deterioration because they are the result of inadequate perfusion. It is this positive feedback loop which accounts for the high mortality rate associated with the shock syndrome.

A simple schematic diagram depicting the relationship between left ventricular work and filling pressure is seen in Fig. 202-2. The upper curve represents the familiar Frank-Starling relationship in the normal heart; the lower curve shows the relation which might be expected in the patient with shock secondary to myocardial infarction. It is obvious that, at all levels of end-diastolic pressure, the left ventricular work of the patient with myocardial infarction is depressed. At point C, the end-diastolic pressure is elevated, but at point B, it may be normal despite the fact that myocardial work is well below that expected of the normal heart at this diastolic pressure, as indicated by point A.

Treatment of pump failure The physiology and ominous prognosis associated with this condition dictate that all patients with shock should, if possible, have continuous monitoring of arterial pressure and of left ventricular filling pressure (as reflected in the pulmonary capillary wedge pressure measured with a pulmonary artery balloon catheter) as well as frequent determinations of cardiac output. When pulmonary edema coexists, endotracheal intubation may be necessary to ensure oxygenation. The relief of pain is important, as some vasodepressor reflex activity may be a response to severe pain. However, narcotics should be used cautiously in view of their propensity to lower arterial pressure.

The primary objective of treatment is to avoid the sequence depicted in Fig. 202-1, by attempting to maintain coronary perfusion

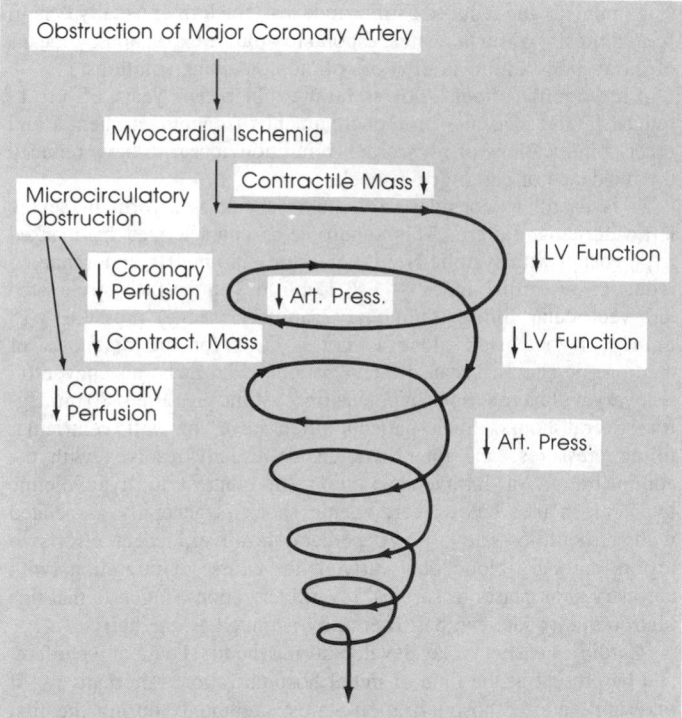

FIGURE 202-1 The sequence of events in the vicious cycle in which coronary artery obstruction leads to cardiogenic shock and progressive circulatory deterioration.

by raising the arterial blood pressure with vasopressors (see below), intraaortic balloon counterpulsation, and manipulation of blood volume to a level that ensures an optimum left ventricular filling pressure (approximately 20 mmHg). The latter may require either infusion of crystalloid or diuresis.

In patients seen within the first 4 to 8 h of the onset of infarction, reperfusion by thrombolytic therapy and/or PTCA (p. 1069) may improve left ventricular function dramatically, thereby interrupting the cycle of hemodynamic deterioration.

Hypovolemia This is an easily corrected condition which may contribute to the hypotension and vascular collapse associated with myocardial infarction in some patients. Hypovolemia may be secondary to previous diuretic use, to reduced fluid intake during the early

FIGURE 202-2 Schematic representation of the Frank-Starling relationship as applied to patients with the shock syndrome in myocardial infarction.

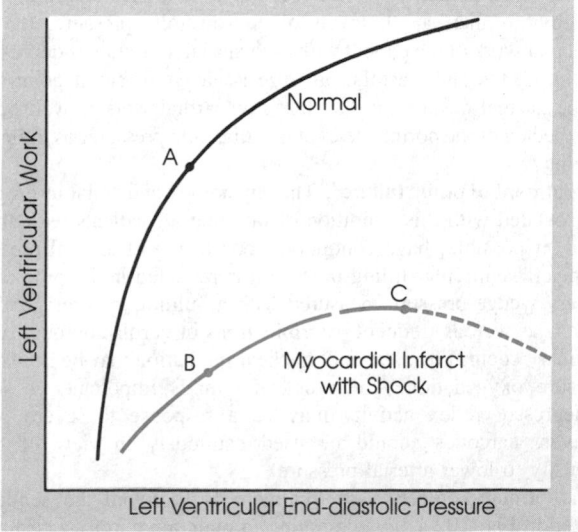

stages of the illness, and/or to vomiting associated with pain or medications. Consequently, hypovolemia should be identified and corrected in patients with acute myocardial infarction and hypotension before embarking upon more vigorous forms of therapy. The optimal left ventricular filling or pulmonary artery wedge pressure may vary considerably among different patients. Each patient's ideal level (generally at approximately 20 mmHg) is reached by cautious fluid administration during careful monitoring of oxygenation and cardiac output. When the cardiac output plateaus (Fig. 202-2, point C), further increases in left ventricular filling pressure will only increase congestive symptoms and decrease systemic oxygenation without raising arterial pressure. Central venous pressure reflects right rather than left ventricular filling pressure and is an inadequate guide for adjustment of blood volume, since left ventricular function is almost always affected much more adversely than right ventricular function in acute myocardial infarction.

Vasopressors A variety of intravenous drugs may be used to augment arterial pressure and cardiac output in patients with cardiogenic shock. Unfortunately, all have important disadvantages or problems associated with their use, and none have been shown to change the outcome in patients with established shock. *Isoproterenol* is a sympathomimetic amine which is now rarely used in the treatment of shock due to myocardial infarction. Although this agent increases contractility, it also produces peripheral vasodilatation and increases heart rate. The resultant increase in myocardial oxygen consumption and reduction of coronary perfusion pressure may extend the area of ischemic injury. *Norepinephrine* (p. 420) is a potent alpha-adrenergic agent with powerful vasoconstrictive properties which also possesses beta-adrenergic activity and therefore enhances contractility. Because the increase in afterload and contractility associated with its use causes a marked increase in myocardial oxygen consumption, it should be reserved for desperate situations or for patients with cardiogenic shock and lowered systemic vascular resistance. It should be started at 2 to 4 μg/min. If pressure cannot be maintained with a dosage of 15 μg/min, it is unlikely that a further increase will be beneficial.

Dopamine (Chap. 68) is useful in many patients with power failure. At low doses [2 to 10 (μg/kg)/min] the drug has positive chronotropic and inotropic effects as a consequence of beta receptor stimulation. At higher doses, a vasoconstrictive effect results from alpha receptor stimulation. At lower doses dopamine [≤2 (μg/kg)/min] also has the unique effect of dilating the renal and splanchnic vascular beds and apparently has little effect on myocardial oxygen consumption. Intravenous dopamine is started at an infusion rate of 2 to 5 (μg/kg)/min with increments in dosage every 2 to 5 min up to a maximum of 20 to 50 (μg/kg)/min. Systolic arterial blood pressure should be maintained at approximately 90 mmHg. *Dobutamine* is a synthetic sympathomimetic amine with positive inotropic action and minimal positive chronotropic or peripheral vasoconstrictive activity in the usual dosage range of 2.5 to 10 (μg/kg)/min. It should not be employed when a vasoconstrictor effect is required. However, in patients with less profound degrees of hypotension, dobutamine may be an extremely useful agent, particularly if positive chronotropy is to be avoided.

Amrinone is a positive inotropic agent without catecholamine structure or activity. It resembles dobutamine in its pharmacologic activity, although it has a more potent vasodilating action. Initially a loading dose of 0.75 mg/kg is given over 2 to 3 min. If effective, this is followed by an infusion of 5 to 10 (μg/kg)/min, followed if necessary 30 min later by an additional bolus of 0.75 mg/kg. If necessary, the dose may then be increased up to 15 (μg/kg)/min for short periods.

Cardiac glycosides (Chap. 195) Controlled studies have failed to demonstrate significant beneficial effects of cardiac glycoside therapy in the early phases (0 to 48 h) of acute myocardial infarction. Hemodynamic improvement has been documented at later times, but this effect, too, is marginal. Since cardiac glycosides cannot improve the function of necrotic myocardium and since pump failure is thought to be related to the total mass of infarcted tissue, digitalis therapy does not usually result in improvement in patients with acute myocardial infarction and sinus rhythm.

Aortic counterpulsation In cardiogenic shock mechanical assistance with an intraaortic balloon pumping system capable of augmenting both diastolic pressure and cardiac output can provide circulatory support. A sausage-shaped balloon at the end of a catheter is introduced percutaneously into the aorta via the femoral artery, and the balloon is automatically inflated during early diastole, thereby enhancing both coronary blood flow and peripheral perfusion. The balloon collapses in early systole, thereby reducing the afterload against which left ventricular ejection takes place. Improvement in hemodynamic status has been observed with balloon pumping in a large number of patients, but, in the absence of early revascularization, long-term survival following this mode of therapy in patients with cardiogenic shock is still disappointing. The balloon counterpulsation system may best be reserved for patients whose condition merits mechanical (surgery or angioplasty) intervention (e.g., patients with continuing ischemia, ventricular septal rupture, or mitral regurgitation) and in whom a successful result is likely to result in the reversal of cardiogenic shock. Intraaortic balloon pumping is contraindicated if aortic regurgitation is present or if aortic dissection is possible or suspected.

There is reason to believe that results of therapy of the shock syndrome secondary to myocardial infarction, while improving gradually as a result of meticulous attention to the details of therapy outlined above, will continue to be disappointing overall because a large fraction of patients with the syndrome have large areas of infarcted myocardium with severe, diffuse coronary atherosclerosis. Emerging evidence suggests that dramatic results can be achieved with emergency revascularization surgery, or, more commonly, coronary angioplasty. However, only a minority of patients developing cardiogenic shock have prompt access to these expensive technologies, and it is hoped that the widespread and early application of thrombolytic therapy will reduce the amount of myocardium which becomes necrotic and thereby reduce the incidence of this syndrome.

Other complications MITRAL REGURGITATION The reported incidence of apical systolic murmurs of mitral regurgitation during the first few days after the onset of a myocardial infarction varies widely (10 to 50 percent of patients) depending on the population studied and the acumen of the observers. In the first hours of infarction, mitral regurgitation can be demonstrated angiographically in approximately 15 percent of patients but is audible in only about one-tenth of those with positive angiograms. Whether audible or angiographically demonstrated, mitral regurgitation is of hemodynamic importance in only a minority of these patients.

The most common cause of mitral regurgitation following myocardial infarction is dysfunction of the papillary muscles of the left ventricle due to ischemia or infarction. Mitral regurgitation may also be the result of alteration in the size or shape of the ventricle due to impaired contractility or to aneurysm formation. Either papillary muscle may rupture, the posterior one twice as frequently as the anterior. Left ventricular function may deteriorate dramatically with superimposition of mitral regurgitation. The differential diagnosis includes perforation of the ventricular septum (see below), and the differentiation from mitral regurgitation is conveniently made at the bedside by color flow Doppler echocardiography. Surgical repair or replacement of the mitral valve may be followed by dramatic improvement in patients in whom acute heart failure results primarily from severe mitral regurgitation due to papillary muscle rupture or dysfunction and in whom myocardial function is relatively well preserved.

If aortic systolic pressure is lowered in patients with mitral regurgitation, a greater fraction of the left ventricular output will be ejected antegrade, thus lessening the regurgitant fraction. To this end, both intraaortic balloon counterpulsation, which lowers the aortic systolic pressure mechanically, and the infusion of sodium nitroprusside or nitroglycerin, which reduce systemic vascular resistance, have

been used with success for the interim management of patients with severe mitral regurgitation in the setting of acute myocardial infarction. Ideally, definitive operative treatment should be postponed for 4 to 6 weeks after the infarct. However, if the patient's hemodynamic and/or clinical condition does not improve or stabilize, surgical treatment should be undertaken, even in the acute stage.

Cardiac rupture Myocardial rupture is a dramatic complication of myocardial infarction most likely to occur during the first week after the onset of symptoms; its frequency increases with the age of the patient. First infarction, a history of hypertension, no history of angina pectoris, and relatively large Q-wave infarcts are associated with a higher incidence of cardiac rupture. The clinical presentation may often be that of a sudden disappearance of the pulse, blood pressure, and consciousness while the electrocardiogram continues to show sinus rhythm (*apparent* electromechanical dissociation). The myocardium continues to contract, but forward flow is not maintained as blood escapes into the pericardium. Cardiac tamponade (Chap. 206) ensues, and closed-chest massage is ineffective. This condition is almost universally fatal.

Septal perforation The pathogenesis of perforation of the ventricular septum is similar to that of external rupture of the myocardium, but the therapeutic potential is greater. Patients with ventricular septal rupture present with severe heart failure in association with the sudden appearance of a pansystolic murmur, often accompanied by a parasternal thrill. It is often impossible to differentiate this condition from rupture of a papillary muscle with resultant mitral regurgitation, and a tall *v* wave in the pulmonary capillary wedge pressure in both conditions further complicates the differentiation. The diagnosis can be established by the demonstration of a left-to-right shunt (i.e., an oxygen step-up at the level of the right ventricle) by limited cardiac catheterization performed at the bedside using a flow-directed balloon catheter. Color flow Doppler echocardiography can be extremely useful for making this diagnosis at the bedside. Rupture of the ventricular septum is amenable to immediate surgical treatment, albeit at a significant risk, but this form of therapy is ordinarily indicated on an urgent basis in patients whose condition cannot be stabilized rapidly. A prolonged period of hemodynamic compromise may produce end-organ damage and other complications that can be avoided by early intervention including nitroprusside infusion and intraaortic balloon counterpulsation.

The physiology of acute mitral regurgitation and acute ventricular septal perforation are similar in that the level of aortic systolic pressure determines in part the regurgitant volume, the principal difference being the chamber into which the regurgitant fraction is ejected. In septal perforation, a fraction of left ventricular output is ejected into the right ventricle. In a manner analogous to mitral regurgitation, lowering of aortic systolic pressure by mechanical (intraaortic balloon counterpulsation) and/or pharmacologic (nitroglycerin or nitroprusside) means can decrease the hemodynamic compromise caused by perforation.

Ventricular aneurysm The term *ventricular aneurysm* is usually used to describe *dyskinesis* or local expansile paradoxical wall motion. Normally functioning myocardial fibers must shorten more if stroke volume and cardiac output are to be maintained in patients with ventricular aneurysm, and if they are unable to do so, overall ventricular function is impaired. Aneurysms are composed of scar tissue and neither predispose to nor are associated with cardiac rupture.

The complications of left ventricular aneurysm do not usually occur for weeks to months following myocardial infarction; they include congestive heart failure, arterial embolism, and ventricular arrhythmias. Apical aneurysms are the most common and the most easily detected by clinical examination. The physical finding of greatest value is a double, diffuse, or displaced apical impulse. The electrocardiographic finding of ST-segment elevation at rest is present in precordial leads in 25 percent of patients with either apical or anterior aneurysms. Ventricular aneurysms are readily detectable by two-dimensional echocardiography, which may also reveal a mural thrombus within an aneurysm. Rarely, myocardial rupture may be contained by a local area of pericardium, along with organizing thrombus and hematoma. Over time this *pseudoaneurysm* enlarges, maintaining communication with the left ventricular cavity via a narrow neck. Because spontaneous rupture of a pseudoaneurysm often occurs, if recognized, it should be surgically repaired.

Right ventricular infarction Approximately one-third of patients with inferoposterior infarction demonstrate at least a minor degree of right ventricular necrosis. An occasional patient with inferoposterior left ventricular infarction also has extensive right ventricular myocardial infarction, and rarely patients present with infarction limited to the right ventricle. These patients often present with signs of severe right ventricular failure (jugular venous distention, Kussmaul's sign, hepatomegaly) with or without hypotension. ST-segment elevations of the right-sided precordial electrocardiographic leads, particularly lead V_4R, are present in the majority of patients with right ventricular infarction. Radionuclide ventriculography and two-dimensional echocardiography are also sensitive in the detection of right ventricular dysfunction associated with acute myocardial infarction. Catheterization of the right side of the heart often reveals a distinctive hemodynamic pattern resembling cardiac tamponade or constrictive pericarditis (Chap. 206). Volume expansion is often successful in treating low cardiac output and hypotension associated with extensive right ventricular infarction.

Postinfarction ischemia and extension Recurrent angina develops in approximately 25 percent of patients hospitalized for acute myocardial infarction. This percentage is even higher in patients undergoing successful thrombolysis. Since recurrent or persistent ischemia often heralds extension of the original infarct and is associated with a doubling of risk following acute myocardial infarction, patients with these symptoms should be considered for prompt coronary arteriography and mechanical revascularization.

Thromboembolism Clinically apparent thromboembolism complicates acute myocardial infarction in approximately 10 percent of cases, but embolic lesions are found in 45 percent of patients in necropsy series, suggesting that thromboembolism is often clinically silent. Thromboembolism is considered to be at least an important contributing cause of death in 25 percent of infarct patients who die following admission to the hospital. Arterial emboli originate from left ventricular mural thrombi, while most pulmonary emboli arise in the leg veins. Thromboembolism most commonly occurs in association with large infarcts in the presence of heart failure. Thromboembolism occurs extremely commonly in patients with echocardiographic evidence of a left ventricular thrombus, but only rarely if a thrombus is not present on the echocardiogram. Although well-controlled trials do not exist, the incidence of embolization appears to be decreased by anticoagulation.

Pericarditis (See also Chap. 206) Pericardial friction rubs and/or pericardial pain are frequently encountered in patients with acute transmural myocardial infarction. This complication can usually be managed with aspirin (650 mg qid). It is important to diagnose the chest pain of pericarditis accurately, since failure to appreciate it may lead to the erroneous diagnosis of recurrent ischemic pain and/or infarct extension with resultant inappropriate use of anticoagulants, nitrates, beta blockers, or coronary arteriography. The possibility exists that anticoagulants can cause tamponade in the presence of acute pericarditis, thus their use is contraindicated in patients with pericarditis, as manifested by either pain or persistent rub, unless there is a compelling indication.

Post-myocardial infarction syndrome—Dressler's syndrome (See also Chap. 206) This syndrome, characterized by fever and pleuropericardial chest pain, is thought to be due to an autoimmune pericarditis, pleuritis, and/or pneumonitis. It may begin from a few days to 6 weeks after myocardial infarction. The occurrence of Dressler's syndrome may be etiologically related to the early use of anticoagulants and appears to have decreased markedly in the last decade as long-term anticoagulants are used less frequently in acute myocardial infarction. The syndrome usually responds promptly to therapy with salicylates. On occasion, glucocorticoids may be required to relieve discomfort of an unusual, refractory nature. Effusions associated with Dressler's syndrome may become hemorrhagic if anticoagulants are administered.

POSTINFARCTION RISK STRATIFICATION AND MANAGEMENT

The goal of preventing reinfarction and death following recovery from myocardial infarction has led to strategies to evaluate risk following infarction. Early after infarction this generally involves use of non-invasive testing. As noted earlier, in stable patients submaximal exercise stress testing should be carried out prior to hospital discharge to detect residual ischemia and ventricular ectopy, and to provide the patient with a guideline for exercise in the early recovery period. Alternatively, or in addition, a maximal (symptom-limited) exercise stress test may be carried out 4 to 6 weeks following infarction. Evaluation of left ventricular function at rest and during exercise is usually warranted as well. Recognition of a depressed left ventricular ejection fraction by echocardiography or radionuclide ventriculography helps the physician with the selection of pharmacologic measures to improve long-term outcome (e.g., beta-blockers and/or ACE inhibitors) (pp. 424 and 1128, respectively). Patients with angina induced at relatively low workloads, those who have a large reversible defect on perfusion imaging or a depressed ejection fraction and demonstrable ischemia, and those in whom exercise provokes symptomatic ventricular arrhythmias should be considered at high risk for recurrent myocardial infarction or death from arrhythmia, and cardiac catheterization with coronary angiography and/or invasive electrophysiologic evaluation is advised, as discussed above.

Many clinical factors have been identified which are associated with an increase in cardiovascular risk following initial recovery from a myocardial infarction. Some of the most important factors, as already noted, include: ongoing symptoms of ischemia, depressed left ventricular ejection fraction (less than 40 percent), rales above the bases on physical examination or congestion on chest radiograph, and symptomatic ventricular arrhythmias. Other features associated with increased risk include history of previous myocardial infarction, age over 70 years, history of diabetes, prolonged sinus tachycardia, hypotension, the occurrence of ST-segment changes at rest without angina ("silent ischemia"), an abnormal signal-averaged electrocardiogram, nonpatency of the infarct-related coronary artery (if angiography is undertaken), and persistent advanced heart block or new intraventricular conduction abnormality on the electrocardiogram. Therapy must be individualized depending on the relative importance of the risk(s) present and the degree of benefit to be achieved by specific therapy including revascularization or the use of pharmacologic agents.

A variety of secondary preventive measures are at least partially responsible for the improved long-term mortality and morbidity following myocardial infarction. The benefits and use of beta blockers, antiplatelet agents and anticoagulants, and ACE inhibitors are discussed above. The relative limitations of calcium antagonists and antiarrhythmic agents have also been noted. Finally, risk factors for atherosclerosis (Table 208-4, p. 1110) should be discussed with the patient, and when possible, favorably modified. In particular, efforts should be made to ensure the cessation of smoking and the control of hypertension and hyperlipidemia. Additionally, regular physical exercise and reduction of emotional stress should be encouraged. Much of the above can be accomplished by referring the patient to a comprehensive cardiac rehabilitation program.

REFERENCES

ACC/AHA: Guidelines for the early management of patients with acute myocardial infarction: A report of the ACC/AHA task force on assessment of diagnostic and therapeutic cardiovascular procedures. Circulation 82:664, 1990

AMERICAN HEART ASSOCIATION: *1992 Heart and Stroke Facts.* Dallas, American Heart Association National Center, 1991, p. 1

ANTMAN EM, BERLIN JA: Declining incidence of ventricular fibrillation in myocardial infarction. Implications for the prophylactic use of lidocaine. Circulation 86:764, 1992

BATES ER: Expanding indications for thrombolytic therapy in acute myocardial infarction. Can J Cardiol 9:152, 1993

BENGTSON JR et al: Prognosis in cardiogenic shock after acute myocardial infarction in the interventional era. J Am Coll Cardiol 20:1482, 1992

EISENBERG MS et al: Thrombolytic therapy. Ann Emerg Med 22:417, 1993

ELDAR M et al: Primary ventricular tachycardia in acute myocardial infarction: Clinical characteristics and mortality. Ann Intern Med 117:31, 1992

FUSTER V et al: The pathogenesis of coronary artery disease and the acute coronary syndromes. N Engl J Med 326:242, 310, 1992

GIBBONS RJ: Technetium 99m sestamibi in the assessment of acute myocardial infarction. Semin Nucl Med 21:213, 1991

GOLDBERG RJ et al: Prognosis of acute myocardial infarction complicated by complete heart block (the Worcester Heart Attack Study). Am J Cardiol 69:1135, 1992

GOMES JA et al: Post-myocardial infarction stratification and the signal-averaged electrocardiogram. Prog Cardiovasc Dis 35:263, 1993

GOTTLIEB S et al: Interrelation of left ventricular ejection fraction, pulmonary congestion and outcome in acute myocardial infarction. Am J Cardiol 69:977, 1992

HORNER SM: Efficacy of intravenous magnesium in acute myocardial infarction in reducing arrhythmias and mortality. Meta-analysis of magnesium in acute myocardial infarction. Circulation 86:774, 1992

JUGDUTT BI: Role of nitrates after acute myocardial infarction. Am J Cardiol 70:82B, 1992

KRONE RJ: The role of risk stratification in the early management of a myocardial infarction. Ann Intern Med 116:223, 1992

LANGE RA, HILLIS LD: Immediate angioplasty for acute myocardial infarction. N Engl J Med 328:726, 1993

LEE L et al: Multicenter Registry of Angioplasty Therapy of Cardiogenic Shock: Initial and Long-term Survival. J Am Coll Cardiol 17:599, 1991

LEE TH, GOLDMAN L: Serum enzyme assays in the diagnosis of acute myocardial infarction. Ann Intern Med 105:221, 1986

LEHMANN KG et al: Mitral regurgitation in early myocardial infarction. Ann Intern Med 117:10, 1992

MAGGIONI AP et al: The risk of stroke in patients with acute myocardial infarction after thrombolytic and antithrombotic treatment. N Engl J Med 327:1, 1992

MUELLER HS et al: Predictors of early morbidity and mortality after thrombolytic therapy of acute myocardial infarction. Analyses of patient subgroups in the Thrombolysis in Myocardial Infarction (TIMI) trial, Phase II. Circulation 85:1254, 1992

MULTICENTER POSTINFARCTION RESEARCH GROUP: Low level exercise testing after myocardial infarction: Usefulness in enhancing clinical risk stratification. Circulation 71:80, 1985

PASTERNAK RC et al: Acute myocardial infarction, in Heart Disease, 4th ed, E Braunwald (ed). Philadelphia, Saunders, 1992, p. 1200

PFEFFER MA et al: Effect of captopril on mortality and morbidity in patients with left ventricular dysfunction after myocardial infarction. Results of the Survival and Ventricular Enlargement Trial. N Engl J Med 327:669, 1992

REEDER GS, GERSH BJ: Modern management of acute myocardial infarction. Curr Probl Cardiol 18:81, 1993

SIEGEL D et al: Risk factor modification after myocardial infarction. Ann Intern Med 109:213, 1988

TCHENG JE et al: Outcome of patients sustaining acute ischemic mitral regurgitation during myocardial infarction. Ann Intern Med 117:18, 1992

TENAGLIA AN, STACK RS: Angioplasty for acute coronary syndromes. Annu Rev Med 44:465, 1993

THIRD INTERNATIONAL STUDY OF INFARCT SURVIVAL COLLABORATIVE GROUP: ISIS-3: A randomized comparison of streptokinase vs tissue plasminogen activator vs anistreplase and of aspirin plus heparin vs aspirin alone among 41,299 cases of suspected acute myocardial infarction. Lancet 339:754, 1992

TIMI STUDY GROUP: Comparison of invasive and conservative strategies after treatment with intravenous tissue plasminogen activator in acute myocardial infarction. Results of the Thrombolysis in Myocardial Infarction (TIMI) Phase II Trial. N Engl J Med 320:618, 1989

TOFLER GH et al: Modifiers of timing and possible triggers of acute myocardial infarction in the Thrombolysis in Myocardial Infarction Phase II (TIMI II) study group. J Am Coll Cardiol 20:1049, 1992

203 ISCHEMIC HEART DISEASE

ANDREW P. SELWYN / EUGENE BRAUNWALD

Ischemia refers to a lack of oxygen due to inadequate perfusion. Ischemic heart disease is a condition of diverse etiologies, all having in common an imbalance between oxygen supply and demand.

ETIOLOGY AND PATHOPHYSIOLOGY

The most common cause of myocardial ischemia is atherosclerotic disease of epicardial coronary arteries. By reducing the lumen of these vessels, atherosclerosis causes an absolute decrease in myocardial perfusion in the basal state or limits appropriate increases in perfusion when the demand for flow is augmented. Coronary blood flow can also be limited by arterial thrombi, spasm, and rarely coronary emboli as well as by ostial narrowing due to luetic aortitis. Congenital abnormalities, such as anomalous origin of the left anterior descending coronary artery from the pulmonary artery, may cause myocardial ischemia and infarction in infancy, but this cause is very rare in adults. Myocardial ischemia can also occur if myocardial oxygen demands are abnormally increased, as in severe ventricular hypertrophy due to hypertension or aortic stenosis. The latter can present with angina that is indistinguishable from that caused by coronary atherosclerosis. A reduction in the oxygen-carrying capacity of the blood, as in extremely severe anemia or in the presence of carboxyhemoglobin, is a rare cause of myocardial ischemia. Not infrequently, two or more causes of ischemia will coexist, such as an increase in oxygen demand due to left ventricular hypertrophy and a reduction in oxygen supply secondary to coronary atherosclerosis.

The normal coronary circulation is dominated and controlled by the myocardial requirements for oxygen. This need is met by the heart's ability to vary coronary vascular resistance (and therefore blood flow) considerably while the myocardium extracts a high and relatively fixed percentage of oxygen (Chap. 12). Normally, intramyocardial resistance arterioles demonstrate an immense capacity for dilation. With exercise and emotional stress, the changing oxygen needs affect coronary vascular resistance and in this manner regulate the supply of blood and oxygen (metabolic regulation). These same vessels adapt to physiologic alterations in blood pressure in order to maintain coronary blood flow at levels appropriate to myocardial needs (autoregulation). Although the large epicardial coronary arteries are capable of constriction and relaxation, in healthy persons they serve as conduits and are referred to as conductance vessels, while the intramyocardial arterioles normally exhibit striking changes in tone and are therefore referred to as resistance vessels. Abnormal constriction or failure of normal dilation of the coronary resistance vessels also can cause ischemia. When it causes angina this condition is sometimes referred to as microvascular angina.

CORONARY ATHEROSCLEROSIS (See also Chap. 208) Epicardial coronary arteries are a major site of atherosclerotic disease. The major risk factors for atherosclerosis (high plasma LDL, low plasma HDL, cigarette smoking, diabetes mellitus, and hypertension) are thought to disturb the normal functions of the vascular endothelium. Dysfunction of vascular endothelium and an abnormal interaction with blood monocytes and platelets lead to subintimal collections of abnormal fat, cells, and debris (i.e., atherosclerotic plaques), which develop at irregular rates in different segments of the epicardial coronary tree and lead eventually to segmental reductions in cross-sectional area. The relationship between pulsatile flow and luminal stenosis is complex, but experiments have shown that when a stenosis reduces the cross-sectional area by approximately 75 percent, a full range of increases in flow to meet increased myocardial demand is not possible. When the luminal area is reduced by more than approximately 80 percent, blood flow at rest may be reduced, and further minor decreases in the stenotic orifice can reduce coronary flow dramatically and cause myocardial ischemia.

Segmental atherosclerotic narrowing of epicardial coronary arteries is caused most commonly by the formation of a plaque, which is subject to fissuring, hemorrhage, and thrombosis. Any of these events can temporarily worsen the obstruction, reduce coronary blood flow, and cause clinical manifestations of myocardial ischemia, as described below. The location of the obstruction will influence the quantity of myocardium rendered ischemic and thus determine the severity of the clinical manifestations. Severe coronary narrowing and myocardial ischemia are frequently accompanied by the development of collateral vessels, especially when the narrowing develops gradually. When well developed, such vessels can provide sufficient blood flow to sustain the viability of the myocardium at rest but not during conditions of increased demand.

Once severe stenosis of a proximal epicardial artery has reduced the cross-sectional area by more than approximately 70 percent, the distal resistance vessels (when they function normally) dilate to reduce vascular resistance and maintain coronary blood flow. A pressure gradient develops across the proximal stenosis, and poststenotic pressure falls. When the resistance vessels are maximally dilated, myocardial blood flow becomes dependent on the pressure in the coronary artery distal to the obstruction. In these circumstances alterations in myocardial oxygenation can be caused by changes in myocardial oxygen demand and changes in the caliber of the stenosed coronary artery due to physiologic vasomotion, pathologic spasm, or small platelet plugs. All these transient events can upset the critical balance between oxygen supply and demand and thus precipitate myocardial ischemia.

EFFECTS OF ISCHEMIA   The inadequate oxygenation induced by coronary atherosclerosis may cause transient disturbances of the mechanical, biochemical, and electrical functions of the myocardium. The abrupt development of ischemia usually affects a segment of left ventricular myocardium with almost instantaneous failure of normal muscle contraction and relaxation. The relatively poor perfusion of the subendocardium causes more intense ischemia of this portion of the wall. Ischemia of large segments of the ventricle will cause transient left ventricular failure, and if the papillary muscles are involved, mitral regurgitation can complicate this event. When ischemic events are transient, they may be associated with angina pectoris; if prolonged, they can lead to myocardial necrosis and scarring with or without the clinical picture of acute myocardial infarction (see Chap. 202). Coronary atherosclerosis is a focal process that usually causes nonuniform ischemia. As a result, regional disturbances of ventricular contractility cause segmental bulging or dyskinesia and can greatly reduce the efficiency of myocardial pump function.

Underlying these mechanical disturbances are a wide range of abnormalities in cell metabolism, function, and structure. When oxygenated, the normal myocardium metabolizes fatty acids and glucose to carbon dioxide and water. With severe oxygen deprivation, fatty acids cannot be oxidized, and glucose is broken down to lactate; intracellular pH is reduced as are the myocardial stores of high-energy phosphates, adenosine triphosphate (ATP), and creatine phosphate. Impaired cell membrane function leads to potassium leakage and the uptake of sodium by myocytes. The severity and duration of the imbalance between myocardial oxygen supply and demand will determine whether the damage is reversible or whether it is permanent, with subsequent myocardial necrosis.

Ischemia also causes characteristic electrocardiographic changes such as repolarization abnormalities, as evidenced by inversion of the T wave and later by displacement of the ST segment (Chap. 189). Transient ST-segment depression often reflects subendocardial ischemia, while transient ST-segment elevation is thought to be caused by more severe transmural ischemia. Another important consequence of myocardial ischemia is electrical instability, since this may lead to ventricular tachycardia or ventricular fibrillation (Chap. 198). Most patients who die suddenly from ischemic heart disease do so as a result of ischemia-induced malignant ventricular tachyarrhythmias (Chap. 35).

CLINICAL MANIFESTATIONS

ASYMPTOMATIC VERSUS SYMPTOMATIC CORONARY ARTERY DISEASE   Postmortem studies on accident victims and military casualties in western countries have shown that coronary atherosclerosis often begins to develop prior to age 20 and is widespread even among adults who were asymptomatic during life. Before the menopause women develop less coronary atherosclerosis and have a much lower incidence of the clinical manifestations of coronary artery disease (angina pectoris, myocardial infarction, and coronary death). This protection is lost progressively after the menopause. When all age groups are considered, ischemic heart disease is the most common cause of death not only in men but also in women (Chap. 5). Exercise stress tests in asymptomatic persons may show evidence of silent myocardial ischemia, i.e., exercise-induced electrocardiographic changes not accompanied by angina; coronary angiographic studies of such persons frequently reveal obstructive coronary artery disease. Postmortem examination of patients with obstructive coronary artery disease who had no history of any clinical manifestations of myocardial ischemia often shows macroscopic scars of myocardial infarction in regions supplied by diseased coronary arteries. According to population studies, approximately 25 percent of patients who survive acute myocardial infarction may not reach medical attention, and these patients carry the same adverse prognosis as those who present with the classic clinical syndrome (Chap. 202). Sudden death may be unheralded and is a common presenting manifestation of ischemic heart disease (Chap. 35). Patients can also present with cardiomegaly and heart failure secondary to ischemic damage of the left ventricular myocardium that caused no symptoms prior to the development of heart failure; this condition is referred to as *ischemic cardiomyopathy*. In contrast to the asymptomatic phase of ischemic heart disease, the symptomatic phase is characterized by chest discomfort due to either angina pectoris or acute myocardial infarction (Chap. 202). Having entered the symptomatic phase, the patient may exhibit a stable or progressive course, revert to the asymptomatic stage, or suddenly die.

CHRONIC STABLE ANGINA PECTORIS   This episodic clinical syndrome is due to transient myocardial ischemia. Various diseases that cause myocardial ischemia as well as the numerous forms of discomfort with which it may be confused are discussed in Chap. 12. Males constitute approximately 70 percent of all patients with angina pectoris and an even greater fraction of those younger than 50 years of age. The typical patient with angina is a 50- to 60-year-old man or 65- to 75-year-old woman who seeks medical help for troublesome or frightening chest discomfort, usually described as heaviness, pressure, squeezing, smothering, or choking and only rarely as frank pain. When the patient is asked to localize the sensation, he or she will typically press on the sternum, sometimes with a clenched fist, to indicate a squeezing, central, substernal discomfort. This symptom is usually crescendo-decrescendo in nature and lasts 1 to 5 min. Angina can radiate to the left shoulder and to both arms, and especially to the ulnar surfaces of the forearm and hand. It can also arise in or radiate to the back, neck, jaw, teeth, and epigastrium.

Although episodes of angina are typically caused by exertion (e.g., exercise, hurrying, or sexual activity) or emotion (e.g., stress, anger, fright, or frustration) and are relieved by rest, they may also occur at rest (see "Unstable Angina Pectoris," below) and at night while the patient is recumbent (angina decubitus). The patient may be awakened at night distressed by typical chest discomfort and dyspnea. The pathophysiology of nocturnal angina is analogous to that of paroxysmal nocturnal dyspnea (Chap. 195), i.e., the expansion of the intrathoracic blood volume that occurs with recumbency causes an increase in cardiac size and myocardial oxygen demand that lead to ischemia and transient left ventricular failure.

The threshold for the development of angina pectoris varies from person to person and may vary by time of day and emotional state. A patient may report symptoms upon minor exertion in the morning (a short walk or shaving) yet by midday may be capable of much greater effort without symptoms. Angina may be precipitated by unfamiliar tasks, a heavy meal, or exposure to cold.

Sharp, fleeting chest pain or prolonged, dull aches localized to the left submammary area are rarely due to myocardial ischemia. However, angina pectoris may be atypical in location and may not be strictly related to provoking factors. In addition, this symptom may exacerbate and remit over days, weeks, or months, and its occurrence can be seasonal.

Systematic questioning of the patient with suspected ischemic heart disease is important to uncover a positive family history of ischemic heart disease, diabetes, hyperlipidemia, hypertension, cigarette smoking, and other risk factors for coronary atherosclerosis.

In *variant (Prinzmetal's) angina,* the chest discomfort characteristically occurs at rest or awakens the patient from sleep. It may be accompanied by palpitations or severe shortness of breath, explosive in onset, severe, and frightening. It may also be brought on by effort, although the workload at which it is precipitated usually varies considerably. Variant angina is caused by focal spasm of proximal epicardial coronary arteries; in approximately three-fourths of the patients atherosclerotic coronary artery obstruction is present, in which case the vasospasm occurs near the stenotic lesion.

Physical examination The physical examination is often normal. The patient's general appearance may reveal signs of risk factors associated with coronary atherosclerosis such as xanthelasma, xanthomas (Chap. 208), or diabetic skin lesions. There may also be signs of anemia, thyroid disease, and nicotine stains on the fingertips from cigarette smoking. Palpation can reveal thickened or absent peripheral arteries, signs of cardiac enlargement, and abnormal contraction of the cardiac impulse (left ventricular akinesia or dyskinesia). Examination of the fundi may reveal increased light reflexes and arteriovenous nicking as evidence of hypertension (an important risk factor for ischemic heart disease), while auscultation can uncover arterial bruits, a third and/or fourth heart sound, and, if acute ischemia or previous infarction has impaired papillary muscle function, a late apical systolic murmur due to mitral regurgitation. These auscultatory signs are best appreciated with the patient in the left decubitus position. Aortic stenosis, aortic regurgitation (Chap. 201), and hypertrophic cardiomyopathy (Chap. 205) must be excluded, since these disorders may cause angina even in the absence of coronary artery disease. Examination during an anginal attack is useful, since ischemia can cause transient left ventricular failure with the appearance of a third and/or fourth heart sound, a dyskinetic cardiac apex, mitral regurgitation, and even pulmonary edema.

Laboratory examination Although the diagnosis of ischemic heart disease can be made with confidence from a typical history, a number of simple laboratory tests can be helpful. The urine should be examined for evidence of diabetes mellitus and renal disease, since both these conditions may accelerate atherosclerosis. Similarly, examination of the blood should include measurements of lipids (cholesterol—total, low density, and high density), glucose, creatinine, hematocrit, and, if indicated based on the physical examination, thyroid function. A chest x-ray is important, since it may show the consequences of ischemic heart disease, i.e., cardiac enlargement, ventricular aneurysm, or signs of heart failure. Calcification of the coronary arteries can sometimes be identified on chest fluoroscopy. These signs can support the diagnosis of coronary artery disease and are important in assessing the degree of cardiac damage and the effects of treatment for heart failure.

Electrocardiogram A normal ECG does not exclude the diagnosis of ischemic heart disease; however, certain characteristic abnormalities in tracings obtained at rest can confirm it. A 12-lead ECG recorded at rest is normal in about half the patients with typical angina pectoris, but there may be signs of an old myocardial infarction (Chap. 189). Serial tracings are particulary useful to look for past or evolving myocardial infarction. Although repolarization abnormalities, i.e., T-wave and ST-segment changes and intraventricular conduction disturbances at rest, are suggestive of ischemic heart disease, they are nonspecific, since they can also occur in pericardial, myocardial, and valvular heart disease or with anxiety, changes in posture, drugs, or esophageal disease. Typical ST-segment and T-wave changes that accompany episodes of angina pectoris and disappear thereafter are more specific. The most characteristic changes include displacement of the ST segment that is similar in every way to that induced during a stress test (see below). The ST segment is usually depressed during angina but may be elevated—sometimes strikingly so—as in the early stages of myocardial infarction and in Prinzmetal's angina.

Stress testing The most widely used test in the diagnosis of ischemic heart disease involves recording the 12-lead ECG before, during, and after exercise on a treadmill or using a bicycle ergometer.

The test consists of a standardized incremental increase in external workload while the patient's ECG, symptoms, and arm blood pressure are continuously monitored. Performance is usually symptom-limited and the test is discontinued upon evidence of chest discomfort, severe shortness of breath, dizziness, fatigue, ST-segment depression of greater than 0.2 mV (2 mm), a fall in systolic blood pressure exceeding 15 mmHg, or the development of a ventricular tachyarrhythmia. This test seeks to discover any limitation in exercise performance and establish the relationship between chest discomfort and the typical electrocardiographic signs of myocardial ischemia. The ischemic ST-segment response is generally defined as flat depression of the ST segment of more than 0.1 mV below the baseline (i.e., the PR segment) and lasting longer than 0.08 s. This type of depression is designated "square wave" or "plateau" and is flat or downsloping. Upsloping or junctional ST-segment changes are not considered characteristic of ischemia and do not constitute a positive test. Although T-wave abnormalities, conduction disturbances, and ventricular arrhythmias that develop during exercise should be noted, they are also not diagnostic. Negative exercise tests in which the target heart rate (85 percent of maximal heart rate for age and sex) is not achieved are considered to be nondiagnostic.

Based on the above criteria, the rate of false-positive diagnoses, using the coronary arteriogram as the gold standard, is approximately 15 percent, and a similar percentage of patients with severe, multivessel coronary artery disease will not have a positive test (false-negative). According to Bayes' theorem, the probability that ischemic heart disease exists in the patient or population under study (pretest probability) must be considered in light of the diagnostic features of the test in order to interpret a positive or negative test result (Fig. 10-2, p. 46). For example, a positive result on exercise indicates that the likelihood of coronary artery disease is 98 percent in males above the age of 50 years with typical angina pectoris, but progressively lower in those with atypical chest pain, nonanginal chest pain, and asymptomatic persons. The incidence of false-positive tests is increased in asymptomatic men under the age of 40 years or premenopausal women without risk factors for premature atherosclerosis, in patients taking cardioactive drugs such as digitalis and quinidine, or in those with intraventricular conduction disturbances, resting abnormalities of the ST segment and the T wave, myocardial hypertrophy, or abnormal serum potassium levels. Obstructive disease limited to the circumflex coronary artery may result in a false-negative stress test since the posterior portion of the heart which this vessel supplies is not well represented on the surface 12-lead ECG.

The physician should be present throughout the exercise test, and it is important to measure total duration of exercise, the time to the onset of ischemic ST-segment change and chest discomfort, the external work performed, and the internal cardiac work performed; the last is represented by the heart rate–blood pressure product. The depth of the ST-segment depression and the time needed for recovery of these electrocardiographic changes are also important. Because the risks of exercise testing are small but real—estimated at one fatality and two nonfatal complications per 10,000 tests—equipment for resuscitation should be available. Modified (heart rate-limited rather than symptom-limited) exercise tests can be performed safely in patients as early as 7 days after myocardial infarction.

The normal response to exercise includes a progressive increase in heart rate and blood pressure. Failure of the blood pressure to increase or an actual decrease in blood pressure with signs of ischemia during the test is an important adverse prognostic sign, since it may reflect ischemia-induced global left ventricular dysfunction. The presence of pain or severe ST-segment depression at a low workload and ST-segment depression that persists for more than 5 min after the termination of exercise will increase the specificity of the test and suggests severe ischemic heart disease.

The exercise test can be enhanced by the intravenous administration of a radioisotope such as thallium 201 or Sesta-Mibi to assess regional myocardial perfusion by means of a gamma camera (p. 971). Technetium 99m can be used to label the blood pool for gated radioisotope angiography. This technique (Fig. 190-8, p. 970) can provide a measure of ventricular volume, ejection fraction, and regional ventricular wall motion at rest and during exercise, and can identify transient global and regional left ventricular dysfunction due to myocardial ischemia at rest or during ischemia. A reduction in ejection fraction during exercise with the appearance of regional wall motion abnormalities is an important sign and suggests the presence of severe ischemia and/or multivessel coronary disease.

An important fraction of patients who need noninvasive stress testing to identify myocardial ischemia and increased risk of coronary events cannot exercise because of peripheral vascular or musculoskeletal disease. In these circumstances intravenous dipyridamole or adenosine can be used in place of exercise. The electrocardiogram with a radionuclide such as thallium 201 is used to detect myocardial ischemia. Ambulatory monitoring of the electrocardiogram can assess myocardial ischemia as episodes of ST-segment depression. These new techniques are sensitive and capable of identifying patients with ischemia who are at increased risk of coronary events. Technetium 99-labeled Sesta-Mibi is a new radionuclide that has advantages over thallium 201.

The severity of ischemia in all of the tests described above has been shown to correlate with risk for future adverse coronary events (myocardial infarction and death).

Two-dimensional echocardiography records cross-sectional images of the left ventricle and can identify regional wall motion abnormalities due to myocardial infarction or persistent ischemia (Chap. 190). In this way, the test can also be used as an aid in the diagnosis of ischemic heart disease.

Coronary arteriography (Chap. 192) This invasive diagnostic method outlines the coronary anatomy and can be used to detect important evidence of coronary atherosclerosis or to exclude this condition. By this means, one can assess the severity of obstructive lesions and when combined with left ventricular angiocardiography can evaluate both global and regional function of the left ventricle. Coronary arteriography is indicated in (1) patients with chronic stable or unstable angina pectoris who are severely symptomatic despite medical therapy and who are being considered for revascularization, i.e., percutaneous transluminal coronary angioplasty or coronary artery bypass graft surgery; (2) patients with troublesome symptoms that present diagnostic difficulties in whom there is need to confirm or rule out the diagnosis of coronary artery disease; and (3) patients suspected of having left main stem or three-vessel coronary artery disease based on signs of severe ischemia on noninvasive testing, regardless of the presence or severity of symptoms.

Examples of other possible clinical situations include:

1 Patients with chest discomfort suggestive of angina pectoris but a negative exercise test who require a definitive diagnosis for guiding medical management, alleviating psychological stress, career or family planning, or insurance purposes.
2 Patients who have been admitted repeatedly to the hospital for suspected acute myocardial infarction but in whom this diagnosis has not been established and in whom the presence or absence of coronary artery disease should be determined.
3 Patients with careers that involve the safety of others (e.g., airline pilots) who have questionable symptoms, suspicious or positive noninvasive tests, and in whom there are reasonable doubts about the state of the coronary arteries.
4 Patients with aortic stenosis or hypertrophic cardiomyopathy and angina in whom the pain could be due to coronary artery disease.
5 Male patients aged 45 and females aged 55 years of age or older who will undergo valve replacement and who may or may not have clinical evidence of myocardial ischemia.
6 Patients who are at high risk after myocardial infarction because of the recurrence of angina, heart failure, frequent ventricular premature contractions, or signs of ischemia in the stress test.
7 Patients with angina pectoris, regardless of severity, in whom noninvasive testing reveals signs of severe ischemia, i.e., early

and/or marked (>2 mm) ST-segment depression, large or multiple perfusion defects and/or increased lung uptake on thallium 201 scintigrams following exercise, global left ventricular dysfunction precipitated by exercise, and/or exercise-induced hypotension.

PROGNOSIS

The principal prognostic indicators in patients with ischemic heart disease are the functional state of the left ventricle, the location and severity of coronary artery narrowing, and the severity or activity of myocardial ischemia. Angina pectoris of recent onset, unstable angina, angina which is unresponsive or poorly responsive to medical therapy or is accompanied by symptoms of congestive heart failure all indicate an increased risk for adverse coronary events. The same is true for the physical signs of heart failure, episodes of pulmonary edema, or roentgenographic evidence of cardiac enlargement. An abnormal resting ECG or positive evidence of myocardial ischemia during a stress test also indicate increased risk. Most importantly, the following signs during noninvasive testing indicate a high risk for coronary events: a strongly positive exercise test showing onset of myocardial ischemia at low workloads, large or multiple perfusion defects or increased lung uptake during stress thallium scanning, a decrease in left ventricular ejection fraction during exercise on radionuclide ventriculography, and hypotension with ischemia during stress testing.

On cardiac catheterization, elevations in left ventricular end-diastolic pressure and ventricular volume and a reduced ejection fraction are the most important signs of left ventricular dysfunction and are associated with a poor prognosis. Patients with chest discomfort but normal left ventricular function and normal coronary arteries have an excellent prognosis. In patients with normal left ventricular function and mild angina but with critical stenoses (≥ 70 percent luminal diameter) of one, two, or three epicardial coronary arteries, the 5-year mortality rates are approximately 2, 8, and 11 percent, respectively. Obstructive lesions of the proximal left anterior descending coronary artery are associated with a greater risk than are lesions of the right or left circumflex coronary artery, since the former vessel usually perfuses a greater quantity of myocardium. Critical stenosis of the left main coronary artery is associated with a mortality of about 15 percent per year.

With any degree of obstructive coronary artery disease, mortality is greatly increased when left ventricular function is impaired; conversely, at any level of left ventricular function, the prognosis is influenced importantly by the extent of myocardium perfused by the critically obstructed vessels. It is useful to consider that coronary atherosclerosis demonstrates its harmful potential by causing transient myocardial ischemia and by leading to myocardial infarction, which characteristically destroys myocardium, thereby reducing cardiac reserve at an unpredictable rate (or causing sudden death). The larger the amount of myocardial necrosis, the less the heart is able to withstand additional damage and the poorer the prognosis. In this light, the various indices of ischemic damage, such as the ECG showing evidence of an old infarction and symptoms or signs of heart failure or cardiac enlargement, should be taken as indications of myocardial damage.

The segmental atherosclerotic plaques in epicardial arteries go through phases of cellular activity, degeneration, endothelial instability, abnormal vasomotion, platelet aggregation, and fissuring or hemorrhage. These factors can temporarily worsen the stenosis and cause abnormal reactivity of the vessel wall thus exacerbating the manifestations of ischemia. The development of unstable angina and/or severe ischemia during stress testing reflects rapid progression.

MANAGEMENT

Each patient must be evaluated individually with respect to life patterns, risk factors, control of symptoms, and prevention of damage to left ventricular myocardium. The degree of the patient's disability and the specific physical and emotional stresses that precipitate pain must all be carefully recorded in order to set the proper goals for treatment. The management plan should consist of (1) explanation and reassurance, (2) reduction of risk factors in an attempt to slow the progression of coronary atherosclerosis, (3) treatment of coexisting conditions capable of aggravating angina, (4) sensible adaptations of activities to minimize anginal attacks, (5) a program of drug therapy, and (6) definition of end points that will indicate the need to consider mechanical revascularization.

EXPLANATION AND REASSURANCE Patients with ischemic heart disease need to understand their condition as best they can and to realize that a long and useful life is possible even though they suffer from angina pectoris or have experienced and recovered from an acute myocardial infarction. Offering case histories of persons in public life who have lived with coronary disease can be of great value when encouraging patients to resume or maintain activity and return to their occupation. A planned program of rehabilitation can encourage patients to lose weight, improve exercise tolerance, and control risk factors with more confidence.

REDUCTION OF RISK FACTORS (SECONDARY PREVENTION) (See also Chap. 208) The discontinuance of cigarette smoking is vital. The risk of coronary events is low when the total plasma cholesterol is less than 200 mg/100 mL, intermediate when it is 200 to 240 mg/100 mL, and abnormally increased when the plasma cholesterol is over 240 mg/100 mL. Clinical trials in selected patients seem to indicate that effective modification of risk factors (e.g., plasma lipid levels) can slow the growth of coronary atherosclerosis and decrease the morbidity and mortality due to coronary artery disease. Ideal weight should be attained and maintained. Aggravating factors (e.g., endocrine disorders, hypertension, and drugs such as glucocorticoids) should be treated and eliminated when possible (see Chaps. 208 and 344). After appropriate diet and exercise, drug therapy should be used in patients in an attempt to reduce the total plasma cholesterol (ideal value <200 mg/100 mL), reduce the plasma LDL fraction (ideal value <130 mg/100 mL) and increase the plasma HDL fraction (ideal value >45 mg/mL). The total cholesterol and LDL fraction are effectively reduced by bile acid binding resins (e.g., cholestyramine) and the HMB CoA reductase inhibitors of cholesterol synthesis (e.g., lovastatin) while the HDL is effectively increased by drugs such as niacin and gemfibrozil (see Chap. 344). Diabetes mellitus and hypertension, when present, should be treated. Unless angina is provoked by strenuous activity, the patient should be encouraged to engage in steady, dynamic exercise such as walking; isometric exercise may be hazardous. By maintaining good physical condition, the patient will be able to perform physical work more efficiently and at a lower pulse rate, thus reducing the frequency of angina pectoris. Patients in good physical condition may also have a better chance of surviving a myocardial infarction. The administration of estrogen to postmenopausal women appears to provide significant protection with a reduction in coronary events. Nevertheless, there is a modest increase in the occurrence of some malignancies and therefore therapy should be individualized.

ELIMINATION OF COEXISTING ILLNESS A number of illnesses that are not primarily cardiac in nature may either increase oxygen demand or decrease oxygen supply to the myocardium and may precipitate or exacerbate angina. In the former category, hypertension and hyperthyroidism may be treated successfully in order to reduce the frequency of anginal attacks. Decreased myocardial oxygen supply may be due to reduced oxygenation of the blood (e.g., in intrinsic pulmonary disease or, when carboxyhemoglobin is present, due to cigarette or cigar smoking) or decreased oxygen-carrying capacity (e.g., in anemia). Correction of these abnormalities, if present, may reduce or even eliminate anginal symptoms.

ADAPTATION OF ACTIVITIES Therapy of angina due to episodes of myocardial ischemia consists of eliminating the discrepancy between the demand of the heart muscle for oxygen and the ability of the coronary circulation to meet this demand. Most patients will understand this fundamental concept and utilize it in the rational programming of activity. Many tasks that ordinarily evoke angina may be accomplished without symptoms simply by reducing the speed at which they are performed. Patients must appreciate the diurnal variation in their tolerance of certain activities and should reduce their energy requirements in the morning and immediately after meals. Sometimes it is helpful to alter the eating pattern, taking small and more frequent meals.

It may be necessary to recommend a change in employment or residence to avoid physical stress; however, with the exception of manual laborers, most patients with ischemic heart disease can usually continue to function merely by allowing more time to complete each task. In some patients, anger and frustration may be the most important factors precipitating myocardial ischemia. If these cannot be avoided, training in stress management may be useful. A treadmill exercise test to determine the approximate heart rate at which ischemic electrocardiographic changes or symptoms develop may be helpful in the development of a specific exercise program. Ambulatory electrocardiography during daily activities may also be helpful in this regard.

DRUG THERAPY The commonly used drugs for angina pectoris are summarized in Table 203-1.

Nitrates This valuable class of drugs in the management of angina pectoris acts by causing systemic venodilation, thereby reducing myocardial wall tension and oxygen requirements, as well as by dilating the epicardial coronary vessels and increasing blood flow in collateral vessels. The absorption of these agents (hence action) is most rapid and complete through the mucous membranes. For this reason, nitroglycerin is administered sublingually in tablets of 0.4 or 0.6 mg. Patients with angina should be instructed to take the

TABLE 203-1 Commonly used drugs for angina pectoris

Drug	Usual Dose	Side Effects	Contraindications
NITRATES			
Sublingual NTG	0.3–0.6 mg	Flushing, headache	Intolerance of side effects
Isosorbide dinitrate SR	40 mg	Flushing, headache, tolerance after 24 h	As above, worsening ischemia on withdrawal
Transdermal NTG	5–100 mg	Flushing, headache, tolerance after 24 h	As above, worsening ischemia on withdrawal
BETA ADRENOCEPTOR BLOCKING DRUGS			
Propranolol	20–80 mg qid	Depression, constipation, impotence, bronchospasm, heart failure, bradycardia	Asthma, AV conduction block, heart failure
Metoprolol	25–200 mg bid	As above	As above
Atenolol	50–150 mg once daily	As above	As above
CALCIUM CHANNEL BLOCKING DRUGS			
Nifedipine XL	30–90 mg once daily	Hypotension, flushing, edema, worsening angina	Hypotension, intolerance of side effects
Diltiazem SR	60–120 mg bid	Constipation, AV conduction block, worsening heart failure	AV conduction block, impaired LV function, bradycardia
Verapamil SR	180–240 mg once daily	Constipation, AV conduction block, worsening heart failure	AV conduction delay, impaired LV function, bradycardia

Abbreviations: SR = slow release, NTG = nitroglycerin, XL = slow release preparation.

medication both to relieve an attack and also in anticipation of stress (exercise or emotional) that is likely to induce an attack. The value of this prophylactic use of the drug cannot be overemphasized.

Headache and a pulsating feeling in the head are the most common side effects of nitroglycerin and fortunately only rarely become disturbing at the doses usually required to relieve or prevent angina. Nitroglycerin deteriorates with exposure to air, moisture, and sunlight, so that if the drug neither relieves discomfort or headache nor produces a slight sensation of burning at the sublingual site of absorption, the preparation may be inactive and a fresh supply should be obtained. If relief is not achieved after the first dose of nitroglycerin, a second or third dose may be given at 5-min intervals. If discomfort continues despite treatment, the patient should consult a physician or report promptly to a hospital emergency room for evaluation of possible unstable angina or acute myocardial infarction (Chap. 202).

Asking the patient with recently diagnosed angina pectoris to record the occurrence of pain relative to activity and other precipitating factors as well as nitroglycerin consumption is often helpful to the physician attempting to tailor a management program. Such a diary may also be valuable for detecting changes in the frequency or severity of discomfort that may signify the development of unstable angina pectoris and/or herald an impending myocardial infarction.

None of the long-acting nitrates is as effective as sublingual nitroglycerin for the acute relief of angina. These preparations can be swallowed, chewed, or administered as a patch or paste by the transdermal route. They can provide effective plasma levels for up to 24 h, but the therapeutic response is highly variable. Different preparations and/or administration during the daytime should be tried only to relieve discomfort in the individual patient while avoiding side effects such as headache and dizziness. Individual dose titration is important in order to prevent side effects. Useful preparations include isosorbide dinitrate (10 to 40 mg PO tid), nitroglycerin ointment (0.5 to 2.0 inches qid), or sustained-release transdermal patches (5 to 25 mg/d). Long-acting nitrates are relatively safe and can be used together with intermittent sublingual nitroglycerin to relieve discomfort and prevent attacks of angina. The nitrates likely bind to guanylate cyclase in vascular smooth muscle cells, oxidize sulfhydryl groups, and are converted to *S*-nitrosothiols. This leads to an increase in cyclic guanosine monophosphate which causes cell relaxation of vascular smooth muscle. Tolerance with loss of efficacy develop with 12 to 24 h of continuous exposure to all of the long-acting nitrates due to depletion of sulfhydryl groups and to counterregulatory alterations in intravascular fluid balance with fluid retention. In order to minimize the effects of tolerance, the minimum effective dose should be used and a minimum of 8 h each day kept free of the drug so as to restore any useful response(s).

Beta-adrenoceptor blockade (See also Chap. 68) Beta-adrenoceptor blockers represent an important component of the pharmacologic treatment of angina pectoris. These drugs reduce myocardial oxygen demand by inhibiting the increases in heart rate and myocardial contractility caused by adrenergic activity. Beta blockage reduces these variables most strikingly during exercise while causing only small reductions in heart rate, cardiac output, and arterial pressure at rest. Propranolol is usually administered in an initial dose of 20 to 40 mg four times a day and is increased as tolerated to 320 mg per day in divided doses. Long-acting beta-blocking drugs (atenolol, 50 to 100 mg/d, and nadolol, 40 to 80 mg/d) offer the advantage of once-a-day dosage (Table 68-1, p. 430). The therapeutic aims include relief of angina and ischemia. These drugs can also reduce mortality and reinfarction when given to patients after myocardial infarction. They can produce fatigue, impotence, cold extremities, intermittent claudication, and bradycardia and can worsen disturbed cardiac conduction, left ventricular failure, and bronchial asthma or intensify the hypoglycemia produced by oral hypoglycemic agents and insulin. Reducing the dose or even discontinuation of the drug may be necessary if these side effects develop and persist.

Calcium antagonists Nifedipine (10 to 40 mg qid), verapamil (80 to 120 mg tid), and diltiazem (30 to 90 mg qid) and other calcium antagonists are all coronary vasodilators that produce variable and dose-dependent reductions in myocardial oxygen demand, contractility, and arterial pressure. These combined pharmacologic effects are advantageous and make these agents quite effective in the treatment of angina pectoris. Verapamil and diltiazem may produce symptomatic disturbances in cardiac conduction and bradyarrhythmias, exert negative inotropic actions, and are more likely to worsen left ventricular failure, particularly when used in combination with beta blockers in patients with underlying left ventricular dysfunction. Although useful effects are usually achieved when calcium antagonists are combined with beta blockers and nitrates, careful individual titration of dose is essential with these potent combinations. Variant (Prinzmetal's) angina responds particularly well to calcium antagonists, supplemented when necessary by nitrates. The calcium antagonists are now formulated as long-acting preparations including nifedipine (30 to 90 mg once daily), diltiazem (60 to 120 mg twice daily), and verapamil (180 to 240 mg once daily). Verapamil should not be combined with beta-adrenoreceptor blocking drugs because of the combined effects on heart rate and contractility. Diltiazem can be combined with beta blockers with caution and only in patients with normal ventricular function and no conduction disturbances. Nifedipine and the beta blockers have complementary actions on coronary blood supply and myocardial oxygen demands. While the former decreases blood pressure and dilates coronary arteries the latter slows heart rate and decreases contractility.

Treatment of angina and heart failure Patients with angina pectoris may also have evidence of elevated left ventricular diastolic pressures and volumes due to transient ischemia. This transient left ventricular failure with angina can be controlled by the judicious use of nitrates, calcium antagonists, and even beta blockers. For patients with established congestive heart failure the increased left ventricular wall tension raises myocardial oxygen demand. Treatment of congestive heart failure with digitalis, angiotensin-converting enzyme inhibitors, and diuretics (Chap. 195) can help to decrease heart size, wall tension, and myocardial oxygen demands, which will help to control angina and ischemia. Nocturnal angina can often be relieved by these agents; however, there is no benefit—and possibly aggravation of angina—when these drugs are used in patients with a normal heart size and no evidence of heart failure. Nitrates are particularly useful and can improve the disturbed hemodynamics of congestive heart failure and relieve angina by preventing or reversing myocardial ischemia. The combination of congestive heart failure and angina in patients with coronary artery disease usually indicates a poor prognosis and warrants serious consideration of cardiac catheterization and mechanical revascularization, if possible.

Aspirin Aspirin is an irreversible inhibitor of platelet cyclooxygenase activity and thereby interferes with platelet activation. Chronic administration of 100 to 325 mg orally per day has been shown to reduce coronary events in asymptomatic adult men, patients with asymptomatic ischemia after myocardial infarction, patients with chronic stable angina, and patients who have survived unstable angina and myocardial infarction. Administration of this drug should be considered in all patients with coronary artery disease in the absence of side effects such as gastrointestinal bleeding, allergy, or dyspepsia.

MECHANICAL REVASCULARIZATION

It is important to appreciate that although the basic management of patients with a lifelong condition such as ischemic heart disease is medical, the years of medical management may be punctuated by mechanical revascularization procedures, as described below. These interventions should not replace the continuing need to ease symptoms and modify risk factors.

PERCUTANEOUS TRANSLUMINAL CORONARY ANGIOPLASTY PTCA is a widely used method to achieve revascularization of the myocardium in patients with symptomatic ischemic heart disease and suitable stenoses of epicardial coronary arteries. Whereas patients with stenosis of the left main coronary artery and those with three-vessel coronary artery disease who require revascularization are best treated with coronary artery bypass surgery, PTCA is widely employed in patients with symptoms and evidence of ischemia due to stenoses of one or two vessels, and even selected patients with three-vessel disease, and may offer many advantages over surgery.

After a flexible guidewire is advanced into a coronary artery and across the stenosis to be dilated, a miniature balloon catheter is advanced over the guidewire and into the stenosis followed by repeated inflations until the stenosis is decreased or relieved. The development of a range of steerable guidewires, low-profile balloon catheters, and balloon catheters that also allow coronary flow during inflation have all helped to decrease complications, reach more distal lesions, and dilate more complex stenoses. (See also Chap. 193.)

Indications and patient selection The most common clinical indication for PTCA is angina pectoris, stable or unstable, which should be accompanied by evidence of ischemia in an exercise test. This symptom should be sufficiently severe to warrant the consideration of bypass graft surgery. PTCA is more effective than medical therapy for the relief of angina in patients with single-vessel coronary artery disease. The value of this procedure in improving outcome has not been established, and therefore it is not generally indicted in asymptomatic or mildly symptomatic patients. PTCA can also be used to dilate stenoses in native coronary arteries and in bypass grafts in patients who have recurrent angina following coronary artery surgery. This is an important indication when the technical difficulties and the increased mortality that accompanies reoperation are considered. Angioplasty has also been carried out in patients with recent total occlusion (within 3 months) of a coronary artery and severe angina; in this group the primary success rate is decreased to approximately 50 percent.

Risks When coronary stenoses are discrete and symmetrical, two and three vessels can be dilated in sequence. However, cautious case selection is essential in order to avoid a prohibitive risk of complications. Female gender, advanced age, the left anterior descending artery, stenoses with thrombus, left ventricular dysfunction, stenosis of an artery perfusing a large segment of myocardium without collaterals, long eccentric or irregular stenoses, and calcified plaques all increase the likelihood of complications. The major complications are usually due to dissection or thrombosis with vessel occlusion, uncontrolled ischemia, and ventricular failure. In experienced hands, the overall mortality rate should be less than 1 percent, the need for emergency coronary surgery less than 3 percent, and myocardial infarction in less than 3 percent of cases. Minor complications occur in 5 to 10 percent of patients and include occlusion of a branch of a coronary artery and complications of arterial catheterization.

Efficacy Primary success, i.e., adequate dilation with relief of angina, is achieved in 85 to 90 percent of cases. Recurrent stenosis of the dilated vessels occurs in 20 to 40 percent of cases within 6 months of the procedure, and angina will recur within 6 to 12 months in 25 percent of cases. This recurrence of symptoms and restenosis is more common in patients with diabetes mellitus, unstable angina, incomplete dilation of the stenosis, dilation of the left anterior descending coronary artery, and stenoses containing thrombi. Dilation of arteries which are totally occluded and of stenotic or occluded vein grafts also exhibit a high incidence of restenosis. It is usual clinical practice to administer aspirin and a calcium channel antagonist for months after the procedure. Although aspirin may help prevent acute coronary thrombosis during and immediately following PTCA, there are no controlled clinical trials that have demonstrated that these medications or any other can clearly reduce the incidence of restenosis.

If patients do not develop restenosis or angina within the first year after angioplasty, the prognosis for maintaining improvement over the subsequent 4 years is excellent. If restenosis occurs, PTCA can be repeated with the same success and risk, but the likelihood of restenosis increases with the third or subsequent attempt.

Between 30 and 50 percent of patients with symptomatic coronary artery disease who require revascularization can be treated by PTCA

and need not undergo coronary artery bypass surgery. Successful angioplasty is less invasive and expensive than coronary artery surgery, usually requires only two days in the hospital, and permits considerable savings in the cost of care. Successful PTCA also allows earlier return to work and the resumption of an active life.

CORONARY ARTERY BYPASS GRAFTING In this procedure, a section of a vein (usually the saphenous) is used to form a connection between the aorta and the coronary artery distal to the obstructive lesion. Alternatively, anastomosis of one or both of the internal mammary arteries to the coronary artery distal to the obstructive lesion may be employed.

Although some indications for coronary artery bypass surgery are controversial, certain areas of agreement exist:

1 The operation is relatively safe, with mortality rates less than 1 percent when the procedure is performed by an experienced surgical team in patients without serious comorbid disease and normal left ventricular function.
2 Intraoperative and postoperative mortality increases with the degree of ventricular dysfunction, comorbidities, and surgical inexperience. The effectiveness and risk of coronary artery bypass grafting vary widely depending on case selection and the skill and experience of the surgical team, so that the latter must be taken into account when a patient is being considered as a candidate for this procedure.
3 Occlusion of *vein grafts* is observed in 10 to 20 percent during the first postoperative year, and the incidence is approximately 2 percent per year during 5- to 7-year follow-up and 5 percent per year thereafter. Long-term patency rates are considerably higher for internal mammary artery implantations; in patients with left anterior descending coronary artery obstruction, survival is better when coronary bypass involves the internal mammary artery rather than a saphenous vein.
4 Angina is abolished or greatly reduced in approximately 85 percent of patients following complete revascularization. Although this is usually associated with graft patency and restoration of blood flow, the pain may also have been alleviated as a result of infarction of the ischemic segment or a placebo effect.
5 Coronary artery bypass grafting does not appear to reduce the incidence of myocardial infarction in patients with chronic ischemic heart disease; perioperative myocardial infarction occurs in 5 to 10 percent of cases, but in most instances these infarcts are small.
6 Mortality is reduced by operation in patients with stenosis of the left main coronary artery as well as in patients with three-vessel coronary artery disease and impaired left ventricular function. However, there is no evidence that coronary artery bypass surgery improves survival in patients with one- or two-vessel disease who have chronic stable angina and normal left ventricular function or in patients with one-vessel disease and impaired left ventricular function. Evidence is conflicting concerning the effects of operation on survival in patients with impaired left ventricular function and obstructive disease of two coronary arteries, one of which is the proximal left anterior descending artery.

Indications for coronary artery bypass grafting are usually based on the severity of symptoms, coronary anatomy, and ventricular function. The ideal candidate is male, less than 70 years of age, has no other complicating disease, has troublesome or disabling symptoms that are not adequately controlled by medical therapy, wishes to lead a more active life, and has severe stenoses of several epicardial coronary arteries with objective evidence of myocardial ischemia as a cause of the chest discomfort. Great symptomatic benefit can be anticipated in such patients. When the patient also has a disturbance of left ventricular function, coronary artery bypass grafting may, in addition, prolong life.

UNSTABLE ANGINA PECTORIS

The following three patient groups may be said to have unstable angina pectoris: (1) patients with new onset (<2 months) angina that is severe and/or frequent (≥3 episodes per day); (2) patients with accelerating angina, i.e., those with chronic stable angina who develop angina that is distinctly more frequent, severe, prolonged, or precipitated by less exertion than previously; (3) those with angina at rest. Unstable angina may be primary, i.e., occur in the absence of an extracardiac condition that has intensified myocardial ischemia, or it may be precipitated by a condition extrinsic to the coronary vascular bed that has intensified myocardial ischemia, such as anemia, fever, infection, tachyarrhythmias, emotional stress, or hypoxemia. Unstable angina may also develop shortly after myocardial infarction. Unstable angina, particularly when it is characterized by rest pain or occurs in the postinfarction state, carries an adverse prognosis, with significant risk of acute myocardial infarction or the development of intractable chronic stable angina.

When unstable angina is accompanied by objective electrocardiographic evidence of transient myocardial ischemia (ST-segment changes and/or T-wave inversions during episodes of chest pain), it is almost always associated with critical stenoses in one or more major epicardial coronary arteries. The atherosclerotic lesions may have a complicated morphology, with evidence of superimposed thrombosis in approximately 25 to 60 percent of cases. Segmental spasm in the vicinity of atherosclerotic plaques may also play a role in the development of unstable angina.

MANAGEMENT   The patient should be admitted promptly to the hospital for observation, further diagnosis, and treatment. It is important to identify and treat concomitant conditions that can intensify ischemia, such as uncontrolled tachycardia, hypertension and diabetes mellitus, cardiomegaly, heart failure, arrhythmias, thyrotoxicosis, and any acute febrile illness. Acute myocardial infarction should be ruled out by means of serial ECGs and measurements of plasma cardiac enzyme activity.

Continuous electrocardiographic monitoring should be carried out and the patients should receive reassurance and sedation. Thrombus formation frequently complicates this condition. Therefore, intravenous heparin should be given for 3 to 5 days to maintain the partial thromboplastin time at 2 to 2.5 times control, together with or followed by oral aspirin at a dose of 325 mg/d. Beta-adrenoceptor blocking drugs and calcium antagonists should be administered, but with caution and an awareness of the possible side effects discussed above. Dosages must be titrated to avoid bradycardia, heart failure, and hypotension. Nitroglycerin should be given by the sublingual route as needed for symptoms. In addition, intravenous nitroglycerin is quite effective, although it requires continuous monitoring of arterial pressure. It is begun at a dosage of 10 μg/min and is raised in 5-μg/min increments to a level at which chest pain is abolished but systolic arterial pressure is maintained or reduced only slightly and other side effects are avoided.

The majority of patients improve with such treatment. However, the clinical outcome is highly variable. If angina and/or electrocardiographic evidence of ischemia do not diminish within 24 to 48 h of the comprehensive treatment described above in patients with no obvious contraindications for revascularization, then cardiac catheterization and coronary arteriography should be performed. If the anatomy is suitable, PTCA can be performed with surgical standby. PTCA in this condition, particularly in the presence of thrombus, is attended by increased risk of acute closure and ischemia. If angioplasty cannot be done, coronary artery bypass grafting should be considered to relieve symptoms and myocardial ischemia and as a means of preventing myocardial damage. If the patient's symptoms and signs are controlled on medical therapy, a diagnostic exercise ECG should be obtained near the time of hospital discharge. If there is evidence of severe myocardial ischemia, serious consideration should be given to catheterization and revascularization. It should be recognized that severe coronary artery disease is often present in patients with unstable angina who respond to medical therapy. Many patients in whom the unstable state is controlled are left with severe chronic stable angina and ultimately require mechanical revascularization.

ASYMPTOMATIC (SILENT) ISCHEMIA

Obstructive coronary artery disease, acute myocardial infarction, and transient myocardial ischemia are frequently asymptomatic. During continuous ambulatory electrocardiographic monitoring, the majority of ambulatory patients with typical chronic stable angina are found to have objective evidence of myocardial ischemia (ST-segment depression) during episodes of chest discomfort while they are active outside the hospital, but many of these patients also appear to have more frequent episodes of asymptomatic ischemia. In addition, there is a large (but as yet unknown) number of totally asymptomatic people with severe coronary atherosclerosis who exhibit ST-segment changes during activity. Evidence of frequent episodes of ischemia (symptomatic and asymptomatic) during daily life appears to indicate an increased likelihood of adverse coronary events such as death and myocardial infarction. The widespread use of exercise electrocardiography during routine examinations has also defined some of these heretofore unrecognized patients with asymptomatic coronary artery disease. Longitudinal studies have demonstrated an increased incidence of coronary events (sudden death, myocardial infarction, and angina) in asymptomatic patients with positive exercise tests. In addition, patients with asymptomatic ischemia after suffering a myocardial infarction are at far greater risk for a second coronary event. Patients who seek evaluation and who have asymptomatic ischemia should be subjected to a detailed noninvasive examination, utilizing stress electrocardiography and radionuclide scintigraphy.

MANAGEMENT   The management of patients with asymptomatic ischemia must be individualized. Thus, the physician should consider the following: (1) the degree of positivity of the exercise test, particularly the stage of exercise at which electrocardiographic signs of ischemia appear, the magnitude and number of the perfusion defect(s) on thallium scintigraphy, and the change in left ventricular ejection fraction which occurs during ischemia and/or during exercise on radionuclide ventriculography; (2) the electrocardiographic leads showing a positive response, with changes in the anterior precordial leads indicating a less favorable prognosis than changes in the inferior leads; and (3) the patient's age, occupation, and general medical condition. Most would agree that an asymptomatic 45-year-old commercial airline pilot with 4-mm ST-segment depression in leads V_1 to V_4 during mild exercise should undergo coronary arteriography, whereas the asymptomatic, sedentary 75-year-old retiree with 1-mm ST-segment depression in leads II and III during maximal activity need not. However, there is no consensus about the appropriate procedure in the large majority of patients for whom the situation is less extreme. Patients with evidence of severe ischemia on noninvasive testing (as outlined earlier) should undergo coronary arteriography. Asymptomatic patients with silent ischemia, three-vessel coronary artery disease, and impaired left ventricular function may be considered appropriate candidates for coronary artery bypass surgery.

The chronic administration of aspirin to patients with asymptomatic ischemia after myocardial infarction has been shown to reduce adverse coronary events. While the incidence of asymptomatic ischemia can be reduced by treatment with beta blockers, calcium channel antagonists, and long-acting nitrates, it is not clear whether this is necessary or desirable in patients who have not suffered a myocardial infarction. However, there is evidence that beta-adrenoceptor blockade begun 7 to 35 days after acute myocardial infarction improves survival (Chap. 202).

REFERENCES

BELLER GA et al: Sensitivity, specificity and prognostic significance of noninvasive testing for occult or known coronary disease. Prog Cardiovasc Dis 24:241, 1987

BRAUNWALD E: Unstable angina—A classification. Circulation 80:410, 1989

———, SOBEL BE et al: Coronary blood flow and myocardial ischemia, in *Heart Disease*, 4th ed, E Braunwald (ed). Philadelphia, Saunders, 1992, pp 1161–1199

DEEDWANIA PC: Asymptomatic ischemia during predischarge Holter monitoring predicts poor prognosis in the postinfarction period. Am J Cardiol 71:859, 1993

————, CARBAJAL EV: Silent ischemia during daily life is an independent predictor of mortality in stable angina. Circulation 81:748, 1990

FAXON D: Percutaneous coronary angioplasty in stable and unstable angina. Cardiol Clin 9:99, 1991

FUSTER V et al: Mechanisms of disease: Pathophysiology of coronary artery disease and the acute coronary syndromes. N Engl J Med 326:24, 1992

GOTTO AM, FARMER JA: Risk factors for coronary artery disease, in *Heart Disease*, 4th ed, E. Braunwald (ed). Philadelphia, Saunders, 1992, pp 1125-1160

HAUDENSCHILD CC: Pathobiology of restenosis after angioplasty. Am J Med 94:40S, 1993

LEUNG WH: Coronary and circulatory support strategies for percutaneous transluminal coronary angioplasty in high-risk patients. Am Heart J 125:1727, 1993

NOBUYOSHI M et al: Restenosis after percutaneous transluminal coronary angioplasty: Pathologic observations in 20 patients 17:433, 1991

NYMAN I et al: Prevention of serious cardiac event by low-dose aspirin in patients with silent myocardial ischemia. Lancet 340:497, 1992

PARISI AF et al: A comparison of angioplasty with medical therapy in the treatment of single-vessel coronary artery disease. N Engl J Med 326:10, 1992

RIDKER PM et al: Low-dose aspirin therapy for chronic stable angina. Ann Intern Med 114:835, 1991

ROCCO MB et al: Prognostic importance of myocardial ischemia detected by ambulatory monitoring in patients with stable coronary artery disease. Circulation 78:877, 1988

RUTHERFORD JD et al: Chronic ischemic heart disease, in *Heart Disease*, 4th ed, E Braunwald (ed). Philadelphia, Saunders, 1992, pp 1292–1364

RYAN TJ et al: Guidelines for percutaneous transluminal coronary angioplasty. A report of the American College of Cardiology/American Heart Association Task Force on assessment of diagnostic and therapeutic cardiovascular procedures (Subcommittee on Percutaneous Transluminal Coronary Angioplasty). Circulation 78:486, 1988

SELWYN AP et al: Pathophysiology of ischemia in patients with coronary artery disease. Progr Cardiovasc Dis 35:1, 1992

Special Report: ACC/AHA guidelines and indications for coronary artery bypass graft surgery. A report of the American College of Cardiology/American Heart Association Task Force on Assessment of Diagnostic and Therapeutic Cardiovascular Procedures (Subcommittee on Coronary Artery Bypass Graft Surgery). Circulation 83:1125, 1991

STAMPFER MJ: Post menopausal estrogen therapy an cardiovascular disease. Ten year follow-up from the Nurses' Health Study. N Engl J Med 325:756, 1991

THEROUX P et al: Aspirin, heparin or both to treat acute unstable angina. N Engl J Med 319:1105, 1988

WILLERSON JT et al: Unstable angina pectoris and the progression to acute myocardial infarction: Role of platelets and platelet-derived mediators. Texas Heart Inst J 18:243, 1991

204 COR PULMONALE

JOHN BUTLER* / EUGENE BRAUNWALD

DEFINITIONS *Cor pulmonale* is enlargement of the right ventricle secondary to diseases of the lung, thorax, or pulmonary circulation. It is sometimes accompanied by right ventricular failure. In right ventricular failure there is an elevation of transmural right ventricular end-diastolic pressure which cannot be accounted for by an increase in right ventricular output. *Chronic* dysfunction of the right ventricular myocardium is rarely a cause of right heart failure but may occur when cor pulmonale and ischemic heart disease coexist. Approximately 20 percent of hospital admissions for heart failure are caused by right ventricular failure associated with cor pulmonale. More than half of the patients with chronic obstructive lung diseases have cor pulmonale, and this condition constitutes between 5 and 10 percent of all adult heart diseases in the United States. It constitutes a higher percentage of all forms of heart disease in countries such as the United Kingdom, where the incidence of obstructive lung disease is higher.

NORMAL FUNCTION OF THE PULMONARY CIRCULATION

The pulmonary circulation is interposed between the right and left ventricles for the purpose of gas exchange, the filtering out of particles, and the chemical "conditioning" of the blood, such as the conversion of angiotensin I to angiotensin II. Normally, flow through the pulmonary vascular bed depends not only on the pumping action of the right ventricle but also on respiratory movements and the

* Deceased

contraction of the left ventricle. Respiratory motion facilitates pulmonary blood flow by aspirating blood into the thorax on inhalation; the blood is then propelled forward by the positive pressure of exhalation acting on a one-way valved system.

The stroke volume of the right ventricle, as of the left, is regulated by its preload, contractility, and afterload (Chap. 194). Since the right ventricle is a compliant reservoir, acute changes in venous return (e.g., an increase with inhalation and decline with exhalation) are accommodated with little change in transmural right ventricular pressure. However, the ability of the right ventricle to increase its systolic pressure is limited. Normally, the right ventricular afterload, which is closely related to the pulmonary artery pressure, is low. The pulmonary artery pressure normally rises slightly when blood is displaced into the chest at the start of exercise, on assuming recumbency, or with cold, anxiety, or pain. A driving pressure of only about 5 cmH$_2$O between the pulmonary artery (15 cmH$_2$O) and the left atrium (10 cmH$_2$O) normally propels the entire cardiac output of approximately 5 L/min at rest through the lungs, and only a modest increase in pressure is necessary to drive a flow of up to 25 L/min through the pulmonary capillary bed during exercise.

The resistance of the pulmonary circulation (R), i.e., the pulmonary vascular resistance (p. 985), is calculated as the intravascular driving pressure (DP), i.e., pulmonary artery pressure minus pulmonary venous or left atrial pressure, divided by the pulmonary blood flow rate ($\dot{Q}$). The caliber of a distensible vessel depends on its transmural pressure. R increases when vessels collapse, narrow, or lengthen, or when the viscosity of the blood increases.

$$R = \frac{Kl\mu}{r^4}$$

where K = constant
l = length
r = radius
μ = viscosity

There is no single value of R which describes the pulmonary vascular bed, because the relationship between driving pressure and flow is not linear; calculated R decreases with increasing pulmonary blood flow because pulmonary vessels are distended and collapsed vessels are recruited (Fig. 204-1).

PATHOPHYSIOLOGY The severity of right ventricular enlargement in cor pulmonale is a function of the magnitude of the increase in afterload. When the pulmonary vascular resistance is increased and relatively fixed, as in pulmonary vascular or parenchymal lung disease, an elevation in cardiac output as occurs with physical exertion can elevate pulmonary artery pressure markedly. Right ventricular afterload is chronically augmented when lung volume is enlarged, as in chronic obstructive lung disease, due to the lengthening of the pulmonary vessels and the compression of the alveolar capillaries. Right ventricular afterload can also increase when lung volume is reduced following extensive pulmonary resection, as well as in restrictive lung diseases in which pulmonary vessels are compressed and distorted. Right ventricular afterload rises with hypoxic pulmonary vasoconstriction, which is an important cause of pulmonary hypertension. Hypoxic vasoconstriction in regions of the lung affected by disease distributes blood flow to normally ventilated regions. The elevation in pulmonary artery pressure becomes a significant stress on the right ventricle when the lung disease is diffuse or when the entire lung becomes hypoxic due to hypoventilation. Hypoxic vasoconstriction results from alveolar, rather than intravascular, hypoxia and is made worse by hypercarbia, probably because of the associated acidosis. When the hematocrit becomes markedly elevated with chronic hypoxemia, the increase in blood viscosity can intensify the pulmonary hypertension.

The elevation of right ventricular afterload responsible for cor pulmonale is caused principally by pulmonary vascular or parenchymal disease. The principal syndromes and their pathophysiologic mechanisms are summarized in Table 204-1.

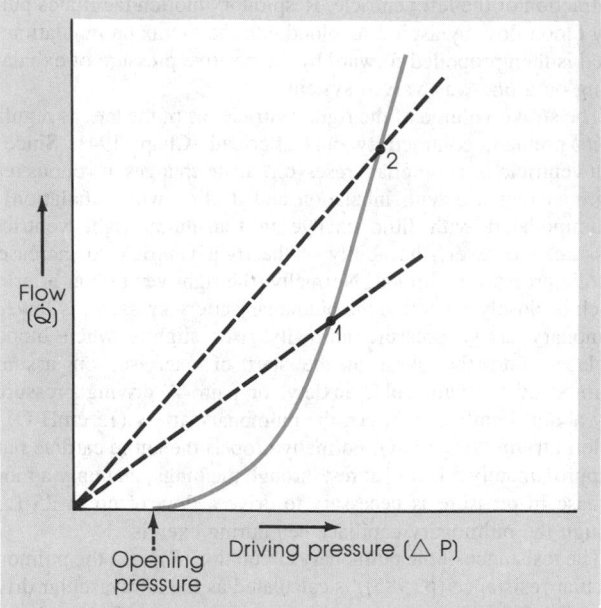

FIGURE 204-1 Relationship between flow and driving pressure ("vascular resistance") in the pulmonary circulation. Note that it does not pass through zero at the origin since an opening pressure must be overcome before flow starts. Thus the calculated vascular resistance (reciprocal of relationship of flow to pressure, dashed lines) falls (1 → 2) as flow increases. (*Modified from Graham et al: Dopamine, dobutamine and phentolamine effects on pulmonary vascular mechanics. J Appl Physiol 54:1277, 1983.*)

PULMONARY VASCULAR DISEASES

In these conditions the right ventricular afterload is elevated as a consequence of the restriction to pulmonary blood flow. In cor pulmonale secondary to pulmonary vascular disease pulmonary hypertension is usually more severe than in pulmonary parenchymal disease. Chronic cor pulmonale secondary to pulmonary vascular disease may result from repeated pulmonary emboli, pulmonary vasculitis, pulmonary vasoconstriction secondary to high altitude, as well as pulmonary venoocclusive disease. Disorders of pulmonary ventilation causing hypoxemia (Chap. 229) may also cause pulmonary hypertension and cor pulmonale. When the cause of elevated pulmonary vascular resistance is unknown the condition is referred to as *primary pulmonary hypertension* (Chap. 225).

COR PULMONALE DUE TO PULMONARY EMBOLI This condition is associated with two distinct syndromes.

Acute cor pulmonale It has been estimated that in the United States about 50,000 people die each year from embolic pulmonary vascular disease (Chap. 226). Probably half die within the first hour from acute right heart failure due to massive or multiple emboli. A large embolic burden causes a sudden, low-output state resulting from the right ventricle's inability to generate the pressure necessary to drive blood through the acutely compromised pulmonary vascular bed. Depression of cardiac output can also occur with a moderate-sized embolism if the pulmonary circulation has been critically compromised by previous pulmonary vascular or parenchymal disease. The right ventricle begins to fail when systolic pressure suddenly exceeds approximately 40 to 45 mmHg. Acute right ventricular failure secondary to pulmonary embolism is suggested by the history of the sudden onset of severe dyspnea and cardiovascular collapse in a patient with, or predisposed to, venous thrombosis. The low cardiac output causes pallor, sweating, hypotension, and a rapid pulse of small amplitude. The neck veins are distended and often exhibit the prominent *v* waves of tricuspid regurgitation. The liver may be pulsatile, distended, and tender. A systolic murmur of tricuspid regurgitation at the left sternal border may be accompanied by a

TABLE 204-1   Cor pulmonale

Mechanisms	Responses	Characteristics
PULMONARY VASCULAR DISEASES		
Emboli, large or multiple	Fall in output due to acute obstruction	Acute cor pulmonale Right ventricular distention Shock
Emboli, small; vasculitis; widespread lung damage (ARDS)	Pulmonary hypertension due to widespread hypoxia and microvascular obstruction High output	Subacute cor pulmonale Right ventricular distention Breathlessness and fever
Emboli, medium and recurrent; primary pulmonary hypertension; diet or drug vasopathy	Pulmonary hypertension due to vascular obstruction Low or normal output	Chronic cor pulmonale Right heart hypertrophy Breathlessness
RESPIRATORY DISEASES		
Obstructive A Chronic bronchitis and emphysema; chronic asthma	Pulmonary hypertension due to hypoxia, vascular stretching and loss Heart beat impeded externally by lung hyperinflation Normal or high output	Chronic cor pulmonale "Blue bloater" Underventilation
Restrictive A Intrinsic: interstitial fibrosis, lung resection	Hypertension due to hypoxia, vascular distortion and loss Normal or low output	Chronic cor pulmonale Breathlessness Overventilation
B Extrinsic: obesity, myxedema, muscle weakness, kyphoscoliosis, upper airway obstruction, diminished respiratory drive, high altitude	Hypertension due to alveolar hypoxia Normal or high output	Chronic cor pulmonale Peripheral edema Underventilation

presystolic (S_4) gallop sound. Arterial blood gases frequently show hypoxemia due to ventilation/perfusion mismatching and a low Pa_{CO_2} due to hyperventilation. If the cardiac output remains adequate to sustain the patient during the critical first two or three hours, the natural lytic response usually results in fragmentation of the clot so that the patient survives. Although it has been shown that treatment with thrombolytic agents lyses clots more rapidly than does heparin (Chap. 226), this therapy is probably indicated only when blood flow is critically reduced and not improving.

Chronic cor pulmonale secondary to pulmonary vascular disease In contrast to acute, massive thromboembolism, when the elevation in pulmonary vascular resistance and the development of right ventricular hypertrophy are gradual, higher pulmonary vascular pressures, sometimes even exceeding systemic arterial levels, may be generated. Chronic cor pulmonale can be caused by recurrent, medium-sized emboli that fail to lyse, but organize and recanalize. Particles from intravenous drug abuse, parasites, or tumor tissue which embolizes into the pulmonary vascular bed also may cause persistent pulmonary hypertension. Chronic cor pulmonale also can be caused by *primary pulmonary hypertension* (Chap. 225) or any chronic widespread vasculitis, such as occurs in association with the collagen vascular disorders, and that affects the pulmonary vascular bed, particularly the CREST syndrome (Chap. 286).

Symptoms and signs Breathlessness is a characteristic feature of pulmonary hypertension due to pulmonary vascular disease. It may be distressing during even mild exertion, and it is *not* relieved by sitting upright. An unproductive cough is another frequent complaint. Anterior chest pain, due to acute dilation of the root of the pulmonary artery or right ventricular ischemia, can occur. The elevation in systemic venous pressure can cause hepatomegaly and ankle edema.

Patients with pulmonary hypertension and cor pulmonale often have tachypnea that is evident both on mild exertion and at rest, and may even persist during sleep. Occasionally there is cyanosis due to arterial hypoxemia and low cardiac output. A right ventricular heave may be palpable along the left sternal border or in the epigastrium and a high-pitched pulmonary ejection click may be audible to the left of the upper sternum. The second (pulmonary) component of the second heart sound is intensified and may be palpable; fixed splitting of the second heart sound may be present and a right ventricular protodiastolic gallop (S_3) which increases during inspiration may be present. A systolic murmur of tricuspid regurgitation, which is augmented by inspiration (p. 952) is often audible; occasionally, a diastolic murmur of pulmonary regurgitation also is heard. Prominent *a* and *v* waves in the jugular venous pulse are evident. The onset of right ventricular failure is reflected by an increase of venous pressure, the development of larger *v* waves associated with worse tricuspid regurgitation, a hepatojugular reflux, and a gallop rhythm with both third and fourth heart sounds. These physical findings of right ventricular failure may be evanescent and can disappear rapidly when pulmonary artery pressure is suddenly reduced by relief of hypoxemia.

Hypocarbia due to alveolar hyperventilation is an important feature of chronic pulmonary hypertension secondary to pulmonary vascular disease. Usually there are no abnormalities on spirometry, but the ratio of dead space to tidal volume may be high, particularly when large-vessel obstruction is present. The diffusing capacity of the lung is reduced when a capillary vasculitis and/or loss of capillary blood volume is associated with pulmonary vascular disease. Typically, exercise causes a marked fall in Pa_{O_2}. The assessment of exercise capacity may be a useful way of following changes in the severity of pulmonary vascular disease in patients with chronic cor pulmonale because exercise ability is limited by cardiac output and the latter, in turn, by the severity of the pulmonary vascular obstruction.

On *radiologic examination* the pulmonary trunk and hilar vessels are enlarged. Widening of the hilum may be judged from the ratio of the distance between the start of the first divisions of the right and left main pulmonary arteries divided by the transverse diameter of the thorax; a ratio >0.36 suggests pulmonary hypertension. Another radiologic indicator of pulmonary hypertension is widening of the descending right pulmonary artery shadow, from a normal value of <16 mm to >20 mm. Ventilation and perfusion lung scans and systemic venography showing deep vein thrombosis are helpful in confirming the diagnosis of embolic pulmonary vascular disease. In the presence of severe pulmonary hypertension, the ECG shows P pulmonale, right axis deviation, and right ventricular hypertrophy.

Echocardiography allows measurement of the thickness of the right ventricular wall and, although volume changes cannot be measured, this technique can show enlargement of the right ventricular cavity in relation to that of the left. The interventricular septum may be displaced leftward. Right ventricular systolic pressure can be estimated from measurement of the peak tricuspid regurgitant flow and pulmonic regurgitant flow with Doppler echocardiography (Chap. 190).

Magnetic resonance imaging (Chap. 191) is useful for measuring right ventricular mass, wall thickness, cavity volume and ejection fraction.

Failure of the right ventricular ejection fraction (measured by radionuclide ventriculography) to increase on exercise appears to be a good indicator of pulmonary hypertension and/or intrinsic right ventricular dysfunction. Myocardial perfusion scintigraphy with thallium 201 or Sesta-Mibi is also useful for diagnosing cor pulmonale (Chap. 190), since the hypertrophied right ventricle is visualized by these radionuclides. (Normally the right ventricle is not imaged because of the much greater uptake by the left ventricle.)

Cardiac catheterization is necessary for the precise measurement of pulmonary vascular pressures, the determination of pulmonary vascular resistance, and its response to oxygen and vasodilators. Catheterization is sometimes indicated in patients with cor pulmonale to exclude congenital and left heart diseases, and it allows pulmonary angiography to be carried out to confirm the nature of the pulmonary vascular obstruction. Measurements of pulmonary vascular pressures and flow should also be made during exercise to look for abnormal pressure increments or poor responses of cardiac output.

Lung biopsy can be useful in demonstrating vasculitis in some types of pulmonary vascular disease such as the collagen vascular diseases, rheumatoid arthritis, and Wegener's granulomatosis.

PARENCHYMAL PULMONARY DISEASES

Cor pulmonale may be caused by both obstructive and restrictive lung diseases, more frequently the former. In these conditions there are usually only modest elevations of pulmonary artery pressure. The development of cor pulmonale confers a poor prognosis on patients with respiratory disease; in patients with cor pulmonale and right ventricular failure, the 3-year survival is approximately 40 percent. Respiratory diseases causing cor pulmonale are usually associated with distortions of the lung which affect the position of the heart, so that cardiac physical signs are altered.

CHRONIC OBSTRUCTIVE LUNG DISEASE (COLD) (See Chap. 223) This is the most common cause of chronic cor pulmonale. The enlargement of the right ventricle is attributed to the mild-to-moderate pulmonary hypertension which is common in severe obstructive bronchitis and emphysema. Pulmonary artery systolic pressure is typically in the range of 40 to 50 mmHg, far below the systemic levels which appear to be tolerated in patients with congenital heart disease and in those with primary pulmonary hypertension. Patients with cor pulmonale due to COLD usually have an advanced form of the disease with FEV_1 <1.0 L (Chap. 214) and Pa_{O_2} ≤60 mmHg. Right ventricular failure secondary to COLD often occurs when there is "acute-on-chronic" respiratory failure with intensification of hypoxemia.

Pulmonary hypertension in COLD is due to the generalized pulmonary vasoconstriction caused by the alveolar hypoxia, acidemia, and hypercarbia; by the mechanical effects of the high lung volume on the pulmonary vessels; by the loss of small vessels in the vascular bed in regions of emphysema; and sometimes by the increased blood viscosity caused by the associated polycythemia. Of these causes hypoxia is undoubtedly the most important. Pulmonary artery pressure rises further on exercise and often falls acutely on inspiration of 100% O_2. Cardiac output tends to be high in the absence of heart failure if hypoxia and hypercarbia are present. Because of the importance of hypoxic pulmonary vasoconstriction in causing pulmonary hypertension, the hypoventilating "blue bloater" with alveolar hypoxia and hypercarbia more frequently suffers from cor pulmonale than does the emphysematous "pink puffer," without alveolar hypoxia (p. 1201). Ischemic left-heart disease is a frequent accompaniment of patients with cor pulmonale secondary to COLD since they usually have a history of heavy cigarette smoking. The elevation of pulmonary artery pressure may be secondary, in part, to the increase in left atrial pressure resulting from left-heart dysfunction. Almost half of all patients who die with cor pulmonale due to COLD also have left ventricular hypertrophy on postmortem examination.

Right ventricular failure often complicates cor pulmonale when patients with COLD develop ventilatory failure with hypoxia and hypercarbia. When there is a worsening of the airflow due to increasing airway obstruction the resulting hypoxia and hypercarbia may increase cardiac output by their vasodilator effect on the systemic arteriolar bed. Hypoxic pulmonary vasoconstriction is intensified and both supraventricular and ventricular arrhythmias may occur. The liver becomes palpable and tender because it is engorged and displaced downward by the low diaphragm; a hepatojugular reflux may be present.

An exacerbation of airway obstruction elevates intrathoracic pressure, which impedes venous return, raises jugular venous pressure, and may cause peripheral edema, even in the absence of heart failure. This elevation of venous pressure secondary to airway obstruction is *not* associated with an increase in the transmural right ventricular pressure, the hallmark of right ventricular failure. The venous hypertension due to airflow obstruction declines, sometimes very rapidly, with relief of the obstruction.

Pathology In COLD right ventricular hypertrophy increases progressively. The main pulmonary arteries are enlarged and the muscular pulmonary arteries show prominent longitudinal muscle, fibrosis, and elastic changes that continue into the arterioles, where the media also becomes muscularized. The small vessels and capillaries are distorted or disappear in regions of lung hyperinflation.

Symptoms and signs A history of a productive cough and dyspnea, perhaps with wheezing, is frequently elicited. Breathlessness limits the patient's ability in the minor stresses of daily living. Frequently there is a history of emergency hospital admissions because of respiratory infection, sometimes necessitating mechanical ventilation. In breathing oxygen, there may be increasing somnolence or other symptoms of hypercarbia such as recurring headaches, confusion, and even vomiting which, when combined with blurred optic discs (also due to cerebral vasodilation), constitutes the "pseudo tumor cerebri" syndrome. Hypoxia due to hypoventilation is usually worse at night, particularly when severe snoring leads to obstructive apnea (Chap. 217).

Physical findings Often there is nicotine staining of the fingers, a tell-tale sign reflecting many years of heavy cigarette smoking. The skin may be warm and the arterial pulse bounding in the high cardiac output state induced by hypoxia and hypercarbia. The distention of the chest due to the airflow obstruction and the rhonchi and wheezes secondary to chronic bronchitis usually make cardiac auscultation difficult. A right-sided protodiastolic gallop sound (S_3) and a systolic murmur of tricuspid regurgitant may be audible. Signs of right-heart failure are, as discussed above, difficult to separate from those due to severe airflow obstruction. However, a sudden worsening of peripheral edema and rise of systemic venous pressure when atrial fibrillation occurs or when pulmonary infection supervenes is usually considered to be evidence of heart failure. This may be confirmed by the presence of a positive hepatojugular reflux. The distinction is important since patients can survive for years with the high systemic venous pressure and edema secondary to airflow obstruction but usually have a poor prognosis after right-heart failure develops.

Laboratory examinations *Pulmonary function studies* show marked airflow obstruction with hypoxemia and hypercarbia. Exercise is limited by ventilatory rather than cardiac dysfunction until right ventricular failure develops. The *chest roentgenogram* reveals hyperinflation, which makes the degree of right-heart enlargement difficult to assess. The central pulmonary arteries are large but the vessels are narrowed and disappear at the periphery, particularly in regions of the lungs which are markedly emphysematous. The ECG is relatively insensitive in demonstrating right-heart enlargement because the enlarged lungs are poor electrical conductors and the inspiratory position of the chest is associated with a vertically positioned heart. Arrhythmias, particularly atrial fibrillation and multifocal atrial tachycardia, are common.

Echocardiographic imaging is often difficult because of the air in the distended lungs but may reveal an increased cross section of the right ventricular cavity and abnormal thickening of the right ventricular wall. Myocardial perfusion scintigraphy shows an abnormally high ratio of right-to-left ventricular uptake.

Right heart catheterization can be carried out at the bedside with a balloon-tipped, flow-directed, multilumen catheter fitted with thermocouples for measuring cardiac output by thermodilution (Chap. 192). The pulmonary artery wedge pressure is usually normal in patients at rest who have uncomplicated cor pulmonale. Cardiac catheterization may be useful in assessing left ventricular function as well as the severity of the pulmonary hypertension and its response to respiring oxygen. Pressure measurements during exercise study may be helpful, particularly in excluding left-heart dysfunction.

Treatment First, medical management of the acute and/or chronic lung disease must be optimal (Chaps. 223 and 230). Alveolar hypoxia should be corrected by improving alveolar ventilation through relieving the airflow obstruction and by judiciously increasing the inspired O_2 concentration. Long-term O_2 therapy is helpful in patients with severe COLD and reduces pulmonary artery pressure and pulmonary vascular resistance. When the lung disease improves and pulmonary vasoconstriction secondary to the alveolar hypoxia and hypercarbia are corrected, tachypnea and the signs attributed to right-heart failure are relieved. Bronchodilators and antibiotics lessen the airflow obstruction and diuretics relieve the edema. Loop diuretics must be used with care since they may cause a metabolic alkalosis and thereby blunt the respiratory drive. Digitalis should be used in the presence of overt right ventricular failure, and phlebotomy should be considered when the hematocrit exceeds 55 percent.

RESTRICTIVE LUNG DISEASES Cor pulmonale in restrictive lung disease is associated with two different clinical syndromes: (1) hyperventilation in patients with a variety of restrictive diseases intrinsic to the lungs (Chap. 224), and (2) hypoventilation in patients with extrinsic diseases, such as obesity, myxedema, musculoskeletal disorder, or neuromuscular dysfunction. Pulmonary hypertension is due to a combination of the hypoxemia and to the increased pulmonary vascular resistance resulting from compression of the pulmonary vessels. Again, oxygen is the main treatment, but specific therapy may be available for some of the underlying lung diseases.

REFERENCES

BEHAR JV et al: Performance of new criteria for right ventricular hypertrophy and myocardial infarction in patients with pulmonary hypertension due to cor pulmonale and mitral stenosis. J Electrocardiog 24:231, 1991

CARTER R et al: Altered exercise gas exchange and cardiac function in patients with mild chronic obstructive pulmonary disease. Chest 103:745, 1993

FERGUSON GT, CHERNIACK RM: Management of chronic obstructive pulmonary disease. N Engl J Med 328:1017, 1993

FISHMAN AP: Pulmonary hypertension and cor pulmonale, in *Pulmonary Diseases and Disorders*, 2d ed., AP Fishman (ed). New York, McGraw Hill, 1988, pp 999–1048

KLINGER JR, HILL NS: Right ventricular dysfunction in chronic obstructive pulmonary disease: Evaluation and management. Chest 99:715–23, 1991

McFADDEN ER, BRAUNWALD E: Cor pulmonale and pulmonary thromboembolism, in *Heart Disease*, 4th ed, E Braunwald (ed). Philadelphia, Saunders, 1992, pp 1581–1601

OLIVER RM et al: Right ventricular function at rest and during exercise in chronic obstructive pulmonary disease. 103:74, 1993

PATTYNAMA PMT et al: Early diagnosis of cor pulmonale with MR imaging of the right ventricle. Radiology 182:375, 1992

TRAMARIN R et al: Doppler echocardiographic evaluation of pulmonary artery pressure in chronic obstructive pulmonary disease. A European multicentre study. Eur Heart J 12:103, 1991

WEITZENBLUM E et al: Benefit from long-term O_2 therapy in chronic obstructive pulmonary disease patients. Respiration 59(suppl I):14–117, 1992

---

205 THE CARDIOMYOPATHIES AND MYOCARDITIDES

JOSHUA WYNNE / EUGENE BRAUNWALD

CARDIOMYOPATHIES

The cardiomyopathies are diseases that involve the myocardium primarily and are not the result of hypertension or congenital, valvular, coronary, arterial, or pericardial abnormalities.* When the

---

* Diffuse myocardial fibrosis secondary to multiple myocardial scars produced by extensive coronary arterial narrowing and occlusion can impair left ventricular function and is frequently referred to as *ischemic cardiomyopathy*. According to the definition given above, however, the term *cardiomyopathy* should be restricted to a condition *primarily* involving heart muscle. In ischemic "cardiomyopathy" the *primary* involvement is in the coronary vessels.

TABLE 205-1 Etiologic classification of cardiomyopathies

PRIMARY MYOCARDIAL INVOLVEMENT

A Idiopathic (D,R,H)
B Familial (D,H)
C Eosinophilic endomyocardial disease (R)
D Endomyocardial fibrosis (R)

SECONDARY MYOCARDIAL INVOLVEMENT

A Infective (D)
   1 Viral myocarditis
   2 Bacterial myocarditis
   3 Fungal myocarditis
   4 Protozoal myocarditis
   5 Metazoal myocarditis
   6 Spirochetal
   7 Rickettsial
B Metabolic (D)
C Familial storage disease (D,R)
   1 Glycogen storage disease
   2 Mucopolysaccharidoses
D Deficiency (D)
   1 Electrolytes
   2 Nutritional
E Connective tissue disorders (D)
   1 Systemic lupus erythematosus
   2 Polyarteritis nodosa
   3 Rheumatoid arthritis
   4 Progressive systemic sclerosis
   5 Dermatomyositis
F Infiltrations and granulomas (R,D)
   1 Amyloidosis
   2 Sarcoidosis
   3 Malignancy
   4 Hemochromatosis
G Neuromuscular (D)
   1 Muscular dystrophy
   2 Myotonic dystrophy
   3 Friedreich's ataxia (H,D)
   4 Refsum's disease
H Sensitivity and toxic reactions (D)
   1 Alcohol
   2 Radiation
   3 Drugs
I Peripartum heart disease (D)
J Endocardial fibroelastosis (R)

NOTE: The principal clinical manifestation(s) of each etiologic grouping is denoted by D (dilated), R (restrictive), or H (hypertrophic) cardiomyopathy.
SOURCE: Adapted from the WHO/ISFC task force report on the definition and classification of cardiomyopathies, 1980.

cardiomyopathies are classified on an etiologic basis, two fundamental forms are recognized: (1) a primary type, consisting of heart muscle disease of unknown cause, and (2) a secondary type, consisting of myocardial disease of known cause or associated with a disease involving other organ systems (Table 205-1). In many cases it is not possible to arrive at a specific etiologic diagnosis, and thus it is often more desirable to classify the cardiomyopathies on the basis of differences in their pathophysiology and clinical presentation (Tables 205-2 and 205-3).

DILATED (CONGESTIVE) CARDIOMYOPATHY In this condition, left and/or right ventricular systolic pump function is impaired, leading to cardiac enlargement and often producing symptoms of congestive heart failure. Mural thrombi are often present, particularly

TABLE 205-2 Clinical classification of cardiomyopathies

1 Dilated (congestive): Left and/or right ventricular enlargement, impaired systolic function, congestive heart failure, arrhythmias, emboli

2 Restrictive: Endomyocardial scarring or myocardial infiltration resulting in restriction to left and/or right ventricular filling

3 Hypertrophic: Disproportionate left ventricular hypertrophy, typically involving septum more than free wall, with or without an intraventricular systolic pressure gradient; usually of a nondilated left ventricular cavity

in the left ventricular apex. Histologic examination reveals extensive areas of interstitial and perivascular fibrosis, with minimal necrosis and cellular infiltration. Although no cause is apparent in many cases, dilated cardiomyopathy probably is the end result of myocardial damage produced by a variety of toxic, metabolic, or infectious agents. There is increasing evidence to suggest that in some patients dilated cardiomyopathy may be the late sequel of acute viral myocarditis, possibly mediated through an immunologic mechanism. Although most commonly a disease of middle-aged men, it may occur in any patient population. A reversible form of dilated cardiomyopathy may be found with alcohol, pregnancy, selenium deficiency, hypophosphatemia, hypocalcemia, and chronic uncontrolled tachycardia. A minority of patients (but probably more than usually suspected) have familial forms of the disease. *Right ventricular dysplasia* is a unique cardiomyopathy marked by progressive replacement of the right ventricular wall with adipose tissue. Often associated with ventricular arrhythmias, the clinical course is variable but sudden death is a constant threat.

Clinical manifestations Symptoms of left- and right-sided congestive failure, manifested by dyspnea on exertion, fatigue, orthopnea, paroxysmal nocturnal dyspnea, peripheral edema, and palpitations, develop gradually in most patients. Some patients have left ventricular dilatation for months or even years before becoming symptomatic. Although vague chest pain may be present, typical angina pectoris is unusual and suggests the presence of concomitant coronary artery disease.

Physical examination Variable degrees of cardiac enlargement and findings of congestive heart failure are noted. In patients with advanced disease, the pulse pressure is narrow, and the jugular venous pressure is elevated. Third and fourth heart sounds are common, and mitral or tricuspid regurgitation may occur. Diastolic murmurs, valvular calcification, and severe hypertension reduce the likelihood of cardiomyopathy.

Laboratory examinations The chest roentgenogram demonstrates left ventricular enlargement, although generalized cardiomegaly often is seen, sometimes due to a concomitant pericardial effusion. The lung fields may demonstrate evidence of pulmonary venous hypertension and interstitial or alveolar edema. The electrocardiogram often shows sinus tachycardia or atrial fibrillation, ventricular arrhythmias, left atrial enlargement, diffuse nonspecific ST-T wave abnormalities, and sometimes intraventricular conduction defects. Echocardiography (see Fig. 190-4) and radionuclide ventriculography (see Fig. 190-8) show left ventricular enlargement, with normal or minimally thickened or thinned walls, and systolic dysfunction (reduced ejection fraction); a pericardial effusion is often noted. Radioisotopic imaging with gallium 67 may identify patients with dilated cardiomyopathy and concomitant myocarditis.

Hemodynamic studies reveal a cardiac output that does not increase normally with exercise. The left ventricular end-diastolic, left atrial, and pulmonary capillary wedge pressures usually are elevated; when failure of the right side of the heart supervenes, the right ventricular end-diastolic, right atrial, and central venous pressures are also elevated. Angiography reveals a dilated, diffusely hypokinetic left ventricle, often with some degree of mitral regurgitation; the coronary arteries are normal, thereby excluding so-called ischemic cardiomyopathy. Transvenous endomyocardial biopsy (Chap. 192) may be helpful in excluding certain conditions such as myocardial infiltration by amyloid; in some patients there is biopsy evidence of myocardial round cell inflammation, suggesting previous viral myocarditis.

Treatment Most patients pursue an inexorably downhill course, and the majority, particularly those over 55 years of age, die within 2 years of the onset of symptoms, but spontaneous improvement or stabilization occurs in a minority. Death is due to either congestive heart failure or ventricular tachy- or bradyarrhythmia; sudden death is a constant threat. Systemic embolization is common, and all patients without contraindications should receive anticoagulants. Strenuous exertion should be interdicted. Treatment of heart failure in dilated cardiomyopathy is directed primarily toward improvement in symp-

TABLE 205-3   Laboratory evaluation of the cardiomyopathies

	Dilated (congestive)	Restrictive	Hypertrophic
Chest roentgenogram	Moderate to marked cardiac enlargement Pulmonary venous hypertension	Mild cardiac enlargement	Mild to moderate cardiac enlargement
Electrocardiogram	ST-segment and T-wave abnormalities	Low voltage, conduction defects	ST-segment and T-wave abnormalities Left ventricular hypertrophy Abnormal Q waves
Echocardiogram	Left ventricular dilatation and dysfunction	Increased left ventricular wall thickness Normal or mildly reduced systolic function	Asymmetric septal hypertrophy (ASH) Systolic anterior motion (SAM) of the mitral valve
Radionuclide studies	Left ventricular dilatation and dysfunction (RVG)	Normal or mildly reduced systolic function (RVG)	Vigorous systolic function (RVG) Asymmetric septal hypertrophy (RVG or ^{201}Tl)
Cardiac catheterization	Left ventricular dilatation and dysfunction Elevated left- and often right-sided filling pressures Diminished cardiac output	Normal or mildly reduced systolic function Elevated left- and right-sided filling pressures	Vigorous systolic function Dynamic left ventricular outflow obstruction Elevated left- and right-sided filling pressures

NOTE: RVG = radionuclide ventriculogram; ^{201}Tl = thallium 201.

toms; an improvement in survival is achieved with angiotensin-converting enzyme inhibitor therapy. Standard therapy of heart failure with salt restriction, diuretics, digitalis, and vasodilators may produce symptomatic improvement. Some patients with dilated cardiomyopathy who have evidence of myocardial inflammation have been treated with immunosuppressive therapy with variable but usually only transient benefit. Others have been treated cautiously with gradually increasing doses of beta-adrenergic blockers with apparent clinical benefit. Antiarrhythmic agents are best avoided for fear of proarrhythmic and other side effects, unless they are needed to treat symptomatic or serious arrhythmias. Alternative therapies, such as surgical interruption of the arrhythmic circuit or implantation of an automatic internal defibrillator, have gained favor. In patients with advanced disease who are refractory to medical therapy and who have no contraindications to the procedure, cardiac transplantation should be considered (Chap. 196).

Alcoholic cardiomyopathy   Individuals who consume large quantities of alcohol over many years may develop a clinical picture identical to idiopathic dilated cardiomyopathy; indeed, alcoholic cardiomyopathy is the major form of secondary dilated cardiomyopathy in the western world. Ceasing alcohol consumption before severe heart failure has developed may halt the progression or even reverse the course of this disease, unlike the idiopathic variety, which is marked by progressive deterioration. Alcoholics with advanced heart failure have a poor prognosis, particularly if they continue to drink; less than one-quarter survive 3 years. The key to the treatment of alcoholic cardiomyopathy is total and permanent abstinence. Although thiamine deficiency may be present in some of these patients, alcoholic cardiomyopathy is associated with a low cardiac output and systemic vasoconstriction. In contrast, beriberi heart disease (Chaps. 77 and 207) is characterized by elevated cardiac output and diminished peripheral vascular resistance, so thiamine deficiency per se does not appear to cause alcoholic cardiomyopathy. The toxic effect of alcohol on striated muscle often extends beyond the heart to cause myopathy in skeletal muscles. A second presentation of alcoholic cardiotoxicity may be found in individuals without overt heart failure and consists of recurrent supraventricular or ventricular tachyarrhythmias. Termed the "holiday heart syndrome," it typically appears after a drinking binge; atrial fibrillation is seen most frequently, followed by atrial flutter and ventricular premature depolarizations. Other patients develop left ventricular hypertrophy, perhaps related to concomitant systemic hypertension; they may present with symptoms of pulmonary congestion due to abnormal diastolic stiffness (diminished compliance) of the left ventricle.

Peripartum cardiomyopathy   Cardiac dilatation and congestive heart failure of unexplained cause may develop during the last month of pregnancy or within the first few months after delivery. The cause of this disorder is unknown but in some patients endomyocardial biopsy has shown evidence of a myocarditis. Necropsy shows cardiac enlargement, often with mural thrombi, along with histologic evidence of myocardial degeneration and fibrosis. The patient who develops peripartum cardiomyopathy typically is multiparous, black, and over the age of 30. While some patients are malnourished, there is no conclusive evidence that dietary deficiencies are etiologically involved. The symptoms, signs, and treatment are similar to those in patients with idiopathic dilated cardiomyopathy; pulmonary and systemic emboli are particularly common. The mortality rate is quite variable but may be as high as 25 to 50 percent. The prognosis in these patients appears to be closely related to whether the heart size returns to normal after the first episode of congestive heart failure. If it does, subsequent pregnancies may sometimes be well tolerated; if the heart remains enlarged, however, further pregnancies frequently produce increasing myocardial damage, ultimately leading to refractory congestive heart failure and death. Those who recover should be encouraged to avoid further pregnancies, particularly if cardiomegaly persists. Some patients with evidence of myocarditis on biopsy appear to respond to immunosuppressive therapy (although there is a high frequency of spontaneous clinical improvement in this condition).

Neuromuscular disease   (See also Chap. 385)   Cardiac involvement is common in many of the muscular dystrophies. In *Duchenne's progressive muscular dystrophy*, myocardial involvement is most frequently indicated by a distinctive and unique electrocardiographic pattern consisting of tall R waves in right precordial leads with an R/S ratio greater than 1.0, often associated with deep Q waves in the limb and lateral precordial leads, and is not found in other forms of muscular dystrophy. These electrocardiographic abnormalities appear to result from selective transmural necrosis of the posterobasal left ventricle and associated papillary muscle. A variety of supraventricular and ventricular arrhythmias is frequently found. Rapidly progressive congestive heart failure may develop despite extended periods of apparent circulatory stability during which the only detectable abnormalities are in the electrocardiogram. *Myotonic dystrophy* is characterized by a variety of electrocardiographic abnormalities, especially disorders of impulse formation and particularly conduction, but other overt clinical evidence of heart disease is uncommon. Because of the abnormalities of impulse generation and conduction, syncope and sudden death are major hazards; in appropriate patients, insertion of a permanent pacemaker may be efficacious. In *limb-girdle* and *fascioscapulohumeral dystrophy*, cardiac involvement is uncommon and seldom severe. Involvement of the heart is very common in *Friedreich's ataxia* (manifested by abnormal electrocardiographic or echocardiographic findings), with as many as half the patients developing cardiac symptoms. The electrocardiogram most commonly demonstrates ST-segment and T-wave abnormalities. The echocardiogram may demonstrate left ventricular hypertrophy, with either symmetric or asymmetric hypertrophy of the left ventricular septum compared with the free wall. Although morphologically similar to some cases of hypertrophic cardiomyopathy, cellular disarray is lacking.

Drugs A variety of pharmacologic agents may damage the myocardium acutely, producing a pattern of inflammation (myocarditis), or they may lead to chronic damage of the type seen with idiopathic dilated cardiomyopathy. Certain drugs produce only electrocardiographic abnormalities, while others may precipitate fulminant congestive heart failure and death. The anthracycline derivatives, particularly *doxorubicin* (Adriamycin), are powerful antineoplastic agents which, when given in high doses (more than 550 mg/m^2 for doxorubicin), may produce fatal heart failure. The incidence of heart failure is related not only to the dose of the drug but also to the presence or absence of several risk factors (cardiac irradiation, age greater than 70 years, underlying heart disease, hypertension, treatment with cyclophosphamide); at any dose patients with these risk factors have an eight- to tenfold greater frequency of developing heart failure than do patients lacking them. Radionuclide ventriculography (Chap. 190) may document preclinical deterioration of left ventricular function and allow appropriate dose adjustments; by so monitoring left ventricular function, it is often possible to continue doxorubicin even in patients at high risk for developing heart failure. Recent efforts to modify the dose schedule by giving the drug more slowly have further reduced the risk of cardiotoxicity.

Some patients with congestive heart failure, even those with severe depression of left ventricular function, have demonstrated recovery of cardiac function with aggressive management with digitalis, diuretics, and vasodilators. In others, late asymptomatic contractile dysfunction is common, even in those without initial cardiotoxicity. Children may demonstrate reduced myocardial hypertrophy and mass over time, presumably due to doxorubicin's inhibition of myocardial cell growth. High-dose *cyclophosphamide* may produce congestive heart failure acutely or within 2 weeks of administration; a characteristic histopathologic feature is myocardial edema and hemorrhagic necrosis. Rarely, patients treated with *5-fluorouracil* will develop chest pain and electrocardiographic changes of myocardial ischemia or infarction. Electrocardiographic changes and arrhythmias may result from treatment with tricyclic antidepressants, the phenothiazines, emetine, lithium, and various aerosol propellants. *Cocaine abuse* is associated with a variety of life-threatening cardiac complications, including sudden death, myocarditis, dilated cardiomyopathy, and acute myocardial infarction (resulting from coronary spasm and/or thrombosis with or without underlying coronary artery stenosis). Thrombolytic therapy has been effective in lysing coronary thrombi in patients with acute myocardial infarction. Nitrates and calcium antagonists have been used as well to treat a variety of cocaine-induced cardiotoxicities.

RESTRICTIVE CARDIOMYOPATHY The hallmark of the restrictive cardiomyopathies is abnormal diastolic function; the ventricular walls are excessively rigid and impede ventricular filling. Myocardial fibrosis, hypertrophy, or infiltration due to a variety of causes is usually responsible. The infiltrative diseases, which represent important causes for secondary restrictive cardiomyopathy, also may show some impairment of systolic function. Myocardial involvement with *amyloid* is a common cause of secondary restrictive cardiomyopathy, although restriction is also seen in hemochromatosis, glycogen deposition, endomyocardial fibrosis, fibroelastosis, the eosinophilias, neoplastic infiltration, and myocardial fibrosis of diverse causes. In many of these conditions, particularly those with substantial concomitant endocardial involvement, partial obliteration of the ventricular cavity by fibrous tissue and thrombus contributes to the abnormally increased resistance to ventricular filling. As a result of persistently elevated venous pressure, these patients commonly have dependent edema, ascites, and an enlarged, tender liver. The jugular venous pressure is elevated and does not fall normally, or it may rise with inspiration (Kussmaul's sign). The heart sounds may be distant, and third and fourth heart sounds are common. In contrast to constrictive pericarditis, which these diseases resemble, the apex impulse is usually easily palpable, and mitral regurgitation is more common. The electrocardiogram shows low-voltage, nonspecific ST-T-wave changes and various arrhythmias. Pericardial calcification on x-ray, which would suggest constrictive pericarditis, is absent. Echocardiography typically reveals symmetrically thickened left ventricular walls and normal or slightly reduced systolic function. Doppler recordings demonstrate accentuated early diastolic filling. Cardiac catheterization shows a decreased cardiac output, elevation of the right and left ventricular end-diastolic pressures, and a dip-and-plateau configuration of the diastolic portion of the ventricular pressure pulse resembling that seen in constrictive pericarditis.

Differentiation from constrictive pericarditis, at the bedside and even after cardiac catheterization, may be difficult or impossible (Chaps. 192 and 206.) This distinction is of importance because the latter condition is potentially curable by operation. Helpful in the differentiation of these two diseases are right ventricular transvenous endomyocardial biopsy (by revealing interstitial infiltration or fibrosis in restrictive cardiomyopathy) and computed tomography or magnetic resonance imaging (by demonstrating a thickened pericardium in constrictive pericarditis).

Endomyocardial fibrosis This is a progressive disease of unknown cause that occurs most commonly in children and young adults residing in tropical and subtropical Africa, particularly Uganda and Nigeria. The disease is characterized by fibrous endocardial lesions of the inflow portion of the right or left ventricle (or both) and often involves the atrioventricular valves, producing valvular regurgitation. The apex of the ventricles may be obliterated by a mass of thrombus and fibrous tissue. In many ways this disease resembles eosinophilic endomyocardial disease, although they occur in quite different geographic areas and age groups. Endomyocardial fibrosis is a frequent cause of heart failure in Africa, accounting for up to one-quarter of deaths due to heart disease.

The clinical picture depends on which ventricle and atrioventricular valve show predominant involvement; left-sided involvement results in symptoms of pulmonary congestion, while predominant right-sided disease presents features of a restrictive cardiomyopathy. Medical treatment is often disappointing, and surgical excision of the fibrotic endocardium and replacement of the involved atrioventricular valve have led to substantial symptomatic improvement in a small number of patients.

Eosinophilic endomyocardial disease Also called *Loeffler's endocarditis* and *fibroplastic endocarditis*, this disease appears to be a subcategory of the hypereosinophilic syndrome in which the heart is predominantly involved, with cardiac damage the apparent result of the toxic effects of eosinophilic proteins. Typically, the endocardium of either or both ventricles thickens markedly, with involvement of the underlying myocardium. Large mural thrombi may develop in either ventricle, thereby compromising the size of the ventricular cavity and serving as a source of pulmonary and systemic emboli. Hepatosplenomegaly and localized eosinophilic infiltration of other organs are usually present. Routine management with digitalis, diuretics, afterload-reducing agents, and anticoagulation as indicated, in conjunction with glucocorticoids and cytotoxic drugs (hydroxyurea in particular), appears to have improved survival substantially.

Differential diagnosis Involvement of the heart is the most frequent cause of death in *primary amyloidosis* (Chap. 281), while clinically significant cardiac involvement is uncommon in the secondary form. Focal deposits of amyloid in elderly patients (*senile cardiac amyloidosis*) are common and usually clinically insignificant. In a minority of patients the clinical cardiac findings are identical to those of primary amyloidosis, the principal difference being the structural composition of the amyloid protein. Aspiration of abdominal fat or biopsy of the rectal mucosa, gingiva, liver, kidney, or myocardium permits the diagnosis to be made before death in over three-quarters of cases. The heart is firm, rubbery, and noncompliant, and four clinical presentations (alone or in combination) are seen: (1) diastolic dysfunction (restrictive cardiomyopathy), (2) systolic dysfunction, (3) arrhythmias, and (4) orthostatic hypotension. The two-dimensional echocardiogram may be helpful in making the diagnosis of amyloidosis and may show a thickened myocardial wall with a distinctive "speckled" appearance. *Hemochromatosis* (Chap. 345) should be suspected if cardiomyopathy occurs in the setting of diabetes mellitus, hepatic cirrhosis, and increased skin pigmentation. Phlebotomy may be of some benefit if employed early in the course of the disease. Continuous subcutaneous administration of deferoxamine may reduce body iron stores and result in clinical improvement. Myocardial *sarcoidosis* (Chap. 292) is generally associated with other manifestations of systemic disease and may have restrictive as well as congestive features, since cardiac infiltration by sarcoid granulomas results not only in increased stiffness of the myocardium but also in diminished systolic contractile function. A variety of arrhythmias, including atrioventricular block, have been noted.

HYPERTROPHIC CARDIOMYOPATHY   This disease is characterized by left ventricular hypertrophy, typically of a nondilated chamber, without obvious antecedent cause. The hypertrophy is thus not secondary to a cardiovascular or systemic disease, such as hypertension or aortic stenosis, that places a hemodynamic burden on the left ventricle. Two commonly found features of the disease have attracted the greatest attention: (1) heterogeneous left ventricular (LV) hypertrophy, often with asymmetric septal hypertrophy (ASH), wherein the upper portion of the interventricular septum is preferentially hypertrophied compared with the posterobasal left ventricular free wall, and (2) a dynamic left ventricular outflow tract pressure gradient, related to a narrowing of the subaortic area as a consequence of the midsystolic apposition of the anterior mitral valve leaflet against the hypertrophied septum, i.e., systolic anterior motion of the mitral valve (SAM). Initial studies of this disease emphasized the dynamic "obstructive" features, and it has been termed *idiopathic hypertrophic subaortic stenosis* (IHSS), *hypertrophic obstructive cardiomyopathy* (HOCM), and *muscular subaortic stenosis*. It has become clear, however, that only about one-quarter of patients with hypertrophic cardiomyopathy demonstrate an outflow tract gradient. The ubiquitous pathophysiologic abnormality is not systolic but rather *diastolic* dysfunction, characterized by increased stiffness of the hypertrophied muscle that results primarily from an abnormality in calcium handling with attendant intracellular calcium overload. This results in elevated diastolic filling pressures and is present despite a hyperdynamic left ventricle.

The pattern of hypertrophy is distinctive in hypertrophic cardiomyopathy and differs from that seen in secondary hypertrophy (as in hypertension). Most patients have striking regional variations in the extent of hypertrophy in different portions of the left ventricle, and the majority demonstrate a ventricular septum whose thickness is disproportionately increased when compared with the free wall. Other patients may demonstrate disproportionate involvement of the apex or left ventricular free wall; 10 percent or more of patients have concentric involvement of the ventricle. All, however, show a bizarre and disorganized arrangement of cardiac muscle cells in the septum, whether or not a gradient is present, along with a variable degree of myocardial fibrosis and abnormalities of the small intramural coronary arteries.

About half of all cases of hypertrophic cardiomyopathy are familially linked, and many are associated with one of several mutations of the beta cardiac myosin heavy chain gene on chromosome 14, with certain mutations associated with more malignant prognoses. The remainder of familial cases presumably are due to mutations of a different gene or genes. Echocardiographic studies have confirmed that about one-third of the first-degree relatives (i.e.,

parents, siblings, and children) of patients with familial hypertrophic cardiomyopathy have evidence of the disease, although in many of these patients the extent of hypertrophy is mild, no outflow tract pressure gradient is present, and symptoms are not prominent. Since the hypertrophic characteristics may not be apparent in childhood and only first appear in adolescence, a single normal echocardiogram in a child does not entirely exclude the presence of the disease. Genetic analysis of peripheral lymphocytes can identify the disease in subjects who demonstrate none of the gross morphologic features of the disease.

In contrast to the obstruction produced by a fixed narrowed orifice, such as valvular aortic stenosis, the pressure gradient in hypertrophic cardiomyopathy, when present, is dynamic and may change between examinations and even from beat to beat. Obstruction appears to result from further narrowing of an already small left ventricular outflow tract by systolic anterior motion of the mitral valve against the hypertrophied septum. While SAM may be found in a variety of other conditions besides hypertrophic cardiomyopathy, it is *always* found when obstruction is present in hypertrophic cardiomyopathy. Three basic mechanisms are involved in the production of the dynamic pressure gradient: (1) increased left ventricular contractility, which reduces ventricular systolic volume and increases the ejection velocity of the blood moving through the outflow tract, thus drawing the anterior mitral valve leaflet against the septum as a result of reduced distending pressure, (2) decreased ventricular volume (preload), which reduces further the size of the outflow tract, and (3) decreased aortic impedance and pressure (afterload), which increases the velocity of flow through the subaortic area and also reduces ventricular systolic volume. Interventions that increase myocardial contractility, such as exercise, isoproterenol, and digitalis glycosides, and those that reduce ventricular volume, such as the Valsalva maneuver, sudden standing, nitroglycerin, amyl nitrite, or tachycardia, all may cause an increase in the gradient and the murmur. Conversely, elevation of arterial pressure by phenylephrine, squatting, sustained handgrip, augmentation of venous return by passive leg raising, and expansion of the blood volume all increase ventricular volume and ameliorate the gradient and murmur.

Clinical features   Many patients with hypertrophic cardiomyopathy are asymptomatic and may be relatives of patients with known disease. Unfortunately, the first clinical manifestation of the disease may be sudden death, frequently occurring in children and young adults, often during or after physical exertion. In symptomatic patients, the most common complaint is dyspnea, largely due to increased stiffness of the left ventricular walls, which impairs ventricular filling and leads to elevated left ventricular diastolic and left atrial pressures. Other symptoms include angina pectoris, fatigue, syncope, and near-syncope ("graying-out spells"). Symptoms are not related to the presence or severity of an outflow gradient. Most patients with gradients demonstrate a double or triple apical impulse, a rapidly rising carotid arterial pulse, and a fourth heart sound. The hallmark of obstructive hypertrophic cardiomyopathy is a systolic murmur, which is typically harsh, diamond-shaped, and usually begins well after the first heart sound, since ejection is unimpeded early in systole. The murmur is best heard at the lower left sternal border as well as at the apex, where it is often more holosystolic and blowing in quality, no doubt due to the mitral regurgitation that usually accompanies obstructive hypertrophic cardiomyopathy.

Laboratory evaluation   The *electrocardiogram* commonly shows left ventricular hypertrophy and widespread, deep, broad Q waves that suggest an old myocardial infarction. Many patients demonstrate arrhythmias, both atrial (supraventricular tachycardia or atrial fibrillation) and ventricular (ventricular tachycardia), during ambulatory (Holter) monitoring. *Chest roentgenography* may be normal, although a mild to moderate increase in the cardiac silhouette is common. The mainstay of the diagnosis of hypertrophic cardiomyopathy is the *echocardiogram*, which demonstrates left ventricular hypertrophy, often with the septum 1.3 or more times the thickness of the high posterior left ventricular free wall. The septum may demonstrate an unusual ground glass appearance, probably related to its abnormal cellular architecture and myocardial fibrosis. Systolic anterior motion of the mitral valve is found in patients with pressure gradients. The left ventricular cavity typically is small in hypertrophic cardiomyopathy, with vigorous posterior wall motion but reduced septal excursion. A rare form of hypertrophic cardiomyopathy, characterized by apical hypertrophy, is often associated with giant negative T waves on the electrocardiogram and a "spade-shaped" left ventricular cavity on angiography, and usually has a benign clinical course. *Radionuclide scintigraphy* with thallium 201 frequently reveals evidence of myocardial perfusion defects even in asymptomatic patients.

The two typical *hemodynamic* features are an elevated left ventricular diastolic pressure due to diminished left ventricular compliance and, when obstruction is present, a systolic pressure gradient between the body of the left ventricle and the subaortic region. When a gradient is not present, it often can be induced by provocative maneuvers such as infusion of isoproterenol, inhalation of amyl nitrite, or the Valsalva maneuver.

Treatment Beta-adrenergic blockers often are used and may ameliorate to some degree the symptoms of angina pectoris and syncope in one-third to one-half of patients. Resting intraventricular pressure gradients usually are unchanged, although these drugs may limit the increase in the gradient that occurs during exercise. It is not known whether beta-adrenergic blockers offer any protection against sudden death, which presumably is arrhythmic in origin. It is not established whether any antiarrhythmic agent is efficacious in this setting. However, amiodarone appears to be effective in reducing the frequency of supraventricular as well as life-threatening ventricular arrhythmias. Verapamil and diltiazem may reduce the stiffness of the ventricle, reduce the elevated diastolic pressures, increase exercise tolerance, and, in some instances, reduce the severity of outflow tract gradients, although adverse side effects occur in about one-quarter of patients. Disopyramide has been used in some patients to reduce left ventricular contractility and the outflow gradient. Dual-chamber permanent pacing recently has gained favor because it improves symptoms and reduces the outflow gradient in patients with severe symptoms, presumably by altering the pattern of ventricular contraction. Surgical myotomy/myectomy of the hypertrophied septum may result in lasting symptomatic improvement in about three-quarters of operated patients, but the mortality of approximately 5 percent limits the operation to severely symptomatic patients with large pressure gradients who are unresponsive to medical management. Digitalis, diuretics, nitrates, and beta-adrenergic agonists are best avoided if possible, particularly in patients with known left ventricular outflow tract pressure gradients.

Prognosis The natural history of hypertrophic cardiomyopathy is variable, although many patients demonstrate an improvement or stabilization of symptoms with time. Atrial fibrillation is common late in the course of the disease; its onset may lead to an increase in symptoms, presumably due to loss of the atrial contribution to filling of the thickened ventricle. Infective endocarditis occurs in less than 10 percent of patients, and endocarditis prophylaxis is indicated, particularly in patients with resting obstruction and mitral regurgitation. Progression of hypertrophic cardiomyopathy to left ventricular dilatation and dysfunction without an outflow gradient has been reported but is unusual; in about 5 to 10 percent of patients, however, some degree of left ventricular systolic impairment, wall thinning, and chamber enlargement occurs over time. The major cause of mortality in hypertrophic cardiomyopathy is sudden death, which may occur in asymptomatic patients or interrupt an otherwise stable course in symptomatic ones. Predictors of sudden death include age less than 30 years, ventricular tachycardia on ambulatory monitoring, marked ventricular hypertrophy, syncope, and a family history of sudden death. There is no correlation between the risk of sudden death and the severity of symptoms or the presence or severity of an outflow tract pressure gradient. Since sudden death often occurs during or just after physical exertion, strenuous exercise should be avoided in all patients, regardless of symptoms. Hemodynamic factors

appear to play a role. It is likely that most deaths, particularly those that are sudden, are due to ventricular arrhythmias.

MYOCARDITIDES

Myocarditis is said to be present when the heart is involved in an inflammatory process. Most commonly the result of an infectious process, myocarditis also may be present in hypersensitivity states such as acute rheumatic fever (Chap. 200) or may be caused by radiation, chemicals, physical agents, and drugs. In an unknown number of cases, acute myocarditis progresses to chronic dilated cardiomyopathy. While almost every infectious agent is capable of producing myocarditis, clinically significant acute myocarditis in the United States is caused most commonly by viruses, especially coxsackievirus B. In most cases the clinical manifestations are nonspecific (fatigue, dyspnea), and the presence of myocarditis is inferred only by the finding of transient electrocardiographic ST-T-wave abnormalities, but arrhythmias, heart failure, and death may occur in fulminant cases, particularly in infants and pregnant women. In some patients myocarditis simulates acute myocardial infarction, with chest pain, electrocardiographic changes, and elevated serum levels of myocardial enzymes.

Physical examination may be normal in patients who have only electrocardiographic abnormalities, although more severe cases may show a muffled first heart sound, along with a third heart sound and a murmur of mitral regurgitation. A pericardial friction rub may be audible in patients with associated pericarditis.

Experimental studies suggest that exercise may be deleterious in patients with myocarditis, and strenuous activity should be proscribed until the electrocardiogram has returned to normal. Patients who develop congestive heart failure respond to the usual measures (digitalis, diuretics, salt restriction), but they appear to be unusually sensitive to digitalis. Arrhythmias are common and are occasionally difficult to manage. Deaths attributed to heart failure, tachyarrhythmias, and heart block have been reported, and it seems prudent to monitor the electrocardiogram of patients with arrhythmias, especially during the acute illness.

Though viral myocarditis is most often self-limited and without sequelae, severe involvement may recur, and it is likely that acute viral myocarditis occasionally progresses to a chronic form. Patients with viral myocarditis often give a history of a preceding upper respiratory febrile illness, and viral nasopharyngitis or tonsillitis may be evident clinically. The isolation of virus from the stool, pharyngeal washings, or other body fluids and changes in specific antibody titers are helpful clinically. Some instances of apparent *idiopathic* dilated cardiomyopathy (p. 1089) appear to arise from mild or subclinical episodes of myocarditis. While glucocorticoids may exacerbate heart damage in animals with acute viral myocarditis, a small number of patients with congestive heart failure and inflammatory myocarditis appear to have responded to immunosuppression. Serial right ventricular endomyocardial biopsies have shown regression of inflammatory infiltrates in some patients so treated. However, such therapy remains experimental at present.

Bacterial myocarditis Bacterial involvement of the heart is uncommon, but when it does occur, it is usually as a complication of bacterial endocarditis (typically due to *Staphylococcus aureus* and enterococci). Myocardial abscess formation may involve the valve rings and interventricular septum. *Diphtheritic myocarditis* develops in over one-quarter of the patients with diphtheria, is one of the most serious complications, and is the most common cause of death due to diphtheria (Chap. 104). Cardiac damage is due to the liberation of a toxin that inhibits protein synthesis and leads to a dilated, flabby, hypocontractile heart; the conducting system is frequently involved as well. Cardiomegaly and severe congestive heart failure typically appear after the first week of illness. Prompt therapy with antitoxin is crucial; antibiotic therapy is also indicated but is of less urgency.

Chagas' disease Chagas' disease, caused by the protozoan *Trypanosoma cruzi* and transmitted by an insect vector (Chap. 176), produces an extensive myocarditis that typically becomes evident years after the initial infection. It is one of the most common causes of heart disease encountered in Central and South America; in rural areas up to 20 percent of the population may be affected. An increasing number of cases are found in the United States as patients migrate from endemic areas. Although only a minority of infected individuals have an acute illness, upwards of one-third develop chronic myocardial damage. Electrocardiographic evidence of cardiac involvement may appear in adolescence, although symptoms often do not appear until adulthood. The chronic form is characterized by dilatation of several cardiac chambers, fibrosis and thinning of the ventricular wall, aneurysm formation in the areas of thinning (especially at the apex), and mural thrombi. Chronic progressive heart failure is the rule and is associated with reduced survival. The electrocardiogram typically shows right bundle branch block and left anterior hemiblock, which may progress to complete atrioventricular block. The echocardiogram may reveal a unique pattern of hypokinesis of the posterior left ventricular wall and relatively preserved septal motion. Ventricular arrhythmias are common and are seen especially during and after exertion; oral amiodarone appears to be particularly effective in treating ventricular tachyarrhythmias. The cause of death is either intractable congestive heart failure or an arrhythmia. Therapy is directed toward amelioration of the congestive heart failure and arrhythmias; progressive conduction system disease and heart block may require implantation of a pacemaker. Medical therapy is often unsatisfactory or unavailable, however, and a more promising tactic has been the institution of public health measures, particularly the use of insecticides to eliminate the vector.

Toxoplasmic myocarditis (See also Chap. 177) This uncommon form of protozoal myocardial involvement occurs most frequently in immunosuppressed adults; congenital toxoplasmal infections are much more common, but myocarditis is not a prominent feature. Myocardial involvement may lead to cardiac dilatation, pericarditis, and pericardial effusion. Heart failure, arrhythmias, and conduction abnormalities may be seen. Because of the difficulty in diagnosing this condition, it may be a more common problem than is usually appreciated. Treatment is with pyrimethamine and sulfonamides, but the response to treatment is variable.

Giant cell myocarditis This rare myocarditis of unknown cause is characterized by the presence of multinucleated giant cells in the myocardium. It usually causes rapidly fatal congestive heart failure and arrhythmia in young to middle-aged adults. At necropsy, the distinctive features include cardiac enlargement, ventricular thrombi, grossly visible serpiginous areas of myocardial necrosis in both ventricles, and microscopic evidence of giant cells within an extensive inflammatory infiltrate. The cause of giant cell myocarditis remains obscure, although it occurs in association with thymoma, systemic lupus erythematosus, and thyrotoxicosis. No therapy has been shown to be efficacious.

Lyme carditis (See also Chap. 137) Lyme disease is caused by a tick-borne spirochete and is most common in the Northeast, upper Midwest and Pacific Coastal regions of the United States during the summer months. About 10 percent of patients develop symptomatic cardiac involvement, with conduction abnormalities the most common manifestations. Concomitant myopericarditis is not uncommon, and mild asymptomatic left ventricular dysfunction may occur. Intravenous ceftriaxone or penicillin is used in all but the mildest forms of Lyme carditis, in which case oral amoxicillin or doxycycline is employed. A temporary pacemaker may be needed for symptomatic heart block; the utility of glucocorticoids in reversing heart block is uncertain, but they are usually employed.

Human immunodeficiency virus myocarditis Many HIV-infected patients have subclinical cardiac involvement, including pericardial effusion, right-sided chamber enlargement, and neoplastic involvement. The most common finding is left ventricular dysfunction, often due to myocarditis, that in some cases appears to be due to infiltration of the myocardium by the virus itself. The clinical manifestations of cardiac involvement may be incorrectly attributed to concurrent noncardiac problems such as pneumonia. This is unfortunate, since the dilated cardiomyopathy of HIV infection may respond at least transiently to standard therapy with digitalis, diuretics, and vasodilators.

REFERENCES

COHN LH et al: Long-term follow-up of patients undergoing myotomy/myectomy for obstructive hypertrophic cardiomyopathy. Am J Cardiol 70:657, 1992

FANANAPAZIR L et al: Impact of dual-chamber permanent pacing in patients with obstructive hypertrophic cardiomyopathy with symptoms refractory to verapamil and β-adrenergic blocker therapy. Circulation 85:2149, 1992

FRIMAN G, FOHLMAN J: The epidemiology of viral heart disease. Scand J Infect Dis Suppl 88:7, 1993

GILBERT EM et al: Beta-adrenergic receptor regulation and left ventricular function in idiopathic dilated cardiomyopathy. Am J Cardiol 71:23C, 1993

GWATHMEY JK et al: Diastolic dysfunction in hypertrophic cardiomyopathy. J Clin Invest 87:1023, 1991

HAGAR JM, RAHIMTOOLA SH: Chagas' heart disease in the United States. N Engl J Med 325:763, 1991

JACOB AJ et al: Effects of abstinence on alcoholic heart muscle disease. Am J Cardiol 68:805, 1991

KLONER RA et al: The effects of acute and chronic cocaine use on the heart. Circulation 85:407, 1992

LARSEN L et al: Sudden death in idiopathic dilated cardiomyopathy: Role of ventricular arrhythmias. PACE Pacing Clin Electrophysiol 16:1051, 1993

MANOLIO TA et al: Prevalence and etiology of idiopathic dilated cardiomyopathy (summary of a National Heart, Lung, and Blood Institute workshop). Am J Cardiol 69:1458, 1992

MIDEI MG et al: Peripartum myocarditis and cardiomyopathy. Circulation 81:922, 1990

NARULA J et al: Recognition of acute myocarditis masquerading as acute myocardial infarction. N Engl J Med 328:100, 1993

WATKINS H et al: Characteristics and prognostic implications of myosin missense mutations in familial hypertrophic cardiomyopathy. N Engl J Med 326:1108, 1992

WYNNE J, BRAUNWALD E: The cardiomyopathies and myocarditides: Toxic, chemical and physical damage to the heart, in *Heart Disease*, 4th ed, E Braunwald (ed). Philadelphia, Saunders, 1992, pp 1394–1450

206 PERICARDIAL DISEASE

EUGENE BRAUNWALD

NORMAL FUNCTIONS OF THE PERICARDIUM The visceral pericardium is a serous membrane which is separated by a small amount (15 to 50 mL) of fluid, an ultrafiltrate of plasma, from a fibrous sac, the parietal pericardium. The pericardium prevents sudden dilatation of the cardiac chambers during exercise and hypervolemia, and as the result of the development of a negative intrapericardial pressure during ejection, it facilitates atrial filling during ventricular systole. The pericardium also restricts the anatomic position of the heart, minimizes friction between the heart and surrounding structures, prevents displacement of the heart and kinking of the great vessels, and probably retards the spread of infections from the lungs and pleural cavities to the heart. Notwithstanding the foregoing, total absence of the pericardium does not produce obvious clinical disease. In partial left pericardial defects the main pulmonary artery and left atrium may bulge through the defect; very rarely, herniation and subsequent strangulation of the left atrium may cause sudden death.

ACUTE PERICARDITIS

It is useful to classify the types of pericarditis both clinically and etiologically (Table 206-1), since this disorder is by far the most common pathologic process involving the pericardium. Pain, a pericardial friction rub, electrocardiographic changes, and pericardial effusion with cardiac tamponade and paradoxic pulse are cardinal

TABLE 206-1 Classification of pericarditis

I **Clinical classification**
  A Acute pericarditis (<6 weeks)
    1 Fibrinous
    2 Effusive (or bloody)
  B Subacute pericarditis (6 weeks to 6 months)
    1 Constrictive
    2 Effusive-constrictive
  C Chronic pericarditis (>6 months)
    1 Constrictive
    2 Effusive
    3 Adhesive (nonconstrictive)
II **Etiologic classification**
  A Infectious pericarditis
    1 Viral
    2 Pyogenic
    3 Tuberculous
    4 Mycotic
    5 Other infections (syphilitic, parasitic)
  B Noninfectious pericarditis
    1 Acute myocardial infarction
    2 Uremia
    3 Neoplasia
      a Primary tumors (benign or malignant)
      b Tumors metastatic to pericardium
    4 Myxedema
    5 Cholesterol
    6 Chylopericardium
    7 Trauma
      a Penetrating chest wall
      b Nonpenetrating
    8 Aortic aneurysm (with leakage into pericardial sac)
    9 Postirradiation
    10 Associated with atrial septal defect
    11 Associated with severe chronic anemia
    12 Infectious mononucleosis
    13 Familial Mediterranean fever
    14 Familial pericarditis
      a Mulibrey nanism*
    15 Sarcoidosis
    16 Acute idiopathic
  C Pericarditis presumably related to hypersensitivity or autoimmunity
    1 Rheumatic fever
    2 Collagen vascular disease
      a Systemic lupus erythematosus
      b Rheumatoid arthritis
      c Scleroderma
    3 Drug-induced
      a Procainamide
      b Hydralazine
      c Other
    4 Postcardiac injury
      a Postmyocardial infarction (Dressler's syndrome)
      b Postpericardiotomy

* An autosomal recessive syndrome, characterized by growth failure, muscle hypotonia, hepatomegaly, ocular changes, enlarged cerebral ventricles, mental retardation, and chronic constrictive pericarditis.

manifestations of many forms of acute pericarditis and will be considered prior to a discussion of the most common forms of the disorder.

Chest pain is an important but not invariable symptom in various forms of acute pericarditis (Chap. 12); it is usually present in the acute infectious types and in many of the forms presumed to be related to hypersensitivity or autoimmunity. Pain is often absent in a slowly developing tuberculous, postirradiation, neoplastic, or uremic pericarditis. The pain of pericarditis is often severe. It is characteristically retrosternal and left precordial, referred to the back and the trapezius ridge. Often the pain is pleuritic consequent to accompanying pleural inflammation, i.e., sharp and aggravated by inspiration, coughing, and changes in body position, but sometimes it is a steady, constrictive pain which radiates into either arm or both arms and resembles that of myocardial ischemia; therefore, confusion with myocardial infarction is common. Characteristically, however, the pericardial pain may be relieved by sitting up and leaning forward. The differentiation of acute myocardial infarction from acute pericarditis becomes even more perplexing when, with acute pericarditis, the serum transaminase and creatine kinase levels rise, presumably

because of concomitant involvement of the epicardium. However, these enzyme elevations, if they occur, are quite modest, given the extensive electrocardiographic ST-segment elevation in pericarditis.

The *pericardial friction rub* is the most important physical sign; it may have up to three components per cardiac cycle and is high-pitched, scratching, and grating, as described in Chap. 188; it can sometimes be elicited only when firm pressure with the diaphragm of the stethoscope is applied to the chest wall at the left lower sternal border. It is heard most frequently during expiration with the patient in the sitting position, but an independent pleural friction rub may be audible during inspiration with the patient leaning forward or in the left lateral decubitus position. The rub is often inconstant and transitory, and a loud to-and-fro leathery sound may disappear within a few hours, possibly to reappear the following day.

Moderate elevations of the MB fraction of creatine phosphokinase may occur and reflect accompanying epimyocarditis.

The *electrocardiogram* in acute pericarditis without massive effusion usually displays changes secondary to acute subepicardial inflammation (see Fig. 189-19, p. 964). There is widespread elevation of the ST segments, involving two or three standard limb leads and V_2 to V_6, with reciprocal depressions only in aVR and sometimes V_1 and without significant changes in QRS complexes, except for some reduction in voltage in patients with large pericardial effusions. After several days, the ST segments return to normal, and only then do the T waves become inverted. In contrast, in acute myocardial infarction, reciprocal depression of ST segments is usually more prominent; QRS changes occur, particularly the development of Q waves, as well as notching and loss of the amplitude of R waves; and T-wave inversions usually occur within hours *before* the ST segments have become isoelectric. Sequential electrocardiograms are useful in distinguishing acute pericarditis from acute myocardial infarction. In the latter, elevated ST segments return to normal within hours. Early repolarization is a normal variant and also may cause widespread ST-segment elevation, most prominent in left precordial leads. However, in this condition the T waves are usually tall and the ST/T ratio is under 0.25, but it exceeds this number in acute pericarditis. Depression of the PQ segment (below the TP segment) also is common and reflects atrial involvement. With large pericardial effusions, the QRS voltage is reduced; atrial premature beats and atrial fibrillation are sometimes noted.

PERICARDIAL EFFUSION Usually associated with pain and/or the above-mentioned electrocardiographic changes characteristic of pericarditis and an enlargement of the cardiac silhouette, pericardial effusion is especially important clinically when it develops within a relatively short time, since it may lead to cardiac tamponade. Differentiation from cardiac enlargement may be difficult, but heart sounds tend to become faint; the friction rub may disappear or remain clearly audible, and the apex impulse may vanish, but sometimes it remains palpable albeit medial to the left border of cardiac dullness. The base of the left lung may be compressed by pericardial fluid, producing Ewart's sign, a patch of dullness beneath the angle of the left scapula. The chest roentgenogram may show a ''water bottle'' configuration of the cardiac silhouette, but it also may be normal or almost so. Lucent pericardial fat lines may be seen deep within the cardiopericardial silhouette. Fluoroscopic examination may show the ventricular pulsations to be diminished.

Diagnosis of pericardial effusion Echocardiography (Chap. 190) is the most effective diagnostic laboratory technique available, since it is sensitive, specific, simple, innocuous, noninvasive, and may be performed at the bedside. The presence of pericardial fluid is recorded by two-dimensional transthoracic echocardiography as a relatively echo-free space between the posterior pericardium and left ventricular epicardium in patients with small effusions and a space between the anterior right ventricle and the parietal pericardium just beneath the anterior chest wall with larger effusions (Fig. 206-1). In patients with large effusions the heart may swing freely within the pericardial sac; when severe, the extent of this motion alternates and may be associated with electrical alternans. Echocardiography

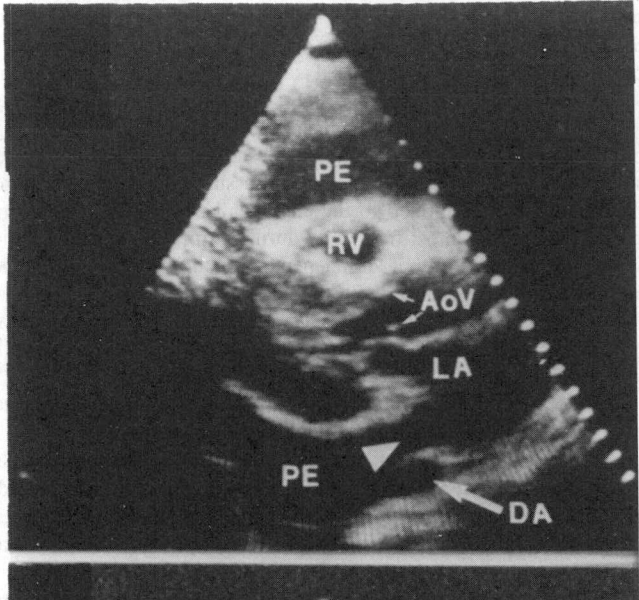

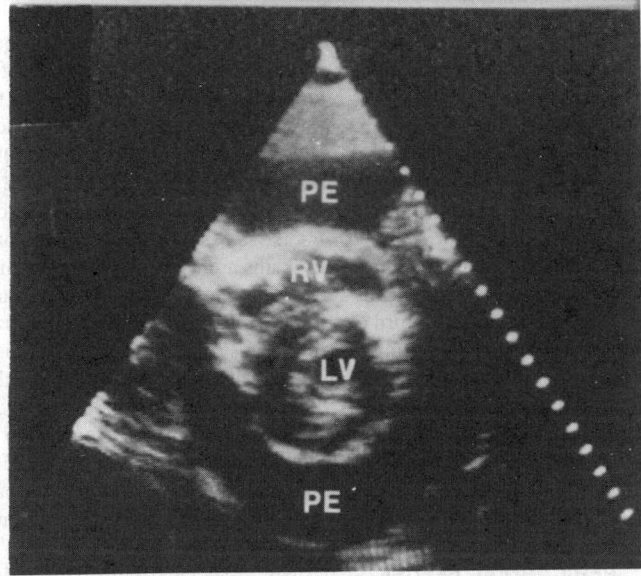

FIGURE 206-1   Two-dimensional (*upper panel*) and short-axis (*lower panel*) parasternal scans in systole in a patient with a large pericardial effusion surrounding the entire heart. Fluid is seen to extend behind the left atrium (*white arrowhead*) and anterior to the descending thoracic aorta (DA). AoV = aortic valve; LA = left atrium; LV = left ventricle; PE = pericardial effusion; RV = right ventricle. (*Modified from PC Come (ed), Diagnostic Cardiology: Noninvasive imaging techniques, Philadelphia, Lippincott, 1985.*)

also allows localization and estimation of the quantity of pericardial fluid. When pericardial effusion causes tamponade, during inspiration right ventricular diameter increases while left ventricular diameter and mitral valve opening decrease. Often the right ventricular cavity is reduced and there is late diastolic inward motion (collapse) of the right ventricular free wall and of the right atrium. Doppler ultrasound shows exaggerated tricuspid and pulmonic flow with reciprocal changes in mitral flow during inspiration. The diagnosis of pericardial fluid or thickening may be confirmed by computed tomography or magnetic resonance imaging (Chap 190); these techniques may be superior to echocardiography in detecting loculated pericardial effusions. At cardiac catheterization the catheter is introduced into the right atrium and rotated so that its tip makes contact with the lateral right atrial wall. In the presence of an effusion or pericardial thickening, the tip of the catheter is separated from the radiolucent lungs by an opaque band. When contrast medium is injected rapidly into the right atrium, the angiocardiogram also shows the lateral wall to be separated from the edge of the cardiac silhouette.

When it is deemed desirable to remove pericardial fluid for diagnostic and/or therapeutic purposes, a needle attached to a properly grounded electrocardiographic lead is inserted into the pericardial space, usually through a subxiphoid approach, and, if possible, using echocardiographic control. Intrapericardial pressure should be measured before fluid is withdrawn. Pericardial effusion nearly always has the physical characteristics of an exudate. Bloody fluid is commonly due to tuberculosis or tumor, but it also may be found in the effusion of rheumatic fever, in post-cardiac injury and post-myocardial infarction, especially following the administration of anticoagulants, and in uremic pericarditis.

CARDIAC TAMPONADE   The accumulation of fluid in the pericardium in an amount sufficient to cause serious obstruction to the inflow of blood to the ventricles results in cardiac tamponade, a grave complication which may be fatal if it is not treated promptly. The three most common causes of tamponade are neoplastic disease, idiopathic pericarditis, and uremia, but it also results from bleeding into the pericardial space following cardiac operations, trauma (including cardiac perforation during diagnostic procedures), tuberculosis, and hemopericardium; the latter may result when a patient with any form of acute pericarditis is treated with anticoagulants. The three principal features of tamponade are elevation of intracardiac pressures, limitation of ventricular filling in diastole, and reduction of cardiac output. The amount of fluid necessary to produce this critical state may be as small as 200 mL when the fluid develops rapidly or over 2000 mL in slowly developing effusions when the pericardium has had the opportunity to stretch and adapt to the increasing volume of fluid. The volume of fluid required to produce tamponade also varies directly with the thickness of the ventricular myocardium and inversely with the thickness of the parietal pericardium.

Table 206-2 lists the features that distinguish cardiac tamponade from constrictive pericarditis. The classic findings of falling arterial pressure, rising venous pressure, and a small, quiet heart with faint heart sounds usually are seen only with severe, acute tamponade, as occurs with cardiac trauma or rupture. Tamponade may also develop more slowly, and the clinical manifestations resemble those of heart failure, including dyspnea, orthopnea, hepatic engorgement, and jugular venous hypertension. A high index of suspicion for cardiac tamponade is required, since, in many instances, no obvious cause for pericardial disease is apparent, and tamponade should be considered in any patient with hypotension and elevation of jugular venous pressure with a prominent x descent; in contrast to constrictive pericarditis, often the y descent is diminutive or absent. A positive Kussmaul sign (see below) is rare in cardiac tamponade, as is a pericardial knock. Their presence suggests that an organizing process and epicardial constriction are present in addition to effusion. A widening of the area of flatness to percussion across the anterior aspect of the chest wall, a paradoxical pulse (see below), relatively clear lung fields, diminished pulsations of the cardiac silhouette on fluoroscopy, enlargement of the cardiac silhouette (especially in subacute or chronic tamponade), reduction in amplitude of the QRS complexes, and *electrical alternans* of the P, QRS, and T waves should raise the suspicion of cardiac tamponade.

Since immediate treatment of tamponade may be lifesaving, prompt measures to establish the diagnosis, i.e., echocardiography sometimes followed by cardiac catheterization, should be undertaken. The latter reveals elevation of the right atrial pressure with prominence of the x but not of the y descent (Table 206-2). When measured, the pericardial pressure is also elevated and equal to the right atrial pressure. There is "equalization" of pressures, i.e., the pulmonary artery wedge is equal, or close, to right atrial, right ventricular, and pulmonary artery diastolic pressures. The "square root" sign in the ventricular pressure pulses and the prominent y descent in atrial and jugular venous pressure are characteristic of constrictive pericarditis (see below) and are usually absent in tamponade. In an emergency, pericardiocentesis may be carried out without cardiac catheterization but preferably after confirmation of the clinical diagnosis by echocardiography.

TABLE 206-2 Features that distinguish constrictive pericarditis from similar clinical disorders

Characteristic	Tamponade	Constrictive pericarditis	Restrictive cardiomyopathy	RVMI*
Clinical				
Pulsus paradoxus	Common	Usually absent	Rare	Rare
Jugular veins				
Prominent y descent	Absent	Usually present	Rare	Rare
Prominent x descent	Present	Usually absent	Present	Rare
Kussmaul's sign	Absent	Present	Absent	Absent
Third heart sound	Absent	Absent	Rare	May be present
Pericardial knock	Absent	Often present	Absent	Absent
Electrocardiogram				
Low ECG voltage	May be present	May be present	May be present	Absent
Electrical alternans	May be present	Absent	Absent	Absent
Echocardiography				
Thickened pericardium	Absent	Present	Absent	Absent
Pericardial calcification	Absent	Often present	Absent	Absent
Pericardial effusion	Present	Absent	Absent	Absent
RV size	Usually small	Usually normal	Usually normal	Enlarged
Myocardial thickness	Normal	Normal	Usually increased	Normal
Right atrial collapse and RVDC	Present	Absent	Absent	Absent
Increased early filling mitral flow velocity	Absent	Present	Present	May be present
Exaggerated respiratory variation in flow velocity	Present	Present	Absent	Absent
Computed tomography, Magnetic resonance imaging				
Thickened/calcific pericardium	Absent	Present	Absent	Absent
Cardiac catheterization				
Equalization of diastolic procedures	Usually present	Usually present	Usually absent	Absent or present
Cardiac biopsy helpful?	No	No	Somewhat	No

* RV = right ventricle, RVMI = right ventricular myocardial infarction, RVDC = right ventricular diastolic collapse, ECG = electrocardiograph
SOURCE: From GM Brockington et al, Cardiol Clin 8:645, 1990.

Paradoxical pulse This important clue to the presence of cardiac tamponade consists of *a greater than normal (10 mmHg) inspiratory decline in systolic arterial pressure.* When severe, it may be detected by palpating weakness or disappearance of the arterial pulse during inspiration, but usually sphygmomanometric measurement of systolic pressure during slow respiration is required (Fig. 206-2).

Since both ventricles share a tight incompressible covering, i.e., the pericardial sac, in cardiac tamponade the inspiratory enlargement of the right ventricle compresses and reduces left ventricular volume substantially; leftward bulging of the interventricular septum further reduces the left ventricular cavity as the right ventricle enlarges during inspiration. Thus in cardiac tamponade the normal inspiratory augmentation of right ventricular volume causes an exaggerated reciprocal reduction in left ventricular volume. Also, respiratory distress increases the fluctuations in intrathoracic pressure, which exaggerates the mechanism just described. Right ventricular infarction (Chap. 202) may resemble cardiac tamponade with hypotension, elevated jugular venous pressure, an absent y descent in the jugular venous pulse, and occasionally pulsus paradoxus. The differentiation between these two conditions is shown in Table 206-2.

Paradoxical pulse, a hallmark of cardiac tamponade, occurs in only approximately one-third of patients with *constrictive pericarditis.* It is important to bear in mind that paradoxical pulse is not pathognomonic of pericardial disease because it may be observed in various forms of restrictive cardiomyopathies (Chap. 205) and in some cases of hypovolemic shock, chronic obstructive airways disease, and severe bronchial asthma.

Low-pressure tamponade refers to mild tamponade in which the intrapericardial pressure is increased from its slightly subatmospheric levels to +5 to +10 mmHg; in some instances hypovolemia coexists. As a consequence, the central venous pressure is normal or only slightly elevated while arterial pressure is unaffected. The patients are asymptomatic or complain of mild weakness and dyspnea. The

diagnosis is aided by echocardiography, and both hemodynamic and clinical manifestations improve following pericardiocentesis.

TREATMENT Patients with acute pericarditis should be placed at bed rest until pain and fever have disappeared. Anticoagulants should be avoided. The patient should be observed frequently for the development of an effusion; if a moderate or large effusion is already present, the patient should be hospitalized and signs of tamponade must be watched for carefully. In the presence of an effusion, arterial and venous pressures and heart rate should be monitored continuously or followed carefully and serial echocardiograms obtained. If manifestations of tamponade appear, pericardiocentesis must be carried out at once, since relief of the intrapericardial pressure may be lifesaving. A small catheter advanced over the needle inserted into the pericardial cavity may be left in place to allow draining of the pericardial space if fluid reaccumulates. When a *diagnostic* pericardiocentesis of a large effusion is carried out, an attempt should be made to remove as much fluid as possible.

VIRAL OR IDIOPATHIC FORM OF ACUTE PERICARDITIS This disorder is an important clinical entity because of its frequency and because it may be confused with other, more serious illnesses. In some cases, an A or B coxsackievirus or the virus of influenza, echovirus type 8, mumps, herpes simplex, chickenpox, or adenovirus has been isolated from pericardial fluid and/or appropriate elevations in viral antibody titers have been noted; in many instances, acute pericarditis has occurred in association with illnesses of known viral origin and, presumably, was caused by the same agent. Commonly, there is an antecedent infection of the respiratory tract, but in many patients such an association is not evident and viral isolation and serologic studies are negative. Most frequently, a viral causation cannot be established, nor can it be excluded; the term *acute idiopathic pericarditis* is then appropriate.

Regardless of the specific causative factor, the clinical manifestations are similar. Acute pericarditis occurs at all ages but is more

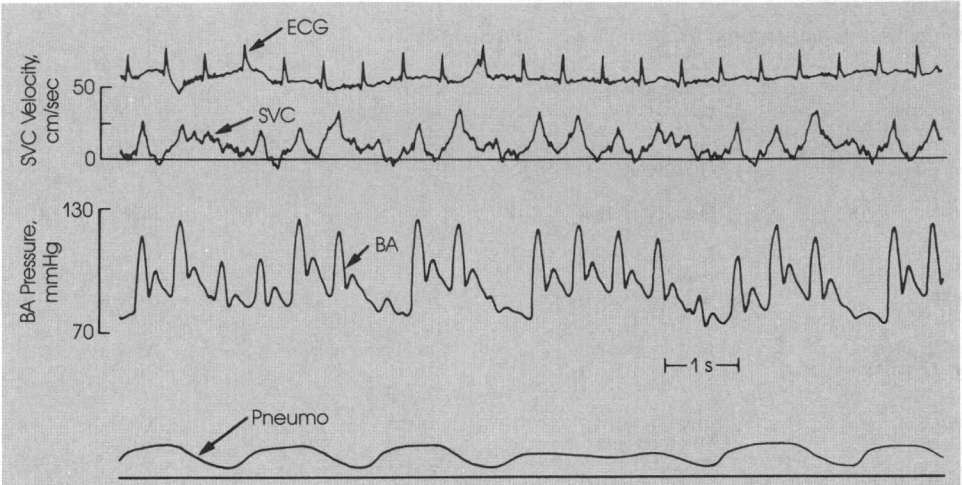

FIGURE 206-2 Simultaneous recording of electrocardiogram (ECG), blood flow velocity in the superior vena cava (SVC), brachial arterial pressure (BA), and the pneumogram (Pneumo) in a patient with cardiac compression and paradoxical pulse. A downward deflection of the pneumogram denotes inspiration, when SVC blood velocity rises and arterial pressure falls (paradoxical pulse). Arterial pressure is maintained during prolonged expiratory pause.

frequent in young adults; it is often associated with pleural effusions and pneumonitis. The appearance of fever and precordial pain at about the same time, often 10 to 12 days after a presumed viral illness, constitutes an important feature in the differentiation of acute pericarditis from myocardial infarction, in which pain precedes fever. The constitutional symptoms are usually mild to moderate, but occasionally the initial symptoms are stormy, the temperature rising to 40°C. The disease ordinarily runs its course in a few days to 4 weeks, but one or more recurrences occur in about one-fourth of patients. Although accumulation of some pericardial fluid is common, tamponade is unusual, and constrictive pericarditis develops rarely. A pericardial friction rub is often audible. The ST-segment alterations in the electrocardiogram are usually transitory, but the abnormal T waves may persist for several years or indefinitely and be a source of confusion in persons without a clear history of pericarditis. Pleuritis and pneumonitis frequently accompany pericarditis. The erythrocyte sedimentation rate is elevated. Granulocytosis followed by lymphocytosis is common.

Management   There is no specific therapy, but bed rest and anti-inflammatory treatment with aspirin, if necessary up to 900 mg qid, may be given. If this is ineffective, one of the nonsteroidal anti-inflammatory agents, such as indomethacin (25 to 75 mg qid) or a glucocorticoid (e.g., prednisone, 20 to 80 mg daily) effectively suppresses the clinical manifestations of the acute illness and may be useful in patients in whom the purulent and tuberculous forms of pericarditis have been excluded. After the patient has been asymptomatic and afebrile for about 1 week, the dose of the anti-inflammatory agent is gradually tapered. Occasionally, tamponade progression to chronic constrictive pericarditis occurs. When recurrences are multiple, frequent, disabling, and continue beyond 2 years, pericardiectomy may be effective in terminating the illness.

POST-CARDIAC INJURY SYNDROME   An acute form of pericarditis may appear under a variety of circumstances which have one common feature: previous injury to the myocardium, with blood in the pericardial cavity. The syndrome has been observed when the injury has been induced in the course of a cardiac operation (postpericardiotomy syndrome). It also may follow myocardial infarction (Dressler's syndrome) (Chap. 202) or develop after trauma of the heart (Chap. 207), e.g., a stab wound, contusions after a nonpenetrating blow to the chest, or perforation of the heart with a catheter.

The principal symptom is the pain of acute pericarditis, which usually develops 1 to 4 weeks following the cardiac injury but sometimes appears only after a lapse of months. Recurrences are common and may occur up to 2 years or more after the injury. Fever to 40°C, pericarditis, pleuritis, and pneumonitis are the outstanding features, the bout of illness usually subsiding in 1 or 2 weeks. The pericarditis, which appears to be the most constant lesion, may be of

the fibrinous variety, or it may be a pericardial effusion, which is often serosanguineous, rarely causes tamponade, and is accompanied by arthralgias. Leukocytosis, an increased sedimentation rate, and electrocardiographic changes typical of acute pericarditis also may occur.

The mechanisms responsible for this syndrome have not been identified, but there is a likelihood that they are the result of a hypersensitivity reaction in which the antigen originates from injured myocardial tissue and/or pericardium; the suggested designation of post-cardiac injury syndrome for this group of disorders implies that they may have a common pathogenetic mechanism. Circulating autoantibodies to myocardium occur frequently, but their precise role in this syndrome has not been defined. Viral infection also may play an etiologic role, since antiviral antibodies are often elevated in patients who develop this syndrome following cardiac surgery.

The clinical picture of the post-cardiac injury syndrome mimics acute viral or acute idiopathic pericarditis. Moreover, it is possible that the recurrences that occur so frequently in the latter condition are not always caused by an exacerbation of the original (presumably viral) infection but that the original injury may have initiated the sequence of events that culminates in the post-cardiac injury syndrome.

Often no treatment is necessary aside from aspirin and analgesics. The management of pericardial effusion and tamponade has already been discussed. When the illness is followed by a series of disabling recurrences, therapy with a nonsteroidal anti-inflammatory agent or a glucocorticoid is usually effective.

DIFFERENTIAL DIAGNOSIS   Since there is no specific test for *acute idiopathic pericarditis* the diagnosis is one of exclusion. Consequently, all other disorders that may be associated with acute fibrinous pericarditis must be considered. When associated with *acute myocardial infarction*, acute fibrinous pericarditis may be confused with acute viral or idiopathic pericarditis; this complication of infarction, described in Chap. 202 is characterized by the occurrence of fever, pain, and a friction rub in the first 4 days following the development of the infarct (to be distinguished from the pericarditis in Dressler's syndrome, which is a form of post-cardiac injury pericarditis and which occurs a week or two following myocardial infarction). Electrocardiographic abnormalities (such as the appearance of Q waves, brief ST-segment elevations with reciprocal changes, and earlier T-wave changes in myocardial infarction), the extent of the elevations of myocardial enzymes, and the total clinical picture are helpful in relating pericarditis to acute myocardial infarction. A common diagnostic error is assuming that acute viral or idiopathic pericarditis represents acute myocardial infarction and vice versa.

Acute pericarditis occurring as a component of the post-cardiac injury syndrome is most likely to be confused with acute idiopathic pericarditis. Pericarditis secondary to post-cardiac injury is differentiated from acute idiopathic pericarditis chiefly by timing. If it occurs within a few weeks of a myocardial infarction or a chest blow, it may be justified to conclude that the two are probably related. If the infarct has been silent or the chest blow forgotten, the relationship to the pericarditis may not be recognized.

It is important to distinguish *pericarditis due to collagen disease* from acute idiopathic pericarditis. Most important in the differential diagnosis is the pericarditis due to systemic lupus erythematosus (Chap. 284); often pain is present, sometimes the pericarditis appears as an asymptomatic effusion, and rarely, tamponade develops. Very rarely, when pericarditis occurs in the absence of other evidence of any underlying disorder, differentiation from acute viral and idiopathic pericarditis or tuberculous pericarditis may be made on discovery of lupus erythematosus (LE) cells, a rise in antinuclear antibodies, or by the specific methods for diagnosing tuberculosis (see below). Acute pericarditis may complicate the viral, pyrogenic, mycobacterial, and fungal infections that occur in AIDS. Acute pericarditis is an occasional complication of *rheumatoid arthritis, scleroderma,* and *polyarteritis nodosa,* but again, other evidence of these diseases is usually obvious. Asymptomatic pericardial effusion is also frequent in these disorders. It is important to question every patient with acute pericarditis about the ingestion of procainamide, hydralazine, isoniazid, cromolyn, and minoxidil, since these drugs can cause this syndrome.

The pericarditis of *acute rheumatic fever* is generally associated with evidence of severe pancarditis and with cardiac murmurs (Chap. 200). *Pyogenic (purulent) pericarditis* is usually secondary to cardiothoracic operations, immunosuppressive therapy, rupture of the esophagus into the pericardial sac, or rupture of a ring abscess in a patient with infective endocarditis and with septicemia complicating aseptic pericarditis. It is now uncommonly due to pneumococcal pneumonia and pleuritis, previously the most common cause. *Tuberculous pericarditis* (see Chap. 130) may present as an acute pericarditis, associated with fever, weight loss, and other clinical manifestations of active systemic tuberculosis; the diagnosis may be aided by a positive tuberculin test and evidence of pulmonary or mediastinal tuberculosis. Tubercle bacilli can be cultured from the pericardial space only infrequently, and a biopsy of the pericardium with bacteriologic and histologic examination may be required. Alternatively, tuberculous pericarditis may present as a chronic asymptomatic effusion, as subacute effusive-constrictive pericarditis (see below), or as frank chronic constrictive pericarditis (see below).

Uremic pericarditis (Chap. 237) occurs in up to one-third of patients with chronic uremia and is seen most frequently in patients undergoing chronic hemodialysis. It may be fibrinous or associated with a bloody effusion. A friction rub is common, but pain is usually absent. Treatment with an anti-inflammatory agent and intensification of hemodialysis is usually adequate. Occasionally, tamponade occurs and pericardiocentesis is required. When uremic pericarditis is recurrent, persistent or very troubling pericardiectomy may be necessary. Pericarditis due to *neoplastic diseases* results from extension or invasion of primary or metastatic tumors (most commonly carcinoma of the lung and breast, malignant melanoma, lymphoma, and leukemia) to the pericardium; pain, atrial arrhythmias, and tamponade are complications which occur occasionally. *Mediastinal irradiation* for neoplasm may cause pericarditis after eradication of the tumor. Unusual causes of acute pericarditis include syphilis, fungal infection (histoplasmosis, blastomycosis, aspergillosis, and candidiasis), and parasitic infestation (amebiasis, toxoplasmosis, echinococcosis, trichinosis).

CHRONIC PERICARDIAL EFFUSIONS   Chronic pericardial effusions are not infrequently encountered in patients without an antecedent history of acute pericarditis. They may cause few symptoms per se, and they may be suspected by finding an enlarged cardiac silhouette on chest roentgenogram which may be obtained in the course of the workup of a patient with symptoms related to the underlying illness.

Tuberculosis   This is a common cause of chronic pericardial effusion, although less so in the United States than in other parts of the world (Chap. 130). The symptoms are often those of a chronic,

systemic illness in an individual with pericardial effusion. It is important to bear this condition in mind when a middle-aged or elderly person with fever has apparent enlargement of the cardiac silhouette of undetermined origin, with or without elevation of venous pressure. Weight loss, fever, and fatigability are sometimes observed. Inasmuch as treatment is quite effective, overlooking a tuberculous pericardial effusion may cause serious consequences. Consequently, no method of examination should be omitted to exclude this diagnosis in such patients. Included are chest roentgenograms for pulmonary tuberculosis and a search for tuberculosis in other organs; tuberculin skin tests, repeated after several weeks; and cultures and smears of gastric washings and of pleural and pericardial fluid. Finally, if the etiology of chronic pericardial effusion is still obscure, a pericardial biopsy, preferably by a limited thoracotomy, should be performed. If definitive evidence is then still lacking but the specimen shows caseation necrosis, antituberculous chemotherapy for at least 24 months is justified (Chap. 130). Pericardiectomy should be carried out in order to prevent the development of constriction if the biopsy specimen shows a thickened pericardium.

Other causes of chronic pericardial effusion   *Myxedema* may be responsible for a pericardial effusion that is sometimes massive but rarely, if ever, causes cardiac tamponade. The other manifestations of myxedema should clarify the diagnosis, but unfortunately, even when they are present, the diagnosis is frequently overlooked. It is important, therefore, to carry out appropriate tests for thyroid function (Chap. 334) in patients with an enlarged cardiac outline of undetermined origin. The cardiac silhouette is markedly enlarged and an echocardiogram is necessary to distinguish cardiomegaly from pericardial effusion. *Cholesterol pericardial disease* produces large pericardial effusions with a high cholesterol content, which may induce an inflammatory response and constrictive pericarditis.

Neoplasms, systemic lupus erythematosus, rheumatoid arthritis, mycotic infections, radiation therapy, pyogenic infections, severe chronic anemia, and chylopericardium also may cause chronic pericardial effusion and should be considered and specifically looked for in such patients.

Aspiration and analysis of the pericardial fluid are often helpful in diagnosis. In infections the organism can often be identified by smear or culture. Grossly sanguineous pericardial fluid results most commonly from a neoplasm, tuberculosis, uremia, or slow leakage from an aortic aneurysm.

CHRONIC CONSTRICTIVE PERICARDITIS

This disorder results when the healing of an acute fibrinous or serofibrinous pericarditis or a chronic pericardial effusion is followed by obliteration of the pericardial cavity with the formation of granulation tissue. This gradually contracts and forms a firm scar, encasing the heart and interfering with filling of the ventricles. In some reports, a high percentage of all cases has been of tuberculous origin. In other series, particularly those reported in the United States in the last two decades, tuberculosis has been an infrequent cause. Chronic constrictive pericarditis also may follow purulent infection, trauma, cardiac operation of any type, mediastinal irradiation, histoplasmosis, neoplastic disease, and acute viral or idiopathic pericarditis, rheumatoid arthritis, lupus erythematosus, and chronic renal failure with uremia treated by chronic dialysis. In many patients the cause of the pericardial disease is undetermined, and in them an asymptomatic or forgotten bout of viral pericarditis, acute or idiopathic, may have been the inciting event. Routine radiographic examination may reveal calcification of the pericardium in a person who is free of all symptoms referable to the heart (calcific, not constrictive, pericarditis). The heart also may be constricted and compressed by malignant tumors or organized blood clot in the pericardial cavity.

The basic physiologic abnormality in symptomatic patients with chronic constrictive pericarditis, as in those with cardiac tamponade, is the inability of the ventricles to fill adequately during diastole because of the limitations imposed by the rigid, thickened pericardium or the tense pericardial fluid. However, in constrictive pericarditis ventricular filling is unimpeded during early diastole but is reduced abruptly when the elastic limit of the pericardium is reached, while in cardiac tamponade ventricular filling is impeded throughout diastole. In chronic constrictive pericarditis stroke volume is reduced, and the end-diastolic pressures in both ventricles and the mean pressures in the atria, pulmonic veins, and systemic veins are all elevated to about the same levels. Despite these hemodynamic changes, myocardial function may actually be normal or only slightly impaired; instead, the ventricles may be considered to be underloaded.

In constrictive pericarditis the central venous and right and left atrial pressure pulses display an M-shaped contour, with prominent x and y descents; the y descent (absent or diminished in cardiac tamponade) is the most prominent deflection and is interrupted by a rapid rise in pressure during early diastole, when ventricular filling is impeded by the constricting pericardium. These characteristic changes are transmitted to the jugular veins, where they may be recognized by inspection or recorded. In constrictive pericarditis, both ventricular pressure pulses exhibit characteristic ''square root'' signs during diastole. These hemodynamic changes, although characteristic, are not pathognomonic of constrictive pericarditis but also may be observed in cardiomyopathies characterized by restriction of ventricular filling, as discussed in Chap. 205.

CLINICAL FINDINGS (See Table 206-2) Weakness, fatigue, weight loss, and anorexia are common. The patient often appears to be chronically ill with decreased skeletal muscle mass and a protuberant abdomen. Contrary to a widely held impression, dyspnea, though absent or slight at rest, is often present on exertion, and orthopnea is common in chronic constrictive pericarditis, although it is not severe. However, attacks of acute left ventricular failure (acute pulmonary edema) practically never occur. The cervical veins are distended and may remain so even after intensive diuretic treatment, and venous pressure may fail to decline during inspiration (Kussmaul's sign). In about one-third of the cases a paradoxical pulse may be observed. Congestive hepatomegaly is pronounced and may impair hepatic function; ascites is common and is usually more prominent than dependent edema. In about half of patients the heart is normal in size; if it is enlarged, the enlargement is rarely extreme. The apical pulse is reduced in intensity, retracts in systole, and moves outward in diastole. The heart sounds may be distant; an early third heart sound, i.e., a pericardial knock, occurring 0.06 to 0.12 s after aortic valve closure which coincides with a sudden deceleration in ventricular filling, is often conspicuous; and murmurs are usually absent. The apex beat is poorly defined, and cardiac pulsations under fluoroscopic examination are diminished. Because of the high sustained venous pressure, congestive splenomegaly may make the spleen palpable. In the absence of infective endocarditis or tricuspid valve disease, splenomegaly in a patient with congestive heart failure should arouse suspicion of constrictive pericarditis. Protein-losing gastroenteropathy due to impaired lymphatic drainage from the small intestine, and the nephrotic syndrome, or marked proteinuria or hypoalbuminemia, may complicate chronic constrictive pericarditis.

The electrocardiogram frequently displays low voltage of the QRS complex and diffuse flattening or inversion of the T waves. P mitrale may be present in patients with sinus rhythm; atrial fibrillation is present in about one-third of patients. The echocardiogram usually, but not invariably, shows pericardial thickening and reduced amplitude of left ventricular wall motion, prominent early diastolic filling, and normal left ventricular size.

Systemic and/or pulmonary venous congestion is initially the result of impaired filling of the ventricles caused by the restrictive action of the inelastic pericardium. However, the fibrotic process may extend into the myocardium and cause myocardial scarring, and venous congestion may then be due to the combined effects of the myocardial and pericardial lesions. The interference with filling reduces the work of the heart, and perhaps this leads to myocardial atrophy. The latter

probably accounts for the delayed beneficial effects of operative treatment observed in some patients with advanced disease.

Inasmuch as the usual physical signs of cardiac disease (murmurs, cardiac enlargement) may be inconspicuous or absent in chronic constrictive pericarditis, hepatic enlargement and dysfunction associated with intractable ascites may lead to a mistaken diagnosis of cirrhosis of the liver. This error can be avoided if the neck veins are inspected carefully in all patients with ascites and hepatomegaly. *Given a clinical picture resembling hepatic cirrhosis, but with the added feature of distended neck veins, careful search for calcification of the pericardium by chest roentgenography, fluoroscopy, and echocardiography should be carried out and may disclose this curable or remediable form of heart disease.* Calcification occurs in only about one-half of these patients, usually in those with long-standing pericardial constriction. Most patients with chronic constrictive pericarditis show pericardial thickening on echocardiographic examination. However, echocardiography cannot definitively exclude the diagnosis. Magnetic resonance imaging and computed tomography are more accurate than echocardiography in establishing or excluding the presence of a thickened pericardium (Chap. 191). Pericardial thickening and even pericardial calcification, however, are not synonymous with constrictive pericarditis since they may occur without seriously impairing ventricular filling.

DIFFERENTIAL DIAGNOSIS Like cor pulmonale (Chap. 204), chronic constrictive pericarditis may be associated with severe systemic venous hypertension but with little or no pulmonary congestion; the heart usually is not enlarged, and a striking inspiratory fall in arterial pressure may be present. However, in cor pulmonale, advanced parenchymal pulmonary disease is usually obvious and venous pressure *falls* during inspiration; i.e., Kussmaul's sign is negative. *Tricuspid stenosis* (p. 1064) also may simulate chronic constrictive pericarditis; congestive hepatomegaly, splenomegaly, ascites, and venous distention may be equally prominent, and the manifestations of left-sided heart failure may be inconspicuous. However, in tricuspid stenosis, the characteristic murmur, the almost universal coexistence of mitral stenosis, the absence of a paradoxic pulse, and the absence, in the jugular venous pulse, of the steep, deep y descent followed by a rapid ascent (manifested by the diastolic shock on palpation and its audible equivalent, the pericardial knock) facilitate the clinical differentiation.

Because constrictive pericarditis can be corrected surgically it is important, though often difficult, to distinguish chronic constrictive pericarditis from various forms of heart disease which are characterized by a similar physiologic abnormality, i.e., restriction of ventricular filling. These restrictive cardiomyopathies, which may resemble pericarditis clinically, are described in Chap. 205 and include endomyocardial fibrosis and infiltrative cardiomyopathies such as amyloidosis, hemochromatosis, sarcoidosis, scleroderma, and idiopathic myocardial hypertrophy. In the last the marked thickening of the ventricular wall is responsible for the diminished compliance (Table 206-2).

The features favoring the diagnosis of one of the above forms of cardiomyopathy are a well-defined apex beat, enlargement of the heart, and pronounced orthopnea with attacks of acute left ventricular failure, left ventricular hypertrophy, gallop sounds (in place of a pericardial knock), bundle branch block, and in some cases significant Q waves in the electrocardiogram. The echocardiogram shows ventricular thickening. At catheterization, patients with chronic constrictive pericarditis usually have left atrial or pulmonary arterial wedge pressure equaling right atrial pressure, the latter often exceeding 15 mmHg despite intensive medical treatment for heart failure. The pulmonary artery systolic pressure is often less than 50 mmHg, and the right ventricular end-diastolic pressure often reaches one-third of the systolic pressure; the cardiac output is slightly depressed. In patients with cardiomyopathy, the left atrial usually exceeds the right atrial pressure by more than 5 mmHg, the mean right atrial pressure is often below 15 mmHg following intensive treatment with diuretics, the pulmonary artery systolic pressure often exceeds 50 mmHg, and the right ventricular end-diastolic pressure is usually less than one-third of the systolic pressure, while the cardiac output is markedly depressed. The volumes of both ventricles, as determined by angiography or echocardiography, are characteristically reduced or normal in constrictive pericarditis, and the ejection fractions are normal or almost so. The left ventricular end-diastolic volume also may be normal in some cardiomyopathies, but it is frequently elevated in others in which the ejection fraction is markedly reduced; the latter finding militates strongly against the diagnosis of constrictive pericarditis. The echocardiogram in chronic constrictive pericarditis characteristically shows pericardial thickening, i.e., a distinct echo posterior to the left ventricular wall, and paradoxical septal motion. The left ventricular wall moves sharply outward in early diastole and then remains flat. The definitive diagnosis of restrictive cardiomyopathy, when it is due to an infiltrative disease such as amyloidosis, can often be established by endomyocardial biopsy. CT scanning and MRI are very useful in distinguishing between restrictive cardiomyopathy and chronic constrictive pericarditis (Chap. 191).

When a patient has progressive, disabling, and unresponsive congestive failure, and if he or she displays any of the phenomena of constrictive heart disease, the most careful and detailed clinical and laboratory studies must be carried out in order to detect or exclude constrictive pericarditis, which is potentially a curable condition. Cardiac catheterization, selective angiocardiography, coronary arteriography, endomyocardial biopsy, and MRI may be required. However, in the very rare instance when even these examinations do not yield a definitive diagnosis, surgical exploration of the pericardium is the only decisive method of determining whether constrictive pericarditis is responsible for the clinical manifestations of heart failure.

Occult constrictive disease Patients with this condition may have unexplained fatigue, dyspnea, and chest pain. No overt manifestations of pericardial disease are present, but following the rapid intravenous infusion of 1 L saline solution, diastolic equilibration of intracardiac atrial and ventricular pressures found in overt constrictive pericarditis occur. Although symptomatic improvement may follow pericardiectomy, this procedure should not be carried out in asymptomatic persons.

TREATMENT Pericardial resection is the only definitive treatment of constrictive pericarditis, but dietary sodium restriction and diuretics are useful during preoperative preparation. Digitalis may be beneficial in the prevention of heart failure when resection of the thickened pericardium permits an increased inflow into the ventricles and hence places an enhanced burden on an atrophic myocardium. The benefits derived from cardiac decortication are often striking, and the improvement, though slight at first, usually is progressive over a period of many months. The risk of this operation depends on the extent of penetration of the myocardium by the calcific process, by the severity of myocardial atrophy, by the extent of secondary impairment of hepatic and/or renal function, and by the patient's general condition. Operative mortality is in the range of 7 to 15 percent; the patients with the most severe and/or advanced disease are at highest risk. Therefore, surgical treatment should be carried out relatively early in the course.

Many cases of constrictive pericarditis are of tuberculous origin. Antituberculous therapy during the phase of effusion may prevent the development of constriction, and such therapy should be carried out before and after operation, if a tuberculous origin is suspected or cannot be excluded in a patient with chronic constrictive pericarditis (Chap. 130).

SUBACUTE EFFUSIVE-CONSTRICTIVE PERICARDITIS This form of pericardial disease is characterized by the combination of a tense effusion in the pericardial space and constriction of the heart by thickened pericardium. It shares a number of features both with pericardial effusion producing cardiac compression and with pericardial constriction. It may be caused by tuberculosis, multiple attacks of acute idiopathic pericarditis, radiation, traumatic pericarditis, uremia, and scleroderma. The heart is generally enlarged, and

there are a paradoxical pulse and a prominent x descent (without a prominent y descent) in the atrial pressure pulse. Following pericardiocentesis, the physiologic findings may change from those of cardiac tamponade to those of pericardial constriction, with a "square root" sign in the ventricular pressure pulse and a prominent y descent in the atrial and jugular venous pressure pulses. Furthermore, the intrapericardial pressure and the central venous pressure may decline, but not to normal. In many patients the condition progresses to the chronic constrictive form of the disease. Wide excision of both the visceral and parietal pericardium is usually effective.

OTHER DISORDERS OF THE PERICARDIUM

Pericardial cysts appear as rounded or lobulated deformities of the cardiac silhouette, most commonly at the right cardiophrenic angle. They do not cause symptoms, and their major clinical significance lies in the possibility of confusion with a tumor, ventricular aneurysm, or massive cardiomegaly. *Tumors* involving the pericardium are most commonly secondary to malignant neoplasms originating in or invading the mediastinum, including carcinoma of the bronchus and breast, lymphoma, and melanoma. The most common *primary* malignant tumor is the mesothelioma. The usual clinical picture of malignant pericardial tumor is an insidiously developing, often bloody, pericardial effusion. Surgical exploration is required to establish a definitive diagnosis and to carry out definitive or, more commonly, palliative treatment.

REFERENCES

ARSENIAN MA: Cardiovascular sequelae of therapeutic thoracic radiation. Prog Cardiovasc Dis 33:299, 1991

DACSO CC: Pericarditis in AIDS. Cardiol Clin 8:697, 1990

FOWLER NO: Cardiac tamponade. A clinical or an echocardiographic diagnosis? 87:1738, 1993

———: Tuberculous pericarditis. JAMA 266:99, 1991

GOLD RG: Post-viral pericarditis. Eur Heart J 9:(G):175, 1988

HANCOCK EW: Subacute effusive-constrictive pericarditis. Circulation 43:183, 1971

KHAN AH: The postcardiac injury syndromes. Clin Cardiol 15:67, 1992

LORELL B, BRAUNWALD E: Pericardial disease, in *Heart Disease*, 4th ed, E Braunwald (ed). Philadelphia, Saunders, 1992, pp 1465–1516

McCAUHGAN BC et al: Early and late results of pericardiectomy for constrictive pericarditis. J Thorac Cardiovasc Surg 89:340, 1985

VAITKUS PT, KUSSMAUL WG: Constrictive versus restrictive cardiomyopathy: A reappraisal and update of diagnostic criteria. Am Heart J 122:1431, 1991

ZISKIND AA et al: Percutaneous balloon pericardiotomy for the treatment of cardiac tamponade and large pericardial effusions; description of technique and report of the first 50 cases. J Am Coll Cardiol 21:1, 1993

207 CARDIAC TUMORS, CARDIAC MANIFESTATIONS OF SYSTEMIC DISEASES, AND TRAUMATIC CARDIAC INJURY

WILSON S. COLUCCI / EUGENE BRAUNWALD

TUMORS OF THE HEART

PRIMARY TUMORS Primary tumors of the heart are rare and are often classified as "benign" histologically (Table 207-1). However, since all cardiac tumors have the potential for causing life-threatening complications, and many are now curable by surgery, it is important that this diagnosis be made whenever possible. Approximately three-quarters are *histologically* benign, and the remainder are malignant, in almost all cases sarcomas.

TABLE 207-1   Relative incidence of primary tumors of the heart

Type	Percent
BENIGN	
Myxoma	30.5
Lipoma	10.5
Papillary fibroelastoma	9.9
Rhabdomyoma	8.5
Fibroma	4.0
Hemangioma	3.5
Teratoma	3.3
Mesothelioma of the AV node	2.8
Other benign tumors	2.1
Total	75.1
MALIGNANT	
Sarcomas	18.6
Lymphoma	1.6
Other malignant tumors	4.7
Total	24.9

source: Modified from HA McAllister, JJ Fenoglio, in *Atlas of Tumor Pathology*, Washington, Armed Forces Institute of Pathology, 1978, fasc 15, 2d series.

TABLE 207-2   Comparison of clinical features of sporadic myxoma and syndrome myxoma

Feature	Sporadic	Syndrome
Age (y) (range)	56 (39–82)	25 (10–56)
Female/male ratio	2·7:1	1·8:1
Patients (no.)	70	44
Cardiac myxomas (no.)	72	103
Distributions of myxomas (%):		
Atrial/ventricular	100/0	87/13
Single/multiple	99/1	50/50
Biatrial	0	23
Recurrent	0	18
Freckling (%)	0	68
Noncardiac tumors (%)	0	57
Endocrine neoplasm (%)	0	30
Familial (%)	0	14

source: HJ Vidaillet et al: "Syndrome myxoma:" A subset of patients with cardiac myxoma associated with pigmented skin lesions and peripheral and endocrine neoplasms. Br Heart J 57:247, 1987

Clinical presentation   Cardiac tumors may present with a wide array of cardiac and noncardiac manifestations. There may be signs and symptoms of all the more common forms of heart disease, including chest pain, syncope, heart failure, murmurs, arrhythmias, conduction disturbances, and pericardial effusion or tamponade. The specific signs and symptoms produced are most closely related to the location of the tumor.

Myxoma   Myxomas are the most common type of primary cardiac tumor for all age groups, accounting for one-third to one-half of all cases at postmortem, and for approximately three-quarters of the tumors that are treated surgically. They occur at all ages and show no sex preference. Although the large majority of myxomas are sporadic, some are familial with autosomal dominant transmission or are part of a syndrome that involves a complex of abnormalities including lentigines or pigmented nevi, primary nodular adrenal cortical disease with or without Cushing's syndrome, myxomatous mammary fibroadenomas, testicular tumors, and/or pituitary adenomas with gigantism or acromegaly. Certain constellations of findings have been referred to as the *NAME syndrome* (nevi, atrial myxoma, myxoid neurofibroma, and ephelides) or the *LAMB syndrome* (lentigines, atrial myxoma, and blue nevi). Approximately 7 percent of cardiac myxomas are familial or part of the *syndrome myxoma* with complex abnormalities described above.

Most authorities consider the myxoma a true neoplasm, while others have suggested that it is formed by organization of an intracardiac thrombus attached to the endocardium. The large majority of sporadic myxomas are solitary and located in the atria, particularly the left, where they arise from the interatrial septum in the vicinity of the fossa ovalis. Sporadic myxomas may also occur in the ventricles or may be found in multiple locations. In contrast to sporadic myxomas, familial or syndrome myxoma tumors tend to occur in younger individuals, are more often multiple in location, and are more likely to have postoperative recurrences, probably reflecting their multicentric nature (Table 207-2). Most are pedunculated on a fibrovascular stalk and average 4 to 8 cm in diameter. The most common clinical presentation resembles that of mitral valve disease, either stenosis as a result of tumor prolapse into the mitral orifice during diastole or regurgitation as a consequence of injury to the valve by tumor-induced trauma. Ventricular myxomas may cause outflow obstruction and may therefore mimic subaortic or subpulmonic stenosis. Characteristically, the symptoms and signs of atrial myxomas are highly dependent on position, intermittent, and sudden in onset as a result of changes in tumor position with gravity. On auscultation,

a characteristic low-pitched sound, termed a "tumor plop," is audible during early or middiastole and is thought to result from the tumor abruptly stopping as it strikes the ventricular wall. Myxomas may also present with peripheral or pulmonary emboli, or any of several noncardiac signs and symptoms including fever, weight loss, cachexia, malaise, arthralgia, rash, clubbing, Raynaud's phenomenon, hypergammaglobulinemia, anemia, polycythemia, leukocytosis, elevated erythrocyte sedimentation rate, thrombocytopenia, or thrombocytosis. Not surprisingly, myxomas are frequently misdiagnosed as endocarditis, collagen vascular disease, or noncardiac tumor.

Both M-mode and two-dimensional echocardiography (Fig. 190-4), are useful in the diagnosis of cardiac myxoma, the latter having the advantage of allowing determination of the site of tumor attachment and tumor size, important considerations in the planning of surgical excision. Computed tomography and particularly magnetic resonance imaging may provide important information regarding the size, shape, and surface characteristics of the tumor. Because myxomas may be familial, echocardiographic screening of first-degree relatives is appropriate, particularly if the patient is young and has multiple tumors or other evidence of syndrome myxoma. While cardiac catheterization and angiography are often performed prior to surgery, catheterization of the chamber from which the tumor originates is attended by the risk of dislodgment of tumor emboli. In many centers catheterization is no longer considered mandatory when adequate noninvasive information is available and other cardiac diseases (e.g., coronary artery disease) are not considered likely.

Surgical excision utilizing cardiopulmonary bypass is indicated and is generally curative. Occasional reports of tumor recurrence are most likely due to inadequate excision of multiple tumor sites not evident at the time of presentation.

Other benign tumors   Cardiac *lipomas*, although relatively common, are usually incidental findings at postmortem examination and seldom result in symptoms. However, they may grow as large as 15 cm and present with symptoms due to mechanical interference with cardiac function, arrhythmias, or conduction disturbances, or as an abnormality of the cardiac silhouette on chest x-ray. *Papillary fibroelastomas*, similarly, are relatively common findings on cardiac valves or the adjacent endothelium at postmortem but seldom result in clinical symptoms. Occasionally, these growths may cause mechanical interference with valvular function. *Rhabdomyomas* and *fibromas*, the most frequent tumors in infants and children, most commonly occur in the ventricles, and therefore produce signs and symptoms by mechanical obstruction which may mimic valvular stenosis, congestive heart failure, restrictive or hypertrophic cardiomyopathy, and pericardial constriction. Rhabdomyomas are probably hamartomatous growths, are multiple in about 90 percent of cases, and may be associated with tuberous sclerosis, adenoma sebaceum, and benign kidney tumors in approximately 30 percent of patients. Calcification of a cardiac tumor strongly suggests that it is a fibroma, although myxomas and sarcomas may also be calcified. *Hemangiomas* and *mesotheliomas* are generally small tumors, most often intramyocardial in location, and may cause atrioventricular conduction disturbances and even sudden death as a result of their propensity for location in the region of the AV node.

Sarcomas Cardiac sarcomas may be of several histologic types, but in general are characterized by a rapidly downhill course leading to the patient's death in weeks to months from the time of presentation as a result of hemodynamic compromise, local invasion, or distant metastases. Sarcomas commonly involve the right side of the heart, and because of their rapid growth, invasion of the pericardial space and obstruction of the cardiac chambers or venae cavae are common. Sarcomas also can occur on the left side of the heart and they may be mistaken for myxomas. At the time of presentation these tumors have often spread too extensively for surgical excision. While there are scattered reports of palliation with surgery, radiotherapy, and/or chemotherapy, the overall experience with cardiac sarcomas is poor. The one exception to this appears to be cardiac lymphosarcomas, which may respond to a combination of chemo- and radiotherapy.

TUMORS METASTATIC TO THE HEART Tumors metastatic to the heart are several times more common than primary tumors, and as the life expectancy of patients with various forms of malignant neoplasms is extended by more effective therapy, it is likely that the frequency of cardiac metastases will also increase. Although cardiac metastases occur in 1 to 20 percent of all tumor types, the incidence is especially high in malignant melanoma, and to a somewhat lesser extent in leukemia and lymphoma. In absolute numbers, cardiac metastases are most common in carcinoma of the breast and lung, reflecting the high incidence of these cancers. Cardiac metastases almost always occur in the setting of widespread primary disease, and most often there is either primary or metastatic disease elsewhere in the thoracic cavity. Nevertheless, occasionally a cardiac metastasis may be the initial presentation of a tumor elsewhere in the body.

Cardiac metastases reach the heart via the bloodstream, lymphatics, or direct invasion and generally are small, firm nodules; diffuse infiltrations may also occur, especially with sarcomas or hematologic neoplasms. The pericardium is most often involved, followed by myocardial involvement of any chamber, and, rarely, by involvement of the endocardium or cardiac valves.

Cardiac metastases result in clinical manifestations only about 10 percent of the time, and rarely are they the cause of death. In most patients they are *not* the cause of the presenting clinical features but occur in the setting of a previously recognized malignant neoplasm. While cardiac metastases may present a large number of nonspecific signs and symptoms, the most common are dyspnea, signs of acute pericarditis, cardiac tamponade, a rapid increase in the cardiac silhouette on chest x-ray, the new onset of an ectopic tachyarrhythmia, AV block, and congestive heart failure. As with primary cardiac tumors, the clinical presentation is more closely related to the location and size of the tumor than to its histologic type. Many of these signs and symptoms may also occur with myocarditis, pericarditis, or cardiomyopathy resulting from radiotherapy or chemotherapy.

The electrocardiographic findings are entirely nonspecific and may include ST-T-wave changes, decreased QRS voltage, arrhythmias, and conduction disturbances. On chest roentgenography the cardiac silhouette is most often normal but may reveal a pericardial effusion or bizarre contour. Echocardiography is useful for the diagnosis of pericardial effusion and the visualization of larger metastases. Computed tomography, magnetic resonance imaging, and radionuclide imaging with gallium or thallium may provide useful anatomic information. Angiography may delineate discrete lesions, and pericardiocentesis can allow a specific cytologic diagnosis. Since most patients with cardiac metastases have widespread disease, therapy generally consists of pericardiocentesis when there is hemodynamic compromise and treatment directed at the primary tumor. The removal of a malignant effusion by pericardiocentesis, with or without concomitant instillation of a sclerosing agent (e.g., tetracycline), or placement of a pericardial window for drainage to the pleural space may palliate symptoms and delay or prevent reaccumulation of the effusion.

CARDIAC EFFECTS OF CANCER THERAPY See Chap. 205.

CARDIOVASCULAR MANIFESTATIONS OF SYSTEMIC DISEASES

DIABETES MELLITUS (See Chap. 337) In patients with insulin-dependent diabetes mellitus there is an increased incidence of large-vessel atherosclerosis and myocardial infarction, and diabetics are more likely to have an abnormal or absent pain response to myocardial ischemia, probably as a result of generalized autonomic nervous system dysfunction. Diabetic patients may also have myocardial dysfunction characteristic of a restrictive cardiomyopathy in the absence of large-vessel coronary artery disease, with abnormal relaxation of the myocardium, and evidenced clinically by elevated left ventricular filling pressures. Histologically, these patients have increased amounts of collagen, glycoprotein, triglycerides, and cholesterol in the myocardial interstitium, and in some cases intimal thickening, hyaline deposition, and inflammatory changes have been observed in small intramural arteries. Diabetic subjects have an increased risk of developing clinical heart failure, even after correction for the presence of coronary artery disease, hypertension, and obesity, and it is likely that diabetic cardiomyopathy contributes to excessive cardiovascular morbidity and mortality of these patients. There is some evidence that insulin therapy results in an amelioration of the myocardial dysfunction.

MALNUTRITION AND THIAMINE DEFICIENCY (BERIBERI) Malnutrition (See Chap. 72) In patients whose intake of protein, calories, or both is severely deficient, the heart may become thin, pale, and flabby with myofibrillar atrophy and interstitial edema. The systolic pressure and cardiac output are low and the pulse pressure narrow. Generalized edema is common and is due to a combination of factors, including reduced serum oncotic pressure and myocardial dysfunction. Such profound states of malnutrition, termed *marasmus* in the case of caloric deficiency or *kwashiorkor* in the case of relative protein deficiency, are most common in underdeveloped countries. However, significant nutritional heart disease may also occur in developed nations, particularly in patients with chronic diseases such as AIDS, in the semistarvation that can occur in anorexia nervosa, or in patients with severe cardiac failure in whom gastrointestinal hypoperfusion and venous congestion may cause anorexia and malabsorption. Open-heart surgery poses an increased risk in such patients, who may benefit from preoperative intensive hyperalimentation. Deficient nutrients and minerals should be replaced gradually since rapid expansion of the intravascular space may stress the weakened heart and result in overt congestive heart failure.

Thiamine deficiency (See Chap. 77) In many cases, malnutrition is accompanied by thiamine deficiency, although this hypovitaminosis may also occur in the presence of an adequate protein and caloric intake, particularly in the Far East, where polished rice deficient in thiamine may be a major dietary component. The widespread use of thiamine-enriched flour in western nations confines this disease primarily to alcoholics and food faddists. Clinically, there is usually evidence of generalized malnutrition, peripheral neuropathy, glossitis, and anemia. The characteristic cardiovascular syndrome is that of high-output heart failure with tachycardia, increased cardiac output, and often elevated filling pressures in the left and right sides of the heart. It appears that the major cause of the high-output state is vasomotor depression, the precise mechanism of which is not understood, but which leads to a reduced systemic vascular resistance. The cardiac examination reveals a wide pulse pressure, tachycardia, a third heart sound, and, frequently, a systolic murmur at the apex. The electrocardiogram may show decreased voltage, a prolonged QT interval, and T-wave abnormalities; the chest x-ray generally shows a large heart with signs of congestive heart failure. The response to thiamine is often dramatic, with an increase in systemic vascular resistance, decrease in cardiac output, clearing of pulmonary congestion, and a reduction in heart size often occurring in 12 to 48 h. Although the response to digitalis and diuretics may be poor prior to thiamine therapy, these agents may be important *after* thiamine is given, since the left ventricle may not be capable of dealing with the increased workload presented by the return of vascular tone.

OBESITY (See Chap. 73) Although not defined as a disease per se, severe obesity, particularly when it occurs in an upper-body distribution, is associated with an increase in cardiovascular morbidity and mortality, due in part to hypertension, glucose intolerance, and atherosclerotic coronary artery disease, all of which are more prevalent in obese patients. In addition, these patients have a distinct abnormality of the cardiovascular system characterized by increases in total and central blood volumes, cardiac output, and left ventricular filling pressure. It appears that cardiac output is elevated in order to help supply the metabolic needs of the excessive adipose tissue. Left ventricular filling pressure is often at the upper limits of normal and rises excessively with exercise. As a result of chronic volume and pressure overload, eccentric cardiac hypertrophy with cardiac dilation and abnormal ventricular function may develop. Pathologically, there is left and, in some cases, right ventricular hypertrophy and generalized cardiac enlargement, which is not due simply to fatty infiltration of the myocardium. Clinically, these patients may develop pulmonary congestion, peripheral edema, and exercise intolerance, findings which may be difficult to recognize in massively obese patients. Weight reduction is the most effective therapy and results in reduction in blood volume and in return of cardiac output toward normal. However, rapid weight reduction may cause cardiac arrhythmias and sudden death due to electrolyte imbalance and may result in cardiac atrophy similar to that seen in malnutrition. Digitalis, sodium restriction, and diuretics may also be useful. This form of heart disease should be distinguished from the Pickwickian syndrome (Chap. 229), which may share several of the cardiovascular features but, in addition, frequently has components of central apnea, hypoxemia, pulmonary hypertension, and cor pulmonale.

THYROID DISEASE (See Chap. 334) Thyroid hormone exerts a major influence on the cardiovascular system by a number of direct and indirect mechanisms, and not surprisingly, cardiovascular effects are prominent in both hypo- and hyperthyroidism. Thyroid hormone causes increases in total-body metabolism and oxygen consumption that indirectly place an increased workload on the heart. In addition, although the exact mechanism has not been defined, thyroid hormone exerts direct inotropic, chronotropic, and dromotropic effects that are similar to those seen with adrenergic stimulation (e.g., tachycardia, increased cardiac output). It has been shown that thyroid hormone increases the synthesis of myosin and of Na^+,K^+-ATPase, as well as the density of myocardial beta-adrenergic receptors.

Hyperthyroidism Excess thyroid hormone results in increases in heart rate, cardiac output, stroke volume, pulse pressure, and measures of left ventricular contractility. Patients may present with palpitations, systolic hypertension, fatigue, or, in patients with underlying heart disease, angina or heart failure. Sinus tachycardia is found in about 40 percent of patients, and atrial fibrillation in about 15 percent. Other findings include a hyperactive precordium, an increase in the intensity of the first heart sound and the pulmonic component of the second heart sound, and a third heart sound. An increased incidence of mitral valve prolapse has been associated with hyperthyroidism, and in some cases there may be a midsystolic murmur heard best at the left sternal border with or without a systolic ejection click. A systolic scratchy sound, the *Means-Lerman scratch*, may occasionally be heard at the left second intercostal space during expiration and is thought to result from the rubbing of the hyperdynamic pericardium against the pleura. Elderly patients with hyperthyroidism may present with only the cardiovascular manifestations of thyrotoxicosis, such as atrial fibrillation, which may be resistant to therapy until the hyperthyroidism is controlled. Angina pectoris and congestive heart failure are unusual unless there is coexistent underlying heart disease, and in many cases will resolve with therapy of the hyperthyroidism.

Hypothyroidism There is a reduction in cardiac output, stroke volume, heart rate, blood pressure, and pulse pressure. In about one-third of patients there is a pericardial effusion which only rarely results in tamponade. Increased capillary permeability results in pleural and pericardial effusions, but only rarely results in tamponade. Other clinical signs include cardiomegaly, bradycardia, weak arterial pulses, and distant heart sounds. As a result of earlier detection and treatment of hypothyroidism, these overt signs are commonly absent, and the major findings may be exertional dyspnea and easy fatigability. Although the signs and symptoms of myxedema may suggest the diagnosis of congestive heart failure, in the absence of other cardiac disease, myocardial failure is uncommon. Biochemical abnormalities, including elevations of creatine kinase, serum glutamic oxaloacetic transaminase, and lactic dehydrogenase, may lead to a mistaken diagnosis of myocardial infarction. The electrocardiogram generally shows sinus bradycardia and low voltage and may show prolongation of the QT interval, decreased P-wave voltage, prolonged AV conduction time, intraventricular conduction disturbances, and nonspecific ST-T-wave abnormalities. Chest x-ray may show cardiomegaly, often with a "water bottle" configuration, pleural effusions, and, in some cases, evidence of congestive heart failure. Pathologically, the heart is pale, dilated, and flabby, often with myofibrillar swelling, loss of striations, and interstitial fibrosis.

Patients with hypothyroidism frequently have elevations of cholesterol and triglycerides and severe atherosclerotic coronary artery disease. Prior to treatment with thyroid hormone, patients with hypothyroidism frequently do not have angina pectoris, presumably because of the low metabolic demands made by their condition. However, such patients, especially when elderly, are prone to angina and myocardial infarction during replacement of thyroid hormone, and this should always be done with extreme care, starting with very low doses which are increased gradually.

MALIGNANT CARCINOID (See Chap. 276) These tumors elaborate a variety of vasoactive amines (e.g., serotonin), kinins, indoles, and other substances which are believed to be responsible for the diarrhea, flushing, and labile blood pressure seen in these patients. The cardiac lesions due to gastrointestinal carcinoids are almost exclusively in the right side of the heart and occur only when there are hepatic metastases, suggesting that the substance responsible for the cardiac lesions is inactivated by passage through the liver and lungs. Similar lesions occur in the left side of the heart when there is a right-to-left shunt or the tumor is located in the lungs. Fibrous plaques are found on the endothelium of the cardiac chambers, valves, and great vessels. These plaques, which result in distortion of the cardiac valves, consist of smooth muscle cells embedded in a stroma of acid mucopolysaccharide and collagen, and presumably result from healing of endothelial injury. The clinical syndrome is most often that of tricuspid regurgitation, pulmonic stenosis, or both. In some cases a high-output state may occur, presumably as a result of a decrease in systemic vascular resistance due to a vasoactive substance released by the tumor. Progression of the cardiac lesions does not appear to be affected by treatment with serotonin antagonists, and in some severely symptomatic patients valve replacement is indicated. Coronary artery spasm, presumably due to a circulating vasoactive substance, may occur in patients with carcinoid syndrome.

PHEOCHROMOCYTOMA (See Chap. 336) In addition to causing hypertension, which may be labile or sustained, the high circulating levels of catecholamines may also cause direct myocardial injury. Focal myocardial necrosis and inflammatory cell infiltration are seen in about 50 percent of patients who die with pheochromocytoma and may contribute to clinically significant left ventricular failure and pulmonary edema. Left ventricular function and congestive heart failure may resolve after removal of the tumor. In addition, hypertension results in left ventricular hypertrophy.

RHEUMATOID ARTHRITIS AND THE COLLAGEN VASCULAR DISEASES Rheumatoid arthritis (See Chap. 285) There may be inflammation of any or all parts of the heart in patients with rheumatoid arthritis. *Pericarditis* is the most common cause of clinically apparent disease and may be found in 30 to 50 percent of all patients with rheumatoid arthritis, particularly those with subcutaneous nodules, if carefully searched for by echocardiography or at postmortem examination. However, only a small fraction of these patients will have clinical evidence of pericarditis, which usually follows a benign course, but occasionally may progress to cardiac tamponade or constrictive pericarditis. The pericardial fluid is generally an exudate, with decreased concentrations of complement and glucose and elevated cholesterol. Treatment is directed at the underlying rheumatoid arthritis and may include glucocorticoids. Pericardiectomy is usually required in cases of tamponade or persistent effusion. *Coronary arteritis* with intimal inflammation and edema is present in about 20 percent of cases but only rarely results in angina pectoris or myocardial infarction. The cardiac valves, most often the mitral and aortic, may be involved by inflammation and granuloma formation which in some cases may cause clinically significant regurgitation due to valve deformity. Myocarditis rarely results in cardiac dysfunction.

Seronegative arthropathies   The seronegative arthropathies (Chaps. 289 and 298), ankylosing spondylitis, Reiter's syndrome, psoriatic arthritis, and the arthritides associated with ulcerative colitis and regional enteritis may be accompanied by a pancarditis and proximal aortitis; the latter may result in aortic regurgitation and may extend into the anterior mitral valve ring and/or AV node. Both aortic regurgitation and AV block are more common in patients with peripheral joint involvement and long-standing disease; treatment with aortic valve replacement and permanent pacemaker placement may be required. Up to one-fifth of patients with peripheral joint involvement and disease for more than 30 years have significant aortic regurgitation. Occasionally, aortic regurgitation precedes the onset of arthritis, and, therefore, the diagnosis of a seronegative arthritis should be considered in young males with isolated aortic regurgitation.

Systemic lupus erythematosus (SLE) (See Chap. 284)   Pericarditis is common, occurring in about two-thirds of patients, and generally pursues a benign course, although rarely tamponade or constriction may result. The characteristic *endocardial lesions* of SLE, described by Libman and Sacks, consist of wartlike lesions most often located at the angles of the AV valves or on the ventricular surface of the mitral valve. Hemodynamically important valvular regurgitation is rare. Patients with SLE and elevated levels of antibody to cardiolipin appear to have a particularly high incidence of valvular disease, which is also more severe than in patients without these antibodies. Myocarditis generally parallels the activity of the disease, and although common histologically, seldom results in clinical heart failure unless associated with hypertension. Although arteritis of large coronary arteries may rarely result in myocardial ischemia, there is also an increased frequency of coronary atherosclerosis which may be related to hypertension or glucocorticoid therapy.

TRAUMATIC HEART DISEASE

Cardiac damage may be due to both penetrating and nonpenetrating injuries. The most frequent cause of a *nonpenetrating injury* is impact of the chest against the steering wheel of an automobile. Serious injury of the heart may ensue even though no external sign of thoracic trauma is evident. Although the commonest injury is myocardial contusion, any structure of the heart may be affected by the trauma. If the valvular apparatus is ruptured, a loud heart murmur produced by valvular regurgitation may appear, followed by the development of rapidly progressive heart failure. The most serious consequence of nonpenetrating injury is rupture, either of the atria or of the ventricles, which is generally fatal. Hemopericardium may also follow tearing of a pericardial vessel or coronary artery.

Myocardial contusion may cause arrhythmias, bundle branch block, or electrocardiographic abnormalities resembling those of infarction, and so it is important to bear trauma in mind as a cause of otherwise unexplained electrocardiographic changes. Similarly, myocardial contusion may produce positive radionuclide scans and regional impairment of ventricular function, as occurs in myocardial infarction (Chap. 190). Pericardial effusion may occur weeks or even months after the accident. In these cases, the pericardial effusion is a manifestation of the postcardiac injury syndrome, which resembles the postpericardiotomy syndrome (Chap. 206).

Acute myocardial failure resulting from rupture of a valve usually requires operative correction. Myocardial infarction due to trauma is treated similarly to that due to ischemic heart disease (Chap. 202). Pericardial hemorrhage often leads to constriction which must be treated by decortication.

Penetrating injuries of the heart, produced by bullets or stab wounds, usually result in immediate or very rapid death because of hemopericardium or massive hemorrhage. However, sometimes the patient survives the acute incident and presents with a cardiac murmur and congestive heart failure. A left-to-right shunt due to traumatic ventricular septal defect, aortopulmonary artery fistula, or coronary arteriovenous fistula may be suspected and confirmed by cardiac catheterization and angiocardiography. Operation is indicated if hemodynamically significant abnormalities are present or if a foreign body, e.g., a bullet, is lodged in the heart. Immediate thoracotomy should be carried out if there is cardiac tamponade and/or shock, whether the trauma was penetrating or nonpenetrating. Pericardiocentesis may be helpful in patients with tamponade, but usually only as a holding maneuver. Patients who suffer penetrating injuries of the heart should be carefully examined several weeks after the event to rule out a ventricular septal defect or mitral regurgitation that may have gone undetected at the time of emergency surgery.

Rupture of the aorta is a common consequence of chest trauma. Indeed, rupture of the aorta at the isthmus or just above the aortic valve is the most common vascular deceleration injury. The clinical presentation is similar to that in aortic dissection (Chap. 210). The arterial pressure and pulse amplitude may be increased in the upper extremities and decreased in the lower extremities, and on chest roentgenogram there may be widening of the mediastinum. Occasionally, the rupture is limited by the aortic adventitia and results in a silent false aneurysm that may be discovered months or years after the injury. When great vessel rupture is due to a penetrating injury, there is usually a hemothorax and, less often, a hemopericardium. Hematoma formation may compress major vessels, and arteriovenous fistulae may be formed, sometimes resulting in high-output congestive heart failure.

REFERENCES

ACTIS DATO GM et al: Long-term follow-up of cardiac myxomas (7–31 years). J Cardiovasc Surg 34:141, 1993

CASTELLS E et al: Cardiac myxomas: Surgical treatment, long-term results and recurrence. J Cardiovasc Surg 34:49, 1993

COHN PF, BRAUNWALD E: Traumatic heart disease, in *Heart Disease*, 4th ed, E Braunwald (ed). Philadelphia, Saunders, 1992, p 1517

COLUCCI WS, BRAUNWALD E: Primary tumors of the heart, in *Heart Disease*, 4th ed, E Braunwald (ed). Philadelphia, Saunders, 1992 p 1451

GALVE E et al: Prevalence, morphologic types, and evolution of cardiac valvular disease in systemic lupus erythematosus. N Engl J Med 319:817, 1988

HARA KS et al: Rheumatoid pericarditis: Clinical features and survival. Medicine (Baltimore) 69:81, 1990

IMPERATO-McGINLEY J et al: Reversibility of catecholamine-induced dilated cardiomyopathy in a child with a pheochromocytoma. N Engl J Med 316:793, 1987

KLEIN I: Thyroid hormone and the cardiovascular system. Am J Med 88:631, 1990

LUNDIN L: Carcinoid heart disease. A cardiologist's viewpoint. Acta Oncol 30:499, 1991

NIHOYANNOPOULOS P et al: Cardiac abnormalities in systemic lupus erythematosus. Association with raised anticardiolipin antibodies. Circulation 82:369, 1990

O'NEILL TW, BRESNIHAN B: The heart in ankylosing spondylitis. Ann Rheum Dis 51:705, 1992

STOLLERMAN GH: Rheumatic fever and other rheumatic diseases of the heart, in *Heart Disease*, 4th ed, E Braunwald (ed). Philadelphia, Saunders, 1992, p 1721

TAZELAAR HD et al: Pathology of surgically excised primary cardiac tumors. Mayo Clin Proc 67:957, 1992

UUSITUPA MI et al: Diabetic heart muscle disease. Ann Med 22:377, 1990

VIDAILLET HR JR: Cardiac tumors associated with hereditary syndromes. Am J Cardiol 61:1355, 1988

section 2 **Disorders of the vascular system**

208 ATHEROSCLEROSIS AND OTHER FORMS OF ARTERIOSCLEROSIS

EDWIN L. BIERMAN

Arteriosclerosis, a generic term for thickening and hardening of the arterial wall, is responsible for the majority of deaths in the United States and most westernized societies. One type of arteriosclerosis is *atherosclerosis*, the disorder of the larger arteries that underlies most *coronary artery disease*, *aortic aneurysm*, and *arterial disease of the lower extremities* and also plays a major role in *cerebrovascular disease*. Atherosclerosis is by far the leading cause of death in the United States, both above and below age 65 and in both sexes (Table 208-1).

Other types of arteriosclerosis include focal calcific arteriosclerosis (*Mönckeberg's sclerosis*) and *arteriolosclerosis*. The major arterial diseases other than arteriosclerosis include *congenital structural defects*, *inflammatory* or granulomatous diseases (e.g., syphilitic aortitis), and disorders affecting mainly the smaller vessels, such as *hypersensitivity* or autoimmune diseases.

THE NORMAL ARTERY

STRUCTURE The normal artery wall consists of three layers: the intima, the media, and the adventitia.

Intima A single continuous layer of *endothelial cells* lines the lumen of all arteries. The intima is delimited on its outer aspect by a perforated tube of elastic tissue, the *internal elastic lamina*. This tube of elastic tissue is particularly prominent in the large elastic arteries and the medium-caliber muscular arteries, and it disappears in capillaries. The endothelial cells are attached to one another by a series of junctional complexes and are also attached, apparently somewhat tenuously, to an underlying meshwork of loose connective tissue, the *basal lamina*. These lining endothelial cells normally form a barrier that controls the entry of substances from the blood into the artery wall. Such substances usually enter the cells by specific transport systems. In addition, endothelial cells secrete a variety of substances that affect blood coagulation and the contraction and relaxation of the subjacent vascular smooth muscle (see below). Normally, no other cell type is present in the intima of most arteries.

Media The media consists of only one cell type, the *smooth-muscle cell*, arranged in either a single layer (as in small muscular arteries) or multiple lamellae (as in elastic arteries). These cells are surrounded by small amounts of collagen and elastic fibers, which they elaborate, and usually take the pattern of diagonal concentric spirals through the vessel wall. They are closely apposed to one another and may be attached by junctional complexes. The smooth-muscle cell appears to be the major connective tissue–forming cell of the artery wall, producing collagen, elastic fibers, and proteoglycans. In this sense it is analogous to the fibroblast in skin, the osteoblast in bone, and the chondroblast in cartilage. The media is bounded on the luminal side by the *internal elastic lamina* and on the abluminal side by a less continuous sheet of elastic tissue, the *external elastic lamina*. In *elastic arteries*, such as the aorta and the

major pulmonary arteries, elastic lamellae are prominent. Such arteries expand and increase their elastic tension with the pulse of systole. In diastole, the elastic fibers recoil, helping to propel the blood distally and progressively damping the pulsatile character of flow toward more terminal vessels. In *muscular arteries*, in which smooth-muscle cells predominate, peripheral flow is regulated, particularly in arterioles, by contraction (vasoconstriction) and relaxation (vasodilatation). Located about midway through the media of most arteries is a "nutritional watershed." The outer portion is nourished from the small blood vessels (vasa vasorum) in the adventitia; the inner layers receive their nutrients from the lumen.

Adventitia The outermost layer of the artery is the adventitia, which is delimited on the luminal aspect by the external elastic lamina. This external coat consists of a loose interwoven admixture of collagen bundles, elastic fibers, smooth-muscle cells, and fibroblasts. This layer also contains the vasa vasorum and nerves.

METABOLISM AND FUNCTION The artery wall is a metabolically active organ that must meet a steady demand for energy to maintain smooth-muscle tension and endothelial cell function and to repair and replenish tissue constituents. The mechanical forces on the arterial wall are complex, and considerable tensile stresses are imposed on it, mainly by hydraulic force. Shear or frictional stresses are especially prominent near the entrance regions of branches. The form and manner in which these forces are dissipated depend on flow, the amount of elastic tension developed, and the tethering or external support provided by surrounding structures. Arteries are also permeable pipes, which constantly exchange fluid and solutes with the blood they carry.

Maintenance of the endothelial cell lining is critical. Endothelial cell turnover occurs at a slow rate but may be accelerated in focal areas by changing patterns of flow along the vessel wall. When intact, these cells selectively control the passage of circulating substances by active transport (endocytosis and exocytosis) through their cytoplasm, and they elaborate connective tissue components to form their own substratum. In addition, intact endothelial cells function to prevent clotting partly by elaboration of a particular prostaglandin (prostacyclin or PGI_2) that inhibits platelet function, thereby enhancing unimpeded flow of blood. When the lining is damaged, platelets adhere to it, in part as the result of production of a different class of prostaglandins, the thromboxanes, and form a clot; endothelial cells

---

TABLE 208-1 Deaths by cause in the United States, 1989

Causes of death	No. of deaths, thousands			
	Below age 65		Age 65 and above	
	Male	Female	Male	Female
All causes	394	217	721	717
All cardiovascular diseases	107	48	345	432
Ischemic heart disease	62	21	197	221
Cerebrovascular disease	10	9	47	78
All infectious disease	5	3	1	2
All cancer	85	77	177	158
Accidents	56	19	14	14

SOURCE: National Center of Health Statistics, *Vital Statistics Report, Final Mortality Statistics, 1989.*

function in the clotting process by elaboration of key substances, including factor VIII.

The metabolism of arteries reflects the biochemistry of smooth-muscle cells. Arterial smooth-muscle cells form abundant collagen, elastic fibers, soluble and insoluble elastin, and glucosaminoglycans (mainly dermatan sulfate). Multiple anabolic and catabolic pathways are present. These cells metabolize glucose by both anaerobic and aerobic glycolysis. A variety of catabolic enzymes are present, including fibrinolysins, mixed-function oxidases, and lysosomal hydrolases. Because of the prominence of lipids in atherosclerotic lesions, much attention has been directed to lipid metabolism in arteries. Arterial wall cells can synthesize fatty acids, cholesterol, phospholipids, and triglycerides from endogenous substrates to satisfy their structural needs (membrane replenishment), but smooth-muscle cells appear preferentially to utilize lipids from plasma lipoproteins transported into the wall. Circulating lipoproteins traverse endothelial cells in pinocytotic vesicles. Smooth-muscle cells possess specific high-affinity surface receptors for certain apoproteins on the surface of lipid-rich lipoproteins, thus facilitating the entry of lipoproteins into the cell by adsorptive endocytosis. As has been shown for cultured skin fibroblasts, in arterial smooth-muscle cells these vesicles fuse with lysosomes, resulting in catabolism of lipoprotein components (Chap. 344). Free cholesterol entering the cell in this manner inhibits endogenous cholesterol synthesis, facilitates its own esterification, and partially limits further entry of cholesterol by regulating the number of lipoprotein receptors. However, lipoprotein cholesterol can gain entry into arterial smooth-muscle cells by unregulated receptor-independent pathways, potentially causing cholesterol ester accumulation. Because of the importance of regulation of arterial smooth-muscle cell proliferation, interest also has focused on the elaboration of growth factors and growth inhibitors by arterial wall cells. Both endothelial cells and smooth-muscle cells are capable of elaborating a variety of growth regulatory molecules, functions that may be altered in disease. Further, endothelial cells can regulate vascular tone by elaboration of molecules that produce vasoconstriction or vasodilation (e.g., nitric oxide) and can elaborate cytokines and adhesion molecules that influence interactions with circulating blood cells.

Thus many complex and interrelated metabolic processes are present in arterial wall cells. Although some of these may play a role in the production of arteriosclerosis, no one biochemical reaction or cellular function can be singled out as culpable. Physiologic factors, such as transfer processes across the endothelial lining, the flux of oxygen and substrates from both the luminal and adventitial sides of the wall, and the reverse flow of catabolic products, need to be considered as well. The ability of the arterial wall to maintain the integrity of its endothelium, prevent platelet aggregation, prevent adherence of blood mononuclear cells, prevent cholesterol accumulation, prevent intimal smooth-muscle cell proliferation, and ensure the nutrition of its middle portion may be the critical determinants of the arteriosclerotic process.

CHANGES WITH AGING   The major change that occurs with normal aging in the arterial wall in humans is a slow, apparently continuous, symmetric increase in the thickness of the intima. This intimal thickening results from a gradual accumulation of smooth-muscle cells surrounded by additional connective tissue. In the nondiseased artery wall, lipid content, mainly cholesterol ester and phospholipid (particularly sphingomyelin), also progressively increases with age. While most of the phospholipid in the normal artery wall appears to be derived from in situ synthesis, the cholesterol ester that accumulates with aging appears to be derived from plasma, since it contains principally linoleic acid, the major plasma cholesterol ester fatty acid. Furthermore, low-density lipoproteins are immunologically detectable in the intima of normal arteries in direct relation to their concentration in plasma. It has been estimated that between the second and sixth decade, the normal intima accumulates approximately 25 μmol (10 mg) cholesterol per gram of tissue. Thus, as the normal artery ages, smooth-muscle cells and connective tissue accumulate

diffusely in the intima, leading to progressive thickening, coupled with progressive accumulation of sphingomyelin and cholesterol linoleate. This diffuse age-related intima thickening is to be distinguished from focal discrete raised fibrous plaques, a characteristic feature of atherosclerosis.

Functionally, these changes with aging result in gradually increasing rigidity of vessels. The larger arteries may become dilated, elongated, and tortuous, and aneurysms may form in areas of an encroaching degenerating arteriosclerotic plaque. Such "wear-and-tear" changes are frequently proportional to the vessel diameter and correlated with branching, curvature, and anatomic points of attachment. The amount of external support also determines the ability of vessels, weakened by loss of elasticity, to withstand hydrostatic pressure. The unsupported cerebral arteries may be particularly vulnerable in this regard. Although senescence is accompanied by the intimal thickening that is a feature of localized atheromatosis, the changes of aging and arteriosclerosis appear to be separate and distinct processes.

NONATHEROMATOUS FORMS OF ARTERIOSCLEROSIS

Atherosclerosis involves primarily the intimal layer and occurs most commonly in the abdominal aorta and its large renal and lower extremity branches, the coronary arteries, and the cerebral vasculature. It may accompany or accelerate the other major forms of arteriosclerosis, *focal calcification* and *arteriolosclerosis* (Table 208-2).

FOCAL CALCIFICATION   Not to be confused with atherosclerosis is focal calcification of the media, particularly in the medium-sized muscular arteries. This type of arteriosclerosis is called *Mönckeberg's sclerosis* and is common in the lower extremities, upper extremities, and the arterial supply of the genital tract in both sexes. This disorder is rare in individuals below age 50 and affects both sexes indiscriminately. The process involves degeneration of smooth-muscle cells followed by calcium deposition. The vessels become hard and tortuous so that palpable vessels such as the radial artery can be felt as rigid tubes. Its characteristic radiologic appearance consists of regular concentric calcifications in cross section and a "railroad track" in longitudinal section, commonly seen in vessels in the pelvis, legs, and feet. The medial changes alone do not narrow the lumen, have little effect on the circulation, and have relatively little clinical significance. However, in the lower extremities, medial arterial calcification is often associated with atherosclerosis, leading to arterial occlusion. These changes are common in the elderly and in patients

TABLE 208-2   Disorders associated with early arteriosclerosis

ATHEROSCLEROSIS

Diabetes mellitus
Hypertension
Familial hypercholesterolemia
Familial combined hyperlipidemia
Familial dysbetalipoproteinemia
Familial hypoalphalipoproteinemia
Hypothyroidism
Cholesterol ester storage disease
Systemic lupus erythematosus
Homocysteinemia

NONATHEROMATOUS ARTERIOSCLEROSIS

Diabetes mellitus
Chronic renal insufficiency
Chronic vitamin D intoxication
Pseudoxanthoma elasticum
Idiopathic arterial calcification in infancy
Aortic valvular calcification in the elderly
Werner's syndrome

on long-term glucocorticoid therapy, but in individuals with diabetes mellitus, focal calcification may be accelerated and severe. It is much more common in diabetics with neuropathy, and sympathetic denervation of medial smooth muscle has been implicated in its cause.

Focal calcification also can produce the arteriosclerotic aortic valve in the elderly. Progressive calcium deposition occurs on the aortic surface of normal trileaflet aortic valves with age, resulting in a spectrum of clinical findings ranging from an innocent systolic murmur to severe calcific aortic stenosis (Chap. 201).

ARTERIOLOSCLEROSIS This disorder involves hyaline and degenerative changes affecting both the intima and media of smooth arteries and arterioles, particularly in the spleen, pancreas, adrenal, and kidney. In the kidney, but not necessarily elsewhere, arteriosclerosis is almost invariably associated with hypertension. Lesser degrees of sustained hypertension characteristically cause *hyalinization* of renal arterioles; more severe or malignant hypertension produces a typical *fibrous and elastic hyperplasia*, and even necrosis, of the media and intima.

ATHEROSCLEROSIS

LESIONS   Morbid anatomy Atherosclerosis is a patchy nodular type of arteriosclerosis. The lesions are commonly classified as *early lesions* (*initial lesions* and *fatty streaks*), *intermediate lesions*, *fibrous plaques*, and *complicated lesions*.

Initial (fatty streak) and *intermediate lesions* are focal, small, and nonobstructive. Initial lesions may be detectable only chemically or microscopically, consist of lipid deposition in intimal macrophages (macrophage foam cells), and represent the first changes that have been found to evolve into lesions associated with clinical disease. Often found in children, they are located in atherosclerosis-susceptible regions of the arterial tree.

Fatty streaks are visible to the naked eye on the endothelial surface of the aorta and coronary arteries. They are still small and nonobstructive and contain a larger accumulation of lipid-filled smooth-muscle cells and macrophages (foam cells) and fibrous tissue in focal areas of the intima. They are stained distinctly by fat-soluble dyes but may be visible without staining as yellowish or whitish patches, streaks, or dots on the intimal surface. The lipid is mainly cholesterol oleate and is mainly intracellular.

Fatty streaks are visible in the aorta and coronary arteries of very young children and increase in the aorta at puberty. Whether or not these lesions progress to advanced lesions at particular sites depends largely on hemodynamic forces and the plasma levels of atherogenic lipoproteins. Those lesions that are prone to progression develop extracellular lipid and debris in the proteoglycan matrix so that lipid pools form among the layers of intimal smooth-muscle cells. At this stage, a single lipid core is not evident, cell death is not apparent, and cholesterol crystals are rarely found. These lesions are considered to be intermediate or preatheromatous, on the way to developing the lipid core characterizing the advanced lesion (atheroma or fibrous plaque).

Fibrous plaques are palpably elevated areas of intimal thickening and represent the most characteristic lesion of advancing atherosclerosis. These atheromatous lesions first appear in the abdominal aorta, coronary arteries, and carotid arteries in the third decade and increase progressively with age. They appear in men before women, in the aorta before the coronary arteries, and much later in the vertebral and intracranial cerebral arteries. Reasons for the difference in susceptibility of various segments of the arterial tree and the nonuniform distribution of lesions are not known. Typically, the fibrous plaque is firm, elevated, and dome-shaped, with an opaque glistening surface that bulges into the lumen. It consists of a central core of extracellular lipid (with cholesterol crystals) and necrotic cell debris ("gruel") covered by a fibromuscular layer or cap containing large numbers of smooth-muscle cells, macrophages, and collagen. Thus the plaque is much thicker than is normal intima. Although the lipid,

like that of fatty streaks, is mainly cholesterol ester, the principal esterified fatty acid is linoleic rather than oleic, reflecting its largely extracellular distribution. Thus plaque cholesterol ester composition differs from fatty streaks but resembles plasma lipoproteins.

The *complicated lesion* is a calcified fibrous plaque containing various degrees of necrosis, thrombosis, and ulceration. These are the lesions frequently associated with symptoms. With increasing necrosis and accumulation of gruel, the arterial wall progressively weakens, and rupture of the intima can occur, causing aneurysm and hemorrhage. Arterial emboli can form when fragments of plaque dislodge into the lumen. Stenosis and impaired organ function result from gradual occlusion as plaques thicken and thrombi form.

Localization Although the term *generalized atherosclerosis* is commonly used clinically, lesions are actually irregularly distributed; different vessels are involved at different ages and to varying degrees. The abdominal aorta is involved earliest and most severely by atherosclerotic lesions, and it is the bellwether of lesions elsewhere. The aorta is usually most heavily involved at or near the orifices of its branches (particularly at the level of the coronary and intercostal arteries), in the aortic arch, and frequently at its bifurcation into the iliac arteries. There is more atherosclerosis in the lower than in the upper limbs. In the legs, the incidence decreases peripherally as the musculoelastic vessels give way to large muscular arteries and these become smaller vessels, such as the plantar or digital arteries. Plaques and thromboses are particularly common in the *femoral* artery, in Hunter's canal, and in the *popliteal* artery just above the knee joint. The *anterior* and *posterior tibial* arteries are often occluded together, but in different sites—the posterior where it rounds the internal malleolus and the anterior where it is superficial and becomes the dorsalis pedis artery. The peroneal artery, which is well embedded in muscle, often escapes when other major vessels are occluded, and it may be the main blood supply to the extremity (*peroneal leg*). Atherosclerosis in abdominal branches, except for the renal and mesenteric arteries, causes less difficulty than in coronary and cerebral vessels.

In the *coronary arteries*, raised lesions are most prominent in the main stems, the highest incidence being a short distance beyond the ostia. Atherosclerosis is nearly always found in the epicardial (extramural) portions of the vessels, while the intramural coronary arteries are spared. Coronary atherosclerosis is often diffuse. The degree to which the lumen is narrowed varies, but once the process is present, all the intima of the extramural portions of the vessel is usually involved. A single tiny plaque occluding an otherwise normal coronary artery is rare. Selective involvement of the coronary arteries may relate to the unique hemodynamic forces, unlike those of other major arteries, resulting from greater flow in diastole than systole. The implications of these flow patterns for atherogenesis are as yet unknown. Typical atheromatous fibrous plaques also develop in saphenous vein aortocoronary bypass grafts.

In the cervical and cerebral arteries the distribution of atherosclerosis is patchy, as it may be in other arteries. It first appears in the base of the brain in the carotid, basilar, and vertebral arteries. The proximal portion of the internal carotid artery in the neck is a site of special predilection. There is a concentration of lesions near bifurcations. Atherosclerosis in the *pulmonary artery* bears no relation to the severity of the disease in the aorta or other systemic arteries. There is some involvement in about half of adults over 50 years of age who have no reason to have pulmonary hypertension. Pulmonary hypertension per se, however, is associated with medial hypertrophy, intimal thickening, and great acceleration of atheroma formation.

THEORIES OF ATHEROGENESIS A generally accepted theory for the pathogenesis of atherosclerosis consistent with a variety of experimental evidence is the *reaction to injury* hypothesis. According to this idea, the endothelial cells lining the intima are exposed to repeated or continuing insults to their integrity. The injury to the endothelium may be subtle or gross, resulting in a loss of the ability of the cells to function normally and act as a permeability barrier. In the extreme, the cells may desquamate. Examples of types of "injury" to the endothelium include metabolic injury, as in chronic hypercholesterolemia or homocysteinemia, mechanical stress associated with hypertension, and immunologic injury, as may be seen after cardiac or renal transplantation. Dysfunctional endothelial cells at susceptible sites in the arterial tree would lead to exposure of the subendothelial tissue to increased concentrations of plasma constituents. This may trigger a sequence of events including monocyte and platelet adherence, migration of monocytes into the intima to become macrophages, platelet aggregation and formation of microthrombi, and release of platelet and macrophage secretory products, including growth factors and cytokines (such as platelet-derived growth factor, interleukin 1, colony stimulating factors), in conjunction with plasma constituents, including lipoproteins and hormones such as insulin. This could stimulate the proliferation of intimal smooth-muscle cells at these sites of injury. These proliferating smooth-muscle cells would deposit a connective tissue matrix and accumulate lipid, a process that would be particularly enhanced with hyperlipidemia. Monocyte-derived macrophages also can accumulate lipids, some of which are in the form of lipid-protein complexes characteristic of oxidized lipoproteins. These cells are also capable of modifying lipoproteins in situ, favoring their uptake by scavenger receptors. Endothelial cells and macrophages can elaborate a chemoattractant protein that sustains accumulation of monocyte-derived macrophages.

Adherence of monocytes to altered endothelial cells and their migration into the arterial wall to become resident macrophages may be the earliest cellular abnormality in atherogenesis. Thus repeated or chronic injury could lead to a slowly progressing lesion involving a gradual increase in intimal smooth-muscle cells, macrophages, connective tissue, and lipid. Areas where the shearing stress on endothelial cells is increased, such as branch points or bifurcation of vessels, would be at greatest risk. As the lesions progress and the intima becomes thicker, blood flow over the sites will be altered and will potentially place the lining endothelial cells at even greater risk for further injury, leading to an inexorable cycle of events culminating in the complicated lesion. However, a single or a few injurious episodes may lead to a proliferative response that could regress, in contrast to continued or chronic injury. This hypothesis of reaction to injury thus is consistent with the known intimal thickening observed during normal aging, would explain how many of the etiologic factors implicated in atherogenesis might enhance lesion formation, might explain how inhibitors of platelet aggregation could interfere with lesion formation, and could elucidate how treatment targeted at risk-factor reduction can interrupt progression or even produce regression of atheromatous lesions.

Other theories of atherogenesis are not mutually exclusive. The *monoclonal hypothesis* suggests, on the basis of single isoenzyme types found in lesions, that the intimal proliferative lesions result from the multiplication of single, individual smooth-muscle cells, as do benign tumors. In this manner, mitogenic, and possibly mutagenic, factors that might stimulate smooth-muscle cell proliferation would act on single cells. Focal *clonal senescence* may explain how intrinsic aging processes contribute to atherosclerosis. According to this hypothesis, the intimal smooth-muscle cells that proliferate to form an atheroma are normally under feedback control by mitosis inhibitors formed by the smooth-muscle cells in the contiguous media, and this feedback control system tends to fail with age as these controlling cells die and are not adequately replaced. This is consistent with the observation that cultured human arterial medial smooth-muscle cells, like fibroblasts, show a decline in their ability to replicate as a function of donor age.

The *lysosomal theory* suggests that altered lysosomal function might contribute to atherogenesis. Since lysosomal enzymes can accomplish the generalized degradation of cellular components required for continuing renewal, this system has been implicated in cellular aging and the accumulation of lipofuscin or "age pigment." It has been suggested that increased deposition of cholesterol esters in arterial smooth-muscle cells may be related in part to a relative deficiency in the activity of lysosomal cholesterol ester hydrolase. Consonant with this idea, some patients with the rare cholesterol ester storage disease caused by a defect in lysosomal cholesterol ester hydrolase may have accelerated atherosclerosis. However, lipid droplets in foam cells are often cytoplasmic rather than lysosomal, and this theory is not now widely held.

RECOGNITION OF ATHEROSCLEROSIS Angiographic visualization of deformity in the lumen of a vessel remains the best presumptive test of silent atherosclerosis. Coronary angiography now permits visualization and assessment of arteries as small as 0.5 mm in diameter. Several sophisticated noninvasive techniques have been developed for demonstrating its presence. Doppler probes for measuring velocity and amount of blood flow have been used noninvasively and adapted to determine vessel outlines. Ultrasonic techniques are not yet clinically useful for detection of plaques in the coronary arteries.

Functional tests based on pathophysiologic or metabolic effects of a narrowed arterial lumen often give indirect clues. Assessment of electrocardiographic changes induced after standardized exercise is a relatively simple noninvasive aid to the diagnosis of coronary atherosclerosis with significant narrowing. Similarly, myocardial perfusion defects demonstrable with imaging techniques using radionuclides are usually attributable to atherosclerosis (Chap. 191). Digital plethysmography with exercise often unmasks significant atherosclerotic involvement of lower extremity arteries.

Radiographic demonstration of calcification in the location of arteries does not always indicate the presence of atherosclerosis. Although calcified coronary vessels usually indicate atherosclerosis, complete luminal obstruction may occur in the absence of any calcification. Calcification or beading of peripheral arteries is not correlated directly with atherosclerosis but more likely reflects medial sclerosis. Abnormalities in retinal arterioles evident on funduscopic examination are not well correlated with atherosclerosis in arteries. Thus, despite the availability of a variety of tests, detection of atherosclerosis usually awaits one of the clinical events attending a critical decrease of blood flow in an involved vessel. As yet there is no blood test for atherosclerosis. Knowledge of the prevalence and incidence of arteriosclerosis and most of the inferences concerning its causes are derived from tabulations of the appearance of its sequelae.

Ischemic heart disease (IHD), synonymous with *coronary heart disease* or *arteriosclerotic heart disease* (Chap. 203), is the most reliable indicator of atherosclerosis available today. Practically all patients with myocardial infarction, as defined by electrocardiographic and enzymatic changes, have coronary atherosclerosis. Rare exceptions are due to congenital anomalies of the coronary vessels, emboli, or ostial occlusion due to the other types of cardiac or vascular disease. Nontraumatic *sudden death* (Chap. 35) makes up a sizable portion of all deaths eventually certified as due to IHD. At autopsy, evidence of fresh myocardial infarction or of *coronary thrombosis* is usually absent. While ventricular fibrillation may have been due to sudden closure of a partially compromised vessel by a small thrombus or embolus or to *spasm*, none of these need have preceded a fatal arrhythmia. The majority of victims of sudden death have had a previous diagnosis of IHD; the number who had diabetes or hypertension is also significant. In epidemiologic studies of IHD, *angina pectoris* and electrocardiographic changes attributable to ischemia without infarction are considered "softer end points" and are treated separately.

Cerebrovascular disease (stroke) is a less reliable criterion for the presence of atherosclerosis. It includes *cerebral thrombosis* and *cerebral hemorrhage* (Chap. 368). Cerebral thrombosis, including infarction or softening without evidence of embolus, is usually due to atherosclerosis. On the other hand, cerebral hemorrhage is most often the result of congenital aneurysms or of vascular defects peculiar to hypertension and diabetes. Dissections of the aorta (Chap. 210), *peripheral vascular disease* (Chap. 211), thrombosis of other major vessels, and ischemic renal disease (Chap. 243) likewise are not used to determine the prevalence of atherosclerosis in a population or as an index of atherosclerosis elsewhere. Therefore, from an epidemiologic standpoint, consideration of atherosclerosis focuses on IHD.

INCIDENCE AND PREVALENCE According to the National Health Examination Survey, about 5 million Americans have IHD. It is the leading cause of death in males after age 35 and in all persons after age 45. Premature deaths from IHD, arbitrarily defined as those appearing before age 65, occur preponderantly in men, and a third of all deaths from IHD in males occur before age 65. In fact, nearly all the excess premature mortality in American males is due to IHD. Between the ages of 35 and 55, the death rate is five times higher in white men than in white women in the United States. The exceptions are women with hypertension, diabetes, hyperlipidemia, or premature (usually iatrogenic) menopause, who are at increased risk and often share the risk of the male. For both sexes, there is more than a fivefold increase in the average annual incidence of myocardial infarction between ages 40 and 60. A higher mortality rate in younger nonwhite women is probably due mainly to a greater incidence of hypertension in blacks. There is less difference between men and women in the prevalence of angina pectoris than in that of myocardial infarction; after age 65, more women than men have angina without a history of infarction.

Changing death rates In the United States death rates from IHD rose appreciably between 1940 and 1960. Mortality peaked in 1963 and started to decline, with the rate of decline accelerating in recent years for all ages, for both sexes, and for whites and nonwhites. This recent decline in mortality from coronary atherosclerosis (Table 208-3) is the first recorded in American history and is almost unique among industrialized countries. In other parts of the world, including Russia and many countries in eastern Europe, IHD death rates are still climbing. By contrast, in the United States, the IHD death rate declined by 57 percent between 1968 and 1990. The trend cannot be attributed to a single cause, but there has been a concurrent change in living habits, including reduced cigarette smoking among middle-aged men, decreased consumption of animal fats and cholesterol, better control of hypertension, and improved treatment of IHD.

International comparisons In most industrialized countries, IHD is the major single cause of premature cardiovascular deaths. There are, however, marked differences in premature death rates among them. The seven having the highest rates in men between 35 and 74 years of age are Finland, Scotland, Northern Ireland, Australia, New Zealand, England, and the United States. Much lower age-adjusted death rates from IHD are found in Latin America and Japan. The rates in Japan are about one-sixth those in the United States. Subsamples obtained in many countries convey the strong impression that upper socioeconomic classes that have adopted the culture of western industrialized countries have far more IHD than do lower socioeconomic classes. Among the most obvious cultural differences between these groups are total calories, fat content of the diet, and amount of physical work. Extensive epidemiologic studies have not revealed the reasons for differences between cultures that are superficially similar. Migrants to the United States tend to have a higher risk of death from premature IHD than do age-matched relatives who remain at home. Although there are many instances in which

TABLE 208-4   Risk factors for atherosclerosis

Male gender
Family history of premature IHD (before age 55 in a parent or sibling)
Hyperlipidemia
Cigarette smoking (currently smoking more than 10 cigarettes per day)
Hypertension
Low HDL cholesterol [below 0.9 mmol/L (35 mg/dL)]
Diabetes mellitus
Hyperinsulinemia
Abdominal obesity
High lipoprotein (a)
Personal history of cerebrovascular disease or occlusive peripheral vascular disease

different ethnic groups in the same locality have widely differing prevalences of IHD, the available data suggest that cultural factors are more important than genetic determination of IHD. Nevertheless, genetic heterogeneity undoubtedly underlies many of the striking differences in susceptibility seen among individuals sharing the same ethnic and cultural setting.

ETIOLOGIC FACTORS A number of conditions and habits present more frequently in individuals who develop atherosclerosis than in the general population; these factors have been termed *risk factors*. The majority of people below age 65 afflicted with atherosclerosis have one or more identifiable risk factors other than aging (Table 208-4). The risk-factor concept implies that a person with at least one risk factor is more likely to develop a clinical atherosclerotic event and is likely to do so earlier than a person with no risk factors. The presence of multiple risk factors further accelerates atherosclerosis. They vary in terms of importance in the population of the United States. Hypercholesterolemia, hypertension, and cigarette smoking may be the most potent factors involved in causation of atherosclerosis. Risk factors also vary in terms of their potential reversibility with current techniques of preventive management.

Thus age, gender, and genetic factors are currently considered to be irreversible risk factors, whereas continually emerging evidence suggests that elimination of cigarette smoking and treatment of hypertension reverses the high risk for atherosclerosis attributable to those factors. A major multicenter trial has shown that reduction of hypercholesterolemia reduces the risk of IHD. Life insurance policyholder data suggest that reduction of obesity reduces total mortality, presumably by diminishing the sequelae of atherosclerosis. Other potentially reversible factors are currently under study.

These factors are not mutually exclusive, since they clearly interact. For example, obesity, particularly of the abdominal type (assessed by the waist/hip circumference ratio), appears to be causally associated with hypertension, hyperglycemia, hypercholesterolemia, hypertriglyceridemia, and low high-density lipoprotein (HDL) cholesterol levels. Genetic factors may play a role by exerting direct effects on arterial wall cell structure and metabolism, or they may act indirectly via such factors as hypertension, hyperlipidemia, diabetes, and obesity. Aging appears to be one of the more complex factors associated with the development of atherosclerosis, since many of the risk factors in themselves are related to aging, e.g., elevated blood pressure, hyperglycemia, and hyperlipidemia. Thus, in addition to the possible involvement of intrinsic aging in atherogenesis (perhaps through effects on arterial wall metabolism), a variety of associated metabolic factors are also age-dependent.

Hyperlipidemia Both *hypercholesterolemia* and *hypertriglyceridemia* appear to be important risk factors for atherosclerosis. While there is no absolute quantitative definition of hyperlipidemia, statistical definitions, based on the upper 5 or 10 percent of the distribution of plasma lipid levels within a population, are often used. Such definitions are likely to detect affected individuals from families with one of the familial hyperlipidemias or having hyperlipidemia associated with other diseases or drugs; they also are useful for prediction of emergence of premature atherosclerosis and institution of preventive measures. However, these upper limits of "normality" are too high

TABLE 208-3   Age-adjusted death rates by cause in the United States, 1968, 1979, and 1990

Cause of death	Rate per 100,000 population		
	1968	1979	1990
All deaths	744	577	520
All cardiovascular diseases	362	254	190
Ischemic heart disease	242	150	103
Cerebrovascular disease	71	42	28
Cancer	129	131	135

SOURCE: The National Center for Health Statistics, *Monthly Vital Statistics Report, Advance Report of Final Mortality Statistics, 1990.*

for defining those cholesterol and triglyceride levels that are correlated with increasing risk of IHD in whole populations. Thus correlations between the cholesterol concentrations in young men in North America and the incidence of premature IHD indicate that an increasing risk can be detected when the cholesterol level is higher than 5.20 mmol/L (200 mg/dL), a value close to the median for men from 40 to 49 years of age in this population. Extrapolation of similar data from other populations suggests that the cholesterol level at birth averages 1.5 mmol/L (60 mg/dL). Within a month the average has risen to about 3 mmol/L (120 mg/dL) and by the first year to 4.5 mmol/L (175 mg/dL). A second rise begins in the third decade and continues to about age 50 in men and somewhat later in women.

A similar age-related increase in plasma triglyceride level is also observed. The increases in cholesterol are associated mainly with a rise in *low-density lipoprotein* (LDL) concentrations; the increases in triglyceride are associated with a rise in *very low density lipoproteins* (VLDL) and *remnants* of their catabolism (mainly intermediate-density lipoprotein, IDL). Adiposity may play a key role in this age-associated rise in triglyceride and cholesterol levels, since the increases in triglyceride, cholesterol, and body weight with age in whole populations occur concurrently. In primitive people who remain thin throughout adulthood, plasma lipids do not increase with age. Metabolic mechanisms have been postulated whereby abdominal obesity, which is associated with insulin resistance of peripheral tissues and compensatory hyperinsulinemia, promotes enhanced production of triglyceride- and cholesterol-rich lipoproteins by the liver and consequent hyperlipidemia, hypertension, and hyperglycemia (the insulin-resistance syndrome). Current concepts of plasma lipoprotein transport suggest that accumulation of cholesterol in the circulation may in part be secondary to excessive production of triglyceride-rich lipoproteins. Particle size of LDL (small, dense LDL or LDL subclass phenotype pattern B) has been implicated as a risk factor for IHD. LDL pattern B may be inherited as a dominant genetic trait and is also associated with high triglyceride and low HDL cholesterol levels, central obesity, and other features of the insulin-resistance syndrome. While closely associated with IHD in cross-sectional studies, LDL pattern B may not be an *independent* indicator of risk.

HYPERCHOLESTEROLEMIA   This is associated unequivocally with increased incidence of premature IHD; however, its importance varies in relation to age. In the Framingham Study, cholesterol levels in men below age 40 were closely related to the future development of IHD; this relation was less pronounced in older individuals. In the Multiple Risk Factor Intervention Trial (MRFIT), men with cholesterol levels above about 6 mmol/L (240 mg/dL) had more than a threefold increase in risk of IHD death compared with men with cholesterol levels below about 5 mmol/L (200 mg/dL). There is a continuous exponential gradient of risk as the cholesterol level ascends. These data are supported by comparisons of the prevalence of IHD and cholesterol (or LDL) in many other populations. The relationship of triglycerides and VLDL to IHD is confounded by a rise in cholesterol as VLDL increases. Nevertheless, in several, but not all, population studies, increased triglycerides (or VLDL) are independently correlated with premature IHD.

HYPERTRIGLYCERIDEMIA   This may be associated with premature atherosclerosis in some specific disorders; this association may not be apparent in studies of whole populations. Patients with high VLDL levels who come from families with familial combined hyperlipidemia appear to be at the same increased risk as those affected members of these families with elevated LDL levels. In contrast, patients with comparably elevated VLDL levels who come from families with pure monogenic familial hypertriglyceridemia do not appear to have an increased risk. In addition, high VLDL levels may increase the risk for premature atherosclerosis when associated with other risk factors for coronary artery disease, such as in diabetics and in patients on chronic hemodialysis who smoke and are hypertensive. Individuals in whom remnant lipoproteins accumulate, with resulting elevations in both cholesterol and triglycerides (Chap. 344), also seem to be at risk for early development of atherosclerosis.

Some of these relationships were clarified in a comprehensive study in Seattle of the role of the genetics of hyperlipidemia in clinical atherosclerosis in which 500 consecutive survivors of myocardial infarction were tested. Hyperlipidemia was present in about one-third of the group. Approximately one-half of the males and two-thirds of the females below age 50 had either hypertriglyceridemia, hypercholesterolemia, or both. On the other hand, in individuals over age 70, the prevalence of atherosclerotic coronary disease was very high, yet virtually no males (and only about one-fourth of the females) had hyperlipidemia. Thus in both sexes there appeared to be a progressive decline with age in the association of hyperlipidemia with myocardial infarction. More than half the hyperlipidemic atherosclerotic survivors appeared to have simple monogenic familial disorders inherited as an autosomal dominant trait (*familial combined hyperlipidemia* was the most common and *familial hypercholesterolemia* was the least common). These simply inherited hyperlipidemias were more frequent in myocardial infarction survivors below age 60 than in those who were older. In contrast, nonmonogenic forms of hyperlipidemia occurred with equal frequency above and below age 60. Thus it appears that genes associated with the simply inherited hyperlipidemias accelerate atherosclerosis. While all studies indicate that hyperlipidemia is a very meaningful risk factor below age 50 and that it operates independently of, and in addition to, hypertension, diabetes, obesity, and other factors, blood lipid levels continue to predict IHD in men and women over age 65.

SCREENING   When the screening of individuals for hyperlipidemia occurs after a myocardial infarction, it is several decades too late, although interruption of further progression of atherosclerosis now appears possible. Screening at birth or in childhood for genetic hyperlipidemia is not practical or useful except in the instance of familial hypercholesterolemia, which may affect about 1 in 1000 children. This is detectable by LDL elevations in cord blood when one already knows that a parent is affected. Other genetic or nongenetic primary hyperlipidemia often is not apparent until the third decade. *Today, screening measurement of blood cholesterol levels (nonfasting) by physicians is recommended for all adult patients. It is especially important in all young persons who have a family history of premature IHD.*

Hyperlipidemia is best confirmed by measurement of the concentration of total cholesterol and triglycerides and of HDL cholesterol in serum or plasma in a sample obtained after an overnight fast. The measurements should be made by a reliable laboratory that follows a program of standardization. Routine use of lipoprotein electrophoresis provides little additional information, is nonspecific, and is not recommended for screening or for management.

MANAGEMENT OF HYPERLIPIDEMIAS   In adults less than 65 years of age, a cholesterol concentration (C) greater than 6 mmol/L (240 mg/dL) or a triglyceride concentration (TG) greater than 2.8 mmol/L (250 mg/dL) clearly indicates hyperlipidemia sufficient to require some attention by the physician to the items listed in Table 208-5. Less severe degrees of hypercholesterolemia nevertheless can impart some degree of risk for IHD. The National Cholesterol Education Program (NCEP) has suggested that total cholesterol (C) > 6.2 mmol/L (240 mg/dL) is "high risk" and should prompt careful evaluation (see Table 208-5), estimation of LDL cholesterol, and some approach to cholesterol lowering. Cholesterol between 5.2 and 6.1 mmol/dL (200 and 239 mg/dL) is borderline high. The presence of two or more risk factors (independent of C or TG levels) listed in Table 208-4 or preexisting IHD puts these patients in the high-risk category. For treatment decisions, and when TG < 4.5 mmol/L (400 mg/dL), LDL cholesterol (LDL-C) levels can be estimated as total C − HDL-C − TG/5. Patients considered at high risk for IHD should be treated aggressively to lower blood cholesterol out of the high-risk range (Table 208-6). If C < 5.2 mmol/L (200 mg/dL), the tests need not be repeated for several years in an adult who maintains body weight and does not otherwise change in health or life-style. If causes of *secondary hyperlipidemia* or offending drugs are absent, attention to the origin of *primary hyperlipidemia* turns mainly to diet and

---

TABLE 208-5 Factors to consider in patients with hyperlipidemia

Disorders to which hyperlipidemia is secondary
  Uncontrolled diabetes mellitus (insulin deficiency)
  Hypothyroidism
  Uremia
  Nephrotic syndrome (hypoproteinemia)
  Obstructive liver disease
  Dysproteinemia (multiple myeloma, lupus erythematosus)
Drugs producing or aggravating hyperlipidemia
  Oral contraceptives
  Glucocorticoids
  Antihypertensives (thiazides and beta blockers)
Dietary factors
  Caloric intake (recent weight gain)
  Content of saturated fats and cholesterol
  Alcohol intake
Genetic disorders (primary hyperlipidemias)
  Family history of hyperlipidemia or xanthomas
  History of pancreatitis or recurrent abdominal pain

---

genetic causes. Severe hyperlipidemia [C > 7.8 mmol/L (300 mg/dL) or TG > 5.6 mmol/L (500 mg/dL)] usually reflects a genetic disorder; when xanthomas are present, it practically always does. Diagnosis always includes examination of first-degree relatives and proceeds according to information contained in Chap. 344.

Reduction of hypercholesterolemia results in a decrease in progression of atherosclerosis in humans and other primates. Several controlled trials of different diets which have been accompanied by a fall in mean cholesterol levels in small test populations have shown a favorable effect on incidence of the overall complications of IHD. The drug clofibrate given to a normal population reduced the incidence of nonfatal myocardial infarctions and was associated with a reduction of cholesterol levels; however, total mortality was not lowered. In the Lipid Research Clinics trial, the drug cholestyramine given to hypercholesterolemic asymptomatic men reduced morbidity and mortality from myocardial infarction in direct relation to the degree of cholesterol lowering; again, however, total mortality was not reduced. Lipid lowering by means of bile acid–binding resins (with niacin and diet therapy) also decreases progression and even induces regression of coronary lesions, as demonstrated by angiography in patients who have had coronary artery bypass graft surgery. Another fibric acid drug, gemfibrozil, has been shown to reduce mortality from IHD (but not total mortality) in association with lowered TG and C and raised HDL-C. Thus the weight of evidence strongly favors conservative measures to reduce cholesterol levels in patients through middle age and aggressive measures in patients who are frankly hypercholesterolemic, have clinical evidence of IHD, or are at high risk for progression of IHD.

Diet The first step in treatment of primary hyperlipidemia is attention to diet. All patients with mild to moderate hyperlipidemia

---

TABLE 208-6 Guidelines for treatment of high blood cholesterol in adults

	Cholesterol, mmol/L (mg/dL)			
	Desirable	Borderline-high	High	Decision
Total C	<5.2 (200)	5.2–6.1 (200–239)*	>6.2 (240)	Estimate LDL-C if total C borderline or high
LDL-C	<3.4 (130)	3.4–4.1 (130–159)*	>4.1 (160)	Diet treatment if LDL-C borderline or high
			>4.9 (190) or >4.1 (160)* or >3.4 (130)†	Drug treatment if LDL-C exceeds cut points after diet

* Becomes high risk if more than two risk factors (see Table 208-4) are present.
† High risk if definite IHD is present
SOURCE: National Cholesterol Education Program.

---

should first be brought to normal weight if they exceed it and then be maintained on a diet emphasizing decreases in intake of saturated fat and cholesterol. If hypertriglyceridemia is present, alcohol intake should be limited or eliminated. A single dietary approach to all forms of hyperlipidemia, including reduced intake of calories, cholesterol (to less than 300 mg/d), and saturated fat (to less than 10 percent of total calories), is appropriate for most patients. The degree of dietary modification would be proportional to the degree and nature of the hyperlipidemia. In practice, such a modification translates into limitation of animal fats and substitution of vegetable oils, fish, and carbohydrates. Increased physical activity is often a useful adjunct to dietary management. The maximum effect of such a regimen will be observed within 3 months after body weight has stabilized.

Drug therapy This often needs to be added for the management of the familial hyperlipidemias (Chap. 344) and for patients with a positive family history of atherosclerosis. Drug therapy is recommended by the NCEP for any adult patient whose LDL cholesterol level remains greater than 4.9 mmol/L (190 mg/dL) or greater than 4.1 mmol/L (160 mg/dL) in the presence of two or more risk factors (see Table 208-4) after an adequate trial of at least 3 months of diet therapy alone. A more aggressive approach is recommended for patients with clinically manifest IHD, with a suggested LDL cholesterol level of 3.4 mmol/L (130 mg/dL) or greater for initiation of drug therapy. A decision to start drug therapy should be made only after careful evaluation, since it usually commits patients to lifelong treatment. Continued follow-up and monitoring are essential. Drugs that act primarily by lowering LDL cholesterol (bile acid–binding resins, nicotinic acid, HMG-CoA reductase inhibitors; Table 208-7) are the drugs of choice for high-risk patients.

The resins act by enhancing sterol excretion and indirectly increasing LDL receptor–mediated catabolism of circulating LDL. They are minimally absorbed and have no systemic toxicity. Since there have been successful trials demonstrating safety and efficacy in primary prevention of IHD, they can be considered for use in children with familial hypercholesterolemia and for primary prevention in young adults. Nicotinic acid usage also has been associated with a reduction in recurrent IHD and total mortality in a secondary prevention trial and with regression of IHD in several angiographic studies. It uniquely lowers LDL and VLDL levels while raising HDL cholesterol (see below). It is the least expensive drug; side effects can be minimized by careful attention to very gradual increases in dosage. By blocking the rate-limiting step in cholesterol synthesis, the HMG-CoA reductase inhibitors (vastatins) enhance LDL receptor–mediated catabolism of LDL and are very effective in lowering LDL cholesterol levels. Side effects are minimal, and these drugs have been associated with regression of IHD in angiographic trials. Long-term efficacy and safety are being studied. Estrogen replacement therapy is effective in postmenopausal women with hypercholesterolemia and may be the first-choice agent in that patient group. Other LDL-lowering drugs (see Table 208-7) have had limited utility thus far. Aside from nicotinic acid, drugs that lower LDL cholesterol may increase VLDL, and conversely, drugs that lower VLDL may increase LDL in some patients. Thus LDL-lowering drugs alone are contraindicated in hypertriglyceridemia.

If TG remains greater than 3.4 mmol/L (300 mg/dL) after diet, a fibric acid derivative or nicotinic acid may be tried (see Table 208-7). Fibrates appear to decrease VLDL synthesis and enhance lipoprotein lipase–mediated catabolism of VLDL, thereby lowering TG and reciprocally raising HDL cholesterol levels. These drugs increase lithogenicity of bile and can produce myopathy. In a group of patients with high VLDL cholesterol, high LDL cholesterol, and low HDL cholesterol levels, gemfibrozil was effective in the primary prevention of IHD.

Two types of drugs may be used simultaneously if both C and TG are high. In patients with familial hypercholesterolemia (Chap. 344), combined therapy with a resin and nicotinic acid has achieved dramatic normalization of LDL cholesterol levels. Further studies are needed to define the long-term efficiency of various lipid-lowering agents in

TABLE 208-7 Drugs available for treatment of the hyperlipidemias

Class of drug	Drugs available	Major lipoprotein decreased	Mechanism	Usual daily dose	Common side effects	Reduces IHD risk
Fibric acid derivates	Clofibrate, gemfibrozil	VLDL	Decreases VLDL synthesis; enhances LPL action*	2 g 1–2 g	Gallstones, myopathy	Yes
Nicotinic acid	Nicotinic acid	VLDL, LDL	Decreases VLDL synthesis	2–6 g	Gastrointestinal symptoms, flushing, hyperglycemia, hepatic dysfunction	Yes
Bile acid–binding resins	Cholestyramine, cholestipol	LDL	Promotes sterol excretion; increases LDL receptor–mediated removal	4–24 g 5–20 g	Gastrointestinal symptoms, high VLDL	Yes
HMG-CoA reductase inhibitors	Lovastatin, simvastatin, pravastatin	LDL	Blocks cholesterol synthesis; increases LDL receptor–mediated removal	10–40 mg 5–20 mg 10–40 mg	Gastrointestinal symptoms, myopathy	Yes
Probucol	Probucol	LDL	Unknown	1 g	Diarrhea, low HDL	Unknown
Estrogens	Premarin, estradiol	LDL	Unknown	0.625 mg 2 mg	High VLDL, endometrial cancer	Yes

* LPL = lipoprotein lipase.

the prevention or reversal of atherosclerosis and its sequelae. The long-term effects of any of these drugs used before puberty are unknown, and their use during pregnancy is not advocated. There is a paucity of data to justify their use in the elderly, although studies are underway. In a revision of the NCEP, it was suggested that elderly individuals should not be excluded from treatment solely on the basis of age, since they are responsive to cholesterol-lowering regimens. As the first approach to this group, attention to multiple risk factors and hygienic measures (diet and physical activity) appears appropriate.

OTHER RISK FACTORS High-density lipoproteins (HDL) The level of HDL, a complex family of particles that carry about 20 percent of the total plasma cholesterol, is inversely associated with the development of premature atherosclerosis and therefore can be considered an "antirisk factor." HDL levels can be assessed simply by measurement of cholesterol in the supernatant fluid after the other lipoproteins in plasma have been precipitated. Thus individuals whose HDL cholesterol is elevated may be less likely to develop IHD; conversely, low HDL cholesterol is associated with increased risk of IHD. In the Framingham Study, low HDL cholesterol was a more potent lipid risk factor than was high total cholesterol or LDL. At least five diverse population studies have confirmed a close correlation between IHD and low HDL, independent of other factors.

Consistent with differences in risk between the sexes, HDL cholesterol averages about 25 percent higher in women than in men. Estrogens tend to raise and androgens tend to lower HDL levels. In women, low HDL, particularly when associated with diabetes and obesity, markedly raises the risk of IHD. Octogenarians tend to have high HDL, which may be partly familial. Of interest for preventive measures, cigarette smoking decreases and regular strenuous exercise increases HDL cholesterol. Regular exercise increases HDL even in individuals after myocardial infarction. A small daily intake of alcohol has been associated with both reduced risk of IHD and high HDL levels. Mechanisms for these effects remain unknown.

The utility of HDL cholesterol measurements as a single determinant of risk in individuals is limited because the analytical error in many laboratories exceeds the differences in HDL levels associated with risk. HDL measurements are most helpful for estimation of LDL cholesterol. Because of the close inverse relationship between plasma triglycerides (or VLDL) and HDL, HDL in most hypertriglyceridemic persons, with or without hypercholesterolemia, will be predictably low. Low HDL cholesterol is one of the factors that can place patients in a high-risk category for IHD (see Table 208-6).

Hypertension (See Chap. 209) High blood pressure is an important risk factor for atherosclerosis, mainly IHD and cerebrovascular disease. The risk increases progressively with increasing blood pressure; in the Framingham Study, IHD incidence in middle-aged

men with blood pressures exceeding 160/95 was more than five times that in normotensive men (blood pressure 140/90 or less). Hypertensive men and women are both affected, with the diastolic pressure perhaps being more important. In industrialized populations, blood pressure appears to increase inexorably with age; however, the nature of this age relation varies among populations, since there are remote primitive populations that age without any changes in blood pressure levels. The age-associated blood pressure increase might be related to physical activity or dietary factors, particularly sodium and total caloric content. Hypertension appears to increase atherosclerosis throughout the age span.

Conversely, the risk for atherosclerosis appears diminished by therapeutic reduction of blood pressure. Recent intervention studies have shown convincingly that reduction of diastolic levels that had been greater than 105 mmHg significantly reduces the incidence of strokes, IHD, and congestive heart failure in men. Even when patients with diastolic pressures between 90 and 105 mmHg are similarly maintained on adequate treatment, the incidence of some of these complications may be reduced. A recent trial of treatment of isolated systolic hypertension in otherwise healthy elderly subjects showed that reduction of blood pressure substantially reduced both IHD and stroke. Special urgency for relief of hypertension obtains when hyperlipidemia, diabetes, or other risk factors are present.

Cigarette smoking Not only is cigarette smoking one of the more potent risk factors for atherosclerosis, it is also one of the factors that when reduced or eliminated clearly decreases the risk of developing atherosclerosis. Ample statistical evidence supports a mean increase of about 70 percent in the death rate and a three- to fivefold increase in risk of IHD in men who smoke one pack of cigarettes per day compared with nonsmokers. In general, the increase in death rate is proportional to the amount smoked and decreases with age. Excess morbidity from myocardial infarction is also present in women smokers, but the relationship is somewhat less firm than in men. However, there is an impressive accentuation of IHD mortality in women over age 35 taking oral contraceptives who in addition smoke cigarettes. In some atherosclerosis-prone populations, such as patients maintained on long-term hemodialysis, cigarette smoking interacts with other risk factors, resulting in a marked enhancement of atherosclerosis mortality. Such interaction is also likely for diabetic and hypertensive populations.

The association of smoking and increased IHD remains unexplained. Pipe and cigar smokers have a lesser increase in risk of IHD, presumably because less smoke is inhaled. Smokers dying of causes other than IHD have been found at autopsy to have more coronary atherosclerosis than nonsmokers. The major influence of smoking is on the incidence of sudden death, however. Those who stop smoking show a prompt decline in risk and may reach the risk level of nonsmokers as early as after 1 year of abstention.

Hyperglycemia and diabetes mellitus (See Chap. 337) Studies in a variety of populations have shown an association of hyperglycemia with clinically evident atherosclerotic disease, suggesting a role of hyperglycemia in atherogenesis. In known diabetics, both insulin-dependent (IDD) and non-insulin-dependent (NIDD) types, there is at least a twofold increase in incidence of myocardial infarction compared with nondiabetics. This risk is markedly increased in younger diabetics; recent data indicate that about one-third of patients with IDD die of IHD by age 55. Diabetic women are even more prone to IHD than are diabetic men. There is an increased tendency toward cerebral thrombosis and infarction but not toward cerebral hemorrhage in diabetes. Gangrene of the lower extremities has been variously estimated to be from 8 to 150 times as frequent in diabetics as in nondiabetics and is most often found in diabetics who smoke. Diabetes mellitus is associated with an increase in atherosclerosis observed at autopsy in a variety of populations worldwide, whether the prevalence of atherosclerosis in a particular population is high or low. Mortality from IHD in diabetes is increased even in populations in which the incidence of IHD is low, such as those in Asia. Data from MRFIT show that while IHD mortality increases as a function of the number and intensity of the major risk factors in diabetics, just as it does in nondiabetics, for every risk-factor level, diabetics have three- to fivefold higher IHD mortality rates.

The risk for atherosclerotic disease, however, does not appear to be grossly related to the degree of hyperglycemia among diabetics. Results in the University Group Diabetes Program Study have suggested that reduction of blood glucose by insulin does not appear to influence mortality from established atherosclerosis during a 5-year period. Thus hyperglycemia and atherosclerosis are associated, since there is an increased prevalence of large-vessel disease in known diabetics and, conversely, an increased prevalence of hyperglycemia in association with atherosclerotic disease. These associations remain unexplained and reversibility undocumented. Clinical and experimental studies also support a role for the insulin-resistance syndrome and high circulating insulin levels in IHD. The capillary microangiopathy, pathognomonic of diabetes mellitus and causing important dysfunction of the kidneys and retina, has unknown clinical significance in relation to atherosclerotic disease in larger arteries.

Obesity In general, morbidity and mortality from IHD are higher in direct relation to the degree of overweight beyond about 30 percent. Furthermore, from data obtained in the Framingham Study, it appears that obesity may accelerate atherosclerosis, since its effect is more apparent before age 50. Nevertheless, some of the major epidemiologic studies of coronary heart disease have not demonstrated an independent relationship between this condition and anything less than very severe obesity. A close relation between type of obesity (i.e., abdominal) and IHD has been identified. Furthermore, abdominal obesity is a disorder closely associated with several other potent risk factors, i.e., hypertriglyceridemia, hypercholesterolemia, hyperglycemia, and hypertension. This cluster defines the insulin-resistance syndrome. The relationship between obesity and atherosclerosis is thus multifaceted; since in practice obesity does not occur "independently," it is of considerable importance as a risk factor, particularly abdominal obesity.

Physical inactivity Study of the relationship of the prevalence of IHD to daily (occupational) physical activity is made difficult because so many variables are involved. Among prospective studies, the Framingham data do indicate that the less sedentary an individual is, the less susceptible that individual is to sudden death. Physical work may be the major determinant of greatly differing incidences of IHD in southern black and white males in the United States and in populations that move from rural areas to urbanized environments. How physical activity may operate to decrease death from IHD, or possibly to decrease atherogenesis, is not known. Beyond the amelioration of hyperlipidemia by increasing caloric expenditure, no mechanism has been demonstrated. The meaning of the physical activity–induced increase in HDL, the antirisk factor for IHD, remains mysterious. Physical training has been shown to improve exercise performance in patients with IHD and angina pectoris. Regular physical activity is supported as a desirable element in a program of preventive health maintenance.

Stress and personality There is a valid clinical impression that psychic or emotional stress and anxiety are associated with precipitation of overt IHD and sudden death. Debate continues as to whether there may be distinct personality types prone to or relatively immune to premature IHD (the so-called personality types A and B) and whether the presumably more deleterious type is amenable to correction beyond elimination of cigarette smoking and adverse dietary patterns and avoidance of stressful life situations. Many social and demographic analyses have so far failed to reach any agreement about the etiologic relationships of occupation and similar situational factors and the incidence of IHD.

Genetic factors Premature atherosclerosis often appears to be familial. In many instances this can be attributed to the inheritance of risk factors such as hypertension, diabetes mellitus, and hyperlipidemia. Occasionally, families with excessive premature vascular disease can be found in which none of the known risk factors appears to be operating. Genetic determinants of protective factors, such as HDL, and of nonlipid risk factors, such as apolipoprotein B and lipoprotein (a), need to be understood; undoubtedly other important determinants remain to be discovered. Nevertheless, family history is one of the more important factors to be weighed in assessment of risk, thereby helping the physician to avoid missing treatable risk factors and in institution of appropriate preventive measures.

ROLE OF DIET IN RISK FOR ATHEROSCLEROSIS The relationship of diet to IHD remains an area of intense interest and persistent controversy. In epidemiologic studies, no population habitually subsisting on a diet low in saturated fat and cholesterol has an appreciable amount of IHD. These populations also tend to have lower plasma lipid concentrations. There is a general upward shift of average cholesterol and triglyceride levels in highly developed countries, which is an effect of change in total culture and life-style as well as in diet. Dietary changes in migrant populations who move from more primitive to more industrialized societies commonly include increased intake of total calories, animal fats, cholesterol, and salt, leading to a diet-accentuated emergence of risk factors such as obesity, hyperlipidemia, diabetes, and hypertension. There is no question that the plasma cholesterol (and LDL) level is sensitive to the amount of saturated fat and cholesterol in the diet. The "average" adult male in the United States eats about 140 g fat per day and about 0.1 mmol (400 mg) cholesterol. The mixture of fats ingested usually contains about three times as much saturated fatty acids (mainly palmitic and stearic) as polyunsaturated fatty acids (mainly linoleic and linolenic). If a healthy young adult switches from this diet to one containing the same amount of total fat in which the ratio of polyunsaturates to saturates is closer to unity and the cholesterol content is less than 0.07 mmol (300 mg) per day, the cholesterol concentration will usually drop by 10 to 15 percent within 2 weeks and remain depressed on continuation of the diet.

The average cholesterol level in most populations is most closely related to the amount of animal fats (meat, eggs, and milk products, major sources of long-chain saturated fatty acids and cholesterol) in the diet. Increased animal fat consumption also tends to be correlated with a greater proportion of dietary fats being saturated and with lesser intake of complex carbohydrates and vegetable fibers; these are dietary changes that may lead to a rise in plasma cholesterol levels. The average triglyceride level is more sensitive to total caloric balance and to alcohol intake. It is important to note that physical activity, emotional stress, smoking, and intake of coffee or tea have only weak or indirect influences on total cholesterol and triglyceride concentrations.

In experimental animals, added dietary cholesterol and fat are essential for the production of atherosclerosis. Typical American diets fed to nonhuman primates produce aortic and coronary atherosclerosis which is reversible when a cholesterol-free diet is fed. Controlled metabolic studies in humans show a direct relation between dietary and plasma cholesterol below intakes of about 0.15 mmol (600 mg) per day; no relation is observed at higher intakes when plasma cholesterol is already high. There appear to be marked genetic variations in the ability of dietary cholesterol to influence plasma cholesterol level among individuals and among populations. The relation between dietary polyunsaturated/saturated fat ratio (P/S) and both cholesterol and triglyceride levels also has been amply established. The unique triglyceride-lowering effects of the particular long-chain polyunsaturated fatty acids in large ocean fish are currently under study.

A definitive prospective study of the effect of diet on IHD in the general population has never been undertaken. Nevertheless, reports of newer studies of alterations of diet in high-risk populations provide strong evidence of a reversible relation among diet, plasma lipids, and IHD. On this basis, numerous authoritative nutrition councils have recommended prudent dietary modifications for the general population of western countries to be instituted early in life and to include a caloric intake adjusted to achieve and maintain ideal body weight, a reduction in total fat calories to 30 to 35 percent of total calories achieved by a substantial reduction in dietary saturated fat to less than 10 percent of total calories, and a reduction in cholesterol intake to less than 300 mg/d. Although a causal relationship in humans between sodium intake and hypertension has not been firmly established, avoidance of excessive dietary sodium also has been recommended.

RISK FACTORS AND MECHANISMS OF ATHEROGENESIS

Adiposity produces insulin resistance in peripheral tissues (mainly muscle and adipose), which leads to compensatory hyperinsulinemia. The liver is not resistant to some effects of insulin, and enhanced production of triglyceride-rich lipoproteins results, leading to elevated plasma triglyceride and cholesterol levels. Thus it has been demonstrated that body weight is related not only to triglyceride levels but also to cholesterol levels. Concomitantly, obesity is associated with increased total-body cholesterol synthesis. Obesity, particularly the abdominal type, produces higher circulating levels of insulin, both in the basal state and after stimulation with glucose or other secretagogues. Since obesity is related to atherosclerosis—both directly and via hypertension, hypertriglyceridemia, hypercholesterolemia, and hyperglycemia—it is not surprising that many studies show a relationship between serum insulin levels, particularly after oral glucose intake, and atherosclerotic disease of the coronary and peripheral arteries. A few studies, however, suggest that this association between insulin and atherosclerosis occurs independently of obesity. It has been postulated that insulin may directly affect arterial wall metabolism, leading to increased endogenous lipid synthesis and thus predisposing to atherosclerosis. Insulin has been shown to stimulate proliferation of arterial smooth-muscle cells, enhance binding of LDL and VLDL, and decrease binding of HDL to cells; it therefore may be one of the plasma factors involved in atheroma formation.

Hypertension may enhance atherogenesis by directly producing injury via mechanical stress on endothelial cells at specific high-pressure sites in the arterial tree. The sequence of events in the chronic injury hypothesis of atherogenesis would follow. In addition, hypertension alters endothelial permeability and markedly increases lysosomal enzyme activity. Experimental hypertension also increases the thickness of the intimal smooth-muscle layer in the arterial wall and increases connective tissue elements. It is still not known if continued high pressure within the artery produces changes in the ability of smooth-muscle cells or stem cells to proliferate.

Diabetes could provide a unique contribution to atherogenesis. Although the fundamental genetic abnormality in either type of human diabetes mellitus remains unknown, it has been suggested that genetic diabetes in humans imparts a primary cellular abnormality intrinsic to all cells, resulting in a decreased life span of individual cells, which in turn results in increased cell turnover in tissues. If arterial endothelial and smooth-muscle cells are intrinsically defective in

diabetes, accelerated atherogenesis can be readily postulated on the basis of any one of the current theories of pathogenesis. Platelet dysfunction in diabetes also may play a role.

The role of glucose in atheroma formation, if any, is poorly understood. Hyperglycemia is known to affect aortic wall metabolism. Sorbitol, a product of the insulin-independent aldose reductase pathway of glucose metabolism (the polyol pathway), accumulates in the arterial wall in the presence of high glucose concentrations, resulting in osmotic effects, including increased cell water content and decreased oxygenation. Increased glucose also appears to stimulate proliferation of cultured arterial smooth-muscle cells. Glycosylation of apolipoproteins and other key proteins intrinsic to the arterial wall producing advanced glycosylated end products also may be involved. When deposited in the artery, these products may influence arterial wall cell function. For example, glycosylated collagen avidly binds and traps LDL. Glycosylated LDL can be formed which may be more susceptible to oxidation and more readily deliver cholesterol to arterial wall cells than native LDL.

The development of atherosclerosis accelerates in approximate quantitative relation to the degree of *hyperlipidemia*. A long-established theory suggests that the higher the circulating levels of lipoprotein, the more likely they are to gain entrance to the arterial wall. By an acceleration of the usual transendothelial transport, large concentrations of lipoproteins within the arterial wall could overwhelm the ability of smooth-muscle cells and monocyte-derived macrophages to metabolize them. Lipoproteins have been immunologically identified in atheroma, and in humans there is a close relationship between plasma cholesterol and arterial lipoprotein cholesterol concentration. High-density lipoproteins may be protective in relation to their ability to promote cholesterol efflux from artery wall cells. Chemically modified or oxidized lipoproteins, possibly produced in hyperlipidemic disorders, could gain access to the scavenger arterial wall macrophages, leading to formation of foam cells. It is possible that the lipid that accumulates in the arterial wall with increasing age results from infiltration of plasma lipoproteins which bind to matrix components. However, atheromatous lesions are associated with a more marked increase in arterial wall lipids, which may result in part from injury to the endothelium produced by chronic hyperlipidemia, as demonstrated in cholesterol-fed monkeys.

The effect of *chronic smoke inhalation* from cigarettes could result in repetitive toxic injury to endothelial cells, thereby accelerating atherogenesis. Hypoxia stimulates proliferation of cultured human arterial smooth-muscle cells; thus, since cigarette smoking is associated with high levels of carboxyhemoglobin and low oxygen delivery to tissues, another mechanism for atherogenesis is suggested. Hypoxia could produce diminished lysosomal enzyme degradative ability, as evidenced by impaired degradation of LDL by smooth-muscle cells, causing LDL-derived cholesterol to accumulate in the cells. Consistent with this suggestion is the fact that aortic lesions that resemble atheroma have been produced in experimental animals by systemic hypoxia, and lipid accumulation in the arterial wall of cholesterol-fed rabbits and monkeys appear to be increased by hypoxia.

RISK FACTOR REVERSAL AND REGRESSION OF ATHEROSCLEROSIS

By removal or reversal of a single risk factor or group of risk factors, the emergence of clinical consequences of atherosclerosis can be lessened, and the regression or interruption of progression of atherosclerosis, determined by direct or indirect examination of lesions, can be accomplished in humans. Recent studies of the size of coronary or peripheral artery atheromatous lesions by sequential arteriograms taken before and after a period of treatment aimed at risk-factor reversal strongly suggest that interruption of lesion progression and even regression of lesions are possible. Treatments that have been successful include lipid-lowering by single drugs, multiple drugs, diet alone, combinations of diet and drug therapy, and ileal bypass surgery. Advanced atherosclerotic lesions appear to respond more favorably when serum LDL cholesterol levels are reduced to the low levels that prevail in populations consuming a low-fat diet. There is also encouraging evidence in animals, most notably in primates, that relatively complicated plaques induced by hyperlipidemia will regress and that further progression of atherosclerosis will cease when hyperlipidemia is removed.

Risk factor reversal is feasible in asymptomatic individuals and should be encouraged. Through mass-media educational efforts, whole communities can be influenced to reduce smoking, change diet, and lower blood pressure levels. Adult males in the United States have lowered cigarette consumption, although increases among teenage girls are disappointing. There has been a trend toward lower cholesterol and saturated fat consumption in the United States, coupled with increasing attention to weight reduction and the use of exercise programs. Concomitantly, and perhaps causally, there has been the noted decline in IHD mortality. Therefore, efforts to prevent atherogenesis, to interrupt progression, and perhaps to promote regression of existing lesions by risk factor reduction seem warranted.

PREVENTION   Although premature IHD is overall the most costly and common of the untimely complications of atherosclerosis, preoccupation with IHD should not obscure the fact that angina pectoris and myocardial infarction are expressions of late-stage atherosclerotic lesions. Factors precipitating these clinical events may be independent of those leading to initiation of plaque formation or its progression to a complicated lesion. Steps taken to prevent recurrence of myocardial infarction or fatal arrhythmia, termed *secondary prevention*, will not necessarily be the same as those taken to delay or prevent formation of atherosclerosis (*primary prevention*). Since atherosclerotic plaques have been detected in the coronary arteries of American males as early as the second decade in autopsy studies of Korean and Vietnam war deaths, primary prevention of atherosclerosis must begin early in life, long before there is any suspicion of IHD.

Thus *prevention of atherosclerosis, rather than treatment, is the goal*. Although an effective program has not been established with certainty, enough is known to act as a guide both in identification of those with a higher risk and in development of conservative measures that probably will reduce that risk. Thus prevention currently is equated with risk-factor reduction.

The decline of American death rates from premature IHD coincides with two trends in health practices. One is the increasing recognition of the importance of detecting and attempting to correct some of the risk factors correlated with atherosclerosis. The other is a greater awareness of the dietary sources of cholesterol and saturated fats and a tendency of the public to restrict their intake somewhat. Whether these trends are causally related to the decline in death rate is not known. While a rigorous approach to changes in life-style for the general population may be debatable, it is desirable to continue finding and helping those most susceptible to early atherosclerosis. The physician's role in risk-factor reduction involves treatment of hypertension and hyperlipidemia and advice regarding diet, body weight, smoking, and exercise. Drug treatment of hyperlipidemia should be limited to those individuals at high risk who do not respond adequately to dietary management. Since pooled data from trials are encouraging, the long-term use of antiplatelet drugs to reduce the incidence of reinfarction or death in individuals with IHD has been advocated.

TREATMENT   There is no agent proven to have any value in "treatment" of atherosclerosis unless it clearly reduces severe hyperlipidemia or obvious hypertension. In fact, there is no treatment of atherosclerosis, only of its complications. While end-stage treatment technology has reduced morbidity, prevention remains the long-term goal of both research and medical practice.

REFERENCES

AUSTIN MA: Plasma triglyceride and coronary heart disease. Arteriosclerosis Thrombosis. 11:2, 1991

AVIRAM M: Modified forms of low density lipoprotein and atherosclerosis. Atherosclerosis 98:1, 1993

BIERMAN EL: Atherogenesis in diabetes. Arteriosclerosis Thrombosis. 12:647, 1992

————: Aging and atherosclerosis, in *Principles of Geriatric Medicine and Gerontology*, 3d ed, WR Hazzard et al (eds). New York, McGraw-Hill, 1993

BROWN G et al: Regression of coronary artery disease as a result of intensive lipid-lowering therapy in men with high levels of apolipoprotein B. N Engl J Med 323:1289, 1990

CLARKE R et al: Hyperhomocysteinemia: An independent risk factor for vascular disease. N Engl J Med 324:1149, 1991

EVERHART JE et al: Medial arterial calcification and its association with mortality and complications of diabetes. Diabetologia 31:16, 1988

LEONE A: Cardiovascular damage from smoking: A fact or a belief? Int J Cardiol 38:113, 1993

NATIONAL CHOLESTEROL EDUCATION PROGRAM: Report of the National Cholesterol Education Program Expert Panel on Detection, Evaluation and Treatment of High Blood Cholesterol in Adults. JAMA 269:3015, 1993

POOTHULLIL JM: Obesity, hyperlipidemia and non-insulin-dependent diabetes: A unified theory. Neurosci Biobehav Rev 17:85, 1993

RIFKIND RB (ed): *Drug Treatment of Hyperlipidemia*. New York, Dekker, 1991

ROSS R: The pathogenesis of atherosclerosis: A perspective for the 1990's. Nature 362:801, 1993

SHARRETT AR: Invasive versus noninvasive studies of risk factors and atherosclerosis. Circulation 87:II48, 1993

STAMPFER MJ et al: Postmenopausal estrogen therapy and cardiovascular disease. N Engl J Med 326:756, 1991

STARY HC et al: A definition of the intima of human arteries and of its atherosclerosis-prone regions. Circulation 85:391, 1992

VOS J et al: Retardation and arrest of progression or regression of coronary artery disease: A review. Prog Cardiovasc Dis 35:435, 1993

WALLACE RB, ANDERSON RA: Blood lipids, lipid-related measures, and the risk of atherosclerotic cardiovascular disease. Epidemiol Rev 9:95, 1987

YLA HERTTUALA S: Biochemistry of the arterial wall in developing atherosclerosis. Ann NY Acad Sci 623:40, 1991

209   HYPERTENSIVE VASCULAR DISEASE

GORDON H. WILLIAMS

An elevated arterial pressure is probably the most important public health problem in developed countries. It is common, asymptomatic, readily detectable, usually easily treatable, and often leads to lethal complications if left untreated. As a result of extensive educational programs in the late 1960s and 1970s by both private and governmental agencies, the number of undiagnosed and/or untreated patients has been significantly reduced to a level of less than 20 percent. This factor may be the most important one responsible for the decline in cardiovascular mortality which has taken place during the past 20 years (Chap. 208). Although our understanding of the pathophysiology of an elevated arterial pressure has increased, in 90 to 95 percent of cases the etiology (and thus potentially the prevention or cure) is still largely unknown. As a consequence, in most cases the hypertension is treated nonspecifically, resulting in a large number of minor side effects and a relatively high (~50 percent) non-compliance rate.

DEFINITION   Since there is no dividing line between normal and high blood pressure, arbitrary levels have been established to define those who have an increased risk of developing a morbid cardiovascular event and/or will clearly benefit from medical therapy. These definitions should consider not only the level of diastolic pressure but also systolic pressure, age, sex, and race. For example, patients with a diastolic pressure greater than 90 mmHg will have a significant reduction in morbidity and mortality with adequate therapy. These, then, are patients who have hypertension and who should be considered for treatment.

The level of *systolic* pressure is also important in assessing arterial pressure's influence on cardiovascular morbidity. Males with normal diastolic pressures (<82 mmHg) but elevated systolic pressures (>158 mmHg) have a $2\frac{1}{2}$-fold increase in their cardiovascular mortality rates when compared with individuals with similar diastolic pressures but whose systolic pressures are normal (<130 mmHg). Reduction in mortality and morbidity with treatment, specifically in the elderly, has been documented in these patients. This beneficial effect is mainly secondary to a reduction in strokes and occurs in women as well. Other significant factors which modify blood pressure's influence on the frequency of morbid cardiovascular events are age, race, and sex, with young black males being most adversely affected by hypertension.

When hypertension is suspected, blood pressure should be measured at least twice during two separate examinations after the initial screening. In adults, a *diastolic* pressure below 85 mmHg is considered to be normal; between 85 and 89 is high normal; 90 to 104 is mild hypertension; 105 to 114 moderate hypertension; 115 or greater is severe hypertension. When the diastolic pressure is below 90 mmHg, a *systolic* pressure below 140 mmHg indicates normal blood pressure; between 140 and 159 is borderline isolated systolic hypertension; 160 or higher is isolated systolic hypertension. Increasing use of 12- or 24-h blood pressure monitoring may provide additional useful information in patients who are difficult to classify. However, normal values for this procedure and their utility in relationship to therapeutic outcomes are not currently available.

Arterial pressure fluctuates in most persons, whether they are normotensive or hypertensive. Those who are classified as having *labile* hypertension are patients who sometimes, but not always, have arterial pressures within the hypertensive range. These patients are often considered to have borderline hypertension.

Sustained hypertension can become accelerated or enter a malignant phase, although this is unusual in treated patients. Though a patient with *malignant hypertension* often has a blood pressure above 200/140, it is papilledema, usually accompanied by retinal hemorrhages and exudates, and not the absolute pressure level, that defines this condition. *Accelerated hypertension* signifies a significant recent increase over previous hypertensive levels associated with evidence of vascular damage on funduscopic examination but without papilledema.

PREVALENCE   The prevalence of hypertension depends on both the racial composition of the population studied and the criteria used to define the condition. In a white suburban population like that in the Framingham Study, nearly one-fifth have blood pressures greater than 160/95, while almost one-half have pressures greater than 140/90. An even higher prevalence has been documented in the nonwhite population.

The prevalence of various forms of secondary hypertension depends on the nature of the population studied and how extensive the evaluation is. There are no available data to define the frequency of secondary hypertension in the general population, although in middle-aged males it has been reported to be 6 percent. On the other hand, in referral centers where patients undergo an extensive evaluation, it has been reported to be as high as 35 percent. The various forms of hypertension are outlined in Table 209-1, and their relative frequencies are given in Table 209-2.

ESSENTIAL HYPERTENSION

Patients with arterial hypertension and no definable cause are said to have *primary*, *essential*, or *idiopathic hypertension*. Undoubtedly, the primary difficulty in uncovering the mechanism(s) responsible for the hypertension in these patients is attributable to the variety of systems that are involved in the regulation of arterial pressure—peripheral and/or central adrenergic, renal, hormonal, and vascular—and to the complexity of the relationships of these systems to one another. Several abnormalities have been described in patients with essential hypertension, often with a claim that one or more of these are primarily responsible for the hypertension. While it is still uncertain whether these individual abnormalities are primary or secondary, varying expressions of a single disease process or reflective of separate disease entities, the accumulating data increasingly support the latter hypothesis. Therefore, just as pneumonia is caused by a variety of infectious agents, even though the clinical picture observed may be similar, so essential hypertension likely has a number of distinct causes. Thus the distinction between primary and secondary hypertension has become blurred, and the approach to both the diagnosis and therapy of hypertensive patients has been modified. For

TABLE 209-1   Classification of arterial hypertension

SYSTOLIC HYPERTENSION WITH WIDE PULSE PRESSURE

A Decreased compliance of aorta (arteriosclerosis)
B Increased stroke volume
  1 Aortic regurgitation
  2 Thyrotoxicosis
  3 Hyperkinetic heart syndrome
  4 Fever
  5 Arteriovenous fistula
  6 Patent ductus arteriosus

SYSTOLIC AND DIASTOLIC HYPERTENSION (INCREASED PERIPHERAL VASCULAR RESISTANCE)

A Renal
  1 Chronic pyelonephritis
  2 Acute and chronic glomerulonephritis
  3 Polycystic renal disease
  4 Renovascular stenosis or renal infarction
  5 Most other severe renal disease (arteriolar nephrosclerosis, diabetic nephropathy, etc.)
  6 Renin-producing tumors
B Endocrine
  1 Oral contraceptives
  2 Adrenocortical hyperfunction
    a Cushing's disease and syndrome
    b Primary hyperaldosteronism
    c Congenital or hereditary adrenogenital syndromes (17α-hydroxylase and 11β-hydroxylase defects)
  3 Pheochromocytoma
  4 Myxedema
  5 Acromegaly
C Neurogenic
  1 Psychogenic
  2 "Diencephalic syndrome"
  3 Familial dysautonomia (Riley-Day)
  4 Polyneuritis (acute porphyria, lead poisoning)
  5 Increased intracranial pressure (acute)
  6 Spinal cord section (acute)
D Miscellaneous
  1 Coarctation of aorta
  2 Increased intravascular volume (excessive transfusion, polycythemia vera)
  3 Polyarteritis nodosa
  4 Hypercalcemia
  5 Medications, e.g., glucocorticoids, cyclosporine
E Unknown etiology
  1 Essential hypertension (>90% of all cases of hypertension)
  2 Toxemia of pregnancy
  3 Acute intermittent porphyria

example, as a group of patients with essential hypertension is separated into a distinct subset (e.g., low-renin essential hypertension), such patients have not been reclassified as having a form of secondary hypertension but rather remain in the essential hypertensive group. In this chapter, those individuals with a specific structural organ defect responsible for hypertension are defined as having a *secondary* form of hypertension. In contrast, individuals who may have general-

TABLE 209-2   Prevalence of various forms of hypertension in the general population and in specialized referral clinics*

Diagnosis	General population, %	Specialty clinic, %
Essential hypertension	92–94	65–85
Renal hypertension:		
Parenchymal	2–3	4–5
Renovascular	1–2	4–16
Endocrine hypertension:		
Primary aldosteronism	0.3	0.5–12
Cushing's syndrome	<0.1	0.2
Pheochromocytoma	<0.1	0.2
Oral contraceptive–induced	2–4	1–2
Miscellaneous	0.2	1

* Estimates based on a number of reports in the literature.

ized or functional abnormalities causing their hypertension, even if discrete, are defined as having *essential* hypertension.

HEREDITY Genetic factors have long been assumed to be important in the genesis of hypertension. Data supporting this view can be found in animal studies as well as in population studies in humans. One approach has been to assess the correlation of blood pressure within families (familial aggregation). From these studies, the minimum size of the genetic factor can be expressed by a correlation coefficient of approximately 0.2. However, the variation in the size of the genetic factor in different studies reemphasizes the likely heterogeneous nature of the essential hypertensive population. Additionally, most studies support the concept that the inheritance is probably multifactorial or that a number of different genetic defects each have as one of their phenotypic expressions an elevated blood pressure. Finally, monogenic defects have now been reported which have as one of their consequences an increased arterial pressure, e.g., glucocorticoid-remediable aldosteronism (see below and Chap. 335).

ENVIRONMENT A number of environmental factors have been specifically implicated in the development of hypertension, including salt intake, obesity, occupation, alcohol intake, family size, and crowding. These factors have all been assumed to be important in the increase in blood pressure with age in more affluent societies, in contrast to the decline in blood pressure with age in more primitive cultures.

SALT SENSITIVITY The environmental factor which has received the greatest attention is salt intake. Even this factor illustrates the heterogeneous nature of the essential hypertensive population in that the blood pressure in only approximately 60 percent of hypertensives is particularly responsive to the level of sodium intake. The cause of this special sensitivity to salt varies, with primary aldosteronism, bilateral renal artery stenosis, renal parenchymal disease, or low-renin essential hypertension accounting for about half the patients. In the remainder, the pathophysiology is still uncertain, but recent postulated contributing factors include chloride, calcium, a generalized cellular membrane defect, insulin resistance, and "nonmodulation" (see below).

Role of renin Renin is an enzyme secreted by the juxtaglomerular cell of the kidney and linked with aldosterone in a negative feedback loop (see Chap. 335). While a variety of factors can modify this secretion, the primary determinant is the volume status of the individual, particularly as related to changes in dietary sodium intake. The end product of the action of renin on its substrate is the generation of the peptide angiotensin II. The response of target tissues to this peptide is uniquely determined by the prior dietary electrolyte intake. For example, sodium intake normally modulates adrenal and renal vascular responses to angiotensin II. With sodium restriction, adrenal responses are enhanced and the renal vascular responses reduced. Sodium loading has the opposite effect. The range of plasma renin activities observed in hypertensive subjects is more broad than in normotensive individuals. Thus some hypertensive patients have been defined as having low-renin and others as having high-renin essential hypertension.

LOW-RENIN ESSENTIAL HYPERTENSION Approximately 20 percent of patients who by all other criteria have essential hypertension have suppressed plasma renin activity. This occurs more frequently in black than in white patients. Though these patients are not hypokalemic, they have been reported to have expanded extracellular fluid volumes, and it is tempting to implicate sodium retention and renin suppression due to excessive production of an unidentified mineralocorticoid. Involvement of the adrenal cortex is suggested by the observation that large doses of spironolactone, the mineralocorticoid antagonist, and the inhibition of steroidogenesis by aminoglutethimide can result in sodium loss and lowering of blood pressure in these patients. A search for other mineralocorticoids has not proven fruitful. Some studies have suggested that the adrenal cortex of many of these patients has an increased sensitivity to angiotensin II as the underlying mechanism. Not only does this hypothesis potentially explain their low plasma renin activity, it also suggests the cause of their

hypertension. On a normal or high-sodium diet, they will not suppress aldosterone production normally, thus leading to a mild degree of hyperaldosteronism with its resultant increased sodium retention, volume expansion, and increase in blood pressure. Since this altered sensitivity has been reported even in patients with normal-renin hypertension, it is likely that patients with low-renin hypertension are not a distinct subset but rather form part of a continuum of patients with essential hypertension.

NONMODULATING ESSENTIAL HYPERTENSION In another subset of the hypertensive population, an adrenal defect the opposite of that observed in low-renin patients is present; i.e., the adrenal response to sodium restriction is reduced. In these individuals, sodium intake does not modulate either adrenal or renal vascular responses to angiotensin II. This subset of hypertensives has been termed *nonmodulators* because of the absence of the sodium-mediated modulation of target tissue responses to angiotensin II. These individuals comprise 25 to 30 percent of the hypertensive population, have normal or high plasma renin activity levels, and have a salt-sensitive form of hypertension because of a defect in the kidney's ability to excrete sodium appropriately. Furthermore, the abnormality appears to be genetically determined and can be corrected by the administration of a converting-enzyme inhibitor.

HIGH-RENIN ESSENTIAL HYPERTENSION Approximately 15 percent of patients with essential hypertension have plasma renin activity levels elevated above the normal range. It has been suggested that plasma renin plays an important role in the pathogenesis of the elevated arterial pressure in these patients. However, most studies have documented that saralasin (a competitive antagonist for angiotensin II) significantly reduces blood pressure in less than half these patients. This has led some investigators to postulate that the elevated renin levels and blood pressure may both be secondary to an increased activity of the adrenergic system. It has been proposed that in patients with angiotensin-dependent high-renin hypertension whose arterial pressures are lowered by saralasin, the mechanism responsible for the increased renin and, therefore, the hypertension is the nonmodulating defect.

Sodium ion vs. chloride or calcium Most studies assessing the role of salt in the hypertensive process have assumed that it is the sodium ion which is important. However, some investigators have suggested that the chloride ion may be equally important. This suggestion is based on the observation that feeding chloride-free sodium salts to salt-sensitive hypertensive animals fails to increase arterial pressure. Calcium also has been implicated in the pathogenesis of some forms of essential hypertension. A low calcium intake has been associated with an increase in blood pressure in epidemiologic studies; an increase in leukocyte cytosolic calcium levels has been reported in some hypertensives; and finally, calcium entry blockers are effective antihypertensive agents. Several studies have reported a potential link between the salt-sensitive forms of hypertension and calcium. It has been postulated that with salt loading and a defect in the kidney's ability to excrete it, a secondary increase in circulating natriuretic factors may occur. One of these, the so-called digitalis-like natriuretic factor, inhibits ouabain-sensitive sodium-potassium ATPase and thereby leads to intracellular calcium accumulation and a hyperreactive vascular smooth muscle.

Cell membrane defect Another postulated explanation for salt-sensitive hypertension is a generalized cell membrane defect. This hypothesis derives most of its data from studies on circulating blood elements, particularly red blood cells, in which abnormalities in the transport of sodium across the cell membrane have been documented. Since both increases and decreases in the activity of different transport systems have been reported, it is likely that some abnormalities are primary and some secondary processes. It has been assumed that this abnormality reflects an undefined alteration in the cellular membrane and that this defect occurs in many, perhaps all, cells of the body, particularly the vascular smooth muscle. Because of this defect, there is then an abnormal accumulation of calcium within vascular smooth muscle, resulting in a heightened vascular responsivity to vasoconstrictor agents. This defect has been proposed to be present in 35 to 50 percent of the essential hypertensive population based on studies using red cells. Other studies suggest that the abnormality in the red cell sodium transport is not a fixed abnormality but can be modified by environmental factors.

Each of these hypotheses has as a common final pathway an increase in cytosolic calcium resulting in increased vascular reactivity. However, as described above, several mechanisms might produce the increase in calcium accumulation.

INSULIN RESISTANCE Insulin resistance and/or hyperinsulinemia have been suggested as being responsible for the increased arterial pressure in some patients with hypertension. While it is clear that a substantial fraction of the hypertensive population has insulin resistance and hyperinsulinemia, it is less certain that this is more than an association. Insulin resistance is common in patients with type II diabetes mellitus or obesity. Both obesity and diabetes mellitus occur more frequently in hypertensive than normotensive subjects. However, several studies have documented that hyperinsulinemia and insulin resistance are present even in lean hypertensive patients free of diabetes mellitus, suggesting that this relationship is more than coincidence.

Hyperinsulinemia can increase arterial pressure by one or more of four mechanisms. An underlying assumption in each is that some, but not all, insulin target tissues are resistant to its effects. Specifically, tissues involved in glucose homeostasis are resistant (thereby producing the hyperinsulinemia), while tissues involved in the hypertensive process are not. First, hyperinsulinemia produces renal sodium retention (at least acutely) and increases sympathetic activity. Either or both of these could lead to an increase in arterial pressure. Another mechanism is vascular smooth-muscle hypertrophy secondary to insulin's mitogenic action. Finally, insulin also modifies ion transport across the cell membrane, thereby potentially increasing the cytosolic calcium levels of insulin-sensitive vascular or renal tissues. Via this mechanism, arterial pressure would be increased for reasons similar to those described above for the membrane-defect hypothesis. It is important to point out, however, that insulin's role in controlling arterial pressure is only vaguely understood, and therefore, its potential as a pathogenic factor in hypertension remains unclear.

FACTORS MODIFYING THE COURSE OF ESSENTIAL HYPERTENSION Age, race, sex, smoking, alcohol intake, serum cholesterol, glucose intolerance, and weight may all alter the prognosis of this disease. The younger the patient when hypertension is first noted, the greater is the reduction in life expectancy if the hypertension is left untreated. In the United States, urban blacks have about twice the prevalence rate for hypertension as whites and more than four times the hypertension-induced morbidity rate. At all ages and in both white and nonwhite populations, females with hypertension fare better than males, and the prevalence of hypertension in premenopausal females is substantially less than in age-matched males or postmenopausal females. Yet females with hypertension run the same relative risk of a morbid cardiovascular event compared with their normotensive counterparts as males do. Accelerated atherosclerosis is an invariable companion of hypertension. Thus it is not surprising that independent risk factors associated with the development of atherosclerosis, e.g., an elevated serum cholesterol, glucose intolerance, and/or cigarette smoking, significantly enhance the effect of hypertension on mortality rates regardless of age, sex, or race (Chap. 208). There also is no question that a positive correlation exists between obesity and arterial pressure. A gain in weight is associated with an increased frequency of hypertension in subjects with normal pressures, and weight loss in obese subjects with hypertension lowers their arterial pressure and, if they are being treated, the intensity of therapy required to maintain them normotensive. Whether these changes are mediated by changes in insulin resistance is unknown. However, there are no convincing data that obesity adversely affects the hypertension-associated mortality rate.

NATURAL HISTORY Because essential hypertension is a heterogeneous disorder, variables in addition to the level of arterial pressure

TABLE 209-3 Factors indicating an adverse prognosis in hypertension

Black race
Youth
Male
Persistent diastolic pressure >115 mmHg
Smoking
Diabetes mellitus
Hypercholesterolemia
Obesity
Excess alcohol intake
Evidence of end organ damage
  A Cardiac
    1 Cardiac enlargement
    2 ECG changes of ischemic or left ventricular strain
    3 Myocardial infarction
    4 Congestive heart failure
  B Eyes
    1 Retinal exudates and hemorrhages
    2 Papilledema
  C Renal: impaired renal function
  D Nervous system: cerebrovascular accident

modify its course. Thus the probability of developing a morbid cardiovascular event with a given arterial pressure may vary by as much as twentyfold depending on whether associated risk factors are present (Table 209-3). Although exceptions have been reported, most untreated adults with hypertension will develop further increases in their arterial pressure with time. Furthermore, both from actuarial data and from experience in the era prior to effective therapy, it has been documented that untreated hypertension is associated with a shortening of life by 10 to 20 years, usually related to an acceleration of the atherosclerotic process, with the rate of acceleration in part related to the severity of the hypertension. Even individuals with relatively mild disease, i.e., without evidence of end organ damage, left untreated for 7 to 10 years have a high risk of developing significant complications. Nearly 30 percent will exhibit atherosclerotic complications, and more than 50 percent will have end organ damage related to the hypertension itself, e.g., cardiomegaly, congestive heart failure, retinopathy, a cerebrovascular accident, and/or renal insufficiency. Thus, even in its mild forms, hypertension is a progressive and lethal disease if left untreated.

SECONDARY HYPERTENSION

As noted earlier, in only a small minority of patients with an elevated arterial pressure can a specific cause be identified. Yet these patients should not be ignored for at least two reasons: (1) with correction of the cause, their hypertension may be cured, and (2) the secondary forms may provide insight into the etiology of essential hypertension. Nearly all the secondary forms are related to an alteration in hormone secretion and/or renal function and are discussed in detail in other chapters.

RENAL HYPERTENSION (See also Chap. 243) Hypertension produced by renal disease is the result of either (1) a derangement in the renal handling of sodium and fluids leading to volume expansion or (2) an alteration in renal secretion of vasoactive materials resulting in a systemic or local change in arteriolar tone. The main subdivisions of renal hypertension are renovascular hypertension, including preeclampsia and eclampsia, and renal parenchymal hypertension. A simple explanation for *renal vascular hypertension* is that decreased perfusion of renal tissue due to stenosis of a main or branch renal artery activates the renin-angiotensin system, described in Chap. 335. Circulating angiotensin II elevates arterial pressure by direct vasoconstriction, by stimulation of aldosterone secretion with resultant sodium retention, and/or by stimulating the adrenergic nervous system. In actual practice, only about one-half of patients with renovascular hypertension have absolute elevations in renin activity in peripheral plasma, although when renin measurements are referenced against an index of sodium balance, a much higher fraction have inappropriately high values.

Activation of the renin-angiotensin system also has been offered as an explanation for the hypertension in both acute and chronic *renal parenchymal disease*. In this formulation, the only difference between renovascular and renal parenchymal hypertension is that the decreased perfusion of renal tissue in the latter case results from inflammatory and fibrotic changes involving multiple small intrarenal vessels. There are enough differences between the two conditions, however, to suggest that other mechanisms are active in renal parenchymal disease: (1) peripheral plasma renin activity is elevated far less frequently in renal parenchymal than in renovascular hypertension; (2) cardiac output is said to be normal in the renal parenchymal type (unless uremia and anemia are present) but slightly elevated in renovascular hypertension; (3) circulatory responses to tilting and to the Valsalva maneuver are exaggerated in the latter condition; and (4) blood volume tends to be high in patients with severe renal parenchymal disease and low in patients with severe renovascular hypertension. Alternative explanations for the hypertension in renal parenchymal disease include the possibilities that the damaged kidneys (1) produce an unidentified vasopressor substance other than renin, (2) fail to produce a necessary humoral vasodilator substance (perhaps prostaglandin or bradykinin), (3) fail to inactivate circulating vasopressor substances, and/or (4) are ineffective in disposing of sodium, and the retained sodium is responsible for the hypertension, as outlined earlier. Though all these explanations, including participation of the renin-angiotensin system, probably have some validity in individual patients, the hypothesis involving sodium retention is particularly attractive. It is supported by the observation that those patients with chronic pyelonephritis or polycystic renal disease who are salt wasters do not develop hypertension and by the observation that removal of salt and water by dialysis or diuretics is effective in controlling arterial pressure in the majority of patients with renal parenchymal disease.

A rare form of renal hypertension results from the excess secretion of renin by juxtaglomerular cell tumors or nephroblastomas. The initial presentation is similar to that of hyperaldosteronism with hypertension, hypokalemia, and overproduction of aldosterone. However, in contrast to primary aldosteronism, peripheral renin activity is *elevated instead of subnormal*. This disease can be distinguished from other forms of secondary aldosteronism by the presence of normal renal function and with unilateral increases in renal vein renin concentration without a renal artery lesion.

ENDOCRINE HYPERTENSION   Adrenal hypertension   Hypertension is a feature of a variety of adrenal cortical abnormalities. In *primary aldosteronism* (Chap. 335) there is a clear relationship between the aldosterone-induced sodium retention and the hypertension. Normal individuals given aldosterone develop hypertension only if they also ingest sodium. Since aldosterone causes sodium retention by stimulating renal tubular exchange of sodium for potassium, hypokalemia is a prominent feature in most patients with primary aldosteronism, and therefore, the measurement of serum potassium provides a simple screening test. The effect of sodium retention and volume expansion in chronically suppressing plasma renin activity is critically important for the definitive diagnosis. In most clinical situations, plasma renin activity and plasma or urinary aldosterone levels parallel each other, but in patients with primary aldosteronism, aldosterone levels are high and relatively fixed because of autonomous aldosterone secretion, while plasma renin activity levels are suppressed and respond sluggishly to sodium depletion. Primary aldosteronism may be secondary either to a tumor or to bilateral adrenal hyperplasia. It is important to distinguish between these two conditions preoperatively, since usually the hypertension in the latter is not modified by operation.

The sodium-retaining effect of large amounts of glucocorticoids also offers an explanation for the hypertension in severe cases of Cushing's syndrome (Chap. 335). Moreover, increased production of mineralocorticoids also has been documented in some patients with Cushing's syndrome. However, the hypertension in many cases of Cushing's syndrome does not seem volume-dependent, leading investigators to speculate that it may be secondary to glucocorticoid-induced production of renin substrate (angiotensin-mediated hypertension) or the increased cortisol levels saturating the 11-hydroxysteroid dehydrogenase enzyme system in the kidney. In the forms of the adrenogenital syndrome due to C-11 or C-17 hydroxylase deficiency (Chap. 335), deoxycorticosterone accounts for the sodium retention and the resultant hypertension, which is accompanied by suppression of plasma renin activity.

In patients with pheochromocytoma (Chap. 336), increased secretion of epinephrine and norepinephrine by a tumor most often located in the adrenal medulla causes excessive stimulation of adrenergic receptors, which results in peripheral vasoconstriction and cardiac stimulation. This diagnosis is confirmed by demonstrating increased urinary excretion of epinephrine and norepinephrine or their metabolites.

Acromegaly (See also Chap. 331)   Hypertension, coronary atherosclerosis, and cardiac hypertrophy are frequent complications of this condition.

Hypercalcemia (See also Chap. 356)   The hypertension which occurs in up to one-third of patients with hyperparathyroidism ordinarily can be attributed to renal parenchymal damage due to nephrolithiasis and nephrocalcinosis. However, increased calcium levels also can have a direct vasoconstrictive effect. In some cases, the hypertension disappears when the hypercalcemia is corrected. Thus, paradoxically, the increased serum calcium level in hyperparathyroidism raises blood pressure, while epidemiologic studies suggest that a high calcium intake lowers blood pressure. To further confuse the issue, calcium entry blocking agents are effective antihypertensive agents. Additional studies are needed to resolve these seemingly conflicting observations.

Oral contraceptives   The most common cause of endocrine hypertension is that resulting from the use of estrogen-containing oral contraceptives. Indeed, this may be the most common form of secondary hypertension. The mechanism producing the hypertension is likely to be secondary to activation of the renin-angiotensin-aldosterone system. Thus both volume (aldosterone) and vasoconstrictor (angiotensin II) factors are important. The estrogen component of oral contraceptive agents stimulates the hepatic synthesis of the renin substrate angiotensinogen, which in turn favors the increased production of angiotensin II and secondary aldosteronism. Women taking oral contraceptives have increased plasma concentrations of angiotensin II and aldosterone with some increase in arterial pressure. However, only about 5 percent actually have an increase in arterial pressure greater than 140/90, and in about half of these the hypertension will remit within 6 months of stopping the drug.

Why some women taking oral contraceptives develop hypertension and others do not is unclear but may be related to (1) increased vascular sensitivity to angiotensin II, (2) the presence of mild renal disease, (3) familial factors (over one-half have a positive family history for hypertension), (4) age (hypertension is significantly more prevalent in women over age 35), and/or (5) obesity. Indeed some investigators have suggested that the oral contraceptives are simply unmasking women with essential hypertension.

COARCTATION OF THE AORTA (See also Chap. 199)   The hypertension associated with coarctation may be caused by the constriction itself or perhaps by the changes in the renal circulation which result in an unusual form of renal arterial hypertension. The diagnosis of coarctation is usually evident from physical examination and routine x-ray findings.

EFFECTS OF HYPERTENSION

Patients with hypertension die prematurely; the most common cause of death is heart disease, with stroke and renal failure also frequent, particularly in those with significant retinopathy.

EFFECTS ON HEART   Cardiac compensation for the excessive work load imposed by increased systemic pressure is at first sustained by concentric left ventricular hypertrophy, characterized by an increase in wall thickness. Ultimately, the function of this chamber deteriorates, the cavity dilates, and the symptoms and signs of heart failure appear (Chap. 195). Angina pectoris also may occur because of the combination of accelerated coronary arterial disease and increased myocardial oxygen requirements as a consequence of the increased myocardial mass (Chap. 203). On physical examination, the heart is enlarged and has a prominent left ventricular impulse. The sound of aortic closure is accentuated, and there may be a faint murmur of aortic regurgitation. Presystolic (atrial, fourth) heart sounds appear frequently in hypertensive heart disease, and a protodiastolic (ventricular, third) heart sound or summation gallop rhythm may be present. Electrocardiographic changes of left ventricular hypertrophy (Chap. 189) may occur, but the electrocardiogram substantially underestimates the frequency of cardiac hypertrophy compared with that observed with the echocardiogram. Evidence of ischemia or infarction may be observed late in the disease. The majority of deaths due to hypertension result from myocardial infarction or congestive heart failure.

NEUROLOGIC EFFECTS The neurologic effects of long-standing hypertension may be divided into retinal and central nervous system changes. Because the retina is the only tissue in which the arteries and arterioles can be examined directly, repeated ophthalmoscopic examination provides the opportunity to observe the progress of the vascular effects of hypertension (Table 209-4). The Keith-Wagener-Barker classification of the *retinal changes* in hypertension has provided a simple and excellent means for serial evaluation of hypertensive patients. Increasing severity of hypertension is associated with focal spasm and progressive general narrowing of the arterioles, as well as the appearance of hemorrhages, exudates, and papilledema. These retinal lesions often produce scotomata, blurred vision, and even blindness, especially in the presence of papilledema or hemorrhages of the macular area. Hypertensive lesions may develop acutely and, if therapy results in significant reduction of blood pressure, may show rapid resolution. Rarely, these lesions resolve without therapy. In contrast, retinal arteriolosclerosis results from endothelial and muscular proliferation, and it accurately reflects similar changes in other organs. Sclerotic changes do not develop as rapidly as hypertensive lesions, nor do they regress appreciably with therapy. As a consequence of increased wall thickness and rigidity, sclerotic arterioles distort and compress the veins as they cross within their common fibrous sheath, and the reflected light streak from the arterioles is changed by the increased opacity of the vessel wall.

Central nervous system dysfunction also occurs frequently in patients with hypertension. Occipital headaches, most often in the morning, are among the most prominent early symptoms of hypertension. Dizziness, light-headedness, vertigo, tinnitus, and dimmed vision or syncope also may be observed, but the more serious manifestations are due to vascular occlusion, hemorrhage, or encephalopathy (Chap. 368). The pathogeneses of the former two disorders are quite different. *Cerebral infarction* is secondary to the increased atherosclerosis observed in hypertensive patients, while *cerebral hemorrhage* is the result of both the elevated arterial pressure and the development of cerebral vascular microaneurysms (Charcot-Bouchard aneurysms). Only age and arterial pressure are known to influence the development of the microaneurysms. Thus it is not surprising that the association of arterial pressure with cerebral hemorrhage is much better than with either cerebral or myocardial infarction.

Hypertensive encephalopathy consists of the following symptom complex: severe hypertension, disordered consciousness, increased intracranial pressure, retinopathy with papilledema, and seizures. The pathogenesis is uncertain but probably not related to arteriolar spasm or cerebral edema. Focal neurologic signs are infrequent and, if present, suggest that infarction, hemorrhage, or transient ischemic attacks are more likely diagnoses. Although some investigators have suggested that prompt lowering of arterial pressure in these patients may adversely affect cerebral blood flow, most studies indicate that this is not the case.

RENAL EFFECTS (See also Chap. 243) Arteriosclerotic lesions of the afferent and efferent arterioles and the glomerular capillary tufts are the most common renal vascular lesions in hypertension and result in decreased glomerular filtration rate and tubular dysfunction. Proteinuria and microscopic hematuria occur because of glomerular lesions, and approximately 10 percent of the deaths secondary to hypertension result from renal failure. Blood loss in hypertension occurs not only from renal lesions; epistaxis, hemoptysis, and metrorrhagia also occur frequently in these patients.

APPROACH TO THE PATIENT WITH HYPERTENSION

In evaluating patients with hypertension, the initial history, physical examination, and laboratory tests should be directed at (1) uncovering correctable secondary forms of hypertension (see Table 209-1), (2) establishing a pretreatment baseline, (3) assessing factors which may influence the type of therapy or which may be adversely modified by therapy, (4) determining if target organ damage is present, and (5) determining whether other risk factors for the development of arteriosclerotic cardiovascular disease are present (see Chap. 208).

TABLE 209-4 Classification of hypertensive and arteriolosclerotic retinopathy

Degree	Hypertension — Arterioles					Arteriolosclerosis	
	General narrowing AV ratio*	Focal spasm†	Hemor-rhages	Exudates	Papilledema	Arteriolar light reflex	AV crossing defects‡
Normal	3:4	1:1	0	0	0	Fine yellow line, red blood column	none
Grade I	1:2	1:1	0	0	0	Broadened yellow line, red blood column	Mild depression of vein
Grade II	1:3	2:3	0	0	0	Broad yellow line, "copper wire," blood column not visible	Depression or humping of vein
Grade III	1:4	1:3	+	+	0	Broad white line, "silver wire," blood column not visible	Right-angle deviation, tapering, and disappearance of vein under arteriole; distal dilatation of vein
Grade IV	Fine, fibrous cords	Obliteration of distal flow	+	+	+	Fibrous cords, blood column not visible	Same as grade III

* This is the ratio of arteriolar to venous diameters.
† This is the ratio of diameters of region of spasm to proximal arteriole.
‡ Arteriolar length and tortuosity increase with severity.

Ideally, this evaluation also would determine the underlying mechanism(s) in essential hypertension, particularly if such information leads to a more specific therapeutic program. Unfortunately, at the present time this aspect of the evaluation is limited either by lack of knowledge of the underlying mechanisms, uncertainty as to the specificity of therapy for a distinct subset even if the underlying mechanisms are known, or the prohibitive expense in defining a subset of hypertensive patients even if specific therapy were available. However, with the accumulation of additional information, a sixth component in the evaluation of patients with hypertension may become increasingly more important.

SYMPTOMS AND SIGNS The majority of patients with hypertension have no specific symptoms referable to their blood pressure elevation and will be identified only in the course of a physical examination. When symptoms do bring the patient to the physician, they fall into three categories. They are related to (1) the elevated pressure itself, (2) the hypertensive vascular disease, and (3) the underlying disease in the case of secondary hypertension. Though popularly considered a symptom of elevated arterial pressure, headache is characteristic only of severe hypertension; most commonly it is localized to the occipital region, is present when the patient awakens in the morning, and subsides spontaneously after several hours. Other possibly related complaints include dizziness, palpitations, easy fatigability, and impotence. Complaints referable to vascular disease include epistaxis, hematuria, blurring of vision owing to retinal changes, episodes of weakness or dizziness due to transient cerebral ischemia, angina pectoris, and dyspnea due to cardiac failure. Pain due to dissection of the aorta or to a leaking aneurysm is an occasional presenting symptom.

Examples of symptoms related to the underlying disease in secondary hypertension are polyuria, polydipsia, and muscle weakness secondary to hypokalemia in patients with primary aldosteronism or weight gain and emotional lability in patients with Cushing's syndrome. The patient with a pheochromocytoma may present with episodic headaches, palpitations, diaphoresis, and postural dizziness.

CLINICAL EVALUATION History A strong family history of hypertension, along with the reported finding of intermittent pressure elevation in the past, favors the diagnosis of essential hypertension. Secondary hypertension often develops before the age of 35 or after 55. The history of use of adrenal steroids or estrogens is of obvious significance. A history of repeated urinary tract infections suggests chronic pyelonephritis, although this condition may occur in the absence of symptoms; nocturia and polydipsia suggest renal or endocrine disease, while trauma to either flank or an episode of acute flank pain may be a clue to the presence of renal injury. A history of weight gain is compatible with Cushing's syndrome, and weight loss with pheochromocytoma. A number of aspects of the history aid in determining whether vascular disease has progressed to dangerous stages. These include angina pectoris and symptoms of cerebrovascular insufficiency, of congestive heart failure, and/or of peripheral vascular insufficiency. Other risk factors that should be elicited include cigarette smoking, diabetes mellitus, lipid disorders, and a family history of early deaths due to cardiovascular disease. Finally, aspects of the patient's lifestyle which could contribute to the hypertension or affect its treatment should be assessed, including diet, physical activity, family status, work, and educational level.

Physical examination The physical examination starts with the patient's general appearance. For instance, are the round face and trunkal obesity of Cushing's syndrome present? Is muscular development in the upper extremities out of proportion to that in the lower extremities, suggesting coarctation of the aorta? The next step is to compare the blood pressures and pulses in both upper extremities and in the supine and standing positions (for at least 2 min). A rise in diastolic pressure when the patient goes from the supine to the standing position is most compatible with essential hypertension; a fall, in the absence of antihypertensive medications, suggests secondary forms of hypertension. The patient's height and weight should be recorded. Detailed examination of the ocular fundi is mandatory,

since funduscopic findings provide one of the best indications of the duration of hypertension and of prognosis. A useful guide is the Keith-Wagener-Barker classification of funduscopic changes (Table 209-4; see also Atlas 8); the specific changes in each fundus should be recorded and a grade assigned. Palpation and auscultation of the carotid arteries for evidence of stenosis or occlusion are important; narrowing of a carotid artery may be a manifestation of hypertensive vascular disease, and it also may be a clue to the presence of a renal arterial lesion, since these two lesions may occur together. In examination of the heart and lungs, one should search for evidence of left ventricular hypertrophy and cardiac decompensation. Is there a left ventricular lift? Are third and fourth heart sounds present? Are there pulmonary rales? A third heart sound and pulmonary rales are unusual in uncomplicated hypertension. Their presence suggests ventricular dysfunction. Chest examination also includes a search for extracardiac murmurs and palpable collateral vessels that may result from coarctation of the aorta.

The most important part of the abdominal examination is auscultation for bruits originating in stenotic renal arteries. Bruits due to renal arterial narrowing nearly always have a diastolic component or may be continuous and are best heard just to the right or left of the midline above the umbilicus or in the flanks; they are present in many patients with renal artery stenosis due to fibrous dysplasia and in 40 to 50 percent of those with functionally significant stenosis due to arteriosclerosis. The abdomen also should be palpated for abdominal aneurysm and for the enlarged kidneys of polycystic renal disease. The femoral pulses must be carefully felt, and if they are decreased and/or delayed in comparison with the radial pulse, the blood pressure in the lower extremities must be measured. Even if the femoral pulse is normal to palpation, arterial pressure in the lower extremities should be recorded at least once in patients in whom hypertension is discovered before the age of 30 years. Finally, examination of the extremities for edema and a search for evidence of a previous cerebrovascular accident and/or other intracranial pathology should be performed.

Laboratory investigation Controversy exists as to what laboratory studies should be performed in patients presenting with hypertension. In general, the disagreement resides in how extensively to evaluate the patient for secondary forms of hypertension or subsets of essential hypertension. In the following discussion, laboratory studies are divided into those which should be performed in all patients with sustained hypertension (basic studies) and those which should be added if (1) from the initial evaluation a secondary form of hypertension is suggested and/or (2) arterial pressure is not controlled after initial therapy (secondary studies).

BASIC STUDIES Renal status is evaluated by assessing the presence of protein, blood, and glucose in the urine and measuring serum creatinine and/or blood urea nitrogen (BUN). Microscopic examination of the urine is also helpful. A serum potassium level is needed both as a screen for mineralocorticoid-induced hypertension and as a baseline prior to initiating diuretic therapy.

Other blood chemistries also may be useful, particularly since they often can be ordered as a battery of automated tests at minimal cost to the patient. For example, a blood glucose determination is helpful both because diabetes mellitus may be associated with accelerated arteriosclerosis, renal vascular disease, and diabetic nephropathy in patients with hypertension and because primary aldosteronism, Cushing's syndrome, and pheochromocytoma all may be associated with hyperglycemia. Furthermore, since antihypertensive therapy with diuretics, for example, can raise the blood glucose level, it is important to establish a baseline. The possibility of hypercalcemia also may be investigated. Serum uric acid determination is useful because of the increased incidence of hyperuricemia in patients with renal and essential hypertension and because, as with blood glucose, the level subsequently may be raised by treatment with diuretics. Serum cholesterol, HDL cholesterol, and triglycerides may be measured to identify other factors which predispose to the development of arteriosclerosis. An electrocardiogram should be obtained in all cases as an assessment of cardiac status, particularly if left ventricular hypertrophy is present, and as a baseline. The echocardiogram is more sensitive than either the electrocardiogram or physical examination in determining if cardiac hypertrophy is present. Thus, in some circumstances, this may be a useful addition in the *baseline* evaluation of a hypertensive patient, particularly since left ventricular hypertrophy is an independent cardiovascular risk factor and its presence suggests the need for vigorous antihypertensive therapy. Furthermore, while substantial increases in arterial pressure usually correlate with the presence or absence of left ventricular hypertrophy, mild increases may not. Thus one cannot use the level of blood pressure per se as a surrogate marker for the presence or absence of left ventricular hypertrophy. On the other hand, because of the cost of an echocardiogram and the uncertainty as to whether the resultant information would modify therapy, it is unclear that routine *follow-up* echocardiograms during therapy are justified. The chest roentgenogram also may be helpful by providing the opportunity to identify aortic dilatation or elongation and the rib notching that occurs in coarctation of the aorta.

SECONDARY STUDIES (Table 209-5)   Certain clues from the history, physical examination, and basic laboratory studies may suggest an unusual cause for the hypertension and dictate the need for special studies. For example, the abrupt onset of severe hypertension and/or the onset of hypertension of any severity under the age of 25 or after the age of 50 years should lead to laboratory tests to exclude renovascular hypertension and pheochromocytoma. A history of headaches, palpitations, anxiety attacks, unusual sweating, hyperglycemia, and weight loss also should lead to tests to exclude pheochromocytoma. The presence of an abdominal bruit should lead to workup for renovascular hypertension, and the finding of bilateral upper abdominal masses on physical examination, consistent with polycystic renal disease, should lead to the performance of an intravenous pyelogram. An elevated creatinine or blood urea nitrogen level, associated with proteinuria and hematuria, should initiate a detailed workup for renal insufficiency (Chap. 235). Special studies for secondary hypertension are also indicated if there is therapeutic failure with the initial drug program. The specific diagnostic measures depend on the most likely causes of secondary hypertension.

Pheochromocytoma   (See also Chap. 336)   The easiest and best screening procedure for pheochromocytoma is the measurement of catecholamines or their metabolites in a 24-h urine collected during the time the patient is hypertensive. Measurement of plasma catecholamine levels also may be useful. These tests may be indicated even in patients who do not have episodic hypertension, since over half the patients with pheochromocytoma have fixed hypertension.

TABLE 209-5   Laboratory tests and special studies for evaluation of hypertension

BASIC STUDIES

A Always included
  1 Urine for protein, blood, and glucose
  2 Hematocrit
  3 Serum potassium
  4 Serum creatinine and/or blood urea nitrogen
  5 Electrocardiogram
B Usually included, depending on cost and other factors
  1 Microscopic urinalysis
  2 White blood cell count
  3 Plasma/blood glucose, cholesterol, HDL cholesterol, and triglycerides
  4 Serum calcium, phosphate, and uric acid
  5 Chest x-ray

SPECIAL STUDIES TO SCREEN FOR SECONDARY HYPERTENSION

A Renovascular: digital subtraction angiogram or rapid sequence IVP
B Pheochromocytoma: 24-h urine for creatinine, metanephrines, and catecholamines or plasma catecholamines
C Cushing's syndrome: overnight dexamethasone suppression test or 24-h urine cortisol

---

Provocative tests are seldom, if ever, indicated, although occasionally a suppressive test may be useful.

Cushing's syndrome   (See also Chap. 335)   A 24-h urine test for cortisol or the administration of 1 mg dexamethasone at bedtime, followed by measurement of plasma cortisol at 7 to 10 A.M., is the best test for the presence of this condition. A urine cortisol level less than 2750 nmol (100 μg) or suppression of the plasma cortisol level to below 140 nmol/L (5 μg/dL) effectively rules out Cushing's syndrome.

Renovascular hypertension   (See also Chap. 243)   The standard screening test for renal vascular hypertension has been the rapid-sequence intravenous pyelogram (IVP). Features suggestive of renal ischemia include (1) unilateral delayed appearance and excretion of contrast material, (2) a difference in kidney size greater than 1.5 cm, (3) irregular contour of the renal silhouette, suggesting partial infarction or atrophy, (4) indentations on the ureter or renal pelvis, possibly due to dilated ureteral arteries (collateral notching), and (5) hyperconcentration of contrast medium in the collecting system of the smaller kidney. When these criteria are used, the false-positive rate is 11 percent and the false-negative rate 12 percent. The digital subtraction angiogram has been received with considerable enthusiasm as a more precise screening test for renal vascular disease. Its ultimate place as a screening test is unclear, however, because of its relatively high cost and the need for an arterial rather than a venous injection. The isotope renogram and saralasin infusion test, both enthusiastically endorsed in the past as screening procedures, are now used infrequently because of either lower sensitivity and specificity or limited availability. However, the captopril-induced renogram may be more useful. This test takes advantage of the dependency of the renal vasculature on angiotensin II. Thus, when individuals with renal artery stenosis are given a converting enzyme inhibitor (captopril) which reduces angiotensin II levels on the stenotic side, there will be renal blood flow pattern demonstrating a reduced uptake and delayed excretion as assessed by the isotope renogram.

The definitive test of surgically correctable renal disease is the combination of a renal angiogram and renal vein renin determinations. The renal arteriogram both establishes the presence of a renal arterial lesion and aids in determining whether the lesion is due to atherosclerosis or to one of the fibrous or fibromuscular dysplasias. It does not, however, prove that the lesion is responsible for the hypertension, nor does it permit prediction of the chances of surgical cure; it must be noted that (1) renal artery stenosis is a frequent finding by angiography and at postmortem in normotensive individuals, and (2) essential hypertension is a common condition and may occur in combination with renal arterial stenosis which actually may not be responsible for the hypertension. Bilateral renal vein catheterization for measurement of plasma renin activity is therefore used to assess the functional significance of any lesion noted on arteriography. When one kidney is ischemic and the other is normal, all the renin released comes from the involved kidney. In the most straightforward situation, the ischemic kidney has a significantly higher venous plasma renin activity than the normal kidney by a factor of 1.5 or more. Moreover, the renal venous blood draining the uninvolved kidney exhibits levels similar to those in the inferior vena cava below the entrance of the renal veins. Significant benefit from operative correction may be anticipated in at least 80 percent of patients with the findings described above if care is taken to prepare the patient properly prior to renal vein blood sampling, i.e., discontinuing renin-suppressing drugs, such as beta blockers, for at least 10 days, placing the patient on a low-sodium intake for 4 days, and/or giving a converting enzyme inhibitor for 24 h. When obstructing lesions in the *branches* of the renal arteries are demonstrated by arteriography, an attempt to obtain blood samples from the main *branches* of the renal vein should be made in an effort to identify a localized intrarenal arterial lesion responsible for the hypertension.

Primary aldosteronism   (See also Chap. 335)   These patients almost always exhibit hypokalemia. Diuretic therapy often complicates the picture when the hypokalemia is first observed and needs to be assessed. Given hypokalemia, the relation between plasma renin activity and the aldosterone level becomes the key to the diagnosis of primary aldosteronism. The aldosterone concentration or excretion is high and plasma renin activity is low in primary aldosteronism, and these levels are relatively unaffected by changes in sodium balance. A critical part of the evaluation after primary aldosteronism has been established is to determine whether unilateral or bilateral disease is present, since surgical removal of the lesion usually reduces arterial pressure only in those with unilateral disease.

Plasma renin activity measurements Some studies have suggested that most hypertensive patients should have a plasma renin level measured and related to a 24-h urine sodium excretion rate to assess whether high, low, or normal levels are present. It has been proposed that this information may be important for both therapeutic and prognostic reasons. However, as noted earlier, it is unclear, on the basis of presently available data and treatment programs, that these random measurements are really useful except in patients with findings suggestive of renal vascular disease or mineralocorticoid excess in whom lateralizing renal vein renin levels or suppressed peripheral renin levels may be of diagnostic and/or therapeutic significance.

TREATMENT

Virtually every patient with a diastolic arterial pressure which persistently exceeds 90 mmHg, or any patient over 65 years of age with a systolic arterial pressure over 160 mmHg, is a candidate for diagnostic studies and for subsequent treatment. Furthermore, at any given level of blood pressure elevation, the ultimate risk of developing hypertensive vascular complications is greater in men than in women and in younger than in older persons. It may be argued, then, that it is hard to justify producing the uncomfortable side effects of therapy in, for example, an asymptomatic woman over 70 years of age with a diastolic pressure of 90 mmHg. On the other hand, it is easy to justify side effects in a man of 30 with a diastolic pressure exceeding 110 mmHg because such a person may be expected to receive the greatest benefit from therapy. Fortunately, the choice of treatment is such that a satisfactory program to control arterial pressure with minimal side effects can be developed for most patients, particularly as more studies assessing the impact of specific therapeutic agents on the patient's quality of life are reported. A reasonable guideline would be that all patients with diastolic pressure repeatedly above 90 mmHg should be treated unless specific contraindications exist. Patients with isolated *systolic* hypertension (levels greater than 160 mmHg) also should be treated if they are over age 65. It is uncertain that individuals under age 65 who have isolated systolic hypertension will benefit from therapy until the results of a well-controlled, perspective study are completed. Patients with labile hypertension or isolated systolic hypertension who are not treated should have regular follow-up examinations at 6-month intervals because of the frequent development of progressive and/or sustained hypertension.

The identification of an operable form of secondary hypertension does not automatically mean that surgical treatment is indicated. The decision depends on the age and general health of the patient, the natural history of the lesion, and the response of the arterial pressure to drug therapy. In patients with renovascular hypertension, the feasibility of renal angioplasty, surgical repair versus nephrectomy, and the degree of overall renal functional impairment must be considered. Age and general health are important in patients with renovascular hypertension due to arteriosclerosis, because there is no evidence that repair of the stenosis increases life expectancy in the elderly patient with other evidence of vascular disease. Knowledge of the natural history of the disease is especially important when approaching the decision in the young patient with renal artery stenosis due to fibrous dysplasia. If the arteriographic appearance suggests that the stenosis is due to intimal or subadventitial fibroplasia, the lesion may be expected to progress, and operation or angioplasty is required. Medial fibroplasia, on the other hand, often remains stable,

and operation or angioplasty may not be necessary if pressure can be controlled by drug therapy. The decision regarding operation also should be considered carefully in patients with primary aldosteronism when bilateral adrenal venography does not demonstrate a tumor, because such patients may prove to have multinodular hyperplasia. This means that bilateral adrenalectomy would be required to eliminate the aldosterone excess, and even then, hypertension usually persists. If hypokalemia can be controlled by spironolactone or other drug therapy and arterial pressure lowered with antihypertensive agents, then it is reasonable to withhold operative treatment.

GENERAL MEASURES Nondrug therapeutic intervention is probably indicated in all patients with sustained hypertension and probably most with labile hypertension. The general measures employed include (1) relief of stress, (2) diet, (3) regular aerobic exercise, (4) weight reduction (if needed), and (5) control of other risk factors contributing to the development of arteriosclerosis. Relief of emotional and environmental stress is one of the reasons for the improvement in hypertension that occurs when a patient is hospitalized. Though it is usually impossible to extricate the hypertensive patient from all internal and external stresses, he or she should be advised to avoid any unnecessary tensions. In rare instances, it may be appropriate to recommend a change of job or of life-style. It has been suggested that relaxation techniques also may lower arterial pressure. However, it is uncertain that these techniques alone have much long-term effect.

Dietary management has three aspects:

1 Because of the documented efficacy of sodium restriction and volume contraction in lowering blood pressure, patients previously were instructed to curtail sodium intake drastically. Some investigators have suggested this is no longer necessary. They base their conclusion on two observations: (a) In many patients the blood pressure is not sensitive to the level of sodium intake, and (b) diuretics provide another method of decreasing body sodium stores in those individuals whose blood pressure may be sodium-sensitive. However, a number of reports have documented that while mild sodium restriction has little, if any, direct action on blood pressure, it significantly potentiates the efficacy of nearly all antihypertensive agents, and thus, by allowing blood pressure control with lower doses of drugs, side effects are reduced. In addition, it is quite clear that in some hypertensive patients, as noted above, the level of sodium intake does influence the blood pressure. Thus, since there is no apparent risk to mild sodium restriction, the most practical approach now is to advise mild dietary sodium restriction (up to 5 g NaCl per day), which can be achieved by eliminating all additions of salt to food which is prepared normally. Some studies also have reported lowering of arterial pressure by *increasing* potassium and/or calcium intake. While the advisability of this form of dietary alteration is still controversial, since a moderately high calcium intake (1.5 g elemental calcium daily) probably also reduces the extent of age-related osteoporosis, it is probably a useful adjunct.

2 Caloric restriction should be urged for the patient who is overweight. Some obese patients will show a significant reduction in pressure simply as a consequence of weight loss.

3 A restriction in intake of cholesterol and saturated fats is recommended, since such a diet may diminish the incidence of arteriosclerotic complications. Reducing or eliminating alcohol intake is also beneficial. Regular exercise is indicated within the limits of the patient's cardiovascular status. Not only is exercise helpful in controlling weight, but also there is evidence that physical conditioning itself may lower arterial pressure. Isotonic exercises (jogging, swimming) are better than isometric exercises (weight lifting) since, if anything, the latter raises arterial pressure. The dietary management outlined above is aimed at the control of other risk factors. Probably the most significant additional step that could be taken in this area would be to convince the smoker to give up cigarettes.

DRUG THERAPY (Table 209-6) To make rational use of antihypertensive drugs, the sites and mechanisms of their action must be understood. In general, there are five classes of drugs: diuretics, antiadrenergic agents, vasodilators, calcium entry blockers, and angiotensin-converting enzyme (ACE) inhibitors.

Diuretics (See also Chap. 195) The thiazides are the most frequently used and most extensively investigated members of this group, and their early effect certainly is related to sodium diuresis and volume depletion. A reduction in peripheral vascular resistance also has been reported by some workers to be important in the long term. Traditionally, thiazide diuretics have formed the cornerstone of most therapeutic programs designed to lower arterial pressure and are usually effective within 3 to 4 days. Furthermore, they have been shown to reduce mortality and morbidity in long-term trials. However, in recent years, increasing resistance to their routine use has occurred primarily because of their adverse metabolic effects, which include hypokalemia due to renal potassium loss, hyperuricemia due to uric acid retention, carbohydrate intolerance, and hyperlipidemia. The more potent loop-acting diuretics furosemide and bumetanide also have been shown to be antihypertensive but have been used less extensively for this purpose primarily because of their shorter duration of action. Spironolactone causes renal sodium loss by blocking the effect of mineralocorticoids, and therefore, it may be more effective in patients whose mineralocorticoids are present in excess, e.g., primary or secondary aldosteronism. Although they do not compete directly with aldosterone, triamterene and amiloride act at the same site as spironolactone to impede sodium reabsorption and are effective in the same situations as spironolactone, except triamterene has little intrinsic antihypertensive effect. Their major disadvantage is that they can produce hyperkalemia, particularly in patients with impaired renal function. Any of these three potassium-sparing diuretics also can be given along with thiazide diuretics to minimize renal potassium loss.

Antiadrenergic agents (See also Chap. 68) These drugs act at one or more sites either centrally on the vasomotor center, in peripheral neurons modifying catecholamine release, or by blocking adrenergic receptor sites on target tissue. Drugs that appear to have predominant *central actions* are *clonidine, methyldopa, guanabenz,* and *guanfacine.* These drugs and their metabolites are predominantly alpha-receptor agonists. Stimulation of alpha$_2$ receptors in the vasomotor centers of the brain *reduces* sympathetic outflow, thereby reducing arterial pressure. Usually a fall in cardiac output and heart rate also occurs, more commonly with clonidine and guanabenz, but the baroreceptor reflex is intact. Thus postural symptoms are absent. However, rebound hypertension may occur rarely when these drugs, particularly clonidine and guanabenz, are stopped. This is probably secondary to the increase in norepinephrine release which had been inhibited by these agents secondary to their agonist effect on presynaptic alpha receptors.

Another class of antiadrenergic agents is the *ganglionic blocking* drugs, which have little effect when the patient is supine but prevent reflex vasoconstriction in the upright position. Ganglionic blocking agents interfere with parasympathetic as well as sympathetic function, and this results in such side effects as impairment of visual accommodation, paralytic ileus, retention of urine, and failure of erection and ejaculation. Because of these problems, ganglionic blocking agents are now usually reserved for the rapid lowering of arterial pressure by parenteral administration of the short-acting agent *trimethaphan* in patients with severe hypertension.

Various drugs act at *postganglionic adrenergic nerve endings.* The *rauwolfia alkaloids* such as reserpine are the oldest members of the group; their long-term effect results from their ability to inhibit the storage of norepinephrine within the vesicles in adrenergic nerve endings, thus leading to depletion of catecholamine stores. The frequent side effects, including depression, nasal congestion, diarrhea, impairment of sexual function, and increased gastric secretion, have limited the use of these drugs. Reserpine is contraindicated in patients with current or past depression. *Guanethidine* and its shorter-acting analogue guanadrel block the release of norepinephrine from adrener-gic nerve endings. They usually reduce cardiac output and lower systolic more than diastolic blood pressure. They also produce a greater postural effect than the other drugs that act at the nerve endings, and orthostatic hypotension is a frequent side effect, particularly if other factors promoting vasodilation are present, e.g., heat, exercise, alcohol ingestion. However, centrally mediated side effects (sedation, depression) are infrequently observed because these drugs are poorly soluble in lipids and therefore do not readily enter the central nervous system.

The last group of drugs affecting the adrenergic system are those which block the *peripheral adrenergic receptors*, alpha, beta, or both (see also Chap. 68). *Phentolamine* and *phenoxybenzamine* block the action of norepinephrine at *alpha*-adrenergic receptor sites. While the preceding two compounds block both presynaptic (alpha$_2$) and postsynaptic (alpha$_1$) alpha receptors, the former action accounts for the tolerance which develops, while *prazosin* is more effective because it selectively blocks only *postsynaptic alpha* receptors, i.e., alpha$_1$ receptors. Thus presynaptic alpha activity remains, suppressing norepinephrine release, and tolerance occurs only infrequently. Accordingly, prazosin produces less tachycardia but more postural hypotension than direct-acting vasodilators, e.g., hydralazine, and rarely can produce substantial hypotension following the first dose.

A number of effective *beta-adrenergic receptor blocking agents* are available which block sympathetic effects on the heart and should be most effective in reducing cardiac output and in lowering arterial pressure when there is increased cardiac sympathetic nerve activity. In addition, they block the adrenergic nerve–mediated release of renin from the renal juxtaglomerular cells, and this action may be an important component of their blood pressure–lowering action. Beta-adrenergic blockers are particularly useful when employed in conjunction with vascular smooth-muscle relaxants, which tend to evoke a reflex increase in heart rate, and with diuretics, the administration of which often results in an elevation of circulating renin activity. In practice, beta blockers appear to be effective even when there is no evidence of increased sympathetic tone, with about one-half or more of all hypertensive patients showing a fall in pressure. Furthermore, like diuretics, they have been shown to reduce morbidity and mortality in long-term clinical trials. However, these agents can precipitate congestive heart failure and asthma in susceptible individuals and must be used with caution in diabetics receiving hypoglycemic therapy because they inhibit the usual sympathetic responses to hypoglycemia. Cardioselective beta-blocking agents (so-called beta$_1$ blockers) have been developed (metoprolol, atenolol) which may be superior to nonselective beta blockers such as propranolol and timolol in patients with bronchospasm. Nadolol, a nonselective beta blocker, unlike other drugs of this class, is excreted unchanged in the urine and has a half-life of 14 to 20 h. Therefore, only one dose a day is required. Atenolol also usually only needs to be given once a day. Pindolol and acebutolol are nonselective beta blockers with partial agonist activity and, therefore, produce less bradycardia. Labetalol exerts both alpha- and beta-adrenergic blocking actions. Thus it lowers arterial pressure by the same complex actions as do beta blockers but also directly by reducing systemic vascular resistance. Usually it has a more rapid onset of action but produces more postural symptoms and chronic sexual dysfunction than the other beta blockers.

Vasodilators *Hydralazine* is the most versatile of the drugs that cause direct relaxation of vascular smooth muscle; it is effective both orally and parenterally, acting mainly on arterial resistance rather than on venous capacitance vessels, as evidenced by lack of postural changes. Unfortunately, the effect of hydralazine on peripheral resistance is partly negated by reflex increases in sympathetic discharge that raise heart rate and cardiac output. This limits the usefulness of hydralazine, especially in patients with severe coronary artery disease. However, the efficacy of hydralazine can be increased if it is given in conjunction with beta blockers or drugs such as methyldopa or clonidine, all of which block reflex sympathetic stimulation of the heart. A serious side effect of doses of hydralazine exceeding 300 mg/d has been the production of a lupus erythematosus–like syndrome.

TABLE 209-6 Drugs used in treatment of hypertension—listed according to site of action

Site of action	Drug	Dosage	Indications	Contraindications	Frequent or peculiar side effects
DIURETICS					
Renal tubule	Thiazides: e.g., hydrochlorothiazide	Depends on specific drug Oral: 12.5–25 mg daily or twice daily	Mild hypertension, as adjunct in treatment of moderate to severe hypertension	Diabetes mellitus, hyperuricemia, primary aldosteronism	Potassium depletion, hyperglycemia, hyperuricemia, hypercholesterolemia, dermatitis, purpura, depression, hypercalcemia
	Loop acting: e.g., furosemide	Oral: 20–80 mg 2 or 3 times a day	Mild hypertension, as adjunct in severe or malignant hypertension particularly with renal failure	Hyperuricemia, primary aldosteronism	Potassium depletion, hyperuricemia, hyperglycemia, hypocalcemia, blood dyscrasias, rash, nausea, vomiting, diarrhea
	Potassium-sparing: Spironolactone	Oral: 25 mg 2 to 4 times daily	Hypertension due to hypermineralocorticoidism, adjunct to thiazide therapy	Renal failure	Hyperkalemia, diarrhea, gynecomastia, menstrual irregularities
	Triamterene	Oral: 50–100 mg 1 or 2 times daily			Hyperkalemia, nausea, vomiting, leg cramps, nephrolithiasis, GI disturbances
	Amiloride	Oral: 5–10 mg daily			
ANTIADRENERGIC AGENTS					
Central	Clonidine	Oral: 0.05–0.6 mg twice daily	Mild to moderate hypertension, renal disease with hypertension		Postural hypotension, drowsiness, dry mouth, rebound hypertension after abrupt withdrawal, insomnia
	Guanabenz	Oral: 4–16 mg twice daily			
	Guanfacine	Oral: 1–3 mg daily			
	Methyldopa (also acts by blocking sympathetic nerves)	Oral: 250–1000 mg twice daily IV: 250–1000 mg every 4–6 h (tolerance may develop)	Mild to moderate hypertension (oral), malignant hypertension (IV)	Pheochromocytoma, active hepatic disease (IV), during MAO inhibitor administration	Postural hypotension, sedation, fatigue, diarrhea, impaired ejaculation, fever, gynecomastia, lactation, positive Coombs' tests (occasionally associated with hemolysis), chronic hepatitis, acute ulcerative colitis, lupus-like syndrome
Autonomic ganglia	Trimethaphan	IV: 1–6 mg/min	Severe or malignant hypertension	Severe coronary artery disease, cerebrovascular insufficiency, diabetes mellitus (on hypoglycemic therapy), glaucoma, prostatism	Postural hypotension, visual symptoms, dry mouth, constipation, urinary retention, impotence
Nerve endings	Rauwolfia alkaloids: Reserpine	Oral: 0.05–0.25 mg daily	Mild to moderate hypertension in young patient	Pheochromocytoma, peptic ulcer, depression, during MAO inhibitor administration	Depression, nightmares, nasal congestion, dyspepsia, diarrhea, impotence
	Guanethidine Guanadrel	Oral: 10–150 mg daily Oral 5–50 mg twice daily	Moderate to severe hypertension	Pheochromocytoma, severe coronary artery disease, cerebrovascular insufficiency, during MAO inhibitor administration	Postural hypotension, bradycardia, dry mouth, diarrhea, impaired ejaculation, fluid retention, asthma
Alpha receptors	Phentolamine	IV: 1–5 mg bolus	Suspected or proved pheochromocytoma	Severe coronary artery disease	Tachycardia weakness, dizziness, flushing
	Phenoxybenzamine	Oral: 10–50 mg once or twice daily (tolerance may develop)	Proven pheochromocytoma		Postural hypotension, tachycardia, miosis, nasal congestion, dry mouth
	Prazosin	Oral: 1–10 mg twice daily	Mild to moderate hypertension	Use with caution in the elderly	Sudden syncope, headache, sedation dizziness, tachycardia anticholinergic effect, fluid retention
	Terazosin	Oral: 1–20 mg daily			
Beta receptors	Propranolol	Oral: 10–120 mg 2 to 4 times daily	Mild to moderate hypertension (especially with evidence for hyperdynamic circulation), adjunct to hydralazine therapy	Congestive heart failure, asthma, diabetes mellitus (on hypoglycemic therapy), during MAO inhibitor administration, COPD, sick sinus syndrome, 2d or 3d degree heart block	Dizziness, depression, bronchospasm, nausea, vomiting, diarrhea, constipation, heart failure, fatigue, Raynaud's phenomenon, hallucinations, hypertriglyceridemia, hypercholesterolemia, psoriasis; sudden withdrawal may precipitate angina or myocardial injury in patients with heart disease
	Metoprolol	Oral: 25–150 mg twice daily			
	Nadolol	Oral: 20–120 mg daily			
	Atenolol	Oral 25–100 mg daily			
	Timolol	Oral: 5–15 mg twice daily			

Site of action	Drug	Dosage	Indications	Contraindications	Frequent or peculiar side effects
ANTIADRENERGIC AGENTS *(continued)*					
	Betaxolol	Oral: 10–20 mg daily			
	Carteolol	Oral: 2.5–10 mg daily			
	Pindolol	Oral: 5–30 mg twice daily			Less resting bradycardia than other beta blockers
	Acebutolol	Oral: 200–600 mg twice daily			
alpha/beta receptor	Labetalol	Oral: 100–600 mg twice daily IV: 2 mg/min			Similar to beta blockers with more postural effects
VASODILATORS					
Vascular smooth muscle	Hydralazine	Oral: 10–75 mg 4 times daily IV or IM: 10–50 mg every 6 h (tolerance may develop)	As adjunct in treatment of moderate to severe hypertension (oral), malignant hypertension (IV or IM), renal disease with hypertension	Lupus erythematosus, severe coronary artery disease	Headache, tachycardia, angina pectoris, anorexia, nausea, vomiting, diarrhea, lupus-like syndrome, rash, fluid retention
	Minoxidil	Oral 2.5–40 mg twice daily	Severe hypertension	Severe coronary artery disease	Tachycardia, aggravates angina, marked fluid retention, hair growth on face and body, coarsening of facial features, possible pericardial effusions
	Diazoxide	IV: 1–3 mg/kg up to 150 mg rapidly	Severe or malignant hypertension	Diabetes mellitus, hyperuricemia, congestive heart failure	Hyperglycemia, hyperuricemia, sodium retention
	Nitroprusside	IV:0.5–8 (µg/kg)/min	Malignant hypertension		Apprehension, weakness, diaphoresis, nausea, vomiting, muscle twitching, cyanide toxicity
ANGIOTENSIN-CONVERTING ENZYME INHIBITORS					
Converting enzyme	Captopril	Oral: 12.5–75 mg twice daily	Mild to severe hypertension, renal artery stenosis	Renal failure (reduction of dose), bilateral renal artery stenosis, pregnancy	Leukopenia, pancytopenia, hypotension, cough, angioedema, urticarial rash, fever, loss of taste, acute renal failure in bilateral renal artery stenosis, hyperkalemia
	Benazepril	Oral: 10–40 mg daily			Same as captopril, but little evidence for leukopenia, but perhaps increased frequency of cough and angioedema. All can be given once daily, but side effects are reduced if one-half dose is given twice daily. Fosinopril is excreted more in bile than others.
	Enalapril	Oral: 2.5–40 mg daily			
	Enalaprilat	IV: 0.625–1.25 mg over 5 minutes every 6–8 h			
	Fosinopril	Oral: 10–40 mg daily			
	Lisinopril	Oral: 5–40 mg daily			
	Quinapril	Oral: 10–80 mg daily			
	Ramipril	Oral: 2.5–20 mg daily			
CALCIUM CHANNEL ANTAGONISTS					
Vascular smooth muscle	Nifedipine	Oral: 10–30 mg 4 times daily or as XL form 30–90 mg daily	Mild to moderate hypertension	Heart failure, 2d or 3d degree heart block	Tachycardia, flushing, gastrointestinal disturbances, hyperkalemia, edema, headache
	Amlodipine	Oral: 2.5–10 mg daily			
	Felodipine XL	Oral: 5–10 mg daily			
	Isradipine	Oral: 2.5–10 mg daily			
	Nicardipine	Oral: 20–40 mg 3 times daily			
	Diltiazem	Oral: 30–90 mg 4 times daily or as CD form 180–300 mg daily			Same as nifedipine, except no tachycardia, but can cause heart block, constipation, and liver dysfunction
	Verapamil	Oral: 30–120 mg 4 times daily or as SR form 120–480 mg daily			

TABLE 209-7   Therapeutic agents used to treat malignant hypertension

Drug	Route	Starting dose	Onset	Peak	Duration	Oral preparation available
			__Time course of action__			
IMMEDIATE ONSET						
Nitroprusside	Continuous IV	0.25 (µg/mg)/min	<1 min	1–2 min	2–5 min	No
Trimethaphan	Continuous IV	0.5 mg/min	<1 min	1–2 min	2–5 min	No
Nitroglycerin	Continuous IV	5 µg/min	1–5 min	2–6 min	3–10 min	No
Diazoxide	IV bolus	50 mg q 5–10 min up to 600 mg	1–5 min	2–4 min	4–12 h	No
DELAYED ONSET						
Enalaprilat	IV	1.25 mg q 6 h	10–15 min	3–4 h	6–24 h	Yes
Hydralazine	IV, IM	5–10 mg q 20 min × 3	10–20 min	20–40 min	4–12 h	Yes
Labetalol	IV	20–80 mg q 10 min up to 300 mg	5 min	20–30 min	3–6 h	Yes
Nifedipine	SL	10–20 mg	5–15 min	30–60 min	3–6 h	Yes

Minoxidil is even more potent but unfortunately produces significant hypertrichosis and fluid retention and, therefore, is mainly limited to patients with severe hypertension and renal insufficiency.

Diazoxide, a thiazide derivative, is restricted in its application to acute situations. It is not a diuretic; in fact, it causes sodium retention. However, like other thiazides, it reduces carbohydrate tolerance. It must be given rapidly intravenously to guarantee effect. It begins to act immediately to lower blood pressure, and its effects may last for several hours. *Nitroprusside* given intravenously also acts as a direct vasodilator, with onset and offset of actions that are almost immediate. *Nitroglycerin* is a third direct-acting vasodilator useful as an intravenous agent. These latter three drugs are useful only for the treatment of hypertensive emergencies (Table 209-7).

ACE inhibitors   Drugs from several of the categories discussed above have been shown to possess an additional action resulting in inhibition of renin secretion. These include clonidine, reserpine, methyldopa, and beta blockers. A second group of drugs in this class compress those which inhibit the enzyme converting angiotensin I into angiotensin II. These agents are useful because they not only inhibit the generation of a potent vasoconstrictor (angiotensin II) but also may retard the degradation of a potent vasodilator (bradykinin), alter prostaglandin production (most notably with captopril), and can modify the activity of the adrenergic nervous system. They are especially useful in renal or renovascular hypertension, as well as in accelerated and malignant hypertension. However, in patients with bilateral renal artery stenosis, rapid deterioration of renal function may occur. They are also as effective in mild, uncomplicated hypertension as beta blockers and thiazides—probably with fewer side effects, particularly those which adversely affect the patient's quality of life.

These drugs should be used with caution when the renin system is activated, e.g., with severe heart failure, prior diuretic therapy, or substantial salt restriction, in order to avoid profound hypotension. Usually diuretics are stopped 2 to 3 days before starting an ACE inhibitor and are added back later if needed.

Calcium channel antagonists   These drugs modify the entry of calcium into cells by blocking the slow or voltage-dependent calcium channels, resulting in vasodilatation and, in the case of nifedipine and nicardipine, usually reflex tachycardia. Diltiazem and verapamil both can slow atrioventricular conduction—a feature not observed with nifedipine. While calcium channel antagonists are also useful in angina pectoris (see Chap. 203), because of their negative inotropic actions, they should be used with caution in hypertensive patients with heart failure.

APPROACH TO DRUG THERAPY (Fig. 209-1)   The aim of drug therapy is to use the agents just described, alone or in combination, to return arterial pressure to normal levels with minimal side effects. Ideally, one would choose a therapeutic program which specifically corrects the underlying defect resulting in the elevated blood pressure,

e.g., spironolactone for patients with primary aldosteronism. As our knowledge of the mechanisms underlying the hypertension in individual patients increases, more specific drug programs will become available. This presumably will result in normalization of blood pressure with fewer side effects. In the absence of this information,

FIGURE 209-1   Schematic approach to the treatment of the patient with hypertension in whom a specific form of therapy is unavailable or unknown and volume expansion is not present.

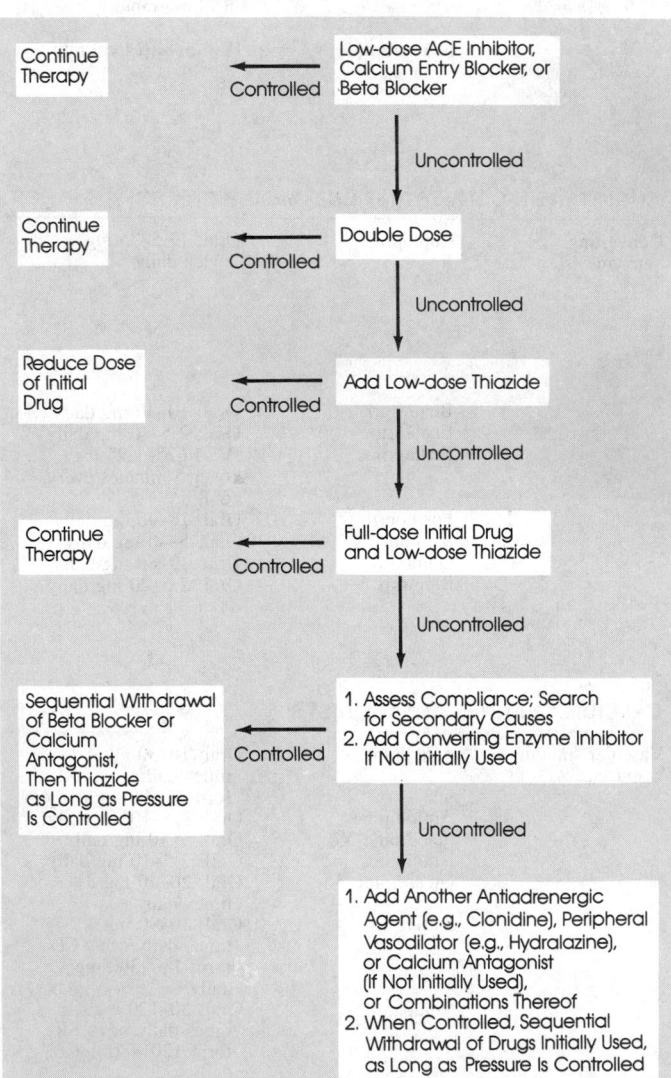

an empirical approach is used, which takes into consideration efficacy, safety, impact on the quality of life, compliance, ease of administration, and cost. When used in combination, drugs are chosen for their different sites of action. However, except for those patients with severe hypertension (average diastolic blood pressure >130 mmHg), in whom intensive therapy with several agents simultaneously usually is required, most patients should be treated *initially* with a single agent. Since many effective antihypertensive agents are available, a number of useful therapeutic regimens have been developed, with the ideal program still unclear. Initial therapy with a diuretic or beta blocker has been the usual first approach, particularly since they are the only agents proven to reduce mortality. However, this does not mean that other effective antihypertensives would fail to have the same beneficial effect if used in similar trials. Thus ACE inhibitors and calcium channel antagonists are also effective as first-line therapy, replacing the old stepped-care approach. The physician is therefore required to choose from four classes of agents for initial therapy with little evidence that one is more effective than another. Some have suggested that an ACE inhibitor or calcium channel blocker be used first, because of their reduced side effects, with a slight preference for ACE inhibitors because of their longer duration of action, potentially fewer adverse effects, and increased compliance rates. I agree with this suggestion. The reason for choosing one drug over the others is empirical, although, in general, older individuals and blacks may be particularly responsive to diuretics, while younger individuals and whites respond well to beta blockers, ACE inhibitors, and calcium channel antagonists.

The schema outlined in Fig. 209-1 takes into account the presently available data on effectiveness, adverse reactions, compliance, impact on quality of life, and economic impact (including cost, usage of health care resources, quality and quantity of work performance) in deciding when to use a given agent. This approach is applicable to all patients in whom an indication for a specific form of therapy is lacking. Because of its lower cost, low-dose thiazide therapy, e.g., 25 mg hydrochlorothiazide (or its equivalent) daily, often has been the first choice. However, three major concerns with widespread thiazide usage have arisen: relatively poor compliance rates (approximately 80 percent) probably reflecting an adverse effect on the patient's quality of life, adverse metabolic effects (hypokalemia, hypomagnesemia, hyperglycemia, and hypercholesterolemia), and potentially an increased frequency of cardiac arrhythmias including sudden death, probably secondary to the electrolyte disturbances. These concerns, coupled with the eight- to tenfold increase in cost associated with the frequent need for potassium supplementation or a potassium-sparing diuretic, have caused some to suggest that thiazides should play a more restricted role in initial antihypertensive therapy, limited to those individuals who are volume-expanded. Thus ACE inhibitors, beta blockers, and calcium channel antagonists are probably the preferred first-line therapy for hypertension, with beta blockers being particularly useful in patients with a hyperactive hemodynamic state, e.g., hypertension with an elevated heart rate.

Under any circumstance, the agent should be started at a low dose, e.g., 25 mg atenolol, 25 mg captopril, 5 mg enalapril, or 120 mg diltiazem (or their equivalents) in divided doses as needed (Table 209-6). If arterial pressure is lowered to less than 140/90 with any of these agents, no further therapy is indicated (see Fig. 209-1). If it is not after 1 to 3 months, the next step is to double the dose of the primary agent. If still not controlled, then 25 mg hydrochlorothiazide (or its equivalent) per day should be added. Thiazides potentiate the action of ACE inhibitors and probably of beta blockers and at least are additive to the antihypertensive effect of calcium channel antagonists. Combining diuretics with ACE inhibitors is particularly appealing because the adverse metabolic effects of the thiazide, in part, will be ameliorated by the ACE inhibitor. This is not true for beta blockers or calcium antagonists. Indeed, beta blockers and thiazides may actually potentiate each other's adverse effects insofar as electrolytes (hypokalemia) and metabolic actions (hypercholesterolemia) are concerned.

If therapy with two drugs does not achieve blood pressure control, the primary agent should be increased to full dose, e.g., 100 mg captopril or atenolol, 20 mg enalapril, or 360 mg diltiazem. While larger doses than these can be used, it is probably advisable to switch to another medication rather than increase the dose further. Occasionally, increasing the thiazide to the equivalent of 50 mg hydrochlorothiazide daily may bring about control of the hypertension; however, thiazide doses higher than this are seldom, if ever, warranted because they almost invariably produce significant side effects. If the blood pressure is still not controlled, then a detailed search for a secondary cause of hypertension, as outlined above, is indicated. If none is found, then a dietary assessment often will reveal a high sodium intake. With reduction in salt intake to 5 g/d or less, blood pressure often is controlled. If the blood pressure is still not controlled, then the primary agent should be switched, maintaining the thiazide. Caution should be used if an ACE inhibitor was not the original agent, since administration of such an agent to a patient who already is taking a diuretic may lead to profound hypotension. If none of the changes produce better control of arterial pressure, then the combination of a calcium channel antagonist and an ACE inhibitor or triple therapy usually with a diuretic, ACE inhibitor, and hydralazine may be effective.

If the blood pressure is controlled, then there should be stepwise reduction in the dose and/or withdrawal of some of the agents in order to determine the minimal therapeutic program that will maintain the blood pressure at 140/90 mmHg or less.

Fewer than 5 percent of patients will still be hypertensive at this point. In them, one first should consider the reasons for therapeutic failure, as shown in Table 209-8. If none can be identified, then one of the other agents such as a vasodilator listed in Table 209-6 (e.g., hydralazine) or an antiadrenergic agent (e.g., prazosin or clonidine) should be added. If blood pressure is controlled, previous drugs are sequentially withdrawn in order to determine the minimal therapeutic program that maintains a normal blood pressure.

While the recommendations outlined above are satisfactory for a large majority of patients, it is important to use a flexible approach, because individual patients may respond differently to individual drugs and drug combinations. For those patients requiring multiple drugs, once the appropriate combination has been found, the use of a single formulation with the appropriate combination of drugs may simplify the regimen and thereby increase compliance. Every effort should be made to reduce the number of times each day the patients must interrupt their schedules for the medication. Pharmacologic treatment of essential hypertension is usually lifelong, and since most patients are asymptomatic, compliance with a complex regimen may be a serious problem, particularly if the therapeutic regimen has a negative impact on the quality of the patient's life. Finally, what level of arterial pressure should be accepted as adequate control remains uncertain. It is clear that reducing diastolic blood pressure to below 90 mmHg is appropriate and beneficial in reducing morbidity and/or mortality. However, whether a reduction below 85 mmHg is warranted, particularly in elderly patients, remains controversial.

TABLE 209-8 Reasons for poor therapeutic response in patients with hypertension

Inadequate patient compliance
Volume expansion
  Excessive sodium intake
  Secondary to nondiuretic antihypertensive agent
Excessive weight gain
Inadequate doses
Drug antagonism
  Cold remedies
  Sympathomimetics
  Oral contraceptives (estrogens)
  Adrenal steroids
Secondary forms of hypertension

Special considerations Five groups of patients with hypertension require special consideration because of associated conditions.

RENAL DISEASE Reduction of arterial pressure in hypertensive patients with impaired renal function is often accompanied initially by an increase in serum creatinine. This change does not represent further structural renal damage and should not deter continuation of therapy, since achievement of blood pressure control may eventually reduce the value toward normal. However, if serum creatinine increases in patients treated with a converting enzyme inhibitor, care needs to be exercised because these patients may have bilateral renal artery disease. Their renal function will continue to deteriorate as long as the converting enzyme inhibitor is given. Thus converting enzyme inhibitors should be used cautiously in patients with impaired renal function, and renal function should be assessed frequently (every 4 to 5 days) for the first 3 weeks. While converting enzyme inhibitors are contraindicated in patients with bilateral renal artery stenosis, these are the drugs of choice in patients with unilateral renal artery stenosis and a normally functioning contralateral kidney and perhaps in patients with chronic renal failure.

CORONARY ARTERY DISEASE In these patients who also may be taking cardiac glycosides, thiazides should be used judiciously, and a reduction in serum potassium levels should be looked for and, if found, should be corrected rapidly. Beta blockers should be withdrawn carefully, if at all, in these patients. Finally, calcium channel antagonists and converting enzyme inhibitors may be useful in these patients because they minimize a number of potential adverse reactions accompanying other therapeutic agents, particularly nonspecific vasodilators.

DIABETES MELLITUS The diabetic patient with hypertension is particularly challenging because many of the agents used to lower blood pressure can affect glucose metabolism adversely. Converting enzyme inhibitors may be particularly useful in these individuals. They have no known adverse effects on glucose or lipid metabolism and may actually minimize the development of diabetic nephropathy by reducing renal vascular resistance and renal perfusion pressure—the primary factor underlying renal deterioration in these patients.

PREGNANCY The patient who is pregnant and hypertensive or who develops hypertension during pregnancy (pregnancy-induced hypertension, preeclampsia, eclampsia) is particularly difficult to treat. Because it is uncertain that autoregulation of uterine blood flow occurs, lowering blood pressure in the pregnant hypertensive may result in reduce placental and fetal perfusion. Thus a conservative approach to lowering blood pressure is usually indicated. In the second and third trimesters, antihypertensives often are not indicated unless the diastolic pressure exceeds 95 mmHg. In general, severe salt restriction and/or diuretics are not given because of the associated increase in fetal wastage. Beta blockers need to be used cautiously for similar reasons. Methyldopa and hydralazine, and to a lesser extent calcium channel antagonists, are the most frequent antihypertensives used because they have no known adverse effects on the fetus. Little is known about the safety of other antihypertensives in pregnancy except that nitroprusside and converting enzyme inhibitors may cause adverse effects on the fetus and are contraindicated.

ELDERLY PATIENTS The hypertensive patient who is over age 65, and particularly those over age 75, offers substantial challenges to the physician. Several recent studies have documented that in healthy elderly patients, whether male or female, there is a substantial reduction in strokes and stroke-related deaths in those treated with relatively modest doses of antihypertensive agents. This is true whether the patient has systolic and diastolic hypertension or isolated systolic hypertension. What is not clear from these studies is how broadly the results can be extrapolated, since they were performed in healthy elderly patients, while many such patients have other diseases. Thus, in the elderly hypertensive patient, individualization of therapy still seems warranted.

Probably fewer than one-third of hypertensive patients in the United States are being treated effectively. Only a small number of these failures are related to drug unresponsiveness. The majority are related to (1) failure to detect hypertension, (2) failure to institute effective treatment of the asymptomatic hypertensive subject, and (3) failure of the asymptomatic hypertensive subject to adhere to therapy. In order to improve this deficiency, patients must be educated to continue treatment once an effective regimen has been identified. Side effects and inconveniences of treatment must be minimized or counteracted in order to obtain the patient's continued cooperation.

MALIGNANT HYPERTENSION

In addition to marked blood pressure elevation in association with papilledema and retinal hemorrhages and exudates, the full-blown picture of malignant hypertension may include manifestations of hypertensive encephalopathy, such as severe headache, vomiting, visual disturbances (including transient blindness), transient paralyses, convulsions, stupor, and coma. These have been attributed to spasm of cerebral vessels and to cerebral edema. In some patients who have died, multiple small thrombi have been found in the cerebral vessels. Cardiac decompensation and rapidly declining renal function are other critical features of malignant hypertension. Oliguria may, in fact, be the presenting feature. The vascular lesion characteristic of malignant hypertension is fibrinoid necrosis of the walls of small arteries and arterioles, and this can be reversed by effective antihypertensive therapy.

The pathogenesis of malignant hypertension is unknown. However, at least two independent processes, dilatation of cerebral arteries and generalized arteriolar fibrinoid necrosis, contribute to the associated signs and symptoms. The cerebral arteries dilate because the normal autoregulation of cerebral blood flow decompensates secondary to the markedly elevated arterial pressure. As a result, cerebral blood flow is excessive, producing the encephalopathy associated with malignant hypertension. Many patients also show evidence of a microangiopathic hemolytic anemia; this secondary phenomenon could contribute to the deterioration of renal function. Most patients also have elevated levels of peripheral plasma renin activity and increased aldosterone production, and these may be involved in causing vascular damage.

About 1 percent of hypertensive patients develop the malignant phase, which occurs in the course of both essential and secondary hypertension. Rarely it is the first recognized manifestation of the blood pressure problem, and it is unusual for it to occur in patients under treatment. The average age at diagnosis is 40, and men are more often affected than women. Prior to the availability of effective therapy, life expectancy after diagnosis of malignant hypertension was less than 2 years, with most deaths being due to renal failure, cerebral hemorrhage, or congestive heart failure. With the advent of effective antihypertensive therapy, at least half the patients survive for more than 5 years.

Malignant hypertension is a medical emergency that requires immediate therapy. However, it needs to be distinguished from severe hypertension, since overly aggressive therapy in malignant hypertension could result in a potentially hazardous reduction in myocardial and cerebral perfusion. The initial aim of therapy should be to reduce diastolic pressure by one-third, but not below 95 mmHg. The drugs available for treatment of malignant hypertension can be divided into two groups on the basis of time of onset of action (see Table 209-7). Those in the first group act within a few minutes but are not satisfactory for long-term management. If the patient is having convulsions, and if arterial pressure must be reduced rapidly, then one from the immediate-acting group should be used. The first three agents in this group require continuous infusion and close monitoring. *Nitroprusside* is given by continuous intravenous infusion at a dose of 0.25 to 8.0 (μg/kg)/min. It is probably the agent of choice in this condition since it dilates both arterioles and veins. It has the advantage over the ganglionic blockers of not being associated with the development of tachyphylaxis and can be utilized for days with few side effects. The dosage must be controlled with an infusion pump. *Trimethaphan*, a ganglionic blocker, is given at a rate of 0.5 to 5 mg/min. It also dilates arterioles and veins. The patient should be in the sitting position, and the pressure should be monitored closely, preferably in an intensive care unit. Monitoring may be more complex than with nitroprusside, but trimethaphan may be better therapy in acute aortic dissection. *Nitroglycerin* affects veins more than arterioles and is given by continuous infusion at a rate of 5 to 100 µg/min. It is particularly useful in treating hypertension following coronary bypass surgery. *Diazoxide* is the easiest to administer, for no individual titration of dosage is required. It primarily affects arteriolar and not venous tone. A dose of 50 to 150 mg is given rapidly intravenously, and the antihypertensive effect is noted in 1 to 5 min. The same dose can be repeated in 5 to 10 min, if necessary, or when the pressure begins to rise, usually after several hours. The total dose should not exceed 600 mg/d. In an occasional patient, pressure may drop below normal levels after diazoxide administration. It should not be used in patients in whom aortic dissection or myocardial infarction is suspected. Because it can increase the force of myocardial contraction, often a beta blocker is given concomitantly. *Enalaprilat*, an intravenous form of the ACE inhibitor *enalapril*, also has proven effective in preliminary studies. Finally, intravenous *labetalol* may be particularly useful in patients with a myocardial infarct or angina because it prevents an increase in heart rate. However, it may be ineffective in patients previously treated with beta blockers and is contraindicated in patients with heart failure, asthma, bradycardia, or heart block. It also may serve as an alternative therapy in patients with eclampsia who are unresponsive to hydralazine.

Patients given any of these agents also should receive other medications effective for long-term control. Those in the second group in Table 209-7 require 30 min or more to obtain full effect but have the advantage of being satisfactory for subsequent oral administration and for long-term management of the patient's hypertension. If such a delay in attainment of full effect is acceptable, intravenous *hydralazine* is effective in many patients within 10 min; an effective protocol involves giving 10-mg doses intravenously every 10 to 15 min until the desired effect has been obtained or until a total of 50 mg has been administered. The total required for response may then be repeated intramuscularly or intravenously every 6 h. Hydralazine should be used with caution in patients with significant coronary artery disease and should be avoided in patients evidencing myocardial ischemia or aortic dissection. It is effective in preeclampsia. Sublingual *nifedipine* has been reported to be useful in some cases, although it may produce tachycardia, and success has not been uniform.

Furosemide is an important adjunct to the therapy just discussed. Given either orally or intravenously, it serves to maintain sodium diuresis in the face of a falling arterial pressure and thus will speed recovery from encephalopathy and congestive heart failure as well as maintain sensitivity to the primary antihypertensive drug. Digitalis (Chap. 195) also may be indicated if there is evidence of cardiac decompensation.

In patients with malignant hypertension in whom the existence of pheochromocytoma is suspected, urine should be collected for measurement of the products of catecholamine metabolism, and drugs which might release additional catecholamines, such as methyldopa, reserpine, and guanethidine, must be avoided. The parenteral drug of choice in these patients is phentolamine, administered with care to avoid a precipitous reduction in arterial pressure.

There is hope even for patients who fail to respond sufficiently to any of the forms of therapy and who show progressive deterioration in renal function. In some, a period of peritoneal dialysis or hemodialysis to deplete extracellular fluid has resulted in better blood pressure control and eventual improvement in renal function. In other patients with refractory hypertension and renal failure who do not respond to volume depletion or hypotensive therapy, including minoxidil, particularly those with marked elevation of plasma renin activity, bilateral nephrectomy has resulted in amelioration of hypertension; subsequently, these patients have been maintained on chronic dialysis or have received renal homografts. However, bilateral nephrectomy should be avoided where possible because (1) the loss of renal erythropoietin will contribute to the associated anemia, (2) vitamin D metabolism may be adversely affected, and (3) all residual renal function will be lost.

REFERENCES

CALHOUN DA et al: Treatment of hypertensive crisis. N Engl J Med 323:1177, 1990

DAHLOF B et al: Morbidity and mortality in the Swedish Trial in Old Patients with Hypertension (STOP-Hypertension). Lancet 338:1281, 1991

DANNENBERG AL et al: Incidence of hypertension in the Framingham study. Am J Publ Health 78:676, 1988

FARNETT L et al: The J-curve phenomenon and the treatment of hypertension: Is there a point beyond which pressure reduction is dangerous? JAMA 265:489, 1991

GIFFORD RW et al: Office evaluation of hypertension: A statement for health professionals by a writing group of the Council for High Blood Pressure Research, American Heart Association. Circulation 79:283, 1989

GOTTDIENER JS et al: Left ventricular hypertrophy in men with normal blood pressure: Relation to exaggerated blood pressure response to exercise. Ann Intern Med 112(3):161, 1990

JOINT NATIONAL COMMITTEE ON DETECTION, EVALUATION AND TREATMENT OF HIGH BLOOD PRESSURE: The fifth report. Arch Intern Med 153:154, 1993

KEANE WF et al: Angiotensin-converting enzyme inhibitors and progressive renal insufficiency: Current experience and future directions. Ann Intern Med 111:503, 1989

KURTZ TW, SPENCE MA: Genetics of essential hypertension. Am J Med 94:77, 1993

LAVIE CJ et al: Regression of increased left ventricular mass by antihypertensives. Drugs 42:945, 1991

LIFTON RP, JEUNEMAITRE X: Finding genes that cause human hypertension. J Hypertens 11:231, 1993

LITTENBERG B et al: Screening for hypertension. Ann Intern Med 112(3):192, 1990

NALLY JV et al: Diagnostic criteria of renovascular hypertension with captopril renography: A consensus statement. Am J Hypertens 4:749S, 1991

OBERMAN A et al: Pharmacologic and nutritional treatment of mild hypertension: Changes in cardiovascular risk status. Ann Intern Med 112(2):89, 1990

PARATI G, MANCIA G: Calcium antagonists in the treatment of arterial hypertension. Am Heart J 125:642, 1993

SALVETTI A: Newer ACE inhibitors: A look at the future. Drugs 40:800, 1990

SHEP COOPERATIVE RESEARCH GROUP: Prevention of stroke by antihypertensive drug treatment in older persons with isolated systolic hypertension: Final results of the Systolic Hypertension in the Elderly Program (SHEP) JAMA 265:3255, 1991

STAMLER J et al: Blood pressure, systolic and diastolic, and cardiovascular risks. US population data. Arch Intern Med 153:598, 1993

SUBCOMMITTEE OF NON-PHARMACOLOGIC THERAPY OF THE JOINT NATIONAL COMMITTEE ON DETECTION, EVALUATION AND TREATMENT OF HIGH BLOOD PRESSURE: Non-pharmacological approaches to the control of high blood pressure: Final report. Hypertension 8:444, 1986

WEIDMANN P et al: Pathogenesis and treatment of hypertension associated with diabetes mellitus. Am Heart J 125:1498, 1993

WEINBERGER MH Racial differences in renal sodium excretion: Relationship to hypertension. Am J Kidney Dis 21:41, 1993

WILLIAMS GH: Quality of life and its impact on hypertensive patients. Am J Med 82:98, 1987

———: Converting enzyme inhibitors in the treatment of hypertension. N Engl J Med 319:1517, 1989

———, HOLLENBERG NK: Pathophysiology of essential hypertension, in *Cardiology*, vol 2, WW Parmley, J Chatterjee (eds). Philadelphia, Lippincott, 1990, chap 22

210 DISEASES OF THE AORTA

VICTOR J. DZAU / MARK A. CREAGER

The aorta is the conduit through which the blood ejected from the left ventricle is delivered to the systemic arterial bed. In adults, its diameter is approximately 3 cm at the origin, 2.5 cm in the descending portion in the thorax, and 1.8 to 2 cm in the abdomen. The aortic wall consists of a thin intima composed of endothelium, subendothelial connective tissue, and an internal elastic lamina; a thick tunica media composed of smooth-muscle cells and extracellular matrix; and an adventitia composed primarily of connective tissue and enclosing the vasa vasorum and nervi vascularis. In addition to its conduit function, the viscoelastic and compliant properties of the aorta also subserve a buffering function. The aorta is distended during systole to enable a

TABLE 210-1 Diseases of the aorta: Classification and etiology

Aortic aneurysm
  Atherosclerosis
  Cystic medial necrosis
  Syphilitic infection
  Mycotic infection
  Rheumatic aortitis
  Trauma
Aortic dissection
  Cystic medial necrosis
  Systemic hypertension
  Atherosclerosis
Aortic occlusion
  Atherosclerosis
  Thromboembolism
Aortitis
  Syphilitic aortitis
  Rheumatic aortitis
  Takayasu's arteritis and aortic arch syndromes
  Giant cell arteritis

portion of the stroke volume to be stored, and it recoils during diastole so that blood continues to flow to the periphery during diastole. Because of its continuous exposure to high pulsatile pressure and shear stress, the aorta is particularly prone to injury and disease resulting from mechanical trauma (Table 210-1). The aorta is also more prone to rupture than any other vessel, especially with the development of aneurysmal dilatation, since its wall tension, as governed by Laplace's law (i.e., proportional to the product of pressure and radius), is intrinsically high.

AORTIC ANEURYSM

An *aneurysm* is defined as a pathologic dilatation of a segment of a blood vessel. A *true* aneurysm involves all three layers of the vessel wall and is distinguished from a *pseudoaneurysm*, in which the intimal and medial layers are disrupted and the dilatation is lined by adventitia only and sometimes by perivascular clot. Aneurysms also may be classified according to their gross appearance. A *fusiform* aneurysm affects the entire circumference of a segment of the vessel, resulting in a diffusely dilated lesion. In contrast, a *saccular* aneurysm involves only a portion of the circumference, resulting in an outpouching of the vessel wall.

The most common pathologic condition associated with aortic aneurysm is atherosclerosis. It is controversial whether atherosclerosis itself actually causes aortic aneurysm or develops as a secondary event in the dilated aorta. Causality is inferred by studies that have shown that many patients with aortic aneurysms have coexisting risk factors and atherosclerosis in other blood vessels. Familial clusterings of abdominal aortic aneurysms occur in 20 percent of patients, suggesting a hereditary basis of the disease. Indeed, a mutation of the gene encoding type III procollagen has been implicated. Additional causes of aortic aneurysm include cystic medial necrosis, syphilis or other bacterial infections, rheumatic aortitis, and trauma. Congenital aortic aneurysms may be primary or associated with other anomalies, such as a bicuspid aortic valve or aortic coarctation.

Aortic aneurysms are also classified according to location, i.e., abdominal versus thoracic. Those in the abdominal aorta are almost always associated with atherosclerosis. Aneurysms of the ascending thoracic aorta may be related to cystic medial necrosis, atherosclerosis, syphilis, bacterial infections, or rheumatoid arthritis. Aneurysms of the descending thoracic aorta are usually contiguous with infradiaphragmatic aneurysms and, as with the latter, are associated with atherosclerosis.

Aortic aneurysms usually do not produce symptoms. However, as they expand, they may become painful. Compression or erosion of adjacent tissue by aneurysms also may cause symptoms. The formation of mural thrombi within the aneurysm may predispose to peripheral embolization. Occasionally, an aneurysm may leak, leading to extravasation of blood into the vessel wall and the periadventitial area and causing acute pain and local tenderness. This is usually a harbinger of rupture and represents a medical emergency. More often, acute rupture occurs without any prior warning, and this complication is always life-threatening.

ATHEROSCLEROTIC ANEURYSMS Seventy-five percent of atherosclerotic aneurysms are located in the distal abdominal aorta below the renal arteries. An abdominal aneurysm commonly produces no symptoms and is usually detected on routine examination as a palpable, pulsatile, and nontender mass, or it is an incidental finding during an abdominal x-ray or ultrasound performed for other reasons. Some patients may complain of strong pulsations in the abdomen, others of lower back pain. Rarely, there is leakage of the aneurysm with severe pain and tenderness. Acute pain and hypotension occur with rupture of the aneurysm, requiring emergency operation.

Abdominal radiography may demonstrate the calcified outline of the aneurysm. However, about 25 percent of aneurysms are not calcified and cannot be visualized by plain x-ray. A more accurate method of detection is ultrasound, which can delineate the transverse and longitudinal dimensions of the aneurysm; mural thrombus may be detected. Ultrasound is useful for serial documentation of aneurysm size. Both computed tomography (CT) with contrast and magnetic resonance imaging (MRI) have been introduced for the detection and follow-up of aortic aneurysm. These relatively expensive but noninvasive techniques provide higher resolution than ultrasound and have replaced the latter in some centers. Abdominal aortography remains the gold standard in evaluating patients with aneurysm for surgery, but this procedure carries a small risk of complications, such as bleeding, allergic reactions, and atheroembolism. This technique is useful in documenting the extent of the aneurysm, especially its upper and lower limits, and the extent of associated atherosclerotic vascular disease. However, since the presence of mural clots may reduce the laminal size, aortography may underestimate the diameter of an aneurysm.

Prognosis is related to both the size of the aneurysm and the severity of coexistent coronary artery and cerebral vascular diseases. The mortality of patients with abdominal aneurysms exceeding 6 cm in diameter who do not undergo surgical treatment is approximately 50 percent in 1 year, while in those with lesions between 4 and 6 cm, it is 25 percent. The risk of rupture increases with the size of the aneurysm. Most of the others succumb to coronary heart disease and stroke.

Operative excision with replacement with a graft is indicated for patients with abdominal aneurysms greater than 6 cm in diameter, as well as in symptomatic patients and in those with rapidly expanding aneurysms irrespective of the absolute diameter. Except for patients with exceptionally high operative risk, operation is also usually recommended in patients with aneurysm diameters of 5 to 6 cm. Serial noninvasive follow-up of smaller (<5 cm) aneurysms is an alternative to immediate surgery. In surgical candidates, careful preoperative cardiac and general medical evaluations (followed by appropriate therapy of complicating conditions) are essential. Preexisting coronary artery disease, congestive heart failure, pulmonary disease, diabetes and advanced age add to the risk of surgery. If clinically indicated, preoperative evaluation should identify high-risk coronary artery disease using an exercise stress test or dipyridamole thallium scanning. Noninvasive tests, such as stress echocardiography or ambulatory electrocardiographic monitoring for silent ischemia, are favored in some institutions. Perioperative management should include the placement of a Swan-Ganz catheter and arterial line to monitor and optimize left ventricular filling pressure, cardiac output, and arterial pressure, especially during clamping and declamping of aorta, as well as during the immediate postoperative period. With careful preoperative cardiac evaluation and postoperative care, which includes Swan-Ganz catheterization, operative mortality approximates

1 to 2 percent. Following acute rupture, the mortality of emergency operation is generally greater than 50 percent.

CYSTIC MEDIAL NECROSIS This is due to the degeneration of collagen and elastic fibers in the media of the aorta, which are replaced by multiple clefts of mucoid material. Cystic medial necrosis characteristically affects the proximal aorta, results in circumferential weakness and dilatation, and leads to the development of fusiform aneurysms involving the ascending aorta and the sinuses of Valsalva. This condition is particularly prevalent in patients with the Marfan syndrome and Ehlers-Danlos syndrome type IV (Chap. 351) but is also seen in pregnancy and hypertension and sometimes as an isolated condition in patients without any other apparent disease. The clinical manifestations include expanding aneurysms, rupture, and aortic regurgitation. Operative repair is indicated in patients in whom the diameter of the aortic root exceeds 6 cm to prevent dissection or rupture. Control of arterial pressure is an important part of the long-term management of this condition.

MYCOTIC ANEURYSM This rare condition develops as the result of staphylococcal, streptococcal, or salmonella infections of the aorta, usually at an atherosclerotic plaque. Blood cultures are usually positive and reveal the nature of the infecting agent. The aneurysms are usually saccular. Treatment requires parenteral antibiotics and surgical excision.

TRAUMA Aortic rupture may develop following penetrating injury or blunt trauma. Deceleration injury may tear the aortic isthmus at the site of insertion of the ligamentum arteriosum. Other causes of arotic aneurysm, such as syphilitic infection and rheumatic vasculitides, are discussed below under "Aortitis."

AORTIC DISSECTION

Aortic dissection is caused by a circumferential or transverse tear of the intima, usually along the right lateral wall of the ascending aorta where the hydraulic shear stress is high. It has been speculated that the initiating event is a medial hemorrhage that dissects into and disrupts the intima. Another common site is the descending thoracic aorta just below the ligamentum arteriosum. The pulsate aortic flow then dissects along the elastic lamellar plates of the aorta and creates a false lumen. The dissection usually propagates distally down the descending aorta and into its major branches, but it also may propagate proximally. In some cases, a secondary distal intimal disruption occurs, resulting in the reentry of blood from the false to the true lumen.

DeBakey and coworkers classified aortic dissections as type I, in which an intimal tear occurs in the ascending aorta but which involves the descending aorta as well, type II, in which the dissection is limited to the ascending aorta, and type III, in which the intimal tear is located in the descending area with distal propagation of the dissection (Fig. 210-1). Another classification (Stanford) is that of type A, in which the dissection involves the ascending aorta (proximal dissection), and type B, in which it is limited to the descending aorta (distal dissection). From a management standpoint, classification into type A or B is more practical and useful, since DeBakey types I and II are managed in a similar manner.

The factors that predispose to aortic dissection include systemic hypertension, a coexisting condition in 70 percent of patients, and cystic medial necrosis. Aortic dissection is the major cause of morbidity and mortality in patients with the Marfan syndrome (Chap. 351). The incidence is also increased in patients with congenital aortic valve anomalies (e.g., bicuspid valve), in those with coarctation of the aorta, and in otherwise normal women during the third trimester of pregnancy.

CLINICAL MANIFESTATIONS The presentations of aortic dissection are the consequences of intimal tear, dissecting hematoma, occlusion of involved arteries, and compression of adjacent tissues. Acute aortic dissection presents with the sudden onset of pain (Chap.

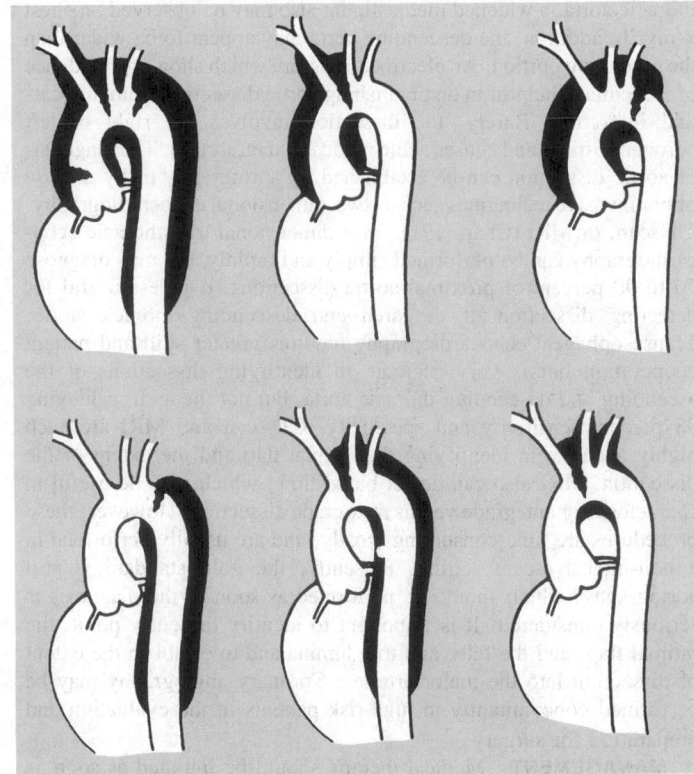

FIGURE 210-1 Classification of aortic dissections. Stanford classification: Top panels illustrate type A dissections that involve the ascending aorta independent of site of tear and distal extension; type B dissections (bottom panels) involve transverse and/or descending aorta without involvement of the ascending aorta. DeBakey classification: Type I dissection involves ascending to descending aorta (top left); type II dissection is limited to ascending or transverse aorta, without descending aorta (top center + top right); type III dissection involves descending aorta only (bottom left). (*From DC Miller, in RM Doroghazi, EE Slater (eds). Aortic Dissection. New York, McGraw-Hill, 1983, with permission.*)

12), which is often described as very severe and tearing and associated with diaphoresis. The pain may be localized to the front or back of the chest, often the interscapular region, and typically migrates with propagation of the dissection. Other symptoms include syncope, dyspnea, and weakness. Physical findings may include hypertension or hypotension, loss of pulses, aortic regurgitation, pulmonary edema, and neurologic findings due to carotid artery obstruction (hemiplegia, hemianesthesia) or spinal cord ischemia (paraplegia). Bowel ischemia, hematuria, and myocardial ischemia have all been observed. These clinical manifestations reflect complications resulting from the dissection occluding the major arteries. Furthermore, clinical manifestations may result from the compression of adjacent structures (e.g., superior cervical ganglia, superior vena cava, bronchus, esophagus) by the expanding dissection aneurysm and include Horner's syndrome, superior vena caval syndrome, hoarseness, dysphagia, and airway compromise. Hemopericardium and cardiac tamponade may complicate a type A lesion with retrograde dissection. Acute aortic regurgitation is an important and common (over 50 percent) complication of proximal dissection. This is the outcome of either a circumferential tear that widens the aortic root or a disruption of the annulus by dissecting hematoma that tears a leaflet(s) or displaces it below the line of closure. Signs of aortic regurgitation include bounding pulses, a wide pulse pressure, a diastolic murmur often radiating to the right sternal border, and evidence of congestive heart failure. The clinical manifestation depends on the severity of the regurgitation.

In dissections involving the ascending aorta, the chest x-ray often reveals a widened superior mediastinum. A pleural effusion (usually left-sided) also may be present. In dissections of the descending thoracic aorta, a widened mediastinum also may be observed on chest x-ray. In addition, the descending aorta may appear to be wider than the ascending portion. An electrocardiogram which shows no evidence of ischemia is helpful in distinguishing aortic dissection from myocardial infarction. Rarely, the dissection involves the right or left coronary ostium and causes acute myocardial infarction. The diagnosis of aortic dissection can be established by aortography or by the use of noninvasive techniques such as two-dimensional echocardiography, CT scan, or MRI (Chap. 191). Two-dimensional transthoracic echocardiography can be performed simply and rapidly and may diagnose 70 to 90 percent of proximal aortic dissections. It is less useful for detecting dissection of the arch and descending thoracic aorta. Transesophageal echocardiography requires greater skill and patient cooperation but is very accurate in identifying dissections of the ascending and descending thoracic aorta, but not the arch, achieving 98 percent sensitivity and specificity. CT scan and MRI are each highly accurate in identifying the intimal flap and the extent of the dissection. MRI also can detect blood flow, which may be useful in characterizing antegrade versus retrograde dissection. However, these procedures are time-consuming, costly, and are usually performed in a non-intensive-care setting. Presently, the gold standard is still aortography, which should be performed as soon as the diagnosis is seriously considered. It is important to identify the entry point, the intimal flap, and the false and true lumina and to establish the extent of dissection into the major arteries. Coronary angiography may be performed concomitantly in high-risk patients in the evaluation and preparation for surgery.

MANAGEMENT Medical therapy should be initiated as soon as the diagnosis is considered. The patient should be admitted to an intensive care unit for monitoring hemodynamics and urine output. Unless hypotension is present, therapy should be aimed at reducing cardiac contractility and systemic arterial pressure, and thereby shear stress. For acute dissection, unless contraindicated, beta-adrenergic blockers should be administered via the parenteral route, using either intravenous propranolol, metoprolol, or the short-acting esmolol to achieve a heart rate of approximately 60 beats per minute. This should be accompanied by sodium nitroprusside infusion to lower systolic blood pressure to 120 mmHg or less. Recently, labetalol (p. 1127), a drug with both beta- and alpha-adrenergic blocking properties, also has been used as a parenteral agent in the acute therapy of dissection. Trimethaphan, a ganglionic blocker, may be used if nitroprusside or labetalol cannot be employed. Experience with calcium antagonists is limited. Direct vasodilators, such as diazoxide and hydralazine, are contraindicated because these agents can increase hydraulic shear and may propagate dissection.

For ascending aortic dissection (type A), surgical correction, which includes reconstruction of the aortic wall, is the preferred treatment. Emergency operation carries a high operative mortality. Thus, if possible, surgery should be deferred for several days, allowing time for stabilization of the patient's clinical status. However, if pain continues and evidence of further dissection develops despite medical therapy, emergency surgery is indicated. The overall in-hospital mortality rate after surgical treatment of patients with aortic dissection is reported to be 15 to 20 percent. The major causes of perioperative mortality and morbidity include myocardial infarction, paraplegia, renal failure, tamponade, hemorrhage, and sepsis. For uncomplicated and stable distal dissection (type B), medical therapy is the preferred treatment unless there is clinical evidence of propagation, compromise of major branches of the aorta, impending rupture, or continued pain. The in-hospital mortality rate of medically treated patients with type B dissection is 15 to 20 percent. Long-term therapy for patients with aortic dissection (with or without surgery) consists of the control of hypertension and reduction of cardiac contractility with the use of beta blockers plus other antihypertensive agents such as angiotensin-converting enzyme inhibitor or calcium antagonist. The long-term prognosis for patients with treated dissections (with the exception of those with the Marfan syndrome) is generally good; the 10-year survival rate is approximately 60 percent.

AORTIC OCCLUSION

CHRONIC ARTERIOSCLEROTIC OCCLUSIVE DISEASE
Chronic occlusive disease usually involves the distal abdominal aorta below the renal arteries. Frequently the disease extends to the common iliac arteries, but it may spare the external iliac arteries. Because of the slowly progressive nature of the atherosclerotic process, the natural history of aortic occlusion is usually chronic and insidious. Claudication characteristically involves the lower back, buttocks, and thighs and may be associated with impotence in males (Leriche syndrome). The severity of the symptoms depends on the adequacy of collaterals. With sufficient collateral blood flow, a complete occlusion of the abdominal aorta may occur without the development of ischemic symptoms. The physical findings include absence of femoral and other distal pulses bilaterally and the detection of an audible bruit over the abdomen (usually at or below the umbilicus) and the common femoral arteries. Atrophic skin, loss of hair, and coolness of the lower extremities are usually observed. In advanced ischemia, rubor on dependency and pallor on elevation can be seen.

The diagnosis is usually established by the physical examination and noninvasive testing, including leg pressure measurements, Doppler velocity analysis, and pulse volume recordings. The anatomy may be defined by abdominal aortography prior to revascularization. Operative treatment is indicated in patients with debilitating symptoms and/or with the development of leg ischemia.

ACUTE OCCLUSION Acute occlusion in the distal abdominal aorta represents a medical emergency because it threatens the viability of the lower extremities. It usually results from an occlusive embolus that almost always originates from the heart. Rarely, acute occlusion may occur as the result of in situ thrombosis in a preexisting severely narrowed segment of the aorta or plaque rupture and hemorrhage into such an area.

The clinical picture is one of acute ischemia of the lower extremities. Severe rest pain, coolness, and pallor of the lower extremities and the absence of distal pulses bilaterally are the usual manifestations. Diagnosis should be established rapidly by aortography. Emergency thrombectomy or revascularization is indicated.

AORTITIS

Aortitis frequently affects the ascending aorta and may result in aneurysmal dilatation and aortic regurgitation; it occasionally obstructs branch vessels of the aorta.

SYPHILITIC AORTITIS This late manifestation of luetic infection (Chap. 133) usually affects the proximal ascending aorta, particularly the aortic root, resulting in aortic dilatation and aneurysm formation. Syphilitic aortitis may occasionally involve the aortic arch or the descending aorta. The aneurysms may be saccular or fusiform and are usually asymptomatic, but compression of and erosion into adjacent structures may result in symptoms; rupture also may occur.

The initial lesion is an obliterative endarteritis of the vasa vasorum, especially in the adventitia. This is an inflammatory response to the invasion of the adventitia by the spirochetes. Destruction of the aortic media occurs as the spirochetes spread into this layer, usually via the lymphatics accompanying the vasa vasorum. Destruction of collagen and elastic tissues leads to dilation of the aorta, scar formation, and calcification. These changes account for the characteristic radiographic appearance of a calcified ascending aortic aneurysm.

The disease typically presents as an incidental radiographic finding 15 to 30 years after initial infection. Symptoms may result from aortic regurgitation, narrowing of coronary ostia due to syphilitic aortitis, compression of adjacent structures (e.g., esophagus), or rupture. Diagnosis is established by a positive serologic test, i.e., VDRL or fluorescent treponemal antibody (see Chap. 133). Treatment includes penicillin and surgical excision and repair.

RHEUMATIC AORTITIS Rheumatoid arthritis (Chap. 285), ankylosing spondylitis (Chap. 289), psoriatic arthritis (Chap. 298), Reiter's syndrome (Chap. 289), Behçet's syndrome (Chap. 290), relapsing polychondritis, and inflammatory bowel disorders may all be associated with aortitis involving the ascending aorta. The inflammatory lesions usually involve the ascending aorta and may extend to the sinuses of Valsalva, the mitral valve leaflets, and adjacent myocardium. The clinical manifestations are aneurysm, aortic regurgitation, and involvement of the cardiac conduction system.

TAKAYASU'S ARTERITIS AND OTHER AORTIC ARCH SYNDROMES Inflammatory diseases of the aortic arch resulting in obstruction of the aorta and its major arteries characterize this major group of diseases. Takayasu's arteritis is also termed *pulseless disease* because of the frequent occlusion of the large arteries originating from the aorta. It also may involve the descending thoracic and abdominal aorta and occlude large branches such as the renal arteries. The pathology is a panarteritis with marked intimal hyperplasia, medial and adventitial thickening, and, in chronic form, fibrotic occlusion. The disease is most prevalent in young females of Asian descent. During the acute stage, fever, malaise, weight loss, and other systemic symptoms may be evident. An elevation of the erythrocyte sedimentation rate is common. The chronic stages of the disease present with symptoms related to large artery occlusion, such as upper extremity claudication, cerebral ischemia, and syncope. The chronic disease is intermittently active. Since the process is progressive and there is no definitive therapy, the prognosis is usually poor. Glucocorticoids and immunosuppressive agents have been reported to be effective in some patients during the acute phase. Occasionally, anticoagulation prevents thrombosis and complete occlusion of a large artery. Surgical bypass of a critically stenotic artery may be necessary.

GIANT CELL ARTERITIS (See Chap. 291) Primarily large and medium-sized arteries are affected. The pathology is that of focal granulomatous lesions involving the entire arterial wall. It may be associated with polymyalgia rheumatica (Chap. 23). Obstruction of medium-sized arteries (e.g., temporal and ophthalmic arteries) and of major branches of the aorta and the development of aortitis and aortic regurgitation are some of the complications of the disease. High-dose glucocorticoid therapy may be effective when given early.

REFERENCES

CIGARROA JE et al: Diagnostic imaging in the evaluation of suspected aortic dissection: Old standards and new directions. N Engl J Med 328:35. 1993

CREAGER MA et al: Aneurysmal disease of the aorta and its branches. in *Vascular Medicine*. J Loscalzo et al (eds). Boston. Little. Brown. 1992. pp 903–930

DESANCTIS RW et al: Medical progress: Aortic dissection. N Engl J Med 317:1060. 1987

EAGLE KA, DESANCTIS RW: Diseases of the aorta. in *Heart Disease*. 4th ed. E Braunwald (ed). Philadelphia. Saunders. 1992. pp 1528–1558

―――― et al: Combining clinical and thallium data optimizes preoperative assessment of cardiac risk before major vascular surgery. Ann Intern Med 110:859. 1989

ERNST CB: Abdominal aortic aneurysm. N Engl J Med 328:1167. 1993

GUILMET D et al: Aortic dissection: Anatomic types and surgical approaches. J Cardiovasc Surg 34:23. 1993

HUNDER GG et al: Pathogenesis of giant cell arteritis. Arthritis Rheum 36:757. 1993

KULVANIEMI H et al: Genetic causes of aortic aneurysms: Unlearning at least part of what the textbooks say. J Clin Invest 88:1441. 1991

NEVITT MP et al: Prognosis of abdominal aortic aneurysys: A population based study. N Engl J Med 321:1009. 1989

NIENABER CA et al: The diagnosis of thoracic aortic dissection by noninvasive imaging procedures. N Engl J Med 328:1. 1993

REED D et al: Are aortic aneurysms caused by atherosclerosis? Circulation 85:205. 1992

211 VASCULAR DISEASES OF THE EXTREMITIES

MARK A. CREAGER / VICTOR J. DZAU

ARTERIAL DISORDERS

ATHEROSCLEROSIS OF THE EXTREMITIES Atherosclerosis (arteriosclerosis obliterans) is the leading cause of occlusive arterial disease of the extremities in patients over 40 years old; the highest incidence occurs in the sixth and seventh decades of life. As in patients with atherosclerosis of the coronary and cerebral vasculature, there is an increased prevalence of peripheral atherosclerotic occlusive disease in individuals with hypertension, hypercholesterolemia, and diabetes mellitus and in cigarette smokers. Atherosclerosis of the extremities is seen most frequently in elderly males.

Pathology (See Chap. 208) Segmental lesions causing stenosis or occlusion are usually localized in large and medium-sized vessels. The pathology of the lesions includes atherosclerotic plaques with calcium deposition, thinning of the media, patchy destruction of muscle and elastic fibers, fragmentation of the internal elastic lamina, and thrombi composed of platelets and fibrin. The primary sites of involvement are the abdominal aorta and iliac arteries in 30 percent of symptomatic patients, the femoral and popliteal arteries in 80 to 90 percent of patients, and the more distal vessels (including the tibial and peroneal arteries) in 40 to 50 percent of patients. Atherosclerotic lesions occur preferentially at arterial branch points, sites of increased turbulence, altered shear stress, and intimal injury. Involvement of the distal vasculature is most common in elderly individuals and patients with diabetes mellitus.

Clinical evaluation The most common *symptom* is intermittent claudication, which is defined as a pain, ache, cramp, numbness, or sense of fatigue in the muscles; it occurs during exercise but is relieved with rest. The site of claudication is distal to the location of the occlusive lesion. For example, buttock, hip, and thigh discomfort occurs in patients with aortoiliac disease (Leriche syndrome), whereas calf claudication develops in patients with femoral-popliteal disease. Symptoms are far more common in the lower than in the upper extremities because of the higher incidence of obstructive lesions. In patients with severe arterial occlusive disease, rest pain may develop. Patients will complain of pain or a feeling of cold or numbness in the foot and toes. Frequently these symptoms occur at night when the legs are in a "neutral" position and improve when the legs are in a dependent position. With severe ischemia, rest pain may be present.

Important *physical findings* of chronic arterial insufficiency include decreased or absent pulses distal to the obstruction, the presence of bruits over the narrowed artery, and muscle atrophy. With more severe disease, hair loss, thickened nails, smooth and shiny skin, reduced skin temperature, and pallor or cyanosis are frequent physical signs. In addition, ulcers or gangrene may occur. Elevation of the legs and repeated flexing of the calf muscles produce pallor of the soles of the feet, whereas rubor, secondary to reactive hyperemia, may develop when the legs are dependent. The duration of time for rubor to develop or for the veins in the foot to fill when the patient's legs are transferred from an elevated to a dependent position is related to the severity of the ischemia and presence of collateral vessels. Patients with severe ischemia may develop peripheral edema, because frequently they keep their legs in a dependent position. Ischemic neuritis can result in numbness and hyporeflexia.

Noninvasive testing The history and physical examination are usually sufficient to establish the diagnosis of peripheral arterial occlusive disease. Objective assessment of the severity of disease is obtained by noninvasive techniques. These include digital pulse volume recordings, Doppler flow velocity waveform analysis, duplex ultrasonography (which combines B-mode imaging and pulse-wave

Doppler examination), segmental pressure measurements, stress testing (usually using a treadmill), and tests of reactive hyperemia. In the presence of significant arterial occlusive disease, the volume displacement in the leg is decreased with each pulse, and the Doppler velocity contour becomes progressively flatter. Duplex ultrasonography is often useful in detecting stenotic lesions in native arteries and bypass grafts.

Arterial pressure can be recorded noninvasively along the legs by serial placement of sphygmomanometric cuffs and use of a Doppler device to auscultate or record blood flow. Normally, blood pressures in the legs and arms are similar. Indeed, ankle pressures may be slightly higher than arm pressures due to pulse-wave reflection. In the presence of hemodynamically significant stenoses, the arterial pressure in the leg is decreased. Thus, if one were to obtain a ratio of the ankle and brachial artery pressures, it would be >1.0 in normal individuals and <1.0 in patients with occlusive disease. A ratio of <0.5 is consistent with severe ischemia.

Treadmill testing allows the physician to assess functional limitations objectively. Decline of the ankle-brachial systolic pressure ratio immediately after exercise may provide further support for the diagnosis of arterial occlusive disease in patients with equivocal symptoms and findings on examination. Exercise testing also allows simultaneous evaluation for the presence of coronary artery disease.

Angiography should not be used for routine diagnostic testing but is performed prior to potential revascularization. It is useful for defining the anatomy to assist operative planning and is also indicated if nonsurgical interventions are being considered, such as percutaneous transluminal angioplasty or thrombolysis.

Prognosis The natural history of patients with peripheral arterial occlusive disease is influenced primarily by the extent of coexistent coronary artery and cerebral vascular disease. Studies utilizing coronary angiography have estimated that approximately one-half of patients with symptomatic peripheral arterial occlusive disease also have significant coronary artery disease. Life-table analysis has indicated that patients with claudication have a 70 percent 5-year and a 50 percent 10-year survival rate. The majority of deaths are either sudden or secondary to myocardial infarction. The likelihood of symptomatic progression of peripheral arterial occlusive disease appears less than the chance of succumbing to coronary artery disease. Approximately 70 percent of nondiabetic patients who present with mild to moderate claudication remain symptomatically stable. Improvement may occur in 10 to 15 percent of these patients; deterioration is likely to occur in the remainder, with approximately 5 percent of the group ultimately undergoing amputation. Prognosis is worse in those patients who continue to smoke cigarettes or have diabetes mellitus.

Management Therapeutic options include supportive measures, pharmacologic treatment, nonoperative interventions, and surgery. Supportive measures include meticulous care of the feet. The feet should be kept clean, and excessive drying should be prevented with the use of moisturizing creams. Well-fitting and protective shoes are advised to reduce trauma. Sandals and shoes made of synthetic materials that do not "breathe" should be avoided. Elastic support hose should be avoided, since these reduce blood flow to the skin. In patients with ischemia at rest, shock blocks under the head of the bed together with a canopy over the feet may improve perfusion pressure and ameliorate some of the rest pain.

Treatment of associated factors that contribute to the development of atherosclerosis should be initiated. The importance of discontinuing cigarette smoking cannot be overemphasized. The physician must assume a major role in this life-style modification. It is important to control blood pressure in hypertensive patients but to avoid hypotensive levels. Treatment of hypercholesterolemia is advocated, although reduction in cholesterol levels has not been shown unequivocally to reverse peripheral atherosclerotic lesions. However, it has been shown to prevent or to slow progression of the disease. Patients with claudication also should be encouraged to exercise regularly and to progressively increasing levels. Supervised exercise training

programs may improve muscle efficiency and prolong walking distance. Patients also should be advised to walk for 30 to 45 minutes daily, stopping at the onset of claudication and resting until the symptoms resolve before resuming ambulation. Other forms of exercise, such as bicycle riding and swimming, provide overall cardiovascular and psychological benefit and often are tolerated better than walking.

PHARMACOLOGIC MANAGEMENT This form of treatment of patients with peripheral arterial occlusive disease has not been as successful as the medical treatment of coronary artery disease (Chap. 203). In particular, vasodilators, as a class, have not proven to be beneficial. During exercise, peripheral vasodilation occurs normally distal to sites of significant arterial stenoses. As a result, perfusion pressure falls, often to levels less than that generated in the interstitial tissue by the exercising muscle. Unless vasodilators are able to improve collateral blood flow, it is unlikely that they would improve perfusion pressure and thereby increase blood supply to the exercising muscle. Drugs such as alpha-adrenergic blocking agents, calcium channel antagonists, papaverine, and other vasodilators have not been shown to be effective in patients with occlusive arterial disease. Pentoxifylline, a substituted xanthine derivative, has been reported to decrease blood viscosity and to increase red cell flexibility, thereby increasing blood flow to the microcirculation and enhancing tissue oxygenation. Several placebo-controlled studies have reported that pentoxifylline increased duration of exercise in patients with claudication, but its efficacy has not been confirmed in all clinical trials. Long-term parenteral administration of vasodilator prostaglandins may decrease pain and facilitate healing of ulcers in patients with severe limb ischemia.

Platelet inhibitors, particularly aspirin, have been reported to decrease progression of atherosclerosis in patients with peripheral arterial occlusive disease. Aspirin also reduces the risk of adverse cardiovascular events in patients with peripheral atherosclerosis. However, no study with aspirin has demonstrated any improvement in exercise capacity. Ticlopidine, a drug that inhibits platelet aggregation via its effect on ADP-dependent activation of glycoprotein IIb/IIIa, also reduces cardiovascular morbidity and mortality in patients with claudication. The anticoagulants heparin and warfarin have not been shown to be effective in patients with chronic arterial occlusive disease but may be useful in acute arterial obstruction secondary to thrombosis or systemic embolism. Similarly, thrombolytic intervention using drugs such as streptokinase, urokinase, or recombinant tissue plasminogen activator may have a role in the treatment of acute thrombotic arterial occlusion but is not effective in patients with chronic arterial occlusion secondary to atherosclerosis.

REVASCULARIZATION Such procedures, including nonoperative as well as operative interventions, are usually reserved for patients with progressive, severe, or disabling symptoms and ischemia at rest, as well as for those individuals who must be symptom-free because of their occupation. Angiography should be performed principally in those patients who are being considered for a revascularization procedure. Nonoperative interventions include percutaneous transluminal angioplasty (PTA), laser angioplasty, atherectomy, and stent placement. PTA of the iliac artery is associated with a higher success rate than PTA of the femoral and popliteal arteries. Approximately 90 to 95 percent of iliac PTAs are initially successful, and the 3-year patency rate is in excess of 75 percent. The initial success rate for femoral-popliteal PTA is approximately 80 percent, with a 60 percent 3-year patency rate. Patency rates are influenced by the severity of pretreatment stenoses; the prognosis of total occlusive lesions is worse than that of nonocclusive stenotic lesions. Laser angioplasty usually is used in conjunction with PTA and results in similar patency rates. The efficacy of percutaneous atherectomy and stent placement is being addressed in clinical trials.

Several operative procedures are available for treating patients with aortoiliac and femoral-popliteal artery disease. The preferred operative procedure depends on the location and extent of the obstruction(s) and general medical condition of the patient. Operative procedures for aortoiliac disease include aortobifemoral bypass, axillofemoral bypass, femoral-femoral bypass, and aortoiliac endarterectomy. The most commonly utilized procedure is the aortobifemoral bypass, using knitted Dacron grafts. Immediate graft patency approaches 99 percent, and 5- and 10-year graft patency in survivors is in excess of 90 and 80 percent, respectively. Operative complications include myocardial infarction and stroke, infection of the graft, peripheral embolization, and sexual dysfunction from interruption of autonomic nerves in the pelvis. Operative mortality ranges from 1 to 3 percent, mostly due to ischemic heart disease.

Operative therapy for femoral-popliteal artery disease includes in situ and reverse autogenous saphenous vein bypass grafts, polytetrafluoroethylene (PTFE) or other synthetic grafts, and thromboendarterectomy. Operative mortality ranges from 1 to 3 percent. Long-term patency rate is dependent on the type of graft utilized, the location of the distal anastomosis, and the patency of runoff vessels beyond the anastomosis. Patency rates of femoral-popliteal saphenous vein bypass grafts at 1 year approach 90 percent and at 5 years 70 to 80 percent. Five-year patency rates of infrapopliteal saphenous vein bypass grafts are 60 to 70 percent. In contrast, 5-year patency rates of infrapopliteal PTFE grafts are less than 30 percent. Lumbar sympathectomy alone or as an adjunct to aortofemoral reconstruction has fallen into disfavor. While this procedure may increase blood flow to the skin, it does not increase blood flow to muscle. There is no good clinical evidence that lumbar sympathectomy increases graft patency or improves limb survival.

Preoperative cardiac risk assessment may identify individuals most likely to experience an adverse cardiac event during the perioperative period. Patients with angina, prior myocardial infarction, ventricular ectopy, or heart failure are among those with increased risk. Noninvasive tests such as treadmill testing, if feasible, dipyridamole thallium or Sesta-MIBI scintigraphy, and ambulatory ischemia monitoring enable further stratification of patient risk. Patients with abnormal tests require close supervision and adjunctive management with antianginal medications. It is not known whether coronary angiography and coronary arterial revascularization reduce overall perioperative mortality in high-risk patients undergoing peripheral vascular surgery, but these procedures should be considered in patients suspected of having left main or three-vessel coronary artery disease.

FIBROMUSCULAR DYSPLASIA This is a hyperplastic disorder affecting medium-sized and small arteries. It occurs predominantly in females and usually involves renal and carotid arteries but can affect extremity vessels such as the iliac and subclavian arteries. The histologic classification includes intimal, medial, and periadventitial dysplasia. Medial dysplasia is the most common type and is characterized by hyperplasia of the media with or without fibrosis of the elastic membrane. It is identified angiographically by a "string of beads" appearance caused by thickened fibromuscular ridges contiguous with thin, less involved portions of the arterial wall. When limb vessels are involved, clinical manifestations are similar to those for atherosclerosis, including claudication and rest pain. PTA and surgical reconstruction have been beneficial in patients with debilitating symptoms or threatened limbs.

THROMBOANGIITIS OBLITERANS Thromboangiitis obliterans (Buerger's disease) is an inflammatory occlusive vascular disorder involving small and medium-sized arteries and veins in the distal upper and lower extremities. Cerebral, visceral, and coronary vessels also may be affected. This disorder develops most frequently in men under age 40. The prevalence is higher in Asians and individuals whose lineage originates in eastern Europe. While the cause of thromboangiitis obliterans is not known, there is a definite relationship to cigarette smoking and an increased incidence of HLA-B5 and -A9 antigens in patients with this disorder.

In the initial stages of thromboangiitis obliterans, polymorphonuclear leukocytes infiltrate the walls of the small and medium-sized arteries and veins. The internal elastic lamina is preserved, and thrombus may develop in the vascular lumen. As the disease progresses, mononuclear cells, fibroblasts, and giant cells replace the

neutrophils. Later stages are characterized by perivascular fibrosis and recanalization.

The clinical features of thromboangiitis obliterans often include a triad of claudication of the affected extremity, Raynaud's phenomenon (see below), and migratory superficial vein thrombophlebitis. Claudication is usually confined to the lower calves and feet or forearms and hands because this disorder primarily affects distal vessels. In the presence of severe digital ischemia, trophic nail changes, ulcerations, and gangrene may develop at the tips of the fingers. The physical examination shows normal brachial and popliteal pulses but reduced or absent radial, ulnar, and/or tibial pulses. Arteriography is helpful in making the diagnosis. Smooth, tapering segmental lesions in the distal vessels are characteristic, as are collateral vessels at sites of vascular occlusion. Proximal atherosclerotic disease is usually absent. The diagnosis can be confirmed by excisional biopsy and pathologic examination of an involved vessel.

There is no specific treatment except abstention from tobacco. The prognosis is worse in individuals who continue to smoke, but results are discouraging even in those who do stop smoking. Arterial bypass of the larger vessels may be used in selected instances, as well as local debridement, depending on symptoms and severity of ischemia. Antibiotics may be useful; anticoagulants and glucocorticoids are not helpful. If these measures fail, amputation may be required.

VASCULITIS Other vasculitides may affect the arteries supplying the upper and lower extremities. Takayasu's arteritis and giant cell (temporal) arteritis are discussed in Chap. 291.

ACUTE ARTERIAL OCCLUSION This results in the sudden cessation of blood flow to an extremity. The severity of ischemia and the viability of the extremity are dependent on the location and extent of the occlusion and the presence and subsequent development of collateral blood vessels. There are two principal causes of acute arterial occlusion: embolism and thrombus in situ.

The most common sources of arterial emboli are the heart, aorta, and large arteries. Cardiac disorders that cause thromboembolism include atrial fibrillation, both chronic and paroxysmal, and acute myocardial infarction, ventricular aneurysm, cardiomyopathy, infectious and marantic endocarditis, prosthetic heart valves, and atrial myxoma. Emboli to the distal vessels also may originate from proximal sites of atherosclerosis and aneurysms of the aorta and large vessels. Less frequently, an arterial occlusion may result paradoxically from a venous thrombus that has entered the systemic circulation via a patent foramen ovale or other septal defect. Arterial emboli tend to lodge at the bifurcation of vessels because the caliber of the vessel decreases at these sites; in the lower extremities, emboli lodge most frequently in the femoral artery, followed by the iliac artery, aorta, and popliteal and tibioperoneal arteries.

Acute arterial thrombosis in situ occurs most frequently in atherosclerotic vessels at the site of a stenosis or aneurysm and in arterial bypass grafts. Trauma to an artery also may result in the formation of an acute arterial thrombus. Arterial occlusion may complicate arterial punctures and placement of catheters. Less frequent causes include the thoracic outlet compression syndrome, causing subclavian artery occlusion, and entrapment of the popliteal artery by abnormal placement of the medial head of the gastrocnemius muscle. Polycythemia and hypercoagulable disorders (Chaps. 309 and 316) are also associated with acute arterial thrombosis.

Clinical features The symptoms of the acute arterial occlusion depend on the location, duration, and severity of the obstruction. Often, severe pain, paresthesias, numbness, and coldness develop in the involved extremity within 1 h. Paralysis may occur with severe and persistent ischemia. Physical findings include loss of pulses distal to the occlusion, cyanosis or pallor, mottling, decreased skin temperature, muscle stiffening, loss of sensation, weakness, and/or absent deep tendon reflexes. If acute arterial occlusion occurs in the presence of an adequate collateral circulation, as is often the case in acute graft occlusion, the symptoms and findings may be less impressive. In this situation, the patient complains about an abrupt decrease in the distance walked before claudication occurs or of modest pain and paresthesias. Pallor and coolness are evident, but sensory and motor functions are generally preserved. The diagnosis of acute arterial occlusion is usually apparent from the clinical presentation. Arteriography is useful for confirming the diagnosis and demonstrating the location and extent of occlusion.

Management Once the diagnosis is made, the patient should be anticoagulated with intravenous heparin to prevent propagation of the clot. In cases of severe ischemia of recent onset and particularly when limb viability is jeopardized, immediate intervention to ensure reperfusion is indicated. Surgical thromboembolectomy or arterial bypass procedures are used to restore blood flow to the ischemic extremity promptly, particularly when a large proximal vessel is occluded.

Intraarterial thrombolytic therapy is effective when acute arterial occlusion is caused by a thrombus in an atherosclerotic vessel or arterial bypass graft. Thrombolytic therapy also may be indicated when the patient's overall condition contraindicates surgical intervention or when smaller distal vessels are occluded, thus preventing surgical access. Intraarterial streptokinase is administered as a bolus injection of 25,000 to 250,000 IU followed by a continuous infusion of 5000 to 15,000 IU/h. One approach for administering intraarterial urokinase is to give a bolus of 60,000 to 120,000 IU followed by 240,000 IU/ h for 2 h, 120,000 IU/h for 2 h, and then 60,000 IU/h. Clinical trials are now in progress to assess the efficacy of intraarterial recombinant tissue plasminogen activator (tPA). Meticulous observation for hemorrhagic complications is required during intraarterial thrombolytic therapy.

If the limb is not in jeopardy, a more conservative approach that includes observation and administration of anticoagulants may be taken. Anticoagulation prevents recurrent embolism and reduces the likelihood of thrombus propagation. It can be initiated with intravenous heparin and followed by oral warfarin. Recommended dosages are the same as those used in deep vein thrombosis (see later). Emboli resulting from infectious endocarditis, prosthetic heart valves, or atrial myxoma often require surgical intervention to remove the cause.

ATHEROEMBOLISM Atheroembolism constitutes a subset of acute arterial occlusion. In this condition, multiple small deposits of fibrin, platelet, and cholesterol debris embolize from proximal atherosclerotic lesions or aneurysmal sites. Atheroembolism may occur after intraarterial procedures. Since the emboli tend to lodge in the small vessels of the muscle and skin and may not occlude the large vessels, distal pulses usually remain palpable. Patients complain of acute pain and tenderness at the site of embolization. Digital vascular occlusion may result in ischemia and the "blue toe" syndrome; digital necrosis and gangrene may develop. Localized areas of tenderness, pallor, and livedo reticularis (see below) occur at sites of emboli. Skin or muscle biopsy may demonstrate cholesterol crystals.

Ischemia resulting from atheroemboli is notoriously difficult to treat. Usually neither surgical revascularization procedures nor thrombolytic therapy is helpful because of the multiplicity, composition, and distal location of the emboli. Some evidence suggests that platelet inhibitors prevent atheroembolism. Surgical intervention to remove or bypass the atherosclerotic vessel or aneurysm that causes the recurrent atheroemboli may be necessary.

THORACIC OUTLET COMPRESSION SYNDROME This refers to a symptom complex resulting from compression of the neurovascular bundle at the thoracic outlet (artery, vein, or nerves) as it courses through the neck and shoulder. Cervical ribs, abnormalities of the scalenus anticus muscle, the proximity of the clavicle to the first rib, or abnormal insertion of the pectoralis minor muscle may compress the subclavian artery and brachial plexus as these structures pass from the thorax to the arm. Patients may develop shoulder and arm pain, weakness, paresthesias, claudication, Raynaud's phenomenon, and even ischemic tissue loss and gangrene. Examination is often normal unless provocative maneuvers are performed. Occasionally, distal pulses are decreased or absent and digital cyanosis and ischemia may be evident. Tenderness may be present in the supraclavicular fossa.

Abducting the affected arm 90° and externally rotating the shoulder may precipitate symptoms. Several additional maneuvers are used to confirm the diagnosis of vascular compression and suggest the location of the abnormality. These include the scalene (extension of the neck and rotation of the head to the side of the symptoms), costoclavicular (posterior rotation of shoulders), and hyperabduction (raising the arm 180°) maneuvers which may cause subclavian bruits and loss of pulses in the arm. A chest x-ray will indicate the presence of cervical ribs. The electromyogram will be abnormal if the brachial plexus is involved.

Most patients can be managed conservatively. They should be advised to avoid those positions that cause symptoms. Many patients benefit from shoulder girdle exercises. Surgical procedures such as removal of the first rib or resection of the scalenus anticus muscle are necessary occasionally for relief of symptoms or treatment of ischemia.

ARTERIOVENOUS FISTULAS These abnormal communications between an artery and a vein, bypassing the capillary bed, may be congenital or acquired. Congenital arteriovenous fistulas are the result of persistent embryonic vessels that fail to differentiate into arteries and veins; these may be associated with birth marks, are located in almost every organ of the body, and frequently occur in the extremities. Acquired arteriovenous fistulas are either created to provide vascular access for hemodialysis or occur as a result of a penetrating injury such as a gunshot or knife wound or as complications of arterial catheterization or surgical dissection. An infrequent cause of arteriovenous fistula is rupture of an arterial aneurysm into a vein.

The clinical features depend on the location and size of the fistula. Frequently, a pulsatile mass is palpable, and a thrill and bruit lasting throughout systole and diastole are present over the fistula. With long-standing fistulas, clinical manifestations of chronic venous insufficiency, including peripheral edema, large tortuous varicose veins, and stasis pigmentation, become apparent because of the high venous pressure. Evidence of ischemia may occur in the distal portion of the extremity. Skin temperature is higher over the arteriovenous fistula. Large arteriovenous fistulas may result in an increased cardiac output with consequent cardiomegaly and high-output heart failure (Chap. 195).

Diagnosis This is often evident from the physical examination. Compression of a large arteriovenous fistula may cause reflex slowing of the heart rate (Nicoladoni-Branham sign). Arteriography can confirm the diagnosis and is useful in demonstrating the site and size of the arteriovenous fistula.

Management This may involve surgery, radiotherapy, or embolization. Congenital arteriovenous fistulas are often difficult to treat because the communications may be numerous and extensive and new ones frequently develop after ligation of the most obvious ones. Many of these lesions are best treated conservatively using elastic support hose to reduce the consequences of venous hypertension. Occasionally, embolization with autologous material, such as fat or muscle, or with hemostatic agents, such as gelatin sponges or silicon spheres, is used to obliterate the fistula. Acquired arteriovenous fistulas are usually amenable to surgical treatment that involves division or excision of the fistula. Occasionally this requires autogenous or synthetic grafting to reestablish continuity of the artery and vein.

RAYNAUD'S PHENOMENON Raynaud's phenomenon is characterized by episodic digital ischemia, manifested clinically by the sequential development of digital blanching, cyanosis, and rubor of the fingers or toes following cold exposure and subsequent rewarming. Emotional stress also may precipitate Raynaud's phenomenon. The color changes are usually well demarcated and are confined to the fingers or toes. Typically, one or more digits will appear white when the patient is exposed to a cold environment or touches a cold object. The blanching, or pallor, represents the ischemic phase of the phenomenon and is secondary to vasospasm of digital arteries. During the ischemic phase, capillaries and venules dilate, and cyanosis results from the deoxygenated blood that is present in these vessels. Sensation of cold, numbness, or paresthesias of the digits often accompany the phases of pallor cyanosis.

With rewarming, the digital vasospasm resolves, and blood flow into the dilated arterioles and capillaries increases dramatically. This "reactive hyperemia" imparts a bright red color to the digits. In addition to rubor and warmth, patients often experience a throbbing, painful sensation during the hyperemic phase. Although the triphasic color response is typical of Raynaud's phenomenon, some patients may develop only pallor and cyanosis; others may experience only cyanosis.

Pathophysiology Raynaud originally proposed that cold-induced episodic digital ischemia was secondary to exaggerated reflex sympathetic vasoconstriction. This theory is supported by the fact that adrenergic blocking drugs as well as sympathectomy decrease the frequency and severity of Raynaud's phenomenon in some patients. An alternative hypothesis is that there is enhanced digital vascular responsiveness to cold or to normal sympathetic stimuli. It is also possible that normal reflex sympathetic vasoconstriction is superimposed on local digital vascular disease or that there is enhanced adrenergic neuroeffector activity.

Raynaud's phenomenon is broadly separated into two categories: the idiopathic variety termed *Raynaud's disease* and the secondary variety, which is associated with other disease states or known causes of vasospasm (Table 211-1).

Raynaud's disease This appellation is applied when the secondary causes of Raynaud's phenomenon have been excluded. Over 50 percent of patients with Raynaud's phenomenon have Raynaud's disease. Women are affected about five times more often than men, and the age of presentation is usually between 20 and 40 years. The fingers are involved more frequently than the toes. Initial episodes may involve only one or two fingertips, but subsequent attacks may involve the entire finger and may include all the fingers. The toes are affected in 40 percent of patients. Although vasospasm of the toes usually occurs in patients with symptoms in the fingers, it may happen alone. Rarely, the earlobes and the tip of the nose are involved. Raynaud's phenomenon occurs frequently in patients who also have migraine headaches or variant angina. These associations suggest that there may be a common predisposing cause for the vasospasm.

The physical examination is often entirely normal; the radial, ulnar, and pedal pulses are normal. The fingers and toes may be cool between attacks and may perspire excessively. Thickening and tightening of the digital subcutaneous tissue, i.e., sclerodactyly, develop in 10 percent of patients. Angiography of the digits for diagnostic purposes is not indicated.

Patients with Raynaud's disease, in general, appear to have the milder forms of Raynaud's phenomenon. Less than 1 percent of these patients lose a part of a digit. After the diagnosis is made, the disease spontaneously improves in approximately 15 percent of patients and progresses in about 30 percent.

Secondary causes of Raynaud's phenomenon Raynaud's phenomenon occurs in 80 to 90 percent of patients with systemic sclerosis

---

TABLE 211-1 Classification of Raynaud's phenomenon

Primary or idiopathic Raynaud's phenomenon: Raynaud's disease
Secondary Raynaud's phenomenon
   Collagen vascular diseases: scleroderma, systemic lupus erythematosus, rheumatoid arthritis, dermatomyositis, polymyositis
   Arterial occlusive diseases: atherosclerosis of the extremities, thromboangiitis obliterans, acute arterial occlusion, thoracic outlet syndrome
   Pulmonary hypertension
   Neurologic disorders: invertebral disk disease, syringomyelia, spinal cord tumors, stroke, poliomyelitis, carpal tunnel syndrome
   Blood dyscrasias: cold agglutinins, cryoglobulinemia, cryofibrinogenemia, myeloproliferative disorders, Waldenström's macroglobulinemia
   Trauma: vibration injury, hammer hand syndrome, electric shock, cold injury, typing, piano playing
   Drugs: ergot derivatives, methysergide, beta-adrenergic receptor blockers, bleomycin, vinblastin, cisplatin

---

(scleroderma) and is the presenting symptom in 30 percent (Chap. 286). It may be the only symptom of scleroderma for many years. Abnormalities of the digital vessels may contribute to the development of Raynaud's phenomenon in this disorder. Ischemic fingertip ulcers may develop and progress to gangrene and autoamputation. About 20 percent of patients with systemic lupus erythematosus (SLE) have Raynaud's phenomenon (Chap. 284). Occasionally, persistent digital ischemia develops and may result in ulcers or gangrene. In most severe cases, the small vessels are occluded by a proliferative endarteritis. Raynaud's phenomenon occurs in about 30 percent of patients with dermatomyositis or polymyositis (Chap. 384). It frequently develops in patients with rheumatoid arthritis and may be related to the intimal proliferation that occurs in the digital arteries.

Atherosclerosis of the extremities is a frequent cause of Raynaud's phenomenon in men over age 50. Thromboangiitis obliterans is an uncommon cause of Raynaud's phenomenon but should be considered in young men, particularly in those who are cigarette smokers. The development of cold-induced pallor in these disorders may be confined to one or two digits of the involved extremity. Occasionally, Raynaud's phenomenon may occur following acute occlusion of large and medium-sized arteries by a thrombus or embolus. Embolization of atheroembolic debris may cause digital ischemia. The latter often involves one or two digits and should not be confused with Raynaud's phenomenon. In patients with the thoracic outlet syndrome, Raynaud's phenomenon may result from diminished intravascular pressure, stimulation of sympathetic fibers in the brachial plexus, or a combination of both. Raynaud's phenomenon occurs in patients with primary pulmonary hypertension (Chap. 225); this is more than coincidental and may reflect a neurohumoral abnormality that affects both the pulmonary and digital circulations.

A variety of blood dyscrasias may be associated with Raynaud's phenomenon. Cold-induced precipitation of plasma proteins, hyperviscosity, and aggregation of red cells and platelets may occur in patients with cold agglutinins, cryoglobulinemia, or cryofibrinogenemia. Hyperviscosity syndromes that accompany myeloproliferative disorders and Waldenström's macroglobulinemia also should be considered in the initial evaluation of patients with Raynaud's phenomenon.

Raynaud's phenomenon occurs often in patients whose vocations require the use of vibrating hand tools such as chain saws or jackhammers. The frequency of Raynaud's phenomenon also seems to be increased in pianists and typists. Electric shock injury to the hands and frostbite may lead to the later development of Raynaud's phenomenon.

Several drugs have been causally implicated in Raynaud's phenomenon. These include ergot preparations, methysergide, beta-adrenergic receptor antagonists, and the chemotherapeutic agents bleomycin, vinblastine, and cisplatin.

Management Most patients with Raynaud's phenomenon experience only mild and infrequent episodes. These patients need reassurance and should be instructed to dress warmly and avoid unnecessary cold exposure. In addition to gloves and mittens, patients should protect the trunk, head, and feet with warm clothing in order to prevent cold-induced reflex vasoconstriction. Tobacco use is contraindicated.

Drug treatment should be reserved for the severe cases. The calcium channel antagonists, especially nifedipine (10 to 30 mg tid) and diltiazem (30 to 90 mg tid), decrease the frequency and severity of Raynaud's phenomenon. Long-acting preparations of these drugs also may be effective. Adrenergic blocking agents, such as reserpine (0.25 to 0.5 mg qd), have been shown to increase nutritional blood flow to the fingers. Some, but not all, patients achieve satisfactory results with long-term reserpine therapy. Moreover, systemic use of this drug is limited by side effects of hypotension, nasal stuffiness, lethargy, and depression. The postsynaptic alpha$_1$-adrenergic antagonist prazosin (1 to 5 mg tid) has been used with favorable responses. Doxazosin and terazosin also may be effective. Other sympatholytic agents such as methyldopa, guanethidine, and phenoxybenzamine may be useful in some patients. Parenteral treatment with vasodilator prostaglandins is under investigation, but its potential utility is applicable more to severe digital ischemia than to episodic Raynaud's phenomenon. Surgical sympathectomy is helpful in some patients who are unresponsive to medical therapy, but benefit is often transient.

ACROCYANOSIS   In this condition, there is arterial vasoconstriction and secondary dilatation of the capillaries and venules with resulting persistent cyanosis of the hands and, less frequently, the feet. Cyanosis may be intensified by exposure to a cold environment. Women are affected much more frequently than men, and the age of onset is usually less than 30 years. Generally patients are asymptomatic but seek medical attention because of the discoloration. Examination reveals normal pulses, peripheral cyanosis, and moist palms. Trophic skin changes and ulcerations do *not* occur. The disorder can be distinguished from Raynaud's phenomenon because it is persistent and not episodic, the discoloration extends proximally from the digits, and blanching does not occur. Ischemia secondary to arterial occlusive disease usually can be excluded by the presence of normal pulses. Central cyanosis and decreased arterial oxygen saturation are not present. Patients should be reassured and advised to dress warmly and avoid cold exposure. Pharmacologic intervention is not indicated.

LIVEDO RETICULARIS   In this condition, localized areas of the extremities develop a mottled or netlike appearance of reddish to blue discoloration. The mottled appearance may be more prominent following cold exposure. The idiopathic form of this disorder occurs equally in men and women, and the most common age of onset is in the third decade. Patients with the idiopathic form usually are asymptomatic and seek attention for cosmetic reasons. Livedo reticularis also occurs following atheroembolism (see above). Rarely, skin ulcerations develop. Patients should be reassured and advised to avoid cold environments. No drug treatment is indicated.

PERNIO (CHILBLAINS)   This is a vasculitic disorder associated with exposure to cold; acute forms have been described. Raised erythematous lesions develop on the lower part of the legs and feet in cold weather. These are associated with pruritus and a burning sensation, and they may blister and ulcerate. Pathologic examination demonstrates angiitis characterized by intimal proliferation and perivascular infiltration of mononuclear and polymorphonuclear leukocytes. Giant cells may be present in the subcutaneous tissue. Patients should avoid exposure to cold, and ulcers should be kept clean and protected with sterile dressings. Sympatholytic drugs may be effective in some patients.

ERYTHROMELALGIA (ERYTHERMALGIA)   This disorder is characterized by burning pain and erythema of the extremities. The feet are involved more frequently than the hands, and males are affected more frequently than females. Erythromelalgia may occur at any age but is most common in middle age. It may be primary or secondary to disorders such as polycythemia vera and hypertension. Patients complain of burning in the extremities, precipitated by exposure to a warm environment and aggravated by the dependent position. The symptoms are relieved by exposing the affected area to cool air or water or by elevation. Erythromelalgia can be distinguished from ischemia secondary to arterial occlusive disorders and peripheral neuropathy because the peripheral pulses are present and the neurologic examination is normal. There is no specific treatment; aspirin may produce relief. Treatment of associated disorders in secondary erythromelalgia may be helpful.

FROSTBITE   In this condition, tissue damage results from severe environmental cold exposure or from direct contact with a very cold object. Tissue injury results from both freezing and vasoconstriction. Frostbite usually affects the distal aspects of the extremities or exposed parts of the face, such as the ears, nose, chin, and cheeks. Superficial frostbite involves the skin and subcutaneous tissue. Patients experience pain or paresthesia, and the skin appears white and waxy. After rewarming, there is cyanosis and erythema, wheal and flare formation, edema, and superficial blisters. Deep frostbite involves muscle, nerves, and deeper blood vessels. It may result in edema of the hand or foot, vesicles and bullae, tissue necrosis, and gangrene.

Initial treatment is rewarming, performed in an environment where reexposure to freezing conditions will not occur. Rewarming is accomplished by immersion of the affected part in a water bath at temperatures of 40 to 44°C (104 to 111°F. Massage, application of ice water, and extreme heat are contraindicated. The injured area should be cleansed with soap or antiseptic and sterile dressings applied. Analgesics are often required during rewarming. Antibiotics are used if there is evidence of infection. The efficacy of sympathetic blocking drugs is not established. Following recovery, the affected extremity may exhibit increased sensitivity to cold.

VENOUS DISORDERS

Veins in the extremities can be broadly classified as either superficial or deep. In the lower extremity, the superficial venous system includes the greater and lesser saphenous veins and their tributaries. The deep veins of the leg accompany the major arteries. Perforating veins connect the superficial and the deep systems at multiple locations. Bicuspid valves are present throughout the venous system to direct the flow of venous blood centrally.

VENOUS THROMBOSIS   The presence of thrombus within a superficial or deep vein and the accompanying inflammatory response in the vessel wall is termed *venous thrombosis* or *thrombophlebitis*. Initially, the thrombus is composed principally of platelets and fibrin. Red cells become interspersed with fibrin, and the thrombus tends to propagate in the direction of blood flow. The inflammatory response in the vessel wall may be minimal or characterized by granulocyte infiltration, loss of endothelium, and edema.

The factors that predispose to venous thrombosis were initially described by Virchow in 1856 and include stasis, vascular damage, and hypercoagulability. Accordingly, a variety of clinical situations are associated with increased risk of venous thrombosis (Table 211-2). Venous thrombosis may occur in more than 50 percent of patients having orthopedic surgical procedures, particularly those involving the hip or knee, and in 10 to 40 percent of patients who undergo abdominal or thoracic operations. The prevalence of venous thrombosis is particularly high in patients with cancer of the pancreas, lungs, genitourinary tract, stomach, and breast. Approximately 10 to 20 percent of patients with idiopathic deep vein thrombosis have or develop clinically overt cancer; there is no consensus on whether these individuals should be subjected to intensive diagnostic workup to search for occult malignancy. Risk of thrombosis is increased following trauma, such as fractures of the spine, pelvis, femur, and tibia. Immobilization, regardless of the underlying disease, is a major predisposing cause of venous thrombosis. This may account for the relatively high incidence in patients with acute myocardial infarction or congestive heart failure. The incidence of venous thrombosis is increased during pregnancy, particularly in the third trimester and in

---

TABLE 211-2   Conditions associated with an increased risk for development of venous thrombosis

Surgery
  Orthopedic, thoracic, abdominal, and genitourinary procedures
Neoplasms
  Pancreas, lung, ovary, testes, urinary tract, breast, stomach
Trauma
  Fractures of spine, pelvis, femur, tibia
Immobilization
  Acute myocardial infarction, congestive heart failure, stroke, postoperative convalescence
Pregnancy
Estrogen use (for replacement or contraception)
Hypercoagulable states
  Deficiencies of antithrombin III, protein C, or protein S; anticardiolipin antibodies; myeloproliferative diseases; dysfibrinogenemia; disseminated intravascular coagulation
Venulitis
  Thromboangiitis obliterans, Behçet's disease, homocysteinuria
Previous deep vein thrombosis

the first month postpartum, and in individuals who use estrogens. A variety of clinical disorders that produce systemic hypercoagulability, including antithrombin II, protein C, and protein S deficiencies, systemic lupus erythematosus, myeloproliferative diseases, dysfibrinogenemia, and disseminated intravascular coagulation, may cause venous thrombosis. Venulitis occurring in thromboangiitis obliterans, Behçet's disease, and homocysteinuria also may cause venous thrombosis.

DEEP VENOUS THROMBOSIS The most important consequences of this disorder are pulmonary embolism (Chap. 226) and the syndrome of chronic venous insufficiency. Deep thrombosis of the iliac, femoral, or popliteal veins is suggested by unilateral leg swelling, warmth, and erythema. Tenderness may be present along the course of the involved veins, and a cord may be palpable. There may be increased tissue turgor, distention of superficial veins, and the appearance of prominent venous collaterals. In some patients, deoxygenated hemoglobin in stagnant veins imparts a cyanotic hue to the limb, a condition called *phlegmasia cerulea dolens*. In markedly edematous legs, the interstitial tissue pressure may exceed the capillary perfusion pressure, causing pallor, a condition designated *phlegmasia alba dolens*.

The diagnosis of deep venous thrombosis of the calf is often difficult to make at the bedside. This is so because only one of multiple veins may be involved, allowing adequate venous return through the remaining patent vessels. The most common complaint is calf pain. Examination may reveal posterior calf tenderness, warmth, increased tissue turgor or modest swelling, and rarely, a cord. Increased resistance or pain during dorsiflexion of the foot, Homan's sign, is an unreliable diagnostic sign.

Deep venous thrombosis occurs less frequently in the upper extremity than in the lower extremity, but the incidence is increasing because of greater utilization of subclavian catheters. The clinical features and complications are similar to those described for the leg.

Diagnosis Various noninvasive tests are used to diagnose deep venous thrombosis, including duplex venous ultrasonography (B-mode, i.e., two-dimensional, imaging and pulse-wave Doppler interrogation), plethysmographic techniques, and ^{125}I-fibrinogen scanning. By imaging the deep veins, the presence of thrombus can be detected by direct visualization or by inference when the vein does not collapse with compressive maneuvers. The Doppler ultrasound measures the velocity of blood flow in veins. This velocity is normally affected by respiration and by manual compression of the foot or calf. Flow abnormalities occur when deep venous obstruction is present. The positive predictive value of duplex venous ultrasonography approaches 95 percent for proximal deep vein thrombosis. Since it is more difficult to visualize calf veins than proximal veins, the sensitivity of this technique is only 50 to 75 percent, although the specificity of this technique for calf vein thrombosis is 95 percent.

Plethysmographic techniques used to measure changes in venous capacitance during physiologic maneuvers include impedance plethysmography (IPG) and phleborheography (PRG). IPG uses skin electrodes, and PRG uses a series of air-filled cuffs to detect changes in leg volume. Venous obstruction blunts the normal changes in venous capacitance that occur during respiration or following inflation and deflation of a thigh cuff. The predictive value of these tests for detecting occlusive thrombi in proximal veins is approximately 90 percent. However, these tests are much less sensitive in the detection of deep venous thrombosis of the calves.

^{125}I-fibrinogen scanning is occasionally used for the diagnosis of deep venous thrombosis. Since this isotope is actively taken up by the propagating venous thrombi, increases in radioactivity detected with a counter imply the presence of a thrombus. Fibrinogen scans detect more than 90 percent of calf vein thrombi but are less specific for proximal venous thrombi. A serious limitation of the technique is that it may take 48 to 72 h after administration of the isotope for a fibrinogen scan to become positive.

Deep venous thrombosis also can be diagnosed by venography. Contrast medium is injected into a superficial vein of the foot and directed to the deep system by the application of tourniquets. The presence of a filling defect or absence of filling of the deep veins is required to make the diagnosis.

Deep vein thrombosis must be differentiated from a variety of disorders that cause unilateral leg pain or swelling, including muscle trauma or hemorrhage, a ruptured popliteal cyst, and lymphedema. It may be difficult to distinguish swelling caused by the postphlebitic syndrome from that due to acute recurrent deep venous thrombosis. Leg pain also may result from nerve compression syndrome, arthritis, tendinitis, fractures, and arterial occlusive disorders. A careful history and physical examination can usually determine the cause of these symptoms.

Management Prevention of pulmonary embolism is the most important reason for treating patients with deep vein thrombosis, since in the early stages the thrombus may be loose and poorly adherent to the vessel wall. Patients should be placed in bed, and the affected extremity should be elevated above the level of the heart until the edema and tenderness subside. Anticoagulants prevent thrombus propagation and allow the endogenous lytic system to operate. Heparin should be administered intravenously as an initial bolus of 5000 to 10,000 IU, followed by a continuous infusion of 1000 to 1500 IU/h. The rate of the heparin infusion should be adjusted so that the activated partial thromboplastin time (APTT) is approximately twice the control value. Intermittent intravenous and subcutaneous injections of heparin have been used as alternative forms of therapy. In less than 5 percent of patients, heparin therapy may cause thrombocytopenia. Infrequently, these patients develop arterial thrombosis and ischemia. Heparin treatment should be maintained for at least 7 to 10 days. Warfarin is administered during the first week of treatment with heparin and may be started as early as the first day of heparin treatment. It is important to overlap heparin treatment with oral anticoagulant therapy for at least 4 to 5 days because the full anticoagulant effect of warfarin is delayed. The dose of warfarin should be adjusted to maintain the prothrombin time by 4 to 7 s beyond control values, equivalent to an international normalized ratio (INR) of 2.0 to 3.0. The use of anticoagulants for isolated deep vein thrombosis of the calf is controversial because the incidence of pulmonary embolism is very low. However, approximately 20 percent of calf thrombi propagate to the thigh, thereby increasing the risk of pulmonary embolism.

The incidence of pulmonary embolism in patients presenting with deep calf vein thrombosis is 5 to 20 percent. Therefore, patients with calf vein thrombosis should either receive anticoagulants or be followed with serial noninvasive tests to determine whether proximal propagation has occurred. Anticoagulant treatment should be continued for 3 to 12 months for patients with acute proximal deep vein thrombosis to decrease the chance of recurrence. The duration of anticoagulant treatment for patients with calf vein thrombosis should be at least 6 weeks. The duration of treatment is indefinite for patients with recurrent deep vein thrombosis and for those in whom associated causes, such as malignancy or hypercoagulability, have not been eliminated. If treatment with anticoagulants is contraindicated because of a bleeding diathesis or risk of hemorrhage, protection from pulmonary embolism can be achieved by mechanically interrupting the flow of blood through the inferior vena cava. Inferior vena cava plication generally has been replaced by percutaneous insertion of a filter.

Thrombolytic drugs such as streptokinase, urokinase, and tissue plasminogen activator also may be used, but there is no evidence that thrombolytic therapy is more effective than anticoagulants in preventing pulmonary embolism. However, early administration of thrombolytic drugs may accelerate clot lysis, preserve venous valves, and decrease the potential for developing postphlebitic syndrome.

Prophylaxis should be considered in clinical situations where the risk of deep vein thrombosis is high. Low-dose heparin (5000 units 2 h prior to surgery and then 5000 units every 8 to 12 h postoperatively), warfarin, and external pneumatic compression are all useful. Low-dose heparin reduces the risk of deep vein thrombosis associated with thoracic and abdominal surgery and in patients placed at prolonged bedrest. Low-molecular-weight heparin (4000 to 5000 Da) has been shown to prevent deep vein thrombosis in patients undergoing abdominal or hip surgery. It is purported to have greater efficacy and a lower incidence of bleeding than conventional heparin. Warfarin, in doses that increase the prothrombin time, equivalent to an INR of 2.0 to 3.0, is effective in preventing deep vein thrombosis associated with bone fractures and orthopedic surgery. Warfarin is started the night before surgery and continued throughout the convalescent period. External pneumatic compression devices applied to the legs are used to prevent deep vein thrombosis when even low doses of heparin or warfarin may cause serious bleeding, such as during neurosurgery or transurethral resection of the prostate.

SUPERFICIAL VEIN THROMBOSIS   Thrombosis of the greater or lesser saphenous veins or their tributaries, i.e., superficial vein thrombosis, does not result in pulmonary embolism or chronic venous insufficiency. It is associated with intravenous catheters and infusions, occurs in varicose veins, and may develop in association with deep vein thrombosis. Migrating superficial vein thrombosis is often a marker for a carcinoma and also may occur in patients with vasculitides, such as thromboangiitis obliterans. The clinical features of superficial vein thrombosis are easily distinguishable from those of deep vein thrombosis. Patients complain of pain localized to the site of the thrombus. Examination reveals a reddened, warm, and tender cord extending along a superficial vein. The surrounding area may be red and edematous.

Therapy is primarily supportive. Initially, patients can be placed at bed rest with leg elevation and application of warm compresses. Nonsteroidal anti-inflammatory drugs may provide analgesia but also may obscure clinical evidence of thrombus propagation. If a thrombosis of the greater saphenous vein develops in the thigh and extends toward the saphenofemoral vein junction, it is reasonable to consider anticoagulant therapy to prevent extension of the thrombus into the deep system and a possible pulmonary embolism.

VARICOSE VEINS   These are dilated tortuous superficial veins that result from defective structure and function of the valves of the saphenous veins, from intrinsic weakness of the vein wall, from high intraluminal pressure, or rarely, from arteriovenous fistulas. Varicose veins can be categorized as primary or secondary. Primary varicose veins originate in the superficial system and occur two to three times as frequently in women as in men. Approximately half of patients have a family history of varicose veins. Secondary varicose veins result from deep venous insufficiency and incompetent perforating veins or from deep venous occlusion causing enlargement of superficial veins that are serving as collaterals.

Patients with venous varicosities are often concerned about the cosmetic appearance of their legs. Symptoms consist of a dull ache or pressure sensation in their legs after prolonged standing; it is relieved with leg elevation. The legs feel heavy, and occasionally, mild ankle edema develops. Extensive venous varicosities may cause skin ulcerations near the ankle. Superficial venous thrombosis may be a recurring problem, and rarely, a varicosity ruptures and bleeds. Visual inspection of the legs in the dependent position usually confirms the presence of varicose veins.

Varicose veins usually can be treated with conservative measures. Symptoms often decrease when the legs are elevated periodically, when prolonged standing is avoided, and when elastic support hose are worn. External compression stockings provide a counterbalance to the hydrostatic pressure within the veins. Small symptomatic varicose veins may be treated with sclerotherapy, in which a sclerosing solution is injected into the involved varicose vein and a compression bandage is applied. Surgical therapy usually involves extensive ligation and stripping of the greater and lesser saphenous veins and should be reserved for those patients who are very symptomatic, suffer recurrent superficial vein thrombosis, and/or develop skin ulceration. Surgical therapy may be indicated for cosmetic reasons.

CHRONIC VENOUS INSUFFICIENCY   This may result from deep vein thrombosis and/or valvular incompetence. Following deep vein thrombosis, the delicate valve leaflets become thickened and contracted so that they are incapable of preventing retrograde flow of blood; the vein becomes rigid and thick-walled. Although most veins recanalize after an episode of thrombosis, the large proximal veins may remain occluded. Secondary incompetence develops in distal valves because high pressures distend the vein and separate the leaflets. Primary deep venous valvular dysfunction also may occur without previous thrombosis. Patients with venous insufficiency often complain of a dull ache in the leg that worsens with prolonged standing and resolves with leg elevation. Examination demonstrates increased leg circumference, edema, and superficial varicose veins. Erythema, dermatitis, and hyperpigmentation develop along the distal aspect of the leg, and skin ulceration may occur near the medial and lateral malleoli. Cellulitis may be a recurring problem. Patients should be advised to avoid prolonged standing or sitting; frequent leg elevation is helpful. Graduated compression stockings should be worn during the day. These efforts should be intensified if skin ulcers develop. Ulcers should be treated with applications of wet to dry dressings and occasionally dilute topical antibiotic solutions. Commercially available dressings comprising antiseptic solutions and compressive bandages may be applied and should be changed weekly until healing occurs. Recurrent ulceration and severe edema may be treated by surgical interruption of incompetent communicating veins. Rarely, surgical valvuloplasty and bypass of venous occlusions are employed.

LYMPHATIC DISORDERS

Lymphatic capillaries are blind-ended tubes formed by a single layer of endothelial cells. The absent or widely fenestrated basement membrane of lymphatic capillaries allows greater access to interstitial proteins and particles. Lymphatic capillaries merge to form larger vessels which contain smooth muscle and are capable of vasomotion. Small and medium-sized lymphatic vessels empty into progressively larger channels which drain into the thoracic duct. The lymphatic circulation is involved in the absorption of interstitial fluid and in the response to infection.

LYMPHEDEMA   Lymphedema may be categorized as primary or secondary (Table 211-3). The prevalence of primary lymphedema is approximately 1 per 10,000 individuals. Primary lymphedema may be secondary to agenesis, hypoplasia, or obstruction of the lymphatic vessels. It may be associated with the Turner syndrome, the Noonan syndrome, the yellow nail syndrome, the intestinal lymphangiectasia syndrome, and lymphangiomyomatosis. Women are affected more frequently than men. There are three clinical subtypes: congenital lymphedema, which appears shortly after birth; lymphedema praecox, which has its onset at the time of puberty; and lymphedema tarda, which usually begins after age 35. Familial forms of congenital lymphedema (Milroy's disease) and lymphedema praecox (Meige's disease) may be inherited in an autosomal dominant manner with variable penetrance; autosomal or sex-linked recessive forms are less common.

Secondary lymphedema is an acquired condition resulting from

TABLE 211-3   Causes of lymphedema

Primary
  Congenital (includes Milroy's disease)
  Lymphedema praecox (includes Meige's disease)
  Lymphedema tarda
Secondary
  Recurrent lymphangitis
  Filariasis
  Tuberculosis
  Neoplasm
  Surgery
  Radiation therapy

damage to or obstruction of previously normal lymphatic channels (see Table 211-3). Recurrent episodes of bacterial lymphangitis, usually caused by streptococci, are a very common cause of lymphedema. The most common cause of secondary lymphedema worldwide is filariasis (Chap. 182). Tumors, such as prostate cancer and lymphoma, also can obstruct lymphatic vessels. Both surgery and radiation therapy for breast carcinoma may cause lymphedema of the upper extremity. Less common causes include tuberculosis, contact dermatitis, lymphogranuloma venereum, rheumatoid arthritis, pregnancy, and self-induced or factitious lymphedema following application of tourniquets.

Lymphedema is generally a painless condition, but patients may experience a chronic dull, heavy sensation in the leg, and most often patients are concerned about the appearance of the leg. Lymphedema of the lower extremity, initially involving the foot, gradually progresses up the leg so that the entire limb becomes edematous. In the early stages of lymphedema, the edema is soft and pits easily with pressure. In the chronic stages, the limb has a woody texture, and the tissues become indurated and fibrotic. At this stage, the edema may no longer be pitting. The limb loses its normal contour, and the toes appear square. Lymphedema should be distinguished from other disorders that cause unilateral leg swelling, such as deep vein thrombosis and chronic venous insufficiency. In the latter, edema is softer and there is often evidence of a stasis dermatitis, hyperpigmentation, and superficial venous varicosities.

The evaluation of patients with lymphedema should include diagnostic studies to clarify the cause. Abdominal and pelvic ultrasound and computed tomography can be used to detect obstructing lesions such as neoplasms. Lymphoscintigraphy and lymphangiography are rarely indicated, but either can be used to confirm the diagnosis or differentiate primary from secondary lymphedema. Lymphoscintigraphy involves the injection of radioactively labeled technetium-containing colloid into the distal subcutaneous tissue of the affected extremity. Lymphangiography requires the isolation and cannulation of a distal lymphatic vessel and subsequent injection of contrast material. In primary lymphedema, lymphatic channels are absent, hypoplastic, or ectatic. In secondary lymphedema, lymphatic channels usually are dilated, and the level of obstruction may be determined.

Management   Patients with lymphedema of the lower extremities must be instructed to take meticulous care of their feet to prevent recurrent lymphangitis. Skin hygiene is important, and emollients can be used to prevent drying. Prophylactic antibiotics are often helpful, and fungal infection should be treated aggressively. Patients should be encouraged to participate in physical activity; frequent leg elevation can reduce the amount of edema. Patients can be fitted with graduated compression hose to reduce the amount of lymphedema that develops with upright posture. Occasionally, intermittent pneumatic compression devices can be applied at home to facilitate reduction of the edema. Diuretics are contraindicated and may cause depletion of intravascular volume and metabolic abnormalities. Recently, microsurgical lymphovenous anastomotic procedures have been performed to rechannel lymph flow from obstructed lymphatic vessels into the venous system.

REFERENCES

ANDERSON FA JR et al: A population-based perspective of the incidence and case fatality rates of venous thrombosis and pulmonary embolism: The Worcester DVT study. Arch Intern Med 151:933, 1991

BLANKENHORN DH et al: Effects of colestipol-niacin therapy on human femoral atherosclerosis. Circulation 83:438, 1991

BROWSE NL: The diagnosis and management of primary lymphedema. J Vasc Surg 3:181, 1986

CAPEK P et al: Femoropopliteal angioplasty: Factors influencing long-term success. Circulation 83:I70, 1991

CLEOPHAS TJ, NIEMEYER MG: Raynaud's syndrome, an enigma after 130 years. Angiology 44:196, 1993

COFFMAN JD: Intermittent claudication and rest pain: Physiologic concepts and therapeutic approaches. Prog Cardiovasc Dis 22:59, 1979

———: Raynaud's Phenomenon. New York, Oxford, 1989

CRIQUI MH et al: Mortality over a period of 10 years in patients with peripheral arterial disease. N Engl J Med 326:381, 1992

EUROPEAN WORKING GROUP ON CRITICAL LEG ISCHEMIA: Second European consensus document on chronic critical leg ischemia. Circulation 84:IV1, 1991

GOLDHABER SZ: Thrombolysis in venous thromboembolism: An international perspective. Chest 94:176S, 1990

GRESHAM CL: Deep venous thrombosis. South Med J 86:438, 1993

LOSCALZO J et al: The Textbook of Vascular Medicine and Biology. Boston, Little, Brown, 1992

OLIN JW et al: The changing clinical spectrum of thromboangiitis obliterans. Circulation 82:IV3, 1990

SMITH GD et al: Intermittent claudication, heart disease risk factors, and mortality: The Whitehall study. Circulation 82:1925, 1990

YOUNG JR et al: Peripheral Vascular Diseases. St. Louis, Mosby–Year Book, 1991

INDEX

INDEX

(Note: Page numbers in **boldface** indicate major topics or principal discussions; numbers preceded by A indicate Atlas plates.)

TOPICAL TABLE OF CONTENTS